# Drug Information Handbook *for* Nursing

*including*

**Assessment, Administration, Monitoring Guidelines, and Patient Education**

***2nd Edition*** 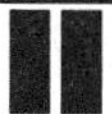 ***1999-2000***

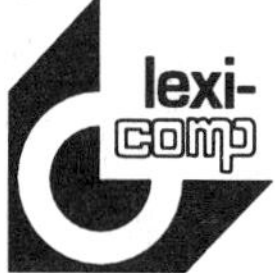

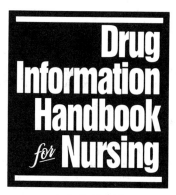


including

**Assessment, Administration, Monitoring Guidelines, and Patient Education**

***2nd Edition*** | ***1999-2000***

**Beatrice B. Turkoski, RN, PhD**
*Assistant Professor*
School of Nursing
Kent State University
Kent, Ohio

**Brenda R. Lance, RN, MSN**
*Nurse Coordinator*
Ritzman Infusion Services
Akron, Ohio

**Mark F. Bonfiglio, BS, PharmD, RPh**
*Director of Pharmacotherapy Resources*
Lexi-Comp, Inc
Hudson, Ohio

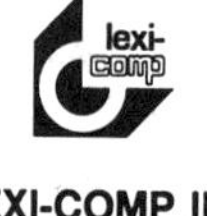


**LEXI-COMP INC**
Hudson (Cleveland)

## NOTICE

Drug information is constantly evolving because of ongoing research and clinical experience and is often subject to interpretation. While great care has been taken to ensure the accuracy of the information presented, the reader is advised that the authors, editors, reviewers, contributors, and publishers cannot be responsible for the continued currency of the information or for any errors, omissions, or the application of this information, or for any consequences arising therefrom. Therefore, the author(s) and/or the publisher shall have no liability to any person or entity with regard to claims, loss, or damage caused, or alleged to be caused, directly or indirectly, by the use of information contained herein. Because of the dynamic nature of drug information, readers are advised that decisions regarding drug therapy must be based on the independent judgment of the clinician, changing information about a drug (eg, as reflected in the literature and manufacturer's most current product information), and changing medical practices. The authors are not responsible for any inaccuracy of quotation or for any false or misleading implication that may arise due to the text or formulas as used or due to the quotation of revisions no longer official. Further, the *Drug Information Handbook for Nursing* is not offered as a guide to dosing. The reader, herewith, is advised that information shown under the heading **Dosing** is provided only as an indication of the amount of the drug typically given or taken during therapy. Actual dosing amount for any specific drug should be based on an in-depth evaluation of the individual patient's therapy requirement and strong consideration given to such issues as contraindications, warnings, precautions, adverse reactions, along with the interaction of other drugs. The manufacturers most current product information or other standard recognized references should always be consulted for such detailed information prior to drug use.

The authors and contributors have written this book in their private capacities. No official support or endorsement by any federal agency or pharmaceutical company is intended or inferred.

If you have any suggestions or questions regarding any information presented in this handbook, please contact our drug information pharmacist at

**1-800-837-LEXI (5394)**



This manual was produced using the FormuLex™ Program —
a complete publishing service of Lexi-Comp Inc.

ISBN 0-916589-82-X

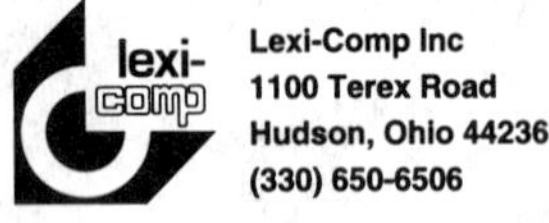


**Lexi-Comp Inc**
**1100 Terex Road**
**Hudson, Ohio 44236**
**(330) 650-6506**

# TABLE OF CONTENTS



## APPENDIX

# PREFACE

The ever-expanding roles of nurses requires them to be informed and knowledgeable about safe pharmacotherapy. Yet, at the same time, there is an expanding number and complexity of pharmacotherapeutic agents used in both outpatient and institutional settings. In addition, there is an increased availability of over-the-counter (OTC) agents and nonregulated biological and herbal products used by the public, whose information about use and safety may or may not be accurate.

The information about current drug therapy is voluminous and the quality of that information varies greatly. Compiling reliable information into a logical guide for nurses, when facing the complexities of diverse disease states and the demands of today's changing healthcare environment, is difficult. The authors of this book have extensively reviewed the available literature and have developed the *Drug Information Handbook for Nursing* with the intent to provide pertinent information related to pharmacotherapeutic agents.

The introductory section of the *Drug Information Handbook for Nursing* includes directions for using the book and a list of common abbreviations, General Nursing Considerations (Assessment, Administration, Monitoring, and Patient Education), Patient Factors That Influence Drug Therapy, and Nursing Management of Common Side Effects.

Each of the monographs presents information in a concise and consistent manner with appropriate referencing to an extensive appendix of helpful information. Each monograph includes pertinent therapeutic purpose, administration guidelines, and possible adverse reactions. The section Additional Nursing Issues, in each monograph, reflects both the therapeutic monitoring recommendations and specific patient teaching information that addresses administration, storage, possible adverse effects, possible interventions, and symptoms the patient should report to the prescriber.

The extensive Appendix includes sections on topical antifungals, over-the-counter medications, and common herbal use. It also includes conversion information, administration guidelines, comparison charts of drugs in specific classes, definitions of selected adverse reactions and drugs associated with specific reactions, maternal and fetal information, OBRA guidelines for long-term care, and overdose guidelines.

The introductory information, the format of the individual monographs, and the valuable appendix information in the *Drug Information Handbook for Nursing* was designed to provide Registered Professional Nurses and upper-division nursing students with information to facilitate safe clinical decision-making.

# ABOUT THE AUTHORS

### Beatrice B. Turkoski, RN, PhD

Dr Turkoski received her BSN from Alverno College in Wisconsin, an MS in Community Health Nursing from the University of Wisconsin-Milwaukee School of Nursing, and a PhD from the University of Wisconsin. Her extensive professional nursing experience includes several years as a clinician in critical care in Wisconsin and Israel, Director of Nursing, clinician, and researcher in gerontology and chronic adult illness in Wisconsin and Ohio, and clinical nurse specialist in family/community practice in Israel.

In her graduate faculty role at Kent State University School of Nursing, Dr Turkoski developed and teaches the Advanced Pharmacology and Applied Therapeutics courses for students in the Nurse Practitioner and Clinical Nurse Specialist programs. Her expertise in this area is highly regarded by both students and faculty. She also conducts continuing education programs and workshops in geriatric pharmacology for healthcare professionals in hospitals, long-term care, and home care.

Dr Turkoski is an active member and officer in several national and international professional organizations. Her impressive list of professional activities includes presentations in the United States, Europe, China, Korea, Canada, and Israel. In recent publications, Dr Turkoski has addressed the subject of biorhythms and medications, behavioral manifestations of adverse drug reactions, and the impact of age on medication response.

### Brenda R. Lance, RN, MSN, DARM

Ms Lance received a diploma in nursing from Methodist Hospital School of Nursing in Lubbock, Texas. She also has earned bachelor's and master's degrees in nursing from Kent State University, Kent, Ohio.

Ms Lance's nursing experiences and expertise are numerous and varied. Her nursing career spans 27 years, having worked in intensive care, emergency room, ambulatory care clinics, home health, and home infusion. She is currently the nurse coordinator for Ritzman Infusion Services, Akron, Ohio.

In addition to many years of direct patient care experience, she is also certified in risk management, has extensive experience in Joint Commission on Accreditation of Healthcare Organizations standards and Medicare regulations for home health, and has been a military nurse for the past 27 years. She holds the rank of Captain (0-6) in the U.S. Naval Reserve Nurse Corps.

Ms Lance is a member of the Sigma Theta Tau (National Honor Society of Nursing), the Association of Military Surgeons of the United States, the Naval Reserve Association, and the Intravenous Nurses Society.

### Mark F. Bonfiglio, BS, PharmD, RPh

Dr Bonfiglio received his BA in Biology and BS in Pharmacy from the University of Toledo. He earned his Doctor of Pharmacy degree from Ohio State University and subsequently completed a Residency in Critical Care Pharmacy at the Ohio State University Hospitals. For the next 8 years he was a faculty member of the Ohio Northern University College of Pharmacy, reaching the rank of Associate Clinical Professor. During this time, his appointment was shared by the institutions where he maintained his clinical practice. Initially, he served for 6 years at Akron City Hospital as a Critical Care Pharmacy Specialist, followed by 2 years in practice as a Pharmacotherapy Specialist in Internal Medicine at the Akron General Medical Center. He conducted research activities and authored numerous publications in addition to his activities in practice and education.

Currently, Dr Bonfiglio works at Lexi-Comp Inc as the Director of Pharmacotherapy Resources and maintains a part-time practice at the Akron General Medical Center. He is an invited lecturer to many professional organizations and is an author of several courseware modules for the Ohio Council of Colleges of Pharmacy nontraditional PharmD initiative. He has also served as a reviewer for *The Annals of Pharmacotherapy* and *Pharmacotherapy.* Professional memberships include the Society of Critical Care Medicine (SCCM), American College of Clinical Pharmacy (ACCP), and American Society of Health System Pharmacists (ASHP).

# EDITORIAL ADVISORY PANEL

**Martin D. Higbee, PharmD**
*Associate Professor*
Department of Pharmacy Practice
The University of Arizona
Tucson, Arizona

**Jane Hurlburt Hodding, PharmD**
*Supervisor, Children's Pharmacy*
Memorial Miller Children's Hospital
Long Beach, California

**Rebecca T. Horvat, PhD**
*Assistant Professor of Pathology and Laboratory Medicine*
University of Kansas Medical Center
Kansas City, Kansas

**Carlos M. Isada, MD**
Department of Infectious Disease
Cleveland Clinic Foundation
Cleveland, Ohio

**David S. Jacobs, MD**
*President, Pathologists Chartered*
Overland Park, Kansas

**Bernard L. Kasten, Jr, MD, FCAP**
*Vice President/Medical Director*
Corning Medical Laboratories
Teterboro, New Jersey

**Donna M. Kraus, PharmD**
*Associate Professor of Pharmacy Practice*
Departments of Pharmacy Practice and Pediatrics
*Clinical Pharmacist*
Pediatric Intensive Care Unit
University of Illinois at Chicago
Chicago, Illinois

**Charles Lacy, RPh, PharmD**
*Drug Information Pharmacist*
Cedars-Sinai Medical Center
Los Angeles, California

**Leonard L. Lance, RPh, BSPharm**
*Pharmacist*
Lexi-Comp Inc
Hudson, Ohio

**Jerrold B. Leikin, MD**
*Associate Director*
Emergency Services
Rush-Presbyterian-St. Luke's Medical Center
Chicago, Illinois

**Timothy F. Meiller, DDS, PhD**
*Professor*
Department of Oral Medicine and Diagnostic Sciences
Baltimore College of Dental Surgery
*Professor of Oncology*
Greenebaum Cancer Center
University of Maryland at Baltimore
Baltimore, Maryland

**Eugene S. Olsowka, MD, PhD**
*Pathologist*
Institute of Pathology PC
Saginaw, Michigan

**Frank P. Paloucek, PharmD**
*Clinical Associate Professor*
University of Illinois
Chicago, Illinois

## EDITORIAL ADVISORY PANEL *(Continued)*

**Christopher J. Papasian, PhD**
*Director of Diagnostic Microbiology and Immunology Laboratories*
Truman Medical Center
Kansas City, Missouri

**Martha Sajatovic, MD**
*Assistant Professor of Psychiatry*
Case Western Reserve University
Cleveland, Ohio

**Todd P. Semla, PharmD**
Department of Clinical Pharmacy
*Project Coordinator and Clinical Pharmacist*
Evanston Hospital
Evanston, Illinois

**Carol K. Taketomo, PharmD**
*Pharmacy Manager*
Children's Hospital of Los Angeles
Los Angeles, California

**Lowell L. Tilzer, MD**
*Associate Medical Director*
Community Blood Center of Greater Kansas
Kansas City, Missouri

**Richard L. Wynn, PhD**
*Professor and Chairman of Pharmacology*
Baltimore College of Dental Surgery
Dental School
University of Maryland at Baltimore
Baltimore, Maryland

# ACKNOWLEDGMENTS

This handbook exists in its present form as the result of the concerted efforts of the following individuals: Robert D. Kerscher, publisher and president of Lexi-Comp, Inc; Lynn D. Coppinger, managing editor; Barbara F. Kerscher, production manager; David C. Marcus, director of information systems; and Kelley K. Engle, RPh.

Other members of the Lexi-Comp staff whose contributions deserve special mention include Diane M. Harbart, MT (ASCP), medical editor; Jeanne E. Wilson, production/systems liaison; Leslie J. Ruggles, Julie A. Katzen, Jennifer L. Rocky, Stacey L. Hurd, Kathleen E. Schleicher, and Linda L. Taylor, project managers; Alexandra J. Hart, composition specialist; Jackie L. Mizer, Ginger S. Conner, and Kathy Smith, production assistants; Tracey J. Reinecke, graphic designer; Cynthia A. Bell, CPhT; Edmund A. Harbart, vice-president, custom publishing division; Jack L. Stones, vice-president, reference publishing division; Jay L. Katzen, director of marketing and business development; Jerry M. Reeves, Marc L. Long, and Patrick T. Grubb, regional sales managers; Brad F. Bolinski, Kristin M. Thompson, Matthew C. Kerscher, Tina L. Collins, Kelene A. Murphy, and Leslie G. Rodia, sales and marketing representatives; Paul A. Rhine and Jason M. Buchwald, academic account managers; Kenneth J. Hughes, manager of authoring systems; Sean M. Conrad and James M. Stacey, system analysts; Thury L. O'Connor, vice-president of technology; David J. Wasserbauer, vice-president, finance and administration; Elizabeth M. Conlon and Rebecca A. Dryhurst, accounting; and Frederick C. Kerscher, inventory and fulfillment manager.

Much of the material contained in this book was a result of pharmacy contributors throughout the United States and Canada. Lexi-Comp has assisted many medical institutions to develop hospital-specific formulary manuals that contain clinical drug information as well as dosing. Working with clinical pharmacists, hospital pharmacy and therapeutics committees, and hospital drug information centers, Lexi-Comp has developed an evolutionary drug database that reflects the practice of pharmacy in these major institutions.

In addition, the authors wish to thank their families, friends, and colleagues who supported them in their efforts to complete this handbook.

# ORGANIZATION OF THE DRUG INFORMATION HANDBOOK FOR NURSING

The *Drug Information Handbook for Nursing* is divided into the following sections.

## Introduction

The introductory text includes guidelines for use of the handbook and a brief overview of General Nursing Issues (Assessment, Administration, Monitoring, and Patient Education), Patient Factors That Influence Drug Therapy, and Nursing Management of Side Effects.

## Individual Drug Monographs

Medications are arranged alphabetically by generic name. Extensive cross-referencing (with easy visibility marked with a diamond ♦) is provided by U.S., Canadian, and Mexican brand names and synonyms. Abbreviated monographs contain unique information, commonly for combination formulations, and a cross-reference to the corresponding individual entity monographs.

## Controlled Substance Index

This index provides a list of drug names and their corresponding controlled substance classification.

## Appendix

The last section is an extensive appendix of useful information that includes conversion and laboratory information, comparison charts for selected classes of drugs, maternal and fetal guidelines, OBRA recommendations for long-term care, and overdose information.

### Drug Monographs

The following table describes the format of the drug monographs and a brief description of each field of information.

| | |
|---|---|
| **Generic Name** | U.S. adopted name. |
| **Pronunciation Guide** | Phonetic pronunciation if the generic name. |
| **U.S. Brand Names** | U.S. trade names (manufacturer specific). |
| **Synonyms** | Other names or accepted abbreviations of the generic drug. |
| **Therapeutic Category** | Systematic classification of medications. |
| **Pregnancy Risk Factor** | Five categories established by the FDA to indicate the potential of a systemically absorbed drug for causing birth defects. |
| **Lactation** | Information describing characteristics of using the drug listed in the monograph while breast-feeding (where recommendation of American Academy of Pediatrics differs, notation is made). The following distinctions are made.<br><br>Does not enter breast milk<br>Compatible<br>Excretion in breast milk unknown<br>Use caution<br>Not recommended<br>Contraindicated<br>Consult prescriber |

*(continued)*

**Use** — Describes information pertaining to appropriate indications of the drug listed in the monograph. Includes FDA approved and non-FDA approved indications.

**Mechanism of Action/Effect** — A brief description of how the drug works.

**Contraindications** — Information pertaining to inappropriate use of the drug, or disease states and patient populations in which the drug should not be used.

**Warnings/Precautions** — Warnings include hazardous conditions related to use of the drug; precautions include disease states or patient populations in which the drug should be used with caution.

**Drug Interactions**

Cytochrome P-450 Effect — Drugs which are involved in possible interactions due to their activity with the hepatic cytochrome P-450 system are identified. Their role as inducers, inhibitors, or substrates for a specific isoenzyme are listed.

Decreased Effect — Drug combinations that result in a decreased therapeutic effect between the drug listed in the monograph and other drugs or drug classes.

Increased Effect/Toxicity — Drug combinations that result in a increased or toxic therapeutic effect between the drug listed in the monograph and other drugs or drug classes.

**Food Interactions** — Information regarding effect or implications of food while taking the drug.

**Effects on Lab Values** — A list of assay interferences when taking the drug.

**Adverse Reactions** — Drug-induced side effects are grouped by percentage of incidence (>10%; 1%-10%) and body system. Adverse reactions for <1% incidence are listed as a group. **Side effects of <1% incidence are included only if important or life-threatening.**

**Overdose/Toxicology** — Comment or considerations with signs or symptoms of excess drug ingestion.

**Pharmacodynamics/Kinetics**

Protein Binding — The percent of drug listed in the monograph bound to circulating proteins (ie, albumin, etc).

Distribution — Includes pharmacokinetic information describing the volume of distribution for the drug and other sites of transfer (ie, placenta, crossing the blood-brain-barrier, CSF, etc).

Half-Life — The reported half-life of elimination for the parent or metabolites of the drug.

Time to Peak — Describes the relative time after ingestion when concentration achieves the highest serum concentration.

Metabolism — Describes the site of metabolism and may include the percentage of active metabolites.

Excretion — Route of drug elimination.

## ORGANIZATION OF THE DRUG INFORMATION HANDBOOK FOR NURSING *(Continued)*

*(continued)*

| | |
|---|---|
| Onset | The time after drug administration when therapeutic effect is observed. May also include time for peak therapeutic effect. |
| Duration | Length of therapeutic effect. |
| **Formulations** | A description of the product including strength and formulation (ie, tablet, capsule, injection, syrup, etc). |
| **Dosing** | |
| Adults | The recommended amount of drug to be given to adult patients. |
| Elderly | A suggested amount of drug to be given to elderly patients which may include adjustments from adult dosing. Lack of information in the monograph may imply that the drug is not used in the elderly patient or no specific adjustments could be identified. |
| Renal Impairment | Suggested dosage adjustments based on compromised renal function, including dosing instructions for patients on dialysis. |
| Hepatic Impairment | Suggested dosage adjustments based on compromised liver function. |
| **Administration** | |
| Oral<br>I.M.<br>I.V.<br>I.V. Detail<br>Inhalation<br>Topical<br>Other | The administration field contains six subfields by route regarding issues relative to appropriately giving a medication. Includes suggestions on final drug concentrations and/or rates of infusion for parenteral medications. Also includes comments regarding the timing of drug administration relative to meals. |
| **Stability** | |
| Storage | Relates to appropriate storage of the medication prior to opening the manufacturers original packaging. Information is only given if recommendations are for storage at other than room temperature. Also includes storage requirements for reconstituted products. |
| Reconstitution | Includes comments on solution choice with time or conditions for the mixture to maintain full potency before administration. |
| Compatibility | Contains information regarding stability of drug combinations when administered together or through Y-site administration sets. Known incompatibilities may also be included. |
| **Monitoring Laboratory Tests** | Suggested laboratory tests to monitor for safety and efficacy of the drug listed in the monographs. |
| **Additional Nursing Issues** | Includes comments suggesting nursing care of a patient and includes the following subfields. |
| Physical Assessment | Monitoring guidelines |

*(continued)*

| | |
|---|---|
| Patient Education/Instruction | Suggested items to discuss with the patient or caregiver when taking the medication. May include issues regarding contraception, self-monitoring, precautions, and administration. |
| Dietary Issues | Includes information on how the medication should be taken relative to meals or food. |
| Geriatric Consideration | Comments or suggestions of drug use in elderly patients. May include monitoring, dose adjustments, precautions, or comments on appropriateness of use. |
| Breast-feeding Issues | Provides further information relating to taking the drug while nursing. |
| Pregnancy Issues | Comments related to safe drug administration during pregnancy are listed if appropriate. |
| Other Issues | Any additional pertinent information regarding nursing issues is provided. |
| **Additional Information** | Included dose equivalents, sodium or potassium content, strength equivalents (mg = mEq), or specific brand information. |
| **Related Information** | Cross-reference with page number to other pertinent drug information found elsewhere in this handbook. |

# SYMBOLS & ABBREVIATIONS USED IN THIS HANDBOOK*

| | |
|---|---|
| °C | degrees Celsius (Centigrade) |
| $<$ | less than |
| $>$ | greater than |
| $\leq$ | less than or equal to |
| $\geq$ | greater than or equal to |
| µg | microgram |
| µmol | micromole |
| AAPC | antibiotic associated pseudomembranous colitis |
| ABG | arterial blood gas |
| ABMT | autologous bone marrow transplant |
| ACE | angiotensin-converting enzyme |
| ACLS | advanced cardiac life support |
| ADH | antidiuretic hormone |
| AED | antiepileptic drug |
| AIDS | acquired immunodeficiency syndrome |
| ALL | acute lymphoblastic leukemia |
| ALT | alanine aminotransferase (formerly called SGPT) |
| AML | acute myeloblastic leukemia |
| ANA | antinuclear antibodies |
| ANC | absolute neutrophil count |
| ANLL | acute nonlymphoblastic leukemia |
| APTT | activated partial thromboplastin time |
| ASA (class I-IV) | American Society of Anesthesiology physical status classification of surgical patients according to their baseline health<br>ASA I: Normal healthy patients<br>ASA II: Patients having controlled disease states (eg, controlled hypertension)<br>ASA III: Patients having a disease which compromises their organ function (eg, decompensated CHF, end stage renal failure)<br>ASA IV: Patients who are extremely critically ill |
| AST | aspartate aminotransferase (formerly called SGOT) |
| AUC | area under the curve (area under the serum concentration-time curve) |
| A-V | atrial-ventricular |
| BMT | bone marrow transplant |
| BUN | blood urea nitrogen |
| cAMP | cyclic adenosine monophosphate |
| CBC | complete blood count |
| CHF | congestive heart failure |
| CI | cardiac index |
| $Cl_{cr}$ | creatinine clearance |
| CMV | cytomegalovirus |
| CNS | central nervous system |
| COPD | chronic obstructive pulmonary disease |
| CSF | cerebrospinal fluid |
| CT | computed tomography |
| CVA | cerebral vascular accident |
| CVP | central venous pressure |
| d | day |
| $D_5W$ | dextrose 5% in water |
| $D_5$/1/2NS | dextrose 5% in sodium chloride 0.45% |
| $D_{10}W$ | dextrose 10% in water |

| | |
|---|---|
| DIC | disseminated intravascular coagulation |
| $DL_{co}$ | pulmonary diffusion capacity for carbon monoxide |
| DNA | deoxyribonucleic acid |
| DVT | deep vein thrombosis |
| ECHO | echocardiogram |
| ECMO | extracorporeal membrane oxygenation |
| EEG | electroencephalogram |
| EKG | electrocardiogram |
| ESR | erythrocyte sedimentation rate |
| E.T. | endotracheal |
| $FEV_1$ | forced expiratory volume exhaled after 1 second |
| FSH | follicle-stimulating hormone |
| FVC | forced vital capacity |
| g | gram |
| G-6-PD | glucose-6-phosphate dehydrogenase |
| GA | gestational age |
| GABA | gamma-aminobutyric acid |
| GE | gastroesophageal |
| GI | gastrointestinal |
| GU | genitourinary |
| h | hour |
| HIV | human immunodeficiency virus |
| HPLC | high performance liquid chromatography |
| IBW | ideal body weight |
| ICP | intracranial pressure |
| IgG | immune globulin G |
| I.M. | intramuscular |
| INR | international normalized ratio |
| int. unit | international units |
| I.O. | intraosseous |
| I & O | input and output |
| IOP | intraocular pressure |
| I.T. | intrathecal |
| I.V. | intravenous |
| IVH | intraventricular hemorrhage |
| IVP | intravenous push |
| JRA | juvenile rheumatoid arthritis |
| kg | kilogram |
| L | liter |
| LDH | lactate dehydrogenase |
| LE | lupus erythematosus |
| LH | luteinizing hormone |
| LP | lumbar puncture |
| LR | lactated Ringer's |
| MAC | *Mycobacterium avium* complex |
| MAO | monoamine oxidase |
| MAP | mean arterial pressure |
| mcg | microgram |
| mg | milligram |
| MI | myocardial infarction |
| min | minute |
| mL | milliliter |
| mo | month |
| mOsm | milliosmoles |
| MRI | magnetic resonance image |
| MRSA | methicillin-resistant *Staphylococcus aureus* |
| NCI | National Cancer Institute |

## SYMBOLS & ABBREVIATIONS USED IN THIS HANDBOOK* *(Continued)*

| | |
|---|---|
| ND | nasoduodenal |
| ng | nanogram |
| NG | nasogastric |
| NMDA | n-methyl-d-aspartate |
| nmol | nanomole |
| NPO | nothing per os (nothing by mouth) |
| NSAID | nonsteroidal anti-inflammatory drug |
| O.R. | operating room |
| OTC | over-the-counter (nonprescription) |
| PABA | para-aminobenzoic acid |
| PALS | pediatric advanced life support |
| PCA | postconceptional age |
| PCP | *Pneumocystis carinii* pneumonia |
| PCWP | pulmonary capillary wedge pressure |
| PDA | patent ductus arteriosus |
| PIP | peak inspiratory pressure |
| PNA | postnatal age |
| PSVT | paroxysmal supraventricular tachycardia |
| PT | prothrombin time |
| PTT | partial thromboplastin time |
| PUD | peptic ulcer disease |
| PVC | premature ventricular contraction |
| PVR | peripheral vascular resistance |
| qsad | add an amount sufficient to equal |
| RAP | right arterial pressure |
| RIA | radioimmunoassay |
| RNA | ribonucleic acid |
| S-A | sino-atrial |
| S.C. | subcutaneous |
| $S_{cr}$ | serum creatinine |
| SIADH | syndrome of inappropriate antidiuretic hormone |
| S.L. | sublingual |
| SLE | systemic lupus erythematosus |
| SVR | systemic vascular resistance |
| SVT | supraventricular tachycardia |
| SWI | sterile water for injection |
| $T_3$ | triiodothyronine |
| $T_4$ | thyroxine |
| TIBC | total iron binding capacity |
| TPN | total parenteral nutrition |
| TSH | thyroid stimulating hormone |
| TT | thrombin time |
| UTI | urinary tract infection |
| $V_d$ | volume of distribution |
| $V_{dss}$ | volume of distribution at steady-state |
| VMA | vanillylmandelic acid |
| w/w | weight for weight |
| y | year |

*Other than drug synonyms

# FDA PREGNANCY CATEGORIES

Throughout this book there is a field labeled Pregnancy Risk Factor (PRF) and the letter A, B, C, D, or X immediately following which signifies a category. The FDA has established these five categories to indicate the potential of a systemically absorbed drug for causing birth defects. The key differentiation among the categories rests upon the reliability of documentation and the risk:benefit ratio. Pregnancy Category X is particularly notable in that if any data exists that may implicate a drug as a teratogen and the risk:benefit ratio is clearly negative, the drug is contraindicated during pregnancy.

These categories are summarized as follows:

A Controlled studies in pregnant women fail to demonstrate a risk to the fetus in the first trimester with no evidence of risk in later trimesters. The possibility of fetal harm appears remote.

B Either animal-reproduction studies have not demonstrated a fetal risk but there are no controlled studies in pregnant women, or animal-reproduction studies have shown an adverse effect (other than a decrease in fertility) that was not confirmed in controlled studies in women in the first trimester and there is no evidence of a risk in later trimesters.

C Either studies in animals have revealed adverse effects on the fetus (teratogenic or embryocidal effects or other) and there are no controlled studies in women, or studies in women and animals are not available. Drugs should be given only if the potential benefits justify the potential risk to the fetus.

D There is positive evidence of human fetal risk, but the benefits from use in pregnant women may be acceptable despite the risk (eg, if the drug is needed in a life-threatening situation or for a serious disease for which safer drugs cannot be used or are ineffective).

X Studies in animals or human beings have demonstrated fetal abnormalities or there is evidence of fetal risk based on human experience, or both, and the risk of the use of the drug in pregnant women clearly outweighs any possible benefit. The drug is contraindicated in women who are or may become pregnant.

# GENERAL NURSING ISSUES (Assessment, Administration, Monitoring, and Patient Education)

## ASSESSMENT

Assessment is the primary action in the nursing process and it is also a vital part of optimal drug therapy. Assessment activities must precede administering any medication. Appropriate assessment includes not just the particulars of the presenting complaint, but also must include what the patient understands or believes about the problem (eg, etiology and prognosis of complaint, impact of lifestyle habits, etc). Information gathered in primary assessment should serve as a guide to patient education and to identify specific areas that need close monitoring. Generally, assessment starts with a thorough patient history that can include:

- Current complaint: History, observation, laboratory results, other treatments, etc
- Other concurrent conditions: Chronic illnesses
- Past health problems and treatments: Resolved, chronic, treatments effective/noneffective
- Current drugs: Prescription, OTC, home remedies, herbs and herbal medicines
- Past drugs: Reason for taking, effectiveness, adverse effects
- Allergies or adverse effects: Drugs, household products, food products, environmental factors
- Health habits: Caffeine, alcohol, nicotine, street drugs, sleep, activity, nutrition, hydration, sexual activity, pregnant, lactating, use of contraceptives (barrier or oral)
- Physical: Vital signs, weight, height; may include particulars (as necessary) about any body system: pulmonary, cardiac, circulatory, hepatic, renal, gastrointestinal, genitourinary, integument, skeletal, or connective tissues systems
- Psychosocial support: Financial, religious, personal, community

## SAFE ADMINISTRATION

Safe administration is grounded in the five "Right" principles: Right Drug, Right Dose, Right Patient, Right Route, Right Time.

**Right drug** – involves checking drug dispensed with the written prescription. Many drugs have similar names (terbutaline/tolbutamine, calciferol/calcitriol); caution must be used to determine the exact drug prescribed. In addition, a nurse must understand why any particular medication is being prescribed.

**Right dose** – requires checking the prescribed dosage, being aware of the "average" or "usual" dosage for that drug, or identifying any particular patient characteristics which may be rational for unusual dosing. Determining the right dose for some medications means titrating dose to monitored physiological parameters determined by hemodynamic or cardiac monitoring, according to kidney or liver function, or calculating dose according to body weight or body surface area.

**Right patient** – means identifying each individual patient. Patients in healthcare institutions most generally wear identifying namebands that can be checked prior to administration. When patients are not wearing namebands (eg, at home, in rehabilitation, in outpatient settings), asking patients to identify themselves will reduce medication misadventures.

**Right route** – includes consideration of traditional routes (P.O., I.V., I.M., or S.C., etc). Right route should also include knowledge about whether the dispensed oral drug form can be changed. Can the drug safely be crushed, chewed, dissolved, administered via a nasogastric or any other type of feeding tube. Extended-release formulations should never be crushed, chewed, or dissolved (see Tablets That Cannot Be Crushed or Altered *on page 1333*). Some intravenous drugs should be administered via a central line because the possibility of peripheral extravasation presents a serious risk for the patient. Some intravenous drugs (eg, ectoposide VP-16, idarubicin, hydroxyzine, ifosfamide, irinotecan, mannitol, mechlorethamine, mitomycin, nafcillin, norepinephrine, phenobarbital, phenylephrine, phenytoin, potassium chloride, vasopressin, etc) are extremely irritating to peripheral veins; this requires their administration via a central line or as dilute solutions at a slow rate given peripherally.

**Right time** – necessitates knowledge of a drug's bioavailability; knowing whether the drug should be given at around-the-clock intervals, or whether doses need to be timed in a specific manner. Are there specific dietary considerations? Food will slow the absorption time of many drugs, however, their overall effect will not be affected. Administering medications with food will often reduce the nausea or vomiting that occurs when medications are given on an empty stomach. The drug monographs clearly identify those drugs that must specifically be administered on an empty stomach or should definitely be administered with food. Some monographs include the recommendation for administering in the early part of the day – to reduce night-time sleep interruptions (diuretics).

## MONITORING

**Additional Nursing Issues** in each monograph address a wide variety of assessment and monitoring activities. Advanced nurse practitioners may be responsible for both prescribing and monitoring. However, at all times the nurse responsible for administering the medication or instructing the patient about administration is also responsible for monitoring effectiveness and adverse effects and communicating details of any untoward or adverse results to the prescriber. Some common monitoring responsibilities are described in the following paragraphs.

**Monitoring laboratory tests results** includes knowing what tests are necessary to monitor drug response and ensuring that ordered tests are done at appropriate times. Communicating laboratory results to the appropriate prescriber is frequently a nursing responsibility.

Some laboratory tests must be completed prior to administering the first dose of a drug (eg, culture and sensitivity tests, tests that indicate premedication status of liver, kidney, or other systems function). Standard peak and trough serum concentration recommendations are available from most laboratories. Since these may change somewhat among laboratories, it is always best to check with the laboratory that will be completing peak and trough assays to identify their exact timing regulations.

**Assessing patient knowledge/teaching** indicates the need to discuss that particular area of concern with a patient (or caregiver) and to identify that the knowledge is correct and complete. If the patient's/caregiver's knowledge is incomplete or incorrect, then it is vital to teach the patient (or caregiver) the necessary information (eg, does a patient know the correct procedure for using inhalators, for instilling ophthalmic medications, for administering injectable medications (and dispensing needles), or inserting a suppository? Is the patient's knowledge about identifying signs and symptoms of opportunistic infections accurate? Is the patient aware of the precautions necessary with antihypertensives (eg, postural hypotension precautions)? Does the patient understand the rationale for contraception, the difference between oral and barrier forms of contraception? Sometime patients need to be referred to other professionals for advanced education pertaining to their disease and the prescribed drugs (eg, drug monographs for medications used to treat diabetics suggest referring the patient to a diabetic educator).

**Monitoring vital signs** means more than just identifying normal or abnormal patient responses. It also means communicating any adverse signs or symptoms to the prescriber. When the patient is in danger it may be necessary to discontinue a medication and notify the prescriber. In other instances, it will mean contacting the prescriber for further instructions. Some monitoring is constant, as with emergency drugs; and some is intermittent, as with patient administered medications. Awareness of the need for monitoring, the rationale behind monitoring instructions, and the type of monitoring required is a nursing responsibility.

## GENERAL NURSING ISSUES (Assessment, Administration, Monitoring, and Patient Education) *(Continued)*

**Monitoring for adverse/toxic response.** Known adverse reactions are identified according to frequency (>10%, 1% to 10%, <1% (limited to important or life-threatening symptoms)) in each drug monograph in the *Drug Information Handbook for Nursing*. The Physical Assessment/Monitoring section of Additional Nursing Issues also includes reminders about the necessity for monitoring the most threatening or severe of those possible side effects.

**Patient education/instruction** sections in each drug monograph include the major points that patients need to know about administration safety, including appropriate timing, dietary precautions, and drug interaction precautions. Patient education content also indicates possible actions the patient may take to reduce unpleasant inherent adverse effects (eg, postural hypotension precautions; caution against driving or engaging in hazardous activity because of confusion, dizziness, or impaired judgment; the need to prevent excessive exposure to sunlight because of photosensitivity; and strategies to reduce or prevent nausea and vomiting. Adverse effects that should be reported to the prescriber are also identified, including the necessity for informing the prescriber if the patient is pregnant or intends to be pregnant. In monographs for drugs classified as C, D, or X pregnancy risk factors, such information is included in both the Monitoring and Education sections.

**Geriatric information** includes considerations that are pertinent for that drug in relation to therapy for older patients. In addition to these precautions or information, it is necessary to remember the general effects of aging on drug response, especially the effects that impaired circulation or renal function may have on pharmacokinetics.

# PATIENT FACTORS THAT INFLUENCE DRUG THERAPY

Many factors related to an individual patient, or a group of similar patients, can impact the pharmacokinetics of drugs and relate to adverse reactions.

## PREGNANCY/LACTATION

The changes that occur during pregnancy may necessitate dosage changes for some drugs. Decreased gastric tract motility, increased blood volume, decreased protein binding sites, and increased glomerular filtration rates may alter the degree of anticipated pharmacotherapeutic response.

Primarily, the concern about drugs during pregnancy is the effect of drugs on the fetus; either teratogenic (causing birth defects) or systemic (causing addiction). Although many drugs cross the placenta, the type of drug, the concentration of that drug, and the gestational age at time of exposure of the fetus are primary determinants of fetal reaction. When prescribing or administering drugs to any child-bearing age female, it is vital to ask when her last menstrual period was and, if necessary, to wait for the results of a pregnancy test before starting any drug therapy. Of course, it is best to avoid all drugs during pregnancy, however, in some cases, the physiological context (ie, cardiac output, renal blood flow, etc) may be altered enough to require the use of drugs that are not needed by the same woman when not pregnant.

Most systematically absorbed drugs have been assigned a pregnancy risk factor based on the drugs potential to cause birth defects. This permits an evaluation of the risk:benefit ratio when prescribing or administering drugs becomes necessary. Drugs in the risk factor class "A" are generally considered to be safe for use during pregnancy, class "X" drugs are never safe and are known to be positively teratogenic.

These categories are summarized as follows:

A Controlled studies in pregnant women fail to demonstrate a risk to the fetus in the first trimester with no evidence of risk in later trimesters. The possibility of fetal harm appears remote.

B Either animal-reproduction studies have not demonstrated a fetal risk but there are no controlled studies in pregnant women, or animal-reproduction studies have shown an adverse effect (other than a decrease in fertility) that was not confirmed in controlled studies in women in the first trimester and there is no evidence of a risk in later trimesters.

C Either studies in animals have revealed adverse effects on the fetus (teratogenic or embryocidal effects or other) and there are no controlled studies in women, or studies in women and animals are not available. Drugs should be given only if the potential benefits justify the potential risk to the fetus.

D There is positive evidence of human fetal risk, but the benefits from use in pregnant women may be acceptable despite the risk (eg, if the drug is needed in a life-threatening situation or for a serious disease for which safer drugs cannot be used or are ineffective).

X Studies in animals or human beings have demonstrated fetal abnormalities or there is evidence of fetal risk based on human experience, or both, and the risk of the use of the drug in pregnant women clearly outweighs any possible benefit. The drug is contraindicated in women who are or may become pregnant.

**Contraception note:** Many drugs will interact with and decrease the effect of oral contraceptives (eg, barbiturates, some antibiotics (minocycline, ampicillin, tetracycline, corticosteroids, and benzodiazepines). When a second drug will decrease the effect of oral contraceptives, the patient needs to be educated about the necessity for using a "barrier" form of contraception. Barrier contraception (alone or in combination with some form of oral contraception) is

## PATIENT FACTORS THAT INFLUENCE DRUG THERAPY *(Continued)*

also often recommended for the patient who must take drugs with pregnancy risk factors "D" (idarubicin) or class "X" (isotretinoin).

Because many drugs and substances used by a mother appear in breast milk, care must be taken to evaluate the drug effects on the lactating woman and the infant. Some drugs are identified as being clearly contraindicated during lactation, others may cross into breast milk but adverse side effects on the fetus have not been identified, and for some drugs the administration times should be distanced from nursing time. Nurses should advise lactating women about the effects that drugs may have on the infant.

### AGE

All pharmacokinetics – absorption, distribution, metabolism, and excretion – are different in infants, young adults, and elderly patients. Elderly patients may have mildly decreased or severely decreased blood flow to all organs, gastric motility may be slowed, kidney function may be reduced, decreased nutrition may result in decreased albumin, and sedentary lifestyles may have an impact on drug response. Slower gastric motility means that absorption is slowed, resulting in longer time periods to clinical response. Decreased blood flow means that distribution is altered, resulting in decreased response or longer response time. Decreased available albumin results in higher levels of drug in circulation – more toxic responses with "normal" doses. Excretion may be altered with decreased glomerular filtration rates or slower gastric emptying which can result in increased levels of drug remaining in the system.

The ratio between total body water and total body fat also changes with age; older persons have decreased amounts of total body water and higher body fat. This aspect of aging also influences the blood concentration of some drugs. In a person with increased body fat, fat-soluble drugs are distributed to tissues more than to plasma; resulting in a longer response time as the drug must then be redistributed from tissue to plasma. The idiosyncratic response incidence also increases with an aging population. Responses to drugs may be both more exaggerated or diminished with the "usual" doses of some drugs.

In addition, and of major concern with elderly patients, is the incidence of polypharmacy; the increased numbers of drugs the patient may be taking. Older patients may have 2, 3, 4, or 5 (or more) chronic conditions for which they are taking medication. In addition, they may be seeing a different prescriber for each of these conditions. Often, it is a nurse who identifies and coordinates the care of these elderly patients, and the nurse must be aware of the possibility for increased incidence of adverse effects.

### BODY WEIGHT/BUILD

Most "recommended" dosages of drugs are based on the average size, young or middle aged adult (usually males). Extremely obese or extremely thin patients may be prone to adverse effects as a result of "nonindividualized" prescribing. Decreased muscle mass can result in reduced creatinine from muscle breakdown which is artificially low or appears normal when dosing is based on "average" or estimated rather than "actual" creatinine clearance.

### SMOKING, ALCOHOL, NUTRITION, AND HYDRATION

Smoking has a direct impact on liver enzyme activity, blood flow, and the central nervous system (see table *on page 1415*) Excessive alcohol intake impacts liver enzymes, renal function, and has an additive effect with most antipsychotic, sedative, or anxiolytic medications, as well as altering responses to many other medications. Nutrition and hydration also play an important part in drug responses and possible adverse reactions. Poor hydration may result in reduced blood flow and excretion. Decreased or prolonged gastric motility can result in slowed excretion and/or prolonged absorption. Poor or inadequate nutrition may result in decreased protein available for binding.

It is vital that a patient's current habits are considered when prescribing, administering, or monitoring drug therapy, but in addition, patients must be aware of the need to inform their professional care provider that they have changed their smoking, alcohol, or dietary patterns. When dosage of theophylline is based on the fact that the patient is a smoker and that the patient stops smoking, the theophylline dosage must be adjusted to prevent overdose. When a patient is on warfarin, drastic increases in the amount of vitamin K intake through increased green leafy vegetables can dramatically alter the dose of warfarin.

## OTHER PATIENT FACTORS THAT INFLUENCE DRUG RESPONSE

Genetic variations, differences in circadian patterns, psychological temperament, and disease states can also impact the incidence of adverse reactions. Genetic differences in enzymes may influence the incidence of adverse effects (fast acetylators or slow acetylators). Circadian rhythms differ among individuals and impact on absorption patterns, hormone secretion, or urinary excretion patterns. Disease states can and do change all aspects of pharmacokinetics: cirrhosis can impair liver enzyme metabolism rate; abnormal thyroid function can influence drug metabolism; diseases which affect blood circulation (eg, hypertension, CHF, Raynaud's phenomena, malignancies, etc) can have an impact on absorption, distribution, and excretion; diabetes impacts response to many drugs; malnutrition commonly associated with disease can drastically reduce albumin levels; and kidney disease will reduce excretion rates for many drugs.

# THERAPEUTIC NURSING MANAGEMENT OF SIDE EFFECTS

## MANAGEMENT OF DRUG-RELATED PROBLEMS

Patients may experience some type of side effect or adverse drug reaction as a result of their drug therapy. The type of effect, the severity, and the frequency of occurrence is dependent on the medication and dose being used, as well as the individual's response to therapy. The following information is presented as helpful tips to assist the patient through these drug-related problems. Pharmacological support may also be required for their management.

### Alopecia

- Your hair loss is temporary. Hair usually will begin to grow within 3-6 months of completing drug therapy.
- Your hair may come back with a different texture, color, or thickness.
- Avoid excessive shampooing and hair combing, or harsh hair care products.
- Avoid excessive drying of hair.
- Avoid use of permanents, dyes, or hair sprays.
- Always cover head in cold weather or sunshine.

### Anemia

- Observe all bleeding precautions (see Thrombocytopenia).
- Get adequate sleep and rest.
- Be alert for potential for dizziness, fainting, or extreme fatigue.
- Maintain adequate nutrition and hydration.
- Have laboratory tests done as recommended.
- If unusual bleeding occurs, notify prescriber.

### Anorexia

- Small frequent meals containing favorite foods may tempt appetite.
- Eat simple foods such as toast, rice, bananas, mashed potatoes, scrambled eggs.
- Eat in a pleasant environment conducive to eating.
- When possible, eat with others.
- Avoid noxious odors when eating.
- Use nutritional supplements high in protein and calories.
- Freezing nutritional supplements sometimes makes them more palatable.
- A small glass of wine (if not contraindicated) may stimulate appetite.
- Mild exercise or short walks may stimulate appetite.
- Request antiemetic medication to reduce nausea or vomiting.

### Diarrhea

- Include fiber, high protein foods, and fruits in dietary intake.
- Drink plenty of liquids.
- Buttermilk, yogurt, or boiled milk may be helpful.
- Antidiarrheal agents may be needed. Consult your prescriber.
- Include regular rest periods in your activities.
- Institute skin care regimen to prevent breakdown and promote comfort.

### Fluid Retention/Edema

- Elevate legs when sitting.
- Wear support hose.
- Increase physical exercise.
- Maintain adequate hydration; avoiding fluids will not reduce edema.
- Weigh yourself regularly.
- If your prescriber has advised you to limit your salt intake, avoid foods such as ham, bacon, processed meats, and canned foods. Many foods are high in salt content. Read labels carefully.

- Report to prescriber if any of the following occur: sudden weight gain, decrease in urination, swelling of hands or feed, increase in waist size, wet cough, or difficulty breathing.

**Headache**

- Lie down.
- Use cool cloth on forehead.
- Avoid caffeine.
- Use mild analgesics. Consult prescriber.

**Leukopenia/Neutropenia**

- Monitor for signs of infections: persistent sore throat, fever, chills, fatigue, headache, flu-like symptoms, vaginal discharge, foul-smelling stools.
- Prevent infection. Maintain strict handwashing at all times. Avoid crowds when possible. Avoid exposure to infected persons.
- Avoid exposure to temperature changes.
- Maintain adequate nutrition and hydration.
- Maintain good personal hygiene.
- Avoid injury or skin breaks.
- Avoid vaccinations (unless recommended by healthcare provider).
- Avoid sunburn.

**Nausea and Vomiting**

- Eat food served cold or at room temperature. Ice chips are sometimes helpful.
- Drink clear liquids in severe cases of nausea. Avoid carbonated beverages.
- Sip liquids slowly.
- Avoid spicy food. Bland foods are easier to digest.
- Rinse mouth with lemon water. Practice good oral hygiene.
- Avoid sweet, fatty, salty foods and foods with strong odors.
- Eat small frequent meals rather than heavy meals.
- Use relaxation techniques and guided imagery.
- Use distractions such as meals, television, reading, games, etc.
- Sleep during intense periods of nausea.
- Chew gum or suck on hard candy or lozenges.
- Eat in an upright (sitting position), rather than semirecumbant.
- Avoid tight constrictive clothing at meal time.
- Use some mild exercise following light meals rather than lying down.
- Request antiemetic medication to reduce nausea or vomiting.

**Postural Hypotension**

- Use care and rise slowly from sitting or lying position to standing.
- Use care when climbing stairs.
- Initiate ambulation slowly. Get your bearings before you start walking.
- Do not bend over; always squat slowly if you must pick up something from floor.
- Use caution when showering or bathing (use secure handrails).

**Stomatitis**

- Perform good oral hygiene frequently, especially before and after meals.
- Avoid use of strong or alcoholic commercial mouthwashes.
- Keep lips well lubricated.
- Avoid tobacco or other products that are irritating to the oral mucosa.
- Avoid hot, spicy, excessively salty foods.
- Eat soft foods and drink adequate fluids.
- Request topical or systemic analgesics for painful ulcerations.
- Be alert for and report signs of oral fungal infections.

**Thrombocytopenia**

- Avoid aspirin and aspirin-containing products.

## THERAPEUTIC NURSING MANAGEMENT OF SIDE EFFECTS *(Continued)*

- Use electric or safety razor and blunt scissors.
- Use soft toothbrush or cotton swabs for oral care. Avoid use of dental floss.
- Avoid use of enemas, cathartics, and suppositories unless approved by prescriber.
- Avoid valsalva maneuvers such as straining at stool.
- Use stool softeners if necessary to prevent constipation. Consult prescriber.
- Avoid blowing nose forcefully.
- Never go barefoot, wear protective foot covering.
- Use care when trimming nails (if necessary).
- Maintain safe environment; arrange furniture to provide safe passageway.
- Maintain adequate lighting in darkened areas to avoid bumping into objects.
- Avoid handling sharp tools or instruments.
- Avoid contact sports or activities that might result in injury.
- Promptly report signs of bleeding; abdominal pain; blood in stool, urine, or vomitus; unusual fatigue; easy bruising; bleeding around gums; or nosebleeds.
- If injection or bloodsticks are necessary, inform healthcare provider that you may have excess bleeding.

**Vertigo**

- Observe postural hypotension precautions.
- Use caution when driving or using any machinery.
- Avoid sudden position shifts; do not "rush".
- Utilize appropriate supports (eg, cane, walker) to prevent injury.

# SELECTED REFERENCES

Bennett WM, Arnoff, GR, Golper TA, et al, *Drug Prescribing in Renal Failure, Dosing Guidelines for Adults*, 3rd ed, Philadelphia, PA: American College of Physicians, 1994.

Briggs GG, Freeman RK, and Yaffe SJ, *Drugs in Pregnancy and Lactation*, 5th ed, Baltimore, MD: Williams and Wilkins, 1998.

*Compendium of Pharmaceuticals and Specialties*, 37th ed, Toronto, Canada: Canadian Pharmaceutical Association, Webcom Limited, 1997.

*Diccionarieo De Especialidades Farmaceuticas*, 41th ed, Versailles, KY: Rand McNally Book Services, 1995.

Donnelly AJ, Cunningham FE, and Baughman VL, *Anesthesiology & Critical Care Drug Handbook*, 2nd ed, Hudson, OH: Lexi-Comp Inc. 1999.

*Drug Interaction Facts*, St Louis, MO: J.B. Lippincott Co (Facts and Comparisons Division), 1998.

*Facts and Comparisons*, St Louis, MO: J.B. Lippincott Co (Facts and Comparisons Division), 1998.

Fuller MA and Sajatovic M, *Drug Information Handbook for Psychiatry*, Hudson, OH: Lexi-Comp Inc, 1999.

Grabenstein JD, *ImmunoFacts Vaccines and Immunologic Drugs*, St Louis, MO: Facts and Comparisons, 1995.

*Handbook of Nonprescription Drugs*, Washington, DC: American Pharmaceutical Association, 1996.

Hansten PD and Horn JR, *Hansten and Horns Drug Interactions Analysis and Management*, Vancouver, WA: Applied Therapeutics, Inc, 1998.

Isada CM, Kasten BL, Goldman MP, et al, *Infectious Disease Handbook*, 3rd ed, Hudson, OH: Lexi-Comp Inc, 1999.

Jacobs DS, DeMott WR, Finley PR, et al, *Laboratory Test Handbook With Key Word Index*, 3rd ed, Hudson, OH: Lexi-Comp Inc, 1996.

Katzung BG, *Basic and Clinical Pharmacology*, 7th ed, Prentice Hall, 1997.

Lacy CF, Armstrong LL, Ingram NB, and Lance LL, *Drug Information Handbook*, 7th ed, Hudson, OH: Lexi-Comp Inc, 1999.

Lance LL, Lacy CF, and Goldman MP, *Drug Information Handbook for the Allied Health Professional*, 6th ed, Hudson, OH: Lexi-Comp Inc, 1999.

Leikin JB and Paloucek FP, *Poisoning & Toxicology Compendium*, 2nd ed, Hudson, OH: Lexi-Comp Inc, 1998.

*Martindale the Extra Pharmacopoeia*, 31st ed, London, England: Royal Pharmaceutical Society of Great Britain, 1996.

McEvoy GK and Litvak K, *AHFS Drug Information*, Bethesda, MD: American Society of Health-System Pharmacists, 1998.

*Physician's Desk Reference*, 52nd ed, Montvale, NJ: Medical Economics Books, 1996.

*Physician's Desk Reference for Ophthalmology*, 26th ed, Montvale, NJ: Medical Economics Books, 1997.

Semla TP, Beizer JL, and Higbee MD, *Geriatric Dosage Handbook*, 4th ed, Hudson, OH: Lexi-Comp Inc, 1998.

Taketomo CK, Hodding JH, and Kraus DM, *Pediatric Dosage Handbook*, 6th ed, Hudson, OH: Lexi-Comp Inc, 1999.

Trissel LA, *Handbook on Injectable Drugs*, 9th ed, Bethesda, MD: American Society of Health-System Pharmacists, Inc, 1996.

*United States Pharmacopeia Dispensing Information (USP DI)*, 18th ed, Rockville, MD: United States Pharmacopeial Convention, Inc, 1998.

Wynn RL, Meiller TF, and Crossley HL, *Drug Information Handbook for Dentistry*, 4th ed, Hudson, OH: Lexi-Comp Inc, 1998.

Zucchero FJ, Hogan MJ, and Schultz CD, *Evaluations of Drug Interactions*, St Louis, MO: First Data Bank, 1995.

# ALPHABETICAL LISTING OF DRUGS

♦ **A-200™ Shampoo** *see page 1294*

♦ **A and D™ Ointment** *see page 1294*

## Abacavir (a BAK a veer)

**U.S. Brand Names** Ziagen®

**Therapeutic Category** Antiretroviral Agent, Reverse Transcriptase Inhibitor (Nucleoside)

**Pregnancy Risk Factor** Unknown

**Lactation** Excretion in breast milk unknown/contraindicated

**Use** Investigational as of 8/1/98; treatment of HIV infections in combination with at least two other antiretroviral agents

**Mechanism of Action/Effect** Nucleoside reverse transcriptase inhibitor which interferes with HIV viral RNA dependent DNA polymerase resulting in inhibition of viral replication

**Contraindications** Hypersensitivity to abacavir or carbovir; do not rechallenge patients who have experienced hypersensitivity to abacavir

**Adverse Reactions**

Central nervous system: Headache

Dermatologic: Rash

Gastrointestinal: Nausea

Neuromuscular & skeletal: Weakness

Miscellaneous: Hypersensitivity reaction [fever, rash (in 50% of patients), nausea (within 4 weeks of initiating therapy)]

**Pharmacodynamics/Kinetics**

**Half-life Elimination:** 0.8-1.5 hours

**Time to Peak:** 0.7-1.7 hours

**Metabolism:** Liver

**Excretion:** Urine

**Dosing**

**Adults:** Oral: 600-1200 mg/day in 2-3 divided doses

**Elderly:** Refer to adult dosing.

**Additional Nursing Issues**

**Physical Assessment:** Assess for previous reaction to abacavir (do not administer if previous reaction). Monitor laboratory tests on a regular basis. Monitor for signs of opportunistic infection (eg, fever, sore throat, easy bruising or bleeding, mouth sores, unhealed sores). **Pregnancy risk factor unknown** - benefits of use should outweigh possible risks. Breast-feeding is contraindicated.

**Patient Information/Instruction:** This is not a cure for AIDS or AIDS complex, nor will it reduce the risk of transmission to others. Long-term effects are not known. You will need frequent blood tests to adjust dosage for maximum therapeutic effect. Take as directed, for full course of therapy; do not discontinue (even if feeling better). You may experience headache or muscle pain or weakness. Report skin rash, acute headache, severe nausea or vomiting, or difficulty breathing. **Pregnancy/breast-feeding precautions:** Inform prescriber if you are or intend to be pregnant. Do not breast-feed.

**Additional Information** Product information was not available at the time of this writing; abacavir expanded access program: 1-800-501-4672.

**Related Information**

Antiretroviral Agents Comparison *on page 1373*

♦ **Abbokinase® Injection** *see* Urokinase *on page 1195*

♦ **Abbreviations & Symbols Commonly Used in Medical Orders** *see page 1242*

♦ **ABCD** *see* Amphotericin B Cholesteryl Sulfate Complex *on page 85*

## Abciximab (ab SIK si mab)

**U.S. Brand Names** ReoPro®

**Synonyms** C7E3

**Therapeutic Category** Antiplatelet Agent, Glycoprotein IIb/IIIa Inhibitor

**Pregnancy Risk Factor** C

**Lactation** Excretion in breast milk unknown

**Use** Adjunct to percutaneous transluminal coronary angioplasty or atherectomy (PTCA) for the prevention of acute cardiac ischemic complications in patients at high risk for abrupt closure of the treated coronary vessel

**Mechanism of Action/Effect** Inhibits fibrinogen binding, platelet aggregation, and prolongs bleeding time.

**Contraindications** Hypersensitivity to abciximab or to murine proteins; active internal hemorrhage or recent (within 6 weeks) clinically significant GI or GU bleeding; history of cerebrovascular accident within 2 years or cerebrovascular accident with significant neurological deficit; clotting abnormalities or administration of oral anticoagulants within 7 days unless prothrombin time (PT) is ≤1.2 times control PT value; thrombocytopenia (<100,000 cells/µL); recent (within 6 weeks) major surgery or trauma; intracranial tumor, arteriovenous malformation, or aneurysm; severe uncontrolled hypertension; history of vasculitis; use of dextran before PTCA or intent to use dextran during PTCA

**Warnings** Administration of abciximab is associated with increased frequency of major bleeding complications including retroperitoneal bleeding, spontaneous GI or GU bleeding, and bleeding at the arterial access site and in the following: patients weighing <75 kilograms, elderly patients (>65 years of age), history of previous GI disease, recent thrombolytic therapy.

Increased risk of hemorrhage during or following angioplasty is associated with unsuccessful PTCA, PTCA procedure >70 minutes duration, or PTCA performed within 12 hours of symptom onset for acute myocardial infarction.

There is no data concerning the safety or efficacy of readministration of abciximab. Administration of abciximab may result in human antichimeric antibody formation that can cause hypersensitivity reactions (including anaphylaxis), thrombocytopenia, or diminished efficacy. Anticoagulation, such as with heparin, may contribute to the risk of bleeding.

Pregnancy factor C.

**Drug Interactions**

**Increased Effect/Toxicity:** Bleeding is increased when given with heparin, other anticoagulants, thrombolytics, or antiplatelet drugs. Allergic reactions may occur when abciximab is taken with diagnostic or therapeutic monoclonal antibodies.

**Adverse Reactions**

>10%:

Cardiovascular: Hypotension
Central nervous system: Pain
Hematologic: Major bleeding episodes

1% to 10%:

Gastrointestinal: Nausea, vomiting
Hematologic: Minor bleeding episodes, thrombocytopenia
Ocular: Abnormal vision

<1% (Limited to important or life-threatening symptoms): Anemia, leukocytosis, bradycardia, peripheral edema, pleural effusion, pneumonia

**Overdose/Toxicology** Since abciximab is a platelet antiaggregate, patients who bleed following administration may be best treated with platelet infusions.

**Pharmacodynamics/Kinetics**

**Metabolism:** Liver and kidney

**Excretion:** Urine, feces, lung

**Formulations** Injection: 2 mg/mL (5 mL)

**Dosing**

**Adults:** I.V.: 0.25 mg/kg bolus 10-60 minutes prior to starting PTCA, followed by a continuous infusion of 10 mcg/minute for 12 hours

**Elderly:** Refer to adult dosing.

**Administration**

**I.V.:** Infuse at a rate of 17 mL/hour (10 mcg/minute) for 12 hours via pump.

**I.V. Detail:** Do not shake vial. Always withdraw abciximab through a 0.22 micron filter. Continuous infusion: Use 4.5 mL (9 mg) of abciximab in 250 mL of NS or $D_5W$ to make a solution with a final concentration of 35 mcg/mL.

**Stability**

**Storage:** Vials should be stored at 2°C to 8°C. Do not freeze.

**Reconstitution:** After admixture, the prepared solution is stable for 12 hours.

**Compatibility:** Abciximab should be administered in a separate intravenous line. No incompatibilities have been observed with glass bottles or PVC bags.

**Monitoring Laboratory Tests** Prothrombin time, activated partial thromboplastin time, hemoglobin, hematocrit, platelet count, fibrinogen, fibrin split products

**Additional Nursing Issues**

**Physical Assessment:** Monitor vital signs and laboratory results prior to, during, and after therapy. Assess infusion insertion site and peripheral pulses during and after therapy (every 15 minutes or as institutional policy). Observe and teach patient bleeding precautions (avoid invasive procedures and activities that could result in injury). Monitor closely for signs of excessive bleeding (CNS changes; blood in urine, stool, or vomitus; unusual bruising or bleeding). **Pregnancy risk factor C.** Note breast-feeding caution.

**Patient Information/Instruction:** This medication can only be administered I.V. You will have a tendency to bleed easily following this medication; use caution to prevent injury (use electric razor, use soft toothbrush, and use caution with sharps). If bleeding occurs, apply pressure to bleeding spot until bleeding stops completely. Report unusual bruising or bleeding; blood in urine, stool, or vomitus; bleeding gums; or changes in vision. **Breast-feeding precautions:** Consult prescriber if breast-feeding.

**Additional Information** Abciximab is intended for coadministration with aspirin postangioplasty and heparin infused and weight adjusted to maintain a therapeutic bleeding time (eg, ACT 300-500 seconds).

- **Abelcet™ Injection** *see* Amphotericin B Lipid Complex *on page 87*
- **Abenol®** *see* Acetaminophen *on page 32*
- **Abitrate®** *see* Clofibrate *on page 285*
- **ABLC** *see* Amphotericin B Lipid Complex *on page 87*
- **Absorbine® Antifungal** *see page 1247*
- **Absorbine® Antifungal Foot Powder [OTC]** *see* Miconazole *on page 767*
- **Absorbine® Jock Itch** *see page 1247*
- **Absorbine Jr.® Antifungal** *see page 1247*
- **Acanol** *see* Loperamide *on page 688*

## Acarbose (AY car bose)

**U.S. Brand Names** Precose®

**Therapeutic Category** Antidiabetic Agent (Miscellaneous)

**Pregnancy Risk Factor** B

(Continued)

## Acarbose *(Continued)*

**Lactation** Excretion in breast milk unknown

**Use** Monotherapy, as indicated as an adjunct to diet to lower blood glucose in patients with noninsulin-dependent diabetes mellitus (NIDDM) whose hyperglycemia cannot be managed on diet alone; in combination with a sulfonylurea, insulin, or metformin when diet plus either agent alone does not result in adequate glycemic control. The effect of acarbose to enhance glycemic control is additive to that of other hypoglycemic agents when used in combination.

**Mechanism of Action/Effect** Delays glucose absorption and lowers postprandial hyperglycemia.

**Contraindications** Hypersensitivity to acarbose or any component; patients with diabetic ketoacidosis or cirrhosis; patients with inflammatory bowel disease, colonic ulceration, partial intestinal obstruction, or in patients predisposed to intestinal obstruction; patients who have chronic intestinal diseases associated with marked disorders of digestion or absorption and in patients who have conditions that may deteriorate as a result of increased gas formation in the intestine

**Warnings** Patients receiving sulfonylureas: Acarbose given in combination with a sulfonylurea will cause a further lowering of blood glucose and may increase the hypoglycemic potential of the sulfonylurea. If hypoglycemia occurs, appropriate adjustments in the dosage of these agents should be made. Oral glucose (dextrose) should be used in the treatment of mild to moderate hypoglycemia.

Elevated serum transaminase levels: Treatment-emergent elevations of serum transaminases (AST and/or ALT) occurred in 15% of acarbose-treated patients in long-term studies. These serum transaminase elevations appear to be dose related and were asymptomatic, reversible, more common in females, and, in general, were not associated with other evidence of liver dysfunction.

**Drug Interactions**

**Decreased Effect:** The effect of acarbose is decreased when taken with diuretics, corticosteroids, phenothiazines, thyroid products, estrogens, oral contraceptives, phenytoin, nicotinic acid, sympathomimetics, calcium channel-blocking drugs, isoniazid, intestinal adsorbents, and digestive enzyme preparations.

**Increased Effect/Toxicity:** See Warnings/Precautions.

**Adverse Reactions**

>10%:

Gastrointestinal: Abdominal pain (21%) and diarrhea (33%) tend to return to pretreatment levels over time, and the frequency and intensity of flatulence (77%) tend to abate with time

Hepatic: Elevated liver transaminases

<1% (Limited to important or life-threatening symptoms): Severe gastrointestinal distress

**Pharmacodynamics/Kinetics**

**Metabolism:** GI tract

**Excretion:** Renal

**Formulations** Tablet: 50 mg, 100 mg

**Dosing**

**Adults:** Oral: Dosage must be individualized on the basis of effectiveness and tolerance while not exceeding the maximum recommended dose of 100 mg 3 times/day.

Initial: 25 mg 3 times/day

Maintenance dose: Should be adjusted at 4- to 8-week intervals based on 1-hour postprandial glucose levels and tolerance until maintenance dose is reached; maintenance dose: 50-100 mg 3 times/day.

Maximum:

≤60 kg: 50 mg 3 times/day

>60 kg: 100 mg 3 times/day

**Elderly:** Refer to adult dosing.

**Renal Impairment:** Use of acarbose in patients with significant renal impairment is not recommended.

**Administration**

**Oral:** Drug should be **taken with the first bite of each main meal.**

**Stability**

**Storage:** Store at <25°C (77°F) and protect from moisture.

**Monitoring Laboratory Tests** Postprandial glucose, glycosylated hemoglobin levels, and serum transaminase levels should be checked every 3 months during the first year of treatment and periodically thereafter.

**Additional Nursing Issues**

**Physical Assessment:** Assess effectiveness and interactions of other medications (see Drug Interactions). See Warnings/Precautions and Contraindications for use cautions. Monitor effectiveness of therapy and monitor laboratory tests every 3 months during therapy (see above). Monitor for adverse response (eg, hypoglycemia - see Adverse Reactions and Overdose/Toxicology). Assess knowledge/teach patient or refer patient to diabetic educator for instruction in appropriate use, possible side effects and appropriate interventions, and adverse symptoms to report. Note breast-feeding caution.

**Patient Information/Instruction:** Take this medication exactly as directed, with the first bite of each main meal. Do not change dosage or discontinue without first consulting prescriber. Do not take other medications with or within 2 hours of this medication unless so advised by prescriber. It is important to follow dietary and lifestyle recommendations of prescriber. You will be instructed in signs of hypo-/hyperglycemia by prescriber or diabetic educator. If combining acarbose with other diabetic medication (eg, sulfonylureas, insulin), keep source of glucose (sugar) on hand in case hypoglycemia occurs. You may experience mild side effects during first weeks of acarbose therapy (eg, bloating, flatulence, diarrhea, abdominal discomfort); these should diminish over time. Report severe or persistent side effects, fever, extended vomiting or flu, or change in color of urine or stool. **Breast-feeding precautions:** Consult prescriber if breast-feeding.

**Geriatric Considerations:** Monitor change in preprandial blood glucose concentrations to account for potential age-related changes in postprandial glucose.

**Related Information**

Antidiabetic Oral Agents Comparison *on page 1370*

♦ **Accolate®** *see* Zafirlukast *on page 1223*

♦ **Accupril®** *see* Quinapril *on page 1001*

♦ **Accutane®** *see* Isotretinoin *on page 637*

## Acebutolol (a se BYOO toe lole)

**U.S. Brand Names** Sectral®

**Therapeutic Category** Antiarrhythmic Agent, Class II; Beta Blocker (with Intrinsic Sympathomimetic Activity)

**Pregnancy Risk Factor** B/D (2nd and 3rd trimesters)

**Lactation** Enters breast milk/use caution (AAP rates "compatible")

**Use** Treatment of hypertension, ventricular arrhythmias, angina

**Mechanism of Action/Effect** Nonselectively blocks beta receptors in heart and kidney; decreases excitability of the heart, cardiac output, and oxygen consumption; release of renin from kidney

**Contraindications** Hypersensitivity to beta-blocking agents. Avoid use in uncompensated congestive heart failure, cardiogenic shock, bradycardia or heart block, sinus node dysfunction, and A-V conduction abnormalities. Although acebutolol primarily blocks $beta_1$-receptors, high doses can result in $beta_2$-receptor blockage. Pregnancy (2nd and 3rd trimesters).

**Warnings** Abrupt withdrawal of drug **should be avoided.** May result in an exaggerated cardiac responsiveness such as tachycardia, hypertension, ischemia, angina, myocardial infarction, and sudden death. It is recommended that patients be tapered gradually off of beta-blockers over a 2-week period rather than via abrupt discontinuation. Use with caution in diabetic patients. Beta-blockers may impair glucose tolerance, potentiate hypoglycemia, and/or mask symptoms of hypoglycemia in a diabetic patient. Use with caution in bronchospastic lung disease and renal dysfunction (especially the elderly). See Dosing - Renal/Hepatic Impairment.

**Drug Interactions**

**Decreased Effect:** Decreased effect of beta-blockers with aluminum salts, barbiturates, calcium salts, cholestyramine, colestipol, NSAIDs, penicillins (ampicillin), rifampin, and salicylates due to decreased bioavailability and plasma levels. Decreased effect of sulfonylureas with beta-blockers. However, the decreased effect has not been shown with tolbutamide.

**Increased Effect/Toxicity:** Increased effect/toxicity of acebutolol with reserpine has been shown to enhance the effect and may present with bradycardia, hypotension, vertigo, syncope or orthostatic changes in blood pressure without compensatory tachycardia. Avoid using with alpha adrenergic stimulants (phenylephrine, epinephrine, etc) which may have exaggerated hypertensive responses. Beta-blockers may affect the action or levels of ethanol, disopyramide, nondepolarizing muscle relaxants and theophylline although the effects are difficult to predict.

**Food Interactions** Peak serum acebutolol levels may be slightly decreased if taken with food.

**Effects on Lab Values** ↑ triglycerides, potassium, uric acid, cholesterol (S), glucose, thyroxine (S); ↓ HDL

**Adverse Reactions**

>10%: Central nervous system: Fatigue

1% to 10%:

- Cardiovascular: Chest pain, edema, bradycardia, hypotension
- Central nervous system: Headache, dizziness, insomnia, depression, abnormal dreams
- Dermatologic: Rash
- Gastrointestinal: Constipation, diarrhea, heartburn, nausea, flatulence
- Genitourinary: Polyuria
- Neuromuscular & skeletal: Arthralgia, myalgia
- Ocular: Abnormal vision
- Respiratory: Dyspnea, bronchospasm, rhinitis, cough

<1% (Limited to important or life-threatening symptoms): Ventricular arrhythmias, heart block, heart failure

**Overdose/Toxicology** Symptoms of intoxication include cardiac disturbances, CNS toxicity, bronchospasm, hypoglycemia, and hyperkalemia. The most common cardiac symptoms include hypotension and bradycardia. Atrioventricular block, intraventricular conduction disturbances, cardiogenic shock, and asystole may occur with severe overdose, especially with membrane-depressant drugs (eg, propranolol). CNS effects include convulsions and coma. Respiratory arrest (commonly seen with propranolol and other membrane-depressant and lipid-soluble drugs). Treat symptomatically. Cardiac and hemodynamic monitoring may be necessary.

(Continued)

## Acebutolol *(Continued)*

**Pharmacodynamics/Kinetics**

**Protein Binding:** 5% to 15%

**Half-life Elimination:** 6-7 hours average

**Time to Peak:** 2-4 hours

**Metabolism:** Liver

**Excretion:** Bile and urine

**Onset:** 1-2 hours

**Duration:** 12-24 hours

**Formulations** Capsule, as hydrochloride: 200 mg, 400 mg

**Dosing**

**Adults:** Oral: 400-800 mg/day twice daily; maximum: 1200 mg/day

**Elderly:** Oral: Initial: 200-400 mg/day; dose reduction due to age-related decrease in $Cl_{cr}$ will be necessary; do not exceed 800 mg/day.

**Renal Impairment:**

$Cl_{cr}$ 25-49 mL/minute/1.73 $m^2$: Reduce dose by 50%.

$Cl_{cr}$ <25 mL/minute/1.73 $m^2$: Reduce dose by 75%.

**Hepatic Impairment:** Use with caution.

**Additional Nursing Issues**

**Physical Assessment:** Assess effectiveness and interactions of other medications (see Drug Interactions). See Warnings/Precautions and Contraindications for use cautions. Monitor effectiveness of therapy, laboratory tests, and adverse response on a regular basis during therapy (see Adverse Reactions and Overdose/Toxicology). When discontinuing therapy, taper dosage over 2 weeks. Assess knowledge/teach patient appropriate use, possible side effects (including altered glucose tolerance for diabetics) and appropriate interventions, and adverse symptoms to report. **Pregnancy Risk Factor B/D - see Pregnancy Risk Factor.** Note breast-feeding caution.

**Patient Information/Instruction:** Take exactly as directed; do not increase, decrease, or adjust dosage without consulting prescriber. Take pulse daily, prior to medication, and follow prescriber's instruction about holding medication. Do not take with antacids. Do not use alcohol and OTC medications such as cold remedies without consulting prescriber. If diabetic, monitor serum sugars closely (may alter glucose tolerance or mask signs of hypoglycemia). May cause fatigue, dizziness (use caution when driving or engaging in tasks that require alertness until response to drug is known); postural hypotension (use caution when changing position from lying or sitting to standing or when climbing stairs); or alteration in sexual performance (reversible). Report chest pain or palpitations, unresolved swelling of extremities or unusual weight gain, difficulty breathing or new cough, skin rash, unresolved fatigue, unresolved constipation or diarrhea, unusual muscle weakness, or CNS disturbances. **Pregnancy/breast-feeding precautions:** Inform prescriber if you are pregnant. Consult prescriber if breast-feeding.

**Geriatric Considerations:** Geriatric patients may require dose reduction due to age related decrease in $Cl_{cr}$. Beta-adrenergic blocking drugs may result in a decreased response as compared to younger adults.

**Related Information**

Beta-Blockers Comparison *on page 1376*


- **ACE Inhibitors and Angiotensin Antagonists Comparison** *see page 1362*
- **Acel-Imune®** *see page 1256*
- **Acenex®** *see page 1294*
- **Aceon®** *see* Perindopril Erbumine *on page 910*
- **Acephen® [OTC]** *see* Acetaminophen *on this page*
- **Aceta® [OTC]** *see* Acetaminophen *on this page*


## Acetaminophen (a seet a MIN oh fen)

**U.S. Brand Names** Acephen® [OTC]; Aceta® [OTC]; Apacet® [OTC]; Dapa® [OTC]; Dorcol® [OTC]; Feverall™ [OTC]; Genapap® [OTC]; Infants Feverall™ [OTC]; Neopap® [OTC]; Panadol® [OTC]; Tempra® [OTC]; Tylenol® [OTC]

**Synonyms** APAP; N-Acetyl-P-Aminophenol; Paracetamol

**Therapeutic Category** Analgesic, Miscellaneous

**Pregnancy Risk Factor** B

**Lactation** Enters breast milk/compatible

**Use** Treatment of mild to moderate pain and fever; does not have anti-inflammatory effects

**Mechanism of Action/Effect** Reduces fever by acting on the hypothalamus to cause vasodilatation and sweating

**Contraindications** Hypersensitivity to acetaminophen or any component; patients with known G-6-PD deficiency

**Warnings** May cause severe hepatic toxicity on overdose. Use with caution in patients with alcoholic liver disease or who consume large amounts of alcohol. Chronic daily dosing in adults of 5-8 g of acetaminophen over several weeks or 3-4 g/day of acetaminophen for 1 year have resulted in liver damage.

**Drug Interactions**

**Cytochrome P-450 Effect:** CYP1A2 enzyme substrate (minor), CYP2E1 and 3A3/4 enzyme substrate

**Decreased Effect:** Rifampin can interact to reduce the analgesic effectiveness of acetaminophen.

**Increased Effect/Toxicity:** Alcohol abuse, barbiturates, carbamazepine, hydantoins, and sulfinpyrazone can increase the hepatotoxic potential of acetaminophen. Warfarin effect may be enhanced.

**Food Interactions** Peak serum acetaminophen levels may be decreased if taken with food.

**Effects on Lab Values** ↑ chloride, bilirubin, uric acid, glucose, ammonia (B), chloride (S), uric acid (S), alkaline phosphatase (S), chloride (S); ↓ sodium, bicarbonate, calcium (S)

**Adverse Reactions** <1% (Limited to important or life-threatening symptoms): Blood dyscrasias (agranulocytosis, thrombocytopenia, neutropenia, pancytopenia, leukopenia), anemia, hepatitis, analgesic nephropathy, nephrotoxicity with chronic overdose, sterile pyuria

**Overdose/Toxicology** Symptoms of overdose include hepatic necrosis, transient azotemia, renal tubular necrosis with acute toxicity, anemia, and GI disturbances with chronic toxicity. Treatment consists of acetylcysteine 140 mg/kg orally (loading) followed by 70 mg/kg every 4 hours for 17 doses; therapy should be initiated based upon laboratory analysis suggesting a high probability of hepatotoxic potential. Activated charcoal is very effective at binding acetaminophen. Intravenous acetylcysteine should be reserved for patients unable to take oral forms.

**Pharmacodynamics/Kinetics**

**Half-life Elimination:** Adults: Normal renal function: 1-3 hours; End-stage renal disease: 1-3 hours

**Time to Peak:** Oral: 10-60 minutes after normal doses, may be delayed in acute overdoses

**Metabolism:** Liver

**Excretion:** Urine

**Onset:** <1 hour

**Duration:** 4-6 hours

**Formulations**

Caplet: 160 mg, 325 mg, 500 mg
Caplet, extended: 650 mg
Capsule: 80 mg
Drops: 48 mg/mL (15 mL); 60 mg/0.6 mL (15 mL); 80 mg/0.8 mL (15 mL); 100 mg/mL (15 mL, 30 mL)
Elixir: 80 mg/5 mL, 120 mg/5 mL, 160 mg/5 mL, 167 mg/5 mL, 325 mg/5 mL
Liquid, oral: 160 mg/5 mL, 500 mg/15 mL
Solution: 100 mg/mL (15 mL); 120 mg/2.5 mL
Suppository, rectal: 80 mg, 120 mg, 125 mg, 300 mg, 325 mg, 650 mg
Suspension, oral: 160 mg/5 mL
Suspension, oral drops: 80 mg/0.8 mL
Tablet: 325 mg, 500 mg, 650 mg
Tablet, chewable: 80 mg, 160 mg

**Dosing**

**Adults:** Oral, rectal: 325-650 mg every 4-6 hours or 1000 mg 3-4 times/day; do **not** exceed 4 g/day. If fever is not controlled with acetaminophen alone, give with full doses of ibuprofen on an every 4- to 6-hour schedule, if not otherwise contraindicated.

**Elderly:** Refer to adult dosing.

**Renal Impairment:**

$Cl_{cr}$ 10-50 mL/minute: Administer every 6 hours.
$Cl_{cr}$ <10 mL/minute: Administer every 8 hours (metabolites accumulate).
Moderately dialyzable (20% to 50%)

**Hepatic Impairment:** Appears to be well tolerated in cirrhosis. Serum levels may need monitoring with long-term use. Use with caution.

**Administration**

**Oral:** Shake suspension well before pouring dose.

**Stability**

**Storage:** Do not freeze suppositories.

**Monitoring Laboratory Tests** Serum APAP levels with long-term use in patients with hepatic disease

**Additional Nursing Issues**

**Physical Assessment: Assess patient for history of liver disease or alcohol abuse** (acetaminophen and excessive alcohol may have adverse liver effects). Assess other medications patient may be taking for additive or adverse interactions (see Drug Interactions). Monitor for therapeutic effectiveness and monitor for signs of overdose (see above). Monitor vital signs and signs of adverse reactions (see Adverse Reactions) at beginning of therapy and at regular intervals with long-term use. Assess knowledge/teach patient appropriate use. Teach patient to monitor for adverse reactions, adverse reactions to report, and appropriate interventions to reduce side effects.

**Patient Information/Instruction:** Take exactly as directed (do not increase dose or frequency); most adverse effects are related to excessive use. Take with food or milk. While using this medication, avoid alcohol and other prescription or OTC medications that contain acetaminophen. Maintain adequate hydration (2-3 L/day of fluids unless instructed to restrict fluid intake). This medication will not reduce inflammation; consult prescriber for anti-inflammatory, if needed. Report unusual bleeding (stool, mouth, urine) or bruising; unusual fatigue and weakness; change in elimination patterns; or change in color of urine or stool.

**Additional Information** Some formulations may contain ethanol.

♦ **Acetaminophen and Aspirin** *see page 1294*

- **Acetaminophen and Butalbital Compound** *see* Butalbital Compound and Acetaminophen *on page 175*

## Acetaminophen and Codeine (a seet a MIN oh fen & KOE deen)

**U.S. Brand Names** Capital® and Codeine; Phenaphen® With Codeine; Tylenol® With Codeine

**Synonyms** Codeine and Acetaminophen

**Therapeutic Category** Analgesic, Combination (Narcotic)

**Pregnancy Risk Factor** C

**Lactation** Enters breast milk/use caution

**Use** Relief of mild to moderate pain

**Formulations**

Capsule:

#2: Acetaminophen 325 mg and codeine phosphate 15 mg (C-III)
#3: Acetaminophen 325 mg and codeine phosphate 30 mg (C-III)
#4: Acetaminophen 325 mg and codeine phosphate 60 mg (C-III)

Elixir: Acetaminophen 120 mg and codeine phosphate 12 mg per 5 mL with alcohol 7% (C-V)

Suspension, oral, alcohol free: Acetaminophen 120 mg and codeine phosphate 12 mg per 5 mL (C-V)

Tablet: Acetaminophen 500 mg and codeine phosphate 30 mg (C-III); acetaminophen 650 mg and codeine phosphate 30 mg (C-III)

Tablet:

#1: Acetaminophen 300 mg and codeine phosphate 7.5 mg (C-III)
#2: Acetaminophen 300 mg and codeine phosphate 15 mg (C-III)
#3: Acetaminophen 300 mg and codeine phosphate 30 mg (C-III)
#4: Acetaminophen 300 mg and codeine phosphate 60 mg (C-III)

**Dosing**

**Adults:** Doses should be adjusted according to severity of pain and response of the patient. Adult doses ≥60 mg codeine fail to give commensurate relief of pain but merely prolong analgesia and are associated with an appreciably increased incidence of side effects. Oral:

Antitussive: Based on codeine (15-30 mg/dose) every 4-6 hours
Analgesic: Based on codeine (30-60 mg/dose) every 4-6 hours
1-2 tablets every 4 hours to a maximum of 12 tablets/24 hours

**Elderly:** Doses should be titrated to appropriate analgesic effect.
1 Tylenol® [#3] or 2 Tylenol® [#2] tablets every 4 hours; do **not** exceed 4 g/day acetaminophen.

**Renal Impairment:** Refer to individual monographs for Acetaminophen and Codeine.

**Additional Nursing Issues**

**Physical Assessment:** See individual components listed in Related Information. **Pregnancy risk factor C** - benefits of use should outweigh possible risks. Note breast-feeding caution.

**Patient Information/Instruction:** See individual components listed in Related Information. **Pregnancy/breast-feeding precautions:** Inform prescriber if you are or intend to be pregnant. Consult prescriber if breast-feeding.

**Additional Information** The elixir formulation contains ethanol.

**Related Information**

Acetaminophen *on page 32*
Codeine *on page 299*

- **Acetaminophen and Dextromethorphan** *see page 1294*
- **Acetaminophen and Diphenhydramine** *see page 1294*
- **Acetaminophen and Hydrocodone** *see* Hydrocodone and Acetaminophen *on page 568*
- **Acetaminophen and Oxycodone** *see* Oxycodone and Acetaminophen *on page 873*
- **Acetaminophen and Phenyltoloxamine** *see page 1294*
- **Acetaminophen and Propoxyphene** *see* Propoxyphene and Acetaminophen *on page 985*
- **Acetaminophen and Pseudoephedrine** *see page 1294*
- **Acetaminophen, Caffeine, Hydrocodone, Chlorpheniramine, and Phenylephrine** *see* Hydrocodone, Chlorpheniramine, Phenylephrine, Acetaminophen, and Caffeine *on page 576*
- **Acetaminophen, Chlorpheniramine, and Pseudoephedrine** *see page 1294*
- **Acetaminophen, Dextromethorphan, and Pseudoephedrine** *see page 1294*
- **Acetasol®** *see page 1291*
- **Acetasol HC®** *see page 1291*
- **Acetazolam®** *see* Acetazolamide *on this page*

## Acetazolamide (a set a ZOLE a mide)

**U.S. Brand Names** Diamox®; Diamox Sequels®

**Therapeutic Category** Anticonvulsant, Miscellaneous; Carbonic Anhydrase Inhibitor; Diuretic, Carbonic Anhydrase Inhibitor; Ophthalmic Agent, Antiglaucoma

**Pregnancy Risk Factor** C

**Lactation** Enters breast milk/compatible

**Use** Lowers intraocular pressure to treat glaucoma; diuretic; adjunct treatment of refractory seizures and acute altitude sickness; centrencephalic epilepsies

**Mechanism of Action/Effect** Reversible inhibition of the enzyme carbonic anhydrase resulting in reduction of hydrogen ion secretion at renal tubule and an increased renal excretion of sodium, potassium, bicarbonate, and water. Decreases production of aqueous humor; also inhibits carbonic anhydrase in central nervous system to retard abnormal and excessive discharge from CNS neurons.

**Contraindications** Hypersensitivity to sulfonamides or acetazolamide; patients with hepatic disease or insufficiency; patients with decreased sodium and/or potassium levels; patients with adrenocortical insufficiency, hyperchloremic acidosis, severe renal disease or dysfunction, or severe pulmonary obstruction; long-term use in noncongestive angle-closure glaucoma

**Warnings** Use in impaired hepatic function may result in coma. Use with caution in patients with respiratory acidosis and diabetes mellitus. Impairment of mental alertness and/or physical coordination may occur. I.M. administration is painful. Drug may cause substantial increase in blood glucose in some diabetic patients. Malaise and complaints of tiredness and myalgia are signs of excessive dosing and acidosis in the elderly. Cross-sensitivity between sulfonamide antibiotics and sulfonamide diuretics including various thiazide diuretics. **Sustained release is not recommended for anticonvulsant use.** Pregnancy factor C.

**Drug Interactions**

**Decreased Effect:** Use of acetazolamide may increase lithium excretion and alter excretion of other drugs by alkalinization of urine (such as amphetamines, quinidine, procainamide, methenamine, phenobarbital, salicylates). Primidone serum concentrations may be decreased.

**Increased Effect/Toxicity:** Concurrent use with diflunisal may increase the effect of acetazolamide causing a significant decrease in intraocular pressure. Increased side effects may result. Cyclosporine trough concentrations may be increased resulting in possible nephrotoxicity and neurotoxicity. Salicylate use may result in carbonic anhydrase inhibitor accumulation and toxicity including CNS depression and metabolic acidosis. Digitalis toxicity may occur if hypokalemia is untreated.

**Effects on Lab Values** May cause false-positive results for urinary protein with Albustix®, Labstix®, Albutest®, Bumintest®.

**Adverse Reactions**

>10%:
- Central nervous system: Malaise, unusual drowsiness or weakness
- Gastrointestinal: Anorexia, weight loss, diarrhea, metallic taste, nausea, vomiting
- Genitourinary: Polyuria
- Neuromuscular & skeletal: Numbness, tingling, or burning in hands, fingers, feet, toes, mouth, tongue, lips, or anus

1% to 10%:
- Central nervous system: Mental depression
- Renal: Renal calculi

<1% (Limited to important or life-threatening symptoms): Convulsions, hyperchloremic metabolic acidosis, hypokalemia, hyperglycemia, bone marrow suppression, blood dyscrasias, cholestatic jaundice

**Overdose/Toxicology** Symptoms of overdose include low blood sugar, tingling of lips and tongue, nausea, yawning, confusion, agitation, tachycardia, sweating, convulsions, stupor, and coma. Hypoglycemia should be managed with 50 mL I.V. dextrose 50% followed immediately with a continuous infusion of 10% dextrose in water (administer at a rate sufficient enough to approach a serum glucose level of 100 mg/dL). The use of corticosteroids to treat hypoglycemia is controversial, however, adding 100 mg of hydrocortisone to the dextrose infusion may prove helpful.

**Pharmacodynamics/Kinetics**

**Half-life Elimination:** 2.4-5.8 hours

**Excretion:** Urine

**Onset:** Extended release capsule: 2 hours; peak effect: 3-6 hours; I.V.: 2 minutes; peak effect: 15 minutes; Tablet, peak effect: 1-4 hours

**Duration:** Extended release capsule: 18-24 hours; Tablet: 8-12 hours; I.V.: 4-5 hours

**Formulations**

Capsule, sustained release: 500 mg
Injection: 500 mg
Tablet: 125 mg, 250 mg

**Dosing**

**Adults: Note:** I.M. administration is not recommended.

Glaucoma:
- Chronic simple (open-angle): Oral: 250 mg 1-4 times/day or 500 mg sustained release capsule twice daily
- Secondary, acute (closed-angle): I.M., I.V.: 250-500 mg, may repeat in 2-4 hours to a maximum of 1 g/day

Edema: Oral, I.M., I.V.: 250-375 mg once daily

Epilepsy: Oral: 8-30 mg/kg/day in 1-4 divided doses, not to exceed 1 g/day. **Sustained release capsule is not recommended for treatment of epilepsy.**

Altitude sickness: Oral: 250 mg every 8-12 hours (or 500 mg extended release capsules every 12-24 hours). Therapy should begin 24-48 hours before and continue during ascent and for at least 48 hours after arrival at the high altitude.

Urine alkalinization: Oral: 5 mg/kg/dose repeated 2-3 times over 24 hours

**Elderly:** Oral: Initial: 250 mg once or twice daily; use lowest effective dose possible.

**Renal Impairment:**

$Cl_{cr}$ 10-50 mL/minute: Administer every 12 hours.

$Cl_{cr}$ <10 mL/minute: Avoid use → ineffective.

Moderately dialyzable (20% to 50%)

(Continued)

## Acetazolamide *(Continued)*

**Administration**

**I.V.:** Recommended rate of administration: 100-500 mg/minute for I.V. push and 4-8 hours for I.V. infusions

**Stability**

**Reconstitution:** Reconstituted solution may be refrigerated (2°C to 8°C) for 1 week.

**Standard diluent:** 500 mg/50 mL $D_5W$

Minimum volume: 50 mL $D_5W$

Stability of IVPB solution is 5 days at room temperature (25°C) and 44 days at refrigeration (5°C). Reconstitute with at least 5 mL sterile water to provide a solution containing not more than 100 mg/mL. Further dilution in 50 mL of either $D_5W$ or NS for I.V. infusion administration.

**Monitoring Laboratory Tests** Intraocular pressure, serum electrolytes, periodic CBC with differential

**Additional Nursing Issues**

**Physical Assessment:** Assess allergy history prior to beginning therapy. Assess effectiveness and interactions of other medications (see Drug Interactions). See Warnings/Precautions and Contraindications for extensive use cautions. Monitor effectiveness of therapy, laboratory tests, including serum glucose (see above) and adverse response (see Adverse Reactions and Overdose/Toxicology). Assess knowledge/teach patient appropriate use, possible side effects and appropriate interventions, and adverse symptoms to report. **Pregnancy risk factor C** - benefits of use should outweigh possible risks.

**Patient Information/Instruction:** Take as directed; do not chew or crush long-acting capsule (contents may be sprinkled on soft food). You will need periodic ophthalmic examinations while taking this medication. You may experience drowsiness, dizziness, or weakness (use caution when driving or engaging in tasks that require alertness until response to drug is known); nausea, loss of appetite, or altered taste (small frequent meals, frequent mouth care, sucking lozenges, or chewing gum may help). Monitor serum glucose closely (may cause altered blood glucose in some diabetic patients, or unusual response to some forms of glucose testing); increased sensitivity to sunlight (use sunblock, protective clothing, and avoid exposure to direct sunlight). Report unusual and persistent tiredness; numbness, burning, or tingling of extremities or around mouth, lips, or anus; muscle weakness; black stool; or excessive depression. **Pregnancy precautions:** Inform prescriber if you are or intend to be pregnant.

**Geriatric Considerations:** Malaise and complaints of tiredness and myalgia are signs of excessive dosing and acidosis in the elderly. Assess blood pressure (orthostatic hypotension can occur).

**Additional Information** pH: 9.2

**Related Information**

Glaucoma Drug Comparison *on page 1385*

- **Acetic Acid and Aluminum Acetate** *see page 1291*
- **Acetic Acid and Hydrocortisone** *see page 1291*
- **Acetic Acid and Propylene Glycol** *see page 1291*
- **Acetic Acid Otic** *see page 1291*
- **Acetoxymethylprogesterone** *see* Medroxyprogesterone *on page 714*
- **Acetylcholine** *see page 1282*

## Acetylcysteine (a se teel SIS teen)

**U.S. Brand Names** Mucomyst®; Mucosil™

**Synonyms** Mercapturic Acid; NAC; *N*-Acetylcysteine; *N*-Acetyl-L-Cysteine

**Therapeutic Category** Antidote; Mucolytic Agent

**Pregnancy Risk Factor** B

**Lactation** Excretion in breast milk unknown/compatible

**Use** Adjunctive mucolytic therapy in patients with abnormal or viscid mucous secretions in acute and chronic bronchopulmonary diseases; pulmonary complications of surgery and cystic fibrosis; diagnostic bronchial studies; antidote for acute acetaminophen toxicity

**Unlabeled use:** Enema to treat bowel obstruction due to meconium ileus or its equivalent

**Mechanism of Action/Effect** Exerts mucolytic action through its free sulfhydryl group which opens up the disulfide bonds in the mucoproteins thus lowering mucous viscosity. The exact mechanism of action in acetaminophen toxicity is unknown. It is thought to act by providing substrate for conjugation with the toxic metabolite.

**Contraindications** Hypersensitivity to acetylcysteine or any component

**Warnings** Since increased bronchial secretions may develop after inhalation, percussion, postural drainage, and suctioning should follow. If bronchospasm occurs, administer a bronchodilator. Discontinue acetylcysteine if bronchospasm progresses.

**Adverse Reactions**

**Inhalation:**

>10%:

Stickiness on face after nebulization

Miscellaneous: Unpleasant odor during administration

1% to 10%:

Central nervous system: Drowsiness, chills, fever

Gastrointestinal: Vomiting, nausea, stomatitis

Local: Irritation

Respiratory: Bronchospasm, rhinorrhea, hemoptysis

Miscellaneous: Clamminess

**Systemic:**

1% to 10%:

Central nervous system: Fever, drowsiness

Gastrointestinal: Nausea, vomiting

<1% (Limited to important or life-threatening symptoms): Bronchospastic allergic reaction

**Overdose/Toxicology** Treatment of acetylcysteine toxicity is usually aimed at reversing anaphylactoid symptoms or controlling nausea and vomiting. The use of epinephrine, antihistamines, and steroids may be beneficial.

**Pharmacodynamics/Kinetics**

**Half-life Elimination:** Oral: Reduced acetylcysteine: 2 hours; Total acetylcysteine: 5.5 hours

**Metabolism:** Liver

**Excretion:** Urine

**Onset:** Oral: Peak plasma levels 1-2 hours; Inhalation: Mucus liquefaction occurs maximally within 5-10 minutes

**Duration:** Oral: Can persist for >1 hour

**Formulations** Solution, as sodium: 10% [100 mg/mL] (4 mL, 10 mL, 30 mL); 20% [200 mg/mL] (4 mL, 10 mL, 30 mL, 100 mL)

**Dosing**

**Adults:**

Acetaminophen poisoning: Loading dose: Oral: 140 mg/kg; followed by 70 mg/kg every 4 hours (for 17 doses); repeat dose if emesis occurs within 1 hour of administration. Therapy should continue until all doses are administered even though the acetaminophen plasma level has dropped below the toxic range.

Inhalation: Acetylcysteine 10% and 20% solution (Mucomyst®) (dilute 20% solution with sodium chloride or sterile water for inhalation); 10% solution may be used undiluted

Nebulization into face-mask, tracheostomy, mouth piece: 1-10 mL of 20% solution or 2-10 mL of 10% solution 3-4 times/day

Closed tent or croupette: Up to 300 mL of 10% or 20% solution treatment

Direct instillation into tracheostomy: 1-2 mL of 10% to 20% solution every 1-4 hours

Percutaneous intratracheal catheter: 1-2 mL of 20% solution or 2-4 mL of 10% solution every 1-4 hours by syringe attached to catheter

Instillation to a particular portion of bronchial tree using small plastic catheter (placed under local anesthesia and with direct visualization): 2-5 mL of 20% solution by syringe attached to catheter

Diagnostic procedures: 2-3 doses of 1-2 mL of 20% solution or 2-4 mL of 10% solution by nebulization or intratracheal instillation before the procedure

**Note:** Patients should receive an aerosolized bronchodilator 10-15 minutes prior to acetylcysteine.

**Elderly:** Refer to adult dosing.

**Administration**

**Oral:** For treatment of acetaminophen overdosage, administer orally as a 5% solution. Dilute the 20% solution 1:3 with a cola, orange juice, or other soft drink. Use within 1 hour of preparation. Unpleasant odor becomes less noticeable as treatment progresses.

**Inhalation:** Acetylcysteine is incompatible with tetracyclines, erythromycin, amphotericin B, iodized oil, chymotrypsin, trypsin, and hydrogen peroxide. Administer separately. Intermittent aerosol treatments are commonly given when patient arises, before meals, and just before retiring at bedtime.

**Stability**

**Storage:** Store opened vials in the refrigerator. Use within 96 hours.

**Reconstitution:** Once diluted for administration, preparation should be used within 1 hour. Light purple color of solution does **not** affect its mucolytic activity.

**Additional Nursing Issues**

**Physical Assessment:** Monitor effectiveness of therapy and advent of adverse/allergic effects. Instruct patient on appropriate use and adverse effects to report.

**Patient Information/Instruction:** Pulmonary treatment: Prepare solution (may dilute with sterile water to reduce concentrate from impeding nebulizer) and use as directed. Clear airway by coughing deeply before using aerosol. Wash face and face-mask after treatment to remove any residual. You may experience drowsiness (use caution when driving) or nausea or vomiting (small frequent meals may help). Report persistent chills or fever, adverse change in respiratory status, palpitations, or extreme anxiety or nervousness.

- **Acetylsalicylic Acid** *see* Aspirin *on page 111*
- **Aches-N-Pain® [OTC]** *see* Ibuprofen *on page 592*
- **Achromycin®** *see page 1282*
- **Achromycin® Ophthalmic** *see* Tetracycline *on page 1111*
- **Achromycin® Topical** *see* Tetracycline *on page 1111*
- **Aciclovir** *see* Acyclovir *on page 39*
- **Acifur** *see* Acyclovir *on page 39*
- **Acimox** *see* Amoxicillin *on page 80*
- **Acloral®** *see* Ranitidine *on page 1008*
- **Aclovate® Topical** *see* Topical Corticosteroids *on page 1152*
- **Acnomel®** *see page 1294*

## Acrivastine and Pseudoephedrine (AK ri vas teen & soo doe e FED rin)

**U.S. Brand Names** Semprex®-D

**Synonyms** Pseudoephedrine and Acrivastine

**Therapeutic Category** Antihistamine

**Pregnancy Risk Factor** B

**Lactation** Enters breast milk/contraindicated

**Use** Temporary relief of allergies, rhinitis, and nasal congestion

**Mechanism of Action/Effect** Refer to Pseudoephedrine monograph; acrivastine is a competitive $H_1$-receptor site blocker.

**Contraindications** Hypersensitivity to pseudoephedrine, acrivastine (or other alkylamine antihistamines), or any component; MAO inhibitor therapy within 14 days of initiating therapy; severe hypertension; severe coronary artery disease; renal impairment ($Cl_{cr}$ <48 mL/minute)

**Warnings** Use with caution in patients >60 years of age. Use with caution in patients with high blood pressure, ischemic heart disease, diabetes, increased intraocular pressure, GI or GU obstruction, asthma, thyroid disease, or prostatic hypertrophy. Not recommended for use in children.

**Drug Interactions**

**Decreased Effect:** Decreased effect of guanethidine, reserpine, methyldopa, and beta-blockers when given in conjunction with acrivastine and pseudoephedrine.

**Increased Effect/Toxicity:** Increased risk of hypertensive crisis when given with MAO inhibitors or sympathomimetics. Increased risk of severe CNS depression when given with CNS depressants and alcohol.

**Adverse Reactions**

>10%: Central nervous system: Drowsiness, headache

1% to 10%:

- Cardiovascular: Tachycardia, palpitations
- Central nervous system: Nervousness, dizziness, insomnia, vertigo, lightheadedness, fatigue
- Gastrointestinal: Nausea, vomiting, dry mouth, diarrhea
- Genitourinary: Dysuria
- Neuromuscular & skeletal: Weakness
- Respiratory: Pharyngitis, cough increase
- Miscellaneous: Sweating

**Overdose/Toxicology** Symptoms of overdose include trembling, tachycardia, stridor, loss of consciousness, and possible convulsions. There is no specific antidote for pseudoephedrine intoxication, and treatment is primarily supportive.

**Pharmacodynamics/Kinetics**

**Half-life Elimination:** 1.5 hours

**Metabolism:** Liver

**Excretion:** Urine

**Duration:** 12 hours

**Formulations** Capsule: Acrivastine 8 mg and pseudoephedrine hydrochloride 60 mg

**Dosing**

**Adults:** 1 capsule 3-4 times/day

**Elderly:** Refer to adult dosing.

**Renal Impairment:** Do not use.

**Additional Nursing Issues**

**Physical Assessment:** Assess effectiveness and interactions of other medications (see Drug Interactions). See Contraindications and Warnings/Precautions for cautious use. Monitor effectiveness of therapy and adverse reactions (see Adverse Reactions) at beginning of therapy and periodically with long-term use. Assess knowledge/teach patient appropriate use, interventions to reduce side effects, and adverse symptoms to report. Breast-feeding is contraindicated.

**Patient Information/Instruction:** Take as directed; do not exceed recommended dose. Avoid use of other depressants, alcohol, or sleep-inducing medications unless approved by prescriber. You may experience drowsiness or dizziness (use caution when driving or engaging in hazardous activity until response to drug is known); or dry mouth, nausea or vomiting (frequent small meals, frequent mouth care, chewing gum, or sucking lozenges may help). Report persistent dizziness, sedation, or agitation; chest pain, rapid heartbeat, or palpitations; difficulty breathing or increased cough; changes in urinary pattern; muscle weakness; or lack of improvement or worsening or condition. **Breast-feeding precautions:** Do not breast-feed.


- ♦ **Acrivastine and Pseudoephedrine** *see page 1294*
- ♦ **Acromicina** *see* Tetracycline *on page 1111*
- ♦ **ACT** *see* Dactinomycin *on page 327*
- ♦ **ACT®** *see page 1294*
- ♦ **Actagen® Syrup** *see page 1294*
- ♦ **Actagen® Tablet** *see page 1294*
- ♦ **Acthar®** *see page 1248*
- ♦ **ActHIB®** *see page 1256*
- ♦ **Acti-B$_{12}$®** *see* Hydroxocobalamin *on page 583*
- ♦ **Acticort 100®** *see* Hydrocortisone *on page 578*
- ♦ **Actidose-Aqua® [OTC]** *see* Charcoal *on page 243*
- ♦ **Actidose® With Sorbitol [OTC]** *see* Charcoal *on page 243*
- ♦ **Actifed® Allergy Tablet (Day) [OTC]** *see* Pseudoephedrine *on page 992*
- ♦ **Actifed® Allergy Tablet (Night)** *see page 1294*

- **Actigall™** *see* Ursodiol *on page 1197*
- **Actimmune®** *see* Interferon Gamma-1b *on page 618*
- **Actinex® Topical** *see* Masoprocol *on page 707*
- **Actinomycin D** *see* Dactinomycin *on page 327*
- **Actiprofen®** *see* Ibuprofen *on page 592*
- **Activase®** *see* Alteplase *on page 58*
- **Activated Carbon** *see* Charcoal *on page 243*
- **Activated Dimethicone** *see page 1294*
- **Activated Ergosterol** *see* Ergocalciferol *on page 432*
- **Activated Methylpolysiloxane** *see page 1294*
- **Activelle™** *see* Estradiol and Norethindrone *on page 443*
- **Actonel®** *see* Risedronate *on page 1026*
- **Actron® [OTC]** *see* Ketoprofen *on page 645*
- **ACU-dyne®** *see page 1294*
- **Acular®** *see page 1282*
- **Acular® Ophthalmic** *see* Ketorolac Tromethamine *on page 646*
- **Acupril** *see* Quinapril *on page 1001*
- **Acutrim® 16 Hours [OTC]** *see* Phenylpropanolamine *on page 922*
- **Acutrim® II, Maximum Strength [OTC]** *see* Phenylpropanolamine *on page 922*
- **Acutrim® Late Day [OTC]** *see* Phenylpropanolamine *on page 922*
- **ACV** *see* Acyclovir *on this page*
- **Acycloguanosine** *see* Acyclovir *on this page*


## Acyclovir (ay SYE kloe veer)

**U.S. Brand Names** Zovirax®

**Synonyms** Aciclovir; ACV; Acycloguanosine

**Therapeutic Category** Antiviral Agent

**Pregnancy Risk Factor** C

**Lactation** Enters breast milk/compatible

**Use** Treatment of initial and prophylaxis of recurrent mucosal and cutaneous herpes simplex (HSV-1, HSV-2) infections, herpes simplex encephalitis, genital herpes simplex infections, herpes zoster (start treatment within 72 hours of appearance of rash), varicella-zoster, varicella pneumonia, ocular herpes simplex infections, herpes simplex proctitis, herpes simplex Whitlow; does not prevent postherpetic neuralgia; prevention of herpes simplex and cytomegalovirus infections following bone marrow or renal transplantation; treatment of disseminated primary eczema herpeticum, herpes simplex-associated erythema multiforme

**Mechanism of Action/Effect** Inhibits DNA synthesis and viral replication

**Contraindications** Hypersensitivity to acyclovir

**Warnings** Use with caution in patients with pre-existing renal disease or in those receiving other nephrotoxic drugs. Maintain adequate urine output (1.5-2 L/m$^2$/24 hours) during treatment with acyclovir. Use intravenous acyclovir with caution in patients with underlying neurologic abnormalities, dehydration, or prerenal azotemia. Pregnancy factor C.

**Drug Interactions**

**Increased Effect/Toxicity:** Increased CNS side effects when taken with zidovudine or probenecid.

**Adverse Reactions**

**Systemic: Oral:**

1% to 10%:

Central nervous system: Lightheadedness, headache

Gastrointestinal: Nausea, vomiting, abdominal pain

**Systemic: Parenteral:**

>10%:

Central nervous system: Lightheadedness

Gastrointestinal: Nausea, vomiting, anorexia

Local: Inflammation at injection site or phlebitis

1% to 10%: Renal: Acute renal failure

<1% (Limited to important or life-threatening symptoms): Coma, confusion, hallucination, seizures, tremors, hallucinations, leukopenia, thrombocytopenia, anemia

**Topical:**

>10%: Mild pain, burning, or stinging

1% to 10%: Itching

**Overdose/Toxicology** Symptoms of overdose include seizures, somnolence, confusion, elevated serum creatinine, and renal failure. In the event of overdose, sufficient urine flow must be maintained to avoid drug precipitation within renal tubules. Hemodialysis has resulted in up to 60% reduction in serum acyclovir levels.

**Pharmacodynamics/Kinetics**

**Protein Binding:** <30%

**Half-life Elimination:** 3 hours (normal renal function)

**Time to Peak:** Oral: Within 1.5-2 hours; I.V.: Within 1 hour

**Metabolism:** Small amount of hepatic metabolism

**Excretion:** Urine

**Formulations**

Capsule: 200 mg

Powder for Injection: 500 mg (10 mL); 1000 mg (20 mL)

Ointment, topical: 5% [50 mg/g] (3 g, 15 g)

Suspension, oral (banana flavor): 200 mg/5 mL

(Continued)

## Acyclovir *(Continued)*

Tablet: 400 mg, 800 mg

**Dosing**

**Adults:** Dosing weight should be based on the smaller of lean body weight or total body weight.

**Treatment of herpes simplex virus infections:**

Mucocutaneous HSV or severe initial herpes genitalis infection: 750 mg/m²/day divided every 8 hours or 5 mg/kg/dose every 8 hours for 5-10 days

HSV encephalitis: 1500 mg/m²/day divided every 8 hours or 10 mg/kg/dose for 10 days

**Treatment of genital herpes simplex virus infections:**

Oral: 200 mg every 4 hours while awake (5 times/day) for 10 days if initial episode; for 5 days if recurrence (begin at earliest signs of disease)

Topical: ½" ribbon of ointment for a 4" square surface area every 3 hours (6 times/day)

**Treatment of varicella-zoster virus (chickenpox) infections:**

Oral: 600-800 mg/dose every 4 hours while awake (5 times/day) for 7-10 days or 1000 mg every 6 hours for 5 days

I.V.: 1500 mg/m²/day divided every 8 hours or 10 mg/kg/dose every 8 hours for 7 days

**Treatment of herpes zoster (shingles) infections:**

Oral (immunocompromised): 800 mg every 4 hours (5 times/day) for 7-10 days

I.V.:

Adult (immunocompromised): 10 mg/kg/dose or 500 mg/m²/dose every 8 hours

Older Adults (immunocompromised): 7.5 mg/kg/dose every 8 hours

If nephrotoxicity occurs: 5 mg/kg/dose every 8 hours

**Prophylaxis in immunocompromised patients:**

Varicella zoster or herpes zoster in HIV-positive patients: Oral: 400 mg every 4 hours (5 times/day) for 7-10 days

Bone marrow transplant recipients: I.V.:

Allogeneic patients who are HSV seropositive: 150 mg/m²/dose (5 mg/kg) every 12 hours; with clinical symptoms of herpes simplex: 150 mg/m²/dose every 8 hours

Allogeneic patients who are CMV seropositive: 500 mg/m²/dose (10 mg/kg) every 8 hours; for clinically symptomatic CMV infection, consider replacing acyclovir with ganciclovir

**Chronic suppressive therapy for recurrent genital herpes simplex virus infections:** 200 mg 3-4 times/day or 400 mg twice daily for up to 12 months, followed by re-evaluation

**Elderly:** Refer to adult dosing.

**Renal Impairment:**

Oral: HSV/varicella-zoster:

$Cl_{cr}$ 10-25 mL/minute: Administer dose every 8 hours.

$Cl_{cr}$ <10 mL/minute: Administer dose every 12 hours.

I.V.:

$Cl_{cr}$ 25-50 mL/minute: 5-10 mg/kg/dose: Administer every 12 hours.

$Cl_{cr}$ 10-25 mL/minute: 5-10 mg/kg/dose: Administer every 24 hours.

$Cl_{cr}$ <10 mL/minute: 2.5-5 mg/kg/dose: Administer every 24 hours.

Dialyzable (50% to 100%); administer dose postdialysis.

Peritoneal dialysis effects: Dose as for $Cl_{cr}$ <10 mL/minute.

Continuous arteriovenous or venovenous hemofiltration (CAVH/CAVHD) effects: Dose as for $Cl_{cr}$ <10 mL/minute.

**Administration**

**I.V.:** For I.V. infusion only. Avoid rapid infusion. Infuse over 1 hour to prevent renal damage.

**Stability**

**Storage:** Reconstituted solutions remain stable for 24 hours at room temperature. Do not refrigerate reconstituted solutions as they may precipitate.

**Reconstitution:** Concentrations >10 mg/mL (usual recommended concentration is <7 mg/mL in $D_5W$) increase the risk of phlebitis.

**Compatibility:** Incompatible with blood products and protein-containing solutions.

**Monitoring Laboratory Tests** Urinalysis, BUN, serum creatinine, liver enzymes, CBC

**Additional Nursing Issues**

**Physical Assessment:** Monitor laboratory tests on a regular basis. Monitor for signs of opportunistic infection (eg, fever, sore throat, easy bruising or bleeding, mouth sores, unhealed sores). Assess/teach necessity of maintaining adequate hydration, appropriate use of acyclovir, and contagion precautions. **Pregnancy risk factor C** - benefits of use should outweigh possible risks.

**Patient Information/Instruction:** This is not a cure for herpes (recurrences tend to appear within 3 months of original infection), nor will this medication reduce the risk of transmission to others when lesions are present. Take as directed for full course of therapy; do not discontinue even if feeling better. Maintain adequate hydration (2-3 L/day of fluids unless instructed to restrict fluid intake) to prevent renal complications. Avoid use of other topical creams, lotions, or ointments unless approved by prescriber. You may experience nausea or vomiting (small frequent meals, frequent mouth care, sucking lozenges, or chewing gum may help); lightheadedness or dizziness (use caution when driving or engaging in tasks that require alertness until response to drug is known); headache, fever, muscle pain (an analgesic may be recommended). Report persistent lethargy, acute headache, severe nausea or vomiting, confusion or hallucinations, rash, or difficulty breathing. **Pregnancy precautions:** Inform prescriber if you are or intend to be pregnant.

**Geriatric Considerations:** Calculate creatinine clearance. Dose adjustment may be necessary depending on renal function.

**Additional Information** Sodium content of 1 g: 4.2 mEq

- **Adalat®** *see* Nifedipine *on page 824*
- **Adalat® CC** *see* Nifedipine *on page 824*
- **Adalat® Oros** *see* Nifedipine *on page 824*
- **Adalat PA®** *see* Nifedipine *on page 824*
- **Adalat® Retard** *see* Nifedipine *on page 824*
- **Adalken®** *see* Penicillamine *on page 894*
- **Adamantanamine Hydrochloride** *see* Amantadine *on page 61*

## Adapalene (a DAP a leen)

**U.S. Brand Names** Differin®

**Therapeutic Category** Acne Products

**Pregnancy Risk Factor** C

**Lactation** Excretion in breast milk unknown

**Use** Topical treatment of acne vulgaris

**Contraindications** Hypersensitivity to adapalene or any component of the gel; avoid use if the patient has sunburn where the drug would be applied.

**Warnings** Use with caution in patients with eczema. Avoid excessive exposure to sunlight and sunlamps. Avoid contact with abraded skin, mucous membranes, eyes, mouth, and angles of the nose. Pregnancy factor C.

**Adverse Reactions** >10%: Dermatologic: Erythema, scaling, dryness, pruritus, burning, pruritus or burning immediately after application

**Overdose/Toxicology** Toxic signs of overdose commonly respond to drug discontinuation, with spontaneous resolution in a few days to weeks. When confronted with signs of increased intracranial pressure, treatment with mannitol (0.25 g/kg I.V. up to 1 g/kg/dose repeated every 5 minutes as needed), dexamethasone (1.5 mg/kg I.V. load followed with 0.375 mg/kg every 6 hours for 5 days), and/or hyperventilation should be employed.

**Formulations** Gel, topical (alcohol free): 0.1% (15 g, 45 g)

**Dosing**

**Adults:** Topical: Apply once daily before bedtime; results appear after 8-12 weeks of therapy.

**Elderly:** Refer to adult dosing.

**Additional Nursing Issues**

**Physical Assessment:** See Contraindications and Warnings/Precautions for use cautions. Monitor effectiveness of therapy and adverse reactions at beginning and periodically during therapy. Assess knowledge/teach patient appropriate use and adverse symptoms to report for prescribed form of drug. **Pregnancy risk factor C** - benefits of use should outweigh possible risks. Note breast-feeding caution.

**Patient Information/Instruction:** For external use only. Apply with gloves in thin film at night to thoroughly clean/dry skin; avoid area around eyes or mouth. Do not apply occlusive dressing. Results make take 8-12 weeks to appear. You may experience transient burning or stinging immediately after applying. Report worsening of condition or skin redness, dryness, peeling, or burning that persists between applications. **Pregnancy/breast-feeding precautions:** Inform prescriber if you are or intend to be pregnant. Consult prescriber if breast-feeding.

- **Adapin® Oral** *see* Doxepin *on page 399*
- **Adeflor®** *see* Vitamin, Multiple *on page 1219*
- **Adena a Ungena** *see* Vidarabine *on page 1210*
- **Adenine Arabinoside** *see* Vidarabine *on page 1210*
- **Adenocard®** *see* Adenosine *on this page*

## Adenosine (a DEN oh seen)

**U.S. Brand Names** Adenocard®

**Synonyms** 9-Beta-D-Ribofuranosyladenine

**Therapeutic Category** Antiarrhythmic Agent, Class IV

**Pregnancy Risk Factor** C

**Lactation** Excretion in breast milk unknown

**Use** Treatment of paroxysmal supraventricular tachycardia (PSVT) including that associated with accessory bypass tracts (Wolff-Parkinson-White syndrome); when clinically advisable, appropriate vagal maneuvers should be attempted prior to adenosine administration; **not effective in atrial flutter, atrial fibrillation, or ventricular tachycardia**

**Mechanism of Action/Effect** Slows conduction time through the A-V node and restores normal sinus rhythm

**Contraindications** Hypersensitivity to adenosine or any component; second or third degree A-V block or sick-sinus syndrome (except in patients with a functioning artificial pacemaker), atrial flutter, atrial fibrillation, and ventricular tachycardia

**Warnings** Patients with pre-existing S-A nodal dysfunction may experience prolonged sinus pauses after adenosine. There have been reports of atrial fibrillation/flutter in patients with PSVT associated with accessory conduction pathways after adenosine. Adenosine decreases conduction through the A-V node and may produce a short-lasting first, second, or third degree heart block. Because of the very short half-life, the effects are generally self-limiting. Rare, prolonged episodes of asystole have been reported,

(Continued)

## Adenosine *(Continued)*

with fatal outcomes in some cases. At the time of conversion to normal sinus rhythm, a variety of new rhythms may appear on the EKG. Adenosine could produce bronchoconstriction in patients with asthma. Pregnancy factor C.

**Drug Interactions**

**Decreased Effect:** Methylxanthines (eg, caffeine, theophylline) antagonize effects.

**Increased Effect/Toxicity:** Dipyridamole potentiates effects of adenosine. Use with carbamazepine may increase heart block.

**Food Interactions** The therapeutic effect of adenosine may be decreased if used concurrently with caffeine.

**Adverse Reactions**

>10%:

Cardiovascular: Facial flushing (18%), palpitations, chest pain, hypotension
Central nervous system: Headache
Respiratory: Shortness of breath/dyspnea (12%)
Miscellaneous: Sweating

1% to 10%:

Central nervous system: Dizziness
Gastrointestinal: Nausea (3%)
Neuromuscular & skeletal: Paresthesia, numbness
Respiratory: Chest pressure (7%)

<1% (Limited to important or life-threatening symptoms): Hypotension, lightheadedness, headache, dizziness, intracranial pressure, hyperventilation

**Overdose/Toxicology** Since adenosine half-life is <10 seconds, adverse effects are rapidly self-limiting. Treatment of prolonged effects requires individualization. Theophylline and other methylxanthines are competitive inhibitors of adenosine and may have a role in reversing its toxic effects.

**Pharmacodynamics/Kinetics**

**Half-life Elimination:** <10 seconds

**Onset:** Clinical effects occur rapidly

**Duration:** Very brief

**Formulations** Injection, preservative free: 3 mg/mL (2 mL)

**Dosing**

**Adults:** Rapid I.V. push (over 1-2 seconds) via peripheral line: 6 mg; if not effective within 1-2 minutes, 12 mg may be given; may repeat 12 mg bolus if needed; maximum single dose: 12 mg

**Note:** Patients who are receiving concomitant theophylline therapy may be less likely to respond to adenosine therapy. Higher doses may be needed for administration via peripheral versus central vein.

**Elderly:** Refer to adult dosing. May be more sensitive to effects of adenosine.

**Administration**

**I.V.:** For rapid bolus I.V. use only. Give I.V. push over 1-2 seconds at port closest to insertion site.

**I.V. Detail:** Follow each bolus with rapid normal saline flush. **Note:** Preliminary results in adults suggest adenosine may be administered via central line at lower doses (eg, adults, initial: 3 mg). Do not mix with any other drugs in syringe or solution.

**Stability**

**Storage:** Do **not** refrigerate, precipitation may occur (may dissolve by warming to room temperature).

**Additional Nursing Issues**

**Physical Assessment:** Assess other medications patient may be taking for effectiveness and interactions (see Drug Interactions). Requires use of infusion pump and continuous cardiac and hemodynamic monitoring during infusion. Be alert for adverse reactions (see Warnings/Precautions and Adverse Reactions). Note that adenosine could produce bronchoconstriction in patients with asthma (see Warnings/Precautions). Note breast-feeding caution.

**Patient Information/Instruction:** Adenosine is administered in emergencies, patient education should be appropriate to the situation.

**Geriatric Considerations:** Geriatric patients may be more sensitive to the effects of this medication.

**Other Issues:** Confirm labeling before administration. **Do not use adenosine phosphate (given I.M. for symptomatic relief of varicose veins complications). Have emergency resuscitation and equipment available when using this drug.**

**Related Information**

Antiarrhythmic Drug Classification Comparison *on page 1366*

- **Adistan** *see* Astemizole *on page 114*
- **Adlone® Injection** *see* Methylprednisolone *on page 754*
- **ADR** *see* Doxorubicin *on page 401*
- **Adrenalin®** *see* Epinephrine *on page 424*
- **Adrenaline** *see* Epinephrine *on page 424*
- **Adriamycin PFS™** *see* Doxorubicin *on page 401*
- **Adriamycin RDF™** *see* Doxorubicin *on page 401*
- **Adrucil® Injection** *see* Fluorouracil *on page 500*
- **Adsorbocarpine® Ophthalmic** *see* Ophthalmic Agents, Glaucoma *on page 853*
- **Adsorbocarpine® Ophthalmic** *see* Pilocarpine *on page 931*
- **Adsorbonac® Ophthalmic** *see page 1294*

- **Adsorbotear® Ophthalmic Solution** *see page 1294*
- **Advanced Formula Oxy® Sensitive Gel** *see page 1294*
- **Advil® [OTC]** *see* Ibuprofen *on page 592*
- **Advil® Cold & Sinus Caplets** *see page 1294*
- **Aeroaid®** *see page 1294*
- **Aerobec** *see* Beclomethasone *on page 135*
- **AeroBid®-M Oral Aerosol Inhaler** *see* Flunisolide *on page 497*
- **AeroBid® Oral Aerosol Inhaler** *see* Flunisolide *on page 497*
- **Aerodine®** *see page 1294*
- **Aerolate III®** *see* Theophylline *on page 1115*
- **Aerolate JR®** *see* Theophylline *on page 1115*
- **Aerolate SR® S** *see* Theophylline *on page 1115*
- **Aerolone®** *see* Isoproterenol *on page 632*
- **AeroZoin®** *see page 1294*
- **A.F. Anacin®** *see* Acetaminophen *on page 32*
- **Afrin® Children's Nose Drops** *see page 1294*
- **Afrin® Nasal Solution** *see page 1294*
- **Afrin® Saline Mist** *see page 1294*
- **Afrin® Tablet [OTC]** *see* Pseudoephedrine *on page 992*
- **Aftate® for Athletes Foot** *see page 1247*
- **Aftate® for Jock Itch** *see page 1247*
- **A.F. Valdecasas®** *see* Folic Acid *on page 515*
- **Agenerase®** *see* Amprenavir *on page 93*
- **Aggrastat®** *see* Tirofiban *on page 1141*
- **$AgNO_3$** *see* Silver Nitrate *on page 1057*
- **AHF** *see* Antihemophilic Factor (Human) *on page 99*
- **A-hydroCort®** *see* Hydrocortisone *on page 578*
- **Airet®** *see* Albuterol *on page 45*
- **Akarpine® Ophthalmic** *see* Ophthalmic Agents, Glaucoma *on page 853*
- **Akarpine® Ophthalmic** *see* Pilocarpine *on page 931*
- **AKBeta® Ophthalmic** *see* Ophthalmic Agents, Glaucoma *on page 853*
- **AK-Chlor®** *see page 1282*
- **AK-Chlor® Ophthalmic** *see* Chloramphenicol *on page 248*
- **AK-Cide®** *see page 1282*
- **AK-Con®** *see page 1282*
- **AK-Con® Ophthalmic** *see page 1294*
- **AK-Dex®** *see* Dexamethasone *on page 346*
- **AK-Dilate®** *see page 1282*
- **AK-Dilate® Ophthalmic Solution** *see* Phenylephrine *on page 920*
- **AK-Fluor® Injection** *see page 1248*
- **AK-Homatropine®** *see page 1282*
- **AK-NaCl®** *see page 1294*
- **AK-Nefrin®** *see page 1282*
- **AK-Nefrin® Ophthalmic Solution** *see* Phenylephrine *on page 920*
- **AK-Neo-Dex®** *see page 1282*
- **AK-Neo-Dex® Ophthalmic** *see* Neomycin and Dexamethasone *on page 816*
- **Akorazol** *see* Ketoconazole *on page 643*
- **AK-Pentolate®** *see page 1248*
- **AK-Pentolate®** *see page 1282*
- **AK-Poly-Bac®** *see page 1282*
- **AK-Poly-Bac® Ophthalmic** *see* Bacitracin and Polymyxin B *on page 130*
- **AK-Pred® Ophthalmic** *see* Prednisolone *on page 960*
- **AKPro® Ophthalmic** *see* Ophthalmic Agents, Glaucoma *on page 853*
- **AK-Spore H.C.® Ophthalmic Ointment** *see* Bacitracin, Neomycin, Polymyxin B, and Hydrocortisone *on page 131*
- **AK-Spore H.C.® Ophthalmic Ointment** *see page 1282*
- **AK-Spore H.C.® Ophthalmic Suspension** *see page 1282*
- **Ak-Spore H.C. Otic®** *see page 1291*
- **AK-Spore® Ophthalmic Ointment** *see* Bacitracin, Neomycin, and Polymyxin B *on page 130*
- **AK-Spore® Ophthalmic Ointment** *see page 1282*
- **AK-Spore® Ophthalmic Solution** *see page 1282*
- **AK-Sulf®** *see page 1282*
- **AK-Sulf® Ophthalmic** *see* Sulfacetamide *on page 1080*
- **AK-Taine®** *see page 1248*
- **AKTob®** *see page 1282*
- **AKTob® Ophthalmic** *see* Tobramycin *on page 1142*
- **AK-Tracin®** *see page 1282*
- **AK-Tracin® Ophthalmic** *see* Bacitracin *on page 129*
- **AK-Trol®** *see page 1282*
- **Akwa Tears® Solution** *see page 1294*
- **Ala-Cort®** *see* Hydrocortisone *on page 578*

- **Ala-Cort®** *see* Topical Corticosteroids *on page 1152*
- **Ala-Quin® Topical** *see* Clioquinol and Hydrocortisone *on page 284*
- **Ala-Scalp®** *see* Hydrocortisone *on page 578*
- **Ala-Scalp®** *see* Topical Corticosteroids *on page 1152*
- **Alatrovafloxacin Mesylate** *see* Trovafloxacin *on page 1189*
- **Alazide®** *see* Hydrochlorothiazide and Spironolactone *on page 568*
- **Alba-Dex®** *see* Dexamethasone *on page 346*
- **Albalon®** *see page 1282*
- **Albalon-A® Ophthalmic Solution** *see page 1294*
- **Albalon® Liquifilm® Ophthalmic** *see page 1294*


## Albendazole (al BEN da zole)

**U.S. Brand Names** Albenza®

**Therapeutic Category** Anthelmintic

**Pregnancy Risk Factor** C

**Lactation** Excretion in breast milk unknown/not recommended

**Use** Treatment of parenchymal neurocysticercosis and cystic hydatid disease of the liver, lung, and peritoneum; treatment of ascariasis, trichuriasis, enterobiasis, hookworm, strongyloidiasis, giardiasis, and microsporidiosis in AIDS

**Contraindications** Hypersensitivity to albendazole or any component

**Warnings** Corticosteroids should be administered 1-2 days before albendazole therapy in patients with neurocysticercosis to minimize inflammatory reactions. Pregnancy factor C.

**Drug Interactions**

**Cytochrome P-450 Effect:** May inhibit CYP1A2 enzyme

**Decreased Effect:** Cimetidine may increase albendazole metabolism.

**Increased Effect/Toxicity:** Albendazole serum levels are increased when taken with dexamethasone, praziquantel.

**Food Interactions** Albendazole serum levels may be increased if taken with food.

**Adverse Reactions**

1% to 10%:

Central nervous system: Dizziness, headache, vertigo, fever
Dermatologic: Alopecia (reversible)
Gastrointestinal: Abdominal pain, nausea, vomiting
Hepatic: Increased LFTs, jaundice

<1% (Limited to important or life-threatening symptoms): Increased intracranial pressure, eosinophilia, granulocytopenia, neutropenia, pancytopenia, leukopenia, acute renal failure

**Pharmacodynamics/Kinetics**

**Protein Binding:** 70% bound to plasma proteins

**Half-life Elimination:** 8-12 hours

**Time to Peak:** Within 2-5 hours

**Metabolism:** Liver

**Excretion:** Bile

**Formulations** Tablet: 200 mg

**Dosing**

**Adults:** Oral:

Neurocysticercosis:

<60 kg: 15 mg/kg/day in 2 divided doses (maximum: 800 mg/day) with meals for 8-30 days

≥60 kg: 400 mg twice daily for 8-30 days

**Note:** Give concurrent anticonvulsant and steroid therapy during first week.

Hydatid:

<60 kg: 15 mg/kg/day in 2 divided doses with meals (maximum: 800 mg/day) for three 28-day cycles with 14-day drug-free interval in-between

≥60 kg: 400 mg twice daily for 3 cycles as above

Strongyloidiasis/tapeworm: 400 mg/day for 3 days; may repeat in 3 weeks

Hookworm, pinworm, roundworm: 400 mg as a single dose; may repeat in 3 weeks

Oral or intravenous corticosteroids should be considered to prevent cerebral hypertensive episodes during the first week of anticysticeral therapy.

**Elderly:** Refer to adult dosing.

**Additional Nursing Issues**

**Physical Assessment:** See Warnings/Precautions for pretreatment suggestions. Monitor effectiveness of therapy and adverse reactions. Instruct patient on appropriate administration and symptoms to report. **Pregnancy risk factor C** - benefits of use must outweigh possible risks. Breast-feeding is not recommended.

**Patient Information/Instruction:** Take according to prescribed dosage schedule with meals. You may experience loss of hair (reversible); dizziness or headaches (use caution when driving or engaging in tasks that require alertness until response to drug is known). Report unusual fever, abdominal pain, unresolved vomiting, yellowing of skin or eyes, darkening of urine, or light colored stools. **Pregnancy/breast-feeding precautions:** Inform prescriber if you are or intend to be pregnant. Breast-feeding is not recommended.


- **Albenza®** *see* Albendazole *on this page*
- **Albert® Docusate** *see* Docusate *on page 392*
- **Albert® Glyburide** *see* Glyburide *on page 538*
- **Albert® Oxybutynin** *see* Oxybutynin *on page 870*
- **Albert® Pentoxifylline** *see* Pentoxifylline *on page 908*

## Albumin (al BYOO min)

**U.S. Brand Names** Albuminar®; Albumisol®; Albutein®; Buminate®; Plasbumin®

**Synonyms** Albumin (Human)

**Therapeutic Category** Blood Product Derivative; Plasma Volume Expander, Colloid

**Pregnancy Risk Factor** C

**Lactation** Excretion in breast milk unknown/compatible

**Use** Plasma volume expansion and maintenance of cardiac output in the treatment of certain types of shock or impending shock; may be useful for burn patients, ARDS, and cardiopulmonary bypass. Other uses considered (but not proven) are retroperitoneal surgery, peritonitis, ascites, and hypoproteinemia. Unless the condition responsible for hypoproteinemia can be corrected, albumin can provide only symptomatic relief or supportive treatment. Albumin is not an appropriate treatment for nutritional protein deficiency.

**Mechanism of Action/Effect** Restores plasma volume

**Contraindications** Hypersensitivity to albumin or any component; patients with severe anemia or cardiac failure

**Warnings** Use with caution in patients with hepatic or renal failure or for whom sodium restriction is necessary. Rapid infusion of albumin solutions may cause vascular overload. Test methods and treatment methods may not totally eradicate HBAg and HIV from pooled plasma used in processing of this product. Pregnancy factor C.

**Effects on Lab Values** ↑ alkaline phosphatase (S)

**Adverse Reactions**

1% to 10%:

Cardiovascular: Precipitation of congestive heart failure, decreased myocardial contractility

Respiratory: Pulmonary edema, dyspnea

Renal: Salt and water retention

<1% (Limited to important or life-threatening symptoms): Hypotension, tachycardia

**Overdose/Toxicology** Symptoms of overdose include hypervolemia, congestive heart failure, and pulmonary edema.

**Formulations** Injection, as human: 5% [50 mg/mL] (50 mL, 250 mL, 500 mL, 1000 mL); 25% [250 mg/mL] (10 mL, 20 mL, 50 mL, 100 mL)

**Dosing**

**Adults:** I.V.:

Use **5%** solution in hypovolemic patients or intravascularly-depleted patients.

Use **25%** solution in patients in whom fluid and sodium intake is restricted.

Usual dose (**depends on patient's condition**): 25 g; no more than 250 g should be administered within 48 hours.

Hypoproteinemia: 0.5-1 g/kg/dose; repeat every 1-2 days as calculated to replace ongoing losses.

Hypovolemia: 0.5-1 g/kg/dose; repeat as needed; maximum: 6 g/kg/day.

**Elderly:** Refer to adult dosing.

**Administration**

**I.V.:** Albumin is best administered at a rate of 2-4 mL/minute; 25% albumin may be given at a rate of 1 mL/minute.

**I.V. Detail:** Do not dilute 5% solution. Use 5-micron or larger filter; do not give through a 0.22 micron filter. Albumin administration must be completed within 4 hours after opening vial (solution does not contain preservative). Rapid infusion may cause vascular overload. Albumin 25% may be given undiluted or diluted in normal saline. May give in combination or through the same administration set as saline or carbohydrates. Do not use with alcohol or protein hydrolysates, precipitation may form.

**Stability**

**Storage:** Do **not** use solution if it is turbid or contains a deposit; solution should be clear amber.

**Reconstitution:** Do not use sterile water as a diluent.

**Additional Nursing Issues**

**Physical Assessment:** Observe patient for signs of hypervolemia. Use with caution in patients requiring sodium restrictions. Rapid infusion may cause hypotension. Monitor vital signs, central venous pressure, intake and output closely during administration. Assess for signs of fluid overload. If fever, tachycardia, or hypotension occurs, stop infusion and notify prescriber. **Pregnancy risk factor C.**

**Patient Information/Instruction:** **Pregnancy precautions:** Inform prescriber if you are pregnant.

**Additional Information**

Sodium content of 1 L: Both 5% and 25% albumin contain 130-160 mEq.

pH: 6.4-7.4

- **Albuminar®** *see* Albumin *on this page*
- **Albumin (Human)** *see* Albumin *on this page*
- **Albumisol®** *see* Albumin *on this page*
- **Albutein®** *see* Albumin *on this page*

## Albuterol (al BYOO ter ole)

**U.S. Brand Names** Airet®; Proventil®; Proventil® HFA; Ventolin®; Ventolin® Rotocaps®; Volmax®

**Synonyms** Salbutamol

**Therapeutic Category** $Beta_2$ Agonist

**Pregnancy Risk Factor** C

**Lactation** Excretion in breast milk unknown

(Continued)

## Albuterol *(Continued)*

**Use** Bronchodilator in reversible airway obstruction due to asthma or COPD; prevention of exercise-induced bronchospasm

**Mechanism of Action/Effect** Relaxes bronchial smooth muscle by action on beta$_2$-receptors with little effect on heart rate

**Contraindications** Hypersensitivity to albuterol, adrenergic amines, or any ingredients

**Warnings** Use with caution in patients with hyperthyroidism, diabetes mellitus, sensitivity to sympathomimetic amines, or with cardiovascular disorders including coronary insufficiency or hypertension. Excessive use may result in tolerance. Pregnancy factor C.

**Drug Interactions**

**Decreased Effect:** When used with beta-adrenergic blockers (eg, propranolol) the effect of albuterol is decreased.

**Increased Effect/Toxicity:** When used with inhaled ipratropium, an increased duration of bronchodilation may occur. Nifedipine may increase FEV-1. Cardiovascular effects are potentiated in patients also receiving MAO inhibitors, tricyclic antidepressants, sympathomimetic agents (eg, amphetamine, dopamine, dobutamine), and inhaled anesthetics (eg, enflurane).

**Effects on Lab Values** ↑ renin (S), aldosterone (S)

**Adverse Reactions**

>10%:

Cardiovascular: Tachycardia, palpitations, pounding heartbeat

Gastrointestinal: GI upset, nausea

1% to 10%:

Cardiovascular: Flushing of face, hypertension or hypotension

Central nervous system: Nervousness, CNS stimulation, hyperactivity, insomnia, dizziness, lightheadedness, drowsiness, headache

Gastrointestinal: Dry mouth, heartburn, vomiting, unusual taste

Genitourinary: Dysuria

Neuromuscular & skeletal: Muscle cramping, tremor, weakness

Respiratory: Coughing

Miscellaneous: Sweating

<1% (Limited to important or life-threatening symptoms): Chest pain, unusual pallor, paradoxical bronchospasm

**Overdose/Toxicology** Symptoms of overdose include hypertension, tachycardia, angina, and hypokalemia. Treatment of hypokalemia and tachyarrhythmias consists of prudent use of a cardioselective beta-adrenergic blocker (eg, atenolol or metoprolol), keeping in mind the potential for induction of bronchoconstriction in an asthmatic individual. Dialysis has not been shown to be of value in the treatment of overdose with albuterol.

**Pharmacodynamics/Kinetics**

**Half-life Elimination:** Inhalation: 3.8 hours; Oral: 3.7-5 hours

**Metabolism:** Liver

**Excretion:** Urine

**Onset:** Peak effect: Oral: 2-3 hours; Nebulization/oral inhalation: Within 0.5-2 hours

**Duration:** Oral: 4-6 hours; Nebulization/oral inhalation: 3-4 hours

**Formulations**

Aerosol: 90 mcg/dose (17 g) [200 doses]

Proventil®, Ventolin®: 90 mcg/dose (17 g) [200 doses]

Aerosol, chlorofluorocarbon free (Proventil® HFA): 90 mcg/dose (17 g)

Capsule for oral inhalation (Ventolin® Rotocaps®): 200 mcg [to be used with Rotahaler® inhalation device]

Solution, inhalation: 0.083% (3 mL); 0.5% (20 mL)

Airet®: 0.083%

Proventil®: 0.083% (3 mL); 0.5% (20 mL)

Ventolin®: 0.5% (20 mL)

Syrup, as sulfate: 2 mg/5 mL (480 mL)

Proventil®, Ventolin®: 2 mg/5 mL (480 mL)

Tablet, as sulfate: 2 mg, 4 mg

Proventil®, Ventolin®: 2 mg, 4 mg

Tablet, extended release:

Proventil® Repetabs®: 4 mg

Volmax®: 4 mg, 8 mg

**Dosing**

**Adults:**

Oral: 2-4 mg/dose 3-4 times/day; maximum dose not to exceed 32 mg/day (divided doses)

Inhalation MDI: 90 mcg/spray:

1-2 inhalations every 4-6 hours although some patients may be controlled on 1 puff every 4 hours; maximum: 12 inhalations/day

Exercise-induced bronchospasm: 2 inhalations 15 minutes before exercising

Inhalation: Nebulization: 2.5 mg = 0.5 mL of the 0.5% inhalation solution to be diluted in 1-2.5 mL of NS delivered over 5-15 minutes; intensive care patients may require more frequent administration; maximum: 1 mL diluted in 1-2 mL normal saline

Rotahaler®: 200 mcg inhaled every 4-6 hours using a Rotahaler® inhalation device

**Elderly:** Refer to adult dosing and Geriatric Considerations.

**Renal Impairment:** Not removed by hemodialysis

**Administration**

**Inhalation:** Shake well before use.

**Monitoring Laboratory Tests** Arterial or capillary blood gases (if patients condition warrants)

**Additional Nursing Issues**

**Physical Assessment:** Assess effectiveness and interactions of other medications (see Drug Interactions). See Contraindications and Warnings/Precautions for use cautions. Monitor effectiveness of therapy (relief of airway obstruction) and adverse reactions (eg, cardiac and CNS changes - see Adverse Reactions) at beginning of therapy and periodically with long-term use. For inpatient care, monitor vital signs and lung sounds prior to and periodically during therapy. Assess knowledge/teach patient appropriate use, interventions to reduce side effects, and adverse symptoms to report. **Pregnancy risk factor C** - benefits of use should outweigh possible risks. Note breast-feeding caution.

**Patient Information/Instruction:** Use exactly as directed (see Administration below). Do not use more often than recommended. Maintain adequate hydration (2-3 L/day of fluids unless instructed to restrict fluid intake). You may experience nervousness, dizziness, or fatigue (use caution when driving or engaging in hazardous activities until response to drug is known); dry mouth, unpleasant taste, stomach upset (frequent small meals, frequent mouth care, chewing gum, or sucking lozenges may help); or difficulty urinating (always void before treatment). Report unresolved GI upset, dizziness or fatigue, vision changes, chest pain or palpitations, persistent inability to void, nervousness or insomnia, muscle cramping or tremor, or unusual cough. **Pregnancy/breast-feeding precautions:** Inform prescriber if you are or intend to be pregnant. Consult prescriber if breast-feeding.

**Administration:** Self-administered inhalation: Store canister upside down; do not freeze. Shake canister before using. Sit when using medication. Close eyes when administering albuterol to avoid spray getting into eyes. Exhale slowly and completely through nose; inhale deeply through mouth while administering aerosol. Hold breath for 1-3 seconds after inhalation. Wait at least 1 full minute between inhalations. Wash mouthpiece between use. If more than one inhalation medication is used, use albuterol first and wait 5 minutes between medications.

Self-administered nebulizer: Wash hands before and after treatment. Wash and dry nebulizer after each treatment. Twist open the top of one unit dose vial and squeeze contents into nebulizer reservoir. Connect nebulizer reservoir to the mouthpiece or face-mask. Connect nebulizer to compressor. Sit in comfortable, upright position. Place mouthpiece in your mouth or put on face mask and turn on compressor. If face-mask is used, avoid leakage around the mask to avoid mist getting into eyes which may cause vision problems. Breath calmly and deeply until no more mist is formed in nebulizer (about 5 minutes). At this point treatment is finished.

**Geriatric Considerations:** Because of its minimal effect on beta$_1$-receptors and its relatively long duration of action, albuterol is a rational choice in the elderly when a beta agonist is indicated. Elderly patients may find it beneficial to utilize a spacer device when using a metered dose inhaler. The Ventolin® Rotahaler® is an alternative for patients who have difficulty using the metered dose inhaler. Oral use should be avoided due to adverse effects.

**Related Information**

Inhalant (Asthma, Bronchospasm) Agents *on page 1388*

- **Alcaine®** *see page 1248*
- **Alclometasone** *see* Topical Corticosteroids *on page 1152*
- **Alcohol** *see page 1291*
- **Alcohol and Hydrocortisone** *see page 1291*
- **Alcohol, Ethyl** *see page 1246*
- **Alconefrin® Nasal Solution [OTC]** *see* Phenylephrine *on page 920*
- **Aldactazide®** *see* Hydrochlorothiazide and Spironolactone *on page 568*
- **Aldactone®** *see* Spironolactone *on page 1070*

## Aldesleukin (al des LOO kin)

**U.S. Brand Names** Proleukin®

**Synonyms** Interleukin-2

**Therapeutic Category** Biological Response Modulator

**Pregnancy Risk Factor** C

**Lactation** Enters breast milk/contraindicated

**Use** Primarily investigated in tumors known to have a response to immunotherapy, such as melanoma and renal cell carcinoma; has been used in conjunction with LAK cells, TIL cells, IL-1, and interferon

**Mechanism of Action/Effect** IL-2 promotes proliferation, differentiation, and recruitment of T and B cells, natural killer (NK) cells, and thymocytes; IL-2 also causes cytolytic activity in a subset of lymphocytes and subsequent interactions between the immune system and malignant cells; IL-2 can stimulate lymphokine-activated killer (LAK) cells and tumor-infiltrating lymphocytes (TIL) cells. LAK cells (which are derived from lymphocytes from a patient and incubated in IL-2) have the ability to lyse cells which are resistant to NK cells; TIL cells (which are derived from cancerous tissue from a patient and incubated in IL-2) have been shown to be 50% more effective than LAK cells.

**Contraindications** Hypersensitivity to interleukin-2 or any component; patients with an abnormal thallium stress test or pulmonary function test; patients who have had an organ

(Continued)

## Aldesleukin *(Continued)*

allograft; retreatment in patients who have experienced sustained ventricular tachycardia (≥5 beats), cardiac rhythm disturbances not controlled or unresponsive to management, recurrent chest pain with EKG changes (consistent with angina or myocardial infarction), intubation required >72 hours, pericardial tamponade; renal dysfunction requiring dialysis >72 hours; coma or toxic psychosis lasting >48 hours; repetitive or difficult to control seizures; bowel ischemia/perforation; GI bleeding requiring surgery

**Warnings** Has been associated with capillary leak syndrome (CLS). CLS results in hypotension and reduced organ perfusion which may be severe and can result in death. Therapy should be restricted to patients with normal cardiac and pulmonary functions as defined by thallium stress and formal pulmonary function testing. Extreme caution should be used in patients with normal thallium stress tests and pulmonary functions tests who have a history of prior cardiac or pulmonary disease.

Intensive aldesleukin treatment is associated with impaired neutrophil function (reduced chemotaxis) and with an increased risk of disseminated infection, including sepsis and bacterial endocarditis, in treated patients. Consequently, pre-existing bacterial infections should be adequately treated prior to initiation of therapy. Additionally, all patients with indwelling central lines should receive antibiotic prophylaxis effective against *S. aureus*. Antibiotic prophylaxis which has been associated with a reduced incidence of staphylococcal infections in aldesleukin studies includes the use of oxacillin, nafcillin, ciprofloxacin, or vancomycin. Disseminated infections acquired in the course of treatment are a major contributor to treatment morbidity and use of antibiotic prophylaxis, and aggressive treatment of suspected and documented infections may reduce the morbidity of aldesleukin treatment.

Pregnancy factor C.

**Drug Interactions**

**Decreased Effect:** Corticosteroids have been shown to decrease toxicity of IL-2, but have not been used since there is concern that they may reduce the efficacy of the lymphokine.

**Increased Effect/Toxicity:** Aldesleukin may affect central nervous function; therefore, interactions could occur following concomitant administration of psychotropic drugs (eg, narcotics, analgesics, antiemetics, sedatives, tranquilizers).

Concomitant administration of drugs possessing nephrotoxic (eg, aminoglycosides, indomethacin), myelotoxic (eg, cytotoxic chemotherapy), cardiotoxic (eg, doxorubicin), or hepatotoxic (eg, methotrexate, asparaginase) effects with aldesleukin may increase toxicity in these organ systems. The safety and efficacy of aldesleukin in combination with chemotherapies has not been established.

Beta-blockers and other antihypertensives may potentiate the hypotension seen with Proleukin®.

**Adverse Reactions**

>10%:

Cardiovascular: Sensory dysfunction, sinus tachycardia, arrhythmias, pulmonary congestion; hypotension (dose-limiting toxicity) which may require vasopressor support and hemodynamic changes resembling those seen in septic shock can be seen within 2 hours of administration; chest pain, acute myocardial infarction, SVT with hypotension has been reported, edema

Central nervous system: Dizziness, pain, fever, chills, cognitive changes, fatigue, malaise, disorientation, somnolence, paranoid delusion, and other behavioral changes; reversible and dose related; however, may continue to worsen for several days even after the infusion is stopped

Dermatologic: Pruritus, erythema, rash, dry skin, exfoliative dermatitis, macular erythema

Gastrointestinal: Nausea, vomiting, weight gain, diarrhea, stomatitis, anorexia, GI bleeding

Hematologic: Anemia, thrombocytopenia, leukopenia, eosinophilia, coagulation disorders

Hepatic: Elevated transaminase and alkaline phosphatase, jaundice

Neuromuscular & skeletal: Weakness, rigors which can be decreased or ameliorated with acetaminophen or a nonsteroidal agent and meperidine

Renal: Oliguria, anuria, proteinuria; renal failure (dose-limiting toxicity) manifested as oliguria noted within 24-48 hours of initiation of therapy; marked fluid retention, azotemia, and increased serum creatinine seen, which may return to baseline within 7 days of discontinuation of therapy; hypophosphatemia

Respiratory: Dyspnea, pulmonary edema

1% to 10%: Cardiovascular: Increase in vascular permeability: Capillary-leak syndrome manifested by severe peripheral edema, ascites, pulmonary infiltration, and pleural effusion; occurs in 2% to 4% of patients and is resolved after therapy ends

<1% (Limited to important or life-threatening symptoms): Congestive heart failure, coma, seizure, alopecia, pancreatitis, polyuria

**Overdose/Toxicology** Side effects following the use of aldesleukin are dose related. Administration of more than the recommended dose has been associated with a more rapid onset of expected dose-limiting toxicities. Adverse reactions generally will reverse when the drug is stopped particularly because of its short serum half-life. Provide supportive treatment of any continuing symptoms. Life-threatening toxicities have been ameliorated by the I.V. administration of dexamethasone, but may result in a less than therapeutic effect of aldesleukin.

**Pharmacodynamics/Kinetics**

**Distribution:** 30% into plasma; 70% into liver, kidney, and lung

**Half-life Elimination:** 20-120 minutes

**Metabolism:** Kidney

**Formulations** Powder for injection, lyophilized: 22 x $10^6$ int. units [18 million int. units/mL = 1.1 mg/mL when reconstituted]

**Dosing**

**Adults:** All orders should be written in million International units (million int. units) (refer to individual protocols).

Metastatic renal cell carcinoma: Treatment consists of two 5-day treatment cycles separated by a rest period. 600,000 units/kg (0.037 mg/kg)/dose administered every 8 hours by a 15-minute I.V. infusion for a total of 14 doses. Following 9 days of rest, the schedule is repeated for another 14 doses, for a maximum of 28 doses per course.

**Investigational regimen:** I.V. continuous infusion: 4.5 million units/m$^2$/day in 250-1000 mL of $D_5W$ for 5 days

**Dose modification:** Hold or interrupt a dose rather than reducing dose; refer to individual protocols.

**Retreatment:** Patients should be evaluated for response ~4 weeks after completion of a course of therapy and again immediately prior to the scheduled start of the next treatment course. Additional courses of treatment may be given to patients only if there is some tumor shrinkage following the last course and retreatment is not contraindicated. Each treatment course should be separated by a rest period of at least 7 weeks from the date of hospital discharge. Tumors have continued to regress up to 12 months following the initiation of therapy.

**Elderly:** Refer to adult dosing.

**Administration**

**I.V.:** Infuse over 15 minutes. Administer in $D_5W$ only; incompatible with sodium chloride solutions.

**I.V. Detail: Management of symptoms related to vascular leak syndrome:**

If actual body weight increases >10% above baseline, or rales or rhonchi are audible:

Administer furosemide at dosage determined by patient response.

Administer dopamine hydrochloride 2-4 mcg/kg/minute to maintain renal blood flow and urine output.

If patient has dyspnea at rest: Give supplemental oxygen by face-mask.

If patient has severe respiratory distress: Intubate patient and provide mechanical ventilation. Administer ranitidine (as the hydrochloride salt), 50 mg I.V. every 8-12 hours as prophylaxis against stress ulcers.

**Stability**

**Storage:** Store vials of lyophilized injection in a refrigerator at 2°C to 8°C (36°F to 46°F).

**Reconstitution:** Reconstituted or diluted solution should be refrigerated. Gently swirl, do not shake.

**Standard aldesleukin I.V. dilutions:** Dose/50-1000 mL $D_5W$

Concentrations <1,000,000 units/mL require the addition of human albumin to PVC bag prior to addition of IL-2.

Concentrations of IL-2 which fall into the unstable range (60-100 mcg/mL **or** 1-1.7 million units/mL) require addition of human serum albumin (final human serum albumin concentration of 0.1%) as shown in the table.

**Volume of Human Serum Albumin to Be Added to IL-2 (Aldesleukin - Proleukin™) Infusions in $D_5W$**

| Volume of I.V. Diluent (mL) | Volume of 5% Human Serum Albumin to Be Added Prior to IL-2 Addition (mL) | Volume of 25% Human Serum Albumin to Be Added Prior to IL-2 Addition (mL) |
|---|---|---|
| 50 | 1 | 0.2 |
| 100 | 2 | 0.4 |
| 150 | 3 | 0.6 |
| 200 | 4 | 0.8 |
| 250 | 5 | 1 |
| 500 | 10 | 2 |

**Recommendations for IL-2 (Aldesleukin - Proleukin™) Dilutions in $D_5W$***

| Concentration (mcg/mL) | Concentration (million units/mL) | Stability Recommendation |
|---|---|---|
| <60 | <1 | Human serum albumin must be added to bag **prior to addition** of IL-2. These solutions are stable for 6 days at room temperature†. |
| 60-100 | 1-1.7 | **These concentrations should not be utilized as they are unstable.** |
| 100-500 | 1.7-8.4 | These solutions are stable for 6 days at room temperature†. |

*1.3 mg of IL-2 (aldesleukin - Proleukin™) is equivalent to 22 million units.

†Although stability is 6 days, IL-2 does not contain a preservative and 23-hour expiration dating should be used.

(Continued)

## Aldesleukin *(Continued)*

**Note:** As with most biological proteins, solutions containing IL-2 should not be filtered; filtration will result in significant loss of bioactivity.

**Compatibility:** Incompatible with NS. Compatible only with $D_5W$.

**Monitoring Laboratory Tests** The following clinical evaluations are recommended for all patients prior to beginning treatment and then daily during drug administration: Standard hematologic tests including CBC, differential, and platelet counts; blood chemistries including electrolytes, renal and hepatic function; chest x-rays.

**Additional Nursing Issues**

**Physical Assessment:** Assess vital signs, cardiac status, respiratory status, CNS status, fluid balance, and laboratory reports daily prior to beginning infusion and for 2 hours following infusion (see Warnings/Precautions, Drug Interactions, and Adverse Reactions). Closely monitor infusion site for extravasation. Assess frequently for development of opportunistic infection. **Pregnancy risk factor C.** Breast-feeding is contraindicated.

**Patient Information/Instruction:** This drug can only be administered by infusion. Avoid alcohol and all OTC or prescription drugs unless approved by your oncologist. You will be sensitive to sunlight; use of sunblock (15 SPF or greater), wear protective clothing, or avoid direct sun exposure. You will be susceptible to infection; avoid crowds or infected persons or persons with contagious diseases. Frequent mouth care and small frequent meals may help counteract any GI effects you may experience and will help maintain adequate nutrition and fluid intake. This drug may result in many side effects; you will be monitored and assessed closely during therapy, however, it is important that you report any changes or problems for evaluation. Report any changes in urination, unusual bruising or bleeding, chest pain or palpitations, acute dizziness, respiratory difficulty, fever or chills, changes in cognition, rash, feelings of pain or numbness in extremities, severe GI upset or diarrhea, vaginal discharge or mouth sores, yellowing of eyes or skin, or any changes in color of urine or stool. **Pregnancy/breast-feeding precautions:** Inform prescriber if you are pregnant. Do not breast-feed.


- **Aldomet®** *see* Methyldopa *on page 750*
- **Aldoril®** *see* Methyldopa and Hydrochlorothiazide *on page 751*
- **Aldoril®-15** *see* Methyldopa and Hydrochlorothiazide *on page 751*
- **Aldoril®-25** *see* Methyldopa and Hydrochlorothiazide *on page 751*


## Alendronate (a LEN droe nate)

**U.S. Brand Names** Fosamax®

**Therapeutic Category** Bisphosphonate Derivative

**Pregnancy Risk Factor** C

**Lactation** Excretion in breast milk unknown

**Use** Treatment of osteoporosis in postmenopausal women, Paget's disease of the bone

**Mechanism of Action/Effect** Inhibits bone resorption via actions on osteoclasts or precursors; decreases the rate of bone resorption, leading to an indirect decrease in bone formation

**Contraindications** Hypersensitivity to bisphosphonates or any component; hypocalcemia; abnormalities of the esophagus which delay esophageal emptying such as stricture or achalasia; inability to stand or sit upright for at least 30 minutes

**Warnings** Use with caution in patients with renal impairment. Use of alendronate in postmenopausal women taking hormone replacement is not recommended. May cause esophageal erosion/ulceration and stricture. Hypocalcemia and vitamin D deficiency must be corrected before starting alendronate. Pregnancy factor C.

**Drug Interactions**

**Decreased Effect:** Calcium supplements, antacids may decrease alendronate absorption.

**Increased Effect/Toxicity:** I.V. ranitidine has been shown to double the bioavailability of alendronate.

**Food Interactions** Coadministration with caffeine may reduce alendronate efficacy. Coadministration with dairy products may decrease alendronate absorption. Beverages (especially orange juice and coffee), food, and medications (eg, antacids, calcium, iron, and multivalent cations) may reduce the absorption of alendronate.

**Adverse Reactions**

**Note:** Incidence of adverse effects increases significantly in patients treated for Paget's disease at 40 mg/day, mostly GI adverse effects

1% to 10%:

Central nervous system: Headache, pain

Gastrointestinal: Flatulence, acid regurgitation, esophagitis ulcer, dysphagia, abdominal distention

<1% (Limited to important or life-threatening symptoms): Erythema (rare), rash, photosensitivity, esophageal stricture

**Overdose/Toxicology** Symptoms of overdose include hypocalcemia, hypophosphatemia, and upper GI adverse affects (eg, upset stomach, heartburn, esophagitis, gastritis, or ulcer). Treat with milk or antacids to bind alendronate. Dialysis would not be beneficial.

**Pharmacodynamics/Kinetics**

**Half-life Elimination:** Estimated to exceed 10 years due to release of alendronate from the skeleton

**Formulations** Tablet, as sodium: 5 mg, 10 mg, 40 mg

**Dosing**

**Adults:**

Osteoporosis in postmenopausal women: 10 mg once daily. Safety studies beyond 4 years of treatment are in progress.

Paget's disease of bone: 40 mg once daily for 6 months

**Elderly:** Oral: See Additional Information.

Prevention of osteoporosis: 5 mg once daily

Osteoporosis: 10 mg once daily. **Note:** Safety studies beyond 4 years of treatment are in progress.

Paget's disease of bone: 40 mg once daily for 6 months; retreatment may be considered after a 6-month period post-treatment in those who relapse as demonstrated by an increase in alkaline phosphatase or in those who fail to decrease alkaline phosphatase to normal.

**Renal Impairment:** $Cl_{cr}$ <35 mL/minute: Alendronate is not recommended.

**Administration**

**Oral:** Take with a full glass of water (6-8 oz) at least 30 minutes before any food, beverage, or medication. Avoid lying down for at least 30 minutes thereafter.

**Monitoring Laboratory Tests** Serum calcium, phosphate, magnesium, potassium, serum creatinine, CBC with differential

**Additional Nursing Issues**

**Physical Assessment:** Monitor for effectiveness of treatment and development of adverse reactions. Assess knowledge/teach lifestyle and dietary changes that will have a beneficial impact of either Paget's disease or osteoporosis. **Pregnancy risk factor C** - benefits of use should outweigh possible risks. Note breast-feeding caution.

**Patient Information/Instruction:** Take as directed, with a full glass of water. Stay in sitting or standing position for 30 minutes following administration to reduce potential for esophageal irritation. Avoid aspirin- or aspirin-containing medications. Consult prescriber to determine necessity of lifestyle changes or dietary supplements of calcium or dietary vitamin D. You may experience GI upset (eg, flatulence, bloating, nausea, acid regurgitation); small frequent meals may help. Report acute headache or gastric pain, unresolved GI upset, or acid stomach. **Pregnancy/breast-feeding precautions:** Inform prescriber if you are or intend to be pregnant. Consult prescriber if breast-feeding.

**Dietary Issues:** Ensure adequate calcium and vitamin D intake to provide for enhanced needs in patients with Paget's disease in whom the pretreatment rate of bone turnover may be greatly elevated.

**Geriatric Considerations:** Since many elderly patients receive diuretics, evaluation of electrolyte status (calcium, phosphate, magnesium, potassium) may need to be done periodically due to the drug class (bisphosphonate). Should assure immobile patients are at least sitting up for 30 minutes after swallowing tablets. Drink a full glass of water with each dose.

**Additional Information** Esophageal irritation and gastric pain have been reported frequently. Proper administration may prevent or decrease this common adverse effect. Patients need to take supplemental calcium while treated with alendronate appropriate for age and hormonal status; vitamin D supplements are suggested if patient is deficient in this vitamin. Patients treated with 10 mg of alendronate daily had significant increases in bone mineral density. Increases were absorbed as early as 3 months and continued throughout the 3 years of study. Mean bone mineral density increases at 3 years were: spine, trochanter 8%; femoral neck 6%; total body bone mineral density 2.5%.


- **Alepsal** *see* Phenobarbital *on page 917*
- **Alersule Forte®** *see page 1306*
- **Alesse™** *see* Oral Contraceptives *on page 859*
- **Aleve® [OTC]** *see* Naproxen *on page 807*
- **Alfotax** *see* Cefotaxime *on page 221*
- **Algitrin®** *see* Acetaminophen *on page 32*


## Alglucerase (al GLOO ser ase)

**U.S. Brand Names** Ceredase®; Cerezyme®

**Synonyms** Glucocerebrosidase

**Therapeutic Category** Enzyme

**Pregnancy Risk Factor** C

**Lactation** Excretion in breast milk unknown/use caution

**Use** Long-term enzyme replacement treatment of Gaucher's disease

**Mechanism of Action/Effect** Replaces the missing enzyme, glucocerebrosidase associated with Gaucher's disease

**Contraindications** Hypersensitivity to alglucerase or any component

**Warnings** Prepared from pooled human placental tissue that may contain the causative agents of some viral diseases. Pregnancy factor C.

**Adverse Reactions**

>10%: Local: Discomfort, burning, and edema at the site of injection

<1% (Limited to important or life-threatening symptoms): Abdominal discomfort, nausea, vomiting

**Overdose/Toxicology** No obvious toxicity has been detected after single doses up to 234 units/kg.

(Continued)

## Alglucerase *(Continued)*

**Formulations** Injection: 10 units/mL (5 mL); 80 units/mL (5 mL)

**Dosing**

**Adults:** Usually administered as a 20-60 units/kg I.V. infusion given with a frequency ranging from 3 times/week to once every 2 weeks. Schedule determined by patient's response to therapy.

**Elderly:** Refer to adult dosing.

**Administration**

**I.V.:** Infuse over 1-2 hours.

**I.V. Detail:** Effective only via I.V. Filter during administration. Do not shake, shaking may render glycoprotein inactive. Do not mix with any other additives. Dilute with NS only.

**Stability**

**Storage:** Refrigerate (4°C), do not freeze. Contains no preservatives. Do not store opened vials for future use.

**Monitoring Laboratory Tests** CBC, platelets, acid phosphatase (AP), plasma glucocerebroside

**Additional Nursing Issues**

**Physical Assessment:** Monitor vital signs, energy level, change in bleeding tendency, reduced joint swelling, or bone pain. **Pregnancy risk factor C** - benefits of use should outweigh possible risks. Note breast-feeding caution.

**Patient Information/Instruction:** Treatment is required for life. **Pregnancy/breast-feeding precautions:** Inform prescriber if you are or intend to be pregnant. Consult prescriber if breast-feeding.

- **Alidol** *see* Ketorolac Tromethamine *on page 646*
- **Alin** *see* Dexamethasone *on page 346*
- **Alin Depot** *see* Dexamethasone *on page 346*

## Alitretinoin (a li TRET i noyn)

**U.S. Brand Names** Panretin®

**Therapeutic Category** Antineoplastic Agent, Miscellaneous; Retinoic Acid Derivative

**Pregnancy Risk Factor** D

**Lactation** Excretion in breast milk unknown/not recommended

**Use** Topical treatment of cutaneous lesions in AIDS-related Kaposi's sarcoma; not indicated when systemic therapy for Kaposi's sarcoma is indicated

**Mechanism of Action/Effect** Binds to retinoid receptors to inhibit growth of Kaposi's sarcoma

**Contraindications** Hypersensitivity to alitretinoin, other retinoids, or any component; pregnancy

**Warnings** May cause fetal harm if absorbed by a woman who is pregnant. Patients with cutaneous T-cell lymphoma have a high incidence of treatment-limiting adverse reactions. May be photosensitizing (based on experience with other retinoids); minimize sun or other UV exposure of treated areas. Do not use concurrently with topical products containing DEET (a common component of insect repellant products); increased toxicity may result. A common component of insect repellant products. Safety in pediatric patients or geriatric patients has not been established. Occlusive dressing should not be used.

**Drug Interactions**

**Increased Effect/Toxicity:** Increased toxicity of DEET may occur if products containing this compound are used concurrently with alitretinoin. Due to limited absorption after topical application, interaction with systemic medications is unlikely.

**Adverse Reactions**

>10%:

Central nervous system: Pain (0% to 34%)
Dermatologic: Rash (25% to 77%), pruritus (8% to 11%)
Neuromuscular & skeletal: Paresthesia (3% to 22%)

5% to 10%:

Cardiovascular: Edema (3% to 8%)
Dermatologic: Exfoliative dermatitis (3% to 9%), skin disorder (0% to 8%)

**Overdose/Toxicology** There has been no experience with human overdosage of alitretinoin, and overdose is unlikely following topical application. Treatment is symptomatic and supportive.

**Formulations** Gel: 0.1%, 60 g tube

**Dosing**

**Adults:** Topical: Apply gel twice daily to cutaneous Kaposi's sarcoma lesions.

**Elderly:** Refer to adult dosing.

**Stability**

**Storage:** Store at room temperature.

**Additional Nursing Issues**

**Physical Assessment:** See Contraindications, Warnings/Precautions, and Drug Interactions for use cautions. Monitor effectiveness of therapy and adverse reactions at beginning and periodically during therapy. Assess knowledge/teach patient appropriate use and adverse symptoms to report. **Pregnancy risk factor D** - assess knowledge/instruct patient on need to use appropriate contraceptive measures and the need to avoid pregnancy (see Pregnancy Issues). Breast-feeding is not recommended.

**Patient Information/Instruction:** For external use only. Use exactly as directed; do not overuse. Avoid use of any product such as insect repellants which contain DEET (check with your pharmacist). Wear protective clothing and or avoid exposure to direct sun or sunlamps. Wash hands thoroughly before applying. Avoid applying skin products that contain alcohol of harsh chemicals during treatment. Do not apply occlusive dressings. Stop treatment and inform prescriber if rash, skin irritation, redness, scaling, or excessive dryness appears. **Pregnancy/breast-feeding precautions:** Do not get pregnant while taking this medication; use appropriate barrier contraceptive measures. Breast-feeding is not recommended.

**Pregnancy Issues:** Potentially teratogenic and/or embryotoxic; limb, craniofacial, or skeletal defects have been observed in animal models. If used during pregnancy or if the patient becomes pregnant while using alitretinoin, the woman should be advised of potential harm to the fetus. Women of childbearing potential should avoid becoming pregnant.

- ♦ **Alkaban-AQ®** *see* Vinblastine *on page 1211*
- ♦ **Alka-Mints® [OTC]** *see* Calcium Supplements *on page 185*
- ♦ **Alka-Seltzer® Plus Cold Liqui-Gels Capsules** *see page 1294*
- ♦ **Alka-Seltzer® Plus Flu & Body Aches Non-Drowsy Liqui-Gels®** *see page 1294*
- ♦ **Alkeran®** *see* Melphalan *on page 718*
- ♦ **Allbee® With C** *see* Vitamin, Multiple *on page 1219*
- ♦ **Allbee® With C** *see page 1294*
- ♦ **Allegra®** *see* Fexofenadine *on page 482*
- ♦ **Aller-Chlor®** *see page 1294*
- ♦ **Allercon® Tablet** *see page 1294*
- ♦ **Allerdryl®** *see* Diphenhydramine *on page 381*
- ♦ **Allerest® [OTC]** *see page 1282*
- ♦ **Allerest® 12 Hour Capsule** *see page 1294*
- ♦ **Allerest® 12 Hour Nasal Solution** *see page 1294*
- ♦ **Allerest® Eye Drops** *see page 1294*
- ♦ **Allerest® Maximum Strength** *see page 1294*
- ♦ **Allerest® No Drowsiness** *see page 1294*
- ♦ **Allerfrin® Syrup** *see page 1294*
- ♦ **Allerfrin® Tablet** *see page 1294*
- ♦ **Allergan®** *see page 1291*
- ♦ **Allergan® Ear Drops** *see page 1306*
- ♦ **AllerMax® Oral [OTC]** *see* Diphenhydramine *on page 381*
- ♦ **Allernix®** *see* Diphenhydramine *on page 381*
- ♦ **Allerphed® Syrup** *see page 1294*

## Allopurinol (al oh PURE i nole)

**U.S. Brand Names** Zyloprim®

**Therapeutic Category** Xanthine Oxidase Inhibitor

**Pregnancy Risk Factor** C

**Lactation** Enters breast milk/compatible

**Use** Prevention of attacks of gouty arthritis and nephropathy; treatment of secondary hyperuricemia which may occur during treatment of tumors or leukemia; prevent recurrent calcium oxalate calculi; cutaneous and visceral leishmaniasis

**Mechanism of Action/Effect** Allopurinol inhibits xanthine oxidase, the enzyme responsible for the conversion of hypoxanthine to xanthine to uric acid. Allopurinol is metabolized to oxypurinol which is also an inhibitor of xanthine oxidase; allopurinol acts on purine catabolism, reducing the production of uric acid without disrupting the biosynthesis of vital purines.

**Contraindications** Hypersensitivity to allopurinol or any component

**Warnings** Do not use to treat asymptomatic hyperuricemia. Discontinue at first signs of rash. Reduce dosage in renal insufficiency. Reinstate with caution in patients who have had a previous mild allergic reaction. Monitor liver function and complete blood counts before initiating therapy and periodically during therapy. Use with caution in patients taking diuretics concurrently. Pregnancy factor C.

**Drug Interactions**

**Cytochrome P-450 Effect:** Hepatic enzyme inhibitor; isoenzyme profile not defined

**Decreased Effect:** Alcohol decreases effectiveness.

**Increased Effect/Toxicity:** Allopurinol inhibits metabolism of azathioprine, mercaptopurine, theophylline, and oral anticoagulants. Use with ampicillin or amoxicillin may increase the incidence of skin rash. Urinary acidification with large amounts of vitamin C may increase kidney stone formation. Thiazide diuretics enhance toxicity; monitor renal function. Allopurinol may compete for excretion in renal tubule with chlorpropamide and increase chlorpropamide's serum half-life. Increased risk of bone marrow suppression when given with myelosuppressive agents.

**Adverse Reactions**

>10%: Dermatologic: Skin rash (usually maculopapular), exfoliative, urticarial or purpuric lesions

1% to 10%:

Central nervous system: Drowsiness, chills, fever

Dermatologic: Alopecia

Gastrointestinal: Nausea, vomiting, diarrhea, abdominal pain, gastritis, heartburn

Hepatic: Increased alkaline phosphatase, AST, and ALT, hepatomegaly, hyperbilirubinemia, and jaundice, hepatic necrosis has been reported

(Continued)

## Allopurinol *(Continued)*

<1% (Limited to important or life-threatening symptoms): Vasculitis, toxic epidermal necrolysis, erythema multiforme, Stevens-Johnson syndrome, bone marrow suppression has been reported in patients receiving allopurinol with other myelosuppressive agents, anemia, agranulocytosis, aplastic anemia, thrombocytopenia, hepatotoxicity, thrombophlebitis, peripheral neuropathy, neuritis, paresthesia, renal impairment, epistaxis; idiosyncratic: Reaction characterized by fever, chills, leukopenia, leukocytosis, eosinophilia, arthralgia, skin rash, pruritus, nausea, and vomiting

**Overdose/Toxicology** If significant amounts of allopurinol have been absorbed, it is theoretically possible that oxypurinol stones could form, but no record of such occurrence exists. Alkalinization of urine and forced diuresis can help prevent potential xanthine stone formation.

**Pharmacodynamics/Kinetics**

**Half-life Elimination:** Parent drug: 1-3 hours; Oxypurinol: 18-30 hours; End-stage renal disease: Half-life prolonged

**Metabolism:** ~75% metabolized to active metabolites, chiefly oxypurinol

**Excretion:** Urine

**Onset:** Decreases in serum uric acid occur in 1-2 days with nadir achieved in 1-2 weeks

**Formulations** Tablet: 100 mg, 300 mg

**Dosing**

**Adults:** Oral:

Gout:

Mild: 200-300 mg/day

Severe: 400-600 mg/day

Myeloproliferative neoplastic disorders: 600-800 mg/day in 2-3 divided doses for prevention of acute uric acid nephropathy for 2-3 days starting 1-2 days before chemotherapy

**Elderly:** Oral: Initial: 100 mg/day; increase until desired uric acid level is obtained.

**Renal Impairment:** Oral:

Must be adjusted due to accumulation of allopurinol and metabolites; see table.

**Adult Maintenance Doses of Allopurinol***

| Creatinine Clearance (mL/min) | Maintenance Dose of Allopurinol (mg) |
|---|---|
| 140 | 400 qd |
| 120 | 350 qd |
| 100 | 300 qd |
| 80 | 250 qd |
| 60 | 200 qd |
| 40 | 150 qd |
| 20 | 100 qd |
| 10 | 100 q2d |
| 0 | 100 q3d |

*This table is based on a standard maintenance dose of 300 mg of allopurinol per day for a patient with a creatinine clearance of 100 mL/min.

Hemodialysis: Administer dose after hemodialysis or administer 50% supplemental dose.

**Administration**

**Oral:** Should be administered after meals.

**Monitoring Laboratory Tests** CBC, serum uric acid levels, hepatic and renal function, especially at start of therapy

**Additional Nursing Issues**

**Physical Assessment:** Assess effectiveness and interactions of other medications patient may be taking (see Contraindications and Drug Interactions). Monitor for therapeutic response (eg, frequency and severity of gouty attacks), laboratory values, and adverse reactions (see Adverse Reactions and Overdose/Toxicology) at beginning of therapy and periodically with long-term use. Assess knowledge/teach patient appropriate use, interventions to reduce side effects, and adverse symptoms to report. **Pregnancy risk factor C** - benefits of use should outweigh possible risks.

**Patient Information/Instruction:** Take as directed. Maintain adequate hydration (2-3 L/day of fluids unless instructed to restrict fluid intake) to avoid possible adverse renal problems. While using this medication, do not use alcohol, other prescription or OTC medications, or vitamin substances without consulting prescriber. You may experience drowsiness (use caution when driving or engaging in tasks requiring alertness until response to drug is known); nausea, vomiting, or heartburn (small frequent meals, frequent mouth care, chewing gum, or sucking lozenges may help); hair loss (reversible). Report skin rash or lesions; painful urination or blood in urine or stool; unresolved nausea or vomiting; numbness of extremities; pain or irritation of the eyes; swelling of lips, mouth, or tongue; unusual fatigue; easy bruising or bleeding; yellowing of skin or eyes; or any change in color of urine or stool. **Pregnancy precautions:** Inform prescriber if you are or intend to be pregnant.

**Geriatric Considerations:** Adjust dose based on renal function.

♦ **All-*trans*-Retinoic Acid** *see* Tretinoin (Oral) *on page 1168*
♦ **Almora®** *see* Magnesium Supplements *on page 703*
♦ **Aloid** *see* Miconazole *on page 767*

- **Alomide®** *see page 1282*
- **Alpha-Baclofen®** *see* Baclofen *on page 131*
- **Alpha-Dextrano"40"** *see* Dextran *on page 351*
- **Alphagan® Ophthalmic** *see* Ophthalmic Agents, Glaucoma *on page 853*
- **Alphamin®** *see* Hydroxocobalamin *on page 583*
- **Alphamul®** *see page 1294*
- **Alpha-Tamoxifen®** *see* Tamoxifen *on page 1095*
- **Alphatrex®** *see* Betamethasone *on page 148*
- **Alphatrex®** *see* Topical Corticosteroids *on page 1152*


## Alprazolam (al PRAY zoe lam)

**U.S. Brand Names** Xanax®

**Therapeutic Category** Benzodiazepine

**Pregnancy Risk Factor** D

**Lactation** Enters breast milk/contraindicated

**Use** Treatment of anxiety disorders; adjunct in the treatment of depression; management of panic attacks; treatment of premenstrual syndrome

**Mechanism of Action/Effect** Binds at stereospecific receptors at several sites within the central nervous system; effects may be mediated through gamma-aminobutyric acid; anxiety effects occur at doses well below those necessary to cause sedation

**Contraindications** Hypersensitivity to alprazolam or any component; may be cross-sensitivity with other benzodiazepines; severe uncontrolled pain, narrow-angle glaucoma, severe respiratory depression, pre-existing CNS depression; pregnancy

**Warnings** Withdrawal symptoms including seizures have occurred 18 hours to 3 days after abrupt discontinuation. When discontinuing therapy, decrease daily dose by no more than 0.5 mg every 3 days. Reduce dose in patients with significant hepatic disease. Not intended for management of anxieties and minor distresses associated with everyday life.

**Drug Interactions**

**Cytochrome P-450 Effect:** CYP3A3/4 enzyme substrate

**Decreased Effect:** Carbamazepine and disulfiram decrease the effect of alprazolam.

**Increased Effect/Toxicity:** Alprazolam potentiates the CNS depressant effects of phenothiazines, narcotics, barbiturates, alcohol, general anesthetics, antihistamines, monoamine oxidase inhibitors, and antidepressants. Oral contraceptives, CNS depressants, cimetidine, and lithium increase toxicity of alprazolam. Potential for serotonin syndrome if combined with other serotonergic drugs.

**Effects on Lab Values** ↑ with alkaline phosphatase

**Adverse Reactions**

>10%:

Central nervous system: Drowsiness, ataxia, lightheadedness, headache, dizziness, impaired coordination, anxiety, fatigue, slurred speech, irritability, nervousness, insomnia, memory impairment, cognitive disorder, dysarthria, anxiety

Gastrointestinal: Decreased salivation (dry mouth)

Genitourinary: Micturition difficulties

1% to 10%:

Cardiovascular: Tachycardia, syncope

Central nervous system: Confusion, increased libido, depersonalization, mental depression, perceptual disturbances, paresthesias, weakness, akathisia, agitation, disinhibition, talkativeness, derealization, dream abnormalities, fear, decreased libido

Gastrointestinal: Abdominal or stomach cramps, increased or decreased appetite, weight gain or loss, nausea, vomiting

Neuromuscular & skeletal: Muscle cramps

Ocular: Photophobia, blurred vision

Otic: Tinnitus

Respiratory: Nasal congestion

Miscellaneous: Sweating

<1% (Limited to important or life-threatening symptoms): Agranulocytosis, anemia, leukopenia, neutropenia, thrombocytopenia, hepatic dysfunction, dystonic extrapyramidal effects, muscle weakness

**Overdose/Toxicology** Symptoms of overdose include somnolence, confusion, coma, and diminished reflexes. Treatment for benzodiazepine overdose is supportive. Flumazenil has been shown to selectively block the binding of benzodiazepines to CNS receptors, resulting in a reversal of benzodiazepine-induced sedation; however, its use may not reverse respiratory depression.

**Pharmacodynamics/Kinetics**

**Protein Binding:** 80%

**Half-life Elimination:** 12-15 hours

**Time to Peak:** Within 1-2 hours

**Metabolism:** Liver

**Excretion:** Urine

**Onset:** Within 1 hour

**Duration:** Variable 8-24 hours

**Formulations** Tablet: 0.25 mg, 0.5 mg, 1 mg, 2 mg

**Dosing**

**Adults:** Oral: 0.25-0.5 mg 2-3 times/day, titrate dose upward; maximum: 4 mg/day

**Note:** Treatment lasting more than 4 months should be re-evaluated to determine the patient's need for the drug.

(Continued)

## Alprazolam *(Continued)*

**Elderly:** Oral: Initial: 0.125-0.25 mg twice daily; increase by 0.125 mg/day as needed.

**Hepatic Impairment:** Oral: Reduce dose by 50% to 60% or avoid in cirrhosis.

**Additional Nursing Issues**

**Physical Assessment:** Assess other medications patient may be taking for effectiveness and interactions (see Drug Interactions). See Contraindications and Warnings/Precautions for cautious use. Assess for history of addiction; long-term use can result in dependence, abuse, or tolerance; periodically evaluate need for continued use. Monitor therapeutic response (eg, mood, affect, anxiety level, sleep pattern) and adverse reactions at beginning of therapy and periodically with long-term use (see Adverse Reactions and Overdose/Toxicology). Taper dosage slowly when discontinuing. Assess knowledge/teach patient appropriate use, interventions to reduce side effects, and adverse symptoms to report. **Pregnancy risk factor D** - assess knowledge/teach appropriate use of barrier contraceptives. Breast-feeding is contraindicated.

**Patient Information/Instruction:** Take exactly as directed (do not increase dose or frequency); may cause physical and/or psychological dependence. Do not use excessive alcohol, or other prescription or OTC medications (especially pain medications, sedatives, antihistamines, or hypnotics) without consulting prescriber. Maintain adequate hydration (2-3 L/day of fluids unless instructed to restrict fluid intake). You may experience drowsiness, lightheadedness, impaired coordination, dizziness, or blurred vision (use caution when driving or engaging in hazardous tasks until response to drug is known); nausea, vomiting, or dry mouth (small frequent meals, frequent mouth care, chewing gum, or sucking lozenges may help); constipation (increased exercise, fluids, or dietary fruit and fiber may help); altered sexual drive or ability (reversible); photosensitivity (use sunscreen, wear protective clothing and eyewear, and avoid direct sunlight). Report persistent CNS effects (eg, confusion, depression, increased sedation, excitation, headache, agitation, insomnia or nightmares, dizziness, fatigue, impaired coordination, changes in personality, or changes in cognition); changes in urinary pattern; muscle cramping, weakness, tremors, or rigidity; ringing in ears or visual disturbances; chest pain, palpitations, or rapid heartbeat; excessive perspiration; excessive GI symptoms (cramping, constipation, vomiting, anorexia); or worsening of condition. **Pregnancy/breast-feeding precautions:** Do not get pregnant while taking this medication; use appropriate barrier contraceptive measures as recommended by your prescriber. Do not breast-feed.

**Geriatric Considerations:** Due to short duration of action, it is considered to be a benzodiazepine of choice in the elderly.

**Related Information**

Antiemetics for Chemotherapy-Induced Nausea and Vomiting *on page 1307*
Anxiolytic/Hypnotic Use in Long-Term Care Facilities *on page 1430*
Benzodiazepines Comparison *on page 1375*

## Alprostadil (al PROS ta dill)

**U.S. Brand Names** Caverject® Injection; Edex®; Muse® Pellet

**Synonyms** $PGE_1$; Prostaglandin $E_1$

**Therapeutic Category** Prostaglandin

**Pregnancy Risk Factor** X

**Lactation** Not indicated for use in women

**Use** Diagnosis and treatment of erectile dysfunction; adjunct in the diagnosis of erectile dysfunction, patent ductus arteriosus in neonate

**Mechanism of Action/Effect** Causes vasodilation by dilation of cavernosal arteries when injected along the penile shaft, allowing blood flow to, and entrapment in, the lacunar spaces of the penis (ie, corporeal veno-occlusive mechanism)

**Contraindications** Hypersensitivity to alprostadil or any component; conditions predisposing patients to priapism (sickle cell anemia, multiple myeloma, leukemia); patients with anatomical deformation of the penis, penile implants; use is contraindicated in males for whom sexual activity is inadvisable

**Warnings** Priapism may occur. Treat immediately to avoid penile tissue damage and permanent loss of potency. Discontinue therapy if signs of penile fibrosis develop (penile angulation, cavernosal fibrosis, or Peyronie's disease). Use with caution in the presence of bleeding tendencies (inhibits platelet aggregation). Hypotension or syncope may occur within 1 hour of administration; avoid driving or hazardous tasks.

**Drug Interactions**

**Increased Effect/Toxicity:** Risk of hypotension and syncope may be increased with antihypertensives.

**Adverse Reactions**

>10%:

- Cardiovascular: Flushing
- Central nervous system: Fever
- Genitourinary: Penile pain
- Respiratory: Apnea

1% to 10%:

- Cardiovascular: Bradycardia, hypotension, hypertension, tachycardia, cardiac arrest, edema
- Central nervous system: Seizures, headache, dizziness
- Endocrine & metabolic: Hypokalemia
- Gastrointestinal: Diarrhea
- Genitourinary: Priapism, penile fibrosis, penis disorder, penile rash, penile edema
- Hematologic: Disseminated intravascular coagulation

Local: Injection site hematoma, injection site bruising
Neuromuscular & skeletal: Back pain
Respiratory: Upper respiratory infection, flu syndrome, sinusitis, nasal congestion, cough
Miscellaneous: Sepsis, localized pain in structures other than the injection site
<1% (Limited to important or life-threatening symptoms): Cerebral bleeding, congestive heart failure, second degree heart block, shock, supraventricular tachycardia, ventricular fibrillation, hyperemia, anuria, balanitis, urethral bleeding, penile numbness, yeast infection, penile pruritus and erythema, abnormal ejaculation, anemia, bleeding, thrombocytopenia, hyperbilirubinemia, bradypnea, bronchial wheezing, peritonitis, leg pain, perineal pain

**Overdose/Toxicology** Symptoms of overdose when treating patent ductus arteriosus include apnea, bradycardia, hypotension, and flushing. If hypotension or pyrexia occurs, the infusion rate should be reduced until symptoms subside. Apnea or bradycardia requires drug discontinuation. If intracavernous overdose occurs, supervise until systemic effects have resolved or until penile detumescence has occurred.

**Pharmacodynamics/Kinetics**

**Half-life Elimination:** 5-10 minutes
**Metabolism:** Lungs
**Excretion:** Urine
**Onset:** Rapid
**Duration:** <1 hour

**Formulations**

Injection:
Caverject®: 5 mcg, 10 mcg, 20 mcg
Edex®: 5 mcg, 10 mcg, 20 mcg, 40 mcg
Pellet, urethral (Muse®): 125 mcg, 250 mcg, 500 mcg, 1000 mcg

**Dosing**

**Adults: Erectile dysfunction**:
Caverject®:
Individualize dose by careful titration. Usual dose: 2.5-60 mcg (doses >60 mcg are not recommended). Initiate dosage titration at 2.5 mcg, increasing by 2.5 mcg to a dose of 5 mcg, and then in increments of 5-10 mcg depending on the erectile response until the dose produces an erection suitable for intercourse, not lasting >1 hour. If there is absolutely no response to initial 2.5 mcg dose, the second dose may increased to 7.5 mcg, followed by increments of 5-10 mcg.
Neurogenic etiology (eg, spinal cord injury): Initiate dosage titration at 1.25 mcg, increasing to a dose of 2.5 mcg, and then 5 mcg. Increase further in increments of 5 mcg until the dose is reached that produces an erection suitable for intercourse, not lasting >1 hour.
**Note:** Patient must stay in the physician's office until complete detumescence occurs. If there is no response, then the next higher dose may be given within 1 hour. If there is still no response, a 1-day interval before giving the next dose is recommended. Increasing the dose or concentration in the treatment of impotence results in increasing pain and discomfort.
Muse® Pellet: Intraurethral: Administer as needed to achieve an erection. Duration of action is about 30-60 minutes; use only two systems per 24-hour period.

**Elderly:** Refer to adult dosing.

**Administration**

**Other:** Erectile dysfunction: Use a ½ inch, 27- to 30-gauge needle. Inject into the dorsolateral aspect of the proximal third of the penis, avoiding visible veins alternate side of the penis for injections.

**Stability**

**Storage:** Refrigerate at 2°C to 8°C until dispensed. After dispensing, stable for up to 3 months at or below 25°C. Do not freeze.

**Reconstitution:** Use only the supplied diluent for reconstitution (ie, bacteriostatic/sterile water with benzyl alcohol 0.945%).

**Additional Nursing Issues**

**Physical Assessment:** After individual dose titration is determined by physician, the Caverject® injection (or Muse®) is generally self-administered by the patient. Assessment and monitoring focus on teaching and evaluating patient knowledge of guidelines for use, appropriate administration and needle disposal, interventions to reduce side effects, and adverse symptoms to report. **Pregnancy risk factor X** - determine that patient and sexual partner(s) are capable of using barrier contraceptive measures during treatment and for 1 month following discontinuance of therapy.

**Patient Information/Instruction:** Use only as directed, no more than 3 times/week, allowing 24 hours between injections. Store in refrigerator and dilute with supplied diluent immediately before use. Use alternate sides of penis with each injection. Dispose of syringes and needle and single dose vials in a safe manner (do not share medication, syringes, or needles). Note that the risk of transmitting blood-borne disease is increased with use of alprostadil injections since a small amount of bleeding at injection site is possible. Stop using alprostadil and contact prescriber immediately if signs of priapism occur, erections last more than 4-6 hours, or you experience moderate to severe penile pain. Report penile problems (eg, nodules, new penile pain, rash, bruising, numbness, swelling, signs of infection, abnormal ejaculations); cardiac symptoms (hypo- or hypertension, chest pain, palpitations, irregular heartbeat); flushing, fever, flu-like symptoms; difficulty breathing, or wheezing; or other adverse reactions. Refer to prescriber every 3 months to ensure proper technique and for dosage evaluation. **Pregnancy precautions:** This drug will cause severe fetal defects. Consult prescriber for appropriate barrier contraception education for you and your

(Continued)

## Alprostadil *(Continued)*

sexual partner(s). Do not give blood while taking this medication and for 1 month following discontinuance.

**Geriatric Considerations:** Elderly may have concomitant diseases which would contraindicate the use of alprostadil. Other forms of attaining penile tumescence are recommended.

- **AL-R®** *see page 1294*
- **Alrex™** *see page 1282*
- **Altace™** *see* Ramipril *on page 1007*

## Alteplase (AL te plase)

**U.S. Brand Names** Activase®

**Synonyms** Alteplase, Recombinant; Tissue Plasminogen Activator, Recombinant; t-PA

**Therapeutic Category** Thrombolytic Agent

**Pregnancy Risk Factor** C

**Lactation** Excretion in breast milk unknown

**Use** Management of acute myocardial infarction for the lysis of thrombi in coronary arteries; management of acute massive pulmonary embolism (PE) in adults

**Acute myocardial infarction (AMI):** Chest pain ≥20 minutes, ≤12-24 hours; S-T elevation ≥0.1 mV in at least two EKG leads

**Acute pulmonary embolism (APE):** Age ≤75 years: As soon as possible within 5 days of thrombotic event. Documented massive pulmonary embolism by pulmonary angiography or echocardiography or high probability lung scan with clinical shock.

**Mechanism of Action/Effect** Dissolves thrombus (clot)

**Contraindications** Intracranial surgery or bleeding; severe uncontrolled hypertension (systolic ≥180 mm Hg, diastolic ≥110 mm Hg); recent (within 1 month): cerebrovascular accident or transient ischemic attack, GI bleeding, trauma, or surgery, prolonged external cardiac massage; intracranial neoplasm; suspected aortic dissection; arteriovenous malformation or aneurysm; bleeding diathesis; severe hepatic or renal disease; hemostatic defects

**Warnings** Doses >150 mg have been associated with an increase of intracranial hemorrhage. **Do not use central venous puncture (CVP line) or noncompressible arterial sticks.** Pregnancy factor C.

**Drug Interactions**

**Increased Effect/Toxicity:** Alteplase increases the effects of anticoagulants. Aspirin, ticlopidine, dipyridamole, and heparin are at least additive to the effect of alteplase.

**Effects on Lab Values** Altered results of coagulation and fibrinolytic agents

**Adverse Reactions**

1% to 10%:

Cardiovascular: Hypotension
Central nervous system: Fever
Dermatologic: Bruising
Gastrointestinal: GI hemorrhage, nausea, vomiting
Genitourinary: GU hemorrhage

<1% (Limited to important or life-threatening symptoms): Retroperitoneal hemorrhage, gingival hemorrhage, intracranial hemorrhage rapid lysis of coronary artery thrombi by thrombolytic agents may be associated with reperfusion-related atrial and/or ventricular arrhythmias, epistaxis

**Overdose/Toxicology** Increased incidence of intracranial bleeding

**Pharmacodynamics/Kinetics**

**Half-life Elimination:** Cleared rapidly by the liver; ~80% is cleared within 10 minutes after infusion is terminated

**Metabolism:** Liver

**Duration:** >50% present in plasma is cleared within 5 minutes after the infusion has been terminated, and ~80% is cleared within 10 minutes

**Formulations** Powder for injection, lyophilized (recombinant): 20 mg [11.6 million units] (20 mL); 50 mg [29 million units] (50 mL); 100 mg [58 million units] (100 mL)

**Dosing**

**Adults:**

Coronary artery thrombi:

Patients >67 kg: I.V.: Front loading dose: Total dose is 100 mg over 1.5 hours. Add this dose to a 100 mL bag of 0.9% sodium chloride for a total volume of 200 mL. Infuse 15 mg (30 mL) over 1-2 minutes; infuse 50 mg (100 mL) over 30 minutes. (Begin heparin 5000-10,000 unit bolus followed by continuous infusion of 1000 units/hour.) Infuse 35 mg/hour (70 mL) for next 60 minutes.

Patients ≤67 kg: Administer 15 mg as an I.V. bolus, then 0.75 mg/kg over 30 minutes, not to exceed 50 mg, and then 0.5 mg/kg over the next 60 minutes not to exceed 35 mg.

Acute pulmonary embolism: 100 mg over 2 hours

Acute ischemic stroke: Doses should be given within the first 3 hours of the onset of symptoms. Load with 0.09 mg/kg as a bolus, followed by 0.81 mg/kg as a continuous infusion over 60 minutes; maximum total dose should not exceed 90 mg.

**Elderly:** Refer to adult dosing.

**Administration**

**I.V.:** Infuse 15 mg (30 mL) over 1-2 minutes. Infuse 50 mg (100 mL) over 30 minutes.

**I.V. Detail:** Reconstituted solution should be clear or pale yellow and transparent. Avoid agitation during dilution.

**Stability**

**Storage:** Refrigerate

**Reconstitution:** Add the dose to a 100 mL bag of 0.9% sodium chloride for a total volume of 200 mL. Use sterile water (preservative free) provided by manufacturer for reconstitution. Do not use bacteriostatic water. Slight foaming may occur with reconstitution but will dissipate after standing for several minutes. Refrigerate; must be used within 8 hours of reconstitution.

**Compatibility:** Compatible with either $D_5W$ or NS. Physically compatible with lidocaine, metoprolol, or propranolol when administered via Y-site. Incompatible with dobutamine, dopamine, heparin, and nitroglycerin infusions. Do not mix other medications into infusion solution.

**Monitoring Laboratory Tests** CBC, PTT

**Additional Nursing Issues**

**Physical Assessment:** Monitor vital signs; laboratory results; and EKG prior to, during, and after therapy. Arrhythmias may occur; have antiarrhythmic drugs available. Assess infusion site and monitor for hemorrhage every 10 minutes (or according to institutional policy) during therapy and for 1 hour following therapy. Maintain strict bedrest. Monitor for excess bleeding and use/teach bleeding precautions (avoid invasive procedures and activities that could cause trauma). **Pregnancy risk factor C.** Note breast-feeding caution.

**Patient Information/Instruction:** This medication can only be administered I.V. You will have a tendency to bleed easily following this medication; use caution to prevent injury - use electric razor, soft toothbrush, and use caution with sharps. Strict bedrest should be maintained to reduce the risk of bleeding. If bleeding occurs, apply pressure to bleeding spot until bleeding stops completely. Report unusual bruising or bleeding; blood in urine, stool, or vomitus; bleeding gums; changes in vision; difficulty breathing; or chest pain.

**Other Issues:** Drug is frequently administered with heparin. Discontinue both if serious bleeding occurs. Avoid invasive procedures.

**Additional Information** pH: 5-7.5

- **Alteplase, Recombinant** *see* Alteplase *on previous page*
- **Alter-$H_2$®** *see* Ranitidine *on page 1008*
- **ALternaGEL® [OTC]** *see* Aluminum Hydroxide *on next page*

## Altretamine (al TRET a meen)

**U.S. Brand Names** Hexalen®

**Synonyms** Hexamethylmelamine

**Therapeutic Category** Antineoplastic Agent, Miscellaneous

**Pregnancy Risk Factor** D

**Lactation** Excretion in breast milk unknown

**Use** Palliative treatment of persistent or recurrent ovarian cancer following first-line therapy with a cisplatin- or alkylating agent-based combination

**Mechanism of Action/Effect** Exact mechanism of action that causes cell death is not known. Metabolism in the liver is required for cytotoxicity. Although altretamine clinical antitumor spectrum resembles that of alkylating agents, the drug has demonstrated activity in alkylator-resistant patients; probably requires hepatic microsomal mixed-function oxidase enzyme activation to become cytotoxic. The drug selectively inhibits the incorporation of radioactive thymidine and uridine into DNA and RNA, inhibiting DNA and RNA synthesis. Metabolized to reactive intermediates which covalently bind to microsomal proteins and DNA. These reactive intermediates can spontaneously degrade to demethylated melamines and formaldehyde which are also cytotoxic.

**Contraindications** Hypersensitivity to altretamine; pre-existing severe bone marrow depression; severe neurologic toxicity; pregnancy

**Warnings** The U.S. Food and Drug Administration (FDA) currently recommends that procedures for proper handling and disposal of antineoplastic agents be considered. Use with caution in patients previously treated with other myelosuppressive drugs or with pre-existing neurotoxicity. Use with caution in patients with renal or hepatic dysfunction. Altretamine may be slightly mutagenic.

**Drug Interactions**

**Decreased Effect:** Phenobarbital may increase metabolism of altretamine which may decrease the effect.

**Increased Effect/Toxicity:** Altretamine may cause severe orthostatic hypotension when administered with MAO inhibitors. Cimetidine may decrease metabolism of altretamine.

**Adverse Reactions**

>10%:

Central nervous system: Peripheral sensory neuropathy, neurotoxicity

Gastrointestinal: Nausea, vomiting

Hematologic: Anemia, thrombocytopenia, leukopenia

1% to 10%:

Central nervous system: Seizures

Gastrointestinal: Anorexia, diarrhea, stomach cramps

Hepatic: Increased alkaline phosphatase

<1% (Limited to important or life-threatening symptoms): Alopecia, myelosuppression, hepatotoxicity, tremor

**Overdose/Toxicology** Symptoms of overdose include nausea, vomiting, peripheral neuropathy, severe bone marrow suppression. Treatment is supportive.

(Continued)

## Altretamine *(Continued)*

**Pharmacodynamics/Kinetics**

**Half-life Elimination:** 13 hours

**Metabolism:** Liver

**Excretion:** Urine

**Formulations** Capsule: 50 mg

**Dosing**

**Adults:** Oral:

4-12 mg/kg/day in 3-4 divided doses for 21-90 days

Alternatively: 240-320 mg/m²/day in 3-4 divided doses per day for 21 days, repeated every 6 weeks

Alternatively: 260 mg/m²/day in 4 divided doses per day for 14-21 days of a 28-day cycle

**Temporarily discontinue** for ≥14 days and restart at 200 mg/m²/day if any of the following occurs: GI intolerance unresponsive to symptom measures, WBC <2000/mm³, granulocyte count <1000/mm³, platelet count <75,000/mm³, progressive neurotoxicity.

**Elderly:** Refer to adult dosing.

**Administration**

**Oral:** Administer total daily dose as 4 divided oral doses after meals and at bedtime.

**Monitoring Laboratory Tests** Peripheral blood counts and neurologic examinations should be done routinely before and after drug therapy.

**Additional Nursing Issues**

**Physical Assessment:** Monitor closely for adverse side effects (blood tests and neurological status)or toxic response (see above). Patients receiving altretamine may be fragile and identification and intervention to reduce adverse side effects is necessary. **Pregnancy risk factor D** - assess knowledge/teach appropriate use of barrier contraceptives. Note breast-feeding caution.

**Patient Information/Instruction:** Take as directed, preferably after meals. Avoid alcohol and aspirin or medications containing aspirin. You may experience nausea or vomiting during therapy or several weeks after therapy is discontinued; small frequent meals may help. You will be more susceptible to infection while taking this medication; avoid crowds or persons with infections or contagious conditions. Report any numbness, tingling, or pain in extremities; unrelieved nausea or vomiting; tremors; yellowing of skin or eyes; fever; chills; easy bruising or unusual bleeding; extreme weakness or increased fatigue. **Pregnancy/breast-feeding precautions:** Do not get pregnant while taking this medication; use appropriate barrier contraceptive measures as recommended by your prescriber. Consult prescriber if breast-feeding.


- ♦ **Alu-Cap® [OTC]** *see* Aluminum Hydroxide *on this page*
- ♦ **Aludrox®** *see page 1294*
- ♦ **Aluminum Acetate and Calcium Acetate** *see page 1294*
- ♦ **Aluminum Carbonate** *see page 1294*


## Aluminum Hydroxide (a LOO mi num hye DROKS ide)

**U.S. Brand Names** ALternaGEL® [OTC]; Alu-Cap® [OTC]; Alu-Tab® [OTC]; Amphojel® [OTC]; Dialume® [OTC]; Nephrox Suspension [OTC]

**Therapeutic Category** Antacid; Antidote

**Pregnancy Risk Factor** C

**Lactation** Excretion in breast milk unknown

**Use** Treatment of hyperacidity; hyperphosphatemia

**Mechanism of Action/Effect** Neutralizes or reduces gastric acidity, resulting in increased gastric pH and inhibition of pepsin activity

**Contraindications** Hypersensitivity to aluminum salts or any component

**Warnings** Binds with phosphate ions. Hypophosphatemia may occur with prolonged administration or large doses. Use with caution in patients with congestive heart failure, renal failure, edema, cirrhosis, and low sodium diets, and patients who have recently suffered GI hemorrhage. Uremic patients not receiving dialysis may develop aluminum intoxication or osteomalacia and osteoporosis due to phosphate depletion. Pregnancy factor C.

**Drug Interactions**

**Decreased Effect:** Aluminum hydroxide decreases the effect of tetracyclines, digoxin, indomethacin, iron salts, isoniazid, allopurinol, benzodiazepines, corticosteroids, penicillamine, phenothiazines, ranitidine, ketoconazole, and itraconazole.

**Effects on Lab Values** ↓ phosphorus, inorganic (S); may interfere with some gastric imaging techniques or gastric acid secretion tests.

**Adverse Reactions**

>10%: Gastrointestinal: Constipation, chalky taste, stomach cramps, fecal impaction

1% to 10%: Gastrointestinal: Nausea, vomiting, discoloration of feces (white speckles)

<1% (Limited to important or life-threatening symptoms): Hypophosphatemia, hypomagnesemia

**Overdose/Toxicology** Aluminum antacids may cause constipation, phosphate depletion, and bezoar or fecalith formation. In patients with renal failure, aluminum may accumulate to toxic levels. Deferoxamine, traditionally used as an iron chelator, has been shown to increase urinary aluminum output. Deferoxamine chelation of aluminum has resulted in improvement of clinical symptoms and bone histology; however, this remains an experimental treatment for aluminum poisoning and has significant potential for adverse effects.

**Formulations**

Capsule:

Alu-Cap®: 400 mg

Dialume®: 500 mg

Liquid: 600 mg/5 mL

ALternaGEL®: 600 mg/5 mL

Suspension, oral: 320 mg/5 mL; 450 mg/5 mL; 675 mg/5 mL

Amphojel®: 320 mg/5 mL

Tablet:

Amphojel®: 300 mg, 600 mg

Alu-Tab®: 500 mg

**Dosing**

**Adults:** Oral:

Antacid: 30 mL 1 and 3 hours postprandial and at bedtime

Hyperphosphatemia: 500-1800 mg, 3-6 times/day, between meals and at bedtime

Acute: 30-60 mL/dose every hour; titrate to maintain the gastric pH >5

Healing phase: 15-45 mL every 3-6 hours or 1 and 3 hours after meals and at bedtime

**Elderly:** Refer to adult dosing.

**Administration**

**Oral:** Dose should be followed with water.

**Monitoring Laboratory Tests** Calcium and phosphate levels periodically when patient is on chronic therapy

**Additional Nursing Issues**

**Physical Assessment:** Monitor appropriate laboratory tests and effectiveness of treatment. Assess for constipation and treat accordingly. **Pregnancy risk factor C** - benefits of use should outweigh possible risks. Note breast-feeding caution.

**Patient Information/Instruction:** Take as directed, preferably 2 hours before or 2 hours after meals and any other medications. Dilute liquid dose with water or juice and shake well. Do not increase sodium intake and maintain adequate hydration (2-3 L/day of fluids unless instructed to restrict fluid intake). Chew tablet thoroughly before swallowing with full glass of water. You may experience constipation (increased exercise or dietary fluids, fiber, and fruit may help). If unrelieved, see prescriber. Report unresolved nausea, malaise, muscle weakness, blood in stool or black stool, or abdominal pain. **Pregnancy/breast-feeding precautions:** Inform prescriber if you are or intend to be pregnant. Consult prescriber if breast-feeding.

**Geriatric Considerations:** Elderly, due to disease and/or drug therapy, may be predisposed to constipation and fecal impaction. This may be managed with a stool softener or laxatives. Careful evaluation of possible drug interactions must be done. Consider renal insufficiency (<30 mL/minute) as predisposition to aluminum toxicity.

- **Aluminum Hydroxide and Magnesium Carbonate** *see page 1294*
- **Aluminum Hydroxide and Magnesium Hydroxide** *see page 1294*
- **Aluminum Hydroxide and Magnesium Trisilicate** *see page 1294*
- **Aluminum Hydroxide, Magnesium Hydroxide, and Simethicone** *see page 1294*
- **Aluminum Sucrose Sulfate, Basic** *see* Sucralfate *on page 1078*
- **Alupent®** *see* Metaproterenol *on page 732*
- **Alu-Tab® [OTC]** *see* Aluminum Hydroxide *on previous page*
- **Alvidina** *see* Ranitidine *on page 1008*

## Amantadine (a MAN ta deen)

**U.S. Brand Names** Symadine®; Symmetrel®

**Synonyms** Adamantanamine Hydrochloride

**Therapeutic Category** Anti-Parkinson's Agent (Dopamine Agonist); Antiviral Agent

**Pregnancy Risk Factor** C

**Lactation** Enters breast milk/use caution

**Use** Symptomatic and adjunct treatment of parkinsonism; prophylaxis and treatment of influenza A viral infection; treatment of drug-induced extrapyramidal symptoms (pseudoparkinsonism)

**Mechanism of Action/Effect** As an antiviral, blocks the uncoating of influenza A virus preventing penetration of virus into host; antiparkinsonian activity may be due to its blocking the reuptake of dopamine into presynaptic neurons and causing direct stimulation of postsynaptic receptors

**Contraindications** Hypersensitivity to amantadine hydrochloride or any component

**Warnings** Use with caution in patients with liver disease, a history of recurrent and eczematoid dermatitis, uncontrolled psychosis or severe psychoneurosis, seizures, and in those receiving CNS stimulant drugs. When treating Parkinson's disease, do not discontinue abruptly. In many patients, the therapeutic benefits of amantadine are limited to a few months. Pregnancy factor C.

**Drug Interactions**

**Increased Effect/Toxicity:** When taken with drugs associated with anticholinergic or CNS stimulants, activity may result in an increased atropine-like effect of amantadine. Hydrochlorothiazide plus triamterene or amiloride can increase the toxicity of amantadine.

**Adverse Reactions**

1% to 10%:

Cardiovascular: Orthostatic hypotension, peripheral edema

Central nervous system: Insomnia, depression, anxiety, irritability, dizziness, hallucinations, ataxia, headache, confusion, somnolence, nervousness, dream abnormality, agitation, fatigue

(Continued)

## Amantadine *(Continued)*

Dermatologic: Livedo reticularis

Gastrointestinal: Nausea, anorexia, constipation, diarrhea, dry mouth

Respiratory: Dry nose

<1% (Limited to important or life-threatening symptoms): Congestive heart failure, hypertension, psychosis, slurred speech, euphoria, amnesia, instances of convulsions, leukopenia, neutropenia, dyspnea

**Overdose/Toxicology** Symptoms of overdose include nausea, vomiting, slurred speech, blurred vision, lethargy, hallucinations, seizures, and myoclonic jerking. Treatment should be directed at reducing CNS stimulation, controlling seizures, and maintaining cardiovascular function.

**Pharmacodynamics/Kinetics**

**Protein Binding:** Normal renal function: ~67%; Hemodialysis patient: ~59%

**Distribution:** Crosses blood brain barrier

**Half-life Elimination:** Normal renal function: 2-7 hours; End-stage renal disease: 7-10 days

**Metabolism:** Not appreciable, small amounts of an acetyl metabolite identified

**Excretion:** Urine

**Onset:** Onset of antidyskinetic action: Within 48 hours

**Formulations**

Amantadine hydrochloride:

Capsule: 100 mg

Syrup: 50 mg/5 mL (480 mL)

**Dosing**

**Adults:**

Parkinson's disease: 100 mg twice daily

Influenza A viral infection: 200 mg/day in 1-2 divided doses

Influenza A prophylaxis: Minimum 10 day course of therapy following exposure if the vaccine has just been given or for 90 days following exposure if the vaccine is unavailable or contraindicated and re-exposure is possible

**Elderly:** Dose is based on renal function. Elderly patients should take the drug in 2 daily doses rather than a single dose to avoid adverse neurologic reactions with improved tolerance.

**Renal Impairment:**

Drug-induced extrapyramidal reactions:

$Cl_{cr}$ 30-50 mL/minute: Administer 100 mg on day 1 and 100 mg every day thereafter.

$Cl_{cr}$ 15-29 mL/minute: Administer 200 mg on day 1 followed by 100 mg on alternate days.

$Cl_{cr}$ <15 mL/minute: Administer 200 every 7 days (includes patient maintained on 3 times/week hemodialysis).

Hemodialysis: Slightly hemodialyzable (5% to 20%); no supplemental dose is needed.

Peritoneal dialysis: No supplemental dose is needed.

Continuous arteriovenous or venous-venous hemofiltration (CAVH/CAVHD): No supplemental dose is needed.

**Stability**

**Storage:** Protect from freezing.

**Monitoring Laboratory Tests** Renal function

**Additional Nursing Issues**

**Physical Assessment:** Assess effectiveness and interactions of other medications patient may be taking (see Contraindications and Drug Interactions). Monitor renal function, therapeutic response (eg, Parkinsonian symptoms), and adverse reactions: opportunistic infections (fever, mouth and vaginal sores or plaques, unhealed wounds, etc) and CNS changes (see Warnings/Precautions, Adverse Reactions, and Overdose/Toxicology) at beginning of therapy and periodically throughout therapy. When treating Parkinson's disease, taper slowly when discontinuing. Assess knowledge/teach patient appropriate use, interventions to reduce side effects, and adverse symptoms to report. **Pregnancy risk factor C** - benefits of use should outweigh possible risks. Note breast-feeding caution.

**Patient Information/Instruction:** Take as directed; do not increase dosage, take more often than prescribed, or discontinue without consulting prescriber. Maintain adequate hydration (2-3 L/day of fluids unless instructed to restrict fluid intake) and void before taking medication. Take last dose of day in the afternoon to reduce incidence of insomnia. Avoid alcohol, sedatives, or hypnotics unless consulting prescriber. You may experience decreased mental alertness or coordination (use caution when driving, climbing stairs, or engaging in tasks requiring alertness until response to drug is known); nausea, or dry mouth (small frequent meals, frequent mouth care, sucking lozenges, or chewing gum may help). Report unusual swelling of extremities, difficulty breathing or shortness of breath, change in gait or increased tremors, or changes in mentation (depression, anxiety, irritability, hallucination, slurred speech). **Pregnancy/breast-feeding precautions:** Inform prescriber if you are pregnant. Consult prescriber if breast-feeding.

**Geriatric Considerations:** Elderly patients may be more susceptible to the CNS effects of amantadine; using 2 divided daily doses may minimize this effect. The syrup may be used to administer doses <100 mg.

♦ **Amaphen®** *see* Butalbital Compound and Acetaminophen *on page 175*

♦ **Amaryl®** *see* Glimepiride *on page 534*

## Ambenonium (am be NOE nee um)

**U.S. Brand Names** Mytelase® Caplets®

**Therapeutic Category** Cholinergic Agonist

**Pregnancy Risk Factor** C

**Lactation** Excretion in breast milk unknown/not recommended

**Use** Symptomatic treatment of myasthenia gravis

**Mechanism of Action/Effect** Action increases acetylcholine concentration at transmission sites in parasympathetic neurons and skeletal muscles by inhibiting acetylcholinesterase

**Contraindications** Hypersensitivity to bromides. Routine administration of atropine or other belladonna alkaloids with ambenonium is contraindicated because they may suppress the muscarinic symptoms of excessive GI stimulation, leaving only the more serious symptoms of muscle fasciculations and paralysis as signs of overdosage. Should not be administered to patients receiving mecamylamine. Usually used only in myasthenia gravis.

**Warnings** Prolonged action after cholinergics, drug should be discontinued until the patient is stabilized. Use with caution in patients with asthma, epilepsy, bradycardia, hyperthyroidism, or peptic ulcer. Differentiation of cholinergic/myasthenia crisis is critical, use edrophonium and clinical judgment. Anticholinergic insensitivity may develop for brief or prolonged periods. Reduce or withhold dosages until the patient becomes sensitive again. May require respiratory support. Pregnancy factor C.

**Drug Interactions**

**Decreased Effect:** Corticosteroids antagonize effects of anticholinesterases in myasthenia gravis. Procainamide or quinidine may reverse ambenonium cholinergic effects on muscle.

**Increased Effect/Toxicity:** Succinylcholine neuromuscular blockade may be prolonged.

**Effects on Lab Values** ↑ aminotransferase [ALT (SGPT)/AST (SGOT)] (S), amylase (S)

**Adverse Reactions**

>10%:

Gastrointestinal: Diarrhea, increased salivation, nausea, stomach cramps, dysphagia
Miscellaneous: Increased diaphoresis

1% to 10%:

Genitourinary: Urge to urinate
Ocular: Small pupils, lacrimation
Respiratory: Increased bronchial secretions

<1% (Limited to important or life-threatening symptoms): Bradycardia, A-V block, seizures, headache, dysphoria, drowsiness, thrombophlebitis, laryngospasm, respiratory paralysis, hypersensitivity, hyper-reactive cholinergic responses

**Overdose/Toxicology** Have atropine on hand to reverse cholinergic crisis or hypersensitivity reaction.

**Formulations** Tablet, as chloride: 10 mg

**Dosing**

**Adults:** Oral: 5-25 mg 3-4 times/day

**Elderly:** Refer to adult dosing.

**Additional Nursing Issues**

**Physical Assessment:** Assess bladder and sphincter adequacy prior to administering medication. Assess other medications patient may be taking for effectiveness and interactions (see Contraindications and Drug Interactions). Monitor therapeutic effects, and adverse reactions: cholinergic crisis (DUMBELS - **d**iarrhea, **u**rination, **m**iosis, **b**ronchospasm/**b**radycardia, **e**xcitability, **l**acrimation, and **s**alivation/excessive **s**weating) (see Warnings/Precautions, Adverse Reactions, and Overdose/Toxicology). Assess knowledge/teach patient appropriate use, interventions to reduce side effects, and adverse symptoms to report. **Pregnancy risk factor C** - benefits of use should outweigh possible risks. Breast-feeding is not recommended.

**Patient Information/Instruction:** This drug will not cure myasthenia gravis, but it may reduce the symptoms. Use as directed; do not increase dose or discontinue without consulting prescriber. Maintain adequate hydration (2-3 L/day of fluids unless instructed to restrict fluid intake). May cause dizziness, drowsiness, or postural hypotension (rise slowly from sitting or lying position and use caution when driving or climbing stairs); vomiting or loss of appetite (frequent small meals, frequent mouth care, sucking lozenges, or chewing gum may help); or diarrhea (boiled milk, yogurt, or buttermilk may help). Report persistent abdominal discomfort; significantly increased salivation, sweating, tearing, or urination; flushed skin; chest pain or palpitations; acute headache; unresolved diarrhea; excessive fatigue, insomnia, dizziness, or depression; increased muscle, joint, or body pain; vision changes or blurred vision; or shortness of breath or wheezing. **Pregnancy/breast-feeding precautions:** Inform prescriber if you are or intend to be pregnant. Breast-feeding is not recommended.


- ♦ **Ambenyl® Cough Syrup** *see page 1306*
- ♦ **Ambi 10®** *see page 1294*
- ♦ **Ambien™** *see* Zolpidem *on page 1232*
- ♦ **Ambi® Skin Tone [OTC]** *see* Hydroquinone *on page 583*
- ♦ **AmBisome®** *see* Amphotericin B (Liposomal) *on page 88*
- ♦ **Ambotetra** *see* Tetracycline *on page 1111*
- ♦ **Amcort®** *see* Triamcinolone *on page 1171*
- ♦ **Ameblin** *see* Metronidazole *on page 763*
- ♦ **Amen®** *see* Medroxyprogesterone *on page 714*
- ♦ **Amerge™** *see* Naratriptan *on page 809*

- **Americaine [OTC]** *see* Benzocaine *on page 141*
- **Americaine®** *see page 1291*
- **Amesec®** *see page 1294*
- **A-methaPred® Injection** *see* Methylprednisolone *on page 754*
- **Amethocaine Hydrochloride** *see* Tetracaine *on page 1110*
- **Amethopterin** *see* Methotrexate *on page 743*
- **Ametop™** *see* Tetracaine *on page 1110*
- **Amfepramone** *see* Diethylpropion *on page 365*
- **Amgenal® Cough Syrup** *see page 1306*
- **Amicar®** *see* Aminocaproic Acid *on page 68*


## Amifostine (am i FOS teen)

**U.S. Brand Names** Ethyol®

**Synonyms** Ethiofos; Gammaphos

**Therapeutic Category** Antidote

**Pregnancy Risk Factor** C

**Lactation** Excretion in breast milk unknown/contraindicated

**Use** Reduces the cumulative renal toxicity associated with repeated administration of cisplatin in patients with advanced ovarian cancer or nonsmall cell lung cancer. In these settings, the clinical data dose not suggest that the effectiveness of cisplatin-based chemotherapy regimens is altered by amifostine.

**Mechanism of Action/Effect** Reduces the toxic effects of cisplatin

**Contraindications** Hypersensitivity to aminothiol compounds or mannitol

**Warnings** The U.S. Food and Drug Administration (FDA) currently recommends that procedures for proper handling and disposal of antineoplastic agents be considered.

Limited data is currently available regarding the preservation of antitumor efficacy when amifostine is administered prior to cisplatin therapy in settings other than advanced ovarian cancer or nonsmall cell lung cancer. Amifostine should therefore not be used in patients receiving chemotherapy for other malignancies in which chemotherapy can produce a significant survival benefit or cure, except in the context of a clinical study.

Patients who are hypotensive or in a state of dehydration should not receive amifostine. Patients receiving antihypertensive therapy that cannot be stopped for 24 hours preceding amifostine treatment also should not receive amifostine. Patients should be adequately hydrated prior to amifostine infusion and kept in a supine position during the infusion. Blood pressure should be monitored every 5 minutes during the infusion. If hypotension requiring interruption of therapy occurs, patients should be placed in the Trendelenburg position and given an infusion of normal saline using a separate I.V. line.

It is recommended that antiemetic medication, including dexamethasone 20 mg I.V. and a serotonin 5-$HT_3$ receptor antagonist be administered prior to and in conjunction with amifostine.

Reports of clinically relevant hypocalcemia are rare, but serum calcium levels should be monitored in patients at risk of hypocalcemia, such as those with nephrotic syndrome.

Pregnancy factor C.

**Drug Interactions**

**Increased Effect/Toxicity:** Special consideration should be given to patients receiving antihypertensive medications or other drugs that could potentiate hypotension.

**Adverse Reactions**

>10%:

Cardiovascular: Flushing; hypotension (62%) (see Additional Information)

Central nervous system: Chills, dizziness, somnolence

Gastrointestinal: Nausea/vomiting (may be severe)

Respiratory: Sneezing

Miscellaneous: Feeling of warmth/coldness, hiccups

<1% (Limited to important or life-threatening symptoms): Mild rashes, hypocalcemia, rigors

**Overdose/Toxicology** Symptoms of overdose include nausea, vomiting, and hypotension. Treatment includes supportive measures as clinically indicated.

**Pharmacodynamics/Kinetics**

**Half-life Elimination:** 9 minutes

**Metabolism:** Hepatic dephosphorylation to two metabolites (WR-33278 and WR-1065)

**Excretion:** Renal; plasma clearance: 2.17 L/minute

**Formulations** Injection: 500 mg

**Dosing**

**Adults:** I.V. (refer to individual protocols): 910 mg/m$^2$ administered once daily as a 15-minute I.V. infusion, starting 30 minutes prior to chemotherapy. A 15-minute infusion is better tolerated than more extended infusions. Further reductions in infusion times have not been systematically investigated. The infusion of amifostine should be interrupted if the systolic blood pressure decreases significantly from the baseline value. See table. If the blood pressure returns to normal within 5 minutes and the patient is asymptomatic, the infusion may be restarted so that the full dose of amifostine may be administered. If the full dose of amifostine cannot be administered, the dose of amifostine for subsequent cycles should be 740 mg/m$^2$.

**Decrease in Systolic Blood Pressure**

| Baseline systolic blood pressure (mm Hg) | <100 | 100–119 | 120–139 | 140–179 | ≥180 |
|---|---|---|---|---|---|
| Decrease in systolic blood pressure during infusion of amifostine (mm Hg) | 20 | 25 | 30 | 40 | 50 |

**Elderly:** Refer to adult dosing.

**Administration**

**I.V.:** Administer over 15 minutes; administration as a longer infusion is associated with a higher incidence of side effects.

**Stability**

**Storage:** Store vials of lyophilized powder at refrigeration, 2°C to 8°C.

**Reconstitution:** Reconstitute with 9.5 mL of sterile 0.9% sodium chloride. The reconstituted solution (500 mg/10 mL) is chemically stable for up to 5 hours at room temperature (25°C) or up to 24 hours under refrigeration 2°C to 8°C. Amifostine should be further diluted in 0.9% sodium chloride to a concentration of 5-40 mg/mL and is chemically stable for up to 5 hours at room temperature (25°C) or up to 24 hours when stored under refrigeration 2°C to 8°C.

**Compatibility:** See the Chemotherapy Compatibility Chart *on page 1311*.

**Additional Nursing Issues**

**Physical Assessment:** Monitor blood pressure closely during infusion (continuously or every 5-7 minutes - see Dosing). Monitor nausea and treat with antiemetic as indicated. **Pregnancy risk factor C.** Breast-feeding is contraindicated.

**Patient Information/Instruction:** This I.V. medication is given to help reduce side effects of your chemotherapy. Report immediately any nausea; you will be given medication. Report chills, severe dizziness, tremors or shaking, or sudden onset of hiccups. **Breast-feeding precautions:** Do not breast-feed.

## Amikacin (am i KAY sin)

**U.S. Brand Names** Amikin® Injection

**Therapeutic Category** Antibiotic, Aminoglycoside

**Pregnancy Risk Factor** C

**Lactation** Enters breast milk/compatible

**Use** Treatment of gram-negative enteric infection resistant to gentamicin and tobramycin (bone infections, respiratory tract infections, endocarditis, and septicemia); infection of mycobacterial organisms susceptible to amikacin including *Pseudomonas*, *Proteus*, *Serratia*, and gram-positive *Staphylococcus*; initial treatment of staph infection when penicillin is contraindicated or in mixed organism injection

**Mechanism of Action/Effect** Inhibits protein synthesis in susceptible bacteria by binding to ribosomal subunits

**Contraindications** Hypersensitivity to amikacin sulfate or any component; cross-sensitivity may exist with other aminoglycosides; dehydration; myasthenia gravis; parkinsonism

**Warnings** Dose and/or frequency of administration must be monitored and modified in patients with renal impairment. Drug should be discontinued if signs of ototoxicity, nephrotoxicity, or hypersensitivity occur. Ototoxicity is proportional to the amount of drug given and the duration of treatment. Tinnitus or vertigo may be indications of vestibular injury and impending bilateral **irreversible** damage. Renal damage is usually reversible. May contain sulfites, use with caution in patients with asthma. Pregnancy factor C.

**Drug Interactions**

**Increased Effect/Toxicity:** Amikacin may increase or prolong effect of depolarizing and nondepolarizing neuromuscular blocking agents. Concurrent use of amphotericin may increase nephrotoxicity or nephrotoxic drugs and may increase ototoxicity with other ototoxic drugs.

**Adverse Reactions**

1% to 10%:

Central nervous system: Neurotoxicity

Otic: Ototoxicity (auditory), ototoxicity (vestibular)

Renal: Nephrotoxicity

<1% (Limited to important or life-threatening symptoms): Eosinophilia, dyspnea

**Overdose/Toxicology** Symptoms of overdose include ototoxicity, nephrotoxicity, and neuromuscular toxicity. Treatment of choice following a single acute overdose appears to be maintenance of urine output of at least 3 mL/kg/hour during the acute treatment phase. Dialysis is of questionable value in enhancing aminoglycoside elimination. If required, hemodialysis is preferred over peritoneal dialysis in patients with normal renal function.

**Pharmacodynamics/Kinetics**

**Half-life Elimination:** Dependent on renal function: Normal renal function: 1.4-2.3 hours; Anuria: End-stage renal disease: 28-86 hours

**Time to Peak:** Serum concentration: I.M.: Within 45-120 minutes; I.V.: Within 30 minutes following a 30-minute infusion

**Excretion:** Urine

**Formulations** Injection, as sulfate: 50 mg/mL (2 mL, 4 mL); 250 mg/mL (2 mL, 4 mL)

(Continued)

## Amikacin *(Continued)*

**Dosing**

**Adults:** Individualization is critical because of the low therapeutic index.

**Use of ideal body weight (IBW) for determining the mg/kg/dose appears to be more accurate than dosing on the basis of total body weight (TBW).**

In morbid obesity, dosage requirement may best be estimated using a dosing weight of IBW + 0.4 (TBW - IBW).

I.M., I.V.: 5-7.5 mg/kg/dose every 8 hours

**Elderly:** Individualized dosing is critical because of the low therapeutic index.

I.M., I.V.: Initial: 15-20 mg/kg/day divided every 12-24 hours; occasionally every 8- or 48-hour dosing may be required. Dosage adjustments should be based on serum concentrations and calculated pharmacokinetic parameters.

Once daily or extended interval: I.V.: 15-20 mg/kg/dose given every 24, 36, or 48 hours depending on $Cl_{cr}$. Check renal impairment dosing suggestions.

**Renal Impairment:** Individualization is critical because of the low therapeutic index. Some patients may require larger or more frequent doses if serum levels document the need (ie, cystic fibrosis or febrile granulocytopenic patients).

$Cl_{cr}$ ≥60 mL/minute: Administer every 8 hours.
$Cl_{cr}$ 40-60 mL/minute: Administer every 12 hours.
$Cl_{cr}$ 20-40 mL/minute: Administer every 24 hours.
$Cl_{cr}$ 10-20 mL/minute: Administer every 48 hours.
$Cl_{cr}$ <10 mL/minute: Administer every 72 hours.
Dialyzable (50% to 100%)

Administer dose postdialysis or administer $^2/_3$ normal dose as a supplemental dose postdialysis and follow levels.

Peritoneal dialysis effects: Dose as $Cl_{cr}$ <10 mL/minute: Follow levels.

Continuous arteriovenous or venovenous hemodiafiltration (CAVH) effects: Dose as $Cl_{cr}$ 10-40 mL/minute: Follow levels.

**Administration**

**I.M.:** Administer I.M. injection in large muscle mass. Administer around-the-clock to promote less variation in peak and trough serum levels. Do not mix with other drugs, administer separately.

**I.V.:** Infuse over 30-60 minutes.

**Stability**

**Reconstitution:** Stable for 24 hours at room temperature and 2 days at refrigeration when mixed in $D_5W$, $D_5{}^1/_4NS$, $D_5{}^1/_2NS$, NS, LR

**Monitoring Laboratory Tests** Perform culture and sensitivity testing prior to initiating therapy. Urinalysis, BUN, serum creatinine, appropriately timed peak and trough concentrations. Aminoglycoside levels measured from blood taken from Silastic® central catheters can sometimes give falsely high readings (draw levels from alternate lumen or peripheral stick, if possible). Initial and periodic peak and trough plasma drug levels should be determined, particularly in critically ill patients with serious infections or in disease states known to significantly alter aminoglycoside pharmacokinetics (eg, cystic fibrosis, burns, or major surgery).

**Additional Nursing Issues**

**Physical Assessment:** Assess effectiveness and interactions of other medications (see Drug Interactions). See Contraindications and Warnings/Precautions for use cautions. Monitor effectiveness of therapy, laboratory tests (see Monitoring Laboratory Tests), and adverse response (eg ototoxicity, nephrotoxicity, neurotoxicity - see Adverse Reactions and Overdose/Toxicology). Assess hearing and renal status before, during, and after therapy. Assess knowledge/teach patient possible side effects/interventions, and adverse symptoms to report. **Pregnancy risk factor C** - benefits of use should outweigh possible risks.

**Patient Information/Instruction:** This drug can only be administered I.V. or I.M. It is important to maintain adequate hydration (2-3 L/day of fluids unless instructed to restrict fluid intake). Report change in hearing acuity, ringing or roaring in ears, alteration in balance, vertigo, feeling of fullness in head; pain, tingling, or numbness of any body part; change in urinary pattern or decrease in urine; signs of opportunistic infection (eg, white plaques in mouth, vaginal discharge, unhealed sores, sore throat, unusual fever, chills); pain, redness, or swelling at injection site; or other adverse reactions. **Pregnancy precautions:** Inform prescriber if you are or intend to be pregnant.

**Geriatric Considerations:** Adjust dose based on renal function.

**Breast-feeding Issues:** No specific recommendations. However, aminoglycosides are not systemically available when taken orally. Therefore, the risk to the infant is minimal if ingested with breast milk.

**Additional Information**

Injection contains sulfites.
Sodium content of 1 g: 29.9 mg (1.3 mEq).
pH: 3.5-5.5

**Related Information**

Peak and Trough Guidelines *on page 1331*
TB Drug Comparison *on page 1402*

- **Amikafur®** *see* Amikacin *on previous page*
- **Amikayect** *see* Amikacin *on previous page*
- **Amikin®** *see* Amikacin *on previous page*
- **Amikin® Injection** *see* Amikacin *on previous page*

## Amiloride (a MIL oh ride)

**U.S. Brand Names** Midamor®

**Therapeutic Category** Diuretic, Potassium Sparing

**Pregnancy Risk Factor** B

**Lactation** Excretion in breast milk unknown/contraindicated

**Use** Counteracts potassium loss induced by other diuretics in the treatment of hypertension or edematous conditions including CHF, hepatic cirrhosis, and hypoaldosteronism; usually used in conjunction with more potent diuretics such as thiazides or loop diuretics

**Investigational use:** Cystic fibrosis; reduction of lithium induced polyuria

**Mechanism of Action/Effect** Decreases potassium and calcium excretion in distal tubule, cortical collecting tubule, and collecting direct by inhibiting sodium, potassium, and ATPase; increases sodium, magnesium, and water excretion

**Contraindications** Hypersensitivity to amiloride or any component; hyperkalemia; potassium supplementation; impaired renal function; diabetes mellitus

**Warnings** Use cautiously in patients with severe hepatic insufficiency, May cause hyperkalemia. Medication should be discontinued if potassium level is >6.5 mEq/L.

**Drug Interactions**

**Decreased Effect:** Decreased effect of amiloride with use of nonsteroidal anti-inflammatory agents.

**Increased Effect/Toxicity:** Increased risk of amiloride-associated hyperkalemia with triamterene, spironolactone, angiotensin-converting enzyme (ACE) inhibitors, potassium preparations, and indomethacin. Increased toxicity with amantadine and lithium by reduction of renal excretion.

**Food Interactions** Hyperkalemia may result if amiloride is taken with potassium-containing foods.

**Effects on Lab Values** ↑ potassium (S)

**Adverse Reactions**

1% to 10%:

Central nervous system: Headache, fatigue, dizziness

Endocrine & metabolic: Hyperkalemia, hyperchloremic metabolic acidosis, dehydration, hyponatremia, gynecomastia

Gastrointestinal: Nausea, diarrhea, vomiting, abdominal pain, gas pain, appetite changes, constipation

Genitourinary: Impotence

Neuromuscular & skeletal: Muscle cramps, weakness

Respiratory: Cough, dyspnea

<1% (Limited to important or life-threatening symptoms): Orthostatic hypotension, arrhythmias, palpitations, chest pain, alopecia, GI bleeding, polyuria, bladder spasms, dysuria, jaundice, increased intraocular pressure, shortness of breath

**Overdose/Toxicology** Clinical signs of toxicity are consistent with dehydration and electrolyte disturbance. Large amounts may result in life-threatening hyperkalemia (>6.5 mEq/L). This can be treated with I.V. glucose (dextrose 25% in water), rapid-acting insulin, concurrent I.V. sodium bicarbonate, and (if needed) Kayexalate® oral or rectal solution in sorbitol. Persistent hyperkalemia may require dialysis.

**Pharmacodynamics/Kinetics**

**Protein Binding:** 23%

**Half-life Elimination:** Normal renal function: 6-9 hours; End-stage renal disease: 8-144 hours

**Metabolism:** No active metabolites

**Excretion:** Urine and feces

**Onset:** 2 hours

**Duration:** 24 hours

**Formulations** Tablet, as hydrochloride: 5 mg

**Dosing**

**Adults:** Oral: Initial: 5-10 mg/day (up to 20 mg)

**Elderly:** Oral: Initial: 5 mg once daily or every other day

**Renal Impairment:** Oral:

$Cl_{cr}$ 10-50 mL/minute: Administer at 50% of normal dose.

$Cl_{cr}$ <10 mL/minute: Avoid use.

**Administration**

**Oral:** Take with food or meals to avoid GI upset.

**Monitoring Laboratory Tests** Serum electrolytes, renal function

**Additional Nursing Issues**

**Physical Assessment:** Monitor for effectiveness of therapy and possible adverse effects. Assess fluid status (I & O, daily weight, blood pressure) and monitor for adverse effects (eg, hyperkalemia, hyperchloremic metabolic acidosis, hyponatremia - see above). Breast-feeding is contraindicated.

**Patient Information/Instruction:** Take as directed, preferably early in day. Do not increase dietary intake of potassium unless instructed by prescriber (too much potassium can be as harmful as too little). You may experience dizziness or fatigue; use caution when driving or engaging in tasks that require alertness until response to drug is known. You may experience constipation (increased dietary fluid, fiber, or fruit may help), impotence (reversible), or loss of head hair (rare). Report muscle cramping or weakness, unresolved nausea or vomiting, palpitations, or difficulty breathing. **Breast-feeding precautions:** Do not breast-feed.

**Geriatric Considerations:** Adjust dose for renal impairment.

## Amiloride and Hydrochlorothiazide

(a MIL oh ride & hye droe klor oh THYE a zide)

**U.S. Brand Names** Moduretic®

**Synonyms** Hydrochlorothiazide and Amiloride

**Therapeutic Category** Diuretic, Combination

**Pregnancy Risk Factor** B

**Lactation** Excretion in breast milk unknown/contraindicated

**Use** Potassium-sparing diuretic, antihypertensive

**Formulations** Tablet: Amiloride hydrochloride 5 mg and hydrochlorothiazide 50 mg

**Dosing**

**Adults:** Oral: Initial: 1 tablet/day, then may be increased to 2 tablets/day if needed; usually given in a single dose

**Elderly:** Oral: Initial: ½ to 1 tablet/day

**Additional Nursing Issues**

**Physical Assessment:** See individual components listed in Related Information. Breast-feeding is contraindicated.

**Patient Information/Instruction:** See individual components listed in Related Information. **Breast-feeding precautions:** Do not breast-feed.

**Geriatric Considerations:** Potassium excretion may be decreased in the elderly, increasing the risk of hyperkalemia with potassium-sparing diuretics such as amiloride.

**Related Information**

Amiloride *on previous page*
Hydrochlorothiazide *on page 566*

♦ **2-Amino-6-Mercaptopurine** *see* Thioguanine *on page 1122*
♦ **2-Amino-6-Trifluoromethoxy-Benzothiazole** *see* Riluzole *on page 1023*
♦ **Aminobenzylpenicillin** *see* Ampicillin *on page 90*

## Aminocaproic Acid (a mee noe ka PROE ik AS id)

**U.S. Brand Names** Amicar®

**Therapeutic Category** Hemostatic Agent

**Pregnancy Risk Factor** C

**Lactation** Excretion in breast milk unknown

**Use** Treatment of excessive bleeding from fibrinolysis; treatment of chronic bleeding tendencies; orphan drug status for topical treatment of traumatic ocular hyphema

**Mechanism of Action/Effect** Competitively inhibits activation of plasminogen to plasmin, also, a lesser antiplasmin effect

**Contraindications** Disseminated intravascular coagulation; evidence of an intravascular clotting process

**Warnings** Rapid I.V. administration of the undiluted drug is not recommended. Aminocaproic acid may accumulate in patients with decreased renal function. Intrarenal obstruction may occur secondary to glomerular capillary thrombosis or clots in the renal pelvis and ureters. Do not use in hematuria of upper urinary tract origin unless possible benefits outweigh risks. Use with caution in patients with cardiac, renal, or hepatic disease. Do not administer without a definite diagnosis of laboratory findings indicative of hyperfibrinolysis. Inhibition of fibrinolysis may promote clotting or thrombosis. Subsequently, use with great caution in patients with or at risk for veno-occlusive disease of the liver. Benzyl alcohol is used as a preservative, therefore, these products should not be used in the neonate. Pregnancy risk C.

**Drug Interactions**

**Increased Effect/Toxicity:** Increased risk of hypercoagulability with oral contraceptives, estrogens.

**Effects on Lab Values** ↑ potassium, creatine phosphokinase [CPK] (S)

**Adverse Reactions**

>10%: Gastrointestinal: Anorexia, nausea

1% to 10%:

Cardiovascular: Hypotension, bradycardia, arrhythmia

Central nervous system: Dizziness, headache, malaise, fatigue

Dermatologic: Rash (measles-like skin rash or itching on face and/or palms of hands); masculinization and hirsutism in females

Endocrine & metabolic: Adrenocortical insufficiency

Gastrointestinal: GI irritation, vomiting, cramps, diarrhea

Hematologic: Decreased platelet function, elevated serum enzymes, leukopenia, agranulocytosis, thrombocytopenia

Neuromuscular & skeletal: Myopathy, weakness

Otic: Tinnitus

Respiratory: Nasal congestion

<1% (Limited to important or life-threatening symptoms): Convulsions, rhabdomyolysis, renal failure

**Overdose/Toxicology** Symptoms of overdose include nausea, diarrhea, delirium, hepatic necrosis, and thromboembolism.

**Pharmacodynamics/Kinetics**

**Distribution:** 5 g oral/I.V., followed by 1-1.25 g/hour, generally yields a steady-state plasma level of 0.13 mg/mL.

**Half-life Elimination:** Oral: 1-2 hours

**Metabolism:** Oral: Minimal hepatic

**Excretion:** Oral: 68% to 86% excreted as unchanged drug in urine within 12 hours

**Onset:** Oral: Peak effect: Within 2 hours; Therapeutic effect: Within 1-72 hours after dose

**Formulations**

Injection: 250 mg/mL (20 mL, 96 mL, 100 mL)

Syrup: 1.25 g/5 mL (480 mL)

Tablet: 500 mg

**Dosing**

**Adults:** In the management of acute bleeding syndromes, oral dosage regimens are the same as the I.V. dosage regimens (see I.V. Administration).

Chronic bleeding: Oral, I.V.: 5-30 g/day in divided doses at 3- to 6-hour intervals

Acute bleeding syndrome: Traumatic hyphema: Oral: 100 mg/kg/dose every 6-8 hours

Elevated fibrinolytic activity: Oral: 5 g during first hour, followed by 1-1.25 g/hour for approximately 8 hours or until bleeding stops

Maximum daily dose: Oral, I.V.: 30 g

**Elderly:** Refer to adult dosing.

**Renal Impairment:** Oliguria or ESRD: Reduce dose by 15% to 25%.

**Administration**

**I.V.:** Administer 4-5 g in 250 mL of diluent during first hour followed by continuous infusion at the rate of 1-1.25 g/hour in 50 mL of diluent, continue for 8 hours or until bleeding stops.

**I.V. Detail:** Administer by infusion using appropriate I.V. solution (dextrose 5%, 0.9% sodium chloride, or lactated Ringer's). Rapid I.V. injection (IVP) should be avoided since hypotension, bradycardia, and arrhythmia may result. Aminocaproic acid may accumulate in patients with decreased renal function. Do not use dextrose in patients with subarachnoid hemorrhage; incompatible with sodium lactate.

**Monitoring Laboratory Tests** Fibrinogen, fibrin split products, creatine phosphokinase (with long-term therapy)

**Additional Nursing Issues**

**Physical Assessment:** Monitor laboratory results on a regular basis during therapy. Monitor (teach patient to monitor and report) signs of adverse reactions: bleeding, clotting, thromboembolism (eg, chest pain, dyspnea, edema, hemoptysis, leg pain, positive Homans' sign), hypotension, or CNS changes (see Adverse Reactions). **Pregnancy risk factor C** - benefits of use should outweigh possible risks. Note breast-feeding caution.

**Patient Information/Instruction:** Take oral medication exactly as directed. This medication may cause dizziness and fatigue (use caution when driving or engaging in tasks that require alertness until response to drug is known); hypotension (use caution when rising from a lying or sitting position or climbing stairs); menstrual irregularities, increased body hair, or sexual dysfunction (should reverse when treatment is completed); or nausea or vomiting (small frequent meals, frequent mouth care, sucking lozenges, or chewing gum may help). Report immediately chest pain; dyspnea; swelling; nosebleed; warmth, swelling, pain, or redness in calves; skin rash; muscle pain or weakness; ringing in ears; or acute abdominal cramping. **Pregnancy/breast-feeding precautions:** Inform prescriber if you are or intend to be pregnant. Consult prescriber if breast-feeding.

**Additional Information** Some formulations may contain benzyl alcohol.

♦ **Amino-Cerv™ Vaginal Cream** *see* Urea *on page 1193*

## Aminoglutethimide (a mee noe gloo TETH i mide)

**U.S. Brand Names** Cytadren®

**Therapeutic Category** Antineoplastic Agent, Miscellaneous

**Pregnancy Risk Factor** D

**Lactation** Excretion in breast milk unknown/contraindicated

**Use** Suppression of adrenal function in selected patients with Cushing's syndrome; used successfully in postmenopausal patients with advanced breast carcinoma and in patients with metastatic prostate carcinoma as third-line hormonal agent

**Mechanism of Action/Effect** Blocks the conversion of cholesterol to delta-5-pregnenolone, thereby reducing the synthesis of adrenal glucocorticoids, mineralocorticoids, estrogens, aldosterone, and androgens. This inhibits growth of tumors that need estrogen to thrive.

**Contraindications** Hypersensitivity to aminoglutethimide, any component, or glutethimide; hypotension; hypothyroidism; pregnancy

**Warnings** Monitor blood pressure in all patients at appropriate intervals. Hypothyroidism may occur. **Mineralocorticoid replacement therapy may be necessary in up to 50% of patients.**

**Drug Interactions**

**Cytochrome P-450 Effect:** Cytochrome P-450 hepatic microsomal enzyme inducer; isoenzymes undefined

**Decreased Effect:** Aminoglutethimide may decrease therapeutic effect of dexamethasone, digitoxin (after 3-8 weeks), theophylline, warfarin, and medroxyprogesterone.

**Effects on Lab Values** ↑ alkaline phosphatase (S), AST (SGOT), TSH; ↓ plasma cortisol, thyroxine (S), and urinary aldosterone

**Adverse Reactions** Most adverse effects will diminish in incidence and severity after the first 2-6 weeks

(Continued)

## Aminoglutethimide *(Continued)*

>10%:

Central nervous system: Headache, dizziness, drowsiness, and lethargy are frequent at the start of therapy, clumsiness
Dermatologic: Skin rash
Gastrointestinal: Nausea, vomiting, anorexia
Hepatic: Cholestatic jaundice
Neuromuscular & skeletal: Myalgia
Renal: Nephrotoxicity
Respiratory: Pulmonary alveolar damage
Miscellaneous: Systemic lupus erythematosus

1% to 10%:

Cardiovascular: Hypotension and tachycardia, orthostatic hypotension
Central nervous system: Headache
Dermatologic: Hirsutism in females
Endocrine & metabolic: Adrenocortical insufficiency
Hematologic: Rare cases of neutropenia, leukopenia, thrombocytopenia, pancytopenia, and agranulocytosis have been reported
Neuromuscular & skeletal: Myalgia

**Overdose/Toxicology** Symptoms of overdose include ataxia, somnolence, lethargy, dizziness, distress, fatigue, coma, hyperventilation, respiratory depression, hypovolemia, and shock. Treatment is supportive.

**Pharmacodynamics/Kinetics**

**Protein Binding:** 20% to 25%

**Half-life Elimination:** 7-15 hours; shorter following multiple administrations than following single doses (induces hepatic enzymes increasing its own metabolism)

**Metabolism:** Liver

**Excretion:** Urine

**Onset:** 3-5 days

**Formulations** Tablet, scored: 250 mg

**Dosing**

**Adults:** Oral:

Cushing disease: 250 mg every 6 hours may be increased at 1- to 2-week intervals to a total of 2 g/day

Cancer therapy: 250 mg twice daily with hydrocortisone 20 mg AM, 20 mg PM, and 60 mg at bedtime for 2 weeks; then 250 mg twice daily with hydrocortisone 10 mg AM, 10 mg PM, and 20 mg at bedtime

**Elderly:** Refer to adult dosing.

**Renal Impairment:** Dose reduction may be necessary.

**Administration**

**Oral:** Give in divided doses, 2-3 times/day to reduce incidence of nausea and vomiting.

**Additional Nursing Issues**

**Physical Assessment:** Monitor appropriate laboratory tests as ordered. Monitor vital signs and for signs or symptoms of adverse reactions identified above with special attention to signs or symptoms of hypothyroidism (eg, slow pulse, lethargy, dry skin, thick tongue) or symptoms of Cushing syndrome (eg, moon face, hump, hypertension, fragility, hirsutism, mood swings, increased susceptibility to infection). **Pregnancy risk factor D** - assess knowledge/teach appropriate use of barrier contraceptives. Breast-feeding is contraindicated.

**Patient Information/Instruction:** May be taken with food to reduce incidence of nausea. You may experience drowsiness or dizziness; avoid driving or engaging in tasks that require alertness until response to drug is known. Small frequent meals may reduce incidence of nausea or vomiting. Masculinization may occur and is reversible when treatment is discontinued. Report rash, unresolved nausea, vomiting, lethargy, yellowing of skin or eyes, easy bruising or bleeding, change in color of urine or stool, increased growth of facial hair, thick tongue, severe mood swings, palpitations, or respiratory difficulty. **Pregnancy/breast-feeding precautions:** Do not get pregnant while taking this medication; use appropriate barrier contraceptive measures. Do not breast-feed.

♦ **Amino-Opti-E® [OTC]** *see* Vitamin E *on page 1218*

♦ **Aminophylline, Amobarbital, and Ephedrine** *see page 1294*

## Aminosalicylate Sodium (a MEE noe sa LIS i late SOW dee um)

**U.S. Brand Names** Sodium P.A.S.

**Synonyms** PAS

**Therapeutic Category** Salicylate

**Pregnancy Risk Factor** C

**Lactation** Enters breast milk/not recommended

**Use** Treatment of tuberculosis with combination drugs

**Mechanism of Action/Effect** Aminosalicylic acid (PAS) is a highly specific bacteriostatic agent active against *M. tuberculosis.* Most strains of *M. tuberculosis* are sensitive to a concentration of 1 mcg/mL. Structurally related to para-aminobenzoic acid (PABA) and its mechanism of action is thought to be similar to the sulfonamides, a competitive antagonism with PABA. Disrupts plate biosynthesis in sensitive organisms.

**Contraindications** Hypersensitivity to aminosalicylate sodium

**Warnings** Use with caution in patients with hepatic or renal dysfunction, patients with gastric ulcer, patients with CHF, and patients who are sodium restricted. Pregnancy factor C.

**Drug Interactions**

**Decreased Effect:** Aminosalicylate sodium may decrease serum levels of digoxin and vitamin $B_{12}$.

**Adverse Reactions**

1% to 10%: Gastrointestinal: Nausea, vomiting, diarrhea, abdominal pain

<1% (Limited to important or life-threatening symptoms): Vasculitis, fever, leukopenia, agranulocytosis, thrombocytopenia, hemolytic anemia, jaundice, hepatitis

**Overdose/Toxicology** Acute overdose results in crystalluria and renal failure, nausea, and vomiting. Alkalinization of urine with sodium bicarbonate and forced diuresis can prevent crystalluria and nephrotoxicity.

**Pharmacodynamics/Kinetics**

**Metabolism:** Liver

**Excretion:** Urine

**Formulations** Tablet: 500 mg

**Dosing**

**Adults:** Oral: 150 mg/kg/day in 2-3 equally divided doses (usually 12-14 g/day)

**Elderly:** Refer to adult dosing.

**Renal Impairment:**

$Cl_{cr}$ 10-50 mL/minute: Administer 50% to 75% of dose.

$Cl_{cr}$ <10 mL/minute: Administer 50% of dose.

Administer after hemodialysis: Administer 50% of dose.

Continuous arteriovenous or venovenous hemofiltration (CAVH): Dose as $Cl_{cr}$ 10-50 mL/minute.

**Hepatic Impairment: Use with caution.**

**Administration**

**Oral:** Do not use tablets that are discolored (ie, brown or purple).

**Additional Nursing Issues**

**Physical Assessment:** Monitor for effectiveness of treatment and indications of adverse effects (see above). **Pregnancy risk factor C** - benefits of use should outweigh possible risks. Breast-feeding is not recommended.

**Patient Information/Instruction:** May be taken with food. Do not take tablets that are discolored (brown or purple); see pharmacist for new prescription. Do not stop taking without consulting prescriber. Report persistent sore throat, fever, unusual bleeding or bruising, persistent nausea or vomiting, or abdominal pain. **Pregnancy/breast-feeding precautions:** Inform prescriber if you are or intend to be pregnant. Breast-feeding is not recommended.

**Geriatric Considerations:** See Warnings/Precautions; elderly may require lower recommended dose.

♦ **5-Aminosalicylic Acid** *see* Mesalamine *on page 727*

## Amiodarone (a MEE oh da rone)

**U.S. Brand Names** Cordarone®; Pacerone®

**Therapeutic Category** Antiarrhythmic Agent, Class III

**Pregnancy Risk Factor** D

**Lactation** Enters breast milk/contraindicated

**Use**

Oral: Management of life-threatening recurrent ventricular fibrillation (VF) or hemodynamically unstable ventricular tachycardia (VT)

I.V.: Initiation of treatment and prophylaxis of frequency recurring VF and unstable VT in patients refractory to other therapy. Also, for patients for whom oral amiodarone is indicated but who are unable to take oral medication.

**Mechanism of Action/Effect** Class III antiarrhythmic agent which inhibits adrenergic stimulation, prolongs the action potential and refractory period in myocardial tissue; decreases A-V conduction and sinus node function

**Contraindications** Hypersensitivity to amiodarone; severe sinus node dysfunction; second and third degree A-V block; marked sinus bradycardia except if pacemaker is placed; thyroid disease; pregnancy; hypokalemia

**Warnings** Not considered first-line antiarrhythmic due to high incidence of significant and potentially fatal toxicity (ie, hypersensitivity pneumonitis or interstitial/alveolar pneumonitis, hepatic failure, heart block, bradycardia or exacerbated arrhythmias), especially with large doses. Reserve for use in arrhythmias refractory to other therapy. Hospitalize patients while loading dose is administered. Use cautiously in the elderly due to predisposition to toxicity. Due to an extensive tissue distribution and prolonged elimination period, the time at which a life-threatening arrhythmia will recur following discontinued therapy or an interaction with subsequent treatment is unpredictable. Patients must be observed carefully and extreme caution taken when other antiarrhythmic agents are substituted after discontinuation of amiodarone. May cause optic neuropathy and/or neuritis.

**Drug Interactions**

**Cytochrome P-450 Effect:** CYP3A3/4 enzyme substrate; CYP2C9, 2D6, and 3A3/4 enzyme inhibitor

**Increased Effect/Toxicity:** May decrease metabolism of anticoagulants, beta-blockers, digoxin, flecainide, tricyclics, phenothiazines, phenytoin, procainamide, and quinidine and lead to significantly increased plasma concentration. Amiodarone may cause increased effects of these drugs and potentially fatal toxicity. Concomitant administration may result in additive effects of amiodarone with calcium channel blockers.

**Effects on Lab Values** Thyroid function tests: Amiodarone partially inhibits the peripheral conversion of thyroxine ($T_4$) to tri-iodothyronine ($T_3$); serum $T_4$ and reverse tri-

(Continued)

## Amiodarone *(Continued)*

iodothyronine ($RT_3$) concentrations may be increased and serum $T_3$ may be decreased. Most patients remain clinically euthyroid, however, clinical hypothyroidism or hyperthyroidism may occur.

**Adverse Reactions** With large dosages (≥400 mg/day), adverse reactions occur in ~75% patients and require discontinuance in 5% to 20%.

>10%:

- Cardiovascular: Hypotension (especially with I.V. form)
- Gastrointestinal: Nausea, vomiting (Oral form)

1% to 10%:

- Cardiovascular: Congestive heart failure, cardiac arrhythmias (atropine-resistant bradycardia, heart block, sinus arrest, paroxysmal
- Central nervous system: Ataxia, fever, fatigue, malaise, dizziness, headache, insomnia, nightmares
- Dermatologic: Photosensitivity
- Endocrine & metabolic: Hypothyroidism or hyperthyroidism (less common), decreased libido
- Gastrointestinal: Constipation, anorexia, abdominal pain, abnormal salivation, abnormal taste (oral form)
- Hematologic: Coagulation abnormalities
- Hepatic: Abnormal liver function tests
- Local: Phlebitis with concentrations >3 mg/mL
- Ocular: Visual disturbances
- Neuromuscular & skeletal: Tremor, paresthesias, muscle weakness
- Respiratory: Pulmonary fibrosis (cough, fever, dyspnea, malaise), interstitial pneumonitis
- Miscellaneous: Alveolitis ventricular tachycardia), myocardial depression, flushing, edema, abnormal smell (oral form)

<1% (Limited to important or life-threatening symptoms): Hypotension (with oral form), vasculitis, atrial fibrillation, increased Q-T interval, ventricular fibrillation, pseudotumor cerebri, rash, alopecia, discoloration of skin (slate blue), Stevens-Johnson syndrome, hyperglycemia, hypertriglyceridemia, thrombocytopenia, cirrhosis, severe hepatic toxicity (potentially fatal hepatitis), increased ALT and AST, optic neuritis, corneal microdeposits, photophobia, peripheral neuropathy, bronchiolitis obliterans organizing pneumonia, pancreatitis, pancytopenia, neutropenia, toxic epidermal necrolysis

**Overdose/Toxicology** Symptoms include extension of pharmacologic effects, sinus bradycardia and/or heart block, hypotension, and Q-T prolongation. Patients should be monitored for several days following ingestion. Intoxication with amiodarone necessitates EKG monitoring. Bradycardia may be atropine resistant. Injectable isoproterenol or a temporary pacemaker may be required.

**Pharmacodynamics/Kinetics**

**Protein Binding:** 96%

**Half-life Elimination:** Oral chronic therapy: 40-55 days (range: 26-107 days)

**Metabolism:** Liver

**Excretion:** Feces

**Onset:** Onset of effect: 3 days to 3 weeks after starting therapy; Peak effect: 1 week to 5 months; Onset of I.V. form may be more rapid

**Duration:** Following discontinuation of therapy: 7-50 days

**Formulations**

Amiodarone hydrochloride:

- Injection: 50 mg/mL with benzyl alcohol (3 mL)
- Tablet, scored: 200 mg

**Dosing**

**Adults:**

Oral: Ventricular arrhythmias: 800-1600 mg/day in 1-2 doses for 1-3 weeks, then 600-800 mg/day in 1-2 doses for 1 month; maintenance: 400 mg/day; lower doses are recommended for supraventricular arrhythmias.

I.V.:

First 24 hours: 1000 mg according to following regimen

- Step 1: 150 mg (10 mL) over first 10 minutes (mix 3 mL in 100 mL $D_5W$)
- Step 2: 360 mg (200 mL) over next 6 hours (mix 18 mL in 500 mL $D_5W$)
- Step 3: 540 mg (300 mL) over next 18 hours

After the first 24 hours: 0.5 mg/minute utilizing concentration of 1-6 mg/mL

Breakthrough VF or VT: 150 mg supplemental doses in 100 mL $D_5W$ over 10 minutes

**Note:** When switching from I.V. to oral therapy, use the following as a guide:

- <1 week I.V. infusion → 800-1600 mg/day
- 1- to 3-week I.V. infusion → 600-800 mg/day
- >3 week I.V. infusion → 400 mg

**Elderly:** Refer to adult dosing.

**Renal Impairment:** Hemodialysis effects: Not removed by hemodialysis or peritoneal dialysis (0% to 5%); no supplemental doses required.

**Hepatic Impairment:** Dosage adjustment is probably necessary in substantial hepatic impairment.

**Administration**

**I.V.:** Infusions >2 hours must be administered in glass or polyolefin bottles.

**Stability**

**Storage:** Store at room temperature and protect from light.

**Compatibility:** Incompatible with aminophylline, cefamandole, cefazolin, heparin, mezlocillin, and sodium bicarbonate.

**Monitoring Laboratory Tests** Thyroid function, pulmonary function

**Additional Nursing Issues**

**Physical Assessment:** Assess other medications patient may be taking for effectiveness and interactions (see Drug Interactions).

I.V.: Requires use of infusion pump and continuous cardiac and hemodynamic monitoring during infusion. Be alert for adverse reactions (see Warnings/Precautions and Adverse Reactions).

Oral: Monitor laboratory tests (see above), therapeutic response (cardiac status), and symptoms of adverse effects (see Warnings/Precautions, Adverse Reactions, and Overdose/Toxicology) at beginning of therapy and regularly during long-term therapy. **Pregnancy risk factor D** - assess knowledge/teach appropriate use of barrier contraceptives. Breast-feeding is contraindicated.

**Patient Information/Instruction:** Emergency use: Patient condition will determine amount of patient education. Oral: May be taken with food to reduce GI disturbance. Do not change dosage or discontinue drug without consulting prescriber. Regular blood work, ophthalmic exams, and cardiac assessment will be necessary while taking this medication on a long-term basis. You may experience dizziness, weakness, or insomnia (use caution when driving, climbing stairs, or engaging in tasks requiring alertness until response to drug is known); hypotension (use caution changing position - rising from sitting or lying); nausea, vomiting, loss of appetite, or stomach discomfort, abnormal taste (small frequent meals, frequent mouth care, chewing gum, or sucking lozenges may help); photosensitivity (use sunscreen, wear protective clothing and eyewear, and avoid direct sunlight); or decreased libido (reversible). Report persistent dry cough or shortness of breath; chest pain, palpitations, irregular or slow heartbeat; unusual bruising or bleeding; blood in urine, feces (black stool), vomitus; pain, swelling, or warmth in calves; muscle tremor, weakness, numbness, or changes in gait; skin rash or irritation; or changes in urinary patterns. **Pregnancy/breast-feeding precautions:** Do not get pregnant while taking this medication; use appropriate barrier contraceptive measures. Do not breast-feed.

**Geriatric Considerations:** Elderly may be predisposed to toxicity (see Drug Interactions). Half-life may be prolonged due to decreased clearance (see Hepatic/Renal Impairment).

**Related Information**

Antiarrhythmic Drug Classification Comparison *on page 1366*

♦ **Ami-Tex LA®** *see* Guaifenesin and Phenylpropanolamine *on page 550*

♦ **Amitone® [OTC]** *see* Calcium Supplements *on page 185*

## Amitriptyline (a mee TRIP ti leen)

**U.S. Brand Names** Elavil®; Enovil®

**Therapeutic Category** Antidepressant, Tricyclic (Tertiary Amine)

**Pregnancy Risk Factor** D

**Lactation** Enters breast milk/not recommended (AAP rates "of concern")

**Use** Treatment of various forms of depression, often in conjunction with psychotherapy; relieves certain chronic and neuropathic pain, prophylaxis against migraine headaches

**Mechanism of Action/Effect** Reverses depression; relieves pain for some chronic pain conditions; prevents migraine headaches; increases the synaptic concentration of serotonin and/or norepinephrine in the central nervous system by inhibition of their reuptake by the presynaptic neuronal membrane

**Contraindications** Hypersensitivity to amitriptyline (cross-sensitivity with other tricyclics may occur); patients receiving MAO inhibitors within past 14 days; narrow-angle glaucoma; pregnancy

**Warnings** Amitriptyline should not be abruptly discontinued in patients receiving therapeutic doses for prolonged periods. Use with caution in patients with cardiac conduction disturbances. An EKG prior to initiation of therapy is advised. Use with caution in patients with a history of hyperthyroidism, renal or hepatic impairment, closed angle glaucoma, seizure disorder, or patients undergoing elective surgery. This is the most anticholinergic and sedating of the antidepressants. Due to pronounced effects on the cardiovascular system (hypotension), many psychiatrists agree it is best to avoid in the elderly. Patients with schizophrenia, paranoia, or bipolar disorder may exhibit worsening of symptoms.

**Drug Interactions**

**Cytochrome P-450 Effect:** CYP1A2, 2C9, 2C18, 2C19, 2D6, and 3A3/4 enzyme substrate

**Decreased Effect:** Phenobarbital may reduce the effect of amitriptyline. Amitriptyline blocks the uptake of guanethidine.

**Increased Effect/Toxicity:** Clonidine taken with amitriptyline may lead to hypertensive crisis. Amitriptyline may be additive with or may potentiate the action of other CNS depressants. Amitriptyline with MAO inhibitors may cause hyperpyrexia, hypertension, tachycardia, confusion, and seizures; **deaths have been reported**. Amitriptyline may increase the prothrombin time in patients stabilized on warfarin. Amitriptyline potentiates the vasopressor and cardiac effects of sympathomimetic agents such as isoproterenol, epinephrine, etc. Cimetidine and methylphenidate may decrease the metabolism of amitriptyline leading to increased serum levels of amitriptyline. Additive

(Continued)

## Amitriptyline *(Continued)*

anticholinergic effects may be seen with amitriptyline and other anticholinergic agents. Potential for serotonin syndrome if combined with other serotonergic drugs.

**Effects on Lab Values** Amitriptyline may increase or decrease serum glucose levels, may elevate liver function tests, and may prolong conduction time.

**Adverse Reactions** Anticholinergic effects may be pronounced; moderate to marked sedation can occur (tolerance to these effects usually occurs).

>10%:
- Central nervous system: Dizziness, drowsiness, headache
- Gastrointestinal: Dry mouth, constipation, increased appetite, nausea, unpleasant taste, weight gain
- Neuromuscular & skeletal: Weakness

1% to 10%:
- Cardiovascular: Hypotension, postural hypotension, arrhythmias, tachycardia
- Central nervous system: Nervousness, restlessness, parkinsonian syndrome, insomnia, sedation, fatigue, anxiety, impaired cognitive function, seizures have occurred occasionally, extrapyramidal symptoms are possible
- Gastrointestinal: Diarrhea, heartburn
- Genitourinary: Sexual dysfunction, urinary retention
- Neuromuscular & skeletal: Tremor
- Ocular: Eye pain, blurred vision
- Miscellaneous: Sweating (excessive)

<1% (Limited to important or life-threatening symptoms): Alopecia, photosensitivity, trouble with gums, decreased lower esophageal sphincter tone may cause GE reflux, testicular edema, leukopenia, eosinophilia, rarely agranulocytosis, cholestatic jaundice, increased liver enzymes, increased intraocular pressure, sudden death

**Overdose/Toxicology** Symptoms of overdose include agitation, confusion, hallucinations, urinary retention, hypothermia, hypotension, ventricular tachycardia, and seizures. Treatment is symptomatic and supportive. Alkalinization by sodium bicarbonate and/or hyperventilation may limit cardiac toxicity.

**Pharmacodynamics/Kinetics**

**Distribution:** Crosses the placenta

**Half-life Elimination:** 9-25 hours (15-hour average)

**Metabolism:** Liver

**Excretion:** Urine

**Onset:** Onset of therapeutic effect: 7-21 days

Desired therapeutic effect (for depression) may take as long as 3-4 weeks, at that point dosage should be reduced to lowest effective level.

When used for migraine headache prophylaxis, therapeutic effect may take as long as 6 weeks. A higher dosage may be required in a heavy smoker, because of increased metabolism.

**Formulations**

Amitriptyline hydrochloride:
- Injection: 10 mg/mL (10 mL)
- Tablet: 10 mg, 25 mg, 50 mg, 75 mg, 100 mg, 150 mg

**Dosing**

**Adults:** Do **not** administer I.V.

Pain management: Initial: <40 kg: 0.3 mg/kg; >50 kg: 10-20 mg increased to desired effect (usually 25-150 mg/day)

Antidepressant:
- Oral: 30-100 mg/day single dose at bedtime or in divided doses. Dose may be gradually increased up to 300 mg/day. Once symptoms are controlled, decrease gradually to lowest effective dose.
- I.M.: 20-30 mg 4 times/day

**Elderly:** Oral: Initial: 10-25 mg at bedtime; dose should be increased in 10-25 mg increments every week if tolerated; dose range: 25-150 mg/day. See Renal/Hepatic Impairment.

**Renal Impairment:** Nondialyzable

**Hepatic Impairment:** Use with caution and monitor plasma levels and patient response.

**Additional Nursing Issues**

**Physical Assessment:** Assess other medications patient may be taking for effectiveness and interactions (see Drug Interactions). See Contraindications and Warnings/Precautions for cautious use. Assess for suicidal tendencies before beginning therapy. May cause physiological or psychological dependence, tolerance, or abuse, evaluate need for continued use periodically. **Note:** Amitriptyline may increase or decrease serum glucose levels. Monitor therapeutic response, and adverse reactions at beginning of therapy and periodically with long-term use (see Adverse Reactions and Overdose/Toxicology). Taper dosage slowly when discontinuing. Assess knowledge/teach patient appropriate use, interventions to reduce side effects, and adverse symptoms to report. **Pregnancy risk factor D** - assess knowledge/teach appropriate use of barrier contraceptives. Breast-feeding is not recommended.

**Patient Information/Instruction:** Take exactly as directed (do not increase dose or frequency); may take several weeks to achieve desired results; may cause physical and/or psychological dependence. Do not use alcohol, excess caffeine, and other prescription or OTC medications not approved by prescriber. Maintain adequate hydration (2-3 L/day of fluids unless instructed to restrict fluid intake). May turn urine blue-green (normal). You may experience drowsiness, lightheadedness, impaired coordination, dizziness, or blurred vision (use caution when driving or engaging in tasks requiring alertness until response to drug is known); constipation (increased exercise, fluids, or dietary fruit and fiber may help); urinary retention (void before taking medication); postural hypotension (use caution climbing stairs or when changing position from lying or sitting to standing); altered sexual drive or ability (reversible); or photosensitivity (use sunscreen, wear protective clothing and eyewear, and avoid direct sunlight). Report persistent CNS effects (eg, nervousness, restlessness, insomnia, anxiety, excitation, headache, agitation, impaired coordination, changes in cognition); muscle cramping, weakness, tremors, or rigidity; ringing in ears or visual disturbances; chest pain, palpitations, or irregular heartbeat; blurred vision; or worsening of condition. **Pregnancy/breast-feeding precautions:** Do not get pregnant while taking this medication; use appropriate barrier contraceptive measures. Breast-feeding is not recommended.

**Geriatric Considerations:** The most anticholinergic and sedating of the antidepressants. Due to pronounced effects on the cardiovascular system (hypotension), many psychiatrists agree it is best to avoid in the elderly.

**Breast-feeding Issues:** Generally, it is not recommended to breast-feed if taking antidepressants because of the long half-life, active metabolites, and the potential for side effects in the infant.

**Related Information**

Antidepressant Agents Comparison *on page 1368*
Peak and Trough Guidelines *on page 1331*

## Amitriptyline and Chlordiazepoxide

(a mee TRIP ti leen & klor dye az e POKS ide)

**U.S. Brand Names** Limbitrol®

**Synonyms** Chlordiazepoxide and Amitriptyline

**Therapeutic Category** Antidepressant, Tricyclic (Tertiary Amine)

**Pregnancy Risk Factor** D

**Lactation** Excretion in breast milk unknown/contraindicated

**Use** Treatment of moderate to severe anxiety and/or agitation and depression

**Formulations**

Tablet:
5-12.5: Amitriptyline hydrochloride 12.5 mg and chlordiazepoxide 5 mg
10-25: Amitriptyline hydrochloride 25 mg and chlordiazepoxide 10 mg

**Dosing**

**Adults:** Oral: Initial: 3-4 tablets in divided doses; this may be increased to 6 tablets/day as required. Some patients respond to smaller doses and can be maintained on 2 tablets.

**Elderly:** Refer to dosing in individual monographs.

**Additional Nursing Issues**

**Physical Assessment:** See individual components listed in Related Information. **Pregnancy risk factor D** - assess knowledge/instruct patient on need to use appropriate contraceptive measures and the need to avoid pregnancy. Breast-feeding is contraindicated.

**Patient Information/Instruction:** See individual components listed in Related Information. **Pregnancy/breast-feeding precautions:** Inform prescriber if you are or intend to be pregnant. Do not breast-feed.

**Related Information**

Amitriptyline *on page 73*
Chlordiazepoxide *on page 250*

## Amitriptyline and Perphenazine (a mee TRIP ti leen & per FEN a zeen)

**U.S. Brand Names** Etrafon®; Triavil®

**Synonyms** Perphenazine and Amitriptyline

**Therapeutic Category** Antidepressant, Tricyclic (Tertiary Amine)

**Pregnancy Risk Factor** D

**Lactation** Enters breast milk/contraindicated

**Use** Treatment of patients with moderate to severe anxiety and depression

**Formulations**

Tablet:
2-10: Amitriptyline hydrochloride 10 mg and perphenazine 2 mg
4-10: Amitriptyline hydrochloride 10 mg and perphenazine 4 mg
2-25: Amitriptyline hydrochloride 25 mg and perphenazine 2 mg
4-25: Amitriptyline hydrochloride 25 mg and perphenazine 4 mg
4-50: Amitriptyline hydrochloride 50 mg and perphenazine 4 mg

**Dosing**

**Adults:** Oral: 1 tablet 2-4 times/day

**Elderly:** Refer to dosing in individual monographs.

**Hepatic Impairment:** Avoid use in severe hepatic failure.

**Additional Nursing Issues**

**Physical Assessment:** See individual components listed in Related Information. **Pregnancy risk factor D** - assess knowledge/instruct patient on need to use appropriate contraceptive measures and the need to avoid pregnancy. Breast-feeding is contraindicated.

**Patient Information/Instruction:** See individual components listed in Related Information. **Pregnancy/breast-feeding precautions:** Inform prescriber if you are or intend to be pregnant. Do not breast-feed.

**Related Information**

Amitriptyline *on page 73*
Perphenazine *on page 912*

## Amlodipine (am LOE di peen)

**U.S. Brand Names** Norvasc®

**Therapeutic Category** Calcium Channel Blocker

**Pregnancy Risk Factor** C

**Lactation** Excretion in breast milk unknown/use caution

**Use** Treatment of hypertension and angina

**Mechanism of Action/Effect** Inhibits calcium ion from entering the "slow channels" or select voltage-sensitive areas of vascular smooth muscle and myocardium during depolarization

**Contraindications** Hypersensitivity to amlodipine; allergy to diltiazem; decreased hepatic function

**Warnings** Use with caution and titrate dosages for patients with impaired renal or hepatic function. Use caution when treating patients with congestive heart failure, sick-sinus syndrome, severe left ventricular dysfunction, hypertrophic cardiomyopathy (especially obstructive), concomitant therapy with beta-blockers or digoxin, edema, or increased intracranial pressure with cranial tumors. Do not abruptly withdraw (may cause chest pain). Pregnancy factor C.

**Drug Interactions**

**Cytochrome P-450 Effect:** CYP3A3/4 enzyme substrate

**Decreased Effect:** Possible increased serum levels and toxicity of cyclosporine if taken concomitantly with amlodipine.

**Adverse Reactions**

>10%: Cardiovascular: Peripheral edema (ankles & feet)

1% to 10%:

Cardiovascular: Edema, palpitations, flushing
Central nervous system: Fatigue, headache, dizziness, somnolence
Dermatologic: Dermatitis, rash
Endocrine & metabolic: Sexual dysfunction
Gastrointestinal: Nausea, abdominal pain, heartburn
Respiratory: Shortness of breath
Neuromuscular & skeletal: Muscle cramps

<1% (Limited to important or life-threatening symptoms): Hypotension, chest pain, bradycardia, arrhythmias, abnormal EKG, ventricular extrasystoles, alopecia, petechiae

**Overdose/Toxicology** Primary cardiac symptoms of calcium channel blocker overdose include hypotension and bradycardia. Noncardiac symptoms include confusion, stupor, nausea, vomiting, metabolic acidosis, and hyperglycemia. Treat other signs and symptoms symptomatically.

**Pharmacodynamics/Kinetics**

**Protein Binding:** 93%

**Distribution:** No data on crossing the placenta

**Half-life Elimination:** 30-50 hours

**Metabolism:** Liver

**Excretion:** Urine

**Onset:** 30-50 minutes; Peak effect: 6-12 hours

**Duration:** 24 hours

**Formulations** Tablet: 2.5 mg, 5 mg, 10 mg

**Dosing**

**Adults:** Oral: Initial: 2.5-5 mg once daily; usual dose: 5-10 mg once daily; maximum: 10 mg once daily

**Elderly:** Oral: Initial: 2.5 mg once daily; increase by 2.5 mg increments at 7- to 14-day intervals; maximum recommended dose: 10 mg/day.

**Hepatic Impairment:** 2.5 mg once daily

**Administration**

**Oral:** May be taken without regard to meals.

**Additional Nursing Issues**

**Physical Assessment:** Monitor blood pressure, cardiac rhythm, I & O ratio, weight, edema, signs or symptoms of adverse reactions (see above) at beginning of therapy or when titrating dose, and periodically throughout long-term therapy. Monitor blood pressure closely if patient is also taking nitrates. **Pregnancy risk factor C** - benefits of use should outweigh possible risks. Note breast-feeding caution.

**Patient Information/Instruction:** Take as prescribed; do not stop abruptly without consulting prescriber. You may experience headache (if unrelieved, consult prescriber), nausea or vomiting (frequent small meals may help), or constipation (increased dietary bulk and fluids may help). May cause drowsiness; use caution when driving or engaging in tasks that require alertness until response to drug is known. Report unrelieved headache, vomiting, constipation, palpitations, peripheral or facial swelling, weight gain >5 lb/week, or respiratory changes. **Pregnancy/breast-feeding precautions:** Inform prescriber if you are or intend to be pregnant. Inform prescriber if breast-feeding.

**Geriatric Considerations:** Elderly or debilitated persons may experience a greater hypotensive response. Theoretically, constipation may be more of a problem with elderly.

**Related Information**

Calcium Channel Blocking Agents Comparison *on page 1378*

## Amlodipine and Benazepril (am LOE di peen & ben AY ze pril)

**U.S. Brand Names** Lotrel®

**Synonyms** Benazepril and Amlodipine

**Therapeutic Category** Antihypertensive Agent, Combination

**Pregnancy Risk Factor** C/D (2nd and 3rd trimesters)

**Lactation**

Amlodipine: Excretion in breast milk unknown

Benazepril: Enters breast milk

**Use** Treatment of hypertension

**Formulations**

Capsule:

- Amlodipine 2.5 mg and benazepril hydrochloride 10 mg
- Amlodipine 5 mg and benazepril hydrochloride 10 mg
- Amlodipine 5 mg and benazepril hydrochloride 20 mg

**Dosing**

**Adults:** Dosage is individualized and adjusted to response: Oral: 1 capsule/day. May be used as a replacement for separate dosing of components or combination when response to single agent is suboptimal.

**Elderly:** Refer to dosing in individual monographs.

**Renal Impairment:** $Cl_{cr}$ <30 mL/minute: Not recommended since the initial dose of benazepril at this level of renal function is 5 mg. Titration of individual agents is preferred.

**Additional Nursing Issues**

**Physical Assessment:** See individual components listed in Related Information. **Pregnancy risk factor C/D** - see Pregnancy Risk Factor - assess knowledge/instruct patient on need to use appropriate contraceptive measures and the need to avoid pregnancy. Note breast-feeding caution.

**Patient Information/Instruction:** See individual components listed in Related Information. **Pregnancy/breast-feeding precautions:** Inform prescriber if you are or intend to be pregnant. Consult prescriber if breast-feeding.

**Related Information**

Amlodipine *on previous page*

Benazepril *on page 139*

♦ **Ammonapse** *see* Sodium Phenylbutyrate *on page 1064*

## Amobarbital (am oh BAR bi tal)

**U.S. Brand Names** Amytal®

**Synonyms** Amylobarbitone

**Therapeutic Category** Barbiturate

**Pregnancy Risk Factor** D

**Lactation** Excretion in breast milk unknown/not recommended

**Use**

Oral: Hypnotic in short-term treatment of insomnia; reduce anxiety and provide sedation preoperatively

I.M., I.V.: Control status epilepticus or acute seizure episodes; used in catatonic, negativistic, or manic reactions

**Mechanism of Action/Effect** Interferes with transmission of impulses from the thalamus to the cortex of the brain resulting in an imbalance in central inhibitory and facilitatory mechanisms

**Contraindications** Marked liver function impairment; latent porphyria; patients with nephritis, respiratory distress, or hypersensitivity to barbiturates. Do not administer in presence of chronic or acute pain, pregnancy, or previous history of addiction to sedative/hypnotic drugs.

**Warnings** Potential for drug dependency exists. Use with caution in patients with CHF, hepatic or renal impairment, or hypovolemic shock. When administered I.V., respiratory depression and hypotension are possible, have equipment and personnel available. I.V. form should be given only to hospitalized patients.

**Drug Interactions**

**Decreased Effect:** Effectiveness of cimetidine, tricyclic antidepressants, beta-blockers, theophylline, quinidine, oral anticoagulants, steroids, oral contraceptives, and doxycycline may be reduced with coadministration of amobarbital.

**Increased Effect/Toxicity:** Increased toxicity of amobarbital when combined with other CNS depressants, antidepressants, antihistamines, MAO inhibitors, or alcohol. Respiratory and CNS depression may be additive.

**Effects on Lab Values** ↑ ammonia (B); ↓ bilirubin (S)

**Adverse Reactions**

>10%: Central nervous system: Dizziness, clumsiness or unsteadiness, lightheadedness, "hangover" effect, drowsiness

1% to 10%:

Central nervous system: Confusion, mental depression, unusual excitement, nervousness, faint feeling, headache, insomnia, nightmares

Gastrointestinal: Nausea, vomiting, constipation

<1% (Limited to important or life-threatening symptoms): Rash, exfoliative dermatitis, urticaria, Stevens-Johnson syndrome, agranulocytosis, megaloblastic anemia, thrombocytopenia, respiratory depression, apnea, laryngospasm

**Overdose/Toxicology** Symptoms of overdose include unsteady gait, slurred speech, confusion, jaundice, hypothermia, fever, and hypotension. Treatment is supportive. Forced alkaline diuresis is of no value in the treatment of intoxications with short-acting

(Continued)

## Amobarbital *(Continued)*

barbiturates. Charcoal hemoperfusion or hemodialysis may be useful in harder-to-treat intoxications, especially in the presence of very high serum barbiturate levels.

**Pharmacodynamics/Kinetics**

**Distribution:** Readily crosses the placenta

**Half-life Elimination:** Biphasic Initial: 40 minutes; Terminal: 20 hours

**Metabolism:** Liver

**Excretion:** Urine

**Onset:** Oral: Within 1 hour; I.V.: Within 5 minutes

**Formulations**

Amobarbital sodium:

- Capsule: 65 mg, 200 mg
- Injection: 250 mg, 500 mg
- Tablet: 30 mg, 50 mg, 100 mg

**Dosing**

**Adults:**

Insomnia: Oral: 65-200 mg at bedtime

Sedation: Oral: 30-50 mg 2-3 times/day

Preanesthetic: Oral: 200 mg 1-2 hours before surgery

Hypnotic:

- Oral: 65-200 mg at bedtime
- I.M., I.V.: 65-500 mg, should not exceed 500 mg I.M. or 1000 mg I.V.

**Elderly:** Not recommended for use in the elderly.

**Renal Impairment:** Use with caution.

**Hepatic Impairment:** Use with caution. No specific recommendations; however, contraindicated in severe hepatic impairment.

**Administration**

**I.M.:** Deep injection to prevent pain, sterile abscess, and sloughing.

**I.V.:** Infuse slowly and titrate slowly to desired effect (may cause arteriospasm, thrombosis, gangrene).

**I.V. Detail:** Do **not** mix with any other drugs. Use large vein to prevent extravasation.

**Stability**

**Reconstitution:** Hydrolyzes when exposed to air. Use contents of vial within 30 minutes after reconstitution. Use only clear solution.

**Additional Nursing Issues**

**Physical Assessment:** Assess effectiveness and interactions of other medications (see Drug Interactions). See Contraindications and Warnings/Precautions for cautious use. Assess for history of addiction; long-term use can result in dependence, abuse, or tolerance. Periodically evaluate the need for continued use. After long-term use, taper dosage slowly when discontinuing.

I.V. (see Administration): Monitor infusion site frequently (keep patient under observation - vital signs, CNS, cardiac and respiratory status), and observe safety/seizure precautions. Monitor effectiveness and adverse reactions (see above).

Oral: Monitor for effectiveness of therapy and adverse reactions (see Adverse Reactions) at beginning of therapy and periodically with long-term use. Assess knowledge/teach patient seizure precautions (if appropriate), appropriate use, interventions to reduce possible side effects, and adverse symptoms to report.

**Pregnancy risk factor D** - assess knowledge/instruct patient to use appropriate contraceptive measures and the need to avoid pregnancy. Breast-feeding is not recommended.

**Patient Information/Instruction:** I.V./I.M.: Patient instructions and information are determined by patient condition and therapeutic purpose. If self-administered, use exactly as directed (do not increase dose or frequency or discontinue without consulting prescriber); may cause physical and/or psychological dependence. While using this medication, do not use alcohol or other prescription or OTC medications (especially pain medications, sedatives, antihistamines, or hypnotics) without consulting prescriber. Maintain adequate hydration (2-3 L/day of fluids unless instructed to restrict fluid intake). You may experience drowsiness, dizziness, or blurred vision (use caution when driving or engaging in tasks requiring alertness until response to drug is known); nausea, vomiting, or loss of appetite (small frequent meals, frequent mouth care, chewing gum, or sucking lozenges may help); constipation (increased exercise, fluids, or dietary fruit and fiber may help). If medication is used to control seizures, wear identification of epileptic status and medication. Report skin rash or irritation; CNS changes (confusion, depression, increased sedation, excitation, headache, insomnia, or nightmares); difficulty breathing or shortness of breath; changes in urinary pattern or menstrual pattern; muscle weakness or tremors; or difficulty swallowing or feeling of tightness in throat. **Pregnancy/breast-feeding precautions:** Do not get pregnant while taking this medication; use appropriate barrier contraceptive measures. Breast-feeding is not recommended.

**Geriatric Considerations:** May cause morning "hangover" effects.

**Related Information**

Antipsychotic Medication Guidelines *on page 1436*

## Amobarbital and Secobarbital (am oh BAR bi tal & see koe BAR bi tal)

**U.S. Brand Names** Tuinal®

**Synonyms** Secobarbital and Amobarbital

**Therapeutic Category** Barbiturate

**Pregnancy Risk Factor** D

**Lactation** Excretion in breast milk unknown/not recommended

**Use** Short-term treatment of insomnia

**Formulations**

Capsule:

100: Amobarbital sodium 50 mg and secobarbital sodium 50 mg

200: Amobarbital sodium 100 mg and secobarbital sodium 100 mg

**Dosing**

**Adults:** Oral: 1-2 capsules at bedtime

**Elderly:** Not recommended for use in the elderly.

**Hepatic Impairment:** Use with caution. Dose should be reduced; however, no specific recommendations.

**Additional Nursing Issues**

**Physical Assessment:** See individual components listed in Related Information. **Pregnancy risk factor D** - assess knowledge/instruct patient on need to use appropriate contraceptive measures and the need to avoid pregnancy. Breast-feeding is not recommended.

**Patient Information/Instruction:** See individual components listed in Related Information. **Pregnancy/breast-feeding precautions:** Inform prescriber if you are or intend to be pregnant. Breast-feeding is not recommended.

**Related Information**

Amobarbital *on page 77*

Antipsychotic Medication Guidelines *on page 1436*

Secobarbital *on page 1049*

♦ **AMO Vitrax®** *see page 1248*

♦ **AMO Vitrax®** *see page 1282*

## Amoxapine (a MOKS a peen)

**U.S. Brand Names** Asendin®

**Therapeutic Category** Antidepressant, Tricyclic (Secondary Amine)

**Pregnancy Risk Factor** C

**Lactation** Enters breast milk/contraindicated (AAP rates "of concern")

**Use** Treatment of neurotic and endogenous depression and mixed symptoms of anxiety and depression; major depression with psychotic features

**Mechanism of Action/Effect** Reduces the reuptake of serotonin and norepinephrine and blocks the response of dopamine receptors to dopamine

**Contraindications** Hypersensitivity to amoxapine or other tricyclics; narrow-angle glaucoma; patients receiving MAO inhibitors within past 14 days

**Warnings** Use with caution in patients with seizures, cardiac conduction disturbances, cardiovascular diseases, urinary retention, impaired hepatic or renal function, paranoia, bipolar disease, hyperthyroidism, or those receiving thyroid replacement. Do not discontinue abruptly in patients receiving high doses. Tolerance develops in 1-3 months in some patients. Close medical follow-up is essential. May exacerbate symptoms in patients with tardive dyskinesia. Pregnancy factor C.

**Drug Interactions**

**Decreased Effect:** Amoxapine decreases the effect of clonidine, guanethidine, other antihypertensives, and indirect-acting sympathomimetics (ephedrine).

**Increased Effect/Toxicity:** Amoxapine increases the effect of CNS depressants, adrenergic agents, anticholinergic agents, cimetidine, and ranitidine. Amoxapine increases toxicity of MAO inhibitors (hyperpyrexia, tachycardia, hypertension, seizures or death may occur). Similar interactions as with other tricyclics may occur. Amoxapine may increase the incidence of cardiac arrhythmias with quinidine or procainamide. Oral contraceptives and estrogens may inhibit amoxapine metabolism, increasing serum levels/toxicity. Potential for serotonin syndrome if combined with other serotonergic drugs.

**Effects on Lab Values** ↑ glucose, liver function tests; ↓ WBC

**Adverse Reactions**

>10%:

Central nervous system: Drowsiness

Gastrointestinal: Dry mouth, constipation, nausea, unpleasant taste, weight gain

1% to 10%:

Central nervous system: Dizziness, headache, confusion, nervousness, restlessness, insomnia, ataxia, excitement

Dermatologic: Edema, skin rash

Endocrine: Elevated prolactin levels

Gastrointestinal: Increased appetite

Neuromuscular & skeletal: Tremor, weakness

Ocular: Blurred vision

Miscellaneous: Sweating

<1% (Limited to important or life-threatening symptoms): Hypotension, tachycardia, anxiety, seizures, neuroleptic malignant syndrome, extrapyramidal symptoms, tardive dyskinesia, breast enlargement, galactorrhea, SIADH, increased or decreased libido, impotence, menstrual irregularity, painful ejaculation, testicular edema, urinary retention, agranulocytosis, leukopenia, elevated liver enzymes, increased intraocular pressure, mydriasis, lacrimation

**Overdose/Toxicology** Symptoms of overdose include grand mal convulsions, acidosis, coma, and renal failure. Following initiation of essential overdose management, toxic symptoms should be treated. Ventricular arrhythmias often respond to phenytoin 15-20 mg/kg (adults) with concurrent systemic alkalinization (sodium bicarbonate 0.5-2 mEq/kg

(Continued)

## Amoxapine *(Continued)*

I.V.). Physostigmine (1-2 mg I.V. slowly for adults) may be indicated for reversing cardiac arrhythmias that are due to vagal blockade, or for anticholinergic effects, but should only be used as a last measure in life-threatening situations.

**Pharmacodynamics/Kinetics**

**Protein Binding:** 80%

**Half-life Elimination:** Parent drug: 11-16 hours; Active metabolite: 30 hours

**Metabolism:** Liver

**Excretion:** Urine

**Onset:** Onset of antidepressant effect: Usually occurs after 1-2 weeks

**Formulations** Tablet: 25 mg, 50 mg, 100 mg, 150 mg

**Dosing**

**Adults:** Once symptoms are controlled, decrease gradually to lowest effective dose. Maintenance dose is usually given at bedtime to reduce daytime sedation.

Oral: Initial: 25 mg 2-3 times/day. If tolerated, dosage may be increased to 100 mg 2-3 times/day. May be given in a single bedtime dose when dosage <300 mg/day.

Maximum daily dose:

Inpatients: 600 mg

Outpatients: 400 mg

**Elderly:** Oral (once symptoms are controlled, decrease gradually to lowest effective dose): Initial: 25 mg at bedtime increased by 25 mg weekly for outpatients and every 3 days for inpatients if tolerated; usual dose: 50-150 mg/day, but doses up to 300 mg may be necessary. See Geriatric Considerations.

**Administration**

**Oral:** May be administered with food to decrease GI distress.

**Additional Nursing Issues**

**Physical Assessment:** Assess other medications patient may be taking for effectiveness and interactions (see Drug Interactions). See Contraindications and Warnings/Precautions for cautious use. Assess for history of addiction; long-term use can result in dependence, abuse, or tolerance; periodically evaluate need for continued use. **Note:** Amoxapine may affect glucose levels. Monitor therapeutic response (eg, mood, affect, anxiety level, sleep pattern) and adverse reactions at beginning of therapy and periodically with long-term use (see Adverse Reactions and Overdose/Toxicology). Taper dosage slowly when discontinuing. Assess knowledge/teach patient appropriate use, interventions to reduce side effects, and adverse symptoms to report. **Pregnancy risk factor C** - benefits of use should outweigh possible risks. Breast-feeding is contraindicated.

**Patient Information/Instruction:** Take exactly as directed (do not increase dose or frequency). Full effect may not occur for 3-5 weeks; may cause physical and/or psychological dependence. Do not use excessive alcohol or other prescription or OTC medications (especially pain medications, sedatives, antihistamines, or hypnotics) without consulting prescriber. Maintain adequate hydration (2-3 L/day of fluids unless instructed to restrict fluid intake). You may experience drowsiness, lightheadedness, impaired coordination, dizziness, or blurred vision (use caution when driving or engaging in tasks requiring alertness until response to drug is known); nausea, vomiting, increased appetite, or dry mouth (small frequent meals, frequent mouth care, chewing gum, or sucking lozenges may help); constipation (increased exercise, fluids, or dietary fruit and fiber may help); or altered sexual drive or ability (reversible). Report persistent CNS effects (confusion, restlessness, anxiety, insomnia, excitation, headache, dizziness, fatigue, impaired coordination); muscle cramping, weakness, tremors, or rigidity; visual disturbances; excessive GI symptoms (cramping, constipation, vomiting); or worsening of condition. **Pregnancy/breast-feeding precautions:** Inform prescriber if you are or intend to be pregnant. Do not breast-feed.

**Geriatric Considerations:** Amoxapine is not the drug of choice in the elderly. Significant anticholinergic and orthostatic effects can occur and there is a risk for tardive dyskinesia and neuroleptic malignant syndrome.

**Other Issues:** Instruct the patient on the signs or symptoms of neuroleptic syndrome and tardive dyskinesia.

**Related Information**

Antidepressant Agents Comparison *on page 1368*

## Amoxicillin (a moks i SIL in)

**U.S. Brand Names** Amoxil®; Biomox®; Polymox®; Trimox®; Wymox®

**Synonyms** Amoxycillin; *p*-Hydroxyampicillin

**Therapeutic Category** Antibiotic, Penicillin

**Pregnancy Risk Factor** B

**Lactation** Enters breast milk/compatible

**Use** Treatment of otitis media, sinusitis, and infections caused by susceptible organisms involving the respiratory tract, skin, and urinary tract; prophylaxis of bacterial endocarditis; in combination with other agents (ie, lansoprazole and clarithromycin) to eradicate *Helicobacter* pylori

**Mechanism of Action/Effect** Interferes with bacterial cell wall synthesis during active multiplication, causing cell wall death and resultant bactericidal activity against susceptible bacteria

**Contraindications** Hypersensitivity to amoxicillin, any component, penicillins, beta-lactams, cephalosporins, or imipenem

**Warnings** In patients with renal impairment, doses and/or frequency of administration should be modified in response to the degree of renal impairment. A high percentage of patients with infectious mononucleosis have developed rash during therapy with amoxicillin.

**Drug Interactions**

**Decreased Effect:** Efficacy of oral contraceptives may be reduced by amoxicillin. Decreased effectiveness with tetracyclines and chloramphenicol.

**Increased Effect/Toxicity:** Disulfiram and probenecid may increase amoxicillin levels. Effects of anticoagulants may be increased. Theoretically, allopurinol taken with amoxicillin has an additive potential for amoxicillin rash.

**Food Interactions** Amoxicillin serum concentrations may be decreased if taken with food.

**Effects on Lab Values** ↑ AST, ALT, protein; altered response to Benedict's reagent in Clinitest®

**Adverse Reactions**

>10%:

Central nervous system: Headache

Gastrointestinal: Nausea (mild), vomiting

Miscellaneous: Oral candidiasis, vaginal candidiasis

1% to 10%:

Dermatologic: Urticaria, exfoliative dermatitis

Miscellaneous: Allergic reactions, specifically anaphylaxis; serum sickness-like reactions

<1% (Limited to important or life-threatening symptoms): Seizures, leukopenia, neutropenia, thrombocytopenia, jaundice, hepatotoxicity, interstitial nephritis, *Clostridium difficile* colitis

**Overdose/Toxicology** Symptoms of penicillin overdose include neuromuscular hypersensitivity (eg, agitation, hallucinations, asterixis, encephalopathy, confusion, and seizures). Electrolyte imbalance may occur if the preparation contains potassium or sodium salts, especially in renal failure. Hemodialysis may be helpful to aid in removal of the drug from blood; otherwise, treatment is symptom directed and supportive.

**Pharmacodynamics/Kinetics**

**Protein Binding:** 17% to 20%

**Half-life Elimination:** Adults with normal renal function: 0.7-1.4 hours; Patients with $Cl_{cr}$ <10 mL/minute: 7-21 hours

**Metabolism:** Liver

**Excretion:** Urine

**Formulations**

Capsule, as trihydrate: 250 mg, 500 mg

Powder for oral suspension, as trihydrate: 125 mg/5 mL (5 mL, 80 mL, 100 mL, 150 mL, 200 mL); 250 mg/5 mL (5 mL, 80 mL, 100 mL, 150 mL, 200 mL)

Powder for oral suspension, drops, as trihydrate: 50 mg/mL (15 mL, 30 mL)

Tablet, chewable, as trihydrate: 125 mg, 250 mg

Tablet, film coated: 500 mg, 875 mg

**Dosing**

**Adults:** Oral: 250-500 mg every 8 hours or 500-875 mg twice daily; maximum: 2-3 g/day

Uncomplicated gonorrhea: 3 g plus probenecid 1 g in a single dose

Endocarditis prophylaxis (standard): 2 g 1 hour before dental procedure

*Helicobacter pylori*: Clinically effective treatment regimens include triple therapy with amoxicillin or tetracycline, metronidazole, and bismuth subsalicylate; amoxicillin, metronidazole, and an $H_2$-receptor antagonist; 250-500 mg 3 times/day or 500-875 mg twice daily

**Elderly:** Refer to adult dosing.

**Renal Impairment:**

$Cl_{cr}$ 10-50 mL/minute: Administer every 12 hours.

$Cl_{cr}$ <10 mL/minute: Administer every 24 hours.

Moderately dialyzable (20% to 50%) by hemodialysis or peritoneal dialysis; approximately 50 mg of amoxicillin per liter of filtrate is removed by continuous arteriovenous or venovenous hemofiltration (CAVH); dose as per $Cl_{cr}$ <10 mL/minute guidelines.

**Administration**

**Oral:** Administer around-the-clock to promote less variation in peak and trough serum levels.

**Stability**

**Reconstitution:** After reconstitution the suspension remains stable for 7 days at room temperature or 14 days if refrigerated. Unit dose antibiotic oral syringes are stable for 48 hours.

**Monitoring Laboratory Tests** Perform culture and sensitivity testing prior to initiating therapy.

**Additional Nursing Issues**

**Physical Assessment:** Monitor appropriate laboratory tests as ordered. Monitor for (teach patient to monitor and report) effectiveness of therapy and adverse reactions as identified above, including development of opportunistic infections (eg, fever, chills, unhealed sores, white plaques in mouth or vagina, purulent vaginal discharge, fatigue). Assess/teach contraceptive measures if appropriate (amoxicillin may reduce effectiveness of oral contraceptives).

**Patient Information/Instruction:** Take entire prescription, even if you are feeling better. Take at equal intervals around-the-clock; may be taken with milk, juice, or food. You may experience nausea or vomiting (small frequent meals, frequent mouth care, sucking lozenges, or chewing gum may help). If diabetic, drug may cause false tests with Clinitest® urine glucose monitoring; use of glucose oxidase methods (Clinistix®) or

(Continued)

## Amoxicillin *(Continued)*

serum glucose monitoring is preferable. This drug may interfere with oral contraceptives; an alternate form of birth control should be used. Report rash; unusual diarrhea; vaginal itching, burning, or pain; unresolved vomiting or constipation; fever or chills; unusual bruising or bleeding; or if condition being treated worsens or does not improve by the time prescription is completed.

**Geriatric Considerations:** Resistance to amoxicillin has been a problem in patients on frequent antibiotics or in nursing homes. Alternative antibiotics may be necessary in these populations. Consider renal function.

## Amoxicillin and Clavulanate Potassium

(a moks i SIL in & klav yoo LAN ate poe TASS ee um)

**U.S. Brand Names** Augmentin®

**Synonyms** Amoxicillin and Clavulanic Acid; Clavulanate Potassium and Amoxicillin

**Therapeutic Category** Antibiotic, Penicillin

**Pregnancy Risk Factor** B

**Lactation** Enters breast milk/compatible

**Use** Treatment of otitis media, sinusitis, and infections caused by susceptible organisms involving the lower respiratory tract, skin and skin structure, and urinary tract. Spectrum is the same as amoxicillin with additional coverage of beta-lactamase producing *B. catarrhalis, H. influenzae, N. gonorrhoeae,* and *S. aureus* (not MRSA). The expanded coverage of this combination makes it a useful alternative when amoxicillin resistance is present and patients cannot tolerate alternative treatments.

**Mechanism of Action/Effect** Interferes with bacterial cell wall synthesis during active multiplication, causing cell wall death and resultant bactericidal activity against susceptible bacteria. Clavulanic acid binds and inhibits beta-lactamases that inactivate amoxicillin resulting in amoxicillin having an expanded spectrum of activity.

**Contraindications** Hypersensitivity to amoxicillin, clavulanic acid, penicillins, cephalosporins, or imipenem; concomitant use of disulfiram

**Warnings** In patients with renal impairment, doses and/or frequency of administration should be modified in response to the degree of renal impairment. A high percentage of patients with infectious mononucleosis have developed rash during therapy. A low incidence of cross-allergy with cephalosporins exists. Incidence of diarrhea is higher than with amoxicillin alone. Hepatic dysfunction, although rare, is more common in elderly and/or males and/or with prolonged treatment.

**Drug Interactions**

**Decreased Effect:** Efficacy of oral contraceptives, tetracyclines, and chloramphenicol may be reduced when taken with Augmentin®.

**Increased Effect/Toxicity:** Disulfiram, probenecid may increase amoxicillin levels. Increased effect of anticoagulants with amoxicillin. Theoretically, allopurinol taken with Augmentin® has an additive potential for rash.

**Effects on Lab Values** Urinary glucose (Benedict's solution, Clinitest®)

**Adverse Reactions**

>10%:
- Central nervous system: Headache
- Gastrointestinal: Nausea (mild), vomiting
- Miscellaneous: Oral candidiasis, vaginal candidiasis

1% to 10%:
- Dermatologic: Urticaria, exfoliative dermatitis
- Miscellaneous: Allergic reactions, specifically anaphylaxis; serum sickness-like reactions

<1% (Limited to important or life-threatening symptoms): Seizures, leukopenia, neutropenia, thrombocytopenia, jaundice, hepatotoxicity, interstitial nephritis, *Clostridium difficile* colitis

**Overdose/Toxicology** Symptoms of penicillin overdose include neuromuscular hypersensitivity (eg, agitation, hallucinations, asterixis, encephalopathy, confusion, and seizures). Electrolyte imbalance may occur if the preparation contains potassium or sodium salts, especially in renal failure. Hemodialysis may be helpful to aid in removal of the drug from blood; otherwise, treatment is supportive or symptom directed.

**Pharmacodynamics/Kinetics**

**Half-life Elimination:** Adults with normal renal function: ~1 hour for both agents; Patients with $Cl_{cr}$ <10 mL/minute: 7-21 hours

**Metabolism:** Liver

**Excretion:** Urine

**Formulations**

Suspension, oral:
- 125 (banana flavor): Amoxicillin trihydrate 125 mg and clavulanate potassium 31.25 mg per 5 mL (75 mL, 150 mL)
- 200: Amoxicillin 200 mg and clavulanate potassium 28.5 mg per 5 mL (50 mL, 75 mL, 100 mL)
- 250 (orange flavor): Amoxicillin trihydrate 250 mg and clavulanate potassium 62.5 mg per 5 mL (75 mL, 150 mL)
- 400: Amoxicillin 400 mg and clavulanate potassium 57 mg per 5 mL (50 mL, 75 mL, 100 mL)

Tablet:
- 250: Amoxicillin trihydrate 250 mg and clavulanate potassium 125 mg
- 500: Amoxicillin trihydrate 500 mg and clavulanate potassium 125 mg
- 875: Amoxicillin trihydrate 875 mg and clavulanate potassium 125 mg

Tablet, chewable:
125: Amoxicillin trihydrate 125 mg and clavulanate potassium 31.25 mg
250: Amoxicillin trihydrate 250 mg and clavulanate potassium 62.5 mg

**Dosing**

**Adults:**

Oral: 250-500 mg every 8 hours or 875 mg every 12 hours

Two 250 mg tablets are not equivalent to a 500 mg tablet (both tablet sizes contain equivalent clavulanate); potassium content: 0.16 mEq of potassium per 31.25 mg of clavulanic acid

**Elderly:** Refer to adult dosing.

**Renal Impairment:** Oral:

$Cl_{cr}$ 10-30 mL/minute: Administer every 12 hours.

$Cl_{cr}$ <10 mL/minute: Administer every 24 hours.

Hemodialysis effects: Moderately dialyzable (20% to 50%)
Amoxicillin/clavulanic acid: Administer dose after dialysis.

Peritoneal dialysis effects: Moderately dialyzable (20% to 50%)
Amoxicillin: Administer 250 mg every 12 hours.
Clavulanic acid: Dose for $Cl_{cr}$ <10 mL/minute.

Continuous arteriovenous or venovenous hemofiltration (CAVH) effects:
Amoxicillin: ~50 mg of amoxicillin/L of filtrate is removed.
Clavulanic acid: Dose for $Cl_{cr}$ <10 mL/minute.

**Administration**

**Oral:** Administer around-the-clock to promote less variation in peak and trough serum levels.

**Stability**

**Reconstitution:** Discard unused suspension after 10 days. Reconstituted oral suspension should be kept in refrigerator. Unit dose antibiotic oral syringes are stable for 48 hours.

**Monitoring Laboratory Tests** Renal, hepatic, and hematologic function periodically with prolonged therapy. Perform culture and sensitivity testing prior to initiating therapy.

**Additional Nursing Issues**

**Physical Assessment:** Monitor appropriate laboratory tests as ordered. Monitor for (teach patient to monitor and report) effectiveness of therapy and adverse reactions as identified above, including development of opportunistic infections (fever, chills, unhealed sores, white plaques in mouth or vagina, purulent vaginal discharge, fatigue). Assess/teach contraceptive measures if appropriate (amoxicillin may reduce effectiveness of oral contraceptives).

**Patient Information/Instruction:** Take entire prescription, even if you are feeling better. Take at equal intervals around-the-clock; may be taken with milk, juice, or food. You may experience nausea or vomiting (small frequent meals, frequent mouth care, sucking lozenges, or chewing gum may help). If using oral contraceptives, use additional contraceptive measures; amoxicillin may reduce effectiveness of your oral contraceptive. Report rash; unusual diarrhea; vaginal itching, burning, or pain; unresolved vomiting or constipation; fever or chills; unusual bruising or bleeding; or if condition being treated worsens or does not improve by the time prescription is completed.

**Geriatric Considerations:** Resistance to amoxicillin has been a problem in patients on frequent antibiotics or in nursing homes. However, expanded coverage of this combination makes it a useful alternative when amoxicillin resistance is present and patients cannot tolerate alternative treatments. Consider renal function. Considered one of the drugs of choice in the outpatient treatment of community-acquired pneumonia in older adults.

**Related Information**

Amoxicillin *on page 80*

- **Amoxicillin and Clavulanic Acid** *see* Amoxicillin and Clavulanate Potassium *on previous page*
- **Amoxicillin, Lansoprazole, and Clarithromycin** *see* Lansoprazole, Amoxicillin, and Clarithromycin *on page 656*
- **Amoxifur** *see* Amoxicillin *on page 80*
- **Amoxil®** *see* Amoxicillin *on page 80*
- **Amoxisol** *see* Amoxicillin *on page 80*
- **Amoxivet** *see* Amoxicillin *on page 80*
- **Amoxycillin** *see* Amoxicillin *on page 80*
- **Amphojel® [OTC]** *see* Aluminum Hydroxide *on page 60*
- **Amphotec™** *see* Amphotericin B Cholesteryl Sulfate Complex *on page 85*

## Amphotericin B (am foe TER i sin bee)

**U.S. Brand Names** Fungizone®

**Synonyms** MPHO

**Therapeutic Category** Antifungal Agent, Parenteral; Antifungal Agent, Topical

**Pregnancy Risk Factor** B

**Lactation** Excretion in breast milk unknown/contraindicated

**Use** Treatment of severe systemic and central nervous system infections caused by susceptible fungi such as *Candida* species, *Histoplasma capsulatum*, *Cryptococcus neoformans*, *Aspergillus* species, *Blastomyces dermatitidis*, *Torulopsis glabrata*, and *Coccidioides immitis*; fungal peritonitis; irrigant for bladder fungal infections; topically for cutaneous and mucocutaneous candidal infections. Low-dose amphotericin B 0.1-0.25 mg/kg/day has been administered after bone marrow transplantation to reduce the risk of
(Continued)

## Amphotericin B *(Continued)*

invasive fungal disease. Alternative routes of administration and extemporaneous preparations have been used when standard antifungal therapy is not available (eg, inhalation, intraocular injection, subconjunctival application, intracavitary administration into various joints and the pleural space).

**Mechanism of Action/Effect** Binds to ergosterol altering cell membrane permeability in susceptible fungi and causing leakage of cell components with subsequent cell death

**Contraindications** Hypersensitivity to amphotericin or any component

**Warnings** Avoid additive toxicity with other nephrotoxic drugs. Monitor BUN and serum creatinine, potassium, and magnesium levels every 2-4 days, and daily in patients at risk for acute renal dysfunction. I.V. amphotericin is used primarily for the treatment of patients with progressive and potentially fatal fungal infections. Topical preparations may stain clothing. The standard dosage of lipid-based amphotericin B formulations, including amphotericin B cholesteryl sulfate (Amphotec®), amphotericin B lipid complex (Abelcet®), and liposomal amphotericin B (AmBisome®) is manyfold greater than the dosage of conventional amphotericin B. To prevent inadvertent overdose, the product name and dosage must be verified for any amphotericin B dosage exceeding 1.5 mg/kg. Amphotericin B has been administered to pregnant women without obvious deleterious effects to the fetus, but the number of cases reported is small. Use during pregnancy only if absolutely necessary.

**Drug Interactions**

**Decreased Effect:** Pharmacologic antagonism may occur with azole antifungal agents (ketoconazole, miconazole)

**Increased Effect/Toxicity:** Toxic effect with other nephrotoxic drugs such as cyclosporine and aminoglycosides may be additive. Corticosteroids may increase potassium depletion caused by amphotericin. Amphotericin B may predispose patients receiving digitalis glycosides or neuromuscular blocking agents to toxicity secondary to hypokalemia.

**Effects on Lab Values** ↑ BUN (S), serum creatinine, alkaline phosphate, bilirubin; ↓ magnesium, potassium (S)

**Adverse Reactions**

**Systemic:**

>10%:

- Cardiovascular: Hypotension, tachypnea
- Central nervous system: Fever, chills, headache (less frequent with I.T.), malaise
- Endocrine & metabolic: Hypokalemia, hypomagnesemia
- Gastrointestinal: Anorexia, nausea (less frequent with I.T.), vomiting (less frequent with I.T.), diarrhea, heartburn, cramping epigastric pain
- Hematologic: Normochromic-normocytic anemia
- Neuromuscular & skeletal: Generalized pain, including muscle and joint pains (less frequent with I.T.)
- Renal: Decreased renal function and renal function abnormalities including: azotemia, renal tubular acidosis, nephrocalcinosis
- Local: Pain at injection site with or without phlebitis or thrombophlebitis (incidence may increase with peripheral infusion of admixtures >0.1 mg/mL)

1% to 10%:

- Cardiovascular: Hypertension, flushing
- Central nervous system: Delirium, arachnoiditis, pain along lumbar nerves (especially I.T. therapy)
- Genitourinary: Urinary retention
- Hematologic: Leukocytosis
- Neuromuscular & skeletal: Paresthesia (especially with I.T. therapy)

<1% (Limited to important or life-threatening symptoms): Cardiac arrest, bone marrow suppression, convulsions, maculopapular rash, coagulation defects, thrombocytopenia, agranulocytosis, leukopenia, acute liver failure, vision changes, hearing loss, anuria, dyspnea, renal tubular acidosis, renal failure

**Overdose/Toxicology** Symptoms of overdose include renal dysfunction, cardiac arrest, anemia, thrombocytopenia, granulocytopenia, fever, nausea, and vomiting. Treatment is supportive.

**Pharmacodynamics/Kinetics**

**Half-life Elimination:** Biphasic: Initial: 15-48 hours; Terminal: 15 days

**Excretion:** Urine

**Formulations**

- Cream: 3% (20 g)
- Lotion: 3% (30 mL)
- Ointment, topical: 3% (20 g)
- Powder for injection, lyophilized: 50 mg
- Suspension, oral: 100 mg/mL (24 mL with dropper)

**Dosing**

**Adults:**

I.V.:

- Test dose (not required): 1 mg infused over 20-30 minutes. Many clinicians believe a test dose is unnecessary.
- Maintenance dose: 0.25-1.5 mg/kg/day. Once therapy is established, 1.0- 1.5 mg/kg may be given over 4-6 hours every other day; do not exceed 1.5 mg/kg/day; cumulative dose: 1-4 g over 4-10 weeks.
- Duration of therapy varies with nature of infection: Histoplasmosis, *Cryptococcus*, aspergillosis, fusariosis, or blastomycosis may be treated with total dose of 2-4 g.

Topical: Apply to affected areas 2-4 times/day for 1-4 weeks of therapy depending on nature and severity of infection.

Administration via bladder irrigation: 50 mg/day in 1 L of sterile water irrigation solution instilled over 24 hours for 2-7 days or until cultures are clear.

**Elderly:** Refer to adult dosing.

**Renal Impairment:**

If renal dysfunction is due to the drug, the daily total can be decreased by 50% or the dose can be given every other day. I.V. therapy may take several months.

Poorly dialyzed; no supplemental dosage is necessary when using hemo- or peritoneal dialysis or CAVH/CAVHD.

Administration in dialysate: 1-2 mg/L of peritoneal dialysis fluid either with or without low-dose I.V. amphotericin B (a total dose of 2-10 mg/kg given over 7-14 days).

**Administration**

**I.V.:** May be infused over 4-6 hours. For a patient who experiences chills, fever, hypotension, nausea or other nonanaphylactic infusion-related reactions, premedication with the following drugs, 30-60 minutes prior to drug administration: A nonsteroidal (ibuprofen, choline magnesium trisalicylate, etc) with or without diphenhydramine; or acetaminophen with diphenhydramine, or hydrocortisone 50-100 mg. If the patient experiences rigors during the infusion, meperidine may be administered. Bolus infusion of normal saline immediately preceding, or immediately preceding and following amphotericin B may reduce drug-induced nephrotoxicity. Risk of nephrotoxicity increases with amphotericin B doses >1 mg/kg/day. Infusion of admixtures more concentrated than 0.25 mg/mL should be limited to patients absolutely requiring volume contraction.

**I.V. Detail:** Precipitate may form in ionic dialysate solutions.

**Topical:** Wear gloves to administer. Amphotericin may stain skin and clothing.

**Stability**

**Storage:** Amphotericin B does not have a bacteriostatic constituent, subsequently admixture expiration is determined by sterility more than chemical stability.

Admixture concentration: Standard admixture concentrations are 0.1 mg/mL (peripheral infusion) and 0.25 mg/mL (central administration). Although 0.8 mg/mL in $D_5W$ is physically compatible and chemically stable, the safety of infusing amphotericin B >0.25 mg/mL has not been formally evaluated (see Adverse Reactions).

**Reconstitution:** Reconstitute only with sterile water without preservatives, not bacteriostatic water. **Benzyl alcohol, sodium chloride, or other electrolyte solutions may cause precipitation.** Short-term exposure (<24 hours) to light during I.V. infusion does **not** appreciably affect potency. Reconstituted solutions with sterile water for injection and kept in the dark remain stable for 24 hours at room temperature and 1 week when refrigerated. Stability of parenteral admixture at room temperature (25°C) is 24 hours; at refrigeration (4°C) is 2 days.

Standard diluent: Dose per 500 mL $D_5W$

**Compatibility:** Admixtures are with glass or plastic containers, including polyvinylchloride, although some sterile evacuated glass containers have small amounts of ionic liquid buffer that may cause precipitation. See the Compatibility of Drugs Chart *on page 1315*.

**Monitoring Laboratory Tests** BUN and serum creatinine levels should be determined every other day when therapy is increased and at least weekly thereafter. Monitor serum electrolytes (especially potassium and magnesium), liver function, and CBC.

**Additional Nursing Issues**

**Physical Assessment:** Assess effectiveness and interactions of other medications (see Drug Interactions). See Warnings/Precautions and Contraindications for use cautions. Monitor effectiveness of therapy and monitor laboratory tests frequently during therapy (see above). Monitor closely for adverse response (eg, anaphylactoid reactions, acute respiratory distress, hypokalemia, and nephrotoxicity - see Warnings/Precautions, Adverse Reactions, and Overdose/Toxicology). Assess knowledge/teach patient appropriate use (outpatient), possible side effects and appropriate interventions, and adverse symptoms to report. Breast-feeding is contraindicated.

**Patient Information/Instruction:** Take/use as directed; complete full regimen of treatment (most skin lesions may take 1-3 weeks of therapy). Maintain adequate hydration (2-3 L/day of fluids unless instructed to restrict fluid intake). You may experience nausea, vomiting, or anorexia (small frequent meals, frequent mouth care, sucking lozenges, or chewing gum may help); generalized muscle or joint paint (mild analgesic may help); hypotension (use caution when rising from sitting or lying position or when climbing stairs). Report severe muscle cramping or weakness, chest pain or palpitations, CNS disturbances, skin rash, change in urinary patterns or difficulty voiding, black stool, or unusual bruising or bleeding; (I.V. report pain at infusion site).

Topical: Amphotericin cream may slightly discolor skin and stain clothing; use gloves when applying. Avoid covering topical application with occlusive bandages. Most skin lesions require 1-3 weeks of therapy. Maintain good personal hygiene to reduce the spread and recurrence of lesions.

**Breast-feeding precautions:** Do not breast-feed.

**Geriatric Considerations:** Caution should be exercised and renal function and desired effect monitored closely in older adults.

## Amphotericin B Cholesteryl Sulfate Complex

(am foe TER i sin bee kole LES te ril SUL fate KOM plecks)

**U.S. Brand Names** Amphotec™

**Synonyms** ABCD; Amphotericin B Colloidal Dispersion

(Continued)

## Amphotericin B Cholesteryl Sulfate Complex *(Continued)*

**Therapeutic Category** Antifungal Agent, Parenteral

**Pregnancy Risk Factor** B

**Lactation** Excretion in breast milk unknown/contraindicated

**Use** Treatment of invasive aspergillosis in patients who have failed amphotericin B deoxycholate treatment, or who have renal impairment or experience unacceptable toxicity which precludes treatment with amphotericin B deoxycholate in effective doses; empiric management of presumed fungal infection during persistent febrile neutropenia in patients at risk for acute renal dysfunction

**Mechanism of Action/Effect** Binds to ergosterol altering cell membrane permeability in susceptible fungi and causing leakage of cell components with subsequent cell death

**Contraindications** Hypersensitivity to amphotericin B or any component

**Warnings** Anaphylaxis has been reported. Facilities for cardiopulmonary resuscitation should be available. Infusion reactions, sometimes severe, usually subside with continued therapy.

**Drug Interactions**

**Decreased Effect:** Pharmacologic antagonism may occur with azole antifungals (ketoconazole, miconazole, etc).

**Increased Effect/Toxicity:** Toxic effect with other nephrotoxic drugs such as cyclosporine and aminoglycosides may be additive. Corticosteroids may increase potassium depletion caused by amphotericin. Amphotericin B may predispose patients receiving digitalis glycosides or neuromuscular blocking agents to toxicity secondary to hypokalemia.

**Adverse Reactions** 1% to 10%:

Cardiovascular: Hypotension, tachycardia
Central nervous system: Headache, chills, fever
Dermatologic: Rash
Endocrine & metabolic: Hypokalemia, hypomagnesemia
Gastrointestinal: Nausea, diarrhea, abdominal pain
Hematologic: Thrombocytopenia
Hepatic: Abnormal LFTs
Neuromuscular & skeletal: Rigors
Respiratory: Dyspnea

**Note:** Amphotericin B colloidal dispersion has an improved therapeutic index compared to conventional amphotericin B, and has been used safely in patients with amphotericin B-related nephrotoxicity; however, continued decline of renal function has occurred in some patients.

**Overdose/Toxicology** Symptoms of overdose include renal dysfunction, anemia, thrombocytopenia, granulocytopenia, fever, nausea, and vomiting. Treatment is supportive.

**Pharmacodynamics/Kinetics**

**Distribution:** $V_d$: Total amphotericin B increases with increasing doses of total amphotericin B (with 4 mg/kg/day = 4 L/kg); predominantly distributed in the liver; concentrations in kidneys and other tissues are lower than observed with conventional amphotericin B

**Half-life Elimination:** 28-29 hours

**Time to Peak:** Plasma concentration: Total amphotericin B remains between 1-3 mcg/mL

**Excretion:** Clearance: 0.1 L/hour/kg (with 4 mg/kg/day)

**Formulations** Suspension for injection: 5 mg/mL (20 mL)

**Dosing**

**Adults:** I.V.: 3-4 mg/kg/day; 6 mg/kg/day has been used for treatment of life-threatening invasive mold infections in immunocompromised patients; maximum: 7.5 mg/kg/day. Initially infuse at 1 mg/kg/hour. Rate of infusion may be increased with subsequent doses to 3 mg/kg/hour as patient tolerance allows. Treatment should continue as patient tolerance allows, until complete resolution of microbiologic and clinical evidence of fungal disease.

**Elderly:** Refer to adult dosing.

**Administration**

**I.V.:** For a patient who experiences chills, fever, hypotension, nausea, or other nonanaphylactic infusion-related reactions, premedication with the following drugs, 30-60 minutes prior to drug administration: A nonsteroidal (ibuprofen, choline magnesium trisalicylate, etc) with or without diphenhydramine; or acetaminophen with diphenhydramine, or hydrocortisone 50-100 mg. If the patient experiences rigors during the infusion, meperidine may be administered. Avoid infusing faster than 1 mg/kg/hour.

**Stability**

**Compatibility:** See the Compatibility of Drugs Chart *on page 1315.*

**Monitoring Laboratory Tests** Monitor serum electrolytes (especially potassium and magnesium), liver function, and CBC.

**Additional Nursing Issues**

**Physical Assessment:** Assess effectiveness and interactions of other medications (see Drug Interactions). See Warnings/Precautions and Contraindications for use cautions. Monitor effectiveness of therapy and monitor laboratory tests frequently during therapy (see above). Monitor closely for adverse response (eg, anaphylactoid reaction, hypokalemia, and nephrotoxicity - see Warnings/Precautions, Adverse Reactions, and Overdose/Toxicology). Assess knowledge/teach patient possible side effects and appropriate interventions and adverse symptoms to report. Breast-feeding is contraindicated.

**Patient Information/Instruction:** This medication can only be administered by infusion and therapy may last several weeks. Maintain good hydration (2-3 L/day of fluids unless instructed to restrict fluid intake). You may experience postural hypotension (use caution when changing from lying or sitting position to standing or when climbing stairs); nausea or vomiting (small frequent meals, frequent mouth care, sucking lozenges, or chewing gum may help). Report chest pain or palpitations; skin rash; chills or fever; persistent nausea, vomiting, or abdominal pain; sore throat; excessive fatigue; swelling of extremities or unusual weight gain; difficulty breathing; pain at infusion site; muscle cramping or weakness; or other adverse reactions. **Breast-feeding precautions:** Do not breast-feed.

**Geriatric Considerations:** The pharmacokinetics and dosing of amphotericin have not been studied in the elderly. It appears that use is similar to young adults. Caution should be exercised and renal function and desired effect monitored closely.

♦ **Amphotericin B Colloidal Dispersion** *see* Amphotericin B Cholesteryl Sulfate Complex *on page 85*

## Amphotericin B Lipid Complex (am foe TER i sin bee LIP id KOM pleks)

**U.S. Brand Names** Abelcet™ Injection

**Synonyms** ABLC

**Therapeutic Category** Antifungal Agent, Parenteral

**Pregnancy Risk Factor** B

**Lactation** Enters breast milk/contraindicated

**Use** Treatment of aspergillosis in patients who are refractory to or intolerant of conventional amphotericin B therapy; orphan drug status for cryptococcal meningitis

**Mechanism of Action/Effect** Mechanism is like amphotericin - includes binding to ergosterol altering cell membrane permeability in susceptible fungi and causing leakage of cell components with subsequent cell death.

**Contraindications** Hypersensitivity to amphotericin or any component

**Warnings** See Warnings/Precautions in Amphotericin B monograph.

**Drug Interactions**

**Decreased Effect:** Pharmacologic antagonism may occur with azole antifungal agents (ketoconazole, miconazole)

**Increased Effect/Toxicity:** See Drug Interactions - Increased Effect/Toxicity in Amphotericin B monograph.

**Effects on Lab Values** ↑ BUN (S), serum creatinine, alkaline phosphate, bilirubin; ↓ magnesium, potassium (S)

**Adverse Reactions** Nephrotoxicity and infusion-related hyperpyrexia, rigor, and chilling are reduced relative to amphotericin deoxycholate.

>10%:

- Central nervous system: Chills, fever
- Renal: Increased serum creatinine
- Miscellaneous: Multiple organ failure

1% to 10%:

- Cardiovascular: Hypotension, cardiac arrest
- Central nervous system: Headache, pain
- Dermatologic: Rash
- Endocrine & metabolic: Bilirubinemia, hypokalemia, acidosis
- Gastrointestinal: Nausea, vomiting, diarrhea, gastrointestinal hemorrhage, abdominal pain
- Renal: Renal failure
- Respiratory: Respiratory failure, dyspnea, pneumonia

**Formulations** Injection: 5 mg/mL (20 mL)

**Dosing**

**Adults:** I.V.: 2.5-5 mg/kg/day as a single infusion. Test dose is not recommended.

**Elderly:** Refer to adult dosing.

**Renal Impairment:** The effects of renal impairment on drug pharmacokinetics or pharmacodynamics are currently unknown. The dose of amphotericin B lipid complex may be adjusted or drug administration may have to be interrupted in patients with acute kidney dysfunction to reduce the magnitude of renal impairment.

Hemodialysis: No supplemental dosage is necessary.

Peritoneal dialysis: No supplemental dosage is necessary.

Continuous arterio-venous or veno-venous hemofiltration (CAVH/CAVHD): No supplemental dosage is necessary.

**Administration**

**I.V.:** For a patient who experiences chills, fever, hypotension, nausea, or other nonanaphylactic infusion-related reactions, premedication with the following drugs, 30-60 minutes prior to drug administration: A nonsteroidal (ibuprofen, choline magnesium trisalicylate, etc) with or without diphenhydramine; or acetaminophen with diphenhydramine, or hydrocortisone 50-100 mg. If the patient experiences rigors during the infusion, meperidine may be administered. If infusion time exceeds 2 hours, mix contents by shaking infusion bag every 2 hours.

**I.V. Detail:** Do not use an inline filter. Flush line with dextrose; normal saline may cause precipitate.

**Stability**

**Storage:** Shake vial gently to disperse yellow sediment at bottom of container. Withdraw correct volume to prepare dose. Inject into appropriate volume of $D_5W$ through 5-micron filter needle provided by manufacturer. Each filter needle may be used to filter the contents of up to four vials. 1 mg/mL in $D_5W$, 48 hours at 2°C to 8°C, then an additional 6 hours at room temperature; 2 mg/mL in $D_5W$ may be used for pediatric

(Continued)

## Amphotericin B Lipid Complex *(Continued)*

patients or adult patients requiring volume reduction. Infuse 2.5 mg/kg/hour. Do not use an in-line filter. Admixture must be inverted several times before infusion, then every 2 hours, to prevent settling or aggregation of lipid particles. Protect from light.

**Compatibility:** Do not admix or Y-site with any blood products, intravenous drugs, or intravenous fluids other than $D_5W$. See the Compatibility of Drugs Chart *on page 1315*.

**Monitoring Laboratory Tests** BUN and serum creatinine levels should be determined every other day while therapy is increased and at least weekly thereafter. Monitor serum electrolytes (especially potassium and magnesium), liver function, and CBC.

**Additional Nursing Issues**

**Physical Assessment:** Assess effectiveness and interactions of other medications (see Drug Interactions). See Warnings/Precautions and Contraindications for use cautions. Monitor effectiveness of therapy and monitor laboratory tests frequently during therapy (see above). Monitor closely for adverse response (see Warnings/Precautions, Adverse Reactions, and Overdose/Toxicology). Assess knowledge/teach patient possible side effects and appropriate interventions, and adverse symptoms to report. Breast-feeding is contraindicated.

**Patient Information/Instruction:** Infusion therapy may take several months. Maintain good personal hygiene to reduce spread and recurrence of lesions. Maintain adequate hydration (2-3 L/day of fluids unless instructed to restrict fluid intake). You may experience postural hypotension (use caution when changing from lying or sitting position to standing or when climbing stairs); nausea or vomiting (small frequent meals, frequent mouth care, sucking lozenges, or chewing gum may help). Report chest pain or palpitations, chills or fever, skin rash, muscle cramping or weakness, alteration in voiding patterns, CNS disturbances, pain at injection site, persistent GI disturbance, or other adverse reactions. **Breast-feeding precautions:** Do not breast-feed.

**Geriatric Considerations:** Caution should be exercised and renal function and desired effect monitored closely in older adults.

## Amphotericin B (Liposomal) (am foe TER i sin bee lye po SO mal)

**U.S. Brand Names** AmBisome®

**Synonyms** L-AmB; Liposomal Amphotericin B

**Therapeutic Category** Antifungal Agent, Parenteral

**Pregnancy Risk Factor** B

**Use** Empirical therapy for presumed fungal infection in febrile, neutropenic patients; treatment of patients with *Aspergillus* species, *Candida* species, and/or *Cryptococcus* species infections refractory to amphotericin B desoxycholate, or in patients where renal impairment or unacceptable toxicity precludes the use of amphotericin B desoxycholate; treatment of visceral leishmaniasis. In immunocompromised patients with visceral leishmaniasis treated with AmBisome®, relapse rates were high following initial clearance of parasites

**Mechanism of Action/Effect** Amphotericin B, the active ingredient, acts by binding to the sterol component of a cell membrane leading to alterations in cell permeability and cell death. While amphotericin B has a higher affinity for the ergosterol component of the fungal cell membrane, it can also bind to the cholesterol component of the mammalian cell leading to cytotoxicity. AmBisome®, the liposomal preparation of amphotericin B, has been shown to penetrate the cell wall of both extracellular and intracellular forms of susceptible fungi.

**Contraindications** Hypersensitivity to amphotericin B or any component unless in the opinion of the treating physician, the benefit of therapy outweighs the risk

**Warnings** Anaphylaxis has been reported with amphotericin B desoxycholate and other amphotericin B-containing drugs. Facilities for cardiopulmonary resuscitation should be available during administration due to the possibility of anaphylactic reaction. As with any amphotericin B-containing product the drug should be administered by medically trained personnel. During the initial dosing period, patients should be under close clinical observation. AmBisome® has been shown to be significantly less toxic than amphotericin B desoxycholate; however, adverse events may still occur. If severe respiratory distress occurs, the infusion should be immediately discontinued and the patient should not receive further infusions. Acute reactions (including fever and chills) may occur 1-2 hours after starting an intravenous infusion. These reactions are usually more common with the first few doses and generally diminish with subsequent doses.

**Drug Interactions**

**Increased Effect/Toxicity:** Drug interactions have not been studied in a controlled manner; however, drugs that interact with conventional amphotericin B may also interact with amphotericin B liposome for injection. The following drug interactions have been described for conventional amphotericin B.

Antineoplastic agents: Concurrent use of antineoplastic agents may enhance the potential for renal toxicity, bronchospasm, and hypotension. Antineoplastic agents should be given concomitantly with caution.

Corticosteroids and corticotropin (ACTH): Concurrent use of corticosteroids and ACTH may potentiate hypokalemia which could predispose the patient to cardiac dysfunction. If used concomitantly, serum electrolytes and cardiac function should be closely monitored.

Digitalis glycosides: Concurrent use may induce hypokalemia and may potentiate digitalis toxicity. When administered concomitantly, serum potassium levels should be closely monitored.

Flucytosine: Concurrent use of flucytosine may increase the toxicity of flucytosine by possibly increasing its cellular uptake and/or impairing its renal excretion.

Azoles (eg, ketoconazole, miconazole, clotrimazole, fluconazole, etc): *In vitro* and *in vivo* animal studies of the combination of amphotericin B and imidazoles suggest that imidazoles may induce fungal resistance to amphotericin B. Combination therapy should be administered with caution, especially in immunocompromised patients.

Leukocyte transfusions: Acute pulmonary toxicity has been reported in patients simultaneously receiving intravenous amphotericin B and leukocyte transfusions.

Other nephrotoxic medications: Concurrent use of amphotericin B and other nephrotoxic medications may enhance the potential for drug-induced renal toxicity. Intensive monitoring of renal function is recommended in patients requiring any combination of nephrotoxic medications.

Skeletal muscle relaxants: Amphotericin B-induced hypokalemia may enhance the curariform effect of skeletal muscle relaxants (eg, tubocurarine) due to hypokalemia. When administered concomitantly, serum potassium levels should be closely monitored.

**Adverse Reactions** Reduced nephrotoxicity as well as frequent infusion related side effects have been reported with this formulation.

>10%:

Central nervous system: Chills, fever

Renal: Increased serum creatinine

1% to 10%:

Cardiovascular: Hypotension, cardiac arrest

Central nervous system: Headache, pain

Dermatologic: Rash

Endocrine & metabolic: Bilirubinemia, hypokalemia, acidosis

Gastrointestinal: Nausea, vomiting, diarrhea, gastrointestinal hemorrhage, abdominal pain

Renal: Renal failure

Respiratory: Respiratory failure, dyspnea, pneumonia

**Overdose/Toxicology** The toxicity due to overdose has not been defined. Repeated daily doses up to 7.5 mg/kg have been administered in clinical trials with no reported dose-related toxicity. If overdosage should occur, cease administration immediately. Symptomatic supportive measures should be instituted. Particular attention should be given to monitoring renal function.

**Pharmacodynamics/Kinetics**

**Half-life Elimination:** Terminal elimination: 174 hours

**Formulations** Injection: 50 mg

**Dosing**

**Adults:** I.V.:

Empirical therapy: Recommended initial dose of 3 mg/kg/day

Systemic fungal infections (*Aspergillus, Candida, Cryptococcus*): Recommended initial dose of 3-5 mg/kg/day

Treatment of visceral leishmaniasis: AmBisome® achieved high rates of acute parasite clearance in immunocompetent patients when total doses of 12-30 mg/kg were administered. Most of these immunocompetent patients remained relapse-free during follow-up periods of 6 months or longer. While acute parasite clearance was achieved in most of the immunocompromised patients who received total doses of 30-40 mg/kg, the majority of these patients were observed to relapse in the 6 months following the completion of therapy.

Dosing and rate of infusion should be individualized to the needs of the specific patient to ensure maximum efficacy while minimizing systemic toxicities or adverse events.

For immunocompetent patients who do not achieve parasitic clearance with the recommended dose, a repeat course of therapy may be useful.

**Elderly:** See adult dosing.

**Renal Impairment:**

**Dosing adjustment in renal impairment:** None necessary; effects of renal impairment are not currently known.

Hemodialysis: No supplemental dosage is necessary.

Peritoneal dialysis effects: No supplemental dosage is necessary.

Continuous arteriovenous or venovenous hemofiltration (CAVH/CAVHD): No supplemental dosage is necessary.

**Administration**

**I.V.:** Should be administered by intravenous infusion, using a controlled infusion device, over a period of approximately 2 hours. Infusion time may be reduced to approximately 1 hour in patients in whom the treatment is well-tolerated. If the patient experiences discomfort during infusion, the duration of infusion may be increased. Administer at a rate of 2.5 mg/kg/hour.

For a patient who experiences chills, fever, hypotension, nausea, or other nonanaphylactic infusion-related reactions, premedication with the following drugs, 30-60 minutes prior to drug administration: A nonsteroidal (ibuprofen, choline magnesium trisalicylate, etc) with or without diphenhydramine; or acetaminophen with diphenhydramine, or hydrocortisone 50-100 mg. If the patient experiences rigors during the infusion, meperidine may be administered.

**I.V. Detail:** Infusion bag or syringe should be shaken before start of infusion. If infusion time exceeds 2 hours, the contents of the infusion bag should be mixed every 2 hours by shaking. Final concentration should be 2 mg/mL.

(Continued)

## Amphotericin B (Liposomal) *(Continued)*

**Stability**

**Reconstitution:** Must be reconstituted using sterile water for injection, USP (without a bacteriostatic agent). Vials containing 50 mg of amphotericin B are prepared as follows.

1. Aseptically add 12 mL of sterile water for injection, USP to each vial to yield a preparation containing 4 mg amphotericin B/mL. **Caution:** Do not reconstitute with saline or add saline to the reconstituted concentration, or mix with other drugs. The use of any solution other than those recommended, or the presence of a bacteriostatic agent in the solution, may cause precipitation.

2. Immediately after the addition of water, **shake the vial vigorously** for 30 seconds to completely disperse the powder, it then forms a yellow, translucent suspension. Visually inspect the vial for particulate matter and continue shaking until completely dispersed.

**Filtration and Dilution:**

3. Calculate the amount of reconstituted (4 mg/mL) to be further diluted.

4. Withdraw this amount of reconstituted powder into a sterile syringe.

5. Attach the 5-micron filter, provided, to the syringe. Inject the syringe contents through the filter, into the appropriate amount of 5% Dextrose Injection. (Use only one filter per vial.)

6. Must be diluted with 5% dextrose injection to a final concentration of 1-2 mg/mL prior to administration. Lower concentrations (0.2-0.5 mg/mL) may be appropriate for infants and small children to provide sufficient volume for infusion. **Discard partially used vials.** Injection should commence within 6 hours of dilution with 5% dextrose injection. An in-line membrane filter may be used for the intravenous infusion; provided, **the mean pore diameter of the filter should not be less than 1 micron.**

**Monitoring Laboratory Tests** BUN and serum creatinine levels should be determined every other day while therapy is increased and at least weekly thereafter. Serum potassium and magnesium should be monitored closely. Monitor for signs of hypokalemia (muscle weakness, cramping, drowsiness, EKG changes, etc). Monitor electrolytes, liver function, hematocrit, and CBC regularly.

**Additional Nursing Issues**

**Patient Information/Instruction:** I.V. therapy may take several months. Personal hygiene is very important to help reduce the spread and recurrence of lesions. Most skin lesions require 1-3 weeks of therapy. Report any hearing loss.

**Additional Information** AmBisome® is a true single bilayer liposomal drug delivery system.

## Ampicillin (am pi SIL in)

**U.S. Brand Names** Marcillin®; Omnipen®; Omnipen®-N; Polycillin®; Polycillin-N®; Principen®; Totacillin®; Totacillin®-N

**Synonyms** Aminobenzylpenicillin

**Therapeutic Category** Antibiotic, Penicillin

**Pregnancy Risk Factor** B

**Lactation** Enters breast milk/compatible

**Use** Treatment of susceptible bacterial infections (nonbeta-lactamase-producing organisms) caused by streptococci, pneumococci, nonpenicillinase-producing staphylococci, *Listeria*, meningococci; some strains of *H. influenzae*, *Salmonella*, *Shigella*, *E. coli*, *Enterobacter*, and *Klebsiella*

**Mechanism of Action/Effect** Interferes with bacterial cell wall synthesis during active multiplication, causing cell wall death and resultant bactericidal activity against susceptible bacteria

**Contraindications** Hypersensitivity to ampicillin, penicillins, cephalosporins, or imipenem

**Warnings** Dosage adjustment may be necessary in patients with renal impairment. A low incidence of cross-allergy with other beta-lactams exists. High percentage of patients with infectious mononucleosis have developed rash during therapy with ampicillin. Appearance of a rash should be carefully evaluated to differentiate a nonallergic ampicillin rash from a hypersensitivity reaction. Ampicillin rash is a generalized dull red, maculopapular rash, generally appearing 3-14 days after the start of therapy. It normally begins on the trunk and spreads over most of the body. It may be most intense at pressure areas, elbows, and knees.

**Drug Interactions**

**Decreased Effect:** Efficacy of oral contraceptives may be reduced with ampicillin.

**Increased Effect/Toxicity:** Ampicillin increases the effect of disulfiram and anticoagulants. Probenecid may increase penicillin levels. Theoretically, allopurinol taken with ampicillin has an additive potential for rash.

**Food Interactions** Ampicillin serum concentrations may be decreased if taken with food.

**Effects on Lab Values** ↑ protein, positive Coombs' [direct]; alters result of urinary glucose (Benedict's solution, Clinitest®)

**Adverse Reactions**

>10%:

Central nervous system: Headache
Gastrointestinal: Nausea (mild), vomiting
Miscellaneous: Oral candidiasis, vaginal candidiasis

1% to 10%:

Dermatologic: Urticaria, exfoliative dermatitis

Miscellaneous: Allergic reactions, specifically anaphylaxis; serum sickness-like reactions

<1% (Limited to important or life-threatening symptoms): Seizures, leukopenia, neutropenia, thrombocytopenia, jaundice, hepatotoxicity, interstitial nephritis, *Clostridium difficile* colitis

**Overdose/Toxicology** Symptoms of penicillin overdose include neuromuscular hypersensitivity (eg, agitation, hallucinations, asterixis, encephalopathy, confusion, and seizures). Electrolyte imbalance may occur if the preparation contains potassium or sodium salts, especially in renal failure. Hemodialysis may be helpful to aid in removal of the drug from blood; otherwise, treatment is supportive or symptom directed.

**Pharmacodynamics/Kinetics**

**Half-life Elimination:** 1-1.8 hours; Anuria/end-stage renal disease: 7-20 hours

**Excretion:** Urine

**Formulations**

Ampicillin anhydrous: Capsule: 250 mg, 500 mg

Ampicillin sodium: Powder for injection: 125 mg, 250 mg, 500 mg, 1 g, 2 g, 10 g

Ampicillin trihydrate:

Capsule: 250 mg, 500 mg

Powder for oral suspension: 125 mg/5 mL (5 mL unit dose, 80 mL, 100 mL, 150 mL, 200 mL); 250 mg/5 mL (5 mL unit dose, 80 mL, 100 mL, 150 mL, 200 mL); 500 mg/5 mL (5 mL unit dose, 100 mL)

Powder for oral suspension, drops,: 100 mg/mL (20 mL)

**Dosing**

**Adults:**

Oral: 250-500 mg every 6 hours

I.M.: 500 mg to 1.5 g every 4-6 hours

I.V.: 500 mg to 3 g every 4-6 hours; maximum: 12 g/day

Sepsis/meningitis: 150-250 mg/kg/24 hours divided every 3-4 hours

**Elderly:** Administer usual adult dose unless renal function is markedly reduced.

**Renal Impairment:**

$Cl_{cr}$ 30-50 mL/minute: Administer every 6-8 hours.

$Cl_{cr}$ 10-30 mL/minute: Administer every 8-12 hours.

$Cl_{cr}$ <10 mL/minute: Administer every 12 hours.

Moderately dialyzable (20% to 50%)

Administer dose after dialysis.

Peritoneal dialysis effects: Moderately dialyzable (20% to 50%)

Administer 250 mg every 12 hours.

Continuous arteriovenous or venovenous hemofiltration (CAVH): Dose as for $Cl_{cr}$ 10-50 mL/minute.

**Administration**

**Oral:** Administer around-the-clock to promote less variation in peak and trough serum levels.

**I.V.:** Administer around-the-clock to promote less variation in peak and trough serum levels. Administer over 3-5 minutes (125-500 mg) or over 10-15 minutes (1-2 g). More rapid infusion may cause seizures.

**Stability**

**Reconstitution:**

Oral: Oral suspension is stable for 7 days at room temperature or for 14 days under refrigeration.

I.V.:

Minimum volume: Concentration should not exceed 30 mg/mL due to concentration-dependent stability restrictions. Manufacturer may supply as either the anhydrous or the trihydrate form.

Solutions for I.M. or direct I.V. should be used within 1 hour. Solutions for I.V. infusion will be inactivated by dextrose at room temperature. If dextrose-containing solutions are to be used, the resultant solution will only be stable for 2 hours versus 8 hours in the 0.9% sodium chloride injection. $D_5W$ has limited stability.

Stability of parenteral admixture in NS at room temperature (25°C) is 8 hours.

Stability of parenteral admixture in NS at refrigeration temperature (4°C) is 2 days.

Standard diluent: 500 mg/50 mL NS; 1 g/50 mL NS; 2 g/100 mL NS

**Compatibility:** Ampicillin and gentamicin should not be mixed in the same I.V. tubing or administered concurrently. See the Compatibility of Drugs Chart *on page 1315*.

**Monitoring Laboratory Tests** Perform culture and sensitivity testing prior to initiating therapy.

**Additional Nursing Issues**

**Physical Assessment:** Monitor appropriate laboratory tests as ordered. Monitor for (teach patient to monitor and report) effectiveness of therapy and adverse reactions as identified above, including development of opportunistic infections (eg, fever, chills, unhealed sores, white plaques in mouth or vagina, purulent vaginal discharge, fatigue).

**Patient Information/Instruction:** Take entire prescription, even if you are feeling better. Take at equal intervals around-the-clock; preferably on an empty stomach with a full glass of water (1 hour before or 2 hours after meals). Maintain adequate hydration (2-3 L/day of fluids unless instructed to restrict fluid intake). You may experience nausea or vomiting (small frequent meals, frequent mouth care, sucking lozenges, or chewing gum may help). If diabetic, drug may cause false tests with Clinitest® urine glucose monitoring; use of glucose oxidase methods (Clinistix®) or serum glucose monitoring is preferable. This drug may interfere with oral contraceptives; an alternate

(Continued)

## Ampicillin *(Continued)*

form of birth control should be used. Report rash; unusual diarrhea; unusual vaginal discharge, itching, burning, or pain; mouth sores; unresolved vomiting or constipation; fever or chills; unusual bruising or bleeding; or if condition being treated worsens or does not improve by the time prescription is completed.

**Geriatric Considerations:** See Drug Interactions and Renal Impairment. Adjust dose for renal impairment.

**Additional Information**

Sodium content of 5 mL suspension (250 mg/5 mL): 10 mg (0.4 mEq)
Sodium content of 1 g: 66.7 mg (3 mEq)
pH: 8-10

## Ampicillin and Sulbactam (am pi SIL in & SUL bak tam)

**U.S. Brand Names** Unasyn®

**Synonyms** Sulbactam and Ampicillin

**Therapeutic Category** Antibiotic, Penicillin

**Pregnancy Risk Factor** B

**Lactation** Enters breast milk/use caution

**Use** Treatment of susceptible bacterial infections involved with skin and skin structure, intra-abdominal infections, gynecologic infections; spectrum is that of ampicillin plus organisms producing beta-lactamases such as *S. aureus, H. influenzae, E. coli, Klebsiella, Acinetobacter, Enterobacter*, and anaerobes

**Mechanism of Action/Effect** Interferes with bacterial cell wall synthesis during active multiplication, causing cell wall death and resultant bactericidal activity against susceptible bacteria. The addition of sulbactam, a beta-lactamase inhibitor, to ampicillin extends the spectrum of ampicillin to include beta-lactamase producing organisms.

**Contraindications** Hypersensitivity to ampicillin, any component, sulbactam, penicillins, cephalosporins, or imipenem

**Warnings** Dosage adjustment may be necessary in patients with renal impairment. A low incidence of cross-allergy with other beta-lactams exists. A high percentage of patients with infectious mononucleosis have developed rash during therapy with ampicillin. Appearance of a rash should be carefully evaluated to differentiate a nonallergic ampicillin rash from a hypersensitivity reaction.

**Drug Interactions**

**Decreased Effect:** Efficacy of oral contraceptives may be reduced with ampicillin and sulbactam.

**Increased Effect/Toxicity:** Disulfiram or probenecid can increase ampicillin levels. Theoretically, allopurinol taken with ampicillin has an additive potential for rash.

**Effects on Lab Values** False-positive urinary glucose levels (Benedict's solution, Clinitest®); may cause temporary decreases in serum estrogens in pregnant women.

**Adverse Reactions**

>10%:

Central nervous system: Headache
Gastrointestinal: Nausea (mild), vomiting
Local: Pain at injection site (I.M.)
Miscellaneous: Oral candidiasis, vaginal candidiasis

1% to 10%:

Dermatologic: Urticaria, exfoliative dermatitis
Miscellaneous: Allergic reactions, specifically anaphylaxis; serum sickness-like reactions

<1% (Limited to important or life-threatening symptoms): Seizures, leukopenia, neutropenia, thrombocytopenia, jaundice, hepatotoxicity interstitial nephritis, *Clostridium difficile* colitis

**Overdose/Toxicology** Symptoms of penicillin overdose include neuromuscular hypersensitivity (eg, agitation, hallucinations, asterixis, encephalopathy, confusion, and seizures). Electrolyte imbalance may occur if the preparation contains potassium or sodium salts, especially in renal failure. Hemodialysis may be helpful to aid in removal of the drug from blood; otherwise, treatment is supportive or symptom directed.

**Pharmacodynamics/Kinetics**

**Protein Binding:** Ampicillin: 28%; Sulbactam: 38%

**Half-life Elimination:** 1-1.8 hours

**Excretion:** Urine

**Formulations** Powder for injection: 1.5 g [ampicillin sodium 1 g and sulbactam sodium 0.5 g]; 3 g [ampicillin sodium 2 g and sulbactam sodium 1 g]

**Dosing**

**Adults:** Recommendations for Unasyn® are based on the ampicillin component.

I.M., I.V.: 1-2 g ampicillin (1.5-3 g Unasyn®) every 6-8 hours; maximum: 8 g ampicillin/day (12 g Unasyn®)

**Elderly:** Refer to adult dosing.

**Renal Impairment:**

$Cl_{cr}$ >50 mL/minute: Administer every 6 hours.
$Cl_{cr}$ 10-50 mL/minute: Administer every 6-12 hours.
$Cl_{cr}$ <10 mL/minute: Administer every 12-24 hours.

**Administration**

**I.V.:** Administer around-the-clock to promote less variation in peak and trough serum levels. Administer by slow injection over 10-15 minutes or I.V. over 15-30 minutes.

**Stability**

**Reconstitution:** I.M. and direct I.V. administration: Use within 1 hour after preparation. Reconstitute with sterile water for injection or 0.5% or 2% lidocaine hydrochloride injection (I.M.). Sodium chloride 0.9% (NS) is the diluent of choice for I.V. piggyback use. Solutions made in NS are stable up to 72 hours when refrigerated whereas dextrose solutions (same concentration) are stable for only 4 hours.

**Compatibility:** Ampicillin and gentamicin should not be mixed in the same I.V. tubing or administered concurrently.

**Monitoring Laboratory Tests** Hematologic, renal, and hepatic function with prolonged therapy. Perform culture and sensitivity testing prior to initiating therapy.

**Additional Nursing Issues**

**Physical Assessment:** Monitor appropriate laboratory tests as ordered. Monitor for (teach patient to monitor and report) effectiveness of therapy and adverse reactions as identified above, including development of opportunistic infections (eg, fever, chills, unhealed sores, white plaques in mouth or vagina, purulent vaginal discharge, fatigue). Note breast-feeding caution.

**Patient Information/Instruction:** Take entire prescription, even if you are feeling better. Take at equal intervals around-the-clock; preferably on an empty stomach with a full glass of water (1 hour before or 2 hours after meals). Maintain adequate hydration (2-3 L/day of fluids unless instructed to restrict fluid intake). You may experience nausea or vomiting (small frequent meals, frequent mouth care, sucking lozenges, or chewing gum may help). If diabetic, drug may cause false tests with Clinitest® urine glucose monitoring; use of glucose oxidase methods (Clinistix®) or serum glucose monitoring is preferable. This drug may interfere with oral contraceptives; an alternate form of birth control should be used. Report rash; unusual diarrhea; vaginal discharge, itching, burning, or pain; mouth sores; unresolved vomiting or constipation; fever or chills; unusual bruising or bleeding; or if condition being treated worsens or does not improve by the time prescription is completed. **Breast-feeding precautions:** Consult prescriber if breast-feeding.

**Geriatric Considerations:** Adjust dose for renal function.

**Additional Information** Each 3 g vial contains 2 g of ampicillin and 1 g of sulbactam. Sulbactam has very little antibacterial activity by itself, but effectively extends the spectrum of ampicillin to include beta-lactamase producing strains that are resistant to ampicillin alone.

Sodium content of 1.5 g (ampicillin 1 g plus sulbactam 0.5 g as trisodium salts): 5 mEq

pH: 8-10

**Related Information**

Ampicillin *on page 90*

♦ **Ampicin® Sodium** *see* Ampicillin *on page 90*

## Amprenavir (am PRE na veer)

**U.S. Brand Names** Agenerase®

**Therapeutic Category** Antiretroviral Agent, Protease Inhibitor

**Pregnancy Risk Factor** Unknown

**Use** Treatment of HIV infections in combination with at least two other antiretroviral agents

**Mechanism of Action/Effect** Binds to the protease activity site and inhibits the activity of the enzyme. HIV protease is required for the cleavage of viral polyprotein precursors into individual functional proteins found in infectious HIV. Inhibition prevents cleavage of these polyproteins, resulting in the formation of immature, noninfectious viral particles.

**Contraindications** Hypersensitivity to amprenavir or any component; concurrent therapy with rifampin, astemizole, bepridil, cisapride, dihydroergotamine, ergotamine, midazolam, and triazolam; severe previous allergic reaction to sulfonamides

**Warnings** Because of hepatic metabolism and effect on cytochrome P-450 enzymes, amprenavir should be used with caution in combination with other agents metabolized by this system (see Contraindications and Drug Interactions). Use with caution in patients with diabetes mellitus, sulfonamide allergy, hepatic impairment, or hemophilia. Redistribution of fat may occur (eg, buffalo hump, peripheral wasting, cushingoid appearance). Additional vitamin E supplements should be avoided. Concurrent use of sildenafil should be avoided.

**Drug Interactions**

**Increased Effect/Toxicity:** CYP3A4 inhibitor and substrate. Abacavir, clarithromycin, indinavir, ketoconazole, and zidovudine increase the AUC of amprenavir. Nelfinavir had no effect on AUC, but increased the $C_{min}$ of amprenavir. Amprenavir increased the AUC of ketoconazole, rifabutin, and zidovudine during concurrent therapy. Amprenavir may enhance the toxicity of astemizole, bepridil, cisapride, dihydroergotamine, ergotamine, midazolam, and triazolam - concurrent therapy with these drugs and amprenavir is contraindicated. May increase serum concentration of HMGCoA reductase inhibitors, diltiazem, nicardipine, nifedipine, nimodipine, alprazolam, clorazepate, diazepam, flurazepam, itraconazole, dapsone, erythromycin, loratadine, sildenafil, carbamazepine, and pimizide. May also increase the toxic effect of amiodarone, lidocaine, quinidine, warfarin, and tricyclic antidepressants. Serum concentration monitoring of these drugs is necessary.

**Adverse Reactions** Protease inhibitors cause dyslipidemia which includes elevated cholesterol and triglycerides and a redistribution of body fat centrally to cause "protease paunch", buffalo hump, facial atrophy, and breast enlargement. These agents also cause hyperglycemia.

>10%:

Gastrointestinal: Nausea (38% to 73%), vomiting (20% to 29%), diarrhea (33% to 56%)

(Continued)

## Amprenavir *(Continued)*

Dermatologic: Rash (28%)
Endocrine & metabolic: Hyperglycemia (37% to 41%), hypertriglyceridemia (38% to 27%)
Miscellaneous: Perioral tingling/numbness
1% to 10%:
Central nervous system: Depression (4% to 15%), headache, paresthesia, fatigue
Gastrointestinal: Taste disorders (1% to 10%)
Dermatologic: Stevens-Johnson syndrome (1% of total, 4% of patients who develop a rash)

**Pharmacodynamics/Kinetics**
**Metabolism:** Hepatic, via cytochrome P-450 isoenzymes (primarily CYP3A4)
**Excretion:** Biliary and urine, as metabolites

**Formulations**
Capsules: 50 mg, 150 mg
Solution: 15 mg/mL

**Dosing**
**Adults:** Oral: Capsules: 1200 mg twice daily
**Elderly:** Refer to adult dosing.
**Hepatic Impairment:**
Child-Pugh score between 5-8: 450 mg twice daily
Child-Pugh score between 9-12: 300 mg twice daily

**Additional Nursing Issues**
**Physical Assessment:** Assess effectiveness and interactions of other medications (see Drug Interactions). See Contraindications and Warnings/Precautions for use cautions. Monitor effectiveness of therapy and adverse reactions at beginning of therapy and periodically with long-term use (see Adverse Reactions). Assess knowledge/teach patient appropriate use, interventions to reduce side effects, and adverse symptoms to report.
**Patient Information/Instruction:** Amprenavir is not a cure for HIV, nor has it been found to reduce transmission of HIV. Take as directed, with or without food. Maintain adequate fluid intake (2-3 L/day of fluids unless instructed to restrict fluid intake) and adequate nutritional intake (small, frequent meals may help). You will be more susceptible to infection (avoid crowds or exposure to contagious diseases or infection). You may experience headache or confusion (use caution when driving or engaging in tasks requiring alertness until response to drug in known); headache (mild analgesic may help); nausea, vomiting, or increase flatulence (small frequent meals, may help); diarrhea (increased dietary fiber, exercise, or boiled milk may help). Inform prescriber if you experience muscle numbness or tingling; unresolved persistent vomiting, diarrhea, or abdominal pain; difficulty breathing or chest pain; unusual skin rash; or change in color of stool or urine. **Pregnancy/breast-feeding precautions:** Inform prescriber if you are or intend to be pregnant or breast-feed.

**Additional Information** Capsules contain 109 int. units of vitamin E per capsule; oral solution contains 46 int. units of vitamin E per mL.

**Related Information**
Antiretroviral Agents Comparison *on page 1373*


- **Amvisc®** *see page 1248*
- **Amvisc®** *see page 1282*
- **Amvisc® Plus** *see page 1248*
- **Amvisc Plus®** *see page 1282*


## Amyl Nitrite (AM il NYE trite)

**Synonyms** Isoamyl Nitrite
**Therapeutic Category** Antidote; Vasodilator
**Pregnancy Risk Factor** X
**Lactation** Excretion in breast milk unknown/not recommended
**Use** Coronary vasodilator in angina pectoris; adjunct in treatment of cyanide poisoning; produce changes in the intensity of heart murmurs
**Mechanism of Action/Effect** Relaxes vascular smooth muscle; decreased venous ratios and arterial blood pressure; reduces left ventricular work; decreases myocardial $O_2$ consumption; in cyanide poisoning, amyl nitrite converts hemoglobin to methemoglobin that binds with cyanide to form cyanate hemoglobin
**Contraindications** Hypersensitivity to nitrates; severe anemia; head injury; pregnancy
**Warnings** Use with caution in patients with increased intracranial pressure, low systolic blood pressure, and coronary artery disease.

**Drug Interactions**
**Increased Effect/Toxicity:** Alcohol taken with amyl nitrite may have additive side effects.

**Adverse Reactions**
1% to 10%:
Cardiovascular: Postural hypotension, cutaneous flushing of head, neck, and clavicular area, tachycardia
Central nervous system: Headache, restlessness
Gastrointestinal: Nausea, vomiting
<1% (Limited to important or life-threatening symptoms): Hemolytic anemia

**Overdose/Toxicology** Symptoms of overdose include hypotension. Treatment includes general supportive measures.

**Pharmacodynamics/Kinetics**

**Onset:** Angina relieved within 30 seconds

**Duration:** 3-15 minutes

**Formulations** Inhalant, crushable glass perles: 0.18 mL, 0.3 mL

**Dosing**

**Adults:**

Angina: 1-6 inhalations from 1 capsule are usually sufficient to produce the desired effect.

Cyanide poisoning: Repeat inhalation every 60 seconds until I.V. sodium nitrate and I.V. sodium thiosulfate infusion are available.

**Elderly:** Refer to adult dosing.

**Administration**

**Oral:** Administer nasally. Keep patient lying down during administration. Crush ampul in woven covering between fingers and then hold under patient's nostrils for 15-30 seconds.

**Stability**

**Storage:** Store in cool place and protect from light.

**Additional Nursing Issues**

**Physical Assessment:** Monitor blood pressure and heart rate closely during and following therapy. **Pregnancy risk factor X.** Breast-feeding is not recommended.

**Patient Information/Instruction:** When this drug is used in emergency situations, patient education should be appropriate to situation (ie, do not change positions or make any sudden moves without asking for assistance). If patient administered, lie down during administration, crush ampul in woven covering between fingers, and then hold under nose and inhale. May repeat in 3-5 minutes if necessary. If no relief after three doses, contact emergency services for transport to hospital immediately. Vapors are highly flammable; do not use where vapors may ignite. **Pregnancy/breast-feeding precautions:** Inform prescriber if you are or intent to be pregnant, may cause severe fetal defects. Breast-feeding is not recommended.


- ♦ **Amylobarbitone** *see* Amobarbital *on page 77*
- ♦ **Amytal®** *see* Amobarbital *on page 77*
- ♦ **Anabolin® Injection** *see* Nandrolone *on page 806*
- ♦ **Anacin® [OTC]** *see* Aspirin *on page 111*
- ♦ **Anadrol®** *see* Oxymetholone *on page 874*
- ♦ **Anafranil®** *see* Clomipramine *on page 287*
- ♦ **Ana-Kit®** *see page 1246*
- ♦ **Analphen** *see* Acetaminophen *on page 32*
- ♦ **Anamine® Syrup** *see page 1294*
- ♦ **Anandron®** *see* Nilutamide *on page 826*
- ♦ **Anapenil** *see* Penicillin V Potassium *on page 900*
- ♦ **Anaplex® Liquid** *see page 1294*
- ♦ **Anapolon®** *see* Oxymetholone *on page 874*
- ♦ **Anaprox®** *see* Naproxen *on page 807*
- ♦ **Anapsique** *see* Amitriptyline *on page 73*
- ♦ **Anaspaz®** *see* Hyoscyamine *on page 590*


## Anastrozole (an AS troe zole)

**U.S. Brand Names** Arimidex®

**Therapeutic Category** Antineoplastic Agent, Miscellaneous

**Pregnancy Risk Factor** C (teratogenic)

**Lactation** Excretion in breast milk unknown

**Use** Treatment of advanced breast cancer in postmenopausal women with disease progression following tamoxifen therapy. Patients with ER-negative disease and patients who did not respond to tamoxifen therapy rarely responded to anastrozole.

**Mechanism of Action/Effect** Potent and selective nonsteroidal aromatase inhibitor. It significantly lowers serum estradiol concentrations and has no detectable effect on formation of adrenal corticosteroids or aldosterone. In postmenopausal women, the principal source of circulating estrogen is conversion of adrenally generated androstenedione to estrone by aromatase in peripheral tissues.

**Contraindications** Hypersensitivity to anastrozole or any component

**Warnings** Use with caution in patients with hyperlipidemias. Mean serum total cholesterol and LDL cholesterol increase in patients receiving anastrozole. Pregnancy factor C.

**Drug Interactions**

**Cytochrome P-450 Effect:** CYP3A3/4 enzyme substrate; CYP1A2, 2C8, 2C9, and 3A3/4 enzyme inhibitor

**Increased Effect/Toxicity:** Anastrozole inhibited *in vitro* metabolic reactions catalyzed by cytochromes P-450 1A2, 2C8/9, and 3A4, but only at relatively high concentrations. It is unlikely that coadministration of anastrozole with other drugs will result in clinically significant inhibition of cytochrome P-450-mediated metabolism of other drugs. Inhibitors of CYP3A4 may increase anastrozole concentrations.

**Effects on Lab Values** Lab test abnormalities: GGT, AST, ALT, alkaline phosphatase, total cholesterol and LDL increased; threefold elevations of mean serum GGT levels have been observed among patients with liver metastases. These changes were likely related to the progression of liver metastases in these patients, although other contributing factors could not be ruled out. Mean serum total cholesterol levels increased by 0.5 mmol/L among patients.

(Continued)

## Anastrozole *(Continued)*

**Adverse Reactions**

>5%:

Central nervous system: Headache, dizziness, depression
Cardiovascular: Flushing, peripheral edema, chest pain
Dermatologic: Rash
Gastrointestinal: Little to mild nausea (10%), vomiting, diarrhea, abdominal pain, anorexia, dry mouth
Genitourinary: Pelvic pain
Neuromuscular & skeletal: Increased bone and tumor pain, muscle weakness, paresthesia
Respiratory: Dyspnea, cough, pharyngitis

2% to 5%:

Cardiovascular: Hypertension
Central nervous system: Somnolence, confusion, insomnia, anxiety, nervousness, fever, malaise, accidental injury
Dermatologic: Hair thinning, pruritus
Endocrine & metabolic: Breast pain
Gastrointestinal: Weight loss
Genitourinary: Urinary tract infection
Hematologic: Anemia, leukopenia
Local: Thrombophlebitis
Neuromuscular & skeletal: Myalgia, arthralgia, pathological fracture, neck pain
Respiratory: Sinusitis, bronchitis, rhinitis
Miscellaneous: Flu-like syndrome, infection

**Overdose/Toxicology** Symptoms of overdose include severe irritation to the stomach (necrosis, gastritis, ulceration, and hemorrhage). There is no specific antidote; treatment must be symptomatic. Dialysis may be helpful because anastrozole is not highly protein bound.

**Pharmacodynamics/Kinetics**

**Half-life Elimination:** 50 hours

**Metabolism:** Liver

**Excretion:** Urine and feces

**Formulations** Tablet: 1 mg

**Dosing**

**Adults:** Breast cancer: Oral (refer to individual protocols): 1 mg once daily

**Elderly:** Refer to adult dosing.

**Renal Impairment:** Because only about 10% is excreted unchanged in the urine, dosage adjustment in patients with renal insufficiency is not necessary.

**Hepatic Impairment:** Plasma concentrations in subjects with hepatic cirrhosis were within the range concentrations in normal subjects across all clinical trials; therefore, no dosage adjustment is needed.

**Additional Nursing Issues**

**Physical Assessment:** Monitor for effectiveness of therapy. Monitor and teach patient about adverse effects to report. Instruct patient on appropriate precautions for postural hypotension. **Pregnancy risk factor C.** Note breast-feeding caution.

**Patient Information/Instruction:** Take as prescribed. Maintain adequate hydration (2-3 L/day of fluids unless instructed to restrict fluid intake) and nutrition. If experiencing nausea, vomiting, or anorexia, small frequent meals, frequent mouth care, sucking lozenges, or chewing gum may help or contact prescriber for relief. This medication may cause dizziness and fatigue (use caution when driving or engaging in tasks that require alertness until response to drug is known); or increased bone pain (contact prescriber for analgesia). Report swelling of extremities, chest pain or palpitations, acute headache or dizziness, increased muscle pain or weakness, CNS changes (eg, confusion, insomnia, nervousness), breast or pelvic pain, unusual bruising or bleeding, flu-like symptoms, or respiratory difficulty. **Pregnancy/breast-feeding precautions:** Consult prescriber if pregnant or breast-feeding.

- **Anatuss® [OTC]** *see* Guaifenesin, Phenylpropanolamine, and Dextromethorphan *on page 551*
- **Anbesol® [OTC]** *see* Benzocaine *on page 141*
- **Anbesol® Maximum Strength [OTC]** *see* Benzocaine *on page 141*
- **Ancef®** *see* Cefazolin *on page 214*
- **Ancobon®** *see* Flucytosine *on page 492*
- **Ancotil®** *see* Flucytosine *on page 492*
- **Androderm® Transdermal System** *see* Testosterone *on page 1108*
- **Android®** *see* Methyltestosterone *on page 756*
- **Andro-L.A.® Injection** *see* Testosterone *on page 1108*
- **Androlone®-D Injection** *see* Nandrolone *on page 806*
- **Androlone® Injection** *see* Nandrolone *on page 806*
- **Andropository® Injection** *see* Testosterone *on page 1108*
- **Anectine® Chloride Injection** *see page 1248*
- **Anectine® Flo-Pack®** *see page 1248*
- **Anestacon®** *see* Lidocaine *on page 674*
- **Aneurine Hydrochloride** *see* Thiamine *on page 1120*
- **Anexate®** *see* Flumazenil *on page 496*
- **Anexsia®** *see* Hydrocodone and Acetaminophen *on page 568*
- **Angiotrofin** *see* Diltiazem *on page 377*

- **Angiotrofin A.P.** *see* Diltiazem *on page 377*
- **Angiotrofin Retard** *see* Diltiazem *on page 377*
- **Anglix** *see* Nitroglycerin *on page 831*
- **Anglopen** *see* Ampicillin *on page 90*
- **Anisoylated Plasminogen Streptokinase Activator Complex** *see* Anistreplase *on this page*
- **Anistal** *see* Ranitidine *on page 1008*


## Anistreplase (a NISS tre plase)

**U.S. Brand Names** Eminase®

**Synonyms** Anisoylated Plasminogen Streptokinase Activator Complex; APSAC

**Therapeutic Category** Thrombolytic Agent

**Pregnancy Risk Factor** C

**Lactation** Excretion in breast milk unknown

**Use** Management of acute myocardial infarction (AMI) in adults; lysis of thrombi obstructing coronary arteries; reduction of infarct size

**Mechanism of Action/Effect** Lysis of thrombi activates the conversion of plasminogen to plasmin; effective both outside and within the formed thrombus/embolus

**Contraindications** Hypersensitivity to anistreplase or other kinases (streptokinase); active internal bleeding; history of CVA; intracranial neoplasma; history of cerebrovascular accident; recent intracranial surgery or trauma; arteriovenous malformation or aneurysm; severe uncontrolled hypertension

**Warnings** This medication is 10 times more potent than streptokinase as a thrombolytic. Pregnancy factor C.

**Drug Interactions**

**Increased Effect/Toxicity:** Increased efficacy and bleeding potential with anticoagulants (heparin, warfarin) and antiplatelet agents (aspirin, ticlopidine).

**Effects on Lab Values** ↓ plasminogen, fibrinogen; ↑ TT, APTT, PT

**Adverse Reactions**

>10%:

- Central nervous system: Fever
- Cardiovascular: Arrhythmias, hypotension, perfusion arrhythmias
- Hematologic: Bleeding or oozing from cuts

<1% (Limited to important or life-threatening symptoms): Anemia, eye hemorrhage, bronchospasm, epistaxis, anaphylactic reaction

**Pharmacodynamics/Kinetics**

**Half-life Elimination:** 70-120 minutes

**Metabolism:** Liver

**Excretion:** Unknown

**Duration:** Fibrinolytic effect persists for 4-6 hours following administration.

**Formulations** Powder for injection, lyophilized: 30 units

**Dosing**

**Adults:** I.V.: 30 units injected over 2-5 minutes as soon as possible after onset of symptoms

**Elderly:** Refer to adult dosing.

**Administration**

**I.V.:** Given as an I.V. bolus over 2-5 minutes.

**Stability**

**Storage:** Store lyophilized powder between 2°C and 8°C (36°F to 46°F).

**Reconstitution:** Discard solution 30 minutes after reconstitution if not administered. Do not shake solution.

**Compatibility:** Do not add to any infusion fluid. Do not add any other medication to vial or syringe.

**Additional Nursing Issues**

**Physical Assessment:** Monitor closely for cardiac arrhythmias with coronary reperfusion. Monitor for symptoms of bleeding or severe hypotension (see Adverse Reactions). Observe bleeding precautions (ie, avoid invasive procedures, protect patient from injury). **Pregnancy risk factor C.** Note breast-feeding caution.

**Patient Information/Instruction:** I.V. administration for cardiac emergencies: Patient instruction should be appropriate to situation. Following infusion, absolute bedrest is important; call for assistance changing position. You will have increased tendency to bleed; avoid razors, scissors or sharps, and use soft toothbrush or cotton swabs. Report back pain, abdominal pain, muscle cramping, acute onset headache, chest pain, or bleeding.

**Other Issues:** Drug should not be used for any condition in which bleeding constitutes a significant hazard or would be particularly difficult to manage. Avoid nonessential handling of patient after administration of drug.

**Additional Information** pH: 7.3


- **Anitrim** *see* Co-trimoxazole *on page 307*
- **Anodynos-DHC®** *see* Hydrocodone and Acetaminophen *on page 568*
- **Anoquan®** *see* Butalbital Compound and Acetaminophen *on page 175*
- **Ansaid® Oral** *see* Flurbiprofen *on page 509*
- **Ansamycin** *see* Rifabutin *on page 1018*
- **Antabuse®** *see* Disulfiram *on page 387*
- **Antagon-1®** *see* Astemizole *on page 114*
- **Antalgin® Dialicels** *see* Indomethacin *on page 606*
- **Antazoline Phosphate and Naphazoline** *see page 1282*

- **Antazoline-V® Ophthalmic Solution** *see page 1294*
- **Antazone®** *see* Sulfinpyrazone *on page 1086*
- **Antepsin** *see* Sucralfate *on page 1078*
- **Anthra-Derm®** *see* Anthralin *on this page*
- **Anthraforte®** *see* Anthralin *on this page*


## Anthralin (AN thra lin)

**U.S. Brand Names** Anthra-Derm®; Drithocreme®; Drithocreme® HP 1%; Dritho-Scalp®

**Synonyms** Dithranol

**Therapeutic Category** Antipsoriatic Agent; Keratolytic Agent

**Pregnancy Risk Factor** C

**Lactation** Excretion in breast milk unknown

**Use** Treatment of psoriasis (quiescent or chronic psoriasis)

**Mechanism of Action/Effect** Inhibits synthesis of nucleic protein from inhibition of DNA synthesis to affected areas

**Contraindications** Hypersensitivity to anthralin or any component; acute psoriasis (acutely or actively inflamed psoriatic eruptions); use on the face

**Warnings** If redness is observed, reduce frequency of dosage or discontinue application. Avoid eye contact. Should generally not be applied to intertriginous skin areas and high strengths should not be used on these sites. Do not apply to face or genitalia. Use caution in patients with renal disease and in those having extensive and prolonged applications. Perform periodic urine tests for albuminuria. Pregnancy factor C.

**Drug Interactions**

**Increased Effect/Toxicity:** Long-term use of topical corticosteroids may destabilize psoriasis and withdrawal may also give rise to a "rebound" phenomenon. Allow an interval of at least 1 week between the discontinuance of topical corticosteroids and the commencement of therapy.

**Adverse Reactions**

1% to 10%: Dermatologic: Transient primary irritation of uninvolved skin; temporary discoloration of hair and fingernails, may stain skin, hair, or fabrics

**Formulations**

Cream: 0.1% (50 g, 65 g); 0.2% (65 g); 0.25% (50 g); 0.4% (65 g); 0.5% (50 g); 1% (50 g, 65 g)

Ointment, topical: 0.1% (42.5 g); 0.25% (42.5 g); 0.4% (60 g); 0.5% (42.5 g); 1% (42.5 g)

**Dosing**

**Adults:** Generally, apply once a day or as directed. The irritant potential of anthralin is directly related to the strength being used and each patient's individual tolerance. Always commence treatment for at least 1 week using the lowest strength possible.

Skin application: Apply sparingly only to psoriatic lesions and rub gently and carefully into the skin until absorbed. Avoid applying an excessive quantity which may cause unnecessary soiling and staining of the clothing or bed linen.

Scalp application: Comb hair to remove scalar debris and, after suitably parting, rub cream well into the lesions, taking care to prevent the cream from spreading onto the forehead.

Remove by washing or showering; optimal period of contact will vary according to the strength used and the patient's response to treatment. Continue treatment until the skin is entirely clear (ie, when there is nothing to feel with the fingers and the texture is normal).

**Elderly:** Refer to adult dosing.

**Additional Nursing Issues**

**Physical Assessment:** See Contraindications and Warnings/Precautions for use cautions. When applied to large areas of skin or for extensive periods of time, monitor for adverse skin or systemic reactions. Assess knowledge/teach patient appropriate application and use and adverse symptoms (see Adverse Reactions) to report. **Pregnancy risk factor C** - systemic absorption may be minimal with appropriate use. Note breast-feeding caution.

**Patient Information/Instruction:** For external use only. Use exactly as directed; do not overuse. Before using, wash and dry area gently. Wear gloves to apply a thin film to affected area and rub in gently. May discolor fabric, skin, or hair. If dressing is necessary, use a porous dressing. Avoid contact with eyes. Avoid exposing treated area to direct sunlight; sunburn can occur. Remove by washing; optimal period of contact will vary according to strength used and response to treatment. Report increased swelling, redness, rash, itching, signs of infection, worsening of condition, or lack of healing. **Pregnancy/breast-feeding precautions:** Inform prescriber if you are or intend to be pregnant. Consult prescriber if breast-feeding.

Scalp: Comb hair to remove scalar debris, part hair, and rub cream into lesions. Do not allow cream to spread to forehead or onto neck. Remove by washing hair.


- **Anthranol®** *see* Anthralin *on this page*
- **Anthrascalp®** *see* Anthralin *on this page*
- **Anthrax Vaccine Adsorbed** *see page 1256*
- **Antiarrhythmic Drug Classification Comparison** *see page 1366*
- **AntibiOtic®** *see page 1291*
- **Anti-CD20 Monoclonal Antibodies** *see* Rituximab *on page 1031*
- **Antidepressant Agents Comparison** *see page 1368*
- **Antidepressant Medication Guidelines** *see page 1435*
- **Antidiabetic Oral Agents Comparison** *see page 1370*
- **Antidigoxin Fab Fragments** *see* Digoxin Immune Fab *on page 372*

- ♦ **Antidiuretic Hormone (ADH)** *see* Vasopressin *on page 1205*
- ♦ **Antidotes, Antivenins, and Antitoxins** *see page 1246*
- ♦ **Antiemetics for Chemotherapy-Induced Nausea and Vomiting** *see page 1307*
- ♦ **Antifungal Agents, Topical** *see page 1247*


## Antihemophilic Factor (Human) (an tee hee moe FIL ik FAK tor HYU man)

**U.S. Brand Names** Hemofil® M; Humate-P®; Koāte®-HP; Koāte®-HS; Monoclate-P®; Profilate® OSD; Profilate® SD

**Synonyms** AHF; Factor VIII

**Therapeutic Category** Antihemophilic Agent; Blood Product Derivative

**Pregnancy Risk Factor** C

**Lactation** Excretion in breast milk unknown/use caution

**Use** Management of hemophilia A in patients whom a deficiency in factor VIII has been demonstrated; can be of significant therapeutic value in patients with acquired factor VII inhibitors not exceeding 10 Bethesda units/mL

**Unlabeled use:** Can be of value in von Willebrand disease

**Mechanism of Action/Effect** Activates factor X in conjunction with activated factor IX; activated factor X converts prothrombin to thrombin, which converts fibrinogen to fibrin and with factor XIII forms a stable clot

**Contraindications** Hypersensitivity to mouse protein (Monoclate-P®, Hemofil® M, Method M, Monoclonal Purified) and antihemophilic factor (human); Method M and Monoclonal Purified contain trace amounts of mouse protein

**Warnings** Risk of viral transmission is not totally eradicated. Because antihemophilic factor is prepared from pooled plasma, it may contain the causative agent of viral hepatitis. Antihemophilic factor contains trace amounts of blood groups A and B isohemagglutinins and when large or frequently repeated doses are given to individuals with blood groups A, B, and AB, the patient should be monitored for signs of progressive anemia and the possibility of intravascular hemolysis should be considered. Test methods and treatment methods may not totally eradicate HBAg and HIV from pooled plasma used in processing of this product. Pregnancy factor C.

**Adverse Reactions** <1% (Limited to important or life-threatening symptoms): Tachycardia, epistaxis

**Overdose/Toxicology** Intravascular hemolysis

**Pharmacodynamics/Kinetics**

**Half-life Elimination:** Biphasic: 4-24 hours with a mean of 12 hours

**Formulations** Injection: 10 mL, 20 mL, 30 mL

**Dosing**

**Adults:**

I.V.: Individualize dosage based on coagulation studies performed prior to and during treatment at regular interval; 1 AHF unit is the activity present in 1 mL of normal pooled human plasma; dosage should be adjusted to actual vial size currently stocked in the pharmacy.

Surgery patients: The factor VIII level should be raised to approximately 100% by giving a preoperative dose of 50 int. units/kg, to maintain hemostatic levels, repeat infusions may be necessary every 6-12 hours initially and for a total of 10-14 days until healing is complete.

Hospitalized patient: 20-50 units/kg/dose; may be higher for special circumstances; dose can be given every 12-24 hours and more frequently in special circumstances.

**Elderly:** Refer to adult dosing.

**Administration**

**I.V.:** For I.V. administration only. Maximum rate of administration is product dependent: Monoclate-P® 2 mL/minute; Humate-P® 4 mL/minute. Administration of other products should not exceed 10 mL/minute.

**I.V. Detail:** Use filter needle to draw product into syringe. Use plastic syringes (solutions may stick to glass).

**Stability**

**Storage:** Dried concentrate should be refrigerated 2°C to 8°C (36°F to 46°F) but may be stored at room temperature for up to 6 months depending upon specific product. If refrigerated, the dried concentrate and diluent should be warmed to room temperature before reconstitution.

**Reconstitution:** Gently agitate or rotate vial after adding diluent, do not shake vigorously. Do **not** refrigerate after reconstitution, a precipitation may occur. Method M, monoclonal purified products should be administered within 1 hour after reconstitution. Stability of parenteral admixture at room temperature 25°C is 24 hours, but it is recommended to administer within 3 hours after reconstitution.

**Monitoring Laboratory Tests** Monitor antihemophilic factor levels prior to and during treatment. In patients with circulating inhibitors, the inhibitor level should be monitored.

**Additional Nursing Issues**

**Physical Assessment:** Monitor vital signs, cardiac status, and CNS status during and following infusion. Reduce rate of administration or temporarily discontinue if tachycardia occurs. **Pregnancy risk factor C** - benefits of use should outweigh possible risks. Note breast-feeding caution.

**Patient Information/Instruction:** This medication can only be given I.V. Report sudden onset headache, rash, chest or back pain, or respiratory difficulties. Future safety: Wear some identification that you have a hemophilic condition. **Pregnancy/breast-feeding precautions:** Inform prescriber if you are or intend to be pregnant. Consult prescriber if breast-feeding.

## Antihemophilic Factor (Recombinant)

(an tee hee moe FIL ik FAK tor ree KOM be nant)

**U.S. Brand Names** Bioclate™; Helixate™; Recombinate®

**Synonyms** Factor VIII Recombinant

**Therapeutic Category** Antihemophilic Agent

**Pregnancy Risk Factor** C

**Lactation** Excretion in breast milk unknown/use caution

**Use** Management of hemophilia A in patients whom a deficiency in factor VIII has been demonstrated

**Contraindications** Hypersensitivity to mouse protein (Monoclate-P®, Hemofil® M, Method M, Monoclonal Purified) and antihemophilic factor (human); Method M and Monoclonal Purified contain trace amounts of mouse protein

**Warnings** Administer with caution using universal precautions. Pregnancy factor C.

**Adverse Reactions** <1% (Limited to important or life-threatening symptoms): Flushing, tachycardia, tightness in neck or chest, slight decrease in BP, headache, nausea, vomiting, paresthesia, allergic vasomotor reactions

**Pharmacodynamics/Kinetics**

**Distribution:** Does not readily cross the placenta

**Half-life Elimination:** 4-24 hours (biphasic)

**Metabolism:** Liver

**Formulations** Injection: 250 units, 500 units, 1000 units

**Dosing**

**Adults:** I.V.: Individualize dosage based on coagulation studies performed prior to and during treatment at regular intervals. One AHF unit is the activity present in 1 mL of normal pooled human plasma; dosage should be adjusted to actual vial size currently stocked in the pharmacy.

Hospitalized patient: 20-50 units/kg/dose; may be higher for special circumstances; dose can be given every 12-24 hours and more frequently in special circumstances.

**Elderly:** Refer to adult dosing.

**Administration**

**I.V.:** For I.V. administration only; maximum rate of administration is product dependent: Monoclate-P® 2 mL/minute; Humate-P® 4 mL/minute; administration of other products should not exceed 10 mL/minute.

**I.V. Detail:** Use filter needle to draw product into syringe. Reduce rate of administration or temporarily discontinue if patient becomes tachycardic.

**Stability**

**Storage:** Helixate™ should be kept refrigerated from 2°C to 8°C (36°F to 48°F), but it can also be stored at room temperature (up to 25°C or 77°F) for up to 3 months. Package should not be frozen as that might result in breakage of the diluent bottle.

**Monitoring Laboratory Tests** Coagulation studies; plasma factor studies before, during, and after therapy

**Additional Nursing Issues**

**Physical Assessment:** Monitor vital signs before, during, and after therapy. Reduce flow rate if acute tachycardia or chest pain occurs. Monitor for acute, hypersensitivity reaction (eg, flushing, backache, headache, hypotension vomiting) - notify prescriber if symptoms occur. **Pregnancy risk factor C.** Note breast-feeding caution.

**Patient Information/Instruction:** Can only be administered I.V. Alert medical or dental personnel of your need for this factor. Immediately report signs of hypersensitivity reaction (eg, hives, tight feeling in chest or wheezing, dizziness, headache, or difficulty breathing). **Pregnancy/breast-feeding precautions:** Inform prescriber if you are or intend to be pregnant. Consult prescriber if breast-feeding.

**Additional Information**

**Formula to approximate percentage increase in plasma antihemophilic factor:**

Units required = desired level increase (desired level - actual level) x plasma volume (mL)

Total blood volume (mL blood/kg) = 70 mL/kg (adults); 80 mL/kg (children)

Plasma volume = total blood volume (mL) x [1 - Hct (in decimals)]

ie, for a 70 kg adult with a Hct = 40% : plasma volume = [70 kg x 70 mL/kg] x [1 - 0.4] = 2940 mL

To calculate number of units of factor VIII needed to increase level to desired range (highly individualized and dependent on patient's condition):

Number of units = desired level increase [desired level - actual level] x plasma volume in mL (ie, for a 100% level in the above patient who has an actual level of 20% the number of units needed = [1 (for a 100% level) - 0.2] x 2940 mL = 2352 units).

♦ **Antihist-1®** *see page 1294*

## Anti-inhibitor Coagulant Complex

(an tee-in HI bi tor coe AG yoo lant KOM pleks)

**U.S. Brand Names** Autoplex T®; Feiba VH Immuno®

**Synonyms** Coagulant Complex Inhibitor

**Therapeutic Category** Antihemophilic Agent; Blood Product Derivative

**Pregnancy Risk Factor** C

**Lactation** Excretion in breast milk unknown/use caution

**Use** Patients with factor VIII inhibitors who are to undergo surgery or those who are bleeding

**Contraindications** DIC; patients with normal coagulation mechanism

**Warnings** Products are prepared from pooled human plasma. Such plasma may contain the causative agents of viral diseases. Test methods and treatment methods may not totally eradicate HBAg and HIV from pooled plasma used in processing of this product. Pregnancy factor C.

**Effects on Lab Values** ↑ ↓ PT, PTT; ↑ fibrin split products; ↓ WBCT, fibrin, platelets

**Adverse Reactions** <1% (Limited to important or life-threatening symptoms): Hypotension, fever, headache, chills, rash, urticaria, disseminated intravascular coagulation

**Overdose/Toxicology** Rapid infusion may cause hypotension. Excessive administration can cause DIC.

**Formulations**

Injection:

Autoplex T®, with heparin 2 units: Each bottle is labeled with correctional units of Factor VIII

Feiba VH Immuno®, heparin free: Each bottle is labeled with correctional units of Factor VIII

**Dosing**

**Adults:** Dosage range: 25-100 factor VIII correctional units per kg depending on the severity of hemorrhage

Tests used to control efficacy such as APTT, WBCT, and TEG do not correlate with clinical efficacy. Dosing to normalize these values may result in DIC. Identification of the clotting deficiency as caused by factor VIII inhibitors is essential prior to starting therapy.

**Elderly:** Refer to adult dosing.

**Hepatic Impairment:** Use with extreme caution.

**Administration**

**I.V.:** I.V. push (maximum rate: 2 units/kg/minute or 2.5-7.5 mL/minutes).

**I.V. Detail:** Do not refrigerate or shake reconstituted solution. Administration must be complete within 3 hours after reconstitution by the blood bank.

**Stability**

**Storage:** Store at 2°C to 8°C (36°F to 46°F)

**Reconstitution:** Do **not** shake or refrigerate after reconstitution. Use within 1-3 hours after reconstitution.

**Additional Nursing Issues**

**Physical Assessment:** Monitor vital signs and hemodynamic status. If hypotension develops, slow the rate of infusion. **Pregnancy risk factor C.** Note breast-feeding caution.

**Patient Information/Instruction:** This medication can only be given I.V. Immediately report backache, itching or rash, difficulty breathing, acute feelings of anxiety, or sudden onset headache. **Pregnancy/breast-feeding precautions:** Inform prescriber if you are pregnant. Consult prescriber if breast-feeding.


- **Antilirium®** *see* Physostigmine *on page 928*
- **Antiminth®** *see page 1294*
- **Antipsychotic Agents Comparison** *see page 1371*
- **Antipsychotic Medication Guidelines** *see page 1436*
- **Antipyrine and Benzocaine** *see page 1291*
- **Antipyrine and Benzocaine** *see page 1306*
- **Antirabies Serum (Equine)** *see page 1256*
- **Antiretroviral Agents Comparison** *see page 1373*
- **Antispas® Injection** *see* Dicyclomine *on page 362*


## Antithrombin III (an tee THROM bin three)

**U.S. Brand Names** ATnativ®; Thrombate III™

**Synonyms** ATIII; Heparin Cofactor I

**Therapeutic Category** Anticoagulant; Blood Product Derivative

**Pregnancy Risk Factor** C

**Lactation** Excretion in breast milk unknown/use caution

**Use** Hereditary antithrombin III deficiency

**Unlabeled use:** Has been used effectively for acquired antithrombin III deficiencies related to DIC, preeclampsia, liver disease, shock and surgery complicated by DIC.

**Mechanism of Action/Effect** Antithrombin III is the primary physiologic inhibitor of *in vivo* coagulation. Its principal actions are the inactivation of thrombin, plasmin, and other active serine proteases of coagulation.

**Contraindications** Hypersensitivity to antithrombin III or any component

**Warnings** Test methods and treatment methods may not totally eradicate HBAg and HIV from pooled plasma used in processing of this product. Pregnancy factor C.

**Drug Interactions**

**Increased Effect/Toxicity:** Anticoagulation effect of heparin is enhanced if given with antithrombin III.

**Adverse Reactions** <1% (Limited to important or life-threatening symptoms): Chest tightness, chest pain, vasodilatory effects, edema, urticaria, fluid overload, hematoma formation, shortness of breath

**Overdose/Toxicology** Levels of 150% to 200% have been documented in patients with no signs or symptoms of complications.

**Formulations** Powder for injection: 500 units (50 mL)

(Continued)

## Antithrombin III *(Continued)*

**Dosing**

**Adults:** After first dose of antithrombin III, level should increase to 120% of normal; thereafter maintain at levels >80%. Generally, achieved by administration of maintenance doses once every 24 hours. Initially and until patient is stabilized, measure antithrombin III level at least twice daily, thereafter once daily and always immediately before next infusion. 1 unit = quantity of antithrombin III in 1 mL of normal pooled human plasma; administration of 1 unit/1 kg raises AT-III level by 1% to 2%; assume plasma volume of 40 mL/kg.

Initial dosage (units) = [desired AT-III level % - baseline AT-III level %] x body weight (kg) divided by 1%/units/kg (eg, if a 70 kg adult patient had a baseline AT-III level of 57%, the initial dose would be (120% - 57%) x 70/1%/units/kg = 4410 units).

Measure antithrombin III preceding and 30 minutes after dose to calculate *in vivo* recovery rate; maintain level within normal range for 2-8 days depending on type of surgery or procedure.

**Elderly:** Refer to adult dosing.

**Administration**

**I.V.:** Infuse over 5-10 minutes. Rate of infusion is 50 units/minute (1 mL/minute) not to exceed 100 units/minute (2 mL/minute).

**Stability**

**Reconstitution:** Reconstitute with 10 mL sterile water for injection, normal saline, or $D_5W$. **Do not shake**. Stability of I.V. admixture is 24 hours at room temperature; do not refrigerate.

**Monitoring Laboratory Tests** Antithrombin III levels during treatment period

**Additional Nursing Issues**

**Physical Assessment:** Monitor vital signs, cardiac status, and CNS status during and following infusion. Reduce rate of administration or temporarily discontinue if tachycardia occurs. **Pregnancy risk factor C** - benefits of use should outweigh possible risks. Note breast-feeding caution.

**Patient Information/Instruction:** This medication can only be given I.V. Report sudden onset headache, rash, chest or back pain, or respiratory difficulties. Future safety: Wear some identification that you have a hemophilic condition. **Pregnancy/breast-feeding precautions:** Consult prescriber if pregnant or breast-feeding.

- **Antithymocyte Globulin (Equine)** *see* Lymphocyte Immune Globulin *on page 700*
- **Anti-Tuss® Expectorant [OTC]** *see* Guaifenesin *on page 548*
- **Antivenin** *see page 1246*
- **Antivert®** *see* Meclizine *on page 712*
- **Antrizine®** *see* Meclizine *on page 712*
- **Anturan®** *see* Sulfinpyrazone *on page 1086*
- **Anturane®** *see* Sulfinpyrazone *on page 1086*
- **Anucort-HC® Suppository** *see* Hydrocortisone *on page 578*
- **Anucort-HC® Suppository** *see* Topical Corticosteroids *on page 1152*
- **Anuprep HC® Suppository** *see* Hydrocortisone *on page 578*
- **Anuprep HC® Suppository** *see* Topical Corticosteroids *on page 1152*
- **Anusol® HC-1 [OTC]** *see* Hydrocortisone *on page 578*
- **Anusol® HC-1 [OTC]** *see* Topical Corticosteroids *on page 1152*
- **Anusol® HC-2.5% [OTC]** *see* Hydrocortisone *on page 578*
- **Anusol® HC-2.5% [OTC]** *see* Topical Corticosteroids *on page 1152*
- **Anusol-HC® Suppository** *see* Hydrocortisone *on page 578*
- **Anusol-HC® Suppository** *see* Topical Corticosteroids *on page 1152*
- **Anusol® Ointment** *see page 1294*
- **Anxanil®** *see* Hydroxyzine *on page 588*
- **Anxiolytic/Hypnotic Use in Long-Term Care Facilities** *see page 1430*
- **Anzemet®** *see* Dolasetron *on page 393*
- **Apacet® [OTC]** *see* Acetaminophen *on page 32*
- **APAP** *see* Acetaminophen *on page 32*
- **Apatate®** *see page 1294*
- **A.P.L.®** *see* Chorionic Gonadotropin *on page 264*
- **Apo®-Acetazolamide** *see* Acetazolamide *on page 34*
- **Apo®-Allopurinol** *see* Allopurinol *on page 53*
- **Apo®-Alpraz** *see* Alprazolam *on page 55*
- **Apo®-Amilzide** *see* Amiloride and Hydrochlorothiazide *on page 68*
- **Apo®-Amitriptyline** *see* Amitriptyline *on page 73*
- **Apo®-Amoxi** *see* Amoxicillin *on page 80*
- **Apo®-Ampi Trihydrate** *see* Ampicillin *on page 90*
- **Apo®-ASA** *see* Aspirin *on page 111*
- **Apo®-Atenol** *see* Atenolol *on page 115*
- **Apo® Bromocriptine** *see* Bromocriptine *on page 162*
- **Apo®-C** *see* Ascorbic Acid *on page 108*
- **Apo®-Capto** *see* Captopril *on page 192*
- **Apo®-Carbamazepine** *see* Carbamazepine *on page 195*
- **Apo®-Cefaclor** *see* Cefaclor *on page 210*
- **Apo®-Cephalex** *see* Cephalexin *on page 237*

♦ **Apo®-Chlorax** *see* Clidinium and Chlordiazepoxide *on page 281*
♦ **Apo®-Chlordiazepoxide** *see* Chlordiazepoxide *on page 250*
♦ **Apo®-Chlorpromazine** *see* Chlorpromazine *on page 256*
♦ **Apo®-Chlorpropamide** *see* Chlorpropamide *on page 259*
♦ **Apo®-Chlorthalidone** *see* Chlorthalidone *on page 260*
♦ **Apo®-Cimetidine** *see* Cimetidine *on page 268*
♦ **Apo®-Clomipramine** *see* Clomipramine *on page 287*
♦ **Apo®-Clonidine** *see* Clonidine *on page 289*
♦ **Apo®-Clorazepate** *see* Clorazepate *on page 292*
♦ **Apo®-Cloxi** *see* Cloxacillin *on page 295*
♦ **Apo®-Diazepam** *see* Diazepam *on page 355*
♦ **Apo®-Diclo** *see* Diclofenac *on page 358*
♦ **Apo®-Diflunisal** *see* Diflunisal *on page 368*
♦ **Apo®-Diltiaz** *see* Diltiazem *on page 377*
♦ **Apo®-Dipyridamole FC** *see* Dipyridamole *on page 383*
♦ **Apo®-Dipyridamole SC** *see* Dipyridamole *on page 383*
♦ **Apo®-Doxepin** *see* Doxepin *on page 399*
♦ **Apo®-Doxy** *see* Doxycycline *on page 406*
♦ **Apo®-Doxy Tabs** *see* Doxycycline *on page 406*
♦ **Apo®-Enalapril** *see* Enalapril *on page 416*
♦ **Apo®-Erythro E-C** *see* Erythromycin *on page 435*
♦ **Apo®-Famotidine** *see* Famotidine *on page 470*
♦ **Apo®-Fenofibrate** *see* Fenofibrate *on page 475*
♦ **Apo®-Ferrous Gluconate** *see* Iron Supplements *on page 627*
♦ **Apo®-Ferrous Sulfate** *see* Iron Supplements *on page 627*
♦ **Apo®-Fluphenazine** *see* Fluphenazine *on page 505*
♦ **Apo®-Flurazepam** *see* Flurazepam *on page 507*
♦ **Apo®-Flurbiprofen** *see* Flurbiprofen *on page 509*
♦ **Apo®-Fluvoxamine** *see* Fluvoxamine *on page 514*
♦ **Apo®-Folic** *see* Folic Acid *on page 515*
♦ **Apo®-Furosemide** *see* Furosemide *on page 523*
♦ **Apo®-Gain** *see page 1294*
♦ **Apo®-Gemfibrozil** *see* Gemfibrozil *on page 530*
♦ **Apo®-Glyburide** *see* Glyburide *on page 538*
♦ **Apo®-Guanethidine** *see* Guanethidine *on page 553*
♦ **Apo®-Hydralazine** *see* Hydralazine *on page 564*
♦ **Apo®-Hydro** *see* Hydrochlorothiazide *on page 566*
♦ **Apo®-Hydroxyzine** *see* Hydroxyzine *on page 588*
♦ **Apo®-Ibuprofen** *see* Ibuprofen *on page 592*
♦ **Apo®-Imipramine** *see* Imipramine *on page 600*
♦ **Apo®-Indapadmide** *see* Indapamide *on page 604*
♦ **Apo®-Indomethacin** *see* Indomethacin *on page 606*
♦ **Apo®-ISDN** *see* Isosorbide Dinitrate *on page 634*
♦ **Apo®-Keto** *see* Ketoprofen *on page 645*
♦ **Apo®-Keto-E** *see* Ketoprofen *on page 645*
♦ **Apo®-Lisinopril** *see* Lisinopril *on page 681*
♦ **Apo®-Lorazepam** *see* Lorazepam *on page 691*
♦ **Apo®-Lovastatin** *see* Lovastatin *on page 695*
♦ **Apo®-Meprobamate** *see* Meprobamate *on page 724*
♦ **Apo®-Methazide** *see* Methyldopa and Hydrochlorothiazide *on page 751*
♦ **Apo®-Methyldopa** *see* Methyldopa *on page 750*
♦ **Apo®-Metoclop** *see* Metoclopramide *on page 758*
♦ **Apo®-Metoprolol (Type L)** *see* Metoprolol *on page 761*
♦ **Apo®-Metronidazole** *see* Metronidazole *on page 763*
♦ **Apo®-Minocycline** *see* Minocycline *on page 774*
♦ **Apo®-Nadol** *see* Nadolol *on page 798*
♦ **Apo®-Naproxen** *see* Naproxen *on page 807*
♦ **Apo®-Nifed** *see* Nifedipine *on page 824*
♦ **Apo®-Nitrofurantoin** *see* Nitrofurantoin *on page 829*
♦ **Apo®-Nizatidine** *see* Nizatidine *on page 834*
♦ **Apo®-Nortriptyline** *see* Nortriptyline *on page 839*
♦ **Apo®-Oxazepam** *see* Oxazepam *on page 868*
♦ **Apo®-Pentoxifylline SR** *see* Pentoxifylline *on page 908*
♦ **Apo®-Pen VK** *see* Penicillin V Potassium *on page 900*
♦ **Apo®-Peram** *see* Amitriptyline and Perphenazine *on page 75*
♦ **Apo®-Perphenazine** *see* Perphenazine *on page 912*
♦ **Apo®-Pindol** *see* Pindolol *on page 934*
♦ **Apo®-Piroxicam** *see* Piroxicam *on page 940*
♦ **Apo®-Prazo** *see* Prazosin *on page 958*
♦ **Apo®-Prednisone** *see* Prednisone *on page 962*
♦ **Apo®-Primidone** *see* Primidone *on page 964*

- **Apo®-Procainamide** *see* Procainamide *on page 967*
- **Apo®-Propranolol** *see* Propranolol *on page 986*
- **Apo®-Ranitidine** *see* Ranitidine *on page 1008*
- **Apo®-Salvent** *see* Albuterol *on page 45*
- **Apo®-Selegiline** *see* Selegiline *on page 1050*
- **Apo®-Spirozide** *see* Hydrochlorothiazide and Spironolactone *on page 568*
- **Apo®-Sulfamethoxazole** *see* Sulfamethoxazole *on page 1082*
- **Apo®-Sulfasalazine** *see* Sulfasalazine *on page 1084*
- **Apo®-Sulfatrim** *see* Co-trimoxazole *on page 307*
- **Apo®-Sulfinpyrazone** *see* Sulfinpyrazone *on page 1086*
- **Apo®-Sulin** *see* Sulindac *on page 1088*
- **Apo®-Tamox** *see* Tamoxifen *on page 1095*
- **Apo®-Temazepam** *see* Temazepam *on page 1100*
- **Apo®-Tetra** *see* Tetracycline *on page 1111*
- **Apothecary/Metric Conversions** *see page 1347*
- **Apo®-Theo LA** *see* Theophylline *on page 1115*
- **Apo®-Thioridazine** *see* Thioridazine *on page 1123*
- **Apo®-Timol** *see* Timolol *on page 1138*
- **Apo®-Timop** *see* Ophthalmic Agents, Glaucoma *on page 853*
- **Apo®-Timop** *see* Timolol *on page 1138*
- **Apo®-Tolbutamide** *see* Tolbutamide *on page 1146*
- **Apo®-Triazide** *see* Hydrochlorothiazide and Triamterene *on page 568*
- **Apo®-Triazo** *see* Triazolam *on page 1174*
- **Apo®-Trihex** *see* Trihexyphenidyl *on page 1179*
- **Apo®-Trimip** *see* Trimipramine *on page 1183*
- **Apo®-Verap** *see* Verapamil *on page 1208*
- **Apo®-Zidovudine** *see* Zidovudine *on page 1227*
- **APPG** *see* Penicillin G Procaine *on page 899*
- **Apraclonidine** *see page 1248*
- **Apraclonidine** *see* Ophthalmic Agents, Glaucoma *on page 853*
- **Apresazide®** *see* Hydralazine and Hydrochlorothiazide *on page 565*
- **Apresolina** *see* Hydralazine *on page 564*
- **Apresoline®** *see* Hydralazine *on page 564*
- **Aprodine® Syrup** *see page 1294*
- **Aprodine® Tablet** *see page 1294*

## Aprotinin (a proe TYE nin)

**U.S. Brand Names** Trasylol®

**Therapeutic Category** Blood Product Derivative; Hemostatic Agent

**Pregnancy Risk Factor** B

**Lactation** Excretion in breast milk unknown

**Use** Reduction or prevention of blood loss in patients undergoing coronary artery bypass surgery when a high risk of excessive bleeding exists, including open heart reoperation, pre-existing coagulopathies, operations on the great vessels, and when a patient's beliefs prohibit blood transfusions

**Mechanism of Action/Effect** Has variety of effects on coagulation system; serine protease inhibitor; inhibits plasmin, kallikrein, and platelet activation producing antifibrinolytic effects; a weak inhibitor of plasma pseudocholinesterase. It also inhibits the contact phase activation of coagulation and preserves adhesive platelet glycoproteins making them resistant to damage from increased circulating plasmin or mechanical injury occurring during bypass

**Contraindications** Hypersensitivity to aprotinin or any component; patients with thromboembolic disease requiring anticoagulants or blood factor administration

**Warnings** Patients with a previous exposure to aprotinin are at an increased risk of hypersensitivity reactions. Test methods and treatment methods may not totally eradicate HBAg and HIV from pooled plasma used in processing of this product.

**Drug Interactions**

**Decreased Effect:** Fibrinolytic effects of streptokinase or anistreplase. Hypotensive response to ACE-inhibitors.

**Increased Effect/Toxicity:** Heparin's whole blood clotting time may be prolonged. Use with succinylcholine or tubocurarine may produce prolonged or recurring apnea.

**Effects on Lab Values** Aprotinin prolongs whole blood clotting time of heparinized blood as determined by the Hemochrom® method or similar surface activation methods. Patients may require additional heparin even in the presence of activated clotting time levels that appear to represent adequate anticoagulation.

**Adverse Reactions**

1% to 10%

Cardiovascular: Atrial fibrillation, myocardial infarction, heart failure, atrial flutter, ventricular tachycardia, hypotension, supraventricular tachycardia

Central nervous system: Fever, mental confusion

Local: Phlebitis

Renal: Increased potential for postoperative renal dysfunction

Respiratory: Dyspnea, bronchoconstriction

<1% (Limited to important or life-threatening symptoms): Cerebral embolism, cerebrovascular events, convulsions, hemolysis, liver damage, pulmonary edema

**Overdose/Toxicology** The maximum amount of aprotinin that can safely be given has not yet been determined. One case report of aprotinin overdose was associated with the development of hepatic and renal failure and eventually death. Autopsy demonstrated severe hepatic necrosis and extensive renal tubular and glomerular necrosis. The relationship between these findings and aprotinin remains unclear.

**Pharmacodynamics/Kinetics**

**Half-life Elimination:** 150 minutes

**Metabolism:** Kidney

**Excretion:** Urine

**Formulations** Injection: 1.4 mg/mL [10,000 units/mL] (100 mL, 200 mL)

**Dosing**

**Adults:**

Test dose: **All** patients should receive a 1 mL I.V. test dose at least 10 minutes prior to the loading dose to assess the potential for allergic reactions

Regimen A (standard dose):

2 million units (280 mg) loading dose I.V. over 20-30 minutes
2 million units (280 mg) into pump prime volume
500,000 units/hour (70 mg/hour) I.V. during operation

Regimen B (low-dose):

1 million units (140 mg) loading dose I.V. over 20-30 minutes
1 million units (140 mg) into pump prime volume
250,000 units/hour (35 mg/hour) I.V. during operation

**Elderly:** Refer to adult dosing.

**Administration**

**I.V.:** Administer through a central line. Infuse loading dose over 20-30 minutes, then continuous infusion at 50 mL/hour.

**I.V. Detail:** Do not infuse any other drug through the same line.

**Stability**

**Storage:** Vials should be stored between 2°C and 25°C and protected from freezing.

**Compatibility:** Aprotinin is incompatible with corticosteroids, heparin, tetracyclines, amino acid solutions, and fat emulsion.

**Monitoring Laboratory Tests** Bleeding times, prothrombin time, activated clotting time, platelet count, red blood cell counts, hematocrit, hemoglobin and fibrinogen degradation products; for toxicity also include renal function.

**Additional Nursing Issues**

**Physical Assessment: Monitor infusion site carefully.** Systemic hemodynamic monitoring is generally in effect when patients receive this drug. Continuous blood pressure monitoring is required. Sudden drops in blood pressure may occur. Observe for adequate fluid balance (I & O ratio) and adequate respiratory function. Note breast-feeding caution.

**Patient Information/Instruction:** You will be unaware of the effects of this drug, however, you will be closely monitored at all times. **Breast-feeding precautions:** Consult prescriber if breast-feeding.


♦ **Aprovel** *see* Irbesartan *on page 623*
♦ **APSAC** *see* Anistreplase *on page 97*
♦ **Aquacare® Topical [OTC]** *see* Urea *on page 1193*
♦ **Aquachloral® Supprettes®** *see* Chloral Hydrate *on page 245*
♦ **AquaMEPHYTON® Injection** *see* Phytonadione *on page 929*
♦ **Aquaphyllin®** *see* Theophylline *on page 1115*
♦ **AquaSite® Ophthalmic Solution** *see page 1294*
♦ **Aquasol A®** *see* Vitamin A *on page 1217*
♦ **Aquasol E® [OTC]** *see* Vitamin E *on page 1218*
♦ **Aquatag®** *see* Benzthiazide *on page 144*
♦ **AquaTar®** *see page 1294*
♦ **Aquatensen®** *see* Methyclothiazide *on page 748*
♦ **Aqueous Procaine Penicillin G** *see* Penicillin G Procaine *on page 899*
♦ **Aqueous Testosterone** *see* Testosterone *on page 1108*
♦ **Aquest®** *see* Estrone *on page 451*
♦ **ARA-A** *see* Vidarabine *on page 1210*
♦ **Arabinofuranosyladenine** *see* Vidarabine *on page 1210*
♦ **Arabinosylcytosine** *see* Cytarabine *on page 322*
♦ **ARA-C** *see* Cytarabine *on page 322*
♦ **Aralen® Phosphate** *see* Chloroquine Phosphate *on page 252*
♦ **Aralen® Phosphate With Primaquine Phosphate** *see* Chloroquine and Primaquine *on page 252*
♦ **Arava™** *see* Leflunomide *on page 657*


## Ardeparin (ar dee PA rin)

**U.S. Brand Names** Normiflo®

**Synonyms** Ardeparin Sodium

**Therapeutic Category** Low Molecular Weight Heparin

**Pregnancy Risk Factor** C

**Lactation** Excretion in breast milk unknown/use caution

**Use** Prevention of deep vein thrombosis (DVT) which may lead to pulmonary embolism following knee replacement surgery

(Continued)

## Ardeparin *(Continued)*

**Mechanism of Action/Effect** A low molecular weight heparin with antithrombotic properties; a partially depolymerized porcine mucosal heparin that has the same molecular subunits as heparin sodium, although its molecular weight is lower; acts at multiple sites in the normal coagulation system; binds to and accelerates the activity of antithrombin III, thereby inhibiting thrombosis by inactivating factor Xa and thrombin; inhibits thrombin by binding to heparin cofactor II

**Contraindications** Hypersensitivity to ardeparin, pork products, or other low-molecular weight heparins; cerebrovascular disease or other active hemorrhage; cerebral aneurysm; severe uncontrolled hypertension; thrombocytopenia associated with a positive *in vitro* test for antiplatelet antibodies in the presence of ardeparin

**Warnings** Not intended for I.M. or I.V. use. Use with extreme caution in patients with history of heparin-induced thrombocytopenia. May cause allergic-type reaction including anaphylactic symptoms and life-threatening or less severe asthmatic episodes in certain susceptible individuals. Sulfite sensitivity is more likely in asthmatics than nonasthmatics. Use with extreme caution in patients with conditions having increased risk of hemorrhage (ie, bacterial endocarditis, congenital or acquired bleeding disorders, active ulcerative or angiodysplastic gastrointestinal disease, severe uncontrolled hypertension, hemorrhagic stroke, or shortly after brain, spinal, or ophthalmologic surgery) or in patients treated concomitantly with platelet inhibitors. Use with caution in patients with hypersensitivity to methylparaben or propylparaben. Use with caution in patients with bleeding diathesis, recent GI bleeding, thrombocytopenia or platelet defects, severe liver disease, hypertensive or diabetic retinopathy, or if undergoing invasive procedure especially if receiving other drugs known to interfere with hemostasis.

Patient should be observed closely for bleeding if ardeparin is administered during or immediately following diagnostic lumbar puncture, epidural anesthesia, or spinal anesthesia. If thromboembolism develops despite ardeparin prophylaxis, ardeparin should be discontinued and appropriate treatment should be initiated.

Carefully monitor patients receiving low molecular weight heparins or heparinoids. These drugs, when used concurrently with spinal or epidural anesthesia or spinal puncture, may cause bleeding or hematomas within the spinal column. Increased pressure on the spinal cord may result in permanent paralysis if not detected and treated immediately.

Pregnancy risk C.

**Drug Interactions**

**Increased Effect/Toxicity:** Use with anticoagulants or platelet inhibitors, including aspirin and NSAIDs, may induce or augment bleeding.

**Adverse Reactions** 1% to 10%:

Central nervous system: Fever, confusion

Dermatologic: Pruritus, rash, ecchymosis

Gastrointestinal: Nausea, constipation, vomiting

Hematologic: Hemorrhage, thrombocytopenia, anemia

Case reports of long-term or permanent paralysis have occurred when used in association with epidural or spinal anesthesia (due to hematoma). Risk is increased by indwelling catheters or concomitant use of other drugs which alter hemostasis (NSAIDs, anticoagulants, or platelet inhibitors).

**Overdose/Toxicology** The main symptom of overdose is bleeding which may first be indicated with bleeding at the surgical site or at the venipuncture site. Other symptoms include epistaxis, hematuria, or blood in stool. Easy bruising or petechiae may precede frank bleeding.

Treatment includes discontinuing the drug and applying pressure to the site, if possible, and replacing volume and hemostatic blood elements (eg, fresh frozen plasma, platelets) as necessary. 1 mg protamine neutralizes approximately 100 anti-Xa units of ardeparin. Anti-IIa activity of I.V. ardeparin is completely neutralized within 10 minutes following I.V. infusion dose of equal weight protamine sulfate (about 1 mg protamine sulfate for each 100 anti-Xa units of ardeparin). The anti-Xa and Heptest® activities of ardeparin are reduced by ~75% within 10 minutes and are almost completely neutralized within 30 minutes after protamine sulfate administration. Protamine sulfate may cause anaphylactoid reactions that can be life-threatening; it should be given only when resuscitation techniques and treatment of anaphylactic shock are available (see Protamine Sulfate for additional information).

**Pharmacodynamics/Kinetics**

**Half-life Elimination:** 3 hours

**Time to Peak:** Peak plasma levels: 2-3 hours (anti-Xa activity). **Note:** Peak anti-Xa plasma levels produced by ardeparin are about twice as high as those produced by heparin, and ardeparin anti-Xa half-life in plasma is longer than that for unfractionated heparin parameters for ardeparin suggest saturable elimination.

**Excretion:** Like other low molecular weight heparins, elimination of ardeparin appears to be via renal excretion as unchanged drug. Pharmacokinetic parameters for ardeparin suggest saturable elimination.

**Duration:** ~12 hours

**Formulations** Injection, as sodium: 5000 anti-Xa units (0.5 mL); 10,000 anti-Xa units (0.5 mL)

**Dosing**

**Adults:** S.C.: 50 anti-Xa units/kg every 12 hours for DVT prophylaxis

If the ardeparin formulation used contains 5000 anti-Xa units/0.5 mL (which is recommended for patients up to 100 kg or 220 lbs), the volume to be administered is calculated as follows:

Patient's weight (kg) x 0.005 mL/kg = volume (mL)

If the ardeparin formulation used contains 10,000 anti-Xa units/0.5 mL (which is recommended for patients >100 kg or 220 lbs), the volume to be administered is calculated as follows:

Patient's weight (kg) x 0.0025 mL/kg = volume (mL)

**Elderly:** Refer to adult dosing.

**Renal Impairment:** No adjustment is necessary. Not dialyzable.

**Administration**

**Other:** Administer by deep S.C. injection; do not give I.M. Patient should be sitting or lying down. May be injected into abdomen (avoid the navel), the anterior aspect of the thighs, or the outer aspect of the upper arms. Vary site with each injection. A skinfold held between the thumb and forefinger must be lifted. Entire length of the needle is inserted into the fold at a 45° to 90° angle. Before injecting, draw back on the plunger to ensure the needle is not in the intravascular space. Do not rub injection site after completing injection. Treatment should begin the evening of the day of surgery or the following morning and is continued for up to 14 days or until patient is fully ambulatory.

**Stability**

**Storage:** Store at room temperature 15°C to 25°C (59°F to 77°F).

**Monitoring Laboratory Tests** Platelets, occult blood, anti-Xa activity, if available; the monitoring of PT and/or PTT is not necessary.

**Additional Nursing Issues**

**Physical Assessment:** Monitor laboratory tests (see Monitoring Laboratory Tests). Patients should be observed closely for bleeding if administered during or immediately following diagnostic lumbar puncture, epidural anesthesia, or spinal anesthesia. If thromboembolism develops despite ardeparin prophylaxis, ardeparin should be discontinued and appropriate treatment should be initiated. See Administration - Other. **Pregnancy risk factor C** - benefits of use should outweigh possible risks. Consult prescriber if breast-feeding.

**Patient Information/Instruction:** Inform prescriber of any over-the-counter or prescription medication you may take including aspirin, warfarin, NSAID (eg, ibuprofen, naproxen). Because this drug can alter the effects of certain laboratory tests, be sure to remind your prescriber that you are taking this medication when you are scheduled for any tests. This medication should not be mixed with, or added to, any other drug in the same syringe. Laboratory tests will be done periodically while taking this medication to monitor its effects and to prevent side effects. Use each dose at the scheduled time. If you miss a dose, use it as soon as remembered; do not use it if it is near the time for the next dose. Instead, skip the missed dose and resume your usual dosing schedule. Do not "double-up" the dose to catch up. **Pregnancy/breast-feeding precautions:** Inform prescriber if you are or intend to be pregnant.

**Geriatric Considerations:** No significant differences in safety in patients >65 years of age vs those <65 years of age.

**Related Information**

Low Molecular Weight Heparins Comparison *on page 1395*

- **Ardeparin Sodium** *see* Ardeparin *on page 105*
- **Arduan®** *see page 1248*
- **Aredia™** *see* Pamidronate *on page 880*
- **Arfonad® Injection** *see page 1248*
- **Argesic®-SA** *see* Salsalate *on page 1042*
- **8-Arginine Vasopressin** *see* Vasopressin *on page 1205*
- **Argyrol® S.S. 20%** *see* Silver Protein, Mild *on page 1058*
- **Aricept®** *see* Donepezil *on page 394*
- **Arimidex®** *see* Anastrozole *on page 95*
- **Aristocort®** *see* Topical Corticosteroids *on page 1152*
- **Aristocort®** *see* Triamcinolone *on page 1171*
- **Aristocort® A** *see* Topical Corticosteroids *on page 1152*
- **Aristocort® A** *see* Triamcinolone *on page 1171*
- **Aristocort® Forte** *see* Triamcinolone *on page 1171*
- **Aristocort® Intralesional** *see* Triamcinolone *on page 1171*
- **Aristospan® Intra-Articular** *see* Triamcinolone *on page 1171*
- **Aristospan® Intralesional** *see* Triamcinolone *on page 1171*
- **Arm-a-Med® Isoetharine** *see* Isoetharine *on page 629*
- **Arm-a-Med® Isoproterenol** *see* Isoproterenol *on page 632*
- **Arm-a-Med® Metaproterenol** *see* Metaproterenol *on page 732*
- **A.R.M.® Caplet** *see page 1294*
- **Armour® Thyroid** *see* Thyroid *on page 1130*
- **Arovit** *see* Vitamin A *on page 1217*
- **Arrestin®** *see* Trimethobenzamide *on page 1180*
- **Artane®** *see* Trihexyphenidyl *on page 1179*
- **Artha-G®** *see* Salsalate *on page 1042*
- **Arthritis Foundation® NightTime Maximum Strength Caplet** *see page 1294*
- **Arthropan®** *see page 1294*

- **Arthrotec®** *see* Diclofenac and Misoprostol *on page 360*
- **Articulose-50® Injection** *see* Prednisolone *on page 960*
- **Artificial Tears** *see page 1294*
- **Artosin** *see* Tolbutamide *on page 1146*
- **Artrenac** *see* Diclofenac *on page 358*
- **Artron** *see* Naproxen *on page 807*
- **Artyflam** *see* Piroxicam *on page 940*
- **A.S.A. [OTC]** *see* Aspirin *on page 111*
- **ASA®** *see* Aspirin *on page 111*
- **ASA** *see* Aspirin *on page 111*
- **5-ASA** *see* Mesalamine *on page 727*
- **Asacol® Oral** *see* Mesalamine *on page 727*
- **Asaphen** *see* Aspirin *on page 111*
- **Ascorbic 500** *see* Ascorbic Acid *on this page*


## Ascorbic Acid (a SKOR bik AS id)

**U.S. Brand Names** Ascorbicap® [OTC]; C-Crystals® [OTC]; Cebid® Timecelles® [OTC]; Cecon® [OTC]; Cevalin® [OTC]; Cevi-Bid® [OTC]; Ce-Vi-Sol® [OTC]; Dull-C® [OTC]; Flavorcee® [OTC]; N'ice® Vitamin C Drops [OTC]; Vita-C® [OTC]

**Synonyms** Vitamin C

**Therapeutic Category** Vitamin, Water Soluble

**Pregnancy Risk Factor** A/C (if dose exceeds RDA recommendation)

**Lactation** Enters breast milk/compatible

**Use** Prevention and treatment of scurvy and to acidify the urine

**Investigational use:** In large doses to decrease the severity of "colds"; dietary supplementation; a 20-year study was recently completed involving 730 individuals which indicates a possible decreased risk of death by stroke when ascorbic acid at doses ≥45 mg/day was administered.

**Mechanism of Action/Effect** Not fully understood; necessary for collagen formation and tissue repair; involved in some oxidation-reduction reactions as well as other metabolic pathways, such as synthesis of carnitine, steroids, and catecholamines and conversion of folic acid to folinic acid

**Warnings** Diabetics and patients prone to recurrent renal calculi (eg, dialysis patients) should not take excessive doses for extended periods of time. Pregnancy factor C (doses exceeding RDA recommendations).

**Drug Interactions**

**Decreased Effect:** Ascorbic acid and fluphenazine may decrease fluphenazine levels. Ascorbic acid and warfarin may decrease anticoagulant effect. Changes in dose of ascorbic acid when taken with oral contraceptives may reduce the contraceptive effect.

**Increased Effect/Toxicity:** Ascorbic acid enhances iron absorption from the GI tract. Concomitant ascorbic acid taken with oral contraceptives may increase contraceptive effect.

**Effects on Lab Values** False-positive urinary glucose with cupric sulfate reagent, false-negative urinary glucose with glucose oxidase method; false-negative stool occult blood 48-72 hours after ascorbic acid ingestion

**Adverse Reactions**

1% to 10%: Renal: Hyperoxaluria (incidence dose-related)

<1% (Limited to important or life-threatening symptoms): Faintness, dizziness, headache, fatigue, flank pain

**Overdose/Toxicology** Symptoms of overdose include renal calculi, nausea, gastritis, and diarrhea. Diuresis with forced fluids may be useful following massive ingestion.

**Pharmacodynamics/Kinetics**

**Distribution:** Widely distributed

**Metabolism:** Liver

**Excretion:** In urine; there is an individual specific renal threshold for ascorbic acid. When blood levels are high, ascorbic acid is excreted in the urine; whereas, when the levels are subthreshold, very little if any ascorbic acid is cleared into the urine.

**Formulations**

Capsule, timed release: 500 mg
Crystals: 4 g/teaspoonful (100 g, 500 g); 5 g/teaspoonful (180 g)
Injection: 250 mg/mL (2 mL, 30 mL); 500 mg/mL (2 mL, 50 mL)
Liquid, oral: 35 mg/0.6 mL (50 mL)
Lozenges: 60 mg
Powder: 4 g/teaspoonful (100 g, 500 g)
Solution, oral: 100 mg/mL (50 mL)
Syrup: 500 mg/5 mL (5 mL, 10 mL, 120 mL, 480 mL)
Tablet: 25 mg, 50 mg, 100 mg, 250 mg, 500 mg, 1000 mg
Tablet:
Chewable: 100 mg, 250 mg, 500 mg
Timed release: 500 mg, 1000 mg, 1500 mg

**Dosing**

**Adults:** Oral, I.M., I.V., S.C.:

Recommended daily allowance (RDA): 60 mg
Scurvy: 100-250 mg 1-2 times/day for at least 2 weeks
Urinary acidification: 4-12 g/day in 3-4 divided doses
Prevention and treatment of colds: 1-3 g/day
Dietary supplement: 50-200 mg/day

Wound healing: 300-500 mg/day; larger amounts have been also recommended; maximum 7-10 days pre- and postoperatively

Burns: 1-2 g/day

Prevention and treatment of cold: 1-3 g/day

**Elderly:** Refer to adult dosing.

**Administration**

**I.V.:** Avoid rapid I.V. injection.

**Stability**

**Storage:** Injectable form should be stored under refrigeration (2°C to 8°C). Protect oral dosage forms from light. Rapidly oxidized when in solution in air and alkaline media.

**Monitoring Laboratory Tests** pH of urine when used as an acidifying agent

**Additional Nursing Issues**

**Physical Assessment:** See Contraindications and Warnings/Precautions for use cautions. Assess effectiveness and interactions of other medications (see Drug Interactions). Note Effects on Lab values (above) - instruct diabetic patients accordingly. Assess knowledge/teach patient appropriate administration according to formulation of drug and purpose for ascorbic acid therapy and adverse symptoms to report. **Pregnancy risk factor A/C** - see Pregnancy Risk Factor for cautious use.

**Patient Information/Instruction:** Take exactly as directed; do not take more than the recommended dose. Do not chew or crush extended release tablets. Take oral doses with 8 ounces of water. Diabetics should use serum glucose monitoring method. Report pain on urination, faintness, or flank pain.

**Geriatric Considerations:** Minimum RDA for elderly is not established. Vitamin C is provided mainly in citrus fruits and tomatoes. The elderly, however, avoid citrus fruits due to cost and difficulty preparing (peeling). Daily replacement through a single multiple vitamin is recommended. Use of natural vitamin C or rose hips offers no advantages. Acidity may produce GI complaints.

**Additional Information** Sodium content of 1 g: ~5 mEq

♦ **Ascorbicap® [OTC]** *see* Ascorbic Acid *on previous page*

♦ **Ascriptin® [OTC]** *see* Aspirin *on page 111*

♦ **Asendin®** *see* Amoxapine *on page 79*

♦ **Asmalix®** *see* Theophylline *on page 1115*

## Asparaginase (a SPIR a ji nase)

**U.S. Brand Names** Elspar®

**Synonyms** Colaspase

**Therapeutic Category** Antineoplastic Agent, Miscellaneous

**Pregnancy Risk Factor** C

**Lactation** Excretion in breast milk unknown

**Use** Treatment of acute lymphocytic leukemia, lymphoma; for induction therapy

**Mechanism of Action/Effect** Asparaginase deprives tumor cells of the amino acid for protein synthesis and inhibits cell (malignant) proliferation. There are two purified preparations of the enzyme: one from *Escherichia coli* and one from *Erwinia carotovora*. These two preparations vary slightly in the gene sequencing and have slight differences in enzyme characteristics. Both are highly specific for asparagine and have <10% activity for the D-isomer. The preparation from *E. coli* has had the most use in clinical and research practice.

**Contraindications** Hypersensitivity to asparaginase or any component; if a reaction occurs to Elspar®, obtain **Erwinia L-asparaginase (must be special ordered from manufacturer)** and use with caution; pancreatitis

**Warnings** The U.S. Food and Drug Administration (FDA) currently recommends that procedures for proper handling and disposal of antineoplastic agents be considered. Monitor for severe allergic reactions. The risk for hypersensitivity increases with successive doses. See Administration. Pregnancy factor C.

**Drug Interactions**

**Decreased Effect:** Asparaginase terminates methotrexate action.

**Increased Effect/Toxicity:** Increased toxicity has been noticed when asparaginase is administered with vincristine (neuropathy) and prednisone (hyperglycemia). Decreased metabolism when used with cyclophosphamide. Increased hepatotoxicity when used with mercaptopurine.

**Effects on Lab Values** ↓ thyroxine and thyroxine-binding globulin

**Adverse Reactions**

>10%:

Immediate effects: Fever, chills, nausea, and vomiting occur in 50% to 60% of patients

Gastrointestinal: Emetic potential: Moderate (30% to 60%)

Hypersensitivity effects: Hypersensitivity and anaphylactic reactions occur in ~10% to 40% of patients and can be fatal. This reaction is more common in patients receiving asparaginase alone or by I.V. administration. Hypersensitivity appears rarely with the first dose and more commonly after the second or third treatment. Hypersensitivity may be treated with antihistamines and/or steroids. If an anaphylactic reaction occurs, a change in treatment to the *Erwinia* preparation may be made, since this preparation does not share antigenic cross-reactivity with the *E. coli* preparation. Note that allergic reactions to the *Erwinia* preparation may also occur and ultimately develop in 5% to 20% of patients.

Pancreatitis: Occur in <15% of patients but may progress to severe hemorrhagic pancreatitis

1% to 10%:

Endocrine & metabolic: Hyperuricemia

Miscellaneous: Mouth sores

(Continued)

## Asparaginase *(Continued)*

<1% (Limited to important or life-threatening symptoms): Seizures, coma which may be due to elevated $NH_4$ levels; hyperthermia, fever, transient diabetes mellitus; increases in serum bilirubin, AST, alkaline phosphatase; hypotension, laryngeal spasm, azotemia

Hematologic: Inhibition of protein synthesis will cause a decrease in production of albumin, insulin (resulting in hyperglycemia), serum lipoprotein, antithrombin III, and clotting factors II, V, VII, VIII, IX, and X. The loss of the later two proteins may result in either thrombotic or hemorrhagic events. These protein losses occur in 100% of patients. Leg vein thrombosis.

Myelosuppressive: Myelosuppression is uncommon; WBC: Mild; Platelets: Mild; Onset (days): 7; Nadir (days): 14; Recovery (days): 21 possible decrease in mobilization of lipids

**Overdose/Toxicology** Symptoms of overdose include nausea and diarrhea

**Pharmacodynamics/Kinetics**

**Half-life Elimination:** 8-30 hours

**Metabolism:** Systemically degraded, only trace amounts are found in the urine

**Excretion:** Clearance unaffected by age, renal function, or hepatic function

**Formulations** Injection: 10,000 units/vial

**Dosing**

**Adults:** Dose must be individualized based upon clinical response and tolerance of the patient. (Refer to individual protocols.)

I.M. administration is **preferred** over I.V. administration; I.M. administration may decrease the risk of anaphylaxis.

Asparaginase is available from two different microbiological sources: One is from *Escherichia coli* and the other is from *Erwinia carotovora*. The *Erwinia* is restricted to patients who have sustained anaphylaxis to the *E. coli* preparation.

I.M., I.V.: 6000 units/m² every other day for 3-4 weeks or daily doses of 1000-20,000 units/m² for 10-20 days; other induction regimens have been utilized.

Desensitization should be performed before administering the first dose of asparaginase to patients who developed a positive reaction to the intradermal skin test or who are being retreated. One schedule begins with a total of 1 unit given I.V. and doubles the dose every 10 minutes until the total amount given in the planned dose for that day.

For example, if a patient was to receive a total dose of 4000 units, he/she would receive injections 1 through 12 during the desensitization

**Asparaginase Desensitization**

| Injection No. | Elspar Dose (IU) | Accumulated Total Dose |
|---|---|---|
| 1 | 1 | 1 |
| 2 | 2 | 3 |
| 3 | 4 | 7 |
| 4 | 8 | 15 |
| 5 | 16 | 31 |
| 6 | 32 | 63 |
| 7 | 64 | 127 |
| 8 | 128 | 255 |
| 9 | 256 | 511 |
| 10 | 512 | 1023 |
| 11 | 1024 | 2047 |
| 12 | 2048 | 4095 |
| 13 | 4096 | 8191 |
| 14 | 8192 | 16,383 |
| 15 | 16,384 | 32,767 |
| 16 | 32,768 | 65,535 |
| 17 | 65,536 | 131,071 |
| 18 | 131,072 | 262,143 |

**Elderly:** Refer to adult dosing.

**Administration**

**I.M.:** Must only be given as a deep intramuscular injection into a large muscle; use two injection sites for I.M. doses >2 mL.

**I.V.:** The following precautions should be taken when administering. Only administer in a hospital setting. Give a small test dose first. Note that a negative skin test does not preclude the possibility of an allergic reaction. Desensitization should be performed in patients who have been found to be hypersensitive by the intradermal skin test or who have received previous courses of therapy with the drug. Have epinephrine, diphenhydramine, and hydrocortisone at the bedside. Have a running I.V. in place. A physician should be readily accessible.

**I.V. Detail:** The intradermal skin test is commonly given prior to the initial injection, using a dose of 0.1 mL of 20 units/mL solution (~2 units). The skin test site should be observed for at least 1 hour for a wheal or erythema.

**Stability**

**Storage:** Intact vials of powder should be refrigerated <8°C; however, the manufacturer states that asparaginase is stable for at least 48 hours at room temperature.

**Reconstitution:** Lyophilized powder should be reconstituted with 1-5 mL sterile water for I.V. administration or NS for I.M. use, reconstituted solutions are stable 1 week at room temperature. Shake well but not too vigorously.

**Standard I.M. dilution:** 5000 units/mL: 2 mL/syringe

**Standard I.V. dilution:** Dose in 50-250 mL NS or $D_5W$

Stable for 8 hours at room temperature or refrigeration after dilution.

**Monitoring Laboratory Tests** Intradermal skin test prior to fist dose and other doses if more than 1 week between doses; CBC, serum amylase, blood glucose, liver function prior to and frequently during therapy

**Additional Nursing Issues**

**Physical Assessment:** Monitor all skin tests and laboratory tests. Assess I.V. site closely for extravasation and monitor blood pressure every 15 minutes for 1 hour. With each dose, monitor closely for immediate signs of hypersensitivity (anaphylactic reaction - chills, respiratory difficulty, rash) (may occur in 10% to 40% of patients - see Adverse Reactions) and monitor for hyperglycemic reaction. In event of hypersensitivity or hyperglycemia, stop drug and notify prescriber immediately. Nausea and vomiting occur in 50% of cases; treatment with appropriate antiemetic may help. Monitor CNS changes (eg, hallucination, agitation, acute depression). Maintain safety precautions. Monitor for signs of infection (eg, fever, chills, unhealed sores, mouth or vaginal plaque, increased vaginal discharge, foul-smelling stools). **Pregnancy risk factor C** - benefits of use should outweigh possible risks. Note breast-feeding caution.

**Patient Information/Instruction:** This medication can only be given I.M. or I.V. It is vital to maintain good hydration (2-3 L/day of fluids unless instructed to restrict fluid intake) and good nutritional status (small frequent meal may help). You may experience acute gastric disturbances (eg, nausea or vomiting); frequent mouth care or lozenges may help or antiemetic may be prescribed. Report any respiratory difficulty, skin rash, or acute anxiety immediately. Report unusual fever or chills, confusion, agitation, depression, yellowing of skin or eyes, unusual bleeding or bruising, unhealed sores, or vaginal discharge. **Pregnancy/breast-feeding precautions:** Inform prescriber if you are or intend to be pregnant. Consult prescriber if breast-feeding.

**Pregnancy Issues:** Based on limited reports in humans, the use of asparaginase does not seem to pose a major risk to the fetus when used in the 2nd and 3rd trimesters, or when exposure occurs prior to conception in either females or males. Because of the teratogenicity observed in animals and the lack of human data after the 1st trimester exposure, asparaginase should be used cautiously, if at all, during this period.

- **A-Spas® S/L** *see* Hyoscyamine *on page 590*
- **Aspergum® [OTC]** *see* Aspirin *on this page*

## Aspirin (AS pir in)

**U.S. Brand Names** Anacin® [OTC]; A.S.A. [OTC]; Ascriptin® [OTC]; Aspergum® [OTC]; Bayer® Aspirin [OTC]; Bufferin® [OTC]; Easprin®; Ecotrin® [OTC]; Empirin® [OTC]; Measurin® [OTC]; Synalgos® [OTC]; ZORprin®

**Synonyms** Acetylsalicylic Acid; ASA

**Therapeutic Category** Antiplatelet Agent; Salicylate

**Pregnancy Risk Factor** C/D (if full-dose aspirin in 3rd trimester)

**Lactation** Enters breast milk/use caution

**Use** Treatment of mild to moderate pain, inflammation, and fever; prophylaxis for myocardial infarction and transient ischemic episodes; management of rheumatoid arthritis, rheumatic fever, osteoarthritis, and gout (high dose)

**Mechanism of Action/Effect** Inhibits prostaglandin synthesis, acts on the hypothalamus heat-regulating center to reduce fever, blocks prostaglandin synthetase action which prevents formation of the platelet-aggregating substance thromboxane $A_2$

**Contraindications** Hypersensitivity to salicylates or other NSAIDs; bleeding disorders (factor VII or IX deficiencies); allergy to tartrazine dye; asthma diagnosis; pregnancy (if full-dose aspirin in 3rd trimester)

**Warnings** Use with caution in patients with platelet and bleeding disorders, renal dysfunction, erosive gastritis, peptic ulcer disease, or vitamin K deficiency. Previous nonreaction does not guarantee future safe taking of medication. Do not use aspirin in children <16 years of age for chickenpox or flu symptoms due to the association with Reye's syndrome.

Otic: Discontinue use if dizziness, tinnitus, or impaired hearing occurs. Surgical patients should avoid ASA if possible, for 1 week prior to surgery because of the possibility of postoperative bleeding. Use with caution in impaired hepatic function.

Elderly are at high risk for adverse effects from nonsteroidal anti-inflammatory agents. See Geriatric Considerations.

Pregnancy factor C/D (if full-dose aspirin in 3rd trimester).

**Drug Interactions**

**Decreased Effect:** Aspirin may cause a decrease of NSAIDs serum concentration. Aspirin may decrease the effects of probenecid. Increased serum salicylate levels when taken with with urine acidifiers (ammonium chloride, methionine). Aspirin may decreased the antihypertensive effect of captopril, or beta-blockers when taken together. Aspirin may decrease antihypertensive and diuretic effects of furosemide and thiazide diuretics.

**Increased Effect/Toxicity:** Aspirin may increase methotrexate serum levels and may displace valproic acid from binding sites which can result in toxicity. NSAIDs and

(Continued)

## Aspirin *(Continued)*

aspirin increase GI adverse effects (ulceration). Aspirin with oral anticoagulants may increase bleeding. There is a greater effect of sulfonylureas when given with ASA. Buspirone increases free fraction *in vitro.* Bleeding times may be additionally prolonged with verapamil.

**Food Interactions** Food may decrease the rate but not the extent of oral absorption. Take with food or or large volume of water or milk to minimize GI upset.

**Effects on Lab Values** False-negative results for glucose oxidase urinary glucose tests (Clinistix®). Interferes with Gerhardt test, VMA determination; 5-HIAA, xylose tolerance test and $T_3$ and $T_4$.

**Adverse Reactions**

>10%: Gastrointestinal: Nausea, vomiting, heartburn, epigastric discomfort, heartburn, stomach pains

1% to 10%:

- Central nervous system: Fatigue
- Dermatologic: Rash, urticaria
- Gastrointestinal: Gastrointestinal ulceration
- Hematologic: Hemolytic anemia
- Neuromuscular & skeletal: Weakness
- Respiratory: Dyspnea
- Miscellaneous: Anaphylactic shock

<1% (Limited to important or life-threatening symptoms): Iron deficiency, occult bleeding, prolongation of bleeding time, leukopenia, thrombocytopenia, anemia, hepatotoxicity, impaired renal function, bronchospasm

**Overdose/Toxicology** Symptoms of overdose include tinnitus, headache, dizziness, confusion, metabolic acidosis, hyperpyrexia, hypoglycemia, and coma. Treatment should be based upon symptomatology.

**Pharmacodynamics/Kinetics**

**Half-life Elimination:** Dose-dependent; 3 hours at low dose, up to 10 hours at higher doses

**Time to Peak:** ~1-2 hours

**Metabolism:** Liver

**Excretion:** Urine

**Duration:** 4-6 hours

**Formulations**

Capsule: 356.4 mg and caffeine 30 mg

Suppository, rectal: 60 mg, 120 mg, 125 mg, 130 mg, 195 mg, 200 mg, 300 mg, 325 mg, 600 mg, 650 mg, 1.2 g

Tablet: 65 mg, 75 mg, 81 mg, 325 mg, 500 mg

Tablet: 400 mg and caffeine 32 mg

Tablet:

- Buffered: 325 mg and magnesium-aluminum hydroxide 150 mg; 325 mg, magnesium hydroxide 75 mg, aluminum hydroxide 75 mg, buffered with calcium carbonate; 325 mg and magnesium-aluminum hydroxide 75 mg
- Chewable: 81 mg
- Controlled release: 800 mg
- Delayed release: 81 mg
- Enteric coated: 81 mg, 325 mg, 500 mg, 650 mg, 975 mg
- Gum: 227.5 mg
- Timed release: 650 mg

**Dosing**

**Adults:**

- Analgesic and antipyretic: Oral, rectal: 325-650 mg every 4-6 hours up to 4 g/day
- Anti-inflammatory: Oral: Initial: 2.4-3.6 g/day in divided doses; usual maintenance: 3.6-5.4 g/day; monitor serum concentrations
- TIA: Oral: 1.3 g/day in 2-4 divided doses
- Myocardial infarction prophylaxis: 160-325 mg/day

**Elderly:** See Geriatric Considerations. Refer to adult dose; adjust if necessary due to decreased renal function.

**Renal Impairment:**

$Cl_{cr}$ <10 mL/minute: Avoid use.

Dialyzable (50% to 100%)

**Hepatic Impairment:** Avoid use in severe liver disease.

**Administration**

**Oral:** Do not crush sustained release or enteric coated tablet. Administer with food or a full glass of water to minimize GI distress.

**Stability**

**Storage:** Keep suppositories in refrigerator; do not freeze. Hydrolysis of aspirin occurs upon exposure to water or moist air, resulting in salicylate and acetate, which possess a vinegar-like odor. Do not use if a strong odor is present.

**Additional Nursing Issues**

**Physical Assessment: Do not use for persons with allergic reaction to salicylate or other NSAIDs** (see Contraindications). Assess other medications patient may be taking for additive or adverse interactions (see Drug Interactions). Do not take longer than 3 days for fever, or 10 days for pain without consulting medical advisor. Monitor therapeutic effectiveness. Monitor for signs of adverse reactions or overdose (see Overdose/Toxicology and Adverse Reactions) at beginning of therapy and periodically with long-term therapy. Assess knowledge/teach patient appropriate use. Teach patient to monitor for adverse reactions, adverse reactions to report, and appropriate interventions to reduce side effects. **Pregnancy risk factor C/D** - see Pregnancy Risk Factor - benefits of use should outweigh possible risks. Note breast-feeding caution.

**Patient Information/Instruction:** If self-administered, use exactly as directed (do not increase dose or frequency); adverse reactions can occur with overuse. Take with food or milk. Do not use aspirin with strong vinegary odor. Do not crush or chew extended release products. While using this medication, avoid alcohol, excessive amounts of vitamin C, or salicylate-containing foods (curry powder, prunes, raisins, tea, or licorice), other prescription or OTC medications containing aspirin or salicylate, or other NSAIDs without consulting prescriber. Maintain adequate hydration (2-3 L/day of fluids unless instructed to restrict fluid intake). You may experience nausea, vomiting, gastric discomfort (frequent mouth care, small frequent meals, sucking lozenges, or chewing gum may help). GI bleeding, ulceration, or perforation can occur with or without pain. May discolor stool (pink/red). Stop taking aspirin and report ringing in ears; persistent pain in stomach; unresolved nausea or vomiting; difficulty breathing or shortness of breath; unusual bruising or bleeding (mouth, urine, stool); or skin rash. **Pregnancy/breast-feeding precautions:** Inform prescriber if you are or intend to be pregnant. Consult prescriber if breast-feeding.

**Geriatric Considerations:** Elderly are at high risk for adverse effects from nonsteroidal anti-inflammatory agents. Elderly with GI complications can develop peptic ulceration and/or hemorrhage asymptomatically. The concomitant use of $H_2$ blockers, omeprazole, and sucralfate is not effective as prophylaxis with the exception of NSAID-induced duodenal ulcers which may be prevented by the use of ranitidine. Misoprostol is the only prophylactic agent proven effective. Also, concomitant disease and drug use contribute to the risk for GI adverse effects. Use lowest effective dose for shortest period possible. Consider renal function decline with age. Use of NSAIDs can compromise existing renal function especially when $Cl_{cr}$ is ≤30 mL/minute. Tinnitus may be a difficult and unreliable indication of toxicity due to age-related hearing loss or eighth cranial nerve damage. CNS adverse effects such as confusion, agitation, and hallucination are generally seen in overdose or high-dose situations, but elderly may demonstrate these adverse effects at lower doses than younger adults.

♦ **Aspirin and Butalbital Compound** *see* Butalbital Compound and Aspirin *on page 176*

## Aspirin and Codeine (AS pir in & KOE deen)

**U.S. Brand Names** Empirin® With Codeine

**Synonyms** Codeine and Aspirin

**Therapeutic Category** Analgesic, Combination (Narcotic)

**Pregnancy Risk Factor** D

**Lactation** Enters breast milk/use caution

**Use** Relief of mild to moderate pain

**Formulations**

Tablet:

#2: Aspirin 325 mg and codeine phosphate 15 mg

#3: Aspirin 325 mg and codeine phosphate 30 mg

#4: Aspirin 325 mg and codeine phosphate 60 mg

**Dosing**

**Adults:** Oral: 1-2 tablets (#3 tablet) every 4-6 hours as needed for pain

**Elderly:** One ASA with codeine 30 mg (#3 tablet), or two ASA with codeine 15 mg (#2 tablet) every 4-6 hours as needed for pain

**Renal Impairment:**

$Cl_{cr}$ 10-50 mL/minute: Administer 75% of dose.

$Cl_{cr}$ <10 mL/minute: Avoid use.

**Hepatic Impairment:** Avoid use in severe liver disease.

**Additional Nursing Issues**

**Physical Assessment:** See individual components listed in Related Information. **Pregnancy risk factor D** - assess knowledge/instruct patient on need to use appropriate contraceptive measures and the need to avoid pregnancy. Note breast-feeding caution.

**Patient Information/Instruction:** See individual components listed in Related Information. **Pregnancy/breast-feeding precautions:** Inform prescriber if you are or intend to be pregnant. Consult prescriber if breast-feeding.

**Related Information**

Aspirin *on page 111*

Codeine *on page 299*

♦ **Aspirin and Hydrocodone** *see* Hydrocodone and Aspirin *on page 570*

## Aspirin and Meprobamate (AS pir in & me proe BA mate)

**U.S. Brand Names** Equagesic®

**Synonyms** Meprobamate and Aspirin

**Therapeutic Category** Antianxiety Agent, Miscellaneous

**Pregnancy Risk Factor** D

**Lactation** Enters breast milk/use caution due to aspirin content

**Use** Adjunct to treatment of skeletal muscular disease in patients exhibiting tension and/or anxiety

**Formulations** Tablet: Aspirin 325 mg and meprobamate 200 mg

(Continued)

## Aspirin and Meprobamate *(Continued)*

**Dosing**

**Adults:** Oral: 1 tablet 3-4 times/day

**Elderly:** Refer to dosing in individual monographs; use with caution.

**Additional Nursing Issues**

**Physical Assessment:** See individual components listed in Related Information. **Pregnancy risk factor D** - assess knowledge/instruct patient on need to use appropriate contraceptive measures and the need to avoid pregnancy. Note breast-feeding caution.

**Patient Information/Instruction:** See individual components listed in Related Information. **Pregnancy/breast-feeding precautions:** Inform prescriber if you are or intend to be pregnant. Consult prescriber if breast-feeding.

**Related Information**

Aspirin *on page 111*
Meprobamate *on page 724*

- **Aspirin and Methocarbamol** *see* Methocarbamol and Aspirin *on page 743*
- **Aspirin and Oxycodone** *see* Oxycodone and Aspirin *on page 873*
- **Aspirin and Propoxyphene** *see* Propoxyphene and Aspirin *on page 985*
- **Aspirin-Free Bayer® Select® Allergy Sinus Caplets** *see page 1294*
- **Aspirin, Orphenadrine, and Caffeine** *see* Orphenadrine, Aspirin, and Caffeine *on page 865*
- **Astemina** *see* Astemizole *on this page*

## Astemizole (a STEM mi zole)

**U.S. Brand Names** Hismanal®

**Therapeutic Category** Antihistamine

**Pregnancy Risk Factor** C

**Lactation** Excretion in breast milk unknown/not recommended

**Use** Perennial and seasonal allergic rhinitis and other allergic symptoms including urticaria

**Mechanism of Action/Effect** Competes with histamine for $H_1$-receptor sites on effector cells in the GI tract, blood vessels, and respiratory tract; binds to lung receptors significantly greater than it binds to cerebellar receptors, resulting in a reduced sedative potential

**Contraindications** Hypersensitivity to astemizole or any component; hepatic dysfunction; concomitant administration of erythromycin, ketoconazole, fluconazole, itraconazole, mibefradil, or clarithromycin with astemizole has severe cardiovascular effects including Q-T interval prolongation, ventricular tachycardia, ventricular fibrillation, death, cardiac arrest, hypotension, and palpitations

**Warnings** Use with caution in patients receiving drugs which prolong QRS or Q-T interval. Rare cases of severe cardiovascular events (cardiac arrest, arrhythmias) have been reported in the following situations: overdose (even as low as 20-30 mg/day) when used in combination with erythromycin, ketoconazole, or itraconazole. Pregnancy factor C.

**Drug Interactions**

**Cytochrome P-450 Effect:** CYP3A3/4 enzyme substrate

**Increased Effect/Toxicity:** Erythromycin, troleandomycin, ciprofloxacin, cimetidine, itraconazole, ketoconazole, fluconazole, miconazole, clarithromycin, quinine (doses >430 mg/day), indinavir, ritonavir, saquinavir, nelfinavir, fluoxetine, fluvoxamine, sertraline, mibefradil, paroxetine, nefazodone, zileuton, and disulfiram reduce hepatic metabolism which has resulted in severe, life-threatening cardiac arrhythmias (See Contraindications). Additive CNS depression with other CNS depressants, alcohol, or procarbazine. Prolonged anticholinergic effects with MAO inhibitors.

**Food Interactions** Astemizole bioavailability may be decreased if taken with food. Do not take with grapefruit juice.

**Adverse Reactions**

1% to 10%:

Central nervous system: Drowsiness, headache, fatigue, nervousness, dizziness

Gastrointestinal: Appetite increase, weight increase, nausea, diarrhea, abdominal pain, dry mouth

Neuromuscular & skeletal: Arthralgia

Respiratory: Pharyngitis

<1% (Limited to important or life-threatening symptoms): Palpitations, edema, depression, angioedema, hepatitis, bronchospasm, epistaxis

**Overdose/Toxicology** Symptoms of overdose include sedation, apnea, diminished mental alertness, ventricular tachycardia, and torsade de pointes. There is no specific treatment for antihistamine overdose. Clinical toxicity is due to blockade of cholinergic receptors. For anticholinergic overdose with severe life-threatening symptoms, physostigmine 1-2 mg S.C. or I.V. slowly, may be given to reverse these effects. Treat symptomatically.

**Pharmacodynamics/Kinetics**

**Protein Binding:** 97%

**Half-life Elimination:** 7-11 days

**Time to Peak:** Oral: Peak plasma levels appear in 1-4 hours following administration

**Metabolism:** Liver

**Excretion:** Feces and urine

**Onset:** <24 hours, but may take 2-3 days; Peak effect: 9-12 days

**Duration:** Long-acting, with steady-state plasma levels seen within 4-8 weeks following initiation of chronic therapy

**Formulations** Tablet: 10 mg

**Dosing**

**Adults:** Oral: 10-30 mg/day; give 30 mg on first day, 20 mg on second day, then 10 mg/day in a single dose

**Elderly:** Oral: 10 mg/day

**Administration**

**Oral:** Give on an empty stomach.

**Additional Nursing Issues**

**Physical Assessment:** Assess effectiveness and interactions of other medications (see Drug Interactions). See Contraindications and Warnings/Precautions for cautious use. Monitor effectiveness of therapy and adverse reactions (eg, excess anticholinergic effects - see Adverse Reactions) at beginning of therapy and periodically with long-term use. Assess knowledge/teach patient appropriate use, interventions to reduce side effects, and adverse symptoms to report. **Pregnancy risk factor C** - benefits of use should outweigh possible risks. Breast-feeding is not recommended.

**Patient Information/Instruction:** Notify prescriber if taking any cardiac medication. Take as directed; do not exceed recommended dose. Take on an empty stomach (1 hour before or 2 hours after meals). Avoid use of other depressants, alcohol, or sleep-inducing medications unless approved by prescriber. You may experience drowsiness or dizziness (use caution when driving or engaging in tasks requiring alertness until response to drug is known); dry nasal membranes (use of humidifier may help); or dry mouth, abdominal pain, or nausea (frequent small meals, frequent mouth care, chewing gum, or sucking hard candy may help). Report persistent sedation, depression, or agitation; difficulty breathing or expectorating (thick secretions); tremors or loss of coordination; lack of improvement or worsening or condition. **Pregnancy/breast-feeding precautions:** Inform prescriber if you are or intend to be pregnant. Breast-feeding is not recommended.

**Geriatric Considerations:** Because of its low incidence of sedation and anticholinergic effects, astemizole would be a rational choice in the elderly when an antihistamine is indicated.


- ♦ **AsthmaHaler®** *see* Epinephrine *on page 424*
- ♦ **AsthmaNefrin® [OTC]** *see* Epinephrine *on page 424*
- ♦ **Astramorph™ PF Injection** *see* Morphine Sulfate *on page 790*
- ♦ **Atacand®** *see* Candesartan *on page 188*
- ♦ **Atarax®** *see* Hydroxyzine *on page 588*
- ♦ **Atasol®** *see* Acetaminophen *on page 32*
- ♦ **Atasol® 8, 15, 30 With Caffeine** *see* Acetaminophen and Codeine *on page 34*
- ♦ **Atemperator-S®** *see* Valproic Acid and Derivatives *on page 1198*


## Atenolol (a TEN oh lole)

**U.S. Brand Names** Tenormin®

**Therapeutic Category** Beta Blocker, $Beta_1$ Selective

**Pregnancy Risk Factor** D

**Lactation** Enters breast milk/use caution (AAP rates "compatible")

**Use** Treatment of hypertension, alone or in combination with other agents; management of angina pectoris, postmyocardial infarction patients

**Unlabeled use:** Acute alcohol withdrawal, supraventricular and ventricular arrhythmias, and migraine headache prophylaxis

**Mechanism of Action/Effect** Competitively blocks response to beta-adrenergic stimulation, selectively blocks $beta_1$-receptors with little or no effect on $beta_2$-receptors except at high doses

**Contraindications** Hypersensitivity to beta-blocking agents; pulmonary edema; cardiogenic shock; bradycardia; heart block without a pacemaker; uncompensated congestive heart failure; sinus node dysfunction; A-V conduction abnormalities; pregnancy

**Warnings** Administer with caution to patients (especially the elderly) with bronchospastic disease, CHF, renal dysfunction, severe peripheral vascular disease, myasthenia gravis, diabetes mellitus, or hyperthyroidism. **Abrupt withdrawal of the drug should be avoided.** Drug should be discontinued over 1-2 weeks. Beta-blockers may impair glucose tolerance, potentiate hypoglycemia, and/or mask signs or symptoms of hypoglycemia in a diabetic patient. Modify dosage in patients with renal impairment.

**Drug Interactions**

**Decreased Effect:** Decreased effect of beta-blockers with aluminum salts, barbiturates, calcium salts, cholestyramine, colestipol, NSAIDs, penicillins (ampicillin), rifampin, salicylates, and sulfinpyrazone due to decreased bioavailability and plasma levels. Beta-blockers may decrease the effect of sulfonylureas.

**Increased Effect/Toxicity:** Beta-blockers may increase the effect/toxicity of flecainide, haloperidol (hypotensive effects), phenothiazines, clonidine (hypertensive crisis after or during withdrawal of either agent), and epinephrine (initial hypertensive episode followed by bradycardia). Calcium channel blockers may have an additive effect when taken with atenolol. Beta-blockers may affect the action or levels of ethanol, disopyramide, nondepolarizing muscle relaxants although the effects are difficult to predict.

**Food Interactions** Atenolol serum concentrations may be decreased if taken with food.

**Effects on Lab Values** ↑ glucose; ↓ HDL

**Adverse Reactions**

1% to 10%:

Cardiovascular: Persistent bradycardia, hypotension, chest pain, edema, heart failure, second or third degree A-V block, Raynaud's phenomenon

(Continued)

## Atenolol *(Continued)*

Central nervous system: Dizziness, fatigue, insomnia, lethargy, confusion, mental impairment, depression, headache, nightmares

Gastrointestinal: Constipation, diarrhea, nausea

Genitourinary: Impotence

Miscellaneous: Cold extremities

<1% (Limited to important or life-threatening symptoms): Dyspnea (especially with large doses), wheezing

**Overdose/Toxicology** Symptoms of toxicity include lethargy, respiratory drive disorder, wheezing, sinus pause and bradycardia. Additional effects associated with any beta-blocker are congestive heart failure, hypotension, bronchospasm, and hypoglycemia. Treatment includes removal of unabsorbed drug by induced emesis, gastric lavage, or administration of activated charcoal and symptomatic treatment of toxic responses. Atenolol can be removed by hemodialysis.

**Pharmacodynamics/Kinetics**

**Protein Binding:** Low at 3% to 15%

**Distribution:** Low lipophilicity; does **not** cross the blood-brain barrier

**Half-life Elimination:** Normal renal function: 6-9 hours (prolonged in renal impairment); End-stage renal disease: 15-35 hours

**Time to Peak:** Oral: Within 1-2 hours; I.V.: More rapid

**Metabolism:** Liver

**Excretion:** Feces and urine

**Duration:** 12-24 hours (normal renal function)

**Formulations**

Injection: 0.5 mg/mL (10 mL)

Tablet: 25 mg, 50 mg, 100 mg

**Dosing**

**Adults:**

Oral:

Hypertension: 50 mg once daily, may increase to 100 mg/day; doses >100 mg are unlikely to produce any further benefit

Angina pectoris: 50 mg once daily, may increase to 100 mg/day; some patients may require 200 mg/day

Postmyocardial infarction: Follow I.V. dose with 100 mg/day or 50 mg twice daily for 6-9 days postmyocardial infarction

I.V.: Postmyocardial infarction: Early treatment: 5 mg slow I.V. over 5 minutes; may repeat in 10 minutes; if both doses are tolerated, may start oral atenolol 50 mg every 12 hours or 100 mg/day for 6-9 days postmyocardial infarction

**Elderly:** Refer to adult dosing.

**Renal Impairment:**

$Cl_{cr}$ 15-35 mL/minute: Administer 50 mg/day maximum.

$Cl_{cr}$ <15 mL/minute: Administer 50 mg every other day maximum.

Hemodialysis effects: Moderately dialyzable (20% to 50%) via hemodialysis; administer dose postdialysis or administer 25-50 mg supplemental dose. Elimination is not enhanced with peritoneal dialysis. Supplemental dose is not necessary.

**Administration**

**I.V.:** Administer I.V. at 1 mg/minute. **Intravenous administration requires a cardiac and blood pressure monitor.**

**Additional Nursing Issues**

**Physical Assessment:** I.V. requires continuous cardiac and hemodynamic monitoring.

Oral: Assess other medications the patient may taking for effectiveness and interactions (see Drug Interactions). Assess blood pressure and heart rate prior to and following first dose, any change in dosage, and periodically thereafter. Monitor or advise patient to monitor weight and fluid balance (I & O), assess for signs of CHF (edema, new cough or dyspnea, unresolved fatigue), and assess therapeutic effectiveness. Monitor serum glucose levels of diabetic patients since beta-blockers may alter glucose tolerance. Use/teach postural hypotension precautions.

**Pregnancy risk factor D** - assess knowledge/instruct patient on need to use appropriate contraceptive measures and the need to avoid pregnancy. Note breast-feeding caution.

**Patient Information/Instruction:** Take exactly as directed. Do not increase, decrease, or adjust dosage without consulting prescriber. Take pulse daily, prior to medication and follow prescriber's instruction about holding medication. Do not take with antacids. Do not use alcohol or OTC medications (eg, cold remedies) without consulting prescriber. If diabetic, monitor serum sugars closely (may alter glucose tolerance or mask signs of hypoglycemia). May cause fatigue, dizziness, or postural hypotension; use caution when changing position from lying or sitting to standing, when driving, or when climbing stairs until response to medication is known. May cause alteration in sexual performance (reversible). Report unresolved swelling of extremities, difficulty breathing or new cough, unresolved fatigue, unusual weight gain, unresolved constipation, or unusual muscle weakness. **Pregnancy/breast-feeding precautions:** Use appropriate contraceptive measures; do not get pregnant while taking this drug. Consult prescriber if breast-feeding.

**Geriatric Considerations:** Due to alterations in the beta-adrenergic autonomic nervous system, beta-adrenergic blockade may result in less hemodynamic response than seen in younger adults.

**Related Information**

Beta-Blockers Comparison *on page 1376*

## Atenolol and Chlorthalidone (a TEN oh lole & klor THAL i done)

**U.S. Brand Names** Tenoretic®

**Synonyms** Chlorthalidone and Atenolol

**Therapeutic Category** Antihypertensive Agent, Combination

**Pregnancy Risk Factor** D

**Lactation** Excretion in breast milk unknown

**Use** Treatment of hypertension with a cardioselective beta-blocker and a diuretic

**Formulations**

Tablet:

50: Atenolol 50 mg and chlorthalidone 25 mg

100: Atenolol 100 mg and chlorthalidone 25 mg

**Dosing**

**Adults:** Initial: 1 (50) tablet once daily, then individualize dose until optimal dose is achieved

**Elderly:** Refer to adult dosing.

**Renal Impairment:**

$Cl_{cr}$ 15-35 mL/minute: Administer 50 mg/day.

$Cl_{cr}$ <15 mL/minute: Administer 50 mg every other day.

**Additional Nursing Issues**

**Physical Assessment:** See individual components listed in Related Information. **Pregnancy risk factor D** - assess knowledge/instruct patient on need to use appropriate contraceptive measures and the need to avoid pregnancy. Note breast-feeding caution.

**Patient Information/Instruction:** See individual components listed in Related Information. **Pregnancy/breast-feeding precautions:** Inform prescriber if you are or intend to be pregnant. Consult prescriber if breast-feeding.

**Related Information**

Atenolol *on page 115*

Chlorthalidone *on page 260*

- **ATG** *see* Lymphocyte Immune Globulin *on page 700*
- **Atgam®** *see* Lymphocyte Immune Globulin *on page 700*
- **Atiflan** *see* Naproxen *on page 807*
- **ATIII** *see* Antithrombin III *on page 101*
- **Atiquim®** *see* Naproxen *on page 807*
- **Atisuril®** *see* Allopurinol *on page 53*
- **Ativan®** *see* Lorazepam *on page 691*
- **ATnativ®** *see* Antithrombin III *on page 101*
- **Atolone®** *see* Triamcinolone *on page 1171*

## Atorvastatin (a TORE va sta tin)

**U.S. Brand Names** Lipitor®

**Therapeutic Category** Antilipemic Agent (HMG-CoA Reductase Inhibitor)

**Pregnancy Risk Factor** X

**Lactation** Enters breast milk/contraindicated

**Use** Adjunct to diet for the reduction of elevated total and LDL cholesterol, apolipoprotein B, and triglyceride levels in patients with hypercholesterolemia (Type IIA, IIB, and IIC); adjunctive therapy to diet for treatment of elevated serum triglyceride levels (Type IV); treatment of primary dysbetalipoproteinemia (Type III) in patients who do not respond adequately to diet. Also may be used in hypercholesterolemic patients without clinically evident heart disease to reduce the risk of myocardial infarction, to reduce the risk for revascularization, and reduce the risk of death due to cardiovascular causes

**Mechanism of Action/Effect** Inhibitor of 3-hydroxy-3-methylglutaryl coenzyme A (HMG-CoA) reductase, the rate limiting enzyme in cholesterol synthesis (reduces the production of mevalonic acid from HMG-CoA); this then results in a compensatory increase in the expression of LDL receptors on hepatocyte membranes and a stimulation of LDL catabolism

**Contraindications** Hypersensitivity to atorvastatin or any component (may have cross-sensitivity with other HMG-CoA reductase inhibitors); patients with active liver disease; pregnancy

**Warnings** Discontinue therapy if symptoms of myopathy or renal failure due to rhabdomyolysis develop. Use with caution in patients with history of liver disease or who consume excessive amounts of alcohol.

**Drug Interactions**

**Cytochrome P-450 Effect:** CYP3A3/4 enzyme substrate

**Decreased Effect:** Colestipol, antacids decreased plasma concentrations but effect on LDL cholesterol was not altered.

**Increased Effect/Toxicity:** Gemfibrozil, azole antifungals, clofibrate, niacin, erythromycin, cyclosporine (musculoskeletal effects such as myopathy, myalgia and/or muscle weakness accompanied by markedly elevated CK concentrations, rash and/or pruritus). Increased effect/toxicity of levothyroxine. Digoxin levels may be increased by 20%. Concentrations of norethindrone (30%) and ethinyl estradiol (20%) may be increased.

**Adverse Reactions**

1% to 10%:

Cardiovascular: Chest pain

(Continued)

## Atorvastatin *(Continued)*

Central nervous system: Headache, insomnia, dizziness
Gastrointestinal: Diarrhea, flatulence, abdominal pain (2% to 3%), nausea
Genitourinary: Urinary tract infection
Neuromuscular & skeletal: Myalgia (1% to 5%)
Respiratory: Bronchitis, rhinitis

<1% (Limited to important or life-threatening symptoms): Euphoria, mild confusion, impaired short-term memory, mild LFT increases, rhabdomyolysis, angioneurotic edema, anaphylaxis, photosensitivity, pancreatitis

**Overdose/Toxicology** Few symptoms are anticipated. Treatment is supportive.

**Pharmacodynamics/Kinetics**

**Protein Binding:** 98%

**Half-life Elimination:** 14 hours (parent)

**Time to Peak:** Serum concentration: 1-2 hours

**Metabolism:** Liver

**Excretion:** Urine

**Onset:** Maximal reduction in plasma cholesterol and triglycerides in 2 weeks; initial changes in 3-5 days

**Formulations** Tablet: 10 mg, 20 mg, 40 mg

**Dosing**

**Adults:** Oral: Initial: 10 mg once daily; titrate up to 80 mg/day if needed.

**Elderly:** Refer to adult dosing.

**Renal Impairment:** No dosage adjustment necessary.

**Hepatic Impairment:** Decrease dosage with severe disease (eg, chronic alcoholic liver disease).

**Monitoring Laboratory Tests** Monitor lipid levels after 2-4 weeks; LFTs prior to initiation and 12 weeks after initiation or first dose or dose elevation, and periodically (semiannually) thereafter; CPK

**Additional Nursing Issues**

**Physical Assessment:** Monitor lab results prior to beginning therapy, at 6 and 12 weeks after initiating dose, and periodically during long-term therapy. Monitor for adverse effects and instruct patient what adverse effects to report. **Pregnancy risk factor X** - determine that patient is not pregnant before starting therapy. Do not give to sexually active patients (male or female) of childbearing age unless capable of complying with barrier contraceptive use. Breast-feeding is contraindicated.

**Patient Information/Instruction:** May take with meals at any time of day. Maintain adequate hydration (2-3 L/day of fluids unless instructed to restrict fluid intake). You will need laboratory evaluation during therapy. May cause headache (mild analgesic may help); diarrhea (yogurt or buttermilk may help); euphoria, giddiness, confusion (use caution when driving or engaging in tasks that require alertness until response to medication is known). Report unresolved diarrhea, excessive or acute muscle cramping or weakness, changes in mood or memory, yellowing of skin or eyes, easy bruising or bleeding, and unusual fatigue. **Pregnancy/breast-feeding precautions:** Inform prescriber if you are pregnant. Do not get pregnant or engage in sexual activity with women of childbearing age during therapy and for 1 month following therapy unless using barrier contraceptive measures. This drug can cause severe fetal defects. Do not donate blood for same period of time. Do not breast-feed.

**Dietary Issues:** Before initiation of therapy, patients should be placed on a standard cholesterol-lowering diet for 3-6 months and the diet should be continued during drug therapy.

**Geriatric Considerations:** The definition of and, therefore, when to treat hyperlipidemia in the elderly is a controversial issue. The National Cholesterol Education Program recommends that all adults 20 years of age and older maintain a plasma cholesterol <200 mg/dL. By this definition, 60% of all elderly would be considered to have a borderline high (200-239 mg/dL) or high (≥240 mg/dL) plasma cholesterol. However, plasma cholesterol has been shown to be a less reliable predictor of coronary heart disease in the elderly. Therefore, it is the authors' belief that pharmacologic treatment be reserved for those who are unable to obtain a desirable plasma cholesterol level by diet alone and for whom the benefits of treatment are believed to outweigh the potential adverse effects, drug interactions, and cost of treatment.

**Related Information**

Lipid-Lowering Agents Comparison *on page 1393*

## Atovaquone (a TOE va kwone)

**U.S. Brand Names** Mepron™

**Therapeutic Category** Antiprotozoal

**Pregnancy Risk Factor** C

**Lactation** Excretion in breast milk unknown/use caution

**Use** Acute oral treatment of mild to moderate *Pneumocystis carinii* pneumonia (PCP) in patients who are intolerant to co-trimoxazole; prevention of PCP in patients who are intolerant of co-trimoxazole. Also has been used for treatment/suppression of *Toxoplasma gondii* encephalitis, primary prophylaxis of HIV-infected persons at high risk for developing *Toxoplasma gondii* encephalitis

**Mechanism of Action/Effect** Has not been fully elucidated; may inhibit electron transport in mitochondria inhibiting metabolic enzymes

**Contraindications** Life-threatening allergic reaction to the drug or formulation

**Warnings** Has only been used in mild to moderate PCP. Use with caution in elderly patients due to potentially impaired renal, hepatic, and cardiac function. Pregnancy factor C.

**Drug Interactions**

**Decreased Effect:** Rifamycins (rifampin) used concurrently decreases the steady-state plasma concentrations of atovaquone.

**Increased Effect/Toxicity:** Possible increased toxicity with other highly protein-bound drugs.

**Adverse Reactions**

>10%:

Central nervous system: Headache, fever, insomnia, anxiety
Dermatologic: Rash
Gastrointestinal: Nausea, diarrhea, vomiting
Respiratory: Cough

1% to 10%:

Central nervous system: Dizziness
Dermatologic: Pruritus
Endocrine & metabolic: Hypoglycemia, hyponatremia
Gastrointestinal: Abdominal pain, constipation, anorexia, heartburn
Hematologic: Anemia, neutropenia, leukopenia
Hepatic: Elevated amylase and liver enzymes
Neuromuscular & skeletal: Weakness
Renal: Elevated BUN/creatinine
Respiratory: Cough
Miscellaneous: Oral *Monilia*

**Pharmacodynamics/Kinetics**

**Protein Binding:** >99.9%

**Distribution:** Enterohepatically recirculated

**Half-life Elimination:** 2.9 days

**Metabolism:** Liver

**Excretion:** Feces

**Formulations** Suspension, oral (citrus flavor): 750 mg/5 mL (210 mL)

**Dosing**

**Adults:** Oral: 750 mg 2 times/day with food for 21 days

**Elderly:** Refer to adult dosing.

**Stability**

**Storage:** Do not freeze.

**Additional Nursing Issues**

**Physical Assessment:** Monitor for CNS and respiratory changes, patient knowledge of adverse reactions (see above). Assess for interactions with other prescription or OTC medications (see above). **Pregnancy risk factor C** - benefits of use should outweigh possible risks. Note breast-feeding caution.

**Patient Information/Instruction:** Take as directed. Take with high-fat meals. You may experience dizziness or lightheadedness; use caution when driving or engaging in tasks that require alertness until response to drug is known. Small meals may help reduce nausea. Report unresolved diarrhea, fever, mouth sores (use good mouth care), unresolved headache or vomiting. **Pregnancy/breast-feeding precautions:** Inform prescriber if you are or intend to be pregnant. Consult prescriber if breast-feeding.

- **Atozine®** *see* Hydroxyzine *on page 588*
- **Atridox™** *see* Doxycycline *on page 406*
- **Atromid-S®** *see* Clofibrate *on page 285*
- **Atropair®** *see page 1282*
- **Atropair® Ophthalmic** *see* Atropine *on this page*

## Atropine (A troe peen)

**U.S. Brand Names** Atropair® Ophthalmic; Atropine-Care® Ophthalmic; Atropisol® Ophthalmic; Isopto® Atropine Ophthalmic; I-Tropine® Ophthalmic; Ocu-Tropine® Ophthalmic

**Therapeutic Category** Anticholinergic Agent; Anticholinergic Agent, Ophthalmic; Antidote; Antispasmodic Agent, Gastrointestinal; Ophthalmic Agent, Mydriatic

**Pregnancy Risk Factor** C

**Lactation** Enters breast milk (trace amounts)/use caution (AAP rates "compatible")

**Use** Preoperative medication to inhibit salivation and secretions; treatment of sinus bradycardia; treatment of exercise-induced bronchospasm; antidote for organophosphate pesticide poisoning; to produce mydriasis and cycloplegia for examination of the retina and optic disc and accurate measurement of refractive errors; uveitis

**Mechanism of Action/Effect** Blocks the action of acetylcholine at parasympathetic sites in smooth muscle, secretory glands and the CNS; increases cardiac output, dries secretions, antagonizes histamine and serotonin

**Contraindications** Hypersensitivity to atropine sulfate or any component; narrow-angle glaucoma; tachycardia; thyrotoxicosis; obstructive disease of the GI tract; obstructive uropathy

**Warnings** Use with caution in elderly patients. Low doses cause a paradoxical decrease in heart rates. Some commercial products contain sodium metabisulfite, which can cause allergic-type reactions. May accumulate with multiple inhalational administration, particularly in the elderly. Heat prostration may occur in hot weather. Use with caution in patients with autonomic neuropathy, prostatic hypertrophy, hyperthyroidism, congestive
(Continued)

## Atropine *(Continued)*

heart failure, cardiac arrhythmias, chronic lung disease, or biliary tract disease. Anticholinergic agents are generally not well tolerated in the elderly and their use should be avoided when possible. Atropine is rarely used except as a preoperative agent or in the acute treatment of bradyarrhythmias. Pregnancy factor C.

**Drug Interactions**

**Decreased Effect:** Phenothiazines, levodopa, antihistamines with cholinergic mechanisms decrease anticholinergic effects of atropine.

**Increased Effect/Toxicity:** Amantadine increases anticholinergic effects.

**Adverse Reactions**

>10%:
- Dermatologic: Dry, hot skin
- Gastrointestinal: Impaired GI motility, constipation, dry throat, dry mouth
- Local: Irritation at injection site
- Respiratory: Dry nose
- Miscellaneous: Sweating (decreased)

1% to 10%:
- Dermatologic: Increased sensitivity to light
- Endocrine & metabolic: Decreased flow of breast milk
- Gastrointestinal: Dysphagia

<1% (Limited to important or life-threatening symptoms): Orthostatic hypotension, tachycardia, palpitations, ventricular fibrillation, confusion, drowsiness, ataxia, fatigue, delirium, headache, loss of memory, restlessness, elderly may be at increased risk for confusion and hallucinations, increased intraocular pain, blurred vision, mydriasis

**Overdose/Toxicology** Symptoms of overdose include dilated, unreactive pupils; blurred vision; hot, dry flushed skin; dryness of mucous membranes; difficulty swallowing; foul breath; diminished or absent bowel sounds; urinary retention; tachycardia; hyperthermia; hypertension; and increased respiratory rate. For anticholinergic overdose with severe life-threatening symptoms, physostigmine 1-2 mg S.C. or I.V. slowly, may be given to reverse these effects.

**Pharmacodynamics/Kinetics**

**Distribution:** Widely distributes throughout the body; crosses the placenta; crosses the blood-brain barrier

**Half-life Elimination:** 2-3 hours

**Metabolism:** Liver

**Excretion:** Urine

**Onset:** I.V.: Rapid

**Formulations**

Atropine sulfate:
- Injection: 0.1 mg/mL (5 mL, 10 mL); 0.3 mg/mL (1 mL, 30 mL); 0.4 mg/mL (1 mL, 20 mL, 30 mL); 0.5 mg/mL (1 mL, 5 mL, 30 mL); 0.8 mg/mL (0.5 mL, 1 mL); 1 mg/mL (1 mL, 10 mL)
- Ointment, ophthalmic: 0.5%, 1% (3.5 g)
- Solution, ophthalmic: 0.5% (1 mL, 5 mL); 1% (1 mL, 2 mL, 5 mL, 15 mL); 2% (1 mL, 2 mL); 3% (5 mL)
- Tablet: 0.4 mg

**Dosing**

**Adults:** Doses <0.5 mg have been associated with paradoxical bradycardia.
- Asystole: I.V.: 1 mg; may repeat every 3-5 minutes as needed; may give intratracheal in 1 mg/10 mL dilution only, intratracheal dose should be 2-2.5 times the I.V. dose.
- Preanesthetic: I.M., I.V., S.C.: 0.4-0.6 mg 30-60 minutes preop and repeat every 4-6 hours as needed.
- Bradycardia: I.V.: 0.5-1 mg every 5 minutes, not to exceed a total of 3 mg or 0.04 mg/kg; may give intratracheal in 1 mg/10 mL dilution only, intratracheal dose should be 2-2.5 times the I.V. dose.
- Neuromuscular blockade reversal: I.V.: 25-30 mcg/kg 30 seconds before neostigmine or 10 mcg/kg 30 seconds before edrophonium
- Organophosphate or carbamate poisoning: I.V.: 1-2 mg/dose every 10-20 minutes until atropine effect (dry flushed skin, tachycardia, mydriasis, fever) is observed, then every 1-4 hours for at least 24 hours; up to 50 mg in first 24 hours and 2 g over several days may be given in cases of severe intoxication.
- Bronchospasm: Inhalation: 0.025-0.05 mg/kg/dose every 4-6 hours as needed (maximum: 5 mg/dose)
- Ophthalmic solution: 1%: Instill 1-2 drops 1 hour before the procedure.
- Uveitis: Instill 1-2 drops 4 times/day.
- Ophthalmic ointment: Apply a small amount in the conjunctival sac up to 3 times/day. Compress the lacrimal sac by digital pressure for 1-3 minutes after instillation.

**Elderly:** Refer to adult dosing.

**Stability**

**Storage:** Store injection at <40°C; avoid freezing.

**Compatibility:** See the Compatibility of Drugs Chart *on page 1315* and the Compatibility of Drugs in Syringe Chart *on page 1317*.

**Additional Nursing Issues**

**Physical Assessment:** Assess other medications patient may be taking for effectiveness and interactions (see Warnings/Precautions and Drug Interactions).

Systemic administration: Monitor therapeutic response and adverse reactions (see above), ensure patient safety (side rails up, call light within reach), have patient void prior to administration, and ensure adequate hydration and environmental temperature control.

Oral, ophthalmic: Monitor therapeutic response according to purpose for use, adverse response (eg, acute atropine toxicity - see Warnings/Precautions, Adverse Reactions, and Overdose/Toxicology). Assess knowledge/teach patient appropriate use, interventions to reduce side effects, and adverse symptoms to report. **Pregnancy risk factor C** - benefits of use should outweigh possible risks. See breast-feeding caution. (Systemic effects have been reported following ophthalmic administration.)

**Patient Information/Instruction:** Take exactly as directed, 30 minutes before meals. Maintain adequate hydration (2-3 L/day of fluids unless instructed to restrict fluid intake). Void before taking medication. You may experience dizziness, blurred vision, sensitivity to light (use caution when driving or engaging in tasks requiring alertness until response to drug is known); dry mouth, nausea, or vomiting (small frequent meals, frequent mouth care, sucking lozenges, or chewing gum may help); orthostatic hypotension (use caution when climbing stairs and when rising from lying or sitting position); constipation (increased exercise, fluid, or dietary fiber may reduce constipation, if not effective consult prescriber); increased sensitivity to heat and decreased perspiration (avoid extremes of heat, reduce exercise in hot weather); decreased milk if breast-feeding. Report hot, dry, flushed skin; blurred vision or vision changes; difficulty swallowing; chest pain, palpitations, or rapid heartbeat; painful or difficult urination; increased confusion, depression, or loss of memory; rapid or difficult respirations; muscle weakness or tremors; or eye pain.

Ophthalmic: Instill as often as recommended. Wash hands before using. Sit or lie down, open eye, look at ceiling, and instill prescribed amount of solution. Do not blink for 30 seconds, close eye and roll eye in all directions, and apply gentle pressure to inner corner of eye for 1-2 minutes. Do not let tip of applicator touch eye or contaminate tip of applicator. Temporary stinging or blurred vision may occur.

**Pregnancy/breast-feeding precautions:** Inform prescriber if you are or intend to be pregnant. Consult prescriber if breast-feeding.

**Geriatric Considerations:** Anticholinergic agents are generally not well tolerated in the elderly and their use should be avoided when possible (see Warnings/Precautions, Adverse Reactions). In the elderly, anticholinergic agents should not be used as prophylaxis against extrapyramidal symptoms.

**Additional Information** Some formulations may contain sulfites.

**Related Information**

Ophthalmic Agents *on page 1282*


- **Atropine and Difenoxin** *see* Difenoxin and Atropine *on page 367*
- **Atropine and Diphenoxylate** *see* Diphenoxylate and Atropine *on page 382*
- **Atropine-Care®** *see page 1282*
- **Atropine-Care® Ophthalmic** *see* Atropine *on page 119*
- **Atropine, Hyoscyamine, Scopolamine, and Phenobarbital** *see* Hyoscyamine, Atropine, Scopolamine, and Phenobarbital *on page 591*
- **Atropisol®** *see page 1282*
- **Atropisol® Ophthalmic** *see* Atropine *on page 119*
- **Atrovent®** *see* Ipratropium *on page 621*
- **Attapulgite** *see page 1294*
- **Attenuvax®** *see page 1256*
- **Augmentin®** *see* Amoxicillin and Clavulanate Potassium *on page 82*
- **Auralgan Otic®** *see page 1291*


## Auranofin (au RANE oh fin)

**U.S. Brand Names** Ridaura®

**Therapeutic Category** Gold Compound

**Pregnancy Risk Factor** C

**Lactation** Enters breast milk/contraindicated

**Use** Management of active stage of classic or definite rheumatoid arthritis in patients that do not respond to or tolerate other agents; psoriatic arthritis; adjunct or alternative therapy for pemphigus

**Mechanism of Action/Effect** Gold is taken up by macrophages which results in inhibition of phagocytosis and lysosomal membrane stabilization; other actions observed are decreased serum rheumatoid factor and alterations in immunoglobulins. Additionally, complement activation is decreased, prostaglandin synthesis is inhibited, and lysosomal enzyme activity is decreased.

**Contraindications** Renal disease; history of blood dyscrasias; congestive heart failure; exfoliative dermatitis; necrotizing enterocolitis; history of anaphylactic reactions; diabetics

**Warnings** Therapy should be discontinued if platelet count falls to <100,000/mm$^3$, WBC <4000, granulocytes <1500/mm$^3$. Explain the possibility of adverse effects and their manifestations before initiating therapy. Use with caution in patients with renal or hepatic impairment. Pregnancy factor C.

**Drug Interactions**

**Decreased Effect:** One case report of elevated phenytoin levels when taken concomitantly.

**Effects on Lab Values** May enhance the response to a tuberculin skin test

**Adverse Reactions**

>10%:

Dermatologic: Itching, rash

Gastrointestinal: Stomatitis, abdominal or stomach cramps, bloated feeling, anorexia, diarrhea, nausea

(Continued)

## Auranofin *(Continued)*

Ocular: Conjunctivitis
Renal: Proteinuria

1% to 10%:

Dermatologic: Urticaria, alopecia
Gastrointestinal: Glossitis, constipation, change in taste
Hematologic: Eosinophilia, leukopenia, thrombocytopenia
Renal: Hematuria

<1% (Limited to important or life-threatening symptoms): Angioedema, ulcerative enterocolitis, GI hemorrhage, gingivitis, dysphagia, metallic taste, agranulocytosis, anemia, aplastic anemia, hepatotoxicity, peripheral neuropathy, interstitial pneumonitis

**Overdose/Toxicology** Symptoms of overdose include hematuria, proteinuria, fever, nausea, vomiting, and diarrhea. Signs of gold toxicity include decrease in hemoglobin, leukocytes, granulocytes, and platelets; proteinuria; hematuria; pruritus; stomatitis; or persistent diarrhea. Metallic taste may indicate stomatitis.

For treatment of mild gold poisoning, dimercaprol 2.5 mg/kg 4 times/day for 2 days, or for more severe forms of gold intoxication, dimercaprol 3 mg/kg every 4 hours for 2 days, should be initiated. After 2 days the initial dose should be repeated twice daily on the third day, and once daily thereafter for 10 days. Other chelating agents have been used with some success.

**Pharmacodynamics/Kinetics**

**Protein Binding:** 60% (82% of binding is to albumin)

**Distribution:** Not well defined, penetrates into synovial fluid, associated with circulating red blood cells

**Half-life Elimination:** Serum: 11-23 days; biologic 30-78 days (longer in chronic dosing)

**Time to Peak:** 2 hours

**Excretion:** Urine (15%) and feces (85% over 6 months)

**Onset:** Delayed; may require as long as 3 months

**Duration:** Prolonged

**Formulations** Capsule: 3 mg [gold 29%]

**Dosing**

**Adults:** Oral: 6 mg/day in 1-2 divided doses; after 3 months may be increased to 9 mg/day in 3 divided doses; if still no response after 3 months at 9 mg/day, discontinue drug

**Elderly:** Refer to adult dosing.

**Renal Impairment:**

$Cl_{cr}$ 50-80 mL/minute: Reduce dose to 50%.
$Cl_{cr}$ <50 mL/minute: Avoid use.

**Stability**

**Storage:** Store in tight, light-resistant containers at 15°C to 30°C.

**Monitoring Laboratory Tests** CBC with differential, platelet count, urinalysis, baseline renal and liver function; may monitor auranofin serum levels. Discontinue therapy if platelet count falls to <100,000/mm$^3$.

**Additional Nursing Issues**

**Physical Assessment:** Monitor laboratory tests (see above), therapeutic response (eg, relief of pain and inflammation, activity tolerance), and adverse reactions at beginning of therapy and periodically throughout therapy (see Warnings/Precautions, Adverse Reactions and Overdose/Toxicology). Assess knowledge/teach patient appropriate use, interventions to reduce side effects, and adverse symptoms to report. **Pregnancy risk factor C** - benefits of use should outweigh possible risks. Breast-feeding is contraindicated.

**Patient Information/Instruction:** Take exactly as directed. Drug effects may not be seen for as long as 3 weeks to 3 months. You may experience metallic taste or mouth sores (frequent mouth care and sucking lozenges may help); gray-blue color or irritation and reddening of skin (avoid excessive exposure to sunlight; use sunscreen, sunglasses, and protective clothing); nausea, bloating, or loss of appetite (small frequent meals, chewing gum, or sucking on lozenges may help); or loss of hair (reversible). Report unusual bruising; blood in mouth, urine, stool, vomitus; persistent fatigue; persistent metallic taste; abdominal cramping, vomiting, diarrhea; sores in mouth; skin rash or itching; or irritated or painful eyes. **Pregnancy/breast-feeding precautions:** Inform prescriber if you are or intend to be pregnant. Do not breast-feed.

**Geriatric Considerations:** Tolerance to gold decreases with advanced age. Use cautiously only after traditional therapy and other disease-modifying antirheumatic drugs (DMARDs) have been attempted.

- **Auro-Dri®** *see page 1291*
- **Auro® Ear Drops** *see page 1291*
- **Auro® Ear Drops** *see page 1294*
- **Aurolate®** *see* Gold Sodium Thiomalate *on page 541*
- **Auroto®** *see page 1306*
- **Auroto Otic®** *see page 1291*
- **Autoplex T®** *see* Anti-inhibitor Coagulant Complex *on page 100*
- **Avandia®** *see* Rosiglitazone *on page 1037*
- **Avapro®** *see* Irbesartan *on page 623*
- **Avapro® HCT** *see* Irbesartan and Hydrochlorothiazide *on page 624*
- **AVC™ Cream** *see* Sulfanilamide *on page 1084*
- **AVC™ Suppository** *see* Sulfanilamide *on page 1084*

- ♦ **Aveeno® Cleansing Bar** *see page 1294*
- ♦ **Aventyl® Hydrochloride** *see* Nortriptyline *on page 839*
- ♦ **A-Vicon** *see* Vitamin A *on page 1217*
- ♦ **Avirax™** *see* Acyclovir *on page 39*
- ♦ **Avitene®** *see page 1248*
- ♦ **A-Vitex** *see* Vitamin A *on page 1217*
- ♦ **Avlosulfon®** *see* Dapsone *on page 334*
- ♦ **Avonex™** *see* Interferon Beta-1a *on page 616*
- ♦ **Axid®** *see* Nizatidine *on page 834*
- ♦ **Axid® AR [OTC]** *see* Nizatidine *on page 834*
- ♦ **Axocet®** *see* Butalbital Compound and Acetaminophen *on page 175*
- ♦ **Ayercillin®** *see* Penicillin G Procaine *on page 899*
- ♦ **Aygestin®** *see* Norethindrone *on page 836*
- ♦ **Ayr® Saline** *see page 1294*
- ♦ **Azactam®** *see* Aztreonam *on page 127*
- ♦ **Azantac** *see* Ranitidine *on page 1008*


## Azatadine (a ZA ta deen)

**U.S. Brand Names** Optimine®

**Therapeutic Category** Antihistamine

**Pregnancy Risk Factor** B

**Lactation** Excretion in breast milk unknown/not recommended

**Use** Treatment of perennial and seasonal allergic rhinitis and chronic urticaria

**Mechanism of Action/Effect** Azatadine has both anticholinergic and antiserotonin activity; has been demonstrated to inhibit mediator release from human mast cells *in vitro*; mechanism of this action is suggested to prevent calcium entry into the mast cell through voltage-dependent calcium channels

**Contraindications** Hypersensitivity to azatadine or to other related antihistamines including cyproheptadine; patients taking monoamine oxidase inhibitors should not use azatadine; antihistamines should not be used to treat lower respiratory tract symptoms

**Warnings** Use with caution in patients with narrow-angle glaucoma, stenosing peptic ulcer, urinary bladder obstruction, prostatic hypertrophy, asthmatic attacks. Sedation and somnolence are the most commonly reported adverse effects.

**Drug Interactions**

**Increased Effect/Toxicity:** Potential for increased side effects when used with procarbazine, CNS depressants, tricyclic antidepressants, and alcohol.

**Adverse Reactions**

>10%:

Central nervous system: Slight to moderate drowsiness

Respiratory: Thickening of bronchial secretions

1% to 10%:

Central nervous system: Headache, fatigue, nervousness, dizziness

Gastrointestinal: Appetite increase, weight gain, nausea, diarrhea, abdominal pain, dry mouth

Neuromuscular & skeletal: Arthralgia

Respiratory: Pharyngitis

<1% (Limited to important or life-threatening symptoms): Hepatitis, bronchospasm, epistaxis

**Overdose/Toxicology** Symptoms of overdose include CNS depression or stimulation, dry mouth, flushed skin, fixed and dilated pupils, apnea. There is no specific treatment for antihistamine overdose; however, anticholinesterase inhibitors may be useful.

**Pharmacodynamics/Kinetics**

**Protein Binding:** Minimally bound to plasma protein

**Distribution:** Crosses the blood brain barrier

**Half-life Elimination:** ~8.7 hours

**Time to Peak:** 4 hours after the dose

**Metabolism:** Liver

**Excretion:** Urine

**Onset:** 1-2 hours

**Formulations** Tablet, as maleate: 1 mg

**Dosing**

**Adults:** Oral: 1-2 mg twice daily

**Elderly:** 1 mg once or twice daily

**Additional Nursing Issues**

**Physical Assessment:** Assess effectiveness and interactions of other medications (see Drug Interactions). See Contraindications and Warnings/Precautions for cautious use. Monitor effectiveness of therapy and adverse reactions (see Adverse Reactions) at beginning of therapy and periodically with long-term use. Assess knowledge/teach patient appropriate use, interventions to reduce side effects, and adverse symptoms to report. Breast-feeding is not recommended.

**Patient Information/Instruction:** Take as directed; do not exceed recommended dose. Avoid use of other depressants, alcohol, or sleep-inducing medications unless approved by prescriber. You may experience drowsiness or dizziness (use caution when driving or engaging in tasks requiring alertness until response to drug is known); or dry mouth, abdominal pain, or nausea (frequent small meals, frequent mouth care, chewing gum, or sucking hard candy may help). Report persistent sore throat, difficulty

(Continued)

## Azatadine *(Continued)*

breathing, or expectorating (thick secretions); excessive sedation or mental stimulation; frequent nosebleeds; unusual joint or muscle pain; or lack of improvement or worsening or condition. **Breast-feeding precautions:** Breast-feeding is not recommended.

**Geriatric Considerations:** Reduce dose in the elderly. Antihistamines are more likely to cause dizziness, excessive sedation, syncope, toxic confusion states, and hypotension in the elderly. See Additional Information and Warnings/Precautions.

## Azatadine and Pseudoephedrine (a ZA ta deen & soo doe e FED rin)

**U.S. Brand Names** Trinalin® Repetabs®

**Synonyms** Pseudoephedrine and Azatadine

**Therapeutic Category** Antihistamine/Decongestant Combination

**Pregnancy Risk Factor** C

**Lactation** Excretion in breast milk unknown/not recommended

**Use** Perennial and seasonal allergic rhinitis and other allergic symptoms including urticaria

**Formulations** Tablet: Azatadine maleate 1 mg and pseudoephedrine sulfate 120 mg

**Dosing**

**Adults:** Oral: 1 tablet twice daily

**Elderly:** Refer to dosing in individual monographs.

**Additional Nursing Issues**

**Physical Assessment:** See individual components listed in Related Information. **Pregnancy risk factor C** - benefits of use should outweigh possible risks. Breast-feeding is not recommended.

**Patient Information/Instruction:** See individual components listed in Related Information. **Pregnancy/breast-feeding precautions:** Inform prescriber if you are or intend to be pregnant. Breast-feeding is not recommended.

**Related Information**

Azatadine *on previous page*
Pseudoephedrine *on page 992*

## Azathioprine (ay za THYE oh preen)

**U.S. Brand Names** Imuran®

**Therapeutic Category** Immunosuppressant Agent

**Pregnancy Risk Factor** D

**Lactation** Excretion in breast milk unknown/not recommended

**Use** Adjunct with other agents in prevention of rejection of solid organ transplants; used in severe active rheumatoid arthritis unresponsive to other agents

**Unlabeled use:** Treatment of chronic ulcerative colitis, generalized myasthenia gravis; controlling the progression of Behçet's syndrome, and Crohn's disease

**Mechanism of Action/Effect** Antagonizes purine metabolism and may inhibit synthesis of DNA, RNA, and proteins; may also interfere with cellular metabolism and inhibit mitosis

**Contraindications** Hypersensitivity to azathioprine or any component; pregnancy

**Warnings** Chronic immunosuppression increases the risk of neoplasia. Has mutagenic potential to both men and women and with possible hematologic toxicities. Use with caution in patients with liver disease, renal impairment. Monitor hematologic function closely.

**Drug Interactions**

**Decreased Effect:** Azathioprine and cyclosporine may result in a decrease in cyclosporine levels. Azathioprine and nondepolarizing neuromuscular blockers may cause the action of the neuromuscular blocker to be decreased or reversed. Azathioprine and anticoagulants may result in decreased action of the anticoagulant.

**Increased Effect/Toxicity:** Azathioprine and allopurinol may result in an increased action and toxic effect of azathioprine (recommendations of lowering the dose of allopurinol to 1/4 to 1/3 of the normal dose). Azathioprine and ACE inhibitors may induce severe leukopenia. Azathioprine and methotrexate may result in elevated levels of the metabolite 6-MP.

**Adverse Reactions** Dose reduction or temporary withdrawal allows reversal

>10%:
- Gastrointestinal: Nausea, vomiting, anorexia, diarrhea
- Hematologic: Leukopenia, megaloblastic anemia
- Miscellaneous: Secondary infection

1% to 10%:
- Central nervous system: Fever, chills
- Dermatologic: Rash
- Hematologic: Thrombocytopenia
- Hepatic: Hepatitis or biliary stasis

<1% (Limited to important or life-threatening symptoms): Hypotension, alopecia, veno-occlusive disease (potentially fatal), pneumonitis

**Overdose/Toxicology** Symptoms of overdose include nausea, vomiting, diarrhea, and hematologic toxicity. Following initiation of essential overdose management, symptomatic and supportive treatment should be instituted. Dialysis has been reported to remove significant amounts of the drug and its metabolites, and should be considered as a treatment option in those patients who deteriorate despite established forms of therapy.

**Pharmacodynamics/Kinetics**

**Protein Binding:** ~30%

**Distribution:** Crosses the placenta

**Half-life Elimination:** Parent drug: 12 minutes; 6-mercaptopurine: 0.7-3 hours; End-stage renal disease: Slightly prolonged

**Metabolism:** Liver

**Excretion:** Urine

**Formulations**

Azathioprine sodium:

Injection: 100 mg (20 mL)

Tablet (scored): 50 mg

**Dosing**

**Adults: I.V. dose is equivalent to oral dose.**

Renal transplantation: Oral, I.V.: 2-5 mg/kg/day to start, then 1-3 mg/kg/day maintenance

Rheumatoid arthritis: Oral: 1 mg/kg/day for 6-8 weeks; increase by 0.5 mg/kg every 4 weeks until response or up to 2.5 mg/kg/day

**Elderly:**

Renal transplantation: Refer to adult dosing.

Rheumatoid arthritis: Oral: 1 mg/kg/day (50-100 mg); titrate gradually by 25 mg/day until response or toxicity (see Renal Impairment for dose adjustments)

**Renal Impairment:**

$Cl_{cr}$ 10-50 mL/minute: Administer 75% of normal dose.

$Cl_{cr}$ <10 mL/minute: Administer 50% of normal dose.

Slightly dialyzable (5% to 20%)

Administer dose posthemodialysis.

CAPD effects: Unknown

CAVH effects: Unknown

**Administration**

**I.V.:** Can be administered IVP over 5 minutes at a concentration not to exceed 10 mg/mL **or** azathioprine can be further diluted with normal saline or $D_5W$ and administered by intermittent infusion over 15-60 minutes.

**Stability**

**Storage:** Stability of parenteral admixture at room temperature (25°C) is 24 hours. Stability of parenteral admixture at refrigeration temperature (4°C) is 16 days.

**Compatibility:** Stable in neutral or acid solutions, but is hydrolyzed to mercaptopurine in alkaline solutions.

**Monitoring Laboratory Tests** CBC, platelet counts, total bilirubin, alkaline phosphatase

**Additional Nursing Issues**

**Physical Assessment:** Assess effectiveness and interactions of other medications patient may be taking (see Drug Interactions). Monitor laboratory tests (see above), therapeutic response (according to purpose for use), and adverse reactions at beginning of therapy and periodically throughout therapy, especially opportunistic infection (see Warnings/Precautions, Adverse Reactions, and Overdose/Toxicology). Assess knowledge/teach patient appropriate use, interventions to reduce side effects, and adverse symptoms to report. **Pregnancy risk factor D** - assess knowledge/instruct patient on the need to use appropriate contraceptive measures and the need to avoid pregnancy. Breast-feeding is not recommended.

**Patient Information/Instruction:** Take as prescribed (may take in divided doses or with food if GI upset occurs).

Rheumatoid arthritis: Response may not occur for up to 3 months; do not discontinue without consulting prescriber.

Organ transplant: Azathioprine will usually be prescribed with other antirejection medications.

You will be susceptible to infection (avoid vaccinations unless approved by prescriber) and avoid crowds or infected persons or persons with contagious diseases. You may experience nausea, vomiting, loss of appetite (small frequent meals, frequent mouth care, chewing gum, or sucking lozenges may help). Report abdominal pain and unresolved gastrointestinal upset (eg, persistent vomiting or diarrhea); unusual fever or chills, bleeding or bruising, sore throat, unhealed sores, or signs of infection; yellowing of skin or eyes; or change in color of urine or stool. **Pregnancy/breast-feeding precautions:** Do not get pregnant while taking this medication; use appropriate barrier contraceptive measures. Breast-feeding is not recommended.

**Geriatric Considerations:** Immunosuppressive toxicity is increased in the elderly. Signs or symptoms of infection may differ in the elderly. Lethargy or confusion may be the first signs of infection.

♦ **Azatrilem** *see* Azathioprine *on previous page*

♦ **Azdone®** *see* Hydrocodone and Aspirin *on page 570*

## Azelaic Acid (a zeh LAY ik AS id)

**U.S. Brand Names** Azelex®

**Therapeutic Category** Topical Skin Product, Acne

**Pregnancy Risk Factor** B

**Lactation** Excretion in breast milk unknown/use caution

**Use** *Acne vulgaris*: Topical treatment of mild to moderate inflammatory acne vulgaris

**Mechanism of Action/Effect** Exact mechanism is not known; *in vitro*, azelaic acid possesses antimicrobial activity against *Propionibacterium acnes* and *Staphylococcus*

(Continued)

## Azelaic Acid *(Continued)*

*epidermidis*; may decrease micromedo formation; dietary content normally found in whole grain cereals, can be formed endogenously

**Contraindications** Hypersensitivity to azelaic acid or any component

**Warnings** For external use only; not for ophthalmic use. There have been isolated reports of hypopigmentation after use. If sensitivity or severe irritation develops, discontinue treatment and institute appropriate therapy.

**Adverse Reactions**

1% to 10%:

Dermatologic: Desquamation, dryness of skin, erythema, mild inflammatory reaction, mild pruritus

Local: Burning, stinging, tingling

<1% (Limited to important or life-threatening symptoms): Erythema, dryness, rash, peeling, dermatitis, contact dermatitis

**Pharmacodynamics/Kinetics**

**Half-life Elimination:** Healthy subjects: 12 hours after topical dosing

**Excretion:** Urine

**Formulations** Cream: 20% (30 g)

**Dosing**

**Adults:** Topical: After skin is thoroughly washed and patted dry, gently but thoroughly massage a thin film of azelaic acid cream into the affected areas twice daily, in the morning and evening. The duration of use can vary and depends on the severity of the acne. In the majority of patients with inflammatory lesions, improvement of the condition occurs within 4 weeks.

**Elderly:** Refer to adult dosing.

**Administration**

**Topical:** Apply with gloves and wash hands following application.

**Additional Nursing Issues**

**Physical Assessment:** See Contraindications and Warnings/Precautions for use cautions. Monitor effectiveness of therapy and adverse reactions at beginning and periodically during therapy. Assess knowledge/teach patient appropriate use and adverse symptoms to report for prescribed form of drug. Note breast-feeding caution.

**Patient Information/Instruction:** Apply with gloves and wash hands following application. Use for the full prescribed treatment period. Avoid the use of occlusive dressings or wrappings. Keep away from the mouth, eyes and other mucous membranes. If it does come in contact with the eyes, wash eyes with large amounts of water and consult prescriber if eye irritation persists. Patients with dark complexion should report changes in skin color. Temporary skin irritation (eg, pruritus, burning or stinging) may occur when azelaic acid is applied to broken or inflamed skin, usually at the start of treatment. However, this irritation commonly subsides if treatment is continued. If it continues, apply only once a day, or stop the treatment until these effects have subsided. If irritation persists, discontinue use and consult prescriber. **Breast-feeding precautions:** Consult prescriber if breast-feeding.

♦ **Azelex®** *see* Azelaic Acid *on previous page*

♦ **Azidothymidine** *see* Zidovudine *on page 1227*

## Azithromycin (az ith roe MYE sin)

**U.S. Brand Names** Zithromax™

**Therapeutic Category** Antibiotic, Macrolide

**Pregnancy Risk Factor** B

**Lactation** Excretion in breast milk unknown

**Use**

Children: Treatment of acute otitis media due to *H. influenzae, M. catarrhalis*, or *S. pneumoniae*; pharyngitis/tonsillitis due to *S. pyogenes*

Adults: Treatment of mild to moderate upper and lower respiratory tract infections, infections of the skin and skin structure, and sexually transmitted diseases due to susceptible strains of *C. trachomatis, M. catarrhalis, H. influenzae, S. aureus, S. pneumoniae, Mycoplasma pneumoniae*, and *C. psittaci*

**Note:** Penicillin I.M. is the usual drug of choice in the treatment of *S. pyogenes* infections and the prophylaxis of rheumatic fever; azithromycin is often effective in its eradication in the nasopharynx; perform susceptibility tests when patients are treated with azithromycin

**Mechanism of Action/Effect** Inhibits RNA-dependent protein synthesis at the chain elongation step; binds to the 50S ribosomal subunit resulting in blockage of transpeptidation

**Contraindications** Hypersensitivity to azithromycin, other macrolide antibiotics, or any components; hepatic impairment; use with pimozide

**Warnings** Use with caution in patients with hepatic dysfunction. Hepatic impairment with or without jaundice has occurred chiefly in older children and adults. It may be accompanied by malaise, nausea, vomiting, abdominal colic, and fever. Discontinue use if these occur. May mask or delay symptoms of incubating gonorrhea or syphilis, so appropriate culture and sensitivity tests should be performed prior to initiating azithromycin. Pseudomembranous colitis has been reported with use of macrolide antibiotics.

**Drug Interactions**

**Cytochrome P-450 Effect:** May inhibit CYP3A3/4 enzymes (weak)

**Decreased Effect:** Decreased peak serum levels with aluminum- and magnesium-containing antacids by 24%. Total absorption is unaffected.

**Increased Effect/Toxicity:** Azithromycin increases levels of tacrolimus, alfentanil, astemizole, terfenadine, loratadine, bromocriptine, carbamazepine, cyclosporine, digoxin, disopyramide, and triazolam. Azithromycin did not affect the response to warfarin or theophylline although caution is advised when administered together.

**Adverse Reactions**

1% to 10%: Gastrointestinal: Diarrhea, nausea, abdominal pain

<1% (Limited to important or life-threatening symptoms): Palpitations, chest pain, vaginitis, eosinophilia, elevated LFTs, cholestatic jaundice, interstitial nephritis (acute)

**Overdose/Toxicology** Symptoms of overdose include nausea, vomiting, diarrhea, and prostration. Treatment is supportive and symptomatic.

**Pharmacodynamics/Kinetics**

**Protein Binding:** 7% to 50% (concentration-dependent)

**Distribution:** Extensive tissue distribution

**Half-life Elimination:** 68 hours

**Time to Peak:** 2.3-4 hours

**Metabolism:** Liver

**Excretion:** Urine and bile

**Formulations** See also Trovafloxacin/Azithromycin Compliance Pack.

Azithromycin dihydrate:

Capsule: 250 mg

Capsule (Z-PAK™): 6 capsules per package: 250 mg

Powder for injection: 500 mg in 10 mL vials

Powder for oral suspension: 100 mg/5 mL (15 mL); 200 mg/5 mL (15 mL, 22.5 mL); 1 g (single-dose packet)

Tablet: 250 mg, 600 mg

**Dosing**

**Adults:**

Oral:

Mild to moderate respiratory tract, skin, and soft tissue infections: 500 mg in a single loading dose on day 1 followed by 250 mg/day as a single dose on days 2-5

Nongonococcal urethritis and cervicitis: 1 g in a single dose, 1 hour before or 2 hours after a meal

Chancroid and *Chlamydia*: 1 g in a single dose

I.V.:

Community-acquired pneumonia: 500 mg as a single dose for at least 2 days, follow I.V. therapy by the oral route with a single daily dose of 500 mg to complete a 7- to 10-day course of therapy.

Pelvic inflammatory disease (PID): 500 mg as a single dose for 1-2 days, follow I.V. therapy by the oral route with a single daily dose of 250 mg to complete a 7-day course of therapy.

**Elderly:** Refer to adult dosing.

**Administration**

**Oral:** Do not take oral suspension with food. Administer 1 hour before or 2 hours after meals. Tablets can be taken without regard for food.

**I.V.:** Administer over at least 60 minutes.

**Monitoring Laboratory Tests** Liver function, CBC with differential

**Additional Nursing Issues**

**Physical Assessment:** Assess any previous allergic reactions to antibiotics or erythromycin, or any macrolide antibiotic. Inform patients being treated for STDs about preventing transmission. Monitor for signs or symptoms of opportunistic infections (eg, unhealed sores in mouth or vagina, excess vaginal discharge, unresolved fever). Note breast-feeding caution.

**Patient Information/Instruction:** Take as directed. Take all of prescribed medication. Do not discontinue until prescription is completed. Take suspension 1 hour before or 2 hours after meals; tablet form may be taken with meals to decrease GI effects. Do not take with aluminum- or magnesium-containing antacids. May cause transient abdominal distress, diarrhea, headache. Report signs of additional infections (eg, sores in mouth or vagina, vaginal discharge, unresolved fever, severe vomiting, or diarrhea). **Breast-feeding precautions:** Consult prescriber if breast-feeding.

**Geriatric Considerations:** Dosage adjustment does not appear to be necessary in the elderly. Considered one of the drugs of choice in the treatment of outpatient treatment of community-acquired pneumonia in older adults.

- **Azithromycin/Trovafloxacin Compliance Pak** *see* Trovafloxacin/Azithromycin Compliance Pak *on page 1191*
- **Azmacort™** *see* Triamcinolone *on page 1171*
- **Azopt® Ophthalmic** *see* Ophthalmic Agents, Glaucoma *on page 853*
- **Azo-Standard® [OTC]** *see* Phenazopyridine *on page 914*
- **Azo Wintomylon** *see* Phenazopyridine *on page 914*
- **AZT** *see* Zidovudine *on page 1227*
- **Azthreonam** *see* Aztreonam *on this page*

## Aztreonam (AZ tree oh nam)

**U.S. Brand Names** Azactam®

**Synonyms** Azthreonam

**Therapeutic Category** Antibiotic, Miscellaneous

**Pregnancy Risk Factor** B

**Lactation** Enters breast milk/use caution (AAP rates "compatible")

(Continued)

## Aztreonam *(Continued)*

**Use** Treatment of patients with documented aerobic gram-negative bacillary infection in which beta-lactam therapy is contraindicated (eg, penicillin or cephalosporin allergy); treatment of urinary tract infections, lower respiratory tract infections, septicemia, skin/skin structure infections, intra-abdominal infections, and gynecologic infections; as part of a multiple-drug regimen for the empirical treatment of neutropenic fever in persons with a history of beta-lactam allergy or with known multidrug-resistant organisms

**Mechanism of Action/Effect** Monobactam which is active only against gram-negative bacilli; inhibits bacterial cell wall synthesis during active multiplication, causing cell wall destruction

**Contraindications** Hypersensitivity to aztreonam or any component

**Warnings** Check hypersensitivity to other beta-lactams. May have cross-allergenicity to penicillins and cephalosporins. Requires dosage reduction in renal impairment.

**Effects on Lab Values** Urine glucose (Clinitest®)

**Adverse Reactions**

1% to 10%:

Dermatologic: Rash

Gastrointestinal: Diarrhea, nausea, vomiting

Local: Thrombophlebitis, pain at injection site

<1% (Limited to important or life-threatening symptoms): Hypotension, transient EKG changes (ventricular bigeminy and PVC), seizures, confusion, headache, vertigo, insomnia, dizziness, fever, toxic epidermal necrolysis, purpura, erythema multiforme, exfoliative dermatitis, urticaria, petechiae, pruritus, sweating, pseudomembranous colitis, abdominal cramps, *C. difficile*-associated diarrhea, mouth ulcer, altered taste, halitosis, vaginitis, vaginal candidiasis, hepatitis, jaundice, elevation of liver enzymes, thrombocytopenia, pancytopenia, leukocytosis, thrombocytopenia, neutropenia, anemia, bronchospasm, anaphylaxis

**Overdose/Toxicology** Symptoms of overdose include seizures. Treatment is supportive. If necessary, dialysis can reduce the drug concentration in the blood.

**Pharmacodynamics/Kinetics**

**Protein Binding:** ~56%

**Distribution:** Relative diffusion of antimicrobial agents from blood into cerebrospinal fluid (CSF): Good only with inflammation (exceeds usual MICs): Ratio of CSF to blood level (%): Inflamed meninges: 8-40; Normal meninges: ~1

**Half-life Elimination:** Normal renal function: 1.7-2.9 hours; End-stage renal disease: 6-8 hours

**Time to Peak:** Within 60 minutes (I.M., I.V. push) and 90 minutes (I.V. infusion)

**Metabolism:** Liver

**Excretion:** Urine and feces

**Formulations** Powder for injection: 500 mg (15 mL, 100 mL); 1 g (15 mL, 100 mL); 2 g (15 mL, 100 mL)

**Dosing**

**Adults:**

Urinary tract infection: I.M., I.V.: 500 mg to 1 g every 8-12 hours

Moderately severe systemic infections: 1 g I.V. or I.M. or 2 g I.V. every 8-12 hours

Severe systemic or life-threatening infections (especially caused by *Pseudomonas aeruginosa*): I.V.: 2 g every 6-8 hours; maximum: 8 g/day

**Elderly:** Refer to adult dosing.

**Renal Impairment:**

$Cl_{cr}$ 30-50 mL/minute: Administer every 12 hours.

$Cl_{cr}$ 10-30 mL/minute: Administer every 24 hours.

$Cl_{cr}$ <10 mL/minute: Administer every 48 hours.

Hemodialysis effects: Moderately dialyzable (20% to 50%); administer dose postdialysis or supplemental dose of 500 mg after dialysis.

Peritoneal dialysis: Administer as for $Cl_{cr}$ <10 mL/minute.

Continuous arteriovenous or venovenous hemofiltration (CAVH/CAVHD): Dose as for $Cl_{cr}$ 10-50 mL/minute

**Administration**

**I.M.:** Inject deep into large muscle mass.

**I.V.:** I.V. route is preferred for doses ≥1 g or in patients with severe life-threatening infections. Administer by IVP over 3-5 minutes or by intermittent infusion over 20-60 minutes at a final concentration not to exceed 20 mg/mL.

**I.V. Detail:** Monitor infusion/injection sites carefully. Administer around-the-clock to promote less variation in peak and trough serum levels.

**Stability**

**Reconstitution:** Reconstituted solutions are colorless to light yellow straw and may turn pink upon standing without affecting potency. Use reconstituted solutions and I.V. solutions (in NS and $D_5W$) within 48 hours if kept at room temperature (25°C) or 7 days if kept in refrigerator (4°C).

**Compatibility:** Incompatible when mixed with nafcillin, metronidazole.

**Monitoring Laboratory Tests** Obtain specimens for culture and sensitivity before the first dose.

**Additional Nursing Issues**

**Physical Assessment:** Assess allergy history before initiating therapy. See Warnings/Precautions and Contraindications for use cautions. Monitor effectiveness of therapy, laboratory tests, and adverse response (see Adverse Reactions and Overdose/Toxicology). Assess knowledge/teach patient possible side effects and adverse symptoms to report. Note breast-feeding caution.

**Patient Information/Instruction:** This medication can only be administered I.M. or I.V. You may experience nausea or GI distress. Frequent mouth care, frequent small meals, sucking lozenges, or chewing gum may help relieve these symptoms. May cause false readings with urine glucose testing. Diabetics should use alternate means of monitoring glucose. Report any unrelieved diarrhea or vomiting, pain at injection sites, unresolved fever, unhealed or new sores in mouth or vagina, vaginal discharge, or acute onset of respiratory difficulty. **Breast-feeding precautions:** Consult prescriber if breast-feeding.

**Geriatric Considerations:** Adjust dose relative to renal function.

**Additional Information** pH: 4.5-7.5; sodium-free


- **Azulfidine®** *see* Sulfasalazine *on page 1084*
- **Azulfidine® EN-tabs®** *see* Sulfasalazine *on page 1084*
- **Babee Teething® [OTC]** *see* Benzocaine *on page 141*
- **Bacid® [OTC]** *see Lactobacillus acidophilus* and *Lactobacillus bulgaricus on page 651*
- **Baciguent® Topical [OTC]** *see* Bacitracin *on this page*
- **Bacigvent** *see* Bacitracin *on this page*
- **Baci-IM® Injection** *see* Bacitracin *on this page*
- **Bacitin** *see* Bacitracin *on this page*


## Bacitracin (bas i TRAY sin)

**U.S. Brand Names** AK-Tracin® Ophthalmic; Baciguent® Topical [OTC]; Baci-IM® Injection

**Therapeutic Category** Antibiotic, Ophthalmic; Antibiotic, Topical; Antibiotic, Miscellaneous

**Pregnancy Risk Factor** C

**Lactation** Excretion in breast milk unknown/use caution

**Use** Treatment of susceptible bacterial infections (staphylococcal pneumonia and empyema); due to toxicity risks, systemic and irrigant uses of bacitracin should be limited to situations where less toxic alternatives would not be effective; oral administration has been successful in antibiotic-associated colitis

**Mechanism of Action/Effect** Inhibits bacterial cell wall synthesis by preventing transfer of mucopeptides into the growing cell wall

**Contraindications** Hypersensitivity to bacitracin or any component; I.M. use is contraindicated in patients with renal impairment

**Warnings** Prolonged use may result in overgrowth of nonsusceptible organisms. I.M. use may cause renal failure due to tubular and glomerular necrosis. **Do not administer intravenously** because severe thrombophlebitis occurs. Pregnancy factor C.

**Drug Interactions**

**Increased Effect/Toxicity:** Nephrotoxic drugs, neuromuscular blocking agents, and anesthetics (increased neuromuscular blockade).

**Adverse Reactions** 1% to 10%:

Cardiovascular: Hypotension, edema of the face/lips, tightness of chest
Central nervous system: Pain
Dermatologic: Rash, itching
Gastrointestinal: Anorexia, nausea, vomiting, diarrhea, rectal itching
Hematologic: Blood dyscrasias
Miscellaneous: Sweating

**Overdose/Toxicology** Symptoms of overdose include nephrotoxicity (parenteral), nausea, and vomiting (oral). Treatment is symptomatic and supportive.

**Pharmacodynamics/Kinetics**

**Protein Binding:** Minimally bound to plasma proteins

**Distribution:** Relative diffusion of bacitracin from blood into cerebrospinal fluid (CSF): Nil even with inflammation

**Time to Peak:** I.M.: Within 1-2 hours

**Excretion:** Urine

**Duration:** 6-8 hours

**Formulations**

Injection: 50,000 units
Ointment:
Ophthalmic: 500 units/g (3.5 g, 3.75 g)
AK-Tracin®: 500 units/g (3.5 g)
Topical: 500 units/g (1.5 g, 3.75 g, 15 g, 30 g, 120 g, 454 g)

**Dosing**

**Adults:** Do not administer I.V.:

Antibiotic-associated colitis: Oral: 25,000 units 4 times/day for 7-10 days
Topical: Apply 1-5 times/day.
Ophthalmic, ointment: Instill ¼" to ½" ribbon every 3-4 hours into conjunctival sac for acute infections, or 2-3 times/day for mild to moderate infections for 7-10 days.
Irrigation, solution: 50-100 units/mL in normal saline, lactated Ringer's, or sterile water for irrigation; soak sponges in solution for topical compresses 1-5 times/day or as needed during surgical procedures.

**Elderly:** Refer to adult dosing.

**Administration**

**Oral:** The injection formulation is extemporaneously prepared and flavored to improve palatability.

**I.M.:** For I.M. administration only. pH of urine should be kept >6 by using sodium bicarbonate. Bacitracin sterile powder should be dissolved in 0.9% sodium chloride

(Continued)

## Bacitracin *(Continued)*

injection containing 2% procaine hydrochloride. Do not use diluents containing parabens.

**I.V.:** Not for I.V. administration.

**Stability**

**Reconstitution:** For I.M. use only. Bacitracin sterile powder should be dissolved in 0.9% sodium chloride injection containing 2% procaine hydrochloride. Once reconstituted, bacitracin is stable for 1 week under refrigeration (2°C to 8°C). Sterile powder should be stored in the refrigerator. Do not use diluents containing parabens.

**Monitoring Laboratory Tests** I.M.: Urinalysis, renal function

**Additional Nursing Issues**

**Physical Assessment:** Do not administer I.V.

Oral, I.M.: Monitor laboratory results and renal function, effectiveness of therapy, and adverse reactions (see above).

Ophthalmic/topical: Instruct patient on appropriate application and use, possible adverse reactions, and symptoms to report.

**Pregnancy risk factor C.** Note breast-feeding caution.

**Patient Information/Instruction:**

Oral, I.M.: Maintain adequate hydration (2-3 L/day of fluids unless instructed to restrict fluid intake). Report rash, redness, or itching; change in urinary pattern; acute dizziness; swelling of face or lips; chest pain or tightness; acute nausea or vomiting; or loss of appetite (small frequent meals or frequent mouth care may help).

Ophthalmic: Instill as many times per day as directed. Wash hands before using. Gently pull lower eyelid forward, instill prescribed amount of ointment into lower eyelid. Close eye and roll eyeball in all directions. May cause blurred vision; use caution when driving or engaging in tasks that require clear vision. Report any adverse reactions such as rash or itching, swelling of face or lips, burning or pain in eye, worsening of condition, or if condition does not improve.

Topical: Apply a thin film as many times as day as prescribed to the affected area. May cover with porous sterile bandage (avoid occlusive dressings). Do not use longer than 1 week unless advised by healthcare provider.

**Pregnancy/breast-feeding precautions:** Inform prescriber if you are or intend to be pregnant. Consult prescriber if breast-feeding.

**Additional Information** 1 unit is equivalent to 0.026 mg

**Related Information**

Ophthalmic Agents *on page 1282*

## Bacitracin and Polymyxin B (bas i TRAY sin & pol i MIKS in bee)

**U.S. Brand Names** AK-Poly-Bac® Ophthalmic; Betadine® First Aid Antibiotics + Moisturizer [OTC]; Polysporin® Ophthalmic; Polysporin® Topical

**Synonyms** Polymyxin B and Bacitracin

**Therapeutic Category** Antibiotic, Ophthalmic; Antibiotic, Topical

**Pregnancy Risk Factor** C

**Lactation** Excretion in breast milk unknown/use caution

**Use** Treatment of superficial infections caused by susceptible organisms

**Formulations**

Ointment:

- Ophthalmic: Bacitracin 500 units and polymyxin B sulfate 10,000 units per g (3.5 g)
- Topical: Bacitracin 500 units and polymyxin B sulfate 10,000 units per g in white petrolatum (15 g, 30 g)

Powder: Bacitracin 500 units and polymyxin B sulfate 10,000 units per g (10 g)

**Dosing**

**Adults:**

Ophthalmic ointment: Instill ½" ribbon in the affected eye(s) every 3-4 hours for acute infections or 2-3 times/day for mild to moderate infections for 7-10 days.

Topical ointment/powder: Apply to affected area 1-4 times/day; may cover with sterile bandage if needed.

**Elderly:** Refer to adult dosing.

**Additional Nursing Issues**

**Physical Assessment:** See individual components listed in Related Information. **Pregnancy risk factor C** - benefits of use should outweigh possible risks. Note breast-feeding caution.

**Patient Information/Instruction:** See individual components listed in Related Information. **Pregnancy/breast-feeding precautions:** Inform prescriber if you are or intend to be pregnant. Consult prescriber if breast-feeding.

**Related Information**

Bacitracin *on previous page*
Ophthalmic Agents *on page 1282*
Polymyxin B Sulfate *on page 946*

## Bacitracin, Neomycin, and Polymyxin B

(bas i TRAY sin, nee oh MYE sin, & pol i MIKS in bee)

**U.S. Brand Names** AK-Spore® Ophthalmic Ointment; Medi-Quick® Topical Ointment [OTC]; Mycitracin® Topical [OTC]; Neomixin® Topical [OTC]; Neosporin® Ophthalmic Ointment; Neosporin® Topical Ointment [OTC]; Ocutricin® Topical Ointment; Septa® Topical Ointment [OTC]; Triple Antibiotic® Topical

**Synonyms** Neomycin, Bacitracin, and Polymyxin B; Polymyxin B, Bacitracin, and Neomycin

**Therapeutic Category** Antibiotic, Ophthalmic; Antibiotic, Topical

**Pregnancy Risk Factor** C

**Lactation** Excretion in breast milk unknown/use caution

**Use** Helps prevent infection in minor cuts, scrapes and burns; short-term treatment of superficial external ocular infections caused by susceptible organisms

**Formulations**

Ointment:

Ophthalmic: Bacitracin 400 units, neomycin sulfate 3.5 mg, and polymyxin B sulfate 10,000 units and per g

Topical: Bacitracin 400 units, neomycin sulfate 3.5 mg, and polymyxin B sulfate 5000 units per g

**Dosing**

**Adults:**

Ophthalmic ointment: Instill ½" ribbon into the conjunctival sac every 3-4 hours for acute infections or 2-3 times/day for mild to moderate infections for 7-10 days.

Topical: Apply 1-4 times/day to affected areas and cover with sterile bandage if necessary.

**Elderly:** Refer to adult dosing.

**Additional Nursing Issues**

**Physical Assessment:** See individual components listed in Related Information. **Pregnancy risk factor C** - benefits of use should outweigh possible risks. Note breast-feeding caution.

**Patient Information/Instruction:** See individual components listed in Related Information. **Pregnancy/breast-feeding precautions:** Inform prescriber if you are or intend to be pregnant. Consult prescriber if breast-feeding.

**Related Information**

Bacitracin *on page 129*
Neomycin *on page 815*
Ophthalmic Agents *on page 1282*
Polymyxin B Sulfate *on page 946*

## Bacitracin, Neomycin, Polymyxin B, and Hydrocortisone

(bas i TRAY sin, nee oh MYE sin, pol i MIKS in bee, & hye droe KOR ti sone)

**U.S. Brand Names** AK-Spore H.C.® Ophthalmic Ointment; Cortisporin® Ophthalmic Ointment; Cortisporin® Topical Ointment; Neotricin HC® Ophthalmic Ointment

**Synonyms** Hydrocortisone, Bacitracin, Neomycin, and Polymyxin B; Neomycin, Bacitracin, Polymyxin B, and Hydrocortisone; Polymyxin B, Bacitracin, Neomycin, and Hydrocortisone

**Therapeutic Category** Antibiotic, Ophthalmic; Antibiotic, Otic; Antibiotic, Topical; Corticosteroid, Ophthalmic; Corticosteroid, Otic; Corticosteroid, Topical

**Pregnancy Risk Factor** C

**Lactation** Excretion in breast milk unknown/use caution

**Use** Prevention and treatment of susceptible superficial topical infections

**Formulations**

Ointment:

Ophthalmic: Bacitracin 400 units, neomycin sulfate 3.5 mg, polymyxin B sulfate 10,000 units, and hydrocortisone 10 mg per g (3.5 g)

Topical: Bacitracin 400 units, neomycin sulfate 3.5 mg, polymyxin B sulfate 10,000 units, and hydrocortisone 10 mg per g (15 g)

**Dosing**

**Adults:**

Ophthalmic ointment: Instill ½" ribbon to inside of lower lid every 3-4 hours until improvement occurs.

Topical: Apply sparingly 2-4 times/day.

**Elderly:** Refer to adult dosing.

**Additional Nursing Issues**

**Physical Assessment:** See individual components listed in Related Information. **Pregnancy risk factor C** - benefits of use should outweigh possible risks. Note breast-feeding caution.

**Patient Information/Instruction:** See individual components listed in Related Information. **Pregnancy/breast-feeding precautions:** Inform prescriber if you are or intend to be pregnant. Consult prescriber if breast-feeding.

**Related Information**

Bacitracin *on page 129*
Hydrocortisone *on page 578*
Neomycin *on page 815*
Ophthalmic Agents *on page 1282*
Polymyxin B Sulfate *on page 946*

♦ **Bacitracin, Neomycin, Polymyxin B, and Lidocaine** *see page 1294*

## Baclofen (BAK loe fen)

**U.S. Brand Names** Lioresal®

**Therapeutic Category** Skeletal Muscle Relaxant

**Pregnancy Risk Factor** C

**Lactation** Enters breast milk (small amounts)/compatible

**Use** Treatment of reversible spasticity associated with multiple sclerosis or spinal cord lesions

(Continued)

## Baclofen *(Continued)*

**Unlabeled use:** Intractable hiccups, intractable pain relief, and bladder spasticity

**Mechanism of Action/Effect** Inhibits the transmission of both monosynaptic and polysynaptic reflexes at the spinal cord level, possibly by hyperpolarization of primary afferent fiber terminals, with resultant relief of muscle spasticity

**Contraindications** Hypersensitivity to baclofen or any component

**Warnings** Use with caution in patients with seizure disorder, impaired renal function. Avoid abrupt withdrawal of the drug. Elderly are more sensitive to the effects of baclofen and are more likely to experience adverse CNS effects at higher doses. Pregnancy factor C.

**Drug Interactions**

**Increased Effect/Toxicity:** Baclofen may decrease the clearance of ibuprofen or other NSAIDs and increase the potential for renal toxicity.

**Effects on Lab Values** ↑ alkaline phosphatase, AST, glucose, ammonia (B); ↓ bilirubin (S)

**Adverse Reactions**

>10%:

Central nervous system: Drowsiness, vertigo, dizziness, psychiatric disturbances, insomnia, slurred speech, ataxia, hypotonia

Neuromuscular & skeletal: Weakness

1% to 10%:

Cardiovascular: Hypotension

Central nervous system: Fatigue, confusion, headache, insomnia

Dermatologic: Rash

Gastrointestinal: Nausea, constipation

Genitourinary: Polyuria

<1% (Limited to important or life-threatening symptoms): Palpitations, chest pain, syncope, enuresis, urinary retention, dysuria, impotence, inability to ejaculate, nocturia, hematuria, dyspnea

**Overdose/Toxicology** Symptoms of overdose include vomiting, muscle hypotonia, salivation, drowsiness, coma, seizures, and respiratory depression. Atropine has been used to improve ventilation, heart rate, blood pressure, and core body temperature. Treatment is symptom directed and supportive.

**Pharmacodynamics/Kinetics**

**Protein Binding:** 30%

**Half-life Elimination:** 3.5 hours

**Time to Peak:** Oral: Within 2-3 hours

**Metabolism:** Liver

**Excretion:** Urine and feces

**Onset:** Muscle relaxation effect requires 3-4 days; Peak effect: Maximal clinical effect is not seen for 5-10 days

**Formulations**

Injection, intrathecal, preservative free: 500 mcg/mL (20 mL); 2000 mcg/mL (5 mL)

Tablet: 10 mg, 20 mg

**Dosing**

**Adults:**

Oral: 5 mg 3 times/day, may increase 5 mg/dose every 3 days to a maximum of 80 mg/day

Intrathecal:

Test dose: 50-100 mcg, doses >50 mcg should be given in 25 mcg increments, separated by 24 hours

Maintenance: After positive response to test dose, a maintenance intrathecal infusion can be administered via an implanted intrathecal pump. Initial dose via pump: Infusion at a 24-hourly rate dosed at twice the test dose.

**Elderly:** Oral (the lowest effective dose is recommended): Initial: 5 mg 2-3 times/day, increasing gradually as needed; if benefits are not seen withdraw the drug slowly.

**Renal Impairment:** May be necessary to reduce dosage.

**Additional Nursing Issues**

**Physical Assessment:** Assess effectiveness and interactions of other medications (see Drug Interactions). See Contraindications and Warnings/Precautions for use cautions. Monitor effectiveness of therapy (according to rational for therapy) and adverse reactions (eg, cardiovascular and CNS status - see Adverse Reactions) at beginning of therapy and periodically with long-term use. Assess knowledge/teach patient appropriate use, interventions to reduce side effects, and adverse symptoms to report. **Pregnancy risk factor C** - benefits of use should outweigh possible risks.

**Patient Information/Instruction:** Take this drug as prescribed. Do not discontinue without consulting prescriber (abrupt discontinuation may cause hallucinations). Do not take any prescription or OTC sleep-inducing drugs, sedatives, antispasmodics without consulting prescriber. Avoid alcohol use. You may experience transient drowsiness, lethargy, or dizziness; use caution when driving or engaging in tasks requiring alertness until response to drug is known. Frequent small meals or lozenges may reduce GI upset. Report unresolved insomnia, painful urination, change in urinary patterns, constipation, or persistent confusion. **Pregnancy precautions:** Inform prescriber if you are or intend to be pregnant.

**Geriatric Considerations:** The elderly are more sensitive to the effects of baclofen and are more likely to experience adverse CNS effects at higher doses. Two cases of encephalopathy were reported after inadvertent high doses (50 mg/day and 90 mg/day) were given to elderly patients.

- ♦ **Bactelan** *see* Co-trimoxazole *on page 307*
- ♦ **Bacticort®** *see page 1291*
- ♦ **Bactocill®** *see* Oxacillin *on page 866*
- ♦ **Bactocin** *see* Ofloxacin *on page 847*
- ♦ **Bactrim™** *see* Co-trimoxazole *on page 307*
- ♦ **Bactrim™ DS** *see* Co-trimoxazole *on page 307*
- ♦ **Bactroban®** *see* Mupirocin *on page 792*
- ♦ **Bactroban® Nasal** *see* Mupirocin *on page 792*
- ♦ **Baker's P&S Topical** *see page 1294*
- ♦ **Baking Soda** *see* Sodium Bicarbonate *on page 1061*
- ♦ **Balanced Salt Solution** *see page 1294*
- ♦ **Balcoran** *see* Vancomycin *on page 1202*
- ♦ **Baldex®** *see* Dexamethasone *on page 346*
- ♦ **BAL in Oil®** *see page 1248*
- ♦ **Balminil® Decongestant** *see* Pseudoephedrine *on page 992*
- ♦ **Balminil® Expectorant** *see* Guaifenesin *on page 548*
- ♦ **Balnetar® Bath Oil** *see page 1294*
- ♦ **Bancap HC®** *see* Hydrocodone and Acetaminophen *on page 568*
- ♦ **Banophen® Decongestant Capsule** *see page 1294*
- ♦ **Banophen® Oral [OTC]** *see* Diphenhydramine *on page 381*
- ♦ **Bapadin®** *see* Bepridil *on page 146*
- ♦ **Barbidonna®** *see* Hyoscyamine, Atropine, Scopolamine, and Phenobarbital *on page 591*
- ♦ **Barbilixir®** *see* Phenobarbital *on page 917*
- ♦ **Barbita®** *see* Phenobarbital *on page 917*
- ♦ **Barc™ Liquid** *see page 1294*
- ♦ **Baridium® [OTC]** *see* Phenazopyridine *on page 914*
- ♦ **Barophen®** *see* Hyoscyamine, Atropine, Scopolamine, and Phenobarbital *on page 591*
- ♦ **Basaljel®** *see page 1294*


## Basiliximab (ba si LIKS i mab)

**U.S. Brand Names** Simulect®

**Therapeutic Category** Immunosuppressant Agent; Monoclonal Antibody

**Pregnancy Risk Factor** B - per Manufacturer (see Pregnancy Issues)

**Lactation** Excretion in breast milk unknown/not recommended

**Use** Prophylaxis of acute organ rejection in renal transplantation

**Mechanism of Action/Effect** Mouse-derived monoclonal IgG antibody which blocks the alpha-chain of the interleukin-2 (IL-2) receptor complex; this receptor is expressed on activated T lymphocytes and is a critical pathway for activating cell-mediated allograft rejection

**Contraindications** Hypersensitivity to murine proteins or any component of this product

**Warnings** To be used as a component of immunosuppressive regimen which includes cyclosporine and corticosteroids. Only physicians experienced in transplantation and immunosuppression should prescribe, and patients should receive the drug in a facility with adequate equipment and staff capable of providing the laboratory and medical support required for transplantation.

The incidence of lymphoproliferative disorders and/or opportunistic infections may be increased by immunosuppressive therapy. Hypersensitivity reactions have not been observed in clinical trials. However, similar medications have been associated with reactions including urticaria, dyspnea, and hypotension. Discontinue the drug if a reaction occurs. Medications for the treatment of hypersensitivity reactions should be available for immediate use. Effects of readministration have not been evaluated in humans. Treatment may result in the development of human antimurine antibodies (HAMA); however, limited evidence suggesting the use of muromonab-CD3 or other murine products is not precluded.

**Drug Interactions**

**Decreased Effect:** Basiliximab is an immunoglobulin; specific drug interactions have not been evaluated, but are not anticipated.

**Increased Effect/Toxicity:** Basiliximab is an immunoglobulin; specific drug interactions have not been evaluated, but are not anticipated.

**Adverse Reactions** Administration of basiliximab did not appear to increase the incidence or severity of adverse effects in clinical trials. Adverse events were reported in 99% of both the placebo and basiliximab groups.

>10%:

Cardiovascular: Edema, peripheral edema, hypertension

Central nervous system: Fever, headache, dizziness, insomnia

Dermatologic: Wound complications, acne

Endocrine and metabolic: Hypokalemia, hyperkalemia, hyperglycemia, hyperuricemia, hypophosphatemia, hypocalcemia, hypercholesterolemia, acidosis

Gastrointestinal: Constipation, nausea, diarrhea, abdominal pain, vomiting, dyspepsia, moniliasis, weight gain

Genitourinary: Dysuria, urinary tract infection

Hematologic: Anemia

Neuromuscular and skeletal: Leg pain, back pain, tremor

Respiratory: Dyspnea, infection (upper respiratory), coughing, rhinitis, pharyngitis

Miscellaneous: Viral infection, asthenia

(Continued)

## Basiliximab *(Continued)*

3% to 10%:

Cardiovascular: Chest pain, cardiac failure, hypotension, arrhythmia, tachycardia, vascular disorder, generalized edema

Central nervous system: Hypoesthesia, neuropathy, agitation, anxiety, depression, malaise, fatigue, rigors

Dermatologic: Cyst, herpes infection, hypertrichosis, pruritus, rash, skin disorder, skin ulceration

Endocrine and metabolic: Dehydration, diabetes mellitus, fluid overload, hypercalcemia, hyperlipidemia, hypoglycemia, hypomagnesemia

Gastrointestinal: Flatulence, gastroenteritis, GI hemorrhage, gingival hyperplasia, melena, esophagitis, stomatitis

Genitourinary: Impotence, genital edema, albuminuria, bladder disorder, hematuria, urinary frequency, oliguria, abnormal renal function, renal tubular necrosis, ureteral disorder, urinary retention

Hematologic: Hematoma, hemorrhage, purpura, thrombocytopenia, thrombosis, polycythemia

Neuromuscular and skeletal: Arthralgia, arthropathy, cramps, fracture, hernia, myalgia, paresthesia

Ocular: Cataract, conjunctivitis, abnormal vision

Renal: Increased BUN

Respiratory: Bronchitis, bronchospasm, pneumonia, pulmonary edema, sinusitis

Miscellaneous: Accidental trauma, facial edema, sepsis, infection, increased glucocorticoids

**Overdose/Toxicology** There have been no reports of overdose.

**Pharmacodynamics/Kinetics**

**Half-life Elimination:** Mean: 7.2 days

**Metabolism:** Clearance (mean): 41 mL/hour

**Duration:** Mean: 36 days (determined by IL-2R alpha saturation)

**Formulations** Powder for injection: 20 mg

**Dosing**

**Adults:** I.V.: Adults: 20 mg within 2 hours prior to transplant surgery, followed by a second 20 mg dose 4 days after transplantation

**Elderly:** Refer to adult dosing.

**Renal Impairment: Dosing adjustment/comments in renal impairment**: No specific dosing adjustment is recommended.

**Hepatic Impairment: Dosing adjustment/comments in hepatic impairment**: No specific dosing adjustment is recommended.

**Administration**

**I.V.:** For central or intravenous administration only. Infuse over 20-30 minutes.

**Stability**

**Storage:** Store vials under refrigeration 2°C to 8°C (36°F to 46°F). Reconstituted vials are stable under refrigeration for 24 hours, but only 4 hours at room temperature.

**Reconstitution:** Reconstitute vials with 5 mL sterile water for injection. Dilute reconstituted contents in 50 mL of normal saline or 5% dextrose.

**Additional Nursing Issues**

**Physical Assessment:** See Contraindications and Warnings/Precautions for use cautions. Monitor infusion site, cardiovascular, respiratory, and renal function during infusion. Monitor for adverse reactions (see Adverse Reactions) during infusion and periodically following infusion. Monitor closely for opportunistic infection (eg, chills, fever, sore throat, easy bruising or bleeding, mouth sores, unhealed sores). Assess knowledge/teach patient possible side effects/interventions and adverse symptoms to report as inpatient or following discharge. Breast-feeding is not recommended (see Breast-feeding Issues).

**Patient Information/Instruction:** This medication, which may help to reduce transplant rejection, can only be given by infusion. You will be monitored and assessed closely during infusion and thereafter, however, it is important that you report any changes or problems for evaluation. You will be susceptible to infection; avoid crowds or infected persons or persons with contagious diseases. Frequent mouth care and small frequent meals may help counteract any GI effects you may experience and will help maintain adequate nutrition and fluid intake. Report any changes in urination; unusual bruising or bleeding; chest pain or palpitations; acute dizziness; respiratory difficulty; fever or chills; changes in cognition; rash; feelings of pain or numbness in extremities; severe GI upset or diarrhea; unusual back or leg pain or muscle tremors; vision changes; or any sign of infection (chills, fever, sore throat, easy bruising or bleeding, mouth sores, unhealed sores, vaginal discharge). **Breast-feeding precautions:** Breast-feeding is not recommended.

**Breast-feeding Issues:** It is not known whether basiliximab is excreted in human milk. Because many immunoglobulins are secreted in milk and the potential for serious adverse reactions exists, a decision should be made whether to discontinue nursing or discontinue the drug, taking into account the importance of the drug to the mother.

**Pregnancy Issues:** IL-2 receptors play an important role in the development of the immune system. Use in pregnant women only when benefit exceeds potential risk to the fetus. Women of childbearing potential should use effective contraceptive measures before beginning treatment and for 2 months after completion of therapy with this agent.

♦ **Batrizol** *see* Co-trimoxazole *on page 307*

♦ **Baycol™** *see* Cerivastatin *on page 241*

- **Bayer® Aspirin [OTC]** *see* Aspirin *on page 111*
- **Bayer® Select® Chest Cold Caplets** *see page 1294*
- **Bayer® Select® Head Cold Caplets** *see page 1294*
- **BCG Vaccine** *see page 1256*
- **BCNU** *see* Carmustine *on page 204*
- **B Complex** *see* Vitamin, Multiple *on page 1219*
- **B Complex With C** *see* Vitamin, Multiple *on page 1219*
- **B-D Glucose®** *see page 1294*
- **Because®** *see page 1294*
- **Beclodisk®** *see* Beclomethasone *on this page*
- **Becloforte®** *see* Beclomethasone *on this page*


## Beclomethasone (be kloe METH a sone)

**U.S. Brand Names** Beclovent® Oral Inhaler; Beconase AQ® Nasal Inhaler; Beconase® Nasal Inhaler; Vancenase® AQ Inhaler; Vancenase® Nasal Inhaler; Vanceril® Oral Inhaler

**Therapeutic Category** Corticosteroid, Oral Inhaler; Corticosteroid, Nasal

**Pregnancy Risk Factor** C

**Lactation** Enters breast milk (oral)/use caution

**Use**

Oral inhalation: Treatment of bronchial asthma in patients who require chronic administration of corticosteroids

Nasal aerosol: Symptomatic treatment of seasonal or perennial rhinitis and nasal polyposis

**Mechanism of Action/Effect** Acts at cellular level to prevent or control inflammation

**Contraindications** Hypersensitivity to beclomethasone or fluorocarbons, oleic acid in the formulation; status asthmaticus; systemic fungal infections

**Warnings** Not to be used in status asthmaticus. Avoid using higher than recommended dosages since suppression of hypothalamic, pituitary, or adrenal function may occur. Pregnancy factor C.

**Adverse Reactions**

1% to 10%:

Dermatologic: Itching, allergic contact dermatitis, erythema, dryness papular rashes, folliculitis, furunculosis, pustules, pyoderma, vesiculation, hyperesthesia, skin infection (secondary)

Local: Burning, irritation

<1% (Limited to important or life-threatening symptoms): Hypertrichosis, acneiform eruptions, hypopigmentation, perioral dermatitis, bruising, maceration of skin, hirsutism, skin atrophy, striae, hypopigmentation, skin laceration, telangiectasia, Cushing's syndrome, hypokalemic syndrome, glaucoma, cataracts (posterior subcapsular)

**Overdose/Toxicology** Symptoms of overdose include irritation and burning of the nasal mucosa, sneezing, intranasal and pharyngeal *Candida* infections, nasal ulceration, epistaxis, rhinorrhea, nasal stuffiness, and headache. When consumed in high doses over prolonged periods, systemic hypercorticism and adrenal suppression may occur. In those cases, discontinuation of the corticosteroid should be done judiciously.

**Pharmacodynamics/Kinetics**

**Protein Binding:** Oral: 87%

**Distribution:** Inhalation: 10% to 25% of dose reaches respiratory tract

**Half-life Elimination:** Oral: Initial: 3 hours; Terminal: 15 hours

**Metabolism:** Liver

**Excretion:** Kidney

**Onset:** Therapeutic effect: Within 1-4 weeks of use

**Formulations**

Beclomethasone dipropionate:

Nasal:

Inhalation: (Beconase®, Vancenase®): 42 mcg/inhalation [200 metered doses] (16.8 g)

Spray (Vancenase® AQ Nasal): 0.084% [120 actuations] (19 g)

Spray, aqueous, nasal (Beconase AQ®, Vancenase® AQ): 42 mcg/inhalation [≥200 metered doses] (25 g); 84 mcg/inhalation [≥200 metered doses] (25 g)

Oral: Inhalation:

Beclovent®, Vanceril®: 42 mcg/inhalation [200 metered doses] (16.8 g)

Vanceril® Double Strength: 84 mcg/inhalation (5.4 g - 40 metered doses, 12.2 g - 120 metered doses)

**Dosing**

**Adults:** Nasal and oral inhalation dosage forms are not to be used interchangeably.

Nasal: 1 spray in each nostril 2-4 times/day

Oral inhalation: 2 inhalations 3-4 times/day; alternatively 2-4 inhalations twice daily; do not exceed 20 inhalations/day. Patients with severe asthma should be started on 12-16 inhalations/day (divided 3-4 times/day) and dose should be adjusted downward according to the patient's response.

**Elderly:** Refer to adult dosing.

**Administration**

**Inhalation:** Shake well before use. Keep oral inhaler clean and unobstructed, wash in warm water and dry thoroughly. Rinse mouth and throat after use to prevent *Candida* infection.

(Continued)

## Beclomethasone *(Continued)*

**Stability**

**Storage:** Do not store near heat or open flame.

**Additional Nursing Issues**

**Physical Assessment:** Not to be used to treat status asthmaticus or fungal infections of nasal passages. Monitor therapeutic effects, and adverse reactions (see Warnings/Precautions, Adverse Reactions, and Overdose/Toxicology). When changing from systemic steroids to inhalational steroids, taper reduction of systemic medication slowly. Assess knowledge/teach patient appropriate use, interventions to reduce side effects, and adverse symptoms to report. **Pregnancy risk factor C** - benefits of use should outweigh possible risks. Note breast-feeding caution.

**Patient Information/Instruction:** Use as directed; do not increase dosage or discontinue abruptly without consulting prescriber. It may take 1-4 weeks for you to realize full effects of treatment. Review use of inhaler or spray with prescriber or follow package insert for directions. Keep oral inhaler clean and unobstructed. Always rinse mouth and throat after use of inhaler to prevent opportunistic infection. If you are also using an inhaled bronchodilator, wait 10 minutes before using this steroid aerosol. Report adverse effects such as skin redness, rash, or irritation; pain or burning of nasal mucosa; white plaques in mouth or fuzzy tongue; unresolved headache; or worsening of condition or lack of improvement. **Pregnancy/breast-feeding precautions:** Inform prescriber if you are or intend to be pregnant. Consult prescriber if breast-feeding.

**Geriatric Considerations:** Older patients may have difficulty with oral metered dose inhalers and may benefit from the use of a spacer or chamber device.

**Related Information**

Inhalant (Asthma, Bronchospasm) Agents *on page 1388*

- **Beclovent® Oral Inhaler** *see* Beclomethasone *on previous page*
- **Beconase AQ® Nasal Inhaler** *see* Beclomethasone *on previous page*
- **Beconase Aqua** *see* Beclomethasone *on previous page*
- **Beconase® Nasal Inhaler** *see* Beclomethasone *on previous page*
- **Becotide 100** *see* Beclomethasone *on previous page*
- **Becotide 250** *see* Beclomethasone *on previous page*
- **Becotide Aerosol** *see* Beclomethasone *on previous page*
- **Becotin® Pulvules®** *see* Vitamin, Multiple *on page 1219*
- **Beepen-VK®** *see* Penicillin V Potassium *on page 900*
- **Beknol** *see* Benzonatate *on page 143*
- **Belix® Oral [OTC]** *see* Diphenhydramine *on page 381*

## Belladonna and Opium (bel a DON a & OH pee um)

**U.S. Brand Names** B&O Supprettes®

**Synonyms** Opium and Belladonna

**Therapeutic Category** Analgesic, Combination (Narcotic); Antispasmodic Agent, Urinary

**Pregnancy Risk Factor** C

**Lactation** Excretion in breast milk unknown/use caution

**Use** Relief of moderate to severe pain associated with rectal or bladder tenesmus that may occur in postoperative states and neoplastic situations; pain associated with ureteral spasms not responsive to non-narcotic analgesics; space intervals between injections of opiates

**Mechanism of Action/Effect** Anticholinergic alkaloids act primarily by competitive inhibition of the muscarinic actions of acetylcholine on structures innervated by postganglionic cholinergic neurons and on smooth muscle; resulting effects include antisecretory activity on exocrine glands and intestinal mucosa and smooth muscle relaxation. Contains many narcotic alkaloids including morphine; its mechanism for gastric motility inhibition is primarily due to this morphine content, resulting in a decrease in digestive secretions, an increase in GI muscle tone, and therefore a reduction in GI propulsion.

**Contraindications** Glaucoma; severe renal or hepatic disease; bronchial asthma; respiratory depression; convulsive disorders; acute alcoholism; premature labor

**Warnings** Usual precautions of opiate agonist therapy should be observed. Use with caution and generally in reduced doses in the very young or geriatric patients. Pregnancy factor C.

**Drug Interactions**

**Decreased Effect:** May decrease effects of drugs with cholinergic mechanisms. Antipsychotic efficacy of phenothiazines may be decreased.

**Increased Effect/Toxicity:** Additive effects with CNS depressants. May increase effects of digoxin and atenolol. Coadministration with other anticholinergic agents (phenothiazines, tricyclic antidepressants, amantadine, and antihistamines) may increase effects such as dry mouth, constipation, and urinary retention.

**Effects on Lab Values** ↑ aminotransferase [ALT (SGPT)/AST (SGOT)] (S)

**Adverse Reactions**

>10%:

Dermatologic: Dry skin

Gastrointestinal: Constipation, dry throat, dry mouth

Local: Irritation at injection site

Respiratory: Dry nose

Miscellaneous: Sweating (decreased)

1% to 10%:

Dermatologic: Increased sensitivity to light

Endocrine & metabolic: Decreased flow of breast milk
Gastrointestinal: Dysphagia

<1% (Limited to important or life-threatening symptoms): Orthostatic hypotension, ventricular fibrillation, tachycardia, palpitations, confusion, drowsiness, headache, loss of memory, fatigue, ataxia, CNS depression, increased intraocular pain, blurred vision, respiratory depression

**Overdose/Toxicology** Primary attention should be directed to ensuring adequate respiratory exchange. Opiate agonist-induced respiratory depression may be reversed with parenteral naloxone hydrochloride. Anticholinergic toxicity may be caused by strong binding of a belladonna alkaloid to cholinergic receptors. Physostigmine 1-2 mg given slowly S.C. or I.V. may be administered to reverse overdose with life-threatening effects.

**Pharmacodynamics/Kinetics**

**Metabolism:** Liver

**Excretion:** Urine

**Onset:** Belladonna: 1-2 hours; Opium: Within 30 minutes

**Formulations**

Suppository:
Belladonna extract 15 mg and opium 30 mg
Belladonna extract 15 mg and opium 60 mg

**Dosing**

**Adults:** Rectal: 1 suppository 1-2 times/day, up to 4 doses/day

**Elderly:** Refer to adult dosing.

**Administration**

**Other:** Prior to rectal insertion, the finger and suppository should be moistened. Assist with ambulation.

**Stability**

**Storage:** Store at 15°C to 30°C; avoid freezing.

**Additional Nursing Issues**

**Physical Assessment:** Assess other medications patient may be taking for additive or adverse interactions (additive adverse effects with all CNS depressants, tricyclic antidepressants, and other anticholinergics - see Warnings/Precautions and Drug Interactions). Monitor for effectiveness of pain relief and monitor for signs of overdose (see above). Monitor blood pressure, CNS and respiratory status, and degree of sedation at beginning of therapy and at regular intervals with long-term use. May cause physical and/or psychological dependence. For inpatients, implement safety measures (eg, side rails up, call light within reach, instructions to call for assistance, etc). Assess knowledge/teach patient appropriate use if self-administered. Teach patient to monitor for adverse reactions (see Adverse Reactions), adverse reactions to report, and appropriate interventions to reduce side effects. **Pregnancy risk factor C** - benefits of use should outweigh possible risks. Note breast-feeding caution.

**Patient Information/Instruction:** If self-administered, use exactly as directed (do not increase dose or frequency); may cause physical and/or psychological dependence. Take with food or milk. While using this medication, do not use alcohol and other prescription or OTC medications (especially sedatives, tranquilizers, antihistamines, or pain medications) without consulting prescriber. Maintain adequate hydration (2-3 L/day of fluids unless instructed to restrict fluid intake). May cause hypotension, dizziness, or drowsiness (use caution when driving, climbing stairs, or changing position (rising from sitting or lying to standing) or when engaging in tasks requiring alertness until response to drug is known); dry mouth or throat (frequent mouth care, frequent sips of fluids, chewing gum, or sucking lozenges may help); constipation (increased exercise, fluids, or dietary fruit and fiber may help - if constipation remains an unresolved problem, consult prescriber about use of stool softeners); photosensitivity (use sunscreen, wear protective clothing and eyewear, and avoid direct sunlight); decreased perspiration (avoid extremes in temperature or excessive activity in hot environments). Report chest pain or palpitations; persistent dizziness; changes in mentation; changes in gait; blurred vision; shortness of breath or difficulty breathing. **Pregnancy/breast-feeding precautions:** Inform prescriber if you are or intend to be pregnant. Consult prescriber if breast-feeding.

## Belladonna, Phenobarbital, and Ergotamine Tartrate

(bel a DON a, fee noe BAR bi tal, & er GOT a meen TAR trate)

**U.S. Brand Names** Bellergal-S®; Bel-Phen-Ergot S®; Phenerbel-S®

**Synonyms** Ergotamine Tartrate, Belladonna, and Phenobarbital; Phenobarbital, Belladonna, and Ergotamine Tartrate

**Therapeutic Category** Ergot Derivative

**Pregnancy Risk Factor** X

**Lactation** Enters breast milk (ergotamine)/contraindicated

**Use** Management and treatment of menopausal disorders, GI disorders and recurrent throbbing headache

**Contraindications** Hypersensitivity to belladonna alkaloids, phenobarbital, ergotamine, or any component; dopamine therapy; hypertension; glaucoma; pregnancy; coronary heart disease and peripheral vascular disease; impaired hepatic or renal function; sepsis; history of manifest or latent porphyria

**Warnings** Total weekly dosage of ergotamine should not exceed 10 mg. May be habit-forming. Use with caution in patients with bronchial asthma or obstructive uropathy. Caution should be used with prolonged use.

**Drug Interactions**

**Decreased Effect:** Phenobarbital may lower plasma levels of dicumarol due to decreased absorption. Possible interaction between ergot alkaloids and beta-blockers.

(Continued)

## Belladonna, Phenobarbital, and Ergotamine Tartrate *(Continued)*

**Increased Effect/Toxicity:** Combined administration of phenobarbital and CNS depressants such as alcohol, tricyclic depressants, phenothiazines, and narcotic analgesics may result in potentiation of depressant actions. **Phenobarbital taken with warfarin induces liver enzymes that enhances clearance of warfarin. A reduction in phenobarbital dose in patients receiving warfarin has resulted in fatal bleeding episodes.** Griseofulvin, quinidine, doxycycline, and estrogen have been shown to be metabolized at an increased rate. Belladonna and concomitant administration of tricyclic antidepressants may result in additive anticholinergic effects. Valproic acid appears to decrease barbiturate metabolism, possible with phenytoin.

**Adverse Reactions**

>10%:

Cardiovascular: Peripheral vascular effects (numbness and tingling of fingers and toes)

Central nervous system: Drowsiness, dizziness,

Dermatologic: Dry skin

Gastrointestinal: Constipation, dry mouth and throat, diarrhea, nausea, vomiting

Respiratory: Dry nose

Miscellaneous: Decreased diaphoresis

1% to 10%:

Cardiovascular: Precordial distress and pain, transient tachycardia or bradycardia

Dermatologic: Photosensitivity

Endocrine & metabolic: Decreased flow of breast milk

Gastrointestinal: Difficulty in swallowing

Neuromuscular & skeletal: Muscle pains in the extremities, weakness in the legs

<1% (Limited to important or life-threatening symptoms): Orthostatic hypotension, ventricular fibrillation, tachycardia, palpitations, confusion, headache, loss of memory, drowsiness, skin rash, increased intraocular pain, blurred vision

**Pharmacodynamics/Kinetics**

**Distribution:** Ergotamine: Crosses blood brain barrier

**Half-life Elimination:** Ergotamine: 21 hours

**Metabolism:** Ergotamine: Liver

**Excretion:** Belladonna: Urine; Ergotamine: Feces and urine (4%)

**Formulations** Tablet, sustained release: l-alkaloids of belladonna 0.2 mg, phenobarbital 40 mg, and ergotamine tartrate 0.6 mg

**Dosing**

**Adults:** Oral: 1 tablet each morning and evening

**Elderly:** Refer to dosing in individual monographs.

**Additional Nursing Issues**

**Physical Assessment:** Monitor (instruct patient to monitor and report) for signs or symptoms of adverse reaction: excessive depression, peripheral vascular effects, dryness (eg, skin, mouth, eyes), and constipation. Closely monitor all other medications (prescriptive and OTC) that the patient may be taking. This combination drug interacts with many commonly prescribed drugs to potentiate adverse/toxic reactions, or to reduce the effectiveness of other drugs. **Pregnancy risk factor X** - determine that patient is not pregnant before beginning treatment and do not give to women of childbearing age or to males who may have intercourse with women of childbearing age unless both male and female are capable of complying with barrier contraceptive measures during therapy and for 1 month following therapy. Breast-feeding is contraindicated.

**Patient Information/Instruction:** Take as directed; do not take more than recommended dose. Maintain adequate nutritional and fluid intake (2-3 L/day of fluids unless instructed to restrict fluid intake) to prevent constipation. May cause drowsiness or dizziness (use caution when driving or engaging in tasks that require alertness until response to drug is known); dry throat or mouth (frequent mouth care or sucking on lozenges may help); dry nose (use humidifier); photosensitivity (use sunblock, wear protective clothing and eyewear, and avoid direct sunlight); nausea or vomiting (small frequent meals, frequent mouth care, sucking lozenges, or chewing gum may help); dry skin (mild skin lotion may help); or orthostatic hypotension (use caution when rising from sitting or lying position or climbing stairs). Report any signs of numbness in extremities (fingers and toes), unusual leg pain or cyanosis of extremities; difficulty swallowing; persistent muscle pain or weakness; pain in eye or vision changes; or chest pain, rapid heartbeat, or palpitations. **Pregnancy/breast-feeding precautions:** Inform prescriber if you are pregnant and do not get pregnant during or for 1 month following therapy. Male: Do not cause a female to become pregnant. Male/female: Consult prescriber for instruction on appropriate contraceptive measures. This drug may cause severe fetal defects. Do not breast-feed.

**Pregnancy Issues:** Potential uterotonic effects.


- ♦ **Bellergal®** *see* Belladonna, Phenobarbital, and Ergotamine Tartrate *on previous page*
- ♦ **Bellergal-S®** *see* Belladonna, Phenobarbital, and Ergotamine Tartrate *on previous page*
- ♦ **Bellergal® Spacetabs®** *see* Belladonna, Phenobarbital, and Ergotamine Tartrate *on previous page*
- ♦ **Bel-Phen-Ergot S®** *see* Belladonna, Phenobarbital, and Ergotamine Tartrate *on previous page*
- ♦ **Benadon** *see* Pyridoxine *on page 997*
- ♦ **Benadryl® Decongestant Allergy Tablet** *see page 1294*
- ♦ **Benadryl® Injection** *see* Diphenhydramine *on page 381*

- **Benadryl® Oral [OTC]** *see* Diphenhydramine *on page 381*
- **Benadryl® Topical** *see* Diphenhydramine *on page 381*
- **Ben-Allergin-50® Injection** *see* Diphenhydramine *on page 381*
- **Ben-Aqua®** *see page 1294*
- **Benaxima** *see* Cefotaxime *on page 221*
- **Benaxona** *see* Ceftriaxone *on page 232*

## Benazepril (ben AY ze pril)

**U.S. Brand Names** Lotensin®

**Therapeutic Category** Angiotensin-Converting Enzyme (ACE) Inhibitors

**Pregnancy Risk Factor** C/D (2nd and 3rd trimesters)

**Lactation** Enters breast milk/compatible

**Use** Treatment of hypertension, either alone or in combination with other antihypertensive agents

**Mechanism of Action/Effect** Competitive inhibitor of angiotensin-converting enzyme (ACE); prevents conversion of angiotensin I to angiotensin II, a potent vasoconstrictor; results in lower levels of angiotensin II which causes an increase in plasma renin activity and a reduction in aldosterone secretion

**Contraindications** Hypersensitivity to benazepril, any component, or other ACE inhibitors; pregnancy (2nd and 3rd trimesters)

**Warnings** Use with caution in patients with collagen vascular disease, hypovolemia, valvular stenosis, hyperkalemia, or recent anesthesia. Modify dosage in patients with renal impairment (especially renal artery stenosis), severe congestive heart failure, or with coadministered diuretic therapy. Severe hypotension may occur in patients who are sodium and/or volume depleted. Initiate lower doses and monitor closely when starting therapy in these patients. Pregnancy factor C/D (2nd and 3rd trimesters).

**Drug Interactions**

**Decreased Effect:** Rifampin may decrease the effect of ACE inhibitors. Antacids may decrease the bioavailability of ACE inhibitors which may be more likely to occur with captopril, separate administration times by 1-2 hours. NSAIDs, specifically indomethacin, may reduce the hypotensive effects of ACE inhibitors. More likely to occur in low renin or volume dependent hypertensive patients.

**Increased Effect/Toxicity:** Diuretics have additive hypotensive effects with ACE inhibitors. Probenecid increases blood levels of captopril which may occur with other ACE inhibitors. Phenothiazines taken with ACE inhibitors may increase the pharmacologic effects of the ACE inhibitor. Allopurinol and ACE inhibitors may cause a higher risk of hypersensitivity reaction when taken concurrently. Digoxin and ACE inhibitors may result in elevated serum digoxin levels. Lithium and ACE inhibitors may result in elevated serum levels of lithium with symptoms of toxicity. Potassium supplements or potassium-sparing diuretics with ACE inhibitors may result in elevated serum potassium levels.

**Adverse Reactions**

1% to 10%:

Central nervous system: Headache, dizziness, fatigue, somnolence, postural dizziness

Gastrointestinal: Nausea

Respiratory: Transient cough

<1% (Limited to important or life-threatening symptoms): Hypotension, tachycardia, palpitations, chest pain pectoris, flushing, anxiety, insomnia, nervousness, rash, photosensitivity, angioedema, pruritus, hyperkalemia, hypertonia, paresthesia, muscle weakness, arthralgia, arthritis, myalgia, weakness, asthma, bronchitis, dyspnea, sinusitis, pancreatitis, Stevens-Johnson syndrome, hemolytic anemia, eosinophilic pneumonia (attributed to other ACE inhibitors)

**Overdose/Toxicology** Mild hypotension has been the primary toxic effect seen with acute overdose. Bradycardia may also occur. Hyperkalemia occurs even with therapeutic doses, especially in patients with renal insufficiency and those taking NSAIDs. Treatment is symptom directed and supportive.

**Pharmacodynamics/Kinetics**

**Half-life Elimination:** Parent drug: 0.6 hour; Metabolite elimination: 22 hours (from 24 hours after dosing onward); Metabolite: 1.5-2 hours after fasting or 2-4 hours after a meal

**Time to Peak:** 1-1.5 hours (unchanged parent drug)

**Metabolism:** Liver

**Excretion:** Urine

**Onset:**

Reduction in plasma angiotensin-converting enzyme activity: Oral: Peak effect: 1-2 hours after administration of 2-20 mg dose

Reduction in blood pressure: Peak effect after single oral dose: 2-6 hours; Maximum response with continuous therapy: 2 weeks

**Duration:** >90% inhibition for 24 hours has been observed after 5-20 mg dose

**Formulations** Tablet, as hydrochloride: 5 mg, 10 mg, 20 mg, 40 mg

**Dosing**

**Adults:** Oral: 20-40 mg/day as a single dose or 2 divided doses; maximum daily dose: 80 mg

**Elderly:** Patients taking diuretics should have them discontinued 2-3 days prior to starting benazepril. If they cannot be discontinued, then initial dose should be 5 mg; restart after blood pressure is stabilized if needed.

Oral: Initial: 5-10 mg/day in single or divided doses; usual range: 20-40 mg/day; adjust for renal function.

(Continued)

## Benazepril *(Continued)*

**Renal Impairment:**

$Cl_{cr}$ <30 mL/minute: Administer 5 mg/day initially; maximum daily dose: 40 mg.

Hemodialysis effects: Moderately dialyzable (20% to 50%); administer dose postdialysis or administer 25% to 35% supplemental dose.

Peritoneal dialysis: Supplemental dose is not necessary.

**Monitoring Laboratory Tests** CBC, renal function tests, electrolytes

**Additional Nursing Issues**

**Physical Assessment:** Assess effectiveness and interactions of other medications (see Drug Interactions). See Warnings/Precautions and Contraindications for use cautions. Monitor effectiveness of therapy, laboratory tests, and adverse response on a regular basis during therapy, eg, postural hypotension (see Adverse Reactions and Overdose/Toxicology). Assess knowledge/teach patient appropriate use, possible side effects and appropriate interventions, and adverse symptoms to report. **Pregnancy risk factor C/D** - see Pregnancy Risk Factor - assess knowledge/teach appropriate use of barrier contraceptives. See Pregnancy Issues.

**Patient Information/Instruction:** Take exactly as directed; do not discontinue without consulting prescriber. Take first dose at bedtime. Take all doses on an empty stomach (30 minutes before or 2 hours after meals). This drug does not eliminate need for diet or exercise regimen as recommended by prescriber. May cause dizziness, fainting, lightheadedness (use caution when driving or engaging in tasks that require alertness until response to drug is known); postural hypotension (use caution when rising from lying or sitting position or climbing stairs); nausea, vomiting, abdominal pain, dry mouth, or transient loss of appetite (small frequent meals, frequent mouth care, sucking lozenges, or chewing gum may help) - report if these persist. Report mouth sores; fever or chills; swelling of extremities, face, mouth, or tongue; difficulty in breathing or unusual cough; or other persistent adverse reactions. **Pregnancy precautions:** Do not get pregnant while taking this medication; use appropriate barrier contraceptive measures.

**Geriatric Considerations:** Due to frequent decreases in glomerular filtration (also creatinine clearance) with aging, elderly patients may have exaggerated responses to ACE inhibitors. Differences in clinical response due to hepatic changes are not observed. ACE inhibitors may be preferred agents in elderly patients with congestive heart failure and diabetes mellitus. Diabetic proteinuria is reduced and insulin sensitivity is enhanced. In general, the side effect profile is favorable in elderly and causes little or no CNS confusion. Use lowest dose recommendations initially.

**Pregnancy Issues:** ACE inhibitors can cause fetal injury or death if taken during the 2nd or 3rd trimester. Discontinue ACE inhibitors as soon as pregnancy is detected. ACE inhibitors should not be used if patient is sexually active and not using contraceptives.

**Related Information**

ACE Inhibitors and Angiotensin Antagonists Comparison *on page 1362*

◆ **Benazepril and Amlodipine** *see* Amlodipine and Benazepril *on page 77*

## Benazepril and Hydrochlorothiazide

(ben AY ze pril & hye droe klor oh THYE a zide)

**U.S. Brand Names** Lotensin HCT®

**Synonyms** Hydrochlorothiazide and Benazepril

**Therapeutic Category** Antihypertensive Agent, Combination

**Pregnancy Risk Factor** C/D (2nd and 3rd trimesters)

**Lactation** Enters breast milk/compatible

**Use** Treatment of hypertension

**Formulations**

Tablet:

Benazepril 5 mg and hydrochlorothiazide 6.25 mg
Benazepril 10 mg and hydrochlorothiazide 12.5 mg
Benazepril 20 mg and hydrochlorothiazide 12.5 mg
Benazepril 20 mg and hydrochlorothiazide 25 mg

**Dosing**

**Adults:** Benazepril: 5-20 mg; hydrochlorothiazide: 6.25-25 mg/day

**Elderly:** Dose is individualized.

**Renal Impairment:** $Cl_{cr}$ <30 mL/minute: Not recommended; loop diuretics preferred

**Additional Nursing Issues**

**Physical Assessment:** See individual components listed in Related Information. **Pregnancy risk factor C/D** - see Pregnancy Risk Factor - assess knowledge/instruct patient on need to use appropriate contraceptive measures and the need to avoid pregnancy.

**Patient Information/Instruction:** See individual components listed in Related Information. **Pregnancy precautions:** Inform prescriber if you are or intend to be pregnant.

**Related Information**

Benazepril *on previous page*
Hydrochlorothiazide *on page 566*

◆ **Benecid Probenecida Valdecasas** *see* Probenecid *on page 966*

◆ **Benemid®** *see* Probenecid *on page 966*

◆ **Benoxyl®** *see page 1294*

◆ **Bentiromide** *see page 1248*

◆ **Bentyl® Hydrochloride Injection** *see* Dicyclomine *on page 362*

- **Bentyl® Hydrochloride Oral** *see* Dicyclomine *on page 362*
- **Bentylol®** *see* Dicyclomine *on page 362*
- **Benuryl™** *see* Probenecid *on page 966*
- **Benylin® Cough Syrup [OTC]** *see* Diphenhydramine *on page 381*
- **Benylin DM®** *see page 1294*
- **Benylin® Expectorant [OTC]** *see* Guaifenesin and Dextromethorphan *on page 549*
- **Benza®** *see page 1294*
- **Benzac AC® Gel** *see page 1294*
- **Benzac AC® Wash** *see page 1294*
- **Benzac W® Gel** *see page 1294*
- **Benzac W® Wash** *see page 1294*
- **5-Benzagel®** *see page 1294*
- **10-Benzagel®** *see page 1294*
- **Benzalkonium Chloride** *see page 1294*
- **Benzalkonium Chloride, Benzocaine, Butyl Aminobenzoate, Tetracaine** *see* Benzocaine, Butyl Aminobenzoate, Tetracaine, and Benzalkonium Chloride *on next page*
- **Benzamycin®** *see* Erythromycin and Benzoyl Peroxide *on page 437*
- **Benzanil** *see* Penicillin G, Parenteral, Aqueous *on page 897*
- **Benzashave® Cream** *see page 1294*
- **Benzathine Benzylpenicillin** *see* Penicillin G Benzathine *on page 896*
- **Benzathine Penicillin G** *see* Penicillin G Benzathine *on page 896*
- **Benzedrex® Inhaler** *see page 1294*
- **Benzene Hexachloride** *see* Lindane *on page 678*
- **Benzetacil** *see* Penicillin G Benzathine *on page 896*
- **Benzhexol Hydrochloride** *see* Trihexyphenidyl *on page 1179*
- **Benzilfan** *see* Penicillin G Benzathine *on page 896*

## Benzocaine (BEN zoe kane)

**U.S. Brand Names** Americaine [OTC]; Anbesol® [OTC]; Anbesol® Maximum Strength [OTC]; Babee Teething® [OTC]; Benzocol® [OTC]; Benzodent® [OTC]; Chigger-Tox® [OTC]; Cylex® [OTC]; Dermoplast® [OTC]; Foille® [OTC]; Foille® Medicated First Aid [OTC]; Hurricaine®; Lanacane® [OTC]; Maximum Strength Anbesol® [OTC]; Maximum Strength Orajel® [OTC]; Mycinettes® [OTC]; Numzitdent® [OTC]; Numzit Teething® [OTC]; Orabase®-B [OTC]; Orabase®-O [OTC]; Orajel® Brace-Aid Oral Anesthetic [OTC]; Orajel® Maximum Strength [OTC]; Orajel® Mouth-Aid [OTC]; Orasept® [OTC]; Orasol® [OTC]; Rhulicaine® [OTC]; Rid-A-Pain® [OTC]; Slim-Mint® [OTC]; Solarcaine® [OTC]; Spec-T® [OTC]; Tanac® [OTC]; Trocaine® [OTC]; Unguentine® [OTC]; Vicks® Children's Chloraseptic® [OTC]; Vicks® Chloraseptic® Sore Throat [OTC]; Zilactin-B® Medicated [OTC]; ZilaDent® [OTC]

**Synonyms** Ethyl Aminobenzoate

**Therapeutic Category** Local Anesthetic

**Pregnancy Risk Factor** C

**Lactation** Excretion in breast milk unknown

**Use** Local anesthetic (ester derivative); temporary relief of pain associated with local anesthetic for pruritic dermatosis, pruritus, minor burns, acute congestive and serous otitis media, swimmer's ear, otitis externa, toothache, minor sore throat pain, canker sores, hemorrhoids, rectal fissures, anesthetic lubricant for passage of catheters and endoscopic tubes; nonprescription diet aid

**Mechanism of Action/Effect** Benzocaine blocks both the initiation and conduction of nerve impulses by decreasing the neuronal membrane's permeability to sodium ions, which results in inhibition of depolarization with resultant blockade of conduction. As a diet aide, the anesthetic effect appears to decrease the ability to detect degrees of sweetness by taste perception.

**Contraindications** Hypersensitivity to benzocaine, other ester-type local anesthetics, or any component; ophthalmic use

**Warnings** Not intended for use when infections are present. Pregnancy factor C.

**Adverse Reactions** Dose-related and may result in high plasma levels

1% to 10%:
- Dermatologic: Angioedema, contact dermatitis
- Local: Burning, stinging

<1% (Limited to important or life-threatening symptoms): Edema, urticaria, urethritis, methemoglobinemia in infants

**Pharmacodynamics/Kinetics**

**Metabolism:** Plasma and liver

**Excretion:** Urine

**Formulations**

Topical for mucous membranes:
- Gel: 6% (7.5 g); 20% (2.5 g, 3.75 g, 7.5 g, 30 g)
- Liquid: 20% (3.75 mL, 9 mL, 13.3 mL, 30 mL)

Topical for skin disorders:
- Aerosol, external use: 5% (92 mL, 105 g); 20% (82.5 mL, 90 mL, 92 mL, 150 mL)
- Cream: (30 g, 60 g); 5% (30 g, 1 lb); 6% (28.4 g)
- Lotion: (120 mL); 8% (90 mL)
- Ointment: 5% (3.5 g, 28 g)
- Spray: 5% (97.5 mL); 20% (20 g, 60 g, 120 g, 13.3 mL, 120 mL)

Mouth/throat preparations:
- Cream: 5% (10 g)

(Continued)

## Benzocaine *(Continued)*

Gel: 6.3% (7.5 g); 7.5% (7.2 g, 9.45 g, 14.1 g); 10% (6 g, 9.45 g, 10 g, 15 g); 15% (10.5 g); 20% (9.45 g, 14.1 g)
Liquid: 20% (3.7 mL); 5% (8.8 mL); 6.3% (9 mL, 22 mL, 14.79 mL); 10% (13 mL); 20% (13.3 mL)
Lotion: 0.2% (15 mL); 2.5% (15 mL)
Lozenges: 5 mg, 6 mg, 10 mg, 15 mg
Ointment: 20% (30 g)
Paste: 20% (5 g, 15 g)

Nonprescription diet aid:
Candy: 6 mg
Gum: 6 mg

**Dosing**

**Adults:**

Mucous membranes: Dosage varies depending on area to be anesthetized and vascularity of tissues.

Oral mouth/throat preparations: Do not administer for >2 days unless directed by a physician; refer to specific package labeling.

Topical: Apply to affected area as needed.

Oral: Nonprescription diet aid: 6-15 mg just prior to food consumption, not to exceed 45 mg/day

**Elderly:** Refer to adult dosing.

**Administration**

**Topical:** Do not eat for 1 hour after application to oral mucosa. Chemical burns should be neutralized before application of benzocaine. Avoid application to large areas of broken skin, especially in children.

**Additional Nursing Issues**

**Physical Assessment:** Monitor for effectiveness of application and adverse reactions (see Adverse Reactions). Oral: Use caution to prevent gagging or choking and avoid food or drink for 1 hour. Teach patient adverse reactions to report; use and teach appropriate interventions to promote safety. **Pregnancy risk factor C** - benefits of use should outweigh possible risks. Note breast-feeding caution.

**Patient Information/Instruction:** Use as directed; do not overuse. Do not apply when infections are present and do not apply to large areas of broken skin. Do not eat or drink for 1 hour following oral application. Discontinue application and report if swelling of mouth, lips, tongue, or throat occurs; or if skin irritation occurs at application site. **Pregnancy/breast-feeding precautions:** Inform prescriber if you are pregnant. Consult prescriber if breast-feeding.

**Related Information**

Otic Agents *on page 1291*

♦ **Benzocaine, Antipyrine, and Phenylephrine** *see page 1291*

## Benzocaine, Butyl Aminobenzoate, Tetracaine, and Benzalkonium Chloride

(BEN zoe kane, BYOO til a meen oh BENZ oh ate, TET ra kane, & benz al KOE nee um KLOR ide)

**U.S. Brand Names** Cetacaine®

**Synonyms** Benzalkonium Chloride, Benzocaine, Butyl Aminobenzoate, Tetracaine; Butyl Aminobenzoate, Benzocaine, Tetracaine, and Benzalkonium Chloride; Tetracaine Hydrochloride, Benzocaine, Butyl Aminobenzoate, and Benzalkonium Chloride

**Therapeutic Category** Local Anesthetic

**Pregnancy Risk Factor** C

**Lactation** For topical use

**Use** Topical anesthetic to control pain or gagging

**Formulations** Aerosol: Benzocaine 14%, butyl aminobenzoate 2%, tetracaine 2%, and benzalkonium chloride 0.5% (56 g)

**Dosing**

**Adults:** Apply to affected area for approximately 1 second

**Elderly:** Refer to adult dosing.

**Additional Nursing Issues**

**Physical Assessment:** Instruct patient on appropriate precautions. **Pregnancy risk factor C** - benefits of use should outweigh possible risks.

**Patient Information/Instruction:** This spray may help control pain or gagging. If mouth or throat is numb, use caution with food and fluids. Your sensation to heat may be disturbed, your ability to swallow may be disturbed; use caution when swallowing to prevent choking. **Pregnancy precautions:** Inform prescriber if you are or intend to be pregnant.

**Related Information**

Benzocaine *on previous page*
Tetracaine *on page 1110*

♦ **Benzocaine, Gelatin, Pectin, and Sodium Carboxymethylcellulose** *see page 1294*

♦ **Benzocol® [OTC]** *see* Benzocaine *on previous page*

♦ **Benzodent® [OTC]** *see* Benzocaine *on previous page*

♦ **Benzodiazepines Comparison** *see page 1375*

♦ **Benzoic Acid and Salicylic Acid** *see page 1294*

♦ **Benzoin** *see page 1294*

## Benzonatate (ben ZOE na tate)

**U.S. Brand Names** Tessalon® Perles

**Therapeutic Category** Antitussive

**Pregnancy Risk Factor** C

**Lactation** Excretion in breast milk unknown

**Use** Symptomatic relief of nonproductive cough

**Mechanism of Action/Effect** Suppresses cough by topical anesthetic action on the respiratory stretch receptors

**Contraindications** Hypersensitivity to benzonatate or related compounds (such as tetracaine)

**Warnings** Pregnancy factor C.

**Adverse Reactions**

1% to 10%:

Central nervous system: Sedation, headache, dizziness, mental confusion, visual hallucinations, vague "chilly" sensation

Dermatologic: Rash

Gastrointestinal: Constipation, nausea, vomiting, GI upset

Neuromuscular & skeletal: Numbness in chest

Ocular: Burning sensation in eyes

Respiratory: Stuffy nose

**Overdose/Toxicology** Symptoms of overdose include restlessness, tremor, and CNS stimulation. Benzonatate's local anesthetic activity can reduce the patient's gag reflex and, therefore, may contradict the use of ipecac following ingestion. Treatment is supportive and symptomatic.

**Pharmacodynamics/Kinetics**

**Onset:** Therapeutic: Within 15-20 minutes

**Duration:** 3-8 hours

**Formulations** Capsule: 100 mg

**Dosing**

**Adults:** Oral: 100 mg 3 times/day or every 4 hours up to 600 mg/day

**Elderly:** Refer to adult dosing.

**Administration**

**Oral:** Swallow capsule whole (do not break or chew).

**Additional Nursing Issues**

**Physical Assessment:** Monitor effectiveness of therapy (relief of cough, lung sounds, and respiratory pattern) and adverse reactions (eg, CNS changes - see Adverse Reactions) at beginning of therapy and periodically with long-term use. Assess knowledge/teach patient appropriate use, interventions to reduce side effects, and adverse symptoms to report. **Pregnancy risk factor C** - benefits of use should outweigh possible risks. Note breast-feeding caution.

**Patient Information/Instruction:** Take only as prescribed; do not exceed prescribed dose or frequency. Do not break or chew tablet. Maintain adequate hydration (2-3 L/day of fluids unless instructed to restrict fluid intake). Avoid use of other depressants, alcohol, or sleep-inducing medications unless approved by prescriber. You may experience drowsiness, impaired coordination, blurred vision, or increased anxiety (use caution when driving or engaging in tasks requiring alertness until response to drug is known); or upset stomach or nausea (frequent small meals, frequent mouth care, chewing gum, or sucking hard candy may help). Report persistent CNS changes (dizziness, sedation, tremor, or agitation), numbness in chest or feeling of chill, visual changes or burning in eyes, numbness of mouth or difficulty swallowing, or lack of improvement or worsening or condition. **Pregnancy/breast-feeding precautions:** Inform prescriber if you are or intend to be pregnant. Consult prescriber if breast-feeding.

**Geriatric Considerations:** No specific geriatric information is available about benzonatate. Avoid use in patients with impaired gag reflex or who cannot swallow the capsule whole.

♦ **Benzoyl Peroxide** *see page 1294*

♦ **Benzoyl Peroxide and Erythromycin** *see* Erythromycin and Benzoyl Peroxide *on page 437*

## Benzoyl Peroxide and Hydrocortisone

(BEN zoe il peer OKS ide & hye droe KOR ti sone)

**U.S. Brand Names** Vanoxide-HC®

**Synonyms** Hydrocortisone and Benzoyl Peroxide

**Therapeutic Category** Acne Products

**Pregnancy Risk Factor** C

**Lactation** For topical use

**Use** Treatment of acne vulgaris and oily skin

**Formulations** Lotion: Benzoyl peroxide 5% and hydrocortisone alcohol 0.5% (25 mL)

**Dosing**

**Adults:** Shake well; apply thin film 1-3 times/day, gently massage into skin

**Elderly:** Refer to adult dosing.

**Additional Nursing Issues**

**Physical Assessment:** See individual components listed in Related Information. **Pregnancy risk factor C** - benefits of use should outweigh possible risks.

**Patient Information/Instruction:** See individual components listed in Related Information. **Pregnancy precautions:** Inform prescriber if you are or intend to be pregnant.

(Continued)

## Benzoyl Peroxide and Hydrocortisone *(Continued)*

**Related Information**

Hydrocortisone *on page 578*

## Benzthiazide (benz THYE a zide)

**U.S. Brand Names** Aquatag®; Exna®; Hydrex®; Marazide®; Proaqua®

**Therapeutic Category** Diuretic, Thiazide

**Pregnancy Risk Factor** D

**Lactation** Excretion in breast milk unknown/use caution©

**Use** Management of mild to moderate hypertension; treatment of edema in congestive heart failure and nephrotic syndrome

**Contraindications** Hypersensitivity to benzthiazide or any component; cross-sensitivity with other thiazides and sulfonamide derivatives; anuria; renal decompensation; pregnancy

**Warnings** Use with caution with hypokalemia, hepatic disease, gout, lupus erythematosus, diabetes mellitus, and severe renal diseases.

**Drug Interactions**

**Decreased Effect:** Decreased effect of oral hypoglycemics. Decreased absorption of benzthiazide with cholestyramine and colestipol.

**Increased Effect/Toxicity:** Increased effect of benzthiazide with furosemide and other loop diuretics. Benzthiazide Increases toxicity/levels of lithium.

**Adverse Reactions**

1% to 10%:

Cardiovascular: Orthostatic hypotension
Endocrine & metabolic: Hypokalemia
Dermatologic: Photosensitivity
Gastrointestinal: Anorexia, epigastric distress

<1% (Limited to important or life-threatening symptoms): Purpura, rash, urticaria, necrotizing angiitis, vasculitis, cutaneous vasculitis, hyperuricemia or gout, hyponatremia, sexual ability (decreased), hyperglycemia, glycosuria, nausea, vomiting, cholecystitis, pancreatitis, diarrhea or constipation, aplastic anemia, hemolytic anemia, leukopenia, agranulocytosis, thrombocytopenia, hepatic function impairment, uremia

**Overdose/Toxicology** Symptoms of overdose include hypermotility, diuresis, lethargy, confusion, and muscle weakness. Treatment is supportive.

**Pharmacodynamics/Kinetics**

**Onset:** Within 2 hours

**Duration:** 12 hours

**Formulations** Tablet: 50 mg

**Dosing**

**Adults:** Oral: 50-200 mg/day

**Elderly:** Refer to adult dosing.

**Additional Nursing Issues**

**Physical Assessment:** Monitor blood pressure standing and lying down. Monitor fluid balance (I & O ratio), weight, and signs or symptoms of edema. **Pregnancy risk factor D** - assess knowledge/teach appropriate use of barrier contraceptives. Note breast-feeding caution.

**Patient Information/Instruction:** Take early in the day and take last dose in early evening to avoid frequent night urination. Take with food to reduce GI upset. Weigh yourself on a regular basis (same time, same clothes). Report unresolved weight gain (more than 3-5 pounds in 3 days). You may experience dizziness or drowsiness; change positions slowly and use caution when driving or engaging in tasks that require alertness until response to drug is known. May cause photosensitivity; use sunscreen wear protective clothing and eyewear, and avoid direct sunlight. You may experience decreased sexual function; this will resolve when medication is discontinued. Report increased swelling of ankles, fingers, dizziness or trembling, cramps, or muscle pain. **Pregnancy/breast-feeding precautions:** Do not get pregnant while taking this medication; use appropriate barrier contraceptive measures. Consult prescriber if breast-feeding.

## Benztropine (BENZ troe peen)

**U.S. Brand Names** Cogentin®

**Therapeutic Category** Anticholinergic Agent; Anti-Parkinson's Agent (Anticholinergic)

**Pregnancy Risk Factor** C

**Lactation** Excretion in breast milk unknown

**Use** Adjunctive treatment of Parkinson's disease; treatment of drug-induced extrapyramidal effects (except tardive dyskinesia)

**Mechanism of Action/Effect** Thought to partially block striatal cholinergic receptors to help balance cholinergic and dopaminergic activity

**Contraindications** Narrow-angle glaucoma; pyloric or duodenal obstruction; stenosing peptic ulcers; bladder neck obstructions; achalasia; myasthenia gravis

**Warnings** Use with caution in hot weather or during exercise. Elderly patients frequently develop increased sensitivity and require strict dosage regulation - side effects may be more severe in elderly patients with atherosclerotic changes. Use with caution in patients with tachycardia, cardiac arrhythmias, hypertension, hypotension, prostatic hypertrophy (especially in the elderly) or any tendency toward urinary retention, liver or kidney disorders, and obstructive disease of the GI or GU tract. When given in large doses or to susceptible patients, may cause weakness and inability to move particular muscle groups. Pregnancy factor C.

**Drug Interactions**

**Decreased Effect:** Gastric degradation of levodopa may increase due to benztropine effect of delayed gastric emptying which reduces the amount of levodopa that can be absorbed.

**Increased Effect/Toxicity:** Central anticholinergic syndrome can occur when administered with narcotic analgesics, phenothiazines and other antipsychotics, tricyclic antidepressants, antihistamines, quinidine and some other antiarrhythmics.

**Adverse Reactions**

>10%:

Dermatologic: Dry skin

Gastrointestinal: Constipation, dry throat, dry mouth

Respiratory: Dry nose

Miscellaneous: Sweating (decreased)

1% to 10%:

Dermatologic: Increased sensitivity to light

Endocrine & metabolic: Decreased flow of breast milk

Gastrointestinal: Dysphagia

<1% (Limited to important or life-threatening symptoms): Tachycardia, orthostatic hypotension, ventricular fibrillation, palpitations, coma, drowsiness, nervousness, hallucinations; the elderly may be at increased risk for confusion and hallucinations, headache, loss of memory, fatigue, ataxia, false sense of well-being (especially with elderly or with high doses), loss of memory (elderly), hyperthermia, fever, heat stroke, toxic psychosis, dysuria, blurred vision, mydriasis, increased intraocular pain

**Overdose/Toxicology** Symptoms of overdose include CNS depression, confusion, nervousness, hallucinations, dizziness, blurred vision, nausea, vomiting, and hyperthermia. For anticholinergic overdose with severe life-threatening symptoms, physostigmine 1-2 mg S.C. or I.V. slowly, may be given to reverse these effects.

**Pharmacodynamics/Kinetics**

**Metabolism:** Liver

**Excretion:** Urine

**Onset:** Oral: Within 1 hour; Parenteral: Within 15 minutes

**Duration:** 6-48 hours (wide range)

**Formulations**

Benztropine mesylate:

Injection: 1 mg/mL (2 mL)

Tablet: 0.5 mg, 1 mg, 2 mg

**Dosing**

**Adults:**

Drug-induced extrapyramidal reaction: Oral, I.M., I.V.: 1-4 mg/dose 1-2 times/day

Acute dystonia: I.M., I.V.: 1-2 mg

Parkinsonism: Oral: 0.5-6 mg/day in 1-2 divided doses; if one dose is greater, give at bedtime. Titrate dose in 0.5 mg increments at 5- to 6-day intervals.

**Elderly:** Oral: Initial: 0.5 mg once or twice daily; titrate dose in 0.5 mg increments at every 5-6 days; maximum: 6 mg/day.

**Additional Nursing Issues**

**Physical Assessment:** Assess effectiveness and interactions of other medications patient may be taking (see Contraindications and Drug Interactions). Monitor renal function, therapeutic response (eg, Parkinsonian symptoms), and adverse reactions such as anticholinergic syndrome (dry mouth and mucous membranes, constipation, epigastric distress, CNS disturbances, paralytic ileus) at beginning of therapy and periodically throughout therapy (see Warnings/Precautions, Adverse Reactions, and Overdose/Toxicology). Assess knowledge/teach patient appropriate use, interventions to reduce side effects, and adverse symptoms to report. **Pregnancy risk factor C** - benefits of use should outweigh possible risks. Note breast-feeding caution.

**Patient Information/Instruction:** Take exactly as directed; do not increase, decrease, or discontinue without consulting prescriber. Take at the same time each day. Do not use alcohol and all prescription or OTC sedatives or CNS depressants without consulting prescriber. You may experience drowsiness, dizziness, confusion, and blurred vision (use caution when driving, climbing stairs, or engaging in tasks requiring alertness until response to drug is known); increased susceptibility to heat stroke, decreased perspiration (use caution in hot weather - maintain adequate fluids and reduce exercise activity); constipation (increased exercise, fluids, or dietary fruit and fiber may help). Report unresolved nausea, vomiting, or gastric disturbances; rapid or pounding heartbeat, chest pain or palpitation; difficulty breathing; CNS changes (hallucination, loss of memory, nervousness, etc); eye pain; prolonged fever; painful or difficult urination; unresolved constipation; increased muscle spasticity or rigidity; skin rash; or significant worsening of condition. **Pregnancy/breast-feeding precautions:** Inform prescriber if you are or intend to be pregnant. Consult prescriber if breast-feeding.

**Geriatric Considerations:** Anticholinergic agents are generally not well tolerated in the elderly and their use should be avoided when possible (see Warnings/Precautions and Adverse Reactions). In the elderly, anticholinergic agents should not be used as prophylaxis against extrapyramidal symptoms.

- **Benzylpenicillin Benzathine** *see* Penicillin G Benzathine *on page 896*
- **Benzylpenicillin Potassium** *see* Penicillin G, Parenteral, Aqueous *on page 897*
- **Benzylpenicillin Sodium** *see* Penicillin G, Parenteral, Aqueous *on page 897*

## Bepridil (BE pri dil)

**U.S. Brand Names** Vascor®

**Therapeutic Category** Calcium Channel Blocker

**Pregnancy Risk Factor** C

**Lactation** Enters breast milk/compatible

**Use** Treatment of chronic stable angina; due to side effect profile, reserve for patients who have been intolerant of other antianginal therapy; may be used alone or in combination with nitrates or beta-blockers

**Mechanism of Action/Effect** Bepridil, a Type 4 calcium antagonist, possesses characteristics of the traditional calcium antagonists, inhibiting calcium ion from entering the "slow channels" or select voltage-sensitive areas of vascular smooth muscle and myocardium during depolarization and producing a relaxation of coronary vascular smooth muscle and coronary vasodilation. However, bepridil may also inhibit fast sodium channels (inward), which may account for some of its side effects (eg, arrhythmias); a direct bradycardia effect of bepridil has been postulated via direct action on the S-A node. Bepridil also has Type 1 antiarrhythmic properties.

**Contraindications** History of hypersensitivity to bepridil or any component; history of serious ventricular or atrial arrhythmias (especially tachycardia or those associated with accessory conduction pathways); sick-sinus syndrome; second or third degree A-V block (without a functioning pacemaker); cardiogenic shock; hypotension; uncompensated cardiac insufficiency; congenital Q-T interval prolongation; patients taking other drugs that prolong the Q-T interval; calcium channel blockers or adenosine

**Warnings** Use with caution in patients with sick-sinus syndrome, severe left ventricular dysfunction, and sinus bradycardia. Use with care in patients with hepatic or renal impairment, hypertrophic cardiomyopathy (especially obstructive), concomitant therapy with beta-blockers or digoxin, edema, or congestive heart failure. Do not abruptly withdraw (chest pain may result). Elderly patients may have a greater hypotensive effect. Pregnancy factor C.

**Drug Interactions**

**Cytochrome P-450 Effect:** CYP3A3/4 enzyme substrate

**Increased Effect/Toxicity:** Use with $H_2$ blockers may increase bioavailability of bepridil. Use with beta-blockers may increase cardiac depressant effects on A-V conduction. Use with carbamazepine may increase carbamazepine levels. Use with cyclosporine may increase cyclosporine levels. Use with fentanyl may increase hypotension. Use with digitalis may increase digitalis levels. Use with quinidine may increase quinidine levels (hypotension, bradycardia). Use with theophylline may increase pharmacologic actions of theophylline.

**Effects on Lab Values** ↑ aminotransferases, CPK, LDH

**Adverse Reactions**

>10%:

Central nervous system: Dizziness or lightheadedness

Gastrointestinal: Diarrhea, nausea

1% to 10%:

Cardiovascular: Arrhythmias, including torsade de pointes; bradycardia, congestive heart failure or pulmonary edema

Central nervous system: Headache, unusual drowsiness or weakness

Gastrointestinal: Constipation

<1% (Limited to important or life-threatening symptoms): Hypotension, peripheral edema, agranulocytosis, gynecomastia

**Overdose/Toxicology** Primary cardiac symptoms of calcium blocker overdose include hypotension and bradycardia. In addition, bepridil may also cause Q-T prolongation and torsade de pointes. Noncardiac symptoms include confusion, stupor, nausea, vomiting, metabolic acidosis, and hyperglycemia. Following initial gastric decontamination, if possible, repeated calcium administration may promptly reverse depressed cardiac contractility (but not sinus node depression or peripheral vasodilation). Glucagon, epinephrine, and amrinone may treat refractory hypotension. Glucagon and epinephrine also increase the heart rate (outside the U.S., 4-aminopyridine may be available as an antidote). Dialysis and hemoperfusion are not effective in enhancing elimination although repeat-dose activated charcoal may serve as an adjunct with sustained-release preparations. Large doses of calcium chloride may be required to treat initially refractory hypotension and bradycardia.

**Pharmacodynamics/Kinetics**

**Protein Binding:** >99%

**Half-life Elimination:** 24 hours

**Time to Peak:** 2-3 hours

**Metabolism:** Liver

**Excretion:** Urine

**Onset:** 1 hour

**Formulations** Tablet, as hydrochloride: 200 mg, 300 mg, 400 mg

**Dosing**

**Adults:** Oral: Initial: 200 mg/day, then adjust dose at 10-day intervals until optimal response is achieved; maximum daily dose: 400 mg.

**Elderly:** Elderly require frequent monitoring due to side effect profile (cardiac) (see Geriatric Considerations and Additional Information).

**Administration**

**Oral:** May be taken with food or at bedtime if nausea occurs.

**Monitoring Laboratory Tests** EKG required prior to beginning therapy; hospitalization is generally required for initiation or escalation of therapy.

**Additional Nursing Issues**

**Physical Assessment:** Monitor cardiac status and blood pressure during initiation or escalation of therapy and at regular intervals during long-term therapy. Carefully assess all other medications (prescription and OTC) the patient may be taking (see Drug interactions). **Pregnancy risk factor C** - benefits of use should outweigh possible risks.

**Patient Information/Instruction:** Take as directed (may be taken with food to reduce gastric side effects). Do not discontinue without consulting prescriber. Regular EKGs and follow-up with prescriber may be required. If taking potassium supplements or potassium-sparing diuretics, serum potassium monitoring will be required. May cause dizziness, shakiness, visual disturbances, or headache; use caution when driving or engaging in tasks that require alertness until response to drug is known. Report irregular or pounding heartbeat, respiratory difficulty, swelling of hands or feet, unresolved headache, dizziness, constipation, or any unusual bleeding or bruising. **Pregnancy precautions:** Inform prescriber if you are or intend to be pregnant.

**Geriatric Considerations:** Elderly may experience a greater hypotensive response. Theoretically, constipation may be more of a problem in the elderly.

**Additional Information** This agent is not considered the drug of first choice, but is used for cases refractory to other calcium channel blockers.

**Related Information**

Calcium Channel Blocking Agents Comparison *on page 1378*

- **Berocca®** *see* Vitamin, Multiple *on page 1219*
- **Berocca®** *see page 1294*
- **Berubigen®** *see* Cyanocobalamin *on page 311*
- **Beta-2®** *see* Isoetharine *on page 629*
- **Beta-Blockers Comparison** *see page 1376*

## Beta-Carotene (BAY tah KARE oh teen)

**Therapeutic Category** Vitamin, Fat Soluble

**Pregnancy Risk Factor** C

**Lactation** Excretion in breast milk unknown/use caution

**Use** Reduces severity of photosensitivity reactions in patients with erythropoietic protoporphyria (EPP)

**Mechanism of Action/Effect** The exact mechanism of action in erythropoietic protoporphyria has not as yet been elucidated; although patient must become carotenemic before effects are observed, there appears to be more than a simple internal light screen responsible for the drug's action. A protective effect was achieved when beta-carotene was added to blood samples. The concentrations of solutions used were similar to those achieved in treated patients. Topically applied beta-carotene is considerably less effective than systemic therapy.

**Contraindications** Hypersensitivity to beta-carotene

**Warnings** Use with caution in patients with renal or hepatic impairment. Not proven effective as a sunblock. Pregnancy factor C.

**Drug Interactions**

**Increased Effect/Toxicity:** Fulfills vitamin A requirements, do not prescribe additional vitamin A

**Adverse Reactions**

>10%: Dermatologic: Carotenodermia (yellowing of palms, hands, or soles of feet, and to a lesser extent the face)

<1% (Limited to important or life-threatening symptoms): Bruising

**Pharmacodynamics/Kinetics**

**Metabolism:** Prior to absorption, converted to vitamin A in the wall of the small intestine and then further oxidized to retinoic acid and retinol in the presence of fat and bile acids; small amounts are then stored in the liver; retinol (active) is conjugated with glucuronic acid

**Excretion:** Urine and feces

**Formulations** Capsule: 15 mg, 30 mg

**Dosing**

**Adults:** Oral: 30-300 mg/day

**Elderly:** Refer to adult dosing.

**Monitoring Laboratory Tests** Hepatic and renal function

**Additional Nursing Issues**

**Physical Assessment:** Monitor lab tests with long-term use. Assess knowledge/teach patient appropriate use, possible side effects, and adverse symptoms to report. **Pregnancy risk factor C** - benefits of use should outweigh possible risks. Note breast-feeding caution.

**Patient Information/Instruction:** Take exactly as directed; do not take more than the recommended dose. Take with meals. Skin may appear slightly yellow-orange. Not a proven sunblock. **Pregnancy/breast-feeding precautions:** Inform prescriber if you are or intend to be pregnant. Consult prescriber if breast-feeding.

- **Betachron E-R®** *see* Propranolol *on page 986*
- **Betadine®** *see page 1294*
- **Betadine® 5% Sterile Ophthalmic Prep Solution** *see page 1294*
- **Betadine® First Aid Antibiotics + Moisturizer [OTC]** *see* Bacitracin and Polymyxin B *on page 130*
- **9-Beta-D-Ribofuranosyladenine** *see* Adenosine *on page 41*
- **Betaferon®** *see* Interferon Beta-1b *on page 617*

- **Betagan® Liquifilm® Ophthalmic** *see* Ophthalmic Agents, Glaucoma *on page 853*
- **Betagen** *see page 1294*
- **Betaloc®** *see* Metoprolol *on page 761*
- **Betaloc® Durules®** *see* Metoprolol *on page 761*


## Betamethasone (bay ta METH a sone)

**U.S. Brand Names** Alphatrex®; Betatrex®; Beta-Val®; Betnovate; Celestoderm®; Celestone®; Celestone® Soluspan®; Cel-U-Jec®; Diprolene®; Diprolene® AF; Diprosone®; Ectosone; Luxiq®; Maxivate®; Psorion® Cream; Teladar®; Valisone®

**Synonyms** Flubenisolone

**Therapeutic Category** Corticosteroid, Oral; Corticosteroid, Parenteral; Corticosteroid, Topical

**Pregnancy Risk Factor** C

**Lactation** Excretion in breast milk unknown/use caution

**Use** Inflammatory dermatoses such as seborrheic or atopic dermatitis, neurodermatitis, anogenital pruritus, psoriasis, inflammatory phase of xerosis

**Mechanism of Action/Effect** Binds to corticosteroid receptors in cell and acts to prevent or control inflammation

**Contraindications** Hypersensitivity to betamethasone or any component; systemic fungal infections

**Warnings** Fatalities have occurred due to adrenal insufficiency in asthmatic patients during and after transfer from systemic corticosteroids to aerosol steroids. Several months may be required for this process. During this period, aerosol steroids do **not** provide the systemic steroid needed to treat patients having trauma, surgery, or infections. Use with caution in patients with hypothyroidism, cirrhosis, ulcerative colitis. Do not use occlusive dressings on weeping or exudative lesions and general caution with occlusive dressings should be observed. Discontinue if skin irritation or contact dermatitis should occur. Do not use in patients with decreased skin circulation. Pregnancy factor C.

**Drug Interactions**

**Cytochrome P-450 Effect:** CYP3A enzyme substrate, may induce metabolism by CYP isoenzymes.

**Decreased Effect:** May induce cytochrome P-450 enzymes, which may lead to decreased effect of any drug metabolized by P-450 (ie, barbiturates, phenytoin, rifampin). Decreased effectiveness of salicylates when taken with betamethasone.

**Increased Effect/Toxicity:** Inhibitors of CYP3A4 may decrease metabolism of betamethasone.

**Adverse Reactions**

**Systemic:**

>10%:

Central nervous system: Insomnia, nervousness
Gastrointestinal: Increased appetite, indigestion

1% to 10%:

Central nervous system: Dizziness or lightheadedness, headache
Dermatologic: Hirsutism, hypopigmentation
Endocrine & metabolic: Diabetes mellitus
Neuromuscular & skeletal: Arthralgia
Ocular: Cataracts, glaucoma
Respiratory: Epistaxis
Miscellaneous: Sweating

<1% (Limited to important or life-threatening symptoms): Vertigo, seizures, psychoses, pseudotumor cerebri, mood swings, delirium, hallucinations, euphoria, Cushing's syndrome, pituitary-adrenal axis suppression, growth suppression, glucose intolerance, hypokalemia, alkalosis, amenorrhea, sodium and water retention, hyperglycemia

**Ophthalmic:**

1% to 10%: Ocular: Temporary mild blurred vision

<1% (Limited to important or life-threatening symptoms): Watering of eyes, corneal thinning and/or globe perforation, glaucoma, ocular hypertension, optic nerve damage, visual acuity and field defects, secondary ocular infection

**Topical:**

1% to 10%:

Dermatologic: Itching, allergic contact dermatitis, erythema, dryness papular rashes, folliculitis, furunculosis, pustules, pyoderma, vesiculation, hyperesthesia, skin infection (secondary)
Local: Burning, irritation

<1% (Limited to important or life-threatening symptoms): Cushing's syndrome, hypokalemic syndrome, glaucoma, cataracts (posterior subcapsular)

**Overdose/Toxicology** When consumed in high doses for prolonged periods, systemic hypercorticism and adrenal suppression may occur. In those cases, discontinuation of the corticosteroid should be done judiciously.

**Pharmacodynamics/Kinetics**

**Protein Binding:** 64%

**Half-life Elimination:** 6.5 hours

**Time to Peak:** I.V.: Within 10-36 minutes

**Metabolism:** Liver

**Excretion:** Urine

**Formulations**

Betamethasone base (Celestone®), Oral:

Syrup: 0.6 mg/5 mL (118 mL)

Tablet: 0.6 mg
Betamethasone dipropionate (Diprosone®)
Aerosol: 0.1% (85 g)
Cream: 0.05% (15 g, 45 g)
Lotion: 0.05% (20 mL, 30 mL, 60 mL)
Ointment: 0.05% (15 g, 45 g)
Betamethasone dipropionate augmented (Diprolene®)
Cream: 0.05% (15 g, 45 g)
Gel: 0.05% (15 g, 45 g)
Lotion: 0.05% (30 mL, 60 mL)
Ointment, topical: 0.05% (15 g, 45 g)
Betamethasone valerate (Betatrex®, Valisone®)
Cream: 0.01% (15 g, 60 g); 0.1% (15 g, 45 g, 110 g, 430 g)
Lotion: 0.1% (20 mL, 60 mL)
Foam (Luxiq®): 0.12% (100 gm)
Ointment: 0.1% (15 g, 45 g)
Injection: Sodium phosphate (Celestone Phosphate®, Cel-U-Jec®): 4 mg betamethasone phosphate/mL (equivalent to 3 mg betamethasone/mL) (5 mL)
Injection, suspension: Sodium phosphate and acetate (Celestone® Soluspan®): 6 mg/mL (3 mg of betamethasone sodium phosphate and 3 mg of betamethasone acetate per mL) (5 mL)

**Dosing**

**Adults:** Base dosage on severity of disease and patient response.
Oral: 2.4-4.8 mg/day in 2-4 doses; range: 0.6-7.2 mg/day
I.M.: Betamethasone sodium phosphate and betamethasone acetate: 0.6-9 mg/day (generally, 1/3 to 1/2 of oral dose) divided every 12-24 hours
Intrabursal, intra-articular, intradermal: 0.25-2 mL
Intralesional: Rheumatoid arthritis/osteoarthritis:
Very large joints: 1-2 mL
Large joints: 1 mL
Medium joints: 0.5-1 mL
Small joints: 0.25-0.5 mL
Topical: Apply thin film 2-4 times/day
Foam: Massage small amounts of foam into scalp until foam disappears; repeat until entire affected scalp area is treated.

**Elderly:** Refer to adult dosing. Use the lowest effective dose.

**Administration**

**Oral:** Not for alternate day therapy; once daily doses should be given in the morning.

**I.M.:** Do **not** give injectable sodium phosphate/acetate suspension I.V.

**Topical:** Apply topical sparingly to areas. Not for use on broken skin or in areas of infection. Do not apply to wet skin unless directed. Do not apply to face or inguinal area. Do not cover with occlusive dressing.

**Additional Nursing Issues**

**Physical Assessment:** Assess other medications patient may be taking for effectiveness and interactions (see Drug Interactions). Note Warnings/Precautions and Contraindications for cautious use. Monitor therapeutic response, and adverse effects according to indications for therapy, dose, route (systemic or topical), and duration of therapy (see Dosing, Warnings/Precautions, Adverse Reactions). With systemic administration, diabetics should monitor glucose levels closely (corticosteroids may alter glucose levels). Instruct patient on appropriate application of particular form of betamethasone, advise about appropriate interventions for side effects, and instruct about symptoms to report. When used for long-term therapy (longer than 10-14 days) do not discontinue abruptly; decrease dosage incrementally. **Pregnancy risk factor C** - benefits of use should outweigh possible risks. Note breast-feeding caution.

**Patient Information/Instruction:** Take exactly as directed; do not increase dose or discontinue abruptly, consult prescriber. Take oral medication with or after meals. Limit intake of caffeine or stimulants. Prescriber may recommend increased dietary vitamins, minerals, or iron. Diabetics should monitor glucose levels closely (antidiabetic medication may need to be adjusted). Inform prescriber if you are experiencing greater than normal levels of stress (medication may need adjustment). Some forms of this medication may cause GI upset (oral medication may be taken with meals to reduce GI upset; small frequent meals and frequent mouth care may reduce GI upset). You may be more susceptible to infection (avoid crowds and persons with contagious or infective conditions). Report promptly excessive nervousness or sleep disturbances; signs of infection (sore throat, unhealed injuries); excessive growth of body hair or loss of skin color; changes in vision; excessive or sudden weight gain (>3 lb/week); swelling of face or extremities; difficulty breathing; muscle weakness; change in color of stools (tarry) or persistent abdominal pain; or worsening of condition or failure to improve. **Pregnancy/breast-feeding precautions:** Inform prescriber if you are or intend to be pregnant. Consult prescriber if breast-feeding.

Topical: For external use only, Not for eyes or mucous membranes or open wounds. Apply in a thin layer (may rub in lightly). Apply light dressing (if necessary) to area being treated. Do not use occlusive dressing unless so advised by prescriber. Avoid prolonged or excessive use around sensitive tissues, genital, or rectal areas. Inform prescriber if condition worsens (redness, swelling, irritation, open sores) or fails to improve.

**Geriatric Considerations:** Because of the risk of adverse effects, systemic corticosteroids should be used cautiously in the elderly, in the smallest possible dose, and for the shortest possible time.

**Additional Information** Sodium phosphate formulation contains sulfites.

◆ **Betamethasone** *see* Topical Corticosteroids *on page 1152*

## Betamethasone and Clotrimazole

(bay ta METH a sone & kloe TRIM a zole)

**U.S. Brand Names** Lotrisone®

**Synonyms** Clotrimazole and Betamethasone

**Therapeutic Category** Antifungal Agent, Topical

**Pregnancy Risk Factor** C

**Lactation** Excretion in breast milk unknown/use caution

**Use** Topical treatment of various dermal fungal infections

**Formulations** Cream: Betamethasone dipropionate 0.05% and clotrimazole 1% (15 g, 45 g)

**Dosing**

**Adults:** Topical: Apply twice daily for 2 weeks in tinea cruris and tinea corporis; 4 weeks in tinea pedis.

**Elderly:** Refer to adult dosing.

**Additional Nursing Issues**

**Physical Assessment:** See individual components listed in Related Information. **Pregnancy risk factor C** - benefits of use should outweigh possible risks. Note breast-feeding caution.

**Patient Information/Instruction:** See individual components listed in Related Information. **Pregnancy/breast-feeding precautions:** Inform prescriber if you are or intend to be pregnant. Consult prescriber if breast-feeding.

**Related Information**

Betamethasone *on page 148*
Clotrimazole *on page 294*

◆ **Betapace®** *see* Sotalol *on page 1066*
◆ **Betapen®-VK** *see* Penicillin V Potassium *on page 900*
◆ **Betaseron®** *see* Interferon Beta-1b *on page 617*
◆ **Betatrex®** *see* Betamethasone *on page 148*
◆ **Betatrex®** *see* Topical Corticosteroids *on page 1152*
◆ **Beta-Val®** *see* Betamethasone *on page 148*
◆ **Beta-Val®** *see* Topical Corticosteroids *on page 1152*
◆ **Betaxin®** *see* Thiamine *on page 1120*

## Betaxolol (be TAKS oh lol)

**U.S. Brand Names** Betoptic® Ophthalmic; Betoptic® S Ophthalmic; Kerlone® Oral

**Therapeutic Category** Beta Blocker, Beta$_1$ Selective; Ophthalmic Agent, Antiglaucoma

**Pregnancy Risk Factor** C (1st trimester)/D (2nd trimester)

**Lactation** Oral: Enters breast milk/use caution

**Use** Treatment of chronic open-angle glaucoma and ocular hypertension; management of hypertension

**Mechanism of Action/Effect** Competitively blocks beta$_1$-receptors, with little or no effect on beta$_2$-receptors; ophthalmic reduces intraocular pressure by reducing the production of aqueous humor

**Contraindications** Hypersensitivity to betaxolol or any component; bronchial asthma; sinus bradycardia; second and third degree A-V block; cardiac failure (unless a functioning pacemaker is present); cardiogenic shock; pregnancy (2nd trimester)

**Warnings** Some products contain sulfites which can cause allergic reactions. Diminished response occurs over time. Use with caution in patients with decreased renal or hepatic function (dosage adjustment required). Patients with a history of asthma, congestive heart failure, diabetes mellitus, or bradycardia appear to be at a higher risk for adverse effects. Pregnancy factor C/D (3rd trimester).

**Drug Interactions**

**Cytochrome P-450 Effect:** CYP1A2 and 2D6 enzyme substrate

**Decreased Effect:** Decreased effect of betaxolol with aluminum salts, barbiturates, calcium salts, cholestyramine, colestipol, NSAIDs, penicillins (ampicillin), rifampin, salicylates, and sulfinpyrazone due to decreased bioavailability and plasma levels. Beta-blockers may decrease the effect of sulfonylureas.

**Increased Effect/Toxicity:** Increased effect/toxicity of betaxolol with calcium blockers (diltiazem, felodipine, nicardipine). Concomitant use of betaxolol (or any other beta-blocker) may increase the effect/toxicity of flecainide, haloperidol (hypotensive effects), hydralazine, phenothiazines, clonidine (hypertensive crisis after or during withdrawal of either agent), epinephrine (initial hypertensive episode followed by bradycardia), nifedipine and verapamil, lidocaine, ergots (peripheral ischemia). Beta-blockers may affect the action or levels of ethanol, disopyramide, nondepolarizing muscle relaxants, and theophylline although the effects are difficult to predict.

**Adverse Reactions**

**Ophthalmic:**

>10%: Ocular: Conjunctival hyperemia

1% to 10%:

Ocular: Anisocoria, corneal punctate keratitis, keratitis, corneal staining, decreased corneal sensitivity, eye pain, vision disturbances

**Systemic:**

>10%:

Central nervous system: Drowsiness, insomnia

Endocrine & metabolic: Decreased sexual ability

1% to 10%:

Cardiovascular: Bradycardia, palpitations, edema, congestive heart failure, reduced peripheral circulation

Central nervous system: Mental depression

Gastrointestinal: Diarrhea or constipation, nausea, vomiting, stomach discomfort

Respiratory: Bronchospasm

Miscellaneous: Cold extremities

<1% (Limited to important or life-threatening symptoms): Chest pain, thrombocytopenia

**Overdose/Toxicology** Symptoms of significant overdose include bradycardia, hypotension, A-V block, CHF, bronchospasm, hypoglycemia. Treat initially with fluids. Sympathomimetics (eg, epinephrine or dopamine), glucagon, or a pacemaker can be used to treat toxic bradycardia, asystole, and/or hypotension.

**Pharmacodynamics/Kinetics**

**Protein Binding:** Oral: 50%

**Half-life Elimination:** Oral: 12-22 hours

**Time to Peak:** Ophthalmic: Within 2 hours

**Metabolism:** Liver

**Excretion:** Urine

**Onset:** Ophthalmic: 30 minutes; Oral: 1-1.5 hours

**Duration:** Ophthalmic: 12 hours

**Formulations**

Betaxolol hydrochloride:

Solution, ophthalmic (Betoptic®): 0.5% (2.5 mL, 5 mL, 10 mL)

Suspension, ophthalmic (Betoptic® S): 0.25% (2.5 mL, 10 mL, 15 mL)

Tablet (Kerlone®): 10 mg, 20 mg

**Dosing**

**Adults:**

Ophthalmic: Instill 1 drop twice daily.

Oral: 10 mg/day; may increase dose to 20 mg/day after 7-14 days if desired response is not achieved; initial dose in elderly patient: 5 mg/day.

**Elderly:**

Ophthalmic: Refer to adult dosing.

Oral: Initial: 5 mg/day

**Administration**

**Other:** Ophthalmic: Shake well before using. Tilt head back and instill in eye. Keep eye open and do not blink for 30 seconds. Apply gentle pressure to lacrimal sac for 1 minute. Wipe away excess from skin. Do not touch applicator to eye and do not contaminate tip of applicator.

**Stability**

**Storage:** Avoid freezing.

**Monitoring Laboratory Tests** Ophthalmic: Intraocular pressure

**Additional Nursing Issues**

**Physical Assessment:** Assess other medications patient may be taking for effectiveness and interactions (see Warnings/Precautions and Drug Interactions). Monitor laboratory tests, therapeutic response, and adverse reactions (see Adverse Reactions and Overdose/Toxicology) periodically throughout therapy. Assess knowledge/teach patient appropriate use, interventions to reduce side effects, and adverse symptoms to report. **Pregnancy risk factor C/D** - see Pregnancy Risk Factor - benefits of use should outweigh possible risks. Note breast-feeding caution. Systemic absorption from ophthalmic instillation is minimal.

**Patient Information/Instruction:**

Oral: Use as directed; do not increase dose unless directed by prescriber. You may experience dizziness or blurred vision (use caution when driving engaging in tasks requiring alertness until response to drug is known); nausea or vomiting (small frequent meals, frequent mouth care, sucking lozenges, or chewing gum may help). Report persistent GI response (nausea, vomiting, diarrhea, or constipation); chest pain or palpitations; unusual cough, difficulty breathing, swelling or coolness of extremities; or unusual mental depression. **Pregnancy/breast-feeding precautions:** Inform prescriber if you are or intend to be pregnant. Consult prescriber if breast-feeding.

Ophthalmic: Shake well before using. Tilt head back and instill in eye. Keep eye open; do not blink for 30 seconds. Apply gentle pressure to corner of eye for 1 minute. Wipe away excess from skin. Do not touch applicator to eyes or contaminate tip of applicator. Report if condition does not improve or if you experience eye pain, vision disturbances, or other adverse eye response.

**Geriatric Considerations:** Oral: Due to alterations in the beta-adrenergic autonomic nervous system, beta-adrenergic blockade may result in less hemodynamic response than seen in younger adults.

♦ **Betaxolol** *see* Ophthalmic Agents, Glaucoma *on page 853*

## Bethanechol (be THAN e kole)

**U.S. Brand Names** Duvoid®; Myotonachol™; Urabeth®; Urecholine®

**Therapeutic Category** Cholinergic Agonist

**Pregnancy Risk Factor** C

**Lactation** Excretion in breast milk unknown/contraindicated

**Use** Nonobstructive urinary retention and retention due to neurogenic bladder; treatment and prevention of bladder dysfunction caused by phenothiazines; diagnosis of flaccid or atonic neurogenic bladder; gastroesophageal reflux

(Continued)

## Bethanechol *(Continued)*

**Mechanism of Action/Effect** Stimulates cholinergic receptors in the smooth muscle of the urinary bladder and GI tract resulting in increased peristalsis, increased GI and pancreatic secretions, bladder muscle contraction, and increased ureteral peristaltic waves

**Contraindications** Hypersensitivity to bethanechol; do not use in patients with mechanical obstruction of the GI or GU tract or when the strength or integrity of the GI or bladder wall is in question. It is also contraindicated in patients with hyperthyroidism, peptic ulcer disease, epilepsy, obstructive pulmonary disease, bradycardia, vasomotor instability, atrioventricular conduction defects, hypotension, or parkinsonism. **Contraindicated for I.M. or I.V. use due to a likely severe cholinergic reaction.**

**Warnings** Potential for reflux infection if the sphincter fails to relax as bethanechol contracts the bladder. Syringe containing atropine should be readily available for treatment of serious side effects. For S.C. injection only; do not give I.M. or I.V. Pregnancy factor C.

**Drug Interactions**

**Decreased Effect:** Procainamide, quinidine may decrease the effects of bethanechol.

**Increased Effect/Toxicity:** Bethanechol and ganglionic blockers may cause a critical fall in blood pressure. Cholinergic drugs or anticholinesterase agents may have additive effects with bethanechol.

**Effects on Lab Values** ↑ lipase, AST, amylase (S), bilirubin, aminotransferase [ALT (SGPT)/AST (SGOT)] (S)

**Adverse Reactions**

**Oral:**

<1% (Limited to important or life-threatening symptoms): Hypotension with reflex tachycardia, flushed skin, malaise, headache, belching, abdominal cramps, nausea, diarrhea, excessive salivation, borborygmi, urinary frequency, shortness of breath, wheezing, blurred vision, miosis, sweating, vasomotor response

**Subcutaneous:**

1% to 10%:

Cardiovascular: Hypotension with reflex tachycardia, flushed skin
Central nervous system: Malaise, headache
Gastrointestinal: Belching, abdominal cramps, nausea, diarrhea, excessive salivation, borborygmi
Genitourinary: Urinary frequency
Respiratory: Shortness of breath, wheezing
Ocular: Blurred vision, miosis
Miscellaneous: Sweating, vasomotor response

**Overdose/Toxicology** Symptoms of overdose include nausea, vomiting, abdominal cramps, diarrhea, involuntary defecation, flushed skin, hypotension, and bronchospasm. Treat symptomatically; atropine for severe muscarinic symptoms, epinephrine to reverse severe cardiovascular or pulmonary sequelae.

**Pharmacodynamics/Kinetics**

**Onset:** Oral: 30-90 minutes; S.C.: 5-15 minutes

**Duration:** Oral: Up to 6 hours; S.C.: 2 hours

**Formulations**

Bethanechol chloride:
Injection: 5 mg/mL (1 mL)
Tablet: 5 mg, 10 mg, 25 mg, 50 mg

**Dosing**

**Adults:**

Oral: 10-50 mg 2-4 times/day
S.C.: 2.5-5 mg 3-4 times/day, up to 7.5-10 mg every 4 hours for neurogenic bladder

**Elderly:** Use the lowest effective dose.

**Administration**

**I.M.:** Do **not** administer I.V. or I.M., a severe cholinergic reaction may occur.

**I.V.:** Do **not** administer I.V. or I.M., a severe cholinergic reaction may occur.

**Other:** Administer injection by S.C. route only. Adverse reactions are more common with injection formulation.

**Additional Nursing Issues**

**Physical Assessment:** Assess bladder and sphincter adequacy prior to administering medication. Assess other medications patient may be taking for effectiveness and interactions (see Drug Interactions). See Contraindications and Warnings/Precautions for cautious use. Monitor laboratory tests, therapeutic effect, and adverse reactions (eg, cholinergic crisis - DUMBELS - **d**iarrhea, **u**rination, **m**iosis, **b**ronchospasm/**b**radycardia, **e**xcitability, **l**acrimation, and **s**alivation/excessive **s**weating) (see Warnings/Precautions, Adverse Reactions, and Overdose/Toxicology). Assess knowledge/teach patient appropriate use, interventions to reduce side effects, and adverse symptoms to report. **Pregnancy risk factor C** - benefits of use should outweigh possible risks. Breast-feeding is contraindicated.

**Patient Information/Instruction:** Oral: Take as directed, on an empty stomach to avoid nausea or vomiting. Do not discontinue without consulting prescriber. Maintain adequate hydration (2-3 L/day of fluids unless instructed to restrict fluid intake). May cause dizziness or hypotension (rise slowly from sitting or lying position and use caution when driving or climbing stairs); vomiting or loss of appetite (frequent small meals, frequent mouth care, sucking lozenges, or chewing gum may help). Report persistent abdominal discomfort; significantly increased salivation, sweating, tearing, or urination; flushed skin; chest pain or palpitations; acute headache; unresolved diarrhea; excessive fatigue, insomnia, dizziness, or depression; increased muscle, joint, or body pain; vision changes or blurred vision; or respiratory difficulty or wheezing. **Pregnancy/breast-feeding precautions:** Inform prescriber if you are or intend to be pregnant. Do not breast-feed.

**Geriatric Considerations:** Urinary incontinence in an elderly patient should be investigated. Bethanechol may be used for overflow incontinence (dribbling) caused by an atonic or hypotonic bladder, but clinical efficacy is variable (see Contraindications, Warnings/Precautions, and Adverse Reactions).

- **Betimol® Ophthalmic** *see* Ophthalmic Agents, Glaucoma *on page 853*
- **Betimol® Ophthalmic** *see* Timolol *on page 1138*
- **Betnesol® [Disodium Phosphate]** *see* Betamethasone *on page 148*
- **Betnovate** *see* Betamethasone *on page 148*
- **Betnovate** *see* Topical Corticosteroids *on page 1152*
- **Betoptic® Ophthalmic** *see* Betaxolol *on page 150*
- **Betoptic® Ophthalmic** *see* Ophthalmic Agents, Glaucoma *on page 853*
- **Betoptic® S Ophthalmic** *see* Betaxolol *on page 150*
- **Betoptic® S Ophthalmic** *see* Ophthalmic Agents, Glaucoma *on page 853*
- **Bewon®** *see* Thiamine *on page 1120*
- **Bexophene®** *see* Propoxyphene and Aspirin *on page 985*
- **Biavax® II** *see page 1256*
- **Biaxin™** *see* Clarithromycin *on page 279*

## Bicalutamide (bye ka LOO ta mide)

**U.S. Brand Names** Casodex®

**Therapeutic Category** Androgen

**Pregnancy Risk Factor** X

**Lactation** Excretion in breast milk unknown

**Use** In combination therapy with LHRH agonist analogues in treatment of advanced prostatic carcinoma

**Mechanism of Action/Effect** Nonsteroidal antiandrogen that inhibits androgen uptake or inhibits binding of androgen in target tissues

**Contraindications** Hypersensitivity to bicalutamide or any component; pregnancy

**Drug Interactions**

**Increased Effect/Toxicity:** Bicalutamide may displace warfarin from protein binding sites which may result in an increased anticoagulant effect, especially when bicalutamide therapy is started after the patient is already on warfarin.

**Adverse Reactions**

10%:

Cardiovascular: Flushing (hot flashes), chest pain
Gastrointestinal: Abdominal pain, constipation, nausea
Neuromuscular & skeletal: Weakness
Miscellaneous: Pain (general)

1% to 10%:

Cardiovascular: Hypertension, chest pain pectoris, congestive heart failure, edema, peripheral edema
Central nervous system: Anxiety, headache, dizziness, depression, confusion, somnolence, nervousness, fever, chills, insomnia
Dermatologic: Dry skin, pruritus, alopecia, rash
Endocrine & metabolic: Breast pain, diabetes mellitus (hyperglycemia), decreased libido, dehydration, gout, impotency
Gastrointestinal: Diarrhea, vomiting, anorexia, heartburn, rectal hemorrhage, dry mouth, melena, weight gain or loss
Genitourinary: Polyuria, urinary impairment, dysuria, urinary retention, urinary urgency
Hematologic: Anemia
Hepatic: Alkaline phosphatase increased
Neuromuscular & skeletal: Muscle weakness, arthritis, myalgia, leg cramps, pathological fracture, neck pain, hypertonia, neuropathy
Renal: Creatinine increased
Respiratory: Cough increased, dyspnea, pharyngitis, bronchitis, pneumonia, rhinitis, lung disorder
Miscellaneous: Sepsis, neoplasma

**Overdose/Toxicology** Symptoms of overdose include hypoactivity, ataxia, anorexia, vomiting, slow respiration, and lacrimation. Management is supportive. Dialysis is of no benefit.

**Pharmacodynamics/Kinetics**

**Half-life Elimination:** Active enantiomer is 5.8 days

**Metabolism:** Liver

**Excretion:** Urine

**Formulations** Tablet: 50 mg

**Dosing**

**Adults:** Oral: 1 tablet once daily (morning or evening). Start treatment at the same time as treatment with an LHRH analog.

**Elderly:** Refer to adult dosing.

**Renal Impairment:** None necessary as renal impairment has no significant effect on elimination.

**Hepatic Impairment:** Use with caution in patients with moderate to severe hepatic impairment.

(Continued)

## Bicalutamide *(Continued)*

**Administration**

**Oral:** Dose should be taken at the same time each day with or without food.

**Stability**

**Storage:** Store at room temperature.

**Monitoring Laboratory Tests** Periodic liver function, prostate specific antigen (PSA) levels at regular intervals

**Additional Nursing Issues**

**Physical Assessment:** Assess effectiveness and interactions of other medications (see Drug Interactions, eg, anticoagulants and hypoglycemic agents). See Warnings/Precautions and Contraindications for use cautions. Monitor effectiveness of therapy, laboratory tests, and adverse response (see Adverse Reactions and Overdose/Toxicology). Assess knowledge/teach patient appropriate use, possible side effects and appropriate interventions, and adverse symptoms to report. **Pregnancy risk factor X** - instruct patient on absolute need for barrier contraceptives. Note breast-feeding caution.

**Patient Information/Instruction:** Take as directed and do not alter dose or discontinue without consulting prescriber. Take at the same time each day with or without food. Void before taking medication. Diabetics should monitor serum glucose closely and notify prescriber of changes; this medication can alter hypoglycemic requirements. You may lose your hair and experience impotency. May cause dizziness, confusion, or drowsiness (use caution when driving or engaging in tasks that require alertness until response to drug is known); nausea or vomiting (small frequent meals, frequent mouth care, sucking lozenges, or chewing gum may help); or constipation (increased dietary fiber, fruit, or fluid and increased exercise may help). Report easy bruising or bleeding; yellowing of skin or eyes; change in color of urine or stool; unresolved changes in CNS (nervousness, chills, insomnia, somnolence); skin rash, redness, or irritation; chest pain or palpitations; difficulty breathing; urinary retention or inability to void; muscle weakness, tremors, or pain; persistent nausea, vomiting, diarrhea, or constipation; or other unusual signs or adverse reactions. **Pregnancy precautions/breast-feeding:** This drug will cause fetal abnormalities - use barrier contraceptives. Inform prescriber if breast-feeding.

**Geriatric Considerations:** Renal impairment has no clinically significant changes in elimination of the parent compound or active metabolite; therefore, no dosage adjustment is needed in the elderly. In dosage studies, no difference was found between young adults and elderly with regard to steady-state serum concentrations for bicalutamide and its active R-enantiomer metabolite.


- **Bicillin® L-A** *see* Penicillin G Benzathine *on page 896*
- **Bicitra®** *see* Sodium Citrate and Citric Acid *on page 1063*
- **Biclin** *see* Amikacin *on page 65*
- **BiCNU®** *see* Carmustine *on page 204*
- **Bilem** *see* Tamoxifen *on page 1095*
- **Biltricide®** *see* Praziquantel *on page 957*
- **Binotal** *see* Ampicillin *on page 90*
- **Biocef** *see* Cephalexin *on page 237*
- **Bioclate™** *see* Antihemophilic Factor (Recombinant) *on page 100*
- **Bioderm®** *see* Bacitracin and Polymyxin B *on page 130*
- **Biodine** *see page 1294*
- **Biomox®** *see* Amoxicillin *on page 80*
- **Bion® Tears Solution** *see page 1294*
- **Biosint®** *see* Cefotaxime *on page 221*
- **Biozyme-C®** *see* Collagenase *on page 303*
- **Bisac-Evac®** *see page 1294*
- **Bisacodyl** *see page 1294*
- **Bisacodyl Uniserts®** *see page 1294*
- **Bisco-Lax®** *see page 1294*
- **Bismatrol® [OTC]** *see* Bismuth Subsalicylate *on this page*
- **Bismuth Subgallate** *see page 1294*


## Bismuth Subsalicylate (BIZ muth sub sa LIS i late)

**U.S. Brand Names** Bismatrol® [OTC]; Pepto-Bismol® [OTC]

**Therapeutic Category** Antidiarrheal

**Pregnancy Risk Factor** C/D (3rd trimester)

**Lactation** Enters breast milk/use caution

**Use** Symptomatic treatment of mild, nonspecific diarrhea; control of traveler's diarrhea (enterotoxigenic *Escherichia coli*); as an adjunct in the treatment of *Helicobacter pylori*-associated peptic ulcer disease

**Mechanism of Action/Effect** Bismuth subsalicylate exhibits both antisecretory, antacid, and antimicrobial action. This agent may provide some anti-inflammatory action as well.

**Contraindications** Hypersensitivity to salicylates; history of severe GI bleeding; history of coagulopathy; pregnancy (3rd trimester)

**Warnings** Subsalicylate should be used with caution if patient is taking aspirin, additive toxicity. Beware of salicylate content when prescribing. Pregnancy factor C/D (3rd trimester).

**Drug Interactions**

**Decreased Effect:** Bismuth subsalicylate may decrease absorption of tetracyclines, decrease effectiveness of corticosteroids, sulfinpyrazone.

**Increased Effect/Toxicity:** Increased toxicity when taken with aspirin, warfarin, or sulfonylureas.

**Effects on Lab Values** ↑ uric acid, AST; may interfere with radiologic tests since bismuth is radiopaque.

**Adverse Reactions**

>10%: Gastrointestinal: Discoloration of the tongue (darkening), grayish black stools

<1% (Limited to important or life-threatening symptoms): Anxiety, confusion, slurred speech, headache, mental depression, impaction may occur in infants and debilitated patients, hearing loss, buzzing in ears

**Pharmacodynamics/Kinetics**

**Metabolism:** Liver

**Excretion:** Urine

**Formulations**

Caplet, swallowable: 262 mg

Liquid: 262 mg/15 mL (120 mL, 240 mL, 360 mL, 480 mL); 524 mg/15 mL (120 mL, 240 mL, 360 mL)

Tablet, chewable: 262 mg

**Dosing**

**Adults:** Oral:

Nonspecific diarrhea: Subsalicylate: 2 tablets or 30 mL every 30 minutes to 1 hour as needed up to 8 doses/24 hours

Prevention of traveler's diarrhea: 2.1 g/day or 2 tablets 4 times/day before meals and at bedtime

Subgallate: 1-2 tablets 3 times/day with meals

**Elderly:** Refer to adult dosing.

**Renal Impairment:** Should probably be avoided in patients with renal failure

**Additional Nursing Issues**

**Physical Assessment:** Monitor for causes of diarrhea before prescribing. Monitor for tinnitus. May aggravate or cause gout attack. May enhance bleeding if used with anticoagulants. Monitor for concurrent medications (eg, corticosteroids and antihyperglycemics). **Pregnancy risk factor C/D** - see Pregnancy Risk Factor - assess knowledge/teach appropriate use of barrier contraceptives. Note breast-feeding caution.

**Patient Information/Instruction:** Should be taken before meals. Chew tablet well or shake suspension well before using. May blacken stools or turn tongue black. If diarrhea persists for more than 2 days, consult prescriber. If ringing in ears occurs, stop medication and notify prescriber (may indicate toxic reaction). **Pregnancy/breast-feeding precautions:** Inform prescriber if you are or intend to be pregnant. Consult prescriber if breast-feeding.

**Geriatric Considerations:** Tinnitus and CNS side effects (confusion, dizziness, high tone deafness, delirium, psychosis) may be difficult to assess in some elderly. Limit use of this agent in the elderly.

**Additional Information** Sodium content: <2 mg/262 mg tablet; liquid 262 mg/15 mL, 5 mg sodium; liquid 524 mg/15 mL, <5 mg sodium

## Bisoprolol (bis OH proe lol)

**U.S. Brand Names** Zebeta®

**Therapeutic Category** Beta Blocker, $Beta_1$ Selective

**Pregnancy Risk Factor** C/D (2nd and 3rd trimesters)

**Lactation** Enters breast milk/use caution

**Use** Treatment of hypertension, alone or in combination with other agents

**Unlabeled use:** Angina pectoris, supraventricular arrhythmias, PVCs

**Mechanism of Action/Effect** Selective inhibitor of $beta_1$-adrenergic receptors; little or no effect on $beta_2$-receptors at doses <10 mg

**Contraindications** Hypersensitivity to beta-blocking agents; uncompensated congestive heart failure; cardiogenic shock; bradycardia or heart block; sinus node dysfunction; A-V conduction abnormalities; pregnancy (2nd and 3rd trimesters)

**Warnings** Use with caution in patients with inadequate myocardial function, bronchospastic disease, hyperthyroidism, diabetes, congestive heart failure, undergoing anesthesia, and in those with impaired hepatic function. Acute withdrawal may exacerbate symptoms (gradually taper over a 2-week period). High doses can result in $beta_2$-receptor blockage; therefore, use with caution in patients (especially elderly) with bronchospastic lung disease and renal dysfunction. Beta-blockers may impair glucose tolerance, potentiate hypoglycemia, and/or mask symptoms of hypoglycemia in a diabetic patient. Pregnancy factor C/D (2nd and 3rd trimesters).

**Drug Interactions**

**Cytochrome P-450 Effect:** CYP2D6 enzyme substrate

**Decreased Effect:** Decreased effect/levels of bisoprolol with rifampin which may or may not require dose adjustment.

**Increased Effect/Toxicity:** Increased effect/toxicity/levels of antiarrhythmics (ie, disopyramide), calcium channel blockers (verapamil, diltiazem), anticholinergics and other beta-blockers, reserpine, or guanethidine. Increased chance of postural hypotension with other antihypertensives. Possible increased effect of insulin.

**Effects on Lab Values** ↑ thyroxine (S), cholesterol (S), glucose, triglycerides, uric acid; ↓ HDL; possible false glucose tolerance tests

**Adverse Reactions**

>10%:

(Continued)

## Bisoprolol *(Continued)*

Central nervous system: Drowsiness, insomnia
Endocrine & metabolic: Decreased sexual ability

1% to 10%:

Cardiovascular: Bradycardia, palpitations, edema, congestive heart failure, reduced peripheral circulation
Central nervous system: Mental depression
Gastrointestinal: Diarrhea or constipation, nausea, vomiting, stomach discomfort
Ocular: Mild ocular stinging and discomfort, tearing, photophobia, decreased corneal sensitivity, keratitis
Respiratory: Bronchospasm
Miscellaneous: Cold extremities

<1% (Limited to important or life-threatening symptoms): Chest pain, arrhythmias, orthostatic hypotension, nervousness, headache, depression, hallucinations, confusion (especially in the elderly), psoriasiform eruption, itching, thrombocytopenia, leukopenia, shortness of breath

**Overdose/Toxicology** Symptoms of overdose include severe hypotension, bradycardia, heart failure, bronchospasm, and hypoglycemia. Treat initially with I.V. fluids. Sympathomimetics (eg, epinephrine or dopamine), glucagon, or a pacemaker can be used to treat the toxic bradycardia, asystole, and/or hypotension. Bisoprolol may be removed by hemodialysis. Other treatment is symptomatic and supportive.

**Pharmacodynamics/Kinetics**

**Protein Binding:** 26% to 33%

**Distribution:** Distributed widely to body tissues; highest concentrations in heart, liver, lungs, and saliva; crosses the blood-brain barrier

**Half-life Elimination:** 9-12 hours

**Time to Peak:** 1.7-3 hours

**Metabolism:** Liver

**Excretion:** Urine

**Onset:** 1-2 hours

**Formulations** Tablet, as fumarate: 5 mg, 10 mg

**Dosing**

**Adults:** Oral: 5 mg once daily, may be increased to 10 mg, and then up to 20 mg once daily, if necessary

**Elderly:** Oral: Initial: 2.5 mg/day; may be increased by 2.5-5 mg/day; maximum recommended dose: 20 mg/day

**Renal Impairment:** Oral: Initial: 2.5 mg/day; increase cautiously
Not dialyzable

**Monitoring Laboratory Tests** Serum glucose regularly

**Additional Nursing Issues**

**Physical Assessment:** Assess effects and interactions with other medications patient may be taking (see Drug Interactions). Assess blood pressure and heart rate prior to and following first doses and any change in dosage. Monitor or advise patient to monitor weight and fluid balance (I & O) and assess for signs of CHF (eg, edema, new cough or dyspnea, unresolved fatigue), and assess therapeutic effectiveness. Monitor serum glucose levels of diabetic patients since beta-blockers may alter glucose tolerance. Use/teach postural hypotension precautions. **Pregnancy risk factor C/D** - see Pregnancy Risk Factor - benefits of use should outweigh possible risks. Note breast-feeding caution.

**Patient Information/Instruction:** Take exactly as directed. Do not increase, decrease, or adjust dosage without consulting prescriber. Do not take with antacids and do not use alcohol or OTC medications (eg, cold remedies) without consulting prescriber. If diabetic, monitor serum sugars closely (may alter glucose tolerance or mask signs of hypoglycemia). May cause fatigue, dizziness, or postural hypotension; use caution when changing position from lying or sitting to standing, or when driving or climbing stairs until response to medication is known. May cause alteration in sexual performance (reversible). Report palpitations, unresolved swelling of extremities, difficulty breathing or new cough, unresolved fatigue, unusual weight gain, unresolved constipation, or unusual muscle weakness. **Pregnancy/breast-feeding precautions:** Inform prescriber if you are or intend to be pregnant. Consult prescriber if breast-feeding.

**Geriatric Considerations:** Due to alterations in the beta-adrenergic autonomic nervous system, beta-adrenergic blockade may result in less hemodynamic response than seen in younger adults.

**Related Information**

Beta-Blockers Comparison *on page 1376*

## Bisoprolol and Hydrochlorothiazide

(bis OH proe lol & hye droe klor oh THYE a zide)

**U.S. Brand Names** Ziac™

**Synonyms** Hydrochlorothiazide and Bisoprolol

**Therapeutic Category** Antihypertensive Agent, Combination

**Pregnancy Risk Factor** C/D (2nd and 3rd trimesters)

**Lactation** Enters breast milk/use caution

**Use** Treatment of hypertension

**Formulations** Tablet:

Bisoprolol fumarate 2.5 mg and hydrochlorothiazide 6.25 mg
Bisoprolol fumarate 5 mg and hydrochlorothiazide 6.25 mg
Bisoprolol fumarate 10 mg and hydrochlorothiazide 6.25 mg

**Dosing**

**Adults:** Oral: Dose is individualized, given once daily

**Elderly:** Refer to adult dosing.

**Hepatic Impairment:** Caution should be used in dosing/titrating patients.

**Additional Nursing Issues**

**Physical Assessment:** See individual components listed in Related Information. **Pregnancy risk factor C/D** - see Pregnancy Risk Factor - benefits of use should outweigh possible risks. Note breast-feeding caution.

**Patient Information/Instruction:** See individual components listed in Related Information. **Pregnancy/breast-feeding precautions:** Inform prescriber if you are on intend to get pregnant. Consult prescriber if breast-feeding.

**Related Information**

Bisoprolol *on page 155*
Hydrochlorothiazide *on page 566*

## Bitolterol (bye TOLE ter ole)

**U.S. Brand Names** Tornalate®

**Therapeutic Category** $Beta_2$ Agonist

**Pregnancy Risk Factor** C

**Lactation** Excretion in breast milk unknown

**Use** Prevention and treatment of bronchial asthma and bronchospasm

**Mechanism of Action/Effect** Selectively stimulates $beta_2$-adrenergic receptors in the lungs producing bronchial smooth muscle relaxation; minor $beta_1$ activity

**Contraindications** Hypersensitivity to bitolterol or any component

**Warnings** Use with caution in patients with unstable vasomotor symptoms, diabetes, hyperthyroidism, prostatic hypertrophy or a history of seizures. Also use caution in the elderly and those patients with cardiovascular disorders such as coronary artery disease, arrhythmias, and hypertension. Excessive use may result in cardiac arrest and death. Do not use concurrently with other sympathomimetic bronchodilators. Pregnancy factor C.

**Drug Interactions**

**Decreased Effect:** Decreased effect with beta-adrenergic blockers (eg, propranolol).

**Increased Effect/Toxicity:** Increased toxicity with MAO inhibitors, tricyclic antidepressants, sympathomimetic agents (eg, amphetamine, dopamine, dobutamine), inhaled anesthetics (eg, enflurane). Increased toxicity (cardiotoxicity) with aminophylline, theophylline, or oxtriphylline.

**Adverse Reactions**

>10%: Neuromuscular & skeletal: Trembling

1% to 10%:

- Cardiovascular: Flushing of face, hypertension, pounding heartbeat
- Central nervous system: Dizziness, lightheadedness, nervousness, headache
- Gastrointestinal: Dry mouth, nausea
- Respiratory: Bronchial irritation, coughing

<1% (Limited to important or life-threatening symptoms): Chest pain, arrhythmias, tachycardia, paradoxical bronchospasm

**Overdose/Toxicology** Symptoms of overdose include tremor, dizziness, nervousness, headache, nausea, coughing. Treatment is symptomatic/supportive. Prudent use of a cardioselective beta-adrenergic blocker (eg, atenolol or metoprolol) should be considered, keeping in mind the potential for induction of bronchoconstriction in an asthmatic individual. Dialysis has not been shown to be of value in the treatment of overdose with bitolterol.

**Pharmacodynamics/Kinetics**

**Half-life Elimination:** 3 hours

**Time to Peak:** Inhalation: Within 1 hour

**Metabolism:** Liver

**Excretion:** Urine and feces

**Onset:** Rapid

**Duration:** 4-8 hours

**Formulations**

Bitolterol mesylate:

- Aerosol, oral: 0.8% [370 mcg/metered spray, 300 inhalations] (15 mL)
- Solution, inhalation: 0.2% (10 mL, 30 mL, 60 mL)

**Dosing**

**Adults:**

- Bronchospasm: 2 inhalations at an interval of at least 1-3 minutes, followed by a third inhalation if needed
- Prevention of bronchospasm: 2 inhalations every 8 hours; do not exceed 3 inhalations every 6 hours or 2 inhalations every 4 hours

**Elderly:** Refer to adult dosing.

**Administration**

**Inhalation:** Administer around-the-clock to promote less variation in peak and trough serum levels.

**Additional Nursing Issues**

**Physical Assessment:** Assess effectiveness and interactions of other medications (see Drug Interactions). See Contraindications and Warnings/Precautions for use cautions. Monitor effectiveness of therapy (relief of airway obstruction) and adverse reactions (eg, cardiac and CNS changes - see Adverse Reactions) at beginning of therapy and periodically with long-term use. For inpatient care, monitor vital signs and lung sounds prior to and periodically during therapy. Assess knowledge/teach patient appropriate use, interventions to reduce side effects, and adverse symptoms to report.

(Continued)

## Bitolterol *(Continued)*

**Pregnancy risk factor C** - benefits of use should outweigh possible risks. Note breast-feeding caution.

**Patient Information/Instruction:** Use exactly as directed (see Administration below). Do not use more often than recommended. Maintain adequate hydration (2-3 L/day of fluids unless instructed to restrict fluid intake). You may experience nervousness, dizziness, or fatigue (use caution when driving or engaging in tasks requiring alertness until response to drug is known); or dry mouth, stomach upset (frequent small meals, frequent mouth care, chewing gum, or sucking hard candy may help). Report unresolved GI upset; dizziness or fatigue; vision changes; chest pain, rapid heartbeat, or palpitations; nervousness or insomnia; muscle cramping or tremor; or unusual cough. **Pregnancy/breast-feeding precautions:** Inform prescriber if you are or intend to be pregnant. Consult prescriber if breast-feeding.

**Administration:** Self-administered inhalation: Store canister upside down; do not freeze. Shake canister before using. Sit when using medication. Close eyes when administering bitolterol to avoid spray getting into eyes. Exhale slowly and completely through nose; inhale deeply through mouth while administering aerosol. Hold breath for 1-3 seconds after inhalation. Wait at least 1 full minute between inhalations. Wash mouthpiece between use. If more than one inhalation medication is used, use bitolterol first and wait 5 minutes between medications.

Self-administered nebulizer: Wash hands before and after treatment. Wash and dry nebulizer after each treatment. Twist open the top of one unit dose vial and squeeze contents into nebulizer reservoir. Connect nebulizer reservoir to the mouthpiece or face-mask. Connect nebulizer to compressor. Sit in comfortable, upright position. Place mouthpiece in your mouth or put on face-mask and turn on compressor. If face-mask is used, avoid leakage around the mask to avoid mist getting into eyes which may cause vision problems. Breath calmly and deeply until no more mist is formed in nebulizer (about 5 minutes). At this point treatment is finished.

**Geriatric Considerations:** Elderly patients may find it beneficial to utilize a spacer device when using a metered dose inhaler. Difficulty in using the inhaler often limits its effectiveness (see Adverse Reactions).

**Additional Information** Some formulations may contain ethanol.

**Related Information**

Inhalant (Asthma, Bronchospasm) Agents *on page 1388*

- **Black Draught®** *see page 1294*
- **Blastocarb** *see* Carboplatin *on page 199*
- **Blastolem** *see* Cisplatin *on page 273*
- **BlemErase® Lotion** *see page 1294*
- **Blenoxane®** *see* Bleomycin *on this page*
- **Bleolem** *see* Bleomycin *on this page*

## Bleomycin (blee oh MYE sin)

**U.S. Brand Names** Blenoxane®

**Synonyms** BLM

**Therapeutic Category** Antineoplastic Agent, Antibiotic

**Pregnancy Risk Factor** D

**Lactation** Excretion in breast milk unknown/not recommended

**Use** Treatment of squamous cell carcinomas, melanomas, sarcomas, testicular carcinomas, Hodgkin's lymphoma, and non-Hodgkin's lymphoma; sclerosing agent for malignant pleural effusion

**Mechanism of Action/Effect** Inhibits synthesis of DNA

**Contraindications** Hypersensitivity to bleomycin sulfate or any component; severe pulmonary disease; pregnancy

**Warnings** The U.S. Food and Drug Administration (FDA) currently recommends that procedures for proper handling and disposal of antineoplastic agents be considered. Occurrence of pulmonary fibrosis is higher in elderly patients and in those receiving >400 units total and in smokers and patients with prior radiation therapy. A severe idiosyncratic reaction consisting of hypotension, mental confusion, fever, chills, and wheezing is possible. Check lungs prior to each treatment for crackles.

**Drug Interactions**

**Decreased Effect:** Bleomycin and digitalis glycosides may decrease plasma levels of digoxin. Concomitant therapy with phenytoin results in decreased phenytoin levels, possibly due to decreased oral absorption.

**Increased Effect/Toxicity:** Bleomycin with digoxin may result in elevated serum digoxin levels due to decreased renal clearance. CCNU increases severity of leukopenia. Results in delayed bleomycin elimination due to a decrease in creatinine clearance secondary to cisplatin.

**Adverse Reactions**

>10%:

Cardiovascular: Raynaud's phenomenon

Central nervous system: Mild febrile reaction, fever, chills, patients may become febrile after intracavitary administration

Dermatologic: Pruritic erythema

Integument: ~50% of patients will develop erythema, induration, and hyperkeratosis and peeling of the skin; hyperpigmentation, alopecia, nailbed changes may occur; this appears to be dose-related and is reversible after cessation of therapy

Gastrointestinal: Mucocutaneous toxicity, stomatitis, nausea, vomiting, anorexia

Emetic potential: Moderately low (10% to 30%)
Local: Phlebitis, pain at tumor site
**Irritant chemotherapy**
Respiratory: Pneumonitis
1% to 10%:
Dermatologic: Alopecia
Gastrointestinal: Weight loss
Respiratory: Pulmonary fibrosis and death
Miscellaneous: Idiosyncratic: Similar to anaphylaxis and occurs in 1% of lymphoma patients; may include hypotension, confusion, fever, chills, and wheezing. May be immediate or delayed for several hours; symptomatic treatment includes volume expansion, vasopressor agents, antihistamines, and steroids
<1% (Limited to important or life-threatening symptoms): Myocardial infarction, cerebrovascular accident, hepatotoxicity, renal toxicity
Hematologic: Myelosuppressive:
WBC: Rare
Platelets: Rare
Onset (days): 7
Nadir (days): 14
Recovery (days): 21
Dose-related when total dose is >400 units or with single doses >30 units; pathogenesis is poorly understood, but may be related to damage of pulmonary, vascular, or connective tissue; manifested as an acute or chronic interstitial pneumonitis with interstitial fibrosis, hypoxia, and death; symptoms include cough, dyspnea, and bilateral pulmonary infiltrates noted on CXR; it is controversial whether steroids improve symptoms of bleomycin pulmonary toxicity; tachypnea, rales

**Overdose/Toxicology** Symptoms of overdose include chills, fever, pulmonary fibrosis, and hyperpigmentation. Treatment is supportive.

**Pharmacodynamics/Kinetics**

**Protein Binding:** 1%

**Distribution:** Highest concentrations are seen in skin, kidney, lung, heart tissues. Low concentrations are seen in testes and GI tract; does not cross blood-brain barrier

**Half-life Elimination:** Half-life (biphasic): Dependent upon renal function:
Normal renal function: Initial: 1.3 hours; Terminal: 9 hours
End-stage renal disease: Initial: 2 hours; Terminal: 30 hours

**Time to Peak:** I.M.: Within 30 minutes

**Metabolism:** Liver, GI tract, skin, lungs, kidney, and serum

**Excretion:** Urine

**Formulations** Powder for injection, as sulfate: 15 units

**Dosing**

**Adults:** Refer to individual protocols; 1 unit = 1 mg; may be administered I.M., I.V., S.C., or intracavitary.

Test dose for lymphoma patient: I.M., I.V., S.C.: 1-5 units of bleomycin before the first dose; monitor vital signs every 15 minutes; wait a minimum of 1 hour before administering remainder of dose.

**Single agent therapy:**
I.M./I.V./S.C.: Squamous cell carcinoma, lymphosarcoma, reticulum cell sarcoma, testicular carcinoma: 0.25-0.5 units/kg (10-20 units/m$^2$) 1-2 times/week
Continuous intravenous infusion: 15 units/m$^2$ over 24 hours/day for 4 days

**Combination agent therapy:**
I.M./I.V.: 3-4 units/m$^2$
I.V.: ABVD: 10 units/m$^2$ on days 1 and 15
Maximum cumulative lifetime dose: 400 units
Intracavitary injection for malignant pleural effusion: 60 units in 50-100 mL SWI

**Elderly:** Refer to adult dosing.

**Renal Impairment:**
$Cl_{cr}$ 10-50 mL/minute: Administer 75% of normal dose.
$Cl_{cr}$ <10 mL/minute: Administer 50% of normal dose.
Hemodialysis: None
CAPD effects: None
CAVH effects: None

**Administration**

**I.M.:** May cause pain at injection site.

**I.V.:** May be an irritant. I.V. doses should be administered slowly (≤1 unit/minute).

**Other:** S.C.: May cause pain at injection site.

**Stability**

**Storage:** Refrigerate intact vials of powder.

**Reconstitution:** Reconstitute powder with 1-5 mL SWI or NS which is stable at room temperature for 28 days or in refrigerator for 14 days. May use bacteriostatic agent if prolonged storage is necessary.

**Standard I.V. dilution:** Dose/50-1000 mL NS or $D_5W$
Stable for 96 hours at room temperature and 14 days under refrigeration.

**Compatibility:** Incompatible with amino acid solutions, ascorbic acid, cefazolin, furosemide, diazepam, hydrocortisone, mitomycin, nafcillin, penicillin G, and aminophylline. Compatible with cyclophosphamide, doxorubicin, mesna, vinblastine, and vincristine. See the Chemotherapy Compatibility Chart *on page 1311*.

**Monitoring Laboratory Tests** Pulmonary function (total lung volume, forced vital capacity, carbon monoxide diffusion), renal function, chest x-ray, CBC with differential and platelet count, liver function

(Continued)

## Bleomycin *(Continued)*

**Additional Nursing Issues**

**Physical Assessment:** Monitor laboratory results prior to, during, and following therapy. Assess respiratory status (eg, lung sounds, chest x-ray, pulmonary function) and fluid balance ( I & O, weight) prior to instituting each dose; consult prescriber with adverse changes (see Warnings/Precautions and Adverse Reactions). **Pregnancy risk factor D.** Breast-feeding is not recommended.

**Patient Information/Instruction:** You may experience loss of appetite, nausea, vomiting, mouth sores; small frequent meals, frequent mouth care with soft swab, frequent mouth rinses, sucking lozenges, or chewing gum may help. If unresolved notify prescriber. You may experience fever or chills (will usually resolve); redness, peeling, or increased color of skin, or loss of hair (reversible after cessation of therapy). Report any change in respiratory status; difficulty breathing; wheezing; air hunger; increased secretions; difficulty expectorating secretions; confusion; unresolved fever or chills; sores in mouth; vaginal itching, burning, or discharge; sudden onset of dizziness; or acute headache. **Breast-feeding precautions:** Breast-feeding is not recommended.

- **Bleph®-10** *see page 1282*
- **Bleph®-10 Ophthalmic** *see* Sulfacetamide *on page 1080*
- **Blephamide®** *see page 1282*
- **Blis-To-Sol®** *see page 1247*
- **BLM** *see* Bleomycin *on page 158*
- **Blocadren® Oral** *see* Timolol *on page 1138*
- **Blocan** *see* Cimetidine *on page 268*
- **Bluboro®** *see page 1294*
- **Body Surface Area of Adults and Children** *see page 1348*
- **Bonine® [OTC]** *see* Meclizine *on page 712*
- **Boric Acid** *see page 1291*
- **Boric Acid** *see page 1294*
- **Borofax® Topical** *see page 1294*
- **Boropak®** *see page 1294*
- **B&O Supprettes®** *see* Belladonna and Opium *on page 136*
- **Botox®** *see page 1282*
- **Botulinum Toxin Type A** *see page 1282*
- **BQ® Tablet** *see page 1294*
- **Braccoprial®** *see* Pyrazinamide *on page 994*
- **Braxan** *see* Amiodarone *on page 71*
- **Breathe Free®** *see page 1294*
- **Breezee® Mist Antifungal [OTC]** *see* Miconazole *on page 767*
- **Breezee® Mist Antifungal** *see page 1247*
- **Breonesin® [OTC]** *see* Guaifenesin *on page 548*
- **Brethaire® Inhalation Aerosol** *see* Terbutaline *on page 1105*
- **Brethine® Injection** *see* Terbutaline *on page 1105*
- **Brethine® Oral** *see* Terbutaline *on page 1105*
- **Bretylate®** *see* Bretylium *on this page*

## Bretylium (bre TIL ee um)

**Therapeutic Category** Antiarrhythmic Agent, Class III

**Pregnancy Risk Factor** C

**Lactation** Excretion in breast milk unknown

**Use** Treatment of ventricular tachycardia and fibrillation; treatment of other serious ventricular arrhythmias resistant to lidocaine

**Mechanism of Action/Effect** Class III antiarrhythmic; after an initial release of norepinephrine at the peripheral adrenergic nerve terminals, bretylium inhibits further release by postganglionic nerve endings in response to sympathetic nerve stimulation

**Contraindications** Hypersensitivity to bretylium or any component; digitalis intoxication-induced arrhythmias

**Warnings** Hypotension, patients with fixed cardiac output (severe pulmonary hypertension or aortic stenosis) may experience severe hypotension due to decrease in peripheral resistance without ability to increase cardiac output. Reduce dose in renal failure patients. May have prolonged half-life with aging, and elderly may be more prone to experience hypotension. Pregnancy factor C.

**Drug Interactions**

**Increased Effect/Toxicity:** Other antiarrhythmic agents may potentiate or antagonize cardiac effects. Toxic effects may be additive. The vasopressor effects of catecholamines may be enhanced by bretylium. May potentiate digitalis toxicity.

**Adverse Reactions**

>10%: Cardiovascular: Hypotension (both postural and supine)

1% to 10%: Gastrointestinal: Nausea, vomiting

<1% (Limited to important or life-threatening symptoms): Transient initial hypertension, increase in premature ventricular contractions (PVCs), bradycardia, chest pain, flushing, syncope, postural hypotension, renal impairment, respiratory depression, nasal congestion, shortness of breath

**Overdose/Toxicology** Symptoms of overdose include significant hypertension followed by severe hypotension. Administration of a short-acting hypotensive agent should be used for the hypertensive response. Treatment is symptomatic and supportive. Dialysis is not useful.

**Pharmacodynamics/Kinetics**

**Protein Binding:** 1% to 6%

**Half-life Elimination:** 7-11 hours; average: 4-17 hours; End-stage renal disease: 16-32 hours

**Time to Peak:** 6-9 hours

**Metabolism:** Not metabolized

**Excretion:** Urine

**Onset:** Onset of antiarrhythmic effect: I.M.: May require 2 hours; I.V.: Within 6-20 minutes

**Duration:** 6-24 hours

**Formulations**

Bretylium tosylate:

Infusion, premixed in $D_5W$: 1 mg/mL (500 mL); 2 mg/mL (250 mL); 4 mg/mL (250 mL, 500 mL)

Injection: 50 mg/mL (10 mL, 20 mL)

**Dosing**

**Adults:** (**Note**: Patients should undergo defibrillation/cardioversion before and after bretylium doses as necessary.)

Immediate life-threatening ventricular arrhythmias, ventricular fibrillation, unstable ventricular tachycardia: Initial: I.V.: 5 mg/kg (undiluted) over 1 minute; if arrhythmia persists, give 10 mg/kg (undiluted) over 1 minute and repeat as necessary (usually at 15- to 30-minute intervals) up to a total dose of 30-35 mg/kg

Other life-threatening ventricular arrhythmias:

Initial: I.M., I.V.: 5-10 mg/kg, may repeat every 1-2 hours if arrhythmia persist; give I.V. dose (diluted) over 8-10 minutes

Maintenance dose: I.M.: 5-10 mg/kg every 6-8 hours; I.V. (diluted): 5-10 mg/kg every 6 hours; I.V. infusion (diluted): 1-2 mg/minute (little experience with doses >40 mg/kg/day)

**Elderly:** Refer to adult dosing.

**Renal Impairment:**

$Cl_{cr}$ 10-50 mL/minute: Administer 25% to 50% of dose.

$Cl_{cr}$ <10 mL/minute: Administer 25% of dose.

Not dialyzable

**Administration**

**I.M.:** I.M. injection in adults should not exceed 5 mL volume in any one site.

**I.V.:** 2 g/250 mL $D_5W$ (infusion pump should be used for I.V. infusion)

Bolus, emergency: Infuse rapidly (1 minute).

Bolus, nonemergency: May be given over 8-10 minutes.

Suggested rate of I.V. infusion: 1-4 mg/minute.

1 mg/minute = 7 mL/hour
2 mg/minute = 15 mL/hour
3 mg/minute = 22 mL/hour
4 mg/minute = 30 mL/hour

**I.V. Detail:** An initial worsening of arrhythmia, as well as nausea, may occur with bolus. During continuous infusions, hypotension may occur.

**Stability**

**Storage:** The premix infusion should be stored at room temperature and protected from freezing.

**Reconstitution:** Standard diluent: 2 g/250 mL $D_5W$

**Additional Nursing Issues**

**Physical Assessment:** Assess other medications patient may be taking for effectiveness and interactions (see Drug Interactions). I.V.: Requires use of infusion pump and continuous cardiac and hemodynamic monitoring during infusion. Be alert for adverse reactions (see Warnings/Precautions and Adverse Reactions). **Pregnancy risk factor C.** Note breast-feeding caution.

**Patient Information/Instruction:** Emergency use: Patient education is determined by patient condition. You may experience nausea or vomiting (call for assistance if this occurs, do not try to get out of bed or change position on your own). Report chest pain, acute dizziness, or difficulty breathing immediately. **Breast-feeding precautions:** Consult prescriber if breast-feeding.

**Geriatric Considerations:** See Warnings/Precautions and Adverse Reactions.

**Related Information**

Antiarrhythmic Drug Classification Comparison *on page 1366*


- **Brevibloc® Injection** *see* Esmolol *on page 438*
- **Brevicon®** *see* Oral Contraceptives *on page 859*
- **Brevoxyl® Gel** *see page 1294*
- **Bricanyl® Injection** *see* Terbutaline *on page 1105*
- **Bricanyl® Oral** *see* Terbutaline *on page 1105*
- **Brimonidine** *see* Ophthalmic Agents, Glaucoma *on page 853*
- **Brinzolamide** *see* Ophthalmic Agents, Glaucoma *on page 853*
- **Brispen** *see* Dicloxacillin *on page 361*
- **Brofed® Elixir** *see page 1294*
- **Bromaline® Elixir** *see page 1294*
- **Bromanate DC®** *see* Brompheniramine, Phenylpropanolamine, and Codeine *on page 163*
- **Bromanate® Elixir** *see page 1294*

- **Bromanyl® Cough Syrup** *see page 1306*
- **Bromarest®** *see page 1294*
- **Bromatapp®** *see page 1294*
- **Brombay®** *see page 1294*
- **Bromfed® Syrup** *see page 1294*
- **Bromfed® Tablet** *see page 1294*
- **Bromfenex® PD** *see page 1294*

## Bromocriptine (broe moe KRIP teen)

**U.S. Brand Names** Parlodel®

**Therapeutic Category** Anti-Parkinson's Agent (Dopamine Agonist); Ergot Derivative

**Pregnancy Risk Factor** B

**Lactation** Enters breast milk/contraindicated

**Use** Usually used with levodopa or levodopa/carbidopa to treat Parkinson's disease - treatment of parkinsonism in patients unresponsive or allergic to levodopa; treatment of prolactin-secreting pituitary adenomas, acromegaly, amenorrhea/galactorrhea secondary to hyperprolactinemia in the absence of primary tumor; neuroleptic malignant syndrome; **the indication for prevention of postpartum lactation has been withdrawn** voluntarily by the manufacturer

**Mechanism of Action/Effect** Semisynthetic ergot alkaloid derivative with dopaminergic properties; inhibits prolactin secretion and can improve symptoms of Parkinson's disease by directly stimulating dopamine receptors in the corpus stratum

**Contraindications** Hypersensitivity to bromocriptine or any component; severe ischemic heart disease or peripheral vascular disorders

**Warnings** Use with caution in patients with impaired renal or hepatic function.

**Drug Interactions**

**Cytochrome P-450 Effect:** CYP3A3/4 enzyme substrate

**Decreased Effect:** Amitriptyline, butyrophenones, imipramine, methyldopa, phenothiazines, reserpine, may decrease bromocriptine's efficacy at reducing prolactin.

**Increased Effect/Toxicity:** Increased cardiovascular toxicity when bromocriptine is taken with ergot alkaloids. Potential for serotonin syndrome if combined with other serotonergic drugs.

**Adverse Reactions** Incidence of adverse effects is high, especially at beginning of treatment and with dosages >20 mg/day.

1% to 10%:
- Cardiovascular: Hypotension, Raynaud's phenomenon
- Central nervous system: Mental depression, confusion, hallucinations
- Gastrointestinal: Nausea, constipation or diarrhea, anorexia, dry mouth
- Neuromuscular & skeletal: Leg cramps
- Respiratory: Nasal congestion

<1% (Limited to important or life-threatening symptoms): Hypertension, myocardial infarction, syncope, dizziness, drowsiness, fatigue, insomnia, headache, seizures

**Overdose/Toxicology** Symptoms of overdose include nausea, vomiting, and hypotension. Treatment is symptomatic and supportive.

**Pharmacodynamics/Kinetics**

**Protein Binding:** 90% to 96%

**Half-life Elimination:** Half-life (biphasic): Initial: 6-8 hours; Terminal: 50 hours

**Time to Peak:** 1-2 hours

**Metabolism:** Liver

**Excretion:** Urine

**Formulations**

Bromocriptine mesylate:
- Capsule: 5 mg
- Tablet: 2.5 mg

**Dosing**

**Adults:** Oral:
- Parkinsonism: 1.25 mg 2 times/day, increased by 2.5 mg/day in 2- to 4-week intervals (usual dose range is 30-90 mg/day in 3 divided doses), though elderly patients can usually be managed on lower doses
- Hyperprolactinemia: 2.5 mg 2-3 times/day
- Acromegaly: Initial: 1.25-2.5 mg increasing as necessary every 3-7 days; usual dose: 20-30 mg/day

**Elderly:** Refer to adult dosing; however, elderly patients can usually be managed on lower doses.

**Hepatic Impairment:** No guidelines are available, however, adjustment may be necessary.

**Additional Nursing Issues**

**Physical Assessment:** Assess effectiveness and interactions of other medications patient may be taking (see Contraindications and Drug Interactions). Monitor laboratory tests, therapeutic response (eg, mental status, involuntary movements), and adverse reactions at beginning of therapy and periodically throughout therapy (see Warnings/Precautions, Adverse Reactions, and Overdose/Toxicology). Assess knowledge/teach patient appropriate use, interventions to reduce side effects, and adverse symptoms to report. Breast-feeding is contraindicated.

**Patient Information/Instruction:** Take exactly as directed (may be prescribed in conjunction with levodopa/carbidopa); do not change dosage or discontinue without consulting prescriber. Therapeutic effects may take several weeks or months to achieve and you may need frequent monitoring during first weeks of therapy. Take with meals if GI upset occurs, before meals if dry mouth occurs, after eating if drooling or if nausea occurs. Take at the same time each day. Maintain adequate hydration (2-3 L/day of fluids unless instructed to restrict fluid intake); void before taking medication. Do not use alcohol and prescription or OTC sedatives or CNS depressants without consulting prescriber. Urine or perspiration may appear darker. You may experience drowsiness, dizziness, confusion, or vision changes (use caution when driving, climbing stairs, or engaging in tasks requiring alertness until response to drug is known); orthostatic hypotension (use caution when changing position - rising to standing from sitting or lying); constipation (increased exercise, fluids, or dietary fruit and fiber may help); nasal congestion (consult prescriber for appropriate relief); nausea, vomiting, loss of appetite, or stomach discomfort (small frequent meals, frequent mouth care, chewing gum, or sucking lozenges may help). Report unresolved constipation or vomiting; chest pain or irregular heartbeat; acute headache or dizziness; CNS changes (hallucination, loss of memory, seizures, acute headache, nervousness, etc); painful or difficult urination; increased muscle spasticity, rigidity, or involuntary movements; skin rash; or significant worsening of condition. **Breast-feeding precautions:** Do not breast-feed.

**Geriatric Considerations:** See Adverse Reactions; elderly patients are usually managed on lower doses.

- **Bromodiphenhydramine and Codeine** *see page 1306*
- **Bromotuss® w/Codeine Cough Syrup** *see page 1306*
- **Bromphen®** *see page 1294*
- **Bromphen DC® w/Codeine** *see* Brompheniramine, Phenylpropanolamine, and Codeine *on this page*
- **Brompheniramine** *see page 1294*
- **Brompheniramine and Phenylephrine** *see page 1294*
- **Brompheniramine and Phenylpropanolamine** *see page 1294*
- **Brompheniramine and Pseudoephedrine** *see page 1294*

## Brompheniramine, Phenylpropanolamine, and Codeine

(brome fen IR a meen, fen il proe pa NOLE a meen, & KOE deen)

**U.S. Brand Names** Bromanate DC®; Bromphen DC® w/Codeine; Dimetane®-DC; Myphetane DC®; Poly-Histine CS®

**Synonyms** Codeine, Brompheniramine, and Phenylpropanolamine; Phenylpropanolamine, Brompheniramine, and Codeine

**Therapeutic Category** Antihistamine/Decongestant/Antitussive

**Pregnancy Risk Factor** C

**Lactation** Excretion in breast milk unknown/contraindicated

**Use** Relief of coughs and upper respiratory symptoms, including nasal congestion, associated with allergy or the common cold

**Formulations** Liquid: Brompheniramine maleate 2 mg, phenylpropanolamine hydrochloride 12.5 mg, and codeine phosphate 10 mg per 5 mL with alcohol 0.95% (480 mL)

**Dosing**

**Adults:** Oral: 10 mL every 4 hours

**Elderly:** Refer to adult dosing.

**Additional Nursing Issues**

**Physical Assessment:** See individual components listed in Related Information. **Pregnancy risk factor C** - benefits of use should outweigh possible risks. Breast-feeding is contraindicated.

**Patient Information/Instruction:** See individual components listed in Related Information. **Pregnancy/breast-feeding precautions:** Inform prescriber if you are or intend to be pregnant. Do not breast-feed.

**Related Information**

Codeine *on page 299*
Phenylpropanolamine *on page 922*

- **Bromphen® Tablet** *see page 1294*
- **Bronalide®** *see* Flunisolide *on page 497*
- **Bronchial®** *see* Theophylline and Guaifenesin *on page 1118*
- **Bronitin®** *see* Epinephrine *on page 424*
- **Bronkaid® Mist [OTC]** *see* Epinephrine *on page 424*
- **Bronkodyl®** *see* Theophylline *on page 1115*
- **Bronkometer®** *see* Isoetharine *on page 629*
- **Bronkosol®** *see* Isoetharine *on page 629*
- **Brontex® Liquid** *see* Guaifenesin and Codeine *on page 549*
- **Brontex® Tablet** *see* Guaifenesin and Codeine *on page 549*
- **Brotane®** *see page 1294*
- **BSS® Ophthalmic** *see page 1294*
- **Bucladin®-S Softab®** *see* Buclizine *on this page*

## Buclizine (BYOO kli zeen)

**U.S. Brand Names** Bucladin®-S Softab®; Vibazine®

**Therapeutic Category** Antihistamine

**Pregnancy Risk Factor** C

**Lactation** Excretion in breast milk unknown/contraindicated

**Use** Prevention and treatment of nausea, vomiting, and dizziness associated with motion sickness; symptomatic treatment of vertigo

(Continued)

## Buclizine *(Continued)*

**Mechanism of Action/Effect** Buclizine acts centrally to suppress nausea and vomiting. It also has CNS depressant, anticholinergic, antispasmodic, and local anesthetic effects, and suppresses labyrinthine activity and conduction in vestibular-cerebellar nerve pathways.

**Contraindications** Hypersensitivity to buclizine or any component

**Warnings** Product contains tartrazine. Use with caution in patients with angle-closure glaucoma, peptic ulcer, urinary tract obstruction, hyperthyroidism, bronchial asthma, and cardiac arrhythmias (conditions that can all be aggravated by anticholinergics). Some preparations contain sodium bisulfite; syrup contains alcohol. Pregnancy factor C.

**Drug Interactions**

**Increased Effect/Toxicity:** Increased toxicity with CNS depressants, MAO inhibitors, and tricyclic antidepressants.

**Adverse Reactions**

>10%: Central nervous system: Drowsiness

<1% (Limited to important or life-threatening symptoms): Headache, nervousness, restlessness

**Overdose/Toxicology** Symptoms of overdose include CNS stimulation or depression; overdose may result in death in infants and children. There is no specific treatment for antihistamine overdose. Clinical toxicity is due to blockade of cholinergic receptors. For anticholinergic overdose with severe life-threatening symptoms, physostigmine 1-2 mg I.V. slowly, may be given to reverse these effects.

**Pharmacodynamics/Kinetics**

**Metabolism:** Liver

**Excretion:** Urine

**Formulations** Tablet, chewable, as hydrochloride: 50 mg

**Dosing**

**Adults:** Oral:

Motion sickness (prophylaxis): 50 mg 30 minutes prior to traveling; may repeat 50 mg after 4-6 hours

Vertigo: 50 mg twice daily, up to 150 mg/day

**Elderly:** Refer to adult dosing; use lowest effective dose.

**Administration**

**Oral:** Bucladin®-S Softab® may be chewed, swallowed whole, or allowed to dissolve in mouth.

**Additional Nursing Issues**

**Physical Assessment:** Assess interactions of other medications (see Drug Interactions). See Warnings/Precautions and Contraindications for use cautions. Monitor effectiveness of therapy, adverse response (eg, CNS changes - see Adverse Reactions and Overdose/Toxicology). Assess knowledge/teach patient possible side effects and appropriate interventions, and adverse symptoms to report. **Pregnancy risk factor C** - benefits of use should outweigh possible risks. Breast-feeding is contraindicated.

**Patient Information/Instruction:** Take as directed. Do not increase dose or take more often than recommended. May cause drowsiness; use caution when driving or engaging in tasks that require alertness until response to drug is known. May cause dry mouth; lozenges, gum, or liquids may help. May cause headache or feelings of jitteriness or anxiety; these will go away when drug is discontinued. **Pregnancy/breast-feeding precautions:** Inform prescriber if you are or intend to be pregnant. Do not breast-feed.

**Geriatric Considerations:** Due to anticholinergic action, use lowest dose in divided doses to avoid side effects and their inconvenience. Limit use if possible. May cause confusion or aggravate symptoms of confusion in those with dementia.

## Budesonide (byoo DES oh nide)

**U.S. Brand Names** Pulmicort Turbuhaler®; Rhinocort®

**Therapeutic Category** Corticosteroid, Oral Inhaler; Corticosteroid, Nasal; Corticosteroid, Topical

**Pregnancy Risk Factor** C

**Lactation** Excretion in breast milk unknown/use caution

**Use** Management of symptoms of seasonal or perennial rhinitis in adults and nonallergic perennial rhinitis in adults

**Mechanism of Action/Effect** Anti-inflammatory effect on nasal tissues

**Warnings** Use with caution in patients with hypothyroidism, cirrhosis, hypertension, congestive heart failure, ulcerative colitis, or thromboembolic disorders. Do not stop medication abruptly if on prolonged therapy. Fatalities have occurred due to adrenal insufficiency in asthmatic patients during and after transfer from systemic corticosteroids to aerosol steroids. Several months may be required to slowly taper systemic corticosteroid therapy when transferring to inhaled treatment. During this period, aerosol steroids do **not** provide the systemic steroid needed to treat patients having trauma, surgery, or infections. When consumed in excessive quantities, systemic hypercorticism and adrenal suppression may occur. Withdrawal and discontinuation of the corticosteroid should be done carefully. Pregnancy factor C.

**Drug Interactions**

**Cytochrome P-450 Effect:** CYP3A3/4 enzyme substrate

**Decreased Effect:** Although there have been no reported drug interactions to date, one would expect budesonide could potentially interact with drugs known to interact with other corticosteroids.

**Adverse Reactions**

>10%:

Cardiovascular: Pounding heartbeat

Central nervous system: Nervousness, headache, dizziness

Dermatologic: Itching, rash

Gastrointestinal: GI irritation, bitter taste, oral candidiasis

Respiratory: Coughing, upper respiratory tract infection, bronchitis, hoarseness

Miscellaneous: Increased susceptibility to infections, sweating

1% to 10%:

Central nervous system: Insomnia, psychic changes

Dermatologic: Acne, urticaria

Endocrine & metabolic: Menstrual problems

Gastrointestinal: Anorexia, increase in appetite, dry mouth, dry throat, loss of taste perception

Ocular: Cataracts

Respiratory: Epistaxis

Miscellaneous: Loss of smell

<1% (Limited to important or life-threatening symptoms): Bronchospasm, shortness of breath

**Pharmacodynamics/Kinetics**

**Metabolism:** Hepatic

**Excretion:** Urine

**Formulations**

Aerosol: 32 mcg per actuation (7 g)

Turbuhaler®: 200 mcg per inhalation (160 mcg delivered to patient) (200 doses)

**Dosing**

**Adults:**

Intranasal: 256 mcg/day, given as either 2 sprays in each nostril in the morning and evening or as 4 sprays in each nostril in the morning

Inhalation: 1- to 4-inhalations twice daily using Turbuhaler® device; maintenance therapy may be gradually reduced to a single daily inhalation. See table.

**Budesonide**

| Previous Therapy | Recommended Starting Dose | Highest Recommended Dose |
|---|---|---|
| Bronchodilators alone | 200-400 mcg twice daily | 400 mcg twice daily |
| Inhaled corticosteroids* | 200-400 mcg twice daily | 800 mcg twice daily |
| Oral corticosteroids | 400-800 mcg twice daily | 800 mcg twice daily |

*In patients with mild to moderate asthma who are well controlled on inhaled corticosteroids, dosing with Pulmicort® Turbuhaler 200 mcg or 400 mcg once daily may be considered. Pulmicort Turbuhaler® can be administered once daily either in the morning or in the evening.

**Elderly:** Refer to adult dosing.

**Administration**

**Inhalation:** For intranasal use only. Shake well before using.

**Additional Nursing Issues**

**Physical Assessment:** Monitor therapeutic effects and adverse reactions (see Warnings/Precautions, Adverse Reactions, and Overdose/Toxicology). When changing from systemic steroids to inhalational steroids, taper reduction of systemic medication slowly (may take several months). Assess knowledge/teach patient appropriate use, interventions to reduce side effects, and adverse symptoms to report. **Pregnancy risk factor C** - benefits of use should outweigh possible risks. Note breast-feeding caution.

**Patient Information/Instruction:** Use as directed; do not increase dosage or discontinue abruptly without consulting prescriber. It may take several days for you to realize full effects of treatment. If you are also using an inhaled bronchodilator, wait 10 minutes before using this steroid aerosol. You may experience dizziness, anxiety, or blurred vision (rise slowly from sitting or lying position and use caution when driving or engaging in tasks requiring alertness until response to drug is known); or taste disturbance or aftertaste (frequent mouth care and mouth rinses may help). Report pounding heartbeat or chest pain; acute nervousness or inability to sleep; severe sneezing or nosebleed; difficulty breathing, sore throat, hoarseness, or bronchitis; respiratory difficulty or bronchospasms; disturbed menstrual pattern; vision changes; loss of taste or smell perception; or worsening of condition or lack of improvement. **Pregnancy/breast-feeding precautions:** Inform prescriber if you are or intend to be pregnant. Consult prescriber if breast-feeding.

**Administration:** Take 3-5 deep breaths. Use inhaler on inspiration. Allow 1 full minute between inhalations. Rinse mouth with water after use to reduce aftertaste and incidence of candidiasis.

**Geriatric Considerations:** Ensure that patients can correctly use nasal inhaler.

**Additional Information** Each 7 g canister contains 200 metered doses.

- **Bufferin® [OTC]** *see* Aspirin *on page 111*
- **Bufigen** *see* Nalbuphine *on page 801*
- **Bulfacetamide and Phenylephrine** *see page 1282*
- **Bumedyl®** *see* Bumetanide *on this page*

## Bumetanide (byoo MET a nide)

**U.S. Brand Names** Bumex®

**Therapeutic Category** Diuretic, Loop

(Continued)

## Bumetanide *(Continued)*

**Pregnancy Risk Factor** C

**Lactation** Excretion in breast milk unknown/use caution

**Use** Management of edema secondary to congestive heart failure or hepatic or renal disease including nephrotic syndrome; may be used alone or in combination with antihypertensives in the treatment of hypertension; can be used in furosemide-allergic patients

**Mechanism of Action/Effect** Inhibits reabsorption of sodium and chloride in the ascending loop of Henle and proximal renal tubule, causing increased excretion of water, sodium, chloride, magnesium, phosphate and calcium

**Contraindications** Hypersensitivity to bumetanide or any component; anuria or increasing azotemia

**Warnings** Loop diuretics are potent diuretics. Excess amounts can lead to profound diuresis with fluid and electrolyte loss. Close medical supervision and dose evaluation is required. Pregnancy factor C.

**Drug Interactions**

**Decreased Effect:** Bumetanide may reduce the effect of indomethacin and other NSAIDs, or probenecid when taken in combination. Decreased diuresis and natriuresis with NSAIDs.

**Increased Effect/Toxicity:** Increased effect of other antihypertensive agents. Lithium's excretion may be decreased resulting in increased serum levels and toxicity. Increased risk of ototoxicity with aminoglycoside antibiotics or cisplatin.

**Adverse Reactions**

>10%:

Cardiovascular: Orthostatic hypotension

1% to 10%:

Cardiovascular: Chest pain

Central nervous system: Headache

Gastrointestinal: Diarrhea, anorexia, stomach cramps

Endocrine & metabolic: Hyponatremia, hypochloremic alkalosis, hypokalemia, premature ejaculation or difficulty in keeping an erection

Optic: Blurred vision

<1% (Limited to important or life-threatening symptoms): Gout, leukopenia, agranulocytosis, thrombocytopenia, hepatic dysfunction

**Overdose/Toxicology** Symptoms of overdose include electrolyte depletion and volume depletion. Treatment is symptomatic and supportive.

**Pharmacodynamics/Kinetics**

**Protein Binding:** 95%

**Half-life Elimination:** Adults: 1-1.5 hours

**Metabolism:** Liver

**Excretion:** Urine

**Onset:** Oral, I.M.: 0.5-1 hour I.V.: 2-3 minutes

**Duration:** 6 hours

**Formulations**

Injection: 0.25 mg/mL (2 mL, 4 mL, 10 mL)

Tablet: 0.5 mg, 1 mg, 2 mg

**Dosing**

**Adults:**

Oral: 0.5-2 mg/dose 1-2 times/day; maximum: 10 mg/day

I.M., I.V.: 0.5-1 mg/dose; maximum: 10 mg/day

Continuous I.V. infusions of 0.9-1 mg/hour may be more effective than bolus dosing

**Elderly:** Initial: Oral: 0.5 mg once daily, increase as necessary.

**Administration**

**I.V.:** Give I.V. slowly, over 1-2 minutes.

**Stability**

**Storage:** I.V. infusion solutions should be used within 24 hours after preparation. Light sensitive - discoloration may occur when exposed to light.

**Monitoring Laboratory Tests** Serum electrolytes, renal function

**Additional Nursing Issues**

**Physical Assessment:** Monitor blood pressure and weight at beginning of therapy and periodically during long-term use. Assess I & O ratios and for signs of fluid retention. Monitor carefully for development of adverse side effects (see above). **Pregnancy risk factor C** - benefits should outweigh possible risks. Note breast-feeding caution.

**Patient Information/Instruction:** May be taken with food to reduce GI effects. Take single dose early in day (single dose) or last dose early in afternoon (twice daily) to prevent sleep interruptions. Include orange juice or bananas (or other sources of potassium-rich foods) in your daily diet but do not take supplemental potassium without consulting prescriber. You may experience dizziness, hypotension, lightheadedness, or weakness; use caution when changing position (rising from sitting or lying position), when driving, exercising, climbing stairs, or performing hazardous tasks, and avoid excessive exercise in hot weather. Report swelling of ankles or feet, weight increase or decrease more than 3 pounds in any one day, increased fatigue, muscle cramps or trembling, and any changes in hearing. **Pregnancy/breast-feeding precautions:** Inform prescriber if you are or intend to be pregnant; contraceptives may be recommended. Consult prescriber if breast-feeding.

**Geriatric Considerations:** See Warnings/Precautions. Severe loss of sodium and/or increases in BUN can cause confusion. For any change in mental status in patients on bumetanide, monitor electrolytes and renal function.

**Additional Information** 1 mg bumetanide = 40 mg furosemide


- **Bumex®** *see* Bumetanide *on page 165*
- **Buminate®** *see* Albumin *on page 45*
- **Buphenyl®** *see* Sodium Phenylbutyrate *on page 1064*


## Bupivacaine (byoo PIV a kane)

**U.S. Brand Names** Marcaine®; Sensorcaine®; Sensorcaine®-MPF

**Therapeutic Category** Local Anesthetic

**Pregnancy Risk Factor** C

**Lactation** Enters breast milk/contraindicated

**Use** Local anesthetic (injectable) for peripheral nerve block, infiltration, sympathetic block, caudal or epidural block, retrobulbar block

**Mechanism of Action/Effect** Blocks both the initiation and conduction of nerve impulses by decreasing the neuronal membrane's permeability to sodium ions, which results in inhibition of depolarization with resultant blockade of conduction

**Contraindications** Hypersensitivity to bupivacaine or any component; para-aminobenzoic acid or parabens; heart block; hypotension; history of malignant hyperthermia

**Warnings** Use with caution in patients with liver disease. Some commercially available formulations contain sodium metabisulfite, which may cause allergic-type reactions. Pending further data, should not be used in children <12 years of age and the solution for spinal anesthesia should not be used in children <18 years of age. **Do not use solutions containing preservatives for caudal or epidural block.** Convulsions due to systemic toxicity leading to cardiac arrest have been reported, presumably following unintentional intravascular injection. 0.75% is **not** recommended for obstetrical anesthesia. Pregnancy factor C.

**Drug Interactions**

**Increased Effect/Toxicity:** Increased effect if used with hyaluronidase. Bupivacaine used in conjunction with epinephrine in patients on beta-blockers, ergot-type oxytocics, MAO inhibitors, tricyclic antidepressants, phenothiazines, vasopressors, isoproterenol may result in prolonged hypotension or hypertension.

**Adverse Reactions** 1% to 10%:

Cardiovascular: Cardiac arrest, hypotension, bradycardia, palpitations
Central nervous system: Seizures, restlessness, anxiety, dizziness
Gastrointestinal: Nausea, vomiting
Neuromuscular & skeletal: Weakness
Ocular: Blurred vision
Otic: Tinnitus
Respiratory: Apnea

**Overdose/Toxicology** Treatment is symptomatic and supportive. Termination of anesthesia by pneumatic tourniquet inflation should be attempted when bupivacaine is administered by infiltration or regional injection. Treatment is symptomatic and supportive. Methemoglobinemia should be treated with methylene blue 1-2 mg/kg in a 1% sterile aqueous solution by I.V. push over 4-6 minutes, repeated up to a total dose of 7 mg/kg.

**Pharmacodynamics/Kinetics**

**Half-life Elimination:** 1.5-5.5 hours

**Metabolism:** Liver

**Excretion:** Small amounts in urine

**Onset:** Onset of anesthesia (dependent on route administered): Within 4-10 minutes generally

**Duration:** 1.5-8.5 hours

**Formulations**

Bupivacaine hydrochloride:

Injection: 0.25% (10 mL, 20 mL, 30 mL, 50 mL); 0.5% (10 mL, 20 mL, 30 mL, 50 mL); 0.75% (2 mL, 10 mL, 20 mL, 30 mL)

Injection with epinephrine (1:200,000): 0.25% (10 mL, 30 mL, 50 mL); 0.5% (1.8 mL, 3 mL, 5 mL, 10 mL, 30 mL, 50 mL); 0.75% (30 mL)

**Dosing**

**Adults:** Dose varies with procedure, depth of anesthesia, vascularity of tissues, duration of anesthesia and condition of patient. Do not use solutions containing preservatives for caudal or epidural block.

Caudal block (with or without epinephrine): 15-30 mL of 0.25% or 0.5%

Epidural block (other than caudal block): 10-20 mL of 0.25% or 0.5%

Peripheral nerve block: 5 mL dose of 0.25% or 0.5% (12.5-25 mg); maximum: 2.5 mg/kg (plain); 3 mg/kg (with epinephrine); up to a maximum of 400 mg/day

Sympathetic nerve block: 20-50 mL of 0.25% (no epinephrine) solution

**Elderly:** Refer to adult dosing.

**Stability**

**Storage:** Solutions with epinephrine should be protected from light.

**Additional Nursing Issues**

**Physical Assessment:** Assess other medications patient may be taking for additive or adverse interactions (see Drug Interactions). Monitor for effectiveness of anesthesia, and adverse reactions (see Adverse Reactions). Monitor for return of sensation. Teach patient adverse reactions to report; use and teach appropriate interventions to promote safety. **Pregnancy risk factor C** - benefits of use should outweigh possible risks. Breast-feeding is contraindicated.

(Continued)

## Bupivacaine *(Continued)*

**Patient Information/Instruction:** This medication is given to reduce sensation in the injected area. You will experience decreased sensation to pain, heat, or cold in the area and/or decreased muscle strength (depending on area of application) until the effects wear off; use necessary caution to reduce incidence of possible injury until full sensation returns. If used in mouth, do not eat or drink until full sensation returns. Immediately report chest pain or palpitations; increased restlessness, anxiety, or dizziness; skeletal or muscle weakness; difficulty breathing; ringing in ears; or changes in vision. **Pregnancy/breast-feeding precautions:** Inform prescriber if you are pregnant. Do not breast-feed.

**Additional Information** Metabisulfites in epinephrine-containing injection.

♦ **Buprenex®** *see* Buprenorphine *on this page*

## Buprenorphine (byoo pre NOR feen)

**U.S. Brand Names** Buprenex®

**Therapeutic Category** Analgesic, Narcotic

**Pregnancy Risk Factor** C

**Lactation** Excretion in breast milk unknown

**Use** Management of moderate to severe pain; heroin withdrawal

**Mechanism of Action/Effect** Opiate agonist/antagonist that produces analgesia by binding to kappa and mu opiate receptors in the CNS

**Contraindications** Hypersensitivity to buprenorphine or any component

**Warnings** Use with caution in patients with hepatic dysfunction, decreased respiratory function, increased intracranial pressure, Addison's disease, urethral stricture, hepatic or renal dysfunction, or possible neurologic injury. May precipitate abstinence syndrome in narcotic-dependent patients. Pregnancy factor C.

**Drug Interactions**

**Increased Effect/Toxicity:** Increased toxicity with barbiturates, benzodiazepines (increase CNS and respiratory depression), tranquilizers, narcotic analgesics, and phenothiazines.

**Adverse Reactions**

>10%: Central nervous system: Drowsiness

1% to 10%:

Cardiovascular: Hypotension

Central nervous system: Dizziness, headache

Gastrointestinal: Vomiting, nausea

Respiratory: Respiratory depression (mild)

<1% (Limited to important or life-threatening symptoms): Hypertension, increased or decreased heart rate, urinary retention, respiratory depression (severe)

**Overdose/Toxicology** Symptoms of overdose include CNS depression, pinpoint pupils, hypotension, and bradycardia. Treatment is supportive. Naloxone, 2 mg I.V. with repeat administration as necessary up to a total of 10 mg, can also be used to reverse toxic effects of the opiate.

**Pharmacodynamics/Kinetics**

**Protein Binding:** High

**Half-life Elimination:** 2.2-3 hours (range: 1.2-7.2 hours)

**Metabolism:** Liver

**Excretion:** Bile and urine

**Onset:** Onset of analgesia: Within 10-30 minutes

**Duration:** 6-8 hours

**Formulations** Injection, as hydrochloride: 0.3 mg/mL (1 mL)

**Dosing**

**Adults:** I.M., slow I.V.: 0.3-0.6 mg every 6 hours as needed. **Long-term use is not recommended.**

**Elderly:** I.M., slow I.V.: 0.15 mg every 6 hours; elderly patients are more likely to suffer from confusion and drowsiness compared to younger patients. **Long-term use is not recommended.**

**Administration**

**I.V.:** Administer I.V. dose slowly.

**Stability**

**Storage:** Protect from excessive heat >40°C (104°F) and light.

**Compatibility:** Compatible with 0.9% sodium chloride, lactated Ringer's solution, 5% dextrose in water, scopolamine, haloperidol, glycopyrrolate, droperidol, and hydroxyzine. Incompatible with diazepam and lorazepam.

**Monitoring Laboratory Tests** LFTs

**Additional Nursing Issues**

**Physical Assessment:** Assess other medications patient may be taking for possible additive or adverse interactions (see Drug Interactions). Monitor for effectiveness of pain relief and monitor for signs of overdose (see above). Monitor blood pressure, CNS and respiratory status, and degree of sedation at beginning of therapy and at regular intervals with long-term use. For inpatients, implement safety measures (eg, side rails up, call light within reach, instructions to call for assistance, etc). Assess knowledge/teach patient appropriate use (if self-administered). Teach patient to monitor for adverse reactions (see Adverse Reactions), adverse reactions to report, and appropriate interventions to reduce side effects. **Pregnancy risk factor C** - benefits of use should outweigh possible risks. Note breast-feeding caution.

**Patient Information/Instruction:** If self-administered, use exactly as directed (do not increase dose or frequency). While using this medication, do not use alcohol and other prescription or OTC medications (especially sedatives, tranquilizers, antihistamines, or pain medications) without consulting prescriber. May cause dizziness, drowsiness, confusion, or blurred vision (use caution when driving, climbing stairs, or changing position - rising from sitting or lying to standing, or when engaging in tasks requiring alertness until response to drug is known). You may experience nausea or vomiting (frequent mouth care, small frequent meals, sucking lozenges, or chewing gum may help). Report unresolved nausea or vomiting; difficulty breathing or shortness of breath; excessive sedation or unusual weakness; rapid heartbeat or palpitations. **Pregnancy/breast-feeding precautions:** Inform prescriber if you are or intend to be pregnant. Consult prescriber if breast-feeding.

**Additional Information** 0.3 mg buprenorphine = 10 mg morphine injection or 75 mg meperidine injection; has longer duration of action than either agent.

**Related Information**

Narcotic/Opioid Analgesic Comparison *on page 1396*

## Bupropion (byoo PROE pee on)

**U.S. Brand Names** Wellbutrin®; Zyban™

**Therapeutic Category** Antidepressant, Dopamine-Reuptake Inhibitor

**Pregnancy Risk Factor** B

**Lactation** Enters breast milk/not recommended

**Use** Treatment of depression; smoking cessation (Zyban™)

**Mechanism of Action/Effect** Antidepressant structurally different from all other previously marketed antidepressants; weak blocker of serotonin and norepinephrine reuptake, inhibits neuronal dopamine reuptake and is **not** a monoamine oxidase A or B inhibitor

**Contraindications** Hypersensitivity to bupropion or any component; seizure disorder; prior diagnosis of bulimia or anorexia nervosa; concurrent use of a monoamine oxidase (MAO) inhibitor; head injury; CNS tumor

**Warnings** The estimated seizure potential is increased many fold with doses in the 450-600 mg/day range. Giving a single dose <150 mg will lessen the seizure potential. Use in patients with renal or hepatic impairment increases possible toxic effects. Pregnancy factor C.

**Drug Interactions**

**Cytochrome P-450 Effect:** CYP2B6 and 2D6 enzyme substrate, CYP3A3/4 enzyme substrate (minor)

**Decreased Effect:** Increased clearance which reduces the effect of the following agents: carbamazepine, phenytoin, cimetidine, phenobarbital.

**Increased Effect/Toxicity:** Bupropion in combination with levodopa and MAO inhibitors has potential for increased toxicity and adverse reactions. Increased risk of seizures.

**Effects on Lab Values** Decreased prolactin levels

**Adverse Reactions**

**Depression:**

>10%:

Central nervous system: Agitation, insomnia, fever, headache, psychosis, confusion, anxiety, restlessness, dizziness, seizures, chills, akathisia

Gastrointestinal: Nausea, vomiting, dry mouth, constipation, weight loss

Genitourinary: Impotence

Neuromuscular & skeletal: Tremor

1% to 10%:

Central nervous system: Hallucinations, drowsiness

Dermatologic: Rash

Ocular: Blurred vision

<1% (Limited to potentially life-threatening symptoms): Chest pain, abnormal EKG, myocardial infarction, GI bleeding, stomach ulcer, intestinal perforation, elevated LFTs, jaundice, dyspnea, epistaxis, pulmonary embolism

**Smoking cessation:**

>10%:

Central nervous system: Insomnia

Gastrointestinal: Dry mouth

1% to 10%:

Cardiovascular: Hot flashes, hypertension

Central nervous system: Dizziness, tremor, somnolence

Dermatologic: Pruritus, rash, dry skin, urticaria, acne

Gastrointestinal: Increased appetite, anorexia, taste perversion

Neuromuscular & skeletal: Arthralgia, myalgia, cramps

Respiratory: Bronchitis

Hematologic: Ecchymosis

<1% (limited to life-threatening or severe): Angioedema, exfoliative dermatitis, rhabdomyolysis, anemia, pancytopenia, thrombocytopenia, hyperglycemia, hypoglycemia, SIADH

**Overdose/Toxicology** Symptoms of overdose include labored breathing, salivation, arched back, ataxia, and convulsions. Dialysis may be of limited value after drug absorption because of slow tissue-to-plasma diffusion. Treatment is symptomatic and supportive.

(Continued)

## Bupropion *(Continued)*

**Pharmacodynamics/Kinetics**

**Protein Binding:** 82% to 88%

**Half-life Elimination:** 14 hours

**Time to Peak:** Oral: Within 3 hours

**Metabolism:** Liver

**Excretion:** Urine and feces

**Onset:** >2 weeks to therapeutic effect

**Formulations**

Tablet: 75 mg, 100 mg

Tablet, sustained release: 100 mg, 150 mg

Tablet, sustained release (Zyban™): 150 mg

**Dosing**

**Adults:** Oral:

Depression: 100 mg 3 times/day; begin at 100 mg twice daily; may increase to a maximum dose of 450 mg/day; dose should not be increased by more than 50 mg/day once weekly to minimize the risk of seizures.

Smoking cessation: Initial: 150 mg/day for the first 3 days, then increase dose to 150 mg twice a day for 7-12 weeks; maximum: 300 mg/day.

**Elderly:**

Depression: Oral: 50-100 mg/day, increase by 50-100 mg every 3-4 days as tolerated; there is evidence that the elderly respond at 150 mg/day in divided doses, but some may require a higher dose.

Smoking cessation: Refer to adult dosing.

**Renal Impairment:** Patients with renal failure should receive a reduced dosage initially and be closely monitored.

**Hepatic Impairment:** Patients with hepatic failure should receive a reduced dosage initially and be closely monitored.

**Additional Nursing Issues**

**Physical Assessment:** Assess other medications patient may be taking for effectiveness and interactions (see Drug Interactions). See Contraindications and Warnings/Precautions for cautious use. Monitor therapeutic response, and adverse reactions at beginning of therapy and periodically with long-term use (see Adverse Reactions and Overdose/Toxicology). Taper dosage slowly when discontinuing. Assess knowledge/teach patient appropriate use, interventions to reduce side effects, and adverse symptoms to report. **Pregnancy risk factor C** - benefits of use should outweigh possible risks. Breast-feeding is not recommended.

**Patient Information/Instruction:**

Depression: Take as directed, in equally divided doses, do not take in larger dose or more often than recommended. Do not discontinue without consulting prescriber. Do not use excessive alcohol or OTC medications not approved by prescriber. May cause drowsiness, clouded sensorium, restlessness, or agitation (use caution when driving or engaging in tasks requiring alertness until response to drug is known); nausea, vomiting, or dry mouth (small frequent meals, frequent mouth care, chewing gum, or sucking lozenges may help); constipation (increased exercise, fluids, or dietary fruit and fiber may help); or impotence (reversible). Report persistent CNS effects (agitation, confusion, anxiety, restlessness, insomnia, psychosis, hallucinations, seizures); muscle weakness or tremor; skin rash or irritation; chest pain or palpitations, abdominal pain or blood in stools; yellowing of skin or eyes; difficulty breathing, bronchitis, or unusual cough.

Smoking cessation: Use as directed, do not take extra doses. Do not combine narcotic patches with use of Zyban™ unless approved by prescriber. May cause dry mouth and insomnia (these may resolve with continued use). Report any difficulty breathing, unusual cough, dizziness, or muscle tremors.

**Pregnancy/breast-feeding precautions:** Inform prescriber if you are or intend to be pregnant. Breast-feeding is not recommended.

**Geriatric Considerations:** Limited data is available about the use of bupropion in the elderly. Two studies have found it equally effective when compared to imipramine. Its side effect profile (minimal anticholinergic and blood pressure effects) may make it useful in persons who do not tolerate traditional cyclic antidepressants.

**Breast-feeding Issues:** Generally, it is not recommended to breast-feed if taking antidepressants because of the long half-life, active metabolites, and the potential for side effects in the infant.

**Related Information**

Antidepressant Agents Comparison *on page 1368*

- **Burinex®** *see* Bumetanide *on page 165*
- **Burrow's Otic®** *see page 1291*
- **BuSpar®** *see* Buspirone *on this page*

## Buspirone (byoo SPYE rone)

**U.S. Brand Names** BuSpar®

**Therapeutic Category** Antianxiety Agent, Miscellaneous

**Pregnancy Risk Factor** B

**Lactation** Excretion in breast milk unknown/not recommended

**Use** Management of anxiety

**Unlabeled use:** major depression, panic attacks

**Mechanism of Action/Effect** Selectively antagonizes CNS serotonin 5-$HT_{1A}$ receptors without affecting benzodiazepine-GABA receptors; may down-regulate postsynaptic 5-$HT_2$ receptors as do antidepressants

**Contraindications** Hypersensitivity to buspirone or any component

**Warnings** Use in hepatic or renal impairment is not recommended. Does not prevent or treat withdrawal from benzodiazepines.

**Drug Interactions**

**Cytochrome P-450 Effect:** CYP3A3/4 enzyme substrate

**Decreased Effect:** Decreased effect with fluoxetine.

**Increased Effect/Toxicity:** Increased effects with cimetidine and food. Increased toxicity with MAO inhibitors, phenothiazines, CNS depressants, digoxin, and haloperidol. Aspirin and digoxin increase free concentration *in vitro*. Potential for serotonin syndrome if combined with other serotonergic drugs.

**Food Interactions** Food may decrease the absorption of buspirone, but it may also decrease the first-pass metabolism, thereby increasing the bioavailability of buspirone.

**Effects on Lab Values** ↑ AST, ALT, growth hormone(s), prolactin (S)

**Adverse Reactions**

>10%:

Central nervous system: Dizziness, lightheadedness, headache, restlessness

Gastrointestinal: Nausea

1% to 10%: Central nervous system: Drowsiness

≤1% (Limited to important or life-threatening symptoms): Chest pain, tachycardia, confusion, insomnia, nightmares, sedation, disorientation, excitement, fever, ataxia, drowsiness, leukopenia, eosinophilia, angioedema, serotonin syndrome, visual changes

**Overdose/Toxicology** Symptoms of overdose include dizziness, drowsiness, pinpoint pupils, nausea, and vomiting. There is no known antidote for buspirone. Treatment is supportive.

**Pharmacodynamics/Kinetics**

**Protein Binding:** 95%

**Half-life Elimination:** 2-3 hours

**Time to Peak:** Oral: Within 1 hour

**Metabolism:** Liver

**Excretion:** Urine

**Formulations** Tablet, as hydrochloride: 5 mg, 10 mg

**Dosing**

**Adults:** Oral: 15 mg/day (5 mg 3 times/day); may increase in increments of 5 mg/day every 2-4 days to a maximum of 60 mg/day.

**Elderly:** Oral: Initial: 5 mg twice daily, increase by 5 mg/day every 2-3 days as needed up to 20-30 mg/day; maximum daily dose: 60 mg/day (see Geriatric Considerations).

**Renal Impairment:** Generally not recommended, however, anuric patients may be dosed at 25% to 50% of the usual dose and monitored closely. Patients with creatinine clearance of 10-70 mL/minute demonstrate up to fourfold accumulation.

**Hepatic Impairment:** Dosage should be decreased in patients with severe hepatic insufficiency and the patient should be monitored closely.

**Additional Nursing Issues**

**Physical Assessment:** Assess other medications patient may be taking for effectiveness and interactions (see Drug Interactions). See Contraindications and Warnings/Precautions for cautious use. Monitor therapeutic response and adverse reactions (see Adverse Reactions above) at beginning of therapy and periodically with long-term use. Assess knowledge/teach patient appropriate use, interventions to reduce side effects, and adverse symptoms to report. Breast-feeding is not recommended.

**Patient Information/Instruction:** Take only as directed; do not increase dose or take more often than prescribed. May take 2-3 weeks to see full effect; do not discontinue without consulting prescriber. Do not use excessive alcohol or other prescription or OTC medications (especially pain medications, sedatives, antihistamines, or hypnotics) without consulting prescriber. Maintain adequate hydration (2-3 L/day of fluids unless instructed to restrict fluid intake). You may experience drowsiness, lightheadedness, impaired coordination, dizziness, or blurred vision (use caution when driving or engaging in tasks requiring alertness until response to drug is known); or upset stomach, nausea (small frequent meals, frequent mouth care, chewing gum, or sucking lozenges may help). Report persistent vomiting, chest pain or rapid heartbeat, persistent CNS effects (eg, confusion, restlessness, anxiety, insomnia, excitation, headache, dizziness, fatigue, impaired coordination), or worsening of condition. **Breast-feeding precautions:** Breast-feeding is not recommended.

**Geriatric Considerations:** Because buspirone is less sedating than other anxiolytics, it may be a useful agent in geriatric patients when an anxiolytic is indicated.

## Busulfan (byoo SUL fan)

**U.S. Brand Names** Busulfex®; Myleran®

**Therapeutic Category** Antineoplastic Agent, Alkylating Agent

**Pregnancy Risk Factor** D

**Lactation** Contraindicated

**Use** Palliative treatment of chronic myelogenous leukemia and bone marrow disorders, such as polycythemia vera and myeloid metaplasia; conditioning regimens for bone marrow transplantation

**Mechanism of Action/Effect** Interferes with DNA function; cytotoxic

**Contraindications** Hypersensitivity to busulfan or any component; failure to respond to previous courses; pregnancy; chronic lymphocytic leukemia, acute leukemia

(Continued)

## Busulfan *(Continued)*

**Warnings** The U.S. Food and Drug Administration (FDA) currently recommends that procedures for proper handling and disposal of antineoplastic agents be considered. May induce severe bone marrow hypoplasia. Reduce or discontinue dosage at first sign, as reflected by an abnormal decrease in any of the formed elements of the blood. Use with caution in patients recently given other myelosuppressive drugs or radiation treatment. If white blood count is high, hydration and allopurinol should be employed to prevent hyperuricemia. Avoid I.M. injections if platelet count falls to <100,000/mm³.

**Drug Interactions**

**Cytochrome P-450 Effect:** CYP3A3/4 enzyme substrate

**Adverse Reactions**

>10%:

- Dermatologic: Skin hyperpigmentation (busulfan tan), urticaria, erythema, alopecia
- Endocrine & metabolic: Ovarian suppression, amenorrhea, sterility
- Genitourinary: Azoospermia, testicular atrophy; malignant tumors have been reported in patients on busulfan therapy
- Hematologic: Severe pancytopenia, leukopenia, thrombocytopenia, anemia, and bone marrow suppression are common and patients should be monitored closely while on therapy; since this is a delayed effect (busulfan affects the stem cells), the drug should be discontinued temporarily at the first sign of a large or rapid fall in any blood element; some patients may develop bone marrow fibrosis or chronic aplasia which is probably due to the busulfan toxicity; in large doses, busulfan is myeloablative and is used for this reason in BMT
- Myelosuppressive:
  - WBC: Moderate
  - Platelets: Moderate
  - Onset (days): 7-10
  - Nadir (days): 14-21
  - Recovery (days): 28

1% to 10%:

- Cardiovascular: Hypotension
- Central nervous system: Confusion,
- Dermatologic: Hyperpigmentation
- Endocrine & metabolic: Amenorrhea, hyperuricemia
- Gastrointestinal: Nausea, stomatitis, anorexia, vomiting, diarrhea; drug has little effect on the GI mucosal lining
  - Emetic potential: Low (<10%)
- Hepatic: Elevated LFTs
- Neuromuscular & skeletal: Weakness
- Ocular: Cataracts
- Respiratory: Bronchopulmonary dysplasia

<1% (Limited to important or life-threatening symptoms): Adrenal suppression, gynecomastia, isolated cases of hemorrhagic cystitis have been reported, hepatic dysfunction; after long-term or high-dose therapy, a syndrome known as busulfan lung may occur; this syndrome is manifested by a diffuse interstitial pulmonary fibrosis and persistent cough, fever, rales, and dyspnea. May be relieved by corticosteroids.

**BMT:**

- Central nervous system: Generalized or myoclonic seizures and loss of consciousness, abnormal electroencephalographic findings
- Gastrointestinal: Mucositis, anorexia, moderately emetogenic
- Hepatic: Veno-occulsive disease (VOD), hyperbilirubinemia
- Miscellaneous: Transient pain at tumor sites, transient autoimmune disorders

**Overdose/Toxicology** Symptoms of overdose include leukopenia and thrombocytopenia. Induction of vomiting or gastric lavage with charcoal is indicated for recent ingestion; the effects of dialysis are unknown.

**Pharmacodynamics/Kinetics**

**Protein Binding:** ~14%

**Distribution:** Distributed into the CSF and saliva with levels similar to plasma

**Half-life Elimination:** After first dose: 3.4 hours; After last dose: 2.3 hours

**Time to Peak:** Oral: Within 4 hours; I.V.: Within 5 minutes

**Metabolism:** Liver

**Excretion:** Urine

**Duration:** 28 days

**Formulations**

Oral: Tablet: 2 mg

Injection (Busulfex®): 6 mg/mL (10 mL)

**Dosing**

**Adults:** Oral (refer to individual protocols):

- BMT marrow-ablative conditioning regimen: 1 mg/kg/dose (ideal body weight) every 6 hours for 16 doses
- High dose BMT:
  - 0.875-1 mg/kg/dose every 6 hours for 16 doses; total dose: 12-16 mg/kg
  - 37.5 mg/m² every 6 hours for 16 doses; total dose: 600 mg/m²
- Remission:
  - Induction of CML: 4-8 mg/day (may be as high as 12 mg/day)
  - Maintenance doses: Controversial, range from 1-4 mg/day to 2 mg/week; treatment is continued until WBC reaches 10,000-20,000 cells/mm³ at which time drug is discontinued; when WBC reaches 50,000/mm³, maintenance dose is resumed.

Unapproved uses:

Polycythemia vera: 2-6 mg/day

Thrombocytosis: 4-6 mg/day

I.V.: 0.8 mg/kg (ideal body weight or actual body weight, whichever is lower) every 6 hours for 4 days (a total of 16 doses)

I.V. dosing in morbidly obese patients: Dosing should be based on adjusted ideal body weight (AIBW) which should be calculated as ideal body weight (IBW) + 0.25 times (actual weight minus ideal body weight)

AIBW = IBW + 0.25 x (AW - IBW)

Cyclophosphamide, in combination with busulfan, is given on each of two days as a 1-hour infusion at a dose of 160 mg/m$^2$ beginning on day 3, 6 hours following the 16th dose of busulfan

**Elderly:** Oral (refer to individual protocols): Start with lowest recommended doses for adults.

**Administration**

**Oral: BMT only:** Phenytoin or clonazepam should be administered prophylactically during and for at least 48 hours following completion of busulfan. Risk of seizures is increased in patients with sickle cell disease. Increased risk of VOD when busulfan AUC >3000 μmol(min)/L (mean AUC, 2012 μmol(min)/L). To facilitate ingestion of high doses, insert multiple tablets into clear gel capsules.

**I.M.:** Avoid I.M. injection if platelet count falls to <100,000/mm$^3$.

**I.V.:** Intravenous busulfan should be administered via a CENTRAL venous catheter as a 2-hour infusion - every 6 hours for 4 consecutive days for a total of 16 doses

**Stability**

**Storage:** Store unopened ampules (injection) under refrigeration (2-8\°C) Final solution is stable for up to 8 hours at room temperature (25°C) but the infusion must also be completed within that 8-hour time frame. Dilution of busulfan injection in 0.9% sodium chloride is stable for up to 12 hours at refrigeration (2°C to 8°C) but the infusion must also be completed within that 12-hour time frame.

**Reconstitution:** Store unopened ampuls under refrigeration at 2°C to 8°C/36°F to 46°F. Dilute busulfan injection in 0.9% sodium chloride injection or dextrose 5% in water. The dilution volume should be ten times the volume of busulfan injection, ensuring that the final concentration of busulfan is ≥0.5 mg/mL.

**Monitoring Laboratory Tests** CBC with differential and platelet count, hemoglobin, liver function

**Additional Nursing Issues**

**Physical Assessment:** Monitor for effectiveness of therapy and development of adverse reactions (pulmonary fibrosis may occur 4-5 months after therapy begins - see Adverse Reactions). Observe bleeding precaution (avoid invasive procedures and instruct patient on safety measures). Instruct patient on use, possible side effects, and symptoms to report. **Pregnancy risk factor D** - assess knowledge/teach appropriate use of barrier contraceptives. Breast-feeding is contraindicated.

**Patient Information/Instruction:** Take oral medication as directed with chilled liquids. Maintain adequate hydration (2-3 L/day of fluids unless instructed to restrict fluid intake) to help prevent kidney complications. Avoid alcohol, acidic or spicy foods, aspirin or OTC medications unless approved by prescriber. Brush teeth with soft toothbrush or cotton swab. You may lose head hair or experience darkening of skin color (reversible when medication is discontinued), amenorrhea, sterility, or skin rash. You may experience nausea, vomiting, anorexia, or constipation (small frequent meals, increased exercise, and increased dietary fruit or fiber may help). You will be more susceptible to infection (avoid crowds or contagious persons, and do not receive any vaccinations unless approved by prescriber). Report palpitations or chest pain, excessive dizziness, confusion, respiratory difficulty, numbness or tingling of extremities, unusual bruising or bleeding, pain or changes in urination, or other adverse effects. **Pregnancy/breast-feeding precautions:** Do not get pregnant while taking this medication; use appropriate barrier contraceptive measures. Do not breast-feed.

**Geriatric Considerations:** Toxicity to immunosuppressives is increased in the elderly. Start with lowest recommended adult doses. Signs of infection, such as fever and rise in WBCs, may not occur. Lethargy and confusion may be more prominent signs of infection.

♦ **Busulfex®** *see* Busulfan *on page 171*

## Butabarbital Sodium (byoo ta BAR bi tal SOW dee um)

**U.S. Brand Names** Butalan®; Buticaps®; Butisol Sodium®

**Therapeutic Category** Barbiturate

**Pregnancy Risk Factor** D

**Lactation** Enters breast milk/contraindicated

**Use** Sedative, hypnotic (short-term)

**Mechanism of Action/Effect** Interferes with transmission of impulses from the thalamus to the cortex of the brain resulting in an imbalance in central inhibitory and facilitatory mechanisms

**Contraindications** Hypersensitivity to butabarbital or any component; presence of acute or chronic pain; latent porphyria; marked liver impairment; nephritis; impaired respiratory function; history of narcotic and hypnotic drug addiction; pregnancy

**Warnings** Use cautiously in the presence of acute or chronic pain, seizure disorders, hyperthyroidism, diabetes, severe pulmonary or respiratory disease, or status asthmaticus.

(Continued)

## Butabarbital Sodium *(Continued)*

**Drug Interactions**

**Decreased Effect:** Decreased effect with phenothiazines, haloperidol, quinidine, cyclosporine, tricyclic antidepressants, corticosteroids, theophylline, ethosuximide, warfarin, oral contraceptives, chloramphenicol, griseofulvin, doxycycline, and beta-blockers.

**Increased Effect/Toxicity:** Increased effect/toxicity when taken in combination with propoxyphene, benzodiazepines, CNS depressants, valproic acid, methylphenidate, and chloramphenicol.

**Effects on Lab Values** ↑ ammonia (B); ↓ bilirubin (S)

**Adverse Reactions**

>10%:

Central nervous system: Dizziness, clumsiness or unsteadiness, lightheadedness, "hangover" effect, drowsiness

1% to 10%:

Central nervous system: Confusion, mental depression, unusual excitement, nervousness, faint feeling, headache, insomnia, nightmares

Gastrointestinal: Nausea, vomiting, constipation

<1% (Limited to important or life-threatening symptoms): Hypotension, rash, exfoliative dermatitis, urticaria, Stevens-Johnson syndrome, agranulocytosis, megaloblastic anemia, thrombocytopenia, respiratory depression, apnea, laryngospasm

**Overdose/Toxicology** Symptoms of overdose include slurred speech, confusion, nystagmus, tachycardia, and hypotension. Treatment is symptomatic and supportive. Forced alkaline diuresis is of no value in the treatment of intoxications with short-acting barbiturates. Charcoal hemoperfusion or hemodialysis may be useful in harder-to-treat intoxications, especially in the presence of very high serum barbiturate levels.

**Pharmacodynamics/Kinetics**

**Half-life Elimination:** 40-140 hours

**Time to Peak:** Oral: Within 40-60 minutes

**Metabolism:** Liver

**Excretion:** Urine

**Formulations**

Capsule: 15 mg, 30 mg

Elixir, with alcohol 7%: 30 mg/5 mL (480 mL, 3780 mL); 33.3 mg/5 mL (480 mL, 3780 mL)

Tablet: 15 mg, 30 mg, 50 mg, 100 mg

**Dosing**

**Adults:** Oral:

Sedative: 15-30 mg 3-4 times/day

Hypnotic: 50-100 mg

Preop: 50-100 mg 1-1½ hours before surgery

**Elderly:** Not recommended for use in the elderly.

**Additional Nursing Issues**

**Physical Assessment:** Assess effectiveness and interactions of other medications (see Drug Interactions). See Contraindications and Warnings/Precautions for cautious use. Assess for history of addiction; long-term use can result in dependence, abuse, or tolerance. Evaluate periodically for need for continued use. After long-term use, taper dosage slowly when discontinuing. For inpatient use, institute safety measures (side rails, night light, call bell, assistance with ambulation) and monitor effectiveness and adverse reactions. For outpatient use, monitor effectiveness and adverse reactions (see Adverse Reactions) at beginning of therapy and periodically with long-term use. Assess knowledge/teach patient appropriate use, interventions to reduce side effects, and adverse symptoms to report. **Pregnancy risk factor D** - assess knowledge/teach appropriate use of barrier contraceptives. Breast-feeding is contraindicated.

**Patient Information/Instruction:** Use exactly as directed (do not increase dose or frequency or discontinue without consulting prescriber); may cause physical and/or psychological dependence. While using this medication, do not use alcohol or other prescription or OTC medications (especially, pain medications, sedatives, antihistamines, or hypnotics) without consulting prescriber. Maintain adequate hydration (2-3 L/day of fluids unless instructed to restrict fluid intake). You may experience drowsiness, dizziness, or blurred vision (use caution driving or engaging in tasks requiring alertness until response to drug is known); nausea or vomiting (small frequent meals, frequent mouth care, chewing gum, or sucking lozenges may help); constipation (increased exercise, fluids, or dietary fruit and fiber may help). Report skin rash or irritation; CNS changes (confusion, depression, increased sedation, excitation, headache, insomnia, or nightmares); difficulty breathing or shortness of breath; difficulty swallowing or feeling of tightness in throat; unusual weakness or unusual bleeding in mouth, urine, or stool; or other unanticipated adverse effects. **Pregnancy/breast-feeding precautions:** Do not get pregnant while taking this medication; use appropriate contraceptive measures. Do not breast-feed.

**Additional Information** Some formulations may contain ethanol or tartrazine.

**Related Information**

Antipsychotic Medication Guidelines *on page 1436*

♦ **Butacortelone** *see* Ibuprofen *on page 592*

♦ **Butalan®** *see* Butabarbital Sodium *on previous page*

## Butalbital Compound and Acetaminophen

(byoo TAL bi tal KOM pound & a seet a MIN oh fen)

**U.S. Brand Names** Amaphen®; Anoquan®; Axocet®; Endolor®; Esgic®; Esgic-Plus®; Femcet®; Fioricet®; G-1®; Medigesic®; Phrenilin®; Phrenilin Forte®; Repan®; Sedapap-10®; Triapin®; Two-Dyne®

**Synonyms** Acetaminophen and Butalbital Compound

**Therapeutic Category** Barbiturate

**Pregnancy Risk Factor** D

**Lactation** Enters breast milk/contraindicated

**Use** Relief of the symptomatic complex of tension or muscle contraction headache

**Contraindications** Hypersensitivity to butalbital or any component; patients with porphyria; pregnancy

**Warnings** Administer with caution, if at all, to patients who are mentally depressed, have suicidal tendencies, or a history of drug abuse. May be habit-forming.

**Drug Interactions**

**Decreased Effect:** Butalbital may diminish effects of uricosuric agents such as probenecid and sulfinpyrazone.

**Increased Effect/Toxicity:** MAO inhibitors may enhance CNS effects of butalbital. Increased effect (CNS depression) with narcotic analgesics, alcohol, general anesthetics, tranquilizers such as chlordiazepoxide, sedative hypnotics, or other CNS depressants.

**Effects on Lab Values** Acetaminophen may produce false-positive test results for urinary 5-hydroxyindoleacetic acid.

**Adverse Reactions**

>10%:

- Central nervous system: Dizziness, lightheadedness, drowsiness
- Gastrointestinal: Nausea, heartburn, stomach pains, dyspepsia, epigastric discomfort

1% to 10%:

- Central nervous system: Confusion, mental depression, unusual excitement, nervousness, faint feeling, insomnia, nightmares, intoxicated feeling
- Dermatologic: Rash
- Gastrointestinal: Constipation, GI ulceration

<1% (Limited to important or life-threatening symptoms): Tachycardia, chest pain, palpitations, syncope, hallucinations, nervousness, jitters, exfoliative dermatitis, Stevens-Johnson syndrome, agranulocytosis, megaloblastic anemia, thrombocytopenia, occult bleeding, prolongation of bleeding time, leukopenia, iron deficiency anemia, hepatotoxicity, thrombophlebitis, impaired renal function, respiratory depression, bronchospasm, epistaxis, allergic reaction

**Overdose/Toxicology** Symptoms of barbiturate overdose include unsteady gait, slurred speech, confusion, respiratory depression, hypotension, and coma. Treatment is supportive.

Symptoms of acetaminophen overdose include hepatic necrosis, transient azotemia, renal tubular necrosis with acute toxicity, anemia, and GI disturbances with chronic toxicity. Treatment consists of acetylcysteine 140 mg/kg orally (loading) followed by 70 mg/kg every 4 hours for 17 doses; therapy should be initiated based upon laboratory analysis suggesting a high probability of hepatotoxic potential. Activated charcoal is very effective at binding acetaminophen. Intravenous acetylcysteine should be reserved for patients unable to take oral forms.

**Pharmacodynamics/Kinetics**

**Half-life Elimination:** 61 hours in healthy volunteers

**Formulations**

Capsule:

- Amaphen®, Anoquan®, Endolor®, Esgic®, Femcet®, G-1®, Medigesic®, Repan®, Two-Dyne®: Butalbital 50 mg, caffeine 40 mg, and acetaminophen 325 mg
- Axocet®; Phrenilin Forte®: Butalbital 50 mg and acetaminophen 650 mg
- Triapin®: Butalbital 50 mg and acetaminophen 325 mg

Tablet:

- Esgic®, Fioricet®, Repan®: Butalbital 50 mg, caffeine 40 mg, and acetaminophen 325 mg
- Phrenilin®: Butalbital 50 mg and acetaminophen 325 mg
- Sedapap-10®: Butalbital 50 mg and acetaminophen 650 mg

**Dosing**

**Adults:** Oral: 1-2 tablets or capsules every 4 hours; not to exceed 6 tablets or capsules/day

**Elderly:** Not recommended for use in the elderly.

**Renal Impairment:** Dosage should be reduced.

**Hepatic Impairment:** Dosage should be reduced.

**Stability**

**Storage:** Store at room temperature below 30°C (86°F). Protect from moisture.

**Additional Nursing Issues**

**Physical Assessment: Assess patient for history of liver disease or alcohol abuse** (acetaminophen and excessive alcohol may have adverse liver effects). Assess other medications patient may be taking for additive or adverse interactions (see Drug Interactions). Monitor for therapeutic effectiveness and monitor for signs of overdose. Monitor vital signs and signs of adverse reactions (see Adverse Reactions) at beginning of therapy and at regular intervals with long-term use. Assess knowledge/teach patient appropriate use. Teach patient to monitor for adverse reactions, adverse reactions to report, and appropriate interventions to reduce side effects. **Pregnancy risk**

(Continued)

## Butalbital Compound and Acetaminophen *(Continued)*

**factor D** - assess knowledge/teach appropriate use of barrier contraceptives. Breast-feeding is contraindicated.

**Patient Information/Instruction:** If self-administered, use exactly as directed (do not increase dose or frequency); may cause physical and/or psychological dependence. Take with food or milk. While using this medication, do not use alcohol and other prescription or OTC medications (especially sedatives, tranquilizers, antihistamines, or pain medications) without consulting prescriber. Maintain adequate hydration (2-3 L/day of fluids unless instructed to restrict fluid intake). May cause dizziness, lightheadedness, confusion, or drowsiness (use caution when driving, climbing stairs, or changing position - rising from sitting or lying to standing, or when engaging in tasks requiring alertness until response to drug is known); heartburn or epigastric discomfort (frequent mouth care, frequent sips of fluids, chewing gum, or sucking lozenges may help); constipation (increased exercise, fluids, or dietary fruit and fiber may help). Report chest pain or palpitations; persistent dizziness; confusion, nightmares, excitation, or changes in mentation; shortness of breath or difficulty breathing; skin rash; unusual bleeding or bruising; or unusual fatigue and weakness. **Pregnancy/breast-feeding precautions:** Do not get pregnant while taking this medication; use appropriate barrier contraceptive measures. Do not breast-feed.

**Geriatric Considerations:** Elderly may react to barbiturates with marked excitement, depression, and confusion.

## Butalbital Compound and Aspirin

(byoo TAL bi tal KOM pound & AS pir in)

**U.S. Brand Names** Fiorgen PF®; Fiorinal®; Isollyl Improved®; Lanorinal®; Marnal®

**Synonyms** Aspirin and Butalbital Compound

**Therapeutic Category** Barbiturate

**Pregnancy Risk Factor** C/D (if used for long periods or in high doses near end of pregnancy)

**Lactation** Enters breast milk/use caution due to aspirin content

**Use** Relief of the symptomatic complex of tension or muscle contraction headache

**Contraindications** Hypersensitivity to butalbital or any component; patients with porphyria; pregnancy (extended use or high doses near term)

**Warnings** Use with extreme caution in the presence of peptic ulcer or coagulation abnormality - can produce psychological/physical drug dependence. Children and teenagers should not use this product. Pregnancy factor C (D if extended use, high doses, or late in pregnancy).

**Drug Interactions**

**Decreased Effect:** May decrease the effect of uricosuric agents (probenecid and sulfinpyrazone) reducing their effect on gout.

**Increased Effect/Toxicity:** Enhanced effect/toxicity with oral anticoagulants (warfarin), oral antidiabetic agents, insulin, 6-mercaptopurine, methotrexate, NSAIDs, narcotic analgesics (propoxyphene, meperidine, etc), benzodiazepines, sedative-hypnotics, other CNS depressants. The CNS effects of butalbital may be enhanced by MAO inhibitors.

**Effects on Lab Values** Aspirin may interfere with serum amylase, fasting blood glucose, cholesterol, protein, AST (SGOT), uric acid, PT, and bleeding time. Aspirin may interfere with laboratory results in urine of glucose, 5-hydroxyindoleacetic acid, Gerhardt ketone, VMA, uric acid, diacetic acid, and spectrophotometric detection of barbiturates.

**Adverse Reactions**

>10%:

Central nervous system: Dizziness, drowsiness

Gastrointestinal: Nausea, heartburn, stomach pains, dyspepsia, epigastric discomfort

1% to 10%:

Central nervous system: Lightheadedness

Gastrointestinal: Nausea, vomiting, flatulence

<1% (Limited to important or life-threatening symptoms): Exfoliative dermatitis, Stevens-Johnson syndrome, toxic epidermal necrosis, bone marrow suppression (one case report)

**Pharmacodynamics/Kinetics**

**Half-life Elimination:** 61 hours in healthy volunteers

**Formulations**

Capsule: (Fiorgen PF®, Fiorinal®, Isollyl Improved®, Lanorinal®, Marnal®): Butalbital 50 mg, caffeine 40 mg, and aspirin 325 mg

Tablet:

Fiorinal®, Isollyl Improved®, Lanorinal®, Marnal®: Butalbital 50 mg, caffeine 40 mg, and aspirin 325 mg

**Dosing**

**Adults:** Oral: 1-2 tablets or capsules every 4 hours; not to exceed 6 tablets or capsules/day

**Elderly:** Not recommended for use in the elderly.

**Renal Impairment:** Dosage should be reduced.

**Hepatic Impairment:** Dosage should be reduced.

**Stability**

**Storage:** Store below 25°C (77°F).

**Additional Nursing Issues**

**Physical Assessment:** Monitor for effectiveness of pain relief. Monitor CNS status, heart rate, blood pressure, fluid balance (I & O), and elimination regularly. Combination drug contains aspirin; assess for aspirin sensitivity and see Warnings/Precautions and

Drug Interactions. **Pregnancy risk factor C/D** - see Pregnancy Risk Factor for cautious use. Note breast-feeding caution.

**Patient Information/Instruction:** Take as directed; do not exceed prescribed amount. Avoid alcohol, aspirin or aspirin-containing medications, or any OTC medications unless approved by prescriber. Maintain adequate hydration (2-3 L/day of fluids unless instructed to restrict fluid intake) to prevent constipation. You may experience drowsiness, impaired judgment or coordination; use caution when driving or engaging in tasks that require alertness until response to drug is known. Small frequent meals may help reduce GI upset. Report any ringing in ears; abdominal pain; easy bruising or bleeding; blood in urine; severe weakness; acute unresolved dizziness or confusion, nervousness, nightmares, insomnia; or skin rash. **Pregnancy/breast-feeding precautions:** Inform prescriber if you are or intend to be pregnant. Consult prescriber if breast-feeding.

**Geriatric Considerations:** Elderly may react to barbiturates with marked excitement, depression, and confusion.

## Butalbital Compound and Codeine

(byoo TAL bi tal KOM pound & KOE deen)

**U.S. Brand Names** Fiorinal® With Codeine

**Synonyms** Codeine and Butalbital Compound

**Therapeutic Category** Analgesic, Combination (Narcotic); Barbiturate

**Pregnancy Risk Factor** C/D (if used for prolonged periods or in high doses at term)

**Lactation** Excretion in breast milk unknown/use caution

**Use** Mild to moderate pain when sedation is needed

**Contraindications** Hypersensitivity to butalbital, codeine, aspirin, or any component; opium derivatives; patients with a hemorrhagic diathesis (eg, hemophilia, hypoprothrombinemia, von Willebrand disease, the thrombocytopenias, thrombasthenia, and other ill-defined hereditary platelet dysfunctions, severe vitamin K deficiency, and severe liver damage); patients with peptic ulcer or other serious GI lesions; patients with porphyria; pregnancy (if used for prolonged periods or in high doses at term)

**Warnings** Habit-forming, potentially abusable; patients on anticoagulant therapy. Pregnancy factor C/D (extended use or high doses near term).

**Drug Interactions**

**Decreased Effect:** Aspirin/butalbital/caffeine/codeine may diminish effects of uricosuric agents such as probenecid and sulfinpyrazone.

**Increased Effect/Toxicity:** MAO inhibitors may enhance CNS effects of butalbital. Patients receiving concomitant corticosteroids and chronic use of ASA, withdrawal of corticosteroids may result in salicylism. ASA/butalbital/caffeine/codeine may enhance effects of oral anticoagulants. Increased effect with oral antidiabetic agents and insulin, 6-mercaptopurine and methotrexate, NSAIDs, other narcotic analgesics, alcohol, general anesthetics, tranquilizers such as chlordiazepoxide, sedative hypnotics, or other CNS depressants.

**Effects on Lab Values**

Aspirin: Serum amylase, fasting blood glucose, cholesterol, protein, AST (SGOT), uric acid, PT and bleeding time; urine glucose, 5-hydroxy indoleacetic acid, Gerhardt ketone; vanillylmandelic acid, urine-uric acid, diacetic acid, and spectrophotometric detection of barbiturates

Codeine: Increased serum amylase

**Adverse Reactions**

>10%:

Central nervous system: Dizziness, lightheadedness, drowsiness

Gastrointestinal: Nausea, heartburn, stomach pains, dyspepsia, epigastric discomfort

1% to 10%:

Central nervous system: Confusion, mental depression, unusual excitement, nervousness, faint feeling, insomnia, nightmares, intoxicated feeling

Dermatologic: Rash

Gastrointestinal: Constipation, GI ulceration

<1% (Limited to important or life-threatening symptoms): Tachycardia, chest pain, palpitations, syncope, hallucinations, nervousness, jitters, exfoliative dermatitis, Stevens-Johnson syndrome, agranulocytosis, megaloblastic anemia, thrombocytopenia, occult bleeding, prolongation of bleeding time, leukopenia, iron deficiency anemia, hepatotoxicity, thrombophlebitis, impaired renal function, respiratory depression, bronchospasm, epistaxis, allergic reaction

**Overdose/Toxicology** Symptoms of overdose include unsteady gait, slurred speech, confusion, respiratory depression, hypotension, and coma. Opioid symptoms may be reversed by naloxone, 2 mg I.V., with repeated doses as necessary up to a total of 10 mg. Barbiturate treatment is symptomatic and supportive.

**Pharmacodynamics/Kinetics**

**Half-life Elimination:** 35-88 hours

**Formulations** Capsule: Butalbital 50 mg, caffeine 40 mg, aspirin 325 mg and codeine phosphate 30 mg

**Dosing**

**Adults:** Oral: 1-2 capsules every 4 hours as needed for pain; up to 6 capsules/day

**Elderly:** Not recommended for use in the elderly.

**Stability**

**Storage:** Store below 25°C (77°F).

**Additional Nursing Issues**

**Physical Assessment: Do not use for persons with allergic reaction to aspirin, opium, or codeine** (see Contraindications). Assess other medications patient may be

(Continued)

## Butalbital Compound and Codeine *(Continued)*

taking for additive or adverse interactions (see Drug Interactions). Monitor for effectiveness of pain relief and monitor for signs of overdose (see above). Monitor vital signs and signs of adverse reactions - especially gastrointestinal bleeding (see Adverse Reactions) at beginning of therapy and at regular intervals with long-term use. May cause physical and/or psychological dependence. Discontinue slowly after long-term use. For inpatients, implement safety measures (eg, side rails up, call light within reach, instructions to call for assistance, etc). Assess knowledge/teach patient appropriate use if self-administered. Teach patient to monitor for adverse reactions, adverse reactions to report, and appropriate interventions to reduce side effects. **Pregnancy risk factor C/D** - see Pregnancy Risk Factor - benefits of use should outweigh possible risks. Note breast-feeding caution.

**Patient Information/Instruction:** If self-administered, use exactly as directed (do not increase dose or frequency); may cause physical and/or psychological dependence. Take with food or milk. While using this medication, do not use alcohol and other prescription or OTC medications (especially sedatives, tranquilizers, antihistamines, or pain medications) without consulting prescriber. Maintain adequate hydration (2-3 L/day of fluids unless instructed to restrict fluid intake). May cause dizziness, lightheadedness, confusion, or drowsiness (use caution when driving, climbing stairs, or changing position - rising from sitting or lying to standing, or when engaging in tasks requiring alertness until response to drug is known); heartburn or epigastric discomfort (frequent mouth care, frequent sips of fluids, chewing gum, or sucking lozenges may help); constipation (increased exercise, fluids, or dietary fruit and fiber may help - if constipation remains an unresolved problem, consult prescriber about use of stool softeners). Report chest pain or palpitations; persistent dizziness; confusion, nightmares, excitation, or changes in mentation; shortness of breath or difficulty breathing; skin rash, unusual bleeding or bruising; or unusual fatigue and weakness. **Pregnancy/breast-feeding precautions:** Inform prescriber if you are or intend to be pregnant. Consult prescriber if breast-feeding.

**Pregnancy Issues:** Not known whether this drug causes fetal harm or can affect reproduction capacity; only given if clearly needed.

**Other Issues:** Abrupt discontinuation after sustained use (generally >10 days) may cause withdrawal symptoms.


- ♦ **Butenafine** *see page 1247*
- ♦ **Buticaps®** *see* Butabarbital Sodium *on page 173*
- ♦ **Butisol Sodium®** *see* Butabarbital Sodium *on page 173*


## Butorphanol (byoo TOR fa nole)

**U.S. Brand Names** Stadol®; Stadol® NS

**Therapeutic Category** Analgesic, Narcotic

**Pregnancy Risk Factor** B/D (if used for prolonged periods or in high doses at term)

**Lactation** Enters breast milk/use caution (AAP rates "compatible")

**Use** Management of moderate to severe pain

**Mechanism of Action/Effect** Mixed narcotic agonist-antagonist with central analgesic actions; binds to opiate receptors in the CNS, causing inhibition of ascending pain pathways, altering the perception of and response to pain; produces generalized CNS depression

**Contraindications** Hypersensitivity to butorphanol or any component; avoid use in opiate-dependent patients who have not been detoxified, may precipitate opiate withdrawal; pregnancy (if used for prolonged periods or in high doses at term)

**Warnings** Use with caution in patients with hepatic/renal dysfunction, may elevate CSF pressure, may increase cardiac workload. Tolerance or drug dependence may result from extended use. May impair mental and physical abilities for varying periods of time.

**Drug Interactions**

**Increased Effect/Toxicity:** Increased toxicity with CNS depressants, phenothiazines, barbiturates, skeletal muscle relaxants, alfentanil, guanabenz, and MAO inhibitors.

**Adverse Reactions**

>10%: Central nervous system: Drowsiness

1% to 10%:

Cardiovascular: Flushing of the face, hypotension

Central nervous system: Dizziness, lightheadedness, headache

Gastrointestinal: Anorexia, nausea, vomiting

Genitourinary: Decreased urination

Miscellaneous: Physical and psychological dependence, sweating, withdrawal syndrome

<1% (Limited to important or life-threatening symptoms): Bradycardia or tachycardia, hypertension, paradoxical CNS stimulation, confusion, hallucinations, mental depression, false sense of well being, malaise, restlessness, nightmares, CNS depression, shortness of breath, dyspnea, respiratory depression

**Overdose/Toxicology** Symptoms of overdose include respiratory depression, cardiac and CNS depression. Treatment is supportive. Naloxone, 2 mg I.V. with repeat administration as necessary up to a total of 10 mg, can also be used to reverse toxic effects of the opiate.

**Pharmacodynamics/Kinetics**

**Protein Binding:** 80%

**Half-life Elimination:** 2.5-4 hours

**Time to Peak:** I.M.: Within 0.5-1 hour; I.V.: Within 4-5 minutes

**Metabolism:** Liver

**Excretion:** Urine and bile

**Onset:** I.M.: 5-10 minutes; I.V.: <10 minutes; Nasal: Within 15 minutes

**Duration:** I.M./I.V.: 3-4 hours; Nasal: 4-5 hours

**Formulations**

Butorphanol tartrate:

Injection: 1 mg/mL (1 mL); 2 mg/mL (1 mL, 2 mL, 10 mL)

Spray, nasal: 10 mg/mL [14-15 doses] (2.5 mL)

**Dosing**

**Adults:**

I.M.: 1-4 mg every 3-4 hours as needed

I.V.: 0.5-2 mg every 3-4 hours as needed

Nasal spray: Headache: 1 spray in 1 nostril; if adequate pain relief is not achieved within 60-90 minutes, an additional 1 spray in 1 nostril may be given (each spray gives ~1 mg of butorphanol). May repeat 3-4 hours following last dose, as needed.

**Elderly:**

I.M., I.V.: 0.5-2 mg every 6-8 hours, increase as necessary.

Nasal: 1 mg (1 spray in one nostril); after 90-120 minutes, assess whether a second dose is needed; may repeat 3-4 hours following last dose, as needed.

**Renal Impairment:**

$Cl_{cr}$ 10-50 mL/minute: Administer 75% of dose.

$Cl_{cr}$ <10 mL/minute: Administer 50% of dose.

**Administration**

**Inhalation:** See Dosing.

**Stability**

**Storage:** Store at room temperature; protect from freezing.

**Compatibility:** Incompatible when mixed in the same syringe with diazepam, dimenhydrinate, methohexital, pentobarbital, secobarbital, or thiopental. See the Compatibility of Drugs in Syringe Chart *on page 1317.*

**Additional Nursing Issues**

**Physical Assessment:** Assess other medications patient may be taking for possible additive or adverse interactions (see Warnings/Precautions and Drug Interactions). Monitor for effectiveness of pain relief and monitor for signs of overdose (see above). Monitor blood pressure, CNS and respiratory status, and degree of sedation at beginning of therapy and at regular intervals with long-term use. For inpatients, implement safety measures (eg, side rails up, call light within reach, instructions to call for assistance, etc). May cause physical and/or psychological dependence. Assess knowledge/teach patient appropriate use (if self-administered). Teach patient to monitor for adverse reactions (see Adverse Reactions), adverse reactions to report, and appropriate interventions to reduce side effects. **Pregnancy risk factor B/D** - see Pregnancy Risk Factor for cautious use. Note breast-feeding caution.

**Patient Information/Instruction:** If self-administered, use exactly as directed (do not increase dose or frequency); may cause physical and/or psychological dependence. While using this medication, do not use alcohol and other prescription or OTC medications (especially sedatives, tranquilizers, antihistamines, or pain medications) without consulting prescriber. May cause dizziness, drowsiness, confusion, or blurred vision (use caution when driving, climbing stairs, or changing position - rising from sitting or lying to standing, or when engaging in tasks requiring alertness until response to drug is known); nausea or vomiting, or loss of appetite (frequent mouth care, small frequent meals, sucking lozenges, or chewing gum may help). Report unresolved nausea or vomiting; difficulty breathing or shortness of breath; restlessness, insomnia, euphoria, or nightmares; excessive sedation or unusual weakness; facial flushing, rapid heartbeat, or palpitations; urinary difficulty; or vision changes. **Pregnancy/breast-feeding precautions:** Inform prescriber if you are or intend to be pregnant. If you are breast-feeding, take dose immediately after breast-feeding or 3-4 hours prior to next feeding.

**Geriatric Considerations:** Adjust dose for renal function in the elderly.

**Related Information**

Narcotic/Opioid Analgesic Comparison *on page 1396*

- **Butyl Aminobenzoate, Benzocaine, Tetracaine, and Benzalkonium Chloride** *see* Benzocaine, Butyl Aminobenzoate, Tetracaine, and Benzalkonium Chloride *on page 142*
- **Buvacaina** *see* Bupivacaine *on page 167*
- **Byclomine® Injection** *see* Dicyclomine *on page 362*
- **Bydramine® Cough Syrup [OTC]** *see* Diphenhydramine *on page 381*
- **C2B8 Monoclonal Antibody** *see* Rituximab *on page 1031*
- **C7E3** *see* Abciximab *on page 28*
- **Cafatine®** *see* Ergotamine Derivatives *on page 434*
- **Cafatine-PB®** *see* Ergotamine Derivatives *on page 434*
- **Cafergot®** *see* Ergotamine Derivatives *on page 434*
- **Cafetrate®** *see* Ergotamine Derivatives *on page 434*

## Caffeine and Sodium Benzoate (KAF een & sow dee um BEN zoe ate)

**Synonyms** Sodium Benzoate and Caffeine

**Therapeutic Category** Diuretic, Miscellaneous

**Pregnancy Risk Factor** C

(Continued)

## Caffeine and Sodium Benzoate *(Continued)*

**Lactation** Caffeine: Enters breast milk/use caution (AAP rates "compatible")

**Use** Emergency stimulant in acute circulatory failure; as a diuretic; and to relieve spinal puncture headache

**Formulations** Injection: Caffeine 125 mg and sodium benzoate 125 mg per mL (2 mL)

**Dosing**

**Adults:** I.M., I.V.: 500 mg, maximum single dose: 1 g

Spinal puncture headaches: 500 mg in 1000 mL NS infused over 1 hour, followed by 1000 mL NS infused over 1 hour; a second course of caffeine can be given for unrelieved headache pain in 4 hours.

**Elderly:** Refer to adult dosing.

**Additional Nursing Issues**

**Physical Assessment:** See individual components listed in Related Information. **Pregnancy risk factor C** - benefits of use should outweigh possible risks. Note breast-feeding caution.

**Patient Information/Instruction:** See individual components listed in Related Information. **Pregnancy/breast-feeding precautions:** Inform prescriber if you are or intend to be pregnant. Consult prescriber if breast-feeding.

- **Caffeine, Hydrocodone, Chlorpheniramine, Phenylephrine, and Acetaminophen** *see* Hydrocodone, Chlorpheniramine, Phenylephrine, Acetaminophen, and Caffeine *on page 576*
- **Caffeine, Orphenadrine, and Aspirin** *see* Orphenadrine, Aspirin, and Caffeine *on page 865*
- **Calan®** *see* Verapamil *on page 1208*
- **Calan® SR** *see* Verapamil *on page 1208*
- **Cal Carb-HD® [OTC]** *see* Calcium Supplements *on page 185*
- **Calci-Chew™ [OTC]** *see* Calcium Supplements *on page 185*
- **Calciday-667® [OTC]** *see* Calcium Supplements *on page 185*

## Calcifediol (kal si fe DYE ole)

**U.S. Brand Names** Calderol®

**Synonyms** 25-$D_3$; 25-Hydroxycholecalciferol; 25-Hydroxyvitamin $D_3$

**Therapeutic Category** Vitamin D Analog

**Pregnancy Risk Factor** A/D (if dose exceeds RDA recommendation)

**Lactation** Enters breast milk/compatible

**Use** Treatment and management of metabolic bone disease associated with chronic renal failure

**Mechanism of Action/Effect** Vitamin D analog that (along with calcitonin and parathyroid hormone) regulates serum calcium homeostasis by promoting absorption of calcium and phosphorus in the small intestine; promotes renal tubule resorption of phosphate; increases rate of accumulation and resorption in bone minerals

**Contraindications** Hypersensitivity to calcifediol or any component; hypercalcemia; malabsorption syndrome; hypervitaminosis D; significantly decreased renal function; pregnancy (if dose exceeds RDA recommendation)

**Warnings** Adequate (supplemental) dietary calcium is necessary for clinical response to vitamin D. Calcium-phosphate product (serum calcium times phosphorus) must not exceed 70. Avoid hypercalcemia.

**Drug Interactions**

**Decreased Effect:** The effect of calcifediol is decreased when taken with cholestyramine or colestipol.

**Increased Effect/Toxicity:** Increased effect with thiazide diuretics. Additive effect with antacids (magnesium).

**Effects on Lab Values** ↑ calcium (S), cholesterol (S), magnesium, BUN, AST, ALT; ↓ alk phos

**Adverse Reactions**

1% to 10%:

Cardiovascular: Hypotension, cardiac arrhythmias, hypertension
Central nervous system: Irritability, headache
Dermatologic: Pruritus
Endocrine & metabolic: Polydipsia, hypermagnesemia
Gastrointestinal: Nausea, vomiting, constipation, anorexia, pancreatitis, metallic taste
Genitourinary: Polyuria
Neuromuscular & skeletal: Myalgia, bone pain
Ocular: Conjunctivitis, photophobia

<1% (Limited to important or life-threatening symptoms): Overt psychosis, seizures, elevated AST/ALT

**Overdose/Toxicology** Symptoms of overdose include hypercalcemia and hypercalciuria. Following withdrawal of the drug, treatment consists of bedrest, liberal intake of fluids, reduced calcium intake, and cathartic administration. Severe hypercalcemia requires I.V. hydration and forced diuresis. Urine output should be monitored and maintained at >3 mL/kg/hour during the acute treatment phase. I.V. saline can quickly and significantly increase excretion of calcium into urine. Calcitonin, cholestyramine, prednisone, sodium EDTA, biphosphonates, and mithramycin have all been used successfully to treat the more resistant cases of vitamin D-induced hypercalcemia.

**Pharmacodynamics/Kinetics**

**Distribution:** Activated in the kidneys; stored in liver and fat depots

**Half-life Elimination:** 12-22 days

**Time to Peak:** Oral: Within 4 hours

**Excretion:** Bile and feces

**Formulations** Capsule: 20 mcg, 50 mcg

**Dosing**

**Adults:** Oral: Hepatic osteodystrophy: 20-100 mcg/day or every other day; titrate to obtain normal serum calcium/phosphate levels; increase dose at 4-week intervals

**Elderly:** Daily supplement for elderly (800 int. units): 20 mcg

Hepatic osteodystrophy: Refer to adult dosing (see Additional Information).

**Monitoring Laboratory Tests** Serum calcium levels frequently when starting therapy and regularly thereafter

**Additional Nursing Issues**

**Physical Assessment:** See Contraindications and Warnings/Precautions for use cautions. Assess effectiveness and interactions of other medications (see Drug Interactions). Note Effects on Lab Values (above). Monitor lab tests for effectiveness of therapy and adverse effects (see Adverse Reactions and Overdose/Toxicology). Assess knowledge/teach patient appropriate administration, possible side effects/interventions, and adverse symptoms to report. **Pregnancy risk factor A/D** - see Pregnancy Risk Factor for cautious use.

**Patient Information/Instruction:** Take exact dose as prescribed; do not increase dose. Maintain recommended diet and calcium supplementation. Avoid taking magnesium-containing antacids. You may experience nausea, vomiting, or metallic taste (frequent small meals, frequent mouth care, chewing gum, or sucking lozenges may help) or hypotension (use caution when rising from sitting or lying position or when climbing stairs or bending over). Report chest pain or palpitations, acute headache, skin rash, change in vision or eye irritation, CNS changes, weakness or lethargy.

**Geriatric Considerations:** Recommended daily allowances (RDA) have not been developed for persons >65 years of age.

**Additional Information** 1000 mcg = 40,000 units of vitamin D activity; this product is not generally recommended for daily supplementation due to dosage forms, strengths, and cost.


♦ **Calciferol™ Injection** *see* Ergocalciferol *on page 432*

♦ **Calciferol™ Oral** *see* Ergocalciferol *on page 432*

♦ **Calcijex™** *see* Calcitriol *on page 183*

♦ **Calcimar® Injection** *see* Calcitonin *on next page*

♦ **Calci-Mix™ [OTC]** *see* Calcium Supplements *on page 185*


## Calcipotriene (kal si POE try een)

**U.S. Brand Names** Dovonex®

**Therapeutic Category** Topical Skin Product; Vitamin, Fat Soluble

**Pregnancy Risk Factor** C

**Lactation** Excretion in breast milk unknown

**Use** Treatment of moderate plaque psoriasis

**Mechanism of Action/Effect** Synthetic vitamin $D_3$ analog which regulates skin cell production and proliferation

**Contraindications** Hypersensitivity to calcipotriene or any component; patients with demonstrated hypercalcemia or evidence of vitamin D toxicity; use on the face

**Warnings** Use may cause irritations of lesions and surrounding uninvolved skin. If irritation develops, discontinue use. Transient, rapidly reversible elevation of serum calcium has occurred during use. If elevation in serum calcium occurs above the normal range, discontinue treatment until calcium levels are normal. For external use only; not for ophthalmic, oral, or intravaginal use. Pregnancy factor C.

**Adverse Reactions**

>10%: Dermatologic: Burning, itching, skin irritation, erythema, dry skin, peeling, rash, worsening of psoriasis

1% to 10%: Dermatologic: Hyperpigmentation

**Formulations**

Cream: 0.005% (30 g, 60 g, 100 g)

Ointment, topical: 0.005% (30 g, 60 g, 100 g)

**Dosing**

**Adults:** Topical: Apply in a thin film to the affected skin twice daily and rub in gently and completely.

**Elderly:** Refer to adult dosing.

**Administration**

**Topical:** For external use only; apply with gloves.

**Monitoring Laboratory Tests** Serum calcium

**Additional Nursing Issues**

**Physical Assessment:** See Contraindications and Warnings/Precautions for use cautions. When applied to large areas of skin or for extensive periods of time, monitor for adverse skin or systemic reactions. Assess knowledge/teach patient appropriate application and use and adverse symptoms (see Adverse Reactions) to report. **Pregnancy risk factor C** - systemic absorption may be minimal with appropriate use. Note breast-feeding caution.

**Patient Information/Instruction:** For external use only. Use exactly as directed; do not overuse. Before using, wash and dry area gently. Wear gloves to apply a thin film to affected area and rub in gently. If dressing is necessary, use a porous dressing.

(Continued)

## Calcipotriene *(Continued)*

Avoid contact with eyes. Avoid exposing treated area to direct sunlight; sunburn can occur. Report increased swelling, redness, rash, itching, signs of infection, worsening of condition, or lack of healing. **Pregnancy/breast-feeding precautions:** Inform prescriber if you are or intend to be pregnant. Consult prescriber if breast-feeding.

## Calcitonin (kal si TOE nin)

**U.S. Brand Names** Calcimar® Injection; Cibacalcin® Injection; Miacalcin® Injection; Miacalcin® Nasal Spray; Osteocalcin® Injection; Salmonine® Injection

**Synonyms** Calcitonin (Human); Calcitonin (Salmon)

**Therapeutic Category** Antidote

**Pregnancy Risk Factor** C (human); B (salmon)

**Lactation** Excretion in breast milk unknown

**Use**

Calcitonin (salmon): Treatment of Paget's disease of bone and as adjunctive therapy for hypercalcemia; postmenopausal osteoporosis and osteogenesis imperfecta

Calcitonin (human): Treatment of Paget's disease of bone

**Mechanism of Action/Effect** Structurally similar to human calcitonin; it directly inhibits osteoclastic bone resorption; promotes the renal excretion of calcium, phosphate, sodium, magnesium and potassium by decreasing tubular reabsorption; increases the jejunal secretion of water, sodium, potassium, and chloride

**Contraindications** Hypersensitivity to salmon protein or gelatin diluent with the salmon product

**Warnings** A skin test should be performed prior to initiating therapy of calcitonin salmon. Have epinephrine immediately available for a possible hypersensitivity reaction. Use caution with renal insufficiency, pernicious anemia. Pregnancy factor C (human).

**Drug Interactions**

**Decreased Effect:** Calcitonin may be antagonized by calcium and vitamin D in treating hypercalcemia.

**Adverse Reactions**

>10%:
- Cardiovascular: Facial flushing
- Gastrointestinal: Nausea, diarrhea, anorexia
- Local: Edema at injection site

1% to 10%:
- Genitourinary: Polyuria
- Neuromuscular & skeletal: Back/joint pain

Respiratory: Nasal bleeding/crusting (following intranasal administration)

<1% (Limited to important or life-threatening symptoms): Shortness of breath

**Overdose/Toxicology** Symptoms of overdose include nausea, vomiting, hypocalcemia, and hypocalcemic tetany. Treat symptomatically.

**Pharmacodynamics/Kinetics**

**Distribution:** Does not cross into the placenta

**Half-life Elimination:** S.C.: 1.2 hours

**Metabolism:** Rapidly by the kidneys

**Excretion:** As inactive metabolites in urine

**Onset:** Hypercalcemia: Onset of reduction in calcium: 2 hours

**Duration:** Hypercalcemia: 6-8 hours

**Formulations**

Injection:
- Human (Cibacalcin®): 0.5 mg/vial
- Salmon: 200 units/mL (2 mL)

Spray, nasal: 200 units/activation (0.09 mL/dose) (2 mL glass bottle with pump)

**Dosing**

**Adults:**

Paget's disease: Salmon calcitonin:
- I.M., S.C.: 100 units/day to start, 50 units/day or 50-100 units every 1-3 days maintenance dose
- Intranasal: 200-400 units (1-2 sprays)/day
- Human calcitonin: S.C.: Initial: 0.5 mg/day (maximum: 0.5 mg twice daily); maintenance: 0.5 mg 2-3 times/week or 0.25 mg/day

Hypercalcemia: Initial: Salmon calcitonin: I.M., S.C.: 4 units/kg every 12 hours; may increase up to 8 units/kg every 12 hours to a maximum of every 6 hours

Osteogenesis imperfecta: Salmon calcitonin: I.M., S.C.: 2 units/kg 3 times/week

Postmenopausal osteoporosis: Salmon calcitonin:
- I.M., S.C.: 100 units/day
- Intranasal: 200 units (1 spray)/day

**Elderly:** Refer to adult dosing.

**Administration**

**I.M.:** I.M. route is preferred if volume exceeds 2 mL. Taking medication in the evening may minimize the problems of flushing, nausea, and vomiting.

**Other:** Skin test should be performed prior to administration of salmon calcitonin

**Stability**

**Storage:**

Salmon calcitonin: Injection: Store under refrigeration at 2°C to 6°C (36°F to 43°F); stable for up to 2 weeks at room temperature.

Salmon calcitonin: Nasal: Store unopened bottle under refrigeration at 2°C to 8°C. Once the pump has been activated, store at room temperature.

Human calcitonin: Store at <25°C (77°F) and protect from light.

**Reconstitution:** Salmon calcitonin: Injection: NS has been recommended for the dilution to prepare a skin test. Use reconstituted human calcitonin within 6 hours.

**Monitoring Laboratory Tests** Serum electrolytes and calcium, alkaline phosphatase and 24-hour urine collection for hydroxyproline excretion (Paget's disease)

**Additional Nursing Issues**

**Physical Assessment:** Monitor skin test after 15 minutes for local inflammatory reaction before initiating therapy (increased erythema or skin wheal indicates positive reaction and allergy - greater with salmon calcitonin). Monitor appropriate laboratory tests as ordered. Monitor for signs or symptoms of adverse or toxic effects as indicated above, especially signs of hypocalcemic tetany (eg, muscular twitching, tetanic spasms, convulsions) and signs of hypercalcemia (eg, thirst, anorexia, polyuria, nausea, vomiting). Teach and monitor patient for appropriate administration of subcutaneous or I.M. injections or proper use of nasal spray. If the patient is taking calcitonin for hypercalcemia, give instructions on an appropriate low calcium diet and monitor adherence. **Pregnancy risk factor B/C** - see Pregnancy Risk Factor - benefits of use should outweigh possible risks. Note breast-feeding caution.

**Patient Information/Instruction:** When this drug is given subcutaneously or I.M. it will be necessary for you or a significant other to learn to prepare and give the injections (keep drug vials in a refrigerator - do not freeze). Report significant nasal irritation if using calcitonin nasal spray. Follow directions exactly. Increased warmth and flushing may be experienced with this drug and should only last about 1 hour after administration (taking drug in the evening may minimize these discomforts). Immediately report twitching, muscle spasm, dark colored urine, hives, significant skin rash, palpitations, or difficulty breathing. **Pregnancy/breast-feeding precautions:** Inform prescriber if you are or intend to be pregnant. Consult prescriber if breast-feeding.

**Dietary Issues:** Adequate vitamin D and calcium intake is essential for osteoporosis. Patients with Paget's disease and hypercalcemia should follow a low calcium diet as prescribed.

**Geriatric Considerations:** Calcitonin may be the drug of choice for postmenopausal women unable to take estrogens to increase bone density and reduce fractures. Calcium and vitamin D supplements should also be given. Calcitonin may also be effective in steroid-induced osteoporosis and other states associated with high bone turnover.

- **Calcitonin (Human)** *see* Calcitonin *on previous page*
- **Calcitonin (Salmon)** *see* Calcitonin *on previous page*

## Calcitriol (kal si TRYE ole)

**U.S. Brand Names** Calcijex™; Rocaltrol®

**Synonyms** 1,25 Dihydroxycholecalciferol

**Therapeutic Category** Vitamin D Analog

**Pregnancy Risk Factor** A/D (if dose exceeds RDA recommendation)

**Lactation** Enters breast milk/compatible

**Use** Management of hypocalcemia in patients on chronic renal dialysis; reduce elevated parathyroid hormone levels (including predialysis patients); decrease severity of psoriatic lesions in psoriatic vulgaris

**Mechanism of Action/Effect** Promotes absorption of calcium in the intestines and retention at the kidneys thereby increasing calcium levels in the serum; decreases excessive serum phosphatase levels, parathyroid hormone levels, and decreases bone resorption; increases renal tubule phosphate resorption

**Contraindications** Hypercalcemia; vitamin D toxicity; abnormal sensitivity to the effects of vitamin D; malabsorption syndrome; pregnancy (if dose exceeds RDA recommendation)

**Warnings** Adequate dietary (supplemental) calcium is necessary for clinical response to vitamin D. Maintain adequate fluid intake. Calcium-phosphate product (serum calcium times phosphorus) must not exceed 70. Avoid hypercalcemia or use with renal function impairment and secondary hyperparathyroidism.

**Drug Interactions**

**Decreased Effect:** Cholestyramine and colestipol decrease absorption/effect of calcitriol.

**Increased Effect/Toxicity:** Risk of hypercalcemia with thiazide diuretics. Risk of hypermagnesemia with magnesium-containing antacids.

**Effects on Lab Values** ↑ calcium, cholesterol, magnesium, BUN, AST, ALT, calcium (S), cholesterol (S); ↓ alkaline phosphatase

**Adverse Reactions**

1% to 10%:

Cardiovascular: Hypotension, cardiac arrhythmias, hypertension
Central nervous system: Irritability, headache
Dermatologic: Pruritus
Endocrine & metabolic: Polydipsia
Gastrointestinal: Nausea, vomiting, constipation, anorexia, pancreatitis, metallic taste
Genitourinary: Polyuria
Neuromuscular & skeletal: Myalgia, bone pain
Ocular: Conjunctivitis, photophobia

<1% (Limited to important or life-threatening symptoms): Increased LFTs

**Overdose/Toxicology** Symptoms of overdose include hypercalcemia and hypercalciuria. Following withdrawal of the drug, treatment consists of bedrest, liberal intake of fluids, reduced calcium intake, and cathartic administration. Severe hypercalcemia

(Continued)

## Calcitriol *(Continued)*

requires I.V. hydration and forced diuresis. Urine output should be monitored and maintained at >3 mL/kg/hour during the acute treatment phase. I.V. saline can quickly and significantly increase excretion of calcium into urine. Calcitonin, cholestyramine, prednisone, sodium EDTA, biphosphonates, and mithramycin have all been used successfully to treat the more resistant cases of vitamin D-induced hypercalcemia.

**Pharmacodynamics/Kinetics**

**Half-life Elimination:** 3-8 hours

**Metabolism:** Liver

**Excretion:** Feces

**Onset:** ~2-6 hours

**Duration:** 3-5 days

**Formulations**

Capsule: 0.25 mcg, 0.5 mcg
Oral Solution: 1 mcg/mL (15 mL)
Injection: 1 mcg/mL (1 mL); 2 mcg/mL (1 mL)

**Dosing**

**Adults:** Individualize dosage to maintain calcium levels of 9-10 mg/dL.

Renal failure:

Oral: 0.25 mcg/day or every other day (may require 0.5-1 mcg/day)

I.V.: 0.5 mcg (0.01 mcg/kg) 3 times/week; most doses in the range of 0.5-3 mcg (0.01-0.05 mcg/kg) 3 times/week

Hypoparathyroidism/pseudohypoparathyroidism: Oral: 0.5-2 mcg/day

Vitamin D-dependent rickets: Oral: 1 mcg once daily

Vitamin D-resistant rickets (familial hypophosphatemia): Oral: Initial: 0.015-0.02 mcg/kg once daily; maintenance: 0.03-0.06 mcg/kg once daily; maximum dose: 2 mcg once daily

**Elderly:** Refer to adult dosing. Individualize dosage to maintain calcium levels of 9-10 mg/dL (adjust for low albumin).

**Administration**

**Oral:** Can be administered without regard to food. Give with meals to reduce GI problems.

**Stability**

**Storage:** Store in tight, light-resistant container. Calcitriol degrades upon prolonged exposure to light.

**Monitoring Laboratory Tests** Serum calcium and phosphorus, and renal function. The serum calcium times phosphate product should not be allowed to exceed 70.

**Additional Nursing Issues**

**Physical Assessment:** See Contraindications and Warnings/Precautions for use cautions. Assess effectiveness and interactions of other medications (see Drug Interactions). Monitor lab tests, effectiveness of therapy, and adverse effects at beginning of therapy and regularly with long-term use (see Adverse Reactions and Overdose/Toxicology). Assess knowledge/teach patient appropriate use, appropriate nutritional counseling, possible side effects/interventions, and adverse symptoms to report. **Pregnancy risk factor A/D** - see Pregnancy Risk Factor for cautious use.

**Patient Information/Instruction:** Take exact dose as prescribed; do not increase dose. Maintain recommended diet and calcium supplementation. Avoid taking magnesium-containing antacids. You may experience nausea, vomiting, loss of appetite, or metallic taste (frequent small meals, frequent mouth care, chewing gum, or sucking lozenges may help); or hypotension (use caution when rising from sitting or lying position or when climbing stairs or bending over). Report chest pain or palpitations; acute headache; skin rash; change in vision or eye irritation; CNS changes; unusual weakness or fatigue; persistent nausea, vomiting, cramps, or diarrhea; or muscle or bone pain.

**Geriatric Considerations:** Appetite and caloric requirements may decrease with advanced age. Assess diet for adequate nutrient intake with regard to vitamins and minerals. (Daily vitamin supplements are sometimes recommended). Persons >65 years of age have decreased absorption and may have decreased intake of vitamin D. This may require supplement with daily vitamin D intake, especially for those with high risk for osteoporosis.

**Additional Information** Not used as a daily supplement due to dosage forms, strengths, and cost. 1 mcg = 40,000 units.

- **Calcium Acetate** *see* Calcium Supplements *on next page*
- **Calcium Carbonate** *see* Calcium Supplements *on next page*
- **Calcium Carbonate and Simethicone** *see page 1294*
- **Calcium Channel Blocking Agents Comparison** *see page 1378*
- **Calcium Chloride** *see* Calcium Supplements *on next page*
- **Calcium Citrate** *see* Calcium Supplements *on next page*
- **Calcium Citrate** *see page 1294*
- **Calcium Glubionate** *see* Calcium Supplements *on next page*
- **Calcium Gluceptate** *see* Calcium Supplements *on next page*
- **Calcium Gluconate** *see* Calcium Supplements *on next page*
- **Calcium Lactate** *see* Calcium Supplements *on next page*
- **Calcium Lactate** *see page 1294*
- **Calcium Leucovorin** *see* Leucovorin *on page 662*
- **Calcium Phosphate, Dibasic** *see page 1294*
- **Calcium Phosphate, Tribasic** *see* Calcium Supplements *on next page*

♦ **Calcium Polycarbophil** *see page 1294*
♦ **Calcium Rich [OTC]** *see* Calcium Supplements *on this page*

## Calcium Supplements (KAL see um SUP la ments)

**U.S. Brand Names** Alka-Mints® [OTC]; Amitone® [OTC]; Cal Carb-HD® [OTC]; Calci-Chew™ [OTC]; Calciday-667® [OTC]; Calci-Mix™ [OTC]; Calcium Rich [OTC]; Calphron®; Cal-Plus® [OTC]; Caltrate® 600 [OTC]; Caltrate, Jr.® [OTC]; Chooz® [OTC]; Citracal® [OTC]; Dicarbosil® [OTC]; Equilet® [OTC]; Florical® [OTC]; Gencalc® 600 [OTC]; Kalcinate® Cal Plus®; Mallamint® [OTC]; Mylanta® Soothing Antacids [OTC]; Neo-Calglucon® [OTC]; Nephro-Calci® [OTC]; Os-Cal® 500 [OTC]; Oyst-Cal 500 [OTC]; Oystercal® 500; Phos-Ex®; PhosLo®; Posture® [OTC]; Quick Dissolve Maalox® Maximum Strength; Rolaids®; Titralac® [OTC]; Tums® [OTC]; Tums® E-X Extra Strength Tablet [OTC]; Tums® Extra Strength Liquid [OTC]; Tums® Ultra® [OTC]

**Synonyms** Calcium Acetate; Calcium Carbonate; Calcium Chloride; Calcium Citrate; Calcium Glubionate; Calcium Gluceptate; Calcium Gluconate; Calcium Lactate; Calcium Phosphate, Tribasic

**Therapeutic Category** Electrolyte Supplement; Electrolyte Supplement, Parenteral

**Pregnancy Risk Factor** C

**Lactation** Excretion in breast milk unknown/use caution

**Use** Treatment and prevention of calcium depletion; relief of acid indigestion, heartburn; emergency treatment of hypocalcemic tetany; treatment of hypermagnesemia, cardiac disturbances of hyperkalemia, hypocalcemia, or calcium channel blocking agent toxicity

**Mechanism of Action/Effect** Moderates nerve and muscle performance via action potential excitation threshold regulation; neutralizes acidity of stomach (carbonate salt)

**Contraindications** Hypercalcemia, renal calculi, ventricular fibrillation

**Warnings** Use cautiously in patients with sarcoidosis, respiratory failure, acidosis, renal or cardiac disease. Avoid too rapid I.V. administration. Avoid extravasation. Use with caution in digitalized patients. Quick Dissolve Maalox® Maximum Strength tablets contain aspartame. Avoid or use with caution in phenylketonuria. Pregnancy factor C.

**Drug Interactions**

**Decreased Effect:** May antagonize the effects of calcium channel blockers (eg, verapamil). When administered orally, calcium decreases the absorption of tetracycline, atenolol, iron, quinolone antibiotics, alendronate, sodium fluoride, and zinc. Decreases potassium-binding ability of polystyrene sulfonate.

**Increased Effect/Toxicity:** May potentiate digoxin toxicity. High doses of calcium with thiazide diuretics may result in milk-alkali syndrome and hypercalcemia.

**Adverse Reactions**

Cardiovascular: Vasodilation, hypotension, bradycardia, cardiac arrhythmias, ventricular fibrillation, syncope
Central nervous system: Headache, mental confusion, dizziness, lethargy, coma
Dermatologic: Erythema
Endocrine & metabolic: Hypercalcemia, milk-alkali syndrome, hypophosphatemia, hypercalciuria, hypomagnesemia
Gastrointestinal: Constipation, nausea, vomiting, xerostomia, elevated serum amylase
Local: Tissue necrosis (I.V. administration)
Neuromuscular & skeletal: Muscle weakness

**Pharmacodynamics/Kinetics**

**Excretion:** Feces (unabsorbed) and via renal mechanisms under hormonal control

**Formulations** Elemental calcium listed in brackets

**Calcium acetate:**
- Capsule: Phos-Ex® 125: 500 mg [125 mg]
- Tablet:
  - Calphron®: 667 mg [169 mg]
  - Phos-Ex® 62.5: 250 mg [62.5 mg]
  - Phos-Ex® 167: 668 mg [167 mg]
  - Phos-Ex® 250: 1000 mg [250 mg]
  - PhosLo®: 667 mg [169 mg]

**Calcium carbonate:**
- Capsule: 1500 mg [600 mg]
  - Calci-Mix™: 1250 mg [500 mg]
  - Florical®: 364 mg [145.6 mg] with sodium fluoride 8.3 mg
- Liquid (Tums® Extra Strength): 1000 mg/5 mL [400 mg/5 mL] (360 mL)
- Lozenge (Mylanta® Soothing Antacids): 600 mg [240 mg]
- Powder (Cal Carb-HD®): 6.5 g/packet [2.6 g]
- Suspension, oral: 1250 mg/5 mL [500 mg]
- Tablet: 650 mg [260 mg], 1500 mg [600 mg]
  - Calciday-667®: 667 mg [267 mg]
  - Os-Cal® 500, Oyst-Cal 500, Oystercal® 500: 1250 mg [500 mg]
  - Cal-Plus®, Caltrate® 600, Gencalc® 600, Nephro-Calci®: 1500 mg [600 mg]
- Tablet, chewable:
  - Alka-Mints®: 850 mg [340 mg]
  - Amitone®: 350 mg [140 mg] ®
  - Caltrate, Jr.®: 750 mg [300 mg]
  - Calci-Chew™, Os-Cal®: 750 mg [300 mg]
  - Chooz®, Dicarbosil®, Equilet®, Tums®: 500 mg [200 mg]
  - Mallamint®: 420 mg [168 mg]
  - Quick Dissolve Maalox® Maximum Strength: 1000 mg [400 mg]
  - Rolaids® Calcium Rich: 550 mg [220 mg]
  - Tums® E-X Extra Strength: 750 mg [300 mg]
  - Tums® Ultra®: 1000 mg [400 mg]

(Continued)

## Calcium Supplements *(Continued)*

Florical®: 364 mg [145.6 mg] with sodium fluoride 8.3 mg

**Calcium chloride:**

Injection: 10% 100 mg/mL [27.2 mg/mL] (10 mL) (1.4 mEq calcium/mL)

**Calcium citrate:**

Tablet: 950 mg [200 mg]

Tablet, effervescent: 2376 mg [500 mg]

**Calcium glubionate:** Syrup: 1.8 g/5 mL [115 mg/5mL] (480 mL) (1.2 mEq calcium/mL)

**Calcium gluceptate:** Injection: 220 mg/mL [18 mg/mL] (5 mL, 50 mL) (0.9 mEq/mL)

**Calcium gluconate:**

Injection: 10% 100 mg/mL [9 mg/mL] (10 mL, 50 mL, 100 mL, 200 mL) (0.45 mEq/mL)

Tablet: 500 mg [45 mg], 650 mg [58.5 mg], 975 mg [87.75 mg], 1 g [90 mg]

**Calcium lactate:** Tablet: 325 mg [42.25 mg], 650 mg [84.5 mg]

**Calcium phosphate, tribasic:** Tablet, sugar free: 1565.2 mg [600 mg]

### Dosing

**Adults: Note:** Multiple salt forms of calcium exist; close attention must be paid to the salt form when ordering and administering calcium; incorrect selection or substitution of one salt for another without proper dosage adjustment may result in serious over- or underdosing.

Oral: **Note:** For comparison information of calcium salts, see table.

**Elemental Calcium Content of Calcium Salts**

| Calcium Salt | Elemental Calcium (mg/1 g of salt form) | mEq calcium per gram | Approximate Equivalent Doses (mg of calcium salt) |
|---|---|---|---|
| Calcium acetate | 250 | 12.7 | 354 |
| Calcium carbonate | 400 | 20 | 225 |
| Caclium chloride | 270 | 13.5 | 330 |
| Calcium citrate | 211 | 10.6 | 425 |
| Calcium glubionate | 64 | 3.2 | 1400 |
| Calcium gluceptate | 82 | 4.1 | 1100 |
| Calcium gluconate | 90 | 4.5 | 1000 |
| Calcium lactate | 130 | 6.5 | 700 |
| Calcium phosphate, tribasic | 390 | 19.3 | 233 |

**Recommended daily allowance (RDA): Dosage is in terms of elemental calcium:**

Adults >24 years: 800 mg/day

**Adequate intake** (1997 National Academy of Science Recommendations): **Dosage is in terms of elemental calcium:**

19-50 years: 1000 mg/day

>50 years: 1200 mg/day

**Prevention of osteoporosis**

Oral calcium supplementation: 1000-1500 mg of **elemental calcium** daily (divided in 500 mg increments)

Women > 65 years of age receiving estrogen supplements: 1000 mg/day in divided doses

Women > 65 years of age who are NOT receiving estrogen supplements or men > 55 years of age: 1500 mg/day in divided doses

**Hypocalcemia** (dose depends on clinical condition and serum calcium level): **Oral:**

Dose expressed in mg of **elemental calcium**: 1-2 g or more per day in 3-4 divided doses

Dose expressed in mg of **calcium gluconate:** 10-20 g daily in 3-4 divided doses

Dose expressed in mg of **calcium glubionate:** 6-18 g/day in divided doses

Dose expressed in mg of **calcium lactate:** 1.5-3 g divided every 8 hours

**Hypocalcemia: I.V.:**

Dosage expressed in mg of **calcium chloride:** 500 mg to 1 g/dose every 6 hours

Dose expressed in mg of **calcium gluceptate:** 500 mg to 1.1 g/dose as needed

Dose expressed in mg of **calcium gluconate:** 2-15 g/day as a continuous infusion or in divided doses

**Cardiac arrest in the presence of hyperkalemia or hypocalcemia, magnesium toxicity, or calcium antagonist toxicity: I.V.:**

Dosage expressed in mg of **calcium chloride:** 2-4 mg/kg; may repeat in 10 minutes if necessary

Dose expressed in mg of **calcium gluceptate:** 1.1-1.54 g/dose

Dosage expressed in mg of **calcium gluconate:** 500-800 mg (maximum 3 g/dose)

**Hypocalcemia secondary to citrated blood infusion: I.V.:** Give 0.45 mEq **elemental** calcium for each 100 mL citrated blood infused

**Tetany: I.V.:**

Dose expressed in mg of **calcium chloride:** 1 g over 10-30 minutes; may repeat after 6 hours

Dose expressed in mg of **calcium gluconate:** 1-3 g may be administered until therapeutic response occurs

**Antacid (calcium carbonate):**

Adults: 0.5 - 1.5 g orally as needed

**Administration**

**Oral:** Administer with plenty of fluids with or following meals.

**I.M.:** Do not inject calcium salts I.M. or administer S.C. since severe necrosis and sloughing may occur; extravasation of calcium can result in severe necrosis and tissue sloughing. Do not use scalp vein or small hand or foot veins for I.V. administration. Not for endotracheal administration.

**I.V.:**

For direct I.V. injection, infuse at a maximum rate of 50-100 mg/mL of calcium salt (gluconate, chloride or gluceptate)

I.V. infusion: Dilute to a maximum concentration and infuse over 1 hour or at a maximum rate of infusion as follows:

Salt form (Maximum dilution; Maximum rate of infusion)

Calcium **chloride:** 20 mg/mL; 45-90 mg/kg/hour; 0.6-1.2 mEq/kg/hour

Calcium **gluceptate:** 55 mg/mL: 150-300 mg/kg/hour; 0.6-1.2 mEq/kg/hour

Calcium **gluconate:** 50 mg/mL; 120-240 mg/kg/hour; 0.6-1.2 mEq/kg/hour

**Stability**

**Compatibility:** Incompatible with bicarbonates, phosphates, and sulfates.

**Monitoring Laboratory Tests** Serum calcium (ionized calcium preferred if available, see Additional Information), phosphate, magnesium

**Additional Nursing Issues**

**Physical Assessment:** Assess other medications patient may be taking for effectiveness and interactions (especially calcium channel blockers or cardiac glycosides - see Warnings/Precautions and Drug Interactions). Monitor laboratory tests, therapeutic effect, adverse or toxic effects as noted above with attention to changes in cardiac rhythm and bowel pattern (may cause severe constipation). Assess knowledge/teach patient appropriate use, interventions to reduce side effects, and adverse symptoms to report. If administered I.V., monitor EKG, vital signs, and CNS status during infusion and regularly after infusion is completed. Assess I.V. site for extravasation (see Administration). **Pregnancy risk factor C** - benefits of use should outweigh possible risks. Note breast-feeding caution.

**Patient Information/Instruction:** Follow instructions for dosing. Take with a full glass of water or juice, 1-3 hours after meals and other medications and 1-2 hours before any iron supplements. Avoid alcohol, other antacids, caffeine, or other calcium supplements unless approved by prescriber. You may experience constipation (increasing exercise or dietary fluid, fiber, or fruits may help). Report severe, unresolved GI disturbances and unusual emotional lability (mood swings). **Pregnancy/breast-feeding precautions:** Inform prescriber if you are or intend to be pregnant. Consult prescriber if breast-feeding.

**Dietary Issues:** Do not give orally with bran, foods high in oxalates, or whole grain cereals which may decrease calcium absorption. Avoid foods high in oxalates (eg, spinach, rhubarb).

**Geriatric Considerations:** Constipation and gas can be significant in the elderly, but are usually mild and may be resolved by switching to another calcium salt form. Achlorhydria is common in the elderly, calcium carbonate may not be the ideal calcium supplement for dietary or treatment use (administration with food will help). Citrate salts may be better absorbed. When using in the elderly, check albumin status and make appropriate decisions concerning reference serum concentrations. Elderly, especially the ill, often have low albumin due to malnutrition.

**Additional Information** Due to a poor correlation between the serum ionized calcium (free) and total serum calcium, particularly in states of low albumin or acid/base imbalances, direct measurement of ionized calcium is recommended. If ionized calcium is unavailable, in low albumin states, the corrected **total** serum calcium may be estimated by this equation (assuming a normal albumin of 4 g/dL); corrected total calcium = total serum calcium + 0.8 (4 - measured serum albumin).

- **Calculations/Conversions/Laboratory Values** *see page 1347*
- **CaldeCORT®** *see* Hydrocortisone *on page 578*
- **CaldeCORT®** *see* Topical Corticosteroids *on page 1152*
- **CaldeCORT® Anti-Itch Spray** *see* Hydrocortisone *on page 578*
- **CaldeCORT® Anti-Itch Spray** *see* Topical Corticosteroids *on page 1152*
- **Calderol®** *see* Calcifediol *on page 180*
- **Caldesene® Topical** *see page 1247*
- **Calm-X® Oral** *see page 1294*
- **Calmylin Expectorant** *see* Guaifenesin *on page 548*
- **Calphron®** *see* Calcium Supplements *on page 185*
- **Cal-Plus® [OTC]** *see* Calcium Supplements *on page 185*
- **Caltine®** *see* Calcitonin *on page 182*
- **Caltrate® 600 [OTC]** *see* Calcium Supplements *on page 185*
- **Caltrate, Jr.® [OTC]** *see* Calcium Supplements *on page 185*
- **Cam-ap-es®** *see* Hydralazine, Hydrochlorothiazide, and Reserpine *on page 565*
- **Campho-Phenique® Liquid** *see page 1294*
- **Camphor and Phenol** *see page 1294*
- **Camphorated Tincture of Opium** *see* Paregoric *on page 885*
- **Camphor, Menthol, and Phenol** *see page 1294*
- **Camptosar®** *see* Irinotecan *on page 624*

## Candesartan (kan de SAR tan)

**U.S. Brand Names** Atacand®

**Therapeutic Category** Angiotensin II Antagonists

**Pregnancy Risk Factor** C/D (2nd and 3rd trimesters)

**Lactation** Enters breast milk/contraindicated

**Use** Treatment of hypertension; alone or in combination with other antihypertensive agents

**Mechanism of Action/Effect** Blocks the vasoconstrictor and aldosterone-secreting effects of angiotensin II by binding of angiotensin II at the AT1 receptor in many tissues, such as vascular smooth muscle and the adrenal gland. Independent of pathways for angiotensin II synthesis. Does not affect the response to bradykinin; does not bind to block other hormone receptors or ion channels known to be important in cardiovascular regulation.

**Contraindications** Hypersensitivity to candesartan or any component; sensitivity to other A-II receptor antagonists; pregnancy (2nd and 3rd trimesters); hyperaldosteronism (primary); renal artery stenosis (bilateral)

**Warnings** Avoid use or use smaller dose in volume-depleted patients. Drugs which alter renin-angiotensin system have been associated with deterioration in renal function, including oliguria, acute renal failure, and progressive azotemia. Use with caution in patients with renal artery stenosis (unilateral or bilateral) to avoid decrease in renal function. Use caution in patients with pre-existing renal insufficiency (may decrease renal perfusion). Pregnancy factor C/D (2nd and 3rd trimesters).

**Drug Interactions**

**Increased Effect/Toxicity:** Potassium salts/supplements; candesartan is not metabolized by cytochrome P-450.

**Food Interactions** Food reduces the time to maximal concentration and increases the $C_{max}$.

**Adverse Reactions**

1% to 10%:

- Cardiovascular: Flushing, chest pain, peripheral edema
- Central nervous system: Dizziness, lightheadedness, drowsiness, fatigue, headache
- Dermatologic: Rash
- Gastrointestinal: Nausea, diarrhea, vomiting
- Neuromuscular & skeletal: Back pain, arthralgia
- Respiratory: Upper respiratory tract infection, pharyngitis, rhinitis, bronchitis, cough, sinusitis

<1% (Limited to important or life-threatening symptoms): Angina, myocardial infarction, dyspnea

**Overdose/Toxicology** Symptoms of overdose include hypotension and tachycardia. Treatment is supportive.

**Pharmacodynamics/Kinetics**

**Protein Binding:** 99%

**Half-life Elimination:** Dose-dependent: 5-9 hours

**Time to Peak:** 3-4 hours

**Metabolism:** Candesartan cilexetil is metabolized to candesartan by the intestinal wall cells

**Excretion:** Total body clearance: 0.37 mL/kg/minute; renal clearance: 0.19 mL/kg/minute; 26% renal excretion

**Onset:** 2-3 hours; peak effect: 6-8 hours

**Duration:** >24 hours

**Formulations** Tablet, as cilexetil: 4 mg, 8 mg, 16 mg, 32 mg

**Dosing**

**Adults:** Oral: 4-32 mg once daily. Dosage must be individualized. Blood pressure response is dose-related over the range of 2-32 mg. The usual recommended starting dose is 16 mg once daily when it is used as monotherapy in patients who are not volume depleted. It can be administered once or twice daily with total daily doses ranging from 8-32 mg; larger doses do not appear to have a greater effect and there is relatively little experience with such doses.

**Elderly:** See Adult Dosing. No initial dosage adjustment is necessary for elderly patients (although higher concentrations ($C_{max}$) and AUC were observed in these populations), for patients with mildly impaired renal function, or for patients with mildly impaired hepatic function.

**Monitoring Laboratory Tests** Electrolytes, serum creatinine, BUN, urinalysis

**Additional Nursing Issues**

**Physical Assessment:** See Warnings/Precautions, Dosing, and Adverse Reactions. Monitor blood pressure (standing and sitting), cardiac rate and rhythm, weight, and fluid balance at beginning of therapy, when adjusting dosage, and regularly with long-term therapy. Use and teach postural hypotension precautions and need for regular blood pressure monitoring. **Pregnancy risk factor C/D** - see Pregnancy Risk Factor - benefits of use must outweigh possible risks. Breast-feeding is contraindicated.

**Patient Information/Instruction:** Take exactly as directed; do not miss doses, alter dosage, or discontinue without consulting prescriber. Do not alter salt or potassium intake without consulting prescriber. Change position slowly when rising from sitting or lying or when climbing stairs. May cause transient drowsiness, dizziness, or headache; avoid driving or engaging in tasks requiring alertness until response to drug is known. Small frequent meals may help reduce any nausea or vomiting. Report unusual weight gain or swelling of ankles and hands; persistent fatigue; unusual flu or cold symptoms or dry cough; difficulty breathing; chest pain or palpitations; swelling of eyes, face, or lips; skin rash; muscle pain or weakness; unusual bleeding (in urine, stool, or gums); or excessive sweating. **Pregnancy/breast-feeding precautions:** Inform prescriber if you are or intend to be pregnant - contraceptives may be recommended. Do not breast-feed.

**Geriatric Considerations:** High concentrations occur in the elderly compared to younger subjects. AUC may be doubled in patients with renal impairment.

**Pregnancy Issues:** The drug should be discontinued as soon as possible when pregnancy is detected. Drugs which act directly on renin-angiotensin can cause fetal and neonatal morbidity and death.

**Related Information**

ACE Inhibitors and Angiotensin Antagonists Comparison *on page 1362*

♦ ***Candida albicans* (*Monilia*)** *see page 1248*

♦ **Capastat® Sulfate** *see* Capreomycin *on page 191*

## Capecitabine (ka pe SITE a been)

**U.S. Brand Names** Xeloda™

**Therapeutic Category** Antineoplastic Agent, Antimetabolite

**Pregnancy Risk Factor** D

**Lactation** Excretion in breast milk unknown/contraindicated

**Use** Treatment of patients with metastatic breast cancer resistant to both paclitaxel and an anthracycline-containing chemotherapy regimen or resistant to paclitaxel and for whom further anthracycline therapy is not indicated (eg, patients who have received cumulative doses of 400 mg/m$^2$ of doxorubicin or doxorubicin equivalents). Resistance is defined as progressive disease while on treatment, with or without an initial response, or relapse within 6 months of completing treatment with an anthracycline-containing adjuvant regimen.

**Mechanism of Action/Effect** Capecitabine is a prodrug of fluorouracil. It undergoes hydrolysis in the liver and tissues to form fluorouracil. It interferes with DNA (and to a lesser degree RNA) synthesis. Appears to be specific for G and S Phases of the cell cycle.

**Contraindications** Hypersensitivity to capecitabine, fluorouracil, or any component; pregnancy

**Warnings** The U.S. Food and Drug Administration (FDA) currently recommends that procedures for proper handling and disposal of antineoplastic agents be considered. Use with caution in patients with bone marrow suppression, poor nutritional status, or renal or hepatic dysfunction. The drug should be discontinued if intractable diarrhea, stomatitis, bone marrow suppression, or myocardial ischemia develop. Use with caution in patients who have received extensive pelvic radiation or alkylating therapy.

Capecitabine can cause severe diarrhea. Median time to first occurrence is 31 days. Subsequent doses should be reduced after grade 3 or 4 diarrhea.

Hand-and-foot syndrome (palmar-plantar erythrodysesthesia or chemotherapy-induced acral erythema) is characterized by numbness, dysesthesia/paresthesia, tingling, painless or painful swelling, erythema, desquamation, blistering, and severe pain. If grade 2 or 3 hand-and-foot syndrome occurs, interrupt administration of capecitabine until the event resolves or decreases in intensity to grade 1. Following grade 3 hand-and-foot syndrome, decrease subsequent doses of capecitabine.

There has been cardiotoxicity associated with fluorinated pyrimidine therapy, including myocardial infarction, angina, dysrhythmias, cardiogenic shock, sudden death, and EKG changes. These adverse events may be more common in patients with a history of coronary artery disease.

**Drug Interactions**

**Increased Effect/Toxicity:** Taking capecitabine immediately before an aluminum hydroxide/magnesium hydroxide antacid, or a meal, increases the absorption of capecitabine. The concentration of 5-fluorouracil is increased and its toxicity may be enhanced by leucovorin. Deaths from severe enterocolitis, diarrhea, and dehydration have been reported in elderly patients receiving weekly leucovorin and fluorouracil. Altered coagulation parameters have been noted in patients receiving coumarin derivatives (warfarin) with capecitabine.

**Food Interactions** Food reduced the rate and extent of absorption of capecitabine. Because current safety and efficacy data are based upon administration with food, it is recommended that capecitabine be administered with food. In all clinical trials, patients were instructed to administer capecitabine within 30 minutes after a meal.

**Adverse Reactions**

>10%:

- Central nervous system: Fatigue (41%), fever (12%)
- Gastrointestinal: Diarrhea (57%), may be dose limiting; mild to moderate nausea (53%), vomiting (37%), stomatitis (24%), anorexia (23%), abdominal pain (20%), constipation (15%)
- Dermatologic: Palmar-plantar erythrodysesthesia (hand-and-foot syndrome) (57%), may be dose limiting; dermatitis (37%)
- Hematologic: Lymphopenia (94%), anemia (72%), neutropenia (26%), thrombocytopenia (24%)
- Hepatic: Increased bilirubin (22%)
- Neuromuscular & skeletal: Paresthesia (21%)
- Ocular: Eye irritation (15%)

1% to 10%:

- Central nervous system: Headache (9%), dizziness (8%), insomnia (8%)
- Dermatologic: Nail disorders (7%)
- Gastrointestinal: Intestinal obstruction (1.1%)
- Endocrine & metabolic: Dehydration (7%)

(Continued)

## Capecitabine *(Continued)*

Neuromuscular & skeletal: Myalgia (9%)

<1% (Limited to important or life-threatening symptoms): Alopecia, necrotizing enterocolitis, hematemesis, GI hemorrhage, photosensitization, radiation recall, chest pain, ataxia, encephalopathy, bronchospasm, respiratory distress, bone pain, cardiomyopathy, hypotension, DVT, lymphedema, PE, CVA, ITP, pancytopenia, hepatic fibrosis, cholestasis, hepatitis, hypersensitivity

**Overdose/Toxicology** Symptoms of overdose include myelosuppression, nausea, vomiting, diarrhea, and alopecia. No specific antidote exists. Monitor hematologically for at least 4 weeks. Treatment is supportive.

**Pharmacodynamics/Kinetics**

**Protein Binding:** <60% (35% to albumin)

**Half-life Elimination:** Elimination: 0.5-1 hour

**Metabolism:**

Hepatic: Inactive metabolites: 5′-deoxy-5-fluorocytidine, 5′-deoxy-5-fluorouridine

Tissues: Active metabolite: 5-fluorouracil

**Excretion:** Renal: 70%, 50% as α-fluoro-β-alanine

**Formulations** Tablet: 150 mg, 500 mg

**Dosing**

**Adults:** Oral: 2500 mg/m²/day in 2 divided doses (~12 hours apart) at the end of a meal for 2 weeks followed by a 1-week rest period given as 3-week cycles

**Capecitabine Dose Calculation According to BSA Table**

| Dose Level 2500 mg/m²/day | | # of tablets per dose (morning and evening) | |
|---|---|---|---|
| **Surface Area (m²)** | **Total Daily Dose (mg)** | **150 mg** | **500 mg** |
| ≤1.24 | 3000 | 0 | 3 |
| 1.25-1.36 | 3300 | 1 | 3 |
| 1.37-1.51 | 3600 | 2 | 3 |
| 1.52-1.64 | 4000 | 0 | 4 |
| 1.65-1.76 | 4300 | 1 | 4 |
| 1.77-1.91 | 4600 | 2 | 4 |
| 1.92-2.04 | 5000 | 0 | 5 |
| 2.05-2.17 | 5300 | 1 | 5 |
| ≥2.18 | 5600 | 2 | 5 |

**Recommended Dose Modifications**

| Toxicity NCI Grades | During a Course of Therapy | Dose Adjustment for Next Cycle (% of starting dose) |
|---|---|---|
| Grade 1 | Maintain dose level | Maintain dose level |
| Grade 2 | | |
| 1st appearance | Interrupt until resolved to grade 0-1 | 100% |
| 2nd appearance | Interrupt until resolved to grade 0-1 | 75% |
| 3rd appearance | Interrupt until resolved to grade 0-1 | 50% |
| 4th appearance | Discontinue treatment permanently | |
| Grade 3 | | |
| 1st appearance | Interrupt until resolved to grade 0-1 | 75% |
| 2nd appearance | Interrupt until resolved to grade 0-1 | 50% |
| 3rd appearance | Discontinue treatment permanently | |
| Grade 4 | | |
| 1st appearance | Discontinue permanently OR If physician deems it to be in the patient's best interest to continue, interrupt until resolved to grade 0-1 | 50% |

Dosage modification guidelines: Carefully monitor patients for toxicity. Toxicity caused by capecitabine administration may be managed by symptomatic treatment, dose interruptions, and adjustment of dose. Once the dose has been reduced, it should not be increased at a later time.

**Elderly:** The elderly may be pharmacodynamically more sensitive to the toxic effects of 5-fluorouracil. Use with caution in monitoring the effects of capecitabine. Insufficient data are available to provide dosage modifications.

**Hepatic Impairment:**

Mild to moderate impairment: No starting dose adjustment is necessary; however, carefully monitor patients.

Severe hepatic impairment: Patients have not been studied.

**Administration**

**Oral:** Capecitabine is administered orally, usually in two divided doses taken 12 hours apart. Doses should be taken after meals with water.

**Stability**

**Storage:** Tablets are stored at room temperature.

**Monitoring Laboratory Tests** CBC with differential, hepatic function, renal function

**Additional Nursing Issues**

**Physical Assessment:** Patient will require close monitoring; note Warnings/Precautions, Dosing, and Adverse Reactions. Monitor laboratory tests closely. Monitor cardiac, CNS, respiratory, and respiratory status frequently during therapy. Assess for fluid imbalance (eg, I & O, edema, weight gain), opportunistic infection, or acute gastrointestinal disturbances. **Pregnancy risk factor D** - assess knowledge/teach both male and female appropriate use of barrier contraceptives during and for 1 month following therapy. See Warnings/Precautions. Breast-feeding is contraindicated.

**Patient Information/Instruction:** Take with food or within 30 minutes after meal. Avoid use of antacids within 2 hours of taking capecitabine. Do not crush, chew, or dissolve tablets. You will need frequent blood tests while taking this medication. Maintain adequate hydration (2-3 L/day of fluids unless instructed to restrict fluid intake). You may experience lethargy, dizziness, visual changes, confusion, anxiety (avoid driving or engaging in tasks requiring alertness until response to drug is known). For nausea, vomiting, loss of appetite, or dry mouth small, frequent meals, chewing gum, or sucking lozenges may help. You may experience loss of hair (will grow back when treatment is discontinued). You may experience photosensitivity (use sunscreen, wear protective clothing and eyewear, and avoid direct sunlight). You may experience dry, itchy, skin, and dry or irritated eyes (avoid contact lenses). You will be more susceptible to infection; avoid crowds or infected persons. Report chills or fever, confusion, persistent or violent vomiting or stomach pain, persistent diarrhea, respiratory difficulty, chest pain or palpitations, unusual bleeding or bruising, bone pain, muscle spasms/tremors, or vision changes immediately. **Pregnancy/breast-feeding precautions:** Do not get pregnant while taking this medication - both male and female should use appropriate barrier contraceptive measures. Do not give blood during this therapy or for 1 month following discontinuation of therapy. Do not breast-feed.

**Additional Information** This drug is enzymatically converted to 5-fluorouracil (5-FU) *in vivo.*

**Related Information**

Antiemetics for Chemotherapy-Induced Nausea and Vomiting *on page 1307*

- **Capital® and Codeine** *see* Acetaminophen and Codeine *on page 34*
- **Capitral®** *see* Captopril *on next page*
- **Capitrol® Shampoo** *see page 1294*
- **Capoten®** *see* Captopril *on next page*
- **Capotena** *see* Captopril *on next page*
- **Capozide®** *see* Captopril and Hydrochlorothiazide *on page 194*

## Capreomycin (kap ree oh MYE sin)

**U.S. Brand Names** Capastat® Sulfate

**Therapeutic Category** Antibiotic, Miscellaneous; Antitubercular Agent

**Pregnancy Risk Factor** C

**Lactation** Excretion in breast milk unknown

**Use** Treatment of tuberculosis (not responsive to first line antituberculosis agents) in conjunction with at least one other antituberculosis agent

**Mechanism of Action/Effect** Polypeptide antibiotic. The antimicrobial mechanism of action of capreomycin is not well understood. Mycobacterial species that have become resistant to other agents are usually still sensitive to the action of capreomycin. However, significant cross-resistance with viomycin, kanamycin, and neomycin occurs.

**Contraindications** Hypersensitivity to capreomycin sulfate or any component

**Warnings** The use of capreomycin in patients with renal insufficiency, pre-existing auditory impairment, and other oto- and nephrotoxic drug (especially other parenteral antituberculous agents) must be undertaken with great caution. The risk of additional eighth nerve impairment or renal injury should be weighed against the benefits to be derived from therapy. Pregnancy factor C.

**Drug Interactions**

**Increased Effect/Toxicity:** Capreomycin increases effect/duration of nondepolarizing neuromuscular blocking agents. Capreomycin has additive nephro- and ototoxicity, respiratory paralysis with aminoglycosides (eg, streptomycin).

**Effects on Lab Values** ↑ BUN, leukocytosis; ↓ potassium (S), platelets

**Adverse Reactions**

>10%:

Renal: Nephrotoxicity (increased thirst, anorexia, nausea, vomiting, greatly increased or decreased frequency of urination)

Otic: Ototoxicity

1% to 10%:

Hematologic: Eosinophilia

<1% (Limited to important or life-threatening symptoms): Vertigo, fever, rash, leukocytosis, thrombocytopenia; pain, induration, and bleeding at injection site; tinnitus, hypersensitivity reactions

**Overdose/Toxicology** Symptoms of overdose include renal failure, ototoxicity, and thrombocytopenia. Treatment is supportive.

**Pharmacodynamics/Kinetics**

**Half-life Elimination:** Dependent upon renal function and varies with creatinine clearance; 4-6 hours

(Continued)

## Capreomycin *(Continued)*

**Time to Peak:** I.M.: Within 1 hour

**Excretion:** Essentially excreted unchanged in the urine; no significant accumulation after ≥30 day of 1 g/day dosing in patients with normal renal function

**Formulations** Injection, as sulfate: 100 mg/mL (10 mL)

**Dosing**

**Adults:** I.M.: 15-30 mg/kg/day up to 1 g/day for 60-120 days, followed by 1 g 2-3 times/week

**Elderly:** Refer to adult dosing.

**Renal Impairment:** $Cl_{cr}$ <10 mL/minute: Decrease dose to ~33% of usual and administer every 48 hours. See table.

**Capreomycin Sulfate**

| $Cl_{cr}$ (mL/min) | Dose (mg/kg) for each dosing interval | | |
|---|---|---|---|
| | **24 h** | **48 h** | **72 h** |
| 0 | 1.29 | 2.58 | 3.87 |
| 10 | 2.43 | 4.87 | 7.3 |
| 20 | 3.58 | 7.16 | 10.7 |
| 30 | 4.72 | 9.45 | 14.2 |
| 40 | 5.87 | 11.7 | |
| 50 | 7.01 | 14 | |
| 60 | 8.16 | | |
| 80 | 10.4 | | |
| 100 | 12.7 | | |
| 110 | 13.9 | | |

**Administration**

**I.M.:** The solution for injection may acquire a pale straw color and darken with time. This is not associated with a loss of potency or development of toxicity. Administer deep I.M. into large muscle mass.

**Stability**

**Reconstitution:** Wait 2-3 minutes after reconstituting to allow for complete dissolution of the drug, then draw up dose.

**Monitoring Laboratory Tests** Renal function, CBC

**Additional Nursing Issues**

**Physical Assessment:** Assess effectiveness and interactions of other medications (see Drug Interactions). See Warnings/Precautions and Contraindications for use cautions. Monitor effectiveness of therapy, laboratory tests, and adverse response (see Adverse Reactions and Overdose/Toxicology). Assess knowledge/teach patient the need for regular laboratory and audiometry testing, possible side effects and adverse symptoms to report. **Pregnancy risk factor C** - benefits of use should outweigh possible risks. Note breast-feeding caution.

**Patient Information/Instruction:** Take as prescribed; do not discontinue without consulting prescriber. Maintain adequate hydration (2-3 L/day of fluids unless instructed to restrict fluid intake) to reduce incidence of nephrotoxicity. While taking this medication, routine blood tests and auditory tests will be necessary. Report any hearing loss, dizziness or vertigo, persistent nausea or vomiting, loss of appetite, or increased frequency of urination. **Pregnancy/breast-feeding precautions:** Inform prescriber if you are or intend to be pregnant. Consult prescriber if breast-feeding.

**Geriatric Considerations:** Adjust dose for renal function.

**Related Information**

TB Drug Comparison *on page 1402*

♦ **Capsaicin** *see page 1294*

♦ **Capsin®** *see page 1294*

## Captopril (KAP toe pril)

**U.S. Brand Names** Capoten®

**Therapeutic Category** Angiotensin-Converting Enzyme (ACE) Inhibitors

**Pregnancy Risk Factor** C/D (2nd and 3rd trimesters)

**Lactation** Enters breast milk/compatible

**Use** Management of hypertension; treatment of congestive heart failure, diabetic nephropathy

**Unlabeled use:** Treatment of hypertensive crisis, rheumatoid arthritis; diagnosis of anatomic renal artery stenosis, hypertension secondary to scleroderma renal crisis; diagnosis of aldosteronism, idiopathic edema, Bartter's syndrome, postmyocardial infarction for prevention of ventricular failure; increase circulation in Raynaud's phenomenon, hypertension secondary to Takayasu's disease

**Mechanism of Action/Effect** Competitive inhibitor of angiotensin-converting enzyme (ACE); prevents conversion of angiotensin I to angiotensin II, a potent vasoconstrictor; results in lower levels of angiotensin II which causes an increase in plasma renin activity and a reduction in aldosterone secretion

**Contraindications** Hypersensitivity to captopril, other ACE inhibitors, or any component; pregnancy (2nd or 3rd trimester)

**Warnings** Use with caution and modify dosage in patients with renal impairment (decrease dosage) (especially renal artery stenosis), severe congestive heart failure, or with coadministered diuretic therapy. Severe hypotension may occur in patients who are sodium and/or volume depleted, initiate lower doses and monitor closely when starting therapy in these patients. ACE inhibitors may be preferred agents in elderly patients with congestive heart failure and diabetes mellitus (diabetic proteinuria is reduced, minimal CNS effects, and enhanced insulin sensitivity); however, due to decreased renal function, tolerance must be carefully monitored. Pregnancy factor C/D (2nd and 3rd trimesters)..

**Drug Interactions**

**Cytochrome P-450 Effect:** CYP2D6 enzyme substrate

**Decreased Effect:** Rifampin may decrease the effect of ACE inhibitors. Antacids may decrease the bioavailability of captopril, separate administration times by 1-2 hours. NSAIDs, specifically indomethacin, may reduce the hypotensive effects of ACE inhibitors. More likely to occur in low renin or volume dependent hypertensive patients.

**Increased Effect/Toxicity:** Probenecid increases blood levels of captopril. Diuretics have additive hypotensive effects with ACE inhibitors. Phenothiazines taken with ACE inhibitors may increase the pharmacologic effects of the ACE inhibitor. Allopurinol and ACE inhibitors may cause a higher risk of hypersensitivity reaction when taken concurrently. Digoxin and ACE inhibitors may result in elevated serum digoxin levels. Lithium and ACE inhibitors may result in elevated serum levels of lithium with symptoms of toxicity. Potassium supplements or potassium-sparing diuretics with ACE inhibitors may result in elevated serum potassium levels.

**Food Interactions** Captopril serum concentrations may be decreased if taken with food.

**Effects on Lab Values** ↑ BUN, creatinine, potassium, positive Coombs' [direct]; ↓ cholesterol (S); may cause false-positive results in urine acetone determinations using sodium nitroprusside reagent

**Adverse Reactions**

1% to 10%:

- Cardiovascular: Tachycardia, chest pain, palpitations
- Central nervous system: Insomnia, headache, dizziness, fatigue, malaise
- Dermatologic: Rash, pruritus, alopecia
- Gastrointestinal: Abdominal pain, vomiting, nausea, diarrhea, anorexia, constipation, abnormal taste, dry mouth, peptic ulcer
- Neuromuscular & skeletal: Paresthesias
- Renal: Oliguria
- Respiratory: Transient cough, dyspnea

<1% (Limited to important or life-threatening symptoms): Hypotension, cardiac arrest, syncope, vasculitis, drowsiness, ataxia, confusion, depression, nervousness, muscle weakness, fever, angioedema, erythema multiforme, exfoliative dermatitis, photosensitivity, Stevens-Johnson syndrome, hyperkalemia, heartburn, glossitis, pancreatitis, aphthous ulcer, impotence, polyuria, interstitial nephritis, anemia, eosinophilia, neutropenia/agranulocytosis, thrombocytopenia, hepatitis, myalgia, arthralgia, proteinuria, increased BUN/serum creatinine, nephrotic syndrome, asthma, bronchospasm

**Overdose/Toxicology** Mild hypotension has been the primary toxic effect seen with acute overdose. Bradycardia may also occur. Hyperkalemia occurs even with therapeutic doses, especially in patients with renal insufficiency and those taking NSAIDs. Treatment is symptom directed and supportive.

**Pharmacodynamics/Kinetics**

**Protein Binding:** 25% to 30%

**Half-life Elimination:** Dependent upon renal and cardiac function: Adults, normal: 1.9 hours; Congestive heart failure: 2.06 hours; Anuria: 20-40 hours

**Time to Peak:** 1-2 hours

**Metabolism:** Liver

**Excretion:** Urine

**Onset:** Maximal decrease in blood pressure 1-1.5 hours after dose

**Duration:** Dose related, may require several weeks of therapy before full hypotensive effect is seen

**Formulations** Tablet: 12.5 mg, 25 mg, 50 mg, 100 mg

**Dosing**

**Adults: Note:** Dosage must be titrated according to patient's response; use lowest effective dose. Oral:

Hypertension:

- Initial: 12.5-25 mg 2-3 times/day; may increase by 12.5-25 mg/dose at 1- to 2-week intervals up to 50 mg 3 times/day. Add diuretic before further dosage increases.
- Maximum: 150 mg 3 times/day

Congestive heart failure:

- Initial: 6.25-12.5 mg 3 times/day in conjunction with cardiac glycoside and diuretic therapy. Initial dose depends upon patient's fluid/electrolyte status.
- Target: 50 mg 3 times/day
- Maximum: 100 mg 3 times/day

Diabetic nephropathy:

- 25 mg 3 times/day. May be taken with other antihypertensive therapy if required to further lower blood pressure.

**Elderly: Note:** Dosage must be titrated according to patient's response; use lowest effective dose.

**Renal Impairment:**

$Cl_{cr}$ 10-50 mL/minute: Administer at 75% of normal dose.

$Cl_{cr}$ <10 mL/minute: Administer at 50% of normal dose.

(Continued)

## Captopril *(Continued)*

**Note:** Smaller dosages given every 8-12 hours are indicated in patients with renal dysfunction. Renal function and leukocyte count should be carefully monitored during therapy.

Hemodialysis effects: Moderately dialyzable (20% to 50%); administer dose postdialysis or administer 25% to 35% supplemental dose.

Peritoneal dialysis: Supplemental dose is not necessary.

**Monitoring Laboratory Tests** BUN, serum creatinine, urine dipstick for protein, CBC, electrolytes

**Additional Nursing Issues**

**Physical Assessment:** Assess effectiveness and interactions of other medications (see Drug Interactions). See Warnings/Precautions and Contraindications for use cautions. Monitor effectiveness of therapy, laboratory tests, and adverse response on a regular basis during therapy (eg, postural hypotension - see Adverse Reactions and Overdose/Toxicology). Assess knowledge/teach patient appropriate use, possible side effects and appropriate interventions, and adverse symptoms to report. **Pregnancy risk factor C/D** - see Pregnancy Risk Factor - assess knowledge/teach appropriate use of barrier contraceptives. See Pregnancy Issues.

**Patient Information/Instruction:** Take exactly as directed; do not discontinue without consulting prescriber. Take first dose at bedtime. Take all doses on an empty stomach (30 minutes before or 2 hours after meals). This drug does not eliminate need for diet or exercise regimen as recommended by prescriber. Do not use potassium supplements or salt substitutes containing potassium without consulting prescriber. May cause dizziness, fainting, lightheadedness (use caution when driving or engaging in tasks that require alertness until response to drug is known); postural hypotension (use caution when rising from lying or sitting position or climbing stairs); nausea, vomiting, abdominal pain, dry mouth, or transient loss of appetite (small frequent meals, frequent mouth care, sucking lozenges, or chewing gum may help) - report if these persist. Report chest pain or palpitations; mouth sores; fever or chills; swelling of extremities, face, mouth, or tongue; skin rash; numbness, tingling, or pain in muscles; difficulty in breathing or unusual cough; other persistent adverse reactions. **Pregnancy precautions:** Do not get pregnant while taking this medication; use appropriate barrier contraceptive measures.

**Geriatric Considerations:** Due to frequent decreases in glomerular filtration (also creatinine clearance) with aging, elderly patients may have exaggerated responses to ACE inhibitors. Differences in clinical response due to hepatic changes are not observed.

**Pregnancy Issues:** ACE inhibitors can cause fetal injury or death if taken during the 2nd or 3rd trimester. Discontinue ACE inhibitors as soon as pregnancy is detected. ACE inhibitors should not be used if patient is sexually active and not using contraceptives.

**Related Information**

ACE Inhibitors and Angiotensin Antagonists Comparison *on page 1362*

## Captopril and Hydrochlorothiazide

(KAP toe pril & hye droe klor oh THYE a zide)

**U.S. Brand Names** Capozide®

**Synonyms** Hydrochlorothiazide and Captopril

**Therapeutic Category** Antihypertensive Agent, Combination

**Pregnancy Risk Factor** C/D (2nd and 3rd trimesters)

**Lactation** Enters breast milk/compatible

**Use** Management of hypertension and treatment of congestive heart failure

**Formulations**

Tablet:

25/15: Captopril 25 mg and hydrochlorothiazide 15 mg
25/25: Captopril 25 mg and hydrochlorothiazide 25 mg
50/15: Captopril 50 mg and hydrochlorothiazide 15 mg
50/25: Captopril 50 mg and hydrochlorothiazide 25 mg

**Dosing**

**Adults:** Oral:

Hypertension: Initial: 25 mg 2-3 times/day; may increase at 1- to 2-week intervals up to 150 mg 3 times/day (captopril dosages)

Congestive heart failure: 6.25-25 mg 3 times/day (maximum: 450 mg/day) (captopril dosages)

**Elderly:** Refer to dosing in individual monographs.

**Renal Impairment:** May respond to smaller or less frequent doses.

**Additional Nursing Issues**

**Physical Assessment:** See individual components listed in Related Information. **Pregnancy risk factor C/D** - see Pregnancy Risk Factor - assess knowledge/instruct patient on need to use appropriate contraceptive measures and the need to avoid pregnancy.

**Patient Information/Instruction:** See individual components listed in Related Information. **Pregnancy precautions:** Inform prescriber if you are or intend to be pregnant.

**Related Information**

Captopril *on page 192*
Hydrochlorothiazide *on page 566*

- **Capzasin-P®** *see page 1294*
- **Carafate®** *see* Sucralfate *on page 1078*

## Caramiphen and Phenylpropanolamine

(kar AM i fen & fen il proe pa NOLE a meen)

**U.S. Brand Names** Detuss®; Ordrine AT® Extended Release Capsule; Rescaps-D® S.R. Capsule; Tuss-Allergine® Modified T.D. Capsule; Tuss-Genade® Modified Capsule; Tussogest® Extended Release Capsule

**Synonyms** Phenylpropanolamine and Caramiphen

**Therapeutic Category** Antihistamine

**Pregnancy Risk Factor** C

**Lactation** Excretion in breast milk unknown

**Use** Symptomatic relief of cough and nasal congestion associated with the common cold

**Formulations**

Capsule, timed release: Caramiphen edisylate 40 mg and phenylpropanolamine hydrochloride 75 mg

Liquid: Caramiphen edisylate 6.7 mg and phenylpropanolamine hydrochloride 12.5 mg per 5 mL

**Dosing**

**Adults:** Oral: 1 capsule every 12 hours or 2 teaspoonfuls every 4 hours; do not exceed 12 teaspoonfuls in 24 hours.

**Elderly:** Refer to dosing in individual monographs.

**Additional Nursing Issues**

**Physical Assessment:** See individual components listed in Related Information. **Pregnancy risk factor C** - benefits of use should outweigh possible risks. Note breast-feeding caution.

**Patient Information/Instruction:** See individual components listed in Related Information. **Pregnancy/breast-feeding precautions:** Inform prescriber if you are or intend to be pregnant. Consult prescriber if breast-feeding.

**Related Information**

Phenylpropanolamine *on page 922*

♦ **Carbac** *see* Loracarbef *on page 689*

♦ **Carbachol** *see* Ophthalmic Agents, Glaucoma *on page 853*

## Carbamazepine (kar ba MAZ e peen)

**U.S. Brand Names** Epitol®; Tegretol®; Tegretol®-XR

**Therapeutic Category** Anticonvulsant, Miscellaneous

**Pregnancy Risk Factor** D

**Lactation** Enters breast milk/compatible

**Use** Prophylaxis of generalized tonic-clonic, partial (especially complex partial), and mixed partial or generalized seizure disorder

**Unlabeled use:** Treatment of bipolar disorders and other affective disorders; treatment of resistant schizophrenia, alcohol withdrawal, restless leg syndrome, and psychotic behavior associated with dementia; may be used to relieve pain in trigeminal neuralgia or diabetic neuropathy

**Mechanism of Action/Effect** In addition to anticonvulsant effects, carbamazepine has anticholinergic, antineuralgic, antidiuretic, muscle relaxant and antiarrhythmic properties; stimulates the release of ADH and potentiates its action in promoting reabsorption of water; chemically related to tricyclic antidepressants

**Contraindications** Hypersensitivity to carbamazepine or any component; **may have cross-sensitivity with tricyclic antidepressants**; should not be used in any patient with bone marrow depression; MAO inhibitor use; pregnancy

**Warnings** MAO inhibitors should be discontinued for a minimum of 14 days before carbamazepine is begun. Administer with caution to patients with history of cardiac damage or hepatic disease. Potentially fatal blood cell abnormalities have been reported following treatment. Carbamazepine is not effective in absence, myoclonic, or akinetic seizures. Elderly may have increased risk of SIADH-like syndrome.

**Drug Interactions**

**Cytochrome P-450 Effect:** CYP2C8 and CYP3A3/4 enzyme substrate; CYP1A2, 2C, 2C9, 2C18, 2C19, 2D6, and 3A3/4 enzyme inducer

**Decreased Effect:** Carbamazepine may induce the metabolism of warfarin, cyclosporine, doxycycline, oral contraceptives, phenytoin, theophylline, benzodiazepines, ethosuximide, valproic acid, corticosteroids, and thyroid hormones. Do not mix suspension with other liquid medicinal agents or diluents.

**Increased Effect/Toxicity:** Erythromycin, isoniazid, propoxyphene, verapamil, danazol, isoniazid, diltiazem, and cimetidine may inhibit hepatic metabolism of carbamazepine resulting in an increase of carbamazepine serum concentrations and toxicity. Potential for serotonin syndrome if combined with other serotonergic drugs.

**Food Interactions** Carbamazepine serum levels may be increased if taken with food.

**Effects on Lab Values** ↑ BUN, AST, ALT, bilirubin, alkaline phosphatase (S); ↓ calcium, $T_3$, $T_4$, sodium (S)

**Adverse Reactions**

>10%:

Central nervous system: Sedation, dizziness, fatigue, drowsiness, ataxia, confusion, lightheadedness

Gastrointestinal: Nausea, vomiting

Ocular: Blurred vision, nystagmus

1% to 10%:

Dermatologic: Stevens-Johnson syndrome, toxic epidermal necrolysis

Endocrine & metabolic: Hyponatremia, SIADH

Gastrointestinal: Diarrhea

(Continued)

## Carbamazepine *(Continued)*

Miscellaneous: Sweating, systemic lupus erythematosus (SLE)-like syndrome

<1% (Limited to important or life-threatening symptoms): Edema, congestive heart failure, syncope, bradycardia, hypertension or hypotension, A-V block, arrhythmias, slurred speech, mental depression, hypocalcemia, hyponatremia, urinary retention, sexual problems in males, neutropenia (can be transient), aplastic anemia, agranulocytosis, eosinophilia, leukopenia, pancytopenia, thrombocytopenia, bone marrow suppression, hepatitis, peripheral neuritis, diplopia, pancreatitis

**Overdose/Toxicology** Symptoms of overdose include dizziness ataxia, drowsiness, nausea, vomiting, tremor, agitation, nystagmus, urinary retention, dysrhythmias, coma, seizures, twitches, respiratory depression, and neuromuscular disturbances. Activated charcoal is effective at binding certain chemicals and this is especially true for carbamazepine. Other treatment is supportive and symptomatic.

**Pharmacodynamics/Kinetics**

**Protein Binding:** 75% to 90%; may be decreased in newborns

**Half-life Elimination:** Initial: 18-55 hours; Multiple dosing: 12-17 hours

**Time to Peak:** Unpredictable, within 4-8 hours

**Metabolism:** Liver

**Excretion:** Urine

**Onset:** Requires several days to reach steady-state concentrations

**Formulations**

Suspension, oral (citrus-vanilla flavor): 100 mg/5 mL (450 mL)

Tablet: 200 mg

Tablet, chewable: 100 mg

Tablet, extended release: 100 mg, 200 mg, 400 mg

**Dosing**

**Adults:** Oral (dosage must be adjusted according to patient's response and serum concentrations): 200 mg twice daily to start, increase by 200 mg/day at weekly intervals until therapeutic levels achieved; usual dose: 800-1200 mg/day in 3-4 divided doses; some patients have required up to 1.6-2.4 g/day

Trigeminal or glossopharyngeal neuralgia: Initial: 100 mg twice daily with food, gradually increasing in increments of 100 mg twice daily as needed usual maintenance: 400-800 mg daily in 2 divided doses

**Elderly:** Refer to adult dosing.

**Renal Impairment:** $Cl_{cr}$ <10 mL/minute: Administer 75% of dose.

**Administration**

**Oral:** Suspension dosage form must be given on a 3-4 times/day schedule versus tablets which can be given 2-4 times/day. When carbamazepine suspension has been combined with chlorpromazine or thioridazine solutions a precipitate forms which may result in loss of effect. Therefore, it is recommended that the carbamazepine suspension dosage form not be administered at the same time with other liquid medicinal agents or diluents.

**Monitoring Laboratory Tests** Serum carbamazepine levels, CBC, LFTs, platelets, reticulocyte count, iron level

**Additional Nursing Issues**

**Physical Assessment:** Assess effectiveness and interactions of other medications patient may be taking (see Contraindications, Warnings/Precautions, and Drug Interactions). Monitor for therapeutic response (seizure activity, force, type, duration), laboratory values, and adverse reactions (see Adverse Reactions) at beginning of therapy and periodically with long-term use. Taper dosage slowly when discontinuing. Observe and teach seizure/safety precautions. Assess knowledge/teach patient appropriate use, interventions to reduce side effects, and adverse symptoms to report. **Pregnancy risk factor D** - (carbamazepine may reduce effects of oral contraceptives) may cause fetal harm; benefits of use should outweigh possible risks.

**Patient Information/Instruction:** Take exactly as directed (do not increase dose or frequency or discontinue without consulting prescriber). While using this medication, do not use alcohol and other prescription or OTC medications (especially pain medications, sedatives, antihistamines, or hypnotics) without consulting prescriber. Maintain adequate hydration (2-3 L/day of fluids unless instructed to restrict fluid intake). You may experience drowsiness, dizziness, or blurred vision (use caution when driving or engaging in tasks requiring alertness until response to drug is known); nausea, vomiting, loss of appetite, or dry mouth (small frequent meals, frequent mouth care, chewing gum, or sucking lozenges may help). Wear identification of epileptic status and medications. Report CNS changes, mentation changes, or changes in cognition; muscle cramping, weakness, tremors, changes in gait; persistent GI symptoms (cramping, constipation, vomiting, anorexia); rash or skin irritations; unusual bruising or bleeding (mouth, urine, stool); worsening of seizure activity, or loss of seizure control. **Pregnancy precautions:** Inform prescriber if you are or intend to be pregnant.

**Geriatric Considerations:** Elderly may have increased risk of SIADH-like syndrome.

**Other Issues:**

Timing of serum samples: Absorption is slow, peak levels occur 6-8 hours after ingestion of the first dose. The half-life ranges from 8-60 hours; therefore, steady-state is achieved in 2-5 days.

Therapeutic levels: 6-12 μg/mL (SI: 25-51 μmol/L)

Toxic concentration: >15 μg/mL. Patients who require higher levels of 8-12 μg/mL (SI: 34-51 μmol/L) should be watched closely. Side effects including CNS effects occur commonly at higher dosage levels. If other anticonvulsants are given therapeutic range is 4-8 μg/mL.

**Related Information**
Peak and Trough Guidelines *on page 1331*

- **Carbamide** *see* Urea *on page 1193*
- **Carbamide Peroxide** *see page 1291*
- **Carbamide Peroxide** *see page 1294*
- **Carbastat® Ophthalmic** *see* Ophthalmic Agents, Glaucoma *on page 853*
- **Carbazep** *see* Carbamazepine *on page 195*
- **Carbazina** *see* Carbamazepine *on page 195*
- **Carbecin Inyectable** *see* Carbenicillin *on this page*

## Carbenicillin (kar ben i SIL in)

**U.S. Brand Names** Geocillin®

**Synonyms** Carindacillin

**Therapeutic Category** Antibiotic, Penicillin

**Pregnancy Risk Factor** B

**Lactation** Enters breast milk/use caution

**Use** Treatment of serious urinary tract infections and prostatitis caused by susceptible gram-negative aerobic bacilli or mixed aerobic-anaerobic bacterial infections excluding those secondary to *Klebsiella* sp and *Serratia marcescens*

**Mechanism of Action/Effect** Interferes with bacterial cell wall synthesis during active multiplication

**Contraindications** Hypersensitivity to carbenicillin, any component, penicillins, cephalosporins, or imipenem

**Warnings** Avoid use in patients with severe renal impairment ($Cl_{cr}$ <10 mL/minute). Dosage modification is required in patients with impaired renal and/or hepatic function. Use with caution in patients with history of hypersensitivity to cephalosporins.

**Drug Interactions**

**Decreased Effect:** Decreased efficacy of oral contraceptives is possible with carbenicillin. Decreased effectiveness with tetracyclines.

**Increased Effect/Toxicity:** Increased bleeding effects if taken with high doses of heparin or oral anticoagulants.

**Effects on Lab Values** ↑ AST (SGOT), ALT (SGPT)

**Adverse Reactions**

>10%: Gastrointestinal: Diarrhea

1% to 10%: Gastrointestinal: Nausea, bad taste, vomiting, flatulence, glossitis

<1% (Limited to important or life-threatening symptoms): Headache, hyperthermia, rash, urticaria, hypokalemia, furry tongue, epigastric distress, anemia, thrombocytopenia, leukopenia, neutropenia, eosinophilia, elevated LFTs, hematuria, hypersensitivity reactions

**Overdose/Toxicology** Symptoms of overdose include neuromuscular hypersensitivity and convulsions. Hemodialysis may be helpful to aid in removal of the drug from blood; otherwise, treatment is supportive or symptom directed.

**Pharmacodynamics/Kinetics**

**Protein Binding:** 50%

**Distribution:** Crosses the placenta; distributes into bile; low concentrations attained in CSF

**Half-life Elimination:** 1-1.5 hours, prolonged to 10-20 hours with renal insufficiency

**Time to Peak:** Within 0.5-2 hours in patients with normal renal function; serum concentrations following oral absorption are inadequate for treatment of systemic infections

**Excretion:** Urine

**Formulations** Tablet, film coated, as sodium: 382 mg [base]

**Dosing**

**Adults:** Oral: 1-2 tablets every 6 hours for urinary tract infections or 2 tablets every 6 hours for prostatitis

**Renal Impairment:**

$Cl_{cr}$ 10-50 mL/minute: Administer every 12-24 hours.

$Cl_{cr}$ <10 mL/minute: Administer every 24-48 hours.

Moderately dialyzable (20% to 50%)

**Administration**

**Oral:** Administer around-the-clock to promote less variation in peak and trough serum levels. Give at least 1 hour before aminoglycosides.

**Stability**

**Compatibility:** See the Compatibility of Drugs Chart *on page 1315.*

**Monitoring Laboratory Tests** Renal and hepatic function, CBC, serum potassium, bleeding times. Perform culture and sensitivity testing prior to initiating therapy.

**Additional Nursing Issues**

**Physical Assessment:** Monitor for effectiveness of therapy. Monitor or instruct patient to monitor and report signs of opportunistic infection (eg, sore throat, fever, chills, fatigue, thrush, vaginal discharge, diarrhea), edema, dehydration, or hypersensitivity reactions (see above). Note breast-feeding caution.

**Patient Information/Instruction:** Take as prescribed, at equal intervals around-the-clock, with a full glass of water, and preferably on an empty stomach (1 hour before or 2 hours after meals). Do not skip doses and take full course of treatment even if feeling better. Frequent mouth care will help relieve dry mouth and bitter aftertaste. Report swelling, respiratory difficulty, easy bruising or bleeding, or signs of opportunistic infection (eg, sore throat, fever, chills, fatigue, thrush, vaginal discharge, diarrhea). If diabetic, drug may cause false tests with Clinitest® urine glucose monitoring; use of

(Continued)

## Carbenicillin *(Continued)*

glucose oxidase methods (Clinistix®) or serum glucose monitoring is preferable. **Pregnancy/breast-feeding precautions:** This drug may interfere with oral contraceptives; an alternate form of birth control should be used. Consult prescriber if breast-feeding.

**Geriatric Considerations:** Has not been studied in the elderly.

♦ **Carbidopa and Levodopa** *see* Levodopa and Carbidopa *on page 667*

## Carbinoxamine and Pseudoephedrine

(kar bi NOKS a meen & soo doe e FED rin)

**U.S. Brand Names** Carbiset® Tablet; Carbiset-TR® Tablet; Carbodec® Syrup; Carbodec® Tablet; Carbodec TR® Tablet; Cardec-S® Syrup; Rondec® Drops; Rondec® Filmtab®; Rondec® Syrup; Rondec-TR®

**Synonyms** Pseudoephedrine and Carbinoxamine

**Therapeutic Category** Adrenergic Agonist Agent; Antihistamine, $H_1$ Blocker; Decongestant

**Pregnancy Risk Factor** C

**Lactation** Excretion in breast milk unknown/contraindicated

**Use** Temporary relief of nasal congestion, running nose, sneezing, itching of nose or throat, and itchy, watery eyes due to the common cold, hay fever, or other respiratory allergies

**Mechanism of Action/Effect** Carbinoxamine competes with histamine for $H_1$-receptor sites on effector cells in the GI tract, blood vessels, and respiratory tract

**Contraindications** Hypersensitivity to carbinoxamine or pseudoephedrine or any component; severe hypertension or coronary artery disease, MAO inhibitor therapy, GI or GU obstruction, narrow-angle glaucoma; avoid use in premature or term infants due to a possible association with SIDS

**Warnings** Narrow-angle glaucoma, bladder neck obstruction, symptomatic prostatic hypertrophy, asthmatic attack, and stenosing peptic ulcer. Pregnancy factor C.

**Drug Interactions**

**Increased Effect/Toxicity:** Barbiturates, tricyclic antidepressants, MAO inhibitors, ethanolamine antihistamines

**Adverse Reactions**

>10%:

Central nervous system: Slight to moderate drowsiness

Respiratory: Thickening of bronchial secretions

1% to 10%:

Central nervous system: Headache, fatigue, nervousness, dizziness

Gastrointestinal: Appetite increase, weight gain, nausea, diarrhea, abdominal pain, dry mouth

Neuromuscular & skeletal: Arthralgia

Respiratory: Pharyngitis

<1% (Limited to important or life-threatening symptoms): Edema, palpitations, depression, angioedema, photosensitivity, rash, hepatitis, bronchospasm, epistaxis

**Overdose/Toxicology** Symptoms of overdose include dry mouth, flushed skin, dilated pupils, and CNS depression. There is no specific treatment for antihistamine overdose. Clinical toxicity is due to blockade of cholinergic receptors. For anticholinergic overdose with severe life-threatening symptoms, physostigmine 1-2 mg I.V. slowly, may be given to reverse these effects.

**Formulations**

Drops: Carbinoxamine maleate 2 mg and pseudoephedrine hydrochloride 25 mg per mL (30 mL with dropper)

Syrup: Carbinoxamine maleate 4 mg and pseudoephedrine hydrochloride 60 mg per 5 mL (120 mL, 480 mL)

Tablet:

Film-coated: Carbinoxamine maleate 4 mg and pseudoephedrine hydrochloride 60 mg

Sustained release: Carbinoxamine maleate 8 mg and pseudoephedrine hydrochloride 120 mg

**Dosing**

**Adults:** Oral:

Liquid: 5 mL 4 times/day

Tablets: 1 tablet 4 times/day

**Elderly:** Refer to adult dosing.

**Additional Nursing Issues**

**Physical Assessment:** Assess effectiveness and interactions of other medications (see Drug Interactions). See Contraindications and Warnings/Precautions for cautious use. Monitor effectiveness of therapy and adverse reactions (see Adverse Reactions) at beginning of therapy and periodically with long-term use. Assess knowledge/teach patient appropriate use, interventions to reduce side effects, and adverse symptoms to report. **Pregnancy risk factor C** - benefits of use should outweigh possible risks. Breast-feeding is contraindicated.

**Patient Information/Instruction:** Take as directed; do not exceed recommended dose. Maintain adequate hydration (2-3 L/day of fluids unless instructed to restrict fluid intake). Avoid use of other depressants, alcohol, or sleep-inducing medications unless approved by prescriber. You may experience drowsiness, impaired coordination, blurred vision, or increased anxiety (use caution when driving or engaging in tasks requiring alertness until response to drug is known); or dry mouth or nausea (frequent small meals, frequent mouth care, chewing gum, or sucking hard candy may help). Report persistent dizziness, sedation, or agitation; difficulty breathing or increased cough; changes in urinary pattern; muscle weakness; or lack of improvement or worsening or condition. **Pregnancy/breast-feeding precautions:** Inform prescriber if you are or intend to be pregnant. Do not breast-feed.

**Geriatric Considerations:** Elderly are more predisposed to adverse effects of sympathomimetics since they frequently have cardiovascular diseases and diabetes mellitus as well as multiple drug therapies. It may be advisable to treat with a short-acting/immediate-release formulation before initiating sustained-release/long-acting formulations.

**Related Information**

Pseudoephedrine *on page 992*

- **Carbiset® Tablet** *see* Carbinoxamine and Pseudoephedrine *on previous page*
- **Carbiset-TR® Tablet** *see* Carbinoxamine and Pseudoephedrine *on previous page*
- **Carbocaine®** *see* Mepivacaine *on page 723*
- **Carbodec® Syrup** *see* Carbinoxamine and Pseudoephedrine *on previous page*
- **Carbodec® Tablet** *see* Carbinoxamine and Pseudoephedrine *on previous page*
- **Carbodec TR® Tablet** *see* Carbinoxamine and Pseudoephedrine *on previous page*
- **Carbolit®** *see* Lithium *on page 683*
- **Carboplat** *see* Carboplatin *on this page*

## Carboplatin (KAR boe pla tin)

**U.S. Brand Names** Paraplatin®

**Synonyms** CBDCA

**Therapeutic Category** Antineoplastic Agent, Alkylating Agent

**Pregnancy Risk Factor** D

**Lactation** Excretion in breast milk unknown/contraindicated

**Use** Monotherapy or combination therapy for ovarian carcinoma, cervical, small cell lung carcinoma, esophageal cancer, testicular, bladder cancer, mesothelioma, pediatric brain tumors, sarcoma, neuroblastoma

**Mechanism of Action/Effect** Analogue of cisplatin which covalently binds to DNA; possible cross-linking and interference with the function of DNA

**Contraindications** Hypersensitivity to carboplatin or any component (anaphylactic-like reactions may occur) or to mannitol; severe bone marrow depression; excessive bleeding; pregnancy

**Warnings** The U.S. Food and Drug Administration (FDA) currently recommends that procedures for proper handling and disposal of antineoplastic agents be considered. Bone marrow suppression is more severe in patients receiving other bone marrow suppressing therapies or who have had previous radiation therapy.

Carboplatin preparation should be performed in a Class II laminar flow biologic safety cabinet and personnel should be wearing surgical gloves and a closed front surgical gown with knit cuffs. Appropriate safety equipment is recommended for preparation, administration, and disposal of antineoplastics. If carboplatin contacts the skin, wash and flush thoroughly with water.

**Drug Interactions**

**Increased Effect/Toxicity:** Nephrotoxic drugs; aminoglycosides increase risk of ototoxicity.

**Adverse Reactions**

>10%:

- Endocrine & metabolic: Electrolyte abnormalities such as hypocalcemia and hypomagnesemia, hyponatremia, hypokalemia
- Gastrointestinal: Nausea, vomiting, stomatitis
  - Emetic potential: Moderate
  - Time course for nausea and vomiting: Onset: 2-6 hours; Duration: 1-48 hours
- Hematologic: Neutropenia, leukopenia, thrombocytopenia, anemia
- Myelosuppressive: Dose-limiting toxicity
  - WBC: Severe (dose-dependent)
  - Platelets: Severe
  - Nadir: 21-24 days
  - Recovery: 28-35 days
- Hepatic: Abnormal liver function tests
- Local: Pain at injection site
- Neuromuscular & skeletal: Weakness

1% to 10%:

- Dermatologic: Alopecia
- Gastrointestinal: Diarrhea, anorexia
- Hematologic: Hemorrhagic complications
- Neuromuscular & skeletal: Peripheral neuropathy
- Otic: Ototoxicity

<1% (Limited to important or life-threatening symptoms): Neurotoxicity has only been noted in patients previously treated with cisplatin; urticaria; rash; nephrotoxicity (uncommon)

**BMT:**

- Dermatologic: Alopecia
- Endocrine & metabolic: Hypokalemia, hypomagnesemia
- Gastrointestinal: Nausea, vomiting, mucositis
- Hepatic: Elevated liver function tests
- Renal: Nephrotoxicity

**Overdose/Toxicology** Symptoms of overdose include bone marrow suppression and hepatic toxicity. Treatment is symptomatic and supportive.

(Continued)

## Carboplatin *(Continued)*

**Pharmacodynamics/Kinetics**

**Protein Binding:** 0%

**Half-life Elimination:** 22-40 hours; 2.5-5.9 hours in patients with $Cl_{cr}$ >60 mL/minute

**Metabolism:** Liver

**Excretion:** Urine

**Formulations** Powder for injection, lyophilized: 50 mg, 150 mg, 450 mg

**Dosing**

**Adults:** IVPB, I.V. infusion, intraperitoneal (refer to individual protocols):

Ovarian cancer: Usual doses range from 360 mg/m² I.V. every 3 weeks single agent therapy to 300 mg/m² every 4 weeks as combination therapy.

In general, however, single intermittent courses of carboplatin should not be repeated until the neutrophil count is at least 2000/mm³ and the platelet count is at least 100,000/mm³.

The dose adjustments in the table are modified from a controlled trial in previously treated patients with ovarian carcinoma. Blood counts were done weekly, and the recommendations are based on the lowest post-treatment platelet or neutrophil value.

**Carboplatin Dosage Adjustment Based on Pretreatment Platelet Counts**

| Platelets (cells/mm³) | Neutrophils (cells/mm³) | Adjusted Dose (From Prior Course) |
|---|---|---|
| >100,000 | >2000 | 125% |
| 50-100,000 | 500-2000 | No adjustment |
| <50,000 | <500 | 75% |

**Dosage adjustment based on the Egorin formula** (based on platelet counts):

Previously untreated patients:

$$\text{dosage (mg/m}^2) = (0.091)\,\frac{(Cl_{cr})}{(BSA)}\,\frac{(\text{Pretreat Plt count} - \text{Plt nadir count desired} \times 100)}{(\text{Pretreatment Plt count})} + 86$$

Previously treated patients with heavily myelosuppressive agents:

$$\text{dosage (mg/m}^2) = (0.091)\,\frac{(Cl_{cr})}{(BSA)}\,\frac{[(\text{Pretreat Plt count} - \text{Plt nadir count desired} \times 100) - 17]}{(\text{Pretreatment Plt count})} + 86$$

High dose: I.V.: 1.2-2.4 g/m² administered as 3-4 divided doses; generally infused over at least 60 minutes; 400 mg/m² has been infused over 15-30 minutes; generally combined with other high-dose chemotherapeutic drugs.

Autologous BMT: I.V.: 1600 mg/m² (total dose) divided over 4 days **requires BMT (ie, FATAL without BMT)**

**Elderly:** Refer to adult dosing.

**Renal Impairment:** These dosing recommendations apply to the initial course of treatment. Subsequent dosages should be adjusted according to the patient's tolerance based on the degree of bone marrow suppression.

$Cl_{cr}$ <60 mL/minute are at increased risk of severe bone marrow suppression. In renally impaired patients who received single agent carboplatin therapy, the incidence of severe leukopenia, neutropenia, or thrombocytopenia has been about 25% when the following dosage modifications have been used:

$Cl_{cr}$ 41-59 mL/minute: Recommended dose on day 1 is 250 mg/m².

$Cl_{cr}$ 16-40 mL/minute: Recommended dose on day 1 is 200 mg/m².

$Cl_{cr}$ <15 mL/minute: The data available for patients with severely impaired kidney function is too limited to permit a recommendation for treatment.

**or**

Calvert formula (GFR = glomerular filtration rate)

Total dose (mg) = Target AUC x (GFR + 25)

**Note:** The dose of carboplatin calculated is total mg dose **not** mg/m². AUC is the area under the concentration versus time curve.

Target AUC value will vary depending upon:

Number of agents in the regimen

Treatment status (ie, previously untreated or treated)

Single Agent Carboplatin/No Prior Chemotherapy

Total dose (mg) = 6-8 (GFR + 25)

Single Agent Carboplatin/Prior Chemotherapy

Total dose (mg) = 4-6 (GFR + 25)

Combination Chemotherapy/No Prior Chemotherapy

Total dose (mg) = 4.5-6 (GFR + 25)

Combination Chemotherapy/Prior Chemotherapy

**Note:** A reasonable approach for these patients would be to use a target AUC value <5 for the initial cycle.

Intraperitoneal: 200-650 mg/m² in 2 L of dialysis fluid have been administered into the peritoneum of ovarian cancer patients.

**Hepatic Impairment:** There are no published studies available on the dosing of carboplatin in patients with impaired liver function. Human data regarding the biliary elimination of carboplatin are not available; however, pharmacokinetic studies in rabbits and rats reflect a biliary excretion of 0.4% to 0.7% of the dose (ie, 0.05 mL/minute/kg biliary clearance).

**Administration**

**I.V.:** Administer as IVPB over 15 minutes up to a continuous intravenous infusion over 24 hours. May also be administered intraperitoneally.

**I.V. Detail:** Do not use needles or I.V. administration sets containing aluminum parts that may come in contact with carboplatin (aluminum can react causing precipitate formation and loss of potency).

**BMT only:** Observe serum creatinine. Carboplatin is nephrotoxic and drug accumulation occurs with decreased creatinine clearance.

**Stability**

**Storage:** Store intact vials at room temperature 15°C to 30°C (59°F to 86°F).

**Reconstitution:** Reconstitute powder to yield a final concentration of 10 mg/mL which is stable for 5 days at room temperature (25°C). Aluminum needles should not be used for administration due to binding with the platinum ion.

**Standard I.V. dilution:** Dose/250-1000 mL $D_5W$ or NS

Further dilution to a concentration up to 0.5 mg/mL is stable at room temperature (25°C) for 24 hours in $D_5W$ or NS.

**Compatibility:** Incompatible with aluminum, fluorouracil (5FU), mesna, sodium bicarbonate. Should be considered incompatible in a syringe of solution with any other drug because of toxicity and specific use. See the Chemotherapy Compatibility Chart *on page 1311.*

**Monitoring Laboratory Tests** CBC with differential and platelet count, serum electrolytes, urinalysis, creatinine clearance, liver function

**Additional Nursing Issues**

**Physical Assessment:** Monitor laboratory tests and auditory evaluation prior to each infusion and on a regular basis throughout therapy. Assess for and teach patient to recognize major adverse reactions: peripheral neuropathy (numbness, pain, or tingling of extremities, and muscle weakness), electrolyte or metabolic disturbances, ototoxicity, fluid imbalance (I & O, edema), nutritional status (anorexia, weight loss), hearing loss, etc (see Adverse Reactions). **Pregnancy risk factor D** - assess knowledge/teach appropriate use of barrier contraceptives. Breast-feeding is contraindicated.

**Patient Information/Instruction:** Maintain adequate nutrition (frequent small meals may help) and adequate hydration (2-3 L/day of fluids unless instructed to restrict fluid intake). Nausea and vomiting may be severe; request antiemetic. You will be susceptible to infection; avoid crowds or exposure to infection. Report sore throat, fever, chills, unusual fatigue or unusual bruising/bleeding, difficulty breathing, muscle cramps or twitching, or change in hearing acuity. **Pregnancy/breast-feeding precautions:** Do not get pregnant while taking this medication; use appropriate barrier contraceptive measures. Do not breast-feed.

**Other Issues:** Carboplatin is sometimes confused with cisplatin. Institute measures to prevent mix-ups.

## Carboprost Tromethamine (KAR boe prost tro METH a meen)

**U.S. Brand Names** Hemabate™

**Therapeutic Category** Abortifacient; Prostaglandin

**Pregnancy Risk Factor** X

**Lactation** Excretion in breast milk unknown/opportunity for use is minimal

**Use** Termination of pregnancy and refractory postpartum uterine bleeding

**Investigational use:** Hemorrhagic cystitis

**Mechanism of Action/Effect** Carboprost tromethamine is a prostaglandin similar to prostaglandin $F_2$. Carboprost tromethamine stimulates the gravid uterus to contract, which usually results in expulsion of the products of conception. Used to induce abortion between 13-20 weeks of pregnancy.

**Contraindications** Hypersensitivity to carboprost tromethamine or any component; acute pelvic inflammatory disease; pregnancy

**Warnings** Use with caution in patients with history of asthma, hypotension or hypertension, cardiovascular, adrenal, renal or hepatic disease, anemia, jaundice, diabetes, epilepsy, or compromised uterus.

**Adverse Reactions**

>10%: Gastrointestinal: Diarrhea, vomiting, nausea

1% to 10%:

Cardiovascular: Flushing

Central nervous system: Dizziness, headache

Gastrointestinal: Stomach cramps

<1% (Limited to important or life-threatening symptoms): Hypertension, hypotension, bradycardia or tachycardia, drowsiness, vertigo, nervousness, fever, dystonia, vasovagal syndrome, breast tenderness, dry mouth, hematemesis, abnormal taste, bladder spasms, myalgia, blurred vision, coughing, asthma, respiratory distress, septic shock, hiccups

**Pharmacodynamics/Kinetics**

**Metabolism:** Liver

**Excretion:** Urine

**Formulations** Injection: Carboprost 250 mcg and tromethamine 83 mcg per mL (1 mL)

(Continued)

## Carboprost Tromethamine *(Continued)*

**Dosing**

**Adults:** I.M.:

Abortion: 250 mcg to start, 250 mcg at 1½-hour to 3½-hour intervals depending on uterine response; a 500 mcg dose may be given if uterine response is not adequate after several 250 mcg doses; do not exceed 12 mg total dose

Refractory postpartum uterine bleeding: Initial: 250 mcg; may repeat at 15- to 90-minute intervals to a total dose of 2 mg

Bladder irrigation for hemorrhagic cystitis (refer to individual protocols): [0.4-1.0 mg/dL as solution] 50 mL instilled into bladder 4 times/day for 1 hour

**Elderly:** Refer to adult dosing.

**Administration**

**I.M.:** Give deep I.M.. Rotate site if repeat injections are required.

**I.V.:** Do not inject I.V.; may result in bronchospasm, hypertension, vomiting, and anaphylaxis.

**Stability**

**Storage:** Refrigerate ampuls.

**Reconstitution:** Bladder irrigation: Dilute immediately prior to administration in NS; stability unknown.

**Additional Nursing Issues**

**Physical Assessment:** See Contraindications and Warnings/Precautions for cautious use. Note that nausea or vomiting may be significant; premedication with an antiemetic may be considered. Monitor effectiveness (eg, uterine contractions) and adverse reactions (eg, hypertension, hemorrhage, or respiratory effects, prolonged or excessively elevated temperature - see Adverse Reactions). Report contractions lasting longer than 1 minute or absence of contractions. Assess for complete expulsion of uterine contents (fetal tissue). Assess knowledge/instruct patient on adverse symptoms to report. If used to treat hemorrhagic cystitis (bladder irrigation). **Pregnancy risk factor X.**

**Patient Information/Instruction:** This medication is used to stimulate expulsion of uterine contents (fetal tissue) or stimulate uterine contractions to reduce uterine bleeding. Report increased blood loss, acute abdominal cramping, persistent elevation of temperature, foul-smelling vaginal discharge. Increased temperature (elevated temperature) may occur 1-16 hours after therapy and last for several hours. **Pregnancy precautions:** If being treated for hemorrhagic cystitis, inform prescriber if pregnant.

- **Carboptic® Ophthalmic** *see* Ophthalmic Agents, Glaucoma *on page 853*
- **Carboxymethylcellulose Sodium** *see page 1294*
- **Cardec-S® Syrup** *see* Carbinoxamine and Pseudoephedrine *on page 198*
- **Cardene®** *see* Nicardipine *on page 820*
- **Cardene® I.V.** *see* Nicardipine *on page 820*
- **Cardene® SR** *see* Nicardipine *on page 820*
- **Cardinit** *see* Nitroglycerin *on page 831*
- **Cardio-Green®** *see page 1248*
- **Cardioquin®** *see* Quinidine *on page 1002*
- **Cardiorona** *see* Amiodarone *on page 71*
- **Cardipril®** *see* Captopril *on page 192*
- **Cardizem® CD** *see* Diltiazem *on page 377*
- **Cardizem® Injectable** *see* Diltiazem *on page 377*
- **Cardizem® SR** *see* Diltiazem *on page 377*
- **Cardizem® Tablet** *see* Diltiazem *on page 377*
- **Cardura®** *see* Doxazosin *on page 398*
- **Carexan** *see* Itraconazole *on page 639*
- **Carindacillin** *see* Carbenicillin *on page 197*
- **Carisoprodate** *see* Carisoprodol *on this page*

## Carisoprodol (kar i soe PROE dole)

**U.S. Brand Names** Rela®; Sodol®; Soma®; Soprodol®; Soridol®

**Synonyms** Carisoprodate; Isobamate

**Therapeutic Category** Skeletal Muscle Relaxant

**Pregnancy Risk Factor** C

**Lactation** Enters breast milk (high concentrations)/not recommended

**Use** Skeletal muscle relaxant

**Mechanism of Action/Effect** Precise mechanism is not yet clear, but many effects have been ascribed to its central depressant actions.

**Contraindications** Hypersensitivity to carisoprodol, meprobamate, or any component; acute intermittent porphyria

**Warnings** Use with caution in renal and hepatic dysfunction. Pregnancy factor C.

**Drug Interactions**

**Cytochrome P-450 Effect:** CYP2C19 enzyme substrate

**Increased Effect/Toxicity:** Alcohol, CNS depressants, psychotropic drugs, and phenothiazines may increase toxicity.

**Adverse Reactions**

>10%: Central nervous system: Drowsiness

1% to 10%:

Cardiovascular: Tachycardia, tightness in chest, flushing of face, syncope

Central nervous system: Mental depression, allergic fever, dizziness, lightheadedness, headache, paradoxical CNS stimulation
Dermatologic: Angioedema, dermatitis (allergic)
Gastrointestinal: Nausea, vomiting, stomach cramps
Neuromuscular & skeletal: Trembling
Ocular: Burning eyes
Respiratory: Shortness of breath
Miscellaneous: Hiccups

<1% (Limited to important or life-threatening symptoms): Rash, urticaria, erythema multiforme, aplastic anemia, leukopenia, eosinophilia, clumsiness

**Overdose/Toxicology** Symptoms of overdose include CNS depression, stupor, coma, shock, and respiratory depression. Treatment is supportive.

**Pharmacodynamics/Kinetics**
**Distribution:** Crosses the placenta
**Half-life Elimination:** 8 hours
**Metabolism:** Liver
**Excretion:** Kidneys
**Onset:** Within 30 minutes
**Duration:** 4-6 hours

**Formulations** Tablet: 350 mg

**Dosing**
**Adults:** Oral: 350 mg 3-4 times/day; take last dose at bedtime; compound: 1-2 tablets 4 times/day
**Elderly:** Not recommended for use in the elderly; see Geriatric Considerations.

**Administration**
**Oral:** Give with food to decrease GI upset.

**Additional Nursing Issues**
**Physical Assessment:** Assess effectiveness and interactions of other medications (see Drug Interactions). See Contraindications and Warnings/Precautions for use cautions. Monitor effectiveness of therapy (according to rational for therapy) and adverse reactions (eg, cardiovascular and CNS status - see Adverse Reactions) at beginning of therapy and periodically with long-term use. Do not discontinue abruptly; taper dosage slowly (withdrawal symptoms such as abdominal cramping, headache, insomnia may occur). Assess knowledge/teach patient appropriate use, interventions to reduce side effects (postural hypotension precautions), and adverse symptoms to report. **Pregnancy risk factor C** - benefits of use should outweigh possible risks. Breast-feeding is not recommended.

**Patient Information/Instruction:** Take exactly as directed with food. Do not increase dose or discontinue without consulting prescriber. Do not use alcohol, prescriptive or OTC antidepressants, sedatives, and pain medications without consulting prescriber. You may experience drowsiness, dizziness, lightheadedness (avoid driving or engaging in tasks requiring alertness until response to drug is known); nausea, vomiting, or cramping (small, frequent meals, frequent mouth care, or sucking hard candy may help); or postural hypotension (change position slowly when rising from sitting or lying or when climbing stairs). Report excessive drowsiness or mental agitation; palpitations, rapid heartbeat, or chest pain; skin rash; muscle cramping or tremors; or respiratory difficulty. **Pregnancy/breast-feeding precautions:** Inform prescriber if you are or intend to be pregnant. Breast-feeding is not recommended.

**Geriatric Considerations:** Because of the risk of orthostatic hypotension and CNS depression, avoid or use with caution in the elderly. Not considered a drug of choice in the elderly.

## Carisoprodol and Aspirin (kar i soe PROE dole & AS pir in)

**U.S. Brand Names** Soma® Compound
**Therapeutic Category** Skeletal Muscle Relaxant
**Pregnancy Risk Factor** C
**Lactation** Enters breast milk/contraindicated
**Use** Skeletal muscle relaxant
**Formulations** Tablet: Carisoprodol 200 mg and aspirin 325 mg

**Dosing**
**Adults:** Oral: 1 or 2 tablets 4 times/day
**Elderly:** Avoid use in the elderly due to risk of orthostatic hypotension and CNS depression.

**Additional Nursing Issues**
**Physical Assessment:** See individual components listed in Related Information. **Pregnancy risk factor C** - benefits of use should outweigh possible risks. Breast-feeding is contraindicated.

**Patient Information/Instruction:** See individual components listed in Related Information. **Pregnancy/breast-feeding precautions:** Inform prescriber if you are or intend to be pregnant. Do not breast-feed.

**Related Information**
Aspirin *on page 111*
Carisoprodol *on previous page*

## Carisoprodol, Aspirin, and Codeine

(kar i soe PROE dole, AS pir in, and KOE deen)

**U.S. Brand Names** Soma® Compound w/Codeine
**Synonyms** Isobamate
**Therapeutic Category** Skeletal Muscle Relaxant

(Continued)

## Carisoprodol, Aspirin, and Codeine *(Continued)*

**Pregnancy Risk Factor** C

**Lactation** Enters breast milk/contraindicated

**Use** Skeletal muscle relaxant

**Formulations** Tablet: Carisoprodol 200 mg, aspirin 325 mg, and codeine phosphate 16 mg

**Dosing**

**Adults:** Oral: 1 or 2 tablets 4 times/day

**Elderly:** Avoid use in the elderly due to the risk of orthostatic hypotension and CNS depression.

**Additional Nursing Issues**

**Physical Assessment:** See individual components listed in Related Information. **Pregnancy risk factor C** - benefits of use should outweigh possible risks. Breast-feeding is contraindicated.

**Patient Information/Instruction:** See individual components listed in Related Information. **Pregnancy/breast-feeding precautions:** Inform prescriber if you are or intend to be pregnant. Do not breast-feed.

**Additional Information** Some formulations may contain sulfites.

**Related Information**

Aspirin *on page 111*
Carisoprodol *on page 202*
Codeine *on page 299*

♦ **Carmol-HC® Topical Cream** *see page 1306*
♦ **Carmol® Topical [OTC]** *see* Urea *on page 1193*

## Carmustine (kar MUS teen)

**U.S. Brand Names** BiCNU®

**Synonyms** BCNU

**Therapeutic Category** Antineoplastic Agent, Alkylating Agent

**Pregnancy Risk Factor** D

**Lactation** Excretion in breast milk unknown/contraindicated

**Use** Treatment of brain tumors, multiple myeloma, Hodgkin's disease and non-Hodgkin's lymphomas, melanoma, lung cancer, colon cancer

**Mechanism of Action/Effect** Interferes with the normal function of DNA by alkylation and cross-linking the strands of DNA, and by possible protein modification

**Contraindications** Hypersensitivity to carmustine or any component; myelosuppression from previous chemotherapy or other causes; pregnancy

**Warnings** The U.S. Food and Drug Administration (FDA) currently recommends that procedures for proper handling and disposal of antineoplastic agents be considered. Administer with caution to patients with depressed platelet, leukocyte or erythrocyte counts, renal or hepatic impairment. Bone marrow depression, notably thrombocytopenia and leukopenia, may lead to bleeding and overwhelming infections in an already compromised patient. Will last for at least 6 weeks after a dose, do not give courses more frequently than every 6 weeks because the toxicity is cumulative.

**Drug Interactions**

**Increased Effect/Toxicity:** Carmustine given in combination with cimetidine is reported to cause bone marrow depression. Carmustine given in combination with etoposide is reported to cause severe hepatic dysfunction with hyperbilirubinemia, ascites, and thrombocytopenia.

**Adverse Reactions**

>10%:

Cardiovascular: Hypotension is associated with **high-dose** administration secondary to the high alcohol content of the diluent

Central nervous system: Dizziness and ataxia

Dermatologic: Hyperpigmentation of skin

Gastrointestinal: Nausea and vomiting occur within 2-4 hours after drug injection; dose-related

Emetic potential:

<200 mg: Moderately high (60% to 90%)

≥200 mg: High (>90%)

Time course of nausea/vomiting: Onset: 2-6 hours; Duration: 4-6 hours

Hematologic: Myelosuppressive: Delayed, occurs 4-6 weeks after administration and is dose-related; usually persists for 1-2 weeks; thrombocytopenia is usually more severe than leukopenia. Myelofibrosis and preleukemic syndromes have been reported.

WBC: Moderate

Platelets: Severe

Onset (days): 14

Nadir (days): 21-35

Recovery (days): 42-50

Local: Burning at injection site

**Irritant chemotherapy:** Pain at injection site

Ocular: Ocular toxicity, and retinal hemorrhages

1% to 10%:

Dermatologic: Facial flushing is probably due to the ethanol used in reconstitution, alopecia

Gastrointestinal: Stomatitis, diarrhea, anorexia

Hematologic: Anemia

<1% (Limited to important or life-threatening symptoms): Reversible toxicity; increased LFTs in 20%; fibrosis occurs mostly in patients treated with prolonged total doses >1400 mg/m$^2$ or with bone marrow transplantation doses; risk factors include a history of lung disease, concomitant bleomycin, or radiation therapy; PFTs should be conducted prior to therapy and monitored; patients with predicted FVC or DLCO <70% are at a higher risk; azotemia; decrease in kidney size; renal failure

**BMT:**

Cardiovascular: Hypotension (infusion-related), arrhythmias (infusion-related)

Central nervous system: Encephalopathy, ethanol intoxication, seizures, fever

Endocrine & metabolic: Hyperprolactinemia and hypothyroidism in patients with brain tumors treated with radiation

Gastrointestinal: Severe nausea and vomiting

Hepatic Hepatitis, hepatic veno-occlusive disease

Pulmonary: Dyspnea

**Overdose/Toxicology** Symptoms of overdose include nausea, vomiting, thrombocytopenia, and leukopenia. Treatment is symptomatic and supportive.

**Pharmacodynamics/Kinetics**

**Distribution:** Readily crosses the blood-brain barrier producing CSF levels equal to 15% to 70% of blood plasma levels

**Half-life Elimination:** Biphasic: Initial: 1.4 minutes; Secondary: 20 minutes (active metabolites may persist for days and have a plasma half-life of 67 hours)

**Metabolism:** Rapid

**Excretion:** Urine

**Formulations** Powder for injection: 100 mg/vial packaged with 3 mL of absolute alcohol for use as a sterile diluent

**Dosing**

**Adults:** I.V. (refer to individual protocols): 80 mg/m$^2$ for 3 days every 6-8 weeks; 75-200 mg/m$^2$ every 6-8 weeks

High dose BMT: I.V.: 300-600 mg/m$^2$ infused over at least 2 hours; may be divided into two doses administered every 12 hours; maximum single-dose agent: 1200 mg/m$^2$; generally combined with other high-dose chemotherapeutic drugs.

**Elderly:** Refer to adult dosing.

**Hepatic Impairment:** Dosage adjustment may be necessary; however, no specific guidelines are available.

**Administration**

**I.V.:** Irritant (alcohol-based diluent). Significant absorption to PVC containers - should be administered in either glass or Excel® container. Infusion of drug over 1 hour is recommended.

High-dose carmustine: Maximum rate of infusion ≤3 mg/m$^2$/minute to avoid excessive flushing, agitation, and hypotension. Infusions should run over at least 2 hours.

**Fatal doses if not followed by bone marrow or peripheral stem cell infusions.**

**I.V. Detail:** To minimize severe burning, vein irritation, flushing of the skin, and suffusion of conjunctiva.

**Extravasation management:** Elevate extremity. Inject long-acting dexamethasone (Decadron® LA) or by hyaluronidase (Wydase®) throughout tissue with a 25- to 37-gauge needle. Apply warm, moist compresses.

**BMT only:** Vital signs must be monitored frequently during the infusion of high-dose carmustine. Carmustine 100 mg must be dissolved in absolute ethanol 3 mL diluent provided by the manufacturer.

**BMT only:** Patients receiving high-dose carmustine must be supine and may require the Trendelenburg position, fluid support, and vasopressor support.

Administration of carmustine 300, 450, and 600 mg/m$^2$ respectively, delivers ethanol 11, 17, and 23 g/m$^2$ I.V. Infusion-related cardiovascular effects are primarily due to concomitant ethanol and acetaldehyde. Use with great caution in patients with aldehyde dehydrogenase-2 deficiency or history of "alcohol flushing syndrome". Acute lung injury tends to occur 1-3 months following carmustine infusion. Patients must be counseled to contact their BMT physician for dyspnea, cough, or fever following carmustine. Acute lung injury is managed with a course of corticosteroids.

**Stability**

**Storage:** Store intact vials under refrigeration; vials are stable for 7 days at room temperature.

**Reconstitution:** Initially dilute with 3 mL of absolute alcohol diluent. Further dilute with 27 mL SWI to result in a concentration of 3.3 mg/mL with 10% ethanol. Initial solutions are stable for 8 hours at room temperature (25°C) and 24 hours at refrigeration (2°C to 8°C) and protected from light. Further dilution in $D_5W$ or NS is stable for 8 hours at room temperature (25°C) and 48 hours at refrigeration (4°C) in glass or Excel® protected from light.

**Standard I.V. dilution:** Dose/150-500 mL $D_5W$ or NS

Must use glass or Excel® containers for administration. Protect from light. Stable for 8 hours at room temperature (25°C) and 48 hours under refrigeration (4°C).

**Compatibility:** Incompatible with sodium bicarbonate. Compatible with cisplatin. See the Chemotherapy Compatibility Chart *on page 1311.*

**Monitoring Laboratory Tests** CBC with differential, platelet count, pulmonary function, liver and renal function

**Additional Nursing Issues**

**Physical Assessment:** Closely monitor infusion site for extravasation; acute cellulitis may occur. Assess vital signs, cardiac status, respiratory status, CNS status, fluid

(Continued)

## Carmustine *(Continued)*

balance, and laboratory reports prior to beginning each infusion and periodically during therapy (see Warnings/Precautions and Adverse Reactions). Administer antiemetic prior to therapy. Assess for and teach adverse reactions to report and appropriate comfort interventions. **Pregnancy risk factor D** - assess knowledge/teach appropriate use of barrier contraceptives. Breast-feeding is contraindicated.

**Patient Information/Instruction:** This drug can only be administered by infusion. Limit oral intake for 4-6 hours before therapy. Do not use of alcohol, aspirin-containing products, and OTC medications without consulting prescriber. It is important to maintain adequate nutrition and hydration during therapy (2-3 L/day of fluids unless instructed to restrict fluid intake); frequent small meals may help. Take 2-3 L/day of fluids. You may experience nausea or vomiting (frequent small meals, frequent mouth care, sucking lozenges, or chewing gum may help). If this is ineffective, consult prescriber for antiemetic medication. You may experience loss of hair (reversible). You will be more susceptible to infection (avoid crowds and exposure to infection as much as possible). You will be more sensitive to sunlight; use sunblock, wear protective clothing and dark glasses, or avoid direct exposure to sunlight. Frequent mouth care with soft toothbrush or cotton swabs and frequent mouth rinses may help relieve mouth sores. Report fever, chills, unusual bruising or bleeding, signs of infection, excessive fatigue, yellowing of eyes or skin, or change in color of urine or stool. **Pregnancy/breast-feeding precautions:** Do not get pregnant while taking this medication, use appropriate barrier contraceptive measures. Do not breast-feed.

- **Carnotprim Primperan®** *see* Metoclopramide *on page 758*
- **Carnotprim Primperan® Retard** *see* Metoclopramide *on page 758*

## Carteolol (KAR tee oh lole)

**U.S. Brand Names** Cartrol® Oral; Ocupress® Ophthalmic

**Therapeutic Category** Beta Blocker (with Intrinsic Sympathomimetic Activity); Ophthalmic Agent, Antiglaucoma

**Pregnancy Risk Factor** C/D (2nd and 3rd trimesters)

**Lactation** Excretion in breast milk unknown/use caution

**Use**

Oral: Management of hypertension

Ophthalmic: Treatment of chronic open-angle glaucoma and intraocular hypertension

**Mechanism of Action/Effect** Blocks both beta$_1$- and beta$_2$-receptors and has mild intrinsic sympathomimetic activity; has negative inotropic and chronotropic effects and can significantly slow A-V nodal conduction

**Contraindications** Hypersensitivity to betaxolol or any component; bronchial asthma; sinus bradycardia; second and third degree A-V block; cardiac failure (unless a functioning pacemaker present); cardiogenic shock; pregnancy (2nd and 3rd trimesters)

**Warnings** Some products contain sulfites which can cause allergic reactions. Diminished response over time. May increase muscle weakness. Use with a miotic in angle-closure glaucoma. Use with caution in patients with decreased renal or hepatic function (dosage adjustment required) or patients with a history of asthma, congestive heart failure, or bradycardia. Severe CNS, cardiovascular, and respiratory adverse effects have been seen following ophthalmic use. Use with caution in diabetics. Beta-blockers may impair glucose tolerance, potentiate hypoglycemia, and/or mask symptoms or hypoglycemia in a diabetic patient. Pregnancy factor C/D (2nd and 3rd trimesters).

**Drug Interactions**

**Decreased Effect:** Decreased effect of beta-blockers with aluminum salts, barbiturates, calcium salts, cholestyramine, colestipol, NSAIDs, penicillins (ampicillin), rifampin, salicylates, and sulfinpyrazone due to decreased bioavailability and plasma levels. Beta-blockers may decrease the effect of sulfonylureas (possibly hyperglycemia).

**Increased Effect/Toxicity:** Increased effect/toxicity of beta-blockers with calcium blockers (diltiazem, felodipine, nicardipine). Beta-blockers may increase the effect/toxicity of catecholamine-depleting drugs (reserpine) resulting in hypotension or bradycardia; flecainide, haloperidol (hypotensive effects), hydralazine, phenothiazines, acetaminophen, clonidine (hypertensive crisis after or during withdrawal of either agent), epinephrine (initial hypertensive episode followed by bradycardia), nifedipine and verapamil lidocaine, ergots (peripheral ischemia). Beta-blockers may affect the action or levels of ethanol, disopyramide, nondepolarizing muscle relaxants and theophylline although the effects are difficult to predict. May increase response to insulin.

**Adverse Reactions**

**Ophthalmic:**

>10%: Ocular: Conjunctival hyperemia

1% to 10%:

Ocular: Anisocoria, corneal punctate keratitis, corneal staining, decreased corneal sensitivity, eye pain, vision disturbances

**Systemic:**

>10%:

Central nervous system: Drowsiness, insomnia

Endocrine & metabolic: Decreased sexual ability

1% to 10%:

Cardiovascular: Bradycardia, palpitations, edema, congestive heart failure, reduced peripheral circulation

Central nervous system: Mental depression

Gastrointestinal: Diarrhea or constipation, nausea, vomiting, stomach discomfort

Respiratory: Bronchospasm

Miscellaneous: Cold extremities

<1% (Limited to important or life-threatening symptoms): Chest pain, arrhythmias, orthostatic hypotension, nervousness, headache, depression, hallucinations, confusion (especially in the elderly), psoriasiform eruption, itching, polyuria, thrombocytopenia, leukopenia, shortness of breath

**Overdose/Toxicology** Symptoms of intoxication include cardiac disturbances, CNS toxicity, bronchospasm, hypoglycemia, and hyperkalemia. The most common cardiac symptoms include hypotension and bradycardia. Atrioventricular block, intraventricular conduction disturbances, cardiogenic shock, and asystole may occur with severe overdose, especially with membrane-depressant drugs (eg, propranolol). CNS effects include convulsions, coma, and respiratory arrest (commonly seen with propranolol and other membrane-depressant and lipid-soluble drugs). Treatment is symptomatic and supportive.

**Pharmacodynamics/Kinetics**

**Protein Binding:** 23% to 30%

**Half-life Elimination:** 6 hours

**Metabolism:** 30% to 50%

**Excretion:** Renally excreted metabolites

**Onset:** Onset of effect: Oral: 1-1.5 hours; Peak effect: 2 hours

**Duration:** 12 hours

**Formulations**

Carteolol hydrochloride:

Solution, ophthalmic (Ocupress®): 1% (5 mL, 10 mL)

Tablet (Cartrol®): 2.5 mg, 5 mg

**Dosing**

**Adults:**

Oral: 2.5 mg as a single daily dose, with a maintenance dose normally 2.5-5 mg once daily; maximum daily dose: 10 mg; doses >10 mg do not increase response and may in fact decrease effect

Ophthalmic: Instill 1 drop in affected eye(s) twice daily

**Elderly:** Refer to adult dosing.

**Renal Impairment:** Oral:

$Cl_{cr}$ >60 mL/minute/1.73 $m^2$: Administer every 24 hours.

$Cl_{cr}$ 20-60 mL/minute/1.73 $m^2$: Administer every 48 hours.

$Cl_{cr}$ <20 mL/minute/1.73 $m^2$: Administer every 72 hours.

**Administration**

**Oral:** Take with meals.

**Other:** Ophthalmic: Intended for twice daily dosing. Keep eye open and do not blink for 30 seconds after instillation. Wear sunglasses to avoid photophobic discomfort. Apply gentle pressure to lacrimal sac during and immediately following instillation (1 minute).

**Additional Nursing Issues**

**Physical Assessment:** Assess effects and interactions with other medications patient may be taking (see Drug Interactions).

Oral: Assess blood pressure and heart rate prior to and following first doses and any change in dosage. Monitor or advise patient to monitor weight and fluid balance (I & O). Assess for signs of CHF (eg, edema, new cough or dyspnea, unresolved fatigue) and assess therapeutic effectiveness. Monitor serum glucose levels of diabetic patients since beta-blockers may alter glucose tolerance. Use/teach postural hypotension precautions.

Ophthalmic: Instruct patient on appropriate instillation.

**Pregnancy risk factor C/D** - benefits of use should outweigh possible risks. Note breast-feeding caution.

**Patient Information/Instruction:**

Oral: Take exactly as directed. Do not increase, decrease, or adjust dosage without consulting prescriber. Take pulse daily, prior to medication; follow prescriber's instruction about holding medication. Do not take with antacids and avoid alcohol or OTC medications (eg, cold remedies) without consulting prescriber. If diabetic, monitor serum blood glucose closely (may alter glucose tolerance or mask signs of hypoglycemia). May cause fatigue, dizziness, or postural hypotension; use caution when changing position from lying or sitting to standing, when driving, or climbing stairs until response to medication is known. May cause alteration in sexual performance (reversible). Report unresolved swelling of extremities, difficulty breathing or new cough, unresolved fatigue, unusual weight gain, unresolved constipation, or unusual muscle weakness. **Pregnancy/breast-feeding precautions:** Inform prescriber if you are or intend to be pregnant. Consult prescriber if breast-feeding.

Ophthalmic: Wash hands before instilling. Sit or lie down to instill. Open eye, look at ceiling, and instill prescribed amount of medication. Close eye and apply gentle pressure to inner corner of eye. Do not let tip of applicator touch eye or contaminate tip of applicator. Temporary stinging or burning may occur. Report persistent pain, burning, vision disturbances, swelling, itching, or worsening of condition.

**Geriatric Considerations:** Oral: Due to alterations in the beta-adrenergic autonomic nervous system, beta-adrenergic blockade may result in less hemodynamic response than seen in younger adults.


- **Carteolol** *see* Ophthalmic Agents, Glaucoma *on page 853*
- **Carter's Little Pills®** *see page 1294*
- **Cartia® XT** *see* Diltiazem *on page 377*
- **Cartrol® Oral** *see* Carteolol *on previous page*

## Carvedilol (KAR ve dil ole)

**U.S. Brand Names** Coreg®

**Therapeutic Category** Alpha-/Beta- Blocker; Beta Blocker, Nonselective

**Pregnancy Risk Factor** C/D (2nd and 3rd trimesters)

**Lactation** Excretion in breast milk unknown/contraindicated

**Use** Management of hypertension; can be used alone or in combination with other agents, especially thiazide-type diuretics

**Unlabeled use:** Clinical trials of carvedilol indicate a potential indication for congestive heart failure, angina pectoris, or idiopathic cardiomyopathy

**Mechanism of Action/Effect** As a racemic mixture, carvedilol has nonselective beta-adrenoreceptor and alpha-adrenergic blocking activity at equal potency. No intrinsic sympathomimetic activity has been documented. Associated effects include reduction of cardiac output, exercise- or beta agonist-induced tachycardia, reduction of reflex orthostatic tachycardia, vasodilation, decreased peripheral vascular resistance (especially in standing position), decreased renal vascular resistance, reduced plasma renin activity, and increased levels of atrial natriuretic peptide.

**Contraindications** Hypersensitivity to carvedilol or any component; uncompensated congestive heart failure (NYHA Class IV); asthma or bronchospastic disease (status asthmaticus may result); cardiogenic shock; severe bradycardia or second or third degree heart block; symptomatic hepatic disease; pregnancy (2nd and 3rd trimesters)

**Warnings** Use with caution in patients with congestive heart failure treated with digitalis, diuretic, or ACE inhibitor since A-V conduction may be slowed. Discontinue therapy if any evidence of liver injury occurs. Use caution in patients with peripheral vascular disease, those undergoing anesthesia, in hyperthyroidism and diabetes mellitus. If no other antihypertensive is tolerated, very small doses may be cautiously used in patients with bronchospastic disease. Abrupt withdrawal of the drug should be avoided, drug should be discontinued over 1-2 weeks. Beta-blockers may impair glucose tolerance, potentiate hypoglycemia, and/or mask signs or symptoms of hypoglycemia in a diabetic patient. Pregnancy factor C/D (2nd and 3rd trimesters).

**Drug Interactions**

**Cytochrome P-450 Effect:** CYP2C, 2C9, and 2D6 enzyme substrate

**Decreased Effect:** Rifampin may reduce the plasma concentration of carvedilol by up to 70%. Decreased effect of beta-blockers has also occurred with aluminum salts, barbiturates, calcium salts, cholestyramine, colestipol, NSAIDs, penicillins (ampicillin), salicylates, and sulfinpyrazone due to decreased bioavailability and plasma levels. Beta-blockers may decrease the effect of sulfonylureas.

**Increased Effect/Toxicity:** Carvedilol may enhance the action of antidiabetic agents, calcium channel blockers, and digoxin. Clonidine and cimetidine increase the effect and AUC of carvedilol, respectively.

**Effects on Lab Values** ↑ hepatic enzymes, BUN, NPN, alkaline phosphatase; ↓ HDL

**Adverse Reactions**

1% to 10%:

- Cardiovascular: Bradycardia, postural hypotension, edema
- Central nervous system: Dizziness, somnolence, insomnia, fatigue
- Gastrointestinal: Diarrhea, abdominal pain
- Neuromuscular & skeletal: Back pain
- Respiratory: Rhinitis, pharyngitis, dyspnea

<1% (Limited to important or life-threatening symptoms): A-V block, extrasystoles, hypertension, hypotension, palpitations, peripheral ischemia, syncope, ataxia, vertigo, depression, nervousness, malaise, decreased male libido, hypercholesterolemia, hyperglycemia, hyperuricemia, constipation, dry mouth, impotence, anemia, leukopenia, hyperbilirubinemia, increased LFTs, paresthesia, myalgia, weakness, asthma, cough, aplastic anemia (only reported when administered with other associated medications)

**Overdose/Toxicology** Symptoms of intoxication include cardiac disturbances, CNS toxicity, bronchospasm, hypoglycemia, and hyperkalemia. The most common cardiac symptoms include hypotension and bradycardia. Atrioventricular block, intraventricular conduction disturbances, cardiogenic shock, and asystole may occur with severe overdose, especially with membrane-depressant drugs (eg, propranolol). CNS effects include convulsions, coma, and respiratory arrest (commonly seen with propranolol and other membrane-depressant and lipid-soluble drugs). Treatment is symptom directed and supportive.

**Pharmacodynamics/Kinetics**

**Half-life Elimination:** 7-10 hours

**Metabolism:** First-pass metabolism; extensively metabolized primarily by aromatic ring oxidation and glucuronidation (2% excreted unchanged); three active metabolites (4-hydroxphenyl metabolite is 13 times more potent than parent drug); plasma concentrations in the elderly and those with cirrhotic liver disease are 50% and 4-7 times higher, respectively

**Excretion:** Primarily via bile into feces

**Onset:** 1-2 hours

**Formulations** Tablet: 6.25 mg, 12.5 mg, 25 mg

**Dosing**

**Adults:** Oral:

Hypertension: 6.25 mg twice daily; if tolerated, dose should be maintained for 1-2 weeks, then increased to 12.5 mg twice daily. Dosage may be increased to a maximum of 25 mg twice daily after 1-2 weeks. Reduce dosage if heart rate drops to <55 beats/minute.

Congestive heart failure: Dosage must be individualized, and adjustment of other heart failure medications may be necessary. Initial: 3.125 mg twice daily for 2 weeks; if tolerated, may be increased to 6.25 mg twice daily. Thereafter, the dose may be increased by doubling the dose every 2 weeks to the highest dose tolerated by the patient. Patients should be observed for 1 hour after the initial dose of each dosage increase to assess lightheadedness or dizziness. The maximum dose in patients <85 kg is 25 mg twice daily, in patients >85 kg the maximum dose is 50 mg twice daily. Doses should be taken with food to slow absorption. (Prior to initiation, other heart failure medications should be stabilized)

Angina pectoris: 25-50 mg twice daily

**Note:** Minimize risk of bradycardia with initiation of treatment with a low dose, slow upward titration, and administration with food. Full antihypertensive effect is usually seen within 7-14 days.

**Elderly:** Refer to adult dosing.

**Hepatic Impairment:** Use is contraindicated in liver dysfunction.

**Administration**

**Oral:** Take with food.

**Monitoring Laboratory Tests** Renal studies, BUN, liver function

**Additional Nursing Issues**

**Physical Assessment:** Assess effects and interactions with other medications patient may be taking (see Drug Interactions). Assess blood pressure and heart rate prior to and following first doses and any change in dosage. Monitor or advise patient to monitor weight and fluid balance (I & O). Assess for signs of CHF (eg, edema, new cough or dyspnea, unresolved fatigue) and assess therapeutic effectiveness (eg, hypertension, reduction of angina). Monitor serum glucose levels of diabetic patients closely since beta-blockers may alter glucose tolerance. Use/teach postural hypotension precautions. **Pregnancy risk factor C/D** - benefits of use should outweigh possible risks. Breast-feeding is contraindicated.

**Patient Information/Instruction:** Take exactly as directed. Do not increase, decrease, or adjust dosage without consulting prescriber. Take pulse daily, prior to medication; follow prescriber's instruction about holding medication. Do not take with antacids and avoid alcohol or OTC medications (eg, cold remedies) without consulting prescriber. If diabetic, monitor serum glucose closely (may alter glucose tolerance or mask signs of hypoglycemia). May cause fatigue, dizziness, or postural hypotension; use caution when changing position from lying or sitting to standing, when driving, or climbing stairs until response to medication is known. May cause alteration in sexual performance (reversible). Report unresolved swelling of extremities, difficulty breathing or new cough, unresolved fatigue, unusual weight gain, unresolved constipation, or unusual muscle weakness. **Pregnancy/breast-feeding precautions:** Inform prescriber if you are or intend to be pregnant. Do not breast-feed.

**Geriatric Considerations:** Due to alterations in the beta-adrenergic autonomic nervous system, beta-adrenergic blockade may result in less hemodynamic response than seen in younger adults.

**Related Information**

Beta-Blockers Comparison *on page 1376*

## Cascara Sagrada (kas KAR a sah GRAH dah)

**Therapeutic Category** Laxative, Stimulant

**Pregnancy Risk Factor** C

**Lactation** Enters breast milk/use caution - see Breast-feeding Issues. (AAP rates "compatible")

**Use** Temporary relief of constipation; sometimes used with milk of magnesia ("black and white" mixture)

**Mechanism of Action/Effect** Direct chemical irritation of the intestinal mucosa resulting in an increased rate of colonic motility and change in fluid and electrolyte secretion

**Contraindications** Nausea; vomiting; abdominal pain; fecal impaction; intestinal obstruction; GI bleeding; appendicitis; congestive heart failure

**Warnings** Excessive use can lead to electrolyte imbalance, fluid imbalance, vitamin deficiency, steatorrhea, osteomalacia, cathartic colon, and dependence. Pregnancy factor C.

**Drug Interactions**

**Decreased Effect:** Decreased effect of oral anticoagulants.

**Effects on Lab Values** ↓ calcium (S), potassium (S)

**Adverse Reactions** 1% to 10%:

Central nervous system: Faintness

Endocrine & metabolic: Electrolyte and fluid imbalance

Gastrointestinal: Abdominal cramps, nausea, diarrhea

Genitourinary: Discoloration of urine (reddish pink or brown)

**Pharmacodynamics/Kinetics**

**Metabolism:** Liver

**Onset:** 6-10 hours

**Formulations**

Aromatic fluid extract: 120 mL, 473 mL

Tablet: 325 mg

**Dosing**

**Adults: Note:** Cascara sagrada fluid extract is 5 times more potent than cascara sagrada aromatic fluid extract.

Oral (aromatic fluid extract): 5 mL/day (range: 2-6 mL) as needed at bedtime (1 tablet as needed at bedtime)

(Continued)

## Cascara Sagrada *(Continued)*

**Elderly:** Refer to adult dosing.

**Additional Nursing Issues**

**Physical Assessment:** Identify cause of constipation if possible. Assess for abdominal distention, bowel sounds, abdominal pain. Assess for cramping, rectal pain, rectal bleeding, nausea, vomiting; discontinue if these symptoms occur. Monitor fluid status - evaluate I & O ratio. Monitor for electrolyte imbalance (eg, muscle cramps, pain, weakness, dizziness, excessive thirst). **Pregnancy risk factor C** - benefits of use should outweigh possible risks. Note breast-feeding caution.

**Patient Information/Instruction:** Take with water on an empty stomach for better absorption. Do not take within 1 hour of antacids, milk, or cimetidine. Evacuation will usually occur 6-12 hours after taking. Cascara should not be used regularly for more than 1 week. A regular toileting routine, adequate fluids, regular exercise, and a diet that includes roughage and bulk will help to prevent constipation. May discolor urine (black/brown). **Pregnancy/breast-feeding precautions:** Inform prescriber if you are or intend to be pregnant. Consult prescriber if breast-feeding.

**Geriatric Considerations:** Elderly are often predisposed to constipation due to disease, immobility, drugs, low residue diets, and a decreased "thirst reflex" with age. Avoid stimulant cathartic use on a chronic basis if possible. Use osmotic, lubricant, stool softeners, and bulk agents as prophylaxis. Patients should be instructed for proper dietary fiber and fluid intake as well as regular exercise. Monitor closely for fluid/electrolyte imbalance, CNS signs of fluid/electrolyte loss, and hypotension.

**Breast-feeding Issues:** Cascara sagrada should be avoided if nursing because it may have a laxative effect on the infant.

**Related Information**

Laxatives: Classification and Properties Comparison *on page 1392*

- **Casodex®** *see* Bicalutamide *on page 153*
- **Castor Oil** *see page 1294*
- **Cataflam® Oral** *see* Diclofenac *on page 358*
- **Catapresan-100®** *see* Clonidine *on page 289*
- **Catapres® Oral** *see* Clonidine *on page 289*
- **Catapres-TTS® Transdermal** *see* Clonidine *on page 289*
- **Cauteridol®** *see* Ranitidine *on page 1008*
- **Caverject® Injection** *see* Alprostadil *on page 56*
- **CBDCA** *see* Carboplatin *on page 199*
- **CCNU** *see* Lomustine *on page 686*
- **C-Crystals® [OTC]** *see* Ascorbic Acid *on page 108*
- **2-CdA** *see* Cladribine *on page 278*
- **CDDP** *see* Cisplatin *on page 273*
- **Cebid® Timecelles® [OTC]** *see* Ascorbic Acid *on page 108*
- **Ceclor®** *see* Cefaclor *on this page*
- **Ceclor® CD** *see* Cefaclor *on this page*
- **Cecon® [OTC]** *see* Ascorbic Acid *on page 108*
- **Cedax®** *see* Ceftibuten *on page 229*
- **Cedocard®-SR** *see* Isosorbide Dinitrate *on page 634*
- **CeeNU®** *see* Lomustine *on page 686*
- **Ceepryn®** *see page 1294*

## Cefaclor (SEF a klor)

**U.S. Brand Names** Ceclor®; Ceclor® CD

**Therapeutic Category** Antibiotic, Cephalosporin (Second Generation)

**Pregnancy Risk Factor** B

**Lactation** Enters breast milk (small amounts)/use caution

**Use** Infections caused by susceptible organisms including *Staphylococcus aureus* and *H. influenzae*; treatment of otitis media, sinusitis, and infections involving the respiratory tract, skin and skin structure, bone and joint, and urinary tract

**Mechanism of Action/Effect** Inhibits bacterial cell wall synthesis by binding to one or more of the penicillin-binding proteins (PBPs)

**Contraindications** Hypersensitivity to cefaclor, any component, other cephalosporins, or penicillins

**Warnings** Modify dosage in patients with severe renal impairment. Prolonged use may result in superinfection. Cross-sensitivity to penicillins exists (~10%).

**Drug Interactions**

**Increased Effect/Toxicity:** Probenecid may decrease cephalosporin elimination. Furosemide, aminoglycosides when taken with cefaclor may result in additive nephrotoxicity. Bleeding may occur when administered with anticoagulants.

**Food Interactions** Cefaclor serum levels may be decreased if taken with food.

**Effects on Lab Values** Positive Coombs' [direct], false-positive urine glucose (Clinitest®)

**Adverse Reactions**

1% to 10%:

Gastrointestinal: Diarrhea (1.5%)

Hematologic: Eosinophilia (2%)

Hepatic: Elevated transaminases (2.5%)

Dermatologic: Rash (maculopapular, erythematous, or morbilliform) (1% to 1.5%)

<1% (Limited to important or life-threatening symptoms): Anaphylaxis, urticaria, pruritus, angioedema, serum-sickness, arthralgia, hepatitis, cholestatic jaundice, Stevens-

Johnson syndrome, nausea, vomiting, pseudomembranous colitis, vaginitis, hemolytic anemia, neutropenia, interstitial nephritis, CNS irritability, hyperactivity, agitation, nervousness, insomnia, confusion, dizziness, hallucinations, somnolence, seizures, prolonged PT

Reactions reported with other cephalosporins include fever, abdominal pain, superinfection, renal dysfunction, toxic nephropathy, hemorrhage, cholestasis

**Overdose/Toxicology** Symptoms of overdose include neuromuscular hypersensitivity and convulsions. Many beta-lactam containing antibiotics have the potential to cause neuromuscular hyperirritability or convulsive seizures. Hemodialysis may be helpful to aid in removal of the drug from blood; otherwise, treatment is supportive or symptom directed.

**Pharmacodynamics/Kinetics**

**Protein Binding:** 25%

**Distribution:** Crosses the placenta

**Half-life Elimination:** 0.5-1 hour (prolonged in renal impairment)

**Time to Peak:** Capsule: 60 minutes; Suspension: 45 minutes

**Metabolism:** Partially

**Excretion:** Urine

**Formulations**

Capsule: 250 mg, 500 mg

Powder for oral suspension (strawberry flavor): 125 mg/5 mL (75 mL, 150 mL); 187 mg/5 mL (50 mL, 100 mL); 250 mg/5 mL (75 mL, 150 mL); 375 mg/5 mL (50 mL, 100 mL)

Tablet, extended release: 375 mg, 500 mg

**Dosing**

**Adults:** Oral: 250-500 mg every 8 hours or daily dose can be given in 2 divided doses

**Elderly:** Refer to adult dosing.

**Renal Impairment:**

$Cl_{cr}$ <50 mL/minute: Administer 50% of dose.

Moderately dialyzable (20% to 50%)

**Administration**

**Oral:** Administer around-the-clock to promote less variation in peak and trough serum levels. Shake well for oral suspension.

**Stability**

**Reconstitution:** Refrigerate suspension after reconstitution. Discard after 14 days. Do not freeze.

**Monitoring Laboratory Tests** AST (SGOT), ALT (SGPT), CBC, bilirubin, LDH, alkaline phosphatase, Coombs' test monthly if on long-term therapy; perform culture and sensitivity studies prior to initiating drug therapy.

**Additional Nursing Issues**

**Physical Assessment:** Assess for previous history of reactions to other cephalosporins or penicillins. Monitor for adverse reactions (see above); these can occur a few days after therapy is initiated. Assess for potential nephrotoxicity (see Drug Interactions). Assess bowel function (if severe diarrhea occurs, discontinue drug). Monitor urine output (if decreased, notify prescriber). Assess for opportunistic infection (eg, fever, malaise, rash, diarrhea, itching, fever, chills, or increased cough). Note breast-feeding caution.

**Patient Information/Instruction:** Take as directed, at regular intervals around-the-clock (with or without food). Chilling oral suspension improves flavor (do not freeze). Do not chew or crush extended release tablets. Complete full course of medication, even if you feel better. Drink 2-3 L fluid/day. Small frequent meals, frequent mouth care, sucking lozenges, or chewing gum may reduce nausea or vomiting. If diarrhea occurs, yogurt or buttermilk may help. May cause false-positive test with Clinitest®; use another form of testing. May interfere with oral contraceptives; additional contraceptive measures are necessary. Report severe, unresolved diarrhea; vaginal itching or drainage; sores in mouth; blood, pus, or mucus in stool or urine; easy bleeding or bruising; unusual fever or chills; rash; or respiratory difficulty. **Breast-feeding precautions:** Consult prescriber if breast-feeding.

**Breast-feeding Issues:** Theoretically, drug absorbed by nursing infant may change bowel flora or affect fever work-up result. **Note:** As a class, cephalosporins are used to treat infections in infants.

## Cefadroxil (sef a DROKS il)

**U.S. Brand Names** Duricef®; Ultracef®

**Therapeutic Category** Antibiotic, Cephalosporin (First Generation)

**Pregnancy Risk Factor** B

**Lactation** Enters breast milk (small amounts)/use caution (AAP rates "compatible")

**Use** Treatment of susceptible bacterial infections, including those caused by group A beta-hemolytic *Streptococcus*

**Mechanism of Action/Effect** Inhibits bacterial cell wall synthesis by binding to one or more of the penicillin-binding proteins (PBPs)

**Contraindications** Hypersensitivity to cefadroxil or other cephalosporins

**Warnings** Modify dosage in patients with severe renal impairment. Prolonged use may result in superinfection. Cross-sensitivity to penicillins exists (~10%).

**Drug Interactions**

**Increased Effect/Toxicity:** Bleeding may occur when administered with anticoagulants.

**Effects on Lab Values** Positive Coombs' [direct], glucose, protein; ↓ glucose

(Continued)

## Cefadroxil *(Continued)*

**Adverse Reactions**

1% to 10%: Gastrointestinal: Diarrhea

<1% (Limited to important or life-threatening symptoms): Anaphylaxis, rash (maculopapular and erythematous), erythema multiforme, Stevens-Johnson syndrome, serum sickness, arthralgia, urticaria, pruritus, angioedema, pseudomembranous colitis, abdominal pain, dyspepsia, nausea, vomiting, elevated transaminases, cholestasis, vaginitis, neutropenia, agranulocytosis, thrombocytopenia, fever

Reactions reported with other cephalosporins include toxic epidermal necrolysis, abdominal pain, superinfection, renal dysfunction, toxic nephropathy, aplastic anemia, hemolytic anemia, hemorrhage, prolonged prothrombin time, increased BUN, increased creatinine, eosinophilia, pancytopenia, seizures

**Overdose/Toxicology** Symptoms of overdose include neuromuscular hypersensitivity and convulsions. Many beta-lactam containing antibiotics have the potential to cause neuromuscular hyperirritability or convulsive seizures. Hemodialysis may be helpful to aid in removal of the drug from blood; otherwise, treatment is supportive or symptom directed.

**Pharmacodynamics/Kinetics**

**Protein Binding:** 20%

**Distribution:** Crosses the placenta

**Half-life Elimination:** 1-2 hours; 20-24 hours in renal failure

**Time to Peak:** Within 70-90 minutes

**Excretion:** Urine

**Formulations**

Cefadroxil monohydrate:

Capsule: 500 mg

Suspension, oral: 125 mg/5 mL, 250 mg/5 mL, 500 mg/5 mL (50 mL, 100 mL)

Tablet: 1 g

**Dosing**

**Adults:** Oral: 1-2 g/day in 2 divided doses

**Elderly:** Refer to adult dosing.

**Renal Impairment:**

$Cl_{cr}$ 10-25 mL/minute: Administer every 24 hours.

$Cl_{cr}$ <10 mL/minute: Administer every 36 hours.

**Administration**

**Oral:** Administer around-the-clock to promote less variation in peak and trough serum levels.

**Stability**

**Reconstitution:** Refrigerate suspension after reconstitution. Discard after 14 days.

**Monitoring Laboratory Tests** AST (SGOT), ALT (SGPT), CBC, bilirubin, LDH, alkaline phosphatase, Coombs' test monthly if on long-term therapy; perform culture and sensitivity studies prior to initiating drug therapy.

**Additional Nursing Issues**

**Physical Assessment:** Assess for previous history of reactions to other cephalosporins or penicillins. Monitor for allergic reactions (see above); these can occur a few days after therapy is initiated. Assess for potential nephrotoxicity (see Drug Interactions). Assess bowel function (if severe diarrhea occurs, discontinue drug). Monitor urine output (if decreased, notify prescriber). Assess for opportunistic infection (eg, fever, malaise, rash, diarrhea, itching, redness, fever, chills, or increased cough). Note breast-feeding caution.

**Patient Information/Instruction:** Take as directed, at regular intervals around-the-clock (with or without food). Chilling oral suspension improves flavor (do not freeze). Complete full course of medication, even if you feel better. Drink 2-3 L fluid/day. If diarrhea occurs, yogurt or buttermilk may help. May cause false-positive test with Clinitest®; use another form of testing. May interfere with oral contraceptives; additional contraceptive measures are necessary. Report severe, unresolved diarrhea; vaginal itching or drainage; sores in mouth; blood, pus, or mucus in stool or urine; easy bleeding or bruising; unusual fever or chills; rash; or respiratory difficulty. **Breast-feeding precautions:** Consult prescriber if breast-feeding.

**Geriatric Considerations:** Adjust dose for renal function in the elderly.

**Breast-feeding Issues:** Theoretically, drug absorbed by nursing infant may change bowel flora or affect fever work-up result. **Note:** As a class, cephalosporins are used to treat infections in infants.

♦ **Cefadyl®** *see* Cephapirin *on page 238*

## Cefamandole (sef a MAN dole)

**U.S. Brand Names** Mandol®

**Therapeutic Category** Antibiotic, Cephalosporin (Second Generation)

**Pregnancy Risk Factor** B

**Lactation** Enters breast milk/use caution

**Use** Treatment of susceptible bacterial infection; mainly respiratory tract, skin and skin structure, bone and joint, urinary tract and gynecologic, as well as, septicemia

**Mechanism of Action/Effect** Inhibits bacterial cell wall synthesis by binding to one or more of the penicillin-binding proteins (PBPs)

**Contraindications** Hypersensitivity to cefamandole nafate, any component, or other cephalosporins

**Warnings** Modify dosage in patients with severe renal impairment. Prolonged use may result in superinfection. Cross-sensitivity to penicillins exists (~10%). Hypoprothrombinemia has been reported rarely which is promptly reversed by vitamin K administration. Episodes more commonly occur in the elderly or medically compromised patients who may have a vitamin K deficiency. Monitor PT in these patients.

**Drug Interactions**

**Increased Effect/Toxicity:** Disulfiram-like reaction has been reported when taken within 72 hours of alcohol consumption. Increased cefamandole plasma levels when taken with probenecid. Aminoglycosides, furosemide when taken with cefamandole may increased nephrotoxicity. Increase in hypoprothrombinemic effect with warfarin or heparin and cefamandole.

**Effects on Lab Values** ↑ alkaline phosphatase, AST, ALT, BUN, creatinine, prothrombin time (S), glucose, protein; ↓ glucose; positive Coombs' [direct]

**Adverse Reactions** Contains MTT side chain which may lead to increased risk of hypoprothrombinemia and bleeding.

1% to 10%:

Gastrointestinal: Diarrhea

Local: Thrombophlebitis

<1% (Limited to important or life-threatening symptoms): Anaphylaxis, rash (maculopapular and erythematous), urticaria, pseudomembranous colitis, nausea, vomiting, elevated transaminases, cholestasis, eosinophilia, neutropenia, thrombocytopenia, increased BUN, increased creatinine, fever, prolonged PT

Reactions reported with other cephalosporins include toxic epidermal necrolysis, Stevens-Johnson syndrome, abdominal pain, superinfection, renal dysfunction, toxic nephropathy, aplastic anemia, hemolytic anemia, hemorrhage, pancytopenia, vaginitis, seizures

**Overdose/Toxicology** Symptoms of overdose include neuromuscular hypersensitivity, and convulsions. Many beta-lactam containing antibiotics have the potential to cause neuromuscular hyperirritability or convulsive seizures. Hemodialysis may be helpful to aid in removal of the drug from blood; otherwise, treatment is supportive or symptom directed.

**Pharmacodynamics/Kinetics**

**Protein Binding:** 56% to 78%

**Distribution:** Distributes well throughout body, except CSF; poor penetration even with inflamed meninges; extensive enterohepatic circulation; high concentrations in the bile

**Half-life Elimination:** 30-60 minutes (prolonged in renal impairment)

**Time to Peak:** I.M.: Within 1-2 hours; I.V.: Within 10 minutes

**Excretion:** Urine and bile

**Formulations** Powder for injection, as nafate: 500 mg (10 mL); 1 g (10 mL, 100 mL); 2 g (20 mL, 100 mL); 10 g (100 mL)

**Dosing**

**Adults:** I.M., I.V.: 4-12 g/24 hours divided every 4-6 hours or 500-1000 mg every 4-8 hours; maximum: 2 g/dose

**Elderly:** Refer to adult dosing.

**Renal Impairment:**

$Cl_{cr}$ 50-80 mL/minute: Administer 750-2000 mg every 6 hours.

$Cl_{cr}$ 25-50 mL/minute: Administer 750-2000 mg every 8 hours.

$Cl_{cr}$ 10-25 mL/minute: Administer 500-1250 mg every 8 hours or 1 g every 6 hours.

$Cl_{cr}$ 2-10 mL/minute: Administer 500-1000 mg every 12 hours.

$Cl_{cr}$ <2 mL/minute: Administer 250-750 mg every 12 hours.

Moderately dialyzable (20% to 50%)

**Administration**

**I.M.:** Inject deep I.M. into large muscle mass.

**I.V.:** Inject direct I.V. over 3-5 minutes. Infuse intermittent infusion over 15-30 minutes.

**Stability**

**Reconstitution:** After reconstitution, $CO_2$ gas is liberated which allows solution to be withdrawn without injecting air. Solution is stable for 24 hours at room temperature and 96 hours when refrigerated. For I.V., infusion in NS and $D_5W$ is stable for 24 hours at room temperature, 1 week when refrigerated, or 26 weeks when frozen.

**Compatibility:** Discontinue other solutions at the same site to avoid compatibility problems.

**Monitoring Laboratory Tests** Prothrombin times; perform culture and sensitivity studies prior to initiating drug therapy.

**Additional Nursing Issues**

**Physical Assessment:** Assess for previous history of reactions to other cephalosporins or penicillins. Monitor for allergic reactions (see above). These can occur a few days after therapy is initiated. Assess for potential nephrotoxicity (see Drug Interactions). Assess bowel function (if severe diarrhea occurs, discontinue drug). Monitor urine output (if decreased, notify prescriber). Assess for opportunistic infection (eg, fever, malaise, rash, diarrhea, itching, redness, fever, chills, or increased cough). Note breast-feeding caution.

**Patient Information/Instruction:** This medication is administered I.M. or I.V. Drink 2-3 L fluid/day. Avoid alcohol during therapy and for 72 hours after last dose (may cause severe disulfiram-like reactions). If diarrhea occurs, yogurt or buttermilk may help. May cause false-positive test with Clinitest®; use another form of testing. May interfere with oral contraceptives; additional contraceptive measures are necessary. Report severe, unresolved diarrhea; vaginal itching or drainage; sores in mouth; blood, pus, or mucus

(Continued)

## Cefamandole *(Continued)*

in stool or urine; easy bleeding or bruising; unusual fever or chills; rash; or respiratory difficulty. **Breast-feeding precautions:** Consult prescriber if breast-feeding.

**Geriatric Considerations:** The risk of coagulation abnormalities (increased PT) limits the use of cefamandole in the elderly. Adjust dose for renal function in the elderly.

**Breast-feeding Issues:** Theoretically, drug absorbed by nursing infant may change bowel flora or affect fever work-up result. **Note:** As a class, cephalosporins are used to treat infections in infants.

**Additional Information** Each gram contains 3.3 mEq of sodium.

- **Cefamezin** *see* Cefazolin *on this page*
- **Cefamox** *see* Cefadroxil *on page 211*
- **Cefaxim** *see* Cefotaxime *on page 221*
- **Cefaxona** *see* Ceftriaxone *on page 232*

## Cefazolin (sef A zoe lin)

**U.S. Brand Names** Ancef®; Kefzol®; Zolicef®

**Therapeutic Category** Antibiotic, Cephalosporin (First Generation)

**Pregnancy Risk Factor** B

**Lactation** Enters breast milk (small amounts)/use caution (AAP rates "compatible")

**Use** Treatment of gram-positive bacilli and cocci (except enterococcus); some gram-negative bacilli including *E. coli*, *Proteus*, and *Klebsiella* may be susceptible

**Mechanism of Action/Effect** Inhibits bacterial cell wall synthesis by binding to one or more of the penicillin-binding proteins (PBPs)

**Contraindications** Hypersensitivity to cefazolin sodium, any component, or other cephalosporins

**Warnings** Modify dosage in patients with severe renal impairment. Prolonged use may result in superinfection. Cross-sensitivity to penicillins exists (~10%).

**Drug Interactions**

**Increased Effect/Toxicity:** High-dose probenecid decreases clearance and increases effect of cefazolin. Aminoglycosides increase nephrotoxic potential when taken with cefazolin.

**Effects on Lab Values** False-positive urine glucose using Clinitest®, positive Coombs' [direct], false increase serum or urine creatinine

**Adverse Reactions**

1% to 10%:

Gastrointestinal: Diarrhea

Local: Pain at injection site

<1% (Limited to important or life-threatening symptoms): Anaphylaxis, rash, pruritus, Stevens-Johnson syndrome, oral candidiasis, nausea, vomiting, abdominal cramps, anorexia, pseudomembranous colitis, eosinophilia, neutropenia, leukopenia, thrombocytopenia, thrombocytosis, elevated transaminases, phlebitis, vaginitis, fever, seizures

Other reactions with cephalosporins include toxic epidermal necrolysis, abdominal pain, cholestasis, superinfection, renal dysfunction, toxic nephropathy, aplastic anemia, hemolytic anemia, hemorrhage, prolonged prothrombin time, pancytopenia

**Overdose/Toxicology** Symptoms of overdose include neuromuscular hypersensitivity and convulsions. Many beta-lactam containing antibiotics have the potential to cause neuromuscular hyperirritability or convulsive seizures. Hemodialysis may be helpful to aid in the removal of drug from blood; otherwise, treatment is supportive or symptom directed.

**Pharmacodynamics/Kinetics**

**Protein Binding:** 74% to 86%

**Distribution:** Crosses the placenta; CSF penetration is poor

**Half-life Elimination:** 90-150 minutes (prolonged in renal impairment); End-stage renal disease: 40-70 hours

**Time to Peak:** I.M.: Within 0.5-2 hours; I.V.: Within 5 minutes

**Metabolism:** Hepatic is minimal

**Excretion:** Urine

**Formulations**

Cefazolin sodium:

Infusion, premixed in $D_5W$ (frozen) (Ancef®): 500 mg (50 mL); 1 g (50 mL)

Injection (Kefzol®): 500 mg, 1 g

Powder for injection (Ancef®, Zolicef®): 250 mg, 500 mg, 1 g, 5 g, 10 g, 20 g

**Dosing**

**Adults:** I.M., I.V.: 1-2 g every 8 hours, depending on severity of infection; maximum: 12 g/day

**Elderly:** Refer to adult dosing.

**Renal Impairment:**

$Cl_{cr}$ 10-30 mL/minute: Administer every 12 hours.

$Cl_{cr}$ <10 mL/minute: Administer every 24 hours.

Moderately dialyzable (20% to 50%); administer dose postdialysis or administer supplemental dose of 0.5-1 g after dialysis.

Peritoneal dialysis: Administer 0.5 g every 12 hours.

Continuous arteriovenous or venovenous hemofiltration (CAVH/CAVHD): Dose as for $Cl_{cr}$ 10-30 ml/min. Removes 30 mg of cefazolin per liter of filtrate per day.

**Administration**

**I.M.:** Inject deep I.M. into large muscle mass.

**I.V.:** Inject direct I.V. over 5 minutes. Infuse intermittent infusion over 30-60 minutes.

**Stability**

**Storage:** Store intact vials at room temperature and protect from temperatures exceeding 40°C. Protection from light is recommended for the powder and for the reconstituted solutions.

**Reconstitution:** Reconstituted solutions of cefazolin are light yellow to yellow. Reconstituted solutions are stable for 24 hours at room temperature and 10 days under refrigeration. Stability of parenteral admixture at room temperature (25°C) is 48 hours. Stability of parenteral admixture at refrigeration temperature (4°C) is 14 days.

Standard diluent: 1 g/50 mL $D_5W$; 2 g/50 mL $D_5W$

**Compatibility:** Discontinue other solutions at the same site to avoid compatibility problems. See the Compatibility of Drugs Chart *on page 1315.*

**Monitoring Laboratory Tests** Prothrombin times; perform culture and sensitivity studies prior to initiating drug therapy.

**Additional Nursing Issues**

**Physical Assessment:** Assess for previous history of reactions to other cephalosporins or penicillins. Monitor for allergic reactions (see above). These can occur a few days after therapy is initiated. Assess for potential nephrotoxicity (see Drug Interactions). Assess bowel function (if severe diarrhea occurs, discontinue drug). Monitor urine output (if decreased, notify prescriber). Assess for opportunistic infection (eg, fever, malaise, rash, diarrhea, itching, redness, fever, chills, or increased cough). Note breast-feeding caution.

**Patient Information/Instruction:** This drug is administered I.V. or I.M. Drink 2-3 L fluid/day. If diarrhea occurs, yogurt or buttermilk may help. May cause false-positive test with Clinitest®; use another form of testing. May interfere with oral contraceptives; additional contraceptive measures are necessary. Report severe, unresolved diarrhea; vaginal itching or drainage; sores in mouth; blood, pus, or mucus in stool or urine; easy bleeding or bruising; unusual fever or chills; rash; or respiratory difficulty. **Breast-feeding precautions:** Consult prescriber if breast-feeding.

**Geriatric Considerations:** Adjust dose for renal function.

**Breast-feeding Issues:** Theoretically, drug absorbed by nursing infant may change bowel flora or affect fever work-up result. **Note:** As a class, cephalosporins are used to treat infections in infants.

**Additional Information**

Each gram contains 2 mEq of sodium.

pH: 4.5-6

## Cefepime (SEF e pim)

**U.S. Brand Names** Maxipime®

**Therapeutic Category** Antibiotic, Cephalosporin (Fourth Generation)

**Pregnancy Risk Factor** B

**Lactation** Enters breast milk/use caution

**Use** Treatment of respiratory tract infections (including bronchitis and pneumonia), cellulitis and other skin and soft tissue infections, and urinary tract infections; considered a fourth generation cephalosporin because it has good gram-negative coverage similar to third generation cephalosporins, but better gram-positive coverage; complicated intra-abdominal infections (combination with metronidazole)

**Mechanism of Action/Effect** Inhibits bacterial cell wall synthesis by binding to one or more of the penicillin-binding proteins (PBPs)

**Contraindications** Hypersensitivity to cefepime, any component, or other cephalosporins

**Warnings** Modify dosage in patients with severe renal impairment. Prolonged use may result in superinfection. Cross-sensitivity to penicillins exists (~10%).

**Drug Interactions**

**Increased Effect/Toxicity:** High-dose probenecid decreases clearance and increases effect of cefepime. Aminoglycosides increase nephrotoxic potential when taken with cefepime.

**Effects on Lab Values** As with other cephalosporins; false-positive Coombs' test; may falsely elevate creatinine values when Jaffé reaction is used; may cause false-positive results in urine glucose tests when using cupric sulfate (Benedict's solution, Clinitest®), false-positive urinary proteins and steroids

**Adverse Reactions**

>10%: Hematologic: Positive Coombs' test without hemolysis

1% to 10%:

Dermatologic: Rash, pruritus

Gastrointestinal: : Diarrhea, nausea, vomiting

Central nervous system: Fever (1%), headache (1%)

Local: Pain, erythema at injection site

<1% (Limited to important or life-threatening symptoms): Leukopenia, neutropenia, agranulocytosis, thrombocytopenia, myoclonus, seizures, encephalopathy, neuromuscular excitability

Other reactions with cephalosporins include toxic epidermal necrolysis, Stevens-Johnson syndrome, erythema multiforme, renal dysfunction, toxic nephropathy, aplastic anemia, hemolytic anemia, hemorrhage, prolonged PT, pancytopenia, vaginitis, superinfection

**Overdose/Toxicology** Symptoms of overdose include neuromuscular hypersensitivity and convulsions. Many beta-lactam containing antibiotics have the potential to cause

(Continued)

## Cefepime *(Continued)*

neuromuscular hyperirritability or convulsive seizures. Hemodialysis may be helpful to aid in removal of the drug from blood; otherwise, treatment is supportive and symptom directed.

**Pharmacodynamics/Kinetics**

**Protein Binding:** Plasma: 16% to 19%

**Distribution:** Penetrates into inflammatory fluid at concentrations ~80% of serum levels and into bronchial mucosa at levels ~60% of those reached in the plasma

**Half-life Elimination:** 2 hours (prolonged in renal impairment)

**Metabolism:** Very little

**Excretion:** Urine

**Formulations** Powder for injection, as hydrochloride: 500 mg, 1 g, 2 g

**Dosing**

**Adults:** I.V., I.M.:

Most infections: 1-2 g every 12 hours for 5-10 days; higher doses or more frequent administration may be required in pseudomonal infections

Urinary tract infections, uncomplicated: 500 mg every 12 hours

**Elderly:** I.V., I.M.: Should be based on renal function and severity of infection.

**Renal Impairment:**

$Cl_{cr}$ 10-30 mL/minute: Administer 500 mg every 24 hours.

$Cl_{cr}$ <10 mL/minute: Administer 250 mg every 24 hours.

Hemodialysis effects: Removed by dialysis; administer supplemental dose of 250 mg after each dialysis session.

Peritoneal dialysis effects: Removed to a lesser extent than hemodialysis; administer 250 mg every 48 hours.

Continuous a-v hemofiltration: Dose as $Cl_{cr}$ >30 mL/minute.

**Administration**

**I.M.:** Inject deep I.M. into large muscle mass.

**I.V.:** Inject direct I.V. over 5 minutes. Infuse intermittent infusion over 30-60 minutes.

**Stability**

**Compatibility:** Discontinue other solutions at the same site to avoid compatibility problems.

**Monitoring Laboratory Tests** Prothrombin times; perform culture and sensitivity studies prior to initiating drug therapy.

**Additional Nursing Issues**

**Physical Assessment:** Assess for previous history of reactions to other cephalosporins or penicillins. Monitor for allergic reactions (see above). These can occur a few days after therapy is initiated. Assess for potential nephfotoxicity (see Drug Interactions). Assess bowel function (if severe diarrhea occurs, discontinue drug). Monitor urine output (if decreased, notify prescriber). Assess for opportunistic infection (eg, fever, malaise, rash, diarrhea, itching, redness, fever, chills, or increased cough). Note breast-feeding caution.

**Patient Information/Instruction:** This drug is administered I.V. or I.M. Drink 2-3 L fluid/day. If diarrhea occurs, yogurt or buttermilk may help. May cause false-positive test with Clinitest®; use another form of testing. May interfere with oral contraceptives; additional contraceptive measures are necessary. Report severe, unresolved diarrhea; vaginal itching or drainage; sores in mouth; blood, pus, or mucus in stool or urine; easy bleeding or bruising; unusual fever or chills; rash; or respiratory difficulty. **Breast-feeding precautions:** Consult prescriber if breast-feeding.

**Geriatric Considerations:** Adjust dose for changes in renal function.

**Breast-feeding Issues:** Theoretically, drug absorbed by nursing infant may change bowel flora or affect fever work-up result. **Note:** As a class, cephalosporins are used to treat infections in infants.

**Additional Information**

Each gram contains 2 mEq of sodium.

pH: 4-6

## Cefixime (sef IKS eem)

**U.S. Brand Names** Suprax®

**Therapeutic Category** Antibiotic, Cephalosporin (Third Generation)

**Pregnancy Risk Factor** B

**Lactation** Excretion in breast milk unknown/use caution

**Use** Treatment of urinary tract infections, otitis media, respiratory infection due to susceptible organisms including *S. pneumoniae* and *pyogenes*, *H. influenzae*, *M. catarrhalis*, and many *Enterobacteriaceae*; documented poor compliance with other oral antimicrobials; outpatient therapy of serious soft tissue or skeletal infections due to susceptible organisms; single-dose oral treatment of uncomplicated cervical/urethral gonorrhea due to *N. gonorrhoeae*; treatment of shigellosis in areas with a high rate of resistance to TMP-SMX

**Mechanism of Action/Effect** Inhibits bacterial cell wall synthesis by binding to one or more of the penicillin-binding proteins (PBPs)

**Contraindications** Hypersensitivity to cefixime or other cephalosporins

**Warnings** Cross-sensitivity to penicillins exists (~10%).

**Drug Interactions**

**Increased Effect/Toxicity:** Probenecid increases cefixime concentration. Cefixime may increase carbamazepine.

**Effects on Lab Values** False-positive reaction for urine glucose using Clinitest®; false-positive urine ketones using tests with nitroprusside

**Adverse Reactions**

>10%: Gastrointestinal: Diarrhea (16%)

1% to 10%: Gastrointestinal: Abdominal pain, nausea, dyspepsia, flatulence

<1% (Limited to important or life-threatening symptoms): Rash, urticaria, pruritus, erythema multiforme, Stevens-Johnson syndrome, serum sickness -like reaction, fever, vomiting, pseudomembranous colitis, transaminase elevations, increased BUN, increased creatinine, headache, dizziness, thrombocytopenia, leukopenia, eosinophilia, prolonged PT, vaginitis, candidiasis

Other reactions with cephalosporins include anaphylaxis, seizures, toxic epidermal necrolysis, renal dysfunction, toxic nephropathy, interstitial nephritis, cholestasis, aplastic anemia, hemolytic anemia, hemorrhage, pancytopenia, neutropenia, agranulocytosis, colitis, superinfection

**Overdose/Toxicology** Symptoms of overdose include neuromuscular hypersensitivity and convulsions. Many beta-lactam containing antibiotics have the potential to cause neuromuscular hyperirritability or convulsive seizures. Hemodialysis may be helpful to aid in the removal of drug from blood; otherwise, treatment is supportive or symptom directed.

**Pharmacodynamics/Kinetics**

**Protein Binding:** 65%

**Distribution:** Into bile, sputum, middle ear discharge; crosses the placenta

**Half-life Elimination:** Normal renal function: 3-4 hours; Renal failure: Up to 11.5 hours

**Time to Peak:** Within 2-6 hours; peak serum concentrations are 15% to 50% higher for the oral suspension versus tablets

**Excretion:** Urine

**Formulations**

Powder for oral suspension (strawberry flavor): 100 mg/5 mL (50 mL, 100 mL)

Tablet, film coated: 200 mg, 400 mg

**Dosing**

**Adults:** Oral:

400 mg/day divided every 12-24 hours

Uncomplicated cervical/urethral gonorrhea due to *N. gonorrhoeae*: 400 mg as a single dose

**Elderly:** Refer to adult dosing.

**Renal Impairment:**

$Cl_{cr}$ 21-60 mL/minute: Administer 75% of the standard dose.

$Cl_{cr}$ <20 mL/minute: Administer 50% of the standard dose.

10% removed by hemodialysis

**Administration**

**Oral:** Oral: Shake well or oral suspension before use. May be administered with or without food. Administer with food to decrease GI distress.

**Stability**

**Reconstitution:** After reconstitution, suspension may be stored for 14 days at room temperature.

**Monitoring Laboratory Tests** Prothrombin times; perform culture and sensitivity studies prior to initiating drug therapy.

**Additional Nursing Issues**

**Physical Assessment:** Assess for previous history of reactions to other cephalosporins or penicillins. Monitor for allergic reactions (see above). These can occur a few days after therapy is initiated. Assess for potential nephrotoxicity (see Drug Interactions). Assess bowel function (if severe diarrhea occurs, discontinue drug). Monitor urine output (if decreased, notify prescriber). Assess for opportunistic infection (eg, fever, malaise, rash, diarrhea, itching, redness, fever, chills, or increased cough). Note breast-feeding caution.

**Patient Information/Instruction:** Take as directed, at regular intervals around-the-clock (with or without food). Chilling oral suspension improves flavor (do not freeze). Complete full course of medication, even if you feel better. Drink 2-3 L fluid/day. If diarrhea occurs, yogurt or buttermilk may help. May cause false-positive test with Clinitest®; use another form of testing. May interfere with oral contraceptives; additional contraceptive measures are necessary. Report severe, unresolved diarrhea; vaginal itching or drainage; sores in mouth; blood, pus, or mucus in stool or urine; easy bleeding or bruising; unusual fever or chills,; rash; or respiratory difficulty. **Breast-feeding precautions:** Consult prescriber if breast-feeding.

**Geriatric Considerations:** Adjust dose for renal function.

**Breast-feeding Issues:** Theoretically, drug absorbed by nursing infant may change bowel flora or affect fever work-up result. **Note:** As a class, cephalosporins are used to treat infections in infants.

**Other Issues:** Otitis media should be treated with the suspension since it results in higher peak blood levels than the tablet.

♦ **Cefizox®** *see* Ceftizoxime *on page 231*

## Cefmetazole (sef MET a zole)

**U.S. Brand Names** Zefazone®

**Therapeutic Category** Antibiotic, Cephalosporin (Second Generation)

**Pregnancy Risk Factor** B

**Lactation** Excretion in breast milk unknown/use caution

**Use** Second generation cephalosporin with an antibacterial spectrum similar to cefoxitin, useful on many aerobic and anaerobic gram-positive and gram-negative bacteria

(Continued)

## Cefmetazole *(Continued)*

**Mechanism of Action/Effect** Inhibits bacterial cell wall synthesis by binding to one or more of the penicillin-binding proteins (PBPs)

**Contraindications** Hypersensitivity to cefmetazole, any component, or other cephalosporins

**Warnings** Cross-sensitivity to penicillins exists (~10%).

**Drug Interactions**

**Increased Effect/Toxicity:** Probenecid may decrease cephalosporin elimination. Furosemide, aminoglycosides in combination with cefmetazole may result in additive nephrotoxicity.

**Effects on Lab Values** May cause false-positive Coombs' test, false-positive results in urine glucose tests when using cupric sulfate (Benedict's solution, Clinitest®), urinary 17-ketosteroids.

**Adverse Reactions** Contains MTT side chain which may lead to increased risk of hypoprothrombinemia and bleeding.

1% to 10%:
- Dermatologic: Rash
- Gastrointestinal: Diarrhea

<1% (Limited to important or life-threatening symptoms): Pain at injection site, phlebitis, pseudomembranous colitis, epigastric pain, candidiasis, bleeding, shock, hypotension, headache, hot flashes, dyspnea, epistaxis, respiratory distress, fever, vaginitis

Other reactions with cephalosporins include anaphylaxis, seizures, toxic epidermal necrolysis, erythema multiforme, Stevens-Johnson syndrome, renal dysfunction, interstitial nephritis, toxic nephropathy, cholestasis, aplastic anemia, hemolytic anemia, hemorrhage, pancytopenia, neutropenia, agranulocytosis, colitis, superinfection

**Overdose/Toxicology** Symptoms of overdose include neuromuscular hypersensitivity and convulsions. Many beta-lactams containing antibiotics have the potential to cause neuromuscular hyperirritability or convulsive seizures. Hemodialysis may be helpful to aid in removal of the drug from blood; otherwise, treatment is supportive or symptom directed.

**Pharmacodynamics/Kinetics**

**Protein Binding:** 65%

**Half-life Elimination:** 72 minutes (prolonged in renal impairment)

**Metabolism:** <15%

**Excretion:** Renal

**Formulations** Powder for injection, as sodium: 1 g, 2 g

**Dosing**

**Adults:** I.V.:

Infections: 2 g every 6-12 hours for 5-14 days

Prophylaxis: 2 g 30-90 minutes before surgery **or** 1 g 30-90 minutes before surgery; repeat 8 and 16 hours later

**Elderly:** Refer to adult dosing.

**Renal Impairment:**

$Cl_{cr}$ >50 mL/minute: Administer every 16 hours.

$Cl_{cr}$ 10-50 mL/minute: Administer every 24 hours.

$Cl_{cr}$ <10 mL/minute: Administer every 48 hours.

**Administration**

**I.M.:** Inject deep I.M. into large muscle mass.

**I.V.:** Inject direct I.V. over 3-5 minutes. Infuse intermittent infusion over 15-30 minutes.

**Stability**

**Reconstitution:** Reconstituted solution and I.V. infusion in NS or $D_5W$ solution are stable for 24 hours at room temperature, 7 days when refrigerated, or 6 weeks when frozen. After freezing, thawed solution is stable for 24 hours at room temperature or 7 days when refrigerated.

**Compatibility:** Discontinue other solutions at the same site to avoid compatibility problems.

**Monitoring Laboratory Tests** Prothrombin times; perform culture and sensitivity studies prior to initiating drug therapy.

**Additional Nursing Issues**

**Physical Assessment:** Assess for previous history of reactions to other cephalosporins or penicillins. Monitor for allergic reactions (see above). These can occur a few days after therapy is initiated. Assess for potential nephrotoxicity (see Drug Interactions). Assess bowel function (if severe diarrhea occurs, discontinue drug). Monitor urine output (if decreased, notify prescriber). Assess for opportunistic infection (eg, fever, malaise, rash, diarrhea, itching, redness, fever, chills, or increased cough). Note breast-feeding caution.

**Patient Information/Instruction:** This drug is administered I.V. or I.M. Drink 2-3 L fluid/day. Avoid alcohol during therapy and for 72 hours after last dose (may cause severe disulfiram-like reactions). If diarrhea occurs, yogurt or buttermilk may help. May cause false-positive test with Clinitest®; use another form of testing. May interfere with oral contraceptives; additional contraceptive measures are necessary. Report severe, unresolved diarrhea; vaginal itching or drainage; sores in mouth; blood, pus, or mucus in stool or urine; easy bleeding or bruising; unusual fever or chills; rash; or respiratory difficulty. **Breast-feeding precautions:** Consult prescriber if breast-feeding.

**Geriatric Considerations:** Cefmetazole has not been studied in the elderly. Adjust dose for renal function.

**Breast-feeding Issues:** Theoretically, drug absorbed by nursing infant may change bowel flora or affect fever work-up result. **Note:** As a class, cephalosporins are used to treat infections in infants.

**Additional Information**

Each gram contains 2 mEq of sodium.

pH: 4.2-6.2

- **Cefobid®** *see* Cefoperazone *on next page*
- **Cefoclin** *see* Cefotaxime *on page 221*
- **Cefol® Filmtab®** *see* Vitamin, Multiple *on page 1219*

## Cefonicid (se FON i sid)

**U.S. Brand Names** Monocid®

**Therapeutic Category** Antibiotic, Cephalosporin (Second Generation)

**Pregnancy Risk Factor** B

**Lactation** Enters breast milk (small amounts)/use caution

**Use** Treatment of susceptible bacterial infection; mainly respiratory tract, skin and skin structure, bone and joint, urinary tract and gynecologic, as well as, septicemia; second generation cephalosporin

**Mechanism of Action/Effect** Inhibits bacterial cell wall synthesis by binding to one or more of the penicillin-binding proteins (PBPs)

**Contraindications** Hypersensitivity to cefonicid sodium, any component, or other cephalosporins

**Warnings** Cross-sensitivity to penicillins exists (~10%).

**Drug Interactions**

**Increased Effect/Toxicity:** Probenecid may decrease cephalosporin elimination. Furosemide, aminoglycosides in combination with cefonicid may result in additive nephrotoxicity.

**Effects on Lab Values** May cause false-positive Coombs' test, false-positive results in urine glucose tests when using cupric sulfate (Benedict's solution, Clinitest®), urinary 17-ketosteroids.

**Adverse Reactions**

1% to 10%:

Hematologic: Increased eosinophils (2.9%), increased platelets (1.7%)

Hepatic: Altered liver function tests (increased transaminases, LDH, alkaline phosphatase) (1.6%)

Local: Pain, burning at injection site (5.7%)

<1% (Limited to important or life-threatening symptoms): Fever, rash, pruritus, erythema, anaphylactoid reactions, diarrhea, pseudomembranous colitis, abdominal pain, increased transaminases, increased BUN, increased creatinine, interstitial nephritis, neutropenia, decreased WBC, thrombocytopenia

Other reactions with cephalosporins include anaphylaxis, seizures, Stevens-Johnson syndrome, toxic epidermal necrolysis, renal dysfunction, toxic nephropathy, cholestasis, aplastic anemia, hemolytic anemia, hemorrhage, pancytopenia, agranulocytosis, colitis, superinfection

**Overdose/Toxicology** Symptoms of overdose include neuromuscular hypersensitivity and convulsions. Many beta-lactam containing antibiotics have the potential to cause neuromuscular hyperirritability or convulsive seizures. Hemodialysis may be helpful to aid in the removal of drug from blood; otherwise, treatment is supportive or symptom directed.

**Pharmacodynamics/Kinetics**

**Protein Binding:** 98%

**Half-life Elimination:** 6-7 hours (prolonged in renal impairment)

**Metabolism:** None

**Excretion:** Renal

**Formulations** Powder for injection, as sodium: 500 mg, 1 g, 10 g

**Dosing**

**Adults:**

I.M., I.V.: 0.5-2 g every 24 hours

Prophylaxis: Preop: 1 g/hour

**Elderly:** Refer to adult dosing.

**Renal Impairment:** See table.

**Cefonicid Sodium**

| $Cl_{cr}$ (mL/min/1.73 $m^2$) | Dose (mg/kg) for each dosing interval |
|---|---|
| 60-79 | 10-24 q24h |
| 40-59 | 8-20 q24h |
| 20-39 | 4-15 q24h |
| 10-19 | 4-15 q48h |
| 5-9 | 4-15 q3-5d |
| <5 | 3-4 q3-5d |

(Continued)

## Cefonicid *(Continued)*

**Administration**

**I.M.:** Inject deep I.M. into large muscle mass.

**I.V.:** Inject direct I.V. over 3-5 minutes. Infuse intermittent infusion over 30 minutes.

**Stability**

**Reconstitution:** Reconstituted solution and I.V. infusion in NS or $D_5W$ solution are stable for 24 hours at room temperature or 72 hours if refrigerated.

**Compatibility:** Discontinue other solutions at the same site to avoid compatibility problems.

**Monitoring Laboratory Tests** Prothrombin times; perform culture and sensitivity studies prior to initiating drug therapy.

**Additional Nursing Issues**

**Physical Assessment:** Assess for previous history of reactions to other cephalosporins or penicillins. Monitor for allergic reactions (see above). These can occur a few days after therapy is initiated. Assess for potential nephrotoxicity (see Drug Interactions). Assess bowel function (if severe diarrhea occurs, discontinue drug). Monitor urine output (if decreased, notify prescriber). Assess for opportunistic infection (eg, fever, malaise, rash, diarrhea, itching, redness, fever, chills, or increased cough). Note breast-feeding caution.

**Patient Information/Instruction:** This medication is administered I.M. or I.V. Drink 2-3 L fluid/day. If diarrhea occurs, yogurt or buttermilk may help. May cause false-positive test with Clinitest®; use another form of testing. May interfere with oral contraceptives; additional contraceptive measures are necessary. Report severe, unresolved diarrhea; vaginal itching or drainage; sores in mouth; blood, pus, or mucus in stool or urine; easy bleeding or bruising; unusual fever or chills; rash; or respiratory difficulty. **Breast-feeding precautions:** Consult prescriber if breast-feeding.

**Geriatric Considerations:** Adjust dose for renal function (estimated $Cl_{cr}$). I.M. administration should be avoided in patients with limited muscle mass.

**Breast-feeding Issues:** Theoretically, drug absorbed by nursing infant may change bowel flora or affect fever work-up result. **Note:** As a class, cephalosporins are used to treat infections in infants.

**Additional Information**

Each gram contains 3.7 mEq of sodium.

pH: 3.5-6.5

## Cefoperazone (sef oh PER a zone)

**U.S. Brand Names** Cefobid®

**Therapeutic Category** Antibiotic, Cephalosporin (Third Generation)

**Pregnancy Risk Factor** B

**Lactation** Enters breast milk (small amounts)/use caution

**Use** Treatment of susceptible bacterial infection; mainly respiratory tract, skin and skin structure, bone and joint, urinary tract and gynecologic, as well as, septicemia

**Mechanism of Action/Effect** Inhibits bacterial cell wall synthesis by binding to one or more of the penicillin-binding proteins (PBPs)

**Contraindications** Hypersensitivity to cefoperazone, any component, or other cephalosporins

**Warnings** Cefoperazone may decrease vitamin K synthesis by suppressing GI flora. Monitor prothrombin time and administer vitamin K as needed. Only reported rarely, especially with cefoperazone and cefamandole. Modify dosage in patients with severe renal impairment. Prolonged use may result in superinfection. Cross-sensitivity to penicillins exists (~10%).

**Drug Interactions**

**Increased Effect/Toxicity:** Probenecid may decrease cephalosporin elimination resulting in increased levels. Furosemide, aminoglycosides in combination with cefoperazone may result in additive nephrotoxicity.

**Effects on Lab Values** May cause false-positive Coombs' test, false-positive results in urine glucose tests when using cupric sulfate (Benedict's solution, Clinitest®), urinary 17-ketosteroids.

**Adverse Reactions** Contains MTT side chain which may lead to increased risk of hypoprothrombinemia and bleeding.

1% to 10%:

- Dermatologic: Rash (maculopapular or erythematous) (2%)
- Gastrointestinal: Diarrhea (3%)
- Hematologic: Decreased neutrophils (2%), decreased hemoglobin or hematocrit (5%), eosinophilia (10%)
- Hepatic: Increased transaminases (5% to 10%)

<1% (Limited to important or life-threatening symptoms): Hypoprothrombinemia, bleeding, pseudomembranous colitis, nausea, vomiting, elevated BUN, elevated creatinine, pain at injection site, induration at injection site, phlebitis, drug fever

Other reactions with cephalosporins include anaphylaxis, seizures, Stevens-Johnson syndrome, toxic epidermal necrolysis, renal dysfunction, toxic nephropathy, cholestasis, aplastic anemia, hemolytic anemia, pancytopenia, agranulocytosis, colitis, superinfection

**Overdose/Toxicology** Symptoms of overdose include neuromuscular hypersensitivity and convulsions. Many beta-lactam containing antibiotics have the potential to cause neuromuscular hyperirritability or convulsive seizures. Hemodialysis may be helpful to aid in removal of the drug from blood; otherwise, treatment is supportive or symptom directed.

**Pharmacodynamics/Kinetics**

**Distribution:** Widely distributed in most body tissues and fluids; highest concentrations in bile; low penetration in CSF; variable when meninges are inflamed; crosses the placenta

**Half-life Elimination:** 2 hours, higher with hepatic disease or biliary obstruction

**Time to Peak:** I.M.: Within 1-2 hours; I.V.: Within 15-20 minutes (serum levels 2-3 times the serum levels following I.M. administration)

**Excretion:** Bile and feces

**Formulations**

Cefoperazone sodium:

Injection, premixed (frozen): 1 g (50 mL); 2 g (50 mL)

Powder for injection: 1 g, 2 g

**Dosing**

**Adults:** I.M., I.V.: 2-4 g/day in divided doses every 12 hours; up to 12 g/day

**Elderly:** Refer to adult dosing.

**Hepatic Impairment:** Reduce dose 50% in patients with advanced liver cirrhosis; maximum daily dose: 4 g.

**Administration**

**I.M.:** Inject deep I.M. into large muscle mass.

**I.V.:** Inject direct I.V. over 3-5 minutes. Infuse intermittent infusion over 30 minutes.

**Stability**

**Reconstitution:** Reconstituted solution and I.V. infusion in NS or $D_5W$ solution are stable for 24 hours at room temperature, 5 days when refrigerated or 3 weeks, when frozen. After freezing, thawed solution is stable for 48 hours at room temperature or 10 days when refrigerated.

**Compatibility:** Discontinue other solutions at the same site to avoid compatibility problems.

**Monitoring Laboratory Tests** Prothrombin times; perform culture and sensitivity studies prior to initiating drug therapy.

**Additional Nursing Issues**

**Physical Assessment:** Assess for previous history of reactions to other cephalosporins or penicillins. Monitor for allergic reactions (see above). These can occur a few days after therapy is initiated. Assess prothrombin time and assess for nephrotoxicity (see Warnings/Precautions and Drug Interactions). Assess bowel function (if severe diarrhea occurs, discontinue drug). Assess for opportunistic infection (eg, fever, malaise, rash, diarrhea, itching, redness, fever, chills, or increased cough). Note breast-feeding caution.

**Patient Information/Instruction:** This drug is administered I.M. or I.V. Drink 2-3 L fluid/day. Avoid alcohol during therapy and for 72 hours after last dose (may cause severe disulfiram-like reactions). If diarrhea occurs, yogurt or buttermilk may help. May cause false-positive test with Clinitest®; use another form of testing. May interfere with oral contraceptives; additional contraceptive measures are necessary. Report severe, unresolved diarrhea; vaginal itching or drainage; sores in mouth; blood, pus, or mucus in stool or urine; easy bleeding or bruising; unusual fever or chills; rash; or respiratory difficulty. **Breast-feeding precautions:** Consult prescriber if breast-feeding.

**Geriatric Considerations:** No dose adjustment necessary for renal impairment.

**Breast-feeding Issues:** Theoretically, drug absorbed by nursing infant may change bowel flora or affect fever work-up result. **Note:** As a class, cephalosporins are used to treat infections in infants.

**Additional Information**

Each gram contains 1.5 mEq of sodium.

pH: 4.5-6.5

♦ **Cefotan®** *see* Cefotetan *on page 223*

## Cefotaxime (sef oh TAKS eem)

**U.S. Brand Names** Claforan®

**Therapeutic Category** Antibiotic, Cephalosporin (Third Generation)

**Pregnancy Risk Factor** B

**Lactation** Enters breast milk/use caution (AAP rates "compatible")

**Use** Treatment of susceptible infection in respiratory tract, skin and skin structure, bone and joint, urinary tract, gynecologic as well as septicemia, and documented or suspected meningitis

**Mechanism of Action/Effect** Inhibits bacterial cell wall synthesis by binding to one or more of the penicillin-binding proteins (PBPs)

**Contraindications** Hypersensitivity to cefotaxime, any component, or other cephalosporins

**Warnings** Modify dosage in patients with severe renal impairment. Prolonged use may result in superinfection. Cross-sensitivity to penicillins exists (~10%).

**Drug Interactions**

**Increased Effect/Toxicity:** Probenecid may decrease cephalosporin elimination resulting in increased levels. Furosemide, aminoglycosides in combination with cefotaxime may result in additive nephrotoxicity.

**Effects on Lab Values** False-positive Coombs' test, false-positive reaction for urine glucose tests using Clinitest® or Benedict's solution, false elevation of creatinine using Jaffé test

**Adverse Reactions**

1% to 10%:

Dermatologic: Rash, pruritus

(Continued)

## Cefotaxime *(Continued)*

Gastrointestinal: Diarrhea, nausea, vomiting, colitis
Local: Pain at injection site

<1% (Limited to important or life-threatening symptoms): Anaphylaxis, urticaria, arrhythmias (after rapid IV injection via central catheter), pseudomembranous colitis, neutropenia, thrombocytopenia, eosinophilia, headache, fever, transaminase elevations, interstitial nephritis, increased BUN, increased creatinine, increased transaminases, phlebitis, candidiasis, vaginitis,

Other reactions with cephalosporins include seizures, Stevens-Johnson syndrome, toxic epidermal necrolysis, renal dysfunction, toxic nephropathy, cholestasis, aplastic anemia, hemolytic anemia, hemorrhage, pancytopenia, agranulocytosis, colitis, superinfection

**Overdose/Toxicology** Symptoms of overdose include neuromuscular hypersensitivity and convulsions. Many beta-lactam containing antibiotics have the potential to cause neuromuscular hyperirritability or convulsive seizures. Hemodialysis may be helpful to aid in removal of the drug from blood; otherwise, treatment is supportive or symptom directed.

**Pharmacodynamics/Kinetics**

**Distribution:** Widely distributed to body tissues and fluids including aqueous humor, ascitic and prostatic fluids, and bone; penetrates CSF when meninges are inflamed; crosses the placenta

**Half-life Elimination:**

Cefotaxime: 1-1.5 hours (prolonged with renal and/or hepatic impairment)
Desacetylcefotaxime: 1.5-1.9 hours (prolonged in renal impairment)

**Time to Peak:** I.M.: Within 30 minutes

**Metabolism:** Liver

**Excretion:** Urine

**Formulations**

Cefotaxime sodium:

Infusion, premixed in $D_5W$ (frozen): 1 g (50 mL); 2 g (50 mL)
Powder for injection: 500 mg, 1 g, 2 g, 10 g

**Dosing**

**Adults:**

Gonorrhea: I.M.: 1 g as a single dose
Uncomplicated infections: I.M., I.V.: 1 g every 12 hours
Moderate/severe infections: I.M., I.V.: 1-2 g every 8 hours
Infections commonly needing higher doses (eg, septicemia): I.V.: 2 g every 6-8 hours
Life-threatening infections: I.V.: 2 g every 4 hours
Preop: I.M., I.V.: 1 g 30-90 minutes before surgery
C-section: 1 g as soon as the umbilical cord is clamped, then 1 g I.M., I.V. at 6- and 12-hours intervals.

**Elderly:** Refer to adult dosing.

**Renal Impairment:**

$Cl_{cr}$ 10-50 mL/minute: Administer every 8-12 hours.
$Cl_{cr}$ <10 mL/minute: Administer every 24 hours.
Moderately dialyzable (20% to 50%)
Continuous a-v hemofiltration (CAVH): 1 gm every 12 hours.

**Hepatic Impairment:** Moderate dosage reduction is recommended in severe liver disease.

**Administration**

**I.M.:** Inject deep I.M. into large muscle mass.

**I.V.:** Inject direct I.V. over 3-5 minutes. Infuse intermittent infusion over 30 minutes.

**Stability**

**Reconstitution:** Reconstituted solution is stable for 24 hours at room temperature and 10 days when refrigerated. For I.V. infusion in NS or $D_5W$, solution is stable for 24 hours at room temperature, 5 days when refrigerated, or 13 weeks when frozen. After freezing, thawed solution is stable for 24 hours at room temperature or 10 days when refrigerated.

**Compatibility:** Discontinue other solutions at the same site to avoid compatibility problems.

**Monitoring Laboratory Tests** Prothrombin times; perform culture and sensitivity studies prior to initiating drug therapy.

**Additional Nursing Issues**

**Physical Assessment:** Assess for previous history of reactions to other cephalosporins or penicillins. Monitor for allergic reactions (see above). These can occur a few days after therapy is initiated. Assess for potential nephrotoxicity (see Drug Interactions). Assess bowel function (if severe diarrhea occurs, discontinue drug). Monitor urine output (if decreased, notify prescriber). Assess for opportunistic infection (eg, fever, malaise, rash, diarrhea, itching, redness, fever, chills, or increased cough). Note breast-feeding caution.

**Patient Information/Instruction:** This medication is administered I.M. or I.V. Drink 2-3 L fluid/day. If diarrhea occurs, yogurt or buttermilk may help. May cause false-positive test with Clinitest®; use another form of testing. May interfere with oral contraceptives; additional contraceptive measures are necessary. Report severe, unresolved diarrhea; vaginal itching or drainage; sores in mouth; blood, pus, or mucus in stool or urine; easy bleeding or bruising; unusual fever or chills; rash; or respiratory difficulty. **Breast-feeding precautions:** Consult prescriber if breast-feeding.

**Geriatric Considerations:** Adjust dose for renal function.

**Breast-feeding Issues:** Theoretically, drug absorbed by nursing infant may change bowel flora or affect fever work-up result. **Note:** As a class, cephalosporins are used to treat infections in infants.

**Additional Information**

Each gram contains 2.2 mEq of sodium.

pH: 5-7.5

## Cefotetan (SEF oh tee tan)

**U.S. Brand Names** Cefotan®

**Therapeutic Category** Antibiotic, Cephalosporin (Second Generation)

**Pregnancy Risk Factor** B

**Lactation** Enters breast milk (small amounts)/use caution

**Use** Treatment of susceptible bacterial infection; mainly respiratory tract, skin and skin structure, bone and joint, urinary tract and gynecologic, as well as, septicemia, similar spectrum to cefoxitin

**Mechanism of Action/Effect** Inhibits bacterial cell wall synthesis by binding to one or more of the penicillin-binding proteins (PBPs)

**Contraindications** Hypersensitivity to cefotetan, any component, or other cephalosporins

**Warnings** Modify dosage in patients with severe renal impairment. Prolonged use may result in superinfection. Cross-sensitivity to penicillins exists (~10%).

**Drug Interactions**

**Increased Effect/Toxicity:** Probenecid may decrease cephalosporin elimination. Furosemide, aminoglycosides in combination with cefotetan may result in additive nephrotoxicity. May cause disulfiram-like reaction with concomitant alcohol use.

**Effects on Lab Values** ↑ alkaline phosphatase, AST, ALT, BUN, creatinine, glucose, protein; ↓ glucose; may cause false-positive Coombs' test, false-positive results in urine glucose tests when using cupric sulfate (Benedict's solution, Clinitest®), urinary 17-ketosteroids.

**Adverse Reactions** Contains MTT side chain which may lead to increased risk of hypoprothrombinemia and bleeding.

1% to 10%:

Gastrointestinal: Diarrhea (1.3%)

Hepatic: Increased transaminases (1.2%)

Miscellaneous: Hypersensitivity reactions (1.2%)

<1% (Limited to important or life-threatening symptoms): Anaphylaxis, urticaria, rash, pruritus, pseudomembranous colitis, nausea, vomiting, eosinophilia, thrombocytosis, agranulocytosis, hemolytic anemia, leukopenia, thrombocytopenia, prolonged PT, bleeding, elevated BUN, elevated creatinine, nephrotoxicity, phlebitis, fever

Other reactions with cephalosporins include: Seizures, Stevens-Johnson syndrome, toxic epidermal necrolysis, renal dysfunction, toxic nephropathy, cholestasis, aplastic anemia, hemolytic anemia, hemorrhage, pancytopenia, agranulocytosis, colitis, superinfection

**Overdose/Toxicology** Symptoms of overdose include neuromuscular hypersensitivity and convulsions. Many beta-lactam containing antibiotics have the potential to cause neuromuscular hyperirritability or convulsive seizures. Hemodialysis may be helpful to aid in removal of the drug from blood; otherwise, treatment is supportive or symptom directed.

**Pharmacodynamics/Kinetics**

**Protein Binding:** 76% to 90%

**Distribution:** Widely distributed to body tissues and fluids including bile, sputum, prostatic and peritoneal fluids; low concentrations enter CSF; crosses the placenta

**Half-life Elimination:** 1.5-3 hours (prolonged in severe renal impairment)

**Time to Peak:** I.M.: Within 1.5-3 hours

**Excretion:** Urine

**Formulations** Powder for injection, as disodium: 1 g (10 mL, 100 mL); 2 g (20 mL, 100 mL); 10 g (100 mL)

**Dosing**

**Adults:** I.M., I.V.: 1-6 g/day in divided doses every 12 hours; 1-2 g may be given every 24 hours for urinary tract infection

**Elderly:** Refer to adult dosing.

**Renal Impairment:**

$Cl_{cr}$ 10-30 mL/minute: Administer every 24 hours.

$Cl_{cr}$ <10 mL/minute: Administer every 48 hours.

Slightly dialyzable (5% to 20%)

Continuous a-v hemofiltration (CAVH): 750 mg every 12 hours.

**Administration**

**I.M.:** Inject deep I.M. into large muscle mass.

**I.V.:** Inject direct I.V. over 3-5 minutes. Infuse intermittent infusion over 30 minutes.

**Stability**

**Reconstitution:** Reconstituted solution is stable for 24 hours at room temperature and 96 hours when refrigerated. For I.V. infusion in NS or $D_5W$ solution and after freezing, thawed solution is stable for 24 hours at room temperature or 96 hours when refrigerated. Frozen solution is stable for 12 weeks.

**Compatibility:** Discontinue other solutions at the same site to avoid compatibility problems.

(Continued)

## Cefotetan *(Continued)*

**Monitoring Laboratory Tests** Prothrombin time; perform culture and sensitivity studies prior to initiating drug therapy.

**Additional Nursing Issues**

**Physical Assessment:** Assess for previous history of reactions to other cephalosporins or penicillins. Monitor for allergic reactions (see above). These can occur a few days after therapy is initiated. Assess for potential nephrotoxicity (see Drug Interactions). Assess bowel function (if severe diarrhea occurs, discontinue drug). Monitor urine output (if decreased, notify prescriber). Assess for opportunistic infection (eg, fever, malaise, rash, diarrhea, itching, redness, fever, chills, or increased cough). Note breast-feeding caution.

**Patient Information/Instruction:** This medication is administered I.V. or I.M. Drink 2-3 L fluid/day. Avoid alcohol during therapy and for 72 hours after last dose (may cause severe disulfiram-like reactions). If diarrhea occurs, yogurt or buttermilk may help. May cause false-positive test with Clinitest®; use another form of testing. May interfere with oral contraceptives; additional contraceptive measures are necessary. Report severe, unresolved diarrhea; vaginal itching or drainage; sores in mouth; blood, pus, or mucus in stool or urine; easy bleeding or bruising; unusual fever or chills; rash; or respiratory difficulty. **Breast-feeding precautions:** Consult prescriber if breast-feeding.

**Geriatric Considerations:** Cefotetan has not been studied in the elderly. Adjust dose for renal function in the elderly.

**Breast-feeding Issues:** Theoretically, drug absorbed by nursing infant may change bowel flora or affect fever work-up result. **Note:** As a class, cephalosporins are used to treat infections in infants.

**Additional Information**

Each gram contains 3.5 mEq of sodium.

pH: 4.5-6.5

## Cefoxitin (se FOKS i tin)

**U.S. Brand Names** Mefoxin®

**Therapeutic Category** Antibiotic, Cephalosporin (Second Generation)

**Pregnancy Risk Factor** B

**Lactation** Enters breast milk (small amounts)/use caution (AAP rates "compatible")

**Use** Less active against staphylococci and streptococci than first generation cephalosporins, but active against anaerobes including *Bacteroides fragilis*; active against gram-negative enteric bacilli including *E. coli*, *Klebsiella*, and *Proteus*; used predominantly for respiratory tract, skin and skin structure, bone and joint, urinary tract and gynecologic as well as septicemia; surgical prophylaxis; intra-abdominal infections and other mixed infections

**Mechanism of Action/Effect** Inhibits bacterial cell wall synthesis by binding to one or more of the penicillin-binding proteins (PBPs)

**Contraindications** Hypersensitivity to cefoxitin, any component, or other cephalosporins

**Warnings** Use with caution in patients with history of colitis. Cefoxitin may increase resistance of organisms by inducing beta-lactamase. Modify dosage in patients with severe renal impairment. Prolonged use may result in superinfection. Cross-sensitivity to penicillins exists (~10%).

**Drug Interactions**

**Increased Effect/Toxicity:** Probenecid may decrease cephalosporin elimination. Furosemide, aminoglycosides in combination with cefoxitin may result in additive nephrotoxicity.

**Effects on Lab Values** ↑ BUN, AST (SGOT), ALT (SGPT), LDH, alkaline phosphatase. May cause falsely elevated serum and urine creatinine concentrations. May cause false-positive Coombs' test, false-positive results in urine glucose tests when using cupric sulfate (Benedict's solution, Clinitest®).

**Adverse Reactions**

1% to 10%: Gastrointestinal: Diarrhea

<1% (Limited to important or life-threatening symptoms): Anaphylaxis, dyspnea, fever, rash, exfoliative dermatitis, toxic epidermal necrolysis, pruritus, angioedema, nausea, hypotension, vomiting, dyspnea, pseudomembranous colitis, phlebitis, interstitial nephritis, increased BUN, increased creatinine, leukopenia, thrombocytopenia, hemolytic anemia, bone marrow suppression, eosinophilia, increased transaminases, jaundice, thrombophlebitis, increased nephrotoxicity (with aminoglycosides), exacerbation of myasthenia gravis, prolonged PT

Other reactions with cephalosporins include: Seizures, Stevens-Johnson syndrome, toxic epidermal necrolysis, erythema multiforme, urticaria, serum-sickness reactions, renal dysfunction, toxic nephropathy, cholestasis, aplastic anemia, hemolytic anemia, hemorrhage, pancytopenia, agranulocytosis, colitis, vaginitis, superinfection

**Overdose/Toxicology** Symptoms of overdose include neuromuscular hypersensitivity and convulsions. Many beta-lactam containing antibiotics have the potential to cause neuromuscular hyperirritability or convulsive seizures. Hemodialysis may be helpful to aid in removal of the drug from blood; otherwise, treatment is supportive or symptom directed.

**Pharmacodynamics/Kinetics**

**Protein Binding:** 65% to 79%

**Distribution:** Widely distributed to body tissues and fluids including pleural, synovial, ascitic fluid, and bile; poorly penetrates into CSF even with inflammation of the meninges; crosses the placenta

**Half-life Elimination:** 45-60 minutes, increases significantly with renal insufficiency

**Time to Peak:** I.M.: Within 20-30 minutes; I.V.: Within 5 minutes

**Excretion:** Urine

**Formulations**

Cefoxitin sodium:

Infusion, premixed in $D_5W$ (frozen): 1 g (50 mL); 2 g (50 mL)

Powder for injection: 1 g, 2 g, 10 g

**Dosing**

**Adults:** I.M., I.V.: 1-2 g every 6-8 hours (I.M. injection is painful); up to 12 g/day

**Elderly:** I.M., I.V.: Usual adult dose adjusted for estimated $Cl_{cr}$.

**Renal Impairment:** I.M., I.V.:

$Cl_{cr}$ 30-50 mL/minute: Administer 1-2 g every 8-12 hours.

$Cl_{cr}$ 10-29 mL/minute: Administer 1-2 g every 12-24 hours.

$Cl_{cr}$ 5-9 mL/minute: Administer 0.5-1 g every 12-24 hours.

$Cl_{cr}$ <5 mL/minute: Administer 0.5-1 g every 24-48 hours.

Moderately dialyzable (20% to 50%)

Continuous a-v hemofiltration (CAVH): Dose as for $Cl_{cr}$ 10-50 mL/minute

**Administration**

**I.M.:** Inject deep I.M. into large muscle mass.

**I.V.:** Inject direct I.V. over 3-5 minutes. Infuse intermittent infusion over 30 minutes.

**Stability**

**Reconstitution:** Reconstituted solution is stable for 24 hours at room temperature and 48 hours when refrigerated. I.V. infusion in NS or $D_5W$, solution is stable for 24 hours at room temperature, 1 week when refrigerated, or 26 weeks when frozen. After freezing, thawed solution is stable for 24 hours at room temperature or 5 days when refrigerated.

**Compatibility:** Discontinue other solutions at the same site to avoid compatibility problems.

**Monitoring Laboratory Tests** Prothrombin times; perform culture and sensitivity studies prior to initiating drug therapy.

**Additional Nursing Issues**

**Physical Assessment:** Assess for previous history of reactions to other cephalosporins or penicillins. Monitor for allergic reactions (see above). These can occur a few days after therapy is initiated. Assess for potential nephrotoxicity (see Drug Interactions). Assess bowel function (if severe diarrhea occurs, discontinue drug). Monitor urine output (if decreased, notify prescriber). Assess for opportunistic infection (eg, fever, malaise, rash, diarrhea, itching, redness, fever, chills, or increased cough). Note breast-feeding caution.

**Patient Information/Instruction:** This medication is administered I.M. or I.V. Drink 2-3 L fluid/day. If diarrhea occurs, yogurt or buttermilk may help. May cause false-positive test with Clinitest®; use another form of testing. May interfere with oral contraceptives; additional contraceptive measures are necessary. Report severe, unresolved diarrhea; vaginal itching or drainage; sores in mouth; blood, pus, or mucus in stool or urine; easy bleeding or bruising; unusual fever or chills; rash; or respiratory difficulty. **Breast-feeding precautions:** Consult prescriber if breast-feeding.

**Geriatric Considerations:** Adjust dose for renal function in the elderly.

**Breast-feeding Issues:** Theoretically, drug absorbed by nursing infant may change bowel flora or affect fever work-up result. **Note:** As a class, cephalosporins are used to treat infections in infants.

**Additional Information**

Each gram contains 2.3 mEq of sodium.

pH: 4.2-7

## Cefpodoxime (sef pode OKS eem)

**U.S. Brand Names** Vantin®

**Therapeutic Category** Antibiotic, Cephalosporin (Second Generation)

**Pregnancy Risk Factor** B

**Lactation** Enters breast milk (small amounts)/use caution

**Use** Treatment of susceptible acute, community-acquired pneumonia caused by *S. pneumoniae* or nonbeta-lactamase producing *H. influenzae*; acute uncomplicated gonorrhea caused by *N. gonorrhoeae*; uncomplicated skin and skin structure infections caused by *S. aureus* or *S. pyogenes*; acute otitis media caused by *S. pneumoniae*, *H. influenzae*, or *M. catarrhalis*; pharyngitis or tonsillitis; and uncomplicated urinary tract infections caused by *E. coli*, *Klebsiella*, and *Proteus*

**Mechanism of Action/Effect** Inhibits bacterial cell wall synthesis by binding to one or more of the penicillin-binding proteins (PBPs)

**Contraindications** Hypersensitivity to cefpodoxime or other cephalosporins

**Warnings** Modify dosage in patients with severe renal impairment. Prolonged use may result in superinfection. Cross-sensitivity to penicillins exists (~10%).

**Drug Interactions**

**Decreased Effect:** Antacids and $H_2$-receptor antagonists reduce absorption and serum concentration of cefpodoxime.

**Increased Effect/Toxicity:** Probenecid may decrease cephalosporin elimination. Furosemide, aminoglycosides in combination with cefpodoxime may result in additive nephrotoxicity.

**Food Interactions** Cefpodoxime serum levels may be increased if taken with food.

**Effects on Lab Values** May cause false-positive Coombs' test, false-positive results in urine glucose tests when using cupric sulfate (Benedict's solution, Clinitest®). May cause falsely elevated serum and urine creatinine concentrations.

(Continued)

## Cefpodoxime *(Continued)*

**Adverse Reactions**

>10%:

Dermatologic: Diaper rash (12.1%)

Gastrointestinal: Diarrhea in infants and toddlers (15.4%)

1% to 10%:

Central nervous system: Headache (1.1%)

Dermatologic: Rash (1.4%)

Gastrointestinal: Diarrhea (7.2%), nausea (3.8%), abdominal pain (1.6%), vomiting (1.1% to 2.1%)

Genitourinary: Vaginal infections (3.1%)

<1% (Limited to important or life-threatening symptoms): Anaphylaxis, chest pain, hypotension, fungal skin infection, pseudomembranous colitis, vaginal candidiasis, pruritus, flatulence, decreased salivation, malaise, fever, decreased appetite, cough, epistaxis, dizziness, fatigue, anxiety, insomnia, flushing, weakness, nightmares, taste alteration, eye itching, tinnitus, purpuric nephritis

Other reactions with cephalosporins include seizures, Stevens-Johnson syndrome, toxic epidermal necrolysis, erythema multiforme, urticaria, serum-sickness reactions, renal dysfunction, interstitial nephritis toxic nephropathy, cholestasis, aplastic anemia, hemolytic anemia, hemorrhage, pancytopenia, agranulocytosis, colitis, vaginitis, superinfection

**Overdose/Toxicology** Symptoms of overdose include neuromuscular hypersensitivity and convulsions. Many beta-lactam containing antibiotics have the potential to cause neuromuscular hyperirritability or convulsive seizures. Hemodialysis may be helpful to aid in removal of the drug from blood; otherwise, treatment is supportive or symptom directed.

**Pharmacodynamics/Kinetics**

**Protein Binding:** 18% to 23%

**Distribution:** Good tissue penetration, including lung and tonsils; penetrates into pleural fluid

**Half-life Elimination:** 2.2 hours (prolonged in renal impairment)

**Time to Peak:** Within 1 hour (oral)

**Metabolism:** GI tract

**Excretion:** Urine

**Formulations**

Cefpodoxime proxetil:

Granules for oral suspension (lemon creme flavor): 50 mg/5 mL (100 mL); 100 mg/5 mL (100 mL)

Tablet, film coated: 100 mg, 200 mg

**Dosing**

**Adults:** Oral:

Acute community-acquired pneumonia and bacterial exacerbations of chronic bronchitis: 200 mg every 12 hours for 14 days and 10 days, respectively

Skin and skin structure: 400 mg every 12 hours for 7-14 days

Uncomplicated gonorrhea (male/female) and rectal gonococcal infections (female): 200 mg as a single dose

Pharyngitis/tonsillitis: 100 mg every 12 hours for 10 days

Uncomplicated urinary tract infection: 100 mg every 12 hours for 7 days

**Elderly:** Refer to adult dosing.

**Renal Impairment:**

$Cl_{cr}$ <30 mL/minute: Administer every 24 hours.

Hemodialysis: Dose 3 times/week following dialysis.

**Hepatic Impairment:** Dose adjustment is not necessary in patients with cirrhosis.

**Administration**

**Oral:** Administer around-the-clock to promote less variation in peak and trough serum levels.

**Stability**

**Reconstitution:** After mixing, keep suspension in refrigerator, shake well before using. Discard unused portion after 14 days.

**Monitoring Laboratory Tests** Prothrombin times; perform culture and sensitivity studies prior to initiating drug therapy.

**Additional Nursing Issues**

**Physical Assessment:** Assess for previous history of reactions to other cephalosporins or penicillins. Monitor for allergic reactions (see above). These can occur a few days after therapy is initiated. Assess for potential nephrotoxicity (see Drug Interactions). Assess bowel function (if severe diarrhea occurs, discontinue drug). May cause hypoprothrombinemia (monitor for bleeding, easy bruising or bleeding, blood in stool or urine). Monitor urine output (if decreased, notify prescriber). Assess for opportunistic infection (eg, fever, malaise, rash, diarrhea, itching, redness, fever, chills, or increased cough). Note breast-feeding caution.

**Patient Information/Instruction:** Take as directed, at regular intervals around-the-clock (with or without food). Chilling oral suspension improves flavor (do not freeze). Complete full course of medication, even if you feel better. Drink 2-3 L fluid/day. If diarrhea occurs, yogurt or buttermilk may help. May cause false-positive test with Clinitest®; use another form of testing. May interfere with oral contraceptives; additional contraceptive measures are necessary. Report severe, unresolved diarrhea; vaginal itching or drainage; sores in mouth; blood, pus, or mucus in stool or urine; easy bleeding or bruising; unusual fever or chills; rash; or respiratory difficulty. **Breast-feeding precautions:** Consult prescriber if breast-feeding.

**Geriatric Considerations:** Considered one of the drugs of choice for outpatient treatment of community-acquired pneumonia in older adults. Adjust dosage with renal impairment.

**Breast-feeding Issues:** Theoretically, drug absorbed by nursing infant may change bowel flora or affect fever work-up result. **Note:** As a class, cephalosporins are used to treat infections in infants.

**Additional Information** Each gram contains 2.3 mEq of sodium.

## Cefprozil (sef PROE zil)

**U.S. Brand Names** Cefzil®

**Therapeutic Category** Antibiotic, Cephalosporin (Second Generation)

**Pregnancy Risk Factor** B

**Lactation** Enters breast milk/use caution

**Use** Infections causes by susceptible organisms including *S. pneumoniae, S. aureus, S. pyogenes*; treatment of otitis media and infections involving the respiratory tract and skin and skin structure

**Mechanism of Action/Effect** Inhibits bacterial cell wall synthesis by binding to one or more of the penicillin-binding proteins (PBPs)

**Contraindications** Hypersensitivity to cefprozil, any component, or other cephalosporins

**Warnings** Modify dosage in patients with severe renal impairment. Prolonged use may result in superinfection. Cross-sensitivity to penicillins exists (~10%).

**Drug Interactions**

**Increased Effect/Toxicity:** Probenecid may decrease cephalosporin elimination. Furosemide, aminoglycosides in combination with cefprozil may result in additive nephrotoxicity.

**Effects on Lab Values** May cause false-positive Coombs' test, false-positive results in urine glucose tests when using cupric sulfate (Benedict's solution, Clinitest®). May cause falsely elevated serum and urine creatinine concentrations.

**Adverse Reactions**

1% to 10%:

Central nervous system: Dizziness (1%)
Dermatologic: Diaper rash (1.5%)
Gastrointestinal: Diarrhea (2.9%), nausea (3.5%), vomiting (1%), abdominal pain (1%)
Genitourinary: Vaginitis, genital pruritus (1.6%)
Hepatic: Increased transaminases (2%)
Miscellaneous: Superinfection

<1% (Limited to important or life-threatening symptoms): Anaphylaxis, angioedema, pseudomembranous colitis, rash, urticaria, erythema multiforme, serum sickness, Stevens-Johnson syndrome, hyperactivity, headache, insomnia, confusion, somnolence, leukopenia, eosinophilia, thrombocytopenia, elevated BUN, elevated creatinine, arthralgia, cholestatic jaundice, fever

Other reactions with cephalosporins include: Seizures, toxic epidermal necrolysis, renal dysfunction, interstitial nephritis, toxic nephropathy, aplastic anemia, hemolytic anemia, hemorrhage, pancytopenia, agranulocytosis, colitis, vaginitis, superinfection

**Overdose/Toxicology** Symptoms of overdose include neuromuscular hypersensitivity and convulsions. Many beta-lactam containing antibiotics have the potential to cause neuromuscular hyperirritability or convulsive seizures. Hemodialysis may be helpful to aid in removal of the drug from blood; otherwise, treatment is supportive or symptom directed.

**Pharmacodynamics/Kinetics**

**Protein Binding:** 35% to 45%

**Half-life Elimination:** 1.3 hours (normal renal function)

**Time to Peak:** 1.5 hours (fasting state)

**Excretion:** Urine

**Formulations**

Powder for oral suspension, as anhydrous: 125 mg/5 mL (50 mL, 75 mL, 100 mL); 250 mg/5 mL (50 mL, 75 mL, 100 mL)

Tablet, as anhydrous: 250 mg, 500 mg

**Dosing**

**Adults:**

Pharyngitis/tonsillitis: 500 mg every 24 hours for 10 days

Uncomplicated skin and skin structure infections: 250 mg every 12 hours, or 500 mg every 12-24 hours for 10 days

Secondary bacterial infection of acute bronchitis or acute bacterial exacerbation of chronic bronchitis: 500 mg every 12 hours for 10 days

**Elderly:** Refer to adult dosing.

**Renal Impairment:**

$Cl_{cr}$ <30 mL/minute: Reduce dose by 50%

Hemodialysis effects: 55% reduced by hemodialysis

**Administration**

**Oral:** Administer around-the-clock to promote less variation in peak and trough serum levels.

**Stability**

**Reconstitution:** Chilling improves flavor (do not freeze).

**Monitoring Laboratory Tests** Prothrombin time; perform culture and sensitivity studies prior to initiating drug therapy.

(Continued)

## Cefprozil *(Continued)*

**Additional Nursing Issues**

**Physical Assessment:** Assess for previous history of reactions to other cephalosporins or penicillins. Monitor for allergic reactions (see above). These can occur a few days after therapy is initiated. Assess for potential nephrotoxicity (see Drug Interactions). Assess bowel function (if severe diarrhea occurs, discontinue drug). May cause hypoprothrombinemia (monitor for bleeding, easy bruising or bleeding, blood in stool or urine). Monitor urine output (if decreased, notify prescriber). Assess for opportunistic infection (eg, fever, malaise, rash, diarrhea, itching, redness, fever, chills, or increased cough). Note breast-feeding caution.

**Patient Information/Instruction:** Take as directed, at regular intervals around-the-clock (with or without food). Chilling oral suspension improves flavor (do not freeze). Complete full course of medication, even if you feel better. Drink 2-3 L fluid/day. If diarrhea occurs, yogurt or buttermilk may help. May cause false-positive test with Clinitest®; use another form of testing. May interfere with oral contraceptives; additional contraceptive measures are necessary. Report severe, unresolved diarrhea; vaginal itching or drainage; sores in mouth; blood, pus, or mucus in stool or urine; easy bleeding or bruising; unusual fever or chills; rash; or respiratory difficulty. **Breast-feeding precautions:** Consult prescriber if breast-feeding.

**Geriatric Considerations:** Has not been studied exclusively in the elderly. Adjust dose for estimated renal function.

**Breast-feeding Issues:** Theoretically, drug absorbed by nursing infant may change bowel flora or affect fever work-up result. **Note:** As a class, cephalosporins are used to treat infections in infants.

**Additional Information** Each gram contains 2.3 mEq of sodium.

## Ceftazidime (SEF tay zi deem)

**U.S. Brand Names** Ceptaz™; Fortaz®; Tazicef®; Tazidime®

**Therapeutic Category** Antibiotic, Cephalosporin (Third Generation)

**Pregnancy Risk Factor** B

**Lactation** Enters breast milk (small amounts)/use caution (AAP rates "compatible")

**Use** Treatment of documented susceptible *Pseudomonas aeruginosa* infection; *Pseudomonas* infection in patients at risk of developing aminoglycoside-induced nephrotoxicity and/or ototoxicity; empiric therapy of febrile, granulocytopenic patients

**Mechanism of Action/Effect** Inhibits bacterial cell wall synthesis by binding to one or more of the penicillin-binding proteins (PBPs)

**Contraindications** Hypersensitivity to ceftazidime, any component, or other cephalosporins

**Warnings** Modify dosage in patients with severe renal impairment. Prolonged use may result in superinfection. Cross-sensitivity to penicillins exists (~10%).

**Drug Interactions**

**Increased Effect/Toxicity:** Probenecid may decrease cephalosporin elimination. Aminoglycosides: *in vitro* studies indicate additive or synergistic effect against some strains of Enterobacteriaceae and *Pseudomonas aeruginosa*. Furosemide, aminoglycosides in combination with ceftazidime may result in additive nephrotoxicity.

**Effects on Lab Values** May cause false-positive Coombs' test, false-positive results in urine glucose tests when using cupric sulfate (Benedict's solution, Clinitest®), urinary 17-ketosteroids

**Adverse Reactions**

1% to 10%:

Gastrointestinal: Diarrhea (1.3%)

Local: Pain at injection site (1.4%)

Miscellaneous: Hypersensitivity reactions (2%)

<1% (Limited to important or life-threatening symptoms): Anaphylaxis, fever, headache, dizziness, paresthesia, pruritus, rash, Stevens-Johnson syndrome, toxic epidermal necrolysis, erythema multiforme, angioedema, nausea, vomiting, pseudomembranous colitis, eosinophilia, thrombocytosis, leukopenia, hemolytic anemia, elevated transaminases, increased BUN, increased creatinine, phlebitis, candidiasis, vaginitis, encephalopathy, asterixis, neuromuscular excitability

Other reactions with cephalosporins include seizures, urticaria, serum-sickness reactions, renal dysfunction, interstitial nephritis, toxic nephropathy, elevated BUN, elevated creatinine, cholestasis, aplastic anemia, hemolytic anemia, pancytopenia, agranulocytosis, colitis, prolonged PT, hemorrhage, superinfection

**Overdose/Toxicology** Symptoms of overdose include neuromuscular hypersensitivity and convulsions. Many beta-lactam containing antibiotics have the potential to cause neuromuscular hyperirritability or convulsive seizures. Hemodialysis may be helpful to aid in removal of the drug from blood; otherwise, treatment is supportive or symptom directed.

**Pharmacodynamics/Kinetics**

**Protein Binding:** 17%

**Distribution:** Widely distributes throughout the body including bone, bile, skin, CSF (diffuses into CSF with higher concentrations when the meninges are inflamed), endometrium, heart, pleural and lymphatic fluids

**Half-life Elimination:** 1-2 hours (prolonged in renal impairment)

**Time to Peak:** I.M.: Within 1 hour

**Excretion:** Urine

**Formulations**

Infusion, premixed (frozen) (Fortaz®): 1 g (50 mL); 2 g (50 mL)

Powder for injection: 500 mg, 1 g, 2 g, 6 g

**Dosing**

**Adults:**

I.M., I.V.: 1-2 g every 8-12 hours

Urinary tract infections: 250-500 mg every 12 hours

**Elderly:** I.M., I.V.: Dosage should be based on renal function with a dosing interval not more frequent then every 12 hours.

**Renal Impairment:**

$Cl_{cr}$ 31-50 mL/minute: Administer 1 g every 12 hours.

$Cl_{cr}$ 16-30 mL/minute: Administer 1 g every 24 hours.

$Cl_{cr}$ 6-15 mL/minute: Administer 500 mg every 24 hours.

$Cl_{cr}$ <5 mL/minute: Administer 500 mg every 48 hours.

Dialyzable (50% to 100%)

Continuous a-v hemofiltration (CAVH): Dose as $Cl_{cr}$ 30-50 mL/minute

**Administration**

**I.M.:** Inject deep I.M. into large mass muscle.

**I.V.:** Ceftazidime can be administered IVP over 3-5 minutes, or I.V. retrograde, or I.V. intermittent infusion over 15-30 minutes.

**I.V. Detail:** Any carbon dioxide bubbles that may be present in the withdrawn solution should be expelled prior to injection. Administer around-the-clock to promote less variation in peak and trough serum levels.

**Stability**

**Reconstitution:** Any carbon dioxide bubbles that may be present in the withdrawn solution should be expelled prior to injection. Final concentration for I.V. administration should not exceed 100 mg/mL. Reconstituted solution and I.V. infusion in NS or $D_5W$ solution are stable for 24 hours at room temperature, 10 days when refrigerated, or 12 weeks when frozen. After freezing, thawed solution is stable for 24 hours at room temperature or 4 days when refrigerated. After mixing for 96 hours refrigerated.

**Compatibility:** Do not admix with aminoglycosides in same bottle/bag. Discontinue other solutions at the same site to avoid compatibility problems.

**Monitoring Laboratory Tests** Prothrombin times; perform culture and sensitivity studies prior to initiating drug therapy.

**Additional Nursing Issues**

**Physical Assessment:** Assess for previous history of reactions to other cephalosporins or penicillins. Monitor for allergic reactions (see above). These can occur a few days after therapy is initiated. Assess for potential nephrotoxicity (see Drug Interactions). Assess bowel function (if severe diarrhea occurs, discontinue drug). Monitor urine output (if decreased, notify prescriber). Assess for opportunistic infection (eg, fever, malaise, rash, diarrhea, itching, redness, fever, chills, or increased cough). Note breast-feeding caution.

**Patient Information/Instruction:** This medication is administered I.M. or I.V. Drink 2-3 L fluid/day. If diarrhea occurs, yogurt or buttermilk may help. May cause false-positive test with Clinitest®; use another form of testing. May interfere with oral contraceptives; additional contraceptive measures are necessary. Report severe, unresolved diarrhea; vaginal itching or drainage; sores in mouth; blood, pus, or mucus in stool or urine; easy bleeding or bruising; unusual fever or chills; rash; or respiratory difficulty. **Breast-feeding precautions:** Consult prescriber if breast-feeding.

**Geriatric Considerations:** Changes in renal function associated with aging and corresponding alterations in pharmacokinetics result in every 12-hour dosing being an adequate dosing interval. Adjust dose based on renal function.

**Breast-feeding Issues:** Theoretically, drug absorbed by nursing infant may change bowel flora or affect fever work-up result. **Note:** As a class, cephalosporins are used to treat infections in infants.

**Additional Information** With some organisms, resistance may develop during treatment (including *Enterobacter* spp, *Pseudomonas* spp, and *Serratia* spp). Consider combination therapy or periodic susceptibility testing for organisms with inducible resistance (see Warnings/Precautions).

Each gram contains 2.3 mEq of sodium.

pH: 5-8

♦ **Ceftazim** *see* Ceftazidime *on previous page*

## Ceftibuten (sef TYE byoo ten)

**U.S. Brand Names** Cedax®

**Therapeutic Category** Antibiotic, Cephalosporin (Third Generation)

**Pregnancy Risk Factor** B

**Lactation** Excretion in breast milk unknown/use caution

**Use** Oral cephalosporin for bronchitis, otitis media, and pharyngitis/tonsillitis due to *H. influenzae* (highly sensitive) and *M. catarrhalis* (moderately sensitive), both beta-lactamase-producing and nonproducing strains, as well as *S. pneumoniae* (weak) and *S. pyogenes*. **Note:** Documented sensitivity of *S. pneumoniae* to ceftibuten should be present before use, since resistance is known to penicillin-resistant strains (up to 25% of strains in the U.S.). It is highly active against group A streptococci, *N. gonorrhoeae* and *N. meningitidis*, as well. It has the broadest gram-negative spectrum of any oral cephalosporin, active against most strains of Enterobacteriaceae, including *E. coli*, *Salmonella*, *Shigella*, and *Yersinia*. Although ceftibuten may eradicate *S. pyogenes* from the oropharynx, proof of efficacy for prophylaxis of rheumatic fever is not available.

**Mechanism of Action/Effect** Inhibits bacterial cell wall synthesis by binding to one or more of the penicillin-binding proteins (PBPs)

**Contraindications** Hypersensitivity to ceftibuten or other cephalosporins

(Continued)

## Ceftibuten *(Continued)*

**Warnings** Modify dosage in patients with severe renal impairment. Prolonged use may result in superinfection. Cross-sensitivity to penicillins exists (~10%).

**Drug Interactions**

**Increased Effect/Toxicity:** High-dose probenecid decreases clearance. Aminoglycosides in combination with ceftibuten may increase nephrotoxic potential.

**Effects on Lab Values** May cause false-positive Coombs' test, false-positive results in urine glucose tests when using cupric sulfate (Benedict's solution, Clinitest®). May cause falsely elevated serum and urine creatinine concentrations.

**Adverse Reactions**

1% to 10%:

Central nervous system: Headache (3%), dizziness (1%)

Gastrointestinal: Nausea (4%), diarrhea (3%), dyspepsia (2%), vomiting (1%), abdominal pain (1%)

Hematologic: Increased eosinophils (3%), decreased hemoglobin (2%), thrombocytosis

Hepatic: Increased ALT (1%), increased bilirubin (1%)

Renal: Increased BUN (4%)

<1% (Limited to important or life-threatening symptoms): Anorexia, agitation, constipation, diaper rash, dry mouth, dyspnea, dysuria, fatigue, candidiasis, rash, urticaria, irritability, paresthesia, nasal congestion, insomnia, rigors, increased transaminases, increased creatinine, leukopenia

Other reactions with cephalosporins include anaphylaxis, fever, paresthesia, pruritus, Stevens-Johnson syndrome, toxic epidermal necrolysis, erythema multiforme, angioedema, pseudomembranous colitis, hemolytic anemia, candidiasis, vaginitis, encephalopathy, asterixis, neuromuscular excitability, seizures, serum-sickness reactions, renal dysfunction, interstitial nephritis, toxic nephropathy, cholestasis, aplastic anemia, hemolytic anemia, pancytopenia, agranulocytosis, colitis, prolonged PT, hemorrhage, superinfection

**Overdose/Toxicology** Symptoms of overdose include neuromuscular hypersensitivity and convulsions. Many beta-lactam containing antibiotics have the potential to cause neuromuscular hyperirritability or convulsive seizures. Hemodialysis may be helpful to aid in the removal of drug from blood; otherwise, treatment is supportive or symptom directed.

**Pharmacodynamics/Kinetics**

**Distribution:** Crosses the placenta

**Half-life Elimination:** 2 hours

**Excretion:** Urine

**Formulations**

Capsule: 400 mg

Powder for oral suspension (cherry flavor): 90 mg/5 mL (30 mL, 60 mL, 120 mL); 180 mg/5 mL (30 mL, 60 mL, 120 mL)

**Dosing**

**Adults:** Oral: 400 mg once daily for 10 days; maximum: 400 mg

**Elderly:** Refer to adult dosing.

**Renal Impairment:**

$Cl_{cr}$ 30-49 mL//minute: Administer 4.5 mg/kg or 200 mg every 24 hours.

$Cl_{cr}$ 5-29 mL/minute: Administer 2.25 mg/kg or 100 mg every 24 hours.

**Administration**

**Oral:** Administer at the same time each day to maintain adequate blood levels.

**Stability**

**Reconstitution:** Reconstituted suspension is stable for 14 days in the refrigerator.

**Monitoring Laboratory Tests** Renal, hepatic, and hematologic function periodically with prolonged therapy; prothrombin time; perform culture and sensitivity studies prior to initiating drug therapy.

**Additional Nursing Issues**

**Physical Assessment:** Assess for previous history of reactions to other cephalosporins or penicillins. Monitor for allergic reactions (see above). These can occur a few days after therapy is initiated. Assess for potential nephrotoxicity (see Drug Interactions). Assess bowel function (if severe diarrhea occurs, discontinue drug). May cause hypoprothrombinemia (monitor for bleeding, easy bruising or bleeding, blood in stool or urine). Monitor urine output (if decreased, notify prescriber). Assess for opportunistic infection (eg, fever, malaise, rash, diarrhea, itching, redness, fever, chills, or increased cough). Note breast-feeding caution.

**Patient Information/Instruction:** Take as directed, at regular intervals around-the-clock (with or without food). Chilling oral suspension improves flavor (do not freeze). Complete full course of medication, even if you feel better. Drink 2-3 L fluid/day. If diarrhea occurs, yogurt or buttermilk may help. May cause false-positive test with Clinitest®; use another form of testing. May interfere with oral contraceptives; additional contraceptive measures are necessary. Report severe, unresolved diarrhea; vaginal itching or drainage; sores in mouth; blood, pus, or mucus in stool or urine; easy bleeding or bruising; unusual fever or chills; rash; or respiratory difficulty. **Breast-feeding precautions:** Consult prescriber if breast-feeding.

**Geriatric Considerations:** Has not been studied specifically in the elderly. Adjust dose for renal function.

**Breast-feeding Issues:** Theoretically, drug absorbed by nursing infant may change bowel flora or affect fever work-up result. **Note:** As a class, cephalosporins are used to treat infections in infants.

**Additional Information** Each gram contains 2.3 mEq of sodium.

♦ **Ceftin® Oral** *see* Cefuroxime *on page 233*

## Ceftizoxime (sef ti ZOKS eem)

**U.S. Brand Names** Cefizox®

**Therapeutic Category** Antibiotic, Cephalosporin (Third Generation)

**Pregnancy Risk Factor** B

**Lactation** Enters breast milk (small amounts)/use caution

**Use** Treatment of susceptible nonpseudomonal gram-negative rod infections or mixed gram-negative and anaerobic infections; predominantly respiratory tract, skin and skin structure, bone and joint, urinary tract and gynecologic, as well as septicemia

**Mechanism of Action/Effect** Inhibits bacterial cell wall synthesis by binding to one or more of the penicillin-binding proteins (PBPs)

**Contraindications** Hypersensitivity to ceftizoxime, any component, or other cephalosporins

**Warnings** Modify dosage in patients with severe renal impairment. Prolonged use may result in superinfection. Cross-sensitivity to penicillins exists (~10%).

**Drug Interactions**

**Increased Effect/Toxicity:** Probenecid may decrease cephalosporin elimination. Furosemide, aminoglycosides in combination with ceftizoxime may result in additive nephrotoxicity.

**Effects on Lab Values** May cause false-positive Coombs' test, false-positive results in urine glucose tests when using cupric sulfate (Benedict's solution, Clinitest®), urinary 17-ketosteroids.

**Adverse Reactions**

1% to 10%:

Central nervous system: Fever
Dermatologic: Rash, pruritus
Hematologic: Eosinophilia, thrombocytosis
Hepatic: Elevated transaminases, alkaline phosphatase
Local: Pain, burning at injection site

<1% (Limited to important or life-threatening symptoms): Anaphylaxis, diarrhea, nausea, vomiting, injection site reactions, phlebitis, paresthesia, numbness, increased bilirubin, increased BUN, increased creatinine, anemia, leukopenia, neutropenia, thrombocytopenia, vaginitis

Other reactions reported with cephalosporins include Stevens-Johnson syndrome, toxic epidermal necrolysis, erythema multiforme, pseudomembranous colitis, angioedema, hemolytic anemia, candidiasis, encephalopathy, asterixis, neuromuscular excitability, seizures, serum-sickness reactions, renal dysfunction, interstitial nephritis, toxic nephropathy, cholestasis, aplastic anemia, hemolytic anemia, pancytopenia, agranulocytosis, colitis, prolonged PT, hemorrhage, superinfection

**Overdose/Toxicology** Symptoms of overdose include neuromuscular hypersensitivity and convulsions. Many beta-lactam containing antibiotics have the potential to cause neuromuscular hyperirritability or convulsive seizures. Hemodialysis may be helpful to aid in removal of the drug from blood; otherwise, treatment is supportive or symptom directed.

**Pharmacodynamics/Kinetics**

**Protein Binding:** 30%

**Distribution:** Widely distributed into most body tissues and fluids including gallbladder, liver, kidneys, bone, sputum, bile, and pleural and synovial fluids; has good CSF penetration; crosses the placenta

**Half-life Elimination:** 1.6 hours, increases to 25 hours when $Cl_{cr}$ falls to <10 mL/minute

**Time to Peak:** I.M.: Within 0.5-1 hour

**Excretion:** Urine

**Formulations**

Ceftizoxime sodium:

Injection in $D_5W$ (frozen): 1 g (50 mL); 2 g (50 mL)
Powder for injection: 500 mg, 1 g, 2 g, 10 g

**Dosing**

**Adults:** I.M., I.V.: 1-2 g every 8-12 hours, up to 2 g every 4 hours or 4 g every 8 hours for life-threatening infections

**Elderly:** Refer to adult dosing.

**Renal Impairment:**

$Cl_{cr}$ 50-79 mL/minute: Administer 500-1500 mg every 8 hours.
$Cl_{cr}$ 5-49 mL/minute: Administer 250-1000 mg every 12 hours.
$Cl_{cr}$ 0-4 mL/minute: Administer 500-1000 mg every 48 hours or 250-500 mg every 24 hours.
Moderately dialyzable (20% to 50%)
Continuous a-v hemofiltration (CAVH): Dose as for $Cl_{cr}$ 10-50 mL/minute

**Administration**

**I.M.:** Inject deep I.M. into large muscle mass.

**I.V.:** Inject direct I.V. over 3-5 minutes. Infuse intermittent infusion over 30 minutes.

**Stability**

**Reconstitution:** Reconstituted solution is stable for 24 hours at room temperature and 96 hours when refrigerated. For I.V. infusion in NS or $D_5W$, solution is stable for 24 hours at room temperature, 96 hours when refrigerated or 12 weeks when frozen. After

(Continued)

## Ceftizoxime *(Continued)*

freezing, thawed solution is stable for 24 hours at room temperature or 10 days when refrigerated.

**Compatibility:** Discontinue other solutions at the same site to avoid compatibility problems.

**Monitoring Laboratory Tests** Prothrombin times; perform culture and sensitivity studies prior to initiating drug therapy.

**Additional Nursing Issues**

**Physical Assessment:** Assess for previous history of reactions to other cephalosporins or penicillins. Monitor for allergic reactions (see above). These can occur a few days after therapy is initiated. Assess for potential nephrotoxicity (see Drug Interactions). Assess bowel function (if severe diarrhea occurs, discontinue drug). May cause hypoprothrombinemia (monitor for bleeding, easy bruising or bleeding, blood in stool or urine). Monitor urine output (if decreased, notify prescriber). Assess for opportunistic infection (eg, fever, malaise, rash, diarrhea, itching, redness, fever, chills, or increased cough). Note breast-feeding caution.

**Patient Information/Instruction:** This medication is administered I.M. or I.V. Drink 2-3 L fluid/day. If diarrhea occurs, yogurt or buttermilk may help. May cause false-positive test with Clinitest®; use another form of testing. May interfere with oral contraceptives; additional contraceptive measures are necessary. Report severe, unresolved diarrhea; vaginal itching or drainage; sores in mouth; blood, pus, or mucus in stool or urine; easy bleeding or bruising; unusual fever or chills; rash; or respiratory difficulty. **Breast-feeding precautions:** Consult prescriber if breast-feeding.

**Geriatric Considerations:** Adjust dose for renal function in the elderly.

**Breast-feeding Issues:** Theoretically, drug absorbed by nursing infant may change bowel flora or affect fever work-up result. **Note:** As a class, cephalosporins are used to treat infections in infants.

**Additional Information**

Each gram contains 2.6 mEq of sodium.

pH: 5.5-8

## Ceftriaxone (sef trye AKS one)

**U.S. Brand Names** Rocephin®

**Therapeutic Category** Antibiotic, Cephalosporin (Third Generation)

**Pregnancy Risk Factor** B

**Lactation** Enters breast milk/use caution (AAP rates "compatible")

**Use** Treatment of lower respiratory tract infections, skin and skin structure infections, bone and joint infections, intra-abdominal and urinary tract infections, sepsis and meningitis due to susceptible organisms; documented or suspected infection due to susceptible organisms in home care patients and patients without I.V. line access; treatment of documented or suspected gonococcal infection or chancroid; emergency room management of patients at high risk for bacteremia, periorbital or buccal cellulitis, salmonellosis or shigellosis, and pneumonia of unestablished etiology (<5 years of age)

**Mechanism of Action/Effect** Inhibits bacterial cell wall synthesis by binding to one or more of the penicillin-binding proteins (PBPs)

**Contraindications** Hypersensitivity to ceftriaxone sodium, any component, or other cephalosporins

**Warnings** Modify dosage in patients with severe renal impairment. Prolonged use may result in superinfection with yeasts, enterococci, *B. fragilis*, or *P. aeruginosa*. Cross-sensitivity to penicillins exists (~10%).

**Drug Interactions**

**Increased Effect/Toxicity:** Aminoglycosides may result in synergistic antibacterial activity. High-dose probenecid decreases clearance. Aminoglycosides increase nephrotoxic potential.

**Effects on Lab Values** May cause false-positive Coombs' test, false-positive results in urine glucose tests when using cupric sulfate (Benedict's solution, Clinitest®), urinary 17-ketosteroids.

**Adverse Reactions**

1% to 10%:

Dermatologic: Rash (1.7%)
Gastrointestinal: Diarrhea (2.7%)
Hematologic: Eosinophilia (6%), thrombocytosis (5.1%), leukopenia (2.1%)
Hepatic: Elevated transaminases (3.1% to 3.3%)
Local: Pain, induration at injection site (1%)
Renal: Increased BUN (1.2%)

<1% (Limited to important or life-threatening symptoms): Phlebitis, pruritus, fever, chills, anemia, hemolytic anemia, neutropenia, lymphopenia, thrombocytopenia, prolonged PT, nausea, vomiting, dysgeusia, increased alkaline phosphatase, increased bilirubin, increased creatinine, urinary casts, headache, dizziness, candidiasis, vaginitis, diaphoresis, flushing

Other reactions with cephalosporins include anaphylaxis, paresthesia, Stevens-Johnson syndrome, toxic epidermal necrolysis, erythema multiforme, angioedema, pseudomembranous colitis, hemolytic anemia, encephalopathy, asterixis, neuromuscular excitability, seizures, serum-sickness reactions, renal dysfunction, interstitial nephritis, toxic nephropathy, cholestasis, aplastic anemia, hemolytic anemia, pancytopenia, agranulocytosis, colitis, hemorrhage, superinfection

**Overdose/Toxicology** Symptoms of overdose include neuromuscular hypersensitivity and convulsions. Many beta-lactam containing antibiotics have the potential to cause neuromuscular hyperirritability or convulsive seizures. Hemodialysis may be helpful to aid in removal of the drug from blood; otherwise, treatment is supportive or symptom directed.

**Pharmacodynamics/Kinetics**

**Protein Binding:** 85% to 95%

**Distribution:** Widely distributes throughout the body including gallbladder, lungs, bone, bile, CSF (diffuses into the CSF at higher concentrations when the meninges are inflamed)

**Half-life Elimination:** Normal renal and hepatic function: 5-9 hours

**Time to Peak:** I.M.: Within 1-2 hours; I.V.: Within minutes

**Excretion:** Urine

**Formulations**

Ceftriaxone sodium:

Infusion, premixed (frozen): 1 g in $D_{3.8}W$ (50 mL); 2 g in $D_{2.4}W$ (50 mL)

Injection: 350 mg/mL

Powder for injection: 250 mg, 500 mg, 1 g, 2 g, 10 g

**Dosing**

**Adults:**

I.M., I.V.: 1-2 g every 12-24 hours (depending on the type and severity of infection); maximum: 2 g every 12 hours for treatment of meningitis

Uncomplicated gonorrhea: I.M.: 250 mg as a single dose necessary

**Elderly:** Refer to adult dosing.

**Renal Impairment:**

No change necessary

Not dialyzable (0% to 5%)

Administer dose postdialysis.

Peritoneal dialysis effects: Administer 750 mg every 12 hours.

Continuous arteriovenous or venovenous hemofiltration (CAVH/CAVHD): Removes 10 mg of ceftriaxone of liter of filtrate per day.

**Hepatic Impairment:** No change necessary

**Administration**

**I.M.:** Inject deep I.M. into large muscle mass.

**I.V.:** Infuse intermittent infusion over 15-30 minutes.

**Stability**

**Reconstitution:** Reconstituted solution (100 mg/mL) is stable for 3 days at room temperature and 3 days when refrigerated. For I.V. infusion in NS or $D_5W$, solution is stable for 3 days at room temperature, 10 days when refrigerated, or 26 weeks when frozen. After freezing, thawed solution is stable for 3 days at room temperature or 10 days when refrigerated.

**Compatibility:** Discontinue other solutions at the same site to avoid compatibility problems.

**Monitoring Laboratory Tests** Prothrombin times; perform culture and sensitivity studies prior to initiating drug therapy.

**Additional Nursing Issues**

**Physical Assessment:** Assess for previous history of reactions to other cephalosporins or penicillins. Monitor for allergic reactions (see above). These can occur a few days after therapy is initiated. Assess for potential nephrotoxicity (see Drug Interactions). Assess bowel function (if severe diarrhea occurs, discontinue drug). Monitor urine output (if decreased, notify prescriber). Assess for opportunistic infection (eg, fever, malaise, rash, diarrhea, itching, redness, fever, chills, or increased cough). Note breast-feeding caution.

**Patient Information/Instruction:** This medication is administered I.M. or I.V. Drink 2-3 L fluid/day. If diarrhea occurs, yogurt or buttermilk may help. May cause false-positive test with Clinitest®; use another form of testing. May interfere with oral contraceptives; additional contraceptive measures are necessary. Report severe, unresolved diarrhea; vaginal itching or drainage; sores in mouth; blood, pus, or mucus in stool or urine; easy bleeding or bruising; unusual fever or chills; rash; or respiratory difficulty. **Breast-feeding precautions:** Consult prescriber if breast-feeding.

**Geriatric Considerations:** No adjustment for changes in renal function necessary.

**Breast-feeding Issues:** Theoretically, drug absorbed by nursing infant may change bowel flora or affect fever work-up result. **Note:** As a class, cephalosporins are used to treat infections in infants.

**Additional Information**

Each gram contains 3.6 mEq of sodium.

pH: 6.6-6.7

## Cefuroxime (se fyoor OKS eem)

**U.S. Brand Names** Ceftin® Oral; Kefurox® Injection; Zinacef® Injection

**Therapeutic Category** Antibiotic, Cephalosporin (Second Generation)

**Pregnancy Risk Factor** B

**Lactation** Enters breast milk/use caution

**Use** Treatment of infections caused by staphylococci, group B streptococci, *H. influenzae* (Type A and B), *E. coli*, *Enterobacter*, *Salmonella*, and *Klebsiella*; treatment of susceptible infections of the lower respiratory tract, otitis media, urinary tract, skin and soft tissue, bone and joint, sepsis and gonorrhea

**Mechanism of Action/Effect** Inhibits bacterial cell wall synthesis by binding to one or more of the penicillin-binding proteins (PBPs)

**Contraindications** Hypersensitivity to cefuroxime, any component, or other cephalosporins

(Continued)

## Cefuroxime *(Continued)*

**Warnings** Modify dosage in patients with severe renal impairment. Prolonged use may result in superinfection. Cross-sensitivity to penicillins exists (~10%).

**Drug Interactions**

**Increased Effect/Toxicity:** High-dose probenecid decreases clearance. Aminoglycosides in combination with cefuroxime may result in additive nephrotoxicity.

**Food Interactions** Cefuroxime serum levels may be increased if taken with food or dairy products.

**Effects on Lab Values** May cause false-positive Coombs' test, false-positive results in urine glucose tests when using cupric sulfate (Benedict's solution, Clinitest®), urinary 17-ketosteroids.

**Adverse Reactions**

1% to 10%:

Hematologic: Eosinophilia (7%), decreased hemoglobin and hematocrit (10%)

Hepatic: Increased transaminases (4%), increased alkaline phosphatase (2%)

Local: Thrombophlebitis (1.7%)

<1% (Limited to important or life-threatening symptoms): Anaphylaxis, erythema multiforme, toxic epidermal necrolysis, Stevens-Johnson syndrome, interstitial nephritis, dizziness, fever, headache, rash, nausea, vomiting, diarrhea, stomach cramps, GI bleeding, colitis, neutropenia, leukopenia, increased creatinine, increased BUN, pain at injection site, vaginitis, seizures, angioedema, pseudomembranous colitis

Other reactions with cephalosporins include toxic nephropathy, cholestasis, agranulocytosis, colitis, pancytopenia, aplastic anemia, hemolytic anemia, hemorrhage, prolonged PT, encephalopathy, asterixis, neuromuscular excitability, serum-sickness reactions, superinfection

**Overdose/Toxicology** Symptoms of overdose include neuromuscular hypersensitivity and convulsions. Many beta-lactam containing antibiotics have the potential to cause neuromuscular hyperirritability or convulsive seizures. Hemodialysis may be helpful to aid in removal of the drug from blood; otherwise, treatment is supportive or symptom directed.

**Pharmacodynamics/Kinetics**

**Protein Binding:** 33% to 50%

**Distribution:** Widely distributed to body tissues and fluids; crosses the blood-brain barrier; therapeutic concentrations achieved in CSF even when meninges are not inflamed; crosses placenta

**Half-life Elimination:** 1-2 hours (prolonged in renal impairment)

**Time to Peak:** I.M.: Within 15-60 minutes; I.V.: 2-3 minutes

**Excretion:** Urine

**Formulations**

Cefuroxime sodium:

Infusion, premixed (frozen) (Zinacef®): 750 mg (50 mL); 1.5 g (50 mL)

Powder for injection: 750 mg, 1.5 g, 7.5 g

Powder for injection (Kefurox®, Zinacef®): 750 mg, 1.5 g, 7.5 g

Cefuroxime axetil:

Powder for oral suspension (tutti-frutti flavor) (Ceftin®): 125 mg/5 mL (50 mL, 100 mL, 200 mL)

Tablet (Ceftin®): 125 mg, 250 mg, 500 mg

**Dosing**

**Adults:**

Oral: 250-500 mg every 12 hours; uncomplicated urinary tract infection: 125-250 mg every 12 hours

I.M., I.V.: 750 mg to 1.5 g/dose every 8 hours or 100-150 mg/kg/day in divided doses every 6-8 hours; maximum: 6 g/24 hours

**Elderly:** Refer to adult dosing.

**Renal Impairment:**

$Cl_{cr}$ >20 mL/minute: Administer 750-1500 mg every 8 hours.

$Cl_{cr}$ 10-20 mL/minute: Administer 750 mg every 12 hours.

$Cl_{cr}$ <10 mL/minute: Administer 750 mg every 24 hours.

Hemodialysis: Administer doses following dialysis.

Dialyzable (25%)

Continuous a-v hemofiltration (CAVH): Dose as $Cl_{cr}$ 10-20 mL/minute

**Administration**

**Oral:** Administer around-the-clock to promote less variation in peak and trough serum levels. Oral suspension: Administer with food. Shake well before use.

**I.M.:** Inject deep I.M. into large muscle mass.

**I.V.:** Inject direct I.V. over 3-5 minutes. Infuse intermittent infusion over 15-30 minutes.

**Stability**

**Reconstitution:**

Injectable: Reconstituted solution is stable for 24 hours at room temperature and 48 hours when refrigerated. I.V. infusion in NS or $D_5W$ solution is stable for 24 hours at room temperature, 7 days when refrigerated, or 26 weeks when frozen. After freezing, thawed solution is stable for 24 hours at room temperature or 21 days when refrigerated.

Oral suspension: Store in refrigerator or at room temperature. Discard after 10 days.

**Compatibility:** Discontinue other solutions at the same site to avoid compatibility problems.

**Monitoring Laboratory Tests** Prothrombin time; perform culture and sensitivity studies prior to initiating therapy.

**Additional Nursing Issues**

**Physical Assessment:** Assess for previous history of reactions to other cephalosporins or penicillins. Monitor for allergic reactions (see above). These can occur a few days after therapy is initiated. Assess for potential nephrotoxicity (see Drug Interactions). Assess bowel function (if severe diarrhea occurs, discontinue drug). May cause hypoprothrombinemia (monitor for bleeding, easy bruising or bleeding, blood in stool or urine). Monitor urine output (if decreased, notify prescriber). Assess for opportunistic infection (eg, fever, malaise, rash, diarrhea, itching, redness, fever, chills, or increased cough). Note breast-feeding caution.

**Patient Information/Instruction:** Take as directed, at regular intervals around-the-clock (with or without food). Chilling oral suspension improves flavor (do not freeze). Complete full course of medication, even if you feel better. Drink 2-3 L fluid/day. If diarrhea occurs, yogurt or buttermilk may help. May cause false-positive test with Clinitest®; use another form of testing. May interfere with oral contraceptives; additional contraceptive measures are necessary. Report severe, unresolved diarrhea; vaginal itching or drainage; sores in mouth; blood, pus, or mucus in stool or urine; easy bleeding or bruising; unusual fever or chills; rash; or respiratory difficulty. **Breast-feeding precautions:** Consult prescriber if breast-feeding.

**Geriatric Considerations:** Adjust dose for renal function in the elderly. Considered one of the drugs of choice for outpatient treatment of community-acquired pneumonia in the older adult.

**Breast-feeding Issues:** Theoretically, drug absorbed by nursing infant may change bowel flora or affect fever work-up result. **Note:** As a class, cephalosporins are used to treat infections in infants.

**Additional Information**

Each gram contains 2.4 mEq of sodium.

pH: 5-8.5

- **Cefzil®** *see* Cefprozil *on page 227*
- **Celebrex®** *see* Celecoxib *on this page*

## Celecoxib (ce le COX ib)

**U.S. Brand Names** Celebrex®

**Therapeutic Category** Nonsteroidal Anti-Inflammatory Agent (NSAID)

**Pregnancy Risk Factor** C (D after 34 weeks gestation or close to delivery)

**Lactation** Excretion in breast milk unknown

**Use** Relief of the signs and symptoms of osteoarthritis; relief of the signs and symptoms of rheumatoid arthritis in adults

**Mechanism of Action/Effect** Inhibits prostaglandin synthesis by decreasing the activity of the enzyme, cyclo-oxygenase-2 (COX-2), which results in decreased formation of prostaglandin precursors. Celecoxib does not inhibit cyclo-oxygenase-1 (COX-1) at therapeutic concentrations.

**Contraindications** Hypersensitivity to celecoxib or any component, sulfonamides, aspirin, or other nonsteroidal anti-inflammatory drugs (NSAIDs); pregnancy (after 34 weeks gestation or close to delivery)

**Warnings** Gastrointestinal irritation, ulceration, bleeding, and perforation may occur with NSAIDs (it is unclear whether celecoxib is associated with rates of these events which are similar to nonselective NSAIDs). Use with caution in patients with a history of GI disease (bleeding or ulcers), decreased renal function, hepatic disease, congestive heart failure, hypertension, or asthma. Anaphylactoid reactions may occur, even with no prior exposure to celecoxib. Use caution in patients with known or suspected deficiency of cytochrome P-450 isoenzyme 2C9. Pregnancy risk factor C (before 34 weeks gestation)/ D (after 34 weeks).

**Drug Interactions**

**Cytochrome P-450 Effect:** Celecoxib may be a CYP2C9 enzyme substrate and an inhibitor of CYP2D6

**Decreased Effect:** Efficacy of thiazide diuretics, loop diuretics (furosemide), or ACE-inhibitors may be diminished by celecoxib.

**Increased Effect/Toxicity:** Inhibitors of isoenzyme 2C9 may result in significant increases in celecoxib concentrations. Coadministration of drugs by 2D6 may result in increased serum concentrations of these agents. Fluconazole increases celecoxib concentrations two-fold. Lithium concentrations may be increased by celecoxib. Celecoxib may be used with low-dose aspirin, however rates of gastrointestinal bleeding may be increased with coadministration. Celecoxib has not been shown to alter warfarin effects, although bleeding complications may be increased.

**Adverse Reactions**

>10%: Central nervous system: Headache (15.8%)

2% to 10%:

- Cardiovascular: Peripheral edema (2.1%)
- Central nervous system: Insomnia (2.3%), dizziness (2%)
- Dermatologic : Skin rash (2.2%)
- Gastrointestinal: Dyspepsia (8.8%), diarrhea (5.6%), abdominal pain (4.1%), nausea (3.5%), flatulence (2.2%)
- Neuromuscular & skeletal: Back pain (2.8%)
- Respiratory: Upper respiratory tract infection (8.1%), sinusitis (5%), pharyngitis (2.3%), rhinitis (2%)
- Miscellaneous: Accidental injury (2.9%)

0.1% to 2%:

- Cardiovascular: Hypertension (aggravated), chest pain, myocardial infarction, palpitation, tachycardia, facial edema, peripheral edema

(Continued)

## Celecoxib *(Continued)*

Central nervous system: Migraine, vertigo, hypoesthesia, fatigue, fever, pain, hypotonia, anxiety, depression, nervousness, somnolence

Dermatologic: Alopecia, dermatitis, photosensitivity, pruritus, rash (maculopapular), rash (erythematous), dry skin, urticaria

Endocrine & metabolic: Hot flashes, diabetes mellitus, hyperglycemia, hypercholesterolemia, breast pain, dysmenorrhea, menstrual disturbances, hypokalemia

Gastrointestinal: Constipation, tenesmus, diverticulitis, eructation, esophagitis, gastroenteritis, vomiting, gastroesophageal reflux, hemorrhoids, hiatal hernia, melena, stomatitis, anorexia, increased appetite, taste disturbance, dry mouth, tooth disorder, weight gain

Genitourinary: Prostate disorder, vaginal bleeding, vaginitis, monilial vaginitis, dysuria, cystitis, urinary frequency, incontinence, urinary tract infection,

Hepatic: Elevated transaminases, increased alkaline phosphatase

Hematologic: Anemia, thrombocytopenia, ecchymosis

Neuromuscular & skeletal: Leg cramps, increased CPK, neck stiffness, arthralgia, myalgia, bone disorder, fracture, synovitis, tendonitis, neuralgia, paresthesia, neuropathy, weakness

Ocular: Glaucoma, blurred vision, cataract, conjunctivitis, eye pain

Otic: Deafness, tinnitus, earache, otitis media

Renal: Increased BUN, increased creatinine, albuminuria, hematuria, renal calculi

Respiratory: Bronchitis, bronchospasm, cough, dyspnea, laryngitis, pneumonia, epistaxis

Miscellaneous: Allergic reactions, flu-like syndrome, breast cancer, herpes infection, bacterial infection, moniliasis, viral infection, increased diaphoresis

<0.1% (Limited to important or life-threatening symptoms): Congestive heart failure, ventricular fibrillation, pulmonary embolism, syncope, cerebrovascular accident, gangrene, thrombophlebitis, thrombocytopenia, ataxia, acute renal failure, intestinal obstruction, pancreatitis, intestinal perforation, gastrointestinal bleeding, colitis, esophageal perforation, sepsis, sudden death

**Overdose/Toxicology** Symptoms of overdose may include epigastric pain, drowsiness, lethargy, nausea, and vomiting; gastrointestinal bleeding may occur. Rare manifestations include hypertension, respiratory depression, coma, and acute renal failure. Treatment is symptomatic and supportive. Forced diuresis, hemodialysis and/or urinary alkalinization may not be useful.

**Pharmacodynamics/Kinetics**

**Protein Binding:** 97% (albumin)

**Half-life Elimination:** 11 hours

**Time to Peak:** 3 hours

**Metabolism:** Metabolized by cytochrome P-450 isoenzyme 2C9 (CYP2C9)

**Excretion:** In urine as metabolites (<3% unchanged drug)

**Formulations** Capsule: 100 mg, 200 mg

**Dosing**

**Adults:** Oral:

Osteoarthritis: 200 mg/day as a single dose or in divided dose twice daily

Rheumatoid arthritis: 100-200 mg twice daily

**Elderly:** Oral: No specific adjustment is recommended; however, the AUC in elderly patients may be increased by 50% as compared to younger subjects. Use the lowest recommended dose in patients weighing <50 kg.

**Renal Impairment:** No specific dosage adjustment is recommended (AUC decreased by 40%).

**Hepatic Impairment:** Reduced dosage is recommended (AUC may be increased by 40% to 180%).

**Additional Nursing Issues**

**Physical Assessment:** See Contraindications and Warnings/Precautions for use cautions. Assess effectiveness and interactions of other medications (see Drug Interactions, ie, monitor patients taking lithium closely). Assess allergy history (aspirin, NSAIDS, salicylates). Monitor effectiveness of therapy (pain, range of motion, mobility, ADL function, inflammation). Assess knowledge/teach patient appropriate use, possible side effects/interventions, and adverse symptoms to report (see Adverse Reaction and Overdose/Toxicology). **Pregnancy risk factor C/D** - see Pregnancy Risk Factor for cautious use. Note breast-feeding caution.

**Patient Information/Instruction:** Do not take more than recommended dose. May be taken with food to reduce GI upset. Do not take with antacids. Avoid alcohol, aspirin, and OTC medication unless approved by prescriber. You may experience dizziness, confusion, or blurred vision (avoid driving or engaging in tasks requiring alertness until response to drug is known); anorexia, nausea, vomiting, taste disturbance, gastric distress (small frequent meals, frequent mouth care, sucking lozenges, or chewing gum may help). GI bleeding, ulceration, or perforation can occur with or without pain; it is unclear whether celecoxib has rates of these events which are similar to nonselective NSAIDs. Stop taking medication and report immediately stomach pain or cramping, unusual bleeding or bruising, or blood in vomitus, stool, or urine. Report persistent insomnia; skin rash; unusual fatigue or easy bruising or bleeding; muscle pain, tremors, or weakness; sudden weight gain; changes in hearing (ringing in ears); changes in vision; changes in urination pattern; or respiratory difficulty. **Pregnancy/breast-feeding precautions:** Inform prescriber if you are or intend to be pregnant. Consult prescriber if breast-feeding.

**Breast-feeding Issues:** In animal studies, celecoxib has been found to be excreted in milk; it is not known whether celecoxib is excreted in human milk. Because many drugs are excreted in milk, and the potential for serious adverse reactions exists, a decision should be made whether to discontinue nursing or discontinue the drug, taking into account the importance of the drug to the mother.

**Pregnancy Issues:** In late pregnancy may cause premature closure of the ductus arteriosus.

**Related Information**

Nonsalicylate/Nonsteroidal Anti-inflammatory Comparison *on page 1401*

- **Celek® 20** *see* Potassium Supplements *on page 952*
- **Celestoderm®** *see* Betamethasone *on page 148*
- **Celestoderm®** *see* Topical Corticosteroids *on page 1152*
- **Celestone®** *see* Betamethasone *on page 148*
- **Celestone® Soluspan®** *see* Betamethasone *on page 148*
- **Celexa®** *see* Citalopram *on page 276*
- **CellCept®** *see* Mycophenolate *on page 795*
- **Cellufresh® Ophthalmic Solution** *see page 1294*
- **Cellulose, Oxidized** *see page 1248*
- **Celluvisc® Ophthalmic Solution** *see page 1294*
- **Cel-U-Jec®** *see* Betamethasone *on page 148*
- **Cenafed® [OTC]** *see* Pseudoephedrine *on page 992*
- **Cenafed® Plus Tablet** *see page 1294*
- **Cena-K®** *see* Potassium Supplements *on page 952*
- **Cenestin™** *see* Estrogens, Conjugated (Synthetic) *on page 448*
- **Cēpacol® Anesthetic Troche** *see page 1294*
- **Cēpacol® Troches** *see page 1294*
- **Cēpastat®** *see page 1294*

## Cephalexin (sef a LEKS in)

**U.S. Brand Names** Biocef; Keflex®; Keftab®

**Therapeutic Category** Antibiotic, Cephalosporin (First Generation)

**Pregnancy Risk Factor** B

**Lactation** Enters breast milk (small amounts)/use caution

**Use** Treatment of susceptible bacterial infections, including those caused by group A beta-hemolytic *Streptococcus, Staphylococcus, Klebsiella pneumoniae, E. coli, Proteus mirabilis*, and *Shigella*; predominantly used for lower respiratory tract, urinary tract, skin and soft tissue, and bone and joint

**Mechanism of Action/Effect** Inhibits bacterial cell wall synthesis by binding to one or more of the penicillin-binding proteins (PBPs)

**Contraindications** Hypersensitivity to cephalexin, any component, or other cephalosporins

**Warnings** Modify dosage in patients with severe renal impairment. Prolonged use may result in superinfection. Cross-sensitivity to penicillins exists (~10%).

**Drug Interactions**

**Increased Effect/Toxicity:** High-dose probenecid may decrease clearance of cephalexin. Aminoglycosides in combination with cephalexin may result in additive nephrotoxicity.

**Food Interactions** Cephalexin serum levels may be decreased if taken with food.

**Effects on Lab Values** May cause false-positive Coombs' test, false-positive results in urine glucose tests when using cupric sulfate (Benedict's solution, Clinitest®)

**Adverse Reactions**

1% to 10%: Gastrointestinal: Diarrhea

<1% (Limited to important or life-threatening symptoms): Dizziness, fatigue, headache, rash, urticaria, angioedema, anaphylaxis, erythema multiforme, toxic epidermal necrolysis, Stevens-Johnson syndrome, serum-sickness reaction, nausea, vomiting, dyspepsia, gastritis, abdominal pain, pseudomembranous colitis, interstitial nephritis, agitation, hallucinations, confusion, arthralgia, eosinophilia, neutropenia, thrombocytopenia, anemia, increased transaminases, hepatitis, cholestasis

Other reactions with cephalosporins include anaphylaxis, vomiting, agranulocytosis, colitis, pancytopenia, aplastic anemia, hemolytic anemia, hemorrhage, prolonged PT, encephalopathy, asterixis, neuromuscular excitability, seizures, superinfection

**Overdose/Toxicology** Symptoms of overdose include neuromuscular hypersensitivity and convulsions. Many beta-lactam containing antibiotics have the potential to cause neuromuscular hyperirritability or convulsive seizures. Hemodialysis may be helpful to aid in removal of the drug from blood; otherwise, treatment is supportive or symptom directed.

**Pharmacodynamics/Kinetics**

**Protein Binding:** 6% to 15%

**Distribution:** Widely distributed into most body tissues and fluids, including gallbladder, liver, kidneys, bone, sputum, bile, and pleural and synovial fluids; CSF penetration is poor; crosses the placenta

**Half-life Elimination:** 0.5-1.2 hours (prolonged in renal impairment)

**Time to Peak:** Oral: Within 1 hour

**Excretion:** 80% to 100% of dose excreted as unchanged drug in urine within 8 hours

**Formulations**

Cephalexin monohydrate:

Capsule: 250 mg, 500 mg

(Continued)

## Cephalexin *(Continued)*

Powder for oral suspension: 125 mg/5 mL (5 mL unit dose, 60 mL, 100 mL, 200 mL); 250 mg/5 mL (5 mL unit dose, 100 mL, 200 mL)
Suspension, oral, pediatric: 100 mg/mL [5 mg/drop] (10 mL)
Tablet: 250 mg, 500 mg, 1 g
Cephalexin hydrochloride: Tablet: 500 mg

**Dosing**

**Adults:** Oral: 250-1000 mg every 6 hours; maximum: 4 g/day

**Elderly:** Refer to adult dosing.

**Renal Impairment:**

$Cl_{cr}$ >50 mL/minute: Administer every 8 hours.
$Cl_{cr}$ 10-50 mL/minute: Administer every 12 hours.
$Cl_{cr}$ <10 mL/minute: Administer every 12-24 hours.
Moderately dialyzable (20% to 50%)

**Administration**

**Oral:** Administer on an empty stomach (ie, 1 hour prior to, or 2 hours after meals) to increase total absorption. Give around-the-clock to promote less variation in peak and trough serum levels.

**Stability**

**Reconstitution:** Refrigerate suspension after reconstitution; discard after 14 days.

**Monitoring Laboratory Tests** Renal, hepatic, and hematologic function periodically with prolonged therapy; perform culture and sensitivity studies prior to initiating drug therapy.

**Additional Nursing Issues**

**Physical Assessment:** Assess for previous history of reactions to other cephalosporins or penicillins. Monitor for allergic reactions (see above). These can occur a few days after therapy is initiated. Assess for potential nephrotoxicity (see Drug Interactions). Assess bowel function (if severe diarrhea occurs, discontinue drug). Monitor urine output (if decreased, notify prescriber). Assess for opportunistic infection (eg, fever, malaise, rash, diarrhea, itching, redness, fever, chills, or increased cough). Note breast-feeding caution.

**Patient Information/Instruction:** Take as directed, at regular intervals around-the-clock (with or without food). Chilling oral suspension improves flavor (do not freeze). Complete full course of medication, even if you feel better. Drink 2-3 L fluid/day. If diarrhea occurs, yogurt or buttermilk may help. May cause false-positive test with Clinitest®; use another form of testing. May interfere with oral contraceptives; additional contraceptive measures are necessary. Report severe, unresolved diarrhea; vaginal itching or drainage; sores in mouth; blood, pus, or mucus in stool or urine; easy bleeding or bruising; unusual fever or chills; rash; or respiratory difficulty. **Breast-feeding precautions:** Consult prescriber if breast-feeding.

**Geriatric Considerations:** Adjust dose for renal function.

**Breast-feeding Issues:** Theoretically, drug absorbed by nursing infant may change bowel flora or affect fever work-up result. **Note:** As a class, cephalosporins are used to treat infections in infants.

## Cephapirin (sef a PYE rin)

**U.S. Brand Names** Cefadyl®

**Therapeutic Category** Antibiotic, Cephalosporin (First Generation)

**Pregnancy Risk Factor** B

**Lactation** Enters breast milk (small amounts)/use caution

**Use** Treatment of infections when caused by susceptible strains including group A beta-hemolytic *Streptococcus*; used in serious respiratory, genitourinary, gastrointestinal, skin and soft tissue, bone and joint infections; septicemia; endocarditis; identical to cephalothin

**Mechanism of Action/Effect** Inhibits bacterial cell wall synthesis by binding to one or more of the penicillin-binding proteins (PBPs)

**Contraindications** Hypersensitivity to cephapirin sodium, any component, or other cephalosporins

**Warnings** Modify dosage in patients with severe renal impairment. Prolonged use may result in superinfection. Cross-sensitivity to penicillins exists (~10%).

**Drug Interactions**

**Increased Effect/Toxicity:** High-dose probenecid decreases clearance of cephapirin. Aminoglycosides in combination with cephapirin may result in additive nephrotoxicity.

**Effects on Lab Values** May cause false-positive Coombs' test, false-positive results in urine glucose tests when using cupric sulfate (Benedict's solution, Clinitest®), urinary 17-ketosteroids.

**Adverse Reactions**

1% to 10%: Gastrointestinal: Diarrhea

<1% (Limited to important or life-threatening symptoms): CNS irritation, seizures, fever, rash, urticaria, leukopenia, thrombocytopenia, increased transaminases

Other reactions with cephalosporins include anaphylaxis, erythema multiforme, toxic epidermal necrolysis, Stevens-Johnson syndrome, dizziness, fever, headache, encephalopathy, asterixis, neuromuscular excitability, seizures, nausea, vomiting, pseudomembranous colitis, decreased hemoglobin, agranulocytosis, pancytopenia, aplastic anemia, hemolytic anemia, interstitial nephritis, toxic nephropathy, pain at injection site, vaginitis, angioedema, cholestasis, hemorrhage, prolonged PT, serum-sickness reactions, superinfection

**Overdose/Toxicology** Symptoms of overdose include neuromuscular hypersensitivity and convulsions. Many beta-lactam containing antibiotics have the potential to cause neuromuscular hyperirritability or convulsive seizures. Hemodialysis may be helpful to aid in removal of the drug from blood; otherwise, treatment is supportive or symptom directed.

**Pharmacodynamics/Kinetics**

**Protein Binding:** 22% to 25%

**Distribution:** Widely distributed into most body tissues and fluids including gallbladder, liver, kidneys, bone, sputum, bile, and pleural and synovial fluids; CSF penetration is poor; crosses the placenta

**Half-life Elimination:** 36-60 minutes (prolonged in renal impairment)

**Time to Peak:** I.M.: Within 30 minutes; I.V.: Within 5 minutes

**Metabolism:** Partially in the liver, kidney, and plasma to metabolites (50% active)

**Excretion:** Urine

**Formulations** Powder for injection, as sodium: 500 mg, 1 g, 2 g, 4 g, 20 g

**Dosing**

**Adults:** I.M., I.V.: 500 mg to 1 g every 6 hours up to 12 g/day

**Elderly:** Refer to adult dosing.

**Renal Impairment:**

$Cl_{cr}$ 10-50 mL/minute: Administer every 6-8 hours.

$Cl_{cr}$ <10 mL/minute: Administer every 12 hours.

Continuous a-v hemofiltration (CAVH): 1 gram every 8 hours

**Administration**

**I.M.:** Inject deep I.M. into large muscle mass.

**I.V.:** Inject direct I.V. over 3-5 minutes. Infuse intermittent infusion over 15-30 minutes.

**Stability**

**Reconstitution:** Reconstituted solution is stable for 24 hours at room temperature and 10 days when refrigerated. For I.V. infusion in NS or $D_5W$, solution is stable for 24 hours at room temperature, 10 days when refrigerated or 14 days when frozen. After freezing, thawed solution is stable for 12 hours at room temperature or 10 days when refrigerated.

**Compatibility:** Discontinue other solutions at the same site to avoid compatibility problems.

**Monitoring Laboratory Tests** Prothrombin time; perform culture and sensitivity studies prior to initiating drug therapy.

**Additional Nursing Issues**

**Physical Assessment:** Assess for previous history of reactions to other cephalosporins or penicillins. Monitor for allergic reactions (see above). These can occur a few days after therapy is initiated. Assess for potential nephrotoxicity (see Drug Interactions). Assess bowel function (if severe diarrhea occurs, discontinue drug). May cause hypoprothrombinemia (monitor for bleeding, easy bruising or bleeding, blood in stool or urine). Monitor urine output (if decreased, notify prescriber). Assess for opportunistic infection (eg, fever, malaise, rash, diarrhea, itching, redness, fever, chills, or increased cough). Note breast-feeding caution.

**Patient Information/Instruction:** This drug is administered I.M. or I.V. Drink 2-3 L fluid/day. If diarrhea occurs, yogurt or buttermilk may help. May cause false-positive test with Clinitest®; use another form of testing. May interfere with oral contraceptives; additional contraceptive measures are necessary. Report severe, unresolved diarrhea; vaginal itching or drainage; sores in mouth; blood, pus, or mucus in stool or urine; easy bleeding or bruising; unusual fever or chills; rash; or respiratory difficulty. **Breast-feeding precautions:** Consult prescriber if breast-feeding.

**Geriatric Considerations:** Cephapirin has not been studied in the elderly. Adjust dose for renal function.

**Breast-feeding Issues:** Theoretically, drug absorbed by nursing infant may change bowel flora or affect fever work-up result. **Note:** As a class, cephalosporins are used to treat infections in infants.

**Additional Information**

Each gram contains 2.4 mEq of sodium.

pH: 6.5-8.5

## Cephradine (SEF ra deen)

**U.S. Brand Names** Velosef®

**Therapeutic Category** Antibiotic, Cephalosporin (First Generation)

**Pregnancy Risk Factor** B

**Lactation** Enters breast milk/use caution

**Use** Treatment of susceptible bacterial infections, including those caused by group A beta-hemolytic *Streptococcus*; used in in respiratory, genitourinary, gastrointestinal, skin and soft tissue, bone and joint infections

**Mechanism of Action/Effect** Inhibits bacterial cell wall synthesis by binding to one or more of the penicillin-binding proteins (PBPs)

**Contraindications** Hypersensitivity to cephradine, any component, or other cephalosporins

**Warnings** Prolonged use may result in superinfection. Use with caution in patients with a history of colitis. Reduce dose in patients with renal dysfunction. Cross-sensitivity to penicillins exists (~10%).

**Drug Interactions**

**Increased Effect/Toxicity:** High-dose probenecid decreases clearance of cephradine. Aminoglycosides in combination with cephradine may result in additive nephrotoxicity.

(Continued)

## Cephradine *(Continued)*

**Food Interactions** Cephradine serum levels may be decreased if taken with food.

**Effects on Lab Values** May cause false-positive Coombs' test, false-positive results in urine glucose tests when using cupric sulfate (Benedict's solution, Clinitest®)

**Adverse Reactions**

1% to 10%: Gastrointestinal: Diarrhea

<1% (Limited to important or life-threatening symptoms): Rash, nausea, vomiting, pseudomembranous colitis, increased BUN, increased creatinine

Other reactions with cephalosporins include anaphylaxis, erythema multiforme, toxic epidermal necrolysis, Stevens-Johnson syndrome, dizziness, fever, headache, encephalopathy, asterixis, neuromuscular excitability, seizures, neutropenia, leukopenia, agranulocytosis, pancytopenia, aplastic anemia, hemolytic anemia, interstitial nephritis, toxic nephropathy, vaginitis, angioedema, cholestasis, hemorrhage, prolonged PT, serum-sickness reactions, superinfection

**Overdose/Toxicology** Symptoms of overdose include neuromuscular hypersensitivity and convulsions. Many beta-lactam containing antibiotics have the potential to cause neuromuscular hyperirritability or convulsive seizures. Hemodialysis may be helpful to aid in removal of the drug from blood; otherwise, treatment is supportive or symptom directed.

**Pharmacodynamics/Kinetics**

**Protein Binding:** 18% to 20%

**Distribution:** Widely distributed into most body tissues and fluids including gallbladder, liver, kidneys, bone, sputum, bile, and pleural and synovial fluids; CSF penetration is poor; crosses the placenta

**Half-life Elimination:** 1-2 hours (prolonged in renal impairment)

**Time to Peak:** Oral, I.M.: Within 1-2 hours

**Excretion:** Urine

**Formulations**

Capsule: 250 mg, 500 mg

Powder for injection: 250 mg, 500 mg, 1 g, 2 g (in ready to use infusion bottles)

Powder for oral suspension: 125 mg/5 mL (5 mL, 100 mL, 200 mL); 250 mg/5 mL (5 mL, 100 mL, 200 mL)

**Dosing**

**Adults:**

Oral: 250-500 mg every 6-12 hours

I.V.: 2-4 g daily divided into 4 doses; severe infections can be treated up to 8 g daily

**Elderly:** Refer to adult dosing.

**Renal Impairment:**

$Cl_{cr}$ 10-50 mL/minute: Administer 50% of dose.

$Cl_{cr}$ <10 mL/minute: Administer 25% of dose.

**Administration**

**Oral:** Administer around-the-clock to promote less variation in peak and trough serum levels. Shake oral suspension well.

**I.V.:** I.V. push over 3-5 minutes

**I.V. Detail:** Do not admix with aminoglycosides in same bottle/bag.

**Stability**

**Reconstitution:**

Oral suspension: Refrigerated storage maintains potency for 14 days. Room temperature storage maintains potency for 7 days.

I.V., I.M.: Reconstituted solution is stable for 2 hours at room temperature and 24 hours when refrigerated. For I.V. infusion in NS or $D_5W$, solution is stable for 10 hours at room temperature, 48 hours when refrigerated or 6 weeks when frozen. After freezing, thawed solution is stable for 10 hours at room temperature or 48 hours when refrigerated.

**Compatibility:** Do not mix with other antibiotics. Incompatible with lactated Ringer's.

**Monitoring Laboratory Tests** Prothrombin time; perform culture and sensitivity studies prior to initiating drug therapy.

**Additional Nursing Issues**

**Physical Assessment:** Assess for previous history of reactions to other cephalosporins or penicillins. Monitor for allergic reactions (see above). These can occur a few days after therapy is initiated. Assess for potential nephrotoxicity (see Drug Interactions). Assess bowel function (if severe diarrhea occurs, discontinue drug). May cause hypoprothrombinemia (monitor for bleeding, easy bruising or bleeding, blood in stool or urine). Monitor urine output (if decreased, notify prescriber). Assess for opportunistic infection (eg, fever, malaise, rash, diarrhea, itching, redness, fever, chills, or increased cough). Note breast-feeding caution.

**Patient Information/Instruction:** Oral: Take as directed, at regular intervals around-the-clock (with or without food). Chilling oral suspension improves flavor (do not freeze). Complete full course of medication, even if you feel better. Drink 2-3 L fluid/day. If diarrhea occurs, yogurt or buttermilk may help. May cause false-positive test with Clinitest®; use another form of testing. May interfere with oral contraceptives; additional contraceptive measures are necessary. Report severe, unresolved diarrhea; vaginal itching or drainage; sores in mouth; blood, pus, or mucus in stool or urine; easy bleeding or bruising; unusual fever or chills; rash; or respiratory difficulty. **Breast-feeding precautions:** Consult prescriber if breast-feeding.

**Geriatric Considerations:** Cephradine has not been studied in the elderly. Adjust dose for renal function in the elderly.

**Breast-feeding Issues:** Theoretically, drug absorbed by nursing infant may change bowel flora or affect fever work-up result. **Note:** As a class, cephalosporins are used to treat infections in infants.

- **Cephulac®** *see* Lactulose *on page 651*
- **Ceporex** *see* Cephalexin *on page 237*
- **Ceptaz™** *see* Ceftazidime *on page 228*
- **Cerebyx®** *see* Fosphenytoin *on page 520*
- **Ceredase®** *see* Alglucerase *on page 51*
- **Cerezyme®** *see* Alglucerase *on page 51*

## Cerivastatin (se ree va STAT in)

**U.S. Brand Names** Baycol™

**Therapeutic Category** Antilipemic Agent (HMG-CoA Reductase Inhibitor)

**Pregnancy Risk Factor** X

**Lactation** Enters breast milk/contraindicated

**Use** Reduces total LDL serum cholesterol concentrations in primary hypercholesterolemia in conjunction with diet

**Mechanism of Action/Effect** Cerivastatin acts by competitively inhibiting 3-hydroxy-3-methylglutaryl-coenzyme A (HMG-CoA) reductase, the enzyme that catalyzes the rate-limiting step in cholesterol synthesis.

**Contraindications** Hypersensitivity to cerivastatin or any component; patients with active liver disease; unexplained elevated serum transaminases; pregnancy

**Warnings** Use with caution in patients with ALT and AST elevations after the start of therapy. Monitor LFTs which usually return to normal after the first 6 weeks of therapy. HMG-CoA reductase inhibitors have been associated with cases of rhabdomyolysis and acute renal failure secondary to the myoglobinuria usually with creatine kinase levels >10 times the normal limit.

**Drug Interactions**

**Cytochrome P-450 Effect:** CYP3A3/4 enzyme substrate

**Decreased Effect:** Cholestyramine and cerivastatin: when cerivastatin is taken within 1 before or up to 2 hours after cholestyramine, a decrease in absorption of cerivastatin can occur.

**Effects on Lab Values** Elevated transaminases, alkaline phosphatase, gamma-glutamyl transpeptidase, and bilirubin; abnormal thyroid function tests

**Adverse Reactions**

>10%

Central nervous system: Headache (11.8%)
Respiratory: Rhinitis, pharyngitis

1% to 10%:

Cardiovascular: Chest pain, peripheral edema (2%)
Central nervous system: Back pain, asthenia, dizziness, insomnia
Dermatologic: Rash
Gastrointestinal: Abdominal pain, dyspepsia, diarrhea, flatulence, nausea, constipation
Genitourinary: Urinary tract infection
Neuromuscular & skeletal: Arthralgia, myalgia
Respiratory: Sinusitis, cough

<1% (Limited to life-threatening or important symptoms): Elevated serum aminotransferase (>3 times normal), elevated creatinine kinase, myalgia, muscle weakness, anaphylaxis, angioedema, lupus erythematosus-like syndrome, thrombocytopenia, leukopenia, hemolytic anemia, toxic epidermal necrolysis, erythema multiforme including Stevens-Johnson syndrome

**Pharmacodynamics/Kinetics**

**Protein Binding:** 99% bound to plasma proteins; 80% bound to albumin

**Half-life Elimination:** 2-3 hours

**Time to Peak:** 1-3 hours

**Metabolism:** Liver

**Excretion:** Feces and to a lesser extent urine

**Onset:** Maximal reductions in ~2-3 weeks

**Formulations** Tablet, as sodium: 0.2 mg, 0.3 mg

**Dosing**

**Adults:** Oral: 0.3 mg daily in the evening with or without food

**Elderly:** Refer to adult dosing.

**Renal Impairment:** $Cl_{cr}$: ≤60 mL/minute: Reduce dose to 0.2 mg daily in the evening with or without food.

**Hepatic Impairment:** Patients with a history of liver disease or heavy alcohol ingestion should start therapy at the 0.2 mg dose and be monitored closely.

**Administration**

**Oral:** Take with or without food.

**Monitoring Laboratory Tests** Serum cholesterol, liver function tests; test liver function prior to initiation, at then 6 and 12 weeks after initiation or first dose, and periodically thereafter.

**Additional Nursing Issues**

**Physical Assessment:** Monitor laboratory results before beginning therapy, at 6 and 12 weeks after initiating dose, and periodically during long-term therapy (see Monitoring Laboratory Tests). Monitor and instruct patient on appropriate use, possible adverse effects (see above), and symptoms to report. **Pregnancy risk factor X** - determine that patient is not pregnant before beginning treatment and do not give to women of childbearing age or to males who may have intercourse with women of

(Continued)

## Cerivastatin *(Continued)*

childbearing age unless both male and female are capable of complying with barrier contraceptive measures during therapy and for 1 month following therapy. Breast-feeding is contraindicated.

**Patient Information/Instruction:** Take prescribed dose in the evening (with or without food). You will need laboratory evaluation during therapy. Maintain adequate hydration (2-3 L/day of fluids unless instructed to restrict fluid intake). May cause headache (mild analgesic may help); drowsiness, dizziness, or blurred vision (use caution when driving or engaging in tasks that require alertness until response to medication is known). Report chest pain; swelling of extremities; weight gain (>5 lb/week); respiratory difficulty; persistent vomiting or abdominal pain; muscle weakness or pain; persistent cough; swelling of mouth, lips, or face; unusual bruising or bleeding; or skin rash. **Pregnancy/breast-feeding precautions:** Inform prescriber if you are pregnant. Do not get pregnant during or for 1 month following therapy. Male: Do not cause a pregnancy. Male/female: Consult prescriber for instruction on appropriate contraceptive measures. This drug may cause severe fetal defects. Do not breast-feed.

**Geriatric Considerations:** The definition of and, therefore, when to treat hyperlipidemia in the elderly is a controversial issue. The National Cholesterol Education Program recommends that all adults 20 years of age and older maintain a plasma cholesterol <200 mg/dL. By this definition, 60% of all elderly would be considered to have a borderline high (200-239 mg/dL) or high (≥240 mg/dL) plasma cholesterol. However, plasma cholesterol has been shown to be a less reliable predictor of coronary heart disease in the elderly. Therefore, it is the authors' belief that pharmacologic treatment be reserved for those who are unable to obtain a desirable plasma cholesterol level by diet alone and for whom the benefits of treatment are believed to outweigh the potential adverse effects, drug interactions, and cost of treatment.

**Related Information**

Lipid-Lowering Agents Comparison *on page 1393*


- ♦ **Cerose-DM® Liquid** *see page 1294*
- ♦ **Cerubidine®** *see* Daunorubicin Hydrochloride *on page 336*
- ♦ **Cerumenex®** *see page 1291*
- ♦ **Cervidil® Vaginal Insert** *see* Dinoprostone *on page 379*
- ♦ **C.E.S.™** *see* Estrogens, Conjugated (Equine) *on page 446*
- ♦ **CES** *see* Estrogens, Conjugated (Equine) *on page 446*
- ♦ **Cetacaine®** *see* Benzocaine, Butyl Aminobenzoate, Tetracaine, and Benzalkonium Chloride *on page 142*
- ♦ **Cetacort®** *see* Hydrocortisone *on page 578*
- ♦ **Cetacort®** *see* Topical Corticosteroids *on page 1152*
- ♦ **Cetamide®** *see page 1282*
- ♦ **Cetamide® Ophthalmic** *see* Sulfacetamide *on page 1080*
- ♦ **Cetapred®** *see page 1282*
- ♦ **Cetina** *see* Chloramphenicol *on page 248*


## Cetirizine (se TI ra zeen)

**U.S. Brand Names** Zyrtec®

**Synonyms** P-071; UCB-P071

**Therapeutic Category** Antihistamine

**Pregnancy Risk Factor** B

**Lactation** Enters breast milk/not recommended

**Use** Perennial and seasonal allergic rhinitis and other allergic symptoms including urticaria

**Mechanism of Action/Effect** Competes with histamine for $H_1$-receptor sites on effector cells in the GI tract, blood vessels, and respiratory tract

**Contraindications** Hypersensitivity to cetirizine, hydroxyzine, or any component

**Warnings** Cetirizine should be used cautiously in patients with hepatic or renal dysfunction, or the elderly. Doses >10 mg/day may cause significant drowsiness.

**Drug Interactions**

**Increased Effect/Toxicity:** Increased toxicity with CNS depressants and anticholinergics.

**Adverse Reactions**

>10%: Central nervous system: Headache has been reported to occur in 10% to 12% of patients, drowsiness has been reported in as much as 26% of patients on high doses

1% to 10%:

Central nervous system: Somnolence, fatigue, dizziness

Gastrointestinal: Dry mouth

**Overdose/Toxicology** Symptoms of overdose include seizures, sedation, and hypotension. There is no specific treatment for antihistamine overdose. Clinical toxicity is due to blockade of cholinergic receptors. For anticholinergic overdose with severe life-threatening symptoms, physostigmine 1-2 mg I.V. slowly, may be given to reverse these effects.

**Pharmacodynamics/Kinetics**

**Half-life Elimination:** 8-11 hours

**Time to Peak:** Within 30-60 minutes

**Metabolism:** Exact fate is unknown, limited first pass hepatic metabolism

**Excretion:** 50% in urine unchanged

**Onset:** Within 15-30 minutes

**Formulations**

Cetirizine hydrochloride:
- Syrup: 5 mg/5 mL (120 mL)
- Tablet: 5 mg, 10 mg

**Dosing**

**Adults:** Oral: 5-10 mg once daily, depending upon symptom severity

**Elderly:** Oral: Initial: 5 mg once daily; may increase to 10 mg/day; adjust for renal impairment.

**Renal Impairment:**

$Cl_{cr}$ ≤31 mL/minute: Administer 5 mg once daily.
Hemodialysis: 5 mg once daily

**Hepatic Impairment:** Administer 5 mg once daily.

**Administration**

**Oral:** Take without regard to meals.

**Additional Nursing Issues**

**Physical Assessment:** Assess effectiveness and interactions of other medications (see Drug Interactions). See Contraindications and Warnings/Precautions for cautious use. Monitor effectiveness of therapy and adverse reactions (see Adverse Reactions) at beginning of therapy and periodically with long-term use. Assess knowledge/teach patient appropriate use, interventions to reduce side effects, and adverse symptoms to report. Breast-feeding is not recommended.

**Patient Information/Instruction:** Take as directed; do not exceed recommended dose. Avoid use of other depressants, alcohol, or sleep-inducing medications unless approved by prescriber. You may experience drowsiness or dizziness (use caution when driving or engaging in tasks requiring alertness until response to drug is known); or dry mouth, (frequent small meals, frequent mouth care, chewing gum, or sucking hard candy may help). Report persistent sedation, confusion, or agitation; persistent nausea or vomiting; changes in urinary pattern; blurred vision; chest pain or palpitations; or lack of improvement or worsening or condition. **Breast-feeding precautions:** Breast-feeding is not recommended.

**Geriatric Considerations:** Adjust dose for renal function.


- ♦ **Cetylpyridinium** *see page 1294*
- ♦ **Cetylpyridinium and Benzocaine** *see page 1294*
- ♦ **Cevalin® [OTC]** *see* Ascorbic Acid *on page 108*
- ♦ **Cevi-Bid® [OTC]** *see* Ascorbic Acid *on page 108*
- ♦ **Ce-Vi-Sol® [OTC]** *see* Ascorbic Acid *on page 108*
- ♦ **CG** *see* Chorionic Gonadotropin *on page 264*
- ♦ **Charcoaid® [OTC]** *see* Charcoal *on this page*


## Charcoal (CHAR kole)

**U.S. Brand Names** Actidose-Aqua® [OTC]; Actidose® With Sorbitol [OTC]; Charcoaid® [OTC]; Charcocaps® [OTC]; Insta-Char® [OTC]; Liqui-Char® [OTC]

**Synonyms** Activated Carbon; Liquid Antidote; Medicinal Carbon

**Therapeutic Category** Antidiarrheal; Antidote; Antiflatulent

**Pregnancy Risk Factor** C

**Lactation** Does not enter breast milk/compatible

**Use** Emergency treatment in poisoning by drugs and chemicals; repetitive doses for gastric dialysis in uremia to adsorb various waste products, and repetitive doses have proven useful to enhance the elimination of certain drugs (eg, theophylline, phenobarbital, and aspirin)

**Mechanism of Action/Effect** Adsorbs toxic substances or irritants, thus inhibiting GI absorption; adsorbs intestinal gas; the addition of sorbitol results in hyperosmotic laxative action causing catharsis

**Contraindications** Not effective for cyanide, mineral acids, caustic alkalis, organic solvents, iron, ethanol, methanol poisoning, lithium; do not use charcoal with sorbitol in patients with fructose intolerance

**Warnings** When using ipecac with charcoal, induce vomiting with ipecac before administering activated charcoal since charcoal adsorbs ipecac syrup. Charcoal may cause vomiting which is hazardous in petroleum distillate and caustic ingestions. If charcoal in sorbitol is administered, doses should be limited to prevent excessive fluid and electrolyte losses. Do not mix charcoal with milk, ice cream, or sherbet. Pregnancy factor C.

**Drug Interactions**

**Decreased Effect:** Charcoal decreases the effect of ipecac syrup. Also charcoal effect is reduced when taken with milk, ice cream, or sherbet.

**Adverse Reactions** >10%:

Gastrointestinal: Vomiting, diarrhea with sorbitol, constipation
Miscellaneous: Stools will turn black

**Pharmacodynamics/Kinetics**

**Metabolism:** Not metabolized

**Excretion:** As charcoal in feces

**Formulations**

Capsule (Charcocaps®): 260 mg

(Continued)

## Charcoal *(Continued)*

Liquid, activated:
- Actidose-Aqua®: 12.5 g (60 mL); 25 g (120 mL)
- Liqui-Char®: 12.5 g (60 mL); 15 g (75 mL); 25 g (120 mL); 30 g (120 mL); 50 g (240 mL)
- SuperChar®: 30 g (240 mL)

Liquid, activated, with propylene glycol: 12.5 g (60 mL); 25 g (120 mL)

Liquid, activated, with sorbitol:
- Actidose® With Sorbitol: 25 g (120 mL); 50 g (240 mL)
- Charcoaid®: 30 g (150 mL)

Powder for suspension, activated: 15 g, 30 g, 40 g, 120 g, 240 g

**Dosing**

**Adults:** Oral:

Acute poisoning:
- Charcoal with sorbitol: Single-dose: 30-100 g
- Charcoal in water:
  - Single-dose: 30-100 g or 1-2 g/kg
  - Multiple-dose: 20-60 g or 0.5-1 g/kg every 2-6 hours

Gastric dialysis: 20-50 g every 6 hours for 1-2 days

Intestinal gas, diarrhea, GI distress: 520-975 mg after meals or at first sign of discomfort; repeat as needed to a maximum dose of 4.16 g/day

**Elderly:** Refer to adult dosing.

**Administration**

**Oral:** Too concentrated of mixture may clog airway. Flavoring agents (eg, chocolate) and sorbitol can enhance charcoal's palatability. Marmalade, milk, ice cream, and sherbet should be avoided since they can reduce charcoal's effectiveness. If treatment includes ipecac syrup, induce vomiting prior to administration of charcoal.

**Stability**

**Storage:** Adsorbs gases from air, store in closed container.

**Additional Nursing Issues**

**Physical Assessment:** Monitor for active bowel sounds prior to administration. If antidote treatment includes ipecac syrup, induce vomiting before administering charcoal. May be administered with sorbitol or chocolate to improve palatability; do not administer with milk products. **Pregnancy risk factor C.**

**Patient Information/Instruction:** Charcoal will cause your stools to turn black. Do not self-administer as an antidote before calling the poison control center, hospital emergency room, or physician for instructions (charcoal is not the antidote for all poisons). **Pregnancy precautions:** Inform prescriber if you are pregnant.


- ♦ **Charcocaps® [OTC]** *see* Charcoal *on previous page*
- ♦ **Chelated Manganese®** *see page 1294*
- ♦ **Chemet®** *see page 1246*
- ♦ **Chemotherapy Compatibility** *see page 1311*
- ♦ **Chenix®** *see* Chenodiol *on this page*
- ♦ **Chenodeoxycholic Acid** *see* Chenodiol *on this page*


## Chenodiol (kee noe DYE ole)

**U.S. Brand Names** Chenix®

**Synonyms** Chenodeoxycholic Acid

**Therapeutic Category** Bile Acid

**Pregnancy Risk Factor** X

**Lactation** Excretion in breast milk unknown/not recommended

**Use** Oral dissolution of cholesterol gallstones in selected patients

**Mechanism of Action/Effect** Reduces the synthesis of cholesterol and choline acid in the liver; this leads to cholesterol in bile and results in breakdown of cholesterol gallstones

**Contraindications** Presence of known hepatocyte dysfunction or bile ductal abnormalities; a gallbladder confirmed as nonvisualizing after two consecutive single doses of dye; radiopaque stones; gallstone complications or compelling reasons for gallbladder surgery; inflammatory bowel disease or active gastric or duodenal ulcer; pregnancy

**Warnings** Chenodiol is hepatotoxic in animal models including subhuman Primates. Chenodiol should be discontinued if aminotransferases exceed 3 times the upper normal limit. Chenodiol may contribute to colon cancer in otherwise susceptible individuals.

**Drug Interactions**

**Decreased Effect:** Antacids, cholestyramine, colestipol, and oral contraceptives exhibit decreased effectiveness when taken with chenodiol.

**Effects on Lab Values** ↑ aminotransferases, cholesterol, LDL cholesterol, bilirubin (I); ↓ triglycerides

**Adverse Reactions**

>10%: Gastrointestinal: Diarrhea (mild and transient)

<1% (Limited to important or life-threatening symptoms): Hypertransaminasemia (transient), diarrhea (severe), frequent urge for bowel movement, anorexia, cramps, nausea, vomiting, constipation

**Overdose/Toxicology** Symptoms of overdose include diarrhea. A rise in liver function tests has been observed. There is no specific antidote, institute supportive therapy.

**Formulations** Tablet, film coated: 250 mg

**Dosing**

**Adults:** Oral: 13-16 mg/kg/day in 2 divided doses, starting with 250 mg twice daily the first 2 weeks and increasing by 250 mg/day each week thereafter until the recommended or maximum tolerated dose is achieved

**Elderly:** Refer to adult dosing.

**Hepatic Impairment:** Contraindicated for use in the presence of known hepatic dysfunction or bile ductal abnormalities.

**Monitoring Laboratory Tests** Serum aminotransferase, cholesterol

**Additional Nursing Issues**

**Physical Assessment:** Assess for abdominal pain, diarrhea, or jaundice prior to therapy and periodically during therapy (dosage may need to be adjusted). Instruct patient on use, possible adverse reactions, and symptoms to report. **Pregnancy risk factor X** - determine that patient is not pregnant before beginning treatment and do not give to women of childbearing age or to males who may have intercourse with women of childbearing age unless both male and female are capable of complying with barrier contraceptive measures during therapy and for 1 month following therapy. Breast-feeding is not recommended.

**Patient Information/Instruction:** Take as directed, for entire length of therapy. Medication may need to be taken for 24 months before dissolution will occur. Avoid aluminum-based antacids during entire course of therapy. Blood studies and x-rays studies will be necessary during therapy. Report persistent diarrhea and gallstone attacks (abdominal pain, nausea and vomiting, yellowing of skin or eyes). **Pregnancy/breast-feeding precautions:** Inform prescriber if you are pregnant and do not get pregnant during or for 1 month following therapy. Male: Do not cause a female to become pregnant. Male/female: Consult prescriber for instruction on appropriate contraceptive measures. This drug may cause severe fetal defects. Do not donate blood during or for 1 month following therapy. Breast-feeding is not recommended.


- ♦ **Cheracol®** *see* Guaifenesin and Codeine *on page 549*
- ♦ **Cheracol® D [OTC]** *see* Guaifenesin and Dextromethorphan *on page 549*
- ♦ **Chibroxin™ Ophthalmic** *see* Norfloxacin *on page 837*
- ♦ **Chickenpox Vaccine** *see page 1256*
- ♦ **Chigger-Tox® [OTC]** *see* Benzocaine *on page 141*
- ♦ **Children's Advil® Oral Suspension [OTC]** *see* Ibuprofen *on page 592*
- ♦ **Children's Hold®** *see page 1294*
- ♦ **Children's Kaopectate®** *see page 1294*
- ♦ **Children's Motrin® Oral Suspension [OTC]** *see* Ibuprofen *on page 592*
- ♦ **Children's Silfedrine® [OTC]** *see* Pseudoephedrine *on page 992*
- ♦ **Children's Vitamins** *see* Vitamin, Multiple *on page 1219*
- ♦ **Chlo-Amine®** *see page 1294*
- ♦ **Chlorafed® Liquid** *see page 1294*
- ♦ **Chloral** *see* Chloral Hydrate *on this page*


## Chloral Hydrate (KLOR al HYE drate)

**U.S. Brand Names** Aquachloral® Supprettes®

**Synonyms** Chloral; Trichloroacetaldehyde Monohydrate

**Therapeutic Category** Hypnotic, Miscellaneous

**Pregnancy Risk Factor** C

**Lactation** Enters breast milk/compatible

**Use** Short-term sedative and hypnotic (<2 weeks), sedative/hypnotic for dental and diagnostic procedures; sedative prior to EEG evaluations

**Mechanism of Action/Effect** Central nervous system depressant effects are due to its active metabolite trichloroethanol, mechanism unknown

**Contraindications** Hypersensitivity to chloral hydrate or any component; hepatic or renal impairment; gastritis or ulcers; severe cardiac disease

**Warnings** Use with caution in patients with porphyria. Use with caution in neonates, drug may accumulate with repeated use, prolonged use in neonates associated with hyperbilirubinemia. Tolerance to hypnotic effect develops, therefore, not recommended for use longer than 2 weeks. Taper dosage to avoid withdrawal with prolonged use. Trichloroethanol (TCE), a metabolite of chloral hydrate, is a carcinogen in mice; there is no data in humans. Chloral hydrate is considered a second line hypnotic agent in the elderly. Recent interpretive guidelines from the Health Care Financing Administration (HCFA) discourage the use of chloral hydrate in residents of long-term care facilities. Pregnancy factor C.

**Drug Interactions**

**Cytochrome P-450 Effect:** CYP1E2 enzyme substrate

**Increased Effect/Toxicity:** Chloral hydrate may potentiate effects of warfarin, central nervous system depressants, and alcohol when taken together. Vasodilation reaction (flushing, tachycardia, etc) may occur with concurrent use of alcohol. Concomitant use of furosemide (I.V.) may result in flushing, diaphoresis, and blood pressure changes.

**Effects on Lab Values** False-positive urine glucose using Clinitest® method; may interfere with fluorometric urine catecholamine and urinary 17-hydroxycorticosteroid tests

**Adverse Reactions**

>10%:

Central nervous system: Drowsiness

Gastrointestinal: Gastric irritation, nausea, vomiting, unpleasant taste in mouth

(Continued)

## Chloral Hydrate *(Continued)*

1% to 10%:

Central nervous system: Ataxia, dizziness, "hangover" effect, dizziness or lightheadedness, paranoid behavior, mental confusion

Dermatologic: Rash, urticaria

Gastrointestinal: Diarrhea

Hematologic: Leukopenia, eosinophilia

<1% (Limited to important or life-threatening symptoms): Disorientation, sedation, ataxia, excitement (paradoxical), fever, hallucinations, confusion, gastric irritation, ketonuria

**Overdose/Toxicology** Symptoms of overdose include hypotension, respiratory depression, coma, hypothermia, and cardiac arrhythmias. Treatment is supportive and symptomatic.

**Pharmacodynamics/Kinetics**

**Distribution:** Crosses the placenta

**Half-life Elimination:** Active metabolite: 8-11 hours

**Time to Peak:** Within 0.5-1 hour

**Metabolism:** Liver

**Excretion:** Kidney

**Duration:** 4-8 hours

**Formulations**

Capsule: 250 mg, 500 mg

Suppository, rectal: 324 mg, 500 mg, 648 mg

Syrup: 250 mg/5 mL (10 mL); 500 mg/5 mL (5 mL, 10 mL, 480 mL)

**Dosing**

**Adults:** Oral, rectal:

Sedation, anxiety: 250 mg 3 times/day

Hypnotic: 500-1000 mg at bedtime or 30 minutes prior to procedure, not to exceed 2 g/24 hours

**Note:** Withdraw gradually over 2 weeks if patient has been maintained on high doses for prolonged period of time. Do not stop drug abruptly.

**Elderly:** Hypnotic: Initial: Oral: 250 mg at bedtime; adjust for renal impairment. See Geriatric Considerations.

**Renal Impairment:**

$Cl_{cr}$ <50 mL/minute: Avoid use.

Hemodialysis effects: Supplemental dose is not necessary; dialyzable (50% to 100%).

**Hepatic Impairment:** Avoid use in patients with severe hepatic impairment.

**Administration**

**Oral:** Chilling the syrup may help to mask unpleasant taste.

**Stability**

**Storage:** Sensitive to light. Exposure to air causes volatilization. Store in light-resistant, airtight container.

**Additional Nursing Issues**

**Physical Assessment:** For short-term use. Assess effectiveness and interactions of other medications (see Drug Interactions). See Contraindications and Warnings/Precautions for cautious use. Assess for history of addiction; long-term use can result in dependence, abuse, or tolerance. Evaluate periodically for need for continued use (symptoms of dependence may resemble alcoholism, but usually there is more gastritis). After long-term use, taper dosage slowly when discontinuing. For inpatient use, institute safety measures (side rails, night light, call bell, assistance with ambulation) and monitor effectiveness and adverse reactions. For outpatients, monitor for effectiveness of therapy and adverse reactions (see Adverse Reactions) at beginning of therapy and periodically with long-term use. Assess knowledge/teach patient appropriate use, interventions to reduce side effects, and adverse symptoms to report. **Pregnancy risk factor C** - benefits of use should outweigh possible risks.

**Patient Information/Instruction:** Use exactly as directed (do not increase dose or frequency or discontinue without consulting prescriber); may cause physical and/or psychological dependence. While using this medication, do not use alcohol and other prescription or OTC medications (especially, pain medications, sedatives, antihistamines, or hypnotics) without consulting prescriber. Maintain adequate hydration (2-3 L/day of fluids unless instructed to restrict fluid intake). You may experience drowsiness, dizziness, or blurred vision (use caution when driving or engaging in tasks requiring alertness until response to drug is known); nausea, vomiting, unpleasant taste (small frequent meals, frequent mouth care, chewing gum, or sucking lozenges may help); diarrhea (buttermilk, boiled milk, yogurt may help). Report skin rash or irritation, CNS changes (confusion, depression, increased sedation, excitation, headache, insomnia, or nightmares), unresolved gastrointestinal distress, chest pain or palpitations, or ineffectiveness of medication. **Pregnancy precautions:** Inform prescriber if you are or intend to be pregnant.

**Geriatric Considerations:** Chloral hydrate is considered a second- or third-line hypnotic agent in the elderly. Interpretive guidelines from the Health Care Financing Administration (HCFA) discourage the use of chloral hydrate in residents of long-term care facilities.

**Related Information**

Anxiolytic/Hypnotic Use in Long-Term Care Facilities *on page 1430*

## Chlorambucil (klor AM byoo sil)

**U.S. Brand Names** Leukeran®

**Therapeutic Category** Antineoplastic Agent, Alkylating Agent

**Pregnancy Risk Factor** D

**Lactation** Excretion in breast milk unknown

**Use** Management of chronic lymphocytic leukemia, Hodgkin's and non-Hodgkin's lymphoma; breast and ovarian carcinoma; Waldenström's macroglobulinemia, testicular carcinoma, thrombocythemia, choriocarcinoma

**Mechanism of Action/Effect** Interferes with DNA replication and RNA transcription by alkylation and cross-linking the strands of DNA

**Contraindications** Hypersensitivity to chlorambucil, any component, or other alkylating agents; previous resistance; pregnancy

**Warnings** The U.S. Food and Drug Administration (FDA) currently recommends that procedures for proper handling and disposal of antineoplastic agents be considered. Use with caution in patients with seizure disorder and bone marrow suppression. Reduce initial dosage if patient has received radiation therapy, myelosuppressive drugs, or has a depressed baseline leukocyte or platelet count within the previous 4 weeks. Can severely suppress bone marrow function; effects human fertility; is carcinogenic in humans and probably mutagenic and teratogenic as well. Chromosomal damage has been documented. Secondary AML may be associated with chronic therapy.

**Adverse Reactions**

>10%:

- Hematologic: Myelosuppressive: Use with caution when receiving radiation; bone marrow suppression frequently occurs and occasionally bone marrow failure has occurred; blood counts should be monitored closely while undergoing treatment; leukopenia, thrombocytopenia, anemia
  - WBC: Moderate
  - Platelets: Moderate
  - Onset (days): 7
  - Nadir (days): 10-14
  - Recovery (days): 28

1% to 10%:

- Dermatologic: Skin rashes
- Endocrine & metabolic: Hyperuricemia, menstrual changes
- Gastrointestinal: Nausea, vomiting, diarrhea, oral ulceration are all infrequent
  - Emetic potential: Low (<10%)

<1% (Limited to important or life-threatening symptoms): Confusion, agitation, drug fever, ataxia, hallucination; rarely generalized or focal seizures, erythema multiforme, epidermal necrolysis, Stevens-Johnson syndrome, fertility impairment (has caused chromosomal damage in men, both reversible and permanent sterility have occurred in both sexes; can produce amenorrhea in females), oral ulceration, hepatotoxicity, hepatic necrosis weakness, tremors, muscular twitching, peripheral neuropathy, pulmonary fibrosis, secondary malignancies, increased incidence of AML, skin hypersensitivity

**Overdose/Toxicology** Symptoms of overdose include vomiting, ataxia, coma, seizures, and pancytopenia. There are no known antidotes for chlorambucil intoxication. Treatment is mainly supportive and symptomatic.

**Pharmacodynamics/Kinetics**

**Protein Binding:** ~99% bound to albumin; extensive binding to tissues and plasma proteins

**Half-life Elimination:** 90 minutes to 2 hours

**Metabolism:** In the liver to an active metabolite

**Excretion:** 60% excreted in urine within 24 hours, principally as metabolites

**Duration:** ~4 weeks

**Formulations** Tablet, sugar coated: 2 mg

**Dosing**

**Adults:** Oral (refer to individual protocols): 0.1-0.2 mg/kg/day **or** 3-6 mg/m²/day for 3-6 weeks, then adjust dose on basis of blood counts. Pulse dosing has been used in CLL as intermittent, biweekly, or monthly doses of 0.4 mg/kg and increased by 0.1 mg/kg until the disease is under control or toxicity ensues. An alternate regimen is 14 mg/m²/day for 5 days, repeated every 21-28 days.

**Elderly:** Oral (refer to individual protocols): Use lowest recommended doses for adults; usual dose for elderly is 2-4 mg/day, particularly for use in treatment of rheumatoid arthritis.

**Administration**

**Oral:** May divide single daily dose if nausea and vomiting occur. Take 1 hour before or 2 hours after meals.

**Stability**

**Storage:** Protect from light.

**Monitoring Laboratory Tests** Liver function, CBC, platelet count, serum uric acid

**Additional Nursing Issues**

**Physical Assessment:** Monitor for effectiveness of therapy and adverse reactions (see Adverse Reactions) with special attention to hematologic myelosuppression, CNS changes, adverse GI effects, and dermatologic effects. Avoid invasive procedures (including rectal thermometers). Teach patient/caregiver adverse symptoms to report. **Pregnancy risk factor D** - assess knowledge/teach appropriate use of barrier contraceptives. Note breast-feeding caution.

**Patient Information/Instruction:** Take exactly as directed (may be taken with chilled liquids). Maintain adequate hydration (2-3 L/day of fluids unless instructed to restrict fluid intake). Avoid alcohol, acidic, spicy, or hot foods, aspirin, or OTC medications unless approved by prescriber. Hair may be lost during treatment (reversible). You may experience menstrual irregularities and/or sterility. You will be more susceptible to infection; avoid crowds and exposure to infection. Frequent mouth care with soft

(Continued)

## Chlorambucil *(Continued)*

toothbrush or cotton swab may reduce occurrence of mouth sores. Report easy bruising or bleeding; fever or chills; numbness, pain, or tingling of extremities; muscle cramping or weakness; unusual swelling of extremities; menstrual irregularities; or any difficulty breathing. **Pregnancy/breast-feeding precautions:** Do not get pregnant while taking this medication; use appropriate barrier contraceptive measures (male/female). Consult prescriber if breast-feeding.

**Geriatric Considerations:** Toxicity to immunosuppressives is increased in the elderly. Start with lowest recommended adult doses (Dosage). Signs of infection, such as fever and rise in WBCs, may not occur. Lethargy and confusion may be more prominent signs of infection.

**Pregnancy Issues:** Carcinogenic and mutagenic in humans.

## Chloramphenicol (klor am FEN i kole)

**U.S. Brand Names** AK-Chlor® Ophthalmic; Chloromycetin®; Chloroptic® Ophthalmic

**Therapeutic Category** Antibiotic, Ophthalmic; Antibiotic, Otic; Antibiotic, Miscellaneous

**Pregnancy Risk Factor** C

**Lactation** Enters breast milk/not recommended (AAP rates "of concern")

**Use** Treatment of serious infections due to organisms resistant to other less toxic antibiotics or when its penetrability into the site of infection is clinically superior to other antibiotics to which the organism is sensitive; useful in infections caused by *Bacteroides*, *H. influenzae*, *Neisseria meningitidis*, *Salmonella*, and *Rickettsia*

**Mechanism of Action/Effect** Reversibly binds to 50S ribosomal subunits of susceptible organisms preventing amino acids from being transferred to growing peptide chains thus inhibiting protein synthesis

**Contraindications** Hypersensitivity to chloramphenicol or any component

**Warnings** Use with caution in patients with impaired renal or hepatic function and in neonates. Reduce dose with impaired liver function. Use with care in patients with glucose 6-phosphate dehydrogenase deficiency. Serious and fatal blood dyscrasias have occurred after both short-term and prolonged therapy. Should not be used when less potentially toxic agents are effective. Prolonged use may result in superinfection. Pregnancy factor C.

**Drug Interactions**

**Cytochrome P-450 Effect:** CYP2C9 enzyme inhibitor

**Decreased Effect:** Phenobarbital and rifampin may decrease serum concentrations of chloramphenicol.

**Increased Effect/Toxicity:** Chloramphenicol inhibits the metabolism of chlorpropamide, phenytoin, and oral anticoagulants resulting in increased levels.

**Effects on Lab Values** May cause false-positive results in urine glucose tests when using cupric sulfate (Benedict's solution, Clinitest®).

**Adverse Reactions**

**Ophthalmic:**

1% to 10%:

- Local: Burning or stinging
- Ocular: Blurred vision
- Miscellaneous: Hypersensitivity reactions

<1% (Limited to important or life-threatening symptoms): Blood dyscrasias

**Systemic:**

1% to 10%:

- Gastrointestinal: Diarrhea, nausea, vomiting
- Hematologic: Blood dyscrasias

<1% (Limited to important or life-threatening symptoms): Nightmares, headache, stomatitis, enterocolitis, bone marrow suppression, aplastic anemia, peripheral neuropathy, optic neuritis, gray baby syndrome

**Three major toxicities associated with chloramphenicol include:**

Aplastic anemia, an idiosyncratic reaction which can occur with any route of administration; usually occurs 3 weeks to 12 months after initial exposure to chloramphenicol

Bone marrow suppression is thought to be dose-related with serum concentrations >25 µg/mL and reversible once chloramphenicol is discontinued; anemia and neutropenia may occur during the first week of therapy

Gray baby syndrome is characterized by circulatory collapse, cyanosis, acidosis, abdominal distention, myocardial depression, coma, and death; reaction appears to be associated with serum levels ≥50 µg/mL; may result from drug accumulation in patients with impaired hepatic or renal function

**Topical:**

>10%: Miscellaneous: Hypersensitivity reactions

<1% (Limited to important or life-threatening symptoms): Blood dyscrasias

**Overdose/Toxicology** Symptoms of overdose include anemia, metabolic acidosis, hypotension, and hypothermia. Treatment is supportive.

**Pharmacodynamics/Kinetics**

**Protein Binding:** 60%

**Distribution:** Readily crosses the placenta; distributes to most tissues and body fluids

Ratio of CSF to blood level (%): Normal meninges: 66; Inflamed meninges: 66+

**Half-life Elimination:** Prolonged with markedly reduced liver function or combined liver/kidney dysfunction:

Normal renal function: 1.6-3.3 hours; End-stage renal disease: 3-7 hours; Cirrhosis: 10-12 hours

**Time to Peak:** Oral: Within 0.5-3 hours

**Metabolism:** Liver

**Excretion:** Urine

**Formulations**

Capsule: 250 mg

Ointment, ophthalmic: 1% [10 mg/g] (3.5 g)

AK-Chlor®, Chloroptic® S.O.P.: 1% [10 mg/g] (3.5 g)

Powder for injection, as sodium succinate: 1 g

Powder for ophthalmic solution (Chloromycetin®): 25 mg/vial (15 mL)

Solution: 0.5% [5 mg/mL] (7.5 mL, 15 mL)

Ophthalmic (AK-Chlor®, Chloroptic®): 0.5% [5 mg/mL] (2.5 mL, 7.5 mL, 15 mL)

Otic (Chloromycetin®): 0.5% (15 mL)

**Dosing**

**Adults:**

Oral, I.V.: 50-100 mg/kg/day in divided doses every 6 hours; maximum daily dose: 4 g/day.

Ophthalmic: Instill 1-2 drops or 1.25 cm (1/2" of ointment every 3-4 hours); increase interval between applications after 48 hours to 2-3 times/day.

Otic solution: Instill 2-3 drops into ear 3 times/day.

Topical: Gently rub into the affected area 1-4 times/day.

**Elderly:** Refer to adult dosing.

**Renal Impairment:** Slightly dialyzable (5% to 20%) via hemo- and peritoneal dialysis; no supplemental doses are needed in dialysis or continuous arteriovenous or venovenous hemofiltration (CAVH/CAVHD).

**Hepatic Impairment:** Avoid use in severe liver impairment as increased toxicity may occur.

**Administration**

**Oral:** Administer around-the-clock to promote less variation in peak and trough serum levels.

**I.V.:** Infuse via direct I.V. over 3-5 minutes; intermittent infusion over 30-60 minutes.

**Other:** Do not warm ear drops above body temperature. Will decrease its potency.

**Stability**

**Storage:** Refrigerate ophthalmic solution.

**Reconstitution:** Constituted solutions remain stable for 30 days. Use only clear solutions. Frozen solutions remain stable for 6 months.

**Monitoring Laboratory Tests** CBC with reticulocyte and platelet counts, periodic liver and renal function, serum drug concentration; culture and sensitivity specimen should be taken prior to initiating therapy.

**Additional Nursing Issues**

**Physical Assessment:** Assess effectiveness and interactions of other medications patient may be taking (see Drug Interactions). Monitor laboratory tests (see above), therapeutic response, and adverse reactions (eg, CNS disturbances, opportunistic infection), bone marrow depression, aplastic anemia (petechiae, sore throat, fatigue, unusual bleeding or bruising, abdominal or bone pain - see Adverse Reactions). Assess knowledge/teach patient appropriate use, interventions to reduce side effects, and adverse symptoms to report. **Pregnancy risk factor C** - benefits of use should outweigh possible risks. Breast-feeding is not recommended.

**Patient Information/Instruction:**

Oral: Take as directed, at regular intervals around-the-clock, with a large glass of water. Maintain adequate hydration (2-3 L/day of fluids unless instructed to restrict fluid intake). During I.V. administration, a bitter taste may occur; this will pass. Diabetics: Drug may cause false-positive test with Clinitest® glucose monitoring; use alternative glucose monitoring. This drug may interfere with effectiveness of oral contraceptives. You may experience nausea, vomiting (frequent small meals, frequent mouth care, sucking lozenges, or chewing gum may help). Report persistent rash, diarrhea; pain, burning, or numbness of extremities; petechiae; sore throat; fatigue; unusual bleeding or bruising; vaginal itching or discharge; mouth sores; yellowing of skin or eyes; dark urine or stool discoloration (blue); CNS disturbances (nightmares acute headache); or lack or improvement or worsening of condition.

Ophthalmic: Wash hands before instilling. Sit or lie down to instill. Open eye, look at ceiling, and instill prescribed amount of medication. Close eye and apply gentle pressure to inner corner of eye. Do not let tip of applicator touch eye or contaminate tip of applicator. Temporary stinging or burning may occur. Report persistent pain, burning, vision disturbances, swelling, itching, rash, or worsening of condition.

Otic: Wash hands before instilling. Tilt head with affected ear upward. Gently grasp ear lobe and lift back and upward. Instill prescribed drops into ear canal. Do not push dropper into ear. Remain with head tilted for 2 minutes. Report ringing in ears, discharge, or worsening of condition.

Topical: Wash hands before applying or wear gloves. Apply thin film to affected area. May apply porous dressing. Report persistent burning, swelling, itching, or worsening of condition.

**Pregnancy/breast-feeding precautions:** Inform prescriber if you are or intend to be pregnant. Breast-feeding is not recommended.

**Dietary Issues:** May decrease intestinal absorption of vitamin $B_{12}$. May have increased dietary need for riboflavin, pyridoxine, and vitamin $B_{12}$. Consult prescriber.

**Geriatric Considerations:** Chloramphenicol has not been studied in the elderly. It is not necessary to adjust the dose based upon the decrease in renal function associated

(Continued)

## Chloramphenicol *(Continued)*

with age. Chloramphenicol should be reserved for serious infections and the oral form avoided.

**Breast-feeding Issues:** Contraindicated due to potential bone marrow suppression to the infant.

**Additional Information** Each gram contains 2.25 mEq sodium.

**Related Information**

Ophthalmic Agents *on page 1282*
Otic Agents *on page 1291*

- **Chloramphenicol and Prednisolone** *see page 1282*
- **Chloraseptic® Oral** *see page 1294*
- **Chlorate®** *see page 1294*

## Chlordiazepoxide (klor dye az e POKS ide)

**U.S. Brand Names** Libritabs®; Librium®; Mitran® Oral; Reposans-10® Oral

**Synonyms** Methaminodiazepoxide Hydrochloride

**Therapeutic Category** Benzodiazepine

**Pregnancy Risk Factor** D

**Lactation** Enters breast milk/not recommended

**Use** Approved for anxiety; may be useful for acute alcohol withdrawal symptoms

**Contraindications** Hypersensitivity to chlordiazepoxide or any component; pre-existing CNS depression; severe uncontrolled pain; pregnancy

**Warnings** Use with caution in patients with respiratory depression, CNS impairment, liver dysfunction, or a history of drug dependence. Taper gradually over 2 weeks if patient has been maintained on high doses for a prolonged period of time. Do not stop drug abruptly.

**Drug Interactions**

**Cytochrome P-450 Effect:** Possibly a CYP2C8, 2C19, and 3A4 enzyme substrate

**Increased Effect/Toxicity:** Increased toxicity (CNS depression) when combined with alcohol, tricyclic antidepressants, and sedative-hypnotics. MAO inhibitors in combination with chlordiazepoxide may increase the incidence of edema.

**Effects on Lab Values** ↑ triglycerides (S); ↓ HDL

**Adverse Reactions**

>10%:

Central nervous system: Ataxia, dizziness, lightheadedness, drowsiness, slurred speech

1% to 10%:

Central nervous system: Euphoria, headache, mental depression
Endocrine & metabolic: Changes in libido
Gastrointestinal: Abdominal cramps, constipation, diarrhea, dry mouth
Neuromuscular & skeletal: Muscle spasm
Ocular: Blurred vision

<1% (Limited to important or life-threatening symptoms): Tachycardia, phlebitis, hallucinations, convulsions, paranoid symptoms, anemia, agranulocytosis, neutropenia, leukopenia, thrombocytopenia, liver dysfunction, dystonic reactions

**Overdose/Toxicology** Symptoms of overdose include hypotension, respiratory depression, coma, hypothermia, and cardiac arrhythmias. Treatment for benzodiazepine overdose is supportive. Flumazenil has been shown to selectively block the binding of benzodiazepines to CNS receptors, resulting in a reversal of benzodiazepine-induced CNS depression. Respiratory depression may not be reversed.

**Pharmacodynamics/Kinetics**

**Protein Binding:** 90% to 98%

**Distribution:** Crosses the placenta

**Half-life Elimination:** 6.6-25 hours; End-stage renal disease: 5-30 hours; Cirrhosis: 30-63 hours

**Time to Peak:** Oral: Within 2 hours; I.M.: Results in lower peak plasma levels than oral

**Metabolism:** Liver

**Excretion:** Urine

**Duration:** 48 hours to 1 week

**Formulations**

Chlordiazepoxide hydrochloride:

Capsule: 5 mg, 10 mg, 25 mg
Powder for injection: 100 mg
Tablet: 5 mg, 10 mg, 25 mg

**Dosing**

**Adults:**

Anxiety:

Oral: 15-100 mg divided 3-4 times/day
I.M., I.V.: Initial: 50-100 mg followed by 25-50 mg 3-4 times/day as needed

Preoperative anxiety: I.M.: 50-100 mg prior to surgery

Alcohol withdrawal symptoms: Oral, I.V.: 50-100 mg to start, dose may be repeated in 2-4 hours as necessary to a maximum of 300 mg/24 hours

**Elderly:** Anxiety: Oral: 5 mg 2-4 times/day; adjust for renal impairment. Avoid use if possible. See Geriatric Considerations.

**Renal Impairment:**

$Cl_{cr}$ <10 mL/minute: Administer 50% of dose.
Not dialyzable (0% to 5%)

**Hepatic Impairment:** Avoid use.

**Administration**

**I.V.:** Do not infuse into small veins. Infuse 100 mg or any fraction thereof over a minimum of 1 minute.

**I.V. Detail:** Rapid administration may cause symptoms of overdose.

**Stability**

**Storage:** Refrigerate injection and protect from light.

**Compatibility:** Incompatible when mixed with Ringer's solution, normal saline, ascorbic acid, benzquinamide, heparin, phenytoin, promethazine, or secobarbital.

**Additional Nursing Issues**

**Physical Assessment:** Assess other medications patient may be taking for effectiveness and interactions (see Drug Interactions). See Contraindications and Warnings/Precautions for cautious use. Assess for history of addiction; long-term use can result in dependence, abuse, or tolerance; periodically evaluate need for continued use. Monitor therapeutic response (eg, mood, affect, anxiety level, sleep pattern) and adverse reactions at beginning of therapy and periodically with long-term use (see Adverse Reactions and Overdose/Toxicology). Taper dosage slowly when discontinuing. Assess knowledge/teach patient appropriate use, interventions to reduce side effects, and adverse symptoms to report.

I.V.: Monitor vital signs frequently during infusion, observe safety precautions (side rails up, etc), and maintain bedrest for 2-3 hours following infusion. **Pregnancy risk factor D** - assess knowledge/teach appropriate use of barrier contraceptives. Breast-feeding is not recommended.

**Patient Information/Instruction:** Oral: Take exactly as directed (do not increase dose or frequency); may cause physical and/or psychological dependence. Do not use excessive alcohol or other prescription or OTC medications (especially pain medications, sedatives, antihistamines, or hypnotics) without consulting prescriber. Maintain adequate hydration (2-3 L/day of fluids unless instructed to restrict fluid intake). You may experience drowsiness, lightheadedness, impaired coordination, dizziness, or blurred vision (use caution when driving or engaging in tasks requiring alertness until response to drug is known); or dry mouth (small frequent meals, frequent mouth care, chewing gum, or sucking lozenges may help); constipation (increased exercise, fluids, or dietary fruit and fiber may help); or altered sexual drive or ability (reversible). Report persistent CNS effects (eg, euphoria, confusion, increased sedation, depression); chest pain, palpitations, or rapid heartbeat; muscle cramping, weakness, tremors, rigidity, or altered gait; or worsening of condition. **Pregnancy/breast-feeding precautions:** Do not get pregnant while taking this medication; use appropriate barrier contraceptive measures. Breast-feeding is not recommended.

**Geriatric Considerations:** Due to its long-acting metabolite, chlordiazepoxide is not considered a drug of choice in the elderly.

**Breast-feeding Issues:** There is no significant data for chlordiazepoxide, but a related compound diazepam has been shown to accumulate in nursing infants. It is recommended to discontinue nursing or the drug.

**Additional Information** Some formulations may contain benzyl alcohol.

**Related Information**

Anxiolytic/Hypnotic Use in Long-Term Care Facilities *on page 1430*
Benzodiazepines Comparison *on page 1375*

♦ **Chlordiazepoxide and Amitriptyline** *see* Amitriptyline and Chlordiazepoxide *on page 75*

♦ **Chlordiazepoxide and Clidinium** *see* Clidinium and Chlordiazepoxide *on page 281*

♦ **Chloresium®** *see page 1294*

♦ **2-Chlorodeoxyadenosine** *see* Cladribine *on page 278*

♦ **Chloromycetin®** *see* Chloramphenicol *on page 248*

♦ **Chlorophyll** *see page 1294*

## Chloroprocaine (klor oh PROE kane)

**U.S. Brand Names** Nesacaine®; Nesacaine®-MPF

**Therapeutic Category** Local Anesthetic

**Pregnancy Risk Factor** C

**Lactation** Excretion in breast milk unknown

**Use** Infiltration anesthesia and peripheral and epidural anesthesia

**Mechanism of Action/Effect** Reduces sodium flux into nerve cells and prevents propagation of depolarization and conduction of nerve impulses

**Contraindications** Hypersensitivity to chloroprocaine or other ester type anesthetics; myasthenia gravis; concurrent use of bupivacaine; do not use for subarachnoid administration

**Warnings** Use with caution in patients with cardiac disease, renal disease, and hyperthyroidism. Convulsions and cardiac arrest have been reported presumably due to intravascular injection. Pregnancy factor C.

**Drug Interactions**

**Decreased Effect:** The para-aminobenzoic acid metabolite of chloroprocaine may decrease the efficacy of sulfonamide antibiotics.

**Adverse Reactions** <1% (Limited to important or life-threatening symptoms): Myocardial depression, hypotension, bradycardia, cardiovascular collapse, edema, anxiety, restlessness, disorientation, confusion, seizures, drowsiness, unconsciousness, chills, nausea, vomiting, tremor, tinnitus, respiratory arrest, anaphylactoid reactions, shivering

(Continued)

## Chloroprocaine *(Continued)*

**Overdose/Toxicology** Symptoms may include seizures, bradyarrhythmias, metabolic acidosis, and methemoglobinemia. Treatment is symptomatic and supportive. Termination of anesthesia by pneumatic tourniquet inflation should be attempted when chloroprocaine is administered by infiltration or regional injection.

**Pharmacodynamics/Kinetics**

**Metabolism:** Plasma cholinesterases

**Excretion:** Renal

**Onset:** 6-12 minutes

**Duration:** 30-60 minutes

**Formulations**

Chloroprocaine hydrochloride: Injection:

Preservative free (Nesacaine®-MPF): 2% (30 mL); 3% (30 mL)

With preservative (Nesacaine®): 1% (30 mL); 2% (30 mL)

**Dosing**

**Adults:** Dosage varies with anesthetic procedure, the area to be anesthetized, the vascularity of the tissues, depth of anesthesia required, degree of muscle relaxation required, and duration of anesthesia; range: 1.5-25 mL of 2% to 3% solution; single adult dose should not exceed 800 mg.

Infiltration and peripheral nerve block: 1% to 2%

Infiltration, peripheral and central nerve block, including caudal and epidural block: 2% to 3%, without preservatives

**Elderly:** Refer to adult dosing.

**Administration**

**I.V.:** Administer 0.5 g or fraction thereof over 5 minutes.

**Additional Nursing Issues**

**Physical Assessment:** Monitor for effectiveness of anesthesia, and adverse reactions (see Adverse Reactions). Monitor for return of sensation. Teach patient adverse reactions to report; use and teach appropriate interventions to promote safety. **Pregnancy risk factor C** - benefits of use should outweigh possible risks. Note breast-feeding caution.

**Patient Information/Instruction:** This medication is given to reduce sensation in the injected area. You will experience decreased sensation to pain, heat, or cold in the area and/or decreased muscle strength (depending on area of application) until the effects wear off; use necessary caution to reduce incidence of possible injury until full sensation returns. Immediately report chest pain or palpitations; increased restlessness, confusion, anxiety, or dizziness; difficulty breathing; chills, shivering, or tremors; ringing in ears; or changes in vision. **Pregnancy/breast-feeding precautions:** Inform prescriber if you are pregnant. Consult prescriber if breast-feeding.

**Additional Information** Some formulations may contain sulfites.

- **Chlor-optic®** *see page 1282*
- **Chloroptic® Ophthalmic** *see* Chloramphenicol *on page 248*
- **Chloroptic-P®** *see page 1282*

## Chloroquine and Primaquine (KLOR oh kwin & PRIM a kween)

**U.S. Brand Names** Aralen® Phosphate With Primaquine Phosphate

**Synonyms** Primaquine and Chloroquine

**Therapeutic Category** Antimalarial Agent

**Pregnancy Risk Factor** C

**Lactation** Enters breast milk/contraindicated

**Use** Prophylaxis of malaria, regardless of species, in all areas where the disease is endemic

**Formulations** Tablet: Chloroquine phosphate 500 mg [base 300 mg] and primaquine phosphate 79 mg [base 45 mg]

**Dosing**

**Adults:** Oral: Start at least 1 day before entering the endemic area; continue for 8 weeks after leaving the endemic area; 1 tablet/week on the same day each week

**Elderly:** Refer to adult dosing.

**Additional Nursing Issues**

**Physical Assessment:** See individual components listed in Related Information. **Pregnancy risk factor C** - benefits of use should outweigh possible risks. Breast-feeding is contraindicated.

**Patient Information/Instruction:** See individual components listed in Related Information. **Pregnancy/breast-feeding precautions:** Inform prescriber if you are on intend to get pregnant. Do not breast-feed.

**Related Information**

Chloroquine Phosphate *on this page*

Primaquine *on page 963*

## Chloroquine Phosphate (KLOR oh kwin FOS fate)

**U.S. Brand Names** Aralen® Phosphate

**Therapeutic Category** Aminoquinoline (Antimalarial)

**Pregnancy Risk Factor** C

**Lactation** Enters breast milk/compatible

**Use** Suppression or chemoprophylaxis of malaria; treatment of uncomplicated or mild-moderate malaria; extraintestinal amebiasis; rheumatoid arthritis; discoid lupus erythematosus, scleroderma, pemphigus

**Mechanism of Action/Effect** Chloroquine concentrates within parasite acid vesicles and raises internal pH resulting in inhibition of parasite growth

**Contraindications** Hypersensitivity to chloroquine or any component; retinal or visual field changes; patients with psoriasis

**Warnings** Use with caution in patients with liver disease, G-6-PD deficiency, alcoholism or in conjunction with hepatotoxic drugs, psoriasis, porphyria. Pregnancy factor C.

**Drug Interactions**

**Decreased Effect:** Decreased absorption if administered concomitantly with kaolin and magnesium trisilicate.

**Increased Effect/Toxicity:** Chloroquine serum concentrations may be elevated with concomitant cimetidine use.

**Adverse Reactions**

>10%:

Central nervous system: Headache
Dermatologic: Itching (especially in black patients)
Gastrointestinal: Nausea, diarrhea, anorexia, stomach cramps
Ocular: Ciliary muscle dysfunction (difficulty in reading)

1% to 10%:

Dermatologic: Hair bleaching, skin discoloration (blue-black), rash
Ocular: Corneal opacities, blurred vision, retinopathy, keratopathy

<1% (Limited to important or life-threatening symptoms): Hypotension, EKG changes (prolonged QRS interval), fatigue, personality changes, seizures, anorexia, vomiting, stomatitis, blood dyscrasias (agranulocytosis, neutropenia, thrombocytopenia)

**Overdose/Toxicology** Symptoms of overdose include headache, visual changes, cardiovascular collapse, seizures, abdominal cramps, vomiting, cyanosis, methemoglobinemia, leukopenia, and respiratory and cardiac arrest. Following initial measures (immediate GI decontamination), treatment is supportive and symptomatic.

**Pharmacodynamics/Kinetics**

**Distribution:** Widely distributed in body tissues such as eyes, heart, kidneys, liver, and lungs where retention is prolonged; crosses the placenta

**Half-life Elimination:** 3-5 days

**Time to Peak:** Within 1-2 hours

**Metabolism:** Partial hepatic metabolism occurs

**Excretion:** ~70% excreted unchanged in urine; acidification of the urine increases elimination of drug; small amounts of drug may be present in urine months following discontinuation of therapy

**Formulations** Tablet: 250 mg [150 mg base]; 500 mg [300 mg base]

**Dosing**

**Adults:** Oral (**dosage expressed in terms of mg of base**):

Suppression or prophylaxis of malaria: 300 mg/week (base) on the same day each week; begin 1-2 weeks prior to exposure; continue for 4-6 weeks after leaving endemic area. If suppressive therapy is not begun prior to exposure, double the initial loading dose to 600 mg (base) and give in 2 divided doses 6 hours apart, followed by the usual dosage regimen.

Acute attack: 600 mg (base) on day 1, followed by 300 mg (base) 6 hours later, followed by 300 mg (base) on days 2 and 3

Extraintestinal amebiasis: 600 mg base/day for 2 days followed by 300 mg base/day for at least 2-3 weeks

**Elderly:** Refer to adult dosing.

**Renal Impairment:**

$Cl_{cr}$ <10 mL/minute: Administer 50% of dose.

Hemodialysis effects: Minimally removed by hemodialysis

**Monitoring Laboratory Tests** Periodic CBC

**Additional Nursing Issues**

**Physical Assessment:** Assess effectiveness and interactions of other medications (see Drug Interactions). See Contraindications and Warnings/Precautions for use cautions. Monitor effectiveness of therapy (according to purpose for therapy), laboratory tests (see Monitoring Laboratory Tests), and adverse response (see Adverse Reactions and Overdose/Toxicology). Assess knowledge/teach patient appropriate use, possible side effects/interventions, and adverse symptoms to report. **Pregnancy risk factor C** - benefits of use should outweigh possible risks.

**Patient Information/Instruction:** It is important to complete full course of therapy which may take up to 6 months for full effect. May be taken with meals to decrease GI upset and bitter aftertaste. Avoid alcohol. You should have regular ophthalmic exams (every 4-6 months) if using this medication over extended periods. You may experience skin discoloration (blue/black), hair bleaching, or skin rash. If you have psoriasis, you may experience exacerbation. May turn urine black/brown (normal). You may experience nausea, vomiting, or loss of appetite (small frequent meals, frequent mouth care, sucking lozenges, or chewing gum may help) or increased sensitivity to sunlight (wear dark glasses and protective clothing, use sunblock, and avoid direct exposure to sunlight). Report vision changes, rash or itching, persistent diarrhea or GI disturbances, change in hearing acuity or ringing in the ears, chest pain or palpitation, CNS changes, unusual fatigue, easy bruising or bleeding, or any other persistent adverse reactions. **Pregnancy precautions:** Inform prescriber if you are or intend to be pregnant.

## Chlorothiazide (klor oh THYE a zide)

**U.S. Brand Names** Diurigen®; Diuril®

**Therapeutic Category** Diuretic, Thiazide

(Continued)

## Chlorothiazide *(Continued)*

**Pregnancy Risk Factor** D

**Lactation** Enters breast milk/use caution (AAP rates "compatible")

**Use** Management of mild to moderate hypertension, or edema associated with congestive heart failure, pregnancy, or nephrotic syndrome in patients unable to take oral hydrochlorothiazide; when a thiazide is the diuretic of choice

**Mechanism of Action/Effect** Inhibits sodium reabsorption in the distal tubules causing increased excretion of sodium and water as well as potassium and hydrogen ions, magnesium, phosphate, calcium

**Contraindications** Hypersensitivity to chlorothiazide or any component; cross-sensitivity with other thiazides or sulfonamides; anuric patients; pregnancy

**Warnings** Injection must not be administered S.C. or I.M. May cause hyperbilirubinemia, hypokalemia, alkalosis, hyperglycemia, and hyperuricemia. Chlorothiazide is minimally effective in patients with a $Cl_{cr}$ <40 mL/minute. This may limit the usefulness of chlorothiazide in the elderly.

**Drug Interactions**

**Decreased Effect:** NSAIDs + chlorothiazide may lead to decreased antihypertensive effect. Decreased absorption of thiazides with cholestyramine resins. Chlorothiazide causes a decreased effect of oral hypoglycemics.

**Increased Effect/Toxicity:** Chlorothiazide reduces clearance and increases drug levels of digitalis, lithium, and probenecid when taken together.

**Food Interactions** Chlorothiazide serum levels may be increased if taken with food.

**Effects on Lab Values** ↑ creatine phosphokinase [CPK] (S), ammonia (B), amylase (S), calcium (S), chloride (S), cholesterol (S), glucose, acid (S); ↓ chloride (S), magnesium, potassium (S), sodium (S)

**Adverse Reactions**

1% to 10%:

Cardiovascular: Orthostatic hypotension
Endocrine & metabolic: Hypokalemia
Dermatologic: Photosensitivity
Gastrointestinal: Anorexia, epigastric distress

<1% (Limited to important or life-threatening symptoms): Dizziness, headache, weakness, restlessness, purpura, rash, urticaria, necrotizing angiitis, vasculitis, cutaneous vasculitis, alopecia, exfoliative dermatitis (I.I.), toxic epidermal necrolysis (I.V.), Stevens-Johnson syndrome, hyperuricemia or gout, hyponatremia, sexual ability (decreased), hyperglycemia, glycosuria, electrolyte imbalance, nausea, vomiting, cholecystitis, pancreatitis, diarrhea or constipation, polyuria, aplastic anemia, hemolytic anemia, leukopenia, agranulocytosis, thrombocytopenia, hematuria (I.V.), paresthesia, muscle cramps or spasm, uremia, renal failure, pulmonary edema

**Overdose/Toxicology** Symptoms of overdose include hypermotility, diuresis, lethargy, confusion, muscle weakness, and coma. Treatment is supportive.

**Pharmacodynamics/Kinetics**

**Half-life Elimination:** 1-2 hours

**Time to Peak:** Within 4 hours

**Onset:** Onset of diuresis: Oral: 2 hours

**Duration:** Oral: 6-12 hours; I.V.: ~2 hours

**Formulations**

Powder for injection, lyophilized, as sodium: 500 mg
Suspension, oral: 250 mg/5 mL (237 mL)
Tablet: 250 mg, 500 mg

**Dosing**

**Adults:** I.V. form should only be used in adults if unable to take oral in emergency situations:

Oral: 500 mg to 2 g/day divided in 1-2 doses
I.V.: 100-500 mg/day

**Elderly:**

I.V. form should only be used in adults if unable to take oral in emergency situations.
Oral: 500 mg once daily **or** 1 g 3 times/week

**Renal Impairment:** Minimally effective when $Cl_{cr}$ is <20 mL/minute.

**Administration**

**I.M.:** Do **not** administer injection via I.M. or S.C. route.

**I.V.:** Administer 0.5 g or fraction thereof over 5 minutes.

**I.V. Detail:** Avoid extravasation of parenteral solution since it is extremely irritating to tissues.

**Stability**

**Reconstitution:** Reconstituted solution is stable for 24 hours at room temperature. Precipitation will occur in <24 hours in pH <7.4.

**Monitoring Laboratory Tests** Serum electrolytes, renal function

**Additional Nursing Issues**

**Physical Assessment:** Monitor appropriate laboratory tests as ordered. Monitor blood pressure, I & O ratio, weight, and peripheral edema (eg, swelling of feet, ankles, and hands). If patient is taking a cardiac glycoside they will be at increased risk for digitalis toxicity due to potassium-depleting effect of drug. Assess for anorexia, nausea, vomiting, muscle cramps, paresthesis, and confusion. **Pregnancy risk factor D** - assess knowledge/teach appropriate use of barrier contraceptives. Note breast-feeding caution.

**Patient Information/Instruction:** Take once daily dose of chlorothiazide in morning or last of daily doses in early evening to avoid night-time disturbances. Additional potassium may be recommended; follow dietary suggestions of prescriber. You will be more sensitive to sunlight; use sunblock, wear protective clothing, or avoid direct sunlight. You may experience dizziness, weakness, or drowsiness; use caution when driving or engaging in tasks that require alertness until response to drug is known. You may experience postural hypotension; use caution when rising from sitting or lying position or when climbing stairs. Report muscle twitching or cramps; acute loss of appetite; GI distress; severe rash, redness, or itching of skin; sexual dysfunction; palpitations; or respiratory difficulty. **Pregnancy/breast-feeding precautions:** Do not get pregnant while taking this medication; use appropriate barrier contraceptive measures. Consult prescriber if breast-feeding.

**Geriatric Considerations:** Chlorothiazide is minimally effective in patients with a $Cl_{cr}$ <30 mL/minute. This may limit the usefulness of chlorothiazide in the elderly.

**Additional Information** Each 500 mg contains 2 mEq sodium.

## Chlorotrianisene (klor oh trye AN i seen)

**U.S. Brand Names** TACE®

**Therapeutic Category** Estrogen Derivative

**Pregnancy Risk Factor** X

**Lactation** Enters breast milk/use caution

**Use** Treat inoperable prostatic cancer; management of atrophic vaginitis, female hypogonadism, vasomotor symptoms of menopause

**Mechanism of Action/Effect** Diethylstilbestrol derivative with similar estrogenic actions

**Contraindications** Thrombophlebitis; breast cancer; undiagnosed abnormal vaginal bleeding; known or suspected pregnancy (do not use estrogens during pregnancy)

**Warnings** Estrogens have been reported to increase the risk of endometrial carcinoma.

**Adverse Reactions**

>10%:

Cardiovascular: Peripheral edema

Endocrine & metabolic: Enlargement of breasts (female and male), breast tenderness

Gastrointestinal: Nausea, anorexia, bloating

1% to 10%:

Central nervous system: Headache, migraine headache

Endocrine & metabolic: Increased libido (female), decreased libido (male)

Gastrointestinal: Vomiting, diarrhea

<1% (Limited to important or life-threatening symptoms): Hypertension, thromboembolism, myocardial infarction, edema, depression, dizziness, anxiety, stroke, chloasma, melasma, rash, amenorrhea, alterations in frequency and flow of menses, breast tumors, decreased glucose tolerance, increased triglycerides and LDL, nausea, GI distress, gallbladder obstruction, hepatitis, intolerance to contact lenses, increased susceptibility to *Candida* infection

**Overdose/Toxicology** Serious adverse effects have not been reported following ingestion of large doses of estrogen-containing oral contraceptives. Overdosage of estrogen may cause nausea. Withdrawal bleeding may occur in females.

**Pharmacodynamics/Kinetics**

**Distribution:** Stored in fat tissues and slowly released

**Metabolism:** Liver

**Onset:** Commonly occurs within 14 days of therapy

**Formulations** Capsule: 12 mg, 25 mg

**Dosing**

**Adults:** Oral:

Atrophic vaginitis: 12-25 mg/day in 28-day cycles (21 days on and 7 days off)

Female hypogonadism: 12-25 mg cyclically for 21 days. May be followed by I.M. progesterone 100 mg or 5 days of oral progestin; next course may begin on day 5 of induced uterine bleeding.

Postpartum breast engorgement: 12 mg 4 times/day for 7 days or 50 mg every 6 hours for 6 doses; give first dose within 8 hours after delivery

Vasomotor symptoms associated with menopause: 12-25 mg cyclically for 30 days; one or more courses may be prescribed

Prostatic cancer (inoperable/progressing): 12-25 mg/day

**Elderly:** Refer to adult dosing.

**Monitoring Laboratory Tests** Liver function

**Additional Nursing Issues**

**Physical Assessment:** Monitor for effectiveness of therapy periodically during therapy. Monitor (teach patient to monitor and report) adverse reactions. **Pregnancy risk factor X** - determine that patient is not pregnant before beginning treatment and do not give to women of childbearing age or to males who may have intercourse with women of childbearing age unless both male and female are capable of complying with barrier contraceptive measures during therapy and for 1 month following therapy. Note breast-feeding caution.

**Patient Information/Instruction:** Take as directed. May cause enlargement of breast (male/female), menstrual irregularity, increased libido (female), decreased libido (male), nausea or vomiting (small frequent meals, frequent mouth care, sucking lozenges, or chewing gum may help), or acute headache (mild analgesic may help). Report persistent diarrhea; swelling of feet, hands, or legs; sudden severe headache; disturbance of speech or vision; warmth, swelling, or pain in calves; severe abdominal pain; rash; emotional lability; chest pain or palpitations; or signs of vaginal infection. **Pregnancy/breast-feeding precautions:** Inform prescriber if you are pregnant. Do not get pregnant during or for 1 month following therapy. Male: Do not cause a female to become pregnant. Male/female: Consult prescriber for instruction on appropriate

(Continued)

## Chlorotrianisene *(Continued)*

barrier contraceptive measures. This drug may cause severe fetal defects. Do not donate blood during or for 1 month following therapy. Consult prescriber if breast-feeding.

- **Chloroxine** *see page 1294*
- **Chlorphed®** *see page 1294*
- **Chlorphed®-LA Nasal Solution** *see page 1294*
- **Chlorpheniramine** *see page 1294*
- **Chlorpheniramine and Acetaminophen** *see page 1294*
- **Chlorpheniramine and Hydrocodone** *see* Hydrocodone and Chlorpheniramine *on page 571*
- **Chlorpheniramine and Phenylephrine** *see page 1294*
- **Chlorpheniramine and Phenylpropanolamine** *see page 1294*
- **Chlorpheniramine and Pseudoephedrine** *see page 1294*
- **Chlorpheniramine, Ephedrine, Phenylephrine, and Carbetapentane** *see page 1294*
- **Chlorpheniramine, Hydrocodone, Phenylephrine, Acetaminophen, and Caffeine** *see* Hydrocodone, Chlorpheniramine, Phenylephrine, Acetaminophen, and Caffeine *on page 576*
- **Chlorpheniramine, Phenindamine, and Phenylpropanolamine** *see page 1306*
- **Chlorpheniramine, Phenylephrine, and Codeine** *see page 1306*
- **Chlorpheniramine, Phenylephrine, and Dextromethorphan** *see page 1294*
- **Chlorpheniramine, Phenylephrine, and Methscopolamine** *see page 1306*
- **Chlorpheniramine, Phenylephrine, and Phenylpropanolamine** *see page 1294*
- **Chlorpheniramine, Phenylephrine, and Phenyltoloxamine** *see page 1294*
- **Chlorpheniramine, Phenylpropanolamine, and Acetaminophen** *see page 1294*
- **Chlorpheniramine, Phenylpropanolamine, and Dextromethorphan** *see page 1294*
- **Chlorpheniramine, Phenyltoloxamine, Phenylpropanolamine, and Phenylephrine** *see page 1306*
- **Chlorpheniramine, Pseudoephedrine, and Codeine** *see page 1306*
- **Chlorpheniramine, Pyrilamine, and Phenylephrine** *see page 1306*
- **Chlorpheniramine, Pyrilamine, Phenylephrine, and Phenylpropanolamine** *see page 1306*
- **ChlorPro®** *see page 1294*
- **Chlorprom®** *see* Chlorpromazine *on this page*
- **Chlorpromanyl®** *see* Chlorpromazine *on this page*

## Chlorpromazine (klor PROE ma zeen)

**U.S. Brand Names** Ormazine; Thorazine®

**Therapeutic Category** Antipsychotic Agent, Phenothiazine, Aliphatic

**Pregnancy Risk Factor** C

**Lactation** Enters breast milk/not recommended (AAP rates "of concern")

**Use** Treatment of nausea and vomiting, psychoses, Tourette's syndrome, mania, intractable hiccups (adults), behavioral problems (children)

**Mechanism of Action/Effect** Blocks postsynaptic mesolimbic dopaminergic receptors in the brain; exhibits a strong alpha-adrenergic blocking effect and depresses the release of hypothalamic and hypophyseal hormones; believed to depress the reticular-activating system, thus affecting basal metabolism, body temperature, wakefulness, vasomotor tone, and emesis

**Contraindications** Hypersensitivity to chlorpromazine or any component (cross reactivity between phenothiazines may occur); severe CNS depression; coma

**Warnings** Significant hypotension may occur, particularly with parenteral administration. Injection contains sulfites and benzyl alcohol; use with caution. Highly sedating, use with caution in disorders where CNS depression is a feature. Use with caution in Parkinson's disease. Use with caution in patients with hemodynamic instability; bone marrow suppression; predisposition to seizures; subcortical brain damage; or severe cardiac, hepatic, renal, or respiratory disease. May cause swallowing difficulties. Use caution in breast cancer or other prolactin-dependent tumors (may elevate prolactin levels). May alter temperature regulation or mask toxicity of other drugs due to antiemetic effects. May alter cardiac conduction - life-threatening arrhythmias have occurred with therapeutic doses of neuroleptics. May cause orthostatic hypotension.

Phenothiazines may cause anticholinergic effects (eg, confusion, agitation, constipation, dry mouth, blurred vision, urinary retention); therefore, use with caution in patients with decreased gastrointestinal motility, urinary retention, BPH, xerostomia, or visual problems. Conditions which also may be exacerbated by cholinergic blockade include narrow-angle glaucoma (screening is recommended) and worsening of myasthenia gravis. Relative to other neuroleptics, chlorpromazine has a moderate potency of cholinergic blockade.

May cause extrapyramidal reactions including pseudoparkinsonism, acute dystonic reactions, akathisia, and tardive dyskinesia (risk of these reactions is moderate relative to other neuroleptics). May be associated with neuroleptic malignant syndrome (NMS) or pigmentary retinopathy.

Pregnancy factor C.

**Drug Interactions**

**Cytochrome P-450 Effect:** CYP1A2, 2D6, and 3A3/4 enzyme substrate; CYP2D6 enzyme inhibitor

**Increased Effect/Toxicity:** Additive effects with other CNS depressants; epinephrine (hypotension). Chlorpromazine may increase valproic acid serum concentrations.

**Effects on Lab Values** False-positives for phenylketonuria, amylase, uroporphyrins, urobilinogen. May cause false-positive pregnancy test.

**Adverse Reactions**

>10%:

Cardiovascular: Hypotension (especially with I.V. use), tachycardia, arrhythmias, orthostatic hypotension

Central nervous system: Pseudoparkinsonism, akathisia, dystonias, tardive dyskinesia (persistent), dizziness

Gastrointestinal: Constipation

Ocular: Pigmentary retinopathy

Respiratory: Nasal congestion

Miscellaneous: Sweating (decreased)

1% to 10%:

Dermatologic: Pruritus, rash, increased sensitivity to sun

Endocrine & metabolic: Amenorrhea, galactorrhea, gynecomastia, changes in libido, pain in breasts

Gastrointestinal: GI upset, nausea, vomiting, stomach pain, weight gain, dry mouth

Genitourinary: Dysuria, ejaculatory disturbances, urinary retention

Neuromuscular & skeletal: Trembling of fingers

Ocular: Blurred vision

<1% (Limited to important or life-threatening symptoms): Sedation, drowsiness, restlessness, anxiety, extrapyramidal reactions, seizures, altered central temperature regulation, lowering of seizures threshold, neuroleptic malignant syndrome (NMS), discoloration of skin (blue-gray), photosensitivity galactorrhea, priapism, agranulocytosis (more often in women between 4th and 10th weeks of therapy), leukopenia (usually in patients with large doses for prolonged periods), cholestatic jaundice, hepatotoxicity, cornea and lens changes

**Overdose/Toxicology** Symptoms of overdose include deep sleep, coma, extrapyramidal symptoms, abnormal involuntary muscle movements, and hypotension. Following initiation of essential overdose management, toxic symptom treatment and supportive treatment should be initiated.

**Pharmacodynamics/Kinetics**

**Distribution:** Crosses the placenta

**Half-life Elimination:** Half-life, biphasic: Initial: 2 hours; Terminal: 30 hours

**Time to Peak:** Oral: 1-2 hours

**Metabolism:** Liver

**Excretion:** <1% excreted in urine as unchanged drug within 24 hours

**Formulations**

Chlorpromazine hydrochloride:

Capsule, sustained action: 30 mg, 75 mg, 150 mg, 200 mg, 300 mg

Concentrate, oral: 30 mg/mL (120 mL); 100 mg/mL (60 mL, 240 mL)

Injection: 25 mg/mL (1 mL, 2 mL, 10 mL)

Syrup: 10 mg/5 mL (120 mL)

Tablet: 10 mg, 25 mg, 50 mg, 100 mg, 200 mg

Suppository, rectal, as base: 25 mg, 100 mg

**Dosing**

**Adults:**

Psychosis:

Oral: Range: 30-800 mg/day in 1-4 divided doses, initiate at lower doses and titrate as needed; usual dose: 200 mg/day; some patients may require 1-2 g/day

I.M., I.V.: Initial: 25 mg, may repeat (25-50 mg) in 1-4 hours, gradually increase to a maximum of 400 mg/dose every 4-6 hours until patient is controlled; usual dose: 300-800 mg/day

Intractable hiccups: Oral, I.M.: 25-50 mg 3-4 times/day

Nausea and vomiting:

Oral: 10-25 mg every 4-6 hours

I.M., I.V.: 25-50 mg every 4-6 hours

Rectal: 50-100 mg every 6-8 hours

**Elderly:** Nonpsychotic patient; dementia behavior: Initial: 10-25 mg 1-2 times/day; increase at 4- to 7-day intervals by 10-25 mg/day. Increase dose intervals (bid, tid, etc) as necessary to control behavior response or side effects; maximum daily dose: 800 mg; gradual increases (titration) may prevent some side effects or decrease their severity.

**Renal Impairment:** Not dialyzable (0% to 5%)

**Hepatic Impairment:** Avoid use in severe hepatic dysfunction.

**Administration**

**Oral:** Dilute oral concentrate solution in juice before administration.

**I.V.:** Direct of intermittent infusion: Infuse 1 mg or portion thereof over 1 minute.

**Stability**

**Storage:** Protect from light. A slightly yellowed solution does not indicate potency loss, but a markedly discolored solution should be discarded. Diluted injection (1 mg/mL) with NS and stored in 5 mL vials remains stable for 30 days.

**Reconstitution:** Diluted injection (1 mg/mL) with NS and stored in 5 mL vials remains stable for 30 days.

(Continued)

## Chlorpromazine *(Continued)*

**Compatibility:** See the Compatibility of Drugs in Syringe Chart *on page 1317.*

**Monitoring Laboratory Tests** Renal function, CBC, ophthalmic screening

**Additional Nursing Issues**

**Physical Assessment:** Assess other medications patient is taking for effectiveness and interactions (see Drug Interactions). See Contraindications and Warnings/Precautions for cautious use. Has potential for psychological or physiological dependence, abuse, and tolerance. Review ophthalmic exam and monitor laboratory results (see above), therapeutic response (eg, mental status, mood, affect, gait), and adverse reactions at beginning of therapy and periodically with long-term use (eg, excess sedation, extrapyramidal effects, CNS changes - see Adverse Reactions and Overdose). I.V./I.M.: Significant hypotension may occur. Initiate at lower doses (see Dosing) and taper dosage slowly when discontinuing. Assess knowledge/teach patient appropriate use, interventions to reduce side effects, and adverse symptoms to report. **Note:** Chlorpromazine may cause false-positive pregnancy test. **Pregnancy risk factor C** - benefits of use should outweigh possible risks. Breast-feeding is not recommended.

**Patient Information/Instruction:** Use exactly as directed (do not increase dose or frequency); may cause physical and/or psychological dependence. Do not discontinue without consulting prescriber. Tablets/capsules may be taken with food. Mix oral solution with 2-4 ounces of liquid (eg, juice, milk, water). Do not take within 2 hours of any antacid. Store away from light. Avoid excess alcohol or caffeine and other prescription or OTC medications not approved by prescriber. Maintain adequate hydration (2-3 L/day of fluids unless instructed to restrict fluid intake). May turn urine red-brown (normal). You may experience excess drowsiness, lightheadedness, dizziness, or blurred vision (use caution driving or when engaging in tasks requiring alertness until response to drug is known); dry mouth, upset stomach, nausea, vomiting, anorexia (small frequent meals, frequent mouth care, sucking lozenges, or chewing gum may help); constipation (increased exercise, fluids, or dietary fruit and fiber may help); postural hypotension (use caution climbing stairs or when changing position from lying or sitting to standing); urinary retention (void before taking medication); ejaculatory dysfunction (reversible); decreased perspiration (avoid strenuous exercise in hot environments); or photosensitivity (use sunscreen, wear protective clothing and eyewear, and avoid direct sunlight). Report persistent CNS effects (trembling fingers, altered gait or balance, excessive sedation, seizures, unusual movements, anxiety, abnormal thoughts, confusion, personality changes); chest pain, palpitations, rapid heartbeat, or severe dizziness; unresolved urinary retention or changes in urinary pattern; altered menstrual pattern, change in libido, swelling or pain in breasts (male or female); vision changes, skin rash, irritation, or changes in color of skin (gray-blue); or worsening of condition. **Pregnancy/breast-feeding precautions:** Inform prescriber if you are or intend to be pregnant. Breast-feeding is not recommended.

**Dietary Issues:** Interferes with riboflavin metabolism and may induce depletion. Some may recommend increasing riboflavin in diet. May also decrease absorption of vitamin $B_{12}$. Undiluted oral concentrate may precipitate tube feeding.

**Geriatric Considerations:** (See Warnings/Precautions, Adverse Reactions, and Overdose/Toxicology.) Elderly patients have an increased risk of adverse response to side effects or adverse reactions to antipsychotics. These can include but are not limited to the following.

Anticholinergic effects: CNS toxicity with confusion, memory loss, psychotic behavior, and agitation.

Extrapyramidal effects (EPS): Parkinson's syndrome and akathisia may occur as often as 50% in patients >60 years of age. Tardive dyskinesia (motor restlessness) may be 40% in elderly; may be related to duration and total accumulated dose over time; may be somewhat reversible if diagnosed early enough.

Orthostatic hypotension: Increased risk for falls.

Sedation: In nonpsychotic patients this may result in feelings of depersonalization, derealization, and dysphoria.

Cardiac toxicity: Cardiac arrhythmias have occurred with therapeutic doses of antipsychotics.

Malignant neuroleptic syndrome: Development of hyperthermia, muscular rigidity, autonomic instability, and altered mental status.

Many elderly patients receive antipsychotic medications for inappropriate nonpsychotic behavior. Before initiating antipsychotic medication, all possible reversible causes should be investigated. Stress may cause acute "confusion" or worsening of baseline nonpsychotic behaviors; any changes in disease state (in any organ) may result in behavioral changes. Common acute changes in behavior may be also due to increases in drug dose addition or addition of a new drug to the regimen; fluid/electrolyte alterations; infections; or changes in the environment.

Meta-analysis of controlled trials of antipsychotic (phenothiazines, butyrophenones) use with agitated, demented, elderly patients has concluded that the use of neuroleptics results in a response rate of 18%. Clearly, neuroleptic therapy for behavior control should be limited, with frequent attempts to withdraw the agent for behavior control. When use is indicated, initial doses should be lower to start and monitored closely.

**Additional Information** Some formulations may contain benzyl alcohol. Thorazine® injection contains sulfites.

**Related Information**

Antiemetics for Chemotherapy-Induced Nausea and Vomiting *on page 1307*

Antipsychotic Agents Comparison *on page 1371*
Antipsychotic Medication Guidelines *on page 1436*

## Chlorpropamide (klor PROE pa mide)

**U.S. Brand Names** Diabinese®

**Therapeutic Category** Antidiabetic Agent (Sulfonylurea)

**Pregnancy Risk Factor** C

**Lactation** Enters breast milk/contraindicated

**Use** Control blood sugar in adult onset, noninsulin-dependent diabetes (Type II)

**Unlabeled use:** Nephrogenic diabetes insipidus

**Mechanism of Action/Effect** Stimulates insulin release from the pancreatic beta cells; reduces glucose output from the liver; insulin sensitivity is increased at peripheral target sites

**Contraindications** Cross-sensitivity may exist with other hypoglycemics or sulfonamides; do not use with Type I diabetes or with severe renal, hepatic, thyroid, or other endocrine disease, diabetes complicated by ketoacidosis; patients with reduced renal function; dietary noncompliance or irregular meals; alcohol abusers

**Warnings** Patients should be properly instructed in the early detection and treatment of hypoglycemia. Long half-life may complicate recovery from excess effects. Because of chlorpropamide's long half-life, duration of action, and the increased risk for hypoglycemia, it is not considered a hypoglycemic agent of choice in the elderly. Pregnancy factor C.

**Drug Interactions**

**Decreased Effect:** Thiazides and hydantoins (eg, phenytoin) decrease chlorpropamide effectiveness and may increase blood glucose.

**Increased Effect/Toxicity:** Chlorpropamide may cause alcohol associated disulfiram reactions. Chlorpropamide may increase oral anticoagulant effects. Salicylates may cause increased chlorpropamide effects and lower blood glucose more than expected. Sulfonamides may decrease chlorpropamide clearance and enhance blood glucose lowering effects. Chloramphenicol may increase the half-life of chlorpropamide.

**Food Interactions** Chlorpropamide serum levels may be decreased if taken with food.

**Adverse Reactions**

>10%:
- Central nervous system: Headache, dizziness
- Endocrine & metabolic: Hypoglycemia (mild)
- Gastrointestinal: Constipation, diarrhea, heartburn, weight gain, anorexia, epigastric fullness, changes in sensation of taste
- Renal: Polyuria

1% to 10%:
- Dermatologic: Rash, urticaria, photosensitivity
- Endocrine & metabolic: Hypoglycemia (severe)

<1% (Limited to important or life-threatening symptoms): Photosensitivity, aplastic anemia, hemolytic anemia, bone marrow suppression, thrombocytopenia, agranulocytosis, cholestatic jaundice, hepatic porphyria

**Overdose/Toxicology** Symptoms of overdose include low blood glucose levels, tingling of lips and tongue, tachycardia, convulsions, stupor, and coma. The antidote is glucose. Prolonged effects lasting up to 1 week may occur with chlorpropamide.

**Pharmacodynamics/Kinetics**

**Protein Binding:** 60% to 90%

**Half-life Elimination:** 30-42 hours; prolonged in the elderly or with renal disease; End-stage renal disease: 50-200 hours

**Time to Peak:** Within 3-4 hours

**Metabolism:** Liver

**Excretion:** Urine

**Onset:** Oral: Within 6-8 hours

**Formulations** Tablet: 100 mg, 250 mg

**Dosing**

**Adults:** Oral: The dosage of chlorpropamide is variable and should be individualized based upon the patient's response. Initial: 250 mg/day in mild to moderate diabetes in middle-aged, stable diabetic.

**Elderly:** Initial: 100 mg once daily; increase by 50-125 mg/day at 3- to 5-day intervals; severe diabetics may require 500 mg/day; maximum daily dose: 750 mg.

**Renal Impairment:**

$Cl_{cr}$ <50 mL/minute: Avoid use.

Peritoneal dialysis effects: Supplemental dose is not necessary.

**Hepatic Impairment:** Dosage reduction is recommended.

**Administration**

**Oral:** Usually taken before breakfast.

**Monitoring Laboratory Tests** Fasting blood glucose, Hb $A_{1c}$, fructosamine levels

**Additional Nursing Issues**

**Physical Assessment:** Assess effectiveness and interactions of other medications (see Drug Interactions). See Warnings/Precautions and Contraindications for use cautions. Monitor effectiveness of therapy and monitor laboratory tests frequently during therapy (see above). Monitor for adverse response (eg, hypoglycemia - see Adverse Reactions and Overdose/Toxicology). Assess knowledge/teach patient or refer patient to diabetic educator for instruction in appropriate use, possible side effects and appropriate interventions, and adverse symptoms to report. **Pregnancy risk factor C** - benefits of use should outweigh possible risks. Breast-feeding is contraindicated.

(Continued)

## Chlorpropamide *(Continued)*

**Patient Information/Instruction:** This medication is used to control diabetes; it is not a cure. Other components of treatment plan are important: follow prescribed diet, medication, and exercise regimen. Take exactly as directed, at the same time each day. Do not change dose or discontinue without consulting prescriber. Avoid alcohol while taking this medication; could cause severe reaction. Inform prescriber of all other prescription or OTC medications you are taking; do not introduce new medication without consulting prescriber. If you experience hypoglycemic reaction, contact prescriber immediately. Maintain regular dietary intake and exercise routine and always carry quick source of sugar with you. You may experience side effects during first weeks of therapy (headache, constipation or diarrhea, bloating or loss of appetite); consult prescriber if these persist. Report severe or persistent side effects, including fever, extended vomiting or flu-like symptoms, skin rash, easy bruising or bleeding, or change in color of urine or stool. **Pregnancy/breast-feeding precautions:** Inform prescriber if you are or intend to be pregnant. Do not breast-feed.

**Geriatric Considerations:** Because of chlorpropamide's long half-life, duration of action, drug interactions, and the increased risk for hypoglycemia, it is not considered a hypoglycemic agent of choice in the elderly.

**Related Information**

Antidiabetic Oral Agents Comparison *on page 1370*

♦ **Chlor-Rest® Tablet** *see page 1294*

## Chlorthalidone (klor THAL i done)

**U.S. Brand Names** Hygroton®; Thalitone®

**Therapeutic Category** Diuretic, Thiazide

**Pregnancy Risk Factor** D

**Lactation** Enters breast milk/use caution

**Use** Management of mild to moderate hypertension when used alone or in combination with other agents; treatment of edema associated with congestive heart failure, nephrotic syndrome, or pregnancy. Recent studies have found chlorthalidone effective in the treatment of isolated systolic hypertension in the elderly.

**Mechanism of Action/Effect** Sulfonamide-derived diuretic that inhibits sodium and chloride reabsorption in the cortical-diluting segment of the ascending loop of Henle

**Contraindications** Hypersensitivity to chlorthalidone or any component; cross-sensitivity with other thiazides or sulfonamides; do not use in anuric patients; pregnancy

**Warnings** Use with caution in patients with hypokalemia, renal disease, hepatic disease, gout, lupus erythematosus, or diabetes mellitus. Use with caution in severe renal diseases.

**Drug Interactions**

**Decreased Effect:** NSAIDs + thiazide diuretics may decrease the antihypertensive effect. Decreased absorption of thiazides with cholestyramine resins.

**Increased Effect/Toxicity:** Increased effect when taken with furosemide and other loop diuretics. Increased toxicity when chlorthalidone is taken with digitalis glycosides, lithium (decreased clearance and then elevated digitalis or lithium levels).

**Effects on Lab Values** ↑ creatine phosphokinase [CPK] (S), ammonia (B), amylase (S), calcium (S), chloride (S), cholesterol (S), glucose, acid (S); ↓ chloride (S), magnesium, potassium (S), sodium (S)

**Adverse Reactions**

1% to 10%:

Endocrine & metabolic: Hypokalemia
Dermatologic: Photosensitivity
Gastrointestinal: Anorexia, epigastric distress

<1% (Limited to important or life-threatening symptoms): Dizziness, headache, weakness, restlessness, insomnia, purpura, rash, urticaria, necrotizing angiitis, vasculitis, cutaneous vasculitis, hyperuricemia or gout, hyponatremia, sexual ability (decreased), hyperglycemia, glycosuria, nausea, vomiting, cholecystitis, pancreatitis, diarrhea or constipation, polyuria, aplastic anemia, leukopenia, agranulocytosis, thrombocytopenia, hepatic function impairment, paresthesia, muscle cramps or spasm

**Overdose/Toxicology** Symptoms of overdose include hypermotility, diuresis, lethargy, confusion, muscle weakness, and coma. Treatment is supportive.

**Pharmacodynamics/Kinetics**

**Distribution:** Crosses the placenta

**Half-life Elimination:** 35-55 hours (may be prolonged in renal impairment); Anuria: 81 hours

**Metabolism:** Liver

**Excretion:** ~50% to 65% excreted unchanged in urine

**Onset:** Peak effect: 2-6 hours

**Formulations**

Tablet: 25 mg, 50 mg, 100 mg
Hygroton®: 25 mg, 50 mg, 100 mg
Thalitone®: 15 mg, 25 mg

**Dosing**

**Adults:** Oral: 25-100 mg/day or 100 mg 3 times/week

**Elderly:** Oral: Initial: 12.5-25 mg/day or every other day; there is little advantage to using doses >25 mg/day.

**Renal Impairment:** $Cl_{cr}$ <10 mL/minute: Administer every 48 hours.

**Monitoring Laboratory Tests** Serum electrolytes, renal function

**Additional Nursing Issues**

**Physical Assessment:** Monitor laboratory results, blood pressure (standing, sitting, lying), fluid status (I & O, edema, weight), and electrolyte balance (hypokalemia - nausea, vomiting, muscle cramps, confusion, parasthesia). Assess patients taking cardiac glycosides carefully; depleted potassium will increase risk of digitalis toxicity. **Pregnancy risk factor D** - assess knowledge/teach appropriate use of barrier contraceptives. Note breast-feeding caution.

**Patient Information/Instruction:** Take prescribed dose with food early in the day. Include orange juice or bananas in your diet, but do not take potassium supplements without consulting prescriber. You may experience postural hypotension (use caution when rising from lying or sitting position, when climbing stairs, or when driving); photosensitivity (use sunblock, wear protective clothing and eyewear, and avoid direct sunlight); decreased accommodation to heat (avoid excessive exercise in hot weather). Report muscle weakness, tremors, or cramping; persistent nausea or vomiting; swelling of extremities; significant increase in weight; respiratory difficulty; rash; unusual weakness or fatigue; or easy bruising or bleeding. **Pregnancy/breast-feeding precautions:** Do not get pregnant while taking this medication; use appropriate barrier contraceptive measures. Consult prescriber if breast-feeding.

**Geriatric Considerations:** Studies have found chlorthalidone effective in the treatment of isolated systolic hypertension in the elderly.

- **Chlorthalidone and Atenolol** *see* Atenolol and Chlorthalidone *on page 117*
- **Chlorthalidone and Clonidine** *see* Clonidine and Chlorthalidone *on page 291*
- **Chlor-Trimeton®** *see page 1294*
- **Chlor-Trimeton® 4 Hour Relief Tablet** *see page 1294*
- **Chlor-Tripolon® N.D.** *see* Loratadine and Pseudoephedrine *on page 690*

## Chlorzoxazone (klor ZOKS a zone)

**U.S. Brand Names** Flexaphen®; Paraflex®; Parafon Forte™ DSC

**Therapeutic Category** Skeletal Muscle Relaxant

**Pregnancy Risk Factor** C

**Lactation** Excretion in breast milk unknown/not recommended

**Use** Symptomatic treatment of muscle spasm and pain associated with acute musculoskeletal conditions

**Mechanism of Action/Effect** Acts on the spinal cord and subcortical levels by depressing polysynaptic reflexes

**Contraindications** Hypersensitivity to chlorzoxazone or any component; impaired liver function

**Warnings** Pregnancy factor C.

**Drug Interactions**

**Cytochrome P-450 Effect:** CYP2E1 enzyme substrate

**Increased Effect/Toxicity:** Increased effect/toxicity when taken with alcohol or CNS depressants.

**Adverse Reactions**

>10%: Central nervous system: Drowsiness, dizziness, lightheadedness

1% to 10%:

Central nervous system: Headache, paradoxical stimulation

Gastrointestinal: Nausea, vomiting, stomach cramps, constipation, diarrhea, heartburn

<1% (Limited to important or life-threatening symptoms): Rash, hives, angioedema, anemia, agranulocytosis

**Overdose/Toxicology** Symptoms of overdose include nausea, vomiting, diarrhea, drowsiness, dizziness, headache, absent tendon reflexes, and hypotension. Treatment is supportive following attempts to enhance drug elimination. Dialysis, hemoperfusion, and osmotic diuresis have all been useful in reducing serum drug concentrations. The patient should be observed for possible relapses due to incomplete gastric emptying.

**Pharmacodynamics/Kinetics**

**Metabolism:** Liver

**Excretion:** Urine

**Onset:** Within 1 hour

**Duration:** 6-12 hours

**Formulations**

Caplet (Parafon Forte™ DSC): 500 mg

Capsule (Flexaphen®): 250 mg with acetaminophen 300 mg

Tablet: Paraflex®: 250 mg

**Dosing**

**Adults:** Oral: 250-500 mg 3-4 times/day up to 750 mg 3-4 times/day

**Elderly:** Oral: Initial: 250 mg 2-4 times/day; increase as necessary to 750 mg 3-4 times/day.

**Monitoring Laboratory Tests** Periodic liver functions

**Additional Nursing Issues**

**Physical Assessment:** Monitor results of laboratory tests (see above), effectiveness of therapy (according to rational for therapy), and adverse reactions (see Adverse Reactions) at beginning of therapy and periodically with long-term use. Do not discontinue abruptly; taper dosage slowly. Assess knowledge/teach patient appropriate use, interventions to reduce side effects (postural hypotension precautions), and adverse symptoms to report. **Pregnancy risk factor C** - benefits of use should outweigh possible risks. Breast-feeding is not recommended.

**Patient Information/Instruction:** Take exactly as directed, with food. Do not increase dose or discontinue without consulting prescriber. Do not use alcohol, prescriptive or

(Continued)

## Chlorzoxazone *(Continued)*

OTC antidepressants, sedatives, or pain medications without consulting prescriber. May turn urine orange or red (normal). You may experience drowsiness, dizziness, lightheadedness (avoid driving or engaging in tasks that require alertness until response to drug is known); nausea, vomiting, or cramping (small, frequent meals, frequent mouth care, or sucking hard candy may help); postural hypotension (change position slowly when rising from sitting or lying or when climbing stairs); or constipation (increased dietary fluids and fibers or increased exercise may help). Report excessive drowsiness or mental agitation; palpitations, rapid heartbeat, or chest pain; skin rash or swelling of mouth or face; persistent diarrhea or constipation; or unusual weakness or bleeding. **Pregnancy/breast-feeding precautions:** Inform prescriber if you are or intend to be pregnant. Breast-feeding is not recommended.

**Geriatric Considerations:** Start dosing low and increase as necessary. The FDA recently approved a stronger warning about hepatotoxicity in the labeling of chlorzoxazone. Because it can cause unpredictable, fatal hepatic toxicity, the use of chlorzoxazone should be avoided.

- **Cholac®** *see* Lactulose *on page 651*
- **Cholera Vaccine** *see page 1256*

## Cholestyramine Resin (koe LES tir a meen REZ in)

**U.S. Brand Names** LoCHOLEST®; LoCHOLEST® Light; Prevalite®; Questran®; Questran® Light

**Therapeutic Category** Antilipemic Agent (Bile Acid Seqestrant)

**Pregnancy Risk Factor** C

**Lactation** Excretion in breast milk unknown/not recommended

**Use** Adjunct in the management of primary hypercholesterolemia; pruritus associated with elevated levels of bile acids; diarrhea associated with excess fecal bile acids; binding toxicologic agents; pseudomembraneous colitis

**Mechanism of Action/Effect** Forms a nonabsorbable complex with bile acids in the intestine, releasing chloride ions in the process; inhibits enterohepatic reuptake of intestinal bile salts and thereby increases the fecal loss of bile salt-bound low density lipoprotein cholesterol

**Contraindications** Hypersensitivity to cholestyramine or any component; avoid using in complete biliary obstruction; hypolipoproteinemia Types III, IV, V

**Warnings** Use with caution in patients with constipation (GI dysfunction). Caution patients with phenylketonuria (Questran® Light contains aspartame). Overdose may result in GI obstruction. Cholestyramine (especially high doses or long-term therapy) may decrease the absorption of fat-soluble vitamins (vitamins A, D, E, and K), folic acid, calcium, and iron. Deficiencies may occur including hypoprothrombinemia and increased bleeding from vitamin K deficiency. Supplementation of vitamins A, D, E, and K, folic acid, and iron may be required with high-dose, long-term therapy. Pregnancy factor C.

**Drug Interactions**

**Decreased Effect:** Decreased absorption (oral) of digitalis glycosides, warfarin, thyroid hormones, thiazide diuretics, propranolol, phenobarbital, amiodarone, methotrexate, NSAIDs, and other drugs by binding to the drug before absorption from the intestine.

**Effects on Lab Values** ↑ prothrombin time (S); ↓ cholesterol (S), iron (B)

**Adverse Reactions**

>10%: Gastrointestinal: Constipation, heartburn, nausea, vomiting, stomach pain

1% to 10%:

Central nervous system: Headache

Gastrointestinal: Belching, bloating, diarrhea

<1% (Limited to important or life-threatening symptoms): Hyperchloremic acidosis, gallstones or pancreatitis, GI bleeding, peptic ulcer, steatorrhea or malabsorption syndrome, hypoprothrombinemia (secondary to vitamin K deficiency)

**Overdose/Toxicology** Symptoms of overdose include GI obstruction. Treatment is supportive.

**Pharmacodynamics/Kinetics**

**Metabolism:** Not metabolized

**Excretion:** Feces

**Onset:** Peak effect: 21 days

**Formulations**

Powder: 4 g of resin/9 g of powder (378 g) and 9 g (60s)

Powder, for oral suspension, with aspartame: 4 g of resin/5 g of powder (210 g) and 5 g (60s)

**Dosing**

**Adults:** Oral (dosages are expressed in terms of anhydrous resin):

Powder: 4 g 1-6 times/day to a maximum of 16-32 g/day

Tablet: Initial: 4 g once or twice daily; maintenance: 8-16 g/day in 2 divided doses

**Elderly:** Refer to adult dosing.

**Renal Impairment:** Not removed by hemo- or peritoneal dialysis. Supplemental doses not necessary with dialysis or continuous arteriovenous or venovenous hemofiltration effects.

**Administration**

**Oral:** Mix contents of 1 packet or 1 level scoop of powder with 4-6 oz of beverage. Allow to stand 1-2 minutes prior to mixing. May also be mixed with highly fluid soups, cereals, applesauce, etc.

**Monitoring Laboratory Tests** Serum cholesterol and triglyceride levels should be obtained before initiating drug treatment and periodically throughout treatment.

**Additional Nursing Issues**

**Physical Assessment:** Assess other medications patient may be taking for effectiveness and interactions (see Drug Interactions). Monitor laboratory results, therapeutic response, and adverse reactions (eg, GI effects and nutritional status - see Adverse Reactions and Overdose/Toxicology) periodically throughout therapy. Assess knowledge/teach patient appropriate use, interventions to reduce side effects, and adverse symptoms to report. **Pregnancy risk factor C** - benefits of use should outweigh possible risks. Breast-feeding is not recommended.

**Patient Information/Instruction:** Take once or twice a day as directed. Do not take the powder in its dry form; mix with fluid, applesauce, pudding, or jello. Chew bars thoroughly. Take other medications 2 hours before or 4 hours after cholestyramine. Ongoing medical follow-up and laboratory tests may be required. You may experience GI effects (these should resolve after continued use); nausea and vomiting (small frequent meals, frequent mouth care, sucking lozenges, or chewing gum may help); constipation (increased exercise, dietary fluid, fiber, or fruit may help - consult prescriber about use of stool softener or laxative). Report unusual stomach cramping, pain or blood in stool; unresolved nausea, vomiting, or constipation. **Pregnancy/breast-feeding precautions:** Inform prescriber if you are or intend to be pregnant. Breast-feeding is not recommended.

**Geriatric Considerations:** The definition of and, therefore, when to treat hyperlipidemia in the elderly is a controversial issue. Treatment is best reserved for those who are unable to obtain a desirable plasma cholesterol level by diet alone and for whom the benefits of treatment are believed to outweigh the potential adverse effects, drug interactions, and cost of treatment.

**Additional Information**

Questran® Light: Each 5 g dose contains 16.8 mg phenylalanine
Questran® cans 378 g contain 42 doses
Questran® light cans 210 g contain 42 doses

**Related Information**

Lipid-Lowering Agents Comparison *on page 1393*

## Choline Magnesium Trisalicylate

(KOE leen mag NEE zhum trye sa LIS i late)

**U.S. Brand Names** Tricosal®; Trilisate®

**Therapeutic Category** Salicylate

**Pregnancy Risk Factor** C/D (3rd trimester or near term)

**Lactation** Enters breast milk/use caution

**Use** Management of osteoarthritis, rheumatoid arthritis, and other arthritis; salicylate salts may not inhibit platelet aggregation and, therefore, should not be substituted for aspirin in the prophylaxis of thrombosis

**Mechanism of Action/Effect** Inhibits prostaglandin synthesis; acts on the hypothalamus heat-regulating center to reduce fever; blocks the generation of pain impulses

**Contraindications** Hypersensitivity to salicylates or other nonacetylated salicylates or other NSAIDs; tartrazine dye hypersensitivity; bleeding disorders; asthma; pregnancy (3rd trimester or near term)

**Warnings** Use with caution in patients with impaired renal function, erosive gastritis, or peptic ulcer. Avoid use in patients with suspected varicella or influenza (salicylates have been associated with Reye's syndrome in children <16 years of age when used to treat symptoms of chickenpox or the flu). Tinnitus or impaired hearing may indicate toxicity; discontinue use 1 week prior to surgical procedures. Pregnancy factor C/D (3rd trimester or near term).

**Drug Interactions**

**Decreased Effect:** Antacids and choline magnesium trisalicylate may decrease salicylate concentration.

**Increased Effect/Toxicity:** Warfarin and choline magnesium trisalicylate may possibly increase hypoprothrombinemic effect.

**Food Interactions** Salicylate serum levels may be altered if taken with food.

**Effects on Lab Values** False-negative results for glucose oxidase urinary glucose tests (Clinistix®); false-positives using the cupric sulfate method (Clinitest®); also, interferes with Gerhardt test (urinary ketone analysis), VMA determination; 5-HIAA, xylose tolerance test, and $T_3$ and $T_4$; increased PBI; increased uric acid

**Adverse Reactions**

>10%: Gastrointestinal: Nausea, heartburn, stomach pains, heartburn, epigastric discomfort

1% to 10%:

Central nervous system: Fatigue
Dermatologic: Rash
Gastrointestinal: Gastrointestinal ulceration
Hematologic: Hemolytic anemia
Neuromuscular & skeletal: Weakness
Respiratory: Dyspnea
Miscellaneous: Anaphylactic shock

<1% (Limited to important or life-threatening symptoms): Insomnia, nervousness, jitters, occult bleeding, prolongation of bleeding time, leukopenia, thrombocytopenia, iron deficiency anemia, hepatotoxicity, impaired renal function, bronchospasm, increased uric acid

**Overdose/Toxicology** Symptoms of overdose include tinnitus, vomiting, acute renal failure, hyperthermia, irritability, seizures, coma, and metabolic acidosis. For acute ingestion, determine serum salicylate levels 6 hours after ingestion. Nomograms, such as the "Done" nomogram, may be helpful for estimating the severity of aspirin poisoning

(Continued)

## Choline Magnesium Trisalicylate *(Continued)*

and directing treatment using serum salicylate levels. Treatment is based upon symptomatology.

**Pharmacodynamics/Kinetics**

**Distribution:** Readily distributes into most body fluids and tissues; crosses the placenta

**Half-life Elimination:** Dose-dependent ranging from 2-3 hours at low doses to 30 hours at high doses

**Time to Peak:** Oral: ~2 hours

**Formulations**

Liquid: 500 mg/5 mL [choline salicylate 293 mg and magnesium salicylate 362 mg per 5 mL] (237 mL)

Tablet:
500 mg: Choline salicylate 293 mg and magnesium salicylate 362 mg
750 mg: Choline salicylate 440 mg and magnesium salicylate 544 mg
1000 mg: Choline salicylate 587 mg and magnesium salicylate 725 mg

**Dosing**

**Adults:** Oral (based on total salicylate content): 500 mg to 1.5 g 2-3 times/day; usual maintenance dose: 1-4.5 g/day

**Elderly:** Refer to adult dosing.

**Renal Impairment:** Avoid use in severe renal impairment.

**Administration**

**Oral:** Liquid may be mixed with fruit juice just before drinking. Do not administer with antacids. Take with a full glass of water and remain in an upright position for 15-30 minutes after administration.

**Monitoring Laboratory Tests** Serum magnesium with high-dose therapy or in patients with impaired renal function, serum salicylate levels, renal function

**Additional Nursing Issues**

**Physical Assessment: Do not use for persons with allergic reaction to salicylates or other NSAIDs** (see Contraindications). Assess other medications patient may be taking for additive or adverse interactions (see Drug Interactions). Do not take longer than 3 days for fever, or 10 days for pain without consulting medical advisor. Monitor for effectiveness of pain relief. Monitor for signs of adverse reactions or overdose (see Overdose/Toxicology and Adverse Reactions) at beginning of therapy and periodically during long-term therapy. Assess knowledge/teach patient appropriate use. Teach patient to monitor for adverse reactions, adverse reactions to report, and appropriate interventions to reduce side effects. **Pregnancy risk factor C/D** - benefits of use should outweigh possible risks. Note breast-feeding caution.

**Patient Information/Instruction:** If self-administered, use exactly as directed (do not increase dose or frequency); adverse reactions can occur with overuse. Take with food or milk. While using this medication, do not use alcohol, excessive amounts of vitamin C, or salicylate-containing foods (curry powder, prunes, raisins, tea, or licorice), other prescription or OTC medications containing aspirin or salicylate, or other NSAIDs without consulting prescriber. Maintain adequate hydration (2-3 L/day of fluids unless instructed to restrict fluid intake). You may experience nausea, vomiting, gastric discomfort (frequent mouth care, small frequent meals, sucking lozenges, or chewing gum may help). GI bleeding, ulceration, or perforation can occur with or without pain. Stop taking medication and report ringing in ears; persistent pain in stomach; unresolved nausea or vomiting; difficulty breathing or shortness of breath; unusual bruising or bleeding (mouth, urine, stool); or skin rash. **Pregnancy/breast-feeding precautions:** Inform prescriber if you are or intend to be pregnant. Consult prescriber if breast-feeding.

**Geriatric Considerations:** Elderly are at high risk for adverse effects from nonsteroidal anti-inflammatory agents. As much as 60% of elderly can develop peptic ulceration and/or hemorrhage asymptomatically.

**Related Information**

Nonsalicylate/Nonsteroidal Anti-inflammatory Comparison *on page 1401*


- **Choline Salicylate** *see page 1294*
- **Chondroitin Sulfate-Sodium Hyaluronate** *see page 1248*
- **Chondroitin Sulfate - Sodium Hyaluronate** *see page 1282*
- **Chooz® [OTC]** *see* Calcium Supplements *on page 185*
- **Chorex®** *see* Chorionic Gonadotropin *on this page*


## Chorionic Gonadotropin (kor ee ON ik goe NAD oh troe pin)

**U.S. Brand Names** A.P.L.®; Chorex®; Choron®; Follutein®; Glukor®; Gonic®; Pregnyl®; Profasi® HP

**Synonyms** CG; HCG

**Therapeutic Category** Ovulation Stimulator

**Lactation** Excretion in breast milk unknown/unlikely to be used

**Use** Induces ovulation and pregnancy in anovulatory, infertile females; treatment of hypogonadotropic hypogonadism, prepubertal cryptorchidism

**Mechanism of Action/Effect** Stimulates production of gonadal steroid hormones by causing production of androgen by the testis; as a substitute for luteinizing hormone (LH) to stimulate ovulation

**Contraindications** Hypersensitivity to chorionic gonadotropin or any component; precocious puberty; prostatic carcinoma or similar neoplasms

**Warnings** Use with caution in asthma, seizure disorders, migraine, cardiac or renal disease. **Not** effective in the treatment of obesity.

**Adverse Reactions**

>10%: Endocrine & metabolic: Ovarian cysts, uncomplicated ovarian enlargement, pelvic pain

1% to 10%:

Central nervous system: Mental depression, fatigue, headache, irritability, restlessness

Endocrine & metabolic: Enlargement of breasts, precocious puberty

Local: Pain at the injection site

<1% (Limited to important or life-threatening symptoms): Peripheral edema, ovarian hyperstimulation syndrome, gynecomastia

**Pharmacodynamics/Kinetics**

**Half-life Elimination:** Half-life, biphasic: Initial: 11 hours; Terminal: 23 hours

**Excretion:** Excreted unchanged in urine within 3-4 days

**Formulations** Powder for injection: 200 units/mL (10 mL, 25 mL); 500 units/mL (10 mL); 1000 units/mL (10 mL); 2000 units/mL (10 mL)

**Dosing**

**Adults:** I.M.:

Use with menotropins to stimulate spermatogenesis: 5000 units 3 times/week for 4-6 months. With the beginning of menotropins therapy, hCG dose is continued at 2000 units 2 times/week.

Induction of ovulation and pregnancy: 5000-10,000 units 1 day following last dose of menotropins

**Administration**

**I.M.:** I.M. administration only

**Stability**

**Reconstitution:** Following reconstitution with the provided diluent, solutions are stable for 30-90 days, depending on the specific preparation, when stored at 2°C to 15°C.

- **Choron®** *see* Chorionic Gonadotropin *on previous page*
- **Chromagen® OB [OTC]** *see* Vitamin, Multiple *on page 1219*
- **Chronulac®** *see* Lactulose *on page 651*
- **Chymex®** *see page 1248*
- **Chymodiactin®** *see page 1248*
- **Chymopapain** *see page 1248*
- **Cibacalcin® Injection** *see* Calcitonin *on page 182*
- **Ciclopirox** *see page 1247*

## Cidofovir (si DOF o veer)

**U.S. Brand Names** Vistide®

**Therapeutic Category** Antiviral Agent

**Pregnancy Risk Factor** C

**Lactation** Entry into breast milk unknown/contraindicated

**Use** Treatment of CMV retinitis in patients with acquired immunodeficiency syndrome (AIDS)

**Mechanism of Action/Effect** Nucleotide analog that selectively inhibits viral DNA polymerase, suppressing viral DNA synthesis

**Contraindications** Hypersensitivity to cidofovir or clinically severe hypersensitivity to probenecid or other sulfa-containing medications; serum creatinine > 1.5 mg/dL, calculated creatinine clearance of 55 mL/min or urine protein greater to or equal to 100 mg/dL. Direct intraocular injection of cidofovir is contraindicated.

**Warnings** Dose-dependent nephrotoxicity is a major dose-limiting toxicity related to cidofovir. Acute renal failure resulting in dialysis and/or contributing to death have occurred (after as few as 1-2 doses). In patients with renal impairment, potential benefits vs risks should be considered. Dose adjustment or discontinuation may be required for changes in renal failure while on therapy. Renal function secondary to cidofovir is not always reversible. Neutropenia and metabolic acidosis (Fanconi syndrome) have been reported. May decrease intraocular pressure, resulting in decreased visual acuity. Administration of cidofovir must be accompanied by oral probenecid and intravenous saline prehydration. Pregnancy factor C.

**Drug Interactions**

**Increased Effect/Toxicity:** Avoid concomitant administration with other nephrotoxic agents.

**Adverse Reactions**

>10%:

Central nervous system: Infection, chills, fever, headache, amnesia, anxiety, confusion, seizures, insomnia

Dermatologic: Alopecia, rash, acne, skin discoloration

Gastrointestinal: Nausea, vomiting, diarrhea, anorexia, abdominal pain, constipation, heartburn, gastritis

Hematologic: Thrombocytopenia, neutropenia, anemia

Neuromuscular & skeletal: Weakness, paresthesia

Ocular: Amblyopia, conjunctivitis, ocular hypotony

Renal: Tubular damage, proteinuria, Cr elevations

Respiratory: Asthma, bronchitis, coughing, dyspnea, pharyngitis

1% to 10%:

Cardiovascular: Hypotension, pallor, syncope, tachycardia

Central nervous system: Dizziness, hallucinations, depression, somnolence, malaise

Dermatologic: Pruritus, urticaria

(Continued)

## Cidofovir *(Continued)*

Endocrine & metabolic: Hyperglycemia, hyperlipidemia, hypocalcemia, hypokalemia, dehydration
Gastrointestinal: Abnormal taste, stomatitis
Genitourinary: Glycosuria, urinary incontinence, urinary tract infections
Neuromuscular & skeletal: Skeletal pain
Ocular: Retinal detachment, iritis, uveitis, decreased intraocular pressure, abnormal vision
Renal: Hematuria
Respiratory: Pneumonia, rhinitis, sinusitis
Miscellaneous: Sweating, allergic reactions

<1% (Limited to life-threatening or significant reactions): Fanconi syndrome, increased bicarbonate excretion, metabolic acidosis, hepatic failure, pancreatitis, uveitis, iritis

**Overdose/Toxicology** No reports of acute toxicity have been reported, however, hemodialysis and hydration may reduce drug plasma concentrations. Probenecid may assist in decreasing active tubular secretion.

**Pharmacodynamics/Kinetics**

**Protein Binding:** <6%

**Half-life Elimination:** ~2.6 hours (when administered with probenecid)

**Excretion:** Kidney (when administered with probenecid)

**Formulations** Injection: 75 mg/mL (5 mL)

**Dosing**

**Adults:**

Induction treatment: 5 mg/kg once weekly for 2 consecutive weeks
Maintenance treatment: 5 mg/kg administered once every 2 weeks
**Probenecid must be administered orally with each dose of cidofovir.**
Probenecid dose: 2 g 3 hours prior to cidofovir dose, 1 g 2 hours and 8 hours after completion of the infusion; patients should also receive 1 L of normal saline intravenously prior to each infusion of cidofovir; saline should be infused over 1-2 hours.

**Elderly:** Refer to adult dosing.

**Renal Impairment:**

$Cl_{cr}$ 41-55 mL/minute:
Induction (weekly x 2 doses): 2 mg/kg
Maintenance (every other week): 2 mg/kg

$Cl_{cr}$ 30-40 mL/minute:
Induction (weekly x 2 doses): 1.5 mg/kg
Maintenance (every other week): 1.5 mg/kg

$Cl_{cr}$ 20-29 mL/minute:
Induction (weekly x 2 doses): 1 mg/kg
Maintenance (every other week): 1 mg/kg

$Cl_{cr}$ <19 mL/minute:
Induction (weekly x 2 doses): 0.5 mg/kg
Maintenance (every other week): 0.5 mg/kg

Patients with clinically significant changes in serum creatinine during therapy: Cidofovir dose should be reduced to 3 mg/kg and discontinued if creatinine rise is >0.5 mg/dL.
Hemodialysis with high-flux filters may reduce serum concentration by as much as 75%.

**Administration**

**I.V.:** For I.V. infusion only. Infuse over 1 hour.

**Stability**

**Storage:** Store at controlled room temperature 20°C to 25°C (68°F to 77°F).

**Reconstitution:** Cidofovir infusion admixture should be administered within 24 hours of preparation at room temperature or refrigerated. Admixtures should be allowed to equilibrate to room temperature prior to use.

**Monitoring Laboratory Tests** Serum creatinine, serum bicarbonate, acid-base status, urine protein, WBC should be monitored with each dose; monitor intraocular pressure frequently.

**Additional Nursing Issues**

**Physical Assessment:** Monitor laboratory results. Monitor infusion site for extravasation (severe cellulitis and tissue necrosis may result). Monitor for effectiveness of therapy and adverse effects (see above), especially CNS status, fluid balance (I & O, edema, lung sounds, weight), visual changes (acuity, intraocular pressure), acute GI effects, renal damage, opportunistic infection, or adverse respiratory response. Check serum glucose closely for diabetic patients (may cause hyperglycemia). **Pregnancy risk factor C** - women should use effective barrier contraception during and for 1 month following treatment. Males should use barrier contraception during and for 3 months following treatment. Breast-feeding is contraindicated.

**Patient Information/Instruction:** This drug can only be administered I.V. You may experience hair loss (reversible). You may be more susceptible to infection; avoid crowds and infectious situations. You may experience headache, anxiety, confusion; use caution when driving or engaging in tasks that require alertness until response to drug is known. You may experience GI upset (buttermilk or yogurt may help relieve diarrhea); frequent small meals, frequent mouth care, sucking lozenges, or chewing gum may relieve nausea, heartburn, or vomiting; and increased exercise and increased dietary fruit, fluids, or fiber may reduce constipation. You may experience postural hypotension; use caution changing from lying to sitting or standing position and when climbing stairs. Report severe unresolved vomiting, constipation or diarrhea, chills, fever, signs of infection, difficulty breathing or coughing, palpitations, chest pain, syncope, CNS changes (eg, hallucinations, depression, excessive sedation, amnesia, seizures, insomnia), or other severe side effects. **Pregnancy/breast-feeding precautions:** Inform prescriber if you are or intend to be sexually active or pregnant. Do not breast-feed.

**Geriatric Considerations:** Since elderly individuals frequently have reduced kidney function, particular attention should be paid to assessing renal function before and frequently during administration.

**Breast-feeding Issues:** The CDC recommends **not** to breast-feed if diagnosed with HIV to avoid postnatal transmission of the virus.

- **Cigarette Smoking and Effects on Drugs/Toxins** *see page 1415*
- **Cilag®** *see* Acetaminophen *on page 32*
- **Cilastatin and Imipenem** *see* Imipenem and Cilastatin *on page 599*

## Cilostazol (sil OH sta zol)

**U.S. Brand Names** Pletal®

**Therapeutic Category** Antiplatelet Agent

**Pregnancy Risk Factor** C

**Lactation** Excretion in breast milk unknown/not recommended

**Use** Symptomatic management of peripheral vascular disease, primarily intermittent claudication

**Mechanism of Action/Effect** Cilostazol and its metabolites are inhibitors of phosphodiesterase III leading to inhibition of platelet aggregation and vasodilation. Other effects of phosphodiesterase III inhibition include increased cardiac contractility, accelerated AV nodal conduction, increased ventricular automaticity, heart rate, and coronary blood flow.

**Contraindications** Hypersensitivity to cilostazol or any component; heart failure (of any severity)

**Warnings** Use with caution in patients receiving platelet aggregation inhibitors (effects are unknown), hepatic impairment (not studied). Use with caution in patients receiving inhibitors hepatic cytochrome P-450 enzymes, particularly CYP3A4 (such as ketoconazole or erythromycin) or inhibitors of CYP2C19 (such as omeprazole). Pregnancy factor C.

**Drug Interactions**

**Increased Effect/Toxicity:** Cilastazol is a CYP3A4 and CYP2C19 substrate. Increased concentrations of cilostazol have been observed during concurrent therapy with erythromycin and diltiazem, which are inhibitors of CYP3A4 and omeprazole, which is an inhibitor of CYP2C19. Increased concentrations of cilostazol may be anticipated during concurrent therapy with other inhibitors of CYP3A4 (ie, clarithromycin, ketoconazole, itraconazole, fluconazole, miconazole, fluvoxamine, fluoxetine, nefazodone, and sertraline) or inhibitors of CYP2C19. Platelet aggregation with aspirin is further inhibited during concurrent cilastazol. The effect on platelet aggregation with other antiplatelet drugs is unknown.

**Food Interactions** Taking cilostazol with a high-fat meal may increase peak concentration by 90%.

**Adverse Reactions**

>10%:

Central nervous system: Headache (27% to 34%)

Gastrointestinal: Abnormal stools (12% to 15%), diarrhea (12% to 19%)

Miscellaneous: Infection (10% to 14%)

2% to 10%:

Cardiovascular: Peripheral edema (7% to 9%), palpitation (5% to 10%), tachycardia (4%)

Central nervous system: Dizziness (9% to 10%)

Gastrointestinal: Dyspepsia (6%), nausea (6% to 7%), abdominal pain (4% to 5%), flatulence (2% to 3%)

Neuromuscular & skeletal: Back pain (6% to 7%), myalgia (2% to 3%)

Respiratory: Rhinitis (7% to 12%), pharyngitis (7% to 10%), cough (3% to 4%)

<2%: Chills, facial edema, fever, edema, malaise, nuchal rigidity, pelvic pain, retroperitoneal hemorrhage, cerebral infarction/ischemia, congestive heart failure, cardiac arrest, hemorrhage, hypotension, myocardial infarction/ischemia, postural hypotension, ventricular arrhythmia, supraventricular arrhythmia, syncope, anorexia, cholelithiasis, colitis, duodenitis, peptic ulcer, duodenal ulcer, esophagitis, esophageal hemorrhage, gastritis, hematemesis, melena, tongue edema, diabetes mellitus, anemia, ecchymosis, polycythemia, purpura, increased creatinine, gout, hyperlipidemia, hyperuricemia, arthralgia, bone pain, bursitis, anxiety, insomnia, neuralgia, dry skin, urticaria, amblyopia, blindness, conjunctivitis, diplopia, retinal hemorrhage, cystitis, albuminuria, vaginitis, vaginal hemorrhage, urinary frequency

**Overdose/Toxicology** Experience with overdosage in humans is limited. Headache, diarrhea, hypotension, tachycardia, and/or cardiac arrhythmias may occur. Treatment is symptomatic and supportive. Hemodialysis is unlikely to be of value. In some animal models, high-dose or long-term administration was associated with a variety of cardiovascular lesions, including endocardial hemorrhage, hemosiderin deposition and left ventricular fibrosis, coronary arteritis, and periarteritis.

**Pharmacodynamics/Kinetics**

**Distribution:** 97% to 98% protein bound

**Half-life Elimination:** 11-13 hours

**Metabolism:** Hepatic, via CYP3A4 and CYP2C19; at least one metabolite has significant activity

**Excretion:** Urine and feces, as metabolites

**Onset:** 2-4 weeks; treatment for up to 12 weeks may be required before benefit is experienced

**Formulations** Tablet: 50 mg, 100 mg

(Continued)

## Cilostazol *(Continued)*

**Dosing**

**Adults:** Oral: 100 mg twice daily taken at least 30 minutes before or 2 hours after breakfast and dinner; dosage should be reduced to 50 mg twice daily during concurrent therapy with inhibitors of CYP3A4 or CYP2C19 (see Drug Interactions).

**Elderly:** Refer to adult dosing.

**Additional Nursing Issues**

**Physical Assessment:** Assess effectiveness and interactions of other medications (see Drug Interactions, eg, other drugs that inhibit platelet aggregation). See Contraindications and Warnings/Precautions for use cautions (eg, heart failure of any severity). Monitor effectiveness of therapy and adverse reactions at beginning of therapy and periodically with long-term use (see Adverse Reactions). Assess knowledge/teach patient appropriate use, interventions to reduce side effects, and adverse symptoms to report. **Pregnancy risk factor C** - benefits of use should outweigh possible risks. Breast-feeding is not recommended.

**Patient Information/Instruction:** Use exactly as directed; do not discontinue without consulting prescriber. Beneficial effect may take between 2-12 weeks. Take on empty stomach (30 minutes before or 2 hours after meals). Do not take with grapefruit juice. You may experience nervousness, dizziness, or fatigue (use caution when driving or engaging in tasks requiring alertness until response to treatment is known); nausea, vomiting, or flatulence (frequent small meals, frequent mouth care, chewing gum or sucking hard candy may help); or postural hypotension (change position slowly when rising from sitting or lying position or climbing stairs). Report chest pain, palpitations, unusual heart beat, or swelling of extremities; unusual bleeding; unresolved GI upset or pain; dizziness, nervousness, sleeplessness, or fatigue; muscle cramping or tremor; unusual cough; or other adverse effects. **Pregnancy/breast-feeding precautions:** Inform prescriber if you are or intend to be pregnant. Breast-feeding is not recommended.

**Dietary Issues:** Avoid concurrent ingestion of grapefruit juice due to the potential to inhibit CYP3A4. Avoid administration with meals.


- **Ciloxan™** *see page 1282*
- **Ciloxan™ Ophthalmic** *see* Ciprofloxacin *on page 270*
- **Cimetase®** *see* Cimetidine *on this page*


## Cimetidine (sye MET i deen)

**U.S. Brand Names** Tagamet®; Tagamet® HB [OTC]

**Therapeutic Category** Histamine $H_2$ Antagonist

**Pregnancy Risk Factor** B

**Lactation** Enters breast milk/compatible

**Use** Short-term treatment of active duodenal ulcers and benign gastric ulcers; long-term prophylaxis of duodenal ulcer; gastric hypersecretory states; gastroesophageal reflux; prevention of upper GI bleeding in critically ill patients.

**Mechanism of Action/Effect** Competitive inhibition of histamine at $H_2$-receptors of the gastric parietal cells resulting in reduced gastric acid secretion, gastric volume and hydrogen ion concentration reduced

**Contraindications** Hypersensitivity to cimetidine, any component, or other $H_2$ antagonists

**Warnings** Adjust dosages in renal/hepatic impairment or patients receiving drugs metabolized through the cytochrome P-450 system.

**Drug Interactions**

**Cytochrome P-450 Effect:** CYP3A3/4 enzyme substrate; CYP1A2, 2C9, 2C18, 2C19, 2D6, and 3A3/4 enzyme inhibitor

**Increased Effect/Toxicity:** Decreased elimination of lidocaine, theophylline, phenytoin, metronidazole, triamterene, procainamide, quinidine, and propranolol resulting in elevated blood levels with increased effect or toxicity. Inhibition of warfarin metabolism, tricyclic antidepressant metabolism, diazepam elimination and cyclosporine elimination resulting in elevated blood levels and increased toxicity.

**Food Interactions** Cimetidine may increase serum caffeine levels if taken with caffeine. Cimetidine peak serum levels may be decreased if taken with food.

**Effects on Lab Values** ↑ creatinine (S), AST, ALT

**Adverse Reactions**

1% to 10%:

Central nervous system: Headache, dizziness, agitation, drowsiness

Gastrointestinal: Diarrhea, nausea, vomiting

<1% (Limited to important or life-threatening symptoms): Bradycardia, hypotension, tachycardia, neutropenia, agranulocytosis, thrombocytopenia, elevated AST and ALT, elevated creatinine

**Overdose/Toxicology** Treatment is symptomatic and supportive. There is no reported experience with intentional overdose. Reported ingestion of 20 g have had transient side effects seen with recommended doses. Animal data has shown respiratory failure, tachycardia, muscle tremor, vomiting, restlessness, hypotension, salivation, emesis, and diarrhea.

**Pharmacodynamics/Kinetics**

**Protein Binding:** 20%

**Distribution:** Crosses the placenta

**Half-life Elimination:** Normal renal function: 2 hours

**Time to Peak:** Oral: ~1 hour

**Metabolism:** Liver

**Excretion:** Urine

**Onset:** 1 hour

**Duration:** 6 hours

**Formulations**

Infusion, as hydrochloride, in NS: 300 mg (50 mL)

Injection, as hydrochloride: 150 mg/mL (2 mL, 8 mL)

Liquid, oral, as hydrochloride (mint-peach flavor): 300 mg/5 mL with alcohol 2.8% (5 mL, 240 mL)

Tablet: 200 mg, 300 mg, 400 mg, 800 mg

**Dosing**

**Adults:**

Short-term treatment of active ulcers:

Oral: 300 mg 4 times/day or 800 mg at bedtime or 400 mg twice daily for up to 8 weeks

I.M., I.V.: 300 mg every 6 hours or 37.5 mg/hour by continuous infusion; I.V. dosage should be adjusted to maintain an intragastric pH ≥5

Patients with an active bleed: Give cimetidine as a continuous infusion (see above)

Duodenal ulcer prophylaxis: Oral: 400-800 mg at bedtime

Gastric hypersecretory conditions: Oral, I.M., I.V.: 300-600 mg every 6 hours; dosage not to exceed 2.4 g/day

**Elderly:** Refer to adult dosing.

**Renal Impairment:**

$Cl_{cr}$ 10-50 mL/minute: Administer 50% of normal dose.

$Cl_{cr}$ <10 mL/minute: Administer 25% of normal dose.

Slightly dialyzable (5% to 20%)

**Hepatic Impairment:** Usual dose is safe in mild liver disease but use with caution and in reduced dosage in severe liver disease. Increased risk of CNS toxicity in cirrhosis suggested by enhanced penetration of CNS.

**Administration**

**Oral:** Give with meals so that the drug's peak effect occurs at the proper time (peak inhibition of gastric acid secretion occurs at 1 and 3 hours after dosing in fasting subjects and approximately 2 hours in nonfasting subjects. This correlates well with the time food is no longer in the stomach offering a buffering effect). Stagger doses of antacids with cimetidine.

**I.V.:** Administer each 300 mg or fraction thereof over a minimum of 5 minutes when giving I.V. push. Give intermittent infusion over 15-30 minutes for each 300 mg dose.

**I.V. Detail:** Rapid infusion may cause cardiac arrhythmias and hypotension.

**Stability**

**Storage:** Intact vials of cimetidine should be stored at room temperature and protected from light. Cimetidine may precipitate from solution upon exposure to cold but can be redissolved by warming without degradation.

Stability at room temperature for premixed bags: Manufacturer expiration dating and out of overwrap stability: 15 days.

**Reconstitution:** Stability at room temperature for prepared bags is 7 days. Stable in parenteral nutrition solutions for up to 7 days when protected from light.

**Compatibility:** Physically incompatible with barbiturates, amphotericin B, and cephalosporins. See the Compatibility of Drugs Chart *on page 1315* and the Compatibility of Drugs in Syringe Chart *on page 1317.*

**Monitoring Laboratory Tests** CBC, gastric pH, occult blood with GI bleeding; monitor renal function to correct dose.

**Additional Nursing Issues**

**Physical Assessment:** Monitor closely all other prescriptive or OTC medications the patient may be taking (see Drug Interactions). Monitor for signs of peptic ulcer disease (eg, abdominal pain, frank or occult blood in stool, bloody or coffee grounds emesis, or gastric aspirate). Monitor changes in CNS (eg, agitation, severe headache, confusion - especially in elderly patients).

**Patient Information/Instruction:** Take with meals. Limit xanthine-containing foods and beverages which may decrease iron absorption. To be effective, continue to take for the prescribed time (possibly 4-8 weeks) even though symptoms may have improved. Smoking decreases the effectiveness of cimetidine; stop smoking if possible. Avoid use of caffeine or aspirin products. Report diarrhea, black tarry stools, coffee ground like emesis, dizziness, confusion, rash, unusual bleeding or bruising, sore throat, and fever.

**Geriatric Considerations:** Patients diagnosed with PUD should be evaluated for *Helicobacter pylori.* When $H_2$-blockers are indicated, they are the preferred drugs for treating PUD in the elderly due to cost and ease of administration and reduced side effects.

**Additional Information** pH: 3.8-6

- **Cimetigal** *see* Cimetidine *on previous page*
- **Cimogal** *see* Ciprofloxacin *on next page*
- **Cinobac® Pulvules®** *see* Cinoxacin *on next page*

## Cinoxacin (sin OKS a sin)

**U.S. Brand Names** Cinobac® Pulvules®

**Therapeutic Category** Antibiotic, Quinolone

**Pregnancy Risk Factor** B

**Lactation** Excretion in breast milk unknown/contraindicated

**Use** Treatment of urinary tract infections

**Mechanism of Action/Effect** Inhibits microbial synthesis of DNA with resultant inhibition of protein synthesis

**Contraindications** Hypersensitivity to cinoxacin, any component, or other quinolones; history of convulsive disorders

**Warnings** CNS stimulation may occur (tremor, restlessness, confusion, and very rarely hallucinations or seizures). Use with caution in patients with known or suspected CNS disorders or renal impairment. Prolonged use may result in superinfection. Modify dosage in patients with renal impairment.

**Drug Interactions**

**Decreased Effect:** Decreased urine levels occur with probenecid. Decreased absorption with aluminum-, magnesium-, and calcium-containing antacids.

**Increased Effect/Toxicity:** Increased serum levels of cinoxacin when taking probenecid concomitantly.

**Food Interactions** Cinoxacin serum levels may be decreased if taken with food.

**Adverse Reactions**

1% to 10%:

Dermatologic: Skin rash, itching, redness or swelling

Gastrointestinal: Anorexia, diarrhea, nausea, stomach cramps, vomiting

<1% (Limited to important or life-threatening symptoms): Headache, dizziness, photosensitivity

**Overdose/Toxicology** Symptoms of overdose include acute renal failure and seizures. Treatment is supportive. The drug is not removed by peritoneal or hemodialysis.

**Pharmacodynamics/Kinetics**

**Protein Binding:** 60% to 80%

**Distribution:** Crosses the placenta; concentrates in prostate tissue

**Half-life Elimination:** 1.5 hours (prolonged in renal impairment)

**Time to Peak:** Oral: Within 2-3 hours

**Excretion:** ~60% excreted as unchanged drug in urine

**Formulations** Capsule: 250 mg, 500 mg

**Dosing**

**Adults:** Oral: 1 g/day in 2-4 doses for 7-14 days

**Elderly:** Refer to adult dosing.

**Renal Impairment:**

$Cl_{cr}$ 10-50 mL/minute: Administer 250 mg twice daily.

$Cl_{cr}$ <10 mL/minute: Avoid use.

**Administration**

**Oral:** Administer around-the-clock to promote less variation in peak and trough serum levels. Hold antacids for 3-4 hours after giving.

**Monitoring Laboratory Tests** Perform culture and sensitivity studies prior to initiating therapy to determine the causative organism and its susceptibility to cinoxacin. Monitor renal and liver function with prolonged therapy.

**Additional Nursing Issues**

**Physical Assessment:** Monitor effectiveness of therapy. Assess knowledge/instruct patient on use, possible side effects, and symptoms to report. Breast-feeding is contraindicated.

**Patient Information/Instruction:** Take prescribed dose with food. Maintain adequate hydration (2-3 L/day of fluids unless instructed to restrict fluid intake). Avoid antacid use. May cause dizziness; avoid driving or engaging in tasks that require alertness until response to drug is known. Small frequent meals, frequent mouth care, sucking lozenges, or chewing gum may reduce nausea or vomiting. Report skin rash, itching, redness, or swelling; pain, inflammation, or rupture of tendon; pain or burning on urination; or persistent diarrhea or vomiting. **Breast-feeding precautions:** Do not breast-feed.

**Geriatric Considerations:** Adjust dose for renal function in the elderly.

- **Cipro™** *see* Ciprofloxacin *on this page*
- **Ciproflox** *see* Ciprofloxacin *on this page*

## Ciprofloxacin (sip roe FLOKS a sin)

**U.S. Brand Names** Ciloxan™ Ophthalmic; Cipro™

**Therapeutic Category** Antibiotic, Ophthalmic; Antibiotic, Quinolone

**Pregnancy Risk Factor** C

**Lactation** Enters breast milk/contraindicated

**Use** Treatment of documented or suspected infections of the lower respiratory tract, skin and skin structure, bone/joints, and urinary tract due to susceptible bacterial strains; especially indicated for Pseudomonal infections (eg, home care patients) and those due to multidrug resistant gram-negative organisms, documented infectious diarrhea due to *E. coli* (enteropathic strains), *Campylobacter jejuni* or *Shigella*, typhoid fever due to *Salmonella typhi* (although eradication of the chronic typhoid carrier state has not been proven), osteomyelitis when parenteral therapy is not feasible, and sexually transmitted diseases such as uncomplicated cervical and urethral gonorrhea due to *Neisseria gonorrhoeae*; used ophthalmically for superficial ocular infections (corneal ulcers, conjunctivitis) due to susceptible strains; used for otic instillation to treat infection by susceptible strains; acute sinusitis due to *Haemophilus influenzae*, *Streptococcus pneumoniae*, or *Moraxella catarrhalis*; chronic bacterial prostatitis caused by *E. coli* or *Proteus mirabilis*

**Mechanism of Action/Effect** Inhibits DNA-gyrase in susceptible organisms; inhibits relaxation of supercoiled DNA and promotes breakage of double-stranded DNA

**Contraindications** Hypersensitivity to ciprofloxacin, any component, or other quinolones

**Warnings** CNS stimulation may occur (tremor, restlessness, confusion, and very rarely hallucinations or seizures). Use with caution in patients with known or suspected CNS disorder. Prolonged use may result in superinfection. Pregnancy factor C.

**Drug Interactions**

**Cytochrome P-450 Effect:** CYP1A2 enzyme inhibitor

**Decreased Effect:** Decreased absorption with antacids containing aluminum, magnesium, and/or calcium (by up to 98% if given at the same time).

**Increased Effect/Toxicity:** Quinolones cause increased levels of caffeine, warfarin, cyclosporine, and theophylline. Azlocillin, cimetidine, and probenecid increase quinolone levels. An increased incidence of seizures may occur with foscarnet and ciprofloxacin taken in combination.

**Food Interactions** Ciprofloxacin serum levels may be decreased if taken with dairy products. Ciprofloxacin may increase serum caffeine levels if taken with caffeine.

**Adverse Reactions**

**Ophthalmic:**

>10%: Ocular: Burning or other discomfort of the eye, crusting or crystals in corner of eye

1% to 10%:

Gastrointestinal: Bad taste instillation

Ocular: Foreign body sensation, conjunctival hyperemia, itching of eye

**Systemic:**

>10%:

Central nervous system: Dizziness or lightheadedness, headache, nervousness, drowsiness, insomnia

Gastrointestinal: Nausea, diarrhea, vomiting, abdominal pain

1% to 10%: Dermatologic: Photosensitivity

<1% (Limited to important or life-threatening symptoms): Acute psychosis, agitation, hallucinations, tremors, skin rash, itching or redness, Stevens-Johnson syndrome, anemia, increased liver enzymes, ruptured tendons or tendonitis, interstitial nephritis, shortness of breath

**Overdose/Toxicology** Symptoms of overdose include acute renal failure and seizures. Treatment is supportive. The drug is not removed by peritoneal or hemodialysis.

**Pharmacodynamics/Kinetics**

**Protein Binding:** 16% to 43%

**Distribution:** Crosses the placenta; distributes widely throughout body; tissue concentrations often exceed serum concentrations especially in the kidneys, gallbladder, liver, lungs, gynecologic tissue, and prostatic tissue; CSF concentrations reach 10% with noninflamed meninges and 14% to 37% with inflamed meninges

**Half-life Elimination:** Adults with normal renal function: 3-5 hours

**Metabolism:** Liver

**Excretion:** Urine and feces

**Formulations**

Ciprofloxacin hydrochloride:

Infusion in $D_5W$: 400 mg (200 mL)

Infusion in NS or $D_5W$: 200 mg (100 mL)

Injection: 200 mg (20 mL); 400 mg (40 mL)

Ointment, ophthalmic: 3.5 g (0.3%)

Solution, ophthalmic: 3.5 mg/mL (2.5 mL, 5 mL)

Suspension, oral: 250 mg/5 mL (100 mL); 500 mg/5 mL (100 mL)

Tablet: 100 mg, 250 mg, 500 mg, 750 mg

**Dosing**

**Adults:**

Oral:

Urinary tract infection: 250-500 mg every 12 hours for 7-10 days, depending on severity of infection and susceptibility; (3 investigations (n=975) indicate the minimum effective dose for women with acute, uncomplicated urinary tract infection may be 100 mg twice daily for 3 days)

Lower respiratory tract, skin/skin structure infections: 500-750 mg twice daily for 7-14 days depending on severity and susceptibility

Bone/joint infections: 500-750 mg twice daily for 4-6 weeks, depending on severity and susceptibility

Infectious diarrhea: 500 mg every 12 hours for 5-7 days

Typhoid fever: 500 mg every 12 hours for 10 days

Urethral/cervical gonococcal infections: 250-500 mg as a single dose (CDC recommends concomitant doxycycline)

Disseminated gonococcal infection: 500 mg twice daily to complete 7 days of therapy (initial treatment with ceftriaxone 1 g I.M./I.V. daily for 24-48 hours after improvement begins)

Chancroid: 500 mg twice daily for 3 days

I.V.:

Acute sinusitis and chronic bacterial prostatitis: 400 mg every 12 hours

Urinary tract infection: 200-400 mg every 12 hours for 7-10 days

Lower respiratory tract, skin/skin structure infection (mild-moderate): 400 mg every 12 hours for 7-14 days

(Continued)

## Ciprofloxacin *(Continued)*

Ophthalmic:

Solution: Instill 1-2 drops in eye(s) every 2 hours while awake for 2 days and 1-2 drops every 4 hours while awake for the next 5 days

Ointment: Instill one-half inch ribbon into the lower conjunctival sac three times a day for the first two days, then two times a day for the next five days

Otic suspension:

**Elderly:** Refer to adult dosing.

**Renal Impairment:**

$Cl_{cr}$ <30 mL/minute: Administer every 18 hours (oral) and every 18-24 hours (I.V.).

Dialysis: Only small amounts of ciprofloxacin are removed by hemo- or peritoneal dialysis (<10%); usual dose: 250-500 mg every 24 hours following dialysis.

Continuous arteriovenous or venovenous hemofiltration (CAVH): 200-400 mg every 12 hours

**Hepatic Impairment:** Adjustment should be considered in severe hepatic dysfunction.

**Administration**

**Oral:** Administer 2 hours after a meal. May administer with food to minimize GI upset. Avoid antacid use. Drink plenty of fluids to maintain proper hydration and urine output. Hold antacids for 2 hours after giving.

**I.V.:** Administer by slow I.V. infusion over 60 minutes into a large vein.

**I.V. Detail:** Administer slowly to reduce the risk of venous irritation (burning, pain, erythema, and swelling).

**Stability**

**Storage:** Refrigeration and room temperature: Premixed bags: Manufacturer expiration dating; Prepared bags: 14 days.

**Reconstitution:** Final concentration for administration should not exceed 2 mg/mL.

**Compatibility:** Incompatible with aminophylline, amoxicillin sodium, amoxicillin sodium/potassium clavulanate, clindamycin, and mezlocillin. Temporarily discontinue other solutions infusing at the same site.

**Monitoring Laboratory Tests** Patients receiving concurrent ciprofloxacin, theophylline, or cyclosporine should have serum theophylline or cyclosporine levels monitored. Culture and sensitivity specimen should be taken prior to initiating therapy.

**Additional Nursing Issues**

**Physical Assessment:** Assess allergy history before initiating therapy. Assess effectiveness and interactions of other medications (see Drug Interactions). See Warnings/Precautions (CNS stimulation) and Contraindications for use cautions. Monitor effectiveness of therapy, laboratory tests, and adverse response (see Adverse Reactions and Overdose/Toxicology). Assess knowledge/teach patient appropriate use, possible side effects and appropriate interventions, and adverse symptoms to report. **Pregnancy risk factor C** - benefits of use should outweigh possible risks. Breast-feeding is contraindicated.

**Patient Information/Instruction:** Take as directed, preferably on an empty stomach (30 minutes before or 2 hours after meals). Take entire prescription even if feeling better. Maintain adequate hydration (2-3 L/day of fluids unless instructed to restrict fluid intake) to avoid concentrated urine and crystal formation. You may experience nausea, vomiting, or anorexia (small frequent meals, frequent mouth care, sucking lozenges, or chewing gum may help). Report immediately any signs of skin rash, joint or back pain, or difficulty breathing. Report unusual fever or chills; vaginal itching or foul-smelling vaginal discharge; easy bruising or bleeding; or pain, inflammation, or rupture of a tendon.

**Pregnancy/breast-feeding precautions:** Inform prescriber if you are or intend to be pregnant. Do not breast-feed.

**Geriatric Considerations:** Ciprofloxacin should not be used as first-line therapy unless the culture and sensitivity findings show resistance to usual therapy. The interactions with caffeine and theophylline can result in serious toxicity in the elderly. Adjust dose for renal function.

**Additional Information** pH: 3.3-4.6

**Related Information**

Ophthalmic Agents *on page 1282*

TB Drug Comparison *on page 1402*

- **Ciprofloxacin and Hydrocortisone** *see page 1291*
- **Ciprofur** *see* Ciprofloxacin *on page 270*
- **Cipro® HC Otic** *see page 1291*
- **Ciproxina** *see* Ciprofloxacin *on page 270*

## Cisapride (SIS a pride)

**U.S. Brand Names** Propulsid®

**Therapeutic Category** Gastrointestinal Agent, Prokinetic

**Pregnancy Risk Factor** C

**Lactation** Enters breast milk/use caution (AAP rates "compatible")

**Use** Treatment of nocturnal symptoms of gastroesophageal reflux disease (GERD), also demonstrated effectiveness for gastroparesis, refractory constipation, and nonulcer dyspepsia

**Mechanism of Action/Effect** Enhances the release of acetylcholine at the myenteric plexus. *In vitro* studies have shown cisapride to have serotonin-4 receptor agonistic properties which may increase GI motility and cardiac rate; increases lower esophageal sphincter pressure and lower esophageal peristalsis; accelerates gastric emptying of both liquids and solids.

**Contraindications** Hypersensitivity to cisapride or any component; GI hemorrhage, mechanical obstruction, GI perforation, or other situations when GI motility stimulation is dangerous; patients with congestive heart failure, COPD, cancer, multiple organ failure, hypokalemia, or hypomagnesemia; known family history of congenital long QT syndrome and clinically significant bradycardia; patients with prolonged Q-T interval; patients with history of torsade de pointes, sinus node dysfunction; with drugs which prolong Q-T

**Warnings** Serious cardiac ventricular arrhythmias, including ventricular tachycardia, torsade de pointes, and Q-T prolongation have been reported in patients taking cisapride with other drugs that inhibit P-450 3A4 (eg, clarithromycin, erythromycin, fluconazole, itraconazole, ketoconazole, miconazole injection, troleandomycin). Avoid other medications which may prolong Q-T (including antiarrhythmics, some antidepressants, and antipsychotics). Use when stimulation of GI motility may be dangerous (eg, obstruction, perforation, hemorrhage). Pregnancy factor C.

**Drug Interactions**

**Cytochrome P-450 Effect:** CYP3A3/4 enzyme substrate

**Decreased Effect:** Cisapride may decrease the effect of atropine and digoxin.

**Increased Effect/Toxicity:** Cisapride may increase blood levels of warfarin, diazepam, cimetidine, ranitidine, and CNS depressants. Erythromycin, other macrolide antibiotics (troleandomycin, clarithromycin), and the -azole antifungal agents such as fluconazole, ketoconazole, miconazole I.V., itraconazole, indinavir, ritonavir, nefazodone have increased cisapride levels, which has been associated with prolonged Q-T intervals and the potential for torsade de pointes. Diltiazem may also cause this effect. Electrocardiographic toxicity may be additive with other medications which prolong Q-T interval.

**Food Interactions** Coadministration of grapefruit juice with cisapride increases the bioavailability of cisapride and concomitant use should be avoided.

**Adverse Reactions**

>10%:
- Central nervous system: Headache
- Gastrointestinal: Diarrhea (dose dependent)

1% to 10%:
- Cardiovascular: Tachycardia
- Central nervous system: Extrapyramidal effects, somnolence, fatigue, insomnia, anxiety
- Dermatologic: Rash
- Gastrointestinal: Abdominal cramping, constipation, nausea
- Respiratory: Sinusitis, rhinitis, coughing, upper respiratory tract infection, increased incidence of viral infection

<1% (Limited to important or life-threatening symptoms): Seizures (have been reported only in patients with a history of seizures), psychiatric disturbances, bronchospasm, gynecomastia, hyperprolactinemia, methemoglobinemia, apnea, photosensitivity

**Pharmacodynamics/Kinetics**

**Protein Binding:** 97.5% to 98%

**Half-life Elimination:** 6-12 hours

**Metabolism:** Extensively to norcisapride, which is eliminated in urine and feces

**Excretion:** <10% of dose excreted into feces and urine

**Onset:** 0.5-1 hour

**Formulations**

Suspension, oral (cherry cream flavor): 1 mg/mL (450 mL)

Tablet, scored: 10 mg, 20 mg

**Dosing**

**Adults:** Oral: Initial: 5-10 mg 4 times/day at least 15 minutes before meals and at bedtime; in some patients the dosage will need to be increased to 20 mg to obtain a satisfactory result.

**Elderly:** Refer to adult dosing.

**Hepatic Impairment:** Initiate at 50% usual dose.

**Additional Nursing Issues**

**Physical Assessment:** Assess GI function. The increased rate of emptying of the stomach may affect the rate of absorption of other drugs. Carefully monitor the patient's response to all drugs being taken (see Drug Interactions). **Pregnancy risk factor C** - benefits of use should outweigh possible risks. Note breast-feeding caution.

**Patient Information/Instruction:** Take before meals. Avoid alcohol and other CNS depressants. May cause increased sedation. Report severe abdominal pain, prolonged diarrhea, weight loss, or extreme fatigue. **Pregnancy/breast-feeding precautions:** Inform prescriber if you are or intend to be pregnant. Consult prescriber if breast-feeding.

**Geriatric Considerations:** Steady-state serum concentrations are higher than those in younger adults; however, the therapeutic dose and pharmacologic effects are the same as those in younger adults and no adjustment in dose recommended for elderly.

## Cisplatin (SIS pla tin)

**U.S. Brand Names** Platinol®; Platinol®-AQ

**Synonyms** CDDP

**Therapeutic Category** Antineoplastic Agent, Alkylating Agent

**Pregnancy Risk Factor** D

**Lactation** Enters breast milk/contraindicated (AAP rates "compatible")

**Use** Treatment of head and neck, breast, testicular, and ovarian cancer; Hodgkin's and non-Hodgkin's lymphoma; sarcomas, bladder, gastric, lung, esophageal, cervical, and prostate cancer; myeloma, melanoma, mesothelioma, small cell lung cancer, and osteosarcoma

(Continued)

## Cisplatin *(Continued)*

**Mechanism of Action/Effect** Inhibits DNA synthesis

**Contraindications** Hypersensitivity to cisplatin, other platinum-containing compounds, or any component (anaphylactic-like reactions have been reported); pre-existing renal insufficiency; myelosuppression; hearing impairment; pregnancy

**Warnings** The U.S. Food and Drug Administration (FDA) currently recommends that procedures for proper handling and disposal of antineoplastic agents be considered. All patients should receive adequate hydration prior to and for 24 hours after cisplatin administration, with or without mannitol and/or furosemide, to ensure good urine output and decrease the chance of nephrotoxicity. Reduce dosage in renal impairment. Cumulative renal toxicity may be severe. Dose-related toxicities include myelosuppression, nausea, and vomiting. Ototoxicity, especially pronounced in children, is manifested by tinnitus or loss of high frequency hearing and occasionally, deafness. **Serum magnesium, as well as other electrolytes, should be monitored both before and within 48 hours after cisplatin therapy.** Patients who are magnesium depleted should receive replacement therapy before the cisplatin is administered.

Cisplatin preparation should be performed in a Class II laminar flow biologic safety cabinet and personnel should be wearing surgical gloves and a closed front surgical gown with knit cuffs. Appropriate safety equipment is recommended for preparation, administration, and disposal of antineoplastics. If cisplatin contacts the skin, wash and flush thoroughly with water.

**Drug Interactions**

**Decreased Effect:** Sodium thiosulfate theoretically inactivates drug systemically; has been used clinically to reduce systemic toxicity with intraperitoneal administration of cisplatin.

**Increased Effect/Toxicity:** Cisplatin and ethacrynic acid have resulted in severe ototoxicity in animals. Delayed bleomycin elimination with decreased glomerular filtration rate.

**Adverse Reactions**

>10%:

Endocrine & metabolic: Hyperuricemia

Gastrointestinal: Cisplatin is one of the most emetogenic agents used in cancer chemotherapy; nausea and vomiting occur in 76% to 100% of patients and is dose related. **Prophylactic antiemetics should always be prescribed**; nausea and vomiting may last up to 1 week after therapy. Antiemetics should be included in discharge medications.

Emetic potential:
<75 mg: Moderately high (60% to 90%)
≥75 mg: High (>90%)
Time course of nausea/vomiting: Onset: 1-4 hours; Duration: 12-96 hours

Hematologic: Myelosuppressive: Mild with moderate doses, mild to moderate with high-dose therapy
WBC: Mild
Platelets: Mild
Onset (days): 10
Nadir (days): 14-23
Recovery (days): 21-39

Anemia: Can be chronic, when high-dose cisplatin is given for multiple cycles which is responsive to epoetin alfa.

Neuromuscular & skeletal: Neurotoxicity: Peripheral neuropathy is dose- and duration-dependent. The mechanism is through axonal degeneration with subsequent damage to the long sensory nerves. Toxicity can first be noted at doses of 200 mg/m$^2$, with measurable toxicity at doses >350 mg/m$^2$. This process is irreversible and progressive with continued therapy. Ototoxicity occurs in 10% to 30%, and is manifested as high frequency hearing loss. Baseline audiography should be performed.

Otic: Ototoxicity (especially pronounced in children)

Renal: Nephrotoxicity: Related to elimination, protein binding, and uptake of cisplatin; two types of nephrotoxicity: acute renal failure and chronic renal insufficiency

Acute renal failure and azotemia is a dose-dependent process and can be minimized with proper administration and prophylaxis. Damage to the proximal tubules by unbound cisplatin is suspected to cause the toxicity. Proper preplatinum hydration with a chloride containing intravenous fluid is believed to minimize the production of the more nephrotoxic aqua products. It is manifested as increased BUN and creatinine, oliguria, protein wasting, and potassium, calcium, and magnesium wasting.

Chronic renal dysfunction can develop in patients receiving multiple courses of cisplatin. Slow release of tissue-bound cisplatin may contribute to chronic nephrotoxicity. Manifestations of this toxicity are varied, and can include sodium and water wasting, nephropathy, decreased $Cl_{cr}$, and magnesium wasting.

Recommendations for minimizing nephrotoxicity include:
Prepare cisplatin in saline-containing vehicles
Infuse dose over 24 hours
Vigorous hydration with saline-containing intravenous fluids (125-150 mL/hour) before, during, and after cisplatin administration
Simultaneous administration of either mannitol or furosemide
Pretreatment with amifostine
Avoid other nephrotoxic agents (aminoglycosides, amphotericin, etc).

Miscellaneous: Anaphylactic reaction occurs within minutes after administration and can be controlled with epinephrine, antihistamines, and steroids.

1% to 10%:

Gastrointestinal: Anorexia

Local: **Irritant chemotherapy**

<1% (Limited to important or life-threatening symptoms): Bradycardia, arrhythmias, mild alopecia, mouth sores, elevation of liver enzymes, hemolytic anemia, optic neuritis, blurred vision, papilledema, cerebral blindness

**BMT:**

Central nervous system: Peripheral and autonomic neuropathy, ototoxicity

Gastrointestinal: Highly emetogenic

Hematologic: Myelosuppression

Endocrine & metabolic: Hypokalemia, hypomagnesemia

Renal: Acute renal failure, increased serum creatinine, azotemia

Miscellaneous: Transient pain at tumor, transient autoimmune disorders

**Overdose/Toxicology** Symptoms of overdose include severe myelosuppression, intractable nausea and vomiting, kidney and liver failure, deafness, ocular toxicity, and neuritis. There is no known antidote. Hemodialysis appears to have little effect. Treatment is supportive.

**Pharmacodynamics/Kinetics**

**Protein Binding:** >90%

**Distribution:** Rapidly distributes into tissue following administration; found in high concentrations in the kidneys, liver, ovaries, uterus, and lungs

**Half-life Elimination:** Half-life: Initial: 20-30 minutes; Beta: 1 hour; Terminal: ~24 hours; Secondary half-life: 44-73 hours

**Metabolism:** Cellular

**Excretion:** Urine

**Formulations**

Injection, aqueous: 1 mg/mL (50 mL, 100 mL)

Powder for injection: 10 mg, 50 mg

**Dosing**

**Adults:** I.V. (refer to individual protocols):

An estimated $Cl_{cr}$ should be on all cisplatin chemotherapy orders along with other patient parameters (eg, patient's height, weight, and body surface area). Pharmacy and nursing staff should check the $Cl_{cr}$ on the order and determine the appropriateness of cisplatin dosing.

It is recommended that a 24-hour urine creatinine clearance be checked prior to a patient's first dose of cisplatin and periodically thereafter (ie, after every 2-3 cycles of cisplatin).

Pretreatment hydration with 1-2 L of fluid is recommended prior to cisplatin administration. Adequate hydration and urinary output (>100 mL/hour) should be maintained for 24 hours after administration.

**If the dose prescribed is a reduced dose, then this should be indicated on the chemotherapy order.**

Head and neck cancer: 100-150 mg/m$^2$ every 3-4 weeks

Testicular cancer: 10-20 mg/m$^2$/day for 5 days repeated every 3-4 weeks

Metastatic ovarian cancer: 50 mg/m$^2$ every 3 weeks

Intraperitoneal: Cisplatin has been administered intraperitoneal with systemic sodium thiosulfate for ovarian cancer. Doses up to 90-270 mg/m$^2$ have been administered and retained for 4 hours before draining.

High dose BMT: Continuous I.V.: 55 mg/m$^2$/24 hours for 72 hours; total dose: 165 mg/m$^2$

**Elderly:** Refer to adult dosing.

**Renal Impairment:**

$Cl_{cr}$ 10-50 mL/minute: Administer 75% of normal dose.

$Cl_{cr}$ <10 mL/minute: Administer 50% of normal dose.

Hemodialysis: Partially cleared by hemodialysis

Administer dose posthemodialysis

CAPD effects: Unknown

CAVH effects: Unknown

**Administration**

**I.V.:** Irritant. Perform pretreatment hydration (see Dosage).

I.V.: Rate of administration has varied from a 15- to 120-minute infusion, 1 mg/minute infusion, 6- to 8-hour infusion, 24-hour infusion, or per protocol.

Maximum rate of infusion: 1 mg/minute in patients with CHF

**I.V. Detail:** Needles, syringes, catheters, or I.V. administration sets that contain aluminum parts should not be used for administration of drug.

**Extravasation management:** Large extravasations (>20 mL) of concentrated solutions (>0.5 mg/mL) produce tissue necrosis. **Treatment is not recommended unless a large amount of highly concentrated solution is extravasated.** Mix 4 mL of 10% sodium thiosulfate with 6 mL sterile water for injection: Inject 1-4 mL through existing I.V. line cannula. Administer 1 mL for each mL extravasated; inject S.C. if needle is removed.

**Stability**

**Storage:** Store intact vials at room temperature 15°C to 25°C (59°F to 77°F) and protect from light. Do not refrigerate solution as a precipitate may form. If inadvertently refrigerated, the precipitate will slowly dissolve within hours to days, when placed at room temperature. The precipitate may be dissolved without loss of potency by warming solution to 37°C (98.6°F).

(Continued)

## Cisplatin *(Continued)*

Multidose (preservative-free) vials: After initial entry into the vial, solution is stable for 28 days protected from light or for at least 7 days under fluorescent room light at room temperature.

**Reconstitution:** Further dilution stability is dependent on the chloride ion concentration and should be mixed in solutions of NS (at least 0.3% NaCl). Further dilution in NS, $D_5$/0.45% NaCl or $D_5$/NS to a concentration of 0.05-2 mg/mL are stable for 72 hours at 4°C to 25°C in combination with mannitol; may administer 12.5-50 g mannitol/L.

**Standard I.V. dilution:** Dose/250-1000 mL NS, $D_5$/NS or $D_5$/0.45% NaCl; stable for 72 hours at 4°C to 25°C (in combination with mannitol).

**Compatibility:** Incompatible with $D_5$W or other chloride-lacking solutions due to nephrotoxicity. Aluminum-containing I.V. infusion sets and needles should **not** be used due to binding with the platinum. Incompatible with sodium bicarbonate.

**Monitoring Laboratory Tests** Renal function (serum creatinine, BUN, $Cl_{cr}$), electrolytes (particularly magnesium, calcium, potassium), hearing test, neurologic exam (with high dose), liver function periodically, CBC with differential and platelet count, urine output, urinalysis

**Additional Nursing Issues**

**Physical Assessment:** Monitor closely for early signs of anaphylactoid reaction. Monitor laboratory tests prior to each infusion. Monitor infusion site closely for extravasation (see above). Administer antiemetic prior to every treatment and as needed between infusions (see emetic potential above). Monitor closely for adverse reactions which can affect virtually every system (see Adverse Reactions). Teach patient/caregiver appropriate interventions to reduce side effects and necessity of promptly reporting adverse side effects. **Pregnancy risk factor D** - assess knowledge/teach appropriate use of barrier contraceptives. Breast-feeding is contraindicated.

**Patient Information/Instruction:** This drug can only be given I.V. and numerous adverse side effects can occur. Maintaining adequate hydration is extremely important to help avoid kidney damage (2-3 L/day of fluids unless instructed to restrict fluid intake). Nausea and vomiting can be severe and can be delayed for up to 48 hours after infusion and last for 1 week; consult prescriber immediately for appropriate antiemetic medication. May cause hair loss (reversible). You will be susceptible to infection; avoid crowds or infectious situations (do not have any vaccinations without consulting prescriber). Report all unusual symptoms promptly to prescriber. **Pregnancy/breast-feeding precautions:** Do not get pregnant while taking this medication; use appropriate barrier contraceptive measures. Do not breast-feed until prescriber advises it is safe.

**Additional Information**

Sodium content: 9 mg/mL (equivalent to 0.9% sodium chloride solution)
Osmolality of Platinol®-AQ = 285-286 mOsm

- **13-*cis*-Retinoic Acid** *see* Isotretinoin *on page 637*
- **Cisticid** *see* Praziquantel *on page 957*

## Citalopram (sye TAL oh pram)

**U.S. Brand Names** Celexa®

**Synonyms** Nitalapram

**Therapeutic Category** Antidepressant, Selective Serotonin Reuptake Inhibitor

**Pregnancy Risk Factor** C

**Lactation** Enters breast milk/contraindicated

**Use** Treatment of depression; currently being evaluated for use in the treatment of dementia, smoking cessation, alcohol abuse, obsessive-compulsive disorder, and diabetic neuropathy

**Mechanism of Action/Effect** Inhibits CNS neuronal reuptake of serotonin.

**Contraindications** Hypersensitivity to citalopram; hypersensitivity or other adverse sequelae during therapy with other SSRIs; concomitant use with MAO inhibitors or within 2 weeks of discontinuing MAO inhibitors. Potential for severe reaction when used with MAO inhibitors. Serotonin syndrome (hyperthermia, muscular rigidity, mental status changes/agitation, autonomic instability) may occur, possibly resulting in death. Do not use citalopram and MAO inhibitors within 14 days of each other.

**Warnings** As with all antidepressants, use with caution in patients with a history of mania (may activate hypomania/mania). Use with caution in patients with a history of seizures and patients at high risk of suicide. Has potential to impair cognitive/motor performance - should use caution operating hazardous machinery. Elderly and patients with hepatic insufficiency should receive lower dosages. Use with caution in renal insufficiency and other concomitant illness (due to limited drug experience). May cause hyponatremia/SIADH. Pregnancy factor C.

**Drug Interactions**

**Cytochrome P-450 Effect:** CYP3A4 and 2C19 enzyme substrate; weak inhibitor of CYP1A2, 2D6, 2C19 enzymes

**Decreased Effect:** Carbamazepine may increase clearance of citalopram via enzyme induction.

**Increased Effect/Toxicity:** Decreases in citalopram clearance are possible when used with inhibitors of CYP isoenzymes 3A4 and 2C19 (including ketoconazole, itraconazole, fluconazole, and erythromycin).

Caution when used with other CNS active agents. See Contraindications and Warnings/Precautions regarding the use of MAO inhibitors. Cimetidine increases AUC by 43%, lithium may enhance serotonergic effects, and carbamazepine may increase clearance of citalopram via enzyme induction. Potential for serotonin syndrome if combined with other serotonergic drugs. Citalopram may increase the serum concentration of metoprolol. Serum concentrations of imipramine metabolite (desipramine) may be increased.

**Adverse Reactions**

>10%:

Central nervous system: Somnolence (18%), insomnia (15%)

Gastrointestinal: Nausea (21%), dry mouth (20%)

Miscellaneous: Increased diaphoresis (11%)

1% to 10%:

Central nervous system: Fatigue (5%), anxiety (4%), agitation (3%), yawning (2%), fever (2%)

Endocrine/metabolic: Dysmenorrhea (3%), decreased libido (males 3.8%, females 1.3%), anorgasmia (females 1.1%)

Gastrointestinal: Diarrhea (8%), dyspepsia (5%), vomiting (4%), anorexia (4%), abdominal pain (3%)

Genitourinary: Ejaculation disorder (6%), impotence (3%)

Neuromuscular/skeletal: Tremor (8%), arthralgia (2%), myalgia (2%)

Respiratory: Upper respiratory tract infection (5%), rhinitis (5%), sinusitis (3%)

The following events had an incidence >2% in clinical trials but the incidence on placebo was greater than or equal to the incidence on citalopram: Headache, asthenia, dizziness, constipation, palpitation, abnormal vision, sleep disorder, nervousness, pharyngitis, micturition disorder, back pain.

The following emergent effects were also noted at a frequency ≥1% in premarketing trials: Migraine, impaired concentration, confusion, hypotension, postural hypotension, tachycardia, suicide attempt, rash, pruritus, weight gain or loss, abnormal taste, increased appetite, amenorrhea, paresthesia, abnormal accommodation, and cough.

Several cases of hyponatremia and SIADH have been reported with citalopram. As with other antidepressants, hypomania/mania may be activated in a small proportion of patients with major affective disorders.

**Overdose/Toxicology** Symptoms of overdose include dizziness, nausea, vomiting, sweating, tremor, somnolence, and sinus tachycardia. Rare symptoms have included amnesia, confusion, coma, seizures, hyperventilation, and EKG changes (including $Q\text{-}T_c$ prolongation, ventricular arrhythmia, and torsade de pointes). Management is supportive and symptomatic.

**Pharmacodynamics/Kinetics**

**Protein Binding:** Plasma: ~80%

**Half-life Elimination:** 24-48 hours (average 35 hours - doubled in patients with hepatic impairment)

**Time to Peak:** 1-6 hours (average within 4 hours)

**Metabolism:** Extensive hepatic metabolism, including cytochrome P-450 oxidase system, to N-demethylated, N-oxide, and deaminated metabolites

**Excretion:** 10% recovered unchanged in urine; systemic clearance: 330 mL/minute (20% renal)

**Onset:** Usually >2 weeks

**Formulations** Tablet, as hydrobromide: 20 mg, 40 mg

**Dosing**

**Adults:** Oral: 20 mg once daily, in the morning or evening. Dose is generally increased to 40 mg once daily. Doses should be increased by 20 mg at intervals of not less than 1 week. Doses >40 mg/day are not generally recommended, although some patients may respond to doses up to 60 mg/day.

Maintenance: Generally, patients are maintained on the dose required for acute stabilization. If side effects are bothersome, dose reduction by 20 mg/day may be considered.

**Elderly:** Elderly or hepatically impaired patients: Initial dose of 20 mg is recommended; increase dose to 40 mg/day only in nonresponders.

Maintenance: Generally, patients are maintained on the dose required for acute stabilization. If side effects are bothersome, dose reduction by 20 mg/day may be considered.

**Renal Impairment:** None necessary in mild-moderate renal impairment; best avoided in severely impaired renal function ($Cl_{cr}$ <20 mL/minute).

**Stability**

**Storage:** Store at <25°C.

**Monitoring Laboratory Tests** Liver function tests and CBC with continued therapy

**Additional Nursing Issues**

**Physical Assessment:** Assess other medications patient may be taking for possible interaction (especially MAO inhibitors, P-450 inhibitors, and other CNS active agents - see Warnings/Precautions and Drug Interactions). Monitor for adverse reactions (see Adverse Reactions and Overdose/Toxicology) and effectiveness of therapy. Monitor patient periodically for symptom resolution. Assess and monitor for suicidal ideation. Use/teach postural hypotension precautions. **Pregnancy risk factor C** - benefits of use should outweigh possible risks. Breast-feeding is contraindicated.

**Patient Information/Instruction:** The effects of this medication may take up to 3 weeks. Take as directed; do not alter dose or frequency without consulting prescriber. Avoid alcohol, caffeine, and CNS stimulants. You may experience sexual dysfunction (reversible). May cause dizziness, anxiety, or blurred vision (rise slowly from sitting or lying position and use caution when driving or engaging in tasks requiring alertness until response to drug is known); nausea or dry mouth (frequent small meals, frequent mouth care, chewing gum, or sucking lozenges may help). Report confusion or

(Continued)

## Citalopram *(Continued)*

impaired concentration, severe headache, palpitations, rash, insomnia or nightmares, changes in personality, muscle weakness or tremors, altered gait pattern, signs and symptoms of respiratory infection, or excessive perspiration. **Pregnancy/breast-feeding precautions:** Inform prescriber if you are or intend to be pregnant. Do not breast-feed.

**Geriatric Considerations:** Clearance was decreased, while AUC and half-life were significantly increased in elderly patients and in patients with hepatic impairment. Mild to moderate renal impairment may reduce clearance of citalopram (17% reduction noted in trials). No pharmacokinetic information is available concerning patients with severe renal impairment.

**Pregnancy Issues:** Animal reproductive studies have revealed adverse effects on fetal and postnatal development (at doses higher than human therapeutic doses). Should be used in pregnancy only if potential benefit justifies potential risk.

**Related Information**

Antidepressant Agents Comparison *on page 1368*


- ♦ **Citax** *see* Immune Globulin, Intravenous *on page 602*
- ♦ **Citoken** *see* Piroxicam *on page 940*
- ♦ **Citomid** *see* Vincristine *on page 1213*
- ♦ **Citracal® [OTC]** *see* Calcium Supplements *on page 185*
- ♦ **Citracal®** *see page 1294*
- ♦ **Citrate of Magnesia (Magnesium Citrate)** *see* Magnesium Supplements *on page 703*
- ♦ **Citric Acid and Potassium Citrate** *see* Potassium Citrate and Citric Acid *on page 950*
- ♦ **Citric Acid and Sodium Citrate** *see* Sodium Citrate and Citric Acid *on page 1063*
- ♦ **Citrovorum Factor** *see* Leucovorin *on page 662*
- ♦ **Citrucel® Powder** *see page 1294*
- ♦ **CI-719** *see* Gemfibrozil *on page 530*
- ♦ **CLA** *see* Clarithromycin *on next page*


## Cladribine (KLA dri been)

**U.S. Brand Names** Leustatin™

**Synonyms** 2-CdA; 2-Chlorodeoxyadenosine

**Therapeutic Category** Antineoplastic Agent, Antimetabolite

**Pregnancy Risk Factor** D

**Lactation** Enters breast milk/contraindicated

**Use** Treatment of hairy cell and chronic lymphocytic leukemias

**Mechanism of Action/Effect** Incorporates into susceptible cells and into DNA breakage of DNA strand and shutdown of DNA synthesis Cladribine is able to kill resting as well as dividing cells, unlike most other cytotoxic drugs.

**Contraindications** Hypersensitivity to cladribine; pregnancy

**Warnings** The U.S. Food and Drug Administration (FDA) currently recommends that procedures for proper handling and disposal of antineoplastic agents be considered. Because of its myelosuppressive properties, cladribine should be used with caution in patients with pre-existing hematologic or immunologic abnormalities. Prophylactic administration of allopurinol should be considered in patients receiving cladribine because of the potential for hyperuricemia secondary to tumor lysis. Appropriate antibiotic therapy should be administered promptly in patients exhibiting signs or symptoms of neutropenia and infection.

Cladribine preparation should be performed in a Class II laminar flow biologic safety cabinet. Personnel should be wearing surgical gloves and a closed front surgical gown with knit cuffs. Appropriate safety equipment is recommended for preparation, administration, and disposal of antineoplastics. If cladribine contacts the skin, wash and flush thoroughly with water.

**Adverse Reactions**

>10%:

Central nervous system: Fatigue, headache, fever (temperature ≥101°F has been associated with the use of cladribine in approximately 66% of patients in the first month of therapy. Although 69% of patients developed fevers, <33% of febrile events were associated with documented infection)

Dermatologic: Rash

Gastrointestinal: Nausea and vomiting are not severe with cladribine at any dose level. Most cases of nausea were mild, not accompanied by vomiting and did not require treatment with antiemetics; in patients requiring antiemetics, nausea was easily controlled most often by chlorpromazine; anorexia

Hematologic: Anemia (severe); thrombocytopenia; neutropenia; bone marrow suppression commonly observed in patients treated with cladribine, especially at high doses; at the initiation of treatment, however, most patients in clinical studies had hematologic impairment as a result of HCL. During the first 2 weeks after treatment initiation, mean platelet counts decline and subsequently increased with normalization of mean counts by day 12. Absolute neutrophil counts and hemoglobin declined and subsequently increased with normalization of mean counts by week 5 and week 6. CD4 counts nadir at approximately 270, 4-6 months after treatments. Mean CD4 counts after 15 months were <500/mm$^3$. Patients should be considered immunosuppressed for up to 1 year after cladribine therapy.

1% to 10%:

Cardiovascular: Edema, tachycardia, phlebitis

Central nervous system: Dizziness, insomnia, pain, chills, malaise

Dermatologic: Pruritus, erythema
Gastrointestinal: Constipation, diarrhea, abdominal pain
Local: Injection site reactions
Neuromuscular & skeletal: Myalgia, arthralgia, weakness
Respiratory: Coughing, shortness of breath
Miscellaneous: Sweating, trunk pain

**Pharmacodynamics/Kinetics**

**Protein Binding:** 20% to plasma proteins

**Half-life Elimination:** Half-life: Biphasic: Alpha: 25 minutes; Beta: 6.7 hours; Terminal, mean (normal renal function): 5.4 hours

**Formulations** Injection, preservative free: 1 mg/mL (10 mL)

**Dosing**

**Adults:** I.V.:

Hairy cell leukemia:

Continuous intravenous infusion: 0.09-0.1 mg/kg/day continuous infusion for 7 consecutive days

Continuous intravenous infusion: 4 mg/m²/day for 7 days

Non-Hodgkin's lymphoma: Continuous intravenous infusion: 0.1 mg/kg/day for 7 days

**Elderly:** Refer to adult dosing.

**Administration**

**I.V.: Single daily infusion:** Administer diluted in an infusion bag containing 500 mL of 0.9% sodium chloride and repeated for a total of 7 consecutive days.

**Stability**

**Storage:** Store intact vials under refrigeration (2°C to 8°C).

**Reconstitution: 7-day infusion:** Prepare with bacteriostatic 0.9% sodium chloride. Both cladribine and diluent should be passed through a sterile 0.22 micron hydrophilic filter as it is being introduced into the infusion reservoir. The calculated dose of cladribine (7 days x 0.09 mg/kg) should first be added to the infusion reservoir through a filter then the bacteriostatic 0.9% sodium chloride should be added to the reservoir to obtain a total volume of 100 mL.

Further dilution in 100-1000 mL NS is stable for 72 hours. Stable in PVC containers for 24 hours at room temperature and 7 days in Pharmacia Deltec® medication cassettes at room temperature. For 7-day infusion, dilute with bacteriostatic NS and filter through 0.22 micron filter prior to addition into infusion reservoir.

**Standard I.V. 24-hour infusion dilution:** 24-hour dose/500 mL NS
24-hour infusion solution is stable for 24 hours at room temperature.

**Standard I.V. 7-day infusion dilution:** 7-day dose/qs to 100 mL with bacteriostatic NS
7-day infusion solution is stable for 7 days at room temperature.

**Compatibility:** Incompatible with $D_5W$.

**Monitoring Laboratory Tests** Liver and renal function tests, CBC with differential, platelets

**Additional Nursing Issues**

**Physical Assessment:** Closely monitor infusion site for extravasation. Assess vital signs (especially temperature), cardiac status, respiratory status, CNS status, fluid balance, and laboratory reports prior to beginning each infusion and periodically during therapy (see Warnings/Precautions and Adverse Reactions). Assess for and teach adverse reactions to report and appropriate comfort interventions. **Pregnancy risk factor D** - assess knowledge/teach appropriate use of barrier contraceptives. Breast-feeding is contraindicated.

**Patient Information/Instruction:** This drug can only be administered by infusion. Do not use alcohol, aspirin-containing products, and OTC medications without consulting prescriber. It is important to maintain adequate hydration (2-3 L/day of fluids unless instructed to restrict fluid intake) and nutrition during therapy; frequent small meals may help. You may experience nausea or vomiting (frequent small meals, frequent mouth care, sucking lozenges, or chewing gum may help). You will be more susceptible to infection (avoid crowds and exposure to infection). You may experience muscle weakness or pain (mild analgesics may help). Frequent mouth care with soft toothbrush or cotton swabs and frequent mouth rinses may help relieve mouth sores. Report rash; fever; chills; unusual bruising or bleeding; signs of infection; excessive fatigue; yellowing of eyes or skin; change in color of urine or stool; swelling, warmth, or pain in extremities; or difficult respirations. **Pregnancy/breast-feeding precautions:** Do not get pregnant while taking this medication; use appropriate barrier contraceptive measures. Do not breast-feed until prescriber advises it is safe.

- **Claforan®** *see* Cefotaxime *on page 221*
- **Clanda®** *see* Vitamin, Multiple *on page 1219*
- **Claripex®** *see* Clofibrate *on page 285*

## Clarithromycin (kla RITH roe mye sin)

**U.S. Brand Names** Biaxin™

**Synonyms** CLA

**Therapeutic Category** Antibiotic, Macrolide

**Pregnancy Risk Factor** C

**Lactation** Excretion in breast milk unknown/use caution

**Use** Treatment of pharyngitis/tonsillitis, acute maxillary sinusitis, acute exacerbation of chronic bronchitis, pneumonia, uncomplicated skin/skin structure infections due to (eg, *S. pyogenes, S. pneumoniae, S. agalactiae,* viridans *Streptococcus, M. catarrhalis, C. trachomatis, Legionella* sp, *Mycoplasma pneumoniae, S. aureus, H. influenzae*) (MICs
(Continued)

## Clarithromycin *(Continued)*

≤0.25 mcg/mL); has activity against *M. avium* and *M. intracellulare* infection and is indicated for treatment of and prevention of disseminated mycobacterial infections due to *M. avium* complex disease (eg, patients with advanced HIV infection). Exhibits the same spectrum of *in vitro* activity as erythromycin, but with significantly increased potency against those organisms; treatment of peptic ulcer disease with omeprazole and amoxicillin; eradicate *H. pylori* in patients with duodenal ulcer

**Mechanism of Action/Effect** Exerts its antibacterial action by binding to 50S ribosomal subunit resulting in inhibition of protein synthesis. The 14-OH metabolite of clarithromycin is twice as active as the parent compound against some organisms.

**Contraindications** Hypersensitivity to clarithromycin, erythromycin, or any macrolide antibiotic; use with pimozide

**Warnings** In presence of severe renal impairment with or without coexisting hepatic impairment, decreased dosage or prolonged dosing interval may be appropriate. Antibiotic associated colitis has been reported with use of clarithromycin. Elderly patients have experienced increased incidents of adverse effects due to known age-related decreases in renal function. Pregnancy factor C.

**Drug Interactions**

**Cytochrome P-450 Effect:** CYP3A3/4 enzyme substrate; CYP1A2 and 3A3/4 enzyme inhibitor

**Increased Effect/Toxicity:** Clarithromycin increases serum theophylline levels by as much as 20%; significantly increases carbamazepine levels and those of cyclosporine, digoxin, ergot alkaloid, tacrolimus, and triazolam. Peak levels (but not AUC) of zidovudine are often increased. Astemizole should be avoided with use of clarithromycin in cardiac patients or those with electrolyte disturbance since plasma levels may be increased by >3 times. Serious arrhythmias have occurred with cisapride and other drugs which inhibit cytochrome P-450 3A4 (eg, clarithromycin). Fluconazole increases clarithromycin levels and AUC by ~25%. May increase concentrations of HMG-CoA reductase inhibitors (lovastatin and simvastatin).

**Note:** While other drug interactions (bromocriptine, disopyramide, phenytoin, pimozide, and valproate) known to occur with erythromycin have not been reported in clinical trials with clarithromycin, concurrent use of these drugs should be monitored closely.

**Adverse Reactions**

1% to 10%:

Central nervous system: Headache

Gastrointestinal: Diarrhea, nausea, abnormal taste, heartburn, abdominal pain

<1% (Limited to important or life-threatening symptoms): Ventricular tachycardia, torsade de pointes, *Clostridium difficile* colitis, decreased white blood count, elevated prothrombin time, thrombocytopenia; elevated AST, alkaline phosphatase, and bilirubin; elevated BUN/serum creatinine, shortness of breath, leukopenia, neutropenia, manic behavior, tremor, hypoglycemia

**Overdose/Toxicology** Symptoms of overdose include nausea, vomiting, diarrhea, prostration, reversible pancreatitis, hearing loss with or without tinnitus, or vertigo. Treatment includes symptomatic and supportive care.

**Pharmacodynamics/Kinetics**

**Distribution:** Widely distributes into most body tissues with the exception of the CNS

**Half-life Elimination:** 5-7 hours

**Metabolism:** Partially converted to the microbiologically active metabolite, 14-OH clarithromycin

**Excretion:** Primarily renal excretion; clearance approximates normal GFR

**Formulations**

Granules for oral suspension: 125 mg/5 mL (100 mL, 200 mL); 250 mg/5 mL (100 mL, 200 mL)

Tablet, film coated: 250 mg, 500 mg

**Dosing**

**Adults:** Oral:

Usual dose: 250-500 mg every 12 hours for 7-14 days

Upper respiratory tract: 250-500 mg every 12 hours for 10-14 days

Pharyngitis/tonsillitis: 250 mg every 12 hours for 10 days

Acute maxillary sinusitis: 500 mg every 12 hours for 14 days

Lower respiratory tract: 250-500 mg every 12 hours for 7-14 days

Acute exacerbation of chronic bronchitis due to:

*M. catarrhalis* and *S. pneumoniae*: 250 mg every 12 hours for 7-14 days

*H. influenzae*: 500 mg every 12 hours for 7-14 days

Pneumonia due to *M. pneumoniae* and *S. pneumoniae*: 250 mg every 12 hours for 7-14 days

Uncomplicated skin and skin structure: 250 mg every 12 hours for 7-14 days

*Helicobacter pylori*: Combination regimen with bismuth subsalicylate, tetracycline, clarithromycin, and an $H_2$ receptor antagonist; or combination of omeprazole and clarithromycin; 250 mg twice daily to 500 mg 3 times/day

**Elderly:** Refer to adult dosing.

**Renal Impairment:**

$Cl_{cr}$ 10-50 mL/minute: Administer 75% of normal dose.

$Cl_{cr}$ <10 mL/minute: Administer 50% to 75% of normal dose.

Hemodialysis: Administer dose after dialysis.

**Administration**

**Oral:** Clarithromycin may be given with or without meals. Give every 12 hours rather than twice daily to avoid peak and trough variation.

**Monitoring Laboratory Tests** Perform culture and sensitivity studies prior to initiating drug therapy.

**Additional Nursing Issues**

**Physical Assessment:** Assess other medications the patient may be taking for effectiveness and interactions (see Drug Interactions). Monitor for adverse reactions and patient response to therapy. Assess for opportunistic infections. **Pregnancy risk factor C** - benefits of use should outweigh possible risks. Note breast-feeding caution.

**Patient Information/Instruction:** Take full course of therapy; do not discontinue without consulting prescriber. Maintain adequate hydration (2-3 L/day of fluids unless instructed to restrict fluid intake). You may experience nausea (small frequent meals, or sucking lozenges may help); abnormal taste (frequent mouth care or chewing gum may help); diarrhea, headache, or abdominal cramps (medication may be ordered). Report persistent fever or chills, easy bruising or bleeding, or joint pain. Report severe persistent diarrhea, skin rash, sores in mouth, foul-smelling urine, rapid heartbeat or palpitations, or difficulty breathing. Do not refrigerate oral suspension (more palatable at room temperature). **Pregnancy/breast-feeding precautions:** Inform prescriber if you are or intend to be pregnant. Consult prescriber if breast-feeding.

**Geriatric Considerations:** Considered one of the drugs of choice in the outpatient treatment of community-acquired pneumonia in older adults. After doses of 500 mg every 12 hours for 5 days, 12 healthy elderly had significantly increased $C_{max}$ and $C_{min}$, elimination half-lives of clarithromycin and 14-OH clarithromycin compared to 12 healthy young subjects. These changes were attributed to a significant decrease in renal clearance. At a dose of 1000 mg twice daily, 100% of 13 older adults experienced an adverse event compared to only 10% taking 500 mg twice daily.

**Breast-feeding Issues:** No data reported; however, erythromycins may be taken while breast-feeding.

- **Clarithromycin, Lansoprazole, and Amoxicillin** *see* Lansoprazole, Amoxicillin, and Clarithromycin *on page 656*
- **Claritin®** *see* Loratadine *on page 689*
- **Claritin-D®** *see* Loratadine and Pseudoephedrine *on page 690*
- **Claritin-D® 24-Hour** *see* Loratadine and Pseudoephedrine *on page 690*
- **Claritin® Extra** *see* Loratadine and Pseudoephedrine *on page 690*
- **Clarityne®** *see* Loratadine *on page 689*
- **Clavulanate Potassium and Amoxicillin** *see* Amoxicillin and Clavulanate Potassium *on page 82*
- **Clavulanic Acid and Ticarcillin** *see* Ticarcillin and Clavulanate Potassium *on page 1134*
- **Clavulin®** *see* Amoxicillin and Clavulanate Potassium *on page 82*
- **Clear Away® Disc** *see page 1294*
- **Clear By Design® Gel** *see page 1294*
- **Clear Eyes® [OTC]** *see page 1282*
- **Clear Eyes®** *see page 1294*
- **Clearsil® Maximum Strength** *see page 1294*
- **Clear Tussin® 30** *see* Guaifenesin and Dextromethorphan *on page 549*
- **Clemastine** *see page 1294*
- **Clemastine and Phenylpropanolamine** *see page 1294*
- **Cleocin HCl®** *see* Clindamycin *on next page*
- **Cleocin Pediatric®** *see* Clindamycin *on next page*
- **Cleocin Phosphate®** *see* Clindamycin *on next page*
- **Cleocin T®** *see* Clindamycin *on next page*

## Clidinium and Chlordiazepoxide (kli DI nee um & klor dye az e POKS ide)

**U.S. Brand Names** Clindex®; Clinoxide®; Clipoxide®; Librax®; Lidox®

**Synonyms** Chlordiazepoxide and Clidinium

**Therapeutic Category** Antispasmodic Agent, Gastrointestinal

**Pregnancy Risk Factor** D

**Lactation** Enters breast milk/contraindicated

**Use** Adjunct treatment of peptic ulcer; treatment of irritable bowel syndrome

**Contraindications** Hypersensitivity to clidinium, chlordiazepoxide, or any component; glaucoma; prostatic hypertrophy; benign bladder neck obstruction; pregnancy

**Warnings** Use with caution with alcohol or other CNS depressants because of possible combined effects. Do not abruptly discontinue this medication after prolonged use; taper dose gradually.

**Drug Interactions**

**Increased Effect/Toxicity:** Additive effects may result from concomitant benzodiazepine and/or anticholinergic therapy.

**Adverse Reactions**

1% to 10%:

Central nervous system: Drowsiness ataxia, confusion, anticholinergic side effects

Gastrointestinal: Dry mouth, constipation, nausea

<1% (Limited to important or life-threatening symptoms): Syncope, extrapyramidal symptoms, blood dyscrasias, agranulocytosis, jaundice, hepatic dysfunction

**Formulations** Capsule: Clidinium bromide 2.5 mg and chlordiazepoxide hydrochloride 5 mg

**Dosing**

**Adults:** Oral: 1-2 capsules 3-4 times/day, before meals or food and at bedtime. **Caution:** Do not abruptly discontinue after prolonged use; taper dose gradually.

(Continued)

## Clidinium and Chlordiazepoxide *(Continued)*

**Elderly:** Refer to Chlordiazepoxide monograph. Limit dosage to smallest effective amount to preclude the development of ataxia, oversedation, or confusion (not more than 2 capsules/day initially to be increased gradually as needed and tolerated).

**Administration**

**Oral: Caution:** Do not abruptly discontinue after prolonged use; taper dose gradually.

**Monitoring Laboratory Tests** CBC, liver function

**Additional Nursing Issues**

**Physical Assessment:** Assess effectiveness and interactions of other medications (see Drug Interactions). See Warnings/Precautions and Contraindications for use cautions. Monitor effectiveness of therapy, laboratory tests, and adverse response (see Adverse Reactions and Overdose/Toxicology). Assess knowledge/teach patient appropriate use, possible side effects and appropriate interventions, and adverse symptoms to report. **Pregnancy risk factor D** - assess knowledge/teach appropriate use of barrier contraceptives. Breast-feeding is contraindicated.

**Patient Information/Instruction:** Take as directed before meals; do not increase dose and do not discontinue without consulting prescriber first. Avoid alcohol and other CNS depressant medications (antihistamines, sleeping aids, antidepressants) unless approved by prescriber. Void before taking medication. This drug may impair mental alertness (use caution when driving or engaging in tasks that require alertness until response to drug is known). Report excessive and persistent anticholinergic effects (blurred vision, headache, flushing, tachycardia, nervousness, constipation, dizziness, insomnia, mental confusion or excitement, dry mouth, altered taste perception, dysphagia, palpitations, bradycardia, urinary hesitancy or retention, impotence, decreased sweating), or change in color of urine or stools. **Pregnancy/breast-feeding precautions:** Do not get pregnant while taking this medication; use appropriate barrier contraceptive measures. Do not breast-feed.

**Pregnancy Issues:** An increased risk of congenital malformations has been associated with the use of minor tranquilizers during the 1st trimester. Because use of these drugs is rarely a matter of urgency, their use should be avoided during this period.

**Other Issues:** After extended therapy, abrupt discontinuation should be avoided and a gradual dose tapering schedule followed.

**Related Information**

Chlordiazepoxide *on page 250*


- ♦ **Climaderm** *see* Estradiol *on page 441*
- ♦ **Climara® Transdermal** *see* Estradiol *on page 441*
- ♦ **Clinda-Derm® Topical Solution** *see* Clindamycin *on this page*


## Clindamycin (klin da MYE sin)

**U.S. Brand Names** Cleocin HCl®; Cleocin Pediatric®; Cleocin Phosphate®; Cleocin T®; Clinda-Derm® Topical Solution; C/T/S® Topical Solution

**Therapeutic Category** Antibiotic, Miscellaneous

**Pregnancy Risk Factor** B

**Lactation** Enters breast milk/compatible

**Use** Treatment against aerobic and anaerobic streptococci (except enterococci), most staphylococci, *Bacteroides* sp and *Actinomyces*; topically for treatment of severe acne, vaginally for *Gardnerella vaginalis*, alternate treatment for toxoplasmosis, PCP

**Mechanism of Action/Effect** Reversibly binds to 50S ribosomal subunits preventing peptide bond formation thus inhibiting bacterial protein synthesis; bacteriostatic or bactericidal depending on drug concentration, infection site, and organism

**Contraindications** Hypersensitivity to clindamycin or any component; previous pseudomembranous colitis; hepatic impairment

**Warnings** Oral: Dosage adjustment may be necessary in patients with severe hepatic dysfunction. No change necessary with renal insufficiency. Can cause severe and possibly fatal colitis. Use with caution in patients with a history of pseudomembranous colitis. Discontinue drug if significant diarrhea, abdominal cramps, or passage of blood and mucus occurs.

**Drug Interactions**

**Cytochrome P-450 Effect:** CYP3A3/4 enzyme substrate

**Increased Effect/Toxicity:** Increased duration of neuromuscular blockade when given in conjunction with tubocurarine and pancuronium.

**Food Interactions** Peak concentrations may be delayed with food.

**Adverse Reactions**

**Systemic:**

>10%: Gastrointestinal: Pseudomembranous colitis, nausea, vomiting, diarrhea, abdominal pain

1% to 10%:

Cardiovascular: Hypotension
Dermatologic: Urticaria, rashes, Stevens-Johnson syndrome
Hematologic: Neutropenia, thrombocytopenia
Local: Thrombophlebitis, sterile abscess at I.M. injection site
Neuromuscular & skeletal: Polyarthritis
Miscellaneous: Fungal overgrowth, hypersensitivity

**Topical:**

>10%: Dermatologic: Dryness, scaliness, or peeling of skin (lotion)

1% to 10%:

Dermatologic: Contact dermatitis, irritation
Gastrointestinal: Diarrhea (mild), abdominal pain

Miscellaneous: Hypersensitivity

<1% (Limited to important or life-threatening symptoms): Pseudomembranous colitis, nausea, vomiting, diarrhea (severe)

**Vaginal:**

>10%: Genitourinary: Vaginitis or vulvovaginal pruritus (from *Candida albicans*), painful intercourse

1% to 10%:

Central nervous system: Dizziness, headache

Gastrointestinal: Diarrhea, nausea, vomiting, stomach cramps

**Overdose/Toxicology** Symptoms of overdose include diarrhea, nausea, and vomiting. Treatment is supportive.

**Pharmacodynamics/Kinetics**

**Distribution:** No significant levels are seen in CSF, even with inflamed meninges; crosses the placenta; high concentrations in bone, bile, and urine

**Half-life Elimination:** 1.6-5.3 hours, average: 2-3 hours

**Time to Peak:** Oral: Within 60 minutes; I.M.: Within 1-3 hours

**Metabolism:** Hepatic

**Formulations**

Clindamycin hydrochloride:

Capsule: 75 mg, 150 mg, 300 mg

Clindamycin palmitate:

Granules for oral solution: 75 mg/5 mL (100 mL)

Clindamycin phosphate:

Cream, vaginal: 2% (40 g)

Gel, topical: 1% [10 mg/g] (7.5 g, 30 g)

Infusion in $D_5W$: 300 mg (50 mL); 600 mg (50 mL)

Injection: 150 mg/mL (2 mL, 4 mL, 6 mL, 50 mL, 60 mL)

Solution, topical: 1% [10 mg/mL] (30 mL, 60 mL, 480 mL)

Lotion, topical: 1% [10 mg/mL] (60 mL)

**Dosing**

**Adults:**

Oral: 150-450 mg/dose every 6-8 hours; maximum: 1.8 g/day

I.M., I.V.: 1.2-1.8 g/day in 2-4 divided doses; maximum: 4.8 g/day

*Pneumocystis carinii* pneumonia:

Oral: 300-450 mg 4 times/day with primaquine

I.M., I.V.: 1200-2400 mg/day with pyrimethamine

I.V.: 600 mg 4 times/day with primaquine

Topical: Apply a thin film twice daily.

Vaginal: 1 full applicator (100 mg) inserted intravaginally once daily before bedtime for 3 or 7 consecutive days in nonpregnant patients for 7 consecutive days in pregnant patients

**Elderly:** Refer to adult dosing.

**Hepatic Impairment:** Systemic use: Adjustment is recommended in patients with severe hepatic disease.

**Administration**

**Oral:** Administer oral dosage form with a full glass of water to minimize esophageal ulceration. Give around-the-clock to promote less variation in peak and trough serum levels.

**I.M.:** Deep I.M. sites, rotate sites. Do not exceed 600 mg in a single injection.

**I.V.:** Never give as bolus. Do not exceed 1200 mg/day.

**Stability**

**Reconstitution:** Oral: Do **not** refrigerate reconstituted oral solution because it will thicken. Oral solution is stable for 2 weeks at room temperature following reconstitution. I.V. infusion solution in NS or $D_5W$ solution is stable for 16 days at room temperature.

**Compatibility:** See the Compatibility of Drugs Chart *on page 1315*.

**Monitoring Laboratory Tests** CBC, liver and renal function periodically with prolonged therapy

**Additional Nursing Issues**

**Physical Assessment:** Assess effectiveness and interactions of other medications patient may be taking (see Drug Interactions). Monitor laboratory tests (see above), therapeutic response, and adverse reactions (eg, colitis - see Warnings/Precautions and Adverse Reactions) according to dose, route of administration, and purpose of therapy. Assess knowledge/teach patient appropriate use, interventions to reduce side effects, and adverse symptoms to report.

I.V.: Monitor cardiac status and blood pressure. Keep patient recumbent after infusion until blood pressure is stabilized.

**Patient Information/Instruction:**

Oral: Take each dose with a full glass of water. Complete full prescription, even if feeling better. You may experience nausea or vomiting (small frequent meals, frequent mouth care, chewing gum, or sucking lozenges may help). Report dizziness; persistent gastrointestinal effects (pain, diarrhea, vomiting); skin redness, rash, or burning; fever; chills; unusual bruising or bleeding; signs of infection; excessive fatigue; yellowing of eyes or skin; change in color of urine or blackened stool; swelling, warmth, or pain in extremities; difficult respirations; bloody or fatty stool (do not take antidiarrheal without consulting prescriber); or lack or improvement or worsening of condition.

Topical: Wash hands before applying or wear gloves. Apply thin film of gel, lotion, or solution to affected area. May apply porous dressing. Report persistent burning, swelling, itching, or worsening of condition.

(Continued)

## Clindamycin *(Continued)*

Vaginal: Wash hands before using. At bedtime, gently insert full applicator into vagina and expel cream. Wash applicator with soap and water following use. Remain lying down for 30 minutes following administration. Avoid intercourse during 7 days of therapy. Report adverse reactions (dizziness, nausea, vomiting, stomach cramps, or headache) or lack of improvement or worsening of condition.

**Geriatric Considerations:** Elderly patients are often at a higher risk for developing serious colitis and require close monitoring.

**Additional Information** Some formulations may contain benzyl alcohol or tartrazine.

- **Clindex®** *see* Clidinium and Chlordiazepoxide *on page 281*
- **Clinoril®** *see* Sulindac *on page 1088*
- **Clinoxide®** *see* Clidinium and Chlordiazepoxide *on page 281*
- **Clioquinol** *see page 1247*

## Clioquinol and Hydrocortisone

(klye oh KWIN ole & hye droe KOR ti sone)

**U.S. Brand Names** Ala-Quin® Topical; Corque® Topical; Cortin® Topical; Hysone® Topical; Lanvisone® Topical; Pedi-Cort V® Topical; Racet® Topical; UAD® Topical

**Synonyms** Hydrocortisone and Clioquinol; Iodochlorhydroxyquin and Hydrocortisone

**Therapeutic Category** Antifungal Agent, Topical

**Pregnancy Risk Factor** C

**Lactation** Excretion in breast milk unknown

**Use** Treatment of contact or atopic dermatitis, eczema, neurodermatitis, anogenital pruritus, mycotic dermatoses, moniliasis

**Formulations**

Cream: Clioquinol 3% and hydrocortisone 0.5% (15 g, 30 g); clioquinol 3% and hydrocortisone 1% (15 g, 30 g)

Ointment, topical: Clioquinol 3% and hydrocortisone 1% (20 g, 480 g)

**Dosing**

**Adults:** Topical: Apply in a thin film 3-4 times/day.

**Elderly:** Refer to adult dosing.

**Additional Nursing Issues**

**Physical Assessment:** See individual components listed in Related Information. **Pregnancy risk factor C** - benefits of use should outweigh possible risks. Note breast-feeding caution.

**Patient Information/Instruction:** See individual components listed in Related Information. **Pregnancy/breast-feeding precautions:** Inform prescriber if you are on intend to get pregnant. Consult prescriber if breast-feeding.

**Related Information**

Hydrocortisone *on page 578*

- **Clipoxide®** *see* Clidinium and Chlordiazepoxide *on page 281*
- **Clobetasol** *see* Topical Corticosteroids *on page 1152*
- **Clocort® Maximum Strength** *see* Hydrocortisone *on page 578*
- **Clocortolone** *see* Topical Corticosteroids *on page 1152*
- **Cloderm® Topical** *see* Topical Corticosteroids *on page 1152*

## Clofazimine (kloe FA zi meen)

**U.S. Brand Names** Lamprene®

**Therapeutic Category** Leprostatic Agent

**Pregnancy Risk Factor** C

**Lactation** Enters breast milk/contraindicated

**Use** Treatment of dapsone-resistant leprosy; multibacillary dapsone-sensitive leprosy; erythema nodosum leprosum; *Mycobacterium avium-intracellulare* (MAI) infections

**Mechanism of Action/Effect** Binds preferentially to mycobacterial DNA to inhibit mycobacterial growth; also has some anti-inflammatory activity through an unknown mechanism

**Contraindications** Hypersensitivity to clofazimine or any component

**Warnings** Use with caution in patients with GI problems. Dosages >100 mg/day should be used for as short a duration as possible. Skin discoloration resulting from clofazimine treatment may lead to depression. Pregnancy factor C.

**Drug Interactions**

**Decreased Effect:** Combined use may decrease effect with dapsone (unconfirmed).

**Food Interactions** The presence of food increases the extent of absorption.

**Effects on Lab Values** ↑ ESR, glucose (S), albumin, bilirubin, AST

**Adverse Reactions**

>10%:

Dermatologic: Dry skin, skin rash, itching

Gastrointestinal: Abdominal pain, nausea, vomiting, diarrhea, anorexia

Miscellaneous: Pink to brownish-black discoloration of the skin and conjunctiva

1% to 10%:

Endocrine & metabolic: Elevated blood sugar

Gastrointestinal: Change in taste

Ocular: Irritation of the eyes, dryness, burning, itching, photosensitivity

Miscellaneous: Discoloration of sputum, sweat

<1% (Limited to important or life-threatening symptoms): Dizziness, drowsiness, fatigue, headache, giddiness, mental depression, taste disorder, fever, hypokalemia, eosinophilia, anemia, hepatitis, jaundice, enlarged liver, elevated albumin, serum bilirubin and AST, lymphadenopathy

**Overdose/Toxicology** Treatment is supportive.

**Pharmacodynamics/Kinetics**

**Distribution:** Remains in tissues for prolonged periods; highly lipophilic; deposited primarily in fatty tissue and cells of the reticuloendothelial system; taken up by macrophages throughout the body; also distributed to breast milk, mesenteric lymph nodes, adrenal glands, subcutaneous fat, liver, bile, gallbladder, spleen, small intestine, muscles, bones, and skin; does not appear to cross blood-brain barrier

**Half-life Elimination:** Terminal: 8 days; Tissue: 70 days

**Time to Peak:** 1-6 hours with chronic therapy

**Metabolism:** Liver

**Excretion:** Feces

**Formulations** Capsule, as palmitate: 50 mg

**Dosing**

**Adults:** Oral:

Dapsone-resistant leprosy: 100 mg/day in combination with one or more antileprosy drugs for 3 years; then alone 100 mg/day

Dapsone-sensitive multibacillary leprosy: 100 mg/day in combination with two or more antileprosy drugs for at least 2 years and continue until negative skin smears are obtained, then institute single drug therapy with appropriate agent.

Erythema nodosum leprosum: 100-200 mg/day for up to 3 months or longer then taper dose to 100 mg/day when possible

Pyoderma gangrenosum: 300-400 mg/day for up to 12 months

**Elderly:** Refer to adult dosing.

**Hepatic Impairment:** Should be considered in severe hepatic dysfunction.

**Additional Nursing Issues**

**Physical Assessment:** Monitor for Type 2 reaction state (onset of tender skin nodules with joint and lymph gland swelling or visual disturbances). Monitor for adverse GI reactions (eg, GI bleeding, constipation), epistaxis. **Pregnancy risk factor C** - benefits of use should outweigh possible risks. Breast-feeding is contraindicated.

**Patient Information/Instruction:** May be taken with meals. Drug may cause a pink to brownish-black discoloration of the skin, conjunctiva, tears, sweat, urine, feces, and nasal secretions. Although reversible, it may take months to years for skin discoloration to disappear after therapy is complete. Report promptly bone or joint pain, GI disturbance, or vision disturbances. **Pregnancy/breast-feeding precautions:** Inform prescriber if you are or intend to be pregnant. Do not breast-feed.

**Geriatric Considerations:** No specific studies in the elderly. Use with caution in diabetics.

**Related Information**

TB Drug Comparison *on page 1402*

## Clofibrate (kloe FYE brate)

**U.S. Brand Names** Atromid-S®

**Therapeutic Category** Antilipemic Agent (Fibric Acid)

**Pregnancy Risk Factor** C

**Lactation** Excretion in breast milk unknown/contraindicated

**Use** Adjunct to dietary therapy in the management of hyperlipidemias associated with high triglyceride levels (Types III, IV, V); primarily lowers triglycerides and very low density lipoprotein

**Mechanism of Action/Effect** Increases breakdown of VLDL to LDL. Decreases liver synthesis of VLDL. Inhibits cholesterol formation, lowering serum lipid levels. Has antiplatelet effect.

**Contraindications** Hypersensitivity to clofibrate or any component; severe hepatic or renal impairment; primary biliary cirrhosis; peptic ulcer

**Warnings** Clofibrate has been shown to be tumorigenic in animal studies. Increased risk of cholelithiasis, cholecystitis. Discontinue if lipid response is not obtained. Pregnancy factor C.

**Drug Interactions**

**Cytochrome P-450 Effect:** CYP3A3/4 enzyme substrate

**Increased Effect/Toxicity:** Clofibrate may increase effects of warfarin, insulin, and sulfonylureas. Clofibrate's levels may be increased with probenecid.

**Effects on Lab Values** ↑ creatine phosphokinase [CPK] (S); ↓ alkaline phosphatase (S), cholesterol (S), glucose, uric acid (S)

**Adverse Reactions**

>10%: Gastrointestinal: Nausea, diarrhea

1% to 10%:

Central nervous system: Headache, dizziness, fatigue

Gastrointestinal: Vomiting, heartburn, flatulence, abdominal distress, stomatitis

Genitourinary: Impotence

Neuromuscular & skeletal: Muscle cramping, aching, weakness, myalgia

<1% (Limited to important or life-threatening symptoms): Chest pain, cardiac arrhythmias, rash, urticaria, pruritus, alopecia, gallstones or pancreatitis, leukopenia, anemia, eosinophilia, agranulocytosis, increased liver function test, renal toxicity, rhabdomyolysis-induced renal failure

**Overdose/Toxicology** Symptoms of overdose include nausea, vomiting, diarrhea, and GI distress. Treatment is supportive.

(Continued)

## Clofibrate *(Continued)*

**Pharmacodynamics/Kinetics**

**Protein Binding:** 95%

**Half-life Elimination:** 6-24 hours, increases significantly with reduced renal function; with anuria: 110 hours

**Time to Peak:** Within 3-6 hours

**Metabolism:** Liver

**Excretion:** Urine

**Formulations** Capsule: 500 mg

**Dosing**

**Adults:** Oral: 500 mg 4 times/day; some patients may respond to lower doses.

**Elderly:** Refer to adult dosing.

**Renal Impairment:**

$Cl_{cr}$ >50 mL/minute: Administer every 6-12 hours.

$Cl_{cr}$ 10-50 mL/minute: Administer every 12-18 hours.

$Cl_{cr}$ <10 mL/minute: Avoid use.

**Administration**

**Oral:** Administer with meals or milk if GI upset occurs.

**Monitoring Laboratory Tests** Periodic lipid panels

**Additional Nursing Issues**

**Physical Assessment:** Monitor appropriate laboratory tests as ordered. Monitor weight on a regular basis. Monitor for signs or symptoms of adverse effects as indicated above. Assess patients knowledge of and adherence to program of reducing other cardiac risk factors (eg, weight reductions, smoking cessation, low fat/salt diet, increased physical activity, etc). **Pregnancy risk factor C** - benefits of use should outweigh possible risks. Breast-feeding is contraindicated.

**Patient Information/Instruction:** This drug will have to be taken long-term and ongoing follow-up is essential. Adherence to a cardiac risk reduction program, including adherence to prescribed diet, is of major importance. This drug may cause stomach upset; if this occurs, take medication with food or milk. Report chest pain, shortness of breath, irregular heartbeat, palpitations, severe stomach pain with nausea and vomiting, persistent fever, sore throat, or unusual bleeding or bruising. **Pregnancy/breast-feeding precautions:** Inform prescriber if you are or intend to be pregnant. Do not breast-feed.

**Geriatric Considerations:** The definition of, and therefore, when to treat hyperlipidemia in the elderly is a controversial issue. Therefore, treatment may be better reserved for those who are unable to obtain a desirable plasma cholesterol level by diet alone and for whom the benefits of treatment are believed to outweigh the potential adverse effects, drug interactions, and cost of treatment. Adjust dose for renal function.

**Related Information**

Lipid-Lowering Agents Comparison *on page 1393*

♦ **Clomid®** *see* Clomiphene *on this page*

## Clomiphene (KLOE mi feen)

**U.S. Brand Names** Clomid®; Milophene®; Serophene®

**Therapeutic Category** Ovulation Stimulator

**Pregnancy Risk Factor** X

**Lactation** Excretion in breast milk unknown/contraindicated

**Use** Treatment of ovulatory failure in patients desiring pregnancy

**Unlabeled use:** Male infertility

**Mechanism of Action/Effect** Induces ovulation by stimulating the release of pituitary gonadotropins

**Contraindications** Hypersensitivity to clomiphene or any component; liver disease; abnormal uterine bleeding; pregnancy; enlargement or development of ovarian cyst; uncontrolled thyroid or adrenal dysfunction or in the presence of an organic intracranial lesion (ie, pituitary tumor)

**Warnings** Use with caution in patients sensitive to pituitary gonadotropins (eg, polycystic ovary disease). Clomiphene may induce multiple pregnancies, ovarian enlargement, ovarian hyperstimulation syndrome, or abdominal pain, blurring or other visual symptoms.

**Effects on Lab Values** Clomiphene may increase levels of serum thyroxine and thyroxine-binding globulin (TBG)

**Adverse Reactions**

>10%: Endocrine & metabolic: Hot flashes, ovarian enlargement

1% to 10%:

Cardiovascular: Thromboembolism

Central nervous system: Mental depression, headache

Endocrine & metabolic: Breast enlargement (males), breast discomfort (females), abnormal menstrual flow, ovarian cyst formation, ovarian enlargement, premenstrual syndrome, uterine fibroid enlargement

Gastrointestinal: Distention, bloating, nausea, vomiting

Hepatic: Hepatotoxicity

Ocular: Blurring of vision, diplopia, floaters, after-images, phosphenes, photophobia, scotoma

<1% (Limited to important or life-threatening symptoms): Alopecia (reversible), polyuria

**Pharmacodynamics/Kinetics**

**Half-life Elimination:** 5-7 days

**Excretion:** Feces

**Formulations** Tablet, as citrate: 50 mg

**Dosing**

**Adults:** Oral:

Female (ovulatory failure): 50 mg/day for 5 days (first course); start the regimen on or about the fifth day of cycle; if ovulation occurs do not increase dosage; if not, increase next course to 100 mg/day for 5 days. Three courses of therapy are an adequate therapeutic trial. Further treatment is not recommended in patients who do not exhibit ovulation. Long-term therapy is not recommended beyond a total of 6 cycles.

Male (infertility): 25 mg/day for 25 days with 5 days rest, or 100 mg every Monday, Wednesday, Friday

**Stability**

**Storage:** Protect from light.

**Monitoring Laboratory Tests** Urine estrogens and estriol levels; normal levels indicate appropriateness for clomiphene therapy.

**Additional Nursing Issues**

**Physical Assessment:** Female: Assess knowledge/teach appropriate method for measuring basal body temperature to indicate ovulation. Stress importance of following prescriber's instructions for timing intercourse. Instruct patient on schedule of dosing, possible adverse effects (see above), and symptoms to report. **Pregnancy risk factor X** - determine that patient is not pregnant before beginning treatment. Breast-feeding is contraindicated.

**Patient Information/Instruction:** Follow recommended schedule of dosing. You may experience hot flashes (cool clothes and cool environment may help). Report acute sudden headache; difficulty breathing; warmth, pain, redness, or swelling in calves; breast enlargement (male) or breast discomfort (female); abnormal menstrual bleeding; vision changes (blurring, diplopia, photophobia, floaters); acute abdominal discomfort; or fever. **Breast-feeding precautions:** Do not breast-feed.

## Clomipramine (kloe MI pra meen)

**U.S. Brand Names** Anafranil®

**Therapeutic Category** Antidepressant, Tricyclic (Tertiary Amine)

**Pregnancy Risk Factor** C

**Lactation** Enters breast milk/contraindicated (AAP rates "compatible")

**Use** Treatment of obsessive-compulsive disorder (OCD); may also relieve depression, panic attacks, and chronic pain

**Mechanism of Action/Effect** Clomipramine appears to affect serotonin uptake while its active metabolite, desmethylclomipramine, affects norepinephrine uptake

**Contraindications** Patients in acute recovery stage of recent myocardial infarction; not to be used within 14 days of MAO inhibitors; not to be used to treat depression

**Warnings** Seizures are likely and are dose-related. Use with caution in patients with asthma, bladder outlet obstruction, and narrow-angle glaucoma. Pregnancy factor C.

**Drug Interactions**

**Cytochrome P-450 Effect:** CYP1A2, 2C9, 2C18, 2C19, 2D6, and 3A3/4 enzyme substrate; CYP2D6 enzyme inhibitor

**Decreased Effect:** Decreased effects of sympathomimetic drugs when taken with clomipramine. When taken in combination there may be a decreased effect with barbiturates, carbamazepine, and phenytoin.

**Increased Effect/Toxicity:** Increased effect of alcohol, thyroid medications, benzodiazepines, CNS depressants, anticholinergics, and sympathomimetics when given in conjunction with clomipramine. Increased toxicity with MAO inhibitors (increased temperature, seizures, coma, or death). Clomipramine effects increase with concomitant use of cimetidine, fluoxetine, phenothiazines, or oral contraceptives. Can observe additive effects when coadministered with other drugs that can lower the seizure threshold. Potential for serotonin syndrome if combined with other serotonergic drugs.

**Effects on Lab Values** ↑ glucose

**Adverse Reactions**

>10%:

- Central nervous system: Dizziness, drowsiness, headache
- Gastrointestinal: Dry mouth, constipation, increased appetite, nausea, unpleasant taste, weight gain
- Neuromuscular & skeletal: Weakness

1% to 10%:

- Cardiovascular: Arrhythmias, hypotension
- Central nervous system: Confusion, delirium, hallucinations, nervousness, restlessness, parkinsonian syndrome, insomnia
- Gastrointestinal: Diarrhea, heartburn
- Genitourinary: Dysuria, sexual dysfunction
- Neuromuscular & skeletal: Fine muscle tremors
- Ocular: Blurred vision, eye pain
- Miscellaneous: Sweating (excessive)

<1% (Limited to important or life-threatening symptoms): Anxiety, seizures, alopecia, photosensitivity, agranulocytosis, leukopenia, eosinophilia, cholestatic jaundice, increased liver enzymes, increased intraocular pressure

**Overdose/Toxicology** Symptoms of overdose include agitation, confusion, hallucinations, urinary retention, hypothermia, hypotension, tachycardia, ventricular tachycardia,

(Continued)

## Clomipramine *(Continued)*

seizures, and coma. Following initiation of essential overdose management, toxic symptoms should be treated.

**Pharmacodynamics/Kinetics**

**Half-life Elimination:** 20-30 hours

**Metabolism:** Extensive first-pass metabolism; metabolized to desmethylclomipramine (active) in the liver

**Onset:** Usually >2 weeks to therapeutic effect

**Formulations** Capsule, as hydrochloride: 25 mg, 50 mg, 75 mg

**Dosing**

**Adults:** Oral: Initial: 25 mg/day and gradually increase, as tolerated, to 100 mg/day the first 2 weeks, may then be increased to a total of 250 mg/day maximum

**Elderly:** Refer to adult dosing.

**Additional Nursing Issues**

**Physical Assessment:** Assess other medications patient may be taking for effectiveness and interactions (see Drug Interactions). See Contraindications and Warnings/Precautions for cautious use. Monitor therapeutic response, and adverse reactions at beginning of therapy and periodically with long-term use (see Adverse Reactions and Overdose/Toxicology). Taper dosage slowly when discontinuing. Assess knowledge/teach patient appropriate use, interventions to reduce side effects, and adverse symptoms to report. **Pregnancy risk factor C** - benefits of use should outweigh possible risks. Breast-feeding is contraindicated.

**Patient Information/Instruction:** Take multiple dose medication with meals to reduce side effects. Take single daily dose at bedtime to reduce daytime sedation. The effect of this drug may take several weeks to appear. Do not use excessive alcohol, caffeine, and other prescriptive or OTC medications without consulting prescriber. May cause dizziness, drowsiness, headache, or seizures (use caution when driving or engaging in tasks that require alertness until response to drug is known); dry mouth or unpleasant aftertaste (sucking lozenges and frequent mouth care may help); constipation (increased fluids, dietary fiber and fruits, or exercise may help); or orthostatic hypotension (use caution when rising from lying or sitting to standing position or when climbing stairs). Report unresolved constipation or GI upset, unusual muscle weakness, palpitations, or persistent CNS disturbances (hallucinations, delirium, insomnia, or impaired gait). **Pregnancy/breast-feeding precautions:** Inform prescriber if you are or intend to be pregnant. Do not breast-feed.

**Geriatric Considerations:** Not approved as an antidepressant, clomipramine's anticholinergic and hypotensive effects limit its use versus other preferred antidepressants. Elderly patients were found to have higher dose-normalized plasma concentrations as a result of decreased demethylation (decreased 50%) and hydroxylation (25%).

**Breast-feeding Issues:** Generally, it is not recommended to breast-feed if taking antidepressants because of the long half-life, active metabolites, and the potential for side effects in the infant.

**Related Information**

Antidepressant Agents Comparison *on page 1368*

♦ **Clomycin®** *see page 1294*

## Clonazepam (kloe NA ze pam)

**U.S. Brand Names** Klonopin™

**Therapeutic Category** Benzodiazepine

**Pregnancy Risk Factor** C

**Lactation** Enters breast milk/not recommended

**Use** Prophylaxis of petit mal, petit mal variant (Lennox-Gastaut), akinetic, and myoclonic seizures

**Unlabeled use:** Restless legs syndrome, neuralgia, multifocal tic disorder, parkinsonian dysarthria, acute manic episodes, and adjunct therapy for schizophrenia

**Mechanism of Action/Effect** Suppresses the spike-and-wave discharge in absence seizures by depressing nerve transmission in the motor cortex

**Contraindications** Hypersensitivity to clonazepam, any component, or other benzodiazepines; severe liver disease; acute narrow-angle glaucoma

**Warnings** Use with caution in patients with chronic respiratory disease or impaired renal function. Abrupt discontinuance may precipitate withdrawal symptoms, status epilepticus, or seizures in patients with a history of substance abuse. Clonazepam-induced behavioral disturbances may be more frequent in mentally handicapped patients. Pregnancy factor C.

**Drug Interactions**

**Cytochrome P-450 Effect:** CYP3A3/4 enzyme substrate

**Decreased Effect:** Decreased effect of clonazepam by theophylline, phenytoin, or barbiturates due to increased clonazepam clearance.

**Increased Effect/Toxicity:** CNS depressants may increase sedation when taken with clonazepam. Increased effect with cimetidine, contraceptives, and omeprazole.

**Adverse Reactions**

>10%:

Central nervous system: Drowsiness, ataxia, lightheadedness, headache, dizziness, impaired coordination, anxiety, fatigue, slurred speech, irritability, nervousness, insomnia, memory impairment, cognitive disorder, dysarthria, anxiety

Gastrointestinal: Decreased salivation (dry mouth)

Genitourinary: Micturition difficulties

1% to 10%:

Cardiovascular: Tachycardia, syncope

Central nervous system: Confusion, increased libido, depersonalization, mental depression, perceptual disturbances, parethesias, weakness, akathisia, agitation, disinhibition, talkativeness, derealization, dream abnormalities, fear, decreased libido

Gastrointestinal: Abdominal or stomach cramps, increased or decreased appetite, weight gain or loss, nausea, vomiting

Neuromuscular & skeletal: Muscle cramps

Ocular: Photophobia, blurred vision

Otic: Tinnitus

Respiratory: Nasal congestion

Miscellaneous: Sweating

<1% (Limited to important or life-threatening symptoms): Hypotension, agranulocytosis, anemia, leukopenia, neutropenia, thrombocytopenia, hepatic dysfunction

**Overdose/Toxicology** May produce somnolence, confusion, ataxia, diminished reflexes, or coma. Treatment for benzodiazepine overdose is supportive. Flumazenil has been shown to selectively block the binding of benzodiazepines to CNS receptors, resulting in a reversal of benzodiazepine-induced CNS depression, but not respiratory depression.

**Pharmacodynamics/Kinetics**

**Protein Binding:** 85%

**Half-life Elimination:** 19-50 hours

**Time to Peak:** Oral: 1-3 hours; Steady-state: 5-7 days

**Metabolism:** Liver

**Excretion:** Urine

**Onset:** 20-60 minutes

**Duration:** Up to 12 hours

**Formulations** Tablet: 0.5 mg, 1 mg, 2 mg

**Dosing**

**Adults:** Oral:

Initial daily dose not to exceed 1.5 mg given in 3 divided doses; may increase by 0.5-1 mg every third day until seizures are controlled or adverse effects seen

Usual maintenance dose: 0.05-0.2 mg/kg; do not exceed 20 mg/day

**Elderly:** Refer to adult dosing.

**Monitoring Laboratory Tests** Renal function

**Additional Nursing Issues**

**Physical Assessment:** Assess effectiveness and interactions of other medications patient may be taking (see Contraindications, Warnings/Precautions, and Drug Interactions). Assess for history of addiction - long-term use can result in dependence, abuse, or tolerance; periodically evaluate need for continued use. For inpatients, observe safety/seizure precautions. Monitor for therapeutic response, laboratory values, and adverse reactions (see Adverse Reactions) at beginning of therapy and periodically with long-term use. Taper dosage slowly when discontinuing. Assess knowledge/teach patient seizure precautions (if administered for seizures), appropriate use, interventions to reduce side effects, and adverse symptoms to report. **Pregnancy risk factor C** - benefits of use should outweigh possible risks. Breast-feeding is not recommended.

**Patient Information/Instruction:** Take exactly as directed (do not increase dose or frequency); may cause physical and/or psychological dependence. While using this medication, do not use alcohol and other prescription or OTC medications (especially pain medications, sedatives, antihistamines, or hypnotics) without consulting prescriber. Maintain adequate hydration (2-3 L/day of fluids unless instructed to restrict fluid intake). You may experience drowsiness, dizziness, or blurred vision (use caution when driving or engaging in tasks requiring alertness until response to drug is known); nausea, vomiting, loss of appetite, or dry mouth (small frequent meals, frequent mouth care, chewing gum, or sucking lozenges may help); constipation (increased exercise, fluids, or dietary fruit and fiber may help). If medication is used to control seizures, wear identification that you are taking an antiepileptic medication. Report excessive drowsiness, dizziness, fatigue, or impaired coordination; CNS changes (confusion, depression, increased sedation, excitation, headache, agitation, insomnia, or nightmares) or changes in cognition; difficulty breathing or shortness of breath; changes in urinary pattern, changes in sexual activity; muscle cramping, weakness, tremors, or rigidity; ringing in ears or visual disturbances, excessive perspiration, or excessive GI symptoms (cramping, constipation, vomiting, anorexia); worsening of seizure activity, or loss of seizure control. **Pregnancy/breast-feeding precautions:** Inform prescriber if you are or intend to be pregnant. Breast-feeding is not recommended.

**Geriatric Considerations:** Hepatic clearance may be decreased allowing accumulation of active drug. Observe for signs of CNS and pulmonary toxicity.

**Related Information**

Anxiolytic/Hypnotic Use in Long-Term Care Facilities *on page 1430*

Benzodiazepines Comparison *on page 1375*

## Clonidine (KLOE ni deen)

**U.S. Brand Names** Catapres® Oral; Catapres-TTS® Transdermal

**Therapeutic Category** $Alpha_2$ Agonist

**Pregnancy Risk Factor** C

**Lactation** Enters breast milk/not recommended

**Use** Management of mild to moderate hypertension; used alone or in combination with other antihypertensives; not recommended for first-line therapy for hypertension; as a

(Continued)

## Clonidine *(Continued)*

second line agent for decreasing heroin or nicotine withdrawal symptoms in patients with severe symptoms; other uses may include prophylaxis of migraines, glaucoma, and diabetes-associated diarrhea

**Mechanism of Action/Effect** Reduces sympathetic outflow from CNS, producing a decrease in vasomotor tone and heart rate

**Contraindications** Hypersensitivity to clonidine hydrochloride or any component

**Warnings** Use with caution in cerebrovascular disease, coronary insufficiency, renal impairment, sinus node dysfunction. Do not abruptly discontinue as rapid increase in blood pressure, and symptoms of sympathetic overactivity (eg, increased heart rate, tremor, agitation, anxiety, insomnia, sweating, palpitations) may occur. **If need to discontinue, taper dose gradually over 1 week or more.** Adjust dosage in patients with renal dysfunction (especially the elderly). Pregnancy factor C.

**Drug Interactions**

**Decreased Effect:** Tricyclic antidepressants antagonize hypotensive effects of clonidine.

**Increased Effect/Toxicity:** Beta-blockers may potentiate bradycardia in patients receiving clonidine and may increase the rebound hypertension of withdrawal. Discontinue beta-blocker several days before clonidine is tapered. Tricyclic antidepressants may enhance the hypertensive response associated with abrupt clonidine withdrawal.

**Effects on Lab Values** ↑ sodium (S), transient serum glucose; ↓ catecholamines (U); positive Coombs'

**Adverse Reactions**

>10%:

- Cardiovascular: Orthostatic hypotension (especially with epidural route), rebound hypertension, bradycardia
- Central nervous system: Drowsiness (oral use), dizziness (oral use), confusion, anxiety
- Dermatologic: Itching or redness of skin (transdermal systems only)
- Gastrointestinal: Dry mouth (oral use), constipation, nausea
- Genitourinary: Urinary tract infection

1% to 10%:

- Central nervous system: Mental depression, headache, fatigue, hyperaesthesia, pain, nervousness
- Dermatologic: Rash, skin ulcer, darkening of skin (transdermal)
- Respiratory: Dyspnea, hypoventilation
- Cardiovascular: Chest pain
- Endocrine & metabolic: Decreased sexual activity, loss of libido
- Gastrointestinal: Vomiting, constipation, anorexia
- Genitourinary: Nocturia, impotence
- Hepatic: Abnormal liver function tests
- Neuromuscular & skeletal: Weakness
- Otic: Tinnitus

<1% (Limited to important or life-threatening symptoms): Palpitations, tachycardia, Raynaud's phenomenon, congestive heart failure, pruritus, urticaria, alopecia, urinary retention, dysuria

**Overdose/Toxicology** Symptoms of overdose include bradycardia, CNS depression, hypothermia, diarrhea, respiratory depression, and apnea. Treatment is supportive and symptomatic. Naloxone may be utilized in treating CNS depression and/or apnea and should be given I.V., 0.4-2 mg, with repeated doses as needed up to a total of 10 mg, or as an infusion.

**Pharmacodynamics/Kinetics**

**Half-life Elimination:** Normal renal function: 6-20 hours; Renal impairment: 18-41 hours

**Metabolism:** Liver

**Excretion:** Urine and feces

**Onset:** Oral: 0.5-1 hour; $T_{max}$: 2-4 hours

**Duration:** >24 hours

**Formulations**

Clonidine hydrochloride:

- Injection, preservative free: 100 mcg/mL (10 mL)
- Patch, transdermal: 1, 2, and 3 (0.1, 0.2, 0.3 mg/day, 7-day duration)
- Tablet: 0.1 mg, 0.2 mg, 0.3 mg

**Dosing**

**Adults:**

Oral: Initial: 0.1 mg twice daily, usual maintenance dose: 0.2-1.2 mg/day in 2-4 divided doses; maximum recommended dose: 2.4 mg/day

Nicotine withdrawal symptoms: 0.1 mg twice daily to maximum of 0.4 mg/day for 3-4 weeks

Transdermal: Apply once every 7 days; for initial therapy start with 0.1 mg and increase by 0.1 mg at 1- to 2-week intervals; dosages >0.6 mg do not improve efficacy.

Conversion from oral to transdermal:

- Day 1: Place Catapres-TTS® 1; administer 100% of oral dose.
- Day 2: Administer 50% of oral dose.
- Day 3: Administer 25% of oral dose.
- Day 4: Patch remains, no further oral supplement necessary.

**Elderly:** Oral: Initial: 0.1 mg once daily at bedtime, increase gradually as needed.

**Renal Impairment:**

$Cl_{cr}$ <10 mL/minute: Administer 50% to 75% of normal dose initially.

Not dialyzable (0% to 5%) via hemo- or peritoneal dialysis; supplemental dose is not necessary.

**Administration**

**Oral:** Do not discontinue clonidine abruptly.

**Topical:** Patches should be applied weekly at bedtime to a clean, hairless area of the upper outer arm or chest. Rotate patch sites weekly. Redness under patch may be reduced if a topical corticosteroid spray is applied to the area before placement of the patch. If needed, gradually reduce dose over 2-4 days to avoid rebound hypertension.

**Monitoring Laboratory Tests** Liver function tests

**Additional Nursing Issues**

**Physical Assessment:** Assess effectiveness and interactions of other medications (see Drug Interactions). See Contraindications and Warnings/Precautions for use cautions. Monitor for effectiveness of therapy (blood pressure supine and standing) and adverse effects (see Adverse Reactions and Overdose/Toxicology) at beginning of therapy and on a regular basis with long-term therapy. Assess knowledge/teach patient appropriate use, possible side effects/interventions, and adverse symptoms to report. When discontinuing, monitor blood pressure and taper dose and frequency slowly over 1 week or more. **Pregnancy risk factor C** - benefits of use should outweigh possible risks. Breast-feeding is not recommended.

**Patient Information/Instruction:** Take as directed, at bedtime. Do not skip doses or discontinue without consulting prescriber. If using patch, check daily for correct placement. Do not use OTC medications which may affect blood pressure (eg, cough or cold remedies, diet pills, stay-awake medications) without consulting prescriber. This medication may cause drowsiness, dizziness, or impaired judgment (use caution when driving or engaging in tasks that require alertness until response is known); decreased libido or sexual function (will resolve when drug is discontinued); postural hypotension (use caution when rising from sitting or lying position or when climbing stairs); constipation (increase roughage, bulk in diet); or dry mouth or nausea (frequent mouth care or sucking lozenges may help). Report difficulty, pain, or burning on urination; increased nervousness or depression; sudden weight gain (weigh yourself in the same clothes at the same time of day once a week); unusual or persistent swelling of ankles, feet, or extremities; wet cough or respiratory difficulty; chest pain or palpitations; muscle weakness, fatigue, or pain; or other persistent side effects. **Pregnancy/breast-feeding precautions:** Inform prescriber if you are or intend to be pregnant. Breast-feeding is not recommended.

**Geriatric Considerations:** Because of its potential CNS adverse effects, clonidine may not be considered a drug of choice in the elderly. If the decision is to use clonidine, adjust dose based on response and adverse reactions.

## Clonidine and Chlorthalidone (KLOE ni deen & klor THAL i done)

**U.S. Brand Names** Combipres®

**Synonyms** Chlorthalidone and Clonidine

**Therapeutic Category** Antihypertensive Agent, Combination

**Pregnancy Risk Factor** C

**Lactation**

Clonidine: Enters breast milk/not recommended

Chlorthalidone: Enters breast milk/compatible

**Use** Management of mild to moderate hypertension

**Formulations**

Tablet:

0.1: Clonidine 0.1 mg and chlorthalidone 15 mg

0.2: Clonidine 0.2 mg and chlorthalidone 15 mg

0.3: Clonidine 0.3 mg and chlorthalidone 15 mg

**Dosing**

**Adults:** Oral: 1 tablet 1-2 times/day

**Elderly:** May benefit from lower initial dose; refer to individual monographs.

**Additional Nursing Issues**

**Physical Assessment:** See individual components listed in Related Information. **Pregnancy risk factor C** - benefits of use should outweigh possible risks. Breast-feeding is not recommended.

**Patient Information/Instruction:** See individual components listed in Related Information. **Pregnancy/breast-feeding precautions:** Inform prescriber if you are on intend to get pregnant. Breast-feeding is not recommended.

**Related Information**

Chlorthalidone *on page 260*

Clonidine *on page 289*

♦ **Clonodifen®** *see* Diclofenac *on page 358*

## Clopidogrel (kloh PID oh grel)

**U.S. Brand Names** Plavix®

**Therapeutic Category** Antiplatelet Agent

**Pregnancy Risk Factor** B

**Lactation** Excretion in breast milk unknown/not recommended

**Use** Reduce atherosclerotic events (myocardial infarction, stroke, vascular deaths) in patients with atherosclerosis documented by recent myocardial infarction, recent stroke, or established peripheral arterial disease

(Continued)

## Clopidogrel *(Continued)*

**Mechanism of Action/Effect** Clopidogrel blocks the ADP receptor and in so doing, prevents the binding of fibrinogen to that site. Clopidogrel, however, does not alter the receptor, which suggests that it prevents the binding of fibrinogen in an indirect manner. This drug reduces the number of functional ADP receptors. The effect of clopidogrel continues for several days after discontinuing the drug and it effects decrease proportionally to platelet renewal.

**Contraindications** Hypersensitivity to clopidogrel or any component; patients with active pathologic bleeding, coagulation disorders; patients with severe liver disease

**Warnings** Use with caution in patients with hypertension, hepatic or renal impairment, history of bleeding or drug-induced hematologic disorders, or patients scheduled for surgery.

**Drug Interactions**

**Increased Effect/Toxicity:** At high concentrations *in vitro*, clopidogrel inhibits cytochrome P-450 2C9 enzymes. Therefore, it may interfere with the metabolism of phenytoin, tamoxifen, tolbutamide, warfarin, torsemide, fluvastatin, and some NSAIDs which may result in toxicity. Clopidogrel and naproxen resulted in an increase of GI occult blood loss. Clopidogrel prolongs bleeding time. Use with caution with warfarin.

**Adverse Reactions**

1% to 10%:

- Cardiovascular: Chest pain, edema, hypertension
- Central nervous system: Headache, dizziness
- Dermatologic: Rash, pruritus
- Gastrointestinal: Abdominal pain, dyspepsia, diarrhea, nausea, GI hemorrhage
- Hematologic: Purpura
- Neuromuscular & skeletal: Arthralgia, back pain
- Respiratory: Epistaxis, upper respiratory tract infection, dyspnea, rhinitis, bronchitis, cough

<1% (Limited to important or life-threatening symptoms): Neutropenia, agranulocytosis, bleeding, elevated LFTs

**Pharmacodynamics/Kinetics**

**Half-life Elimination:** 7-8 hours

**Metabolism:** Liver, cytochrome P1A to active metabolite

**Formulations** Tablet, as bisulfate: 75 mg

**Dosing**

**Adults:** Oral: 75 mg once daily

**Elderly:** Refer to adult dosing.

**Hepatic Impairment:** Dose adjustment may be necessary for patients with moderate to severe hepatic disease.

**Additional Nursing Issues**

**Physical Assessment:** Assess effectiveness or interactions of other medications patient may be taking. Clopidogrel is a P-450 enzyme inhibitor (see Drug Interactions). Monitor effectiveness of therapy and instruct patient what symptoms to report. Breastfeeding is not recommended.

**Patient Information/Instruction:** Take as directed. May cause headache or dizziness; use caution when driving or engaging in tasks that require alertness until response to drug is known. Small frequent meals, frequent mouth care, sucking lozenges, or chewing gum may reduce nausea or vomiting. Mild analgesics may reduce arthralgia or back pain. Report immediately unusual or acute chest pain or respiratory difficulties, skin rash, unresolved diarrhea or gastrointestinal distress, nosebleed, or acute headache. **Breast-feeding precautions:** Breast-feeding is not recommended.

**Geriatric Considerations:** Plasma levels of the primary clopidogrel metabolite were significantly higher in the elderly (≥75 years). This was not associated with changes in bleeding time or platelet aggregation. No dosage adjustment is recommended.

♦ **Clopra®** *see* Metoclopramide *on page 758*
♦ **Clorafen** *see* Chloramphenicol *on page 248*

## Clorazepate (klor AZ e pate)

**U.S. Brand Names** Gen-XENE®; Tranxene®

**Therapeutic Category** Benzodiazepine

**Pregnancy Risk Factor** D

**Lactation** Excretion in breast milk unknown/not recommended

**Use** Treatment of generalized anxiety and panic disorders; management of alcohol withdrawal; adjunct anticonvulsant in management of partial seizures

**Mechanism of Action/Effect** Facilitates gamma aminobutyric acid (GABA)-mediated transmission inhibitory neurotransmitter action, depresses subcortical levels of CNS

**Contraindications** Hypersensitivity to clorazepate dipotassium or any component; cross-sensitivity with other benzodiazepines may exist; avoid using in patients with pre-existing CNS depression, severe uncontrolled pain, or narrow-angle glaucoma; pregnancy

**Warnings** Use with caution in patients with hepatic or renal disease. Abrupt discontinuation may cause withdrawal symptoms or seizures.

**Drug Interactions**

**Increased Effect/Toxicity:** Increased effect when used in conjunction with cimetidine, CNS depressants, and alcohol. Clorazepate may increase digoxin level.

**Effects on Lab Values** ↓ hematocrit; abnormal liver and renal function tests

**Adverse Reactions**

>10%:

Central nervous system: Drowsiness, ataxia, lightheadedness, headache, dizziness, impaired coordination, anxiety, fatigue, slurred speech, irritability, nervousness, insomnia, memory impairment, cognitive disorder, dysarthria, anxiety

Gastrointestinal: Decreased salivation (dry mouth)

Genitourinary: Micturition difficulties

1% to 10%:

Cardiovascular: Tachycardia, syncope

Central nervous system: Confusion, increased libido, depersonalization, mental depression, perceptual disturbances, parethesias, weakness, akathisia, agitation, disinhibition, talkativeness, derealization, dream abnormalities, fear, decreased libido

Gastrointestinal: Abdominal or stomach cramps, increased or decreased appetite, weight gain or loss, nausea, vomiting

Neuromuscular & skeletal: Muscle cramps

Ocular: Photophobia, blurred vision

Otic: Tinnitus

Respiratory: Nasal congestion

Miscellaneous: Sweating

<1% (Limited to important or life-threatening symptoms): Hypotension, abnormal LFTs, decreased hematocrit, abnormal kidney function tests

**Overdose/Toxicology** May produce somnolence, confusion, ataxia, diminished reflexes, and coma. Treatment for benzodiazepine overdose is supportive. Rarely is mechanical ventilation required. Flumazenil has been shown to selectively block the binding of benzodiazepines to CNS receptors, resulting in a reversal of benzodiazepine-induced CNS depression, but not respiratory depression.

**Pharmacodynamics/Kinetics**

**Distribution:** Crosses the placenta; appears in urine

**Half-life Elimination:** Desmethyldiazepam: 48-96 hours; Oxazepam: 6-8 hours

**Time to Peak:** Oral: Within 1 hour

**Metabolism:** Liver

**Excretion:** Urine

**Onset:** ~1 hour

**Duration:** Variable 8-24 hours

**Formulations**

Clorazepate dipotassium:

Capsule: 3.75 mg, 7.5 mg, 15 mg

Tablet: 3.75 mg, 7.5 mg, 15 mg

Tablet, single dose: 11.25 mg, 22.5 mg

**Dosing**

**Adults:** Oral:

Anxiety: 7.5-15 mg 2-4 times/day, or given as single dose of 11.25 or 22.5 mg at bedtime

Alcohol withdrawal: Initial: 30 mg, then 15 mg 2-4 times/day on first day; maximum daily dose: 90 mg; gradually decrease dose over subsequent days.

**Elderly:** Oral: Anxiety: 7.5 mg 1-2 times/day; use is not recommended in the elderly.

**Stability**

**Compatibility:** Unstable in water.

**Additional Nursing Issues**

**Physical Assessment:** Assess other medications patient may be taking for effectiveness and interactions (see Drug Interactions). See Contraindications and Warnings/Precautions for cautious use. Assess for history of addiction; long-term use can result in dependence, abuse, or tolerance; periodically evaluate need for continued use. Monitor therapeutic response (eg, mood, affect, anxiety level, sleep pattern) and adverse reactions at beginning of therapy and periodically with long-term use (see Adverse Reactions and Overdose/Toxicology). Taper dosage slowly when discontinuing. Assess knowledge/teach patient appropriate use, interventions to reduce side effects, and adverse symptoms to report **Pregnancy risk factor D** - assess knowledge/teach appropriate use of barrier contraceptives. Breast-feeding is not recommended.

**Patient Information/Instruction:** Take exactly as directed (do not increase dose or frequency); may cause physical and/or psychological dependence. Do not use excessive alcohol and other prescription or OTC medications (especially pain medications, sedatives, antihistamines, or hypnotics) without consulting prescriber. Maintain adequate hydration (2-3 L/day of fluids unless instructed to restrict fluid intake). You may experience drowsiness, lightheadedness, impaired coordination, dizziness, or blurred vision (use caution when driving or engaging in tasks requiring alertness until response to drug is known); nausea, vomiting, or dry mouth (small frequent meals, frequent mouth care, chewing gum, or sucking lozenges may help); constipation (increased exercise, fluids, or dietary fruit and fiber may help); altered sexual drive or ability (reversible); or photosensitivity (use sunscreen, wear protective clothing and eyewear, and avoid direct sunlight). Report persistent CNS effects (eg, confusion, depression, increased sedation, excitation, headache, agitation, insomnia or nightmares, dizziness, fatigue, impaired coordination, changes in personality, or changes in cognition); changes in urinary pattern; muscle cramping, weakness, tremors, or rigidity; ringing in ears or visual disturbances; chest pain, palpitations, or rapid heartbeat; excessive perspiration; excessive GI symptoms (cramping, constipation,

(Continued)

## Clorazepate *(Continued)*

vomiting, anorexia); or worsening of condition. **Pregnancy/breast-feeding precautions:** Do not get pregnant while using this medication; use appropriate barrier contraceptive measures. Breast-feeding is not recommended.

**Geriatric Considerations:** Clorazepate is not considered a drug of choice in the elderly. Long-acting benzodiazepines have been associated with falls in the elderly.

**Breast-feeding Issues:** No specific data for clorazepate; however, other benzodiazepines have been shown to be excreted in breast milk. Therefore, it is recommended not to nurse while taking clorazepate.

**Related Information**

Anxiolytic/Hypnotic Use in Long-Term Care Facilities *on page 1430*

Benzodiazepines Comparison *on page 1375*

- **Clor-K-Zaf®** *see* Potassium Supplements *on page 952*
- **Cloruro® De Potasio Kaliolite®** *see* Potassium Supplements *on page 952*

## Clotrimazole (kloe TRIM a zole)

**U.S. Brand Names** Femizole-7® [OTC]; Gyne-Lotrimin® [OTC]; Gyne-Lotrimin®-3; Lotrimin®; Lotrimin® AF Cream [OTC]; Lotrimin® AF Lotion [OTC]; Lotrimin® AF Solution [OTC]; Mycelex®; Mycelex®-7; Mycelex®-G

**Therapeutic Category** Antifungal Agent, Oral Nonabsorbed; Antifungal Agent, Topical; Antifungal Agent, Vaginal

**Pregnancy Risk Factor** B (topical)/C (troches)

**Lactation** Excretion in breast milk unknown

**Use** Treatment of susceptible fungal infections, including oropharyngeal candidiasis, dermatophytoses, superficial mycoses, and cutaneous candidiasis, as well as vulvovaginal candidiasis; limited data suggests that the use of clotrimazole troches may be effective for prophylaxis against oropharyngeal candidiasis in neutropenic patients

**Mechanism of Action/Effect** Binds to phospholipids in the fungal cell membrane altering cell wall permeability resulting in loss of essential intracellular elements

**Contraindications** Hypersensitivity to clotrimazole or any component

**Warnings** Clotrimazole should not be used for treatment of ocular or systemic fungal infection. Use with caution with hepatic impairment. Safety and effectiveness of clotrimazole lozenges (troches) in children <3 years of age have not been established. Pregnancy risk factor C (troches).

**Drug Interactions**

**Cytochrome P-450 Effect:** CYP3A3/4 and 3A5-7 enzyme inhibitor

**Adverse Reactions**

**Oral:**

>10%: Hepatic: Abnormal liver function tests

1% to 10%:

Gastrointestinal: Nausea and vomiting may occur in patients on clotrimazole troches

Local: Mild burning, irritation, stinging to skin or vaginal area

**Vaginal:**

1% to 10%: Genitourinary: Vulvar/vaginal burning

<1% (Limited to important or life-threatening symptoms): Vulvar itching, soreness, edema, or discharge; polyuria; burning or itching of penis of sexual partner

**Pharmacodynamics/Kinetics**

**Time to Peak:**

Oral topical administration: Salivary levels occur within 3 hours following 30 minutes of dissolution time in the mouth.

Vaginal cream: High vaginal levels occur within 8-24 hours.

Vaginal tablet: High vaginal levels occur within 1-2 days.

**Excretion:** As metabolites via bile

**Formulations**

Combination pack (Mycelex-7®): Vaginal tablet 100 mg (7's) and vaginal cream 1% (7 g)

Cream:

Topical (Lotrimin®, Lotrimin® AF, Mycelex®, Mycelex® OTC) : 1% (15 g, 30 g, 45 g, 90 g)

Vaginal (Femizole-7®, Gyne-Lotrimin®, Mycelex®-G): 1% (45 g, 90 g)

Vaginal (Gyne-Lotrimin-3®): 2% (21 g)

Lotion (Lotrimin®): 1% (30 mL)

Solution, topical (Lotrimin®, Lotrimin® AF, Mycelex®, Mycelex® OTC): 1% (10 mL, 30 mL)

Tablet, vaginal (Gyne-Lotrimin®, Mycelex®-G): 100 mg (7s); 500 mg (1s)

Troche (Mycelex®): 10 mg

Twin pack (Mycelex®): Vaginal tablet 500 mg (1's) and vaginal cream 1% (7 g)

**Dosing**

**Adults:**

Oral:

Prophylaxis: 10 mg troche dissolved 3 times/day for the duration of chemotherapy or until steroids are reduced to maintenance levels

Treatment: 10 mg troche dissolved slowly 5 times/day for 14 consecutive days

Topical: Apply twice daily; if no improvement occurs after 4 weeks of therapy, reevaluate diagnosis.

Vaginal:

Cream (1%): Insert 1 applicatorful of 1% vaginal cream daily (preferably at bedtime) for 7 consecutive days.

Cream (2%): Insert 1 applicatorful of 2% vaginal cream daily (preferably at bedtime) for 3 consecutive days

Tablet: Insert 100 mg/day for 7 days or 500 mg single dose.

Topical: Apply to affected area twice daily (morning and evening) for 7 consecutive days.

**Elderly:** Refer to adult dosing.

**Administration**

**Oral:** Allow to dissolve slowly over 15-30 minutes.

**Topical:** For external use only. Apply sparingly. Protect hands with latex gloves. Do not use occlusive dressings.

**Other:** Avoid contact with eyes.

**Monitoring Laboratory Tests** Periodic liver function during oral therapy with clotrimazole lozenges

**Additional Nursing Issues**

**Physical Assessment:** Monitor for appropriate use and effectiveness of treatment. **Pregnancy risk factor B/C** - see Pregnancy Risk Factor. Assess for opportunistic infections. Note breast-feeding caution.

**Patient Information/Instruction:**

Oral: Do not swallow oral medication whole; allow to dissolve slowly in mouth. You may experience nausea or vomiting (small frequent meals, frequent mouth care, chewing gum, or sucking lozenges may help). Report signs of opportunistic infection (eg, white plaques in mouth, fever, chills, perianal itching or vaginal discharge, fatigue, unhealed wounds or sores).

Topical: Wash hands before applying or wear gloves. Apply thin film of gel, lotion, or solution to affected area. May apply porous dressing. Report persistent burning, swelling, itching, worsening of condition, or lack of response to therapy.

Vaginal: Wash hands before using. Insert full applicator into vagina gently and expel cream, or insert tablet into vagina, at bedtime. Wash applicator with soap and water following use. Remain lying down for 30 minutes following administration. Avoid intercourse during therapy (sexual partner may experience penile burning or itching). Report adverse reactions (eg, vulvular itching, frequent urination), worsening of condition, or lack of response to therapy.

**Pregnancy/breast-feeding precautions:** Inform prescriber if pregnant. Consult prescriber if breast-feeding.

**Geriatric Considerations:** Localized fungal infections frequently follow broad spectrum antimicrobial therapy. Specifically, oral and vaginal infections due to *Candida*.

♦ **Clotrimazole and Betamethasone** *see* Betamethasone and Clotrimazole *on page 150*

## Cloxacillin (kloks a SIL in)

**U.S. Brand Names** Cloxapen®; Tegopen®

**Therapeutic Category** Antibiotic, Penicillin

**Pregnancy Risk Factor** B

**Lactation** Excretion in breast milk unknown

**Use** Treatment of susceptible bacterial infections, notably penicillinase-producing staphylococci causing respiratory tract, skin and skin structure, bone and joint, urinary tract infections, endocarditis, septicemia, and meningitis

**Mechanism of Action/Effect** Inhibits bacterial cell wall synthesis

**Contraindications** Hypersensitivity to cloxacillin, any component, penicillins, cephalosporins, or imipenem

**Warnings** Use with caution in patients allergic to cephalosporins due to a low incidence of cross-hypersensitivity.

**Drug Interactions**

**Decreased Effect:** Efficacy of oral contraceptives may be reduced when taken with cloxacillin.

**Increased Effect/Toxicity:** Disulfiram and probenecid may increase penicillin levels. Cloxacillin may increase effect of anticoagulants.

**Effects on Lab Values** May interfere with urinary glucose tests using cupric sulfate (Benedict's solution, Clinitest®); may inactivate aminoglycosides *in vitro*; false-positive urine and serum proteins; false-positive in uric acid, urinary steroids

**Adverse Reactions**

>10%:

Central nervous system: Headache

Gastrointestinal: Nausea (mild), vomiting

Miscellaneous: Oral candidiasis, vaginal candidiasis

1% to 10%:

Dermatologic: Urticaria, exfoliative dermatitis

Miscellaneous: Allergic reactions, specifically anaphylaxis; serum sickness-like reactions

<1% (Limited to important or life-threatening symptoms): Seizures, anxiety, confusion, hallucinations, depression, leukopenia, neutropenia, thrombocytopenia, jaundice, hepatotoxicity, interstitial nephritis, *Clostridium difficile* colitis

**Overdose/Toxicology** Symptoms of penicillin overdose include neuromuscular hypersensitivity (eg, agitation, hallucinations, asterixis, encephalopathy, confusion, and seizures). Electrolyte imbalance may occur if the preparation contains potassium or sodium salts, especially in renal failure. Hemodialysis may be helpful to aid in removal of the drug from blood; otherwise, treatment is supportive or symptom directed.

(Continued)

## Cloxacillin *(Continued)*

**Pharmacodynamics/Kinetics**

**Protein Binding:** 90% to 98%

**Distribution:** Crosses the placenta; distributed widely to most body fluids and bone; penetration into cells, into the eye, and across normal meninges is poor; inflammation increased amount that crosses the blood-brain barrier

**Half-life Elimination:** 0.5-1.5 hours (prolonged in renal impairment and in neonates)

**Time to Peak:** Oral: Within 0.5-2 hours

**Metabolism:** Liver

**Excretion:** Urine and bile

**Formulations**

Cloxacillin sodium:

Capsule: 250 mg, 500 mg

Powder for oral suspension: 125 mg/5 mL (100 mL, 200 mL)

**Dosing**

**Adults:** Oral: 250-500 mg every 6 hours

**Elderly:** Refer to adult dosing.

**Renal Impairment:** Elimination of drug is slow in renally impaired.

Not dialyzable (0% to 5%)

**Administration**

**Oral:** Administer around-the-clock to reduce variation between peak and trough concentrations. Suspension: Shake well before use. Take on an empty stomach.

**Stability**

**Storage:** Refrigerate suspension.

**Reconstitution:** Refrigerate oral solution after reconstitution. Discard after 14 days Stable for 3 days at room temperature.

**Monitoring Laboratory Tests** PT if patient is concurrently on warfarin. Perform culture and sensitivity testing prior to initiating therapy.

**Additional Nursing Issues**

**Physical Assessment:** Monitor for adverse effects, especially anaphylactic reactions. Monitor for signs or symptoms of superinfection. Note breast-feeding caution.

**Patient Information/Instruction:** Take 1 hour before or 2 hours after meals with water. Finish all medication; do not skip doses. Take around-the-clock. If diabetic, drug may cause false tests with Clinitest® urine glucose monitoring; use of glucose oxidase methods (Clinistix®) or serum glucose monitoring is preferable. This drug may interfere with oral contraceptives; an alternate form of birth control should be used. Immediately report any signs or symptoms of anaphylactic reactions (eg, chills, fever, wheezing, tightness in chest), excessive GI side effects, or signs or symptoms of opportunistic infection (eg, white spots or sores in mouth, vaginal discharge or sores, fever, fatigue, unhealed sores or wounds). **Breast-feeding precautions:** Inform prescriber if breast-feeding.

♦ **Cloxapen®** *see* Cloxacillin *on previous page*

## Clozapine (KLOE za peen)

**U.S. Brand Names** Clozaril®

**Therapeutic Category** Antipsychotic Agent, Dibenzodiazepine

**Pregnancy Risk Factor** B

**Lactation** Enters breast milk/contraindicated

**Use** Management of treatment-refractory schizophrenic patients; schizoaffective disorder; treatment of refractory bipolar disorder

**Mechanism of Action/Effect** Clozapine is a weak dopamine$_1$ and dopamine$_2$ receptor blocker; in addition, it blocks the serotonin$_2$, alpha-adrenergic, and histamine $H_1$ central nervous system receptors

**Contraindications** In patients with WBC ≤3500 cells/mm$^3$ before therapy; if WBC falls to <3000 cells/mm$^3$ during therapy the drug should be withheld and patient monitored for signs or symptoms of infection to disappear. Clozapine can be restarted if WBC rises to >3000 cells/mm$^3$ and ANC returns to levels >1500/mm$^3$. Contraindicated in bone marrow suppression, myeloproliferative disease, or with history of clozapine-induced agranulocytosis.

**Warnings** Medication should not be stopped abruptly. Taper off over 1-2 weeks. WBC testing should occur weekly for the duration of therapy. Select patients who have received clozapine chronically (>6 months) may have biweekly CBCs; also for 4 weeks after drug discontinuation. Significant risk of agranulocytosis, potentially life-threatening. Use with caution in patients receiving other marrow suppressive agents, patients with renal impairment, history of seizures, narrow angle glaucoma, or respiratory disorders. Risk of extrapyramidal reactions, neuroleptic malignant syndrome or tardive dyskinesia appears to be very low relative to other antipsychotics.

**Drug Interactions**

**Cytochrome P-450 Effect:** CYP1A2, 2C, 2E1, 3A3/4 enzyme substrate, CYP2D6 enzyme substrate (minor)

**Decreased Effect:** Clozapine decreases effect of epinephrine. Decreased effect of clozapine with phenytoin.

**Increased Effect/Toxicity:** Increased effect of other CNS depressants, guanabenz, anticholinergics. Increased toxicity of clozapine when taken with cimetidine, MAO inhibitors, neuroleptics, tricyclic antidepressants. Fluvoxamine and possibly paroxetine and sertraline may elevate clozapine concentrations. Dosage reduction should be considered, particularly with fluvoxamine.

**Adverse Reactions**

>10%:

Cardiovascular: Tachycardia, hypotension or orthostatic hypotension
Central nervous system: Fever, headache, drowsiness
Gastrointestinal: Constipation, nausea, vomiting, unusual weight gain

1% to 10%:

Cardiovascular: EKG changes, hypertension, syncope
Central nervous system: Agitation, akathisia, confusion
Gastrointestinal: Abdominal discomfort, heartburn, dry mouth
Ocular: Blurred vision
Miscellaneous: Sweating (increased)

<1% (Limited to important or life-threatening symptoms): Insomnia, seizures, tardive dyskinesia, mental depression, neuroleptic malignant syndrome, agranulocytosis, eosinophilia, granulocytopenia, leukopenia, thrombocytopenia

**Overdose/Toxicology** Symptoms of overdose include altered states of consciousness, tachycardia, hypotension, hypersalivation, and respiratory depression. Following initiation of essential overdose management, toxic symptom treatment and supportive treatment should be initiated.

**Pharmacodynamics/Kinetics**

**Protein Binding:** 97%

**Half-life Elimination:** Mean half-life: 12 hours (range: 4-66 hours)

**Time to Peak:** 2.5 hours (range: 1-6 hours)

**Metabolism:** Undergoes extensive metabolism primarily to unconjugated forms

**Excretion:** Urine and feces

**Formulations** Tablet: 25 mg, 100 mg

**Dosing**

**Adults:** Available only through a distribution system which ensures WBC monitoring.

Oral: 25 mg once or twice daily initially, and increased as tolerated to a target dose of 300-450 mg/day after 2 weeks, but may require doses as high as 600-900 mg/day

**Elderly:** Oral: Experience in the elderly is limited; initial dose should be 25 mg/day; increase as tolerated by 25 mg/day to desired response. Maximum daily dose in the elderly should probably be 450 mg. Dose titration to 300-450 mg/day may be attained in 2 weeks if tolerated; however, elderly may require slower titration and daily increases may not be tolerated.

**Monitoring Laboratory Tests** Weekly CBC, ophthalmic screening

**Additional Nursing Issues**

**Physical Assessment:** Assess other medications patient is taking for effectiveness and interactions (see Drug Interactions). See Contraindications and Warnings/Precautions for cautious use. Has potential for psychological or physiological dependence, abuse, and tolerance. Review ophthalmic exam and monitor laboratory results weekly (see above), therapeutic response (mental status, mood, affect), and adverse reactions at beginning of therapy and periodically with long-term use (especially orthostatic hypotension, EKG changes, anticholinergic and extrapyramidal effects - see Adverse Reactions and Overdose/Toxicology). Initiate at lower doses (see Dosing) and taper dosage slowly when discontinuing. Assess knowledge/teach patient appropriate use, interventions to reduce side effects, and adverse symptoms to report (see below). Breast-feeding is contraindicated.

**Patient Information/Instruction:** Use exactly as directed (do not increase dose or frequency); may cause physical and/or psychological dependence. Do not discontinue without consulting prescriber. Avoid excess alcohol or caffeine and other prescription or OTC medications not approved by prescriber. Maintain adequate hydration (2-3 L/day of fluids unless instructed to restrict fluid intake). You may experience headache, excess drowsiness, dizziness, or blurred vision (use caution driving or when engaging in tasks requiring alertness until response to drug is known); dry mouth, nausea, vomiting (small frequent meals, frequent mouth care, sucking lozenges, or chewing gum may help); or postural hypotension (use caution climbing stairs or when changing position from lying or sitting to standing). Report persistent CNS effects (insomnia, depression, altered consciousness); palpitations, rapid heartbeat, severe dizziness; vision changes; hypersalivation, tearing, sweating; difficulty breathing; or worsening of condition. **Breast-feeding precautions:** Do not breast-feed.

**Geriatric Considerations:** Not recommended for use in nonpsychotic patients.

**Related Information**

Antipsychotic Agents Comparison *on page 1371*
Antipsychotic Medication Guidelines *on page 1436*

♦ **Clozaril®** *see* Clozapine *on previous page*
♦ **Clysodrast®** *see page 1294*
♦ **CMV-IGIV** *see* Cytomegalovirus Immune Globulin Intravenous, Human *on page 324*
♦ **Coagulant Complex Inhibitor** *see* Anti-inhibitor Coagulant Complex *on page 100*
♦ **Coal Tar** *see page 1294*
♦ **Coal Tar and Salicylic Acid** *see page 1294*
♦ **Coal Tar, Lanolin, and Mineral Oil** *see page 1294*
♦ **Cobex®** *see* Cyanocobalamin *on page 311*

## Cocaine (koe KANE)

**Therapeutic Category** Local Anesthetic

**Pregnancy Risk Factor** C/X (if nonmedicinal use)

**Lactation** Enters breast milk/contraindicated

**Use** Topical anesthesia for mucous membranes

(Continued)

## Cocaine *(Continued)*

**Mechanism of Action/Effect** Blocks both the initiation and conduction of nerve impulses

**Contraindications** Hypersensitivity to cocaine or any component; systemic use; pregnancy (nonmedicinal use)

**Warnings** Use with caution in patients with hypertension, severe cardiovascular disease, thyrotoxicosis, or a history of drug abuse. Use with caution in patients with severely traumatized mucosa and sepsis in the region of intended application. Repeated topical application can result in psychic dependence and tolerance. May cause cornea to become clouded or pitted, therefore, normal saline should be used to irrigate and protect cornea during surgery. Not for injection. Pregnancy factor C/X (nonmedicinal use).

**Drug Interactions**

**Cytochrome P-450 Effect:** CYP3A3/4 enzyme substrate

**Increased Effect/Toxicity:** Increased toxicity with MAO inhibitors. Use with epinephrine may cause extreme hypertension and/or cardiac arrhythmias.

**Adverse Reactions**

>10%:

Central nervous system: CNS stimulation

Gastrointestinal: Loss of taste perception

Respiratory: Rhinitis, nasal congestion

Miscellaneous: Loss of smell

1% to 10%:

Cardiovascular: Heart rate (decreased) with low doses, tachycardia with moderate doses, hypertension, cardiomyopathy, cardiac arrhythmias, myocarditis, QRS prolongation, Raynaud's phenomenon, cerebral vasculitis, thrombosis, fibrillation (atrial), flutter (atrial), sinus bradycardia, congestive heart failure, pulmonary hypertension, sinus tachycardia, tachycardia (supraventricular), arrhythmias (ventricular), vasoconstriction

Central nervous system: Fever, nervousness, restlessness, euphoria, excitation, headache, psychosis, hallucinations, agitation, seizures, slurred speech, hyperthermia, dystonic reactions, cerebral vascular accident, vasculitis, clonic-tonic reactions, paranoia, sympathetic storm

Dermatologic: Skin infarction, pruritus, madarosis

Gastrointestinal: Nausea, anorexia, colonic ischemia, spontaneous bowel perforation

Genitourinary: Priapism, uterine rupture

Hematologic: Thrombocytopenia

Neuromuscular & skeletal: Chorea (extrapyramidal), paresthesia, tremors, fasciculations

Ocular: Mydriasis (peak effect at 45 minutes; may last up to 12 hours), sloughing of the corneal epithelium, ulceration of the cornea, iritis, mydriasis, chemosis

Renal: Myoglobinuria, necrotizing vasculitis

Respiratory: Tachypnea, nasal mucosa damage (when snorting), hyposmia, bronchiolitis obliterans organizing pneumonia

Miscellaneous: "Washed-out" syndrome

**Overdose/Toxicology** Symptoms of overdose include anxiety, excitement, confusion, nausea, vomiting, headache, rapid pulse, irregular respiration, delirium, fever, seizures, respiratory arrest, hallucinations, dilated pupils, muscle spasms, sensory aberrations, and cardiac arrhythmias.

Fatal dose: Oral: 500 mg to 1.2 g; severe toxic effects have occurred with doses as low as 20 mg.

Since no specific antidote for cocaine exists, serious toxic effects are treated symptomatically.

**Pharmacodynamics/Kinetics**

**Half-life Elimination:** Following topical administration to mucosa: 75 minutes

**Metabolism:** Liver

**Excretion:** Urine

**Onset:** Onset of action: Within 1 minute; Peak action: Within 5 minutes

**Duration:** ≥30 minutes, depending on dosage administered

**Formulations**

Cocaine hydrochloride:

Powder: 5 g, 25 g

Solution, topical: 4% [40 mg/mL] (2 mL, 4 mL, 10 mL); 10% [100 mg/mL] (4 mL, 10 mL)

Solution, topical, viscous: 4% [40 mg/mL] (4 mL, 10 mL); 10% [100 mg/mL] (4 mL, 10 mL)

Tablet, soluble, for topical solution: 135 mg

**Dosing**

**Adults:** Dosage depends on the area to be anesthetized, tissue vascularity, technique of anesthesia, and individual patient tolerance. The lowest dose necessary to produce adequate anesthesia should be used, not to exceed 1 mg/kg.

Topical application (ear, nose, throat, bronchoscopy): Concentrations of 1% to 4% are used. Concentrations >4% are not recommended because of potential for increased incidence and severity of systemic toxic reactions.

**Elderly:** Refer to adult dosing; use with caution.

**Administration**

**Topical:** Use only on mucous membranes of the oral, laryngeal, and nasal cavities. Do not use on extensive areas of broken skin.

**Stability**

**Storage:** Store in well-closed, light-resistant containers.

**Additional Nursing Issues**

**Physical Assessment:** Assess other medications the patient may be taking for effectiveness and interactions (see Drug Interactions). Monitor adverse effects (eg, cardiovascular, CNS, and respiratory effects) and teach patient adverse symptoms to report (see Adverse Reactions and Overdose/Toxicology). **Pregnancy risk factor C/X (if nonmedicinal use).** Breast-feeding is contraindicated.

**Patient Information/Instruction:** When used orally, do not take anything by mouth until full sensation returns. Ocular: Use caution when driving or engaging in tasks that require alert vision (mydriasis may last for several hours). At time of use or immediately thereafter, report any unusual cardiovascular, CNS, or respiratory symptoms immediately. Following use, report skin irritation or eruption; alterations in vision, eye pain or irritation; persistent gastrointestinal effects; muscle or skeletal tremors, numbness, or rigidity; urinary or genital problems; or persistent fatigue. When used orally, do not take anything by mouth until full sensation returns. **Pregnancy/breast-feeding precautions:** Inform prescriber if you are pregnant. Do not breast-feed.

**Related Information**

Hallucinogenic Drugs Comparison *on page 1386*

- ♦ **Coccidioidin Skin Test** *see page 1248*
- ♦ **Codafed® Expectorant** *see* Guaifenesin, Pseudoephedrine, and Codeine *on page 552*
- ♦ **Codamine®** *see* Hydrocodone and Phenylpropanolamine *on page 574*
- ♦ **Codamine® Pediatric** *see* Hydrocodone and Phenylpropanolamine *on page 574*
- ♦ **Codehist® DH Liquid** *see page 1306*

## Codeine (KOE deen)

**Synonyms** Methylmorphine

**Therapeutic Category** Analgesic, Narcotic; Antitussive

**Pregnancy Risk Factor** C/D (if used for prolonged periods or in high doses at term)

**Lactation** Enters breast milk/use caution (AAP rates "compatible")

**Use** Treatment of mild to moderate pain; antitussive in lower doses

**Mechanism of Action/Effect** Inhibits perception of and response to pain; causes cough supression; produces generalized CNS depression

**Contraindications** Hypersensitivity to codeine or any component; premature infants or during premature labor; pregnancy (if used for prolonged periods or in high doses at term)

**Warnings** Use with caution in patients with hypersensitivity reactions to other phenanthrene derivative opioid agonists (morphine, hydrocodone, hydromorphone, levorphanol, oxycodone, oxymorphone); respiratory diseases including asthma, emphysema, and COPD; or severe liver or renal insufficiency. Some preparations contain sulfites which may cause allergic reactions. May be habit-forming.

Not recommended for use for cough control in patients with a productive cough. The elderly may be particularly susceptible to CNS depression, confusion, and constipating effects of narcotics.

Pregnancy factor C/D (if used for prolonged periods or in high doses at term).

**Drug Interactions**

**Cytochrome P-450 Effect:** CYP2D6 and 3A3/4 enzyme substrate; CYP2D6 enzyme inhibitor

**Decreased Effect:** Decreased effect with cigarette smoking.

**Increased Effect/Toxicity:** May cause severely increased toxicity of codeine when taken with CNS depressants, phenothiazines, tricyclic antidepressants, other narcotic analgesics, guanabenz, MAO inhibitors, and neuromuscular blockers.

**Effects on Lab Values** ↑ aminotransferase [ALT (SGPT)/AST (SGOT)] (S)

**Adverse Reactions**

>10%:

Central nervous system: Drowsiness

Gastrointestinal: Constipation

1% to 10%:

Cardiovascular: Tachycardia or bradycardia, hypotension

Central nervous system: Dizziness, lightheadedness, false feeling of well being, malaise, headache, restlessness, paradoxical CNS stimulation, confusion

Dermatologic: Rash, urticaria

Gastrointestinal: Dry mouth, anorexia, nausea, vomiting

Hepatic: Increased transaminases

Genitourinary: Decreased urination, ureteral spasm

Local: Burning at injection site

Ocular: Blurred vision

Neuromuscular & skeletal: Weakness

Respiratory: Shortness of breath, dyspnea

Miscellaneous: Physical and psychological dependence, histamine release

<1% (Limited to important or life-threatening symptoms): Convulsions, hallucinations, mental depression, nightmares, insomnia

**Overdose/Toxicology** Symptoms of overdose include CNS and respiratory depression, GI cramping, and constipation. Naloxone, 2 mg I.V. with repeat administration as necessary up to a total of 10 mg, can also be used to reverse toxic effects of the opiate.

(Continued)

## Codeine *(Continued)*

**Pharmacodynamics/Kinetics**

**Protein Binding:** 7%

**Distribution:** Crosses the placenta

**Half-life Elimination:** 2.5-3.5 hours

**Metabolism:** Liver

**Excretion:** Urine

**Onset:**

Onset of action: Oral: 0.5-1 hour; I.M.: 10-30 minutes

Peak action: Oral: 1-1.5 hours; I.M.: 0.5-1 hour

**Duration:** 4-6 hours

**Formulations**

Codeine phosphate:

Injection: 30 mg (1 mL, 2 mL); 60 mg (1 mL, 2 mL)

Tablet, soluble: 30 mg, 60 mg

Codeine sulfate:

Tablet: 15 mg, 30 mg, 60 mg

Tablet, soluble: 15 mg, 30 mg, 60 mg

**Dosing**

**Adults:** Doses should be titrated to appropriate analgesic effect. When changing routes of administration, note that oral dose is $^2/_3$ as effective as parenteral dose.

Analgesic: Oral, I.M., I.V., S.C.: 30 mg/dose; range: 15-60 mg every 4-6 hours as needed; maximum: 360 mg/24 hours

Antitussive: Oral (for nonproductive cough): 10-20 mg/dose every 4-6 hours as needed; maximum: 120 mg/day

**Elderly:** Refer to adult dosing.

**Renal Impairment:**

$Cl_{cr}$ 10-50 mL/minute: Administer 75% of dose.

$Cl_{cr}$ <10 mL/minute: Administer 50% of dose.

**Hepatic Impairment:** Dosing adjustment is probably necessary in hepatic insufficiency.

**Stability**

**Storage:** Store injection between 15°C to 30°C, avoid freezing. Do not use if injection is discolored or contains a precipitate. Protect injection from light.

**Additional Nursing Issues**

**Physical Assessment:** Assess other medications patient may be taking for possible additive or adverse interactions (see Warnings/Precautions and Drug Interactions). Monitor for effectiveness of pain relief and monitor for signs of overdose (see above). Monitor blood pressure, CNS and respiratory status, and degree of sedation at beginning of therapy and at regular intervals with long-term use. May cause physical and/or psychological dependence. For inpatients, implement safety measures (eg, side rails up, call light within reach, instructions to call for assistance, etc). Assess knowledge/teach patient appropriate use (if self-administered). Teach patient to monitor for adverse reactions (see Adverse Reactions), adverse reactions to report, and appropriate interventions to reduce side effects. **Pregnancy risk factor C/D** - see Pregnancy Risk Factor - assess knowledge/teach patient use of barrier contraceptives if appropriate. Note breast-feeding caution.

**Patient Information/Instruction:** If self-administered, use exactly as directed (do not increase dose or frequency); may cause physical and/or psychological dependence. While using this medication, do not use alcohol and other prescription or OTC medications (especially sedatives, tranquilizers, antihistamines, or pain medications) without consulting prescriber. Maintain adequate hydration (2-3 L/day of fluids unless instructed to restrict fluid intake). May cause dizziness, drowsiness, confusion, agitation, impaired coordination, or blurred vision (use caution when driving, climbing stairs, or changing position - rising from sitting or lying to standing, or when engaging in tasks requiring alertness until response to drug is known); nausea or vomiting, or loss of appetite (frequent mouth care, small frequent meals, sucking lozenges, or chewing gum may help); constipation (increased exercise, fluids, or dietary fruit and fiber may help - if constipation remains an unresolved problem, consult prescriber about use of stool softeners). Report confusion, insomnia, excessive nervousness, excessive sedation or drowsiness, or shakiness; acute GI upset; difficulty breathing or shortness of breath; facial flushing, rapid heartbeat or palpitations; urinary difficulty; unusual muscle weakness; or vision changes. **Pregnancy/breast-feeding precautions:** Inform prescriber if you are or intend to be pregnant. If you are breast-feeding, take medication immediately after breast-feeding or 3-4 hours prior to next feeding.

**Geriatric Considerations:** The elderly may be particularly susceptible to CNS depression and confusion as well as the constipating effects of narcotics.

**Additional Information** Codeine phosphate contains sulfites.

**Related Information**

Controlled Substances Comparison *on page 1379*

Narcotic/Opioid Analgesic Comparison *on page 1396*

◆ **Codeine and Acetaminophen** *see* Acetaminophen and Codeine *on page 34*

◆ **Codeine and Aspirin** *see* Aspirin and Codeine *on page 113*

◆ **Codeine and Butalbital Compound** *see* Butalbital Compound and Codeine *on page 177*

◆ **Codeine and Guaifenesin** *see* Guaifenesin and Codeine *on page 549*

◆ **Codeine and Promethazine** *see* Promethazine and Codeine *on page 980*

- **Codeine, Brompheniramine, and Phenylpropanolamine** *see* Brompheniramine, Phenylpropanolamine, and Codeine *on page 163*
- **Codeine Contin®** *see* Codeine *on page 299*
- **Codeine, Guaifenesin, and Pseudoephedrine** *see* Guaifenesin, Pseudoephedrine, and Codeine *on page 552*
- **Codeine, Promethazine, and Phenylephrine** *see* Promethazine, Phenylephrine, and Codeine *on page 981*
- **Codiclear® DH** *see* Hydrocodone and Guaifenesin *on page 571*
- **Codoxy®** *see* Oxycodone and Aspirin *on page 873*
- **Codroxomin®** *see* Hydroxocobalamin *on page 583*
- **Cogentin®** *see* Benztropine *on page 144*
- **Co-Gesic®** *see* Hydrocodone and Acetaminophen *on page 568*
- **Cognex®** *see* Tacrine *on page 1092*
- **Co-Hist®** *see page 1294*
- **Colace® [OTC]** *see* Docusate *on page 392*
- **Colaspase** *see* Asparaginase *on page 109*
- **Colax-C®** *see* Docusate *on page 392*
- **Colax® Tablet** *see page 1294*
- **ColBENEMID®** *see* Colchicine and Probenecid *on next page*

## Colchicine (KOL chi seen)

**Therapeutic Category** Colchicine

**Pregnancy Risk Factor** C (oral); D (parenteral)

**Lactation** Enters breast milk/use caution (AAP rates "compatible")

**Use** Treat acute gouty arthritis attacks and to prevent recurrences of such attacks; management of familial Mediterranean fever

**Mechanism of Action/Effect** Reduces the deposition of urate crystals that perpetuates the inflammatory response

**Contraindications** Hypersensitivity to colchicine or any component; serious renal, gastrointestinal, hepatic, or cardiac disorders; blood dyscrasias; pregnancy (parenteral)

**Warnings** Severe local irritation can occur following S.C. or I.M. administration. Use with caution in debilitated patients or elderly patients or patients with severe GI, renal, or liver disease. Pregnancy factor C (oral)/D (parenteral).

**Drug Interactions**

**Decreased Effect:** Vitamin $B_{12}$ absorption may be decreased with colchicine. Acidifying agents inhibit action of colchicine.

**Increased Effect/Toxicity:** Increased toxicity may be seen when taken with sympathomimetic agents or CNS depressant (effects are enhanced). Alkalizing agents potentiate effects of colchicine.

**Effects on Lab Values** May cause false-positive results in urine tests for erythrocytes or hemoglobin

**Adverse Reactions**

>10%: Gastrointestinal: Nausea, vomiting, diarrhea, abdominal pain

1% to 10%:

Dermatologic: Alopecia

Gastrointestinal: Anorexia

<1% (Limited to important or life-threatening symptoms): Arrhythmias (with intravenous administration), agranulocytosis, aplastic anemia, bone marrow suppression, hepatotoxicity

**Overdose/Toxicology** Symptoms of overdose include acute nausea, vomiting, abdominal pain, shock, kidney damage, muscle weakness, burning in throat, watery to bloody diarrhea, hypotension, anuria, cardiovascular collapse, delirium, convulsions, and respiratory paralysis. Treatment includes gastric lavage and measures to prevent shock, hemodialysis or peritoneal dialysis. Atropine and morphine may relieve abdominal pain.

**Pharmacodynamics/Kinetics**

**Protein Binding:** 10% to 31%

**Distribution:** Concentrates in leukocytes, kidney, spleen, and liver; does not distribute in heart, skeletal muscle, and brain

**Half-life Elimination:** 12-30 minutes; End-stage renal disease: 45 minutes

**Time to Peak:** Oral: Within 0.5-2 hours declining for the next 2 hours before increasing again due to enterohepatic recycling

**Metabolism:** Liver

**Excretion:** Bile

**Onset:** Relief of pain and inflammation occurs within 12 hours if adequately dosed

**Formulations**

Injection: 0.5 mg/mL (2 mL)

Tablet: 0.5 mg, 0.6 mg

**Dosing**

**Adults:**

Prophylaxis of familial Mediterranean fever: Oral: 1-2 mg/day in 2-3 divided doses

Gouty arthritis, acute attacks:

Oral: Initial: 0.5-1.2 mg, then 0.5-0.6 mg every 1-2 hours or 1-1.2 mg every 2 hours until relief or GI side effects (nausea, vomiting, or diarrhea) occur to a maximum total dose of 8 mg; wait 3 days before initiating another course of therapy.

I.V.: Initial: 1-3 mg, then 0.5 mg every 6 hours until response, not to exceed 4 mg/day. If pain recurs, it may be necessary to administer a daily dose of 1-2 mg for several days, however, do not give more colchicine by any route for at least 7 days

(Continued)

## Colchicine *(Continued)*

after a full course of I.V. therapy (4 mg). Transfer to oral colchicine in a dose similar to that being given I.V.

Gouty arthritis, prophylaxis of recurrent attacks: Oral: 0.5-0.6 mg/day or every other day

**Elderly:** Refer to adult dosing.

**Renal Impairment:**

$Cl_{cr}$ <50 mL/minute: Avoid chronic use or administration.

$Cl_{cr}$ <10 mL/minute: Decrease dose by 50% for treatment of acute attacks.

Hemodialysis effects: Not dialyzable (0% to 5%)

Supplemental dose is not necessary.

**Administration**

**I.V.:** Injection should be made over 2-5 minutes into tubing of free-flowing I.V. with compatible fluid. Do not give I.M. or S.C.

**Stability**

**Storage:** Protect tablets from light.

**Compatibility:** I.V. colchicine is incompatible with dextrose or I.V. solutions with preservatives.

**Monitoring Laboratory Tests** CBC and renal function on a regular basis

**Additional Nursing Issues**

**Physical Assessment:** Assess effectiveness and interactions of other medications patient may be taking (see Contraindications and Drug Interactions). I.V. (see Dosing and Administration): Monitor for therapeutic response (frequency and severity of gouty attacks), laboratory values, and adverse reactions (see Adverse Reactions and Overdose/Toxicology) at beginning of therapy and periodically with long-term use. Assess knowledge/teach patient appropriate use, interventions to reduce side effects, and adverse symptoms to report. **Pregnancy risk factor C/D** - see Pregnancy Risk Factor - assess knowledge/teach patient on the need to use appropriate contraceptive measures and the need to avoid pregnancy. Note breast-feeding caution.

**Patient Information/Instruction:** Take as directed; do not exceed recommended dosage. Consult prescriber about a low-purine diet. Maintain adequate hydration (2-3 L/day of fluids unless instructed to restrict fluid intake). Do not use alcohol or aspirin-containing medication without consulting prescriber. You may experience nausea, vomiting, or anorexia (small frequent meals, frequent mouth care, chewing gum, or sucking lozenges may help); hair loss (reversible). Stop medication and report to prescriber if severe vomiting, watery or bloody diarrhea, or abdominal pain occurs. Report muscle tremors or weakness; fatigue; easy bruising or bleeding; yellowing of eyes or skin; or pale stool or dark urine. **Pregnancy/breast-feeding precautions:** Inform prescriber if you are or intend to be pregnant. Consult prescriber if breast-feeding.

**Geriatric Considerations:** Colchicine appears to be more toxic in the elderly, particularly in the presence of renal, gastrointestinal, or cardiac disease. The most predictable oral side effects are (gastrointestinal) vomiting, abdominal pain, and nausea. If colchicine is stopped at this point, other more severe adverse effects may be avoided, such as bone marrow suppression, peripheral neuritis, etc.

## Colchicine and Probenecid (KOL chi seen & proe BEN e sid)

**U.S. Brand Names** ColBENEMID®; Proben-C®

**Synonyms** Probenecid and Colchicine

**Therapeutic Category** Antigout Agent

**Pregnancy Risk Factor** C (oral); D (parenteral)

**Lactation**

Colchicine: Compatible

Probenecid: Excretion in breast milk unknown

**Use** Treatment of chronic gouty arthritis when complicated by frequent, recurrent acute attacks of gout

**Formulations** Tablet: Colchicine 0.5 mg and probenecid 0.5 g

**Dosing**

**Adults:** Oral: 1 tablet/day for 1 week, then 1 tablet twice daily thereafter

**Elderly:** Refer to dosing in individual monographs; adjust for renal impairment.

**Renal Impairment:** Probenecid may not be effective in patients with chronic renal insufficiency particularly when $Cl_{cr}$ is ≤30 mL/minute.

**Additional Nursing Issues**

**Physical Assessment:** See individual components listed in Related Information. **Pregnancy risk factor C/D** - see Pregnancy Risk Factor - assess knowledge/instruct patient on need to use appropriate contraceptive measures and the need to avoid pregnancy. Note breast-feeding caution.

**Patient Information/Instruction:** See individual components listed in Related Information. **Pregnancy/breast-feeding precautions:** Inform prescriber if you are or intend to be pregnant. Consult prescriber if breast-feeding.

**Related Information**

Colchicine *on previous page*

Probenecid *on page 966*

♦ **Colchiquim** *see* Colchicine *on previous page*

♦ **Colchiquim-30** *see* Colchicine *on previous page*

♦ **Cold & Allergy® Elixir** *see page 1294*

♦ **Cold-eze® [OTC]** *see* Zinc Supplements *on page 1230*

♦ **Coldloc®** *see* Guaifenesin, Phenylpropanolamine, and Phenylephrine *on page 552*

- **Coldloc-LA®** *see* Guaifenesin and Phenylpropanolamine *on page 550*
- **Coldrine®** *see page 1294*
- **Colestid®** *see* Colestipol *on this page*

## Colestipol (koe LES ti pole)

**U.S. Brand Names** Colestid®

**Therapeutic Category** Antilipemic Agent (Bile Acid Seqestrant)

**Pregnancy Risk Factor** C

**Lactation** Not recommended

**Use** Adjunct in management of primary hypercholesterolemia; regression of arteriolosclerosis; relief of pruritus associated with elevated levels of bile acids; possibly used to decrease plasma half-life of digoxin in toxicity

**Mechanism of Action/Effect** Increases fetal loss of low density lipoprotein cholesterol

**Contraindications** Hypersensitivity to colestipol or any component; avoid using in complete biliary obstruction

**Warnings** Avoid in patients with high triglycerides, GI dysfunction (constipation). May be associated with increased bleeding tendency as a result of hypothrombinemia secondary to vitamin K deficiency. May cause depletion of vitamins A, D, E. Pregnancy factor C.

**Drug Interactions**

**Decreased Effect:** Decreased absorption of tetracycline, penicillin G, vitamins A, D, E, and K, digitalis glycosides, warfarin, thyroid hormones, thiazide diuretics, propranolol, phenobarbital, amiodarone, methotrexate, NSAIDs, and other drugs by binding to the drug in the intestine.

**Effects on Lab Values** ↑ prothrombin time (S); ↓ cholesterol (S)

**Adverse Reactions**

>10%: Gastrointestinal: Constipation

1% to 10%:

Central nervous system: Headache, dizziness, anxiety, vertigo, drowsiness, fatigue

Gastrointestinal: Abdominal pain and distention, belching, flatulence, nausea, vomiting, diarrhea

<1% (Limited to important or life-threatening symptoms): Peptic ulceration, gallstones, GI irritation and bleeding, anorexia, steatorrhea or malabsorption syndrome, cholelithiasis, cholecystitis, shortness of breath

**Overdose/Toxicology** Symptoms of overdose include GI obstruction, nausea, and GI distress. Treatment is supportive.

**Pharmacodynamics/Kinetics**

**Excretion:** Bile

**Formulations**

Colestipol hydrochloride:

Granules: 5 g packet, 300 g, 500 g

Tablet: 1 g

**Dosing**

**Adults:** Oral: 5-30 g/day in divided doses 2-4 times/day

**Elderly:** Refer to adult dosing.

**Administration**

**Oral:** Dry powder should be added to at least 90 mL of liquid and stirred until completely mixed. Other drugs should be administered at least 1 hour before or 4 hours after colestipol.

**Additional Nursing Issues**

**Physical Assessment:** Assess other medications the patient may be taking for effectiveness and interactions (see Drug Interactions). Monitor knowledge/teach patient appropriate preparation and use, possible adverse reactions, and symptoms to report. **Pregnancy risk factor C** - benefits of use should outweigh possible risks. Breast-feeding is not recommended.

**Patient Information/Instruction:** Take with 38-45 ounces of water or fruit juice. Rinse glass with small amount of water to ensure full dose is taken. Other medications should be taken 2 hours before or 2 hours after colestipol. You may experience constipation (increased exercise, increased dietary fluids, fruit, fiber, or stool softener may help) or drowsiness or dizziness (use caution when driving or engaging in tasks that require alertness until response to drug is known). Report acute gastric pain, tarry stools, or difficulty breathing. **Pregnancy/breast-feeding precautions:** Inform prescriber if you are or intend to be pregnant. Breast-feeding is not recommended.

**Geriatric Considerations:** Pharmacologic treatment should be reserved for those who are unable to obtain a desirable plasma cholesterol level by diet alone and for whom the benefits of treatment are believed to outweigh the potential adverse effects, drug interactions, and cost of treatment.

**Related Information**

Lipid-Lowering Agents Comparison *on page 1393*

- **Colistin, Neomycin, and Hydrocortisone** *see page 1291*

## Collagenase (KOL la je nase)

**U.S. Brand Names** Biozyme-C®; Santyl®

**Therapeutic Category** Enzyme, Topical Debridement

**Pregnancy Risk Factor** C

**Lactation** Excretion in breast milk unknown

**Use** Promotes debridement of necrotic tissue in dermal ulcers and severe burns; indicated for stage 3, 4 decubitus ulcers

(Continued)

## Collagenase *(Continued)*

**Mechanism of Action/Effect** Digests collagen in injured tissue. Collagenase will not attack collagen in healthy tissue or newly formed granulation tissue. In addition, it does not act on fat, fibrin, keratin, or muscle.

**Contraindications** Hypersensitivity to collagenase

**Warnings** For external use only. Avoid contact with eyes. Monitor debilitated patients for systemic bacterial infections because debriding enzymes may increase the risk of bacteremia. Pregnancy factor C.

**Drug Interactions**

**Decreased Effect:** Enzymatic activity is inhibited by detergents, benzalkonium chloride, hexachlorophene, nitrofurazone, tincture of iodine, and heavy metal ions (silver and mercury).

**Adverse Reactions** 1% to 10%: Local: Irritation

**Overdose/Toxicology** Action of enzyme may be stopped by applying Burow's solution.

**Formulations** Ointment, topical: 250 units/g (15 g, 30 g)

**Dosing**

**Adults:** Topical: Apply once daily.

**Elderly:** Refer to adult dosing.

**Administration**

**Topical:** For external use only. Clean target area of all interfering agents listed above. If infection is persistent, apply powdered antibiotic first. Do not introduce into major body cavities. Monitor debilitated patients for systemic bacterial infections.

**Additional Nursing Issues**

**Physical Assessment:** See Contraindications and Warnings/Precautions for use cautions. See application directions above. When applied to large areas or for extensive periods of time, monitor for adverse reactions. Assess knowledge/teach patient appropriate application and use and adverse symptoms to report. **Pregnancy risk factor C.** Note breast-feeding caution.

**Patient Information/Instruction:** Use exactly as directed; do not overuse. Wear gloves to apply a thin film to affected area. If dressing is necessary, use a porous dressing. Avoid contact with eyes. Report increased swelling, redness, rash, itching, signs of infection, worsening of condition, or lack of healing. **Pregnancy/breast-feeding precautions:** Inform prescriber if you are or intend to be pregnant. Consult prescriber if breast-feeding.

**Geriatric Considerations:** Preventive skin care should be instituted in all older patients at high risk for pressure ulcers. Collagenase is indicated in stage 3 and 4 pressure ulcers.

- **Collyrium Fresh® Ophthalmic** *see page 1294*
- **Colovage®** *see* Polyethylene Glycol-Electrolyte Solution *on page 945*
- **Columina** *see* Cimetidine *on page 268*
- **Coly-Mycin® S Otic Drops** *see page 1291*
- **Colyte®** *see* Polyethylene Glycol-Electrolyte Solution *on page 945*
- **CombiPatch®** *see* Oral Contraceptives *on page 859*
- **CombiPatch®** *see* Estradiol and Norethindrone *on page 443*
- **Combipres®** *see* Clonidine and Chlorthalidone *on page 291*
- **Combivent®** *see* Ipratropium and Albuterol *on page 622*
- **Comfort® [OTC]** *see page 1282*
- **Comfort® Ophthalmic** *see page 1294*
- **Comfort® Tears Solution** *see page 1294*
- **Comhist® LA Capsule** *see page 1294*
- **Comhist® Tablet** *see page 1294*
- **Compatibility of Drugs** *see page 1315*
- **Compatibility of Drugs in Syringe** *see page 1317*
- **Compazine®** *see* Prochlorperazine *on page 971*
- **Complan** *see* Vitamin, Multiple *on page 1219*
- **Compound E** *see* Cortisone *on next page*
- **Compound F** *see* Hydrocortisone *on page 578*
- **Compound S** *see* Zidovudine *on page 1227*
- **Compound W®** *see page 1294*
- **Compoz® Gel Caps [OTC]** *see* Diphenhydramine *on page 381*
- **Compoz® Nighttime Sleep Aid [OTC]** *see* Diphenhydramine *on page 381*
- **Comprecin** *see* Enoxacin *on page 420*
- **Comtrex® Maximum Strength Non-Drowsy** *see page 1294*
- **Conazol** *see* Ketoconazole *on page 643*
- **Conex® [OTC]** *see* Guaifenesin and Phenylpropanolamine *on page 550*
- **Congess® Jr** *see* Guaifenesin and Pseudoephedrine *on page 551*
- **Congess® Sr** *see* Guaifenesin and Pseudoephedrine *on page 551*
- **Congest** *see* Estrogens, Conjugated (Equine) *on page 446*
- **Congestac®** *see* Guaifenesin and Pseudoephedrine *on page 551*
- **Congestant D®** *see page 1294*
- **Conjugated Estrogens** *see* Estrogens, Conjugated (Equine) *on page 446*
- **Constilac®** *see* Lactulose *on page 651*
- **Constulose®** *see* Lactulose *on page 651*
- **Consupren** *see* Cyclosporine *on page 317*

- **Contac® Cough Formula Liquid [OTC]** *see* Guaifenesin and Dextromethorphan *on page 549*
- **Contergan®** *see* Thalidomide *on page 1113*
- **Control® [OTC]** *see* Phenylpropanolamine *on page 922*
- **Controlled Substances Comparison** *see page 1379*
- **Contuss®** *see* Guaifenesin, Phenylpropanolamine, and Phenylephrine *on page 552*
- **Contuss® XT** *see* Guaifenesin and Phenylpropanolamine *on page 550*
- **Cophene-B®** *see page 1294*
- **Cophene XP®** *see* Hydrocodone, Pseudoephedrine, and Guaifenesin *on page 577*
- **Coptin®** *see* Sulfadiazine *on page 1081*
- **Co-Pyronil® 2 Pulvules®** *see page 1294*
- **Coradur®** *see* Isosorbide Dinitrate *on page 634*
- **Corax®** *see* Chlordiazepoxide *on page 250*
- **Cordarone®** *see* Amiodarone *on page 71*
- **Cordran®** *see* Topical Corticosteroids *on page 1152*
- **Cordran® SP** *see* Topical Corticosteroids *on page 1152*
- **Coreg®** *see* Carvedilol *on page 208*
- **Corgard®** *see* Nadolol *on page 798*
- **Coricidin D®** *see page 1294*
- **Coricidin® Tablet** *see page 1294*
- **Corium®** *see* Clidinium and Chlordiazepoxide *on page 281*
- **Corogal** *see* Nifedipine *on page 824*
- **Cor-Oticin®** *see page 1282*
- **Corotrend** *see* Nifedipine *on page 824*
- **Corotrend Retard** *see* Nifedipine *on page 824*
- **Corque® Topical** *see* Clioquinol and Hydrocortisone *on page 284*
- **CortaGel® [OTC]** *see* Hydrocortisone *on page 578*
- **CortaGel® [OTC]** *see* Topical Corticosteroids *on page 1152*
- **Cortaid® Maximum Strength [OTC]** *see* Hydrocortisone *on page 578*
- **Cortaid® Maximum Strength [OTC]** *see* Topical Corticosteroids *on page 1152*
- **Cortaid® With Aloe [OTC]** *see* Hydrocortisone *on page 578*
- **Cortaid® With Aloe [OTC]** *see* Topical Corticosteroids *on page 1152*
- **Cortatrigen®** *see page 1291*
- **Cort-Dome®** *see* Hydrocortisone *on page 578*
- **Cort-Dome®** *see* Topical Corticosteroids *on page 1152*
- **Cortef®** *see* Hydrocortisone *on page 578*
- **Cortef®** *see* Topical Corticosteroids *on page 1152*
- **Cortef® Feminine Itch** *see* Hydrocortisone *on page 578*
- **Cortef® Feminine Itch** *see* Topical Corticosteroids *on page 1152*
- **Cortenema®** *see* Hydrocortisone *on page 578*
- **Cortenema®** *see* Topical Corticosteroids *on page 1152*
- **Corticaine®** *see* Hydrocortisone *on page 578*
- **Corticaine®** *see* Topical Corticosteroids *on page 1152*
- **Corticaine® Topical Cream** *see page 1294*
- **Corticosteroids Comparison, Systemic Equivalencies** *see page 1383*
- **Corticosteroids Comparison, Topical** *see page 1384*
- **Corticosteroids, Topical** *see* Topical Corticosteroids *on page 1152*
- **Corticotropin** *see page 1248*
- **Cortifoam®** *see* Hydrocortisone *on page 578*
- **Cortifoam®** *see* Topical Corticosteroids *on page 1152*
- **Cortin® Topical** *see* Clioquinol and Hydrocortisone *on page 284*

## Cortisone (KOR ti sone)

**U.S. Brand Names** Cortone® Acetate

**Synonyms** Compound E

**Therapeutic Category** Corticosteroid, Oral; Corticosteroid, Parenteral

**Pregnancy Risk Factor** D

**Lactation** Enters breast milk/use caution

**Use** Management of adrenocortical insufficiency, hypercalcemia response to cancer; short-term treatment of inflammatory and allergic disorders

**Mechanism of Action/Effect** Decreases inflammation through glucocorticoid and mineralcorticoid activity

**Contraindications** Serious infections, except septic shock or tuberculous meningitis; idiopathic thrombocytopenia purpura (I.M. use); administration of live virus vaccines; fungal infections; pregnancy

**Warnings** Use with caution in patients with hypothyroidism, cirrhosis, hypertension, congestive heart failure, ulcerative colitis, thromboembolic disorders, osteoporosis, convulsive disorders, peptic ulcer, diabetes mellitus, and myasthenia gravis, hypothyroidism, inflammatory bowel disease. Prolonged therapy (>5 days) of pharmacologic doses of corticosteroids may lead to hypothalamic-pituitary-adrenal suppression, the degree of adrenal suppression varies with the degree and duration of glucocorticoid therapy. This must be taken into consideration when taking patients off steroids.

(Continued)

## Cortisone *(Continued)*

**Drug Interactions**

**Cytochrome P-450 Effect:** CYP3A3/4 enzyme substrate

**Decreased Effect:** Barbiturates, phenytoin, and rifampin may decrease cortisone effects. Live virus vaccines, diuretics (potassium-depleting) may decrease cortisone effects. Anticholinesterase agents may decrease effect of cortisone. Cortisone may decrease effects of warfarin or salicylates.

**Increased Effect/Toxicity:** Estrogens may (increase cortisone effects). Cortisone + NSAIDs may increase ulcerogenic potential. Cortisone may increase potassium depletion due to diuretics.

**Effects on Lab Values** Suppression of reactions to skin tests

**Adverse Reactions** In chronic, long-term use, may result in cushingoid appearance, osteoporosis, muscle weakness (proximal), and suppression of the adrenal-hypothalmic pituitary axis.

>10%:

Central nervous system: Insomnia, nervousness
Gastrointestinal: Increased appetite, indigestion

1% to 10%:

Central nervous system: Dizziness or lightheadedness, headache
Dermatologic: Hirsutism, hypopigmentation
Endocrine & metabolic: Diabetes mellitus
Neuromuscular & skeletal: Arthralgia
Ocular: Cataracts, glaucoma
Respiratory: Epistaxis
Miscellaneous: Sweating

<1% (Limited to important or life-threatening symptoms): Edema, hypertension, seizures, psychoses, pseudotumor cerebri, delirium, hallucinations, euphoria, Cushing's syndrome, pituitary-adrenal axis suppression, growth suppression, glucose intolerance, hypokalemia, alkalosis, amenorrhea, sodium and water retention, hyperglycemia

**Overdose/Toxicology** When consumed in high doses for prolonged periods, systemic hypercorticism and adrenal suppression may occur. In those cases, discontinuation of the corticosteroid should be done judiciously.

**Pharmacodynamics/Kinetics**

**Distribution:** Crosses the placenta; distributes to muscles, liver, skin, intestines, and kidneys

**Half-life Elimination:** 30 minutes to 2 hours; End-stage renal disease: 3.5 hours

**Excretion:** Bile and urine

**Onset:** Peak effect: Oral: Within 2 hours; I.M.: Within 20-48 hours

**Formulations**

Cortisone acetate:

Injection: 50 mg/mL (10 mL)
Tablet: 5 mg, 10 mg, 25 mg

**Dosing**

**Adults:** If possible, administer glucocorticoids before 9 AM to minimize adrenocortical suppression. Dosing depends upon the condition being treated and the response of the patient. Supplemental doses may be warranted during times of stress in the course of withdrawing therapy.

Oral, I.M.: 25-300 mg/day in divided doses every 12-24 hours
Taper off when discontinuing drug.

**Elderly:** Use lowest effective dose.

**Renal Impairment:** Hemodialysis effects: Supplemental dose is not necessary.

**Administration**

**I.M.:** Administer I.M. daily dose before 9 AM to minimize adrenocortical suppression. I.M. use only. Shake vial before measuring out dose.

**Stability**

**Compatibility: Note:** Insoluble in water; supplemental doses may be warranted during times of stress in the course of withdrawing therapy.

**Additional Nursing Issues**

**Physical Assessment:** Assess effectiveness and interactions of other medications (see Drug Interactions). See Contraindications and Warnings/Precautions for use cautions. Monitor for effectiveness of therapy and adverse reactions according to dose, route, and length of therapy. Assess knowledge/teach patient appropriate use, possible side effects/interventions, and adverse symptoms to report (ie, opportunistic infection, adrenal suppression - see Adverse Reactions and Overdose/Toxicology). Diabetics: Monitor serum glucose levels closely; corticosteroids can alter hypoglycemic requirements. Dose may need to be increased if patient is experiencing higher than normal levels of stress. When discontinuing, taper dose and frequency slowly. **Pregnancy risk factor D** - assess knowledge/teach appropriate use of barrier contraceptives. Note breast-feeding caution.

**Patient Information/Instruction:** Take oral formulation as directed, with food or milk in the morning. Do not take more than prescribed or discontinue without consulting prescriber. Maintain adequate nutritional intake; consult prescriber for possibility of special dietary instructions. If diabetic, monitor serum glucose closely and notify prescriber of any changes; this medication can alter hypoglycemic requirements. Inform prescriber if you are experiencing unusual stress; dosage may need to be adjusted. You will be susceptible to infection; avoid crowds or infected persons or persons with contagious diseases. You may experience insomnia or nervousness; use caution when driving or engaging in tasks requiring alertness until response to drug is known. Report excessive or sudden weight gain, swelling of extremities, difficulty breathing, muscle pain or weakness, change in menstrual pattern, vision changes, signs of hyperglycemia, signs of infection (eg, fever, chills, mouth sores, perianal itching, vaginal discharge), other persistent side effects, or worsening of condition. **Pregnancy/breast-feeding precautions:** Do not get pregnant while taking this medication; use appropriate barrier contraceptive measures. Consult prescriber if breast-feeding.

**Geriatric Considerations:** Because of the risk of adverse effects, systemic corticosteroids should be used cautiously in the elderly, in the smallest possible dose, and for the shortest possible time.

**Additional Information** Insoluble in water

**Related Information**

Corticosteroids Comparison, Systemic Equivalencies *on page 1383*

- **Cortisporin® Ophthalmic Ointment** *see* Bacitracin, Neomycin, Polymyxin B, and Hydrocortisone *on page 131*
- **Cortisporin® Ophthalmic Ointment** *see page 1282*
- **Cortisporin® Ophthalmic Suspension** *see page 1282*
- **Cortisporin® Otic** *see page 1291*
- **Cortisporin® Topical Ointment** *see* Bacitracin, Neomycin, Polymyxin B, and Hydrocortisone *on page 131*
- **Cortizone®-5 [OTC]** *see* Hydrocortisone *on page 578*
- **Cortizone®-5 [OTC]** *see* Topical Corticosteroids *on page 1152*
- **Cortizone®-10 [OTC]** *see* Hydrocortisone *on page 578*
- **Cortizone®-10 [OTC]** *see* Topical Corticosteroids *on page 1152*
- **Cortone® Acetate** *see* Cortisone *on page 305*
- **Cortrosyn® Injection** *see page 1248*
- **Corvert®** *see* Ibutilide *on page 594*
- **Coryphen® Codeine** *see* Aspirin and Codeine *on page 113*
- **Cosmegen®** *see* Dactinomycin *on page 327*
- **Cosyntropin** *see page 1248*
- **Cotazym®** *see* Pancrelipase *on page 882*
- **Cotazym-S®** *see* Pancrelipase *on page 882*
- **Cotrim®** *see* Co-trimoxazole *on this page*
- **Cotrim® DS** *see* Co-trimoxazole *on this page*

## Co-trimoxazole (koe trye MOKS a zole)

**U.S. Brand Names** Bactrim™; Bactrim™ DS; Cotrim®; Cotrim® DS; Septra®; Septra® DS; Sulfatrim®

**Synonyms** SMX-TMP; SMZ-TMP; Sulfamethoxazole and Trimethoprim; TMP-SMX; TMP-SMZ; Trimethoprim and Sulfamethoxazole

**Therapeutic Category** Antibiotic, Sulfonamide Derivative

**Pregnancy Risk Factor** C/D (near term)

**Lactation** Enters breast milk/compatible

**Use**

Oral treatment of urinary tract infections; acute otitis media in children; acute exacerbations of chronic bronchitis in adults; prophylaxis of *Pneumocystis carinii* pneumonitis (PCP)

I.V. treatment of documented PCP, empiric treatment of PCP in immune compromised patients; treatment of documented or suspected shigellosis, typhoid fever, *Nocardia asteroides* infection, or other infections caused by susceptible bacterial

**Mechanism of Action/Effect** Sulfamethoxazole interferes with bacterial folic acid synthesis; trimethoprim inhibits enzymes of the folic acid pathway

**Contraindications** Hypersensitivity to any sulfa drug or any component; porphyria; megaloblastic anemia due to folate deficiency; severe renal insufficiency; marked hepatic dysfunction; pregnancy (3rd trimester)

**Warnings** Use with caution in patients with G-6-PD deficiency, impaired renal or hepatic function. Adjust dosage in patients with renal impairment. Injection vehicle contains benzyl alcohol and sodium metabisulfite. Fatalities associated with severe reactions including Stevens-Johnson syndrome, toxic epidermal necrolysis, hepatic necrosis, agranulocytosis, aplastic anemia, and other blood dyscrasias. Discontinue use at first sign of rash. Elderly patients appear at greater risk for more severe adverse reactions. May cause hypoglycemia (particularly in malnourished, renal, or hepatic impairment). Use caution in patients with porphyria or thyroid dysfunction. May cause hyperkalemia. Slow acetylators may be more prone to adverse reactions. Pregnancy factor C/D (near term).

**Drug Interactions**

**Cytochrome P-450 Effect:** CYP2C9 enzyme inhibitor

**Decreased Effect:** Co-trimoxazole causes decreased effect of cyclosporines and tricyclic antidepressants. Procaine and indomethacin may cause decreased effect of co-trimoxazole.

**Increased Effect/Toxicity:** Co-trimoxazole may cause an increased effect of sulfonylureas and oral anticoagulants. Co-trimoxazole may displace highly protein-bound drugs like methotrexate, phenytoin, or cyclosporine causing increased free serum concentrations of the highly bound drugs and lead to associated toxicity common with those agents. May compete for renal secretion of methotrexate. May enhance nephrotoxicity of cyclosporine. May increase digoxin concentrations.

(Continued)

## Co-trimoxazole *(Continued)*

**Effects on Lab Values** ↑ creatinine (Jaffé alkaline picrate reaction); increased serum methotrexate by dihydrofolate reductase method; does not interfere with RAI method

**Adverse Reactions**

>10%:

Dermatologic: Allergic skin reactions including rashes and urticaria, photosensitivity
Gastrointestinal: Nausea, vomiting, anorexia

1% to 10%:

Dermatologic: Stevens-Johnson syndrome, toxic epidermal necrolysis
Hematologic: Blood dyscrasias
Hepatic: Hepatitis

<1% (Limited to important or life-threatening symptoms): Confusion, depression, hallucinations, seizures, fever, ataxia, erythema multiforme, stomatitis, diarrhea, pseudomembranous colitis, pancreatitis, thrombocytopenia, megaloblastic anemia, granulocytopenia, aplastic anemia, hemolysis (with G-6-PD deficiency), cholestatic jaundice, kernicterus in neonates, interstitial nephritis, pancytopenia, rhabdomyolysis

**Overdose/Toxicology** Symptoms of overdose include nausea, vomiting, GI distress, hematuria, and crystalluria. Bone marrow suppression may occur. Treatment is supportive. Adequate fluid intake is essential. Peritoneal dialysis is not effective and hemodialysis is only moderately effective in removing co-trimoxazole. Leucovorin 5-15 mg/day may accelerate hematologic recovery.

**Pharmacodynamics/Kinetics**

**Protein Binding:** SMX: 68%; TMP: 68%

**Distribution:** Crosses the placenta

**Half-life Elimination:** SMX: 9 hours; TMP: 6-17 hours, both are prolonged in renal failure

**Time to Peak:** Within 1-4 hours

**Metabolism:** Liver

**Excretion:** Urine

**Formulations** The 5:1 ratio (SMX to TMP) remains constant in all dosage forms:

Injection: Sulfamethoxazole 80 mg and trimethoprim 16 mg per mL (5 mL, 10 mL, 20 mL, 30 mL, 50 mL)

Suspension, oral: Sulfamethoxazole 200 mg and trimethoprim 40 mg per 5 mL (20 mL, 100 mL, 150 mL, 200 mL, 480 mL)

Tablet: Sulfamethoxazole 400 mg and trimethoprim 80 mg

Tablet, double strength: Sulfamethoxazole 800 mg and trimethoprim 160 mg

**Dosing**

**Adults:** Dosage recommendations are based on the trimethoprim component.

Urinary tract infection/chronic bronchitis: Oral: 1 double strength tablet every 12 hours for 10-14 days

Sepsis: I.V.: 20 TMP/kg/day divided every 6 hours

*Pneumocystis carinii*:

Prophylaxis: Oral: 1 double strength tablet daily or 3 times weekly

Treatment: Oral, I.V.: 15-20 mg TMP/kg/day divided in 3-4 doses daily

**Elderly:** Refer to adult dosing.

**Renal Impairment:**

$Cl_{cr}$ 15-30 mL/minute: Reduce dose by 50%.

$Cl_{cr}$ <15 mL/minute: Not recommended

**Administration**

**I.V.:** Infuse over 60-90 minutes, must dilute well before giving.

**I.V. Detail:** May be given less diluted in a central line. Not for I.M. injection. Maintain adequate fluid intake to prevent crystalluria. Administer around-the-clock every 6-12 hours.

**Stability**

**Storage:** Do not refrigerate injection. Less soluble in more alkaline pH. Protect from light.

**Reconstitution:** Do not refrigerate injection. Do not use NS as a diluent. Injection vehicle contains benzyl alcohol and sodium metabisulfite.

Stability of parenteral admixture at room temperature (25°C):

5 mL/125 mL $D_5W$ = 6 hours
5 mL/100 mL $D_5W$ = 4 hours
5 mL/75 mL $D_5W$ = 2 hours

**Monitoring Laboratory Tests** Perform culture and sensitivity testing prior to initiating therapy.

**Additional Nursing Issues**

**Physical Assessment:** Monitor for signs or symptoms of adverse reactions, respiratory distress, CNS changes, acute GI upset, photosensitivity. Monitor I & O ratios; encourage fluids. **Pregnancy risk factor C/D** - benefits of use should outweigh possible risks.

**Patient Information/Instruction:** Take oral medication with 8 oz of water on an empty stomach (1 hour before or 2 hours after meals) for best absorption. Finish all medication; do not skip doses. You may experience increased sensitivity to sunlight; use sunblock, wear protective clothing and dark glasses, or avoid direct exposure to sunlight. Small frequent meals, frequent mouth care, sucking lozenges, or chewing gum may reduce nausea or vomiting. Report skin rash, sore throat, blackened stool, or unusual bruising or bleeding immediately. **Pregnancy precautions:** Inform prescriber if you are or intend to be pregnant.

**Geriatric Considerations:** Elderly patients appear at greater risk for more severe adverse reactions. Adjust dose based on renal function.

**Additional Information** Some formulations may contain benzyl alcohol or ethanol. Bactrim™ injection contains sulfites.

**Related Information**

Sulfamethoxazole *on page 1082*

- **Coumadin®** *see* Warfarin *on page 1220*
- **Covera-HS®** *see* Verapamil *on page 1208*
- **Cozaar®** *see* Losartan *on page 693*
- **CP-99,219-27** *see* Trovafloxacin *on page 1189*
- **CPM** *see* Cyclophosphamide *on page 313*
- **Creatinine Clearance Estimating Methods in Patients With Stable Renal Function** *see page 1349*
- **Credaxol** *see* Ranitidine *on page 1008*
- **Crema Blanca Bustillos** *see* Hydroquinone *on page 583*
- **Creon 10®** *see* Pancrelipase *on page 882*
- **Creon 20®** *see* Pancrelipase *on page 882*
- **Creo-Terpin®** *see page 1294*
- **Cresyl Acetate** *see page 1291*
- **Cresylate®** *see page 1291*
- **Crinone™** *see* Progesterone *on page 974*
- **Crinone V** *see* Progesterone *on page 974*
- **Crixivan®** *see* Indinavir *on page 605*
- **Crolom™** *see page 1282*
- **Crolom® Ophthalmic Solution** *see* Cromolyn Sodium *on this page*
- **Cromoglicic Acid** *see* Cromolyn Sodium *on this page*

## Cromolyn Sodium (KROE moe lin SOW dee um)

**U.S. Brand Names** Crolom® Ophthalmic Solution; Gastrocrom® Oral; Intal® Nebulizer Solution; Intal® Oral Inhaler; Nasalcrom® Nasal Solution; Opticrom® Ophthalmic Solution

**Synonyms** Cromoglicic Acid; Disodium Cromoglycate; DSCG

**Therapeutic Category** Mast Cell Stabilizer; Ophthalmic Agent

**Pregnancy Risk Factor** B

**Lactation** Excretion in breast milk unknown/no data available

**Use** Adjunct in the prophylaxis of allergic disorders, including rhinitis, giant papillary conjunctivitis, and asthma; inhalation product may be used for prevention of exercise-induced bronchospasm; systemic mastocytosis, food allergy, and treatment of inflammatory bowel disease; **cromolyn is a prophylactic drug with no benefit for acute situations**

**Mechanism of Action/Effect** Prevents the mast cell release of histamine, leukotrienes and slow-reacting substance of anaphylaxis

**Contraindications** Hypersensitivity to cromolyn or any component; acute asthma attacks

**Warnings** Severe anaphylactic reactions may occur rarely. Cromolyn is a prophylactic drug with no benefit for acute situations. Do not use in patients with severe renal or hepatic impairment. Caution should be used when withdrawing the drug or tapering the dose as symptoms may recur. Use with caution in patients with a history of cardiac arrhythmias. Avoid contact lens use during treatment with ophthalmic solution.

**Adverse Reactions**

**Inhalation:**

>10%: Gastrointestinal: Unpleasant taste in mouth

**Nasal:**

>10%: Respiratory: Increase in sneezing, burning, stinging, or irritation inside of nose

1% to 10%:

Central nervous system: Headache

Gastrointestinal: Unpleasant taste

Respiratory: Hoarseness, coughing, postnasal drip

<1% (Limited to important or life-threatening symptoms): Anaphylactic reactions, epistaxis

**Ophthalmic:**

>10%: Ocular: Burning or stinging of eye

1% to 10%: Ocular: Dryness or puffiness around the eye, watering or itching of eye

<1% (Limited to important or life-threatening symptoms): Chemosis, conjunctival injection, styes (or other eye irritation not present before therapy)

**Systemic:**

>10%:

Central nervous system: Headache

Gastrointestinal: Diarrhea

1% to 10%:

Central nervous system: Insomnia

Dermatologic: Rash

Gastrointestinal: Abdominal pain, nausea

Neuromuscular: Myalgia

**Overdose/Toxicology** Symptoms of overdose include bronchospasm, laryngeal edema, and dysuria. Treat symptomatically.

(Continued)

## Cromolyn Sodium *(Continued)*

**Pharmacodynamics/Kinetics**

**Half-life Elimination:** 80-90 minutes

**Time to Peak:** Inhalation: Within 15 minutes

**Excretion:** Urine and feces

**Formulations**

Capsule:
Oral (Gastrocrom®): 100 mg
Inhalation, oral (Intal®): 800 mcg/spray (8.1 g)
Solution, for nebulization:
10 mg/mL (2 mL)
Intal®: 10 mg/mL (2 mL)
Solution, nasal (Nasalcrom®): 40 mg/mL (13 mL)
Solution, ophthalmic (Crolom®, Opticrom®): 4% (2.5 mL, 10 mL)

**Dosing**

**Adults:** Not effective for immediate relief of symptoms in acute asthmatic attacks; must be used at regular intervals for 2-4 weeks to be effective.

Oral: 200 mg 4 times/day 15-20 minutes before meal, up to 400 mg 4 times/day
Inhalation: Metered spray: 2 inhalations 4 times/day
Nasal: Instill 1 spray in each nostril 3-4 times/day
Ophthalmic: Instill 1-2 drops 4-6 times/day into each eye
Nebulization solution: Single dose of 20 mg

**Elderly:** Refer to adult dosing.

**Stability**

**Storage:** Store nebulizer solution protected from direct light.

**Compatibility:** Nebulizer solution is compatible with metaproterenol sulfate, isoproterenol hydrochloride, 0.25% isoetharine hydrochloride, epinephrine hydrochloride, terbutaline sulfate, and 20% acetylcysteine solution for at least 1 hour after their admixture. Store nebulizer solution protected from direct light.

**Monitoring Laboratory Tests** Periodic pulmonary function

**Additional Nursing Issues**

**Physical Assessment:** This is prophylactic therapy, not to be used for acute situations (see Contraindications and Warnings/Precautions). Monitor laboratory tests (long-term use) and adverse reactions (see Warnings/Precautions, Adverse Reactions, and Overdose/Toxicology). Assess knowledge/teach patient appropriate use, interventions to reduce side effects, and adverse symptoms to report. Note breast-feeding caution.

**Patient Information/Instruction:** Oral: Use as directed; do not increase dosage or discontinue abruptly without consulting prescriber. You may experience dizziness or nervousness (use caution when driving or engaging in tasks requiring alertness until response to drug is known); diarrhea (boiled milk, yogurt, or buttermilk may help); or headache or muscle pain (mild analgesic may offer relief). Report persistent insomnia; skin rash or irritation; abdominal pain or difficulty swallowing; unusual cough, bronchospasm, or difficulty breathing; decreased urination; or if condition worsens or fails to improve.

Nebulizer: Store nebulizer solution away from light. Prepare nebulizer according to package instructions. Clear as much mucus as possible before use. Rinse mouth following each use to prevent opportunistic infection and reduce unpleasant aftertaste. Report if symptoms worsen or condition fails to improve.

Nasal: Instill 1 spray into each nostril 3-4 times a day. You may experience unpleasant taste (rinsing mouth and frequent oral care may help); or headache (mild analgesic may help). Report increased sneezing, burning, stinging, or irritation inside of nose; sore throat, hoarseness, nosebleed; anaphylactic reaction (skin rash, fever, chills, backache, difficulty breathing, chest pain); or worsening of condition or lack of improvement.

Ophthalmic: For ophthalmic use only. Wash hands before using. Tilt head back and look upward. Put drops of suspension or apply thin ribbon of ointment inside lower eyelid. Close eye and roll eyeball in all directions. Do not blink for ½ minute. apply gentle pressure to inner corner of eye for 30 seconds. Do not use any other eye preparation for at least 10 minutes. Do not let tip of applicator touch eye or contaminate tip of applicator. Do not share medication with anyone else. Temporary stinging or blurred vision may occur. Inform prescriber if condition worsens or fails to improve or if you experience eye pain, redness, burning, watering, dryness, double vision, puffiness around eye, vision disturbances, or other adverse eye response; or worsening of condition or lack of improvement.

**Geriatric Considerations:** Assess the patient's ability to empty capsules via the Spinhaler®. Older persons often have difficulty with inhaled and ophthalmic dosage forms.

**Related Information**

Inhalant (Asthma, Bronchospasm) Agents *on page 1388*
Ophthalmic Agents *on page 1282*

♦ ***Crotalidae* Polyvalent** *see page 1246*

## Crotamiton (kroe TAM i tonn)

**U.S. Brand Names** Eurax® Topical

**Therapeutic Category** Scabicidal Agent

**Pregnancy Risk Factor** C

**Lactation** Excretion in breast milk unknown

**Use** Treatment of scabies and symptomatic treatment of pruritus

**Mechanism of Action/Effect** Mechanism of action unknown

**Contraindications** Hypersensitivity to crotamiton or any component; patients who manifest a primary irritation response to topical medications; avoid use when skin is inflamed or irritated

**Warnings** Avoid contact with face, eyes, mucous membranes, and urethral meatus. Do not apply to acutely inflamed or raw skin. For external use only. Pregnancy factor C.

**Adverse Reactions** <1% (Limited to important or life-threatening symptoms): Irritation, pruritus, contact dermatitis, warm sensation

**Overdose/Toxicology** Symptoms of ingestion include burning sensation in mouth, irritation of the buccal, esophageal and gastric mucosa, nausea, vomiting, and abdominal pain. There is no specific antidote. General measures to eliminate the drug and reduce its absorption, combined with symptomatic treatment, are recommended.

**Formulations**

Cream: 10% (60 g)

Lotion: 10% (60 mL, 454 mL)

**Dosing**

**Adults:** Topical:

Scabicide: Wash thoroughly and scrub away loose scales, then towel dry; apply a thin layer and massage drug onto skin of the entire body from the neck to the toes (with special attention to skin folds, creases, and interdigital spaces). Repeat application in 24 hours. Take a cleansing bath 48 hours after the final application. Treatment may be repeated after 7-10 days if live mites are still present.

Pruritus: Massage into affected areas until medication is completely absorbed; repeat as necessary

**Elderly:** Refer to adult dosing.

**Administration**

**Topical:** For external use only. Shake lotion well before using. Avoid contact with face, eyes, mucous membranes, and urethral meatus.

**Additional Nursing Issues**

**Physical Assessment:** Assess knowledge/teach patient appropriate application and use and adverse symptoms to report (see Adverse Reactions). **Pregnancy risk factor C.** Note breast-feeding caution.

**Patient Information/Instruction:** For topical use only. Apply lotion to whole body from the chin down being sure to cover all skin folds and creases. Apply a second application 24 hours later. Avoid eyes. Take a bath 48 hours after application. All contaminated clothing and bed linen should be washed to avoid reinfestation. If cure is not achieved after 2 doses, use alternative therapy. **Pregnancy/breast-feeding precautions:** Inform prescriber if you are or intend to be pregnant. Consult prescriber if breast-feeding.

- **Cruex® Topical** *see page 1247*
- **Cryocriptina** *see* Bromocriptine *on page 162*
- **Cryopril** *see* Captopril *on page 192*
- **Cryosolona** *see* Methylprednisolone *on page 754*
- **Cryoval** *see* Valproic Acid and Derivatives *on page 1198*
- **Cryoxifeno** *see* Tamoxifen *on page 1095*
- **Crystalline Penicillin** *see* Penicillin G, Parenteral, Aqueous *on page 897*
- **Crystamine®** *see* Cyanocobalamin *on this page*
- **Crysticillin® A.S.** *see* Penicillin G Procaine *on page 899*
- **C/T/S® Topical Solution** *see* Clindamycin *on page 282*
- **CTX** *see* Cyclophosphamide *on page 313*
- **Cuprimine®** *see* Penicillamine *on page 894*
- **Curretab®** *see* Medroxyprogesterone *on page 714*
- **Cutivate™** *see* Fluticasone *on page 511*
- **Cutivate™** *see* Topical Corticosteroids *on page 1152*
- **CYA** *see* Cyclosporine *on page 317*
- **Cyanide Antidote Kit** *see page 1246*

## Cyanocobalamin (sye an oh koe BAL a min)

**U.S. Brand Names** Berubigen®; Cobex®; Crystamine®; Cyanoject®; Cyomin®; Ener-B® [OTC]; Kaybovite-1000®; Nascobal®; Redisol®; Rubramin-PC®; Sytobex®

**Synonyms** Vitamin $B_{12}$

**Therapeutic Category** Vitamin, Water Soluble

**Pregnancy Risk Factor** A/C (if dose exceeds RDA recommendation)

**Lactation** Enters breast milk/compatible

**Use** Treatment of pernicious anemia; vitamin $B_{12}$ deficiency; increased $B_{12}$ requirements due to pregnancy, thyrotoxicosis, hemorrhage, malignancy, liver or kidney disease

**Mechanism of Action/Effect** Coenzyme for various metabolic functions, including fat and carbohydrate metabolism and protein synthesis, used in cell replication and hematopoiesis

**Contraindications** Hypersensitivity to cyanocobalamin, any component, or cobalt; patients with hereditary optic nerve atrophy, gout, Leber's disease

**Warnings** I.M. route used to treat pernicious anemia. Vitamin $B_{12}$ deficiency for >3 months results in irreversible degenerative CNS lesions. Treatment of vitamin $B_{12}$ megaloblastic anemia may result in severe hypokalemia, sometimes, fatal, when anemia corrects due to cellular potassium requirements. $B_{12}$ deficiency masks signs of polycythemia vera. Vegetarian diets may result in $B_{12}$ deficiency. Pernicious anemia occurs (Continued)

## Cyanocobalamin *(Continued)*

more often in gastric carcinoma than in general population. Pregnancy factor C (if dose exceeds RDA recommendation).

**Drug Interactions**

**Decreased Effect:** Alcohol decreases $B_{12}$ absorption. Chloramphenicol, cholestyramine, cimetidine, colchicine, neomycin, PAS, potassium may reduce absorption and/or effect of cyanocobalamin.

**Effects on Lab Values** Methotrexate, pyrimethamine, and most antibiotics invalidate folic acid and vitamin $B_{12}$ diagnostic microbiological blood assays

**Adverse Reactions**

1% to 10%:

Dermatologic: Itching

Gastrointestinal: Diarrhea

<1% (Limited to important or life-threatening symptoms): Peripheral vascular thrombosis

**Pharmacodynamics/Kinetics**

**Protein Binding:** Bound to transcobalamin II

**Distribution:** Principally stored in the liver, also stored in the kidneys and adrenals

**Metabolism:** Converted in the tissues to active coenzymes methylcobalamin and deoxyadenosylcobalamin

**Formulations**

Gel, nasal:

Ener-B®: 400 mcg/0.1 mL

Nascobal®: 500 mcg/0.1 mL (5 mL)

Injection: 30 mcg/mL (30 mL); 100 mcg/mL (1 mL, 10 mL, 30 mL); 1000 mcg/mL (1 mL, 10 mL, 30 mL)

Tablet [OTC]: 25 mcg, 50 mcg, 100 mcg, 250 mcg, 500 mcg, 1000 mcg

**Dosing**

**Adults:** I.M. or deep S.C.:

Recommended daily allowance (RDA): 2 mcg

Pernicious anemia, congenital (if evidence of neurologic involvement): 1000 mcg/day for at least 2 weeks; maintenance: 50 mcg/month

Adults: 100 mcg/day for 6-7 days; if improvement, give same dose on alternate days for 7 doses; then every 3-4 days for 2-3 weeks; once hematologic values have returned to normal, maintenance dosage: 100 mcg/month. **Note:** Use only parenteral therapy as oral therapy is not dependable.

Vitamin $B_{12}$ deficiency: Initial: 30 mcg/day for 5-10 days; maintenance: 100-200 mcg/month

Schilling test: I.M.: 1000 mcg

**Elderly:** Refer to adult dosing.

**Administration**

**Oral:** Not recommended

**I.M.:** I.M. or deep S.C. are preferred routes of administration.

**I.V.:** Not recommended

**Stability**

**Storage:** Clear pink to red solutions are stable at room temperature. Protect from light.

**Compatibility:** Incompatible with chlorpromazine, phytonadione, prochlorperazine, warfarin, ascorbic acid, dextrose, heavy metals, oxidizing or reducing agents.

**Monitoring Laboratory Tests** Erythrocyte and reticulocyte count, hemoglobin, hematocrit; monitor potassium concentrations during early therapy.

**Additional Nursing Issues**

**Physical Assessment:** See Contraindications and Warnings/Precautions for use cautions. Assess effectiveness and interactions of other medications (see Drug Interactions). Monitor laboratory tests at beginning of therapy and periodically with long-term therapy (see above). Assess knowledge/teach patient appropriate administration (injection technique and needle disposal), appropriate nutritional counseling, and adverse symptoms to report. **Pregnancy risk factor A/C** - see Pregnancy Risk Factor for cautious use.

**Patient Information/Instruction:** Use exactly as directed. Pernicious anemia may require monthly injections for life. Report skin rash; swelling, pain, or redness of extremities; or acute persistent diarrhea.

**Geriatric Considerations:** There exists evidence that people, particularly elderly whose serum cobalamin concentrations <500 pg/mL, should receive replacement parenteral therapy.

♦ **Cyanoject®** *see* Cyanocobalamin *on previous page*

♦ **Cyclizine** *see page 1294*

## Cyclobenzaprine (sye kloe BEN za preen)

**U.S. Brand Names** Flexeril®

**Therapeutic Category** Skeletal Muscle Relaxant

**Pregnancy Risk Factor** B

**Lactation** Excretion in breast milk unknown/not recommended

**Use** Treatment of muscle spasm associated with acute painful musculoskeletal conditions; supportive therapy in tetanus

**Mechanism of Action/Effect** Centrally acting skeletal muscle relaxant pharmacologically related to tricyclic antidepressants; reduces tonic somatic motor activity influencing both alpha and gamma motor neurons

**Contraindications** Hypersensitivity to cyclobenzaprine or any component; do not use concomitantly or within 14 days of MAO inhibitors; hyperthyroidism, congestive heart failure, arrhythmias

**Warnings** Cyclobenzaprine shares the toxic potentials of the tricyclic antidepressants and the usual precautions of tricyclic antidepressant therapy and cholinergic blockage should be observed. Use with caution in patients with urinary hesitancy or angle-closure glaucoma.

**Drug Interactions**

**Cytochrome P-450 Effect:** CYP1A2, 2D6 and 3A3/4 enzyme substrate

**Decreased Effect:** Cyclobenzaprine may block effect of guanethidine.

**Increased Effect/Toxicity:** Do not use concomitantly or within 14 days after MAO inhibitors; combination may cause hypertensive crisis, severe convulsions. Because of cyclobenzaprine similarities to the tricyclic antidepressants, there may be additive toxicities and side effects similar to tricyclic antidepressants. Because of cyclobenzaprine's anticholinergic action, use with caution in patients receiving those agents since effects may be additive. Cyclobenzaprine may enhance effects of alcohol, barbiturates, and other CNS depressants.

**Adverse Reactions**

>10%:

Central nervous system: Drowsiness, dizziness, lightheadedness

Gastrointestinal: Dry mouth

1% to 10%:

Cardiovascular: Edema of the face/lips, syncope

Gastrointestinal: Bloated feeling

Genitourinary: Problems in urinating, polyuria

Neuromuscular & skeletal: Problems in speaking, muscle weakness

Ocular: Blurred vision

Otic: Tinnitus

<1% (Limited to important or life-threatening symptoms): Syncope, rash, dermatitis, angioedema, dysuria, hepatitis

**Overdose/Toxicology** Symptoms of overdose include troubled breathing, drowsiness, syncope, seizures, tachycardia, hallucinations, and vomiting. Following initiation of essential overdose management, treatment is supportive and symptomatic.

**Pharmacodynamics/Kinetics**

**Half-life Elimination:** 1-3 days

**Time to Peak:** Within 3-8 hours

**Metabolism:** Liver

**Excretion:** Urine and bile

**Onset:** Commonly occurs within 1 hour

**Duration:** 8->24 hours

**Formulations** Tablet, as hydrochloride: 10 mg

**Dosing**

**Adults:** Oral: 20-40 mg/day in 2-4 divided doses; maximum: 60 mg/day. Do not use longer than 2-3 weeks.

**Elderly:** See Geriatric Considerations.

**Additional Nursing Issues**

**Physical Assessment:** Assess effectiveness and interactions of other medications (see Drug Interactions). See Contraindications and Warnings/Precautions for use cautions. Monitor effectiveness of therapy (according to rational for therapy), and adverse reactions (see Adverse Reactions) at beginning and periodically during therapy. Assess knowledge/teach patient appropriate use, interventions to reduce side effects (postural hypotension precautions), and adverse symptoms to report. Breast-feeding is not recommended.

**Patient Information/Instruction:** Take exactly as directed. Do not increase dose or discontinue without consulting prescriber. Do not use alcohol, prescriptive or OTC antidepressants, sedatives, or pain medications without consulting prescriber. You may experience drowsiness, dizziness, lightheadedness (avoid driving or engaging in tasks that require alertness until response to drug is known); or urinary retention (void before taking medication). Report excessive drowsiness or mental agitation, chest pain, skin rash, swelling of mouth/face, difficulty speaking, ringing in ears, or blurred vision. **Breast-feeding precautions:** Breast-feeding is not recommended.

**Geriatric Considerations:** High doses in the elderly caused drowsiness and dizziness; therefore, use the lowest dose possible. Because cyclobenzaprine causes anticholinergic effects, it may not be the skeletal muscle relaxant of choice in the elderly.


- ♦ **Cyclogyl®** *see page 1248*
- ♦ **Cyclogyl®** *see page 1282*
- ♦ **Cyclomen®** *see* Danazol *on page 332*
- ♦ **Cyclomydril® Ophthalmic** *see page 1248*
- ♦ **Cyclopentolate** *see page 1248*
- ♦ **Cyclopentolate** *see page 1282*
- ♦ **Cyclopentolate and Phenylephrine** *see page 1248*


## Cyclophosphamide (sye kloe FOS fa mide)

**U.S. Brand Names** Cytoxan® Injection; Cytoxan® Oral; Neosar® Injection

**Synonyms** CPM; CTX; CYT

**Therapeutic Category** Antineoplastic Agent, Alkylating Agent

**Pregnancy Risk Factor** D

**Lactation** Enters breast milk/contraindicated

(Continued)

## Cyclophosphamide *(Continued)*

**Use** Treatment of Hodgkin's and non-Hodgkin's lymphoma, Burkitt's lymphoma, chronic lymphocytic leukemia, chronic granulocytic leukemia, AML, ALL, mycosis fungoides, breast cancer, multiple myeloma, neuroblastoma, retinoblastoma, rhabdomyosarcoma, Ewing's sarcoma; testicular, endometrium and ovarian, and lung cancer, and as a conditioning regimen for BMT; prophylaxis of rejection for kidney, heart, liver, and BMT transplants, severe rheumatoid disorders, nephrotic syndrome, Wegener's granulomatosis, idiopathic pulmonary hemosideroses, myasthenia gravis, multiple sclerosis, systemic lupus erythematosus, lupus nephritis, autoimmune hemolytic anemia, idiopathic thrombocytic purpura, macroglobulinemia, and antibody-induced pure red cell aplasia

**Mechanism of Action/Effect** Interferes with the normal function of DNA by alkylation and cross-linking the strands of DNA, and by possible protein modification; cyclophosphamide also possesses potent immunosuppressive activity; note that cyclophosphamide must be metabolized to its active form in the liver

**Contraindications** Hypersensitivity to cyclophosphamide or any component; pregnancy

**Warnings** The U.S. Food and Drug Administration (FDA) currently recommends that procedures for proper handling and disposal of antineoplastic agents be considered. Dosage adjustment needed for renal or hepatic failure. Use with caution in patients with bone marrow depression.

Cyclophosphamide preparation should be performed in a Class II laminar flow biologic safety cabinet. Personnel should be wearing surgical gloves and a closed front surgical gown with knit cuffs. Appropriate safety equipment is recommended for preparation, administration, and disposal of antineoplastics. If cyclophosphamide contacts the skin, wash and flush thoroughly with water.

**Drug Interactions**

**Cytochrome P-450 Effect:** CYP2B6, 2D6, and 3A3/4 enzyme substrate

**Decreased Effect:** Cyclophosphamide may decrease digoxin serum levels.

**Increased Effect/Toxicity:**

Increased toxicity:

- Allopurinol may cause an increase in bone marrow depression and may result in significant elevations of cyclophosphamide cytotoxic metabolites.
- Anesthetic agents: Cyclophosphamide reduces serum pseudocholinesterase concentrations and may prolong the neuromuscular blocking activity of succinylcholine. Use with caution with halothane, nitrous oxide, and succinylcholine.
- Chloramphenicol causes prolonged cyclophosphamide half-life and increased toxicity.
- Cimetidine inhibits hepatic metabolism of drugs and may decrease the activation of cyclophosphamide.
- Doxorubicin: Cyclophosphamide may enhance cardiac toxicity of anthracyclines.
- Phenobarbital and phenytoin induce hepatic enzymes and cause a more rapid production of cyclophosphamide metabolites with a concurrent decrease in the serum half-life of the parent compound.
- Tetrahydrocannabinol results in enhanced immunosuppression in animal studies.
- Thiazide diuretics: Leukopenia may be prolonged.

**Effects on Lab Values** ↑ uric acid in serum and urine; false-positive Pap test; suppression of some skin tests

**Adverse Reactions**

>10%:

- Dermatologic: Alopecia is frequent, but hair will regrow although it may be of a different color or texture; alopecia usually occurs 3 weeks after therapy; darkening of skin/fingernails
- Endocrine & metabolic: Fertility: May cause sterility; interferes with oogenesis and spermatogenesis; may be irreversible in some patients; gonadal suppression (amenorrhea)
- Gastrointestinal: Nausea and vomiting occur more frequently with larger doses, usually beginning 6-10 hours after administration; also seen are anorexia, stomatitis; mucositis
- Hematologic: Leukopenia or infection (usually asymptomatic)
  - Emetic potential:
  - Oral: Low (<10%)
  - <1 g: Moderate (30% to 60%)
  - ≥1 g: High (>90%)
  - Time course of nausea/vomiting: Onset: 6-8 hours; Duration: 8-24 hours
- Hepatic: Jaundice seen occasionally

1% to 10%:

- Central nervous system: Headache
- Dermatologic: Skin rash, facial flushing, myxedema
- Gastrointestinal: Diarrhea or stomach pain
- Hematologic: Myelosuppressive: Thrombocytopenia occurs less frequently than with mechlorethamine, anemia
  - WBC: Moderate
  - Platelets: Moderate
  - Onset (days): 7
  - Nadir (days): 10-14
  - Recovery (days): 21

<1% (Limited to important or life-threatening symptoms): High-dose therapy may cause cardiac dysfunction manifested as congestive heart failure; cardiac necrosis or hemorrhagic myocarditis has occurred rarely, but is fatal. Cyclophosphamide may also

potentiate the cardiac toxicity of anthracyclines. Hyperglycemia, hypokalemia, distortion, hyperuricemia, SIADH has occurred with I.V. doses >50 mg/kg, stomatitis, hemorrhagic colitis, acute hemorrhagic cystitis is believed to be a result of chemical irritation of the bladder by acrolein, a cyclophosphamide metabolite. Acute hemorrhagic cystitis occurs in 7% to 12% of patients, and has been reported in up to 40% of patients. Hemorrhagic cystitis can be severe and even fatal. Patients should be encouraged to drink plenty of fluids (3-4 L/day) during therapy, void frequently, and avoid taking the drug at night-time. If large I.V. doses are being administered, I.V. hydration should be given during therapy. The administration of mesna or continuous bladder irrigation may also be warranted. Hepatic toxicity, renal tubular necrosis has occurred, but usually resolves after the discontinuation of therapy. Nasal congestion occurs when given in large I.V. doses via 30-60 minute infusion; patients experience runny eyes, nasal burning, rhinorrhea, sinus congestion, and sneezing during or immediately after the infusion; interstitial pulmonary fibrosis with prolonged high dosage has occurred. Secondary malignancy: Has developed with cyclophosphamide alone or in combination with other antineoplastics; both bladder carcinoma and acute leukemia are well documented; rare instances of anaphylaxis have been reported.

**BMT:**

Cardiovascular: Heart failure, cardiac necrosis, pericardial tamponade
Endocrine & metabolic: Hyponatremia
Gastrointestinal: Severe nausea and vomiting
Miscellaneous: Hemorrhagic cystitis, secondary malignancy

**Overdose/Toxicology** Symptoms of overdose include myelosuppression, alopecia, nausea, and vomiting. Treatment is supportive.

**Pharmacodynamics/Kinetics**

**Distribution:** Widely distributed including brain; crosses placenta

**Metabolism:** Liver

**Excretion:** Urine

**Formulations**

Powder for injection: 100 mg, 200 mg, 500 mg, 1 g, 2 g
Powder for injection, lyophilized: 100 mg, 200 mg, 500 mg, 1 g, 2 g
Tablet: 25 mg, 50 mg

**Dosing**

**Adults:** Refer to individual protocols. Patients with compromised bone marrow function may require a 33% to 50% reduction in initial loading dose.

- Oral: 50-100 mg/m²/day as continuous therapy or 400-1000 mg/m² in divided doses over 4-5 days as intermittent therapy
- I.V.:
  - Single doses: 400-1800 mg/m² (30-50 mg/kg) per treatment course (1-5 days) which can be repeated at 2- to 4-week intervals
  - Maximum single dose without BMT is 7 g/m² (190 mg/kg) single agent therapy
  - Continuous daily doses: 60-120 mg/m² (1-2.5 mg/kg) per day
- High dose BMT:
  - I.V.:
    - 60 mg/kg/day for 2 days (total dose: 120 mg/kg)
    - 50 mg/kg/day for 4 days (total dose: 200 mg/kg)
    - 1.8 g/m²/day for 4 days (total dose: 7.2 g/m²)
  - Continuous I.V.:
    - 1.5 g/m²/24 hours for 96 hours (total dose: 6 g/m²)
    - 1875 mg/m²/24 hours for 72 hours (total dose: 5625 mg/m²)
    - Duration of infusion is 1-24 hours; generally combined with other high-dose chemotherapeutic drugs, lymphocyte immune globulin, or total body irradiation (TBI).
- Nephrotic syndrome: Oral: 2-3 mg/kg/day every day for up to 12 weeks when corticosteroids are unsuccessful

**Elderly:** Refer to individual protocols: Initial and maintenance for induction: 1-2 mg/kg/day; adjust for renal clearance.

**Renal Impairment:** A large fraction of cyclophosphamide is eliminated by hepatic metabolism; some authors recommend no dose adjustment unless severe renal insufficiency ($Cl_{cr}$ <20 mL/minute).

$Cl_{cr}$ >10 mL/minute: Administer 100% of normal dose.
$Cl_{cr}$ <10 mL/minute: Administer 75% of normal dose.
Hemodialysis effects: Moderately dialyzable (20% to 50%)
Administer dose posthemodialysis or administer supplemental 50% dose.
CAPD effects: Unknown
CAVH effects: Unknown

**Hepatic Impairment:** Some authors recommend dosage reductions (of up to 30%); however, the pharmacokinetics of cyclophosphamide are not significantly altered in the presence of hepatic insufficiency.

**Administration**

**I.V.:** May be administered I.M., I.P., intrapleurally, IVPB, or continuous intravenous infusion. I.V. infusions may be administered over 1-2 hours. Doses >500 mg to approximately 1 g may be administered over 20-30 minutes.

**I.V. Detail:** May be administered slow IVP in lower doses. Force fluids up to 2 L/day to minimize bladder toxicity; high-dose regimens should be accompanied by vigorous hydration with or without mesna therapy.

**BMT only:** Approaches to reduction of hemorrhagic cystitis include infusion of 0.9% NaCl 3 L/m²/24 hours, infusion of 0.9% NaCl 3 L/m²/24 hours with continuous 0.9% NaCl bladder irrigation 300-1000 mL/hour, and infusion of 0.9% NaCl 1.5-3 L/m²/24

(Continued)

## Cyclophosphamide *(Continued)*

hours with intravenous mesna. Hydration should begin at least 4 hours before cyclophosphamide and continue at least 24 hours after completion of cyclophosphamide. The dose of daily mesna used should equal the daily dose of cyclophosphamide. Mesna can be administered as a continuous 24-hour intravenous infusion or be given in divided doses every 4 hours. Mesna should begin at the start of treatment, and continue at least 24 hours following the last dose of cyclophosphamide.

**Stability**

**Storage:** Store intact vials of powder at room temperature (25°C to 35°C).

**Reconstitution:** Reconstitute vials with SWI to a concentration of 20 mg/mL as follows below; reconstituted solutions are stable for 24 hours at room temperature (25°C) and 6 days at refrigeration (5°C).

100 mg vial = 5 mL
200 mg vial = 10 mL
500 mg vial = 25 mL
1 g vial = 50 mL
2 g vial = 100 mL

Further dilutions in $D_5W$ or NS are stable for 24 hours at room temperature (25°C) and 6 days at refrigeration (5°C)

Maximum concentration of cyclophosphamide is limited to 20 mg/mL due to solubility of cyclophosphamide

**Standard I.V. push dilution:** Dose up to 500 mg/30 mL syringe

Maximum syringe size for IVP is a 30 mL syringe. Syringe should be ≤75% full.

**Standard IVPB dilution:** May further dilute in $D_5W$ or NS after initial reconstitution with SWI

Doses up to 2 g/250 mL volume
Doses up to 4 g/500 mL volume

**Compatibility:** See the Chemotherapy Compatibility Chart *on page 1311.*

**Monitoring Laboratory Tests** CBC with differential, platelet count, ESR, BUN, UA, serum electrolytes, serum creatinine

**Additional Nursing Issues**

**Physical Assessment:** Monitor results of all laboratory tests prior to each I.V. treatment or frequently during oral therapy. Monitor for effect and/or interactions of other prescription and OTC medications (see Drug Interactions). Know and monitor for adverse effects of this medication (see Adverse Reactions). Instruct patient about appropriate interventions to reduce side effects and symptoms to report. **Pregnancy risk factor D** - assess knowledge/teach appropriate use of barrier contraceptives. Breast-feeding is contraindicated.

**Patient Information/Instruction:** Tablets may be taken during or after meals to reduce GI effects. Maintain adequate fluid balance (2-3 L/day of fluids unless instructed to restrict fluid intake). Void frequently and report any difficulty or pain with urination. May cause hair loss (reversible after treatment) or sterility or amenorrhea (sometimes reversible). If you are diabetic, you will need to monitor serum glucose closely to avoid hypoglycemia. You may be more susceptible to infection; avoid crowds and unnecessary exposure to infection. Report unusual bleeding or bruising; persistent fever or sore throat; blood in urine, stool (black stool), or vomitus; delayed healing of any wounds; skin rash; yellowing of skin or eyes; or changes in color of urine or stool. **Pregnancy/breast-feeding precautions:** Do not get pregnant while taking this medication; use appropriate barrier contraceptive measures. Do not breast-feed.

**Geriatric Considerations:** Toxicity to immunosuppressives is increased in the elderly. Start with lowest recommended adult doses. Signs of infection, such as fever and WBC rise, may not occur. Lethargy and confusion may be more prominent signs of infection; adjust dose for renal function in the elderly.

## Cycloserine (sye kloe SER een)

**U.S. Brand Names** Seromycin® Pulvules®

**Therapeutic Category** Antibiotic, Miscellaneous; Antitubercular Agent

**Pregnancy Risk Factor** C

**Lactation** Enters breast milk/compatible

**Use** Adjunctive treatment in pulmonary or extrapulmonary tuberculosis; retreatment of acute urinary tract infections caused by *E. coli* or *Enterobacter* sp when less toxic conventional therapy has failed or is contraindicated

**Mechanism of Action/Effect** Inhibits bacterial cell wall synthesis by competing with amino acid (D-alanine) for incorporation into the bacterial cell wall; bacteriostatic or bactericidal

**Contraindications** Hypersensitivity to cycloserine or any component

**Warnings** Epilepsy, depression, severe anxiety, psychosis, severe renal insufficiency, chronic alcoholism. Pregnancy factor C.

**Drug Interactions**

**Increased Effect/Toxicity:** Alcohol, isoniazid, and ethionamide increase toxicity of cycloserine. Cycloserine inhibits the hepatic metabolism of phenytoin and may increase risk of epileptic seizures.

**Adverse Reactions**

>10%: Central nervous system: Drowsiness, headache, restlessness, mental depression, nightmares, speech problems, thoughts of suicide

1% to 10%:

Cardiovascular: Congestive heart failure
Central nervous system: Seizures
Dermatologic: Rash

Hepatic: Elevated liver enzymes

Neuromuscular & skeletal: Tremor

**Overdose/Toxicology** Symptoms of overdose include confusion, CNS depression, psychosis, coma, and seizures. Decontaminate with activated charcoal. Can be hemodialyzed. Management is supportive. Administer 100-300 mg/day of pyridoxine to reduce neurotoxic effects. Acute toxicity can occur with ingestion >1 g.

**Pharmacodynamics/Kinetics**

**Distribution:** Crosses the placenta; distributed widely to most body fluids and tissues including CSF, breast milk, bile, sputum, lymph tissue, lungs, and ascitic, pleural, and synovial fluids

**Half-life Elimination:** 10 hours in patients with normal renal function

**Time to Peak:** Oral: Within 3-4 hours

**Metabolism:** Liver

**Excretion:** Urine

**Formulations** Capsule: 250 mg

**Dosing**

**Adults:** Some of the neurotoxic effects may be relieved or prevented by the concomitant administration of pyridoxine.

Tuberculosis: Oral: Initial: 250 mg every 12 hours for 14 days, then give 500 mg to 1 g/day in 2 divided doses for 18-24 months (maximum daily dose: 1 g)

**Elderly:** Refer to adult dosing.

**Renal Impairment:**

$Cl_{cr}$ 10-50 mL/minute: Administer every 12-24 hours.

$Cl_{cr}$ <10 mL/minute: Administer every 24 hours.

**Monitoring Laboratory Tests** Periodic renal, hepatic, hematological tests, plasma cycloserine concentrations

**Additional Nursing Issues**

**Physical Assessment:** Assess effectiveness and interactions of other medications (see Drug Interactions). See Warnings/Precautions and Contraindications for use cautions. Monitor effectiveness of therapy, laboratory tests, and adverse response (see Adverse Reactions and Overdose/Toxicology). Assess knowledge/teach patient possible side effects and adverse symptoms to report. **Pregnancy risk factor C** - benefits of use should outweigh possible risks.

**Patient Information/Instruction:** Take as prescribed; do not discontinue without consulting prescriber. Avoid alcohol. Maintain recommended diet and adequate hydration (2-3 L/day of fluids unless instructed to restrict fluid intake). You may experience drowsiness or restlessness (use caution when driving or engaging in tasks that require alertness until response to drug is known). Report skin rash, acute headache, tremors or changes in mentation (confusion, nightmares, depression, or suicide ideation), or fluid retention (respiratory difficulty, swelling of extremities, unusual weight gain). **Pregnancy precautions:** Inform prescriber if you are or intend to be pregnant.

**Geriatric Considerations:** Adjust dose for renal function.

**Related Information**

TB Drug Comparison *on page 1402*

♦ **Cyclosporin A** *see* Cyclosporine *on this page*

## Cyclosporine (SYE kloe spor een)

**U.S. Brand Names** Neoral® Oral; Sandimmune® Injection; Sandimmune® Oral; Sang CyA®

**Synonyms** CYA; Cyclosporin A

**Therapeutic Category** Immunosuppressant Agent

**Pregnancy Risk Factor** C

**Lactation** Enters breast milk/contraindicated

**Use** Immunosuppressant which may be used with azathioprine and/or corticosteroids to prolong organ and patient survival in kidney, liver, and heart transplants; used in allogeneic bone marrow transplants for prevention and treatment of graft-versus-host disease; also used in some cases of severe autoimmune disease that are resistant to corticosteroids and other therapy.

**Investigation use:** Short-term high-dose cyclosporine as a modulator of multidrug resistance in cancer treatment

**Mechanism of Action/Effect** Inhibition of production and release of interleukin II and inhibits interleukin II-induced activation of resting T-lymphocytes

**Contraindications** Hypersensitivity to cyclosporine, Cremophor® EL (I.V. solution), or any other I.V. component (ie, polyoxyl 35 castor oil is an ingredient of the parenteral formulation, and polyoxyl 40 hydrogenated castor oil is an ingredient of cyclosporine capsules and solution for microemulsion)

**Warnings** Infection and possible development of lymphoma may result. Make dose adjustments to avoid toxicity or possible organ rejection using cyclosporine blood levels because absorption is erratic and elimination is highly variable. Administer with adrenal corticosteroids but not with other immunosuppressive agents. Adjustment of dose should only be made under the direct supervision of an experienced physician. Reserve I.V. use for patients who cannot take oral form. Maintain patent airway; other supportive measures and agents for treating anaphylaxis should be present when I.V. drug is given. Nephrotoxic: If possible avoid concomitant use of other potentially nephrotoxic drugs (eg, acyclovir, aminoglycoside antibiotics, amphotericin B, ciprofloxacin). Injectable form contains ethanol. Pregnancy factor C.

(Continued)

## Cyclosporine *(Continued)*

**Drug Interactions**

**Cytochrome P-450 Effect:** CYP3A3/4 enzyme substrate

**Decreased Effect:** Rifampin, phenytoin, and phenobarbital decrease plasma concentration of cyclosporine.

**Increased Effect/Toxicity:** Ketoconazole, fluconazole, itraconazole, corticosteroids increase plasma concentration of cyclosporine and toxicity associated with elevated levels.

**Food Interactions** Cyclosporine peak serum levels may be elevated if taken with food. Renal toxicity may result if cyclosporine is taken with grapefruit juice.

**Effects on Lab Values** Specific whole blood, HPLC assay for cyclosporine may be falsely elevated if sample is drawn from the same line through which dose was administered (even if flush has been administered and/or dose was given hours before).

**Adverse Reactions**

>10%:

- Cardiovascular: Hypertension
- Dermatologic: Hirsutism
- Endocrine & metabolic: Hypomagnesemia, hyperkalemia
- Gastrointestinal: Gingival hyperplasia
- Neuromuscular & skeletal: Tremor
- Renal: Nephrotoxicity

1% to 10%:

- Central nervous system: Seizure, headache
- Dermatologic: Acne
- Gastrointestinal: Abdominal discomfort, nausea, vomiting
- Hepatic: Hepatotoxicity
- Neuromuscular & skeletal: Leg cramps
- Miscellaneous: Increased susceptibility to infection

<1% (Limited to important or life-threatening symptoms): Hypotension, tachycardia, warmth, flushing, hyperkalemia, hypomagnesemia, hyperuricemia, renal toxicity, respiratory distress

**Overdose/Toxicology** Symptoms of overdose include hepatotoxicity, nephrotoxicity, nausea, vomiting, and tremor. CNS toxicity, secondary to direct action of the drug, may not be reflected in serum concentrations, and may be more predictable by renal magnesium loss. Treatment is supportive.

**Pharmacodynamics/Kinetics**

**Protein Binding:** 90% to 98% of cyclosporine in blood is bound to lipoproteins

**Distribution:** Widely distributed in tissues and body fluids including liver, pancreas, and lungs; crosses the placenta

**Half-life Elimination:**

Solution or soft gelatin capsule (Sandimmune®): Biphasic, alpha phase: 1.4 hours and terminal phase 6-24 hours

Solution or soft gelatin capsule in a microemulsion (Neoral®): 8.4 hours

**Time to Peak:**

Oral solution or capsule (Sandimmune®): 2-6 hours; some patients have a second peak at 5-6 hours

Oral solution or capsule in a microemulsion (Neoral®): 1.5-2 hours (in renal transplant patients)

**Metabolism:** Liver

**Excretion:** Bile

**Formulations**

- Capsule (Sandimmune®): 25 mg, 100 mg
- Capsule, soft gel (Sandimmune®): 50 mg
- Capsule, soft gel for microemulsion (Neoral®): 25 mg, 100 mg
- Injection (Sandimmune®): 50 mg/mL (5 mL)
- Solution, oral (Sandimmune®): 100 mg/mL (50 mL)
- Solution, oral for microemulsion (Neoral®): 100 mg/mL (50 mL)

**Dosing**

**Adults:** Oral dosage is ~3 times the I.V. dosage; **dosage should be based on ideal body weight.**

**Cyclosporine**

| Condition | Cyclosporine |
|---|---|
| Switch from I.V. to oral therapy | Threefold increase in dose |
| T-tube clamping | Decrease dose; increase availability of bile facilitates absorption of CsA |
| Pediatric patients | About 2-3 times higher dose compared to adults |
| Liver dysfunction | Decrease I.V. dose; increase oral dose |
| Renal dysfunction | Decrease dose to decrease levels if renal dysfunction is related to the drug |
| Dialysis | Not removed |
| Inhibitors of hepatic metabolism | Decrease dose |
| Inducers of hepatic metabolism | Monitor drug level; may need to increase dose |

I.V.:

Initial: 5-6 mg/kg/day beginning 4-12 hours prior to organ transplantation; patients should be switched to oral cyclosporine as soon as possible; dose should be infused over 2-24 hours

Maintenance: 2-10 mg/kg/day in divided doses every 8-12 hours; dose should be adjusted to maintain whole blood HPLC trough concentrations in the reference range

Oral: Solution or soft gelatin capsule (Sandimmune®):

Initial: 14-18 mg/kg/day, beginning 4-12 hours prior to organ transplantation

Maintenance: 5-15 mg/kg/day divided every 12-24 hours; maintenance dose is usually tapered to 3-10 mg/kg/day

Focal segmental glomerulosclerosis: Initial: 3 mg/kg/day divided every 12 hours

Dosing considerations of cyclosporine, see table.

Oral: Solution or soft gelatin capsule in a microemulsion (Neoral®): Based on the organ transplant population:

Initial: Same as the initial dose for solution or soft gelatin capsule (listed above)

**or**

Renal: 9 mg/kg/day (range: 6-12 mg/kg/day)

Liver: 8 mg/kg/day (range: 4-12 mg/kg/day)

Heart: 7 mg/kg/day (range: 4-10 mg/kg/day)

**Note:** A 1:1 ratio conversion from Sandimmune® to Neoral® has been recommended initially; however, lower doses of Neoral® may be required after conversion to prevent overdose. Total daily doses should be adjusted based on the cyclosporine trough blood concentration and clinical assessment of organ rejection. Cyclosporine blood trough levels should be determined prior to conversion. After conversion to Neoral®, cyclosporine trough levels should be monitored every 4-7 days

**Elderly:** Refer to adult dosing (**Note:** Sandimmune® and Neoral® are not bioequivalent and cannot be used interchangeably without physician supervision).

**Renal Impairment:** Adjustment for cyclosporine therapy for severe psoriasis:

**Serum creatinine levels ≥25% above pretreatment levels:** Take another sample within 2 weeks. If the level remains ≥25% above pretreatment levels, decrease dosage of cyclosporine microemulsion by 25% to 50%. If 2 dosage adjustments do not reverse the increase in serum creatinine levels, treatment should be discontinued.

**Serum creatinine ≥50% above pretreatment levels:** Decrease cyclosporine dosage by 25% to 50%. If 2 dosage adjustments do not reverse the increase in serum creatinine levels, treatment should be discontinued.

**Note:** Increase the frequency of blood pressure monitoring after each alteration in dosage of cyclosporine. Cyclosporine dosage should be decreased by 25% to 50% in patients with no history of hypertension who develop sustained hypertension during therapy and, if hypertension persists, treatment with cyclosporine should be discontinued.

**Hepatic Impairment:** Dosage adjustment is probably necessary, monitor levels closely.

## Administration

**Oral:** Do not administer liquid from plastic or styrofoam cup. Mixing with milk, chocolate milk, or orange juice preferably at room temperature, improves palatability. Stir well. Do not allow to stand before drinking. Rinse with more diluent to ensure that the total dose is taken; after use, dry outside of pipette. Do not rinse with water or other cleaning agents.

## Stability

**Storage:** Cyclosporine injection is a clear, faintly brown-yellow solution which should be stored at <30°C and protected from light.

**Reconstitution:** Cyclosporine concentrate for injection should be further diluted [1 mL (50 mg) of concentrate in 20-100 mL of $D_5W$ or NS] for administration by intravenous infusion. Light protection is not required for intravenous admixtures of cyclosporine.

Stability of injection of parenteral admixture at room temperature (25°C) is 6 hours in PVC; 24 hours in Excel®, PAB® containers, or glass.

Polyoxyethylated castor oil (Cremophor® EL) surfactant in cyclosporin injection may leach phthalate from PVC containers such as bags and tubing. The actual amount of diethylhexyl phthalate (DEHP) plasticizer leached from PVC containers and administration sets may vary in clinical situations, depending on surfactant concentration, bag size, and contact time.

Doses <250 mg should be prepared in 100 mL of $D_5W$ or NS

Doses >250 mg should be prepared in 250 mL of $D_5W$ or NS

Minimum volume: 100 mL $D_5W$ or NS

Do not refrigerate oral or I.V. solution

**Oral solution:** Use the contents of the oral solution within 2 months after opening. Should be mixed in glass containers.

**Monitoring Laboratory Tests** Cyclosporine levels, serum electrolytes, renal function, hepatic function

## Additional Nursing Issues

### Physical Assessment:

I.V.: Monitor closely for first 30-60 minutes of infusion and frequently thereafter to assess for adverse reactions (CNS changes or hypertension).

Oral: Teach patient appropriate administration, possible side effects, and symptoms to report (see above).

**Pregnancy risk factor C** - benefits of use should outweigh possible risks. Breast-feeding is contraindicated.

(Continued)

## Cyclosporine *(Continued)*

**Patient Information/Instruction:** Use glass container for liquid solution (do not use plastic or styrofoam cup). Mixing with milk, chocolate milk, or orange juice at room temperature improves flavor. Mix thoroughly and drink at once. Take dose at the same time each day. You will be susceptible to infection; avoid crowds and exposure to any infectious diseases. Do not have any vaccinations without consulting prescriber. Practice good oral hygiene to reduce gum inflammation; see dentist regularly during treatment. Report acute headache; unusual hair growth or deepening of voice; mouth sores or swollen gums; persistent nausea, vomiting, or abdominal pain; muscle pain or cramping; unusual swelling of extremities, weight gain, or change in urination; or chest pain or rapid heartbeat. **Pregnancy/breast-feeding precautions:** Inform prescriber if you are or intend to be pregnant. Do not breast-feed.

**Related Information**

Peak and Trough Guidelines *on page 1331*


- **Cycrin®** *see* Medroxyprogesterone *on page 714*
- **Cylert®** *see* Pemoline *on page 892*
- **Cylex® [OTC]** *see* Benzocaine *on page 141*
- **Cymevene** *see* Ganciclovir *on page 526*
- **Cyomin®** *see* Cyanocobalamin *on page 311*


## Cyproheptadine (si proe HEP ta deen)

**U.S. Brand Names** Periactin®

**Therapeutic Category** Antihistamine

**Pregnancy Risk Factor** B

**Lactation** Excretion in breast milk unknown/contraindicated

**Use** Perennial and seasonal allergic rhinitis and other allergic symptoms including urticaria; its off-labeled uses have included appetite stimulation, blepharospasm, cluster headaches, migraine headaches, Nelson's syndrome, pruritus, schizophrenia, spinal cord damage associated spasticity, and tardive dyskinesia

**Mechanism of Action/Effect** A potent antihistamine and serotonin antagonist

**Contraindications** Hypersensitivity to cyproheptadine or any component; narrow-angle glaucoma, bladder neck obstruction, acute asthmatic attack, stenosing peptic ulcer, GI tract obstruction, those on MAO inhibitors; avoid use in premature and term newborns due to potential association with SIDS

**Warnings** Do not use in the presence of symptomatic prostate hypertrophy. Antihistamines are more likely to cause dizziness, excessive sedation, syncope, toxic confusion states, and hypotension in the elderly. In case reports, cyproheptadine has promoted weight gain in anorexic adults, though it has not been specifically studied in the elderly. All cases of weight loss or decreased appetite should be adequately assessed.

**Drug Interactions**

**Increased Effect/Toxicity:** MAO inhibitors may cause hallucinations when taken with cyproheptadine.

**Effects on Lab Values** Diagnostic antigen skin tests; ↑ amylases (S); ↓ fasting glucose (S)

**Adverse Reactions**

>10%:

Central nervous system: Slight to moderate drowsiness
Respiratory: Thickening of bronchial secretions

1% to 10%:

Central nervous system: Headache, fatigue, nervousness, dizziness
Gastrointestinal: Appetite stimulation, nausea, diarrhea, abdominal pain, dry mouth
Neuromuscular & skeletal: Arthralgia
Respiratory: Pharyngitis

<1% (Limited to important or life-threatening symptoms): Tachycardia, palpitations, edema, sedation, CNS stimulation, seizures, depression, hemolytic anemia, leukopenia, thrombocytopenia, hepatitis, bronchospasm, epistaxis

**Overdose/Toxicology** Symptoms of overdose include CNS depression or stimulation, dry mouth, flushed skin, fixed and dilated pupils, and apnea. There is no specific treatment for antihistamine overdose. Clinical toxicity is due to blockade of cholinergic receptors. For anticholinergic overdose with severe life-threatening symptoms, physostigmine 1-2 mg I.V. slowly, may be given to reverse these effects.

**Pharmacodynamics/Kinetics**

**Metabolism:** Liver

**Excretion:** Urine

**Formulations**

Cyproheptadine hydrochloride:

Syrup: 2 mg/5 mL with alcohol 5% (473 mL)
Tablet: 4 mg

**Dosing**

**Adults:** Oral: 4-20 mg/day divided every 8 hours (not to exceed 0.5 mg/kg/day)

**Elderly:** Oral: Initial: 4 mg twice daily

**Hepatic Impairment:** Dosage should be reduced in patients with significant hepatic dysfunction.

**Additional Nursing Issues**

**Physical Assessment:** Assess effectiveness and interactions of other medications (see Drug Interactions). See Contraindications and Warnings/Precautions for cautious use. Monitor effectiveness of therapy and adverse reactions (eg, excess anticholinergic effects - see Adverse Reactions) at beginning of therapy and periodically with long-term use. Assess knowledge/teach patient appropriate use, interventions to reduce side effects, and adverse symptoms to report. Breast-feeding is contraindicated.

**Patient Information/Instruction:** Take as directed; do not exceed recommended dose. Avoid use of other depressants, alcohol, or sleep-inducing medications unless approved by prescriber. You may experience drowsiness or dizziness (use caution when driving or engaging in tasks requiring alertness until response to drug is known); or dry mouth, nausea, or abdominal pain (frequent small meals, frequent mouth care, chewing gum, or sucking hard candy may help). Report persistent sedation, confusion, or agitation; changes in urinary pattern; blurred vision; chest pain or palpitations; sore throat difficulty breathing or expectorating (thick secretions); or lack of improvement or worsening or condition. **Breast-feeding precautions:** Do not breast-feed.

**Geriatric Considerations:** Elderly may not tolerate anticholinergic effects.

**Additional Information** Some formulations may contain ethanol.

♦ **Cystagon®** *see* Cysteamine *on this page*

## Cysteamine (sis TEE a meen)

**U.S. Brand Names** Cystagon®

**Therapeutic Category** Anticystine Agent; Urinary Tract Product

**Pregnancy Risk Factor** C

**Lactation** Excretion in breast milk unknown

**Use** Management of nephropathic cystinosis; approved as orphan drug 8/15/94

**Mechanism of Action/Effect** Lowers cystine levels in cells of clients with cystinosis, an inherited defect that results in abnormal cystine transport formation of crystals that damage the kidneys

**Contraindications** Hypersensitivity to cysteamine or penicillamine

**Warnings** Withhold cysteamine if a mild rash develops. Restart at a lower dose and titrate to therapeutic dose. Adjust cysteamine dose if CNS symptoms due to the drug develop. Adjust cysteamine dose downward if severe GI symptoms develop (most common during initiation of therapy). Pregnancy factor C.

**Effects on Lab Values** Abnormal liver function tests

**Adverse Reactions**

>10%:

- Central nervous system: Fever, lethargy
- Dermatologic: Rash
- Gastrointestinal: Vomiting, anorexia, diarrhea

1% to 10%:

- Central nervous system: Confusion, dizziness, mental depression
- Neuromuscular & skeletal: Trembling
- Gastrointestinal: Sore throat, bad breath, constipation

<1% (Limited to important or life-threatening symptoms): Seizures, dehydration, anemia, leukopenia

**Overdose/Toxicology** Symptoms may include vomiting, reduction of motor activity, GI or renal hemorrhage. Treatment is generally supportive. Hemodialysis may be appropriate.

**Formulations** Capsule, as bitartrate: 50 mg, 150 mg

**Dosing**

**Adults:** Initiate therapy with $^1/_4$ to $^1/_8$ of maintenance dose; titrate slowly upward over 4-6 weeks.

Adults (>110 lb): 2 g/day in 4 divided doses; dosage may in increased to 1.95 g/m$^2$/day if cystine levels are <1 nmol/$^1/_2$ cystine/mg protein, although intolerance and incidence of adverse events may be increased.

**Elderly:** Refer to adult dosing.

**Administration**

**Oral:** Sprinkle capsule contents over food if unable to swallow capsule

**Monitoring Laboratory Tests** Blood counts and LFTs during therapy; monitor leukocyte cystine measurements every 3 months to determine adequate dosage and compliance (measure 5-6 hours after administration); monitor more frequently when switching salt forms

**Additional Nursing Issues**

**Physical Assessment:** Monitor all laboratory results. Monitor or instruct patient to monitor for adverse reactions; especially CNS changes, GI disturbances, or rash. If reactions are noted, medication should be held until reactions clear, and medication started at a lower dose. **Pregnancy risk factor C** - benefits of use should outweigh possible risks. Note breast-feeding caution.

**Patient Information/Instruction:** Take as directed. Maintain adequate hydration (2-3 L/day of fluids unless instructed to restrict fluid intake). It may be necessary to include other medication in treatment regimen. Periodic blood tests will need to be performed. You may experience dizziness, confusion, or lethargy; use caution with tasks that require alertness until response to drug is known. Report fever, gastric disturbances, or rash. **Pregnancy/breast-feeding precautions:** Inform prescriber if you are or intend to be pregnant. Consult prescriber if breast-feeding.

♦ **Cystospaz®** *see* Hyoscyamine *on page 590*
♦ **Cystospaz-M®** *see* Hyoscyamine *on page 590*
♦ **CYT** *see* Cyclophosphamide *on page 313*
♦ **Cytadren®** *see* Aminoglutethimide *on page 69*

## Cytarabine (sye TARE a been)

**U.S. Brand Names** Cytosar-U®

**Synonyms** Arabinosylcytosine; ARA-C; Cytosine Arabinosine Hydrochloride

**Therapeutic Category** Antineoplastic Agent, Antimetabolite

**Pregnancy Risk Factor** D

**Lactation** Excretion in breast milk unknown/not recommended

**Use** Ara-C is one of the most active agents in leukemia; also active against lymphoma, meningeal leukemia, and meningeal lymphoma; has little use in the treatment of solid tumors

**Mechanism of Action/Effect** Inhibition of DNA synthesis in S Phase of cell division; degree of its cytotoxicity correlates linearly with its incorporation into DNA, therefore, incorporation into the DNA is responsible for drug activity and toxicity

**Contraindications** Hypersensitivity to cytarabine or any component; pregnancy (do not use unless benefits outweigh risks)

**Warnings** Use with caution in patients with impaired hepatic function. The U.S. Food and Drug Administration (FDA) currently recommends that procedures for proper handling and disposal of antineoplastic agents be considered. Must monitor drug tolerance, protect and maintain a patient compromised by drug toxicity that includes bone marrow depression with leukopenia, thrombocytopenia and anemia along with nausea, vomiting, diarrhea, abdominal pain, oral ulceration, and hepatic impairment. Marked bone marrow depression necessitates dosage reduction in the number of days of administration.

Cytarabine preparation should be performed in a Class II laminar flow biologic safety cabinet. Personnel should be wearing surgical gloves and a closed front surgical gown with knit cuffs. Appropriate safety equipment is recommended for preparation, administration, and disposal of antineoplastics. If cytarabine contacts the skin, wash and flush thoroughly with water.

**Drug Interactions**

**Decreased Effect:** Decreased effect of gentamicin, flucytosine. Decreased digoxin oral tablet absorption.

**Increased Effect/Toxicity:** Alkylating agents and radiation, purine analogs, and methotrexate when coadministered with cytarabine result in increased toxic effects.

**Adverse Reactions**

>10%:

**High-dose therapy toxicities:** Cerebellar toxicity, conjunctivitis (make sure the patient is on steroid eye drops during therapy), corneal keratitis, hyperbilirubinemia, pulmonary edema, pericarditis, and tamponade

Central nervous system: Has produced seizures when given I.T.; cerebellar syndrome (or cerebellar toxicity), manifested as ataxia, dysarthria, and dysdiadochokinesia, has been reported to be dose-related. This may or may not be reversible.

Dermatologic: Oral/anal ulceration, rash

Gastrointestinal: Nausea, vomiting, anorexia, stomatitis/mucositis which subside quickly after discontinuing the drug; GI effects may be more pronounced with divided I.V. bolus doses than with continuous infusion

Emetic potential:

<500 mg: Moderately low (10% to 30%)

500 mg to 1500 mg: Moderately high (60% to 90%)

>1-1.5 g: High (>90%)

Time course of nausea/vomiting: Onset: 1-3 hours; Duration: 3-8 hours

Hematologic: Bleeding, leukopenia, thrombocytopenia

Myelosuppressive: Occurs within the first week of treatment and lasts for 10-14 days; primarily manifested as granulocytopenia, but anemia can also occur

WBC: Severe

Platelets: Severe

Onset (days): 4-7

Nadir (days): 14-18

Recovery (days): 21-28

Hepatic: Hepatic dysfunction, mild jaundice, and acute increase in transaminases can be produced

1% to 10%:

Cardiovascular: Cardiomegaly

Central nervous system: Dizziness, headache, somnolence, confusion, neuritis, malaise

Dermatologic: Skin freckling, itching, alopecia, cellulitis at injection site

Endocrine and metabolic: Hyperuricemia or uric acid nephropathy

Gastrointestinal: Esophagitis, diarrhea

Genitourinary: Urinary retention

Hematologic: Megaloblastic anemia

Hepatic: Hepatotoxicity

Local: Thrombophlebitis

Neuromuscular & skeletal: Myalgia, bone pain, peripheral neuropathy

Respiratory: Syndrome of sudden respiratory distress progressing to pulmonary edema, pneumonia

Miscellaneous: Sepsis

<1% (Limited to important or life-threatening symptoms): Pancreatitis

**BMT:**

Dermatologic: Rash, desquamation may occur following cytarabine and TBI

Gastrointestinal: Severe nausea and vomiting, mucositis, diarrhea

Neurologic:

Cerebellar toxicity: Nystagmus, dysarthria, dysdiadochokinesis, slurred speech

Cerebral toxicity: Somnolence, confusion

Ocular: Photophobia, excessive tearing, blurred vision, local discomfort, chemical conjunctivitis

Respiratory: Noncardiogenic pulmonary edema (onset 22-27 days following completion of therapy)

**Overdose/Toxicology** Symptoms of overdose include myelosuppression, megaloblastosis, nausea, vomiting, respiratory distress, and pulmonary edema. A syndrome of sudden respiratory distress progressing to pulmonary edema and cardiomegaly has been reported following high doses. Treatment is symptomatic and supportive.

**Pharmacodynamics/Kinetics**

**Distribution:** Widely and rapidly distributed since it enters the cells readily; crosses the blood-brain barrier, and CSF levels of 40% to 50% of the plasma level are reached

**Half-life Elimination:** Initial: 7-20 minutes; Terminal: 0.5-2.6 hours

**Metabolism:** Liver

**Excretion:** Urine

**Formulations**

Cytarabine hydrochloride:

Powder for injection: 100 mg, 500 mg, 1 g, 2 g

Powder for injection (Cytosar-U®): 100 mg, 500 mg, 1 g, 2 g

**Dosing**

**Adults:** I.V. bolus, IVPB, and continuous intravenous infusion doses of cytarabine are very different. Bolus doses are relatively well tolerated since the drug is rapidly metabolized. Continuous infusion uniformly results in myelosuppression. Refer to individual protocols.

Induction remission:

I.V.: 200 mg/m$^2$/day for 5 days at 2-week intervals

100-200 mg/m$^2$/day for 5- to 10-day therapy course or every day until remission

I.T.: 5-75 mg/m$^2$ every 2-7 days until CNS findings normalize

**or**

Maintenance remission:

I.V.: 70-200 mg/m$^2$/day for 2-5 days at monthly intervals

I.M., S.C.: 1-1.5 mg/kg single dose for maintenance at 1- to 4-week intervals

High-dose therapies:

Doses as high as 1-3 g/m$^2$ have been used for refractory or secondary leukemias or refractory non-Hodgkin's lymphoma.

Doses of 3 g/m$^2$ every 12 hours for up to 12 doses have been used

Bone marrow transplant: 1.5 g/m$^2$ continuous infusion over 48 hours

**Elderly:** Refer to adult dosing.

**Renal Impairment:** In one study, 76% of patients with a $Cl_{cr}$ <60 mL/minute experienced neurotoxicity. Dosage adjustment of high-dose therapy should be considered in patients with renal insufficiency.

**Hepatic Impairment:** Dose may need to be adjusted in patients with liver failure since cytarabine is partially detoxified in the liver.

**Administration**

**I.V.:** Can be administered I.M., IVP, I.V. infusion, or S.C. at a concentration not to exceed 100 mg/mL. I.V. may be administered either as a bolus, IVPB (high doses >500 mg/m$^2$) or continuous intravenous infusion (doses of 100-200 mg/m$^2$).

**I.V. Detail:** I.V. doses >200 mg/m$^2$ may produce conjunctivitis which can be ameliorated with prophylactic use of corticosteroid (0.1% dexamethasone) eye drops. Dexamethasone eye drops should be administered at 1-2 drops every 6 hours for 2-7 days after cytarabine is done.

**BMT only:** Risk of cerebellar toxicity increases with creatinine clearance <60 mL/minute, age older than 50 years, pre-existing CNS lesion, and alkaline phosphatase levels exceeding 3 times the upper limit of normal. Conjunctivitis is prevented and treated with saline or corticosteroid eye drops. As prophylaxis, eye drops should be started 6-12 hours before initiation of cytarabine and continued 24 hours following the last dose.

**Stability**

**Storage:** Store intact vials of powder at room temperature 15°C to 30°C (59°F to 86°F).

**Reconstitution: Warning:** Bacteriostastic diluent should **not** be used for the preparation of either high doses or intrathecal doses of cytarabine. Reconstitute with SWI, $D_5W$ or NS. Dilute to a concentration of 100 mg/mL as follows. Reconstituted solutions are stable for 48 hours at 15°C to 30°C.

100 mg vial = 1 mL

500 mg vial = 5 mL

1 g vial = 10 mL

2 g vial = 20 mL

Further dilution in $D_5W$ or NS is stable for 8 days at room temperature (25°C)

**Standard I.V. dilution:**

I.V. push: Dose/syringe (concentration: 100 mg/mL)

Maximum syringe size for IVP is 30 mL syringe and syringe should be ≤75% full

IVPB: Dose/100 mL $D_5W$ or NS

Continuous intravenous infusion: Dose/250-1000 mL $D_5W$ or NS

**Standard intrathecal dilutions:**

Dose/3-5 mL lactated Ringer's ± methotrexate (12 mg) ± hydrocortisone (15-50 mg)

Intrathecal solutions in 3-20 mL lactated Ringer's are stable for 7 days at room temperature (30°C); however, should be used within 24 hours due to sterility concerns.

(Continued)

## Cytarabine *(Continued)*

**Compatibility:**

**Standard I.V. dilution:**

Compatible with vincristine, potassium chloride, calcium, magnesium, and idarubicin.

Incompatible with 5-FU, gentamicin, heparin, insulin, methylprednisolone, nafcillin, oxacillin, and penicillin G sodium.

**Standard intrathecal dilutions:**

Compatible with methotrexate and hydrocortisone in lactated Ringer's or NS for 24 hours at room temperature (25°C).

See the Chemotherapy Compatibility Chart *on page 1311*.

**Monitoring Laboratory Tests** Liver function, CBC with differential and platelet count, serum creatinine, BUN, serum uric acid

**Additional Nursing Issues**

**Physical Assessment:** Monitor laboratory results prior to therapy and frequently during therapy. Monitor closely for adverse reactions (see Adverse Reactions, especially CNS changes that indicate cerebellar toxicity), ocular inflammation, respiratory or cardiac changes, acute pancreatitis, and thrombosis at site of infusion. **Pregnancy risk factor D** - assess knowledge/teach appropriate use of barrier contraceptives and the need to avoid pregnancy during therapy and 4 months following therapy. Breast-feeding is not recommended.

**Patient Information/Instruction:** This drug can only be given by infusion or injection. During therapy maintain adequate hydration (2-3 L/day of fluids unless instructed to restrict fluid intake). You will be more susceptible to infection; avoid crowds and exposure to infection. Do not have any vaccinations without consulting prescriber. Small frequent meals, frequent mouth care, sucking lozenges, or chewing gum may reduce incidence of nausea or vomiting or loss of appetite. If these measures are ineffective, consult prescriber for antiemetic medication. Report immediately any signs of CNS changes or change in gait, easy bruising or bleeding, yellowing of eyes or skin, change in color of urine or blackened stool, respiratory difficulty, or palpitations. **Pregnancy/breast-feeding precautions:** Do not get pregnant while taking this medication; use appropriate barrier contraceptive measures during and 4 months after therapy to prevent possible harm to the fetus. Breast-feeding is not recommended.

**Additional Information** Supplied with diluent containing benzyl alcohol, which should not be used when preparing either high-dose or I.T. doses.

♦ **Cytochrome P-450 Enzymes and Drug Metabolism** *see page 1405*

♦ **CytoGam™** *see* Cytomegalovirus Immune Globulin Intravenous, Human *on this page*

## Cytomegalovirus Immune Globulin Intravenous, Human

(sye toe meg a low VYE rus i MYUN GLOB yoo lin in tra VEE nus, HYU man)

**U.S. Brand Names** CytoGam™

**Synonyms** CMV-IGIV

**Therapeutic Category** Immune Globulin

**Pregnancy Risk Factor** C

**Lactation** Excretion in breast milk unknown

**Use** Attenuation of primary CMV disease associated with kidney transplantation

**Mechanism of Action/Effect** CMV-IGIV is a preparation of immunoglobulin G derived from pooled healthy blood donors with a high titer of CMV antibodies; administration provides a passive source of antibodies against cytomegalovirus

**Contraindications** Hypersensitivity to this or any other human immunoglobulin preparations; patients with selective immunoglobulin A deficiency (↑ potential for anaphylaxis)

**Warnings** Studies indicate that product carries little or no risk for transmission of HIV. Pregnancy factor C.

**Drug Interactions**

**Decreased Effect:** May inactivate live virus vaccines (eg, measles, mumps, rubella). Defer live virus vaccines during therapy and for 3 months following therapy.

**Adverse Reactions**

1% to 10%:

Cardiovascular: Flushing of the face

Gastrointestinal: Nausea, vomiting

Neuromuscular & skeletal: Muscle cramps, back pain

Respiratory: Wheezing

Miscellaneous: Sweating

<1% (Limited to important or life-threatening symptoms): Tightness in the chest

**Formulations** Powder for injection, lyophilized, detergent treated: 2500 mg ± 250 mg (50 mL)

**Dosing**

**Adults:** I.V.: Dosing schedule:

Initial (within 72 hours after transplant): 150 mg/kg/dose

2 weeks after transplant: 100 mg/kg/dose

4, 6, 8 weeks after transplant: 100 mg/kg/dose

12 and 16 weeks after transplant: 50 mg/kg/dose

**Elderly:** Refer to adult dosing.

**Administration**

**I.V.:** For I.V. use only. Administer as separate infusion. Infuse beginning at 15 mg/kg/hour, then increase to 30 mg/kg/hour after 30 minutes if no untoward reactions. May titrate up to 60 mg/kg/hour. Do not administer faster than 75 mL/hour.

**Stability**

**Reconstitution:** Use reconstituted product within 6 hours.

**Additional Nursing Issues**

**Physical Assessment:** Assess for history of previous allergic reactions (see Contraindications). See Administration for safe infusion. Monitor vital signs during infusion and observe for adverse or allergic reactions (see Adverse Reactions). Teach patient adverse symptoms to report. **Pregnancy risk factor C** - benefits of use should outweigh possible risks. Note breast-feeding caution.

**Patient Information/Instruction:** This medication can only be administered by infusion. You will be monitored closely during the infusion. If you experience nausea ask for assistance, do not get up alone. Do not have any vaccination for the next 3 months without consulting prescriber. Immediately report chills, muscle cramping, low back pain, chest pain or tightness, or difficulty breathing. **Pregnancy/breast-feeding precautions:** Inform prescriber if you are or intend to be pregnant. Consult prescriber if breast-feeding.

- **Cytomel® Oral** *see* Liothyronine *on page 679*
- **Cytosar-U®** *see* Cytarabine *on page 322*
- **Cytosine Arabinosine Hydrochloride** *see* Cytarabine *on page 322*
- **Cytotec®** *see* Misoprostol *on page 776*
- **Cytovene®** *see* Ganciclovir *on page 526*
- **Cytoxan® Injection** *see* Cyclophosphamide *on page 313*
- **Cytoxan® Oral** *see* Cyclophosphamide *on page 313*
- **25-$D_3$** *see* Calcifediol *on page 180*
- **D-3-Mercaptovaline** *see* Penicillamine *on page 894*
- **D4T** *see* Stavudine *on page 1073*
- **Dabex** *see* Metformin *on page 734*

## Dacarbazine (da KAR ba zeen)

**U.S. Brand Names** DTIC-Dome®

**Synonyms** DIC; Imidazole Carboxamide

**Therapeutic Category** Antineoplastic Agent, Alkylating Agent

**Pregnancy Risk Factor** C

**Lactation** Excretion in breast milk unknown/not recommended

**Use** Treatment of malignant melanoma, Hodgkin's disease, soft-tissue sarcomas, fibrosarcomas, rhabdomyosarcoma, islet cell carcinoma, medullary carcinoma of the thyroid, and neuroblastoma

**Mechanism of Action/Effect** Inhibits DNA/RNA and protein synthesis; cytotoxic

**Contraindications** Hypersensitivity to dacarbazine or any component

**Warnings** The U.S. Food and Drug Administration (FDA) currently recommends that procedures for proper handling and disposal of antineoplastic agents be considered. Use with caution in patients with bone marrow depression. In patients with renal and/or hepatic impairment, dosage reduction may be necessary. Avoid extravasation of the drug. Pregnancy factor C.

Dacarbazine preparation should be performed in a Class II laminar flow biologic safety cabinet. Personnel should be wearing surgical gloves and a closed front surgical gown with knit cuffs. Appropriate safety equipment is recommended for preparation, administration, and disposal of antineoplastics. If dacarbazine contacts the skin, wash and flush thoroughly with water.

**Adverse Reactions**

>10%:

Local: Pain and burning at infusion site

**Irritant chemotherapy**

Gastrointestinal: Anorexia; moderate to severe nausea and vomiting in 90% of patients and lasting up to 12 hours after administration; nausea and vomiting are dose-related and occur more frequently when given as a one-time dose, as opposed to a less intensive 5-day course; diarrhea may also occur

Hematologic: Anemia, leukopenia, thrombocytopenia

Emetic potential:

<500 mg: Moderately high (60% to 90%)

≥500 mg: High (>90%)

Time course of nausea/vomiting: Onset: 1-2 hours; Duration: 2-4 hours

1% to 10%:

Cardiovascular: Facial flushing

Central nervous system: Headache

Dermatologic: Alopecia, rash

Flu-like effects: Fever, malaise, headache, myalgia, and sinus congestion may last up to several days after administration

Gastrointestinal: Anorexia, metallic taste

Hematologic: Myelosuppressive: Mild to moderate is common and dose-related dose-limiting toxicity

WBC: Mild (primarily leukocytes)

Platelets: Mild

Onset (days): 7

Nadir (days): 21-25

Recovery (days): 21-28

Neuromuscular & skeletal: Paresthesias

Respiratory: Sinus congestion

(Continued)

## Dacarbazine *(Continued)*

<1% (Limited to important or life-threatening symptoms): Orthostatic hypotension, polyneuropathy, headache, seizures, photosensitivity reactions, alopecia, elevated LFTs, hepatic vein thrombosis and hepatocellular necrosis

**BMT:**

Cardiovascular: Hypotension (infusion-related)

Gastrointestinal: Severe nausea and vomiting

**Overdose/Toxicology** Symptoms of overdose include myelosuppression and diarrhea. There are no known antidotes and treatment is symptomatic and supportive.

**Pharmacodynamics/Kinetics**

**Protein Binding:** Minimal (5%)

**Distribution:** Exceeding total body water and suggesting binding to some tissue (probably the liver)

**Half-life Elimination:** Half-life (biphasic): Initial: 20-40 minutes; Terminal: 5 hours

**Metabolism:** Extensive in the liver, and hepatobiliary excretion is probably of some importance; metabolites may also have an antineoplastic effect

**Excretion:** Hepatobiliary; ~30% to 50% of dose excreted unchanged in the urine by tubular secretion

**Onset:** I.V.: 18-24 days

**Formulations** Injection: 100 mg (10 mL, 20 mL); 200 mg (20 mL, 30 mL); 500 mg (50 mL)

**Dosing**

**Adults:** I.V. (refer to individual protocols):

Malignant melanoma: 2-4.5 mg/kg/day for 10 days, repeat in 4 weeks **or** may use 250 mg/m$^2$/day for 5 days, repeat in 3 weeks

Hodgkin's disease: 150 mg/m$^2$/day for 5 days, repeat every 4 weeks **or** 375 mg/m$^2$ on day 1, repeat in 15 days of each 28-day cycle in combination with other agents **or** 375 mg/m$^2$ repeated in 15 days of each 28-day cycle

High dose BMT: I.V.: 1-3 g/m$^2$; maximum dose as a single agent: 3.38 g/m$^2$; generally combined with other high-dose chemotherapeutic drugs.

**Elderly:** Refer to adult dosing.

**Renal Impairment:** Adjustment is warranted.

**Hepatic Impairment:** Monitor closely for signs of toxicity.

**Administration**

**I.V.:** Irritant. Infuse over 30-60 minutes.

**I.V. Detail:** Rapid infusion may cause severe venous irritation.

**Extravasation management:** Local pain, burning sensation, and irritation at the injection site may be relieved by local application of hot packs. If extravasation occurs, apply cold packs. Protect exposed tissue from light following extravasation.

**BMT only:** Doses of 6591 mg/m$^2$ have been administered, although hypotension is considered the nonhematologic dose-limiting side effect for doses >3380 mg/m$^2$. Infusion-related hypotension may be secondary to calcium chelation by citric acid in formulation.

**Stability**

**Storage:** Store intact vials under refrigeration (2°C to 8°C) and protect from light. Vials are stable for 4 weeks at room temperature.

**Reconstitution:** Reconstitute with a minimum of 2 mL (100 mg vial) or 4 mL (200 mg vial) of SWI, $D_5W$, or NS. Dilute to a concentration of 10 mg/mL as follows. Reconstituted solution is stable for 24 hours at room temperature (20°C) and 96 hours under refrigeration (4°C):

100 mg vial = 9.9 mL

200 mg vial = 19.7 mL

500 mg vial = 49.5 mL

Further dilution in 200-500 mL of $D_5W$ or NS is stable for 24 hours at room temperature and protected from light. Decomposed drug turns pink.

**Standard I.V. dilution:** Dose/250-500 mL $D_5W$ or NS

Stable for 24 hours at room temperature and refrigeration (4°C) when protected from light.

**Compatibility:** See the Chemotherapy Compatibility Chart *on page 1311*.

**Monitoring Laboratory Tests** CBC with differential, platelet count, liver function

**Additional Nursing Issues**

**Physical Assessment:** Monitor laboratory results prior to therapy and frequently during therapy. Monitor I.V. site closely for extravasation. Stop infusion immediately if extravasation occurs. Monitor for and teach patient to monitor for adverse reactions as identified above. Emetic potential is moderately high; restrict oral intake 4-6 hours prior to infusion and start antiemetic medication before starting infusion. Monitor nutritional and hydration status frequently during therapy. Instruct patient on appropriate interventions to reduce adverse effects and symptoms to report. **Pregnancy risk factor C** - benefits of use should outweigh possible risks. Breast-feeding is not recommended.

**Patient Information/Instruction:** Limit oral intake for 4-6 hours before therapy. Do not use alcohol, aspirin-containing products, and OTC medications without consulting prescriber. It is important to maintain adequate nutrition and hydration (2-3 L/day of fluids unless instructed to restrict fluid intake) during therapy; frequent small meals may help. You may experience nausea or vomiting (frequent small meals, frequent mouth care, sucking lozenges, or chewing gum may help). If this is ineffective, consult prescriber for antiemetic medication. You may experience loss of hair (reversible); you will be more susceptible to infection (avoid crowds and exposure to infection as much as possible); you will be more sensitive to sunlight; use sunblock, wear protective clothing and dark glasses, or avoid direct exposure to sunlight. Flu-like symptoms (eg, malaise, fever, myalgia) may occur 1 week after infusion and persist for 1-3 weeks; consult prescriber for severe symptoms. Report fever, chills, unusual bruising or bleeding, signs of infection, excessive fatigue, yellowing of eyes or skin, or change in color of urine or stool. **Pregnancy/breast-feeding precautions:** Inform prescriber if you are or intend to be pregnant. Breast-feeding is not recommended.

♦ **Dacodyl®** *see page 1294*

## Dactinomycin (dak ti noe MYE sin)

**U.S. Brand Names** Cosmegen®

**Synonyms** ACT; Actinomycin D

**Therapeutic Category** Antineoplastic Agent, Antibiotic

**Pregnancy Risk Factor** C

**Lactation** Excretion in breast milk unknown/contraindicated

**Use** Treatment of testicular tumors, melanoma, choriocarcinoma, Wilms' tumor, neuroblastoma, retinoblastoma, rhabdomyosarcoma, uterine sarcomas, Ewing's sarcoma, Kaposi's sarcoma, and soft tissue sarcoma

**Mechanism of Action/Effect** Causes cell death by inhibiting messenger RNA

**Contraindications** Hypersensitivity to dactinomycin or any component; patients with chickenpox or herpes zoster

**Warnings** The U.S. Food and Drug Administration (FDA) currently recommends that procedures for proper handling and disposal of antineoplastic agents be considered. Drug is extremely irritating to tissues and must be administered I.V. If extravasation occurs during I.V. use, severe damage to soft tissues will occur. Use with caution in patients who have received radiation therapy or in the presence of hepatobiliary dysfunction. Reduce dosage in patients who are receiving radiation therapy simultaneously. Pregnancy factor C.

Dactinomycin preparation should be performed in a Class II laminar flow biologic safety cabinet. Personnel should be wearing surgical gloves and a closed front surgical gown with knit cuffs. Appropriate safety equipment is recommended for preparation, administration, and disposal of antineoplastics. If dactinomycin contacts the skin, wash and flush thoroughly with water.

**Drug Interactions**

**Increased Effect/Toxicity:** Dactinomycin potentiates the effects of radiation therapy. Radiation may cause skin erythema which may become severe. Also associated with GI toxicity.

**Adverse Reactions**

>10%:

- Central nervous system: Unusual fatigue, malaise, fever
- Dermatologic: Alopecia (reversible), skin eruptions, acne, increased pigmentation of previously irradiated skin
- Endocrine & metabolic: Hypocalcemia
- Gastrointestinal: **Highly emetogenic**
  - Severe nausea and vomiting occurs in most patients and persists for up to 24 hours; stomatitis, anorexia, abdominal pain, esophagitis, diarrhea
  - Time course of nausea/vomiting: Onset: 2-5 hours; Duration: 4-24 hours
- Hematologic: Myelosuppressive: Dose-limiting toxicity; anemia, aplastic anemia, agranulocytosis, pancytopenia, leukopenia, thrombocytopenia
  - WBC: Moderate
  - Platelets: Moderate
  - Onset (days): 7
  - Nadir (days): 14-21
  - Recovery (days): 21-28
- Local: **Vesicant chemotherapy**

1% to 10%: Gastrointestinal: Diarrhea, mucositis

<1% (Limited to important or life-threatening symptoms): Hepatitis, liver function tests abnormalities

**Overdose/Toxicology** Symptoms of overdose include myelosuppression, nausea, vomiting, glossitis, and oral ulceration. There are no known antidotes and treatment is symptomatic and supportive.

**Pharmacodynamics/Kinetics**

**Distribution:** Poor penetration into CSF; crosses the placenta; high concentrations found in bone marrow and tumor cells, submaxillary gland, liver, and kidney

**Half-life Elimination:** 36 hours

**Time to Peak:** I.V.: Within 2-5 minutes

**Metabolism:** Minimal

**Excretion:** Urine

**Formulations** Powder for injection, lyophilized: 0.5 mg

**Dosing**

**Adults:** Refer to individual protocols.

**Calculation of the dosage for obese or edematous patients should be on the basis of surface area in an effort to relate dosage to lean body mass.**

I.V.:

15 mcg/kg/day **or** 400-600 mcg/m$^2$/day (maximum: 500 mcg) for 5 days, may repeat every 3-6 weeks **or**

2.5 mg/m$^2$ given in divided doses over 1-week period and repeated at 2-week intervals **or**

0.75-2 mg/m$^2$ as a single dose given at intervals of 1-4 weeks have been used

(Continued)

## Dactinomycin *(Continued)*

**Elderly:** Refer to adult dosing.

**Administration**

**I.V.:** Vesicant. Infuse over 10-15 minutes.

**I.V. Detail:** Care should be taken to avoid extravasation. Administer slow I.V. push over 10-15 minutes. An in-line cellulose membrane filter should not be used during administration of dactinomycin solutions. Do not give I.M. or S.C. Avoid extravasation. Extremely damaging to soft tissue and will cause a severe local reaction if extravasation occurs.

**Extravasation management:** Apply ice immediately for 30-60 minutes, then alternate off/on every 15 minutes for 1 day. Data is not currently available regarding potential antidotes for dactinomycin.

**Stability**

**Storage:** Store intact vials at room temperature (30°C) and protect from light. Storage at high temperatures (up to 50°C) for up to 2 weeks is permissible.

**Reconstitution:** Dilute with 1.1 mL of preservative-free SWI to yield a final concentration of 500 mcg/mL. Do not use preservative diluent as precipitation may occur. Solution is chemically stable for 24 hours at room temperature (25°C). Significant binding of the drug occurs with micrometer nitrocellulose filter materials.

**Standard I.V. dilution:**

I.V. push: Dose/syringe (500 mcg/mL)

IVPB: Dose/50 mL $D_5W$ or NS

Stable for 24 hours at room temperature.

**Compatibility:** Compatible with $D_5W$ or NS. See the Chemotherapy Compatibility Chart *on page 1311.*

**Monitoring Laboratory Tests** CBC with differential and platelet count, liver and renal function

**Additional Nursing Issues**

**Physical Assessment:** Monitor laboratory results prior to therapy and frequently during therapy. Monitor I.V. site closely for extravasation. Stop infusion immediately if extravasation occurs. Monitor for and teach patient to monitor for adverse reactions as identified above. Emetic potential is very high; restrict oral intake 4-6 hours prior to infusion and start antiemetic medication before starting infusion. Monitor nutritional and hydration status frequently during therapy. Instruct patient on appropriate interventions to reduce adverse effects and symptoms to report. **Pregnancy risk factor C** - benefits of use should outweigh possible risks. Breast-feeding is contraindicated.

**Patient Information/Instruction:** Limit oral intake for 4-6 hours before therapy. Do not use alcohol, aspirin-containing products and OTC medications without consulting prescriber. It is important to maintain adequate nutrition and hydration (2-3 L/day of fluids unless instructed to restrict fluid intake) during therapy; frequent small meals may help. You may experience nausea or vomiting (frequent small meals, frequent mouth care, sucking lozenges, or chewing gum may help). If this is ineffective consult prescriber for antiemetic medication. You may experience loss of hair (reversible); you will be more susceptible to infection (avoid crowds and exposure to infection as much as possible); you will be more sensitive to sunlight; use sunblock, wear protective clothing and dark glasses, or avoid direct exposure to sunlight. Flu-like symptoms (eg, malaise, fever, myalgia) may occur 1 week after infusion and persist for 1-3 weeks; consult prescriber for severe symptoms. Report fever, chills, unusual bruising or bleeding, signs of infection, excessive fatigue, yellowing of eyes or skin, or change in color of urine or stool. **Pregnancy/breast-feeding precautions:** Inform prescriber if you are or intend to be pregnant. Do not breast-feed.

- **Dafloxen®** *see* Naproxen *on page 807*
- **D.A.II® Tablet** *see page 1306*
- **Dairy Ease®** *see page 1294*
- **Dakin's Solution** *see* Sodium Hypochlorite Solution *on page 1063*
- **Dakrina® Ophthalmic Solution** *see page 1294*
- **Daktarin** *see* Miconazole *on page 767*
- **Dalacin® C [Hydrochloride]** *see* Clindamycin *on page 282*
- **Dalacin® C** *see* Clindamycin *on page 282*
- **Dalalone L.A.®** *see* Dexamethasone *on page 346*
- **Dallergy®** *see page 1306*
- **Dallergy-D® Syrup** *see page 1294*
- **Dalmane®** *see* Flurazepam *on page 507*
- ***d*-Alpha Tocopherol** *see* Vitamin E *on page 1218*

## Dalteparin (dal TE pa rin)

**U.S. Brand Names** Fragmin®

**Therapeutic Category** Low Molecular Weight Heparin

**Pregnancy Risk Factor** B

**Lactation** Excretion in breast milk unknown/use caution

**Use** Prevention of deep vein thrombosis which may lead to pulmonary embolism, in patients requiring abdominal surgery who are at risk for thromboembolism complications (ie, patients >40 years of age, obese, patients with malignancy, history of deep vein thrombosis or pulmonary embolism, and surgical procedures requiring general anesthesia and lasting longer than 30 minutes). Prevention of DVT in patients undergoing hip surgery.

**Mechanism of Action/Effect** Low molecular weight heparin analog; the commercial product contains 3% to 15% heparin; has been shown to inhibit both factor Xa and factor IIa (thrombin), however, the antithrombotic effect of dalteparin is characterized by a higher ratio of antifactor Xa to antifactor IIa activity (ratio = 4)

**Contraindications** Hypersensitivity to dalteparin or other low-molecular weight heparins, heparin, or pork products; cerebrovascular disease or other active hemorrhage; cerebral aneurysm; severe uncontrolled hypertension

**Warnings** Use with caution in patients with pre-existing thrombocytopenia, recent childbirth, subacute bacterial endocarditis, peptic ulcer disease, pericarditis or pericardial effusion, liver or renal function impairment, recent lumbar puncture, vasculitis, concurrent use of aspirin (increased bleeding risk), previous hypersensitivity to heparin, or heparin-associated thrombocytopenia. Patients with recent or anticipated epidural or spinal anesthesia are at risk of developing spinal or epidural hematoma; paralysis may result.

**Drug Interactions**

**Increased Effect/Toxicity:** Caution should be used when using aspirin, other platelet inhibitors, and oral anticoagulants in combination with dalteparin due to an increased risk of bleeding.

**Effects on Lab Values** ↑ AST, ALT levels

**Adverse Reactions**

1% to 10%:

- Central nervous system: Allergic fever
- Dermatologic: Pruritus, rash, bullous eruption, skin necrosis
- Hematologic: Bleeding, wound hematoma
- Local: Pain at injection site, injection site hematoma, injection site reactions
- Miscellaneous: Anaphylactoid reactions, allergic reactions

<1% (Limited to important or life-threatening symptoms): Thrombocytopenia

Case reports of long-term or permanent paralysis have occurred when used in association with epidural or spinal anesthesia (due to hematoma). Risk is increased by indwelling catheters or concomitant use of other drugs which alter hemostasis (NSAIDs, anticoagulants, or platelet inhibitors).

**Pharmacodynamics/Kinetics**

**Metabolism:** Liver

**Excretion:** Urine

**Onset:** 1-2 hours

**Duration:** >12 hours

**Formulations** Injection: Prefilled syringe: 2500 units (16 mg) in 0.2 mL

**Dosing**

**Adults:** S.C.:

Abdominal surgery:

- Low-moderate risk patient: 2500 units 1-2 hours prior to surgery, then once daily for 5-10 days postoperatively
- High risk patient: 5000 units 1-2 hours prior to surgery and then once daily for 5-10 days postoperatively

Hip surgery:

- 2500 units 2 hours prior to surgery followed by 2500 units on the evening of the day of surgery (at least 6 hours after the first dose - omit evening dose if surgery if performed in the evening). Begin dose of 5000 units once daily on the first postoperative day. Usual duration 5-10 days (up to 14 days).
- Alternatively, a dose of 5000 units may be administered on the evening before surgery, followed by 5000 units once daily, starting on the evening of the day of surgery. Usual duration 5-10 days (up to 14 days).

**Elderly:** Refer to adult dosing.

**Administration**

**I.M.: Do not give I.M.**

**Other:** Administer deep S.C. only, alternate injection site R → L anterolateral/posterolateral abdominal wall. Do not give I.M. Apply pressure to injection site. Do not massage.

**Stability**

**Storage:** Store at temperatures ≤25°C.

**Monitoring Laboratory Tests** Periodic CBC including platelet count, stool occult blood; monitoring of PT and PTT is not necessary.

**Additional Nursing Issues**

**Physical Assessment:** Assess effectiveness and interactions of other medications (see Drug Interactions). See Warnings/Precautions and Contraindications for use cautions. Monitor effectiveness of therapy, laboratory tests (see above) and adverse response (eg, thrombolytic reactions - see Adverse Reactions and Overdose/Toxicology). Assess knowledge/teach patient appropriate use, possible side effects and appropriate interventions (eg, bleeding precautions), and adverse symptoms to report. Note breast-feeding caution.

**Patient Information/Instruction:** This drug can only be administered by injection. You may have a tendency to bleed easily while taking this drug; brush teeth with soft brush, floss with waxed floss, use electric razor, avoid scissors or sharp knives and potentially harmful activities. Report unusual fever; unusual bleeding or bruising (bleeding gums, nosebleed, blood in urine, dark stool); pain in joints or back; severe head pain; skin rash; or redness, swelling, or pain at injection site. **Breast-feeding precautions:** Consult prescriber if breast-feeding.

**Pregnancy Issues:** Multiple-dose vials contain benzyl alcohol (avoid in pregnant women due to association with fatal syndrome in premature infants).

**Related Information**

Low Molecular Weight Heparins Comparison *on page 1395*

♦ **Damason-P®** *see* Hydrocodone and Aspirin *on page 570*

## Danaparoid (da NAP a roid)

**U.S. Brand Names** Orgaran®

**Therapeutic Category** Anticoagulant; Low Molecular Weight Heparin

**Pregnancy Risk Factor** B

**Lactation** Excretion in breast milk unknown/compatible

**Use**

Unlabeled use: Systemic anticoagulation for patients with heparin-induced Prevention of postoperative deep vein thrombosis following elective hip replacement surgery

**Unlabeled use:** System anticoagulation for patients with heparin-induced thrombocytopenia: Factor Xa inhibition is used to monitor degree of anticoagulation if necessary

**Contraindications** Hypersensitivity to danaparoid or known hypersensitivity to pork products; patients with severe hemorrhagic diathesis including active major bleeding, hemorrhagic stroke in the acute phase, hemophilia, and idiopathic thrombocytopenic purpura; Type II thrombocytopenia associated with a positive *in vitro* test for antiplatelet antibody in the presence of danaparoid

**Warnings** Do not administer intramuscularly. Use with extreme caution in patients with a history of bacterial endocarditis, hemorrhagic stroke, recent CNS or ophthalmological surgery, bleeding diathesis, uncontrolled arterial hypertension, or a history of recent GI ulceration and hemorrhage. Danaparoid shows a low cross-sensitivity with antiplatelet antibodies in individuals with Type II heparin-induced thrombocytopenia. This product contains sodium sulfite which may cause allergic-type reactions, including anaphylactic symptoms and life-threatening asthmatic episodes in susceptible people; this is seen more frequently in asthmatics. Patients with recent or anticipated epidural or spinal anesthesia are at risk of developing spinal or epidural hematoma; paralysis may result.

**Drug Interactions**

**Increased Effect/Toxicity:** Increased toxicity with oral anticoagulants and platelet inhibitors.

**Adverse Reactions** 1% to 10%:

Cardiovascular: Peripheral edema, generalized edema
Central nervous system: Fever, insomnia, headache, dizziness
Dermatologic: Rash, pruritus
Gastrointestinal: Nausea, constipation, vomiting
Genitourinary: Urinary tract infections, urinary retention
Hematologic: Anemia, hemorrhage, hematoma
Local: Injection site pain
Neuromuscular & skeletal: Joint disorder, weakness

Case reports of long-term or permanent paralysis have occurred when used in association with epidural or spinal anesthesia (due to hematoma). Risk is increased by indwelling catheters or concomitant use of other drugs which alter hemostasis (NSAIDs, anticoagulants, or platelet inhibitors).

**Overdose/Toxicology** Symptoms of overdose include hemorrhage. Protamine zinc has been used to reverse effects, but the effects of danaproid are not effectively antagonized.

**Adult Danaparoid Treatment Dosing Regimens**

| | Body Weight (kg) | I.V. Bolus aFXaU | Long–Term Infusion aFXaU | Level of aFXaU/mL | Monitoring |
|---|---|---|---|---|---|
| **Deep Vein Thrombosis OR Acute Pulmonary Embolism** | <55<br>55-90<br>>90 | 1250<br>2500<br>3750 | 400 units/h over 4 h then 300 units/h over 4 h, then 150-200 units/h maintenance dose | 0.5-0.8 | Days 1-3 daily, then every alternate day |
| **Deep Vein Thrombosis OR Pulmonary Embolism >5 d old** | <90<br>>90 | 1250<br>1250 | S.C.: 3 x 750/d<br>S.C.: 3 x 1250/d | <0.5 | Not necessary |
| **Embolectomy** | <90 | 2500 preoperatively | S.C.: 2 x 1250/d postoperatively | <0.4 | Not necessary |
| | >90 and high risk | 2500 preoperatively | 750 units/20 mL NaCl perioperatively, arterial irrigation if necessary | 0.5-0.8 | Days 1-3 daily, then every alternate day |
| **Peripheral Arterial Bypass** | | 2500 preoperatively | 150-200 units/h | 0.5-0.8 | Days 1-3 daily, then every alternate day |
| **Cardiac Catheter** | <90<br>>90 | 2500 preoperatively<br>3750 preoperatively | | | |
| **Surgery (excluding vascular)** | | | S.C.: 750, 1-4 h preoperatively<br>S.C.: 750, 2-5 h postoperatively, then 2 x 750/d | <0.35 | Not necessary |

**Pharmacodynamics/Kinetics**

**Half-life Elimination:** Plasma: Mean terminal half-life: ~24 hours

**Excretion:** Urine

**Onset:** Maximum antifactor Xa and antithrombin (antifactor IIa) activities occur 2-5 hours after S.C. administration

**Formulations** Injection, as sodium: 750 anti-Xa units/0.6 mL

**Dosing**

**Adults:** S.C.:

Adults: 750 anti-Xa units twice daily; beginning 1-4 hours before surgery and then not sooner than 2 hours after surgery and every 12 hours until the risk of DVT has diminished, the average duration of therapy is 7-10 days

Treatment: See table.

S.C.: 750 anti-Xa units twice daily; beginning 1-4 hours before surgery and then not sooner than 2 hours after surgery and every 12 hours until the risk of DVT has diminished; the average duration of therapy is 7-10 days.

**Elderly:** Dose adjustment may be necessary in elderly patients with severe renal impairment.

**Renal Impairment:** Adjustment may be necessary in patients with severe renal impairment. Patients with serum creatinine levels ≥2.0 mg/dL should be carefully monitored.

S.C.:

Hemodialysis: See table

**Haemodialysis With Danaparoid Sodium**

| **Dialysis on alternate days** | **Dosage prior to dialysis in aFXaU (dosage for body wt <55 kg)** | |
|---|---|---|
| First dialysis | 3750 (2500) | |
| Second dialysis | 3750 (2000) | |
| **Further dialysis:** | | |
| **aFXa level before dialysis (eg, day 5)** | **Bolus before next dialysis, aFXaU (eg, day 7)** | **aFXa level during dialysis** |
| <0.3 | 3000 (<55 kg 2000) | 0.5-0.8 |
| 0.3-0.35 | 2500 (2000) | |
| 0.35-0.4 | 2000 (1500) | |
| >0.4 | 0 | |
| | if fibrin strands occur, 1500 aFXaU I.V. | |
| **Monitoring: 30 minutes before dialysis and after 4 hours of dialysis** | | |
| **Daily Dialysis** | | |
| First dialysis | 3750 (2500) | |
| Second dialysis | 2500 (2000) | |
| Further dialyses | See above | |
| As with "dialysis on alternate days", always take the aFXa activity preceding the previous dialysis as a basis for the current dosage. | | |

**Administration**

**I.M.:** Do not administer I.M.

**Other:** Administer by subcutaneous injection, **not** I.M. Have patient lie down and administer by deep S.C. injection using a fine needle (25- to 26-gauge). Rotate sites of injection.

**Stability**

**Storage:** Store intact vials or ampuls under refrigeration

**Monitoring Laboratory Tests** Platelets, occult blood, anti-Xa activity, if available; the monitoring of PT and/or PTT is not necessary.

**Additional Nursing Issues**

**Physical Assessment:** Assess effectiveness and interactions of other medications (see Drug Interactions). See Warnings/Precautions and Contraindications for use cautions. Monitor effectiveness of therapy, laboratory tests (see above) and adverse response (eg, thrombolytic reactions - see Adverse Reactions and Overdose/Toxicology). Assess knowledge/teach patient appropriate use, possible side effects and appropriate interventions (eg, bleeding precautions), and adverse symptoms to report.

**Patient Information/Instruction:** This drug can only be administered by injection. You may have a tendency to bleed easily while taking this drug; brush teeth with soft brush, floss with waxed floss, use electric razor, avoid scissors or sharp knives and potentially harmful activities. Report unusual swelling of extremities or sudden increase in weight; unusual fever; persistent nausea, vomiting, or GI upset; unusual bleeding or bruising (bleeding gums, nosebleed, blood in urine, dark stool); pain in joints or back; pain or itching on urination; skin rash; or redness, swelling, or pain at injection site.

**Geriatric Considerations:** Evaluation of elderly's creatinine serum concentrations is important before initiating therapy.

**Related Information**

Low Molecular Weight Heparins Comparison *on page 1395*

## Danazol (DA na zole)

**U.S. Brand Names** Danocrine®

**Therapeutic Category** Androgen

**Pregnancy Risk Factor** X

**Lactation** Enters breast milk/not recommended

**Use** Treatment of endometriosis, fibrocystic breast disease, and hereditary angioedema

**Mechanism of Action/Effect** Suppresses pituitary output of follicle-stimulating hormone and luteinizing hormone that causes regression and atrophy of normal and ectopic endometrial tissue; decreases rate of growth of abnormal breast tissue; reduces attacks associated with hereditary angioedema by increasing levels of C4 component of complement

**Contraindications** Hypersensitivity to danazol or any component; undiagnosed genital bleeding; significant renal, hepatic, or cardiac impairment; pregnancy

**Warnings** Use with caution in patients with seizure disorders, migraine, impaired hepatic function, renal, or cardiac disease.

**Drug Interactions**

**Cytochrome P-450 Effect:** CYP3A3/4 enzyme inhibitor

**Increased Effect/Toxicity:** When used with insulin, the glucose lowering effects of insulin may be enhanced requiring a dose reduction of insulin. Warfarin and danazol may enhance the anticoagulant effects of warfarin leading to toxicity. Carbamazepine and danazol may result in increased carbamazepine toxicity.

**Adverse Reactions**

>10%:

Cardiovascular: Edema

Dermatologic: Oily skin, acne, hirsutism

Endocrine & metabolic: Fluid retention, breakthrough bleeding, irregular menstrual periods, decreased breast size

Gastrointestinal: Weight gain

Hepatic: Hepatic impairment

Miscellaneous: Voice deepening

1% to 10%:

Endocrine & metabolic: Virilization, androgenic effects, amenorrhea, hypoestrogenism

Neuromuscular & skeletal: Weakness

<1% (Limited to important or life-threatening symptoms): Benign intracranial hypertension, skin rashes, photosensitivity; Stevens-Johnson syndrome leukocytosis, cholestatic jaundice, hepatic dysfunction

**Pharmacodynamics/Kinetics**

**Half-life Elimination:** 4.5 hours (variable)

**Time to Peak:** Within 2 hours

**Metabolism:** Liver

**Excretion:** Urine

**Onset:** Within 4 weeks following daily doses

**Formulations** Capsule: 50 mg, 100 mg, 200 mg

**Dosing**

**Adults:** Oral:

Endometriosis: 100-400 mg twice daily for 3-6 months (may extend to 9 months)

Fibrocystic breast disease: 50-200 mg twice daily for 2-6 months

Hereditary angioedema: 400-600 mg/day in 2-3 divided doses

**Monitoring Laboratory Tests** Liver and renal function

**Additional Nursing Issues**

**Physical Assessment:** Assess effectiveness and interactions of other medications (see Drug Interactions, eg, anticoagulants and hypoglycemic agents). See Warnings/Precautions and Contraindications for use cautions. Monitor effectiveness of therapy, laboratory tests, and adverse response (see Adverse Reactions and Overdose/Toxicology). Assess knowledge/teach patient appropriate use, possible side effects and appropriate interventions, and adverse symptoms to report. **Pregnancy risk factor X** - determine that patient is not pregnant before beginning treatment and do not give to women of childbearing age or male having intercourse with women of childbearing age unless capable of complying with barrier contraceptive measures 1 month prior to therapy, during therapy, and for 1 month following therapy. Teach patients good breast exam technique. Breast-feeding is not recommended during therapy and for 1 month following therapy.

**Patient Information/Instruction:** Take as directed; do not discontinue without consulting prescriber. Therapy may take up to several months depending on purpose for therapy. Diabetics should monitor serum glucose closely and notify prescriber of changes; this medication can alter hypoglycemic requirements. You may experience acne, growth of body hair, deepening of voice, loss of libido, impotence, or menstrual irregularity (usually reversible). Report changes in menstrual pattern; deepening of voice or unusual growth of body hair; persistent penile erections; fluid retention (swelling of ankles, feet, or hands, difficulty breathing, or sudden weight gain); change in color of urine or stool; yellowing of eyes or skin; unusual bruising or bleeding; or other adverse reactions.

**Pregnancy/breast-feeding precautions:** Female: Inform prescriber if you are pregnant. Do not get pregnant during therapy of for 1 month following therapy. Male: Do not cause pregnancy. Male/female: Consult prescriber for appropriate barrier contraceptive measures. This drug may cause severe fetal defects. Do not donate blood during or for 1 month following therapy (same reason). Breast-feeding is not recommended during and for 1 month following therapy.

♦ **Danocrine®** *see* Danazol *on previous page*

♦ **Dantrium®** *see* Dantrolene *on this page*

## Dantrolene (DAN troe leen)

**U.S. Brand Names** Dantrium®

**Therapeutic Category** Skeletal Muscle Relaxant

**Pregnancy Risk Factor** C

**Lactation** Excretion in breast milk unknown/not recommended

**Use** Treatment of spasticity associated with spinal cord injury, stroke, cerebral palsy, or multiple sclerosis; treatment of malignant hyperthermia

**Mechanism of Action/Effect** Acts directly on skeletal muscle by interfering with release of calcium ion from the sarcoplasmic reticulum; prevents or reduces the increase in myoplasmic calcium ion concentration that activates the acute catabolic processes associated with malignant hyperthermia

**Contraindications** Active hepatic disease; should not be used where spasticity is used to maintain posture or balance

**Warnings** Use with caution in patients with impaired cardiac function or impaired pulmonary function. Has potential for hepatotoxicity. Overt hepatitis has been most frequently observed between the third and twelfth month of therapy. Hepatic injury appears to be greater in females and in patients >35 years of age. Pregnancy factor C.

**Drug Interactions**

**Increased Effect/Toxicity:** Increased toxicity with estrogens (hepatotoxicity), CNS depressants (sedation), MAO inhibitors, phenothiazines, clindamycin (increased neuromuscular blockade), verapamil (hyperkalemia and cardiac depression), warfarin, clofibrate, and tolbutamide.

**Effects on Lab Values** ↑ aminotransferase [ALT (SGPT)/AST (SGOT)] (S), alkaline phosphatase, LDH, BUN, and total serum bilirubin

**Adverse Reactions**

>10%:

- Central nervous system: Drowsiness, dizziness, lightheadedness, fatigue
- Dermatologic: Rash
- Gastrointestinal: Diarrhea (mild), vomiting
- Neuromuscular & skeletal: Muscle weakness

1% to 10%:

- Cardiovascular: Pleural effusion with pericarditis
- Central nervous system: Chills, fever, headache, insomnia, nervousness, mental depression
- Gastrointestinal: Diarrhea (severe), constipation, anorexia, stomach cramps
- Ocular: Blurred vision
- Respiratory: Respiratory depression

<1% (Limited to important or life-threatening symptoms): Seizures, confusion, hepatitis

**Overdose/Toxicology** Symptoms of overdose include CNS depression, hypotension, nausea, and vomiting. For decontamination, lavage with activated charcoal and administer a cathartic. Do not use ipecac. Other treatment is supportive and symptomatic.

**Pharmacodynamics/Kinetics**

**Half-life Elimination:** 8.7 hours

**Metabolism:** Liver

**Excretion:** Urine and feces

**Formulations**

Dantrolene sodium:

- Capsule: 25 mg, 50 mg, 100 mg
- Powder for injection: 20 mg

**Dosing**

**Adults:**

Spasticity: Oral: 25 mg/day to start, increase frequency to 2-4 times/day, then increase dose by 25 mg every 4-7 days to a maximum of 100 mg 2-4 times/day or 400 mg/day

Malignant hyperthermia:

- Oral: 4-8 mg/kg/day in 4 divided doses
  - Preoperative prophylaxis: Begin 1-2 days prior to surgery with last dose 3-4 hours prior to surgery
- I.V.: 1 mg/kg; may repeat dose up to cumulative dose of 10 mg/kg (mean effective dose is 2.5 mg/kg), then switch to oral dosage
  - Preoperative: 2.5 mg/kg ~1¼ hours prior to anesthesia and infused over 1 hour with additional doses as needed and individualized

**Elderly:** Refer to adult dosing.

**Administration**

**I.V.:** Therapeutic or emergency dose can be administered with rapid continuous I.V. push. Follow-up doses should be administered over 2-3 minutes.

**I.V. Detail:** Avoid extravasation; tissue irritant. 36 vials are needed for adequate hyperthermia therapy.

**Stability**

**Reconstitution:** Reconstitute vial by adding 60 mL of sterile water for injection USP (**not bacteriostatic water for injection**). Protect from light. Use within 6 hours. Avoid glass bottles for I.V. infusion.

**Monitoring Laboratory Tests** Liver function for potential hepatotoxicity

**Additional Nursing Issues**

**Physical Assessment:** Assess effectiveness and interactions of other medications (see Drug Interactions). See Contraindications and Warnings/Precautions for use

(Continued)

## Dantrolene *(Continued)*

cautions. I.V.: Monitor vital signs, cardiac function, respiratory status and I.V. site (extravasation very irritating to tissues) frequently during infusion. Monitor effectiveness of therapy (according to rational for therapy) and adverse reactions (see Adverse Reactions) at beginning and periodically during therapy. Assess knowledge/teach patient appropriate use, interventions to reduce side effects, and adverse symptoms to report. **Pregnancy risk factor C** - benefits of use should outweigh possible risks. Breast-feeding is not recommended.

**Patient Information/Instruction:** Take exactly as directed. Do not increase dose or discontinue without consulting prescriber. Do not use alcohol, prescriptive or OTC antidepressants, sedatives, or pain medications without consulting prescriber. You may experience drowsiness, dizziness, lightheadedness (avoid driving or engaging in tasks that require alertness until response to drug is known); nausea or vomiting (small, frequent meals, frequent mouth care, or sucking hard candy may help); or diarrhea (buttermilk, boiled milk, or yogurt may help). Report excessive confusion; drowsiness or mental agitation; chest pain, palpitations, or difficulty breathing; skin rash; or vision disturbances. **Pregnancy/breast-feeding precautions:** Inform prescriber if you are or intend to be pregnant. Breast-feeding is not recommended.

♦ **Daonil** *see* Glyburide *on page 538*
♦ **Dapa® [OTC]** *see* Acetaminophen *on page 32*
♦ **Dapacin® Cold Capsule** *see page 1294*
♦ **Dapiprazole** *see page 1248*

## Dapsone (DAP sone)

**U.S. Brand Names** Avlosulfon®

**Synonyms** DDS; Diaminodiphenylsulfone

**Therapeutic Category** Antibiotic, Miscellaneous

**Pregnancy Risk Factor** C

**Lactation** Enters breast milk/not recommended (AAP rates "compatible")

**Use** Treatment of leprosy and dermatitis herpetiformis; alternative agent for *Pneumocystis carinii* pneumonia prophylaxis (given alone) and in combination with trimethoprim for treatment

**Mechanism of Action/Effect** Dapsone is a sulfone antimicrobial that prevents normal bacterial utilization of PABA for the synthesis of folic acid.

**Contraindications** Hypersensitivity to dapsone or any component

**Warnings** Use with caution in patients with severe anemia, G-6-PD deficiency, hypersensitivity to other sulfonamides, or restricted hepatic function. Pregnancy factor C.

**Drug Interactions**

**Cytochrome P-450 Effect:** CYP2C9, 2E1, and 3A3/4 enzyme substrate

**Decreased Effect:** Para-aminobenzoic acid and rifampin levels are decreased when given with dapsone.

**Increased Effect/Toxicity:** Increased toxicity with folic acid antagonists (methotrexate).

**Adverse Reactions**

>10%:
- Hematologic: Hemolytic anemia, methemoglobinemia with cyanosis
- Dermatologic: Skin rash

1% to 10%:
- Central nervous system: Reactional states
- Hematologic: Dose-related hemolysis,

<1% (Limited to important or life-threatening symptoms): Exfoliative dermatitis, leukopenia, agranulocytosis, hepatitis, cholestatic jaundice, peripheral neuropathy

**Overdose/Toxicology** Symptoms of overdose include nausea, vomiting, hyperexcitability, methemoglobin-induced depression, seizures, cyanosis, and hemolysis. Following decontamination, methylene blue 1-2 mg/kg I.V. is the treatment of choice.

**Pharmacodynamics/Kinetics**

**Distribution:** Throughout total body water and present in all tissues, especially liver and kidney

**Half-life Elimination:** 30 hours (range: 10-50 hours)

**Metabolism:** Liver

**Excretion:** Urine

**Formulations** Tablet: 25 mg, 100 mg

**Dosing**

**Adults:** Oral:
- Leprosy: 50-100 mg/day for 3-10 years
- Dermatitis herpetiformis: Start at 50 mg/day, increase to 300 mg/day, or higher to achieve full control, reduce dosage to minimum level as soon as possible
- Treatment of *Pneumocystis carinii* pneumonia: 100 mg/day in combination with trimethoprim (15-20 mg/kg/day) for 21 days

**Elderly:** Refer to adult dosing.

**Renal Impairment:** No specific guidelines are available

**Administration**

**Oral:** May give with meals if GI upset occurs.

**Stability**

**Storage:** Protect from light.

**Monitoring Laboratory Tests** Liver function, CBC

**Additional Nursing Issues**

**Physical Assessment:** Monitor drug adherence on a regular basis. Assess for adverse reactions. Teach patient appropriate use, possible side effects, and symptoms to report. **Pregnancy risk factor C** - benefits of use should outweigh possible risks. Breast-feeding is not recommended.

**Patient Information/Instruction:** Take as directed, for full term of therapy (treatment for leprosy may take 3-10 years). Do not take with antacids, alkaline foods, or drugs (may decrease dapsone absorption). Frequent blood tests may be required during therapy. Discontinue if rash develops and notify prescriber. Report persistent sore throat, fever, chills; constant fatigue; yellowing of skin or eyes; or easy bruising or bleeding. **Pregnancy/breast-feeding precautions:** Inform prescriber if you are or intend to be pregnant. Breast-feeding is not recommended.

- **Daraprim®** *see* Pyrimethamine *on page 998*
- **Darvocet-N®** *see* Propoxyphene and Acetaminophen *on page 985*
- **Darvocet-N® 100** *see* Propoxyphene and Acetaminophen *on page 985*
- **Darvon®** *see* Propoxyphene *on page 984*
- **Darvon® Compound-65 Pulvules®** *see* Propoxyphene and Aspirin *on page 985*
- **Darvon-N®** *see* Propoxyphene *on page 984*
- **Darvon-N® Compound (contains caffeine)** *see* Propoxyphene and Aspirin *on page 985*
- **Darvon-N® With ASA** *see* Propoxyphene and Aspirin *on page 985*
- **Daunomycin** *see* Daunorubicin Hydrochloride *on next page*

## Daunorubicin Citrate (Liposomal)

(daw noe ROO bi sin SI trate lip po SOE mal)

**U.S. Brand Names** DaunoXome®

**Therapeutic Category** Antineoplastic Agent, Antibiotic

**Pregnancy Risk Factor** D

**Lactation** Excretion in breast milk unknown/not recommended

**Use** Advanced HIV-associated Kaposi's sarcoma

**Mechanism of Action/Effect** Binds to DNA and inhibits DNA synthesis causing cell death

**Contraindications** Hypersensitivity to daunorubicin or any component; pregnancy

**Warnings** The U.S. Food and Drug Administration (FDA) currently recommends that procedures for proper handling and disposal of antineoplastic agents be considered.

The primary toxicity is myelosuppression, especially off the granulocytic series, which may be severe, with much less marked effects on platelets and erythroid series. Potential cardiac toxicity, particularly in patients who have received prior anthracyclines or who have pre-existing cardiac disease, may occur. Refer to Daunorubicin monograph.

Although grade 3-4 injection site inflammation has been reported in patients treated with the liposomal daunorubicin, no instances of local tissue necrosis were observed with extravasation. However, refer to Daunorubicin monograph and avoid extravasation.

Reduce dosage in patients with impaired hepatic function. Hyperuricemia can be induced secondary to rapid lysis of leukemic cells. As a precaution, administer allopurinol prior to initiating antileukemic therapy.

Use with caution in patients with systemic infection and cardiac disease.

Daunorubicin (liposomal) preparation should be performed in a Class II laminar flow biologic safety cabinet. Personnel should be wearing surgical gloves and a closed front surgical gown with knit cuffs. Appropriate safety equipment is recommended for preparation, administration, and disposal of antineoplastics. If daunorubicin (liposomal) contacts the skin, wash and flush thoroughly with water.

**Adverse Reactions**

>10%:

- Dermatologic: Alopecia (reversible)
- Gastrointestinal: Mild nausea or vomiting occurs in 50% of patients within the first 24 hours; esophagitis or stomatitis may occur 3-7 days after administration, but is not as severe as that caused by doxorubicin
  - Time course for nausea/vomiting: Onset: 1-3 hours; Duration: 4-24 hours
- Genitourinary: Discoloration of urine (red)

1% to 10%:

- Cardiovascular: Congestive heart failure; maximum lifetime dose: Refer to Warnings/Precautions
- Dermatologic: Darkening or redness of skin
- Endocrine & metabolic: Hyperuricemia
- Gastrointestinal: GI ulceration, diarrhea
- Hematologic: Myelosuppressive: Dose-limiting toxicity; occurs in all patients; leukopenia is more significant than thrombocytopenia
  - WBC: Severe
  - Platelets: Severe
  - Onset (days): 7
  - Nadir (days): 14
  - Recovery (days): 21-28
- Local: **Vesicant chemotherapy**

<1% (Limited to important or life-threatening symptoms): Pericarditis, myocarditis; elevation in serum bilirubin, AST, and alkaline phosphatase

(Continued)

## Daunorubicin Citrate (Liposomal) *(Continued)*

**Overdose/Toxicology** Symptoms of acute overdose are increased severity of the observed dose-limiting toxicities of therapeutic doses, myelosuppression (especially granulocytopenia), fatigue, nausea, and vomiting. Treatment is symptomatic.

**Pharmacodynamics/Kinetics**

**Half-life Elimination:** 4.4 hours

**Formulations** Injection: 2 mg/mL equivalent to 50 mg daunorubicin base

**Dosing**

**Adults:** I.V. (dosage varies with protocol used): 30-60 mg/m$^2$/day for 3-5 days; repeat dose in 3-4 weeks; total cumulative dose should not exceed 400-600 mg/m$^2$

**Elderly:** Refer to adult dosing.

**Renal Impairment:**

$S_{cr}$ 1.2-3 mg/dL: Reduce dose to 75% of normal.

$S_{cr}$ >3 mg/dL: Reduce dose to 50% of normal.

**Hepatic Impairment:**

Serum bilirubin 1.2-3 mg/dL: Reduce to 75% of normal dose.

Serum bilirubin >3 mg/dL: Reduce to 50% of normal dose.

**Administration**

**I.V.:** Vesicant. Infuse over 1 hour; do not mix with other drugs.

**I.V. Detail: Extravasation management:** Daunorubicin is a vesicant; infiltration can cause severe inflammation, tissue necrosis, and ulceration. If the drug is infiltrated, consult institutional policy, apply ice to the area, and elevate the limb.

**Stability**

**Storage:** Store in refrigerator 2°C to 8°C (37°F to 45°F); do not freeze. Protect from light.

**Reconstitution:** Only fluid which may be mixed with DaunoXome® is $D_5W$. Must not be mixed with saline, bacteriostatic agents such as benzyl alcohol, or any other solution.

**Compatibility:** Incompatible with sodium bicarbonate and 5-FU, heparin, and dexamethasone. See the Chemotherapy Compatibility Chart *on page 1311*.

**Monitoring Laboratory Tests** Cardiac function, WBC, hematologic monitoring, liver and renal function prior to each course of treatment; repeat blood counts prior to each dose and withhold if the absolute granulocyte count is <750 cells/mm$^3$. Monitor serum uric acid levels.

**Additional Nursing Issues**

**Physical Assessment:** Monitor laboratory tests as ordered. Drug is a vesicant; assess infusion site frequently for extravasation which may result in cellulitis and tissue necrosis. Emetic potential is moderate; restrict oral intake 4-6 hours prior to infusion and start antiemetic medication before starting infusion. Monitor for adverse effects as indicated above; especially for signs of congestive heart failure, hypertension, palpitations, tachycardia, edema, respiratory changes, or fluid imbalance (weight gain/loss, edema), or opportunistic infection (fever, chills, easy bruising or bleeding, fatigue, purulent vaginal drainage, unhealed mouth sores). **Pregnancy risk factor D** - assess knowledge/teach appropriate use of barrier contraceptives to both male and female patients (nonhormonal birth control is recommended). Breast-feeding is not recommended.

**Patient Information/Instruction:** This medication can only be administered I.V. During therapy, do not use alcohol, aspirin-containing products, and OTC medications without consulting prescriber. It is important to maintain adequate nutrition and hydration (2-3 L/day of fluids unless instructed to restrict fluid intake) during therapy; frequent small meals may help. You may experience nausea or vomiting (frequent small meals, frequent mouth care, sucking lozenges, or chewing gum may help); you may experience loss of hair (reversible); you will be more susceptible to infection (avoid crowds and exposure to infection as much as possible). Urine may turn red-brown (normal). Yogurt or buttermilk may help reduce diarrhea (if unresolved, contact prescriber for medication relief). Report fever, chills, unusual bruising or bleeding, signs of infection, excessive fatigue, yellowing of eyes or skin, darkening in color of urine (red/pink), abdominal pain or blood in stools, swelling of extremities, difficulty breathing, or unresolved diarrhea. **Pregnancy/breast-feeding precautions:** Do not get pregnant or cause a pregnancy (males) while taking this medication; use appropriate barrier contraceptive measures during and for 1 month following therapy. Breast-feeding is not recommended.

## Daunorubicin Hydrochloride (daw noe ROO bi sin hye droe KLOR ide)

**U.S. Brand Names** Cerubidine®

**Synonyms** Daunomycin; DNR; Rubidomycin Hydrochloride

**Therapeutic Category** Antineoplastic Agent, Antibiotic

**Pregnancy Risk Factor** D

**Lactation** Excretion in breast milk unknown/not recommended

**Use** Treatment of ANLL and myeloblastic leukemia; questionable results in neuroblastoma

**Mechanism of Action/Effect** Inhibition of DNA and RNA synthesis; is not cell cycle-specific for the S Phase of cell division; daunomycin is preferred over doxorubicin for the treatment of ANLL because of its dose-limiting toxicity (myelosuppression) is not of concern in the therapy of this disease; has less mucositis associated with its use

**Contraindications** Hypersensitivity to daunorubicin or any component; congestive heart failure or arrhythmias; pre-existing bone marrow suppression; pregnancy

**Warnings** The U.S. Food and Drug Administration (FDA) currently recommends that procedures for proper handling and disposal of antineoplastic agents be considered. I.V. use only, severe local tissue necrosis will result if extravasation occurs. Reduce dose in patients with impaired hepatic, renal, or biliary function. Severe myelosuppression is possible when used in therapeutic doses. Total cumulative dose should take into account previous or concomitant treatment with cardiotoxic agents or irradiation of chest.

**Irreversible myocardial toxicity may occur as total dosage approaches:**

550 mg/m$^2$ in adults
400 mg/m$^2$ in patients receiving chest radiation
300 mg/m$^2$ in children >2 years of age or
10 mg/kg in children <2 years; this may occur during therapy or several months after therapy.

Daunorubicin preparation should be performed in a Class II laminar flow biologic safety cabinet. Personnel should be wearing surgical gloves and a closed front surgical gown with knit cuffs. Appropriate safety equipment is recommended for preparation, administration, and disposal of antineoplastics. If daunorubicin contacts the skin, wash and flush thoroughly with water.

**Effects on Lab Values** ↑ potassium (S)

**Adverse Reactions**

>10%:

Dermatologic: Alopecia (reversible)
Gastrointestinal: Mild nausea or vomiting occurs in 50% of patients within the first 24 hours; esophagitis or stomatitis may occur 3-7 days after administration, but is not as severe as that caused by doxorubicin
Time course for nausea/vomiting: Onset: 1-3 hours; Duration: 4-24 hours
Genitourinary: Discoloration of urine (red)

1% to 10%:

Cardiovascular: Congestive heart failure; maximum lifetime dose: Refer to Warnings/ Precautions
Dermatologic: Darkening or redness of skin
Endocrine & metabolic: Hyperuricemia
Gastrointestinal: GI ulceration, diarrhea
Hematologic: Myelosuppressive: Dose-limiting toxicity; occurs in all patients; leukopenia is more significant than thrombocytopenia
WBC: Severe
Platelets: Severe
Onset (days): 7
Nadir (days): 14
Recovery (days): 21-28
Local: **Vesicant chemotherapy**

<1% (Limited to important or life-threatening symptoms): Pericarditis, myocarditis; elevation in serum bilirubin, AST, and alkaline phosphatase

**Overdose/Toxicology** Symptoms of overdose include myelosuppression, nausea, vomiting, and stomatitis. There are no known antidotes. Treatment is symptomatic and supportive.

**Pharmacodynamics/Kinetics**

**Distribution:** Crosses the placenta; distributed to many body tissues, particularly the liver, kidneys, lung, spleen, and heart; does not distribute into the CNS

**Half-life Elimination:** Distribution: 2 minutes; Elimination: 14-20 hours; Terminal: 18.5 hours; Daunorubicinol plasma half-life: 24-48 hours

**Metabolism:** Liver

**Excretion:** Urine and bile (may turn urine red)

**Formulations** Powder for injection, lyophilized: 20 mg

**Dosing**

**Adults:** I.V. (refer to individual protocols): 30-60 mg/m$^2$/day for 3-5 days, repeat dose in 3-4 weeks
Single agent induction for AML: 60 mg/m$^2$/day for 3 days; repeat every 3-4 weeks
Combination therapy induction for AML: 45 mg/m$^2$/day for 3 days of the first course of induction therapy; subsequent courses: Every day for 2 days
ALL combination therapy: 45 mg/m$^2$/day for 3 days
Cumulative dose should not exceed 400-600 mg/m$^2$

**Elderly:** Refer to adult dosing.

**Renal Impairment:**

$Cl_{cr}$ <10 mL/minute: Administer 75% of normal dose.
$S_{cr}$ >3 mg/dL: Administer 50% of normal dose.

**Hepatic Impairment:**

Serum bilirubin 1.2-3 mg/dL or AST 60-180 int. units: Reduce dose to 75%.
Serum bilirubin 3.1-5 mg/dL or AST >180 int. units: Reduce dose to 50%.
Serum bilirubin >5 mg/dL: Omit use.

**Administration**

**I.V.:** Vesicant. **Never** be administered I.M. or S.C. Administer IVP over 1-5 minutes.

**I.V. Detail:** Administer into the tubing of a rapidly infusing I.V. solution of $D_5W$ or NS; daunorubicin has also been diluted in 100 mL of $D_5W$ or NS and infused over 15-30 minutes. Avoid extravasation, can cause severe tissue damage. Flush with 5-10 mL of I.V. solution before and after drug administration.

**Extravasation management:** Apply ice immediately for 30-60 minutes; then alternate off/on every 15 minutes for 1 day. Topical cooling may be achieved using ice packs or cooling pad with circulating ice water. Cooling of site for 24 hours as tolerated by the patient. Elevate and rest extremity 24-48 hours, then resume normal activity as tolerated. Application of cold inhibits vesicant's cytotoxicity. Application of heat or sodium bicarbonate can be harmful and is contraindicated. If pain, erythema, and/or swelling

(Continued)

## Daunorubicin Hydrochloride *(Continued)*

persist beyond 48 hours, refer patient immediately to plastic surgeon for consultation and possible debridement.

**Stability**

**Storage:** Store intact vials at room temperature and protect from light.

**Reconstitution:** Dilute vials with 4 mL SWI for a final concentration of 5 mg/mL. Reconstituted solution is stable for 4 days at 15°C to 25°C. Protect from direct sunlight or fluorescent light to decrease photo-inactivation after storage in solution for several days. Decomposed drug turns purple. For I.V. push administration, desired dose is withdrawn into a syringe containing 10-15 mL NS. Further dilution in $D_5W$, LR, or NS is stable for 24 hours at room temperature (25°C) and up to 4 weeks if protected from light.

**Standard I.V. dilution:**

I.V. push: Dose/syringe (initial concentration is 5 mg/mL; however, qs to 10-15 mL with NS)

Maximum syringe size for IVP is a 30 mL syringe and syringe should be <75% full.

IVPB: Dose/50-100 mL NS or $D_5W$

Stable for 24 hours at room temperature (25°C).

**Compatibility:** Incompatible with heparin, sodium bicarbonate, 5-FU, and dexamethasone. See the Chemotherapy Compatibility Chart *on page 1311*.

**Monitoring Laboratory Tests** CBC with differential, platelet count, liver function, EKG, ventricular ejection fraction, renal function

**Additional Nursing Issues**

**Physical Assessment:** Monitor laboratory tests as ordered. Drug is a vesicant; assess infusion site frequently for extravasation which may result in cellulitis and tissue necrosis. Emetic potential is moderate; restrict oral intake 4-6 hours prior to infusion and start antiemetic medication before starting infusion. Monitor for adverse effects as indicated above; especially for signs of cardiac toxicity (congestive heart failure, tachycardia), edema, respiratory changes, fluid imbalance (weight gain/loss, edema), or opportunistic infection (eg, fever, chills, easy bruising or bleeding, fatigue, purulent vaginal drainage, unhealed mouth sores). **Pregnancy risk factor D** - assess knowledge/teach appropriate use of barrier contraceptives to both male and female patients (nonhormonal birth control is recommended). Breast-feeding is not recommended.

**Patient Information/Instruction:** This medication can only be administered I.V. During therapy, do not use alcohol, aspirin-containing products, and OTC medications without consulting prescriber. It is important to maintain adequate nutrition and hydration (2-3 L/day of fluids unless instructed to restrict fluid intake) during therapy; frequent small meals may help. You may experience nausea or vomiting (frequent small meals, frequent mouth care, sucking lozenges, or chewing gum may help). You may experience loss of hair (reversible); you will be more susceptible to infection (avoid crowds and exposure to infection as much as possible). Urine may turn red-pink (normal). Yogurt or buttermilk may help reduce diarrhea (if unresolved, contact prescriber for medication relief). Report fever, chills, unusual bruising or bleeding, signs of infection, abdominal pain or blood in stools, excessive fatigue, yellowing of eyes or skin, swelling of extremities, difficulty breathing, or unresolved diarrhea. **Pregnancy/breast-feeding precautions:** Do not get pregnant or cause a pregnancy (males) while taking this medication; use appropriate barrier contraceptive measures during and for 1 month following therapy. Breast-feeding is not recommended.


- **DaunoXome®** *see* Daunorubicin Citrate (Liposomal) *on page 335*
- **Daypro™** *see* Oxaprozin *on page 867*
- **DC 240® Softgels® [OTC]** *see* Docusate *on page 392*
- **DCF** *see* Pentostatin *on page 906*
- **DDAVP® Nasal Spray** *see* Desmopressin *on page 345*
- **ddC** *see* Zalcitabine *on page 1225*
- **ddI** *see* Didanosine *on page 363*
- **DDS** *see* Dapsone *on page 334*
- **1-Deamino-8-D-Arginine Vasopressin** *see* Desmopressin *on page 345*
- **Deavynfar** *see* Chlorpropamide *on page 259*
- **Debrisan® [OTC]** *see* Dextranomer *on page 352*
- **Debrox® Otic** *see page 1291*
- **Debrox® Otic** *see page 1294*
- **Decadron®** *see* Dexamethasone *on page 346*
- **Decadronal®** *see* Dexamethasone *on page 346*
- **Decadron®-LA** *see* Dexamethasone *on page 346*
- **Decadron Turbinaire®** *see* Dexamethasone *on page 346*
- **Deca-Durabolin® Injection** *see* Nandrolone *on page 806*
- **Decaject-L.A.®** *see* Dexamethasone *on page 346*
- **Decaris** *see* Levamisole *on page 665*
- **Decaspray®** *see* Dexamethasone *on page 346*
- **Decaspray®** *see* Topical Corticosteroids *on page 1152*
- **Declomycin®** *see* Demeclocycline *on page 341*
- **Decofed® Syrup [OTC]** *see* Pseudoephedrine *on page 992*
- **Decohistine® DH Liquid** *see page 1306*
- **Decohistine® Expectorant** *see* Guaifenesin, Pseudoephedrine, and Codeine *on page 552*

- ♦ **Deconamine® SR** *see page 1294*
- ♦ **Deconamine® Syrup** *see page 1294*
- ♦ **Deconamine® Tablet** *see page 1294*
- ♦ **Deconsal® II** *see* Guaifenesin and Pseudoephedrine *on page 551*
- ♦ **Decorex** *see* Dexamethasone *on page 346*
- ♦ **Defen-LA®** *see* Guaifenesin and Pseudoephedrine *on page 551*


## Deferoxamine (de fer OKS a meen)

**U.S. Brand Names** Desferal® Mesylate

**Therapeutic Category** Antidote

**Pregnancy Risk Factor** C

**Lactation** Excretion in breast milk unknown/contraindicated

**Use** Acute iron intoxication; chronic iron overload secondary to multiple transfusions; diagnostic test for iron overload; iron overload secondary to congenital anemias; hemochromatosis; removal of corneal rust rings following surgical removal of foreign bodies

**Investigational use:** Treatment of aluminum accumulation in renal failure

**Mechanism of Action/Effect** Complexes with trivalent ions (ferric ions) to form ferrioxamine, which are removed by the kidneys

**Contraindications** Patients with anuria, primary hemochromatosis

**Warnings** Use with caution in patients with severe renal disease, pyelonephritis. May increase susceptibility to *Yersinia enterocolitica*. Pregnancy factor C.

**Adverse Reactions**

>10%:

Cardiovascular: Flushing, hypotension, tachycardia, shock, edema
Central nervous system: Convulsions
Ocular: Blurred vision
Otic: Hearing loss
Respiratory: Respiratory distress syndrome

1% to 10%:

Central nervous system: Fever
Dermatologic: Erythema, urticaria, pruritus, rash, cutaneous wheal formation
Endocrine and metabolic: Hypocalcemia
Gastrointestinal: Abdominal discomfort, diarrhea
Hematologic: Thrombocytopenia
Local: Pain and induration at injection site
Neuromuscular & skeletal: Leg cramps
Miscellaneous: Anaphylaxis

**Overdose/Toxicology** Symptoms of overdose include hypotension, blurring of vision, diarrhea, leg cramps, and tachycardia. Treatment is symptomatic and supportive.

**Pharmacodynamics/Kinetics**

**Half-life Elimination:** Parent drug: 6.1 hours; Ferrioxamine: 5.8 hours

**Metabolism:** Liver

**Excretion:** Urine

**Formulations** Powder for injection, as mesylate: 500 mg

**Dosing**

**Adults:**

Acute iron toxicity: I.V. route is preferred in all cases: 15 mg/kg/hour (although rates up to 40-50 mg/kg/hour have been given in patients with massive iron intoxication); maximum recommended dose: 6 g/day.

End points: Loss of vin rosé-colored urine and serum iron level <350 μ/dL and resolution of clinical signs of intoxication.

**Note:** Test dose I.M. injection is not recommended due to risk of sterile abscess formation and hypotension, however, usual dose is 50 mg/kg; observe for vin rosé-colored urine

Chronic iron overload:

I.M.: 0.5-1 g every day
I.V.: 2 g after each unit of blood infusion at 15 mg/kg/hour
S.C.: 1-2 g every day over 8-24 hours

Has been used investigationally as a single 40 mg/kg I.V. dose over 2 hours, to promote mobilization of aluminum from tissue stores as an aid in the diagnosis of aluminum-associated osteodystrophy.

**Elderly:** Refer to adult dosing.

**Renal Impairment:** $Cl_{cr}$ <10 mL/minute: Administer 50% of dose.

**Administration**

**I.M.:** I.M. is the preferred route. Add 2 mL sterile water to 500 mg vial. For I.M. or S.C. administration, no further dilution is required.

**I.V.:** I.M. is preferred route; maximum I.V. rate is 15 mg/kg/hour.

**I.V. Detail:** Urticaria, hypotension, and shock have occurred following rapid I.V. administration; for I.V. infusion, dilute in dextrose, normal saline, or lactated Ringer's; 10 mg/mL (maximum: 25 mg/mL); maximum rate of infusion: 15 mg/kg/hour.

**Stability**

**Storage:** Protect from light.

**Reconstitution:** Reconstituted solutions (sterile water) may be stored at room temperature for 7 days.

**Monitoring Laboratory Tests** Serum iron, total iron binding capacity, ophthalmologic exam and audiometry with chronic therapy

(Continued)

## Deferoxamine *(Continued)*

**Additional Nursing Issues**

**Physical Assessment:** Monitor laboratory tests (see above). I.V.: Infuse slowly (see Administration) and monitor infusion site. Monitor for acute reactions; urticaria, hypotension and shock can occur following rapid I.V. administration. Monitor for adverse reactions (eg, cardiac, respiratory, or CNS symptoms - see Adverse Reactions) and teach patient importance of reporting adverse symptoms promptly. **Pregnancy risk factor C** - benefits of use should outweigh possible risks. Breast-feeding is contraindicated.

**Patient Information/Instruction:** I.V.: Instructions depend on patient condition. You will be monitored closely for effects of this medication and frequent blood or urine tests may be necessary. Report chest pain, rapid heartbeat, headache, pain, swelling, or irritation at infusion site; skin rash; changes or loss of hearing or vision; or acute abdominal or leg cramps. **Pregnancy/breast-feeding precautions:** Inform prescriber if you are or intend to be pregnant. Do not breast-feed.

**Additional Information** Iron chelate colors urine salmon pink.


- ♦ **Deficol®** *see page 1294*
- ♦ **Degas®** *see page 1294*
- ♦ **Degest® [OTC]** *see page 1282*
- ♦ **Degest® 2 Ophthalmic** *see page 1294*
- ♦ **Dehydral™** *see* Methenamine *on page 739*
- ♦ **Dehydrobenzperidol** *see* Droperidol *on page 409*
- ♦ **Dekasol-L.A.®** *see* Dexamethasone *on page 346*
- ♦ **Del Aqua-5® Gel** *see page 1294*
- ♦ **Del Aqua-10® Gel** *see page 1294*
- ♦ **Delatest® Injection** *see* Testosterone *on page 1108*
- ♦ **Delatestryl® Injection** *see* Testosterone *on page 1108*


## Delavirdine (de la VIR deen)

**U.S. Brand Names** Rescriptor®

**Synonyms** U-90152S

**Therapeutic Category** Antiretroviral Agent, Reverse Transcriptase Inhibitor (Non-Nucleoside)

**Pregnancy Risk Factor** C

**Lactation** Enters breast milk/contraindicated

**Use** Treatment of HIV-1 infection in combination with appropriate antiretrovirals

**Mechanism of Action/Effect** Delavirdine binds directly to reverse transcriptase, blocking RNA-dependent and DNA-dependent DNA polymerase activities

**Contraindications** Hypersensitivity to delavirdine or any components

**Warnings** Avoid use with terfenadine, astemizole, benzodiazepines, clarithromycin, dapsone, cisapride, rifabutin, and rifampin. Use with caution in patients with hepatic or renal dysfunction. Due to rapid emergence of resistance, delavirdine should not be used as monotherapy. Cross-resistance may be conferred to other non-nucleoside reverse transcriptase inhibitors, although potential for cross-resistance with protease inhibitors is low. Long-term effects of delavirdine are not known. Safety and efficacy have not been established in children. Rash, which occurs frequently, may require discontinuation of therapy; usually occurs within 1-3 weeks and lasts <2 weeks. Most patients may resume therapy following a treatment interruption. Pregnancy factor C.

**Drug Interactions**

**Cytochrome P-450 Effect:** CYP2D6 and 3A3/4 enzyme substrate; CYP2D6 and 3A3/4 enzyme inhibitor

**Decreased Effect:** Decreased plasma concentrations of delavirdine with carbamazepine, phenobarbital, phenytoin, rifabutin, rifampin, didanosine, and saquinavir. Decreased absorption of delavirdine with antacids, histamine-2 receptor antagonists, and didanosine. Delavirdine decreases plasma concentrations of didanosine.

**Increased Effect/Toxicity:** Increased plasma concentrations of delavirdine with clarithromycin, ketoconazole, and fluoxetine. Delavirdine increases plasma concentrations of indinavir, saquinavir, terfenadine, astemizole, clarithromycin, dapsone, rifabutin, ergot derivatives, alprazolam, midazolam, triazolam, dihydropyridine calcium channel blockers, cisapride, quinidine, and warfarin.

**Adverse Reactions**

1% to 10%:

Central nervous system: Headache, fatigue
Dermatologic: Rash, pruritus
Gastrointestinal: Nausea, diarrhea, vomiting
Metabolic: Increased ALT (SGPT), increased AST (SGOT)

<1% (Limited to important or life-threatening symptoms): Allergic reaction, chest pain, edema, malaise, neck rigidity, bradycardia, palpitation, postural hypotension, syncope, tachycardia, vasodilation, abnormal coordination, confusion, hallucination, neuropathy, nystagmus, paralysis, paranoid symptoms, vertigo, angioedema, dermal leukocytoblastic vasculitis, desquamation, erythema multiforme, alopecia, Stevens-Johnson syndrome, vesiculobullous rash, nonspecific hepatitis, calculi of kidney, hematuria, proteinuria, kidney pain, hemospermia, anemia, ecchymosis, eosinophilia, granulocytosis, neutropenia, pancytopenia, thrombocytopenia, alcohol intolerance, hyperkalemia, hyperuricemia, hyponatremia, hypophosphatemia, hypocalcemia, increased serum creatinine, phosphokinase, increased serum alkaline phosphatase, myalgia, dyspnea, epistaxis, increased lipase

**Overdose/Toxicology** Reports of human overdose with delavirdine are not available. GI decontamination and supportive measures are recommended. Dialysis is unlikely to be of benefit in removing this drug since it is extensively metabolized by the liver and is highly protein bound.

**Pharmacodynamics/Kinetics**

**Protein Binding:** ~98%, primarily albumin

**Distribution:** Not reported

**Half-life Elimination:** 2-11 hours

**Time to Peak:** 1 hour

**Metabolism:** Hepatic; extensively metabolized by the cytochrome P-450 3A or possibly 2D6

**Excretion:** Feces and urine (**Note:** May reduce CYP3A activity and inhibit its own metabolism.)

**Formulations** Tablet: 100 mg

**Dosing**

**Adults:** Oral: 400 mg 3 times/day

**Elderly:** Refer to adult dosing.

**Administration**

**Oral:** Patients with achlorhydria should take the drug with an acidic beverage. Antacids and delavirdine should be separated by 1 hour. A dispersion of delavirdine may be prepared by adding 4 tablets to at least 3 oz of water. Allow to stand for a few minutes and stir until uniform dispersion. Drink immediately. Rinse glass and mouth following ingestion to ensure total dose administered.

**Monitoring Laboratory Tests** Liver function tests if administered with saquinavir

**Additional Nursing Issues**

**Physical Assessment:** Monitor laboratory results on a regular basis. Assess effectiveness of other medications patient may be taking for possible decreased or toxic effects (see Drug Interactions). Monitor for effectiveness of therapy and adverse reactions (see Warnings/Precautions and Adverse Reactions). **Pregnancy Risk Factor C.** Contraindicated for breast-feeding women - delavirdine is only used to treat patients with HIV and the CDC recommends that women with HIV not breast-feed in order to prevent transmission of HIV.

**Patient Information/Instruction:** Delavirdine is not a cure for HIV nor has it been found to reduce transmission of HIV. Take as directed, with food. Do not take antacids within 1 hour of delavirdine. Mix 4 tablets in 3-5 ounces of water, allow to stand a few minutes, and stir; drink immediately. You may experience nausea or vomiting (small frequent meals, frequent mouth care, sucking lozenges, or chewing gum may help - consult prescriber if nausea or vomiting persists). Report mouth sores; skin rash or irritation; muscle weakness or tremors; easy bruising or bleeding, fever or chills; CNS changes (eg, hallucinations, confusion, dizziness, altered coordination); swelling of face, lips, or tongue; yellowing of eyes or skin; or dark urine or pale stools. **Pregnancy/ breast-feeding precautions:** Inform prescriber if you are or intend to be pregnant. Do not breast-feed.

**Breast-feeding Issues:** The CDC recommends that women with HIV **not** breast-feed in order to prevent transmission of HIV.

**Additional Information** Rescriptor®, a non-nucleoside reverse transcriptase inhibitor, should be used as second line therapy in combination with two nucleoside reverse transcriptase inhibitors. Potential compliance problems, frequency of administration and adverse effects should be discussed with patients before initiating therapy to help prevent the emergence of resistance.

**Related Information**

Antiretroviral Agents Comparison *on page 1373*

- **Delaxin®** *see* Methocarbamol *on page 742*
- **Delcort®** *see* Hydrocortisone *on page 578*
- **Delestrogen® Injection** *see* Estradiol *on page 441*
- **Delfen®** *see page 1294*
- **Delsym®** *see page 1294*
- **Delta-Cortef® Oral** *see* Prednisolone *on page 960*
- **Deltacortisone** *see* Prednisone *on page 962*
- **Deltadehydrocortisone** *see* Prednisone *on page 962*
- **Deltahydrocortisone** *see* Prednisolone *on page 960*
- **Deltasone®** *see* Prednisone *on page 962*
- **Delta-Tritex®** *see* Topical Corticosteroids *on page 1152*
- **Delta-Tritex®** *see* Triamcinolone *on page 1171*
- **Del-Vi-A®** *see* Vitamin A *on page 1217*
- **Demadex®** *see* Torsemide *on page 1159*
- **Demazin® Syrup** *see page 1294*

## Demeclocycline (dem e kloe SYE kleen)

**U.S. Brand Names** Declomycin®

**Synonyms** Demethylchlortetracycline

**Therapeutic Category** Antibiotic, Tetracycline Derivative

**Pregnancy Risk Factor** D

**Lactation** Enters breast milk/use caution

**Use** Treatment of susceptible bacterial infections (acne, gonorrhea, pertussis and urinary tract infections) caused by both gram-negative and gram-positive organisms; used when

(Continued)

## Demeclocycline *(Continued)*

penicillin is contraindicated (other agents are preferred); treatment of chronic syndrome of inappropriate secretion of antidiuretic hormone (SIADH)

**Mechanism of Action/Effect** Inhibits protein synthesis by binding with the 30S and possibly the 50S ribosomal subunit(s) of susceptible bacteria; may also cause alterations in the cytoplasmic membrane; inhibits actions of ADH in patients with SAIDH

**Contraindications** Hypersensitivity to demeclocycline, tetracyclines, or any component; pregnancy

**Warnings** Photosensitivity reactions occur frequently with this drug.

**Drug Interactions**

**Decreased Effect:** Decreased effect with antacids (aluminum, calcium, zinc, or magnesium), bismuth salts, sodium bicarbonate, barbiturates, carbamazepine, and hydantoins. Decreased effect of oral contraceptives, penicillins.

**Increased Effect/Toxicity:** Increased effect of warfarin, digoxin when taken with demeclocycline.

**Food Interactions** Demeclocycline serum levels may be decreased if taken with food.

**Effects on Lab Values** May interfere with tests for urinary glucose (false-negative urine glucose using Clinistix®).

**Adverse Reactions**

>10%:

Central nervous system: Dizziness, lightheadedness, unsteadiness
Dermatologic: Photosensitivity
Gastrointestinal: Nausea, diarrhea

Miscellaneous: Discoloration of teeth in children

1% to 10%:

Endocrine & metabolic: Diabetes insipidus syndrome
Gastrointestinal: Pancreatitis, hypertrophy of the papilla
Hepatic: Hepatotoxicity
Miscellaneous: Superinfections (fungal overgrowth)

<1% (Limited to important or life-threatening symptoms): Pericarditis increased intracranial pressure, bulging fontanels in infants, dermatologic effects, pruritus, exfoliative dermatitis, acute renal failure, azotemia

**Overdose/Toxicology** Symptoms of overdose include diabetes insipidus, nausea, anorexia, and diarrhea. Treatment is supportive.

**Pharmacodynamics/Kinetics**

**Protein Binding:** 41% to 50%

**Half-life Elimination:** Reduced renal function: 10-17 hours

**Time to Peak:** Oral: Within 3-6 hours

**Metabolism:** Liver

**Excretion:** Urine and feces

**Onset:** Onset of action for diuresis in SIADH: Several days

**Formulations**

Demeclocycline hydrochloride:

Capsule: 150 mg
Tablet: 150 mg, 300 mg

**Dosing**

**Adults:** Oral: 150 mg 4 times/day or 300 mg twice daily

Uncomplicated gonorrhea (penicillin sensitive): 600 mg stat, 300 mg every 12 hours for 4 days (3 g total)

SIADH: 900-1200 mg/day or 13-15 mg/kg/day divided every 6-8 hours initially, then decrease to 600-900 mg/day

**Elderly:** Refer to adult dosing.

**Renal Impairment:** Should be avoided in patients with renal dysfunction.

**Hepatic Impairment:** Should be avoided in patients with hepatic dysfunction.

**Administration**

**Oral:** Administer 1 hour before or 2 hours after food or milk with plenty of fluid.

**Monitoring Laboratory Tests** CBC, renal and hepatic function; perform culture and sensitivity studies prior to initiating therapy to determine the causative organism and its susceptibility to demeclocycline.

**Additional Nursing Issues**

**Physical Assessment:** Assess effectiveness or interactions of other medications patient may be taking (see Drug Interactions). Monitor laboratory test results. Monitor for adverse reactions (see above). Teach patient appropriate administration, possible adverse reactions, and symptoms to report. **Pregnancy risk factor D** - assess knowledge/teach appropriate use of barrier contraceptives. Note breast-feeding caution.

**Patient Information/Instruction:** Preferable to take on an empty stomach (1 hour before or 2 hours after meals). Take at regularly scheduled times around-the-clock. Avoid antacids, iron, or dairy products within 2 hours of taking demeclocycline. You may experience photosensitivity (use sunscreen, wear protective clothing and eyewear, and avoid direct sunlight); dizziness or lightheadedness (use caution when driving or engaging in tasks that require alertness until response to drug is known); nausea/vomiting (frequent small meals, frequent mouth care, sucking lozenges, or chewing gum may help); or diarrhea (buttermilk, yogurt, or boiled milk may help). If diabetic, drug may cause false tests with Clinitest® urine glucose monitoring; use of glucose oxidase methods (Clinistix®) or serum glucose monitoring is preferable. Report rash or intense itching; yellowing of skin or eyes; change in color of urine or stools; fever or chills; dark urine or pale stools; vaginal itching or discharge; foul-smelling stools; excessive thirst or urination; acute headache; unresolved diarrhea; or difficulty breathing. **Pregnancy/breast-feeding precautions:** Do not get pregnant while taking this medication - Oral contraceptives effectiveness may be reduced; use appropriate barrier contraceptive measures. Consult prescriber if breast-feeding.

**Geriatric Considerations:** Has not been studied exclusively in the elderly.

- **Demercarium** *see* Ophthalmic Agents, Glaucoma *on page 853*
- **Demerol®** *see* Meperidine *on page 721*
- **4-Demethoxydaunorubicin** *see* Idarubicin *on page 595*
- **Demethylchlortetracycline** *see* Demeclocycline *on page 341*
- **Demolox** *see* Amoxapine *on page 79*
- **Demulen®** *see* Oral Contraceptives *on page 859*
- **Denavir™** *see* Penciclovir *on page 894*
- **Denorex® DHS® Tar** *see page 1294*
- **Denvar** *see* Cefixime *on page 216*
- **Deodorized Opium Tincture** *see* Opium Tincture *on page 857*
- **2′-Deoxycoformycin** *see* Pentostatin *on page 906*
- **Depacon®** *see* Valproic Acid and Derivatives *on page 1198*
- **Depakene®** *see* Valproic Acid and Derivatives *on page 1198*
- **Depakote®** *see* Valproic Acid and Derivatives *on page 1198*
- **depAndro® Injection** *see* Testosterone *on page 1108*
- **Depen®** *see* Penicillamine *on page 894*
- **depGynogen® Injection** *see* Estradiol *on page 441*
- **depMedalone® Injection** *see* Methylprednisolone *on page 754*
- **Depo®-Estradiol Injection** *see* Estradiol *on page 441*
- **Depogen® Injection** *see* Estradiol *on page 441*
- **Depoject® Injection** *see* Methylprednisolone *on page 754*
- **Depo-Medrol® Injection** *see* Methylprednisolone *on page 754*
- **Deponit® Patch** *see* Nitroglycerin *on page 831*
- **Depopred® Injection** *see* Methylprednisolone *on page 754*
- **Depo-Provera® Injection** *see* Medroxyprogesterone *on page 714*
- **Depot-3® Month** *see* Leuprolide *on page 663*
- **Depotest® Injection** *see* Testosterone *on page 1108*
- **Depo®-Testosterone Injection** *see* Testosterone *on page 1108*
- **Depot-Ped™** *see* Leuprolide *on page 663*
- **Deprenyl** *see* Selegiline *on page 1050*
- **Deproic** *see* Valproic Acid and Derivatives *on page 1198*
- **Deproist® Expectorant With Codeine** *see* Guaifenesin, Pseudoephedrine, and Codeine *on page 552*
- **Derifil®** *see page 1294*
- **Dermacort®** *see* Hydrocortisone *on page 578*
- **Dermaflex® Gel** *see* Lidocaine *on page 674*
- **Dermarest Dricort®** *see* Hydrocortisone *on page 578*
- **Dermarest Dricort®** *see* Topical Corticosteroids *on page 1152*
- **Derma-Smoothe/FS®** *see* Topical Corticosteroids *on page 1152*
- **Dermatop®** *see* Topical Corticosteroids *on page 1152*
- **Dermatophytin® Injection** *see page 1248*
- **Dermatophytin-O** *see page 1248*
- **Dermazin™** *see* Silver Sulfadiazine *on page 1059*
- **DermiCort®** *see* Hydrocortisone *on page 578*
- **DermiCort®** *see* Topical Corticosteroids *on page 1152*
- **Dermifun** *see* Miconazole *on page 767*
- **Dermolate® [OTC]** *see* Hydrocortisone *on page 578*
- **Dermolate® [OTC]** *see* Topical Corticosteroids *on page 1152*
- **Dermoplast® [OTC]** *see* Benzocaine *on page 141*
- **Dermtex® HC With Aloe** *see* Hydrocortisone *on page 578*
- **Dermtex® HC With Aloe** *see* Topical Corticosteroids *on page 1152*
- **DES** *see* Diethylstilbestrol *on page 366*
- **Deserpidine and Methyclothiazide** *see* Methyclothiazide and Deserpidine *on page 749*
- **Desferal® Mesylate** *see* Deferoxamine *on page 339*
- **Desiccated Thyroid** *see* Thyroid *on page 1130*

## Desipramine (des IP ra meen)

**U.S. Brand Names** Norpramin®

**Synonyms** Desmethylimipramine Hydrochloride

**Therapeutic Category** Antidepressant, Tricyclic (Secondary Amine)

**Pregnancy Risk Factor** C

**Lactation** Enters breast milk/not recommended (AAP rates "of concern")

**Use** Treatment of various forms of depression, often in conjunction with psychotherapy; analgesic adjunct in chronic pain, peripheral neuropathies

**Unlabeled use:** Cocaine withdrawal

**Mechanism of Action/Effect** Traditionally believed to increase the synaptic concentration of norepinephrine in the central nervous system by inhibition of its reuptake by the presynaptic neuronal membrane. However, additional receptor effects have been found

(Continued)

## Desipramine *(Continued)*

including desensitization of adenyl cyclase, down regulation of beta-adrenergic receptors, and down regulation of serotonin receptors.

**Contraindications** Hypersensitivity to desipramine (cross-sensitivity with other tricyclic antidepressants may occur); patients receiving MAO inhibitors within past 14 days; narrow-angle glaucoma

**Warnings** Use with caution in patients with cardiovascular disease, conduction disturbances, urinary retention, seizure disorders, hyperthyroidism, or those receiving thyroid replacement. Some formulations contain tartrazine which may cause an allergic reaction. Do not discontinue abruptly in patients receiving long-term high-dose therapy. Pregnancy factor C.

**Drug Interactions**

**Cytochrome P-450 Effect:** CYP1A2 and 2D6 enzyme substrate; CYP2D6 inhibitor

**Decreased Effect:** Decreased effects of antihypertensive agents (guanethidine, clonidine, guanabenz, guanfacine). Desipramine may also lower carbamazepine serum levels.

**Increased Effect/Toxicity:** Sympathomimetics (norepinephrine) taken with desipramine have an increased risk of adverse reactions. Increased toxicity with anticholinergics, alcohol, CNS depressants, MAO inhibitors (phenelzine). (Hyperpyrexia, tachycardia, hypertension, seizures, or death may occur.) Increased risk of bleeding with oral anticoagulants. Fluoxetine, paroxetine, cimetidine, and ritonavir enhance the effects of desipramine by elevating serum desipramine levels. Potential for serotonin syndrome if combined with other serotonergic drugs.

**Effects on Lab Values** ↑ glucose; ↓ glucose has also been reported

**Adverse Reactions**

>10%:

Central nervous system: Dizziness, drowsiness, headache

Gastrointestinal: Dry mouth, constipation, increased appetite, nausea, unpleasant taste, weight gain

Neuromuscular & skeletal: Weakness

1% to 10%:

Cardiovascular: Arrhythmias, hypotension

Central nervous system: Confusion, delirium, hallucinations, nervousness, restlessness, parkinsonian syndrome, insomnia

Gastrointestinal: Diarrhea, heartburn

Genitourinary: Dysuria, sexual dysfunction

Neuromuscular & skeletal: Fine muscle tremors

Ocular: Blurred vision, eye pain

Miscellaneous: Sweating (excessive)

<1% (Limited to important or life-threatening symptoms): Anxiety, seizures, alopecia, photosensitivity, agranulocytosis, leukopenia, eosinophilia, cholestatic jaundice, increased liver enzymes, increased intraocular pressure, sudden death

**Overdose/Toxicology** Symptoms of overdose include agitation, confusion, hallucinations, hyperthermia, urinary retention, CNS depression, cyanosis, dry mucous membranes, cardiac arrhythmias, and seizures. Treatment is supportive. Ventricular arrhythmias and EKG changes (eg, QRS widening) often respond with concurrent systemic alkalinization (sodium bicarbonate 0.5-2 mEq/kg I.V. or hyperventilation). Arrhythmias unresponsive to phenytoin 15-20 mg/kg (adults) may respond to lidocaine. Physostigmine (1-2 mg I.V. slowly for adults) may be indicated for reversing life-threatening cardiac arrhythmias.

**Pharmacodynamics/Kinetics**

**Half-life Elimination:** 7-60 hours

**Time to Peak:** Within 4-6 hours

**Metabolism:** Liver

**Excretion:** Urine

**Onset:** 1-3 weeks (maximum antidepressant effects: after >2 weeks)

**Formulations** Tablet (Norpramin®), as hydrochloride: 10 mg, 25 mg, 50 mg, 75 mg, 100 mg, 150 mg

**Dosing**

**Adults:** Oral: Initial: 75 mg/day in divided doses; increase gradually to 150-200 mg/day in divided or single dose; maximum: 300 mg/day

**Elderly:** Oral: Initial: 10-25 mg/day; increase by 10-25 mg every 3 days for inpatients and every week for outpatients if tolerated; usual maintenance dose: 75-100 mg/day, but doses up to 150 mg/day may be necessary.

**Renal Impairment:** Hemodialysis/peritoneal dialysis effects: Supplemental dose is not necessary.

**Additional Nursing Issues**

**Physical Assessment:** Assess other medications patient may be taking for effectiveness and interactions (see Drug Interactions). See Contraindications and Warnings/Precautions for cautious use. Assess for suicidal tendencies before beginning therapy. May cause physiological or psychological dependence, tolerance, or abuse; periodically evaluate need for continued use. **Note:** Desipramine may increase or decrease serum glucose levels. Monitor therapeutic response, and adverse reactions at beginning of therapy and periodically with long-term use (see Adverse Reactions and Overdose/Toxicology). Taper dosage slowly when discontinuing. Assess knowledge/teach patient appropriate use, interventions to reduce side effects, and adverse symptoms to report. **Pregnancy risk factor C** - contraceptive education may be appropriate. Breast-feeding is not recommended.

**Patient Information/Instruction:** Take exactly as directed (do not increase dose or frequency); may take several weeks to achieve desired results; may cause physical and/or psychological dependence. Avoid excessive alcohol, excess caffeine, and other prescription or OTC medications not approved by prescriber. Maintain adequate hydration (2-3 L/day of fluids unless instructed to restrict fluid intake). You may experience drowsiness, lightheadedness, impaired coordination, dizziness, or blurred vision (use caution when driving or engaging in tasks requiring alertness until response to drug is known); constipation (increased exercise, fluids, or dietary fruit and fiber may help); urinary retention (void before taking medication); postural hypotension (use caution climbing stairs or when changing position from lying or sitting to standing); altered sexual drive or ability (reversible); or photosensitivity (use sunscreen, wear protective clothing and eyewear, and avoid direct sunlight). Report persistent CNS effects (eg, nervousness, restlessness, insomnia, anxiety, excitation, headache, agitation, impaired coordination, changes in cognition); muscle cramping, weakness, tremors, or rigidity; chest pain, palpitations, or irregular heartbeat; blurred vision or eye pain; yellowing of skin or eyes; or worsening of condition. **Pregnancy/breast-feeding precautions:** Inform prescriber if you are or intend to be pregnant; contraceptives may be recommended. Breast-feeding is not recommended.

**Geriatric Considerations:** Preferred agent because of its milder side effect profile; patients may experience excitation or stimulation, in such cases, give as a single morning dose or divided dose.

**Breast-feeding Issues:** Generally, it is not recommended to breast-feed if taking antidepressants because of the long half-life, active metabolites, and the potential for side effects in the infant.

**Additional Information** Some formulations may contain tartrazine.

**Related Information**

Antidepressant Agents Comparison *on page 1368*
Peak and Trough Guidelines *on page 1331*

♦ **Desitin® Ointment** *see page 1294*

♦ **Desmethylimipramine Hydrochloride** *see* Desipramine *on page 343*

## Desmopressin (des moe PRES in)

**U.S. Brand Names** DDAVP® Nasal Spray; Stimate® Nasal

**Synonyms** 1-Deamino-8-D-Arginine Vasopressin

**Therapeutic Category** Vasopressin Analog, Synthetic

**Pregnancy Risk Factor** B

**Lactation** Enters breast milk/use caution

**Use** Treatment of diabetes insipidus and controlling bleeding in mild hemophilia, von Willebrand disease, and thrombocytopenia (eg, uremia); primary nocturnal enuresis

**Mechanism of Action/Effect** Enhances reabsorption of water in the kidneys by increasing cellular permeability of the collecting ducts; possibly causes smooth muscle constriction with resultant vasoconstriction; raises plasma levels of von Willebrand factor and factor VIII

**Contraindications** Hypersensitivity to desmopressin or any component; avoid using in patients with Type IIB or platelet-type von Willebrand disease or patients with <5% factor VIII activity level

**Warnings** Avoid overhydration especially when drug is used for its hemostatic effect.

**Drug Interactions**

**Decreased Effect:** Demeclocycline and lithium may decrease ADH response.

**Increased Effect/Toxicity:** Chlorpropamide, fludrocortisone may increase ADH response.

**Adverse Reactions**

1% to 10%:

- Cardiovascular: Facial flushing
- Central nervous system: Headache, dizziness
- Gastrointestinal: Nausea, abdominal cramps
- Genitourinary: Vulval pain
- Local: Pain at the injection site
- Respiratory: Nasal congestion (intranasal use)

<1% (Limited to important or life-threatening symptoms): Increase in blood pressure

**Overdose/Toxicology** Symptoms of overdose include drowsiness, headache, confusion, anuria, and water intoxication.

**Pharmacodynamics/Kinetics**

**Half-life Elimination:** I.V. infusion: Elimination (terminal): 75 minutes

**Onset:**

Intranasal administration: Onset of ADH effects: Within 1 hour; Peak effect: Within 1-5 hours

I.V. infusion: Onset of increased factor VIII activity: Within 15-30 minutes; Peak effect: 90 minutes to 3 hours

**Duration:** Intranasal administration: 5-21 hours

**Formulations**

Desmopressin acetate:

- Injection (DDAVP®): 4 mcg/mL (1 mL)
- Solution, nasal:
  - DDAVP®: 100 mcg/mL (2.5 mL, 5 mL)
  - Stimate®: 1.5 mg/mL (2.5 mL)
- Tablet (DDAVP®): 0.1 mg, 0.2 mg

(Continued)

## Desmopressin *(Continued)*

**Dosing**

**Adults:**

Diabetes insipidus: I.V., S.C.: 2-4 mcg/day in 2 divided doses or 1/10 of the maintenance intranasal dose; intranasal: Initial: 0.1 mL (10 mcg) divided 1-2 times/day; range: 0.1-0.4 mL/day in 1-3 divided doses

Primary nocturnal enuresis: 20 mcg intranasally at bedtime. Administer 50% of the dose per nostril. Adjust dose to response (range: 10-40 mcg).

von Willebrand disease, thrombocytopathies, hemophilia:

Intranasal: 2-4 mcg/kg/dose

I.V.: 0.3 mcg/kg by slow infusion over 15-30 minutes; usually tachyphylaxis occurs after 2-3 doses in 24 hours; recovery of responsiveness may take 48-72 hours

Oral: Begin therapy 12 hours after the last intranasal dose for patients previously on intranasal therapy; 0.05 mg twice daily; adjust individually to optimal therapeutic dose. Total daily dose should be increased or decreased (range: 0.1-1.2 mg divided 2-3 times/day) as needed to obtain adequate antidiuresis.

**Elderly:** Refer to adult dosing.

**Administration**

**I.V.:** Infuse over 15-30 minutes.

**I.V. Detail:** Dilute in 10-50 mL 0.9% sodium chloride.

**Other:** Nasal pump spray delivers 0.1 mL (10 mcg); for other doses which are not multiples, use rhinal tube.

**Stability**

**Storage:** Keep in refrigerator, avoid freezing. Discard discolored solutions. Nasal solution is stable for 3 weeks at room temperature. Injection is stable for 2 weeks at room temperature.

**Monitoring Laboratory Tests**

Diabetes insipidus: Urine volume, specific gravity, plasma and urine osmolality, serum electrolytes

Hemophilia: Factor VIII antigen levels, APTT, bleeding time (for von Willebrand disease and thrombocytopathies)

**Additional Nursing Issues**

**Physical Assessment:** Monitor laboratory results (see above) according to diagnosis. Monitor effectiveness of therapy and for adverse effects as identified above. I.V. infusion: Monitor vital sign and cardiac status. Teach patients appropriate administration techniques, precautions, and symptoms to report. Note breast-feeding caution.

**Patient Information/Instruction:** Use specific product as directed. Diabetes insipidus: Avoid overhydration. Weigh yourself daily at the same time in the same clothes. Report increased weight or swelling of extremities. If using intranasal product, inspect nasal membranes regularly. Report swelling or increased nasal congestion. All uses: Report unresolved headache, difficulty breathing, acute heartburn or nausea, abdominal cramping, or vulval pain. **Breast-feeding precautions:** Consult prescriber if breast-feeding.

**Geriatric Considerations:** Elderly patients should be cautioned not to increase their fluid intake beyond that sufficient to satisfy their thirst in order to avoid water intoxication and hyponatremia.

- **Desogen®** *see* Oral Contraceptives *on page 859*
- **Desogestrel and Ethinyl Estradiol** *see* Oral Contraceptives *on page 859*
- **Desonide** *see* Topical Corticosteroids *on page 1152*
- **DesOwen® Topical** *see* Topical Corticosteroids *on page 1152*
- **Desoximetasone** *see* Topical Corticosteroids *on page 1152*
- **Desoxyephedrine Hydrochloride** *see* Methamphetamine *on page 737*
- **Desoxyn®** *see* Methamphetamine *on page 737*
- **Desoxyn Gradumet®** *see* Methamphetamine *on page 737*
- **Desoxyphenobarbital** *see* Primidone *on page 964*
- **Desoxyribonuclease and Fibrinolysin** *see* Fibrinolysin and Desoxyribonuclease *on page 483*
- **Desquam-E® Gel** *see page 1294*
- **Desquam-X® Gel** *see page 1294*
- **Desquam-X® Wash** *see page 1294*
- **Desyrel®** *see* Trazodone *on page 1167*
- **Detensol®** *see* Propranolol *on page 986*
- **Detrol™** *see* Tolterodine *on page 1151*
- **Detuss®** *see* Caramiphen and Phenylpropanolamine *on page 195*
- **Detussin® Expectorant** *see* Hydrocodone, Pseudoephedrine, and Guaifenesin *on page 577*
- **Devrom® Chewable Tablet** *see page 1294*
- **Dexacidin®** *see page 1282*
- **Dexair®** *see* Dexamethasone *on this page*

## Dexamethasone (deks a METH a sone)

**U.S. Brand Names** AK-Dex®; Alba-Dex®; Baldex®; Dalalone L.A.®; Decadron®; Decadron®-LA; Decadron Turbinaire®; Decaject-L.A.®; Decaspray®; Dekasol-L.A.®; Dexair®; Dexasone L.A.®; Dexone®; Dexone L.A.®; Dezone®; Hexadrol®; I-Methasone®; Maxidex®; Ocu-Dex®; Solurex L.A.®

**Therapeutic Category** Corticosteroid, Oral; Corticosteroid, Oral Inhaler; Corticosteroid, Nasal; Corticosteroid, Ophthalmic; Corticosteroid, Parenteral; Corticosteroid, Topical

**Pregnancy Risk Factor** C

**Lactation** Excretion in breast milk unknown

**Use** Systemically and locally for chronic inflammation, allergic, hematologic, neoplastic, and autoimmune diseases; management of cerebral edema, septic shock; diagnostic agent; antiemetic

**Mechanism of Action/Effect** Decreases inflammation by suppression of migration of polymorphonuclear leukocytes and reversal of increased capillary permeability; suppresses normal immune response

**Contraindications**

Ophthalmic: Use in viral, fungal, or tuberculosis diseases of the eye

Systemic or topical: Active untreated infections

**Warnings** Fatalities have occurred due to adrenal insufficiency in asthmatic patients during and after transfer from systemic corticosteroids to aerosol steroids. Aerosol steroids do not provide the systemic steroid needed to treat patients having trauma, surgery, or infections. Use with caution in patients with hypothyroidism, cirrhosis, hypertension, congestive heart failure, ulcerative colitis, or thromboembolic disorders. Because of the risk of adverse effects, systemic corticosteroids should be used cautiously in the elderly in the smallest possible dose and for the shortest possible time. Pregnancy factor C.

**Drug Interactions**

**Cytochrome P-450 Effect:** CYP3A3/4 enzyme substrate; CYP3A3/4 enzyme inducer; CYP3A3/4 enzyme inhibitor

**Decreased Effect:** Barbiturates, phenytoin, and rifampin may cause decreased dexamethasone effects. Dexamethasone decreases effect of salicylates, vaccines, and toxoids.

**Adverse Reactions**

**Systemic:**

>10%:

Central nervous system: Insomnia, nervousness

Gastrointestinal: Increased appetite, indigestion

1% to 10%:

Dermatologic: Hirsutism

Endocrine & metabolic: Diabetes mellitus

Neuromuscular & skeletal: Arthralgia

Ocular: Cataracts

Respiratory: Epistaxis

<1% (Limited to important or life-threatening symptoms): Seizures, mood swings, headache, delirium, hallucinations, euphoria, skin atrophy, bruising, hyperpigmentation, acne, amenorrhea, sodium and water retention, Cushing's syndrome, hyperglycemia, bone growth suppression, abdominal distention, ulcerative esophagitis, pancreatitis, muscle wasting, hypersensitivity reactions

**Topical:** <1% (Limited to important or life-threatening symptoms): Itching, dryness, folliculitis, hypertrichosis, acneiform eruptions, hypopigmentation, perioral dermatitis, allergic contact dermatitis, skin maceration, skin atrophy, striae, miliaria, burning, irritation, secondary infection

**Overdose/Toxicology** When consumed in high doses over prolonged periods, systemic hypercorticism and adrenal suppression may occur. In these cases, discontinuation of the corticosteroid should be done judiciously.

**Pharmacodynamics/Kinetics**

**Half-life Elimination:** Normal renal function: 1.8-3.5 hours; Biological half-life: 36-54 hours

**Time to Peak:** Oral: Within 1-2 hours; I.M.: Within 8 hours

**Metabolism:** Liver

**Excretion:** Urine and bile

**Duration:** Duration of metabolic effect: Can last for 72 hours; acetate is a long-acting repository preparation with a prompt onset of action.

**Formulations**

Dexamethasone acetate:

Injection:

Suspension: 8 mg/mL (1 mL, 5 mL); 16 mg/mL (1 mL, 5 mL)

Dexamethasone sodium phosphate:

Aerosol:

Oral: 84 mcg dexamethasone per activation (12.6 g)

Nasal: 84 mcg dexamethasone/spray (12.6 g)

Injection:

Sodium phosphate: 4 mg/mL (1 mL, 5 mL, 10 mL, 25 mL, 30 mL); 10 mg/mL (1 mL, 10 mL); 20 mg/mL (5 mL); 24 mg/mL (5 mL, 10 mL)

Ophthalmic:

Ointment: 0.05% (3.5 g)

Suspension: 0.1% with methylcellulose 0.5% (5 mL, 15 mL)

Oral:

Concentrate: 0.5 mg/0.5 mL (30 mL) (30% alcohol)

Elixir: 0.5 mg/5 mL (5 mL, 20 mL, 100 mL, 120 mL, 237 mL, 240 mL, 500 mL)

Solution: 0.5 mg/5 mL (5 mL, 20 mL, 500 mL)

Tablet: 0.25 mg, 0.5 mg, 0.75 mg, 1 mg, 1.5 mg, 2 mg, 4 mg, 6 mg

Tablet, therapeutic pack: 6 x 1.5 mg; 8 x 0.75 mg

Topical, aerosol: 0.01% (58 g); 0.04% (25 g)

(Continued)

## Dexamethasone *(Continued)*

**Dosing**

**Adults:**

Acute nonlymphoblastic leukemia (ANLL) protocol: I.V.: 2 $mg/m^2$/dose every 8 hours for 12 doses

Antiemetic (prior to chemotherapy): Oral/I.V. (should be given as sodium phosphate): 10 $mg/m^2$/dose (usually 20 mg) for first dose then 5 $mg/m^2$/dose every 6 hours as needed

Anti-inflammatory:

Oral, I.M., I.V. (injections should be given as sodium phosphate): 0.75-9 mg/day in divided doses every 6-12 hours

I.M. (as acetate): 8-16 mg; may repeat in 1-3 weeks

Intralesional (as acetate): 0.8-1.6 mg

Intra-articular/soft tissue (as acetate): 4-16 mg; may repeat in 1-3 weeks

Intra-articular, intralesional, or soft tissue (as sodium phosphate): 0.4-6 mg/day

Cerebral edema: I.V. 10 mg stat, 4 mg I.M./I.V. (should be given as sodium phosphate) every 6 hours until response is maximized, then switch to oral regimen, then taper off if appropriate. Dosage may be reduced after 24 days and gradually discontinued over 5-7 days.

Diagnosis for Cushing's syndrome: Oral: 1 mg at 11 PM, draw blood at 8 AM the following day for plasma cortisol determination.

Physiological replacement: Oral, I.M., I.V. (should be given as sodium phosphate): 0.03-0.15 mg/kg/day **or** 0.6-0.75 $mg/m^2$/day in divided doses every 6-12 hours

Shock therapy: Addisonian crisis/shock (ie, adrenal insufficiency/responsive to steroid therapy): I.V. (given as sodium phosphate): 4-10 mg as a single dose, which may be repeated if necessary

Unresponsive shock (ie, unresponsive to steroid therapy): I.V. (given as sodium phosphate): 1-6 mg/kg as a single I.V. dose or up to 40 mg initially followed by repeat doses every 2-6 hours while shock persists

Ophthalmic:

Ointment: Apply thin coating into conjunctival sac 3-4 times/day; gradually taper dose to discontinue.

Suspension: Instill 2 drops into conjunctival sac every hour during the day and every other hour during the night; gradually reduce dose to every 3-4 hours, then to 3-4 times/day.

Topical: Apply 1-4 times/day.

**Elderly:** Refer to adult dosing. Use cautiously in the elderly in the smallest possible dose.

**Renal Impairment:** Hemodialysis or peritoneal dialysis: Supplemental dose is not necessary.

**Administration**

**Oral:** Administer oral formulation with meals to decrease GI upset.

**I.M.:** Acetate injection is **not** for I.V. use.

**Topical:** Topical formation is for external use. Do not use on open wounds. Apply sparingly to occlusive dressings. Should not be used in the presence of open or weeping lesions.

**Stability**

**Storage:** Dexamethasone 4 mg/mL injection solution is clear and colorless. Dexamethasone 24 mg/mL injection solution is clear and colorless to light yellow. Injection solution should be protected from light and freezing.

**Reconstitution:** Stability of injection of parenteral admixture at room temperature (25°C) is 24 hours. Stability of injection of parenteral admixture at refrigeration temperature (4°C) is 2 days. Protect from light and freezing. Standard diluent: 4 mg/50 mL $D_5W$; 10 mg/50 mL $D_5W$. Minimum volume: 50 mL $D_5W$.

**Monitoring Laboratory Tests** Hemoglobin, occult blood loss, serum potassium, glucose

Dexamethasone suppression test, overnight: 8 AM cortisol <6 mg/100 mL (dexamethasone 1 mg). Plasma cortisol determination should be made on the day after giving dose.

**Additional Nursing Issues**

**Physical Assessment:** Assess other medications patient may be taking for effectiveness and interactions (see Drug Interactions). Note Contraindications and Warnings/Precautions for cautious use. Monitor laboratory tests, therapeutic response, and adverse effects according to indications for therapy, dose, route (systemic or topical), and duration of therapy (see Dosing, Warnings/Precautions, Adverse Reactions). With systemic administration, diabetics should monitor glucose levels closely (corticosteroids may alter glucose levels). Instruct patient on appropriate application of particular form of dexamethasone. Advise about appropriate interventions for side effects and instruct about symptoms to report. When used for long-term therapy (longer than 10-14 days) do not discontinue abruptly; decrease dosage incrementally. **Pregnancy risk factor C** - benefits of use should outweigh possible risks. Note breast-feeding caution.

**Patient Information/Instruction:** Take exactly as directed; do not increase dose or discontinue abruptly without consulting prescriber. Take oral medication with or after meals. Limit intake of caffeine or stimulants. Prescriber may recommend increased dietary vitamins, minerals, or iron. Diabetics should monitor glucose levels closely (antidiabetic medication may need to be adjusted). Inform prescriber if you are experiencing greater than normal levels of stress (medication may need adjustment). Some forms of this medication may cause GI upset (oral medication may be taken with meals to reduce GI upset; small frequent meals and frequent mouth care may reduce GI upset). You may be more susceptible to infection (avoid crowds and persons with contagious or infective conditions). Report promptly excessive nervousness or sleep disturbances; any signs of infection (sore throat, unhealed injuries); excessive growth of body hair or loss of skin color; changes in vision; excessive or sudden weight gain (>3 lb/week); swelling of face or extremities; difficulty breathing; muscle weakness; change in color of stools (tarry) or persistent abdominal pain; or worsening of condition or failure to improve. **Pregnancy/breast-feeding precautions:** Inform prescriber if you are or intend to be pregnant. Consult prescriber if breast-feeding.

Ophthalmic: For ophthalmic use only. Wash hands before using. Tilt head back and look upward. Put drops of suspension or apply thin ribbon of ointment inside lower eyelid. Close eye and roll eyeball in all directions. Do not blink for ½ minute. Apply gentle pressure to inner corner of eye for 30 seconds. Do not use any other eye preparation for at least 10 minutes. Do not touch tip of applicator to eye or contaminate tip of applicator. Do not share medication with anyone else. Wear sunglasses when in sunlight; you may be more sensitive to bright light. Inform prescriber if condition worsens or fails to improve or if you experience eye pain, disturbances of vision, or other adverse eye response.

Topical: For external use only. Not for eyes or mucous membranes or open wounds. Apply in very thin layer to occlusive dressing. Apply dressing to area being treated. Avoid prolonged or excessive use around sensitive tissues, genital, or rectal areas. Inform prescriber if condition worsens (swelling, redness, irritation, pain, open sores) or fails to improve.

Aerosol: Not for use during acute asthmatic attack. Follow directions that accompany product. Rinse mouth and throat after use to prevent candidiasis. Do not use intranasal product if you have a nasal infection, nasal injury, or recent nasal surgery. If using two products, consult prescriber in which order to use the two products. Inform prescriber if condition worsens or does not improve.

**Geriatric Considerations:** Because of the risk of adverse effects, systemic corticosteroids should be used cautiously in the elderly in the smallest possible dose, and for the shortest possible time.

**Pregnancy Issues:** Dexamethasone has been used in patients with premature labor (26-34 weeks gestation) to stimulate fetal lung maturation. Effects on the fetus: Crosses the placenta; transient leukocytosis has been reported. Available evidence suggests safe use during pregnancy.

**Additional Information** Some formulations may contain sulfites.


- ♦ **Dexamethasone** *see* Topical Corticosteroids *on page 1152*
- ♦ **Dexamethasone and Neomycin** *see* Neomycin and Dexamethasone *on page 816*
- ♦ **Dexasone L.A.®** *see* Dexamethasone *on page 346*
- ♦ **Dexatrim® Pre-Meal [OTC]** *see* Phenylpropanolamine *on page 922*
- ♦ **Dexbrompheniramine and Pseudoephedrine** *see page 1294*
- ♦ **Dexchlor®** *see* Dexchlorpheniramine *on this page*


## Dexchlorpheniramine (deks klor fen EER a meen)

**U.S. Brand Names** Dexchlor®; Poladex®; Polaramine®

**Therapeutic Category** Antihistamine

**Pregnancy Risk Factor** B

**Lactation** Excretion in breast milk unknown/not recommended

**Use** Perennial and seasonal allergic rhinitis and other allergic symptoms including urticaria

**Mechanism of Action/Effect** Competes with histamine for $H_1$-receptor sites on effector cells in the GI tract, blood vessels, and respiratory tract

**Contraindications** Hypersensitivity to dexchlorpheniramine or any component; narrow-angle glaucoma

**Warnings** Bladder neck obstruction, symptomatic prostatic hypertrophy, asthmatic attack, and stenosing peptic ulcer

**Drug Interactions**

**Increased Effect/Toxicity:** Increased effect/toxicity with CNS depressants, MAO inhibitors, tricyclic antidepressants, phenothiazines, and guanabenz.

**Effects on Lab Values** May interfere with a methacholine bronchial challenge.

**Adverse Reactions**

>10%:

Central nervous system: Slight to moderate drowsiness

Respiratory: Thickening of bronchial secretions

1% to 10%:

Central nervous system: Headache, fatigue, nervousness, dizziness

Gastrointestinal: Appetite increase, weight gain, nausea, diarrhea, abdominal pain, dry mouth

Neuromuscular & skeletal: Arthralgia

Respiratory: Pharyngitis

<1% (Limited to important or life-threatening symptoms): Palpitations, hepatitis, bronchospasm, epistaxis

**Overdose/Toxicology** Symptoms of overdose include dry mouth, flushed skin, dilated pupils, CNS depression. There is no specific treatment for antihistamine overdose. Clinical toxicity is due to blockade of cholinergic receptors. For anticholinergic overdose with severe life-threatening symptoms, physostigmine 1-2 mg I.V. slowly, may be given to reverse these effects.

(Continued)

## Dexchlorpheniramine *(Continued)*

**Pharmacodynamics/Kinetics**

**Time to Peak:** Peak effect: Oral: Within 3 hours

**Metabolism:** Liver

**Excretion:** Urine

**Onset:** ~1 hour

**Duration:** 3-6 hours

**Formulations**

Dexchlorpheniramine maleate:

Syrup (orange flavor): 2 mg/5 mL with alcohol 6% (480 mL)

Tablet: 2 mg

Tablet, sustained action: 4 mg, 6 mg

**Dosing**

**Adults:** Oral: 2 mg every 4-6 hours or 4-6 mg timed release at bedtime or every 8-10 hours

**Elderly:** Refer to adult dosing.

**Additional Nursing Issues**

**Physical Assessment:** Assess effectiveness and interactions of other medications (see Drug Interactions). See Contraindications and Warnings/Precautions for cautious use. Monitor effectiveness of therapy and adverse reactions (eg, excess anticholinergic effects - see Adverse Reactions) at beginning of therapy and periodically with long-term use. Assess knowledge/teach patient appropriate use, interventions to reduce side effects, and adverse symptoms to report. Breast-feeding is not recommended.

**Patient Information/Instruction:** Take as directed; do not exceed recommended dose. Do not chew or crush sustained release tablet. Avoid use of other depressants, alcohol, or sleep-inducing medications unless approved by prescriber. You may experience drowsiness or dizziness (use caution when driving or engaging in tasks requiring alertness until response to drug is known); or dry mouth, nausea, or abdominal pain (frequent small meals, frequent mouth care, chewing gum, or sucking hard candy may help). Report persistent sedation, confusion, or agitation; changes in urinary pattern; blurred vision; sore throat, difficulty breathing or expectorating (thick secretions); or lack of improvement or worsening or condition. **Breast-feeding precautions:** Breast-feeding is not recommended.

**Geriatric Considerations:** Anticholinergic action may cause significant confusional symptoms, constipation, or problems voiding urine.

**Additional Information** Some formulations may contain ethanol.

◆ **Dexedrine®** *see* Dextroamphetamine *on page 353*

◆ **Dexone®** *see* Dexamethasone *on page 346*

◆ **Dexone L.A.®** *see* Dexamethasone *on page 346*

## Dexrazoxane (deks ray ZOKS ane)

**U.S. Brand Names** Zinecard®

**Synonyms** ICRF-187

**Therapeutic Category** Cardioprotectant

**Pregnancy Risk Factor** C

**Lactation** Excretion in breast milk unknown

**Use** Reduction of the incidence and severity of cardiomyopathy associated with doxorubicin administration in women with metastatic breast cancer who have received a cumulative doxorubicin dose of 300 mg/m$^2$ and who would benefit from continuing therapy with doxorubicin. It is not recommended for use with the initiation of doxorubicin therapy.

**Mechanism of Action/Effect** Derivative of EDTA and potent intracellular chelating agent. The mechanism of cardioprotectant activity is not fully understood. Appears to be converted intracellularly to a ring-opened chelating agent that interferes with iron-mediated free radical generation thought to be responsible, in part, for anthracycline-induced cardiomyopathy.

**Contraindications** Do not use with chemotherapy regimens that do not contain an anthracycline.

**Warnings** Dexrazoxane may add to the myelosuppression caused by chemotherapeutic agents. There is some evidence that the use of dexrazoxane concurrently with the initiation of fluorouracil, doxorubicin, and cyclophosphamide (FAC) therapy interferes with the antitumor efficacy of the regimen, and this use is not recommended. Dexrazoxane should only be used in those patients who have received a cumulative doxorubicin dose of 300 mg/m$^2$ and are continuing with doxorubicin therapy. Dexrazoxane does not eliminate the potential for anthracycline-induced cardiac toxicity. Carefully monitor cardiac function. Pregnancy factor C.

**Drug Interactions**

**Decreased Effect:** There is some evidence that the use of dexrazoxane concurrently with the initiation of FAC therapy interferes with the antitumor efficacy of the regimen, and this use is not recommended.

**Adverse Reactions** Adverse experiences are likely attributable to the FAC regimen, with the exception of pain on injection that was observed mainly with dexrazoxane. Patients receiving FAC with dexrazoxane experienced more severe leukopenia, granulocytopenia, and thrombocytopenia at nadir than patients receiving FAC without dexrazoxane; but recovery counts were similar for the two groups.

1% to 10%: Dermatologic: Urticaria, recall skin reaction, extravasation

**Overdose/Toxicology** Management includes supportive care until resolution of myelosuppression and related conditions is complete. Retention of a significant dose fraction of unchanged drug in the plasma pool, minimal tissue partitioning or binding, and availability of >90% of systemic drug levels in the unbound form suggest that dexrazoxane could be removed using conventional peritoneal or hemodialysis.

**Pharmacodynamics/Kinetics**

**Distribution:** Not bound to plasma proteins

**Half-life Elimination:** 2.1-2.5 hours

**Excretion:** 42% of dose excreted in the urine; renal clearance: 3.35 L/hour/$m^2$; plasma clearance: 6.25-7.88 L/hour/$m^2$

**Formulations** Powder for injection, lyophilized: 250 mg, 500 mg (10 mg/mL when reconstituted)

**Dosing**

**Adults:** I.V.: The recommended dosage ratio of dexrazoxane:doxorubicin is 10:1 (eg, 500 mg/$m^2$ dexrazoxane:50 mg/$m^2$ doxorubicin).

**Elderly:** Refer to adult dosing.

**Administration**

**I.V.:** Doxorubicin should not be given prior to the I.V. injection of dexrazoxane. Give dexrazoxane by slow I.V. push or rapid drip I.V. infusion from a bag. Give doxorubicin within 30 minutes after beginning the infusion with dexrazoxane.

**Stability**

**Storage:** Store intact vials at controlled room temperature (15°C to 30°C/59°F to 86°F).

**Reconstitution:** Caution should be exercised in the handling and preparation of the reconstituted solution; the use of gloves is recommended. If dexrazoxane powder or solutions contact the skin or mucosae, immediately wash with soap and water.

Reconstituted and diluted solutions are stable for 6 hours at controlled room temperature or under refrigeration (2°C to 8°C/36°F to 46°F). Must be reconstituted with 0.167 Molar (M/6) sodium lactate injection to a concentration of 10 mg dexrazoxane/mL sodium lactate. Reconstituted dexrazoxane solution may be diluted with either 0.9% sodium chloride injection or 5% dextrose injection to a concentration of 1.3-5 mg/mL in intravenous infusion bags.

**Monitoring Laboratory Tests** Since dexrazoxane will always be used with cytotoxic drugs, and since it may add to the myelosuppressive effects of cytotoxic drugs, frequent complete blood counts are recommended. Monitor LFTs.

**Additional Nursing Issues**

**Physical Assessment:** Monitor for effectiveness of therapy and adverse effects. **Pregnancy risk factor C** - benefits of use should outweigh possible risks. Note breast-feeding caution.

**Patient Information/Instruction:** This I.V. medication is given to reduce incidence of cardiac complications with doxorubicin. Report promptly any pain at infusion site. **Pregnancy/breast-feeding precautions:** Inform prescriber if pregnant. Consult prescriber if breast-feeding.

**Other Issues:** Follow guidelines for handling cytotoxic agents. If drug comes in contact with skin or mucosa, wash immediately with soap and water.

## Dextran (DEKS tran)

**U.S. Brand Names** Gentran®; LMD®; Macrodex®; Rheomacrodex®

**Synonyms** Dextran, High Molecular Weight; Dextran, Low Molecular Weight

**Therapeutic Category** Plasma Volume Expander

**Pregnancy Risk Factor** C

**Lactation** Excretion in breast milk unknown

**Use** Blood volume expander used in treatment of shock or impending shock when blood or blood products are not available

**Mechanism of Action/Effect** Produces plasma volume expansion by virtue of its highly colloidal starch structure, similar to albumin

**Contraindications** Hypersensitivity to dextrans or any component (see Dextran 1)

**Warnings** Use caution in patients with CHF, renal insufficiency, thrombocytopenia, or active hemorrhage. **Observe patients closely during the first minute of infusion and have other means of maintaining circulation with epinephrine and diphenhydramine available should dextran therapy result in an anaphylactoid reaction.** Patients should be well hydrated at the start of therapy. Discontinue dextran if urine specific gravity is low and/or if oliguria or anuria occurs or if there is a precipitous rise in central venous pressure and signs of circulatory overload. Pregnancy factor C.

**Adverse Reactions**

<1% (Limited to important or life-threatening symptoms): Mild hypotension, tightness of chest, wheezing

**Overdose/Toxicology** Symptoms of overdose include fluid overload, pulmonary edema, increased bleeding time, and decreased platelet function. Treatment is supportive. Blood products containing clotting factors may be necessary.

**Pharmacodynamics/Kinetics**

**Excretion:** ~75% excreted in urine within 24 hours

**Onset:** I.V.: Within minutes to 1 hour (depending upon the molecular weight polysaccharide administered), infusion volume expansion occurs

**Formulations**

Injection:

High molecular weight:

6% dextran 75 in dextrose 5% (500 mL)

Gentran®: 6% dextran 75 in sodium chloride 0.9% (500 mL)

(Continued)

## Dextran *(Continued)*

Gentran®, Macrodex®: 6% dextran 70 in sodium chloride 0.9% (500 mL)
Macrodex®: 6% dextran 70 in dextrose 5% (500 mL)
Low molecular weight: Gentran®, LMD®, Rheomacrodex®:
10% dextran 40 in dextrose 5% (500 mL)
10% dextran 40 in sodium chloride 0.9% (500 mL)

**Dosing**

**Adults:** I.V.: 500-1000 mL; if therapy continues beyond 24 hours, total daily dosage should not exceed 10 mL/kg and therapy should not continue beyond 5 days.

**Elderly:** Use with extreme caution in patients with renal or hepatic impairment.

**Renal Impairment:** Use with extreme caution.

**Hepatic Impairment:** Use with extreme caution.

**Administration**

**I.V.:** For I.V. infusion only (use an infusion pump). Infuse initial 500 mL at a rate of 20-40 mL/minute if hypervolemic. Reduce rate for additional infusion to 4 mL/minute. **Observe patients closely for anaphylactic reaction.**

**I.V. Detail:** Have other means of maintaining circulation with epinephrine and diphenhydramine available should dextran therapy result in an anaphylactoid reaction.

**Stability**

**Storage:** Store at room temperature. Discard partially used containers. If crystals have formed, can heat in a water bath at 100°C or autoclave at 110°C for 15 minutes.

**Compatibility:** Do not add any drugs to dextran solution. To prevent coagulation of blood, flush tubing well or change I.V. tubing before infusing blood after dextran.

**Monitoring Laboratory Tests** Hemoglobin and hematocrit, electrolytes, serum protein

**Additional Nursing Issues**

**Physical Assessment:** Monitor closely during first minute of infusion (see Warnings/Precautions and Administration). Continue to monitor pulse, blood pressure, and central venous pressure every 5-15 minutes for the first hour and then periodically thereafter. Observe for increased bleeding.

**Patient Information/Instruction:** Since this medication is generally used in emergency situations, patient education should be appropriate.

**Additional Information**

Sodium content of 500 mL: 77 mEq
pH: 3.0-7.0

## Dextran 1 (DEKS tran won)

**U.S. Brand Names** Promit®

**Therapeutic Category** Plasma Volume Expander

**Pregnancy Risk Factor** C

**Lactation** Excretion in breast milk unknown

**Use** Prophylaxis of serious anaphylactic reactions to I.V. infusion of dextran

**Mechanism of Action/Effect** Binds to dextran-reactive immunoglobulin without bridge formation and no formation of large immune complexes

**Contraindications** Hypersensitivity to dextrans or any component

**Warnings** If immune adverse reactions occur, do not administer large volumes of dextran solutions for clinical use. Pregnancy factor C.

**Adverse Reactions** <1% (Limited to important or life-threatening symptoms): Mild hypotension, tightness of chest, wheezing

**Formulations** Injection: 150 mg/mL (20 mL)

**Dosing**

**Adults:** Administer 1 dose only prior to dextran. Give 1-2 minutes before I.V. infusion of dextran. Time between dextran 1 and dextran solution should not exceed 15 minutes.

**Elderly:** Refer to adult dosing.

**Administration**

**I.V.:** Infuse over 1 minute.

**Stability**

**Storage:** Protect from freezing.

**Compatibility:** Do not dilute or admix with dextrans.

- **Dextran, High Molecular Weight** *see* Dextran *on previous page*
- **Dextran, Low Molecular Weight** *see* Dextran *on previous page*

## Dextranomer (deks TRAN oh mer)

**U.S. Brand Names** Debrisan® [OTC]

**Therapeutic Category** Topical Skin Product

**Pregnancy Risk Factor** C

**Lactation** For external use

**Use** Clean exudative wounds; no controlled studies have found dextranomer to be more effective than conventional therapy

**Mechanism of Action/Effect** Dextranomer is a network of dextran-sucrose beads possessing a great many exposed hydroxy groups. When this network is applied to an exudative wound surface, the exudate is drawn by capillary forces generated by the swelling of the beads, with vacuum forces producing an upward flow of exudate into the network.

**Contraindications** Hypersensitivity to dextranomer or any component; deep fistulas; sinus tracts

**Warnings** Do not use in deep fistulas or any area where complete removal is not assured. Do not use on dry wounds (ineffective). Avoid contact with eyes. Pregnancy factor C.

**Adverse Reactions** 1% to 10%:
Local: Transitory pain, blistering
Dermatologic: Maceration may occur, erythema
Hematologic: Bleeding

**Formulations**
Beads: 4 g, 25 g, 60 g, 120 g
Paste: 10 g foil packets

**Dosing**
**Adults:** Apply to affected area every 12 hours or more frequent as needed. Removal should be done by irrigation.
**Elderly:** Refer to adult dosing.

**Administration**
**Topical:** For external use only. Debride and clean wound before application. Sprinkle beads into ulcer (or apply paste) to 1/4" thickness. Change dressings 1-4 times/day depending on drainage. Change dressing before it is completely dry to facilitate removal.

**Additional Nursing Issues**
**Physical Assessment:** See Contraindications and Warnings/Precautions for use cautions. See application directions above. When applied to large areas or for extensive periods of time, monitor for adverse reactions. Assess knowledge/teach patient appropriate application and use and adverse symptoms to report. **Pregnancy risk factor C.**
**Patient Information/Instruction:** Use exactly as directed; do not overuse. Clean wound as directed. Sprinkle beads into or apply paste to 1/4" thickness. Change dressing 1-4 times/day before dressing is completely dry to facilitate removal. Wash hands carefully following application. Avoid contact with eyes or other nonulcerous tissue. Report increased swelling, redness, rash, itching, signs of infection, worsening of condition, or lack of healing. **Pregnancy precautions:** Inform prescriber if you are or intend to be pregnant.
**Geriatric Considerations:** Debrisan® is indicated in stage 3 and 4 decubitus ulcers.

## Dextroamphetamine (deks troe am FET a meen)

**U.S. Brand Names** Dexedrine®; Oxydess® II; Spancap® No. 1

**Therapeutic Category** Stimulant

**Pregnancy Risk Factor** C

**Lactation** Enters breast milk/contraindicated

**Use** Treatment of narcolepsy, exogenous obesity, abnormal behavioral syndrome in children (minimal brain dysfunction), attention-deficit/hyperactivity disorder (ADHD)

**Mechanism of Action/Effect** Blocks reuptake of dopamine and norepinephrine from the synapse, thus increasing the amount of circulating dopamine and norepinephrine in the cerebral cortex to reticular activating system. Inhibits the action of monoamine oxidase and causes catecholamines to be released.

**Contraindications** Hypersensitivity to dextroamphetamine or any component; advanced arteriosclerosis; hypertension; hyperthyroidism; glaucoma; MAO inhibitors

**Warnings** Use with caution in patients with psychopathic personalities, cardiovascular disease, hypertension, angina, and glaucoma. Has high potential for abuse. Prolonged administration may lead to drug dependence. Use in weight reduction programs only when alternative therapy has been ineffective. Pregnancy factor C.

**Drug Interactions**
**Decreased Effect:** Methyldopa decreases antihypertensive efficacy. Decreased effect with acidifiers and psychotropics may occur.
**Increased Effect/Toxicity:** May precipitate arrhythmias in patients receiving general anesthetics. Amphetamines taken with MAO inhibitors (phenelzine, tranylcypromine) have resulted in severe hypertensive reactions. The same hypertensive reaction may also occur with related drugs, isocarboxazid, or furazolidone. May increase the effect/toxicity of tricyclic antidepressants, phenytoin, phenobarbital, propoxyphene, norepinephrine, and meperidine.

**Food Interactions** Dextroamphetamine serum levels may be altered if taken with acidic food, juices, or vitamin C.

**Adverse Reactions**
>10%:
Cardiovascular: Arrhythmia
Central nervous system: False feeling of well being, nervousness, restlessness, insomnia

1% to 10%:
Cardiovascular: Hypertension
Central nervous system: Mood or mental changes, dizziness, lightheadedness, headache
Endocrine & metabolic: Changes in libido
Gastrointestinal: Diarrhea, nausea, vomiting, stomach cramps, constipation, anorexia, weight loss, dry mouth
Ocular: Blurred vision
Miscellaneous: Sweating (increased)

<1% (Limited to important or life-threatening symptoms): Chest pain, CNS stimulation (severe), Tourette's syndrome, hyperthermia, seizures, paranoia

**Overdose/Toxicology** Symptoms of overdose include restlessness, tremor, confusion, hallucinations, panic, dysrhythmias, nausea, and vomiting. There is no specific antidote for dextroamphetamine intoxication and treatment is primarily supportive. Hyperactivity
(Continued)

## Dextroamphetamine *(Continued)*

and agitation usually respond to reduced sensory input; however, with extreme agitation, haloperidol (2-5 mg I.M. for adults) may be required.

**Pharmacodynamics/Kinetics**

**Half-life Elimination:** 34 hours (urine pH dependent)

**Time to Peak:** Oral: Within 3 hours

**Metabolism:** Liver

**Excretion:** Urine

**Onset:** 1-1.5 hours

**Formulations**

Dextroamphetamine sulfate:

Capsule, sustained release: 5 mg, 10 mg, 15 mg

Tablet: 5 mg, 10 mg (5 mg tablets contain tartrazine)

**Dosing**

**Adults:** Oral:

Narcolepsy: Initial: 10 mg/day, may increase at 10 mg increments in weekly intervals until side effects appear; maximum: 60 mg/day

Exogenous obesity: 5-30 mg/day in divided doses of 5-10 mg 30-60 minutes before meals

**Elderly:** Refer to adult dosing; start with lowest dose. Use with caution.

**Administration**

**Oral:** Do not crush sustained release drug product. Administer as single dose in morning or as divided doses with breakfast and lunch. Should be administered 30 minutes before meals and at least 6 hours before bedtime.

**Stability**

**Storage:** Protect from light.

**Additional Nursing Issues**

**Physical Assessment:** Assess effectiveness and interactions of other medications patient may be taking (see Drug Interactions). Assess for history of psychopathology, homicidal or suicidal tendencies, or addiction; long-term use can result in dependence, abuse, or tolerance. Periodically evaluate the need for continued use. Monitor blood pressure, vital signs, and adverse reactions at start of therapy, when changing dosage, and at regular intervals during therapy (see Adverse Reactions). Monitor serum glucose closely with diabetic patients (amphetamines may alter antidiabetic requirements). Taper dosage slowly when discontinuing. Assess knowledge/teach patient appropriate use, possible side effects, and symptoms to report. **Pregnancy risk factor C** - contraceptive education may be appropriate - benefits of use should outweigh possible risks. Breast-feeding is contraindicated.

**Patient Information/Instruction:** Take exactly as directed (do not increase dose or frequency without consulting prescriber); may cause physical and/or psychological dependence. Take early in day to avoid sleep disturbance, 30 minutes before meals. Avoid alcohol, caffeine, or OTC medications that act as stimulants. You may experience restlessness, false sense of euphoria, or impaired judgment (use caution when driving or engaging in tasks requiring alertness until response to drug is known); dry mouth (frequent mouth care, sucking lozenges, or chewing gum may help); nausea or vomiting (small frequent meals, frequent mouth care may help); constipation (increased exercise, dietary fiber, fruit, or fluid may help); diarrhea (buttermilk, boiled milk, or yogurt may help); or altered libido (reversible). Diabetics need to monitor serum glucose closely (may alter antidiabetic medication requirements). Report chest pain, palpitations, or irregular heartbeat; extreme fatigue or depression; CNS changes (aggressiveness, restlessness, euphoria, sleep disturbances); severe unremitting abdominal distress or cramping; blackened stool; changes in sexual activity; or blurred vision. **Pregnancy/breast-feeding precautions:** Inform prescriber if you are or intend to be pregnant. Do not breast-feed.

**Additional Information** Some formulations may contain ethanol or tartrazine.

- **Dextromethorphan** *see page 1294*
- **Dextromethorphan and Guaifenesin** *see* Guaifenesin and Dextromethorphan *on page 549*
- **Dextromethorphan and Promethazine** *see* Promethazine and Dextromethorphan *on page 980*
- **Dextromethorphan, Guaifenesin, and Phenylpropanolamine** *see* Guaifenesin, Phenylpropanolamine, and Dextromethorphan *on page 551*
- **Dextropropoxyphene** *see* Propoxyphene *on page 984*
- **Dey-Dose® Isoproterenol** *see* Isoproterenol *on page 632*
- **Dey-Dose® Metaproterenol** *see* Metaproterenol *on page 732*
- **Dey-Drop® Ophthalmic Solution** *see* Silver Nitrate *on page 1057*
- **Dey-Lute® Isoetharine** *see* Isoetharine *on page 629*
- **Dezone®** *see* Dexamethasone *on page 346*
- **DHAD** *see* Mitoxantrone *on page 780*
- **DHC Plus®** *see* Dihydrocodeine Compound *on page 373*
- **D.H.E. 45® Injection** *see* Dihydroergotamine *on page 374*
- **DHPG Sodium** *see* Ganciclovir *on page 526*
- **DHS® Tar** *see page 1294*
- **DHS Zinc®** *see page 1294*
- **DHT™** *see* Dihydrotachysterol *on page 375*
- **Diaβeta®** *see* Glyburide *on page 538*

- ♦ **Diabetic Tussin DM® [OTC]** *see* Guaifenesin and Dextromethorphan *on page 549*
- ♦ **Diabetic Tussin EX® [OTC]** *see* Guaifenesin *on page 548*
- ♦ **Diabinese®** *see* Chlorpropamide *on page 259*
- ♦ **Diagnostics and Surgical Aids** *see page 1248*
- ♦ **Dialose® Plus Capsule** *see page 1294*
- ♦ **Dialose® Plus Tablet** *see page 1294*
- ♦ **Dialume® [OTC]** *see* Aluminum Hydroxide *on page 60*
- ♦ **Diamine T.D.®** *see page 1294*
- ♦ **Diaminodiphenylsulfone** *see* Dapsone *on page 334*
- ♦ **Diamox®** *see* Acetazolamide *on page 34*
- ♦ **Diamox Sequels®** *see* Acetazolamide *on page 34*
- ♦ **Diaparene®** *see page 1294*
- ♦ **Diapid® Nasal Spray** *see* Lypressin *on page 701*
- ♦ **Diar-Aid® [OTC]** *see* Loperamide *on page 688*
- ♦ **Diasorb®** *see page 1294*
- ♦ **Diastat® Gel** *see* Diazepam *on this page*
- ♦ **Diatex** *see* Diazepam *on this page*
- ♦ **Diaval** *see* Tolbutamide *on page 1146*
- ♦ **Diazemuls®** *see* Diazepam *on this page*
- ♦ **Diazemuls® Injection** *see* Diazepam *on this page*


## Diazepam (dye AZ e pam)

**U.S. Brand Names** Diastat® Gel; Diazemuls® Injection; Emulsified Dizac® Injection; Emulsified Valium®

**Therapeutic Category** Benzodiazepine

**Pregnancy Risk Factor** D

**Lactation** Enters breast milk/contraindicated (AAP rates "of concern")

**Use** Management of general anxiety disorders, panic disorders, and provide preoperative sedation, light anesthesia, and amnesia; treatment of status epilepticus, alcohol withdrawal symptoms; skeletal muscle relaxant

**Mechanism of Action/Effect** Depresses all levels of the CNS, including the limbic and reticular formation, probably through the increased action of gamma-aminobutyric acid (GABA), which is a major inhibitory neurotransmitter in the brain

**Contraindications** Hypersensitivity to diazepam or any component; there may be a cross-sensitivity with other benzodiazepines; do not use in a comatose patient, in those with pre-existing CNS depression, respiratory depression, narrow-angle glaucoma, or severe uncontrolled pain; pregnancy

**Warnings** Use with caution in patients receiving other CNS depressants, patients with low albumin, hepatic dysfunction, and in the elderly and young infants. Due to its long-acting metabolite, diazepam is not considered a drug of choice in the elderly. Long-acting benzodiazepines have been associated with falls in the elderly.

**Drug Interactions**

**Cytochrome P-450 Effect:** CYP1A2, 2C8, and 2C9 enzyme substrate, CYP3A3/4 enzyme substrate (minor), and diazepam and desmethyldiazepam are CYP2C19 enzyme substrates

**Decreased Effect:** Enzyme inducers may increase the metabolism and result in a decreased effect of diazepam.

**Increased Effect/Toxicity:** CNS depressants (alcohol, barbiturates, opioids) may enhance sedation and respiratory depression. Cimetidine may decrease the metabolism of diazepam resulting in enhanced effect. Cisapride can significantly increase diazepam levels. Valproic acid may displace diazepam from binding sites which may result in an increase in sedative effects. Selective serotonin reuptake inhibitors (eg, fluoxetine, sertraline, paroxetine) have greatly increased diazepam levels by altering its clearance.

**Food Interactions** Diazepam serum levels may be increased if taken with food.

**Effects on Lab Values** False-negative urinary glucose determinations when using Clinistix® or Diastix®

**Adverse Reactions**

>10%:

Central nervous system: Drowsiness, ataxia, lightheadedness, headache, dizziness, impaired coordination, anxiety, fatigue, slurred speech, irritability, nervousness, insomnia, memory impairment, cognitive disorder, dysarthria, anxiety

Gastrointestinal: Decreased salivation (dry mouth)

Genitourinary: Micturition difficulties

1% to 10%:

Cardiovascular: Syncope

Central nervous system: Confusion, increased libido, depersonalization, mental depression, perceptual disturbances, parethesias, weakness, akathisia, agitation, disinhibition, talkativeness, derealization, dream abnormalities, fear, decreased libido

Gastrointestinal: Abdominal or stomach cramps, increased or decreased appetite, weight gain or loss, nausea, vomiting

Neuromuscular & skeletal: Muscle cramps

Ocular: Photophobia, blurred vision

Otic: Tinnitus

Respiratory: Nasal congestion

Miscellaneous: Sweating

(Continued)

## Diazepam *(Continued)*

<1% (Limited to important or life-threatening symptoms): Tachycardia, phlebitis, hallucinations, convulsions, paranoid symptoms, anemia, agranulocytosis, neutropenia, leukopenia, thrombocytopenia, liver dysfunction, dystonic reactions

**Overdose/Toxicology** Symptoms of overdose include somnolence, confusion, coma, hypoactive reflexes, dyspnea, hypotension, slurred speech, or impaired coordination. Treatment for benzodiazepine overdose is supportive. Flumazenil has been shown to selectively block the binding of benzodiazepines to CNS receptors, resulting in a reversal of benzodiazepine-induced CNS depression, but not respiratory depression.

**Pharmacodynamics/Kinetics**

**Protein Binding:** 98%

**Half-life Elimination:**

Parent drug: 20-50 hours; increased half-life in the elderly and those with severe hepatic disorders

Active major metabolite (desmethyldiazepam): 50-100 hours

**Metabolism:** Liver

**Onset:** I.V. for status epilepticus: Almost immediate

**Duration:** I.V. for status epilepticus: Short, 20-30 minutes

**Formulations**

Gel, rectal (Diastat®): 2.5 mg, 5 mg, 10 mg, 15 mg, 20 mg
Injection: 5 mg/mL (1 mL, 2 mL, 5 mL, 10 mL)
Injection, emulsified (Dizac®): 5 mg/mL (3 mL)
Injection, emulsified (Diazemuls®): 5 mg/mL (2 mL)
Solution, oral (wintergreen-spice flavor): 5 mg/5 mL (5 mL, 10 mL, 500 mL)
Solution, oral concentrate: 5 mg/mL (30 mL)
Tablet: 2 mg, 5 mg, 10 mg

**Dosing**

**Adults: Oral absorption is more reliable than I.M.**

Anxiety/sedation/skeletal muscle relaxation:

Oral: 2-10 mg 2-4 times/day

I.M., I.V.: 2-10 mg, may repeat in 3-4 hours if needed

Status epilepticus: I.V.: 5-10 mg every 10-20 minutes, up to 30 mg in an 8-hour period; may repeat in 2-4 hours if necessary

**Elderly: Oral absorption is more reliable than I.M.**

Oral: Initial:

Anxiety: 1-2 mg 1-2 times/day; increase gradually as needed, rarely need to use >10 mg/day

Skeletal muscle relaxant: 2-5 mg 2-4 times/day

**Renal Impairment:** Hemodialysis effects: Not dialyzable (0% to 5%); supplemental dose is **not** necessary.

**Hepatic Impairment:** Reduce dose by 50% in cirrhosis and avoid in severe/acute liver disease.

**Administration**

**I.V.:** Continuous infusion is not recommended because of precipitation in I.V. fluids and absorption of drug into infusion bags and tubing. Administer each 5 mg I.V. push over at least 1 minute.

**Stability**

**Storage:** Protect parenteral dosage form from light. Potency is retained for up to 3 months when kept at room temperature.

**Reconstitution:** Most stable at pH 4-8, hydrolysis occurs at pH <3.

**Compatibility:** Do not mix I.V. product with other medications. See the Compatibility of Drugs Chart *on page 1315*.

**Additional Nursing Issues**

**Physical Assessment:** Assess effectiveness and interactions of other medications patient may be taking (see Contraindications, Warnings/Precautions, and Drug Interactions). Assess for history of addiction - long-term use can result in dependence, abuse, or tolerance; periodically evaluate need for continued use. Monitor for therapeutic response, laboratory values, and adverse reactions (see Adverse Reactions) at beginning of therapy and periodically with long-term use. Taper dosage slowly when discontinuing. Assess knowledge/teach patient seizure precautions (if administered for seizures), appropriate use, interventions to reduce side effects, and adverse symptoms to report. **Pregnancy risk factor D** - assess knowledge/teach appropriate use of barrier contraceptives. Breast-feeding is not recommended.

**Patient Information/Instruction:** Take exactly as directed (do not increase dose or frequency); may cause physical and/or psychological dependence. While using this medication, do not use alcohol and other prescription or OTC medications (especially pain medications, sedatives, antihistamines, or hypnotics) without consulting prescriber. Maintain adequate hydration (2-3 L/day of fluids unless instructed to restrict fluid intake). You may experience drowsiness, dizziness, or blurred vision (use caution when driving or engaging in tasks requiring alertness until response to drug is known); nausea, vomiting, loss of appetite, or dry mouth (small frequent meals, frequent mouth care, chewing gum, or sucking lozenges may help); constipation (increased exercise, fluids, or dietary fruit and fiber may help). If medication is used to control seizures, wear identification that you are taking an antiepileptic medication. Report CNS changes (confusion, depression, increased sedation, excitation, headache, agitation, insomnia or nightmares, dizziness, fatigue, or impaired coordination) or changes in cognition; difficulty breathing or shortness of breath; changes in urinary pattern; changes in sexual activity; muscle cramping, weakness, tremors, or rigidity; ringing in ears or visual disturbances, excessive perspiration, or excessive GI symptoms (cramping, constipation, vomiting, anorexia); worsening of seizure activity, or loss of seizure control. **Pregnancy/breast-feeding precautions:** Do not get pregnant while taking this medication; use appropriate barrier contraceptive measures. Breast-feeding is not recommended.

**Geriatric Considerations:** Due to its long-acting metabolite, diazepam is not considered a drug of choice in the elderly. Long-acting benzodiazepines have been associated with falls in the elderly. Interpretive guidelines from the Health Care Financing Administration (HCFA) discourage the use of this agent in residents of long-term care facilities.

**Additional Information** Some formulations may contain benzyl alcohol or ethanol.

**Related Information**

Anxiolytic/Hypnotic Use in Long-Term Care Facilities *on page 1430*
Benzodiazepines Comparison *on page 1375*

## Diazoxide (dye az OKS ide)

**U.S. Brand Names** Hyperstat® I.V.; Proglycem® Oral

**Therapeutic Category** Antihypoglycemic Agent; Vasodilator

**Pregnancy Risk Factor** C

**Lactation** Excretion in breast milk unknown

**Use**

Oral: Hypoglycemia related to islet cell adenoma, carcinoma, hyperplasia, or adenomatosis, nesidioblastosis, leucine sensitivity, or extrapancreatic malignancy

I.V.: Emergency lowering of blood pressure

**Mechanism of Action/Effect** Inhibits insulin release from the pancreas; produces direct smooth muscle relaxation of the peripheral arterioles which results in decrease in blood pressure and reflex increase in heart rate and cardiac output

**Contraindications** Hypersensitivity to diazoxide, thiazides, or other sulfonamide derivatives; aortic coarctation, arteriovenous shunts, dissecting aortic aneurysm

**Warnings** Use diazoxide with caution since it may cause hypotension. Do not administer by S.C. route since diazoxide can cause tissue irritation or necrosis. Use with care in patients with impaired cerebral or cardiac circulation where an abrupt drop in blood pressure may cause further complications. Avoid prolonged hypotension in patients with renal failure. Patients may require a diuretic with repeated I.V. doses. Pregnancy factor C.

**Drug Interactions**

**Decreased Effect:** Diazoxide may increase phenytoin metabolism or the free fraction resulting in a decreased effect of phenytoin.

**Increased Effect/Toxicity:** Diuretics and hypotensive agents may potentiate diazoxide adverse effects. Diazoxide may decrease warfarin protein binding increasing the anticoagulant effect.

**Effects on Lab Values** False-negative insulin response to glucagon

**Adverse Reactions**

**Systemic: Oral:**

>10%: Cardiovascular: Edema

1% to 10%:

- Cardiovascular: Tachycardia
- Gastrointestinal: Changes in ability to taste; constipation, anorexia, nausea, stomach pain, vomiting

<1% (Limited to important or life-threatening symptoms): Chest pain, myocardial infarction or myocardial ischemia, transient focal cerebral ischemic attacks, thrombocytopenia

**Systemic: Parenteral:**

>10%:

- Cardiovascular: Edema
- Endocrine and metabolic: Sodium and water retention

1% to 10%:

- Cardiovascular: Hypotension, tachycardia
- Endocrine and metabolic: Hyperglycemia
- Gastrointestinal: Changes in ability to taste, constipation, anorexia, nausea, vomiting, stomach pain

<1% (Limited to important or life-threatening symptoms): Cerebral ischemia, myocardial ischemia, chest pain pectoris, myocardial infarction, orthostatic hypotension, hyperosmolar coma, thrombocytopenia

**Overdose/Toxicology** Symptoms of overdose include hyperglycemia, ketoacidosis, and hypotension. Treatment includes insulin and supportive measures.

**Pharmacodynamics/Kinetics**

**Protein Binding:** 90%

**Half-life Elimination:** Normal renal function: 20-36 hours; End-stage renal disease: >30 hours

**Excretion:** 50% excreted unchanged in urine

**Onset:** Hyperglycemic effect: Oral: Onset of action: Within 1 hour; Hypotensive effect: I.V.: Peak: Within 5 minutes

**Duration:** Hyperglycemic effect: Oral: Duration (normal renal function): 8 hours; Hypotensive effect: I.V.: Duration: Usually 3-12 hours

**Formulations**

Capsule (Proglycem®): 50 mg

Injection (Hyperstat®): 15 mg/mL (1 mL, 20 mL)

Suspension, oral (chocolate-mint flavor) (Proglycem®): 50 mg/mL (30 mL)

(Continued)

## Diazoxide *(Continued)*

**Dosing**

**Adults:**

Hyperinsulinemic hypoglycemia: Oral: **Note:** Use lower dose listed as initial dose; 3-8 mg/kg/day in divided doses every 8-12 hours.

Hypertension: I.V.: 1-3 mg/kg up to a maximum of 150 mg in a single injection; repeat dose in 5-15 minutes until blood pressure adequately reduced; repeat administration at intervals of 4-24 hours. Monitor the blood pressure closely. Do not use longer than 10 days.

**Elderly:** Refer to adult dosing.

**Renal Impairment:**

No dosing adjustment required.

Elimination is not enhanced via hemo- or peritoneal dialysis; supplemental dose is not necessary.

**Administration**

**Oral:** Shake suspension well before using.

**I.V.:** Diazoxide is given undiluted by rapid I.V. injection over a period of 30 seconds or less but may also be given by continuous infusion.

**I.V. Detail:** Avoid extravasation. Do not administer dark solution.

**Stability**

**Storage:** Protect from light, heat, and freezing. Avoid using darkened solutions.

**Monitoring Laboratory Tests** Blood glucose daily in patients receiving I.V. therapy, serum uric acid

**Additional Nursing Issues**

**Physical Assessment:** Monitor laboratory tests on a regular basis according to diagnosis. I.V.: Monitor infusion site closely for extravasation. Monitor effectiveness of therapy and adverse reactions according to diagnosis and form of medication (see above). Teach patient appropriate monitoring, interventions for adverse effects, and symptoms to report. **Pregnancy risk factor C** - benefits of use should outweigh possible risks. Note breast-feeding caution.

**Patient Information/Instruction:**

I.V. emergency treatment of hypertension: Remain lying down for at least 1 hour following infusion. When up, change positions from sitting or lying to standing slowly.

Oral treatment of hypoglycemia: Monitor serum glucose as directed by prescriber. Report significant changes in serum glucose levels, increased swelling of extremities, increased weight, unresolved constipation, GI upset (eg, nausea, vomiting, constipation, anorexia), chest pain, or palpitations.

**Pregnancy/breast-feeding precautions:** Inform prescriber if you are or intend to be pregnant. Consult prescriber if breast-feeding.

**Additional Information** Some formulations may contain ethanol.


- **Dibacilina** *see* Ampicillin *on page 90*
- **Dibasona** *see* Dexamethasone *on page 346*
- **Dibent® Injection** *see* Dicyclomine *on page 362*
- **Dibucaine** *see page 1294*
- **Dibucaine and Hydrocortisone** *see page 1294*
- **Dibufen** *see* Ibuprofen *on page 592*
- **DIC** *see* Dacarbazine *on page 325*
- **Dicarbosil® [OTC]** *see* Calcium Supplements *on page 185*
- **Dichysterol** *see* Dihydrotachysterol *on page 375*


## Diclofenac (dye KLOE fen ak)

**U.S. Brand Names** Cataflam® Oral; Voltaren® Ophthalmic; Voltaren® Oral; Voltaren-XR® Oral

**Therapeutic Category** Nonsteroidal Anti-Inflammatory Agent (NSAID); Ophthalmic Agent

**Pregnancy Risk Factor** B/D (3rd trimester or near term)

**Lactation** Enters breast milk/use caution

**Use** Acute treatment of mild to moderate pain; acute and chronic treatment of rheumatoid arthritis, ankylosing spondylitis, and osteoarthritis; used for juvenile rheumatoid arthritis, gout, dysmenorrhea; ophthalmic solution for postoperative inflammation after cataract extraction

**Mechanism of Action/Effect** Inhibits prostaglandin synthesis by decreasing activity of the enzyme, cyclo-oxygenase, which results in decreased formation of prostaglandin precursors

**Contraindications** Hypersensitivity to diclofenac, any component, aspirin or other nonsteroidal anti-inflammatory drugs (NSAIDs); porphyria; pregnancy (3rd trimester or near term)

**Warnings** Use with caution in patients with congestive heart failure, hypertension, decreased renal or hepatic function, history of GI disease, or those receiving anticoagulants.

**Drug Interactions**

**Cytochrome P-450 Effect:** CYP2C8 and 2C9 enzyme substrate; CYP2C9 enzyme inhibitor

**Decreased Effect:** Decreased effect of diclofenac with aspirin. Decreased effect of thiazides, furosemide.

**Increased Effect/Toxicity:** Increased toxicity of digoxin, methotrexate, cyclosporine, lithium, insulin, sulfonylureas, potassium-sparing diuretics, warfarin and aspirin.

**Adverse Reactions**

**Ophthalmic:**

>10%: Ocular: Ocular irritation (burning, stinging, itching, mild discomfort)

1% to 10%: Ocular: Allergic reaction (tearing)

**Systemic:**

1% to 10%:

Cardiovascular: Chest pain, arrhythmias, fluid retention/edema

Central nervous system: Dizziness, nervousness, headache

Dermatologic: Rash, itching

Gastrointestinal: GI ulceration, vomiting, abdominal distention, abdominal cramps, constipation, diarrhea, indigestion, abdominal cramps, heartburn, indigestion, nausea

Genitourinary: Vaginal bleeding

Otic: Tinnitus

<1% (Limited to important or life-threatening symptoms): Chest pain, congestive heart failure, hypertension, tachycardia, convulsions, forgetfulness, mental depression, drowsiness, insomnia, nervousness, urticaria, exfoliative dermatitis, erythema multiforme, Stevens-Johnson syndrome, angioedema, stomatitis, colitis, GI hemorrhage, bitter taste, agranulocytosis, anemia, pancytopenia, leukopenia, thrombocytopenia, ecchymosis, hepatitis, peripheral neuropathy, trembling, weakness, interstitial nephritis, nephrotic syndrome, renal impairment, wheezing, laryngeal edema, shortness of breath, epistaxis

**Overdose/Toxicology** Symptoms of overdose include acute renal failure, vomiting, drowsiness, and leukocytosis. Management of nonsteroidal anti-inflammatory (NSAID) intoxication is supportive and symptomatic.

**Pharmacodynamics/Kinetics**

**Protein Binding:** 99%

**Half-life Elimination:** 2 hours

**Time to Peak:** Cataflam®: Within 1 hour; Voltaren®: Within 2 hours

**Metabolism:** Liver

**Excretion:** Urine

**Onset:** Cataflam® has a more rapid onset of action than does the sodium salt (Voltaren®), because it is absorbed in the stomach instead of the duodenum.

**Formulations**

Diclofenac sodium:

Solution, ophthalmic (Voltaren®): 0.1% (2.5 mL, 5 mL)

Tablet, delayed release (Voltaren®): 25 mg, 50 mg, 75 mg

Tablet, extended release, as sodium (Voltaren-XR®): 100 mg

Diclofenac potassium:

Tablet (Cataflam®): 50 mg

**Dosing**

**Adults:**

Oral:

Analgesia: Starting dose: 50 mg 3 times/day

Rheumatoid arthritis: 150-200 mg/day in 2-4 divided doses (100 mg/day of sustained release product)

Osteoarthritis: 100-150 mg/day in 2-3 divided doses (100-200 mg/day of sustained release product)

Ankylosing spondylitis: 100-125 mg/day in 4-5 divided doses

Ophthalmic: Instill 1 drop into affected eye 4 times/day beginning 24 hours after cataract surgery and continuing for 2 weeks

**Elderly:** Refer to adult dosing.

**Administration**

**Oral:** Do not crush tablets. Administer with food or milk to avoid gastric distress. Take with full glass of water to enhance absorption.

**Other:** Ophthalmic: Wait at least 5 minutes before administering other types of eye drops.

**Monitoring Laboratory Tests** CBC, liver enzymes, urine output and BUN/serum creatinine in patients receiving diuretics, occult blood loss

**Additional Nursing Issues**

**Physical Assessment:** Assess other medications patient may be taking for effectiveness and interactions (see Drug Interactions). See Contraindications and Warnings/Precautions for cautious use. Monitor laboratory tests and therapeutic response (eg, relief of pain and inflammation, increased activity tolerance), and adverse reactions (systemic or ophthalmic) at beginning of therapy and periodically throughout therapy (see Adverse Reactions and Overdose/Toxicology). Schedule ophthalmic evaluations for patients who develop eye complaints during long-term NSAID therapy. Assess knowledge/teach patient appropriate use (oral, ophthalmic), interventions to reduce side effects, and adverse symptoms to report. **Pregnancy risk factor B/D.** Note breast-feeding caution.

**Patient Information/Instruction:**

Oral: Take this medication exactly as directed; do not increase dose without consulting prescriber. Do not crush or chew tablets. Take with 8 ounces of water, along with food or milk products to reduce GI distress. Maintain adequate fluid intake (2-3 L/day of fluids unless instructed to restrict fluid intake). Avoid excessive alcohol, aspirin and aspirin-containing medication, and all other anti-inflammatory medications unless consulting prescriber. You may experience dizziness, nervousness, or headache (use caution when driving or engaging in tasks requiring alertness until response to drug is

(Continued)

## Diclofenac *(Continued)*

known); nausea, vomiting, dry mouth, or heartburn (frequent small meals, frequent mouth care, sucking lozenges, or chewing gum may help); or constipation (increased exercise, fluids, or dietary fruit and fiber may help). GI bleeding, ulceration, or perforation can occur with or without pain; discontinue medication and contact prescriber if persistent abdominal pain or cramping, or blood in stool occurs. Report chest pain or palpitations; breathlessness or difficulty breathing; unusual bruising/bleeding or blood in urine, stool, mouth, or vomitus; unusual fatigue; skin rash or itching; unusual weight gain or swelling of extremities; change in urinary pattern; change in vision or hearing; or ringing in ears. **Pregnancy/breast-feeding precautions:** Consult prescriber if pregnant or breast-feeding.

Ophthalmic: For ophthalmic use only. Apply prescribed amount as often as directed. Wash hands before using and do not let tip of applicator touch eye or contaminate tip of applicator. Tilt head back and look upward. Gently pull down lower lid and put drop(s) in inner corner of eye. Close eye and roll eyeball in all directions. Do not blink for ½ minute. Apply gentle pressure to inner corner of eye for 30 seconds. Wipe away excess from skin around eye. Do not use any other eye preparation for at least 10 minutes. Do not touch tip of applicator to eye or contaminate tip of applicator. Do not share medication with anyone else. May cause sensitivity to bright light (dark glasses may help); temporary stinging or blurred vision may occur. Inform prescriber if you experience eye pain, redness, burning, watering, dryness, double vision, puffiness around eye, vision disturbances, or other adverse eye response; worsening of condition or lack of improvement. Consult prescriber if pregnant or breast-feeding.

**Geriatric Considerations:** Elderly are at high risk for adverse effects from nonsteroidal anti-inflammatory agents.

**Pregnancy Issues:** In late pregnancy, as with other NSAIDs, avoid diclofenac since it may cause premature closure of ductus arteriosus.

**Additional Information**

Diclofenac potassium = Cataflam®; potassium content: 5.8 mg (0.15 mEq) per 50 mg tablet

Diclofenac sodium = Voltaren®

Diclofenac sodium (extended release) = Voltaren-XR®

**Related Information**

Nonsalicylate/Nonsteroidal Anti-inflammatory Comparison *on page 1401*

Ophthalmic Agents *on page 1282*

## Diclofenac and Misoprostol (dye KLOE fen ak & mye soe PROST ole)

**U.S. Brand Names** Arthrotec®

**Synonyms** Misoprostol and Diclofenac

**Therapeutic Category** Nonsteroidal Anti-Inflammatory Agent (NSAID); Prostaglandin

**Pregnancy Risk Factor** X

**Lactation** Enters breast milk/contraindicated

**Use** The diclofenac component is indicated for the treatment of osteoarthritis and rheumatoid arthritis; the misoprostol component is indicated for the prophylaxis of NSAID-induced gastric and duodenal ulceration

**Formulations** Tablet:

Diclofenac 50 mg and misoprostol 200 mcg

Diclofenac 75 mg and misoprostol 200 mcg

**Dosing**

**Adults:** Oral:

Arthrotec® 50:

Osteoarthritis: 1 tablet 2-3 times/day

Rheumatoid arthritis: 1 tablet 3-4 times/day

For both regimens, if not tolerated by patient, the dose may be reduced to 1 tablet twice daily.

Arthrotec® 75: Patients who cannot tolerate full daily Arthrotec® 50 regimens: 1 tablet twice daily

**Note:** The use of these tablets may not be as effective at preventing GI ulceration.

**Elderly:** Refer to adult dosing.

**Renal Impairment:** In renal insufficiency, diclofenac should be used with caution due to potential detrimental effects on renal function, and misoprostol dosage reduction may be required if adverse effects occur (misoprostol is renally eliminated).

**Additional Nursing Issues**

**Physical Assessment:** See individual components listed in Related Information. **Pregnancy risk factor X** - determine that patient is not pregnant before beginning treatment and do not give to women of childbearing age or to males who may have intercourse with women of childbearing age unless both male and female are capable of complying with barrier contraceptive measures during therapy and for 1 month following therapy. Breast-feeding is contraindicated.

**Patient Information/Instruction:** See individual components listed in Related Information. **Pregnancy/breast-feeding precautions:** Inform prescriber if you are pregnant. Do not get pregnant during or for 1 month following therapy. Male: Do not cause a female to become pregnant. Male/female: Consult prescriber for instruction on appropriate contraceptive measures. This drug may cause severe fetal defects. Do not breast-feed.

**Related Information**

Diclofenac *on page 358*

Misoprostol *on page 776*

♦ **Diclotride®** *see* Hydrochlorothiazide *on page 566*

## Dicloxacillin (dye kloks a SIL in)

**U.S. Brand Names** Dycill®; Dynapen®; Pathocil®

**Therapeutic Category** Antibiotic, Penicillin

**Pregnancy Risk Factor** B

**Lactation** Excretion in breast milk unknown (probably similar to penicillin G)

**Use** Treatment of systemic infections such as pneumonia, skin and soft tissue infections, and osteomyelitis caused by penicillinase-producing staphylococci

**Mechanism of Action/Effect** Interferes with bacterial cell wall synthesis; causes cell wall death

**Contraindications** Hypersensitivity to dicloxacillin, any component, penicillins, cephalosporins, or imipenem

**Warnings** Monitor PT if patient concurrently on warfarin. Use with caution in patients allergic to cephalosporins. Bad taste of suspension may make compliance difficult.

**Drug Interactions**

**Decreased Effect:** Efficacy of oral contraceptives may be reduced when taken with dicloxacillin.

**Increased Effect/Toxicity:** Disulfiram, probenecid may increase penicillin levels. Increased effect of (warfarin) anticoagulants.

**Effects on Lab Values** Positive Coombs' test [direct]

**Adverse Reactions**

>10%:

Central nervous system: Headache

Gastrointestinal: Nausea (mild), vomiting

Miscellaneous: Oral candidiasis, vaginal candidiasis

1% to 10%:

Dermatologic: Urticaria, exfoliative dermatitis

Miscellaneous: Allergic reactions, specifically anaphylaxis; serum sickness-like reactions

<1% (Limited to important or life-threatening symptoms): Seizures, anxiety, confusion, hallucinations, depression, leukopenia, neutropenia, thrombocytopenia, jaundice, hepatotoxicity, interstitial nephritis, *Clostridium difficile* colitis

**Overdose/Toxicology** Symptoms of penicillin overdose include neuromuscular hypersensitivity (eg, agitation, hallucinations, asterixis, encephalopathy, confusion, and seizures). Electrolyte imbalance may occur if the preparation contains potassium or sodium salts, especially in renal failure. Hemodialysis may be helpful to aid in removal of the drug from blood; otherwise, treatment is supportive or symptom directed.

**Pharmacodynamics/Kinetics**

**Protein Binding:** 96%

**Distribution:** Crosses the placenta

**Half-life Elimination:** 0.6-0.8 hours (slightly prolonged in renal impairment)

**Time to Peak:** Within 0.5-2 hours

**Excretion:** Partially eliminated by the liver and excreted in bile, 56% to 70% is eliminated in urine as unchanged drug

**Formulations**

Dicloxacillin sodium:

Capsule: 125 mg, 250 mg, 500 mg

Powder for oral suspension: 62.5 mg/5 mL (80 mL, 100 mL, 200 mL)

**Dosing**

**Adults:** Oral: 125-500 mg every 6 hours

**Elderly:** Refer to adult dosing.

**Renal Impairment:**

Dosage adjustment not necessary

Not dialyzable (0% to 5%); supplemental dosage not necessary

Peritoneal dialysis effects: Supplemental dosage not necessary

Continuous arteriovenous or venovenous hemofiltration (CAVH/CAVHD): Supplemental dosage not necessary

**Administration**

**Oral:** Administer 1 hour before or 2 hours after meals. Administer around-the-clock to promote less variation in peak and trough serum levels.

**Stability**

**Reconstitution:** Refrigerate suspension after reconstitution. Discard after 14 days if refrigerated or 7 days if kept at room temperature. Unit dose antibiotic oral syringes are stable for 48 hours.

**Monitoring Laboratory Tests** Perform culture and sensitivity studies prior to initiating therapy. Monitor prothrombin time if patient concurrently on warfarin.

**Additional Nursing Issues**

**Physical Assessment:** Assess for previous allergic reaction to penicillins and cephalosporins. Monitor laboratory results and assess effectiveness of therapy. Instruct patient on appropriate use, possible adverse reactions (see above), and symptoms to report. Note breast-feeding caution.

**Patient Information/Instruction:** Take medication as directed, with a large glass of water 1 hour before or 2 hours after meals. Take at regular intervals around-the-clock and take for length of time prescribed. You may experience some gastric distress (small frequent meals may help) and diarrhea (if this persists, consult prescriber). If diabetic, drug may cause false tests with Clinitest® urine glucose monitoring; use of glucose oxidase methods (Clinistix®) or serum glucose monitoring is preferable. This drug may interfere with oral contraceptives; an alternate form of birth control should be

(Continued)

## Dicloxacillin *(Continued)*

used. Report fever, vaginal itching, sores in the mouth, loose foul-smelling stools, yellowing of skin or eyes, and change in color of urine or stool. **Breast-feeding precautions:** Consult prescriber if breast-feeding.

**Additional Information**

Sodium content of 250 mg capsule: 13 mg (0.6 mEq)
Sodium content of suspension 65 mg/5 mL: 27 mg (1.2 mEq)

## Dicyclomine (dye SYE kloe meen)

**U.S. Brand Names** Antispas® Injection; Bentyl® Hydrochloride Injection; Bentyl® Hydrochloride Oral; Byclomine® Injection; Dibent® Injection; Dilomine® Injection; Di-Spaz® Injection; Di-Spaz® Oral; Or-Tyl® Injection

**Synonyms** Dicycloverine Hydrochloride

**Therapeutic Category** Anticholinergic Agent

**Pregnancy Risk Factor** B

**Lactation** Enters breast milk/contraindicated

**Use** Treatment of functional disturbances of GI motility such as irritable bowel syndrome

**Unlabeled use:** Urinary incontinence

**Mechanism of Action/Effect** Blocks the action of acetylcholine at parasympathetic sites in smooth muscle, secretory glands and the CNS

**Contraindications** Hypersensitivity to any anticholinergic drug; narrow-angle glaucoma; myasthenia gravis; should not be used in infants <6 months of age

**Warnings** Use with caution in patients with hepatic or renal disease, ulcerative colitis, hyperthyroidism, cardiovascular disease, hypertension, tachycardia, GI obstruction, obstruction of the urinary tract. The elderly are at increased risk for anticholinergic effects, confusion and hallucinations.

**Drug Interactions**

**Decreased Effect:** Decreased effect with phenothiazines, anti-Parkinson's drugs, haloperidol, sustained release dosage forms, and with antacids.

**Increased Effect/Toxicity:** Dicyclomine taken with anticholinergics, amantadine, narcotic analgesics, Type I antiarrhythmics, antihistamines, phenothiazines, tricyclic antidepressants may result in increased toxicity.

**Adverse Reactions**

>10%:
- Dermatologic: Dry skin
- Gastrointestinal: Constipation, dry throat, dry mouth
- Local: Injection site reactions
- Respiratory: Dry nose
- Miscellaneous: Sweating (decreased)

1% to 10%:
- Dermatologic: Increased sensitivity to light
- Endocrine & metabolic: Decreased flow of breast milk
- Gastrointestinal: Dysphagia
- Ocular: Blurred vision

<1% (Limited to important or life-threatening symptoms): Orthostatic hypotension, tachycardia, palpitations, confusion, drowsiness, headache, lightheadedness, loss of memory, fatigue, seizures, coma, nervousness, excitement, insomnia, bloated feeling, nausea, vomiting, dysuria, urinary retention, muscular hypotonia, weakness, increased intraocular pain, asphyxia, respiratory distress

**Overdose/Toxicology** Symptoms of overdose include CNS stimulation followed by depression, confusion, delusions, nonreactive pupils, tachycardia, and hypertension.

**Pharmacodynamics/Kinetics**

**Half-life Elimination:** Initial phase: 1.8 hours; Terminal phase: 9-10 hours

**Metabolism:** Extensive

**Excretion:** Urine

**Onset:** 1-2 hours

**Duration:** Up to 4 hours

**Formulations**

Dicyclomine hydrochloride:
- Capsule: 10 mg, 20 mg
- Injection: 10 mg/mL (2 mL, 10 mL)
- Syrup: 10 mg/5 mL (118 mL, 473 mL, 946 mL)
- Tablet: 20 mg

**Dosing**

**Adults:**

Oral: Begin with 80 mg/day in 4 equally divided doses, then increase up to 160 mg/day
I.M. **(should not be used I.V.)**: 80 mg/day in 4 divided doses (20 mg/dose)

**Elderly:** 10-20 mg 4 times/day; increasing as necessary to 160 mg/day

**Administration**

**Oral:** Administer 30-60 minutes before a meal.

**I.M.:** Administer as I.M. injection only.

**I.V.:** Do not administer I.V.

**Additional Nursing Issues**

**Physical Assessment:** Assess effectiveness and interactions of other medications (see Drug Interactions). See Warnings/Precautions and Contraindications for use cautions. Monitor effectiveness of therapy, laboratory tests, and adverse response (see Adverse Reactions and Overdose/Toxicology). Assess knowledge/teach patient appropriate use, possible side effects and appropriate interventions, and adverse symptoms to report. Breast-feeding is contraindicated.

**Patient Information/Instruction:** Take as directed before meals; do not increase dose and do not discontinue without consulting prescriber. Avoid alcohol and other CNS depressant medications (antihistamines, sleeping aids, antidepressants) unless approved by prescriber. Void before taking medication. This drug may impair mental alertness (use caution when driving or engaging in tasks that require alertness until response to drug is known); constipation (increased dietary fluid, fruit, or fiber and increased exercise may help). Report excessive and persistent anticholinergic effects (blurred vision, headache, flushing, tachycardia, nervousness, dizziness, insomnia, mental confusion or excitement, dry mouth, altered taste perception, dysphagia, palpitations, bradycardia, urinary hesitancy or retention, impotence, decreased sweating), change in color of urine or stools, or irritation or redness at injection site. **Breast-feeding precautions:** Do not breast-feed.

**Geriatric Considerations:** Long-term use of antispasmodics should be avoided in the elderly. The potential for a toxic reaction is greater than the potential benefit. In addition, the anticholinergic effects of dicyclomine are not well tolerated in the elderly.

♦ **Dicycloverine Hydrochloride** *see* Dicyclomine *on previous page*

## Didanosine (dye DAN oh seen)

**U.S. Brand Names** Videx®

**Synonyms** ddI

**Therapeutic Category** Antiretroviral Agent, Reverse Transcriptase Inhibitor (Nucleoside)

**Pregnancy Risk Factor** B

**Lactation** Excretion in breast milk unknown/contraindicated

**Use** Treatment of advanced HIV infection in patients who are intolerant of zidovudine therapy or who have demonstrated significant clinical or immunologic deterioration during zidovudine therapy

**Mechanism of Action/Effect** Didanosine, a purine nucleoside analogue and the deamination product of dideoxyadenosine (ddA), inhibits HIV replication *in vitro* in both T cells and monocytes. Didanosine is converted within the cell to the mono-, di-, and triphosphates of ddA. These ddA triphosphates act as substrate and inhibitor of HIV reverse transcriptase substrate and inhibitor of HIV reverse transcriptase thereby blocking viral DNA synthesis and suppressing HIV replication.

**Contraindications** Hypersensitivity to didanosine or any component

**Warnings** Didanosine is indicated for treatment of HIV infection only in patients intolerant of zidovudine or who have failed zidovudine. Patients receiving didanosine may still develop opportunistic infections. Peripheral neuropathy occurs in ~35% of patients receiving the drug; pancreatitis (sometimes fatal) occurs in ~9%. Risk factors for developing pancreatitis include a previous history of the condition, concurrent cytomegalovirus or *Mycobacterium avium-intracellulare* infection, and concomitant use of pentamidine or co-trimoxazole. Discontinue didanosine if clinical signs of pancreatitis occur. Lactic acidosis and severe hepatomegaly have occurred with antiretroviral nucleoside analogues. Didanosine may cause retinal depigmentation in children receiving doses >300 mg/m$^2$/day. Patients should undergo retinal examination every 6-12 months. Use with caution in patients with decreased renal or hepatic function, phenylketonuria, sodium-restricted diets, or with edema, congestive heart failure, or hyperuricemia. In high concentrations, didanosine is mutagenic. Due to overlapping toxicity or virologically undesirable combination, it is not recommended to combine DDI with ddC (zalcitabine) therapy.

**Drug Interactions**

**Decreased Effect:** Didanosine may decrease absorption of quinolones, indinavir or tetracyclines. Didanosine should be held during PCP treatment with pentamidine. Drugs whose absorption depends on the level of acidity in the stomach such as ketoconazole, itraconazole, and dapsone will have lower levels and a decreased effect.

**Increased Effect/Toxicity:** Concomitant administration of other drugs which have the potential to cause peripheral neuropathy or pancreatitis may increase the risk of these toxicities. Ganciclovir and allopurinol may increase concentrations.

**Food Interactions** Didanosine serum levels may be decreased by 55% if taken with food.

**Adverse Reactions**

>10%:

Central nervous system: Anxiety, headache, irritability, insomnia, restlessness

Gastrointestinal: Abdominal pain, nausea, diarrhea

Neuromuscular & skeletal: Peripheral neuropathy

1% to 10%:

Central nervous system: Depression

Dermatologic: Rash, pruritus

Gastrointestinal: Pancreatitis

<1% (Limited to important or life-threatening symptoms): Seizures, anemia, granulocytopenia, leukopenia, thrombocytopenia, hepatitis, retinal depigmentation, renal impairment, alopecia, anaphylactoid reaction, lactic acidosis, diabetes mellitus, optic neuritis

**Overdose/Toxicology** Chronic overdose may cause pancreatitis, peripheral neuropathy, diarrhea, hyperuricemia, and hepatic impairment. There is no known antidote for didanosine overdose. Treatment is symptomatic.

(Continued)

## Didanosine *(Continued)*

**Pharmacodynamics/Kinetics**

**Protein Binding:** <5%

**Half-life Elimination:**

Normal renal function: 1.5 hours; however, its active metabolite ddATP has an intracellular half-life >12 hours *in vitro*. This permits the drug to be dosed at 12-hour intervals; total body clearance averages 800 mL/minute.

Impaired renal function: Half-life is increased, with values ranging from 2.5-5 hours.

**Metabolism:** Has not been evaluated in man. Studies conducted in dogs, shows didanosine extensively metabolized with allantoin, hypoxanthine, xanthine, and uric acid being the major metabolites found in the urine.

**Excretion:** Urine

**Formulations**

Powder for oral solution:

Buffered (single dose packet): 100 mg, 167 mg, 250 mg, 375 mg

Pediatric: 2 g, 4 g

Tablet, buffered, chewable (mint flavor): 25 mg, 50 mg, 100 mg, 150 mg

**Dosing**

**Adults:** Oral (administer on an empty stomach):

Dosing is based on patient weight:

<60 kg: 125 mg tablets or 167 mg buffered powder twice daily

≥60 kg: 200 mg tablets or 250 mg buffered powder twice daily

**Note:** Adults should receive 2 tablets per dose for adequate buffering and absorption; tablets should be chewed.

**Elderly:** Refer to adult dosing.

**Renal Impairment:** See table.

**Dosing Adjustment in Renal Impairment**

| $Cl_{cr}$ | >60 kg | | <60 kg | | Interval (h) |
|---|---|---|---|---|---|
| | Tablet | Solution | Tablet | Solution | |
| <10 | 100 | 100 | 75 | 100 | 24 |
| 10-29 | 150 | 167 | 100 | 100 | 24 |
| 30-59 | 100 | 100 | 75 | 100 | 12 |
| 60 | 200 | 250 | 125 | 167 | 12 |

**Hepatic Impairment:** Dosing adjustment should be considered.

**Administration**

**Oral:** Drugs whose absorption depends on the level of acidity in the stomach such as ketoconazole, itraconazole, and dapsone should be administered at least 2 hours prior to didanosine. Administer liquified powder immediately after dissolving. Avoid creating dust if powder spilled, use wet mop or damp sponge. Use a 12-hour dosing interval.

**Stability**

**Storage:** Tablets should be stored in tightly closed bottles at 15°C to 30°C.

**Reconstitution:** Undergoes rapid degradation when exposed to an acidic environment. Tablets dispersed in water are stable for 1 hour at room temperature. Reconstituted buffered solution is stable for 4 hours at room temperature. Reconstituted pediatric solution is stable for 30 days if refrigerated. Unbuffered powder for oral solution must be reconstituted and mixed with an equal volume of antacid at time of preparation.

**Monitoring Laboratory Tests** Serum potassium, uric acid, creatinine, hemoglobin, CBC with neutrophil, platelet count, CD4 cells, liver function, amylase

**Additional Nursing Issues**

**Physical Assessment:** Monitor appropriate laboratory tests. Assess for peripheral neuropathy (eg, numbness or tingling of hands, feet), pancreatitis (eg, abdominal pain or distension, nausea), anemia (eg, fatigue, headache, difficulty breathing). Monitor for signs or symptoms of opportunistic infection (eg, mouth sores, vaginal sores, foul-smelling urine). Breast-feeding is contraindicated.

**Patient Information/Instruction:** Take as directed, 1 hour before or 2 hours after eating. Chew tablets thoroughly and/or dissolve in water. Pour powder into 4 oz of liquid, stir, and drink immediately. Do not mix with fruit juice or other acid-containing liquids. You may experience dizziness; use caution when driving or engaging in tasks that require alertness until response to drug is known. You will be susceptible to infection; avoid crowds. Report numbness or tingling of fingers, toes, or feet; abdominal pain; or persistent nausea or vomiting. Should have a retinal exam every 6-12 months. **Breast-feeding precautions:** Do not breast-feed.

**Geriatric Considerations:** Since the elderly often have a creatinine clearance <60 mL/minute, monitor closely for adverse reactions and adjust dose accordingly to maintain efficacy (CD4 counts).

**Breast-feeding Issues:** The CDC recommends **not** to breast-feed if diagnosed with HIV to avoid postnatal transmission of the virus.

**Additional Information** A recent study (n=245) indicated that a change from AZT to ddI in clinically stable HIV-infected patients with CD4 cell counts of 200-500, resulted in a slowed disease progression rate, a sustained increase in CD4 counts, and a decreased probability of developing a high level of resistance to AZT.

**Related Information**

Antiretroviral Agents Comparison *on page 1373*

♦ **Dideoxycytidine** *see* Zalcitabine *on page 1225*

## Dienestrol (dye en ES trole)

**U.S. Brand Names** DV® Vaginal Cream; Ortho® Dienestrol Vaginal

**Therapeutic Category** Estrogen Derivative

**Pregnancy Risk Factor** X

**Lactation** Excretion in breast milk unknown/contraindicated

**Use** Symptomatic management of atrophic vaginitis or kraurosis vulvae in postmenopausal women

**Mechanism of Action/Effect** Increases the synthesis of DNA, RNA, and various proteins in target tissues; reduces the release of gonadotropin-releasing hormone from the hypothalamus; reduces FSH and LH release from the pituitary

**Contraindications** Pregnancy; should not be used during undiagnosed vaginal bleeding

**Warnings** Use with caution in patients with a history of thromboembolism, stroke, myocardial infarction (especially age >40 who smoke), liver tumor, hypertension, cardiac, or renal or hepatic insufficiency.

**Adverse Reactions**

1% to 10%:

Cardiovascular: Peripheral edema

Endocrine & metabolic: Breast tenderness, breast enlargement

Gastrointestinal: Anorexia, abdominal cramping

<1% (Limited to important or life-threatening symptoms): Hypertension, thromboembolism, myocardial infarction, stroke, migraine, dizziness, anxiety, depression, headache, decreased glucose tolerance, alterations in frequency and flow of menses, breast tenderness or enlargement, increased triglycerides and LDL, cholestatic jaundice, increased susceptibility to *Candida* infection

**Pharmacodynamics/Kinetics**

**Time to Peak:** Topical: Within 3-4 hours

**Metabolism:** Liver

**Formulations** Cream, vaginal: 0.01% (30 g, 78 g)

**Dosing**

**Adults:** Vaginal: Insert 1 applicatorful once or twice daily for 1-2 weeks and then ½ of that dose for 1-2 weeks; maintenance dose: 1 applicatorful 1-3 times/week for 3-6 months

**Elderly:** Refer to adult dosing.

**Administration**

**Other:** Insert applicator high into vagina.

**Additional Nursing Issues**

**Physical Assessment:** See Contraindications and Warnings/Precautions for use cautions. Assess knowledge/teach patient appropriate administration, possible side effects/interventions, and adverse symptoms to report. **Pregnancy risk factor X** - while this medication is generally used postmenopausal, it is necessary to determine that patient is not pregnant before starting therapy. Breast-feeding is contraindicated.

**Patient Information/Instruction:** Use as directed. Insert cream high in vagina. Remain lying down for 30 minutes following insertion. Use of sanitary napkin following administration will protect clothing; do not use a tampon. May cause breast tenderness or enlargement (consult prescriber for relief). Discontinue use and report promptly any pain, redness, warmth, or swelling in calves; sudden onset difficulty breathing; headache; loss of vision; difficulty speaking; sharp or sudden chest pain; severe abdominal pain; or unusual bleeding. **Pregnancy/breast-feeding precautions:** Inform prescriber if pregnant. Do not breast-feed.

## Diethylpropion (dye eth il PROE pee on)

**U.S. Brand Names** Tenuate®; Tenuate® Dospan®

**Synonyms** Amfepramone

**Therapeutic Category** Anorexiant

**Pregnancy Risk Factor** B

**Lactation** Enters breast milk/not recommended

**Use** Short-term adjunct in exogenous obesity

**Mechanism of Action/Effect** Diethylpropion is used as an anorexiant possessing pharmacological and chemical properties similar to those of amphetamines. The mechanism of action of diethylpropion in reducing appetite appears to be secondary to CNS effects, specifically stimulation of the hypothalamus to release catecholamines into the central nervous system. Anorexiant effects are mediated via norepinephrine and dopamine metabolism. An increase in physical activity and metabolic effects (inhibition of lipogenesis and enhancement of lipolysis) may also contribute to weight loss.

**Contraindications** Hypersensitivity to diethylpropion; advanced arteriosclerosis; hyperthyroidism; glaucoma; severe hypertension; hypersensitivity to sympathomimetic amines. Avoid use in patients with a history of drug abuse or agitated states. Use during or within 14 days of MAO inhibitor therapy is contraindicated.

**Warnings** Prolonged administration may lead to dependence. Use with caution in patients with mental illness, diabetes mellitus, cardiovascular disease, nephritis, angina pectoris, hypertension, glaucoma, and patients with a history of drug abuse.

**Drug Interactions**

**Decreased Effect:** Diethylpropion may decrease the effect of antihypertensives (ie, guanethidine, methyldopa). Concomitant use with phenothiazines may have a decreased effect of diethylpropion. Diethylpropion may affect insulin requirements in diabetic patients.

(Continued)

## Diethylpropion *(Continued)*

**Increased Effect/Toxicity:** Increased effect/toxicity with MAO inhibitors (hypertensive crisis), CNS depressants, general anesthetics (arrhythmias), and sympathomimetics (additive vasopressor effects).

**Adverse Reactions**

>10%:

Cardiovascular: Hypertension

Central nervous system: Euphoria, nervousness, insomnia

1% to 10%:

Central nervous system: Confusion, mental depression

Endocrine & metabolic: Changes in libido

Gastrointestinal: Nausea, vomiting, restlessness, constipation

Hematologic: Blood dyscrasias

Neuromuscular & skeletal: Tremor

Ocular: Blurred vision

<1% (Limited to important or life-threatening symptoms): Tachycardia, arrhythmias, depression, headache, alopecia, dysuria, polyuria, dyspnea

**Overdose/Toxicology** There is no specific antidote for amphetamine intoxication and treatment is primarily supportive. Hyperactivity and agitation usually respond to reduced sensory input; however, with extreme agitation, haloperidol (2-5 mg I.M. for adults) may be required.

**Pharmacodynamics/Kinetics**

**Onset:** 1 hour

**Duration:** 12-24 hours

**Formulations**

Diethylpropion hydrochloride:

Tablet: 25 mg

Tablet, controlled release: 75 mg

**Dosing**

**Adults:** Oral:

Tablet: 25 mg 3 times/day before meals or food

Tablet, controlled release: 75 mg at midmorning

**Administration**

**Oral:** Do not crush 75 mg controlled release tablets. Dose should not be given in evening or at bedtime. Take tablets 1 hour before meals. Take controlled-release tablet at midmorning.

**Additional Nursing Issues**

**Physical Assessment:** Assess effectiveness and interactions of other medications patient may be taking (see Drug Interactions). Assess for history of psychopathology, homicidal or suicidal tendencies, or addiction; long-term use can result in dependence, abuse, or tolerance. Periodically evaluate the need for continued use. Monitor blood pressure, vital signs, and adverse reactions at start of therapy, when changing dosage, and at regular intervals during therapy (see Adverse Reactions). Monitor serum glucose closely with diabetic patients (amphetamines may alter antidiabetic requirements). Taper dosage slowly when discontinuing. Assess knowledge/teach patient appropriate use, possible side effects, and symptoms to report. Breast-feeding is not recommended.

**Patient Information/Instruction:** Take exactly as directed (do not increase dose or frequency without consulting prescriber); may cause physical and/or psychological dependence. Do not crush or chew extended release tablets. Take early in day to avoid sleep disturbance, 1 hour before meals. Avoid alcohol, caffeine, or OTC medications that act as stimulants. You may experience restlessness, false sense of euphoria, or impaired judgment (use caution when driving or engaging in tasks requiring alertness until response to drug is known); dry mouth (frequent mouth care, sucking lozenges, or chewing gum may help); nausea or vomiting (small frequent meals, frequent mouth care may help); constipation (increased exercise, dietary fiber, fruit, or fluid may help); diarrhea (buttermilk, boiled milk, or yogurt may help); or altered libido (reversible). Diabetics need to monitor serum glucose closely (may alter antidiabetic medication requirements). Report chest pain, palpitations, or irregular heartbeat; muscle weakness or tremors; extreme fatigue or depression; CNS changes (aggressiveness, restlessness, euphoria, sleep disturbances); severe unremitting abdominal distress or cramping; changes in sexual activity; changes in urinary pattern; or blurred vision. **Breast-feeding precautions:** Breast-feeding is not recommended.

## Diethylstilbestrol (dye eth il stil BES trole)

**U.S. Brand Names** Stilphostrol®

**Synonyms** DES; Diethylstilbestrol Diphosphate Sodium; Stilbestrol

**Therapeutic Category** Estrogen Derivative

**Pregnancy Risk Factor** X

**Lactation** Excretion in breast milk unknown/contraindicated

**Use** Palliative treatment of inoperable metastatic prostatic carcinoma and postmenopausal inoperable, progressing breast cancer

**Mechanism of Action/Effect** Competes with estrogenic and androgenic compounds for binding onto tumor cells and thereby inhibits their effects on tumor growth

**Contraindications** Undiagnosed vaginal bleeding; pregnancy

**Warnings** Use with caution in patients with a history of thromboembolism, stroke, myocardial infarction (especially >40 of age who smoke), liver tumor, hypertension, cardiac, renal or hepatic insufficiency, hypercalcemia, epilepsy, migraine, and metabolic bone disease. Estrogens have been reported to increase the risk of endometrial carcinoma.

**Drug Interactions**

**Decreased Effect:** Barbiturates, phenytoin, and rifampin may decrease steroids.

**Effects on Lab Values** ↑ prothrombin and factors VII, VIII, IX, X; ↑ platelet aggregability; ↑ thyroid binding globulin; ↑ total thyroid hormone ($T_4$); ↑ serum triglycerides/phospholipids; ↓ antithrombin III; ↓ serum folate concentration

**Adverse Reactions**

>10%:

Cardiovascular: Peripheral edema

Endocrine & metabolic: Enlargement of breasts (female and male), breast tenderness

Gastrointestinal: Nausea, anorexia, bloating

1% to 10%:

Central nervous system: Headache, migraine headache

Endocrine & metabolic: Increased libido (female), decreased libido (male)

Gastrointestinal: Vomiting, diarrhea

<1% (Limited to important or life-threatening symptoms): Hypertension, thromboembolism, myocardial infarction, edema, depression, dizziness, anxiety, stroke, amenorrhea, alterations in frequency and flow of menses, breast tumors, decreased glucose tolerance, increased triglycerides and LDL, nausea, GI distress, gallbladder obstruction, hepatitis, intolerance to contact lenses, increased susceptibility to *Candida* infection

**Overdose/Toxicology** Nausea

**Pharmacodynamics/Kinetics**

**Metabolism:** Liver

**Excretion:** Urine and feces

**Formulations**

Injection, as diphosphate sodium (Stilphostrol®): 0.25 g (5 mL)

Tablet: 1 mg, 2.5 mg, 5 mg

Tablet, as diphosphate (Stilphostrol®): 50 mg

**Dosing**

**Adults:**

Male:

Prostate carcinoma (inoperable, progressing): Oral: 1-3 mg/day

Diphosphate: Inoperable progressing prostate cancer:

Oral: 50 mg 3 times/day; increase up to 200 mg or more 3 times/day; maximum daily dose: 1 g

I.V.: Give 0.5 g, dissolved in 250 mL of saline or $D_5W$; administer slowly the first 10-15 minutes then adjust rate so that the entire amount is given in 1 hour. Repeat for ≥5 days depending on patient response, then repeat 0.25-0.5 g 1-2 times for 1 week or change to oral therapy.

Female: Postmenopausal inoperable, progressing breast carcinoma: Oral: 15 mg/day

**Elderly:** Refer to adult dosing.

**Stability**

**Storage:** Intravenous solution should be stored at room temperature and away from direct light. Solution is stable for 3 days as long as cloudiness or precipitation has not occurred.

**Reconstitution:** NS or $D_5W$

**Additional Nursing Issues**

**Physical Assessment:** Monitor appropriate laboratory tests (hypercalcemia). Monitor effectiveness of therapy, adverse effects, and patient knowledge of interventions to reduce adverse effects and symptoms to report. **Pregnancy risk factor X** - determine that patient is not pregnant before beginning treatment and do not give to women of childbearing age or male having intercourse with women of childbearing age unless both male and female are capable of complying with barrier contraceptive measures 1 month prior to therapy, during therapy, and for 1 month following therapy. Breast-feeding is contraindicated during therapy and for 1 month following therapy.

**Patient Information/Instruction:** Use as directed with or after meals (sustained release may be taken at midmorning - do not crush or chew). May cause breast tenderness or enlargement (consult prescriber for relief). You may be more sensitive to sunlight; use sunblock, wear protective clothing and dark glasses, or avoid direct exposure to sunlight. If you are diabetic, monitor serum glucose closely; antidiabetic agent may need to be adjusted. Discontinue use and report promptly any pain, redness, warmth, or swelling in calves; sudden onset difficulty breathing; headache; loss of vision; difficulty speaking; sharp or sudden chest pain; severe abdominal pain; or unusual bleeding or speech. **Pregnancy/breast-feeding precautions:** Inform prescriber if you are pregnant. Do not get pregnant while taking this drug and for 1 month following therapy. Consult prescriber for instruction on appropriate contraceptive measures. This drug may cause severe fetal defects. Do not donate blood during or for 1 month following therapy (same reason). Do not breast-feed.

**Geriatric Considerations:** The benefits of postmenopausal estrogen therapy may be substantial for some women. Diethylstilbestrol is not the drug of choice for vasomotor symptoms, to prevent bone loss, or to treat vaginal atrophy or urinary incontinence secondary to estrogen deficiency. Diethylstilbestrol does have a role in the treatment of inoperable, progressive prostatic carcinoma and inoperable, progressive breast cancer in select men and women.

- **Diethylstilbestrol Diphosphate Sodium** *see* Diethylstilbestrol *on previous page*

## Difenoxin and Atropine (dye fen OKS in & A troe peen)

**U.S. Brand Names** Motofen®

**Synonyms** Atropine and Difenoxin

(Continued)

## Difenoxin and Atropine *(Continued)*

**Therapeutic Category** Antidiarrheal

**Pregnancy Risk Factor** C

**Lactation** Enters breast milk/contraindicated

**Use** Treatment of diarrhea

**Mechanism of Action/Effect** Slows intestinal motility

**Contraindications** Hypersensitivity to difenoxin, atropine, or any component; severe liver disease, jaundice, dehydrated patient, and angle-closure glaucoma; diarrhea associated with organisms that penetrate the intestinal mucosa (toxigenic *E. coli*, *Salmonella* sp, *Shigella*), and pseudomembranous colitis associated with broad spectrum antibiotics

**Warnings** Dosage recommendations should be strictly adhered to. If severe dehydration or electrolyte imbalance is manifested, withhold until appropriate corrective therapy has been initiated. Patients with acute ulcerative colitis should be carefully observed. Use with caution in patients with advanced hepatorenal disease. Pregnancy factor C.

**Drug Interactions**

**Increased Effect/Toxicity:** Concurrent use with MAO inhibitors may precipitate hypertensive crisis. May potentiate action of barbiturates, tranquilizers, narcotics, and alcohol. Difenoxin has the potential to prolong biological half-life of drugs for which the rate of elimination is dependent on the microsomal drug metabolizing enzyme system.

**Adverse Reactions**

1% to 10%:

Central nervous system: Dizziness, drowsiness, lightheadedness, headache

Gastrointestinal: Nausea, vomiting, dry mouth, epigastric distress

<1% (Limited to important or life-threatening symptoms): Tachycardia, confusion, constipation, blurred vision, anaphylaxis

**Pharmacodynamics/Kinetics**

**Time to Peak:** Plasma concentrations within 40-60 minutes

**Metabolism:** Liver

**Excretion:** Urine

**Formulations** Tablet: Difenoxin hydrochloride 1 mg and atropine sulfate 0.025 mg

**Dosing**

**Adults:** Oral: Initial: 2 tablets, then 1 tablet after each loose stool; 1 tablet every 3-4 hours, up to 8 tablets in a 24-hour period; if no improvement after 48 hours, continued administration is not indicated

**Elderly:** Refer to adult dosing; use with caution.

**Stability**

**Storage:** Store at room temperature 15°C to 30°C (59°C to 86°C).

**Additional Nursing Issues**

**Physical Assessment:** Assess effects and interactions of other prescription and OTC medications the patient may be taking (see Drug Interactions). Monitor for effectiveness and adverse CNS effects. **Pregnancy risk factor C** - benefits of use should outweigh possible risks. Breast-feeding is contraindicated.

**Patient Information/Instruction:** Take as directed; do not exceed recommended dose. If no relief in 48 hours, contact prescriber. Avoid alcohol. Keep out of reach of children; can cause severe and fatal respiratory depression if accidentally ingested. You may experience lightheadedness, depression, dizziness, or weakness; use caution when driving or engaging in tasks that require alertness until response to drug is known. Report acute dizziness, headache, or gastrointestinal symptoms. **Pregnancy/breast-feeding precautions:** Inform prescriber if you are or intend to be pregnant. Do not breast-feed.

**Breast-feeding Issues:** Potential for serious adverse reactions in nursing infants.

**Related Information**

Atropine *on page 119*

♦ **Differin®** *see* Adapalene *on page 41*

♦ **Diflorasone** *see* Topical Corticosteroids *on page 1152*

♦ **Diflucan®** *see* Fluconazole *on page 491*

## Diflunisal (dye FLOO ni sal)

**U.S. Brand Names** Dolobid®

**Therapeutic Category** Nonsteroidal Anti-Inflammatory Agent (NSAID)

**Pregnancy Risk Factor** C/D (3rd trimester)

**Lactation** Enters breast milk/use caution

**Use** Management of inflammatory disorders usually including rheumatoid arthritis and osteoarthritis; analgesic for treatment of mild to moderate pain

**Mechanism of Action/Effect** Inhibits prostaglandin synthesis by decreasing the activity of the enzyme, cyclo-oxygenase, which results in decreased formation of prostaglandin precursors

**Contraindications** Hypersensitivity to diflunisal or any component; may be a cross-sensitivity with other nonsteroidal anti-inflammatory agents including aspirin; should not be used in patients with active GI bleeding; pregnancy (3rd trimester)

**Warnings** Peptic ulceration and GI bleeding have been reported. Platelet function and bleeding time are inhibited. Ophthalmologic effects. Use lower dosages in impaired renal function. Peripheral edema, possibility of Reye's syndrome. Pregnancy factor C/D (3rd trimester).

**Drug Interactions**

**Decreased Effect:** Decreased effect with antacids, aspirin.

**Increased Effect/Toxicity:** May cause increased toxicity of cyclosporine, digoxin, methotrexate, anticoagulants, phenytoin, sulfonylureas, sulfonamides, lithium, indomethacin, hydrochlorothiazide, and acetaminophen (levels) when coadministered with diflunisal.

**Effects on Lab Values** ↑ prothrombin time (S), liver tests; ↓ uric acid (S)

**Adverse Reactions**

1% to 10%:

Cardiovascular: Chest pain, arrhythmias

Central nervous system: Dizziness, headache

Dermatologic: Rash

Endocrine & metabolic: Fluid retention

Gastrointestinal: Abdominal cramps, bloated feeling, constipation, diarrhea, indigestion, nausea, vomiting, mouth soreness

Genitourinary: Vaginal bleeding

Otic: Tinnitus

<1% (Limited to important or life-threatening symptoms): Chest pain, vasculitis, tachycardia, fluid retention/edema, convulsions, confusion, hallucinations, mental depression, drowsiness, nervousness, insomnia, disorientation, toxic epidermal necrolysis, urticaria, exfoliative dermatitis, itching, erythema multiforme, Stevens-Johnson syndrome, angioedema, hemolytic anemia, agranulocytosis, thrombocytopenia, hepatitis, interstitial nephritis, nephrotic syndrome, renal impairment, wheezing, shortness of breath, hearing loss

**Overdose/Toxicology** Symptoms of overdose include drowsiness, nausea, vomiting, hyperventilation, tachycardia, tinnitus, stupor, coma, renal failure, and leukocytosis. Management of nonsteroidal anti-inflammatory (NSAID) intoxication is supportive and symptomatic.

**Pharmacodynamics/Kinetics**

**Half-life Elimination:** 8-12 hours (prolonged in renal impairment)

**Time to Peak:** Oral: Within 2-3 hours

**Metabolism:** Liver

**Excretion:** Urine

**Onset:** Onset of analgesia: Within 1 hour

**Duration:** 8-12 hours

**Formulations** Tablet: 250 mg, 500 mg

**Dosing**

**Adults:** Oral:

Pain: Initial: 500-1000 mg followed by 250-500 mg every 8-12 hours; maximum daily dose: 1.5 g

Inflammatory condition: 500-1000 mg/day in 2 divided doses; maximum daily dose: 1.5 g

**Elderly:** Refer to adult dosing.

**Renal Impairment:** $Cl_{cr}$ <50 mL/minute: Administer 50% of normal dose.

**Additional Nursing Issues**

**Physical Assessment: Assess patient for allergic reaction to salicylates or other NSAIDs** (see Contraindications). Assess other medications patient may be taking for additive or adverse interactions (see Drug Interactions). Monitor for effectiveness of pain relief. Monitor for signs of adverse reactions or overdose (see Overdose/Toxicology Adverse Reactions) at beginning of therapy and periodically during long-term therapy. Assess knowledge/teach patient appropriate use. Teach patient to monitor for adverse reactions, adverse reactions to report, and appropriate interventions to reduce side effects. **Pregnancy risk factor C/D** - see Pregnancy Risk Factor - benefits of use should outweigh possible risks. Note breast-feeding caution.

**Patient Information/Instruction:** If self-administered, use exactly as directed (do not increase dose or frequency); adverse reactions can occur with overuse. Do not take longer than 3 days for fever, or 10 days for pain without consulting medical advisor. Take with food or milk. While using this medication, do not use alcohol, excessive amounts of vitamin C, or salicylate-containing foods (curry powder, prunes, raisins, tea, or licorice), other prescription or OTC medications containing aspirin or salicylate, or other NSAIDs without consulting prescriber. Maintain adequate hydration (2-3 L/day of fluids unless instructed to restrict fluid intake). You may experience nausea, vomiting, gastric discomfort (frequent mouth care, small frequent meals, chewing gum, or sucking lozenges may help). GI bleeding, ulceration, or perforation can occur with or without pain. Stop taking medication and report ringing in ears; persistent pain in stomach; unresolved nausea or vomiting; difficulty breathing or shortness of breath; unusual bruising or bleeding (mouth, urine, stool); skin rash; unusual swelling of extremities; chest pain; or palpitations. **Pregnancy/breast-feeding precautions:** Inform prescriber if you are or intend to be pregnant. Consult prescriber if breast-feeding.

**Geriatric Considerations:** Elderly are at high risk for adverse effects from nonsteroidal anti-inflammatory agents.

**Additional Information** Diflunisal is a salicylic acid derivative which is chemically different than aspirin and is not metabolized to salicylic acid. Diflunisal 500 mg is equal in analgesic efficacy to aspirin 650 mg, acetaminophen 650 mg, and acetaminophen 650 mg/propoxyphene napsylate 100 mg, but has a longer duration of effect (8-12 hours). Not recommended as an antipyretic. Not found to be clinically useful to treat fever; at doses of ≥2 g/day, platelets are reversibly inhibited in function. Diflunisal is uricosuric at 500-750 mg/day; causes less GI and renal toxicity than aspirin and other NSAIDs; fecal blood loss is ½ that of aspirin at 2.6 g/day.

(Continued)

## Diflunisal *(Continued)*

**Related Information**

Nonsalicylate/Nonsteroidal Anti-inflammatory Comparison *on page 1401*

- **Di-Gel®** *see page 1294*
- **Digibind®** *see* Digoxin Immune Fab *on page 372*

## Digoxin (di JOKS in)

**U.S. Brand Names** Lanoxicaps®; Lanoxin®

**Therapeutic Category** Antiarrhythmic Agent, Class IV; Cardiac Glycoside

**Pregnancy Risk Factor** C

**Lactation** Enters breast milk (small amounts)/compatible

**Use** Treatment of congestive heart failure and to slow the ventricular rate in tachyarrhythmias such as atrial fibrillation, atrial flutter, and supraventricular tachycardia (paroxysmal atrial tachycardia); cardiogenic shock

**Mechanism of Action/Effect**

Congestive heart failure: Inhibition of the sodium/potassium ATPase pump which acts to increase the intracellular sodium-calcium exchange to increase intracellular calcium leading to increased contractility

Supraventricular arrhythmias: Direct suppression of the A-V node conduction to increase effective refractory period and decrease conduction velocity - positive inotropic effect, enhanced vagal tone, and decreased ventricular rate to fast atrial arrhythmias. Atrial fibrillation may decrease sensitivity and increase tolerance to higher serum digoxin concentrations.

**Contraindications** Hypersensitivity to digoxin or any component; A-V block; idiopathic hypertrophic subaortic stenosis; constrictive pericarditis; ventricular tachycardia or fibrillation; acute MI; electrolyte imbalance

**Warnings** Use with caution in patients with hypoxia, myxedema, hypothyroidism, acute myocarditis. Patients with incomplete A-V block (Stokes-Adams attack) may progress to complete block with digitalis drug administration. Use with caution in patients with acute myocardial infarction, severe pulmonary disease, advanced heart failure, idiopathic hypertrophic subaortic stenosis, Wolff-Parkinson-White syndrome, sick-sinus syndrome (bradyarrhythmias), amyloid heart disease, and constrictive cardiomyopathies. Adjust dose with renal impairment or age. Exercise will reduce serum concentrations of digoxin due to increased skeletal muscle uptake. Recent studies indicate photopsia, chromatopsia, and decreased visual acuity may occur even with therapeutic serum drug levels. Pregnancy factor C.

**Drug Interactions**

**Decreased Effect:**

Decreased effect/levels of digoxin: Antacids (magnesium, aluminum)•, penicillamine•, dietary bran fiber•, radiotherapy⁺, antineoplastic drugs⁺, sucralfate⁺, sulfasalazine⁺, thiazide and loop diuretics⁺, aminosalicylic acid⁺, neomycin⁺⁺, phenytoin⁺⁺, cholestyramine/colestipol/kaolin-pectin⁺⁺, aminoglutethimide⁺⁺

**Note:**

- • = improbable clinical importance
- ⁺ = uncertain clinical significance
- ⁺⁺ = interaction proven needing monitoring for possible dosage adjustments

**Increased Effect/Toxicity:**

Increased effect/toxicity/levels of digoxin: Diltiazem•, spironolactone/triamterene•, ibuprofen•, cimetidine•, omeprazole•, flecainide⁺, acetylsalicylic acid⁺, indomethacin⁺, benzodiazepines⁺, bepridil⁺⁺, reserpine⁺⁺, amphotericin B⁺⁺, erythromycin⁺⁺, quinine sulfate⁺⁺, tetracycline⁺⁺, cyclosporin⁺⁺, amiodarone••, propafenone••, quinidine••, verapamil••, calcium preparations••, itraconazole••

Increased effect/toxicity/levels of digitoxin: Diltiazem•, spironolactone•, amphotericin B⁺⁺, quinidine••, calcium preparations••

**Note:**

- • = improbable clinical importance
- ⁺ = uncertain clinical significance
- ⁺⁺ = interaction proven needing monitoring for possible dosage adjustments
- •• = important interaction needing monitoring, dosage adjustments are likely.

**Food Interactions** Digoxin peak serum levels may be decreased if taken with food. Meals containing increased fiber (bran) or foods high in pectin may decrease oral absorption of digoxin.

**Adverse Reactions**

1% to 10%: Gastrointestinal: Anorexia, nausea, vomiting

<1% (Limited to important or life-threatening symptoms): Sinus bradycardia, A-V block, S-A block, atrial or nodal ectopic beats, ventricular arrhythmias, bigeminy, trigeminy, atrial tachycardia with A-V block

**Overdose/Toxicology** Manifested by a wide variety of signs and symptoms difficult to distinguish from effects associated with cardiac disease. Nausea and vomiting are common early signs of toxicity and may precede or follow evidence of cardiotoxicity. Other symptoms include anorexia, diarrhea, abdominal discomfort, headache, weakness, drowsiness, visual disturbances, mental depression, confusion, restlessness, disorientation, seizures, and hallucinations. Cardiac abnormalities include ventricular tachycardia, unifocal or multifocal PVCs (bigeminal, trigeminal), paroxysmal nodal rhythms, A-V dissociation, excessive slowing of the pulse, A-V block of varying degree, P-R prolongation, S-T depression, and occasional atrial fibrillation. Ventricular fibrillation is a common cause of death (alterations in cardiac rate and rhythm can result in any type of known arrhythmia).

Antidote: Life-threatening digoxin toxicity is treated with Digibind®. Administer potassium except in cases of complete heart block or renal failure. Digitalis-induced arrhythmias not responsive to potassium may be treated with phenytoin or lidocaine. Cholestyramine and colestipol may decrease absorption. Other agents to consider, based on EKG and clinical assessment, include atropine, quinidine, procainamide, and propranolol. **Note:** Other antiarrhythmics appear more dangerous to use in toxicity.

**Pharmacodynamics/Kinetics**

**Protein Binding:** 30% (in uremic patients, digoxin is displaced from plasma protein binding sites)

**Distribution:**

Normal renal function: 6-7 L/kg

$V_d$: Extensive to peripheral tissues, with a distinct distribution phase which lasts 6-8 hours; concentrates in heart, liver, kidney, skeletal muscle and intestines. Heart/serum concentration is 70:1. Pharmacologic effects are delayed and do not correlate well with serum concentrations during distribution phase.

Hyperthyroidism: Increased $V_d$

Hyperkalemia, hyponatremia: Decreased digoxin distribution to heart and muscle

Hypokalemia: Increased digoxin distribution to heart and muscles

Concomitant quinidine therapy: Decreased $V_d$

Chronic renal failure: 4-6 L/kg

Decreased sodium/potassium ATPase activity - decreased tissue binding

**Half-life Elimination:**

Dependent upon age, renal and cardiac function: Adults: 38-48 hours; Adults, anephric: 4-6 days

Half-life: Parent drug: 38 hours; Metabolites: Digoxigenin: 4 hours; Monodigitoxoside: 3-12 hours

**Time to Peak:** Oral: Within 1 hour

**Metabolism:** Stomach; metabolism is reduced in patients with CHF.

**Excretion:** Urine

**Onset:** Oral: 1-2 hours; I.V.: 5-30 minutes; Peak effect: Oral: 2-8 hours; I.V.: 1-4 hours

**Duration:** 3-4 days both forms

**Formulations**

Capsule: 50 mcg, 100 mcg, 200 mcg

Elixir: 50 mcg/mL with alcohol 10% (60 mL)

Injection: 250 mcg/mL (1 mL, 2 mL)

Injection, pediatric: 100 mcg/mL (1 mL)

Tablet: 125 mcg, 250 mcg, 500 mcg

**Dosing**

**Adults:** When changing from oral (tablets or liquid) or I.M. to I.V. therapy, dosage should be reduced by 20% to 25%.

Total digitalizing dose: Give one-half of the total digitalizing dose (TDD) in the initial dose, then give one-quarter of the TDD in each of two subsequent doses at 9- to 12-hour intervals. Obtain EKG 6 hours after each dose to assess potential toxicity.

Oral: 0.75-1.5 mg

I.V. or I.M.: 0.5-1 mg

Daily maintenance dose: Give once daily to children >10 years of age and adults.

Oral: 0.125-0.5 mg

I.V. or I.M.: 0.1-0.4 mg

**Elderly:** Elderly dose is based on lean body weight and normal renal function for age. Decrease dose in patients with decreased renal function (see Renal Impairment).

**Renal Impairment:**

$Cl_{cr}$ 10-50 mL/minute: Administer 25% to 75% of dose or every 36 hours.

$Cl_{cr}$ <10 mL/minute: Administer 10% to 25% of dose or every 48 hours.

Reduce loading dose by 50% in ESRD.

Not dialyzable (0% to 5%)

**Administration**

**I.M.:** Inject no more than 2 mL per injection site. May cause intense pain.

**I.V.:** Inject slowly 1-5 minutes for undiluted form. May dilute up to fourfold with, SWI, $D_5W$, or NS.

**Stability**

**Storage:** Protect elixir and injection from light.

**Compatibility:** Compatible with $D_5W$, $D_{10}W$, NS, and sterile water for injection (when diluted fourfold or greater).

**Monitoring Laboratory Tests**

When to draw serum digoxin concentrations: Digoxin serum concentrations are monitored because digoxin possesses a narrow therapeutic serum range; the therapeutic endpoint is difficult to quantify and digoxin toxicity may be life threatening. Digoxin serum levels should be drawn **at least 4 hours after an intravenous dose** and **at least 6 hours after an oral dose (optimally 12-24 hours after a dose).**

Initiation of therapy:

**If a loading dose is given:** Digoxin serum concentration may be drawn within 12-24 hours after the initial loading dose administration. Levels drawn this early may confirm the relationship of digoxin plasma levels and response but are of little value in determining maintenance doses.

**If a loading dose is not given:** Digoxin serum concentration should be obtained after 3-5 days of therapy.

Maintenance monitoring:

Trough concentrations should be followed just prior to the next dose or at a minimum of 4 hours after an I.V. dose and at least 6 hours after an oral dose.

(Continued)

## Digoxin *(Continued)*

Digoxin serum concentrations should be obtained within 5-7 days (approximate time to steady-state) after any dosage changes. Continue to obtain digoxin serum concentrations 7-14 days after any change in maintenance dose. **Note:** In patients with end-stage renal disease, it may take 15-20 days to reach steady-state.

Patients who are receiving potassium-depleting medications such as diuretics, should be monitored for potassium, magnesium, and calcium levels.

Digoxin serum concentrations should be obtained whenever any of the following conditions occur:

- Questionable patient compliance or to evaluate clinical deterioration following an initial good response
- Changing renal function
- Suspected digoxin toxicity
- Initiation or discontinuation of therapy with drugs (amiodarone, quinidine, verapamil) which potentially interact with digoxin; if quinidine therapy is started; digoxin levels should be drawn within the first 24 hours after starting quinidine therapy, then 7-14 days later or empirically skip one day's digoxin dose and decrease the daily dose by 50%.
- Any disease changes (hypothyroidism)

**Additional Nursing Issues**

**Physical Assessment:** Closely assess effects and interactions with other prescription and OTC medications patient may be taking (see Drug Interactions). Appropriate laboratory tests should be monitored when beginning or changing therapy (especially with I.V. administration) or when patients are receiving diuretics or amphotericin (see Monitoring Laboratory Tests).

I.V.: Monitor EKG continuously.

Oral: Monitor apical pulse before administering any dose. Monitor and teach patient necessity of monitoring for noncardiac signs of toxicity (eg, anorexia, blurred vision, "yellow" vision, confusion).

**Pregnancy risk factor C** - benefits of use should outweigh possible risks.

**Patient Information/Instruction:** Take as directed; do not discontinue without consulting prescriber. Maintain adequate dietary intake of potassium (do not increase without consulting prescriber). Adequate dietary potassium will reduce risk of digoxin toxicity. Take pulse at the same time each day; follow prescriber instructions for holding medication if pulse is below 50. Notify prescriber of acute changes in pulse. Report loss of appetite, nausea, vomiting, persistent diarrhea, swelling of extremities, palpitations, "yellowing" or blurred vision, mental confusion or depression, or unusual fatigue. **Pregnancy precautions:** Inform prescriber if you are or intend to be pregnant.

**Geriatric Considerations:** Elderly may develop exaggerated serum/tissue concentrations due to age-related alterations in clearance and pharmacodynamic differences. Elderly are at risk for toxicity due to age-related changes

**Additional Information** Some formulations may contain ethanol.

**Related Information**

Antiarrhythmic Drug Classification Comparison *on page 1366*
Peak and Trough Guidelines *on page 1331*

## Digoxin Immune Fab (di JOKS in i MYUN fab)

**U.S. Brand Names** Digibind®

**Synonyms** Antidigoxin Fab Fragments

**Therapeutic Category** Antidote

**Pregnancy Risk Factor** C

**Lactation** Excretion in breast milk unknown

**Use** Digoxin immune antigen-binding fragments (Fab) are specific antibodies for the treatment of digitalis intoxication in carefully selected patients; used in life-threatening ventricular arrhythmias secondary to digoxin, acute digoxin ingestion (ie, >10 mg in adults or >4 mg in children), hyperkalemia (serum potassium >5 mEq/L) in the setting of digoxin toxicity

**Mechanism of Action/Effect** Binds with molecules of digoxin or digitoxin and then is excreted by the kidneys and removed from the body

**Contraindications** Hypersensitivity to sheep products

**Warnings** Use with caution in renal or cardiac failure. Allergic reactions are possible; (sheep product)-skin testing is not routinely recommended. Epinephrine should be immediately available. Fab fragments may be eliminated more slowly in patients with renal failure. Heart failure may be exacerbated as digoxin level is reduced. Total serum digoxin concentration may rise precipitously following administration of Digibind®, but this will be almost entirely bound to the Fab fragment and not able to react with receptors in the body. Digibind® will interfere with digitalis immunoassay measurements - this will result in clinically misleading serum digoxin concentrations until the Fab fragment is eliminated from the body (several days to >1 week after Digibind® administration). Hypokalemia has been reported to occur following reversal of digitalis intoxication as has exacerbation of underlying heart failure. Serum digoxin levels drawn prior to therapy may be difficult to evaluate if 6-8 hours have not elapsed after the last dose of digoxin (time to equilibration between serum and tissue). Redigitalization should not be initiated until Fab fragments have been eliminated from the body, which may occur over several days or greater than a week in patients with impaired renal function. Pregnancy factor C.

**Effects on Lab Values** Digibind® will interfere with digitalis immunoassay measurements - this will result in clinically misleading serum digoxin concentrations fragment is eliminated from the body (several days to >1 week after Digibind® administration).

**Adverse Reactions** <1% (Limited to important or life-threatening symptoms): Worsening of low cardiac output or congestive heart failure, rapid ventricular response in patients with atrial fibrillation as digoxin is withdrawn, facial edema and redness, hypokalemia

**Overdose/Toxicology** Symptoms of overdose include delayed serum sickness. Treatment of serum sickness includes acetaminophen, $histamine_1$ and possibly $histamine_2$ blockers, and corticosteroids.

**Pharmacodynamics/Kinetics**

**Half-life Elimination:** 15-20 hours (prolonged in renal impairment)

**Excretion:** Urine

**Onset:** I.V.: Improvement in signs or symptoms occur within 2-30 minutes

**Formulations** Powder for injection, lyophilized: 40 mg

**Dosing**

**Adults:** Each vial of Digibind® will bind approximately 0.6 mg of digoxin or digitoxin.

I.V.: To determine the dose of digoxin immune Fab, first determine the total body load of digoxin (TBL using either an approximation of the amount ingested or a postdistribution serum digoxin concentration). If neither ingestion amount or serum level is known: Dosage is 20 vials (800 mg) I.V. infusion.

**Elderly:** Refer to adult dosing.

**Administration**

**I.V.:** Continuous I.V. infusion over 15-30 minutes is preferred.

**I.V. Detail:** Digoxin immune Fab is reconstituted by adding 4 mL sterile water, resulting in 10 mg/mL for I.V. infusion. The reconstituted solution may be further diluted with NS to a convenient volume (eg, 1 mg/mL).

**Stability**

**Storage:** Should be refrigerated at 2°C to 8°C.

**Reconstitution:** Digoxin immune Fab is reconstituted by adding 4 mL sterile water, resulting in 10 mg/mL for I.V. infusion. The reconstituted solution may be further diluted with NS to a convenient volume (eg, 1 mg/mL). Reconstituted solutions should be used within 4 hours if refrigerated.

**Monitoring Laboratory Tests** Serum potassium, serum digoxin concentration prior to first dose of digoxin immune Fab, subsequent to start of Digibind® therapy; **digoxin levels will greatly increase and are not an accurate determination of body stores.**

**Additional Nursing Issues**

**Physical Assessment:** Note Warnings/Precautions. Monitor lab values (see Effects on Lab Values and Monitoring Laboratory Tests), cardiac status, vital signs, blood pressure, and adverse reactions during and following infusion (see Adverse Reactions). **Pregnancy risk factor C.** Note breast-feeding caution.

**Patient Information/Instruction:** Patient education and instruction will be determined by patient condition and ability to understand. Immediately report dizziness, palpitations, cramping, or difficulty breathing. **Pregnancy/breast-feeding precautions:** Inform prescriber if you are pregnant. Consult prescriber if breast-feeding.

- ♦ **Dihistine® DH Liquid** *see page 1306*
- ♦ **Dihistine® Expectorant** *see* Guaifenesin, Pseudoephedrine, and Codeine *on page 552*
- ♦ **Dihydrex® Injection** *see* Diphenhydramine *on page 381*

## Dihydrocodeine Compound (dye hye droe KOE deen KOM pound)

**U.S. Brand Names** DHC Plus®; Synalgos®-DC

**Therapeutic Category** Analgesic, Narcotic

**Pregnancy Risk Factor** B/D (if used for prolonged periods or in high doses at term)

**Lactation** Excretion in breast milk unknown/use caution

**Use** Management of mild to moderate pain that requires relaxation

**Mechanism of Action/Effect** Binds to opiate receptors in the CNS, causing inhibition of ascending pain pathways, altering the perception of and response to pain; causes cough suppression by direct central action in the medulla; produces generalized CNS depression

**Contraindications** Hypersensitivity to dihydrocodeine or any component; pregnancy (if used for prolonged periods or in high doses at term)

**Warnings** Use with caution in patients with hypersensitivity reactions to other phenanthrene derivative opioid agonists (morphine, hydrocodone, hydromorphone, levorphanol, oxycodone, oxymorphone); respiratory diseases including asthma, emphysema, COPD; or severe liver or renal insufficiency. Some preparations contain sulfites which may cause allergic reactions. May be habit-forming. Dextromethorphan has equivalent antitussive activity but has much lower toxicity in accidental overdose.

**Drug Interactions**

**Cytochrome P-450 Effect:** CYP2D6 enzyme substrate

**Increased Effect/Toxicity:** MAO inhibitors may increase adverse symptoms.

**Adverse Reactions**

>10%:

Central nervous system: Lightheadedness, dizziness, drowsiness, sedation
Dermatologic: Pruritus, skin reactions
Gastrointestinal: Nausea, vomiting, constipation

1% to 10%:

Cardiovascular: Hypotension, palpitations, bradycardia, peripheral vasodilation
Central nervous system: Increased intracranial pressure
Endocrine & metabolic: Antidiuretic hormone release
Gastrointestinal: Biliary tract spasm
Genitourinary: Urinary tract spasm
Ocular: Miosis

(Continued)

## Dihydrocodeine Compound *(Continued)*

Respiratory: Respiratory depression

Miscellaneous: Histamine release, physical and psychological dependence with prolonged use

**Overdose/Toxicology** Symptoms of overdose include CNS depression, pinpoint pupils, hypotension, and bradycardia. Treatment is supportive. Naloxone, 2 mg I.V. with repeat administration as necessary up to a total of 10 mg, can also be used to reverse toxic effects of the opiate.

**Pharmacodynamics/Kinetics**

**Half-life Elimination:** 3.5-4.5 hours

**Time to Peak:** 1.6-1.8 hours

**Metabolism:** Liver

**Onset:** 4-5 hours

**Formulations**

Capsule:

DHC Plus®: Dihydrocodeine bitartrate 16 mg, acetaminophen 356.4 mg, and caffeine 30 mg

Synalgos®-DC: Dihydrocodeine bitartrate 16 mg, aspirin 356.4 mg, and caffeine 30 mg

**Dosing**

**Adults:** Oral: 1-2 capsules every 4-6 hours as needed for pain

**Additional Nursing Issues**

**Physical Assessment:** Assess for history of allergy (aspirin) and other medications patient may be taking for additive or adverse interactions. Monitor for effectiveness of pain relief and monitor for signs of overdose (see above). Monitor blood pressure, CNS and respiratory status, and degree of sedation at beginning of therapy and at regular intervals with long-term use. May cause physical and/or psychological dependence. For inpatients, implement safety measures (eg, side rails up, call light within reach, instructions to call for assistance, etc). Assess knowledge/teach patient appropriate use (if self-administered). Teach patient to monitor for adverse reactions (see Adverse Reactions), adverse reactions to report, and appropriate interventions to reduce side effects. **Pregnancy risk factor B/D** - see Pregnancy Risk Factor for cautious use. Note breast-feeding caution.

**Patient Information/Instruction:** If self-administered, use exactly as directed (do not increase dose or frequency); may cause physical and/or psychological dependence. While using this medication, do not use alcohol and other prescription or OTC medications (especially sedatives, tranquilizers, antihistamines, or pain medications) without consulting prescriber. Maintain adequate hydration (2-3 L/day of fluids unless instructed to restrict fluid intake). May cause dizziness, drowsiness, impaired coordination, or blurred vision (use caution when driving, climbing stairs, or changing position - rising from sitting or lying to standing or when engaging in tasks requiring alertness until response to drug is known); nausea or vomiting (frequent mouth care, small frequent meals, chewing gum, or sucking lozenges may help); constipation (increased exercise, fluids, or dietary fruit and fiber may help - if constipation remains an unresolved problem, consult prescriber about use of stool softeners). Report chest pain or rapid heartbeat; acute headache; swelling of extremities or unusual weight gain; changes in urinary elimination; acute headache; back or flank pain or spasms; or other adverse reactions. **Pregnancy/breast-feeding precautions:** Inform prescriber if you are or intend to be pregnant. Consult prescriber if breast-feeding.

**Related Information**

Aspirin *on page 111*

## Dihydroergotamine (dye hye droe er GOT a meen)

**U.S. Brand Names** D.H.E. 45® Injection; Migranal® Nasal Spray

**Therapeutic Category** Ergot Derivative

**Pregnancy Risk Factor** X

**Lactation** Likely to enter breast milk/contraindicated

**Use** Abort or prevent migraine headaches; an adjunct for DVT prophylaxis for hip surgery, for orthostatic hypotension, xerostomia secondary to antidepressant use, and pelvic congestion with pain

**Mechanism of Action/Effect** Ergot alkaloid alpha-adrenergic blocker directly stimulates vascular smooth muscle to vasoconstrict peripheral and cerebral vessels; also has effects on serotonin receptors

**Contraindications** Hypersensitivity to dihydroergotamine or any component; high-dose aspirin therapy; pregnancy

**Warnings** Use with caution in hypertension, peripheral vascular disease, angina, peripheral vascular disease, impaired renal or hepatic function, sepsis, or malnutrition.

**Drug Interactions**

**Increased Effect/Toxicity:** Increased effect of heparin. Increased toxicity with erythromycin, clarithromycin, nitroglycerin, propranolol, and troleandomycin. Potential for serotonin syndrome if combined with other serotonergic drugs.

**Adverse Reactions**

>10%:

Cardiovascular: Localized edema, peripheral vascular effects (numbness and tingling of fingers and toes)

Central nervous system: Drowsiness, dizziness

Gastrointestinal: Dry mouth, diarrhea, nausea, vomiting

1% to 10%:

Cardiovascular: Precordial distress and pain, transient tachycardia or bradycardia

Neuromuscular & skeletal: Muscle pain in the extremities, weakness in the legs

**Overdose/Toxicology** Symptoms of overdose include peripheral ischemia, paresthesia, headache, nausea, and vomiting. Treatment is supportive. Activated charcoal is effective at binding ergot alkaloids.

**Pharmacodynamics/Kinetics**

**Protein Binding:** 90%

**Half-life Elimination:** 1.3-3.9 hours

**Time to Peak:** I.M.: Within 15-30 minutes

**Metabolism:** Liver

**Excretion:** Bile and feces

**Onset:** Within 15-30 minutes

**Duration:** 3-4 hours

**Formulations** Dihydroergotamine mesylate:

Injection: 1 mg/mL (1 mL)

Spray, nasal: 4 mg/mL [0.5 mg/spray] (1 mL)

**Dosing**

**Adults:**

I.M.: 1 mg at first sign of headache; repeat hourly to a maximum dose of 3 mg total

I.V.: Up to 2 mg maximum dose for faster effects; maximum: 6 mg/week

Intranasal: 1 spray (0.5 mg) of nasal spray should be administered into each nostril. If the condition has not sufficiently improved ~15 minutes later, an additional spray should be administered to each nostril. The usual dosage required to obtain optimal efficacy is a total dosage of 4 sprays (2 mg). Nasal spray is exclusively indicated for the symptomatic treatment of migraine attacks; no more than 4 sprays (2 mg) should be administered for any single migraine attack. An interval of at least 6-8 hours should be observed before treating another migraine attack with the nasal spray or any drug containing dihydroergotamine or ergotamine; no more than 8 sprays (4 mg) (corresponding to the use of 2 ampuls) should be administered during any 24-hour period; maximum weekly dosage: 24 sprays (12 mg).

**Elderly:** Refer to adult dosing.

**Hepatic Impairment:** Dosage reductions are probably necessary but specific guidelines are not available.

**Stability**

**Storage:** Store in refrigerator.

**Additional Nursing Issues**

**Physical Assessment:** Monitor for effectiveness of therapy and patient's knowledge of appropriate administration and needle disposal. **Pregnancy risk factor X** - determine that patient is not pregnant before beginning treatment and do not give to women of childbearing age or to males who may have intercourse with women of childbearing age unless both male and female are capable of complying with barrier contraceptive measures during therapy and for 1 month following therapy. Breast-feeding is contraindicated.

**Patient Information/Instruction:** Take this drug as rapidly as possible when first symptoms occur. Rare feelings of numbness or tingling of fingers, toes, or face may occur; use caution and avoid injury. May cause drowsiness; avoid activities requiring alertness until effects of medication are known. Report heart palpitations, severe nausea or vomiting, or severe numbness of fingers or toes. **Pregnancy/breast-feeding precautions:** Inform prescriber if you are pregnant. Do not get pregnant during or for 1 month following therapy. Male: Do not cause a female to become pregnant. Male/female: Consult prescriber for instruction on appropriate contraceptive measures. This drug may cause severe fetal defects. Do not breast-feed.

**Geriatric Considerations:** Monitor cardiac and peripheral effects closely in the elderly since they often have cardiovascular disease and peripheral vascular impairment (ie, diabetes mellitus, PVD) that will complicate therapy and monitoring for adverse effects.

**Additional Information** The injection formulation contains ethanol.

♦ **Dihydrohydroxycodeinone** *see* Oxycodone *on page 871*

♦ **Dihydromorphinone** *see* Hydromorphone *on page 581*

## Dihydrotachysterol (dye hye droe tak IS ter ole)

**U.S. Brand Names** DHT™; Hytakerol®

**Synonyms** Dichysterol

**Therapeutic Category** Vitamin D Analog

**Pregnancy Risk Factor** A/D (if dose exceeds RDA recommendation)

**Lactation** Enters breast milk/compatible

**Use** Treatment of hypocalcemia associated with hypoparathyroidism; prophylaxis of hypocalcemic tetany following thyroid surgery

**Mechanism of Action/Effect** Synthetic analogue of vitamin D with a faster onset of action; stimulates calcium and phosphate absorption from the small intestine, promotes secretion of calcium from bone to blood; promotes renal tubule resorption of phosphate

**Contraindications** Hypersensitivity to dihydrotachysterol; hypercalcemia; pregnancy (if dose exceeds RDA recommendation)

**Warnings** Calcium-phosphate product (serum calcium and phosphorus) must not exceed 70. Avoid hypercalcemia. Use with caution in coronary artery disease, decreased renal function (especially with secondary hyperparathyroidism), renal stones, and elderly.

**Drug Interactions**

**Decreased Effect:** Decreased effect/levels of vitamin D if taken with cholestyramine, colestipol, or mineral oil. Phenytoin and phenobarbital may inhibit activation leading to decreased effectiveness.

(Continued)

## Dihydrotachysterol *(Continued)*

**Increased Effect/Toxicity:** Thiazide diuretics may increase calcium levels.

**Adverse Reactions**

1% to 10%:

Cardiovascular: Hypotension, cardiac arrhythmias, hypertension
Central nervous system: Irritability, headache
Dermatologic: Pruritus
Endocrine & metabolic: Polydipsia, hypermagnesemia
Gastrointestinal: Nausea, vomiting, constipation, anorexia, pancreatitis, metallic taste
Genitourinary: Polyuria
Neuromuscular & skeletal: Myalgia, bone pain
Ocular: Conjunctivitis, photophobia

<1% (Limited to important or life-threatening symptoms): Overt psychosis, seizures, elevated AST/ALT

**Overdose/Toxicology** Symptoms of overdose include hypercalcemia, anorexia, nausea, weakness, constipation, diarrhea, vague aches, mental confusion, tinnitus, ataxia, depression, hallucinations, syncope, coma, polyuria, polydypsia, nocturia, hypercalciuria, irreversible renal insufficiency or proteinuria, and azotemia. Will spread tissue calcifications, hypertension. Following withdrawal of the drug, treatment consists of bedrest, liberal intake of fluids, reduced calcium intake, and cathartic administration. Severe hypercalcemia requires I.V. hydration and forced diuresis. Urine output should be monitored and maintained at >3 mL/kg/hour during the acute treatment phase. I.V. saline can quickly and significantly increase excretion of calcium into the urine. Calcitonin, cholestyramine, prednisone, sodium EDTA, and mithramycin have all been used successfully to treat the more resistant cases of vitamin D-induced hypercalcemia.

**Pharmacodynamics/Kinetics**

**Excretion:** In bile and feces; stored in liver, fat, skin, muscle, and bone

**Onset:** Peak hypercalcemic effect: Within 2-4 weeks

**Duration:** Can be as long as 9 weeks

**Formulations**

Capsule (Hytakerol®): 0.125 mg

Solution:

Oral Concentrate (DHT™): 0.2 mg/mL (30 mL)
Oral, in oil (Hytakerol®): 0.25 mg/mL (15 mL)

Tablet (DHT™): 0.125 mg, 0.2 mg, 0.4 mg

**Dosing**

**Adults:** Oral:

Hypoparathyroidism: Initial: 0.8-2.4 mg/day for several days followed by maintenance doses of 0.2-1 mg/day
Nutritional rickets: 0.5 mg as a single dose or 13-50 mcg/day until healing occurs
Renal osteodystrophy: Maintenance: 0.25-0.6 mg/24 hours adjusted as necessary to achieve normal serum calcium levels and promote bone healing

**Elderly:** Refer to adult dosing.

**Stability**

**Storage:** Protect from light.

**Monitoring Laboratory Tests** Renal function, serum calcium, nd phosphate concentrations. If hypercalcemia is encountered, discontinue agent until serum calcium returns to normal.

**Additional Nursing Issues**

**Physical Assessment:** See Contraindications and Warnings/Precautions for use cautions. Assess effectiveness and interactions of other medications (see Drug Interactions). Monitor lab tests, effectiveness of therapy, and adverse effects at beginning of therapy and regularly with long-term use (see Adverse Reactions and Overdose/Toxicology). Assess knowledge/teach patient appropriate use, appropriate nutritional counseling, possible side effects/interventions, and adverse symptoms to report. **Pregnancy risk factor A/D** - see Pregnancy Risk Factor for cautious use.

**Patient Information/Instruction:** Take exact dose prescribed; do not take more than recommended. Your prescriber may recommend a special diet. Do not increase calcium intake without consulting prescriber. Avoid magnesium supplements or magnesium-containing antacids. You may experience nausea, vomiting, or metallic taste (frequent small meals, frequent mouth care, or sucking hard candy may help); hypotension (use caution when rising from sitting or lying position or when climbing stairs or bending over). Report chest pain or palpitations; acute headache, dizziness, or feeling of weakness; unresolved nausea or vomiting; persistent metallic taste; unrelieved muscle or bone pain; or CNS irritability.

**Geriatric Considerations:** Recommended daily allowances (RDA) have not been developed for persons >65 years of age; vitamin D, folate, and $B_{12}$ (cyanocobalamin) have decreased absorption with age, but the clinical significance is yet unknown. Calorie requirements decrease with age and therefore, nutrient density must be increased to ensure adequate nutrient intake, including vitamins and minerals. Therefore, the use of a daily supplement with a multiple vitamin with minerals is recommended. Elderly consume less vitamin D, absorption may be decreased, and many elderly have decreased sun exposure; therefore, elderly should receive supplementation with 800 units of vitamin D (20 mcg)/day. This is a recommendation of particular need to those with high risk for osteoporosis.

♦ **Dihydroxyaluminum Sodium Carbonate** *see page 1294*
♦ **1,25 Dihydroxycholecalciferol** *see* Calcitriol *on page 183*
♦ **Diiodohydroxyquin** *see* Iodoquinol *on page 619*

- **Dilacoran** *see* Verapamil *on page 1208*
- **Dilacoran HTA** *see* Verapamil *on page 1208*
- **Dilacoran Retard** *see* Verapamil *on page 1208*
- **Dilacor™ XR** *see* Diltiazem *on this page*
- **Dilafed** *see* Nifedipine *on page 824*
- **Dilantin®** *see* Phenytoin *on page 923*
- **Dilatrate®-SR** *see* Isosorbide Dinitrate *on page 634*
- **Dilaudid®** *see* Hydromorphone *on page 581*
- **Dilaudid-HP®** *see* Hydromorphone *on page 581*
- **Dilocaine®** *see* Lidocaine *on page 674*
- **Dilomine® Injection** *see* Dicyclomine *on page 362*

## Diltiazem (dil TYE a zem)

**U.S. Brand Names** Cardizem® CD; Cardizem® Injectable; Cardizem® SR; Cardizem® Tablet; Cartia® XT; Dilacor™ XR; Tiazac™

**Therapeutic Category** Calcium Channel Blocker

**Pregnancy Risk Factor** C

**Lactation** Enters breast milk/compatible

**Use**

Capsule: Essential hypertension (alone or in combination) - sustained release only; chronic stable angina or angina from coronary artery spasm

Injection: Atrial fibrillation or atrial flutter; paroxysmal supraventricular tachycardia (PSVT)

**Mechanism of Action/Effect** Inhibits calcium ion from entering the "slow channels" or select voltage-sensitive areas of vascular smooth muscle and myocardium during depolarization, producing a relaxation of coronary vascular smooth muscle and coronary vasodilation; increases myocardial oxygen delivery in patients with vasospastic angina

**Contraindications** Hypersensitivity to other diltiazem; severe hypotension; second and third degree heart block except with a functioning pacemaker; atrial and ventricular arrhythmias; acute myocardial infarction and pulmonary congestion evident on x-ray; patients with sick-sinus syndrome except with a functioning pacemaker

**Warnings** Use with caution and titrate dosages for patients with impaired renal or hepatic function. Use caution when treating patients with congestive heart failure, concomitant therapy with beta-blockers or digoxin, presence or worsening of edema. Do not abruptly withdraw (may cause chest pain). Elderly may experience excessive hypotension due to prolonged half-life. Pregnancy factor C.

**Drug Interactions**

**Cytochrome P-450 Effect:** CYP3A3/4 enzyme substrate; CYP1A2, 2D6, and 3A3/4 enzyme inhibitor

**Decreased Effect:** Rifampin reduces diltiazem serum levels resulting in decreased diltiazem effect.

**Increased Effect/Toxicity:** Cimetidine may increase bioavailability of diltiazem. Beta-blockers may increase cardiac depressant effects on A-V conduction. Diltiazem may increase serum levels/toxicity of carbamazepine. Digoxin levels may increase with the addition of diltiazem. Beta-blockers may cause an enhanced cardiac depressant effect on A-V conduction when combined with diltiazem. Diltiazem combined with cyclosporine may elevate serum cyclosporine levels and result in renal toxicity. The toxicity of cisapride (Q-T prolongation) may be increased.

**Food Interactions** Diltiazem serum levels may be elevated if taken with food.

**Adverse Reactions**

1% to 10%:

Cardiovascular: Congestive heart failure, hypotension, peripheral edema, flushing, feeling of warmth

Central nervous system: Headache, dizziness or lightheadedness

Gastrointestinal: Nausea, constipation, diarrhea

Neuromuscular & skeletal: Weakness

Miscellaneous: Allergic reaction

<1% (Limited to important or life-threatening symptoms): Chest pain, A-V block (second degree), bradycardia, hypotension (excessive), tachycardia, thrombocytopenia

**Overdose/Toxicology** Primary cardiac symptoms of calcium blocker overdose include hypotension and bradycardia. Noncardiac symptoms include confusion, stupor, nausea, vomiting, metabolic acidosis, and hyperglycemia.

Following initial gastric decontamination, if possible, repeated calcium administration may promptly reverse depressed cardiac contractility (but not sinus node depression or peripheral vasodilation). Glucagon, epinephrine, and amrinone may treat refractory hypotension. Glucagon and epinephrine also increase heart rate (outside the U.S., 4-aminopyridine may be available as an antidote). Dialysis and hemoperfusion are not effective in enhancing elimination although repeat-dose activated charcoal may serve as an adjunct with sustained-release preparations.

**Pharmacodynamics/Kinetics**

**Protein Binding:** 77% to 85%

**Half-life Elimination:** 4-6 hours (may be prolonged in renal impairment); 5-7 hours with sustained release

(Continued)

## Diltiazem *(Continued)*

**Time to Peak:** Short-acting tablets: Within 2-3 hours; Sustained release: 6-11 hours
**Metabolism:** Liver (metabolites active)
**Excretion:** Urine and bile
**Onset:** Oral: 30-60 minutes (including sustained release)

### Formulations

Capsule, extended release (Cartia® XT): 120 mg, 180 mg, 240 mg, 300 mg
Capsule, sustained release:
Cardizem® CD: 120 mg, 180 mg, 240 mg, 300 mg
Cardizem® SR: 60 mg, 90 mg, 120 mg
Dilacor™ XR: 180 mg, 240 mg
Tiazac™: 120 mg, 180 mg, 240 mg, 300 mg, 360 mg
Injection: 5 mg/mL (5 mL, 10 mL)
Cardizem®: 5 mg/mL (5 mL, 10 mL)
Tablet (Cardizem®): 30 mg, 60 mg, 90 mg, 120 mg

### Dosing

**Adults:** Oral:

Tablets: 30-120 mg 3-4 times/day; dosage should be increased gradually, at 1- to 2-day intervals until optimum response is obtained; usual maintenance dose: 240-360 mg/day

Sustained-release capsules:

**Cardizem SR®:** Initial: 60-120 mg twice daily; adjust to maximum antihypertensive effect (usually within 14 days); usual range: 240-360 mg/day

**Cardizem® CD, Tiazac™:** Hypertension: Total daily dose of short-acting administered once daily or initially 180 or 240 mg once daily; adjust to maximum effect (usually within 14 days); maximum: 480 mg/day; usual range: 240-360 mg/day

**Cardizem® CD:** Angina: Initial: 120-180 mg once daily; maximum: 480 mg once/day

**Dilacor XR®:**

Hypertension: 180-240 mg once daily; maximum: 540 mg/day; usual range: 180-480 mg/day; use lower dose in the elderly

Angina: Initial: 120 mg/day; titrate slowly over 7-14 days up to 480 mg/day, as needed

I.V. (requires an infusion pump): See table.

**Diltiazem — I.V. Dosage and Administration**

| | |
|---|---|
| **Initial Bolus Dose** | 0.25 mg/kg actual body weight over 2 min (average adult dose: 20 mg) |
| **Repeat Bolus Dose** May be administered after 15 min if the response is inadequate | 0.35 mg/kg actual body weight over 2 min (average adult dose: 25 mg) |
| **Continuous Infusion** Infusions >24 h or infusion rates >15 mg/h are not recommended | Initial infusion rate of 10 mg/h; rate may be increased in 5 mg/h increments up to 15 mg/h as needed; some patients may respond to an initial rate of 5 mg/h |

If Cardizem® injectable is administered by continuous infusion for >24 hours, the possibility of decreased diltiazem clearance, prolonged elimination half-life, and increased diltiazem and/or diltiazem metabolite plasma concentrations should be considered.

**Conversion from I.V. diltiazem to oral diltiazem:** Start oral approximately 3 hours after bolus dose

**Oral dose (mg/day) is approximately equal to [rate (mg/hour) x 3 + 3] x 10**

3 mg/hour = 120 mg/day
5 mg/hour = 180 mg/day
7 mg/hour = 240 mg/day
11 mg/hour = 360 mg/day
15 mg/hour = 480 mg/day

**Elderly:** Refer to adult dosing.

**Renal Impairment:** Use with caution as diltiazem is extensively metabolized by the liver and excreted in the kidneys and bile. Not removed by hemo- or peritoneal dialysis; supplemental dose is not necessary.

**Hepatic Impairment:** Use with caution as diltiazem is extensively metabolized by the liver and excreted in the kidneys and bile.

### Administration

**Oral:** Do not crush sustained release capsules.

**I.V.:** Bolus doses given over 2 minutes with continuous EKG and blood pressure monitoring. Continuous infusion should be via infusion pump.

**I.V. Detail:** Response to bolus may require several minutes to reach maximum. Response may persist for several hours after infusion is discontinued.

### Additional Nursing Issues

**Physical Assessment:** Assess other medications patient may be taking for effectiveness and interactions (see Drug Interactions). I.V. requires use of infusion pump and continuous cardiac and hemodynamic monitoring. Monitor therapeutic response (cardiac status) and adverse reactions (see Warnings/Precautions, Adverse Reactions, and Overdose/Toxicology) when beginning therapy, when titrating dosage, and periodically during long-term therapy. Assess knowledge/teach patient appropriate use (oral), interventions to reduce side effects, and adverse symptoms to report. **Pregnancy risk factor C** - benefits of use should outweigh possible risks.

**Patient Information/Instruction:** Oral: Take as directed; do not alter dosage or discontinue therapy without consulting prescriber. Do not crush or chew extended release form. Avoid (or limit) alcohol and caffeine. You may experience dizziness or lightheadedness (use caution when driving or engaging in tasks requiring alertness until response to drug is known); nausea or vomiting (small frequent meals, frequent mouth care, chewing gum, or sucking lozenges may help); constipation (increased exercise, dietary fiber, fruit, or fluid may help); diarrhea (buttermilk, boiled milk, or yogurt may help). Report chest pain, palpitations, irregular heartbeat, unusual cough, difficulty breathing, swelling of extremities, muscle tremors or weakness, confusion or acute lethargy, or skin rash. **Pregnancy precautions:** Inform prescriber if you are or intend to be pregnant.

**Geriatric Considerations:** Elderly may experience a greater hypotensive response.

**Related Information**

Antiarrhythmic Drug Classification Comparison *on page 1366*
Calcium Channel Blocking Agents Comparison *on page 1378*

- **Dimantil** *see* Warfarin *on page 1220*
- **Dimaphen® Elixir** *see page 1294*
- **Dimaphen® Tablets** *see page 1294*
- **Dimenhydrinate** *see page 1294*
- **Dimercaprol** *see page 1248*
- **Dimetabs® Oral** *see page 1294*
- **Dimetane®-DC** *see* Brompheniramine, Phenylpropanolamine, and Codeine *on page 163*
- **Dimetane® Decongestant Elixir** *see page 1294*
- **Dimetane® Extentabs®** *see page 1294*
- **Dimetapp® 4-Hour Liqui-Gel Capsule** *see page 1294*
- **Dimetapp® Elixir** *see page 1294*
- **Dimetapp® Extentabs** *see page 1294*
- **Dimetapp® Sinus Caplets** *see page 1294*
- **Dimetapp® Tablet** *see page 1294*
- **Dimethoxyphenyl Penicillin Sodium** *see* Methicillin *on page 740*
- **β,β-Dimethylcysteine** *see* Penicillamine *on page 894*

## Dimethyl Sulfoxide (dye meth il sul FOKS ide)

**U.S. Brand Names** Rimso®-50

**Synonyms** DMSO

**Therapeutic Category** Urinary Tract Product

**Pregnancy Risk Factor** C

**Lactation** Excretion in breast milk unknown

**Use** Symptomatic relief of interstitial cystitis

**Formulations** Solution: 50% [500 mg/mL] (50 mL)

**Dosing**

**Adults:** Not for I.M. or I.V. administration; only for bladder instillation. Instill 50 mL of solution directly into bladder and allow to remain for 15 minutes. Repeat in 2 weeks or until symptoms are relieved, then increase intervals between treatments.

**Elderly:** Refer to adult dosing.

- **Dimodan** *see* Disopyramide *on page 386*

## Dinoprostone (dye noe PROST one)

**U.S. Brand Names** Cervidil® Vaginal Insert; Prepidil® Vaginal Gel; Prostin $E_2$® Vaginal Suppository

**Synonyms** $PGE_2$; Prostaglandin $E_2$

**Therapeutic Category** Abortifacient; Prostaglandin

**Pregnancy Risk Factor** C

**Use**

Gel: Promote cervical ripening prior to labor induction; usage for gel includes any patient undergoing induction of labor with an unripe cervix, most commonly for preeclampsia, eclampsia, postdates, diabetes, intrauterine growth retardation, and chronic hypertension

Suppositories: Terminate pregnancy from 12th through 28th week of gestation; evacuate uterus in cases of missed abortion or intrauterine fetal death; manage benign hydatidiform mole

**Mechanism of Action/Effect** A synthetic prostaglandin $E_2$ abortifacient that stimulates uterine contractions similar to those seen during natural labor

**Contraindications**

Gel: Hypersensitivity to prostaglandins or any constituents of the cervical gel, history of asthma, contracted pelvis, malpresentation of the fetus

Gel: The following are "relative" contraindications and should only be considered under these circumstances: Patients in whom vaginal delivery is not indicated (ie, herpes genitalia with a lesion at the time of delivery), prior uterine surgery, breech presentation, multiple gestation, polyhydramnios, premature rupture of membranes

Suppository: Hypersensitivity to dinoprostone, acute pelvic inflammatory disease, uterine fibroids, cervical stenosis

**Warnings** Dinoprostone should be used only by medically trained personnel in a hospital. Caution in patients with cervicitis, infected endocervical lesions, acute vaginitis, compromised (scarred) uterus or history of asthma, hypertension or hypotension, epilepsy, diabetes mellitus, anemia, jaundice, or cardiovascular, renal, or hepatic disease.
(Continued)

## Dinoprostone *(Continued)*

Oxytocin should not be used simultaneously with Prepidil™ (>6 hours of the last dose of Prepidil™). Pregnancy factor C.

**Drug Interactions**

**Increased Effect/Toxicity:** Increased effect of oxytocics.

**Adverse Reactions**

>10%:

Central nervous system: Headache, fever, chills or shivering
Gastrointestinal: Vomiting (67%), diarrhea, nausea, abdominal or stomach cramps

1% to 10%:

Cardiovascular: Bradycardia, peripheral vasoconstriction, substernal pressure or pain
Endocrine & metabolic: Uterine hypertonus, increased uterine pain
Neuromuscular & skeletal: Back pain
Respiratory: Wheezing, dyspnea, coughing, bronchospasm

<1% (Limited to important or life-threatening symptoms): Hypotension, cardiac arrhythmias, syncope, flushing, tightness of the chest

**Overdose/Toxicology** Symptoms of overdose include vomiting, bronchospasm, hypotension, chest pain, abdominal cramps, and uterine contractions. Treatment is symptomatic.

**Pharmacodynamics/Kinetics**

**Metabolism:** In many tissues including the kidney, lungs, and spleen
**Excretion:** Urine and feces
**Onset:** Onset of effect (uterine contractions): Within 10 minutes
**Duration:** Up to 2-3 hours

**Formulations**

Insert, vaginal (Cervidil®): 10 mg
Gel, vaginal: 0.5 mg in 3 g syringes [each package contains a 10-mm and 20-mm shielded catheter]
Suppository, vaginal: 20 mg

**Dosing**

**Adults:**

Abortifacient: Insert 1 suppository high in vagina, repeat at 3- to 5-hour intervals until abortion occurs up to 240 mg (maximum); continued administration for longer than 2 days is not advisable.

Cervical ripening:

Gel:

Intracervical: 0.25-1 mg
Intravaginal: 2.5 mg

Vaginal insert: Intracervical: 10 mg; remove upon onset of active labor or after 12 hours.

**Elderly:** Refer to adult dosing.

**Administration**

**Other:** Intracervically: Bring suppository to room temperature just prior to use. Patient should remain supine for 10 minutes following insertion.

**Stability**

**Storage:** Suppositories must be kept frozen, store in freezer not above -4°C (-20°F). Bring to room temperature just prior to use. Cervical gel should be stored under refrigeration 2°C to 8°C (36°F to 46°F).

**Additional Nursing Issues**

**Physical Assessment:** Monitor temperature closely. Monitor uterine tone and vaginal discharge closely throughout procedure and postprocedure. Monitor abortion for completeness (other measures may be necessary if incomplete).

**Patient Information/Instruction:** Nausea and vomiting, cramping or uterine pain, or fever may occur. Report acute pain, respiratory difficulty, or skin rash. Closely monitor for vaginal discharge for several days. Report vaginal bleeding, itching, malodorous or bloody discharge, or severe cramping.

- **Dinoprost Tromethamine** *see page 1248*
- **Diochloram** *see* Chloramphenicol *on page 248*
- **Diocto® [OTC]** *see* Docusate *on page 392*
- **Diocto C®** *see page 1294*
- **Diocto-K® [OTC]** *see* Docusate *on page 392*
- **Diocto-K Plus®** *see page 1294*
- **Dioctolose Plus®** *see page 1294*
- **Dioctyl Calcium Sulfosuccinate** *see* Docusate *on page 392*
- **Dioctyl Potassium Sulfosuccinate** *see* Docusate *on page 392*
- **Dioctyl Sodium Sulfosuccinate** *see* Docusate *on page 392*
- **Diodoquin®** *see* Iodoquinol *on page 619*
- **Dioeze® [OTC]** *see* Docusate *on page 392*
- **Diomycin** *see* Erythromycin *on page 435*
- **Dionephrine** *see* Phenylephrine *on page 920*
- **Dioval® Injection** *see* Estradiol *on page 441*
- **Diovan™** *see* Valsartan *on page 1201*
- **Dipedyne** *see* Zidovudine *on page 1227*
- **Dipentum®** *see* Olsalazine *on page 850*
- **Diphenacen-50® Injection** *see* Diphenhydramine *on next page*
- **Diphen® Cough [OTC]** *see* Diphenhydramine *on next page*

♦ **Diphenhist [OTC]** *see* Diphenhydramine *on this page*

## Diphenhydramine (dye fen HYE dra meen)

**U.S. Brand Names** AllerMax® Oral [OTC]; Banophen® Oral [OTC]; Belix® Oral [OTC]; Benadryl® Injection; Benadryl® Oral [OTC]; Benadryl® Topical; Ben-Allergin-50® Injection; Benylin® Cough Syrup [OTC]; Bydramine® Cough Syrup [OTC]; Compoz® Gel Caps [OTC]; Compoz® Nighttime Sleep Aid [OTC]; Dihydrex® Injection; Diphenacen-50® Injection; Diphen® Cough [OTC]; Diphenhist [OTC]; Dormarex® 2 Oral [OTC]; Dormin® Oral [OTC]; Genahist® Oral; Hydramyn® Syrup [OTC]; Hyrexin-50® Injection; Maximum Strength Nytol® [OTC]; Miles Nervine® Caplets [OTC]; Nordryl® Injection; Nordryl® Oral; Nytol® Oral [OTC]; Phendry® Oral [OTC]; Siladryl® Oral [OTC]; Silphen® Cough [OTC]; Sleep-eze 3® Oral [OTC]; Sleepinal® [OTC]; Sleepwell 2-nite® [OTC]; Sominex® Oral [OTC]; Tusstat® Syrup; Twilite® Oral [OTC]; Uni-Bent® Cough Syrup; 40 Winks® [OTC]

**Therapeutic Category** Antihistamine

**Pregnancy Risk Factor** B

**Lactation** Enters breast milk/contraindicated

**Use** Symptomatic relief of allergic symptoms caused by histamine release which include nasal allergies and allergic dermatosis; can be used for mild night-time sedation; prevention of motion sickness and as an antitussive; has antinauseant and topical anesthetic properties; treatment of antipsychotic-induced dystonic reactions

**Mechanism of Action/Effect** Competes with histamine for $H_1$-receptor sites on effector cells in the GI tract, blood vessels, and respiratory tract

**Contraindications** Hypersensitivity to diphenhydramine or any component; should not be used in acute attacks of asthma

**Warnings** Use with caution in patients with angle-closure glaucoma, peptic ulcer, urinary tract obstruction, and hyperthyroidism. Some preparations contain sodium bisulfite. Syrup contains alcohol. Diphenhydramine has high sedative and anticholinergic properties, so it may not be considered the antihistamine of choice for prolonged use in the elderly.

**Drug Interactions**

**Cytochrome P-450 Effect:** CYP2D6 enzyme substrate

**Increased Effect/Toxicity:** CNS depressants worsen CNS and respiratory depression. Monoamine oxidase inhibitors may increase anticholinergic effects. Syrup should not be given to patients taking drugs that can cause disulfiram reactions (eg, metronidazole, chlorpropamide) due to high alcohol content.

**Effects on Lab Values** May suppress the wheal and flare reactions to skin test antigens.

**Adverse Reactions**

>10%:

- Central nervous system: Slight to moderate drowsiness
- Respiratory: Thickening of bronchial secretions

1% to 10%:

- Central nervous system: Headache, fatigue, nervousness
- Gastrointestinal: Nausea, vomiting, diarrhea, abdominal pain, dry mouth, appetite increase, weight gain, dry mucous membranes
- Neuromuscular & skeletal: Arthralgia
- Respiratory: Pharyngitis

<1% (Limited to important or life-threatening symptoms): Hypotension, palpitations, edema, hepatitis, bronchospasm, epistaxis

**Overdose/Toxicology** Symptoms of overdose include CNS stimulation or depression; overdose may result in death in infants and children. There is no specific treatment for antihistamine overdose. Clinical toxicity is due to blockade of cholinergic receptors. For anticholinergic overdose with life-threatening symptoms, physostigmine 1-2 mg S.C. or I.V. slowly may be given to reverse these effects.

**Pharmacodynamics/Kinetics**

**Protein Binding:** 78%

**Half-life Elimination:** 2-8 hours; elderly: 13.5 hours

**Time to Peak:** 2-4 hours

**Metabolism:** Liver

**Excretion:** Urine

**Onset:** Maximum sedative effect: 1-3 hours; I.V.: More rapid

**Duration:** 4-7 hours

**Formulations**

Diphenhydramine hydrochloride:

- Capsule: 25 mg, 50 mg
- Cream: 1%, 2%
- Elixir: 12.5 mg/5 mL (5 mL, 10 mL, 20 mL, 120 mL, 480 mL, 3780 mL)
- Injection: 10 mg/mL (10 mL, 30 mL); 50 mg/mL (1 mL, 10 mL)
- Lotion: 1% (75 mL)
- Solution, topical spray: 1% (60 mL)
- Syrup: 12.5 mg/5 mL (5 mL, 120 mL, 240 mL, 480 mL, 3780 mL)
- Tablet: 25 mg, 50 mg

**Dosing**

**Adults:**

Oral: 25-50 mg every 6-8 hours

Night-time sleep aid: 50 mg at bedtime

I.M., I.V.: 10-50 mg in a single dose every 2-4 hours, not to exceed 400 mg/day

Topical: For external application, not longer than 7 days

(Continued)

## Diphenhydramine *(Continued)*

**Elderly:** Initial: 25 mg 2-3 times/day increasing as needed

**Administration**

**Oral:** Swallow whole, do not crush or chew sustained release product.

**Stability**

**Storage:** Injection: Protect from light.

**Compatibility:** The following drugs are incompatible with diphenhydramine when mixed in the same syringe: Amobarbital, amphotericin B, cephalothin, diatrizoate, foscarnet, heparin, hydrocortisone, hydroxyzine, pentobarbital, phenobarbital, phenytoin, prochlorperazine, promazine, promethazine, tetracycline, and thiopental. See the Compatibility of Drugs in Syringe Chart *on page 1317*.

**Additional Nursing Issues**

**Physical Assessment:** Assess effectiveness and interactions of other medications (see Drug Interactions). See Contraindications and Warnings/Precautions for cautious use. Monitor effectiveness of therapy and adverse reactions (eg, excess anticholinergic effects - see Adverse Reactions) at beginning of therapy and periodically with long-term use. Assess knowledge/teach patient appropriate use, interventions to reduce side effects, and adverse symptoms to report. Breast-feeding is contraindicated.

**Patient Information/Instruction:** Take as directed; do not exceed recommended dose. Avoid use of other depressants, alcohol, or sleep-inducing medications unless approved by prescriber. You may experience drowsiness or dizziness (use caution when driving or engaging in tasks requiring alertness until response to drug is known); or dry mouth, nausea, or vomiting (frequent small meals, frequent mouth care, chewing gum, or sucking hard candy may help). Report persistent sedation, confusion, or agitation; changes in urinary pattern; blurred vision; sore throat, difficulty breathing, or expectorating (thick secretions); or lack of improvement or worsening or condition. **Breast-feeding precautions:** Do not breast-feed.

**Geriatric Considerations:** Diphenhydramine has high sedative and anticholinergic properties, so it may not be considered the antihistamine of choice for prolonged use in the elderly. Its use as a sleep aid is discouraged due to its anticholinergic effects.

**Breast-feeding Issues:** Infants may be more sensitive to the effects of antihistamines.

**Additional Information** Some formulations may contain ethanol.

**Related Information**

Antiemetics for Chemotherapy-Induced Nausea and Vomiting *on page 1307*
Anxiolytic/Hypnotic Use in Long-Term Care Facilities *on page 1430*

♦ **Diphenhydramine and Pseudoephedrine** *see page 1294*

## Diphenoxylate and Atropine (dye fen OKS i late & A troe peen)

**U.S. Brand Names** Lofene®; Logen®; Lomanate®; Lomodix®; Lomotil®; Lonox®; Low-Quel®

**Synonyms** Atropine and Diphenoxylate

**Therapeutic Category** Antidiarrheal

**Pregnancy Risk Factor** C

**Lactation** Use caution

**Use** Treatment of diarrhea

**Mechanism of Action/Effect** Diphenoxylate inhibits excessive GI motility and GI propulsion; commercial preparations contain a subtherapeutic amount of atropine to discourage abuse

**Contraindications** Hypersensitivity to diphenoxylate, atropine, or any component; severe liver disease; jaundice; dehydrated patient; narrow-angle glaucoma; it should not be used for children <2 years of age

**Warnings** High doses may cause physical and psychological dependence with prolonged use. Use with caution in patients with ulcerative colitis, dehydration, and hepatic dysfunction. Reduction of intestinal motility may be deleterious in diarrhea resulting from *Shigella*, *Salmonella*, toxigenic strains of *E. coli*, and from pseudomembranous enterocolitis associated with broad spectrum antibiotics. If there is no response within 48 hours, the drug is unlikely to be effective and should be discontinued. If chronic diarrhea is not improved symptomatically within 10 days at maximum dosage of 20 mg/day, control is unlikely with further use. Pregnancy factor C.

**Drug Interactions**

**Increased Effect/Toxicity:** MAO inhibitors (hypertensive crisis), CNS depressants when taken with diphenoxylate may result in increased adverse effects, antimuscarinics (paralytic ileus). May prolong half-life of drugs metabolized in liver.

**Adverse Reactions**

1% to 10%:

Central nervous system: Nervousness, restlessness, dizziness, drowsiness, headache, mental depression
Gastrointestinal: Paralytic ileus, dry mouth, megacolon
Genitourinary: Urinary retention and difficult urination
Ocular: Blurred vision
Respiratory: Respiratory depression

<1% (Limited to important or life-threatening symptoms): Tachycardia, nausea, vomiting, abdominal discomfort, pancreatitis, stomach cramps

**Overdose/Toxicology** Symptoms of overdose include drowsiness, hypotension, blurred vision, flushing, dry mouth, and miosis. Administration of activated charcoal will reduce bioavailability of diphenoxylate. Naloxone, 2 mg I.V. with repeat administration as necessary up to a total of 10 mg, can also be used to reverse toxic effects of the opiate. For anticholinergic overdose with severe life-threatening symptoms, physostigmine 1-2 mg S.C. or I.V. slowly, may be given to reverse these effects.

**Pharmacodynamics/Kinetics**

**Half-life Elimination:** Diphenoxylate: 2.5 hours

**Time to Peak:** 2 hours

**Metabolism:** Liver

**Excretion:** Feces

**Onset:** Onset of action: Within 45-60 minutes; Peak effect: Within 2 hours

**Duration:** 3-4 hours

**Formulations**

Solution, oral: Diphenoxylate hydrochloride 2.5 mg and atropine sulfate 0.025 mg per 5 mL (4 mL, 10 mL, 60 mL)

Tablet: Diphenoxylate hydrochloride 2.5 mg and atropine sulfate 0.025 mg

**Dosing**

**Adults:** Oral: 15-20 mg/day of diphenoxylate in 3-4 divided doses; maintenance: 5-15 mg/day in 2-3 divided doses

**Elderly:** Refer to adult dosing.

**Stability**

**Storage:** Protect from light.

**Additional Nursing Issues**

**Physical Assessment:** Ascertain etiology of diarrhea before beginning treatment. Monitor effectiveness of treatment. Monitor for adverse effects (see above) and atropine toxicity (redman syndrome, dry flushed skin, and tachycardia). Potential for physical and psychological dependence. Assess knowledge/teach patient appropriate use, possible side effects, symptoms to report. **Pregnancy risk factor C** - benefits of use should outweigh possible risks. Note breast-feeding caution.

**Patient Information/Instruction:** Take as directed; do not exceed recommended dosage. If no response within 48 hours, notify prescriber. Avoid alcohol or other prescriptive or OTC sedatives or depressants. You may experience drowsiness, blurred vision, impaired coordination; use caution when driving or engaging in tasks that require alertness until response to drug is known. Sucking on lozenges or chewing gum may reduce dry mouth. Report difficulty urinating, persistent diarrhea, respiratory difficulties, fever, or palpitations. **Pregnancy/breast-feeding precautions:** Inform prescriber if you are or intend to be pregnant. Consult prescriber if breast-feeding.

**Geriatric Considerations:** Elderly are particularly sensitive to fluid and electrolyte loss. Maintaining hydration and electrolyte balance is vital.

**Additional Information** If there is no response within 48 hours, the drug is unlikely to be effective and should be discontinued. If chronic diarrhea is not improved symptomatically within 10 days at maximum dosage of 20 mg/day, control is unlikely with further use. Diarrhea should also be treated with dietary measures (ie, clear liquids), and avoid milk products and high sodium foods such as bouillon and soups.

**Related Information**

Atropine *on page 119*

- **Diphenylan Sodium®** *see* Phenytoin *on page 923*
- **Diphenylhydantoin** *see* Phenytoin *on page 923*
- **Diphtheria and Tetanus Toxoid** *see page 1256*
- **Diphtheria Antitoxin** *see page 1246*
- **Diphtheria, Tetanus Toxoids, and Acellular Pertussis Vaccine** *see page 1256*
- **Diphtheria, Tetanus Toxoids, and Whole-Cell Pertussis Vaccine** *see page 1256*
- **Diphtheria, Tetanus Toxoids, Whole-Cell Pertussis Vaccine, and *Haemophilus* B Conjugate Vaccine** *see page 1256*
- **Dipiverin** *see* Ophthalmic Agents, Glaucoma *on page 853*
- **Diprolene®** *see* Betamethasone *on page 148*
- **Diprolene®** *see* Topical Corticosteroids *on page 1152*
- **Diprolene® AF** *see* Betamethasone *on page 148*
- **Diprolene® AF** *see* Topical Corticosteroids *on page 1152*
- **Diprolene® Glycol [Dipropionate]** *see* Betamethasone *on page 148*
- **Diprolene® Glycol [Dipropionate]** *see* Topical Corticosteroids *on page 1152*
- **Dipropylacetic Acid** *see* Valproic Acid and Derivatives *on page 1198*
- **Diprosone®** *see* Betamethasone *on page 148*
- **Diprosone®** *see* Topical Corticosteroids *on page 1152*

## Dipyridamole (dye peer ID a mole)

**U.S. Brand Names** Persantine®

**Therapeutic Category** Antiplatelet Agent; Vasodilator

**Pregnancy Risk Factor** B

**Lactation** Enters breast milk (low concentrations)/use caution

**Use** Maintains patency after surgical grafting procedures including coronary artery bypass; used with warfarin to decrease thrombosis in patients after artificial heart valve replacement; used with aspirin to prevent coronary artery thrombosis; in combination with aspirin or warfarin to prevent other thromboembolic disorders. Dipyridamole may also be given 2 days prior to open heart surgery to prevent platelet activation by extracorporeal bypass pump and as a diagnostic agent in CAD.

**Mechanism of Action/Effect** Inhibits platelet aggregation and may cause vasodilation. May also stimulate release of prostacyclin or $PGD_2$ resulting in coronary vasodilation.

**Contraindications** Hypersensitivity to dipyridamole or any component

(Continued)

## Dipyridamole *(Continued)*

**Warnings** May further decrease blood pressure in patients with hypotension due to peripheral vasodilation; use with caution in patients taking other drugs which affect platelet function or coagulation and in patients with hemostatic defects. Since evidence suggests that clinically used doses are **ineffective for prevention of platelet aggregation**, consideration for low-dose aspirin (81-325 mg/day) alone may be necessary; this will decrease cost as well as inconvenience.

**Drug Interactions**

**Decreased Effect:** Decreased vasodilation from I.V. dipyridamole when given to patients taking theophylline.

**Increased Effect/Toxicity:** Enhances bleeding of anticoagulated patients receiving aspirin, heparin, and warfarin (Coumadin®).

**Adverse Reactions**

>10%:

Cardiovascular: Exacerbation of chest pain pectoris (I.V.), flushing (oral)
Central nervous system: Headache (I.V.), dizziness
Gastrointestinal: Abdominal cramping, diarrhea

1% to 10%:

Cardiovascular: Hypotension, flushing (I.V.), hypertension, tachycardia, extrasystoles, ST-T segment changes,
Central nervous system: Headache (oral)
Dermatologic: Rash
Respiratory: Dyspnea

<1% (Limited to important or life-threatening symptoms): Vasodilatation, syncope, edema, cardiomyopathy

**Overdose/Toxicology** Symptoms of overdose include hypotension and peripheral vasodilation. Dialysis is not effective. Treatment is symptomatic and supportive.

**Pharmacodynamics/Kinetics**

**Protein Binding:** 91% to 99%
**Half-life Elimination:** 10-12 hours
**Time to Peak:** 2-2.5 hours
**Metabolism:** Liver
**Excretion:** Feces

**Formulations**

Injection: 10 mg/2 mL, 50 mg/10 mL
Tablet: 25 mg, 50 mg, 75 mg

**Dosing**

**Adults:**

Oral: 75-400 mg/day in 3-4 divided doses
I.V.: 0.14 mg/kg/minute for 4 minutes; maximum: 60 mg

**Elderly:** Refer to adult dosing.

**Stability**

**Storage:** I.V.: Do not freeze, protect from light.

**Additional Nursing Issues**

**Physical Assessment:** Assess effectiveness and interactions of other medications patient may be taking (see Warnings/Precautions and Drug Interactions). Monitor therapeutic response (dependent on purpose for use) and adverse reactions (see Adverse Reactions and Overdose/Toxicology). Observe and teach bleeding precautions. Note breast-feeding caution.

Oral: Monitor blood pressure on a regular basis.

I.V.: Continuous EKG and blood pressure monitoring during infusion. Assess knowledge/teach patient appropriate use, interventions to reduce side effects, and adverse symptoms to report.

**Patient Information/Instruction:** Oral: Take exactly as directed, with or without food. You may experience mild headache, transient diarrhea, or temporary dizziness (sit or lie down when taking medication). You may have a tendency to bleed easy; use caution with sharps, needles, or razors. Report chest pain, redness around mouth, acute abdominal cramping or severe diarrhea, acute and persistent headache or dizziness, rash, difficulty breathing, or swelling of extremities. **Breast-feeding precautions:** Consult prescriber if breast-feeding.

**Geriatric Considerations:** Since evidence suggests that clinically used doses are ineffective for prevention of platelet aggregation, consideration for low-dose aspirin (81-325 mg/day) alone may be necessary. This will decrease cost as well as inconvenience.

♦ **Dirinol** *see* Dipyridamole *on previous page*

## Dirithromycin (dye RITH roe mye sin)

**U.S. Brand Names** Dynabac®

**Therapeutic Category** Antibiotic, Macrolide

**Pregnancy Risk Factor** C

**Lactation** Excretion in breast milk unknown/use caution

**Use** Treatment of mild to moderate upper and lower respiratory tract infections due to *Moraxella catarrhalis, Streptococcus pneumoniae, Haemophilus influenzae, Legionella pneumophila*, or *S. pyogenes*, and uncomplicated infections of the skin and skin structure due to *Staphylococcus aureus*

**Note:** Serum levels of dirithromycin are not adequate to treat bacteremias due to other sensitive strains. **Empiric** treatment of acute bacterial exacerbations of chronic or secondary bronchitis is not recommended since resistance of the frequently causative agent, *H. influenzae*, occurs.

**Mechanism of Action/Effect** After being converted during intestinal absorption to its active form, erythromycylamine, dirithromycin inhibits protein synthesis by binding to the 50S ribosomal subunits of susceptible microorganisms.

**Contraindications** Hypersensitivity to any macrolide or component of dirithromycin; patients receiving pimozide which when given together predisposes the patient to a possible arrhythmia or sudden death

**Warnings** Contrary to potential serious consequences with other macrolides (eg, cardiac arrhythmias), the combination of terfenadine and dirithromycin has not shown alteration of terfenadine metabolism; however, caution should be taken during coadministration of dirithromycin and terfenadine. Pseudomembranous colitis has been reported and should be considered in patients presenting with diarrhea subsequent to therapy with dirithromycin. Pregnancy factor C.

**Drug Interactions**

**Cytochrome P-450 Effect:** CYP3A3/4 enzyme inhibitor

**Increased Effect/Toxicity:** Absorption of dirithromycin is slightly enhanced with concomitant antacids and $H_2$ antagonists. Dirithromycin may, like erythromycin, increase the effect of alfentanil, anticoagulants, bromocriptine, carbamazepine, cyclosporine, digoxin, disopyramide, ergots, methylprednisolone, cisapride, astemizole, and triazolam.

**Note:** Interactions with nonsedating antihistamines (eg, astemizole and terfenadine) or theophylline are not known to occur; however, caution is advised with coadministration.

**Adverse Reactions**

1% to 10%:

Central nervous system: Headache, dizziness, vertigo, insomnia
Dermatologic: Rash, pruritus, urticaria
Endocrine & metabolic: Hyperkalemia, increased CPK
Gastrointestinal: Abdominal pain, nausea, diarrhea, vomiting, heartburn, flatulence
Hematologic: Thrombocytosis, eosinophilia, segmented neutrophils
Neuromuscular & skeletal: Weakness, pain
Respiratory: Increased cough, dyspnea

<1% (Limited to important or life-threatening symptoms): Palpitations; vasodilation; syncope; edema; neutropenia; thrombocytopenia; decreased hemoglobin/hematocrit; increased alkaline phosphatase, bands, basophils; leukocytosis; monocytosis; increased ALT, AST, GGT; hyperbilirubinemia; increased creatinine; phosphorus; epistaxis; hemoptysis; hyperventilation

**Overdose/Toxicology** Symptoms of overdose include nausea, vomiting, abdominal pain, and diarrhea. Treatment is supportive. Dialysis has not been found effective.

**Pharmacodynamics/Kinetics**

**Protein Binding:** 14% to 30%

**Distribution:** Rapidly and widely distributed (higher levels in tissues than plasma)

**Half-life Elimination:** 8 hours (range: 2-36 hours)

**Metabolism:** Liver

**Excretion:** Hepatic

**Formulations** Tablet, enteric coated: 250 mg

**Dosing**

**Adults:** Oral: 500 mg once daily for 5-14 days (14 days required for treatment of community-acquired pneumonia due to *Legionella*, *Mycoplasma*, or *S. pneumoniae*; 10 days is recommended for treatment of *S. pyogenes* pharyngitis/tonsillitis).

**Elderly:** Refer to adult dosing.

**Renal Impairment:** No adjustment necessary.

**Hepatic Impairment:** No adjustment necessary for mildly impaired hepatic function. Use is not recommended for severe hepatic impairment.

**Administration**

**Oral:** Do not alter (chew or crush) enteric coated dosage form.

**Monitoring Laboratory Tests** CBC; perform culture and sensitivity studies prior to initiating therapy.

**Additional Nursing Issues**

**Physical Assessment:** Monitor for effectiveness of therapy and adverse reactions (see above). Instruct patient on appropriate use, possible adverse reactions (see above), and symptoms to report. **Pregnancy risk factor C** - benefits of use should outweigh possible risks. Note breast-feeding caution.

**Patient Information/Instruction:** Take with food or after meals around-the-clock. Do not chew, cut, or crush tablets. Take complete prescription even if you are feeling better. You may experience dizziness or drowsiness (use caution when driving or engaging in tasks that require alertness until response to drug is known); nausea or vomiting (small frequent meals, frequent mouth care, sucking lozenges, or chewing gum may help); constipation (increased exercise, dietary fiber, fruit, or fluid may help); or diarrhea (buttermilk, boiled milk, or yogurt may help). Report skin rash or itching, easy bruising or bleeding, unhealed sores of mouth, itching or vaginal discharge, fever or chills, unusual cough, muscle cramping or weakness, or palpitations or chest pain. **Pregnancy/breast-feeding precautions:** Inform prescriber if you are or intend to be pregnant. Consult prescriber if breast-feeding.

(Continued)

## Dirithromycin *(Continued)*

**Geriatric Considerations:** Dosage adjustment does not appear to be necessary in the elderly. Considered an appropriate choice in the outpatient treatment of community-acquired pneumonia in older adults.

- **Disalcid®** *see* Salsalate *on page 1042*
- **Disalicylic Acid** *see* Salsalate *on page 1042*
- **Disanthrol®** *see page 1294*
- **Discoloration of Feces Due to Drugs** *see page 1344*
- **Discoloration of Urine Due to Drugs** *see page 1344*
- **Disobrom®** *see page 1294*
- **Disodium Cromoglycate** *see* Cromolyn Sodium *on page 309*
- ***D*-Isoephedrine Hydrochloride** *see* Pseudoephedrine *on page 992*
- **Disolan® Capsule** *see page 1294*
- **Disonate® [OTC]** *see* Docusate *on page 392*
- **Disophrol® Chronotabs®** *see page 1294*
- **Disophrol® Tablet** *see page 1294*

## Disopyramide (dye soe PEER a mide)

**U.S. Brand Names** Norpace®

**Therapeutic Category** Antiarrhythmic Agent, Class I-A

**Pregnancy Risk Factor** C

**Lactation** Enters breast milk/compatible

**Use** Suppression and prevention of unifocal and multifocal atrial and premature, ventricular premature complexes, coupled ventricular tachycardia; effective in the conversion of atrial fibrillation, atrial flutter, and paroxysmal atrial tachycardia to normal sinus rhythm and prevention of the recurrence of these arrhythmias after conversion by other methods

**Mechanism of Action/Effect** Decreases myocardial excitability and conduction velocity; reduces disparity in refractoriness between normal and infarcted myocardium; possesses anticholinergic, peripheral vasoconstrictive, and negative inotropic effects

**Contraindications** Hypersensitivity to disopyramide; pre-existing second or third degree A-V block; cardiogenic shock

**Warnings** Pre-existing urinary retention, family history, or existing angle-closure glaucoma, myasthenia gravis, hypotension during initiation of therapy, congestive heart failure unless caused by an arrhythmias, widening of QRS complex during therapy or Q-T interval (>25% to 50% of baseline QRS complex or Q-T interval), sick-sinus syndrome or Wolfe-Parkinson-White syndrome (WPW), renal or hepatic impairment require decrease in dosage. Disopyramide is ineffective in hypokalemia and potentially toxic with hyperkalemia. Due to changes in total clearance (decreased) in the elderly, monitor closely. The anticholinergic action may be intolerable and require discontinuation. Pregnancy factor C.

**Drug Interactions**

**Cytochrome P-450 Effect:** CYP3A3/4 enzyme substrate

**Decreased Effect:** Hepatic microsomal enzyme inducing agents (eg, phenytoin, phenobarbital, rifampin) may increase metabolism of disopyramide leading to a decreased effect. Anticoagulants may have decreased prothrombin times after discontinuation of disopyramide.

**Increased Effect/Toxicity:** May elevate disopyramide levels. Erythromycin and clarithromycin may increase disopyramide serum concentrations, thus having an increased effect or toxicity, including widening Q-T interval. Digoxin and quinidine serum concentrations may be increased, thus having an increased effect or toxicity. Drugs with anticholinergic effects will be augmented with possibly severe anticholinergic effect.

**Adverse Reactions**

>10%: Genitourinary: Difficult urination

1% to 10%:

Cardiovascular: Chest pains, congestive heart failure, hypotension
Endocrine & metabolic: Hypokalemia
Gastrointestinal: Stomach pain, bloating, dry mouth, anorexia
Neuromuscular & skeletal: Muscle weakness
Ocular: Blurred vision

<1% (Limited to important or life-threatening symptoms): Syncope and conduction disturbances including A-V block, widening QRS complex and lengthening of Q-T interval, hypoglycemia, may initiate contractions of pregnant uterus, hyperkalemia may enhance toxicities, increased cholesterol and triglycerides, agranulocytosis, hepatic cholestasis, elevated liver enzymes, dry eyes, aggravation of glaucoma, dyspnea

**Overdose/Toxicology** Has a low toxic:therapeutic ratio and may easily produce fatal intoxication (acute toxic dose: 1 g in adults). Symptoms of overdose include sinus bradycardia, sinus node arrest or asystole, P-R, QRS, or Q-T interval prolongation, torsade de pointes (polymorphous ventricular tachycardia) and depressed myocardial contractility, which along with alpha-adrenergic or ganglionic blockade, may result in hypotension and pulmonary edema. Other effects are anticholinergic (dry mouth, dilated pupils, and delirium), as well as seizures, coma, and respiratory arrest.

Treatment is symptomatic and effects usually respond to conventional therapies. **Note:** Do not use other Type 1A or 1C antiarrhythmic agents to treat ventricular tachycardia. Sodium bicarbonate may treat wide QRS intervals or hypotension. Markedly impaired conduction or high degree A-V block, unresponsive to bicarbonate, indicates consideration of a pacemaker.

**Pharmacodynamics/Kinetics**

**Protein Binding:** Concentration dependent, ranges from 20% to 60%

**Half-life Elimination:** 4-10 hours, increased half-life with hepatic or renal disease

**Metabolism:** Liver

**Excretion:** Urine

**Onset:** 0.5-3.5 hours

**Duration:** 1.5-8.5 hours

**Formulations**

Disopyramide phosphate:

Capsule: 100 mg, 150 mg

Capsule, sustained action: 100 mg, 150 mg

**Dosing**

**Adults:** Oral:

<50 kg: 100 mg every 6 hours or 200 mg every 12 hours (controlled release)

>50 kg: 150 mg every 6 hours or 300 mg every 12 hours (controlled release); if no response, may increase to 200 mg every 6 hours; maximum dose required for patients with severe refractory ventricular tachycardia is 400 mg every 6 hours.

**Elderly:** Refer to adult dosing.

**Renal Impairment:** 100 mg (nonsustained release) given as follows: See table.

| Creatinine Clearance (mL/min) | Dosage Interval |
|---|---|
| 30-40 | q8h |
| 15-30 | q12h |
| <15 | q24h |

Or alter the dose as follows:

$Cl_{cr}$ 30-40 mL/minute: Reduce dose 50%.

$Cl_{cr}$ 15-30 mL/minute: Reduce dose 75%.

Not dialyzable (0% to 5%) by hemo- or peritoneal methods; supplemental dose is not necessary.

**Hepatic Impairment:** Administer 100 mg every 6 hours or 200 mg every 12 hours (controlled release).

**Administration**

**Oral:** Do not break or chew sustained release capsules. Administer around-the-clock to promote less variation in peak and trough serum levels.

**Monitoring Laboratory Tests** EKG, disopyramide drug level

**Additional Nursing Issues**

**Physical Assessment:** Assess other medications patient may be taking for effectiveness and interactions (see Drug Interactions). See Warnings/Precautions and Contraindications for cautious use. Monitor laboratory tests (see above), therapeutic response (cardiac status), and adverse reactions (eg, excessive anticholinergic effects, electrolyte imbalance - see Warnings, Adverse Reactions) when beginning therapy, when titrating dosage, and periodically during long-term therapy. **Note:** Disopyramide has a low toxic:therapeutic ratio and overdose may easily produce severe and life threatening reactions (see Overdose/Toxicology). **Pregnancy risk factor C** - benefits of use should outweigh possible risks.

**Patient Information/Instruction:** Take as directed, at regular intervals around-the-clock. Do not alter dosage or discontinue therapy without consulting prescriber. Do not crush or chew extended release form. Avoid (or limit) alcohol and caffeine. You may experience dizziness or blurred vision (use caution when driving or engaging in tasks requiring alertness until response to drug is known); or dry mouth (frequent mouth care or sucking on lozenges may help). Report any change in urinary pattern or difficulty urinating; chest pain, palpitations, irregular heartbeat; unusual cough, difficulty breathing, swelling of extremities; muscle tremors or weakness; confusion or acute lethargy; or skin rash. **Pregnancy precautions:** Inform prescriber if you are or intend to be pregnant.

**Geriatric Considerations:** Due to changes in total clearance (decreased) in the elderly, monitor closely. The anticholinergic action may be intolerable and require discontinuation. Monitor for CNS anticholinergic effects (confusion, agitation, hallucinations, etc). **Note:** Dose needs to be altered with $Cl_{cr}$ <40 mL/minute which may be found frequently in the elderly.

**Related Information**

Antiarrhythmic Drug Classification Comparison *on page 1366*

- **Di-Spaz® Injection** *see* Dicyclomine *on page 362*
- **Di-Spaz® Oral** *see* Dicyclomine *on page 362*
- **Dispos-a-Med® Isoproterenol** *see* Isoproterenol *on page 632*
- **Distaval®** *see* Thalidomide *on page 1113*

## Disulfiram (dye SUL fi ram)

**U.S. Brand Names** Antabuse®

**Therapeutic Category** Aldehyde Dehydrogenase Inhibitor

**Pregnancy Risk Factor** C

**Lactation** Excretion in breast milk unknown

**Use** Management of chronic alcoholism

**Mechanism of Action/Effect** When taken concomitantly with alcohol, there is an increase in serum acetaldehyde levels. Increased acetaldehyde causes uncomfortable

(Continued)

## Disulfiram *(Continued)*

symptoms including flushing, nausea, thirst, palpitations, chest pain, vertigo, and hypotension. This reaction is the basis for disulfiram use in postwithdrawal long-term care of alcoholism.

**Contraindications** Hypersensitivity to disulfiram (or other thiuram derivatives) or any component; severe myocardial disease and coronary occlusion; patient receiving alcohol, paraldehyde, alcohol-containing preparations like cough syrup or tonics

**Warnings** Use with caution in patients with diabetes, hypothyroidism, seizure disorders, hepatic cirrhosis, or insufficiency. Should never be administered to a patient when he/she is in a state of alcohol intoxication, or without his/her knowledge. Pregnancy factor C.

**Drug Interactions**

**Cytochrome P-450 Effect:** CYP2C9 and 2E1 enzyme inhibitor, both disulfiram and diethyldithiocarbamate (disulfiram metabolite) are CYP3A3/4 enzyme inhibitors

**Increased Effect/Toxicity:** Use with diazepam or chlordiazepoxide may result in an increased effect. Use with tricyclic antidepressants, metronidazole, or isoniazid may cause encephalopathy. Use with phenytoin may result in increased serum levels and toxicity. Use with warfarin may result in prolonged prothrombin times.

**Adverse Reactions**

>10%: Central nervous system: Drowsiness

1% to 10%:

Central nervous system: Headache, fatigue, mood changes, neurotoxicity, peripheral neuritis

Dermatologic: Rash

Gastrointestinal: Metallic or garlic-like aftertaste

Genitourinary: Impotence

<1% (Limited to important or life-threatening symptoms): Encephalopathy, hepatitis

**Disulfiram reaction with alcohol**: Flushing, sweating, cardiovascular collapse, myocardial infarction, vertigo, seizures, headache, nausea, vomiting, dyspnea, chest pain, death

**Overdose/Toxicology** Management of disulfiram reaction: Institute support measures to restore blood pressure (vasopressors and fluids). Monitor for hypokalemia.

**Pharmacodynamics/Kinetics**

**Metabolism:** Liver

**Excretion:** Feces and lungs

**Onset:** Full effect: 12 hours

**Duration:** May persist for 1-2 weeks after last dose

**Formulations** Tablet: 250 mg, 500 mg

**Dosing**

**Adults:**

Oral: Do not administer until the patient has abstained from alcohol for at least 12 hours.

Initial: 500 mg/day as a single dose for 1-2 weeks; maximum daily dose is 500 mg.

Average maintenance dose: 250 mg/day; range: 125-500 mg; duration of therapy is to continue until the patient is fully recovered socially and a basis for permanent self control has been established. Maintenance therapy may be required for months or even years.

**Administration**

**Oral:** Administration of any medications containing alcohol, including topicals, is contraindicated. Do not administer disulfiram if alcohol has been consumed within the prior 12 hours.

**Monitoring Laboratory Tests** Monitor liver function before, 10-14 days after beginning therapy, and every 6 months during therapy.

**Additional Nursing Issues**

**Physical Assessment:** Assess for adverse drug interactions with other prescription or OTC drugs (see Drug Interactions). Do not administer until the patient has abstained from alcohol for 12 hours. Monitor for CNS changes (eg, sedation, restlessness, peripheral neuropathy, and optic or retrobulbar neuritis). Advise patient about disulfiram reaction if alcohol is ingested. **Pregnancy risk factor C** - benefits of use should outweigh possible risks. Note breast-feeding caution.

**Patient Information/Instruction:** Tablets can be crushed or mixed with water or juice. Metallic aftertaste may occur; this will go away. Do not drink any alcohol, including products containing alcohol (cough and cold syrups), or use alcohol-containing skin products for at least 3 days and preferably 14 days after stopping this medication or while taking this medication. Drowsiness, tiredness, or visual changes may occur. Use care when driving or engaging in tasks requiring alertness until response to drug is known. Report yellow color in eyes or skin and any respiratory difficulty. **Pregnancy/breast-feeding precautions:** Inform prescriber if you are or intend to be pregnant. Consult prescriber if breast-feeding.

- **Dithranol** *see* Anthralin *on page 98*
- **Ditropan®** *see* Oxybutynin *on page 870*
- **Ditropan XL®** *see* Oxybutynin *on page 870*
- **Diuchlor®** *see* Hydrochlorothiazide *on page 566*
- **Diurigen®** *see* Chlorothiazide *on page 253*
- **Diuril®** *see* Chlorothiazide *on page 253*
- **Divalproex Sodium** *see* Valproic Acid and Derivatives *on page 1198*
- **Dixaparine** *see* Heparin *on page 558*
- **Dixarit®** *see* Clonidine *on page 289*

- ♦ **Dixonal** *see* Piroxicam *on page 940*
- ♦ **Dizmiss® [OTC]** *see* Meclizine *on page 712*
- ♦ ***dl*-Alpha Tocopherol** *see* Vitamin E *on page 1218*
- ♦ ***dl*-Norephedrine Hydrochloride** *see* Phenylpropanolamine *on page 922*
- ♦ ***D*-Mannitol** *see* Mannitol *on page 706*
- ♦ **4-DMDR** *see* Idarubicin *on page 595*
- ♦ **D-Med® Injection** *see* Methylprednisolone *on page 754*
- ♦ **DMSO** *see* Dimethyl Sulfoxide *on page 379*
- ♦ **DNase** *see* Dornase Alfa *on page 397*
- ♦ **DNR** *see* Daunorubicin Hydrochloride *on page 336*
- ♦ **Dobuject** *see* Dobutamine *on this page*


## Dobutamine (doe BYOO ta meen)

**U.S. Brand Names** Dobutrex® Injection

**Therapeutic Category** Adrenergic Agonist Agent; Sympathomimetic

**Pregnancy Risk Factor** B (note Pregnancy comments)

**Lactation** Excretion in breast milk unknown

**Use** Short-term management of patients with cardiac decompensation

**Mechanism of Action/Effect** Stimulates $beta_1$-adrenergic receptors, causing increased contractility and heart rate, with little effect on $beta_2$- or alpha-receptors

**Contraindications** Hypersensitivity to sulfites (commercial preparation contains sodium bisulfite); patients with idiopathic hypertrophic subaortic stenosis, atrial fibrillation, or atrial flutter

**Warnings** Hypovolemia should be corrected prior to use. Infiltration causes local inflammatory changes, extravasation may cause dermal necrosis. Use with extreme caution following myocardial infarction. This is a potent drug, it must be diluted prior to use. Experience in controlled trials is limited beyond 48 hours.

**Drug Interactions**

**Decreased Effect:** Beta-adrenergic blockers may decrease effect of dobutamine and increase risk of severe hypotension.

**Increased Effect/Toxicity:** General anesthetics (eg, halothane or cyclopropane) and usual doses of dobutamine have resulted in ventricular arrhythmias in animals. Bretylium and tricyclic antidepressants may potentiate dobutamine's effects.

**Effects on Lab Values** May affect serum assay of chloramphenicol.

**Adverse Reactions**

>10%:

Central nervous system: Headache
Gastrointestinal: Nausea, vomiting

1% to 10%:

Cardiovascular: Premature ventricular beats, bradycardia, hypertension, hypotension, chest pain, palpitations, tachycardia, ventricular arrhythmias
Central nervous system: Nervousness or restlessness
Respiratory: Dyspnea

<1% (Limited to important or life-threatening symptoms): Hypokalemia

**Overdose/Toxicology** Symptoms of overdose include fatigue, nervousness, tachycardia, hypertension, and arrhythmias. Reduce rate of administration or discontinue infusion until condition stabilizes.

**Pharmacodynamics/Kinetics**

**Half-life Elimination:** 2 minutes

**Metabolism:** Liver

**Excretion:** Urine

**Onset:** I.V.: 1-10 minutes; Peak effect: Within 10-20 minutes

**Formulations** Infusion, as hydrochloride: 12.5 mg/mL (20 mL)

**Dosing**

**Adults:** I.V. infusion: 2.5-15 mcg/kg/minute; maximum: 40 mcg/kg/minute, titrate to desired response

**Infusion Rates of Various Dilutions of Dobutamine**

| Desired Delivery Rate (mcg/kg/min) | Infusion Rate (mL/kg/min) | |
|---|---|---|
| | 500 mcg/mL* | 1000 mcg/mL† |
| 2.5 | 0.005 | 0.0025 |
| 5.0 | 0.01 | 0.005 |
| 7.5 | 0.015 | 0.0075 |
| 10.0 | 0.02 | 0.01 |
| 12.5 | 0.025 | 0.0125 |
| 15.0 | 0.03 | 0.015 |

*500 mg per liter or 250 mg per 500 mL of diluent.

†1000 mg per liter or 250 mg per 250 mL of diluent.

**Elderly:** Refer to adult dosing.

**Administration**

**I.V.:** Always administer via infusion device; administer into large vein.

**I.V. Detail: Extravasation management:** Phentolamine: Mix 5 mg with 9 mL of NS; inject a small amount of this dilution into extravasated area. Blanching should reverse

(Continued)

## Dobutamine *(Continued)*

immediately. Monitor site. If blanching should recur, additional injections of phentolamine may be needed.

**Stability**

**Reconstitution:** Remix solution every 24 hours. Store reconstituted solution under refrigeration for 48 hours or 6 hours at room temperature. Pink discoloration of solution indicates slight oxidation but **no** significant loss of potency. Stability of parenteral admixture at room temperature (25°C) is 48 hours; at refrigeration (4°C) stability is 7 days.

Standard adult diluent: 250 mg/500 mL $D_5W$; 500 mg/500 mL $D_5W$

**Compatibility:** Do not give through same I.V. line as heparin, hydrocortisone, sodium succinate, cefazolin, or penicillin. Incompatible with heparin, sodium bicarbonate, cefazolin, and penicillin. Incompatible in alkaline solutions (sodium bicarbonate). Compatible with dopamine, epinephrine, isoproterenol, and lidocaine.

**Monitoring Laboratory Tests** Serum glucose, renal function

**Additional Nursing Issues**

**Physical Assessment:** Assess other medications patient may be taking for effectiveness and interactions (see Drug Interactions). See Warnings/Precautions and Contraindications for cautious use. Infusion pump and continuous cardiac and hemodynamic monitoring are required. Monitor therapeutic response (cardiac status) and adverse reactions (see Warnings/Precautions and Adverse Reactions). Instruct patient on adverse symptoms to report. Note breast-feeding caution.

**Patient Information/Instruction:** When administered in emergencies, patient education should be appropriate to the situation. If patient is aware, instruct to promptly report chest pain, palpitations, rapid heartbeat, headache, nervousness, or restlessness, nausea or vomiting, or difficulty breathing. **Breast-feeding precautions:** Consult prescriber if breast-feeding.

**Geriatric Considerations:** A recent study demonstrated beneficial hemodynamic effects in elderly patients; monitor closely.

**Pregnancy Issues:** Since dobutamine has not been given to pregnant women, benefits of use should outweight risks.

**Additional Information** Some formulations may contain sulfites.

**Related Information**

Inotropic and Vasoconstrictor Comparison *on page 1391*

♦ **Dobutrex® Injection** *see* Dobutamine *on previous page*

## Docetaxel (doe se TAKS el)

**U.S. Brand Names** Taxotere®

**Therapeutic Category** Antineoplastic Agent, Natural Source (Plant) Derivative

**Pregnancy Risk Factor** D

**Lactation** Excretion in breast milk unknown/contraindicated

**Use** Treatment of patients with locally advanced or metastatic breast cancer who have progressed during anthracycline-based therapy or have relapsed during anthracycline-based adjuvant therapy; ovarian cancer

**Investigational use:** Treatment of nonsmall cell lung cancer, gastric, pancreatic, head and neck, soft tissue sarcoma, and melanoma

**Mechanism of Action/Effect** Inhibits cancer cell division by acting on the microtubules

**Contraindications** Hypersensitivity to docetaxel or any component; patients with neutrophil counts <1500 cells/$mm^3$; severe impaired liver function; pregnancy

**Warnings** Early studies reported severe hypersensitivity reactions characterized by hypotension, bronchospasms, or minor reactions with generalized rash/erythema. The overall incidence was 25% in patients who did not receive premedication.

Fluid retention syndrome characterized by pleural effusions, ascites, edema, and weight gain (2-15 kg) has also been reported. It has not been associated with cardiac, pulmonary, renal, hepatic, or endocrine dysfunction. The incidence and severity of the syndrome increase sharply at cumulative doses ≥400 mg/$m^2$. Treatment with corticosteroids (oral dexamethasone 8 mg twice daily for 5 days starting 1 day prior to docetaxel) is necessary to reduce severe fluid retention and hypersensitivity.

Neutropenia was the dose-limiting toxicity; however, this rarely resulted in treatment delays. Patients with increased liver function tests experienced more episodes of neutropenia with a greater number of severe infections. Patients with an absolute neutrophil count <1500 cells/$mm^3$ should not receive docetaxel.

Should generally not be given to patients with bilirubin greater than the upper limit of normal or to patients with AST (SGOT) and/or ALT (SGPT) greater than 1.5x the upper limit of normal concomitantly with alkaline phosphatase greater than 2.5x the upper limit of normal. Obtain baseline levels prior to administration.

Docetaxel preparation should be performed in a Class II laminar flow biologic safety cabinet. Personnel should be wearing surgical gloves and a closed front surgical gown with knit cuffs. Appropriate safety equipment is recommended for preparation, administration, and disposal of antineoplastics. If docetaxel contacts the skin, wash and flush thoroughly with water.

**Drug Interactions**

**Cytochrome P-450 Effect:** CYP3A3/4 enzyme substrate

**Increased Effect/Toxicity:** Increased toxicity with cytochrome P-450 substrate agents. Possibility of an inhibition of metabolism of docetaxel in patients treated with ketoconazole, erythromycin, terfenadine, astemizole, or cyclosporine.

**Adverse Reactions**

Local: **Irritant chemotherapy**

>10%:

Central nervous system: Fever

Dermatologic: Alopecia

Gastrointestinal: Nausea, vomiting, diarrhea, stomatitis

Hematologic: Neutropenia, leukopenia, thrombocytopenia, anemia

Neuromuscular & skeletal: Myalgia

1% to 10%: Cardiovascular: Severe fluid retention: poorly tolerated peripheral edema, generalized edema, pleural effusion requiring urgent drainage, dyspnea at rest, cardiac tamponade or pronounced abdominal distention (due to ascites), myocardial infarction, gastrointestinal perforation, neutropenic enterocolitis

**Pharmacodynamics/Kinetics**

**Protein Binding:** 94%

**Metabolism:** Liver

**Excretion:** Urine and feces

**Formulations** Injection: 40 mg/mL (0.5 mL, 2 mL)

**Dosing**

**Adults:** Corticosteroids (oral dexamethasone 8 mg twice daily for 5 days starting 1 day prior to docetaxel administration) are necessary to reduce the potential for hypersensitivity and severe fluid retention.

I.V. infusion (refer to individual protocol):

Locally advanced or metastatic carcinoma of the breast: 60-100 mg/m² over 1 hour every 3 weeks

**Dosage adjustment in patients who are initially started at 100 mg/m²** (>1 week), cumulative cutaneous reactions, or severe peripheral neuropathy: 75 mg/m²

**Note:** If the patient continues to experience these adverse reactions, the dosage should be reduced to 55 mg/m² or therapy should be discontinued.

**Suggested Docetaxel Maximum Dosages**

| Maximum Dosages | Adults |
|---|---|
| Maximum standard single dose | 100 mg/m² |
| Minimum time between courses | 3 weeks |
| Maximum dose per course | 100 mg/m² |

**Elderly:** Refer to adult dosing.

**Hepatic Impairment:** Total bilirubin ≥ the upper limit of normal (ULN), or AST (SGOT)/ALT (SGPT) >1.5 times the ULN concomitant with alkaline phosphatase >2.5 times the ULN: Docetaxel **should not be administered** secondary to increased incidence of treatment-related mortality.

**Administration**

**I.V.:** Irritant. Anaphylactoid-like reactions have been reported: Premedication with dexamethasone (8 mg orally twice daily for 5 days starting 1 prior to administration of docetaxel). Administer I.V. infusion over 1-hour.

**I.V. Detail:** Follow guidelines for handling cytotoxic agents.

**Stability**

**Storage:** Docetaxel is available in 20 mg and 80 mg vials prepackaged with a special diluent and formulated in polysorbate 80. Docetaxel is diluted with 13% (w/w) ethanol in water giving a final concentration of 10 mg/mL. Docetaxel is slightly more water soluble than paclitaxel. Intact vials should stored under refrigeration 2°C to 8°C (36°F to 46°F) and protected from light. Vials should be stored at room temperature for approximately 5 minutes before using. Freezing does not adversely affect the product.

**Reconstitution:** Compatible with 0.9% sodium chloride or 5% dextrose in water diluted to a final concentration of 0.3-0.9 mg/mL. Diluted solutions are stable for 8 hours at either room temperature 15°C to 25°C (59°F to 77°F) or refrigeration 2°C to 8°C (36°F to 46°F). Solutions must be prepared in a glass bottle, polypropylene, or polyolefin plastic bag to prevent leaching of plasticizers. Nonpolyvinyl chloride tubing should be used.

**Monitoring Laboratory Tests** Peripheral blood counts; liver function especially bilirubin, AST, ALT, and alkaline phosphatase

**Additional Nursing Issues**

**Physical Assessment:** Monitor laboratory tests as ordered. Assess infusion site frequently for extravasation which may result in cellulitis and tissue necrosis. Anaphylactoid-like reactions have been reported; premedication with dexamethasone may be advisable (see Warnings/Precautions and Administration). Monitor for adverse effects as indicated above; especially severe fluid retention, edema, pleural effusion, and opportunistic infection (eg, fever, chills, easy bruising or bleeding, fatigue, purulent vaginal drainage, unhealed mouth sores). **Pregnancy risk factor D.** Breast-feeding is contraindicated.

**Patient Information/Instruction:** This medication can only be administered I.V. During therapy, do not use alcohol, aspirin-containing products, and OTC medications without consulting prescriber. It is important to maintain adequate nutrition and hydration (2-3 L/day of fluids unless instructed to restrict fluid intake) during therapy; frequent small meals may help. You may experience nausea or vomiting (frequent small meals, frequent mouth care, sucking lozenges, or chewing gum may help); you may experience loss of hair (reversible); you will be more susceptible to infection (avoid crowds and exposure to infection as much as possible). Urine may turn red-brown (normal). Yogurt or buttermilk may help reduce diarrhea (if unresolved, contact

(Continued)

## Docetaxel *(Continued)*

prescriber for medication relief). Report swelling of extremities, difficulty breathing, unusual weight gain, abdominal distention, fever, chills, unusual bruising or bleeding, signs of infection, excessive fatigue, or unresolved diarrhea. **Breast-feeding precautions:** Do not breast-feed.

**Other Issues:** Nadir usually occurs at about day 8.

♦ **Docucal-P® Capsule** *see page 1294*

## Docusate (DOK yoo sate)

**U.S. Brand Names** Colace® [OTC]; DC 240® Softgels® [OTC]; Diocto® [OTC]; Diocto-K® [OTC]; Dioeze® [OTC]; Disonate® [OTC]; DOK® [OTC]; DOS® Softgel® [OTC]; D-S-S® [OTC]; Kasof® [OTC]; Modane® Soft [OTC]; Pro-Cal-Sof® [OTC]; Regulax SS® [OTC]; Sulfalax® [OTC]; Surfak® [OTC]

**Synonyms** Dioctyl Calcium Sulfosuccinate; Dioctyl Potassium Sulfosuccinate; Dioctyl Sodium Sulfosuccinate; DOSS; DSS

**Therapeutic Category** Stool Softener

**Pregnancy Risk Factor** C

**Lactation** Excretion in breast milk unknown/compatible

**Use** Stool softener in patients who should avoid straining during defecation and constipation associated with hard, dry stools; prophylaxis for straining (valsalva) following myocardial infarction

**Mechanism of Action/Effect** Reduces surface tension of the oil-water interface of the stool resulting in enhanced incorporation of water and fat allowing for stool softening

**Contraindications** Hypersensitivity to docusate or any component; concomitant use of mineral oil; intestinal obstruction; acute abdominal pain; nausea; vomiting

**Warnings** Prolonged, frequent, or excessive use may result in dependence or electrolyte imbalance. Pregnancy factor C.

**Drug Interactions**

**Decreased Effect:** Decreased effect of warfarin with high doses of docusate.

**Increased Effect/Toxicity:** Increased toxicity with mineral oil, phenolphthalein.

**Effects on Lab Values** ↓ potassium (S), chloride (S)

**Adverse Reactions** 1% to 10%:

Gastrointestinal: Intestinal obstruction, diarrhea, abdominal cramping

Miscellaneous: Throat irritation

**Overdose/Toxicology** Symptoms of overdose include abdominal cramps, diarrhea, fluid loss, and hypokalemia. Treatment is symptomatic.

**Pharmacodynamics/Kinetics**

**Metabolism:** Liver

**Excretion:** Urine

**Onset:** 12-72 hours

**Formulations**

Capsule, as calcium:
- DC 240® Softgels®, Pro-Cal-Sof®, Sulfalax®: 240 mg
- Surfak®: 50 mg, 240 mg

Capsule, as potassium:
- Diocto-K®: 100 mg
- Kasof®: 240 mg

Capsule, as sodium:
- Colace®: 50 mg, 100 mg
- Dioeze®: 250 mg
- Disonate®: 100 mg, 240 mg
- DOK®: 100 mg, 250 mg
- DOS® Softgel®: 100 mg, 250 mg
- D-S-S®: 100 mg
- Modane® Soft: 100 mg
- Regulax SS®: 100 mg, 250 mg

Liquid, as sodium (Diocto®, Colace®, Disonate®, DOK®): 150 mg/15 mL (30 mL, 60 mL, 480 mL)

Syrup, as sodium:
- 50 mg/15 mL (15 mL, 30 mL)
- Colace®, Diocto®, Disonate®, DOK®: 60 mg/15 mL (240 mL, 480 mL, 3780 mL)

Tablet, as sodium (Dialose®): 100 mg

**Dosing**

**Adults:** Docusate salts are interchangeable; the amount of sodium, calcium, or potassium per dosage unit is clinically insignificant.

Oral: 50-500 mg/day in 1-4 divided doses

Rectal: Add 50-100 mg of docusate liquid to enema fluid (saline or water); give as retention or flushing enema

**Elderly:** Refer to adult dosing.

**Administration**

**Oral:** Docusate liquid should be given with milk, or fruit juice, to mask the bitter taste. Capsules should be administered with a full glass of water, milk, or fruit juice.

**Additional Nursing Issues**

**Physical Assessment:** Monitor for effectiveness and/or overuse. **Pregnancy risk factor C** - benefits of use should outweigh possible risks.

**Patient Information/Instruction:** Docusate should be taken with a full glass of water, milk, or fruit juice. Do not use if abdominal pain, nausea, or vomiting are present. Laxative use should be used for a short period of time (<1 week). Prolonged use may result in abuse, dependence, as well as fluid and electrolyte loss. Report bleeding or if constipation occurs. **Pregnancy precautions:** Inform prescriber if you are or intend to be pregnant.

**Geriatric Considerations:** A safe agent to be used in the elderly. Some evidence that doses <200 mg are ineffective.

**Related Information**

Laxatives: Classification and Properties Comparison *on page 1392*

- **Docusate and Casanthranol** *see page 1294*
- **Docusate and Phenolphthalein** *see page 1294*
- **DOK® [OTC]** *see* Docusate *on previous page*
- **Doktors® Nasal Solution [OTC]** *see* Phenylephrine *on page 920*
- **Dolacet®** *see* Hydrocodone and Acetaminophen *on page 568*
- **Dolac Inyectable** *see* Ketorolac Tromethamine *on page 646*
- **Dolac Oral** *see* Ketorolac Tromethamine *on page 646*
- **Dolaren (Carisoprodol With Diclofenac)** *see* Carisoprodol *on page 202*

## Dolasetron (dol A se tron)

**U.S. Brand Names** Anzemet®

**Therapeutic Category** Selective 5-$HT_3$ Receptor Antagonist

**Pregnancy Risk Factor** B

**Lactation** Excretion in breast milk unknown

**Use** Prevention of nausea and vomiting associated with emetogenic cancer chemotherapy, including initial and repeat courses; prevention of postoperative nausea and vomiting and treatment of postoperative nausea and vomiting (injectable form only)

**Mechanism of Action/Effect** Selective 5-$HT_3$ receptor antagonist, blocking serotonin, both peripherally on vagal nerve terminals and centrally in the chemoreceptor trigger zone

**Contraindications** Hypersensitivity to dolasetron

**Warnings** Administer with caution in patients who have or may develop prolongation of cardiac conduction intervals, particularly Q-$T_c$ intervals. These include patients with hypokalemia, hypomagnesemia, patients taking diuretics which may cause electrolyte disturbances, patients with congenital Q-T syndrome, patients taking antiarrhythmic drugs or drug which prolong Q-T interval, and cumulative high-dose anthracycline therapy.

**Drug Interactions**

**Cytochrome P-450 Effect:** CYP2D6 and 3A3/4 enzyme substrate

**Decreased Effect:** Blood levels of active metabolite are decreased during coadministration of rifampin.

**Increased Effect/Toxicity:** Increased blood levels of active metabolite may occur during concurrent administration of cimetidine and atenolol. Inhibitors of this isoenzyme may increase blood levels of active metabolite. Due to the potential to potentiate Q-$T_c$ prolongation, drugs which may prolong Q-T interval directly (eg, antiarrhythmics) or by causing alterations in electrolytes (eg, diuretics) should be used with caution.

**Adverse Reactions** Dolasetron may cause EKG changes which are directly related to the concentration of hydrodolasetron, its active metabolite. Other adverse effects include:

Cancer patients:

>10%

Central nervous system: Headache (24%)

Gastrointestinal: Diarrhea (15%)

1% to 10% - occurring >2% and > placebo:

Central nervous system: Fever (4.3%), fatigue (3.6%), pain (2.4%), dizziness (2.2%), chills (2.0%)

Gastrointestinal: Increased transaminase levels (3.6%), abdominal pain (3.2%)

Cardiovascular: Hypertension (2.9%)

Postoperative patients:

1% to 10% - occurring >2% and > placebo:

Central nervous system: Headache (9.4%), dizziness (5.5%), drowsiness (2.4%), pain (2.4%)

Genitourinary: Urinary retention (2.4%)

<1% (Limited to important or life-threatening symptoms):

Patients in clinical trials involving either cancer patients or surgery: Arrhythmias, hypotension, anaphylaxis, bronchospasm

**Overdose/Toxicology** Prolongation of Q-T, A-V block, severe hypotension, and dizziness have been reported. Treatment is supportive, and continuous EKG monitoring (telemetry) is recommended.

**Pharmacodynamics/Kinetics**

**Protein Binding:** 69% to 77%

**Half-life Elimination:** Dolasetron: <10 minutes; hydrodolasetron 7.3 hours

**Metabolism:** Activated to hydrodolasetron by carbonyl reductase. Hydrodolasetron is metabolized by cytochrome P-450 isoenzyme 2D6.

**Excretion:** Urine and feces

**Formulations** Dolasetron mesylate:

Injection: 20 mg/mL

Tablet: 50 mg, 100 mg

(Continued)

## Dolasetron *(Continued)*

**Dosing**

**Adults:**

Nausea and vomiting associated with cancer chemotherapy:

Oral: 100 mg within 1 hour before chemotherapy (doses of 200 mg have been used)

I.V.: 1.8 mg/kg ~30 minutes before chemotherapy (maximum 100 mg)

Prevention of postoperative nausea and vomiting;

Oral: 100 mg within 2 hours before surgery (doses of 25-200 mg have been used)

I.V.: 12.5 mg ~15 minutes before stopping anesthesia

**Elderly:** Refer to adult dosing.

**Administration**

**Oral:** May be diluted in apple or apple-grape juice.

**I.V.:** May be given either undiluted IVP over 30 seconds or diluted to 50 mL and administered as an IVPB over 15 minutes.

**Stability**

**Reconstitution:** After dilution, stable at room temperature for 24 hours or under refrigeration for 48 hours.

**Additional Nursing Issues**

**Physical Assessment:** Assess other medications the patient may be taking for effectiveness and interactions (see Drug Interactions). Monitor blood pressure and for adverse cardiac conduction defects, anaphylaxis, and other adverse reactions (see Warnings/Precautions and Adverse Reactions). Note breast-feeding caution.

**Patient Information/Instruction:** This drug is given to reduce the incidence of nausea and vomiting. You may experience headache, drowsiness, or dizziness; request assistance when getting up or changing position and do not perform activities requiring alertness. Report immediately unusual pain, chills, or fever; severe headache or diarrhea; chest pain, palpitations, or tightness; swelling of throat or feeling of tightness in throat; or difficulty urinating. **Breast-feeding precautions:** Consult prescriber if breast-feeding.

♦ **Dolene®** *see* Propoxyphene *on page 984*

♦ **Dolobid®** *see* Diflunisal *on page 368*

♦ **Dolo Pangavit-D** *see* Diclofenac *on page 358*

♦ **Dolophine®** *see* Methadone *on page 735*

♦ **Domeboro® Topical** *see page 1294*

## Donepezil (don EH pa zil)

**U.S. Brand Names** Aricept®

**Synonyms** E2020

**Therapeutic Category** Acetylcholinesterase Inhibitor (Central)

**Pregnancy Risk Factor** C

**Lactation** Excretion in breast milk unknown/not recommended

**Use** Treatment of mild to moderate dementia of the Alzheimer's type

**Mechanism of Action/Effect** Enhances CNS cholinergic function by reversibly inhibiting acetylcholinesterase

**Contraindications** Hypersensitivity to donepezil or piperidine derivatives

**Warnings** Use with caution in patients with sick-sinus syndrome or other supraventricular cardiac conduction abnormalities, in patients with seizures or asthma. Pregnancy factor C.

**Drug Interactions**

**Cytochrome P-450 Effect:** CYP2D6 and 3A3/4 enzyme substrate

**Increased Effect/Toxicity:** Increased effects of succinylcholine, cholinesterase inhibitors, or cholinergic agonists (bethanechol). Concomitant NSAIDs may increase the risk of GI bleeding.

**Adverse Reactions**

>10%:

Central nervous system: Headache

Gastrointestinal: Nausea, diarrhea

1% to 10%:

Cardiovascular: Syncope, chest pain

Central nervous system: Fatigue, insomnia, dizziness, depression, abnormal dreams, somnolence

Dermatologic: Bruising

Gastrointestinal: Anorexia, vomiting, weight loss

Genitourinary: Polyuria

Neuromuscular & skeletal: Muscle cramps, arthritis, body pain

<1% (Limited to important or life-threatening symptoms): Cholecystitis, pancreatitis, seizures, rash, hallucinations, hemolytic anemia

**Overdose/Toxicology** Implement general supportive measures. Donepezil can cause a cholinergic crisis characterized by severe nausea, vomiting, salivation, sweating, bradycardia, hypotension, collapse, and convulsions. Increased muscle weakness is a possibility and may result in death if respiratory muscles are involved.

Tertiary anticholinergics, such as atropine, may be used as an antidote for overdose. I.V. atropine sulfate titrated to effect is recommended with an initial dose of 1-2 mg I.V., with subsequent doses based upon clinical response. Atypical increases in blood pressure and heart rate have been reported with other cholinomimetics when coadministered with quaternary anticholinergics such as glycopyrrolate.

**Pharmacodynamics/Kinetics**

**Protein Binding:** 96% mainly to albumin (75%) and alpha$_1$ acid glycoprotein (21%)

**Half-life Elimination:** 70 hours

**Time to Peak:** Plasma concentration: 3-4 hours

**Metabolism:** By CYP450 isoenzymes 2D6 and 3A4 and undergoes glucuronidation

**Excretion:** Unchanged in urine and extensively metabolized to four major metabolites, two of which are active

**Onset:** May require extended treatment

**Duration:** May be prolonged, particularly in older patients

**Formulations** Tablet: 5 mg, 10 mg

**Dosing**

**Adults:** Initial: 5 mg/day at bedtime; may increase to 10 mg/day at bedtime after 4-6 weeks.

**Elderly:** Refer to adult dosing.

**Additional Nursing Issues**

**Physical Assessment:** Assess bladder adequacy prior to administering medication. Assess other medications patient may be taking for effectiveness and interactions (see Drug Interactions). Monitor laboratory tests, therapeutic effect, and adverse reactions: cholinergic crisis (DUMBELS - **d**iarrhea, **u**rination, **m**iosis, **b**ronchospasm/**b**radycardia, **e**xcitability, **l**acrimation, and **s**alivation/excessive **s**weating) (see Warnings/Precautions, Adverse Reactions, and Overdose/Toxicology). Assess knowledge/teach patient appropriate use, interventions to reduce side effects, and adverse symptoms to report. **Pregnancy risk factor C** - benefits of use should outweigh possible risks. Breast-feeding is not recommended.

**Patient Information/Instruction:** This medication will not cure the disease, but may help reduce symptoms. Use as directed; do not increase dose or discontinue without consulting prescriber. Maintain adequate hydration (2-3 L/day of fluids unless instructed to restrict fluid intake). May cause dizziness, sedation, or hypotension (rise slowly from sitting or lying position and use caution when driving or climbing stairs); vomiting or loss of appetite (frequent small meals, frequent mouth care, chewing gum, or sucking lozenges may help); or diarrhea (boiled milk, yogurt, or buttermilk may help). Report persistent abdominal discomfort; significantly increased salivation, sweating, tearing, or urination; flushed skin; chest pain or palpitations; acute headache; unresolved diarrhea; excessive fatigue, insomnia, dizziness, or depression; increased muscle, joint, or body pain; vision changes or blurred vision; or shortness of breath or wheezing. **Pregnancy/breast-feeding precautions:** Inform prescriber if you are or intend to be pregnant. Breast-feeding is not recommended.

**Geriatric Considerations:** Donepezil is a new anticholinesterase for the treatment of Alzheimer's disease. It has been shown to cause an improvement in the ADAS-cog scores. As compared to tacrine, donepezil does **not** cause elevations in liver function tests and does not require routine laboratory monitoring. In addition, it is dosed once a day versus tacrine's four doses per day. For these reasons, donepezil may be preferred over tacrine in the treatment of mild to moderate dementia of the Alzheimer's type.


- **Donnagel®-PG Capsule** *see* Kaolin and Pectin With Opium *on page 642*
- **Donnagel®-PG Suspension** *see* Kaolin and Pectin With Opium *on page 642*
- **Donnamar®** *see* Hyoscyamine *on page 590*
- **Donnapine®** *see* Hyoscyamine, Atropine, Scopolamine, and Phenobarbital *on page 591*
- **Donna-Sed®** *see* Hyoscyamine, Atropine, Scopolamine, and Phenobarbital *on page 591*
- **Donnatal®** *see* Hyoscyamine, Atropine, Scopolamine, and Phenobarbital *on page 591*
- **Dopamet®** *see* Methyldopa *on page 750*


## Dopamine (DOE pa meen)

**U.S. Brand Names** Intropin® Injection

**Therapeutic Category** Adrenergic Agonist Agent; Sympathomimetic

**Pregnancy Risk Factor** C

**Lactation** Excretion in breast milk unknown

**Use** Adjunct in the treatment of shock (eg, MI, open heart surgery, renal failure, cardiac decompensation, etc) which persists after adequate fluid volume replacement

**Mechanism of Action/Effect** Stimulates both adrenergic and dopaminergic receptors, lower doses are mainly dopaminergic stimulating and produce renal and mesenteric vasodilation, higher doses also are both dopaminergic and beta$_1$-adrenergic stimulating and produce cardiac stimulation and renal vasodilation; large doses stimulate alpha-adrenergic receptors

**Contraindications** Hypersensitivity to sulfites (commercial preparation contains sodium bisulfite); pheochromocytoma; ventricular fibrillation

**Warnings** Use with caution in patients with cardiovascular disease or cardiac arrhythmias or patients with occlusive vascular disease. Pregnancy factor C.

**Drug Interactions**

**Decreased Effect:** Tricyclic antidepressants may have a decreased effect when coadministered with dopamine.

**Increased Effect/Toxicity:** Dopamine's effects are prolonged and intensified by MAO inhibitors, alpha- and beta-adrenergic blockers, general anesthetics, phenytoin.

**Adverse Reactions Vesicant chemotherapy**

>10%:

Central nervous system: Headache

Gastrointestinal: Nausea, vomiting

(Continued)

## Dopamine *(Continued)*

1% to 10%:

Cardiovascular: Premature ventricular beats, bradycardia, hypertension, hypotension, chest pain, palpitations, tachycardia, ventricular arrhythmias

Central nervous system: Nervousness or restlessness

Neuromuscular & skeletal: Mild leg cramps, paresthesia, tingling sensation

Respiratory: Dyspnea

<1% (Limited to important or life-threatening symptoms): Polyuria

**Overdose/Toxicology** Symptoms of overdose include severe hypertension, cardiac arrhythmias, acute renal failure. Treat symptomatically.

**Important:** Antidote for peripheral ischemia: To prevent sloughing and necrosis in ischemic areas, the area should be infiltrated as soon as possible with 10-15 mL of saline solution containing 5-10 mg of Regitine® (brand of phentolamine), an adrenergic blocking agent. A syringe with a fine hypodermic needle should be used, and the solution liberally infiltrated throughout the ischemic area. Sympathetic blockade with phentolamine causes immediate and conspicuous local hyperemic changes if the area is infiltrated within 12 hours. Therefore, phentolamine should be given as soon as possible after extravasation is noted.

**Pharmacodynamics/Kinetics**

**Half-life Elimination:** 2 minutes

**Metabolism:** Plasma, kidneys, and liver

**Excretion:** Urine

**Onset:** 5 minutes

**Duration:** <10 minutes

**Formulations**

Dopamine hydrochloride:

Infusion in $D_5W$: 0.8 mg/mL (250 mL, 500 mL); 1.6 mg/mL (250 mL, 500 mL); 3.2 mg/mL (250 mL, 500 mL)

Injection: 40 mg/mL (5 mL, 10 mL, 20 mL); 80 mg/mL (5 mL, 20 mL); 160 mg/mL (5 mL)

**Dosing**

**Adults:** I.V. infusion:

1-5 mcg/kg/minute up to 50 mcg/kg/minute, titrate to desired response; infusion may be increased by 1-4 mcg/kg/minute at 10- to 30-minute intervals until optimal response is obtained

If dosages >20-30 mcg/kg/minute are needed, a more direct-acting vasopressor may be more beneficial (ie, epinephrine, norepinephrine)

Hemodynamic effects of dopamine are dose-dependent:

Low-dose: 1-5 mcg/kg/minute, increased renal blood flow and urine output

Intermediate-dose: 5-15 mcg/kg/minute, increased renal blood flow, heart rate, cardiac contractility, and cardiac output

High-dose: >15 mcg/kg/minute, alpha-adrenergic effects begin to predominate, vasoconstriction, increased blood pressure

**Elderly:** Refer to adult dosing. Monitor closely, especially due to increase in cardiovascular disease with age.

**Administration**

**I.V.:** Vesicant. **Must be diluted prior to use.**

**I.V. Detail:** Monitor continuously for free flow. Administration into an umbilical arterial catheter is not recommended; central line administration.

**Extravasation management:** Due to short half-life, withdrawal of drug is often only necessary treatment. Use phentolamine as antidote. Mix 5 mg with 9 mL of NS; inject a small amount of this dilution into extravasated area. Blanching should reverse immediately. Monitor site. If blanching should recur, additional injections of phentolamine may be needed.

**Stability**

**Storage:** Protect from light. Solutions that are darker than slightly yellow should not be used.

**Compatibility:** Incompatible with alkaline solutions or iron salts. Compatible when coadministered with dobutamine, epinephrine, isoproterenol, and lidocaine. See the Compatibility of Drugs Chart *on page 1315*.

**Monitoring Laboratory Tests** Continuous hemodynamic monitoring; serum glucose, renal function

**Additional Nursing Issues**

**Physical Assessment:** Assess other medications patient may be taking for effectiveness and interactions (see Drug Interactions). See Warnings/Precautions and Contraindications for cautious use. Infusion pump and continuous cardiac and hemodynamic monitoring are required for inpatient therapy. Assess I.V. site frequently (see Administration for extravasation antidote instructions). Monitor therapeutic response (cardiac status, renal function) and adverse reactions including peripheral ischemia (see antidote above) (see Warnings/Precautions and Adverse Reactions). Instruct patient on adverse symptoms to report. Note breast-feeding caution.

Low dose home infusion therapy requires frequent monitoring of cardiac and renal status, and adverse reactions.

**Patient Information/Instruction:** When administered in emergencies, patient education should be appropriate to the situation. If patient is aware, instruct to promptly report chest pain, palpitations, rapid heartbeat, headache, nervousness or restlessness, nausea or vomiting, or difficulty breathing.

**Geriatric Considerations:** Has not been specifically studied in the elderly.

**Additional Information** The injection formulation contains sulfites.

**Related Information**

Inotropic and Vasoconstrictor Comparison *on page 1391*

- **Dopar®** *see* Levodopa *on page 666*
- **Dopram® Injection** *see* Doxapram *on next page*
- **Dorcol® [OTC]** *see* Acetaminophen *on page 32*
- **Dormarex® 2 Oral [OTC]** *see* Diphenhydramine *on page 381*
- **Dormicum** *see* Midazolam *on page 769*
- **Dormin® Oral [OTC]** *see* Diphenhydramine *on page 381*

## Dornase Alfa (DOOR nase AL fa)

**U.S. Brand Names** Pulmozyme®

**Synonyms** DNase; Recombinant Human Deoxyribonuclease

**Therapeutic Category** Enzyme

**Pregnancy Risk Factor** B

**Lactation** Excretion in breast milk unknown

**Use** Cystic fibrosis; reduce the frequency of respiratory infection that requires parenteral antibiotics, and to improve pulmonary function

**Mechanism of Action/Effect** The hallmark of cystic fibrosis lung disease is the presence of abundant, purulent airway secretions composed primarily of highly polymerized DNA. Dornase selectively cleaves DNA, thus reducing mucous viscosity and as a result, airflow in the lung is improved and the risk of bacterial infection may be decreased.

**Contraindications** Hypersensitivity to dornase alfa, Chinese hamster ovary cell products (eg, epoetin alfa), or any component

**Warnings** No clinical trials have been conducted to demonstrate safety and effectiveness of dornase in children <5 years of age, in patients with pulmonary function <40% of normal, or in patients for longer treatment periods >12 months.

**Adverse Reactions**

>10%:

Cardiovascular: Chest pain

Respiratory: Pharyngitis

Miscellaneous: Voice alteration

1% to 10%:

Dermatologic: Rash

Ocular: Conjunctivitis

Respiratory: Laryngitis, cough, dyspnea, hemoptysis, rhinitis, hoarse throat, wheezing

**Pharmacodynamics/Kinetics**

**Half-life Elimination:** Following nebulization, enzyme levels are measurable in the sputum within 15 minutes and decline rapidly thereafter.

**Formulations** Solution, inhalation: 1 mg/mL (2.5 mL)

**Dosing**

**Adults:** Inhalation: 2.5 mg once daily through selected nebulizers in conjunction with a Pulmo-Aide® or a Pari-Proneb® compressor

**Elderly:** Refer to adult dosing.

**Stability**

**Storage:** Must be stored in the refrigerator at 2°C to 8°C (36°F to 46°F) and protected from strong light. Should not be exposed to room temperature for a total of 24 hours.

**Compatibility:** Should not be diluted or mixed with any other drugs in the nebulizer, this may inactivate the dornase alfa.

**Additional Nursing Issues**

**Physical Assessment:** See Contraindications and Warnings/Precautions for use cautions. Monitor effectiveness of therapy (respiratory rate, lung sounds, characteristics of cough and sputum) and adverse reactions (see Adverse Reactions) at beginning of therapy and periodically with long-term use. Assess knowledge/teach patient appropriate use, interventions to reduce side effects, and adverse symptoms to report. Note breast-feeding caution.

**Patient Information/Instruction:** Use exactly as directed by prescriber (see Administration below). Report any signs of adverse response, skin rash, sore throat, respiratory wheezing, cough, or difficulty breathing. **Breast-feeding precautions:** Consult prescriber if breast-feeding.

**Administration:** Self-administered nebulizer: Store in refrigerator, away from light. Do not combine with any other medications in the nebulizer. Wash hands before and after treatment. Wash and dry nebulizer after each treatment. Twist open the top of one unit dose vial and squeeze contents into nebulizer reservoir. Connect nebulizer reservoir to the mouthpiece or face-mask. Connect nebulizer to compressor. Sit in comfortable, upright position. Put on face-mask and turn on compressor. Avoid leakage around the mask to avoid mist getting into eyes. Breath calmly and deeply until no more mist is formed in nebulizer (about 5 minutes). At this point treatment is finished.

- **Doryx®** *see* Doxycycline *on page 406*
- **Dorzolamide** *see* Ophthalmic Agents, Glaucoma *on page 853*
- **DOSS** *see* Docusate *on page 392*
- **DOS® Softgel® [OTC]** *see* Docusate *on page 392*
- **Dovonex®** *see* Calcipotriene *on page 181*
- **Doxacurium** *see page 1248*

## Doxapram (DOKS a pram)

**U.S. Brand Names** Dopram® Injection

**Therapeutic Category** Respiratory Stimulant; Stimulant

**Pregnancy Risk Factor** B

**Lactation** Excretion in breast milk unknown

**Use** Respiratory and CNS stimulant; stimulates respiration in patients with drug-induced CNS depression or postanesthesia respiratory depression; in hospitalized patients with COPD associated with acute hypercapnia

**Mechanism of Action/Effect** Stimulates respiration through action on respiratory center in medulla or indirectly on peripheral carotid chemoreceptors

**Contraindications** Hypersensitivity to doxapram or any component; epilepsy; cerebral edema; head injury; severe pulmonary disease; pheochromocytoma; cardiovascular disease; hypertension; hyperthyroidism

**Warnings** May cause severe CNS toxicity, seizures. Should be used with caution in newborns as the U.S. product contains benzyl alcohol (0.9%). Doxapram is neither a nonspecific CNS depressant antagonist nor an opiate antagonist.

**Drug Interactions**

**Increased Effect/Toxicity:** Increased toxicity (elevated blood pressure) with sympathomimetics, MAO inhibitors. Halothane, cyclopropane, and enflurane may sensitize the myocardium to catecholamine and epinephrine which is released at the initiation of doxapram, hence, separate discontinuation of anesthetics and start of doxapram by at least 10 minutes.

**Adverse Reactions** 1% to 10%:

Cardiovascular: Chest pain, tachycardia
Central nervous system: Confusion, dizziness or lightheadedness, headache,
Gastrointestinal: Diarrhea, nausea, vomiting,
Genitourinary: Urination problems
Hematologic: Hemolysis
Respiratory: Coughing, wheezing, troubled breathing
Local: Thrombophlebitis
Miscellaneous: Sweating, feeling of warmth

**Overdose/Toxicology** Symptoms of overdose include excessive increases in blood pressure, tachycardia, arrhythmias, muscle spasticity, and dyspnea. Supportive care is the preferred treatment. Seizures are unlikely and can be treated with benzodiazepines. **Doxapram is not dialyzable.**

**Pharmacodynamics/Kinetics**

**Half-life Elimination:** 3.4 hours (mean half-life)

**Metabolism:** Liver

**Excretion:** Urine

**Onset:** Respiratory stimulation begins: I.V.: Within 20-40 seconds; Peak effect: Within 1-2 minutes

**Duration:** 5-12 minutes

**Formulations** Injection, as hydrochloride: 20 mg/mL (20 mL)

**Dosing**

**Adults:** Respiratory depression following anesthesia: I.V.:

Initial: 0.5-1 mg/kg; may repeat at 5-minute intervals; maximum total dose: 2 mg/kg

I.V. infusion: Initial: 5 mg/minute until adequate response or adverse effects seen; decrease to 1-3 mg/minute; usual total dose: 0.5-4 mg/kg; maximum: 300 mg

Drug-induced CNS depression: Priming dose of 2 mg/kg and repeat in 5 minutes; repeat every 1-2 hours until patient wakes up; if patient relapses, then resume injections every 1-2 hours until patient awakens or maximum daily dose of 3 g is given.

COPD with acute hypercapnia: Start an infusion of 1-2 mg/minute and increase to a maximum of 3 mg/minute.

**Elderly:** Refer to adult dosing.

**Renal Impairment:** Not dialyzable

**Administration**

**I.V.:** Dilute to 1 mg/mL in $D_5W$ or NS for continuous infusion.

**Stability**

**Compatibility:** Incompatible with aminophylline, thiopental, or sodium bicarbonate (alkali drugs).

**Additional Nursing Issues**

**Physical Assessment:** Avoid extravasation, rapid infusion may cause hemolysis. Monitor heart rate, blood pressure, reflexes, CNS status, and apnea episodes on a continuous basis. Discontinue and notify prescriber if sudden severe hypotension or dyspnea occurs. Note breast-feeding caution.

**Patient Information/Instruction:** This drug is generally used in an emergency. Teaching should be appropriate to patient education. Someone will be observing response at all times. **Breast-feeding precautions:** Consult prescriber if breast-feeding.

**Geriatric Considerations:** Has not been studied in the elderly.

**Additional Information** Some formulations may contain benzyl alcohol.

## Doxazosin (doks AYE zoe sin)

**U.S. Brand Names** Cardura®

**Therapeutic Category** Alpha$_1$ Blockers

**Pregnancy Risk Factor** C

**Lactation** Excretion in breast milk unknown

**Use** Treatment of hypertension alone or in conjunction with diuretics, cardiac glycosides, ACE inhibitors or calcium antagonists (particularly appropriate for those with hypertension and other cardiovascular risk factors such as hypercholesterolemia and diabetes mellitus); treatment of urinary outflow obstruction and/or obstructive and irritative symptoms associated with benign prostatic hyperplasia (particularly useful in patients with troublesome symptoms who are unable or unwilling to undergo invasive procedures, but who require rapid symptomatic relief)

**Mechanism of Action/Effect** Competitively inhibits postsynaptic alpha-adrenergic receptors which results in vasodilation of veins and arterioles and a decrease in total peripheral resistance and blood pressure; approximately 50% as potent on a weight by weight basis as prazosin

**Contraindications** Hypersensitivity to doxazosin or any component

**Warnings** Use with caution in patients with renal impairment. Can cause marked hypotension and syncope with sudden loss of consciousness with the first dose. Anticipate a similar effect if therapy is interrupted for a few days, if dosage is increased rapidly, or if another antihypertensive drug is introduced. Pregnancy factor C.

**Drug Interactions**

**Decreased Effect:** Decreased hypotensive effect with NSAIDs.

**Increased Effect/Toxicity:** Increased hypotensive effect with diuretics and antihypertensive medications (especially beta-blockers).

**Effects on Lab Values** Increased urinary VMA 17%, norepinephrine metabolite 42%

**Adverse Reactions**

>10%: Central nervous system: Dizziness, headache, drowsiness

1% to 10%:

Cardiovascular: Palpitations, arrhythmia, tachycardia

Central nervous system: Orthostatic hypotension

Dermatologic: Pruritus, rash

Gastrointestinal: Nausea, vomiting, dry mouth, diarrhea, constipation, flatulence

Respiratory: Rhinitis, dyspnea, epistaxis

**Overdose/Toxicology** Symptoms of overdose include severe hypotension, drowsiness, and tachycardia. Treatment is supportive and symptomatic.

**Pharmacodynamics/Kinetics**

**Time to Peak:** 1-2 hours

**Metabolism:** Liver

**Excretion:** Urine and feces

**Duration:** >24 hours

**Formulations** Tablet: 1 mg, 2 mg, 4 mg, 8 mg

**Dosing**

**Adults:** Oral: 1 mg once daily in morning or evening; may be increased to 2 mg once daily; thereafter titrate upwards, if needed, over several weeks, balancing therapeutic benefit with doxazosin-induced postural hypotension; maximum dose for **hypertension**: 16 mg/day, for **BPH**: 8 mg/day.

**Elderly:** Oral: Initial: 0.5 mg once daily

**Administration**

**Oral:** Syncope may occur usually within 90 minutes of the initial dose.

**Monitoring Laboratory Tests** White blood count

**Additional Nursing Issues**

**Physical Assessment:** Assess effectiveness and interactions of other medications (see Drug Interactions). See Contraindications and Warnings/Precautions for use cautions. Monitor for effectiveness of therapy (blood pressure supine and standing) and adverse reactions (see Adverse Reactions and Overdose/Toxicology) at beginning of therapy and on a regular basis with long-term therapy. Assess knowledge/teach patient appropriate use, possible side effects/interventions, and adverse symptoms to report. When discontinuing, monitor blood pressure and taper dose and frequency slowly over 1 week or more. **Pregnancy risk factor C** - benefits of use should outweigh possible risks. Note breast-feeding caution.

**Patient Information/Instruction:** Take as directed, at bedtime. Do not skip dose or discontinue without consulting prescriber. Follow recommended diet and exercise program. Do not use OTC medications which may affect blood pressure (eg, cough or cold remedies, diet pills, stay-awake medications) without consulting prescriber. This medication may cause drowsiness, dizziness, or impaired judgment (use caution when driving or engaging in tasks that require alertness until response to drug is known); postural hypotension (use caution when rising from sitting or lying position or when climbing stairs); or dry mouth or nausea (frequent mouth care or sucking lozenges may help). Report increased nervousness or depression; sudden weight gain (weigh yourself in the same clothes at the same time of day once a week); unusual or persistent swelling of ankles, feet, or extremities; palpitations or rapid heartbeat; muscle weakness, fatigue, or pain; or other persistent side effects. **Pregnancy/breast-feeding precautions:** Inform prescriber if you are or intend to be pregnant. Consult prescriber if breast-feeding.

**Geriatric Considerations:** Adverse reactions such as dry mouth and urinary problems can be particularly bothersome in the elderly.

## Doxepin (DOKS e pin)

**U.S. Brand Names** Adapin® Oral; Sinequan® Oral; Zonalon® Topical Cream

**Therapeutic Category** Antidepressant, Tricyclic (Tertiary Amine); Topical Skin Product

**Pregnancy Risk Factor** C

**Lactation** Excretion in breast milk unknown/not recommended (AAP rates "of concern")

(Continued)

## Doxepin *(Continued)*

**Use**

Oral: Treatment of various forms of depression, usually in conjunction with psychotherapy; treatment of anxiety disorders

**Unlabeled use:** Analgesic for certain chronic and neuropathic pain

Topical: Short-term (<8 days) management of moderate pruritus in adults with atopic dermatitis or lichen simplex chronicus

**Mechanism of Action/Effect** Increases the synaptic concentration of serotonin and/or norepinephrine in the central nervous system by inhibition of their reuptake by the presynaptic neuronal membrane

**Contraindications** Hypersensitivity to doxepin or any component (cross-sensitivity with other tricyclic antidepressants may occur); narrow-angle glaucoma

**Warnings** Use with caution in patients with cardiovascular disease, conduction disturbances, seizure disorders, urinary retention, hyperthyroidism, or those receiving thyroid replacement. Use with caution in pregnancy. Do not discontinue abruptly in patients receiving chronic high-dose therapy. Pregnancy factor C.

**Drug Interactions**

**Cytochrome P-450 Effect:** CYP2D6 enzyme substrate

**Decreased Effect:** Decreased effect of bretylium, guanethidine, clonidine, levodopa. Decreased effect of doxepin with ascorbic acid, cholestyramine.

**Increased Effect/Toxicity:** Increased effect/toxicity of carbamazepine, amphetamines, sympathomimetics, fluoxetine (seizures), thyroid preparations, MAO inhibitors (convulsions, hypertensive crisis). CNS depressants (ie, benzodiazepines, opiate analgesics, phenothiazines, alcohol), anticholinergics, cimetidine, famotidine may increase doxepin toxicity when used in concomitantly. Potential for serotonin syndrome if combined with other serotonergic drugs.

**Effects on Lab Values** ↑ glucose

**Adverse Reactions**

**Systemic:**

>10%:

- Central nervous system: Sedation, drowsiness, dizziness, headache
- Gastrointestinal: Dry mouth, constipation, increased appetite, nausea, unpleasant taste, weight gain
- Neuromuscular & skeletal: Weakness

1% to 10%:

- Cardiovascular: Hypotension, arrhythmias
- Central nervous system: Confusion, delirium, hallucinations, nervousness, restlessness, parkinsonian syndrome, insomnia
- Gastrointestinal: Diarrhea, heartburn
- Genitourinary: Sexual dysfunction, dysuria
- Neuromuscular & skeletal: Fine muscle tremors
- Ocular: Blurred vision, eye pain
- Miscellaneous: Sweating (excessive)

<1% (Limited to important or life-threatening symptoms): Seizures, alopecia, photosensitivity, breast enlargement, galactorrhea, SIADH, agranulocytosis, leukopenia, eosinophilia, hepatitis, cholestatic jaundice and increased liver enzymes, increased intraocular pressure

**Topical:**

>10%:

- Central nervous system: Drowsiness
- Dermatologic: Burning at site of application
- Gastrointestinal: Changes in taste

1% to 10%:

- Central nervous system: Emotional changes, headache, fatigue
- Dermatologic: Edema at site of application, exacerbation of pruritus or eczema, dryness of skin
- Gastrointestinal: Dry mouth, thirst
- Neuromuscular & skeletal: Parethesias

**Overdose/Toxicology** Symptoms of overdose include confusion, hallucinations, seizures, urinary retention, hypothermia, hypotension, tachycardia, and cyanosis. Following initiation of essential overdose management, toxic symptoms should be treated symptomatically.

**Pharmacodynamics/Kinetics**

**Protein Binding:** 80% to 85%

**Distribution:** Crosses the placenta

**Half-life Elimination:** 6-8 hours

**Metabolism:** Liver

**Excretion:** Urine

**Onset:** Peak antidepressant effect: Usually more than 2 weeks; anxiolytic effects may occur sooner

**Formulations**

Doxepin hydrochloride:

- Capsule: 10 mg, 25 mg, 50 mg, 75 mg, 100 mg, 150 mg
- Concentrate, oral: 10 mg/mL (120 mL)
- Cream (Zonalon®): 5% (30 g)

**Dosing**

**Adults:**

Oral (entire daily dose may be given at bedtime): Initial: 30-150 mg/day at bedtime or in 2-3 divided doses; may gradually increase up to 300 mg/day; single dose should not exceed 150 mg; select patients may respond to 25-50 mg/day.

Topical: Apply a thin film 4 times/day with at least 3- to 4-hour interval between applications.

**Elderly:** Oral: Initial: 10-25 mg at bedtime; increase by 10-25 mg every 3 days for inpatients and weekly for outpatients if tolerated. Rarely does the maximum dose required exceed 75 mg/day; a single bedtime dose is recommended.

**Hepatic Impairment:** Use a lower dose and adjust gradually.

**Administration**

**Oral:** Do not mix oral concentrate with carbonated beverages (physically incompatible).

**Stability**

**Storage:** Protect from light.

**Additional Nursing Issues**

**Physical Assessment:** Assess other medications patient may be taking for effectiveness and interactions (see Drug Interactions). See Contraindications and Warnings/Precautions for cautious use. Monitor laboratory tests, therapeutic response, and adverse reactions at beginning of therapy and periodically with long-term use (see Adverse Reactions and Overdose/Toxicology). Taper dosage slowly when discontinuing. Assess knowledge/teach patient appropriate use (oral, topical), interventions to reduce side effects, and adverse symptoms to report. **Pregnancy risk factor C** - benefits of use should outweigh possible risks. Breast-feeding is not recommended.

**Patient Information/Instruction:**

Oral: Take exactly as directed (do not increase dose or frequency); may take several weeks to achieve desired results; may cause physical and/or psychological dependence. Avoid excessive alcohol, caffeine, and other prescription or OTC medications not approved by prescriber. Maintain adequate hydration (2-3 L/day of fluids unless instructed to restrict fluid intake). You may experience drowsiness, lightheadedness, impaired coordination, dizziness, or blurred vision (use caution when driving or engaging in tasks requiring alertness until response to drug is known); constipation (increased exercise, fluids, or dietary fruit and fiber may help); urinary retention (void before taking medication); postural hypotension (use caution climbing stairs or when changing position from lying or sitting to standing); altered sexual drive or ability (reversible); or photosensitivity (use sunscreen, wear protective clothing and eyewear, and avoid direct sunlight). Report persistent CNS effects (eg, nervousness, restlessness, insomnia, anxiety, excitation, headache, agitation, impaired coordination, changes in cognition); muscle cramping, weakness, tremors, or rigidity; chest pain, palpitations, or irregular heartbeat; blurred vision or eye pain; yellowing of skin or eyes; or worsening of condition. **Pregnancy/breast-feeding precautions:** Inform prescriber if you are or intend to be pregnant. Breast-feeding is not recommended.

Topical: Use as directed. Apply in thin layer; do not overuse. Report increased skin irritation, worsening of condition or lack of improvement.

**Geriatric Considerations:** Preferred agent when sedation is a desired property. Less potential for anticholinergic effects than amitriptyline and less orthostatic hypotension than imipramine.

**Breast-feeding Issues:** Generally, it is not recommended to breast-feed if taking antidepressants because of the long half-life, active metabolites, and the potential for side effects in the infant.

**Related Information**

Antidepressant Agents Comparison *on page 1368*

- **Doxidan® Capsule** *see page 1294*
- **Doxil®** *see* Doxorubicin (Liposomal) *on page 404*
- **Doxolem** *see* Doxorubicin *on this page*

## Doxorubicin (doks oh ROO bi sin)

**U.S. Brand Names** Adriamycin PFS™; Adriamycin RDF™; Rubex®

**Synonyms** ADR; Hydroxydaunomycin Hydrochloride

**Therapeutic Category** Antineoplastic Agent, Antibiotic

**Pregnancy Risk Factor** D

**Lactation** Enters breast milk/contraindicated

**Use** Treatment of leukemias, lymphomas, multiple myeloma, osseous and nonosseous sarcomas, mesotheliomas, germ cell tumors of the ovary or testis, and carcinomas of the head and neck, thyroid, lung, breast, stomach, pancreas, liver, ovary, bladder, prostate, and uterus, neuroblastoma, osteosarcoma

**Mechanism of Action/Effect** Inhibits DNA and RNA synthesis of susceptible bacteria, active throughout cell cycle, results in cell death.

**Contraindications** Hypersensitivity to doxorubicin or any component; severe congestive heart failure; cardiomyopathy; cardiac disease (may lead to cardiac toxicity); pre-existing myelosuppression; patients with impaired cardiac function; patients who received previous treatment with complete cumulative doses of doxorubicin and/or daunorubicin; large bowel carcinoma; brain tumors; pregnancy

**Warnings** The U.S. Food and Drug Administration (FDA) currently recommends that procedures for proper handling and disposal of antineoplastic agents be considered. Total dose should not exceed 550 mg/m$^2$ or 400 mg/m$^2$ in patients with previous or concomitant treatment (with daunorubicin, cyclophosphamide, or irradiation of the cardiac region). Irreversible myocardial toxicity may occur as total dosage approaches 550 mg/m$^2$. I.V. use only, severe local tissue necrosis will result if extravasation occurs.
(Continued)

## Doxorubicin *(Continued)*

Elderly and pediatric patients are at higher risk of cardiotoxicity (delayed). Reduce dose in patients with impaired hepatic function. Severe myelosuppression is also possible. Administration of live vaccines to immunosuppressed patients may be hazardous. Heart failure may occur during therapy or months to years after therapy. Treatment may increase the risk of other neoplasms.

Doxorubicin preparation should be performed in a Class II laminar flow biologic safety cabinet. Personnel should be wearing surgical gloves and a closed front surgical gown with knit cuffs. Appropriate safety equipment is recommended for preparation, administration, and disposal of antineoplastics. If doxorubicin contacts the skin, wash and flush thoroughly with water.

**Drug Interactions**

**Cytochrome P-450 Effect:** CYP3A3/4 enzyme substrate; CYP2D6 enzyme inhibitor

**Decreased Effect:** Doxorubicin may decrease plasma levels and effectiveness of digoxin and phenytoin. Phenobarbital increases elimination (decreases effect) of doxorubicin.

**Increased Effect/Toxicity:** Allopurinol may enhance the antitumor activity of doxorubicin (animal data only). Cyclosporine may decrease clearance of parent and metabolite and may induce coma or seizures and enhance hematologic toxicity. Cyclophosphamide enhances the cardiac toxicity of doxorubicin by producing additional myocardial cell damage. Mercaptopurine increases toxicities. Streptozocin greatly enhances leukopenia and thrombocytopenia. Verapamil alters the cellular distribution of doxorubicin and may result in increased cell toxicity by inhibition of the P-glycoprotein pump. Paclitaxel reduces doxorubicin clearance and increases toxicity if administered prior to doxorubicin. High doses of progesterone enhance toxicity (neutropenia and thrombocytopenia). Based on mouse studies, cardiotoxicity may be enhanced by verapamil. Concurrent therapy with actinomycin-D may result in recall pneumonitis following radiation.

**Adverse Reactions**

>10%:

Dermatologic: Alopecia

Gastrointestinal: Acute nausea and vomiting may be seen in 21% to 55% of patients; mucositis, ulceration, and necrosis of the colon, anorexia, and diarrhea, stomatitis, esophagitis

Emetic potential:

≤20 mg: Moderately low (10% to 30%)

>20 mg or < 60 mg: Moderate (30% to 60%)

≥60 mg: Moderately high (60% to 90%)

Time course for nausea/vomiting: Onset: 1-3 hours; Duration 4-24 hours

Genitourinary: Discoloration of urine (red)

Hematologic: Myelosuppressive: 60% to 80% of patients will have leukopenia; dose-limiting toxicity

WBC: Moderate

Platelets: Moderate

Onset (days): 7

Nadir (days): 10-14

Recovery (days): 21-28

Local: **Vesicant chemotherapy**

1% to 10%:

Cardiac toxicity: Dose-limiting and related to cumulative dose; usually a maximum total lifetime dose of 450-550 mg/m$^2$ is administered; although, it has been demonstrated that if given by continuous infusion in breast cancer patients, higher doses may be tolerated. Patients may present with acute toxicity (arrhythmias, heart block, pericarditis-myocarditis) which may be fatal. More commonly, chronic toxicity is seen, in which patients present with signs of congestive heart failure. Treatment includes aggressive management of CHF with digoxin, diuretics and peripheral vasodilators. Several methods of monitoring cardiac toxicity have been utilized, including myocardial biopsy (expensive and hazardous procedure).

Cardiovascular: Facial flushing

Dermatologic: Hyperpigmentation of nail beds, erythematous streaking along the vein if administered rapidly

Endocrine & metabolic: Hyperuricemia

<1% (Limited to important or life-threatening symptoms):

Pediatric patients may be at increased risk of later neoplastic disease, particularly acute myeloid leukemia (pediatric patients). Prepubertal growth failure may result from intensive chemotherapy regimens.

Radiation recall: Noticed in patients who have had prior irradiation; reactions include redness, warmth, erythema, and dermatitis in the radiation port. Can progress to severe desquamation and ulceration. Occurs 5-7 days after doxorubicin administration; local therapy with topical corticosteroids and cooling have given the best relief.

**Overdose/Toxicology** Symptoms of overdose include myelosuppression, nausea, vomiting, and myocardial toxicity. Treatment of acute overdose consists of treatment of the severely myelosuppressed patient with hospitalization, antibiotics, platelet and granulocyte transfusions, and symptomatic treatment of mucositis.

**Pharmacodynamics/Kinetics**

**Protein Binding:** 70% bound to plasma proteins

**Distribution:** Rapidly distributed into the liver, spleen, kidney, lung, and heart

**Half-life Elimination:** Triphasic:

Primary: 30 minutes

Secondary: 3-3.5 hours for metabolites
Terminal: 17-30 hours for doxorubicin and its metabolites
Male: 54 hours; female: 35 hours
Creatinine clearance: Male: 113 L/hour; female: 44 L/hour

**Metabolism:** In both the liver and in plasma to both active and inactive metabolites

**Excretion:** 80% eventually excreted in bile and feces

**Formulations**

Doxorubicin hydrochloride:
- Aqueous injection with NS: 2 mg/mL (5 mL, 10 mL, 25 mL)
- Preservative free injection: 2 mg/mL (5 mL, 10 mL, 25 mL, 100 mL)
- Powder for injection, lyophilized: 10 mg, 20 mg, 50 mg, 100 mg
- Powder for injection, lyophilized, rapid dissolution formula: 10 mg, 20 mg, 50 mg, 150 mg

**Dosing**

**Adults:** Refer to individual protocols.

I.V. (patient's ideal weight should be used to calculate body surface area):

60-75 mg/m$^2$ as a single dose, repeat every 21 days **or** other dosage regimens like 20-30 mg/m$^2$/day for 2-3 days, repeat in 4 weeks **or** 20 mg/m$^2$ once weekly.

The lower dose regimen should be given to patients with decreased bone marrow reserve, prior therapy or marrow infiltration with malignant cells.

Currently the maximum cumulative dose is 550 mg/m$^2$ or 450 mg/m$^2$ in patients who have received RT to the mediastinal areas; a baseline MUGA should be performed prior to initiating treatment. If the LVEF is <30% to 40%, therapy should not be instituted; LVEF should be monitored during therapy.

Doxorubicin has also been administered intraperitoneal (Phase I in refractory ovarian cancer patients) and intra-arterially.

**Elderly:** Refer to adult dosing.

**Renal Impairment:**

Adjustments are not required.
Hemodialysis effects: Supplemental dose is not necessary.

**Hepatic Impairment:**

Bilirubin 1.5-3 mg/dL: Administer 50% of dose.
Bilirubin 3.1-5 mg/dL: Administer 25% of dose.

**Administration**

**I.V.:** Vesicant. Administer I.V. push over 1-2 minutes or IVPB.

**I.V. Detail:** May be further diluted in either NS of $D_5W$ for I.V. administration. Avoid extravasation associated with severe ulceration and soft tissue necrosis. Flush with 5-10 mL of I.V. solution before and after drug administration.

**Extravasation management:** Apply ice immediately for 30-60 minutes; then alternate off/on every 15 minutes for 1 day. Topical cooling may be achieved using ice packs or cooling pad with circulating ice water. Cooling of site for 24 hours as tolerated by the patient. Elevate and rest extremity 24-48 hours, then resume normal activity as tolerated. Application of cold inhibits vesicant's cytotoxicity. **Application of heat or sodium bicarbonate can be harmful and is contraindicated.** If pain, erythema, and/or swelling persist beyond 48 hours, refer patient immediately to plastic surgeon for consultation and possible debridement.

**Stability**

**Storage:** Store intact vials of solution under refrigeration at 2°C to 8°C and protected from light. Store intact vials of lyophilized powder at room temperature (15°C to 30°C).

**Reconstitution:** Reconstitute lyophilized powder with SWI or NS to a final concentration of 2 mg/mL as follows. Reconstituted solution is stable for 7 days at room temperature (25°C) and 15 days under refrigeration (5°C) when protected from light.

10 mg vial = 5 mL
20 mg vial = 10 mL
50 mg vial = 25 mL

Further dilution in $D_5W$ or NS is stable for 48 hours at room temperature (25°C) when protected from light

Unstable in solutions with a pH <3 or >7. Avoid aluminum needles and bacteriostatic diluents as precipitation occurs. Decomposing drug turns purple. Protect from direct sunlight.

**Standard I.V. dilution:**

I.V. push: Dose/syringe (concentration: 2 mg/mL)

Maximum syringe size for IVP is a 30 mL syringe and syringe should be ≤75% full. Syringes are stable for 7 days at room temperature (25°C) and 15 days under refrigeration (5°C) when protected from light.

IVPB: Dose/50-100 mL $D_5W$ or NS

IVPB solutions are stable for 48 hours at room temperature (25°C) when protected from light.

**Compatibility:** Incompatible with hydrocortisone, fluorouracil, sodium bicarbonate, aminophylline, heparin, cephalothin, dexamethasone, furosemide, dexamethasone, and diazepam. Y-site compatible with vincristine, cyclophosphamide, dacarbazine, bleomycin, and vinblastine. See the Chemotherapy Compatibility Chart *on page 1311.*

**Monitoring Laboratory Tests** CBC with differential, platelet count, echocardiogram, liver function

**Additional Nursing Issues**

**Physical Assessment:** Monitor I.V. site for extravasation. Monitor for local erythematous streaking along vein and/or facial flushing (may indicate rapid infusion rate). Monitor for acute GI reactions, diarrhea (administer antiemetics 30-45 minutes before therapy and around-the-clock if needed). Monitor food and fluid intake (encourage

(Continued)

## Doxorubicin *(Continued)*

small frequent meals and a minimum of 2-3 L water/day). Monitor closely for cardiac or respiratory changes which may indicate cardiac toxicity. **Pregnancy risk factor D** - assess knowledge/teach appropriate use of barrier contraceptives. Breast-feeding is contraindicated.

**Patient Information/Instruction:** This medication can only be administered I.V. During therapy, do not use alcohol, aspirin-containing products, and OTC medications without consulting prescriber. It is important to maintain adequate nutrition and hydration (2-3 L/day of fluids unless instructed to restrict fluid intake) during therapy; frequent small meals may help. You may experience nausea or vomiting (frequent small meals, frequent mouth care, sucking lozenges, or chewing gum may help). You may experience loss of hair (reversible); you will be more susceptible to infection (avoid crowds and exposure to infection as much as possible). Urine may turn red-brown (normal). Yogurt or buttermilk may help reduce diarrhea (if unresolved, contact prescriber for medication relief). Frequent mouth care and use of a soft toothbrush or cotton swabs may reduce mouth sores. May discolor urine (red/pink). Report fever, chills, unusual bruising or bleeding, signs of infection, abdominal pain or blood in stools, excessive fatigue, yellowing of eyes or skin, swelling of extremities, difficulty breathing, or unresolved diarrhea. **Pregnancy/breast-feeding precautions:** Do not get pregnant or cause a pregnancy (males) while taking this medication; use appropriate barrier contraceptive measures for at least 1 month following therapy. Do not breast-feed.

## Doxorubicin (Liposomal) (doks oh ROO bi sin lip pah SOW mal)

**U.S. Brand Names** Doxil®

**Therapeutic Category** Antineoplastic Agent, Anthracycline; Antineoplastic Agent, Antibiotic

**Pregnancy Risk Factor** D

**Lactation** Enters breast milk/contraindicated

**Use** Treatment of AIDS-related Kaposi's sarcoma in patients with disease that has progressed on prior combination chemotherapy or in patients who are intolerant to such therapy

**Mechanism of Action/Effect** Inhibits DNA and RNA synthesis of susceptible bacteria, active throughout cell cycle, results in cell death

**Contraindications** Hypersensitivity to doxorubicin or any component; pregnancy

**Warnings** The U.S. Food and Drug Administration (FDA) currently recommends that procedures for proper handling and disposal of antineoplastic agents be considered. Total dose should not exceed 550 mg/m$^2$ or 400 mg/m$^2$ in patients with previous or concomitant treatment (with daunorubicin, cyclophosphamide, or irradiation of the cardiac region). Irreversible myocardial toxicity may occur as total dosage approaches 550 mg/m$^2$. I.V. use only, severe local tissue necrosis will result if extravasation occurs. Reduce dose in patients with impaired hepatic function. Severe myelosuppression is also possible.

Doxorubicin (liposomal) preparation should be performed in a Class II laminar flow biologic safety cabinet. Personnel should be wearing surgical gloves and a closed front surgical gown with knit cuffs. Appropriate safety equipment is recommended for preparation, administration, and disposal of antineoplastics. If doxorubicin contacts the skin, wash and flush thoroughly with water.

**Drug Interactions**

**Cytochrome P-450 Effect:** CYP3A3/4 enzyme substrate; CYP2D6 enzyme inhibitor

**Decreased Effect:** No formal drug interaction studies have been conducted with doxorubicin hydrochloride liposome injection; however, it may interact with drugs known to interact with the conventional formulation of doxorubicin hydrochloride. Doxorubicin may decrease plasma levels and effectiveness of digoxin and phenytoin. Phenobarbital increases elimination (decreases effect) of doxorubicin.

**Increased Effect/Toxicity:** No formal drug interaction studies have been conducted with doxorubicin hydrochloride liposome injection; however, it may interact with drugs known to interact with the conventional formulation of doxorubicin hydrochloride. Allopurinol may enhance the antitumor activity of doxorubicin (animal data only). Cyclosporine may induce coma or seizures. Cyclophosphamide enhances the cardiac toxicity of doxorubicin by producing additional myocardial cell damage. Mercaptopurine increases toxicities. Streptozocin greatly enhances leukopenia and thrombocytopenia. Verapamil alters the cellular distribution of doxorubicin and may result in increased cell toxicity by inhibition of the P-glycoprotein pump.

**Adverse Reactions** Information on adverse events is based on the experience reported in 753 patients with AIDS-related Kaposi's sarcoma enrolled in four studies.

>10%:

- Gastrointestinal: Nausea; emetic potential:
  - ≤20 mg: Moderately low (10% to 30%)
  - >20 mg or <75 mg: Moderate (30% to 60%)
  - ≥75 mg: Moderately high (49%)
- Hematologic: Myelosuppressive: 60% to 80% of patients will have leukopenia; dose-limiting toxicity
  - WBC: Moderate
  - Platelets: Moderate
  - Onset (days): 7
  - Nadir (days): 10-14
  - Recovery (days): 21-28
- Local: **Irritant chemotherapy**

1% to 10%:

Cardiovascular: Cardiac toxicity (9.7%): Cardiomyopathy, congestive heart failure, arrhythmia, pericardial effusion, tachycardia, facial flushing

Dermatologic: Hyperpigmentation of nail beds, erythematous streaking along the vein if administered rapidly

Endocrine & metabolic: Hyperuricemia

**Overdose/Toxicology** Symptoms of overdose include increases in mucositis, leukopenia, and thrombocytopenia. For acute overdose, treatment of the severely myelosuppressed patient consists of hospitalization, antibiotics, platelet and granulocyte transfusion, and symptomatic treatment of mucositis.

**Pharmacodynamics/Kinetics**

**Protein Binding:** Doxorubicin: 70% bound to plasma proteins

**Metabolism:** Liver and in plasma to both active and inactive metabolites

**Excretion:** Mean clearance value of 0.041 L/hour/$m^2$

**Formulations** Injection, as hydrochloride: 2 mg/mL (10 mL)

**Dosing**

**Adults:** Refer to individual protocols.

I.V. (patient's ideal weight should be used to calculate body surface area): 20 mg/$m^2$ over 30 minutes, once every 3 weeks, for as long as patients respond satisfactorily and tolerate treatment

**Elderly:** Refer to adult dosing.

**Hepatic Impairment:**

Bilirubin 1.2-3 mg/dL: Administer 50% of dose.

Bilirubin >3 mg/dL: Administer 25% of dose.

**Administration**

**I.V.:** Irritant. Administer IVPB over 30 minutes. Further dilute in $D_5W$. Do not administer as a bolus injection or undiluted solution. **Do not administer intramuscular or subcutaneous.**

**I.V. Detail:** Avoid extravasation associated with severe ulceration and soft tissue necrosis. Flush with 5-10 mL of $D_5W$ solution before and after drug administration.

**Extravasation management:** Apply ice immediately for 30-60 minutes; then alternate off/on every 15 minutes for 1 day. Topical cooling may be achieved using ice packs or cooling pad with circulating ice water. Cooling of site for 24 hours as tolerated by the patient. Elevate and rest extremity 24-48 hours, then resume normal activity as tolerated. Application of cold inhibits vesicant's cytotoxicity. **Application of heat or sodium bicarbonate can be harmful and is contraindicated.** If pain, erythema, and/or swelling persist beyond 48 hours, refer patient immediately to plastic surgeon for consultation and possible debridement.

**Stability**

**Storage:** Store intact vials of solution under refrigeration at 2°C to 8°C and avoid freezing. Prolonged freezing may adversely affect liposomal drug products, however, short-term freezing (<1 month) does not appear to have a deleterious effect.

**Reconstitution:** The appropriate dose (up to a maximum of 90 mg) must be diluted in 250 mL of dextrose 5% in water prior to administration. Diluted doxorubicin hydrochloride liposome injection is stable when refrigerated at 2°C to 8°C for 48 hours. When stored at room temperature, remains stable for 24 hours. **Do not use with in-line filters.**

**Compatibility:** Incompatible with heparin or fluorouracil. See the Chemotherapy Compatibility Chart *on page 1311*.

**Monitoring Laboratory Tests** CBC with differential, platelet count, echocardiogram, liver function

**Additional Nursing Issues**

**Physical Assessment:** Monitor I.V. site for extravasation. Monitor for local erythematous streaking along vein and/or facial flushing (may indicate rapid infusion rate). Monitor for acute GI reactions, diarrhea (administer antiemetics 30-45 minutes before therapy and around-the-clock if needed). Monitor food and fluid intake (encourage small frequent meals and a minimum of 2-3 L water/day). Monitor closely for cardiac or respiratory changes which may indicate cardiac toxicity. **Pregnancy risk factor D** - assess knowledge/teach appropriate use of barrier contraceptives. Breast-feeding is contraindicated.

**Patient Information/Instruction:** This medication can only be administered I.V. During therapy, do not use alcohol, aspirin-containing products, and OTC medications without consulting prescriber. It is important to maintain adequate nutrition and hydration (2-3 L/day of fluids unless instructed to restrict fluid intake) during therapy; frequent small meals may help. You may experience nausea or vomiting (frequent small meals, frequent mouth care, sucking lozenges, or chewing gum may help). You may experience loss of hair (reversible); you will be more susceptible to infection (avoid crowds and exposure to infection as much as possible). Urine may turn red-brown (normal). Yogurt or buttermilk may help reduce diarrhea (if unresolved, contact prescriber for medication relief). Frequent mouth care and use of a soft toothbrush or cotton swabs may reduce mouth sores. Report fever, chills, unusual bruising or bleeding, signs of infection, abdominal pain or blood in stools, excessive fatigue, yellowing of eyes or skin, darkening in color of urine or pale colored stools, swelling of extremities, difficulty breathing, or unresolved diarrhea. **Pregnancy/breast-feeding precautions:** Do not get pregnant or cause a pregnancy (males) while taking this medication; use appropriate barrier contraceptive measures for at least 1 month following therapy. Do not breast-feed.

♦ **Doxy®** *see* Doxycycline *on next page*

♦ **Doxychel®** *see* Doxycycline *on next page*

♦ **Doxycin** *see* Doxycycline *on this page*

## Doxycycline (doks i SYE kleen)

**U.S. Brand Names** Atridox™; Doryx®; Doxy®; Doxychel®; Periostat™; Vibramycin®; Vibra-Tabs®

**Therapeutic Category** Antibiotic, Tetracycline Derivative

**Pregnancy Risk Factor** D

**Lactation** Enters breast milk/not recommended

**Use**

Dental: Treatment of periodontitis associated with presence of *Actinobacillus actinomycetemcomitans* (AA)

Atridox™ gel and Periostat™ capsules are indicated for the treatment of adult periodontitis

Medical: Principally in the treatment of infections caused by susceptible *Rickettsia*, *Chlamydia*, and *Mycoplasma* along with uncommon susceptible gram-negative and gram-positive organisms; alternative to mefloquine for malaria prophylaxis

**Unapproved use:** Treatment for syphilis in penicillin-allergic patients; sclerosing agent for pleural effusions

**Mechanism of Action/Effect** Inhibits protein synthesis by binding with the 30S and possibly the 50S ribosomal subunit(s) of susceptible bacteria; may also cause alterations in the cytoplasmic membrane

Doxycycline inhibits collagenase *in vitro* and has been shown to inhibit collagenase in the gingival crevicular fluid in adults with periodontitis

**Contraindications** Hypersensitivity to doxycycline, tetracycline, or any component; children <8 years of age; severe hepatic dysfunction; pregnancy

**Warnings** Do not use during pregnancy - use of tetracyclines during tooth development may cause permanent discoloration of the teeth and enamel hypoplasia. Prolonged use may result in superinfection, including oral or vaginal candidiasis. Photosensitivity reaction may occur with this drug; avoid prolonged exposure to sunlight or tanning equipment.

**Drug Interactions**

**Cytochrome P-450 Effect:** CYP3A3/4 enzyme substrate

**Decreased Effect:** Decreased effect when taken with antacids containing aluminum, calcium, or magnesium. Decreased bioavailability or half-life when taken with iron, bismuth subsalicylate, barbiturates, phenytoin, and carbamazepine. Tetracyclines decrease the contraceptive effect of oral contraceptives. Concurrent use of tetracycline and Penthrane has been reported to result in fatal renal toxicity.

**Increased Effect/Toxicity:** Increased digoxin toxicity when taken with digoxin. Increased prothrombin time with warfarin.

**Food Interactions** Doxycycline serum levels may be decreased if taken with food.

**Effects on Lab Values** False-negative urine glucose using Clinistix®

**Adverse Reactions**

>10%:

- Central nervous system: Dizziness, lightheadedness, unsteadiness
- Dermatologic: Photosensitivity
- Gastrointestinal: Nausea, diarrhea
- Miscellaneous: Discoloration of teeth in children

1% to 10%:

- Gastrointestinal: Pancreatitis, hypertrophy of the papilla
- Hepatic: Hepatotoxicity
- Miscellaneous: Superinfections (fungal overgrowth)

<1% (Limited to important or life-threatening symptoms): Pericarditis, increased intracranial pressure, bulging fontanels in infants, exfoliative dermatitis, acute renal failure, azotemia

**Overdose/Toxicology** Symptoms of overdose include nausea, anorexia, and diarrhea. Treatment is supportive.

**Pharmacodynamics/Kinetics**

**Protein Binding:** 90%

**Half-life Elimination:** 12-15 hours (usually increases to 22-24 hours with multiple dosing); End-stage renal disease: 18-25 hours

**Time to Peak:** Within 1.5-4 hours

**Metabolism:** Partially inactivated in the GI tract

**Excretion:** Urine and feces

**Formulations**

Capsule, as hyclate:

- Periostat™: 20 mg
- Doxychel®, Vibramycin®: 50 mg
- Doxy®, Doxychel®, Vibramycin®: 100 mg

Capsule, coated pellets, as hyclate (Doryx®): 100 mg

Gel, for subgingival application: Atridox™: 50 mg in each 500 mg of blended formulation; 2-syringe system contains doxycycline syringe (50 mg) and delivery system syringe (450 mg) along with a blunt cannula

Powder for injection, as hyclate (Doxy®, Doxychel®, Vibramycin® IV): 100 mg, 200 mg

Powder for oral suspension, as monohydrate (raspberry flavor) (Vibramycin®): 25 mg/5 mL (60 mL)

Syrup, as calcium (raspberry-apple flavor) (Vibramycin®): 50 mg/5 mL (30 mL, 473 mL)

Tablet, as hyclate

- Doxychel®: 50 mg
- Doxychel®, Vibra-Tabs®: 100 mg

**Dosing**

**Adults:** Oral, I.V.:

Acute gonococcal infection: 200 mg immediately, then 100 mg at bedtime on the first day followed by 100 mg twice daily for 3 days **or** 300 mg immediately followed by 300 mg in 1 hour

Primary and secondary syphilis: 300 mg/day in divided doses for ≥10 days

Uncomplicated chlamydial infections: 100 mg twice daily for ≥7 days

Endometritis, salpingitis, parametritis, or peritonitis: 100 mg I.V. twice daily with cefoxitin 2 g every 6 hours for 4 days and for ≥48 hours after patient improves; then continue with oral therapy 100 mg twice daily to complete a 10- to 14-day course of therapy

Sclerosing agent for pleural effusion injection: 500 mg as a single dose in 30-50 mL of NS or SWI

Dental: As adjunctive treatment for periodontitis: 20 mg twice daily at least 1 hour before morning and evening meals for up to 9 months

Subgingival application: Dose depends on size, shape and number of pockets treated. Contains 50 mg doxycycline per 500 mg of formulation in each final blended syringe product. Application may be repeated 4 months after initial treatment.

**Elderly:** Refer to adult dosing.

**Renal Impairment:**

No change is necessary.

Not dialyzable; 0% to 5% by hemo- and peritoneal methods or by continuous arteriovenous or venovenous hemofiltration (CAVH/CAVHD); no supplemental dosage is necessary.

**Administration**

**Oral:** May give with meals to decrease GI upset.

**I.V.:** Infuse slowly, usually over 1-4 hours.

**I.V. Detail:** Avoid extravasation.

**Other:** See manufacturer's information for administration procedures for Atridox™ gel.

**Stability**

**Storage:** Protect solution from direct sunlight. Store dental gel at 2°C to 8°C (36°F to 46°F). After mixing, coupled syringes may be stored for a maximum of 3 days at room temperature.

**Monitoring Laboratory Tests** Perform culture and sensitivity testing prior to initiating therapy.

**Additional Nursing Issues**

**Physical Assessment:** Monitor effectiveness of therapy and patient's knowledge of administration guidelines. Monitor I.V. closely; can be very irritating. Avoid extravasation. **Pregnancy risk factor D** - assess knowledge/teach appropriate use of barrier contraceptives. Breast-feeding is not recommended.

**Patient Information/Instruction:** Take as directed, for the entire prescription, even if you are feeling better. Avoid alcohol and maintain adequate hydration (2-3 L/day of fluids unless instructed to restrict fluid intake). You may be very sensitive to sunlight; use sunblock, wear protective clothing and eyewear, or avoid exposure to direct sunlight. You may experience lightheadedness, dizziness, or drowsiness (use caution when driving or engaging in tasks that require alertness until response to drug is known); nausea or vomiting (small frequent meals, frequent mouth care, sucking lozenges, or chewing gum may help); or diarrhea (buttermilk, boiled milk, or yogurt may help). If diabetic, drug may cause false tests with Clinitest® urine glucose monitoring; use of glucose oxidase methods (Clinistix®) or serum glucose monitoring is preferable. Report skin rash or itching, easy bruising or bleeding, yellowing of skin or eyes, pale stool or dark urine, unhealed sores of mouth, itching or vaginal discharge, fever or chills, or unusual cough. **Pregnancy/breast-feeding precautions:** Do not get pregnant while taking this medication - Oral contraceptives effectiveness may be reduced; use appropriate barrier contraceptive measures. Breast-feeding is not recommended.

**Dietary Issues:** Administration with iron, calcium, milk or other dairy products may decrease doxycycline absorption. May decrease absorption of calcium, iron, magnesium, zinc, and amino acids,

**Additional Information** pH: 1.8-3.3


- **Doxytec** *see* Doxycycline *on previous page*
- **DPA** *see* Valproic Acid and Derivatives *on page 1198*
- **D-Penicillamine** *see* Penicillamine *on page 894*
- **DPH** *see* Phenytoin *on page 923*
- **DPT** *see page 1256*
- **Dramamine® II [OTC]** *see* Meclizine *on page 712*
- **Dramamine® Oral** *see page 1294*
- **Dri/Ear®** *see page 1291*
- **Dri-Ear® Otic** *see page 1294*
- **Driken** *see* Iron Dextran Complex *on page 626*
- **Drisdol® Oral** *see* Ergocalciferol *on page 432*
- **Dristan® Cold Caplets** *see page 1294*
- **Dristan® Long Lasting Nasal Solution** *see page 1294*
- **Dristan® Saline Spray** *see page 1294*
- **Dristan® Sinus Caplets** *see page 1294*
- **Drithocreme®** *see* Anthralin *on page 98*
- **Drithocreme® HP 1%** *see* Anthralin *on page 98*

- **Dritho-Scalp®** *see* Anthralin *on page 98*
- **Drixomed®** *see page 1294*
- **Drixoral®** *see page 1294*
- **Drixoral® Cough & Congestion Liquid Caps** *see page 1294*
- **Drixoral® Cough Liquid Caps** *see page 1294*
- **Drixoral® Cough & Sore Throat Liquid Caps** *see page 1294*
- **Drixoral® Nasal** *see page 1294*
- **Drixoral® Non-Drowsy [OTC]** *see* Pseudoephedrine *on page 992*
- **Drixoral® Syrup** *see page 1294*


## Dronabinol (droe NAB i nol)

**U.S. Brand Names** Marinol®

**Synonyms** Tetrahydrocannabinol; THC

**Therapeutic Category** Antiemetic

**Pregnancy Risk Factor** C

**Lactation** Enters breast milk/contraindicated

**Use** When conventional antiemetics fail to relieve the nausea and vomiting associated with cancer chemotherapy, AIDS-related anorexia

**Mechanism of Action/Effect** Not well defined, probably inhibits the vomiting center in the medulla oblongata

**Contraindications** Hypersensitivity to dronabinol or any component; use only for cancer chemotherapy-induced nausea; patients with a history of schizophrenia

**Warnings** Use with caution in patients with heart disease, hepatic disease, or seizure disorders. Reduce dosage in patients with severe hepatic impairment. May have potential for abuse; drug is psychoactive substance in marijuana. Monitor for possible psychotic reaction with first dose. Pregnancy factor C.

**Drug Interactions**

**Cytochrome P-450 Effect:** CYP2C18 and 3A3/4 enzyme substrate

**Increased Effect/Toxicity:** Increased toxicity (drowsiness) with alcohol, barbiturates, and benzodiazepines.

**Effects on Lab Values** ↓ FSH, LH, growth hormone, testosterone

**Adverse Reactions** >10%:

Central nervous system: Drowsiness, dizziness, anxiety, trouble thinking

Gastrointestinal: Nausea, vomiting

Neuromuscular & skeletal: Clumsiness or unsteadiness

Cardiovascular: Orthostatic hypotension, tachycardia

Central nervous system: Depression, restlessness headache, hallucinations, mood change

Gastrointestinal: Dry mouth

Neuromuscular & skeletal: Paresthesia, weakness

**Overdose/Toxicology** Symptoms of overdose include tachycardia, hyper- and hypotension. Treatment is symptomatic.

**Pharmacodynamics/Kinetics**

**Protein Binding:** 97% to 99%

**Half-life Elimination:** 19-24 hours

**Time to Peak:** Within 2-3 hours

**Metabolism:** Liver

**Excretion:** Feces and urine

**Onset:** Within 1 hour

**Formulations** Capsule: 2.5 mg, 5 mg, 10 mg

**Dosing**

**Adults:** Oral: 5 mg/m$^2$ 1-3 hours before chemotherapy, then give 5 mg/m$^2$/dose every 2-4 hours after chemotherapy for a total of 4-6 doses/day; dose may be increased up to a maximum of 15 mg/m$^2$/dose if needed (dosage may be increased by 2.5 mg/m$^2$ increments).

Appetite stimulant (AIDS-related): Initial: 2.5 mg twice daily (before lunch and dinner); titrate up to a maximum of 20 mg/day.

**Elderly:** Refer to adult dosing.

**Hepatic Impairment:** Usual dose should be reduced in patients with severe liver failure.

**Stability**

**Storage:** Store in a cool place.

**Additional Nursing Issues**

**Physical Assessment:** Assess interactions of other medications (see Drug Interactions). See Warnings/Precautions and Contraindications for use cautions. Monitor effectiveness of therapy, adverse response (eg, severe psychotic reactions - this drug is the psychoactive substance in marijuana) (see Adverse Reactions and Overdose/Toxicology). Assess knowledge/teach patient appropriate use, possible side effects and appropriate interventions, and adverse symptoms to report. **Pregnancy risk factor C** - benefits of use should outweigh possible risks. Breast-feeding is contraindicated.

**Patient Information/Instruction:** Take exactly as directed; do not increase dose or take more often than prescribed. Do not use alcohol or other depressant medications without consulting prescriber. You may experience psychotic reaction, impaired coordination or judgment, faintness, dizziness, or drowsiness (do not drive or engage in activities that require alertness and coordination until response to drug is known); clumsiness, unsteadiness, or muscular weakness (change position slowly and use caution when climbing stairs). Report excessive or persistent CNS changes (euphoria, anxiety, depression, memory lapse, bizarre though patterns, excitability, inability to control thoughts or behavior, fainting), respiratory difficulties, rapid heartbeat, or other adverse reactions. **Pregnancy/breast-feeding precautions:** Inform prescriber if you are or intend to be pregnant. Do not breast-feed.

**Related Information**

Antiemetics for Chemotherapy-Induced Nausea and Vomiting *on page 1307*

## Droperidol (droe PER i dole)

**U.S. Brand Names** Inapsine®

**Therapeutic Category** Antiemetic

**Pregnancy Risk Factor** C

**Lactation** Excretion in breast milk unknown

**Use** Tranquilizer and antiemetic in surgical and diagnostic procedures; antiemetic for cancer chemotherapy; preoperative medication; has good antiemetic effect as well as sedative and antianxiety effects

**Mechanism of Action/Effect** Alters the action of dopamine in the CNS, at subcortical levels, to produce sedation; reduces emesis by blocking dopamine stimulation of the chemotrigger zone

**Contraindications** Hypersensitivity to droperidol or any component

**Warnings** Use with caution in patients with seizures, bone marrow depression, severe liver disease, or respiratory disorders. Significant hypotension may occur, especially when the drug is administered parenterally. (Injection contains benzyl alcohol and sulfites which may cause allergic reactions). Antipsychotic related sedation in nonpsychotic patients is extremely unpleasant due to feelings of depersonalization, derealization, and dysphoria. Life-threatening arrhythmias have occurred at therapeutic doses of antipsychotics.

Pregnancy factor C.

**Elderly:** Development of tardive dyskinesia (TD) may be 40% in the elderly. Development of the syndrome and the irreversible nature are related to duration and total cumulative dose over time. TD syndrome may be somewhat reversible if diagnosed early enough. Drug induced **Parkinson's syndrome** and **akathisia** may occur as often as 50% in patients older than 60 years. Increased confusion, memory loss, psychotic behavior, and agitation frequently occur as a consequence of anticholinergic effects. The elderly are also at a much greater risk for orthostatic hypotension.

**Drug Interactions**

**Increased Effect/Toxicity:** Other CNS depressants may cause additive effects (CNS or respiratory depression, etc). Droperidol plus fentanyl or other analgesics may increase blood pressure. Induction anesthesia may increase hypotension. Droperidol plus epinephrine may decrease blood pressure due to alpha-adrenergic blockade effects of droperidol. Droperidol plus atropine may cause tachycardia.

**Adverse Reactions**

>10%:
- Cardiovascular: Mild to moderate hypotension, tachycardia
- Central nervous system: Postoperative drowsiness

1% to 10%:
- Cardiovascular: Hypertension
- Central nervous system: Extrapyramidal reactions
- Respiratory: Respiratory depression

<1% (Limited to important or life-threatening symptoms): Laryngospasm, bronchospasm

**Overdose/Toxicology** Symptoms of overdose include hypotension, tachycardia, hallucinations, and extrapyramidal symptoms. Following initiation of essential overdose management, toxic symptom treatment and supportive treatment should be initiated.

**Pharmacodynamics/Kinetics**

**Half-life Elimination:** 2.3 hours

**Metabolism:** Liver

**Excretion:** Urine and feces

**Onset:** Following parenteral administration: Peak effect: Within 30 minutes

**Duration:** Following parenteral administration: 2-4 hours, may extend to 12 hours

**Formulations** Injection: 2.5 mg/mL (1 mL, 2 mL, 5 mL, 10 mL)

**Dosing**

**Adults:** Titrate carefully to desired effect
- Premedication: I.M.: 2.5-10 mg 30 minutes to 1 hour preoperatively
- Adjunct to general anesthesia: I.V. induction: 0.22-0.275 mg/kg; maintenance: 1.25-2.5 mg/dose
- Alone in diagnostic procedures: I.M.: Initial: 2.5-10 mg 30 minutes to 1 hour before; then 1.25-2.5 mg if needed
- Nausea and vomiting: I.M., I.V.: 2.5-5 mg/dose every 3-4 hours as needed

**Elderly:** Elderly patients should be started on lowest dose recommendations for adults; titrate carefully to desired effect.

**Administration**

**I.V.:** I.V. should be administered slow IVP (over 2-5 minutes) or IVPB.

**Stability**

**Storage:** Droperidol ampuls/vials should be stored at room temperature and protected from light.

**Reconstitution:**
- Standard diluent: 2.5 mg/50 mL $D_5W$
- Stability of parenteral admixture at room temperature (25°C): 7 days

(Continued)

## Droperidol *(Continued)*

**Compatibility:** Incompatible with barbiturates.

**Additional Nursing Issues**

**Physical Assessment:** Assess other medications the patient may be taking for effectiveness and interactions (see Drug Interactions). See Contraindications and Warnings/Precautions for cautious use. Monitor vital signs and respiratory status on a frequent basis immediately following administration and for several hours afterward. Monitor for extrapyramidal effects for 24-48 hours after therapy (see Adverse Reactions and Overdose/Toxicology). Use orthostatic hypotension precautions until the patient is stable. **Pregnancy risk factor C** - benefits of use should outweigh possible risks. Note breast-feeding caution.

**Patient Information/Instruction:** This drug may cause you to feel very sleepy; do not attempt to get up without assistance. Immediately report any difficulty breathing, confusion, loss of thought processes, or palpitations. **Pregnancy/breast-feeding precautions:** Inform prescriber if you are pregnant. Consult prescriber if breast-feeding.

**Geriatric Considerations:** Use of droperidol in the elderly may result in severe and often irreversible undesirable effects. Before initiating antipsychotic therapy, the clinician should investigate possible reversible causes.

**Related Information**

Antiemetics for Chemotherapy-Induced Nausea and Vomiting *on page 1307*

## Droperidol and Fentanyl (droe PER i dole & FEN ta nil)

**U.S. Brand Names** Innovar®

**Synonyms** Fentanyl and Droperidol

**Therapeutic Category** Analgesic, Combination (Narcotic)

**Pregnancy Risk Factor** C

**Lactation** Excretion in breast milk unknown

**Use** Produce and maintain analgesia and sedation during diagnostic or surgical procedures (neuroleptanalgesia and neuroleptanesthesia); adjunct to general anesthesia

**Formulations** Injection: Droperidol 2.5 mg and fentanyl 50 mcg per mL (2 mL, 5 mL)

**Dosing**

**Adults:**

Premedication: I.M.: 0.5-2 mL 30-60 minutes prior to surgery

Adjunct to general anesthesia: I.V.: 0.09-0.11 mL/kg as slow infusion (1 mL/1-2 minutes) until sleep occurs

**Elderly:** Refer to adult dosing.

**Additional Nursing Issues**

**Physical Assessment:** See individual components listed in Related Information. **Pregnancy risk factor C** - benefits of use should outweigh possible risks. Note breast-feeding caution.

**Patient Information/Instruction:** See individual components listed in Related Information. **Pregnancy/breast-feeding precautions:** Inform prescriber if you are on intend to get pregnant. Consult prescriber if breast-feeding.

**Related Information**

Droperidol *on previous page*

Fentanyl *on page 478*

- **Drotic®** *see page 1291*
- **Droxia™** *see* Hydroxyurea *on page 586*
- **Dr Scholl's® Athlete's Foot** *see page 1247*
- **Dr Scholl's® Cracked Heel Relief Cream [OTC]** *see* Lidocaine *on page 674*
- **Dr Scholl's® Disk** *see page 1294*
- **Dr Scholl's® Maximum Strength Tritin** *see page 1247*
- **Dr Scholl's® Wart Remover** *see page 1294*
- **Dry Eyes® Solution** *see page 1294*
- **Dry Eye® Therapy Solution** *see page 1294*
- **Dryox® Gel** *see page 1294*
- **Dryox® Wash** *see page 1294*
- **DSCG** *see* Cromolyn Sodium *on page 309*
- **DSMC Plus®** *see page 1294*
- **D-S-S® [OTC]** *see* Docusate *on page 392*
- **DSS** *see* Docusate *on page 392*
- **D-S-S Plus®** *see page 1294*
- **DTIC-Dome®** *see* Dacarbazine *on page 325*
- **DTO** *see* Opium Tincture *on page 857*
- **Duadacin® Capsule** *see page 1294*
- **Dulcolax®** *see page 1294*
- **Dull-C® [OTC]** *see* Ascorbic Acid *on page 108*
- **DuoCet™** *see* Hydrocodone and Acetaminophen *on page 568*
- **DuoFilm®** *see page 1294*
- **Duofilm® Solution** *see page 1294*
- **Duo-Medihaler® Aerosol** *see* Isoproterenol and Phenylephrine *on page 634*
- **DuoPlant® Gel** *see page 1294*
- **Duo-Trach®** *see* Lidocaine *on page 674*
- **DuP 753** *see* Losartan *on page 693*
- **Duphalac®** *see* Lactulose *on page 651*

- **Duplex® T** *see page 1294*
- **Durabolin® Injection** *see* Nandrolone *on page 806*
- **Duracef®** *see* Cefadroxil *on page 211*
- **Duradoce®** *see* Hydroxocobalamin *on page 583*
- **Duradyne DHC®** *see* Hydrocodone and Acetaminophen *on page 568*
- **Dura-Estrin® Injection** *see* Estradiol *on page 441*
- **Durafuss-G®** *see* Guaifenesin *on page 548*
- **Duragen® Injection** *see* Estradiol *on page 441*
- **Duragesic® Transdermal** *see* Fentanyl *on page 478*
- **Dura-Gest®** *see* Guaifenesin, Phenylpropanolamine, and Phenylephrine *on page 552*
- **Duralone® Injection** *see* Methylprednisolone *on page 754*
- **Duramist® Plus** *see page 1294*
- **Duramorph® Injection** *see* Morphine Sulfate *on page 790*
- **Durater** *see* Famotidine *on page 470*
- **Duratest® Injection** *see* Testosterone *on page 1108*
- **Durathate® Injection** *see* Testosterone *on page 1108*
- **Duration® Nasal Solution** *see page 1294*
- **Dura-Vent®** *see* Guaifenesin and Phenylpropanolamine *on page 550*
- **Dura-Vent/DA®** *see page 1306*
- **Duricef®** *see* Cefadroxil *on page 211*
- **Durogesic** *see* Fentanyl *on page 478*
- **Durrax®** *see* Hydroxyzine *on page 588*
- **Duvoid®** *see* Bethanechol *on page 151*
- **DV® Vaginal Cream** *see* Dienestrol *on page 365*
- **Dwelle® Ophthalmic Solution** *see page 1294*
- **D-Xylose** *see page 1248*
- **Dyazide®** *see* Hydrochlorothiazide and Triamterene *on page 568*
- **Dycill®** *see* Dicloxacillin *on page 361*
- **Dyclone®** *see* Dyclonine *on this page*

## Dyclonine (DYE kloe neen)

**U.S. Brand Names** Dyclone®; Sucrets® [OTC]

**Therapeutic Category** Local Anesthetic; Local Anesthetic, Oral

**Pregnancy Risk Factor** C

**Lactation** Excretion in breast milk unknown

**Use** Local anesthetic prior to laryngoscopy, bronchoscopy, or endotracheal intubation; use topically for temporary relief of pain associated with oral mucosa or anogenital lesions

**Mechanism of Action/Effect** Blocks impulses at peripheral nerve endings in skin and mucous membranes by altering cell membrane permeability to ionic transfer

**Contraindications** Contraindicated in patients allergic to chlorobutanol (preservative used in dyclonine) or dyclonine

**Warnings** Use with caution in patients with sepsis or traumatized mucosa in the area of application to avoid rapid systemic absorption. May impair swallowing and enhance the danger of aspiration. Use with caution in patients with shock or heart block. Resuscitative equipment, oxygen, and resuscitative drugs should be immediately available when dyclonine topical solution is administered to mucous membranes. **Not for injection or ophthalmic use.** Pregnancy factor C.

**Adverse Reactions** Dose-related and may result in high plasma levels

1% to 10%:

Dermatologic: Angioedema, contact dermatitis

Local: Burning, stinging

**Overdose/Toxicology** Symptoms of overdose are CNS (seizures, excitation) and cardiovascular (hypotension, myocardial depression). Treatment is supportive and symptomatic.

**Pharmacodynamics/Kinetics**

**Onset:** Onset of local anesthesia: 2-10 minutes

**Duration:** 30-60 minutes

**Formulations**

Dyclonine hydrochloride:

Lozenges: 1.2 mg, 3 mg

Solution, topical: 0.5% (30 mL); 1% (30 mL)

**Dosing**

**Adults:** Topical solution (use lowest dose needed to provide effective anesthesia):

Mouth sores: 5-10 mL of 0.5% or 1% to oral mucosa (swab or swish and then spit) 3-4 times/day as needed; maximum single dose: 200 mg (40 mL of 0.5% solution or 20 mL of 1% solution)

Bronchoscopy: Use 2 mL of the 1% solution or 4 mL of the 0.5% solution sprayed onto the larynx and trachea every 5 minutes until the reflex has been abolished

**Elderly:** Refer to adult dosing.

**Stability**

**Storage:** Store in tight, light-resistant containers.

**Additional Nursing Issues**

**Physical Assessment:** Observe condition of mucous membranes in area to be treated; avoid use in traumatized areas (see Warnings/Precautions). Monitor for effectiveness of anesthesia and for adverse or toxic reactions (seizures, hypotension, cardiac depression). Monitor for return of sensation (swallowing). Teach patient

(Continued)

## Dyclonine *(Continued)*

adverse reactions to report; use and teach appropriate interventions to promote safety. **Pregnancy risk factor C** - benefits of use should outweigh possible risks. Note breast-feeding caution.

**Patient Information/Instruction:** This medication is given to reduce sensation in the injected area. When used in mouth or throat; do not eat or drink anything for at least 1 hour following treatment. Take small sips of water at first to ensure that you can swallow without difficulty. Your tongue and mouth may be numb - use caution to avoid biting yourself. Immediately report swelling of face, lips, tongue; chest pain or palpitations; increased restlessness, confusion, anxiety, or dizziness. **Pregnancy/breast-feeding precautions:** Inform prescriber if you are or intend to be pregnant. Consult prescriber if breast-feeding.

- ♦ **Dynabac®** *see* Dirithromycin *on page 384*
- ♦ **Dynacin® Oral** *see* Minocycline *on page 774*
- ♦ **DynaCirc®** *see* Isradipine *on page 638*
- ♦ **DynaCirc SRO®** *see* Isradipine *on page 638*
- ♦ **Dynafed® Maximum Strength** *see page 1294*
- ♦ **Dynapen®** *see* Dicloxacillin *on page 361*
- ♦ **Dyrenium®** *see* Triamterene *on page 1173*
- ♦ **E2020** *see* Donepezil *on page 394*
- ♦ **Ear-Dri®** *see page 1291*
- ♦ **Ear Eze®** *see page 1291*
- ♦ **Ear-Sol®** *see page 1291*
- ♦ **Ear-Sol® H.C.** *see page 1291*
- ♦ **Easprin®** *see* Aspirin *on page 111*
- ♦ **E-Base®** *see* Erythromycin *on page 435*
- ♦ **Ecapresan** *see* Captopril *on page 192*
- ♦ **Ecaten** *see* Captopril *on page 192*
- ♦ **Echothiophate** *see* Ophthalmic Agents, Glaucoma *on page 853*
- ♦ **E-Complex-600® [OTC]** *see* Vitamin E *on page 1218*

## Econazole (e KONE a zole)

**U.S. Brand Names** Spectazole™ Topical

**Therapeutic Category** Antifungal Agent, Topical

**Pregnancy Risk Factor** C - see Pregnancy Issues

**Lactation** Excretion in breast milk unknown

**Use** Topical treatment of tinea pedis (athlete's foot), tinea cruris (jock itch), tinea corporis (ringworm), tinea versicolor, and cutaneous candidiasis

**Mechanism of Action/Effect** Alters fungal cell wall membrane permeability; may interfere with RNA and protein synthesis, and lipid metabolism of susceptible fungi; may be fungistatic or fungicidal

**Contraindications** Hypersensitivity to econazole, miconazole, or any component

**Warnings** Discontinue drug if sensitivity or chemical irritation occurs. Not for ophthalmic or intravaginal use. Pregnancy factor C.

**Adverse Reactions**

1% to 10%: Genitourinary: Vulvar/vaginal burning

<1% (Limited to important or life-threatening symptoms): Vulvar itching, soreness, edema, or discharge; polyuria; burning or itching of penis of sexual partner

**Pharmacodynamics/Kinetics**

**Metabolism:** Liver

**Excretion:** Urine and feces

**Formulations** Cream, as nitrate: 1% (15 g, 30 g, 85 g)

**Dosing**

**Adults:** Topical:

Tinea pedis, tinea cruris, tinea corporis, tinea versicolor: Apply sufficient amount to cover affected areas once daily.

Cutaneous candidiasis: Apply sufficient quantity twice daily (morning and evening).

Duration of treatment: Candidal infections and tinea cruris, versicolor, and corporis should be treated for 2 weeks and tinea pedis for 1 month; occasionally, longer treatment periods may be required.

**Elderly:** Refer to adult dosing.

**Administration**

**Topical:** Duration of treatment: Candidal infections and tinea cruris, versicolor, and corporis should be treated for 2 weeks and tinea pedis for 1 month. Occasionally, longer treatment periods may be required. For external use only. Avoid eye contact.

**Additional Nursing Issues**

**Physical Assessment:** Assess knowledge/teach patient appropriate application and use and adverse symptoms to report (see Adverse Reactions). **Pregnancy risk factor C.** Note breast-feeding caution.

**Patient Information/Instruction:** For external use only. Apply exactly as directed and for the length of time prescribed. Report if conditions worsens or persists or if infection occurs. **Pregnancy/breast-feeding precautions:** Inform prescriber if you are or intend to be pregnant. Consult prescriber if breast-feeding.

**Pregnancy Issues:** Should not be used during the 1st trimester of pregnancy, unless essential to patient's welfare. Use during the 2nd and 3rd trimesters only if necessary.

- ♦ **Econopred® Ophthalmic** *see* Prednisolone *on page 960*

- **Econopred® Plus Ophthalmic** *see* Prednisolone *on page 960*
- **Ecostatin®** *see* Econazole *on previous page*
- **Ecotrin® [OTC]** *see* Aspirin *on page 111*
- **Ectaprim®** *see* Co-trimoxazole *on page 307*
- **Ectaprim®-F** *see* Co-trimoxazole *on page 307*
- **Ectosone** *see* Betamethasone *on page 148*
- **Ectosone** *see* Topical Corticosteroids *on page 1152*
- **Ed A-Hist® Liquid** *see page 1294*
- **Edecrin®** *see* Ethacrynic Acid *on page 455*
- **Edenol** *see* Furosemide *on page 523*
- **Edex®** *see* Alprostadil *on page 56*
- **Edmar** *see* Astemizole *on page 114*


## Edrophonium (ed roe FOE nee um)

**U.S. Brand Names** Enlon® Injection; Reversol® Injection; Tensilon® Injection

**Therapeutic Category** Antidote; Cholinergic Agonist; Diagnostic Agent, Myasthenia Gravis

**Pregnancy Risk Factor** C

**Lactation** Excretion in breast milk unknown

**Use** Diagnosis of myasthenia gravis; differentiation of cholinergic from myasthenic crises; reversal of nondepolarizing neuromuscular blockers; treatment of paroxysmal atrial tachycardia

**Mechanism of Action/Effect** Inhibits destruction of acetylcholine by acetylcholinesterase. This facilitates transmission of impulses across myoneural junction and results in increased cholinergic responses such as miosis, increased tonus of intestinal and skeletal muscles, bronchial and ureteral constriction, bradycardia, and increased salivary and sweat gland secretions.

**Contraindications** Hypersensitivity to edrophonium or any component; GI or GU obstruction; hypersensitivity to sulfite agents

**Warnings** Use with caution in patients with bronchial asthma and those receiving a cardiac glycoside. Atropine sulfate should always be readily available as an antagonist. Overdosage can cause cholinergic crisis which may be fatal (DUMBELS - **d**iarrhea, **u**rination, **m**iosis, **b**ronchospasm/**b**radycardia, **e**xcitability, **l**acrimation, **s**alivation/excessive **s**weating), and acute muscle weakness. I.V. atropine should be readily available for treatment of cholinergic reactions. Pregnancy factor C.

**Drug Interactions**

**Decreased Effect:** Atropine, nondepolarizing muscle relaxants, procainamide, and quinidine may antagonize the effects of edrophonium.

**Increased Effect/Toxicity:** Digoxin may enhance bradycardia potential of edrophonium. Succinylcholine, decamethonium, nondepolarizing muscle relaxants (eg, pancuronium, vecuronium) effects are prolonged by edrophonium. I.V. acetazolamide, neostigmine, physostigmine, and acute muscle weakness may increase the effects of edrophonium.

**Effects on Lab Values** ↑ aminotransferase [ALT (SGPT)/AST (SGOT)] (S), amylase (S)

**Adverse Reactions**

>10%:

Gastrointestinal: Nausea, vomiting, diarrhea, excessive salivation, stomach cramps

Miscellaneous: Increased sweating

1% to 10%:

Genitourinary: Urinary frequency

Ocular: Small pupils, lacrimation

Respiratory: Increased bronchial secretions

<1% (Limited to important or life-threatening symptoms): Bradycardia, A-V block, seizures, laryngospasm, bronchospasm, respiratory paralysis

**Overdose/Toxicology** Symptoms of overdose include muscle weakness, nausea, vomiting, miosis, bronchospasm, and respiratory paralysis. Maintain an adequate airway. Antidote is atropine for muscarinic symptoms. Pralidoxime (2-PAM) may also be needed to reverse severe muscle weakness or paralysis. Skeletal muscle effects of edrophonium are not alleviated by atropine.

**Pharmacodynamics/Kinetics**

**Half-life Elimination:** 1.8 hours

**Onset:** I.M.: Within 2-10 minutes; I.V.: Within 30-60 seconds

**Duration:** I.M.: 5-30 minutes; I.V.: 10 minutes

**Formulations** Injection, as chloride: 10 mg/mL (1 mL, 10 mL, 15 mL)

**Dosing**

**Adults:** Usually administered I.V., however, if not possible, I.M. or S.C. may be used.

Diagnosis:

I.V.: 2 mg test dose administered over 15-30 seconds; 8 mg given 45 seconds later if no response is seen. Test dose may be repeated after 30 minutes.

I.M.: Initial: 10 mg; if no cholinergic reaction occurs, give 2 mg 30 minutes later to rule out false-negative reaction.

Titration of oral anticholinesterase therapy: 1-2 mg given 1 hour after oral dose of anticholinesterase; if strength improves, an increase in neostigmine or pyridostigmine dose is indicated.

Reversal of nondepolarizing neuromuscular blocking agents (neostigmine with atropine usually preferred): I.V.: 10 mg over 30-45 seconds; may repeat every 5-10 minutes up to 40 mg.

Termination of paroxysmal atrial tachycardia: I.V. rapid injection: 5-10 mg

(Continued)

## Edrophonium *(Continued)*

Differentiation of cholinergic from myasthenic crisis: I.V.: 1 mg; may repeat after 1 minute. **Note:** Intubation and controlled ventilation may be required if patient has cholinergic crisis.

**Elderly:** Refer to adult dosing.

**Renal Impairment:** Dose may need to be reduced in patients with chronic renal failure.

**Additional Nursing Issues**

**Physical Assessment:** While administration of edrophonium for MG diagnosis is supervised by a neurologist and use as a neuromuscular blocking agent is supervised by an anesthesiologist. Nursing responsibilities include careful monitoring of the patient. Monitor for cholinergic crisis; keep atropine at hand for antidote. Patients receiving the medication for MG testing will have been advised by their neurologist about drug effects. Those patients receiving medication for neuromuscular block will be unaware of drug effects. Teaching is unnecessary. Patient should not be left alone until all drug effects and the possibility of cholinergic crisis have passed. **Pregnancy risk factor C** - benefits of use should outweigh possible risks. Note breast-feeding caution.

**Patient Information/Instruction: Pregnancy/breast-feeding precautions:** Inform prescriber if you are or intend to be pregnant. Consult prescriber if breast-feeding.

**Geriatric Considerations:** Many elderly will have diseases which may influence the use of edrophonium. Also, many elderly will need doses reduced 50% due to creatinine clearances in the 10-50 mL/minute range (common in the aged). Side effects or concomitant disease may warrant use of pyridostigmine.

- **ED-SPAZ®** *see* Hyoscyamine *on page 590*
- **E.E.S.®** *see* Erythromycin *on page 435*

## Efavirenz (e FAV e renz)

**U.S. Brand Names** Sustiva™

**Therapeutic Category** Antiretroviral Agent, Reverse Transcriptase Inhibitor (Non-Nucleoside)

**Pregnancy Risk Factor** C

**Lactation** Enters breast milk/contraindicated

**Use** Treatment of HIV-1 infections in combination with at least two other antiretroviral agents; has some activity against hepatitis B virus and herpes viruses

**Contraindications** Hypersensitivity to efavirenz or any component

**Warnings** Do not use as single-agent therapy. Do not administer with other agents metabolized by cytochrome P-450 isoenzyme 3A4 including astemizole, cisapride, midazolam, triazolam, or ergot alkaloids (potential for life-threatening adverse effects). History of mental illness/drug abuse (predisposition to psychological reactions). Discontinue if severe rash (involving blistering, desquamation, mucosal involvement, or fever) develops. Use caution in patients with known or suspected hepatitis B or C infection (monitoring of liver function is recommended); hepatic impairment. Persistent elevations of serum transaminases greater than five times the upper limit of normal should prompt evaluation - benefit of continued therapy should be weighed against possible risk of hepatotoxicity. Children are more susceptible to development of rash; prophylactic antihistamines may be used. Pregnancy factor C. Women of childbearing potential should undergo pregnancy testing prior to initiation of therapy.

**Drug Interactions**

**Cytochrome P-450 Effect:** Increased effect: CYP3A4, 2C9, 2C19 enzyme inhibitor; CYP3A4 enzyme inducer

**Decreased Effect:** Other inducers of this enzyme (including phenobarbital, rifampin, and rifabutin) may decrease serum concentrations of efavirenz. Concentrations of indinavir may be reduced; dosage increase to 1000 mg three times a day is recommended. Concentrations of saquinavir may be decreased (use as sole protease inhibitor is not recommended). Plasma concentrations of clarithromycin are decreased (clinical significance unknown). May decrease effect of warfarin.

**Increased Effect/Toxicity:** Coadministration with medications metabolized by these enzymes may lead to increased concentration-related effects. Coadministration with astemizole, cisapride, midazolam, triazolam, and ergot alkaloids may result in life-threatening toxicities. The AUC of nelfinavir is increased (20%); AUC of both ritonavir and efavirenz are increased by 20% during concurrent therapy. The AUC of ethinyl estradiol is increased 37% by efavirenz (clinical significance unknown). May increase effect of warfarin.

**Food Interactions** High fat meals increase the absorption of efavirenz.

**Adverse Reactions**

1% to 10%

Central nervous system: Dizziness (2% to 10%), inability to concentrate (0% to 9%), insomnia (0% to 7%), headache (5% to 6%) abnormal dreams (0% to 4%), somnolence (0% to 3%), depression (0% to 2%), anorexia (0% to 5%), nervousness (0% to 2%), fatigue (2% to 7%), hypoesthesia (1% to 2%)

Dermatologic: Rash (5% to 20%), pruritus (0% to 2%)

Gastrointestinal: Nausea (0% to 12%), vomiting (0% to 7%), diarrhea (2% to 12%), dyspepsia (0% to 4%), elevated transaminases (2% to 3%), abdominal pain (0% to 3%), flatulence (0% to 1%)

Genitourinary: Renal calculus (0% to 1%), hematuria (0% to 1%)

Miscellaneous: Increased sweating (0% to 2%)

<2%:

Cardiovascular: Edema (peripheral), syncope, flushing, palpitations, tachycardia

Central nervous system: Fever, pain, malaise, ataxia, depression, seizures, hallucinations, psychosis, depersonalization, amnesia, anxiety, apathy, emotional lability, agitation, confusion, euphoria, impaired coordination, migraine, speech disorder, vertigo
Dermatologic: Hot flashes, alopecia, eczema, folliculitis, skin exfoliation, urticaria
Endocrine & metabolic: Cholesterol and triglycerides (increased)
Gastrointestinal: Pancreatitis, dry mouth, taste disturbance
Genitourinary:
Hepatic: Hepatitis
Local: Thrombophlebitis
Neuromuscular & skeletal: Asthenia, neuralgia, paresthesia, peripheral neuropathy, tremor, arthralgia, myalgia
Ocular: Abnormal vision, diplopia
Otic: Tinnitus
Respiratory: Asthma
Miscellaneous: Alcohol intolerance, allergic reaction, parosmia

**Overdose/Toxicology** Increased central nervous system symptoms and involuntary muscle contractions have been reported in accidental overdose. Treatment is supportive. Activated charcoal may enhance elimination; dialysis is unlikely to remove the drug.

**Pharmacodynamics/Kinetics**

**Distribution:** Highly protein bound (>99%) primarily to albumin; CSF concentrations exceed free fraction in serum

**Half-life Elimination:** Single dose: 52-76 hours; after multiple doses: 40-55 hours

**Time to Peak:** 3-8 hours

**Metabolism:** Hepatic via cytochrome P-450 isoenzymes 3A4 and 2B6; may induce enzymes and therefore its own metabolism

**Excretion:** Urine and feces

**Formulations** Capsule: 50 mg, 100 mg, 200 mg

**Dosing**

**Adults:** Dosing at bedtime is recommended to limit central nervous system effects; should not be used as single-agent therapy.

Oral: 600 mg once daily

**Elderly:** Refer to adult dosing.

**Renal Impairment:** No dosage adjustment is recommended.

**Hepatic Impairment:** Limited clinical experience - use with caution.

**Stability**

**Storage:** Store below 25°C (77°F).

**Monitoring Laboratory Tests** False-positive test for cannabinoids have been reported when the CEDIA DAU Multi-Level THC assay is used. False-positive results with other assays for cannabinoids have not been observed. Monitor serum transaminases (discontinuation of treatment should be considered for persistent elevations greater than five times the upper limit of normal), cholesterol, and triglycerides.

**Additional Nursing Issues**

**Physical Assessment:** Assess other medications patient may be taking for effectiveness and interactions (see Warnings/Precautions and Drug Interactions). Monitor laboratory tests (see above), therapeutic effects, and adverse reactions (eg, CNS effects - see Warnings/Precautions and Adverse Reactions). Assess knowledge/instruct patient on appropriate use, interventions to reduce side effects, and adverse symptoms to report. **Pregnancy risk factor C** - benefits of use should outweigh possible risks. Breast-feeding is contraindicated.

**Patient Information/Instruction:** Efavirenz is not a cure for HIV, nor will it reduce transmission of HIV. Take as directed (usually at bedtime to reduce CNS effects), with or without food. Do not alter dose or discontinue without consulting prescriber. Avoid high fat meals when taking this medication. Maintain adequate hydration (2-3 L/day of fluids unless instructed to restrict fluid intake). Avoid excessive alcohol (severe reaction), prescription, and OTC sedatives unless consulting prescriber. You may experience dry mouth, taste disturbances, nausea, or vomiting (small frequent meals or sucking hard candy may help - consult prescriber if nausea or vomiting persists); diarrhea (buttermilk, boiled milk, or yogurt may help); or dizziness, anxiety, tremor, impaired coordination (use caution when driving or engaging in tasks requiring alertness until response to drug is known); Report CNS changes (acute headache, abnormal dreams, sleepiness or fatigue, seizures, hallucinations, amnesia, emotional lability, confusion); sense of fullness or ringing in ears; vision changes or double vision; muscle pain, weakness, tremors, numbness, spasticity, or change in gait; skin rash or irritation; chest pain or palpitations; or other unusual effects related to this medication. **Pregnancy/breast-feeding precautions:** Inform prescriber if you are or intend to be pregnant. Do not breast-feed.

**Dietary Issues:** Avoid high-fat meals when taking this medication. May be taken with or without food

**Related Information**

Antiretroviral Agents Comparison *on page 1373*

- **Effer-K™** *see* Potassium Supplements *on page 952*
- **Effer-Syllium® [OTC]** *see* Psyllium *on page 993*
- **Effexor®** *see* Venlafaxine *on page 1206*
- **Efidac/24® [OTC]** *see* Pseudoephedrine *on page 992*
- **Efodine®** *see page 1294*
- **Efudex® Topical** *see* Fluorouracil *on page 500*
- **Efudix** *see* Fluorouracil *on page 500*

- ♦ **E-IPV** *see page 1256*
- ♦ **Elantan** *see* Isosorbide Mononitrate *on page 635*
- ♦ **Elase-Chloromycetin® Topical** *see* Fibrinolysin and Desoxyribonuclease *on page 483*
- ♦ **Elase® Topical** *see* Fibrinolysin and Desoxyribonuclease *on page 483*
- ♦ **Elavil®** *see* Amitriptyline *on page 73*
- ♦ **Elavil Plus®** *see* Amitriptyline and Perphenazine *on page 75*
- ♦ **Eldecort®** *see* Hydrocortisone *on page 578*
- ♦ **Eldepryl®** *see* Selegiline *on page 1050*
- ♦ **Eldercaps® [OTC]** *see* Vitamin, Multiple *on page 1219*
- ♦ **Eldopaque® [OTC]** *see* Hydroquinone *on page 583*
- ♦ **Eldopaque Forte®** *see* Hydroquinone *on page 583*
- ♦ **Eldoquin® [OTC]** *see* Hydroquinone *on page 583*
- ♦ **Eldoquin® Forte®** *see* Hydroquinone *on page 583*
- ♦ **Electrolyte Lavage Solution** *see* Polyethylene Glycol-Electrolyte Solution *on page 945*
- ♦ **Elequine** *see* Levofloxacin *on page 669*
- ♦ **Elimite™ Cream** *see* Permethrin *on page 911*
- ♦ **Elixicon®** *see* Theophylline *on page 1115*
- ♦ **Elixophyllin®** *see* Theophylline *on page 1115*
- ♦ **Elocon® Topical** *see* Topical Corticosteroids *on page 1152*
- ♦ **Elspar®** *see* Asparaginase *on page 109*
- ♦ **Eltor®** *see* Pseudoephedrine *on page 992*
- ♦ **Eltroxin®** *see* Levothyroxine *on page 673*
- ♦ **Emcyt®** *see* Estramustine *on page 444*
- ♦ **Emecheck® Liquid** *see page 1294*
- ♦ **Emetrol® Liquid** *see page 1294*
- ♦ **Eminase®** *see* Anistreplase *on page 97*
- ♦ **Emko®** *see page 1294*
- ♦ **EMLA®** *see* Lidocaine and Prilocaine *on page 677*
- ♦ **Empirin® [OTC]** *see* Aspirin *on page 111*
- ♦ **Empirin® With Codeine** *see* Aspirin and Codeine *on page 113*
- ♦ **Empracet® 30, 60** *see* Acetaminophen and Codeine *on page 34*
- ♦ **Emtec-30®** *see* Acetaminophen and Codeine *on page 34*
- ♦ **Emulsan 20%** *see* Fat Emulsion *on page 471*
- ♦ **Emulsified Dizac® Injection** *see* Diazepam *on page 355*
- ♦ **Emulsified Valium®** *see* Diazepam *on page 355*
- ♦ **Emulsoil®** *see page 1294*
- ♦ **E-Mycin®** *see* Erythromycin *on page 435*
- ♦ **Enaladil** *see* Enalapril *on this page*


## Enalapril (e NAL a pril)

**U.S. Brand Names** Vasotec®; Vasotec® I.V.

**Therapeutic Category** Angiotensin-Converting Enzyme (ACE) Inhibitors

**Pregnancy Risk Factor** C/D (2nd and 3rd trimesters)

**Lactation** Enters breast milk/compatible

**Use** Management of mild to severe hypertension and congestive heart failure

**Unlabeled use:** Hypertensive crisis, diabetic nephropathy, rheumatoid arthritis, diagnosis of anatomic renal artery stenosis, hypertension secondary to scleroderma renal crisis, diagnosis of aldosteronism, idiopathic edema, Bartter's syndrome, postmyocardial infarction for prevention of ventricular failure

**Investigational:** Severe congestive heart failure in infants, neonatal hypertension, acute pulmonary edema

**Mechanism of Action/Effect** Competitive inhibitor of angiotensin-converting enzyme (ACE); prevents conversion of angiotensin I to angiotensin II, a potent vasoconstrictor; results in lower levels of angiotensin II which causes an increase in plasma renin activity and a reduction in aldosterone secretion

**Contraindications** Hypersensitivity to enalapril, enalaprilat, other ACE inhibitors, or any component; pregnancy (2nd and 3rd trimesters)

**Warnings** Use with caution and modify dosage in patients with renal impairment (especially renal artery stenosis), severe congestive heart failure, or with coadministered diuretic therapy, valvular stenosis, hyperkalemia (>5.7 mEq/L). Severe hypotension may occur in patients who are sodium and/or volume depleted. Initiate lower doses and monitor closely when starting therapy in these patients. Pregnancy factor C/D (2nd and 3rd trimesters).

**Drug Interactions**

**Cytochrome P-450 Effect:** CYP3A3/4 enzyme substrate

**Decreased Effect:** Rifampin may decrease the effect of ACE inhibitors. Antacids may decrease the bioavailability of ACE inhibitors, may be more likely to occur with captopril, separate administration times by 1-2 hours. NSAIDs, specifically indomethacin, may reduce the hypotensive effects of ACE inhibitors. More likely to occur in low renin or volume dependent hypertensive patients.

**Increased Effect/Toxicity:** Diuretics have additive hypotensive effects with ACE inhibitors. Probenecid increases blood levels of captopril which may occur in other ACE inhibitors. Phenothiazines taken with ACE inhibitors may increase the pharmacologic effects of the ACE inhibitor. Allopurinol and ACE inhibitors may cause a higher risk of hypersensitivity reaction when taken concurrently. Digoxin and ACE inhibitors may result in elevated serum digoxin levels. Lithium and ACE inhibitors may result in elevated serum levels of lithium with symptoms of toxicity. Potassium supplements or potassium-sparing diuretics with ACE inhibitors may result in elevated serum potassium levels.

**Effects on Lab Values** Positive Coombs' [direct]; may cause false-positive results in urine acetone determinations using sodium nitroprusside reagent

**Adverse Reactions**

1% to 10%:

Cardiovascular: Chest pain, hypotension, orthostatic hypotension, tachycardia, chest pain pectoris, syncope

Central nervous system: Headache, dizziness, fatigue, vertigo, muscle weakness

Dermatologic: Rash

Gastrointestinal: Abdominal pain, vomiting, nausea, diarrhea

Genitourinary: Urinary tract infection

Neuromuscular & skeletal: Paresthesia, weakness

Respiratory: Bronchitis, cough, dyspnea

<1% (Limited to important or life-threatening symptoms): Chest pain, flushing, palpitations, cardiac arrest, myocardial infarction, cerebrovascular accident, tachycardia, vasculitis, atrial fibrillation, bradycardia, alopecia, erythema multiforme, pruritus, Stevens-Johnson syndrome, urticaria, angioedema, photosensitivity, pemphigus, hypoglycemia, hyperkalemia, impotence, eosinophilia, bone marrow depression, neutropenia, thrombocytopenia, hemolytic anemia, hepatitis, hepatic failure, oliguria, renal dysfunction, asthma, bronchospasm, upper respiratory infection, pulmonary embolism, pulmonary edema

**Overdose/Toxicology** Mild hypotension has been the primary toxic effect seen with acute overdose. Bradycardia may also occur. Hyperkalemia occurs even with therapeutic doses, especially in patients with renal insufficiency and those taking NSAIDs. Following initiation of essential overdose management, toxic symptom treatment and supportive treatment should be initiated.

**Pharmacodynamics/Kinetics**

**Protein Binding:** 50% to 60%

**Half-life Elimination:**

Enalapril: Healthy: 2 hours; With congestive heart failure: 3.4-5.8 hours

Enalaprilat: 35-38 hours

**Time to Peak:** Oral: Enalapril: Within 0.5-1.5 hours; Enalaprilat (active): Within 3-4.5 hours

**Metabolism:** Liver

**Excretion:** Urine

**Onset:** Oral: ~1 hour

**Duration:** Oral: 12-24 hours

**Formulations**

Enalaprilat: Injection: 1.25 mg/mL (1 mL, 2 mL)

Enalapril maleate: Tablet: 2.5 mg, 5 mg, 10 mg, 20 mg

**Dosing**

**Adults:** Use lower listed initial dose in patients with hyponatremia, hypovolemia, severe congestive heart failure, decreased renal function, or in those receiving diuretics.

Oral: Enalapril:

Hypertension: 2.5-5 mg/day then increase as required, usual therapeutic dose for hypertension: 10-40 mg/day in 1-2 divided doses; usual therapeutic dose for heart failure: 5-20 mg/day

Heart failure: As adjunct with diuretics and digitalis, initiate with 2.5 mg once or twice daily (usual range: 5-20 mg/day in 2 divided doses; maximum: 40 mg)

Asymptomatic left ventricular dysfunction: 2.5 mg twice daily, titrated as tolerated to 20 mg/day

I.V.: Enalaprilat:

Hypertension: 1.25 mg/dose, given over 5 minutes every 6 hours; doses as high as 5 mg/dose every 6 hours have been tolerated for up to 36 hours. **Note:** If patients are concomitantly receiving diuretic therapy, begin with 0.625 mg I.V. over 5 minutes; if the effect is not adequate after 1 hour, repeat the dose and administer 1.25 mg at 6-hour intervals thereafter; if adequate, administer 0.625 mg I.V. every 6 hours.

Has been used investigationally in acute pulmonary edema.

**Conversion from I.V. to oral therapy if not concurrently on diuretics:** 5 mg once daily; subsequent titration as needed; if concurrently receiving diuretics and responding to 0.625 mg I.V. every 6 hours, initiate with 2.5 mg/day.

**Elderly:** Refer to adult dosing.

**Renal Impairment:**

Oral: Enalapril: Hypertension:

$Cl_{cr}$ 30-80 mL/minute: Administer 5 mg/day titrated upwards to maximum of 40 mg.

$Cl_{cr}$ <30 mL/minute: Administer 2.5 mg day titrated upward until blood pressure is controlled up to a maximum of 40 mg.

For heart failure patients with sodium <130 mEq/L or serum creatinine >1.6 mg/dL, initiate dosage with 2.5 mg/day, increasing to twice daily as needed; increase further in increments of 2.5 mg/dose at >4-day intervals to a maximum daily dose of 40 mg.

I.V.: Enalaprilat:

$Cl_{cr}$ >30 mL/minute: Initiate with 1.25 mg every 6 hours and increase dose based on response.

$Cl_{cr}$ <30 mL/minute: Initiate with 0.625 mg every 6 hours and increase dose based on response.

(Continued)

## Enalapril *(Continued)*

Moderately dialyzable (20% to 50%)

Administer dose postdialysis (eg, 0.625 mg I.V. every 6 hours) or administer 20% to 25% supplemental dose following dialysis; Clearance: 62 mL/minute

Peritoneal dialysis effects: Supplemental dose is not necessary, although some removal of drug occurs.

**Hepatic Impairment:** Hydrolysis of enalapril to enalaprilat may be delayed and/or impaired in patients with severe hepatic impairment, but the pharmacodynamic effects of the drug do not appear to be significantly altered. No dosage adjustment is necessary.

**Administration**

**I.V.:** Give direct IVP over at least 5 minutes or dilute up to 50 mL and infuse.

**Stability**

**Storage:** Enalaprilat: Clear, colorless solution which should be stored at <30°C.

**Reconstitution:** Enalaprilat: I.V. is stable for 24 hours at room temperature in $D_5W$ or NS.

**Monitoring Laboratory Tests** CBC, renal function tests, electrolytes

**Additional Nursing Issues**

**Physical Assessment:** Assess effectiveness and interactions of other medications (see Drug Interactions). See Warnings/Precautions and Contraindications for use cautions. Monitor effectiveness of therapy, laboratory tests, and adverse response on a regular basis during therapy (eg, postural hypotension - see Adverse Reactions and Overdose/Toxicology). Assess knowledge/teach patient appropriate use according to drug form and purpose of therapy, possible side effects and appropriate interventions, and adverse symptoms to report. **Pregnancy risk factor C/D** - see Pregnancy Risk Factor - assess knowledge/instruct patient on use of barrier contraceptive measures; danger of use during pregnancy must outweigh risk to fetus. See Pregnancy Issues.

**Patient Information/Instruction:** Take exactly as directed; do not discontinue without consulting prescriber. Take first dose at bedtime. Take all doses on an empty stomach (30 minutes before or 2 hours after meals). This drug does not eliminate need for diet or exercise regimen as recommended by prescriber. Do not use potassium supplements or salt substitutes containing potassium without consulting prescriber. May cause dizziness, fainting, lightheadedness (use caution when driving or engaging in tasks that require alertness until response to drug is known); postural hypotension (use caution when rising from lying or sitting position or climbing stairs); nausea, vomiting, abdominal pain, dry mouth, or transient loss of appetite (small frequent meals, frequent mouth care, sucking lozenges, or chewing gum may help) - report if these persist. Report chest pain or palpitations; mouth sores; fever or chills; swelling of extremities, face, mouth, or tongue; skin rash; numbness, tingling, or pain in muscles; difficulty in breathing or unusual cough; or other persistent adverse reactions. **Pregnancy precautions:** Do not get pregnant while taking this medication; use appropriate barrier contraceptive measures.

**Geriatric Considerations:** Due to frequent decreases in glomerular filtration (also creatinine clearance) with aging, elderly patients may have exaggerated responses to ACE inhibitors.

**Pregnancy Issues:** ACE inhibitors can cause fetal injury or death if taken during the 2nd or 3rd trimester. Discontinue ACE inhibitors as soon as pregnancy is detected. ACE inhibitors should not be used if patient is sexually active and not using contraceptives.

**Related Information**

ACE Inhibitors and Angiotensin Antagonists Comparison *on page 1362*

## Enalapril and Diltiazem (e NAL a pril & dil TYE a zem)

**U.S. Brand Names** Teczem®

**Therapeutic Category** Antihypertensive Agent, Combination

**Pregnancy Risk Factor** C/D (2nd and 3rd trimesters)

**Lactation** Enters breast milk/use caution

**Use** Treatment of hypertension, however, not indicated for initial treatment of hypertension; replacement therapy in patients receiving separate dosage forms (for patient convenience); when monotherapy with one component fails to achieve desired antihypertensive effect, or when dose-limiting adverse effects limit upward titration of monotherapy

**Formulations** Tablet, extended release: Enalapril maleate 5 mg and diltiazem maleate 180 mg

**Dosing**

**Adults:** Oral: 1 tablet (5 mg enalapril/180 mg diltiazem) daily; individualize dose to achieve optimal effect.

**Elderly:** Overall safety and efficacy are not different in elderly patients, although a greater sensitivity to effects may be observed in some older individuals. See adult dosing.

**Renal Impairment:** Usual regimen need not be adjusted unless patient's creatinine clearance is <30 mL/minute. Titration of individual components must be done prior to switching to combination product.

**Additional Nursing Issues**

**Physical Assessment:** See individual components listed in Related Information. **Pregnancy risk factor C/D** - see Pregnancy Risk Factor - assess knowledge/instruct patient on need to use appropriate contraceptive measures and the need to avoid pregnancy. Note breast-feeding caution.

**Patient Information/Instruction:** See individual components listed in Related Information. **Pregnancy/breast-feeding precautions:** Inform prescriber if you are or intend to be pregnant. Consult prescriber if breast-feeding.

**Related Information**

Diltiazem *on page 377*
Enalapril *on page 416*

## Enalapril and Felodipine (e NAL a pril & fe LOE di peen)

**U.S. Brand Names** Lexxel™

**Therapeutic Category** Antihypertensive Agent, Combination

**Pregnancy Risk Factor** C/D (2nd and 3rd trimesters)

**Lactation** Enters breast milk/use caution

**Use** Treatment of hypertension, however, not indicated for initial treatment of hypertension; replacement therapy in patients receiving separate dosage forms (for patient convenience); when monotherapy with one component fails to achieve desired antihypertensive effect, or when dose-limiting adverse effects limit upward titration of monotherapy

**Formulations** Tablet, extended release: Enalapril maleate 5 mg and felodipine 5 mg

**Dosing**

**Adults:** Oral: 1 tablet/day, individualize dose to achieve optimal effect. In some patients, the effect of enalapril may diminish toward the end of the dosing interval. Twice daily dosing may be considered.

**Elderly:** Recommended initial dose of felodipine is 2.5 mg daily. Titration of individual components is preferred.

**Renal Impairment:** $Cl_{cr}$ <30 mL/minute: Recommended initial dose of enalapril is 2.5 mg/day. Titration of individual components is preferred.

**Hepatic Impairment:** Recommended initial dose of felodipine is 2.5 mg daily. Titration of individual components is preferred.

**Additional Nursing Issues**

**Physical Assessment:** See individual components listed in Related Information. **Pregnancy risk factor C/D** - see Pregnancy Risk Factor - assess knowledge/instruct patient on need to use appropriate contraceptive measures and the need to avoid pregnancy. Note breast-feeding caution.

**Patient Information/Instruction:** See individual components listed in Related Information. **Pregnancy/breast-feeding precautions:** Inform prescriber if you are or intend to be pregnant. Consult prescriber if breast-feeding.

**Related Information**

Enalapril *on page 416*
Felodipine *on page 474*

## Enalapril and Hydrochlorothiazide

(e NAL a pril & hye droe klor oh THYE a zide)

**U.S. Brand Names** Vaseretic® 10-25; Vaseretic® 5-12.5

**Synonyms** Hydrochlorothiazide and Enalapril

**Therapeutic Category** Antihypertensive Agent, Combination

**Pregnancy Risk Factor** C/D (2nd and 3rd trimesters)

**Lactation** Enters breast milk (both ingredients)/compatible

**Use** Treatment of hypertension

**Formulations**

Tablet:
- Enalapril maleate 5 mg and hydrochlorothiazide 12.5 mg
- Enalapril maleate 10 mg and hydrochlorothiazide 25 mg

**Dosing**

**Adults:** Enalapril:
- Oral: 10-40 mg/day in single dose or two divided doses
- Monotherapy (patients not on diuretics): Initial: 5 mg/day

**Elderly:** Refer to dosing in individual monographs; adjust for renal impairment.

**Renal Impairment:**
- $Cl_{cr}$ >30 mL/minute: Usual dose
- Severe renal failure: Avoid; loop diuretics are recommended.

**Additional Nursing Issues**

**Physical Assessment:** See individual components listed in Related Information. **Pregnancy risk factor C/D** - see Pregnancy Risk Factor - assess knowledge/instruct patient on need to use appropriate contraceptive measures and the need to avoid pregnancy.

**Patient Information/Instruction:** See individual components listed in Related Information. **Pregnancy precautions:** Inform prescriber if you are or intend to be pregnant.

**Related Information**

Enalapril *on page 416*
Hydrochlorothiazide *on page 566*


- ♦ **Enbrel®** *see* Etanercept *on page 453*
- ♦ **Encare®** *see page 1294*
- ♦ **Endantadine®** *see* Amantadine *on page 61*
- ♦ **End Lice® Liquid** *see page 1294*
- ♦ **Endocet®** *see* Oxycodone and Acetaminophen *on page 873*
- ♦ **Endodan®** *see* Oxycodone and Aspirin *on page 873*
- ♦ **Endolor®** *see* Butalbital Compound and Acetaminophen *on page 175*
- ♦ **Enduron®** *see* Methyclothiazide *on page 748*

- **Enduronyl®** *see* Methyclothiazide and Deserpidine *on page 749*
- **Enduronyl® Forte** *see* Methyclothiazide and Deserpidine *on page 749*
- **Ener-B® [OTC]** *see* Cyanocobalamin *on page 311*
- **Engerix-B®** *see page 1256*
- **Eni** *see* Ciprofloxacin *on page 270*
- **Enlon® Injection** *see* Edrophonium *on page 413*
- **Enomine®** *see* Guaifenesin, Phenylpropanolamine, and Phenylephrine *on page 552*
- **Enovil®** *see* Amitriptyline *on page 73*


## Enoxacin (en OKS a sin)

**U.S. Brand Names** Penetrex™

**Therapeutic Category** Antibiotic, Quinolone

**Pregnancy Risk Factor** C

**Lactation** Excretion in breast milk unknown/contraindicated

**Use** Treatment of complicated and uncomplicated urinary tract infections caused by susceptible gram-negative and gram-positive bacteria

**Mechanism of Action/Effect** Disrupts DNA replication in susceptible bacteria; broad spectrum bactericidal effect

**Contraindications** Hypersensitivity to enoxacin, any component, or other quinolones

**Warnings** Use with caution in patients with a history of convulsions or epilepsy, renal dysfunction, psychosis, syphilis, elevated intracranial pressure, and prepubertal children. Nalidixic acid and ciprofloxacin (related compounds) have been associated with erosions of the cartilage in weight-bearing joints and other signs of arthropathy in immature animals and children. Similar precautions are advised for enoxacin although no data is available. Pregnancy factor C.

**Drug Interactions**

**Cytochrome P-450 Effect:** CYP1A2 enzyme inhibitor

**Decreased Effect:** Decreased effect with antacids (magnesium, aluminum), iron and zinc salts, sucralfate, and bismuth salts.

**Increased Effect/Toxicity:** Enoxacin increases toxicity/levels of warfarin, cyclosporine, digoxin, and caffeine. Increased levels of enoxacin with cimetidine.

**Food Interactions** Enoxacin serum caffeine levels may be increased if taken with caffeine.

**Adverse Reactions**

>10%:

Central nervous system: Dizziness or lightheadedness, headache, nervousness, drowsiness, insomnia

Gastrointestinal: Nausea, diarrhea, vomiting, abdominal pain

1% to 10%: Dermatologic: Photosensitivity

<1% (Limited to important or life-threatening symptoms): Skin rash, itching or redness, Stevens-Johnson syndrome, anemia, increased liver enzymes, interstitial nephritis, shortness of breath

**Overdose/Toxicology** Symptoms of overdose include acute renal failure and seizures. Treatment is supportive; diazepam may be used for seizures. Not removed by peritoneal or hemodialysis.

**Pharmacodynamics/Kinetics**

**Distribution:** Penetrates well into tissues and body secretions

**Half-life Elimination:** 3-6 hours (average)

**Metabolism:** Liver

**Excretion:** Urine and feces

**Formulations** Tablet: 200 mg, 400 mg

**Dosing**

**Adults:** Oral: 400 mg twice daily

**Elderly:** Refer to adult dosing.

**Renal Impairment:** $Cl_{cr}$ <50 mL/minute: Administer 50% of dose.

**Monitoring Laboratory Tests** Perform culture and sensitivity studies prior to starting treatment. During prolonged therapy, monitor CBC and renal and hepatic function periodically.

**Additional Nursing Issues**

**Physical Assessment:** Monitor response to therapy and monitor or instruct patient to monitor for signs of opportunistic infection (eg, fever, fatigue, furry tongue, thrush, perineal itching or vaginal discharge, loose foul-smelling stools, unhealed sores). **Pregnancy risk factor C** - benefits of use should outweigh possible risks. Breast-feeding is contraindicated.

**Patient Information/Instruction:** Take as prescribed and for as long as directed. Take on an empty stomach (1 hour prior to or after meals). Do not use antacids within 2 hours of medication. Maintain adequate hydration (2-3 L/day of fluids unless instructed to restrict fluid intake). You may experience stomach discomfort (eat small, frequent meals) and dizziness or blurred vision (use caution when driving). May cause photosensitivity (use sunscreen, wear protective clothing and eyewear, and avoid direct sunlight). Report skin rash; visual changes; severe gastric upset; weakness; pain, inflammation, or rupture of tendon; or signs or symptoms of opportunistic infection (eg, white spots or sores in mouth or perineal area, itching or vaginal discharge, unhealed sores, fever). **Pregnancy/breast-feeding precautions:** Inform prescriber if you are or intend to be pregnant. Do not breast-feed.

**Geriatric Considerations:** Adjust dose for renal function.

## Enoxaparin (e noks ah PAIR in)

**U.S. Brand Names** Lovenox® Injection

**Therapeutic Category** Anticoagulant; Low Molecular Weight Heparin

**Pregnancy Risk Factor** B

**Lactation** Excretion in breast milk unknown (probably safe - see Breast-feeding)

**Use** Prevention of deep vein thrombosis following hip or knee replacement surgery or abdominal surgery in patients at risk for thromboembolic complications; inpatient treatment of acute deep vein thrombosis with and without pulmonary embolism when administered in conjunction with warfarin sodium; outpatient treatment of acute deep vein thrombosis without pulmonary embolism when administered in conjunction with warfarin sodium; prevention of ischemic complications of unstable angina and non-Q wave myocardial infarction (when administered with aspirin)

**Mechanism of Action/Effect** Low molecular weight heparin that blocks factor Xa and IIa to prevent thrombus and clot formation

**Contraindications** Hypersensitivity to enoxaparin, heparin, or pork products; patients with active major bleeding; thrombocytopenia associated with a positive *in vitro* test for antiplatelet antibody or enoxaparin-induced platelet aggregation

**Warnings** Do not administer intramuscularly. Use with extreme caution in patients with a history of heparin-induced thrombocytopenia, bacterial endocarditis, hemorrhagic stroke, recent CNS or ophthalmological surgery, bleeding diathesis, uncontrolled arterial hypertension, or a history of recent GI ulceration and hemorrhage. Patients with recent or anticipated epidural or spinal anesthesia are at risk of developing spinal or epidural hematoma; paralysis may result.

**Drug Interactions**

**Increased Effect/Toxicity:** Increased toxicity with oral anticoagulants, platelet inhibitors, cephalosporins, and penicillins.

**Effects on Lab Values** ↑ AST, ALT levels

**Adverse Reactions**

1% to 10%:

- Central nervous system: Fever, confusion, pain
- Dermatologic: Erythema, bruising
- Gastrointestinal: Nausea
- Hematologic: Hemorrhage, thrombocytopenia, hypochromic anemia, hematoma
- Local: Irritation

<1% (limited to severe or life-threatening): Hyperlipidemia, hypertriglyceridemia

Case reports of long-term or permanent paralysis have occurred when used in association with epidural or spinal anesthesia (due to hematoma). Risk is increased by indwelling catheters or concomitant use of other drugs which alter hemostasis (NSAIDs, anticoagulants, or platelet inhibitors).

At the recommended doses, single injections of enoxaparin do not significantly influence platelet aggregation or affect global clotting time (ie, prothrombin time or activated partial thromboplastin time).

**Overdose/Toxicology** Symptoms of overdose include hemorrhage. Protamine zinc has been used to reverse effects.

**Pharmacodynamics/Kinetics**

**Protein Binding:** Low molecular weight heparins do not bind to heparin binding proteins.

**Half-life Elimination:** Half-life, plasma: Low molecular weight heparin is 2-4 times longer than standard heparin independent of the dose.

**Metabolism:** Liver

**Excretion:** Urine

**Onset:** Maximum antifactor Xa and antithrombin (antifactor IIa) activities occur 3-5 hours after S.C. administration.

**Duration:** Following a 40 mg dose, significant antifactor Xa activity persists in plasma for ~12 hours.

**Formulations**

Ampul: 30 mg

Injection, preservative free, as sodium: 30 mg/0.3 mL

Prefilled syringes: 30 mg/0.3 mL; 40 mg/0.4 mL

Graduated prefilled syringes: 60 mg/0.6 mL; 80 mg/o.8 mL; 100 mg/1.0 mL

**Dosing**

**Adults:** S.C.:

Hip or knee replacement surgery: 30 mg twice daily; first dose 12-24 hours after surgery provided hemostasis has been established; usual duration after knee replacement is 7-10 days (up to 14 days). Alternative dosing for hip replacement surgery: 40 mg once daily, initial dose given 12 hours prior to surgery. Following hip surgery, after the initial phase of prophylaxis (either twice daily or once daily regimen), patients should be continued on 40 mg S.C. once daily for 3 weeks.

Abdominal surgery: 40 mg once daily; initial dose given 2 hours prior to surgery; usual duration is 7-10 days (up to 12 days)

Treatment of deep vein thrombosis and pulmonary embolism:

Outpatients: 1 mg per kilogram every 12 hours. Warfarin treatment should be initiated when appropriate (usually within 72 hours of initiating enoxaparin).

Inpatients: 1 mg/kg every 12 hours or 1.5 mg/kg once daily. Warfarin treatment should be initiated when appropriate (usually within 72 hours of initiating enoxaparin).

(Continued)

## Enoxaparin *(Continued)*

Unstable angina and non-Q wave myocardial infarction: 1 mg/kg every 12 hours (in conjunction with oral aspirin). Usual duration 2-8 days (2 days minimum). Should not be given within 6-8 hours of vascular sheath removal. Sheath should remain in place for 6-8 hours after dose of enoxaparin.

**Elderly:** Refer to adult dosing.

**Renal Impairment:** Adjustment may be necessary in the elderly and patients with severe renal impairment.

**Administration**

**I.M.:** Do not administer I.M.

**Other:** Give deep S.C. injection, alternate sites. Apply pressure following injection. Do **not** massage site.

**Monitoring Laboratory Tests** Platelets, occult blood, anti-Xa activity, if available; the monitoring of PT and/or PTT is not necessary.

**Additional Nursing Issues**

**Physical Assessment:** Assess effectiveness and interactions of other medications (see Drug Interactions). See Warnings/Precautions and Contraindications for use cautions. Monitor effectiveness of therapy, laboratory tests (see above) and adverse response (eg, thrombolytic reactions - see Adverse Reactions and Overdose/Toxicology). Assess knowledge/teach patient appropriate use, possible side effects and appropriate interventions (eg, bleeding precautions), and adverse symptoms to report.

**Patient Information/Instruction:** This drug can only be administered by injection. You may have a tendency to bleed easily while taking this drug; brush teeth with soft brush, floss with waxed floss, use electric razor, avoid scissors or sharp knives, and potentially harmful activities. Report chest pain; persistent constipation; persistent erection; unusual bleeding or bruising (bleeding gums, nosebleed, blood in urine, dark stool); pain in joints or back; or numbness, tingling, swelling, or pain at injection site.

**Geriatric Considerations:** No specific recommendations. Treatment of DVT is not an approved indication, but clinical trials show comparable efficacy to unfractionated heparin.

**Breast-feeding Issues:** This drug has a high molecular weight that would minimize excretion in breast milk and is inactivated by the GI tract which further reduces the risk to the infant.

**Related Information**

Low Molecular Weight Heparins Comparison *on page 1395*


- **Enterobacticel** *see* Co-trimoxazole *on page 307*
- **Enteropride** *see* Cisapride *on page 272*
- **Entex®** *see* Guaifenesin, Phenylpropanolamine, and Phenylephrine *on page 552*
- **Entex® LA** *see* Guaifenesin and Phenylpropanolamine *on page 550*
- **Entex® PSE** *see* Guaifenesin and Pseudoephedrine *on page 551*
- **Entocort®** *see* Budesonide *on page 164*
- **Entoplus** *see* Albendazole *on page 44*
- **Entrophen®** *see* Aspirin *on page 111*
- **Enulose®** *see* Lactulose *on page 651*
- **E Pam®** *see* Diazepam *on page 355*
- **EPEG** *see* Etoposide *on page 463*


## Ephedrine (e FED rin)

**U.S. Brand Names** Kondon's Nasal® [OTC]; Pretz-D® [OTC]

**Therapeutic Category** Alpha/Beta Agonist

**Pregnancy Risk Factor** C

**Lactation** Enters breast milk/not recommended

**Use** Treatment of bronchial asthma, nasal congestion, acute bronchospasm, idiopathic orthostatic hypotension (no longer a preferred agent for asthma or acute bronchospasm with the availability of less toxic $\beta_2$ agents).

**Mechanism of Action/Effect** Releases tissue stores of epinephrine and thereby produces an alpha- and beta-adrenergic stimulation; longer-acting and less potent than epinephrine

**Contraindications** Hypersensitivity to ephedrine or any component; cardiac arrhythmias; angle-closure glaucoma; patients on other sympathomimetic agents

**Warnings** Blood volume depletion should be corrected before ephedrine therapy is instituted. Use caution in patients with unstable vasomotor symptoms, diabetes, hyperthyroidism, prostatic hypertrophy, or a history of seizures. Also use caution in the elderly and those patients with cardiovascular disorders such as coronary artery disease, arrhythmias, and hypertension. Ephedrine may cause hypertension resulting in intracranial hemorrhage. Long-term use may cause anxiety and symptoms of paranoid schizophrenia. Avoid using ephedrine as a bronchodilator. Generally not used as a bronchodilator since new $\beta_2$ agents are less toxic. Use with caution in the elderly, since it crosses the blood-brain barrier and may cause confusion. Pregnancy factor C.

**Drug Interactions**

**Decreased Effect:** Alpha- and beta-adrenergic blocking agents decrease ephedrine vasopressor effects.

**Increased Effect/Toxicity:** Increased (toxic) cardiac stimulation with other sympathomimetic agents, theophylline, cardiac glycosides, or general anesthetics. Increased blood pressure with atropine or MAO inhibitors.

**Effects on Lab Values** Can cause a false-positive amphetamine EMIT assay

**Adverse Reactions**

**Oral:**

>10%: Central nervous system: Nervousness, insomnia

1% to 10%:

Cardiovascular: Flushing of face, hypertension, pounding heartbeat, paleness
Central nervous system: Dizziness, lightheadedness, headache
Gastrointestinal: Dry mouth, nausea, anorexia, vomiting
Neuromuscular & skeletal: Trembling, weakness
Respiratory: Bronchial irritation, coughing
Miscellaneous: Sweating (increased)

<1% (Limited to important or life-threatening symptoms): Chest pain, arrhythmias, tachycardia, paradoxical bronchospasm

**Parenteral** (cardiovascular use):

>10%:

Central nervous system: Headache
Gastrointestinal: Nausea, vomiting

1% to 10%:

Cardiovascular: Premature ventricular beats, bradycardia, hypertension, hypotension, chest pain, palpitations, tachycardia, ventricular arrhythmias
Central nervous system: Nervousness or restlessness
Respiratory: Dyspnea

**Overdose/Toxicology** Symptoms of overdose include dysrhythmias, CNS excitation, respiratory depression, vomiting, and convulsions. There is no specific antidote for ephedrine intoxication and treatment is primarily supportive.

**Pharmacodynamics/Kinetics**

**Distribution:** Crosses the placenta
**Half-life Elimination:** 2.5-3.6 hours
**Metabolism:** Hepatic
**Excretion:** Urine
**Onset:** Oral: Onset of bronchodilation: Within 0.25-1 hour
**Duration:** Oral: 3-6 hours

**Formulations**

Ephedrine sulfate:

Injection: 25 mg/mL (1 mL); 50 mg/mL (1 mL, 10 mL)
Jelly (Kondon's Nasal®): 1% (20 g)
Spray (Pretz-D®): 0.25% (15 mL)

**Dosing**

**Adults:**

I.M., S.C.: 25-50 mg, parenteral adult dose should not exceed 150 mg in 24 hours
I.V.: 5-25 mg/dose slow I.V. push repeated after 5-10 minutes as needed, then every 3-4 hours not to exceed 150 mg/24 hours

**Elderly:** Not recommended for use in the elderly.

**Administration**

**I.V.:** Do not administer unless solution is clear.

**Stability**

**Storage:** Protect all dosage forms from light.

**Additional Nursing Issues**

**Physical Assessment:** Assess other medications patient may be taking for effectiveness and interactions (see Drug Interactions). See Warnings/Precautions and Contraindications for cautious use. Monitor therapeutic response (according to purpose for use) and adverse reactions (eg, hypertension, CNS excitability, urinary retention, dysarrhythmias, respiratory depression - Warnings/Precautions, Adverse Reactions, and Overdose/Toxicology). Assess knowledge/teach patient appropriate use, interventions to reduce side effects, and adverse symptoms to report.

I.V. (cardiovascular therapy): Use infusion pump, continuous cardiac/hemodynamic monitoring, and assess infusion site frequently for extravasation (see Administration for extravasation instructions).

**Pregnancy risk factor C** - benefits of use should outweigh possible risks. Breast-feeding is not recommended.

**Patient Information/Instruction:** Use this medication exactly as directed; do not take more than recommended dosage. Avoid other stimulant prescriptive or OTC medications to avoid serious overdose reactions. Store this medication away from light. You may experience dizziness, blurred vision, restlessness (use caution when driving or engaging in tasks requiring alertness until response to drug is known); or difficulty urinating (empty bladder immediately before taking this medication). Report excessive nervousness or excitation, inability to sleep, facial flushing, pounding heartbeat, muscle tremors or weakness, chest pain or palpitations, bronchial irritation or coughing, or increased sweating. **Pregnancy/breast-feeding precautions:** Inform prescriber if you are or intend to be pregnant. Breast-feeding is not recommended.

**Geriatric Considerations:** Oral formulation was recently removed from the market; avoid as a bronchodilator. Use caution since it crosses the blood-brain barrier and may cause confusion (see Warnings/Precautions, Adverse Reactions).

- **Ephedrine, Theophylline, and Hydroxyzine** *see* Theophylline, Ephedrine, and Hydroxyzine *on page 1118*
- **Ephedrine, Theophylline, and Phenobarbital** *see* Theophylline, Ephedrine, and Phenobarbital *on page 1118*
- **Epifrin®** *see* Epinephrine *on next page*
- **Epifrin®** *see* Ophthalmic Agents, Glaucoma *on page 853*

♦ **E-Pilo®** *see* Pilocarpine and Epinephrine *on page 932*
♦ **E-Pilo-x® Ophthalmic** *see* Pilocarpine and Epinephrine *on page 932*
♦ **Epimorph®** *see* Morphine Sulfate *on page 790*
♦ **Epinal®** *see* Ophthalmic Agents, Glaucoma *on page 853*

## Epinephrine (ep i NEF rin)

**U.S. Brand Names** Adrenalin®; AsthmaHaler®; AsthmaNefrin® [OTC]; Bronitin®; Bronkaid® Mist [OTC]; Epifrin®; EpiPen® Auto-Injector; EpiPen® Jr Auto-Injector; Glaucon®; microNefrin®; Primatene® Mist [OTC]; Sus-Phrine®; Vaponefrin®

**Synonyms** Adrenaline

**Therapeutic Category** Alpha/Beta Agonist; Antidote; Ophthalmic Agent, Antiglaucoma

**Pregnancy Risk Factor** C

**Lactation** Excretion in breast milk unknown

**Use** Treatment of bronchospasms, anaphylactic reactions, cardiac arrest, management of open-angle (chronic simple) glaucoma

**Mechanism of Action/Effect** Stimulates alpha-, $beta_1$-, and $beta_2$-adrenergic receptors resulting in relaxation of smooth muscle of the bronchial tree, cardiac stimulation, and dilation of skeletal muscle vasculature; small doses can cause vasodilation via $beta_2$-vascular receptors; large doses may produce constriction of skeletal and vascular smooth muscle; decreases production of aqueous humor and increases aqueous outflow; dilates the pupil by contracting the dilator muscle

**Contraindications** Hypersensitivity to epinephrine or any component; cardiac arrhythmias; angle-closure glaucoma

**Warnings** Use with caution in elderly patients, patients with diabetes mellitus, cardiovascular diseases (angina, tachycardia, prostatic hypertrophy, history of seizures, renal dysfunction, myocardial infarction), thyroid disease, cerebral arteriosclerosis, or Parkinson's. Some products contain sulfites as preservatives. Rapid I.V. infusion may cause death from cerebrovascular hemorrhage or cardiac arrhythmias. Oral inhalation of epinephrine is **not** the preferred route of administration. Pregnancy factor C.

**Drug Interactions**

**Decreased Effect:** Decreased bronchodilation with β-blockers. Decreases antihypertensive effects of methyldopa or guanethidine.

**Increased Effect/Toxicity:** Increased cardiac irritability if administered concurrently with halogenated inhalation anesthetics, beta-blocking agents, or alpha-blocking agents.

**Effects on Lab Values** ↑ bilirubin (S), catecholamines (U), glucose, uric acid (S)

**Adverse Reactions**

**Parenteral** (cardiovascular use):

>10%:
- Central nervous system: Headache
- Gastrointestinal: Nausea, vomiting

1% to 10%:
- Cardiovascular: Premature ventricular beats, bradycardia, hypertension, hypotension, chest pain, palpitations, tachycardia, ventricular arrhythmias
- Central nervous system: Nervousness or restlessness
- Respiratory: Dyspnea

**Systemic:**

<1% (Limited to important or life-threatening symptoms): Hypokalemia

>10%:
- Cardiovascular: Pounding heartbeat
- Central nervous system: Nervousness

1% to 10%:
- Cardiovascular: Flushing of face, hypertension, paleness
- Central nervous system: Dizziness, lightheadedness, headache, insomnia
- Gastrointestinal: Nausea, vomiting
- Neuromuscular & skeletal: Trembling, weakness
- Respiratory: Bronchial irritation, coughing
- Miscellaneous: Sweating (increased)

<1% (Limited to important or life-threatening symptoms): Chest pain, arrhythmias, tachycardia, paradoxical bronchospasm

**Overdose/Toxicology** Symptoms of overdose include hypertension, which may result in subarachnoid hemorrhage and hemiplegia; arrhythmias; unusually large pupils; pulmonary edema; renal failure; and metabolic acidosis. There is no specific antidote for epinephrine intoxication and treatment is primarily supportive.

**Pharmacodynamics/Kinetics**

**Distribution:** Crosses the placenta

**Metabolism:** Neural/hepatic

**Excretion:** Urine

**Onset:**

Onset of bronchodilation: Subcutaneous: Within 5-10 minutes; Inhalation: Within 1 minute

Conjunctival instillation: Intraocular pressure falls within 1 hour; Peak effect: Within 4-8 hours

**Duration:** Conjunctival instillation: Duration of ocular effect: 12-24 hours

**Formulations**

Aerosol, oral:

Bitartrate (AsthmaHaler®, Bronitin®): 0.3 mg/spray [epinephrine base 0.16 mg/spray] (10 mL, 15 mL, 22.5 mL)

Bronkaid®: 0.5% (10 mL, 15 mL, 22.5 mL)

Primatene® Mist: 0.2 mg/spray (15 mL, 22.5 mL)
Auto-injector:
EpiPen®: Delivers 0.3 mg I.M. of epinephrine 1:1000 (2 mL)
EpiPen® Jr.: Delivers 0.15 mg I.M. of epinephrine 1:2000 (2 mL)
Solution:
Inhalation:
Adrenalin®: 1% [10 mg/mL, 1:100] (7.5 mL)
Injection:
Adrenalin®: 0.01 mg/mL [1:100,000] (5 mL); 0.1 mg/mL [1:10,000] (3 mL, 10 mL); 1 mg/mL [1:1000] (1 mL, 2 mL, 30 mL)
Suspension (Sus-Phrine®): 5 mg/mL [1:200] (0.3 mL, 5 mL)
Nasal (Adrenalin®): 0.1% [1 mg/mL, 1:1000] (30 mL)
Ophthalmic, as hydrochloride (Epifrin®, Glaucon®): 0.1% (1 mL, 30 mL); 0.5% (15 mL); 1% (1 mL, 10 mL, 15 mL); 2% (10 mL, 15 mL)
Topical (Adrenalin®): 0.1% [1 mg/mL, 1:1000] (10 mL, 30 mL)

## Dosing

**Adults:**
Bronchodilator:
I.M., S.C. (1:1000): 0.1-0.5 mg every 10-15 minutes to 4 hours
Suspension (1:200) S.C.: 0.1-0.3 mL (0.5-1.5 mg)
I.V.: 0.1-0.25 mg (single dose maximum: 1 mg)
Asystole:
I.V.: 1 mg every 3-5 minutes; if this approach fails, alternative regimens include: Intermediate: 2-5 mg every 3-5 minutes; Escalating: 1 mg, 3 mg, 5 mg at 3-minute intervals; High: 0.1 mg/kg every 3-5 minutes.
Intratracheal: Although optimal dose is unknown, doses of 2-2.5 times the I.V. dose may be needed
Refractory hypotension (refractory to dopamine/dobutamine): I.V. infusion administration requires the use of an infusion pump: I.V. infusion: 1 mg in 250 mL NS/$D_5W$ at 0.1-1 mcg/kg/minute; titrate to desired effect.
Hypersensitivity reaction: I.M., S.C.: 0.2-0.5 mg every 20 minutes to 4 hours (single dose maximum: 1 mg)
Nebulization: Instill 8-15 drops into nebulizer reservoirs; administer 1-3 inhalations 4-6 times/day.
Ophthalmic: Instill 1-2 drops in eye(s) once or twice daily.
Intranasal: Apply locally as drops or spray or with sterile swab.

**Elderly:** Refer to adult dosing.

## Administration

**I.M.:** I.M. administration into the buttocks should be avoided.

**I.V.:** Central line administration only. Intravenous infusions require an infusion pump.
Endotracheal: Doses (2-2.5 times the I.V. dose) should be diluted to 10 mL with NS or distilled water prior to administration.
Epinephrine can be administered S.C., I.M. (Sus-Phrine®), I.V.

**I.V. Detail: Extravasation management:** Use phentolamine as antidote. Mix 5 mg with 9 mL of NS. Inject a small amount of this dilution into extravasated area. Blanching should reverse immediately. Monitor site. If blanching should recur, additional injections of phentolamine may be needed.

## Stability

**Storage:** Epinephrine is sensitive to light and air. Protection from light is recommended. Oxidation turns drug pink, then a brown color. **Solutions should not be used if they are discolored or contain a precipitate.**

**Reconstitution:**

**Standard diluent:** 1 mg/250 mL NS

**Preparation of adult I.V. infusion:** Dilute 1 mg in 250 mL of $D_5W$ or NS (4 mcg/mL). Administer at an initial rate of 1 mcg/minute and increase to desired effects. At 20 mcg/minute pure alpha effects occur.
1 mcg/minute: 15 mL/hour
2 mcg/minute: 30 mL/hour
3 mcg/minute: 45 mL/hour, etc

Stability of injection of parenteral admixture at room temperature (25°C) or refrigeration (4°C) is 24 hours.

**Compatibility:** Compatible with dopamine, dobutamine, diltiazem. Incompatible with aminophylline, sodium bicarbonate, or other alkaline solutions. See the Compatibility of Drugs Chart *on page 1315.*

## Additional Nursing Issues

**Physical Assessment:** Assess other medications patient may be taking for effectiveness and interactions (see Drug Interactions). See Warnings/Precautions and Contraindications for cautious use. Monitor therapeutic response (according to purpose for use) and adverse reactions (eg, hypertension, CNS excitability, urinary retention, dysarrhythmias, respiratory depression - see Warnings/Precautions, Adverse Reactions, and Overdose/Toxicology). Assess knowledge/teach patient appropriate use, interventions to reduce side effects, and adverse symptoms to report.

I.V. (cardiovascular therapy): Use infusion pump, continuous cardiac/hemodynamic monitoring, and assess infusion site frequently for extravasation (see Administration for extravasation instructions).

**Pregnancy risk factor C** - benefits of use should outweigh possible risks. Note breast-feeding caution.

(Continued)

## Epinephrine *(Continued)*

**Patient Information/Instruction:** Use this medication exactly as directed; do not take more than recommended dosage. Avoid other stimulant prescriptive or OTC medications to avoid serious overdose reactions. You may experience dizziness, blurred vision, restlessness (use caution when driving or engaging in tasks requiring alertness until response to drug is known); or difficulty urinating (empty bladder immediately before taking this medication). Report excessive nervousness or excitation, inability to sleep, facial flushing, pounding heartbeat, muscle tremors or weakness, chest pain or palpitations, bronchial irritation or coughing, or increased sweating.

Ophthalmic: Wash hands before instilling. Sit or lie down to instill. Open eye, look at ceiling, and instill prescribed amount of medication. Close eye and roll eye in all directions, and apply gentle pressure to inner corner of eye. Do not let tip of applicator touch eye or contaminate tip of applicator. Temporary stinging or burning may occur. Report persistent pain, burning, vision disturbances, swelling, itching, or worsening of condition.

Aerosol: Use aerosol or nebulizer as per instructions. Clear as much mucus as possible before use. Rinse mouth following each use. If more than one inhalation is necessary, wait 1 minute between inhalations. May cause restlessness or nervousness; use caution when driving or engaging in hazardous activities until response to medication is known. Report persistent nervousness, restlessness, sleeplessness, palpitations, tachycardia, chest pain, muscle tremors, dizziness, flushing, or if breathing difficulty persists.

Nasal: Instill 1 spray into each nostril 3-4 times a day. Report if symptoms worsen or nasal passages become irritated.

**Pregnancy/breast-feeding precautions:** Inform prescriber if you are or intend to be pregnant. Consult prescriber if breast-feeding.

**Geriatric Considerations:** The use of epinephrine in the treatment of acute exacerbations of asthma was studied in older adults. A dose of 0.3 mg S.C. every 20 minutes for three doses was well tolerated in older patients with no history of angina or recent myocardial infarction. There was no significant difference in the incidence of ventricular arrhythmias in older adults versus younger adults.

**Additional Information** Some formulations may contain ethanol. The solution formulation contains sulfites.

Epinephrine: Primatene® Mist, Bronkaid® Mist, Sus-Phrine®
Epinephrine bitartrate: AsthmaHaler®, Bronitin®, Primatene® Mist
Epinephrine hydrochloride: Adrenalin®, Epifrin®, EpiPen®, EpiPen® Jr
Racemic epinephrine: AsthmaHaler®, microNefrin®, Vaponefrin®
Epinephryl borate: Epinal®


- **Epinephrine** *see* Ophthalmic Agents, Glaucoma *on page 853*
- **Epinephrine and Lidocaine** *see* Lidocaine and Epinephrine *on page 677*
- **Epinephrine and Pilocarpine** *see* Pilocarpine and Epinephrine *on page 932*
- **EpiPen® Auto-Injector** *see* Epinephrine *on page 424*
- **EpiPen® Jr Auto-Injector** *see* Epinephrine *on page 424*
- **Epitol®** *see* Carbamazepine *on page 195*
- **Epival®** *see* Valproic Acid and Derivatives *on page 1198*
- **Epivir®, Epivir® HBV** *see* Lamivudine *on page 652*
- **EPO** *see* Epoetin Alfa *on this page*


## Epoetin Alfa (e POE e tin AL fa)

**U.S. Brand Names** Epogen®; Procrit®

**Synonyms** EPO; Erythropoietin; *r*HuEPO-α

**Therapeutic Category** Colony Stimulating Factor

**Pregnancy Risk Factor** C

**Lactation** Excretion in breast milk unknown

**Use** Anemia associated with end-stage renal disease; anemia related to AIDS and therapy with AZT-treated in HIV-infected patients; endogenous serum erythropoietin (EPO) level which are inappropriately low for hemoglobin level (eg, anemia of neoplasia)

**Note:** Not appropriate for emergency treatment of anemia; onset or response takes 7-10 days

**Unlabeled use:** Patients undergoing autologous blood donation prior to surgery - EPO may accelerate recovery of hemoglobin level and, in some cases, permit more units of blood to be donated

**Mechanism of Action/Effect** Induces red blood cell production in the bone marrow to be released into the blood stream where they mature to erythrocytes; results in rise in hematocrit and hemoglobin levels

**Contraindications** Hypersensitivity to albumin (human) or mammalian cell-derived products; uncontrolled hypertension

**Warnings** Use with caution in patients with porphyria, hypertension, or a history of seizures; prior to and during therapy, iron stores must be evaluated. It is recommended that the epoetin dose be decreased if the hematocrit increase exceeds 4 points in any 2-week period.

**Pretherapy parameters:**

Serum ferritin >300 ng/dL
Transferrin saturation (serum iron/iron binding capacity x 100) of 20% to 30%
Iron supplementation (usual oral dosing of 325 mg 2-3 times/day) should be given during therapy to provide for increased requirements during expansion of the red cell

mass secondary to marrow stimulation by EPO unless iron stores are already in excess.

For patients with endogenous serum EPO levels which are inappropriately low for hemoglobin level, documentation of the serum EPO level will help indicate which patients may benefit from EPO therapy. Serum EPO levels can be ordered routinely from Clinical Chemistry (red top serum separator tube).

See table.

**Factors Limiting Response to Epoetin Alfa**

| Factor | Mechanism |
|---|---|
| Iron deficiency | Limits hemoglobin synthesis |
| Blood loss/hemolysis | Counteracts epoetin alfa-stimulated erythropoiesis |
| Infection/inflammation | Inhibits iron transfer from storage to bone marrow<br>Suppresses erythropoiesis through activated macrophages |
| Aluminum overload | Inhibits iron incorporation into heme protein |
| Bone marrow replacement<br>Hyperparathyroidsm<br>Metastatic, neoplastic | Limits bone marrow volume |
| Folic acid/vitamin $B_{12}$ deficiency | Limits hemoglobin synthesis |
| Patient compliance | Self-administered epoetin alfa or iron therapy |

Increased mortality has occurred when aggressive dosing is used in CHF or anginal patients undergoing hemodialysis. An Amgen-funded study determined that when patients were targeted for a hematocrit of 42% versus a less aggressive 30%, mortality was higher (35% versus 29%).

Pregnancy factor C.

## Adverse Reactions

>10%:
- Cardiovascular: Hypertension
- Central nervous system: Fatigue, headache, fever

1% to 10%:
- Cardiovascular: Edema, chest pain, polycythemia
- Central nervous system: Dizziness, seizures
- Gastrointestinal: Nausea, vomiting, diarrhea
- Hematologic: Clotted access
- Neuromuscular & skeletal: Arthralgia, weakness

<1% (Limited to important or life-threatening symptoms): Myocardial infarction, CVA/TIA

**Overdose/Toxicology** Symptoms of overdose include erythrocytosis. Maintain adequate airway and provide other supportive measures and agents for treating anaphylaxis when the I.V. drug is given.

## Pharmacodynamics/Kinetics

**Distribution:** Rapid in the plasma compartment; majority of drug is taken up by the liver, kidneys, and bone marrow.

**Half-life Elimination:** Circulating: 4-13 hours in patients with chronic renal failure; 20% shorter in patients with normal renal function

**Time to Peak:** S.C.: 2-8 hours

**Metabolism:** Minimal

**Excretion:** Minimal/urine

**Onset:** Several days; Peak effect: 2-3 weeks

## Formulations

1 mL single-dose vials: Preservative-free solution
- 2000 units/mL
- 3000 units/mL
- 4000 units/mL
- 10,000 units/mL

2 mL multidose vials: Preserved solution: 10,000 units/mL

## Dosing

**Adults:** Individuals with anemia due to iron deficiency, sickle cell disease, autoimmune hemolytic anemia, and bleeding, generally have appropriate endogenous EPO levels to drive erythropoiesis and would not ordinarily be candidates for EPO therapy.

**Dosing recommendations:**

Dosing schedules need to be individualized and careful monitoring of patients receiving the drug is mandatory.

*r*HuEPO-α may be ineffective if other factors such as iron or $B_{12}$/folate deficiency limit marrow response.

**Initial:** I.V., S.C.: 50-150 units/kg 3 times/week

**Dose should be reduced** when the hematocrit reaches the target range of 30% to 36% or a hematocrit increase >4 points over any 2-week period.

**Dose should be held** if the hematocrit exceeds 36% and until the hematocrit decreases to the target range (30% to 36%).

**Dose should be increased** by 25-50 units/kg 3 times/week if the hematocrit does not increase by 5-6 points after 8 weeks of therapy and hematocrit is below the target range; further increases of 25 units/kg 3 times/week may be made at 4- to 6-week intervals until the desired response is obtained. Doses exceeding 300 units/kg 3 times/week are not recommended because a greater biological response is not usually observed.

(Continued)

## Epoetin Alfa *(Continued)*

Maintenance dose: Should be individualized to maintain the hematocrit within the 30% to 36% target range

**Elderly:** Refer to adult dosing.

**Renal Impairment:**

Dialysis patient: Usually administered as I.V. bolus 3 times/week. While administration is independent of the dialysis procedure, it may be administered into the venous line at the end of the dialysis procedure to obviate the need for additional venous access.

Chronic renal failure patients not on dialysis: May be given either as an I.V. or S.C. injection.

Hemodialysis: Supplemental dose is not necessary.

Peritoneal dialysis: Supplemental dose is not necessary.

**Stability**

**Storage:** Vials should be stored at 2°C to 8°C (36°F to 46°F). **Do not freeze or shake.** Vials are stable 2 weeks at room temperature.

**Single-dose 1 mL vial** contains no preservative. Use one dose per vial. Do not re-enter vial. Discard unused portions.

**Multidose 2 mL vial** contains preservative. Store at 2°C to 8°C after initial entry and between doses. Discard 21 days after initial entry.

**Reconstitution:** For minimal dilution, mix with bacteriostatic 0.9% sodium chloride, containing 20 mL of 0.9% sodium chloride and benzyl alcohol as the bacteriostatic agent. Dilutions of 1:10 and 1:20 (1 part epoetin:19 parts sodium chloride) are stable for 18 hours at room temperature. Results showed no loss of epoetin alfa after a 1:20 dilution. 250 mcg/mL albumin remaining after a 1:10 dilution of formulated epoetin alfa should be sufficient to prevent it from binding to commonly encountered containers.

**Monitoring Laboratory Tests** Hematocrit should be determined twice weekly until stabilization within the target range (30% to 36%), and twice weekly for at least 2-6 weeks after a dose increase. See table.

| Test | Initial Phase Frequency | Maintenance Phase Frequency |
|---|---|---|
| Hematocrit/hemoglobin | 2 x/week | 2-4 x/month |
| Blood pressure | 3 x/week | 3 x/week |
| Serum ferritin | Monthly | Quarterly |
| Transferrin saturation | Monthly | Quarterly |
| Serum chemistries including CBC with differential, creatinine, blood urea nitrogen, potassium, phosphorous | Regularly per routine | Regularly per routine |

**Additional Nursing Issues**

**Physical Assessment:** Monitor appropriate laboratory tests to determine effectiveness of therapy. Monitor all I.V. lines for clotting. Monitor vital signs (blood pressure, pulse rate) prior to and during initial therapy, fluid ratio intake/output (edema), CNS response (eg, dizziness, seizures). Monitor other medications and dietary intake for iron intake or changes in iron intake that might influence effectiveness of therapy or laboratory results. Instruct patient/caregiver in appropriate self-administration procedures and disposal of syringes or needles, if necessary. **Pregnancy risk factor C** - benefits of use should outweigh possible risks. Note breast-feeding caution.

**Patient Information/Instruction:** You will require frequent blood tests to determine appropriate dosage. Do not take other medications, vitamin or iron supplements, or make significant changes in your diet without consulting prescriber. Report signs or symptoms of edema (eg, swollen extremities, difficulty breathing, rapid weight gain), onset of severe headache, acute back pain, chest pain, or muscular tremors or seizure activity. **Pregnancy/breast-feeding precautions:** Inform prescriber if you are or intend to be pregnant. Consult prescriber if breast-feeding.

**Geriatric Considerations:** There is limited information about the use of epoetin alfa in the elderly. Endogenous erythropoietin secretion has been reported to be decreased in older adults with normocytic or iron deficiency anemias or those with a serum hemoglobin concentration <12 g/dL; one study did not find such a relationship in the elderly with chronic anemia. A blunted erythropoietin response to anemia has been reported in patients with cancer, rheumatoid arthritis, and AIDS.

**Pregnancy Issues:** Epoetin alpha has been shown to have adverse effects in rats when given in doses 5 times the human dose. Use only if potential benefit justifies the potential risk to the fetus.

**Additional Information**

Reimbursement Hotline (Epogen®): 1-800-272-9376
Professional Services [Amgen]: 1-800-77-AMGEN
Reimbursement Hotline (Procrit®): 1-800-553-3851
Professional services [Ortho Biotech]: 1-800-325-7504

♦ **Epogen®** *see* Epoetin Alfa *on page 426*

## Epoprostenol (e poe PROST en ole)

**U.S. Brand Names** Flolan® Injection

**Therapeutic Category** Plasma Volume Expander, Colloid; Prostaglandin

**Pregnancy Risk Factor** B

**Lactation** Excretion in breast milk unknown

**Use** Treatment of primary pulmonary hypertension in patients not responsive to other treatment; other potential uses include pulmonary hypertension associated with adult respiratory distress syndrome (ARDS), systemic lupus erythematosus (SLE), or congestive heart failure (CHF), neonatal pulmonary hypertension, cardiopulmonary bypass surgery, hemodialysis, atherosclerosis, peripheral vascular disorders, neonatal purpura fulminans, and refractory congestive heart failure

**Mechanism of Action/Effect** Naturally occur ring prostacyclin (PG12) which acts as a strong vasodilator in all vascular beds; inhibits platelet aggregation

**Contraindications** Hypersensitivity to epoprostenol or any component; hyaline membrane disease or persistent fetal circulation and when a dominant left-to-right shunt is present; respiratory distress syndrome

**Warnings** Abrupt interruptions or large sudden reductions in dosage may result in rebound pulmonary hypertension. Some patients with primary pulmonary hypertension have developed pulmonary edema during dose ranging, which may be associated with pulmonary veno-occlusive disease. During chronic use, unless contraindicated, anticoagulants should be coadministered to reduce the risk of thromboembolism. Use cautiously with patients who have bleeding tendencies (inhibits platelet aggregation).

**Drug Interactions**

**Increased Effect/Toxicity:** The hypotensive effects of epoprostenol may be exacerbated by other vasodilators or by using acetate in dialysis fluids. Patients treated with anticoagulants and epoprostenol should be monitored for increased bleeding risk because of shared effects on platelet aggregation.

**Adverse Reactions**

>10%:

- Central nervous system: Fever, chills, anxiety, nervousness, dizziness, headache, hyperesthesia, pain
- Cardiovascular: Flushing, tachycardia, syncope, heart failure,
- Gastrointestinal: Diarrhea, nausea, vomiting
- Neuromuscular & skeletal: Jaw pain, myalgia, tremor, paresthesia
- Respiratory: Hypoxia
- Miscellaneous: Sepsis, flu-like symptoms

1% to 10%:

- Cardiovascular: Bradycardia, chest pain pectoris, edema, arrhythmias, pallor, cyanosis, palpitations, cerebrovascular accident, myocardial ischemia, chest pain
- Central nervous system: Seizures, confusion, depression, insomnia, muscle weakness
- Dermatologic: Pruritus, rash
- Endocrine & metabolic: Hypokalemia, weight change
- Gastrointestinal: Abdominal pain, anorexia, constipation
- Hematologic: Hemorrhage
- Hepatic: Ascites
- Neuromuscular & skeletal: Arthralgias, bone pain
- Hematologic: Disseminated intravascular coagulation
- Ocular: Amblyopia
- Respiratory: Cough increase, dyspnea, epistaxis, pleural effusion
- Miscellaneous: Sweating

<1% (Limited to important or life-threatening symptoms): Thrombocytopenia

**Overdose/Toxicology** Symptoms of overdose include headache, hypotension, tachycardia, nausea, vomiting, diarrhea, and flushing. If any of these symptoms occur, reduce the infusion rate until symptoms subside. If symptoms do not subside, consider drug discontinuation. No fatal events have been reported following overdose with epoprostenol.

**Pharmacodynamics/Kinetics**

**Half-life Elimination:** 2.7-6 minute; steady-state levels are reached in about 15 minutes with continuous infusions

**Metabolism:** Blood

**Excretion:** Urine

**Formulations** Injection, as sodium: 0.5 mg/vial and 1.5 mg/vial, each supplied with 50 mL of sterile diluent

**Dosing**

**Adults:** I.V.:

**Acute dose ranging:** The initial infusion rate should be 2 ng/kg/minute by continuous I.V. and increased in increments of 2 ng/kg/minute every 15 minutes or longer until dose-limiting effects are elicited (such as chest pain, anxiety, dizziness, changes in heart rate, dyspnea, nausea, vomiting, headache, hypotension and/or flushing).

**Continuous chronic infusion:** Initial: 4 ng/kg/minute **less** than the maximum-tolerated infusion rate determined during acute dose ranging.

If maximum-tolerated infusion rate is <5 ng/kg/minute the chronic infusion rate should be ½ the maximum-tolerated acute infusion rate.

**Dosage adjustments:** Dose adjustments in the chronic infusion rate should be based on persistence, recurrence, or worsening of patient symptoms of pulmonary hypertension. If symptoms persist or reoccur after improving, the infusion rate should be increased by 1-2 ng/kg/minute increments, every 15 minutes or more. Following establishment of a new chronic infusion rate, the patient should be observed and vital signs monitored.

**Elderly:** Refer to adult dosing.

**Administration**

**I.V. Detail:** Epoprostenol must be reconstituted with manufacturer-supplied sterile diluent only (see Preparation of Infusion table) and when given on an ongoing basis it must be infused through a central venous catheter. Infuse using an infusion pump.

(Continued)

## Epoprostenol *(Continued)*

**Stability**

**Storage:** Refrigerate ampuls. Protect from freezing.

**Reconstitution:** Prepare fresh solutions every 24 hours. Reconstitute with sterile diluent for epoprostenol.

**Compatibility:** Compatible in $D_5W$, $D_{10}W$, and NS solutions. Do not mix or administer with any other drugs prior to or during administration. Stable for 8 hours at room temperature.

**Preparation of Infusion**

| To Make 100 mL of Solution With Concentration | Directions |
|---|---|
| 3000 ng/mL | Dissolve one 0.5 mg vial with 6 mL supplied diluent, withdraw 3 mL and add to sufficient diluent to make a total of 100 mL. |
| 5000 ng/mL | Dissolve one 0.5 mg vial with 5 mL supplied diluent, withdraw entire vial contents and add a sufficient volume of diluent to make a total of 100 mL. |
| 10,000 ng/mL | Dissolve two 0.5 mg vials each with 5 mL supplied diluent, withdraw entire vial contents and add a sufficient volume of diluent to make a total of 100 mL. |
| 15,000 ng/mL | Dissolve one 1.5 mg vial with 5 mL supplied diluent, withdraw entire vial contents and add a sufficient volume of diluent to make a total of 100 mL. |

**Additional Nursing Issues**

**Physical Assessment:**

Institutional: Continuous pulmonary and hemodynamic arterial monitoring, protimes

Noninstitutional: Avoid sudden rate reduction or abrupt withdrawal or interruption of therapy (see Warnings/Precautions). When adjustment in rate is made, monitor blood pressure (standing and supine) and pulse for several hours to ensure tolerance to new rate. Monitor for bleeding. Monitor (or teach appropriate caregiver or patient to monitor) vital signs on 3 times/day basis. Monitor for improved pulmonary function (decreased exertional dyspnea, fatigue, syncope, chest pain) and improved quality of life. Be alert for any infusion pump malfunction. Assess for signs of overdose (eg, hypoxia, flushing, tachycardia, fever, chills, anxiety, acute headache, tremor, vomiting, diarrhea).

Note breast-feeding caution.

**Patient Information/Instruction:** Therapy on this drug will probably be prolonged, possibly for years. You may experience mild headache, nausea or vomiting, and some muscular pains (use of a mild analgesia may be recommended by your prescriber). Report immediately any signs or symptoms of acute or severe headache, back pain, increased difficult breathing, flushing, fever or chills, any unusual bleeding or bruising, or any onset of unresolved diarrhea. **Breast-feeding precautions:** Consult prescriber if breast-feeding.

**Additional Information** All orders for epoprostenol are distributed only by Quantum Healthcare, Inc. To order the drug or to request reimbursement assistance, call 1-800-622-1820.

pH: 10.2-10.8

♦ **Eprex®** *see* Epoetin Alfa *on page 426*
♦ **Epsom Salts (Magnesium Sulfate)** *see* Magnesium Supplements *on page 703*
♦ **EPT** *see* Teniposide *on page 1101*

## Eptifibatide (ep TIF i ba tide)

**U.S. Brand Names** Integrilin®

**Synonyms** Intrifiban

**Therapeutic Category** Antiplatelet Agent, Glycoprotein IIb/IIIa Inhibitor

**Pregnancy Risk Factor** B

**Lactation** Excretion in breast milk unknown/not recommended

**Use** Treatment of patients with acute coronary syndrome (UA/NQMI), including patients who are to be managed medically and those undergoing percutaneous coronary intervention (PCI including PTCA)

**Mechanism of Action/Effect** Eptifibatide is a IIb/IIa antagonist that reversibly blocks platelet aggregation and prevents thrombosis.

**Contraindications** Hypersensitivity to eptifibatide or related compounds, tirofiban, lamifiban; history of bleeding diathesis or abnormal bleeding (within 30 days); severe hypertension, major surgery within preceding 6 weeks, history of stroke (within 30 days) or any hemorrhagic stroke, platelet count <100,000/mm$^3$; dependence on renal dialysis; renal impairment - serum creatinine >2.0 (180 mcg/kg bolus), >4.0 (135 mcg/kg bolus); concomitant or anticipated other parenteral glycoprotein IIb/IIIa inhibitors

**Warnings** Bleeding is the most common complication encountered during eptifibatide therapy. Most major bleeding has been at the arterial access site for cardiac catheterization or from the gastrointestinal or genitourinary tract. To minimize bleeding complications, care must be taken in sheath insertion/removal. Sheath hemostasis should be achieved at least 4 hours before hospital discharge. Use with caution when administered with other anticoagulants; minimize vascular trauma and other trauma. Avoid obtaining intravenous access via noncompressible sites (eg, subclavian or jugular vein) or I.M. injections.

**Drug Interactions**

**Increased Effect/Toxicity:** Drugs which affect hemostasis include thrombolytics, oral anticoagulants, nonsteroidal anti-inflammatory agents, dipyridamole, ticlopidine, and clopidogrel. Avoid concomitant use of other IIb/IIIa inhibitors.

**Adverse Reactions** Bleeding is the major drug-related adverse effect. Major bleeding was reported in 4.4% to 10.5%; minor bleeding was reported in 10.5% to 14.2%; requirement for transfusion was reported in 5.5% to 12.8%.

Cardiovascular: Hypotension
Local: Injection site reaction
Neuromuscular & skeletal: Back pain

1% to 10%: Hematologic: Thrombocytopenia (2.8% to 3.2%)

<1% (Limited to important or life-threatening symptoms): Intracranial hemorrhage (0.5% to 0.7%), anaphylaxis (0.4% to 0.6%)

**Overdose/Toxicology** Two cases of human overdose have been reported; neither case was eventful or associated with major bleeding. Symptoms of overdose in animal studies include loss of righting reflex, dyspnea, ptosis, decreased muscle tone, and petechial hemorrhage. Treatment is supportive.

**Pharmacodynamics/Kinetics**

**Protein Binding:** ~25%

**Half-life Elimination:** 2.5 hours

**Metabolism:** Total body clearance: 55-58 mL/kg/hour; renal clearance is ~50% of total in healthy subjects

**Excretion:** Renal excretion of eptifibatide and metabolites accounts for majority of drug elimination; significant renal impairment is expected to alter the disposition of this compound

Reversibility: Platelet function is restored in about 4 hours following discontinuation.

**Onset:** Within 1 hour

**Formulations** Injection: 0.75 mg/mL (100 mL); 2 mg/mL (10 mL)

**Dosing**

**Adults:** I.V.:

Acute coronary syndrome: Bolus of 180 mcg/kg over 1-2 minutes begun as soon as possible following diagnosis, followed by a continuous infusion of 2 mcg/kg/minute (maximum: 15 mg/hour) until hospital discharge or initiation of CABG surgery, up to 72 hours. If a patient is to undergo a percutaneous coronary intervention (PCI) while receiving eptifibatide, consideration can be given to decreasing the infusion rate to 0.5 mcg/kg/minute at the time of the procedure. Infusion should be continued for an additional 20-24 hours after the procedure, allowing for up to 96 hours of therapy.

Percutaneous coronary intervention (PCI) in patients not presenting with an acute coronary syndrome: Bolus of 135 mcg/kg administered immediately before the initiation of PCI followed by a continuous infusion of 0.5 mcg/kg/minute for 20-24 hours.

**Elderly:** Refer to adult dosing.

**Administration**

**I.V.:** Administer by I.V. push over 1-2 minutes. Begin continuous infusion immediately following bolus administration, administered directly from the 100 mL vial.

**I.V. Detail:** Visually inspect for discoloration or particulate matter prior to administration. The bolus dose should be withdrawn from the 10 mL vial into a syringe. The 100 mL vial should be spiked with a vented infusion set.

**Stability**

**Storage:** Vials should be stored refrigerated at 2°C to 8°C (36°F to 46°F). Protect from light until administration. Do not use beyond the expiration date. Discard any unused portion left in the vial.

**Monitoring Laboratory Tests** Laboratory tests at baseline and monitoring during therapy: hematocrit and hemoglobin, platelet count, serum creatinine, PT/aPTT, and ACT with PCI (maintain ACT between 300-350 seconds).

**Additional Nursing Issues**

**Physical Assessment:** Monitor vital signs and laboratory results prior to, during, and after therapy. Assess infusion insertion site during and after therapy (every 15 minutes or as institutional policy). Observe and teach patient bleeding precautions (avoid invasive procedures and activities that could result in injury). Monitor closely for signs of excessive bleeding (CNS changes, blood in urine, stool, or vomitus; unusual bruising or bleeding). Breast-feeding is not recommended.

**Patient Information/Instruction:** Emergency use may dictate depth of patient education. This medication can only be administered I.V. You will have a tendency to bleed easily following this medication. Use caution to prevent injury (use electric razor, use soft toothbrush, use caution with sharps). If bleeding occurs, apply pressure to bleeding spot until bleeding stops completely. Report unusual bruising or bleeding (eg, blood in urine, stool, or vomitus, bleeding gums), dizziness or changes in vision, or back pain. **Breast-feeding precautions:** Breast-feeding is not recommended.


- ♦ **Equagesic®** *see* Aspirin and Meprobamate *on page 113*
- ♦ **Equalactin® Chewable Tablet** *see page 1294*
- ♦ **Equanil®** *see* Meprobamate *on page 724*
- ♦ **Equilet® [OTC]** *see* Calcium Supplements *on page 185*
- ♦ **Eramycin®** *see* Erythromycin *on page 435*
- ♦ **Ercaf®** *see* Ergotamine Derivatives *on page 434*
- ♦ **Ergamisol®** *see* Levamisole *on page 665*

♦ **Ergocaf** *see* Ergotamine Derivatives *on page 434*

## Ergocalciferol (er goe kal SIF e role)

**U.S. Brand Names** Calciferol™ Injection; Calciferol™ Oral; Drisdol® Oral

**Synonyms** Activated Ergosterol; Viosterol; Vitamin $D_2$

**Therapeutic Category** Vitamin D Analog

**Pregnancy Risk Factor** A/C (if dose exceeds RDA recommendation)

**Lactation** Enters breast milk/compatible

**Use** Treatment of refractory rickets, hypophosphatemia, hypoparathyroidism

**Mechanism of Action/Effect** Stimulates calcium and phosphate absorption from the small intestine, promotes secretion of calcium from bone to blood; promotes renal tubule phosphate resorption

**Contraindications** Hypersensitivity to ergocalciferol or any component; hypercalcemia; malabsorption syndrome; evidence of vitamin D toxicity

**Warnings** Administer with extreme caution in patients with impaired renal function, heart disease, renal stones, or arteriosclerosis. Must give concomitant calcium supplementation. Maintain adequate fluid intake. Avoid hypercalcemia. Renal function impairment with secondary hyperparathyroidism. Pregnancy factor C (if dose exceeds RDA recommendation).

**Drug Interactions**

**Decreased Effect:** Cholestyramine, colestipol, mineral oil may decrease oral absorption.

**Increased Effect/Toxicity:** Thiazide diuretics may increase vitamin D effects. Cardiac glycosides may increase toxicity.

**Adverse Reactions**

1% to 10%:

- Cardiovascular: Hypotension, cardiac arrhythmias, hypertension
- Central nervous system: Irritability, headache
- Dermatologic: Pruritus
- Endocrine & metabolic: Polydipsia, hypermagnesemia
- Gastrointestinal: Nausea, vomiting, constipation, anorexia, pancreatitis, metallic taste
- Genitourinary: Polyuria
- Neuromuscular & skeletal: Myalgia, bone pain
- Ocular: Conjunctivitis, photophobia

<1% (Limited to important or life-threatening symptoms): Overt psychosis, seizures, elevated AST/ALT

**Overdose/Toxicology** Symptoms of chronic overdose include hypercalcemia, weakness, fatigue, lethargy, and anorexia. Following withdrawal of the drug and oral decontamination, treatment consists of bedrest, liberal intake of fluids, reduced calcium intake, and cathartic administration. Severe hypercalcemia requires I.V. hydration and forced diuresis with I.V. furosemide. Urine output should be monitored and maintained at >3 mL/kg/hour during the acute treatment phase. I.V. saline can quickly and significantly increase excretion of calcium into urine. Calcitonin, mithramycin, and biphosphonates have all been used successfully to treat the more resistant cases of vitamin D-induced hypercalcemia.

**Pharmacodynamics/Kinetics**

**Metabolism:** Inactive until hydroxylated in the liver and the kidney to calcifediol and then to calcitriol (most active form)

**Onset:** Peak effect: ~1 month following daily doses

**Formulations**

- Capsule (Drisdol®): 50,000 units [1.25 mg]
- Injection (Calciferol™): 500,000 units/mL [12.5 mg/mL] (1 mL)
- Liquid (Calciferol™, Drisdol®): 8000 units/mL [200 mcg/mL] (60 mL)
- Tablet (Calciferol™): 50,000 units [1.25 mg]

**Dosing**

**Adults:** Oral dosing is preferred

- Dietary supplementation (each mcg = 40 USP units): 10 mcg/day (400 units)
- Renal failure: 500 mcg/day (20,000 units)
- Hypoparathyroidism: 625 mcg to 5 mg/day (25,000-200,000 units) and calcium supplements
- Vitamin D-dependent rickets: 250 mcg to 1.5 mg/day (10,000-60,000 units)
- Nutritional rickets and osteomalacia:
  - With normal absorption: 25-125 mcg/day (1000-5000 units)
  - With malabsorption: 250-7500 mcg/day (10,000-300,000 units)
- Vitamin D-resistant rickets: 250-1500 mcg/day (10,000-60,000 units) with phosphate supplements

**Elderly:** Refer to adult dosing (see Geriatric Considerations and Additional Information).

**Administration**

**I.M.:** Parenteral injection is for I.M. use only.

**Stability**

**Storage:** Protect from light.

**Monitoring Laboratory Tests** Serum calcium, BUN, phosphorus every 1-2 weeks

**Additional Nursing Issues**

**Physical Assessment:** See Contraindications and Warnings/Precautions for use cautions. Assess effectiveness and interactions of other medications (see Drug Interactions). Monitor lab tests, effectiveness of therapy, and adverse effects at beginning of therapy and regularly with long-term use (see Adverse Reactions and Overdose/Toxicology). Assess knowledge/teach patient appropriate use (injection technique and needle disposal if I.M. self-administered), appropriate nutritional counseling, possible side effects/interventions, and adverse symptoms to report. **Pregnancy risk factor A/C** - see Pregnancy Risk Factor for cautious use.

**Patient Information/Instruction:** Take exact dose prescribed; do not take more than recommended. Your prescriber may recommend a special diet; do not increase calcium intake without consulting prescriber. Avoid magnesium supplements or magnesium-containing antacids. You may experience nausea, vomiting, or metallic taste (frequent small meals, frequent mouth care, or sucking hard candy may help); hypotension (use caution when rising from sitting or lying position or when climbing stairs or bending over). Report chest pain or palpitations; acute headache, dizziness, or feeling of weakness; unresolved nausea or vomiting; persistent metallic taste; unrelieved muscle or bone pain; or CNS irritability.

**Geriatric Considerations:** Recommended daily allowances (RDA) have not been developed for persons >65 years of age. Vitamin D, folate, and $B_{12}$ (cyanocobalamin) have decreased absorption with age, but the clinical significance is yet unknown. Calorie requirements decrease with age and therefore, nutrient density must be increased to ensure adequate nutrient intake, including vitamins and minerals. Therefore, the use of a daily supplement with a multiple vitamin with minerals is recommended. Elderly consume less vitamin D, absorption may be decreased and many elderly have decreased sun exposure; therefore, elderly should receive supplementation with 800 units (20 mcg)/day. This is a recommendation of particular need to those with high risk for osteoporosis.

**Additional Information** 1.25 mg ergocalciferol provides 50,000 units of vitamin D activity

♦ **Ergomar®** *see* Ergotamine Derivatives *on next page*

## Ergonovine (er goe NOE veen)

**Therapeutic Category** Ergot Derivative

**Pregnancy Risk Factor** X

**Lactation** Excretion in breast milk unknown/not recommended

**Use** Prevention or management of postpartum or postabortion uterine hemorrhage; diagnose Prinzmetal's angina

**Mechanism of Action/Effect** Ergot alkaloid alpha-adrenergic agonist directly stimulates vascular smooth muscle to vasoconstrict peripheral and cerebral vessels; may also have antagonist effects on serotonin

**Contraindications** Allergy to ergonovine; induction of labor; threatened spontaneous abortion; pregnancy

**Warnings** Use caution with documented hypertension, chronic heart disease, mitral valve stenosis, peripheral vascular disease, renal or hepatic impairment

**Drug Interactions**

**Increased Effect/Toxicity:** Concomitant use with beta-adrenergic blockers may result in toxic peripheral ischemia, gangrene.

**Adverse Reactions**

>10%:

Cardiovascular: Hypertension (especially with rapid I.V. administration)
Central nervous system: Headache
Gastrointestinal: Nausea or vomiting (especially with I.V.)
Endocrine and metabolic: Uterine cramping

1% to 10%:

Cardiovascular: Bradycardia
Central nervous system: Dizziness
Gastrointestinal: Stomach pain, diarrhea, unpleasant taste
Otic: Tinnitus
Respiratory: Nasal congestion
Miscellaneous: Sweating

<1% (Limited to important or life-threatening symptoms): Cardiac arrest or ventricular arrhythmias, including fibrillation and tachycardia; myocardial infarction, dyspnea, allergic reaction, including shock

**Overdose/Toxicology** Symptoms of overdose include gangrene, seizures, chest pain, numbness in extremities, weak pulse, confusion, excitement, delirium, and hallucinations. Treatment is supportive based on symptomatology.

**Pharmacodynamics/Kinetics**

**Metabolism:** Liver

**Excretion:** Urine and feces

**Onset:** Oral: Within 5-15 minutes; I.M.: Within 2-5 minutes

**Duration:** Uterine effects persist for 3 hours, except when given I.V., then effects persist for ~45 minutes.

**Formulations** Injection, as maleate: 0.2 mg/mL (1 mL)

**Dosing**

**Adults:**

Oral: 1-2 tablets (0.2-0.4 mg) every 6-12 hours for up to 48 hours
I.M., I.V. (**I.V. should be reserved for emergency use only**): 0.2 mg, repeat dose in 2-4 hours as needed

**Elderly:** Refer to adult dosing.

**Administration**

**I.V.:** I.V. use should be limited to patients with severe uterine bleeding or other life-threatening emergency situations. I.V. doses should be administered over a period of not <1 minute.

(Continued)

## Ergonovine *(Continued)*

**I.V. Detail:** Dilute in NS to 5 mL for I.V. administration.

**Stability**

**Storage:** Refrigerate injection. Protect from light. Store intact ampuls in refrigerator, stable for 60-90 days. Do not use if discoloration occurs.

**Additional Nursing Issues**

**Physical Assessment:** Monitor blood pressure (especially with I.V. use). For postpartum use, monitor character and amount of vaginal bleeding. Monitor for ergotamine toxicity (headache, ringing in ears, nausea and vomiting, diarrhea, numbness or coldness of extremities, confusion, hallucinations, dyspnea, chest pain, convulsions). When used to test for Prinzmetal's angina during coronary arteriography, emergency equipment including nitroglycerin must be on hand. **Pregnancy risk factor X** - determine that patient is not pregnant when testing for Prinzmetal's angina. Breast-feeding is not recommended.

**Patient Information/Instruction:** For angina diagnosis cardiologist will instruct patient about what to expect. For postpartum hemorrhage (an emergency situation) patient needs to know why the drug is being given and what side effects she might experience (eg, mild nausea and vomiting, dizziness, headache, ringing ears) and instructed to report difficulty breathing, acute headache, or numbness and cold feeling in extremities, or severe abdominal cramping. **Breast-feeding precautions:** Breast-feeding is not recommended.

## Ergotamine Derivatives (er GOT a meen dah RIV ah tives)

**U.S. Brand Names** Cafatine®; Cafatine-PB®; Cafergot®; Cafetrate®; Ercaf®; Ergomar®; Wigraine®

**Therapeutic Category** Ergot Derivative

**Pregnancy Risk Factor** X

**Lactation** Enters breast milk/contraindicated

**Use** Abort or prevent vascular headaches, such as migraine or cluster

**Mechanism of Action/Effect** Ergot alkaloid alpha-adrenergic blocker directly stimulates vascular smooth muscle to vasoconstrict peripheral and cerebral vessels; also has antagonist effects on serotonin

**Contraindications** Hypersensitivity to ergotamine, caffeine, or any component; peripheral vascular disease; hepatic or renal disease; hypertension; peptic ulcer disease; sepsis; pregnancy

**Warnings** Avoid prolonged administration or excessive dosage because of the danger of ergotism and gangrene. Patients who take ergotamine for extended periods of time may become dependent on it. May be harmful due to reduction in cerebral blood flow. May precipitate angina, myocardial infarction, or aggravate intermittent claudication; therefore, not considered a drug of choice in the elderly.

**Drug Interactions**

**Increased Effect/Toxicity:**

Propranolol: One case of severe vasoconstriction with pain and cyanosis has been reported.

Erythromycin, troleandomycin and other macrolide antibiotics: Monitor for signs of ergot toxicity.

**Adverse Reactions**

>10%:

Cardiovascular: Tachycardia, bradycardia, arterial spasm, claudication and vasoconstriction; rebound headache may occur with sudden withdrawal of the drug in patients on prolonged therapy; localized edema, peripheral vascular effects (numbness and tingling of fingers and toes)

Central nervous system: Drowsiness, dizziness

Gastrointestinal: Nausea, vomiting, diarrhea, dry mouth

1% to 10%:

Cardiovascular: Transient tachycardia or bradycardia, precordial distress and pain

Neuromuscular & skeletal: Weakness in the legs, abdominal or muscle pain, muscle pains in the extremities, paresthesia

**Overdose/Toxicology** Symptoms of overdose include vasospastic effects, nausea, vomiting, lassitude, impaired mental function, hypotension, hypertension, unconsciousness, seizures, shock, and death. Treatment includes general supportive therapy. Activated charcoal is effective at binding ergot alkaloids. Vasodilators should be used with caution to avoid exaggerating any pre-existing hypotension.

**Pharmacodynamics/Kinetics**

**Time to Peak:** Within 0.5-3 hours following coadministration with caffeine

**Metabolism:** Liver

**Excretion:** Bile

**Formulations**

Suppository, rectal (Cafatine®, Cafergot®, Cafetrate®, Wigraine®): Ergotamine tartrate 2 mg and caffeine 100 mg (12s)

Tablet (Ercaf®, Wigraine®): Ergotamine tartrate 1 mg and caffeine 100 mg

Tablet:

Extended release:

Bellergal-S®: Ergotamine tartrate 0.6 mg with belladonna alkaloids 0.2 mg, and phenobarbital 40 mg

Cafatine-PB®: Ergotamine tartrate 1 mg with belladonna alkaloids 0.125 mg, caffeine 100 mg, and pentobarbital 30 mg

Sublingual (Ergomar®): Ergotamine tartrate 2 mg

**Dosing**

**Adults:**

Oral:

Cafergot®: 2 tablets at onset of attack; then 1 tablet every 30 minutes as needed; maximum: 6 tablets per attack; do not exceed 10 tablets/week.

Ergostat®: 1 tablet under tongue at first sign, then 1 tablet every 30 minutes, 3 tablets/24 hours, 5 tablets/week

Rectal (Cafergot® suppositories, Wigraine® suppositories, Cafatine® suppositories): 1 at first sign of an attack; follow with second dose after 1 hour, if needed; maximum: 2 per attack; do not exceed 5/week.

**Elderly:** Not recommended for use in the elderly (see Geriatric Considerations).

**Administration**

**Other:** Do not crush sublingual tablets.

**Additional Nursing Issues**

**Physical Assessment:** Assess patient medication for products which may add to the peripheral vasoconstricting properties. Monitor effectiveness of drug and instruct patient carefully about need to promptly report signs or symptoms of ergotism and toxic effects. **Pregnancy risk factor X** - determine that patient is not pregnant before beginning treatment and do not give to women of childbearing age unless woman is capable of complying with barrier contraceptive measures 1 month prior to therapy, during therapy, and for 1 month following therapy. Breast-feeding is contraindicated.

**Patient Information/Instruction:** Take this drug as directed; do not increase dose or use more often than prescribed. If relief is not obtained, contact your prescriber. Avoid caffeine-containing products (eg, tea, coffee, colas, cocoa); caffeine increases GI absorption of ergotamines. May cause drowsiness (avoid activities requiring alertness until effects of medication are known). You may experience mild nausea/vomiting (you may have an antiemetic prescribed), mild weakness or numbness of extremities (avoid injury). Inspect your extremities for coldness, numbness, or injury. Report immediately extreme numbness, pain, tingling or weakness in extremities (toes, fingers), severe unresolved nausea or vomiting, difficulty breathing or irregular heartbeat.

Inhaler: Follow directions for use on package insert. If more than one inhalation is necessary, wait 5 minutes between inhalations (maximum dose of 6 inhalations/24 hours or 15 inhalations/week)

**Pregnancy/breast-feeding precautions:** Inform prescriber if you are pregnant. Do not get pregnant 1 month before, during, or for 1 month following therapy. Consult prescriber for instruction on appropriate contraceptive measures. This drug may cause severe fetal defects. Do not donate blood during or for 1 month following therapy (same reason). Do not breast-feed.

**Geriatric Considerations:** May be harmful due to reduction in cerebral blood flow. May precipitate angina, myocardial infarction, or aggravate intermittent claudication (see Contraindications and Warnings/Precautions).

**Additional Information** Ergotamine tartrate and caffeine: Cafergot®

- **Ergotamine Tartrate, Belladonna, and Phenobarbital** *see* Belladonna, Phenobarbital, and Ergotamine Tartrate *on page 137*
- **Eritroquim** *see* Erythromycin *on this page*
- **ERO Ear** *see page 1291*
- **E•R•O Ear** *see page 1294*
- **Erybid™** *see* Erythromycin *on this page*
- **Eryc®** *see* Erythromycin *on this page*
- **EryPed®** *see* Erythromycin *on this page*
- **Ery-Tab®** *see* Erythromycin *on this page*
- **Erythro-Base®** *see* Erythromycin *on this page*
- **Erythrocin®** *see* Erythromycin *on this page*

## Erythromycin (er ith roe MYE sin)

**U.S. Brand Names** E-Base®; E.E.S.®; E-Mycin®; Eramycin®; Eryc®; EryPed®; Ery-Tab®; Erythrocin®; Ilosone®; Ilotycin®; PCE®

**Therapeutic Category** Antibiotic, Macrolide; Antibiotic, Ophthalmic

**Pregnancy Risk Factor** B

**Lactation** Enters breast milk/compatible

**Use** Treatment of susceptible bacterial infections including *M. pneumoniae*, *Legionella pneumophila*, diphtheria, pertussis, chancroid, *Chlamydia*, and *Campylobacter* gastroenteritis; used in conjunction with neomycin for decontaminating the bowel

**Unlabeled use:** Gastroparesis

**Mechanism of Action/Effect** Inhibits RNA-dependent protein synthesis

**Contraindications** Hypersensitivity to erythromycin or any component; hepatic impairment; use with pimozide

**Warnings** Hepatic impairment with or without jaundice has occurred with erythromycin use. It may be accompanied by malaise, nausea, vomiting, abdominal colic, and fever. Discontinue use if these occur.

**Drug Interactions**

**Cytochrome P-450 Effect:** CYP3A3/4 enzyme substrate; CYP1A2 and 3A3/4 enzyme inhibitor

**Increased Effect/Toxicity:** Erythromycin decreases clearance of carbamazepine, cyclosporine, and triazolam. Erythromycin may decrease theophylline clearance and increase theophylline's half-life by up to 60% (patients on high-dose theophylline and erythromycin or who have received erythromycin for >5 days may be at higher risk).

(Continued)

## Erythromycin *(Continued)*

Astemizole, and terfenadine increases Q-T interval, may also occur with cisapride. May potentiate anticoagulant effect of warfarin. May decrease clearance of protease inhibitors

**Food Interactions** Erythromycin serum levels may be altered if taken with food.

**Effects on Lab Values** False-positive urinary catecholamines

**Adverse Reactions**

**Ophthalmic:** <1% (Limited to important or life-threatening symptoms): Eye irritation not present before therapy

**Systemic:**

>10%: Gastrointestinal: Abdominal pain, cramping, nausea, vomiting

1% to 10%:

Gastrointestinal: Oral candidiasis
Genitourinary: Vaginal candidiasis
Hepatic: Cholestatic jaundice
Local: Phlebitis at the injection site (injections only)
Miscellaneous: Hypersensitivity reactions

<1% (Limited to important or life-threatening symptoms): Cardiac toxicity, especially Q-T prolongation and torsade de pointes
Gastrointestinal: Pancreatitis

**Topical:**

>10%: Dermatologic: Dry or scaly skin, itching, irritation, stinging, burning (solution or gel)

1% to 10%: Dermatologic: Peeling, redness

**Overdose/Toxicology** Symptoms of overdose include nausea, vomiting, diarrhea, prostration, reversible pancreatitis, hearing loss with or without tinnitus or vertigo. Care is general and supportive only.

**Pharmacodynamics/Kinetics**

**Protein Binding:** 75% to 90%

**Distribution:**

Crosses the placenta

Relative diffusion of antimicrobial agents from blood into cerebrospinal fluid (CSF): Minimal even with inflammation

Ratio of CSF to blood level: Normal meninges: 1% to 12%; Inflamed meninges: 7% to 25%

**Half-life Elimination:** 1.5-2 hours (peak); End-stage renal disease: 5-6 hours

**Time to Peak:** Four hours for the base, 30 minutes to 2.5 hours for the ethylsuccinate; delayed in the presence of food. Due to differences in absorption, **200 mg erythromycin ethylsuccinate produces the same serum levels as 125 mg of erythromycin base.**

**Metabolism:** Liver

**Excretion:** Urine and feces

**Formulations**

**Erythromycin base:**

Capsule, delayed release: 250 mg
Capsule, delayed release, enteric coated pellets (Eryc®): 250 mg
Tablet, delayed release: 333 mg
Tablet, enteric coated (E-Mycin®, Ery-Tab®, E-Base®): 250 mg, 333 mg, 500 mg
Tablet, film coated: 250 mg, 500 mg
Tablet, polymer coated particles (PCE®): 333 mg, 500 mg
Ophthalmic ointment (Ilotycin®): 0.5% (3.5 g)

**Erythromycin estolate:**

Capsule (Ilosone® Pulvules®): 250 mg
Suspension, oral (Ilosone®): 125 mg/5 mL (480 mL); 250 mg/5 mL (480 mL)
Tablet (Ilosone®): 500 mg

**Erythromycin ethylsuccinate:**

Granules for oral suspension (EryPed®): 400 mg/5 mL (60 mL, 100 mL, 200 mL)
Powder for oral suspension (E.E.S.®): 200 mg/5 mL (100 mL, 200 mL)
Suspension, oral (E.E.S.®, EryPed®): 200 mg/5 mL (5 mL, 100 mL, 200 mL, 480 mL); 400 mg/5 mL (5 mL, 60 mL, 100 mL, 200 mL, 480 mL)
Suspension, oral [drops] (EryPed®): 100 mg/2.5 mL (50 mL)
Tablet (E.E.S.®): 400 mg
Tablet, chewable (EryPed®): 200 mg

**Erythromycin gluceptate:**

Injection: 1000 mg (30 mL)

**Erythromycin lactobionate:**

Powder for injection: 500 mg, 1000 mg

**Erythromycin stearate:**

Tablet, film coated (Eramycin®, Erythrocin®): 250 mg, 500 mg

**Dosing**

**Adults:** Erythromycin has been used as a prokinetic agent to improve gastric emptying time and intestinal motility. In adults, 200 mg was infused I.V. initially followed by 250 mg orally 3 times/day 30 minutes before meals.

Oral:

Base: 250-500 mg every 6-12 hours
Ethylsuccinate: 400-800 mg every 6-12 hours
Endocarditis prophylaxis in penicillin-allergic patient: 1 g 2 hours before procedure and 500 mg 6 hours later

Preop bowel preparation: 1 g erythromycin base at 1, 2, and 11 PM on the day before surgery combined with mechanical cleansing of the large intestine and oral neomycin

I.V.: Lactobionate: 15-20 mg/kg/day divided every 6 hours or 500 mg to 1 g every 6 hours, or given as a continuous infusion over 24 hours (maximum: 4 g/24 hours)

Ophthalmic: Instill ½" (1.25 cm) 2-8 times/day depending on the severity of the infection

**Elderly:** Refer to adult dosing.

**Renal Impairment:** Slightly dialyzable (5% to 20%); no supplemental dosage necessary in hemo- or peritoneal dialysis or in continuous arteriovenous or venovenous hemofiltration (CAVH/CAVHD)

**Administration**

**Oral:** Do not crush enteric coated drug product. GI upset, including diarrhea, is common. Can be given with food to decrease GI upset. Do not give with milk or acidic beverages.

**I.V.:** Infuse 1 g over 20-60 minutes.

**I.V. Detail:** Some formulations may contain benzyl alcohol as a preservative. I.V. infusion may be very irritating to the vein. If phlebitis/pain occurs with used dilution, consider diluting further (eg, 1:5) if fluid status of the patient will tolerate, or consider administering in larger available vein. The addition of lidocaine or bicarbonate does not decrease the irritation of erythromycin infusions.

**Stability**

**Storage:** Refrigerate oral suspension.

**Reconstitution:** Erythromycin lactobionate should be reconstituted with sterile water for injection without preservatives to avoid gel formation. The reconstituted solution is stable for 2 weeks when refrigerated for 24 hours at room temperature.

Erythromycin I.V. infusion solution is stable at pH 6-8. Stability of lactobionate is pH dependent. I.V. form has the longest stability in 0.9% sodium chloride (NS) and should be prepared in this base solution whenever possible. Do not use $D_5W$ as a diluent unless sodium bicarbonate is added to solution. If I.V. must be prepared in $D_5W$, 0.5 mL of the 8.4% sodium bicarbonate solution should be added per each 100 mL of $D_5W$.

Stability of parenteral admixture at room temperature (25°C) and at refrigeration temperature (4°C) is 24 hours.

Standard diluent: 500 mg/250 mL $D_5W$/NS; 750 mg/250 mL $D_5W$/NS; 1 g/250 mL $D_5W$/NS.

**Compatibility:** See the Compatibility of Drugs Chart *on page 1315*.

**Monitoring Laboratory Tests** Perform culture and sensitivity studies prior to initiating drug therapy.

**Additional Nursing Issues**

**Physical Assessment:** Assess effectiveness and interactions of other medications patient may be taking (see Drug Interactions - P-450 inhibitor). Monitor for effectiveness of therapy and adverse reactions; especially hearing loss, CNS changes, hypersensitivity reactions, and opportunistic infections (see Adverse Reactions). Monitor liver function with long-term use. Instruct patient on appropriate use, possible adverse reactions (see above), and symptoms to report.

**Patient Information/Instruction:** Take as directed, around-the-clock, with a full glass of water (not juice or milk), preferably on an empty stomach (1 hour before or 2 hours after meals). Take complete prescription even if you are feeling better. You may experience nausea, vomiting, or mouth sores (small frequent meals, frequent mouth care may help). Report skin rash or itching; easy bruising or bleeding; unhealed sores of mouth; itching or vaginal discharge; watery or bloody diarrhea; unresolved vomiting; yellowing of skin or eyes; easy fatigue; pale stool or dark urine; skin rash or itching; white plaques, sores, or fuzziness in mouth; or any change in hearing.

Ophthalmic: Wash hands before applying. Pull down lower eyelid gently, instill thin ribbon of ointment into lower lid, close eye, roll eyeball in all directions. Blurred vision and stinging is temporary. Report persistent pain, burning, vision disturbances, swelling, itching, or worsening of condition.

**Geriatric Considerations:** Dose of erythromycin does not need to be adjusted in the elderly unless there is severe renal impairment or hepatic dysfunction. Has not been studied in the elderly.

**Additional Information** The lactobionate formulation contains benzyl alcohol.

**Related Information**

Ophthalmic Agents *on page 1282*

## Erythromycin and Benzoyl Peroxide

(er ith roe MYE sin & BEN zoe il per OKS ide)

**U.S. Brand Names** Benzamycin®

**Synonyms** Benzoyl Peroxide and Erythromycin

**Therapeutic Category** Acne Products

**Pregnancy Risk Factor** C

**Lactation** Excretion in breast milk unknown/use caution

**Use** Topical control of acne vulgaris

**Formulations** Gel: Erythromycin 30 mg and benzoyl peroxide 50 mg per g

(Continued)

## Erythromycin and Benzoyl Peroxide *(Continued)*

**Dosing**

**Adults:** Apply twice daily, morning and evening

**Additional Nursing Issues**

**Physical Assessment:** See individual components listed in Related Information. **Pregnancy risk factor C** - benefits of use should outweigh possible risks. Note breast-feeding caution.

**Patient Information/Instruction:** See individual components listed in Related Information. **Pregnancy/breast-feeding precautions:** Inform prescriber if you are on intend to get pregnant. Consult prescriber if breast-feeding.

**Related Information**

Erythromycin *on page 435*

## Erythromycin and Sulfisoxazole (er ith roe MYE sin & sul fi SOKS a zole)

**U.S. Brand Names** Eryzole®; Pediazole®

**Synonyms** Sulfisoxazole and Erythromycin

**Therapeutic Category** Antibiotic, Macrolide Combination; Antibiotic, Macrolide; Antibiotic, Sulfonamide Derivative

**Pregnancy Risk Factor** C

**Lactation** Enters breast milk/compatible

**Use** Treatment of susceptible bacterial infections of the upper and lower respiratory tract, otitis media in children caused by susceptible strains of *Haemophilus influenzae*, and other infections in patients allergic to penicillin

**Formulations** Suspension, oral: Erythromycin ethylsuccinate 200 mg and sulfisoxazole acetyl 600 mg per 5 mL (100 mL, 150 mL, 200 mL, 250 mL)

**Dosing**

**Adults:** Oral (dosage recommendation is based on the product's erythromycin content): 400 mg erythromycin and 1200 mg sulfisoxazole every 6 hours

**Elderly:** Not recommended for use in the elderly.

**Renal Impairment:**

Sulfisoxazole must be adjusted in renal impairment.

$Cl_{cr}$ 10-50 mL/minute: Administer every 8-12 hours.

$Cl_{cr}$ <10 mL/minute: Administer every 12-24 hours.

**Additional Nursing Issues**

**Physical Assessment:** See individual components listed in Related Information. **Pregnancy risk factor C** - benefits of use should outweigh possible risks.

**Patient Information/Instruction:** See individual components listed in Related Information. **Pregnancy precautions:** Inform prescriber if you are on intend to get pregnant.

**Related Information**

Erythromycin *on page 435*
Sulfisoxazole *on page 1086*


- **Erythropoietin** *see* Epoetin Alfa *on page 426*
- **Eryzole®** *see* Erythromycin and Sulfisoxazole *on this page*
- **Esclim® Transdermal** *see* Estradiol *on page 441*
- **Eserine Salicylate** *see* Physostigmine *on page 928*
- **Eserine Sulfate** *see* Ophthalmic Agents, Glaucoma *on page 853*
- **Esgic®** *see* Butalbital Compound and Acetaminophen *on page 175*
- **Esgic-Plus®** *see* Butalbital Compound and Acetaminophen *on page 175*
- **Esidrix®** *see* Hydrochlorothiazide *on page 566*
- **Eskalith®** *see* Lithium *on page 683*
- **Eskalith CR®** *see* Lithium *on page 683*
- **Eskazole** *see* Albendazole *on page 44*


## Esmolol (ES moe lol)

**U.S. Brand Names** Brevibloc® Injection

**Therapeutic Category** Antiarrhythmic Agent, Class II; Beta Blocker, $Beta_1$ Selective

**Pregnancy Risk Factor** C

**Lactation** Excretion in breast milk unknown

**Use** Treatment of supraventricular tachycardia, atrial fibrillation/flutter (primarily to control ventricular rate), and hypertension (especially perioperatively)

**Mechanism of Action/Effect** Class II antiarrhythmic: $Beta_1$ adrenergic receptor blocking agent that competes with $beta_1$ adrenergic agonists for available beta receptor sites; it is a selective $beta_1$ antagonist with a very short duration of action; has little if any intrinsic sympathomimetic activity; and lacks membrane stabilizing action; it is administered intravenously and is used when beta blockade of short duration is desired or in critically ill patients in whom adverse effects of bradycardia, heart failure or hypotension may necessitate rapid withdrawal of the drug

**Contraindications** Hypersensitivity to esmolol, any component, or other beta-blockers; sinus bradycardia or heart block; uncompensated congestive heart failure; cardiogenic shock

**Warnings** Must be diluted for continuous I.V. infusion. Use with extreme caution in patients with hyper-reactive airway disease. Use lowest dose possible and discontinue infusion if bronchospasm occurs. Use with caution in diabetes mellitus, hypoglycemia, or renal failure. Avoid extravasation. Caution should be exercised when discontinuing esmolol infusions to avoid withdrawal effects. Esmolol shares the toxic potentials of beta-adrenergic blocking agents and the usual precautions of these agents should be observed. Pregnancy factor C.

**Drug Interactions**

**Decreased Effect:** Decreased effect of beta-blockers with aluminum salts, barbiturates, calcium salts, cholestyramine, colestipol, NSAIDs, penicillins (ampicillin), rifampin, salicylates, and sulfinpyrazone due to decreased bioavailability and plasma levels. Beta-blockers may decrease the effect of sulfonylureas. Xanthines (eg, theophylline, caffeine) may decrease effects of esmolol.

**Increased Effect/Toxicity:** Esmolol may increase the effect/toxicity of verapamil, clonidine (hypertensive crisis after or during withdrawal of either agent) and extend the effect of neuromuscular blocking agents (succinylcholine). Esmolol may increase digoxin serum levels by 10% to 20%. Morphine may increase esmolol blood concentrations. Esmolol may increase theophylline serum concentrations.

**Effects on Lab Values** Increases cholesterol (S), glucose

**Adverse Reactions**

>10%:

Cardiovascular: Asymptomatic and symptomatic hypotension

Miscellaneous: Sweating

1% to 10%:

Cardiovascular: Peripheral ischemia

Central nervous system: Dizziness, somnolence, confusion, headache, agitation, fatigue

Gastrointestinal: Nausea, vomiting

Local: Infusion site reactions

<1% (Limited to important or life-threatening symptoms): Pallor, flushing, bradycardia, chest pain, syncope, heart block, edema, depression, abnormal thinking, anxiety, fever, lightheadedness, seizures, bronchospasm, wheezing, dyspnea, nasal congestion, pulmonary edema

**Overdose/Toxicology** Symptoms of overdose include hypotension, bradycardia, and heart block. Initially, fluids may be the best treatment for hypotension. Sympathomimetics (eg, epinephrine or dopamine), glucagon, or a pacemaker can be used to treat the toxic bradycardia, asystole, and/or hypotension.

**Pharmacodynamics/Kinetics**

**Protein Binding:** 55%

**Half-life Elimination:** 9 minutes

**Metabolism:** In blood by esterases

**Excretion:** Urine

**Onset:** Onset of beta blockade: I.V.: Within 2-10 minutes (onset of effect is quickest when loading doses are administered)

**Duration:** Short, 10-30 minutes; prolonged following higher cumulative doses, extended duration of use

**Formulations** Injection, hydrochloride: 10 mg/mL (10 mL); 250 mg/mL (10 mL)

**Dosing**

**Adults: I.V. administration requires an infusion pump** (must be adjusted to individual response and tolerance):

Loading dose: 500 mcg/kg over 1 minute; follow with a 50 mcg/kg/minute infusion for 4 minutes; if response is inadequate, rebolus with another 500 mcg/kg loading dose over 1 minute, and increase the maintenance infusion to 100 mcg/kg/minute. Repeat this process until a therapeutic effect has been achieved or to a maximum recommended maintenance dose of 200 mcg/kg/minute. Usual dosage range: 50-200 mcg/kg/minute with average dose of 100 mcg/kg/minute.

Esmolol: Hemodynamic effects of beta blockade return to baseline within 20-30 minutes after discontinuing esmolol infusions.

Guidelines for withdrawal of therapy: Transfer to alternative antiarrhythmic drug (propranolol, digoxin, verapamil). Infusion should be reduced by 50% 30 minutes following the first dose of the alternative agent. Following the second dose of the alternative drug, patient's response should be monitored and if control is adequate for the first hours, esmolol may be discontinued.

**Elderly:** Refer to adult dosing.

**Renal Impairment:** Not removed by hemo- or peritoneal dialysis. Supplemental dose is not necessary.

**Administration**

**I.V.:** The 250 mg/mL ampul is **not** for direct I.V. injection, but rather must first be diluted to a final concentration of 10 mg/mL (ie, 2.5 g in 250 mL or 5 g in 500 mL).

**I.V. Detail:** Decrease or discontinue infusion if hypotension, congestive heart failure occur.

**Stability**

**Storage:** Clear, colorless to light yellow solution should be stored at room temperature and protected from temperatures >40°C.

**Reconstitution:** Stability of parenteral admixture at room temperature (25°C) and at refrigeration temperature (4°C) is 24 hours.

**Standard diluent:** 5 g/500 mL NS

**Additional Nursing Issues**

**Physical Assessment:** Assess other medications patient may be taking for effectiveness and interactions (see Drug Interactions). See Warnings/Precautions and Contraindications for cautious use. See Dosing and Warnings/Precautions for withdrawal guidelines. Requires continuous cardiac, hemodynamic, and infusion site monitoring (extravasation). Monitor therapeutic response (cardiac status) and adverse reactions

(Continued)

## Esmolol *(Continued)*

(see Warnings/Precautions and Adverse Reactions). **Pregnancy risk factor C** - benefits of use should outweigh possible risks. Note breast-feeding caution.

**Patient Information/Instruction:** Esmolol is administered in emergencies, patient education should be appropriate to the situation.

**Geriatric Considerations:** Due to alterations in the beta-adrenergic autonomic nervous system, beta-adrenergic blockade may result in less hemodynamic response than seen in younger adults.

**Additional Information** Some formulations may contain ethanol.

**Related Information**

Antiarrhythmic Drug Classification Comparison *on page 1366*

Beta-Blockers Comparison *on page 1376*

- **Esoterica® Facial [OTC]** *see* Hydroquinone *on page 583*
- **Esoterica® Regular [OTC]** *see* Hydroquinone *on page 583*
- **Esoterica® Sensitive Skin Formula [OTC]** *see* Hydroquinone *on page 583*
- **Esoterica® Sunscreen [OTC]** *see* Hydroquinone *on page 583*
- **Estar®** *see page 1294*

## Estazolam (es TA zoe lam)

**U.S. Brand Names** ProSom™

**Therapeutic Category** Benzodiazepine

**Pregnancy Risk Factor** X

**Lactation** Enters breast milk/contraindicated

**Use** Short-term management of insomnia

**Mechanism of Action/Effect** Benzodiazepines may exert their pharmacologic effect through potentiation of the inhibitory activity of GABA.

**Contraindications** Hypersensitivity to estazolam; cross-sensitivity with other benzodiazepines may occur; patients with pre-existing CNS depression; sleep apnea; pregnancy; narrow-angle glaucoma

**Warnings** Abrupt discontinuance may precipitate withdrawal or rebound insomnia. Use with caution in patients receiving other CNS depressants, patients with low albumin, hepatic dysfunction, and in the elderly. May cause drug dependency.

**Drug Interactions**

**Cytochrome P-450 Effect:** Likely to be a substrate for cytochrome isoenzymes (profile not defined)

**Decreased Effect:** Enzyme inducers (phenytoin, phenobarbital, cimetidine, etc) may decrease effect of estazolam.

**Increased Effect/Toxicity:** CNS depressants may increase CNS adverse effects. Cimetidine may decrease metabolism of estazolam and increase risk of toxic effect.

**Adverse Reactions**

>10%: Cardiovascular: Somnolence (42%), muscle weakness (11%)

1% to 10%:

Cardiovascular: Syncope, hypotension

Central nervous system: Hypokinesia (8%), hangover (3%), abnormal thinking (2%), anxiety (1%)

Gastrointestinal: Heartburn

Respiratory: Cold symptoms, pharyngitis, asthma, cough, dyspnea, rhinitis

<1% (Limited to important or life-threatening symptoms): Syncope, seizures, hematuria, agranulocytosis, elevated AST

**Overdose/Toxicology** Symptoms of overdose include respiratory depression, hypoactive reflexes, unsteady gait, and hypotension. Treatment for benzodiazepine overdose is supportive. Flumazenil has been shown to selectively block the binding of benzodiazepines to CNS receptors, resulting in a reversal of benzodiazepine-induced sedation; however, its use may not reverse respiratory depression.

**Pharmacodynamics/Kinetics**

**Metabolism:** Hepatic

**Excretion:** Urine

**Onset:** Within 1 hour

**Duration:** Variable

**Formulations** Tablet: 1 mg, 2 mg

**Dosing**

**Adults:** Oral: 1 mg at bedtime, some patients may require 2 mg; start at doses of 0.5 mg in debilitated patients

**Elderly:** Initial: 0.5-1 mg at bedtime (start at doses of 0.5 mg in small elderly patients).

**Hepatic Impairment:** Adjustment may be necessary.

**Administration**

**Oral:** Avoid abrupt discontinuance in patients with prolonged therapy or seizure disorders.

**Monitoring Laboratory Tests** CBC, liver function with long-term therapy

**Additional Nursing Issues**

**Physical Assessment:** For short-term use. Assess effectiveness and interactions of other medications (see Drug Interactions). See Contraindications and Warnings/Precautions for cautious use. Assess for history of addiction; long-term use can result in dependence, abuse, or tolerance. Evaluate periodically for need for continued use. After long-term use, taper dosage slowly when discontinuing. For inpatient use, institute safety measures (side rails, night light, call bell, assistance with ambulation) and monitor effectiveness and adverse reactions. For outpatients, monitor for effectiveness of therapy and adverse reactions (see Adverse Reactions) at beginning of therapy and periodically with long-term use. Assess knowledge/teach patient appropriate use, interventions to reduce side effects, and adverse symptoms to report. **Pregnancy risk factor X** - determine that patient is not pregnant before beginning treatment and do not give to women of childbearing age or to males who may have intercourse with women of childbearing age unless both male and female are capable of complying with barrier contraceptive measures during therapy and for 1 month following therapy. Breast-feeding is contraindicated.

**Patient Information/Instruction:** Use exactly as directed (do not increase dose or frequency or discontinue without consulting prescriber); may cause physical and/or psychological dependence. While using this medication, do not use alcohol or other prescription or OTC medications (especially, pain medications, sedatives, antihistamines, or hypnotics) without consulting prescriber. Maintain adequate hydration (2-3 L/day of fluids unless instructed to restrict fluid intake). You may experience drowsiness, dizziness, or blurred vision (use caution when driving or engaging in tasks requiring alertness until response to drug is known); GI upset (take with water or milk). Report CNS changes (confusion, depression, increased sedation, excitation, headache, abnormal thinking, insomnia, or nightmares), altered voiding patterns or blood in urine, difficulty breathing, chest pain or palpitations, altered gait pattern, or ineffectiveness of medication. **Pregnancy/breast-feeding precautions:** Inform prescriber if you are pregnant. Do not get pregnant during therapy or for 1 month following therapy. Male: Do not cause a female to become pregnant. Male/female: Consult prescriber for instruction on appropriate contraceptive measures. This drug may cause severe fetal defects. Do not breast-feed.

**Geriatric Considerations:** There has been little experience with this drug in the elderly, but because of its lack of active metabolites, estazolam would be a reasonable choice for elderly patients when a benzodiazepine hypnotic is indicated.

**Related Information**

Anxiolytic/Hypnotic Use in Long-Term Care Facilities *on page 1430*
Benzodiazepines Comparison *on page 1375*

- **Esteprim** *see* Co-trimoxazole *on page 307*
- **Esterified Estrogens** *see* Estrogens, Esterified *on page 449*
- **Estinyl®** *see* Ethinyl Estradiol *on page 458*
- **Estivin II®** *see page 1282*
- **Estivin® II Ophthalmic** *see page 1294*
- **Estrace® Oral** *see* Estradiol *on this page*
- **Estraderm® Transdermal** *see* Estradiol *on this page*
- **Estra-D® Injection** *see* Estradiol *on this page*

## Estradiol (es tra DYE ole)

**U.S. Brand Names** Climara® Transdermal; Delestrogen® Injection; depGynogen® Injection; Depo®-Estradiol Injection; Depogen® Injection; Dioval® Injection; Dura-Estrin® Injection; Duragen® Injection; Esclim® Transdermal; Estrace® Oral; Estraderm® Transdermal; Estra-D® Injection; Estra-L® Injection; Estro-Cyp® Injection; Gynogen L.A.® Injection; Vivelle® Transdermal

**Therapeutic Category** Estrogen Derivative

**Pregnancy Risk Factor** X

**Lactation** Enters breast milk/compatible

**Use** Treatment of atrophic vaginitis, atrophic dystrophy of vulva, menopausal symptoms, female hypogonadism, ovariectomy, primary ovarian failure, inoperable breast cancer, inoperable prostatic cancer, mild to severe vasomotor symptoms associated with menopause

**Mechanism of Action/Effect** Increases the synthesis of DNA, RNA, and various proteins in target tissues; reduces the release of gonadotropin-releasing hormone from the hypothalamus; reduces FSH and LH release from the pituitary

**Contraindications** Pregnancy; undiagnosed genital bleeding; carcinoma of the breast (except in patients treated for metastatic disease); estrogen-dependent tumors; history of thrombophlebitis, thrombosis, or thromboembolic disorders associated with estrogen use

**Warnings** Use with caution in patients with renal or hepatic insufficiency. Estrogens may cause premature closure of epiphyses in young individuals, in patients with a history of thromboembolism, stroke, myocardial infarction (especially >40 years of age who smoke), liver tumor, or hypertension.

Estrogens have been reported to increase the risk of endometrial carcinoma; do not use estrogens during pregnancy. Before prescribing estrogen therapy to postmenopausal women, the risks and benefits must be weighed for each patient. Women should be informed of these risks and benefits, as well as possible side effects and the return of menstrual bleeding (when cycled with a progestin), and be involved in the decision to prescribe. Oral therapy may be more convenient for vaginal atrophy and stress incontinence.

**Drug Interactions**

**Cytochrome P-450 Effect:** CYP1A2 and 3A3/4 enzyme substrate

**Decreased Effect:** Rifampin decreases estrogen serum concentrations.

**Increased Effect/Toxicity:** Estradiol with hydrocortisone increases corticosteroid toxic potential. Anticoagulants and estradiol increase the potential for thromboembolic events.

**Effects on Lab Values** ↑ Prothrombin and factors VII, VIII, IX, X; ↑ platelet aggregability, thyroid binding globulin, total thyroid hormone ($T_4$), serum triglycerides/phospholipids; ↓ antithrombin III, serum folate concentration

(Continued)

## Estradiol *(Continued)*

### Adverse Reactions

**Systemic:**

>10%:

Cardiovascular: Peripheral edema

Endocrine & metabolic: Enlargement of breasts (female and male), breast tenderness

Gastrointestinal: Nausea, anorexia, bloating

1% to 10%:

Central nervous system: Headache, migraine headache

Endocrine & metabolic: Increased libido (female), decreased libido (male)

Gastrointestinal: Vomiting, diarrhea

<1% (Limited to important or life-threatening symptoms): Hypertension, thromboembolism, myocardial infarction, edema, depression, dizziness, anxiety, stroke, amenorrhea, alterations in frequency and flow of menses, breast tumors, decreased glucose tolerance, increased triglycerides and LDL, hepatitis, increased susceptibility to *Candida* infection

**Vaginal:**

1% to 10%:

Cardiovascular: Peripheral edema

Endocrine & metabolic: Breast tenderness, breast enlargement

Gastrointestinal: Anorexia, abdominal cramping

<1% (Limited to important or life-threatening symptoms): Hypertension, thromboembolism, myocardial infarction, decreased glucose tolerance, alterations in frequency and flow of menses, breast tenderness or enlargement, increased triglycerides and LDL, cholestatic jaundice, increased susceptibility to *Candida* infection

**Overdose/Toxicology** Symptoms of overdose include fluid retention, jaundice, thrombophlebitis, nausea, and vomiting. Toxicity is unlikely following single exposure of excessive doses. Treatment following emesis and charcoal administration should be supportive and symptomatic.

### Pharmacodynamics/Kinetics

**Protein Binding:** 80%

**Distribution:** Crosses the placenta

**Half-life Elimination:** 50-60 minutes

**Metabolism:** Liver

**Excretion:** Urine and feces

### Formulations

Cream, vaginal (Estrace®): 0.1 mg/g (42.5 g)

Injection, as cypionate (depGynogen®, Depo®-Estradiol, Depogen®, Dura-Estrin®, Estra-D®, Estro-Cyp®): 5 mg/mL (5 mL, 10 mL)

Injection, as valerate:

Delestrogen®: 10 mg/mL (5 mL, 10 mL); 20 mg/mL (1 mL, 5 mL, 10 mL); 40 mg/mL (5 mL, 10 mL)

Dioval®, Duragen®, Estra-L®, Gynogen L.A.®: 20 mg/mL (10 mL); 40 mg/mL (10 mL)

Tablet, micronized (Estrace®): 1 mg, 2 mg

Tablet: 0.5 mg, 1 mg, 2 mg

Transdermal system

Climara®:

0.05 mg/24 hours [12.5 $cm^2$], total estradiol 3.9 mg

0.1 mg/24 hours [25 $cm^2$], total estradiol 7.8 mg

Esclim®:

0.025 mg/day

0.0375 mg/day

0.05 mg/day

0.075 mg/day

0.1 mg/day

Estraderm®:

0.05 mg/24 hours [10 $cm^2$], total estradiol 4 mg

0.1 mg/24 hours [20 $cm^2$], total estradiol 8 mg

Fempatch®: 0.025 mg/day

Vivelle®:

0.0375 mg/day

0.05 mg/day

0.075 mg/day

0.1 mg/day

Vaginal ring (Estring®): 2 mg gradually released over 90 days

### Dosing

**Adults:** All dosage needs to be adjusted based upon the patient's response:

Male:

Prostate cancer: Valerate: I.M.: ≥30 mg or more every 1-2 weeks

Prostate cancer (androgen-dependent, inoperable, progressing): Oral: 10 mg 3 times/day for at least 3 months

Female:

Breast cancer (inoperable, progressing): Oral: 10 mg 3 times/day for at least 3 months

Osteoporosis prevention: Oral: 0.5 mg/day in a cyclic regimen (3 weeks on and 1 week off of drug)

Hypogonadism, moderate to severe vasomotor symptoms: Oral: 1-2 mg/day in a cyclic regimen for 3 weeks on drug, then 1 week off drug

Moderate to severe vasomotor symptoms: I.M.:

Cypionate: 1-5 mg every 3-4 weeks

Valerate: 10-20 mg every 4 weeks

Postpartum breast engorgement: I.M.: Valerate: 10-25 mg at end of first stage of labor

Transdermal: Apply 0.05 mg patch initially (titrate dosage to response) applied twice weekly in a cyclic regimen, for 3 weeks on drug and 1 week off drug in patients with an intact uterus and continuously in patients without a uterus.

Atrophic vaginitis, kraurosis vulvae: Vaginal: Insert 2-4 g/day for 2 weeks then gradually reduce to 1/2 the initial dose for 2 weeks followed by a maintenance dose of 1 g 1-3 times/week.

**Elderly:** Refer to adult dosing.

**Administration**

**I.M.:** Injection for intramuscular administration only.

**Topical:** Aerosol topical corticosteroids applied under the patch may reduce allergic reactions. Do not apply transdermal system to breasts, but place on trunk of body (preferably abdomen). Rotate application sites.

**Additional Nursing Issues**

**Physical Assessment:** Monitor closely for adverse reactions (see above) and therapeutic response (dependent on rationale for use). Assess knowledge/teach appropriate use and application, adverse signs to report, and need for annual gynecologic exam and breast exam with long-term use. **Pregnancy risk factor X.**

**Patient Information/Instruction:** Use this drug in cycles or term as prescribed. Periodic gynecologic exam and breast exams are important. You may experience nausea or vomiting (small frequent meals may help); dizziness or mental depression (use caution when driving); photosensitivity (use sunscreen, wear protective clothing and eyewear, and avoid direct sunlight); rash; loss of scalp hair; enlargement/tenderness of breasts; increased/decreased libido. Report sudden acute pain in legs or calves, chest, or abdomen; shortness of breath; severe headache or vomiting; weakness or numbness of arms or legs; unusual vaginal bleeding; yellowing of skin or eyes; change in color of urine or stool; or easy bruising or bleeding. **Pregnancy precautions:** Inform prescriber if you are pregnant.

Transdermal patch: Apply to clean dry skin. Do not apply transdermal patch to breasts. Apply to trunk of body (preferably abdomen). Rotate application sites. Aerosol topical corticosteroids may reduce allergic skin reaction; report persistent skin reaction.

Intravaginal cream: Insert high in vagina. Wash hands and applicator before and after use.

**Dietary Issues:** Larger doses of vitamin C (eg, 1 g/day in adults) may increase serum concentrations and adverse effects of estradiol. Vitamin C supplements are not recommended, but their effect may be decreased if vitamin C supplement is administered 2-3 hours after estrogen. Dietary intake of folate and pyridoxine may need to be increased.

**Geriatric Considerations:** Before prescribing estrogen therapy to postmenopausal women, the risks and benefits must be weighed for each patient. Data in women 80 years and older is minimal and it is unclear if reduced risk is applicable to women in this age group. Women should be informed of risks and benefits, as well as possible side effects and the return of menstrual bleeding (when cycled with a progestin), and should be involved in the prescribing options. Oral therapy may be more convenient for vaginal atrophy and urinary incontinence.

**Additional Information**

Estradiol: Estraderm®, Estrace®

Estradiol cypionate: Depo®-Estradiol, depGynogen®, Depogen®, Dura-Estrin®, Estra-D®, Estro-Cyp®

Estradiol valerate: Delestrogen®, Dioval®, Duragen®, Estra-L®

## Estradiol and Norethindrone (es tra DYE ole & nor eth IN drone)

**U.S. Brand Names** Activelle™; CombiPatch®

**Therapeutic Category** Estrogen Derivative

**Use** Treatment of moderate to severe vasomotor symptoms associated with the menopause; treatment of vulvar and vaginal atrophy; transdermal patch used in women with an intact uterus; treatment of hypoestrogenism due to hypogonadism, castration, or primary ovarian failure

**Contraindications** Hypersensitivity to any of the components; known or suspected pregnancy; known or suspected breast cancer; known or suspected estrogen-dependent neoplasia (ie, endometrial cancer); abnormal genital bleeding of unknown etiology; known or suspected active deep venous thrombosis, thromboembolic disorders or stroke, or past history of these conditions associated with estrogen use; liver dysfunction or disease

**Warnings** Use with caution in patients with renal or hepatic insufficiency. Estrogens may cause premature closure of epiphyses in young individuals. Use caution in patients with a history of thromboembolism, stroke, myocardial infarction (especially age >40 who smoke), liver tumor, or hypertension.

Estrogens have been reported to increase the risk of endometrial carcinoma; do not use estrogens during pregnancy. Before prescribing estrogen therapy to postmenopausal women, the risks and benefits must be weighed for each patient. Women should be informed of these risks and benefits, as well as possible side effects and the return of menstrual bleeding (when cycled with a progestin), and be involved in the decision to prescribe. Oral therapy may be more convenient for vaginal atrophy and stress incontinence.

**Adverse Reactions**

>10%:

Cardiovascular: Peripheral edema

(Continued)

## Estradiol and Norethindrone *(Continued)*

Central nervous system: Headache
Endocrine & metabolic: Enlargement of breasts, breast tenderness
Gastrointestinal: Nausea, anorexia, bloating
Respiratory: Upper respiratory tract infection

1% to 10%:
Central nervous system: Insomnia, depression, nervousness, weakness, pain
Respiratory: Sinusitis, pharyngitis
Endocrine & metabolic: Increased libido, postmenopausal bleeding, uterine fibroid, ovarian cyst, menstrual disorder, leukorrhea, abnormal PAP smear
Gastrointestinal: Vomiting, diarrhea, abdominal pain, flatulence
Musculoskeletal: Back pain
Dermatologic: Application site reaction (transdermal patch only), rash
Miscellaneous: Flu-like syndrome

<1% (Limited to important or life-threatening symptoms): Hypertension, thromboembolism, stroke, myocardial infarction, dizziness, decreased glucose tolerance, breast tumors, amenorrhea, hypercalcemia, alterations in frequency and flow of menses, increased triglycerides and LDL, gallstones, cholestatic jaundice, intolerance to contact lenses, increased susceptibility to *Candida* infection

**Formulations**

Tablet (Activelle™): Estradiol 1 mg and norethindrone acetate 0.5 mg (28s)
Transdermal system (CombiPatch™):
9 sq cm: Estradiol 0.05 mg and norethindrone acetate 0.14 mg per day
16 sq cm: Estradiol 0.05 mg and norethindrone acetate 0.25 mg per day

**Dosing**

**Adults:**
Oral: Take 1 tablet daily.
Transdermal (women currently using continuous estrogen or combination estrogen/progestin therapy should complete current cycle prior to initiation):
Continuous combined regimen: 0.05 mg estradiol/0.14 mg norethindrone patch applied twice weekly during a 28-day cycle (the 0.05 mg estradiol/0/25 norethindrone patch may be used if a greater progestin dose is desired)
Continuous sequential regimen: A 0.05 mg estradiol patch is applied twice weekly for 14 days, followed by the 0.05 mg estradiol/0.14 mg norethindrone patch twice weekly for the remaining 14 days of a 28-day cycle

**Elderly:** Refer to adult dosing.

♦ **Estra-L® Injection** *see* Estradiol *on page 441*

## Estramustine (es tra MUS teen)

**U.S. Brand Names** Emcyt®

**Therapeutic Category** Antineoplastic Agent, Alkylating Agent

**Pregnancy Risk Factor** C

**Lactation** Excretion in breast milk unknown/contraindicated

**Use** Palliative treatment of prostatic carcinoma (progressive or metastatic)

**Mechanism of Action/Effect** Mechanism is not completely clear, thought to act as an alkylating agent and as estrogen

**Contraindications** Hypersensitivity to estramustine or any component, estradiol, or nitrogen mustard; active thrombophlebitis or thromboembolic disorders

**Warnings** The U.S. Food and Drug Administration (FDA) currently recommends that procedures for proper handling and disposal of antineoplastic agents be considered. Glucose tolerance may be decreased; elevated blood pressure may occur. Exacerbation of peripheral edema or congestive heart disease may occur. Use with caution in patients with impaired liver function, renal insufficiency, or metabolic bone diseases. Pregnancy factor C.

**Drug Interactions**

**Decreased Effect:** Milk products and calcium-rich foods/drugs may impair the oral absorption of estramustine phosphate sodium

**Food Interactions** Estramustine serum levels may be decreased if taken with dairy products.

**Adverse Reactions**

>10%:
Cardiovascular: Edema
Gastrointestinal: Diarrhea, nausea
Endocrine & metabolic: Sodium retention, decreased libido, breast tenderness, breast enlargement
Respiratory: Dyspnea

1% to 10%:
Cardiovascular: Myocardial infarction
Central nervous system: Insomnia, lethargy
Gastrointestinal: Anorexia, flatulence, vomiting
Local: Thrombophlebitis
Neuromuscular & skeletal: Leg cramps
Respiratory: Pulmonary embolism

<1% (Limited to important or life-threatening symptoms): Cardiac arrest, anemia, leukopenia, thrombocytopenia

**Overdose/Toxicology** Symptoms of overdose include nausea, vomiting, and myelosuppression. There are no known antidotes; treatment is symptomatic and supportive.

**Pharmacodynamics/Kinetics**

**Half-life Elimination:** 20 hours

**Time to Peak:** Within 2-3 hours

**Metabolism:** Dephosphorylated in the intestines and eventually oxidized and hydrolyzed to estramustine, estrone, estradiol, and nitrogen mustard

**Excretion:** Feces via bile

**Formulations** Capsule, as sodium: 140 mg

**Dosing**

**Adults:** Oral: 14 mg/kg/day (range: 10-16 mg/kg/day) in 3-4 divided doses for 30-90 days; some patients have been maintained for >3 years on therapy

**Stability**

**Storage:** Refrigerate at 2°C to 8°C (36°F to 46°F). Capsules may be stored outside of refrigerator for up to 24-48 hours without affecting potency.

**Additional Nursing Issues**

**Physical Assessment:** Monitor closely for adverse reactions (eg, CNS changes, hypertension, thromboembolism), fluid retention (eg, edema, CHF, respiratory changes). Monitor therapeutic response (dependent on rationale for use). Monitor diabetic patients for altered glucose tolerance. Assess knowledge/teach adverse signs to report. **Pregnancy risk factor C** - barrier contraception is recommended for male patients.

**Patient Information/Instruction:** It may take several weeks to manifest effects of this medication. Store capsules in refrigerator. Do not take with milk or milk products. Preferable to take on empty stomach (1 hour before or 2 hours after meals). Small frequent meals, frequent mouth care may reduce incidence of nausea or vomiting. You may experience flatulence, diarrhea, decreased libido (reversible), breast tenderness or enlargement. Report sudden acute pain or cramping in legs or calves, chest pain, shortness of breath, weakness or numbness of arms or legs, difficulty breathing, or edema (increased weight, swelling of legs or feet).

♦ **Estratab®** *see* Estrogens, Esterified *on page 449*

♦ **Estro-Cyp® Injection** *see* Estradiol *on page 441*

♦ **Estrogenic Substance Aqueous** *see* Estrone *on page 451*

## Estrogens and Medroxyprogesterone

(ES troe jenz & me DROKS ee proe JES te rone)

**U.S. Brand Names** Premphase™; Prempro™

**Synonyms** Medroxyprogesterone and Estrogens

**Therapeutic Category** Estrogen Derivative

**Pregnancy Risk Factor** X

**Lactation** Excretion in breast milk unknown/use caution - see Breast-feeding Issues.

**Use** Treatment of women with an intact uterus for moderate to severe vasomotor symptoms associated with menopause; treatment of vulvar and vaginal atrophy; primary ovarian failure; osteoporosis prophylactic

**Contraindications** Hypersensitivity to estrogens, medroxyprogesterone, or any component; pregnancy; thrombophlebitis; cerebral apoplexy; undiagnosed vaginal bleeding; liver disease; carcinoma of the breast; estrogen dependent tumor

**Warnings** Use with caution in patients with asthma, epilepsy, migraine, diabetes, cardiac or renal dysfunction. Estrogens may cause premature closure of the epiphyses in young individuals. Estrogens have been reported to increase the risk of endometrial carcinoma. Pretreatment exams should include Pap smear, physical exam of breasts and pelvic areas. May increase serum cholesterol and LDL, decrease HDL and triglycerides. Use of any progestin during the first 4 months of pregnancy is not recommended. May lead to severe hypercalcemia in patients with breast cancer and bone metastases. Occasional blood pressure increases during estrogen replacement therapy have been attributed to idiosyncratic reactions to estrogens.

**Drug Interactions**

**Cytochrome P-450 Effect:** Estrogen may induce and is a substrate for CYP isoenzymes

**Decreased Effect:** Rifampin, barbiturates, phenytoin, carbamazepine decrease estrogen serum concentrations. Estrogens may decrease effect of sulfonylureas. Aminoglutethimide may decrease effect by increasing hepatic metabolism.

**Increased Effect/Toxicity:** Estrogens may increase metabolism of some benzodiazepines (lorazepam, oxazepam, temazepam), but decrease metabolism of others. Hydrocortisone taken with estrogen may cause corticosteroid induced toxicity. Increased potential for thromboembolic events with anticoagulants.

**Effects on Lab Values** Accelerated PT, partial thromboplastin time, and platelet aggregation time; ↑ platelet count; ↑ HDL; ↑ factors II, VII antigen, VIII coagulant activity, IX, X, XII, XII-X complex, II-VII-X complex, and beta-thromboglobulin; ↑ levels of fibrinogen and fibrinogen activity; ↑ plasminogen antigen and activity; ↑ thyroid-binding globulin; ↑ triglycerides; impaired glucose tolerance; reduced response to metyrapone test; reduced serum folate concentration; other binding proteins may be elevated; ↓ LDL; ↓ levels of antifactor Xa and antithrombin III; ↓ antithrombin III activity

**Adverse Reactions**

>10%:

Cardiovascular: Edema, peripheral edema

Endocrine & metabolic: Breakthrough bleeding, spotting, changes in menstrual flow, amenorrhea, enlargement of breasts, breast tenderness, bloating

Gastrointestinal: Anorexia, nausea

Neuromuscular & skeletal: Weakness

(Continued)

## Estrogens and Medroxyprogesterone *(Continued)*

1% to 10%:

Cardiovascular: Embolism, central thrombosis and embolism
Central nervous system: Mental depression, fever, insomnia, headache
Dermatologic: Melasma, chloasma, allergic rash with or without pruritus
Endocrine & metabolic: changes in cervical erosion and secretions, increased libido
Gastrointestinal: Weight gain or loss, vomiting, diarrhea
Hepatic: Cholestatic jaundice

<1% (Limited to important or life-threatening symptoms): Hypertension, thromboembolism, myocardial infarction, stroke, anxiety, rash, decreased glucose tolerance, increased triglycerides and LDL, breast tumors, cholestatic jaundice, pancreatitis, increased susceptibility to *Candida* infection

**Pharmacodynamics/Kinetics**

**Metabolism:** Liver

**Excretion:** Kidney

**Formulations**

Premphase™: Two separate tablets in therapy pack: Conjugated estrogens 0.625 mg [Premarin®] (28s) taken orally for 28 days and medroxyprogesterone acetate [Cycrin®] 5 mg (14s) which are taken orally with a Premarin® tablet on days 15 through 28

Prempro™: Conjugated estrogens 0.625 mg and medroxyprogesterone acetate 2.5 mg (14s)

**Dosing**

**Adults:** Oral:

Premphase™: 1 maroon tablet/day for 28 days and 1 light purple tablet to be taken with the maroon tablet on days 15-28; for patients with moderate to severe vasomotor symptoms and vulvar and vaginal atrophy associated with menopause, re-evaluate patients at 3- and 6-month intervals to determine if treatment is still necessary.

Prempro™: Dosage as above with the exception that the white 2.5 mg Cycrin® tablet (medroxyprogesterone acetate) is taken on a daily basis with the maroon Premarin® tablet (conjugated estrogen) and not just on days 15-28.

**Elderly:** Refer to adult dosing.

**Stability**

**Storage:** Store at room temperature 20°C to 25°C (68°F to 77°F).

**Monitoring Laboratory Tests** Serum cholesterol, HDL, LDL triglycerides, Pap smear

**Additional Nursing Issues**

**Physical Assessment:** Assess effectiveness/interactions of other medications patient may be taking (see Drug Interactions and Warnings/Precautions). Monitor closely for adverse reactions (eg, CNS changes, hypertension, thromboembolism, fluid retention, edema, CHF, respiratory changes). Monitor therapeutic response (dependent on rationale for use). Monitor diabetic patients for altered glucose tolerance. Assess knowledge/teach adverse signs to report. **Pregnancy risk factor X** - determine that patient is not pregnant before beginning treatment and do not give to women of childbearing age unless female is capable of complying with barrier contraceptive measures during therapy and for 1 month following therapy. Note breast-feeding caution.

**Patient Information/Instruction:** Take this as prescribed; maintain schedule. If also taking supplemental calcium as part of osteoporosis prevention, consult prescriber for recommended amounts. Periodic gynecologic exam and breast exams are important. You may experience nausea or vomiting (small frequent meals may help); dizziness or mental depression (use caution when driving); rash, loss of scalp hair, enlargement/tenderness of breasts, or increased/decreased libido. Report significant swelling of extremities; sudden acute pain in legs or calves, chest or abdomen; shortness of breath; severe headache or vomiting; sudden blindness; weakness or numbness of arm or leg; unusual vaginal bleeding; yellowing of skin or eyes; or unusual bruising or bleeding. **Pregnancy/breast-feeding precautions:** Inform prescriber if you are pregnant. Do not get pregnant during or for 1 month following therapy. Consult prescriber for instruction on appropriate contraceptive measures. Consult prescriber if breast-feeding.

**Breast-feeding Issues:** Has been shown to decrease quantity and quality of milk.

**Pregnancy Issues:** Increased risk of congenital defects in the reproductive organs of the fetus, and possibly other birth defects.

## Estrogens, Conjugated (Equine)

(ES troe jenz KON joo gate ed, EE kwine)

**U.S. Brand Names** Premarin®

**Synonyms** CES; Conjugated Estrogens

**Therapeutic Category** Estrogen Derivative

**Pregnancy Risk Factor** X

**Lactation** Enters breast milk/use caution - Breast-feeding Issues (APP rates "compatible")

**Use** Atrophic vaginitis; hypogonadism; primary ovarian failure; vasomotor symptoms of menopause; prostatic carcinoma; osteoporosis prophylaxis

**Mechanism of Action/Effect** Increases the synthesis of DNA, RNA, and various proteins in target tissues; reduces the release of gonadotropin-releasing hormone from the hypothalamus; reduces FSH and LH release from the pituitary

**Contraindications** Hypersensitivity to estrogens or any component; undiagnosed vaginal bleeding; thrombophlebitis; liver disease; pregnancy; carcinoma of the breast; estrogen dependent tumor

**Warnings** Use with caution in patients with asthma, epilepsy, migraine, diabetes, cardiac or renal dysfunction. Estrogens may cause premature closure of the epiphyses in young individuals. Safety and efficacy in children have not been established. Estrogens have been reported to increase the risk of endometrial carcinoma. Patients with risk factors for thromboembolism should be closely monitored.

**Drug Interactions**

**Cytochrome P-450 Effect:** May be a substrate for cytochrome isoenzymes (profile not defined)

**Decreased Effect:** Rifampin, barbiturates, phenytoin, carbamazepine decrease estrogen serum concentrations. Estrogens may decrease effect of sulfonylureas. Aminoglutethimide may decrease effect by increasing hepatic metabolism.

**Increased Effect/Toxicity:** Hydrocortisone taken with estrogen may cause corticosteroid induced toxicity. Increased potential for thromboembolic events with anticoagulants. Estrogen may increase the effect of carbamazepine, tricyclic antidepressants, and corticosteroids. Increased thromboembolic potential when estrogen is taken with oral anticoagulants.

**Effects on Lab Values** ↑ Prothrombin and factors VII, VIII, IX, X; ↑ platelet aggregability, thyroid binding globulin, total thyroid hormone ($T_4$), serum triglycerides/phospholipids; ↓ antithrombin III, serum folate concentration

**Adverse Reactions**

>10%:

Cardiovascular: Peripheral edema

Endocrine & metabolic: Enlargement of breasts (female and male), breast tenderness

Gastrointestinal: Nausea, anorexia, bloating

1% to 10%:

Central nervous system: Headache, migraine headache

Endocrine & metabolic: Increased libido (female), decreased libido (male)

Gastrointestinal: Vomiting, diarrhea

<1% (Limited to important or life-threatening symptoms): Hypertension, thromboembolism, myocardial infarction, edema, depression, dizziness, anxiety, stroke, amenorrhea, alterations in frequency and flow of menses, breast tumors, decreased glucose tolerance, increased triglycerides and LDL, hepatitis, pancreatitis, increased susceptibility to *Candida* infection

**Overdose/Toxicology** Symptoms of overdose include fluid retention, jaundice, and thrombophlebitis. Toxicity is unlikely following single exposure of excessive doses. Treatment should be supportive and symptomatic.

**Pharmacodynamics/Kinetics**

**Metabolism:** Liver

**Excretion:** Bile and urine

**Formulations**

Cream, vaginal: 0.625 mg/g (42.5 g)

Injection: 25 mg (5 mL)

Tablet: 0.3 mg, 0.625 mg, 0.9 mg, 1.25 mg, 2.5 mg

**Dosing**

**Adults:**

Male: Prostate cancer: Oral: 1.25-2.5 mg 3 times/day

Female:

Hypogonadism: Oral: 2.5-7.5 mg/day for 20 days, off 10 days and repeat until menses occur

Abnormal uterine bleeding:

Oral: 2.5-5 mg/day for 7-10 days; then decrease to 1.25 mg/day for 2 weeks

I.M., I.V.: 25 mg every 6-12 hours until bleeding stops

Moderate to severe vasomotor symptoms: Oral: 0.625-1.25 mg/day

Postpartum breast engorgement: Oral: 3.75 mg every 4 hours for 5 doses, then 1.25 mg every 4 hours for 5 days

Atrophic vaginitis, kraurosis vulvae: Vaginal: Instill 2-4 g/day 3 weeks on and 1 week off.

Osteoporosis: Oral: 0.625 mg/day chronically

Uremic bleeding: I.V.: 0.6 mg/kg/dose daily for 5 days

Vaginal atrophy/urinary continence:

Oral: 0.3-0.625 mg/day; treat for 3 months and repeat as necessary

Cream: 2-4 g/day (½ to 1 applicatorful)

Vasomotor symptoms: 0.3-1.25 mg/day; recommended duration: 5 years

**Elderly:** Refer to adult dosing.

**Hepatic Impairment:**

Mild to moderate liver impairment: Dosage reduction of estrogens is recommended.

Severe liver impairment: **Not recommended.**

**Administration**

**Oral:** Give at bedtime to minimize adverse effects.

**I.M.:** May be administered intramuscularly.

**I.V.:** Administer I.V. doses slowly to avoid a flushing reaction.

**Stability**

**Storage:** Refrigerate injection. At room temperature, the injection is stable for 24 months.

**Reconstitution:** Reconstituted solution is stable for 60 days at refrigeration.

**Compatibility:** Compatible with normal saline, dextrose, and inert sugar solution. Incompatible with proteins, ascorbic acid, or solutions with acidic pH.

**Additional Nursing Issues**

**Physical Assessment:** Assess other medications patient may be taking for effectiveness and interactions (see Drug Interactions). Note Warnings/Precautions and Contraindications for cautious use. Monitor therapeutic response (dependent on rationale for

(Continued)

## Estrogens, Conjugated (Equine) *(Continued)*

use) and adverse effects (eg, CNS, respiratory, fluid status changes, and thromboembolism - see Dosing, Warnings/Precautions, Adverse Reactions). Diabetic patients should monitor glucose levels closely (estrogens may alter glucose levels). Assess knowledge/teach patient appropriate use, interventions to reduce side effects, and adverse symptoms to report. **Pregnancy risk factor X** - determine that patient is not pregnant before beginning treatment and do not give to women of childbearing age unless both male and female are capable of complying with barrier contraceptive measures during therapy and for 1 month following therapy. Note breast-feeding caution.

**Patient Information/Instruction:** Follow prescribed schedule and dose. Periodic gynecologic exam and breast exams are important with long-term use. Consult prescriber for specific dietary recommendations. You may experience nausea or vomiting (small frequent meals may help); dizziness or mental depression (use caution when driving); photosensitivity (use sunscreen, wear protective clothing and eyewear, and avoid direct sunlight); rash, loss of scalp hair (reversible); enlargement/tenderness of breasts (both male and female); increased (female)/decreased (male) libido; or headache (use of mild analgesic may help). Report swelling of extremities or unusual weight gain; chest pain or palpitations; sudden acute pain, warmth, or weakness in legs or calves; shortness of breath; severe headache or vomiting; or unusual vaginal bleeding, amenorrhea, or alterations in frequency and flow of menses.

Intravaginal cream: Insert high in vagina; wash hands and applicator before and after application.

**Pregnancy/breast-feeding precautions:** Inform prescriber if you are pregnant. Do not get pregnant during or for 1 month following therapy. Male/female: Consult prescriber for instruction on appropriate barrier contraceptive measures. This drug may cause severe fetal defects. Consult prescriber if breast-feeding.

**Dietary Issues:** Larger doses of vitamin C (eg, 1 g/day in adults) may increase serum concentrations and adverse effects of estrogens. Vitamin C supplements are not recommended, but their effect/interaction may be decreased if vitamin C supplement is administered 2-3 hours after estrogen. Dietary intake of folate and pyridoxine may need to be increased.

**Geriatric Considerations:** Before prescribing estrogen therapy to postmenopausal women, the risks and benefits must be weighed for each patient. Data in women 80 years and older is minimal and it is unclear if reduced risk is applicable to women in this age group. Women should be informed of risks and benefits, as well as possible side effects and the return of menstrual bleeding (when cycled with a progestin), and should be involved in prescribing options. Oral therapy may be more convenient for vaginal atrophy and urinary incontinence.

**Breast-feeding Issues:** Estrogens have been shown to decrease milk production. The AAP considers ethinyl estradiol which is an estrogen derivative, compatible with breast-feeding and to monitor the growth of the infant closely.

**Additional Information** Contains 50% to 65% sodium estrone sulfate and 20% to 35% sodium equilin sulfate

## Estrogens, Conjugated (Synthetic)

(ES troe jenz, KON joo gate ed, sin THET ik)

**U.S. Brand Names** Cenestin™

**Therapeutic Category** Estrogen Derivative

**Pregnancy Risk Factor** X

**Lactation** Enters breast milk/use caution - Breast-feeding Issues (APP rates "compatible")

**Use** Treatment of moderate to severe vasomotor symptoms of menopause

**Mechanism of Action/Effect** Increases the synthesis of DNA, RNA, and various proteins in target tissues; reduces the release of gonadotropin-releasing hormone from the hypothalamus; reduces FSH and LH release from the pituitary

**Contraindications** Hypersensitivity to estrogens or any component; undiagnosed vaginal bleeding; thrombophlebitis; liver disease; known or suspected pregnancy; carcinoma of the breast; estrogen dependent tumor; thromboembolic disorders

**Warnings** Use with caution in patients with a history of hypercalcemia, cardiac disease, and gallbladder disease. The addition of progestins may attenuate estrogen's effects on raising HDL and lowering LDL cholesterol. May increase blood pressure and serum triglycerides (in patients with familial dyslipidemias). Use caution in patients with hepatic disease or renal dysfunction; may increase risk of venous thromboembolism. Estrogens have been reported to increase the risk of endometrial carcinoma and may increase the risk of breast cancer. Safety and efficacy in children have not been established. Do not use estrogens during pregnancy.

**Drug Interactions**

**Decreased Effect:** Specific drug interactions have not been conducted for the synthetic preparation, however the following interactions have been noted for conjugated estrogens. Rifampin decreases estrogen serum concentrations (other enzyme inducers may share this effect).

**Increased Effect/Toxicity:** Specific drug interactions have not been conducted for the synthetic preparation, however the following interactions have been noted for conjugated estrogens. Hydrocortisone increases corticosteroid toxic potential. Increased potential for thromboembolic events with anticoagulants.

**Adverse Reactions**

>10%:

Cardiovascular: Palpitation (21%), peripheral edema (10%)

Endocrine & metabolic: Breast pain (29%), menorrhagia (14%)
Central nervous system; Headache (68%), insomnia (42%), paresthesia (33%), nervousness (28%), depression (28%), pain (11%), dizziness (11%)
Gastrointestinal: Abdominal pain (28%), flatulence (29%), nausea (18%), dyspepsia (10%)
Musculoskeletal: Myalgia (28%), arthralgia (25%), back pain (14%)
Miscellaneous: Weakness (33%), infection (14%)

1% to 10%:
Gastrointestinal: Vomiting (7%), constipation (6%), diarrhea (6%)
Central nervous system: Hypertonia (6%), fever (1%)
Musculoskeletal: Leg cramps (10%)
Respiratory: Pharyngitis (8%), rhinitis (8%), cough (6%)

Additional adverse reactions associated with estrogen therapy include: Increase in blood pressure, hypercalcemia, thromboembolic disorder, myocardial infarction, hypertension, anxiety, stroke, chorea chloasma, melasma, rash, erythema multiforme, erythema nodosum, alopecia, hirsuitism, breast tumors, amenorrhea, alterations in frequency and flow of menses, changes in cervical secretions, pancreatitis, decreased glucose tolerance, weight gain, weight loss, increased triglycerides and LDL, GI distress, cholestatic jaundice, aggravation of porphyria, breast tenderness, breast enlargement, changes in libido, intolerance to contact lenses, changes in corneal curvature, increased susceptibility to *Candida* infection

**Overdose/Toxicology** Symptoms of overdose include fluid retention, jaundice, and thrombophlebitis. Toxicity is unlikely following single exposures of excessive doses, any treatment following emesis and charcoal administration should be supportive and symptomatic.

**Pharmacodynamics/Kinetics**

**Metabolism:** To inactive compounds in the liver

**Excretion:** Bile and urine

**Formulations** Oral: Tablet: 0.625 mg, 1.25 mg

**Dosing**

**Adults:** Moderate to severe vasomotor symptoms: Oral: 0.625 mg/day; may be titrated up to 1.25 mg daily. Attempts to discontinue medication should be made at 3-6 month intervals.

**Additional Nursing Issues**

**Physical Assessment:** Assess other medications patient may be taking for effectiveness and interactions (see Drug Interactions). Note Warnings/Precautions and Contraindications for cautious use. Monitor therapeutic response (dependent on rationale for use) and adverse effects (eg, CNS, respiratory, fluid status changes, and thromboembolism - see Dosing, Warnings/Precautions, Adverse Reactions). Diabetic patients should monitor glucose levels closely (estrogens may alter glucose levels). Assess knowledge/teach patient appropriate use, interventions to reduce side effects, and adverse symptoms to report. **Pregnancy risk factor X** - determine that patient is not pregnant before beginning treatment and do not give to women of childbearing age unless both male and female are capable of complying with barrier contraceptive measures during therapy and for 1 month following therapy. Note breast-feeding caution.

**Patient Information/Instruction:** Follow prescribed schedule and dose. Periodic gynecologic exam and breast exams are important with long-term use. Consult prescriber for specific dietary recommendations. You may experience nausea or vomiting (small frequent meals may help); dizziness or mental depression (use caution when driving); photosensitivity (use sunscreen, wear protective clothing and eyewear, and avoid direct sunlight); rash, loss of scalp hair (reversible); enlargement/tenderness of breasts (both male and female); increased (female)/decreased (male) libido; or headache (use of mild analgesic may help). Report swelling of extremities or unusual weight gain; chest pain or palpitations; sudden acute pain, warmth, or weakness in legs or calves; shortness of breath; severe headache or vomiting; or unusual vaginal bleeding, amenorrhea, or alterations in frequency and flow of menses.

**Pregnancy/breast-feeding precautions:** Inform prescriber if you are pregnant. Do not get pregnant during or for 1 month following therapy. Male/female: Consult prescriber for instruction on appropriate barrier contraceptive measures. This drug may cause severe fetal defects. Consult prescriber if breast-feeding.

**Additional Information** Not biologically equivalent to conjugated estrogens from equine source. Contains 9 unique estrogenic compounds (equine source contains at least 10 active estrogenic compounds).

## Estrogens, Esterified (ES troe jenz, es TER i fied)

**U.S. Brand Names** Estratab®; Menest®

**Synonyms** Esterified Estrogens

**Therapeutic Category** Estrogen Derivative

**Pregnancy Risk Factor** X

**Lactation** Use caution - see Breast-feeding Issues (AAP rates "compatible")

**Use** Atrophic vaginitis; hypogonadism; primary ovarian failure; vasomotor symptoms of menopause; prostatic carcinoma; osteoporosis prophylactic

**Mechanism of Action/Effect** Primary effects on the interphase DNA-protein complex (chromatin) by binding to a receptor (usually located in the cytoplasm of a target cell) and initiating translocation of the hormone-receptor complex to the nucleus

**Contraindications** Known or suspected cancer of the breast, except in appropriately selected patients being treated for metastatic disease; known or suspected estrogen-dependent neoplasia; known or suspected pregnancy; undiagnosed abnormal genital

(Continued)

## Estrogens, Esterified *(Continued)*

bleeding; active thrombophlebitis or thromboembolic disorders; past history of thrombophlebitis, thrombosis, or thromboembolic disorders associated with previous estrogen use except when used in the treatment of breast or prostatic malignancy

**Warnings** Use with caution in patients with asthma, epilepsy, migraine, diabetes, cardiac or renal dysfunction. Estrogens may cause premature closure of the epiphyses in young individuals. Safety and efficacy in children have not been established. Estrogens have been reported to increase the risk of endometrial carcinoma.

**Drug Interactions**

**Cytochrome P-450 Effect:** May induce and is a substrate for cytochrome isoenzymes (profile not defined)

**Decreased Effect:** Rifampin, barbiturates, phenytoin, carbamazepine decrease estrogen serum concentrations. Estrogens may decrease effect of sulfonylureas. Aminoglutethimide may decrease effect by increasing hepatic metabolism.

**Increased Effect/Toxicity:** Hydrocortisone taken with estrogen may cause corticosteroid induced toxicity. Increased potential for thromboembolic events with anticoagulants. Estrogens may increase the effect of carbamazepine, tricyclic antidepressants, and corticosteroids. Increased thromboembolic potential when estrogens are taken with oral anticoagulants.

**Effects on Lab Values** Endocrine function test may be altered; ↑ prothrombin and factors VII, VIII, IX, X; ↑ platelet aggregability, thyroid binding globulin, total thyroid hormone ($T_4$), serum triglycerides/phospholipids; ↓ antithrombin III, serum folate concentration

**Adverse Reactions**

>10%:

Cardiovascular: Peripheral edema

Endocrine & metabolic: Enlargement of breasts (female and male), breast tenderness

Gastrointestinal: Nausea, anorexia, bloating

1% to 10%:

Central nervous system: Headache, migraine headache

Endocrine & metabolic: Increased libido (female), decreased libido (male)

Gastrointestinal: Vomiting, diarrhea

<1% (Limited to important or life-threatening symptoms): Hypertension, thromboembolism, myocardial infarction, edema, depression, dizziness, anxiety, stroke, amenorrhea, alterations in frequency and flow of menses, breast tumors, decreased glucose tolerance, increased triglycerides and LDL, hepatitis, pancreatitis, increased susceptibility to *Candida* infection

**Overdose/Toxicology** Symptoms of overdose include fluid retention, jaundice, and thrombophlebitis. Toxicity is unlikely following single exposure of excessive doses. Treatment should be supportive and symptomatic.

**Pharmacodynamics/Kinetics**

**Metabolism:** Liver

**Excretion:** Urine

**Formulations** Tablet: 0.3 mg, 0.625 mg, 1.25 mg, 2.5 mg

**Dosing**

**Adults:** Oral:

Male: Prostate cancer (inoperable, progressing): 1.25-2.5 mg 3 times/day

Female:

Hypogonadism: 2.5-7.5 mg/day for 20 days, off 10 days and repeat until menses occur.

Moderate to severe vasomotor symptoms: 0.3-1.25 mg/day

Breast cancer (inoperable, progressing): 10 mg 3 times/day for at least 3 months

**Elderly:** Refer to adult dosing.

**Additional Nursing Issues**

**Physical Assessment:** Monitor closely for adverse reactions (eg, CNS changes, hypertension, thromboembolism), fluid retention (eg, edema, CHF, respiratory changes). Monitor therapeutic response (dependent on rationale for use). Monitor diabetic patients for altered glucose tolerance. Assess knowledge/teach adverse signs to report. **Pregnancy risk factor X** - determine that patient is not pregnant before beginning treatment and do not give to women of childbearing age unless both male and female are capable of complying with barrier contraceptive measures during therapy and for 1 month following therapy. Note breast-feeding caution.

**Patient Information/Instruction:** Use this drug in cycles or term as prescribed. Take each day at the same time with food. Periodic gynecologic exam and breast exams are important. You may experience nausea or vomiting (small frequent meals may help); dizziness or mental depression (use caution when driving); rash; loss of scalp hair; enlargement/tenderness of breasts; or increased/decreased libido. Report significant swelling of extremities, sudden acute pain in legs or calves, chest, or abdomen; shortness of breath; severe headache or vomiting; weakness or numbness of arms or legs; or unusual vaginal bleeding. **Pregnancy/breast-feeding precautions:** Inform prescriber if you are pregnant. Do not get pregnant during or for 1 month following therapy. Male/female: Consult prescriber for instruction on appropriate barrier contraceptive measures. This drug may cause severe fetal defects. Consult prescriber if breast-feeding.

**Breast-feeding Issues:** Estrogens have been shown to decrease milk production. The AAP considers ethinyl estradiol which is an estrogen derivative, compatible with breast-feeding and to monitor the growth of the infant closely.

**Additional Information** Esterified estrogens are a combination of the sodium salts of the sulfate esters of estrogenic substances. The principal component is estrone, with preparations containing 75% to 85% sodium estrone sulfate and 6% to 15% sodium equilin sulfate such that the total is not <90%.

## Estrone (ES trone)

**U.S. Brand Names** Aquest®; Kestrone®

**Synonyms** Estrogenic Substance Aqueous

**Therapeutic Category** Estrogen Derivative

**Pregnancy Risk Factor** X

**Lactation** Excretion in breast milk unknown

**Use** Hypogonadism; primary ovarian failure; vasomotor symptoms of menopause; prostatic carcinoma; inoperable breast cancer, kraurosis vulvae, abnormal uterine bleeding due to hormone imbalance

**Mechanism of Action/Effect** Estrone is a natural ovarian estrogenic hormone that is available as an aqueous mixture of water insoluble estrone and water soluble estrone potassium sulfate; all estrogens, including estrone, act in a similar manner; there is no evidence that there are biological differences among various estrogen preparations other than their ability to bind to cellular receptors inside the target cells

**Contraindications** Hypersensitivity to estrogens or any component; thrombophlebitis; undiagnosed vaginal bleeding; pregnancy

**Warnings** Use with caution in patients with asthma, epilepsy, migraine, diabetes, cardiac or renal dysfunction. Estrogens may cause premature closure of the epiphyses in young individuals. Safety and efficacy in children have not been established. Estrogens have been reported to increase the risk of endometrial carcinoma.

**Drug Interactions**

**Decreased Effect:** Rifampin decreases estrogen serum concentrations.

**Increased Effect/Toxicity:** Hydrocortisone taken with estrogen may cause corticosteroid induced toxicity. Increased potential for thromboembolic events with anticoagulants. Estrone may increase the effect of carbamazepine, tricyclic antidepressants, and corticosteroids. Increased thromboembolic potential when estrone is taken with oral anticoagulants.

**Effects on Lab Values** ↑ Prothrombin and factors VII, VIII, IX, X; ↑ platelet aggregability, thyroid binding globulin, total thyroid hormone ($T_4$), serum triglycerides/phospholipids; ↓ antithrombin III, serum folate concentration

**Adverse Reactions**

**Systemic:**

>10%:
- Cardiovascular: Peripheral edema
- Endocrine & metabolic: Enlargement of breasts (female and male), breast tenderness
- Gastrointestinal: Nausea, anorexia, bloating

1% to 10%:
- Central nervous system: Headache, migraine headache
- Endocrine & metabolic: Increased libido (female), decreased libido (male)
- Gastrointestinal: Vomiting, diarrhea

<1% (Limited to important or life-threatening symptoms): Hypertension, thromboembolism, myocardial infarction, edema, depression, dizziness, anxiety, stroke, chloasma, melasma, rash, amenorrhea, alterations in frequency and flow of menses, breast tumors, decreased glucose tolerance, increased triglycerides and LDL, nausea, GI distress, gallbladder obstruction, hepatitis, intolerance to contact lenses, increased susceptibility to *Candida* infection

**Vaginal:**

1% to 10%:
- Cardiovascular: Peripheral edema
- Endocrine & metabolic: Breast tenderness, breast enlargement
- Gastrointestinal: Anorexia, abdominal cramping

<1% (Limited to important or life-threatening symptoms): Hypertension, thromboembolism, myocardial infarction, stroke, migraine, dizziness, anxiety, depression, headache, chloasma, melasma, rash, decreased glucose tolerance, alterations in frequency and flow of menses, breast tenderness or enlargement, increased triglycerides and LDL, nausea, GI distress, cholestatic jaundice, increased susceptibility to *Candida* infection

**Overdose/Toxicology** Symptoms of overdose include fluid retention, jaundice, and thrombophlebitis. Toxicity is unlikely following single exposure of excessive doses. Treatment should be supportive and symptomatic.

**Pharmacodynamics/Kinetics**

**Metabolism:** Liver

**Excretion:** Bile and urine

**Formulations** Injection: 2 mg/mL (10 mL, 30 mL); 5 mg/mL (10 mL)

**Dosing**

**Adults:** I.M.:
- Male: Prostatic carcinoma: 2-4 mg 2-3 times/week
- Female:
  - Senile vaginitis and kraurosis vulvae: 0.1-0.5 mg 2-3 times/week
  - Breast cancer (inoperable, progressing): 5 mg 3 or more times/week
  - Primary ovarian failure, hypogonadism: 0.1-1 mg/week, up to 2 mg/week in single or divided doses
  - Abnormal uterine bleeding: 2.5 mg/day for several days

(Continued)

## Estrone *(Continued)*

**Elderly:** Refer to adult dosing.

**Hepatic Impairment:**

Mild to moderate liver impairment: Dosage reduction of estrogens is recommended.
Severe liver impairment: **Not recommended.**

**Administration**

**I.M.:** Intramuscular injection only.

**I.V.: Not** for I.V. administration.

**Additional Nursing Issues**

**Physical Assessment:** Monitor closely for adverse reactions (eg, CNS changes, hypertension, thromboembolism), fluid retention (eg, edema, CHF, respiratory changes). Monitor therapeutic response (dependent on rationale for use). Monitor diabetic patients for altered glucose tolerance. Assess knowledge/teach adverse signs to report. **Pregnancy risk factor X** - determine that patient is not pregnant before beginning treatment and do not give to women of childbearing age unless both male and female are capable of complying with barrier contraceptive measures during therapy and for 1 month following therapy. Note breast-feeding caution.

**Patient Information/Instruction:** This drug can only be given I.M. It is important to maintain schedule of drug days and drug-free days. Periodic gynecologic exam and breast exams are important. You may experience nausea or vomiting (small frequent meals may help); dizziness or mental depression (use caution when driving); rash; loss of scalp hair; enlargement/tenderness of breasts; or increased/decreased libido. Report significant swelling of extremities, sudden acute pain in legs or calves, chest, or abdomen; shortness of breath; severe headache or vomiting; weakness or numbness of arms or legs; or unusual vaginal bleeding. **Pregnancy/breast-feeding precautions:** Inform prescriber if you are pregnant. Do not get pregnant during or for 1 month following therapy. Male/female: Consult prescriber for instruction on appropriate barrier contraceptive measures. This drug may cause severe fetal defects. Consult prescriber if breast-feeding.

## Estropipate (ES troe pih pate)

**U.S. Brand Names** Ogen® Oral; Ogen® Vaginal; Ortho-Est® Oral

**Synonyms** Piperazine Estrone Sulfate

**Therapeutic Category** Estrogen Derivative

**Pregnancy Risk Factor** X

**Lactation** Excretion in breast milk unknown

**Use** Atrophic vaginitis; hypogonadism; primary ovarian failure; vasomotor symptoms of menopause; osteoporosis prophylactic

**Mechanism of Action/Effect** Crystalline estrone that has been solubilized as the sulfate and stabilized with piperazine. Primary effects on the interphase DNA-protein complex (chromatin) by binding to a receptor (usually located in the cytoplasm of a target cell) and initiating translocation of the hormone receptor complex to the nucleus.

**Contraindications** Hypersensitivity to estrogens or any component; thrombophlebitis; undiagnosed vaginal bleeding; pregnancy

**Warnings** Use with caution in patients with asthma, epilepsy, migraine, diabetes, cardiac or renal dysfunction. Estrogens may cause premature closure of the epiphyses in young individuals. Safety and efficacy in children have not been established. Estrogens have been reported to increase the risk of endometrial carcinoma.

**Drug Interactions**

**Decreased Effect:** Rifampin decreases estrogen serum concentrations.

**Increased Effect/Toxicity:** Hydrocortisone taken with estrogen may cause corticosteroid induced toxicity. Increased potential for thromboembolic events with anticoagulants. Estrogens may increase the effect of carbamazepine, tricyclic antidepressants, and corticosteroids. Increased thromboembolic potential when estrogens are taken with oral anticoagulants.

**Effects on Lab Values** ↑ prothrombin and factors VII, VIII, IX, X; platelet aggregability, thyroid binding globulin, total thyroid hormone ($T_4$), serum triglycerides/phospholipids; ↓ antithrombin III, serum folate concentration

**Adverse Reactions**

**Systemic:**

>10%:

Cardiovascular: Peripheral edema
Endocrine & metabolic: Enlargement of breasts (female and male), breast tenderness
Gastrointestinal: Nausea, anorexia, bloating

1% to 10%:

Central nervous system: Headache, migraine headache
Endocrine & metabolic: Increased libido (female), decreased libido (male)
Gastrointestinal: Vomiting, diarrhea

<1% (Limited to important or life-threatening symptoms): Hypertension, thromboembolism, myocardial infarction, edema, depression, dizziness, anxiety, stroke, amenorrhea, alterations in frequency and flow of menses, breast tumors, decreased glucose tolerance, increased triglycerides and LDL, hepatitis, intolerance to contact lenses, increased susceptibility to *Candida* infection

**Vaginal:**

1% to 10%:

Cardiovascular: Peripheral edema
Endocrine & metabolic: Breast tenderness, breast enlargement
Gastrointestinal: Anorexia, abdominal cramping

<1% (Limited to important or life-threatening symptoms): Hypertension, thromboembolism, myocardial infarction, stroke, migraine, dizziness, anxiety, depression, headache, decreased glucose tolerance, alterations in frequency and flow of menses, breast tenderness or enlargement, increased triglycerides and LDL, cholestatic jaundice, increased susceptibility to *Candida* infection

**Overdose/Toxicology** Symptoms of overdose include fluid retention, jaundice, and thrombophlebitis. Toxicity is unlikely following single exposure of excessive doses. Treatment following emesis and charcoal administration should be supportive and symptomatic.

**Formulations**

Cream, vaginal: 0.15% [estropipate 1.5 mg/g] (42.5 g tube)

Tablet: 0.625 mg [estropipate 0.75 mg]; 1.25 mg [estropipate 1.5 mg]; 2.5 mg [estropipate 3 mg]; 5 mg [estropipate 6 mg]

**Dosing**

**Adults:** Female:

Moderate to severe vasomotor symptoms: Oral: 0.625-5 mg/day

Hypogonadism or primary ovarian failure: Oral: 1.25-7.5 mg/day for 3 weeks followed by an 8- to 10-day rest period

Osteoporosis prevention: Oral: 0.625 mg/day for 25 days of a 31-day cycle

Atrophic vaginitis or kraurosis vulvae: Vaginal: Instill 2-4 g/day 3 weeks on and 1 week off.

**Elderly:** Refer to adult dosing.

**Hepatic Impairment:**

Mild to moderate liver impairment: Dosage reduction of estrogens is recommended.

Severe liver impairment: **Not recommended.**

**Additional Nursing Issues**

**Physical Assessment:** Monitor closely for adverse reactions (eg, CNS changes, hypertension, thromboembolism), fluid retention (eg, edema, CHF, respiratory changes). Monitor therapeutic response (dependent on rationale for use). Monitor diabetic patients for altered glucose tolerance. Assess knowledge/teach adverse signs to report. **Pregnancy risk factor X** - determine that patient is not pregnant before beginning treatment and do not give to women of childbearing age unless female is capable of complying with barrier contraceptive measures during therapy and for 1 month following therapy. Note breast-feeding caution.

**Patient Information/Instruction:** It is important to maintain schedule of drug days and drug-free days. Periodic gynecologic exam and breast exams are important. You may experience nausea or vomiting (small frequent meals may help); dizziness or mental depression (use caution when driving); rash; loss of scalp hair; enlargement/tenderness of breasts; or increased/decreased libido. Report significant swelling of extremities, sudden acute pain in legs or calves, chest or abdomen; shortness of breath; severe headache or vomiting; weakness or numbness of arms or legs; or unusual vaginal bleeding.

Intravaginal cream: Insert high in vagina, wash hands and applicator before and after application.

**Pregnancy/breast-feeding precautions:** Inform prescriber if you are pregnant. Do not get pregnant during or for 1 month following therapy. Consult prescriber for instruction on appropriate barrier contraceptive measures. This drug may cause severe fetal defects. Consult prescriber if breast-feeding.

- **Estrostep®** *see* Oral Contraceptives *on page 859*
- **Estrostep® Fe** *see* Oral Contraceptives *on page 859*
- **Estrouis®** *see* Estropipate *on previous page*

## Etanercept (et a NER cept)

**U.S. Brand Names** Enbrel®

**Therapeutic Category** Antirheumatic, Disease Modifying

**Pregnancy Risk Factor** B

**Lactation** Excretion in breast milk unknown

**Use** Reduction in signs and symptoms of moderately to severely active rheumatoid arthritis in patients who have had an inadequate response to one or more disease-modifying antirheumatic drugs (DMARDs)

**Mechanism of Action/Effect** Etanercept is a recombinant DNA-derived protein composed of tumor necrosis factor receptor (TNFR) linked to the Fc portion of human IgG1. Etanercept binds tumor necrosis factor (TNF) and blocks its interaction with cell surface receptors. TNF plays an important role in the inflammatory processes of rheumatoid arthritis (RA) and the resulting joint pathology.

**Contraindications** Hypersensitivity to etanercept or any component; patients with sepsis (mortality may be increased)

**Warnings** Etanercept may affect defenses against infections and malignancies. Safety and efficacy in patients with immunosuppression or chronic infections have not been evaluated. Discontinue administration if patient develops a serious infection. Impact on the development and course of malignancies is not fully defined. Treatment may result in the formation of autoimmune antibodies; cases of autoimmune disease have not been described. Non-neutralizing antibodies to etanercept may also be formed. No correlation of antibody development to clinical response or adverse events has been observed. The long-term immunogenicity, carcinogenic potential, or effect on fertility are unknown. No evidence of mutagenic activity has been observed *in vitro* or *in vivo*. The safety of etanercept has not been studied in children <4 years of age.

(Continued)

## Etanercept *(Continued)*

Allergic reactions may occur (<0.5%), but anaphylaxis has not been observed. If an anaphylactic reaction or other serious allergic reaction occurs, administration of etanercept should be discontinued immediately and appropriate therapy initiated.

Patients should be brought up to date with all immunizations before initiating therapy. No data are available concerning the effects of etanercept on vaccination. Live vaccines should not be given concurrently. No data are available concerning secondary transmission of live vaccines in patients receiving etanercept. Patients with a significant exposure to varicella virus should temporarily discontinue etanercept. Treatment with varicella-zoster immune globulin should be considered.

**Drug Interactions**

**Decreased Effect:** Specific drug interaction studies have not been conducted with etanercept.

**Increased Effect/Toxicity:** Specific drug interaction studies have not been conducted with etanercept.

**Adverse Reactions** Events reported include those >3% with incidence higher than placebo.

>10%:

Central nervous system: Headache (17%)

Local: Injection site reaction (37%)

Respiratory: Respiratory tract infection (38%), upper respiratory tract infection (29%), rhinitis (12%)

Miscellaneous: Infection (35%), positive ANA (11%), positive antidouble-stranded DNA antibodies (15% by RIA, 3% by *Crithidia lucilae* assay)

>3% to 10%:

Central nervous system: Dizziness (7%)

Dermatologic: Rash (5%)

Gastrointestinal: Abdominal pain (5%), dyspepsia (4%)

Neuromuscular and skeletal: Weakness (5%)

Respiratory: Pharyngitis (7%), respiratory disorder (5%), sinusitis (3%)

<3%: Malignancies, serious infection, heart failure, myocardial infarction, myocardial ischemia, cerebral ischemia, hypertension, hypotension, cholecystitis, pancreatitis, gastrointestinal hemorrhage, bursitis, depression, dyspnea

**Overdose/Toxicology** No dose-limiting toxicities have been observed during clinical trials. Single I.V. doses up to 60 mg/m$^2$ have been administered to healthy volunteers in an endotoxemia study without evidence of dose-limiting toxicities.

**Pharmacodynamics/Kinetics**

**Half-life Elimination:** 115 hours (98-300 hours)

**Time to Peak:** 72 hours (48-96 hours)

**Metabolism:** Clearance: 89 mL/hour (52 mL/hour/m$^2$)

**Onset:** Within 2-3 weeks

**Formulations** Powder for injection: 25 mg

**Dosing**

**Adults:** S.C.: 25 mg given twice weekly; if the physician determines that it is appropriate, patients may self-inject after proper training in injection technique.

**Elderly:** S.C.: Although greater sensitivity of some elderly patients cannot be ruled out, no overall differences in safety or effectiveness were observed.

**Administration**

**Other: Note:** The needle cover of the diluent syringe contains dry natural rubber (latex), which should not be handled by persons sensitive to this substance. New injections should be given at least one inch from an old site and never into areas where the skin is tender, bruised, red, or hard.

**Stability**

**Storage:** The dose tray containing Enbrel® (sterile powder) must be refrigerated at 2°C to 8°C (36°F to 46°F). Do not freeze. Reconstituted solutions of Enbrel® should be administered as soon as possible after reconstitution. If not administered immediately after reconstitution, Enbrel® may be stored in the vial at 2°C to 8°C (36°F to 46°F) for up to 6 hours.

**Reconstitution:** Reconstitute aseptically with 1 mL sterile bacteriostatic water for injection, USP (supplied). To avoid excessive foaming, inject diluent slowly into the vial. Swirl gently during dissolution, do not shake or vigorously agitate. Do not filter reconstituted solution during preparation or administration. Injection sites should be rotated. **Note:** The needle cover of the diluent syringe contains dry natural rubber (latex), which should not be handled by persons sensitive to this substance.

**Additional Nursing Issues**

**Physical Assessment:** See Contraindications and Warnings/Precautions for use cautions. Monitor effectiveness of therapy (eg, pain, range of motion, mobility, ADL function, inflammation). Assess knowledge/teach patient appropriate administration (injection technique and needle disposal if self-administered), possible side effects/ interventions, and adverse symptoms to report (see Adverse Reactions). Note breast-feeding caution.

**Patient Information/Instruction:** If self-injecting, follow instructions for injection and disposal of needles exactly. If redness, swelling, or irritation appears at the injection site, contact prescriber. Do not have any vaccinations while using this medication without consulting prescriber first. You may experience headache or dizziness (use caution when driving or engaging in tasks requiring alertness until response to drug is known). If stomach pain or cramping, unusual bleeding or bruising, blood in vomitus, stool, or urine occurs, stop taking medication and contact prescriber. Report skin rash, unusual muscle or bone weakness, or signs of respiratory flu or other infection (eg, chills, fever, sore throat, easy bruising or bleeding, mouth sores, unhealed sores). **Breast-feeding precautions:** Consult prescriber if breast-feeding.

**Breast-feeding Issues:** It is not known whether etanercept is excreted in human milk or absorbed systemically after ingestion. Because many immunoglobulins are excreted in human milk, and because of the potential for serious adverse reactions in nursing infants from Enbrel®, a decision should be made whether to discontinue nursing or to discontinue the drug.

**Pregnancy Issues:** Developmental toxicity studies performed in animals have revealed no evidence of harm to the fetus. There are no studies in pregnant women; this drug should be used during pregnancy only if clearly needed.

## Ethacrynic Acid (eth a KRIN ik AS id)

**U.S. Brand Names** Edecrin®

**Synonyms** Sodium Ethacrynate

**Therapeutic Category** Diuretic, Loop

**Pregnancy Risk Factor** B

**Lactation** Considered contraindicated by manufacturer

**Use** Management of edema associated with congestive heart failure; hepatic cirrhosis or renal disease; short-term management of ascites due to malignancy, idiopathic edema, and lymphedema

**Mechanism of Action/Effect** Inhibits reabsorption of sodium and chloride in the ascending loop of Henle and distal renal tubule, interfering with the chloride-binding cotransport system, thus causing increased excretion of water, sodium, chloride, magnesium, and calcium

**Contraindications** Hypersensitivity to ethacrynic acid or any component; anuria; hypotension; dehydration with low serum sodium concentrations; metabolic alkalosis with hypokalemia; history of severe, watery diarrhea from ethacrynic acid

**Warnings** Use with caution in patients with advanced hepatic cirrhosis, diabetes mellitus, hypotension, dehydration, history of watery diarrhea from ethacrynic acid, or hearing impairment. Ototoxicity occurs more frequently than with other loop diuretics. Safety and efficacy in infants have not been established.

**Drug Interactions**

**Decreased Effect:** Probenecid decreases diuretic effects of ethacrynic acid. Ethacrynic acid may decrease the effectiveness of antidiabetic agents.

**Increased Effect/Toxicity:** Hypotensive agents → additive decreased blood pressure. Drugs affected by or causing potassium depletion → additive decreased potassium. Increased nephrotoxic potential with aminoglycosides. Digoxin increases cardiotoxic potential → arrhythmias. Increased warfarin anticoagulant effects; increased lithium levels.

**Adverse Reactions**

>10%:
- Cardiovascular: Orthostatic hypotension
- Gastrointestinal: Diarrhea, anorexia

1% to 10%:
- Central nervous system: Headache, confusion, nervousness
- Gastrointestinal: Stomach cramps
- Endocrine & metabolic: Hyponatremia, hypochloremic alkalosis, hypokalemia
- Ocular: Blurred vision
- Otic: Ototoxicity

<1% (Limited to important or life-threatening symptoms): GI bleeding, pancreatitis, hematuria, hepatic dysfunction, abnormal LFTs, leukopenia, agranulocytosis, thrombocytopenia, renal injury, hematuria

**Overdose/Toxicology** Symptoms of overdose include electrolyte depletion, volume depletion, dehydration, and circulatory collapse. Treatment is supportive.

**Pharmacodynamics/Kinetics**

**Protein Binding:** >90%

**Half-life Elimination:** Normal renal function: 2-4 hours

**Metabolism:** Liver

**Excretion:** Bile and urine

**Onset:**
- Onset of diuretic effect: Oral: Within 30 minutes; I.V.: 5 minutes
- Peak effect: Oral: 2 hours; I.V.: 30 minutes

**Duration:** Oral: 12 hours; I.V.: 2 hours

**Formulations**

Powder for injection, as ethacrynate sodium: 50 mg (50 mL)

Tablet: 25 mg, 50 mg

**Dosing**

**Adults:** I.V. formulation should be diluted in $D_5W$ or NS (1 mg/mL) and infused over several minutes.

Oral: 50-100 mg/day in 1-2 divided doses; may increase in increments of 25-50 mg at intervals of several days to a maximum of 400 mg/24 hours.

I.V.: 0.5-1 mg/kg/dose (maximum: 100 mg/dose); repeat doses not routinely recommended; however, if indicated, repeat doses every 8-12 hours.

**Elderly:** Oral: Initial: 25-50 mg/day

**Renal Impairment:**

$Cl_{cr}$ <10 mL/minute: Avoid use.

Not removed by hemo- or peritoneal dialysis; supplemental dose is not necessary.

(Continued)

## Ethacrynic Acid *(Continued)*

**Administration**

**I.V.:** Injection should **not** be given S.C. or I.M. due to local pain and irritation. Single I.V. doses should not exceed 100 mg. Administer each 10 mg over a minute.

**I.V. Detail:** If a second dose is needed, it is recommended to use a new injection site to avoid possible thrombophlebitis.

**Stability**

**Compatibility:** Do not mix with whole blood or its derivatives.

**Monitoring Laboratory Tests** Renal function, serum electrolytes

**Additional Nursing Issues**

**Physical Assessment:** Assess for effectiveness of therapy, interactions with other medications, and adverse reactions. Monitor blood pressure, weight, I & O ratio, and signs of fluid retention. Breast-feeding is contraindicated.

**Patient Information/Instruction:** Take prescribed dose with food early in day. Include orange juice or bananas (or other potassium-rich foods) in your diet, but do not take potassium supplements without consulting prescriber. You may experience postural hypotension (use caution when rising from lying or sitting position, when climbing stairs, or when driving); lightheadedness, dizziness, or drowsiness (use caution driving or when engaging in hazardous activities); diarrhea (buttermilk, boiled milk, or yogurt may help); or decreased accommodation to heat (avoid excessive exercise in hot weather). Diabetics should monitor serum glucose closely (this medication may interfere with antidiabetic medications). Report changes in hearing or ringing in ears, persistent headache, unusual confusion or nervousness, abdominal pain or blood stool (black stool), palpitations, chest pain, rapid heartbeat, joint or muscle soreness or weakness, flu-like symptoms, skin rash or itching, or blurred vision. Report swelling of ankles or feet, weight changes of more than 3 lb/day, increased fatigue, or muscle cramping or trembling. **Breast-feeding precautions:** Do not breast-feed.

**Geriatric Considerations:** Ethacrynic acid is rarely used because of its increased incidence of ototoxicity as compared to the other loop diuretics (see Additional Information).

**Additional Information** Injection form may be given orally while hospitalized. Ethacrynic acid should be saved for patients who are either allergic or resistant to furosemide or bumetanide.

PH: 6.3-7.7

## Ethambutol (e THAM byoo tole)

**U.S. Brand Names** Myambutol®

**Therapeutic Category** Antitubercular Agent

**Pregnancy Risk Factor** B

**Lactation** Enters breast milk/compatible

**Use** Treatment of tuberculosis and other mycobacterial diseases in conjunction with other antituberculosis agents; only indicated when patients are from areas where drug-resistant *M. tuberculosis* is endemic, in HIV-infected elderly patients, and when drug-resistant *M. tuberculosis* is suspected

**Mechanism of Action/Effect** Suppresses mycobacteria multiplication by interfering with RNA synthesis

**Contraindications** Hypersensitivity to ethambutol or any component; optic neuritis

**Warnings** Use only in children whose visual acuity can accurately be determined and monitored (not recommended for use in children <13 years of age). Dosage modification required in patients with renal insufficiency.

**Drug Interactions**

**Decreased Effect:** Ethambutol absorption is decreased when taken with aluminum salts.

**Effects on Lab Values** ↑ uric acid (S)

**Adverse Reactions**

1% to 10%:

- Central nervous system: Headache, confusion, disorientation
- Endocrine & metabolic: Acute gout or hyperuricemia
- Gastrointestinal: Abdominal pain, anorexia, nausea, vomiting
- Neuromuscular & skeletal: Acute gouty arthritis

<1% (Limited to important or life-threatening symptoms): Abnormal liver function tests, peripheral neuritis

**Overdose/Toxicology** Symptoms of overdose include decrease in visual acuity, anorexia, joint pain, and numbness of extremities. Treatment is supportive.

**Pharmacodynamics/Kinetics**

**Protein Binding:** 20% to 30%

**Distribution:** Well distributed throughout the body with high concentrations in kidneys, lungs, saliva, and red blood cells

Relative diffusion of antimicrobial agents from blood into CSF: Adequate with or without inflammation (exceeds usual MICs)

Ratio of CSF to blood level (%): Normal meninges: 0; Inflamed meninges: 25

**Half-life Elimination:** 2.5-3.6 hours; End-stage renal disease: 7-15 hours

**Metabolism:** Liver

**Excretion:** Urine and feces

**Formulations** Tablet, hydrochloride: 100 mg, 400 mg

**Dosing**

**Adults:** Oral: **Note:** A four-drug regimen (isoniazid, rifampin, pyrazinamide, and either streptomycin or ethambutol) is preferred for the initial, empiric treatment of TB. When the drug susceptibility results are available, the regimen should be altered as appropriate.

**Patients with tuberculosis and without HIV infection:**

**OPTION 1:** Isoniazid resistance rate <4%: Administer daily isoniazid, rifampin, and pyrazinamide for 8 weeks followed by isoniazid and rifampin daily or directly observed therapy (DOT) 2-3 times/week for 16 weeks. If isoniazid resistance rate is not documented, ethambutol or streptomycin should also be administered until susceptibility to isoniazid or rifampin is demonstrated. Continue treatment for at least 6 months or 3 months beyond culture conversion.

**OPTION 2:** Administer daily isoniazid, rifampin, pyrazinamide, and either streptomycin or ethambutol for 2 weeks followed by DOT 2 times/week administration of the same drugs for 6 weeks, and subsequently, with isoniazid and rifampin DOT 2 times/week administration for 16 weeks

**OPTION 3:** Administer isoniazid, rifampin, pyrazinamide, and either ethambutol or streptomycin by DOT 3 times/week for 6 months

**Patients with TB and with HIV infection:** Administer any of the above OPTIONS 1, 2 or 3; however, treatment should be continued for a total of 9 months and at least 6 months beyond culture conversion.

**Note:** Some experts recommend that the duration of therapy should be extended to 9 months for patients with disseminated disease, miliary disease, disease involving the bones or joints, or tuberculosis lymphadenitis

Daily therapy: 15-25 mg/kg/day (maximum: 2.5 g/day)

Directly observed therapy (DOT): Twice weekly: 50 mg/kg (maximum: 2.5 g)

DOT: 3 times/week: 25-30 mg/kg (maximum: 2.5 g)

**Elderly:** Refer to adult dosing.

**Renal Impairment:**

$Cl_{cr}$ 10-50 mL/minute: Administer every 24-36 hours.

$Cl_{cr}$ <10 mL/minute: Administer every 48 hours.

Slightly dialyzable (5% to 20%); Administer dose postdialysis.

Peritoneal dialysis: Dose for $Cl_{cr}$ <10 mL/minute.

Continuous arteriovenous or venovenous hemofiltration: Administer every 24-36 hours.

**Monitoring Laboratory Tests** Periodic visual testing in patients receiving >15 mg/kg/day; periodic renal, hepatic, and hematopoietic tests

**Additional Nursing Issues**

**Physical Assessment:** Monitor for adverse reactions. Note dosing recommendations above and monitor patient adherence to dosing program.

**Patient Information/Instruction:** Take as scheduled, with meals. Avoid missing doses and do not discontinue without consulting prescriber. You may experience GI distress (frequent small meals and good oral care may help), dizziness, disorientation, drowsiness (avoid driving or engaging in tasks that require alertness until response to drug is known). You will need to have frequent ophthalmic exams and periodic medical check-ups to evaluate drug effects. Report changes in vision, numbness or tingling of extremities, or persistent loss of appetite.

**Geriatric Considerations:** Since most elderly patients acquired their tuberculosis before current antituberculin regimens were available, ethambutol is only indicated when patients are from areas where drug resistant *M. tuberculosis* is endemic, in HIV-infected elderly patients, and when drug resistant *M. tuberculosis* is suspected (see dose adjustments for renal impairment).

**Related Information**

TB Drug Comparison *on page 1402*

## Ethchlorvynol (eth klor VI nole)

**U.S. Brand Names** Placidyl®

**Therapeutic Category** Hypnotic, Miscellaneous

**Pregnancy Risk Factor** C

**Lactation** Excretion in breast milk unknown/not recommended

**Use** Short-term management of insomnia

**Mechanism of Action/Effect** Causes nonspecific depression of the reticular activating system

**Contraindications** Hypersensitivity to ethchlorvynol or any component; porphyria

**Warnings** Administer with caution to depressed or suicidal patients or to patients with a history of drug abuse. Intoxication symptoms may appear with prolonged daily doses of as little as 1 g. Withdrawal symptoms may be seen upon abrupt discontinuation. Use with caution in the elderly and in patients with hepatic or renal dysfunction. Use with caution in patients who have a history of paradoxical restlessness to barbiturates or alcohol. Some products may contain tartrazine. Pregnancy factor C.

**Drug Interactions**

**Decreased Effect:** Decreased effect of oral anticoagulants.

**Increased Effect/Toxicity:** Increased toxicity (CNS depression) with alcohol, CNS depressants, MAO inhibitors, and tricyclic antidepressants (delirium).

**Adverse Reactions**

>10%:

Central nervous system: Dizziness

Gastrointestinal: Indigestion, nausea, stomach pain, unpleasant aftertaste

Neuromuscular & skeletal: Weakness

Ocular: Blurred vision

(Continued)

## Ethchlorvynol *(Continued)*

1% to 10%:

Central nervous system: Nervousness, excitement, clumsiness, confusion, drowsiness (daytime)

Dermatologic: Rash

<1% (Limited to important or life-threatening symptoms): Bradycardia, cholestatic jaundice, shortness of breath

**Overdose/Toxicology** Symptoms of overdose include prolonged deep coma, respiratory depression, hypothermia, bradycardia, hypotension, and nystagmus. Treatment is supportive. Hemoperfusion may be helpful in enhancing elimination.

**Pharmacodynamics/Kinetics**

**Half-life Elimination:** 10-20 hours

**Time to Peak:** 2 hours

**Metabolism:** Liver

**Excretion:** Urine

**Onset:** 15-60 minutes

**Duration:** 5 hours

**Formulations** Capsule: 200 mg, 500 mg, 750 mg

**Dosing**

**Adults:** Oral: 500-1000 mg at bedtime

**Elderly:** Not recommended for use in the elderly; see Geriatric Considerations.

**Renal Impairment:** $Cl_{cr}$ <50 mL/minute: Avoid use.

**Administration**

**Oral:** Swallow capsules whole; do **not** chew or crush.

**Stability**

**Storage:** Capsules should **not** be refrigerated.

**Monitoring Laboratory Tests** Cardiac and respiratory function

**Additional Nursing Issues**

**Physical Assessment:** For short-term use. Assess effectiveness and interactions of other medications (see Drug Interactions). See Contraindications and Warnings/Precautions for cautious use. Assess for history of addiction; long-term use can result in dependence, abuse, or tolerance. Evaluate periodically for need for continued use. After long-term use, taper dosage slowly when discontinuing. For inpatient use, institute safety measures (side rails, night light, call bell, assistance with ambulation) and monitor effectiveness and adverse reactions. For outpatients, monitor for effectiveness of therapy and adverse reactions (see Adverse Reactions) at beginning of therapy and periodically with long-term use. Assess knowledge/teach patient appropriate use, interventions to reduce side effects, and adverse symptoms to report. **Pregnancy risk factor C** - benefits must outweigh possible risks. Breast-feeding is not recommended.

**Patient Information/Instruction:** Use exactly as directed (do not increase dose or frequency or discontinue without consulting prescriber); may cause physical and/or psychological dependence. While using this medication, do not use alcohol or other prescription or OTC medications (especially, pain medications, sedatives, antihistamines, or hypnotics) without consulting prescriber. Maintain adequate hydration (2-3 L/day of fluids unless instructed to restrict fluid intake). You may experience drowsiness, dizziness, or blurred vision (use caution when driving or engaging in tasks requiring alertness until response to drug is known); or nausea, vomiting, unpleasant taste (small frequent meals, good mouth care, chewing gum, or sucking lozenges may help). Report rash or skin irritation, CNS changes (confusion, depression, increased sedation, excitation, headache, abnormal thinking, insomnia, or nightmares), muscle pain or weakness, difficulty breathing, chest pain or palpitations, yellow skin or change in color of urine or stool, or ineffectiveness of medication. **Pregnancy/breast-feeding precautions:** Inform prescriber if you are or intend to be pregnant. Breast-feeding is not recommended.

**Geriatric Considerations:** This medication should be avoided in the elderly. The addiction potential, withdrawal problems, and side effect profile is undesirable for use in the elderly. Also, many elderly have creatinine clearances <50 mL/minute. Less problematic agents are available for sleep induction. If used, use lowest effective dose for not more than 7 days.

**Related Information**

Antipsychotic Medication Guidelines *on page 1436*

## Ethinyl Estradiol (ETH in il es tra DYE ole)

**U.S. Brand Names** Estinyl®

**Therapeutic Category** Estrogen Derivative

**Pregnancy Risk Factor** X

**Lactation** Enters breast milk/use caution - see Breast-feeding Issues (AAP rates "compatible")

**Use** Hypogonadism; primary ovarian failure; vasomotor symptoms of menopause; prostatic carcinoma; breast cancer

**Mechanism of Action/Effect** Increases the synthesis of DNA, RNA, and various proteins in target tissues; reduces the release of gonadotropin-releasing hormone from the hypothalamus; reduces FSH and LH release from the pituitary

**Contraindications** Hypersensitivity to ethinyl estradiol or any component; thrombophlebitis; undiagnosed vaginal bleeding; known or suspected pregnancy; carcinoma of the breast; estrogen-dependent tumor

**Warnings** Use with caution in patients with asthma, seizure disorders, migraine, cardiac, renal or hepatic impairment, cerebrovascular disorders or history of breast cancer, past or present thromboembolic disease, and smokers >35 years of age.

**Drug Interactions**

**Cytochrome P-450 Effect:** CYP3A3/4 and 3A5-7 enzyme substrate; CYP1A2 enzyme inhibitor

**Decreased Effect:** Rifampin decreases estrogen serum concentrations.

**Increased Effect/Toxicity:** Hydrocortisone taken with estrogen may cause corticosteroid induced toxicity. Increased potential for thromboembolic events with anticoagulants. Estrogens may increase the effect of carbamazepine, tricyclic antidepressants, and corticosteroids. Increased thromboembolic potential when estrogens are taken with oral anticoagulants.

**Effects on Lab Values** ↑ prothrombin and factors VII, VIII, IX, X; ↑ platelet aggregability, thyroid binding globulin, total thyroid hormone ($T_4$), serum triglycerides/phospholipids; ↓ antithrombin III, serum folate concentration

**Adverse Reactions**

>10%:

Cardiovascular: Peripheral edema
Endocrine & metabolic: Enlargement of breasts (female and male), breast tenderness
Gastrointestinal: Nausea, anorexia, bloating

1% to 10%:

Central nervous system: Headache, migraine headache
Endocrine & metabolic: Increased libido (female), decreased libido (male)
Gastrointestinal: Vomiting, diarrhea

<1% (Limited to important or life-threatening symptoms): Hypertension, thromboembolism, myocardial infarction, edema, amenorrhea, alterations in frequency and flow of menses, breast tumors, decreased glucose tolerance, increased triglycerides and LDL, hepatitis, increased susceptibility to *Candida* infection

**Overdose/Toxicology** Symptoms of overdose include fluid retention, jaundice, thrombophlebitis, and nausea. Toxicity is unlikely following single exposure of excessive doses. Treatment should be supportive and symptomatic.

**Pharmacodynamics/Kinetics**

**Protein Binding:** 50% to 80%

**Metabolism:** Inactivated by liver

**Excretion:** Urine

**Formulations** Tablet: 0.02 mg, 0.05 mg, 0.5 mg

**Dosing**

**Adults:** Oral:

Male: Prostatic cancer (inoperable, progressing): 0.15-2 mg/day for palliation
Female:

Hypogonadism: 0.05 mg 1-3 times/day for 2 weeks of a theoretical menstrual cycle followed by progesterone for 3-6 months
Vasomotor symptoms: 0.02-0.05 mg for 21 days, off 7 days and repeat
Breast cancer (inoperable, progressing): 1 mg 3 times/day for palliation

**Elderly:** Refer to adult dosing.

**Hepatic Impairment:**

Mild to moderate liver impairment: Dosage reduction of estrogens is recommended.
Severe liver impairment: **Not recommended.**

**Administration**

**Oral:** Give at bedtime to minimize occurrence of adverse effects.

**Additional Nursing Issues**

**Physical Assessment:** Assess effectiveness/interactions with other medications patient may be taking (see Drug Interactions). Monitor closely for adverse reactions (eg, CNS changes, hypertension, thromboembolism), fluid retention (eg, edema, CHF, respiratory changes). Monitor therapeutic response (dependent on rationale for use). Assess knowledge/teach adverse signs to report. **Pregnancy risk factor X** - determine that patient is not pregnant before beginning treatment and do not give to women of childbearing age unless both male and female are capable of complying with barrier contraceptive measures during therapy and for 1 month following therapy. Note breast-feeding caution.

**Patient Information/Instruction:** Take according to recommended schedule. It is important to maintain schedule of drug days and drug-free days. Periodic gynecologic exam and breast exams for females are important. You may experience nausea or vomiting (small frequent meals may help); dizziness or mental depression (use caution when driving); rash; loss of scalp hair; enlargement/tenderness of breasts; or increased/decreased libido. Report significant swelling in extremities, sudden acute pain in legs or calves, chest, or abdomen; shortness of breath; severe headache or vomiting; weakness or numbness of arms or legs; or unusual vaginal bleeding. **Pregnancy/breast-feeding precautions:** Inform prescriber if you are pregnant. Do not get pregnant during or for 1 month following therapy. Male/female: Consult prescriber for instruction on appropriate barrier contraceptive measures. This drug may cause severe fetal defects. Consult prescriber if breast-feeding.

**Geriatric Considerations:** Before prescribing estrogen therapy to postmenopausal women, the risks and benefits must be weighed for each patient. Data in women 80 years and older is minimal and it is unclear if the reduced risk is applicable to women in this age group. Women should be informed of these risks and benefits, as well as possible side effects and the return of menstrual bleeding (when cycled with a progestin), and be involved in the decision to prescribe. Oral therapy may be more convenient for vaginal atrophy and urinary incontinence.

(Continued)

## Ethinyl Estradiol *(Continued)*

**Breast-feeding Issues:** Estrogens have been shown to decrease milk production. The AAP considers ethinyl estradiol compatible with breast-feeding and to monitor the growth of the infant closely.

- **Ethinyl Estradiol and Ethynodiol Diacetate** *see* Oral Contraceptives *on page 859*
- **Ethinyl Estradiol and Levonorgestrel** *see* Oral Contraceptives *on page 859*
- **Ethinyl Estradiol and Norethindrone** *see* Oral Contraceptives *on page 859*
- **Ethinyl Estradiol and Norgestrel** *see* Oral Contraceptives *on page 859*
- **Ethiofos** *see* Amifostine *on page 64*

## Ethionamide (e thye on AM ide)

**U.S. Brand Names** Trecator®-SC

**Therapeutic Category** Antitubercular Agent

**Pregnancy Risk Factor** C

**Lactation** Excretion in breast milk unknown

**Use** Treatment of tuberculosis and other mycobacterial diseases, in conjunction with other antituberculosis agents, when first-line agents have failed or resistance has been demonstrated

**Mechanism of Action/Effect** Inhibits peptide synthesis

**Contraindications** Hypersensitivity to ethionamide or any component; severe hepatic impairment

**Warnings** Use with caution in patients receiving cycloserine or isoniazid and with diabetics. Pregnancy factor C.

**Effects on Lab Values** ↓ thyroxine (S)

**Adverse Reactions**

>10%: Gastrointestinal: Anorexia, nausea, vomiting

1% to 10%:

Cardiovascular: Postural hypotension
Central nervous system: Psychiatric disturbances
Gastrointestinal: Metallic taste
Hepatic: Hepatitis, jaundice
Neuromuscular & skeletal: Peripheral neuritis

<1% (Limited to important or life-threatening symptoms): Seizures, rash, hypothyroidism or goiter, hypoglycemia, gynecomastia, thrombocytopenia, optic neuritis

**Overdose/Toxicology** Symptoms of overdose include peripheral neuropathy, anorexia, and joint pain. Treatment is supportive. Pyridoxine may be given to prevent peripheral neuropathy.

**Pharmacodynamics/Kinetics**

**Protein Binding:** 10%
**Distribution:** Crosses the placenta
**Half-life Elimination:** 2-3 hours
**Time to Peak:** Oral: Within 3 hours
**Metabolism:** Hepatic
**Excretion:** Urine

**Formulations** Tablet, sugar coated: 250 mg

**Dosing**

**Adults:** Oral: 500-1000 mg/day in 1-3 divided doses
**Elderly:** Refer to adult dosing.
**Renal Impairment:** $Cl_{cr}$ <50 mL/minute: Administer 50% of dose.

**Administration**

**Oral:** Neurotoxic effects may be relieved by the administration of pyridoxine (6-100 mg daily, lower doses are more common).

**Monitoring Laboratory Tests** Initial and periodic serum ALT and AST

**Additional Nursing Issues**

**Physical Assessment:** Monitor for adverse reactions. Note dosing recommendations above and monitor patient adherence to dosing regimen. Monitor for adverse reactions, especially neurotoxic, hepatic, and CNS alterations (see Adverse Reactions). Instruct patient on appropriate use, possible side effects, and symptoms to report. **Pregnancy risk factor C** - benefits of use should outweigh possible risks. Note breast-feeding caution.

**Patient Information/Instruction:** Take this medication as prescribed; avoid missing doses and do not discontinue without contacting prescriber. You will need to schedule regular medical checkups which will include blood tests. You may experience GI upset (small frequent meals may help), metallic taste and increased salivation (lozenges, frequent mouth care), dizziness, blurred vision (use caution when driving or engaging in tasks that require alertness until response to drug is known), postural hypotension (change position slowly), impotence and/or menstrual difficulties (these will go away when drug is discontinued). Report acute unresolved GI upset, changes in vision, numbness or pain in extremities, or unusual bleeding or bruising. **Pregnancy/breast-feeding precautions:** Inform prescriber if you are or intend to be pregnant. Consult prescriber if breast-feeding.

**Dietary Issues:** Prescriber may recommend an increase in dietary intake of pyridoxine to prevent neurotoxic effects of ethionamide.

**Geriatric Considerations:** Since many elderly have $Cl_{cr}$ <50 mL/minute, adjust dose for renal function.

**Related Information**

TB Drug Comparison *on page 1402*

♦ **Ethmozine®** *see* Moricizine *on page 788*

## Ethosuximide (eth oh SUKS i mide)

**U.S. Brand Names** Zarontin®

**Therapeutic Category** Anticonvulsant, Succinimide

**Pregnancy Risk Factor** C

**Lactation** Enters breast milk/compatible

**Use** Management of absence (petit mal) seizures, myoclonic seizures, and akinetic epilepsy; considered to be drug of choice for simple absence seizures

**Mechanism of Action/Effect** Increases the seizure threshold and suppresses paroxysmal spike-and-wave pattern in absence seizures; depresses nerve transmission in the motor cortex

**Contraindications** Hypersensitivity to ethosuximide or any component

**Warnings** Use with caution in patients with hepatic or renal disease. Abrupt withdrawal of the drug may precipitate absence status. Ethosuximide may increase tonic-clonic seizures in patients with mixed seizure disorders. Ethosuximide must be used in combination with other anticonvulsants in patients with both absence and tonic-clonic seizures. Pregnancy factor C.

**Drug Interactions**

**Cytochrome P-450 Effect:** CYP3A3/4 enzyme substrate; CYP3A3/4 enzyme inducer

**Decreased Effect:** Phenytoin, carbamazepine, primidone, and phenobarbital may increase the hepatic metabolism and decrease the effectiveness of ethosuximide.

**Increased Effect/Toxicity:** Isoniazid may inhibit hepatic metabolism with a resultant increase in ethosuximide serum concentrations.

**Effects on Lab Values** ↑ alkaline phosphatase (S); positive Coombs' [direct]; ↓ calcium (S)

**Adverse Reactions**

>10%:

- Central nervous system: Ataxia, drowsiness, sedation, dizziness, lethargy, euphoria, hallucinations, insomnia, agitation, behavioral changes, headache
- Dermatologic: Stevens-Johnson syndrome
- Gastrointestinal: Weight loss
- Gastrointestinal: Nausea, vomiting, anorexia, abdominal pain
- Miscellaneous: Hiccups, SLE syndrome

1% to 10%:

- Central nervous system: Aggressiveness, mental depression, nightmares
- Neuromuscular & skeletal: Weakness
- Central nervous system: Paranoid psychosis
- Dermatologic: Exfoliative dermatitis
- Hematologic: Leukopenia, aplastic anemia, thrombocytopenia, agranulocytosis, pancytopenia

**Overdose/Toxicology** Acute overdose can cause CNS depression, ataxia, stupor, coma, hypotension. Chronic overdose can cause skin rash, confusion, ataxia, proteinuria, hepatic dysfunction, and hematuria. Treatment is supportive. Hemoperfusion and hemodialysis may be useful.

**Pharmacodynamics/Kinetics**

**Half-life Elimination:** 50-60 hours

**Time to Peak:** Capsule: Within 2-4 hours; Syrup: <2-4 hours

**Metabolism:** Liver

**Excretion:** Urine

**Formulations**

Capsule: 250 mg

Syrup (raspberry flavor): 250 mg/5 mL (473 mL)

**Dosing**

**Adults:** Oral: Initial: 250 mg twice daily; increase by 250 mg as needed every 4-7 days up to 1.5 g/day in 2 divided doses; usual maintenance dose: 20-40 mg/kg/day in 2 divided doses

**Elderly:** Refer to adult dosing.

**Renal Impairment:** Use with caution.

**Hepatic Impairment:** Use with caution.

**Monitoring Laboratory Tests** Trough serum concentrations, CBC, platelets, liver enzymes, urinalysis

**Additional Nursing Issues**

**Physical Assessment:** Assess effectiveness and interactions of other medications patient may be taking (see Contraindications, Warnings/Precautions, and Drug Interactions). Monitor for therapeutic response (seizure activity, force, type, duration), laboratory values, and adverse reactions (see Adverse Reactions) at beginning of therapy and periodically with long-term use. Observe and teach seizure/safety precautions. Taper dosage slowly when discontinuing. Assess knowledge/teach patient appropriate use, interventions to reduce side effects, and adverse symptoms to report. **Pregnancy risk factor C** - benefits of use should outweigh possible risks.

**Patient Information/Instruction:** Take exactly as directed (do not increase dose or frequency or discontinue without consulting prescriber). While using this medication, do not use alcohol and other prescription or OTC medications (especially pain medications, sedatives, antihistamines, or hypnotics) without consulting prescriber. Maintain adequate hydration (2-3 L/day of fluids unless instructed to restrict fluid intake). You may experience drowsiness, dizziness, or blurred vision (use caution when driving or engaging in tasks requiring alertness until response to drug is known); nausea, vomiting, loss of appetite, or dry mouth (small frequent meals, frequent mouth care,

(Continued)

## Ethosuximide *(Continued)*

chewing gum, or sucking lozenges may help); constipation (increased exercise, fluids, or dietary fruit and fiber may help). Wear identification of epileptic status and medications. Report CNS changes, mentation changes, or changes in cognition; muscle cramping, weakness, tremors, or changes in gait; persistent GI symptoms (cramping, constipation, vomiting, anorexia); rash or skin irritations; unusual bruising or bleeding (mouth, urine, stool); worsening of seizure activity, or loss of seizure control. **Pregnancy precautions:** Inform prescriber if you are or intend to be pregnant.

**Geriatric Considerations:** No specific studies with the use of this medication in the elderly. Consider renal function and proceed slowly with dosing increases; monitor closely.

**Related Information**

Peak and Trough Guidelines *on page 1331*

- **Ethoxynaphthamido Penicillin Sodium** *see* Nafcillin *on page 800*
- **Ethyl Aminobenzoate** *see* Benzocaine *on page 141*
- **Ethynodiol Diacetate and Ethinyl Estradiol** *see* Oral Contraceptives *on page 859*
- **Ethyol®** *see* Amifostine *on page 64*
- **Etibi®** *see* Ethambutol *on page 456*

## Etodolac (ee toe DOE lak)

**U.S. Brand Names** Lodine®; Lodine® XL

**Synonyms** Etodolic Acid

**Therapeutic Category** Nonsteroidal Anti-Inflammatory Agent (NSAID)

**Pregnancy Risk Factor** C

**Lactation** Excretion in breast milk unknown/contraindicated

**Use** Acute and long-term use in the management of signs or symptoms of osteoarthritis, rheumatoid arthritis, and management of pain

**Mechanism of Action/Effect** Inhibits prostaglandin synthesis which results in decreased formation of prostaglandin precursors

**Contraindications** Hypersensitivity to etodolac, aspirin, or other NSAIDs; active gastric ulcers/inflammation

**Warnings** Use with caution in patients with congestive heart failure, hypertension, decreased renal or hepatic function, history of GI disease, or those receiving anticoagulants. Pregnancy factor C.

**Drug Interactions**

**Decreased Effect:** Decreased effect with aspirin. May reduce effect of some diuretics and antihypertensive effect of β-blockers.

**Increased Effect/Toxicity:** Etodolac may increase effect/toxicity of aspirin (GI irritation), lithium, methotrexate, digoxin, cyclosporin (nephrotoxicity), and warfarin (bleeding). See Geriatric Considerations.

**Food Interactions** Etodolac peak serum levels may be decreased if taken with food.

**Effects on Lab Values** False-positive for urinary bilirubin and ketone increase bleeding time. Etodolac may cause a lowering of serum uric acid levels.

**Adverse Reactions**

1% to 10%:

Central nervous system: Headache, nervousness

Dermatologic: Itching, rash

Endocrine & metabolic: Fluid retention

Gastrointestinal: Abdominal cramps, heartburn, indigestion, nausea, vomiting, gastritis, GI hemorrhage, GI ulceration

Otic: Tinnitus

<1% (Limited to important or life-threatening symptoms): Congestive heart failure, hypertension, arrhythmia, tachycardia, syncope, urticaria, erythema multiforme, toxic epidermal necrolysis, Stevens-Johnson syndrome, angioedema, exfoliative dermatitis, agranulocytosis, anemia, hemolytic anemia, bone marrow suppression, leukopenia, thrombocytopenia, hepatitis, peripheral neuropathy, toxic amblyopia, acute renal failure, shortness of breath

**Overdose/Toxicology** Symptoms of overdose include acute renal failure, vomiting, drowsiness, leukocytosis. Management of nonsteroidal anti-inflammatory (NSAID) intoxication is supportive and symptomatic.

**Pharmacodynamics/Kinetics**

**Protein Binding:** High

**Half-life Elimination:** 7 hours

**Time to Peak:** 1 hour

**Metabolism:** Liver

**Excretion:** Urine

**Onset:** 2-4 hours (analgesia)

**Duration:** A few days (anti-inflammatory)

**Formulations**

Capsule: 200 mg, 300 mg

Tablet: 400 mg, 500 mg

Tablet, extended release: 400 mg, 600 mg

**Dosing**

**Adults:** Single dose of 76-100 mg is comparable to the analgesic effect of aspirin 650 mg. In patients ≥65 years, no substantial differences in the pharmacokinetics or side-effects profile were seen compared with the general population.

Oral:

Acute pain: 200-400 mg every 6-8 hours, as needed, not to exceed total daily doses of 1200 mg; for patients weighing <60 kg, total daily dose should not exceed 20 mg/kg/day.

Osteoarthritis and Rheumatoid Arthritis: Initial: 800-1200 mg/day given in divided doses: 400 mg 2 or 3 times/day; 300 mg 2, 3 or 4 times/day; 200 mg 3 or 4 times/day; total daily dose should not exceed 1200 mg; for patients weighing <60 kg, total daily dose should not exceed 20 mg/kg/day.

**Elderly:** Refer to adult dosing.

**Stability**

**Storage:** Protect from moisture.

**Monitoring Laboratory Tests** CBC, liver enzymes; in patients receiving diuretics, monitor BUN/serum creatinine.

**Additional Nursing Issues**

**Physical Assessment:** Systemic: Assess effectiveness and interactions of other medications patient may be taking (see Contraindications, Warnings/Precautions, and Drug Interactions). Monitor laboratory tests (see above) and therapeutic response (eg, relief of pain and inflammation, activity tolerance), and adverse reactions (eg, gastrointestinal effects or ototoxicity) at beginning of therapy and periodically throughout therapy (see Warnings/Precautions, Adverse Reactions, and Overdose/Toxicology). Assess knowledge/teach patient appropriate use, interventions to reduce side effects, and adverse symptoms to report. **Pregnancy risk factor C** - benefits of use should outweigh possible risks. Breast-feeding is contraindicated.

**Patient Information/Instruction:** Take this medication exactly as directed; do not increase dose without consulting prescriber. Do not crush tablets or break capsules. Take with food or milk to reduce GI distress. Maintain adequate fluid intake (2-3 L/day of fluids unless instructed to restrict fluid intake). Do not use alcohol, aspirin, or aspirin-containing medication, and all other anti-inflammatory medications without consulting prescriber. You may experience anorexia, nausea, vomiting, or heartburn (frequent small meals, frequent mouth care, sucking lozenges, or chewing gum may help); drowsiness, dizziness, nervousness, or headache (use caution when driving or engaging in tasks requiring alertness until response to drug is known); fluid retention (weigh yourself weekly and report unusual (3-5 lb/week) weight gain). GI bleeding, ulceration, or perforation can occur with or without pain; discontinue medication and contact prescriber if persistent abdominal pain or cramping, or blood in stool occurs. Report breathlessness, difficulty breathing, or unusual cough; chest pain, rapid heartbeat, palpitations; unusual bruising/bleeding; blood in urine, stool, mouth, or vomitus; swollen extremities; skin rash or itching; acute fatigue; or changes in hearing or ringing in ears. **Pregnancy/breast-feeding precautions:** Inform prescriber if you are or intend to be pregnant. Do not breast-feed.

**Geriatric Considerations:** Elderly are at high risk for adverse effects from nonsteroidal anti-inflammatory agents. As much as 60% of elderly who experience GI side effects can develop peptic ulceration and/or hemorrhage asymptomatically.

**Related Information**

Nonsalicylate/Nonsteroidal Anti-inflammatory Comparison *on page 1401*

- **Etodolic Acid** *see* Etodolac *on previous page*
- **Etopophos®** *see* Etoposide Phosphate *on page 466*
- **Etopophos® Injection** *see* Etoposide *on this page*
- **Etopos** *see* Etoposide *on this page*
- **Etopos** *see* Etoposide Phosphate *on page 466*

## Etoposide (e toe POE side)

**U.S. Brand Names** Etopophos® Injection; Toposar® Injection; VePesid® Injection; VePesid® Oral

**Synonyms** EPEG; VP-16

**Therapeutic Category** Antineoplastic Agent, Natural Source (Plant) Derivative

**Pregnancy Risk Factor** D

**Lactation** Enters breast milk/contraindicated

**Use** Treatment of lymphomas, ANLL, lung, testicular, bladder, and prostate carcinoma, hepatoma, rhabdomyosarcoma, uterine carcinoma, neuroblastoma, mycosis fungoides, Kaposi's sarcoma, histiocytosis, gestational trophoblastic disease, Ewing's sarcoma, Wilms' tumor, and brain tumors

**Mechanism of Action/Effect** Inhibits DNA synthesis leading to cell death.

**Contraindications** Hypersensitivity to etoposide or any component; **intrathecal administration**; pregnancy

**Warnings** The U.S. Food and Drug Administration (FDA) currently recommends that procedures for proper handling and disposal of antineoplastic agents be considered. Severe myelosuppression with resulting infection or bleeding may occur. Administer I.V. infusions over a period of at least 30-60 minutes. **Must be diluted - do not give IVP.** Dosage should be adjusted in patients with hepatic or renal impairment.

Etoposide preparation should be performed in a Class II laminar flow biologic safety cabinet. Personnel should be wearing surgical gloves and a closed front surgical gown with knit cuffs. Appropriate safety equipment is recommended for preparation, administration, and disposal of antineoplastics. If etoposide contacts the skin, wash and flush thoroughly with water.

(Continued)

## Etoposide *(Continued)*

**Drug Interactions**

**Cytochrome P-450 Effect:** CYP3A3/4 enzyme substrate

**Increased Effect/Toxicity:**

Cyclosporine: Additive cytotoxic effects on tumor cells and decreased clearance of etoposide.

Methotrexate: Alteration of MTX transport has been found as a slow efflux of MTX and its polyglutamated form out of the cell, leading to intracellular accumulation of MTX.

Calcium antagonists: Increase the rate of VP-16-induced DNA damage and cytotoxicity *in vitro*.

Carmustine: Reports of frequent hepatic dysfunction with hyperbilirubinemia, ascites, and thrombocytopenia.

Warfarin: May increase prothrombin time with concurrent use.

**Adverse Reactions**

>10%:

Dermatologic: Alopecia (reversible)

Gastrointestinal: Occasional diarrhea and infrequent nausea and vomiting at standard doses; severe mucositis occurs with high (BMT) doses, anorexia

Emetic potential: Moderately low (10% to 30%)

Hematologic: Anemia, leukopenia; Myelosuppressive: Principal dose-limiting toxicity of VP-16. White blood cell count nadir is 5-15 days after administration and is more frequent than thrombocytopenia. Recovery is usually within 24-28 days and cumulative toxicity has not been noted with VP-16 as a single agent. No difference in toxicity is seen when VP-16 is administered over a 24-hour period or over 2 hours on 5 consecutive days.

WBC: Mild to severe

Platelets: Mild

Onset (days): 10

Nadir (days): granulocytes 7-14 days; platelets 9-16 days

Recovery (days): 21-28

1% to 10%:

Cardiovascular: Hypotension: Related to drug infusion time; may be related to vehicle used in the I.V. preparation (polysorbate 80 plus polyethylene glycol). Best to administer the drug over 1 hour.

Central nervous system: Unusual fatigue

Gastrointestinal: Stomatitis, diarrhea, abdominal pain, hepatitic dysfunction

<1% (Limited to important or life-threatening symptoms): Tachycardia, neurotoxicity, toxic hepatitis (with high-dose therapy), reports of flushing or bronchospasm which did not recur in one report if patients were pretreated with corticosteroids and antihistamines, peripheral neuropathy

**Irritant chemotherapy**, thrombophlebitis has been reported

**BMT:**

Cardiovascular: Hypotension (infusion-related)

Dermatologic: Skin lesions resembling Stevens-Johnson syndrome, alopecia

Endocrine & metabolic: Metabolic acidosis

Gastrointestinal: Severe nausea and vomiting, mucositis

Hepatic: Hepatitis

Miscellaneous: Secondary malignancy, ethanol intoxication

**Overdose/Toxicology** Symptoms of overdose include bone marrow suppression, leukopenia, thrombocytopenia, nausea, and vomiting. Treatment is supportive.

**Pharmacodynamics/Kinetics**

**Protein Binding:** 94% to 97%

**Distribution:** Poor penetration across blood-brain barrier, with concentrations in the CSF being <10% that of plasma

**Half-life Elimination:** Terminal: 4-15 hours

**Time to Peak:** Oral: 1-1.5 hours

**Metabolism:** Liver

**Excretion:** Urine and feces

**Formulations**

Capsule: 50 mg

Injection: 20 mg/mL (5 mL, 10 mL, 25 mL)

Powder for injection, lyophilized, as phosphate: 119.3 mg (100 mg base)

**Dosing**

**Adults:** Refer to individual protocols.

Oral: Twice the I.V. dose rounded to the nearest 50 mg given once daily if total dose ≤400 mg or in divided doses if >400 mg

Small cell lung cancer:

I.V.: 35 mg/m²/day for 4 days or 50 mg/m²/day for 5 days every 3-4 weeks total dose ≤400 mg/day or in divided doses if >400 mg/day

IVPB: 200-250 mg/m² repeated every 7 weeks

Continuous intravenous infusion: 500 mg/m² over 24 hours every 3 weeks

Testicular cancer:

IVPB: 50-100 mg/m²/day for 5 days repeated every 3-4 weeks

I.V.: 100 mg/m² every other day for 3 doses repeated every 3-4 weeks

BMT/relapsed leukemia: I.V.: 2.4-3.5 g/m² or 25-70 mg/kg administered over 4-36 hours

BMT high dose: I.V.: 750-2400 mg/m²; 10-60 mg/kg; duration of infusion is 1-4 hours to 24 hours; generally combined with other high-dose chemotherapeutic drugs or total body irradiation (TBI).

**Elderly:** Refer to adult dosing.

**Renal Impairment:**

$Cl_{cr}$ 10-50 mL/minute: Administer 75% of normal dose.
$Cl_{cr}$ <10 mL minute: Administer 50% of normal dose.
Hemodialysis effects: Supplemental dose is not necessary.
CAPD effects: Unknown
CAVH effects: Unknown

**Hepatic Impairment:**

Bilirubin 1.5-3 mg/dL or AST 60-180 units: Reduce dose by 50%.
Bilirubin >3 mg/dL or AST >180 units: Reduce by 75%.

**Administration**

**I.M.:** Do not administer I.V. or S.C. (severe tissue necrosis).

**I.V.:** Irritant. Administer lower doses IVPB over at least 30 minutes to minimize the risk of hypotensive reactions.

**I.V. Detail:** Administer high doses (>1 g/dose) via the 2-channel pump method. An in-line 0.22 micron filter should be attached to **all** etoposide infusions due to the high potential for precipitation.

**Extravasation management:** Inject 150-900 units of hyaluronidase S.C. clockwise into the infiltrated area using a 25-gauge needle. Change the needle with each injection. Apply heat immediately for 1 hour, repeat 4 times/day for 3-5 days. **Application of cold or hydrocortisone is contraindicated.**

If necessary, the injection may be used for oral administration. Mix with orange juice, apple juice, or lemonade to a concentration of 0.4 mg/mL or less, and use within a 3-hour period.

**BMT only:** The etoposide formulation contains ethanol 30.3% (v/v). Etoposide 2.4 mg/$m^2$ delivers ethanol 45 g/$m^2$ I.V. Adverse effects may be increased with administration of etoposide to patients with decreased creatinine clearance.

**Stability**

**Storage:** Store intact vials of injection at room temperature and protected from light. Injection solution contains polyethylene glycol vehicle with absolute alcohol. Store oral capsules under refrigeration. Capsules are stable for 3 months at room temperature.

**Reconstitution:** VP-16 should be further diluted in $D_5W$ or NS for administration. Diluted solutions have concentration-dependent stability: More concentrated solutions have shorter stability times.

At room temperature in $D_5W$ or NS in polyvinyl chloride, the concentration is stable as follows:

0.2 mg/mL: 96 hours
0.4 mg/mL: 48 hours
0.6 mg/mL: 8 hours
1 mg/mL: 2 hours
2 mg/mL: 1 hour
20 mg/mL (undiluted): 24 hours

**Standard I.V. dilution:**

**Lower dose regimens (<1 g/dose):**

Doses may be diluted in 100-1000 mL of $D_5W$ or NS

If the concentration is less than or equal to 0.6 mg/mL, the bag should be mixed with the appropriate expiration dating.

If the concentration is >0.6 mg/mL, the concentration is highly unstable and a syringe of undiluted etoposide accompanied with the appropriate volume of diluent will be sent to the nursing unit to be mixed at the bedside just prior to administration.

**High-dose regimens (>1g/dose):**

Total dose should be drawn into an empty Viaflex® container and the appropriate amount of diluent (for a final concentration of 1 mg/mL) will be sent.

Use the **2-Channel Pump Method**: Instill all of the etoposide dose into one Viaflex® container (concentration = 20 mg/mL). Infuse this into one channel (Baxter Flow-Guard 6300 Dual Channel Volumetric Infusion Pump - or any 2-channel infusion pump that does not require a "hard" plastic cassette). Infuse the indicated diluent (ie, $D_5W$ or NS) at a rate of at least 20 times the infusion rate of the etoposide to simulate a 1 mg/mL concentration in the line. The etoposide should be Y-sited into the port most proximal to the patient. A 0.22 micron filter should be attached to the line after the Y-site and before entry into the patient.

**Compatibility:** Y-site compatible with carboplatin, cytarabine, mesna, and daunorubicin. See the Chemotherapy Compatibility Chart *on page 1311.*

**Monitoring Laboratory Tests** CBC with differential, platelet count, bilirubin, renal function

**Additional Nursing Issues**

**Physical Assessment:** Monitor appropriate laboratory tests as ordered prior to each dose. Closely monitor infusion site for extravasation . Monitor BP during infusions. Monitor for adverse effects as noted above, especially peripheral neuropathy, I & O ratio, edema, or respiratory changes. Assess frequently for development of opportunistic infection (see Warnings/Precautions above for avoiding skin contact). **Pregnancy risk factor D** - assess knowledge/teach appropriate use of barrier contraceptives. Advise patient (male/female) on the need for barrier contraceptive measures during and for several weeks following treatment. Breast-feeding is contraindicated.

(Continued)

## Etoposide *(Continued)*

**Patient Information/Instruction:** During therapy, do not use alcohol, aspirin-containing products, and OTC medications without consulting prescriber. It is important to maintain adequate nutrition and hydration (2-3 L/day of fluids unless instructed to restrict fluid intake) during therapy; frequent small meals may help. You may experience mild nausea or vomiting (frequent small meals, frequent mouth care, sucking lozenges, or chewing gum may help). You may experience loss of hair (reversible); you will be more susceptible to infection (avoid crowds and exposure to infection as much as possible). Yogurt or buttermilk may help reduce diarrhea. Frequent mouth care and use of a soft toothbrush or cotton swabs may help prevent mouth sores. This drug may cause sterility or birth defects. Report extreme fatigue, pain or numbness in extremities, severe GI upset or diarrhea, bleeding or bruising, fever, chills, sore throat, vaginal discharge, difficulty breathing, yellowing of eyes or skin, and any changes in color of urine or stool. **Pregnancy/breast-feeding precautions:** Do not get pregnant while taking this medication; use appropriate barrier contraceptive measures. Do not breast-feed while taking this medication and for several weeks after last dose.

**Additional Information** Some formulations may contain benzyl alcohol.

## Etoposide Phosphate (e toe POE side FOS fate)

**U.S. Brand Names** Etopophos®

**Therapeutic Category** Antineoplastic Agent, Irritant; Antineoplastic Agent, Podophyllotoxin Derivative; Vesicant

**Pregnancy Risk Factor** D

**Lactation** Enters breast milk/contraindicated

**Use** Treatment of refractory testicular tumors and small cell lung cancer

**Mechanism of Action/Effect** Etoposide phosphate is converted *in vivo* to the active moiety, etoposide, by dephosphorylation. Etoposide inhibits mitotic activity; inhibits cells from entering prophase; inhibits DNA synthesis. Initially thought to be mitotic inhibitors similar to podophyllotoxin, but actually have no effect on microtubule assembly. However, later shown to induce DNA strand breakage and inhibition of topoisomerase II (an enzyme which breaks and repairs DNA); etoposide acts in late S or early G2 phases.

**Contraindications** Hypersensitivity to etoposide, etoposide phosphate, or any component; **I.T. administration is contraindicated**; pregnancy

**Warnings** The U.S. Food and Drug Administration (FDA) currently recommends that procedures for proper handling and disposal of antineoplastic agents be considered. Severe myelosuppression with resulting infection or bleeding may occur. Dosage should be adjusted in patients with hepatic or renal impairment.

Etoposide phosphate preparation should be performed in a Class II laminar flow biologic safety cabinet. Personnel should be wearing surgical gloves and a closed front surgical gown with knit cuffs. Appropriate safety equipment is recommended for preparation, administration, and disposal of antineoplastics. If etoposide phosphate contacts the skin, wash and flush thoroughly with water.

**Drug Interactions**

**Increased Effect/Toxicity:** Etoposide taken with warfarin may result in prolongation of bleeding times. Alteration of MTX transport has been found as a slow efflux of MTX and its polyglutamated form out of the cell, leading to intercellular accumulation of MTX. Calcium antagonists increase the rate of VP-16-induced DNA damage and cytotoxicity *in vitro*. Use with carmustine has shown reports of frequent hepatic dysfunction with hyperbilirubinemia, ascites, and thrombocytopenia. Cyclosporine may cause additive cytotoxic effects on tumor cells.

**Adverse Reactions**

>10%:

Dermatologic: Alopecia (reversible)

Gastrointestinal: Occasional diarrhea and infrequent nausea and vomiting at standard doses; severe mucositis occurs with high (BMT) doses, anorexia

Emetic potential: Moderately low (10% to 30%)

Hematologic: Myelosuppressive: Principal dose-limiting toxicity of VP-16. White blood cell count nadir is 5-15 days after administration and is more frequent than thrombocytopenia. Recovery is usually within 24-28 days and cumulative toxicity has not been noted with VP-16 as a single agent. No difference in toxicity is seen when VP-16 is administered over a 24-hour period or over 2 hours on 5 consecutive days.

WBC: Mild to severe

Platelets: Mild

Onset (days): 10

Nadir (days): granulocytes 7-14 days; platelets 9-16 days

Recovery (days): 21-28

1% to 10%:

Cardiovascular: Hypotension: Related to drug infusion time; may be related to vehicle used in the I.V. preparation (polysorbate 80 plus polyethylene glycol). Best to administer the drug over 1 hour.

Central nervous system: Unusual fatigue

Gastrointestinal: Stomatitis, abdominal pain, hepatitic dysfunction

<1% (Limited to important or life-threatening symptoms): Tachycardia, neurotoxicity, fever, toxic hepatitis (with high-dose therapy), reports of flushing or bronchospasm which did not recur in one report if patients were pretreated with corticosteroids and antihistamines, peripheral neuropathy

**BMT:** Gastrointestinal: Nausea, vomiting, mucositis

**Overdose/Toxicology** Symptoms of overdose include bone marrow suppression, leukopenia, thrombocytopenia, nausea, and vomiting. Treatment is supportive.

**Pharmacodynamics/Kinetics**

**Protein Binding:** 94% to 97%

**Distribution:** Poor penetration across blood-brain barrier, with concentrations in the CSF being <10% that of plasma

**Half-life Elimination:** 4-15 hours

**Metabolism:** Liver

**Excretion:** Urine and feces

**Formulations** Powder for injection, lyophilized: 119.3 mg (100 mg base)

**Dosing**

**Adults:** Refer to individual protocols.

Small cell lung cancer:

I.V. (in combination with other approved chemotherapeutic drugs): **Equivalent doses of etoposide phosphate to an etoposide dosage** range of 35 mg/m$^2$/day for 4 days to 50 mg/m$^2$/day for 5 days. Courses are repeated at 3- to 4-week intervals after adequate recovery from any toxicity.

Testicular cancer:

I.V. (in combination with other approved chemotherapeutic agents): **Equivalent dose of etoposide phosphate to etoposide dosage** range of 50-100 mg/m$^2$/day on days 1-5 to 100 mg/m$^2$/day on days 1, 3, and 5. Courses are repeated at 3- to 4-week intervals after adequate recovery from any toxicity.

BMT high dose: I.V.: 0.5-2 g/m$^2$ in 2 divided doses; maximum single-dose agent: 3.2 g/m$^2$; generally combined with other high-dose chemotherapeutic drugs.

**Elderly:** Refer to adult dosing.

**Renal Impairment:**

$Cl_{cr}$ 15-50 mL/minute: Administer 75% of normal dose.

$Cl_{cr}$ <15 mL minute: Data is not available and further dose reduction should be considered in these patients.

Hemodialysis: Supplemental dose is not necessary.

Peritoneal dialysis: Supplemental dose is not necessary.

CAPD effects: Unknown

CAVH effects: Unknown

**Hepatic Impairment:**

Bilirubin 1.5-3 mg/dL or AST 60-180 units: Reduce dose by 50%.

Bilirubin 3-5 mg/dL or AST >180 units: Reduce by 75%.

Bilirubin >5 mg/dL: Do not administer.

**Administration**

**I.V.:** Etoposide phosphate solutions should be administered over 30-60 minutes.

**I.V. Detail:** Hypotension may occur with rapid infusion.

**BMT only:** In contrast to etoposide, metabolic acidosis is not a frequent adverse effect of high-dose etoposide phosphate.

**Stability**

**Storage:** Store intact vials of injection under refrigeration 2°C to 8°C (36°F to 46°F). Protect from light. Store capsules in refrigerator.

**Reconstitution:** Reconstituted vials with 5 mL or 10 mL SWI, $D_5W$, NS, bacteriostatic SWI, or bacteriostatic NS to a concentration of 20 mg/mL or 10 mg/mL etoposide (22.7 mg/mL or 11.4 mg/mL etoposide phosphate), respectively. These solutions may be administered without further dilution or may be further diluted to a concentration as low as 0.1 mg/mL etoposide with either $D_5W$ or NS. Solutions are stable in glass or plastic containers at room temperature 20°C to 25°C (68°F to 77°F) or under refrigeration 2°C to 8°C (36°F to 47°F) for up to 24 hours.

**Compatibility:** See the Chemotherapy Compatibility Chart *on page 1311.*

**Monitoring Laboratory Tests** CBC with differential, platelet count, hemoglobin, bilirubin, renal function

**Additional Nursing Issues**

**Physical Assessment:** Monitor appropriate laboratory tests as ordered prior to each I.V. dose and frequently during oral therapy. Closely monitor infusion site for extravasation. Monitor blood pressure during infusions. Monitor for adverse effects as noted above, especially peripheral neuropathy, I & O ratio, edema, or respiratory changes. Assess frequently for development of opportunistic infection (see Warnings/Precautions for avoiding skin contact). **Pregnancy risk factor D** - assess knowledge/teach appropriate use of barrier contraceptives. Instruct patients (male/female) in need for barrier contraceptive measures during and for several weeks following treatment. Breast-feeding is contraindicated.

**Patient Information/Instruction:** This drug can only be administered by infusion. During therapy, do not use alcohol, aspirin-containing products, and OTC medications without consulting prescriber. It is important to maintain adequate nutrition and hydration (2-3 L/day of fluids unless instructed to restrict fluid intake) during therapy; frequent small meals may help. You may experience mild nausea or vomiting (frequent small meals, frequent mouth care, sucking lozenges, or chewing gum may help). You may experience loss of hair (reversible); you will be more susceptible to infection (avoid crowds and exposure to infection as much as possible). Yogurt or buttermilk may help reduce diarrhea. Frequent mouth care and use of a soft toothbrush or cotton swabs may help prevent mouth sores. This drug may cause sterility or birth defects. Report extreme fatigue, pain or numbness in extremities, severe GI upset or diarrhea, bleeding or bruising, fever, chills, sore throat, vaginal discharge, difficulty breathing, yellowing of eyes or skin, and any changes in color of urine or stool. **Pregnancy/breast-feeding precautions:** Do not get pregnant; use appropriate barrier contraceptive measures and avoid breast-feeding while on this drug and for several weeks after last dose. Do not breast-feed.

♦ **Etrafon®** *see* Amitriptyline and Perphenazine *on page 75*

## Etretinate (e TRET i nate)

**U.S. Brand Names** Tegison®

**Therapeutic Category** Antipsoriatic Agent

**Pregnancy Risk Factor** X

**Lactation** Excretion in breast milk unknown/contraindicated

**Use** Treatment of severe recalcitrant psoriasis in patients intolerant of or unresponsive to standard therapies

**Mechanism of Action/Effect** Unknown; related to retinoic acid and retinol (vitamin A)

**Contraindications** Hypersensitivity to etretinate; pregnancy (because of the high likelihood of long-lasting teratogenic effects, do not prescribe etretinate for women who are or who are likely to become pregnant while or after using the drug)

**Warnings** Not to be used in severe obesity or women of childbearing potential unless they are capable of complying with effective contraceptive measures. Therapy is normally begun on the second or third day of the next normal menstrual period. Effective contraception must be used for at least 1 month before beginning therapy, during therapy, and for 1 month after discontinuation of therapy. Pregnancy test must be performed prior to starting therapy.

**Drug Interactions**

**Increased Effect/Toxicity:** Milk increases absorption of etretinate. Additive toxicity with vitamin A.

**Food Interactions** Etretinate serum levels may be increased if taken with food or dairy products.

**Adverse Reactions**

>10%:

- Central nervous system: Fatigue, headache, fever
- Dermatologic: Chapped lips, alopecia
- Endocrine & metabolic: Hypercholesterolemia, hypertriglyceridemia
- Gastrointestinal: Appetite change, dry mouth, sore tongue, unusual thirst
- Neuromuscular & skeletal: Muscle cramps, bone pain, arthralgia
- Ocular: Eyelid abnormalities, increased sensitivity to contact lenses
- Respiratory: Epistaxis

1% to 10%:

- Cardiovascular: Edema
- Central nervous system: Dizziness, lethargy, fever
- Dermatologic: Redness or soreness around fingernails
- Gastrointestinal: Dryness of mouth, nausea
- Hepatic: Hepatitis
- Neuromuscular & skeletal: Myalgia
- Ocular: Blurred vision, conjunctivitis
- Otic: Otitis externa
- Respiratory: Dyspnea

<1% (Limited to important or life-threatening symptoms): Syncope

**Pharmacodynamics/Kinetics**

**Protein Binding:** 99%

**Half-life Elimination:** 4-8 days (with multiple doses)

**Metabolism:** Liver

**Excretion:** Feces

**Formulations** Capsule: 10 mg, 25 mg

**Dosing**

**Adults:** Oral: Individualized; Initial: 0.75-1 mg/kg/day in divided doses, increase by 0.25 mg/kg/day at weekly intervals up to 1.5 mg/kg/day; maintenance dose established after 8-10 weeks of therapy 0.5-0.75 mg/kg/day

**Elderly:** Refer to adult dosing.

**Monitoring Laboratory Tests** Hepatic function prior to treatment, frequently for 1-3 months, and at regular intervals during therapy (every 3-4 months)

**Additional Nursing Issues**

**Physical Assessment:** Etretinate may remain in serum as long as 2-3 years after treatment is discontinued. Monitor laboratory tests (see above) throughout therapy. Monitor for adverse effects as indicated above. Caution patients to avoid donating blood during therapy and for indefinite period following therapy. **Pregnancy risk factor X** - determine that patient is not pregnant before beginning therapy and do not give to women of childbearing age or male having intercourse with women of childbearing age unless both are capable of complying with barrier contraceptive measures for 1 month prior to, during, and for 1 month following therapy. Breast-feeding is contraindicated.

**Patient Information/Instruction:** Take with food. Do not take additional vitamin A supplements. You may experience dizziness, blurred vision, or fatigue; use caution when driving or engaging in tasks that require alertness until response to drug is known. Report persistent severe nausea, abdominal pain, visual disturbances, yellowing of skin or eyes, unusual bruising or bleeding, muscle pain or cramping, or unusual nosebleeds. **Pregnancy/breast-feeding precautions:** Inform prescriber if you are pregnant. Do not get pregnant or cause a pregnancy (males) for 1 month following therapy. Consult prescriber for instruction on appropriate contraceptive measures. This drug cause severe fetal defects. Do not donate blood during therapy or for an indefinite period following therapy. Do not breast-feed.

♦ **Eudal-SR®** *see* Guaifenesin and Pseudoephedrine *on page 551*
♦ **Euglucon®** *see* Glyburide *on page 538*
♦ **Eulexin®** *see* Flutamide *on page 510*

- **Eumetinex** *see* Amoxicillin and Clavulanate Potassium *on page 82*
- **Eurax® Topical** *see* Crotamiton *on page 310*
- **Eutirox** *see* Levothyroxine *on page 673*
- **Eutron®** *see* Methyclothiazide and Pargyline *on page 749*
- **Evac-Q-Mag®** *see* Magnesium Supplements *on page 703*
- **Evalose®** *see* Lactulose *on page 651*
- **Everone® Injection** *see* Testosterone *on page 1108*
- **Evista®** *see* Raloxifene *on page 1006*
- **E-Vitamin® [OTC]** *see* Vitamin E *on page 1218*
- **Exact® Cream** *see page 1294*
- **Excedrin®, Extra Strength** *see page 1294*
- **Excedrin® IB [OTC]** *see* Ibuprofen *on page 592*
- **Excedrin® P.M.** *see page 1294*
- **Exelderm®** *see page 1247*
- **Ex-Lax®, Extra Gentle Pills** *see page 1294*
- **Exna®** *see* Benzthiazide *on page 144*
- **Exsel®** *see page 1294*
- **Extendryl® SR** *see page 1306*
- **Extra Action Cough Syrup [OTC]** *see* Guaifenesin and Dextromethorphan *on page 549*
- **Extravasation Management of Chemotherapeutic Agents** *see page 1319*
- **Extravasation Treatment of Other Drugs** *see page 1321*
- **Eye-Lube-A® Solution** *see page 1294*
- **Eye-Sed® [OTC]** *see* Zinc Supplements *on page 1230*
- **Eye-Sed® Ophthalmic** *see page 1294*
- **Eyesine® Ophthalmic** *see page 1294*
- **Ezide®** *see* Hydrochlorothiazide *on page 566*
- **$F_3T$** *see* Trifluridine *on page 1178*
- **Facicam** *see* Piroxicam *on page 940*
- **Factor VIII** *see* Antihemophilic Factor (Human) *on page 99*
- **Factor VIII Recombinant** *see* Antihemophilic Factor (Recombinant) *on page 100*
- **Factrel®** *see* Gonadorelin *on page 542*
- **Fahrenheit/Centigrade Conversion** *see page 1351*


## Famciclovir (fam SYE kloe veer)

**U.S. Brand Names** Famvir™

**Therapeutic Category** Antiviral Agent

**Pregnancy Risk Factor** B

**Lactation** Excretion in breast milk unknown/contraindicated

**Use** Management of acute herpes zoster (shingles); treatment of recurrent herpes simplex in immunocompetent patients; treatment of recurrent mucocutaneous herpes simplex in HIV-infected patients

**Mechanism of Action/Effect** The prodrug famciclovir undergoes rapid biotransformation to the active compound, penciclovir, then intracellular conversion to triphosphate which is active against HSV-1, HSV-2, VZV, and EBV infected cells.

**Contraindications** Hypersensitivity to famciclovir

**Warnings** Has not been studied in immunocompromised patients or patients with ophthalmic or disseminated zoster. Dosage adjustment is required in patients with renal insufficiency ($Cl_{cr}$ <60 mL/minute) and in patients with noncompensated hepatic disease. Safety and efficacy have not been established in children <18 years of age. Animal studies indicated increases in incidence of carcinomas, mutagenic changes, and decreases in fertility with extremely large doses.

**Drug Interactions**

**Increased Effect/Toxicity:**

Cimetidine: Penciclovir AUC may increase due to impaired metabolism

Digoxin: $C_{max}$ of digoxin increases by ~19%

Probenecid: Penciclovir serum levels significantly increase

Theophylline: Penciclovir AUC/$C_{max}$ may increase and renal clearance decrease, although not clinically significant

**Food Interactions** Rate of absorption and/or conversion to penciclovir and peak concentration are reduced with food, but bioavailability is not affected.

**Adverse Reactions**

>10%: Central nervous system: Headache

1% to 10%:

Central nervous system: Fatigue, fever, dizziness, somnolence

Dermatologic: Pruritus

Gastrointestinal: Diarrhea, nausea, vomiting, constipation, anorexia, abdominal pain

Neuromuscular & skeletal: Rigors, paresthesia

**Overdose/Toxicology** Supportive and symptomatic care is recommended. Hemodialysis may enhance elimination.

**Pharmacodynamics/Kinetics**

**Protein Binding:** 20%

**Half-life Elimination:** Penciclovir: 2-3 hours (10, 20, and 7 hours in HSV-1, HSV-2, and VZV-infected cells); linearly decreased with reductions in renal failure

**Metabolism:** Rapidly deacetylated and oxidized to penciclovir (not by cytochrome P-450)

(Continued)

## Famciclovir *(Continued)*

**Excretion:** >90% of penciclovir is eliminated unchanged in urine; $C_{max}$ and $T_{max}$ are decreased and prolonged, respectively in patients with noncompensated hepatic impairment

**Formulations** Tablet: 125 mg, 250 mg, 500 mg

**Dosing**

**Adults:** Oral:

Acute herpes zoster: 500 mg every 8 hours for 7 days

Recurrent herpes simplex in immunocompetent patient: 125 mg twice daily for 5 days

**Elderly:** Refer to adult dosing.

**Renal Impairment:**

Herpes zoster:

- $Cl_{cr}$ ≥60 mL/minute: Administer 500 mg every 8 hours.
- $Cl_{cr}$ 40-59 mL/minute: Administer 500 mg every 12 hours.
- $Cl_{cr}$ 20-39 mL/minute: Administer 500 mg every 24 hours.
- $Cl_{cr}$ <20 mL/minute: Administer 250 mg every 48 hours.

Recurrent genital herpes:

- $Cl_{cr}$ ≥40 mL/minute: Administer 125 mg every 12 hours.
- $Cl_{cr}$ 20-39 mL/minute: Administer 125 mg every 24 hours.
- $Cl_{cr}$ <20 mL/minute: Administer 125 mg every 48 hours.

**Administration**

**Oral:** Initiate therapy as soon as herpes zoster is diagnosed

**Monitoring Laboratory Tests** Periodic CBC during long-term therapy

**Additional Nursing Issues**

**Physical Assessment:** Assess/teach necessity of maintaining adequate hydration, appropriate use of famciclovir, and contagion precautions. Breast-feeding is contraindicated.

**Patient Information/Instruction:** Take for prescribed length of time, even if condition improves. Do not discontinue without consulting prescriber. This is not a cure for genital herpes. You may experience mild GI disturbances (eg, nausea, vomiting, constipation, or diarrhea), fatigue, headaches, or muscle aches and pains. If these are severe, contact prescriber. **Breast-feeding precautions:** Do not breast-feed.

**Geriatric Considerations:** For herpes zoster (shingles) infections, famciclovir should be started within 72 hours of the appearance of the rash to be effective. Famciclovir has been shown to accelerate healing, reduce the duration of viral shedding, and resolve posthepatic neuralgia faster than placebo. Comparison trials to acyclovir or valacyclovir are not available. Adjust dose for estimated renal function.

**Breast-feeding Issues:** There is no specific data describing the excretion of famciclovir in breast milk and for its associated tumorigenicity. Discontinue nursing or the drug during lactation; however, acyclovir is a possible alternative for the nursing mother.

**Additional Information** Most effective if therapy is initiated within 72 hours of initial lesion.

## Famotidine (fa MOE ti deen)

**U.S. Brand Names** Pepcid®; Pepcid® AC Acid Controller [OTC]

**Therapeutic Category** Histamine $H_2$ Antagonist

**Pregnancy Risk Factor** B

**Lactation** Enters breast milk/compatible

**Use**

Pepcid®: Therapy and treatment of duodenal ulcer, gastric ulcer, control gastric pH in critically ill patients, symptomatic relief in gastritis, gastroesophageal reflux, active benign ulcer, and pathological hypersecretory conditions

Pepcid® AC Acid Controller: Relieves heartburn, acid indigestion and sour stomach

**Mechanism of Action/Effect** Competitive inhibition of histamine at $H_2$ receptors of the gastric parietal cells, which inhibits gastric acid secretion

**Contraindications** Hypersensitivity to famotidine or other $H_2$ antagonists

**Warnings** Modify dose in patients with renal impairment.

**Drug Interactions**

**Decreased Effect:** Decreased effect of ketoconazole and itraconazole.

**Food Interactions** Famotidine bioavailability may be increased if taken with food.

**Adverse Reactions**

1% to 10%:

Central nervous system: Headache, dizziness

Gastrointestinal: Constipation, diarrhea

<1% (Limited to important or life-threatening symptoms): Bradycardia, tachycardia, palpitations, hypertension, seizures, agranulocytosis, neutropenia, thrombocytopenia, increases in AST/ALT, increases in BUN/creatinine or proteinuria, bronchospasm

**Overdose/Toxicology** Symptoms of overdose include hypotension, tachycardia, vomiting, and drowsiness. Treatment is symptomatic and supportive.

**Pharmacodynamics/Kinetics**

**Protein Binding:** 15% to 20%

**Half-life Elimination:** 2.5-3.5 hours (prolonged in renal impairment); Oliguric patient: 20 hours

**Time to Peak:** Oral: Within 1-3 hours

**Excretion:** In urine as unchanged drug

**Onset:** Onset of GI effect: Oral: Within 1 hour

**Duration:** 10-12 hours

**Formulations**

Infusion, premixed in NS: 20 mg (50 mL)

Injection: 10 mg/mL (2 mL, 4 mL)

Powder for oral suspension (cherry-banana-mint flavor): 40 mg/5 mL (50 mL)

Tablet, film coated: 20 mg, 40 mg

Tablet, orally disintegrating: 20 mg, 40 mg

Pepcid® AC Acid Controller [OTC]: 10 mg

Pepcid® AC Chewable [OTC]: 10 mg

**Dosing**

**Adults:**

Oral:

Duodenal ulcer, gastric ulcer: 40 mg/day at bedtime for 4-8 weeks; 20 mg twice a day is also effective;

Duodenal ulcer maintenance therapy: 20 mg once daily at bedtime

Hypersecretory conditions: Initial: 20 mg every 6 hours, may increase up to 160 mg every 6 hours for some patients

GERD: 20 mg twice daily for 6 weeks

Esophagitis induced by GERD: 20 mg or 40 mg twice daily for up to 12 weeks

I.V.: 20 mg every 12 hours

**Elderly:** Refer to adult dosing.

**Renal Impairment:**

$Cl_{cr}$ 30-50 mL/minute: Administer every 24 hours or 50% of dose.

$Cl_{cr}$ <30 mL/minute: Administer every 36-48 hours or 25% of dose.

**Administration**

**I.V.:** Administer over 15-30 minutes; may be given undiluted I.V. push. Inject no faster than 10 mg/minute.

**Stability**

**Reconstitution:**

I.V. Reconstituted I.V. solution is stable for 48 hours at room temperature. I.V. infusion in NS or $D_5W$ solution is stable for 48 hours at room temperature.

Oral: Reconstituted oral suspension is stable for 30 days at room temperature. Do not freeze.

**Additional Nursing Issues**

**Physical Assessment:** Monitor for effectiveness of therapy based on patient diagnosis and response (ie, epigastric or abdominal pain, hematemesis, blood in stool). Monitor for adverse effects identified above. Teach patient symptoms to monitor, interventions for adverse effects, and symptoms to report.

**Patient Information/Instruction:** Take as directed, for full dose as prescribed, even if feeling better. Avoid alcohol and smoking (smoking decreases effectiveness of medication). You may experience some drowsiness or dizziness; use caution when driving or engaging in tasks that require alertness until response to drug is known. Increased exercise, increased dietary fluids, fruits, or fiber may reduce constipation; yogurt or buttermilk may help relieve diarrhea. Report acute headache, unresolved constipation or diarrhea, palpitations, black tarry stools, abdominal pain, rash, worsening of condition being treated, or recurrence of symptoms after therapy is completed.

**Geriatric Considerations:** $H_2$ blockers are the preferred drugs for treating PUD in the elderly due to cost and ease of administration. These agents are no less or more effective than any other therapy. Famotidine is on of the preferred agents (due to side effects, drug interaction profile, and pharmacokinetics). Treatment for PUD in the elderly is recommended for 12 weeks since their lesions are larger; therefore, take longer to heal. Always adjust dose based upon creatinine clearance.

**Breast-feeding Issues:** Famotidine is excreted in breast milk to a lesser degree than cimetidine another $H_2$-antagonist which is considered compatible with nursing.

**Additional Information** pH: 5.7-6.4

- **Famoxal** *see* Famotidine *on previous page*
- **Famvir™** *see* Famciclovir *on page 469*
- **Faraxen** *see* Naproxen *on page 807*
- **Fareston®** *see* Toremifene *on page 1158*
- **Farmotex®** *see* Famotidine *on previous page*

## Fat Emulsion (fat e MUL shun)

**U.S. Brand Names** Intralipid®; Liposyn®; Nutrilipid®; Soyacal®

**Synonyms** Intravenous Fat Emulsion

**Therapeutic Category** Caloric Agent

**Pregnancy Risk Factor** B/C

**Lactation** Excretion in breast milk unknown/compatible

**Use** Source of calories and essential fatty acids for patients requiring parenteral nutrition of extended duration

**Mechanism of Action/Effect** Essential for normal structure and function of cell membranes

**Contraindications** Hypersensitivity to fat emulsion and severe egg or legume (soybean) allergies; pancreatitis with hyperlipemia; pathologic hyperlipidemia; lipoid nephrosis

(Continued)

## Fat Emulsion *(Continued)*

**Warnings** Use caution in patients with severe liver damage, pulmonary disease, anemia, or blood coagulation disorder. Use with caution in jaundiced, premature, and low birth weight children. Pregnancy factor B/C.

**Adverse Reactions**

>10%:

Local: Thrombophlebitis

Miscellaneous: Sepsis

1% to 10%:

Cardiovascular: Cyanosis, flushing, chest pain

Gastrointestinal: Nausea, vomiting, diarrhea

<1% (Limited to important or life-threatening symptoms): Anemia, thrombocytopenia, jaundice, chest pain or back pain

**Overdose/Toxicology** Rapid administration results in fluid or fat overload causing dilution of serum electrolytes, overhydration, pulmonary edema, impaired pulmonary diffusion capacity, and metabolic acidosis. Treatment is supportive.

**Pharmacodynamics/Kinetics**

**Half-life Elimination:** 0.5-1 hour

**Metabolism:** Undergoes lipolysis to free fatty acids, which are utilized by reticuloendothelial cells

**Formulations** Injection: 10% [100 mg/mL] (100 mL, 250 mL, 500 mL); 20% [200 mg/mL] (100 mL, 250 mL, 500 mL)

**Dosing**

**Adults:** Fat emulsion should not exceed 60% of the total daily calories.

Initial: 1 g/kg/day, increase by 0.5-1 g/kg/day to a maximum of 2.5 g/kg/day of 10% and 3 g/kg/day of 20%; maximum rate of infusion: 0.25 g/kg/hour (1.25 mL/kg/hour of 20% solution); do not exceed 50 mL/hour (20%) or 100 mL/hour (10%)

Prevention of fatty acid deficiency (8% to 10% of total caloric intake): 0.5-1 g/kg/24 hours

500 mL twice weekly at rate of 1 mL/minute for 30 minutes, then increase to 500 mL over 4-6 hours

Can be used on a daily basis as a caloric source in TPN

**Elderly:** Refer to adult dosing.

**Administration**

**I.V.:** At the onset of therapy, the patient should be observed for any immediate allergic reactions such as dyspnea, cyanosis, and fever. Infuse for 10-15 minutes at a slower rate. Infuse 10% at 1 mL/minute. If no untoward effects, may increase rate to 500 mL over 4-6 hours. Infuse 20% at 0.5 mL/minute initially; increase to rate of 250 mL over 4-6 hours.

**I.V. Detail:** Change tubing after each infusion. May be simultaneously infused with amino acid dextrose mixtures by means of Y-connector located near infusion site. Hang fat emulsion higher than other fluids (has low specific gravity and could run up into other lines). Infuse via pump using either peripheral or central venous line. Do not use filter in line.

**Stability**

**Storage:** May be stored at room temperature. Do not store partly used bottles for later use. Do not use if emulsion appears to be oiling out.

**Monitoring Laboratory Tests** Serum triglycerides before initiation of therapy and at least weekly during therapy

**Additional Nursing Issues**

**Physical Assessment:** Inspect emulsion before administering. Do not administer if oil separation or oiliness is noted. Assess nutritional status and monitor weight. Assess for allergy to eggs prior to initiating therapy. Pruritic urticaria can occur in patients allergic to eggs. Monitor for fluid overload, thrombosis or sepsis. **Pregnancy risk factor B/C.**

**Patient Information/Instruction:** Report pain at infusion site, difficulty breathing, chest pain, calf pain, or excessive sweating.

♦ **5-FC** *see* Flucytosine *on page 492*
♦ **FDA Pregnancy Categories** *see page 15*
♦ **Febrin®** *see* Acetaminophen *on page 32*
♦ **Fedahist®** *see* Guaifenesin and Phenylpropanolamine *on page 550*
♦ **Fedahist® Expectorant [OTC]** *see* Guaifenesin and Pseudoephedrine *on page 551*
♦ **Fedahist® Tablet** *see page 1294*
♦ **Federal OBRA Regulations Recommended Maximum Doses** *see page 1432*
♦ **Feen-a-Mint® Pills** *see page 1294*
♦ **Feiba VH Immuno®** *see* Anti-inhibitor Coagulant Complex *on page 100*

## Felbamate (FEL ba mate)

**U.S. Brand Names** Felbatol®

**Therapeutic Category** Anticonvulsant, Miscellaneous

**Pregnancy Risk Factor** C

**Lactation** Enters breast milk/not recommended

**Use** Not a first-line agent; reserved for patients who do not adequately respond to alternative agents and whose epilepsy is so severe that benefit outweighs risk of liver failure or aplastic anemia; monotherapy and adjunctive therapy in patients ≥14 years of age with partial seizures with and without secondary generalization

**Contraindications** Hypersensitivity to felbamate or any component; it should be used with caution in those patients who have demonstrated hypersensitivity reactions to other carbamates (eg, meprobamate); patients with a history of previous bone marrow depression; avoid use in patients with pre-existing liver pathology

**Warnings** Antiepileptic drugs should not be suddenly discontinued because of the possibility of increasing seizure frequency. **Reported 10 cases of aplastic anemia in the U.S. after 2½ to 6 months of therapy.** Carter Wallace and the FDA recommended the use of this agent be suspended unless withdrawal of the product would place a patient at greater risk as compared to the frequently fatal form of anemia. Pregnancy factor C.

**Drug Interactions**

**Cytochrome P-450 Effect:** CYP2C19 enzyme inhibitor

**Decreased Effect:** Decreased effect with phenytoin and carbamazepine. Valproate does not significantly effect felbamate levels. Felbamate may decrease carbamazepine levels and increase levels of active metabolite of carbamazepine (these changes may offset each other).

**Increased Effect/Toxicity:** Increased effect/toxicity of phenytoin, valproate. Serum phenobarbital concentrations may be increased.

**Food Interactions** Food does not affect absorption.

**Effects on Lab Values** Blood urea nitrogen is slightly lower (1.25 mg/dL). May cause slightly elevated serum cholesterol level (about 7 mg/dL) in patients receiving about 2.6 g/day.

**Adverse Reactions**

>10%:

- Central nervous system: Headache, fatigue, dizziness, insomnia, somnolence, nervousness
- Gastrointestinal: Anorexia, nausea, vomiting, dyspepsia, constipation

1% to 10%:

- Cardiovascular: Palpitation, tachycardia, facial edema
- Central nervous system: Anxiety, abnormal gait, ataxia, depression, tremor, paresthesia, stupor
- Dermatologic: Acne, rash, pruritus,
- Gastrointestinal: Weight loss or gain, diarrhea, dry mouth, abdominal pain, taste perversion,
- Hematologic: Leukopenia, purpura,
- Hepatic: Elevated ALT (SGPT), elevated AST (SGOT)
- Neuromuscular & skeletal: Myalgia
- Ocular: Miosis, diplopia, abnormal vision
- Respiratory: Cough, pharyngitis, upper respiratory tract infection, rhinitis, sinusitis

<1% (Limited to important or life-threatening symptoms): Hallucinations, euphoria, migraine, suicide attempt, photosensitivity, urticaria, bullous eruption, Stevens-Johnson syndrome, leukocytosis, thrombocytopenia, granulocytopenia, agranulocytosis, dystonia

**Overdose/Toxicology** Symptoms of overdose include sedation, gastrointestinal upset, and tachycardia. Provide general supportive care.

**Pharmacodynamics/Kinetics**

**Protein Binding:** 22% to 25%

**Half-life Elimination:** Cleared renally 40% to 50% as unchanged drug and 40% as inactive metabolites in the urine

**Time to Peak:** Serum concentrations: Within 3 hours

**Formulations**

Suspension, oral: 600 mg/5 mL (240 mL, 960 mL)

Tablet: 400 mg, 600 mg

**Dosing**

**Adults:**

Monotherapy:

Initial: 1200 mg/day in divided doses 3 or 4 times/day; titrate previously untreated patients under close clinical supervision, increasing the dosage in 600 mg increments every 2 weeks to 2400 mg/day based on clinical response and thereafter to 3600 mg/day in clinically indicated.

Conversion to monotherapy: Initiate at 1200 mg/day in divided doses 3 or 4 times/day, reduce the dosage of the concomitant anticonvulsant(s) by 20% to 33% at the initiation of felbamate therapy. At week 2, increase the felbamate dosage to 2400 mg/day while reducing the dosage of the other anticonvulsant(s) up to an additional 33% of their original dosage. At week 3, increase the felbamate dosage up to 3600 mg/day and continue to reduce the dosage of the other anticonvulsant(s) as clinically indicated.

Adjunctive therapy:

Week 1:

Felbamate: 1200 mg/day initial dose

Concomitant anticonvulsant(s): Reduce original dosage by 20% to 33%.

Week 2:

Felbamate: 2400 mg/day (therapeutic range)

Concomitant anticonvulsant(s): Reduce original dosage by up to an additional 33%.

Week 3:

Felbamate: 3600 mg/day (therapeutic range)

Concomitant anticonvulsant(s): Reduce original dosage as clinically indicated.

(Continued)

## Felbamate *(Continued)*

**Elderly:** Refer to adult dosing; start at lowest dose (see Geriatric Considerations).

**Administration**

**Oral:** Give on empty stomach for best absorption.

**Stability**

**Storage:** Store medication in tightly closed container at room temperature away from excessive heat.

**Monitoring Laboratory Tests** Monitor serum levels of concomitant anticonvulsant therapy monitor AST, ALT, and bilirubin on a weekly basis. Hematologic evaluations before therapy begins, frequently during therapy, and for a significant period after discontinuation.

**Additional Nursing Issues**

**Physical Assessment:** Assess effectiveness and interactions of other medications patient may be taking (see Contraindications, Warnings/Precautions, and Drug Interactions). Monitor for therapeutic response (seizure activity, force, type, duration), laboratory values, and adverse reactions (see Adverse Reactions) at beginning of therapy and periodically with long-term use. Taper dosage slowly when discontinuing. Use and teach seizure/safety precautions. Assess knowledge/teach patient appropriate use, interventions to reduce side effects, and adverse symptoms to report. **Pregnancy risk factor C** - benefits of use should outweigh possible risks. Breast-feeding is not recommended.

**Patient Information/Instruction:** Take exactly as directed (do not increase dose or frequency or discontinue without consulting prescriber). While using this medication, do not use alcohol and other prescription or OTC medications (especially pain medications, sedatives, antihistamines, or hypnotics) without consulting prescriber. Maintain adequate hydration (2-3 L/day of fluids unless instructed to restrict fluid intake). You may experience drowsiness, dizziness, or blurred vision (use caution when driving or engaging in tasks requiring alertness until response to drug is known); nausea, vomiting, loss of appetite, or dry mouth (small frequent meals, frequent mouth care, chewing gum, or sucking lozenges may help). Wear identification of epileptic status and medications. Report CNS changes, mentation changes, or changes in cognition; muscle cramping, weakness, tremors, changes in gait; persistent GI symptoms (cramping, constipation, vomiting, anorexia); rash or skin irritations; unusual bruising or bleeding (mouth, urine, stool); cough, runny nose, sore throat, or difficulty breathing; worsening of seizure activity, or loss of seizure control. **Pregnancy/breast-feeding precautions:** Inform prescriber if you are or intend to be pregnant. Breast-feeding is not recommended.

**Geriatric Considerations:** Clinical studies have not included large numbers of patients >65 years of age. Due to decreased hepatic and renal function, dosing should start at the lower end of the dosage range.

**Additional Information** Monotherapy has not been associated with gingival hyperplasia, impaired concentration, weight gain, or abnormal thinking.


- ♦ **Felbatol®** *see* Felbamate *on page 472*
- ♦ **Feldene®** *see* Piroxicam *on page 940*


## Felodipine (fe LOE di peen)

**U.S. Brand Names** Plendil®

**Therapeutic Category** Calcium Channel Blocker

**Pregnancy Risk Factor** C

**Lactation** Excretion in breast milk unknown

**Use** Treatment of hypertension, congestive heart failure

**Mechanism of Action/Effect** Inhibits calcium ions from entering the "slow channels" or select voltage-sensitive areas of vascular smooth muscle and myocardium during depolarization

**Contraindications** Hypersensitivity to felodipine, any component, or other calcium channel blocker; severe hypotension or second and third degree heart block

**Warnings** Use with caution and titrate dosages for patients with impaired renal or hepatic function. Use caution when treating patients with congestive heart failure, sick-sinus syndrome, severe left ventricular dysfunction, hypertrophic cardiomyopathy (especially obstructive), concomitant therapy with beta-blockers or digoxin, edema, or increased intracranial pressure with cranial tumors. Do not abruptly withdraw (may cause chest pain). Elderly may experience hypotension and constipation more readily. Pregnancy factor C.

**Drug Interactions**

**Cytochrome P-450 Effect:** CYP3A3/4 enzyme substrate

**Decreased Effect:** Carbamazepine taken with felodipine may decrease felodipine effect. Felodipine and theophylline may decrease pharmacologic actions of theophylline.

**Increased Effect/Toxicity:** Felodipine and metoprolol may increase cardiac depressant effects on A-V conduction. Felodipine and erythromycin inhibit felodipine and other dihydropyridine calcium antagonist metabolism resulting in a twofold increase in levels and consequent toxicity.

**Food Interactions** Increased therapeutic and vasodilator side effects, including severe hypotension and myocardial ischemia, may occur if felodipine is taken with grapefruit juice. High fat/carbohydrate meals will increase $C_{max}$ by 60%; grapefruit juice by twofold.

**Adverse Reactions**

>10%: Cardiovascular: Peripheral edema

1% to 10%:
Cardiovascular: Chest pain, tachycardia
Central nervous system: Dizziness, lightheadedness
Dermatologic: Rash
Gastrointestinal: Constipation, diarrhea
Miscellaneous: Allergic reaction
<1% (Limited to important or life-threatening symptoms): Hypotension, arrhythmia, bradycardia, palpitations, marked elevations in liver function tests, shortness of breath, gynecomastia

**Overdose/Toxicology** Primary cardiac symptoms of calcium blocker overdose include hypotension and bradycardia. Noncardiac symptoms include confusion, stupor, nausea, vomiting, metabolic acidosis, and hyperglycemia. Treat symptomatically.

**Pharmacodynamics/Kinetics**
**Protein Binding:** >99%
**Half-life Elimination:** 11-16 hours
**Metabolism:** Liver
**Excretion:** Urine
**Onset:** 2-5 hours
**Duration:** 16-24 hours

**Formulations** Tablet, extended release: 2.5 mg, 5 mg, 10 mg

**Dosing**
**Adults:** Oral: 5-10 mg once daily; increase by 5 mg at 2-week intervals, as needed, to a maximum of 20 mg/day.
**Elderly:** Oral: Initial 2.5 mg/day
**Hepatic Impairment:** Begin with 2.5 mg/day; do not use doses >10 mg/day.

**Additional Nursing Issues**
**Physical Assessment:** Monitor blood pressure, cardiac rhythm, I & O ratio, weight, edema, signs or symptoms of adverse reactions (see above) at beginning of therapy or when titrating dose, and periodically throughout long-term therapy. Monitor closely if patient is also taking beta blockers, nitrates or other antihypertensive medications (see Warnings/Precautions). When discontinuing, taper gradually (over 2 weeks). **Pregnancy risk factor C** - benefits of use should outweigh possible risks. Note breast-feeding caution.
**Patient Information/Instruction:** Take without food. Take as prescribed; do not stop abruptly without consulting prescriber immediately. Swallow whole; do not crush or chew. You may experience headache (if unrelieved, consult prescriber), nausea or vomiting (frequent small meals may help), constipation (increased dietary bulk and fluids may help), depression (should resolve when drug is discontinued). May cause dizziness or drowsiness; use caution when driving or engaging in tasks that require alertness until response to drug is known. Report any chest pain or swelling of hands or feet, respiratory distress, sudden weight gain, or unresolved constipation. **Pregnancy/breast-feeding precautions:** Inform prescriber if you are or intend to be pregnant. Consult prescriber if breast-feeding.
**Geriatric Considerations:** Elderly may experience a greater hypotensive response. Theoretically, constipation may be more of a problem in the elderly.

**Related Information**
Calcium Channel Blocking Agents Comparison *on page 1378*

- **Femara™** *see* Letrozole *on page 661*
- **Femcet®** *see* Butalbital Compound and Acetaminophen *on page 175*
- **Femilax® Tablet** *see page 1294*
- **Femiron® [OTC]** *see* Iron Supplements *on page 627*
- **Femizole-7® [OTC]** *see* Clotrimazole *on page 294*
- **Femizol-M® [OTC]** *see* Miconazole *on page 767*
- **Femogen®** *see* Estrone *on page 451*
- **Fenesin™** *see* Guaifenesin *on page 548*
- **Fenesin DM®** *see* Guaifenesin and Dextromethorphan *on page 549*

## Fenofibrate (fen oh FYE brate)

**U.S. Brand Names** Tricor®
**Synonyms** Procetofene; Proctofene
**Therapeutic Category** Antilipemic Agent (Fibric Acid)
**Pregnancy Risk Factor** C
**Lactation** Excretion in breast milk unknown
**Use** Adjunct to dietary therapy for the treatment of adults with very high elevations of serum triglyceride levels (Types IV and V hyperlipidemia) who are at risk of pancreatitis and who do not respond adequately to a determined dietary effort; its efficacy can be enhanced by combination with other hypolipidemic agents that have a different mechanism of action; safety and efficacy may be greater than that of clofibrate
**Mechanism of Action/Effect** Fenofibric acid is believed to increase VLDL catabolism by enhancing the synthesis of lipoprotein lipase; as a result of a decrease in VLDL levels, total plasma triglycerides are reduced by 30% to 60%. Modest increase in HDL occurs in some hypertriglyceridemic patients.
**Warnings** The hypoprothrombinemic effect of anticoagulants is significantly increased with concomitant fenofibrate administration. Use with caution in patients with severe renal dysfunction. Pregnancy factor C.
**Drug Interactions**
**Increased Effect/Toxicity:** Increased hypolipidemic effect when used with cholestyramine or colestipol. Increased hypoprothrombinemic effect when used with warfarin.

(Continued)

## Fenofibrate *(Continued)*

**Adverse Reactions**

>10%: Gastrointestinal: Nausea, gastric discomfort

1% to 10%:

Dermatologic: Skin reactions

Gastrointestinal: Constipation, diarrhea

<1% (Limited to important or life-threatening symptoms): Dizziness, headache, fatigue, insomnia, transient increases in LFTs, arthralgia, myalgia

**Overdose/Toxicology** Symptoms of overdose include nausea, vomiting, diarrhea, and GI distress. Treatment is supportive.

**Pharmacodynamics/Kinetics**

**Protein Binding:** >99%

**Distribution:** Distributes well to most tissues except brain or eye; concentrates in liver, kidneys, and gut

**Half-life Elimination:** Fenofibrate: 21 hours (30 hours in the elderly, 44-54 hours in hepatic impairment)

**Time to Peak:** 4-6 hours

**Metabolism:** Metabolized to its active form, fenofibric acid, by tissue and plasma esterases; then undergoes inactivation by glucuronidation in the liver or kidneys

**Excretion:** 60% to 93% excreted in metabolized form; 5% to 25% excreted fecally; hemodialysis has no effect on removal of fenofibric acid from the plasma.

**Formulations** Capsule: 67 mg

**Dosing**

**Adults:** Initial: 67 mg/day, up to 3 capsules (201 mg)

**Elderly:** Refer to adult dosing.

**Renal Impairment:** Decrease dose or increase dosing interval for patients with renal failure.

**Administration**

**Oral:** 6-8 weeks of therapy is required to determine efficacy.

**Monitoring Laboratory Tests** Total serum cholesterol and triglyceride concentration and CLDL, LDL, and HDL levels should be measured periodically; if only marginal changes are noted in 6-8 weeks, the drug should be discontinued. Serum transaminases should be measured every 3 months; if ALT values increase >100 units/L, therapy should be discontinued. Monitor LFTs prior to initiation, at 6 and 12 weeks after initiation or first dose, then periodically thereafter.

**Additional Nursing Issues**

**Physical Assessment:** Assess other medications patient may be taking for effectiveness and/or interactions (see Drug Interactions). Assess knowledge/instruct patient on appropriate use, possible side effects (see Adverse Reactions), and symptoms to report. **Pregnancy risk factor C** - benefits of use should outweigh possible risks. Note breast-feeding caution.

**Patient Information/Instruction:** Take with food. Do not change dosage without consulting prescriber. Maintain diet and exercise program as prescribed. You may experience mild GI disturbances (eg, gas, diarrhea, constipation, nausea); inform prescriber if these are severe. Report skin rash or irritation, insomnia, unusual muscle pain or tremors, or persistent dizziness. **Pregnancy/breast-feeding precautions:** Inform prescriber if you are or intend to be pregnant. Consult prescriber if breast-feeding.

**Pregnancy Issues:** Although teratogenicity and mutagenicity tests in animals have been negative, significant risk has been identified with clofibrate. Use should be avoided, if possible, in pregnant women since the neonatal glucuronide conjugation pathways are immature.

**Related Information**

Lipid-Lowering Agents Comparison *on page 1393*

## Fenoprofen (fen oh PROE fen)

**U.S. Brand Names** Nalfon®

**Therapeutic Category** Nonsteroidal Anti-Inflammatory Agent (NSAID)

**Pregnancy Risk Factor** B/D (3rd trimester or near delivery)

**Lactation** Enters breast milk/not recommended

**Use** Symptomatic treatment of acute and chronic rheumatoid arthritis and osteoarthritis; relief of mild to moderate pain

**Mechanism of Action/Effect** Inhibits prostaglandin synthesis by decreasing the activity of the enzyme, cyclo-oxygenase, which results in decreased formation of prostaglandin precursors

**Contraindications** Hypersensitivity to fenoprofen, other NSAIDs, or aspirin; pregnancy (3rd trimester or near delivery)

**Warnings** Use with caution in patients with congestive heart failure, hypertension, decreased renal or hepatic function, history of GI disease, or those receiving anticoagulants.

**Drug Interactions**

**Decreased Effect:** Decreased effect with phenobarbital.

**Increased Effect/Toxicity:** Increased effect/toxicity of phenytoin, sulfonamides, sulfonylureas, salicylates, and oral anticoagulants.

**Food Interactions** Fenoprofen peak serum levels may be decreased if taken with food.

**Effects on Lab Values** ↑ chloride (S), sodium (S)

**Adverse Reactions**

1% to 10%:

Central nervous system: Headache, nervousness, dizziness
Dermatologic: Itching, rash
Endocrine & metabolic: Fluid retention
Gastrointestinal: Abdominal cramps, heartburn, indigestion, nausea, vomiting
Otic: Ringing in ears

<1% (Limited to important or life-threatening symptoms): Congestive heart failure, hypertension, arrhythmias, tachycardia, erythema multiforme, toxic epidermal necrolysis, Stevens-Johnson syndrome, angioedema, GI ulceration, agranulocytosis, anemia, hemolytic anemia, bone marrow depression, leukopenia, thrombocytopenia, hepatitis, polyuria, acute renal failure, dyspnea

**Overdose/Toxicology** Symptoms of overdose include acute renal failure, vomiting, drowsiness, and leukocytosis. Management of nonsteroidal anti-inflammatory (NSAID) intoxication is supportive and symptomatic.

**Pharmacodynamics/Kinetics**

**Protein Binding:** 99%
**Distribution:** Does not cross the placenta
**Half-life Elimination:** 2.5-3 hours
**Time to Peak:** Within 2 hours
**Metabolism:** Liver
**Excretion:** Urine and feces
**Onset:** Begins in a few days

**Formulations**

Fenoprofen calcium:
Capsule: 200 mg, 300 mg
Tablet: 600 mg

**Dosing**

**Adults:** Oral:
Rheumatoid arthritis and osteoarthritis: 300-600 mg 3-4 times/day up to 3.2 g/day
Mild to moderate pain: 200 mg every 4-6 hours as needed

**Elderly:** Refer to adult dosing.

**Administration**

**Oral:** Do not crush tablets. Swallow whole with a full glass of water. Take with food to minimize stomach upset.

**Monitoring Laboratory Tests** CBC, liver enzymes; urine output and BUN/serum creatinine in patients receiving diuretics

**Additional Nursing Issues**

**Physical Assessment:** Systemic: Assess effectiveness and interactions of other medications patient may be taking (see Contraindications, Warnings/Precautions, and Drug Interactions). Monitor laboratory tests (see above) and therapeutic response (eg, relief of pain and inflammation, activity tolerance), and adverse reactions (eg, gastrointestinal effects or ototoxicity) at beginning of therapy and periodically throughout therapy (see Warnings/Precautions, Adverse Reactions, and Overdose/Toxicology). Assess knowledge/teach patient appropriate use, interventions to reduce side effects, and adverse symptoms to report. **Pregnancy risk factor B/D** - see Pregnancy Risk Factor for cautious use. Breast-feeding is not recommended. Ophthalmic absorption is probably minimal.

**Patient Information/Instruction:** Take this medication exactly as directed; do not increase dose without consulting prescriber. Do not crush tablets or break capsules. Take with food or milk to reduce GI distress. Maintain adequate fluid intake (2-3 L/day of fluids unless instructed to restrict fluid intake). Do not use alcohol, aspirin, or aspirin-containing medication, and all other anti-inflammatory medications without consulting prescriber. You may experience drowsiness, dizziness, nervousness, or headache (use caution when driving or engaging in tasks requiring alertness until response to drug is known); anorexia, nausea, vomiting, or heartburn (frequent small meals, frequent mouth care, sucking lozenges, or chewing gum may help); fluid retention (weigh yourself weekly and report unusual (3-5 lb/week) weight gain). GI bleeding, ulceration, or perforation can occur with or without pain; discontinue medication and contact prescriber if persistent abdominal pain or cramping, or blood in stool occurs. Report breathlessness, difficulty breathing, or unusual cough; chest pain, rapid heartbeat, palpitations; unusual bruising/bleeding; blood in urine, stool, mouth, or vomitus; swollen extremities; skin rash or itching; acute fatigue; or changes in hearing or ringing in ears. **Pregnancy/breast-feeding precautions:** Inform prescriber if you are or intend to be pregnant. Breast-feeding is not recommended.

**Geriatric Considerations:** Elderly are at high risk for adverse effects from nonsteroidal anti-inflammatory agents. As much as 60% of elderly can develop peptic ulceration and/or hemorrhage asymptomatically. The concomitant use of $H_2$ blockers, omeprazole, and sucralfate is not effective as prophylaxis with the exception of NSAID-induced duodenal ulcers which may be prevented by the use of ranitidine. Misoprostol is the only prophylactic agent proven effective. Also, concomitant disease and drug use contribute to the risk for GI adverse effects. Use lowest effective dose for shortest period possible. Consider renal function decline with age. Use of NSAIDs can compromise existing renal function especially when $Cl_{cr}$ is ≤30 mL/minute. Tinnitus may be a difficult and unreliable indication of toxicity due to age-related hearing loss or eighth cranial nerve damage. CNS adverse effects such as confusion, agitation, and hallucination are generally seen in overdose or high-dose situations, but elderly may demonstrate these adverse effects at lower doses than younger adults.

**Related Information**

Nonsalicylate/Nonsteroidal Anti-inflammatory Comparison *on page 1401*

◆ **Fentanest** *see* Fentanyl *on this page*

## Fentanyl (FEN ta nil)

**U.S. Brand Names** Duragesic® Transdermal; Fentanyl Oralet®; Sublimaze® Injection

**Therapeutic Category** Analgesic, Narcotic; General Anesthetic

**Pregnancy Risk Factor** B/D (if used for prolonged periods or in high doses at term)

**Lactation** Enters breast milk/use caution (AAP rates "compatible")

**Use** Sedation, relief of pain, preoperative medication, adjunct to general or regional anesthesia, management of chronic pain (transdermal product)

**Mechanism of Action/Effect** Binds with stereospecific receptors at many sites within the CNS, increases pain threshold, alters pain reception, inhibits ascending pain pathways

**Contraindications** Hypersensitivity to fentanyl or any component; increased intracranial pressure; severe respiratory depression; severe liver or renal insufficiency; transmucosal route is contraindicated in unmonitored settings where a risk of unrecognized hypoventilation exists or in treating acute or chronic pain; pregnancy (if used for prolonged periods or in high doses at term)

**Warnings** Fentanyl shares the toxic potentials of opiate agonists, and precautions of opiate agonist therapy should be observed. Use with caution in patients with bradycardia. Rapid I.V. infusion may result in skeletal muscle and chest wall rigidity → impaired ventilation → respiratory distress → apnea, bronchoconstriction, laryngospasm. Inject slowly over 3-5 minutes. Nondepolarizing skeletal muscle relaxant may be required.

Transmucosal fentanyl: Fentanyl Oralet® is not indicated for use in unmonitored settings where there is a risk of unrecognized hypoventilation or in treating acute or chronic pain. Patients should be monitored by direct visual observation and by some means of measuring respiratory function, such as pulse oximetry, until they are recovered. Facilities for the administration of fluids, opioid antagonists, oxygen, and resuscitation equipment (including facilities for endotracheal intubation) should be readily available.

Topical patches: Serum fentanyl concentrations may increase approximately 33% for patients with a body temperature of 40°C secondary to a temperature-dependent increase in fentanyl release from the system and increased skin permeability. Patients who experience adverse reactions should be monitored for at least 12 hours after removal of the patch.

The elderly may be particularly susceptible to the CNS depressant and constipating effects of narcotics.

**Drug Interactions**

**Cytochrome P-450 Effect:** CYP3A3/4 enzyme substrate

**Increased Effect/Toxicity:** Increased toxicity with CNS depressants, phenothiazines. Tricyclic antidepressants may potentiate fentanyl's adverse effects. Potential for serotonin syndrome if combined with other serotonergic drugs.

**Adverse Reactions**

>10%:

- Cardiovascular: Bradycardia, hypotension, peripheral vasodilation
- Central nervous system: Drowsiness, sedation, increased intracranial pressure
- Gastrointestinal: Nausea, vomiting
- Endocrine & metabolic: Antidiuretic hormone release
- Ocular: Miosis
- Neuromuscular & skeletal: Chest wall rigidity

1% to 10%:

- Cardiovascular: Cardiac arrhythmias, orthostatic hypotension
- Central nervous system: Confusion, CNS depression
- Gastrointestinal: Constipation
- Ocular: Blurred vision
- Respiratory: Apnea, postoperative respiratory depression

<1% (Limited to important or life-threatening symptoms): Convulsions, respiratory depression, bronchospasm, laryngospasm, hypercarbia

**Overdose/Toxicology** Symptoms of overdose include CNS depression, respiratory depression, and miosis. Treatment is supportive. Naloxone, 2 mg I.V. with repeat administration as necessary up to a total of 10 mg, can also be used to reverse toxic effects of the opiate.

**Pharmacodynamics/Kinetics**

**Distribution:** Highly lipophilic, redistributes into muscle and fat

**Half-life Elimination:** 2-4 hours; Transmucosal: 6.6 hours (range: 5-15 hours)

**Metabolism:** Liver

**Excretion:** Urine

**Onset:** Respiratory depressant effect may last longer than analgesic effect

- I.M.: 7-15 minutes
- I.V.: Almost immediate
- Transmucosal: 5-15 minutes with a maximum reduction in activity/apprehension; Peak analgesia: Within 20-30 minutes

**Duration:** Respiratory depressant effect may last longer than analgesic effect.

I.M.: 1-2 hours; I.V.: 0.5-1 hour; Transmucosal: Related to blood level of the drug

**Formulations**

Injection, as citrate: 0.05 mg/mL (2 mL, 5 mL, 10 mL, 20 mL, 50 mL)

Lozenge, oral transmucosal (raspberry flavored): 200 mcg, 300 mcg, 400 mcg, 600 mcg, 800 mcg, 1200 mcg, 1600 mcg

Transdermal system: 25 mcg/hour [10 $cm^2$]; 50 mcg/hour [20 $cm^2$]; 75 mcg/hour [30 $cm^2$]; 100 mcg/hour [40 $cm^2$] (all available in 5s)

**Dosing**

**Adults:** Doses should be titrated to appropriate effects; wide range of doses, dependent upon desired degree of analgesia/anesthesia.

Sedation for minor procedures/analgesia:

I.M., I.V.: 0.5-1 mcg/kg/dose; higher doses are used for major procedures.

Transmucosal: 5 mcg/kg, suck on lozenge vigorously approximately 20-40 minutes before the start of procedure, drug effect begins within 10 minutes, with sedation beginning shortly thereafter.

Preoperative sedation, adjunct to regional anesthesia, postoperative pain: I.M., I.V.: 50-100 mcg/dose

Adjunct to general anesthesia: I.M., I.V.: 2-50 mcg/kg

General anesthesia without additional anesthetic agents: I.V. 50-100 mcg/kg with $O_2$ and skeletal muscle relaxant

Pain control:

Transdermal: Initial: 25 mcg/hour system

Equianalgesic conversion: If currently receiving opiates, convert to fentanyl equivalent and administer equianalgesic dosage titrated to minimize adverse effects and provide analgesia. To convert patients from oral or parenteral opioids to Duragesic®, the previous 24-hour analgesic requirement should be calculated. This analgesic requirement should be converted to the equianalgesic oral morphine dose. See Equianalgesic Doses of Opioid Agonists table.

**Equianalgesic Doses of Opioid Agonists**

| Drug | Equianalgesic Dose (mg) | |
|---|---|---|
| | I.M. | P.O. |
| Codeine | 130 | 200 |
| Hydromorphone | 1.5 | 7.5 |
| Levorphanol | 2 | 4 |
| Meperidine | 75 | — |
| Methadone | 10 | 20 |
| Morphine | 10 | 60 |
| Oxycodone | 15 | 30 |
| Oxymorphone | 1 | 10 (PR) |

From *N Engl J Med*, 1985, 313:84-95.

Convert the morphine doses to the Duragesic® dose equivalent. See table.

**Corresponding Doses of Oral/Intramuscular Morphine and Duragesic™**

| Oral 24-Hour Morphine (mg/d) | I.M. 24-Hour Morphine (mg/d) | Duragesic™ Dose (mcg/h) |
|---|---|---|
| 45-134 | 8-22 | 25 |
| 135-224 | 28-37 | 50 |
| 225-314 | 38-52 | 75 |
| 315-404 | 53-67 | 100 |
| 405-494 | 68-82 | 125 |
| 495-584 | 83-97 | 150 |
| 585-674 | 98-112 | 175 |
| 675-764 | 113-127 | 200 |
| 765-854 | 128-142 | 225 |
| 855-944 | 143-157 | 250 |
| 945-1034 | 158-172 | 275 |
| 1035-1124 | 173-187 | 300 |

Product information, Duragesic™ — Janssen Pharmaceutica, January, 1991.

The dosage should not be titrated more frequently than every 3 days after the initial dose or every 6 days thereafter. The majority of patients are controlled on every 72-hour administration, however, a small number of patients require every 48-hour administration.

**Elderly:** Elderly have been found to be twice as sensitive as younger patients to the effects of fentanyl. A wide range of doses may be used; when choosing a dose, take into consideration the following patient factors; age, weight, physical status, underlying disease states, other drugs used, type of anesthesia used, and the surgical procedure to be performed.

Transmucosal: Dose should be reduced to 2.5-5 mcg/kg; suck on lozenge vigorously approximately 20-40 minutes before the start of procedure.

**Renal Impairment:**

$Cl_{cr}$ 10-50 mL/minute: Administer at 75% of normal dose.

$Cl_{cr}$ <10 mL/minute: Administer at 50% of normal dose.

(Continued)

## Fentanyl *(Continued)*

### Administration

**Oral:** Transmucosal product should begin 20-40 minutes prior to the anticipated start of surgery, diagnostic, or therapeutic procedure. Foil overwrap should be removed just prior to administration. Once removed, patient should place the unit in mouth and allow it to dissolve. Do **not** chew; unit should be removed after it is consumed or if patient has achieved an adequate sedation and anxiolytic level, and/or shows signs of respiratory depression. For patients who have received transmucosal product within 6-12 hours, it is recommended that if other narcotics are required, they should be used at starting doses $^1/_4$ to $^1/_3$ those usually recommended.

**Topical:** Patients with an elevated temperature may have increased fentanyl absorption transdermally. Observe for adverse effects; dosage adjustment may be needed. Pharmacologic and adverse effects can be seen after discontinuation of transdermal system. Observe patients for at least 12 hours after transdermal product is removed. Keep transdermal product (both used and unused) out of the reach of children. Do **not** use soap, alcohol, or other solvents to remove transdermal gel if it accidentally touches skin, as they may increase transdermal absorption; use copious amounts of water.

### Stability

**Storage:** Protect from light. Store transmucosal product at controlled room temperature of 15°C to 30°C (59°F to 86°F).

**Compatibility:** Incompatible when mixed in the same syringe with pentobarbital. See the Compatibility of Drugs Chart *on page 1315* and the Compatibility of Drugs in Syringe Chart *on page 1317.*

### Additional Nursing Issues

**Physical Assessment:** Assess other medications patient may be taking for additive or adverse interactions (see Drug Interactions). Note Warnings/Precautions and Administration. Monitor for effectiveness of pain relief and monitor for signs of overdose (see above). Monitor blood pressure, CNS and respiratory status, and degree of sedation at beginning of therapy and at regular intervals with long-term use. May cause physical and/or psychological dependence. For inpatients, implement safety measures (eg, side rails up, call light within reach, instructions to call for assistance, etc). Note Warnings/Precautions and assess knowledge/teach patient appropriate use (if self-administered). Teach patient to monitor for adverse reactions (see Adverse Reactions), adverse reactions to report, and appropriate interventions to reduce side effects. **Pregnancy risk factor B/D** - see Pregnancy Risk Factor for cautious use. Note breast-feeding caution.

**Patient Information/Instruction:** While using this medication, do not use alcohol and other prescription or OTC medications (especially sedatives, tranquilizers, antihistamines, or pain medications) without consulting prescriber. Maintain adequate hydration (2-3 L/day of fluids unless instructed to restrict fluid intake). May cause hypotension, dizziness, drowsiness, impaired coordination, or blurred vision (use caution when driving, climbing stairs, or changing position - rising from sitting or lying to standing, or when engaging in tasks requiring alertness until response to drug is known); nausea or vomiting (frequent mouth care, small frequent meals, chewing gum, or sucking lozenges may help); constipation (increased exercise, fluids, or dietary fruit and fiber may help - if constipation remains an unresolved problem, consult prescriber about use of stool softeners). Report acute dizziness, chest pain, slow or rapid heartbeat, acute headache; confusion or changes in mentation; changes in voiding frequency or amount, swelling of extremities, or unusual weight gain; shortness of breath or difficulty breathing; or changes in vision. **Pregnancy/breast-feeding precautions:** Inform prescriber if you are or intend to be pregnant. Consult prescriber if breast-feeding.

**Administration:** Transdermal: Apply to clean, dry skin, immediately after removing from package. Firmly press in place and hold for 20 seconds.

**Geriatric Considerations:** The elderly may be particularly susceptible to the CNS depressant and constipating effects of narcotics; therefore, use with caution.

### Related Information

Controlled Substances Comparison *on page 1379*
Narcotic/Opioid Analgesic Comparison *on page 1396*

- **Fentanyl and Droperidol** *see* Droperidol and Fentanyl *on page 410*
- **Fentanyl Oralet®** *see* Fentanyl *on page 478*
- **Feosol® [OTC]** *see* Iron Supplements *on page 627*
- **Feostat® [OTC]** *see* Iron Supplements *on page 627*
- **Ferancee®** *see page 1294*
- **Feratab® [OTC]** *see* Iron Supplements *on page 627*
- **Fergon® [OTC]** *see* Iron Supplements *on page 627*
- **Fer-In-Sol® [OTC]** *see* Iron Supplements *on page 627*
- **Fer-Iron® [OTC]** *see* Iron Supplements *on page 627*
- **Fermalac®** *see Lactobacillus acidophilus* and *Lactobacillus bulgaricus on page 651*
- **Fero-Grad 500®** *see page 1294*
- **Fero-Gradumet® [OTC]** *see* Iron Supplements *on page 627*
- **Ferospace® [OTC]** *see* Iron Supplements *on page 627*
- **Ferralet® [OTC]** *see* Iron Supplements *on page 627*
- **Ferralyn® Lanacaps® [OTC]** *see* Iron Supplements *on page 627*
- **Ferra-TD® [OTC]** *see* Iron Supplements *on page 627*

## Ferric Gluconate (FER ik GLOO koe nate)

**U.S. Brand Names** Ferrlecit®

**Synonyms** Sodium Ferric Gluconate

**Therapeutic Category** Iron Salt

**Pregnancy Risk Factor** B

**Lactation** Use caution

**Use** Repletion of total body iron content in patients with iron deficiency anemia who are undergoing hemodialysis in conjunction with erythropoietin therapy

**Mechanism of Action/Effect** Supplies a source to elemental iron necessary to the function of hemoglobin, myoglobin and specific enzyme systems; allows transport of oxygen via hemoglobin

**Contraindications** Hypersensitivity to ferric gluconate, benzyl alcohol or any component; use in any anemia not caused by iron deficiency; heart failure (of any severity)

**Warnings** Potentially serious hypersensitivity reactions may occur. Fatal immediate hypersensitivity reactions have occurred with other iron carbohydrate complexes. Avoid rapid administration - flushing and hypotension may occur. Administration rate should not exceed 2.1 mg/minute. Do not administer to patients with iron overload. Use with caution in elderly patients.

**Adverse Reactions** Major adverse reactions which are likely to be related ferrous gluconate include hypotension and hypersensitivity reactions. Hypersensitivity reactions have included pruritus, chest pain, hypotension, nausea, abdominal pain, flank pain, fatigue and rash. Fatal hypersensitivity reactions have occurred with other iron polysaccharide complexes. A test dose is recommended.

1% to 10%:

- Cardiovascular: Hypotension (serious hypotension in 1.3%), chest pain, hypertension, syncope, tachycardia, angina, myocardial infarction, pulmonary edema, hypovolemia, peripheral edema
- Central nervous system: Headache, fatigue, fever, malaise, dizziness, paresthesia, insomnia, agitation, somnolence
- Dermatologic: Pruritus, rash
- Endocrine & metabolic: Hyperkalemia, hypoglycemia, hypokalemia
- Gastrointestinal: Abdominal pain, nausea, vomiting, diarrhea, rectal disorder, dyspepsia, flatulence, melena
- Genitourinary: Urinary tract infection
- Hematologic: Anemia, abnormal erythrocytes, lymphadenopathy
- Local: Injection site reactions, pain
- Neuromuscular & skeletal: Weakness, back pain, leg cramps, myalgia, arthralgia, paresthesia
- Ocular: Blurred vision, conjunctivitis
- Respiratory: Dyspnea, cough, rhinitis, upper respiratory infection, pneumonia
- Miscellaneous: Hypersensitivity reactions (3%), infection, rigors, chills, flu-like syndrome, sepsis, carcinoma, increased sweating, diaphoresis (increased)

<1% (Limited to important or life-threatening symptoms): Epigastric pain, groin pain

**Overdose/Toxicology** Symptoms of iron overdose include CNS toxicity, acidosis, hepatic and renal impairment, hematemesis, and lethargy. A serum iron level ≥300 µg/mL requires treatment due to severe toxicity. Treatment is generally symptomatic and supportive, but severe overdoses may be treated with deferoxamine. Deferoxamine may be administered I.V. (80 mg/kg over 24 hours) or I.M. (40-90 mg/kg every 8 hours). Usual toxic dose of elemental iron: ≥35 mg/kg.

**Formulations** Injection: 12.5 mg/mL (5 mL ampules)

**Dosing**

**Adults:**

- Test dose (recommended): 2 mL diluted in 50 mL 0.9% sodium chloride over 60 minutes
- Repletion of iron in hemodialysis patients: I.V.: 125 mg (10 mL) in 100 mL 0.9% sodium chloride over 1 hour during hemodialysis. Most patients will require a cumulative dose of 1 g elemental iron over approximately 8 sequential dialysis treatments to achieve a favorable response.

**Elderly:** Refer to adult dosing.

**Administration**

**I.V.:** Dilute prior to administration; avoid rapid administration. Infusion rate should not exceed 2.1 mg/minute. Monitor patient for hypotension or hypersensitivity reactions during infusion.

**Monitoring Laboratory Tests** Hemoglobin and hematocrit, serum ferritin, iron saturation

**Additional Nursing Issues**

**Physical Assessment:** Assess effectiveness and interactions of other medications (see Drug Interactions). Monitor results of test dose (see Dosage), infusion rate, effectiveness of therapy (Laboratory results), and adverse reactions at beginning of therapy and periodically during therapy (see Adverse Reactions, laboratory monitoring, and Overdose/Toxicology). Assess knowledge/teach patient adverse symptoms to report. Note breast-feeding caution.

**Patient Information/Instruction:** This medication will be administered by I.V. in conjunction with your dialysis treatment. Report at once chest pain, rapid heart beat, or palpitations; difficulty breathing; headache dizziness, agitation, or inability to sleep; nausea, vomiting, abdominal or flank pain; or skin rash, itching, or redness. **Breast-feeding precautions:** Consult prescriber if breast-feeding.

**Additional Information** The total body iron content normally ranges from 2-4 g of elemental iron. Contains benzyl alcohol 9 mg/mL.

- **Ferrlecit®** *see* Ferric Gluconate *on previous page*
- **Ferromar®** *see page 1294*
- **Ferro-Sequels® [OTC]** *see* Iron Supplements *on page 627*
- **Ferrous Fumarate** *see* Iron Supplements *on page 627*
- **Ferrous Gluconate** *see* Iron Supplements *on page 627*
- **Ferrous Salt and Ascorbic Acid** *see page 1294*
- **Ferrous Salts** *see* Iron Supplements *on page 627*
- **Ferrous Sulfate** *see* Iron Supplements *on page 627*
- **Ferrous Sulfate, Ascorbic Acid, Vitamin B Complex, and Folic Acid** *see page 1306*
- **Fertinorm® H.P.** *see* Urofollitropin *on page 1195*
- **Ferval® Ferroso** *see* Iron Supplements *on page 627*
- **$FeSO_4$ (Ferrous Sulfate)** *see* Iron Supplements *on page 627*
- **Feverall™ [OTC]** *see* Acetaminophen *on page 32*
- **Fever Due to Drugs** *see page 1344*


## Fexofenadine (feks oh FEN a deen)

**U.S. Brand Names** Allegra®

**Therapeutic Category** Antihistamine

**Pregnancy Risk Factor** C

**Lactation** Excretion in breast milk unknown/contraindicated

**Use** Antihistamine indicated for the relief of seasonal allergic rhinitis

**Mechanism of Action/Effect** Fexofenadine is an active metabolite of terfenadine and like terfenadine it competes with histamine for $H_1$-receptor sites on effector cells in the GI tract, blood vessels, and respiratory tract; binds to lung receptors significantly greater than it binds to cerebellar receptors, resulting in a greatly reduced sedative potential

**Contraindications** Hypersensitivity to fexofenadine or any component

**Warnings** Fexofenadine and ketoconazole have been shown to increase peak plasma concentrations of fexofenadine, although this increase has not led to Q-$T_c$ prolongation or cardiac arrhythmias. Pregnancy factor C.

**Drug Interactions**

**Cytochrome P-450 Effect:** CYP3A3/4 enzyme substrate

**Increased Effect/Toxicity:** Erythromycin and ketoconazole increased the $C_{max,ss}$ and $AUC_{ss}$ of fexofenadine when given concomitantly; however, neither drug significantly affected adverse events or Q-$T_c$ intervals. The mechanism of action is unknown and the effect on other macrolide agents or azoles have not been investigated.

**Adverse Reactions** 1% to 10%:

Central nervous system: Drowsiness (1.3%), fatigue (1.3%)
Endocrine & metabolic: Dysmenorrhea (1.5%)
Gastrointestinal: Nausea (1.6%), heartburn (1.3%)
Miscellaneous: Viral infection (cold, flu) (2.5%)

**Overdose/Toxicology** Limited information from overdose describes dizziness, drowsiness, and dry mouth. Not effectively removed by hemodialysis. Doses up to 690 mg twice daily were administered for 1 month without significant adverse effects. Treatment is supportive.

**Pharmacodynamics/Kinetics**

**Half-life Elimination:** 14.4 hours

**Time to Peak:** Plasma concentration: ~2.6 hours after oral administration

**Metabolism:** ~5% mostly by gut flora; only 0.5% to 1.5% metabolized by cytochrome P-450 enzymes

**Excretion:** Primarily in feces (~80%) and in urine (~11%) as unchanged drug

**Onset:** 1 hour

**Duration:** Antihistaminic effect: At least 12 hours

**Formulations** Capsule, hydrochloride: 60 mg

**Dosing**

**Adults:** Oral: 1 capsule (60 mg) twice daily

**Elderly:** Starting dose: 60 mg once daily; adjust for renal impairment.

**Renal Impairment:** $Cl_{cr}$ <40 mL/minute: 60 mg once daily; not effectively removed by hemodialysis

**Stability**

**Storage:** Capsules should be stored at controlled room temperature 20°C to 25°C and protected from excessive moisture.

**Additional Nursing Issues**

**Physical Assessment:** Assess effectiveness and interactions of other medications (see Drug Interactions above). Monitor effectiveness of therapy and adverse reactions (see Adverse Reactions) at beginning of therapy and periodically with long-term use. Assess knowledge/teach patient appropriate use, interventions to reduce side effects, and adverse symptoms to report. **Pregnancy risk factor C** - benefits of use should outweigh possible risks. Breast-feeding is contraindicated.

**Patient Information/Instruction:** Take as directed; do not exceed recommended dose. Store at room temperature in a dry place. Avoid use of other depressants, alcohol, or sleep-inducing medications unless approved by prescriber. You may experience mild drowsiness or dizziness (use caution when driving or engaging in tasks requiring alertness until response to drug is known); or nausea (frequent small meals, frequent mouth care, chewing gum, or sucking hard candy may help). Report persistent sedation or drowsiness, menstrual irregularities, or lack of improvement or worsening or condition. **Pregnancy/breast-feeding precautions:** Inform prescriber if you are or intend to be pregnant. Do not breast-feed.

**Geriatric Considerations:** Plasma levels in the elderly are generally higher than those observed in other age groups. Once daily dosing is recommended when starting therapy in elderly patients or patients with decreased renal function.

- **Fiberall® Chewable Tablet** *see page 1294*
- **Fiberall® Powder [OTC]** *see* Psyllium *on page 993*
- **Fiberall® Wafer [OTC]** *see* Psyllium *on page 993*
- **FiberCon® Tablet** *see page 1294*
- **Fiber-Lax® Tablet** *see page 1294*
- **Fibrepur®** *see* Psyllium *on page 993*

## Fibrinolysin and Desoxyribonuclease

(fye brin oh LYE sin & des oks i rye boe NOO klee ase)

**U.S. Brand Names** Elase-Chloromycetin® Topical; Elase® Topical

**Synonyms** Desoxyribonuclease and Fibrinolysin

**Therapeutic Category** Enzyme

**Pregnancy Risk Factor** C

**Lactation** Excretion in breast milk unknown

**Use** Debriding agent; cervicitis; and irrigating agent in infected wounds

**Formulations**

Ointment, topical:

Elase®: Fibrinolysin 1 unit and desoxyribonuclease 666.6 units per g (10 g, 30 g)

Elase-Chloromycetin®: Fibrinolysin 1 unit and desoxyribonuclease 666.6 units per g with chloramphenicol 10 mg per g (10 g, 30 g)

Powder, dry: Fibrinolysin 25 units and desoxyribonuclease 15,000 units per 30 g

**Dosing**

**Adults:**

Ointment: 2-3 times/day

Wet dressing: 3-4 times/day

**Elderly:** Refer to adult dosing.

## Filgrastim (fil GRA stim)

**U.S. Brand Names** Neupogen® Injection

**Synonyms** G-CSF; Granulocyte Colony Stimulating Factor

**Therapeutic Category** Colony Stimulating Factor

**Pregnancy Risk Factor** C

**Lactation** Excretion in breast milk unknown

**Use**

Patients with nonmyeloid malignancies receiving myelosuppressive anticancer drugs associated with a significant incidence of neutropenia (FDA-approved indication)

Bone marrow transplant - to reduce the duration of neutropenia and neutropenia-related clinical sequelae in patients with nonmyeloid malignancies undergoing myeloablative chemotherapy followed by marrow transplantation (FDA-approved indication)

Severe chronic neutropenia - chronic administration to reduce the incidence and duration of sequelae of neutropenia in symptomatic patients with congenital neutropenia, cyclic neutropenia or idiopathic neutropenia (FDA-approved indication)

**Unlabeled use:** AIDS, aplastic anemia, hairy cell leukemia, myelodysplasia

**Mechanism of Action/Effect** Stimulates the production, maturation, and activation of neutrophils, G-CSF activates neutrophils to increase both their migration and cytotoxicity. Natural proteins which stimulate hematopoietic stem cells to proliferate, prolong cell survival, stimulate cell differentiation, and stimulate functional activity of mature cells. CSFs are produced by a wide variety of cell types. Specific mechanisms of action are not yet fully understood, but possibly work by a second-messenger pathway with resultant protein production. See table.

| Proliferation/Differentiation | G-CSF (Filgrastim) | GM-CSF (Sargramostim) |
|---|---|---|
| Neutrophils | Yes | Yes |
| Eosinophils | No | Yes |
| Macrophages | No | Yes |
| Neutrophil migration | Enhanced | Inhibited |

**Contraindications** Hypersensitivity to *E. coli*-derived proteins or G-CSF

**Warnings** Complete blood count and platelet count should be obtained prior to chemotherapy. Do not use G-CSF in the period 24 hours before to 24 hours after administration of cytotoxic chemotherapy because of the potential sensitivity of rapidly dividing myeloid cells to cytotoxic chemotherapy. Precaution should be exercised in the usage of G-CSF in any malignancy with myeloid characteristics. G-CSF can potentially act as a growth factor for any tumor type, particularly myeloid malignancies. Tumors of nonhematopoietic origin may have surface receptors for G-CSF. Pregnancy factor C.

**Adverse Reactions** Effects are generally mild and dose related

>10%:

Central nervous system: Neutropenic fever, fever

Dermatologic: Alopecia

(Continued)

## Filgrastim *(Continued)*

Gastrointestinal: Nausea, vomiting, diarrhea, mucositis,

Splenomegaly: This occurs more commonly in patients with cyclic neutropenia/congenital agranulocytosis who received S.C. injections for a prolonged (>14 days) period of time; ~33% of these patients experience subclinical splenomegaly (detected by MRI or CT scan); ~3% of these patients experience clinical splenomegaly

Neuromuscular & skeletal: Medullary bone pain (24% incidence): This occurs most commonly in lower back pain, posterior iliac crest, and sternum and is controlled with non-narcotic analgesics

1% to 10%:

Cardiovascular: Chest pain, fluid retention

Central nervous system: Headache

Dermatologic: Skin rash

Gastrointestinal: Anorexia, stomatitis, constipation

Hematologic: Leukocytosis

Local: Pain at injection site

Neuromuscular & skeletal: Weakness

Respiratory: Dyspnea, cough, sore throat

<1% (Limited to important or life-threatening symptoms): Transient supraventricular arrhythmia, pericarditis, thrombophlebitis

**Overdose/Toxicology** No clinical adverse effects have been seen with high doses producing ANC >10,000/mm$^3$. After discontinuing the drug there is a 50% decrease in circulating levels of neutrophils within 1-2 days, and return to pretreatment levels within 1-7 days.

**Pharmacodynamics/Kinetics**

**Distribution:** No evidence of drug accumulation over a 11- to 20-day period

**Half-life Elimination:** 1.8-3.5 hours

**Time to Peak:** S.C.: Within 2-6 hours

**Metabolism:** Systemically

**Onset:** Rapid elevation in neutrophil counts within the first 24 hours, reaching a plateau in 3-5 days

**Duration:** ANC decreases by 50% within 2 days after discontinuing G-CSF; white counts return to the normal range in 4-7 days

**Formulations** Injection, preservative free: 300 mcg/mL (1 mL, 1.6 mL)

**Dosing**

**Adults:** Administered S.C. or I.V. as a single daily infusion over 20-30 minutes.

**Myelosuppressive chemotherapy** 5 mcg/kg/day S.C. or I.V.

Doses may be increased in increments of 5 mcg/kg for each chemotherapy cycle, according to the duration and severity of the absolute neutrophil count (ANC) nadir. In Phase III trials, efficacy was observed at doses of 4-6 mcg/kg/day. Discontinue therapy if the ANC count is >10,000/mm$^3$ after the ANC nadir has occurred following the expected chemotherapy-induced neutrophil nadir. Some cancer centers are stopping therapy at an ANC of 2500/mm$^3$. Duration of therapy needed to attenuate chemotherapy-induced neutropenia may be dependent on the myelosuppressive potential of the chemotherapy regimen employed. Duration of therapy in clinical studies has ranged from 2 weeks to 3 years.

**Bone marrow transplant patient:** 10 mcg/kg/day as an I.V. infusion of 4 or 24 hours or as continuous 24-hour S.C. infusion. Administer first dose at least 24 hours after cytotoxic chemotherapy and at least 24 hours after bone marrow infusion.

**Filgrastim Dose Based on Neutrophil Response**

| Absolute Neutrophil Count | Filgrastim Dose Adjustment |
|---|---|
| When ANC >1000/mm$^3$ for 3 consecutive days | Reduce to 5 mcg/kg/day |
| If ANC remains >1000/mm$^3$ for 3 more consecutive days | Discontinue filgrastim |
| If ANC decreases to <1000/mm$^3$ | Resume at 5 mcg/kg/day |

**Severe chronic neutropenia:**

Congenital neutropenia: 6 mcg/kg twice daily S.C.

Idiopathic/cyclic neutropenia: 5 mcg/kg/day S.C.

Chronic daily administration is required to maintain clinical benefit. Adjust dose based on the patients' clinical course as well as ANC. In Phase III studies, the target ANC was 1500-10,000/mm$^3$. Reduce the dose if the ANC is persistently >10,000/mm$^3$.

Premature discontinuation of G-CSF therapy prior to the time of recovery from the expected neutrophil is generally not recommended. A transient increase in neutrophil counts is typically seen 1-2 days after initiation of therapy.

**Elderly:** Refer to adult dosing.

**Administration**

**I.V.:** May be administered undiluted by S.C. or IVP administration. May also be administered by I.V. infusion over 15-60 minutes in $D_5W$.

**Stability**

**Storage:** Filgrastim is a clear, colorless solution and should be stored under refrigeration at 2°C to 8°C (36°F to 46°F) and protected from direct sunlight. Filgrastim should be protected from freezing and temperatures >30°C to avoid aggregation. The solution should not be shaken since bubbles and/or foam may form. If foaming occurs, the solution should be left undisturbed for a few minutes until bubbles dissipate.

Filgrastim is stable for 24 hours at 9°C to 30°C, however, the manufacturer recommends discarding after 6 hours because of microbiological concerns. The product is packaged as single-use vial without a preservative.

Undiluted filgrastim is stable for 24 hours at 15°C to 30°C and 7 days at 2°C to 8°C in tuberculin syringes. However, refrigeration and use within 24 hours are recommended because of concern for bacterial contamination.

**Reconstitution:** Filgrastim may be diluted in dextrose 5% in water to a concentration ≥15 mcg/mL for I.V. infusion administration. Minimum concentration is 15 mcg/mL Concentrations <15 mcg/mL require addition of albumin (1 mL of 5%) to the bag to prevent absorption to plastics/PVC. This diluted solution is stable for 7 days under refrigeration or at room temperature.

**Compatibility:** Standard diluent: ≥375 mcg/25 mL $D_5W$. Filgrastim is incompatible with 0.9% sodium chloride (normal saline).

**Monitoring Laboratory Tests** CBC and platelet count should be obtained twice weekly. Leukocytosis (white blood cell counts ≥100,000/$mm^3$) has been observed in ~2% of patients receiving G-CSF at doses >5 mcg/kg/day. Monitor platelets and hematocrit regularly.

**Additional Nursing Issues**

**Physical Assessment:** Assess for hypersensitivity to *E. coli* products. Monitor laboratory results. Monitor adverse effects and teach patient adverse effects to monitor and symptoms to report. Assess knowledge/teach patient or caregiver proper storage and administration of medication (see above) and proper disposal of needles and syringes. **Pregnancy risk factor C** - benefits of use should outweigh possible risks. Note breast-feeding caution.

**Patient Information/Instruction:** Follow directions for proper storage and administration of S.C. medication. Never reuse syringes or needles. You may experience bone pain (request analgesic); nausea or vomiting (small frequent meals may help); hair loss (reversible); or sore mouth (frequent mouth care with soft toothbrush or cotton swab may help). Report unusual fever or chills; unhealed sores; severe bone pain; pain, redness, or swelling at injection site; unusual swelling of extremities or difficulty breathing; or chest pain and palpitations. **Pregnancy/breast-feeding precautions:** Inform prescriber if you are or intend to be pregnant. Consult prescriber if breast-feeding.

**Additional Information**

Reimbursement Hotline: 1-800-272-9376

Professional Services [AMGEN]: 1-800-77-AMGEN

♦ **Filibon® [OTC]** *see* Vitamin, Multiple *on page 1219*

## Finasteride (fi NAS teer ide)

**U.S. Brand Names** Propecia®; Proscar®

**Therapeutic Category** Antiandrogen

**Pregnancy Risk Factor** X

**Lactation** Not indicated for use in women

**Use**

Propecia®: Treatment of male pattern hair loss in **men only**. Safety and efficacy were demonstrated in men between 18-41 years of age.

Proscar®: Treatment of symptomatic benign prostatic hyperplasia (BPH)

**Unlabeled use:** Adjuvant monotherapy after radical prostatectomy in the treatment of prostatic cancer

**Mechanism of Action/Effect** Finasteride is a 4-azo analog of testosterone and is a competitive inhibitor of both tissue and hepatic 5-alpha reductase. This results in inhibition of the conversion of testosterone to dihydrotestosterone and markedly suppresses serum dihydrotestosterone levels. Depending on dose and duration, serum testosterone concentrations may or may not increase. Testosterone-dependent processes such as fertility, muscle strength, potency, and libido are not affected by finasteride.

**Contraindications** Hypersensitivity to finasteride; pregnancy; children

**Warnings** A minimum of 6 months of treatment may be necessary to determine whether an individual will respond to finasteride. Use with caution in those patients with liver function abnormalities. Carefully monitor patients with a large residual urinary volume or severely diminished urinary flow for obstructive uropathy. These patients may not be candidates for finasteride therapy.

**Drug Interactions**

**Cytochrome P-450 Effect:** CYP3A3/4 enzyme substrate

**Adverse Reactions** 1% to 10%:

Endocrine & metabolic: Decreased libido

Genitourinary: Impotence, decreased volume of ejaculate

**Pharmacodynamics/Kinetics**

**Protein Binding:** 90%

**Half-life Elimination:**

Half-life, serum: Parent drug: ~5-17 hours (mean: 1.9 fasting, 4.2 with breakfast)

Half-life: Adults: 6 hours (3-16); Elderly: 8 hours

**Time to Peak:** Oral: 2-6 hours

**Metabolism:** Unchanged finasteride is major circulating component; two active metabolites have been identified.

(Continued)

## Finasteride *(Continued)*

**Excretion:** Urine and feces; elimination rate decreased in the elderly

**Onset:** Onset of clinical effect: Within 12 weeks to 6 months of ongoing therapy

**Duration:**

After a single oral dose as small as 0.5 mg: 65% depression of plasma dihydrotestosterone levels persists 5-7 days.

After 6 months of treatment with 5 mg/day: Circulating dihydrotestosterone levels are reduced to castrate levels without significant effects on circulating testosterone. Levels return to normal within 14 days of discontinuation of treatment.

**Formulations**

Tablet, film coated:

Propecia®: 1 mg

Proscar®: 5 mg

**Dosing**

**Adults:** Oral:

Proscar®: Benign prostatic hyperplasia: 5 mg/day as a single dose; clinical responses occur within 12 weeks to 6 months of initiation of therapy. Long-term administration is recommended for maximal response.

Propecia®: 1 mg daily

**Elderly:** Refer to adult dosing.

**Administration**

**Oral:** Administration with food may delay the rate and reduce the extent of oral absorption.

**Additional Nursing Issues**

**Physical Assessment:** See Warnings/Precautions and Contraindications for use cautions. Monitor effectiveness of therapy and adverse response (see Adverse Reactions). Assess knowledge/teach patient appropriate use, possible side effects and adverse symptoms to report. **Pregnancy risk factor X** - instruct patient on absolute need for barrier contraceptives. Childbearing age women should not touch or handle this medication.

**Patient Information/Instruction:** Results of therapy may take several months. Take as directed, with fluids, 30 minutes before or 2 hours after meals. You may experience decreased libido or impotence during therapy. Report any increase in urinary volume or voiding patterns occurs. **Pregnancy precautions:** This drug will cause fetal abnormalities - use barrier contraceptives and do not allow childbearing age women to touch or handle drug.

**Geriatric Considerations:** Clearance of finasteride is decreased in the elderly, but no dosage reductions are necessary.

**Additional Information**

Proscar®: Finasteride may be useful in men with moderately symptomatic BPH who either refuse a TURP, prostatectomy, or are poor surgical candidates. Risk to benefit ratio and cost must be explained to the patient. Currently, there is not way to predict which men will respond to finasteride. A recent study found finasteride to be no more effective than placebo in men with BPH. When added to terazosin (an alpha antagonist), the combination was no more effective than terazosin alone.

Propecia®: Daily use for 3 or more months is necessary before benefit is observed. Withdrawal of treatment leads to reversal of effect within 12 months.

- **Fiorgen PF®** *see* Butalbital Compound and Aspirin *on page 176*
- **Fioricet®** *see* Butalbital Compound and Acetaminophen *on page 175*
- **Fiorinal®** *see* Butalbital Compound and Aspirin *on page 176*
- **Fiorinal®-C ¼, ½** *see* Butalbital Compound and Codeine *on page 177*
- **Fiorinal® With Codeine** *see* Butalbital Compound and Codeine *on page 177*
- **Fisalamine** *see* Mesalamine *on page 727*
- **Fisopred®** *see* Prednisolone *on page 960*
- **FK506** *see* Tacrolimus *on page 1093*
- **Flagenase®** *see* Metronidazole *on page 763*
- **Flagyl® Oral** *see* Metronidazole *on page 763*
- **Flamazine®** *see* Silver Sulfadiazine *on page 1059*
- **Flamicina** *see* Ampicillin *on page 90*
- **Flanax** *see* Naproxen *on page 807*
- **Flarex®** *see* Fluorometholone *on page 499*
- **Flatulex®** *see page 1294*
- **Flavorcee® [OTC]** *see* Ascorbic Acid *on page 108*

## Flavoxate (fla VOKS ate)

**U.S. Brand Names** Urispas®

**Therapeutic Category** Antispasmodic Agent, Urinary

**Pregnancy Risk Factor** B

**Lactation** Excretion in breast milk unknown

**Use** Antispasmodic used to provide symptomatic relief of dysuria, nocturia, suprapubic pain, urgency, and incontinence

**Mechanism of Action/Effect** Exerts a direct relaxant effect on smooth muscles via phosphodiesterase inhibition, providing relief to a variety of smooth muscle spasms; it is especially useful for the treatment of bladder spasticity, whereby it produces an increase in urinary capacity

**Contraindications** Pyloric or duodenal obstruction, GI hemorrhage, GI obstruction, obstructive uropathies of the lower urinary tract

**Warnings** May cause drowsiness, vertigo, and ocular disturbances. Give cautiously in patients with suspected glaucoma.

**Adverse Reactions**

>10%:

Central nervous system: Drowsiness

Gastrointestinal: Dry mouth, dry throat

1% to 10%:

Cardiovascular: Tachycardia, palpitations,

Central nervous system: Nervousness, fatigue, vertigo, headache, hyperpyrexia

Gastrointestinal: Constipation, nausea, vomiting

<1% (Limited to important or life-threatening symptoms): Confusion (especially in the elderly), leukopenia, increased intraocular pressure

**Overdose/Toxicology** Symptoms of overdose include clumsiness, dizziness, drowsiness, flushing, hallucinations, and irritability. Treatment is supportive.

**Pharmacodynamics/Kinetics**

**Metabolism:** To methyl; flavone carboxylic acid active

**Excretion:** Urine

**Onset:** 55-60 minutes

**Formulations** Tablet, film coated, as hydrochloride: 100 mg

**Dosing**

**Adults:** Oral: 100-200 mg 3-4 times/day; reduce the dose when symptoms improve

**Elderly:** Refer to adult dosing.

**Administration**

**Oral:** Should be administered with water on an empty stomach.

**Additional Nursing Issues**

**Physical Assessment:** See Contraindications and Warnings/Precautions for use cautions. Assess kidney function, voiding pattern, incontinent episodes, frequency, urgency/retention, and ophthalmic assessment for glaucoma prior to starting therapy and periodically with long-term therapy. Assess knowledge/teach patient appropriate use, possible side effects/interventions, and adverse symptoms to report. Note breast-feeding caution.

**Patient Information/Instruction:** Take exactly as directed, with water, preferably on an empty stomach (1 hour before or 2 hours after meals). Do not use alcohol or OTC medications without consulting prescriber. You may experience mild drowsiness, nervousness, or dizziness (use caution when driving or engaging in tasks requiring alertness until response to drug is known); nausea, vomiting, dry mouth (small frequent meals, frequent oral care, chewing gum, or sucking hard candy may help); decreased ability to perspire (avoid extremes of heat); constipation (increased exercise or dietary fluid and fiber may help). Report vision changes (blurred vision); rapid heartbeat; or unresolved nausea, vomiting, or constipation. **Breast-feeding precautions:** Consult prescriber if breast-feeding.

**Geriatric Considerations:** Caution should be used in the elderly due to anticholinergic activity (eg, confusion, constipation, blurred vision, and tachycardia).

♦ **Flebocortid [Sodium Succinate]** *see* Hydrocortisone *on page 578*

## Flecainide (fle KAY nide)

**U.S. Brand Names** Tambocor™

**Therapeutic Category** Antiarrhythmic Agent, Class I-C

**Pregnancy Risk Factor** C

**Lactation** Enters breast milk/compatible

**Use** Prevention and suppression of documented life-threatening ventricular arrhythmias (eg, sustained ventricular tachycardia); controlling symptomatic, disabling supraventricular tachycardias in patients without structural heart disease in whom other agents fail

**Mechanism of Action/Effect** Class I-C antiarrhythmic; slows conduction in cardiac tissue by altering transport of ions across cell membranes; causes slight prolongation of refractory periods; decreases the rate of rise of the action potential without affecting its duration; increases electrical stimulation threshold of ventricle, HIS-Purkinje system; possesses local anesthetic and moderate negative inotropic effects

**Contraindications** Hypersensitivity to flecainide or any component; pre-existing second or third degree A-V block; right bundle-branch block associated with left hemiblock (bifascicular block) or trifascicular block; cardiogenic shock, myocardial depression

**Warnings** Pre-existing sinus node dysfunction, sick-sinus syndrome, history of congestive heart failure or myocardial dysfunction; increases in P-R interval ≥300 MS, QRS ≥180 MS, Q-$T_c$ interval increases, and/or new bundle-branch block; patients with pacemakers, renal impairment, and/or hepatic impairment.

The manufacturer and FDA recommend that this drug be reserved for life-threatening ventricular arrhythmias unresponsive to conventional therapy. Its use for symptomatic nonsustained ventricular tachycardia, frequent premature ventricular complexes (PVCs), unifocal and multifocal PVCs and/or coupled PVCs is no longer recommended. Flecainide can worsen or cause arrhythmias with an associated risk of death. Proarrhythmic effects range from an increased number of PVCs to more severe ventricular tachycardias (eg, tachycardias that are more sustained or more resistant to conversion to sinus rhythm).

Pregnancy factor C.

(Continued)

## Flecainide *(Continued)*

**Drug Interactions**

**Cytochrome P-450 Effect:** CYP2D6 enzyme substrate

**Decreased Effect:** Smoking and acid urine increase flecainide clearance.

**Increased Effect/Toxicity:** Digoxin, amiodarone may increase plasma concentrations. Beta-adrenergic blockers, disopyramide, verapamil may enhance negative inotropic effects. Alkalinizing agents (ie, high-dose antacids, cimetidine, carbonic anhydrase inhibitors or sodium bicarbonate) may decrease flecainide clearance.

**Food Interactions** Clearance may be decreased in patients following strict vegetarian diets due to urinary pH ≥8.

**Adverse Reactions**

>10%:

Central nervous system: Dizziness or lightheadedness

Ocular: Visual disturbances

1% to 10%:

Cardiovascular: Palpitations, chest pain, edema, tachycardia, bradycardia, heart block, increased P-R, QRS duration, worsening ventricular arrhythmias, congestive heart failure

Central nervous system: Headache, fatigue, fever, nervousness, hypoesthesia

Dermatologic: Rash

Gastrointestinal: Nausea, anorexia, constipation, abdominal pain

Neuromuscular & skeletal: Tremor, weakness, paresthesia

Respiratory: Dyspnea

<1% (Limited to important or life-threatening symptoms): Possible hepatic dysfunction

**Overdose/Toxicology** Flecainide has a narrow therapeutic index and severe toxicity may occur slightly above the therapeutic range, especially if combined with other antiarrhythmic drugs. (Acute single ingestion of twice the daily therapeutic dose is life-threatening). Symptoms of overdose include increase in P-R, QRS, or Q-T intervals and amplitude of the T wave, A-V block, bradycardia, hypotension, ventricular arrhythmias (monomorphic or polymorphic ventricular tachycardia), and asystole. Other symptoms include dizziness, blurred vision, headache, and GI upset. Treatment is supportive.

**Pharmacodynamics/Kinetics**

**Protein Binding:** 40% to 50% ($alpha_1$ glycoprotein)

**Half-life Elimination:** 7-22 hours, increased with congestive heart failure or renal dysfunction; End-stage renal disease: 19-26 hours

**Time to Peak:** Within 1.5-3 hours

**Metabolism:** Liver

**Excretion:** Urine

**Formulations** Tablet, as acetate: 50 mg, 100 mg, 150 mg

**Dosing**

**Adults:** Oral:

Life-threatening ventricular arrhythmias:

Initial: 100 mg every 12 hours

Increase by 50-100 mg/day (given in 2 doses/day) every 4 days; maximum: 400 mg/day

For patients receiving 400 mg/day who are not controlled and have trough concentrations <0.6 μg/mL, dosage may be increased to 600 mg/day.

Prevention of paroxysmal supraventricular arrhythmias in patients with disabling symptoms but no structural heart disease:

Initial: 50 mg every 12 hours

Increase by 50 mg twice daily at 4-day intervals; maximum: 300 mg/day

**Elderly:** Refer to adult dosing.

**Renal Impairment:**

$Cl_{cr}$ <10 mL/minute: Decrease usual dose by 25% to 50% in severe renal impairment.

Not dialyzable (0% to 5%) via hemo- or peritoneal dialysis; no supplemental dose is necessary.

**Hepatic Impairment:** Monitoring of plasma levels is recommended because half-life is significantly increased. When transferring from another antiarrhythmic agent, allow for 2-4 half-lives of the agent to pass before initiating flecainide therapy.

**Administration**

**Oral:** Administer around-the-clock to promote less variation in peak and trough serum levels.

**Monitoring Laboratory Tests** Periodic serum concentrations, especially in patients with renal or hepatic impairment

**Additional Nursing Issues**

**Physical Assessment:** Assess other medications patient may be taking for effectiveness and interactions (see Drug Interactions). See Warnings/Precautions and Contraindications for cautious use. Monitor laboratory tests (see above), therapeutic response (cardiac status), and adverse reactions (see Warnings/Precautions and Adverse Reactions) when beginning therapy, when titrating dosage, and periodically during long-term therapy. **Note:** Flecainide has a low toxic:therapeutic ratio and overdose may easily produce severe and life-threatening reactions (see Overdose/Toxicology). Assess knowledge/teach patient appropriate use, interventions to reduce side effects, and adverse symptoms to report. **Pregnancy risk factor C** - benefits of use should outweigh possible risks.

**Patient Information/Instruction:** Take exactly as directed, around-the-clock. Do not discontinue without consulting prescriber. You will require frequent monitoring while taking this medication. You may experience lightheadedness, nervousness, dizziness, visual disturbances (use caution when driving or engaging in tasks requiring alertness until response to drug is known); or nausea, vomiting, or loss of appetite (small frequent meals may help). Report palpitations, chest pain, excessively slow or rapid heartbeat; acute nervousness, headache, or fatigue; unusual weight gain; unusual cough; difficulty breathing; swelling of hands or ankles; or muscle tremor, numbness, or weakness. **Pregnancy precautions:** Inform prescriber if you are or intend to be pregnant.

**Related Information**

Antiarrhythmic Drug Classification Comparison *on page 1366*

- **Fleet® Babylax® Rectal** *see page 1294*
- **Fleet® Enema [OTC]** *see* Phosphate Supplements *on page 926*
- **Fleet® Enema** *see page 1294*
- **Fleet® Flavored Castor Oil** *see page 1294*
- **Fleet® Laxative** *see page 1294*
- **Fleet® Mineral Oil Enema** *see page 1294*
- **Fleet® Pain Relief** *see page 1294*
- **Fleet® Phospho®-Soda [OTC]** *see* Phosphate Supplements *on page 926*
- **Fleet® Phospho®-Soda** *see page 1294*
- **Flemoxon** *see* Amoxicillin *on page 80*
- **Flexaphen®** *see* Chlorzoxazone *on page 261*
- **Flexen** *see* Naproxen *on page 807*
- **Flexeril®** *see* Cyclobenzaprine *on page 312*
- **Flodine®** *see* Folic Acid *on page 515*
- **Flogen** *see* Naproxen *on page 807*
- **Flogosan®** *see* Piroxicam *on page 940*
- **Flolan® Injection** *see* Epoprostenol *on page 428*
- **Flomax®** *see* Tamsulosin *on page 1097*
- **Flonase®** *see* Fluticasone *on page 511*
- **Florical® [OTC]** *see* Calcium Supplements *on page 185*
- **Florinef® Acetate** *see* Fludrocortisone *on page 495*
- **Florone®** *see* Topical Corticosteroids *on page 1152*
- **Florone E®** *see* Topical Corticosteroids *on page 1152*
- **Floropryl® Ophthalmic** *see* Ophthalmic Agents, Glaucoma *on page 853*
- **Florvite®** *see* Vitamin, Multiple *on page 1219*
- **Flovent®** *see* Fluticasone *on page 511*
- **Floxacin®** *see* Norfloxacin *on page 837*
- **Floxil** *see* Ofloxacin *on page 847*
- **Floxin®** *see* Ofloxacin *on page 847*
- **Floxin®** *see page 1291*
- **Floxstat** *see* Ofloxacin *on page 847*

## Floxuridine (floks YOOR i deen)

**U.S. Brand Names** FUDR®

**Synonyms** Fluorodeoxyuridine

**Therapeutic Category** Antineoplastic Agent, Antimetabolite

**Pregnancy Risk Factor** D

**Lactation** Excretion in breast milk unknown/contraindicated

**Use** Palliative management of carcinomas of head, neck, and brain as well as liver, gallbladder, and bile ducts; treatment of GI adenocarcinoma metastatic to the liver

**Contraindications** Poor nutritional status; depressed (leukocyte count <5000/mm$^3$ or platelet count <100,000/mm$^3$); bone marrow function; potentially serious infections; pregnancy

**Warnings** The U.S. Food and Drug Administration (FDA) currently recommends that procedures for proper handling and disposal of antineoplastic agents be considered.

Impaired kidney or liver function; the drug should be discontinued if intractable vomiting or diarrhea, precipitous fall in leukocyte or platelet counts, or myocardial ischemia occur.

Use with caution in patients who have had high-dose pelvic radiation or previous use of alkylating agents. Patient should be hospitalized during initial course of therapy.

Use of floxuridine with pentastatin has been associated with a high incidence of fatal pulmonary toxicity; this combination is not recommended.

Floxuridine preparation should be performed in a Class II laminar flow biologic safety cabinet. Personnel should be wearing surgical gloves and a closed front surgical gown with knit cuffs. Appropriate safety equipment is recommended for preparation, administration, and disposal of antineoplastics. If floxuridine contacts the skin, wash and flush thoroughly with water.

**Drug Interactions**

**Decreased Effect:** Patients may experience impaired immune response to vaccines; possible infection after administration of live vaccines in patients receiving immunosuppressants.

**Increased Effect/Toxicity:** Any form of therapy which adds to the stress of the patient, interferes with nutrition, or depresses bone marrow function will increase the toxicity of floxuridine. Pentostatin and floxuridine administered together has resulted in fatal pulmonary toxicity.

**Effects on Lab Values** ↑ potassium (S)

(Continued)

## Floxuridine *(Continued)*

**Adverse Reactions**

>10%:

Central nervous system: Fever, chills, fatigue, pain

Gastrointestinal: GI hemorrhage, stomatitis, esophagopharyngitis, diarrhea, gastritis, nausea, vomiting

Hematologic: Severe hematologic toxicity, neutropenia, thrombocytopenia

Respiratory: Pneumonia

1% to 10%:

Cardiovascular: Edema

Central nervous system: Headache

Dermatologic: Alopecia, dermatitis, rash

Gastrointestinal: Anorexia, glossitis

Genitourinary: Dysuria, urinary tract infection, hematuria, proteinuria

Neuromuscular & skeletal: Myalgia, osteonecrosis, arthralgia

Respiratory: Cough, dyspnea, sinusitis, epistaxis, hemoptysis, hypoxia, bronchitis, upper respiratory infection

<1% (Limited to important or life-threatening symptoms): Myocardial ischemia, angina, hepatic necrosis, anaphylaxis

**Pharmacodynamics/Kinetics**

**Half-life Elimination:** As metabolites in the urine and as respiratory carbon dioxide

**Metabolism:** Following infusion of small doses, most of the drug appears to be metabolized in the liver (as 5-FU) to the active metabolite FUDR-MP. Following rapid administration of single doses, the drug appears to be rapidly catabolized to fluorouracil. Metabolic degradation is less when floxuridine is given by continuous infusion than by single injections.

**Formulations**

Injection, preservative free: 100 mg/mL (5 mL)

Powder for injection: 500 mg (5 mL, 10 mL)

**Dosing**

**Adults:** Refer to individual protocols.

Intra-arterial: Primarily by an implantable pump: 0.1-0.6 mg/kg/day continuous intra-arterial administration for 14 days then heparinized saline is given for 14 days; toxicity requires dose reduction.

I.V.: 25 mg/m$^2$ over 30 minutes daily for 5 consecutive days every 28 days; adjust dose based on the level of hematologic toxicity; delay or discontinue floxuridine if neurotoxicity occurs.

**Elderly:** Adjust dose since elderly patients are prone to toxicity.

**Renal Impairment:** Adjust dose relative to toxicity; patients with renal insufficiency are prone to toxicity.

**Administration**

**I.V.:** Infused for intra-arterial use, use infusion pump, either external or implanted.

**Stability**

**Storage:** Store intact vials at room temperature.

**Reconstitution:** Dilute with 5 mL SWI for a final concentration of 100 mg/mL which is stable for 2 weeks under refrigeration (15°C to 30°C). Contains no preservative. Recommend use within 8 hours of reconstitution.

**Compatibility:** Further dilution in 500-1000 mL $D_5W$ or NS is stable for 2 weeks at room temperature.

Compatible with heparin

**Standard I.V. dilution:** Dose (per day)/500-1000 mL $D_5W$ or NS

**Standard Intra-arterial pump dilution:**

14 day dose/60 mL Infusaid®

Stable for 2 weeks at room temperature.

See the Chemotherapy Compatibility Chart *on page 1311*.

**Monitoring Laboratory Tests** White blood count, platelet count

**Additional Nursing Issues**

**Physical Assessment:** Monitor appropriate laboratory tests as ordered (WBC, platelet count). Monitor for signs or symptoms of adverse effects as noted above especially I & O ratio, CNS changes, increased stress level, and acute GI response. Monitor for opportunistic infections (eg, thrush, open unhealed sores, vaginal discharge, foul-smelling pus, itching or burning on urination, fatigue, bone pain, fever). Instruct patient/caregiver in use of implantable pump. **Pregnancy risk factor D** - assess knowledge/teach appropriate use of barrier contraceptives. Advise patient of the need to refrain from breast-feeding (women should use effective contraception during and after treatment with floxuridine; men should use barrier contraceptive methods during and after treatment). Breast-feeding is contraindicated.

**Patient Information/Instruction:** This drug can only be administered by infusion. Follow instructions of prescriber for care of implantable pump. During therapy, do not use alcohol, aspirin-containing products, and OTC medications without consulting prescriber. It is important to maintain adequate nutrition and hydration (2-3 L/day of fluids unless instructed to restrict fluid intake) during therapy; frequent small meals may help. You may experience mild nausea or vomiting (frequent small meals, frequent mouth care, sucking lozenges, or chewing gum may help); you may experience loss of hair (reversible); you will be more susceptible to infection (avoid crowds and exposure to infection as much as possible). Yogurt or buttermilk may help reduce diarrhea. Frequent mouth care and use of a soft toothbrush or cotton swabs may help prevent mouth sores. This drug may cause sterility or birth defects. Increased emotional or physical stress will adversely affect the response to this medication.

Notify prescriber if you are experiencing unusual or elevated levels of stress. Report extreme fatigue, pain or numbness in extremities, severe GI upset or diarrhea, bleeding or bruising, fever, chills, sore throat, vaginal discharge, or signs of fluid retention (eg, swelling extremities, difficulty breathing, unusual weight gain). **Pregnancy/breast-feeding precautions:** Do not get pregnant; use appropriate barrier contraceptive measures. Do not breast-feed while on this drug and for several weeks after last dose. Male: Use barrier contraceptive measures when having intercourse with women of childbearing age. Do not breast-feed.

♦ **Flubenisolone** *see* Betamethasone *on page 148*

## Fluconazole (floo KOE na zole)

**U.S. Brand Names** Diflucan®

**Therapeutic Category** Antifungal Agent, Oral; Antifungal Agent, Parenteral

**Pregnancy Risk Factor** C

**Lactation** Excretion in breast milk unknown/use caution

**Use** Oral fluconazole should be used in persons able to tolerate oral medications. Parenteral fluconazole should be reserved for patients who are both unable to take oral medications and are unable to tolerate amphotericin B (eg, due to hypersensitivity or renal insufficiency).

**Indications for use in adult patient:**

Oral or vaginal candidiasis unresponsive to nystatin or clotrimazole
Nonlife-threatening *Candida* infections (eg, cystitis, esophagitis)
Treatment of hepatosplenic candidiasis
Treatment of certain *Candida* infections in persons unable to tolerate amphotericin B
Treatment of cryptococcal infections
Secondary prophylaxis for cryptococcal meningitis in persons with AIDS
Antifungal prophylaxis in allogenic bone marrow transplant recipients

**Mechanism of Action/Effect** Interferes with cytochrome P-450 activity, decreasing ergosterol synthesis (principal sterol in fungal cell membrane) and inhibiting cell membrane formation

**Contraindications** Hypersensitivity to fluconazole or other azoles

**Warnings** Should be used with caution in patients with renal and hepatic dysfunction or previous hepatotoxicity from other azole derivatives. Patients who develop abnormal liver function tests during fluconazole therapy should be monitored closely and discontinued if symptoms consistent with liver disease develop. Pregnancy factor C.

**Drug Interactions**

**Cytochrome P-450 Effect:** CYP2C9 enzyme inducer; CYP2C9, 2C18, and 2C19 enzyme inhibitor and CYP3A3/4 enzyme inhibitor (weak)

**Decreased Effect:** Rifampin decreases concentrations of fluconazole.

**Increased Effect/Toxicity:** May increase cyclosporine levels when high doses are used. May increase cisapride levels which has been associated with prolonged Q-T intervals and the potential for torsade de pointes. May increase serum concentrations or AUC of phenytoin, theophylline, sulfonylureas, and zidovudine. Fluconazole may also inhibit warfarin metabolism.

**Adverse Reactions**

1% to 10%:

Central nervous system: Headache, dizziness, drowsiness
Dermatologic: Rash
Gastrointestinal: Nausea, vomiting, abdominal pain, diarrhea

<1% (Limited to important or life-threatening symptoms): Exfoliative skin disorders including Stevens-Johnson syndrome, hypokalemia, agranulocytosis, thrombocytopenia, hepatotoxicity (elevated AST, ALT, or alkaline phosphatase)

**Overdose/Toxicology** Symptoms of overdose include decreased lacrimation, salivation, respiration and motility, urinary incontinence, and cyanosis. Treatment includes supportive measures. A 3-hour hemodialysis will remove 50%.

**Pharmacodynamics/Kinetics**

**Protein Binding:** 11% to 12%

**Distribution:** Relative diffusion of antimicrobial agents from blood into CSF:

Adequate with or without inflammation (exceeds usual MICs)
Ratio of CSF to blood level: Normal meninges: 70% to 80%; Inflamed meninges: >80%

**Half-life Elimination:** 25-30 hours with normal renal function

**Time to Peak:** Oral: Within 2-4 hours

**Excretion:** Urine

**Formulations**

Injection: 2 mg/mL (100 mL, 200 mL in glass bottles and PVC bags)
Powder for oral suspension: 10 mg/mL (35 mL); 40 mg/mL (35 mL)
Tablet: 50 mg, 100 mg, 150 mg, 200 mg

**Dosing**

**Adults:** The daily dose of fluconazole is the same for oral and I.V. administration. Fluconazole 800 mg/day has been used for treatment of *Coccidioides immitis* CNS infections.

Oral, I.V.: See table for once daily dosing.

**Elderly:** Refer to adult dosing.

**Renal Impairment:**

$Cl_{cr}$ 21-50 mL/minute: Administer 50% of recommended dose or administer every 48 hours.

$Cl_{cr}$ <20 mL/minute: Administer 25% of recommended dose or administer every 72 hours.

(Continued)

## Fluconazole *(Continued)*

Hemodialysis effects: 50% removed by hemodialysis

Continuous arteriovenous or venovenous hemofiltration (CAVH): Dose as for $Cl_{cr}$ 10-50 mL/minute.

**Administration**

**I.M.:** For I.V. only; do not administer I.M. or S.C.

**I.V.:** Administer maximum rate of infusion: 200 mg/hour.

**I.V. Detail:** Do not use if cloudy or precipitated. Parenteral fluconazole must be administered by I.V. infusion over approximately 1-2 hours.

**Stability**

**Storage:** Fluconazole for injection should be stored between 5°C to 30°C (glass bottles) or 5°C to 25°C (PVC).

**Reconstitution:** Standard diluent: 200 mg/100 mL NS (premixed); 400 mg/200 mL NS (premixed)

**Compatibility:** Incompatible with ampicillin, calcium gluconate, ceftazidime, cefotaxime, cefuroxime, ceftriaxone, clindamycin, furosemide, imipenem, ticarcillin, and piperacillin.

**Monitoring Laboratory Tests** Culture prior to beginning therapy, periodic liver function (AST, ALT, alkaline phosphatase) and renal function, potassium

**Additional Nursing Issues**

**Physical Assessment:** Assess effectiveness and serious interactions of other medications (see Drug Interactions - P-450 inhibitor). See Use, Warnings/Precautions, and Contraindications for use cautions. Monitor effectiveness of therapy and monitor laboratory tests frequently during therapy (see above). Monitor for adverse response (see Warnings/Precautions, Adverse Reactions, and Overdose/Toxicology). Assess knowledge/teach patient possible side effects and appropriate interventions, and adverse symptoms to report. **Pregnancy risk factor C** - benefits of use should outweigh possible risks. Note breast-feeding caution.

**Patient Information/Instruction:** Take as directed, around-the-clock. Take full course of medication as ordered. Follow good hygiene measures to prevent reinfection. Frequent blood tests may be required. Maintain adequate hydration (2-3 L/day of fluids unless instructed to restrict fluid intake). You may experience headache, dizziness, drowsiness (use caution when driving or engaging in tasks that require alertness until response to drug is known); nausea, vomiting, or diarrhea (small frequent meals, frequent mouth care, sucking lozenges, or chewing gum may help). Report skin rash, redness, or irritation; persistent GI upset; urinary pattern changes; excessively dry eyes or mouth; changes in color of stool or urine. **Pregnancy/breast-feeding precautions:** Inform prescriber if you are or intend to be pregnant. Consult prescriber if breast-feeding.

**Geriatric Considerations:** Fluconazole has not been specifically studied in the elderly population. Dose may need adjustment based on changes of renal function.

## Flucytosine (floo SYE toe seen)

**U.S. Brand Names** Ancobon®

**Synonyms** 5-FC; 5-Flurocytosine

**Therapeutic Category** Antifungal Agent, Oral

**Pregnancy Risk Factor** C

**Lactation** Excretion in breast milk unknown/not recommended

**Use** Adjunctive treatment of susceptible fungal infections (usually *Candida* or *Cryptococcus*); in combination with amphotericin B, fluconazole, or itraconazole; synergy with amphotericin B for fungal infections (*Aspergillus*)

**Mechanism of Action/Effect** Penetrates fungal cells and interferes with fungal RNA and protein synthesis

**Contraindications** Hypersensitivity to flucytosine or any component

**Warnings** Use with extreme caution in patients with renal impairment or bone marrow depression. Dosage modification is required in patients with impaired renal function. Pregnancy factor C.

**Drug Interactions**

**Increased Effect/Toxicity:** Increased effect with amphotericin B. Amphotericin B-induced renal dysfunction may predispose patient to flucytosine accumulation and myelosuppression.

**Food Interactions** Food decreases the rate, but not the extent of absorption.

**Effects on Lab Values** Flucytosine causes markedly false elevations in serum creatinine values when the Ektachem® analyzer is used.

**Adverse Reactions**

1% to 10%:

Dermatologic: Rash

Gastrointestinal: Abdominal pain, diarrhea, anorexia, nausea, vomiting

Hematologic: Anemia, leukopenia, thrombocytopenia

Hepatic: Hepatitis, jaundice

<1% (Limited to important or life-threatening symptoms): Cardiac arrest, bone marrow suppression, elevated liver enzymes, respiratory arrest, anaphylaxis

**Overdose/Toxicology** Symptoms of overdose include nausea, vomiting, diarrhea, and bone marrow suppression. Treatment is supportive.

**Pharmacodynamics/Kinetics**

**Protein Binding:** 2% to 4%

**Distribution:** Into CSF and bronchial secretions

**Half-life Elimination:** 3-8 hours; Anuria: May be as long as 200 hours; End-stage renal disease: 75-200 hours

**Time to Peak:** Within 2-6 hours

**Metabolism:** Minimal

**Excretion:** Urine

**Formulations** Capsule: 250 mg, 500 mg

**Dosing**

**Adults:** Oral: 50-150 mg/kg/day in divided doses every 6 hours

**Elderly:** Refer to adult dosing.

**Renal Impairment:**

$Cl_{cr}$ >50 mL/minute: Administer every 12 hours.

$Cl_{cr}$ 10-50 mL/minute: Administer every 16 hours.

$Cl_{cr}$ <10 mL/minute: Administer every 24 hours.

Hemodialysis effects: Dialyzable (50% to 100%); administer dose posthemodialysis. Administer 0.5-1 g every 24 hours during peritoneal dialysis (adults).

Continuous arteriovenous or venovenous hemofiltration (CAVH): Dose as for $Cl_{cr}$ 10-50 mL/minute.

**Administration**

**Oral:** Administer around-the-clock to promote less variation in peak and trough serum levels.

**Stability**

**Storage:** Protect from light.

**Monitoring Laboratory Tests** Culture prior to first dose, serum creatinine, BUN, alkaline phosphatase, AST, ALT, CBC, serum flucytosine concentrations

**Additional Nursing Issues**

**Physical Assessment:** See Warnings/Precautions and Contraindications for use cautions. Monitor effectiveness of therapy and monitor laboratory tests during therapy (see above). Monitor for adverse response (see Adverse Reactions and Overdose/Toxicology). Assess knowledge/teach patient possible side effects and appropriate interventions, and adverse symptoms to report. **Pregnancy risk factor C** - benefits of use should outweigh possible risks. Breast-feeding is not recommended.

**Patient Information/Instruction:** Take capsules one at a time over a few minutes with food to reduce GI upset. Take full course of medication as ordered. Do not discontinue without consulting prescriber. Practice good hygiene measures to prevent reinfection. Frequent blood tests may be required. You may experience nausea and vomiting (small, frequent meals may help). Report rash, respiratory difficulty, CNS changes (eg, confusion, hallucinations, ataxia, acute headache), yellowing of skin or eyes, and changes in color of stool or urine, unresolved diarrhea or anorexia, or unusual bleeding or fatigue and weakness. **Pregnancy/breast-feeding precautions:** Inform prescriber if you are or intend to be pregnant. Breast-feeding is not recommended.

**Geriatric Considerations:** Adjust for renal function.

♦ **Fludara®** *see* Fludarabine *on this page*

## Fludarabine (floo DARE a been)

**U.S. Brand Names** Fludara®

**Therapeutic Category** Antineoplastic Agent, Antimetabolite

**Pregnancy Risk Factor** D

**Lactation** Excretion in breast milk unknown/contraindicated

**Use** Treatment of chronic lymphocytic leukemia (B-cell) in patients who have not responded to other alkylating agent regimen

**Mechanism of Action/Effect** Inhibits DNA synthesis by inhibition of DNA polymerase and ribonucleotide reductase.

**Contraindications** Hypersensitivity of fludarabine; patients with severe infections; pregnancy

**Warnings** The U.S. Food and Drug Administration (FDA) currently recommends that procedures for proper handling and disposal of antineoplastic agents be considered. Use with caution with renal insufficiency, patients with a fever documented infection or pre-existing hematological disorders (particularly granulocytopenia) or in patients with pre-existing central nervous system disorder (epilepsy), spasticity, or peripheral neuropathy.

Fludarabine preparation should be performed in a Class II laminar flow biologic safety cabinet. Personnel should be wearing surgical gloves and a closed front surgical gown with knit cuffs. Appropriate safety equipment is recommended for preparation, administration, and disposal of antineoplastics. If fludarabine contacts the skin, wash and flush thoroughly with water.

**Drug Interactions**

**Increased Effect/Toxicity:** Cytarabine when administered with or prior to a fludarabine dose competes for deoxycytidine kinase decreasing the metabolism of F-ara-A to the active F-ara-ATP (inhibits the antineoplastic effect of fludarabine); however, administering fludarabine prior to cytarabine may stimulate activation of cytarabine.

**Adverse Reactions**

>10%:

Central nervous system: Fever, chills, fatigue, pain

Dermatologic: Rash

(Continued)

## Fludarabine *(Continued)*

Gastrointestinal: Mild nausea, vomiting, diarrhea, stomatitis, GI bleeding
Genitourinary: Urinary infection
Hematologic: Anemia, thrombocytopenia, leukopenia; Myelosuppression: Dose-limiting toxicity; myelosuppression may not be related to cumulative dose
Granulocyte nadir: 13 days (3-25)
Platelet nadir: 16 days (2-32)
WBC nadir: 8 days
Recovery: 5-7 weeks
Neuromuscular & skeletal: Paresthesia, myalgia, weakness
Respiratory: Manifested as dyspnea and a nonproductive cough; lung biopsy has shown pneumonitis in some patients, pneumonia
Miscellaneous: Infection

1% to 10%:
Cardiovascular: Congestive heart failure, edema
Central nervous system: Malaise, headache
Dermatologic: Alopecia
Endocrine & metabolic: Hyperglycemia
Gastrointestinal: Anorexia
Ocular: Blurred vision
Otic: Hearing loss

<1% (Limited to important or life-threatening symptoms): Reported with higher dose levels; most patients shown to have CNS demyelination; somnolence, blindness, coma, and death also occurred; severe neurotoxicity; metabolic acidosis; life-threatening and sometimes fatal autoimmune hemolytic anemia; often recurs on rechallenge; steroid treatment may or may not be beneficial; reversible hepatotoxicity; renal failure; hematuria; increased serum creatinine; interstitial pneumonitis; tumor lysis syndrome

**Overdose/Toxicology** There are clear dose-dependent toxic neurologic effects associated with fludarabine. Doses of 96 mg/m²/day for 5-7 days are associated with a syndrome characterized by delayed blindness, coma, and death. Symptoms have appeared from 21-60 days following the last dose. Central nervous system toxicity has distinctive features of delayed onset and progressive encephalopathy resulting in fatality. CNS toxicity is reported at an incidence rate of 36% at high doses (≥96 mg/m²/day for 5-7 days) and <0.2% for low doses (≤125 mg/m²/course).

**Pharmacodynamics/Kinetics**

**Distribution:** Widely distributed with extensive tissue binding

**Half-life Elimination:** 9 hours

**Metabolism:** Serum

**Excretion:** Urine

**Formulations** Powder for injection, lyophilized, as phosphate: 50 mg (6 mL)

**Dosing**

**Adults:** I.V.:
Chronic lymphocytic leukemia: 20-25 mg/m²/day over a 30-minute period for 5 days; 5-day courses are repeated every 28-35 days days
Non-Hodgkin's lymphoma: Loading dose: 20 mg/m² followed by 30 mg/m²/day for 48 hours

**Elderly:** Refer to adult dosing.

**Renal Impairment:** $Cl_{cr}$ <50 mL/minute: Monitor closely for toxicity.

**Administration**

**I.V.:** Administer I.V. over 15-30 minutes or continuous infusion.

**Stability**

**Storage:** Store intact vials under refrigeration (2°C to 8°C).

**Reconstitution:** Reconstitute vials with 2 mL SWI to result in a concentration of 25 mg/mL. Solution is stable for 16 days at room temperature (22°C to 25°C) and under refrigeration (2°C to 8°C). Further dilution in 100 mL $D_5W$ or NS is stable for 48 hours at room temperature or refrigeration.

**Standard I.V. dilution:** Dose/100 mL $D_5W$ or NS
Stable for 48 hours at 4°C to 25°C

**Compatibility:** See the Chemotherapy Compatibility Chart *on page 1311.*

**Monitoring Laboratory Tests** CBC with differential, platelet count, AST, ALT, creatinine, serum albumin, uric acid

**Additional Nursing Issues**

**Physical Assessment:** Assess other prescription and OTC medications (see Drug Interactions). Monitor appropriate laboratory tests as ordered. Observe infusion site for extravasation. Monitor for adverse effects as noted above especially signs or symptoms of congestive heart failure, hypertension, and respiratory changes, I & O ratio, signs of edema, or weight gain or loss. Monitor for opportunistic infection (especially UTI). **Pregnancy risk factor D** - assess knowledge/instruct patient on appropriate barrier contraceptive measures. Breast-feeding is contraindicated.

**Patient Information/Instruction:** This drug can only be administered by infusion. During therapy, do not use alcohol, aspirin-containing products, and OTC medications without consulting prescriber. It is important to maintain adequate nutrition and hydration (2-3 L/day of fluids unless instructed to restrict fluid intake) during therapy; frequent small meals may help. You may experience mild nausea or vomiting (frequent small meals, frequent mouth care, sucking lozenges, or chewing gum may help). You may experience loss of hair (reversible); you will be more susceptible to infection (avoid crowds and exposure to infection as much as possible). Yogurt or buttermilk may help reduce diarrhea. Frequent mouth care and use of a soft toothbrush or cotton swabs may help prevent mouth sores. Report extreme fatigue, pain or numbness in extremities, severe GI upset or diarrhea, bleeding or bruising, fever, chills, sore throat, vaginal discharge, difficulty or pain on urination, muscle pain or weakness, unusual cough or difficulty breathing, or other unusual side effects. **Pregnancy/breast-feeding precautions:** Do not get pregnant; use appropriate contraceptive measures. Do not breast-feed while on this drug and for several weeks after last dose. Male: Use barrier contraceptive measures when having intercourse with women of childbearing age. Do not breast-feed.

## Fludrocortisone (floo droe KOR ti sone)

**U.S. Brand Names** Florinef® Acetate

**Synonyms** Fluohydrocortisone Acetate; 9α-Fluorohydrocortisone Acetate

**Therapeutic Category** Corticosteroid, Oral

**Pregnancy Risk Factor** C

**Lactation** Excretion in breast milk unknown

**Use** Partial replacement therapy for primary and secondary adrenocortical insufficiency in Addison's disease; treatment of salt-losing adrenogenital syndrome

**Mechanism of Action/Effect** Promotes increased reabsorption of sodium and loss of potassium from renal distal tubules

**Contraindications** Hypersensitivity to fludrocortisone; systemic fungal infections

**Warnings** Taper dose gradually when therapy is discontinued. Patients with Addison's disease are more sensitive to the action of the hormone and may exhibit side effects in an exaggerated degree. Pregnancy factor C.

**Drug Interactions**

**Decreased Effect:** Anticholinesterases effects are antagonized. Decreased corticosteroid effects by rifampin, barbiturates, and hydantoins. May decrease salicylate levels.

**Adverse Reactions** 1% to 10%:

Cardiovascular: Hypertension, edema, congestive heart failure

Central nervous system: Convulsions, headache, dizziness

Dermatologic: Acne, rash, bruising

Endocrine & metabolic: Hypokalemic alkalosis, suppression of growth, hyperglycemia, HPA suppression

Gastrointestinal: Peptic ulcer

Neuromuscular & skeletal: Muscle weakness

Ocular: Cataracts

Miscellaneous: Sweating, anaphylaxis (generalized)

**Overdose/Toxicology** Symptoms of overdose include hypertension, edema, hypokalemia, excessive weight gain. When consumed in excessive quantities, systemic hypercorticism and adrenal suppression may occur. In those cases, discontinuation of the corticosteroid should be done judiciously.

**Pharmacodynamics/Kinetics**

**Protein Binding:** 42%

**Half-life Elimination:** Plasma: 30-35 minutes; Biological: 18-36 hours

**Time to Peak:** Within 1.7 hours

**Metabolism:** Liver

**Formulations** Tablet, as acetate: 0.1 mg

**Dosing**

**Adults:** Oral: 0.05-0.2 mg/day with ranges of 0.1 mg 3 times/week to 0.2 mg/day

**Elderly:** Refer to adult dosing.

**Administration**

**Oral:** Administration in conjunction with a glucocorticoid is preferable.

**Monitoring Laboratory Tests** Serum electrolytes, serum renin activity

**Additional Nursing Issues**

**Physical Assessment:** Assess effectiveness and interactions of other medications (see Drug Interactions). See Contraindications and Warnings/Precautions for use cautions. Monitor for effectiveness of therapy and adverse reactions according to dose and length of therapy. Assess knowledge/teach patient appropriate use, possible side effects/interventions, and adverse symptoms to report (ie, opportunistic infection, adrenal suppression - see Adverse Reactions and Overdose/Toxicology). Diabetics: Monitor serum glucose levels closely; corticosteroids can alter hypoglycemic requirements. Dose may need to be increased if patient is experiencing higher than normal levels of stress. When discontinuing, taper dose and frequency slowly. **Pregnancy risk factor C** - benefits of use should outweigh possible risks. Note breast-feeding caution.

**Patient Information/Instruction:** Take exactly as directed. Do not take more than prescribed dose and do not discontinue abruptly; consult prescriber. Take with or after meals. Take once-a-day dose with food in the morning. Limit intake of caffeine or stimulants. Maintain adequate nutrition; consult prescriber for possibility of special dietary recommendations. If diabetic, monitor serum glucose closely and notify prescriber of changes; this medication can alter hypoglycemic requirements. Notify prescriber if you are experiencing higher than normal levels of stress; medication may need adjustment. Periodic ophthalmic examinations will be necessary with long-term use. You will be susceptible to infection; avoid crowds or infected persons or persons with contagious diseases. You may experience insomnia or nervousness; use caution when driving or engaging in tasks requiring alertness until response to drug is known. Report weakness, change in menstrual pattern, vision changes, signs of hyperglycemia, signs of infection (eg, fever, chills, mouth sores, perianal itching, vaginal discharge), other persistent side effects, or worsening of condition. **Pregnancy/**

(Continued)

## Fludrocortisone *(Continued)*

**breast-feeding precautions:** Inform prescriber if you are or intend to be pregnant. Consult prescriber if breast-feeding.

**Dietary Issues:** Systemic use of mineralocorticoids/corticosteroids may require a diet with increased potassium, vitamins A, $B_6$, C, D, folate, calcium, zinc, and phosphorus, and decreased sodium. With fludrocortisone a decrease in dietary sodium is often not required as the increased retention of sodium is usually the desired therapeutic effect.

**Geriatric Considerations:** The most common use of fludrocortisone in the elderly is orthostatic hypotension that is unresponsive to more conservative measures. Attempt nonpharmacologic measures (hydration, support stockings etc) before starting drug therapy.

**Related Information**

Corticosteroids Comparison, Systemic Equivalencies *on page 1383*

- **Flu-Imune®** *see page 1256*
- **Fluken** *see* Flutamide *on page 510*
- **Flulem** *see* Flutamide *on page 510*
- **Flumadine®** *see* Rimantadine *on page 1025*

## Flumazenil (FLO may ze nil)

**U.S. Brand Names** Romazicon™ Injection

**Therapeutic Category** Antidote

**Pregnancy Risk Factor** C

**Lactation** Excretion in breast milk unknown/use caution

**Use** Benzodiazepine antagonist - reverses sedative effects of benzodiazepines used in general anesthesia; management of benzodiazepine overdose

**Mechanism of Action/Effect** Antagonizes the effect of benzodiazepines on the GABA/benzodiazepine receptor complex. Flumazenil is benzodiazepine specific and does **not** antagonize other nonbenzodiazepine GABA agonists (including ethanol, barbiturates, general anesthetics); flumazenil does **not** reverse the effects of opiates.

**Contraindications** Hypersensitivity to flumazenil or benzodiazepines; patients given benzodiazepines for control of potentially life-threatening conditions (eg, control of intracranial pressure or status epilepticus); patients who are showing signs of serious cyclic-antidepressant overdosage

**Warnings** Use with caution in overdosage involving multiple drug combinations. Risk of seizures with high-risk patients including the following: patients on benzodiazepines for long-term sedation, tricyclic antidepressant overdose patients, concurrent major sedative-hypnotic drug withdrawal, recent therapy with repeated doses of parenteral benzodiazepines, or myoclonic jerking or seizure activity prior to flumazenil administration.

Does not reverse respiratory depression/hypoventilation or cardiac depression. Resedation: Occurs more frequently in patients where a large single dose or cumulative dose of a benzodiazepine is administered along with a neuromuscular blocking agent and multiple anesthetic agents. **Flumazenil should be used with caution in the intensive care unit because of increased risk of unrecognized benzodiazepine dependence in such settings.**

Pregnancy factor C.

**Drug Interactions**

**Increased Effect/Toxicity:** Toxic effects may emerge (especially with cyclic antidepressants) with attempts of benzodiazepine reversal by flumazenil.

**Adverse Reactions**

>10%: Gastrointestinal: Vomiting, nausea

1% to 10%:

Central nervous system: Dizziness, headache, malaise, anxiety, nervousness, insomnia, abnormal crying, euphoria, depression paranoia, dysphoria, paresthesia

Dermatologic: Rash

Endocrine & metabolic: Hot flashes

Gastrointestinal: Dry mouth

Local: Thrombophlebitis

Ocular: Abnormal vision, diplopia

Otic: Tinnitus

Local: Pain at injection site

Neuromuscular & skeletal: Muscle weakness, tremor

Respiratory: Dyspnea, hyperventilation

Miscellaneous: Increased sweating disorders

<1% (Limited to important or life-threatening symptoms): Arrhythmia, bradycardia, tachycardia, chest pain, hypertension, ventricular extrasystoles, convulsions

**Pharmacodynamics/Kinetics**

**Protein Binding:** 40% to 50%

**Half-life Elimination:** Alpha: 7-15 minutes; Terminal: 41-79 minutes

**Excretion:** Liver; clearance dependent upon hepatic blood flow, 0.2% unchanged in urine

**Onset:** 1-3 minutes; 80% response within 3 minutes; Peak effect: 6-10 minutes

**Duration:** Resedation occurs usually within 1 hour. Duration is related to dose given and benzodiazepine plasma concentrations. Reversal effects of flumazenil may wear off before effects of benzodiazepine.

**Formulations** Injection: 0.1 mg/mL (5 mL, 10 mL)

**Dosing**

**Adults:** See table.

**Flumazenil**

| Adult dosage for **reversal of conscious sedation:** Intravenously through a freely running intravenous infusion into a large vein to minimize pain at the injection site | |
|---|---|
| Initial dose | 0.2 mg intravenously over 15 seconds |
| Repeat doses | If desired level of consciousness is not obtained, 0.2 mg may be repeated at 1-minute intervals |
| Maximum total cumulative dose | 1 mg (usual dose 0.6-1 mg)<br>**In the event of resedation:** repeat doses may be given at 20-minute intervals with maximum of 1 mg/dose and 3 mg/hour |
| Adult dosage for **suspected benzodiazepine overdose:** Intravenously through a freely running intravenous infusion into a large vein to minimize pain at the injection site | |
| Initial dose | 0.2 mg intravenously over 30 seconds |
| Repeat doses | 0.5 mg over 30 seconds repeated at 1-minute intervals |
| Maximum total cumulative dose | 3 mg (usual dose 1-3 mg)<br>Patients with a partial response at 3 mg may require additional titration up to a total dose of 5 mg. If a patient has not responded 5 minutes after cumulative dose of 5 mg, the major cause of sedation is not likely due to benzodiazepines. **In the event of resedation:** may repeat doses at 20-minute intervals with maximum of 1 mg/dose and 3 mg/hour |

Resedation: Repeated doses may be given at 20-minute intervals as needed; repeat treatment doses of 1 mg (at a rate of 0.5 mg/minute) should be given at any time and no more than 3 mg should be given in any hour. After intoxication with high doses of benzodiazepines, the duration of a single dose of flumazenil is not expected to exceed 1 hour; if desired, the period of wakefulness may be prolonged with repeated low intravenous doses of flumazenil, or by an infusion of 0.1-0.4 mg/hour. Most patients with benzodiazepine overdose will respond to a cumulative dose of 1-3 mg and doses >3 mg do not reliably produce additional effects. Rarely, patients with a partial response at 3 mg may require additional titration up to a total dose of 5 mg. **If a patient has not responded 5 minutes after receiving a cumulative dose of 5 mg, the major cause of sedation is not likely to be due to benzodiazepines.**

**Elderly:** Refer to adult dosing.

**Renal Impairment:** Not significantly affected by renal failure ($Cl_{cr}$ <10 mL/minute) or hemodialysis beginning 1 hour after drug administration

**Hepatic Impairment:** Initial dose of flumazenil used for initial reversal of benzodiazepine effects is not changed; however, subsequent doses in liver disease patients should be reduced in amount or frequency.

**Administration**

**I.V.:** Administer in freely running I.V. into large vein. Inject over 15 seconds for general anesthesia and over 30 seconds for overdose.

**Stability**

**Reconstitution:** For I.V. use only. Once drawn up in the syringe or mixed with solution use within 24 hours. Discard any unused solution after 24 hours.

**Compatibility:** Compatible with $D_5W$, lactated Ringer's, or normal saline.

**Additional Nursing Issues**

**Physical Assessment:** Assess level of consciousness frequently. Monitor vital signs and airway closely. EKG monitoring and oxygenation via pulse oximetry is highly recommended. Observe continually for resedation, respiratory depression, preseizure activity, or other residual benzodiazepine effects. May require pain medication sooner after reversal. Assess for nausea and vomiting. **Pregnancy risk factor C** - benefits of use should outweigh possible risks. Note breast-feeding caution.

**Patient Information/Instruction:** Avoid driving or activities requiring alertness for 18-24 hours after drug use. Memory and judgment may be impaired for 24-48 hours. Avoid alcohol or other CNS depressants for 2-3 days after treatment. **Pregnancy/breast-feeding precautions:** Inform prescriber if you are or intend to be pregnant. Consult prescriber if breast-feeding.

## Flunisolide (floo NIS oh lide)

**U.S. Brand Names** AeroBid®-M Oral Aerosol Inhaler; AeroBid® Oral Aerosol Inhaler; Nasalide® Nasal Aerosol; Nasarel™

**Therapeutic Category** Corticosteroid, Oral Inhaler; Corticosteroid, Nasal

**Pregnancy Risk Factor** C

**Lactation** Excretion in breast milk unknown/use caution

**Use** Oral inhaler: Steroid-dependent asthma; nasal solution is used for seasonal or perennial rhinitis

**Mechanism of Action/Effect** Decreases inflammation by suppression of migration of polymorphonuclear leukocytes and reversal of increased capillary permeability; does not depress hypothalamus

**Contraindications** Hypersensitivity to flunisolide; acute status asthmaticus; viral, tuberculosis, fungal, or bacterial respiratory infection; infections of nasal mucosa

**Warnings** Use with caution in patients with hypothyroidism, cirrhosis, hypertension, congestive heart failure, ulcerative colitis, or thromboembolic disorders. Do not stop medication abruptly if on prolonged therapy. Fatalities have occurred due to adrenal insufficiency in asthmatic patients during and after transfer from systemic corticosteroids to aerosol steroids. Several months may be required to slowly taper systemic corticosteroid therapy when transferring to inhaled treatment. During this period, aerosol steroids do **not** provide the systemic steroid needed to treat patients having trauma, surgery, or

(Continued)

## Flunisolide *(Continued)*

infections. When consumed in excessive quantities, systemic hypercorticism and adrenal suppression may occur. Withdrawal and discontinuation of the corticosteroid should be done carefully. Pregnancy factor C.

**Adverse Reactions**

>10%:

Cardiovascular: Pounding heartbeat
Central nervous system: Dizziness, headache, nervousness
Dermatologic: Itching, rash
Endocrine & metabolic: Adrenal suppression, menstrual problems
Gastrointestinal: GI irritation, anorexia, sore throat, bitter taste
Local: Nasal burning, *Candida* infections of the nose or pharynx, atrophic rhinitis
Respiratory: Sneezing, coughing, upper respiratory tract infection, bronchitis, nasal congestion, nasal dryness
Miscellaneous: Increased susceptibility to infections

1% to 10%:

Central nervous system: Insomnia, psychic changes
Dermatologic: Acne, urticaria
Gastrointestinal: Increase in appetite, dry mouth, dry throat, loss of taste perception
Ocular: Cataracts
Respiratory: Epistaxis
Miscellaneous: Sweating, loss of smell

<1% (Limited to important or life-threatening symptoms): Bronchospasm, shortness of breath

**Overdose/Toxicology** When consumed in high doses over prolonged periods, systemic hypercorticism and adrenal suppression may occur. In those cases, discontinuation of the corticosteroid should be done judiciously.

**Pharmacodynamics/Kinetics**

**Half-life Elimination:** 1.8 hours

**Metabolism:** Liver

**Excretion:** Equally in urine and feces

**Formulations**

Inhalant:

Nasal (Nasalide®): 25 mcg/actuation [200 sprays] (25 mL)
Nasal (Nasarel™): 25 mcg/actuation [200 sprays] (25 mL)
Oral:
AeroBid®: 250 mcg/actuation [100 metered doses] (7 g)
AeroBid-M® (menthol flavor): 250 mcg/actuation [100 metered doses] (7 g)

Solution, spray: 0.025% [200 actuations] (25 mL)

**Dosing**

**Adults:**

Oral inhalation: 2 inhalations twice daily (morning and evening) up to 8 inhalations/day maximum
Nasal: 2 sprays in each nostril twice daily (morning and evening); maximum: 8 sprays/day in each nostril

**Elderly:** Refer to adult dosing.

**Administration**

**Inhalation:** Shake well before using. Do not use Nasalide® or Nasarel™ orally. Throw out product after it has been opened for 3 months.

**Additional Nursing Issues**

**Physical Assessment:** Note Contraindications and Warnings/Precautions for cautious use. Not to be used to treat status asthmaticus or fungal infections of nasal passages. Monitor therapeutic effects and adverse reactions (see Warnings/Precautions, Adverse Reactions, and Overdose/Toxicology). When changing from systemic steroids to inhalational steroid, taper reduction of systemic medication slowly (see Warnings/Precautions). Assess knowledge/teach patient appropriate use, interventions to reduce side effects, and adverse symptoms to report. **Pregnancy risk factor C** - benefits of use should outweigh possible risks. Note breast-feeding caution.

**Patient Information/Instruction:** Use as directed; do not use nasal preparations for oral inhalation. Do not increase dosage or discontinue abruptly without consulting prescriber. Review use of inhaler or spray with prescriber or follow package insert for directions. Keep oral inhaler clean and unobstructed. Always rinse mouth and throat after use of inhaler to prevent opportunistic infection. If you are also using an inhaled bronchodilator, wait 10 minutes before using this steroid aerosol. You may experience dizziness, anxiety, or blurred vision (rise slowly from sitting or lying position and use caution when driving or engaging in tasks requiring alertness until response to drug is known); or taste disturbance or aftertaste (frequent mouth care and mouth rinses may help). Report pounding heartbeat or chest pain; acute nervousness or inability to sleep; severe sneezing or nosebleed; difficulty breathing, sore throat, hoarseness, or bronchitis; respiratory difficulty or bronchospasms; disturbed menstrual pattern; vision changes; loss of taste or smell perception; or worsening of condition or lack of improvement. **Pregnancy/breast-feeding precautions:** Inform prescriber if you are or intend to be pregnant. Consult prescriber if breast-feeding.

**Administration:** Inhaler: Sit when using. Take deep breaths for 3-5 minutes, and clear nasal passages before administration (use decongestant as needed). Hold breath for 5-10 seconds after use, and wait 1-3 minutes between inhalations. Follow package insert instructions for use. Do not exceed maximum dosage. If also using inhaled bronchodilator, use before flunisolide. Rinse mouth and throat after use to reduce aftertaste and prevent candidiasis.

**Geriatric Considerations:** Many elderly patients have difficulty using metered dose inhalers, which can limit their effectiveness. Assess technique in all older patients. A spacer device may be beneficial for the oral inhaler.

**Additional Information** Does not contain fluorocarbons; contains polyethylene glycol vehicle.

**Related Information**

Inhalant (Asthma, Bronchospasm) Agents *on page 1388*


- **Fluocinolone** *see* Topical Corticosteroids *on page 1152*
- **Fluocinonide** *see* Topical Corticosteroids *on page 1152*
- **Fluogen®** *see page 1256*
- **Fluohydrocortisone Acetate** *see* Fludrocortisone *on page 495*
- **Fluonid®** *see* Topical Corticosteroids *on page 1152*
- **Fluoracaine® Ophthalmic** *see page 1248*
- **Fluorescein Sodium** *see page 1248*
- **Fluorescite® Injection** *see page 1248*
- **Fluorets® Ophthalmic Strips** *see page 1248*
- **Fluoride** *see page 1294*
- **Fluorigard®** *see page 1294*
- **Fluorinse®** *see page 1294*
- **Fluor-I-Strip®** *see page 1248*
- **Fluor-I-Strip-AT®** *see page 1248*
- **Fluoritab®** *see page 1294*
- **Fluorodeoxyuridine** *see* Floxuridine *on page 489*
- **9α-Fluorohydrocortisone Acetate** *see* Fludrocortisone *on page 495*


## Fluorometholone (flure oh METH oh lone)

**U.S. Brand Names** Flarex®; Fluor-Op®; FML®; FML® Forte

**Therapeutic Category** Corticosteroid, Ophthalmic; Corticosteroid, Topical

**Pregnancy Risk Factor** C

**Lactation** Excretion in breast milk unknown/use caution

**Use** Inflammatory conditions of the eye, including keratitis, iritis, cyclitis, and conjunctivitis

**Mechanism of Action/Effect** Decreases inflammation by suppression of migration of polymorphonuclear leukocytes and reversal of increased capillary permeability

**Contraindications** Hypersensitivity to fluorometholone or any component; herpes simplex; keratitis; fungal diseases of ocular structures; most viral diseases

**Warnings** Not recommended in children <2 years of age. Prolonged use may result in glaucoma, elevated intraocular pressure, or other ocular damage. Some products contain sulfites. Pregnancy factor C.

**Adverse Reactions**

1% to 10%: Ocular: Blurred vision

<1% (Limited to important or life-threatening symptoms): Stinging, burning eyes, increased intraocular pressure, open-angle glaucoma, defect in visual acuity and field of vision, cataracts

**Overdose/Toxicology** When consumed in high doses over prolonged periods, systemic hypercorticism and adrenal suppression may occur. In those cases, discontinuation of the corticosteroid should be done judiciously.

**Formulations**

Ophthalmic:

Ointment (FML®): 0.1% (3.5 g)

Suspension:

Flarex®, Fluor-Op®, FML®: 0.1% (2.5 mL, 5 mL, 10 mL)

FML® Forte: 0.25% (2 mL, 5 mL, 10 mL, 15 mL)

**Dosing**

**Adults:** Ophthalmic:

Ointment: May be applied every 4 hours in severe cases; 1-3 times/day in mild to moderate cases.

Solution: Instill 1-2 drops into conjunctival sac every hour during day, every 2 hours at night until favorable response is obtained, then use 1 drop every 4 hours. For mild to moderate inflammation, instill 1-2 drops into conjunctival sac 2-4 times/day.

**Elderly:** Refer to adult dosing.

**Additional Nursing Issues**

**Physical Assessment:** See Contraindications, Warnings/Precautions, and Overdose/Toxicology for cautious use. Assess knowledge/teach patient appropriate use, interventions to reduce side effects, and adverse symptoms to report (see Adverse Reactions). **Pregnancy risk factor C.** Note breast-feeding caution.

**Patient Information/Instruction:** For ophthalmic use only. Store solution in refrigerator. Apply prescribed amount as often as directed. Wash hands before using and do not let tip of applicator touch eye or contaminate tip of applicator. Tilt head back and look upward. Gently pull down lower lid and put drop(s) in inner corner of eye. Close eye and roll eyeball in all directions. Do not blink for ½ minute. Apply gentle pressure to inner corner of eye for 30 seconds. Wipe away excess from skin around eye. Do not use any other eye preparation for at least 10 minutes. Do not touch tip of applicator to eye or contaminate tip of applicator. Do not share medication with anyone else. May cause sensitivity to bright light (dark glasses may help); temporary stinging or blurred vision may occur. Inform prescriber if you experience eye pain, redness, burning, watering, dryness, double vision, puffiness around eye, vision disturbances, or other adverse eye response; worsening of condition or lack of improvement within 3-4 days.

(Continued)

## Fluorometholone *(Continued)*

**Pregnancy/breast-feeding precautions:** Inform prescriber if you are pregnant. Consult prescriber if breast-feeding.

- **Fluor-Op®** *see* Fluorometholone *on previous page*
- **Fluoroplex® Topical** *see* Fluorouracil *on this page*

## Fluorouracil (flure oh YOOR a sil)

**U.S. Brand Names** Adrucil® Injection; Efudex® Topical; Fluoroplex® Topical

**Synonyms** 5-Fluorouracil; 5-FU

**Therapeutic Category** Antineoplastic Agent, Antimetabolite

**Pregnancy Risk Factor** D (injection); X (topical)

**Lactation** Excretion in breast milk unknown/not recommended

**Use** Treatment of carcinoma of stomach, colon, rectum, breast, and pancreas; topically for management of multiple actinic keratoses and superficial basal cell carcinomas

**Mechanism of Action/Effect** Interferes with DNA synthesis by blocking the methylation of deoxyuricytic acid.

**Contraindications** Hypersensitivity to fluorouracil or any component; patients with poor nutritional status; bone marrow depression; pregnancy

**Warnings** The U.S. Food and Drug Administration (FDA) currently recommends that procedures for proper handling and disposal of antineoplastic agents be considered. Use with caution in patients who have had high-dose pelvic radiation or previous use of alkylating agents. Patient should be hospitalized during initial course of therapy. Use with caution in patients with impaired kidney or liver function. The drug should be discontinued if intractable vomiting or diarrhea, precipitous fall in leukocyte or platelet counts or myocardial ischemia occurs.

Preparation of fluorouracil should be performed in a Class II laminar flow biologic safety cabinet. Personnel should be wearing surgical gloves and a closed front surgical gown with knit cuffs. Appropriate safety equipment is recommended for preparation, administration, and disposal of antineoplastics. If fluorouracil contacts the skin, wash and flush thoroughly with water.

**Drug Interactions**

**Decreased Effect:** Methotrexate: This interaction is schedule dependent; **5-FU should be given following MTX, not prior to.**

If MTX is given first: The cells exposed to MTX before 5-FU have a depleted reduced folate pool which inhibits the binding of the 5dUMP to TS. However, it does not interfere with FUTP incorporation into RNA. Polyglutamines, which accumulate in the presence of MTX may be substituted for the folates and allow binding of FdUMP to TS. MTX given prior to 5-FU may actually activate 5-FU due to MTX inhibition of purine synthesis.

If 5-FU is given first: 5-FU inhibits the TS binding and thus the reduced folate pool is not depleted, thereby negating the effect of MTX

**Increased Effect/Toxicity:** Leucovorin increases the folate pool and in certain tumors, may promote TS inhibition and increase 5-FU activity. Leucovorin must be given before or with the 5-FU to prime the cells; it is not used as a rescue agent in this case. Allopurinol inhibits thymidine phosphorylase (an enzyme that activates 5-FU). The antitumor effect of 5-FU appears to be unaltered, but the toxicity is increased. Cimetidine results in increased plasma levels of 5-FU due to drug metabolism inhibition and reduction of liver blood flow induced by cimetidine.

**Adverse Reactions** Toxicity depends on route and duration of infusion

>10%:

Dermatologic: Dermatitis, pruritic maculopapular rash, alopecia

Gastrointestinal (route and schedule dependent): Heartburn, nausea, vomiting, anorexia, stomatitis, esophagitis, anorexia, stomatitis, and diarrhea; bolus dosing produces milder GI problems, while continuous infusion tends to produce severe mucositis and diarrhea; vomiting is moderate, occurring in 30% to 60% of patients, and responds well to phenothiazines and dexamethasone

Emetic potential:
<1000 mg: Moderately low (10% to 30%)
≥1000 mg: Moderate (30% to 60%)

Hematologic: Leukopenia; Myelosuppressive: Granulocytopenia occurs around 9-14 days after 5-FU and thrombocytopenia around 7-17 days. The marrow recovers after 22 days. Myelosuppression tends to be more pronounced in patients receiving bolus dosing of 5-FU.

WBC: Moderate
Platelets: Mild to moderate
Onset (days): 7-10
Nadir (days): 14
Recovery (days): 21

Local: **Irritant chemotherapy**

1% to 10%:

Dermatologic: Dry skin
Gastrointestinal: GI ulceration

<1% (Limited to important or life-threatening symptoms):

Hypotension, chest pain, EKG changes similar to ischemic changes, and possibly cardiac enzyme abnormalities. Usually occurs within the first 2 days of therapy, and may resolve with nitroglycerin and calcium channel blockers. May be due to coronary vessel vasospasm induced by 5-FU. Hyperpigmentation of nailbeds, face, hands, and veins used in infusion; photosensitization with UV light; palmar-plantar syndrome (hand-foot syndrome), coagulopathy, hepatotoxicity, shortness of breath.

Cerebellar ataxia, headache, somnolence, ataxia are seen primarily in intracarotid arterial infusions for head and neck tumors. This is believed to be caused by fluorocitrate, a neurotoxic metabolite of the parent compound.

**Overdose/Toxicology** Symptoms of overdose include myelosuppression, nausea, vomiting, diarrhea, and alopecia. No specific antidote exists. Monitor hematologically for at least 4 weeks. Treatment is supportive.

**Pharmacodynamics/Kinetics**

**Distribution:** Penetrates the extracellular fluid, CSF, and third space fluids (such as pleural effusions and ascitic fluid)

**Half-life Elimination:** Biphasic: Initial: 6-20 minutes; doses of 400-600 mg/m$^2$ produce drug concentrations above the threshold for cytotoxicity for normal tissue and remain there for 6 hours; two metabolites, FdUMP and FUTP, have prolonged half-lives depending on the type of tissue; the clinical effect of these metabolites has not been determined

**Metabolism:** Liver; must be metabolized to be active

**Excretion:** Urine

**Duration:** ~3 weeks

**Formulations**

Cream, topical:
- Efudex®: 5% (25 g)
- Fluoroplex®: 1% (30 g)

Injection (Adrucil®): 50 mg/mL (10 mL, 20 mL, 50 mL, 100 mL)

Solution, topical:
- Efudex®: 2% (10 mL); 5% (10 mL)
- Fluoroplex®: 1% (30 mL)

**Dosing**

**Adults:** Refer to individual protocols.

**All dosages are based on the patient's actual weight. However, the estimated lean body mass (dry weight) is used if the patient is obese or if there has been a spurious weight gain due to edema, ascites or other forms of abnormal fluid retention.**

I.V.:

Initial: 400-500 mg/m$^2$/day (12 mg/kg/day; maximum: 800 mg/day) for 4-5 days either as a single daily I.V. push or 4-day continuous intravenous infusion

Maintenance dose regimens:
- 200-250 mg/m$^2$ (6 mg/kg) every other day for 4 days repeated in 4 weeks
- 500-600 mg/m$^2$ (15 mg/kg) weekly as a continuous intravenous infusion or I.V. push

Concomitant with leucovorin:
- 370 mg/m$^2$/day for 5 days
- 500-1000 mg/m$^2$ every 2 weeks
- 600 mg/m$^2$/week for 6 weeks
- Although the manufacturer recommends no daily dose >800 mg, higher doses of up to 2 g/day are routinely administered by continuous intravenous infusion. By continuous intravenous infusion, higher daily doses have been successfully used.

Topical:
- Actinic or solar keratosis: Apply twice daily for 2-6 weeks.
- Superficial basal cell carcinomas: Apply 5% twice daily for at least 3-6 weeks and up to 10-12 weeks.

**Renal Impairment:** Hemodialysis: Administer dose posthemodialysis.

**Hepatic Impairment:** Bilirubin >5 mg/dL: Omit use.

**Administration**

**Oral:** I.V. formulation may be given orally mixed in water, grape juice, or carbonated beverage.

**I.V.:** Irritant. Direct I.V. push injection (50 mg/mL solution needs no further dilution) or by I.V. infusion. Toxicity may be reduced by giving the drug as a constant infusion. Bolus doses may be administered by slow IVP or IVPB.

**I.V. Detail:** Warm to body temperature before using. After vial has been entered, any unused portion should be discarded within 1 hour. Continuous infusions may be administered in $D_5W$ or NS. Solution should be protected from direct sunlight. 5-FU may also be administered intra-arterially or intrahepatically (refer to specific protocols).

**Topical:** Wash hands immediately after topical application of the 5% cream; for external use only.

**Stability**

**Storage:** Store intact vials at room temperature and protect from light. Slight discoloration does not usually denote decomposition.

**Reconstitution:** Further dilution in $D_5W$ or NS at concentrations of 0.5-10 mg/mL are stable for 72 hours at 4°C to 25°C.

**Standard I.V. dilution:**

I.V. push: Dose/syringe (concentration: 50 mg/mL)

Maximum syringe size for IVP is a 30 mL syringe and syringe should be <75% full.

Continuous intravenous infusion/IVPB: Dose/50-1000 mL $D_5W$ or NS

Syringe and solution are stable for 72 hours at 4°C to 25°C.

**Compatibility:** Compatible with vincristine, methotrexate, potassium chloride, and magnesium sulfate. Incompatible with cytarabine, diazepam, doxorubicin, and methotrexate. Concentrations >25 mg/mL of fluorouracil and >2 mg/mL of leucovorin are

(Continued)

## Fluorouracil *(Continued)*

incompatible (precipitation occurs). See the Chemotherapy Compatibility Chart *on page 1311.*

**Monitoring Laboratory Tests** CBC with differential, platelet count, renal and liver function

**Additional Nursing Issues**

**Physical Assessment:** Assess other prescription and OTC medications patient may be taking (see Drug Interactions). I.V.: Closely monitor infusion site for extravasation. Monitor laboratory tests prior to each infusion with I.V. use and regularly with topical use. Monitor cardiovascular, respiratory, and renal function frequently during entire cycle of therapy (see Warnings/Precautions, Drug Interactions, and Adverse Reactions). Assess frequently for development of opportunistic infection. Wash hands thoroughly before and after applying topical preparation. Instruct patient on appropriate interventions to reduce side effects and adverse symptoms to report. **Pregnancy risk factor D/X** - see Pregnancy Risk Factor - determine that patient is not pregnant before beginning treatment and do not give to women of childbearing age or to males who may have intercourse with women of childbearing age unless both male and female are capable of complying with barrier contraceptive measures 1 month during therapy and for 1 month following therapy. Breast-feeding is not recommended.

**Patient Information/Instruction:** Avoid alcohol and all OTC drugs unless approved by your oncologist. Maintain adequate hydration (2-3 L/day of fluids unless instructed to restrict fluid intake) and nutrition (small frequent meals may help). You may experience sensitivity to sunlight (use sunblock, wear protective clothing, or avoid direct sunlight); susceptibility to infection (avoid crowds or infected persons or persons with contagious diseases); nausea, vomiting, diarrhea, or loss of appetite (frequent small meals may help - request medication); weakness, lethargy, dizziness, decreased vision (use caution when driving or engaging in tasks requiring alertness until response to drug is known); headache (request medication). Report signs and symptoms of infection (eg, fever, chills, sore throat, burning urination, vaginal itching or discharge, fatigue, mouth sores); bleeding (eg, black or tarry stools, easy bruising, unusual bleeding); vision changes; unremitting nausea, vomiting, or abdominal pain; CNS changes; respiratory difficulty; chest pain or palpitations; severe skin reactions to topical application; or any other adverse reactions.

Topical: Use as directed; do not overuse. Wash hands thoroughly before and after applying medication. Avoid contact with eyes and mouth. Avoid occlusive dressings; use a porous dressing. May cause local reaction (pain, burning, or swelling); if severe contact prescriber.

**Pregnancy/breast-feeding precautions:** Inform prescriber if you are pregnant. Do not get pregnant during or for 1 month following therapy. Male: Do not cause a pregnancy. Male/female: Consult prescriber for instruction on appropriate contraceptive measures. This drug may cause severe fetal defects. Breast-feeding is not recommended.

- **Fluoro-uracil** *see* Fluorouracil *on page 500*
- **5-Fluorouracil** *see* Fluorouracil *on page 500*
- **Fluoxac** *see* Fluoxetine *on this page*

## Fluoxetine (floo OKS e teen)

**U.S. Brand Names** Prozac®

**Therapeutic Category** Antidepressant, Selective Serotonin Reuptake Inhibitor

**Pregnancy Risk Factor** B

**Lactation** Enters breast milk/not recommended (AAP rates "of concern")

**Use** Treatment of depression, obsessive-compulsive disorder, obesity, or bulimia nervosa

**Mechanism of Action/Effect** Inhibits CNS neuron serotonin uptake; minimal or no effect on reuptake of norepinephrine or dopamine; does not significantly bind to alpha-adrenergic, histamine or cholinergic receptors; may therefore be useful in patients at risk from sedation, hypotension, and anticholinergic effects of tricyclic antidepressants

**Contraindications** Hypersensitivity to fluoxetine; patients receiving MAO inhibitors currently or in past 2 weeks

**Warnings** Use with caution in patients with hepatic impairment, history of seizures. MAO inhibitors should be discontinued at least 14 days before initiating fluoxetine therapy. Add or initiate other antidepressants with caution for up to 5 weeks after stopping fluoxetine.

**Drug Interactions**

**Cytochrome P-450 Effect:** CYP2D6 enzyme substrate (minor), CYP2C enzyme substrate (minor), CYP3A3/4 enzyme substrate; CYP2C9 enzyme inducer; CYP1A2, 2C9, 2C18, 2C19, 2D6, and 3A3/4 enzyme inhibitor

**Decreased Effect:** Fluoxetine taken with lithium may increase or decrease serum lithium levels.

**Increased Effect/Toxicity:** Increased effect with tricyclics (2 times ↑ plasma level). Fluoxetine taken with lithium may increase or decrease serum lithium levels. Increased toxicity of diazepam, trazodone via decreased clearance. Increased toxicity with MAO inhibitors (hyperpyrexia, tremors, seizures, delirium, coma). Fluoxetine displaces protein-bound drugs. Potential for serotonin syndrome if combined with other serotonergic drugs.

**Effects on Lab Values** ↑ albumin in urine

**Adverse Reactions** Predominant adverse effects are CNS and GI

>10%:

Central nervous system: Headache, nervousness, insomnia, drowsiness

Gastrointestinal: Nausea, diarrhea, dry mouth

1% to 10%:
- Central nervous system: Anxiety, dizziness, fatigue, sedation
- Dermatologic: Rash, pruritus
- Endocrine & metabolic: SIADH, hypoglycemia, hyponatremia (elderly or volume-depleted patients)
- Gastrointestinal: Anorexia, heartburn, constipation
- Neuromuscular & skeletal: Tremor
- Miscellaneous: Excessive sweating

**Overdose/Toxicology** Symptoms of overdose include ataxia, sedation, and coma. Respiratory depression may occur, especially with coingestion of alcohol or other drugs. Seizures rarely occur. Treatment is supportive.

**Pharmacodynamics/Kinetics**

**Half-life Elimination:** 2-3 days; due to long half-life, resolution of adverse reactions after discontinuation may be slow

**Time to Peak:** Within 4-8 hours

**Metabolism:** Liver

**Excretion:** Urine

**Onset:** 2-4 weeks (therapeutic effects)

**Formulations**

Fluoxetine hydrochloride:
- Capsule: 10 mg, 20 mg
- Liquid (mint flavor): 20 mg/5 mL (120 mL)

**Dosing**

**Adults:** Oral: 20 mg/day in the morning; may increase after several weeks by 20 mg/day increments; maximum: 80 mg/day; doses >20 mg should be divided into morning and noon doses.

Usual dosage range:
- 20-80 mg/day for depression and OCD
- 20-60 mg/day for obesity
- 60-80 mg/day for bulimia nervosa

**Note:** Lower doses of 5 mg/day have been used for initial treatment.

**Elderly:** Oral: Some patients may require an initial dose of 10 mg/day with dosage increases of 10 and 20 mg every several weeks as tolerated; should not be taken at night unless patient experiences sedation.

**Renal Impairment:**

Single dose studies: Pharmacokinetics of fluoxetine and norfluoxetine were similar among subjects with all levels of impaired renal function, including anephric patients on chronic hemodialysis.

Chronic administration: Additional accumulation of fluoxetine or norfluoxetine may occur in patients with severely impaired renal function.

Not removed by hemodialysis.

**Hepatic Impairment:** Elimination half-life of fluoxetine is prolonged in patients with hepatic impairment. A lower or less frequent dose of fluoxetine should be used in these patients.

Cirrhosis patient: Administer a lower dose or less frequent dosing interval.

Compensated cirrhosis without ascites: Administer 50% of normal dose.

**Monitoring Laboratory Tests** Baseline liver and renal function before beginning drug therapy

**Additional Nursing Issues**

**Physical Assessment:** Assess other medications patient may be taking for effectiveness and interactions (see Drug Interactions). See Contraindications and Warnings/Precautions for cautious use. Has potential for psychological or physiological dependence, abuse, or tolerance. Monitor laboratory tests, therapeutic response (ie, mental status, mode, affect, suicidal ideation), and adverse reactions at beginning of therapy and periodically with long-term use (eg, CNS, and gastrointestinal - see Adverse Reactions and Overdose/Toxicology). Taper dosage slowly when discontinuing (see Warnings/Precautions about timing when discontinuing Prozac® and starting another antidepressant). Assess knowledge/teach patient appropriate use, interventions to reduce side effects and adverse symptoms to report. Breast-feeding is not recommended.

**Patient Information/Instruction:** Take exactly as directed (do not increase dose or frequency); may take 2-3 weeks to achieve desired results; may cause physical and/or psychological dependence. Take once-a-day dose in the morning to reduce incidence of insomnia. Avoid excessive alcohol, caffeine, and other prescription or OTC medications not approved by prescriber. Maintain adequate hydration (2-3 L/day of fluids unless instructed to restrict fluid intake). You may experience drowsiness, lightheadedness, impaired coordination, dizziness, or blurred vision (use caution when driving or engaging in tasks requiring alertness until response to drug is known); constipation (increased exercise, fluids, or dietary fruit and fiber may help); anorexia (maintain regular dietary intake to avoid excessive weight loss); or postural hypotension (use caution when climbing stairs or changing position from lying or sitting to standing). If diabetic, monitor serum glucose closely (may cause hypoglycemia). Report persistent CNS effects (nervousness, restlessness, insomnia, anxiety, excitation, headache, sedation); rash or skin irritation; muscle cramping, tremors, or change in gait; respiratory depression or difficulty breathing; or worsening of condition. **Breast-feeding precautions:** Breast-feeding is not recommended.

**Geriatric Considerations:** Fluoxetine's favorable side effect profile makes it a useful alternative to the traditional tricyclic antidepressants. Its potential stimulating and anorexic effects may be bothersome to some patients. Has not been shown to be

(Continued)

## Fluoxetine *(Continued)*

superior in efficacy to the traditional tricyclic antidepressants or other SSRIs. The long half-life in the elderly makes it less attractive compared to other SSRIs. Data from a clinical trial comparing fluoxetine to tricyclics suggests that fluoxetine is significantly less effective than nortriptyline in hospitalized elderly patients with unipolar major affective disorder, especially those with melancholia and concurrent cardiovascular diseases.

**Related Information**

Antidepressant Agents Comparison *on page 1368*

## Fluoxymesterone (floo oks i MES te rone)

**U.S. Brand Names** Halotestin®

**Therapeutic Category** Androgen

**Pregnancy Risk Factor** X

**Lactation** Excretion in breast milk unknown/contraindicated

**Use** Replacement of endogenous testicular hormone; in females, used as palliative treatment of breast cancer, postpartum breast engorgement

**Mechanism of Action/Effect** Synthetic androgenic anabolic hormone responsible for the normal growth and development of male sex organs and maintenance of secondary sex characteristics; stimulates RNA polymerase activity resulting in an increase in protein production; increases bone development

**Contraindications** Hypersensitivity to fluoxymesterone or any component; serious cardiac disease; liver or kidney disease; pregnancy

**Drug Interactions**

**Decreased Effect:** Decreased blood glucose concentrations and insulin requirements in patients with diabetes.

**Increased Effect/Toxicity:** May increase the effect of oral anticoagulants.

**Effects on Lab Values** Decreased levels of thyroxine-binding globulin; decreased total $T_4$ serum levels; increased resin uptake of $T_3$ and $T_4$

**Adverse Reactions**

>10%:
- Male: Priapism
- Female: Menstrual problems (amenorrhea), virilism, breast soreness
- Cardiovascular: Edema
- Dermatologic: Acne

1% to 10%:
- Male: Prostatic carcinoma, hirsutism (increase in pubic hair growth), impotence, testicular atrophy
- Cardiovascular: Edema
- Gastrointestinal: GI irritation, nausea, vomiting
- Genitourinary: Prostatic hypertrophy
- Hepatic: Hepatic dysfunction

<1% (Limited to important or life-threatening symptoms): Leukopenia, polycythemia, hepatic necrosis, cholestatic hepatitis

**Overdose/Toxicology** Symptoms of overdose include water retention. Abnormal liver function tests have been observed.

**Pharmacodynamics/Kinetics**

**Protein Binding:** 98%

**Half-life Elimination:** 10-100 minutes

**Metabolism:** Liver

**Excretion:** Enterohepatic circulation and urinary excretion (90%)

**Formulations** Tablet: 2 mg, 5 mg, 10 mg

**Dosing**

**Adults:** Oral:

Male:
- Hypogonadism: 5-20 mg/day
- Delayed puberty: 2.5-20 mg/day for 4-6 months

Female:
- Inoperable breast carcinoma: 10-40 mg/day in divided doses for 1-3 months
- Breast engorgement: 2.5 mg after delivery, 5-10 mg/day in divided doses for 4-5 days

**Elderly:** Refer to adult dosing.

**Stability**

**Storage:** Protect from light.

**Additional Nursing Issues**

**Physical Assessment:** Assess effectiveness and interactions of other medications (see Drug Interactions, eg, hypoglycemic agents). See Warnings/Precautions and Contraindications for use cautions. Monitor effectiveness of therapy and adverse response (see Adverse Reactions and Overdose/Toxicology). Assess knowledge/teach patient appropriate use, possible side effects and appropriate interventions, and adverse symptoms to report. **Pregnancy risk factor X** - determine that female patient is not pregnant before beginning therapy and do not give to women of childbearing age or to males having intercourse with women of childbearing age unless both male and female are capable of complying with barrier contraceptive measures during therapy and for 1 month following therapy. Breast-feeding is contraindicated during therapy and for 1 month following therapy.

**Patient Information/Instruction:** Take as directed; do not discontinue without consulting prescriber. Diabetics should monitor serum glucose closely and notify prescriber of changes; this medication can alter hypoglycemic requirements. You may experience acne, growth of body hair, loss of libido, impotence, or menstrual irregularity (usually reversible); nausea or vomiting (small frequent meals, frequent mouth care, sucking lozenges, or chewing gum may help). Report changes in menstrual pattern; deepening of voice or unusual growth of body hair; fluid retention (swelling of ankles, feet, or hands, difficulty breathing, or sudden weight gain); change in color of urine or stool; yellowing of eyes or skin; unusual bruising or bleeding; or other adverse reactions. **Pregnancy/breast-feeding precautions:** Inform prescriber if you are pregnant and do not get pregnant during or for 1 month following therapy. Male: Do not cause a female to become pregnant. Male/female: Consult prescriber for instruction on appropriate barrier contraceptive measures. This drug may cause severe fetal defects. Do not breast-feed.

**Additional Information** Halogenated derivative of testosterone with up to 5 times the activity of methyltestosterone

♦ **Flupazine** *see* Trifluoperazine *on page 1176*

## Fluphenazine (floo FEN a zeen)

**U.S. Brand Names** Permitil® Oral; Prolixin Decanoate® Injection; Prolixin Enanthate® Injection; Prolixin® Injection; Prolixin® Oral

**Therapeutic Category** Antipsychotic Agent, Phenothazine, Piperazine

**Pregnancy Risk Factor** C

**Lactation** Enters breast milk/not recommended

**Use** Management of manifestations of psychotic disorders

**Mechanism of Action/Effect** Blocks postsynaptic mesolimbic dopaminergic $D_1$ and $D_2$ receptors in the brain; exhibits a strong alpha-adrenergic blocking and anticholinergic effect, depresses the release of hypothalamic and hypophyseal hormones; believed to depress the reticular activating system thus affecting basal metabolism, body temperature, wakefulness, vasomotor tone, and emesis

**Contraindications** Hypersensitivity to fluphenazine or any component (cross reactivity between phenothiazines may occur); severe CNS depression; coma; subcortical brain damage; blood dyscrasias; hepatic disease

**Warnings** Hypotension may occur, particularly with I.M. administration. May be sedating; use with caution in disorders where CNS depression is a feature. Use with caution in Parkinson's disease. Use caution in patients with hemodynamic instability; bone marrow suppression; predisposition to seizures; or severe cardiac, renal, or respiratory disease. May cause swallowing difficulties. Use with caution in breast cancer or other prolactin-dependent tumors (may elevate prolactin levels). May alter temperature regulation or mask toxicity of other drugs due to antiemetic effects. May alter cardiac conduction - life-threatening arrhythmias have occurred with therapeutic doses of phenothiazines. May cause orthostatic hypotension. Adverse effects of depot injections may be prolonged.

Phenothiazines may cause anticholinergic effects (eg, confusion, agitation, constipation, dry mouth, blurred vision, urinary retention); therefore, use with caution in patients with decreased gastrointestinal motility, urinary retention, BPH, xerostomia, or visual problems. Conditions which also may be exacerbated by cholinergic blockade include narrow-angle glaucoma (screening is recommended) and worsening of myasthenia gravis. Relative to other antipsychotics, fluphenazine has a low potency of cholinergic blockade.

May cause extrapyramidal reactions including pseudoparkinsonism, acute dystonic reactions, akathisia and tardive dyskinesia (risk of these reactions is high relative to other antipsychotics). May be associated with neuroleptic malignant syndrome (NMS) or pigmentary retinopathy.

Pregnancy factor C.

**Drug Interactions**

**Cytochrome P-450 Effect:** CYP2D6 enzyme substrate; CYP2D6 enzyme inhibitor

**Decreased Effect:** Barbiturate levels and fluphenazine effectiveness are decreased when given together.

**Increased Effect/Toxicity:** Increased toxicity with alcohol, effects of both drugs may be increased. Extrapyramidal symptoms and other CNS effects may be increased when coadministered with lithium. May potentiate the effects of narcotics including respiratory depression.

**Effects on Lab Values** ↑ cholesterol (S), glucose; ↓ uric acid (S)

**Adverse Reactions**

>10%:

Cardiovascular: Orthostatic hypotension, hypotension, tachycardia, arrhythmias

Central nervous system: Parkinsonian symptoms, akathisia, dystonias, tardive dyskinesia (persistent), dizziness

Gastrointestinal: Constipation

Ocular: Pigmentary retinopathy

Respiratory: Nasal congestion

Miscellaneous: Decreased sweating

1% to 10%:

Dermatologic: Photosensitivity, rash

Endocrine & metabolic: Changes in menstrual cycle, breast pain, amenorrhea, galactorrhea, gynecomastia, changes in libido

Gastrointestinal: Weight gain, nausea, vomiting, stomach pain

Genitourinary: Difficulty in urination, ejaculatory disturbances

Neuromuscular & skeletal: Trembling of fingers

(Continued)

## Fluphenazine *(Continued)*

<1% (Limited to important or life-threatening symptoms): Extrapyramidal reactions, pseudoparkinsonian signs and symptoms, seizures, altered central temperature regulation, agranulocytosis (more often in women between 4th and 10th weeks of therapy), leukopenia (usually in patients with large doses for prolonged periods), cholestatic jaundice, hepatotoxicity

**Overdose/Toxicology** Symptoms of overdose include deep sleep, hypo- or hypertension, dystonia, seizures, extrapyramidal symptoms, and respiratory failure. Following initiation of essential overdose management, toxic symptom treatment and supportive treatment should be initiated.

**Pharmacodynamics/Kinetics**

**Protein Binding:** 91% and 99%

**Distribution:** Widely distributed; crosses the placenta

**Half-life Elimination:** Derivative dependent: Enanthate: 84-96 hours; Hydrochloride: 33 hours; Decanoate: 163-232 hours

**Metabolism:** Liver

**Excretion:** Liver and kidneys

**Onset:**

Following I.M. or S.C. administration (derivative dependent):

Decanoate (lasts the longest and requires 24-72 hours for onset of action): Onset of action: 24-72 hours; Peak neuroleptic effect: Within 48-96 hours

Hydrochloride salt (acts quickly and persists briefly): Onset of activity: Within 1 hour

**Duration:** Hydrochloride salt: 6-8 hours

**Formulations**

Concentrate, as hydrochloride:

Permitil®: 5 mg/mL with alcohol 1% (118 mL)

Prolixin®: 5 mg/mL with alcohol 14% (120 mL)

Elixir, as hydrochloride (Prolixin®): 2.5 mg/5 mL with alcohol 14% (60 mL, 473 mL)

Injection, as decanoate (Prolixin Decanoate®): 25 mg/mL (1 mL, 5 mL)

Injection, as enanthate (Prolixin Enanthate®): 25 mg/mL (5 mL)

Injection, as hydrochloride (Prolixin®): 2.5 mg/mL (10 mL)

Tablet, as hydrochloride

Permitil®: 2.5 mg, 5 mg, 10 mg

Prolixin®: 1 mg, 2.5 mg, 5 mg, 10 mg

**Dosing**

**Adults:**

Oral: 0.5-10 mg/day in divided doses at 6- to 8-hour intervals; some patients may require up to 40 mg/day

I.M.: 2.5-10 mg/day in divided doses at 6- to 8-hour intervals (parenteral dose is $^1/_3$ to $^1/_2$ the oral dose for the hydrochloride salts)

I.M., S.C. (decanoate): 12.5 mg every 3 weeks

Conversion from hydrochloride to decanoate I.M. 0.5 mL (12.5 mg) decanoate every 3 weeks is approximately equivalent to 10 mg hydrochloride/day

I.M., S.C. (enanthate): 12.5-25 mg every 3 weeks

**Elderly:** Initial (nonpsychotic patient; dementia behavior): 1-2.5 mg/day; increase dose at 4- to 7-day intervals by 1-2.5 mg/day; increase dosing intervals (bid, tid) as necessary to control response or side effects. Maximum daily dose: 20 mg; gradual increases (titration) may prevent some side effects or decrease their severity.

**Renal Impairment:** Use with caution; not dialyzable (0% to 5%).

**Hepatic Impairment:** Use with caution.

**Administration**

**Oral:** Avoid contact of oral solution or injection with skin (contact dermatitis). Oral liquid should be diluted in the following **only**: water, saline, 7-UP®, homogenized milk, carbonated orange beverages, pineapple, apricot, prune, orange, V8® juice, tomato, and grapefruit juices. Do **not** dilute in beverages containing caffeine, tannics, or pactinate.

**I.M.:** Watch for hypotension when administering I.M.

**Monitoring Laboratory Tests** Liver and kidney function, CBC prior to and regularly during therapy, ophthalmic screening

**Additional Nursing Issues**

**Physical Assessment:** Assess other medications patient is taking for effectiveness and interactions (see Drug Interactions). See Contraindications and Warnings/Precautions for cautious use. Has potential for psychological or physiological dependence, abuse, and tolerance. Review ophthalmic screening and monitor laboratory tests (see above), therapeutic response (mental status, mood, affect), and adverse reactions at beginning of therapy and periodically with long-term use (especially anticholinergic and extrapyramidal effects - see Adverse Reactions and Overdose/Toxicology). With I.M. or S.C. use, monitor closely for hypotension. **Note:** Avoid skin contact with oral or injection medication; may cause contact dermatitis (wash immediately with warm, soapy water). Initiate at lower doses (see Dosing) and taper dosage slowly when discontinuing. Assess knowledge/teach patient appropriate use, interventions to reduce side effects, and adverse symptoms to report (see below). **Pregnancy risk factor C** - benefits of use should outweigh possible risks. Breast-feeding is not recommended.

**Patient Information/Instruction:** Use exactly as directed (do not increase dose or frequency); may cause physical and/or psychological dependence. Do not discontinue without consulting prescriber. Dilute with water, milk, orange or grapefruit juice; do not dilute with beverages containing caffeine, tannin, or pactinate (eg, coffee, colas, tea, or apple juice). Do not take within 2 hours of any antacid. Avoid excess alcohol or caffeine and other prescription or OTC medications not approved by prescriber. Avoid skin contact with medication; may cause contact dermatitis (wash immediately with warm, soapy water). Maintain adequate hydration (2-3 L/day of fluids unless instructed to restrict fluid intake). You may experience excess drowsiness, lightheadedness, dizziness, or blurred vision (use caution driving or when engaging in tasks requiring alertness until response to drug is known); dry mouth, upset stomach, nausea, vomiting (small frequent meals, frequent mouth care, chewing gum, or sucking lozenges may help); constipation (increased exercise, fluids, or dietary fruit and fiber may help); postural hypotension (use caution climbing stairs or when changing position from lying or sitting to standing); urinary retention (void before taking medication); ejaculatory dysfunction (reversible); decreased perspiration (avoid strenuous exercise in hot environments); or photosensitivity (use sunscreen, wear protective clothing and eyewear, and avoid direct sunlight). Report persistent CNS effects (eg, trembling fingers, altered gait or balance, excessive sedation, seizures, unusual movements, anxiety, abnormal thoughts, confusion, personality changes); chest pain, palpitations, rapid heartbeat, severe dizziness; unresolved urinary retention or changes in urinary pattern; altered menstrual pattern, change in libido, swelling or pain in breasts (male or female); vision changes; skin rash or irritation or yellowing of skin; or worsening of condition. **Pregnancy/breast-feeding precautions:** Inform prescriber if you are or intend to be pregnant. Breast-feeding is not recommended.

**Geriatric Considerations:** (See Warnings/Precautions, Adverse Reactions, and Overdose/Toxicology.) Elderly patients have an increased risk of adverse response to side effects or adverse reactions to antipsychotics. These can include but are not limited to the following.

Anticholinergic effects: CNS toxicity with confusion, memory loss, psychotic behavior, and agitation.

Extrapyramidal effects (EPS): Parkinson's syndrome and akathisia may occur as often as 50% in patients >60 years of age. Tardive dyskinesia (motor restlessness) may be 40% in elderly; may be related to duration and total accumulated dose over time; may be somewhat reversible if diagnosed early enough.

Orthostatic hypotension: Increased risk for falls.

Sedation: In nonpsychotic patients, may result in feelings of depersonalization, derealization, and dysphoria.

Cardiac toxicity: Cardiac arrhythmias have occurred with therapeutic doses of antipsychotics.

Malignant neuroleptic syndrome: Development of hyperthermia, muscular rigidity, autonomic instability, and altered mental status.

Many elderly patients receive antipsychotic medications for inappropriate nonpsychotic behavior. Before initiating antipsychotic medication, all possible reversible causes should be investigated. Stress may cause acute "confusion" or worsening of baseline nonpsychotic behaviors; any changes in disease state (in any organ) may result in behavioral changes. Common acute changes in behavior may be due also to increases in drug dose addition, or addition of a new drug to the regimen; fluid/electrolyte alterations; infections; or changes in the environment.

Meta-analysis of controlled trials of antipsychotic (phenothiazines, butyrophenones) use with agitated, demented, elderly patients has concluded that the use of neuroleptics results in a response rate of 18%. Clearly, neuroleptic therapy for behavior control should be limited, with frequent attempts to withdraw the agent for behavior control. When use is indicated, initial doses should be lower to start and monitored closely.

**Additional Information** The hydrochloride formulations contain tartrazine and/or ethanol. The decanoate and enanthate injections contain benzyl alcohol.

**Related Information**

Antipsychotic Agents Comparison *on page 1371*
Antipsychotic Medication Guidelines *on page 1436*

♦ **Flura®** *see page 1294*
♦ **Flura-Drops®** *see page 1294*
♦ **Flura-Loz®** *see page 1294*
♦ **Flurandrenolide** *see* Topical Corticosteroids *on page 1152*
♦ **Flurate® Ophthalmic Solution** *see page 1248*

## Flurazepam (flure AZ e pam)

**U.S. Brand Names** Dalmane®

**Therapeutic Category** Benzodiazepine

**Pregnancy Risk Factor** X

**Lactation** Excretion in breast milk unknown/not recommended

**Use** Short-term treatment of insomnia

**Mechanism of Action/Effect** Depresses all levels of the CNS, including the limbic and reticular formation, probably through the increased action of gamma-aminobutyric acid (GABA), which is a major inhibitory neurotransmitter in the brain

**Contraindications** Hypersensitivity to flurazepam or any component; there may be cross-sensitivity with other benzodiazepines; pregnancy; pre-existing CNS depression; respiratory depression; acute angle-closure glaucoma

**Warnings** Use with caution in patients receiving other CNS depressants, patients with low albumin, renal or hepatic dysfunction, and in the elderly. May cause drug dependency.

(Continued)

## Flurazepam *(Continued)*

**Drug Interactions**

**Cytochrome P-450 Effect:** May be a substrate for cytochrome isoenzymes.

**Decreased Effect:** Decreased effect of flurazepam with oral contraceptives (combination products). Cigarette smoking may decrease the sedative effect. Decreased effect of levodopa.

**Increased Effect/Toxicity:** Increased toxicity with alcohol, CNS depressants, morphine, MAO inhibitors, loxapine, cimetidine.

**Effects on Lab Values** Elevated alkaline phosphatase, AST, ALT, and bilirubin (total and direct)

**Adverse Reactions**

>10%:

Central nervous system: Drowsiness, ataxia, lightheadedness, headache, dizziness, impaired coordination, anxiety, fatigue, slurred speech, irritability, nervousness, insomnia, memory impairment, cognitive disorder, dysarthria, anxiety

Gastrointestinal: Decreased salivation (dry mouth)

Genitourinary: Micturition difficulties

1% to 10%:

Cardiovascular: Tachycardia, syncope

Central nervous system: Confusion, depersonalization, mental depression, perceptual disturbances, parethesias, weakness, akathisia, agitation, disinhibition, talkativeness, derealization, dream abnormalities, fear

Endocrine & metabolic: Increased libido, decreased libido

Gastrointestinal: Abdominal or stomach cramps, increased or decreased appetite, weight gain or loss, nausea, vomiting

Neuromuscular & skeletal: Muscle cramps

Ocular: Photophobia, blurred vision

Otic: Tinnitus

Respiratory: Nasal congestion

Miscellaneous: Sweating

<1% (Limited to important or life-threatening symptoms): Hypotension, leukopenia, granulocytopenia; elevated SGOT, SGPT, bilirubin, alkaline phosphatase; dyspnea

**Overdose/Toxicology** Symptoms of overdose include respiratory depression, hypoactive reflexes, unsteady gait, and hypotension. Treatment for benzodiazepine overdose is supportive. Flumazenil has been shown to selectively block the binding of benzodiazepines to CNS receptors, resulting in a reversal of benzodiazepine-induced CNS depression. Respiratory depression may not be reversed.

**Pharmacodynamics/Kinetics**

**Half-life Elimination:** 40-114 hours

**Metabolism:** In the liver to N-desalkylflurazepam (active)

**Onset:** Onset of hypnotic effect: 15-20 minutes; Peak: 3-6 hours

**Duration:** 7-8 hours

**Formulations** Capsule, as hydrochloride: 15 mg, 30 mg

**Dosing**

**Adults:** Oral: 15-30 mg at bedtime

**Elderly:** Oral: 15 mg at bedtime. Avoid use if possible.

**Administration**

**Oral:** Give 30 minutes to 1 hour before bedtime on empty stomach with full glass of water. Can be taken with food if GI distress occurs.

**Stability**

**Storage:** Store in light-resistant containers.

**Additional Nursing Issues**

**Physical Assessment:** For short-term use. Assess effectiveness and interactions of other medications (see Drug Interactions). See Contraindications and Warnings/Precautions for cautious use. Assess for history of addiction; long-term use can result in dependence, abuse, or tolerance. Evaluate periodically for need for continued use. After long-term use, taper dosage slowly when discontinuing. For inpatient use, institute safety measures (side rails, night light, call bell, assistance with ambulation) and monitor effectiveness and adverse reactions. For outpatients, monitor for effectiveness of therapy and adverse reactions (see Adverse Reactions) at beginning of therapy and periodically with long-term use. Assess knowledge/teach patient appropriate use, interventions to reduce side effects, and adverse symptoms to report. **Pregnancy risk factor X** - Determine that patient is not pregnant before beginning treatment and do not give to women of childbearing age or to males who may have intercourse with women of childbearing age unless both male and female are capable of complying with barrier contraceptive measures during therapy and for 1 month following therapy. Breast-feeding is not recommended.

**Patient Information/Instruction:** Use exactly as directed (do not increase dose or frequency or discontinue without consulting prescriber); may cause physical and/or psychological dependence. May take with food to decrease GI upset. While using this medication, do not use alcohol or other prescription or OTC medications (especially, pain medications, sedatives, antihistamines, or hypnotics) without consulting prescriber. Maintain adequate hydration (2-3 L/day of fluids unless instructed to restrict fluid intake). You may experience drowsiness, dizziness, lightheadedness, or blurred vision (use caution when driving or engaging in tasks requiring alertness until response to drug is known); dry mouth, nausea or vomiting (small frequent meals, frequent mouth care, chewing gum, or sucking lozenges may help); difficulty urinating (void before taking medication); or altered libido (resolves when medication is discontinued).

Report CNS changes (confusion, depression, increased sedation, excitation, headache, abnormal thinking, insomnia, or nightmares, memory impairment, impaired coordination); muscle pain or weakness; difficulty breathing; persistent dizziness, chest pain, or palpitations; alterations in normal gait; vision changes; ringing in ears; or ineffectiveness of medication. **Pregnancy/breast-feeding precautions:** Inform prescriber if you are pregnant. Do not get pregnant during or for 1 month following therapy. Male: Do not cause a female to become pregnant. Male/female: Consult prescriber for instruction on appropriate barrier contraceptive measures. This drug may cause severe fetal defects. Breast-feeding is not recommended.

**Geriatric Considerations:** Due to its long-acting metabolite, flurazepam is not considered a drug of choice in the elderly. Long-acting benzodiazepines have been associated with falls in the elderly. Interpretive guidelines from the Health Care Financing. Administration (HCFA) discourage the use of this agent in residents of long-term care facilities.

**Related Information**

Anxiolytic/Hypnotic Use in Long-Term Care Facilities *on page 1430*
Benzodiazepines Comparison *on page 1375*

## Flurbiprofen (flure BI proe fen)

**U.S. Brand Names** Ansaid® Oral; Ocufen® Ophthalmic

**Therapeutic Category** Nonsteroidal Anti-Inflammatory Agent (NSAID); Ophthalmic Agent

**Pregnancy Risk Factor** C

**Lactation** Excretion in breast milk unknown

**Use**

Ophthalmic: Inhibition of intraoperative miosis; prevention and management of postoperative ocular inflammation and postoperative cystoid macular edema remains to be determined

Oral: Acute or long-term treatment of signs and symptoms of rheumatoid arthritis and osteoarthritis

**Mechanism of Action/Effect** Inhibits prostaglandin synthesis by decreasing the activity of the enzyme, cyclo-oxygenase, which results in decreased formation of prostaglandin precursors

**Contraindications** Hypersensitivity to flurbiprofen or any component; hypersensitivity to other NSAIDs or aspirin; dendritic keratitis

**Warnings** Should be used with caution in patients with a history of herpes simplex, keratitis, and patients who might be affected by inhibition of platelet aggregation. Slowing of corneal wound healing; patients in whom asthma, rhinitis, or urticaria is precipitated by aspirin or other NSAIDs. Pregnancy factor C.

**Drug Interactions**

**Cytochrome P-450 Effect:** CYP2C9 enzyme substrate; CYP2C9 enzyme inhibitor

**Decreased Effect:** Ophthalmic: When used with concurrent administration of flurbiprofen, with acetylcholine chloride and carbachol have been shown to be ineffective. Reports of acetylcholine chloride and carbachol being ineffective when used with flurbiprofen.

**Food Interactions** Food may decrease the rate but not the extent of absorption.

**Adverse Reactions**

**Ophthalmic:**

>10%: Ocular: Slowing of corneal wound healing, mild ocular stinging, itching and burning eyes, ocular irritation

1% to 10%: Ocular: Eye redness

**Systemic:**

1% to 10%:

Central nervous system: Headache, nervousness, dizziness
Dermatologic: Itching, rash
Endocrine & metabolic: Fluid retention
Gastrointestinal: Abdominal cramps, heartburn, indigestion, nausea, vomiting
Otic: Tinnitus

<1% (Limited to important or life-threatening symptoms): Congestive heart failure, hypertension, arrhythmias, tachycardia, confusion, hallucinations, aseptic meningitis, mental depression, drowsiness, insomnia, urticaria, erythema multiforme, toxic epidermal necrolysis, Stevens-Johnson syndrome, angioedema, polydipsia, hot flashes, gastritis, GI ulceration, cystitis, polyuria, agranulocytosis, anemia, hemolytic anemia, bone marrow suppression, leukopenia, thrombocytopenia, hepatitis, peripheral neuropathy, toxic amblyopia, blurred vision, conjunctivitis, dry eyes, decreased hearing, acute renal failure, shortness of breath, allergic rhinitis, epistaxis

**Overdose/Toxicology** Symptoms of overdose include apnea, metabolic acidosis, coma, nystagmus, leukocytosis, and renal failure. Management of nonsteroidal anti-inflammatory (NSAID) intoxication is supportive and symptomatic. Since many NSAIDs undergo enterohepatic cycling, multiple doses of charcoal may be needed to reduce the potential for delayed toxicities.

**Pharmacodynamics/Kinetics**

**Half-life Elimination:** 5.7 hours

**Time to Peak:** 1.5 hours

**Metabolism:** Hepatic biotransformation

**Excretion:** Kidney

**Formulations**

Flurbiprofen sodium:

Solution, ophthalmic (Ocufen®): 0.03% (2.5 mL, 5 mL, 10 mL)
Tablet (Ansaid®): 50 mg, 100 mg

(Continued)

## Flurbiprofen *(Continued)*

**Dosing**

**Adults:**

Oral: Rheumatoid arthritis and osteoarthritis: Initial: 50 mg 4 times/day to 100 mg 3 times/day; do not administer more than 100 mg for any single dose; maximum: 300 mg/day.

Ophthalmic: Instill 1 drop every 30 minutes, 2 hours prior to surgery (total of 4 drops to each affected eye)

**Elderly:** Refer to adult dosing.

**Administration**

**Oral:** Take with a full glass of water.

**Additional Nursing Issues**

**Physical Assessment:** Systemic: Assess effectiveness and interactions of other medications patient may be taking (see Contraindications, Warnings/Precautions, and Drug Interactions). Monitor laboratory tests (see above) and therapeutic response (eg, relief of pain and inflammation, activity tolerance), and adverse reactions (eg, GI effects, hepatotoxicity, or ototoxicity) at beginning of therapy and periodically throughout therapy (see Warnings/Precautions, Adverse Reactions, and Overdose/Toxicology). Assess knowledge/teach patient appropriate use, interventions to reduce side effects, and adverse symptoms to report. **Pregnancy risk factor C** - benefits of use should outweigh possible risks. Note breast-feeding caution. Ophthalmic absorption is probably minimal.

**Patient Information/Instruction:**

Oral: Take this medication exactly as directed; do not increase dose without consulting prescriber. Do not crush tablets or break capsules. Take with food or milk to reduce GI distress. Maintain adequate fluid intake (2-3 L/day of fluids unless instructed to restrict fluid intake). Do not use alcohol, aspirin, or aspirin-containing medication, and all other anti-inflammatory medications without consulting prescriber. You may experience drowsiness, dizziness, nervousness, or headache (use caution when driving or engaging in tasks requiring alertness until response to drug is known); anorexia, nausea, vomiting, or heartburn (frequent small meals, frequent mouth care, sucking lozenges, or chewing gum may help); fluid retention (weigh yourself weekly and report unusual (3-5 lb/week) weight gain). GI bleeding, ulceration, or perforation can occur with or without pain; discontinue medication and contact prescriber if persistent abdominal pain or cramping, or blood in stool occurs. Report breathlessness, difficulty breathing, or unusual cough; chest pain, rapid heartbeat, palpitations; unusual bruising/bleeding; blood in urine, stool, mouth, or vomitus; swollen extremities; skin rash or itching; acute fatigue; changes in hearing or ringing in ears. **Pregnancy/breast-feeding precautions:** Inform prescriber if you are or intend to be pregnant. Consult prescriber if breast-feeding.

Ophthalmic: Wash hands before instilling. Sit or lie down to instill. Open eye, look at ceiling, and instill prescribed amount of medication. Close eye and roll eye in all directions, and apply gentle pressure to inner corner of eye. Do not let tip of applicator touch eye or contaminate tip of applicator. Use protective dark eyewear until healed; avoid direct sunlight. Temporary stinging or burning may occur. Report persistent pain, burning, redness, vision disturbances, swelling, itching, or worsening of condition.

**Geriatric Considerations:** Elderly are at high risk for adverse effects from nonsteroidal anti-inflammatory agents. As much as 60% of elderly can develop peptic ulceration and/or hemorrhage asymptomatically. The concomitant use of $H_2$ blockers, omeprazole, and sucralfate is not effective as prophylaxis with the exception of NSAID-induced duodenal ulcers which may be prevented by the use of ranitidine. Misoprostol is the only prophylactic agent proven effective. Also, concomitant disease and drug use contribute to the risk for GI adverse effects. Use lowest effective dose for shortest period possible. Consider renal function decline with age. Use of NSAIDs can compromise existing renal function especially when $Cl_{cr}$ is ≤30 mL/minute. Tinnitus may be a difficult and unreliable indication of toxicity due to age-related hearing loss or eighth cranial nerve damage. CNS adverse effects such as confusion, agitation, and hallucination are generally seen in overdose or high-dose situations, but elderly may demonstrate these adverse effects at lower doses than younger adults.

**Related Information**

Nonsalicylate/Nonsteroidal Anti-inflammatory Comparison *on page 1401*
Ophthalmic Agents *on page 1282*

♦ **Fluress® Ophthalmic Solution** *see page 1248*
♦ **5-Flurocytosine** *see* Flucytosine *on page 492*
♦ **Flurosyn®** *see* Topical Corticosteroids *on page 1152*

## Flutamide (FLOO ta mide)

**U.S. Brand Names** Eulexin®

**Therapeutic Category** Antiandrogen

**Pregnancy Risk Factor** D

**Lactation** Not indicated for use in women

**Use** In combination therapy with LHRH agonist analogues in treatment of metastatic prostatic carcinoma. A study has shown that the addition of flutamide to leuprolide therapy in patients with advanced prostatic cancer increased median actuarial survival time to 34.9 months versus 27.9 months with leuprolide alone. To achieve benefit to combination therapy, both drugs need to be started simultaneously.

**Mechanism of Action/Effect** Nonsteroidal antiandrogen that inhibits androgen uptake or inhibits binding of androgen in target tissues

**Contraindications** Hypersensitivity to flutamide; pregnancy

**Warnings** Gynecomastia occurs in approximately 9% of patients taking flutamide. Patients, who have taken flutamide, with glucose-6 phosphate dehydrogenase deficiency or hemoglobin M disease or smokers are at risk of toxicities associated aniline exposure, including methemoglobinemia, hemolytic anemia, and cholestatic jaundice. Monitor methemoglobin levels. Liver injury including abnormal LFTs, jaundice, hepatic necrosis and hepatic encephalopathy have been reported in patients taking flutamide.

**Drug Interactions**

**Cytochrome P-450 Effect:** CYP3A3/4 enzyme substrate

**Adverse Reactions**

>10%:

Gastrointestinal: Nausea, vomiting, diarrhea

Genitourinary: Impotence

Endocrine & metabolic: Loss of libido, hot flashes

1% to 10%:

Endocrine & metabolic: Gynecomastia

Gastrointestinal: Anorexia

Neuromuscular & skeletal: Numbness in extremities

<1% (Limited to important or life-threatening symptoms): Hypertension, edema, hepatitis

**Overdose/Toxicology** Symptoms of overdose include hypoactivity, ataxia, anorexia, vomiting, slow respiration, and lacrimation. Induce vomiting. Management is supportive. Dialysis is of no benefit.

**Pharmacodynamics/Kinetics**

**Half-life Elimination:** 5-6 hours

**Metabolism:** Liver

**Excretion:** Urine

**Formulations** Capsule: 125 mg

**Dosing**

**Adults:** Oral: 2 capsules every 8 hours for a total daily dose of 750 mg

**Elderly:** Refer to adult dosing.

**Administration**

**Oral:** Contents of capsule may be opened and mixed with applesauce, pudding, or other soft foods. Mixing with a beverage is not recommended.

**Stability**

**Storage:** Store at room temperature.

**Monitoring Laboratory Tests** LFTs, tumor reduction, testosterone/estrogen, phosphatase serum levels, prostate specific antigen

**Additional Nursing Issues**

**Physical Assessment:** See Warnings/Precautions and Contraindications for use cautions. Monitor effectiveness of therapy, laboratory tests, and adverse response (see Adverse Reactions and Overdose/Toxicology). Assess knowledge/teach patient appropriate use, possible side effects, and adverse symptoms to report. **Pregnancy risk factor D** - instruct patient on absolute need for barrier contraceptives.

**Patient Information/Instruction:** Take as directed; do not discontinue without consulting prescriber. You may experience decreased libido, impotence, swelling of breasts, or decreased appetite (small frequent meals may help). Report chest pain or palpitation; acute abdominal pain; pain, tingling, or numbness of extremities; swelling of extremities or unusual weight gain; difficulty breathing; or other persistent adverse effects. **Pregnancy precautions:** This drug will cause fetal abnormalities - use barrier contraceptives.

**Geriatric Considerations:** A study has shown that the addition of flutamide to leuprolide therapy in patients with advanced prostatic cancer increased median actuarial survival time to 34.9 months versus 27.9 months with leuprolide alone. No specific dose alterations are necessary in the elderly.

♦ **Flutex®** *see* Topical Corticosteroids *on page 1152*

♦ **Flutex®** *see* Triamcinolone *on page 1171*

## Fluticasone (floo TIK a sone)

**U.S. Brand Names** Cutivate™; Flonase®; Flovent®

**Therapeutic Category** Corticosteroid, Oral Inhaler; Corticosteroid, Nasal

**Pregnancy Risk Factor** C

**Lactation** Excretion in breast milk unknown

**Use**

Intranasal: Management of seasonal and perennial allergic rhinitis in patients ≥4 years of age

Topical: Relief of inflammation and pruritus associated with corticosteroid-responsive dermatoses [medium potency topical corticosteroid]

**Mechanism of Action/Effect** Fluticasone belongs to a new group of corticosteroids which utilizes a fluorocarbothioate ester linkage at the 17 carbon position; extremely potent vasoconstrictive and anti-inflammatory activity; has a weak hypothalamic -pituitary- adrenocortical axis (HPA) inhibitory potency when applied topically, which gives the drug a high therapeutic index. The mechanism of action for all topical corticosteroids is not well defined, however, is believed to be a combination of three important properties: anti-inflammatory activity, immunosuppressive properties, and antiproliferative actions.

**Contraindications** Hypersensitivity to fluticasone or any component; bacterial infections; ophthalmic use

**Warnings** Adverse systemic effects may occur when used on large areas of the body, denuded areas, for prolonged periods of time, with an occlusive dressing, and/or in

(Continued)

## Fluticasone *(Continued)*

infants or small children. Has been associated with eosinophilic vasculitis (Churg-Strauss syndrome), usually related to decrease or withdrawal of oral corticosteroids. Pregnancy factor C.

**Adverse Reactions**

**Inhalation:**

1% to 10%:

Central nervous system: Headache

Respiratory: Epistaxis, nasal burning, nasal irritation, pharyngitis

<1% (Limited to important or life-threatening symptoms): Bronchospasm, eosinophilic vasculitis (Churg-Strauss syndrome)

**Topical:** <1% (Limited to important or life-threatening symptoms): HPA suppression, Cushing's syndrome, secondary infection

**Overdose/Toxicology** When consumed in high doses over prolonged periods, systemic hypercorticism and adrenal suppression may occur. In those cases, discontinuation of the corticosteroid should be done judiciously.

**Formulations**

Fluticasone propionate:

Spray, aerosol, oral inhalation (Flovent®): 44 mcg/actuation (7.9 g = 60 actuations or 13 g = 120 actuations), 110 mcg/actuation (13 g = 120 actuations); 220 mcg/actuation (13 g = 120 actuations)

Spray, intranasal (Flonase®): 50 mcg/actuation (9 g = 60 actuations, 16 g = 120 actuations)

Topical (Cutivate™):

Cream: 0.05% (15 g, 30 g, 60 g)

Ointment: 0.005% (15 g, 60 g)

**Dosing**

**Adults:**

Topical: Apply sparingly in a thin film twice daily

Intranasal: Initially 2 sprays (50 mcg/spray) (1 spray for children) per nostril once daily. After the first few days, dosage may be reduced to 1 spray per nostril once daily for maintenance therapy. Maximum total daily dose should not exceed 4 sprays (200 mcg)/day.

**Elderly:** Refer to adult dosing.

**Administration**

**Inhalation:** Nasal inhalation: Shake gently before use. For intranasal use only.

**Topical:** Apply sparingly in a thin film of cream or ointment. Rub in lightly.

**Additional Nursing Issues**

**Physical Assessment:** Monitor effectiveness of therapy and adverse reactions (see Adverse Reactions) at beginning of therapy and periodically with long-term use. Assess knowledge/teach patient appropriate use, interventions to reduce side effects, and adverse symptoms to report. **Pregnancy risk factor C** - benefits of use should outweigh possible risks. Note breast-feeding caution.

**Patient Information/Instruction:** Use as directed; do not overuse and use only for length of time prescribed. **Pregnancy/breast-feeding precautions:** Inform prescriber if you are or intend to be pregnant. Consult prescriber if breast-feeding.

Topical: For external use only. Apply thin film of cream to affected area only; rub in lightly. Do not apply occlusive covering unless advised by prescriber. Wash hand thoroughly after use; avoid contact with eyes. Notify prescriber if skin condition persists or worsens.

Nasal spray: Shake gently before use. Use at regular intervals, no more frequently than directed. Report unusual cough or spasm; persistent nasal bleeding, burning, or irritation; or worsening of condition.

**Geriatric Considerations:** No specific information for the elderly patient is available.

♦ **Fluticasone** *see* Topical Corticosteroids *on page 1152*

## Fluvastatin (FLOO va sta tin)

**U.S. Brand Names** Lescol®

**Therapeutic Category** Antilipemic Agent (HMG-CoA Reductase Inhibitor)

**Pregnancy Risk Factor** X

**Lactation** Enters breast milk/not recommended

**Use** Adjunct to dietary therapy to decrease elevated serum total and LDL cholesterol concentrations in primary hypercholesterolemia

**Mechanism of Action/Effect** Acts by competitively inhibiting 3-hydroxyl-3-methylglutaryl-coenzyme A (HMG-CoA) reductase, the enzyme that catalyzes the reduction of HMG-CoA to mevalonate; this is an early rate-limiting step in cholesterol biosynthesis. HDL is increased while total, LDL and VLDL cholesterols, apolipoprotein B, and plasma triglycerides are decreased.

**Contraindications** Hypersensitivity to fluvastatin; active liver disease; elevated serum transaminases; myopathy or marked elevations of CPK; pregnancy

**Warnings** Avoid combination of clofibrate and fluvastatin due to possible myopathy. Consider temporarily withholding therapy in patients with risk of developing renal failure. Avoid prolonged exposure to the sun or other ultraviolet light.

**Drug Interactions**

**Cytochrome P-450 Effect:** CYP2C9 enzyme substrate; CYP2C9, 2C18, and 2C19 enzyme inhibitor

**Decreased Effect:** Administration of cholestyramine at the same time with fluvastatin reduces absorption and clinical effect of fluvastatin.

**Increased Effect/Toxicity:** Anticoagulant effect of warfarin may be increased. Cholestyramine effect will be additive with fluvastatin if administration times are separated. Concurrent use of erythromycin and HMG-CoA reductase inhibitors may increase the risk of rhabdomyolysis.

**Effects on Lab Values** ↑ serum transaminases, CPK, alkaline phosphatase, and bilirubin and thyroid function tests

**Adverse Reactions**

1% to 10%:

Central nervous system: Headache, dizziness, insomnia
Dermatologic: Rash
Gastrointestinal: Heartburn, diarrhea, nausea, constipation, flatulence, abdominal pain
Neuromuscular & skeletal: Back pain, muscle pain, arthropathy
Miscellaneous:

<1% (Limited to important or life-threatening symptoms): Toxic epidermal necrolysis, erythema multiforme, Stevens-Johnson syndrome, angioedema, thrombocytopenia, leukopenia, hemolytic anemia, elevated ESR, elevated serum transaminases, cirrhosis, hepatic necrosis, hepatoma, dyspnea, lupus erythematosus-like syndrome

**Overdose/Toxicology** No symptomatology has been reported in cases of significant overdose; however, supportive measure should be instituted, as required. Usefulness of dialysis is unknown.

**Pharmacodynamics/Kinetics**

**Protein Binding:** >98%

**Half-life Elimination:** 1.2 hours

**Metabolism:** Liver; undergoes extensive first pass hepatic extraction; metabolized to inactive and active metabolites although the active forms do not circulate systemically

**Excretion:** Urine and feces

**Formulations** Capsule: 20 mg, 40 mg

**Dosing**

**Adults:** Oral:

Initial: 20 mg at bedtime
Usual dose: 20-40 mg at bedtime

**Note:** Splitting the 40 mg dose into a twice daily regimen may provide a modest improvement in LDL response. Maximum response occurs within 4-6 weeks. Adjust dosage as needed in response to periodic lipid determinations during the first 4 weeks after a dosage change.

**Elderly:** Refer to adult dosing.

**Hepatic Impairment:** Decrease dose and monitor effects carefully in patients with hepatic insufficiency.

**Administration**

**Oral:** Fluvastatin may be taken without regard to meals; best if taken at bedtime. Lipid-lowering effects are additive when fluvastatin is combined with a bile-acid binding resin or niacin; however, it must be administered at least 2 hours following these drugs.

**Monitoring Laboratory Tests** Obtain baseline LFTs and total cholesterol profile. Repeat tests at 12 weeks after initiation of therapy or elevation in dose and periodically thereafter.

**Additional Nursing Issues**

**Physical Assessment:** Monitor laboratory tests as ordered. **Pregnancy risk factor X** - determine that patient is not pregnant before beginning therapy and do not give to women of childbearing age or male having intercourse with women of childbearing age unless both are capable of complying with barrier contraceptive measures for 1 month prior to, during, and for 1 month following therapy. Breast-feeding is not recommended during therapy and for 1 month following therapy.

**Patient Information/Instruction:** Take at bedtime since highest rate of cholesterol synthesis occurs between midnight and 5 AM. Follow diet and exercise regimen as prescribed. Have periodic ophthalmic exam to check for cataract development. Avoid prolonged exposure to the sun and other ultraviolet light. Report unexplained muscle pain or weakness, especially if accompanied by fever or malaise. **Pregnancy/breast-feeding precautions:** Do not get pregnant during therapy or for 1 month following therapy. Consult prescriber for appropriate barrier contraceptive measures. Breast-feeding is not recommended while on this drug and for several weeks after last dose. Male: Consult prescriber for barrier contraceptive measures when having intercourse with women of childbearing age. This drug may cause severe fetal defects. Male/female: Do not donate blood during or for 1 month following therapy. Breast-feeding is not recommended.

**Dietary Issues:** Before initiation of therapy, patients should be placed on a standard cholesterol-lowering diet for 3-6 months and the diet should be continued during drug therapy.

**Geriatric Considerations:** The definition of and, therefore, when to treat hyperlipidemia in the elderly is a controversial issue. The National Cholesterol Education Program recommends that all adults 20 years of age and older maintain a plasma cholesterol <200 mg/dL. By this definition, 60% of all elderly would be considered to have a borderline high (200-239 mg/dL) or high (≥240 mg/dL) plasma cholesterol. However, plasma cholesterol has been shown to be a less reliable predictor of coronary heart disease in the elderly. Therefore, it is the authors' belief that pharmacologic treatment be reserved for those who are unable to obtain a desirable plasma cholesterol level by diet alone and for whom the benefits of treatment are believed to outweigh the potential adverse effects, drug interactions, and cost of treatment.

(Continued)

## Fluvastatin *(Continued)*

**Pregnancy Issues:** Skeletal malformations have occurred in animals following agents with similar structure. Avoid use in women of childbearing age. Discontinue if pregnancy occurs.

**Related Information**

Lipid-Lowering Agents Comparison *on page 1393*

## Fluvoxamine (floo VOKS ah meen)

**U.S. Brand Names** Luvox®

**Therapeutic Category** Antidepressant, Selective Serotonin Reuptake Inhibitor

**Pregnancy Risk Factor** C

**Lactation** Enters breast milk/not recommended (AAP rates "of concern")

**Use** Approved for the treatment of obsessive-compulsive disorder (OCD)

**Mechanism of Action/Effect** Inhibits CNS neuron serotonin uptake; minimal or no effect on reuptake of norepinephrine or dopamine; does not significantly bind to alpha-adrenergic, histamine or cholinergic receptors

**Contraindications** Hypersensitivity to fluvoxamine or any congeners (eg, fluoxetine); concomitant use with terfenadine, astemizole, or cisapride; use during or within 14 days of MAO inhibitors

**Warnings** Use with caution in patients with liver dysfunction, suicidal tendencies, history of seizures, mania, or drug abuse, ECT, cardiovascular disease, and the elderly. Pregnancy factor C.

**Drug Interactions**

**Cytochrome P-450 Effect:** CYP1A2 enzyme substrate; CYP1A2, 2C9, 2C19, 2D6, and 3A3/4 enzyme inhibitor

**Increased Effect/Toxicity:** Because fluvoxamine inhibits cytochrome P-450 isozymes, it is associated with numerous significant drug interactions.

Increased toxicity: Astemizole is metabolized by the cytochrome P-450 3A4 isozyme, increased levels of these drugs have been associated with prolongation of the Q-T interval and potentially fatal, torsade de pointes ventricular arrhythmias. Since fluvoxamine inhibits the enzyme responsible for their clearance, the concomitant use of these agents is contraindicated.

Potentiates triazolam and alprazolam (dose should be reduced by at least 50%), hypertensive crisis with MAO inhibitors, theophylline (doses should be reduced by $^1/_3$ and plasma levels monitored), warfarin (reduce its dose and monitor PT/INR), carbamazepine (monitor levels), tricyclic antidepressants (monitor effects and reduce doses accordingly), methadone, beta-blockers (reduce dose of propranolol or metoprolol), diltiazem, and tacrine. Caution with other benzodiazepines, phenytoin, lithium, clozapine, alcohol, other CNS drugs, quinidine, ketoconazole. Potential for serotonin syndrome if combined with other serotonergic drugs.

**Adverse Reactions**

>10%: Gastrointestinal: Nausea

1% to 10%:

- Cardiovascular: Palpitations
- Central nervous system: Somnolence, muscle weakness, headache, insomnia, dizziness, nervousness, mania, hypomania, vertigo, abnormal thinking, agitation, anxiety, malaise, amnesia
- Endocrine & metabolic: Decreased libido
- Gastrointestinal: Dry mouth, abdominal pain, vomiting, heartburn, constipation, diarrhea, dysgeusia, anorexia
- Neuromuscular & skeletal: Tremors
- Miscellaneous: Sweating

<1% (Limited to important or life-threatening symptoms): Seizures, toxic epidermal necrolysis, thrombocytopenia, hepatic dysfunction, elevated serum creatinine

**Overdose/Toxicology** Symptoms of overdose include drowsiness, nausea, vomiting, abdominal pain, tremor, sinus bradycardia, and seizures. A specific antidote does not exist. Treatment is supportive.

**Pharmacodynamics/Kinetics**

**Protein Binding:** ~80% (mostly albumin)

**Half-life Elimination:** ~15 hours

**Time to Peak:** 3-8 hours

**Metabolism:** Liver

**Excretion:** Urine

**Onset:** >2 weeks (therapeutic effects)

**Formulations** Tablet: 50 mg, 100 mg

**Dosing**

**Adults:** Oral: Initial: 50 mg at bedtime; adjust in 50 mg increments at 4- to 7-day intervals; usual dose range: 100-300 mg/day; divide total daily dose into 2 doses; give larger portion at bedtime.

**Elderly:** Reduce dose, titrate slowly. See Geriatric Considerations.

**Hepatic Impairment:** Reduce dose, titrate slowly.

**Monitoring Laboratory Tests** Liver and kidney function assessment prior to beginning drug therapy

**Additional Nursing Issues**

**Physical Assessment:** Assess other medications patient may be taking for effectiveness and interactions (see Drug Interactions). See Contraindications and Warnings/Precautions for cautious use. Has potential for psychological or physiological dependence, abuse, or tolerance. Monitor laboratory tests, therapeutic response (ie, mental status, mood, affect, suicidal ideation), and adverse reactions at beginning of therapy and periodically with long-term use (eg, CNS, and gastrointestinal - see Adverse Reactions and Overdose/Toxicology). Taper dosage slowly when discontinuing (allow 3-4 weeks between discontinuing Luvox® and starting another antidepressant). Assess knowledge/teach patient appropriate use, interventions to reduce side effects, and adverse symptoms to report. **Pregnancy risk factor C** - benefits of use should outweigh possible risks. Breast-feeding is not recommended.

**Patient Information/Instruction:** Take exactly as directed (do not increase dose or frequency); may take 2-3 weeks to achieve desired results; may cause physical and/or psychological dependence. Take once-a-day dose at bedtime. Avoid excessive alcohol, caffeine, and other prescription or OTC medications not approved by prescriber. Maintain adequate hydration (2-3 L/day of fluids unless instructed to restrict fluid intake). You may experience drowsiness, lightheadedness, impaired coordination, dizziness, or blurred vision (use caution when driving or engaging in tasks requiring alertness until response to drug is known); nausea, vomiting, or anorexia (small frequent meals, frequent mouth care, chewing gum, or sucking lozenges may help); constipation (increased exercise, fluids, or dietary fruit and fiber may help); diarrhea (buttermilk, yogurt, or boiled milk may help); postural hypotension (use caution when climbing stairs or changing position from lying or sitting to standing); or decreased sexual function or libido (reversible). Report persistent CNS effects (nervousness, restlessness, insomnia, anxiety, excitation, headache, sedation, seizures, mania, abnormal thinking); rash or skin irritation; muscle cramping, tremors, or change in gait; chest pain or palpitations; change in urinary pattern; or worsening of condition. **Pregnancy/breast-feeding precautions:** Inform prescriber if you are or intend to be pregnant. Breast-feeding is not recommended.

**Geriatric Considerations:** It may be best to select a different agent when treating depression in the elderly.

**Related Information**

Antidepressant Agents Comparison *on page 1368*

- **Fluzone®** *see page 1256*
- **Flynoken A** *see* Leucovorin *on page 662*
- **FML®** *see* Fluorometholone *on page 499*
- **FML® Forte** *see* Fluorometholone *on page 499*
- **FML-S® Ophthalmic Suspension** *see page 1282*
- **Foille® [OTC]** *see* Benzocaine *on page 141*
- **Foille® Medicated First Aid [OTC]** *see* Benzocaine *on page 141*
- **Folacin** *see* Folic Acid *on this page*
- **Folate** *see* Folic Acid *on this page*
- **Folbesyn®** *see page 1294*
- **Folex® PFS** *see* Methotrexate *on page 743*

## Folic Acid (FOE lik AS id)

**U.S. Brand Names** Folvite®

**Synonyms** Folacin; Folate; Pteroylglutamic Acid

**Therapeutic Category** Vitamin, Water Soluble

**Pregnancy Risk Factor** A/C (if dose exceeds RDA recommendation)

**Lactation** Enters breast milk/compatible

**Use** Treatment of megaloblastic and macrocytic anemias due to folate deficiency; dietary supplement to prevent neural tube defects in the developing fetus

**Mechanism of Action/Effect** Folic acid is necessary for formation of a number of coenzymes in many metabolic systems, particularly for purine and pyrimidine synthesis; required for nucleoprotein synthesis and maintenance in erythropoiesis; stimulates WBC and platelet production in folate deficiency anemia

**Contraindications** Pernicious, aplastic, or normocytic anemias

**Warnings** Doses >0.1 mg/day may obscure pernicious anemia with continuing irreversible nerve damage progression. Resistance to treatment may occur with depressed hematopoiesis, alcoholism, deficiencies of other vitamins. Injection contains benzyl alcohol (1.5%) as preservative (use care in administration to neonates). Pregnancy factor C (if dose exceeds RDA recommendation).

**Drug Interactions**

**Decreased Effect:** In folate-deficient patients, folic acid therapy may increase phenytoin metabolism which may lead to a decrease in the effect of phenytoin. Phenytoin, primidone, para-aminosalicylic acid, and sulfasalazine may decrease serum folate concentrations resulting in a folic acid deficiency. Concurrent administration of chloramphenicol and folic acid may result in antagonism of the hematopoietic response to folic acid.

**Effects on Lab Values** Falsely low serum concentrations may occur with the *Lactobacillus casei* assay method in patients on anti-infectives (eg, tetracycline).

**Adverse Reactions** <1% (Limited to important or life-threatening symptoms): Bronchospasm

**Pharmacodynamics/Kinetics**

**Onset:** Peak effect: Oral: Within 0.5-1 hour

**Formulations**

Injection, as sodium folate: 5 mg/mL (10 mL); 10 mg/mL (10 mL)

Folvite®: 5 mg/mL (10 mL)

Tablet: 0.1 mg, 0.4 mg, 0.8 mg, 1 mg

Folvite®: 1 mg

(Continued)

## Folic Acid *(Continued)*

**Dosing**

**Adults:** Oral, I.M., I.V., S.C.: Initial: 1 mg/day
Deficiency: 1-3 mg/day
Maintenance dose: 0.5 mg/day
Women of childbearing age, pregnant, and lactating women: 0.8 mg/day

**Elderly:** Refer to adult dosing.

**Administration**

**Oral:** A diluted solution for oral administration may be prepared by diluting 1 mL of folic acid injection (5 mg/mL), with 49 mL sterile water for injection. Resulting solution is 0.1 mg folic acid per 1 mL.

**I.M.:** May also be administered by deep I.M. injection.

**I.V.:** May also be administered by I.V. injection by diluting 1 mL of folic acid injection (5 mg/mL), with 49 mL sterile water for injection. Resulting solution is 0.1 mg folic acid per 1 mL.

**Stability**

**Compatibility:** Incompatible with oxidizing and reducing agents and heavy metal ions.

**Additional Nursing Issues**

**Physical Assessment:** See Pregnancy Risk Factor for cautious use.

**Patient Information/Instruction:** Take as prescribed. Toxicity can occur from elevated doses. Do not self medicate. Increase intake of foods high in folic acid (eg, dried beans, nuts, bran, vegetables, fruits) as recommended by prescriber. Excessive use of alcohol increases requirement for folic acid. May turn urine more intensely yellow. Report skin rash.

**Geriatric Considerations:** Elderly frequently have combined nutritional deficiencies. Must rule out vitamin $B_{12}$ deficiency before initiating folate therapy. Elderly RDA requirements from 1989 RDA are 200 mcg minimum (0.2 mg). Elderly, due to decreased nutrient intake, may benefit from daily intake of a multiple vitamin with minerals.

♦ **Folinic Acid** *see* Leucovorin *on page 662*
♦ **Folitab** *see* Folic Acid *on previous page*
♦ **Follutein®** *see* Chorionic Gonadotropin *on page 264*
♦ **Folvite®** *see* Folic Acid *on previous page*
♦ **Food/Antibiotic Interactions** *see page 1322*
♦ **Food/Water Drug Administration Recommendations** *see page 1323*
♦ **Formula E** *see* Guaifenesin *on page 548*
♦ **Formula Q®** *see* Quinine *on page 1004*
♦ **Formulex®** *see* Dicyclomine *on page 362*
♦ **5-Formyl Tetrahydrofolate** *see* Leucovorin *on page 662*
♦ **Fortaz®** *see* Ceftazidime *on page 228*
♦ **Fortovase®** *see* Saquinavir *on page 1043*
♦ **Fortum** *see* Ceftazidime *on page 228*
♦ **Fosamax®** *see* Alendronate *on page 50*

## Foscarnet (fos KAR net)

**U.S. Brand Names** Foscavir® Injection

**Synonyms** PFA; Phosphonoformic Acid

**Therapeutic Category** Antiviral Agent

**Pregnancy Risk Factor** C

**Lactation** Excretion in breast milk unknown/contraindicated

**Use** Treatment of herpesvirus infections suspected to be caused by acyclovir (HSV, VZV) or ganciclovir (CMV) resistant strains (this occurs almost exclusively in immunocompromised persons with immunocompromised (eg, advanced AIDS), who have received prolonged treatment for a herpesvirus infection); CMV retinitis in persons with AIDS; other CMV infections in persons unable to tolerate ganciclovir

**Mechanism of Action/Effect** Pyrophosphate analogue which acts as a noncompetitive inhibitor of many viral RNA and DNA polymerases as well as HIV reverse transcriptase. Inhibitory effects occur at concentrations which do not affect host cellular DNA polymerases; however, some human cell growth suppression has been observed with high *in vitro* concentrations. Similar to ganciclovir, foscarnet is a virostatic agent. Foscarnet does not require activation by thymidine kinase.

**Contraindications** Hypersensitivity to foscarnet; $Cl_{cr}$ <0.4 mL/minute/kg during therapy is not recommended

**Warnings** Renal impairment occurs to some degree in the majority of patients treated with foscarnet. Renal impairment may occur at any time and is usually reversible within 1 week following dose adjustment or discontinuation of therapy, however, several patients have died with renal failure within 4 weeks of stopping foscarnet. Therefore, renal function should be closely monitored. Foscarnet is deposited in teeth and bone of young, growing animals. It has adversely affected tooth enamel development in rats. Safety and effectiveness in children have not been studied. Imbalance of serum electrolytes or minerals occurs in 6% to 18% of patients (hypocalcemia, low ionized calcium, hypo- or hyperphosphatemia, hypomagnesemia or hypokalemia). Patients with a low ionized calcium may experience perioral tingling, numbness, paresthesias, tetany, and seizures. Seizures have been experienced by up to 10% of AIDS patients. Risk factors for seizures include a low baseline absolute neutrophil count (ANC), impaired baseline renal function and low total serum calcium. Some patients who have experienced seizures have died, while others have been able to continue or resume foscarnet treatment after their mineral or electrolyte abnormality has been corrected, their underlying disease state treated, or their dose decreased. Foscarnet has been shown to be mutagenic *in vitro* and in mice at very high doses. Pregnancy factor C.

**Drug Interactions**

**Increased Effect/Toxicity:** Pentamidine increases hypocalcemia. Concurrent use with ciprofloxacin increases seizure potential.

**Adverse Reactions**

>10%:
- Central nervous system: Fever, headache, seizures
- Gastrointestinal: Nausea, diarrhea, vomiting
- Hematologic: Anemia
- Renal: Nephrotoxicity (abnormal renal function, decreased creatinine clearance)

1% to 10%:
- Central nervous system: Fatigue, malaise, dizziness, hypoesthesia, depression, confusion, anxiety
- Dermatologic: Rash
- Endocrine & metabolic: Electrolyte imbalance
- Gastrointestinal: Anorexia
- Hematologic: Granulocytopenia, leukopenia
- Local: Injection site pain
- Neuromuscular & skeletal: Paresthesia, involuntary muscle contractions, rigors, neuropathy (peripheral), weakness
- Ocular: Vision abnormalities
- Respiratory: Coughing, dyspnea
- Miscellaneous: Sepsis, sweating (increased)

<1% (Limited to important or life-threatening symptoms): Cardiac failure, bradycardia, arrhythmias, cerebral edema, leg edema, peripheral edema, syncope, substernal chest pain, cholecystitis, cholelithiasis, hepatitis, hepatosplenomegaly, ascites, vocal cord paralysis

**Overdose/Toxicology** Symptoms of overdose include seizures, renal dysfunction, perioral or limb paresthesia, and hypocalcemia. Treatment is supportive.

**Pharmacodynamics/Kinetics**

**Distribution:** Up to 28% of cumulative I.V. dose may be deposited in bone

**Half-life Elimination:** ~3 hours

**Metabolism:** Biotransformation does not occur

**Excretion:** Urine

**Formulations** Injection: 24 mg/mL (250 mL, 500 mL)

**Dosing**

**Adults:** I.V.:

CMV retinitis:
- Induction treatment: 60 mg/kg/dose every 8 hours for 14-21 days
- Maintenance therapy: 90-120 mg/kg/day as a single infusion

Acyclovir-resistant HSV induction treatment: 40 mg/kg/dose every 8-12 hours for 14-21 days

**Elderly:** Refer to adult dosing.

**Renal Impairment:** See table.

**Dose Adjustment for Renal Impairment**

Adjust induction dose of foscarnet according to creatinine clearance as follows:

| Creatinine Clearance (mL/min/kg) | Foscarnet Induction Dose (mg/kg q8h) |
|---|---|
| 1.6 | 60 |
| 1.5 | 57 |
| 1.4 | 53 |
| 1.3 | 49 |
| 1.2 | 46 |
| 1.1 | 42 |
| 1 | 39 |
| 0.9 | 35 |
| 0.8 | 32 |
| 0.7 | 28 |
| 0.6 | 25 |
| 0.5 | 21 |
| 0.4 | 18 |

Adjust maintenance dose of foscarnet according to creatinine clearance as follows:

| Creatinine Clearance (mL/min/kg) | Foscarnet Maintenance Dose (mg/kg/day) |
|---|---|
| 1.4 | 90-120 |
| 1.2-1.4 | 78-104 |
| 1-1.2 | 75-100 |
| 0.8-1 | 71-94 |
| 0.6-0.8 | 63-84 |
| 0.4-0.6 | 57-75 |

(Continued)

## Foscarnet *(Continued)*

**Administration**

**I.V.:** Use an infusion pump, at a rate not exceeding 1 mg/kg/minute. Adult induction doses of 60 mg/kg are administered over 1 hour. Adult maintenance doses of 90-120 mg/kg are infused over 2 hours.

**I.V. Detail:** Undiluted (24 mg/mL) solution can be administered without further dilution when using a central venous catheter for infusion. For peripheral vein administration, the solution **must** be diluted to a final concentration **not to exceed** 12 mg/mL. The recommended dosage, frequency, and rate of infusion should not be exceeded.

**Stability**

**Storage:** Foscarnet injection is a clear, colorless solution. It should be stored at room temperature and protected from temperatures >40°C and from freezing.

**Reconstitution:** Foscarnet should be diluted in $D_5W$ or NS and transferred to PVC containers. It is stable for 24 hours at room temperature or refrigeration. For peripheral line administration, foscarnet **must** be diluted to 12 mg/mL with $D_5W$ or NS. For central line administration, foscarnet may be administered undiluted.

**Compatibility:** Incompatible with dextrose 30%, I.V. solutions containing calcium, magnesium, vancomycin, and TPN.

**Monitoring Laboratory Tests** Renal function, CBC, electrolytes

**Additional Nursing Issues**

**Physical Assessment:** Monitor laboratory results on a regular basis. Monitor effectiveness of therapy and adverse reactions as indicated in Warnings/Precautions and Adverse Reactions. Be alert for possibility of seizures. Monitor renal function carefully. Be alert to electrolyte imbalance. Monitor infusion site for irritation. **Pregnancy risk factor C** - benefits of use should outweigh possible risks. Use of barrier contraceptives has been recommended to reduce transmission of disease. Breast-feeding is contraindicated.

**Patient Information/Instruction:** Foscarnet is not a cure for the disease; progression may occur during or following therapy. Regular ophthalmic examinations will be necessary. While on the therapy it is important to maintain adequate nutrition and hydration (2-3 L/day of fluids unless instructed to restrict fluid intake); small frequent meals may help. Do not use alcohol or OTC medications without consulting prescriber. You may experience dizziness or confusion; use caution when driving or engaging in tasks that require alertness until response to drug is known. Report unresolved diarrhea or vomiting, unusual fever, chills, sore throat, unhealed sores, swollen lymph glands or extreme, or malaise. Barrier contraceptives are recommended to reduce transmission of disease. **Breast-feeding precautions:** Do not breast-feed.

**Geriatric Considerations:** Information on the use of foscarnet is lacking in the elderly. Dose adjustments and proper monitoring must be performed because of the decreased renal function common in older patients.

**Breast-feeding Issues:** The CDC recommends **not** to breast-feed if diagnosed with HIV to avoid postnatal transmission of the virus.

♦ **Foscavir® Injection** *see* Foscarnet *on page 516*

## Fosinopril (foe SIN oh pril)

**U.S. Brand Names** Monopril®

**Therapeutic Category** Angiotensin-Converting Enzyme (ACE) Inhibitors

**Pregnancy Risk Factor** C/D (2nd and 3rd trimesters)

**Lactation** Excretion in breast milk unknown

**Use** Treatment of hypertension, either alone or in combination with other antihypertensive agents; congestive heart failure

**Mechanism of Action/Effect** Competitive inhibitor of angiotensin-converting enzyme (ACE); prevents conversion of angiotensin I to angiotensin II, a potent vasoconstrictor; results in lower levels of angiotensin II which causes an increase in plasma renin activity and a reduction in aldosterone secretion; a CNS mechanism may also be involved in hypotensive effect as angiotensin II increases adrenergic outflow from CNS; vasoactive kallikreins may be decreased in conversion to active hormones by ACE inhibitors, thus reducing blood pressure

**Contraindications** Hypersensitivity to fosinopril, any component, or other angiotensin-converting enzyme inhibitors; collagen vascular disease; pregnancy (2nd and 3rd trimesters)

**Warnings** Use with caution and modify dosage in patients with renal impairment (decrease dosage) (especially renal artery stenosis), severe congestive heart failure or with coadministered diuretic therapy; experience in children is limited. Severe hypotension may occur in patients who are sodium and/or volume depleted. Initiate lower doses and monitor closely when starting therapy in these patients. Pregnancy factor C/D (2nd and 3rd trimesters).

**Drug Interactions**

**Decreased Effect:** Rifampin may decrease the effect of ACE inhibitors. Antacids may decrease the bioavailability of ACE inhibitors, may be more likely to occur with captopril, separate administration times by 1-2 hours. NSAIDs, specifically indomethacin, may reduce the hypotensive effects of ACE inhibitors. More likely to occur in low renin or volume dependent hypertensive patients.

**Increased Effect/Toxicity:** Diuretics have additive hypotensive effects with ACE inhibitors. Probenecid increases blood levels of captopril which may occur with other ACE inhibitors. Phenothiazines taken with ACE inhibitors may increase the pharmacologic effects of the ACE inhibitor. Allopurinol and ACE inhibitors may cause a higher risk of hypersensitivity reaction when taken concurrently.

**Effects on Lab Values** Positive Coombs' (direct); may cause false-positive results in urine acetone determinations using sodium nitroprusside reagent; may cause false low serum digoxin levels with the Digi-Tab RIA kit for digoxin.

**Adverse Reactions**

1% to 10%:

Cardiovascular: Orthostatic hypotension

Central nervous system: Headache, dizziness, fatigue

Endocrine & metabolic: Sexual dysfunction

Gastrointestinal: Diarrhea, nausea, vomiting

Respiratory: Cough

<1% (Limited to important or life-threatening symptoms): Chest pain, hypotension, palpitations, chest pain pectoris, cerebrovascular accident, myocardial infarction, flushing, syncope, hypertensive crisis, claudication, hypoglycemia, hyperkalemia, neutropenia, agranulocytosis, anemia, hepatitis, deterioration in renal function, oliguria, asthma, bronchospasm

**Overdose/Toxicology** Mild hypotension has been the primary toxic effect seen with acute overdose. Bradycardia may also occur; hyperkalemia occurs even with therapeutic doses, especially in patients with renal insufficiency and those taking NSAIDs. Treatment is symptom directed and supportive.

**Pharmacodynamics/Kinetics**

**Protein Binding:** ~95%

**Half-life Elimination:** Serum (fosinoprilat): 12 hours

**Time to Peak:** ~3 hours

**Metabolism:** Intestine and liver

**Excretion:** Urine and bile

**Onset:** 1 hour

**Duration:** 24 hours

**Formulations** Tablet: 10 mg, 20 mg

**Dosing**

**Adults:** Oral:

Hypertension: Initial: 10 mg/day; increase to a maximum dose of 80 mg/day. Most patients are maintained on 20-40 mg/day. May need to divide the dose into two if trough effect is inadequate. Discontinue the diuretic, if possible 2-3 days before initiation of therapy. Resume diuretic therapy carefully, if needed.

Heart failure: Initial: 10 mg/day (5 mg if renal dysfunction present) and increase, as needed, to a maximum of 40 mg once daily over several weeks. Usual dose: 20-40 mg/day. If hypotension, orthostasis, or azotemia occurs during titration, consider decreasing concomitant diuretic dose, if any.

**Elderly:** Refer to adult dosing.

**Renal Impairment:** Decrease dose and monitor effects carefully in patients with hepatic insufficiency.

Moderately dialyzable (20% to 50%)

**Monitoring Laboratory Tests** CBC, renal function tests, electrolytes

**Additional Nursing Issues**

**Physical Assessment:** Assess effectiveness and interactions of other medications (see Drug Interactions). See Warnings/Precautions and Contraindications for use cautions. Monitor effectiveness of therapy, laboratory tests, and adverse response on a regular basis during therapy, eg, postural hypotension (see Adverse Reactions and Overdose/Toxicology). Assess knowledge/teach patient appropriate use, possible side effects and appropriate interventions, and adverse symptoms to report. **Pregnancy risk factor C/D** - see Pregnancy Risk Factor - assess knowledge/instruct patient on use of barrier contraceptive measures. See Pregnancy Issues. Note breast-feeding caution.

**Patient Information/Instruction:** Take exactly as directed; do not discontinue without consulting prescriber. Take first dose at bedtime. This drug does not eliminate need for diet or exercise as recommended by prescriber. Do not use potassium supplements or salt substitutes containing potassium without consulting prescriber. May cause dizziness, fainting, lightheadedness (use caution when driving or engaging in tasks that require alertness until response to drug is known); postural hypotension (use caution when rising from lying or sitting position or climbing stairs); nausea, dry cough, diarrhea, or transient loss of appetite (small frequent meals, frequent mouth care, sucking lozenges, or chewing gum may help) - report if these persist; sexual dysfunction (will usually resolve). Report chest pain or palpitations; difficulty breathing or unusual cough; acute headache; or other persistent adverse reactions. **Pregnancy/breast-feeding precautions:** Do not get pregnant while taking this medication; use appropriate barrier contraceptive measures. Consult prescriber if breast-feeding.

**Geriatric Considerations:** Due to frequent decreases in glomerular filtration (also creatinine clearance) with aging, elderly patients may have exaggerated responses to ACE inhibitors. Differences in clinical response due to hepatic changes are not observed. ACE inhibitors may be preferred agents in elderly patients with congestive heart failure and diabetes mellitus. Diabetic proteinuria is reduced and insulin sensitivity is enhanced. In general, the side effect profile is favorable in the elderly and causes little or no CNS confusion; use lowest dose recommendations initially.

**Pregnancy Issues:** ACE inhibitors can cause fetal injury or death if taken during the 2nd or 3rd trimester. Discontinue ACE inhibitors as soon as pregnancy is detected. ACE inhibitors should not be used if patient is sexually active and not using contraceptives.

**Related Information**

ACE Inhibitors and Angiotensin Antagonists Comparison *on page 1362*

## Fosphenytoin (FOS fen i toyn)

**U.S. Brand Names** Cerebyx®

**Therapeutic Category** Anticonvulsant, Hydantoin

**Pregnancy Risk Factor** D

**Lactation** Enters breast milk/compatible (if serum level is within mother's therapeutic range)

**Use** Indicated for short-term parenteral administration when other means of phenytoin administration are unavailable, inappropriate or deemed less advantageous; the safety and effectiveness of fosphenytoin in this use has not been systematically evaluated for more than 5 days; may be used for the control of generalized convulsive status epilepticus and prevention and treatment of seizures occurring during neurosurgery

**Contraindications** Hypersensitivity to phenytoin, other hydantoins, or any component; patients with sinus bradycardia, sinoatrial block, second and third degree A-V block, or Adams-Stokes syndrome; pregnancy

**Warnings** Doses of fosphenytoin are expressed as their phenytoin sodium equivalent. Antiepileptic drugs should not be abruptly discontinued. Hypotension may occur, especially after I.V. administration at high doses and high rates of administration. Administration of phenytoin has been associated with atrial and ventricular conduction depression and ventricular fibrillation. Careful cardiac monitoring is needed when administering I.V. loading doses of fosphenytoin. Use with caution in patients with hypotension and severe myocardial insufficiency. Discontinue if skin rash or lymphadenopathy occurs. Acute hepatotoxicity associated with a hypersensitivity syndrome characterized by fever, skin eruptions, and lymphadenopathy has been reported to occur within the first 2 months of treatment.

**Drug Interactions**

**Cytochrome P-450 Effect:** CYP2C9 and 2C19 enzyme substrate; CYP1A2, 2B6, 2C, 2C9, 2C18, 2C19, 2D6, 3A3/4, and 3A5-7 enzyme inducer

**Decreased Effect:** No drugs are known to interfere with the conversion of fosphenytoin to phenytoin. Phenytoin may decrease the serum concentration or effectiveness of valproic acid, ethosuximide, felbamate, benzodiazepines, carbamazepine, lamotrigine, primidone, warfarin, oral contraceptives, corticosteroids, cyclosporine, theophylline, chloramphenicol, rifampin, doxycycline, quinidine, mexiletine, disopyramide, dopamine, or nondepolarizing skeletal muscle relaxants. Serum phenytoin concentrations may be decreased by rifampin, cisplatin, vinblastine, bleomycin, folic acid.

**Increased Effect/Toxicity:** Phenytoin may increase phenobarbital and primidone levels. Protein binding of phenytoin can be affected by valproic acid or salicylates. Serum phenytoin concentrations may be increased by cimetidine, felbamate, ethosuximide, methsuximide, chloramphenicol, disulfiram, fluconazole, omeprazole, isoniazid, trimethoprim, or sulfonamides.

**Effects on Lab Values** May decrease serum concentrations of thyroxine; may produce artifactually low results in dexamethasone or metyrapone tests; may cause increased serum concentrations of glucose, alkaline phosphatase, and gamma glutamyl transpeptidase (GGT)

**Adverse Reactions** The more important adverse clinical events caused by the I.V. use of fosphenytoin or phenytoin are cardiovascular collapse and/or central nervous system depression. Hypotension can occur when either drug is administered rapidly by the I.V. route. Do not exceed a rate of 150 mg phenytoin equivalent/minute when administering fosphenytoin.

The adverse clinical events most commonly observed with the use of fosphenytoin in clinical trials were nystagmus, dizziness, pruritus, paresthesia, headache, somnolence, and ataxia. Paresthesia and pruritus were seen more often following fosphenytoin (versus phenytoin) administration and occurred more often with I.V. fosphenytoin than with I.M. administration. These events were dose- and rate-related (doses ≥15 mg/kg at a rate of 150 mg/minute). These sensations, generally described as itching, burning, or tingling are usually not at the infusion site. The location of the discomfort varied with the groin mentioned most frequently. The paresthesia and pruritus were transient events that occurred within several minutes of the start of infusion and generally resolved within 10 minutes after completion of infusion.

Transient pruritus, tinnitus, nystagmus, somnolence, and ataxia occurred 2-3 times more often at doses ≥15 mg/kg and rates ≥150 mg/minute.

**I.V. administration** (maximum dose/rate):

>10%:

Central nervous system: Nystagmus, dizziness, somnolence, ataxia

Dermatologic: Pruritus

1% to 10%:

Cardiovascular: Hypotension, vasodilation, tachycardia

Central nervous system: Stupor, incoordination, paresthesia, extrapyramidal syndrome, tremor, agitation, hypesthesia, dysarthria, vertigo, brain edema, headache

Gastrointestinal: Nausea, tongue disorder, dry mouth, vomiting

Ocular: Diplopia, amblyopia

Otic: Tinnitus, deafness

Neuromuscular & skeletal: Pelvic pain, muscle weakness, back pain

Miscellaneous: Taste perversion

**I.M. administration** (substitute for oral phenytoin):

1% to 10%:

Central nervous system: Nystagmus, tremor, ataxia, headache, incoordination, somnolence, dizziness, paresthesia, reflexes decreased

Dermatologic: Pruritus
Gastrointestinal: Nausea, vomiting
Hematologic/lymphatic: Ecchymosis
Neuromuscular & skeletal: Muscle weakness

**Other:** <1% (Limited to important or life-threatening symptoms): Hypertension, cardiac arrest, syncope, cerebral hemorrhage, palpitations, sinus bradycardia, atrial flutter, bundle branch block, cardiomegaly, cerebral infarct, postural hypotension, pulmonary embolus, Q-T interval prolongation, thrombophlebitis, ventricular extrasystoles, congestive heart failure, hypokalemia, hyperglycemia, hypophosphatemia, alkalosis, acidosis, dehydration, hyperkalemia, ketosis, thrombocytopenia, anemia, leukocytosis, cyanosis, hypochromic anemia, leukopenia, lymphadenopathy, acute hepatotoxicity, acute hepatic failure

**Overdose/Toxicology** Symptoms of overdose include unsteady gait, tremor, hyperglycemia, chorea (extrapyramidal), gingival hyperplasia, gynecomastia, myoglobinuria, nephrotic syndrome, slurred speech, mydriasis, myoclonus, confusion, encephalopathy, hyperthermia, drowsiness, nausea, hypothermia, fever, hypotension, respiratory depression, leukopenia, neutropenia, agranulocytosis, granulocytopenia, hyper-reflexia, coma, systemic lupus erythematosus (SLE), and ophthalmoplegia. Treatment is supportive for hypotension.

**Pharmacodynamics/Kinetics**

**Protein Binding:**

Fosphenytoin: 95% to 99% (albumin), can displace phenytoin and increase free fraction (up to 30% unbound) during the period required for conversion of fosphenytoin to phenytoin

Phenytoin: 90% to 95%; increased free fraction can occur in patients with hyperbilirubinemia, hypoalbuminemia, uremia

**Excretion:** Urine

**Formulations** Injection, as sodium: 150 mg [equivalent to phenytoin sodium 100 mg]; 750 mg, [equivalent to phenytoin sodium 500 mg]

**Dosing**

**Adults: The dose, concentration in solutions, and infusion rates for fosphenytoin are expressed as phenytoin sodium equivalents. Fosphenytoin should always be prescribed and dispensed in phenytoin sodium equivalents.**

Status epilepticus: I.V.: Adults: Loading dose: Phenytoin equivalent 15-20 mg/kg I.V. administered at 100-150 mg/minute

Nonemergent loading and maintenance dosing: I.V. or I.M.:

Loading dose: Phenytoin equivalent 10-20 mg/kg I.V. or I.M. (max I.V. rate 150 mg/minute)

Initial daily maintenance dose: Phenytoin equivalent 4-6 mg/kg/day I.V. or I.M.

I.M. or I.V. substitution for oral phenytoin therapy: May be substituted for oral phenytoin sodium at the same total daily dose, however, Dilantin® capsules are ~90% bioavailable by the oral route. Phenytoin, supplied as fosphenytoin, is 100% bioavailable by both the I.M. and I.V. routes. For this reason, plasma phenytoin concentrations may increase when I.M. or I.V. fosphenytoin is substituted for oral phenytoin sodium therapy. In clinical trials I.M. fosphenytoin was administered as a single daily dose utilizing either 1 or 2 injection sites. Some patients may require more frequent dosing.

**Elderly:** Refer to adult dosing.

**Renal Impairment:** Free phenytoin levels should be monitored closely in patients with renal disease or in those with hypoalbuminemia; furthermore, fosphenytoin clearance to phenytoin may be increased without a similar increase in phenytoin clearance in these patients leading to increase frequency and severity of adverse events.

**Hepatic Impairment:** Phenytoin clearance may be substantially reduced in cirrhosis and plasma level monitoring with dose adjustment advisable. Free phenytoin levels should be monitored closely in patients with hepatic disease or in those with hypoalbuminemia; furthermore, fosphenytoin clearance to phenytoin may be increased without a similar increase in phenytoin clearance in these patients leading to increase frequency and severity of adverse events.

**Administration**

**I.M.:** I.M. may be administered as a single daily dose using either 1 or 2 injection sites.

**I.V.:** I.V. administration rate should not exceed 150 mg/minute.

**Stability**

**Storage:** Refrigerate at 2°C to 8°C (36°F to 46°F). Do not store at room temperature for more than 48 hours. Do not use vials that develop particulate matter.

**Compatibility:** See I.V. Administration.

**Additional Nursing Issues**

**Physical Assessment:** See Indications and Warnings/Precautions. Assess all other medications (prescription and OTC) patient may be taking; see Drug Interactions. Continuous hemodynamic monitoring and respiratory status are essential during infusion and for 30 minutes following infusion. Do not draw phenytoin levels until 2 hours following I.V. or 4 hours following I.M. administration. Monitor fluid balance (I & O ratio), diabetic status (see Drug Interactions). **Pregnancy risk factor D** - determine pregnancy status; benefits of use should outweigh possible risks.

**Patient Information/Instruction:** Patients may not be in a position to evaluate their response. If conscious or alert, advise patient to report signs or symptoms of palpitations, racing or falling heartbeat, difficulty breathing, acute faintness, or CNS disturbances (eg, somnolence, ataxia), and visual disturbances. **Pregnancy precautions: Inform prescriber if you are pregnant.**

**Geriatric Considerations:** No significant changes in fosphenytoin pharmacokinetics with age have been noted. Phenytoin clearance is decreased in the elderly and lower

(Continued)

## Fosphenytoin *(Continued)*

doses may be needed. Elderly may have reduced hepatic clearance due to age decline in Phase I metabolism. Elderly may have low albumin which will increase free fraction and, therefore, pharmacologic response. Monitor closely in those who are hypoalbuminemic. Free fraction measurements advised, also elderly may display a higher incidence of adverse effects (cardiovascular) when using the I.V. loading regimen; therefore, recommended to decrease loading I.V. dose to 25 mg/minute.

**Additional Information** 1.5 mg fosphenytoin is approximately equivalent to 1 mg phenytoin. Equimolar fosphenytoin dose is 375 mg (75 mg/mL solution) to phenytoin 250 mg (50 mg/mL).

Water solubility: 142 mg/mL at pH of 9

- **Fostex®** *see page 1294*
- **Fostex® 10% BPO Gel** *see page 1294*
- **Fostex® 10% Wash** *see page 1294*
- **Fostex® Bar** *see page 1294*
- **Fotexina** *see* Cefotaxime *on page 221*
- **Fototar®** *see page 1294*
- **Fragmin®** *see* Dalteparin *on page 328*
- **Fraxiparine** *see* Heparin *on page 558*
- **Freezone® Solution** *see page 1294*
- **Froben®** *see* Flurbiprofen *on page 509*
- **Froben-SR®** *see* Flurbiprofen *on page 509*
- **Froxal** *see* Cefuroxime *on page 233*
- **Frusemide** *see* Furosemide *on next page*
- **FS Shampoo®** *see* Topical Corticosteroids *on page 1152*
- **5-FU** *see* Fluorouracil *on page 500*
- **FUDR®** *see* Floxuridine *on page 489*
- **Ful-Glo® Ophthalmic Strips** *see page 1248*
- **Fulvicin® P/G** *see* Griseofulvin *on page 546*
- **Fulvicin-U/F®** *see* Griseofulvin *on page 546*
- **Fulvina® P/G** *see* Griseofulvin *on page 546*
- **Fumasorb® [OTC]** *see* Iron Supplements *on page 627*
- **Fumerin® [OTC]** *see* Iron Supplements *on page 627*
- **Funduscein® Injection** *see page 1248*
- **Fungiquim** *see* Miconazole *on page 767*
- **Fungistat** *see* Terconazole *on page 1106*
- **Fungistat Dual** *see* Terconazole *on page 1106*
- **Fungizone®** *see* Amphotericin B *on page 83*
- **Fungoid®** *see page 1294*
- **Fungoid® Creme** *see* Miconazole *on page 767*
- **Fungoid® Tincture** *see* Miconazole *on page 767*
- **Fungoid® Topical Solution** *see page 1247*
- **Furacin® Topical** *see* Nitrofurazone *on page 830*
- **Furadantin®** *see* Nitrofurantoin *on page 829*
- **Furadantina** *see* Nitrofurantoin *on page 829*
- **Furalan®** *see* Nitrofurantoin *on page 829*
- **Furan®** *see* Nitrofurantoin *on page 829*
- **Furanite®** *see* Nitrofurantoin *on page 829*

## Furazolidone (fyoor a ZOE li done)

**U.S. Brand Names** Furoxone®

**Therapeutic Category** Antiprotozoal

**Pregnancy Risk Factor** C

**Lactation** Excretion in breast milk unknown

**Use** Treatment of bacterial or protozoal diarrhea and enteritis caused by susceptible organisms *Giardia lamblia* and *Vibrio cholerae*

**Mechanism of Action/Effect** Inhibits several vital enzymatic reactions causing antibacterial and antiprotozoal action

**Contraindications** Hypersensitivity to furazolidone; concurrent use of alcohol; patients <1 month of age because of the possibility of producing hemolytic anemia

**Warnings** Use caution in patients with G-6-PD deficiency when administering large doses for prolonged periods. Furazolidone inhibits monoamine oxidase. Pregnancy factor C.

**Drug Interactions**

**Increased Effect/Toxicity:** Increased effect with sympathomimetic amines, tricyclic antidepressants, tyramine-containing foods, MAO inhibitors, meperidine, anorexiants, dextromethorphan, fluoxetine, paroxetine, sertraline, and trazodone. Increased effect/toxicity of levodopa. Disulfiram-like reaction with alcohol.

**Food Interactions** Clinically severe elevated blood pressure may occur if furazolidone is taken with tyramine-containing foods.

**Effects on Lab Values** False-positive results for urine glucose with Clinitest®

**Adverse Reactions**

>10%: Genitourinary: Discoloration of urine (dark yellow to brown)

1% to 10%:

Central nervous system: Headache

Gastrointestinal: Abdominal pain, diarrhea, nausea, vomiting

<1% (Limited to important or life-threatening symptoms): Orthostatic hypotension, hypoglycemia, disulfiram-like reaction after alcohol ingestion, leukopenia, agranulocytosis, hemolysis in patients with G-6-PD deficiency

**Overdose/Toxicology** Symptoms of overdose include nausea, vomiting, and serotonin crisis. Treatment is supportive.

**Pharmacodynamics/Kinetics**

**Excretion:** Urine

**Formulations**

Liquid: 50 mg/15 mL (60 mL, 473 mL)

Tablet: 100 mg

**Dosing**

**Adults:** Oral: 100 mg 4 times/day; not more than 8.8 mg/kg/day; treatment duration: 7 days

**Elderly:** Refer to adult dosing.

**Monitoring Laboratory Tests** Perform culture and sensitivity studies prior to initiating drug therapy.

**Additional Nursing Issues**

**Physical Assessment:** Monitor other medications patient may be taking for effectiveness and interactions (see Drug Interactions). Avoid use of Clinitest® for diabetics. Monitor for adequate hydration. Assess/teach patient the importance of appropriate diet. Patient should be cautioned against eating foods high in tyramine. See Tyramine Foods List *on page 1422*. **Pregnancy risk factor C** - benefits of use should outweigh possible risks. Note breast-feeding caution.

**Patient Information/Instruction:** Take as directed. Avoid alcohol and tyramine-containing foods during and for 4 days following therapy. Do not take any other prescription or OTC medications without consulting prescriber. Your urine may turn dark brown or yellow (normal). If diabetic, use something other than Clinitest® for urine glucose testing. Report acute GI pain, unresolved diarrhea, unresolved nausea or vomiting, fever, dizziness, or unusual joint pain. Consult prescriber if condition is not resolved at the end of therapy. **Pregnancy/breast-feeding precautions:** Inform prescriber if you are or intend to be pregnant. Consult prescriber if breast-feeding.

**Related Information**

Tyramine Foods List *on page 1422*

♦ **Furazosin** *see* Prazosin *on page 958*

## Furosemide (fyoor OH se mide)

**U.S. Brand Names** Lasix®

**Synonyms** Frusemide

**Therapeutic Category** Diuretic, Loop

**Pregnancy Risk Factor** C

**Lactation** Enters breast milk/use caution

**Use** Management of edema associated with congestive heart failure and hepatic or renal disease; alone or in combination with antihypertensives in treatment of hypertension

**Mechanism of Action/Effect** Inhibits reabsorption of sodium and chloride in the ascending loop of Henle and distal renal tubule, interfering with the chloride-binding cotransport system, thus causing increased excretion of water, sodium, chloride, magnesium, and calcium

**Contraindications** Hypersensitivity to furosemide, any component, or other sulfonamides

**Warnings** Loop diuretics are potent diuretics. Close medical supervision and dose evaluation is required to prevent fluid and electrolyte imbalance. Use caution with other nephrotoxic or ototoxic drugs. Pregnancy factor C.

**Drug Interactions**

**Decreased Effect:** Furosemide may reduce the hypoglycemic effect of antidiabetic agents. Indomethacin, aspirin and other NSAIDs may reduce natriuretic and hypotensive effects of furosemide. Sucralfate may reduce the effect of furosemide, separate administration by 2 hours. Furosemide may antagonize the effect of skeletal muscle relaxants (tubocurarine).

**Increased Effect/Toxicity:** Effects of antihypertensive agents may be enhanced. Lithium renal clearance may be decreased which may result in higher concentrations and toxicity. Concomitant use of furosemide with aminoglycoside antibiotics or other ototoxic drugs should be avoided. Combined use with ethacrynic acid may contribute to ototoxicity. Furosemide may induce salicylate toxicity when combined with high-dose salicylates used for rheumatic disease. Furosemide may potentiate the therapeutic effect of antihypertensives.

**Food Interactions** Furosemide serum levels may be decreased if taken with food.

**Adverse Reactions**

>10%:

Cardiovascular: Orthostatic hypotension

1% to 10%:

Central nervous system: Headache

Dermatologic: Photosensitivity

Endocrine & metabolic: Hypokalemia, hyponatremia, hypochloremic alkalosis

Gastrointestinal: Diarrhea, anorexia, stomach cramps or pain

Ocular: Blurred vision

<1% (Limited to important or life-threatening symptoms): Hepatic dysfunction, agranulocytosis, leukopenia, thrombocytopenia, xanthopsia

(Continued)

## Furosemide *(Continued)*

**Overdose/Toxicology** Symptoms of overdose include electrolyte depletion, volume depletion, hypotension, dehydration, and circulatory collapse. Treatment is supportive.

**Pharmacodynamics/Kinetics**

**Protein Binding:** >98%

**Half-life Elimination:** Normal renal function: 0.5-1.1 hours; End-stage renal disease: 9 hours

**Metabolism:** Liver

**Excretion:** Urine and feces

**Onset:**

Onset of diuresis: Oral: Within 30-60 minutes; I.M.: 30 minutes; I.V.: Within 5 minutes
Peak effect: Oral: Within 1-2 hours

**Duration:** Oral: 6-8 hours; I.V.: 2 hours

**Formulations**

Injection: 10 mg/mL (2 mL, 4 mL, 5 mL, 6 mL, 8 mL, 10 mL, 12 mL)
Solution, oral: 10 mg/mL (60 mL, 120 mL); 40 mg/5 mL (5 mL, 10 mL, 500 mL)
Tablet: 20 mg, 40 mg, 80 mg

**Dosing**

**Adults:**

Oral: 20-80 mg/dose initially increased in increments of 20-40 mg/dose at intervals of 6-8 hours; usual maintenance dose interval is twice daily or every day

I.M., I.V.: 20-40 mg/dose, may be repeated in 1-2 hours as needed and increased by 20 mg/dose with each succeeding dose up to 1000 mg/day; usual dosing interval: 6-12 hours

Continuous I.V. infusion: Initial I.V. bolus dose of 0.1 mg/kg followed by continuous I.V. infusion doses of 0.1 mg/kg/hour doubled every 2 hours to a maximum of 0.4 mg/kg/hour if urine output is <1 mL/kg/hour have been found to be effective and result in a lower daily requirement of furosemide than with intermittent dosing. Other studies have used 20-160 mg/hour continuous I.V. infusion.

**Elderly:** Oral, I.M., I.V.: Initial: 20 mg/day; increase slowly to desired response.

**Renal Impairment:**

Acute renal failure: Doses up to 1-3 g/day may be necessary to initiate desired response; avoid use in oliguric states.

Not removed by hemo- or peritoneal dialysis; supplemental dose is not necessary.

**Hepatic Impairment:** Diminished natriuretic effect with increased sensitivity to hypokalemia and volume depletion in cirrhosis. Monitor effects, particularly with high doses.

**Administration**

**I.V.:** I.V. injections should be given slowly over 1-2 minutes; maximum rate of administration for IVPB or infusion: 4 mg/minute; replace parenteral therapy with oral therapy as soon as possible

**I.V. Detail:** As a general guideline, I.V. bolus doses may be infused at a rate ≤20 mg/minute.

**Stability**

**Storage:** Furosemide injection should be stored at controlled room temperature and protected from light. Exposure to light may cause discoloration. Do not use furosemide solutions if they have a yellow color. Refrigeration may result in precipitation or crystallization, however, resolubilization at room temperature or warming may be performed without affecting the drugs stability.

**Reconstitution:** I.V. infusion solution mixed in NS or $D_5W$ solution is stable for 24 hours at room temperature.

**Compatibility:** Incompatible with amiodarone, buprenorphine, chlorpromazine, diazepam, dobutamine, erythromycin, gentamicin, isoproterenol, meperidine, metoclopramide, netilmicin, prochlorperazine, and promethazine. See the Compatibility of Drugs Chart *on page 1315*.

**Monitoring Laboratory Tests** Serum electrolytes, renal function

**Additional Nursing Issues**

**Physical Assessment:** Monitor appropriate laboratory results, blood pressure, pulse, weight, and hydration status on a regular basis. Monitor/teach patient orthostatic hypotension precautions. Monitor serum glucose for diabetics and lithium levels for appropriate patients until response is established and stable; avoid ototoxic medications (see Drug Interactions). **Pregnancy risk factor C** - benefits of use should outweigh possible risks. Note breast-feeding caution.

**Patient Information/Instruction:** Take as directed, with food or milk early in the day (daily), or if twice daily, take last dose in late afternoon in order to avoid sleep disturbance and achieve maximum therapeutic effect. Keep medication in original container, away from light; do not use discolored medication. Include bananas or orange juice (or other potassium-rich foods) in daily diet; do not take potassium supplements without advice of prescriber. Weigh yourself each day, at the same time, in the same clothes when beginning therapy, and weekly on long-term therapy; report unusual or unanticipated weight gain or loss. You may experience dizziness, blurred vision, or drowsiness; use caution when driving or engaging in tasks that require alertness until response to drug is known. Use caution when rising or changing position. You may experience sensitivity to sunlight; use sunblock or wear protective clothing and sunglasses. Report signs of edema (eg, weight gains, swollen ankles, feet or hands), trembling, numbness or fatigue, any cramping or muscle weakness, palpitations, or unresolved nausea or vomiting. **Pregnancy/breast-feeding precautions:** Inform prescriber if you are or intend to be pregnant. Consult prescriber if breast-feeding.

**Geriatric Considerations:** Severe loss of sodium and/or increase in BUN can cause confusion. For any change in mental status in patients on furosemide, monitor electrolytes and renal function.

**Additional Information**

Sodium content of 1 mL (injection): 0.162 mEq

pH: 8-9.3

- **Furoside®** *see* Furosemide *on page 523*
- **Furoxona Gotas** *see* Furazolidone *on page 522*
- **Furoxona Tabletas** *see* Furazolidone *on page 522*
- **Furoxone®** *see* Furazolidone *on page 522*
- **Fustaren Retard** *see* Diclofenac *on page 358*
- **Fuxen** *see* Naproxen *on page 807*
- **Fuxol** *see* Furazolidone *on page 522*
- **G-1®** *see* Butalbital Compound and Acetaminophen *on page 175*

## Gabapentin (GA ba pen tin)

**U.S. Brand Names** Neurontin®

**Therapeutic Category** Anticonvulsant, Miscellaneous

**Pregnancy Risk Factor** C

**Lactation** Excretion in breast milk unknown/not recommended

**Use** Adjunct for treatment of drug-refractory partial and secondarily generalized seizures in adults with epilepsy; adjunctive treatment of partial seizures with and without secondary generalization; not effective for absence seizures. Unlabeled use: neuropathic pain, bipolar disorders

**Mechanism of Action/Effect** Exact mechanism of action is not known, but does have properties in common with other anticonvulsants; although structurally related to GABA, it does not interact with GABA receptors

**Contraindications** Hypersensitivity to gabapentin or any component

**Warnings** Avoid abrupt withdrawal, may precipitate seizures. May be associated with a slight incidence (0.6%) of status epilepticus and sudden deaths (0.0038 deaths/patient year). Use cautiously in patients with severe renal dysfunction. Rat studies demonstrated an association with pancreatic adenocarcinoma in male rats; clinical implication unknown. Pregnancy factor C.

**Drug Interactions**

**Decreased Effect:** Gabapentin does not modify plasma concentrations of standard anticonvulsant medications (eg, valproic acid, carbamazepine, phenytoin, or phenobarbital). Antacids reduce the bioavailability of gabapentin by 20%.

**Increased Effect/Toxicity:** Cimetidine may decrease clearance of gabapentin. Gabapentin may increase levels of norethindrone by 13%.

**Adverse Reactions**

>10%:

Cardiovascular: Peripheral edema

Central nervous system: Somnolence, dizziness, ataxia, fatigue

Ocular: Nystagmus, blurred vision, diplopia

1% to 10%:

Cardiovascular: Hypotension

Central nervous system: Nervousness, amnesia, depression, anxiety, abnormal coordination, headache, insomnia

Dermatologic: Pruritus

Gastrointestinal: Heartburn, dry throat, dry mouth, nausea, constipation, appetite stimulation (weight gain)

Genitourinary: Impotence, frequent urination

Hematologic: Leukopenia

Neuromuscular & skeletal: Back pain, myalgia, dysarthria, tremor

Otic: Tinnitus

Respiratory: Rhinitis, bronchospasm

Miscellaneous: Hiccups

**Overdose/Toxicology** Symptoms of overdose include somnolence, fatigue, ataxia, and tremors. Treatment is supportive. Enhancement of elimination: Multiple dosing of activated charcoal may be useful. Hemodialysis may be useful.

**Pharmacodynamics/Kinetics**

**Protein Binding:** 0%

**Half-life Elimination:** 5-6 hours

**Excretion:** Urine

**Formulations** Capsule: 100 mg, 300 mg, 400 mg, 600 mg, 800 mg

**Dosing**

**Adults:** If gabapentin is discontinued or if another anticonvulsant is added to therapy, it should be done slowly over a minimum of 1 week.

Oral:

Initial: 300 mg on day 1 (at bedtime to minimize sedation), then 300 mg twice daily on day 2, and then 300 mg 3 times/day on day 3

Total daily dosage range: 900-1800 mg/day administered in 3 divided doses at 8-hour intervals. Doses up to 2400 mg have been tolerated in long-term studies. Up to 3600 mg/day have been given for relatively brief periods.

**Elderly:** Refer to adult dosing.

**Renal Impairment:**

$Cl_{cr}$ >60 mL/minute: Administer 1200 mg/day.

$Cl_{cr}$ 30-60 mL/minute: Administer 600 mg/day.

(Continued)

## Gabapentin *(Continued)*

$Cl_{cr}$ 15-30 mL/minute: Administer 300 mg/day.

$Cl_{cr}$ <15 mL/minute: Administer 150 mg/day.

Hemodialysis: 200-300 mg after each 4-hour dialysis following a loading dose of 300-400 mg.

**Administration**

**Oral:** Administer first dose on first day at bedtime to avoid somnolence and dizziness. Dosage must be adjusted for renal function.

**Monitoring Laboratory Tests** Monitor serum levels of concomitant anticonvulsant therapy. Routine monitoring of gabapentin levels is not mandatory.

**Additional Nursing Issues**

**Physical Assessment:** Assess effectiveness and interactions of other medications patient may be taking (see Drug Interactions). Monitor for therapeutic response (seizure activity, force, type, duration), laboratory values, and adverse reactions (see Adverse Reactions) at beginning of therapy and periodically with long-term use. Taper dosage slowly when discontinuing. Observe and teach seizure/safety precautions. Assess knowledge/teach patient appropriate use, interventions to reduce side effects, and adverse symptoms to report. **Pregnancy risk factor C** - benefits of use should outweigh possible risks. Breast-feeding is not recommended.

**Patient Information/Instruction:** Take exactly as directed (do not increase dose or frequency or discontinue without consulting prescriber). While using this medication, do not use alcohol and other prescription or OTC medications (especially pain medications, sedatives, antihistamines, or hypnotics) without consulting prescriber. Maintain adequate hydration (2-3 L/day of fluids unless instructed to restrict fluid intake). You may experience drowsiness, dizziness, or blurred vision (use caution when driving or engaging in tasks requiring alertness until response to drug is known); nausea, vomiting, loss of appetite, or dry mouth (small frequent meals, frequent mouth care, chewing gum, or sucking lozenges may help). Wear identification of epileptic status. Report CNS changes, mentation changes, or changes in cognition; muscle cramping, weakness, tremors, changes in gait; persistent GI symptoms (cramping, constipation, vomiting, anorexia); difficulty breathing; impotence or changes in urinary pattern; worsening of seizure activity, or loss of seizure control. **Pregnancy/breast-feeding precautions:** Inform prescriber if you are or intend to be pregnant. Breast-feeding is not recommended.

**Geriatric Considerations:** No clinical studies to specifically evaluate this drug in the elderly have been performed; however, in premarketing studies, patients >65 years of age did not demonstrate any difference in side effect profiles from younger adults. Since gabapentin is eliminated renally, dose **must** be adjusted for creatinine clearance in the elderly patient.


- **Gabitril®** *see* Tiagabine *on page 1132*
- **Galecin** *see* Clindamycin *on page 282*
- **Galedol** *see* Diclofenac *on page 358*
- **Galidrin** *see* Ranitidine *on page 1008*
- **Gamikal** *see* Amikacin *on page 65*
- **Gamimune® N** *see* Immune Globulin, Intravenous *on page 602*
- **Gamma Benzene Hexachloride** *see* Lindane *on page 678*
- **Gammagard® S/D** *see* Immune Globulin, Intravenous *on page 602*
- **Gammaphos** *see* Amifostine *on page 64*
- **Gammar®-P I.V.** *see* Immune Globulin, Intravenous *on page 602*
- **Gamulin®** *see page 1256*


## Ganciclovir (gan SYE kloe veer)

**U.S. Brand Names** Cytovene®; Vitrasert®

**Synonyms** DHPG Sodium; GCV Sodium; Nordeoxyguanosine

**Therapeutic Category** Antiviral Agent

**Pregnancy Risk Factor** C

**Lactation** Excretion in breast milk unknown/contraindicated

**Use** Treatment of CMV retinitis in immunocompromised individuals, including patients with acquired immunodeficiency syndrome; treatment of CMV pneumonia in marrow transplant recipients, AIDS patients and organ transplant recipients with CMV colitis, pneumonitis, and multiorgan involvement; bone marrow transplant patients when given in combination with IVIG or CMV hyperimmune globulin

Oral: Alternative to the I.V. formulation for maintenance treatment of CMV retinitis in immunocompromised patients, including patients with AIDS, in whom retinitis is stable following appropriate induction therapy and for whom the risk of more rapid progression is balanced by the benefit associated with avoiding daily I.V. infusions

**Mechanism of Action/Effect** Ganciclovir is phosphorylated to a substrate which competitively inhibits the binding of deoxyguanosine triphosphate to DNA polymerase resulting in inhibition of viral DNA synthesis.

**Contraindications** Hypersensitivity to ganciclovir or acyclovir; absolute neutrophil count <500/mm$^3$; platelet count <25,000/mm$^3$

**Warnings** Dosage adjustment or interruption of ganciclovir therapy may be necessary in patients with neutropenia and/or thrombocytopenia and patients with impaired renal function. Use with extreme caution in children since long-term safety has not been determined and due to ganciclovir's potential for long-term carcinogenic and adverse reproductive effects. Ganciclovir may adversely affect spermatogenesis and fertility. Due to its mutagenic potential, contraceptive precautions for female and male patients need to be followed during and for at least 90 days after therapy with the drug. Take care to administer only into veins with good blood flow. Pregnancy factor C.

**Drug Interactions**

**Decreased Effect:** A decrease in steady-state ganciclovir AUC may occur when used with didanosine.

**Increased Effect/Toxicity:** Zidovudine, immunosuppressive agents may increase hematologic toxicity. Imipenem/cilastatin may increase seizure potential. Oral ganciclovir increased the AUC of zidovudine. Ganciclovir increased didanosine AUC and increases the risk of toxicity (eg, peripheral neuropathy, pancreatitis). Since both drugs have the potential to cause neutropenia and anemia, some patients may not tolerate concomitant therapy with these drugs at full dosage. Risk of nephrotoxicity may be enhanced with concomitant cyclosporine or tacrolimus. The renal clearance of ganciclovir is decreased in the presence of probenecid.

**Adverse Reactions**

>10%:
- Central nervous system: Headache
- Hematologic: Granulocytopenia, thrombocytopenia

1% to 10%:
- Central nervous system: Confusion, fever
- Dermatologic: Rash, pruritus
- Hematologic: Anemia
- Hepatic: Abnormal liver function values
- Miscellaneous: Sepsis

<1% (Limited to important or life-threatening symptoms): Arrhythmia, hypertension, hypotension, edema, alopecia, eosinophilia, hemorrhage, paresthesia, tremor, retinal detachment, dyspnea, coma, seizures, visual loss, hyphema, uveitis (intravitreal implant), increased serum creatinine

**Overdose/Toxicology** Symptoms of overdose include neutropenia, vomiting, hypersalivation, bloody diarrhea, cytopenia, and testicular atrophy. Treatment is supportive. Hemodialysis removes 50% of the drug. Hydration may be of some benefit.

**Pharmacodynamics/Kinetics**

**Protein Binding:** 1% to 2%

**Half-life Elimination:** 1.7-5.8 hours; increases with impaired renal function; End-stage renal disease: 3.6 hours

**Excretion:** Urine

**Formulations**

Capsule: 250 mg

Implant, intravitreal: 4.5 mg released gradually over 5-8 months

Powder for injection, lyophilized: 500 mg (10 mL)

**Dosing**

**Adults:**

Slow I.V. infusion (dosing is based on total body weight):
- Induction therapy: 5 mg/kg/dose every 12 hours for 14-21 days followed by maintenance therapy
- Maintenance therapy: 5 mg/kg/day as a single daily dose for 7 days/week or 6 mg/kg/day for 5 days/week

Oral: 1000 mg 3 times/day with food **or** 500 mg 6 times/day with food

**Elderly:** Refer to adult dosing.

**Renal Impairment:**

I.V. (Induction):
- $Cl_{cr}$ ≥70 mL/minute: No adjustment necessary.
- $Cl_{cr}$ 50-69 mL/minute: Administer 2.5 mg/kg/dose every 12 hours.
- $Cl_{cr}$ 25-49 mL/minute: Administer 2.5 mg/kg/dose every 24 hours.
- $Cl_{cr}$ 10-24 mL/minute: Administer 1.25 mg/kg/dose every 24 hours.
- $Cl_{cr}$ <10 mL/minute: Administer 1.25 mg/kg/dose 3 times a week following hemodialysis.

I.V. (Maintenance):
- $Cl_{cr}$ ≥70 mL/minute: No adjustment necessary.
- $Cl_{cr}$ 50-69 mL/minute: Administer 2.5 mg/kg/dose every 24 hours.
- $Cl_{cr}$ 25-49 mL/minute: Administer 1.25 mg/kg/dose every 24 hours.
- $Cl_{cr}$ 10-24 mL/minute: Administer 0.625 mg/kg/dose every 24 hours.
- $Cl_{cr}$ <10 mL/minute: Administer 0.625 mg/kg/dose 3 times a week following hemodialysis.

Oral:
- $Cl_{cr}$ 50-69 mL/minute: Administer 1500 mg/day or 500 mg 3 times/day.
- $Cl_{cr}$ 25-49 mL/minute: Administer 1000 mg/day or 500 mg twice daily.
- $Cl_{cr}$ 10-24 mL/minute: Administer 500 mg/day.
- $Cl_{cr}$ <10 mL/minute: Administer 500 mg 3 times/week following hemodialysis.

Hemodialysis effects: Dialyzable (50%) following hemodialysis; administer dose postdialysis. During peritoneal dialysis, dose as for $Cl_{cr}$ <10 mL/minute. During continuous arteriovenous or venovenous hemofiltration (CAVH/CAVHD), administer 2.5 mg/kg/dose every 24 hours.

**Administration**

**Oral:** Oral ganciclovir should be administered with food.

**I.V.:** The same precautions utilized with antineoplastic agents should be followed with ganciclovir administration. Ganciclovir should not be administered by I.M., S.C., or rapid IVP. Administer by slow I.V. infusion over at least 1 hour at a final concentration for administration not to exceed 10 mg/mL.

**I.V. Detail:** An **IN-LINE filter** of 0.22-5 micron is recommended during the infusion of all ganciclovir solutions.

(Continued)

## Ganciclovir *(Continued)*

**Stability**

**Storage:** Intact vials should be stored at room temperature and protected from temperatures >40°C.

**Reconstitution:** Preparation should take place in a vertical laminar flow hood with the same precautions as antineoplastic agents. Drug product should be reconstituted immediately before use and any unused portion should be discarded appropriately. Reconstitute powder with sterile water **not** bacteriostatic water because parabens may cause precipitation. Reconstituted solution is stable for 12 hours at room temperature, however, conflicting data indicates that reconstituted solution is stable for 60 days under refrigeration (4°C). Stability of parenteral admixture at room temperature (25°C) and at refrigeration temperature (4°C) is 5 days.

**Compatibility:** Incompatible: Bacteriostatic water for inject contains parabens and may cause precipitation.

**Monitoring Laboratory Tests** CBC with differential and platelet count, serum creatinine before beginning therapy, CBC, and serum creatinine on a regular basis thereafter; liver function tests

**Additional Nursing Issues**

**Physical Assessment:** Monitor laboratory tests as ordered. Assess patient response to ganciclovir or combination treatment. Monitor fluid balance and ensure adequate hydration (2-3 L/day of fluids unless instructed to restrict fluid intake). Instruct patient about necessity for periodic ophthalmic exams. **Pregnancy risk factor C** - ascertain appropriateness of use; barrier contraceptive use is appropriate during therapy and for 60-90 days after therapy for both male and female. Breast-feeding is contraindicated.

**Patient Information/Instruction:** Ganciclovir is not a cure for CMV retinitis. For oral administration, take as directed and maintain adequate hydration (2-3 L/day of fluids unless instructed to restrict fluid intake). You will need frequent blood tests and regular ophthalmic exams while taking this drug. You may experience increased susceptibility to infection; avoid crowds or exposure to infectious persons. You may experience photosensitivity; use sunscreen, wear protective clothing and eyewear, and avoid direct sunlight. Report fever, chills, unusual bleeding or bruising, infection, or unhealed sores or white plaques in mouth. **Pregnancy/breast-feeding precautions:** Inform prescriber if you are pregnant. Males and females should use appropriate barrier contraceptive measures during and for 60-90 days following end of therapy. Do not breast-feed.

**Geriatric Considerations:** Adjust dose based upon renal function.

**Breast-feeding Issues:** The CDC recommends **not** to breast-feed if diagnosed with HIV to avoid postnatal transmission of the virus.

**Additional Information** Sodium content of 500 mg vial: 46 mg. Ganciclovir is very alkaline (pH ~11). Avoid direct contact to skin and mucous membranes. If exposure occurs, rinse with water and wash with soap immediately.


- **Gantanol®** *see* Sulfamethoxazole *on page 1082*
- **Garalen** *see* Gentamicin *on page 531*
- **Garamicina®** *see* Gentamicin *on page 531*
- **Garamycin®** *see* Gentamicin *on page 531*
- **Gas-Ban DS®** *see page 1294*
- **Gastrec** *see* Ranitidine *on page 1008*
- **Gastrocrom® Oral** *see* Cromolyn Sodium *on page 309*
- **Gastrosed™** *see* Hyoscyamine *on page 590*
- **Gas-X®** *see page 1294*
- **Gaviscon®-2 Tablet** *see page 1294*
- **Gaviscon® Liquid** *see page 1294*
- **Gaviscon® Tablet** *see page 1294*
- **G-CSF** *see* Filgrastim *on page 483*
- **GCV Sodium** *see* Ganciclovir *on page 526*
- **Gee Gee® [OTC]** *see* Guaifenesin *on page 548*
- **Gelatin, Absorbable** *see page 1248*
- **Gelatin, Pectin, and Methylcellulose** *see page 1294*
- **Gelfilm® Ophthalmic** *see page 1248*
- **Gelfoam® Topical** *see page 1248*
- **Gel Kam®** *see page 1294*
- **Gelpirin® Geltabs** *see page 1294*
- **Gel-Tin®** *see page 1294*
- **Gelusil®** *see page 1294*


## Gemcitabine (jem SIT a been)

**U.S. Brand Names** Gemzar®

**Therapeutic Category** Antineoplastic Agent, Antimetabolite

**Pregnancy Risk Factor** D

**Lactation** Excretion in breast milk unknown/contraindicated

**Use** Treatment of patients with inoperable pancreatic cancer, locally advanced or metastatic nonsmall cell lung cancer

**Contraindications** Hypersensitivity to gemcitabine; severe thrombocytopenia; acute infection; pregnancy

**Warnings** Use caution in patients with myelosuppression, renal or hepatic dysfunction. Gemcitabine preparation should be performed in a Class II laminar flow biologic safety cabinet. Personnel should be fully trained and wearing surgical gloves and a closed front surgical gown with knit cuffs. Appropriate safety equipment is recommended for preparation, administration, and disposal of etoposide. Accidental exposure to skin should be thoroughly washed with soap and water immediately.

**Drug Interactions**

**Decreased Effect:** No confirmed interactions have been reported. No specific drug interaction studies have been conducted.

**Adverse Reactions** >10%:

Cardiovascular: Peripheral edema
Central nervous system: Fever
Dermatologic: Rash, alopecia
Gastrointestinal: Nausea, vomiting, constipation, diarrhea, stomatitis
Hematologic: Anemia, leukopenia, neutropenia, thrombocytopenia
Hepatic: Elevated liver enzymes (ALT, AST, alkaline phosphatase) and bilirubin
Neuromuscular & skeletal: Pain
Renal: Proteinuria, hematuria, elevated BUN
Respiratory: Dyspnea
Miscellaneous: Infection

**Overdose/Toxicology** Symptoms of overdose include myelosuppression, paresthesia, and severe rash. The principle toxicities were seen when a single dose as high as 5700 mg/m$^2$ was administered by I.V. infusion over 30 minutes every 2 weeks. Monitor blood counts and administer supportive therapy as needed.

**Formulations** Powder for injection, lyophilized, as hydrochloride: 20 mg/mL (10 mL, 50 mL)

**Dosing**

**Adults:** I.V.:

Nonsmall-cell lung cancer: 1000 mg/m$^2$ over 30 minutes administered once weekly for 3 consecutive doses per cycle

Pancreatic cancer: 1000 mg/m$^2$ over 30 minutes administered once weekly for 7 consecutive doses per cycle

**Elderly:** Refer to adult dosing.

**Stability**

**Storage:** Unopened vials are stable until the expiration date indicated on the package when stored at controlled room temperature of 20°C to 25°C (68°F to 77°F).

**Reconstitution:** Stable for 24 hours at controlled room temperature of 20°C to 25°C. Recommended diluent for reconstitution is 0.9% sodium chloride injection without preservatives. Maximum concentration is 40 mg/mL. Reconstitution at concentrations greater than that may cause incomplete dissolution.

**Compatibility:** Compatibility with other drugs has not been studied. No incompatibilities have been observed with infusion bottles or polyvinyl chloride bags and administration sets.

**Monitoring Laboratory Tests** Monitor CBC, including differential and platelet count, prior to each dose. Renal and hepatic function should be performed prior to initiation of therapy and periodically thereafter.

**Additional Nursing Issues**

**Physical Assessment:** Monitor appropriate laboratory tests as ordered (WBC, platelet count, liver and kidney function) prior to each dose. Monitor for signs or symptoms of adverse effects as noted above, increased edema, increased stress level, and acute GI response. Monitor for opportunistic infections (eg, thrush, open unhealed sores, vaginal discharge, foul-smelling pus, itching or burning on urination, fatigue, bone pain, fever). **Pregnancy risk factor D** - assess knowledge/teach appropriate use of barrier contraceptives. Breast-feeding is contraindicated.

**Patient Information/Instruction:** This drug can only be administered by infusion. During therapy, do not use alcohol, aspirin-containing products, and OTC medications without consulting prescriber. It is important to maintain adequate nutrition and hydration (2-3 L/day of fluids unless instructed to restrict fluid intake) during therapy; frequent small meals may help. You may experience mild nausea or vomiting (frequent small meals, frequent mouth care, sucking lozenges, or chewing gum may help); loss of hair (reversible); mouth sores (frequent mouth care and use of a soft toothbrush or cotton swabs may help). You will be more susceptible to infection (avoid crowds and exposure to infection as much as possible). Yogurt or buttermilk may help reduce diarrhea. This drug may cause sterility or birth defects. Report extreme fatigue; severe GI upset or diarrhea; bleeding or bruising, fever, chills, sore throat, vaginal discharge; signs of fluid retention (swelling extremities, difficulty breathing, unusual weight gain); yellowing of skin or eyes or change in color of urine or stool. This drug can only be administered by infusion. During therapy, do not use alcohol, aspirin-containing products, and OTC medications without consulting prescriber. It is important to maintain adequate nutrition and hydration during therapy; frequent small meals may help. Take 2-3 L fluid/day. You may experience mild nausea or vomiting (frequent small meals, frequent mouth care, and sucking on lozenges may help); loss of hair (reversible); mouth sores (frequent mouth care and use of a soft toothbrush or cotton swabs may help). You will be more susceptible to infection (avoid crowds and exposure to infection as much as possible). Yogurt or buttermilk may help reduce diarrhea. This drug may cause sterility or birth defects. Report extreme fatigue; severe GI upset or diarrhea; bleeding or bruising, fever, chills, sore throat, vaginal discharge; signs of fluid retention (swelling extremities, difficulty breathing, unusual weight gain); yellowing of skin or eyes or change in color of urine or stool. **Pregnancy/breast-feeding precautions:** Do not get pregnant while taking this medication; use appropriate barrier contraceptive measures. Do not breast-feed.

(Continued)

## Gemcitabine *(Continued)*

**Geriatric Considerations:** Clearance is affected by age. There is no evidence; however, that unusual dose adjustment is necessary in patients older than 65 years of age. In general, adverse reaction rates were similar to patients older and younger than 65 years. Grade 3/4 thrombocytopenia was more common in the elderly.

**Pregnancy Issues:** It is embryotoxic causing fetal malformations (cleft palate, incomplete ossification, fused pulmonary artery, absence of gallbladder) in animals. There are no studies in pregnant women. If patient becomes pregnant she should be informed of risks.

♦ **Gemcor®** *see* Gemfibrozil *on this page*

## Gemfibrozil (jem FI broe zil)

**U.S. Brand Names** Gemcor®; Lopid®

**Synonyms** CI-719

**Therapeutic Category** Antilipemic Agent (Fibric Acid)

**Pregnancy Risk Factor** C

**Lactation** Excretion in breast milk unknown/contraindicated

**Use** Treatment of hypertriglyceridemia in Types IV and V hyperlipidemia for patients who are at greater risk for pancreatitis and who have not responded to dietary intervention

**Mechanism of Action/Effect** Inhibits lipolysis and decreases subsequent hepatic fatty acid uptake and hepatic secretion of VLDL; decreases serum levels of VLDL and increases HDL levels

**Contraindications** Hypersensitivity to gemfibrozil or any component; renal or hepatic dysfunction; gallbladder disease

**Warnings** Abnormal elevation of AST, ALT, LDH, bilirubin, and alkaline phosphatase has occurred. If no appreciable triglyceride- or cholesterol-lowering effect occurs after 3 months, the drug should be discontinued. Not useful for Type I hyperlipidemia. Myositis may be more common in patients with poor renal function. Pregnancy factor C.

**Drug Interactions**

**Cytochrome P-450 Effect:** CYP3A3/4 enzyme substrate

**Increased Effect/Toxicity:** May potentiate the effects of warfarin. Manufacturer warns against the use of gemfibrozil with concomitant lovastatin therapy; has been reported to result in rhabdomyolysis.

**Adverse Reactions**

>10%:

Gastrointestinal: Heartburn, abdominal pain

Hepatic: Cholelithiasis

1% to 10%:

Central nervous system: Fatigue, vertigo, headache

Dermatologic: Eczema, rash

Gastrointestinal: Diarrhea, nausea, vomiting, constipation, acute appendicitis

<1% (Limited to important or life-threatening symptoms): Atrial fibrillation

**Overdose/Toxicology** Symptoms of overdose include abdominal pain, diarrhea, nausea, and vomiting. Treatment is supportive.

**Pharmacodynamics/Kinetics**

**Protein Binding:** 99%

**Half-life Elimination:** 1.4 hours

**Time to Peak:** Within 1-2 hours

**Metabolism:** Liver

**Excretion:** Urine

**Onset:** May require several days

**Formulations**

Capsule: 300 mg

Tablet, film coated: 600 mg

**Dosing**

**Adults:** Oral: 1200 mg/day in 2 divided doses, 30 minutes before breakfast and dinner

**Elderly:** Refer to adult dosing.

**Renal Impairment:** Hemodialysis effects: Not removed by hemodialysis; supplemental dose is not necessary.

**Monitoring Laboratory Tests** Serum cholesterol, LFTs

**Additional Nursing Issues**

**Physical Assessment:** Monitor appropriate laboratory tests for drug effectiveness. Ensure that patient understands need for follow-up assessment, appropriate use, side effects, and symptoms to report. **Pregnancy risk factor C** - benefits of use should outweigh possible risks. Breast-feeding is contraindicated.

**Patient Information/Instruction:** You must return to provider for assessment of drug effectiveness. Should be taken 30 minutes before meals. Take with milk or meals if GI upset occurs. You may experience loss of appetite and flatulence (frequent small meals may help), muscle aches (mild, temporary pain relievers may be required), dizziness, faintness, or blurred vision (use caution when driving or engaging in tasks that require alertness until response to drug is known). Report severe stomach pain, nausea, vomiting, chills, sore throat, headache, and any vision changes. **Pregnancy/breast-feeding precautions:** Inform prescriber if you are or intend to be pregnant. Do not breast-feed.

**Dietary Issues:** Before initiation of therapy, patients should be placed on a standard cholesterol-lowering diet for 3-6 months and the diet should be continued during drug therapy.

**Geriatric Considerations:** Gemfibrozil is the drug of choice for the treatment of hypertriglyceridemia and hypoalphaproteinemia in the elderly; it is usually well tolerated; myositis may be more common in patients with poor renal function.

**Related Information**

Lipid-Lowering Agents Comparison *on page 1393*

- **Gemzar®** *see* Gemcitabine *on page 528*
- **Genabid®** *see* Papaverine *on page 883*
- **Genac® Tablet** *see page 1294*
- **Genagesic®** *see* Propoxyphene and Acetaminophen *on page 985*
- **Genahist® Oral** *see* Diphenhydramine *on page 381*
- **Genamin® Cold Syrup** *see page 1294*
- **Genamin® Expectorant [OTC]** *see* Guaifenesin and Phenylpropanolamine *on page 550*
- **Genapap® [OTC]** *see* Acetaminophen *on page 32*
- **Genasoft® Plus** *see page 1294*
- **Genaspor® NP-27®** *see page 1247*
- **Genatap® Elixir** *see page 1294*
- **Genatuss® [OTC]** *see* Guaifenesin *on page 548*
- **Genatuss DM® [OTC]** *see* Guaifenesin and Dextromethorphan *on page 549*
- **Gencalc® 600 [OTC]** *see* Calcium Supplements *on page 185*
- **Genenicina®** *see* Gentamicin *on this page*
- **General Nursing Issues** *see page 16*
- **Geneye® Ophthalmic** *see page 1294*
- **Gen-Glybe** *see* Glyburide *on page 538*
- **Gen-K®** *see* Potassium Supplements *on page 952*
- **Genkova** *see* Gentamicin *on this page*
- **Gen-Minoxidil®** *see page 1294*
- **Gen-Nifedipine** *see* Nifedipine *on page 824*
- **Genoptic®** *see page 1282*
- **Genoptic® Ophthalmic** *see* Gentamicin *on this page*
- **Genoptic® S.O.P.** *see page 1282*
- **Genoptic® S.O.P. Ophthalmic** *see* Gentamicin *on this page*
- **Genora® 0.5/35** *see* Oral Contraceptives *on page 859*
- **Genora® 1/35** *see* Oral Contraceptives *on page 859*
- **Genora® 1/50** *see* Oral Contraceptives *on page 859*
- **Genoxal** *see* Cyclophosphamide *on page 313*
- **Gen-Pindolol** *see* Pindolol *on page 934*
- **Genpril® [OTC]** *see* Ibuprofen *on page 592*
- **Genrex** *see* Gentamicin *on this page*
- **Gentab-LA®** *see* Guaifenesin and Phenylpropanolamine *on page 550*
- **Gentacidin®** *see page 1282*
- **Gentacidin® Ophthalmic** *see* Gentamicin *on this page*
- **Gentacin** *see* Gentamicin *on this page*
- **Gentak®** *see page 1282*
- **Gentak® Ophthalmic** *see* Gentamicin *on this page*

## Gentamicin (jen ta MYE sin)

**U.S. Brand Names** Garamycin®; Genoptic® Ophthalmic; Genoptic® S.O.P. Ophthalmic; Gentacidin® Ophthalmic; Gentak® Ophthalmic; G-myticin® Topical; Jenamicin® Injection

**Therapeutic Category** Antibiotic, Aminoglycoside; Antibiotic, Ophthalmic; Antibiotic, Topical

**Pregnancy Risk Factor** C

**Lactation** Enters breast milk (small amounts)/use caution

**Use** Treatment of susceptible bacterial infections, normally gram-negative organisms including *Proteus*, *Serratia*, and gram-positive *Staphylococcus*; treatment of bone infections, respiratory tract infections, skin and soft tissue infections, as well as abdominal and urinary tract infections, endocarditis, and septicemia; topically to treat superficial infections of the skin or ophthalmic infections caused by susceptible bacteria

**Mechanism of Action/Effect** Bactericidal; interferes with bacterial protein synthesis resulting in cell death

**Contraindications** Hypersensitivity to gentamicin or other aminoglycosides

**Warnings** Not intended for long-term therapy due to toxic hazards associated with extended administration. Pre-existing renal insufficiency, vestibular or cochlear impairment, myasthenia gravis, hypocalcemia, conditions which depress neuromuscular transmission.

Parenteral aminoglycosides have been associated with significant nephrotoxicity or ototoxicity. Ototoxicity may be directly proportional to the amount of drug given and the duration of treatment and may not be reversible. Tinnitus or vertigo are indications of vestibular injury and impending hearing loss. Renal damage is usually reversible.

Pregnancy factor C.

**Drug Interactions**

**Increased Effect/Toxicity:** Penicillins, cephalosporins, amphotericin B, loop diuretics may increase nephrotoxic potential. Neuromuscular blocking agents may increase neuromuscular blockade.

(Continued)

## Gentamicin *(Continued)*

**Effects on Lab Values** ↑ protein, BUN, AST, GPT, alkaline phosphatase, serum creatinine; ↓ magnesium potassium, sodium, calcium

**Adverse Reactions**

**Systemic:**

>10%:

Central nervous system: Neurotoxicity (vertigo, ataxia)
Neuromuscular & skeletal: Gait instability
Otic: Ototoxicity (auditory), ototoxicity (vestibular)
Renal: Nephrotoxicity, decreased creatinine clearance

1% to 10%:

Cardiovascular: Edema
Dermatologic: Skin itching, reddening of skin, rash

<1% (Limited to important or life-threatening symptoms): Granulocytopenia, agranulocytosis, thrombocytopenia, elevated LFTs, dyspnea

**Overdose/Toxicology** Symptoms of overdose include ototoxicity, nephrotoxicity, and neuromuscular toxicity. Serum level monitoring is recommended. The treatment of choice, following a single acute overdose, appears to be maintenance of urine output of at least 3 mL/kg/hour during the acute treatment phase. Dialysis is of questionable value in enhancing aminoglycoside elimination.

**Pharmacodynamics/Kinetics**

**Protein Binding:** <30%

**Distribution:**

Crosses the placenta; increased by edema, ascites, fluid overload; decreased in patients with dehydration. See table.

**Aminoglycoside Penetration Into Various Tissues**

| Site | Extent of Distribution |
|---|---|
| Eye | Poor |
| CNS | Poor (<25%) |
| Pleural | Excellent |
| Bronchial secretions | Poor |
| Sputum | Fair (10%-50%) |
| Pulmonary tissue | Excellent |
| Ascitic fluid | Variable (43%-132%) |
| Peritoneal fluid | Poor |
| Bile | Variable (25%-90%) |
| Bile with obstruction | Poor |
| Synovial fluid | Excellent |
| Bone | Poor |
| Prostate | Poor |
| Urine | Excellent |
| Renal tissue | Excellent |

Relative diffusion of antimicrobial agents from blood into cerebrospinal fluid (CSF): Minimal even with inflammation

Ratio of CSF to blood level (%): Normal meninges: Nil; Inflamed meninges: 10-30

**Half-life Elimination:** 1.5-3 hours; end-stage renal disease: 36-70 hours

**Metabolism:** Liver

**Excretion:** Urine

**Formulations**

Gentamicin sulfate:

Cream, topical (Garamycin®, G-myticin®): 0.1% (15 g)
Infusion, in $D_5W$: 60 mg, 80 mg, 100 mg
Infusion, in NS: 40 mg, 60 mg, 80 mg, 90 mg, 100 mg, 120 mg
Injection: 40 mg/mL (1 mL, 1.5 mL, 2 mL)
  Pediatric: 10 mg/mL (2 mL)
  Intrathecal, preservative free (Garamycin®): 2 mg/mL (2 mL)
Ointment:
  Ophthalmic: 0.3% [3 mg/g] (3.5 g)
    Garamycin®, Genoptic® S.O.P., Gentacidin®, Gentak®: 0.3% [3 mg/g] (3.5 g)
  Topical (Garamycin®, G-myticin®): 0.1% (15 g)
Solution, ophthalmic: 0.3% (5 mL, 15 mL)
  Garamycin®, Genoptic®, Gentacidin®, Gentak®: 0.3% (1 mL, 5 mL, 15 mL)

**Dosing**

**Adults:** Individualization is critical because of the low therapeutic index. **Use of ideal body weight (IBW) for determining the mg/kg/dose appears to be more accurate than dosing on the basis of total body weight (TBW).** In morbid obesity, dosage requirement may best be estimated using a dosing weight of IBW + 0.4 (TBW - IBW). Initial and periodic peak and trough plasma drug levels should be determined, particularly in critically ill patients with serious infections or in disease states known to significantly alter aminoglycoside pharmacokinetics (eg, cystic fibrosis, burns, or major surgery).

I.M., I.V.:

Severe life-threatening infections: 2-2.5 mg/kg/dose

Urinary tract infections: 1.5 mg/kg/dose
Synergy (for gram-positive infections): 1 mg/kg/dose
High-dose, once-daily regimens: 5-7 mg/kg/dose once daily
Intrathecal: 4-8 mg/day
Ophthalmic:
Ointment: Instill 1/2" (1.25 cm) 2-3 times/day to every 3-4 hours.
Solution: Instill 1-2 drops every 2-4 hours, up to 2 drops every hour for severe infections.
Topical: Apply 3-4 times/day to affected area.
Some clinicians suggest a daily dose of 4-7 mg/kg for all patients with normal renal function. This dose is at least as efficacious with similar, if not less, toxicity than conventional dosing.

**Elderly:** Refer to adult dosing.

**Renal Impairment:**
$Cl_{cr}$ ≥60 mL/minute: Administer every 8 hours.
$Cl_{cr}$ 40-60 mL/minute: Administer every 12 hours.
$Cl_{cr}$ 20-40 mL/minute: Administer every 24 hours.
$Cl_{cr}$ 10-20 mL/minute: Administer every 48 hours.
$Cl_{cr}$ <10 mL/minute: Administer every 72 hours.
Hemodialysis effects: Dialyzable; removal by hemodialysis: 30% removal of aminoglycosides occurs during 4 hours of HD; administer dose after dialysis and follow levels
Removal by continuous ambulatory peritoneal dialysis (CAPD):
Administration via CAPD fluid:
Gram-negative infection: 4-8 mg/L (4-8 mcg/mL) of CAPD fluid
Gram-positive infection (ie, synergy): 3-4 mg/L (3-4 mcg/mL) of CAPD fluid
Administration via I.V., I.M. route during CAPD: Dose as for $Cl_{cr}$ <10 mL/minute and follow levels.
Removal via continuous arteriovenous or venovenous hemofiltration (CAVH/CAVHD): Dose as for $Cl_{cr}$ 10-40 mL/minute and follow levels.

**Hepatic Impairment:** Monitor plasma concentrations.

**Administration**

**I.M.:** Administer by deep I.M. route if possible. Slower absorption and lower peak concentrations, probably due to poor circulation in the atrophic muscle, may occur following I.M. injection; in paralyzed patients, suggest I.V. route.

**I.V.:** Administer other antibiotics at least 1 hour before or 1 hour after gentamicin.

**Other:** Administer any other ophthalmics 10 minutes before or after gentamicin preparations.

**Stability**

**Storage:** Gentamicin is a colorless to slightly yellow solution which should be stored between 2°C to 30°C, but refrigeration is not recommended.

**Reconstitution:** I.V. infusion solutions mixed in NS or $D_5W$ solution are stable for 24 hours at room temperature and refrigeration.
Premixed bag: Manufacturer expiration date; remove from overwrap stability: 30 days

**Compatibility:** See the Compatibility of Drugs Chart *on page 1315*.

**Monitoring Laboratory Tests** Monitor urinalysis, BUN, serum creatinine, and hearing test before, during, and after treatment, particularly in those at risk for ototoxicity or those receiving prolonged therapy (>2 weeks). **Note:** Serum levels (peak and trough), aminoglycoside levels measured in blood taken from silastic central catheters have been known to give falsely high reading (draw via separate lumen or peripheral site, or flush well).

**Additional Nursing Issues**

**Physical Assessment:** Assess effectiveness and interactions of other medications patient may be taking (see Contraindications and Drug Interactions). Assess patient's hearing level before, during, and following therapy; report changes to prescriber immediately. Monitor for therapeutic response, laboratory values (see above) and adverse reactions: neurotoxicity (vertigo, ataxia), opportunistic infections (fever, mouth and vaginal sores or plaques, unhealed wounds, etc) (see Warnings/Precautions, Adverse Reactions, and Overdose/Toxicology) at beginning of therapy and periodically throughout therapy. Assess knowledge/teach patient appropriate use, interventions to reduce side effects, and adverse symptoms to report. **Pregnancy risk factor C** - benefits of use should outweigh possible risks. Note breast-feeding caution.

**Patient Information/Instruction:** Take exactly as directed and when prescribed. Drink adequate amounts of water (2-3 L/day of fluids unless instructed to restrict fluid intake). You may experience headaches, ringing in ears, dizziness, blurred vision (use caution when driving or engaging in tasks requiring alertness until response to drug is known); GI upset, loss of appetite (small frequent meals and frequent mouth care may help); photosensitivity (use sunscreen wear protective clothing and eyewear, and avoid direct sunlight). Report severe headache, changes in hearing acuity or ringing in ears, changes in urine pattern, difficulty breathing, rash, fever, unhealed sores, sores in mouth, vaginal drainage, muscle or bone pain, change in gait, or worsening of condition. **Pregnancy/breast-feeding precautions:** Inform prescriber if you are or intend to be pregnant. Consult prescriber if breast-feeding.

Ophthalmic: Wash hands before instilling. Sit or lie down to instill. Open eye, look at ceiling, and instill prescribed amount of solution (Ointment: Pull lower lid down gently, instill thin ribbon of ointment inside lid.) Close eye and roll eye in all directions, and apply gentle pressure to inner corner of eye. Do not let tip of applicator touch eye or contaminate tip of applicator. Temporary stinging or blurred vision may occur. Report

(Continued)

## Gentamicin *(Continued)*

persistent pain, burning, vision disturbances, swelling, itching, or worsening of condition.

Topical: Apply thin film of ointment to affected area as often as recommended. May apply porous dressing. Report persistent burning, swelling, itching, worsening of condition, or lack of response to therapy.

**Geriatric Considerations:** Aminoglycosides are important therapeutic interventions for susceptible organisms and as empiric therapy in seriously ill patients. Their use is not without risk of toxicity, however. Additional studies comparing high-dose, once-daily aminoglycosides to traditional dosing regimens in the elderly are needed before once-daily aminoglycoside dosing can be routinely adopted to this patient population.

**Additional Information** Some formulations may contain sulfites.

**Related Information**

Ophthalmic Agents *on page 1282*
Peak and Trough Guidelines *on page 1331*


- ♦ **Gentarim** *see* Gentamicin *on page 531*
- ♦ **Gen-Timolol** *see* Timolol *on page 1138*
- ♦ **Gentran®** *see* Dextran *on page 351*
- ♦ **Gen-Triazolam** *see* Triazolam *on page 1174*
- ♦ **Gen-XENE®** *see* Clorazepate *on page 292*
- ♦ **Geocillin®** *see* Carbenicillin *on page 197*
- ♦ **Geopen®** *see* Carbenicillin *on page 197*
- ♦ **Geref® Injection** *see page 1248*
- ♦ **Geridium®** *see* Phenazopyridine *on page 914*
- ♦ **German Measles Vaccine** *see page 1256*
- ♦ **Gevrabon®** *see page 1294*
- ♦ **GG** *see* Guaifenesin *on page 548*
- ♦ **GG-Cen® [OTC]** *see* Guaifenesin *on page 548*
- ♦ **Gimalxina** *see* Amoxicillin *on page 80*
- ♦ **Ginedisc®** *see* Estradiol *on page 441*
- ♦ **Glaucoma Drug Comparison** *see page 1385*
- ♦ **Glaucon®** *see* Epinephrine *on page 424*
- ♦ **Glaucon®** *see* Ophthalmic Agents, Glaucoma *on page 853*
- ♦ **GlaucTabs®** *see* Methazolamide *on page 738*
- ♦ **Glibenclamide** *see* Glyburide *on page 538*
- ♦ **Glibenil** *see* Glyburide *on page 538*


## Glimepiride (GLYE me pye ride)

**U.S. Brand Names** Amaryl®

**Therapeutic Category** Antidiabetic Agent (Sulfonylurea)

**Pregnancy Risk Factor** C

**Lactation** Excretion in breast milk unknown/contraindicated

**Use** Management of noninsulin-dependent diabetes mellitus (Type II) as an adjunct to diet and exercise to lower blood glucose; in combination with insulin to lower blood glucose in patients whose hyperglycemia cannot be controlled by diet and exercise in conjunction with an oral hypoglycemic agent

**Mechanism of Action/Effect** Stimulates insulin release from the pancreatic beta cells; reduces glucose output from the liver; insulin sensitivity is increased at peripheral target sites

**Contraindications** Hypersensitivity to glimepiride or any component, other sulfonamides; diabetic ketoacidosis (with or without coma)

**Warnings** The administration of oral hypoglycemic drugs (eg, tolbutamide) has been reported to be associated with increased cardiovascular mortality as compared to treatment with diet alone or diet plus insulin. All sulfonylurea drugs are capable of producing severe hypoglycemia. Hypoglycemia is more likely to occur when caloric intake is deficient, after severe or prolonged exercise, when alcohol is ingested, or when more than one glucose-lowering drug is used. Pregnancy factor C.

**Drug Interactions**

**Cytochrome P-450 Effect:** CYP2C9 enzyme substrate

**Decreased Effect:** There may be a decreased effect of glimepiride with corticosteroids, cholestyramine, estrogens, oral contraceptives, phenytoin, rifampin, thiazide and other diuretics, phenothiazines, NSAIDs, thyroid products, nicotinic acid, isoniazid, sympathomimetics, urinary alkalinizers, and charcoal. **Note:** However, data from pooled data did **not** demonstrate drug interactions with calcium channel blockers, estrogens, NSAIDs, HMG CoA reductase inhibitors, sulfonamides, or thyroid hormone.

**Increased Effect/Toxicity:** Anticoagulants, androgens, fluconazole, miconazole, salicylates, gemfibrozil, sulfonamides, tricyclic antidepressants, probenecid, MAO inhibitors, beta-blockers, methyldopa, digitalis glycosides, urinary acidifiers, may increase hypoglycemic effects of glimepiride.

**Adverse Reactions**

1% to 10%:

Central nervous system: Headache, dizziness
Gastrointestinal: Nausea

<1% (Limited to important or life-threatening symptoms): Hypoglycemia, hyponatremia, blood dyscrasias, aplastic anemia, hemolytic anemia, bone marrow suppression, thrombocytopenia, agranulocytosis, cholestatic jaundice

**Overdose/Toxicology** Symptoms of overdose include low blood sugar, tingling of lips and tongue, nausea, yawning, confusion, agitation, tachycardia, sweating, convulsions, stupor, and coma. Intoxication with sulfonylureas can cause hypoglycemia and are best managed with glucose administration (oral for milder hypoglycemia or by injection in more severe forms). Patients should be monitored for a minimum of 24-48 hours after ingestion.

**Pharmacodynamics/Kinetics**

**Protein Binding:** 99.5%

**Half-life Elimination:** 5-9 hours

**Metabolism:** Liver

**Excretion:** Urine and feces

**Onset:** Peak blood glucose reductions: Within 2-3 hours

**Duration:** 24 hours

**Formulations** Tablet: 1 mg, 2 mg, 4 mg

**Dosing**

**Adults:** Oral (allow several days between dose titrations): Initial: 1-2 mg once daily, administered with breakfast or the first main meal; usual maintenance dose: 1-4 mg once daily. After a dose of 2 mg once daily, increase in increments of 2 mg at 1- to 2-week intervals based upon the patient's blood glucose response to a maximum of 8 mg once daily.

**Elderly:** Oral (allow several days between dose titrations): Initial: 1 mg/day; adjust for renal impairment.

**Renal Impairment:** $Cl_{cr}$ <22 mL/minute: Initial starting dose should be 1 mg and dosage increments should be based on fasting blood glucose levels.

**Administration**

**Oral:** May be taken with a meal or food.

**Monitoring Laboratory Tests** Urine for glucose and ketones, fasting blood glucose, hemoglobin $A_{1c}$, fructosamine

**Additional Nursing Issues**

**Physical Assessment:** Assess effectiveness and interactions of other medications (see Drug Interactions). See Warnings/Precautions and Contraindications for use cautions. Monitor effectiveness of therapy and monitor laboratory tests frequently during therapy (see above). Monitor for adverse response (eg, hypoglycemia - see Adverse Reactions and Overdose/Toxicology). Assess knowledge/teach patient or refer patient to diabetic educator for instruction in appropriate use, possible side effects and appropriate interventions, and adverse symptoms to report. **Pregnancy risk factor C** - benefits of use should outweigh possible risks. Breast-feeding is contraindicated.

**Patient Information/Instruction:** This medication is used to control diabetes; it is not a cure. Other components of treatment plan are important: follow prescribed diet, medication, and exercise regimen. Take exactly as directed; 30 minutes before meal(s) at the same time each day. Do not change dose or discontinue without consulting prescriber. Avoid alcohol while taking this medication; could cause severe reaction. Inform prescriber of all other prescription or OTC medications you are taking; do not introduce new medication without consulting prescriber. Do not take other medication within 2 hours of this medication unless so advised by prescriber. If you experience hypoglycemic reaction, contact prescriber immediately. Maintain regular dietary intake and exercise routine and always carry quick source of sugar with you. You may experience side effects during first weeks of therapy (headache, nausea); consult prescriber if these persist. Report severe or persistent side effects, extended vomiting or flu-like symptoms, skin rash, easy bruising or bleeding, or change in color of urine or stool. **Pregnancy/breast-feeding precautions:** Inform prescriber if you are or intend to be pregnant. Do not breast-feed.

**Geriatric Considerations:** Rapid and prolonged hypoglycemia (>12 hours) despite hypertonic glucose injections have been reported; age, hepatic, and renal impairment are independent risk factors for hypoglycemia; dosage titration should be made at weekly intervals. How "tightly" a geriatric patient's blood glucose should be controlled is controversial; however, a fasting blood sugar <150 mg/dL is now an acceptable end point. Such a decision should be based on the patient's functional and cognitive status, how well they recognize hypoglycemic or hyperglycemic symptoms, and how to respond to them and their other disease states.

**Related Information**

Antidiabetic Oral Agents Comparison *on page 1370*

♦ **Glioten** *see* Enalapril *on page 416*

## Glipizide (GLIP i zide)

**U.S. Brand Names** Glucotrol®; Glucotrol® XL

**Synonyms** Glydiazinamide

**Therapeutic Category** Antidiabetic Agent (Sulfonylurea)

**Pregnancy Risk Factor** C

**Lactation** Excretion in breast milk unknown/contraindicated

**Use** Management of noninsulin-dependent diabetes mellitus (Type II)

**Mechanism of Action/Effect** Stimulates insulin release from the pancreatic beta cells; reduces glucose output from the liver; insulin sensitivity is increased at peripheral target sites

**Contraindications** Hypersensitivity to glipizide, any component, other sulfonamides; Type I diabetes mellitus

(Continued)

## Glipizide *(Continued)*

**Warnings** Use with caution in patients with severe hepatic disease. A useful agent since few drug to drug interactions and not dependent upon renal elimination of active drug. Pregnancy factor C.

**Drug Interactions**

**Decreased Effect:** Decreased effect of glipizide with beta-blockers, cholestyramine, hydantoins, rifampin, thiazide diuretics, urinary alkalinizers, and charcoal.

**Increased Effect/Toxicity:** Increased effects/hypoglycemic effects with $H_2$ antagonists, anticoagulants, androgens, cimetidine, fluconazole, salicylates, gemfibrozil, sulfonamides, tricyclic antidepressants, probenecid, MAO inhibitors, methyldopa, digitalis glycosides, and urinary acidifiers.

**Food Interactions** A delayed release of insulin may occur if glipizide is taken with food. Should be administered 30 minutes before meals to avoid erratic absorption.

**Adverse Reactions**

>10%:

- Central nervous system: Headache, dizziness
- Endocrine & metabolic: Hypoglycemia (mild)
- Gastrointestinal: Constipation, diarrhea, heartburn, weight gain, anorexia, epigastric fullness, changes in sensation of taste
- Renal: Polyuria

1% to 10%:

- Dermatologic: Rash, urticaria, photosensitivity
- Endocrine & metabolic: Hypoglycemia (severe)

<1% (Limited to important or life-threatening symptoms): Aplastic anemia, hemolytic anemia, bone marrow suppression, thrombocytopenia, agranulocytosis, cholestatic jaundice, hepatic porphyria

**Overdose/Toxicology** Symptoms of overdose include low blood sugar, tingling of lips and tongue, nausea, yawning, confusion, agitation, tachycardia, sweating, convulsions, stupor, and coma. Intoxication with sulfonylureas can cause hypoglycemia and are best managed with glucose administration (oral for milder hypoglycemia or by injection in more severe forms).

**Pharmacodynamics/Kinetics**

**Protein Binding:** 92% to 99%

**Half-life Elimination:** 2-4 hours

**Metabolism:** Liver

**Excretion:** Urine and feces

**Onset:** Peak blood glucose reductions: Within 1.5-2 hours

**Duration:** 12-24 hours

**Formulations**

Tablet: 5 mg, 10 mg

Tablet, extended release: 5 mg, 10 mg

**Dosing**

**Adults:** Oral (allow several days between dose titrations): 2.5-40 mg/day; doses >15-20 mg/day should be divided and given twice daily. Maximum daily dose 40 mg.

**Elderly:** Oral (allow several days between dose titrations): Initial: 2.5-5 mg/day; increase by 2.5-5 mg/day at 1- to 2-week intervals. Maximum daily dose 40 mg.

**Renal Impairment:** $Cl_{cr}$ <10 mL/minute: Some investigators recommend not using.

**Hepatic Impairment:** Initial dosage should be 2.5 mg/day.

**Administration**

**Oral:** Administer 30 minutes before a meal to achieve greatest reduction in postprandial hyperglycemia. Patients who are NPO may need to have their dose held to avoid hypoglycemia.

**Monitoring Laboratory Tests** Urine for glucose and ketones, fasting blood glucose, hemoglobin $A_{1c}$, fructosamine

**Additional Nursing Issues**

**Physical Assessment:** Assess effectiveness and interactions of other medications (see Drug Interactions). See Warnings/Precautions and Contraindications for use cautions. Monitor effectiveness of therapy and monitor laboratory tests frequently during therapy (see above). Monitor for adverse response (eg, hypoglycemia - see Adverse Reactions and Overdose/Toxicology). Assess knowledge/teach patient or refer patient to diabetic educator for instruction in appropriate use, possible side effects and appropriate interventions, and adverse symptoms to report. **Pregnancy risk factor C** - benefits of use should outweigh possible risks. Breast-feeding is contraindicated.

**Patient Information/Instruction:** This medication is used to control diabetes; it is not a cure. Other components of treatment plan are important: follow prescribed diet, medication, and exercise regimen. Take exactly as directed; 30 minutes before meal(s) at the same time each day. Do not chew or crush extended release tablets. Do not change dose or discontinue without consulting prescriber. Avoid alcohol while taking this medication; could cause severe reaction. Inform prescriber of all other prescription or OTC medications you are taking; do not introduce new medication without consulting prescriber. Do not take other medication within 2 hours of this medication unless so advised by prescriber. If you experience hypoglycemic reaction, contact prescriber immediately. Maintain regular dietary intake and exercise routine and always carry quick source of sugar with you. You may be more sensitive to sunlight (use sunscreen, wear protective clothing and eyewear, and avoid direct sunlight). You may experience side effects during first weeks of therapy (headache, nausea); consult prescriber if these persist. Report severe or persistent side effects, extended vomiting, diarrhea, or constipation; flu-like symptoms; skin rash; easy bruising or bleeding; or change in color of urine or stool. **Pregnancy/breast-feeding precautions:** Inform prescriber if you are or intend to be pregnant. Do not breast-feed.

**Geriatric Considerations:** Glipizide is a useful agent since there are few drug to drug interactions and elimination of the active drug is not dependent upon renal function. How "tightly" a geriatric patient's blood glucose should be controlled is controversial; however, a fasting blood sugar <150 mg/dL is now an acceptable end point. Such a decision should be based on the patient's functional and cognitive status, how well they recognize hypoglycemic or hyperglycemic symptoms, and how to respond to them and their other disease states.

**Related Information**

Antidiabetic Oral Agents Comparison *on page 1370*

- **GlucaGen®** *see* Glucagon *on this page*

## Glucagon (GLOO ka gon)

**U.S. Brand Names** GlucaGen®; Glucagon (rDNA origin)

**Therapeutic Category** Antidote; Diagnostic Agent, Gastrointestinal

**Pregnancy Risk Factor** B

**Lactation** Excretion in breast milk unknown/compatible

**Use** Management of hypoglycemia; diagnostic aid in the radiologic examination of GI tract when a hypnotic state is needed; used with some success as a cardiac stimulant in management of severe cases of beta-adrenergic blocking agent overdosage

**Mechanism of Action/Effect** Stimulates adenylate cyclase to produce increased cyclic AMP, which promotes hepatic glycogenolysis and gluconeogenesis, causing a raise in blood glucose levels

**Contraindications** Hypersensitivity to glucagon or any component

**Warnings** Use with caution in patients with a history of insulinoma and/or pheochromocytoma.

**Drug Interactions**

**Increased Effect/Toxicity:** Glucagon and warfarin - hypoprothrombinemic effects may be increased, possibly with bleeding.

**Adverse Reactions** 1% to 10%:

Cardiovascular: Hypotension

Dermatologic: Urticaria

Gastrointestinal: Nausea, vomiting

Respiratory: Respiratory distress

**Overdose/Toxicology** Symptoms of overdose include hypokalemia, nausea, and vomiting.

**Pharmacodynamics/Kinetics**

**Half-life Elimination:** Plasma: 3-10 minutes

**Metabolism:** Liver, kidneys, and plasma

**Onset:** Peak effect on blood glucose levels: Parenteral: Within 5-20 minutes

**Duration:** 60-90 minutes

**Formulations** Powder for injection, lyophilized: 1 mg [1 unit]; 10 mg [10 units]

**Dosing**

**Adults:**

Hypoglycemia or insulin shock therapy: I.M., I.V., S.C.: 0.5-1 mg, may repeat in 20 minutes as needed. **If patient fails to respond to glucagon, I.V. dextrose must be given.**

Diagnostic aid: I.M., I.V.: 0.25-2 mg 10 minutes prior to procedure

**Elderly:** Refer to adult dosing.

**Administration**

**I.V.:** Bolus may be associated with nausea and vomiting. Continuous infusions may be used in beta-blocker overdose/toxicity.

**Stability**

**Reconstitution:** Reconstitute powder for injection by adding 1 or 10 mL of sterile diluent to a vial containing 1 or 10 units of the drug, respectively, to provide solutions containing 1 mg of glucagon/mL. If dose to be administered is <2 mg of the drug, then use only the diluent provided by the manufacturer. If >2 mg, use sterile water for injection. Use immediately after reconstitution. After reconstitution, use immediately. May be kept at 5°C for up to 48 hours if necessary.

**Monitoring Laboratory Tests** Blood glucose

**Additional Nursing Issues**

**Physical Assessment:** Arouse patient from hypoglycemic or insulin shock as soon as possible and administer carbohydrates. Evaluate insulin dosage and patient's ability to administer appropriate dose. Instruct patient (or significant other) in appropriate administration procedures for emergency use of glucagon. If home glucose monitoring device is available, check blood sugar as soon as possible.

**Patient Information/Instruction:** Identify appropriate support person to administer glucagon if necessary. Follow prescribers instructions for administering glucagon. Review diet, insulin administration, and testing procedures with prescriber or diabetic educator.

**Additional Information** 1 unit = 1 mg

- **Glucagon (rDNA origin)** *see* Glucagon *on this page*
- **Glucal** *see* Glyburide *on next page*
- **Glucocerebrosidase** *see* Alglucerase *on page 51*
- **Glucophage®** *see* Metformin *on page 734*
- **Glucophage® Forte** *see* Metformin *on page 734*

- ♦ **Glucose, Instant** *see page 1294*
- ♦ **Glucose Polymers** *see page 1294*
- ♦ **Glucotrol®** *see* Glipizide *on page 535*
- ♦ **Glucotrol® XL** *see* Glipizide *on page 535*
- ♦ **Glukor®** *see* Chorionic Gonadotropin *on page 264*
- ♦ **Glutose®** *see page 1294*
- ♦ **Glyate® [OTC]** *see* Guaifenesin *on page 548*


## Glyburide (GLYE byoor ide)

**U.S. Brand Names** Diaβeta®; Glynase™ PresTab™; Micronase®

**Synonyms** Glibenclamide

**Therapeutic Category** Antidiabetic Agent (Sulfonylurea)

**Pregnancy Risk Factor** C

**Lactation** Excretion in breast milk unknown/contraindicated

**Use** Management of noninsulin-dependent diabetes mellitus (Type II)

**Mechanism of Action/Effect** Stimulates insulin release from the pancreatic beta cells; reduces glucose output from the liver; insulin sensitivity is increased at peripheral target sites

**Contraindications** Hypersensitivity to glyburide, any component, or other sulfonamides; Type I diabetes mellitus; diabetic ketoacidosis with or without coma

**Warnings** Use with caution in patients with hepatic impairment. Elderly: Rapid and prolonged hypoglycemia (>12 hours) despite hypertonic glucose injections have been reported. Age, malnourished or debilitated conditions, adrenal or pituitary insufficiency, and hepatic and renal impairment are independent risk factors for hypoglycemia. Dosage titration should be made at weekly intervals. Use with caution in patients with renal and hepatic impairment. Pregnancy factor C.

**Drug Interactions**

**Cytochrome P-450 Effect:** CYP3A3/4 enzyme substrate

**Decreased Effect:** Thiazides and other diuretics, corticosteroids may decrease effectiveness of glyburide.

**Increased Effect/Toxicity:** Since this agent is highly protein bound, the toxic potential is increased when given concomitantly with other highly protein-bound drugs (ie, oral anticoagulants, warfarin, phenytoin, other hydantoins, salicylates, NSAIDs, sulfonamides, beta-blockers) resulting in an increased hypoglycemic effect. Alcohol ingestion may cause disulfiram reactions.

**Adverse Reactions**

>10%:

Central nervous system: Headache, dizziness

Endocrine & metabolic: Hypoglycemia (mild)

Gastrointestinal: Constipation, diarrhea, heartburn, weight gain, anorexia, epigastric fullness, changes in sensation of taste

Renal: Polyuria

1% to 10%:

Dermatologic: Rash, urticaria, photosensitivity

Endocrine & metabolic: Hypoglycemia (severe)

<1% (Limited to important or life-threatening symptoms): Aplastic anemia, hemolytic anemia, bone marrow suppression, thrombocytopenia, agranulocytosis, cholestatic jaundice, hepatic porphyria

**Overdose/Toxicology** Symptoms of overdose include severe hypoglycemia, seizures, cerebral damage, tingling of lips and tongue, nausea, yawning, confusion, agitation, tachycardia, sweating, convulsions, stupor, and coma. Intoxication with sulfonylureas can cause hypoglycemia and is best managed with glucose administration (oral for milder hypoglycemia or by injection in more severe forms).

**Pharmacodynamics/Kinetics**

**Protein Binding:** High >99%

**Half-life Elimination:** 5-16 hours; may be prolonged with renal insufficiency or hepatic insufficiency

**Time to Peak:** Within 2-4 hours

**Metabolism:** Liver

**Excretion:** Urine and feces

**Onset:** Oral: Insulin levels in the serum begin to increase within 15-60 minutes after a single dose

**Duration:** Up to 24 hours

**Formulations**

Tablet (Diaβeta®, Micronase®): 1.25 mg, 2.5 mg, 5 mg

Tablet, micronized (Glynase™ PresTab™): 1.5 mg, 3 mg, 6 mg

**Dosing**

**Adults:** Oral (Diaβeta®, Micronase®): 1.25-5 mg to start then increase at weekly intervals to 1.25-20 mg maintenance dose/day divided in 1-2 doses. Maximum: 20 mg/day.

Glynase™ PresTab™: Initial: 0.75-3 mg/day, increase by 1.5 mg/day in weekly intervals, maximum: 12 mg/day.

**Elderly:** Oral (Diaβeta®, Micronase®): Initial: 1.25-2.5 mg/day, increase by 1.25-2.5 mg/day every 1-3 weeks. Maximum: 20 mg/day.

**Renal Impairment:**

$Cl_{cr}$ 10-50 mL/minute: Use conservative initial and maintenance doses.

$Cl_{cr}$ <10 mL/minute: Avoid use.

Hemodialysis effects: Supplemental dose is not necessary.

Peritoneal dialysis effects: Supplemental dose is not necessary.

Continuous arteriovenous or venovenous hemofiltration effects: Supplemental dose is not necessary.

**Hepatic Impairment:** Use conservative initial and maintenance doses and avoid use in severe disease.

**Administration**

**Oral:** Administer before breakfast.

**Monitoring Laboratory Tests** Fasting blood glucose, hemoglobin $A_{1c}$, fructosamine

**Additional Nursing Issues**

**Physical Assessment:** Assess effectiveness and interactions of other medications (see Drug Interactions). See Warnings/Precautions and Contraindications for use cautions. Monitor effectiveness of therapy and monitor laboratory tests frequently during therapy (see above). Monitor for adverse response (eg, hypoglycemia - see Adverse Reactions and Overdose/Toxicology). Assess knowledge/teach patient or refer patient to diabetic educator for instruction in appropriate use, possible side effects and appropriate interventions, and adverse symptoms to report. **Pregnancy risk factor C** - benefits of use should outweigh possible risks. Breast-feeding is contraindicated.

**Patient Information/Instruction:** This medication is used to control diabetes; it is not a cure. Other components of treatment plan are important: follow prescribed diet, medication, and exercise regimen. Take exactly as directed; 30 minutes before meal(s) at the same time each day. Do not change dose or discontinue without consulting prescriber. Avoid alcohol while taking this medication; could cause severe reaction. Inform prescriber of all other prescription or OTC medications you are taking; do not introduce new medication without consulting prescriber. Do not take other medication within 2 hours of this medication unless so advised by prescriber. If you experience hypoglycemic reaction, contact prescriber immediately. Maintain regular dietary intake and exercise routine and always carry quick source of sugar with you. You may be more sensitive to sunlight (use sunscreen, wear protective clothing and eyewear, and avoid direct sunlight). You may experience side effects during first weeks of therapy (headache, nausea); consult prescriber if these persist. Report severe or persistent side effects, extended vomiting or flu-like symptoms, skin rash, easy bruising or bleeding, or change in color of urine or stool. **Pregnancy/breast-feeding precautions:** Inform prescriber if you are or intend to be pregnant. Do not breast-feed.

**Geriatric Considerations:** Rapid and prolonged hypoglycemia (>12 hours) despite hypertonic glucose injections have been reported; age, hepatic, and renal impairment are independent risk factors for hypoglycemia; dosage titration should be made at weekly intervals.

**Related Information**

Antidiabetic Oral Agents Comparison *on page 1370*

- **Glycerin** *see page 1294*
- **Glycerin, Lanolin, and Peanut Oil** *see page 1294*
- **Glycerol** *see page 1294*
- **Glycerol Guaiacolate** *see* Guaifenesin *on page 548*
- **Glycerol-T®** *see* Theophylline and Guaifenesin *on page 1118*
- **Glycerol Triacetate** *see page 1294*
- **Glyceryl Trinitrate** *see* Nitroglycerin *on page 831*
- **Glycofed®** *see* Guaifenesin and Pseudoephedrine *on page 551*

## Glycopyrrolate (glye koe PYE roe late)

**U.S. Brand Names** Robinul®; Robinul® Forte

**Synonyms** Glycopyrronium Bromide

**Therapeutic Category** Anticholinergic Agent

**Pregnancy Risk Factor** B

**Lactation** Excretion in breast milk unknown

**Use** Adjunct in treatment of peptic ulcer disease; inhibit salivation and excessive secretions of the respiratory tract preoperatively; reversal of neuromuscular blockade; control of upper airway secretions

**Mechanism of Action/Effect** Blocks the action of acetylcholine at parasympathetic sites in smooth muscle, secretory glands, and the CNS

**Contraindications** Hypersensitivity to glycopyrrolate or any component; narrow-angle glaucoma; acute hemorrhage; tachycardia; ulcerative colitis may predispose megacolon; obstructive uropathy; paralytic ileus; obstructive disease of GI tract

**Warnings** Not recommended in children <12 years of age. Use caution in the elderly; or in patients with autonomic neuropathy, hepatic or renal disease, hyperthyroidism, CAD, CHF, arrhythmias, BPH, hiatal hernia, or reflux.

**Drug Interactions**

**Decreased Effect:** Decreased effect of levodopa.

**Increased Effect/Toxicity:** Increased toxicity with amantadine and cyclopropane.

**Adverse Reactions**

>10%:

Dermatologic: Dry skin
Gastrointestinal: Constipation, dry throat, dry mouth
Local: Irritation at injection site
Respiratory: Dry nose
Miscellaneous: Sweating (decreased)

1% to 10%:

Dermatologic: Increased sensitivity to light

(Continued)

## Glycopyrrolate *(Continued)*

Endocrine & metabolic: Decreased flow of breast milk
Gastrointestinal: Dysphagia

<1% (Limited to important or life-threatening symptoms): Orthostatic hypotension, ventricular fibrillation, tachycardia, palpitations, increased intraocular pain

**Overdose/Toxicology** Symptoms of overdose include blurred vision, urinary retention, tachycardia, and absent bowel sounds. For anticholinergic overdose with severe life-threatening symptoms, physostigmine 1-2 mg S.C. or I.V. slowly, may be given to reverse these effects.

**Pharmacodynamics/Kinetics**

**Half-life Elimination:** <10 minutes

**Metabolism:** Liver

**Excretion:** Urine

**Onset:**

Oral: Onset of action: Within 50 minutes; Peak effect: Within 1 hour
I.M.: 20-40 minutes
I.V.: 1 minute

**Duration:** Vagal effects: 2-3 hours; Inhibition of salivation: Up to 7 hours; Anticholinergic effects (after oral administration): 8-12 hours

**Formulations**

Injection, as bromide: 0.2 mg/mL (1 mL, 2 mL, 5 mL, 20 mL)
Robinul®: 0.2 mg/mL (1 mL, 2 mL, 5 mL, 20 mL)

Tablet, as bromide:
Robinul®: 1 mg
Robinul® Forte: 2 mg

**Dosing**

**Adults:**

Reverse neuromuscular blockade: I.V.: 0.2 mg for each 1 mg of neostigmine or 5 mg of pyridostigmine administered
Intraoperative: I.V.: 0.1 mg repeated as needed at 2- to 3-minute intervals
Preoperative: I.M.: 4.4 mcg/kg 30-60 minutes before procedure
Peptic ulcer:
Oral: 1-2 mg 2-3 times/day
I.M., I.V.: 0.1-0.2 mg 3-4 times/day

**Elderly:** Refer to adult dosing.

**Administration**

**I.V.:** Administer at a rate of 0.2 mg over 1-2 minutes.

**I.V. Detail:** For I.V. administration, glycopyrrolate may be administered by I.M. or I.V. without dilution. May also be administered via the tubing of a running I.V. infusion of a compatible solution.

**Stability**

**Storage:** Unstable at pH >6.

**Compatibility:** Incompatible with secobarbital (immediate precipitation), sodium bicarbonate (gas evolves), thiopental (immediate precipitation), methylprednisolone sodium, chloramphenicol sodium succinate, dexamethasone sodium phosphate, diazepam, dimenhydrinate, methohexital sodium, and pentobarbital. See the Compatibility of Drugs Chart *on page 1315* and the Compatibility of Drugs in Syringe Chart *on page 1317.*

**Additional Nursing Issues**

**Physical Assessment:** Assess effectiveness and interactions of other medications (see Drug Interactions). See Warnings/Precautions and Contraindications for use cautions (eg, GI or GU obstructions). Have patient void before I.V. or I.M. administration. Monitor effectiveness of therapy and adverse response (see Adverse Reactions and Overdose/Toxicology). Assess knowledge/teach patient appropriate use, possible side effects and appropriate interventions, and adverse symptoms to report. Note breast-feeding caution.

**Patient Information/Instruction:** Take as directed before meals; do not increase dose and do not discontinue without consulting prescriber. Void before taking medication. You may experience dizziness or blurred vision (use caution when driving or engaging in tasks that require alertness until response to drug is known); dry mouth (sucking on lozenges may help); photosensitivity (wear dark glasses in bright sunlight); or impotence (temporary). Report excessive and persistent anticholinergic effects (blurred vision, headache, flushing, tachycardia, nervousness, constipation, dizziness, insomnia, mental confusion or excitement, dry mouth, altered taste perception, dysphagia, palpitations, bradycardia, urinary hesitancy or retention, impotence, decreased sweating). **Breast-feeding precautions:** Consult prescriber if breast-feeding.

**Geriatric Considerations:** Anticholinergic agents are generally not well tolerated in the elderly and their use should be avoided when possible.

**Additional Information**

Some formulations may contain benzyl alcohol.
pH: 2-3

- **Glycopyrronium Bromide** *see* Glycopyrrolate *on previous page*
- **Glycotuss® [OTC]** *see* Guaifenesin *on page 548*
- **Glycotuss-dM® [OTC]** *see* Guaifenesin and Dextromethorphan *on page 549*
- **Glydiazinamide** *see* Glipizide *on page 535*
- **Glynase™ PresTab™** *see* Glyburide *on page 538*
- **Gly-Oxide® Oral: Mollifene® Ear Wax Removing Formula** *see page 1294*

- **Glyset®** *see* Miglitol *on page 771*
- **Glytuss® [OTC]** *see* Guaifenesin *on page 548*
- **GM-CSF** *see* Sargramostim *on page 1045*
- **G-myticin® Topical** *see* Gentamicin *on page 531*
- **GnRH** *see* Gonadorelin *on next page*


## Gold Sodium Thiomalate (gold SOW dee um thye oh MAL ate)

**U.S. Brand Names** Aurolate®

**Therapeutic Category** Gold Compound

**Pregnancy Risk Factor** C

**Lactation** Enters breast milk/compatible (monitor closely)

**Use** Treatment of progressive rheumatoid arthritis

**Mechanism of Action/Effect** Unknown, may decrease prostaglandin synthesis or may alter cellular mechanisms by inhibiting sulfhydryl systems

**Contraindications** Hypersensitivity to gold compounds or any component; systemic lupus erythematosus; history of blood dyscrasias; congestive heart failure; exfoliative dermatitis; colitis

**Warnings** Nonsteroidal anti-inflammatory drugs (NSAIDs) and corticosteroids may be discontinued after initiating gold therapy. Do not inject I.V. Use with caution in patients with liver or renal disease. Pregnancy factor C.

**Drug Interactions**

**Decreased Effect:** Decreased effect with penicillamine and acetylcysteine.

**Adverse Reactions**

>10%:
- Dermatologic: Itching, rash
- Gastrointestinal: Stomatitis, gingivitis, glossitis, metallic taste

1% to 10%:
- Dermatologic: Urticaria, alopecia
- Renal: Proteinuria

<1% (Limited to important or life-threatening symptoms): Agranulocytosis, anemia, aplastic anemia, eosinophilia, thrombocytopenia, hepatotoxicity, hematuria, nephrotic syndrome, interstitial pneumonitis, bronchitis, pulmonary fibrosis

**Overdose/Toxicology** Symptoms of overdose include hematuria, proteinuria, fever, nausea, vomiting, and diarrhea. For treatment of mild gold poisoning, dimercaprol 2.5 mg/kg 4 times/day for 2 days, or for more severe forms of gold intoxication, dimercaprol 3-5 mg/kg every 4 hours for 2 days should be initiated. After 2 days, the initial dose should be repeated twice daily on the third day, and once daily thereafter for 10 days. Other chelating agents have been used with some success.

**Pharmacodynamics/Kinetics**

**Protein Binding:** 95% to 99%

**Half-life Elimination:** Single dose: 3-27 days; usual is approximately 5 days; After third dose: 14-40 days; After eleventh dose: Up to 168 days

**Time to Peak:** Within 4-6 hours

**Excretion:** Urine and feces

**Onset:** Delayed; may require up to 3 months

**Formulations** Injection: 25 mg/mL (1 mL); 50 mg/mL (1 mL, 2 mL, 10 mL)

**Dosing**

**Adults:** I.M.: 10 mg first week; 25 mg second week; then 25-50 mg/week until 1 g cumulative dose has been given. If improvement occurs without adverse reactions, give 25-50 mg every 2-3 weeks for 2-20 weeks, then every 3-4 weeks indefinitely. If no response after cumulative dose of 1 g is administered, discontinue therapy.

**Elderly:** Refer to adult dosing.

**Renal Impairment:**
- $Cl_{cr}$ 50-80 mL/minute: Administer 50% of normal dose.
- $Cl_{cr}$ <50 mL/minute: Avoid use.

**Administration**

**I.V.:** Do not administer intravenously, only for I.M. injection.

**Stability**

**Storage:** Should not be used if solution is darker than pale yellow.

**Monitoring Laboratory Tests** CBC with differential, platelet count, urinalysis

**Additional Nursing Issues**

**Physical Assessment:** Monitor laboratory tests (see above), therapeutic response (eg, relief of pain and inflammation, increased activity tolerance) and adverse reactions (eg, gold toxicity) at beginning of therapy and periodically throughout therapy (see Warnings/Precautions, Adverse Reactions, and Overdose/Toxicology). Assess knowledge/teach patient appropriate interventions to reduce side effects, and adverse symptoms to report. **Pregnancy risk factor C** - benefits of use should outweigh possible risks. Note breast-feeding caution.

**Patient Information/Instruction:** This medication can only be administered I.M. Drug effects may not be seen for as long as 3 weeks to 3 months. Metallic taste or mouth sores may occur (frequent mouth care and lozenges may help); gray-blue color or irritation and reddening of skin may occur (avoid excessive exposure to sunlight, use sunscreen, sunglasses, and protective clothing). Report acute headache, fever; chest pain, palpitations, or irregular heartbeat; unusual bruising, blood in mouth, urine, stool, vomitus; persistent fatigue; persistent metallic taste; abdominal cramping, vomiting, diarrhea; sores in mouth; unresolved skin rash or itching. **Pregnancy/breast-feeding precautions:** Inform prescriber if you are or intend to be pregnant. Consult prescriber if breast-feeding.

(Continued)

## Gold Sodium Thiomalate *(Continued)*

**Geriatric Considerations:** Tolerance to gold decreases with advanced age. Use cautiously only after traditional therapy and other disease-modifying antirheumatic drugs (DMARDs) have been attempted.

**Additional Information** Approximately 50% gold

♦ **GoLYTELY®** *see* Polyethylene Glycol-Electrolyte Solution *on page 945*

## Gonadorelin (goe nad oh REL in)

**U.S. Brand Names** Factrel®; Lutrepulse®

**Synonyms** GnRH; Gonadotropin Releasing Hormone; LH-RH; LRH; Luteinizing Hormone Releasing Hormone

**Therapeutic Category** Diagnostic Agent, Gonadotrophic Hormone; Gonadotropin

**Pregnancy Risk Factor** B

**Lactation** Excretion in breast milk unknown

**Use** Evaluation of the functional capacity and response of gonadotropic hormones; evaluate abnormal gonadotropin regulation as in precocious puberty and delayed puberty. Lutrepulse®: Induction of ovulation in females with hypothalamic amenorrhea.

**Mechanism of Action/Effect** Stimulates the release of luteinizing hormone (LH) from the anterior pituitary gland

**Contraindications** Hypersensitivity to gonadorelin; women with any condition that could be exacerbated by pregnancy; patients who have ovarian cysts or causes of anovulation other than those of hypothalamic origin; any condition that may be worsened by reproductive hormones

**Warnings** Hypersensitivity and anaphylactic reactions have occurred following multiple-dose administration. Use with caution in women in whom pregnancy could worsen pre-existing conditions (eg, pituitary prolactinemia). Multiple pregnancy is a possibility with gonadorelin.

**Drug Interactions**

**Decreased Effect:** Decreased levels/effect with oral contraceptives, digoxin, phenothiazines, and dopamine antagonists.

**Increased Effect/Toxicity:** Increased levels/effect with androgens, estrogens, progestins, glucocorticoids, spironolactone, and levodopa.

**Adverse Reactions** 1% to 10%: Local: Pain at injection site

**Overdose/Toxicology** Symptoms of overdose include abdominal discomfort, nausea, headache, and flushing. Treatment is symptomatic.

**Pharmacodynamics/Kinetics**

**Half-life Elimination:** 4 minutes

**Time to Peak:** Maximal LH release occurs within 20 minutes

**Duration:** 3-5 hours

**Formulations**

Injection, as acetate (Lutrepulse®): 0.8 mg, 3.2 mg

Injection, as hydrochloride (Factrel®): 100 mcg, 500 mcg

**Dosing**

**Adults:**

Diagnostic test: I.V., S.C. hydrochloride salt: 100 mcg administered in women during early phase of menstrual cycle (day 1-7)

Primary hypothalamic amenorrhea: Acetate: I.V.: 5 mcg every 90 minutes via Lutrepulse® pump kit at treatment intervals of 21 days (pump will pulsate every 90 minutes for 7 days)

**Administration**

**I.V.:**

Factrel®: Give I.V. push over 30 seconds

Lutrepulse®: A presterilized reservoir bag with the infusion catheter set supplied with the kit should be filled with the reconstituted solution and administered I.V. using the Lutrepulse® pump. Set the pump to deliver 25-50 mL of solution, based upon the dose, over a pulse period of 1 minute and at a pulse frequency of 90 minutes.

**I.V. Detail:** Factrel®: Dilute in 3 mL of normal saline.

**Stability**

**Reconstitution:**

Factrel®: Prepare immediately prior to use. After reconstitution, store at room temperature and use within 1 day. Discard unused portion.

Lutrepulse®: Reconstitute with diluent immediately prior to use and transfer to plastic reservoir. The solution will supply 90-minute pulsatile doses for 7 consecutive days (Lutrepulse® pump).

**Monitoring Laboratory Tests** LH, FSH

**Additional Nursing Issues**

**Physical Assessment:** Assess other medications patient may be taking for effectiveness and interactions (see Warnings/Precautions and Drug Interactions). When used for induction of ovulation, monitor laboratory tests and therapeutic response. Monitor injection site and instruct patient on use of pulsating pump (if applicable).

**Patient Information/Instruction:** If receiving this drug via pulsating pump, check all procedures with prescriber. Report any rash, pain, or inflammation at injection site, and any change in respiratory status.

♦ **Gonadotropin Releasing Hormone** *see* Gonadorelin *on this page*

♦ **Gonak™** *see page 1248*

♦ **Gonic®** *see* Chorionic Gonadotropin *on page 264*

♦ **Goniosol®** *see page 1248*

- **Goody's® Headache Powders** *see page 1294*
- **Gordofilm® Liquid** *see page 1294*
- **Gormel® Creme [OTC]** *see* Urea *on page 1193*

## Goserelin (GOE se rel in)

**U.S. Brand Names** Zoladex® Implant

**Therapeutic Category** Antineoplastic Agent, Miscellaneous; Gonadotropin Releasing Hormone Analog; Luteinizing Hormone-Releasing Hormone Analog

**Pregnancy Risk Factor** X

**Lactation** Enters breast milk/contraindicated

**Use** Palliative treatment of advanced prostate cancer; management of locally confined (Stage T2b-T4) prostate cancer; induce ovulation or to treat endometriosis

**Mechanism of Action/Effect** LHRH synthetic analog of luteinizing hormone-releasing hormone also known as gonadotropin-releasing hormone (GnRH)

**Contraindications** Hypersensitivity to goserelin or any component; pregnancy

**Warnings** Initially, goserelin transiently increases serum levels of testosterone. Transient worsening of signs or symptoms, usually manifested by an increase in cancer-related pain which was managed symptomatically, may develop during the first few weeks of treatment. Isolated cases of ureteral obstruction and spinal cord compression have been reported. Patient's symptoms may initially worsen temporarily during first few weeks of therapy, cancer-related pain can usually be controlled by analgesics.

**Effects on Lab Values** Serum alkaline phosphatase, serum acid phosphatase, serum testosterone, serum LH and FSH, serum estradiol

**Adverse Reactions**

General: Hormone replacement therapy may decrease vasomotor symptoms and loss of bone mineral density. Worsening of signs and symptoms may occur during the first few weeks of therapy and are usually manifested by an increase in bone pain, increased difficulty in urinating, hot flashes, injection site irritation, and weakness; this will subside, but patients should be aware.

>10%:
- Endocrine & metabolic: Gynecomastia, postmenopausal symptoms, sexual dysfunction, loss of libido, hot flashes
- Genitourinary: Impotence, decreased erection

1% to 10%:
- Cardiovascular: Edema, congestive heart failure
- Central nervous system: Headache, spinal cord compression (possible result of tumor flare), lethargy, dizziness, insomnia
- Dermatologic: Rash
- Endocrine & metabolic: Swelling and increased tenderness of breasts
- Gastrointestinal: Nausea and vomiting, anorexia, diarrhea, weight gain, constipation,
- Genitourinary: Vaginal spotting and breakthrough bleeding
- Local: Pain on injection
- Neuromuscular & skeletal: Bone loss, increased bone pain
- Respiratory: Chronic obstructive pulmonary disease (COPD); upper respiratory infection
- Miscellaneous: Sweating

**Overdose/Toxicology** Symptomatic management

**Pharmacodynamics/Kinetics**

**Half-life Elimination:** Following a bolus S.C. dose: ~5 hours; prolonged in impaired renal function ~12 hours

**Time to Peak:** S.C.: 12-15 days

**Excretion:** Kidney

**Formulations** Injection, implant, as acetate: 3.6 mg, 10.8 mg

**Dosing**

**Adults:**

Subcutaneous injection:
- Monthly implant: 3.6 mg injected into upper abdomen every 28 days. Do not try to aspirate with the goserelin syringe. If the needle is in a large vessel, blood will immediately appear in syringe chamber. While a delay of a few days is permissible, attempt to adhere to the 28-day schedule.
- 3-month implant: 10.8 mg injected into upper abdomen every 12 weeks. While a delay of a few days is permissible, attempt to adhere to the 12-week schedule.

Prostate carcinoma: Intended for long-term administration

Endometriosis: Recommended duration is 6 months; retreatment is not recommended since safety data is not available.

**Elderly:** Refer to adult dosing.

**Administration**

**Other:** Subcutaneous: Do not remove the sterile syringe until immediately before use. Do not aspirate with goserelin syringe.

**Stability**

**Storage:** Zoladex® should be stored at room temperature not to exceed 25°C (77°F). Must be dispensed in an amber bag.

**Additional Nursing Issues**

**Physical Assessment:** Assess pregnancy status prior to insertion of implant. Monitor for adverse reactions (see Adverse Reactions). **Pregnancy risk factor X** - determine that patient is not pregnant before beginning treatment and do not give to women of childbearing age unless female is capable of complying with barrier contraceptive measures 1 month prior to therapy, during therapy, and 1 month following therapy. Breast-feeding is contraindicated.

(Continued)

## Goserelin *(Continued)*

**Patient Information/Instruction:** This drug must be implanted into your stomach every 28 days; it is important to maintain appointment schedule. You may experience systemic hot flashes (cool clothes and temperatures may help), headache (analgesic may help), constipation (increased bulk and water in diet or stool softener may help), sexual dysfunction (decreased libido, decreased erection). Symptoms may worsen temporarily during first weeks of therapy. Report unusual nausea or vomiting, any chest pain, respiratory difficulty, unresolved dizziness, or constipation. **Pregnancy/breast-feeding precautions:** Inform prescriber if you are pregnant; do not get pregnant 1 month before, during, or for 1 month following therapy. Consult prescriber for instruction on appropriate contraceptive measures. This drug may cause severe fetal defects. Do not donate blood during or for 1 month following therapy (same reason). Do not breast-feed.

♦ **Graneodin-B** *see* Benzocaine *on page 141*

## Granisetron (gra NI se tron)

**U.S. Brand Names** Kytril™

**Therapeutic Category** Selective 5-$HT_3$ Receptor Antagonist

**Pregnancy Risk Factor** B

**Lactation** Excretion in breast milk unknown/opportunity for use is minimal

**Use** Prophylaxis and treatment of chemotherapy-related emesis; may be prescribed for patients who are refractory to or have severe adverse reactions to standard antiemetic therapy. Granisetron may be prescribed for young patients (ie, <45 years of age who are more likely to develop extrapyramidal reactions to high-dose metoclopramide) who are to receive highly emetogenic chemotherapeutic agents. Granisetron should not be prescribed for chemotherapeutic agents with a low emetogenic potential (eg, bleomycin, busulfan, cyclophosphamide <1000 mg, etoposide, 5-fluorouracil, vinblastine, vincristine).

**Mechanism of Action/Effect** Selective 5-$HT_3$ receptor antagonist, blocking serotonin, both peripherally on vagal nerve terminals and centrally in the chemoreceptor trigger zone.

**Contraindications** Hypersensitivity to granisetron

**Warnings** Use with caution in patients with liver disease or in pregnant patients.

**Drug Interactions**

**Cytochrome P-450 Effect:** CYP3A3/4 enzyme substrate

**Adverse Reactions**

>10%

Central nervous system: Headache, muscle weakness

Gastrointestinal: Constipation

1% to 10%:

Cardiovascular: Hypertension, Arrhythmias

Central nervous system: Dizziness, insomnia, anxiety, somnolence

Gastrointestinal: Abdominal pain, diarrhea

Hepatic: Elevated LFTs

<1% (Limited to important or life-threatening symptoms): Chest pain, hypotension, atrial fibrillation, syncope, dyspnea

**Pharmacodynamics/Kinetics**

**Protein Binding:** 65%

**Distribution:** Widely distributed throughout the body

**Half-life Elimination:** Cancer patient: 10-12 hours; Healthy volunteer: 3-4 hours

**Metabolism:** Liver

**Excretion:** Feces and urine

**Onset:** Commonly controls emesis within 1-3 minutes of administration

**Duration:** Effects generally last no more than a maximum of 24 hours

**Formulations**

Injection: 1 mg/mL

Tablet: 1 mg (2s), (20s)

**Dosing**

**Adults:**

I.V.: 10 mcg/kg for 1-3 doses. Doses should be administered as a single IVPB over 5 minutes, given just prior to chemotherapy (15-60 minutes before). As intervention therapy for breakthrough nausea and vomiting, during the first 24 hours following chemotherapy, 2 or 3 repeat infusions (same dose) have been administered, separated by at least 10 minutes.

Oral: 1 mg twice daily; the first 1 mg dose should be given up to 1 hour before chemotherapy, and the second tablet, 12 hours after the first dose; or 2 mg once daily; two 1 mg tablets are given up to 1 hour before chemotherapy.

**Note: Granisetron should only be given on the day(s) of chemotherapy.**

**Elderly:** Refer to adult dosing.

**Renal Impairment:** Creatinine clearance values have no relationship to granisetron clearance.

**Hepatic Impairment:** Kinetic studies in patients with hepatic impairment showed that total clearance was approximately halved; however, standard doses were very well tolerated.

**Administration**

**I.V.:** Doses should be given at least 15 minutes prior to initiation of chemotherapy.

**Stability**

**Storage:** I.V.: Do not freeze vials.

**Reconstitution:** I.V.: Stable when mixed in NS or $D_5W$ for 24 hours at room temperature.

**Additional Nursing Issues**

**Physical Assessment:** Monitor blood pressure and cardiac status. Monitor and treat acute headache response. Instruct patient on appropriate measures to relieve constipation. Note breast-feeding caution.

**Patient Information/Instruction:** This drug will be administered on days when you receive chemotherapy to reduce nausea and vomiting. If outpatient chemotherapy, you may be given oral medication to take after return home; take as directed. You may experience drowsiness; use caution when driving. For persistent acute headache request analgesic from prescriber. Frequent mouth care, chewing gum, or sucking on lozenges may relieve persistent nausea. Report unrelieved headache, fever, diarrhea, or constipation. **Breast-feeding precautions:** Consult prescriber if breast-feeding.

**Geriatric Considerations:** Clinical trials with patients older than 65 years of age are limited; however, the data indicates that safety and efficacy are similar to that observed in younger adults. No adjustment in dose necessary for elderly.

**Additional Information** pH: 4.7-7.3

**Related Information**

Antiemetics for Chemotherapy-Induced Nausea and Vomiting *on page 1307*

- **Granulocyte Colony Stimulating Factor** *see* Filgrastim *on page 483*
- **Granulocyte-Macrophage Colony Stimulating Factor** *see* Sargramostim *on page 1045*
- **Graten** *see* Morphine Sulfate *on page 790*

## Grepafloxacin (grep a FLOX a sin)

**U.S. Brand Names** Raxar®

**Synonyms** OPC-17116

**Therapeutic Category** Antibiotic, Quinolone

**Pregnancy Risk Factor** C

**Lactation** Enters breast milk/contraindicated

**Use** Treatment of acute bacterial exacerbations of chronic bronchitis caused by *Haemophilus influenzae*, *Streptococcus pneumoniae*, or *Moraxella catarrhalis*; community-acquired pneumonia caused by *Mycoplasma pneumoniae* or the organisms previously mentioned; uncomplicated gonorrhea caused by *Neisseria gonorrhoeae*, and nongonococcal cervicitis and urethritis caused by *Chlamydia trachomatis*

*In vitro* studies suggest similar or lesser activity against *Enterobacteriaceae* and *P. aeruginosa* but greater activity against gram-positive cocci, especially *S. pneumoniae*, and some anaerobes and *Chlamydia* spp.

**Unlabeled use:** Skin/skin structure infections

**Mechanism of Action/Effect** Inhibits DNA gyrase (topoisomerase II) and topoisomerase I.V. in susceptible organisms; blocks relaxation of supercoiled DNA and promoted breakage of double-stranded DNA. Activity *in vitro* includes atypical, gram-negative, gram-positive (including penicillin-resistant pneumococci), intra- and extracellular aerobic organisms. Bactericidal at concentrations equal to or slightly above MICs.

**Contraindications** Hypersensitivity to grepafloxacin or other quinolone derivatives; patients with hepatic failure; patients with Q-$T_c$ prolongation and use with drugs which prolong Q-$T_c$ interval. Do not use concomitantly with Class I and III antiarrhythmics or bepridil due to the potential risk of cardiac arrhythmias (including torsade de pointes).

**Warnings** CNS stimulation (eg, tremor, paranoia, depression, insomnia, lightheadedness), seizures, increase intracranial pressure, and psychosis may occur with quinolones. Use with caution in patients with known or suspected CNS disease, including atherosclerosis, epilepsy, or other disorders which may lower seizure threshold. Avoid concomitant use of drugs which prolong Q-$T_c$ interval or on-going pro-arrhythmic conditions. Discontinue if rash develops, or if pain, inflammation, or rupture to a tendon occurs. May cause photosensitivity or severe hypersensitivity (anaphylactic or anaphylactoid) reactions. Superinfection, including *C. difficile* colitis may occur due to elimination of normal GI flora. Safety and efficacy in pregnancy and pediatric patients <18 years of age have not been established. Although the significance in humans is unknown, animal studies have demonstrated skeletal deformities when quinolones are administered to immature animals. Pregnancy factor C.

**Drug Interactions**

**Cytochrome P-450 Effect:** CYP1A2 enzyme inhibitor and substrate (also CYP3A4)

**Decreased Effect:** Coadministration with metal cations, including antacids containing aluminum, magnesium, sucralfate, multivitamins with zinc or iron salts markedly reduces absorption. Separate oral administration by at least 4 hours. May decrease (or augment) effect of oral hypoglycemics.

**Increased Effect/Toxicity:** Caffeine and theophylline levels increased during concurrent therapy (reduce dose of theophylline by 50%). Concomitant nonsteroidal anti-inflammatory drugs may increase risk of CNS stimulation/seizures. May augment (or decrease) effects of oral hypoglycemics. Use with caution in patients receiving warfarin - some quinolones enhance effect.

**Adverse Reactions** Patients receiving quinolones have experienced tendon rupture - discontinue if inflammation, pain or rupture of a tendon occurs.

(Continued)

## Grepafloxacin *(Continued)*

>10% (range reported in clinical trials):

Gastrointestinal: Nausea (11.1% to 15.8%), taste perversion (9.0% to 17.8%)

1% to 10%:

Central nervous system: Dizziness (4.3% to 4.9%), headache (4.6% to 4.9%), insomnia (1.3% to 2.1%), anorexia (0.8% to 1.8%), somnolence (1.0% to 1.5%), nervousness (0.6% to 1.7%), pain (0.6% to 1.0%)

Dermatologic: Rash (1.1% to 1.9%), pruritus (1.2% to 1.6%), photosensitivity (0.7% to 1.8%)

Gastrointestinal: Vomiting (1.7% to 5.7%), diarrhea (3.5% to 4.2%), abdominal pain (2.1% to 2.2%), dyspepsia (1.5% to 3.1%), constipation (0.7% to 2.2%), dry mouth (0.8% to 1.1%)

Genitourinary: Vaginitis (1.4% to 3.3%), leukorrhea (0.0% to 1.4%)

Neuromuscular or skeletal: Asthenia (1.4% to 2.3%)

Miscellaneous: Infection (0.4% to 1.3%)

<1% (Limited to important or life-threatening symptoms): Arrhythmia, anaphylactoid/anaphylactic reaction, shock, angioedema, hallucinations, paresthesia, agitation, epidermal necrolysis, amblyopia

**Pharmacodynamics/Kinetics**

**Protein Binding:** 50%

**Distribution:** Approximately 5 L/kg; tissue concentrations generally exceed serum

**Half-life Elimination:** 15.7 hours (average)

**Time to Peak:** Within 2-3 hours of oral dose

**Metabolism:** Hepatic, metabolized by cytochrome P-450 isoenzymes 1A2 and 3A4 (final metabolism to glucuronide conjugates and oxidative metabolites)

**Excretion:** Feces and urine

**Formulations** Tablet, as hydrochloride: 200 mg, 400 mg, 600 mg

**Dosing**

**Adults:**

Acute bacterial exacerbations of chronic bronchitis: 400-600 mg daily for 10 days

Community-acquired pneumonia: 600 mg daily for 10 days

Nongonococcal urethritis or cervicitis: 400 mg daily for 7 days

Uncomplicated gonococcal infection: 400 mg as a single dose

**Elderly:** Refer to adult dosing.

**Hepatic Impairment:** Metabolism/excretion are reduced in hepatic impairment. No specific recommendations on dosage adjustment are provided. Contraindicated in hepatic failure.

**Monitoring Laboratory Tests** Perform culture and sensitivity studies prior to initiating therapy.

**Additional Nursing Issues**

**Physical Assessment:** Assess allergy history before initiating therapy. Assess effectiveness and interactions of other medications (see Drug Interactions). See Warnings/Precautions and Contraindications for use cautions. Monitor effectiveness of therapy, laboratory tests, and adverse response (see Adverse Reactions and Overdose/Toxicology). Assess knowledge/teach patient appropriate use, possible side effects and appropriate interventions, and adverse symptoms to report. **Pregnancy risk factor C** - benefits of use should outweigh possible risks. Breast-feeding is contraindicated.

**Patient Information/Instruction:** Take per recommended schedule; complete full course of therapy and do not skip doses. Take on an empty stomach (1 hour before or 2 hours after meals, dairy products, antacids, or other medications). Maintain adequate hydration (2-3 L/day of fluids unless instructed to restrict fluid intake). Diabetics should monitor glucose levels closely; this medication may alter effect of oral hypoglycemic agents. You may experience dizziness, lightheadedness, anxiety, insomnia, or confusion (use caution when driving or engaging in tasks that require alertness until response to drug is known); photosensitivity (use sunscreen, wear protective clothing and eyewear, and avoid direct sunlight). Report immediately any CNS disturbances (hallucinations, agitation, confusion, seizures), chest pain, or palpitations. Report persistent GI disturbances; muscle or tendon pain, swelling, or redness; signs of opportunistic infection (sore throat, chills, fever, burning, itching on urination, vaginal discharge, white plaques in mouth); or worsening of condition. **Pregnancy/breast-feeding precautions:** Inform prescriber if you are or intend to be pregnant. Do not breast-feed.

**Pregnancy Issues:** Quinolones have been associated with an increase in skeletal malformations in animal models. Use during pregnancy only if potential benefit outweighs possible risks.

♦ **Grifulvin® V** *see* Griseofulvin *on this page*

♦ **Grisactin-500®** *see* Griseofulvin *on this page*

♦ **Grisactin® Ultra** *see* Griseofulvin *on this page*

## Griseofulvin (gri see oh FUL vin)

**U.S. Brand Names** Fulvicin® P/G; Fulvicin-U/F®; Grifulvin® V; Grisactin-500®; Grisactin® Ultra; Gris-PEG®

**Synonyms** Griseofulvin Microsize; Griseofulvin Ultramicrosize

**Therapeutic Category** Antifungal Agent, Oral

**Pregnancy Risk Factor** C

**Lactation** Excretion in breast milk unknown

**Use** Treatment of susceptible tinea infections of the skin, hair, and nails

**Mechanism of Action/Effect** Inhibits fungal cell mitosis at metaphase; binds to human keratin making it resistant to fungal invasion

**Contraindications** Hypersensitivity to griseofulvin or any component; severe liver disease; porphyria (interferes with porphyrin metabolism)

**Warnings** During long-term therapy, periodic assessment of hepatic, renal, and hematopoietic functions should be performed. Hypersensitivity cross reaction between penicillins and griseofulvin is possible. Avoid exposure to intense sunlight to prevent photosensitivity reactions. Pregnancy factor C.

**Drug Interactions**

**Decreased Effect:** Barbiturates may decrease levels. Decreased warfarin activity. Decreased oral contraceptive effectiveness.

**Increased Effect/Toxicity:** Increased toxicity with alcohol, may cause tachycardia and flushing.

**Food Interactions** Griseofulvin concentrations may be increased if taken with food, especially with high fat meals.

**Effects on Lab Values** False-positive urinary VMA levels

**Adverse Reactions**

>10%: Central nervous system: Headache

1% to 10%:

- Central nervous system: Fatigue, confusion, dizziness, insomnia, mental confusion
- Dermatologic: Photosensitivity, rash, urticaria
- Gastrointestinal: Nausea, vomiting, epigastric distress, diarrhea
- Neuromuscular & skeletal: Peripheral neuritis
- Miscellaneous: Oral thrush

<1% (Limited to important or life-threatening symptoms): Angioneurotic edema, GI bleeding, leukopenia, granulocytopenia, hepatitis, proteinuria, nephrosis

**Overdose/Toxicology** Symptoms of overdose include lethargy, vertigo, blurred vision, nausea, vomiting, and diarrhea. Treatment is supportive.

**Pharmacodynamics/Kinetics**

**Distribution:** Crosses the placenta

**Half-life Elimination:** 9-22 hours

**Metabolism:** Liver

**Excretion:** Urine, feces, and perspiration

**Formulations**

Microsize:
- Capsule (Grisactin®): 125 mg, 250 mg
- Suspension, oral (Grifulvin® V): 125 mg/5 mL with alcohol 0.2% (120 mL)
- Tablet:
  - Fulvicin-U/F®, Grifulvin® V: 250 mg
  - Fulvicin-U/F®, Grifulvin® V, Grisactin-500®: 500 mg

Ultramicrosize:
- Tablet:
  - Fulvicin® P/G: 165 mg, 330 mg
  - Fulvicin® P/G, Grisactin® Ultra, Gris-PEG®: 125 mg, 250 mg
  - Grisactin® Ultra: 330 mg

**Dosing**

**Adults:** Oral:
- Microsize: 500-1000 mg/day in single or divided doses
- Ultramicrosize: 330-375 mg/day in single or divided doses; doses up to 750 mg/day have been used for infections more difficult to eradicate such as tinea unguium and tinea pedis.
- Duration of therapy depends on the site of infection:
  - Tinea corporis: 2-4 weeks
  - Tinea capitis: 4-6 weeks or longer
  - Tinea pedis: 4-8 weeks
  - Tinea unguium: 4-6 months

**Elderly:** Refer to adult dosing.

**Monitoring Laboratory Tests** Periodic renal, hepatic, and hematopoietic function especially with long-term use

**Additional Nursing Issues**

**Physical Assessment:** Assess allergy history before beginning therapy (see Drug Interactions). See Warnings/Precautions and Contraindications for use cautions. Monitor effectiveness of therapy and monitor laboratory tests during therapy (see above). Monitor for adverse response (see Adverse Reactions and Overdose/Toxicology). Assess knowledge/teach patient possible side effects and appropriate interventions and adverse symptoms to report. **Pregnancy risk factor C** - benefits of use should outweigh possible risks. **Note:** Oral contraceptives may have decreased effectiveness with griseofulvin. Note breast-feeding caution.

**Patient Information/Instruction:** Take as directed; around-the-clock with food. Take full course of medication; do not discontinue without notifying prescriber. Avoid alcohol while taking this drug (disulfiram reactions). Practice good hygiene measures to prevent reinfection. Frequent blood tests may be required with prolonged therapy. You may experience nausea and vomiting (small, frequent meals may help); confusion, dizziness, drowsiness (use caution when driving or engaging in tasks that require alertness until response to drug is known); nausea, vomiting, or diarrhea (small frequent meals, frequent mouth care, sucking lozenges, or chewing gum may help); increased sensitivity to sun (use sunscreen, wear protective clothing and eyewear, and avoid excessive exposure to direct sunlight). Report skin rash, respiratory difficulty, CNS changes (confusion, dizziness, acute headache), changes in color of stool or

(Continued)

## Griseofulvin *(Continued)*

urine, white plaques in mouth, or worsening of condition. **Breast-feeding precautions:** Inform prescriber if pregnant. Consult prescriber if breast-feeding.

**Additional Information**

Microsize: Fulvicin-U/F®, Grifulvin® V, Grisactin®

Ultramicrosize: Fulvicin® P/G, Grisactin® Ultra, Gris-PEG®; GI absorption of ultramicrosize is ~1.5 times that of microsize

- **Griseofulvin Microsize** *see* Griseofulvin *on page 546*
- **Griseofulvin Ultramicrosize** *see* Griseofulvin *on page 546*
- **Grisovin®-FP** *see* Griseofulvin *on page 546*
- **Grisovin-FP** *see* Griseofulvin *on page 546*
- **Gris-PEG®** *see* Griseofulvin *on page 546*
- **Grunicina** *see* Amoxicillin *on page 80*
- **Guaifed® [OTC]** *see* Guaifenesin and Pseudoephedrine *on page 551*
- **Guaifed-PD®** *see* Guaifenesin and Pseudoephedrine *on page 551*

## Guaifenesin (gwye FEN e sin)

**U.S. Brand Names** Anti-Tuss® Expectorant [OTC]; Breonesin® [OTC]; Diabetic Tussin EX® [OTC]; Durafuss-G®; Fenesin™; Gee Gee® [OTC]; Genatuss® [OTC]; GG-Cen® [OTC]; Glyate® [OTC]; Glycotuss® [OTC]; Glytuss® [OTC]; Guaifenex LA®; GuiaCough® Expectorant [OTC]; Guiatuss® [OTC]; Halotussin® [OTC]; Humibid® L.A.; Humibid® Sprinkle; Hytuss® [OTC]; Hytuss-2X® [OTC]; Liquibid®; Medi-Tuss® [OTC]; Monafed®; Muco-Fen-LA®; Mytussin® [OTC]; Naldecon® Senior EX [OTC]; Organidin® NR; Pneumomist®; Respa-GF®; Robitussin® [OTC]; Scot-Tussin® [OTC]; Siltussin® [OTC]; Sinumist®-SR Capsulets®; Touro Ex®; Tusibron® [OTC]; Uni-Tussin® [OTC]

**Synonyms** GG; Glycerol Guaiacolate

**Therapeutic Category** Expectorant

**Pregnancy Risk Factor** C

**Lactation** Excretion in breast milk unknown/use caution

**Use** Temporary control of nonproductive cough due by increasing bronchial secretions

**Mechanism of Action/Effect** Thought to act as an expectorant by irritating the gastric mucosa and stimulating respiratory tract secretions, thereby increasing respiratory fluid volumes and decreasing phlegm viscosity

**Contraindications** Hypersensitivity to guaifenesin or any component

**Warnings** Do not use for persistent cough, such as occurs with smoking, asthma, or emphysema or cough accompanied by excessive secretions. Pregnancy factor C.

**Effects on Lab Values** Possible color interference with determination of 5-HIAA and VMA

**Adverse Reactions** 1% to 10%:

Central nervous system: Drowsiness, headache

Dermatologic: Rash

Gastrointestinal: Nausea, vomiting, stomach pain

**Overdose/Toxicology** Symptoms of overdose include vomiting, lethargy, coma, and respiratory depression. Treatment is supportive.

**Pharmacodynamics/Kinetics**

**Half-life Elimination:** Approximately 1 hour

**Metabolism:** Liver

**Excretion:** Urine

**Formulations**

Caplet, sustained release (Touro Ex®): 600 mg

Capsule (Breonesin®, GG-Cen®, Hytuss-2X®): 200 mg

Capsule, sustained release (Humibid® Sprinkle): 300 mg

Liquid:

Diabetic Tussin EX®, Organidin® NR, Tusibron®: 100 mg/5 mL (118 mL)

Naldecon® Senior EX: 200 mg/5 mL (118 mL, 480 mL)

Syrup (Anti-Tuss® Expectorant, Genatuss®, Glyate®, GuiaCough® Expectorant, Guiatuss®, Halotussin®, Medi-Tuss®, Mytussin®, Robitussin®, Scot-Tussin®, Siltussin®, Tusibron®, Uni-Tussin®): 100 mg/5 mL with alcohol 3.5% (30 mL, 120 mL, 240 mL, 473 mL, 946 mL)

Tablet:

Duratuss-G®: 1200 mg

Gee Gee®, Glytuss®, Organidin® NR: 200 mg

Glycotuss®, Hytuss®: 100 mg

Sustained release (Fenesin™, Guaifenex LA®, Humibid® L.A., Liquibid®, Monafed®, Muco-Fen-LA®, Pneumomist®, Respa-GF®, Sinumist®-SR Capsulets®): 600 mg

**Dosing**

**Adults:** Oral: 200-400 mg every 4 hours to a maximum of 2.4 g/day

**Elderly:** Refer to adult dosing.

**Stability**

**Storage:** Protect from light.

**Additional Nursing Issues**

**Physical Assessment:** Monitor effectiveness of therapy (relief of cough, lung sounds, and respiratory pattern) and adverse reactions (see Adverse Reactions) at beginning of therapy and periodically with long-term use. Assess knowledge/teach patient appropriate use, interventions to reduce side effects, and adverse symptoms to report. **Pregnancy risk factor C** - benefits of use should outweigh possible risks. Note breast-feeding caution.

**Patient Information/Instruction:** Take only as prescribed; do not exceed prescribed dose or frequency. Do not chew or crush timed release capsule. Maintain adequate hydration (2-3 L/day of fluids unless instructed to restrict fluid intake). You may experience some drowsiness (use caution when driving or engaging in tasks requiring alertness until response to drug is known). Report excessive drowsiness, difficulty breathing, or lack of improvement or worsening or condition. **Pregnancy/breast-feeding precautions:** Inform prescriber if you are or intend to be pregnant. Consult prescriber if breast-feeding.

**Additional Information** Syrup contains 3.5% alcohol

## Guaifenesin and Codeine (gwye FEN e sin & KOE deen)

**U.S. Brand Names** Brontex® Liquid; Brontex® Tablet; Cheracol®; Guaituss AC®; Guiatussin® With Codeine; Mytussin® AC; Robafen® AC; Robitussin® A-C; Tussi-Organidin® NR

**Synonyms** Codeine and Guaifenesin

**Therapeutic Category** Antitussive; Cough Preparation; Expectorant

**Pregnancy Risk Factor** C

**Lactation** Excretion in breast milk unknown/use caution

**Use** Temporary control of cough due to minor throat and bronchial irritation

**Formulations**

Liquid [C-V] (Brontex®): Guaifenesin 75 mg and codeine phosphate 2.5 mg per 5 mL

Syrup [C-V] (Cheracol®, Guaituss AC®, Guiatussin® with Codeine, Mytussin® AC, Robafen® AC, Robitussin® A-C, Tussi-Organidin® NR): Guaifenesin 100 mg and codeine phosphate 10 mg per 5 mL (60 mL, 120 mL, 480 mL)

Tablet [C-III] (Brontex®): Guaifenesin 300 mg and codeine phosphate 10 mg

**Dosing**

**Adults:** Oral: 5-10 mL every 4-8 hours not to exceed 60 mL/24 hours

**Elderly:** Refer to adult dosing.

**Additional Nursing Issues**

**Physical Assessment:** See individual components listed in Related Information. **Pregnancy risk factor C** - benefits of use should outweigh possible risks. Note breast-feeding caution.

**Patient Information/Instruction:** See individual components listed in Related Information. **Pregnancy/breast-feeding precautions:** Inform prescriber if you are on intend to get pregnant. Consult prescriber if breast-feeding.

**Related Information**

Codeine *on page 299*

Guaifenesin *on previous page*

## Guaifenesin and Dextromethorphan

(gwye FEN e sin & deks troe meth OR fan)

**U.S. Brand Names** Benylin® Expectorant [OTC]; Cheracol® D [OTC]; Clear Tussin® 30; Contac® Cough Formula Liquid [OTC]; Diabetic Tussin DM® [OTC]; Extra Action Cough Syrup [OTC]; Fenesin DM®; Genatuss DM® [OTC]; Glycotuss-dM® [OTC]; Guaifenex DM®; GuiaCough® [OTC]; Guiatuss-DM® [OTC]; Halotussin®-DM [OTC]; Humibid® DM [OTC]; Iobid DM®; Kolephrin® GG/DM [OTC]; Monafed® DM; Muco-Fen-DM®; Mytussin® DM [OTC]; Naldecon® Senior DX [OTC]; Phanatuss® Cough Syrup [OTC]; Phenadex® Senior [OTC]; Queltuss®; Respa-DM®; Rhinosyn-DMX® [OTC]; Robafen DM® [OTC]; Robitussin®-DM [OTC]; Safe Tussin® 30 [OTC]; Scot-Tussin® Senior Clear [OTC]; Siltussin DM® [OTC]; Synacol® CF [OTC]; Syracol-CF® [OTC]; Tolu-Sed® DM [OTC]; Tusibron-DM® [OTC]; Tuss-DM® [OTC]; Tussi-Organidin® DM NR; Uni-Tussin® DM [OTC]; Vicks® 44E [OTC]; Vicks® Pediatric Formula 44E [OTC]

**Synonyms** Dextromethorphan and Guaifenesin

**Therapeutic Category** Antitussive; Cough Preparation; Expectorant

**Pregnancy Risk Factor** C

**Lactation** Excretion in breast milk unknown

**Use** Temporary control of cough due to minor throat and bronchial irritation

**Formulations**

Syrup:

Benylin® Expectorant: Guaifenesin 100 mg and dextromethorphan hydrobromide 5 mg per 5 mL (118 mL, 236 mL)

Cheracol® D, Clear Tussin® 30, Genatuss DM®, Mytussin® DM, Robitussin®-DM, Siltussin DM®, Tolu-Sed® DM, Tussi-Organidin® DM NR: Guaifenesin 100 mg and dextromethorphan hydrobromide 10 mg per 5 mL (5 mL, 10 mL, 120 mL, 240 mL, 360 mL, 480 mL, 3780 mL)

Contac® Cough Formula Liquid: Guaifenesin 67 mg and dextromethorphan hydrobromide 10 mg per 5 mL (120 mL)

Extra Action Cough Syrup, GuiaCough®, Guiatuss DM®, Halotussin® DM, Rhinosyn-DMX®, Tusibron-DM®, Uni-tussin® DM: Guaifenesin 100 mg and dextromethorphan hydrobromide 15 mg per 5 mL (120 mL, 240 mL, 480 mL)

Kolephrin® GG/DM: Guaifenesin 150 mg and dextromethorphan hydrobromide 10 mg per 5 mL (120 mL)

Naldecon® Senior DX: Guaifenesin 200 mg and dextromethorphan hydrobromide 15 mg per 5 mL (118 mL, 480 mL)

Phanatuss®: Guaifenesin 85 mg and dextromethorphan hydrobromide 10 mg per 5 mL

Vicks® 44E: Guaifenesin 66.7 mg and dextromethorphan hydrobromide 6.7 mg per 5 mL

Tablet:

Extended release

(Continued)

## Guaifenesin and Dextromethorphan *(Continued)*

Guaifenex DM®, Iobid DM®, Fenesin DM®, Humibid® DM, Monafed® DM, Respa-DM®: Guaifenesin 600 mg and dextromethorphan hydrobromide 30 mg
Glycotuss-dM®: Guaifenesin 100 mg and dextromethorphan hydrobromide 10 mg
Queltuss®: Guaifenesin 100 mg and dextromethorphan hydrobromide 15 mg
Syracol-CF®: Guaifenesin 200 mg and dextromethorphan hydrobromide 15 mg
Tuss-DM®: Guaifenesin 200 mg and dextromethorphan hydrobromide 10 mg

**Dosing**

**Adults:** Oral: 5 mL every 4 hours or 10 mL every 6-8 hours not to exceed 40 mL/24 hours

**Elderly:** Refer to adult dosing.

**Additional Nursing Issues**

**Physical Assessment:** See individual components listed in Related Information. **Pregnancy risk factor C** - benefits of use should outweigh possible risks. Note breast-feeding caution.

**Patient Information/Instruction:** See individual components listed in Related Information. **Pregnancy/breast-feeding precautions:** Inform prescriber if you are on intend to get pregnant. Consult prescriber if breast-feeding.

**Related Information**

Guaifenesin *on page 548*

♦ **Guaifenesin and Hydrocodone** *see* Hydrocodone and Guaifenesin *on page 571*

## Guaifenesin and Phenylpropanolamine

(gwye FEN e sin & fen il proe pa NOLE a meen)

**U.S. Brand Names** Ami-Tex LA®; Coldloc-LA®; Conex® [OTC]; Contuss® XT; Dura-Vent®; Entex® LA; Fedahist®; Genamin® Expectorant [OTC]; Gentab-LA®; Guaifenex® PPA 75; Guaipax®; Myminic® Expectorant [OTC]; Naldecon-EX® Children's Syrup [OTC]; Nolex® LA; Partuss® LA; Phenylfenesin® L.A.; Profen II®; Profen-LA®; Rymed-TR®; Silaminic® Expectorant [OTC]; Sildicon-E® [OTC]; Snaplets-EX® [OTC]; Theramine® Expectorant [OTC]; Triaminic® Expectorant [OTC]; Tri-Clear® Expectorant [OTC]; Triphenyl® Expectorant [OTC]; ULR-LA®; Vanex-LA®; Vicks® DayQuil® Sinus Pressure & Congestion Relief [OTC]

**Synonyms** Phenylpropanolamine and Guaifenesin

**Therapeutic Category** Decongestant; Expectorant

**Pregnancy Risk Factor** C

**Lactation** Excretion in breast milk unknown

**Use** Symptomatic relief of those respiratory conditions where tenacious mucous plugs and congestion complicate the problem such as sinusitis, pharyngitis, bronchitis, asthma, and as an adjunctive therapy in serous otitis media

**Formulations**

Caplet:

Vicks® DayQuil® Sinus Pressure & Congestion Relief: Guaifenesin 200 mg and phenylpropanolamine hydrochloride 25 mg
Gentab-LA®, Rymed-TR®: Guaifenesin 400 mg and phenylpropanolamine hydrochloride 75 mg

Drops:

Fedahist® Expectorant Pediatric: Guaifenesin 40 mg and phenylpropanolamine hydrochloride 7.5 mg per mL (30 mL)
Sildicon-E®: Guaifenesin 30 mg and phenylpropanolamine hydrochloride 6.25 mg per mL (30 mL)

Granules (Snaplets-EX®): Guaifenesin 50 mg and phenylpropanolamine hydrochloride 6.25 mg (pack)

Liquid:

Conex®, Genamin® Expectorant, Myminic® Expectorant, Silaminic® Expectorant, Theramine® Expectorant, Triaminic® Expectorant, Tri-Clear® Expectorant, Triphenyl® Expectorant: Guaifenesin 100 mg and phenylpropanolamine hydrochloride 12.5 mg per 5 mL (120 mL, 240 mL, 480 mL, 3780 mL)
Naldecon-EX® Children's Syrup: Guaifenesin 100 mg and phenylpropanolamine hydrochloride 6.25 mg per 5 mL (120 mL)

Tablet, extended release:

Ami-Tex LA®, Contuss® XT, Entex® LA, Guaipax®, Nolex® LA, Partuss® LA, Phenylfenesin® L.A., ULR-LA®: Guaifenesin 400 mg and phenylpropanolamine hydrochloride 75 mg
Dura-Vent®, Profen-LA®: Guaifenesin 600 mg and phenylpropanolamine hydrochloride 75 mg
Coldloc-LA®, Guaifenex® PPA 75, Profen II®: Guaifenesin 600 mg and phenylpropanolamine hydrochloride 37.5 mg

**Dosing**

**Adults:** Oral:

Syrup: 10 mL syrup every 4 hours
Tablet: 1 tablet every 12 hours

**Elderly:** Refer to adult dosing; use with caution.

**Additional Nursing Issues**

**Physical Assessment:** See individual components listed in Related Information. **Pregnancy risk factor C** - benefits of use should outweigh possible risks. Note breast-feeding caution.

**Patient Information/Instruction:** See individual components listed in Related Information. **Pregnancy/breast-feeding precautions:** Inform prescriber if you are on intend to get pregnant. Consult prescriber if breast-feeding.

**Related Information**
Guaifenesin *on page 548*
Phenylpropanolamine *on page 922*

## Guaifenesin and Pseudoephedrine

(gwye FEN e sin & soo doe e FED rin)

**U.S. Brand Names** Congess® Jr; Congess® Sr; Congestac®; Deconsal® II; Defen-LA®; Entex® PSE; Eudal-SR®; Fedahist® Expectorant [OTC]; Glycofed®; Guaifed® [OTC]; Guaifed-PD®; Guaifenex PSE®; GuaiMax-D®; Guaitab®; Guai-Vent™; Guai-Vent/PSE™; Guiatuss PE® [OTC]; Halotussin® PE [OTC]; Histalet® X; Nasabid®; Respa-1st®; Respaire®-60 SR; Respaire®-120 SR; Robitussin-PE® [OTC]; Robitussin® Severe Congestion Liqui-Gels® [OTC]; Ru-Tuss® DE; Rymed®; Sinufed® Timecelles®; Sudex®; Touro LA®; Tuss-LA®; V-Dec-M®; Versacaps®; Zephrex®; Zephrex LA®

**Synonyms** Pseudoephedrine and Guaifenesin

**Therapeutic Category** Decongestant; Expectorant

**Pregnancy Risk Factor** C

**Lactation** Excretion in breast milk unknown

**Use** Enhance the output of respiratory tract fluid and reduce mucosal congestion and edema in the nasal passage

**Formulations**

Capsule:
- Guai-Vent™: Guaifenesin 250 mg and pseudoephedrine hydrochloride 120 mg
- Robitussin® Severe Congestion Liqui-Gels®: Guaifenesin 200 mg and pseudoephedrine hydrochloride 30 mg
- Rymed®: Guaifenesin 250 mg and pseudoephedrine hydrochloride 30 mg

Capsule, extended release:
- Congess® Jr: Guaifenesin 125 mg and pseudoephedrine hydrochloride 60 mg
- Nasabid®: Guaifenesin 250 mg and pseudoephedrine hydrochloride 90 mg
- Congess® Sr, Guaifed®, Respaire®-120 SR: Guaifenesin 250 mg and pseudoephedrine hydrochloride 120 mg
- Guaifed-PD®, Sinufed® Timecelles®, Versacaps®: Guaifenesin 300 mg and pseudoephedrine hydrochloride 60 mg
- Respaire®-60 SR: Guaifenesin 200 mg and pseudoephedrine hydrochloride 60 mg
- Tuss-LA® Capsule: Guaifenesin 500 mg and pseudoephedrine hydrochloride 120 mg

Drops, oral (Fedahist® Expectorant Pediatric): Guaifenesin 40 mg and pseudoephedrine hydrochloride 7.5 mg per mL (30 mL)

Syrup:
- Fedahist® Expectorant, Guaifed®: Guaifenesin 200 mg and pseudoephedrine hydrochloride 30 mg per 5 mL (120 mL, 240 mL)
- Guiatuss® PE, Halotussin® PE, Robitussin-PE®, Rymed®: Guaifenesin 100 mg and pseudoephedrine hydrochloride 30 mg per 5 mL (120 mL, 240 mL, 480 mL)
- Histalet® X: Guaifenesin 200 mg and pseudoephedrine hydrochloride 45 mg per 5 mL (473 mL)

Tablet:
- Congestac®, Guiatab®, Zephrex®: Guaifenesin 400 mg and pseudoephedrine hydrochloride 60 mg
- Glycofed®: Guaifenesin 100 mg and pseudoephedrine hydrochloride 30 mg

Tablet, extended release:
- Deconsal® II, Defen-L.A.®, Respa-1st®: Guaifenesin 600 mg and pseudoephedrine hydrochloride 60 mg
- Entex® PSE, Guaifenex PSE®, GuaiMax-D®, Guai-Vent/PSE™, Ru-Tuss® DE, Sudex®, Zephrex LA®: Guaifenesin 600 mg and pseudoephedrine hydrochloride 120 mg
- Eudal-SR®, Histalet® X, Touro LA®: Guaifenesin 400 mg and pseudoephedrine hydrochloride 120 mg
- Tuss-LA® Tablet, V-Dec-M®: Guaifenesin 5 mg and pseudoephedrine hydrochloride 120 mg

**Dosing**

**Adults:** 10 mL syrup every 4 hours; maximum: 60 mL daily

**Elderly:** Refer to adult dosing; use with caution.

**Additional Nursing Issues**

**Physical Assessment:** See individual components listed in Related Information. **Pregnancy risk factor C** - benefits of use should outweigh possible risks. Note breast-feeding caution.

**Patient Information/Instruction:** See individual components listed in Related Information. **Pregnancy/breast-feeding precautions:** Inform prescriber if you are on intend to get pregnant. Consult prescriber if breast-feeding.

**Related Information**
Guaifenesin *on page 548*
Pseudoephedrine *on page 992*

- **Guaifenesin and Theophylline** *see* Theophylline and Guaifenesin *on page 1118*
- **Guaifenesin, Hydrocodone, and Pseudoephedrine** *see* Hydrocodone, Pseudoephedrine, and Guaifenesin *on page 577*

## Guaifenesin, Phenylpropanolamine, and Dextromethorphan

(gwye FEN e sin, fen il proe pa NOLE a meen, & deks troe meth OR fan)

**U.S. Brand Names** Anatuss® [OTC]; Guiatuss CF® [OTC]; Naldecon® DX Adult Liquid [OTC]; Robafen® CF [OTC]; Robitussin-CF® [OTC]; Siltussin-CF® [OTC]

**Synonyms** Dextromethorphan, Guaifenesin, and Phenylpropanolamine; Phenylpropanolamine, Guaifenesin, and Dextromethorphan

(Continued)

## Guaifenesin, Phenylpropanolamine, and Dextromethorphan *(Continued)*

**Therapeutic Category** Cough Preparation; Decongestant; Expectorant

**Pregnancy Risk Factor** C

**Lactation** Excretion in breast milk unknown/not recommended

**Use** Temporarily relieves nasal congestion and controls cough due to minor throat and bronchial irritation; helps loosen phlegm and thin bronchial secretions to make coughs more productive

**Formulations**

Syrup:

Anatuss®: Guaifenesin 100 mg, phenylpropanolamine hydrochloride 25 mg, and dextromethorphan hydrobromide 15 mg per 5 mL (120 mL, 473 mL)

Guiatuss® CF, Robafen® CF, Robitussin-CF®: Guaifenesin 100 mg, phenylpropanolamine hydrochloride 12.5 mg, and dextromethorphan hydrobromide 10 mg per 5 mL (120 mL, 240 mL, 360 mL, 480 mL)

Naldecon® DX Adult: Guaifenesin 200 mg, phenylpropanolamine hydrochloride 12.5 mg, and dextromethorphan hydrobromide 10 mg per 5 mL (120 mL, 473 mL)

Siltussin-CF®: Guaifenesin 100 mg, phenylpropanolamine hydrochloride 12.5 mg, and dextromethorphan hydrobromide 10 mg per 5 mL

Tablet: (Anatuss®): Guaifenesin 100 mg, phenylpropanolamine hydrochloride 25 mg, and dextromethorphan hydrobromide 15 mg

**Dosing**

**Adults:** 10 mL syrup every 4 hours; maximum: 60 mL daily

**Elderly:** Refer to adult dosing; use with caution.

**Additional Nursing Issues**

**Physical Assessment:** See individual components listed in Related Information. **Pregnancy risk factor C** - benefits of use should outweigh possible risks. Breast-feeding is not recommended.

**Patient Information/Instruction:** See individual components listed in Related Information. **Pregnancy/breast-feeding precautions:** Inform prescriber if you are on intend to get pregnant. Breast-feeding is not recommended.

**Related Information**

Guaifenesin *on page 548*
Phenylpropanolamine *on page 922*

## Guaifenesin, Phenylpropanolamine, and Phenylephrine

(gwye FEN e sin, fen il proe pa NOLE a meen, & fen il EF rin)

**U.S. Brand Names** Coldloc®; Contuss®; Dura-Gest®; Enomine®; Entex®; Guaifenex®; Guiatex®; Respinol-G®; ULR®

**Synonyms** Phenylephrine, Guaifenesin, and Phenylpropanolamine; Phenylpropanolamine, Guaifenesin, and Phenylephrine

**Therapeutic Category** Decongestant; Expectorant

**Pregnancy Risk Factor** C

**Lactation** Excretion in breast milk unknown

**Use** Temporary relief of nasal congestion, running nose, sneezing, itching of nose and throat, and itchy, watery eyes due to common cold, hay fever, or other upper respiratory allergies

**Formulations**

Capsule (Contuss®, Dura-Gest®, Enomine®, Entex®, Guiatex®, ULR®): Guaifenesin 200 mg, phenylpropanolamine hydrochloride 45 mg, and phenylephrine hydrochloride 5 mg

Liquid (Coldloc®, Contuss®, Entex®, Guaifenex®): Guaifenesin 100 mg, phenylpropanolamine hydrochloride 20 mg, and phenylephrine hydrochloride 5 mg per 5 mL (118 mL, 480 mL)

Tablet (Respinol-G®): Guaifenesin 200 mg, phenylpropanolamine hydrochloride 45 mg, and phenylephrine hydrochloride 5 mg

**Dosing**

**Adults:** Oral: 1 capsule 4 times daily

**Elderly:** Refer to adult dosing; use with caution.

**Additional Nursing Issues**

**Physical Assessment:** See individual components listed in Related Information. **Pregnancy risk factor C** - benefits of use should outweigh possible risks. Note breast-feeding caution.

**Patient Information/Instruction:** See individual components listed in Related Information. **Pregnancy/breast-feeding precautions:** Inform prescriber if you are on intend to get pregnant. Consult prescriber if breast-feeding.

**Related Information**

Guaifenesin *on page 548*
Phenylephrine *on page 920*
Phenylpropanolamine *on page 922*

## Guaifenesin, Pseudoephedrine, and Codeine

(gwye FEN e sin, soo doe e FED rin, & KOE deen)

**U.S. Brand Names** Codafed® Expectorant; Decohistine® Expectorant; Deproist® Expectorant With Codeine; Dihistine® Expectorant; Guiatuss DAC®; Guiatussin® DAC; Halotussin® DAC; Isoclor® Expectorant; Mytussin® DAC; Novahistine® Expectorant; Nucofed®; Nucofed® Pediatric Expectorant; Nucotuss®; Phenhist® Expectorant; Robitussin®-DAC; Ryna-CX®; Tussar® SF Syrup

**Synonyms** Codeine, Guaifenesin, and Pseudoephedrine; Pseudoephedrine, Guaifenesin, and Codeine

**Therapeutic Category** Antitussive/Decongestant/Expectorant

**Pregnancy Risk Factor** C

**Lactation** Excretion in breast milk unknown/use caution

**Use** Temporarily relieves nasal congestion and controls cough due to minor throat and bronchial irritation; helps loosen phlegm and thin bronchial secretions to make coughs more productive

**Formulations**

Liquid:

C-III: Nucofed®, Nucotuss®: Guaifenesin 200 mg, pseudoephedrine hydrochloride 60 mg, and codeine phosphate 20 mg per 5 mL (480 mL)

C-V: Codafed® Expectorant, Decohistine® Expectorant, Deproist® Expectorant with Codeine, Dihistine® Expectorant, Guiatuss DAC®, Guiatussin® DAC, Halotussin® DAC, Isoclor® Expectorant, Mytussin® DAC, Nucofed® Pediatric Expectorant, Phenhist® Expectorant, Robitussin®-DAC, Ryna-CX®, Tussar® SF: Guaifenesin 100 mg, pseudoephedrine hydrochloride 30 mg, and codeine phosphate 10 mg per 5 mL (120 mL, 480 mL, 4000 mL)

**Dosing**

**Adults:** 10 mL syrup every 4 hours

**Elderly:** Refer to adult dosing; use with caution.

**Additional Nursing Issues**

**Physical Assessment:** See individual components listed in Related Information. **Pregnancy risk factor C** - benefits of use should outweigh possible risks. Note breast-feeding caution.

**Patient Information/Instruction:** See individual components listed in Related Information. **Pregnancy/breast-feeding precautions:** Inform prescriber if you are on intend to get pregnant. Consult prescriber if breast-feeding.

**Related Information**

Codeine *on page 299*
Guaifenesin *on page 548*
Pseudoephedrine *on page 992*

♦ **Guaifenex®** *see* Guaifenesin, Phenylpropanolamine, and Phenylephrine *on previous page*
♦ **Guaifenex DM®** *see* Guaifenesin and Dextromethorphan *on page 549*
♦ **Guaifenex LA®** *see* Guaifenesin *on page 548*
♦ **Guaifenex® PPA 75** *see* Guaifenesin and Phenylpropanolamine *on page 550*
♦ **Guaifenex PSE®** *see* Guaifenesin and Pseudoephedrine *on page 551*
♦ **GuaiMax-D®** *see* Guaifenesin and Pseudoephedrine *on page 551*
♦ **Guaipax®** *see* Guaifenesin and Phenylpropanolamine *on page 550*
♦ **Guaitab®** *see* Guaifenesin and Pseudoephedrine *on page 551*
♦ **Guaituss AC®** *see* Guaifenesin and Codeine *on page 549*
♦ **Guai-Vent™** *see* Guaifenesin and Pseudoephedrine *on page 551*
♦ **Guai-Vent/PSE™** *see* Guaifenesin and Pseudoephedrine *on page 551*

## Guanethidine (gwahn ETH i deen)

**U.S. Brand Names** Ismelin®

**Therapeutic Category** False Neurotransmitter

**Pregnancy Risk Factor** C

**Lactation** Excretion in breast milk unknown

**Use** Treatment of moderate to severe hypertension

**Mechanism of Action/Effect** Acts as a false neurotransmitter that blocks the adrenergic actions of norepinephrine

**Contraindications** Hypersensitivity to guanethidine or any component; pheochromocytoma; patients taking MAO inhibitors

**Warnings** Orthostatic hypotension can occur frequently. Use with caution in patients with CHF, in patients with regional vascular disease, and in patients with asthma or active peptic ulcer. Withdraw therapy 2 weeks prior to surgery to decrease chance of vascular collapse and cardiac arrest during anesthesia. Pregnancy factor C.

**Drug Interactions**

**Decreased Effect:** Decreased effect of guanethidine with tricyclic antidepressants, indirect-acting amines (ephedrine, phenylpropanolamine), and phenothiazines.

**Increased Effect/Toxicity:** Increased toxicity of direct-acting amines (epinephrine, norepinephrine). Increased effect of beta-blockers, vasodilators, and other antihypertensives.

**Adverse Reactions**

>10%:

Cardiovascular: Palpitations, bradycardia, chest pain, peripheral edema, orthostatic hypotension

Central nervous system: Fatigue, headache, faintness, drowsiness, confusion

Gastrointestinal: Increased bowel movements, gas pain, constipation, anorexia, weight gain/loss

Genitourinary: Nocturia, polyuria, impotence, ejaculation disturbances

Neuromuscular & skeletal: Paresthesia, aching limbs, leg cramps, backache, arthralgia

Ocular: Visual disturbances

Respiratory: Shortness of breath, coughing

1% to 10%:

Central nervous system: Psychological problems, depression, sleep disorders

Gastrointestinal: Glossitis, nausea, vomiting, dry mouth

(Continued)

## Guanethidine *(Continued)*

Renal: Hematuria

<1% (Limited to important or life-threatening symptoms): Syncope

**Overdose/Toxicology** Symptoms of overdose include hypotension, blurred vision, dizziness, and syncope. Treatment is supportive and symptomatic.

**Pharmacodynamics/Kinetics**

**Half-life Elimination:** 5-10 days

**Metabolism:** Liver

**Excretion:** Urine and feces

**Onset:** Within 0.5-2 hours; Peak antihypertensive effect: Within 6-8 hours

**Duration:** 24-48 hours

**Formulations** Tablet, as monosulfate: 10 mg, 25 mg

**Dosing**

**Adults:** Oral:

Ambulatory patient: Initial: 10 mg/day, increase at 5- to 7-day intervals to a maximum of 25-50 mg/day

Hospitalized patient: Initial: 25-50 mg/day, increase by 25-50 mg/day or every other day to desired therapeutic response

**Elderly:** Oral: Initial: 5 mg once daily; adjust for renal impairment. Avoid use if possible.

**Renal Impairment:** $Cl_{cr}$ <10 mL/minute: Administer every 24-36 hours.

**Administration**

**Oral:** Tablet may be crushed.

**Monitoring Laboratory Tests** Renal function

**Additional Nursing Issues**

**Physical Assessment:** Assess effectiveness and interactions of other medications (see Drug Interactions). See Contraindications and Warnings/Precautions for use cautions. Monitor for effectiveness of therapy (blood pressure supine and standing) and adverse reactions (see Adverse Reactions and Overdose/Toxicology) at beginning of therapy and on a regular basis with long-term therapy. Assess knowledge/teach patient appropriate use, possible side effects/interventions, and adverse symptoms to report. When discontinuing, monitor blood pressure and taper dose and frequency slowly over 1 week or more. **Pregnancy risk factor C** - benefits of use should outweigh possible risks. Note breast-feeding caution.

**Patient Information/Instruction:** Take as directed. Do not skip dose or discontinue without consulting prescriber. Store medication container away from light. Follow recommended diet and exercise program. Do not use OTC medications which may affect blood pressure (eg, cough or cold remedies, diet pills, stay-awake medications) without consulting prescriber. This medication may cause drowsiness, dizziness, or impaired judgment (use caution when driving or engaging in tasks that require alertness until response to drug is known); decreased libido or sexual function (will resolve when drug is discontinued); postural hypotension (use caution when rising from sitting or lying position or when climbing stairs - this may be worse in early morning, during hot weather, following exercise, or with alcohol use); or dry mouth or nausea (frequent mouth care or sucking lozenges may help). Report difficulty, pain, or burning on urination; increased nervousness or depression; sudden weight gain (weigh yourself in the same clothes at the same time of day once a week); unusual or persistent swelling of ankles, feet, or extremities; wet cough or respiratory difficulty; chest pain or palpitations; muscle weakness, fatigue, or pain; or other persistent side effects. **Pregnancy/breast-feeding precautions:** Inform prescriber if you are or intend to be pregnant. Consult prescriber if breast-feeding.

**Geriatric Considerations:** Because of its CNS adverse effects and high incidence of orthostatic hypotension, guanethidine is not considered a drug of choice for treatment of hypertension in the elderly. If used, adjust dose for renal function and monitor patient closely.

- **Gugecin** *see* Cinoxacin *on page 270*
- **GuiaCough® [OTC]** *see* Guaifenesin and Dextromethorphan *on page 549*
- **GuiaCough® Expectorant [OTC]** *see* Guaifenesin *on page 548*
- **Guiatex®** *see* Guaifenesin, Phenylpropanolamine, and Phenylephrine *on page 552*
- **Guiatuss® [OTC]** *see* Guaifenesin *on page 548*
- **Guiatuss CF® [OTC]** *see* Guaifenesin, Phenylpropanolamine, and Dextromethorphan *on page 551*
- **Guiatuss DAC®** *see* Guaifenesin, Pseudoephedrine, and Codeine *on page 552*
- **Guiatuss-DM® [OTC]** *see* Guaifenesin and Dextromethorphan *on page 549*
- **Guiatussin® DAC** *see* Guaifenesin, Pseudoephedrine, and Codeine *on page 552*
- **Guiatussin® With Codeine** *see* Guaifenesin and Codeine *on page 549*
- **Guiatuss PE® [OTC]** *see* Guaifenesin and Pseudoephedrine *on page 551*
- **G-well®** *see* Lindane *on page 678*
- **Gynecort® [OTC]** *see* Hydrocortisone *on page 578*
- **Gynecort® [OTC]** *see* Topical Corticosteroids *on page 1152*
- **Gyne-Lotrimin® [OTC]** *see* Clotrimazole *on page 294*
- **Gyne-Lotrimin®-3** *see* Clotrimazole *on page 294*
- **Gynergen®** *see* Ergotamine Derivatives *on page 434*
- **Gyne-Sulf®** *see* Sulfabenzamide, Sulfacetamide, and Sulfathiazole *on page 1079*
- **Gyno-Daktarin** *see* Miconazole *on page 767*
- **Gyno-Daktarin V** *see* Miconazole *on page 767*
- **Gynogen L.A.® Injection** *see* Estradiol *on page 441*

- ♦ **Gynol II®** *see page 1294*
- ♦ **Habitrol™ Patch** *see* Nicotine *on page 822*
- ♦ ***Haemophilus* B Conjugate Vaccine** *see page 1256*
- ♦ **Halcinolide** *see* Topical Corticosteroids *on page 1152*
- ♦ **Halcion®** *see* Triazolam *on page 1174*
- ♦ **Haldol®** *see* Haloperidol *on this page*
- ♦ **Haldol® Decanoate** *see* Haloperidol *on this page*
- ♦ **Haley's M-O®** *see* Magnesium Supplements *on page 703*
- ♦ **Haley's M-O® Oral Suspension** *see page 1294*
- ♦ **Hallucinogenic Drugs Comparison** *see page 1386*
- ♦ **Halobetasol** *see* Topical Corticosteroids *on page 1152*
- ♦ **Halog®** *see* Topical Corticosteroids *on page 1152*
- ♦ **Halog®-E** *see* Topical Corticosteroids *on page 1152*


## Haloperidol (ha loe PER i dole)

**U.S. Brand Names** Haldol®; Haldol® Decanoate

**Therapeutic Category** Antipsychotic Agent, Butyrophenone

**Pregnancy Risk Factor** C

**Lactation** Enters breast milk/not recommended

**Use** Treatment of psychoses, Tourette's disorder, and severe behavioral problems in children; emergency sedation of severely agitated or delirious patients; may be effective in infantile autism and has been commonly used to reduce disabling choreiform movements associated with Huntington's disease

**Mechanism of Action/Effect** Blocks postsynaptic mesolimbic dopaminergic $D_1$ and $D_2$ receptors in the brain; exhibits a strong alpha-adrenergic blocking and anticholinergic effect, depresses the release of hypothalamic and hypophyseal hormones; believed to depress the reticular activating system thus affecting basal metabolism, body temperature, wakefulness, vasomotor tone, and emesis

**Contraindications** Hypersensitivity to haloperidol or any component; Parkinson's disease; severe CNS depression; bone marrow suppression; severe cardiac or hepatic disease; coma

**Warnings** Hypotension may occur, particularly with parenteral administration. Decanoate form should never be administered I.V. Avoid in thyrotoxicosis. May be sedating; use with caution in disorders where CNS depression is a feature. Use caution in patients with hemodynamic instability, predisposition to seizures, subcortical brain damage, renal or respiratory disease. May cause swallowing difficulties. Use with caution in breast cancer or other prolactin-dependent tumors (may elevate prolactin levels). May alter temperature regulation or mask toxicity of other drugs due to antiemetic effects. May alter cardiac conduction - life-threatening arrhythmias have occurred with therapeutic doses of antipsychotics. Adverse effects of decanoate may be prolonged. May result in orthostatic hypotension. Some tablets contain tartrazine.

May cause anticholinergic effects (eg, confusion, agitation, constipation, dry mouth, blurred vision, urinary retention); therefore, use with caution in patients with decreased gastrointestinal motility, urinary retention, BPH, xerostomia, or visual problems. Conditions which also may be exacerbated by cholinergic blockade include narrow-angle glaucoma (screening is recommended) and worsening of myasthenia gravis. Relative to other neuroleptics, haloperidol has a low potency of cholinergic blockade.

May cause extrapyramidal reactions including pseudoparkinsonism, acute dystonic reactions, akathisia, and tardive dyskinesia (risk of these reactions is high relative to other neuroleptics). May be associated with neuroleptic malignant syndrome (NMS) or pigmentary retinopathy.

Pregnancy factor C.

**Drug Interactions**

**Cytochrome P-450 Effect:** CYP1A2 enzyme substrate, CYP2D6 enzyme substrate (minor); CYP2D6 enzyme inhibitor

**Decreased Effect:** Carbamazepine and phenobarbital may increase metabolism and decrease effectiveness of haloperidol.

**Increased Effect/Toxicity:** CNS depressants may increase adverse effects. Epinephrine may cause hypotension. Haloperidol and anticholinergic agents may increase intraocular pressure. Concurrent use with lithium has occasionally caused acute encephalopathy-like syndrome.

**Effects on Lab Values** ↓ cholesterol (S)

**Adverse Reactions** Sedation and anticholinergic effects are more pronounced than extrapyramidal effects. EKG changes, retinal pigmentation are more common than with chlorpromazine.

>10%:

- Central nervous system: Sedation, drowsiness, restlessness, anxiety, extrapyramidal reactions, dystonic reactions, pseudoparkinsonian signs and symptoms, tardive dyskinesia, neuroleptic malignant syndrome (NMS), seizures, altered central temperature regulation, akathisia
- Endocrine & metabolic: Swelling of breasts
- Gastrointestinal: Weight gain, constipation

1% to 10%:

- Cardiovascular: Hypotension (especially orthostatic), tachycardia, arrhythmias, abnormal T waves with prolonged ventricular repolarization
- Central nervous system: Hallucinations
- Gastrointestinal: Nausea, vomiting

(Continued)

## Haloperidol *(Continued)*

Genitourinary: Difficult urination

<1% (Limited to important or life-threatening symptoms): Tardive dystonia, agranulocytosis, leukopenia (usually inpatients with large doses for prolonged periods,) cholestatic jaundice, obstructive jaundice, laryngospasm, respiratory depression

**Overdose/Toxicology** Symptoms of overdose include deep sleep, dystonia, agitation, dysrhythmias, and extrapyramidal symptoms. Treatment is supportive and symptomatic.

**Pharmacodynamics/Kinetics**

**Protein Binding:** 90%

**Distribution:** Crosses the placenta

**Half-life Elimination:** 20 hours

**Time to Peak:** 20 minutes

**Metabolism:** Liver

**Excretion:** Liver and feces

**Onset:** Onset of sedation: I.V.: Within 1 hour

**Duration:** ~3 weeks for decanoate form

**Formulations**

Haloperidol lactate:

Concentrate, oral: 2 mg/mL (5 mL, 10 mL, 15 mL, 120 mL, 240 mL)

Injection: 5 mg/mL (1 mL, 2 mL, 2.5 mL, 10 mL)

Haloperidol decanoate:

Injection: 50 mg/mL (1 mL, 5 mL); 100 mg/mL (1 mL, 5 mL)

Tablet: 0.5 mg, 1 mg, 2 mg, 5 mg, 10 mg, 20 mg

**Dosing**

**Adults:** Taper drug when therapy is to be discontinued.

Oral: 0.5-5 mg 2-3 times/day; usual maximum: 30 mg/day; some patients may require up to 100 mg/day.

I.M. (as lactate): 2-5 mg every 4-8 hours as needed

I.M. (as decanoate): Initial: 10-15 times the daily oral dose administered at 3- to 4-week intervals

Sedation in the Intensive Care Unit:

I.M./IVP/IVPB: May repeat bolus doses after 30 minutes until calm achieved then administer 50% of the maximum dose every 6 hours

Mild agitation: 0.5-2 mg

Moderate agitation: 2-5 mg

Severe agitation: 10-20 mg

Continuous intravenous infusion (100 mg/100 mL $D_5W$): Rates of 1-40 mg/hour have been used.

**Elderly:** Taper drug when therapy is to be discontinued.

Nonpsychotic patients, dementia behavior: Oral:

Initial: 0.25-0.5 mg 1-2 times/day; increase dose at 4- to 7-day intervals by 0.25-0.5 mg/day; increase dosing intervals (twice daily, 3 times/day, etc) as necessary to control response or side effects

Maximum daily dose: 50 mg; gradual increases (titration) may prevent side effects or decrease their severity

**Renal Impairment:** Hemodialysis/peritoneal dialysis effects: Supplemental dose is not necessary.

**Administration**

**Oral:** Dilute the oral concentrate with water or juice before administration. **Note:** Avoid skin contact with oral medication; may cause contact dermatitis.

**I.M.:** The decanoate injectable formulation should be administered I.M. only; **do not give decanoate I.V.**

**I.V.:**

Decanoate: Do **not** administer I.V.

Lactate: Although not an FDA-approved route of administration, Haldol® has been administered by this route in many acute care settings.

**I.V. Detail:** The response to I.V. Haldol® may be delayed by several minutes.

**Stability**

**Storage:** Protect oral dosage forms from light. Haloperidol lactate injection should be stored at controlled room temperature and protected from light, freezing, and temperatures >40°C. Exposure to light may cause discoloration and the development of a grayish-red precipitate over several weeks.

**Reconstitution:** Haloperidol lactate may be administered IVPB or I.V. infusion in $D_5W$ solutions. NS solutions should not be used due to reports of decreased stability and incompatibility.

Standardized dose: 0.5-100 mg/50-100 mL $D_5W$

Stability of standardized solutions is 38 days at room temperature (24°C).

**Monitoring Laboratory Tests** Ophthalmic screening

**Additional Nursing Issues**

**Physical Assessment:** Assess other medications patient is taking for effectiveness and interactions (especially drugs metabolized by P-450 enzymes, see Drug Interactions). See Contraindications and Warnings/Precautions for cautious use. Has potential for psychological or physiological dependence, abuse, and tolerance. Review ophthalmic screening (see Monitoring Laboratory Tests) and monitor therapeutic response (mental status, mood, affect) and adverse reactions at beginning of therapy and periodically with long-term use (sedation, anticholinergic, and extrapyramidal effects - see Adverse Reactions and Overdose/Toxicology). With I.M. or I.V. use, monitor closely for hypotension. Initiate at lower doses (see Dosing) and taper dosage slowly when discontinuing. **Note:** Avoid skin contact with oral medication; may cause contact dermatitis (wash immediately with warm, soapy water). Assess knowledge/teach patient appropriate use, interventions to reduce side effects, and adverse symptoms to report (see below). **Pregnancy risk factor C** - benefits of use should outweigh possible risks. Breast-feeding is not recommended.

**Patient Information/Instruction:** Use exactly as directed (do not increase dose or frequency); may cause physical and/or psychological dependence. It may take 2-3 weeks to achieve desired results; do not discontinue without consulting prescriber. Dilute oral concentration with water or juice. Do not take within 2 hours of any antacid. Store away from light. Avoid excess alcohol or caffeine and other prescription or OTC medications not approved by prescriber. Maintain adequate hydration (2-3 L/day of fluids unless instructed to restrict fluid intake). Avoid skin contact with medication; may cause contact dermatitis (wash immediately with warm, soapy water). You may experience excess drowsiness, restlessness, dizziness, or blurred vision (use caution driving or when engaging in tasks requiring alertness until response to drug is known); nausea, vomiting (small frequent meals, frequent mouth care, chewing gum, or sucking lozenges may help); constipation (increased exercise, fluids, or dietary fruit and fiber may help); postural hypotension (use caution climbing stairs or when changing position from lying or sitting to standing); urinary retention (void before taking medication); decreased perspiration (avoid strenuous exercise in hot environments). Report persistent CNS effects (eg, trembling fingers, altered gait or balance, excessive sedation, seizures, unusual movements, anxiety, abnormal thoughts, confusion, personality changes); chest pain, palpitations, rapid heartbeat, severe dizziness; unresolved urinary retention or changes in urinary pattern; vision changes; skin rash or yellowing of skin; difficulty breathing; or worsening of condition. **Pregnancy/breast-feeding precautions:** Inform prescriber if you are or intend to be pregnant. Breast-feeding is not recommended.

**Geriatric Considerations:** (See Warnings/Precautions, Adverse Reactions, and Overdose/Toxicology.) Elderly patients have an increased risk of adverse response to side effects or adverse reactions to antipsychotics. These can include but are not limited to the following.

Anticholinergic effects: CNS toxicity with confusion, memory loss, psychotic behavior, and agitation.

Extrapyramidal effects (EPS): Parkinson's syndrome and akathisia may occur as often as 50% in patients >60 years of age. Tardive dyskinesia (motor restlessness) may be 40% in elderly; may be related to duration and total accumulated dose over time; may be somewhat reversible if diagnosed early enough.

Orthostatic hypotension: Increased risk for falls.

Sedation: In nonpsychotic patients, may result in feelings of depersonalization, derealization, and dysphoria.

Cardiac toxicity: Cardiac arrhythmias have occurred with therapeutic doses of antipsychotics.

Malignant neuroleptic syndrome: Development of hyperthermia, muscular rigidity, autonomic instability, and altered mental status.

Many elderly patients receive antipsychotic medications for inappropriate nonpsychotic behavior. Before initiating antipsychotic medication, all possible reversible causes should be investigated. Stress may cause acute "confusion" or worsening of baseline nonpsychotic behaviors; any changes in disease state (in any organ) may result in behavioral changes. Common acute changes in behavior may be due also to increases in drug dose addition, or addition of a new drug to the regimen; fluid/electrolyte alterations; infections; or changes in the environment.

Meta-analysis of controlled trials of antipsychotic (phenothiazines, butyrophenones) use with agitated, demented, elderly patients has concluded that the use of neuroleptics results in a response rate of 18%. Clearly, neuroleptic therapy for behavior control should be limited, with frequent attempts to withdraw the agent for behavior control. When use is indicated, initial doses should be lower to start and monitored closely.

**Additional Information** Some formulations may contain tartrazine.

**Related Information**

Antiemetics for Chemotherapy-Induced Nausea and Vomiting *on page 1307*
Antipsychotic Agents Comparison *on page 1371*
Antipsychotic Medication Guidelines *on page 1436*

♦ **Haloperil** *see* Haloperidol *on page 555*
♦ **Haloprogin** *see page 1247*
♦ **Halotestin®** *see* Fluoxymesterone *on page 504*
♦ **Halotex®** *see page 1247*
♦ **Halotussin® [OTC]** *see* Guaifenesin *on page 548*
♦ **Halotussin® DAC** *see* Guaifenesin, Pseudoephedrine, and Codeine *on page 552*
♦ **Halotussin®-DM [OTC]** *see* Guaifenesin and Dextromethorphan *on page 549*
♦ **Halotussin® PE [OTC]** *see* Guaifenesin and Pseudoephedrine *on page 551*
♦ **Haltran® [OTC]** *see* Ibuprofen *on page 592*
♦ **Havrix®** *see page 1256*
♦ **Hayfebrol® Liquid** *see page 1294*
♦ **H-BIG®** *see page 1256*
♦ **HCFA Guidelines for Unnecessary Drugs in Long-Term Care Facilities** *see page 1434*

- ♦ **HCG** *see* Chorionic Gonadotropin *on page 264*
- ♦ **HCTZ** *see* Hydrochlorothiazide *on page 566*
- ♦ **Head & Shoulders® Intensive Treatment** *see page 1294*
- ♦ **Head & Shoulders® Shampoo** *see page 1294*
- ♦ **Healon®** *see page 1248*
- ♦ **Healon®** *see page 1282*
- ♦ **Healon® GV** *see page 1248*
- ♦ **Healon GV®** *see page 1282*
- ♦ **Helberina** *see* Heparin *on this page*
- ♦ **Helistat®** *see page 1248*
- ♦ **Helixate™** *see* Antihemophilic Factor (Recombinant) *on page 100*
- ♦ **Helminzole** *see* Mebendazole *on page 709*
- ♦ **Hemabate™** *see* Carboprost Tromethamine *on page 201*
- ♦ **Hemobion® 200** *see* Iron Supplements *on page 627*
- ♦ **Hemobion® 400 (Mexico)** *see* Iron Supplements *on page 627*
- ♦ **Hemocyte® [OTC]** *see* Iron Supplements *on page 627*
- ♦ **Hemofil® M** *see* Antihemophilic Factor (Human) *on page 99*
- ♦ **Hemotene®** *see page 1248*
- ♦ **Hemril-HC® Uniserts®** *see* Hydrocortisone *on page 578*
- ♦ **Hemril-HC® Uniserts®** *see* Topical Corticosteroids *on page 1152*
- ♦ **Henexal** *see* Furosemide *on page 523*


## Heparin (HEP a rin)

**U.S. Brand Names** Hep-Lock®; Liquaemin®

**Synonyms** Heparin Lock Flush

**Therapeutic Category** Anticoagulant

**Pregnancy Risk Factor** C

**Lactation** Does not enter breast milk/compatible

**Use** Prophylaxis and treatment of thromboembolic disorders

**Mechanism of Action/Effect** Potentiates the action of antithrombin III and thereby inactivates thrombin (as well as activated coagulation factors IX, X, XI, XII, and plasmin) and prevents the conversion of fibrinogen to fibrin; heparin also stimulates release of lipoprotein lipase (lipoprotein lipase hydrolyzes triglycerides to glycerol and free fatty acids)

**Contraindications** Hypersensitivity to heparin or any component; severe thrombocytopenia; subacute bacterial endocarditis; suspected intracranial hemorrhage; uncontrollable bleeding (unless secondary to disseminated intravascular coagulation)

**Warnings** Use with caution as hemorrhaging may occur. Risk factors for hemorrhage include I.M. injections, peptic ulcer disease, increased capillary permeability, menstruation, or severe renal, hepatic, or biliary disease. Use with caution in patients with shock or severe hypotension. Some preparations contain sulfite which may cause allergic reactions. Heparin does not possess fibrinolytic activity and, therefore, cannot lyse established thrombi. Discontinue heparin if hemorrhage occurs. Severe hemorrhage or overdosage may require protamine. Use caution with white clot syndrome (new thrombus associated with thrombocytopenia) and heparin resistance. Pregnancy factor C.

**Drug Interactions**

**Decreased Effect:** Decreased effect with digoxin, tetracycline, nicotine, antihistamine, I.V. nitroglycerine.

**Increased Effect/Toxicity:** Increased toxicity of heparin with NSAIDs, aspirin, dipyridamole, dextran, and hydroxychloroquine.

**Effects on Lab Values** ↑ thyroxine (S) (competitive protein binding methods), PT, PTT, bleeding time. A volume of at least 10 mL of blood should be removed and discarded from a heparinized line before blood samples are sent for coagulation testing.

**Adverse Reactions**

>10%:

Dermatologic: Unexplained bruising

Gastrointestinal: Constipation, vomiting of blood, bleeding from gums

Hematologic: Hemorrhage, blood in urine

1% to 10%:

Cardiovascular: Chest pain

Genitourinary: Frequent or persistent erection

Neuromuscular & skeletal: Peripheral neuropathy

Miscellaneous: Allergic reactions

<1% (Limited to important or life-threatening symptoms): Elevated liver enzymes; thrombocytopenia (heparin-associated thrombocytopenia occurs in <1% of patients, immune thrombocytopenia occurs with progressive fall in platelet counts and, in some cases, thromboembolic complications; daily platelet counts for 5-7 days at initiation of therapy may help detect the onset of this complication)

**Overdose/Toxicology** The primary symptom of overdose is bleeding. Antidote is protamine; dose 1 mg neutralizes 1 mg (100 units) of heparin. Discontinue all heparin if evidence of progressive immune thrombocytopenia occurs.

**Pharmacodynamics/Kinetics**

**Distribution:** Does not cross placenta

**Half-life Elimination:**

Mean: 1.5 hours

Range: 1-2 hours; affected by obesity, renal function, hepatic function, malignancy, presence of pulmonary embolism, and infections

**Metabolism:** Liver

**Excretion:** Urine

**Onset:** Onset of anticoagulation: I.V.: Immediate with use; S.C.: Within 20-30 minutes

**Formulations**

Heparin sodium:

Lock flush injection:

Beef lung source: 10 units/mL (1 mL, 2 mL, 2.5 mL, 3 mL, 5 mL, 10 mL, 30 mL); 100 units/mL (1 mL, 2 mL, 2.5 mL, 3 mL, 5 mL, 10 mL, 30 mL)

Porcine intestinal mucosa source: 10 units/mL (1 mL, 2 mL, 10 mL, 30 mL); 100 units/mL (1 mL, 2 mL, 10 mL, 30 mL)

Porcine intestinal mucosa source, preservative free: 10 units/mL (1 mL); 100 units/mL (1 mL)

Multiple-dose vial injection:

Beef lung source, with preservative: 1000 units/mL (5 mL, 10 mL, 30 mL); 5000 units/mL (10 mL); 10,000 units/mL (4 mL, 5 mL, 10 mL); 20,000 units/mL (2 mL, 5 mL, 10 mL); 40,000 units/mL (5 mL)

Porcine intestinal mucosa source, with preservative: 1000 units/mL (10 mL, 30 mL); 5000 units/mL (10 mL); 10,000 units/mL (4 mL); 20,000 units/mL (2 mL, 5 mL)

Single-dose vial injection:

Beef lung source: 1000 units/mL (1 mL); 5000 units/mL (1 mL); 10,000 units/mL (1 mL); 20,000 units/mL (1 mL); 40,000 units/mL (1 mL)

Porcine intestinal mucosa: 1000 units/mL (1 mL); 5000 units/mL (1 mL); 10,000 units/mL (1 mL); 20,000 units/mL (1 mL); 40,000 units/mL (1 mL)

Unit dose injection:

Porcine intestinal mucosa source, with preservative: 1000 units/dose (1 mL, 2 mL); 2500 units/dose (1 mL); 5000 units/dose (0.5 mL, 1 mL); 7500 units/dose (1 mL); 10,000 units/dose (1 mL); 15,000 units/dose (1 mL); 20,000 units/dose (1 mL)

Heparin sodium infusion, porcine intestinal mucosa source:

$D_5W$: 40 units/mL (500 mL); 50 units/mL (250 mL, 500 mL); 100 units/mL (100 mL, 250 mL)

NaCl 0.45%: 2 units/mL (500 mL, 1000 mL); 50 units/mL (250 mL); 100 units/mL (250 mL)

NaCl 0.9%: 2 units/mL (500 mL, 1000 mL); 5 units/mL (1000 mL); 50 units/mL (250 mL, 500 mL, 1000 mL)

Heparin calcium:

Unit dose injection, porcine intestinal mucosa, preservative free: 5000 units/dose (0.2 mL); 12,500 units/dose (0.5 mL); 20,000 units/dose (0.8 mL)

**Dosing**

**Adults:** Line flushing: When using heparin to maintain patency of venous access devices, 10 units/mL is commonly used for younger infants (eg, <10 kg) while 100 units/mL is used for older infants, children, and adults. Volume of heparin flush is usually similar to volume of catheter (or slightly greater). See manufacturer's recommendation for specific line used. Additional flushes should be given when stagnant blood is observed in catheter, after catheter is used for drug or blood administration, and after blood withdrawal from catheter.

Arterial lines are heparinized with a final concentration of 1 unit/mL.

Prophylaxis (low-dose heparin): S.C.: 5000 units every 8-12 hours

Intermittent I.V.: Initial: 10,000 units, then 50-70 units/kg (5000-10,000 units) every 4-6 hours

I.V. infusion: 50 units/kg to start, then 15-25 units/kg/hour as continuous infusion; increase dose by 5 units/kg/hour every 4 hours as required according to PTT results, usual range: 10-30 units/hour

Weight-based protocol: Follow institutional protocols. For example: 80 units/kg I.V. push followed by continuous infusion of 18 units/kg/hour.

**Elderly:** Refer to adult dosing.

**Administration**

**I.M.:** Do not administer I.M. due to pain, irritation, and hematoma formation.

**I.V.:**

Continuous infusion: Infuse via infusion pump.

Heparin lock: Inject via injection cap using positive pressure flushing technique.

**Stability**

**Storage:** Heparin solutions are colorless to slightly yellow. Minor color variations do not affect therapeutic efficacy. Heparin should be stored at controlled room temperature and protected from freezing and temperatures >40°C.

**Reconstitution:** Stability at room temperature and refrigeration:

Prepared bag: 24 hours

Premixed bag: After seal is broken 4 days

Out of overwrap stability: 30 days

Standard diluent: 25,000 units/500 mL $D_5W$ (premixed)

Minimum volume: 250 mL $D_5W$

**Compatibility:** See the Compatibility of Drugs Chart *on page 1315* and the Compatibility of Drugs in Syringe Chart *on page 1317.*

**Monitoring Laboratory Tests** Platelet counts, PTT, hemoglobin, hematocrit, signs of bleeding. For intermittent I.V. injections, PTT is measured 3.5-4 hours after I.V. injection. **Note:** Continuous I.V. infusion is preferred vs I.V. intermittent injections. For full-dose heparin (ie, nonlow-dose), the dose should be titrated according to PTT results. For anticoagulation, an APTT 1.5-2.5 times normal is usually desired. APTT is usually measured prior to heparin therapy, 6-8 hours after initiation of a continuous infusion

(Continued)

## Heparin *(Continued)*

(following a loading dose), and 6-8 hours after changes in the infusion rate; increase or decrease infusion by 2-4 units/kg/hour dependent on PTT. See table.

**Heparin Infusion Dose Adjustment**

| APTT | Adjustment |
|---|---|
| >3 x control | ↓ Infusion rate 50% |
| 2-3 x control | ↓ Infusion rate 25% |
| 1.5-2 x control | No change |
| <1.5 x control | ↑ Rate of infusion 25%; max 2500 units/h |

**Additional Nursing Issues**

**Physical Assessment:** Assess effectiveness and interactions of other medications (see Drug Interactions). See Warnings/Precautions and Contraindications for use cautions. Monitor effectiveness of therapy, laboratory tests (see above), and adverse response (eg, thrombolytic reactions - see Adverse Reactions and Overdose/Toxicology). Assess knowledge/teach patient appropriate use, possible side effects and appropriate interventions (eg, bleeding precautions), and adverse symptoms to report. **Pregnancy risk factor C** - benefits of use should outweigh possible risks.

**Patient Information/Instruction:** This drug can only be administered by injection. You may have a tendency to bleed easily while taking this drug; brush teeth with soft brush, floss with waxed floss, use electric razor, avoid scissors or sharp knives, and potentially harmful activities. May discolor urine or stool. Report CNS changes (fever, confusion), unusual fever, persistent nausea or GI upset, unusual bleeding or bruising (bleeding gums, nosebleed, blood in urine, dark stool), pain in joints or back, swelling or pain at injection site. **Pregnancy precautions:** Inform prescriber if you are pregnant.

**Geriatric Considerations:** In the clinical setting, age has not been shown to be a reliable predictor of a patient's anticoagulant response to heparin. However, it is common for older patients to have a "standard" response for the first 24-48 hours after a loading dose (5000 units) and a maintenance infusion of 800-1000 units/hour. After this period, they then have an exaggerated response (eg, elevated PTT), requiring a lower infusion rate. Hence, monitor closely during this period of therapy. Older women are more likely to have bleeding complications and osteoporosis may be a problem when used >3 months or total daily dose exceeds 30,000 units.

**Additional Information** Some formulations may contain benzyl alcohol. Heparin sodium formulations may contain sulfites.

**Related Information**

Protamine Sulfate *on page 989*


- **Heparin Cofactor I** *see* Antithrombin III *on page 101*
- **Heparin Lock Flush** *see* Heparin *on page 558*
- **Hepatitis A Vaccine** *see page 1256*
- **Hepatitis B Immune Globulin** *see page 1256*
- **Hepatitis B Vaccine** *see page 1256*
- **Hep-Lock®** *see* Heparin *on page 558*
- **Heptalac®** *see* Lactulose *on page 651*
- **Herceptin®** *see* Trastuzumab *on page 1165*
- **Herklin** *see* Lindane *on page 678*
- **HES** *see* Hetastarch *on this page*
- **Hespan®** *see* Hetastarch *on this page*


## Hetastarch (HET a starch)

**U.S. Brand Names** Hespan®

**Synonyms** HES; Hydroxyethyl Starch

**Therapeutic Category** Plasma Volume Expander, Colloid

**Pregnancy Risk Factor** C

**Lactation** Excretion in breast milk unknown/compatible

**Use** Blood volume expander used in treatment of shock or impending shock when blood or blood products are not available; does not have oxygen-carrying capacity and is not a substitute for blood or plasma

**Mechanism of Action/Effect** Produces plasma volume expansion by virtue of its highly colloidal starch structure, similar to albumin

**Contraindications** Severe bleeding disorders; renal failure with oliguria or anuria; severe congestive heart failure

**Warnings** Anaphylactoid reactions have occurred. Use with caution in patients with thrombocytopenia (may interfere with platelet function). Large volume may cause drops in hemoglobin concentrations. Use with caution in patients at risk from overexpansion of blood volume, including the very young or aged patients, those with congestive heart failure or pulmonary edema. Large volumes may interfere with platelet function and prolong PT and PTT times. Pregnancy factor C.

**Adverse Reactions** <1% (Limited to important or life-threatening symptoms): Peripheral edema; heart failure; circulatory overload bleeding; prolongation of PT, PTT, clotting time, and bleeding time

**Overdose/Toxicology** Symptoms of overdose include heart failure, nausea, vomiting, circulatory overload, and bleeding. Treatment is supportive.

**Pharmacodynamics/Kinetics**

**Metabolism:** Molecules >50,000 daltons require enzymatic degradation by the reticuloendothelial system or amylases in the blood prior to urinary and fecal excretion.

**Excretion:** Urine

**Onset:** Onset of volume expansion: I.V.: Within 30 minutes

**Duration:** 24-36 hours

**Formulations** Infusion, in sodium chloride 0.9%: 6% (500 mL)

**Dosing**

**Adults:** I.V. only: 500-1000 mL (up to 1500 mL/day) or 20 mL/kg/day (up to 1500 mL/day); larger volumes (15,000 mL/24 hours) have been used safely in small numbers of patients.

**Elderly:** Refer to adult dosing.

**Renal Impairment:** $Cl_{cr}$ <10 mL/minute: Initial dose is the same but subsequent doses should be reduced by 20% to 50% of normal.

**Administration**

**I.V.:** Administer I.V. only. May administer up to 1.2 g/kg/hour (20 mL/kg/hour). Infusion pump is required.

**I.V. Detail:** Do not use if crystalline precipitate forms or is turbid deep brown.

**Stability**

**Storage:** Store at room temperature; do not freeze.

**Reconstitution:** Do not use if crystalline precipitate forms or is turbid deep brown.

**Compatibility:** Change I.V. tubing or flush copiously with normal saline before adding blood.

**Additional Nursing Issues**

**Physical Assessment:** Monitor closely for possible acute reaction; see Adverse Reactions. Monitor blood pressure, pulse, central venous pressure, and urine output every 5-15 minutes for the first hour and closely thereafter. Observe closely for fluid overload. **Pregnancy risk factor C.**

**Patient Information/Instruction:** Report immediately any respiratory difficulty, acute headache, muscle pain, or abdominal cramping. **Pregnancy precautions:** Inform prescriber if you are pregnant.

**Additional Information** pH: 3.5-7


- **Hexachlorocyclohexane** *see* Lindane *on page 678*
- **Hexadrol®** *see* Dexamethasone *on page 346*
- **Hexalen®** *see* Altretamine *on page 59*
- **Hexamethylenetetramine** *see* Methenamine *on page 739*
- **Hexamethylmelamine** *see* Altretamine *on page 59*
- **Hexavitamin** *see* Vitamin, Multiple *on page 1219*
- **Hexit®** *see* Lindane *on page 678*
- **H.H.R.®** *see* Hydralazine, Hydrochlorothiazide, and Reserpine *on page 565*
- **Hib Polysaccharide Conjugate** *see page 1256*
- **HibTITER®** *see page 1256*
- **Hi-Cor-1.0®** *see* Hydrocortisone *on page 578*
- **Hi-Cor-1.0®** *see* Topical Corticosteroids *on page 1152*
- **Hi-Cor-2.5®** *see* Hydrocortisone *on page 578*
- **Hi-Cor-2.5®** *see* Topical Corticosteroids *on page 1152*
- **Hidramox®** *see* Amoxicillin *on page 80*
- **Higroton 50** *see* Chlorthalidone *on page 260*
- **Hipokinon** *see* Trihexyphenidyl *on page 1179*
- **Hiprex®** *see* Methenamine *on page 739*
- **Hip-Rex™** *see* Methenamine *on page 739*
- **Hismanal®** *see* Astemizole *on page 114*
- **Histalet Forte® Tablet** *see page 1306*
- **Histalet® Syrup** *see page 1294*
- **Histalet® X** *see* Guaifenesin and Pseudoephedrine *on page 551*
- **Histatab® Plus Tablet** *see page 1294*
- **Hista-Vadrin® Tablet** *see page 1294*
- **Histerone® Injection** *see* Testosterone *on page 1108*
- **Histolyn-CYL® Injection** *see page 1248*
- **Histoplasmin** *see page 1248*
- **Histor-D® Syrup** *see page 1294*
- **Histor-D® Timescelles®** *see page 1306*


## Histrelin (his TREL in)

**U.S. Brand Names** Supprelin™ Injection

**Therapeutic Category** Gonadotropin Releasing Hormone Analog; Luteinizing Hormone-Releasing Hormone Analog

**Pregnancy Risk Factor** X

**Lactation** Enters breast milk/contraindicated

**Use** Treatment of central idiopathic precocious puberty; treatment of estrogen-associated gynecologic disorders such as acute intermittent porphyria, endometriosis, leiomyomata uteri, and premenstrual syndrome

**Mechanism of Action/Effect** Histrelin is a synthetic long-acting gonadotropin-releasing hormone analog; with daily administration, it desensitizes the pituitary to endogenous gonadotropin-releasing hormone (ie, suppresses gonadotropin release by causing down

(Continued)

## Histrelin *(Continued)*

regulation of the pituitary); this results in a decrease in gonadal sex steroid production which stops the secondary sexual development

**Contraindications** Hypersensitivity to histrelin; pregnancy

**Warnings** The site of injection should be varied daily. The dose should be administered at the same time each day. In precocious puberty, changing the dosage schedule or noncompliance may result in inadequate control of the pubertal process.

**Adverse Reactions**

>10%:

Cardiovascular: Vasodilation
Central nervous system: Headache
Gastrointestinal: Abdominal pain
Genitourinary: Vaginal bleeding, vaginal dryness
Local: Skin reaction at injection site

1% to 10%:

Central nervous system: Mood swings, headache, pain
Dermatologic: Rashes, urticaria
Endocrine & metabolic: Breast tenderness, hot flashes
Gastrointestinal: Nausea, vomiting
Genitourinary: Increased urinary calcium excretion
Neuromuscular & skeletal: Joint stiffness

**Pharmacodynamics/Kinetics**

**Onset:**

Precocious puberty: Onset of hormonal responses: Within 3 months of initiation of therapy

Acute intermittent porphyria associated with menses: Amelioration of symptoms: After 1-2 months of therapy

Treatment of endometriosis or leiomyomata uteri: Onset of responses: After 3-6 months of treatment

**Formulations** Injection: 7-day kits of single use: 120 mcg/0.6 mL; 300 mcg/0.6 mL; 600 mcg/0.6 mL

**Dosing**

**Adults:** S.C.:

Central idiopathic precocious puberty: Usual dose is 10 mcg/kg/day given as a single daily dose at the same time each day

Acute intermittent porphyria in women: 5 mcg/day

Endometriosis: 100 mcg/day

Leiomyomata uteri: 20-50 mcg/day or 4 mcg/kg/day

**Administration**

**Other:** Subcutaneous: Injection site should be varied daily. Dose should be administered at the same time each day. Allow vial to reach room temperature before injecting contents.

**Stability**

**Storage:** Refrigerate at 2°C to 8°C (36°F to 46°F) and protect from light.

**Monitoring Laboratory Tests** Precocious puberty: Prior to initiating therapy monitor height and weight, hand and wrist x-rays, total sex steroid levels, beta-hCG level, adrenal steroid level, gonadotropin-releasing hormone stimulation test, pelvic/adrenal/testicular ultrasound/head CT. During therapy, monitor 3 months after initiation and then every 6-12 months; serial levels of sex steroids and gonadotropin-releasing hormone testing.

**Additional Nursing Issues**

**Physical Assessment:** Monitor evaluations for precocious puberty prior to and during therapy. Treatment may be discontinued when patient reaches appropriate age for puberty. Teach patient/caregiver appropriate administration procedures (eg, rotate sites, monitor sites for infection, disposal of syringes). Monitor for adverse reactions (see above) blood pressure, and effectiveness of therapy. **Pregnancy risk factor X** - determine that patient is not pregnant before beginning treatment and do not give to women of childbearing age unless female is capable of complying with barrier contraceptive measures 1 month prior to therapy, during therapy, and 1 month following therapy. Breast-feeding is contraindicated.

**Patient Information/Instruction:** Use as directed - daily at the same time. Maintain regular follow-up schedule. You may experience headache and GI distress (analgesics may help), vaginal bleeding, pain, irritation (during first weeks of therapy), nausea or anorexia (small frequent meals may help), flushing or redness (cold clothes and cool environment may help). Report irregular or rapid heartbeat, unresolved nausea or vomiting, difficulty breathing, or infection at injection sites. **Pregnancy/breast-feeding precautions:** Inform prescriber if you are pregnant. Do not get pregnant 1 month before, during, or for 1 month following therapy. Consult prescriber for instruction on appropriate contraceptive measures. This drug may cause severe fetal defects. Do not donate blood during or for 1 month following therapy (same reason). Do not breast-feed.


- **Histrodrix®** *see page 1294*
- **Hivid®** *see* Zalcitabine *on page 1225*
- **HMS Liquifilm®** *see* Medrysone *on page 715*
- **HN$_2$** *see* Mechlorethamine *on page 710*
- **Hold® DM** *see page 1294*
- **Homatropine** *see page 1282*
- **Homatropine and Hydrocodone** *see* Hydrocodone and Homatropine *on page 572*
- **Honvol®** *see* Diethylstilbestrol *on page 366*

- **Horse Antihuman Thymocyte Gamma Globulin** *see* Lymphocyte Immune Globulin *on page 700*
- **H.P. Acthar® Gel** *see page 1248*
- **Humalog®** *see* Insulin Preparations *on page 609*
- **Humate-P®** *see* Antihemophilic Factor (Human) *on page 99*
- **Humatin®** *see* Paromomycin *on page 887*
- **Humegon™** *see* Menotropins *on page 720*
- **Humibid® DM [OTC]** *see* Guaifenesin and Dextromethorphan *on page 549*
- **Humibid® L.A.** *see* Guaifenesin *on page 548*
- **Humibid® Sprinkle** *see* Guaifenesin *on page 548*
- **HuMist® Nasal Mist** *see page 1294*
- **Humorsol® Ophthalmic** *see* Ophthalmic Agents, Glaucoma *on page 853*
- **Humulin® 50/50** *see* Insulin Preparations *on page 609*
- **Humulin® 70/30** *see* Insulin Preparations *on page 609*
- **Humulin® L** *see* Insulin Preparations *on page 609*
- **Humulin® N** *see* Insulin Preparations *on page 609*
- **Humulin® R** *see* Insulin Preparations *on page 609*
- **Humulin® U** *see* Insulin Preparations *on page 609*
- **Hurricaine®** *see* Benzocaine *on page 141*

## Hyaluronidase (hye al yoor ON i dase)

**U.S. Brand Names** Wydase® Injection

**Therapeutic Category** Antidote

**Pregnancy Risk Factor** C

**Lactation** Excretion in breast milk unknown

**Use** Increases the dispersion and absorption of other drugs; increases rate of absorption of parenteral fluids given by hypodermoclysis; enhances diffusion of locally irritating or toxic drugs in the management of I.V. extravasation

**Mechanism of Action/Effect** Modifies the permeability of connective tissue through hydrolysis of hyaluronic acid, one of the chief ingredients of tissue cement which offers resistance to diffusion of liquids through tissues

**Contraindications** Hypersensitivity to hyaluronidase or any component; do not inject in or around infected, inflamed, or cancerous areas

**Warnings** Drug infiltrates in which hyaluronidase is contraindicated: Dopamine, alpha-adrenergic agonists. An intradermal skin test for sensitivity should be performed before actual administration using 0.02 mL of a 150 units/mL of hyaluronidase solution. Pregnancy factor C.

**Drug Interactions**

**Decreased Effect:** Salicylates, cortisone, ACTH, estrogens, antihistamines

**Adverse Reactions** <1% (Limited to important or life-threatening symptoms): Tachycardia, hypotension

**Overdose/Toxicology** Symptoms of overdose include local edema, urticaria, erythema, chills, nausea, vomiting, and hypotension.

**Pharmacodynamics/Kinetics**

**Onset:** Immediate by the subcutaneous or intradermal routes for the treatment of extravasation

**Duration:** 24-48 hours

**Formulations**

Injection, stabilized solution: 150 units/mL (1 mL, 10 mL)

Powder for injection, lyophilized: 150 units, 1500 units

**Dosing**

**Adults:** Absorption and dispersion of drugs: 150 units are added to the vehicle containing the drug.

**Elderly:** Refer to adult dosing.

**Administration**

**I.V.:** Do **not** administer I.V. Administer hyaluronidase intradermally or subcutaneously within the first few minutes to 1 hour after the extravasation of a necrotizing agent is recognized.

**Stability**

**Reconstitution:** Reconstituted hyaluronidase solution remains stable for only 24 hours when stored in the refrigerator. Do not use discolored solutions.

**Additional Nursing Issues**

**Physical Assessment: Pregnancy risk factor C** - benefits of use should outweigh possible risks. Note breast-feeding caution.

**Patient Information/Instruction:** Report itching, pain, changes in respiration, or excessive dizziness. **Pregnancy/breast-feeding precautions:** Inform prescriber if you are or intend to be pregnant. Consult prescriber if breast-feeding.

**Geriatric Considerations:** The most common use of hyaluronidase in the elderly is in hypodermoclysis. Hypodermoclysis is very useful in dehydrated patients in whom oral intake is minimal and I.V. access is a problem.

**Additional Information** The USP hyaluronidase unit is equivalent to the turbidity-reducing (TR) unit and the International Unit. Each unit is defined as being the activity contained in 100 mcg of the International Standard Preparation.

- **Hybalamin®** *see* Hydroxocobalamin *on page 583*
- **Hybolin™ Decanoate Injection** *see* Nandrolone *on page 806*
- **Hybolin™ Improved Injection** *see* Nandrolone *on page 806*

- ♦ **Hycamptamine** *see* Topotecan *on page 1157*
- ♦ **Hycamtin™** *see* Topotecan *on page 1157*
- ♦ **HycoClear Tuss®** *see* Hydrocodone and Guaifenesin *on page 571*
- ♦ **Hycodan®** *see* Hydrocodone and Homatropine *on page 572*
- ♦ **Hycomine®** *see* Hydrocodone and Phenylpropanolamine *on page 574*
- ♦ **Hycomine® Compound** *see* Hydrocodone, Chlorpheniramine, Phenylephrine, Acetaminophen, and Caffeine *on page 576*
- ♦ **Hycomine® Pediatric** *see* Hydrocodone and Phenylpropanolamine *on page 574*
- ♦ **Hycort®** *see* Hydrocortisone *on page 578*
- ♦ **Hycort®** *see* Topical Corticosteroids *on page 1152*
- ♦ **Hycotuss® Expectorant Liquid** *see* Hydrocodone and Guaifenesin *on page 571*


## Hydralazine (hye DRAL a zeen)

**U.S. Brand Names** Apresoline®

**Therapeutic Category** Vasodilator

**Pregnancy Risk Factor** C

**Lactation** Enters breast milk/compatible

**Use** Management of moderate to severe hypertension, congestive heart failure, hypertension secondary to preeclampsia/eclampsia; treatment of primary pulmonary hypertension

**Mechanism of Action/Effect** Direct vasodilation of arterioles (with little effect on veins) with decreased systemic resistance

**Contraindications** Hypersensitivity to hydralazine or any component; dissecting aortic aneurysm; mitral valve rheumatic heart disease

**Warnings** Discontinue hydralazine in patients who develop systemic lupus erythematosus (SLE)-like syndrome or positive ANA. Use with caution in patients with severe renal disease or cerebral vascular accidents or with known or suspected coronary artery disease. Monitor blood pressure closely with I.V. use. Some formulations may contain tartrazines or sulfites. Slow acetylators, patients with decreased renal function, and patients receiving >200 mg/day (chronically) are at higher risk for SLE. Titrate dosage to patient's response. Usually administered with diuretic and a beta-blocker to counteract side effects of sodium and water retention and reflex tachycardia. Pregnancy factor C.

**Drug Interactions**

**Increased Effect/Toxicity:** MAO inhibitors may cause significant decrease in blood pressure. Indomethacin may decrease hypotensive effects.

**Food Interactions** Hydralazine serum levels may be decreased if taken with food or enteral nutrition.

**Adverse Reactions**

>10%:
- Cardiovascular: Palpitations, flushing, tachycardia, chest pain pectoris
- Central nervous system: Headache
- Gastrointestinal: Nausea, vomiting, diarrhea, anorexia

1% to 10%:
- Cardiovascular: Hypotension
- Gastrointestinal: Constipation
- Ocular: Lacrimation
- Respiratory: Dyspnea, nasal congestion

<1% (Limited to important or life-threatening symptoms): Positive ANA, positive LE cells. **Note:** Because of blunted beta-receptor response, the elderly are less likely to experience reflex tachycardia; this puts them at greater risk for orthostatic hypotension.

**Overdose/Toxicology** Symptoms of overdose include hypotension, tachycardia, and shock. Treatment is supportive and symptomatic.

**Pharmacodynamics/Kinetics**

**Protein Binding:** 85% to 90%

**Distribution:** Crosses the placenta

**Half-life Elimination:** Normal renal function: 2-8 hours; End-stage renal disease: 7-16 hours

**Metabolism:** Liver; large first-pass effect orally

**Excretion:** Urine

**Onset:** Oral: 20-30 minutes; I.V.: 5-20 minutes

**Duration:** Oral: 2-4 hours; I.V.: 2-6 hours

**Formulations**

Hydralazine hydrochloride:
- Injection: 20 mg/mL (1 mL)
- Tablet: 10 mg, 25 mg, 50 mg, 100 mg

**Dosing**

**Adults:**

Oral:
- Hypertension:
  - Initial: 10 mg 4 times/day
  - Increase by 10-25 mg/dose every 2-5 days
  - Maximum: 300 mg/day
- Congestive heart failure:
  - Initial: 10-25 mg 3 times/day
  - Target: 75 mg 3 times/day
  - Maximum: 100 mg 3 times/day

I.M., I.V.:
Hypertensive: Initial: 10-20 mg/dose every 4-6 hours as needed, may increase to 40 mg/dose; change to oral therapy as soon as possible.
Preeclampsia/eclampsia: 5 mg/dose then 5-10 mg every 20-30 minutes as needed

**Elderly:** Oral: Initial: 10 mg 2-3 times/day; increase by 10-25 mg/day every 2-5 days.

**Renal Impairment:**
$Cl_{cr}$ 10-50 mL/minute: Administer every 8 hours.
$Cl_{cr}$ <10 mL/minute: Administer every 8-16 hours in fast acetylators and every 12-24 hours in slow acetylators.
Hemodialysis effects: Supplemental dose is not necessary.
Peritoneal dialysis effects: Supplemental dose is not necessary.

**Administration**
**I.V.:** Inject over 1 minute.

**Stability**
**Storage:** Intact ampuls/vials of hydralazine should not be stored under refrigeration because of possible precipitation or crystallization.
**Reconstitution:** Hydralazine should be diluted in NS for IVPB administration due to decreased stability in $D_5W$. Stability of IVPB solution in NS is 4 days at room temperature.

**Monitoring Laboratory Tests** ANA titer

**Additional Nursing Issues**
**Physical Assessment:** Monitor heart rate and positional blood pressure (standing and sitting/lying): (oral - on a regular basis), (I.V. - frequently during and after infusion). Use/teach orthostatic precautions. Assess for fluid retention (eg, routine weight, I & O, peripheral edema, jugular vein distention, and respiratory difficulties). **Pregnancy risk factor C** - benefits of use should outweigh possible risks.
**Patient Information/Instruction:** Take as directed, with meals. Do not use alcohol or OTC medication without consulting prescriber. Weigh daily at the same time, in the same clothes. Report weight gain >5 lb/week, swelling of feet or ankles. May cause dizziness or weakness; change position slowly when rising from sitting or lying position and avoid driving or activities requiring alertness until response to drug is known. You may experience nausea (small frequent meals may help), impotence (reversible), or constipation (fluids, exercise, dietary fiber may help). This medication does not replace other antihypertensive interventions; follow instructions for diet and lifestyle changes. Report flu-like symptoms, difficulty breathing, skin rash, blackened stool, or numbness and tingling of extremities. **Pregnancy precautions:** Use appropriate contraception and inform prescriber if you are or intend to be pregnant.
**Dietary Issues:** Long-term use of hydralazine may cause pyridoxine deficiency resulting in numbness, tingling, and paresthesias. If symptoms develop, pyridoxine supplements may be needed.

**Additional Information**
Some formulations may contain tartrazine.
pH: 3.4-4

## Hydralazine and Hydrochlorothiazide

(hye DRAL a zeen & hye droe klor oh THYE a zide)

**U.S. Brand Names** Apresazide®; Hydrazide®; Hy-Zide®

**Synonyms** Hydrochlorothiazide and Hydralazine

**Therapeutic Category** Antihypertensive Agent, Combination

**Pregnancy Risk Factor** C

**Lactation** Enters breast milk/compatible

**Use** Management of moderate to severe hypertension and treatment of congestive heart failure

**Formulations**
Capsule:
25/25: Hydralazine hydrochloride 25 mg and hydrochlorothiazide 25 mg
50/50: Hydralazine hydrochloride 50 mg and hydrochlorothiazide 50 mg
100/50: Hydralazine hydrochloride 100 mg and hydrochlorothiazide 50 mg

**Dosing**
**Adults:** Oral: 1 capsule twice daily
**Elderly:** Refer to dosing in individual monographs.

**Additional Nursing Issues**
**Physical Assessment:** See individual components listed in Related Information. **Pregnancy risk factor C** - benefits of use should outweigh possible risks.
**Patient Information/Instruction:** See individual components listed in Related Information. **Pregnancy precautions:** Inform prescriber if you are on intend to get pregnant.

**Related Information**
Hydralazine *on previous page*
Hydrochlorothiazide *on next page*

## Hydralazine, Hydrochlorothiazide, and Reserpine

(hye DRAL a zeen, hye droe klor oh THYE a zide, & re SER peen)

**U.S. Brand Names** Cam-ap-es®; H.H.R.®; Hydrap-ES®; Marpres®; Ser-A-Gen®; Ser-Ap-Es®; Serathide®; Tri-Hydroserpine®

**Synonyms** Hydrochlorothiazide, Hydralazine, and Reserpine; Reserpine, Hydralazine, and Hydrochlorothiazide

**Therapeutic Category** Antihypertensive Agent, Combination

**Pregnancy Risk Factor** C

(Continued)

## Hydralazine, Hydrochlorothiazide, and Reserpine *(Continued)*

**Lactation** Enters breast milk/compatible

**Use** Hypertensive disorders

**Formulations** Tablet: Hydralazine 25 mg, hydrochlorothiazide 15 mg, and reserpine 0.1 mg

**Dosing**

**Adults:** Oral: 1-2 tablets 3 times/day

**Elderly:** Refer to dosing in individual monographs.

**Additional Nursing Issues**

**Physical Assessment:** See individual components listed in Related Information. **Pregnancy risk factor C** - benefits of use should outweigh possible risks.

**Patient Information/Instruction:** See individual components listed in Related Information. **Pregnancy precautions:** Inform prescriber if you are on intend to get pregnant.

**Related Information**

Hydralazine *on page 564*
Hydrochlorothiazide *on this page*
Reserpine *on page 1013*


- **Hydramyn® Syrup [OTC]** *see* Diphenhydramine *on page 381*
- **Hydrap-ES®** *see* Hydralazine, Hydrochlorothiazide, and Reserpine *on previous page*
- **Hydrazide®** *see* Hydralazine and Hydrochlorothiazide *on previous page*
- **Hydrea®** *see* Hydroxyurea *on page 586*
- **Hydrex®** *see* Benzthiazide *on page 144*
- **Hydrocet®** *see* Hydrocodone and Acetaminophen *on page 568*


## Hydrochlorothiazide (hye droe klor oh THYE a zide)

**U.S. Brand Names** Esidrix®; Ezide®; HydroDIURIL®; Hydro-Par®; Oretic®

**Synonyms** HCTZ

**Therapeutic Category** Diuretic, Thiazide

**Pregnancy Risk Factor** B

**Lactation** Enters breast milk/use caution (AAP rates "compatible")

**Use** Management of mild to moderate hypertension; treatment of edema in congestive heart failure and nephrotic syndrome

**Mechanism of Action/Effect** Inhibits sodium reabsorption in the distal tubules causing increased excretion of sodium and water as well as potassium and hydrogen ions

**Contraindications** Hypersensitivity to hydrochlorothiazide or any component; cross-sensitivity with other thiazides and sulfonamide derivatives; anuria; renal decompensation

**Warnings** Use with caution in renal disease, hepatic disease, gout, lupus erythematosus, diabetes mellitus; some products may contain tartrazine. Hydrochlorothiazide is not effective in patients with a $Cl_{cr}$ <30 mL/minute, therefore, it may not be a useful agent in many elderly patients.

**Drug Interactions**

**Decreased Effect:** Hydrochlorothiazide may decrease oral sulfonylurea (antidiabetic) drug efficacy.

**Increased Effect/Toxicity:** Hydrochlorothiazide may increase hypotensive effect of other antihypertensive agents. Digoxin and hydrochlorothiazide may increase digoxin related arrhythmias. Lithium and hydrochlorothiazide may increased lithium levels. Tetracyclines and hydrochlorothiazide may increase uremia.

**Food Interactions** Hydrochlorothiazide peak serum levels may be decreased if taken with food.

**Effects on Lab Values** ↑ creatine phosphokinase [CPK] (S), ammonia (B), amylase (S), calcium (S), chloride (S), cholesterol (S), glucose, acid (S); ↓ chloride (S), magnesium, potassium (S), sodium (S); tyramine and phentolamine tests; histamine tests for pheochromocytoma

**Adverse Reactions**

1% to 10%:

Cardiovascular: Orthostatic hypotension, hypotension
Endocrine & metabolic: Hypokalemia
Dermatologic: Photosensitivity
Gastrointestinal: Anorexia, epigastric distress

<1% (Limited to important or life-threatening symptoms): Allergic myocarditis, alopecia, exfoliative dermatitis, toxic epidermal necrolysis, erythema multiforme, Stevens-Johnson syndrome, aplastic anemia, hemolytic anemia, leukopenia, agranulocytosis, thrombocytopenia, hepatic function impairment, renal failure, interstitial nephritis, respiratory distress, allergic reactions (possibly with life-threatening anaphylactic shock), eosinophilic pneumonitis

**Overdose/Toxicology** Symptoms of overdose include hypermotility, diuresis, lethargy, confusion, and muscle weakness. Treatment is supportive.

**Pharmacodynamics/Kinetics**

**Half-life Elimination:** 5.6-14.8

**Metabolism:** No metabolism

**Excretion:** Urine

**Onset:** Diuretic effect within 2 hours; Peak effect: 4-6 hours

**Duration:** 6-12 hours

**Formulations**

Solution, oral (mint flavor): 50 mg/5 mL (50 mL)

Tablet: 25 mg, 50 mg, 100 mg

**Dosing**

**Adults:** Oral (effect of drug may be decreased when used every day): 25-100 mg/day in 1-2 doses; maximum: 200 mg/day

**Elderly:** Oral: 12.5-25 mg once daily; minimal increase in response and more electrolyte disturbances are seen with doses >50 mg/day.

**Renal Impairment:** $Cl_{cr}$ <50 mL/minute: Dosing adjustment not effective, therefore not generally recommended.

**Administration**

**Oral:** May be taken with food or milk. Take early in day to avoid nocturia. Take the last dose of multiple doses no later than 6 PM unless instructed otherwise.

**Monitoring Laboratory Tests** Serum electrolytes, BUN, creatinine

**Additional Nursing Issues**

**Physical Assessment:** Assess effectiveness/interactions of other medications patient may be taking (see Drug Interactions). Monitor heart rate, blood pressure (sitting, lying, and standing), and fluid status (edema, jugular vein distention, weight, respiratory difficulty) when starting therapy and on a regular basis with long-term therapy. Assess knowledge/teach patient appropriate use, possible side effects (including possibility of hyperglycemia), and symptoms to report. Note breast-feeding caution.

**Patient Information/Instruction:** This medication does not replace other antihypertensive recommendations (diet and lifestyle changes). Take as directed, with meals, early in the day to avoid nocturia. Avoid alcohol or OTC medication unless approved by prescriber. Include bananas and/or orange juice in daily diet; do not take potassium supplements unless recommended by prescriber. May cause dizziness or postural hypotension (use caution when rising from sitting or lying position, when driving, climbing stairs, or engaging in tasks that require alertness until response to drug is known); nausea or vomiting (small frequent meals, frequent mouth care, sucking lozenges, or chewing gum may help); impotence (reversible); constipation (increased exercise or dietary fruit, fiber, or fluids will help); photosensitivity (use sunscreen, wear protective clothing and eyewear, and avoid direct sunlight). If diabetic, monitor serum glucose closely; this medication may increase serum glucose levels. Report persistent flu-like symptoms, chest pain, palpitations, muscle cramping, difficulty breathing, skin rash or itching, unusual bruising or easy bleeding, or excessive fatigue. **Pregnancy/breast-feeding precautions:** Consult prescriber if breast-feeding.

**Geriatric Considerations:** Hydrochlorothiazide is not effective in patients with a $Cl_{cr}$ <30 mL/minute, therefore, it may not be a useful agent in many elderly patients.

- ♦ **Hydrochlorothiazide and Amiloride** *see* Amiloride and Hydrochlorothiazide *on page 68*
- ♦ **Hydrochlorothiazide and Benazepril** *see* Benazepril and Hydrochlorothiazide *on page 140*
- ♦ **Hydrochlorothiazide and Bisoprolol** *see* Bisoprolol and Hydrochlorothiazide *on page 156*
- ♦ **Hydrochlorothiazide and Captopril** *see* Captopril and Hydrochlorothiazide *on page 194*
- ♦ **Hydrochlorothiazide and Enalapril** *see* Enalapril and Hydrochlorothiazide *on page 419*
- ♦ **Hydrochlorothiazide and Hydralazine** *see* Hydralazine and Hydrochlorothiazide *on page 565*
- ♦ **Hydrochlorothiazide and Irbesartan** *see* Irbesartan and Hydrochlorothiazide *on page 624*
- ♦ **Hydrochlorothiazide and Lisinopril** *see* Lisinopril and Hydrochlorothiazide *on page 683*
- ♦ **Hydrochlorothiazide and Losartan** *see* Losartan and Hydrochlorothiazide *on page 694*
- ♦ **Hydrochlorothiazide and Methyldopa** *see* Methyldopa and Hydrochlorothiazide *on page 751*
- ♦ **Hydrochlorothiazide and Propranolol** *see* Propranolol and Hydrochlorothiazide *on page 988*

## Hydrochlorothiazide and Reserpine

(hye droe klor oh THYE a zide & re SER peen)

**U.S. Brand Names** Hydropres®; Hydro-Serp®; Hydroserpine®

**Synonyms** Reserpine and Hydrochlorothiazide

**Therapeutic Category** Antihypertensive Agent, Combination

**Pregnancy Risk Factor** C

**Lactation** Enters breast milk/compatible

**Use** Management of mild to moderate hypertension; treatment of edema in congestive heart failure and nephrotic syndrome

**Formulations**

Tablet:

25: Hydrochlorothiazide 25 mg and reserpine 0.125 mg

50: Hydrochlorothiazide 50 mg and reserpine 0.125 mg

**Dosing**

**Adults:** Oral: 1-2 tablets once or twice daily

**Elderly:** Refer to dosing in individual monographs.

**Additional Nursing Issues**

**Physical Assessment:** See individual components listed in Related Information. **Pregnancy risk factor C** - benefits of use should outweigh possible risks.

(Continued)

## Hydrochlorothiazide and Reserpine *(Continued)*

**Patient Information/Instruction:** See individual components listed in Related Information. **Pregnancy precautions:** Inform prescriber if you are on intend to get pregnant.

**Related Information**

Hydrochlorothiazide *on page 566*

Reserpine *on page 1013*

## Hydrochlorothiazide and Spironolactone

(hye droe klor oh THYE a zide & speer on oh LAK tone)

**U.S. Brand Names** Alazide®; Aldactazide®; Spironazide®; Spirozide®

**Synonyms** Spironolactone and Hydrochlorothiazide

**Therapeutic Category** Antihypertensive Agent, Combination

**Pregnancy Risk Factor** C

**Lactation** Enters breast milk/use caution

**Use** Management of mild to moderate hypertension; treatment of edema in congestive heart failure and nephrotic syndrome, and cirrhosis of the liver accompanied by edema and/or ascites

**Formulations**

Tablet:

25/25: Hydrochlorothiazide 25 mg and spironolactone 25 mg

50/50: Hydrochlorothiazide 50 mg and spironolactone 50 mg

**Dosing**

**Adults:** Oral: 1-8 tablets in 1-2 divided doses

**Elderly:** Oral: Initial: 1 tablet/day; increase as necessary.

**Renal Impairment:** Efficacy of hydrochlorothiazide is limited in patients with $Cl_{cr}$ <30 mL/minute.

**Additional Nursing Issues**

**Physical Assessment:** See individual components listed in Related Information. **Pregnancy risk factor C** - benefits of use should outweigh possible risks. Note breast-feeding caution.

**Patient Information/Instruction:** See individual components listed in Related Information. **Pregnancy/breast-feeding precautions:** Inform prescriber if you are on intend to get pregnant. Consult prescriber if breast-feeding.

**Related Information**

Hydrochlorothiazide *on page 566*

Spironolactone *on page 1070*

## Hydrochlorothiazide and Triamterene

(hye droe klor oh THYE a zide & trye AM ter een)

**U.S. Brand Names** Dyazide®; Maxzide®

**Synonyms** Triamterene and Hydrochlorothiazide

**Therapeutic Category** Antihypertensive Agent, Combination; Diuretic, Potassium Sparing; Diuretic, Thiazide

**Pregnancy Risk Factor** C

**Lactation** Excretion in breast milk unknown/use caution

**Use** Management of mild to moderate hypertension; treatment of edema in congestive heart failure and nephrotic syndrome

**Formulations**

Capsule (Dyazide®): Hydrochlorothiazide 25 mg and triamterene 37.5 mg

Tablet:

Maxzide®-25: Hydrochlorothiazide 25 mg and triamterene 37.5 mg

Maxzide®: Hydrochlorothiazide 50 mg and triamterene 75 mg

**Dosing**

**Adults:** Oral: 1-2 capsules twice daily after meals

**Elderly:** Oral: Initial: 1 capsule/day or every other day

**Additional Nursing Issues**

**Physical Assessment:** See individual components listed in Related Information. **Pregnancy risk factor C** - benefits of use should outweigh possible risks. Note breast-feeding caution.

**Patient Information/Instruction:** See individual components listed in Related Information. **Pregnancy/breast-feeding precautions:** Inform prescriber if you are on intend to get pregnant. Consult prescriber if breast-feeding.

**Related Information**

Hydrochlorothiazide *on page 566*

Triamterene *on page 1173*

- **Hydrochlorothiazide, Hydralazine, and Reserpine** *see* Hydralazine, Hydrochlorothiazide, and Reserpine *on page 565*
- **Hydrocil® [OTC]** *see* Psyllium *on page 993*
- **Hydro-Cobex®** *see* Hydroxocobalamin *on page 583*

## Hydrocodone and Acetaminophen

(hye droe KOE done & a seet a MIN oh fen)

**U.S. Brand Names** Anexsia®; Anodynos-DHC®; Bancap HC®; Co-Gesic®; Dolacet®; DuoCet™; Duradyne DHC®; Hydrocet®; Hydrogesic®; Hy-Phen®; Lorcet®-HD; Lorcet® Plus; Lortab®; Margesic® H; Medipain 5®; Norcet®; Stagesic®; T-Gesic®; Vicodin®; Vicodin® ES; Vicodin® HP; Zydone®

**Synonyms** Acetaminophen and Hydrocodone

**Therapeutic Category** Analgesic, Combination (Narcotic)

**Pregnancy Risk Factor** C

**Lactation** Excretion in breast milk unknown/contraindicated

**Use** Relief of moderate to severe pain

**Mechanism of Action/Effect** See individual agents

**Contraindications** Hypersensitivity to hydrocodone, acetaminophen, or any component; CNS depression; severe respiratory depression

**Warnings** Use with caution in patients with hypersensitivity reactions to other phenanthrene derivative opioid agonists (morphine, hydrocodone, hydromorphone, levorphanol, oxycodone, oxymorphone). Tablets contain metabisulfite which may cause allergic reactions. Pregnancy factor C.

**Drug Interactions**

**Decreased Effect:** Decreased effect with phenothiazines.

**Increased Effect/Toxicity:** Hydrocodone with other narcotic analgesics, CNS depressants, antianxiety agents or antipsychotics may cause enhanced CNS depression. MAO inhibitors or tricyclic antidepressants with hydrocodone may increase the effect of either agent.

**Food Interactions** Rate of absorption of acetaminophen may be decreased when administered with food high in carbohydrates.

**Adverse Reactions**

>10%:

- Cardiovascular: Hypotension
- Central nervous system: Lightheadedness, dizziness, sedation, drowsiness, fatigue
- Neuromuscular & skeletal: Weakness

1% to 10%:

- Cardiovascular: Bradycardia
- Central nervous system: Confusion
- Gastrointestinal: Nausea, vomiting
- Genitourinary: Decreased urination
- Respiratory: Shortness of breath, dyspnea

**Overdose/Toxicology** Symptoms of overdose include hepatic necrosis, blood dyscrasias, and respiratory depression. Treatment consists of acetylcysteine 140 mg/kg orally (loading) followed by 70 mg/kg every 4 hours for 17 doses; therapy should be initiated based upon laboratory analysis suggesting a high probability for hepatotoxic potential. Naloxone, 2 mg I.V. with repeat administration as necessary up to a total of 10 mg, can also be used to reverse toxic effects of the opiate. Activated charcoal is effective at binding certain chemicals, and this is especially true for acetaminophen.

**Pharmacodynamics/Kinetics**

**Distribution:** Crosses the placenta

**Half-life Elimination:** Hydrocodone: 3.8 hours

**Metabolism:** Hydrocodone and APAP: Liver

**Excretion:** Urine

**Onset:** Onset of narcotic analgesia: Within 10-20 minutes

**Duration:** 3-6 hours

**Formulations**

Capsule:

Bancap HC®, Dolacet®, Hydrocet®, Hydrogesic®, Lorcet®-HD, Margesic® H, Medipain 5®, Norcet®, Stagesic®, T-Gesic®, Zydone®: Hydrocodone bitartrate 5 mg and acetaminophen 500 mg

Elixir (tropical fruit punch flavor) (Lortab®): Hydrocodone bitartrate 2.5 mg and acetaminophen 167 mg per 5 mL with alcohol 7% (480 mL)

Solution, oral (tropical fruit punch flavor) (Lortab®): Hydrocodone bitartrate 2.5 mg and acetaminophen 167 mg per 5 mL with alcohol 7% (480 mL)

Tablet: Hydrocodone bitartrate 5 mg and acetaminophen 400 mg; hydrocodone bitartrate 7.5 mg and acetaminophen 400 mg; hydrocodone bitartrate 10 mg and acetaminophen 400 mg; hydrocodone bitartrate 5 mg and acetaminophen 500 mg; hydrocodone bitartrate 7.5 mg and acetaminophen 750 mg; hydrocodone bitartrate 7.5 mg and acetaminophen 500 mg; hydrocodone bitartrate 7.5 mg and acetaminophen 650 mg; hydrocodone bitartrate 10 mg and acetaminophen 650 mg

Lortab® 2.5/500: Hydrocodone bitartrate 2.5 mg and acetaminophen 500 mg

Anexsia® 5/500, Anodynos-DHC®, Co-Gesic®, DuoCet™, DHC®; Hy-Phen®, Lorcet®, Lortab®® 5/500, Vicodin®: Hydrocodone bitartrate 5 mg and acetaminophen 500 mg

Lortab® 7.5/500: Hydrocodone bitartrate 7.5 mg and acetaminophen 500 mg

Anexsia® 7.5/650, Lorcet® Plus: Hydrocodone bitartrate 7.5 mg and acetaminophen 650 mg

Vicodin® ES: Hydrocodone bitartrate 7.5 mg and acetaminophen 750 mg

Norco®: Hydrocodone bitartrate 10 mg and acetaminophen 325 mg

Lortab® 10/500: Hydrocodone bitartrate 10 mg and acetaminophen 500 mg

Lorcet® 10/650: Hydrocodone bitartrate 10 mg and acetaminophen 650 mg

Vicodin® HP: Hydrocodone bitartrate 10 mg and acetaminophen 660 mg

Zydone®: Hydrocodone bitartrate 5 mg and acetaminophen 400 mg; hydrocodone bitartrate 7.5 mg and acetaminophen 400 mg; Hydrocodone bitartrate 10 mg and acetaminophen 400 mg

**Dosing**

**Adults:** Analgesic: Oral (doses should be titrated to appropriate analgesic effect): 1-2 tablets or capsules every 4-6 hours or 5-10 mL solution every 4-6 hours as needed for pain

**Elderly:** Doses should be titrated to appropriate analgesic effect; 2.5-5 mg of the hydrocodone component every 4-6 hours. Do not exceed 4 g/day of acetaminophen.

(Continued)

## Hydrocodone and Acetaminophen *(Continued)*

**Additional Nursing Issues**

**Physical Assessment: Assess patient for history of liver disease or alcohol abuse** (acetaminophen and excessive alcohol may have adverse liver effects). Assess other medications patient may be taking for additive or adverse interactions (see Drug Interactions). Monitor for effectiveness of pain relief and monitor for signs of overdose (see above). Monitor vital signs and signs of adverse reactions (see Adverse Reactions) at beginning of therapy and at regular intervals with long-term use. May cause physical and/or psychological dependence. Discontinue slowly after long-term use. For inpatients, implement safety measures (eg, side rails up, call light within reach, instructions to call for assistance, etc). Assess knowledge/teach patient appropriate use if self-administered. Teach patient to monitor for adverse reactions, adverse reactions to report, and appropriate interventions to reduce side effects. **Pregnancy risk factor C** - benefits of use should outweigh possible risks. Breast-feeding is contraindicated.

**Patient Information/Instruction:** If self-administered, use exactly as directed (do not increase dose or frequency); may cause physical and/or psychological dependence. Take with food or milk. While using this medication, do not use alcohol and other prescription or OTC medications (especially sedatives, tranquilizers, antihistamines, or pain medications) without consulting prescriber. Maintain adequate hydration (2-3 L/day of fluids unless instructed to restrict fluid intake). May cause dizziness, lightheadedness, confusion, or drowsiness (use caution when driving, climbing stairs, or changing position - rising from sitting or lying to standing, or when engaging in tasks requiring alertness until response to drug is known); nausea or vomiting (frequent mouth care, frequent sips of fluids, chewing gum, or sucking lozenges may help). Report chest pain or palpitations; persistent dizziness, shortness of breath, or difficulty breathing; unusual bleeding or bruising; or unusual fatigue and weakness. **Pregnancy/breast-feeding precautions:** Inform prescriber if you are or intend to be pregnant. Do not breast-feed.

**Geriatric Considerations:** The elderly may be particularly susceptible to the CNS depressant action (sedation, confusion) and constipating effects of narcotics. If 1 tablet/dose is used, it may be useful to add an additional 325 mg of acetaminophen to maximize analgesic effect and minimize additional risk of narcotic related adverse effects.

**Related Information**

Acetaminophen *on page 32*

## Hydrocodone and Aspirin (hye droe KOE done & AS pir in)

**U.S. Brand Names** Azdone®; Damason-P®; Lortab® ASA; Panasal® 5/500

**Synonyms** Aspirin and Hydrocodone

**Therapeutic Category** Analgesic, Combination (Narcotic)

**Pregnancy Risk Factor** D

**Lactation** Enters breast milk/contraindicated

**Use** Relief of moderate to moderately severe pain

**Mechanism of Action/Effect** Refer to individual agents.

**Warnings** Use with caution in patients with impaired renal function, erosive gastritis, or peptic ulcer disease. Children and teenagers should not use for chickenpox or flu symptoms before a physician is consulted about Reye's syndrome.

**Drug Interactions**

**Increased Effect/Toxicity:** Increased toxicity with CNS depressants, warfarin (bleeding).

**Effects on Lab Values** Urine glucose, urinary 5-HIAA, serum uric acid

**Adverse Reactions**

>10%:

Cardiovascular: Hypotension
Central nervous system: Lightheadedness, dizziness, sedation, drowsiness, fatigue
Gastrointestinal: Nausea, heartburn, stomach pains, heartburn, epigastric discomfort
Neuromuscular & skeletal: Weakness

1% to 10%:

Cardiovascular: Bradycardia
Central nervous system: Confusion
Dermatologic: Rash
Gastrointestinal: Vomiting, gastrointestinal ulceration
Genitourinary: Decreased urination
Hematologic: Hemolytic anemia
Respiratory: Shortness of breath, dyspnea
Miscellaneous: Anaphylactic shock

<1% (Limited to important or life-threatening symptoms): Occult bleeding, prolongated bleeding time, leukopenia, thrombocytopenia, iron deficiency anemia, hepatotoxicity, impaired renal function, bronchospasm

**Overdose/Toxicology** Naloxone is the antidote for codeine. Naloxone, 2 mg I.V. with repeat administration as necessary up to a total of 10 mg, can also be used to reverse toxic effects of the opiate. Nomograms, such as the "Done" nomogram, can be very helpful for estimating the severity of aspirin poisoning and for directing treatment using serum salicylate levels. Treatment can also be based upon symptomatology; see Aspirin.

**Formulations** Tablet: Hydrocodone bitartrate 5 mg and aspirin 500 mg

**Dosing**

**Adults:** Oral: 1-2 tablets every 4-6 hours as needed for pain

**Elderly:** Refer to dosing in individual monographs.

**Administration**

**Oral:** Administer with food or a full glass of water to minimize GI distress.

**Additional Nursing Issues**

**Physical Assessment: Do not use for persons with allergic reaction to aspirin or aspirin-containing medications.** Assess other medications patient may be taking for additive or adverse interactions (see Drug Interactions). Monitor for effectiveness of pain relief and monitor for signs of overdose (see above). Monitor vital signs and signs of adverse reactions (see Adverse Reactions) at beginning of therapy and at regular intervals with long-term use. May cause physical and/or psychological dependence. Discontinue slowly after long-term use. For inpatients, implement safety measures (eg, side rails up, call light within reach, instructions to call for assistance, etc). Assess knowledge/teach patient appropriate use if self-administered. Teach patient to monitor for adverse reactions, adverse reactions to report, and appropriate interventions to reduce side effects. **Pregnancy risk factor D** - assess knowledge/instruct patient on need to use appropriate contraceptive measures and the need to avoid pregnancy. Breast-feeding is contraindicated.

**Patient Information/Instruction:** If self-administered, use exactly as directed (do not increase dose or frequency); may cause physical and/or psychological dependence. Take with food or milk. While using this medication, do not use alcohol, excessive amounts of vitamin C, or salicylate-containing foods (curry powder, prunes, raisins, tea, or licorice), other aspirin- or salicylate-containing medications, and other prescription or OTC medications (especially sedatives, tranquilizers, antihistamines, or pain medications) without consulting prescriber. Maintain adequate hydration (2-3 L/day of fluids unless instructed to restrict fluid intake). May cause hypotension, dizziness, drowsiness, impaired coordination, or blurred vision (use caution when driving, climbing stairs, or changing position - rising from sitting or lying to standing, or when engaging in tasks requiring alertness until response to drug is known); nausea, vomiting, or dry mouth (frequent mouth care, small frequent meals, chewing gum, or sucking lozenges may help); constipation (increased exercise, fluids, or dietary fruit and fiber may help - if constipation remains an unresolved problem, consult prescriber about use of stool softeners). Report ringing in ears; persistent pain in stomach; unresolved nausea or vomiting; difficulty breathing or shortness of breath; yellowing of skin or eyes; changes in color of stool or urine; or unusual bruising or bleeding. **Pregnancy/breast-feeding precautions:** Use appropriate contraceptive measures; do not get pregnant while taking this drug. Do not breast-feed.

**Related Information**

Aspirin *on page 111*

## Hydrocodone and Chlorpheniramine

(hye droe KOE done & klor fen IR a meen)

**U.S. Brand Names** Tussionex®; Pennkinetic®

**Synonyms** Chlorpheniramine and Hydrocodone

**Therapeutic Category** Antihistamine/Antitussive

**Pregnancy Risk Factor** C

**Lactation** Excretion in breast milk unknown/contraindicated

**Use** Symptomatic relief of cough and allergy

**Adverse Reactions** <1% (Limited to important or life-threatening symptoms): Drowsiness, sedation, lethargy, anxiety, facial pruritus, constipation, nausea, ureteral spasm, respiratory depression, dryness of pharynx

**Pharmacodynamics/Kinetics**

**Half-life Elimination:** Hydrocodone: 3.8 hours

**Time to Peak:** Hydrocodone: 1.3 hours

**Metabolism:** Hydrocodone: Liver

**Excretion:** Hydrocodone: Urine

**Duration:** Hydrocodone: 4-6 hours

**Formulations** Syrup, alcohol free: Hydrocodone polistirex 10 mg and chlorpheniramine polistirex 8 mg per 5 mL (480 mL, 900 mL)

**Dosing**

**Adults:** Oral: 5 mL every 12 hours; do not exceed 10 mL/24 hours.

**Elderly:** Refer to dosing in individual monographs.

**Additional Nursing Issues**

**Physical Assessment: Pregnancy risk factor C** - benefits of use should outweigh possible risks. Breast-feeding is contraindicated.

**Patient Information/Instruction: Pregnancy precautions:** Inform prescriber if you are or intend to be pregnant. Do not breast-feed.

## Hydrocodone and Guaifenesin (hye droe KOE done & gwye FEN e sin)

**U.S. Brand Names** Codiclear® DH; HycoClear Tuss®; Hycotuss® Expectorant Liquid; Kwelcof®

**Synonyms** Guaifenesin and Hydrocodone

**Therapeutic Category** Antitussive/Expectorant

**Pregnancy Risk Factor** C

**Lactation** Excretion in breast milk unknown/contraindicated

**Use** Symptomatic relief of nonproductive coughs associated with upper and lower respiratory tract congestion

(Continued)

## Hydrocodone and Guaifenesin *(Continued)*

**Contraindications** Hypersensitivity to hydrocodone, guaifenesin, or any component; increased intracranial pressure; depressed ventilation

**Warnings** Can produce drug dependence and therefore has potential for abuse. Patients with chronic obstructive pulmonary disease.

**Drug Interactions**

**Increased Effect/Toxicity:** Patients receiving general anesthetics, analgesics, other narcotics, phenothiazines, sedative hypnotics, other CNS depressants (alcohol) or other tranquilizers may exhibit enhanced CNS effects.

**Effects on Lab Values** Increase in urinary 5-hydroxyindoleacetic acid, therefore, may interfere with interpretation of this test for diagnosis of carcinoid syndrome. Discontinue guaifenesin 24 hours prior to collection.

**Adverse Reactions**

Cardiovascular: Hypertension, postural hypotension, palpitations

Central nervous system: Drowsiness, sedation, mental clouding, mental and physical impairment, anxiety, fear, dysphoria, dizziness, psychotic dependence, mood changes

Gastrointestinal: Nausea, vomiting, constipation with prolonged use

Genitourinary: Ureteral spasm, urinary retention

Ocular: Blurred vision

Respiratory: Respiratory depression (dose related)

**Overdose/Toxicology** Symptoms of overdose include respiratory depression, Cheyne-Stokes respiration and cyanosis, extreme somnolence progressing to stupor or coma, skeletal muscle flaccidity, cold clammy skin, sometimes bradycardia and hypotension. Naloxone, 2 mg I.V. with repeat administration as necessary up to a total of 10 mg, can also be used to reverse toxic effects of the opiate.

**Pharmacodynamics/Kinetics**

**Half-life Elimination:** Hydrocodone: 3.8 hours

**Time to Peak:** Hydrocodone: 1.3 hours

**Metabolism:** Hydrocodone: Liver

**Excretion:** Hydrocodone: Urine

**Duration:** Hydrocodone: 4-6 hours

**Formulations** Liquid: Hydrocodone bitartrate 5 mg and guaifenesin 100 mg per 5 mL (120 mL, 480 mL)

**Dosing**

**Adults:** Oral: 5 mL every 4 hours, after meals and at bedtime, not to exceed 30 mL in a 24-hour period; start dose at 5 mL and do not exceed 15 mL for any single dose.

**Elderly:** Refer to dosing in individual monographs.

**Additional Nursing Issues**

**Physical Assessment:** Assess effectiveness and interactions of other medications (see Drug Interactions). See Contraindications and Warnings/Precautions for cautious use. **Note:** May be habit-forming. Monitor effectiveness of therapy (relief of cough, lung sounds, and respiratory pattern) and adverse reactions (eg, cardiac and CNS changes - see Adverse Reactions) at beginning of therapy and periodically with long-term use. Assess knowledge/teach patient appropriate use, interventions to reduce side effects, and adverse symptoms to report. **Pregnancy risk factor C** - benefits of use should outweigh possible risks. Breast-feeding is contraindicated.

**Patient Information/Instruction:** Take only as prescribed; do not exceed prescribed dose or frequency. May be habit-forming. Maintain adequate hydration (2-3 L/day of fluids unless instructed to restrict fluid intake). Avoid use of other depressants, alcohol, or sleep-inducing medications, or tranquilizers or pain medications unless approved by prescriber. You may experience orthostatic hypotension (change position slowly when rising from sitting or lying or when climbing stairs); drowsiness, impaired coordination, or blurred vision (use caution when driving or engaging in tasks requiring alertness until response to drug is known); nausea or vomiting (frequent small meals, frequent mouth care, chewing gum, or sucking hard candy may help); or constipation (increased exercise, fluids, or dietary fruit and fiber may help). Report persistent CNS changes (dizziness, sedation, tremor, or agitation), difficulty breathing, persistent abdominal cramping, visual changes, or lack of improvement or worsening or condition. **Pregnancy/breast-feeding precautions:** Inform prescriber if you are or intend to be pregnant. Do not breast-feed.

**Related Information**

Guaifenesin *on page 548*

## Hydrocodone and Homatropine (hye droe KOE done & hoe MA troe peen)

**U.S. Brand Names** Hycodan®; Hydromet®; Hydropane®; Hydrotropine®; Tussigon®

**Synonyms** Homatropine and Hydrocodone

**Therapeutic Category** Antitussive; Cough Preparation

**Pregnancy Risk Factor** C

**Lactation** Excretion in breast milk unknown/contraindicated

**Use** Symptomatic relief of cough

**Contraindications** Hypersensitivity to hydrocodone, homatropine, or any component; increased intracranial pressure; narrow-angle glaucoma; depressed ventilation

**Warnings** Use with caution in patients with hypersensitivity to other phenanthrene derivatives. Use with caution in patients with respiratory diseases, or severe liver or renal failure. Use with caution in children with spastic paralysis, in the elderly, and in patients with prostatic hypertrophy.

**Effects on Lab Values** ↑ ALT, AST (S)

**Adverse Reactions**

>10%:

Cardiovascular: Hypotension

Central nervous system: Lightheadedness, dizziness, sedation, drowsiness, fatigue

Neuromuscular & skeletal: Weakness

1% to 10%:

Cardiovascular: Bradycardia, tachycardia

Central nervous system: Confusion

Gastrointestinal: Nausea, vomiting

Genitourinary: Decreased urination

Respiratory: Shortness of breath, dyspnea

**Overdose/Toxicology** Symptoms of overdose include CNS and respiratory depression; GI cramping; dilated, unreactive pupils; blurred vision; hot, dry flushed skin; dryness of mucous membranes; difficulty swallowing; foul breath; diminished or absent bowel sounds; urinary retention; tachycardia; hyperthermia; hypertension; and increased respiratory rate. CNS depression is an extension of the pharmacologic effect. Treatment is supportive. Naloxone, 2 mg I.V. with repeat administration as necessary up to a total of 10 mg, can also be used to reverse toxic effects of the opiate.

**Pharmacodynamics/Kinetics**

**Half-life Elimination:** Hydrocodone: 3.8 hours

**Time to Peak:** Hydrocodone: 1.3 hours

**Metabolism:** Hydrocodone: Liver

**Excretion:** Hydrocodone: Urine

**Duration:** Hydrocodone: 4-6 hours

**Formulations**

Syrup (Hycodan®, Hydromet®, Hydropane®, Hydrotropine®): Hydrocodone bitartrate 5 mg and homatropine methylbromide 1.5 mg per 5 mL (120 mL, 480 mL, 4000 mL)

Tablet (Hycodan®, Tussigon®): Hydrocodone bitartrate 5 mg and homatropine methylbromide 1.5 mg

**Dosing**

**Adults:** Oral (based on hydrocodone component): 5-10 mg every 4-6 hours, a single dose should not exceed 15 mg; do not administer more frequently than every 4 hours.

**Elderly:** Refer to dosing in individual monographs.

**Additional Nursing Issues**

**Physical Assessment:** Monitor effectiveness of therapy (relief of cough, lung sounds, and respiratory pattern) and adverse reactions (eg, CNS changes - see Adverse Reactions) at beginning of therapy and periodically with long-term use. **Note:** May be habit-forming. Assess knowledge/teach patient appropriate use, interventions to reduce side effects, and adverse symptoms to report. **Pregnancy risk factor C** - benefits of use should outweigh possible risks. Breast-feeding is contraindicated.

**Patient Information/Instruction:** Take only as prescribed; do not exceed prescribed dose or frequency. May be habit-forming. Maintain adequate hydration (2-3 L/day of fluids unless instructed to restrict fluid intake). Avoid use of other depressants, alcohol, or sleep-inducing medications, or tranquilizers or pain medications unless approved by prescriber. You may experience orthostatic hypotension (change position slowly when rising from sitting or lying or when climbing stairs); drowsiness, impaired coordination, or blurred vision (use caution when driving or engaging in tasks requiring alertness until response to drug is known); nausea or vomiting (frequent small meals, frequent mouth care, chewing gum, or sucking hard candy may help); or constipation (increased exercise, fluids, or dietary fruit and fiber may help). Report persistent CNS changes (dizziness, sedation, tremor, or agitation), difficulty breathing, persistent abdominal cramping, visual changes, or lack of improvement or worsening or condition. **Pregnancy/breast-feeding precautions:** Inform prescriber if you are or intend to be pregnant; contraceptives may be recommended. Do not breast-feed.

## Hydrocodone and Ibuprofen (hye droe KOE done & eye byoo PROE fen)

**U.S. Brand Names** Vicoprofen®

**Synonyms** Ibuprofen and Hydrocodone

**Therapeutic Category** Analgesic, Combination (Narcotic)

**Pregnancy Risk Factor** C

**Lactation** Excretion in breast milk unknown/contraindicated

**Use** Short-term (generally less than 10 days) management of acute pain

**Contraindications** Hypersensitivity to hydrocodone or ibuprofen; patients who have experienced asthma, urticaria, or allergic reactions after taking aspirin or other NSAIDs

**Warnings** Use with caution in patients with asthma or in patients who have experienced hypersensitivity reactions to opioids due to cross sensitivity to hydrocodone. Hydrocodone may produce drug dependence.

**Drug Interactions**

**Decreased Effect:** Ibuprofen may reduce the antihypertensive effect of ACE inhibitors.

**Increased Effect/Toxicity:** Anticholinergic agents taken with hydrocodone may cause paralytic ileus. Aspirin taken concomitantly may enhance adverse effects. Other CNS depressants (eg, antihistamines, alcohol, antipsychotics, etc) taken concomitantly may exhibit additive CNS toxicity. Warfarin taken with ibuprofen may result in additional risk of bleeding. Methotrexate taken with ibuprofen may enhance methotrexate toxicity. Furosemide taken with ibuprofen may reduce the effect of furosemide. Lithium taken with ibuprofen may elevate lithium serum levels.

**Adverse Reactions**

>10%:

Central nervous system: Headache (27%), somnolence (22%), dizziness (14%)

(Continued)

## Hydrocodone and Ibuprofen *(Continued)*

Gastrointestinal: Constipation (22%), nausea (21%), dyspepsia (12%)

3% to 9%:

Cardiovascular: Edema
Central nervous system: Anxiety, insomnia, nervousness
Dermatologic: Pruritus
Gastrointestinal: Diarrhea, dry mouth, flatulence, vomiting
Miscellaneous: Sweating

<3%:

Cardiovascular: Palpitations, vasodilation
Central nervous system: Confusion, hypertonia, paresthesia, thinking abnormalities
Endocrine & metabolic: Weight decrease
Gastrointestinal: Gastritis, melena, mouth ulcers, thirst
Genitourinary: Urinary frequency
Otic: Tinnitus
Respiratory: Dyspnea, hiccups, pharyngitis, rhinitis

<1% (Limited to important or life-threatening symptoms): Allergic reaction, arrhythmia, hypotension, tachycardia, vertigo, elevated liver enzymes, asthma, bronchitis, pulmonary congestion, pneumonia, shallow breathing

**Overdose/Toxicology** Symptoms of toxicity may include respiratory depression, CNS depression, metabolic acidosis, seizures, hypotension, blood loss, coma, meiosis, and renal failure. Naloxone is the antidote for hydrocodone. Naloxone, 2 mg I.V. with repeat administration as necessary up to a total of 10 mg, can also be used to reverse toxic effects of the opiate. Treatment of NSAID overdose is supportive with symptomatic management as necessary.

**Pharmacodynamics/Kinetics**

**Protein Binding:** Ibuprofen: 99%; Hydrocodone: 19% to 45%

**Half-life Elimination:** Ibuprofen: 2.2 hours; Hydrocodone: 4.5 hours

**Time to Peak:** Ibuprofen: 1.8 hours; Hydrocodone: 1.7 hours

**Metabolism:** Liver

**Excretion:** Urine

**Formulations** Tablet: Hydrocodone bitartrate 7.5 mg; ibuprofen 200 mg

**Dosing**

**Adults:** Short-term use is recommended, not to exceed 10 days; Oral: 1 tablet every 4-6 hours, do not exceed 5 tablets during a 24-hour period.

**Elderly:** Refer to dosing in individual monographs.

**Additional Nursing Issues**

**Physical Assessment:** Assess other medications patient may be taking for additive or adverse interactions (see Drug Interactions). Monitor for effectiveness of pain relief and monitor for signs of overdose (see above). Monitor vital signs and signs of adverse reactions (see Adverse Reactions) at beginning of therapy and at regular intervals with long-term use. May cause physical and/or psychological dependence. Discontinue slowly after long-term use. For inpatients, implement safety measures (eg, side rails up, call light within reach, instructions to call for assistance, etc). Assess knowledge/ teach patient appropriate use if self-administered. Teach patient to monitor for adverse reactions, adverse reactions to report, and appropriate interventions to reduce side effects. **Pregnancy risk factor C** - benefits of use should outweigh possible risks. Breast-feeding is contraindicated.

**Patient Information/Instruction:** If self-administered, use exactly as directed (do not increase dose or frequency); may cause physical and/or psychological dependence. Take with food or milk. While using this medication, do not use alcohol and other prescription or OTC medications (especially sedatives, tranquilizers, antihistamines, or pain medications) without consulting prescriber. Maintain adequate hydration (2-3 L/ day of fluids unless instructed to restrict fluid intake). May cause dizziness, drowsiness, confusion, nervousness, or anxiety (use caution when driving, climbing stairs, or changing position - rising from sitting or lying to standing, or when engaging in tasks requiring alertness until response to drug is known); nausea, dry mouth, decreased appetite, or gastric distress (frequent mouth care, frequent sips of fluids, chewing gum, or sucking lozenges may help); constipation (increased exercise, fluids, or dietary fruit and fiber may help - if constipation remains an unresolved problem, consult prescriber about use of stool softeners). Report chest pain or palpitations; persistent dizziness, shortness of breath, or difficulty breathing; unusual bleeding (stool, mouth, urine) or bruising; unusual fatigue and weakness; change in elimination patterns; or change in color of urine or stool. **Pregnancy/breast-feeding precautions:** Inform prescriber if you are or intend to be pregnant. Do not breast-feed.

**Geriatric Considerations:** Elderly patients have been reported to have a higher incidence of constipation and may be more sensitive to the renal effects of ibuprofen. Therefore, consider using lower doses or longer intervals between doses if alternative agents cannot be used.

**Related Information**

Ibuprofen *on page 592*

## Hydrocodone and Phenylpropanolamine

(hye droe KOE done & fen il proe pa NOLE a meen)

**U.S. Brand Names** Codamine®; Codamine® Pediatric; Hycomine®; Hycomine® Pediatric; Hydrocodone PA® Syrup

**Synonyms** Phenylpropanolamine and Hydrocodone

**Therapeutic Category** Antitussive/Decongestant

**Pregnancy Risk Factor** C

**Lactation** Excretion in breast milk unknown/contraindicated

**Use** Symptomatic relief of cough and nasal congestion

**Contraindications** Hypersensitivity to hydrocodone, phenylpropanolamine, or any component; MAO inhibitor therapy; hypertension; hyperthyroidism; increased cranial pressure; heart disease; diabetes; depressed ventilatory function

**Warnings** Avoid use in severe pulmonary or liver disease. Use cautiously in the elderly. May be habit-forming. Administer with same degree of caution appropriate to use of other narcotic drugs. Produces dose-related respiratory depression. Produces adverse reactions which may obscure the clinical course of patients with head injuries. May obscure diagnosis or clinical course of patients with acute abdominal conditions.

**Drug Interactions**

**Increased Effect/Toxicity:** CNS depressants, phenothiazines, tricyclic antidepressants, other narcotics, general anesthetics, other tranquilizers, sedative-hypnotics increase CNS depression. Hypertensive crisis may occur with concurrent use of phenylpropanolamine and MAO inhibitors, indomethacin, beta-blockers, methyldopa.

**Adverse Reactions** Incidence unknown:

Cardiovascular: Hypertension, postural hypotension, tachycardia, palpitations

Central nervous system: Sedation, drowsiness, mental clouding, lethargy, impairment of mental and physical performance, anxiety, fear, dysphoria, dizziness, psychic dependence, mood changes

Dermatologic: Rash, pruritus

Gastrointestinal: Nausea, vomiting, constipation with prolonged use

Genitourinary: Ureteral spasm, spasm of vesical sphincters and urinary retention

Ocular: Blurred vision

Respiratory: Respiratory depression

**Overdose/Toxicology** Symptoms of overdose include respiratory depression, Cheyne-Stokes respiration and cyanosis, extreme somnolence progressing to stupor or coma, skeletal muscle flaccidity, cold clammy skin, sometimes bradycardia and hypotension. Naloxone, 2 mg I.V. with repeat administration as necessary up to a total of 10 mg, can also be used to reverse toxic effects of the opiate.

**Pharmacodynamics/Kinetics**

**Half-life Elimination:** Hydrocodone: 3.8 hours

**Time to Peak:** Hydrocodone: 1.3 hours

**Metabolism:** Hydrocodone: Liver

**Excretion:** Hydrocodone: Urine

**Duration:** Hydrocodone: 4-6 hours

**Formulations**

Syrup:

Codamine®, Hycomine®: Hydrocodone bitartrate 5 mg and phenylpropanolamine hydrochloride 25 mg per 5 mL (480 mL)

Codamine® Pediatric, Hycomine® Pediatric: Hydrocodone bitartrate 2.5 mg and phenylpropanolamine hydrochloride 12.5 mg per 5 mL (480 mL)

**Dosing**

**Adults:** 5 mL every 4 hours; maximum: 30 mL in 24 hours

**Elderly:** Refer to adult dosing; use with caution.

**Stability**

**Storage:** Store at controlled room temperature 15°C to 30°C (59°F to 86°F).

**Additional Nursing Issues**

**Physical Assessment:** Assess effectiveness and interactions of other medications (see Drug Interactions). See Contraindications and Warnings/Precautions for cautious use. **Note:** May be habit-forming. Monitor effectiveness of therapy (relief of cough, lung sounds, and respiratory pattern) and adverse reactions (eg, cardiac and CNS changes - see Adverse Reactions) at beginning of therapy and periodically with long-term use. Assess knowledge/teach patient appropriate use, interventions to reduce side effects, and adverse symptoms to report. **Pregnancy risk factor C** - benefits of use should outweigh possible risks. Breast-feeding is contraindicated.

**Patient Information/Instruction:** Take only as prescribed; do not exceed prescribed dose or frequency. May be habit-forming. Maintain adequate hydration (2-3 L/day of fluids unless instructed to restrict fluid intake). Avoid use of other depressants, alcohol, or sleep-inducing medications, or tranquilizers or pain medications unless approved by prescriber. You may experience orthostatic hypotension (change position slowly when rising from sitting or lying or when climbing stairs); drowsiness, impaired coordination, or blurred vision (use caution when driving or engaging in tasks requiring alertness until response to drug is known); nausea or vomiting (frequent small meals, frequent mouth care, chewing gum, or sucking hard candy may help); or urinary retention (void before taking medication). Report persistent CNS changes (dizziness, sedation, tremor, anxiety, mood changes, or agitation), difficulty breathing, visual changes, pain on urination or inability to void, or lack of improvement or worsening or condition. **Pregnancy/breast-feeding precautions:** Inform prescriber if you are or intend to be pregnant. Do not breast-feed.

**Geriatric Considerations:** Use with caution in the elderly.

**Pregnancy Issues:** Not known whether either of the two components causes fetal harm; give only if clearly needed.

**Related Information**

Phenylpropanolamine *on page 922*

## Hydrocodone, Chlorpheniramine, Phenylephrine, Acetaminophen, and Caffeine

(hye droe KOE done, klor fen IR a meen, fen il EF rin, a seet a MIN oh fen, & KAF een)

**U.S. Brand Names** Hycomine® Compound

**Synonyms** Acetaminophen, Caffeine, Hydrocodone, Chlorpheniramine, and Phenylephrine; Caffeine, Hydrocodone, Chlorpheniramine, Phenylephrine, and Acetaminophen; Chlorpheniramine, Hydrocodone, Phenylephrine, Acetaminophen, and Caffeine; Phenylephrine, Hydrocodone, Chlorpheniramine, Acetaminophen, and Caffeine

**Therapeutic Category** Antitussive

**Pregnancy Risk Factor** C

**Lactation** Excretion in breast milk unknown/contraindicated

**Use** Symptomatic relief of cough and symptoms of upper respiratory infection

**Contraindications** Hypersensitivity to any component; patients on MAO inhibitors; patients with heart disease, hypertension, diabetes, hyperthyroidism, presence of intracranial lesion associated with increased intracranial pressure; depressed ventilatory function

**Warnings** May be habit-forming. Prescribe and administer with the same degree of caution appropriate to the use of other narcotic drugs or prostatic hypertrophy. Produces dose-related respiratory depression. May produce adverse reactions which may obscure the clinical course of patients with head injuries. May obscure the diagnosis or clinical course of patients with acute abdominal conditions.

**Drug Interactions**

**Increased Effect/Toxicity:** Other narcotics, analgesics, general anesthetics, phenothiazines, other tranquilizers, sedative-hypnotics, or other CNS depressants (alcohol) may cause additive CNS depression. MAO inhibitors or other sympathomimetics may elevate blood pressure or increase anticholinergic side effects of antihistamines.

**Adverse Reactions**

Cardiovascular: Hypertension, postural hypotension, tachycardia, palpitations

Central nervous system: Sedation, drowsiness, mental clouding, lethargy, impairment of mental and physical performance, anxiety, fear, dysphoria, dizziness, psychic dependence, mood changes

Dermatologic: Rash, pruritus

Gastrointestinal: Nausea, vomiting, constipation with prolonged use

Genitourinary: Ureteral spasms, spasm of vesical sphincters and urinary retention

Ocular: Blurred vision

Respiratory: Respiratory depression

**Pharmacodynamics/Kinetics**

**Half-life Elimination:** Hydrocodone: 3.8 hours

**Time to Peak:** Hydrocodone: 1.3 hours

**Metabolism:** Hydrocodone: Liver

**Excretion:** Hydrocodone: Urine

**Duration:** Hydrocodone: 4-6 hours

**Formulations** Tablet: Hydrocodone bitartrate 5 mg, chlorpheniramine maleate 2 mg, phenylephrine hydrochloride 10 mg, acetaminophen 250 mg, and caffeine 30 mg

**Dosing**

**Adults:** Oral: 1 tablet every 4 hours, up to 4 times/day; interval should **not** be less than 4 hours.

**Elderly:** Refer to dosing in individual monographs.

**Stability**

**Storage:** Store at controlled room temperature 15°C to 30°C (59°F to 86°F).

**Additional Nursing Issues**

**Physical Assessment:** Assess effectiveness and interactions of other medications (see Drug Interactions). See Contraindications and Warnings/Precautions for cautious use. **Note:** May be habit-forming. Monitor effectiveness of therapy (relief of cough, lung sounds, and respiratory pattern) and adverse reactions (eg, cardiac and CNS changes, respiratory depression - see Adverse Reactions) at beginning of therapy and periodically with long-term use. Assess knowledge/teach patient appropriate use, interventions to reduce side effects, and adverse symptoms to report. **Pregnancy risk factor C** - benefits of use should outweigh possible risks. Breast-feeding is contraindicated.

**Patient Information/Instruction:** Take only as prescribed; do not exceed prescribed dose or frequency. May be habit-forming. Maintain adequate hydration (2-3 L/day of fluids unless instructed to restrict fluid intake). Avoid use of other depressants, alcohol, or sleep-inducing medications, or tranquilizers or pain medications unless approved by prescriber. You may experience orthostatic hypotension (change position slowly when rising from sitting or lying or when climbing stairs); drowsiness, impaired coordination, or blurred vision (use caution when driving or engaging in tasks requiring alertness until response to drug is known); nausea or vomiting (frequent small meals, frequent mouth care, chewing gum, or sucking hard candy may help); urinary retention (void before taking medication); or constipation (increased exercise, fluids or dietary fruit and fiber may help). Report persistent CNS changes (dizziness, sedation, tremor, anxiety, mood changes, or agitation); chest pain, palpitations, rapid heartbeat; difficulty breathing; visual changes; pain on urination or inability to void; or lack of improvement or worsening or condition. **Pregnancy/breast-feeding precautions:** Inform prescriber if you are or intend to be pregnant. Do not breast-feed.

**Geriatric Considerations:** Antihistamines may produce drowsiness or excitation especially in the elderly.

**Pregnancy Issues:** Not known whether any of the components can cause fetal harm; give only if clearly needed.

**Related Information**

Acetaminophen *on page 32*
Phenylephrine *on page 920*

♦ **Hydrocodone PA® Syrup** *see* Hydrocodone and Phenylpropanolamine *on page 574*

## Hydrocodone, Pseudoephedrine, and Guaifenesin

(hye droe KOE done, soo doe e FED rin, & gwye FEN e sin)

**U.S. Brand Names** Cophene XP®; Detussin® Expectorant; SRC® Expectorant; Tussafin® Expectorant

**Synonyms** Guaifenesin, Hydrocodone, and Pseudoephedrine; Pseudoephedrine, Hydrocodone, and Guaifenesin

**Therapeutic Category** Antitussive/Decongestant/Expectorant

**Pregnancy Risk Factor** C

**Lactation** Enters breast milk/contraindicated

**Use** Symptomatic relief of irritating, nonproductive cough associated with respiratory conditions such as bronchitis, bronchial asthma, tracheobronchitis, and the common cold

**Contraindications** Hypersensitivity to any ingredient or component; severe hypertension; severe coronary artery disease; concurrent use with MAO inhibitors

**Warnings** May be habit-forming. Prescribe and administer the same degree of caution as all oral medications containing narcotics. Use caution in patients with hypertension, diabetes, ischemic heart disease, hyperthyroidism, increased intraocular pressure, prostatic hypertrophy. Patients with severe respiratory impairment or patients with impaired respiratory drive.

**Drug Interactions**

**Increased Effect/Toxicity:** Beta-blockers and MAO inhibitors potentiate sympathomimetic effects of pseudoephedrine. Sympathomimetics may reduce the antihypertensive effects of methyldopa, and reserpine. Other narcotics, analgesics, general anesthetics, phenothiazines, other tranquilizers, sedative hypnotics, other CNS depressants (alcohol) may cause increased CNS depression.

**Effects on Lab Values** Guaifenesin interferes with the colorimetric determination of 5-hydroxyindoleacetic acid (5-HIAA) and vanillylmandelic acid (VMS)

**Adverse Reactions** Incidence unknown:

Cardiovascular: Arrhythmias, tachycardia, hypertension

Central nervous system: Drowsiness, fear, anxiety, tenseness, restlessness, pallor, insomnia, hallucinations, CNS depression

Gastrointestinal: GI upset, nausea, constipation with prolonged use

Genitourinary: Dysuria

Hepatic: Slight elevation in serum transaminase levels

Neuromuscular & skeletal: Weakness, tremor

Respiratory: Respiratory difficulty

Patients hyper-reactive to pseudoephedrine may display ephedrine-like reactions such as tachycardia, palpitations, headache, dizziness, or nausea; patient idiosyncrasy to adrenergic agents may be manifested by insomnia, dizziness, weakness, tremor, or arrhythmias.

**Overdose/Toxicology** Overdosage in the elderly may cause hallucinations, convulsions, CNS depression, or death. Naloxone, 2 mg I.V. with repeat administration as necessary up to a total of 10 mg, can also be used to reverse toxic effects of the opiate.

**Pharmacodynamics/Kinetics**

**Half-life Elimination:** Hydrocodone: 3.8 hours

**Time to Peak:** Hydrocodone: 1.3 hours

**Metabolism:** Hydrocodone: Liver

**Excretion:** Hydrocodone: Urine

**Duration:** Hydrocodone: 4-6 hours

**Formulations** Liquid: Hydrocodone bitartrate 5 mg, pseudoephedrine hydrochloride 60 mg, and guaifenesin 200 mg per 5 mL with alcohol 12.5% (480 mL)

**Dosing**

**Adults:** Oral: 5 mL every 6 hours

**Elderly:** Refer to dosing in individual monographs.

**Additional Nursing Issues**

**Physical Assessment:** Assess effectiveness and interactions of other medications (see Drug Interactions). See Contraindications and Warnings/Precautions for cautious use. **Note:** May be habit-forming. Monitor effectiveness of therapy (relief of cough, lung sounds, and respiratory pattern) and adverse reactions (eg, cardiac and CNS changes - see Adverse Reactions) at beginning of therapy and periodically with long-term use. Assess knowledge/teach patient appropriate use, interventions to reduce side effects, and adverse symptoms to report. **Pregnancy risk factor C** - benefits of use should outweigh possible risks. Breast-feeding is contraindicated.

**Patient Information/Instruction:** Take only as prescribed; do not exceed prescribed dose or frequency. May be habit-forming. Maintain adequate hydration (2-3 L/day of fluids unless instructed to restrict fluid intake). Avoid use of other depressants, alcohol, or sleep-inducing medications, or tranquilizers or pain medications unless approved by prescriber. You may experience orthostatic hypotension (change position slowly when rising from sitting or lying or climbing stairs); drowsiness, impaired coordination, or blurred vision (use caution when driving or engaging in tasks requiring alertness until response to drug is known); nausea or vomiting (frequent small meals, frequent mouth

(Continued)

## Hydrocodone, Pseudoephedrine, and Guaifenesin *(Continued)*

care, chewing gum, or sucking hard candy may help); constipation (increased exercise, fluids, or dietary fruit and fiber may help). Report persistent CNS changes (dizziness, sedation, tremor, or agitation), difficulty breathing, persistent abdominal cramping, visual changes, or lack of improvement or worsening or condition. **Pregnancy/breast-feeding precautions:** Inform prescriber if you are or intend to be pregnant. Do not breast-feed.

**Geriatric Considerations:** Elderly are more likely to have adverse reactions.

**Pregnancy Issues:** Not known whether any of three components can cause fetal harm; give only if clearly needed.

**Related Information**

Guaifenesin *on page 548*
Pseudoephedrine *on page 992*

- **Hydrocort®** *see* Hydrocortisone *on this page*
- **Hydrocort®** *see* Topical Corticosteroids *on page 1152*

## Hydrocortisone (hye droe KOR ti sone)

**U.S. Brand Names** Acticort 100®; A-hydroCort®; Ala-Cort®; Ala-Scalp®; Anucort-HC® Suppository; Anuprep HC® Suppository; Anusol® HC-1 [OTC]; Anusol® HC-2.5% [OTC]; Anusol-HC® Suppository; CaldeCORT®; CaldeCORT® Anti-Itch Spray; Cetacort®; Clocort® Maximum Strength; CortaGel® [OTC]; Cortaid® Maximum Strength [OTC]; Cortaid® With Aloe [OTC]; Cort-Dome®; Cortef®; Cortef® Feminine Itch; Cortenema®; Corticaine®; Cortifoam®; Cortizone®-5 [OTC]; Cortizone®-10 [OTC]; Delcort®; Dermacort®; Dermarest Dricort®; DermiCort®; Dermolate® [OTC]; Dermtex® HC With Aloe; Eldecort®; Gynecort® [OTC]; Hemril-HC® Uniserts®; Hi-Cor-1.0®; Hi-Cor-2.5®; Hycort®; Hydrocort®; Hydrocortone® Acetate; Hydrocortone® Phosphate; HydroSKIN®; Hydro-Tex® [OTC]; Hytone®; LactiCare-HC®; Lanacort® [OTC]; Locoid®; Nutracort®; Orabase® HCA; Pandel®; Penecort®; Procort® [OTC]; Proctocort™; Scalpicin®; Solu-Cortef®; S-T Cort®; Synacort®; Tegrin®-HC [OTC]; Texacort®; U-Cort™; Westcort®

**Synonyms** Compound F

**Therapeutic Category** Corticosteroid, Oral; Corticosteroid, Parenteral; Corticosteroid, Rectal

**Pregnancy Risk Factor** C

**Lactation** Excretion in breast milk unknown

**Use** Management of adrenocortical insufficiency; relief of inflammation of corticosteroid-responsive dermatoses (low and medium potency topical corticosteroid); adjunctive treatment for ulcerative colitis

**Mechanism of Action/Effect** Decreases inflammation by suppression of migration of polymorphonuclear leukocytes and reversal of increased capillary permeability

**Contraindications** Hypersensitivity to hydrocortisone; serious infections, except septic shock or tuberculous meningitis; known viral, fungal, or tubercular skin lesions

**Warnings** Use with caution in patients with hyperthyroidism, cirrhosis, nonspecific ulcerative colitis, hypertension, osteoporosis, thromboembolic tendencies, CHF, convulsive disorders, myasthenia gravis, thrombophlebitis, peptic ulcer, and diabetes. Acute adrenal insufficiency may occur with abrupt withdrawal after long-term therapy or with stress. Young pediatric patients may be more susceptible to adrenal axis suppression from topical therapy. Because of the risk of adverse effects, systemic corticosteroids should be used cautiously in the elderly, in the smallest possible dose, and for the shortest possible time. Pregnancy factor C.

**Drug Interactions**

**Cytochrome P-450 Effect:** CYP2D6 and 3A3/4 enzyme substrate

**Decreased Effect:** Hydrocortisone may decrease the hypoglycemic effect of insulin. Phenytoin, phenobarbital, ephedrine, and rifampin increase metabolism of hydrocortisone resulting in a decreased steroid blood level.

**Increased Effect/Toxicity:** Hydrocortisone in combination with oral anticoagulants may increase prothrombin time. Potassium-depleting diuretics increase risk of hypokalemia. Cardiac glycosides increase risk of arrhythmias or digitalis toxicity secondary to hypokalemia.

**Adverse Reactions**

**Systemic:**

>10%:

Central nervous system: Insomnia, nervousness
Gastrointestinal: Increased appetite, indigestion

1% to 10%:

Central nervous system: Dizziness, lightheadedness, headache
Dermatologic: Hirsutism, hypopigmentation
Endocrine & metabolic: Diabetes mellitus
Neuromuscular & skeletal: Arthralgia
Ocular: Cataracts, glaucoma
Respiratory: Epistaxis
Miscellaneous: Sweating

<1% (Limited to important or life-threatening symptoms): Seizures, pseudotumor cerebri, Cushing's syndrome, pituitary-adrenal axis suppression, growth suppression, glucose intolerance, hypokalemia, alkalosis, amenorrhea, sodium and water retention, hyperglycemia,

**Topical:**

1% to 10%:

Dermatologic: Itching, allergic contact dermatitis, erythema, dryness papular rashes, folliculitis, furunculosis, pustules, pyoderma, vesiculation, hyperesthesia, skin infection (secondary)

Local: Burning, irritation

<1% (Limited to important or life-threatening symptoms): Cushing's syndrome, hypokalemic syndrome, glaucoma, cataracts (posterior subcapsular)

**Overdose/Toxicology** When consumed in high doses for prolonged periods, systemic hypercorticism and adrenal suppression may occur. In those cases, discontinuation of the corticosteroid should be done judiciously.

**Pharmacodynamics/Kinetics**

**Half-life Elimination:** Biologic: 8-12 hours

**Metabolism:** Liver

**Excretion:** Renally, mainly as 17-hydroxysteroids and 17-ketosteroids

**Onset:**

Hydrocortisone acetate: Slow onset but long duration of action when compared with more soluble preparations.

Hydrocortisone sodium phosphate: A water soluble salt with a rapid onset but short duration of action.

Hydrocortisone sodium succinate: A water soluble salt which is rapidly active.

**Formulations**

Acetate:

Aerosol, rectal (Cortifoam®): 10% [90 mg/applicatorful] 20 g

Cream:

CaldeCORT®, Corticaine®, Gynecort®, Cortaid® with Aloe, Cortef® Feminine Itch, Lanacort®: 0.5% (15 g, 22.5 g, 30 g)

Anusol-HC-1®, CaldeCORT®, Clocort® Maximum Strength, Cortaid® Maximum Strength, Dermarest Dricort®, U-Cort™: 1% (15 g, 21 g, 30 g, 120 g)

Ointment, topical:

Cortaid® with Aloe, Lanacort® 5: 0.5% (15 g, 30 g)

Gynecort® 10, Lanacort® 10: 1% (15 g, 30 g)

Injection, suspension (Hydrocortone® Acetate): 25 mg/mL (5 mL, 10 mL); 50 mg/mL (5 mL, 10 mL)

Paste (Orabase® HCA): 0.5% (5 g)

Solution, topical (Scalpicin®): 1%

Suppository, rectal (Anucort-HC®, Anuprep HC®, Anusol-HC®, Hemril-HC® Uniserts®): 25 mg

Base:

Aerosol, topical:

CaldeCORT® Anti-Itch Spray, Cortaid®: 0.5% (45 g, 58 g)

Cortaid® Maximum Strength: 1% (45 mL)

Cream:

Cort-Dome®, Corticaine®, Cortizone®-5, DermiCort®, Dermolate®, Dermtex® HC with Aloe, HydroSKIN®, Hydro-Tex®: 0.5% (15 g, 30 g, 120 g, 454 g)

Ala-Cort®, Cort-Dome®, Delcort®, Dermacort®, DermiCort®, Eldecort®, Hi-Cor-1.0®, Hycort®, Hytone®, Nutracort®, Penecort®, Synacort®: 1% (15 g, 20 g, 30 g, 60 g, 120 g, 240 g, 454 g)

Anusol-HC-2.5%®, Eldecort®, Hi-Cor-2.5®, Hydrocort®, Hytone®, Synacort®: 2.5% (15 g, 20 g, 30 g, 60 g, 120 g, 240 g, 454 g)

Rectal (Proctocort™): 1% (30 g)

Gel:

CortaGel®: 0.5% (15 g, 30 g)

CortaGel® Extra Strength: 1% (15 g, 30 g)

Lotion:

Cetacort®, DermiCort®, HydroSKIN®, S-T Cort®: 0.5% (60 mL, 120 mL)

Acticort 100®, Cetacort®, Cortizone-10®, Dermacort®, HydroSKIN® Maximum Strength, Hytone®, LactiCare-HC®, Nutracort®: 1% (60 mL, 120 mL)

Ala-Scalp®: 2% (30 mL)

Hytone®, LactiCare-HC®, Nutracort®: 2.5% (60 mL, 120 mL)

Ointment, topical:

Cortizone®-5, HydroSKIN®: 0.5% (30 g)

Cortizone®-10, Hycort®, HydroSKIN®, Hydro-Tex®, Hytone®, Tegrin®-HC: 1% (15 g, 20 g, 30 g, 60 g, 120 g, 240 g, 454 g)

Hytone®: 2.5% (20 g, 30 g)

Solution:

Pentecort®: 1% (30 mL, 60 mL)

Texacort®: 1% (30 mL)

Suspension, rectal (Cortenema®): 100 mg/60 mL (7s)

Tablet:

Cortef®: 5 mg, 10 mg, 20 mg

Hydrocortone®: 10 mg, 20 mg

Butyrate:

Locoid®:

Cream: 0.1% (15 g, 45 g)

Ointment, topical: 0.1% (15 g, 45 g)

Solution, topical: 0.1% (20 mL, 60 mL)

Pandel®: Cream: 1% (15 g, 45 g)

Cypionate:

Suspension, oral (Cortef®): 10 mg/5 mL (120 mL)

(Continued)

## Hydrocortisone *(Continued)*

Sodium phosphate:
Injection (Hydrocortone® Phosphate): 50 mg/mL (2 mL, 10 mL)
Sodium succinate:
Injection (A-hydroCort®, Solu-Cortef®): 100 mg, 250 mg, 500 mg, 1000 mg
Valerate (Westcort®):
Cream: 0.2% (15 g, 45 g, 60 g)
Ointment, topical: 0.2% (15 g, 45 g, 60 g, 120 g)

### Dosing

**Adults:** Dose should be based on severity of disease and patient response.

Acute adrenal insufficiency: I.M., I.V.: Succinate: 100 mg I.V. bolus, then 300 mg/day in divided doses every 8 hours or as a continuous infusion for 48 hours. Once patient is stable change to oral, 50 mg every 8 hours for 6 doses, then taper to 30-50 mg/day in divided doses.

Chronic adrenal corticoid insufficiency: Oral: 20-30 mg/day

Anti-inflammatory or immunosuppressive: Oral, I.M., I.V.: Succinate: 15-240 mg every 12 hours

Congenital adrenal hyperplasia: Oral: Initial: 30-36 mg/m$^2$/day with $^1/_3$ of dose every morning and $^2/_3$ every evening or $^1/_4$ every morning and mid-day and $^1/_2$ every evening; maintenance: 20-25 mg/m$^2$/day in divided doses

Shock: I.M., I.V.: Succinate: 500 mg to 2 g every 2-6 hours

Status asthmaticus: I.V.: Succinate: 1-2 mg/kg/dose every 6 hours for 24 hours, then maintenance of 0.5-1 mg/kg every 6 hours

Rheumatic diseases:
Intralesional, intra-articular, soft tissue injection: Acetate:
Large joints: 25 mg (up to 37.5 mg)
Small joints: 10-25 mg
Tendon sheaths: 5-12.5 mg
Soft tissue infiltration: 25-50 mg (up to 75 mg)
Bursae: 25-37.5 mg
Ganglia: 12.5-25 mg

Dermatosis: Topical: Apply to affected area 3-4 times/day.

Ulcerative colitis: Rectal: 10-100 mg 1-2 times/day for 2-3 weeks

**Elderly:** Because of the risk of adverse effects, systemic corticosteroids should be used cautiously in the elderly, in the smallest possible dose, and for the shortest possible time.

### Administration

**Oral:** Administer with food or milk to decrease GI upset.

**I.V.:**

Parenteral: Hydrocortisone sodium succinate may be administered by I.M. or I.V. routes.

I.V. bolus: Dilute to 50 mg/mL and give over 30 seconds to several minutes (depending on the dose).

I.V. intermittent infusion: Dilute to 1 mg/mL and give over 20-30 minutes.

**Note:** Should be administered in a 0.1-1 mg/mL concentration due to stability problems.

**Topical:** Apply a thin film to clean, dry skin and rub in gently.

### Stability

**Storage:** Hydrocortisone sodium phosphate and hydrocortisone sodium succinate are clear, light yellow solutions which are heat labile.

**Reconstitution:** After initial reconstitution, hydrocortisone sodium succinate solutions are stable for 3 days at room temperature and refrigeration if protected from light. Stability of parenteral admixture (Solu-Cortef®) at room temperature (25°C) and at refrigeration temperature (4°C) is concentration dependent.

Minimum volume: Concentration should not exceed 1 mg/mL.
Stability of concentration ≤1 mg/mL: 24 hours
Stability of concentration >1 mg/mL to <25 mg/mL: Unpredictable, 4-6 hours
Stability of concentration ≥25 mg/mL: 3 days
Standard diluent (Solu-Cortef®): 50 mg/50 mL $D_5W$; 100 mg/100 mL $D_5W$

**Compatibility:** See the Compatibility of Drugs Chart *on page 1315*.

**Monitoring Laboratory Tests** Serum glucose, electrolytes

### Additional Nursing Issues

**Physical Assessment:** Monitor laboratory results, effects and interactions of other medications patient may be taking, response to therapy and adverse effects according to diagnosis, formulation of hydrocortisone, dosage, and extent of time used (see Drug Interactions, Adverse Reactions, Dosage Forms and Dosing). Systemic administration and long-term use will require close and frequent monitoring, especially for Cushing's syndrome. Assess/teach patient appropriate use, interventions for possible adverse reactions, and symptoms to report. **Pregnancy risk factor C** - benefits of use should outweigh possible risks. (Topical absorption may be minimal.) Note breast-feeding caution.

**Patient Information/Instruction:**

Systemic: Take as directed; do not increase doses and do not stop abruptly without consulting prescribed. Dosage of systemic hydrocortisone is usually tapered off gradually. Take oral dose with food to reduce GI upset. Hydrocortisone may cause immunosuppression and mask symptoms of infection; avoid exposure to contagion and notify prescriber of any signs of infection (eg, fever, chills, sore throat, injury) and notify dentist or surgeon (if necessary) that you are taking this medication. You may experience increased appetite, indigestion, or increased nervousness. Report any sudden weight gain (>5 lb/week), swelling of extremities or difficulty breathing, abdominal pain, severe vomiting, black or tarry stools, fatigue, anorexia, weakness, or unusual mood swings. **Pregnancy precautions:** Inform prescriber if you are or intend to be pregnant. Consult prescriber if breast-feeding.

Topical: Before applying, wash area gently and thoroughly. Apply gel, cream, or ointment in thin film to cleansed area and rub in gently until medication vanishes. Avoid exposing affected area to sunlight; you will be more sensitive and severe sunburn may occur. Consult prescriber if breast-feeding.

Rectal: Insert suppository gently as high as possible with gloved finger while lying down. Avoid injury with long or sharp fingernails. Remain in resting position for 10 minutes after insertion.

**Dietary Issues:** Systemic use of corticosteroids may require a diet with increased potassium, vitamins A, $B_6$, C, D, folate, calcium, zinc, phosphorus, and decreased sodium.

**Additional Information** Some formulations may contain sulfites.

Sodium content of 1 g (sodium succinate injection): 47.5 mg (2.07 mEq)

Hydrocortisone base topical cream, lotion, and ointments in concentrations of 0.25%, 0.5%, and 1% may be OTC or prescriptive depending on the product labeling

- **Hydrocortisone** *see* Topical Corticosteroids *on page 1152*
- **Hydrocortisone and Benzoyl Peroxide** *see* Benzoyl Peroxide and Hydrocortisone *on page 143*
- **Hydrocortisone and Clioquinol** *see* Clioquinol and Hydrocortisone *on page 284*
- **Hydrocortisone and Iodoquinol** *see* Iodoquinol and Hydrocortisone *on page 620*
- **Hydrocortisone and Lidocaine** *see* Lidocaine and Hydrocortisone *on page 677*
- **Hydrocortisone and Neomycin** *see* Neomycin and Hydrocortisone *on page 817*
- **Hydrocortisone, Bacitracin, Neomycin, and Polymyxin B** *see* Bacitracin, Neomycin, Polymyxin B, and Hydrocortisone *on page 131*
- **Hydrocortone® Acetate** *see* Hydrocortisone *on page 578*
- **Hydrocortone® Phosphate** *see* Hydrocortisone *on page 578*
- **Hydro-Crysti-12®** *see* Hydroxocobalamin *on page 583*
- **HydroDIURIL®** *see* Hydrochlorothiazide *on page 566*
- **Hydrogesic®** *see* Hydrocodone and Acetaminophen *on page 568*
- **Hydromagnesium Aluminate** *see* Magaldrate *on page 702*
- **Hydromet®** *see* Hydrocodone and Homatropine *on page 572*
- **Hydromorph Contin®** *see* Hydromorphone *on this page*

## Hydromorphone (hye droe MOR fone)

**U.S. Brand Names** Dilaudid®; Dilaudid-HP®

**Synonyms** Dihydromorphinone

**Therapeutic Category** Analgesic, Narcotic

**Pregnancy Risk Factor** B/D (if used for prolonged periods or in high doses at term)

**Lactation** Excretion in breast milk unknown/not recommended

**Use** Management of moderate to severe pain; antitussive at lower doses

**Mechanism of Action/Effect** Binds to opiate receptors in the CNS, causing inhibition of ascending pain pathways, altering the perception of and response to pain; causes cough supression by direct central action in the medulla; produces generalized CNS depression

**Contraindications** Hypersensitivity to hydromorphone, any component, or other phenanthrene derivative; pregnancy (if used for prolonged periods or in high doses at term)

**Warnings** Tablet and cough syrup contain tartrazine which may cause allergic reactions. Hydromorphone shares toxic potential of opiate agonists, and precaution of opiate agonist therapy should be observed. Extreme caution should be taken to avoid confusing the highly concentrated injection with the less concentrated injectable product. Injection contains benzyl alcohol. Use with caution in patients with hypersensitivity to other phenanthrene opiates, in patients with respiratory disease, or severe liver or renal failure.

**Drug Interactions**

**Increased Effect/Toxicity:** CNS depressants, phenothiazines, and tricyclic antidepressants may potentiate the adverse effects of hydromorphone.

**Effects on Lab Values** ↑ aminotransferase [ALT (SGPT)/AST (SGOT)] (S)

**Adverse Reactions**

>10%:

Cardiovascular: Palpitations, hypotension, peripheral vasodilation

Central nervous system: Dizziness, lightheadedness, drowsiness

Gastrointestinal: Anorexia

Miscellaneous: Physical and psychological dependence

1% to 10%:

Cardiovascular: Tachycardia, bradycardia, flushing of face

Central nervous system: CNS depression, increased intracranial pressure, fatigue, headache, nervousness, restlessness

Endocrine & metabolic: Antidiuretic hormone release

Gastrointestinal: Nausea, vomiting, constipation, stomach cramps, dry mouth, biliary tract spasm

Genitourinary: Decreased urination, ureteral spasm, urinary tract spasm

Hepatic: Increased transaminases

Neuromuscular & skeletal: Trembling, weakness

Ocular: Miosis, blurred vision

Respiratory: Respiratory depression, dyspnea, shortness of breath

(Continued)

## Hydromorphone *(Continued)*

**Overdose/Toxicology** Symptoms of overdose include CNS depression, respiratory depression, miosis, apnea, pulmonary edema, and convulsions. Along with supportive measures, naloxone, 2 mg I.V. with repeat administration as necessary up to a total of 10 mg, can also be used to reverse toxic effects of the opiate.

**Pharmacodynamics/Kinetics**

**Half-life Elimination:** 1-3 hours

**Metabolism:** Liver

**Excretion:** Urine

**Onset:** Analgesic effect: Within 15-30 minutes; Peak effect: Within 0.5-1.5 hours

**Duration:** 4-5 hours

**Formulations**

Hydromorphone hydrochloride:

Injection:

Dilaudid®: 1 mg/mL (1 mL); 2 mg/mL (1 mL, 20 mL); 3 mg/mL (1 mL); 4 mg/mL (1 mL)

Dilaudid-HP®: 10 mg/mL (1 mL, 2 mL, 5 mL)

Liquid: 5 mg/5 mL (480 mL)

Powder for injection: (Dilaudid-HP®): 250 mg

Suppository, rectal: 3 mg (6s)

Tablet: 1 mg, 2 mg, 3 mg, 4 mg, 8 mg

**Dosing**

**Adults:**

Doses should be titrated to appropriate analgesic effects; when changing routes of administration, note that oral doses are <50% as effective as parenteral doses (may be only one-fifth as effective).

Pain:

Oral, I.M., I.V., S.C.: 1-4 mg/dose every 4-6 hours as needed; usual adult dose: 2 mg/dose

Rectal: 3 mg every 6-8 hours

Antitussive: Oral: 1 mg every 3-4 hours as needed

**Elderly:** Doses should be titrated to appropriate analgesic effects. When changing routes of administration, note that oral doses are less than half as effective as parenteral doses (may be only 20% as effective).

Pain: Oral: 1-2 mg every 4-6 hours

Antitussive: Refer to adult dosing.

**Hepatic Impairment:** Dose adjustment should be considered.

**Stability**

**Storage:** Protect tablets from light. Do not store intact ampuls in refrigerator. A slightly yellowish discoloration has not been associated with a loss of potency.

**Compatibility:** I.V. is incompatible when mixed with minocycline, prochlorperazine, sodium bicarbonate, tetracycline, and thiopental.

**Additional Nursing Issues**

**Physical Assessment:** Assess other medications patient may be taking for additive or adverse interactions (see Drug Interactions). Monitor for effectiveness of pain relief and for signs of overdose (see above). Monitor blood pressure, CNS and respiratory status, and degree of sedation at beginning of therapy and at regular intervals with long-term use. May cause physical and/or psychological dependence. For inpatients, implement safety measures (eg, side rails up, call light within reach, instructions to call for assistance, etc). Assess knowledge/teach patient appropriate use (if self-administered). Teach patient to monitor for adverse reactions (see Adverse Reactions), adverse reactions to report, and appropriate interventions to reduce side effects. Discontinue slowly after prolonged use. **Pregnancy risk factor B/D** - see Pregnancy Risk Factor for cautious use. Breast-feeding is not recommended.

**Patient Information/Instruction:** If self-administered, use exactly as directed (do not increase dose or frequency); may cause physical and/or psychological dependence. While using this medication, do not use alcohol and other prescription or OTC medications (especially sedatives, tranquilizers, antihistamines, or pain medications) without consulting prescriber. Maintain adequate hydration (2-3 L/day of fluids unless instructed to restrict fluid intake). May cause dizziness, drowsiness, impaired coordination, or blurred vision (use caution when driving, climbing stairs, or changing position - rising from sitting or lying to standing, or when engaging in tasks requiring alertness until response to drug is known); loss of appetite, nausea, or vomiting (frequent mouth care, small frequent meals, chewing gum, or sucking lozenges may help); constipation (increased exercise, fluids, or dietary fruit and fiber may help - if constipation remains an unresolved problem, consult prescriber about use of stool softeners). Report chest pain, slow or rapid heartbeat, acute dizziness, or persistent headache; swelling of extremities or unusual weight gain; changes in urinary elimination; acute headache; back or flank pain or spasms; or other adverse reactions. **Pregnancy/breast-feeding precautions:** Inform prescriber if you are or intend to be pregnant. Breast-feeding is not recommended.

**Geriatric Considerations:** Elderly may be particularly susceptible to the CNS depressant and constipating effects of narcotics.

**Additional Information** The injection formulation contains benzyl alcohol. Some formulations may contain tartrazine or sulfites.

Equianalgesic doses:

Morphine 10 mg I.M. = hydromorphone 1.5 mg I.M.

Hydromorphone 1.3-1.5 mg I.M.; or 1-1.5 mg S.C. = hydromorphone 7.5 mg oral

**Related Information**
Controlled Substances Comparison *on page 1379*
Narcotic/Opioid Analgesic Comparison *on page 1396*

- **Hydropane®** *see* Hydrocodone and Homatropine *on page 572*
- **Hydro-Par®** *see* Hydrochlorothiazide *on page 566*
- **Hydrophen®** *see* Theophylline, Ephedrine, and Hydroxyzine *on page 1118*
- **Hydropres®** *see* Hydrochlorothiazide and Reserpine *on page 567*
- **Hydroquinol** *see* Hydroquinone *on this page*

## Hydroquinone (HYE droe kwin one)

**U.S. Brand Names** Ambi® Skin Tone [OTC]; Eldopaque® [OTC]; Eldopaque Forte®; Eldoquin® [OTC]; Eldoquin® Forte®; Esoterica® Facial [OTC]; Esoterica® Regular [OTC]; Esoterica® Sensitive Skin Formula [OTC]; Esoterica® Sunscreen [OTC]; Melanex®; Melpaque HP®; Melquin HP®; Nuquin HP®; Porcelana® [OTC]; Porcelana® Sunscreen [OTC]; Solaquin® [OTC]; Solaquin Forte®

**Synonyms** Hydroquinol; Quinol

**Therapeutic Category** Depigmenting Agent

**Pregnancy Risk Factor** C

**Lactation** Excretion in breast milk unknown

**Use** Gradual bleaching of hyperpigmented skin conditions

**Mechanism of Action/Effect** Produces reversible depigmentation of the skin by suppression of melanocyte metabolic processes, in particular the inhibition of the enzymatic oxidation of tyrosine to DOPA (3,4-dihydroxyphenylalanine); sun exposure reverses this effect and will cause repigmentation.

**Contraindications** Hypersensitivity to hydroquinone; sunburn; depilatory usage

**Warnings** Limit application to area no larger than face and neck or hands and arms. Pregnancy factor C.

**Adverse Reactions** 1% to 10%:
Dermatologic: Dermatitis, dryness, erythema, stinging, inflammatory reaction, sensitization
Local: Irritation

**Pharmacodynamics/Kinetics**
**Onset:** Onset of depigmentation produced by hydroquinone varies among individuals.
**Duration:** Duration of depigmentation produced by hydroquinone varies among individuals

**Formulations**
Cream, topical:
Esoterica® Sensitive Skin Formula: 1.5% [OTC] (85 g)
Eldopaque®, Eldoquin®, Esoterica® Facial, Esoterica® Regular, Porcelana®: 2% [OTC] (14.2 g, 28.4 g, 60 g, 85 g, 120 g)
Eldopaque Forte®, Eldoquin® Forte®, Melquin HP®: 4% (14.2 g, 28.4 g)
Cream, topical, with sunblock:
Esoterica® Sunscreen, Porcelana®, Solaquin®: 2% [OTC] (28.4 g, 120 g)
Melpaque HP®, Nuquin HP®, Solaquin Forte®: 4% (14.2 g, 28.4 g)
Gel, topical, with sunscreen (Solaquin Forte®): 4% (14.2 g, 28.4 g)
Solution, topical (Melanex®): 3% (30 mL)

**Dosing**
**Adults:** Topical: Apply a thin layer and rub in twice daily.
**Elderly:** Refer to adult dosing.

**Administration**
**Topical:** For external use only; avoid eye contact.

**Additional Nursing Issues**
**Physical Assessment:** See Contraindications and Warnings/Precautions for use cautions. See application directions above. When applied to large areas or for extensive periods of time, monitor for adverse reactions. Assess knowledge/teach patient appropriate application and use and adverse symptoms to report. **Pregnancy risk factor C** - systemic absorption may be minimal with appropriate use. Note breast-feeding caution.
**Patient Information/Instruction:** Use exactly as directed; do not overuse. Therapeutic effect may take several weeks. Test response by applying to small area of unbroken skin and check in 24 hours; if irritation or blistering occurs do not use. Avoid contact with eyes. Do not apply to open wounds or weeping areas. Before using, wash and dry area gently. Apply a thin film to affected area and rub in gently. Avoid direct sunlight or use sunblock or protective clothing to prevent repigmentation. Report swelling, redness, rash, itching, signs of infection, worsening of condition, or lack of healing. **Pregnancy/breast-feeding precautions:** Inform prescriber if you are or intend to be pregnant. Consult prescriber if breast-feeding.

- **Hydro-Serp®** *see* Hydrochlorothiazide and Reserpine *on page 567*
- **Hydroserpine®** *see* Hydrochlorothiazide and Reserpine *on page 567*
- **HydroSKIN®** *see* Hydrocortisone *on page 578*
- **Hydro-Tex® [OTC]** *see* Hydrocortisone *on page 578*
- **Hydro-Tex® [OTC]** *see* Topical Corticosteroids *on page 1152*
- **Hydrotropine®** *see* Hydrocodone and Homatropine *on page 572*

## Hydroxocobalamin (hye droks oh koe BAL a min)

**U.S. Brand Names** Alphamin®; Codroxomin®; Hybalamin®; Hydro-Cobex®; Hydro-Crysti-12®; LA-12®
(Continued)

## Hydroxocobalamin *(Continued)*

**Synonyms** Vitamin $B_{12a}$

**Therapeutic Category** Vitamin, Water Soluble

**Pregnancy Risk Factor** A/C (if doses exceed RDA recommendation)

**Lactation** Enters breast milk/compatible

**Use** Treatment of pernicious anemia, vitamin $B_{12}$ deficiency, increased $B_{12}$ requirements due to pregnancy, thyrotoxicosis, hemorrhage, malignancy, liver or kidney disease

**Mechanism of Action/Effect** Coenzyme for various metabolic functions, including fat and carbohydrate metabolism and protein synthesis, used in cell replication and hematopoiesis

**Contraindications** Hypersensitivity to cyanocobalamin, cobalt, or any component; patients with hereditary optic nerve atrophy

**Warnings** Some products contain benzoyl alcohol. Avoid use in premature infants. An intradermal test dose should be performed for hypersensitivity. Use only if oral supplementation not possible or when treating pernicious anemia. Pregnancy factor C (if doses exceed RDA recommendation).

**Adverse Reactions**

1% to 10%:

Dermatologic: Itching

Gastrointestinal: Diarrhea

<1% (Limited to important or life-threatening symptoms): Peripheral vascular thrombosis

**Formulations** Injection: 1000 mcg/mL (10 mL, 30 mL)

**Dosing**

**Adults:** Vitamin $B_{12}$ deficiency: I.M.: 30 mcg/day for 5-10 days, followed by 100-200 mcg/month

**Elderly:** Refer to adult dosing.

**Administration**

**I.M.:** Administer I.M. only. May require coadministration of folic acid.

**Monitoring Laboratory Tests** Reticulocyte count, Hct, iron and folic acid, and serum levels before treatment, after first week of treatment, and routinely thereafter

**Additional Nursing Issues**

**Physical Assessment:** See Contraindications and Warnings/Precautions for use cautions. Monitor laboratory tests at beginning of therapy and periodically with long-term therapy. Assess knowledge/teach patient appropriate administration (injection technique and needle disposal), nutritional counseling, and adverse symptoms to report. **Pregnancy risk factor A/C** - see Pregnancy Risk Factor for cautious use.

**Patient Information/Instruction:** Use exactly as directed. Pernicious anemia may require monthly injections for life. Report skin rash; swelling, pain, or redness in extremities; or acute persistent diarrhea.

**Geriatric Considerations:** Evidence exists that people, particularly elderly, whose serum cobalamin concentrations are <500 pg/mL, should receive replacement parenteral therapy. This recommendation is based upon neuropsychiatric disorders and cardiovascular disorders associated with lower sodium cobalamin concentrations.

♦ **Hydroxyamphetamine and Tropicamide** *see page 1248*

♦ **Hydroxycarbamide** *see* Hydroxyurea *on page 586*

## Hydroxychloroquine (hye droks ee KLOR oh kwin)

**U.S. Brand Names** Plaquenil®

**Therapeutic Category** Aminoquinoline (Antimalarial)

**Pregnancy Risk Factor** C

**Lactation** Enters breast milk/compatible

**Use** Suppresses and treats acute attacks of malaria; treatment of systemic lupus erythematosus and rheumatoid arthritis

**Mechanism of Action/Effect** Interferes with digestive vacuole function within sensitive malarial parasites by increasing the pH and interfering with lysosomal degradation of hemoglobin; inhibits locomotion of neutrophils and chemotaxis of eosinophils; impairs complement-dependent antigen-antibody reactions

**Contraindications** Hypersensitivity to hydroxychloroquine, 4-aminoquinoline derivatives, or any component; retinal or visual field changes attributable to 4-aminoquinolines

**Warnings** Use with caution in patients with hepatic disease, G-6-PD deficiency, psoriasis, and porphyria. Long-term use in children is not recommended. Perform baseline and periodic (6 months) ophthalmologic examinations. Test periodically for muscle weakness. Pregnancy factor C.

**Adverse Reactions**

>10%:

Central nervous system: Headache

Dermatologic: Itching

Gastrointestinal: Diarrhea, anorexia, nausea, stomach cramps, vomiting

Ocular: Ciliary muscle dysfunction

1% to 10%:

Central nervous system: Dizziness, lightheadedness, nervousness, restlessness

Dermatologic: Bleaching of hair, rash, discoloration of skin (black-blue)

Ocular: Ocular toxicity, keratopathy, retinopathy

<1% (Limited to important or life-threatening symptoms): Seizures, agranulocytosis, aplastic anemia, neutropenia, thrombocytopenia, neuromyopathy

**Overdose/Toxicology** Symptoms of overdose include headache, drowsiness, visual changes, cardiovascular collapse, and seizures followed by respiratory and cardiac arrest. Treatment is symptomatic. Urinary alkalinization will enhance renal elimination.

**Pharmacodynamics/Kinetics**

**Protein Binding:** 55%

**Half-life Elimination:** 32-50 days

**Metabolism:** Liver

**Excretion:** Urine, may be enhanced by urinary acidification

**Onset:** Rheumatic disease: May require 4-6 weeks to respond (maximum after several months)

**Formulations** Tablet, as sulfate: 200 mg [base 155 mg]

**Dosing**

**Adults:** Oral:

Chemoprophylaxis of malaria: 2 tablets/week on same day each week; begin 2 weeks before exposure; continue for 4-6 weeks after leaving endemic area.

Acute attack: 4 tablets first dose day 1; 2 tablets in 6 hours day 1; 2 tablets in 1 dose day 2; and 2 tablets in 1 dose on day 3.

Rheumatoid arthritis: 2-3 tablets/day to start taken with food or milk; increase dose until optimum response level is reached; usually after 4-12 weeks dose should be reduced by 1/2 and a maintenance dose of 1-2 tablets/day given.

Lupus erythematosus: 2 tablets every day or twice daily for several weeks depending on response; 1-2 tablets/day for prolonged maintenance therapy.

**Elderly:** Refer to adult dosing.

**Hepatic Impairment:** Use with caution, dosage adjustment may be necessary.

**Administration**

**Oral:** Take with food or milk.

**Monitoring Laboratory Tests** CBC, liver function

**Additional Nursing Issues**

**Physical Assessment:** See Contraindications and Warnings/Precautions for use cautions. Monitor effectiveness of therapy (according to purpose for therapy), laboratory tests (see Monitoring Laboratory Tests), and adverse response (see Adverse Reactions and Overdose/Toxicology). Assess knowledge/teach patient appropriate use, possible side effects/interventions, and adverse symptoms to report. Assess deep tendon reflexes; monitor for muscle weakness. **Pregnancy risk factor C** - benefits of use should outweigh possible risks.

**Patient Information/Instruction:** It is important to complete full course of therapy which may take up to 6 months for full effect. May be taken with meals to decrease GI upset and bitter aftertaste. Avoid alcohol. You should have regular ophthalmic exams (every 4-6 months) if using this medication over extended periods. You may experience skin discoloration (blue/black), hair bleaching, or skin rash. If you have psoriasis, you may experience exacerbation. You may experience dizziness, headache, nervousness, or lightheadedness (use caution when driving or engaging in tasks requiring alertness until response to drug is known); nausea, vomiting, or loss of appetite (small frequent meals, frequent mouth care, sucking lozenges, or chewing gum may help); or increased sensitivity to sunlight (wear dark glasses and protective clothing, use sunblock, and avoid direct exposure to sunlight). Report vision changes, rash or itching, persistent diarrhea or GI disturbances, change in hearing acuity or ringing in the ears, chest pain or palpitation, CNS changes, unusual fatigue, easy bruising or bleeding, or any other persistent adverse reactions. **Pregnancy precautions:** Inform prescriber if you are or intend to be pregnant.

**Additional Information**

Hydroxychloroquine sulfate 200 mg = hydroxychloroquine base 155 mg
Hydroxychloroquine sulfate 200 mg = chloroquine phosphate 250 mg

- **25-Hydroxycholecalciferol** *see* Calcifediol *on page 180*
- **Hydroxydaunomycin Hydrochloride** *see* Doxorubicin *on page 401*
- **Hydroxyethyl Starch** *see* Hetastarch *on page 560*

## Hydroxyprogesterone (hye droks ee proe JES te rone)

**U.S. Brand Names** Hylutin® Injection; Hyprogest® 250 Injection

**Therapeutic Category** Progestin

**Pregnancy Risk Factor** D

**Lactation** Excretion in breast milk unknown/use caution

**Use** Treatment of amenorrhea, abnormal uterine bleeding, endometriosis, uterine carcinoma

**Mechanism of Action/Effect** Natural steroid hormone that induces secretory changes in the endometrium, promotes mammary gland development, relaxes uterine smooth muscle, blocks follicular maturation and ovulation and maintains pregnancy

**Contraindications** Hypersensitivity to hydroxyprogesterone or any component; thrombophlebitis; thromboembolic disorders; cerebral hemorrhage; liver impairment; carcinoma of the breast; undiagnosed vaginal bleeding; pregnancy

**Warnings** Use with caution in patients with asthma, seizure disorders, migraine, cardiac or renal impairment, or a history of mental depression. Observe patients closely for signs or symptoms of thrombotic disorders. Use of any progestin during the first 4 months of pregnancy is not recommended.

**Drug Interactions**

**Decreased Effect:** Rifampin may increase clearance of hydroxyprogesterone.

**Effects on Lab Values** Thyroid function tests, liver function tests, and endocrine function tests

**Adverse Reactions**

>10%:

Cardiovascular: Edema

(Continued)

## Hydroxyprogesterone *(Continued)*

Endocrine & metabolic: Breakthrough bleeding, spotting, changes in menstrual flow, amenorrhea
Gastrointestinal: Anorexia
Local: Pain at injection site
Neuromuscular & skeletal: Weakness

1% to 10%:
Central nervous system: Mental depression, insomnia, fever
Dermatologic: Melasma or chloasma, allergic rash with or without pruritus
Gastrointestinal: Weight gain or loss
Genitourinary: Changes in cervical erosion and secretions, increased breast tenderness
Hepatic: Cholestatic jaundice

**Overdose/Toxicology** Toxicity is unlikely following single exposure of excessive doses. Supportive treatment is adequate in most cases.

**Pharmacodynamics/Kinetics**

**Time to Peak:** I.M.: 3-7 days; concentrations are measurable for 3-4 weeks after injection.

**Metabolism:** Liver

**Excretion:** Urine

**Formulations**

Hydroxyprogesterone caproate:
Injection:
125 mg/mL (10 mL)
Hylutin®, Hyprogest®: 250 mg/mL (5 mL)

**Dosing**

**Adults:** I.M.:
Amenorrhea: 375 mg; if no bleeding, begin cyclic treatment with estradiol valerate.
Production of secretory endometrium and desquamation: (Medical D and C): 125-250 mg administered on day 10 of cycle; repeat every 7 days until supression is no longer desired.
Uterine carcinoma: 1 g or more; may repeat one or more times weekly (1-7 g/week) for up to 12 weeks

**Elderly:** Refer to adult dosing.

**Administration**

**I.M.:** Administer deep I.M. only.

**Stability**

**Storage:** Store at <40°C (15°C to 30°C); avoid freezing.

**Monitoring Laboratory Tests** Thyroid, liver, and endocrine function

**Additional Nursing Issues**

**Physical Assessment:** Monitor blood pressure, mammogram, and results of Pap tests before beginning treatment and at least annually. Teach patient injection procedures if appropriate, possible side effects, and symptoms to report. Monitor serum glucose for diabetic patients during first months of therapy. **Pregnancy risk factor D** - assess knowledge/instruct patient on use of barrier contraceptive measures. Note breast-feeding caution.

**Patient Information/Instruction:** Maintain a regular schedule of injections as prescribed. This drug can only be given deep I.M. injection. If diabetic, monitor serum glucose closely. You may experience some sensitivity to sunlight; wear protective clothing, use sunblock, or avoid sunlight. You may experience dizziness; use caution when driving or engaging in tasks that require alertness until response to drug is known. Report rash, alopecia, radically increased weight gain or swelling, anorexia, muscular weakness, fever, or unresolved nausea or vomiting. Report immediately any swelling or warmth in calves, chest pain or respiratory difficulty, severe headache or acute dizziness, numbness and/or tingling in extremities. **Pregnancy/breast-feeding precautions:** Do not get pregnant while taking this medication; use appropriate barrier contraceptive measures (serious fetal damage has occurred). Consult prescriber if breast-feeding.

♦ **Hydroxypropyl Methylcellulose** *see page 1248*

## Hydroxyurea (hye droks ee yoor EE a)

**U.S. Brand Names** Droxia™; Hydrea®

**Synonyms** Hydroxycarbamide

**Therapeutic Category** Antineoplastic Agent, Antimetabolite

**Pregnancy Risk Factor** D

**Lactation** Enters breast milk/contraindicated

**Use** CML in chronic phase; radiosensitizing agent in the treatment of primary brain tumors; head and neck tumors; uterine cervix and nonsmall cell lung cancer; psoriasis; sickle cell anemia and other hemoglobinopathies; resistant chronic myelocytic leukemia; hematologic conditions such as essential thrombocythemia, polycythemia vera, hypereosinophilia, and hyperleukocytosis due to acute leukemia. Has shown activity against renal cell cancer; malignant melanoma; metastatic or inoperable carcinoma of the ovary; head, neck, and lip cancer; and prostate cancer.

Use in sickle cell disease: For patients >18 years of age who have had at least three "painful crises" in the previous year - to reduce frequency of these crises and the need for blood transfusions

**Unlabeled use:** Thrombocythemia; Has been used in combination with antiretroviral agents in the treatment of HIV

**Mechanism of Action/Effect** Interferes with synthesis of DNA, without interfering with RNA synthesis

**Contraindications** Hypersensitivity to hydroxyurea; severe anemia; severe bone marrow depression; WBC <2500/mm$^3$ or platelet count <100,000/mm$^3$; pregnancy

**Warnings** Use with caution in patients with renal impairment, in patients who have received prior irradiation therapy with exacerbation of postirradiation erythema, bone marrow suppression, erythrocytic abnormalities, mucositis, and in the elderly. The U.S. Food and Drug Administration (FDA) currently recommends that procedures for proper handling and disposal of antineoplastic agents be considered.

**Drug Interactions**

**Increased Effect/Toxicity:** Zidovudine, zalcitabine, didanosine may increase synergy. The potential for neurotoxicity may increase with concomitant administration with fluorouracil. Modulation of its metabolism and cytotoxicity → reduction of cytarabine dose is recommended.

**Adverse Reactions**

>10%:

- Central nervous system: Drowsiness
- Gastrointestinal: Mild to moderate nausea and vomiting may occur, as well as diarrhea, constipation, mucositis, ulceration of the GI tract, anorexia
- Hematologic: Anemia, leukopenia; Myelosuppression: Dose-limiting toxicity, causes a rapid drop in leukocyte count (seen in 4-5 days in nonhematologic malignancy and more rapidly in leukemia); thrombocytopenia and anemia occur less often; reversal of WBC count occurs rapidly, but the platelet count may take 7-10 days to recover.
  - WBC: Moderate
  - Platelets: Moderate
  - Onset (days): 7
  - Nadir (days): 10
  - Recovery (days): 21

1% to 10%:

- Dermatologic: Dermatologic changes (hyperpigmentation, erythema of the hands and face, maculopapular rash, or dry skin), alopecia
- Gastrointestinal: Stomatitis
- Hematologic: Thrombocytopenia
- Hepatic: Abnormal LFTs and hepatitis
- Miscellaneous: Carcinogenic potential

<1% (Limited to important or life-threatening symptoms): Neurotoxicity, seizures, elevation of hepatic enzymes, increased creatinine and BUN due to impairment of renal tubular function, acute diffuse pulmonary infiltrates (rare), dyspnea

**Overdose/Toxicology** Symptoms of overdose include myelosuppression, facial swelling, hallucinations, and disorientation. Treatment is supportive.

**Pharmacodynamics/Kinetics**

**Half-life Elimination:** 3-4 hours

**Time to Peak:** Within 2 hours

**Metabolism:** Liver

**Excretion:** Urine

**Formulations**

Capsule: 500 mg

Capsule (Droxia™): 200 mg, 300 mg, 400 mg

**Dosing**

**Adults:** Oral (refer to individual protocols):

Dose should always be titrated to patient response and WBC counts; usual oral doses range from 10-30 mg/kg/day or 500-3000 mg/day; if WBC count falls to <2500 cells/mm$^3$, or the platelet count to <100,000/mm$^3$, therapy should be stopped for at least 3 days and resumed when values rise toward normal.

- Solid tumors:
  - Intermittent therapy: 80 mg/kg as a single dose every third day
  - Continuous therapy: 20-30 mg/kg/day given as a single dose/day
- Concomitant therapy with irradiation: 80 mg/kg as a single dose every third day starting at least 7 days before initiation of irradiation
- Resistant chronic myelocytic leukemia: 20-30 mg/kg/day divided daily
- HIV (in combination with antiretroviral agents): 1000-1500 mg daily in single or divided doses
- Sickle cell anemia (moderate/severe disease): Hydroxyurea administration in adults (age range: 22-42 years) has produced beneficial effects in several small studies.
  - *Acceptable range:*
    - Neutrophils ≥2500 cells/mm$^3$
    - Platelets ≥95,000/mm$^3$
    - Hemoglobin >5.3 g/dL, and
    - Reticulocytes ≥95,000/mm$^3$ if the hemoglobin concentration is <9 g/dL
  - *Toxic range:*
    - Neutrophils <2000 cells/mm$^3$
    - Platelets <80,000/mm$^3$
    - Hemoglobin <4.5 g/dL
    - Reticulocytes <80,000/mm$^3$ if the hemoglobin concentration is <9 g/dL
  - Initial: 15 mg/kg/day, increased by 5 mg/kg every 12 weeks unless toxicity is observed or the maximum tolerated dose of 35 mg/kg/day is achieved.
  - Monitor for toxicity every 2 weeks. If toxicity occurs, stop treatment until the bone marrow recovers. Restart at 2.5 mg/kg/day less than the dose at which toxicity occurs. If no toxicity occurs over the next 12 weeks, then the subsequent dose

(Continued)

## Hydroxyurea *(Continued)*

should be increased by 2.5 mg/kg/day. Reduced dosage of hydroxyurea alternating with erythropoietin may decrease myelotoxicity and increase levels of fetal hemoglobin in patients who have not been helped by hydroxyurea alone.

**Elderly:** Refer to adult dosing.

**Renal Impairment:**

$Cl_{cr}$ 10-50 mL/minute: Administer 50% of normal dose.
$Cl_{cr}$ <10 mL/minute: Administer 20% of normal dose.
Hemodialysis effects: Unknown
CAPD effects: Unknown
CAVH effects: Unknown

**Administration**

**Oral:** Capsules may be opened and emptied into water (will not dissolve completely).

**Stability**

**Storage:** Store capsules at room temperature.

**Monitoring Laboratory Tests** CBC with differential, platelets, renal and liver function, serum uric acid

**Additional Nursing Issues**

**Physical Assessment:** Assess other medications patient may be taking for effectiveness and interactions (see Warnings/Precautions and Drug Interactions). Hydroxyurea therapy requires close supervision; monitor laboratory results before therapy and frequently during therapy (see list of necessary laboratory testing above), therapeutic therapeutic effects, and adverse reactions (eg, hematologic, renal, respiratory response, nutritional status, and opportunistic infection - see Adverse Reactions and Overdose/Toxicology). Observe exposure cautions: people not taking hydroxyurea should not be exposed to it; if powder from capsule is spilled, wipe up with a damp, disposable towel immediately, and discard the towel in a closed container such as a plastic bag and wash hands thoroughly. Assess knowledge/instruct patient (caregiver) appropriate use and handling, interventions to reduce side effects, and adverse symptoms to report. **Pregnancy risk factor D** - assess knowledge/instruct patient on use of barrier contraceptive measures. Breast-feeding is contraindicated.

**Patient Information/Instruction:** Take capsules exactly on schedule directed by prescriber (dosage and timing will be specific to purpose of therapy). Contents of capsule may be emptied into a glass of water and taken immediately. You will require frequent monitoring and blood tests while taking this medication to assess effectiveness and monitor adverse reactions. You will be susceptible to infection; avoid crowds, infected persons, and persons with contagious diseases. You may experience nausea, vomiting, or loss of appetite (small frequent meals, frequent mouth care, sucking lozenges, or chewing gum may help); constipation (increased exercise, fluid, or dietary fiber may help); diarrhea (buttermilk, boiled milk, or yogurt may help); mouth sores (frequent mouth care will help). Report persistent vomiting, diarrhea, constipation, stomach pain, or mouth sores; skin rash, redness, irritation, or sores; painful or difficult urination; increased confusion, depression, hallucinations, lethargy, or seizures; persistent fever or chills, unusual fatigue, white plaques in mouth, vaginal discharge, or unhealed sores; unusual lassitude, weakness, or muscle tremors; easy bruising/bleeding; or blood in vomitus, stool, or urine. People not taking hydroxyurea should not be exposed to it; if powder from capsule is spilled, wipe up with damp, disposable towel immediately, and discard the towel in a closed container, such as a plastic bag. Wash hands thoroughly. **Pregnancy/breast-feeding precautions:** Do not get pregnant while taking this medication; use appropriate barrier contraceptive measures. Do not breast-feed.

**Geriatric Considerations:** Elderly may be more sensitive to the effects of this drug. Advance dose slowly and adjust dose for renal function with careful monitoring.

♦ **25-Hydroxyvitamin $D_3$** *see* Calcifediol *on page 180*

## Hydroxyzine (hye DROKS i zeen)

**U.S. Brand Names** Anxanil®; Atarax®; Atozine®; Durrax®; Hy-Pam®; Hyzine-50®; Neucalm®; Quiess®; Rezine®; Vamate®; Vistacon-50®; Vistaquel®; Vistaril®; Vistazine®

**Therapeutic Category** Antiemetic; Antihistamine

**Pregnancy Risk Factor** C

**Lactation** Excretion in breast milk unknown

**Use** Treatment of anxiety, as a preoperative sedative, an antipruritic, an antiemetic, and in alcohol withdrawal symptoms

**Mechanism of Action/Effect** Competes with histamine for $H_1$-receptor sites on effector cells in the GI tract, blood vessels, and respiratory tract

**Contraindications** Hypersensitivity to hydroxyzine or any component

**Warnings** S.C., intra-arterial, and I.V. administration are **not** recommended since thrombosis and digital gangrene can occur. Extravasation can result in sterile abscess and marked tissue induration. Should be used with caution in patients with narrow-angle glaucoma, prostatic hypertrophy, bladder neck obstruction, and in patients with asthma or COPD. Anticholinergic effects are not well tolerated in the elderly. Hydroxyzine may be useful as a short-term antipruritic, but it is not recommended for use as a sedative or anxiolytic in the elderly. Pregnancy factor C.

**Drug Interactions**

**Decreased Effect:** Epinephrine decreases vasopressor effect.

**Increased Effect/Toxicity:** Increased toxicity with CNS depressants and anticholinergics.

**Adverse Reactions**

Local: **Irritant**

>10%:

Central nervous system: Slight to moderate drowsiness

Respiratory: Thickening of bronchial secretions

1% to 10%:

Central nervous system: Headache, fatigue, nervousness, dizziness

Gastrointestinal: Appetite increase, weight gain, nausea, diarrhea, abdominal pain, dry mouth

Neuromuscular & skeletal: Arthralgia

Respiratory: Pharyngitis

<1% (Limited to important or life-threatening symptoms): Palpitations, hypotension, edema, hepatitis, bronchospasm

**Overdose/Toxicology** Symptoms of overdose include seizures, sedation, and hypotension. There is no specific treatment for antihistamine overdose. Clinical toxicity is due to blockade of cholinergic receptors. For anticholinergic overdose with severe life-threatening symptoms, physostigmine 1-2 mg I.V. slowly, may be given to reverse these effects.

**Pharmacodynamics/Kinetics**

**Half-life Elimination:** 3-7 hours

**Time to Peak:** Within 2 hours

**Metabolism:** Exact fate is unknown

**Onset:** Within 15-30 minutes

**Duration:** 4-6 hours

**Formulations**

Hydroxyzine hydrochloride:

Injection:

Vistaril®: 25 mg/mL (1 mL, 2 mL, 10 mL)

Hyzine-50®, Neucalm®, Quiess®, Vistacon-50®, Vistaquel®, Vistaril®, Vistazine®: 50 mg/mL (1 mL, 2 mL, 10 mL)

Syrup (Atarax®): 10 mg/5 mL (120 mL, 480 mL, 4000 mL)

Tablet:

Anxanil®: 25 mg

Atarax®: 10 mg, 25 mg, 50 mg, 100 mg

Atozine®: 10 mg, 25 mg, 50 mg

Durrax®: 10 mg, 25 mg

Hydroxyzine pamoate:

Capsule:

Hy-Pam®: 25 mg, 50 mg

Vamate®: 25 mg, 50 mg, 100 mg

Vistaril®: 25 mg, 50 mg, 100 mg

Suspension, oral (Vistaril®:) 25 mg/5 mL (120 mL, 480 mL)

**Dosing**

**Adults:**

Antiemetic: I.M.: 25-100 mg/dose every 4-6 hours as needed

Anxiety: Oral: 25-100 mg 4 times/day; maximum: 600 mg/day

Preoperative sedation:

Oral: 50-100 mg

I.M.: 25-100 mg

Management of pruritus: Oral: 25 mg 3-4 times/day

**Elderly:** Management of pruritus: 10 mg 3-4 times/day; increase to 25 mg 3-4 times/day if necessary.

**Hepatic Impairment:** Change dosing interval to every 24 hours in patients with primary biliary cirrhosis.

**Administration**

**I.M.:** Administer deep in large muscle.

**I.V.:** Irritant. Use caution when administering I.V.

**I.V. Detail:** Extravasation can result in sterile abscess and marked tissue induration.

**Stability**

**Storage:** Protect from light. Store at 15°C to 30°C and protected from freezing.

**Compatibility:** I.V. is incompatible when mixed with aminophylline, amobarbital, chloramphenicol, dimenhydrinate, heparin, penicillin G, pentobarbital, phenobarbital, phenytoin, ranitidine, sulfisoxazole, and vitamin B complex with C. See the Compatibility of Drugs Chart *on page 1315.*

**Additional Nursing Issues**

**Physical Assessment:** Assess other medications patient may be taking for effectiveness and possible interactions (see Warnings/Precautions and Drug Interactions).

Systemic: Monitor therapeutic response and adverse reactions (see above); ensure patient safety (side rails up, call light within reach); have patient void prior to administration; and ensure adequate hydration and environmental temperature control.

Oral: Monitor therapeutic response according to purpose for use, adverse reactions (eg, acute atropine toxicity - see Warnings/Precautions, Adverse Reactions, and Overdose/Toxicology).

Assess knowledge/teach patient appropriate use, interventions to reduce side effects, and adverse symptoms to report. **Pregnancy risk factor C** - benefits of use should outweigh possible risks. Note breast-feeding caution.

**Patient Information/Instruction:** Take this drug as prescribed; do not increase dosage or discontinue without consulting prescriber. Store medication away from light.

(Continued)

## Hydroxyzine *(Continued)*

Maintain adequate hydration (2-3 L/day of fluids unless instructed to restrict fluid intake). Void before taking medication. Do not use excessive alcohol or other CNS depressants or sleeping aids without consulting prescriber. May cause dizziness, drowsiness, or blurred vision (use caution when driving or engaging in tasks requiring alertness until response to drug is known); or nausea, dry mouth, appetite disturbances (small frequent meals, frequent mouth care, or sucking hard candy may help). Report unusual weight gain, unresolved nausea or diarrhea, chest pain or palpitations, muscle or joint pain, excess sedation, sore throat, or difficulty breathing. **Pregnancy/ breast-feeding precautions:** Inform prescriber if you are or intend to be pregnant. Consult prescriber if breast-feeding.

**Geriatric Considerations:** Anticholinergic effects are not well tolerated in the elderly. Hydroxyzine may be useful as a short-term antipruritic, but it is not recommended for use as a sedative or anxiolytic in the elderly.

**Additional Information**

Hydroxyzine hydrochloride: Anxanil®, Atarax®, Quiess®, Vistaril® injection, Vistazine®

Hydroxyzine pamoate: Hy-Pam®, Vistaril® capsule and suspension

**Related Information**

Anxiolytic/Hypnotic Use in Long-Term Care Facilities *on page 1430*

- **Hydroxyzine, Theophylline, and Ephedrine** *see* Theophylline, Ephedrine, and Hydroxyzine *on page 1118*
- **Hygroton®** *see* Chlorthalidone *on page 260*
- **Hylutin® Injection** *see* Hydroxyprogesterone *on page 585*
- **Hyoscine** *see* Scopolamine *on page 1047*

## Hyoscyamine (hye oh SYE a meen)

**U.S. Brand Names** Anaspaz®; A-Spas® S/L; Cystospaz®; Cystospaz-M®; Donnamar®; ED-SPAZ®; Gastrosed™; Levbid®; Levsin®; Levsinex®; Levsin/SL®

**Synonyms** *L*-Hyoscyamine Sulfate

**Therapeutic Category** Anticholinergic Agent

**Pregnancy Risk Factor** C

**Lactation** Excretion in breast milk unknown/use caution

**Use** Treatment of GI tract disorders caused by spasm; adjunctive therapy for peptic ulcers, spastic bladder, cystitis, pylorospasm, and associated abdominal cramps; adjunct in the treatment of irritable bowel syndrome or neurogenic bladder

**Mechanism of Action/Effect** Blocks the action of acetylcholine at parasympathetic sites in smooth muscle, secretory glands, and the CNS; increases cardiac output, dries secretions, antagonizes histamine and serotonin

**Contraindications** Hypersensitivity to belladonna alkaloids; narrow-angle glaucoma; obstructive uropathy; obstructive GI tract disease; myasthenia gravis

**Warnings** Use with caution in children with spastic paralysis. Use with caution in elderly patients. Low doses cause a paradoxical decrease in heart rates. Some commercial products contain sodium metabisulfite, which can cause allergic-type reactions. Heat prostration may occur in hot weather. Use with caution in patients with autonomic neuropathy, prostatic hypertrophy, hyperthyroidism, congestive heart failure, cardiac arrhythmias, chronic lung disease, and biliary tract disease. Pregnancy factor C.

**Drug Interactions**

**Decreased Effect:** Decreased effect with antacids.

**Increased Effect/Toxicity:** Increased toxicity with amantadine, antimuscarinics, haloperidol, phenothiazines, tricyclic antidepressants, and MAO inhibitors.

**Adverse Reactions**

>10%:

Dermatologic: Dry skin

Gastrointestinal: Dry throat, dry mouth

Local: Irritation at injection site

Respiratory: Dry nose

Miscellaneous: Sweating (decreased)

1% to 10%:

Dermatologic: Photosensitivity

Gastrointestinal: Constipation, dysphagia

Ocular: Blurred vision, mydriasis

<1% (Limited to important or life-threatening symptoms): Palpitations, orthostatic hypotension, increased intraocular pressure

**Overdose/Toxicology** Symptoms of overdose include dilated, unreactive pupils; blurred vision; hot, dry flushed skin; dryness of mucous membranes; difficulty swallowing; foul breath; diminished or absent bowel sounds; urinary retention; tachycardia; hyperthermia; hypertension; and increased respiratory rate. For anticholinergic overdose with severe life-threatening symptoms, physostigmine 1-2 mg S.C. or I.V. slowly, may be given to reverse these effects.

**Pharmacodynamics/Kinetics**

**Protein Binding:** 50%

**Distribution:** Crosses the placenta

**Half-life Elimination:** 13% to 38%

**Metabolism:** Liver

**Excretion:** Urine

**Onset:** 2-3 minutes

**Duration:** 4-6 hours

**Formulations**

Capsule, as sulfate, timed release (Cystospaz-M®, Levsinex®): 0.375 mg
Elixir, as sulfate (Levsin®): 0.125 mg/5 mL with alcohol 20% (480 mL)
Injection, as sulfate (Levsin®): 0.5 mg/mL (1 mL, 10 mL)
Solution, oral (Gastrosed™, Levsin®): 0.125 mg/mL (15 mL)
Tablet, as sulfate:
Anaspaz®, Gastrosed™, Levsin®: 0.125 mg
Cystospaz®: 0.15 mg

**Dosing**

**Adults:**

Oral or S.L.: 0.125-0.25 mg 3-4 times/day before meals or food and at bedtime
Oral: 0.375-0.75 mg (timed release) every 12 hours
I.M., I.V., S.C.: 0.25-0.5 mg every 6 hours

**Elderly:** Refer to adult dosing.

**Administration**

**I.V.:** Inject over at least 1 minute.

**I.V. Detail:** May be administered undiluted.

**Additional Nursing Issues**

**Physical Assessment:** Assess effectiveness and interactions of other medication (see Drug Interactions). See Warnings/Precautions and Contraindications for use cautions (eg, GI or GU obstructions). Have patient void before I.M. administration. Monitor effectiveness of therapy and adverse response (see Adverse Reactions and Overdose/Toxicology). Assess knowledge/teach patient appropriate use, possible side effects and appropriate interventions, and adverse symptoms to report. **Pregnancy risk factor C** - benefits of use should outweigh possible risks. Note breast-feeding caution.

**Patient Information/Instruction:** Take as directed before meals; do not increase dose and do not discontinue without consulting prescriber. Void before taking medication. You may experience dizziness or blurred vision (use caution when driving or engaging in tasks that require alertness until response to drug is known); dry mouth (sucking on lozenges may help); photosensitivity (wear dark glasses in bright sunlight); or impotence (temporary). Report chest pain or palpitations, or excessive and persistent anticholinergic effects (blurred vision, headache, flushing, tachycardia, nervousness, constipation, dizziness, insomnia, mental confusion or excitement, hyperthermia, dry mouth, altered taste perception, dysphagia, palpitations, bradycardia, urinary hesitancy or retention, impotence, decreased sweating). **Pregnancy/breast-feeding precautions:** Inform prescriber if you are or intend to be pregnant. Consult prescriber if breast-feeding.

**Geriatric Considerations:** Avoid long-term use. The potential for toxic reactions is higher than the potential benefit, elderly are particularly prone to CNS side effects of anticholinergics (eg, confusion, delirium, hallucinations). Side effects often occur before clinical response is obtained. Generally not recommended because of the side effects.

**Additional Information** The injection formulation contains benzyl alcohol. Some formulations may contain ethanol or sulfites.

pH: Levsin®: 3.0-6.5

## Hyoscyamine, Atropine, Scopolamine, and Phenobarbital

(hye oh SYE a meen, A troe peen, skoe POL a meen, & fee noe BAR bi tal)

**U.S. Brand Names** Barbidonna®; Barophen®; Donnapine®; Donna-Sed®; Donnatal®; Hyosophen®; Kinesed®; Malatal®; Relaxadon®; Spaslin®; Spasmolin®; Spasmophen®; Spasquid®; Susano®

**Synonyms** Atropine, Hyoscyamine, Scopolamine, and Phenobarbital; Phenobarbital, Hyoscyamine, Atropine, and Scopolamine; Scopolamine, Hyoscyamine, Atropine, and Phenobarbital

**Therapeutic Category** Anticholinergic Agent; Antispasmodic Agent, Gastrointestinal

**Pregnancy Risk Factor** C

**Lactation** Excretion in breast milk unknown/use caution

**Use** Adjunct in treatment of peptic ulcer disease, irritable bowel, spastic colitis, spastic bladder, and renal colic

**Formulations**

Capsule (Donnatal®, Spasmolin®): Hyoscyamine sulfate 0.1037 mg, atropine sulfate 0.0194 mg, scopolamine hydrobromide 0.0065 mg, and phenobarbital 16.2 mg

Elixir (Barophen®, Donna-Sed®, Donnatal®, Hyosophen®, Spasmophen®, Spasquid®, Susano®): Hyoscyamine sulfate 0.1037 mg, atropine sulfate 0.0194 mg, scopolamine hydrobromide 0.0065 mg, and phenobarbital 16.2 mg per 5 mL (120 mL, 480 mL, 4000 mL)

Tablet:

Barbidonna®: Hyoscyamine hydrobromide 0.1286 mg, atropine sulfate 0.025 mg, scopolamine hydrobromide 0.0074 mg, and phenobarbital 16 mg

(Continued)

## Hyoscyamine, Atropine, Scopolamine, and Phenobarbital *(Continued)*

Barbidonna® No. 2: Hyoscyamine hydrobromide 0.1286 mg, atropine sulfate 0.025 mg, scopolamine hydrobromide 0.0074 mg, and phenobarbital 32 mg

Chewable (Kinesed®): Hyoscyamine hydrobromide 0.12 mg, atropine sulfate 0.12 mg, scopolamine hydrobromide 0.007 mg, and phenobarbital 16 mg

Donnapine®, Donnatal®, Hyosophen®, Malatal®, Relaxadon®, Spaslin®, Susano®: Hyoscyamine sulfate 0.1037 mg, atropine sulfate 0.0194 mg, scopolamine hydrobromide 0.0065 mg, and phenobarbital 16.2 mg

Donnatal® No. 2: Hyoscyamine sulfate 0.1037 mg, atropine sulfate 0.0194 mg, scopolamine hydrobromide 0.0065 mg, and phenobarbital 32.4 mg

Long-acting (Donnatal®): Hyoscyamine sulfate 0.3111 mg, atropine sulfate 0.0582 mg, scopolamine hydrobromide 0.0195 mg, and phenobarbital 48.6 mg

Spasmophen®: Hyoscyamine sulfate 0.1037 mg, atropine sulfate 0.0194 mg, scopolamine hydrobromide 0.0065 mg, and phenobarbital 15 mg

**Dosing**

**Adults:** Oral: 1-2 capsules or tablets 3-4 times/day; or 1 Donnatal® Extentab® in sustained release form every 12 hours; or 5-10 mL elixir 3-4 times/day or every 8 hours

**Elderly:** Refer to adult dosing.

**Additional Nursing Issues**

**Physical Assessment:** See individual components listed in Related Information. **Pregnancy risk factor C** - benefits of use should outweigh possible risks. Note breast-feeding caution.

**Patient Information/Instruction:** See individual components listed in Related Information. **Pregnancy/breast-feeding precautions:** Inform prescriber if you are on intend to get pregnant. Consult prescriber if breast-feeding.

**Related Information**

Atropine *on page 119*
Hyoscyamine *on page 590*
Phenobarbital *on page 917*
Scopolamine *on page 1047*


- **Hyosophen®** *see* Hyoscyamine, Atropine, Scopolamine, and Phenobarbital *on previous page*
- **Hy-Pam®** *see* Hydroxyzine *on page 588*
- **HyperHep®** *see page 1256*
- **Hyperstat® I.V.** *see* Diazoxide *on page 357*
- **Hyper-Tet®** *see page 1256*
- **Hy-Phen®** *see* Hydrocodone and Acetaminophen *on page 568*
- **HypoTears PF Solution** *see page 1294*
- **HypoTears Solution** *see page 1294*
- **HypRho®-D** *see page 1256*
- **HypRho®-D Mini-Dose** *see page 1256*
- **Hyprogest® 250 Injection** *see* Hydroxyprogesterone *on page 585*
- **Hyrexin-50® Injection** *see* Diphenhydramine *on page 381*
- **Hysone® Topical** *see* Clioquinol and Hydrocortisone *on page 284*
- **Hytakerol®** *see* Dihydrotachysterol *on page 375*
- **Hytinic®** *see page 1294*
- **Hytone®** *see* Hydrocortisone *on page 578*
- **Hytone®** *see* Topical Corticosteroids *on page 1152*
- **Hytrin®** *see* Terazosin *on page 1102*
- **Hytuss® [OTC]** *see* Guaifenesin *on page 548*
- **Hytuss-2X® [OTC]** *see* Guaifenesin *on page 548*
- **Hyzaar®** *see* Losartan and Hydrochlorothiazide *on page 694*
- **Hy-Zide®** *see* Hydralazine and Hydrochlorothiazide *on page 565*
- **Hyzine-50®** *see* Hydroxyzine *on page 588*
- **Ibenzmethyzin** *see* Procarbazine *on page 970*
- **Iberet-Folic-500®** *see* Vitamin, Multiple *on page 1219*
- **Iberet-Folic-500® Controlled Release Tablet** *see page 1306*
- **Iberet®-Liquid** *see page 1294*
- **Ibidomide Hydrochloride** *see* Labetalol *on page 649*
- **Ibuprin® [OTC]** *see* Ibuprofen *on this page*


## Ibuprofen (eye byoo PROE fen)

**U.S. Brand Names** Aches-N-Pain® [OTC]; Advil® [OTC]; Children's Advil® Oral Suspension [OTC]; Children's Motrin® Oral Suspension [OTC]; Excedrin® IB [OTC]; Genpril® [OTC]; Haltran® [OTC]; Ibuprin® [OTC]; Ibuprohm® [OTC]; Ibu-Tab®; Junior Strength Motrin® [OTC]; Medipren® [OTC]; Menadol® [OTC]; Midol® 200 [OTC]; Motrin®; Motrin® IB [OTC]; Nuprin® [OTC]; Pamprin IB® [OTC]; PediaProfen™; Saleto-200® [OTC]; Saleto-400®; Trendar® [OTC]; Uni-Pro® [OTC]

**Synonyms** *p*-Isobutylhydratropic Acid

**Therapeutic Category** Nonsteroidal Anti-Inflammatory Agent (NSAID)

**Pregnancy Risk Factor** B/D (3rd trimester)

**Lactation** Enters breast milk/use caution (AAP rates "compatible")

**Use** Treatment of inflammatory diseases, osteoarthritis and rheumatoid arthritis, including juvenile rheumatoid arthritis, mild to moderate pain, fever, primary dysmenorrhea, gout, ankylosing spondylitis, acute migraine headache

**Mechanism of Action/Effect** Inhibits prostaglandin synthesis by decreasing the activity of the enzyme, cyclo-oxygenase, which results in decreased formation of prostaglandin precursors

**Contraindications** Hypersensitivity to ibuprofen, any component, aspirin, or other nonsteroidal anti-inflammatory drugs (NSAIDs); pregnancy (3rd trimester)

**Warnings** Do not exceed 3200 mg/day. Use with caution in patients with congestive heart failure, hypertension, decreased renal or hepatic function, history of GI disease (bleeding or ulcers), or those receiving anticoagulants. Elderly are at a high risk for adverse effects from nonsteroidal anti-inflammatory agents. As much as 60% of elderly can develop peptic ulceration and/or hemorrhage asymptomatically.

Use lowest effective dose for shortest period possible. Use of NSAIDs can compromise existing renal function especially when $Cl_{cr}$ is <30 mL/minute. CNS adverse effects such as confusion, agitation, and hallucination are generally seen in overdose or high-dose situations; however, elderly may demonstrate these adverse effects at lower doses than younger adults.

**Drug Interactions**

**Cytochrome P-450 Effect:** CYP2C8 and 2C9 enzyme substrate

**Decreased Effect:** Aspirin may decrease ibuprofen serum concentrations.

**Increased Effect/Toxicity:** Ibuprofen may increase digoxin, methotrexate, and lithium serum concentrations.

**Food Interactions** Ibuprofen peak serum levels may be decreased if taken with food.

**Effects on Lab Values** ↑ chloride (S), sodium (S), bleeding time

**Adverse Reactions**

1% to 10%:

- Central nervous system: Headache, nervousness, dizziness, fatigue
- Dermatologic: Rash, urticaria, itching
- Endocrine & metabolic: Fluid retention
- Gastrointestinal: Heartburn, vomiting, abdominal pain, peptic ulcer, GI bleeding, GI perforation, abdominal cramps, indigestion, nausea
- Otic: Tinnitus

<1% (Limited to important or life-threatening symptoms): Edema, congestive heart failure, arrhythmias, tachycardia, hypertension, erythema multiforme, toxic epidermal necrolysis, Stevens-Johnson syndrome, lupus erythematosus syndrome, Henoch-Schönlein vasculitis, angioedema, aseptic meningitis with fever and coma, neutropenia, agranulocytosis, aplastic anemia, inhibit platelet aggregation, hemolytic anemia, bone marrow depression, leukopenia, thrombocytopenia, eosinophilia, hepatitis acute renal failure, polyuria, azotemia, hematuria, elevated serum creatinine, dyspnea

**Overdose/Toxicology** Symptoms of overdose include apnea, metabolic acidosis, coma, nystagmus, seizures, leukocytosis, and renal failure. Management of nonsteroidal anti-inflammatory (NSAID) intoxication is supportive and symptomatic. Since many NSAIDs undergo enterohepatic cycling, multiple doses of charcoal may be needed to reduce the potential for delayed toxicities.

**Pharmacodynamics/Kinetics**

**Protein Binding:** 90% to 99%

**Half-life Elimination:** 2-4 hours; End-stage renal disease: Unchanged

**Time to Peak:** Within 1-2 hours

**Metabolism:** Liver

**Excretion:** In urine (1% as free drug); some biliary excretion occurs

**Onset:** Onset of analgesia: 30-60 minutes; Onset of anti-inflammatory effect: Up to 7 days; Peak action: 1-2 weeks

**Duration:** 4-6 hours

**Formulations**

Caplet: 100 mg
Drops, oral (berry flavor): 40 mg/mL (15 mL)
Suspension, oral: 100 mg/5 mL [OTC] (60 mL, 120 mL, 480 mL)
Suspension, oral, drops: 40 mg/mL [OTC]
Tablet: 100 mg [OTC], 200 mg [OTC], 300 mg, 400 mg, 600 mg, 800 mg
Tablet, chewable: 50 mg, 100 mg

**Dosing**

**Adults:** Oral:

- Inflammatory disease: 400-800 mg/dose 3-4 times/day; maximum: 3.2 g/day
- Analgesia/pain/fever/dysmenorrhea: 200-400 mg/dose every 4-6 hours; maximum daily dose: 1.2 g (unless directed by physician)

**Elderly:** Refer to adult dosing.

**Hepatic Impairment:** Avoid use in severe hepatic impairment.

**Administration**

**Oral:** Administer with food.

**Monitoring Laboratory Tests** CBC, periodic liver function, renal function (serum BUN, and creatinine)

**Additional Nursing Issues**

**Physical Assessment: Assess patient for allergic reaction to salicylates or other NSAIDs** (see Contraindications). Assess other medications patient may be taking for additive or adverse interactions (see Warnings/Precautions and Drug Interactions). Monitor for therapeutic effectiveness. Monitor for signs of adverse reactions or overdose (especially - adverse gastrointestinal response - see Overdose/Toxicology and Adverse Reactions) at beginning of therapy and periodically during long-term therapy. With long-term therapy, periodic ophthalmic exams are recommended. Assess knowledge/teach patient appropriate use. Teach patient to monitor for adverse reactions, adverse reactions to report, and appropriate interventions to reduce side effects.

(Continued)

## Ibuprofen *(Continued)*

**Pregnancy risk factor B/D** - see Pregnancy Risk Factor - benefits of use should outweigh possible risks. See breast-feeding caution.

**Patient Information/Instruction:** If self-administered, use exactly as directed (do not increase dose or frequency); adverse reactions can occur with overuse. Do not take longer than 3 days for fever, or 10 days for pain without consulting medical advisor. Take with food or milk. While using this medication, do not use alcohol, excessive amounts of vitamin C, or salicylate containing foods (curry powder, prunes, raisins, tea, or licorice), other prescription or OTC medications containing aspirin or salicylate, or other NSAIDs without consulting prescriber. Maintain adequate hydration (2-3 L/day of fluids unless instructed to restrict fluid intake). May discolor urine (red/pink). You may experience nausea, vomiting, gastric discomfort (frequent mouth care, small frequent meals, chewing gum, sucking lozenges may help). GI bleeding, ulceration, or perforation can occur with or without pain. Stop taking medication and report ringing in ears; persistent cramping or pain in stomach; unresolved nausea or vomiting; difficulty breathing or shortness of breath; unusual bruising or bleeding (mouth, urine, stool); skin rash; unusual swelling of extremities; chest pain; or palpitations. **Pregnancy/breast-feeding precautions:** Inform prescriber if you are or intend to be pregnant. Consult prescriber if breast-feeding.

**Geriatric Considerations:** Elderly are at a high risk for adverse effects from nonsteroidal anti-inflammatory agents. As much as 60% of elderly can develop peptic ulceration and/or hemorrhage asymptomatically. The concomitant use of $H_2$ blockers, omeprazole, and sucralfate is not effective as prophylaxis with the exception of NSAID-induced duodenal ulcers which may be prevented by the use of ranitidine. Misoprostol is the only prophylactic agent proven effective. Also, concomitant disease and drug use contribute to the risk for GI adverse effects. Use lowest effective dose for shortest period possible. Consider renal function decline with age. Use of NSAIDs can compromise existing renal function especially when $Cl_{cr}$ is ≤30 mL/minute. Tinnitus may be a difficult and unreliable indication of toxicity due to age-related hearing loss or eighth cranial nerve damage. CNS adverse effects such as confusion, agitation, and hallucination are generally seen in overdose or high-dose situations, but elderly may demonstrate these adverse effects at lower doses than younger adults.

**Additional Information** Sucrose content of 5 mL (suspension): 2.5 g

**Related Information**

Nonsalicylate/Nonsteroidal Anti-inflammatory Comparison *on page 1401*


- **Ibuprofen and Hydrocodone** *see* Hydrocodone and Ibuprofen *on page 573*
- **Ibuprohm® [OTC]** *see* Ibuprofen *on page 592*
- **Ibu-Tab®** *see* Ibuprofen *on page 592*


## Ibutilide (i BYOO ti lide)

**U.S. Brand Names** Corvert®

**Therapeutic Category** Antiarrhythmic Agent, Class III

**Pregnancy Risk Factor** C

**Lactation** Enters breast milk/contraindicated

**Use** Acute termination of atrial fibrillation or flutter of recent onset; the effectiveness of ibutilide has not been determined in patients with arrhythmias >90 days in duration

**Mechanism of Action/Effect** Exact mechanism of action is unknown; prolongs the action potential in cardiac tissue

**Contraindications** Hypersensitivity to ibutilide or any component

**Warnings** Potentially fatal arrhythmias (eg, polymorphic ventricular tachycardia) can occur with ibutilide, **usually** in association with torsade de pointes (Q-T prolongation). Studies indicate a 1.7% incidence of arrhythmias in treated patients. The drug should be given in a setting of continuous EKG monitoring and by personnel trained in treating arrhythmias particularly polymorphic ventricular tachycardia. Patients with chronic atrial fibrillation may not be the best candidates for ibutilide since they often revert after conversion and the risks of treatment may not be justified when compared to alternative management. Dosing adjustments are not required in patients with renal or hepatic dysfunction since a maximum of only two 10-minute infusions are utilized. Drug distribution, rather than administration, is one of the primary mechanisms responsible for termination of the pharmacologic effect. Safety and efficacy in children have not been established. Pregnancy factor C.

**Drug Interactions**

**Increased Effect/Toxicity:** Class 1A antiarrhythmic drugs (disopyramide, quinidine, and procainamide) and other class III drugs such as amiodarone and sotalol should not be given concomitantly with ibutilide due to their potential to prolong refractoriness. The potential for prolongation of the Q-T interval may occur if ibutilide is given concurrently with phenothiazines, tricyclic and tetracyclic antidepressants, and the nonsedating antihistamines (terfenadine and astemizole). Signs of digoxin toxicity may be masked when coadministered with ibutilide.

**Adverse Reactions**

1% to 10%:

Cardiovascular: Sustained polymorphic ventricular tachycardia (ie, torsade de pointes) often requiring cardioversion, nonsustained polymorphic ventricular tachycardia nonsustained monomorphic ventricular extrasystoles, nonsustained monomorphic VT tachycardia/supraventricular tachycardia, hypotension, bundle branch block, A-V block, bradycardia, Q-T segment prolongation, hypertension, palpitations

Central nervous system: Headache

Gastrointestinal: Nausea

<1% (Limited to important or life-threatening symptoms): Supraventricular extrasystoles, nodal arrhythmia, congestive heart failure, syncope, idioventricular rhythm, sustained monomorphic VT, renal failure

**Overdose/Toxicology** Symptoms of overdose include CNS depression, rapid gasping breathing, and convulsions. Arrhythmias occur. Treatment is supportive. Antiarrhythmics are generally avoided.

**Pharmacodynamics/Kinetics**

**Half-life Elimination:** 2-12 hours (average: 6 hours)

**Metabolism:** Liver

**Excretion:** Urine

**Onset:** Within 90 minutes after start of infusion (1/2 of conversions to sinus rhythm occur during infusion)

**Formulations** Injection, as fumarate: 0.1 mg/mL (10 mL)

**Dosing**

**Adults:** I.V.: Initial:

<60 kg: 0.01 mg/kg over 10 minutes

≥60 kg: 1 mg over 10 minutes

If the arrhythmia does not terminate within 10 minutes after the end of the initial infusion, a second infusion of equal strength may be infused over a 10-minute period.

**Elderly:** Refer to adult dosing.

**Administration**

**I.V.:** Infuse over 10 minutes.

**I.V. Detail:** Observe patient with continuous EKG monitoring for at least 4 hours following infusion or until Q-$T_c$ has returned to baseline. Skilled personnel and proper equipment should be available during administration of ibutilide and subsequent monitoring of the patient.

**Stability**

**Reconstitution:** May be administered undiluted or diluted in 50 mL diluent (0.9% NS or $D_5W$). Admixtures are chemically and physically stable for 24 hours at room temperature and for 48 hours at refrigerated temperatures.

**Monitoring Laboratory Tests** Electrolytes

**Additional Nursing Issues**

**Physical Assessment:** Assess other medications patient may be taking for effectiveness and interactions (see Drug Interactions). See Warnings/Precautions for cautious use. Requires infusion pump and continuous cardiac and hemodynamic monitoring during and for 4 hours following infusion (see Administration). Monitor laboratory tests (see above), therapeutic response, and adverse reactions (see Warnings/Precautions and Adverse Reactions). Teach patient adverse symptoms to report. **Pregnancy risk factor C** - benefits of use should outweigh possible risks. Breast-feeding is contraindicated.

**Patient Information/Instruction:** This drug is only given I.V. and you will be on continuous cardiac monitoring during and for several hours following administration. You may experience headache or irregular heartbeat during infusion. Report chest pain or respiratory difficulty immediately. **Pregnancy/breast-feeding precautions:** Inform prescriber if you are or intend to be pregnant. Do not breast-feed.

**Pregnancy Issues:** Teratogenic and embryocidal in rats; avoid use in pregnancy.

**Related Information**

Antiarrhythmic Drug Classification Comparison *on page 1366*

♦ **ICI 204, 219** *see* Zafirlukast *on page 1223*

♦ **ICRF-187** *see* Dexrazoxane *on page 350*

♦ **Idamycin®** *see* Idarubicin *on this page*

## Idarubicin (eye da ROO bi sin)

**U.S. Brand Names** Idamycin®

**Synonyms** 4-Demethoxydaunorubicin; 4-DMDR

**Therapeutic Category** Antineoplastic Agent, Antibiotic

**Pregnancy Risk Factor** D

**Lactation** Excretion in breast milk unknown

**Use** In combination treatment of acute myeloid leukemia (AML), this includes classifications M1 through M7 of the French-American-British (FAB) classification system and acute lymphocytic leukemia (ALL) in children

**Mechanism of Action/Effect** Similar to daunorubicin, idarubicin exhibits inhibitory effects on DNA and RNA polymerase.

**Contraindications** Hypersensitivity to idarubicin, daunorubicin, or any component; pregnancy

**Warnings** The U.S. Food and Drug Administration (FDA) currently recommends that procedures for proper handling and disposal of antineoplastic agents be considered. Give I.V. slowly into a freely flowing I.V. infusion. Do not give I.M. or S.C.; severe necrosis can result if extravasation occurs. Can cause myocardial toxicity and is more common in patients who have previously received anthracyclines or have pre-existing cardiac disease. Reduce dose in patients with impaired hepatic function. Irreversible myocardial toxicity may occur as total dosage approaches 137.5 mg/m$^2$. Severe myelosuppression is also possible.

Idarubicin preparation should be performed in a Class II laminar flow biologic safety cabinet. Personnel should be wearing surgical gloves and a closed front surgical gown

(Continued)

## Idarubicin *(Continued)*

with knit cuffs. Appropriate safety equipment is recommended for preparation, administration, and disposal of antineoplastics. If idarubicin contacts the skin, wash and flush thoroughly with water.

**Adverse Reactions**

>10%:

Central nervous system: Headache, fever
Dermatologic: Alopecia, rash, urticaria
Gastrointestinal: Mucositis, nausea, vomiting, diarrhea, stomatitis
Genitourinary: Reddish urine
Hematologic: Hemorrhage, anemia
Leukopenia (nadir: 8-29 days)
Thrombocytopenia (nadir: 10-15 days)
Local: Tissue necrosis upon extravasation, erythematous streaking
**Vesicant chemotherapy**
Miscellaneous: Infection

1% to 10%:

Cardiovascular: Arrhythmias, EKG changes, cardiomyopathy, congestive heart failure, myocardial toxicity, acute life-threatening arrhythmias
Central nervous system: Seizures
Endocrine & metabolic: Hyperuricemia
Neuromuscular & skeletal: Peripheral neuropathy
Miscellaneous: Pulmonary allergy

<1% (Limited to important or life-threatening symptoms): Enterocolitis with perforation, elevations in liver enzymes or bilirubin

**Overdose/Toxicology** Symptoms of overdose include severe myelosuppression and increased GI toxicity. Treatment is supportive. It is unlikely that therapeutic efficacy or toxicity would be altered by conventional peritoneal or hemodialysis.

**Pharmacodynamics/Kinetics**

**Protein Binding:** 94% to 97%

**Distribution:** Large volume due to extensive tissue binding and distributes into CSF

**Half-life Elimination:** Oral: 14-35 hours; I.V.: 12-27 hours

**Metabolism:** Liver

**Excretion:** ~15% of an I.V. dose has been recovered in urine as idarubicin and idarubicinol. Similar amounts are excreted via bile.

**Formulations** Powder for injection, lyophilized, as hydrochloride: 5 mg, 10 mg

**Dosing**

**Adults:** I.V.: 12 mg/m²/day for 3 days by slow (10-15 minutes) I.V. injection in combination with Ara-C. The Ara-C may be given as 100 mg/m²/day by continuous infusion for 7 days or as Ara-C 25 mg/m² I.V. bolus followed by Ara-C 200 mg/m²/day for 5 days continuous infusion.

**Elderly:** Refer to adult dosing.

**Renal Impairment:** Dose reduction is recommended.
Serum creatinine ≥2 mg/dL: Reduce dose by 25%.

**Hepatic Impairment:**
Bilirubin 1.5-5.0 mg/dL or AST 60-180 units: Reduce dose 50%.
Bilirubin >5 mg/dL or AST >180 units: Do not administer.

**Administration**

**I.V.:** Vesicant. Administer by intermittent infusion over 10-15 minutes.

**I.V. Detail:** Administer into a free flowing I.V. solution of NS or $D_5W$. Avoid extravasation - potent vesicant. Local erythematous streaking along the vein may indicate rapid administration. Unless specific data is available, do not mix with other drugs.

**Extravasation management:** Topical cooling may be achieved using ice packs or cooling pad with circulating ice water. Cooling of site for 24 hours as tolerated by the patient. Elevate and rest extremity 24-48 hours, then resume normal activity as tolerated. Application of cold inhibits vesicant's cytotoxicity. **Application of heat can be harmful and is contraindicated.** If pain, erythema, and/or swelling persist beyond 48 hours, refer patient immediately to plastic surgeon for consultation and possible debridement.

**Stability**

**Storage:** Store intact vials of lyophilized powder at room temperature and protect from light.

**Reconstitution:** Dilute powder with NS to a concentration of 1 mg/mL as follows: Solution is stable for 72 hours at room temperature and 7 days under refrigeration.
5 mg = 5 mL
10 mg = 10 mL
Further dilution in $D_5W$ or NS is stable for 4 weeks at room temperature and protected from light.

**Standard I.V. dilution:**
I.V. push: Dose/syringe (concentration is 1 mg/mL)
Maximum syringe size for IVP is 30 mL syringe and syringe should be ≤75% full.
IVPB: Dose/100 mL $D_5W$ or NS
Syringe and IVPB solutions are stable for 72 hours at room temperature and 7 days under refrigeration.

**Compatibility:** Incompatible with fluorouracil, etoposide, dexamethasone, heparin, hydrocortisone, methotrexate, and vincristine. See the Chemotherapy Compatibility Chart *on page 1311.*

**Monitoring Laboratory Tests** CBC with differential, platelet count, ECHO, EKG, serum electrolytes, creatinine, uric acid, ALT, AST, bilirubin

**Additional Nursing Issues**

**Physical Assessment:** Monitor infusion site closely; extravasation may result in cellulitis and tissue necrosis (see above). Monitor results of laboratory tests and adverse reactions as noted above, especially hemorrhage, anemia, fluid status (edema, lung sounds, weight), and opportunistic infection. **Pregnancy risk factor D** - assess knowledge/teach patient appropriate use of barrier contraceptives. Note breast-feeding caution.

**Patient Information/Instruction:** This drug can only be administered I.V. Maintain adequate nutrition and hydration (2-3 L/day of fluids unless instructed to restrict fluid intake). May cause hair loss (will grow back); nausea or vomiting (consult prescriber for antiemetic medication); you will be susceptible to infection (avoid crowds and exposure to infection); or urine may turn red-brown (normal). Report immediately any pain, burning, or stinging at infusion site; difficulty breathing; or swelling of extremities. **Pregnancy/breast-feeding precautions:** Use appropriate contraceptive measures; do not get pregnant while taking this drug (serious fetal damage has occurred). Consult prescriber if breast-feeding.

- **Idulamine®** *see* Azatadine *on page 123*
- **Ifex® Injection** *see* Ifosfamide *on this page*
- **IFLrA** *see* Interferon Alfa-2a *on page 612*

## Ifosfamide (eye FOSS fa mide)

**U.S. Brand Names** Ifex® Injection

**Therapeutic Category** Antineoplastic Agent, Alkylating Agent

**Pregnancy Risk Factor** D

**Lactation** Enters breast milk/contraindicated

**Use** In combination with certain other antineoplastics in treatment of lung cancer, Hodgkin's and non-Hodgkin's lymphoma, breast cancer, acute and chronic lymphocytic leukemia, ovarian cancer, testicular cancer, and sarcomas, pancreatic and gastric carcinoma

**Mechanism of Action/Effect** Inhibits protein synthesis and DNA synthesis; an analogue of cyclophosphamide, and like cyclophosphamide, it undergoes activation by microsomal enzymes in the liver. Ifosfamide is metabolized to active compounds, ifosfamide mustard, and acrolein.

**Contraindications** Hypersensitivity to ifosfamide; severely depressed bone marrow function; pregnancy

**Warnings** The U.S. Food and Drug Administration (FDA) currently recommends that procedures for proper handling and disposal of antineoplastic agents be considered. Used in combination with mesna as a prophylactic agent to protect against hemorrhagic cystitis. Use with caution in patients with impaired renal function or those with compromised bone marrow reserve. May require therapy cessation if confusion or coma occurs; carcinogenic in rats.

Preparation of ifosfamide should be performed in a Class II laminar flow biologic safety cabinet. Personnel should be wearing surgical gloves and a closed front surgical gown with knit cuffs. Appropriate safety equipment is recommended for preparation, administration, and disposal of antineoplastics. If ifosfamide contacts the skin, wash and flush thoroughly with water.

**Drug Interactions**

**Cytochrome P-450 Effect:** CYP2B6 and 3A3/4 enzyme substrate

**Increased Effect/Toxicity:** Activation by microsomal enzymes may be enhanced during therapy with enzyme inducers such as phenobarbital, carbamazepine, and phenytoin.

**Adverse Reactions**

>10%:

Central nervous system: Somnolence, confusion, hallucinations (12%) and coma (rare) have occurred and are usually reversible and usually occur with higher doses or in patients with reduced renal function; depressive psychoses, polyneuropathy

Dermatologic: Alopecia occurs in 50% to 83% of patients 2-4 weeks after initiation of therapy, may be as high as 100% in combination therapy

Gastrointestinal: Nausea and vomiting in 58% of patients is dose and schedule related (more common with higher doses and after bolus regimens); nausea and vomiting can persist up to 3 days after therapy; also anorexia, diarrhea, constipation, transient increase in LFTs and stomatitis noted.

Emetic potential: Moderate (58%)

Time course of nausea/vomiting: Onset: 2-3 hours; Duration: 12-72 hours

Genitourinary: Hemorrhagic cystitis has been frequently associated with the use of ifosfamide. A urinalysis prior to each dose should be obtained. **Ifosfamide should never be administered without a uroprotective agent (MESNA).** Hematuria has been reported in 6% to 92% of patients. Renal toxicity occurs in 6% of patients and is manifested as an increase in BUN or serum creatinine and is most likely related to tubular damage. Renal toxicity, including ARF, may occur more frequently with high-dose ifosfamide. Metabolic acidosis may occur in up to 31% of patients.

1% to 10%:

Dermatologic: Phlebitis, dermatitis, nail ridging, skin hyperpigmentation, impaired wound healing

Endocrine & metabolic: SIADH

Hematologic: Myelosuppression: Less of a problem than with cyclophosphamide if used alone. Leukopenia is mild to moderate, thrombocytopenia and anemia are rare.

(Continued)

## Ifosfamide *(Continued)*

However, myelosuppression can be severe when used with other chemotherapeutic agents or with high-dose therapy. Be cautious with patients with compromised bone marrow reserve.
WBC: Moderate
Platelets: Mild
Onset (days): 7
Nadir (days): 10-14
Hepatic: Elevated liver enzymes
Respiratory: Nasal congestion, pulmonary fibrosis
Miscellaneous: Immunosuppression, sterility, possible secondary malignancy, allergic reactions

<1% (Limited to important or life-threatening symptoms): Cardiotoxicity, pulmonary toxicity

**Overdose/Toxicology** Symptoms of overdose include myelosuppression, nausea, vomiting, diarrhea, and alopecia; direct extensions of the drug's pharmacologic effect. Treatment is supportive.

**Pharmacodynamics/Kinetics**

**Protein Binding:** Not appreciably protein bound

**Distribution:** Does penetrate CNS, but not in therapeutic levels

**Half-life Elimination:** Pharmacokinetics are dose-dependent; 11-15 hours with high-dose (3800-5000 mg/m$^2$) or 4-7 hours with lower doses (1800 mg/m$^2$)

**Metabolism:** Liver

**Excretion:** Urine

**Formulations** Powder for injection: 1 g, 3 g

**Dosing**

**Adults:** I.V. (refer to individual protocols):

Doses may be given as 50 mg/kg/day **or** 700-2000 mg/m$^2$/day for 5 days. Alternatives include 2400 mg/m$^2$/day for 3 days **or** 5000 mg/m$^2$ as a single dose.

Doses of 700-900 mg/m$^2$/day for 5 days may be given IVP; courses may be repeated every 3-4 weeks.

To prevent bladder toxicity, ifosfamide should be given with extensive hydration consisting of at least 2 L of oral or I.V. fluid per day. A protector, such as mesna, should also be used to prevent hemorrhagic cystitis. The dose-limiting toxicity is hemorrhagic cystitis and ifosfamide should be used in conjunction with a uroprotective agent.

**Elderly:** Refer to adult dosing.

**Renal Impairment:**

$S_{cr}$ 2.1-3.0 mg/dL: Reduce dose by 25% to 50%.
$S_{cr}$ >3.0 mg/dL: Withhold drug.

**Hepatic Impairment:** Although no specific guidelines are available, it is possible that higher doses are indicated in hepatic disease.

**Administration**

**I.V.:** Administer slow I.V. push, IVPB over 30 minutes or continuous intravenous infusion over 5 days. Mesna should be administered concomitantly (20% of the ifosfamide dose 15 minutes before, 4 hours after and 8 hours after ifosfamide administration).

**I.V. Detail:** Adequate hydration (at least 2 L/day) of the patient before and for 72 hours after therapy is recommended to minimize the risk of hemorrhagic cystitis.

**Stability**

**Storage:** Store intact vials at room temperature or under refrigeration. Syringe and IVPB are stable for 7 days at room temperature and 6 weeks under refrigeration.

**Reconstitution:** Dilute powder with SWI or NS to a concentration of 50 mg/mL as follows. Incompatible with bacteriostatic SWI or NS. Solution is stable for 7 days at room temperature and 3 weeks under refrigeration.
1 g vial = 20 mL
3 g vial = 60 mL
Further dilution in NS, $D_5W$ or LR is stable for 7 days at room temperature
Compatible with mesna in NS for up to 9 days at room temperature.

**Standard I.V. dilution:**
I.V. push: Dose/syringe (concentration = 50 mg/mL)
Maximum syringe size for IVP is a 30 mL syringe and syringe should be ≤75% full
IVPB: Dose/100-1000 mL $D_5W$ or NS

**Compatibility:** Incompatible with bacteriostatic SWI or bacteriostatic NS. Compatible with mesna in NS for up to 9 days at room temperature. See the Chemotherapy Compatibility Chart *on page 1311.*

**Monitoring Laboratory Tests** CBC with differential, platelet count, urine output, urinalysis, liver and renal function

**Additional Nursing Issues**

**Physical Assessment:** Use caution to prevent extravasation. Monitor laboratory tests prior to each infusion. Monitor for extensive adverse reactions as noted above, especially kidney function. Hydrate (2-3 L/day of fluids unless instructed to restrict fluid intake) for 72 hours prior to infusion (see Administration) to minimize risk of hemorrhagic cystitis. Premedicate with antiemetic prior to each infusion. **Pregnancy risk factor D** - assess knowledge/instruct patient on use of barrier contraceptive measures. Breast-feeding is contraindicated.

**Patient Information/Instruction:** This drug can only be administered I.V. Report immediately any pain, stinging, or burning at infusion site. It is vital to maintain adequate hydration (2-3 L/day of fluids unless instructed to restrict fluid intake) for 3 days prior to infusion and each day of therapy. May cause hair loss (will grow back);

nausea or vomiting (consult prescriber for antiemetic medication); and you will be susceptible to infection (avoid crowds and exposure to infection). Report immediately pain or irritation on urination, severe diarrhea, CNS changes (eg, hallucinations, confusion, somnolence), signs of opportunistic infection (eg, fever, chills, easy bruising or unusual bleeding), difficulty breathing, swelling of extremities, or any other adverse effects. **Pregnancy/breast-feeding precautions:** Do not get pregnant or breast-feed while undergoing treatment with ifosfamide until deemed safe by prescriber.

**Related Information**

Mesna *on page 729*


- **Ifoxan** *see* Ifosfamide *on page 597*
- **IGIV** *see* Immune Globulin, Intravenous *on page 602*
- **Ilosone®** *see* Erythromycin *on page 435*
- **Ilotycin®** *see* Erythromycin *on page 435*
- **Ilotycin®** *see page 1282*
- **Ilozyme®** *see* Pancrelipase *on page 882*
- **Imdur™** *see* Isosorbide Mononitrate *on page 635*
- **I-Methasone®** *see* Dexamethasone *on page 346*
- **Imidazole Carboxamide** *see* Dacarbazine *on page 325*
- **Imigran** *see* Sumatriptan Succinate *on page 1090*
- **Imipemide** *see* Imipenem and Cilastatin *on this page*


## Imipenem and Cilastatin (i mi PEN em & sye la STAT in)

**U.S. Brand Names** Primaxin®

**Synonyms** Cilastatin and Imipenem; Imipemide

**Therapeutic Category** Antibiotic, Carbapenem

**Pregnancy Risk Factor** C

**Lactation** Enters breast milk (small amounts)/use caution

**Use** Treatment of documented multidrug resistant gram-negative infection due to organisms proven or suspected to be susceptible to imipenem/cilastatin; treatment of multiple organism infection in which other agents have an insufficient spectrum of activity or are contraindicated due to toxic potential; antibacterial activity includes resistant gram-negative bacilli (*Pseudomonas aeruginosa* and *Enterobacter* sp), gram-positive bacteria (methicillin-sensitive *Staphylococcus aureus* and *Enterococcus* sp) and anaerobes

**Mechanism of Action/Effect** A carbapenem with broad-spectrum antibacterial activity including resistant gram-negative bacilli (*Pseudomonas aeruginosa* and *Enterococcus* sp), gram-positive bacteria (methicillin-sensitive *Staphylococcus aureus* and *Enterococcus* sp) and anaerobes; inhibits cell wall synthesis; cilastatin prevents renal metabolism of imipenem

**Contraindications** Hypersensitivity to imipenem/cilastatin or any component

**Warnings** Dosage adjustment is required in patients with impaired renal function. Prolonged use may result in superinfection. Use with caution in patients with a history of seizures or hypersensitivity to beta-lactams. Elderly patients often require lower doses. Pregnancy factor C.

**Drug Interactions**

**Increased Effect/Toxicity:** Beta-lactam antibiotics and probenecid may increase potential for toxicity.

**Effects on Lab Values** Interferes with urinary glucose determination using Clinitest®

**Adverse Reactions**

>10%:

Central nervous system: Confusion, dizziness, seizures, tremors

Gastrointestinal: Nausea, diarrhea, vomiting

Local: Thrombophlebitis (pain at injection site)

1% to 10%: Miscellaneous: Infusion rate reaction

<1% (Limited to important or life-threatening symptoms): Hypotension, palpitations, pseudomembranous colitis, neutropenia, eosinophilia, emergence of resistant strains of *P. aeruginosa*

**Overdose/Toxicology** Symptoms of overdose include neuromuscular hypersensitivity and seizures. Hemodialysis may be helpful to aid in removal of the drug from blood; otherwise, treatment is supportive or symptom directed.

**Pharmacodynamics/Kinetics**

**Distribution:** Crosses the placenta

**Half-life Elimination:** Imipenem: 1 hour, extended with renal insufficiency; Cilastatin: 1 hour, extended with renal insufficiency

**Metabolism:** Kidney

**Excretion:** Urine

**Formulations**

Powder for injection:

I.M.:

Imipenem 500 mg and cilastatin 500 mg

Imipenem 750 mg and cilastatin 750 mg

I.V.:

Imipenem 250 mg and cilastatin 250 mg

Imipenem 500 mg and cilastatin 500 mg

**Dosing**

**Adults:** I.M. and I.V. (dosing based on imipenem component):

I.V.: 500 mg every 6-8 hours (1 g every 6-8 hours for severe *Pseudomonas* infection); infuse each 250-500 mg dose over 20-30 minutes. Infuse each 1 g dose over 40-60 minutes.

(Continued)

## Imipenem and Cilastatin *(Continued)*

Mild to moderate infection **only**: I.M.: 500-750 mg every 12 hours (**Note:** 750 mg is recommended for intra-abdominal and more severe respiratory, dermatologic, or gynecologic infections. Total daily I.M. dosages >1500 mg are not recommended. Deep I.M. injection should be carefully made into a large muscle mass only).

**Elderly:** Refer to adult dosing.

**Renal Impairment:** See table.

| Creatinine Clearance (mL/min/1.73 m$^2$) | Frequency | % Decrease in Daily Maximum Dose |
|---|---|---|
| 30-70 | q6-8h | 50 |
| 20-30 | q8-12h | 63 |
| 5-20 | q12h | 75 |

Hemodialysis effects: Imipenem (**not cilastatin**) is moderately dialyzable (20% to 50%) by hemodialysis. Administer dose postdialysis. During peritoneal dialysis, dose as for $Cl_{cr}$ <10 mL/minute.

Continuous arteriovenous or venovenous hemofiltration (CAVH/CAVHD): Dose as for $Cl_{cr}$ 20-30 mL/minute; monitor closely for seizure activity (imipenem is removed well but cilastatin is not)

**Administration**

**I.V.:** Do not administer I.V. push. Final concentration should not exceed 5 mg/mL. Infuse over 30-60 minutes.

**I.V. Detail:** Vial contents must be transferred to 100 mL of infusion solution. If nausea and/or vomiting occur during administration, decrease the rate of I.V. infusion. Do not mix with or physically add to other antibiotics; however, may administer concomitantly.

**Stability**

**Storage:** Imipenem/cilastatin powder for injection should be stored at <30°C.

**Reconstitution:** All IVPB should be prepared fresh. Do not use dextrose as a diluent due to limited stability. Reconstituted solutions are stable 10 hours at room temperature and 48 hours at refrigeration (4°C) with NS. If reconstituted with 5% or 10% dextrose injection, 5% dextrose and sodium bicarbonate, 5% dextrose and 0.9% sodium chloride, is stable for 4 hours at room temperature and 24 hours when refrigerated. Imipenem is inactivated at acidic or alkaline pH.

Standard diluent: 500 mg/100 mL NS; 1 g/250 mL NS

**Monitoring Laboratory Tests** Perform culture and sensitivity studies prior to initiating therapy. Periodically monitor renal, hepatic, and hematologic function.

**Additional Nursing Issues**

**Physical Assessment:** Monitor results of appropriate laboratory tests. Monitor vital signs and CNS status (seizures), fluid balance (I & O), liver function, infusion or injection sites. Monitor closely for opportunistic infection (eg, fever, chills, sore throat, vaginal discharge, oral plaques). Maintain adequate nutritional and hydration status. Use serum glucose monitoring for diabetic patients. **Pregnancy risk factor C** - benefits of use should outweigh possible risks. Note breast-feeding caution.

**Patient Information/Instruction:** Report warmth, swelling, irritation at infusion or injection site. Maintain adequate hydration (2-3 L/day of fluids unless instructed to restrict fluid intake) and nutrition. Report unresolved nausea or vomiting (small, frequent meals may help). Diabetics must use serum glucose testing rather than Clinitest®. Report feelings of excessive dizziness, palpitations, visual disturbances, and CNS changes. Report chills, or unusual discharge, or foul-smelling urine. **Pregnancy/breast-feeding precautions:** Inform prescriber if you are or intend to be pregnant. Consult prescriber if breast-feeding.

**Geriatric Considerations:** Many of the seizures attributed to imipenem/cilastatin were in elderly patients. Dose must be adjusted for creatinine clearance.

**Additional Information**

Sodium content of 1 g: 3.2 mEq

pH: 6.5-7.5

## Imipramine (im IP ra meen)

**U.S. Brand Names** Janimine®; Tofranil®; Tofranil-PM®

**Therapeutic Category** Antidepressant, Tricyclic (Tertiary Amine)

**Pregnancy Risk Factor** D

**Lactation** Enters breast milk/not recommended (AAP rates "of concern")

**Use** Treatment of various forms of depression, often in conjunction with psychotherapy; certain types of chronic and neuropathic pain; panic disorder

**Mechanism of Action/Effect** Traditionally believed to increase the synaptic concentration of serotonin and/or norepinephrine in the central nervous system by inhibition of their reuptake by the presynaptic neuronal membrane. However, additional receptor effects have been found including desensitization of adenyl cyclase, down regulation of beta-adrenergic receptors, and down regulation of serotonin receptors.

**Contraindications** Hypersensitivity to imipramine (cross-sensitivity with other tricyclics may occur); patients receiving MAO inhibitors or fluoxetine within past 14 days; narrow-angle glaucoma; pregnancy

**Warnings** Use with caution in patients with cardiovascular disease, conduction disturbances, seizure disorders, urinary retention, hyperthyroidism or those receiving thyroid replacement. Do not discontinue abruptly in patients receiving long-term, high-dose therapy. Some oral preparations contain tartrazine and injection contains sulfites, both of which can cause allergic reactions.

Orthostatic hypotension is a concern with this agent, especially in patients taking other medications that may affect blood pressure. May precipitate arrhythmias in predisposed patients. May aggravate seizures. A less anticholinergic antidepressant may be a better choice.

**Drug Interactions**

**Cytochrome P-450 Effect:** CYP1A2, 2C9, 2C18, 2C19, 2D6, and 3A3/4 enzyme substrate

**Decreased Effect:** Imipramine inhibits the antihypertensive effects of clonidine.

**Increased Effect/Toxicity:** MAO inhibitors may cause hyperpyrexia, hypertension, tachycardia, confusion, seizures, and death. May increase the prothrombin time in patients stabilized on warfarin. May potentiate the action of other CNS depressants. Potentiates the vasopressor and cardiac effects of sympathomimetic agents such as isoproterenol, epinephrine, etc. Additive anticholinergic effects are seen with other anticholinergic agents. Cimetidine reduces the hepatic metabolism of imipramine. Tricyclic antidepressants like imipramine may enhance the hypertensive response associated with abrupt clonidine withdrawal. Potential for serotonin syndrome if combined with other serotonergic drugs.

**Effects on Lab Values** ↑ glucose

**Adverse Reactions** Less sedation and anticholinergic effects than amitriptyline

>10%:

Central nervous system: Dizziness, drowsiness, headache

Gastrointestinal: Increased appetite, nausea, unpleasant taste, weight gain, dry mouth, constipation

Genitourinary: Urinary retention

Neuromuscular & skeletal: Weakness

1% to 10%:

Cardiovascular: Postural hypotension, arrhythmias, tachycardia

Central nervous system: Confusion, delirium, hallucinations, nervousness, restlessness, parkinsonian syndrome, insomnia

Endocrine & metabolic: Sexual dysfunction

Gastrointestinal: Diarrhea, heartburn

Genitourinary: Dysuria

Neuromuscular & skeletal: Fine muscle tremors

Ocular: Blurred vision, eye pain

Miscellaneous: Sweating (excessive)

<1% (Limited to important or life-threatening symptoms): Seizures, alopecia, testicular edema, leukopenia, eosinophilia, rarely agranulocytosis, increased liver enzymes, cholestatic jaundice, increased intraocular pressure, allergic reactions, has been associated with falls, sudden death

**Overdose/Toxicology** Symptoms of overdose include confusion, hallucinations, constipation, cyanosis, tachycardia, urinary retention, ventricular tachycardia, and seizures. Following initiation of essential overdose management, toxic symptoms should be treated. Ventricular arrhythmias often respond to concurrent systemic alkalinization (sodium bicarbonate 0.5-2 mEq/kg I.V.) Physostigmine (1-2 mg I.V. slowly for adults) may be indicated to reverse life-threatening cardiac arrhythmias.

**Pharmacodynamics/Kinetics**

**Distribution:** Crosses the placenta

**Half-life Elimination:** 6-18 hours

**Metabolism:** Liver

**Excretion:** Urine

**Onset:** Peak antidepressant effect: Usually after ≥2 weeks

**Formulations**

Capsule, as pamoate (Tofranil-PM®): 75 mg, 100 mg, 125 mg, 150 mg

Injection, as hydrochloride (Tofranil®): 12.5 mg/mL (2 mL)

Tablet, as hydrochloride (Janimine®, Tofranil®): 10 mg, 25 mg, 50 mg

**Dosing**

**Adults:** Maximum antidepressant effect may not be seen for 2 or more weeks after initiation of therapy.

Oral: Initial: 25 mg 3-4 times/day, increase dose gradually, total dose may be given at bedtime; maximum: 300 mg/day

I.M.: Initial: Up to 100 mg/day in divided doses; change to oral as soon as possible.

**Elderly:** Maximum antidepressant effect may not be seen for 2 or more weeks after initiation of therapy.

Initial: 10-25 mg at bedtime; increase by 10-25 mg every 3 days for inpatients and weekly for outpatients if tolerated; average daily dose to achieve a therapeutic concentration: 100 mg/day; range: 50-150 mg/day.

**Stability**

**Storage:** Solutions are stable at a pH of 4-5. Turns yellowish or reddish on exposure to light. Slight discoloration does not affect potency. Marked discoloration is associated with loss of potency.

**Monitoring Laboratory Tests** EKG, CBC

**Additional Nursing Issues**

**Physical Assessment:** Assess other medications patient may be taking for effectiveness and interactions (see Drug Interactions). See Contraindications and Warnings/Precautions for cautious use. Has potential for psychological or physiological dependence, abuse, and tolerance. Monitor laboratory tests, therapeutic response (ie,

(Continued)

## Imipramine *(Continued)*

mental status, mood, affect, suicidal ideation), and adverse reactions at beginning of therapy and periodically with long-term use (see Adverse Reactions and Overdose/Toxicology). Taper dosage slowly when discontinuing (allow 3-4 weeks between discontinuing Tofranil® and starting another antidepressant). Assess knowledge/teach patient appropriate use, interventions to reduce side effects, and adverse symptoms to report. **Pregnancy risk factor D** - assess knowledge/instruct patient on use of barrier contraceptives. Breast-feeding is not recommended.

**Patient Information/Instruction:** Oral: Take exactly as directed (do not increase dose or frequency); may take 2-3 weeks to achieve desired results; may cause physical and/or psychological dependence. Take in the evening. Avoid excessive alcohol, caffeine, and other prescription or OTC medications not approved by prescriber. Maintain adequate hydration (2-3 L/day of fluids unless instructed to restrict fluid intake). You may experience drowsiness, lightheadedness, impaired coordination, dizziness, or blurred vision (use caution when driving or engaging in tasks requiring alertness until response to drug is known); nausea, vomiting, altered taste, dry mouth (small frequent meals, frequent mouth care, chewing gum, or sucking lozenges may help); constipation (increased exercise, fluids, or dietary fruit and fiber may help); diarrhea (buttermilk, yogurt, or boiled milk may help); postural hypotension (use caution when climbing stairs or changing position from lying or sitting to standing); or urinary retention (void before taking medication). Report persistent insomnia; muscle cramping or tremors; chest pain, palpitations, rapid heartbeat, swelling of extremities, or severe dizziness; unresolved urinary retention; rash or skin irritation; yellowing of eyes or skin; pale stools/dark urine; or worsening of condition. **Pregnancy/breast-feeding precautions:** Do not get pregnant while taking this medication; use appropriate barrier contraceptive measures. Breast-feeding is not recommended.

**Geriatric Considerations:** Orthostatic hypotension is a concern with this agent, especially in patients taking other medications that may affect blood pressure. May precipitate arrhythmias in predisposed patients; may aggravate seizures. A less anticholinergic antidepressant may be a better choice. Data from a clinical trial comparing fluoxetine to tricyclics suggests that fluoxetine is significantly less effective than nortriptyline in hospitalized elderly patients with unipolar major affective disorder, especially those with melancholia and concurrent cardiovascular diseases.

**Additional Information** The pamoate formulation contains tartrazine. The injection formulation contains sulfites.

Imipramine hydrochloride: Tofranil®, Janimine®
Imipramine pamoate: Tofranil-PM®

**Related Information**

Antidepressant Agents Comparison *on page 1368*
Peak and Trough Guidelines *on page 1331*

♦ **Imitrex®** *see* Sumatriptan Succinate *on page 1090*
♦ **Immune Globulin, Intramuscular** *see page 1256*

## Immune Globulin, Intravenous (i MYUN GLOB yoo lin, IN tra VEE nus)

**U.S. Brand Names** Gamimune® N; Gammagard® S/D; Gammar®-P I.V.; Polygam® S/D; Sandoglobulin®; Venoglobulin®-I; Venoglobulin®-S

**Synonyms** IGIV; IVIG

**Intravenous Globulin Product Comparison**

| | Gamimune® N | Sandoglobulin® | Venoglobulin®-I |
|---|---|---|---|
| FDA indication | Primary immunodeficiency, ITP | Primary immunodeficiency, ITP | Primary immunodeficiency, ITP |
| Contraindication | IgA deficiency | IgA deficiency | IgA deficiency |
| IgA content | 270 mcg/mL | 720 mcg/mL | 20-24 mcg/mL |
| Adverse reactions (%) | 5.2 | 2.5-6.6 | 6 |
| Plasma source | >2000 paid donors | 8000-15,000 voluntary donors | 6000-9000 paid donors |
| Half-life | 21 d | 21-23 d | 29 d |
| IgG subclass (%) | | | |
| $IgG_1$ (60-70) | 60 | 60.5 (55.3)[1] | 62.3[2] |
| $IgG_2$ (19-31) | 29.4 | 30.2 (35.7) | 32.8 |
| $IgG_3$ (5-8.4) | 6.5 | 6.6 (6.3) | 2.9 |
| $IgG_4$ (0.7-4) | 4.1 | 2.6 (2.6) | 2 |
| Monomers (%) | >95 | >92 | >98 |
| Gammaglobulin (%) | >98 | >96 | >98 |
| Storage | Refrigerate | Room temp | Room temp |
| Recommendations for initial infusion rate | 0.01-0.02 mL/kg/min | 0.01-0.03 mL/kg/min | 0.01-0.02 mL/kg/min |
| Maximum infusion rate | 0.08 mL/kg/min | 2.5 mL/min | 0.04 mL/kg/min |
| Maximum concentration for infusion (%) | 10 | 12 | 10 |

[1]Skvaril F and Gardi A, "Differences Among Available Immunoglobulin Preparations for Intravenous Use," *Pediatr Infect Dis J*, 1988, 7:543-48.

[2]Roomer J, Morgenthaler JJ, Scherz R, et al, "Characterization of Various Immunoglobulin Preparations for Intravenous Application," *Vox Sang*, 1982, 42:62-73.

[3]ASHP Commission on Therapeutics, ASHP Therapeutic Guidelines for Intravenous Immune Globulin, *Clin Pharm*, 1992, 11:117-36.

[4]Manufacturer's Product Information/Personal Communication.

**Therapeutic Category** Immune Globulin

**Pregnancy Risk Factor** C

**Lactation** Excretion in breast milk unknown

**Use** Treatment of immunodeficiency syndromes (hypogammaglobulinemia, agammaglobulinemia, IgG subclass deficiencies, severe combined immunodeficiency syndromes (SCIDS), Wiskott-Aldrich syndrome), idiopathic thrombocytopenic purpura; in conjunction with appropriate anti-infective therapy to prevent or modify acute bacterial or viral infections in patients with iatrogenically-induced or disease-associated immunodepression; chronic lymphocytic leukemia (CLL) - chronic prophylaxis autoimmune neutropenia, bone marrow transplantation patients, autoimmune hemolytic anemia or neutropenia, refractory dermatomyositis/polymyositis, autoimmune diseases (myasthenia gravis, SLE, bullous pemphigoid, severe rheumatoid arthritis), Kawasaki disease, Guillain-Barré syndrome. Therapy should be guided by clinical observation and serial determination of serum IgG levels.

**Mechanism of Action/Effect** Replacement therapy for primary and secondary immunodeficiencies; interference with $F_c$ receptors on the cells of the reticuloendothelial system for autoimmune cytopenias and ITP; possible role of contained antiviral-type antibodies

**Contraindications** Hypersensitivity to immune globulin or any component; anaphylactic hypersensitivity reactions can occur, especially in IgA-deficient patients

**Warnings** Studies indicate that the currently available products have no discernible risk of transmitting HIV or hepatitis B. Pregnancy factor C.

**Drug Interactions**

**Increased Effect/Toxicity:** Live virus, vaccines (measles, mumps, rubella); do not administer within 3 months after administration of these vaccines.

**Adverse Reactions**

1% to 10%:
- Cardiovascular: Flushing of the face, tachycardia
- Central nervous system: Chills
- Gastrointestinal: Nausea
- Respiratory: Dyspnea

<1% (Limited to important or life-threatening symptoms): Tightness in the chest

**Pharmacodynamics/Kinetics**

**Half-life Elimination:** 21-24 days

**Onset:** I.V. provides immediate antibody levels.

**Formulations**

Injection: Gamimune® N: 5% [50 mg/mL] (10 mL, 50 mL, 100 mL); 10% [100 mg/mL] (50 mL, 100 mL, 200 mL)

Powder for injection, lyophilized:
- Gammar-P®-IV: 1 g, 2.5 g, 5 g
- Sandoglobulin®: 1 g, 3 g, 6 g
- Venoglobulin®-I: 2.5 g, 5 g
- Detergent treated:
  - Gammagard® S/D: 2.5 g, 5 g, 10 g
  - Polygam® S/D: 2.5 g, 5 g, 10 g
- Venoglobulin®-S: 2.5 g, 5 g, 10 g

**Dosing**

**Adults:** I.V.:

**Dosages should be based on ideal body weight** and not actual body weight in morbidly obese patients.

Primary immunodeficiency disorders: 200-400 mg/kg every 4 weeks or as per monitored serum IgG concentrations

Chronic lymphocytic leukemia (CLL): 400 mg/kg/dose every 3 weeks

Idiopathic thrombocytopenic purpura (ITP): Maintenance dose:
- 400 mg/kg/day for 5 consecutive days
- 800 mg/kg/day for 2 consecutive days

Chronic ITP: 400-1000 mg/kg/dose every 7 or 14 days

Kawasaki disease:
- 400 mg/kg/day for 4 days within 10 days of onset of fever
- 800 mg/kg/day for 1-2 days within 10 days of onset of fever
- 2 g/kg for one dose only

Acquired immunodeficiency syndrome (patients must be symptomatic):
- 200-250 mg/kg/dose every 2 weeks
- 400-500 mg/kg/dose every month or every 4 weeks

Autoimmune hemolytic anemia and neutropenia: 1000 mg/kg/dose for 2-3 days

Autoimmune diseases: 400 mg/kg/day for 4 days

Postallogeneic bone marrow transplant: 500 mg/kg/week for 4 months post-transplant

Adjuvant to severe cytomegalovirus infections: 500 mg/kg/dose every other day for 7 doses

Guillain-Barré syndrome:
- 400 mg/kg/day for 4 days
- 1000 mg/kg/day for 2 days
- 2000 mg/kg/day for 1 day

Refractory dermatomyositis: 2 g/kg/dose every month x 3-4 doses

Refractory polymyositis: 1 g/kg/day x 2 days every month x 4 doses

Chronic inflammatory demyelinating polyneuropathy:
- 400 mg/kg/day for 5 doses once each month
- 800 mg/kg/day for 3 doses once each month
- 1000 mg/kg/day for 2 days once each month

(Continued)

## Immune Globulin, Intravenous *(Continued)*

**Elderly:** Refer to adult dosing.

**Renal Impairment:** $Cl_{cr}$ <10 mL/minute: Avoid use.

**Administration**

**I.V.:** For I.V. use only. For initial treatment, a lower concentration and/or a slower rate of infusion should be used.

**Stability**

**Reconstitution:** Stability and dilution is dependent upon the manufacturer and brand.

**Compatibility:** Do not mix with other drugs. See the Compatibility of Drugs Chart *on page 1315.*

**Additional Nursing Issues**

**Physical Assessment:** Assess for history of previous allergic reactions (see Contraindications). See Administration for safe infusion. Monitor vital signs during infusion and observe for adverse or allergic reactions (see Adverse Reactions). Teach patient adverse symptoms to report. **Pregnancy risk factor C** - benefits of use should outweigh possible risks. Note breast-feeding caution.

**Patient Information/Instruction:** This medication can only be administered by infusion. You will be monitored closely during the infusion. If you experience nausea ask for assistance, do not get up alone. Do not have any vaccinations for the next 3 months without consulting prescriber. Immediately report chills; chest pain, tightness, or rapid heartbeat; acute back pain; or difficulty breathing. **Pregnancy/breast-feeding precautions:** Inform prescriber if you are or intend to be pregnant. Consult prescriber if breast-feeding.

- **Immunization Guidelines** *see page 1250*
- **Immunizations (Vaccines)** *see page 1256*
- **Imodium®** *see* Loperamide *on page 688*
- **Imodium® A-D [OTC]** *see* Loperamide *on page 688*
- **Imot Ofteno** *see* Ophthalmic Agents, Glaucoma *on page 853*
- **Imot Ofteno** *see* Timolol *on page 1138*
- **Imuran®** *see* Azathioprine *on page 124*
- **I-Naphline®** *see page 1282*
- **I-Naphline® Ophthalmic** *see page 1294*
- **Inapsine®** *see* Droperidol *on page 409*

## Indapamide (in DAP a mide)

**U.S. Brand Names** Lozol®

**Therapeutic Category** Diuretic, Thiazide

**Pregnancy Risk Factor** B

**Lactation** Excretion in breast milk unknown

**Use** Management of mild to moderate hypertension; treatment of edema in congestive heart failure and nephrotic syndrome

**Mechanism of Action/Effect** Enhances sodium, chloride, and water excretion by interfering with the transport of sodium ions across the renal tubular epithelium

**Contraindications** Hypersensitivity to indapamide or any component; cross-sensitivity with other thiazides and sulfonamide derivatives; anuria

**Warnings** Use with caution in patients with renal or hepatic disease, gout, lupus erythematosus, or diabetes mellitus.

**Drug Interactions**

**Decreased Effect:** Decreased effect of oral hypoglycemics. Decreased absorption with cholestyramine and colestipol when taken together.

**Increased Effect/Toxicity:** Increased effect with furosemide and other loop diuretics. Increased toxicity/levels of lithium. When given with digoxin, diuretic-induced hypokalemia increases the risk of digoxin toxicity.

**Adverse Reactions**

1% to 10%:

Cardiovascular: Orthostatic hypotension, palpitations, flushing

Central nervous system: Dizziness, lightheadedness, vertigo, headache, weakness, restlessness, drowsiness, fatigue, lethargy, malaise, lassitude, anxiety, agitation, depression, nervousness

Gastrointestinal: Anorexia, gastric irritation, nausea, vomiting, abdominal pain, cramping, bloating, diarrhea, constipation, dry mouth, weight loss

Genitourinary: Nocturia, frequent urination, polyuria

Neuromuscular & skeletal: Muscle cramps, spasm

Ocular: Blurred vision

Respiratory: Rhinorrhea

<1% (Limited to important or life-threatening symptoms): Purpura, necrotizing angiitis, vasculitis, cutaneous vasculitis, impotency, reduced libido, hyperglycemia, glycosuria, hyperuricemia

**Overdose/Toxicology** Symptoms of overdose include lethargy, diuresis, hypermotility, confusion, and muscle weakness. Treatment is supportive.

**Pharmacodynamics/Kinetics**

**Protein Binding:** 71% to 79%

**Half-life Elimination:** 14-18 hours

**Time to Peak:** 2-2.5 hours

**Metabolism:** Liver

**Excretion:** Urine and feces

**Onset:** 1-2 hours

**Duration:** Up to 36 hours

**Formulations** Tablet: 1.25 mg, 2.5 mg

**Dosing**

**Adults:** Oral:

Hypertension: 1.25 mg/day; if no response after 4 weeks, increase to 2.5 mg/day; maximum: 5 mg. **Note:** There is little therapeutic benefit to increasing the dose to >5 mg/day; there is, however, an increased risk of electrolyte disturbances.

Congestive heart failure: 2.5 mg/day; if no response after 1 week, increase to 5 mg.

**Elderly:** Refer to adult dosing.

**Administration**

**Oral:** May be taken with food or milk. Take early in day to avoid nocturia. Take the last dose of multiple doses no later than 6 PM unless instructed otherwise.

**Monitoring Laboratory Tests** Serum electrolytes, renal function

**Additional Nursing Issues**

**Physical Assessment:** Monitor appropriate laboratory tests (see above). Monitor blood pressure and cardiac status on a regular basis. Instruct/teach patient or caregiver on orthostatic hypotension precautions and possible side effects and symptoms to report. Monitor fluid balance (I & O) and weight on a regular basis. Assess effectiveness of oral hypoglycemics with diabetic patients. Note breast-feeding caution.

**Patient Information/Instruction:** Take as directed, early in the day (last dose late afternoon). Do not exceed recommended dosage. Noninsulin-dependent diabetics should monitor serum glucose closely (medication may decrease effect of oral hypoglycemics). Monitor weight on a regular basis. Report sudden or excessive weight gain, swelling of ankles or hands, or difficulty breathing. You may experience dizziness, weakness, or drowsiness; use caution when changing position (rising from sitting or lying position) and when driving or engaging in tasks that require alertness until response to drug is known. Use may experience sensitivity to sunlight (use sunblock, wear protective clothing or sunglasses), impotence (reversible), dry mouth or thirst (frequent mouth care, chewing gum or sucking on lozenges may help). Report unusual bleeding, palpitations, numbness or tingling or cramping. **Breast-feeding precautions:** Consult prescriber if breast-feeding.

**Geriatric Considerations:** Thiazide diuretics lose efficacy when $Cl_{cr}$ is <30-35 mL/minute. Many elderly may have $Cl_{cr}$ below this limit. Calculate $Cl_{cr}$ for elderly before initiating therapy. Indapamide has the advantage over thiazide diuretics in that it is effective when $Cl_{cr}$ is <30 mL/minute.


- **Inderal®** *see* Propranolol *on page 986*
- **Inderalici** *see* Propranolol *on page 986*
- **Inderal® LA** *see* Propranolol *on page 986*
- **Inderide®** *see* Propranolol and Hydrochlorothiazide *on page 988*


## Indinavir (in DIN a veer)

**U.S. Brand Names** Crixivan®

**Therapeutic Category** Antiretroviral Agent, Protease Inhibitor

**Pregnancy Risk Factor** C

**Lactation** Enters breast milk/contraindicated

**Use** Treatment of HIV infection, as part of a multidrug regimen (at least three antiretroviral agents)

**Mechanism of Action/Effect** Indinavir is a protease inhibitor which prevents cleavage of protein precursors essential for HIV infection of new cells and viral replication.

**Contraindications** Hypersensitivity to indinavir or any component; avoid use with terfenadine, astemizole, cisapride, ergot alkaloids, or benzodiazepines

**Warnings** Use caution in patients with hepatic insufficiency. Dosage reduction may be needed. Nephrolithiasis may occur with use. If signs or symptoms of nephrolithiasis occur, interrupt therapy for 1-3 days. Ensure adequate hydration. Pregnancy factor C.

**Drug Interactions**

**Cytochrome P-450 Effect:** CYP3A3/4 enzyme substrate; CYP3A3/4 enzyme inhibitor

**Decreased Effect:** Gastric pH is lowered and absorption may be decreased when didanosine and indinavir are taken <1 hour apart. Concurrent use of rifampin may decrease effectiveness. Rifabutin decreases indinavir concentrations (dose increase is recommended).

**Increased Effect/Toxicity:** A reduction of dose is often required when coadministered with ketoconazole. Terfenadine, astemizole, cisapride, ergot alkaloids and benzodiazepines should be avoided with indinavir due to a potentially serious toxicity. Rifabutin concentrations are increased.

**Food Interactions** Indinavir bioavailability may be decreased if taken with food.

**Adverse Reactions**

>10%:

Central nervous system: Headache

Gastrointestinal: Nausea, vomiting

Hepatic: Asymptomatic hyperbilirubinemia

(Continued)

## Indinavir *(Continued)*

1% to 10%:

Central nervous system: Malaise, insomnia, dizziness, somnolence

Gastrointestinal: Abdominal pain, diarrhea, acid regurgitation, anorexia, taste perversion

Hematologic: Decreased hemoglobin, decreased neutrophils

Hepatic: Increased LFTs

Neuromuscular & skeletal: Muscle weakness, flank pain, back pain

Renal: Nephrolithiasis

<1% (Limited to important or life-threatening symptoms): Decreased platelets

Protease inhibitors cause hyperglycemia and dyslipidemia (elevated cholesterol/triglycerides) and a redistribution of fat (protease paunch, buffalo hump, facial atrophy and breast engorgement)

**Pharmacodynamics/Kinetics**

**Protein Binding:** 60% in the plasma

**Half-life Elimination:** 1.8 ± 0.4 hour

**Metabolism:** Liver

**Excretion:** Feces and urine

**Formulations** Capsule: 200 mg, 333 mg, 400 mg

**Dosing**

**Adults:** Oral: 800 mg every 8 hours; if receiving concurrent rifabutin, dose should be increased to 1000 mg every 8 hours.

**Elderly:** Refer to adult dosing.

**Hepatic Impairment:** 600 mg every 8 hours with mild/medium impairment due to cirrhosis or with ketoconazole coadministration

**Administration**

**Oral:** Drink at least 48 oz of water daily. Take the drug with water, 1 hour before or 2 hours after a meal.

**Monitoring Laboratory Tests** Liver function tests, CBC

**Additional Nursing Issues**

**Physical Assessment:** Monitor therapeutic response. Monitor for signs of opportunistic infection (eg, fever, chills, vaginal discharge, oral plaques, foul-smelling urine), and kidney function. **Pregnancy risk factor C** - benefits of use should outweigh possible risks. Breast-feeding is contraindicated.

**Patient Information/Instruction:** Take as directed, around-the-clock, with a large glass of water, preferably 1 hour before or 2 hours after meals. Maintain adequate hydration (2-3 L/day of fluids unless instructed to restrict fluid intake). If indinavir and didanosine are prescribed together, take at least 1 hour apart on an empty stomach. **Pregnancy/breast-feeding precautions:** Inform prescriber if you are or intend to be pregnant. Do not breast-feed.

**Breast-feeding Issues:** The CDC recommends **not** to breast-feed if diagnosed with HIV to avoid postnatal transmission of the virus.

**Pregnancy Issues:** Hyperbilirubinemia may be exacerbated in neonates.

**Additional Information** One study of previously untreated patients with a mean CD4 cell count of 250 cells/mm$^3$ found that indinavir plus zidovudine lowered serum HIV below detectable levels in 56% of 52 patients treated for 24 weeks. Other studies show similar results. Indinavir alone has suppressed serum HIV below detectable levels in 40% to 60% of patients treated up to 48 weeks.

**Related Information**

Antiretroviral Agents Comparison *on page 1373*


- **Indochron E-R®** *see* Indomethacin *on this page*
- **Indocid®** *see* Indomethacin *on this page*
- **Indocid® SR** *see* Indomethacin *on this page*
- **Indocin®** *see* Indomethacin *on this page*
- **Indocin® SR** *see* Indomethacin *on this page*
- **Indocyanine Green** *see page 1248*
- **Indometacin** *see* Indomethacin *on this page*


## Indomethacin (in doe METH a sin)

**U.S. Brand Names** Indochron E-R®; Indocin®; Indocin® SR

**Synonyms** Indometacin

**Therapeutic Category** Nonsteroidal Anti-Inflammatory Agent (NSAID)

**Pregnancy Risk Factor** B/D (if used longer than 48 hours or after 34-week gestation)

**Lactation** Enters breast milk/use caution (AAP rates "compatible")

**Use** Management of inflammatory diseases and rheumatoid disorders; moderate pain; acute gouty arthritis

**Mechanism of Action/Effect** Inhibits prostaglandin synthesis by decreasing the activity of the enzyme, cyclo-oxygenase, which results in decreased formation of prostaglandin precursors

**Contraindications** Hypersensitivity to indomethacin, any component, aspirin, or other nonsteroidal anti-inflammatory drugs (NSAIDs); active GI bleeding, ulcer disease; premature neonates with necrotizing enterocolitis, impaired renal function, active bleeding, thrombocytopenia; pregnancy (if used longer than 48 hours or after 34-week gestation)

**Warnings** Use with caution in patients with cardiac dysfunction, hypertension, renal or hepatic impairment, epilepsy, history of GI bleeding, patients receiving anticoagulants. Elderly are at a high risk for adverse effects from nonsteroidal anti-inflammatory agents.

As much as 60% of elderly can develop peptic ulceration and/or hemorrhage asymptomatically.

Use lowest effective dose for shortest period possible. Use of NSAIDs can compromise existing renal function especially when $Cl_{cr}$ is <30 mL/minute.

CNS adverse effects such as confusion, agitation, and hallucination are generally seen in overdose or high-dose situations; but elderly may demonstrate these adverse effects at lower doses than younger adults.

**Drug Interactions**

**Cytochrome P-450 Effect:** CYP2C9 enzyme substrate

**Decreased Effect:** May decrease antihypertensive effects of beta-blockers, hydralazine and captopril. Indomethacin may decrease the antihypertensive and diuretic effect of thiazides (hydrochlorothiazide, etc) and loop diuretics (furosemide, bumetanide).

**Increased Effect/Toxicity:** Indomethacin may increase serum potassium with potassium-sparing diuretics. Probenecid may increase indomethacin serum concentrations. Other NSAIDs may increase GI adverse effects. May increase nephrotoxicity of cyclosporine. Indomethacin may increase serum concentrations of digoxin, methotrexate, lithium, and aminoglycosides (reported with I.V. use in neonates).

**Food Interactions** Indomethacin peak serum levels may be delayed if taken with food.

**Effects on Lab Values** Positive Coombs' [direct]; ↑ sodium, chloride, bleeding time

**Adverse Reactions**

1% to 10%:

Central nervous system: Dizziness, vertigo, depression, fatigue, headache, somnolence

Endocrine & metabolic: Fluid retention

Gastrointestinal: Nausea, vomiting, heartburn, diarrhea, abdominal distress, constipation

Otic: Tinnitus

<1% (Limited to important or life-threatening symptoms): Hypertension, hypotension, chest pain, congestive heart failure, arrhythmias, tachycardia, palpitations, coma, convulsions, exfoliative dermatitis, erythema nodosum, erythema multiforme, Stevens-Johnson syndrome, toxic epidermal necrolysis, hyperkalemia, dilutional hyponatremia (I.V.), hypoglycemia (I.V.), polydipsia, hyperglycemia, glycosuria, hemolytic anemia, bone marrow depression, agranulocytosis, thrombocytopenic purpura, aplastic anemia, disseminated intravascular coagulation, leukopenia, hepatitis, jaundice, hematuria, proteinuria, nephrotic syndrome, interstitial nephritis, elevated BUN, renal failure, dyspnea

**Overdose/Toxicology** Symptoms of overdose include drowsiness, lethargy, nausea, vomiting, seizures, paresthesia, headache, dizziness, GI bleeding, cerebral edema, tinnitus, leukocytosis, and renal failure. Management of nonsteroidal anti-inflammatory (NSAID) intoxication is supportive and symptomatic.

**Pharmacodynamics/Kinetics**

**Protein Binding:** 90%

**Distribution:** Crosses the placenta

**Half-life Elimination:** 4.5 hours, longer in neonates

**Time to Peak:** Oral: Within 3-4 hours

**Metabolism:** Liver; with significant enterohepatic cycling

**Excretion:** Significant enterohepatic recycling; excreted in urine principally as glucuronide conjugates

**Onset:** Within 30 minutes

**Duration:** 4-6 hours

**Formulations**

Capsule (Indocin®): 25 mg, 50 mg

Capsule, sustained release (Indocin® SR): 75 mg

Suppository, rectal (Indocin®): 50 mg

Suspension, oral (Indocin®): 25 mg/5 mL (5 mL, 10 mL, 237 mL, 500 mL)

**Dosing**

**Adults:** Analgesia: Oral, rectal: 25-50 mg/dose 2-3 times/day; maximum: 200 mg/day; extended release capsule should be given on a 1-2 times/day schedule

**Elderly:** Refer to adult dosing.

**Administration**

**Oral:** Administer with food, milk, or antacids to decrease GI adverse effects. Extended release capsules must be swallowed whole, do not crush.

**Stability**

**Storage:** Suppositories do not require refrigeration.

**Monitoring Laboratory Tests** Renal function (serum creatinine, BUN), CBC, liver function

**Additional Nursing Issues**

**Physical Assessment:** Assess effectiveness and interactions of other medications patient may be taking (see Contraindications and Drug Interactions). Monitor laboratory tests (see above) and therapeutic response (eg, relief of pain and inflammation, increased activity tolerance), and adverse reactions (eg, GI effects, hepatotoxicity, or ototoxicity) at beginning of therapy and periodically throughout therapy (see Warnings/Precautions, Adverse Reactions, and Overdose/Toxicology). Schedule ophthalmic evaluations for patients who develop eye complaints during long-term NSAID therapy. Assess knowledge/teach patient appropriate use, interventions to reduce side effects, and adverse symptoms to report. **Pregnancy risk factor B/D** - see Pregnancy Risk Factor for cautious use. Note breast-feeding caution.

(Continued)

## Indomethacin *(Continued)*

**Patient Information/Instruction:**

Oral: Take this medication exactly as directed; do not increase dose without consulting prescriber. Do not crush, break, or chew capsules. Take with food or milk to reduce GI distress. Maintain adequate fluid intake (2-3 L/day of fluids unless instructed to restrict fluid intake).

Rectal: Suppositories do not need to be refrigerated. Wash hands before inserting unwrapped suppository high up in rectum. Wearing glove is recommended. (Use caution to avoid damage with long fingernails.)

Do not use alcohol, aspirin, or aspirin-containing medication, and all other anti-inflammatory medications without consulting prescriber. You may experience drowsiness, dizziness, nervousness, or headache (use caution when driving or engaging in tasks requiring alertness until response to drug is known); anorexia, nausea, vomiting, or heartburn (frequent small meals, frequent oral care, sucking lozenges, or chewing gum may help); fluid retention (weigh yourself weekly and report unusual (3-5 lb/week) weight gain). May discolor stool (green). GI bleeding, ulceration, or perforation can occur with or without pain; discontinue medication and contact prescriber if persistent abdominal pain or cramping, or blood in stool occurs. Report breathlessness, difficulty breathing, or unusual cough; chest pain, rapid heartbeat, palpitations; unusual bruising/bleeding; blood in urine, stool, gums, or vomitus; swollen extremities; skin rash, irritation, or itching; acute fatigue; or changes in hearing or ringing in ears. **Pregnancy/breast-feeding precautions:** Inform prescriber if you are or intend to be pregnant. Consult prescriber if breast-feeding.

**Geriatric Considerations:** Elderly are at high risk for adverse effects from nonsteroidal anti-inflammatory agents. As much as 60% of elderly can develop peptic ulceration and/or hemorrhage asymptomatically. The concomitant use of $H_2$ blockers, omeprazole, and sucralfate is not effective as prophylaxis with the exception of NSAID-induced duodenal ulcers which may be prevented by the use of ranitidine. Misoprostol is the only prophylactic agent proven effective. Also, concomitant disease and drug use contribute to the risk for GI adverse effects. Use lowest effective dose for shortest period possible. Consider renal function decline with age. Use of NSAIDs can compromise existing renal function especially when $Cl_{cr}$ is $\leq$30 mL/minute. Tinnitus may be a difficult and unreliable indication of toxicity due to age-related hearing loss or eighth cranial nerve damage. CNS adverse effects such as confusion, agitation, and hallucination are generally seen in overdose or high-dose situations, but elderly may demonstrate these adverse effects at lower doses than younger adults. Indomethacin frequently causes confusion at recommended doses in the elderly.

**Additional Information** Some formulations may contain ethanol.

**Related Information**

Nonsalicylate/Nonsteroidal Anti-inflammatory Comparison *on page 1401*


- **INF-Alpha 2** *see* Interferon Alfa-2b *on page 614*
- **Infants Feverall™ [OTC]** *see* Acetaminophen *on page 32*
- **InFed™ Injection** *see* Iron Dextran Complex *on page 626*
- **Inflamase® Forte Ophthalmic** *see* Prednisolone *on page 960*
- **Inflamase® Mild** *see page 1282*
- **Inflamase® Mild Ophthalmic** *see* Prednisolone *on page 960*


## Infliximab (in FLIKS e mab)

**U.S. Brand Names** Remicade™

**Therapeutic Category** Gastrointestinal Agent, Miscellaneous; Monoclonal Antibody

**Pregnancy Risk Factor** C

**Lactation** Excretion in breast milk unknown/not recommended

**Use** Treatment of moderately to severely active Crohn's disease for the reduction of signs and symptoms in patients who have an inadequate response to conventional therapy, or for the treatment of patients with fistulizing Crohn's disease for reduction of the number of draining enterocutaneous fistula(s)

**Contraindications** Hypersensitivity to murine proteins or any component

**Warnings** Hypersensitivity reactions, including urticaria, dyspnea, and hypotension have occurred. Discontinue the drug if a reaction occurs. Medications for the treatment of hypersensitivity reactions should be available for immediate use. Autoimmune antibodies and a lupus-like syndrome have been reported. If antibodies to double-stranded DNA are confirmed in a patient with lupus-like symptoms, treatment should be discontinued. May affect normal immune responses. Affect on the development of lymphoma and infection in Crohn's patients are unknown. Treatment may result in the development of human antichimeric antibodies (HACA). The presence of these antibodies may predispose patients to infusion reactions. Pregnancy factor C.

**Drug Interactions**

**Decreased Effect:** Specific drug interaction studies have not been conducted.

**Increased Effect/Toxicity:** Specific drug interaction studies have not been conducted.

**Adverse Reactions**

>10%:

Central nervous system: Headache (22.6%), fatigue (10.6%), fever (10.1%)
Gastrointestinal: Nausea (16.6%), abdominal pain (12.1%)
Local: Infusion reactions (16%)
Respiratory: Upper respiratory tract infection (16.1%)
Miscellaneous: Infections (21%)

1% to 10%:

Cardiovascular: Chest pain (5.5%)

Central nervous system: Pain (8.5%), dizziness (8%)

Dermatologic: Rash (6%), pruritus (5%)

Gastrointestinal: Vomiting (8.5%)

Neuromuscular & skeletal: Myalgia (5%), back pain (5%)

Respiratory: Pharyngitis (8.5%), bronchitis (7%), rhinitis (6%), cough (5%), sinusitis (5%)

Miscellaneous: Development of antibodies to double-stranded DNA (9%), candidiasis (5%), serious infection (pneumonia, cellulitis, catheter-associated sepsis, cholecystitis, endophthalmitis, furunculosis) (3%)

<1% (Limited to important or life-threatening symptoms): Lupus-like syndrome (2 patients); a proportion of patients (12%) with fistulizing disease developed new abscess 8-16 weeks after the last infusion of infliximab

**Pharmacodynamics/Kinetics**

**Half-life Elimination:** 9.5 days

**Onset:** Within 2 weeks

**Formulations** Powder for injection: 100 mg

**Dosing**

**Adults:**

Moderately to severely active Crohn's disease: I.V.: 5 mg/kg as a single infusion over a minimum of 2 hours

Fistulizing Crohn's disease: 5 mg/kg as an infusion over a minimum of 2 hours, dose repeated at 2 and 6 weeks after the initial infusion

**Elderly:** Refer to adult dosing.

**Renal Impairment:** No specific adjustment is recommended.

**Hepatic Impairment:** No specific adjustment is recommended.

**Administration**

**I.V.:** Infuse over at least 2 hours.

**I.V. Detail:** Do not infuse with other agents. Use in-line filter.

**Stability**

**Storage:** Store vials at 2°C to 8°C (36°F to 46°F); do not freeze. Does not contain preservative.

**Reconstitution:** Reconstitute vials with 10 mL sterile water for injection. Total dose of reconstituted product should be further diluted to 250 mL of 0.9% sodium chloride injection.

**Additional Nursing Issues**

**Physical Assessment:** Monitor therapeutic response (reduction of signs and symptoms of Crohn's disease or reduction in number of Crohn's related fistulas), adverse reactions (eg, hypersensitivity, respiratory effects - see Warnings/Precautions and Adverse Reactions). Teach patient appropriate interventions to reduce side effects and adverse symptoms to report. **Pregnancy risk factor C** - benefits of use should outweigh possible risks. Breast-feeding is not recommended.

**Patient Information/Instruction:** This drug can only be administered by infusion. Report adverse symptoms: headache or unusual fatigue; increased nausea or abdominal pain; cough, runny nose, difficulty breathing; chest pain or persistent dizziness; fatigue, muscle pain or weakness, back pain; fever or chills, mouth sores, vaginal itching or discharge, sore throat, unhealed sores, or frequent infections. **Pregnancy/breast-feeding precautions:** Inform prescriber if you are or intend to be pregnant. Breast-feeding is not recommended.

**Breast-feeding Issues:** It is not known whether infliximab is secreted in human milk. Because many immunoglobulins are secreted in milk and the potential for serious adverse reactions exists, a decision should be made whether to discontinue nursing or discontinue the drug, taking into account the importance of the drug to the mother.


♦ **Influenza Virus Vaccine** *see page 1256*

♦ **Infufer®** *see* Iron Dextran Complex *on page 626*

♦ **INH** *see* Isoniazid *on page 630*

♦ **Inhalant (Asthma, Bronchospasm) Agents** *see page 1388*

♦ **Inhepar** *see* Heparin *on page 558*

♦ **Inhibitron®** *see* Omeprazole *on page 851*

♦ **Innovar®** *see* Droperidol and Fentanyl *on page 410*

♦ **Inotropic and Vasoconstrictor Comparison** *see page 1391*

♦ **Insect Sting Kit** *see page 1246*

♦ **Insogen®** *see* Chlorpropamide *on page 259*

♦ **Insta-Char® [OTC]** *see* Charcoal *on page 243*

♦ **Insta-Glucose®** *see page 1294*

♦ **Insulina Lenta** *see* Insulin Preparations *on this page*

♦ **Insulina NPH** *see* Insulin Preparations *on this page*

♦ **Insulina Regular** *see* Insulin Preparations *on this page*


## Insulin Preparations (IN su lin prep a RAY shuns)

**U.S. Brand Names** Humalog®; Humulin® 50/50; Humulin® 70/30; Humulin® L; Humulin® N; Humulin® R; Humulin® U; Lente® Iletin® I; Lente® Iletin® II; Lente® Insulin; Lente® L; Novolin® 70/30; Novolin® L; Novolin® N; Novolin® R; NPH Iletin® I; NPH Insulin; NPH-N; Pork NPH Iletin® II; Pork Regular Iletin® II; Regular (Concentrated) Iletin® II U-500; Regular Iletin® I; Regular Insulin; Regular Purified Pork Insulin; Velosulin® Human

**Therapeutic Category** Antidiabetic Agent (Insulin); Antidote

(Continued)

## Insulin Preparations *(Continued)*

**Pregnancy Risk Factor** B

**Lactation** Does not enter breast milk/compatible

**Use** Treatment of insulin-dependent diabetes mellitus, also noninsulin-dependent diabetes mellitus unresponsive to treatment with diet and/or oral hypoglycemics; to assure proper utilization of glucose and reduce glucosuria in nondiabetic patients receiving parenteral nutrition whose glucosuria cannot be adequately controlled with infusion rate adjustments or those who require assistance in achieving optimal caloric intakes; hyperkalemia (use with glucose to shift potassium into cells to lower serum potassium levels)

**Mechanism of Action/Effect** The principal hormone required for proper glucose utilization in normal metabolic processes; it is obtained from beef or pork pancreas or a biosynthetic process converting pork insulin to human insulin; insulins are categorized into 3 groups related to promptness, duration, and intensity of action

**Warnings** Any change of insulin should be made cautiously. Changing manufacturers, type and/or method of manufacture, may result in the need for a change of dosage. Human insulin differs from animal-source insulin. Hypoglycemia may result from increased work or exercise without eating. Use with caution in patients with a previous hypersensitivity reaction. S.C. doses used in insulin-resistant patients must be reduced if given I.V., only regular insulin should be given I.V.

**Drug Interactions**

**Decreased Effect:** Decreased hypoglycemic effect of insulin with corticosteroids, dextrothyroxine, diltiazem, dobutamine, epinephrine, niacin, oral contraceptives, thiazide diuretics, thyroid hormone, and smoking.

**Increased Effect/Toxicity:** Increased hypoglycemic effect of insulin with alcohol, alpha blockers, anabolic steroids, beta-blockers (nonselective beta-blockers may delay recovery from hypoglycemic episodes and mask signs/symptoms of hypoglycemia; cardioselective beta-blocker agents may be alternatives), clofibrate, guanethidine, MAO inhibitors, pentamidine, phenylbutazone, salicylates, sulfinpyrazone, and tetracyclines.

**Adverse Reactions**

1% to 10%:

Cardiovascular: Palpitation, tachycardia, pallor

Central nervous system: Fatigue, mental confusion, loss of consciousness, headache, hypothermia

Dermatologic: Urticaria, redness

Endocrine & metabolic: Hypoglycemia

Gastrointestinal: Hunger, nausea, numbness of mouth

Local: Itching, edema, stinging, or warmth at injection site, atrophy or hypertrophy of S.C. fat tissue

Neuromuscular & skeletal: Muscle weakness, paresthesia, tremors

Ocular: Transient presbyopia or blurred vision, blurred vision

Miscellaneous: Sweating, anaphylaxis

**Overdose/Toxicology** Symptoms of overdose include tachycardia, anxiety, hunger, tremor, pallor, headache, motor dysfunction, speech disturbances, sweating, palpitations, coma, and death. Antidote is glucose and glucagon, if necessary.

**Pharmacodynamics/Kinetics**

**Onset:**

Onset and duration of hypoglycemic effects depend upon preparation administered. See table.

**Pharmacokinetics/Pharmacodynamics: Onset and Duration of Hypoglycemic Effects Depend Upon Preparation Administered**

| | Onset (h) | Peak (h) | Duration (h) |
|---|---|---|---|
| Insulin, regular (Novolin® R) | 0.5–1 | 2-3 | 5–7 |
| Isophane insulin suspension (NPH) (Novolin® N) | 1–1.5 | 4–12 | 18–24 |
| Insulin zinc suspension (Lente®) | 1–2.5 | 8–12 | 18–24 |
| Isophane insulin suspension and regular insulin injection (Novolin® 70/30) | 0.5 (0.5) | 4-8 (2-12) | 24 (24) |
| Prompt zinc insulin suspension (PZI) | 4-8 | 14-24 | 36 |
| Extended insulin zinc suspension (Ultralente®) | 4-8 | 16–18 | >36 |

Onset and duration: Insulin lispro may begin to act in 15-30 minutes. Biosynthetic NPH human insulin shows a more rapid onset and shorter duration of action than corresponding porcine insulins; human insulin and purified porcine regular insulin are similarly efficacious following S.C. administration. The duration of action of highly purified porcine insulins is shorter than that of conventional insulin equivalents. Duration depends on type of preparation and route of administration as well as patient related variables. In general, the larger the dose of insulin, the longer the duration of activity.

**Formulations** All insulins are 100 units/mL (10 mL) except where indicated:

RAPID-ACTING:

**Insulin Lispro rDNA Origin:** Humalog® [*Lilly*] (1.5 mL, 3 mL, 10 mL)

**Insulin Injection** (Regular Insulin)

Beef and pork: Regular Iletin® I [*Lilly*]

Human:

rDNA: Humulin® R [*Lilly*], Novolin® R [*Novo Nordisk*]

Semisynthetic: Velosulin® Human [*Novo Nordisk*]

Pork: Regular Insulin [*Novo Nordisk*]

Purified pork:

Pork Regular Iletin® II [*Lilly*], Regular Purified Pork Insulin [*Novo Nordisk*]

Regular (Concentrated) Iletin® II U-500 (*Lilly*): 500 units/mL

INTERMEDIATE-ACTING:

**Insulin Zinc Suspension** (Lente)

Beef and pork: Lente® Iletin® I [*Lilly*]

Human, rDNA: Humulin® L [*Lilly*], Novolin® L [*Novo Nordisk*]

Purified pork: Lente® Iletin® II [*Lilly*], Lente® L [*Novo Nordisk*]

**Isophane Insulin Suspension** (NPH)

Beef and pork: NPH Iletin® I [*Lilly*]

Human, rDNA: Humulin® N [*Lilly*], Novolin® N [*Novo Nordisk*]

Purified pork: Pork NPH Iletin® II [*Lilly*], NPH-N [*Novo Nordisk*]

LONG-ACTING:

**Insulin Zinc Suspension, Extended** (Ultralente®)

Human, rDNA: Humulin® U [Lilly]

COMBINATIONS:

**Isophane Insulin Suspension and Insulin Injection**

Isophane insulin suspension (50%) and insulin injection (50%) human (rDNA): Humulin® 50/50 [*Lilly*]

Isophane insulin suspension (70%) and insulin injection (30%) human (rDNA): Humulin® 70/30 [*Lilly*], Novolin® 70/30 [*Novo Nordisk*]

**Dosing**

**Adults:** Dose requires continuous medical supervision; may administer I.V. (regular), I.M., S.C.

Diabetes mellitus: The number and size of daily doses, time of administration, and diet and exercise require continuous medical supervision. Lispro should be given within 15 minutes of a meal and human regular insulin should be given within 30-60 minutes before a meal. Maintenance doses should be administered subcutaneously and sites should be rotated to prevent lipodystrophy.

0.5-1 unit/kg/day in divided doses

Hyperkalemia: Give calcium gluconate and $NaHCO_3$ first then 50% dextrose at 0.5-1 mL/kg and insulin 1 unit for every 4-5 g dextrose given

Diabetic ketoacidosis: I.V. loading dose: 0.1 unit/kg, then maintenance continuous infusion: 0.1 unit/kg/hour (range: 0.05-0.2 units/kg/hour depending upon the rate of decrease of serum glucose - rapid decrease of serum glucose may lead to cerebral edema).

Optimum rate of decrease (serum glucose): 80-100 mg/dL/hour

**Note:** Newly diagnosed patients with IDDM presenting in DKA and patients with blood sugars <800 mg/dL may be relatively "sensitive" to insulin and should receive loading and initial maintenance doses approximately 1/2 of those indicated above.

**Elderly:** Refer to adult dosing.

**Renal Impairment:**

$Cl_{cr}$ 10-50 mL/minute: Administer at 75% of normal dose.

$Cl_{cr}$ <10 mL/minute: Administer at 25% to 50% of normal dose and monitor glucose closely.

Hemodialysis effects: Because of a large molecular weight (6000 daltons), insulin is not significantly removed by either peritoneal or hemodialysis.

Supplemental dose is not necessary.

Peritoneal dialysis effects: Supplemental dose is not necessary.

Continuous arteriovenous or venovenous hemofiltration effects: Supplemental dose is not necessary.

**Administration**

**I.V.:** Regular insulin may be administered by S.C., I.M., or I.V. routes.

I.V. administration (requires use of an infusion pump): **Only regular insulin** may be administered I.V.

**To be ordered as units/hour:** Example: Standard diluent of regular insulin only: 100 units/100 mL NS (can be given as a more diluted solution, ie, 100 units/250 mL NS)

**I.V. Detail:**

I.V. infusions: To minimize adsorption problems to I.V. solution bag:

If new tubing is **not** needed: Wait a minimum of 30 minutes between the preparation of the solution and the initiation of the infusion.

If new tubing is needed: After receiving the insulin drip solution, the administration set should be attached to the I.V. container and the line should be flushed with the insulin solution. Wait 30 minutes, then flush the line again with the insulin solution prior to initiating the infusion.

If insulin is required prior to the availability of the insulin drip, regular insulin should be administered by I.V. push injection.

Because of adsorption, the actual amount of insulin being administered could be substantially less than the apparent amount. Therefore, adjustment of the insulin

(Continued)

## Insulin Preparations *(Continued)*

drip rate should be based on effect and not solely on the apparent insulin dose. Furthermore, the apparent dose should not be used as the basis for determining the subsequent insulin dose upon discontinuing the insulin drip. Dose requires continuous medical supervision.

Can be given as a more diluted solution, ie, 100 units/250 mL NS.

Insulin rate of infusion (100 units regular/100 mL NS)

1 unit/hour: 1 mL/hour
2 units/hour: 2 mL/hour
3 units/hour: 3 mL/hour
4 units/hour: 4 mL/hour
5 units/hour: 5 mL/hour, etc

**Other:** Cold injections should be avoided. S.C. administration is usually made into the thighs, arms, buttocks, or abdomen, with sites rotated. When mixing regular insulin with other preparations of insulin, regular insulin should be drawn into syringe first.

**Stability**

**Storage:** Bottle in use is stable at room temperature up to 1 month and 3 months refrigerated. Cold (freezing) causes more damage to insulin than room temperatures up to 100°F. Avoid direct sunlight.

**Compatibility:** Isophane insulin suspension (NPH) is compatible with regular insulin. Protamine zinc insulin suspension is compatible with regular insulin.

**Monitoring Laboratory Tests** Urine sugar and acetone, serum glucose, electrolytes

**Additional Nursing Issues**

**Physical Assessment:** Assess effectiveness and interactions of other medications (see Drug Interactions). See Warnings/Precautions and Contraindications for use cautions. Monitor effectiveness of therapy and monitor laboratory tests frequently during therapy (see above). Monitor for adverse response (eg, hypoglycemia - see Adverse Reactions and Overdose/Toxicology). Assess knowledge/teach patient or refer patient to diabetic educator for instruction in appropriate use (including safe disposal of syringes and needles), possible side effects and appropriate interventions, and adverse symptoms to report.

**Patient Information/Instruction:** This medication is used to control diabetes; it is not a cure. Other components of treatment plan are important: follow prescribed diet, medication, and exercise regimen. Take exactly as directed. Do not change dose or discontinue unless so advised by prescriber. Inform prescriber of all other prescription or OTC medications you are taking; do not introduce new medication without consulting prescriber. If you experience hypoglycemic reaction, contact prescriber immediately. Maintain regular dietary intake and exercise routine and always carry quick source of sugar with you. Report adverse side effects, including chest pain or palpitations; persistent fatigue, confusion, headache; skin rash or redness; numbness of mouth, lips, or tongue; muscle weakness or tremors; changes in vision; difficulty breathing; or nausea, vomiting, or flu-like symptoms.

**Geriatric Considerations:** How "tightly" a geriatric patient's blood glucose should be controlled is controversial; however, a fasting blood sugar <150 mg/dL is now an acceptable end point. Such a decision should be based on the patient's functional and cognitive status, how well they recognize hypoglycemic or hyperglycemic symptoms, and how to respond to them and their other disease states. Patients who are unable to accurately draw up their dose will need assistance such as prefilled syringes. Initial doses may require considerations for renal function in the elderly with dosing adjusted subsequently based on blood glucose monitoring.

**Additional Information** The term "purified" refers to insulin preparations containing no more than 10 ppm proinsulin (purified and human insulins are less immunogenic).


- **Intacglobin** *see* Immune Globulin, Intravenous *on page 602*
- **Intal® Nebulizer Solution** *see* Cromolyn Sodium *on page 309*
- **Intal® Oral Inhaler** *see* Cromolyn Sodium *on page 309*
- **Integrilin®** *see* Eptifibatide *on page 430*
- **Intercept™** *see page 1294*
- **α-2-Interferon** *see* Interferon Alfa-2b *on page 614*


## Interferon Alfa-2a (in ter FEER on AL fa too aye)

**U.S. Brand Names** Roferon-A®

**Synonyms** IFLrA; rIFN-A

**Therapeutic Category** Biological Response Modulator

**Pregnancy Risk Factor** C

**Lactation** Enters breast milk/contraindicated

**Use** Patients >18 years of age: Hairy cell leukemia, AIDS-related Kaposi's sarcoma, chronic hepatitis C, chronic myelogenous leukemia (CML), adjuvant treatment to surgery for primary or recurrent malignant melanoma; multiple unlabeled uses; indications and dosage regimens are specific for a particular brand of interferon

**Mechanism of Action/Effect** Alpha interferons are a family of proteins that have antiviral, antiproliferative, and immune-regulating activity. Inhibits cell growth and proliferation and enhances immune response.

**Contraindications** Hypersensitivity to alfa-2a interferon or any component

**Warnings** Use with caution in patients with seizure disorders, brain metastases, compromised CNS, multiple sclerosis, and patients with pre-existing cardiac disease, severe renal or hepatic impairment, or myelosuppression. Higher doses in the elderly or in malignancies other than hairy cell leukemia may result in severe obtundation. Pregnancy factor C.

**Drug Interactions**

**Cytochrome P-450 Effect:** Inhibits metabolism by cytochrome P-450 (isoenzyme profiles not defined)

**Increased Effect/Toxicity:** Cimetidine may augment the antitumor effects of interferon in melanoma. Theophylline clearance has been reported to be decreased in hepatitis patients receiving interferon. Vinblastine enhances interferon toxicity in several patients; increased incidence of paresthesia has also been noted.

**Adverse Reactions**

>10%:

- Central nervous system: Dizziness, fatigue, malaise, fever (usually within 4-6 hours), chills
- Dermatologic: Rash
- Gastrointestinal: Dry mouth, nausea, vomiting, diarrhea, abdominal cramps, weight loss, metallic taste
- Hematologic: Mildly myelosuppressive and well tolerated if used without adjunct antineoplastic agents; thrombocytosis has been reported, leukopenia (mainly neutropenia), anemia, thrombocytopenia, decreased hemoglobin, hematocrit, platelets
- Myelosuppressive:
  - WBC: Mild
  - Platelets: Mild
  - Onset (days): 7-10
  - Nadir (days): 14
  - Recovery (days): 21
- Neuromuscular & skeletal: Rigors, arthralgia
- Miscellaneous: Flu-like syndrome, sweating

1% to 10%:

- Central nervous system: Headache, delirium, somnolence, neurotoxicity
- Dermatologic: Alopecia, dry skin
- Gastrointestinal: Anorexia, stomatitis
- Hepatic: Hepatotoxicity
- Neuromuscular & skeletal: Peripheral neuropathy, leg cramps
- Ocular: Blurred vision
- Miscellaneous: Sweating

<1% (Limited to important or life-threatening symptoms): Tachycardia, arrhythmias, chest pain, hypotension, SVT, edema, increased hepatic transaminase, proteinuria, increased BUN/creatinine, dyspnea

**Overdose/Toxicology** Symptoms of overdose include CNS depression, obtundation, flu-like symptoms, and myelosuppression. Treatment is supportive.

**Pharmacodynamics/Kinetics**

**Distribution:** The $V_d$ of interferon is 31 L; but has been noted to be much greater (370-720 L) in leukemia patients receiving continuous infusion IFN. IFN does not penetrate the CSF.

**Half-life Elimination:** I.M., I.V.: 2 hours after administration; S.C.: 3 hours

**Time to Peak:** I.M., S.C.: ~6-8 hours

**Metabolism:** Kidneys

**Excretion:** Urine

**Formulations**

Injection: 3 million units/mL (1 mL); 6 million units/mL (3 mL); 9 million units/mL (0.9 mL, 3 mL); 36 million units/mL (1 mL)

Powder for injection: 6 million units/mL when reconstituted

**Dosing**

**Adults:** I.M., S.C. (refer to individual protocols):

- Hairy cell leukemia:
  - Induction: 3 million units/day for 16-24 weeks.
  - Maintenance: 3 million units 3 times/week (may be treated for up to 20 consecutive weeks)
- AIDS-related Kaposi's sarcoma:
  - Induction: 36 million units/day for 10-12 weeks
  - Maintenance: 36 million units 3 times/week (may begin with dose escalation from 3-9-18 million units each day over 3 consecutive days followed by 36 million units/day for the remainder of the 10-12 weeks of induction)
  - If severe adverse reactions occur, modify dosage (50% reduction) or temporarily discontinue therapy until adverse reactions abate.

**Elderly:** Refer to adult dosing.

**Administration**

**I.M.:** Reconstitute with recommended amount of bacteriostatic water and agitate gently; do not shake. **Note:** Different vial strengths require different amounts of diluent.

**Other:** S.C. administration is suggested for those who are at risk for bleeding or are thrombocytopenic. Rotate S.C. injection site. Patient should be well hydrated. Reconstitute with recommended amount of bacteriostatic water and agitate gently; do not shake. **Note:** Different vial strengths require different amounts of diluent.

**Stability**

**Storage:** Refrigerate vials at 2°C to 8°C (36°F to 46°F); do not freeze. Do not shake.

**Reconstitution:** After reconstitution, the solution is stable for 24 hours at room temperature and for 1 month when refrigerated.

**Monitoring Laboratory Tests** Baseline chest x-ray, EKG, CBC with differential, liver function, electrolytes, platelets, weight; patients with pre-existing cardiac abnormalities, or in advanced stages of cancer should have EKGs taken before and during treatment.

(Continued)

## Interferon Alfa-2a *(Continued)*

**Additional Nursing Issues**

**Physical Assessment:** Monitor laboratory results on a regular basis (see Monitoring Laboratory Tests). Monitor for effectiveness of therapy and possible adverse reactions (see Warnings/Precautions and Adverse Reactions). Assess knowledge/instruct patient/caregiver on appropriate reconstitution, injection and needle disposal, possible side effects, and symptoms to report. **Pregnancy risk factor C** - barrier contraceptive teaching may be appropriate. Breast-feeding is contraindicated.

**Patient Information/Instruction:** Use as directed; do not change dosage or schedule of administration without consulting prescriber. Maintain adequate hydration (2-3 L/day of fluids unless instructed to restrict fluid intake). You may experience flu-like syndrome (acetaminophen may help); nausea, vomiting, dry mouth, or metallic taste (frequent small meals, frequent mouth care, sucking lozenges, or chewing gum may help); drowsiness, dizziness, agitation, abnormal thinking (use caution when driving or engaging in tasks requiring alertness until response to drug is known). Report unusual bruising or bleeding; persistent abdominal disturbances; unusual fatigue; muscle pain or tremors; chest pain or palpitation; swelling of extremities or unusual weight gain; difficulty breathing; pain, swelling, or redness at injection site; or other unusual symptoms. **Pregnancy/breast-feeding precautions:** Inform prescriber if you are or intend to be pregnant. Do not breast-feed.

**Geriatric Considerations:** No specific data is available for the elderly; however, pay close attention to Warnings/Precautions.

## Interferon Alfa-2b (in ter FEER on AL fa too bee)

**U.S. Brand Names** Intron® A

**Synonyms** INF-Alpha 2; α-2-Interferon; rIFN-α2

**Therapeutic Category** Biological Response Modulator

**Pregnancy Risk Factor** C

**Lactation** Enters breast milk/contraindicated

**Use** Patients >18 years of age: Hairy cell leukemia, condylomata acuminata, AIDS-related Kaposi's sarcoma, chronic hepatitis non-A, non-B(C), chronic hepatitis B; indications and dosage regimens are specific for a particular brand of interferon

**Mechanism of Action/Effect** Alpha interferons are a family of proteins that have antiviral, antiproliferative, and immune-regulating activity. Inhibits cell growth and proliferation and enhances immune response.

**Contraindications** Hypersensitivity to interferon alfa-2b or any component

**Warnings** Use with caution in patients with seizure disorders, brain metastases, compromised CNS, multiple sclerosis, and patients with pre-existing cardiac disease, severe renal or hepatic impairment, or myelosuppression. Higher doses in the elderly or in malignancies other than hairy cell leukemia may result in severe obtundation. Pregnancy factor C.

**Drug Interactions**

**Cytochrome P-450 Effect:** Inhibits metabolism by cytochrome P-450 (isoenzyme profiles not defined)

**Increased Effect/Toxicity:** Cimetidine may augment the antitumor effects of interferon in melanoma. Theophylline clearance has been reported to be decreased in hepatitis patients receiving interferon. Vinblastine enhances interferon toxicity in several patients; increased incidence of paresthesia has also been noted.

**Adverse Reactions**

>10%:

Central nervous system: Dizziness, drowsiness, fatigue, malaise, fever (usually within 4-6 hours), chills

Dermatologic: Rash

Gastrointestinal: Dry mouth, nausea, vomiting, diarrhea, abdominal cramps, weight loss, metallic taste, anorexia

Hematologic: Mildly myelosuppressive and well tolerated if used without adjunct antineoplastic agents; thrombocytosis has been reported, leukopenia (mainly neutropenia), anemia, thrombocytopenia, decreased hemoglobin, hematocrit, platelets

Myelosuppressive: WBC: Mild; Platelets: Mild; Onset (days): 7-10; Nadir (days): 14; Recovery (days): 21

Neuromuscular & skeletal: Rigors, arthralgia

Miscellaneous: Flu-like syndrome, sweating

1% to 10%:

Central nervous system: Neurotoxicity

Dermatologic: Dry skin, alopecia

Gastrointestinal: Stomatitis

Hepatic: Hepatotoxicity

Neuromuscular & skeletal: Peripheral neuropathy, leg cramps

Ocular: Blurred vision

Miscellaneous: Diaphoresis

<1% (Limited to important or life-threatening symptoms): Cardiotoxicity, tachycardia, arrhythmias, hypotension, SVT, chest pain, edema, EEG abnormalities, sensory neuropathy, headache, psychiatric effects, delirium, somnolence, hypothyroidism, increased uric acid level, increased hepatic transaminase, increased ALT and AST, myalgia, proteinuria, increased BUN/creatinine, coughing, dyspnea, nasal congestion, neutralizing antibodies (usually patient can build up a tolerance to side effects)

**Overdose/Toxicology** Symptoms of overdose include CNS depression, obtundation, flu-like symptoms, and myelosuppression. Treatment is supportive.

**Pharmacodynamics/Kinetics**

**Distribution:** The $V_d$ of interferon is 31 L, but has been noted to be much greater (370-720 L) in leukemia patients receiving continuous infusion IFN. IFN does not penetrate the CSF.

**Half-life Elimination:** I.M., I.V.: 2 hours; S.C.: 3 hours

**Time to Peak:** I.M., S.C.: ~6-8 hours

**Metabolism:** Kidneys

**Formulations**

See also Interferon Alfa-2b and Ribavirin Combination Pack monograph.

Injection, albumin free: 3 million units (0.5 mL); 5 million units (0.5 mL); 10 million units (1 mL); 25 million units

Powder for injection, lyophilized: 18 million units, 50 million units

**Dosing**

**Adults:** Refer to individual protocols.

Hairy cell leukemia: I.M., S.C.: 2 million units/m$^2$ 3 times/week for 2 to ≥6 months of therapy

AIDS-related Kaposi's sarcoma: I.M., S.C. (use 50 million unit vial): 30 million units/m$^2$ 3 times/week

Condylomata acuminata: Intralesionally (use 10 million unit vial): 1 million units/lesion 3 times/week for 4-8 weeks; not to exceed 5 million units per treatment (maximum: 5 lesions at one time)

Chronic hepatitis C (non-A/non-B): I.M., S.C.: 3 million units 3 times/week for approximately a 6-month course

Chronic hepatitis B: I.M., S.C.: 5 million units/day or 10 million units 3 times/week for 16 weeks; if severe adverse reactions occur, reduce dosage 50% or temporarily discontinue therapy until adverse reactions abate. When platelet/granulocyte count returns to normal, reinstitute therapy.

**Elderly:** Refer to adult dosing.

**Administration**

**I.M.:** Reconstitute with recommended amount of bacteriostatic water and agitate gently; do not shake. **Note:** Different vial strengths require different amounts of diluent.

**Other:** S.C. administration is suggested for those who are at risk for bleeding or are thrombocytopenic. Rotate S.C. injection site. Patient should be well hydrated. Reconstitute with recommended amount of bacteriostatic water and agitate gently; do not shake. **Note:** Different vial strengths require different amounts of diluent.

**Stability**

**Storage:** Store intact vials at refrigeration (2°C to 8°C).

**Reconstitution:** Reconstitute vials with diluent. Solution is stable for 30 days under refrigeration (2°C to 8°C).

**Standard I.M./S.C. dilution:**

Dose/syringe or dispense vial to floor

Solution is stable for 7 days at room temperature and 30 days under refrigeration (2°C to 8°C).

**Monitoring Laboratory Tests** Baseline chest x-ray, EKG, CBC with differential, liver function, electrolytes, platelets; patients with pre-existing cardiac abnormalities, or in advanced stages of cancer should have EKGs taken before and during treatment.

**Additional Nursing Issues**

**Physical Assessment:** Monitor laboratory results on a regular basis (see Monitoring Laboratory Tests). Monitor for effectiveness of therapy and possible adverse reactions (see Warnings/Precautions and Adverse Reactions). Assess knowledge/instruct patient/caregiver on appropriate reconstitution, injection and needle disposal, possible side effects, and symptoms to report. **Pregnancy risk factor C** - barrier contraceptive teaching may be appropriate. Breast-feeding is contraindicated.

**Patient Information/Instruction:** Use as directed; do not change dosage or schedule of administration without consulting prescriber. Maintain adequate hydration (2-3 L/day of fluids unless instructed to restrict fluid intake). You may experience flu-like syndrome (acetaminophen may help); nausea, vomiting, dry mouth, or metallic taste (frequent small meals, frequent mouth care, sucking lozenges, or chewing gum may help); drowsiness, dizziness, agitation, abnormal thinking (use caution when driving or engaging in tasks requiring alertness until response to drug is known). Report unusual bruising or bleeding; persistent abdominal disturbances; unusual fatigue; muscle pain or tremors; chest pain or palpitation; swelling of extremities or unusual weight gain; difficulty breathing; pain, swelling, or redness at injection site; or other unusual symptoms. **Pregnancy/breast-feeding precautions:** Inform prescriber if you are or intend to be pregnant. Do not breast-feed.

## Interferon Alfa-2b and Ribavirin Combination Pack

(in ter FEER on AL fa too bee)

**U.S. Brand Names** Rebetron™

**Synonyms** Ribavarin and Interferon Alfa-2b Combination Pack

**Therapeutic Category** Antiviral Agent; Biological Response Modulator

**Pregnancy Risk Factor** X

**Use** Treatment of chronic hepatitis C in patients with compensated liver disease who have relapsed following alpha interferon therapy

(Continued)

## Interferon Alfa-2b and Ribavirin Combination Pack *(Continued)*

**Formulations** Combination package:

Patients ≤75 kg:

Each Rebetron™ combination package consists of:

A box containing 6 vials of Intron® A (3 million int. units in 0.5 mL per vial) and 6 syringes and alcohol swabs; two boxes containing 35 Rebetol® capsules each for a total of 70 capsules (5 capsules per blister card)

One 18 million int. units multidose vial of Intron® A injection (22.8 million int. units per 3.8 mL; 3 million int. units/0.5 mL) and 6 syringes and alcohol swabs; two boxes containing 35 Rebetol® capsules each for a total of 70 capsules (5 capsules per blister card)

One 18 million int. units Intron® A injection multidose pen (22.5 million int. units per 1.5 mL; 3 million int. units/0.2 mL) and 6 disposable needles and alcohol swabs; two boxes containing 35 Rebetol® capsules each for a total of 70 capsules (5 capsules per blister card)

Patients >75 kg:

A box containing 6 vials of Intron® A Injection (3 million int. units in 0.5 mL per vial) and 6 syringes and alcohol swabs; two boxes containing 42 Rebetol® capsules each for a total of 84 capsules (6 capsules per blister card)

One 18 million int. units multidose vial of Intron® A injection (22.5 million int. units per 3.8 mL; 3 million int. units/0.5 mL) and 6 syringes and alcohol swabs; two boxes containing 42 Rebetol® capsules each for a total of 84 capsules (6 capsules per blister card)

One 18 million int. units Intron® A Injection multidose pen (22.5 million int. units per 1.5 mL: 3 million int. units/0.2 mL) and 6 disposable needles and alcohol swabs; two boxes containing 42 Rebetol® capsules each for a total of 84 capsules (6 capsules per blister card)

Rebetol® Dose Reduction:

A box containing 6 vials of Intron® A injection (3 million int. units in 0.5 mL per vial) and 6 syringes and alcohol swabs; one box containing 42 Rebetol® capsules (6 capsules per blister card)

One 18 million int. units multidose vial of Intron® A injection (22.8 million int. units per 3.8 mL; 3 million int. units/0.5 mL) and 6 syringes and alcohol swabs; one box containing 42 Rebetol® capsules (6 capsules per blister card)

One 18 million int. units Intron® A injection multidose pen (22.5 million int. units per 1.5 mL; 3 million int. units/0.2 mL) and 6 disposable needles and alcohol swabs; one box containing 42 Rebetol® capsules (6 capsules per blister card)

**Dosing**

**Adults:** The recommended dosage of combination therapy is 3 million int. units of Intron® A injected subcutaneously 3 times/week and 1000-1200 mg of Rebetol® capsules administered orally in a divided daily (morning and evening) dose for 24 weeks. Patients weighing 75 kg (165 pounds) or less should receive 1000 mg of Rebetol® daily (440 mg in the morning, 600 mg in the evening), while patients weighing more than 75 kg should receive 1200 mg of Rebetol® daily (600 mg in the morning and 600 mg in the evening).

**Elderly:** Refer to adult dosing.

**Related Information**

Interferon Alfa-2b *on page 614*
Ribavirin *on page 1016*

## Interferon Beta-1a (in ter FEER on BAY ta won aye)

**U.S. Brand Names** Avonex™

**Synonyms** rIFN-b

**Therapeutic Category** Biological Response Modulator

**Pregnancy Risk Factor** C

**Lactation** Excretion in breast milk unknown/contraindicated

**Use** Treatment of relapsing forms of multiple sclerosis (MS); to slow the accumulation of physical disability and decrease the frequency of clinical exacerbations

**Contraindications** Hypersensitivity to *E. coli* derived products; previous hypersensitivity to interferon beta or human albumin, which is contained in beta interferon

**Warnings** The safety and efficacy of interferon beta in chronic progressive MS have not been evaluated. Flu-like symptom complex (eg, myalgia, fever, chills, malaise, sweating) is reported in 53% of patients who receive interferon beta. Use with caution in patients with depression. Use with caution in patients with pre-existing seizure disorder. Monitor cardiac patients closely for worsening of angina, CHF, or arrhythmias during initiation of therapy. Pregnancy factor C.

**Drug Interactions**

**Cytochrome P-450 Effect:** Inhibits metabolism by cytochrome P-450 (isoenzyme profiles not defined)

**Increased Effect/Toxicity:** Decreases clearance of zidovudine thus increasing zidovudine toxicity.

**Adverse Reactions** 1% to 10%:

Cardiovascular: CHF (rare), tachycardia, syncope

Central nervous system: Headache, lethargy, depression, emotional lability, anxiety, suicidal ideations, somnolence, agitation, confusion

Dermatologic: Alopecia (rare)

Endocrine & metabolic: Hypocalcemia

Gastrointestinal: Nausea, anorexia, vomiting, diarrhea, chronic weight loss

Hematologic: Leukopenia, thrombocytopenia, anemia (frequent, dose-related, but not usually severe)
Hepatic: Elevated liver enzymes (mild, transient)
Local: Pain/redness at injection site (80%)
Neuromuscular & skeletal: Weakness
Ocular: Retinal toxicity/visual changes
Renal: Elevated BUN and $S_{cr}$
Miscellaneous: Flu-like syndrome (fever, nausea, malaise, myalgia) occurs in most patients, but is usually controlled by acetaminophen or NSAIDs; dose-related abortifacient activity was reported in Rhesus monkeys

**Pharmacodynamics/Kinetics**

**Half-life Elimination:** I.M.: 10 hours; S.C.: 8.6 hours

**Time to Peak:** Limited data due to small doses used
Time to peak serum concentration: 3-15 hours
I.M.: 9.8 hours
S.C.: 7.8 hours

**Formulations** Powder for injection, lyophilized: 33 mcg [6.6 million units]

**Dosing**

**Adults:** Adults >18 years: I.M.: 30 mcg once weekly

**Elderly:** Refer to adult dosing.

**Stability**

**Storage:** Do not freeze or expose to high temperatures. Store unreconstituted vial or reconstituted vial at 2°C to 8°C (36°F to 46°F).

**Reconstitution:** Reconstitute with 1.1 mL of diluent and swirl gently to dissolve. The reconstituted product contains no preservative and is for single use only; discard unused portion. Use the reconstituted product within 6 hours.

**Monitoring Laboratory Tests** Hemoglobin, liver function, blood chemistries, complete blood count and differential, WBC, platelet counts, renal function, BUN, creatinine

**Additional Nursing Issues**

**Physical Assessment:** Monitor laboratory results on regular a basis (see Monitoring Laboratory Tests). Monitor for effectiveness of therapy and possible adverse reactions (see Warnings/Precautions and Adverse Reactions). Assess knowledge/instruct patient/caregiver on appropriate reconstitution, injection and needle disposal, possible side effects, and symptoms to report. **Pregnancy risk factor C** - barrier contraceptive teaching may be appropriate. Breast-feeding is contraindicated.

**Patient Information/Instruction:** This is not a cure for MS; you will continue to receive regular treatment and follow-up for MS. Use as directed; do not change dosage or schedule of administration without consulting prescriber. Maintain adequate hydration (2-3 L/day of fluids unless instructed to restrict fluid intake). You may experience flu-like syndrome (acetaminophen may help); nausea, vomiting, or loss of appetite (frequent small meals, frequent mouth care, sucking lozenges, or chewing gum may help); drowsiness, dizziness, agitation, or abnormal thinking (use caution when driving or engaging in tasks requiring alertness until response to drug is known). Report unusual bruising or bleeding; persistent abdominal disturbances; unusual fatigue; muscle pain or tremors; chest pain or palpitations, swelling of extremities; visual disturbances; pain, swelling, or redness at injection site; or other unusual symptoms. **Pregnancy/breast-feeding precautions:** Inform prescriber if you are or intend to be pregnant. Do not breast-feed.

**Breast-feeding Issues:** Potential for serious adverse reactions.

**Pregnancy Issues:** No adequate studies in pregnant women; if a patient becomes pregnant or plans to become pregnant, inform of potential hazards and recommend that therapy be discontinued.

## Interferon Beta-1b (in ter FEER on BAY ta won bee)

**U.S. Brand Names** Betaseron®

**Synonyms** rIFN-b

**Therapeutic Category** Biological Response Modulator

**Pregnancy Risk Factor** C

**Lactation** Excretion in breast milk unknown/contraindicated

**Use** Reduces the frequency of clinical exacerbations in ambulatory patients with relapsing-remitting multiple sclerosis (MS)

**Mechanism of Action/Effect** Alters the expression and response to cell surface antigens and can enhance immune cell activities; mechanism in MS in unknown

**Contraindications** Hypersensitivity to *E. coli* derived products, natural or recombinant interferon beta, albumin human, or any other component

**Warnings** The safety and efficacy of interferon beta-1b in chronic progressive MS have not been evaluated. Flu-like symptom complex (eg, myalgia, fever, chills, malaise, sweating) is reported in 53% of patients who receive interferon beta-1b. Pregnancy factor C.

**Adverse Reactions** Due to the pivotal position of interferon in the immune system, toxicities can affect nearly every organ system: Injection site reactions, injection site necrosis, flu-like symptoms, menstrual disorders, depression (with suicidal ideations), somnolence, palpitations, peripheral vascular disorders, hypertension, blood dyscrasias, dyspnea, laryngitis, cystitis, gastrointestinal complaints, seizures, headache, and liver enzyme elevations

**Overdose/Toxicology** Symptoms of overdose include CNS depression, obtundation, flu-like symptoms, and myelosuppression. Treatment is supportive.

**Formulations** Powder for injection, lyophilized: 0.3 mg [9.6 million units]

(Continued)

## Interferon Beta-1b *(Continued)*

**Dosing**

**Adults:** Adults >18 years: S.C.: 0.25 mg (8 million units) every other day

**Elderly:** Refer to adult dosing.

**Administration**

**Other:** S.C.: Withdraw 1 mL of reconstituted solution from the vial into a sterile syringe fitted with a 27-gauge needle and inject the solution subcutaneously. Sites for self-injection include arms, abdomen, hips, and thighs. S.C. administration is suggested for those who are at risk for bleeding or are thrombocytopenic. Rotate S.C. injection site. Patient should be well hydrated. Reconstitute with recommended amount of bacteriostatic water and agitate gently; do not shake. **Note:** Different vial strengths require different amounts of diluent.

**Stability**

**Storage:** Store solution at 2°C to 8°C (36°F to 46°F). Do not freeze or shake solution.

**Reconstitution:** Use product within 3 hours of reconstitution.

**Monitoring Laboratory Tests** Hemoglobin, liver function, blood chemistries

**Additional Nursing Issues**

**Physical Assessment:** Monitor laboratory results (see above). Monitor closely for adverse reactions (see above) especially patients with psychiatric or suicidal histories. Assess patient/caregiver knowledge and teach proper administration for S.C. injections and disposal of needles if appropriate. Teach the need for adequate hydration. Monitor for opportunistic infection. **Pregnancy risk factor C** - benefits of use should outweigh possible risks. Breast-feeding is contraindicated.

**Patient Information/Instruction:** This is not a cure for MS; you will continue to receive regular treatment and follow-up for MS. Use as directed; do not change dosage or schedule of administration without consulting prescriber. Maintain adequate hydration (2-3 L/day of fluids unless instructed to restrict fluid intake). You may experience flu-like syndrome (acetaminophen may help); nausea, vomiting, or loss of appetite (frequent small meals, frequent mouth care, sucking lozenges, or chewing gum may help); drowsiness, dizziness, agitation, or abnormal thinking (use caution when driving or engaging in tasks requiring alertness until response to drug is known). Report unusual bruising or bleeding; persistent abdominal disturbances; unusual fatigue; muscle pain or tremors; chest pain or palpitations, swelling of extremities; visual disturbances; pain, swelling, or redness at injection site; or other unusual symptoms. **Pregnancy/breast-feeding precautions:** Inform prescriber if you are or intend to be pregnant. Do not breast-feed.

**Additional Information** May be available only in small supplies. For information on availability and distribution, call the patient information line at 800-580-3837.

## Interferon Gamma-1b (in ter FEER on GAM ah won bee)

**U.S. Brand Names** Actimmune®

**Therapeutic Category** Biological Response Modulator

**Pregnancy Risk Factor** C

**Lactation** Excretion in breast milk unknown/contraindicated

**Use** Reduce the frequency and severity of serious infections associated with chronic granulomatous disease

**Unlabeled use:** Alone or as an adjunct in the treatment of basal cell carcinoma, atopic dermatitis, bowenoid papulosis and visceral leishmaniasis. It is also used in nonsmall-cell lung cancer, rheumatoid arthritis, acquired immunodeficiency syndrome, and leukemia, including chronic myelogenous leukemia.

**Contraindications** Hypersensitivity to interferon gamma, *E. coli* derived proteins, or any component

**Warnings** Patients with pre-existing cardiac disease, seizure disorders, CNS disturbances, or myelosuppression should be carefully monitored. Pregnancy factor C.

**Drug Interactions**

**Increased Effect/Toxicity:** Interferon gamma-1b may increase hepatic enzymes or enhance myelosuppression when taken with other myelosuppressive agents. May decrease cytochrome P-450 concentrations leading to increased serum concentrations of drugs metabolized by this pathway.

**Adverse Reactions**

>10%:

Central nervous system: Fever, headache, chills, fatigue
Dermatologic: Rash
Gastrointestinal: Diarrhea, vomiting

1% to 10%:

Central nervous system: Depression
Gastrointestinal: Abdominal pain, weight loss, anorexia
Neuromuscular & skeletal: Myalgia, arthralgia, back pain

<1% (Limited to important or life-threatening symptoms): Hypotension, syncope, tachyarrhythmias, heart block, heart failure, myocardial infarction, deep vein thrombosis, seizure, parkinsonian symptoms, hallucinations, exacerbation of dermatomyositis, hyponatremia, hyperglycemia, GI bleeding, pancreatitis, hepatic insufficiency, reversible renal insufficiency, tachypnea, bronchospasm, interstitial pneumonitis, pulmonary embolism

**Pharmacodynamics/Kinetics**

**Half-life Elimination:** I.V.: 38 minutes; I.M.: 2.9 hours; S.C.: 5.9 hours

**Time to Peak:** Peak plasma concentrations occur 4 hours after I.M. dosing and 7 hours after S.C. dosing.

**Formulations** Injection: 100 mcg [3 million units]

**Dosing**

**Adults:** S.C. (dosing is based on body surface ($m^2$)):

≤0.5: 1.5 mcg/kg/dose

>0.5: 50 mcg/$m^2$ (1.5 million units/$m^2$) 3 times/week

**Elderly:** Refer to adult dosing.

**Stability**

**Storage:** Store refrigerated (2°C to 8°C); do not freeze. Do not shake. Unentered vial should not be left at room temperature for total time exceeding 12 hours prior to use. Vials exceeding 12 hours at room temperature should be discarded.

**Monitoring Laboratory Tests** CBC, platelet counts, renal and liver function, urinalysis (at 3-month intervals during treatment)

**Additional Nursing Issues**

**Physical Assessment:** Monitor closely for effectiveness and/or interactions (see Drug Interactions). Monitor laboratory results on a regular basis (see Monitoring Laboratory Tests). Monitor for effectiveness of therapy and possible adverse reactions (see Warnings/Precautions and Adverse Reactions). Assess knowledge and instruct patient/caregiver on appropriate reconstitution, injection and needle disposal, possible side effects, and symptoms to report. **Pregnancy risk factor C** - benefits of use should outweigh possible risks. Breast-feeding is contraindicated.

**Patient Information/Instruction:** This is not a cure for MS; you will continue to receive regular treatment and follow-up for MS. Use as directed; do not change the dosage or schedule of administration without consulting prescriber. Maintain adequate hydration (2-3 L/day of fluids unless instructed to restrict fluid intake). You may experience flu-like syndrome (acetaminophen may help); nausea, vomiting, or loss of appetite (frequent small meals, frequent mouth care, sucking lozenges, or chewing gum may help); drowsiness, dizziness, agitation, or abnormal thinking (use caution when driving or engaging in tasks requiring alertness until response to drug is known). Report unusual bruising or bleeding; persistent abdominal disturbances; unusual fatigue; muscle pain or tremors; chest pain or palpitations; swelling of extremities; visual disturbances; pain, swelling, or redness at injection site; or other unusual symptoms. **Pregnancy/breast-feeding precautions:** Inform prescriber if you are or intend to be pregnant. Do not breast-feed.

**Breast-feeding Issues:** Potential for serious adverse reactions.

**Pregnancy Issues:** Has shown increased incidence of abortions in primates. There are no adequate studies in pregnant women; use only if potential benefit justifies potential risk to fetus.

**Additional Information** More heat- and acid-labile than alfa interferons; peak serum level after an I.V. dose of 3000 mcg/$m^2$: 7.4-9.6 ng/mL; at 24 hours: 1 ng/mL

♦ **Interleukin-2** *see* Aldesleukin *on page 47*

♦ **Intralipid®** *see* Fat Emulsion *on page 471*

♦ **Intravenous Fat Emulsion** *see* Fat Emulsion *on page 471*

♦ **Intrifiban** *see* Eptifibatide *on page 430*

♦ **Intron® A** *see* Interferon Alfa-2b *on page 614*

♦ **Intropin® Injection** *see* Dopamine *on page 395*

♦ **Invirase®** *see* Saquinavir *on page 1043*

♦ **Iobid DM®** *see* Guaifenesin and Dextromethorphan *on page 549*

♦ **Iodex®** *see page 1294*

♦ **Iodex-p®** *see page 1294*

♦ **Iodochlorhydroxyquin and Hydrocortisone** *see* Clioquinol and Hydrocortisone *on page 284*

## Iodoquinol (eye oh doe KWIN ole)

**U.S. Brand Names** Yodoxin®

**Synonyms** Diiodohydroxyquin

**Therapeutic Category** Amebicide

**Pregnancy Risk Factor** C

**Lactation** Excretion in breast milk unknown

**Use** Treatment of acute and chronic intestinal amebiasis; asymptomatic cyst passers; *Blastocystis hominis* infections; ineffective for amebic hepatitis or hepatic abscess

**Mechanism of Action/Effect** Contact amebicide that works in the lumen of the intestine by an unknown mechanism

**Contraindications** Hypersensitivity to iodine or iodoquinol; hepatic damage; pre-existing optic neuropathy

**Warnings** Optic neuritis, optic atrophy, and peripheral neuropathy have occurred following prolonged use. Avoid long-term therapy. Use with caution in patients with thyroid disease. Pregnancy factor C.

**Effects on Lab Values** May increase protein-bound serum iodine concentrations reflecting a decrease in $^{131}I$ uptake; false-positive ferric chloride test for phenylketonuria

**Adverse Reactions**

>10%: Gastrointestinal: Diarrhea, nausea, vomiting, stomach pain

1% to 10%:

Central nervous system: Fever, chills, agitation, retrograde amnesia, headache

Dermatologic: Rash, urticaria

Endocrine & metabolic: Thyroid gland enlargement

Neuromuscular & skeletal: Peripheral neuropathy, weakness

Ocular: Optic neuritis, optic atrophy, visual impairment

Miscellaneous: Itching of rectal area

(Continued)

## Iodoquinol *(Continued)*

**Overdose/Toxicology** Chronic overdose can result in vomiting, diarrhea, abdominal pain, metallic taste, paresthesia, paraplegia, and loss of vision. Can lead to destruction of long fibers of the spinal cord and optic nerve. Acute overdose may cause delirium, stupor, coma, and amnesia. Treatment is symptomatic.

**Pharmacodynamics/Kinetics**

**Metabolism:** Liver

**Excretion:** Feces

**Formulations**

Powder: 25 g

Tablet: 210 mg, 650 mg

**Dosing**

**Adults:** Oral: 650 mg 3 times/day after meals for 20 days; not to exceed 2 g/day

**Elderly:** This agent is no longer a drug of choice; use only if other therapy is contraindicated or has failed. Due to optic nerve damage, use cautiously in the elderly.

**Administration**

**Oral:** Tablets may be crushed and mixed with applesauce or chocolate syrup. May take with food or milk to reduce stomach upset. Complete full course of therapy.

**Monitoring Laboratory Tests** Ophthalmologic exam

**Additional Nursing Issues**

**Physical Assessment:** See Contraindications and Warnings/Precautions for use cautions. Check allergy status (iodine) prior to beginning therapy. Assess knowledge/teach patient appropriate use, reinfection prevention, possible side effects/interventions, and adverse symptoms to report (see Adverse Reactions and Overdose/Toxicology). **Pregnancy risk factor C** - benefits of use should outweigh possible risks. Note breast-feeding caution.

**Patient Information/Instruction:** Take as directed; complete full course of therapy. Maintain adequate hydration (2-3 L/day of fluids unless instructed to restrict fluid intake) and nutrition. If GI upset occurs, small frequent meals, frequent mouth care, sucking lozenges, or chewing gum may help. Report unresolved or severe nausea or vomiting, skin rash, fever, or fatigue. **Pregnancy/breast-feeding precautions:** Inform prescriber if you are or intend to be pregnant. Consult prescriber if breast-feeding.

## Iodoquinol and Hydrocortisone

(eye oh doe KWIN ole & hye droe KOR ti sone)

**U.S. Brand Names** Vytone® Topical

**Synonyms** Hydrocortisone and Iodoquinol

**Therapeutic Category** Antifungal Agent, Topical; Corticosteroid, Topical

**Pregnancy Risk Factor** C

**Lactation** Excretion in breast milk unknown

**Use** Treatment of eczema, infectious dermatitis, chronic eczematoid otitis externa, mycotic dermatoses

**Formulations** Cream: Iodoquinol 1% and hydrocortisone 1% (30 g)

**Dosing**

**Adults:** Apply 3-4 times/day

**Elderly:** Refer to adult dosing.

**Additional Nursing Issues**

**Physical Assessment:** See individual components listed in Related Information. **Pregnancy risk factor C** - benefits of use should outweigh possible risks. Note breast-feeding caution.

**Patient Information/Instruction:** See individual components listed in Related Information. **Pregnancy/breast-feeding precautions:** Inform prescriber if you are on intend to get pregnant. Consult prescriber if breast-feeding.

**Related Information**

Hydrocortisone *on page 578*

Iodoquinol *on previous page*

♦ **Iopidine®** *see* Ophthalmic Agents, Glaucoma *on page 853*

♦ **Iopidine®** *see page 1248*

♦ **I-Paracaine®** *see page 1248*

## Ipecac Syrup (IP e kak SIR up)

**Therapeutic Category** Antidote

**Pregnancy Risk Factor** C

**Lactation** Excretion in breast milk unknown/use caution

**Use** Treatment of acute oral drug overdosage and in certain poisonings

**Mechanism of Action/Effect** Irritates the gastric mucosa and stimulates the medullary chemoreceptor trigger zone to induce vomiting

**Contraindications** Do not use in unconscious patients, patients with no gag reflex; ingestion of strong bases or acids, volatile oils; seizures

**Warnings** Do not confuse ipecac syrup with ipecac fluid extract, which is 14 times more potent. Use with caution in patients with cardiovascular disease and bulimics. May not be effective in antiemetic overdose. Pregnancy factor C.

**Drug Interactions**

**Decreased Effect:** Activated charcoal, milk, carbonated beverages decrease the effect of ipecac syrup.

**Increased Effect/Toxicity:** Phenothiazines (chlorpromazine has been associated with serious dystonic reactions).

**Adverse Reactions** 1% to 10%:

Cardiovascular: Cardiotoxicity

Central nervous system: Lethargy

Gastrointestinal: Protracted vomiting, diarrhea

Neuromuscular & skeletal: Myopathy

**Overdose/Toxicology** Contains cardiotoxin. Symptoms of overdose include tachycardia, CHF, atrial fibrillation, depressed myocardial contractility, myocarditis, diarrhea, persistent vomiting, and hypotension. Treatment is activated charcoal and gastric lavage.

**Pharmacodynamics/Kinetics**

**Excretion:** Emetine (alkaloid component) may be detected in urine 60 days after excess dose or chronic use.

**Onset:** Within 15-30 minutes

**Duration:** 20-25 minutes; can last longer, 60 minutes in some cases

**Formulations** Syrup: 70 mg/mL (15 mL, 30 mL, 473 mL, 4000 mL)

**Dosing**

**Adults:** Oral: 15-30 mL followed by 200-300 mL of water; repeat dose one time if vomiting does not occur within 20 minutes.

**Elderly:** Refer to adult dosing.

**Administration**

**Oral:** Do **not** administer to unconscious patients. Patients should be kept active and moving following administration of ipecac. If vomiting does not occur after second dose, gastric lavage may be considered to remove ingested substance.

**Additional Nursing Issues**

**Physical Assessment:** The Poison Control Center should be contacted before administration. Administer only to conscious patients. If vomiting does not occur within 30 minutes, contact the Poison Control Center (or prescriber) again. Assess patient's knowledge for home use. Note breast-feeding caution.

**Patient Information/Instruction:** The Poison Control Center should be contacted before administration. Take only as directed; do not take more than recommended or more often than recommended. Follow with 8 oz of water. If vomiting does not occur within 30 minutes, contact the Poison Control Center or emergency services again. Do not administer if vomiting. If vomiting occurs after taking, do not eat or drink until vomiting subsides. **Breast-feeding precautions:** Consult prescriber if breast-feeding.

♦ **I-Pentolate®** *see page 1248*

♦ **I-Pentolate®** *see page 1282*

♦ **I-Phrine®** *see page 1282*

♦ **I-Phrine® Ophthalmic Solution** *see* Phenylephrine *on page 920*

♦ **IPOL™** *see page 1256*

## Ipratropium (i pra TROE pee um)

**U.S. Brand Names** Atrovent®

**Therapeutic Category** Anticholinergic Agent

**Pregnancy Risk Factor** B

**Lactation** Excretion in breast milk unknown/use caution

**Use** Anticholinergic bronchodilator in bronchospasm associated with COPD, bronchitis, and emphysema. Intranasal: Symptomatic relief of rhinorrhea associated with the common cold.

**Mechanism of Action/Effect** Blocks the action of acetylcholine at parasympathetic sites in bronchial smooth muscle causing bronchodilation

**Contraindications** Hypersensitivity to atropine or any component

**Warnings** Not indicated for the initial treatment of acute episodes of bronchospasm. Use with caution in patients with narrow-angle glaucoma, prostatic hypertrophy, or bladder neck obstruction. Ipratropium has not been specifically studied in the elderly, but it is poorly absorbed from the airways and appears to be safe in this population.

**Drug Interactions**

**Increased Effect/Toxicity:** Increased therapeutic effect with albuterol. Increased toxicity with anticholinergics or drugs with anticholinergic properties and dronabinol.

**Adverse Reactions Note:** Ipratropium is poorly absorbed from the lung, so systemic effects are rare

>10%:

Gastrointestinal: Dry mouth, stomach upset, unpleasant taste

Respiratory: Cough

1% to 10%:

Central nervous system: Insomnia

Genitourinary: Urinary retention

Neuromuscular & skeletal: Trembling

Respiratory: Nasal congestion

<1% (Limited to important or life-threatening symptoms): Bronchospasm

**Overdose/Toxicology** Symptoms of overdose include dry mouth, drying of respiratory secretions, cough, nausea, GI distress, blurred vision or impaired visual accommodation, headache, and nervousness. Acute overdose with ipratropium by inhalation is unlikely since it is so poorly absorbed. However, if poisoning occurs, it can be treated like any other anticholinergic toxicity. An anticholinergic overdose with severe life-threatening symptoms may be treated with physostigmine 1-2 mg S.C. or I.V. slowly.

(Continued)

## Ipratropium *(Continued)*

**Pharmacodynamics/Kinetics**

**Distribution:** Inhalation: 15% of dose reaches the lower airways

**Onset:** Onset of bronchodilation: 1-3 minutes after administration; Peak effect: Within 1.5-2 hours

**Duration:** Up to 4-6 hours

**Formulations** Solution, as bromide:

Inhalation: 18 mcg/actuation (14 g)

Nasal spray: 0.03% (30 mL); 0.06% (15 mL)

Nebulizing: 0.02% (2.5 mL)

**Dosing**

**Adults:**

Nebulization: 500 mcg (1 unit-dose vial) administered 3-4 times/day by oral nebulization, with doses 6-8 hours apart

Metered dose inhaler: 2 inhalations 4 times/day every 4-6 hours up to 12 inhalations in 24 hours

Nasal spray: 0.03%: 2 sprays 2 or 3 times/day; 0.06%: 2 sprays 3 or 4 times/day; safety and efficacy of use beyond 4 days in patients with the common cold have not been established.

**Elderly:** Refer to adult dosing.

**Additional Nursing Issues**

**Physical Assessment:** Assess effectiveness and interactions of other medications (especially drugs with anticholinergic activity - see Drug Interactions above). See Contraindications and Warnings/Precautions for cautious use. Monitor effectiveness of therapy and adverse reactions (see Adverse Reactions) at beginning of therapy and periodically with long-term use. Assess knowledge/teach patient appropriate use, interventions to reduce side effects, and adverse symptoms to report. Note breast-feeding caution.

**Patient Information/Instruction:** Use exactly as directed (see below). Do not use more often than recommended. Store solution away from light. Maintain adequate hydration (2-3 L/day of fluids unless instructed to restrict fluid intake). You may experience sensitivity to heat (avoid extremes in temperature); nervousness, dizziness, or fatigue (use caution when driving or engaging in tasks requiring alertness until response to drug is known); dry mouth, unpleasant taste, stomach upset (frequent small meals, frequent mouth care, chewing gum, or sucking hard candy may help); or difficulty urinating (always void before treatment). Report unresolved GI upset, dizziness or fatigue, vision changes, palpitations, persistent inability to void, nervousness, or insomnia. **Breast-feeding precautions:** Consult prescriber if breast-feeding.

**Administration:** Inhaler: Follow instructions for use accompanying the product. Close eyes when administering ipratropium; blurred vision may result if sprayed into eyes. Effects are enhanced by holding breath 10 seconds after inhalation; wait at least 1 full minute between inhalations.

Nebulizer: Wash hands before and after treatment. Wash and dry nebulizer after each treatment. Twist open the top of one unit dose vial and squeeze the contents into the nebulizer resevoir. Connect the nebulizer reservoir to the mouthpiece or face mask. Connect the nebulizer resevoir to the mouthpiece or face mask. Connect nebulizer to compressor. Sit in a comfortable, upright position. Place mouthpiece in your mouth or put on the face mask and turn on the compressor. If a face mask is used, avoid leakage around the mask (temporary blurring of vision, worsening of narrow-angle glaucoma, or eye pain may occur if mist gets into eyes). Breathe calmly and deeply until no more mist is formed in the nebulizer (about 5 minutes). At this point, treatment is finished.

**Geriatric Considerations:** Older patients may find it difficult to use the metered dose inhaler. A spacer device may be useful. Ipratropium has not been specifically studied in the elderly, but it is poorly absorbed from the airways and appears to be safe in this population.

**Related Information**

Inhalant (Asthma, Bronchospasm) Agents *on page 1388*

## Ipratropium and Albuterol (i pra TROE pee um & al BYOO ter ole)

**U.S. Brand Names** Combivent®

**Therapeutic Category** Bronchodilator

**Pregnancy Risk Factor** C

**Lactation** Excretion in breast milk unknown

**Use** Treatment of chronic obstructive pulmonary disease (COPD) in those patients that are currently on a regular bronchodilator who continue to have bronchospasms and require a second bronchodilator

**Formulations** Aerosol: Ipratropium bromide 18 mcg and albuterol sulfate 103 mcg per actuation [200 doses] (14.7 g)

**Dosing**

**Adults:** Inhalation: 2 metered dose inhalations four times daily; may receive additional doses as necessary but total number of doses in 24 hours should not exceed 12 inhalations.

**Additional Nursing Issues**

**Physical Assessment:** See individual components listed in Related Information. **Pregnancy risk factor C** - benefits of use should outweigh possible risks. Note breast-feeding caution.

**Patient Information/Instruction:** See individual components listed in Related Information. **Pregnancy/breast-feeding precautions:** Inform prescriber if you are on intend to get pregnant. Consult prescriber if breast-feeding.

**Related Information**

Albuterol *on page 45*
Ipratropium *on page 621*

- **Iproveratril Hydrochloride** *see* Verapamil *on page 1208*

## Irbesartan (ir be SAR tan)

**U.S. Brand Names** Avapro®

**Therapeutic Category** Angiotensin II Antagonists

**Pregnancy Risk Factor** C/D (2nd and 3rd trimesters)

**Lactation** Excretion in breast milk unknown/contraindicated

**Use** Treatment of hypertension alone or in combination with other antihypertensives

**Mechanism of Action/Effect** Irbesartan is an angiotensin receptor antagonist. Angiotensin II acts as a vasoconstrictor and stimulates the release of aldosterone, which results in reabsorption of sodium and water. These effects result in an elevation in blood pressure. Irbesartan blocks the AT1 angiotensin II receptor, thereby blocking the vasoconstriction and the aldosterone secreting effects of angiotensin II.

**Contraindications** Hypersensitivity to irbesartan or any component; hypersensitivity to other angiotensin-II antagonists; pregnancy (2nd and 3rd trimesters)

**Warnings** Avoid use or use a much smaller dose in patients who are intravascularly volume-depleted. Use caution in patients with unilateral or bilateral renal artery stenosis to avoid a decrease in renal function. AUCs of irbesartan (not the active metabolite) are about 50% greater in patients with $Cl_{cr}$ <30 mL/minute and are doubled in hemodialysis patients. Pregnancy factor C/D (2nd and 3rd trimesters).

**Drug Interactions**

**Cytochrome P-450 Effect:** CYP2C9 enzyme substrate

**Increased Effect/Toxicity:** Blood levels of irbesartan may be increased by inhibitors of cytochrome P-450 isoenzyme 2C9 (eg, sulfafenazole, tolbutamide, nifedipine). Potassium salts/supplements - use with caution.

**Adverse Reactions**

1% to 10%:

Cardiovascular: Edema, chest pain, tachycardia
Central nervous system: Dizziness, headache, fatigue, anxiety, nervousness
Dermatologic: Rash
Gastrointestinal: Diarrhea, dyspepsia/heartburn, nausea, vomiting, abdominal pain
Genitourinary: Urinary tract infection
Neuromuscular & skeletal: Pain, trauma
Respiratory: Upper respiratory infection, cough, sinus disorder, pharyngitis, rhinitis, influenza

<1% (Limited to important or life-threatening symptoms): Angioedema, urticaria

**Overdose/Toxicology** Likely manifestations of overdose include hypotension and tachycardia. Treatment is supportive.

**Pharmacodynamics/Kinetics**

**Protein Binding:** 90%

**Half-life Elimination:** 11-15 hours

**Time to Peak:** 1-2 hours

**Metabolism:** Hepatic, primarily by cytochrome P-450 isoenzyme 2C9 (minimal metabolism also by 3A4)

**Excretion:** Bile and urine

**Duration:** >24 hours

**Formulations** Tablet: 75 mg, 150 mg, 300 mg

**Dosing**

**Adults:** Oral: 150 mg once daily with or without food; patients may be titrated to 300 mg once daily.

**Elderly:** Although AUC and $C_{max}$ values are higher in elderly patients, no specific dosage reduction is recommended. See adult dosing.

**Monitoring Laboratory Tests** Electrolytes, serum creatinine, BUN, urinalysis

**Additional Nursing Issues**

**Physical Assessment:** Assess effectiveness and interactions of other medications (see Drug Interactions). See Warnings/Precautions and Contraindications for use cautions. Monitor effectiveness of therapy, laboratory tests, and adverse response on a regular basis during therapy (see Adverse Reactions and Overdose/Toxicology). Assess knowledge/teach patient appropriate use according to drug form and purpose of therapy, possible side effects and appropriate interventions, and adverse symptoms to report. **Pregnancy risk factor C/D** - see Pregnancy Risk Factor - assess knowledge/teach appropriate contraceptive measures; danger of use during pregnancy must outweigh risk to fetus. Breast-feeding is contraindicated.

**Patient Information/Instruction:** Take exactly as directed; do not discontinue without consulting prescriber. Take first dose at bedtime. This drug does not eliminate need for diet or exercise regimen as recommended by prescriber. May cause dizziness, fainting, lightheadedness (use caution when driving or engaging in tasks that require alertness until response to drug is known); nausea, vomiting, or abdominal pain (small frequent meals, frequent mouth care, sucking lozenges, or chewing gum may help); diarrhea (buttermilk, boiled milk, yogurt may help). Report chest pain or palpitations, skin rash, fluid retention (swelling of extremities), difficulty in breathing or unusual

(Continued)

## Irbesartan *(Continued)*

cough, or other persistent adverse reactions. **Pregnancy/breast-feeding precautions:** Inform prescriber if you are pregnant or if you intend to get pregnant. Do not breast-feed.

**Pregnancy Issues:** The drug should be discontinued as soon as possible after detection of pregnancy. Drugs which act directly on the renin-angiotensin system can cause fetal and neonatal morbidity and death.

**Related Information**

ACE Inhibitors and Angiotensin Antagonists Comparison *on page 1362*

## Irbesartan and Hydrochlorothiazide

(ir be SAR tan & hye droe klor oh THYE a zide)

**U.S. Brand Names** Avapro® HCT

**Synonyms** Hydrochlorothiazide and Irbesartan

**Therapeutic Category** Antihypertensive Agent, Combination

**Pregnancy Risk Factor** C/D (2nd and 3rd trimesters)

**Lactation** Enters breast milk/contraindicated

**Use** Combination therapy for the management of hypertension

**Formulations** Tablet: Irbesartan 150 mg and hydrochlorothiazide 12.5 mg; irbesartan 300 mg and hydrochlorothiazide 12.5 mg

**Dosing**

**Adults:** Dose must be individualized. A patient who is not controlled with either agent alone may be switched to the combination product. Mean effect increases with the dose of each component. The lowest dosage available is 150 mg/12.5 mg. Dose increases should be made not more frequently than every 2-4 weeks.

**Elderly:** Refer to adult dosing.

**Additional Nursing Issues**

**Physical Assessment:** See individual components listed in Related Information. **Pregnancy risk factor C/D** - see Pregnancy Risk Factor. Benefits of use should outweigh possible risks. Breast-feeding is contraindicated.

**Patient Information/Instruction:** See individual components listed in Related Information. **Pregnancy/breast-feeding precautions:** Inform prescriber if you are or intend to be pregnant. Do not breast-feed.

**Related Information**

Hydrochlorothiazide *on page 566*
Irbesartan *on previous page*

♦ **Ircon® [OTC]** *see* Iron Supplements *on page 627*

## Irinotecan (eye rye no TEE kan)

**U.S. Brand Names** Camptosar®

**Therapeutic Category** Antineoplastic Agent, Natural Source (Plant) Derivative

**Pregnancy Risk Factor** D

**Lactation** Enters breast milk/contraindicated

**Use** Treatment of patients with metastatic carcinoma of the colon or rectum whose disease has progressed following 5-FU based therapy

**Contraindications** Hypersensitivity to irinotecan, topotecan, or other camptothecin analogues; acute infection; diarrhea; pregnancy

**Warnings** The U.S. Food and Drug Administration (FDA) currently recommends that procedures for proper handling and disposal of antineoplastic agents be considered.

Irinotecan can induce both early and late forms of diarrhea that appear to be mediated by different mechanisms. Early diarrhea (during or within 24 hours of administration) is cholinergic in nature. It can be preceded by complaints of diaphoresis and abdominal cramping and may be ameliorated by the administration of atropine. The elderly (≥65 years of age) are at particular risk for diarrhea. Late diarrhea (occurring >24 hours after administration) can be prolonged and may lead to dehydration and electrolyte imbalance, and can be life-threatening. Late diarrhea should be treated promptly with loperamide. If grade 3 diarrhea (7-9 stools daily, incontinence, or severe cramping) or grade 4 diarrhea (≥10 stools daily, gross blood in stool, or need for parenteral support), the administration of irinotecan should be delayed until the patient recovers and subsequent doses should be decreased.

Early diarrhea treatment: 0.25-1 mg of intravenous atropine should be considered (unless clinically contraindicated) in patients experiencing diaphoresis, abdominal cramping, or early diarrhea.

Late diarrhea treatment: High-dose loperamide: Oral: 4 mg at the first onset of late diarrhea and then 2 mg every 2 hours until the patient is diarrhea-free for at least 12 hours. During the night, the patient may take 4 mg of loperamide every 4 hours. **Premedication with loperamide is not recommended.**

Deaths due to sepsis following severe myelosuppression have been reported. Therapy should be discontinued if neutropenic fever occurs or if the absolute neutrophil count is <500/mm$^3$. The dose of irinotecan should be reduced if there is a clinically significant decrease in the total WBC (<200/mm$^3$), neutrophil count (<1000/mm$^3$), hemoglobin (<8 g/dL), or platelet count (<100,000/mm$^3$). Routine administration of a colony-stimulating factor is generally not necessary.

Avoid extravasation.

Irinotecan preparation should be performed in a Class II laminar flow biologic safety cabinet. Personnel should be fully trained and wearing surgical gloves and a closed front surgical gown with knit cuffs. Appropriate safety equipment is recommended for preparation, administration, and disposal of irinotecan. Accidental exposure to skin should be thoroughly washed with soap and water immediately.

**Drug Interactions**

**Increased Effect/Toxicity:** Hold diuretics during dosing due to potential risk of dehydration secondary to vomiting and/or diarrhea induced by irinotecan. Prophylactic dexamethasone as an antiemetic may enhance lymphocytopenia. Prochlorperazine may increase incidence of akathisia. Adverse reactions such as myelosuppression and diarrhea would be expected to be exacerbated by other antineoplastic agents.

**Adverse Reactions**

>10%:

Cardiovascular: Vasodilation

Central nervous system: Insomnia, dizziness, fever (45.4%)

Dermatologic: Alopecia (60.5%), rash

Gastrointestinal: Irinotecan therapy may induce two different forms of diarrhea. Onset, symptoms, proposed mechanisms and treatment are different. Overall, 56.9% of patients treated experience abdominal pain and/or cramping during therapy. Anorexia, constipation, flatulence, stomatitis, and heartburn have also been reported.

Diarrhea: Dose-limiting toxicity with weekly dosing regimen

Early diarrhea (50.7% incidence) usually occurs during or within 24 hours of administration. May be accompanied by symptoms of cramping, vomiting, flushing, and sweating. It is thought to be mediated by cholinergic effects which can be successfully managed with atropine (refer to Warnings/Precautions).

Late diarrhea (87.8% incidence) usually occurs >24 hours after treatment. National Cancer Institute (NCI) grade 3 or 4 diarrhea occurs in 30.6% of patients. Late diarrhea generally occurs with a median of 11 days after therapy and lasts approximately 3 days. Patients experiencing grade 3 or 4 diarrhea were noted to have symptoms a total of 7 days. Correlated with irinotecan or SN-38 levels in plasma and bile. Due to the duration, dehydration and electrolyte imbalances are significant clinical concerns. Loperamide therapy is recommended. The incidence of grade 3 or 4 late diarrhea is significantly higher in patients ≥ 65 years of age: close monitoring and prompt initiation of high-dose loperamide therapy is prudent (refer to Warnings/Precautions).

Emetic potential: Moderately high (86.2% incidence, however, only 12.5% grade 3 or 4 vomiting)

Hematologic: Myelosuppressive: Dose-limiting toxicity with 3 week dosing regimen

Grade 1-4 neutropenia occurred in 53.9% of patients. Patients who had previously received pelvic or abdominal radiation therapy or a bilirubin of ≥1.0 mg/dL were noted to have a significantly increased incidence of grade 3 or 4 neutropenia. White blood cell count nadir is 15 days after administration and is more frequent than thrombocytopenia. Recovery is usually within 24-28 days and cumulative toxicity has not been observed.

WBC: Mild to severe

Platelets: Mild

Onset (days): 10

Nadir (days): 14-16

Recovery (days): 21-28

Neuromuscular & skeletal: Weakness (75.7%)

Respiratory: Dyspnea (22%), coughing, rhinitis

Miscellaneous: Sweating

1% to 10%: Local: **Irritant chemotherapy**; thrombophlebitis has been reported

**Overdose/Toxicology** Symptoms of overdose include bone marrow suppression, leukopenia, thrombocytopenia, nausea, and vomiting. Treatment is supportive.

**Pharmacodynamics/Kinetics**

**Half-life Elimination:** Primarily biliary

**Metabolism:** By intestinal flora, plasma, and liver to an active metabolite SN-38

**Formulations** Injection: 20 mg/mL (5 mL)

**Dosing**

**Adults:** I.V.:

6-week cycle: The usual recommended starting dose is 125 mg/m$^2$ (I.V. infusion over 90 minutes) once a week for 4 weeks, followed by a 2-week rest period. Additional 6-week cycles of treatment (4 weeks on therapy, followed by 2 weeks off therapy) may be repeated in patients who remain stable or do not develop intolerable toxicities.

3-week cycle: The usual recommended dose is 350 mg/m$^2$ (I.V. infusion over 90 minutes) once weekly every 3 weeks (300 mg/m$^2$ for patients ≥70 years, prior pelvic/abdominal radiotherapy, or performance status of the two). Subsequent doses should be adjusted to as low as 200 mg/m$^2$ in 50 mg increments based on monitoring for toxicity. Continue as long as tolerated and clinical benefit is seen.

**Elderly:** Refer to adult dosing.

**Hepatic Impairment:** Patients with serum bilirubin of 1-2 mg/dL and prior pelvic/abdominal radiation may be given 100 mg/m$^2$. Further reductions may be warranted at higher bilirubin values.

**Administration**

**I.V.:** Irritant.

**Stability**

**Storage:** Store at controlled room temperature 15°C to 30°C (59°F to 86°F). Protect from light.

**Reconstitution:** Stable for up to 24 hours at room temperature and in ambient fluorescent lighting. Solutions diluted in 5% dextrose injection and stored at refrigerated

(Continued)

## Irinotecan *(Continued)*

temperatures approximately 2°C to 8°C and protected from light are physically and chemically stable for 48 hours.

**Monitoring Laboratory Tests** WBC with differential, hemoglobin, platelet count

**Additional Nursing Issues**

**Physical Assessment:** Monitor appropriate laboratory tests as ordered (CBC, platelet count) on a regular basis. Monitor for acute diarrhea (see Warnings/Precautions). Monitor closely for sepsis (see Warnings/Precautions). Observe infusion site for extravasation which may result in cellulitis and tissue necrosis. **Pregnancy risk factor D** - assess knowledge/teach appropriate use of barrier contraceptives (males and females). Breast-feeding is contraindicated.

**Patient Information/Instruction:** This drug may cause nausea, vomiting, and acute diarrhea. Immediately report these or any signs of dehydration (eg, fainting, dizziness, lightheadedness) to prescriber. Avoid the use of laxatives or food with laxative properties. This drug may cause hair loss; hair will regrow when drug is discontinued. Report difficulty breathing, weight loss, or signs or symptoms of opportunistic infection (eg, fever, fatigue, furry tongue, thrush, perineal itching or vaginal discharge, loose foul-smelling stools). Avoid crowds or exposure to infected persons; you will be susceptible to infection. **Pregnancy/breast-feeding precautions:** Do not get pregnant while taking this medication; use appropriate barrier contraceptive measures (may cause severe fetal abnormalities). Do not breast-feed.

**Pregnancy Issues:** Has shown to be teratogenic in animals. Teratogenic effects include a variety of external, visceral, and skeletal abnormalities. The patient should be warned of potential hazards to the fetus.

**Other Issues:** Diarrhea is dose related. High doses of loperamide can increase tolerated dose of irinotecan. Used in combination with 5-FU and etoposide.

## Iron Dextran Complex (EYE ern DEKS tran KOM pleks)

**U.S. Brand Names** InFed™ Injection

**Therapeutic Category** Iron Salt

**Pregnancy Risk Factor** C

**Lactation** Enters breast milk/contraindicated

**Use** Treatment of microcytic hypochromic anemia resulting from iron deficiency in whom oral administration is infeasible or ineffective

**Mechanism of Action/Effect** The released iron, from the plasma, eventually replenishes the depleted iron stores in the bone marrow where it is incorporated into hemoglobin

**Contraindications** Hypersensitivity to iron dextran; all anemias that are not involved with iron deficiency; hemochromatosis; hemolytic anemia

**Warnings** Use with caution in patients with history of asthma, hepatic impairment, or rheumatoid arthritis. Not recommended in children <4 months of age. Deaths associated with parenteral administration following anaphylactic-type reactions have been reported. Use only in patients where the iron deficient state is not amenable to oral iron therapy. A test dose of 0.5 mL I.V. or I.M. should be given to observe for adverse reactions. Anemia in the elderly is often caused by "anemia of chronic disease" or associated with inflammation rather than blood loss. Iron stores are usually normal or increased, with a serum ferritin >50 ng/mL and a decreased total iron binding capacity. I.V. administration of iron dextran is often preferred over I.M. in the elderly secondary to a decreased muscle mass and the need for daily injections. Pregnancy factor C.

**Drug Interactions**

**Decreased Effect:** Decreased effect with chloramphenicol.

**Food Interactions** Iron bioavailability may be decreased if taken with dairy products.

**Effects on Lab Values** May cause falsely elevated values of serum bilirubin and falsely decreased values of serum calcium.

**Adverse Reactions**

Incidence unknown:

- Cardiovascular: Cardiovascular collapse, hypotension
- Dermatologic: Urticaria
- Hematologic: Leukocytosis

>10%:

- Cardiovascular: Flushing
- Central nervous system: Dizziness, fever, headache, pain
- Gastrointestinal: Nausea, vomiting, metallic taste
- Local: Staining of skin at the site of I.M. injection, phlebitis,
- Miscellaneous: Sweating

1% to 10%:

- Gastrointestinal: Diarrhea
- Genitourinary: Discoloration of urine

<1% (Limited to important or life-threatening symptoms): Respiratory difficulties and cardiovascular collapse have been reported and occur most frequently within the first several minutes of administration.

**Note:** Sweating, urticaria, arthralgia, fever, chills, dizziness, headache, and nausea may be delayed 24-48 hours after I.V. administration or 3-4 days after I.M. administration.

**Overdose/Toxicology** Symptoms of overdose include erosion of GI mucosa, pulmonary edema, hyperthermia, convulsions, tachycardia, hepatic and renal impairment, coma, hematemesis, lethargy, tachycardia, and acidosis. Serum iron level >300 mcg/mL requires treatment of overdose due to severe toxicity. If severe iron overdose (when the serum iron concentration exceeds the total iron-binding capacity) occurs, it may be treated with deferoxamine. Deferoxamine may be administered I.V. (80 mg/kg over 24 hours) or I.M. (40-90 mg/kg every 8 hours).

**Pharmacodynamics/Kinetics**

**Excretion:** Urine and feces (via bile)

**Formulations** Injection: 50 mg/mL (2 mL, 10 mL)

**Dosing**

**Adults:** I.M. (Z-track method should be used for I.M. injection), I.V.:

A 0.5 mL test dose should be given prior to starting iron dextran therapy. Total dose should be divided into a daily schedule for I.M., total dose may be given as a single continuous infusion.

Iron deficiency anemia: Dose (mL) = 0.0476 x wt (kg) x (normal hemoglobin - observed hemoglobin) + (1 mL/5 kg) to maximum of 14 mL for iron stores

Iron replacement therapy for blood loss: Replacement iron (mg) = blood loss (mL) x hematocrit

Maximum daily dose (can give total dose at one time I.V.): Adults >50 kg: 100 mg iron (2 mL)

**Elderly:** Refer to adult dosing.

**Administration**

**I.M.:** Use Z-track technique for I.M. administration (deep into the upper outer quadrant of buttock).

**I.V.:** May be administered I.V. bolus at rate ≤50 mg/minute or diluted in 250-1000 mL NS and infused over 1-6 hours. Infuse initial 25 mL slowly, observe for allergic reactions. Have epinephrine nearby.

**Stability**

**Storage:** Store at room temperature.

**Reconstitution:** Stability of parenteral admixture at room temperature (25°C) is 3 months.

Standard diluent: Dose/250-1000 mL NS
Minimum volume: 250 mL NS

**Monitoring Laboratory Tests** Hemoglobin, hematocrit, reticulocyte count, serum ferritin

**Additional Nursing Issues**

**Physical Assessment:** Monitor laboratory tests regularly. Monitor patient for adverse reactions (see above). Note that adverse response may occur some time (1-4 days) after administration. Assess patients with rheumatoid arthritis for exacerbated swelling and joint pain; adjust medications as needed. **Pregnancy risk factor C.** Breast-feeding is contraindicated.

**Patient Information/Instruction:** You will need frequent blood tests while on this therapy. If you have rheumatoid arthritis you may experience increased swelling or joint pain; consult prescriber for medication adjustment. If you experience dizziness or severe headache, use caution when driving or engaging in tasks that require alertness until response to drug is known. Small frequent meals, frequent mouth care, sucking lozenges, or chewing gum may relieve nausea and metallic taste. You may experience increased sweating. Report acute GI problems, fever, difficulty breathing, rapid heartbeat, yellowing of skin or eyes, or swelling of hands and feet. **Pregnancy/breast-feeding precautions:** Inform prescriber if you are or intend to be pregnant. Do not breast-feed.

**Geriatric Considerations:** Anemia in the elderly is most often caused by "anemia of chronic disease", a result of aging effect in bone marrow, or associated with inflammation rather than blood loss. Iron stores are usually normal or increased, with a serum ferritin >50 ng/mL and a decreased total iron binding capacity. Hence, the anemia is not secondary to iron deficiency but the inability of the reticuloendothelial system to use available iron stores. I.V. administration of iron dextran is often preferred over I.M. in the elderly secondary to a decreased muscle mass and the need for daily injections.

♦ **Iron Sulfate (Ferrous Sulfate)** *see* Iron Supplements *on this page*

## Iron Supplements (EYE ern SUP la ments)

**U.S. Brand Names** Femiron® [OTC]; Feosol® [OTC]; Feostat® [OTC]; Feratab® [OTC]; Fergon® [OTC]; Fer-In-Sol® [OTC]; Fer-Iron® [OTC]; Fero-Gradumet® [OTC]; Ferospace® [OTC]; Ferralet® [OTC]; Ferralyn® Lanacaps® [OTC]; Ferra-TD® [OTC]; Ferro-Sequels® [OTC]; Fumasorb® [OTC]; Fumerin® [OTC]; Hemocyte® [OTC]; Ircon® [OTC]; Mol-Iron® [OTC]; Nephro-Fer™ [OTC]; Simron® [OTC]; Slow FE® [OTC]; Span-FF® [OTC]

**Synonyms** Ferrous Fumarate; Ferrous Gluconate; Ferrous Salts; Ferrous Sulfate; $FeSO_4$ (Ferrous Sulfate); Iron Sulfate (Ferrous Sulfate)

**Therapeutic Category** Iron Salt; Mineral, Oral; Mineral, Parenteral

**Pregnancy Risk Factor** A

**Lactation** Enters breast milk/compatible

**Use** Prevention and treatment of iron deficiency anemias

**Mechanism of Action/Effect** Replaces iron, found in hemoglobin, myoglobin, and other enzymes; allows the transportation of oxygen via hemoglobin

**Contraindications** Hypersensitivity to iron salts; hemochromatosis; hemolytic anemia

**Warnings** Avoid using for longer than 6 months, except in patients with conditions that require prolonged therapy. Avoid in patients with peptic ulcer, enteritis, or ulcerative colitis. Avoid in patients receiving frequent blood transfusions Avoid use in premature infants until the vitamin E stores, deficient at birth, are replenished.

**Drug Interactions**

**Decreased Effect:** Absorption of oral preparation of iron and tetracyclines are decreased when both of these drugs are given together. Absorption of quinolones may

(Continued)

## Iron Supplements *(Continued)*

be decreased due to formation of a ferric ion-quinolone complex. Concurrent administration of antacids and cimetidine may decrease iron absorption. Iron may decrease absorption of penicillamine, methyldopa, and levodopa when given at the same time. Response to iron therapy may be delayed in patients receiving chloramphenicol.

**Increased Effect/Toxicity:** Concurrent administration ≥200 mg vitamin C per 30 mg elemental iron increases absorption of oral iron.

**Food Interactions** Milk, cereals, dietary fiber, tea, coffee, or eggs decrease absorption of iron.

**Effects on Lab Values** False-positive for blood in stool by the guaiac test

**Adverse Reactions**

Gastrointestinal: GI irritation, epigastric pain, nausea, diarrhea, dark stools, constipation
Genitourinary: Discoloration of urine
Miscellaneous: Liquid preparations may temporarily stain the teeth

**Pharmacodynamics/Kinetics**

**Half-life Elimination:** Iron is largely bound to serum transferrin and excreted in the urine, sweat, sloughing of intestinal mucosa, and by menses.

**Time to Peak:** Peak reticulocytosis occurs in 5-10 days, and hemoglobin values increase within 2-4 weeks

**Onset:** Hematologic response to either oral or parenteral iron salts is essentially the same; red blood cell form and color changes within 3-10 days

**Formulations** Amount of **elemental** iron is listed in brackets; most commonly used formulations are bolded

**Ferrous fumarate:**

Capsule, controlled release (Span-FF®): 325 mg [106 mg]
Drops (Feostat®): 45 mg/0.6 mL [15 mg/0.6 mL] (60 mL)
Suspension, oral (Feostat®): 100 mg/5 mL [33 mg/5 mL] (240 mL)
Tablet: 325 mg [106 mg]
  Femiron®: 63 mg [20 mg]
  Fumerin®: 195 mg [64 mg]
  Fumasorb®, Ircon®: 200 mg [66 mg]
  Hemocyte®: 324 mg [106 mg]
  Nephro-Fer™: 350 mg [115 mg]
Tablet, chewable (chocolate flavor): Feostat®: 100 mg [33 mg]
Tablet, timed release:
  Ferro-Sequels®: 150 mg [50 mg] with docusate sodium 100 mg

**Ferrous gluconate:**

Capsule, soft gelatin (Simron®): 86 mg [10 mg]
Elixir (Fergon®): 300 mg/5 mL [34 mg/5 mL] with alcohol 7% (480 mL)
Tablet: **300 mg [34 mg]**; 325 mg [38 mg]
  Fergon®, Ferralet®: 320 mg [37 mg]
Sustained release (Ferralet® Slow Release): 320 mg [37 mg]

**Ferrous sulfate:**

Capsule:
  Exsiccated (Fer-In-Sol®): 190 mg [60 mg]
  Exsiccated, timed release (Feosol®): 159 mg [50 mg]
  Exsiccated, timed release (Ferralyn® Lanacaps®, Ferra-TD®): 250 mg [50 mg]
  Ferospace®: 250 mg [50 mg]
Drops, oral:
  Fer-In-Sol®: **75 mg/0.6 mL [15 mg/0.6 mL]** (50 mL)
  Fer-Iron®: 125 mg/mL [25 mg/mL] (50 mL)
Elixir (Feosol®): 220 mg/5 mL [44 mg/5 mL] with alcohol 5% (473 mL, 4000 mL)
Syrup (Fer-In-Sol®): **90 mg/5 mL [18 mg/5 mL]** with alcohol 5% (480 mL)
Tablet:
  **324 mg [65 mg]**
  Exsiccated (Feosol®) 200 mg [65 mg]
  Exsiccated, timed release (Slow FE®): 160 mg [50 mg]
  Feratab®: **300 mg [60 mg]**
  Mol-Iron®: 195 mg [39 mg]
Timed release (Fero-Gradumet®): 525 mg [105 mg]

**Dosing**

**Adults: Note: Multiple salt forms of iron exist; close attention must be paid to the salt form when ordering and administering iron; incorrect selection or substitution of one salt for another without proper dosage adjustment may result in serious over- or underdosing.**

Oral (dose expressed in terms of **elemental** iron):
  Recommended Daily Allowance, see table.

**Elemental Iron Content of Iron Salts**

| Iron Salt | Elemental Iron Content (% of salt form) | Approximate Equivalent Doses (mg of iron salt) |
|---|---|---|
| Ferrous fumarate | 33 | 197 |
| Ferrous gluconate | 11.6 | 560 |
| Ferrous sulfate | 20 | 324 |

Adults:

Iron deficiency: 60-100 mg elemental iron twice daily up to 60 mg elemental iron 4 times/day, or 50 mg elemental iron (extended release) 1-2 times/day

Prophylaxis: 60-100 mg elemental iron/day; see table

**Administration**

**Oral:** Do not chew or crush sustained release preparations. Administer with water or juice between meals for maximum absorption. May administer with food if GI upset occurs. Do not administer with milk or milk products.

**Monitoring Laboratory Tests** Serum iron, total iron binding capacity, reticulocyte count, hemoglobin, ferritin

**Additional Nursing Issues**

**Physical Assessment:** Assess other medications patient may be taking; instruct patient accordingly about timing of medications. Monitor for adverse side effects and indications of overdose.

**Patient Information/Instruction:** Take this drug as prescribed; do not increase dose. Take at the same time each day. Do not take within 1 hour of other medications or antacids. May be taken with food, but not with milk, eggs, caffeine-containing drinks, cereals, or foods containing dietary fiber. If mixed with liquid (juice or water) use a straw to prevent staining of teeth. You may experience black tarry stools (normal), nausea, vomiting (taking with meals will reduce this), constipation (adequate fluids and exercise may help, may need a stool softener). Report severe unresolved GI irritation, lethargy, rapid respiration, CNS changes, and unrelieved constipation. Keep out of reach of children.

**Geriatric Considerations:** Anemia in the elderly is often caused by "anemia of chronic disease", a result of aging changes in the bone marrow, or associated with inflammation rather than blood loss. Iron stores are usually normal or increased, with a serum ferritin >50 ng/mL and a decreased total iron binding capacity. Hence, the anemia is not secondary to iron deficiency but the inability of the reticuloendothelial system to use available iron stores. Timed release iron preparations should be avoided due to their erratic absorption. Products combined with a laxative or stool softener should not be used unless the need for the combination is demonstrated.

**Additional Information** When treating iron deficiency anemias, treat for 3-4 months after hemoglobin/hematocrit return to normal in order to replenish total body stores. Elemental iron dosages as high as 15 mg/kg/day have been used to supplement neonates receiving concomitant epoetin alpha in the treatment of anemia of prematurity.


- ♦ **ISD** *see* Isosorbide Dinitrate *on page 634*
- ♦ **ISDN** *see* Isosorbide Dinitrate *on page 634*
- ♦ **Ismelin®** *see* Guanethidine *on page 553*
- ♦ **ISMN** *see* Isosorbide Mononitrate *on page 635*
- ♦ **ISMO®** *see* Isosorbide Mononitrate *on page 635*
- ♦ **Ismotic®** *see page 1282*
- ♦ **Isoamyl Nitrite** *see* Amyl Nitrite *on page 94*
- ♦ **Isobac** *see* Co-trimoxazole *on page 307*
- ♦ **Isobamate** *see* Carisoprodol *on page 202*
- ♦ **Isobamate** *see* Carisoprodol, Aspirin, and Codeine *on page 203*
- ♦ **Isocaine® HCl** *see* Mepivacaine *on page 723*
- ♦ **Isoclor® Expectorant** *see* Guaifenesin, Pseudoephedrine, and Codeine *on page 552*
- ♦ **Isodine®** *see page 1294*


## Isoetharine (eye soe ETH a reen)

**U.S. Brand Names** Arm-a-Med® Isoetharine; Beta-2®; Bronkometer®; Bronkosol®; Dey-Lute® Isoetharine

**Therapeutic Category** Adrenergic Agonist Agent; Bronchodilator; Sympathomimetic

**Pregnancy Risk Factor** C

**Lactation** Excretion in breast milk unknown

**Use** Bronchodilator in bronchial asthma and for reversible bronchospasm occurring with bronchitis and emphysema

**Mechanism of Action/Effect** Relaxes bronchial smooth muscle by action on beta$_2$-receptors with very little effect on heart rate

**Contraindications** Hypersensitivity to isoetharine or any component

**Warnings** Excessive or prolonged use may result in decreased effectiveness. Pregnancy factor C.

**Drug Interactions**

**Decreased Effect:** Decreased effect with beta-blockers.

**Increased Effect/Toxicity:** Increased toxicity with other sympathomimetics (eg, epinephrine).

**Effects on Lab Values** ↓ potassium (S)

**Adverse Reactions**

1% to 10%:

Cardiovascular: Tachycardia, hypertension, pounding heartbeat

Central nervous system: Dizziness, lightheadedness, nervousness, headache, insomnia, weakness

Gastrointestinal: Dry mouth, nausea, vomiting

Neuromuscular & skeletal: Trembling

Respiratory: Bronchial irritation, coughing

<1% (Limited to important or life-threatening symptoms): Paradoxical bronchospasm

(Continued)

## Isoetharine *(Continued)*

**Overdose/Toxicology** Symptoms of overdose include nausea, vomiting, hypertension, and tremor. Beta-adrenergic stimulation can cause increased heart rate, decreased blood pressure, and CNS excitation. Treatment is symptomatic.

**Pharmacodynamics/Kinetics**

**Metabolism:** In many tissues including the liver and lungs

**Excretion:** Urine

**Onset:** Peak effect: Inhaler: Within 5-15 minutes

**Duration:** 1-4 hours

**Formulations**

Aerosol, oral, as mesylate: 340 mcg/metered spray

Solution, inhalation, as hydrochloride: 0.062% (4 mL); 0.08% (3.5 mL); 0.1% (2.5 mL, 5 mL); 0.125% (4 mL); 0.167% (3 mL); 0.17% (3 mL); 0.2% (2.5 mL); 0.25% (2 mL, 3.5 mL); 0.5% (0.5 mL); 1% (0.5 mL, 0.25 mL, 10 mL, 14 mL, 30 mL)

**Dosing**

**Adults:** Treatments are usually not repeated more often than every 4 hours, except in severe cases.

Inhalation: Oral: 1-2 inhalations every 4 hours as needed

**Elderly:** Refer to adult dosing.

**Administration**

**Inhalation:** Do not exceed recommended dosage; excessive use may lead to adverse effects or loss of effectiveness. See Patient Education instructions for administration.

**Stability**

**Storage:** Do not use if solution is discolored or a precipitation is present. Protect from light.

**Reconstitution:** Compatible with sterile water, 0.45% sodium chloride, and 0.9% sodium chloride.

**Additional Nursing Issues**

**Physical Assessment:** Monitor heart rate, blood pressure, respiratory rate, and response to treatment. Assess knowledge/teach patient appropriate use, administration, possible side effects, and symptoms to report. **Pregnancy risk factor C** - benefits of use should outweigh possible risks. Note breast-feeding caution.

**Patient Information/Instruction:** Use as directed (see below). Do not use more often than recommended. Store solution away from light. You may experience nervousness, dizziness, or fatigue; use caution when driving or engaging in tasks requiring alertness until response to drug is known. Frequent small meals may reduce incidence of nausea or vomiting. Report unresolved/persistent GI upset, rapid heartbeat or palpitations, dizziness or fatigue, trembling, or difficulty breathing. **Pregnancy/breast-feeding precautions:** Inform prescriber if you are or intend to be pregnant. Consult prescriber if breast-feeding.

**Administration:** Shake canister well before use. Administer pressurized inhalation during the second half of inspiration. If more than one inhalation per dose is necessary, wait at least 1 full minute between inhalations; second inhalation is best delivered after 10 minutes.

**Geriatric Considerations:** Isoetharine has a shorter duration of action than other $beta_2$ selective agonists; therefore, it is usually not considered a first-line drug of choice. The elderly may find it beneficial to utilize a spacer device when using a metered dose inhaler.

**Additional Information** The hydrochloride formulations contain sulfites.

Isoetharine hydrochloride: Arm-a-Med® isoetharine, Beta-2®, Bronkosol®, Dey-Lute® isoetharine

Isoetharine mesylate: Bronkometer®

Isoetharine has a shorter duration of action than other $beta_2$ selective agonists; therefore, it is usually not considered a first-line drug of choice.

**Related Information**

Inhalant (Asthma, Bronchospasm) Agents *on page 1388*

- **Isoflurophate** *see* Ophthalmic Agents, Glaucoma *on page 853*
- **Isoket** *see* Isosorbide Dinitrate *on page 634*
- **Isollyl Improved®** *see* Butalbital Compound and Aspirin *on page 176*

## Isoniazid (eye soe NYE a zid)

**U.S. Brand Names** Laniazid®; Nydrazid®

**Synonyms** INH; Isonicotinic Acid Hydrazide

**Therapeutic Category** Antitubercular Agent

**Pregnancy Risk Factor** C

**Lactation** Enters breast milk/compatible

**Use** Treatment of susceptible tuberculosis infections and prophylactically to those individuals exposed to tuberculosis

**Mechanism of Action/Effect** Unknown, but may include the inhibition of myocolic acid synthesis resulting in disruption of the bacterial cell wall

**Contraindications** Hypersensitivity to isoniazid or any component; acute liver disease; previous history of hepatic damage during isoniazid therapy

**Warnings** Use with caution in patients with renal impairment and chronic liver disease. Severe and sometimes fatal hepatitis may occur or develop even after many months of treatment. Patients must report any prodromal symptoms of hepatitis, such as fatigue, weakness, malaise, anorexia, nausea, or vomiting. Periodic ophthalmic examinations are recommended even when usual symptoms do not occur. Pyridoxine (10-50 mg/day) is recommended in individuals likely to develop peripheral neuropathies. Pregnancy factor C.

**Drug Interactions**

**Cytochrome P-450 Effect:** CYP2E1 enzyme substrate; CYP2E1 enzyme inducer; and CYP1A2, 2C, 2C9, 2C18, 2C19, and 3A3/4 enzyme inhibitor

**Decreased Effect:** Decreased effect/levels of isoniazid with aluminum salts.

**Increased Effect/Toxicity:** Increased toxicity/levels of oral anticoagulants, carbamazepines, cycloserine, hydantoins, and hepatically metabolized benzodiazepines. Reaction with disulfiram.

**Food Interactions** Isoniazid serum levels may be decreased if taken with food. Clinically severe elevated blood pressure may occur if isoniazid is taken with tyramine-containing foods.

**Effects on Lab Values** False-positive urinary glucose with Clinitest®

**Adverse Reactions**

>10%:
- Gastrointestinal: Anorexia, nausea, vomiting, stomach pain
- Hepatic: Hepatitis
- Neuromuscular & skeletal: Weakness, peripheral neuritis

1% to 10%:
- Central nervous system: Dizziness, slurred speech, lethargy
- Neuromuscular & skeletal: Hyper-reflexia

<1% (Limited to important or life-threatening symptoms): Seizures, blood dyscrasias

**Overdose/Toxicology** Symptoms of overdose include nausea, vomiting, slurred speech, dizziness, blurred vision, hallucinations, stupor, coma, and intractable seizures. The onset of metabolic acidosis is within 30 minutes to 3 hours. Because of high morbidity and mortality rates with isoniazid overdose, patients who are asymptomatic after an overdose should be monitored for 4-6 hours. Pyridoxine has been shown to be effective in the treatment of intoxication, especially when seizures occur. Pyridoxine I.V. is administered on a milligram to milligram dose. If the amount of isoniazid ingested is unknown, 5 g of pyridoxine should be given over 3-5 minutes and may be followed by an additional 5 g in 30 minutes. Treatment is supportive. Forced diuresis and hemodialysis can result in more rapid removal.

**Pharmacodynamics/Kinetics**

**Protein Binding:** 10% to 15%

**Half-life Elimination:**
- Fast acetylators: 30-100 minutes
- Slow acetylators: 2-5 hours (prolonged in impaired hepatic function or severe renal impairment)

**Time to Peak:** Within 1-2 hours

**Metabolism:** Liver: with decay rate determined genetically by acetylation phenotype

**Excretion:** Urine, feces, and saliva

**Formulations**

Injection: 100 mg/mL (10 mL)
Syrup (orange flavor): 50 mg/5 mL (473 mL)
Tablet: 50 mg, 100 mg, 300 mg

**Dosing**

**Adults:** Recommendations often change due to resistant strains and newly developed information; consult *MMWR* for current CDC recommendations: **Oral** (intramuscular is available in patients who are unable to either take or absorb oral therapy):

**Note:** A four-drug regimen (isoniazid, rifampin, pyrazinamide, and either streptomycin or ethambutol) is preferred for the initial, empiric treatment of TB. When the drug susceptibility results are available, the regimen should be altered as appropriate.

Adults:
- Prophylaxis: 300 mg/day for 6 months in patients who do not have HIV infection and 12 months in patients who have HIV infection
- Treatment:
  - Daily therapy: 5 mg/kg/day given daily (usual dose: 300 mg/day); 10 mg/kg/day in 1-2 divided doses in patients with disseminated disease
  - Directly observed therapy (DOT): Twice weekly therapy: 15 mg/kg (maximum: 900 mg); 3 times/week therapy: 15 mg/kg (maximum: 900 mg)

**Note:** Concomitant administration of 6-50 mg/day pyridoxine is recommended in malnourished patients or those prone to neuropathy (eg, alcoholics, diabetics).

**Elderly:** Refer to adult dosing.

**Renal Impairment:**
- $Cl_{cr}$ <10 mL/minute: Administer 50% of normal dose.
- Hemodialysis: Dose after dialysis.
- Dialyzable (50% to 100%)

**Hepatic Impairment:** Dose should be reduced in severe hepatic disease.

**Administration**

**Oral:** Should be administered 1 hour before or 2 hours after meals on an empty stomach.

**Stability**

**Storage:** Protect oral dosage forms from light.

**Monitoring Laboratory Tests** Transaminase levels at baseline 1, 3, 6, and 9 months

**Additional Nursing Issues**

**Physical Assessment:** Monitor for signs of adverse or overdose reactions (see above) peripheral neuropathy, CNS changes, and seizures. Diabetic, alcoholic, and malnourished patients will require very close monitoring. Assess/teach necessary dietary precautions. Patient should be cautioned against eating foods high in tyramine.

(Continued)

## Isoniazid *(Continued)*

See Tyramine Foods List *on page 1422*. Arrange for frequent ophthalmic examinations even if no symptoms occur. **Pregnancy risk factor C** - benefits of use should outweigh possible risks.

**Patient Information/Instruction:** Best if taken on an empty stomach (1 hour before or 2 hours after meals). Avoid missing any dose and do not discontinue without notifying prescriber. Avoid alcohol and tyramine-containing foods (eg, fish, preserved meats or sausages, tuna, sauerkraut, aged cheeses, broad beans, liver pate, wine, protein supplements, etc). Increase dietary intake of folate, niacin, magnesium. If diabetic, use serum testing (isoniazid may affect Clinitest® results). You may experience GI distress (taking dose with meals may help). Use caution to prevent injury. You will need to have frequent ophthalmic exams and periodic medical check-ups to evaluate drug effects. Report tingling or numbness in hands or feet, loss of sensation, unusual weakness, fatigue, nausea or vomiting, dark colored urine, change in urinary pattern, yellowing skin or eyes, or change in color of stool. **Pregnancy precautions:** Inform prescriber if you are or intend to be pregnant.

**Geriatric Considerations:** Age has not been shown to affect the pharmacokinetics of INH since acetylation phenotype determines clearance and half-life, acetylation rate does not change significantly with age. Most strains of *M. tuberculosis* found the elderly should be susceptible to INH since most acquired their initial infection prior to INH's introduction.

**Related Information**

TB Drug Comparison *on page 1402*
Tyramine Foods List *on page 1422*

- **Isoniazid and Rifampin** *see* Rifampin and Isoniazid *on page 1021*
- **Isoniazid, Rifampin, and Pyrazinamide** *see* Rifampin, Isoniazid, and Pyrazinamide *on page 1021*
- **Isonicotinic Acid Hydrazide** *see* Isoniazid *on page 630*
- **Isonipecaine Hydrochloride** *see* Meperidine *on page 721*
- **Isoprenaline Hydrochloride** *see* Isoproterenol *on this page*
- **Isopro®** *see* Isoproterenol *on this page*
- **Isopropyl Alcohol** *see page 1291*

## Isoproterenol (eye soe proe TER e nole)

**U.S. Brand Names** Aerolone®; Arm-a-Med® Isoproterenol; Dey-Dose® Isoproterenol; Dispos-a-Med® Isoproterenol; Isopro®; Isuprel®; Medihaler-Iso®; Norisodrine®; Vapo-Iso®

**Synonyms** Isoprenaline Hydrochloride

**Therapeutic Category** $Beta_1$/$Beta_2$ Agonist

**Pregnancy Risk Factor** C

**Lactation** Excretion in breast milk unknown

**Use** Treatment of reversible airway obstruction as in asthma or COPD; parenterally in ventricular arrhythmias due to A-V nodal block; hemodynamically compromised bradyarrhythmias or atropine-resistant bradyarrhythmias; temporary use in third degree A-V block until pacemaker insertion; low cardiac output; vasoconstrictive shock states

**Mechanism of Action/Effect** Stimulates $beta_1$- and $beta_2$-receptors resulting in relaxation of bronchial, GI, and uterine smooth muscle, increased heart rate and contractility, vasodilation of peripheral vasculature

**Contraindications** Angina, pre-existing cardiac arrhythmias (ventricular); tachycardia or A-V block caused by cardiac glycoside intoxication; allergy to sulfites or isoproterenol or other sympathomimetic amines

**Warnings** Use with caution in elderly patients, diabetics, renal or cardiovascular disease, hyperthyroidism. Excessive or prolonged use may result in decreased effectiveness of isoproterenol. Pregnancy factor C.

**Drug Interactions**

**Increased Effect/Toxicity:** Sympathomimetic agents may cause headaches and elevate blood pressure. General anesthetics may cause arrhythmias.

**Adverse Reactions**

>10%:

Central nervous system: Insomnia, restlessness

Gastrointestinal: Dry throat, dry mouth, discoloration of saliva (pinkish-red) [inhalation and sublingual dosage forms]

1% to 10%:

Cardiovascular: Flushing of the face or skin, ventricular arrhythmias, tachycardia, profound hypotension, hypertension, pounding heartbeat

Central nervous system: Nervousness, anxiety, dizziness, headache, lightheadedness

Gastrointestinal: Vomiting, nausea

Neuromuscular & skeletal: Trembling, tremor, weakness

Respiratory: Coughing

Miscellaneous: Sweating

<1% (Limited to important or life-threatening symptoms): Arrhythmias, chest pain, paradoxical bronchospasm

**Parenteral (cardiovascular use):**

>10%:

Central nervous system: Headache

Gastrointestinal: Nausea, vomiting

1% to 10%:

Cardiovascular: Premature ventricular beats, bradycardia, hypertension, hypotension, chest pain, palpitations, tachycardia, ventricular arrhythmias

Central nervous system: Nervousness or restlessness
Respiratory: Dyspnea

**Overdose/Toxicology** Symptoms of overdose include tremor, nausea, vomiting, and hypotension. Beta-adrenergic stimulation can cause increased heart rate, decreased blood pressure, and CNS excitation. Treat symptomatically.

**Pharmacodynamics/Kinetics**

**Half-life Elimination:** 2.5-5 minutes

**Time to Peak:** Oral: Within 1-2 hours

**Metabolism:** By conjugation in many tissues including the liver and lungs

**Excretion:** Urine

**Onset:** Onset of bronchodilation: Oral inhalation: Immediately

**Duration:** Oral inhalation: 1 hour; S.C.: Up to 2 hours

**Formulations**

Inhalation:

Aerosol: 0.2% (1:500) (15 mL, 22.5 mL); 0.25% (1:400) (15 mL)

Solution for nebulization: 0.031% (4 mL); 0.062% (4 mL); 0.25% (0.5 mL, 30 mL); 0.5% (0.5 mL, 10 mL, 60 mL); 1% (10 mL)

Injection: 0.2 mg/mL (1:5000) (1 mL, 5 mL, 10 mL)

Tablet, sublingual: 10 mg, 15 mg

**Dosing**

**Adults:**

Bronchodilation: Inhalation: Metered dose inhaler: 1-2 metered doses 4-6 times/day

Bronchodilation: 1-2 inhalations of a 0.25% solution, no more than 2 inhalations at any one time (1-5 minutes between inhalations); no more than 6 inhalations in any hour during a 24-hour period; maintenance therapy: 1-2 inhalations 4-6 times/day. Alternatively: 0.5% solution via hand bulb nebulizer is 5-15 deep inhalations repeated once in 5-10 minutes if necessary; treatments may be repeated up to 5 times/day.

Sublingual: 10-20 mg every 3-4 hours; not to exceed 60 mg/day

Cardiac arrhythmias: I.V.: 5 mcg/minute initially, titrate to patient response (2-20 mcg/minute).

Shock: I.V.: 0.5-5 mcg/minute; adjust according to response.

**Elderly:** Refer to adult dosing.

**Administration**

**I.V.:** Administer around-the-clock to promote less variation in peak and trough serum levels. I.V. infusion administration requires the use of an infusion pump.

**Stability**

**Storage:** Isoproterenol solution should be stored at room temperature. It should not be used if a color or precipitate is present. Exposure to air, light, or increased temperature may cause a pink to brownish pink color to develop.

**Reconstitution:** Stability of parenteral admixture at room temperature (25°C) or at refrigeration (4°C) is 24 hours.

Standard diluent: 2 mg/500 mL $D_5W$; 4 mg/500 mL $D_5W$

Minimum volume: 1 mg/100 mL $D_5W$

**Compatibility:** Incompatible with alkaline solutions, aminophylline, and furosemide.

**Monitoring Laboratory Tests** EKG, arterial blood gas, arterial blood pressure, CVP

**Additional Nursing Issues**

**Physical Assessment:** Monitor laboratory tests, cardiac, respiratory, and hemodynamic status when used in acute or emergency situations. For inhaler, monitor respiratory and cardiac status after first use and periodically with long-term use. Assess knowledge/teach patient appropriate use and administration procedures. **Pregnancy risk factor C** - benefits of use should outweigh possible risks. Note breast-feeding caution.

**Patient Information/Instruction:**

Sublingual: Do not chew or swallow tables, let them dissolve under the tongue.

Inhalant: Shake canister before use. Administer pressurized inhalation during the second half of inspiration. If more than one dose is necessary, wait at least 1 full minute between inhalations; second inhalation is best delivered after 5-10 minutes. Do not use more often than recommended. Store solution away from light or excess heat or cold.

You may experience nervousness, dizziness, or fatigue. Use caution when driving or engaging in tasks requiring alertness until response to drug is known. Frequent small meals may reduce the incidence of nausea or vomiting. Report chest pain, rapid heartbeat or palpitations, unresolved/persistent GI upset, dizziness, fatigue, trembling, increased anxiety, sleeplessness, or difficulty breathing.

**Pregnancy/breast-feeding precautions:** Inform prescriber if you are pregnant. Consult prescriber if breast-feeding.

**Geriatric Considerations:** The elderly may find it beneficial to utilize a spacer device when using a metered dose inhaler.

**Additional Information** Some formulations may contain ethanol or sulfites.

Isoproterenol hydrochloride: Aerolone®, Dey-Dose® isoproterenol, Dispos-a-Med® isoproterenol, Isopro®, Norisodrine®, Vapo-Iso®

Isoproterenol sulfate: Medihaler-Iso®

**Related Information**

Inhalant (Asthma, Bronchospasm) Agents *on page 1388*
Inotropic and Vasoconstrictor Comparison *on page 1391*

## Isoproterenol and Phenylephrine

(eye soe proe TER e nole & fen il EF rin)

**U.S. Brand Names** Duo-Medihaler® Aerosol

**Synonyms** Phenylephrine and Isoproterenol

**Therapeutic Category** Adrenergic Agonist Agent

**Pregnancy Risk Factor** C

**Lactation** Excretion in breast milk unknown

**Use** Treatment of bronchospasm associated with acute and chronic bronchial asthma, bronchitis, pulmonary emphysema, and bronchiectasis

**Formulations** Aerosol: Each actuation releases isoproterenol hydrochloride 0.16 mg and phenylephrine bitartrate 0.24 mg (15 mL, 22.5 mL)

**Dosing**

**Adults:** Daily maintenance: 1-2 inhalations 4-6 times/day, no more than 2 inhalations at any one time or more than 6 in any 1 hour within 24 hours

**Elderly:** Refer to adult dosing.

**Additional Nursing Issues**

**Physical Assessment:** See individual components listed in Related Information. **Pregnancy risk factor C** - benefits of use should outweigh possible risks. Note breast-feeding caution.

**Patient Information/Instruction:** See individual components listed in Related Information. **Pregnancy/breast-feeding precautions:** Inform prescriber if you are on intend to get pregnant. Consult prescriber if breast-feeding.

**Related Information**

Inhalant (Asthma, Bronchospasm) Agents *on page 1388*
Isoproterenol *on page 632*
Phenylephrine *on page 920*


- **Isoptin®** *see* Verapamil *on page 1208*
- **Isoptin® SR** *see* Verapamil *on page 1208*
- **Isopto® Atropine** *see page 1282*
- **Isopto® Atropine Ophthalmic** *see* Atropine *on page 119*
- **Isopto® Carbachol Ophthalmic** *see* Ophthalmic Agents, Glaucoma *on page 853*
- **Isopto® Carpine Ophthalmic** *see* Ophthalmic Agents, Glaucoma *on page 853*
- **Isopto® Carpine Ophthalmic** *see* Pilocarpine *on page 931*
- **Isopto® Cetamide®** *see page 1282*
- **Isopto® Cetamide® Ophthalmic** *see* Sulfacetamide *on page 1080*
- **Isopto® Cetapred®** *see page 1282*
- **Isopto® Eserine** *see* Ophthalmic Agents, Glaucoma *on page 853*
- **Isopto® Eserine** *see* Physostigmine *on page 928*
- **Isopto® Frin Ophthalmic Solution** *see* Phenylephrine *on page 920*
- **Isopto® Homatropine** *see page 1282*
- **Isopto® Hyoscine Ophthalmic** *see* Scopolamine *on page 1047*
- **Isopto® Plain Solution** *see page 1294*
- **Isopto® Scopolamine** *see page 1282*
- **Isopto® Tears Solution** *see page 1294*
- **Isorbid** *see* Isosorbide Dinitrate *on this page*
- **Isordil®** *see* Isosorbide Dinitrate *on this page*
- **Isosorbide** *see page 1282*


## Isosorbide Dinitrate (eye soe SOR bide dye NYE trate)

**U.S. Brand Names** Dilatrate®-SR; Isordil®; Sorbitrate®

**Synonyms** ISD; ISDN

**Therapeutic Category** Vasodilator

**Pregnancy Risk Factor** C

**Lactation** Excretion in breast milk unknown

**Use** Prevention and treatment of angina pectoris; for congestive heart failure; to relieve pain, dysphagia, and spasm in esophageal spasm with GE reflux

**Mechanism of Action/Effect** Relaxes vascular smooth muscles, decreases arterial resistance and venous return which reduces cardiac oxygen demand. Additionally, coronary artery dilation improves collateral flow to ischemic regions; esophageal smooth muscle is relaxed via the same mechanism.

**Contraindications** Hypersensitivity to isosorbide dinitrate or any component; severe anemia; closed-angle glaucoma; postural hypotension; cerebral hemorrhage; head trauma

**Warnings** Use with caution in patients with increased intracranial pressure, hypotension, hypovolemia, and glaucoma. Sustained release products may be absorbed erratically in patients with GI hypermotility or malabsorption syndrome. Abrupt withdrawal may result in angina. Tolerance may develop. The use of nitrates for angina may occasionally promote reflux esophagitis. This may require dose adjustments or changing therapeutic agents to correct this adverse effect. Pregnancy factor C.

**Drug Interactions**

**Decreased Effect:** Nitrates may decrease the effect of heparin.

**Increased Effect/Toxicity:** Nitrates and alcohol may lead to severe hypotension. Nitrates and aspirin may increase serum nitrate concentrations and therapeutic effect. Nitrates and calcium channel blockers may lead to severe hypotension. Nitrates and dihydroergotamine may lead to elevated blood pressure or decrease antianginal effects. Has been associated with severe reactions and death when sildenafil is given concurrently with nitrates.

**Effects on Lab Values** ↓ cholesterol (S)

**Adverse Reactions**

>10%:

Cardiovascular: Flushing of face and neck, orthostatic hypotension, tachycardia

Central nervous system: Headache, restlessness

Gastrointestinal: Nausea or vomiting

<1% (Limited to important or life-threatening symptoms): Headache (severe or prolonged)

**Overdose/Toxicology** Symptoms of overdose include hypotension, throbbing headache, palpitations, visual disturbances, tachycardia, methemoglobinemia, flushing, diaphoresis, metabolic acidosis, and coma. High levels or methemoglobinemia can cause signs or symptoms of hypoxemia. Treat symptomatically.

**Pharmacodynamics/Kinetics**

**Half-life Elimination:** Parent drug: 1-4 hours; Metabolite (5-mononitrate): 4 hours

**Metabolism:** Liver

**Excretion:** Urine and feces

**Onset:** Sublingual tablet: 2-10 minutes; Chewable tablet: 3 minutes; Oral tablet: 45-60 minutes; Sustained release tablet: 30 minutes

**Duration:** Sublingual tablet: 1-2 hours; Chewable tablet: 0.5-2 hours; Oral tablet: 4-6 hours; Sustained release tablet: 6-12 hours

**Formulations**

Capsule, sustained release: 40 mg

Tablet:

Chewable: 5 mg, 10 mg

Oral: 5 mg, 10 mg, 20 mg, 30 mg

Sublingual: 2.5 mg, 5 mg, 10 mg

Sustained release: 40 mg

**Dosing**

**Adults:**

Angina: Oral: 5-40 mg 4 times/day or 40 mg every 8-12 hours in sustained released dosage form

Congestive heart failure:

Oral:

Initial: 10 mg 3 times/day

Target: 40 mg 3 times/day

Maximum: 80 mg 3 times/day

Sublingual: 2.5-10 mg every 4-6 hours

Chew: 5-10 mg every 2-3 hours

**Note:** Tolerance to nitrate effects develops with chronic exposure. Dose escalation does not overcome this effect. Tolerance can only be overcome by short periods of nitrate absence from the body. Short periods (10-12 hours) or nitrate withdrawal help minimize tolerance.

**Elderly:** Elderly patients should be given lowest recommended adult daily doses initially and titrate upward.

**Renal Impairment:** Hemodialysis: During hemodialysis, administer dose postdialysis or administer supplemental 10-20 mg dose. During peritoneal dialysis, supplemental dose is not necessary.

**Administration**

**Oral:** Do not crush sublingual tablets. Do not administer around-the-clock. The first dose of nitrates should be administered in a physician's office to observe for maximal cardiovascular dynamic effects and adverse effects (orthostatic blood pressure drop, headache).

**Additional Nursing Issues**

**Physical Assessment:** Monitor blood pressure on a regular basis (hypotension). If therapy is being discontinued, reduce dosage gradually. Assess knowledge/teach appropriate use, possible side effects, and symptoms to report. **Pregnancy risk factor C** - benefits of use should outweigh possible risks. Note breast-feeding caution.

**Patient Information/Instruction:** Take as directed, at the same time each day. Do not chew or swallow sublingual tablets; allow them to dissolve under your tongue. Do not change brands without consulting prescriber. Do not discontinue abruptly. Keep medication in original container, tightly closed. Avoid alcohol; combination may cause severe hypotension. Take medication while sitting down and use caution when changing position (rise from sitting or lying position slowly). May cause dizziness; use caution when driving or engaging in hazardous activities until response to drug is known. If chest pain is unresolved in 15 minutes, seek emergency medical help at once. Report acute headache, rapid heartbeat, unusual restlessness or dizziness, muscular weakness, or blurring vision. **Pregnancy/breast-feeding precautions:** Inform prescriber if you are or intend to be pregnant. Consult prescriber if breast-feeding.

## Isosorbide Mononitrate (EYE soe sor bide mon oh NYE trate)

**U.S. Brand Names** Imdur™; ISMO®; Monoket®

**Synonyms** ISMN

**Therapeutic Category** Vasodilator

**Pregnancy Risk Factor** C

**Lactation** Excretion in breast milk unknown

(Continued)

## Isosorbide Mononitrate *(Continued)*

**Use** Long-acting metabolite of the vasodilator isosorbide dinitrate used for the prophylactic treatment of angina pectoris

**Mechanism of Action/Effect** Systemic venodilation, decreasing preload and increasing ingestion function; improves congestive symptoms in heart failure and improves the myocardial perfusion in patients with coronary artery disease

**Contraindications** Hypersensitivity or idiosyncrasy to nitrates; contraindicated due to potential increases in intracranial pressure in patients with head trauma or cerebral hemorrhage

**Warnings** Postural hypotension, transient episodes of weakness, dizziness, or syncope may occur even with small doses. Alcohol accentuates these effects. Tolerance and cross-tolerance to nitrate antianginal and hemodynamic effects may occur during prolonged isosorbide mononitrate therapy (minimized by using the smallest effective dose, by alternating coronary vasodilators or offering drug-free intervals of as little as 12 hours). Increased anginal symptoms may be a result of dosage increases. The use of nitrates for angina may occasionally promote reflux esophagitis and may require dose adjustments or changing therapeutic agents. Pregnancy factor C.

**Drug Interactions**

**Decreased Effect:** Nitrates may decrease the effect of heparin.

**Increased Effect/Toxicity:** Nitrates and alcohol may lead to severe hypotension. Nitrates and aspirin may increase serum nitrate concentrations and therapeutic effect. Nitrates and calcium channel blockers may lead to severe hypotension. Nitrates and dihydroergotamine may lead to elevated blood pressure or decrease antianginal effects. Has been associated with severe reactions and death when sildenafil is given concurrently with nitrates.

**Adverse Reactions**

>10%:

Cardiovascular: Flushing of face and neck, orthostatic hypotension, tachycardia

Central nervous system: Headache, restlessness

Gastrointestinal: Nausea or vomiting

<1% (Limited to important or life-threatening symptoms): Headache (severe or prolonged)

**Overdose/Toxicology** Symptoms of overdose include hypotension, throbbing headache, palpitations, visual disturbances, tachycardia, methemoglobinemia, flushing, diaphoresis, metabolic acidosis, and coma. High levels or methemoglobinemia can cause signs or symptoms of hypoxemia. Treat symptomatically.

**Pharmacodynamics/Kinetics**

**Half-life Elimination:** Mononitrate: ~4 hours (8 times that of dinitrate)

**Metabolism:** Liver

**Excretion:** Urine and feces

**Onset:** Oral: 30-60 minutes

**Formulations**

Tablet (ISMO®, Monoket®): 10 mg, 20 mg

Tablet, extended release (Imdur™): 30 mg, 60 mg, 120 mg

**Dosing**

**Adults:** Oral:

Regular tablet: 20 mg twice daily separated by 7 hours

Extended release tablet (Imdur™): Initial: 30-60 mg once daily; after several days the dosage may be increased to 120 mg/day (given as two 60 mg tablets); maximum: 240 mg/day.

**Elderly:** Start with lowest recommended adult dose.

**Renal Impairment:** Not necessary for elderly or patients with altered renal or hepatic function.

**Administration**

**Oral:** The first dose of nitrates (ie, sublingual, chewable, oral) should be taken in a physician's office to observe for maximal cardiovascular dynamic effects and adverse effects (eg, orthostatic blood pressure drop, headache). Daily dose should be taken in the morning upon arising. Asymmetrical dosing regimen of 7 AM and 3 PM or 9 AM and 5 PM to allow for a nitrate-free dosing interval to minimize nitrate tolerance. Do not administer around-the-clock, an 8- to 12-hour nitrate-free interval is needed each day to prevent tolerance. Extended release tablets should not be chewed or crushed. Should be swallowed with a half-glassful of fluid.

**Stability**

**Storage:** Tablets should be stored in a tight container at room temperature of 15°C to 30°C (59°F to 86°F).

**Monitoring Laboratory Tests** Orthostasis

**Additional Nursing Issues**

**Physical Assessment:** Monitor blood pressure and heart rate on a regular basis (ie, hypotension, arrhythmias). Assess knowledge/teach appropriate use, possible side effects, and symptoms to report. If therapy is being discontinued, reduce dosage gradually. **Pregnancy risk factor C** - benefits of use should outweigh possible risks. Note breast-feeding caution.

**Patient Information/Instruction:** Take as directed, at the same time each day. Do not chew or crush extended release capsules; swallow with 8 oz of water. Do not change brands without consulting prescriber. Do not discontinue abruptly. Keep medication in original container, tightly closed. Avoid alcohol; combination may cause severe hypotension. Take medication while sitting down and use caution when changing position (rise from sitting or lying position slowly). May cause dizziness; use caution when driving or engaging in hazardous activities until response to drug is known. If chest pain is unresolved in 15 minutes, seek emergency medical help at once. Report acute headache, rapid heartbeat, unusual restlessness or dizziness, muscular weakness, or blurring vision. **Pregnancy/breast-feeding precautions:** Inform prescriber if you are or intend to be pregnant. Consult prescriber if breast-feeding.

**Geriatric Considerations:** The first dose of nitrates (sublingual, chewable, oral) should be taken in a physician's office to observe for maximal cardiovascular dynamic effects and adverse effects (orthostatic blood pressure drop, headache). The use of nitrates for angina may occasionally promote reflux esophagitis. This may require dose adjustments or changing therapeutic agents to correct this adverse effect.

## Isotretinoin (eye soe TRET i noyn)

**U.S. Brand Names** Accutane®

**Synonyms** 13-*cis*-Retinoic Acid

**Therapeutic Category** Retinoic Acid Derivative

**Pregnancy Risk Factor** X

**Lactation** Enters breast milk/not recommended

**Use** Treatment of severe recalcitrant cystic and/or conglobate acne unresponsive to conventional therapy

**Investigational use:** Treatment of children with metastatic neuroblastoma or leukemia that does not respond to conventional therapy

**Mechanism of Action/Effect** Reduces sebaceous gland size and reduces sebum production; regulates cell proliferation and differentiation

**Contraindications** Sensitivity to parabens, vitamin A, or other retinoids; pregnancy

**Warnings** Use with caution in patients with diabetes mellitus or hypertriglyceridemia. **Not to be used in women of childbearing potential** unless the woman is capable of complying with effective contraceptive measures because of the high likelihood of teratogenic effects (~20%). Therapy is normally begun on the second or third day of next normal menstrual period. Effective contraception must be used for at least 1 month before beginning therapy, during therapy, and for 1 month after discontinuation of therapy. There have been reports of depression as a possible adverse reaction associated with the use of isotretinoin. It is not clear whether the depression is associated with the drug or the disease.

**Drug Interactions**

**Decreased Effect:** Isotretinoin may increase clearance of carbamazepine resulting in reduced carbamazepine levels.

**Increased Effect/Toxicity:** Avoid other vitamin A products. May interfere with medications used to treat hypertriglyceridemia.

**Food Interactions** Isotretinoin bioavailability may be increased if taken with food.

**Adverse Reactions**

>10%:

Dermatologic: Redness, cheilitis, inflammation of lips, dry skin, pruritus, photosensitivity

Endocrine & metabolic: Increased serum concentration of triglycerides

Gastrointestinal: Dry mouth

Local: Burning

Neuromuscular & skeletal: Bone pain, arthralgia, myalgia

Ocular: Itching eyes

Respiratory: Epistaxis, dry nose

1% to 10%:

Cardiovascular: Facial edema, pallor

Central nervous system: Fatigue, headache, mental depression, hypothermia

Dermatologic: Skin peeling on hands or soles of feet, rash, cellulitis

Endocrine & metabolic: Fluid imbalance, acidosis

Gastrointestinal: Stomach upset

Hepatic: Ascites

Neuromuscular & skeletal: Flank pain

Ocular: Dry eyes, photophobia

Miscellaneous: Lymph disorders

<1% (Limited to important or life-threatening symptoms): Mood changes, pseudomotor cerebri, alopecia, increase in erythrocyte sedimentation rate, decrease in hemoglobin and hematocrit, hepatitis

**Overdose/Toxicology** Symptoms of overdose include headache, vomiting, flushing, abdominal pain, and ataxia. All signs or symptoms have been transient.

**Pharmacodynamics/Kinetics**

**Protein Binding:** 99% to 100%

**Distribution:** Crosses the placenta

**Half-life Elimination:** Parent drug: 10-20 hours; Metabolite: 11-50 hours

**Time to Peak:** Within 3 hours

**Metabolism:** Liver

**Excretion:** Urine and feces

**Formulations** Capsule: 10 mg, 20 mg, 40 mg

**Dosing**

**Adults:** Oral: 0.5-2 mg/kg/day in 2 divided doses (dosages as low as 0.05 mg/kg/day have been reported to be beneficial) for 15-20 weeks or until the total cyst count decreases by 70%.

**Hepatic Impairment:** Empiric dose reductions are recommended in patient with hepatitis.

(Continued)

## Isotretinoin *(Continued)*

**Administration**

**Oral:** Capsules can be swallowed, or chewed and swallowed. The capsule may be opened with a large needle and the contents placed on applesauce or ice cream for patients unable to swallow the capsule. Increased isotretinoin bioavailability when administered with food or milk.

**Stability**

**Storage:** Store at room temperature and protect from light.

**Monitoring Laboratory Tests** **Must have pregnancy test prior to beginning therapy,** CBC with differential and platelet count, baseline sedimentation rate, serum triglycerides, liver enzymes

**Additional Nursing Issues**

**Physical Assessment:** See Contraindications and Warnings/Precautions for use cautions. Assess effectiveness and interactions of other medications (see Drug Interactions). Monitor lab tests, effectiveness of therapy, and adverse effects at beginning of therapy and regularly with long-term use (see Adverse Reactions and Overdose/Toxicology). Monitor diabetic patients closely. Assess knowledge/teach patient appropriate use, possible side effects/interventions, and adverse symptoms to report. **Pregnancy risk factor X** - determine that patient is not pregnant before beginning treatment and do not give to women of childbearing age unless female is capable of complying with barrier contraceptive measures 1 month prior to therapy, during therapy, and 1 month following therapy. Breast-feeding is not recommended.

**Patient Information/Instruction:** Use exactly as directed; do not take more than recommended. Capsule can be chewed and swallowed, swallowed, or opened with a large needle and contents sprinkled on applesauce or ice cream. Do not take any other vitamin A products, limit vitamin A intake, and increase exercise during therapy. Exacerbations of acne may occur during first weeks of therapy. You may experience headache, loss of night vision, lethargy, or visual disturbances (use caution when driving or engaging in tasks requiring alertness until response to drug is known); photosensitivity (use sunscreen, wear protective clothing and eyewear, and avoid direct sunlight); dry mouth or nausea (small frequent meals, sucking hard candy, or chewing gum may may help); dryness, redness, or itching of skin, eye irritation, or increased sensitivity to contact lenses (wear regular glasses). Discontinue therapy and report acute vision changes, rectal bleeding, abdominal cramping, or unresolved diarrhea. **Pregnancy/breast-feeding precautions:** Inform prescriber if you are pregnant. Do not get pregnant 1 month before, during, or for 1 month following therapy. Consult prescriber for instruction on appropriate contraceptive measures. This drug may cause severe fetal defects. Do not donate blood during or for 1 month following therapy (same reason). Breast-feeding is not recommended.

♦ **Isotrex®** *see* Isotretinoin *on previous page*

♦ **Isox** *see* Itraconazole *on next page*

## Isradipine (iz RA di peen)

**U.S. Brand Names** DynaCirc®

**Therapeutic Category** Calcium Channel Blocker

**Pregnancy Risk Factor** C

**Lactation** Excretion in breast milk unknown

**Use** Treatment of hypertension

**Mechanism of Action/Effect** Inhibits calcium ion from entering the "slow channels" or select voltage-sensitive areas of vascular smooth muscle and myocardium during depolarization

**Contraindications** Hypersensitivity to isradipine or any component; hypersensitivity to calcium channel blockers and adenosine

**Warnings** Avoid use in hypotension, congestive heart failure, cardiac conduction defects, PVCs, or idiopathic hypertrophic subaortic stenosis. May cause platelet inhibition. Do not abruptly withdraw (chest pain). May cause hepatic dysfunction or increased angina. Increased intracranial pressure with cranial tumors. Elderly may have greater hypotensive effect. Pregnancy factor C.

**Drug Interactions**

**Cytochrome P-450 Effect:** CYP3A3/4 enzyme substrate

**Decreased Effect:** NSAIDs (diclofenac) and isradipine may decrease the antihypertensive response of isradipine. Lovastatin and isradipine may cause a decrease in lovastatin effect.

**Increased Effect/Toxicity:** Isradipine and beta-blockers may increase cardiovascular adverse effects. Cyclosporine and isradipine may minimally increase cyclosporine levels.

**Food Interactions** Isradipine serum levels may be increased if taken with food.

**Adverse Reactions**

>10%: Central nervous system: Headache

1% to 10%:

- Cardiovascular: Chest pain, hypotension, peripheral edema, tachycardia, flushing
- Central nervous system: Dizziness, fatigue
- Dermatologic: Rash
- Gastrointestinal: Nausea, diarrhea
- Neuromuscular & skeletal: Weakness
- Respiratory: Dyspnea

<1% (Limited to important or life-threatening symptoms): Congestive heart failure, hypotensive (excessive)

**Overdose/Toxicology** Primary cardiac symptoms of calcium blocker overdose include hypotension and bradycardia. Hypotension is caused by peripheral vasodilation, myocardial depression, and bradycardia. Bradycardia results from sinus bradycardia, second- or third-degree atrioventricular block, or sinus arrest with junctional rhythm. Intraventricular conduction is usually not affected so QRS duration is normal (verapamil does prolong the P-R interval and bepridil prolongs the Q-T interval and may cause ventricular arrhythmias, including torsade de pointes).

Noncardiac symptoms include confusion, stupor, nausea, vomiting, metabolic acidosis and hyperglycemia. Repeated calcium administration may promptly reverse the depressed cardiac contractility (but not sinus node depression or peripheral vasodilation).

**Pharmacodynamics/Kinetics**

**Protein Binding:** 95%

**Half-life Elimination:** 8 hours

**Time to Peak:** 1-2 hours

**Metabolism:** Liver

**Excretion:** Renal

**Duration:** 8-16 hours

**Formulations** Capsule: 2.5 mg, 5 mg

**Dosing**

**Adults:** Oral: 2.5 mg twice daily; antihypertensive response is seen in 2-3 hours; maximal response in 2-4 weeks; increase dose at 2- to 4-week intervals at 2.5-5 mg increments; usual dose range: 5-20 mg/day. **Note**: Most patients show no improvement with doses >10 mg/day except adverse reaction rate increases.

**Elderly:** Maximum dose in the elderly should be 10 mg/day; antihypertensive response seen in 2-3 hours; maximal response in 2-4 weeks; increase dose at 2- to 4-week intervals at 2.5-5 mg increments; usual dose range: 5-20 mg/day. **Note**: Most patients show no improvement with doses >10 mg/day except adverse reaction rate increases.

**Additional Nursing Issues**

**Physical Assessment:** Monitor blood pressure, cardiac rhythm, I & O ratio, weight, edema, signs or symptoms of adverse reactions (see above) at beginning of therapy or when titrating dose, and periodically throughout long-term therapy. Monitor blood pressure closely if patient is also taking nitrates or other antihypertensive medications. **Pregnancy risk factor C** - benefits of use should outweigh possible risks. Note breast-feeding caution.

**Patient Information/Instruction:** Take as prescribed; do not stop abruptly without consulting prescriber immediately. You may experience headache (if unrelieved, consult prescriber), nausea or vomiting (frequent small meals may help), constipation (increased dietary bulk and fluids may help), or depression (should resolve when drug is discontinued). May cause dizziness or drowsiness; use caution when driving or engaging in tasks that require alertness until response to drug is known. Report unrelieved headache, vomiting, constipation, palpitations, swelling of hands or feet, or sudden weight gain. **Pregnancy/breast-feeding precautions:** Inform prescriber if you are or intend to be pregnant. Consult prescriber if breast-feeding.

**Geriatric Considerations:** Elderly may experience a greater hypotensive response. Constipation may be more of a problem in the elderly.

**Related Information**

Calcium Channel Blocking Agents Comparison *on page 1378*

- **Isuprel®** *see* Isoproterenol *on page 632*
- **Italnik®** *see* Ciprofloxacin *on page 270*
- **Itch-X®** *see page 1294*

## Itraconazole (i tra KOE na zole)

**U.S. Brand Names** Sporanox®

**Therapeutic Category** Antifungal Agent, Oral; Antifungal Agent, Parenteral

**Pregnancy Risk Factor** C

**Lactation** Enters breast milk/not recommended

**Use** Treatment of susceptible fungal infections in immunocompromised and immunocompetent patients including blastomycosis and histoplasmosis; also indicated for aspergillosis and onychomycosis of the toenail; has activity against *Aspergillus*, *Candida*, *Coccidioides*, *Cryptococcus*, *Sporothrix*, tinea unguium

Intravenous solution is indicated in the treatment of blastomycosis, histoplasmosis (nonmeningeal), aspergillosis (in patients intolerant or refractory to amphotericin B)

**Unlabeled use:** Superficial mycoses including dermatophytoses (eg, tinea capitis), pityriasis versicolor, sebopsoriasis, vaginal and chronic mucocutaneous candidiases; systemic mycoses including candidiasis, meningeal and disseminated cryptococcal infections, paracoccidioidomycosis, coccidioidomycoses; miscellaneous mycoses such as sporotrichosis, chromomycosis, leishmaniasis, fungal keratitis, alternariosis, zygomycosis

**Mechanism of Action/Effect** Interferes with cytochrome P-450 activity, decreasing ergosterol synthesis (principal sterol in fungal cell membrane) and inhibiting cell membrane formation

**Contraindications** Hypersensitivity to itraconazole or other azoles; concomitant use with astemizole, cisapride, lovastatin, midazolam, simvastatin, terfenadine, or triazolam

**Warnings** Rare cases of serious cardiovascular adverse event, including death, ventricular tachycardia, and torsade de pointes have been observed due to increased terfenadine concentrations induced by itraconazole. Patients who develop abnormal liver

(Continued)

## Itraconazole *(Continued)*

function tests during itraconazole therapy should be monitored and therapy discontinued if symptoms of liver disease develop.

**Drug Interactions**

**Cytochrome P-450 Effect:** CYP3A3/4 enzyme substrate; CYP3A3/4 enzyme inhibitor

**Decreased Effect:** Decreased serum levels with carbamazepine, didanosine, isoniazid, phenobarbital, phenytoin, rifabutin, and rifampin. **Should not be administered concomitantly with rifampin.** Absorption requires gastric acidity; therefore, antacids, $H_2$ antagonists (cimetidine, famotidine, nizatidine, and ranitidine), omeprazole, lansoprazole, and sucralfate significantly reduce bioavailability resulting in treatment failures and should not be administered concomitantly. Amphotericin B or fluconazole should be used instead.

**Increased Effect/Toxicity:** May increase cyclosporine or tacrolimus levels (by 50%) when high doses are used. May increase phenytoin serum concentration. May inhibit warfarin metabolism. May increase digoxin serum levels. May increase astemizole, busulfan, cisapride, terfenadine, and vinca alkaloid levels; **concomitant administration is not recommended.** May increase amlodipine, benzodiazepine, buspirone, corticosteroids, and oral hypoglycemic levels. Use with caution in patients prescribed medications eliminated by P-450 3A4 metabolism. Itraconazole increases levels of lovastatin (possibly 20-fold) and other HMG-CoA inhibitors due to inhibition of CYP3A4.

**Food Interactions** Capsules: Enhanced by food and possibly by gastric acidity. Solution: Decreased by food, time to peak concentration prolonged by food.

**Adverse Reactions**

1% to 10%:

Central nervous system: Headache, dizziness, drowsiness

Dermatologic: Rash

Endocrine & metabolic: Hypertriglyceridemia

Gastrointestinal: Abdominal pain, nausea, vomiting, diarrhea, anorexia

Hepatic: Hepatitis

<1% (Limited to important or life-threatening symptoms): Abnormal hepatic function, albuminuria, adrenal suppression, gynecomastia

**Overdose/Toxicology** Overdoses are well tolerated. Treatment is supportive. Dialysis is not effective.

**Pharmacodynamics/Kinetics**

**Protein Binding:** 99.9% bound to plasma proteins; metabolite hydroxy-itraconazole is 99.5% bound to plasma proteins

**Distribution:** Apparent volume averaged 796 ± 185 L or 10 L/kg; highly lipophilic and tissue concentrations are higher than plasma concentrations. The highest itraconazole concentrations are achieved in adipose, omentum, endometrium, cervical, and vaginal mucus, and skin/nails. Aqueous fluids, such as cerebrospinal fluid and urine, contain negligible amounts of itraconazole; steady-state concentrations are achieved in 13 days with multiple administration of itraconazole 100-400 mg/day.

**Half-life Elimination:** After single 200 mg dose: 21 ± 5 hours; steady-state (IV): 35 hours

**Metabolism:** Liver

**Excretion:** Feces and urine

**Formulations**

Capsule: 100 mg

Solution, oral: 100 mg/10 mL (150 mL)

Injection: 10 mg/mL (25 mL ampul)

**Dosing**

**Adults:**

Oral:

Blastomycosis/histoplasmosis: 200 mg once daily, if no obvious improvement or there is evidence of progressive fungal disease, increase the dose in 100 mg increments to a maximum of 400 mg/day. Doses >200 mg/day are given in 2 divided doses. Length of therapy varies from 1 day to >6 months depending on the condition and mycological response.

Aspergillosis: 200-400 mg/day

Onychomycosis: 200 mg once daily for 12 consecutive weeks

Life-threatening infections: Loading dose: 200 mg 3 times/day (600 mg/day) should be given for the first 3 days of therapy.

Oropharyngeal and esophageal candidiasis: Oral solution: 100-200 mg once daily

I.V.: 200 mg twice daily for 4 doses, followed by 200 mg daily

**Elderly:** Refer to adult dosing.

**Renal Impairment:** Not necessary. Itraconazole injection is not recommended in patients with a creatinine clearance <30 mL/minute.

Not dialyzable

**Hepatic Impairment:** May be necessary, but specific guidelines are not available.

**Administration**

**Oral:** Doses >200 mg/day are given in 2 divided doses; do not administer with antacids.

**I.V.:** Use dedicated infusion line. Do not mix with other medications. Infuse over 1 hour.

**Additional Nursing Issues**

**Physical Assessment:** Assess effectiveness and interactions of other medications (see Drug Interactions). See Warnings/Precautions and Contraindications for use cautions. Monitor effectiveness of therapy and and adverse response (see Adverse Reactions and Overdose/Toxicology). Assess knowledge/teach patient possible side effects and appropriate interventions and adverse symptoms to report. **Pregnancy risk factor C** - benefits of use should outweigh possible risks. Breast-feeding is not recommended.

**Patient Information/Instruction:** Take as directed, around-the-clock, with food. Take full course of medication; do not discontinue without notifying prescriber. Practice good hygiene measures to prevent reinfection. If diabetic, test serum glucose regularly (can cause hypoglycemia when given with sulfonylureas). Frequent blood tests may be required with prolonged therapy. You may experience dizziness or drowsiness (use caution when driving or engaging in tasks that require alertness until response to drug is known); nausea, vomiting, or diarrhea (small frequent meals, frequent mouth care, sucking lozenges, or chewing gum may help). Report skin rash or other persistent adverse reactions. **Pregnancy/breast-feeding precautions:** Inform prescriber if you are or intend to be pregnant. Breast-feeding is not recommended.


- **Itranax** *see* Itraconazole *on page 639*
- **I-Tropine®** *see page 1282*
- **I-Tropine® Ophthalmic** *see* Atropine *on page 119*
- **IVIG** *see* Immune Globulin, Intravenous *on page 602*
- **I.V. to Oral Conversion** *see page 1359*
- **Jaa Amp® Trihydrate** *see* Ampicillin *on page 90*
- **Jaa-Prednisone®** *see* Prednisone *on page 962*
- **Janimine®** *see* Imipramine *on page 600*
- **Japanese Encephalitis Virus Vaccine, Inactivated** *see page 1256*
- **Jenamicin® Injection** *see* Gentamicin *on page 531*
- **Jenest-28™** *see* Oral Contraceptives *on page 859*
- **Junior Strength Motrin® [OTC]** *see* Ibuprofen *on page 592*
- **Just Tears® Solution** *see page 1294*
- **K+® 8** *see* Potassium Supplements *on page 952*
- **K+® 10** *see* Potassium Supplements *on page 952*
- **Kabikinase®** *see* Streptokinase *on page 1074*
- **Kadian™** *see* Morphine Sulfate *on page 790*
- **Kalcinate® Cal Plus®** *see* Calcium Supplements *on page 185*


## Kanamycin (kan a MYE sin)

**U.S. Brand Names** Kantrex®

**Therapeutic Category** Antibiotic, Aminoglycoside

**Pregnancy Risk Factor** D

**Lactation** Enters breast milk/compatible

**Use**

Oral: Preoperative bowel preparation in the prophylaxis of infections and adjunctive treatment of hepatic coma (oral kanamycin is not indicated in the treatment of systemic infections); treatment of susceptible bacterial infection including gram-negative aerobes, gram-positive *Bacillus* as well as some mycobacteria

Intraperitoneal: Rarely used in antibiotic irrigations during surgery

**Mechanism of Action/Effect** Interferes with protein synthesis in bacterial cell by binding to ribosomal subunit

**Contraindications** Hypersensitivity to kanamycin, any component, or other aminoglycosides; pregnancy

**Warnings** Use with caution in patients with pre-existing renal insufficiency, vestibular or cochlear impairment, myasthenia gravis, or conditions which depress neuromuscular transmission. Parenteral aminoglycosides are associated with nephrotoxicity or ototoxicity. The ototoxicity may be proportional to the amount of drug given and the duration of treatment. Tinnitus or vertigo are indications of vestibular injury and impending hearing loss. Renal damage is usually reversible.

**Drug Interactions**

**Increased Effect/Toxicity:** Penicillins, cephalosporins, amphotericin B, diuretics may increase nephrotoxicity. Neuromuscular blocking agents may increase neuromuscular blockade.

**Adverse Reactions**

>10%: Renal: Nephrotoxicity

1% to 10%:

Cardiovascular: Edema

Central nervous system: Neurotoxicity

Dermatologic: Skin itching, redness, rash

Otic: Ototoxicity (auditory), ototoxicity (vestibular)

<1% (Limited to important or life-threatening symptoms): Granulocytopenia, agranulocytosis, thrombocytopenia, dyspnea

**Overdose/Toxicology** Symptoms of overdose include ototoxicity, nephrotoxicity, and neuromuscular toxicity. Treatment of choice following a single acute overdose appears to be maintenance of urine output of at least 3 mL/kg/hour during the acute treatment phase. Dialysis is of questionable value for enhancing aminoglycoside elimination.

**Pharmacodynamics/Kinetics**

**Distribution:** Relative diffusion of antimicrobial agents from blood into cerebrospinal fluid (CSF): Good only with inflammation (exceeds usual MICs)

Ratio of CSF to blood level (%): Normal meninges: Nil; Inflamed meninges: 43%

**Half-life Elimination:** 2-4 hours, increases in anuria to 80 hours; End-stage renal disease: 40-96 hours

(Continued)

## Kanamycin *(Continued)*

**Time to Peak:** I.M.: 1-2 hours

**Excretion:** Entirely in the kidney, principally by glomerular filtration

**Formulations**

Kanamycin sulfate:
- Capsule: 500 mg
- Injection:
  - Pediatrics: 75 mg (2 mL)
  - Adults: 500 mg (2 mL); 1 g (3 mL)

**Dosing**

**Adults:**
- Infections: I.M., I.V.: 5-7.5 mg/kg/dose in divided doses every 8-12 hours
- Preoperative intestinal antisepsis: Oral: 1 g every 4-6 hours for 36-72 hours
- Hepatic coma: Oral: 8-12 g/day in divided doses

**Elderly:** I.M., I.V.: Initial dose should be 5-7.5 mg/kg based on ideal body weight (except in obese patients). Maintenance dose and interval should be adjusted for estimated renal function. Dosing interval in most older patients is every 12-24 hours (see Geriatric Considerations).

**Renal Impairment:**
- $Cl_{cr}$ 50-80 mL/minute: Administer 60% to 90% of dose or administer every 8-12 hours.
- $Cl_{cr}$ 10-50 mL/minute: Administer 30% to 70% of dose or administer every 12 hours.
- $Cl_{cr}$ <10 mL/minute: Administer 20% to 30% of dose or administer every 24-48 hours.
- Dialyzable (50% to 100%)

**Administration**

**I.V.:** Dilute to 100-200 mL and infuse over 30 minutes; administer around-the-clock to promote less variation in peak and trough serum levels.

**Stability**

**Storage:** Darkening of vials does not indicate loss of potency.

**Monitoring Laboratory Tests** Perform culture and sensitivity studies prior to initiating therapy to determine the causative organism and its susceptibility to kanamycin. Serum creatinine and BUN every 2-3 days; peak and trough concentrations; aminoglycoside levels in blood taken from Silastic® central catheters can sometime give falsely high readings (sample from alternative lumen or via peripheral stick if possible; otherwise flush very well following administration).

**Additional Nursing Issues**

**Physical Assessment:** Assess effectiveness and interactions of other medications (see Drug Interactions). See Contraindications and Warnings/Precautions for use cautions. Monitor effectiveness of therapy, laboratory tests (see Monitoring Laboratory Tests), and adverse response (eg, ototoxicity, nephrotoxicity, neurotoxicity - see Adverse Reactions and Overdose/Toxicology). Assess hearing and renal status before, during, and after therapy. Assess knowledge/teach patient possible side effects/interventions, and adverse symptoms to report. **Pregnancy risk factor D** - assess knowledge/teach appropriate use of barrier contraceptives.

**Patient Information/Instruction:** It is important to maintain adequate hydration (2-3 L/day of fluids unless instructed to restrict fluid intake). Report change in hearing acuity, ringing or roaring in ears, alteration in balance, vertigo, feeling of fullness in head; pain, tingling, or numbness of any body part; change in urinary pattern or decrease in urine; signs of opportunistic infection (eg, white plaques in mouth, vaginal discharge, unhealed sores, sore throat, unusual fever, chills); pain, redness, or swelling at injection site; skin rash; or other adverse reactions. **Pregnancy precautions:** Do not get pregnant during therapy with this medication; use appropriate barrier contraceptive measures.

**Geriatric Considerations:** Kanamycin is not a drug of choice in the elderly since the elderly may have increased adverse effects (renal).

**Additional Information** The injection formulation contains sulfites.

**Related Information**

TB Drug Comparison *on page 1402*

- ♦ **Kantrex®** *see* Kanamycin *on previous page*
- ♦ **Kaochlor®** *see* Potassium Supplements *on page 952*
- ♦ **Kaochlor-Eff** *see* Potassium Supplements *on page 952*
- ♦ **Kaodene®** *see page 1294*
- ♦ **Kaolin and Pectin** *see page 1294*

## Kaolin and Pectin With Opium (KAY oh lin & PEK tin with OH pee um)

**U.S. Brand Names** Parepectolin®

**Synonyms** Pectin With Opium and Kaolin

**Therapeutic Category** Antidiarrheal

**Pregnancy Risk Factor** C

**Lactation** Excretion in breast milk unknown

**Use** Symptomatic relief of diarrhea

**Formulations** Suspension, oral: Kaolin 5.5 g, pectin 162 mg, and opium 15 mg per 30 mL [3.7 mL paregoric] (240 mL)

**Dosing**

**Adults:** Oral: 15-30 mL with each loose bowel movement, not to exceed 120 mL in 12 hours

**Elderly:** Avoid use in the elderly.

- ♦ **Kaon-Cl®** *see* Potassium Supplements *on page 952*

- **Kaopectate® Advanced Formula** *see page 1294*
- **Kaopectate® II [OTC]** *see* Loperamide *on page 688*
- **Kaopectate® Maximum Strength Caplets** *see page 1294*
- **Kao-Spen®** *see page 1294*
- **Kapectolin®** *see page 1294*
- **Karidium®** *see page 1294*
- **Karigel®** *see page 1294*
- **Karigel®-N** *see page 1294*
- **Kasof® [OTC]** *see* Docusate *on page 392*
- **Kato®** *see* Potassium Supplements *on page 952*
- **Kaybovite-1000®** *see* Cyanocobalamin *on page 311*
- **Kay Ciel®** *see* Potassium Supplements *on page 952*
- **Kayexalate®** *see* Sodium Polystyrene Sulfonate *on page 1064*
- **Kaylixir®** *see* Potassium Supplements *on page 952*
- **K+ Care®** *see* Potassium Supplements *on page 952*
- **K+ Care® ET** *see* Potassium Supplements *on page 952*
- **KCl (Potassium Chloride)** *see* Potassium Supplements *on page 952*
- **K-Dur®** *see* Potassium Supplements *on page 952*
- **Keduril®** *see* Ketoprofen *on page 645*
- **Kedvil** *see* Ibuprofen *on page 592*
- **Keflex®** *see* Cephalexin *on page 237*
- **Keftab®** *see* Cephalexin *on page 237*
- **Kefurox® Injection** *see* Cefuroxime *on page 233*
- **Kefzol®** *see* Cefazolin *on page 214*
- **K-Electrolyte®** *see* Potassium Supplements *on page 952*
- **Kelfiprim** *see* Co-trimoxazole *on page 307*
- **Kemadrin®** *see* Procyclidine *on page 973*
- **Kenacort®** *see* Triamcinolone *on page 1171*
- **Kenaject-40®** *see* Triamcinolone *on page 1171*
- **Kenalog®** *see* Topical Corticosteroids *on page 1152*
- **Kenalog®** *see* Triamcinolone *on page 1171*
- **Kenalog-10®** *see* Triamcinolone *on page 1171*
- **Kenalog-40®** *see* Triamcinolone *on page 1171*
- **Kenalog® H** *see* Topical Corticosteroids *on page 1152*
- **Kenalog® H** *see* Triamcinolone *on page 1171*
- **Kenalog® in Orabase®** *see* Topical Corticosteroids *on page 1152*
- **Kenalog® in Orabase®** *see* Triamcinolone *on page 1171*
- **Kenamil** *see* Zidovudine *on page 1227*
- **Kenaprol** *see* Metoprolol *on page 761*
- **Kenoket** *see* Clonazepam *on page 288*
- **Kenolan** *see* Captopril *on page 192*
- **Kenonel®** *see* Topical Corticosteroids *on page 1152*
- **Kenonel®** *see* Triamcinolone *on page 1171*
- **Kenopril** *see* Enalapril *on page 416*
- **Kentadin** *see* Pentoxifylline *on page 908*
- **Kenzoflex** *see* Ciprofloxacin *on page 270*
- **Keoxifene Hydrochloride** *see* Raloxifene *on page 1006*
- **Keralyt® Gel** *see page 1294*
- **Kerlone® Oral** *see* Betaxolol *on page 150*
- **Kestrone®** *see* Estrone *on page 451*


## Ketoconazole (kee toe KOE na zole)

**U.S. Brand Names** Nizoral®

**Therapeutic Category** Antifungal Agent, Oral; Antifungal Agent, Topical

**Pregnancy Risk Factor** C

**Lactation** Enters breast milk/not recommended

**Use** Treatment of susceptible fungal infections, including candidiasis, oral thrush, blastomycosis, histoplasmosis, paracoccidioidomycosis, chronic mucocutaneous candidiasis, as well as, certain recalcitrant cutaneous dermatophytoses; topically for treatment of tinea corporis, tinea cruris, tinea versicolor, cutaneous candidiasis, and seborrheic dermatitis

**Mechanism of Action/Effect** Inhibits several fungal enzymes that results in a build-up of toxic concentrations of hydrogen peroxide resulting in cell death

**Contraindications** Hypersensitivity to ketoconazole or any component; CNS fungal infections (due to poor CNS penetration); coadministration with astemizole, terfenadine, cisapride, or triazolam is contraindicated due to risk of potentially fatal cardiac arrhythmias

**Warnings** Use with caution in patients with impaired hepatic function. Has been associated with hepatotoxicity, including some fatalities. Perform periodic liver function tests. High doses of ketoconazole may depress adrenocortical function. Pregnancy factor C.

**Drug Interactions**

**Cytochrome P-450 Effect:** CYP3A3/4 enzyme substrate; CYP1A2, 2C, 2C9, 2C18, 2C19, 3A3/4, and 3A5-7 enzyme inhibitor

(Continued)

## Ketoconazole *(Continued)*

**Decreased Effect:** Oral: Decreased ketoconazole serum levels with isoniazid and phenytoin. Decreased/undetectable serum levels with rifampin; **should not be administered concomitantly with rifampin.** Theophylline serum levels may be decreased. Absorption requires gastric acidity; therefore, antacids, $H_2$ antagonists (cimetidine, famotidine, nizatidine, and ranitidine), omeprazole, lansoprazole, and sucralfate significantly reduce bioavailability resulting in treatment failures. Should not be administered concomitantly. Amphotericin B or fluconazole may be used instead.

**Increased Effect/Toxicity:** Oral: May increase cyclosporine levels (by 50%) when high doses are used. Inhibits warfarin metabolism resulting in increased anticoagulant effect. Increases corticosteroid bioavailability and decreases steroid clearance. Increases phenytoin, digoxin, astemizole, terfenadine, and cisapride concentrations. **Concomitant administration with astemizole, terfenadine, or cisapride is contraindicated.**

**Food Interactions** Ketoconazole peak serum levels may be prolonged if taken with food.

**Adverse Reactions**

**Oral:**

1% to 10%:

Dermatologic: Pruritus

Gastrointestinal: Nausea, vomiting, abdominal pain

<1% (Limited to important or life-threatening symptoms): Headache, dizziness, somnolence, fever, chills, bulging fontanelles, gynecomastia, diarrhea, impotence, thrombocytopenia, leukopenia, hemolytic anemia, photophobia

**Cream:** Severe irritation, pruritus, stinging (~5%)

**Shampoo:** Increases in normal hair loss, irritation (<1%), abnormal hair texture, scalp pustules, mild dryness of skin, itching, oiliness/dryness of hair

**Overdose/Toxicology** Oral: Symptoms of overdose include dizziness, headache, nausea, vomiting, diarrhea. Overdoses are well tolerated. Treatment includes supportive measures and gastric decontamination.

**Pharmacodynamics/Kinetics**

**Protein Binding:** 93% to 96%

**Distribution:** Minimal distribution into the CNS

**Half-life Elimination:** Biphasic: Initial: 2 hours; Terminal: 8 hours

**Time to Peak:** 1-2 hours

**Metabolism:** Liver

**Excretion:** Feces and urine

**Formulations**

Cream: 2% (15 g, 30 g, 60 g)

Shampoo: 2% (120 mL)

Tablet: 200 mg

**Dosing**

**Adults:**

Oral: 200-400 mg/day as a single daily dose

Shampoo: Apply twice weekly for 4 weeks with at least 3 days between each shampoo.

Topical: Rub gently into the affected area once daily to twice daily.

**Elderly:** Refer to adult dosing.

**Renal Impairment:** Not dialyzable (0% to 5%)

**Hepatic Impairment:** Dose reductions should be considered in patients with severe liver disease.

**Administration**

**Oral:** Do not take with antacids; take at least 2 hours before antacids.

**Topical:** Cream and shampoo: External use only.

**Monitoring Laboratory Tests** Liver function

**Additional Nursing Issues**

**Physical Assessment:** Assess other medications patient may be taking for effectiveness and/or interactions (see Warnings/Precautions, Drug Interactions). Monitor for effectiveness of therapy and possible adverse reactions (see above). Assess knowledge/teach appropriate application/use, possible side effects, and symptoms to report. **Pregnancy risk factor C** - benefits of use should outweigh possible risks. Breast-feeding is not recommended.

**Patient Information/Instruction:**

Oral: May take with food; at least 2 hours before any antacids. Take full course of medication as directed; some infections may require long periods of therapy. Frequent blood tests may be required with long-term therapy. Practice good hygiene measures to reduce incidence of reinfection. If diabetic, test serum glucose regularly. You may experience nausea and vomiting (small frequent meals, frequent mouth care, sucking lozenges, or chewing gum may help); headache (mild analgesic may be necessary); or dizziness (use caution when driving). Report unresolved headache, rash or itching, yellowing of eyes or skin, changes in color of urine or stool, chest pain or palpitations, or sense of fullness or ringing in ears. **Pregnancy/breast-feeding precautions:** Inform prescriber if you are or intend to be pregnant. Breast-feeding is not recommended.

Topical: Wash and dry area before applying medication thinly. Do not cover with occlusive dressing. Report severe skin irritation or if condition does not improve.

Shampoo: Allow 3 days between shampoos. You may experience some hair loss, scalp irritation, itching, change in hair texture, or scalp pustules. Report severe side effects or if infestation persists.

**Additional Information** Cream formulation contains sulfites.

## Ketoprofen (kee toe PROE fen)

**U.S. Brand Names** Actron® [OTC]; Orudis®; Orudis® KT [OTC]; Oruvail®

**Therapeutic Category** Nonsteroidal Anti-Inflammatory Agent (NSAID)

**Pregnancy Risk Factor** B

**Lactation** Excretion in breast milk unknown/use caution

**Use** Acute or long-term treatment of rheumatoid arthritis and osteoarthritis; primary dysmenorrhea; mild to moderate pain

**Mechanism of Action/Effect** Inhibits prostaglandin synthesis by decreasing the activity of the enzyme, cyclo-oxygenase, which results in decreased formation of prostaglandin precursors

**Contraindications** Hypersensitivity to ketoprofen or other NSAIDs/aspirin

**Warnings** Use with caution in patients with congestive heart failure, hypertension, decreased renal or hepatic function, history of GI disease (bleeding or ulcers), or those receiving anticoagulants.

**Drug Interactions**

**Cytochrome P-450 Effect:** CYP2C and 2C9 enzyme inhibitor

**Decreased Effect:** Decreased effect of diuretics.

**Increased Effect/Toxicity:** Increased effect/toxicity with probenecid, lithium, anticoagulants and methotrexate.

**Food Interactions** Ketoprofen peak serum levels may be decreased if taken with food.

**Effects on Lab Values** ↑ chloride (S), sodium (S), bleeding time

**Adverse Reactions**

1% to 10%:

Central nervous system: Headache, dizziness, drowsiness

Dermatologic: Rash

Gastrointestinal: Nausea, abdominal pain, diarrhea, constipation, flatulence, anorexia, vomiting, stomatitis, heartburn

Otic: Tinnitus

<1% (Limited to important or life-threatening symptoms): Hypertension, palpitation, tachycardia, congestive heart failure, exfoliative dermatitis, bullous rash, hypercoagulability, agranulocytosis, hemolysis, purpura, anemia, thrombocytopenia, hepatic dysfunction, renal failure, hematuria, interstitial nephritis, nephrotic syndrome, dyspnea, bronchospasm

**Overdose/Toxicology** Symptoms of overdose include apnea, metabolic acidosis, coma, nystagmus, seizures, leukocytosis, and renal failure. Management of nonsteroidal anti-inflammatory (NSAID) intoxication is supportive and symptomatic. Since many NSAIDs undergo enterohepatic cycling, multiple doses of charcoal may be needed to reduce the potential for delayed toxicities.

**Pharmacodynamics/Kinetics**

**Half-life Elimination:** 1-4 hours

**Time to Peak:** 1-2 hours

**Metabolism:** Liver

**Excretion:** Renal excretion (60% to 75%)

**Formulations**

Capsule (Orudis®): 25 mg, 50 mg, 75 mg

Actron®, Orudis® KT [OTC]: 12.5 mg

Capsule, extended release (Oruvail®): 100 mg, 200 mg

**Dosing**

**Adults:** Oral:

Rheumatoid arthritis or osteoarthritis: 50-75 mg 3-4 times/day up to a maximum of 300 mg/day

Mild to moderate pain: 25-50 mg every 6-8 hours up to a maximum of 300 mg/day

**Elderly:** Oral: Initial: 25-50 mg 3-4 times/day; increase up to 150-300 mg/day (maximum daily dose: 300 mg).

**Administration**

**Oral:** May take with food to reduce GI upset.

**Monitoring Laboratory Tests** CBC, occult blood loss, periodic liver function; renal function (urine output, serum BUN, creatinine)

**Additional Nursing Issues**

**Physical Assessment:** Assess effectiveness and interactions of other medications patient may be taking (see Contraindications and Drug Interactions). Monitor laboratory tests (see above) and therapeutic response (eg, relief of pain and inflammation, increased activity tolerance), and adverse reactions (eg, GI effects, hepatotoxicity, or ototoxicity) at beginning of therapy and periodically throughout therapy (see Warnings/Precautions, Adverse Reactions, and Overdose/Toxicology). Schedule ophthalmic evaluations for patients who develop eye complaints during long-term NSAID therapy. Assess knowledge/teach patient appropriate use, interventions to reduce side effects, and adverse symptoms to report. Note breast-feeding caution.

**Patient Information/Instruction:** Take this medication exactly as directed; do not increase dose without consulting prescriber. Do not crush tablets or break capsules. Take with food or milk to reduce GI distress. Maintain adequate fluid intake (2-3 L/day of fluids unless instructed to restrict fluid intake). Do not use alcohol, aspirin, or aspirin-containing medication, and all other anti-inflammatory medications without consulting prescriber. You may experience drowsiness, dizziness, nervousness, or headache (use caution when driving or engaging in tasks requiring alertness until response to drug is known); anorexia, nausea, vomiting, or heartburn (frequent small meals, frequent mouth care, sucking lozenges, or chewing gum may help); fluid retention

(Continued)

## Ketoprofen *(Continued)*

(weigh yourself weekly and report unusual (3-5 lb/week) weight gain). GI bleeding, ulceration, or perforation can occur with or without pain; discontinue medication and contact prescriber if persistent abdominal pain or cramping, or blood in stool occurs. Report breathlessness, difficulty breathing, or unusual cough; chest pain, rapid heartbeat, palpitations; unusual bruising/bleeding; blood in urine, stool, mouth, or vomitus; swollen extremities; skin rash or itching; acute fatigue; or changes in hearing or ringing in ears. **Breast-feeding precautions:** Consult prescriber if breast-feeding.

**Geriatric Considerations:** Elderly are at high risk for adverse effects from nonsteroidal anti-inflammatory agents. As much as 60% of elderly can develop peptic ulceration and/or hemorrhage asymptomatically. The concomitant use of $H_2$ blockers, omeprazole, and sucralfate is not effective as prophylaxis with the exception of NSAID-induced duodenal ulcers which may be prevented by the use of ranitidine. Misoprostol is the only prophylactic agent proven effective. Also, concomitant disease and drug use contribute to the risk for GI adverse effects. Use lowest effective dose for shortest period possible. Consider renal function decline with age. Use of NSAIDs can compromise existing renal function especially when $Cl_{cr}$ is ≤30 mL/minute. Tinnitus may be a difficult and unreliable indication of toxicity due to age-related hearing loss or eighth cranial nerve damage. CNS adverse effects such as confusion, agitation, and hallucination are generally seen in overdose or high-dose situations, but elderly may demonstrate these adverse effects at lower doses than younger adults.

**Related Information**

Nonsalicylate/Nonsteroidal Anti-inflammatory Comparison *on page 1401*

## Ketorolac Tromethamine (KEE toe role ak troe METH a meen)

**U.S. Brand Names** Acular® Ophthalmic; Toradol® Injection; Toradol® Oral

**Therapeutic Category** Nonsteroidal Anti-Inflammatory Agent (NSAID); Ophthalmic Agent

**Pregnancy Risk Factor** B/D (3rd trimester)

**Lactation** Enters breast milk/contraindicated (AAP rates "compatible")

**Use** Short-term (<5 days) management of pain; first parenteral NSAID for analgesia; 30 mg provides the analgesia comparable to 12 mg of morphine or 100 mg of meperidine

**Mechanism of Action/Effect** Inhibits prostaglandin synthesis by decreasing the activity of the enzyme, cyclo-oxygenase, which results in decreased formation of prostaglandin precursors

**Contraindications** Hypersensitivity to ketorolac, aspirin, or other NSAIDs; patients who have developed nasal polyps, angioedema, or bronchospastic reactions to other NSAIDs; active peptic ulcer disease; recent GI bleeding or perforation; patients with advanced renal disease or risk of renal failure; labor and delivery; prophylaxis before major surgery; suspected or confirmed cerebrovascular bleeding; hemorrhagic diathesis; concurrent ASA or other NSAIDs; epidural or intrathecal administration; concomitant probenecid; pregnancy (3rd trimester)

**Warnings** Use extra caution and reduce dosages in the elderly because it is cleared renally somewhat slower, and the elderly are also more sensitive to the renal effects of NSAIDs. Use with caution in patients with congestive heart failure, hypertension, decreased renal or hepatic function, history of GI disease (bleeding or ulcers), or those receiving anticoagulants.

**Drug Interactions**

**Decreased Effect:** Decreased effect of diuretics.

**Increased Effect/Toxicity:** May increase levels/effects of lithium, methotrexate, and anticoagulants. Salicylates, probenecid, ACE inhibitors may increase risk of renal impairment.

**Food Interactions** Oral: High-fat meals may delay time to peak (by ~1 hour) and decrease peak concentrations.

**Effects on Lab Values** ↑ chloride (S), sodium (S), bleeding time

**Adverse Reactions** The incidence of these reactions vary with dose and patient age, increasing in frequency with patients older than 65 years.

>10%:
- Central nervous system: Headache
- Gastrointestinal: GI perforation, ulcer, abdominal pain, nausea, heartburn, gastrointestinal pain
- Genitourinary: Acute renal failure
- Hematologic: Wound bleeding (with I.M.)

1% to 10%:
- Cardiovascular: Edema, hypertension
- Central nervous system: Drowsiness, dizziness
- Dermatologic: Pruritus, rash
- Gastrointestinal: Diarrhea, constipation, flatulence, gastrointestinal fullness, vomiting, stomatitis
- Local: Pain at injection site
- Miscellaneous: Sweating

<1% (Limited to important or life-threatening symptoms): Stevens-Johnson syndrome, exfoliative dermatitis, hematuria, proteinuria, eosinophilia, anemia, dyspnea, pulmonary edema

**Ophthalmic:**

>10%: Ocular: Stinging or burning upon instillation

1% to 10%:
- Ocular: Ocular irritation, superficial keratitis
- Miscellaneous: Hypersensitivity reaction

**Overdose/Toxicology** Symptoms of overdose include diarrhea, pallor, vomiting, labored breathing, apnea, metabolic acidosis, leukocytosis, and renal failure. Management of nonsteroidal anti-inflammatory (NSAID) intoxication is supportive and symptomatic.

**Pharmacodynamics/Kinetics**

**Protein Binding:** 99%

**Distribution:** Crosses placenta; poor penetration into CSF

**Half-life Elimination:** 2-8 hours; increased 30% to 50% in the elderly

**Time to Peak:** I.M.: 30-60 minutes

**Metabolism:** Liver

**Excretion:** Renal excretion, 61% appearing in the urine as unchanged drug

**Onset:** Analgesic effect: Onset of action: I.M.: Within 10 minutes; Peak effect: Within 75-150 minutes

**Duration:** Analgesic effect: 6-8 hours

**Formulations**

Injection: 15 mg/mL (1 mL); 30 mg/mL (1 mL, 2 mL)

Solution, ophthalmic: 0.5% (5 mL)

Tablet: 10 mg

**Dosing**

**Adults:** Pain relief usually begins within 10 minutes with parenteral forms:

Oral: 10 mg every 4-6 hours as needed for a maximum of 40 mg/day; on day of transition from I.M. to oral: maximum oral dose: 40 mg (or 120 mg combined oral and I.M.); **maximum 5 days administration**

I.M.: Initial: 30-60 mg, then 15-30 mg every 6 hours as needed for up to 5 days maximum; maximum dose is 120 mg/24 hours for up to 5 days total

I.V.: Initial: 30 mg, then 15-30 mg every 6 hours as needed for up to 5 days **maximum**; maximum daily dose: 120 mg for up to 5 days total

Ophthalmic: Instill 1 drop in eye(s) 4 times/day

**Elderly:** Pain relief usually begins within 10 minutes with parenteral forms:

Elderly >65 years: Renal insufficiency or weight <50 kg:

I.M.: 30 mg, then 15 mg every 6 hours

I.V.: 15 mg every 6 hours as needed for up to 5 days total; maximum daily dose: 60 mg

**Renal Impairment:** Use recommendations under Elderly dosing; use extreme caution.

**Administration**

**Oral:** May take with food to reduce GI upset.

**I.M.:** Administer slowly and deeply into the muscle. Analgesia begins in 30 minutes and maximum effect within 2 hours.

**I.V.:** Administer I.V. bolus over a minimum of 15 seconds; onset within 30 minutes; peak analgesia within 2 hours.

**Stability**

**Storage:** Ketorolac tromethamine injection should be stored at controlled room temperature and protected from light. Injection is clear and has a slight yellow color. Precipitation may occur at relatively low pH values.

**Compatibility:** Compatible with NS, $D_5W$, $D_5NS$, and lactated Ringer's. Incompatible with meperidine, morphine, promethazine, and hydroxyzine.

**Monitoring Laboratory Tests** Renal function (serum creatinine, BUN, urine output), CBC, liver function, platelets

**Additional Nursing Issues**

**Physical Assessment: Assess patient for allergic reaction to salicylates or other NSAIDs** (see Contraindications). Assess other medications patient may be taking for additive or adverse interactions (see Warnings/Precautions and Drug Interactions). I.V./I.M.: See Administration and Dosing. Monitor vital signs on a regular basis during infusion or following injection. Monitor for therapeutic effectiveness. Monitor for signs of adverse reactions or overdose (especially - adverse gastrointestinal response - see Adverse Reactions) at beginning of therapy and periodically during therapy. Assess knowledge/teach patient appropriate use. Teach patient to monitor for adverse reactions, adverse reactions to report, and appropriate interventions to reduce side effects. **Pregnancy risk factor B/D** - see Pregnancy Risk Factor - benefits of use should outweigh possible risks. Breast-feeding is contraindicated.

**Patient Information/Instruction:** If self-administered, use exactly as directed (do not increase dose or frequency); adverse reactions can occur with overuse. Do not take longer than 5 days without consulting medical advisor. Take with food or milk. While using this medication, do not use alcohol, other prescription or OTC medications including aspirin, aspirin-containing medications, or other NSAIDs without consulting prescriber. Maintain adequate hydration (2-3 L/day of fluids unless instructed to restrict fluid intake). You may experience nausea, vomiting, gastric discomfort (frequent mouth care, small frequent meals, chewing gum, or sucking lozenges may help). GI bleeding, ulceration, or perforation can occur with or without pain. Stop taking medication and report ringing in ears; persistent cramping or pain in stomach; unresolved nausea or vomiting; difficulty breathing or shortness of breath; unusual bruising or bleeding (mouth, urine, stool); skin rash; unusual swelling of extremities; chest pain; or palpitations. **Pregnancy/breast-feeding precautions:** Inform prescriber if you are or intend to be pregnant. Do not breast-feed.

Ophthalmic: Instill drops as often as recommended. Wash hands before instilling. Sit or lie down to instill. Open eye, look at ceiling, and instill prescribed amount of solution. Close eye and roll eye in all directions, and apply gentle pressure to inner corner of

(Continued)

## Ketorolac Tromethamine *(Continued)*

eye for 1-2 minutes after instillation. Do not let tip of applicator touch eye or contaminate tip of applicator. Temporary stinging or blurred vision may occur. Report persistent pain, burning, double vision, swelling, itching, worsening of condition. Inform prescriber if you are or intend to be pregnant. Do not breast-feed.

**Geriatric Considerations:** Ketorolac is eliminated more slowly in the elderly. It is recommended to use lower doses in the elderly. The elderly are at high risk for adverse effects from nonsteroidal anti-inflammatory agents. As much as 60% of elderly can develop peptic ulceration and/or hemorrhage asymptomatically. The concomitant use of $H_2$ blockers, omeprazole, and sucralfate is not effective as prophylaxis with the exception of NSAID-induced duodenal ulcers which may be prevented by the use of ranitidine. Misoprostol is the only prophylactic agent proven effective. Also, concomitant disease and drug use contribute to the risk for GI adverse effects. Use lowest effective dose for shortest period possible. Consider renal function decline with age. Use of NSAIDs can compromise existing renal function especially when $Cl_{cr}$ is ≤30 mL/minute. Tinnitus may be a difficult and unreliable indication of toxicity due to age-related hearing loss or eighth cranial nerve damage. CNS adverse effects such as confusion, agitation, and hallucination are generally seen in overdose or high-dose situations, but elderly may demonstrate these adverse effects at lower doses than younger adults.

**Related Information**

Nonsalicylate/Nonsteroidal Anti-inflammatory Comparison *on page 1401*
Ophthalmic Agents *on page 1282*


- **Kevadon®** *see* Thalidomide *on page 1113*
- **Key-Pred® Injection** *see* Prednisolone *on page 960*
- **Key-Pred-SP® Injection** *see* Prednisolone *on page 960*
- **K-G® Elixir** *see* Potassium Supplements *on page 952*
- **K-Gen®** *see* Potassium Supplements *on page 952*
- **KI** *see* Potassium Iodide *on page 951*
- **Kinesed®** *see* Hyoscyamine, Atropine, Scopolamine, and Phenobarbital *on page 591*
- **Kinestase®** *see* Cisapride *on page 272*
- **Kinevac®** *see page 1248*
- **Klaricid** *see* Clarithromycin *on page 279*
- **Klean-Prep®** *see* Polyethylene Glycol-Electrolyte Solution *on page 945*
- **K-Lease®** *see* Potassium Supplements *on page 952*
- **Klerist-D® Tablet** *see page 1294*
- **Klonopin™** *see* Clonazepam *on page 288*
- **K-Lor™** *see* Potassium Supplements *on page 952*
- **Klor-Con®** *see* Potassium Supplements *on page 952*
- **Klor-Con/25®** *see* Potassium Supplements *on page 952*
- **Kloromin®** *see page 1294*
- **Klorvess®** *see* Potassium Supplements *on page 952*
- **Klorvess® Effervescent** *see* Potassium Bicarbonate and Potassium Chloride, Effervescent *on page 949*
- **Klorvess Klyte/Cl** *see* Potassium Supplements *on page 952*
- **Klotrix®** *see* Potassium Supplements *on page 952*
- **Klyndaken** *see* Clindamycin *on page 282*
- **K-Lyte®** *see* Potassium Citrate *on page 949*
- **K-lyte®** *see* Potassium Supplements *on page 952*
- **K-Lyte/Cl®** *see* Potassium Supplements *on page 952*
- **K-Lyte/Cl® Tablet** *see* Potassium Bicarbonate and Potassium Chloride, Effervescent *on page 949*
- **K-lyte DS** *see* Potassium Supplements *on page 952*
- **K-Norm®** *see* Potassium Supplements *on page 952*
- **Koāte®-HP** *see* Antihemophilic Factor (Human) *on page 99*
- **Koāte®-HS** *see* Antihemophilic Factor (Human) *on page 99*
- **Kolephrin® GG/DM [OTC]** *see* Guaifenesin and Dextromethorphan *on page 549*
- **Kolyum®** *see* Potassium Supplements *on page 952*
- **Konakion® Injection** *see* Phytonadione *on page 929*
- **Kondon's Nasal® [OTC]** *see* Ephedrine *on page 422*
- **Kondremul®** *see page 1294*
- **Konsyl® [OTC]** *see* Psyllium *on page 993*
- **Konsyl-D® [OTC]** *see* Psyllium *on page 993*
- **Koromex®** *see page 1294*
- **K-Phos® M.F.** *see* Phosphate Supplements *on page 926*
- **K-Phos® Neutral** *see* Phosphate Supplements *on page 926*
- **K-Phos® No. 2** *see* Phosphate Supplements *on page 926*
- **K-Phos® Original** *see* Phosphate Supplements *on page 926*
- **K-Profen®** *see* Ketoprofen *on page 645*
- **K-Tab®** *see* Potassium Supplements *on page 952*
- **Ku-Zyme® HP** *see* Pancrelipase *on page 882*
- **K-Vescent®** *see* Potassium Supplements *on page 952*
- **Kwelcof®** *see* Hydrocodone and Guaifenesin *on page 571*

- ♦ **Kwellada™** *see* Lindane *on page 678*
- ♦ **Kytril™** *see* Granisetron *on page 544*
- ♦ ***L*-3-Hydroxytyrosine** *see* Levodopa *on page 666*
- ♦ **LA-12®** *see* Hydroxocobalamin *on page 583*



## Labetalol (la BET a lole)

**U.S. Brand Names** Normodyne®; Trandate®

**Synonyms** Ibidomide Hydrochloride

**Therapeutic Category** Alpha-/Beta- Blocker; Beta Blocker, Nonselective

**Pregnancy Risk Factor** C/D (2nd and 3rd trimesters)

**Lactation** Enters breast milk/use caution (AAP rates "compatible")

**Use** Treatment of mild to severe hypertension; I.V. for hypertensive emergencies

**Mechanism of Action/Effect** Blocks alpha-, $beta_1$-, and $beta_2$-adrenergic receptor sites; elevated renins are reduced

**Contraindications** Cardiogenic shock; uncompensated congestive heart failure; bradycardia; pulmonary edema; heart block; pregnancy (2nd and 3rd trimesters)

**Warnings** Paradoxical increase in blood pressure has been reported with treatment of pheochromocytoma or clonidine withdrawal syndrome. Use with caution in patients with hyper-reactive airway disease, congestive heart failure during surgery, diabetes mellitus, or hepatic dysfunction. Orthostatic hypotension may occur with I.V. administration. Patient should remain supine during and for up to 3 hours after I.V. administration. Use with caution in impaired hepatic function (discontinue if signs of liver dysfunction occur). Beta-blockers may impair glucose tolerance, potentiate hypoglycemia, and/or mask the signs or symptoms of hypoglycemia in a diabetic patient. A lower hemodynamic response rate and higher incidence of toxicity may be observed with administration to elderly patients. Use with caution when reducing severely elevated blood pressure (angina and other ischemic events may occur). Pregnancy factor C/D (2nd and 3rd trimesters).

**Drug Interactions**

**Cytochrome P-450 Effect:** CYP2D6 enzyme substrate; CYP2D6 enzyme inhibitor

**Decreased Effect:** Decreased effect of beta-blockers with aluminum salts, barbiturates, calcium salts, cholestyramine, colestipol, NSAIDs, penicillins (ampicillin), rifampin, salicylates, and sulfinpyrazone due to decreased bioavailability and plasma levels. Beta-blockers may decrease the effect of sulfonylureas.

**Increased Effect/Toxicity:** Cimetidine may potentiate labetalol action. Additive hypotensive effects with other hypotensive drugs. Halothane may cause synergistic hypotension. Beta-blockers may affect the action or levels of ethanol, disopyramide, nondepolarizing muscle relaxants, and theophylline although the effects are difficult to predict.

**Food Interactions** Labetalol serum concentrations may be increased if taken with food.

**Effects on Lab Values** False-positive urine catecholamines, VMA if measured by fluorometric or photometric methods; use HPLC or specific catecholamine radioenzymatic technique

**Adverse Reactions**

>10%:

Central nervous system: Drowsiness, insomnia

Endocrine & metabolic: Decreased sexual ability

1% to 10%:

Cardiovascular: Bradycardia, palpitations, edema, congestive heart failure, reduced peripheral circulation

Central nervous system: Mental depression, numbness and/or tingling of fingers, toes, or skin (especially the scalp)

Gastrointestinal: Diarrhea or constipation, nausea, vomiting, stomach discomfort

Respiratory: Bronchospasm

Miscellaneous: Cold extremities

<1% (Limited to important or life-threatening symptoms): Chest pain, arrhythmias, orthostatic hypotension, nervousness, headache, depression, hallucinations, confusion (especially in the elderly), thrombocytopenia, leukopenia, hepatic necrosis, shortness of breath

**Overdose/Toxicology** Symptoms of intoxication include cardiac disturbances, CNS toxicity, bronchospasm, hypoglycemia, and hyperkalemia. The most common cardiac symptoms include hypotension and bradycardia. Atrioventricular block, intraventricular conduction disturbances, cardiogenic shock, and asystole may occur with severe overdose, especially with membrane-depressant drugs (eg, propranolol). CNS effects include convulsions, coma, and respiratory arrest and are commonly seen with propranolol and other membrane-depressant and lipid-soluble drugs. Treatment is symptomatic. Glucagon may be administered to improve cardiac function.

**Pharmacodynamics/Kinetics**

**Protein Binding:** 50%

**Distribution:** Crosses the placenta; moderately lipid soluble, therefore, can enter CNS

**Half-life Elimination:** Normal renal function: 6-8 hours

**Metabolism:** Liver

**Excretion:** Urine

**Onset:**

Oral: 20 minutes to 2 hours

I.V.: 2-5 minutes

Peak effect: Oral: 1-4 hours; I.V.: 5-15 minutes

(Continued)

## Labetalol *(Continued)*

**Duration:** Oral: 8-24 hours (dose-dependent); I.V.: 2-4 hours

**Formulations**

Labetalol hydrochloride:

Injection: 5 mg/mL (20 mL, 40 mL, 60 mL)

Tablet: 100 mg, 200 mg, 300 mg

**Dosing**

**Adults:**

Oral: Initial: 100 mg twice daily, may increase as needed every 2-3 days by 100 mg until desired response is obtained; usual dose: 200-400 mg twice daily; not to exceed 2.4 g/day

I.V.: 20 mg or 1-2 mg/kg whichever is lower, IVP over 2 minutes, may give 40-80 mg at 10-minute intervals, up to 300 mg total dose

I.V. infusion: Initial: 2 mg/minute; titrate to response up to 300 mg total dose. Administration requires the use of an infusion pump.

**I.V. infusion (500 mg/250 mL $D_5$)** rates:

1 mg/minute: 30 mL/hour
2 mg/minute: 60 mL/hour
3 mg/minute: 90 mL/hour
4 mg/minute: 120 mL/hour
5 mg/minute: 150 mL/hour
6 mg/minute: 180 mL/hour

**Elderly:** Oral: Initial: 100 mg 1-2 times/day increasing as needed

**Renal Impairment:** Not removed by hemo- or peritoneal dialysis; supplemental dose is not necessary.

**Hepatic Impairment:** Dosage reduction may be necessary.

**Administration**

**I.V.:** Bolus administered over 2 minutes.

**I.V. Detail:** Loading infusions (2 mg/minute) require close monitoring of heart rate and blood pressure and are terminated after response or cumulative dose of 300 mg. Continuous infusions of 2-6 mg/hour have been used in some settings and should not be confused with loading infusions.

**Stability**

**Storage:** Labetalol should be stored at room temperature or under refrigeration and should be protected from light and freezing. The solution is clear to slightly yellow.

**Reconstitution:** Stability of parenteral admixture at room temperature (25°C) and refrigeration temperature (4°C) is 3 days.

**Standard diluent:** 500 mg/250 mL $D_5W$

Minimum volume: 250 mL $D_5W$

**Compatibility:** Incompatible with sodium bicarbonate, most stable at pH of 2-4. Incompatible with alkaline solutions.

**Additional Nursing Issues**

**Physical Assessment:** Assess effectiveness and interactions of other medications (see Drug Interactions). See Contraindications and Warnings/Precautions for use cautions. Continuous monitoring is recommended for I.V. therapy. Oral therapy: Monitor for effectiveness of therapy (blood pressure supine and standing) and adverse reactions (see Adverse Reactions and Overdose/Toxicology) at beginning of therapy and on a regular basis with long-term therapy. Diabetics: Monitor serum glucose levels closely. Assess knowledge/teach patient appropriate use, possible side effects/interventions, and adverse symptoms to report. When discontinuing, monitor blood pressure and taper dose and frequency. **Pregnancy risk factor C/D** - ascertain pregnancy status and appropriateness of use; benefits should outweigh possible risks. Note breast-feeding caution.

**Patient Information/Instruction:** For I.V. use in emergency situations - patient information is included in general instruction. Oral: Take as directed, with meals. Do not skip dose or discontinue without consulting prescriber. Follow recommended diet and exercise program. Do not use alcohol or OTC medications which may affect blood pressure (eg, cough or cold remedies, diet pills, stay-awake medications) without consulting prescriber. If diabetic, monitor serum glucose closely and notify prescriber of changes; this medication can alter hypoglycemic requirements. You may experience drowsiness, dizziness, or impaired judgment (use caution when driving or engaging in tasks that require alertness until response to drug is known); postural hypotension (use caution when rising from sitting or lying position or when climbing stairs); dry mouth, nausea, or loss of appetite (frequent mouth care or sucking lozenges may help); or sexual dysfunction (reversible, may resolve with continued use). Report altered CNS status (eg, fatigue, depression, numbness or tingling of fingers, toes, or skin); palpitations or slowed heartbeat; difficulty breathing; edema or cold extremities; or other persistent side effects. **Pregnancy/breast-feeding precautions:** Inform prescriber if you are or intend to be pregnant. Consult prescriber if breast-feeding.

**Geriatric Considerations:** Due to alterations in the beta-adrenergic autonomic nervous system, beta-adrenergic blockade may result in less hemodynamic response than seen in younger adults.

**Related Information**

Beta-Blockers Comparison *on page 1376*

◆ **Laboratory Reference Values for Adults** *see page 1352*
◆ **Laboratory Reference Values for Children** *see page 1356*
◆ **Lac-Hydrin® Lotion** *see page 1294*
◆ **Lacril® Ophthalmic Solution** *see page 1294*

- **Lactaid®** *see page 1294*
- **Lactase Enzyme** *see page 1294*
- **Lacteol® Fort** *see Lactobacillus acidophilus* and *Lactobacillus bulgaricus on this page*
- **Lactic Acid and Sodium-PCA** *see page 1294*
- **Lactic Acid With Ammonium Hydroxide** *see page 1294*
- **LactiCare-HC®** *see* Hydrocortisone *on page 578*
- **LactiCare-HC®** *see* Topical Corticosteroids *on page 1152*
- **LactiCare® Lotion** *see page 1294*
- **Lactinex® [OTC]** *see Lactobacillus acidophilus* and *Lactobacillus bulgaricus on this page*

## *Lactobacillus acidophilus* and *Lactobacillus bulgaricus*

(lak toe ba SIL us as i DOF fil us & lak toe ba SIL us bul GAR i cus)

**U.S. Brand Names** Bacid® [OTC]; Lactinex® [OTC]; More-Dophilus® [OTC]

**Therapeutic Category** Antidiarrheal

**Use** Treatment of uncomplicated diarrhea particularly that caused by antibiotic therapy; re-establish normal physiologic and bacterial flora of the intestinal tract

**Mechanism of Action/Effect** Creates an environment unfavorable to potentially pathogenic fungi or bacteria through the production of lactic acid, and favors establishment of an aciduric flora, thereby suppressing the growth of pathogenic microorganisms; helps re-establish normal intestinal flora

**Contraindications** Allergy to milk or lactose

**Warnings** Discontinue if high fever is present. Do not use in children <3 years of age.

**Adverse Reactions** 1% to 10%: Gastrointestinal: Intestinal flatus

**Pharmacodynamics/Kinetics**

**Distribution:** Locally, primarily in the colon

**Excretion:** Feces

**Formulations**

Capsule: 50s, 100s
Granules: 1 g/packet (12 packets/box)
Powder: 12 oz
Tablet, chewable: 50s

**Dosing**

**Adults:** Oral:

Capsules: 2 capsules 2-4 times/day
Granules: 1 packet added to or taken with cereal, food, milk, fruit juice, or water, 3-4 times/day
Powder: 1 teaspoonful daily with liquid
Tablet, chewable: 4 tablets 3-4 times/day; may follow each dose with a small amount of milk, fruit juice, or water

**Elderly:** Refer to adult dosing.

**Stability**

**Storage:** Store in refrigerator.

**Additional Nursing Issues**

**Patient Information/Instruction:** Granules may be added to or taken with cereal, food, milk, fruit juice, or water.

- **Lactoflavin** *see* Riboflavin *on page 1018*
- **Lactrase®** *see page 1294*

## Lactulose (LAK tyoo lose)

**U.S. Brand Names** Cephulac®; Cholac®; Chronulac®; Constilac®; Constulose®; Duphalac®; Enulose®; Evalose®; Heptalac®; Lactulose PSE®

**Therapeutic Category** Ammonium Detoxicant; Laxative, Miscellaneous

**Pregnancy Risk Factor** B

**Lactation** Excretion in breast milk unknown

**Use** Adjunct in the prevention and treatment of portal-systemic encephalopathy (PSE); treatment of chronic constipation

**Mechanism of Action/Effect** The bacterial degradation of lactulose resulting in an acidic pH inhibits the diffusion of $NH_3$ into the blood by causing the conversion of $NH_3$ to $NH_4+$; also enhances the diffusion of $NH_3$ from the blood into the gut where conversion to $NH_4+$ occurs; produces an osmotic effect in the colon with resultant distention promoting peristalsis

**Contraindications** Hypersensitivity to lactulose or any component; patients with galactosemia and require a low galactose diet

**Warnings** Use with caution in patients with diabetes mellitus; monitor periodically for electrolyte imbalance when lactulose is used >6 months or in patients predisposed to electrolyte abnormalities (eg, elderly); patients receiving lactulose and an oral anti-infective agent should be monitored for possible inadequate response to lactulose

**Drug Interactions**

**Decreased Effect:** Oral neomycin, laxatives, antacids

**Adverse Reactions**

>10%: Gastrointestinal: Flatulence, diarrhea (excessive dose)
1% to 10%: Gastrointestinal: Abdominal discomfort, nausea, vomiting

**Overdose/Toxicology** Symptoms of overdose include diarrhea, abdominal pain, hypochloremic alkalosis, dehydration, hypotension, and hypokalemia. Treatment includes supportive care.

(Continued)

## Lactulose *(Continued)*

**Pharmacodynamics/Kinetics**

**Metabolism:** By colonic flora to lactic acid and acetic acid, requires colonic flora for primary drug activation

**Excretion:** Feces and urine

**Formulations** Syrup: 10 g/15 mL (15 mL, 30 mL, 237 mL, 473 mL, 946 mL, 1890 mL)

**Dosing**

**Adults:** Diarrhea may indicate overdosage and responds to dose reduction.

Acute portal-systemic encephalopathy (PSE):

Oral: 20-30 g (30-45 mL) every 1-2 hours to induce rapid laxation; adjust dosage daily to produce 2-3 soft stools; doses of 30-45 mL may be given hourly to cause rapid laxation, then reduce to recommended dose; usual daily dose: 60-100 g (90-150 mL) daily

Rectal administration: 200 g (300 mL) diluted with 700 mL of $H_20$ or NS; administer rectally via rectal balloon catheter and retain 30-60 minutes every 4-6 hours.

Constipation: Oral: 10-20 g/day (15-30 mL/day) increased to 60 mL/day if necessary

**Elderly:** Refer to adult dosing.

**Administration**

**Oral:** Dilute lactulose in water, usually 60-120 mL, prior to administering through a gastric or feeding tube.

**Stability**

**Storage:** Keep solution at room temperature to reduce viscosity. Discard solution if cloudy or very dark.

**Monitoring Laboratory Tests** Serum potassium, serum ammonia

**Additional Nursing Issues**

**Physical Assessment:** See Warnings/Precautions for use cautions. Assess for history of allergies (see Contraindications). Monitor effectiveness of therapy and adverse response (see Adverse Reactions and Overdose/Toxicology). Assess knowledge/teach patient appropriate use, possible side effects/interventions, and adverse symptoms to report. Note breast-feeding caution.

**Patient Information/Instruction:** Not for long-term use. Take as directed, alone, or diluted with water, juice or milk, or take with food. Laxative results may not occur for 24-48 hours; do not take more often than recommended or for a longer time than recommended. Do not use any other laxatives while taking lactulose. Increased fiber, fluids, and exercise may help reduce constipation. Do not use if experiencing abdominal pain, nausea, or vomiting. Diarrhea may indicate overdose. May cause flatulence, belching, or abdominal cramping. Report persistent or severe diarrhea or abdominal cramping. **Breast-feeding precautions:** Consult prescriber if breast-feeding.

**Geriatric Considerations:** Elderly are more likely to show CNS signs of dehydration and electrolyte loss than younger adults. Therefore, monitor closely for fluid and electrolyte loss with chronic use. Sorbitol is equally effective as a laxative and less expensive. However, sorbitol **cannot be substituted** in the treatment of hepatic encephalopathy.

**Related Information**

Laxatives: Classification and Properties Comparison *on page 1392*

- **Lactulose PSE®** *see* Lactulose *on previous page*
- **Ladogal** *see* Danazol *on page 332*
- **L-AmB** *see* Amphotericin B (Liposomal) *on page 88*
- **Lamictal®** *see* Lamotrigine *on page 654*
- **Lamisil®** *see page 1247*
- **Lamisil® Oral** *see* Terbinafine, Oral *on page 1104*

## Lamivudine (la MI vyoo deen)

**U.S. Brand Names** Epivir®, Epivir® HBV

**Synonyms** 3TC

**Therapeutic Category** Antiretroviral Agent, Reverse Transcriptase Inhibitor (Non-Nucleoside)

**Pregnancy Risk Factor** C

**Lactation** Enters breast milk/contraindicated

**Use** In combination with zidovudine for treatment of HIV infection when therapy is warranted based on clinical and/or immunological evidence of disease progression

Epivir®-HBV™: Treatment of chronic hepatitis B associated with evidence of viral replication and active liver inflammation

**Mechanism of Action/Effect** *In vitro*, lamivudine is phosphorylated to its active 5'-triphosphate metabolite (L-TP), which inhibits HIV reverse transcription via viral DNA chain termination; L-TP also inhibits the RNA- and DNA-dependent DNA polymerase activities of reverse transcriptase. The monophosphate form is incorporated into viral DNA by hepatitis B polymerase, resulting in DNA chain termination.

**Contraindications** Hypersensitivity to lamivudine or any component

**Warnings** A decreased dosage is recommended in patients with renal dysfunction since AUC, $C_{max}$, and half-life are increased with diminishing renal function. Lactic acidosis and severe hepatomegaly with steatosis (including fatalities) have been reported. Discontinue therapy in any patient with pronounced hepatotoxicity or lactic acidosis. Pregnancy factor C.

**Drug Interactions**

**Increased Effect/Toxicity:** Zidovudine concentrations increase significantly (~39%) with lamivudine coadministration. Trimethoprim/sulfamethoxazole increases lamivudine's AUC and decreases its renal clearance by 44% and 29%, respectively. Although the AUC was not significantly affected, absorption of lamivudine was slowed and $C_{max}$ was 40% lower when administered to patients who ate a meal versus the fasted state.

**Adverse Reactions**

>10%:

Gastrointestinal: Nausea, diarrhea, vomiting, pancreatitis

Neuromuscular & skeletal: Peripheral neuropathy, paresthesia

1% to 10%:

Central nervous system: Dizziness, depression, fever, chills, insomnia, headache, fatigue

Gastrointestinal: Anorexia, abdominal pain, heartburn, elevated amylase

Hematologic: Neutropenia

Hepatic: Elevated AST, ALT

Neuromuscular & skeletal: Myalgia, arthralgia

Respiratory: Nasal signs and symptoms, cough

<1% (Limited to important or life-threatening symptoms): Lactic acidosis, hepatomegaly, steatosis, hyperglycemia, anaphylaxis, weakness, alopecia, rash, urticaria, pruritus, thrombocytopenia, anemia, hyperbilirubinemia, rhabdomyolysis, peripheral neuropathy

**Overdose/Toxicology** Limited information is available, although there have been no clinical signs or symptoms noted, and hematologic tests remained normal in overdose. No antidote is available. Unknown dialyzability.

**Pharmacodynamics/Kinetics**

**Protein Binding:** Plasma: <36%

**Half-life Elimination:** 5-7 hours

**Metabolism:** 5.6% metabolized to trans-sulfoxide metabolite

**Excretion:** Urine

**Formulations**

Epivir®

Solution, oral: 10 mg/mL (240 mL)

Tablets: 150 mg

Epivir®-HBV™

Solution, oral: 5 mg/mL (240 mL)

Tablets: 100 mg

**Dosing**

**Adults:** Oral:

HIV:

<50 kg: 2 mg/kg twice daily with zidovudine

>50 kg: 150 mg twice daily with zidovudine

Hepatitis B: 100 mg once daily

**Elderly:** Refer to adult dosing.

**Renal Impairment:** Oral:

For HIV patients >16 years:

$Cl_{cr}$ <50 mL/minute: Administer 150 mg twice daily.

$Cl_{cr}$ 30-49 mL/minute: Administer 150 mg once daily.

$Cl_{cr}$ 15-29 mL/minute: Administer 150 mg first dose, then 100 mg once daily.

$Cl_{cr}$ 5-14 mL/minute: Administer 150 mg first dose, then 50 mg once daily.

$Cl_{cr}$ <5 mL/minute: Administer 50 mg first dose, then 25 mg once daily.

Dialysis: No data available.

For treatment of Hepatitis B patients >16 years:

$Cl_{cr}$ <50 mL/minute: Administer 100 mg twice daily.

$Cl_{cr}$ 30-49 mL/minute: Administer 100 mg first dose, then 50 mg once daily.

$Cl_{cr}$ 15-29 mL/minute: Administer 100 mg first dose, then 25 mg once daily.

$Cl_{cr}$ 5-14 mL/minute: Administer 35 mg first dose, then 15 mg once daily.

$Cl_{cr}$ <5 mL/minute: Administer 35 mg first dose, then 25 mg once daily.

Dialysis: No additional dosing is required after routine hemodialysis

**Administration**

**Oral:** Administer on an empty stomach, if possible. Adjust dosage in renal failure.

**Stability**

**Storage:** Store solution at 2°C to 25°C tightly closed.

**Monitoring Laboratory Tests** Amylase, bilirubin, liver enzymes, CBC

**Additional Nursing Issues**

**Physical Assessment:** Monitor laboratory tests on a regular basis. Monitor for signs of opportunistic infection (eg, fever, sore throat, easy bruising or bleeding, mouth sores, unhealed sores). **Pregnancy risk factor C** - benefits of use should outweigh possible risks. Breast-feeding is contraindicated.

**Patient Information/Instruction:** This is not a cure for AIDS or AIDS complex, nor will it reduce the risk of transmission to others. Long-term effects are unknown. You will need frequent blood tests to adjust dosage for maximum therapeutic effect. Take as directed for full course of therapy; do not discontinue (even if feeling better). You may experience loss of appetite; change in taste (sucking on lozenges, chewing gum, or small frequent meals may help); dizziness or numbness (use caution when driving or engaging in tasks that require alertness until response to drug is known); headache, fever, or muscle pain (an analgesic may be recommended). Report persistent lethargy, acute headache, severe nausea or vomiting, difficulty breathing, loss of sensation, or rash. **Pregnancy/breast-feeding precautions:** Inform prescriber if you are or intend to be pregnant. Do not breast-feed.

**Breast-feeding Issues:** The CDC recommends **not** to breast-feed if diagnosed with HIV to avoid postnatal transmission of the virus.

(Continued)

## Lamivudine *(Continued)*

**Pregnancy Issues:** Use only if the potential benefits outweigh the risks although there is no indication of embryolethality in rats at doses up to 130 times the usual adult dose.

**Additional Information** There are, as yet, no results from clinical trials evaluating the effect of lamivudine, in combination with zidovudine, on progression of HIV infection (eg, incidence of opportunistic infections or survival). Patients may continue to develop infections and other complications of HIV infection and should remain under close physician observation.

**Related Information**

Antiretroviral Agents Comparison *on page 1373*

## Lamotrigine (la MOE tri jeen)

**U.S. Brand Names** Lamictal®

**Synonyms** LTG

**Therapeutic Category** Anticonvulsant, Miscellaneous

**Pregnancy Risk Factor** C

**Lactation** Enters breast milk/not recommended

**Use**

Adjunctive therapy: Partial/secondary generalized seizures in adults; generalized seizures associated with Lennox-Gastaut syndrome (pediatric and adult patients); childhood epilepsy (not approved for use in children <2 years of age)

Monotherapy: Conversion to monotherapy only in adults with partial seizures who are receiving treatment with a single enzyme-inducing antiepileptic drug

Unlabeled use: Bipolar disorder

**Mechanism of Action/Effect** A triazine derivative which inhibits release of glutamate (an excitatory amino acid) and inhibits voltage-sensitive sodium channels, which stabilizes neuronal membranes

**Contraindications** Hypersensitivity to lamotrigine or any component

**Warnings** Use caution with impaired renal, hepatic, or cardiac function. Avoid abrupt cessation; taper over at least 2 weeks if possible. Pregnancy factor C.

**Drug Interactions**

**Cytochrome P-450 Effect:** Effects on CYP not characterized, may act as inducer.

**Decreased Effect:** Acetaminophen may increase renal clearance of lamotrigine with decreased or shortened effectiveness. Carbamazepine, phenobarbital, and phenytoin may increase metabolic clearance of lamotrigine resulting in a decreased or shortened term of effectiveness.

**Increased Effect/Toxicity:** Valproic acid increases half-life of lamotrigine with potential for toxicity.

**Adverse Reactions**

>10%:

Central nervous system: Ataxia, dizziness, drowsiness, headache
Dermatologic: Rash, Stevens-Johnson syndrome, angioedema
Gastrointestinal: Nausea, vomiting
Ocular: Blurred vision, diplopia

1% to 10%:

Central nervous system: Confusion, depression, mood changes, tremors, insomnia
Gastrointestinal: Heartburn
Ocular: Nystagmus
Renal: Hematuria

<1% (Limited to important or life-threatening symptoms): Toxic epidermal necrolysis, petechia, anemia, eosinophilia, leukopenia, thrombocytopenia

**Overdose/Toxicology** Symptoms of overdose include QRS prolongation, AV block, dizziness, drowsiness, sedation, and ataxia. Enhancement of elimination: Multiple dosing of activated charcoal may be useful.

**Pharmacodynamics/Kinetics**

**Protein Binding:** 55%

**Half-life Elimination:** 24 hours; increases to 59 hours with concomitant valproic acid therapy; decreases with concomitant phenytoin or carbamazepine therapy to 15 hours

**Time to Peak:** Within 1-4 hours

**Metabolism:** Hepatic and renal

**Excretion:** Urine

**Formulations**

Tablet: 25 mg, 100 mg, 150 mg, 200 mg
Tablet, chewable dispersible: 5 mg, 25 mg

**Dosing**

**Adults:** Oral: Initial: 50-100 mg/day then titrate to daily maintenance dose of 100-400 mg/day in 1-2 divided daily doses.

With concomitant valproic acid therapy: Start initial dose at 25 mg/day then titrate to maintenance dose of 50-200 mg/day in 1-2 divided daily doses.

**Elderly:** Initial:

When administered with other antiepileptic agents **except** valproic acid: 50 mg once daily for 2 weeks; then 50 mg twice daily for 2 weeks; then increase to maintenance dose of 300-500 mg/day in 2 divided doses by 100 mg/day/week.

When administered with valproic acid: 25 mg every other day for 2 weeks; 25 mg daily for 2 weeks; then increase to a maintenance dose of 100-150 mg/day in 2 divided doses per day by increasing daily dose by 25-50 mg/day every 1-2 weeks.

**Monitoring Laboratory Tests** Serum levels of concurrent anticonvulsants, LFTs, renal function

**Additional Nursing Issues**

**Physical Assessment:** Assess effectiveness and interactions of other medications patient may be taking (see Drug Interactions). Monitor for therapeutic response (seizure activity, force, type, duration), laboratory values, and adverse reactions (see Adverse Reactions) at beginning of therapy and periodically with long-term use. Taper dosage slowly when discontinuing. Observe and teach seizure/safety precautions. Assess knowledge/teach patient appropriate use, interventions to reduce side effects, and adverse symptoms to report. **Pregnancy risk factor C** - benefits of use should outweigh possible risks. Breast-feeding is not recommended.

**Patient Information/Instruction:** Take exactly as directed (do not increase dose or frequency or discontinue without consulting prescriber). While using this medication, do not use alcohol and other prescription or OTC medications (especially pain medications, sedatives, antihistamines, or hypnotics) without consulting prescriber. Maintain adequate hydration (2-3 L/day of fluids unless instructed to restrict fluid intake). You may experience drowsiness, dizziness, or blurred vision (use caution when driving or engaging in tasks requiring alertness until response to drug is known); nausea, vomiting, loss of appetite, heartburn, or dry mouth (small frequent meals, frequent mouth care, chewing gum, or sucking lozenges may help). Wear identification of epileptic status and medications. Report CNS changes, mentation changes, or changes in cognition; persistent GI symptoms (cramping, constipation, vomiting, anorexia); skin rash; swelling of face, lips, or tongue; easy bruising or bleeding (mouth, urine, stool); vision changes; worsening of seizure activity, or loss of seizure control. **Pregnancy/breast-feeding precautions:** Inform prescriber if you are or intend to be pregnant. Breast-feeding is not recommended.

**Geriatric Considerations:** Use with caution in the elderly with significant renal impairment.

**Additional Information** Low water solubility

- **Lampicin** *see* Ampicillin *on page 90*
- **Lamprene®** *see* Clofazimine *on page 284*
- **Lanacane® [OTC]** *see* Benzocaine *on page 141*
- **Lanacort® [OTC]** *see* Hydrocortisone *on page 578*
- **Lanacort® [OTC]** *see* Topical Corticosteroids *on page 1152*
- **Lanaphilic® Topical [OTC]** *see* Urea *on page 1193*
- **Lanexat®** *see* Flumazenil *on page 496*
- **Laniazid®** *see* Isoniazid *on page 630*
- **Lanolin, Cetyl Alcohol, Glycerin, and Petrolatum** *see page 1294*
- **Lanophyllin-GG®** *see* Theophylline and Guaifenesin *on page 1118*
- **Lanorinal®** *see* Butalbital Compound and Aspirin *on page 176*
- **Lanoxicaps®** *see* Digoxin *on page 370*
- **Lanoxin®** *see* Digoxin *on page 370*

## Lansoprazole (lan SOE pra zole)

**U.S. Brand Names** Prevacid®

**Therapeutic Category** Proton Pump Inhibitor

**Pregnancy Risk Factor** B

**Lactation** Excretion in breast milk unknown/contraindicated

**Use** Short-term treatment (up to 4 weeks) for healing and symptom relief of active duodenal ulcers (should not be used for maintenance therapy of duodenal ulcers); up to 8 weeks of treatment for all grades of erosive esophagitis (8 additional weeks can be given for incompletely healed esophageal erosions or for recurrence); and long-term treatment of pathological hypersecretory conditions, including Zollinger-Ellison syndrome; short-term treatment of gastroesophageal reflux disease (GERD); in combination with amoxicillin and clarithromycin to eradicate *Helicobacter pylori* in patients with duodenal ulcer

**Contraindications** Hypersensitivity to lansoprazole or any component

**Warnings** Liver disease may require dosage reductions.

**Drug Interactions**

**Cytochrome P-450 Effect:** CYP2C19 enzyme substrate, CYP3A3/4 enzyme substrate (minor)

**Decreased Effect:** Lansoprazole decreases effect of ketoconazole, itraconazole, and other drugs dependent upon acid for absorption. Theophylline clearance is increased slightly. Sucralfate delays and reduces lansoprazole absorption by 30%.

**Food Interactions** Lansoprazole serum concentrations may be decreased if taken with food.

**Adverse Reactions**

>10%

Central nervous system: Dizziness, headache
Dermatologic: Rash
Gastrointestinal: Diarrhea

1% to 10%:

Central nervous system: Fatigue
Gastrointestinal: Abdominal pain, nausea, increased appetite, hypergastrinoma

<1% (Limited to important or life-threatening symptoms): Thrombocytopenia, proteinuria, anaphylactoid reaction

**Overdose/Toxicology** Symptoms of overdose include hypothermia, sedation, and convulsions. Decreased respiratory rate has been demonstrated in animals only. Treatment is supportive. Not dialyzable.

(Continued)

## Lansoprazole *(Continued)*

**Pharmacodynamics/Kinetics**

**Protein Binding:** 97%

**Half-life Elimination:** Healthy patient: 1.5 hours; Elderly: 2.9 hours; Cirrhosis: 7 hours

**Time to Peak:** 1.7 hours

**Metabolism:** Hepatic and parietal cell oxidation to two metabolites (active)

**Excretion:** 33% in urine and 67% in feces

**Duration:** 1 day

**Formulations** Capsule, delayed release: 15 mg, 30 mg

**Dosing**

**Adults:** Oral:

Duodenal ulcer: 15 mg once daily for 4 weeks; maintenance therapy 15 mg once daily.

Gastric ulcer: 30 mg once daily for up to 8 weeks

Erosive esophagitis: 30 mg once daily for up to 8 weeks, continued treatment for an additional 8 weeks may be considered for recurrence or for patients that do not heal after the first 8 weeks of therapy. Maintenance therapy: 15 mg once daily.

Hypersecretory conditions: Initial: 60 mg once daily; adjust dose based upon patient response; dose of 90 mg twice daily have been used; administer doses >120 mg/day in divided doses.

*Helicobacter pylori*-associated antral gastritis: 30 mg daily for 2 weeks (in combination with 1 g amoxicillin and 500 mg clarithromycin given twice daily for 14 days).

**Elderly:** Refer to adult dosing.

**Renal Impairment:** No adjustment necessary

**Hepatic Impairment:** May require a dose reduction.

**Administration**

**Oral:** Administer before food. Do not crush or open capsules. Lansoprazole is unstable in acidic media (eg, stomach contents) and is, therefore, administered as enteric coated granules in capsule form.

**Monitoring Laboratory Tests** Patients with Zollinger-Ellison syndrome should be monitored for gastric acid output, which should be maintained at ≤10 mEq/hour during the last hour before the next lansoprazole dose. Lab monitoring should include CBC, liver function, renal function, and serum gastrin levels.

**Additional Nursing Issues**

**Physical Assessment:** Assess periodic laboratory results. Assess effectiveness of medications that require an acid medium for absorption (eg, ketoconazole, ampicillin, digoxin). Monitor effectiveness of ulcer symptom relief. Breast-feeding is contraindicated.

**Patient Information/Instruction:** Take as directed, before eating. Do not crush or chew capsules. Report unresolved fatigue, diarrhea, or constipation, and appetite changes. **Breast-feeding precautions:** Do not breast-feed.

**Geriatric Considerations:** The clearance of lansoprazole is decreased in the elderly; however, the half-life is only increased by 50% to 100%. This still results in a short half-life and no accumulation is seen in the elderly. The rate of healing and side effects is similar to younger adults; no dosage adjustment is necessary.

## Lansoprazole, Amoxicillin, and Clarithromycin

(lan SOE pra zole, a moks i SIL in, & kla RITH roe mye sin)

**U.S. Brand Names** Prevpac®

**Synonyms** Amoxicillin, Lansoprazole, and Clarithromycin; Clarithromycin, Lansoprazole, and Amoxicillin

**Therapeutic Category** Antibiotic, Macrolide Combination; Antibiotic, Penicillin; Gastrointestinal Agent, Miscellaneous

**Pregnancy Risk Factor** C (clarithromycin)

**Lactation** Excretion in breast milk unknown/contraindicated

**Use** Eradication of *H. pylori* to reduce the risk of recurrent duodenal ulcer

**Formulations** The package contains:

Amoxicillin: 500 mg capsules

Clarithromycin: 500 mg tablets

Lansoprazole: 30 mg capsules

**Dosing**

**Adults:** Lansoprazole 30 mg, amoxicillin 1 g, and clarithromycin 50 mg taken together twice daily

**Elderly:** Refer to adult dosing.

**Additional Nursing Issues**

**Physical Assessment:** See individual components listed in Related Information. **Pregnancy risk factor C** (clarithromycin) - benefits of use should outweigh possible risks. Breast-feeding is contraindicated.

**Patient Information/Instruction:** See individual components listed in Related Information. **Pregnancy/breast-feeding precautions:** Inform prescriber if you are on intend to get pregnant. Do not breast-feed.

**Related Information**

Amoxicillin *on page 80*

Clarithromycin *on page 279*

Lansoprazole *on previous page*

♦ **Lanvisone® Topical** *see* Clioquinol and Hydrocortisone *on page 284*

♦ **Largactil®** *see* Chlorpromazine *on page 256*

♦ **Lariam®** *see* Mefloquine *on page 716*

- ♦ **Larodopa®** *see* Levodopa *on page 666*
- ♦ **Lasix®** *see* Furosemide *on page 523*
- ♦ **Lassar's Zinc Paste** *see page 1294*
- ♦ **Lastet** *see* Etoposide *on page 463*
- ♦ **Latanoprost** *see* Ophthalmic Agents, Glaucoma *on page 853*
- ♦ **Latotryd®** *see* Erythromycin *on page 435*
- ♦ ***Latrodectus mactans*** *see page 1246*
- ♦ **Lauricin** *see* Erythromycin *on page 435*
- ♦ **Laxatives: Classification and Properties Comparison** *see page 1392*
- ♦ **LazerSporin-C®** *see page 1291*
- ♦ **LCR** *see* Vincristine *on page 1213*
- ♦ **L-Deprenyl** *see* Selegiline *on page 1050*
- ♦ ***L*-Dopa** *see* Levodopa *on page 666*
- ♦ **Leche De Magnesia Normex** *see* Magnesium Supplements *on page 703*
- ♦ **Ledercort** *see* Triamcinolone *on page 1171*
- ♦ **Ledermicina** *see* Demeclocycline *on page 341*
- ♦ **Lederpax** *see* Erythromycin *on page 435*
- ♦ **Lederplex®** *see page 1294*
- ♦ **Ledertrexate** *see* Methotrexate *on page 743*
- ♦ **Ledoxina** *see* Cyclophosphamide *on page 313*


## Leflunomide (le FLU no mide)

**U.S. Brand Names** Arava™

**Therapeutic Category** Antimetabolite; Antirheumatic, Disease Modifying

**Pregnancy Risk Factor** X

**Lactation** Excretion in breast milk unknown/contraindicated

**Use** Treatment of active rheumatoid arthritis to reduce signs and symptoms and to retard structural damage, as evidenced by erosions and joint space narrowing seen on x-ray

**Mechanism of Action/Effect** Inhibits pyrimidine synthesis, resulting in antiproliferative and anti-inflammatory effects

**Contraindications** Hypersensitivity to leflunomide or any component; pregnancy

**Warnings** Hepatic disease (including seropositive hepatitis B or C patients) may increase risk of hepatotoxicity. Immunosuppression may increase the risk of lymphoproliferative disorders or other malignancies. Women of childbearing potential should not receive leflunomide until pregnancy has been excluded, patients have been counseled concerning fetal risk, and reliable contraceptive measures have been confirmed. Caution in renal impairment, immune deficiency, bone marrow dysplasia or severe uncontrolled infection. Use of live vaccines is not recommended; will increase uric acid excretion.

**Drug Interactions**

**Cytochrome P-450 Effect:** Cytochrome P-450 2C9 enzyme inhibitor

**Decreased Effect:** Administration of cholestyramine and activated charcoal enhance the elimination of leflunomide's active metabolite.

**Increased Effect/Toxicity:** Theoretically, concomitant use of drugs metabolized by this enzyme, including many NSAIDs, may result in increased serum concentrations and possible toxic effects. Coadministration with methotrexate increases the risk of hepatotoxicity. Leflunomide may also enhance the hepatotoxicity of other drugs. Tolbutamide free fraction may be increased. Rifampin may increase serum concentrations of leflunomide. Leflunomide has uricosuric activity and may enhance activity of other uricosuric agents.

**Food Interactions** No interactions with food have been noted

**Adverse Reactions**

>10%:

Gastrointestinal: Diarrhea (17%)

Respiratory: Respiratory tract infection (15%)

1% to 10%:

Cardiovascular: Hypertension (10%), chest pain (2%), palpitation, tachycardia, vasculitis, vasodilation, varicose vein, edema (peripheral)

Central nervous system: Headache (7%), dizziness (4%), pain (2%), paresthesia (2%), fever, malaise, migraine, anxiety, depression, insomnia, neuralgia, neuritis, sleep disorder

Dermatologic: Alopecia (10%), rash (10%), pruritus (4%), dry skin (2%), eczema (2%), acne, dermatitis, hair discoloration, hematoma, herpes infection, nail disorder, subcutaneous nodule, skin disorder/discoloration, skin ulcer, bruising

Endocrine & metabolic: Hypokalemia (1%), diabetes mellitus, hyperglycemia, hyperlipidemia, hyperthyroidism, menstrual disorder

Gastrointestinal: Nausea (9%), abdominal pain (5%), dyspepsia (5%), weight loss (4%), anorexia (3%), gastroenteritis (3%), stomatitis (3%), vomiting (3%), cholelithiasis, colitis, constipation, esophagitis, flatulence, gastritis, gingivitis, melena, candidiasis (oral), enlarged salivary gland, tooth disorder, xerostomia, taste disturbance

Genitourinary: Urinary tract infection (5%), albuminuria, cystitis, dysuria, hematuria, vaginal candidiasis, prostate disorder, urinary frequency

Hematologic: Anemia

Hepatic: Abnormal liver function tests (5%)

Neuromuscular & skeletal: Back pain (5%), joint disorder (4%), weakness (3%), tenosynovitis (3%), synovitis (2%), arthralgia (1%), muscle cramps (1%), neck pain, pelvic pain, increased CPK, arthrosis, bursitis, myalgia, bone necrosis, bone pain, tendon rupture

(Continued)

## Leflunomide *(Continued)*

Ocular: Blurred vision, cataract, conjunctivitis, eye disorder

Respiratory: Bronchitis (7%), cough (3%), pharyngitis (3%), pneumonia (2%), rhinitis (2%), sinusitis (2%), asthma, dyspnea, epistaxis, lung disorder

Miscellaneous: Infection (4%), accidental injury (5%), allergic reactions (2%), diaphoresis

<1% (Limited to important or life-threatening symptoms): Anaphylaxis, urticaria, eosinophilia, thrombocytopenia, leukopenia

**Overdose/Toxicology** There is no human experience with overdose. Leflunomide is not dialyzable. Cholestyramine and/or activated charcoal enhance elimination of leflunomide's active metabolite (MI). In cases of significant overdose or toxicity, cholestyramine 8 g every 8 hours for 1-3 days may be administered to enhance elimination. Plasma levels are reduced by approximately 40% in 24 hours and 49% to 65% after 48 hours of cholestyramine dosing.

**Pharmacodynamics/Kinetics**

**Half-life Elimination:** Mean 14-15 days; enterohepatic recycling appears to contribute to the long half-life of this agent, since activated charcoal and cholestyramine substantially reduce plasma half-life

**Time to Peak:** 6-12 hours

**Metabolism:** Hepatic, to A77 1726 (MI) which accounts for nearly all pharmacologic activity; further metabolism to multiple inactive metabolites

**Excretion:** Urine and feces

**Formulations** Tablet: 10 mg, 20 mg, 100 mg

**Dosing**

**Adults:**

Oral: Initial: 100 mg/day for 3 days, followed by 20 mg/day; dosage may be decreased to 10 mg/day in patients who have difficulty tolerating the 20 mg dose. Due to the long half-life of the active metabolite, plasma levels may require a prolonged period to decline after dosage reduction.

Guidelines for dosage adjustment or discontinuation based on the severity and persistence of ALT elevation have been developed. For ALT elevations >2 times the upper limit of normal, dosage reduction to 10 mg/day may allow continued administration. Cholestyramine 8 g 3 times/day for 1-3 days may be administered to decrease plasma levels. If elevations >2 times but less than or equal to 3 times the upper limit of normal persist, liver biopsy is recommended. If elevations >3 times the upper limit of normal persist despite cholestyramine administration and dosage reduction, leflunomide should be discontinued and drug elimination should be enhanced with additional cholestyramine as indicated.

**Elderly:** Although hepatic function may decline with age, no specific dosage adjustment is recommended. Patients should be monitored closely for adverse effects which may require dosage adjustment.

**Renal Impairment:** No specific dosage adjustment is recommended. There is no clinical experience in the use of leflunomide in patients with renal impairment. The free fraction of MI is doubled in dialysis patients. Patients should be monitored closely for adverse effects requiring dosage adjustment.

**Hepatic Impairment:** No specific dosage adjustment is recommended. Since the liver is involved in metabolic activation and subsequent metabolism/elimination of leflunomide, patients with hepatic impairment should be monitored closely for adverse effects requiring dosage adjustment.

**Stability**

**Storage:** Protect from light; store at 25°C (77°F).

**Additional Nursing Issues**

**Physical Assessment:** Assess other medications patient may be taking for effectiveness and interactions (see Warnings/Precautions and Drug Interactions). Monitor laboratory tests (see above), therapeutic effects (eg, reduction of rheumatoid arthritis signs and symptoms, structural damage), and adverse reactions (see Warnings/Precautions and Adverse Reactions). Assess knowledge/teach patient appropriate use, interventions to reduce side effects, and adverse symptoms to report. **Pregnancy risk factor X** - determine that patient is not pregnant before beginning treatment and do not give to females or males unless both female or male are capable of complying with barrier contraception during and for 1 month following therapy. Breast-feeding is contraindicated.

**Patient Information/Instruction:** Take as directed; do not increase dose without consulting prescriber. Maintain adequate hydration (2-3 L/day of fluids unless instructed to restrict fluid intake). Store medication away from light. You may experience diarrhea (buttermilk, boiled milk, or yogurt may help); nausea, vomiting, loss of appetite, and flatulence (small frequent meals, frequent mouth care, chewing gum, or sucking lozenges may help); dizziness (use caution when driving or engaging in tasks requiring alertness until response to drug is known). If diabetic, monitor blood sugars closely; this medication may alter glucose levels. Report chest pain, palpitations, rapid heartbeat, or swelling of extremities; persistent gastrointestinal problems; skin rash, redness, irritation, acne, ulcers, or easy bruising; frequency, painful or difficult urination, or genital itching or irritation; depression, acute headache, anxiety, or difficulty sleeping; weakness, muscle tremors, cramping or weakness, back pain, or altered gait; cough, cold symptoms, wheezing, or difficulty breathing; easy bruising/bleeding; blood in vomitus, stool, urine; or other unusual effects related to this medication. **Pregnancy/breast-feeding precautions:** Inform prescriber if you are pregnant. Do not get pregnant or have sex unless using appropriate barrier contraception while on this medication. This drug may cause severe fetal defects. Do not breast-feed.

**Breast-feeding Issues:** It is not known whether leflunomide is secreted in human milk. Because many immunoglobulins are secreted in milk, and the potential for serious adverse reactions exists, a decision should be made whether to discontinue nursing or discontinue the drug, taking into account the importance of the drug to the mother.

**Pregnancy Issues:** Has been associated with teratogenic and embryolethal effects in animal models at low doses. Leflunomide is contraindicated in pregnant women or women of childbearing potential who are not using reliable contraception. Pregnancy must be excluded prior to initiating treatment. Following treatment, pregnancy should be avoided until the drug elimination procedure is completed.

**Additional Information** To enhance elimination, a drug elimination procedure has been developed. Without this procedure, it may take up to 2 years to reach plasma concentrations <0.02 mg/L (a concentration expected to have minimal risk of teratogenicity based on animal models). The procedure consists of the following steps: Administer cholestyramine 8 g 3 times/day for 11 days (the 11 days do not need to be consecutive). Plasma levels <0.02 mg/L should be verified by two separate tests performed at least 14 days apart. If plasma levels are >0.02 mg/L, additional cholestyramine treatment should be considered.


- **Legatrin PM® Caplet** *see page 1294*
- **Lemblastine** *see* Vinblastine *on page 1211*
- **Lenoltec No 1, 2, 3, 4** *see* Acetaminophen and Codeine *on page 34*
- **Lenpryl** *see* Captopril *on page 192*
- **Lente® Iletin® I** *see* Insulin Preparations *on page 609*
- **Lente® Iletin® II** *see* Insulin Preparations *on page 609*
- **Lente® Insulin** *see* Insulin Preparations *on page 609*
- **Lente® L** *see* Insulin Preparations *on page 609*
- **Lentopenil** *see* Penicillin G, Parenteral, Aqueous *on page 897*


## Lepirudin (leh puh ROO din)

**U.S. Brand Names** Refludan®

**Synonyms** Lepirudin (rDNA); Recombinant Hirudin

**Therapeutic Category** Anticoagulant

**Pregnancy Risk Factor** B

**Lactation** Enters breast milk/consult prescriber

**Use** Indicated for anticoagulation in patient with heparin-induced thrombocytopenia (HIT) and associated thromboembolic disease in order to prevent further thromboembolic complications

**Investigational use:** Prevention or reduction of ischemic complications associated with unstable angina

**Mechanism of Action/Effect** Lepirudin is a highly specific direct thrombin inhibitor. Each molecule is capable of binding one molecule of thrombin and inhibiting its thrombogenic activity.

**Contraindications** Hypersensitivity to hirudins; severe renal impairment ($Cl_{cr}$ <15 mL/minute)

**Warnings** Measure baseline APTT prior to initiation. Should not be started in a patient with an initial APTT ratio >2.5. **Intracranial bleeding following concomitant thrombolytic therapy with t-PA or streptokinase may be life-threatening.** Risk of bleeding increased: Recent puncture of large vessels or organ biopsy; vessel or organ anomalies; recent stroke, intracerebral surgery other neuraxial procedures; severe uncontrolled hypertension; bacterial endocarditis, advanced renal impairment, hemorrhagic diathesis, recent major surgery, recent major bleeding (eg, intracranial, gastrointestinal, intraocular, or pulmonary). Dosage adjustment required in renal impairment ($Cl_{cr}$ <60 mL/minute), and lepirudin should be stopped or avoided in patients with $Cl_{cr}$ <15 mL/minute.

Strict monitoring of APTT is required during prolonged therapy - antihirudin antibodies may delay hirudin's renal elimination causing accumulation/exaggerated effects. Caution in hepatic impairment (reduced production of clotting factors). Caution with repeat exposure to hirudin (mild skin rash occurred in 1 of 13 patients).

**Drug Interactions**

**Increased Effect/Toxicity:** Thrombolytics may enhance anticoagulant properties of lepirudin on aPTT and can increase the risk of bleeding complications. Bleeding risk may also be increased by oral anticoagulants (Coumadin®) and platelet function inhibitors (nonsteroidal anti-inflammatory drugs, dipyridamole, ticlopidine, clopidogrel, IIb/IIIa antagonists, and aspirin).

**Adverse Reactions**

**HIT patients:**

>10%: Hematologic: Anemia (12.4%), bleeding from puncture sites (10.6%), hematoma 10.8%

1% to 10%:

Gastrointestinal: GI bleeding/rectal bleeding (5.3%)
Genitourinary: Vaginal bleeding (1.8%)
Renal: Hematuria (4.4%)
Respiratory: Epistaxis (4.4%)

<1%: (Limited to important or life-threatening symptoms): Hemoperitoneum, hemoptysis, liver bleeding, pulmonary bleeding, retroperitoneal bleeding, mouth bleeding

**Non-HIT populations** (including those receiving thrombolytics and/or contrast media):

1% to 10%: Respiratory: Bronchospasm/stridor/dyspnea/cough

<1% (Limited to important or life-threatening symptoms): Angioedema, laryngeal edema, tongue edema, intracranial bleeding (0.6%), allergic reactions (unspecified), anaphylactoid reactions, anaphylaxis

(Continued)

## Lepirudin *(Continued)*

**Overdose/Toxicology** Risk of bleeding is increased, and therefore management is directed towards control of bleeding.

**Pharmacodynamics/Kinetics**

**Distribution:** Primarily to extracellular fluid

**Half-life Elimination:** Variable, 1.3 hours in healthy volunteers; up to 2 days in marked renal insufficiency ($Cl_{cr}$ <15 mL/minute)

**Metabolism:** Unknown, catabolic hydrolysis of amino acids is likely

**Excretion:** Renal; 48% of dose (35% unchanged); systemic clearance is directly proportional to creatinine clearance

**Formulations** Injection: 50 mg

**Dosing**

**Adults:** Maximum dose: Do not exceed 0.21 mg/kg/hour unless an evaluation of coagulation abnormalities limiting response has been completed. **Dosing is weight-based, however patients weighing >110 kg should not receive doses greater than the recommended dose for a patient weighing 110 kg (44 mg bolus and initial maximal infusion rate of 16.5 mg/hour).**

Heparin-induced thrombocytopenia: Bolus dose: 0.4 mg/kg IVP (over 15-20 seconds), followed by continuous infusion at 0.15 mg/kg/hour; bolus and infusion must be reduced in renal insufficiency

Concomitant use with thrombolytic therapy: Bolus dose: 0.2 mg/kg IVP (over 15-20 seconds), followed by continuous infusion at 0.1 mg/kg/hour

Dosing adjustments during infusions: Monitor first APTT 4 hours after the start of the infusion. Subsequent determinations of APTT should be obtained at least once daily during treatment. More frequent monitoring is recommended in renally impaired patients. Any APTT ratio measurement out of range (1.5-2.5) should be confirmed prior to adjusting dose, unless a clinical need for immediate reaction exists. If the APTT is below target range, increase infusion by 20%. If the APTT is in excess of the target range, decrease infusion rate by 50%. A repeat APTT should be obtained 4 hours after any dosing change.

Use in patients scheduled for switch to oral anticoagulants: Reduce lepirudin dose gradually to reach aPTT ratio just above 1.5 before starting warfarin therapy; as soon as INR reaches 2.0, lepirudin therapy should be discontinued.

**Renal Impairment:** Initial: Bolus dose: 0.2 mg/kg IVP (over 15-20 seconds) see table; additional bolus doses of 0.1 mg/kg may be administered every other day (only if APTT falls below lower therapeutic limit).

| $Cl_{cr}$ (mL/min) | Serum Creatinine (mg/dL) | Adjusted Infusion Rate (mg/kg/h) | % of Standard Infusion Rate |
|---|---|---|---|
| 45-60 | 1.6-2.0 | 0.075 | 50% |
| 30-44 | 2.1-3.0 | 0.045 | 30% |
| 15-20 | 3.1-6.0 | 0.0225 | 15% |
| <15 | >6.0 | AVOID USE or STOP infusion | |

**Administration**

**I.V.:** I.V. bolus: Inject slowly for continuous infusion; solutions with 0.2 or 0.4 mg/mL may be used.

**Stability**

**Reconstitution:** Reconstitute 50 mg vials with 1 mL water for injection or 0.9% sodium chloride injection. Bolus dose: Prepare 5 mg/mL solution by transferring contents of 1 reconstituted vial to single use, sterile syringe. Dilute to total volume of 10 mL with 0.9 sodium chloride or 5% dextrose injection. To prepare continuous infusion solutions, either 0.9% sodium chloride or 5% dextrose may be used. Add contents of two reconstituted vials to either 250 mL (to prepare 0.4 mg/mL solution) or 500 mL (to prepare 0.2 mg/mL solution). Once reconstituted, use immediately. Reconstituted solutions remain stable for 24 hours (duration of infusion).

**Monitoring Laboratory Tests** The APTT ratio should be maintained between 1.5 and 2.5. Ratio is calculated by patient's value at a given time divided by reference value (commonly the median of a laboratory normal range).

**Additional Nursing Issues**

**Physical Assessment:** Monitor vital signs and laboratory results prior to, during, and after therapy. Assess infusion insertion site during and after therapy (every 15 minutes or as institutional policy). Observe and teach patient bleeding precautions (avoid invasive procedures and activities that could result in injury). Monitor closely for signs of excessive bleeding (eg, CNS changes, blood in urine, stool, or vomitus; unusual bruising or bleeding). Note breast-feeding caution.

**Patient Information/Instruction:** This medication can only be administered I.V. You will have a tendency to bleed easily following this medication. Use caution to prevent injury (use electric razor, use soft toothbrush, use caution with sharps). If bleeding occurs, apply pressure to bleeding spot until bleeding stops completely. Report unusual bruising or bleeding (eg, blood in urine, stool, or vomitus, bleeding gums, vaginal bleeding, nosebleeds); dizziness or changes in vision; back pain; skin rash; swelling of face, mouth, or throat; or difficulty breathing. **Breast-feeding precautions:** Consult prescriber if breast-feeding.

◆ **Lepirudin (rDNA)** *see* Lepirudin *on previous page*

- **Leponex®** *see* Clozapine *on page 296*
- **Leptilan®** *see* Valproic Acid and Derivatives *on page 1198*
- **Leptopsique** *see* Perphenazine *on page 912*
- **Lertamine** *see* Loratadine *on page 689*
- **Lescol®** *see* Fluvastatin *on page 512*


## Letrozole (LET roe zole)

**U.S. Brand Names** Femara™

**Therapeutic Category** Antineoplastic Agent, Miscellaneous; Aromatase Inhibitor

**Pregnancy Risk Factor** D

**Lactation** Excretion in breast milk unknown/not recommended

**Use** Treatment of advanced breast cancer in postmenopausal women with disease progression following antiestrogen therapy

**Mechanism of Action/Effect** Nonsteroidal, competitive inhibitor of the aromatase enzyme system, which catalyzes conversion of androgens to estrogens. Inhibition leads to a significant reduction in plasma estrogen levels. Approximately 30% of breast cancers are sensitive to estrogen deprivation.

**Contraindications** Hypersensitivity to letrozole or any component; pregnancy

**Warnings** May cause fetal harm when administered to pregnant women (letrozole is indicated in postmenopausal women). Moderate, often (in ~50% of cases) transient, decreases in lymphocyte counts were observed in some patients receiving letrozole 2.5 mg. Two patients on letrozole developed thrombocytopenia (relationship to the drug unclear). Increases in serum transaminases and bilirubin were most often associated with metastatic disease in the liver.

**Drug Interactions**

**Cytochrome P-450 Effect:** CYP3A3/4 and 2A6 enzyme substrate; CYP2A6 and 2C19 enzyme inhibitor

**Increased Effect/Toxicity:** Inhibitors of this enzyme may, in theory, increase letrozole blood levels. Letrozole inhibits cytochrome P-450 isoenzyme 2A6 and 2C19 *in vitro* and may increase blood levels of drugs metabolized by these enzymes. Specific drug interaction studies have not been reported.

**Adverse Reactions** Frequencies reported in clinical trials (regardless of relationship to study drug).

>10%:

Gastrointestinal: Nausea (13% to 15%)

Neuromuscular & skeletal: Musculoskeletal pain (21% to 22%)

1% to 10%:

Central nervous system: Headache (9% to 12%), dizziness (3% to 5%), somnolence (2% to 3%), fatigue (6% to 8%)

Cardiovascular: Chest pain (3% to 6%), hypertension (5% to 7%), peripheral edema (5%)

Dermatologic: Hot flashes (5% to 6%), rash (4% to 5%), pruritus (1% to 2%)

Gastrointestinal: Vomiting (7%), constipation (6% to 7%), diarrhea (5% to 6%), abdominal pain (5% to 6%), anorexia (3% to 5%), dyspepsia (3% to 4%)

Neuromuscular & skeletal: Arthralgia (8%), weakness (4% to 5%)

Respiratory: Dyspnea (7% to 9%), coughing (5% to 6%)

<1% (Limited to important or life-threatening symptoms): Thromboembolic events, fracture, depression, anxiety, pleural effusion

**Overdose/Toxicology** No experience with letrozole overdose has been reported. In single-dose studies, the highest dose used was 30 mg, which was well tolerated. Lethality was observed in animals at doses 50-8000 times the maximum human doses. Toxicity was associated with ataxia, dyspnea, depressed blood pressure, and arrhythmias.

Firm recommendations for treatment are not possible; emesis could be induced if the patient is alert. In general, supportive care and frequent monitoring of vital signs are appropriate.

**Pharmacodynamics/Kinetics**

**Protein Binding:** Weakly bound

**Half-life Elimination:** 2 days

**Metabolism:** Hepatic, by cytochrome P-450 isoenzymes 3A4 and 2A6

**Excretion:** Primarily conjugated metabolites (with ~6% unchanged drug) excreted in urine (~90% of dose)

**Formulations** Tablet: 2.5 mg

**Dosing**

**Adults:** Oral (refer to individual protocols): 2.5 mg once daily without regard to meals; continue treatment until tumor progression is evident. Patients treated with letrozole do not require glucocorticoid or mineralocorticoid replacement therapy.

**Elderly:** Refer to adult dosing.

**Hepatic Impairment:** No dosage adjustment is recommended for patients with mild-to-moderate hepatic impairment. Patients with severe impairment of liver function have not been studied; dose patients with severe impairment of liver function with caution.

**Monitoring Laboratory Tests** Clinical/radiologic evidence of tumor regression in advanced breast cancer patients. Until the toxicity has been defined in larger patient populations, monitor the following laboratory tests periodically during therapy: complete blood counts, thyroid function tests, serum electrolytes, serum transaminases, and serum creatinine.

(Continued)

## Letrozole *(Continued)*

**Additional Nursing Issues**

**Physical Assessment:** Assess pregnancy status prior to administration. Assess other medications patient may be taking for possible interactions (see Drug Interactions). Monitor for adverse reactions (see Adverse Reactions). Instruct patient about signs of adverse reaction to report and possible interventions to reduce side effects. **Pregnancy risk factor D** - assess knowledge/teach appropriate use of barrier contraceptives. Breast-feeding is not recommended.

**Patient Information/Instruction:** Take as directed, without regard to food. You may experience nausea, vomiting, or loss of appetite (frequent mouth care, frequent small meals, chewing gum, or sucking lozenges may help); musculoskeletal pain or headache (mild analgesics may offer relief); sleepiness, fatigue, or dizziness (use caution when driving, climbing stairs, or engaging in tasks that require alertness until response to drug is known); constipation (increased exercise, or dietary fruit or fluids may help); diarrhea (boiled milk or yogurt may help); loss of hair (will grow back). Report chest pain, palpitations, or swollen extremities; vaginal bleeding or hot flashes; unusual coughing or difficulty breathing; severe nausea; muscle pain; or skin rash. **Pregnancy/breast-feeding precautions:** Do not get pregnant while taking this medication; use appropriate barrier contraceptive measures. Breast-feeding is not recommended.

**Pregnancy Issues:** Letrozole may cause fetal harm when administered to pregnant women. Letrozole is embryotoxic and fetotoxic when administered to rats. There are no studies in pregnant women and letrozole is indicated for postmenopausal women.

♦ **Leucomax®** *see* Sargramostim *on page 1045*

## Leucovorin (loo koe VOR in)

**U.S. Brand Names** Wellcovorin®

**Synonyms** Calcium Leucovorin; Citrovorum Factor; Folinic Acid; 5-Formyl Tetrahydrofolate

**Therapeutic Category** Antidote; Vitamin, Water Soluble

**Pregnancy Risk Factor** C

**Lactation** Enters breast milk/compatible

**Use** Antidote for folic acid antagonists (methotrexate [>100 mg/m$^2$], trimethoprim, pyrimethamine); treatment of megaloblastic anemias when folate is deficient as in infancy, sprue, pregnancy, and nutritional deficiency when oral folate therapy is not possible; in combination with fluorouracil in the treatment of malignancy

**Mechanism of Action/Effect** A reduced form of folic acid, but does not require a reduction reaction by an enzyme for activation, allows for purine and thymidine synthesis, a necessity for normal erythropoiesis; leucovorin supplies the necessary cofactor blocked by MTX, enters the cells via the same active transport system as MTX

**Contraindications** Hypersensitivity to leucovorin; pernicious anemia or other megaloblastic anemias where a deficiency of $B_{12}$ is present

**Warnings** Pregnancy factor C.

**Adverse Reactions** <1% (Limited to important or life-threatening symptoms): Seizures, thrombocytosis, wheezing, anaphylactoid reactions

**Pharmacodynamics/Kinetics**

**Half-life Elimination:** Leucovorin: 15 minutes; Metabolite 5MTHF: 33-35 minutes

**Metabolism:** Intestinal mucosa and liver

**Excretion:** Urine and feces

**Onset:** Onset of activity: Oral: Within 30 minutes; I.V.: Within 5 minutes

**Formulations**

Leucovorin calcium:

- Injection: 3 mg/mL (1 mL)
- Powder for injection: 25 mg, 50 mg, 100 mg, 350 mg
- Powder for oral solution: 1 mg/mL (60 mL)
- Tablet: 5 mg, 10 mg, 15 mg, 25 mg

**Dosing**

**Adults:**

Treatment of folic acid antagonist overdosage (eg, pyrimethamine or trimethoprim): Oral: 2-15 mg/day for 3 days or until blood counts are normal or 5 mg every 3 days; doses of 6 mg/day are needed for patients with platelet counts <100,000/mm$^3$.

Folate-deficient megaloblastic anemia: I.M.: 1 mg/day

Megaloblastic anemia secondary to congenital deficiency of dihydrofolate reductase: I.M.: 3-6 mg/day

Rescue dose (rescue therapy should start within 24 hours of MTX therapy): I.V.: 10 mg/m$^2$ to start, then 10 mg/m$^2$ every 6 hours orally for 72 hours until serum MTX concentration is <10$^{-8}$ molar. If serum creatinine 24 hours after methotrexate is elevated 50% or more above the pre-MTX serum creatinine **or** the serum MTX concentration is >5 x 10$^{-6}$ molar (see graph), increase dose to 100 mg/m$^2$/dose every 3 hours until serum methotrexate level is <1 x 10$^{-8}$ molar.

Investigational: Post I.T. methotrexate: Oral, I.V.: 12 mg/m$^2$ as a single dose; post high-dose methotrexate: 100-1000 mg/m$^2$/dose until the serum methotrexate level is less than 1 x 10$^{-7}$ molar.

**The drug should be given parenterally instead of orally in patients with GI toxicity, nausea, vomiting, and when individual doses are >25 mg.**

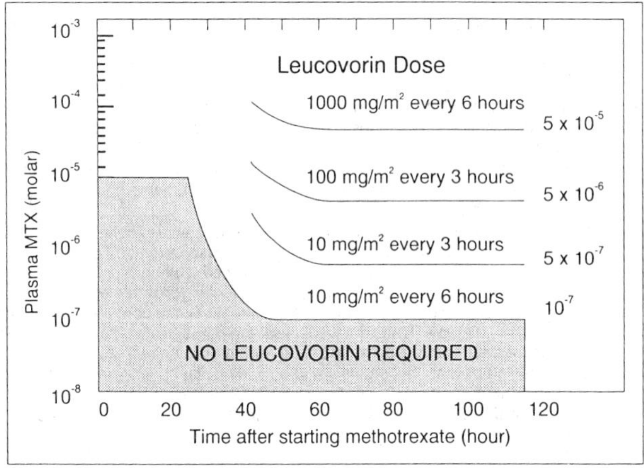


**Elderly:** Refer to adult dosing.

**Administration**

**Oral:** Maximum oral dose: 25 mg

**I.V.:** Leucovorin calcium should be administered I.M. or I.V. I.V. infusion should not exceed 160 mg/minute of leucovorin.

**Stability**

**Storage:** Leucovorin injection should be stored at room temperature and protected from light.

**Reconstitution:** Reconstituted solution is stated to be chemically stable for 7 days. Stability of parenteral admixture at room temperature (25°C) is 24 hours. Stability of parenteral admixture at refrigeration temperature (4°C) is 4 days.

Standard diluent: 50-100 mg/50 mL $D_5W$
Minimum volume: 50 mL $D_5W$

**Compatibility:** Concentrations >2 mg/mL of leucovorin and >25 mg/mL of fluorouracil are incompatible (precipitation occurs). See the Chemotherapy Compatibility Chart *on page 1311.*

**Monitoring Laboratory Tests** Plasma MTX concentration as a therapeutic guide to high-dose MTX therapy with leucovorin factor rescue. Leucovorin is continued until the plasma MTX level is $<1 \times 10^{-7}$ molar. Each dose of leucovorin is increased if the plasma MTX concentration is excessively high (see graph). With 4- to 6-hour high-dose MTX infusions, plasma drug values in excess of $5 \times 10^{-5}$ and $10^{-6}$ molar at 24 and 48 hours after starting the infusion, respectively, are often predictive of delayed MTX clearance; see graph.

**Additional Nursing Issues**

**Physical Assessment:** Monitor for adverse reactions (see above). **Pregnancy risk factor C** - benefits of use should outweigh possible risks.

**Patient Information/Instruction:** Take as directed, at evenly spaced intervals around-the-clock. Maintain hydration (2-3 L of water/day while taking for rescue therapy). For folic acid deficiency, eat foods high in folic acid (eg, meat proteins, bran, dried beans, asparagus, green leafy vegetables). Report respiratory difficulty, lethargy, or rash or itching. **Pregnancy precautions:** Inform prescriber if you are or intend to be pregnant.

**Related Information**

Fluorouracil *on page 500*
Methotrexate *on page 743*
Trimethoprim *on page 1181*

- **Leukeran®** *see* Chlorambucil *on page 246*
- **Leukine™** *see* Sargramostim *on page 1045*
- **Leunase** *see* Asparaginase *on page 109*

## Leuprolide (loo PROE lide)

**U.S. Brand Names** Depot-3® Month; Depot-Ped™; Lupron®; Lupron Depot®; Lupron Depot-Ped™

**Synonyms** Leuprorelin Acetate

**Therapeutic Category** Antineoplastic Agent, Miscellaneous; Luteinizing Hormone-Releasing Hormone Analog

**Pregnancy Risk Factor** X

**Lactation** Excretion in breast milk unknown/not recommended

**Use** Palliative treatment of advanced prostate carcinoma (alternative when orchiectomy or estrogen administration are not indicated or are unacceptable to the patient); combination therapy with flutamide for treating metastatic prostatic carcinoma; endometriosis (3.75 mg depot only); central precocious puberty (may be used as an agent to treat
(Continued)

## Leuprolide *(Continued)*

precocious puberty because of its effect in lowering levels of LH and FSH, testosterone, and estrogen).

**Unlabeled use:** Treatment of breast, ovarian, and endometrial cancer; leiomyoma uteri; infertility; prostatic hypertrophy

**Mechanism of Action/Effect** Continuous daily administration results in suppression of ovarian and testicular steroidogenesis due to decreased levels of LH and FSH with subsequent decrease in testosterone (male) and estrogen (female) levels

**Contraindications** Hypersensitivity to leuprolide; spinal cord compression (orchiectomy suggested); undiagnosed abnormal vaginal bleeding; women who are or may be pregnant should not receive Lupron® Depot®

**Warnings** Use with caution in patients hypersensitive to benzyl alcohol. After 6 months use of Depot® leuprolide, vertebral bone density decreased (average 13.5%). Long-term safety of leuprolide in children has not been established. Urinary tract obstruction may occur upon initiation of therapy. Closely observe patients for weakness, paresthesias, and urinary tract obstruction in first few weeks of therapy. Tumor flare and bone pain may occur at initiation of therapy. Transient weakness and paresthesia of lower limbs, hematuria, and urinary tract obstruction in first week of therapy. Animal studies have shown dose-related benign pituitary hyperplasia and benign pituitary adenomas after 2 years of use. Concurrent hormone replacement therapy reduces loss of bone mineral density.

**Effects on Lab Values** Interferes with pituitary gonadotropic and gonadal function tests during and up to 4-8 weeks after therapy

**Adverse Reactions**

**Female:**

>10%:
- Endocrine & metabolic: Amenorrhea
- Neuromuscular & skeletal: Changes in bone mineral density

1% to 10%:
- Endocrine & metabolic: Decreased libido, breast tenderness
- Miscellaneous: Deepening of voice

**Male/Female:**

>10%: Cardiovascular: Hot flashes

1% to 10%:
- Cardiovascular: Cardiac arrhythmias, palpitations, edema
- Central nervous system: Dizziness, headache, insomnia, paresthesias
- Gastrointestinal: Weight gain, nausea, vomiting
- Ocular: Blurred vision
- Miscellaneous: Pain at injection site

**Male:**

1% to 10%:
- Cardiovascular: Chest pain
- Endocrine & metabolic: Gynecomastia, impotence or decreased libido
- Gastrointestinal: Constipation, anorexia
- Genitourinary: Decreased testicle size

<1% (Limited to important or life-threatening symptoms): Myocardial infarction, thrombophlebitis, pulmonary embolism

**Overdose/Toxicology** Treatment is supportive.

**Pharmacodynamics/Kinetics**

**Half-life Elimination:** 3-4.25 hours

**Excretion:** Not well defined

**Onset:** Serum testosterone levels first increase within 3 days of therapy.

**Duration:** Levels decrease after 2-4 weeks with continued therapy.

**Formulations**

Leuprolide acetate:
- Injection: 5 mg/mL (2.8 mL)
- Powder for injection (depot):
  - Depot®: 3.75 mg, 7.5 mg
  - Depot-3® Month: 11.25 mg
  - Depot-Ped™: 7.5 mg, 11.25 mg, 15 mg

**Dosing**

**Adults:** Requires parenteral administration

Advanced prostatic carcinoma:
- S.C.: 1 mg/day **or**
- I.M., Depot® (suspension): 7.5 mg/dose given monthly (every 28-33 days)

Endometriosis: I.M., Depot® (suspension): 3.75 mg/month for up to 6 months

**Elderly:** Refer to adult dosing.

**Administration**

**I.M.:** When administering the Depot® form, do not use needles smaller than 22-gauge. Reconstitute only with diluent provided.

**Stability**

**Storage:** Store unopened vials of injection in refrigerator. Vial in use can be kept at room temperature (≤30°C/86°F) for several months with minimal loss of potency. Protect from light and store vial in carton until use. Do not freeze. Depot® may be stored at room temperature.

**Reconstitution:** Depot®: Upon reconstitution, the suspension is stable for 24 hours. Does not contain a preservative.

**Monitoring Laboratory Tests** Precocious puberty: GnRH testing (blood LH and FSH levels), testosterone in males and estradiol in females

**Additional Nursing Issues**

**Physical Assessment:** Prostatic carcinoma: Monitor for paresthesia, urinary tract obstruction during first weeks. Monitor all for adverse reactions (see above - cardiac arrhythmias), CNS disturbance, and effectiveness of therapy. Teach patient/caregiver appropriate administration procedures (eg, rotate sites, monitor sites for infection, disposal of syringes). **Pregnancy risk factor X** - do not use if patient is pregnant. Females must use reliable barrier contraceptives during therapy. Breast-feeding is not recommended.

**Patient Information/Instruction:** Use as directed. Do not discontinue abruptly; consult prescriber. You may experience disease flare (increased bone pain) and urinary retention during early treatment (usually resolves), dizziness, headache, lethargy, or faintness (use caution when driving or engaging in tasks that require alertness until response to drug is known), nausea or vomiting (small frequent meals or analgesics may help), hot flashes - flushing or redness (cold clothes and cool environment may help). Report irregular or rapid heartbeat, unresolved nausea or vomiting, numbness of extremities, breast swelling or pain, difficulty breathing, or infection at injection sites. **Pregnancy/breast-feeding precautions:** Do not get pregnant; females must use use barrier contraceptives during and for a time following therapy. Breast-feeding is not recommended.

**Geriatric Considerations:** Leuprolide has the advantage of not increasing risk of atherosclerotic vascular disease, causing swelling of breasts, fluid retention, and thromboembolism as compared to estrogen therapy.

**Additional Information** Some formulations may contain benzyl alcohol.

♦ **Leuprorelin Acetate** *see* Leuprolide *on page 663*

♦ **Leurocristine** *see* Vincristine *on page 1213*

♦ **Leustatin™** *see* Cladribine *on page 278*

## Levamisole (lee VAM i sole)

**U.S. Brand Names** Ergamisol®

**Therapeutic Category** Immune Modulator

**Pregnancy Risk Factor** C

**Lactation** Excretion in breast milk unknown/contraindicated

**Use** Adjuvant treatment with fluorouracil in Dukes stage C colon cancer

**Mechanism of Action/Effect** Clinically, combined therapy with levamisole and 5-fluorouracil has been effective in treating colon cancer patients, whereas demonstrable activity has been demonstrated. Due to the broad range of pharmacologic activities of levamisole, it has been suggested that the drug may act as a biochemical modulator (of fluorouracil, for example, in colon cancer), an effect entirely independent of immune modulation. Further studies are needed to evaluate the mechanisms of action of the drug in cancer patients.

**Contraindications** Hypersensitivity to levamisole or any component

**Warnings** Agranulocytosis can occur asymptomatically and flu-like symptoms can occur without hematologic adverse effects. Frequent hematologic monitoring is necessary. A rare but potentially fatal demyelinating encephalopathy may occur. Pregnancy factor C.

**Drug Interactions**

**Increased Effect/Toxicity:** Increased toxicity/serum levels of phenytoin. Disulfiram-like reaction with alcohol.

**Adverse Reactions**

>10%: Gastrointestinal: Nausea, diarrhea, metallic taste

1% to 10%:

Cardiovascular: Edema

Central nervous system: Fatigue, fever, dizziness, headache, somnolence, depression, nervousness

Dermatologic: Dermatitis, alopecia

Gastrointestinal: Stomatitis, vomiting, anorexia, abdominal pain, constipation

Hematologic: Leukopenia

Neuromuscular & skeletal: Rigors, arthralgia, myalgia, paresthesia

Miscellaneous: Infection

<1% (Limited to important or life-threatening symptoms): Chest pain, seizures, tardive dyskinesia, thrombocytopenia, anemia, granulocytopenia, encephalopathy-like syndrome

**Overdose/Toxicology** Treatment is symptomatic and supportive.

**Pharmacodynamics/Kinetics**

**Half-life Elimination:** 2-6 hours

**Time to Peak:** 1-2 hours

**Metabolism:** Liver

**Excretion:** Urine and feces

**Formulations** Tablet, as base: 50 mg

**Dosing**

**Adults:** Oral: Initial: 50 mg every 8 hours for 3 days, then 50 mg every 8 hours for 3 days every 2 weeks (fluorouracil is always given concomitantly)

**Elderly:** Refer to adult dosing.

**Hepatic Impairment:** May be necessary in patients with liver disease (AUC increased), but no specific guidelines are available. Monitor closely for adverse effects.

**Monitoring Laboratory Tests** CBC with platelet count prior to therapy and weekly prior to treatment, LFTs every 3 months

(Continued)

## Levamisole *(Continued)*

**Additional Nursing Issues**

**Physical Assessment:** See Dosing. Monitor CBC before, during, and after therapy. Monitor and teach patient to monitor for adverse reactions, including opportunistic infections (see above). **Pregnancy risk factor C** - benefits of use should outweigh possible risks. Breast-feeding is contraindicated.

**Patient Information/Instruction:** Take as directed, at regular intervals around-the-clock. Avoid alcohol (may cause disulfiram-like effect). Avoid all aspirin-containing medications. You may experience GI upset (small frequent meals may help); diarrhea (request medication); sensitivity to sun (use sunblock, wear protective clothing, and avoid direct sun); or dizziness, drowsiness, or impaired judgment (use caution when driving, climbing stairs, or engaging in tasks requiring alertness until response to drug is known). You will be more susceptible to infection; avoid crowds or infected persons. Report chills or fever, confusion, persistent or violent vomiting, persistent diarrhea, or respiratory difficulty. **Pregnancy/breast-feeding precautions:** Inform prescriber if you are or intend to be pregnant. Do not breast-feed.

**Related Information**

Fluorouracil *on page 500*


- **Levaquin™** *see* Levofloxacin *on page 669*
- **Levarterenol Bitartrate** *see* Norepinephrine *on page 835*
- **Levate®** *see* Amitriptyline *on page 73*
- **Levatol®** *see* Penbutolol *on page 893*
- **Levbid®** *see* Hyoscyamine *on page 590*
- **Levlen®** *see* Oral Contraceptives *on page 859*
- **Levobunolol** *see* Ophthalmic Agents, Glaucoma *on page 853*
- **Levocabastine** *see page 1282*


## Levodopa (lee voe DOE pa)

**U.S. Brand Names** Dopar®; Larodopa®

**Synonyms** *L*-3-Hydroxytyrosine; *L*-Dopa

**Therapeutic Category** Anti-Parkinson's Agent (Dopamine Agonist)

**Pregnancy Risk Factor** C

**Lactation** Excretion in breast milk unknown

**Use** Treatment of Parkinson's disease; diagnostic agent for growth hormone deficiency

**Mechanism of Action/Effect** Increases dopamine levels in the brain, then stimulates dopaminergic receptors in the basal ganglia to improve the balance between cholinergic and dopaminergic activity

**Contraindications** Hypersensitivity to levodopa or any component; narrow-angle glaucoma; MAO inhibitor therapy; melanomas or any undiagnosed skin lesions

**Warnings** Use with caution in patients with history of myocardial infarction, arrhythmias, asthma, wide-angle glaucoma, or peptic ulcer disease. Sudden discontinuation of levodopa may cause a worsening of Parkinson's disease. Some products may contain tartrazine. Elderly may be more sensitive to CNS effects of levodopa. Pregnancy factor C.

**Drug Interactions**

**Decreased Effect:** Hydantoins (phenytoin, etc) may decrease levodopa effectiveness. Phenothiazines and hypotensive agents may decrease effect of levodopa. Pyridoxine may increase peripheral conversion resulting in decreased levodopa effectiveness.

**Increased Effect/Toxicity:** Increased toxicity with antacids. Monoamine oxidase inhibitors in combination with levodopa may cause hypertensive reactions.

**Food Interactions** Levodopa peak serum concentrations may be decreased if taken with food. High protein diets may decrease the efficacy of levodopa via competition with amino acids in crossing the blood-brain barrier.

**Effects on Lab Values** Levodopa may cause a positive Coombs' test or an elevated uric acid level. See Levodopa and Carbidopa listing.

**Adverse Reactions**

>10%:

- Cardiovascular: Orthostatic hypotension, arrhythmias
- Central nervous system: Dizziness, mental depression, anxiety, confusion, nightmares
- Gastrointestinal: Nausea, vomiting, constipation
- Genitourinary: Dysuria
- Neuromuscular & skeletal: Choreiform and involuntary movements

1% to 10%:

- Central nervous system: Headache
- Gastrointestinal: Anorexia, diarrhea, dry mouth
- Genitourinary: Discoloration of urine
- Neuromuscular & skeletal: Muscle twitching
- Ocular: Eyelid spasms
- Miscellaneous: Discoloration of sweat

<1% (Limited to important or life-threatening symptoms): Duodenal ulcer, GI bleeding, hemolytic anemia

**Overdose/Toxicology** Symptoms of overdose include palpitations, dysrhythmias, spasms, and hypertension. Treatment is supportive. EKG monitoring is warranted.

**Pharmacodynamics/Kinetics**

**Half-life Elimination:** 1.2-2.3 hours

**Time to Peak:** Oral: 1-2 hours

**Metabolism:** Majority of drug is peripherally decarboxylated to dopamine; small amounts of levodopa reach the brain where it is also decarboxylated to active dopamine

**Excretion:** Urine

**Duration:** Variable, usually 6-12 hours

**Formulations**

Capsule: 100 mg, 250 mg, 500 mg

Tablet: 100 mg, 250 mg, 500 mg

**Dosing**

**Adults:** Oral: 500-1000 mg/day in divided doses every 6-12 hours; increase by 100-750 mg/day every 3-7 days until response or total dose of 8000 mg is reached. A significant therapeutic response may not be obtained for 6 months.

**Elderly:** Refer to adult dosing.

**Administration**

**Oral:** Give with meals to decrease GI upset. Sustained release product should not be crushed.

**Additional Nursing Issues**

**Physical Assessment:** Assess effectiveness and interactions of other medications patient may be taking (see Contraindications and Drug Interactions). Monitor therapeutic response (eg, mental status, involuntary movements), and adverse reactions (including levodopa toxicity) at beginning of therapy and periodically throughout therapy (see Warnings/Precautions, Adverse Reactions, and Overdose/Toxicology). Assess knowledge/teach patient appropriate use, interventions to reduce side effects, and adverse symptoms to report. **Pregnancy risk factor C** - benefits of use should outweigh possible risks. Note breast-feeding caution.

**Patient Information/Instruction:** Take exactly as directed; do not change dosage or discontinue without consulting prescriber. Therapeutic effects may take several weeks or months to achieve and you may need frequent monitoring during first weeks of therapy. Take with meals if GI upset occurs, before meals if dry mouth occurs, after eating if drooling or if nausea occurs. Take at the same time each day. Maintain adequate hydration (2-3 L/day of fluids unless instructed to restrict fluid intake); void before taking medication. Do not use alcohol and prescription or OTC sedatives or CNS depressants without consulting prescriber. Urine or perspiration may appear darker. You may experience drowsiness, dizziness, confusion, or vision changes (use caution when driving, climbing stairs, or engaging in tasks requiring alertness until response to drug is known); orthostatic hypotension (use caution when changing position - rising to standing from sitting or lying); increased susceptibility to heat stroke, decreased perspiration (use caution in hot weather - maintain adequate fluids and reduce exercise activity); constipation (increased exercise, fluids, or dietary fruit and fiber may help); dry skin or nasal passages (consult prescriber for appropriate relief); nausea, vomiting, loss of appetite, or stomach discomfort (small frequent meals, frequent mouth care, chewing gum, or sucking lozenges may help). Report unresolved constipation or vomiting; chest pain or irregular heartbeat; difficulty breathing; acute headache or dizziness; CNS changes (hallucination, loss of memory, nervousness, etc); painful or difficult urination; abdominal pain or blood in stool; increased muscle spasticity or rigidity; skin rash; or significant worsening of condition. **Pregnancy/breast-feeding precautions:** Inform prescriber if you are or intend to be pregnant. Consult prescriber if breast-feeding.

**Dietary Issues:** High protein diets may decrease the efficacy of levodopa when used for parkinsonism via competition with amino acids in crossing the blood-brain barrier.

## Levodopa and Carbidopa (lee voe DOE pa & kar bi DOE pa)

**U.S. Brand Names** Sinemet®; Sinemet® CR

**Synonyms** Carbidopa and Levodopa

**Therapeutic Category** Anti-Parkinson's Agent (Dopamine Agonist)

**Pregnancy Risk Factor** C

**Lactation** Excretion in breast milk unknown

**Use** Treatment of parkinsonian syndrome; 50-100 mg/day of carbidopa is needed to block the peripheral conversion of levodopa to dopamine. "On-off" can be managed by giving smaller, more frequent doses of Sinemet® or adding a dopamine agonist or selegiline; when adding a new agent, doses of Sinemet® should usually be decreased.

**Mechanism of Action/Effect** Parkinson's symptoms are due to a lack of striatal dopamine; levodopa circulates in plasma to the blood-brain-barrier (BBB), where it crosses, to be converted by striatal enzymes to dopamine; carbidopa inhibits the peripheral plasma breakdown of levodopa by inhibiting its decarboxylation, and thereby increases available levodopa at the BBB

**Contraindications** Hypersensitivity to levodopa, carbidopa, or any component; narrow-angle glaucoma; MAO inhibitors; do not use in patients with malignant melanoma or undiagnosed skin lesions

**Warnings** Use with caution in patients with history of myocardial infarction, arrhythmias, asthma, wide-angle glaucoma, or peptic ulcer disease. Sudden discontinuation of levodopa may cause a worsening of Parkinson's disease. Some tablets may contain tartrazine. The elderly may be more sensitive to the CNS effects of levodopa. Pregnancy factor C.

(Continued)

## Levodopa and Carbidopa *(Continued)*

**Drug Interactions**

**Decreased Effect:** Decreased effect with hydantoins, pyridoxine. Phenothiazines and hypotensive agents may decrease effects of levodopa.

**Increased Effect/Toxicity:** Increased toxicity with antacids. Monoamine oxidase inhibitors may cause hypertensive reactions. Potential for serotonin syndrome if combined with other serotonergic drugs.

**Effects on Lab Values** False-positive reaction for urinary glucose with Clinitest®; false-negative reaction using Clinistix®; false-positive urine ketones with Acetest®, Ketostix®, Labstix®

**Adverse Reactions**

>10%:

Cardiovascular: Orthostatic hypotension, palpitations, cardiac arrhythmias
Central nervous system: Confusion, nightmares, dizziness, anxiety
Gastrointestinal: Nausea, vomiting, constipation
Neuromuscular & skeletal: Dystonic movements, "on-off", choreiform and involuntary movements
Ocular: Blepharospasm
Renal: Dysuria

1% to 10%:

Central nervous system: Headache
Gastrointestinal: Diarrhea, dry mouth, anorexia
Genitourinary: Discoloration of urine
Neuromuscular & skeletal: Muscle twitching
Ocular: Eyelid spasms
Miscellaneous: Discoloration of sweat

<1% (Limited to important or life-threatening symptoms): Duodenal ulcer, GI bleeding, hemolytic anemia

**Overdose/Toxicology** Symptoms of overdose include palpitations, arrhythmias, spasms; may cause hypertension or hypotension. Treatment is supportive. EKG monitoring is warranted. May precipitate a variety of arrhythmias.

**Pharmacodynamics/Kinetics**

**Protein Binding:** Carbidopa: 36%

**Half-life Elimination:** Carbidopa: 1-2 hours; Levodopa: 1.2-2.3 hours

**Excretion:** Carbidopa: Excreted unchanged; Levodopa: Urine

**Duration:** Variable, 6-12 hours (longer with CR dosage forms)

**Formulations**

Tablet:

10/100: Carbidopa 10 mg and levodopa 100 mg
25/100: Carbidopa 25 mg and levodopa 100 mg
25/250: Carbidopa 25 mg and levodopa 250 mg
Sustained release: Carbidopa 25 mg and levodopa 100 mg; carbidopa 50 mg and levodopa 200 mg

**Dosing**

**Adults:** Oral:

Initial: 25/100 2-4 times/day, increase as necessary to a maximum of 200/2000 mg/day

**Conversion from Sinemet® to Sinemet® CR (50/200):** (Sinemet® [total daily dose of levodopa] / Sinemet® CR)

300-400 mg / 1 tablet twice daily
500-600 mg / 1½ tablets twice daily or one 3 times/day
700-800 mg / 4 tablets in 3 or more divided doses
900-1000 mg / 5 tablets in 3 or more divided doses

Intervals between doses of Sinemet® CR should be 4-8 hours while awake.

**Elderly:** Oral: Initial: 25/100 twice daily, increase as necessary. Sinemet® CR may be used as initial therapy.

**Administration**

**Oral:** Space doses evenly over the waking hours. Give with meals to decrease GI upset. Sustained release product should not be crushed.

**Additional Nursing Issues**

**Physical Assessment:** Assess effectiveness and interactions of other medications patient may be taking (see Contraindications and Drug Interactions). Monitor therapeutic response (eg, mental status, involuntary movements), and adverse reactions (including levodopa toxicity) at beginning of therapy and periodically throughout therapy (see Warnings/Precautions, Adverse Reactions, and Overdose/Toxicology). Assess knowledge/teach patient appropriate use, interventions to reduce side effects, and adverse symptoms to report. **Pregnancy risk factor C** - benefits of use should outweigh possible risks. Note breast-feeding caution.

**Patient Information/Instruction:** Take exactly as directed; do not change dosage or discontinue without consulting prescriber. Therapeutic effects may take several weeks or months to achieve and you may need frequent monitoring during first weeks of therapy. Take with meals if GI upset occurs, before meals if dry mouth occurs, after eating if drooling or if nausea occurs. Take at the same time each day. Maintain adequate hydration (2-3 L/day of fluids unless instructed to restrict fluid intake); void before taking medication. Do not use alcohol and prescription or OTC sedatives or CNS depressants without consulting prescriber. Urine or perspiration may appear darker. You may experience drowsiness, dizziness, confusion, or vision changes (use caution when driving, climbing stairs, or engaging in tasks requiring alertness until response to drug is known); orthostatic hypotension (use caution when changing position - rising to standing from sitting or lying); increased susceptibility to heat stroke, decreased perspiration (use caution in hot weather - maintain adequate fluids and reduce exercise activity); constipation (increased exercise, fluids, or dietary fruit and fiber may help); dry skin or nasal passages (consult prescriber for appropriate relief); nausea, vomiting, loss of appetite, or stomach discomfort (small frequent meals, frequent mouth care, chewing gum, or sucking lozenges may help). Report unresolved constipation or vomiting; chest pain or irregular heartbeat; difficulty breathing; acute headache or dizziness; CNS changes (hallucination, loss of memory, nervousness, etc); painful or difficult urination; abdominal pain or blood in stool; increased muscle spasticity or rigidity; skin rash; or significant worsening of condition. **Pregnancy/ breast-feeding precautions:** Inform prescriber if you are or intend to be pregnant. Consult prescriber if breast-feeding.

**Dietary Issues:** Avoid vitamin products containing vitamin $B_6$ (pyridoxine), which reduces the effectiveness of this medication.

**Geriatric Considerations:** The elderly may be more sensitive to the CNS effects of levodopa.

**Additional Information** 50-100 mg/day of carbidopa is needed to block the peripheral conversion of levodopa to dopamine. "On-off" can be managed by giving smaller, more frequent doses of Sinemet® or adding a dopamine agonist or selegiline; when adding a new agent, doses of Sinemet® should usually be decreased. To avoid fluctuations in levodopa absorption, avoid giving with high protein meals. After a daily levodopa dose of 600-800 mg is reached, some experts recommend adding a dopamine agonist to the regimen, rather than increasing the levodopa dose.

**Related Information**

Levodopa *on page 666*

♦ **Levo-Dromoran®** *see* Levorphanol *on page 671*

## Levofloxacin (lee voe FLOKS a sin)

**U.S. Brand Names** Levaquin™

**Therapeutic Category** Antibiotic, Quinolone

**Pregnancy Risk Factor** C

**Lactation** Enters breast milk/contraindicated

**Use** Acute maxillary sinusitis due to *S. pneumoniae*, *H. influenzae*, or *M. catarrhalis*; acute bacterial exacerbation of chronic bronchitis and community-acquired pneumonia due to *S. aureus*, *S. pneumoniae*, *H. influenzae*, *H. parainfluenzae*, *M. catarrhalis*, *C. pneumoniae*, *L. pneumophila*, *M. pneumoniae*; may be used for uncomplicated skin and skin structure infection due to *S. aureus* or *S. pyogenes*; uncomplicated urinary tract infections caused by susceptible organisms and complicated urinary tract infection due to gram-negative *Enterobacter* sp, including acute pyelonephritis (caused by *E. coli*); although clinical efficacy has been similar between levofloxacin and ofloxacin; levofloxacin is more potent and may be given in lower doses

**Mechanism of Action/Effect** Levofloxacin, a fluorinated quinolone, is a pyridine carboxylic acid derivative which exerts a broad spectrum bactericidal effect. It inhibits DNA gyrase inhibitor, an essential bacterial enzyme that maintains the superhelical structure of DNA. DNA gyrase is required for DNA replication and transcription, DNA repair, recombination, and transposition within the bacteria.

**Contraindications** Hypersensitivity to levofloxacin, any component, or other quinolone

**Warnings** Not recommended in children <18 years of age; other quinolones have caused transient arthropathy in children. CNS stimulation may occur (tremor, restlessness, confusion, and very rarely hallucinations or seizures). Use with caution in patients with known or suspected CNS disorders or renal dysfunction. Prolonged use may result in superinfection. If an allergic reaction (eg, itching, urticaria, dyspnea, pharyngeal or facial edema, loss of consciousness, tingling, cardiovascular collapse) occurs, discontinue the drug immediately. Use caution to avoid possible photosensitivity reactions during and for several days following fluoroquinolone therapy. Pseudomembranous colitis may occur and should be considered in patients who present with diarrhea. Pregnancy factor C.

**Drug Interactions**

**Cytochrome P-450 Effect:** CYP1A2 enzyme inhibitor (minor)

**Decreased Effect:** Decreased absorption with antacids containing aluminum, magnesium, and/or calcium (by up to 98% if given at the same time). Phenytoin serum levels may be reduced by quinolones. Antineoplastic agents may also decrease serum levels of fluoroquinolones.

**Increased Effect/Toxicity:** Minor inhibition of isoenzyme CYP1A2. Quinolones may cause increased levels of caffeine, warfarin, azlocillin, cyclosporine, and theophylline (effect of levofloxacin on theophylline metabolism appears minimal). Azlocillin, cimetidine, and probenecid increases quinolone levels. An increased incidence of seizures may occur with foscarnet.

**Adverse Reactions**

1% to 10%:

Central nervous system: Dizziness, headache, insomnia

Gastrointestinal: Nausea, vomiting, diarrhea, constipation

Neuromuscular & skeletal: Tremor, arthralgia

<1% (Limited to important or life-threatening symptoms): Cardiac failure, hypertension, bradycardia, tachycardia, seizures, elevated transaminases, pseudomembraneous colitis, leukorrhea, granulocytopenia, leukopenia, leukocytosis, thrombocytopenia, jaundice, acute renal failure

**Pharmacodynamics/Kinetics**

**Protein Binding:** 50%

**Distribution:** CSF concentrations ~15% of serum levels; high concentrations are achieved in prostate and gynecologic tissues, sinus, breast milk, and saliva

(Continued)

## Levofloxacin *(Continued)*

**Half-life Elimination:** 6 hours (prolonged in renal impairment)

**Time to Peak:** 1 hour

**Metabolism:** Hepatic, minimal

**Excretion:** Urine

**Formulations**

Infusion, in $D_5W$: 5 mg/mL (50 mL, 100 mL)
Injection: 25 mg/mL (20 mL)
Tablet: 250 mg, 500 mg

**Dosing**

**Adults:** Oral, I.V. (infuse I.V. solution over 60 minutes):

Acute bacterial exacerbation of chronic bronchitis: 500 mg every 24 hours for at least 7 days
Community acquired pneumonia: 500 mg every 24 hours for 7-14 days
Acute maxillary sinusitis: 500 mg every 24 hours for 10-14 days
Uncomplicated skin infections: 500 mg every 24 hours for 7-10 days
Complicated urinary tract infections include acute pyelonephritis: 250 mg every 24 hours for 10 days

**Elderly:** Refer to adult dosing.

**Renal Impairment:**

$Cl_{cr}$ 20-49 mL/minute: Administer 250 mg every 24 hours (initial: 500 mg).
$Cl_{cr}$ 10-19 mL/minute: Administer 250 mg every 48 hours (initial: 500 mg for most infections; 250 mg for renal infections).
Hemodialysis/CAPD: 250 mg every 48 hours (initial: 500 mg)

**Administration**

**I.V.:** Infuse I.V. solution over 60 minutes. Too rapid of infusion can lead to hypotension.

**Stability**

**Storage:** Stable for 72 hours when diluted to 5 mg/mL in a compatible I.V. fluid and stored at room temperature. Stable for 14 days when stored at room temperature. Stable for 6 months when frozen; do not refreeze. Do not thaw in microwave or by bath immersion.

**Compatibility:** Incompatible with mannitol and sodium bicarbonate.

**Monitoring Laboratory Tests** Perform culture and sensitivity studies prior to initiating drug therapy. Monitor CBC periodically during therapy. Monitor renal or hepatic function if therapy is prolonged.

**Additional Nursing Issues**

**Physical Assessment:** Monitor effectiveness of other medications patient may be taking (see Drug Interactions). Monitor adverse reactions and response to therapy. Monitor and teach patient to monitor for signs of opportunistic infection (eg, chills, fever, burning on urination, easy bleeding or bruising, unhealed wounds, vaginal discharge, fuzzy tongue). **Pregnancy risk factor C** - benefits of use should outweigh possible risks. Breast-feeding is contraindicated.

**Patient Information/Instruction:** Oral: Take per recommended schedule, preferably on an empty stomach (1 hour before or 2 hours after meals). Maintain adequate hydration (2-3 L/day of fluids unless instructed to restrict fluid intake). Take complete prescription; do not skip doses. Do not take with antacids. You may experience dizziness, lightheadedness, or confusion; use caution when driving or engaging in tasks that require alertness until response to drug is known. Small frequent meals and frequent mouth care may reduce nausea or vomiting. You may experience photosensitivity; use sunscreen, wear protective clothing and eyewear, and avoid direct sunlight. Report palpitations or chest pain, persistent diarrhea, GI disturbances or abdominal pain, muscle tremor or pain, yellowing of eyes or skin, easy bruising or bleeding, unusual fatigue, fever, chills, signs of infection, or worsening of condition. Report immediately any rash; itching; unusual CNS changes; pain, inflammation, or rupture of tendon; or any facial swelling. **Pregnancy/breast-feeding precautions:** Inform prescriber if you are or intend to get pregnant. Do not breast-feed.

**Geriatric Considerations:** Expanded spectra and once daily dosing. Adjust dose for renal function.

**Additional Information** pH: 3.8-5.8

## Levonorgestrel (LEE voe nor jes trel)

**U.S. Brand Names** Norplant® Implant

**Therapeutic Category** Contraceptive

**Pregnancy Risk Factor** X

**Lactation** Enters breast milk/use caution (AAP rates "compatible")

**Use** Norplant® is a long-term, reversible, method of contraception lasting up to 5 years

**Mechanism of Action/Effect** Ovulation is inhibited and an insufficient luteal phase has also been demonstrated with levonorgestrel administration.

**Contraindications** Women with undiagnosed abnormal uterine bleeding, hemorrhagic diathesis, known or suspected pregnancy, active hepatic disease, active thrombophlebitis, thromboembolic disorders, or known or suspected carcinoma of the breast

**Warnings** Patients presenting with lower abdominal pain should be evaluated for follicular atresia and ectopic pregnancy.

**Drug Interactions**

**Decreased Effect:** The contraceptive effect has been reduced resulting in pregnancy in patients taking carbamazepine or phenytoin.

**Adverse Reactions**

>10%:

Cardiovascular: Swelling of face

Central nervous system: Headache, mood changes, nervousness

Endocrine & metabolic: Amenorrhea, irregular menstrual cycles, menorrhagia, spotting, ovarian enlargement, ovarian cyst formation

Gastrointestinal: Abdominal pain

1% to 10%:

Cardiovascular: Hot flashes

Central nervous system: Dizziness, mental depression, insomnia

Dermatologic: Dermatitis, acne, melasma, loss or gain of body, facial, or scalp hair

Endocrine & metabolic: Hyperglycemia, galactorrhea, breast pain, libido decrease

Gastrointestinal: Nausea, change in appetite, weight gain

Genitourinary: Vaginitis, leukorrhea

Local: Pain or itching at implant site

Neuromuscular & skeletal: Myalgia

<1% (Limited to important or life-threatening symptoms): Thromboembolism

**Overdose/Toxicology** Can result if >6 capsules are *in situ*. Symptoms include uterine bleeding irregularities and fluid retention. Treatment includes removal of all implanted capsules.

**Pharmacodynamics/Kinetics**

**Protein Binding:** Following release from the implant, levonorgestrel enters the blood stream highly bound to sex hormone binding globulin (SHBG), albumin, and alpha$_1$ glycoprotein.

**Half-life Elimination:** 11-45 hours

**Metabolism:** Liver

**Excretion:** Urine

**Formulations** Capsule, subdermal implantation: 36 mg (6s)

**Dosing**

**Adults:** Total administration doses (implanted): 216 mg in 6 capsules which should be implanted during the first 7 days of onset of menses subdermally in the upper arm. Each Norplant® silastic capsule releases 80 mcg of drug/day for 6-18 months, following which a rate of release of 25-30 mcg/day is maintained for ≤5 years. Capsules should be removed by end of 5th year.

**Additional Nursing Issues**

**Physical Assessment:** Monitor for prolonged menstrual bleeding, amenorrhea, irregularity of menses, and other adverse effects (see above). Caution patient about need for annual medical exams. **Pregnancy risk factor X** - ascertain pregnancy status before inserting Norplant®. Note breast-feeding caution.

**Patient Information/Instruction:** Do not attempt to remove implants - see prescriber. You may experience photosensitivity (use sunscreen, wear protective clothing and eyewear, and avoid direct sunlight); dizziness or sleeplessness (use caution when driving or engaging in hazardous tasks until response to drug is known); skin rash, change in skin color, loss of hair, or unusual menses (breakthrough bleeding, irregularity, excessive bleeding - these should resolve after the first month). Report swelling, pain, or excessive feelings of warmth in calves, sudden acute headache, or visual disturbance, unusual nausea or vomiting, and any loss of feeling in arms or legs, unusual menses (if they persist past first month), and irritation at insertion site. **Pregnancy/breast-feeding precautions:** Inform prescriber if pregnant. Consult prescriber if breast-feeding.

♦ **Levonorgestrel and Ethinyl Estradiol** *see* Oral Contraceptives *on page 859*

♦ **Levophed® Injection** *see* Norepinephrine *on page 835*

♦ **Levora®** *see* Oral Contraceptives *on page 859*

## Levorphanol (lee VOR fa nole)

**U.S. Brand Names** Levo-Dromoran®

**Synonyms** Levorphan Tartrate

**Therapeutic Category** Analgesic, Narcotic

**Pregnancy Risk Factor** B/D (if used for prolonged periods or in high doses at term)

**Lactation** Excretion in breast milk unknown/not recommended

**Use** Relief of moderate to severe pain; parenterally for preoperative sedation and as an adjunct to nitrous oxide/oxygen anesthesia; 2 mg levorphanol produces analgesia comparable to that produced by 10 mg of morphine

**Mechanism of Action/Effect** Levorphanol tartrate is a synthetic opioid agonist that is classified as a morphinan derivative. Opioids interact with stereospecific opioid receptors in various parts of the central nervous system and other tissues.

**Contraindications** Hypersensitivity to levorphanol or any component; pregnancy (if used for prolonged periods or in high doses at term)

**Warnings** Use with caution in patients with hypersensitivity reactions to other phenanthrene derivative opioid agonists (morphine, hydrocodone, hydromorphone, levorphanol, oxycodone, oxymorphone); respiratory diseases including asthma, emphysema, COPD or severe liver or renal insufficiency. Some preparations contain sulfites which may cause allergic reactions. May be habit-forming. Dextromethorphan has equivalent antitussive activity but has much lower toxicity in accidental overdose. Elderly may be particularly susceptible to the CNS depressant and constipating effects of narcotics.

**Drug Interactions**

**Increased Effect/Toxicity:** CNS depression is enhanced with coadministration of other CNS depressants.

(Continued)

## Levorphanol *(Continued)*

### Adverse Reactions

>10%:

Cardiovascular: Palpitations, hypotension, peripheral vasodilation
Central nervous system: CNS depression, fatigue, drowsiness, dizziness
Dermatologic: Pruritus
Gastrointestinal: Nausea, vomiting
Neuromuscular & skeletal: Weakness

1% to 10%:

Cardiovascular: Tachycardia or bradycardia
Central nervous system: Nervousness, headache, restlessness, anorexia, malaise, confusion
Gastrointestinal: Stomach cramps, dry mouth, constipation, biliary tract spasm, anorexia
Endocrine & metabolic: Antidiuretic hormone release
Genitourinary: Decreased urination, urinary tract spasm
Local: Pain at injection site
Ocular: Miosis, blurred vision
Respiratory: Respiratory depression

<1% (Limited to important or life-threatening symptoms): Paralytic ileus or toxic megacolon

**Overdose/Toxicology** Symptoms of overdose include CNS depression, respiratory depression, miosis, apnea, pulmonary edema, and convulsions. Naloxone, 2 mg I.V. with repeat administration as necessary up to a total dose of 10 mg, can be used to reverse opiate effects.

### Pharmacodynamics/Kinetics

**Half-life Elimination:** 12-16 hours
**Metabolism:** Liver
**Excretion:** Urine
**Onset:** 10-60 minutes
**Duration:** 4-8 hours

### Formulations

Levorphanol tartrate:
Injection: 2 mg/mL (1 mL, 10 mL)
Tablet: 2 mg

### Dosing

**Adults:**
Oral: 2 mg every 6-24 hours as needed
I.V.: 2-3 mg every 4-6 hours
S.C.: 2 mg, up to 3 mg if necessary, every 6-8 hours

**Elderly:** Refer to adult dosing.

**Hepatic Impairment:** Reduction is necessary in patients with liver disease.

### Administration

**Oral:** For lactating women, administer 4-6 hours prior to breast-feeding.
**I.V.:** Inject 3 mg over 4-5 minutes

### Stability

**Storage:** Store at room temperature. Protect from freezing.

**Compatibility:** I.V. is incompatible when mixed with aminophylline, barbiturates, heparin, methicillin, phenytoin, or sodium bicarbonate.

### Additional Nursing Issues

**Physical Assessment:** Assess other medications patient may be taking for additive or adverse interactions (see Drug Interactions). Monitor for effectiveness of pain relief and monitor for signs of overdose (see above). Monitor blood pressure, CNS and respiratory status, and degree of sedation at beginning of therapy and at regular intervals with long-term use. May cause physical and/or psychological dependence. For inpatients, implement safety measures (eg, side rails up, call light within reach, instructions to call for assistance, etc). Assess knowledge/teach patient appropriate use (if self-administered). Teach patient to monitor for adverse reactions (see Adverse Reactions), adverse reactions to report, and appropriate interventions to reduce side effects. Discontinue slowly after prolonged use. **Pregnancy risk factor B/D** - see Pregnancy Risk Factor for cautious use. Breast-feeding is not recommended.

**Patient Information/Instruction:** If self-administered, use exactly as directed (do not increase dose or frequency); may cause physical and/or psychological dependence. While using this medication, do not use alcohol and other prescription or OTC medications (especially sedatives, tranquilizers, antihistamines, or pain medications) without consulting prescriber. Maintain adequate hydration (2-3 L/day of fluids unless instructed to restrict fluid intake). May cause hypotension, dizziness, drowsiness, impaired coordination, or blurred vision (use caution when driving, climbing stairs, or changing position - rising from sitting or lying to standing, or when engaging in tasks requiring alertness until response to drug is known); loss of appetite, nausea, or vomiting (frequent mouth care, small frequent meals, chewing gum, or sucking lozenges may help); constipation (increased exercise, fluids, or dietary fruit and fiber may help - if constipation remains an unresolved problem, consult prescriber about use of stool softeners). Report chest pain, slow or rapid heartbeat, acute dizziness, or persistent headache; swelling of extremities or unusual weight gain; changes in urinary elimination; acute headache; back or flank pain or spasms; blurred vision; skin rash; or shortness of breath. **Pregnancy/breast-feeding precautions:** Inform prescriber if you are or intend to be pregnant. Breast-feeding is not recommended.

**Geriatric Considerations:** The elderly may be particularly susceptible to the CNS depressant and constipating effects of narcotics.

**Related Information**

Narcotic/Opioid Analgesic Comparison *on page 1396*

- **Levorphan Tartrate** *see* Levorphanol *on page 671*
- **Levo-T™** *see* Levothyroxine *on this page*
- **Levothroid®** *see* Levothyroxine *on this page*

## Levothyroxine (lee voe thye ROKS een)

**U.S. Brand Names** Eltroxin®; Levo-T™; Levothroid®; Levoxyl®; Synthroid®

**Synonyms** *l*-Thyroxine Sodium; $T_4$ Thyroxine Sodium

**Therapeutic Category** Thyroid Product

**Pregnancy Risk Factor** A

**Lactation** Enters breast milk/compatible

**Use** Replacement or supplemental therapy in hypothyroidism

**Mechanism of Action/Effect** It is believed the thyroid hormone exerts its many metabolic effects through control of DNA transcription and protein synthesis

**Contraindications** Hypersensitivity to levothyroxine sodium or any component; recent myocardial infarction or thyrotoxicosis; uncorrected adrenal insufficiency

**Warnings** Ineffective for weight reduction. High doses may produce serious or even life-threatening toxic effects particularly when used with some anorectic drugs. Use with caution and reduce dosage in patients with angina pectoris or other cardiovascular disease. Some formulations of levothyroxine tablets contain tartrazine dye which may cause allergic reactions in susceptible individuals. Use cautiously in the elderly since they may be more likely to have compromised cardiovascular functions. Patients with adrenal insufficiency, myxedema, diabetes mellitus and insipidus may have symptoms exaggerated or aggravated. Thyroid replacement requires periodic assessment of thyroid status. Chronic hypothyroidism predisposes patients to coronary artery disease.

**Drug Interactions**

**Decreased Effect:** Phenytoin may decrease levothyroxine levels. Cholestyramine taken at the same time may decrease absorption of levothyroxine. Levothyroxine may decrease effect of oral sulfonylureas.

**Increased Effect/Toxicity:** Levothyroxine may potentiate the hypoprothrombinemic effect of oral anticoagulants. Tricyclic antidepressants (TCAs) coadministered with levothyroxine may increase potential for toxicity of both drugs.

**Food Interactions** Taking levothyroxine with enteral nutrition may cause reduced bioavailability and may lower serum thyroxine levels leading to signs or symptoms of hypothyroidism.

**Effects on Lab Values** Many drugs may have effects on thyroid function tests: para-aminosalicylic acid, aminoglutethimide, amiodarone, barbiturates, carbamazepine, chloral hydrate, clofibrate, colestipol, corticosteroids, danazol, diazepam, estrogens, ethionamide, fluorouracil, I.V. heparin, insulin, lithium, methadone, methimazole, mitotane, nitroprusside, oxyphenbutazone, phenylbutazone, PTU, perphenazine, phenytoin, propranolol, salicylates, sulfonylureas, and thiazides.

**Adverse Reactions** <1% (Limited to important or life-threatening symptoms): Palpitations, cardiac arrhythmias, tachycardia, chest pain, alopecia, shortness of breath

**Overdose/Toxicology** Chronic overdose is treated by withdrawal of the drug. Massive overdose may require beta-blockers for increased sympathomimetic activity. Chronic overdose may cause hyperthyroidism, weight loss, nervousness, sweating, tachycardia, insomnia, heat intolerance, menstrual irregularities, palpitations, psychosis, and fever. Acute overdose may cause fever, hypoglycemia, CHF, and unrecognized adrenal insufficiency.

Reduce dose or temporarily discontinue therapy. Hypothalamic-pituitary-thyroid axis will return to normal in 6-8 weeks. Serum $T_4$ levels do not correlate well with toxicity. Provide general supportive care.

**Pharmacodynamics/Kinetics**

**Half-life Elimination:** 6-7 days (euthyroid); 9-10 days (hypothyroid); 3-4 days (hyperthyroid)

**Time to Peak:** 2-4 hours

**Metabolism:** Liver

**Excretion:** Feces and urine

**Onset:**

Onset of therapeutic effect: Oral: 3-5 days; I.V. Within 6-8 hours

Peak effect: I.V.: Within 24 hours

**Formulations**

Levothyroxine sodium:

Powder for injection, lyophilized: 200 mcg/vial (6 mL, 10 mL); 500 mcg/vial (6 mL, 10 mL)

Tablet: 25 mcg, 50 mcg, 75 mcg, 88 mcg, 100 mcg, 112 mcg, 125 mcg, 150 mcg, 175 mcg, 200 mcg, 300 mcg

**Dosing**

**Adults:**

Oral: 12.5-50 mcg/day to start, then increase by 25-50 mcg/day at intervals of 2-4 weeks; average adult dose: 100-200 mcg/day

I.M., I.V.: 50% of the oral dose

Myxedema coma or stupor: I.V.: 200-500 mcg one time, then 100-300 mcg the next day if necessary

Thyroid suppression therapy: Oral: 2-6 mcg/kg/day for 7-10 days

(Continued)

## Levothyroxine *(Continued)*

**Elderly:** Dosage should be individualized and response monitored both clinically and with appropriate laboratory (TSH, $T_4$) (see Additional Information).

Oral: 12.5-25 mcg/day to start, then increase by 25-50 mcg/day at intervals of 2-4 weeks; average adult dose: 100-200 mcg/day; many elderly can be safely initiated on 25 mcg/day

I.M., I.V.: Refer to adult dosing.

Myxedema coma or stupor: I.V.: Refer to adult dosing.

Thyroid suppression therapy: Refer to adult dosing.

**Administration**

**I.V.:** Parenteral: Give by direct I.V. infusion over a 2- to 3-minute period.

**I.V. Detail:** Dilute vial with 5 mL normal saline. Use immediately after reconstitution. I.V. form must be prepared immediately prior to administration. Should not be admixed with other solutions.

**Stability**

**Storage:** Protect tablets from light.

**Reconstitution:** Dilute vial with 5 mL normal saline. Use immediately after reconstitution. I.V. form must be prepared immediately prior to administration. Should not be admixed with other solutions. Reconstituted solutions should be used immediately and any unused portions discarded.

**Compatibility:** Do not mix I.V. solution with other I.V. infusion solutions.

**Monitoring Laboratory Tests** Thyroid function (serum thyroxine, thyrotropin concentrations), resin triiodothyronine uptake ($RT_3U$), free thyroxine index (FTI), $T_4$, TSH, TSH may be elevated during the first few months of thyroid replacement despite patients being clinically euthyroid. In cases where $T_4$ remains low and TSH is within normal limits, an evaluation of "free" (unbound) $T_4$ is needed to evaluate further increase in dosage.

**Additional Nursing Issues**

**Physical Assessment:** Assess and adjust other medications patient may be taking, if necessary. Assess appropriate laboratory tests prior to beginning therapy and periodically for long-term therapy. **Important:** See Effects on Lab Values above when considering results of thyroid function tests. Monitor vital signs on a regular basis. Monitor regularly for signs or symptoms of hypo-/hyperthyroidism (be aware of effects of aging on "typical" indications of hyper-/hypothyroidism).

**Patient Information/Instruction:** Thyroid replacement therapy is generally for life. Take as directed, in the morning before breakfast. Do not change brands and do not discontinue without consulting prescriber. Consult prescriber if drastically increasing or decreasing intake of goitrogenic food (eg, asparagus, cabbage, peas, turnip greens, broccoli, spinach, brussels sprouts, lettuce, soybeans). Report chest pain, rapid heart rate, palpitations, heat intolerance, excessive sweating, increased nervousness, agitation, or lethargy.

**Geriatric Considerations:** The elderly do not have a change in serum thyroxine ($T_4$) associated with aging; however, plasma $T_3$ concentrations are decreased 25% to 40% in the elderly. There is not a compensatory rise in thyrotropin suggesting that lower $T_3$ is not reacted upon as a deficiency by the pituitary. This indicates a slightly lower than normal dosage of thyroid hormone replacement is usually sufficient in older patients than in younger adult patients. TSH must be monitored since insufficient thyroid replacement (elevated TSH) is a risk for coronary artery disease and excessive replacement (low TSH) may cause signs of hyperthyroidism and excessive bone loss. Some clinicians suggest levothyroxine is the drug of choice for replacement therapy.

**Additional Information** Levothroid® tablets contain lactose. The 100 mcg tablet may contain tartrazine dye. Check current labeling for formulation ingredients.

To convert doses: Levothyroxine 0.05-0.06 mg is equivalent to 60 mg thyroid USP; 60 mg thyroglobulin; 4.5 mg thyroid strong; 1 grain (60 mg) liotrix.

**Related Information**

Thyroid *on page 1130*


- **Levoxyl®** *see* Levothyroxine *on previous page*
- **Levsin®** *see* Hyoscyamine *on page 590*
- **Levsinex®** *see* Hyoscyamine *on page 590*
- **Levsin/SL®** *see* Hyoscyamine *on page 590*
- **Lexxel™** *see* Enalapril and Felodipine *on page 419*
- **LH-RH** *see* Gonadorelin *on page 542*
- ***L*-Hyoscyamine Sulfate** *see* Hyoscyamine *on page 590*
- **Librax®** *see* Clidinium and Chlordiazepoxide *on page 281*
- **Libritabs®** *see* Chlordiazepoxide *on page 250*
- **Librium®** *see* Chlordiazepoxide *on page 250*
- **Lice-Enz® Shampoo** *see page 1294*
- **Lida-Mantle HC® Topical** *see* Lidocaine and Hydrocortisone *on page 677*
- **Lidex®** *see* Topical Corticosteroids *on page 1152*
- **Lidex-E®** *see* Topical Corticosteroids *on page 1152*


## Lidocaine (LYE doe kane)

**U.S. Brand Names** Anestacon®; Dermaflex® Gel; Dilocaine®; Dr Scholl's® Cracked Heel Relief Cream [OTC]; Duo-Trach®; LidoPen® Auto-Injector; Nervocaine®; Octocaine®; Solarcaine® Aloe Extra Burn Relief [OTC]; Xylocaine®; Zilactin-L® [OTC]

**Synonyms** Lignocaine Hydrochloride

**Therapeutic Category** Analgesic, Topical; Antiarrhythmic Agent, Class I-B; Local Anesthetic

**Pregnancy Risk Factor** C

**Lactation** Enters breast milk (small amounts)/compatible

**Use** Local anesthetic and acute treatment of ventricular arrhythmias due to myocardial infarction, cardiac manipulation, digitalis intoxication; topical local anesthetic; drug of choice for ventricular ectopy, ventricular tachycardia, ventricular fibrillation; for pulseless VT or VF preferably give **after** defibrillation and epinephrine; control of premature ventricular contractions, wide-complex PSVT

**Mechanism of Action/Effect** Class IB antiarrhythmic; suppresses automaticity of conduction tissue by increasing electrical stimulation threshold of ventricles, HIS-Purkinje system, and spontaneous depolarization of ventricles during diastole by direct action on tissues; blocks both initiation and conduction of nerve impulses by decreasing the neuronal membrane's permeability to sodium ions, which results in inhibition of depolarization with resultant blockade of conduction

**Contraindications** Hypersensitivity to amide-type local anesthetics; patients with Adams-Stokes syndrome, or with severe S-A, A-V, or intraventricular heart block (without a pacemaker)

**Warnings** Avoid use of preparations containing preservatives for spinal or epidural (including caudal) anesthesia. Use extreme caution in patients with hepatic disease, heart failure, marked hypoxia, severe respiratory depression, hypovolemia or shock, incomplete heart block or bradycardia, and atrial fibrillation.

Due to decreases in Phase I metabolism and possibly decrease in splanchnic perfusion with age, there may be a decreased clearance or increased half-life in the elderly and increased risk for CNS side effects and cardiac effects.

Pregnancy factor C.

**Drug Interactions**

**Cytochrome P-450 Effect:** CYP3A3/4 enzyme substrate

**Increased Effect/Toxicity:** Concomitant cimetidine or propranolol may result in increased serum concentrations of lidocaine resulting in toxicity. Effect of succinylcholine may be enhanced.

**Adverse Reactions**

**Topical** (dose-related and may result in high plasma levels):

1% to 10%:

Dermatologic: Angioedema, contact dermatitis

Local: Burning, stinging

<1% (Limited to important or life-threatening symptoms): Methemoglobinemia in infants and children

**Parenteral:**

1% to 10%:

Cardiovascular: Hypotension

Central nervous system: Positional headache

Miscellaneous: Shivering

<1% (Limited to important or life-threatening symptoms): Heart block, arrhythmias, cardiovascular collapse, dyspnea, respiratory depression or arrest

**Parenteral: Local:**

1% to 10%:

Cardiovascular: Cardiac arrest, hypotension, bradycardia, palpitations

Central nervous system: Seizures, restlessness, anxiety, dizziness

Gastrointestinal: Nausea, vomiting

Neuromuscular & skeletal: Weakness

Ocular: Blurred vision

Otic: Tinnitus

Respiratory: Apnea

**Overdose/Toxicology** Lidocaine has a narrow therapeutic index. Severe toxicity may occur at doses slightly above the therapeutic range, especially in conjunction with other antiarrhythmic drugs. Symptoms of overdose include sedation, confusion, coma, seizures, respiratory arrest, and cardiac toxicity (sinus arrest, A-V block, asystole, and hypotension). QRS and Q-T intervals are usually normal, although they may be prolonged after massive overdose. Other effects include dizziness, paresthesia, tremor, ataxia, and GI disturbance. Treatment is supportive.

**Pharmacodynamics/Kinetics**

**Protein Binding:** 60% to 80%; binds to $alpha_1$ acid glycoprotein

**Distribution:** $V_d$: Alterable by many patient factors; decreased in CHF and liver disease

**Half-life Elimination:** Biphasic: Increased with CHF, liver disease, shock, severe renal disease; Initial: 7-30 minutes; Terminal: 1.5-2 hours

**Time to Peak:** 0.5-2 hours

**Metabolism:** Liver

**Onset:** Single bolus dose: 45-90 seconds

**Duration:** 10-20 minutes

**Formulations**

Lidocaine hydrochloride:

Cream: 2% (56 g)

Injection: 0.5% [5 mg/mL] (50 mL); 1% [10 mg/mL] (2 mL, 5 mL, 10 mL, 20 mL, 30 mL, 50 mL); 1.5% [15 mg/mL] (20 mL); 2% [20 mg/mL] (2 mL, 5 mL, 10 mL, 20 mL, 30 mL, 50 mL); 4% [40 mg/mL] (5 mL); 10% [100 mg/mL] (10 mL); 20% [200 mg/mL] (10 mL, 20 mL)

Injection:

I.M. use: 10% [100 mg/mL] (3 mL, 5 mL)

(Continued)

## Lidocaine *(Continued)*

Direct I.V.: 1% [10 mg/mL] (5 mL, 10 mL); 20 mg/mL (5 mL)
I.V. admixture, preservative free: 4% [40 mg/mL] (25 mL, 30 mL); 10% [100 mg/mL] (10 mL); 20% [200 mg/mL] (5 mL, 10 mL)
I.V. infusion, in $D_5W$: 0.2% [2 mg/mL] (500 mL); 0.4% [4 mg/mL] (250 mL, 500 mL, 1000 mL); 0.8% [8 mg/mL] (250 mL, 500 mL)
Gel, topical: 2% (30 mL); 2.5% (15 mL)
Liquid, topical: 2.5% (7.5 mL)
Liquid, viscous: 2% (20 mL, 100 mL)
Ointment, topical: 2.5% [OTC], 5% (35 g)
Solution, topical: 2% (15 mL, 240 mL); 4% (50 mL)

**Dosing**

**Adults:**

Topical: Apply to affected area as needed; maximum: 3 mg/kg/dose; do not repeat within 2 hours.

Injectable local anesthetic: Varies with procedure, degree of anesthesia needed, vascularity of tissue, duration of anesthesia required, and physical condition of patient; maximum: 4.5 mg/kg/dose; do not repeat within 2 hours.

Antiarrhythmic:

I.V.: 1-1.5 mg/kg bolus over 2-3 minutes; may repeat doses of 0.5-0.75 mg/kg in 5-10 minutes up to a total of 3 mg/kg; continuous infusion: 1-4 mg/minute

I.V. (2 g/250 mL $D_5W$) infusion rates (infusion pump should be used for I.V. infusion administration):
1 mg/minute: 7 mL/hour
2 mg/minute: 15 mL/hour
3 mg/minute: 21 mL/hour
4 mg/minute: 30 mL/hour

Ventricular fibrillation (after defibrillation and epinephrine): Initial: 1.5 mg/kg, may repeat boluses as above; follow with continuous infusion after return of perfusion.

Prevention of ventricular fibrillation: I.V.: Initial bolus: 0.5 mg/kg; repeat every 5-10 minutes to a total dose of 2 mg/kg

Refractory ventricular fibrillation: Repeat 1.5 mg/kg bolus may be given 3-5 minutes after initial dose.

**Endotracheal: 2-2.5 times the I.V. dose**

**Decrease dose in patients with CHF, shock, or hepatic disease.**

**Elderly:** Refer to adult dosing.

**Renal Impairment:** Not dialyzable (0% to 5%) by hemo- or peritoneal dialysis; supplemental dose is not necessary.

**Hepatic Impairment:** Reduce dose in acute hepatitis and decompensated cirrhosis by 50%.

**Administration**

**I.V.:** Use microdrip (60 gtt/mL) or infusion pump to administer an accurate dose.

**I.V. Detail:** Local thrombophlebitis may occur in patients receiving prolonged I.V. infusions.

**Stability**

**Storage:** Lidocaine injection is stable at room temperature. Stability of parenteral admixture at room temperature (25°C) is the expiration date on premixed bag; out of overwrap stability is 30 days.

**Reconstitution:** Standard diluent: 2 g/250 mL $D_5W$

**Monitoring Laboratory Tests** I.V.: Serum lidocaine levels. Therapeutic levels range from 1.5-5 mcg/mL; >6 mcg/mL is usually toxic.

**Additional Nursing Issues**

**Physical Assessment:** Assess other medications patient may be taking for adverse interactions (see Drug Interactions).

Local anesthetic: Monitor for effectiveness of anesthesia, and adverse reactions (see Adverse Reactions). Dermatologic: Monitor for return of sensation. Oral: Use caution to prevent gagging or choking. Avoid food or drink for 1 hour. Teach patient adverse reactions to report; use and teach appropriate interventions to promote safety.

Antiarrhythmic: I.V.: Monitor EKG, blood pressure, and respirations closely and continually. Keep patient supine to reduce hypotensive effects. Assess frequently for adverse reactions or signs of toxicity (see Adverse Reactions and Overdose/Toxicology). Teach patient adverse reactions to report and appropriate interventions to promote safety.

**Pregnancy risk factor C** - benefits of use should outweigh possible risks.

**Patient Information/Instruction:** I.V.: You will be monitored during infusion. Do not get up without assistance. Report dizziness, numbness, double vision, nausea, pain or burning at infusion site, nightmares, hearing strange noises, seeing unusual visions, or difficulty breathing.

Dermatologic: You will experience decreased sensation to pain, heat, or cold in the area and/or decreased muscle strength (depending on area of application) until effects wear off; use necessary caution to reduce incidence of possible injury until full sensation returns. Report irritation, pain, burning at injection site, persistent numbness, tingling, swelling; restlessness, dizziness, acute weakness; blurred vision; ringing in ears; or difficulty breathing.

Oral: Lidocaine can cause numbness of tongue, cheeks, and throat. Do not eat or drink for 1 hour after use. Take small sips of water at first to ensure that you can swallow without difficulty. Your tongue and mouth may be numb; use caution avoid biting yourself. Immediately report swelling of face, lips, or tongue.

**Pregnancy precautions:** Inform prescriber if you are pregnant.

**Geriatric Considerations:** Due to decreases in Phase I metabolism and possibly decrease in splanchnic perfusion with age, there may be a decreased clearance or increased half-life in the elderly and increased risk for CNS side effects and cardiac effects.

**Related Information**

Antiarrhythmic Drug Classification Comparison *on page 1366*
Peak and Trough Guidelines *on page 1331*

## Lidocaine and Epinephrine (LYE doe kane & ep i NEF rin)

**U.S. Brand Names** Octocaine® With Epinephrine; Xylocaine® With Epinephrine

**Synonyms** Epinephrine and Lidocaine

**Therapeutic Category** Local Anesthetic

**Pregnancy Risk Factor** B

**Lactation** Enters breast milk/compatible

**Use** Local infiltration anesthesia; peripheral nerve block

**Formulations**

Injection with epinephrine:

Epinephrine 1:200,000: Lidocaine hydrochloride 0.5% [5 mg/mL] (50 mL); 1% [10 mg/mL] (30 mL); 1.5% [15 mg/mL] (5 mL, 10 mL, 30 mL); 2% [20 mg/mL] (20 mL)

Epinephrine 1:100,000: Lidocaine hydrochloride 1% [10 mg/mL] (20 mL, 50 mL); 2% [20 mg/mL] (1.8 mL, 20 mL, 50 mL)

Epinephrine 1:50,000: Lidocaine hydrochloride 2% [20 mg/mL] (1.8 mL)

**Dosing**

**Adults:** Dosage varies with the anesthetic procedure, degree of anesthesia needed, vascularity of tissue, duration of anesthesia required, and physical condition of patient.

**Elderly:** Refer to adult dosing.

**Additional Nursing Issues**

**Physical Assessment:** See individual components listed in Related Information.

**Patient Information/Instruction:** See individual components listed in Related Information.

**Additional Information** The injection formulation contains sulfites.

**Related Information**

Epinephrine *on page 424*
Lidocaine *on page 674*

## Lidocaine and Hydrocortisone (LYE doe kane & hye droe KOR ti sone)

**U.S. Brand Names** Lida-Mantle HC® Topical

**Synonyms** Hydrocortisone and Lidocaine

**Therapeutic Category** Anesthetic/Corticosteroid

**Pregnancy Risk Factor** B (lidocaine); C (hydrocortisone)

**Lactation** For topical use

**Use** Topical anti-inflammatory and anesthetic for skin disorders

**Formulations** Cream: Lidocaine 3% and hydrocortisone 0.5% (15 g, 30 g)

**Dosing**

**Adults:** Topical: Apply 2-4 times/day

**Elderly:** Refer to adult dosing.

**Additional Nursing Issues**

**Physical Assessment:** See individual components listed in Related Information. **Pregnancy risk factor C** (hydrocortisone) - benefits of use should outweigh possible risks.

**Patient Information/Instruction:** See individual components listed in Related Information. **Pregnancy precautions:** Inform prescriber if you are on intend to get pregnant.

**Related Information**

Hydrocortisone *on page 578*
Lidocaine *on page 674*

## Lidocaine and Prilocaine (LYE doe kane & PRIL oh kane)

**U.S. Brand Names** EMLA®

**Synonyms** Prilocaine and Lidocaine

**Therapeutic Category** Analgesic, Topical; Anesthetic, Topical; Local Anesthetic

**Pregnancy Risk Factor** B

**Lactation** Enters breast milk/compatible

**Use** Topical anesthetic for use on normal intact skin to provide local analgesia for minor procedures such as I.V. cannulation or venipuncture; useful for painful procedures such as lumbar puncture and skin graft harvesting

**Mechanism of Action/Effect** Local anesthetic action occurs by stabilization of neuronal membranes and inhibiting the ionic fluxes required for the initiation and conduction of impulses

**Contraindications** Hypersensitivity to amide type anesthetic agents (eg, lidocaine, prilocaine, dibucaine, mepivacaine, bupivacaine, etidocaine); hypersensitivity to any components of EMLA® cream or Tegaderm®

(Continued)

## Lidocaine and Prilocaine *(Continued)*

**Drug Interactions**

**Increased Effect/Toxicity:** Class I antiarrhythmic drugs (tocainide, mexiletine): Effects are additive and potentially synergistic. Prilocaine may enhance the effect of other drugs known to induce methemoglobinemia.

**Adverse Reactions**

1% to 10%:

Dermatologic: Angioedema, contact dermatitis

Local: Burning, stinging

<1% (Limited to important or life-threatening symptoms): Bradycardia, hypotension, shock, edema, methemoglobinemia in infants and children, respiratory depression, bronchospasm

**Pharmacodynamics/Kinetics**

**Protein Binding:** Lidocaine: 70%; Prilocaine: 55%

**Distribution:** Both cross the blood-brain barrier

**Half-life Elimination:**

Lidocaine: 65-150 minutes, prolonged with cardiac or hepatic dysfunction

Prilocaine: 10-150 minutes, prolonged in hepatic or renal dysfunction

**Metabolism:** Lidocaine: Liver; Prilocaine: Liver and kidneys

**Onset:** 1 hour for sufficient dermal analgesia; Peak effect: 2-3 hours

**Duration:** 1-2 hours after removal of the cream

**Formulations** Cream: Lidocaine 2.5% and prilocaine 2.5% [2 Tegaderm® dressings] (5 g, 30 g)

**Dosing**

**Adults:** Apply a thick layer (2.5 g/site ~½ of a 5 g tube) of cream to each designated site of intact skin

**Elderly:** Refer to adult dosing.

**Renal Impairment:** Smaller areas of treatment are recommended for patients with renal dysfunction.

**Hepatic Impairment:** Smaller areas of treatment are recommended for patients with hepatic dysfunction.

**Administration**

**Topical:** For external use only. Choose two application sites available for intravenous access. Apply a thick layer (2.5 g/site ~½ of a 5 g tube) of cream to each designated site of intact skin. Cover each site with the occlusive dressing (Tegaderm®). Mark the time on the dressing. **Allow at least 1 hour for optimum therapeutic effect.** Remove the dressing and wipe off excess EMLA® cream (gloves should be worn). **Smaller areas of treatment are recommended for debilitated patients.**

**Stability**

**Storage:** Store at room temperature.

**Additional Nursing Issues**

**Physical Assessment:** Use on intact skin only (see Administration - Topical). Monitor for effectiveness of anesthesia, and adverse reactions (see Adverse Reactions). Monitor for return of sensation.

**Patient Information/Instruction:** This drug will block sensation to the applied area. Report irritation, pain, burning at application site.

**Breast-feeding Issues:** Usual infiltration doses of lidocaine and prilocaine given to nursing mothers has not been shown to affect the health of the nursing infant.

**Related Information**

Lidocaine *on page 674*

- **LidoPen® Auto-Injector** *see* Lidocaine *on page 674*
- **Lidox®** *see* Clidinium and Chlordiazepoxide *on page 281*
- **Lifenal** *see* Diclofenac *on page 358*
- **Lignocaine Hydrochloride** *see* Lidocaine *on page 674*
- **Limbitrol®** *see* Amitriptyline and Chlordiazepoxide *on page 75*
- **Linctus Codeine Blac** *see* Codeine *on page 299*
- **Linctus With Codeine Phosphate** *see* Codeine *on page 299*

## Lindane (LIN dane)

**U.S. Brand Names** G-well®; Scabene®

**Synonyms** Benzene Hexachloride; Gamma Benzene Hexachloride; Hexachlorocyclohexane

**Therapeutic Category** Antiparasitic Agent, Topical; Pediculocide; Scabicidal Agent

**Pregnancy Risk Factor** B - see Pregnancy Issues

**Lactation** Enters breast milk/compatible

**Use** Treatment of scabies (*Sarcoptes scabiei*), *Pediculus capitis* (head lice), and *Pediculus pubis* (crab lice)

**Mechanism of Action/Effect** Directly absorbed by parasites and ova through the exoskeleton; stimulates the nervous system resulting in seizures and death of parasitic arthropods

**Contraindications** Hypersensitivity to lindane or any component

**Warnings** Use with caution in infants and small children, and patients with a history of seizures. Avoid contact with face, eyes, mucous membranes, and urethral meatus. Because of the potential for systemic absorption and CNS side effects, lindane should be used with caution. Not considered a drug of first choice; consider permethrin or crotamiton agent first.

**Drug Interactions**

**Increased Effect/Toxicity:** Oil-based hair dressing may increase potential for toxicity of lindane.

**Adverse Reactions** <1% (Limited to important or life-threatening symptoms): Cardiac arrhythmia, dizziness, restlessness, seizures, headache, ataxia, eczematous eruptions, contact dermatitis, skin and adipose tissue may act as repositories, nausea, vomiting, aplastic anemia, hepatitis, burning and stinging, hematuria, pulmonary edema

**Overdose/Toxicology** Symptoms of overdose include vomiting, restlessness, ataxia, seizures, arrhythmias, pulmonary edema, hematuria, and hepatitis. The drug is absorbed through the skin, mucous membranes, and GI tract, and has occasionally caused serious CNS, hepatic, and renal toxicity when used excessively for prolonged periods, or with accidental ingestion. If ingested, perform gastric lavage and general supportive measures.

**Pharmacodynamics/Kinetics**

**Distribution:** Stored in body fat and accumulates in brain; skin and adipose tissue may act as repositories

**Metabolism:** Liver

**Excretion:** Urine and feces

**Formulations**

Cream: 1% (60 g, 454 g)

Lotion: 1% (60 mL, 473 mL, 4000 mL)

Shampoo: 1% (60 mL, 473 mL, 4000 mL)

**Dosing**

**Adults:** Topical:

Scabies: Apply a thin layer of lotion or cream and massage it on skin from the neck to the toes (head to toe in infants). For adults, bathe and remove the drug after 8-12 hours; repeat treatment in 7 days if lice or nits are still present. For infants, wash off 6 hours after application.

Pediculosis, capitis and pubis: 15-30 mL of shampoo is applied and lathered for 4-5 minutes. Rinse hair thoroughly and comb with a fine tooth comb to remove nits. Repeat treatment in 7 days if lice or nits are still present.

**Elderly:** Refer to adult dosing. Use with caution; see Geriatric Considerations.

**Administration**

**Oral:** Never administer orally.

**Topical:** For topical use only. Apply to dry, cool skin; do not apply to face or eyes.

**Additional Nursing Issues**

**Physical Assessment:** Assess head, hair, and skin surfaces for presence of lice and nits. Assess knowledge/teach patient appropriate application and use and adverse symptoms (see Adverse Reactions) to report.

**Patient Information/Instruction:** For external use only. Do not apply to face and avoid getting in eyes. Do not apply immediately after hot soapy bath. Apply from neck to toes. Bathe to remove drug after 8-12 hours. Repeat in 7 days if lice or nits are still present. Clothing and bedding must be washed in hot water or dry cleaned to kill nits. Wash combs and brushes with lindane shampoo and thoroughly rinse. May need to treat all members of household and all sexual contacts concurrently. Report if condition persists or infection occurs.

**Geriatric Considerations:** Because of the potential for systemic absorption and CNS side effects, lindane should be used with caution. Not considered a drug of first choice; consider permethrin or crotamiton agent first.

**Breast-feeding Issues:** Small amounts are excreted in breast milk; however, the amounts are approximately equal to the amounts absorbed by an infant treated topically.

**Pregnancy Issues:** There are no well controlled studies in pregnant women; treat no more than twice during a pregnancy.

♦ **Lioresal®** *see* Baclofen *on page 131*

## Liothyronine (lye oh THYE roe neen)

**U.S. Brand Names** Cytomel® Oral; Triostat™ Injection

**Synonyms** Sodium *L*-Triiodothyronine; $T_3$ Thyronine Sodium

**Therapeutic Category** Thyroid Product

**Pregnancy Risk Factor** A

**Lactation** Enters breast milk (small amounts)/compatible

**Use** Replacement or supplemental therapy in hypothyroidism, management of nontoxic goiter, chronic lymphocytic thyroiditis, as an adjunct in thyrotoxicosis and as a diagnostic aid; **levothyroxine is recommended for chronic therapy**; although previously thought to benefit cardiac patients with severely reduced fractions, liothyronine injection is no longer considered beneficial

**Mechanism of Action/Effect** Primary active compound is $T_3$ (tri-iodothyronine), which may be converted from $T_4$ (thyroxine) and then circulates throughout the body to influence growth and maturation of various tissues; exact mechanism of action is unknown; however, it is believed the thyroid hormone exerts its many metabolic effects through control of DNA transcription and protein synthesis; involved in normal metabolism, growth, and development; promotes gluconeogenesis, increases utilization and mobilization of glycogen stores, and stimulates protein synthesis, increases basal metabolic rate

**Contraindications** Hypersensitivity to liothyronine sodium or any component; recent myocardial infarction or thyrotoxicosis; undocumented or uncorrected adrenal insufficiency

**Warnings** For I.V. use only. Ineffective for weight reduction. High doses may produce serious or even life-threatening toxic effects particularly when used with some anorectic

(Continued)

## Liothyronine *(Continued)*

drugs. Use with extreme caution in patients with angina pectoris or other cardiovascular disease (including hypertension) or coronary artery disease. Use with caution in elderly patients since they may be more likely to have compromised cardiovascular function. Patients with adrenal insufficiency, myxedema, diabetes mellitus and insipidus may have symptoms exaggerated or aggravated. Thyroid replacement requires periodic assessment of thyroid status. Chronic hypothyroidism predisposes patients to coronary artery disease.

**Drug Interactions**

**Decreased Effect:** Cholestyramine resin may decrease absorption. Oral sulfonylurea requirements are increased. Estrogens may increase thyroid requirements.

**Increased Effect/Toxicity:** Increased oral anticoagulant effects.

**Effects on Lab Values** Many drugs may have effects on thyroid function tests: para-aminosalicylic acid, aminoglutethimide, amiodarone, barbiturates, carbamazepine, chloral hydrate, clofibrate, colestipol, corticosteroids, danazol, diazepam, estrogens, ethionamide, fluorouracil, I.V. heparin, insulin, lithium, methadone, methimazole, mitotane, nitroprusside, oxyphenbutazone, phenylbutazone, PTU, perphenazine, phenytoin, propranolol, salicylates, sulfonylureas, and thiazides.

**Adverse Reactions** <1% (Limited to important or life-threatening symptoms): Palpitations, tachycardia, cardiac arrhythmias, chest pain, alopecia, shortness of breath

**Overdose/Toxicology** Chronic overdose may cause hyperthyroidism, weight loss, nervousness, sweating, tachycardia, insomnia, heat intolerance, menstrual irregularities, palpitations, psychosis, and fever. Acute overdose may cause fever, hypoglycemia, CHF, unrecognized adrenal insufficiency.

Reduce dose or temporarily discontinue therapy. Normal hypothalamic-pituitary-thyroid axis will return to normal in 6-8 weeks. Serum $T_4$ levels do not correlate well with toxicity. In massive acute ingestion, reduce GI absorption and give general supportive care. Excessive adrenergic activity (tachycardia) requires propranolol 1-3 mg I.V. over 10 minutes or 80-160 mg orally/day.

**Pharmacodynamics/Kinetics**

**Half-life Elimination:** 16-49 hours

**Metabolism:** In the liver to inactive compounds

**Excretion:** Urine

**Onset:** Within 24-72 hours

**Duration:** Up to 72 hours

**Formulations**

Liothyronine sodium:

Injection: 10 mcg/mL (1 mL)

Tablet: 5 mcg, 25 mcg, 50 mcg

**Dosing**

**Adults:**

Hypothyroidism: Oral: 25 mcg/day increase by 12.5-25 mcg/day every 1-2 weeks to a maximum of 100 mcg/day

$T_3$ suppression test: Oral: 75-100 mcg/day for 7 days; use lowest dose for elderly

Myxedema coma: I.V.: 25-50 mcg

Patients with known or suspected cardiovascular disease: 10-20 mcg

**Note:** Normally, at least 4 hours should be allowed between doses to adequately assess therapeutic response and no more than 12 hours should elapse between doses to avoid fluctuations in hormone levels. Oral therapy should be resumed as soon as the clinical situation has been stabilized and the patient is able to take oral medication. If levothyroxine rather than liothyronine sodium is used in initiating oral therapy, the prescriber should bear in mind that there is a delay of several days in the onset of levothyroxine activity and that I.V. therapy should be discontinued gradually.

**Elderly:** Hypothyroidism: Oral: Initial: 5 mcg/day, increase by 5 mcg/day every 1-2 weeks; usual maintenance dose: 25-75 mcg/day (see Additional Information).

**Administration**

**Oral:** When switching to tablets, discontinue the injectable, initiate oral therapy at a low dosage, and increase gradually according to response.

**I.V.:** For I.V. use only; **do not administer I.M. or S.C.** Administer doses at least 4 hours, and no more than 12 hours, apart. Resume oral therapy as soon as the clinical situation has been stabilized and the patient is able to take oral medication. If levothyroxine is used for oral therapy, there is a delay of several days in the onset of activity; therefore, discontinue I.V. therapy gradually.

**Stability**

**Storage:** Vials must be stored under refrigeration at 2°C to 8°C (36°F to 46°F).

**Monitoring Laboratory Tests** $T_3$, $T_4$, TSH. TSH may be elevated during the first few months of thyroid replacement despite patients being clinically euthyroid. In cases where $T_4$ remains low and TSH is within normal limits, an evaluation of "free" (unbound) $T_4$ is needed to evaluate further increase in dosage.

**Additional Nursing Issues**

**Physical Assessment:** Monitor laboratory results and vital signs prior to therapy, frequently during early therapy or when changing dosage, and at regular intervals during long-term therapy. Assess and teach patient signs or symptoms of hyper-/hypothyroidism and signs to report.

**Patient Information/Instruction:** Take as directed; do not change brands of medication or discontinue without consulting prescriber. Do not change diet without consulting prescriber. Report chest pain, increased heartbeat, palpitations, excessive weight gain or loss, change in level of energy (increased or decreased), excessive sweating, or intolerance to heat.

**Geriatric Considerations:** Elderly do not have a change in serum thyroxine associated with aging; however, plasma $T_3$ concentrations are decreased 25% to 40% in the elderly. There is not a compensatory rise in thyrotropin suggesting that lower $T_3$ is not reacted upon as a deficiency by the pituitary. This indicates a slightly lower than normal dosage of thyroid hormone replacement is usually sufficient in older patients than in younger adult patients. TSH must be monitored since insufficient thyroid replacement (elevated TSH) is a risk for coronary artery disease and excessive replacement (low TSH) may cause signs of hyperthyroidism and excessive bone loss.

**Additional Information** 15-37.5 mcg is equivalent to 50-60 mcg levothyroxine, 60 mg thyroid USP, 45 mg Thyroid Strong®, and 60 mg thyroglobulin.


- **Liovistin™** *see page 1282*
- **Lipancreatin** *see* Pancrelipase *on page 882*
- **Lipase, Protease, and Amylase** *see* Pancrelipase *on page 882*
- **Lipid-Lowering Agents Comparison** *see page 1393*
- **Lipitor®** *see* Atorvastatin *on page 117*
- **Lipocin** *see* Fat Emulsion *on page 471*
- **Liposomal Amphotericin B** *see* Amphotericin B (Liposomal) *on page 88*
- **Liposyn®** *see* Fat Emulsion *on page 471*
- **Lipovite®** *see page 1294*
- **Liquaemin®** *see* Heparin *on page 558*
- **Liquibid®** *see* Guaifenesin *on page 548*
- **Liqui-Char® [OTC]** *see* Charcoal *on page 243*
- **Liquid Antidote** *see* Charcoal *on page 243*
- **Liquid Pred®** *see* Prednisone *on page 962*
- **Liquifilm®** *see page 1282*
- **Liquifilm® Forte Solution** *see page 1294*
- **Liquifilm® Tears Solution** *see page 1294*
- **Liroken** *see* Diclofenac *on page 358*


## Lisinopril (lyse IN oh pril)

**U.S. Brand Names** Prinivil®; Zestril®

**Therapeutic Category** Angiotensin-Converting Enzyme (ACE) Inhibitors

**Pregnancy Risk Factor** C/D (2nd and 3rd trimesters)

**Lactation** Excretion in breast milk unknown (similar drug captopril is compatible)

**Use** Treatment of hypertension, either alone or in combination with other antihypertensive agents; adjunctive therapy in treatment of CHF (afterload reduction); treatment of hemodynamically stable patients within 24 hours of acute myocardial infarction, to improve survival; treatment of acute myocardial infarction within 24 hours in hemodynamically stable patients to improve survival

**Mechanism of Action/Effect** Competitive inhibitor of angiotensin-converting enzyme (ACE); prevents conversion of angiotensin I to angiotensin II, a potent vasoconstrictor; results in lower levels of angiotensin II which causes an increase in plasma renin activity and a reduction in aldosterone secretion

**Contraindications** Hypersensitivity to lisinopril, any component, or other ACE inhibitors; pregnancy (2nd and 3rd trimesters)

**Warnings** Use with caution and modify dosage in patients with renal impairment (decrease dosage) (especially renal artery stenosis), severe congestive heart failure, or with coadministered diuretic therapy. Severe hypotension may occur in patients who are sodium and/or volume depleted, initiate lower doses and monitor closely when starting therapy in these patients. Pregnancy factor C/D (2nd and 3rd trimesters).

**Drug Interactions**

**Decreased Effect:** Rifampin may decrease the effect of ACE inhibitors. Antacids may decrease the bioavailability of ACE inhibitors, may be more likely to occur with captopril, separate administration times by 1-2 hours. NSAIDs, specifically indomethacin, may reduce the hypotensive effects of ACE inhibitors. More likely to occur in low renin or volume dependent hypertensive patients.

**Increased Effect/Toxicity:** Diuretics have additive hypotensive effects with ACE inhibitors. Probenecid increases blood levels of captopril which may occur in other ACE inhibitors. Phenothiazines taken with ACE inhibitors may increase the pharmacologic effects of the ACE inhibitor. Allopurinol and ACE inhibitors may cause a higher risk of hypersensitivity reaction when taken concurrently. Digoxin and ACE inhibitors may result in elevated serum digoxin levels. Lithium and ACE inhibitors may result in elevated serum levels of lithium with symptoms of toxicity. Potassium supplements or potassium-sparing diuretics with ACE inhibitors may result in elevated serum potassium levels.

**Effects on Lab Values** May cause false-positive results in urine acetone determinations using sodium nitroprusside reagent; ↑ potassium (S), serum creatinine/BUN

**Adverse Reactions**

1% to 10%:

Cardiovascular: Hypotension, chest pain

Central nervous system: Dizziness, headache, fatigue, muscle weakness

Dermatologic: Rash

Gastrointestinal: Diarrhea, vomiting, nausea

Renal: Increased BUN/serum creatinine

Respiratory: Upper respiratory symptoms, cough, dyspnea

(Continued)

## Lisinopril *(Continued)*

<1% (Limited to important or life-threatening symptoms): Flushing, myocardial infarction, chest pain pectoris, orthostatic hypotension, rhythm disturbances, cerebrovascular accident, tachycardia, peripheral edema, vasculitis, palpitations, syncope, neutropenia, bone marrow suppression, anemia, hepatitis, azotemia, bronchitis, sinusitis, pharyngeal pain, asthma, bronchospasm, eosinophilic pneumonitis

**Overdose/Toxicology** Mild hypotension has been the primary toxic effect seen with acute overdose. Bradycardia may also occur; hyperkalemia occurs even with therapeutic doses, especially in patients with renal insufficiency and those taking NSAIDs. Treatment and is symptomatic and supportive.

**Pharmacodynamics/Kinetics**

**Half-life Elimination:** 11-12 hours

**Metabolism:** Liver

**Excretion:** Urine

**Onset:** 1 hour; Peak hypotensive effect: Oral: Within 6 hours

**Duration:** 24 hours

**Formulations** Tablet: 2.5 mg, 5 mg, 10 mg, 20 mg, 40 mg

**Dosing**

**Adults:** Oral:

Initial: 10 mg/day; increase doses 5-10 mg/day at 1- to 2-week intervals; maximum daily dose: 40 mg.

Patients taking diuretics should have them discontinued 2-3 days prior to initiating lisinopril if possible. Restart diuretic after blood pressure is stable if needed. In patients with hyponatremia (<130 mEq/L), start dose at 2.5 mg/day.

Acute myocardial infarction (within 24 hours in hemodynamically stable patients): 5 mg immediately, then 5 mg at 24 hours, 10 mg at 48 hours, and 10 mg every day thereafter for 6 weeks. Patients should continue to receive standard treatments such as thrombolytics, aspirin, and beta-blockers.

**Elderly:** Oral:

Initial: 2.5-5 mg/day; increase doses 2.5-5 mg/day at 1- to 2-week intervals; maximum daily dose: 40 mg.

Patients taking diuretics should have them discontinued 2-3 days prior to initiating lisinopril if possible. Restart diuretic after blood pressure is stable if needed. In patients with hyponatremia (<130 mEq/L), start dose at 2.5 mg/day (see Renal Impairment).

**Renal Impairment:**

$Cl_{cr}$ 10-50 mL/minute: Administer 50% to 75% of normal dose.

$Cl_{cr}$ <10 mL/minute: Administer 25% to 50% of normal dose.

Dialyzable (50%)

**Administration**

**Oral:** Watch for hypotensive effects within 1-3 hours of first dose or new higher dose.

**Monitoring Laboratory Tests** CBC, renal function tests, electrolytes, WBC, potassium

**Additional Nursing Issues**

**Physical Assessment:** Assess effectiveness and interactions of other medications (see Drug Interactions). See Warnings/Precautions and Contraindications for use cautions. Monitor effectiveness of therapy, laboratory tests, and adverse response on a regular basis during therapy, eg, postural (see Adverse Reactions and Overdose/Toxicology). Assess knowledge/teach patient appropriate use, possible side effects and appropriate interventions, and adverse symptoms to report. **Pregnancy risk factor C/D** - see Pregnancy Risk Factor - assess knowledge/teach appropriate use of barrier contraceptives. See Pregnancy Issues.

**Patient Information/Instruction:** Take exactly as directed; do not discontinue without consulting prescriber. Take first dose at bedtime. This drug does not eliminate need for diet or exercise regimen as recommended by prescriber. Do not take potassium supplements or salt substitutes containing potassium without consulting prescriber. May cause dizziness, fainting, lightheadedness (use caution when driving or engaging in tasks that require alertness until response to drug is known); postural hypotension (use caution when rising from lying or sitting position or climbing stairs); nausea, vomiting, abdominal pain, dry mouth, or transient loss of appetite (small frequent meals, frequent mouth care, sucking lozenges, or chewing gum may help) - report if these persist. Report chest pain or palpitations; mouth sores; fever or chills; skin rash; numbness, tingling, or pain in muscles; difficulty in breathing or unusual cough; or other persistent adverse reactions. **Pregnancy precautions:** Do not get pregnant while taking this medication; use appropriate barrier contraceptive measures.

**Geriatric Considerations:** Due to frequent decreases in glomerular filtration (also creatinine clearance) with aging, elderly patients may have exaggerated responses to ACE inhibitors. Differences in clinical response due to hepatic changes are not observed. ACE inhibitors may be preferred agents in elderly patients with congestive heart failure and diabetes mellitus. Diabetic proteinuria is reduced and insulin sensitivity is enhanced. In general, the side effect profile is favorable in the elderly and causes little or no CNS confusion. Use lowest dose recommendations initially.

**Pregnancy Issues:** ACE inhibitors can cause fetal injury or death if taken during the 2nd or 3rd trimester. Discontinue ACE inhibitors as soon as pregnancy is detected. ACE inhibitors should not be used if patient is sexually active and not using contraceptives.

**Related Information**

ACE Inhibitors and Angiotensin Antagonists Comparison *on page 1362*

## Lisinopril and Hydrochlorothiazide

(lyse IN oh pril & hye droe klor oh THYE a zide)

**U.S. Brand Names** Prinzide® 10-12.5; Prinzide® 20-12.5; Prinzide® 20-25; Zestoretic® 10-12.5; Zestoretic® 20-12.5; Zestoretic® 20-25

**Synonyms** Hydrochlorothiazide and Lisinopril

**Therapeutic Category** Antihypertensive Agent, Combination

**Pregnancy Risk Factor** C/D (2nd and 3rd trimesters)

**Lactation**

Hydrochlorothiazide: Compatible

Lisinopril: Excretion in breast milk unknown

**Use** Treatment of hypertension

**Formulations**

Tablet:

Lisinopril 10 mg and hydrochlorothiazide 12.5 mg

[12.5]-Lisinopril 20 mg and hydrochlorothiazide 12.5 mg

[25]-Lisinopril 20 mg and hydrochlorothiazide 25 mg

**Dosing**

**Adults:** Oral: Initial: 10/12.5 or 20/12.5 with further increases of either or both components could depend on clinical response.

**Elderly:** Refer to adult dosing.

**Renal Impairment:** Dosage adjustments should be made with caution. Usual regimens of therapy need not be adjusted as long as patient's $Cl_{cr}$ >30 mL/minute. In patients with more severe renal impairment, loop diuretics are preferred.

**Additional Nursing Issues**

**Physical Assessment:** See individual components listed in Related Information. **Pregnancy risk factor C/D** - see Pregnancy Risk Factor - assess knowledge/instruct patient on need to use appropriate contraceptive measures and the need to avoid pregnancy. Note breast-feeding caution.

**Patient Information/Instruction:** See individual components listed in Related Information. **Pregnancy/breast-feeding precautions:** Inform prescriber if you are or intend to be pregnant. Consult prescriber if breast-feeding.

**Related Information**

Hydrochlorothiazide *on page 566*

Lisinopril *on page 681*

♦ **Listermint® With Fluoride** *see page 1294*

♦ **Lithane®** *see* Lithium *on this page*

♦ **Lithellm® 300** *see* Lithium *on this page*

## Lithium (LITH ee um)

**U.S. Brand Names** Eskalith®; Eskalith CR®; Lithane®; Lithobid®; Lithonate®; Lithotabs®

**Therapeutic Category** Lithium

**Pregnancy Risk Factor** D

**Lactation** Enters breast milk/contraindicated

**Use** Management of acute manic episodes, bipolar disorders, and depression

**Mechanism of Action/Effect** Alters cation transport across cell membrane in nerve and muscle cells and influences reuptake of serotonin and/or norepinephrine

**Contraindications** Hypersensitivity to lithium or any component; severe cardiovascular or renal disease; pregnancy

**Warnings** Lithium toxicity is closely related to serum levels and can occur at therapeutic doses. Serum lithium determinations are required to monitor therapy. Use with caution in patients with cardiovascular or thyroid disease, severe debilitation, dehydration or sodium depletion, or in patients receiving diuretics. Some elderly patients may be extremely sensitive to the effects of lithium. See dosing and therapeutic levels.

**Drug Interactions**

**Decreased Effect:** Decreased effect with xanthines (eg, theophylline, caffeine).

**Increased Effect/Toxicity:** Increased effect/toxicity of CNS depressants, alfentanil, iodide salts. Lithium may induce a hypothyroid effect, more likely to occur in patients receiving thyroid replacement therapy. Increased toxicity with thiazide diuretics (dose may need to be reduced by 30%), NSAIDs, haloperidol, phenothiazines (neurotoxicity), neuromuscular blockers, carbamazepine, fluoxetine, and ACE inhibitors. Potential for serotonin syndrome if combined with other serotonergic drugs.

**Food Interactions** Lithium serum concentrations may be increased if taken with food.

**Effects on Lab Values** ↑ calcium (S), glucose, magnesium, potassium (S); ↓ thyroxine (S)

**Adverse Reactions**

>10%:

Endocrine & metabolic: Polydipsia, stress

Gastrointestinal: Nausea, diarrhea, impaired taste

Neuromuscular & skeletal: Tremor

1% to 10%:

Central nervous system: Drowsiness

Dermatologic: Rash

Gastrointestinal: Bloated feeling, weight gain

Neuromuscular: Muscle twitching, weakness

<1% (Limited to important or life-threatening symptoms): Hypothyroidism, goiter, diabetes insipidus, nonspecific nephron atrophy, renal tubular acidosis, leukocytosis

**Overdose/Toxicology** Symptoms of overdose include sedation, confusion, tremor, joint pain, visual changes, seizures, and coma. There is no specific antidote for lithium

(Continued)

## Lithium *(Continued)*

poisoning. For acute ingestion following initiation of essential overdose management, begin correction of fluid and electrolyte imbalance. Hemodialysis and whole bowel irrigation is the treatment of choice for severe intoxications; charcoal is ineffective.

**Pharmacodynamics/Kinetics**

**Distribution:** Crosses the placenta

**Half-life Elimination:** 18-24 hours; can increase to more than 36 hours in the elderly or in patients with renal impairment

**Time to Peak:** Nonsustained release product: Within 0.5-2 hours following oral absorption

**Metabolism:** Not metabolized

**Excretion:** Urine and feces

**Formulations**

Lithium carbonate:

Capsule: 150 mg, 300 mg, 600 mg

Tablet: 300 mg

Tablet, controlled release: 450 mg (Eskalith CR®)

Tablet, slow release: 300 mg (Lithobid®)

Lithium citrate:

Syrup: 300 mg/5 mL (5 mL, 10 mL, 480 mL)

**Dosing**

**Adults:** Monitor serum concentrations and clinical response (efficacy and toxicity) to determine proper dose.

Oral: 300-600 mg 3-4 times/day; usual maximum maintenance dose: 2.4 g/day or 450-900 mg of sustained release twice daily

**Elderly:** Monitor serum concentrations and clinical response (efficacy and toxicity) to determine proper dose. Adjust for renal impairment.

Oral: Initial: 300 mg twice daily; increase weekly in increments of 300 mg/day, monitoring levels; rarely need to go >900-1200 mg/day.

**Renal Impairment:**

$Cl_{cr}$ 10-50 mL/minute: Administer 50% to 75% of normal dose.

$Cl_{cr}$ <10 mL/minute: Administer 25% to 50% of normal dose.

Dialyzable (50% to 100%)

**Administration**

**Oral:** Give with meals to decrease GI upset.

**Monitoring Laboratory Tests** Serum lithium every 3-4 days during initial therapy. Monitor renal, hepatic, thyroid, and cardiovascular function; fluid status; serum electrolytes; CBC with differential, urinalysis.

Levels should be obtained twice weekly until both patient's clinical status and levels are stable then levels may be obtained every 1-2 months.

Timing of serum samples: Draw trough just before next dose

Therapeutic levels:

Acute mania: 0.6-1.2 mEq/L (SI: 0.6-1.2 mmol/L)

Protection against future episodes in most patients with bipolar disorder: 0.8-1 mEq/L (SI: 0.8-1.0 mmol/L); a higher rate of relapse is described in subjects who are maintained at <0.4 mEq/L (SI: 0.4 mmol/L)

Elderly patients can usually be maintained at lower end of therapeutic range (0.6-0.8 mEq/L)

Toxic concentration: >2 mEq/L (SI: >2 mmol/L)

Adverse effect levels:

GI complaints/tremor: 1.5-2 mEq/L

Confusion/somnolence: 2-2.5 mEq/L

Seizures/death: >2.5 mEq/L

**Additional Nursing Issues**

**Physical Assessment:** Assess effectiveness and interactions of other medications (see Drug Interactions). See Contraindications and Warnings/Precautions for cautious use. Monitor laboratory results at beginning of therapy, when adjusting dose, and periodically thereafter (see above). Monitor effectiveness of therapy and adverse reactions at beginning of therapy and periodically with long-term use. (**Note:** Lithium has a very small window of safety (TI) - see Adverse Reactions). Assess knowledge/teach patient appropriate use, interventions to reduce side effects, and importance of reporting adverse symptoms promptly. **Pregnancy risk factor D** - assess knowledge/teach appropriate use of barrier contraceptives. Breast-feeding is contraindicated.

**Patient Information/Instruction:** Take exactly as directed; do not change dosage without consulting prescriber. Do not crush or chew tablets or capsules. Maintain adequate fluid intake (2-3 L/day of fluids unless instructed to restrict fluid intake) especially in summer. Frequent blood test and monitoring will be necessary. You may experience decreased appetite or altered taste sensation (small frequent meals may help maintain nutrition); or drowsiness or dizziness, especially during early therapy (use caution when driving or engaging in tasks requiring alertness until response to drug is known). Immediately report unresolved diarrhea, abrupt changes in weight, muscular tremors or lack of coordination, fever, or changes in urinary volume. **Pregnancy/breast-feeding precautions:** Do not get pregnant while taking this medication; use appropriate barrier contraceptive measures. Do not breast-feed.

Dietary: Avoid changes in sodium content (eg, low sodium diets); reduction of sodium can increase lithium toxicity. Limit caffeine intake (diuresis can increase lithium toxicity).

**Geriatric Considerations:** Some elderly patients may be extremely sensitive to the effects of lithium. Initial doses need to be adjusted for renal function in the elderly; thereafter, adjust doses based upon serum concentrations and response.

**Additional Information** Lithium carbonate: Eskalith®, Lithane®, Lithobid®, Lithonate®, Lithotabs®

Carbonate 150 mg = 4.06 mEq lithium
Carbonate 300 mg = 8.12 mEq lithium
Carbonate 450 mg = 16.24 mEq lithium
Citrate 300 mg = 8 mEq lithium

**Related Information**

Peak and Trough Guidelines *on page 1331*


- **Lithobid®** *see* Lithium *on page 683*
- **Lithonate®** *see* Lithium *on page 683*
- **Lithotabs®** *see* Lithium *on page 683*
- **LKV-Drops® [OTC]** *see* Vitamin, Multiple *on page 1219*
- **8-*L*-Lysine Vasopressin** *see* Lypressin *on page 701*
- **LMD®** *see* Dextran *on page 351*
- **LoCHOLEST®** *see* Cholestyramine Resin *on page 262*
- **LoCHOLEST® Light** *see* Cholestyramine Resin *on page 262*
- **Locoid®** *see* Hydrocortisone *on page 578*
- **Locoid®** *see* Topical Corticosteroids *on page 1152*
- **Lodimol** *see* Dipyridamole *on page 383*
- **Lodine®** *see* Etodolac *on page 462*
- **Lodine® Retard** *see* Etodolac *on page 462*
- **Lodine® XL** *see* Etodolac *on page 462*
- **Lodoxamide Tromethamine** *see page 1282*
- **Loestrin®** *see* Oral Contraceptives *on page 859*
- **Loestrin® Fe** *see* Oral Contraceptives *on page 859*
- **Lofene®** *see* Diphenoxylate and Atropine *on page 382*
- **Logen®** *see* Diphenoxylate and Atropine *on page 382*
- **Logesic** *see* Diclofenac *on page 358*
- **Logimax** *see* Felodipine *on page 474*
- **Lomanate®** *see* Diphenoxylate and Atropine *on page 382*


## Lomefloxacin (loe me FLOKS a sin)

**U.S. Brand Names** Maxaquin®

**Therapeutic Category** Antibiotic, Quinolone

**Pregnancy Risk Factor** C

**Lactation** Excretion in breast milk unknown/contraindicated

**Use** Quinolone antibiotic for skin and skin structure, lower respiratory and urinary tract infections, and sexually transmitted diseases

**Mechanism of Action/Effect** Inhibits DNA-gyrase in susceptible organisms thereby inhibits relaxation of supercoiled DNA and promotes breakage of DNA strands. DNA gyrase (topoisomerase II), is an essential bacterial enzyme that maintains the superhelical structure of DNA and is required for DNA replication and transcription, DNA repair, recombination, and transposition.

**Contraindications** Hypersensitivity to lomefloxacin or other members of the quinolone group such as nalidixic acid, oxolinic acid, cinoxacin, norfloxacin, ofloxacin, and ciprofloxacin; avoid use in children <18 years of age due to association of other quinolones with transient arthropathies

**Warnings** Use with caution in patients with epilepsy or other CNS diseases which could predispose them to seizures. Pregnancy factor C.

**Drug Interactions**

**Decreased Effect:** Decreased absorption with antacids containing aluminum, magnesium, and/or calcium (by up to 98% if given at the same time).

**Increased Effect/Toxicity:** Quinolones can cause elevated levels of caffeine, warfarin, cyclosporine, and theophylline. Azlocillin, imipenem, cimetidine and probenecid may increase lomefloxacin serum levels.

**Food Interactions** Lomefloxacin peak serum levels may be prolonged if taken with food.

**Adverse Reactions**

>10%:

Central nervous system: Dizziness or lightheadedness, headache, nervousness, drowsiness, insomnia

Gastrointestinal: Nausea, diarrhea, vomiting, abdominal pain

1% to 10%: Dermatologic: Photosensitivity

<1% (Limited to important or life-threatening symptoms): Stevens-Johnson syndrome, anemia, increased liver enzymes, interstitial nephritis, shortness of breath

**Overdose/Toxicology** Symptoms of overdose include acute renal failure and seizures. Treatment is supportive; not removed by peritoneal or hemodialysis.

**Pharmacodynamics/Kinetics**

**Protein Binding:** 20%

**Half-life Elimination:** 5-7.5 hours

**Excretion:** Urine

**Formulations** Tablet, as hydrochloride: 400 mg

(Continued)

## Lomefloxacin *(Continued)*

**Dosing**

**Adults:** Oral:

Lower respiratory and urinary tract infections (UTI): 400 mg once daily for 10-14 days

Urinary tract infection (UTI) due to susceptible organisms:

Uncomplicated cystitis caused by *Eschericia coli*: Female: 400 mg once daily for 3 successive days

Uncomplicated cystitis caused by *Klebsiella pneumoniae, Proteus mirabilis*, or *Staphylococcus saprophyticus*: Female: 400 mg once daily for 10 successive days

Complicated UTI caused by *Eschericia coli, Klebsiella pneumoniae, Proteus mirabilis*, or *Pseudomonas aeruginosa*: 400 mg once daily for 14 successive days

Surgical prophylaxis: 400 mg 2-6 hours before surgery

Uncomplicated gonorrhea: 400 mg as a single dose

**Elderly:** No adjustment necessary for $Cl_{cr}$ ≥40 mL/minute. Follow renal adjustments for patients with reduced renal function.

**Renal Impairment:**

$Cl_{cr}$ 10-40 mL/minute: Initial loading dose = 400 mg; followed by 200 mg once daily maintenance dose

Hemodialysis: Use loading dose of 400 mg; followed by 200 mg once daily for treatment duration.

**Administration**

**Oral:** Take 1 hour before or 2 hours after meals.

**Monitoring Laboratory Tests** Perform culture and sensitivity studies prior to initiating therapy to determine the causative organism and its susceptibility to lomefloxacin. Monitor CBC, renal and hepatic function periodically if therapy is prolonged.

**Additional Nursing Issues**

**Physical Assessment:** Assess for previous history of allergic reactions. Monitor or teach patient to monitor and report allergic reactions (eg, rash, urticaria, pruritus, chills, joint pain, facial edema, respiratory difficulty). These can occur days after therapy is initiated. Monitor or teach patient to monitor and report opportunistic infections (eg, fever, chills, vaginal itching or foul-smelling vaginal discharge, oral thrush, easy bruising). **Pregnancy risk factor C** - benefits of use should outweigh possible risks. Breast-feeding is contraindicated.

**Patient Information/Instruction:** Take as directed, preferably on an empty stomach 1 hour before or 2 hours after meals. Complete entire prescription even if feeling better. Maintain adequate hydration (2-3 L/day of fluids unless instructed to restrict fluid intake). You may experience dizziness or drowsiness; use caution when driving or engaging in tasks that require alertness until response to drug is known. You may experience photosensitivity (use sunscreen, wear protective clothing and eyewear, and avoid direct sunlight). Report any signs of opportunistic infection (eg, fever, chills, vaginal itching or foul-smelling vaginal discharge, oral thrush, easy bruising). Report immediately any signs of allergic reaction (eg, rash, itching or tingling of skin); join pain; difficulty breathing; CNS changes (excitability, seizures); pain, inflammation, or rupture of tendon; or abdominal cramping or pain. **Pregnancy/breast-feeding precautions:** Inform prescriber if you are or intend to be pregnant. Do not breast-feed.

**Geriatric Considerations:** Dosage adjustment is not necessary in patients with normal renal function, $Cl_{cr}$ ≥40 mL/minute; otherwise, follow dosage guidelines for renal impairment. Age-associated increase in half-life and decrease in clearance are thought to be secondary to age-related changes in renal function.

♦ **Lomodix®** *see* Diphenoxylate and Atropine *on page 382*

♦ **Lomotil®** *see* Diphenoxylate and Atropine *on page 382*

## Lomustine (loe MUS teen)

**U.S. Brand Names** CeeNU®

**Synonyms** CCNU

**Therapeutic Category** Antineoplastic Agent, Alkylating Agent

**Pregnancy Risk Factor** D

**Lactation** Enters breast milk/contraindicated

**Use** Treatment of brain tumors, Hodgkin's and non-Hodgkin's lymphomas, melanoma, renal carcinoma, lung cancer, colon cancer

**Mechanism of Action/Effect** Inhibits DNA and RNA synthesis via carbamylation of DNA polymerase, alkylation of DNA, and alteration of RNA, proteins, and enzymes

**Contraindications** Hypersensitivity to lomustine or any component; pregnancy

**Warnings** The U.S. Food and Drug Administration (FDA) currently recommends that procedures for proper handling and disposal for antineoplastic agents be considered. Use with caution in patients with depressed platelet, leukocyte or erythrocyte counts. Bone marrow depression, notably thrombocytopenia and leukopenia, may lead to bleeding and overwhelming infections in an already compromised patient; will last for at least 6 weeks after a dose, do not give courses more frequently than every 6 weeks because the toxicity is cumulative. Use with caution in patients with liver function abnormalities.

**Drug Interactions**

**Cytochrome P-450 Effect:** CYP2D6 enzyme inhibitor

**Decreased Effect:** Decreased effect with phenobarbital, resulting in reduced efficacy of both drugs.

**Increased Effect/Toxicity:** Increased toxicity with cimetidine, reported to cause bone marrow depression or to potentiate the myelosuppressive effects of lomustine.

**Effects on Lab Values** Liver function tests

**Adverse Reactions**

>10%:

Gastrointestinal: Nausea and vomiting occur 3-6 hours after oral administration; this is due to a centrally mediated mechanism, not a direct effect on the GI lining; if vomiting occurs, it is not necessary to replace the dose unless it occurs immediately after drug administration

Emetic potential:

<60 mg: Moderately high (60% to 90%)

≥60 mg: High (>90%)

Time course of nausea/vomiting: Onset: 2-6 hours; Duration: 4-6 hours

Hematologic: Leukopenia; Thrombocytopenia; Myelosuppression: Anemia; effects occur 4-6 weeks after a dose and may persist for 1-2 weeks

WBC: Moderate

Platelets: Severe

Onset (days): 14

Nadir (weeks): 4-5

Recovery (weeks): 6

1% to 10%:

Central nervous system: Neurotoxicity

Dermatologic: Skin rash, alopecia

Gastrointestinal: Stomatitis, diarrhea

Hematologic: Anemia

Renal: Renal failure

<1% (Limited to important or life-threatening symptoms): Hepatotoxicity, pulmonary fibrosis with cumulative doses >600 mg

**Overdose/Toxicology** Symptoms of overdose include nausea, vomiting, and leukopenia. There are no known antidotes. Treatment is symptomatic and supportive.

**Pharmacodynamics/Kinetics**

**Protein Binding:** 50%

**Distribution:** Crosses blood-brain barrier to a greater degree than BNCU and CNS concentrations are equal to that of plasma

**Half-life Elimination:** Parent drug: 16-72 hours; Active metabolite: 1.3-2 days

**Time to Peak:** Active metabolite: Within 3 hours

**Metabolism:** Liver

**Excretion:** Enterohepatically recycled; excreted in the urine, feces, and expired air

**Duration:** Marrow recovery may require 6 weeks

**Formulations**

Capsule: 10 mg, 40 mg, 100 mg

Dose Pack: 10 mg (2s); 100 mg (2s); 40 mg (2s)

**Dosing**

**Adults:** Oral (refer to individual protocols): 100-130 mg/m$^2$ as a single dose every 6 weeks; readjust after initial treatment according to platelet and leukocyte counts.

With compromised marrow function: Initial: 100 mg/m$^2$ as a single dose every 6 weeks

**Subsequent dosing adjustment based on nadir:**

Leukocytes 2000-2900/mm$^3$, platelets 25,000-74,999/mm$^3$: Administer 70% of prior dose.

Leukocytes <2000/mm$^3$, platelets <25,000/mm$^3$: Administer 50% of prior dose.

**Elderly:** Refer to adult dosing.

**Renal Impairment:**

$Cl_{cr}$ 10-50 mL/minute: Administer 75% of normal dose.

$Cl_{cr}$ <10 mL/minute: Administer 50% of normal dose.

Hemodialysis effects: Supplemental dose is not necessary.

**Administration**

**Oral:** Take with fluids on an empty stomach; no food or drink for 2 hours after administration.

**Stability**

**Storage:** Refrigerate (<40°C/<104°F).

**Monitoring Laboratory Tests** CBC with differential, platelet count, hepatic and renal function, pulmonary function

**Additional Nursing Issues**

**Physical Assessment:** Monitor results of all laboratory tests prior to each dose. Know and monitor for adverse effects of this medication (see Adverse Reactions). Instruct patient about appropriate interventions to reduce side effects and symptoms to report. **Pregnancy risk factor D** - assess knowledge/teach appropriate use of barrier contraceptives. Breast-feeding is contraindicated.

**Patient Information/Instruction:** Take with fluids on an empty stomach; do not eat or drink for 2 hours following administration. Do not use alcohol, aspirin, or aspirin-containing medications and OTC medications without consulting prescriber. Maintain adequate fluid balance (2-3 L/day of fluids unless instructed to restrict fluid intake). May cause hair loss (reversible); easy bleeding or bruising (use soft toothbrush or cotton swabs and frequent mouth care, use electric razor, avoid sharp knives or scissors); increased susceptibility to infection (avoid crowds or exposure to infection - do not have any vaccinations unless approved by prescriber). Report unusual bleeding or bruising or persistent fever or sore throat; blood in urine, stool, or vomitus; delayed healing of any wounds; skin rash; yellowing of skin or eyes; changes in color of urine of stool. **Pregnancy/breast-feeding precautions:** Do not get pregnant while taking this medication; use appropriate barrier contraceptive measures. Do not breast-feed.

- **Loniten®** *see page 1294*
- **Lonox®** *see* Diphenoxylate and Atropine *on page 382*

♦ **Lo/Ovral®** *see* Oral Contraceptives *on page 859*

## Loperamide (loe PER a mide)

**U.S. Brand Names** Diar-Aid® [OTC]; Imodium®; Imodium® A-D [OTC]; Kaopectate® II [OTC]; Pepto® Diarrhea Control [OTC]

**Therapeutic Category** Antidiarrheal

**Pregnancy Risk Factor** B

**Lactation** Enters breast milk/compatible

**Use** Treatment of acute diarrhea and chronic diarrhea associated with inflammatory bowel disease; chronic functional diarrhea (idiopathic), chronic diarrhea caused by bowel resection or organic lesions; to decrease the volume of ileostomy discharge

**Unlabeled use:** Treatment of traveler's diarrhea in combination with trimethoprim-sulfamethoxazole (co-trimoxazole) (3 days therapy)

**Mechanism of Action/Effect** Acts directly on intestinal muscles to inhibit peristalsis and prolongs transit time enhancing fluid and electrolyte movement through intestinal mucosa; reduces fecal volume, increases viscosity, and diminishes fluid and electrolyte loss; demonstrates antisecretory activity; exhibits peripheral action

**Contraindications** Hypersensitivity to loperamide or any component; bloody diarrhea; patients who must avoid constipation, diarrhea resulting from some infections, or in patients with pseudomembranous colitis

**Warnings** Large first-pass metabolism, use with caution in hepatic dysfunction. Should not be used if diarrhea accompanied by high fever, blood in stool.

**Drug Interactions**

**Increased Effect/Toxicity:** Loperamide may potentiate the adverse effects of CNS depressants, phenothiazines, tricyclic antidepressants.

**Adverse Reactions** <1% (Limited to important or life-threatening symptoms): Sedation, fatigue, dizziness, drowsiness, nausea, vomiting, constipation, abdominal cramping, dry mouth, abdominal distention, anaphylaxis, shock, toxic epidermal necrolysis, paralytic ileus

**Overdose/Toxicology** Symptoms of overdose include CNS and respiratory depression, GI cramping, constipation, GI irritation, nausea, and vomiting. Overdose is noted when daily doses approximate 60 mg of loperamide. Treatment of overdose includes gastric lavage followed by 100 g activated charcoal through a nasogastric tube. Naloxone, 2 mg I.V. with repeat administration as necessary up to a total dose of 10 mg, can be used to reverse opiate effects.

**Pharmacodynamics/Kinetics**

**Protein Binding:** 97%

**Half-life Elimination:** 7-14 hours

**Metabolism:** Hepatic (>50%) to inactive compounds

**Excretion:** Feces and urine (unchanged drug 30% to 40%)

**Onset:** Oral: Within 0.5-1 hour

**Formulations**

Loperamide hydrochloride:
- Caplet: 2 mg
- Capsule: 2 mg
- Liquid, oral: 1 mg/5 mL (60 mL, 90 mL, 120 mL)
- Tablet: 2 mg

**Dosing**

**Adults:** Oral: Initial: 4 mg (2 capsules), followed by 2 mg after each loose stool, up to 16 mg/day (8 capsules)

**Elderly:** Refer to adult dosing.

**Administration**

**Oral:** Therapy for chronic diarrhea should not exceed 10 days.

**Additional Nursing Issues**

**Physical Assessment:** Assess other medications patient may be taking for effectiveness and/or interactions (see Drug Interactions). Assess for cause of diarrhea before administering first dose. Instruct patient on lifestyle changes which may reduce diarrhea (if appropriate) eg, increased exercise, identifying and avoiding foods that cause diarrhea, safe food preparation and storage, use of buttermilk, yogurt, or boiled milk.

**Patient Information/Instruction:** Do not take more than 8 capsules or 80 mL in 24 hours. May cause drowsiness. If acute diarrhea lasts longer than 48 hours, consult prescriber. Do not take if diarrhea is bloody.

**Geriatric Considerations:** Elderly are particularly sensitive to fluid and electrolyte loss. This generally results in lethargy, weakness, and confusion. Repletion and maintenance of electrolytes and water are essential in the treatment of diarrhea. Drug therapy must be limited in order to avoid toxicity with this agent.

**Additional Information** If clinical improvement is not achieved after 16 mg/day for 10 days, control is unlikely with further use. Continue use if diet or other treatment does not control. Imodium® 2 mg capsules are legend.

**Related Information**

Co-trimoxazole *on page 307*

♦ **Lopid®** *see* Gemfibrozil *on page 530*
♦ **Lopresor** *see* Metoprolol *on page 761*
♦ **Lopressor®** *see* Metoprolol *on page 761*
♦ **Loprox®** *see page 1247*
♦ **Lorabid™** *see* Loracarbef *on next page*

## Loratadine

**Loracarbef** (lor a KAR bef)

**U.S. Brand Names** Lorabid™

**Therapeutic Category** Antibiotic, Carbacephem

**Pregnancy Risk Factor** B

**Lactation** Excretion in breast milk unknown/use caution

**Use** Infections caused by susceptible organisms involving the respiratory tract, acute otitis media, sinusitis, skin and skin structure, bone and joint, and urinary tract and gynecologic

**Mechanism of Action/Effect** Inhibits bacterial cell wall synthesis by binding to one or more of the penicillin binding proteins (PBPs); inhibits the final transpeptidation step of peptidoglycan synthesis in bacterial cell walls, thus inhibiting cell wall biosynthesis.

**Contraindications** Hypersensitivity to loracarbef, cephalosporins, or other beta-lactam antibiotics (eg, penicillins)

**Drug Interactions**

**Increased Effect/Toxicity:** Loracarbef serum levels are increased with coadministered probenecid.

**Food Interactions** Loracarbef peak serum levels may be prolonged if taken with food.

**Adverse Reactions**

>10%: Gastrointestinal: Diarrhea, nausea, vomiting, abdominal pain, anorexia

<1% (Limited to important or life-threatening symptoms): Transient thrombocytopenia, leukopenia, and eosinophilia; transient elevations of ALT, AST, alkaline phosphatase; transient elevations of BUN/creatinine

**Overdose/Toxicology** Symptoms of overdose include abdominal discomfort and diarrhea. Treatment is supportive.

**Pharmacodynamics/Kinetics**

**Half-life Elimination:** ~1 hour (prolonged in renal impairment)

**Time to Peak:** Oral: Within 1 hour

**Excretion:** Plasma clearance: ~200-300 mL/minute

**Formulations**

Capsule: 200 mg, 400 mg

Suspension, oral: 100 mg/5 mL (50 mL, 100 mL); 200 mg/5 mL (50 mL, 100 mL)

**Dosing**

**Adults:** Oral:

Uncomplicated urinary tract infections: 200 mg once daily for 7 days

Skin and soft tissue: 200 mg every 12 hours for 7 days

Uncomplicated pyelonephritis: 400 mg every 12 hours for 14 days

Upper respiratory infection:

Pharyngitis/tonsillitis: 200 mg every 12 hours for 10 days

Sinusitis: 400 mg every 12 hours for 10 days

**Elderly:** Refer to adult dosing.

**Renal Impairment:**

$Cl_{cr}$ ≥50 mL/minute: Administer usual dose.

$Cl_{cr}$ 10-49 mL/minute: Administer 50% of usual dose at usual interval or usual dose given half as often.

$Cl_{cr}$ <10 mL/minute: Administer usual dose every 3-5 days.

Hemodialysis: Doses should be administered after dialysis sessions.

**Administration**

**Oral:** Take on an empty stomach at least 1 hour before or 2 hours after meals. Finish all medication.

**Stability**

**Storage:** Suspension may be kept at room temperature for 14 days.

**Monitoring Laboratory Tests** Perform culture and sensitivity studies prior to initiating therapy.

**Additional Nursing Issues**

**Physical Assessment:** Assess previous history of allergies. Assess effectiveness and interactions of other medications (see Drug Interactions). See Warnings/Precautions and Contraindications for use cautions. Monitor effectiveness of therapy, laboratory tests, and adverse response (see Adverse Reactions and Overdose/Toxicology). Assess knowledge/teach patient appropriate use, possible side effects and appropriate interventions, and adverse symptoms to report (note that allergic reactions can occur days after therapy is initiated). Note breast-feeding caution.

**Patient Information/Instruction:** Take as directed, preferably on an empty stomach (30 minutes before or 2 hours after meals). Take entire prescription even if feeling better. Maintain adequate hydration (2-3 L/day of fluids unless instructed to restrict fluid intake). You may experience nausea, vomiting, or anorexia (small frequent meals, frequent mouth care, sucking lozenges, or chewing gum may help). Report immediately any signs of skin rash, joint or back pain, or difficulty breathing. Report unusual fever, chills, vaginal itching or foul-smelling vaginal discharge, or easy bruising or bleeding. **Breast-feeding precautions:** Consult prescriber if breast-feeding.

**Geriatric Considerations:** Half-life is slightly prolonged with age, presumably due to the reduced creatinine clearance related to aging. Adjust dose for renal function.

**Loratadine** (lor AT a deen)

**U.S. Brand Names** Claritin®

**Therapeutic Category** Antihistamine

**Pregnancy Risk Factor** B

**Lactation** Enters breast milk/not recommended

**Use** Relief of nasal and non-nasal symptoms of seasonal allergic rhinitis

(Continued)

## Loratadine *(Continued)*

**Mechanism of Action/Effect** Long-acting tricyclic antihistamine with selective peripheral histamine $H_1$ receptor antagonistic properties; management of idiopathic chronic urticaria

**Contraindications** Hypersensitivity to loratadine or any component

**Warnings** Patients with liver or renal impairment should start with a lower dose (10 mg every other day), since their ability to clear the drug will be reduced.

**Drug Interactions**

**Cytochrome P-450 Effect:** CYP2D6 and 3A3/4 enzyme substrate

**Increased Effect/Toxicity:** Increased plasma concentrations of loratadine and its active metabolite with ketoconazole. Erythromycin increases the AUC of loratadine and its active metabolite; no change in Q-$T_c$ interval was seen. Increased toxicity with procarbazine, other antihistamines, alcohol.

**Adverse Reactions**

>10%: Central nervous system: Headache

2% to 10%:

- Central nervous system: Somnolence, fatigue
- Gastrointestinal: Dry mouth, nausea, heartburn

<2% (Limited to important or life-threatening symptoms): Chest pain, hypotension, hypertension, palpitations, tachycardia, syncope, seizures, erythema multiforme, angioneurotic edema, jaundice, abnormal LFTs, hepatitis, hepatic necrosis, bronchospasm, dyspnea, epistaxis, hemoptysis, anaphylaxis

**Overdose/Toxicology** Symptoms of overdose include somnolence, tachycardia, and headache. No specific antidote is available. Treatment is symptomatic and supportive. Loratadine is not eliminated by dialysis.

**Pharmacodynamics/Kinetics**

**Half-life Elimination:** 12-15 hours

**Metabolism:** Liver

**Excretion:** Urine and feces

**Onset:** Within 1-3 hours; Peak effect: 8-12 hours

**Duration:** >24 hours

**Formulations**

Solution, oral: 1 mg/mL

Tablet: 10 mg

Rapid-disintegrating tablets: 10 mg (RediTabs®)

**Dosing**

**Adults:** Oral: 10 mg/day

**Elderly:** Refer to adult dosing.

**Hepatic Impairment:** 10 mg every other day to start

**Administration**

**Oral:** Take on an empty stomach.

**Additional Nursing Issues**

**Physical Assessment:** Assess effectiveness and interactions of other medications (see Drug Interactions). See Warnings/Precautions for cautious use. Monitor effectiveness of therapy and adverse reactions (see Adverse Reactions) at beginning of therapy and periodically with long-term use. Assess knowledge/teach patient appropriate use, interventions to reduce side effects, and adverse symptoms to report. Breast-feeding is not recommended.

**Patient Information/Instruction:** Take as directed; do not exceed recommended dose. Avoid use of other depressants, alcohol, or sleep-inducing medications unless approved by prescriber. You may experience drowsiness or dizziness (use caution when driving or engaging in tasks requiring alertness until response to drug is known); or dry mouth or nausea (frequent small meals, frequent mouth care, chewing gum, or sucking hard candy may help). Report persistent dizziness, sedation, or seizures; chest pain, rapid heartbeat, or palpitations; swelling of face, mouth, lips, or tongue; difficulty breathing; changes in urinary pattern; yellowing of skin or eyes, dark urine, or pale stool; or lack of improvement or worsening or condition. **Breast-feeding precautions:** Breast-feeding is not recommended.

**Geriatric Considerations:** Loratadine is one of the newer, nonsedating antihistamines. Because of its low incidence of side effects, it seems to be a good choice in the elderly. However, there is a wide variation in loratadine half-life reported in the elderly and this should be kept in mind when initiating dosing.

## Loratadine and Pseudoephedrine (lor AT a deen & soo doe e FED rin)

**U.S. Brand Names** Claritin-D® 24-Hour; Claritin-D®

**Synonyms** Pseudoephedrine and Loratadine

**Therapeutic Category** Antihistamine/Decongestant Combination

**Pregnancy Risk Factor** B

**Lactation** Enters breast milk/not recommended

**Use** Temporary relief of symptoms of seasonal allergic rhinitis and nasal congestion

**Formulations**

Tablet: Loratadine 5 mg and pseudoephedrine sulfate 120 mg

Tablet, extended release: Loratadine 10 mg and pseudoephedrine sulfate 240 mg

**Dosing**

**Adults:**

Oral: 1 tablet every 12 hours

Extended release: 1 tablet daily

**Elderly:** Refer to adult dosing.

**Renal Impairment:** $Cl_{cr}$ <30 mL/minute: Administer lower initial dose (1 tablet/day) because of reduced clearance.

**Hepatic Impairment:** Should be avoided.

**Additional Nursing Issues**

**Physical Assessment:** See individual components listed in Related Information. Breast-feeding is not recommended.

**Patient Information/Instruction:** See individual components listed in Related Information. **Breast-feeding precautions:** Breast-feeding is not recommended.

**Related Information**

Loratadine *on page 689*
Pseudoephedrine *on page 992*

## Lorazepam (lor A ze pam)

**U.S. Brand Names** Ativan®

**Therapeutic Category** Benzodiazepine

**Pregnancy Risk Factor** D

**Lactation** Enters breast milk/contraindicated (AAP rates "of concern")

**Use** Management of anxiety, status epilepticus; preoperative sedation; for desired amnesia; alcohol detoxification

**Unlabeled use:** Insomnia, psychogenic catatonia, partial complex seizures, and as an antiemetic adjunct

**Mechanism of Action/Effect** Depresses all levels of the CNS, including the limbic and reticular formation, probably through the increased action of gamma-aminobutyric acid (GABA), which is a major inhibitory neurotransmitter in the brain

**Contraindications** Hypersensitivity to lorazepam or any component; there may be a cross-sensitivity with other benzodiazepines; do not use in a comatose patient, those with pre-existing CNS depression, psychosis, acute angle-closure glaucoma, severe uncontrolled pain, or severe hypotension; pregnancy

**Warnings** Use caution in patients with renal or hepatic impairment, organic brain syndrome, myasthenia gravis, or Parkinson's disease. Use with caution in patients with a history of drug dependence. Do **not** inject intra-arterially, arteriospasm and gangrene may occur. Oral doses >0.09 mg/kg produced increased ataxia without increased sedative benefit versus lower doses. Administer with extreme caution to geriatric patients or patients with compromised pulmonary function.

**Drug Interactions**

**Decreased Effect:** Decreased effect of lorazepam with oral contraceptives (combination products). Cigarette smoking may decrease the sedative effect. Decreased effect of levodopa.

**Increased Effect/Toxicity:** Increased effect with morphine. Increased toxicity with alcohol, CNS depressants, MAO inhibitors, loxapine.

**Effects on Lab Values** May result in elevated liver function tests

**Adverse Reactions**

>10%:

- Central nervous system: Drowsiness, ataxia, lightheadedness, headache, dizziness, impaired coordination, anxiety, fatigue, slurred speech, irritability, nervousness, insomnia, memory impairment, cognitive disorder, dysarthria, anxiety
- Gastrointestinal: Decreased salivation (dry mouth)
- Genitourinary: Micturition difficulties

1% to 10%:

- Cardiovascular: Tachycardia, syncope
- Central nervous system: Confusion, increased libido, depersonalization, mental depression, perceptual disturbances, parethesias, weakness, akathisia, agitation, disinhibition, talkativeness, derealization, dream abnormalities, fear, decreased libido
- Gastrointestinal: Abdominal or stomach cramps, increased or decreased appetite, weight gain or loss, nausea, vomiting
- Neuromuscular & skeletal: Muscle cramps
- Ocular: Photophobia, blurred vision
- Otic: Tinnitus
- Respiratory: Nasal congestion
- Miscellaneous: Sweating

<1% (Limited to important or life-threatening symptoms): Agranulocytosis, anemia, leukopenia, neutropenia, thrombocytopenia, hepatic dysfunction

**Overdose/Toxicology** Symptoms of overdose include confusion, coma, hypoactive reflexes, dyspnea, labored breathing. Treatment for benzodiazepine overdose is supportive. Flumazenil has been shown to selectively block the binding of benzodiazepines to CNS receptors, resulting in a reversal of benzodiazepine-induced CNS depression but not respiratory depression.

**Pharmacodynamics/Kinetics**

**Protein Binding:** 85%, free fraction may be significantly higher in the elderly

**Distribution:** Crosses the placenta

**Half-life Elimination:** Adults: 12.9 hours; Elderly: 15.9 hours; End-stage renal disease: 32-70 hours

**Metabolism:** Liver

**Excretion:** Urine and feces

**Onset:** Onset of hypnosis: I.M.: 20-30 minutes; Sedation, anticonvulsant (I.V.): 5 minutes; Oral: 30 minutes to 1 hour

(Continued)

## Lorazepam *(Continued)*

**Duration:** 6-8 hours

### Formulations

Injection: 2 mg/mL (1 mL, 10 mL); 4 mg/mL (1 mL, 10 mL)
Solution, oral concentrated, alcohol and dye free: 2 mg/mL (30 mL)
Tablet: 0.5 mg, 1 mg, 2 mg

### Dosing

**Adults:**

Antiemetic for cancer chemotherapy:
- Oral: 2.5 mg the evening before and just after starting chemotherapy
- I.V.: 1.5 mg/m$^2$ up to a maximum of 3 mg administered over 5 minutes, 45 minutes before starting chemotherapy

Anxiety and sedation: Oral: 1-10 mg/day in 2-3 divided doses; usual dose: 2-6 mg/day in divided doses

Insomnia: Oral: 2-4 mg at bedtime

Preoperative:
- I.M.: 0.05 mg/kg administered 2 hours before surgery; maximum: 4 mg/dose
- I.V.: 0.044 mg/kg 15-20 minutes before surgery; usual maximum: 2 mg/dose

Operative amnesia: I.V.: up to 0.05 mg/kg; maximum: 4 mg/dose

Status epilepticus: I.V.: 4 mg/dose given slowly over 2-5 minutes; may repeat in 10-15 minutes; usual maximum dose: 8 mg

**Elderly:**

Antiemetic for cancer chemotherapy: Refer to adult dosing.
Anxiety and sedation: Oral: Initial: 0.5-1 mg/day in divided doses; initial dose should not exceed 2 mg/day.
Insomnia: Oral: 0.5-1 mg at bedtime
Preoperative: Refer to adult dosing.
Operative amnesia: Refer to adult dosing.
Status epilepticus: Refer to adult dosing.

### Administration

**I.M.:** Should be administered deep into the muscle mass.

**I.V.:** Inadvertent intra-arterial injection may produce arteriospasm resulting in gangrene which may require amputation.

I.V.: Do not exceed 2 mg/minute or 0.05 mg/kg over 2-5 minutes.

**I.V. Detail:** Continuous infusion solutions should have an in-line filter and the solution should be checked frequently for possible precipitation. Emergency resuscitative equipment should be available when administering I.V. Prior to I.V. use, lorazepam injection must be diluted with an equal amount of compatible diluent ($D_5W$, NS, SWI). Injection must be made slowly with repeated aspiration to make sure the injection is not intra-arterial and that perivascular extravasation has not occurred.

### Stability

**Storage:** Intact vials should be refrigerated and protected from light. Do not use discolored or precipitate containing solutions. Injectable vials may be stored at room temperature for up to 60 days.

**Reconstitution:** Stability of parenteral admixture at room temperature (25°C) is 24 hours.

Standard diluent: 1 mg/100 mL $D_5W$

**Compatibility:** I.V. is incompatible when administered in the same line with foscarnet, ondansetron, and sargramostim.

### Additional Nursing Issues

**Physical Assessment:** Assess other medications the patient may be taking for effectiveness and interactions (see Drug Interactions). See Contraindications and Warnings/Precautions for cautious use.

Oral: Assess for history of addiction; long-term use can result in dependence, abuse, or tolerance; periodically evaluate need for continued use. Monitor therapeutic response (eg, mood, affect, anxiety level, sleep pattern) and adverse reactions at beginning of therapy and periodically with long-term use (see Adverse Reactions and Overdose/Toxicology). Taper dosage slowly when discontinuing. Assess knowledge/teach patient appropriate use, interventions to reduce side effects, and adverse symptoms to report.

I.V./I.M.: Monitor cardiac, respiratory, and CNS status (possible retrograde amnesia I.V.), and ability to void. Maintain bedrest for 2-3 hours, and observe when up.

**Pregnancy risk factor D** - assess knowledge/teach appropriate use of barrier contraceptives. Breast-feeding is not recommended.

**Patient Information/Instruction:**

Oral: Take exactly as directed (do not increase dose or frequency); may cause physical and/or psychological dependence. Do not use excessive alcohol or other prescription or OTC medications (especially pain medications, sedatives, antihistamines, or hypnotics) without consulting prescriber. Maintain adequate hydration (2-3 L/day of fluids unless instructed to restrict fluid intake). You may experience drowsiness, lightheadedness, impaired coordination, dizziness, or blurred vision (use caution when driving or engaging in tasks requiring alertness until response to drug is known); nausea, vomiting, or dry mouth (small frequent meals, frequent mouth care, chewing gum, or sucking lozenges may help); constipation (increased exercise, fluids, or dietary fruit and fiber may help); altered sexual drive or ability (reversible); or photosensitivity (use sunscreen, wear protective clothing and eyewear, and avoid direct sunlight). Report persistent CNS effects (eg, confusion, depression, increased sedation, excitation, headache, agitation, insomnia or nightmares, dizziness, fatigue, impaired coordination, changes in personality, or changes in cognition); changes in urinary pattern; chest pain, palpitations, or rapid heartbeat; muscle cramping, weakness, tremors, or rigidity; ringing in ears or visual disturbances; excessive perspiration, or excessive GI symptoms (cramping, constipation, vomiting, anorexia); or worsening of condition. **Pregnancy/breast-feeding precautions:** Do not get pregnant while taking this medication; use appropriate barrier contraceptive measures. Breast-feeding is not recommended.

**Geriatric Considerations:** Because lorazepam is relatively short-acting with an inactive metabolite, it is a preferred agent to use in elderly patients when a benzodiazepine is indicated. Use with caution since elderly patients have decreased pulmonary reserve and are more prone to hypoxia.

**Other Issues:** Taper dosage gradually after long-term therapy, especially in epileptic patients. Abrupt withdrawal may cause tremors, nausea, vomiting, abdominal and/or muscle cramps.

**Additional Information** Some formulations may contain benzyl alcohol.

**Related Information**

Antiemetics for Chemotherapy-Induced Nausea and Vomiting *on page 1307*
Anxiolytic/Hypnotic Use in Long-Term Care Facilities *on page 1430*
Benzodiazepines Comparison *on page 1375*

♦ **Lorcet®-HD** *see* Hydrocodone and Acetaminophen *on page 568*
♦ **Lorcet® Plus** *see* Hydrocodone and Acetaminophen *on page 568*
♦ **Loroxide®** *see page 1294*
♦ **Lortab®** *see* Hydrocodone and Acetaminophen *on page 568*
♦ **Lortab® ASA** *see* Hydrocodone and Aspirin *on page 570*

## Losartan (loe SAR tan)

**U.S. Brand Names** Cozaar®

**Synonyms** DuP 753; MK594

**Therapeutic Category** Angiotensin II Antagonists

**Pregnancy Risk Factor** C/D (2nd and 3rd trimesters)

**Lactation** Excretion in breast milk unknown/contraindicated

**Use** Treatment of hypertension with or without concurrent use of thiazide diuretics

**Mechanism of Action/Effect** As a selective and competitive, nonpeptide angiotensin II receptor antagonist, losartan blocks the vasoconstrictor and aldosterone-secreting effects of angiotensin II. Losartan increases urinary flow rate and in addition to being natriuretic and kaliuretic, increases excretion of chloride, magnesium, uric acid, calcium, and phosphate.

**Contraindications** Hypersensitivity to losartan or any components; pregnancy (2nd and 3rd trimesters)

**Warnings** Avoid use or use a much smaller dose in patients who are intravascularly volume-depleted. Use caution in hepatic impairment and in patients with unilateral or bilateral renal artery stenosis to avoid a decrease in renal function. AUCs of losartan (not the active metabolite) are about 50% greater in patients with $Cl_{cr}$ <30 mL/minute and are doubled in hemodialysis patients. Pregnancy factor C/D (2nd and 3rd trimesters).

**Drug Interactions**

**Cytochrome P-450 Effect:** CYP2C9 and 3A3/4 enzyme substrate

**Decreased Effect:** Phenobarbital caused a reduction of losartan in serum by 20%, clinical effect is unknown.

**Increased Effect/Toxicity:** Cimetidine may increase the amount of losartan by 18% but the clinical effect is unknown.

**Adverse Reactions**

>10%: Central nervous system: Headache

1% to 10%:

- Cardiovascular: Hypotension without reflex tachycardia
- Central nervous system: Dizziness, insomnia
- Endocrine & metabolic: Hyperkalemia
- Gastrointestinal: Diarrhea, heartburn
- Hematologic: Slight decreases in hemoglobin and hematocrit
- Renal: Hypouricemia (with large doses)
- Respiratory: Nasal congestion

<1% (Limited to important or life-threatening symptoms): Angioedema (some patients had previous reactions with ACE inhibitors), orthostatic effects, chest pain, second degree A-V block, CVA, palpitations, sinus bradycardia, tachycardia, flushing, facial edema, alopecia, slight elevations of LFTs and bilirubin, hepatitis, urinary tract infection, mild increases in BUN/creatinine, cough (less than ACE inhibitors), dyspnea, bronchitis

**Overdose/Toxicology** Hypotension and tachycardia may occur with significant overdose. Treatment should be supportive.

**Pharmacodynamics/Kinetics**

**Protein Binding:** 99%

**Distribution:** Does not cross the blood brain barrier

**Half-life Elimination:** Losartan: 1.5-2 hours; Metabolite (E-3174): 6-9 hours

**Time to Peak:** Losartan: 1 hour; Metabolite (E-3174): 3-4 hours

**Metabolism:** Liver

**Excretion:** Urine and feces

**Onset:** 6 hours

**Formulations** Tablet, film coated, as potassium: 25 mg, 50 mg

(Continued)

## Losartan *(Continued)*

**Dosing**

**Adults:**

The usual starting dose is 50 mg once daily; can be administered once or twice daily with total daily doses ranging from 25-100 mg

Usual initial doses in patients receiving diuretics or those with intravascular volume depletion: 25 mg

Patients not receiving diuretics: 50 mg

**Elderly:** Refer to adult dosing.

**Renal Impairment:**

No adjustment necessary.

Hemodialysis effects: Not removed via hemodialysis.

**Hepatic Impairment:** Reduce the initial dose to 25 mg; divide dosage intervals into two.

**Monitoring Laboratory Tests** Electrolytes, serum creatinine, BUN, urinalysis, CBC

**Additional Nursing Issues**

**Physical Assessment:** Assess effectiveness and interactions of other medications (see Drug Interactions). See Warnings/Precautions and Contraindications for use cautions. Monitor effectiveness of therapy, laboratory tests, and adverse response on a regular basis during therapy (see Adverse Reactions and Overdose/Toxicology). Assess knowledge/teach patient appropriate use according to drug form and purpose of therapy, possible side effects and appropriate interventions, and adverse symptoms to report. **Pregnancy risk factor C/D** - see Pregnancy Risk Factor - assess knowledge/teach appropriate use of barrier contraceptives. Breast-feeding is contraindicated.

**Patient Information/Instruction:** Take exactly as directed; do not discontinue without consulting prescriber. Take first dose at bedtime. This drug does not eliminate need for diet or exercise regimen as recommended by prescriber. May cause dizziness, fainting, lightheadedness (use caution when driving or engaging in tasks that require alertness until response to drug is known); diarrhea (buttermilk, boiled milk, yogurt may help). Report chest pain or palpitations; unrelenting headache; swelling of extremities, face, or tongue; difficulty in breathing or unusual cough; flu-like symptoms; or other persistent adverse reactions **Pregnancy/breast-feeding precautions:** Do not get pregnant while taking this medication; use appropriate barrier contraceptive measures. If you are, or plan to be pregnant, notify your prescriber at once. Do not breast-feed.

**Geriatric Considerations:** Serum concentrations of losartan and its metabolites are not significantly different in the elderly patient and no initial dose adjustment is necessary even in low creatinine clearance states (<30 mL/minute).

**Additional Information** Losartan's effect in African-American patients was notably less than in non-African Americans. While dosage adjustments are not needed, plasma levels are twice as high in female hypertensives as male hypertensives.

**Related Information**

ACE Inhibitors and Angiotensin Antagonists Comparison *on page 1362*

## Losartan and Hydrochlorothiazide

(loe SAR tan & hye droe klor oh THYE a zide)

**U.S. Brand Names** Hyzaar®

**Synonyms** Hydrochlorothiazide and Losartan

**Therapeutic Category** Antihypertensive Agent, Combination

**Pregnancy Risk Factor** C/D (2nd and 3rd trimesters)

**Lactation** Enters breast milk/contraindicated

**Use** Treatment of hypertension

**Formulations** Tablet:

Losartan potassium 50 mg and hydrochlorothiazide 12.5 mg

Losartan potassium 100 mg and hydrochlorothiazide 25 mg

**Dosing**

**Adults:** Oral: 1 tablet/day

Titration by clinical effect: Patients not controlled on losartan alone may be switched to losartan HCTZ once daily. If the blood pressure remains uncontrolled after 3 weeks, the dose may be increased to 2 tablets of 50/12.5 mg or 1 tablet of 100/25 mg once daily. More than 2 tablets/day of 50/12.5 mg or 1 tablet of 100/25 mg are not recommended. Maximum antihypertensive effect is attained in about 3 weeks.

**Elderly:** Refer to dosing in individual monographs.

**Renal Impairment:** Usual regimens may be followed as long as $Cl_{cr}$ is ≥30 mL/minute. In patients with more severe renal impairment, loop diuretics are preferred.

**Hepatic Impairment:** Not recommended for titration in patients with hepatic impairment.

**Additional Nursing Issues**

**Physical Assessment:** See individual components listed in Related Information. **Pregnancy risk factor C/D** - see Pregnancy Risk Factor - assess knowledge/instruct patient on need to use appropriate contraceptive measures and the need to avoid pregnancy. Breast-feeding is contraindicated.

**Patient Information/Instruction:** See individual components listed in Related Information. **Pregnancy/breast-feeding precautions:** Inform prescriber if you are or intend to be pregnant. Do not breast-feed.

**Related Information**

Hydrochlorothiazide *on page 566*

Losartan *on previous page*

- **Losec®** *see* Omeprazole *on page 851*
- **Lotemax®** *see page 1282*
- **Lotensin®** *see* Benazepril *on page 139*
- **Lotensin HCT®** *see* Benazepril and Hydrochlorothiazide *on page 140*
- **Loteprednol** *see page 1282*
- **Lotrel®** *see* Amlodipine and Benazepril *on page 77*
- **Lotriderm®** *see* Betamethasone and Clotrimazole *on page 150*
- **Lotrimin®** *see* Clotrimazole *on page 294*
- **Lotrimin® AF Cream [OTC]** *see* Clotrimazole *on page 294*
- **Lotrimin® AF Lotion [OTC]** *see* Clotrimazole *on page 294*
- **Lotrimin® AF Powder [OTC]** *see* Miconazole *on page 767*
- **Lotrimin® AF Solution [OTC]** *see* Clotrimazole *on page 294*
- **Lotrimin® AF Spray Liquid [OTC]** *see* Miconazole *on page 767*
- **Lotrimin® AF Spray Powder [OTC]** *see* Miconazole *on page 767*
- **Lotrisone®** *see* Betamethasone and Clotrimazole *on page 150*


## Lovastatin (LOE va sta tin)

**U.S. Brand Names** Mevacor®

**Synonyms** Mevinolin; Monacolin K

**Therapeutic Category** Antilipemic Agent (HMG-CoA Reductase Inhibitor)

**Pregnancy Risk Factor** X

**Lactation** Enters breast milk/contraindicated

**Use** Adjunct to dietary therapy to decrease elevated serum total and LDL cholesterol concentrations in primary hypercholesterolemia; primary prevention of coronary artery disease (patients without symptomatic disease with average to moderately elevated total and LDL cholesterol and below average HDL cholesterol)

**Mechanism of Action/Effect** Lovastatin acts by competitively inhibiting 3-hydroxyl-3-methylglutaryl-coenzyme A (HMG-CoA) reductase, the enzyme that catalyzes the rate-limiting step in cholesterol biosynthesis.

**Contraindications** Hypersensitivity to lovastatin or any component; active liver disease; pregnancy

**Warnings** May elevate aminotransferases. LFTs should be performed before initiation of therapy, at 6 and 12 weeks after initiation or first dose, and periodically thereafter. Can also cause myalgia and rhabdomyolysis. Use with caution in patients who consume large quantities of alcohol or who have a history of liver disease.

**Drug Interactions**

**Cytochrome P-450 Effect:** CYP3A3/4 and 3A5-7 enzyme substrate

**Decreased Effect:** Cholestyramine taken with lovastatin reduces lovastatin absorption and effect.

**Increased Effect/Toxicity:** Increased toxicity with gemfibrozil (musculoskeletal effects such as myopathy, myalgia, and/or muscle weakness accompanied by markedly elevated CK concentrations, rash, and/or pruritus); clofibrate; niacin, itraconazole, ketoconazole, clarithromycin, nefazodone, erythromycin, cyclosporine (myopathy); and oral anticoagulants (elevated PT). Increased effect/toxicity of levothyroxine.

**Food Interactions** The therapeutic effect of lovastatin may be decreased if taken with food.

**Effects on Lab Values** ↑ liver transaminases (S), altered thyroid function tests

**Adverse Reactions**

1% to 10%:

- Central nervous system: Headache, dizziness
- Dermatologic: Rash, pruritus
- Gastrointestinal: Flatulence, abdominal pain, cramps, diarrhea, constipation, nausea, heartburn
- Neuromuscular & skeletal: Myalgia, elevated creatine phosphokinase (CPK)
- Ocular: Blurred vision

<1% (Limited to important or life-threatening symptoms): Chest pain

**Overdose/Toxicology** Few adverse events have been reported. Treatment is symptomatic.

**Pharmacodynamics/Kinetics**

**Protein Binding:** 95%

**Half-life Elimination:** 1.1-1.7 hours

**Time to Peak:** Oral: 2-4 hours

**Metabolism:** Liver hydrolysis

**Excretion:** ~80% to 85% of dose excreted in feces and 10% in urine

**Onset:** 3 days of therapy required for LDL cholesterol concentration reductions

**Formulations** Tablet: 10 mg, 20 mg, 40 mg

**Dosing**

**Adults:** Oral: Initial: 20 mg with evening meal, then adjust at 4-week intervals; maximum: 80 mg/day. Patients receiving immunosuppressant drugs should start at 10 mg/day and not exceed 20 mg/day. Patients receiving concurrent therapy with niacin or fibrates should not exceed 20 mg lovastatin.

**Elderly:** Refer to adult dosing.

**Renal Impairment:** $Cl_{cr}$ <30 mL/minute: Use with caution and carefully consider doses >20 mg/day.

(Continued)

## Lovastatin *(Continued)*

**Administration**

**Oral:** Administer with meals.

**Monitoring Laboratory Tests** Obtain baseline LFTs and total cholesterol profile. LFTs should be performed before initiation of therapy, at 6 and 12 weeks after initiation or first dose, and periodically thereafter.

**Additional Nursing Issues**

**Physical Assessment:** Assess other medications patient may be taking for effectiveness and/or interactions (see Drug Interactions). Assess knowledge/instruct patient on appropriate use, possible side effects (see Adverse Reactions), and symptoms to report. **Pregnancy risk factor X** - determine that patient is not pregnant before beginning treatment and do not give to women of childbearing age or to males who may have intercourse with women of childbearing age unless both male and female are capable of complying with barrier contraceptive measures during therapy and for 1 month following therapy. Breast-feeding is contraindicated.

**Patient Information/Instruction:** Take with evening meal (highest rate of cholesterol synthesis occurs from midnight to morning). If sleep disturbances occur, take earlier in the day. Do not change dosage without consulting prescriber. Maintain diet and exercise program as identified by prescriber. Have periodic ophthalmic exams while taking lovastatin (check for cataracts). You may experience mild GI disturbances (eg, gas, diarrhea, constipation); inform prescriber if these are severe or if you experience severe muscle pain or tenderness accompanied with malaise, blurred vision, or chest pain. **Pregnancy/breast-feeding precautions:** Inform prescriber if you are pregnant. Do not get pregnant 1 month during or for 1 month following therapy. Male: Do not cause a female to become pregnant. Male/female: Consult prescriber for instruction on appropriate contraceptive measures. This drug may cause severe fetal defects. Do not breast-feed.

**Dietary Issues:** Before initiation of therapy, patients should be placed on a standard cholesterol-lowering diet for 3-6 months and the diet should be continued during drug therapy.

**Geriatric Considerations:** The definition of and, therefore, when to treat hyperlipidemia in the elderly is a controversial issue. The National Cholesterol Education Program recommends that all adults 20 years of age and older maintain a plasma cholesterol <200 mg/dL. By this definition, 60% of all elderly would be considered to have a borderline high (200-239 mg/dL) or high (≥240 mg/dL) plasma cholesterol. However, plasma cholesterol has been shown to be a less reliable predictor of coronary heart disease in the elderly. Therefore, it is the authors' belief that pharmacologic treatment be reserved for those who are unable to obtain a desirable plasma cholesterol level by diet alone and for whom the benefits of treatment are believed to outweigh the potential adverse effects, drug interactions, and cost of treatment.

**Related Information**

Lipid-Lowering Agents Comparison *on page 1393*


- **Lovenox® Injection** *see* Enoxaparin *on page 421*
- **Lowadina** *see* Loratadine *on page 689*
- **Low Molecular Weight Heparins Comparison** *see page 1395*
- **Low-Quel®** *see* Diphenoxylate and Atropine *on page 382*
- **Loxapac®** *see* Loxapine *on this page*


## Loxapine (LOKS a peen)

**U.S. Brand Names** Loxitane®; Loxitane® C; Loxitane® I.M.

**Synonyms** Oxilapine Succinate

**Therapeutic Category** Antipsychotic Agent, Dibenzoxazepine

**Pregnancy Risk Factor** C

**Lactation** Excretion in breast milk unknown/not recommended

**Use** Management of psychotic disorders

**Mechanism of Action/Effect** Unclear, thought to be similar to chlorpromazine

**Contraindications** Hypersensitivity to loxapine or any component (cross reactivity between phenothiazines may occur); severe CNS depression; coma

**Warnings** May cause hypotension, particularly with I.M. administration. Moderately sedating, use with caution in disorders where CNS depression is a feature. Use with caution in Parkinson's disease. Use caution in patients with hemodynamic instability; bone marrow suppression; predisposition to seizures; subcortical brain damage; or severe cardiac, hepatic, renal, or respiratory disease. May cause swallowing difficulties. Use with caution in breast cancer or other prolactin-dependent tumors (may elevate prolactin levels). May alter temperature regulation or mask toxicity of other drugs due to antiemetic effects. May alter cardiac conduction - life-threatening arrhythmias have occurred with therapeutic doses of phenothiazines. May cause orthostatic hypotension.

Phenothiazines may cause anticholinergic effects (eg, confusion, agitation, constipation, dry mouth, blurred vision, urinary retention); therefore, use with caution in patients with decreased gastrointestinal motility, urinary retention, BPH, xerostomia, or visual problems. Conditions which also may be exacerbated by cholinergic blockade include narrow-angle glaucoma (screening is recommended) and worsening of myasthenia gravis. Relative to other antipsychotics, loxapine has a low potency of cholinergic blockade.

May cause extrapyramidal reactions including pseudoparkinsonism, acute dystonic reactions, akathisia, and tardive dyskinesia (risk of these reactions is high relative to other neuroleptics). May be associated with neuroleptic malignant syndrome (NMS) or pigmentary retinopathy.

Pregnancy factor C.

**Drug Interactions**

**Decreased Effect:** Decreased effect of guanethidine and phenytoin.

**Increased Effect/Toxicity:** Increased toxicity with CNS depressants, metrizamide (increased seizure potential), guanabenz, and MAO inhibitors. Respiratory depression and stupor with lorazepam.

**Effects on Lab Values** False-positives for phenylketonuria, amylase, uroporphyrins, urobilinogen; ↑ liver function tests

**Adverse Reactions**

>10%:
- Cardiovascular: Orthostatic hypotension
- Central nervous system: Drowsiness, extrapyramidal effects (parkinsonian), confusion, persistent tardive dyskinesia
- Gastrointestinal: Dry mouth
- Ocular: Blurred vision

1% to 10%:
- Dermatologic: Rash
- Endocrine & metabolic: Gynecomastia
- Gastrointestinal: Constipation, nausea, vomiting

<1% (Limited to important or life-threatening symptoms): Tachycardia, arrhythmias, abnormal T waves with prolonged ventricular repolarization, neuroleptic malignant syndrome (NMS), seizures, adynamic ileus, agranulocytosis (more often in women between fourth and tenth week of therapy), leukopenia (usually in patients with large doses for prolonged periods), cholestatic jaundice

**Overdose/Toxicology** Symptoms of overdose include deep sleep, dystonia, agitation, dysrhythmias, extrapyramidal symptoms, hypotension, and seizures. Treatment is symptomatic and supportive.

**Pharmacodynamics/Kinetics**

**Half-life Elimination:** Half-life, biphasic: Initial: 5 hours; Terminal: 12-19 hours

**Metabolism:** Liver

**Excretion:** Urine and feces

**Onset:** Onset of neuroleptic effect: Oral: Within 20-30 minutes; Peak effect: 1.5-3 hours

**Duration:** ~12 hours

**Formulations**

Loxapine hydrochloride:
- Concentrate, oral: 25 mg/mL (120 mL dropper bottle)
- Injection: 50 mg/mL (1 mL)

Loxapine succinate:
- Capsule: 5 mg, 10 mg, 25 mg, 50 mg

**Dosing**

**Adults:**
- Oral: 10 mg twice daily, increase dose until psychotic symptoms are controlled; usual dose range: 60-100 mg/day in divided doses 2-4 times/day; dosages >250 mg/day are not recommended
- I.M.: 12.5-50 mg every 4-6 hours or longer as needed and change to oral therapy as soon as possible

**Elderly:** Oral: Nonpsychotic patients, dementia behavior: Initial: 5-10 mg 1-2 times/day; increase dose at 4- to 7-day intervals by 5-10 mg/day. Increase dosing intervals (twice daily, 3 times/day, etc) as necessary to control response or side effects. Maximum daily dose: 125 mg; gradual increases (titration) may prevent some side effects or their severity.

**Administration**

**Oral:** Mix oral solution with orange or grapefruit juice 3-5 minutes before administration.

**I.V.: Not** for I.V. administration; injectable is for I.M. use only.

**Monitoring Laboratory Tests** Liver and kidney function, CBC prior to and at regular intervals, ophthalmic screening

**Additional Nursing Issues**

**Physical Assessment:** Assess other medications patient is taking for effectiveness and interactions (See Drug Interactions). See Contraindications and Warnings/Precautions for cautious use. Has potential for psychological or physiological dependence, abuse, and tolerance. Review ophthalmic screening (see Monitoring Laboratory Tests) and monitor laboratory results (see above), therapeutic response (mental status, mood, affect), and adverse reactions at beginning of therapy and periodically with long-term use (orthostatic hypotension, heart rate, fluid balance, anticholinergic response, extrapyramidal effects - see Adverse Reactions and Overdose). I.M.: Monitor closely for hypotension. Initiate at lower doses (see Dosing) and taper dosage slowly when discontinuing. Assess knowledge/teach patient appropriate use, interventions to reduce side effects, and adverse symptoms to report (see below). **Pregnancy risk factor C** - benefits of use should outweigh possible risks. Breast-feeding is not recommended.

**Patient Information/Instruction:** Use exactly as directed (do not increase dose or frequency); may cause physical and/or psychological dependence. It may take 2-3 weeks to achieve desired results; do not discontinue without consulting prescriber. Dilute oral concentration with water or juice. Do not take within 2 hours of any antacid. Avoid excess alcohol or caffeine and other prescription or OTC medications not approved by prescriber. Maintain adequate hydration (2-3 L/day of fluids unless

(Continued)

## Loxapine *(Continued)*

instructed to restrict fluid intake). You may experience excess drowsiness, restlessness, dizziness, or blurred vision (use caution driving or when engaging in tasks requiring alertness until response to drug is known); nausea, vomiting (small frequent meals, frequent mouth care, chewing gum, or sucking lozenges may help); constipation (increased exercise, fluids, or dietary fruit and fiber may help); postural hypotension (use caution climbing stairs or when changing position from lying or sitting to standing); urinary retention (void before taking medication); or decreased perspiration (avoid strenuous exercise in hot environments). Report persistent CNS effects (eg, trembling fingers, altered gait or balance, excessive sedation, seizures, unusual movements, anxiety, abnormal thoughts, confusion, personality changes); chest pain, palpitations, rapid heartbeat, severe dizziness; unresolved urinary retention or changes in urinary pattern; vision changes; skin rash or yellowing of skin; difficulty breathing; or worsening of condition. **Pregnancy/breast-feeding precautions:** Inform prescriber if you are or intend to be pregnant. Breast-feeding is not recommended.

**Geriatric Considerations:** (See Warnings/Precautions, Adverse Reactions, and Overdose/Toxicology.) Elderly patients have an increased risk of adverse response to side effects or adverse reactions to antipsychotics. These can include but are not limited to the following.

Anticholinergic effects: CNS toxicity with confusion, memory loss, psychotic behavior, and agitation.

Extrapyramidal effects (EPS): Parkinson's syndrome and akathisia may occur as often as 50% in patients >60 years of age. Tardive dyskinesia (motor restlessness) may be 40% in elderly; may be related to duration and total accumulated dose over time; may be somewhat reversible if diagnosed early enough.

Orthostatic hypotension: Increased risk for falls.

Sedation: In nonpsychotic patients, may result in feelings of depersonalization, derealization, and dysphoria.

Cardiac toxicity: Cardiac arrhythmias have occurred with therapeutic doses of antipsychotics.

Malignant neuroleptic syndrome: Development of hyperthermia, muscular rigidity, autonomic instability, and altered mental status.

Many elderly patients receive antipsychotic medications for inappropriate nonpsychotic behavior. Before initiating antipsychotic medication, all possible reversible causes should be investigated. Stress may cause acute "confusion" or worsening of baseline nonpsychotic behaviors; any changes in disease state (in any organ) may result in behavioral changes. Common acute changes in behavior may be due also to increases in drug dose addition, or addition of a new drug to the regimen; fluid/electrolyte alterations; infections; or changes in the environment.

Meta-analysis of controlled trials of antipsychotic (phenothiazines, butyrophenones) use with agitated, demented, elderly patients has concluded that the use of neuroleptics results in a response rate of 18%. Clearly, neuroleptic therapy for behavior control should be limited, with frequent attempts to withdraw the agent for behavior control. When use is indicated, initial doses should be lower to start and monitored closely.

**Additional Information**

Loxapine hydrochloride: Loxitane® C oral concentrate, Loxitane® IM
Loxapine succinate: Loxitane® capsule

**Related Information**

Antipsychotic Agents Comparison *on page 1371*
Antipsychotic Medication Guidelines *on page 1436*


- **Loxitane®** *see* Loxapine *on page 696*
- **Loxitane® C** *see* Loxapine *on page 696*
- **Loxitane® I.M.** *see* Loxapine *on page 696*
- **Lozide®** *see* Indapamide *on page 604*
- **Lozol®** *see* Indapamide *on page 604*
- **L-PAM** *see* Melphalan *on page 718*
- **LRH** *see* Gonadorelin *on page 542*
- **L-Sarcolysin** *see* Melphalan *on page 718*
- **LTG** *see* Lamotrigine *on page 654*
- **l-Thyroxine Sodium** *see* Levothyroxine *on page 673*
- **Lubriderm® Lotion** *see page 1294*
- **LubriTears® Solution** *see page 1294*
- **Lucrin** *see* Leuprolide *on page 663*
- **Lucrin Depot** *see* Leuprolide *on page 663*
- **Lugol's Solution** *see* Potassium Iodide *on page 951*
- **Luminal®** *see* Phenobarbital *on page 917*
- **Lupron®** *see* Leuprolide *on page 663*
- **Lupron Depot®** *see* Leuprolide *on page 663*
- **Lupron Depot-Ped™** *see* Leuprolide *on page 663*
- **Lurdex** *see* Albendazole *on page 44*
- **Luride®** *see page 1294*
- **Luride® Lozi-Tab®** *see page 1294*
- **Luride®-SF Lozi-Tab®** *see page 1294*

- **Luritran®** *see* Erythromycin *on page 435*
- **Luteinizing Hormone Releasing Hormone** *see* Gonadorelin *on page 542*
- **Lutrepulse®** *see* Gonadorelin *on page 542*
- **Luvox®** *see* Fluvoxamine *on page 514*
- **Luxiq®** *see* Betamethasone *on page 148*
- **LY170053** *see* Olanzapine *on page 848*


## Lyme Disease Vaccine (LIME dee SEAS vak SEEN)

**U.S. Brand Names** LYMErix®

**Synonyms** Lyme Disease Vaccine (Recombinant OspA)

**Therapeutic Category** Vaccine

**Pregnancy Risk Factor** C

**Lactation** Excretion in breast milk unknown/use caution

**Use** Active immunization against Lyme disease in individuals between 15-70 years of age

**Mechanism of Action/Effect** Lyme disease vaccine is a recombinant, noninfectious lipoprotein (OspA) derived from the outer surface of *Borrelia burgdorferi*, the causative agent of Lyme disease. Vaccination stimulates production of antibodies directed against this organism, including antibodies against the LA-2 epitope, which have bactericidal activity. Since OspA expression is down-regulated after inoculation into the human host, at least part of the vaccine's efficacy may be related to neutralization of bacteria within the midgut of the tick vector, preventing transmission to the human host.

**Contraindications** Hypersensitivity to any component of the vaccine. Vaccination should be postponed during acute moderate to severe febrile illness (minor illness is generally not a contraindication). Safety and efficacy in patients <15 years of age have not been established.

**Warnings** Do not administer to patients with treatment-resistant Lyme arthritis. Will not prevent disease in patients with prior infection and offers no protection against other tick-borne diseases. Immunosuppressed patients or those receiving immunosuppressive therapy (vaccine may not be effective) - defer vaccination until 3 months after therapy. Avoid in patients receiving anticoagulant therapy (due to intramuscular injection). The physician should take all known precautions for prevention of allergic or other reactions. Administer with caution to patients with known or suspected latex allergy (applies only to the LMErix Tip-lok™ syringe, vaccine vial does not contain natural rubber). Duration of immunity has not been established.

**Adverse Reactions** (Limited to overall self-reported events occurring within 30 days following a dose)

>10%: Local: Injection site pain (21.9%)

1% to 10%:

- Central nervous system: Headache (5.6%), fatigue (3.9%), fever (2.6%), chills (2%), dizziness (1%)
- Dermatologic: Rash (1.4%)
- Gastrointestinal: Nausea (1.1%)
- Neuromuscular & skeletal: Arthralgia (6.8%), myalgia (4.8%), muscle aches (2.8%), back pain (1.9%), stiffness (1%)
- Respiratory: Upper respiratory tract infection (4.4%), sinusitis (3.2%), pharyngitis (2.5%), rhinitis (2.4%), cough (1.5%), bronchitis (1.1%)
- Miscellaneous: Viral infection (2.8%), flu-like syndrome (2.5%)

Solicited adverse event rates were higher than unsolicited event rates (above). These included local reactions of soreness (93.5%), redness (41.8%), and swelling (29.9%). In addition, general systemic symptoms included fatigue (40.8%), headache (38.6%), arthralgia (25.6%), rash (11.7%) and fever (3.5%)

Patients with a history of Lyme disease were noted to experience a higher frequency of early musculoskeletal reactions. Other differences in the observed rate of adverse reactions were not significantly different between vaccine and placebo recipients.

**Formulations** Injection:

Vial: 30 mcg/0.5 mL

Prefilled syringe (Tip-Lok™): 30 mcg/0.5 mL

**Dosing**

**Adults:** I.M.: Vaccination with 3 doses of 30 mcg (0.5 mL), administered at 0, 1, and 12 months, is recommended for optimal protection.

**Elderly:** Refer to adult dosing.

**Administration**

**I.M.:** Intramuscular injection into the deltoid region is recommended. Do not administer intravenously, intradermally, or subcutaneously. The vaccine should be used as supplied without dilution.

**Stability**

**Storage:** Store between 2°C and 8°C (36°F and 46°F).

**Monitoring Laboratory Tests** Vaccination will result in a positive *B. burgdorferi* IgG via ELISA (Western blot testing is recommended)

**Additional Nursing Issues**

**Physical Assessment:** See Contraindications and Warnings/Precautions for use cautions. Assess knowledge/teach patient possible side effects/interventions, and adverse symptoms to report (See Adverse Reaction). **Pregnancy risk factor C.** Note breast-feeding caution.

**Patient Information/Instruction:** You will require two more injections over the next 12 months; schedule appointments for those injections as directed by prescriber. You may experience headache, mild nausea, chills, fever, or dizziness following injection. These should subside, if not contact prescriber. Report persistent redness, swelling, or

(Continued)

## Lyme Disease Vaccine *(Continued)*

pain at injection site; skin rash; persistent flu-like symptoms; or muscle aches of stiffness. **Pregnancy/breast-feeding precautions:** Inform prescriber is you are or intend to be pregnant. Consult prescriber if breast-feeding.

**Related Information**

Immunizations (Vaccines) *on page 1256*

- **Lyme Disease Vaccine (Recombinant OspA)** *see* Lyme Disease Vaccine *on previous page*
- **LYMErix®** *see* Lyme Disease Vaccine *on previous page*
- **LYMErix®** *see page 1256*

## Lymphocyte Immune Globulin (LIM foe site i MYUN GLOB yoo lin)

**U.S. Brand Names** Atgam®

**Synonyms** Antithymocyte Globulin (Equine); ATG; Horse Antihuman Thymocyte Gamma Globulin

**Therapeutic Category** Immunosuppressant Agent

**Pregnancy Risk Factor** C

**Lactation** Excretion in breast milk unknown

**Use** Prevention and treatment of renal and other solid organ allograft rejection; treatment of moderate to severe aplastic anemia in patients not considered suitable candidates for bone marrow transplantation; prevention and treatment of graft-versus-host disease following bone marrow transplantation

**Mechanism of Action/Effect** May involve elimination of antigen-reactive T lymphocytes (killer cells) in peripheral blood or alteration of T-cell function

**Contraindications** Hypersensitivity to ATG, thimerosal, or other equine gamma globulins; severe, unremitting leukopenia and/or thrombocytopenia

**Warnings** For I.V. use only. Must be administered via central line due to chemical phlebitis. Should only be used by physicians experienced in immunosuppressive therapy or management of solid organ or bone marrow transplant patients. Adequate laboratory and supportive medical resources must be readily available in the facility for patient management. Rash, dyspnea, hypotension, or anaphylaxis precludes further administration of the drug. Dose must be administered over at least 4 hours. Patient may need to be pretreated with an antipyretic, antihistamine, and/or corticosteroid. Pregnancy factor C.

**Adverse Reactions**

>10%:

Central nervous system: Fever, chills
Dermatologic: Rash
Hematologic: Leukopenia, thrombocytopenia
Miscellaneous: Systemic infection

1% to 10%:

Cardiovascular: Hypotension, hypertension, tachycardia, edema, chest pain
Central nervous system: Headache, malaise, pain
Gastrointestinal: Diarrhea, nausea, stomatitis, GI bleeding
Respiratory: Dyspnea
Local: Edema or redness at injection site, thrombophlebitis
Neuromuscular & skeletal: Myalgia, back pain
Renal: Abnormal renal function tests
Miscellaneous: Sensitivity reactions: Anaphylaxis may be indicated by hypotension, respiratory distress, serum sickness, viral infection

<1% (Limited to important or life-threatening symptoms): Seizures, hemolysis, anemia, acute renal failure, lymphadenopathy

**Pharmacodynamics/Kinetics**

**Distribution:** Poorly distributed into lymphoid tissues; binds to circulating lymphocytes, granulocytes, platelets, bone marrow cells

**Half-life Elimination:** Plasma: 1.5-12 days

**Excretion:** Urine

**Formulations** Injection: 50 mg/mL (5 mL)

**Dosing**

**Adults:** An intradermal skin test is recommended prior to administration of the initial dose of ATG; use 0.1 mL of a 1:1000 dilution of ATG in normal saline. A positive skin reaction consists of a wheal ≥10 mm in diameter. If a positive skin test occurs, the first infusion should be administered in a controlled environment with intensive life support immediately available. A systemic reaction precludes further administration of the drug. The absence of a reaction does **not** preclude the possibility of an immediate sensitivity reaction.

I.V.:

Aplastic anemia protocol: 10-20 mg/kg/day for 8-14 days, then give every other day for 7 more doses **or** 40 mg/kg/day for 4 days.

Rejection prevention: 15 mg/kg/day for 14 days, then give every other day for 7 more doses for a total of 21 doses in 28 days; initial dose should be administered within 24 hours before or after transplantation.

Rejection treatment: 10-15 mg/kg/day for 14 days, then give every other day for 7 more doses.

**Elderly:** Refer to adult dosing.

**Administration**

**I.V.:** Infuse dose over at least 4 hours. Any severe systemic reaction to the skin test such as generalized rash, tachycardia, dyspnea, hypotension, or anaphylaxis should preclude further therapy. **Epinephrine and resuscitative equipment should be nearby.** Patient may need to be pretreated with an antipyretic, antihistamine, and/or corticosteroid. Mild itching and erythema can be treated with antihistamines.

**Stability**

**Storage:** Ampuls must be refrigerated.

**Reconstitution:** Dose must be diluted in 0.45% or 0.9% sodium chloride. Diluted solution is stable for 12 hours (including infusion time) at room temperature and 24 hours (including infusion time) at refrigeration. **The use of dextrose solutions is not recommended (precipitation may occur).**

Standard diluent: Dose/1000 mL NS or 0.45% sodium chloride

Minimum volume: Concentration should not exceed 1 mg/mL for a peripheral line or 4 mg/mL for a central line.

**Monitoring Laboratory Tests** Lymphocyte profile, CBC with differential, platelet count

**Additional Nursing Issues**

**Physical Assessment:** Assess for history of previous allergic reactions (see Contraindications). See Warnings/Precautions and Administration for safe infusion and pretreatment recommendations. Monitor vital signs during infusion and observe for adverse or allergic reactions (see Adverse Reactions). Teach patient adverse symptoms to report. **Pregnancy risk factor C** - benefits of use should outweigh possible risks. Note breast-feeding caution.

**Patient Information/Instruction:** This medication can only be administered by infusion. You will be monitored closely during the infusion. Do not get up alone; ask for assistance if you must get up or change position. Do not have any vaccinations for the next 3 months without consulting prescriber. Immediately report chills; persistent dizziness or nausea; itching or stinging; acute back pain; chest pain or tightness or rapid heartbeat; or difficulty breathing. **Pregnancy/breast-feeding precautions:** Inform prescriber if you are pregnant. Consult prescriber if breast-feeding.

♦ **Lyphocin®** *see* Vancomycin *on page 1202*

♦ **Lyposyn** *see* Fat Emulsion *on page 471*

## Lypressin (lye PRES in)

**U.S. Brand Names** Diapid® Nasal Spray

**Synonyms** 8-*L*-Lysine Vasopressin

**Therapeutic Category** Antidiuretic Hormone Analog

**Pregnancy Risk Factor** C

**Lactation** Enters breast milk/compatible

**Use** Controls or prevents signs and complications of neurogenic diabetes insipidus

**Mechanism of Action/Effect** Increases cyclic adenosine monophosphate (cAMP) which increases water permeability at the renal tubule resulting in decreased urine volume and increased osmolality; causes peristalsis by directly stimulating the smooth muscle in the GI tract

**Contraindications** Hypersensitivity to lypressin or any component

**Warnings** Use with caution in patients with coronary artery disease. Pregnancy factor C.

**Drug Interactions**

**Increased Effect/Toxicity:** Increased effect with chlorpropamide and clofibrate. Carbamazepine may cause prolongation of antidiuretic effects.

**Adverse Reactions** 1% to 10%:

Cardiovascular: Chest tightness

Central nervous system: Dizziness, headache

Gastrointestinal: Abdominal cramping, increased bowel movements

Local: Irritation or burning

Respiratory: Coughing, dyspnea, rhinorrhea, nasal congestion

**Overdose/Toxicology** Symptoms of overdose include drowsiness, headache, confusion, weight gain, and hypertension. Systemic toxicity is unlikely to occur from the nasal spray.

**Pharmacodynamics/Kinetics**

**Half-life Elimination:** 15-20 minutes

**Metabolism:** Liver and kidneys

**Excretion:** Urine

**Onset:** Onset of antidiuretic effect: Intranasal spray: Within 0.5-2 hours

**Duration:** 3-8 hours

**Formulations** Spray: 0.185 mg/mL (equivalent to 50 USP posterior pituitary units/mL) (8 mL)

**Dosing**

**Adults:** Instill 1-2 sprays into one or both nostrils whenever frequency of urination increases or significant thirst develops; usual dosage is 1-2 sprays 4 times/day; range: 1 spray/day at bedtime to 10 sprays each nostril every 3-4 hours

**Elderly:** Refer to adult dosing.

**Administration**

**Inhalation:** Administer intranasally only. Hold bottle upright with patient in vertical position. Spray only 1-2 sprays per nostril.

**Additional Nursing Issues**

**Physical Assessment:** Instruct patient on appropriate administration technique. Inappropriate administration can lead to nasal ulcerations. Monitor nasal passages during long-term therapy. **Pregnancy risk factor C** - benefits of use should outweigh possible risks.

**Patient Information/Instruction:** To control nocturia, an additional dose may be given at bedtime. Notify prescriber if drowsiness, fatigue, headache, shortness of

(Continued)

## Lypressin *(Continued)*

breath, abdominal cramps, or severe nasal irritation occurs. **Pregnancy precautions:** Inform prescriber if you are or intend to be pregnant.

**Geriatric Considerations:** No specific data is available for geriatrics. Given the pathophysiology and treatment response, no specific recommendations are necessary. Treat the elderly as indicated for adults.

**Additional Information** Approximately 2 USP posterior pituitary vasopressor units per spray

- **Lysatec-rt-PA®** *see* Alteplase *on page 58*
- **Lysodren®** *see* Mitotane *on page 779*
- **Maalox®** *see page 1294*
- **Maalox Anti-Gas®** *see page 1294*
- **Maalox® Plus** *see page 1294*
- **Maalox® Therapeutic Concentrate** *see page 1294*
- **Macrobid®** *see* Nitrofurantoin *on page 829*
- **Macrodantin®** *see* Nitrofurantoin *on page 829*
- **Macrodantina** *see* Nitrofurantoin *on page 829*
- **Macrodex®** *see* Dextran *on page 351*
- **Madel** *see* Phenazopyridine *on page 914*

## Mafenide (MA fe nide)

**U.S. Brand Names** Sulfamylon® Topical

**Therapeutic Category** Antibiotic, Topical

**Pregnancy Risk Factor** C

**Lactation** Excretion in breast milk unknown

**Use** Adjunct in the treatment of second and third degree burns to prevent septicemia caused by susceptible organisms such as *Pseudomonas aeruginosa*; prevention of graft loss of meshed autografts on excised burn wounds

**Mechanism of Action/Effect** Interferes with bacterial folic acid synthesis through competitive inhibition of para-aminobenzoic acid

**Contraindications** Hypersensitivity to mafenide, sulfites, or any component

**Warnings** Use with caution in patients with renal impairment and in patients with G-6-PD deficiency. Prolonged use may result in superinfection. Pregnancy factor C.

**Adverse Reactions**

>10%: Local: Pain or burning sensation, excoriation

1% to 10%:
- Cardiovascular: Facial edema
- Dermatologic: Rash
- Miscellaneous: Dyspnea

<1% (Limited to important or life-threatening symptoms): Hyperchloremia, metabolic acidosis, bone marrow suppression, hemolytic anemia, bleeding, porphyria, hyperventilation, tachypnea

**Pharmacodynamics/Kinetics**

**Time to Peak:** Topical: 2-4 hours

**Metabolism:** To para-carboxybenzene sulfonamide which is a carbonic anhydrase inhibitor

**Excretion:** Urine

**Formulations** Cream, topical, as acetate: 85 mg/g (56.7 g, 113.4 g, 411 g)

**Dosing**

**Adults:** Topical: Apply once or twice daily with a sterile gloved hand; apply to a thickness of approximately 16 mm. The burned area should be covered with cream at all times.

**Elderly:** Refer to adult dosing.

**Monitoring Laboratory Tests** Acid-base balance

**Additional Nursing Issues**

**Physical Assessment:** See Warnings/Precautions and Contraindications for use cautions. Assess for effectiveness of therapy and symptoms of infection. Assess knowledge/teach patient appropriate application and use and adverse symptoms (see Adverse Reactions) to report. **Pregnancy risk factor C.** Note breast-feeding caution.

**Patient Information/Instruction:** For external use only. Apply exactly as directed with sterile gloved hand so that burned areas are covered with cream at all times. Avoid getting in eyes. Report facial swelling, skin rash, unusual bleeding, difficulty breathing, or signs of infections. **Pregnancy/breast-feeding precautions:** Inform prescriber if you are or intend to be pregnant. Consult prescriber if breast-feeding.

**Additional Information** Some formulations may contain sulfites.

- **Mag-200** *see* Magnesium Supplements *on next page*

## Magaldrate (MAG al drate)

**U.S. Brand Names** Riopan® [OTC]

**Synonyms** Hydromagnesium Aluminate

**Therapeutic Category** Antacid

**Pregnancy Risk Factor** C

**Lactation** Excretion in breast milk unknown/compatible

**Use** Symptomatic relief of hyperacidity associated with peptic ulcer, gastritis, peptic esophagitis and hiatal hernia

**Warnings** Pregnancy factor C.

**Formulations** Suspension, oral: 540 mg/5 mL (360 mL)

**Dosing**

**Adults:** Oral: 480-1080 mg between meals (1-2 hours after meals and at bedtime)

**Elderly:** Refer to adult dosing.

**Renal Impairment:** $Cl_{cr}$ <30 mL/minute: Not recommended due to risk of hypermagnesemia.

**Additional Nursing Issues**

**Geriatric Considerations:** Elderly, due to disease or drug therapy, may be predisposed to diarrhea or constipation. Diarrhea may result in electrolyte imbalance. Decreased renal function ($Cl_{cr}$ <30 mL/minute) may result in toxicity of aluminum or magnesium. Drug interactions must be considered. If possible, administer antacid 1-2 hours apart from other drugs. When treating ulcers, consider buffer capacity (mEq/mL) antacid.

**Additional Information** Magaldrate is a chemical entity known as hydroxy magnesium aluminate equivalent to magnesium oxide and aluminum oxide. Unlike other magnesium containing antacids, Riopan® is safe to use in renal patients if used cautiously. Magaldrate contains 340-460 mg of magnesium oxide per gram, 210-300 mg aluminum oxide per gram.

## Magaldrate and Simethicone (MAG al drate & sye METH i kone)

**U.S. Brand Names** Riopan Plus® [OTC]

**Synonyms** Simethicone and Magaldrate

**Therapeutic Category** Antacid; Antiflatulent

**Pregnancy Risk Factor** C

**Lactation** Excretion in breast milk unknown/compatible

**Use** Relief of hyperacidity associated with peptic ulcer, gastritis, peptic esophagitis and hiatal hernia which are accompanied by symptoms of gas

**Formulations** Suspension, oral: Magaldrate 480 mg and simethicone 20 mg per 5 mL (360 mL)

**Dosing**

**Adults:** Oral: 5-10 mL between meals and at bedtime

**Elderly:** Refer to adult dosing.

**Additional Nursing Issues**

**Physical Assessment:** See individual components listed in Related Information. **Pregnancy risk factor C** - benefits of use should outweigh possible risks.

**Patient Information/Instruction:** See individual components listed in Related Information. **Pregnancy precautions:** Inform prescriber if you are on intend to get pregnant.

**Related Information**

Magaldrate *on previous page*


- **Magalox Plus®** *see page 1294*
- **Mag-Carb™** *see* Magnesium Supplements *on this page*
- **Magnesia Magma (Magnesium Hydroxide)** *see* Magnesium Supplements *on this page*
- **Magnesium Carbonate** *see* Magnesium Supplements *on this page*
- **Magnesium Chloride** *see* Magnesium Supplements *on this page*
- **Magnesium Chloride** *see page 1294*
- **Magnesium Citrate** *see* Magnesium Supplements *on this page*
- **Magnesium Gluconate** *see* Magnesium Supplements *on this page*
- **Magnesium Gluconate** *see page 1294*
- **Magnesium Hydroxide** *see* Magnesium Supplements *on this page*
- **Magnesium Hydroxide and Mineral Oil Emulsion** *see* Magnesium Supplements *on this page*
- **Magnesium Hydroxide and Mineral Oil Emulsion** *see page 1294*
- **Magnesium Lactate** *see* Magnesium Supplements *on this page*
- **Magnesium Oxide** *see* Magnesium Supplements *on this page*
- **Magnesium Sulfate** *see* Magnesium Supplements *on this page*


## Magnesium Supplements (mag NEE zee um SUP la ments)

**U.S. Brand Names** Almora®; Evac-Q-Mag®; Haley's M-O®; Mag-200; Mag-Carb™; Magonate®; Mag-Ox 400®; Mag-Tab SR®; Magtrate; Maox®; Phillips'® Milk of Magnesia; Slow-Mag®; Uro-Mag®

**Synonyms** Citrate of Magnesia (Magnesium Citrate); Epsom Salts (Magnesium Sulfate); Magnesia Magma (Magnesium Hydroxide); Magnesium Carbonate; Magnesium Chloride; Magnesium Citrate; Magnesium Gluconate; Magnesium Hydroxide; Magnesium Hydroxide and Mineral Oil Emulsion; Magnesium Lactate; Magnesium Oxide; Magnesium Sulfate; Milk of Magnesia (Magnesium Hydroxide); MOM (Magnesium Hydroxide)

**Therapeutic Category** Electrolyte Supplement

**Pregnancy Risk Factor** B

**Lactation** Enters breast milk/compatible

**Use**

Treatment and prevention of hypomagnesemia **(magnesium chloride, magnesium lactate, magnesium carbonate, magnesium sulfate, magnesium gluconate, and magnesium oxide)**

Treatment of hypertension **(magnesium sulfate)**

Treatment of encephalopathy and seizures associated with acute nephritis **(magnesium sulfate)**

(Continued)

## Magnesium Supplements *(Continued)*

Short-term treatment of constipation **(magnesium citrate, magnesium hydroxide, magnesium sulfate, and magnesium oxide)**
Treatment of hyperacidity symptoms **(magnesium hydroxide and magnesium oxide)**
Adjunctive treatment in moderate to severe acute asthma **(magnesium sulfate)**

**Mechanism of Action/Effect** Magnesium is important as a cofactor in many enzymatic reactions in the body. There are at least 300 enzymes which are dependent upon magnesium for normal functioning. Actions on lipoprotein lipase have been found to be important in reducing serum cholesterol. Magnesium is necessary for the maintaining of serum potassium and calcium levels due to its effect on the renal tubule. In the heart, magnesium acts as a calcium channel blocker. It also activates sodium potassium ATPase in the cell membrane to promote resting polarization and produce arrhythmias. Promotes bowel evacuation by causing osmotic retention of fluid which distends the colon and produces increased peristaltic activity when taken orally. To reduce stomach acidity, it reacts with hydrochloric acid in the stomach to form magnesium chloride.

**Contraindications** Serious renal impairment, myocardial damage, heart block; colostomy or ileostomy; intestinal obstruction, impaction, or perforation; appendicitis; abdominal pain

**Warnings** Use with caution in patients with impaired renal function (accumulation of magnesium may lead to magnesium intoxication). Use with caution in digitalized patients (may alter cardiac conduction leading to heart block).

**Drug Interactions**

**Decreased Effect:** Magnesium salts, when given orally, may decrease the absorption of the following: $H_2$ antagonists, phenytoin, iron salts, penicillamine, tetracycline, ciprofloxacin, benzodiazepines, chloroquine, steroids, and glyburide; systemic magnesium may enhance the effects of calcium channel blockers and neuromuscular blockers; may share additive CNS depressant effects with CNS depressants; if sufficient alkalinization of the urine by magnesium salts occurs, the excretion of salicylates is enhanced and the tubular reabsorption of quinidine is enhanced (increased effect)

**Increased Effect/Toxicity:** Magnesium salts, when given orally, may decrease the absorption of the following: $H_2$ antagonists, phenytoin, iron salts, penicillamine, tetracycline, ciprofloxacin, benzodiazepines, chloroquine, steroids, and glyburide; systemic magnesium may enhance the effects of calcium channel blockers and neuromuscular blockers; may share additive CNS depressant effects with CNS depressants; if sufficient alkalinization of the urine by magnesium salts occurs, the excretion of salicylates is enhanced and the tubular reabsorption of quinidine is enhanced (increased effect)

**Adverse Reactions** Adverse effects with magnesium therapy are related to the magnesium serum level

>3 mg/dL: Depressed CNS, blocked peripheral neuromuscular transmission leading to anticonvulsant effects
>5 mg/dL: Depressed deep tendon reflexes, flushing, somnolence
>12 mg/dL: Respiratory paralysis, complete heart block

Other effects:
Cardiovascular: Hypotension
Endocrine & metabolic: Hypermagnesemia
Gastrointestinal: Diarrhea, abdominal cramps, gas formation
Neuromuscular & skeletal: Muscle weakness

**Overdose/Toxicology** See Adverse Reactions.

**Pharmacodynamics/Kinetics**

**Half-life Elimination:** Renal with unabsorbed drug excreted in feces
**Onset:** Anticonvulsant: I.M.: 60 minutes; I.V.: Immediately; Laxative: Oral: 4-8 hours
**Duration:** Anticonvulsant: I.M.: 3-4 hours; I.V.: 30 minutes

**Formulations** Amount of magnesium salt is listed with **elemental** magnesium content in brackets

**Magnesium, amino acid chelate:** Tablet: 500 mg [100 mg]
**Magnesium carbonate:** Capsule, gelatin (Mag-Carb™): 250 mg [5.8 mEq; 70 mg]
**Magnesium chloride:**
Injection: 20% [1.97 mEq/mL] (50 mL)
Tablet, sustained release: 535 mg [5.2 mEq; 63 mg]
**Magnesium citrate:** Solution: 3.85-4.71 mEq/5mL (300 mL)
**Magnesium gluconate:**
Solution: 1000 mg/5 mL [4.8 mEq; 54 mg]
Tablet: 500 mg [2.4 mEq; 27 mg]
**Magnesium hydroxide:**
Liquid: 390 mg/5 mL (10 mL, 15 mL, 20 mL, 30 mL, 100 mL, 120 mL, 180 mL, 360 mL, 720 mL); 400 mg/5 mL; 800 mg/5 mL
Liquid, concentrate: 10 mL equivalent to 30 mL milk of magnesia USP
Suspension, oral: 2.5 g/30 mL (10 mL, 15 mL, 30 mL)
Tablet, chewable: 311 mg
**Magnesium hydroxide and mineral oil:**
Suspension (Haley's M-O®): Each 30 mL contains magnesium hydroxide 24 mL and mineral oil 6 mL
**Magnesium lactate:** Caplet, sustained release (Mag-Tab SR®): 835 mg [7 mEq; 84 mg]
**Magnesium oxide:**
Capsule: 140 mg [7 mEq; 84 mg]
Tablet: 400 mg [20 mEq; 242 mg], 420 mg [21 mEq; 254 mg], 500 mg [25 mEq; 302 mg]
**Magnesium sulfate:**
Granules: ~40 mEq magnesium/5 g (240 g)

Injection: 100 mg/mL (20 mL); 125 mg/mL (8 mL); 250 mg/mL (150 mL); 500 mg/mL (2 mL, 5 mL, 10 mL, 30 mL, 50 mL)

Solution, oral: 50% 500 mg/mL (30 mL) [4.1 mEq/mL; 49.3 mg]

**Dosing**

**Adults: Note:** Multiple salt forms of magnesium exist; close attention must be paid to the salt form when ordering and administering magnesium; incorrect selection or substitution of one salt for another without proper dosage adjustment may result in serious over- or underdosing.

Recommended daily allowance of magnesium: See table.

**Magnesium - Recommended Daily Allowance (RDA) (in terms of elemental magnesium)**

| Age | RDA (mg/day) |
|---|---|
| <5 mo | 40 |
| 5-12 mo | 60 |
| 1-3 y | 80 |
| 4-6 y | 120 |
| 7-10 y | 170 |
| Male | |
| 11-14 y | 270 |
| 15-18 y | 400 |
| >19 y | 350 |
| Female | |
| 11-14 y | 280 |
| 15-18 y | 300 |
| >19 y | 280 |

HYPOMAGNESEMIA:

**Magnesium gluconate:** Oral: 500-1000 mg 3 times/day

**Magnesium sulfate:**

I.M., I.V.: 1 g every 6 hours for 4 doses, or 250 mg/kg over a 4-hour period; for severe hypomagnesemia: 8-12 g/day in divided doses has been used

Oral: 3 g every 6 hours for 4 doses

DAILY MAINTENANCE MAGNESIUM: I.V.:

**Magnesium sulfate or magnesium chloride:** 0.2-0.5 mEq/kg/day or 3-10 mEq/1000 kcal/day (maximum 8-16 mEq/day)

MANAGEMENT OF SEIZURES AND HYPERTENSION: I.M., I.V.:

**Magnesium sulfate:** 1 g every 6 hours for 4 doses as needed

BRONCHODILATION (adjunctive treatment in moderate to severe acute asthma; unlabeled use): I.V.:

**Magnesium sulfate:** 2 g as a single dose

**Note:** Literature evaluating magnesium sulfate's efficacy in the relief of bronchospasm has utilized single dosages in patient's with acute symptomatology who have received aerosol β-agonist therapy.

CATHARTIC: Oral:

**Magnesium citrate** (Citrate of magnesia): 150-300 mL

**Magnesium hydroxide** (Milk of magnesia, MOM): 30-60 mL/day once or in divided doses

**Magnesium hydroxide and mineral oil** (Haley's M-O) (pediatric dosage to provide equivalent dosage of magnesium hydroxide) 30-45 mL once or in divided doses

**Magnesium sulfate:** 10-30 g

**Magnesium oxide:** Adults: 2-4 g at bedtime with full glass of water

ANTACID Oral:

**Magnesium hydroxide:**

Liquid: 5-15 mL/dose, up to 4 times/day

Liquid concentrate: 2.5-7.5 mL/dose, up to 4 times/day

Tablet: 622-1244 mg/dose, up to 4 times/day

**Magnesium oxide:** 140 mg 3-4 times/day or 400-840 mg/day

**Renal Impairment:** Patients in severe renal failure should not receive magnesium due to toxicity from accumulation. Patients with a $Cl_{cr}$ <25 mL/minute receiving magnesium should have serum magnesium levels monitored.

**Administration**

**Oral:**

Solution: Mix with water and administer on an empty stomach; chill **magnesium citrate** prior to administration to improve palatability

Tablet: Take with full glass of water; chew **magnesium hydroxide** chewable tablets thoroughly; do not chew or crush sustained release formulations

**I.V.:** Intermittent infusion: Dilute to a concentration of 0.5 mEq/mL (60 mg/mL of **magnesium sulfate**) (maximum concentration: 1.6 mEq/mL, 200 mg/mL of **magnesium sulfate**) and infuse over 2-4 hours; do not exceed 1 mEq/kg/hour (125 mg/kg/hour of **magnesium sulfate**); in severe circumstances, half of the dosage to be administered may be infused over the first 15-20 minutes; for I.M. administration, dilute **magnesium sulfate** to a maximum concentration of 200 mg/mL prior to injection

**Monitoring Laboratory Tests** Serum magnesium, deep tendon reflexes, renal function

(Continued)

## Magnesium Supplements *(Continued)*

**Additional Nursing Issues**

**Physical Assessment:** Assess patient's knowledge of appropriate administration. If administered I.V., monitor EKG, blood pressure, muscle strength, respiratory effort, CNS status, and deep tendon reflexes. **Note:** MOM concentrate is 3 times as potent as regular strength product. Monitor I & O ratio, edema.

**Patient Information/Instruction:** Take as directed, with water or juice. Shake liquid well before using. Take 1 hour prior to or after other medications. You may experience excessive diarrhea, gastric cramping, dizziness (use fall precautions). Report rectal bleeding, tarry stools, unresolved abdominal cramps, or unrelieved constipation.

**Geriatric Considerations:** Elderly, due to disease or drug therapy, may be predisposed to diarrhea. Diarrhea may result in electrolyte imbalance. Decreased renal function ($Cl_{cr}$ <30 mL/minute) may result in toxicity; monitor for toxicity (see Warnings/Precautions and Contraindications).

**Additional Information** 1 g elemental magnesium = 83.3 mEq = 41.1 mmol

**Related Information**

Antiarrhythmic Drug Classification Comparison *on page 1366*
Laxatives: Classification and Properties Comparison *on page 1392*


- **Magonate®** *see* Magnesium Supplements *on page 703*
- **Magonate®** *see page 1294*
- **Mag-Ox 400®** *see* Magnesium Supplements *on page 703*
- **Mag-Tab SR®** *see* Magnesium Supplements *on page 703*
- **Magtrate** *see* Magnesium Supplements *on page 703*
- **Malatal®** *see* Hyoscyamine, Atropine, Scopolamine, and Phenobarbital *on page 591*
- **Malathion** *see page 1294*
- **Malival** *see* Indomethacin *on page 606*
- **Malival AP** *see* Indomethacin *on page 606*
- **Mallamint® [OTC]** *see* Calcium Supplements *on page 185*
- **Mallazine® Eye Drops** *see page 1294*
- **Mallergan-VC® With Codeine** *see* Promethazine, Phenylephrine, and Codeine *on page 981*
- **Mallisol®** *see page 1294*
- **Malt Soup Extract** *see page 1294*
- **Maltsuprex®** *see page 1294*
- **Mandol®** *see* Cefamandole *on page 212*
- **Mandrake** *see* Podophyllum Resin *on page 944*
- **Manganese** *see page 1294*


## Mannitol (MAN i tole)

**U.S. Brand Names** Osmitrol® Injection; Resectisol® Irrigation Solution

**Synonyms** *D*-Mannitol

**Therapeutic Category** Diuretic, Osmotic

**Pregnancy Risk Factor** C

**Lactation** Excretion in breast milk unknown

**Use** Reduction of increased intracranial pressure associated with cerebral edema; promotion of diuresis in the prevention and/or treatment of oliguria or anuria due to acute renal failure; reduction of increased intraocular pressure; promoting urinary excretion of toxic substances; GU irrigant in transurethral prostatic resection or other transurethral surgical procedures

**Mechanism of Action/Effect** Increases the osmotic pressure of glomerular filtrate, which inhibits tubular reabsorption of water and electrolytes and increases urinary output

**Contraindications** Hypersensitivity to mannitol or any component; severe renal disease (anuria); dehydration; active intracranial bleeding; severe pulmonary edema or congestion

**Warnings** Should not be administered until adequacy of renal function and urine flow is established. Cardiovascular status should also be evaluated. Do not administer electrolyte-free mannitol solutions with blood. Pregnancy factor C.

**Adverse Reactions**

>10%:

Central nervous system: Headache
Gastrointestinal: Nausea, vomiting
Genitourinary: Polyuria

1% to 10%:

Central nervous system: Dizziness
Dermatologic: Rash
Local: **Vesicant chemotherapy**
Ocular: Blurred vision

<1% (Limited to important or life-threatening symptoms): Circulatory overload, congestive heart failure, convulsions, fluid and electrolyte imbalance, water intoxication, dehydration and hypovolemia secondary to rapid diuresis, renal failure, pulmonary edema

**Overdose/Toxicology** Symptoms of overdose include polyuria, hypotension, cardiovascular collapse, pulmonary edema, hyponatremia, hypokalemia, oliguria, and seizures. Increased electrolyte excretion and fluid overload can occur. Hemodialysis will clear mannitol and reduce osmolality.

**Pharmacodynamics/Kinetics**

**Distribution:** Remains confined to extracellular space (except in extreme concentrations) and does not penetrate the blood-brain barrier

**Half-life Elimination:** 1.1-1.6 hours

**Metabolism:** Minimal amounts metabolized in the liver to glycogen

**Excretion:** Urine

**Onset:** Onset of diuresis: Injection: Within 1-3 hours; Onset of reduction in intracerebral pressure: Within 15 minutes

**Duration:** Duration of reduction in intracerebral pressure: 3-6 hours

**Formulations**

Injection: 5% [50 mg/mL] (1000 mL); 10% [100 mg/mL] (500 mL, 1000 mL); 15% [150 mg/mL] (150 mL, 500 mL); 20% [200 mg/mL] (150 mL, 250 mL, 500 mL); 25% [250 mg/mL] (50 mL)

Solution, urogenital: 0.54% [5.4 mg/mL] (2000 mL)

**Dosing**

**Adults:** I.V.:

Test dose (to assess adequate renal function): 12.5 g (200 mg/kg) over 3-5 minutes to produce a urine flow of at least 30-50 mL of urine per hour over the next 2-3 hours.

Initial: 0.5-1 g/kg

Maintenance: 0.25-0.5 g/kg every 4-6 hours; usual adult dose: 20-200 g/24 hours

Intracranial pressure: Cerebral edema: 1.5-2 g/kg/dose I.V. as a 15% to 20% solution over ≥30 minutes; maintain serum osmolality 310-320 mOsm/kg.

Preoperative for neurosurgery: 1.5-2 g/kg administered 1-1.5 hours prior to surgery.

Transurethral irrigation: Use urogenital solution as required for irrigation.

**Elderly:** Refer to adult dosing.

**Administration**

**I.V.:** Vesicant. Do not administer with blood. Crenation and agglutination of red blood cells may occur if administered with whole blood.

**I.V. Detail:** Avoid extravasation.

**Stability**

**Storage:** Should be stored at room temperature (15°C to 30°C) and protected from freezing. Crystallization may occur at low temperatures. Do not use solutions that contain crystals, heating in a hot water bath and vigorous shaking may be utilized for resolubilization. Cool solutions to body temperature before using.

**Monitoring Laboratory Tests** Renal function, serum electrolytes, serum and urine osmolality; for treatment of elevated intracranial pressure, maintain serum osmolality 310-320 mOsm/kg

**Additional Nursing Issues**

**Physical Assessment:** See Dosing and Warnings/Precautions for test dose instructions. Monitor infusion site closely for extravasation (see above). Monitor vital signs, urinary output, and electrolytes. Monitor for effectiveness according to purpose of administration (eg, cerebral edema or trauma - ICP and neurological status; reducing intraocular pressure - eye pain, decreased visual acuity; renal failure - urine specific gravity and urinary output). **Pregnancy risk factor C** - benefits of use should outweigh possible risks. Note breast-feeding caution.

**Patient Information/Instruction:** This medication can only be given by infusion. Report immediately any muscle weakness, numbness, tingling, acute headache, nausea, dizziness, blurred vision, eye pain, difficulty breathing, chest pain, or pain at infusion site. **Pregnancy/breast-feeding precautions:** Inform prescriber if you are pregnant. Consult prescriber if breast-feeding.

**Additional Information** May autoclave or heat to redissolve crystals. Mannitol 20% has an approximate osmolarity of 1100 mOsm/L and mannitol 25% has an approximate osmolarity of 1375 mOsm/L.

pH: 4.5-7


- ♦ **Maox®** *see* Magnesium Supplements *on page 703*
- ♦ **Mapluxin®** *see* Digoxin *on page 370*
- ♦ **Marax®** *see* Theophylline, Ephedrine, and Hydroxyzine *on page 1118*
- ♦ **Marazide®** *see* Benzthiazide *on page 144*
- ♦ **Marbaxin®** *see* Methocarbamol *on page 742*
- ♦ **Marcaine®** *see* Bupivacaine *on page 167*
- ♦ **Marcillin®** *see* Ampicillin *on page 90*
- ♦ **Marezine®** *see page 1294*
- ♦ **Margesic® H** *see* Hydrocodone and Acetaminophen *on page 568*
- ♦ **Marinol®** *see* Dronabinol *on page 408*
- ♦ **Marmine® Oral** *see page 1294*
- ♦ **Marnal®** *see* Butalbital Compound and Aspirin *on page 176*
- ♦ **Marovilina®** *see* Ampicillin *on page 90*
- ♦ **Marpres®** *see* Hydralazine, Hydrochlorothiazide, and Reserpine *on page 565*
- ♦ **Marthritic®** *see* Salsalate *on page 1042*


## Masoprocol (ma SOE pro kole)

**U.S. Brand Names** Actinex® Topical

**Therapeutic Category** Topical Skin Product, Acne

**Pregnancy Risk Factor** B

**Lactation** Excretion in breast milk unknown

**Use** Treatment of actinic keratosis

**Mechanism of Action/Effect** Antiproliferative activity against keratinocytes

**Contraindications** Hypersensitivity to masoprocol or any component

**Warnings** Occlusive dressings should not be used. For external use only.

(Continued)

## Masoprocol *(Continued)*

**Adverse Reactions**

>10%:

Dermatologic: Erythema, flaking, dryness, itching

Local: Burning

1% to 10%:

Dermatologic: Soreness, rash, blistering, excoriation, skin roughness, wrinkling

Neuromuscular & skeletal: Paresthesia

Ocular: Eye irritation

**Formulations** Cream: 10% (30 g)

**Dosing**

**Adults:** Topical: Wash and dry area. Gently massage into affected area every morning and evening for 28 days.

**Administration**

**Topical:** For external use only. Avoid contact with eyes and mucous membranes. Do not use occlusive dressings. Wash hands immediately after use.

**Additional Nursing Issues**

**Physical Assessment:** Monitor effectiveness of therapy and adverse reactions at beginning and periodically during therapy. Assess knowledge/teach patient appropriate use and adverse symptoms to report for prescribed form of drug. Note breast-feeding caution.

**Patient Information/Instruction:** For external use only. Apply with gloves in thin film to thoroughly clean/dry skin; avoid area around eyes or mouth. Do not cover with occlusive dressing. Results make take some time to appear. May stain clothing or fabrics. You may experience transient stinging or burning after application. Report worsening of condition; eye irritation; or skin redness, dryness, peeling, or burning that persists between applications. **Breast-feeding precautions:** Consult prescriber if breast-feeding.

- **Masse® Breast Cream** *see page 1294*
- **Massengill® Medicated Douche w/Cepticin** *see page 1294*
- **Maternal/Fetal Medications** *see page 1423*
- **Maternal/Fetal Toxicology** *see page 1426*
- **Matulane®** *see* Procarbazine *on page 970*
- **Mavik®** *see* Trandolapril *on page 1162*
- **Maxair™ Autohaler™** *see* Pirbuterol *on page 939*
- **Maxair™ Inhalation Aerosol** *see* Pirbuterol *on page 939*
- **Maxalt®** *see* Rizatriptan *on page 1033*
- **Maxalt-MLT™** *see* Rizatriptan *on page 1033*
- **Maxaquin®** *see* Lomefloxacin *on page 685*
- **Maxeran®** *see* Metoclopramide *on page 758*
- **Maxidex®** *see* Dexamethasone *on page 346*
- **Maxiflor®** *see* Topical Corticosteroids *on page 1152*
- **Maximum Strength Anbesol® [OTC]** *see* Benzocaine *on page 141*
- **Maximum Strength Desenex® Antifungal Cream [OTC]** *see* Miconazole *on page 767*
- **Maximum Strength Dex-A-Diet® [OTC]** *see* Phenylpropanolamine *on page 922*
- **Maximum Strength Dexatrim® [OTC]** *see* Phenylpropanolamine *on page 922*
- **Maximum Strength Nytol® [OTC]** *see* Diphenhydramine *on page 381*
- **Maximum Strength Orajel® [OTC]** *see* Benzocaine *on page 141*
- **Maxipime®** *see* Cefepime *on page 215*
- **Maxitrol®** *see page 1282*
- **Maxivate®** *see* Betamethasone *on page 148*
- **Maxivate®** *see* Topical Corticosteroids *on page 1152*
- **Maxolon®** *see* Metoclopramide *on page 758*
- **Maxzide®** *see* Hydrochlorothiazide and Triamterene *on page 568*
- **May Apple** *see* Podophyllum Resin *on page 944*
- **Mazanor®** *see* Mazindol *on this page*
- **Mazepine®** *see* Carbamazepine *on page 195*

## Mazindol (MAY zin dole)

**U.S. Brand Names** Mazanor®; Sanorex®

**Therapeutic Category** Anorexiant

**Pregnancy Risk Factor** C

**Lactation** Enters breast milk/not recommended

**Use** Short-term adjunct in exogenous obesity

**Unlabeled use:** Alone or adjunct in the treatment of narcolepsy and Duchenne's dystrophy

**Mechanism of Action/Effect** Properties similar to amphetamines; also CNS and cardiac prodrug stimulation

**Contraindications** Hypersensitivity to mazindol; glaucoma; agitated states; history of drug abuse; MAO inhibitors

**Warnings** Tolerance may develop within a few weeks. If this occurs, discontinue drug. Do not increase dose. Not recommended for severe hypertensive patients or patients with symptomatic cardiovascular disease including arrhythmias. Pregnancy factor C.

**Drug Interactions**

**Decreased Effect:** Mazindol may decrease the hypotensive effect of guanethidine. Tricyclic antidepressants may decrease the effect of mazindol.

**Increased Effect/Toxicity:** MAO inhibitors or furazolidone may increase the vasopressor effects of anorexiants resulting in hypertensive crisis or intracranial hemorrhage. Insulin and sulfonylurea hypoglycemic effects may be increased when taken with mazindol.

**Adverse Reactions**

>10%:

Cardiovascular: Hypertension
Central nervous system: Euphoria, nervousness, insomnia

1% to 10%:

Central nervous system: Confusion, mental depression, restlessness
Endocrine & metabolic: Changes in libido
Gastrointestinal: Nausea, constipation, vomiting
Hematologic: Blood dyscrasias
Neuromuscular & skeletal: Tremor
Ocular: Blurred vision

<1% (Limited to important or life-threatening symptoms): Tachycardia, arrhythmias, alopecia, testicular pain, dysuria, polyuria, myalgia, dyspnea

**Overdose/Toxicology** Symptoms of overdose include hypertension, tachycardia, and hyperthermia. Treatment is supportive.

**Pharmacodynamics/Kinetics**

**Half-life Elimination:** 33-55 hours

**Excretion:** Urine

**Formulations**

Tablet:

Mazanor®: 1 mg
Sanorex®: 1 mg, 2 mg

**Dosing**

**Adults:** Oral: Initial: 1 mg once daily and adjust to patient response; usual dose is 1 mg 3 times daily, 1 hour before meals, or 2 mg once daily, 1 hour before lunch. Take with meals to avoid GI discomfort.

**Stability**

**Storage:** Store below 77°F (25°C).

**Additional Nursing Issues**

**Physical Assessment:** Assess effectiveness and interactions of other medications patient may be taking (see Drug Interactions). Assess for history of psychopathology, homicidal or suicidal tendencies, or addiction; long-term use can result in dependence, abuse, or tolerance. Periodically evaluate the need for continued use. Monitor blood pressure, vital signs, and adverse reactions at start of therapy, when changing dosage, and at regular intervals during therapy (see Adverse Reactions). Monitor serum glucose closely with diabetic patients (may alter antidiabetic requirements). Taper dosage slowly when discontinuing. Assess knowledge/teach patient appropriate use, possible side effects, and symptoms to report. **Pregnancy risk factor C** - benefits of use should outweigh possible risks (see Pregnancy Issues). Breast-feeding is not recommended.

**Patient Information/Instruction:** Take exactly as directed (do not increase dose or frequency without consulting prescriber). Take 1 hour before meals; if gastric distress occurs may be taken with meals (do not take at bedtime). Avoid alcohol, caffeine, or OTC medications that act as stimulants. You may experience restlessness, false sense of euphoria, or impaired judgment (use caution when driving or engaging in tasks requiring alertness until response to drug is known); nausea or vomiting (small frequent meals, frequent mouth care may help); constipation (increased exercise, dietary fiber, fruit, or fluid may help); diarrhea (buttermilk, boiled milk, or yogurt may help); or altered libido (reversible). Diabetics need to monitor serum glucose closely (may alter antidiabetic medication requirements). Report chest pain, palpitations, or irregular heartbeat; muscle weakness or tremors; CNS changes (aggressiveness, restlessness, euphoria, sleep disturbances); testicular pain or changes in sexual activity; blurred vision; or changes in urinary patterns. **Pregnancy/breast-feeding precautions:** Inform prescriber if you are or intend to be pregnant. Breast-feeding is not recommended.

**Pregnancy Issues:** Increase in neonatal mortality has occurred in animals. Potential benefit should be weighed against possible hazard to mother and infant.

♦ **MCH** *see page 1248*
♦ **MCT Oil®** *see page 1294*
♦ **Measles and Rubella Vaccines, Combined** *see page 1256*
♦ **Measles, Mumps, and Rubella Vaccines, Combined** *see page 1256*
♦ **Measles Virus Vaccine, Live** *see page 1256*
♦ **Measurin® [OTC]** *see* Aspirin *on page 111*

## Mebendazole (me BEN da zole)

**U.S. Brand Names** Vermox®

**Therapeutic Category** Anthelmintic

**Pregnancy Risk Factor** C

**Lactation** Excretion in breast milk unknown/use caution

**Use** Treatment of pinworms, whipworms, roundworms, and hookworms

**Mechanism of Action/Effect** Selectively and irreversibly blocks glucose uptake and other nutrients in susceptible adult intestine-dwelling helminths

(Continued)

## Mebendazole *(Continued)*

**Contraindications** Hypersensitivity to mebendazole or any component

**Warnings** Pregnancy and children <2 years of age are relative contraindications since safety has not been established. Not effective for hydatid disease. Pregnancy factor C.

**Drug Interactions**

**Decreased Effect:** Anticonvulsants such as carbamazepine and phenytoin may increase metabolism of mebendazole

**Food Interactions** Mebendazole serum levels may be increased if taken with food.

**Effects on Lab Values** ↑ LFTs

**Adverse Reactions**

1% to 10%: Gastrointestinal: Abdominal pain, diarrhea, nausea, vomiting

<1% (Limited to important or life-threatening symptoms): Rash, itching, alopecia (with high doses), neutropenia (sore throat, unusual fatigue), angioedema, seizures

**Overdose/Toxicology** Symptoms of overdose include abdominal pain and altered mental status. Treatment is supportive.

**Pharmacodynamics/Kinetics**

**Protein Binding:** 95%

**Half-life Elimination:** 2.8-9 hours

**Time to Peak:** Within 2-4 hours

**Metabolism:** Liver

**Excretion:** Feces and urine

**Formulations** Tablet, chewable: 100 mg

**Dosing**

**Adults:** Oral:

Pinworms: 100 mg as a single dose; may need to repeat after 2 weeks; treatment should include family members in close contact with patient.

Whipworms, roundworms, hookworms: 1 tablet twice daily, morning and evening on 3 consecutive days; if patient is not cured within 3-4 weeks, a second course of treatment may be administered.

Capillariasis: 200 mg twice daily for 20 days

**Elderly:** Refer to adult dosing.

**Renal Impairment:** Not dialyzable (0% to 5%)

**Hepatic Impairment:** Dosage reduction may be necessary in patients with liver dysfunction.

**Administration**

**Oral:** Tablets may be chewed, swallowed whole, or crushed and mixed with food.

**Monitoring Laboratory Tests** Check for helminth ova in feces within 3-4 weeks following the initial therapy. Periodically assess hematologic and hepatic function.

**Additional Nursing Issues**

**Physical Assessment:** Assess effectiveness and interactions of other medications (see Drug Interactions). See Warnings/Precautions and Contraindications for use cautions. Worm infestations are easily transmitted, all close family members should be treated. Instruct patient/caregiver on appropriate use, transmission prevention, possible side effects and appropriate interventions, and adverse symptoms to report. **Pregnancy risk factor C** - benefits of use should outweigh possible risks. Note breast-feeding caution.

**Patient Information/Instruction:** Take exactly as directed for full course of medication. Tablets may be chewed, swallowed whole, or crushed and mixed with food. Increase dietary intake of fruit juices. All family members and close friends should also be treated. To reduce possibility of reinfection, wash hands and scrub nails carefully with soap and hot water before handling food, before eating, and before and after toileting. Keep hands out of mouth. Disinfect toilet daily and launder bed lines, undergarments, and nightclothes daily with hot water and soap. Do not go barefoot and do not sit directly on grass or ground. May cause abdominal pain, nausea, or vomiting (frequent small meals, frequent mouth care, sucking lozenges, or chewing gum may help); hair loss (reversible). Report skin rash or itching, unusual fatigue or sore throat, unresolved diarrhea or vomiting, or CNS changes. **Pregnancy/breast-feeding precautions:** Inform prescriber if you are or intend to be pregnant. Consult prescriber if breast-feeding.

**Breast-feeding Issues:** Since only 2% to 10% of mebendazole is absorbed, it is unlikely that it is excreted in breast milk in significant quantities.

♦ **Mebensole** *see* Mebendazole *on previous page*

## Mechlorethamine (me klor ETH a meen)

**U.S. Brand Names** Mustargen® Hydrochloride

**Synonyms** $HN_2$; Mustine; Nitrogen Mustard

**Therapeutic Category** Antineoplastic Agent, Alkylating Agent

**Pregnancy Risk Factor** D

**Lactation** Excretion in breast milk unknown/not recommended

**Use** Combination therapy of Hodgkin's disease and malignant lymphomas; non-Hodgkin's lymphoma; palliative treatment of bronchogenic, breast and ovarian carcinoma; may be used by intracavitary injection for treatment of metastatic tumors; pleural and other malignant effusions; topical treatment of mycosis fungoides

**Mechanism of Action/Effect** Alkylating agent that inhibits DNA and RNA synthesis via formation of carbonium ions; produces interstrand and intrastrand cross-links in DNA resulting in miscoding, breakage, and failure of replication

**Contraindications** Hypersensitivity to mechlorethamine or any component; pre-existing profound myelosuppression or infection; pregnancy

**Warnings** The U.S. Food and Drug Administration (FDA) currently recommends that procedures for proper handling and disposal of antineoplastic agents be considered.

Preparation of mechlorethamine should be performed in a Class II laminar flow biologic safety cabinet. Personnel should be wearing surgical gloves and a closed front surgical gown with knit cuffs. Appropriate safety equipment is recommended for preparation, administration, and disposal of antineoplastics. If mechlorethamine contacts the skin, wash and flush thoroughly with water. Extravasation of the drug into subcutaneous tissues results in painful inflammation and induration; sloughing may occur. Patients with lymphomas should receive prophylactic allopurinol 2-3 days prior to therapy to prevent complications resulting from tumor lysis.

**Adverse Reactions**

>10%:

Gastrointestinal: Nausea and vomiting usually occur in nearly 100% of patients and onset is within 30 minutes to 2 hours after administration

Emetic potential: High (>90%)

Time course of nausea/vomiting: Onset: 1-3 hours; duration 2-8 hours

Hematologic: Myelosuppressive: Leukopenia and thrombocytopenia can be severe; caution should be used with patients who are receiving radiotherapy, secondary leukemia

WBC: Severe

Platelets: Severe

Onset (days): 4-7

Nadir (days): 14

Recovery (days): 21

Endocrine & metabolic: Delayed menses, oligomenorrhea, temporary or permanent amenorrhea, impaired spermatogenesis; spermatogenesis may return in patients in remission several years after the discontinuation of chemotherapy, chromosomal abnormalities

Genitourinary: Azoospermia

Otic: Ototoxicity

Miscellaneous: Precipitation of herpes zoster

1% to 10%:

Central nervous system: Fever, vertigo

Dermatologic: Alopecia

Endocrine & metabolic: Hyperuricemia

Gastrointestinal: Diarrhea, anorexia, metallic taste

Local: Thrombophlebitis/extravasation: May cause local vein discomfort which may be relieved by warm soaks and pain medication. A brown discoloration of veins may occur. Mechlorethamine is a strong vesicant and can cause tissue necrosis and sloughing.

**Vesicant chemotherapy**

Secondary malignancies: Have been reported after several years in 1% to 6% of patients treated

Neuromuscular & skeletal: Weakness

Otic: Tinnitus

Miscellaneous: Hypersensitivity, anaphylaxis

<1% (Limited to important or life-threatening symptoms): Myelosuppression, hemolytic anemia, hepatotoxicity, peripheral neuropathy

**Overdose/Toxicology** Suppression of all formed elements of blood, uric acid crystals, nausea, vomiting, and diarrhea. Sodium thiosulfate is the specific antidote for nitrogen mustard extravasations. Treatment of systemic overdose is supportive.

**Pharmacodynamics/Kinetics**

**Half-life Elimination:** <1 minute

**Metabolism:** I.V.: Drug undergoes rapid chemical transformation; unchanged drug is undetectable in the blood within a few minutes

**Excretion:** Urine

**Formulations** Powder for injection, hydrochloride: 10 mg

**Dosing**

**Adults:** Refer to individual protocols. Dosage should be based on ideal dry weight. The presence of edema or ascites must be considered so that dosage will be based on actual weight unaugmented by these conditions.

MOPP: I.V.: 6 mg/m$^2$ on days 1 and 8 of a 28-day cycle

I.V.: 0.4 mg/kg **or** 12-16 mg/m$^2$ for one dose **or** divided into 0.1 mg/kg/day for 4 days, repeated at 4- to 6-week intervals

Intracavitary: 10-20 mg diluted in 10 mL of SWI or 0.9% sodium chloride

Intrapericardially: 0.2-0.4 mg/kg diluted in up to 100 mL of 0.9% sodium chloride

Topical mechlorethamine has been used in the treatment of cutaneous lesions of mycosis fungoides. A skin test should be performed prior to treatment with the topical preparation to detect sensitivity and possible irritation (use fresh mechlorethamine 0.1 mg/mL and apply over a 3 x 5 cm area of normal skin).

**Administration**

**I.V.:** Vesicant. Margin of error is very slight. Check dosage carefully before administration. Administer with caution. Administer I.V. push through a free flowing I.V. over 1-3 minutes at a concentration not to exceed 1 mg/mL.

**I.V. Detail:** Mechlorethamine may cause extravasation. Use within 1 hour of preparation. Avoid extravasation since mechlorethamine is a potent vesicant.

**Extravasation management:** Sodium thiosulfate $^1/_6$ molar solution is the specific antidote for nitrogen mustard extravasations and should be used as follows: Mix 4 mL of 10% sodium thiosulfate with 6 mL of sterile water for injection. Inject 5-6 mL of this

(Continued)

## Mechlorethamine *(Continued)*

solution into the existing I.V. line. Remove the needle. Inject 2-3 mL of the solution S.C. clockwise into the infiltrated area using a 25-gauge needle. Change the needle with each new injection. Apply ice immediately for 6-12 hours.

**Stability**

**Storage:** Store intact vials at room temperature.

**Reconstitution:** Must be prepared fresh - solution is stable for only 1 hour after dilution and must be administered within 1 hour. Dilute powder with 10 mL SWI to a final concentration of 1 mg/mL. May be diluted in up to 100 mL NS for intracavitary administration.

**Standard I.V. dilution:** I.V. push: Dose/syringe (concentration is 1 mg/mL)

Maximum syringe for IVP is 30 mL and syringe should be ≤75% full.

**Compatibility:** See the Chemotherapy Compatibility Chart *on page 1311*.

**Monitoring Laboratory Tests** CBC with differential and platelet count

**Additional Nursing Issues**

**Physical Assessment:** Note Administration directions (above) closely. Assess infusion site closely for extravasation (see above). See Dosing for directions for topical use. Monitor appropriate laboratory results prior to beginning each cycle. Antiemetics may be administered prior to injection. Monitor for adverse reactions which may be severe and involve several systems (see Adverse Reactions). Instruct patient/caregiver on appropriate adverse reactions to report and interventions which may reduce systemic effects. **Pregnancy risk factor D** - assess knowledge/teach appropriate use of barrier contraceptives. Breast-feeding is not recommended.

**Patient Information/Instruction:** This medication can only be given by infusion, usually in cycles of therapy. You will need frequent laboratory and medical monitoring during treatment. Do not use alcohol, aspirin or aspirin-containing medications, and OTC medications without consulting prescriber. Maintain adequate fluid balance (2-3 L/day of fluids unless instructed to restrict fluid intake) and adequate nutrition (small frequent meals, frequent mouth care, sucking lozenges, or chewing gum may reduce anorexia and nausea). May cause discoloration (brown color) of veins used for infusion, hair loss (reversible); easy bleeding or bruising (use soft toothbrush or cotton swabs and frequent mouth care, use electric razor, avoid sharp knives or scissors); increased susceptibility to infection (avoid crowds or exposure to infection - do not have any vaccinations unless approved by prescriber). This drug may cause menstrual irregularities, permanent sterility, and birth defects. Report changes in auditory or visual acuity; unusual bleeding or bruising or persistent fever or sore throat; blood in urine, stool, or vomitus; delayed healing of any wounds; skin rash; yellowing of skin or eyes; changes in color of urine of stool; acute or unresolved nausea or vomiting; diarrhea; or loss of appetite. **Pregnancy/breast-feeding precautions:** Do not get pregnant; use appropriate barrier contraceptive measures until prescriber tells you otherwise. Breast-feeding is not recommended.

♦ **Meclan® Topical** *see* Meclocycline *on next page*

## Meclizine (MEK li zeen)

**U.S. Brand Names** Antivert®; Antrizine®; Bonine® [OTC]; Dizmiss® [OTC]; Dramamine® II [OTC]; Meni-D®; Nico-Vert® [OTC]; Ru-Vert-M®; Vergon® [OTC]

**Therapeutic Category** Antihistamine

**Pregnancy Risk Factor** B

**Lactation** Excretion in breast milk unknown/not recommended

**Use** Prevention and treatment of symptoms of motion sickness; management of vertigo with diseases affecting the vestibular system

**Mechanism of Action/Effect** Has central anticholinergic action by blocking chemoreceptor trigger zone; decreases excitability of the middle ear labyrinth and blocks conduction in the middle ear vestibular-cerebellar pathways

**Contraindications** Hypersensitivity to meclizine or any component

**Warnings** Use with caution in patients with angle-closure glaucoma, prostatic hypertrophy, pyloric or duodenal obstruction, or bladder neck obstruction. Use with caution in hot weather, and during exercise. Elderly may be at risk for anticholinergic side effects such as glaucoma, prostatic hypertrophy, constipation, GI obstructive disease. If vertigo does not respond in 1-2 weeks, it is advised to discontinue use. Pregnancy.

**Drug Interactions**

**Increased Effect/Toxicity:** Increased toxicity with CNS depressants, neuroleptics, and anticholinergics.

**Adverse Reactions**

>10%:

Central nervous system: Slight to moderate drowsiness

Respiratory: Thickening of bronchial secretions

1% to 10%:

Central nervous system: Headache, fatigue, nervousness, dizziness

Gastrointestinal: Appetite increase, weight gain, nausea, diarrhea, abdominal pain, dry mouth

Neuromuscular & skeletal: Arthralgia

Respiratory: Pharyngitis

<1% (Limited to important or life-threatening symptoms): Palpitations, hypotension, hepatitis, bronchospasm

**Overdose/Toxicology** Symptoms of overdose include CNS depression, confusion, nervousness, hallucinations, dizziness, blurred vision, nausea, vomiting, and hyperthermia. There is no specific treatment for antihistamine overdose. Clinical toxicity is due to blockade of cholinergic receptors. For anticholinergic overdose with severe life-threatening symptoms, physostigmine 1-2 mg I.V. slowly, may be given to reverse these effects.

**Pharmacodynamics/Kinetics**

**Half-life Elimination:** 6 hours

**Metabolism:** Liver

**Excretion:** Urine and feces

**Onset:** Oral: Within 1 hour

**Duration:** 8-24 hours

**Formulations**

Meclizine hydrochloride:

- Capsule: 15 mg, 25 mg, 30 mg
- Tablet: 12.5 mg, 25 mg, 50 mg
- Tablet:
  - Chewable: 25 mg
  - Film coated: 25 mg

**Dosing**

**Adults:** Oral:

- Motion sickness: 12.5-25 mg 1 hour before travel, repeat dose every 12-24 hours if needed; doses up to 50 mg may be needed
- Vertigo: 25-100 mg/day in divided doses

**Elderly:** Refer to adult dosing; start at lowest dose.

**Additional Nursing Issues**

**Physical Assessment:** Determine cause of vomiting before beginning therapy. Assess effectiveness and interactions of other medications (see Drug Interactions). See Warnings/Precautions and Contraindications for use cautions. Inpatients: Observe safety precautions (eg, bed rails up, call bell at hand). Monitor effectiveness of therapy and adverse response (see Adverse Reactions and Overdose/Toxicology). Assess knowledge/teach patient possible side effects and appropriate interventions and adverse symptoms to report. Breast-feeding is not recommended.

**Patient Information/Instruction:** Take exactly as prescribed; do not increase dose. Avoid alcohol, other CNS depressants, sleeping aids without consulting prescriber. You may experience dizziness, drowsiness, or blurred vision (use caution when driving or engaging in tasks that require alertness until response to drug is known); dry mouth (frequent mouth care, sucking lozenges, or chewing gum may help); constipation (increased dietary fluid, fiber, and fruit and exercise may help); heat intolerance (avoid excessive exercise, hot environments, maintain adequate fluid intake). Report CNS change (hallucination, confusion, nervousness); sudden or unusual weight gain; unresolved nausea or diarrhea; chest pain or palpitations; muscle pain; or changes in urinary pattern. **Breast-feeding precautions:** Breast-feeding is not recommended.

**Geriatric Considerations:** Due to anticholinergic action, use lowest dose in divided doses to avoid side effects and their inconvenience. Limit use if possible. May cause confusion or aggravate symptoms of confusion in those with dementia.

## Meclocycline (me kloe SYE kleen)

**U.S. Brand Names** Meclan® Topical

**Therapeutic Category** Antibiotic, Topical; Topical Skin Product, Acne

**Pregnancy Risk Factor** B

**Lactation** Excretion in breast milk unknown/use caution

**Use** Topical treatment of inflammatory acne vulgaris

**Mechanism of Action/Effect** Inhibits bacterial protein synthesis by binding with the 30S and possibly the 50S ribosomal subunit(s) of susceptible bacteria; may also cause alterations in the cytoplasmic membrane

**Contraindications** Hypersensitivity to tetracyclines or any component

**Warnings** For external use only. Use with caution in patients allergic to formaldehyde.

**Adverse Reactions**

- >10%: Topical: Follicular staining, yellowing of the skin, burning/stinging feeling
- 1% to 10%: Topical: Pain, redness, skin irritation, dermatitis

**Formulations** Cream, topical, as sulfosalicylate: 1% (20 g, 45 g)

**Dosing**

**Adults:** Topical: Apply generously to affected areas twice daily.

**Administration**

**Topical:** Apply generously until skin is wet. Avoid contact with eyes, nose, and mouth.

**Additional Nursing Issues**

**Physical Assessment:** Monitor effectiveness of therapy and adverse reactions at beginning and periodically during therapy. Assess knowledge/teach patient appropriate use and adverse symptoms to report for prescribed form of drug. Note breast-feeding caution.

**Patient Information/Instruction:** For external use only. Apply with gloves to thoroughly clean/dry skin until skin is wet; avoid area around eyes or mouth. Do not cover with occlusive dressing. Results make take some time to appear. May stain clothing or fabrics. You may experience transient stinging or burning after application. If skin turns yellow, washing with soap and water will remove color. Report worsening of condition; eye irritation; or skin redness, dryness, peeling, or burning that persists between applications. **Breast-feeding precautions:** Consult prescriber if breast-feeding.

♦ **Meclomid** *see* Metoclopramide *on page 758*

♦ **Medicinal Carbon** *see* Charcoal *on page 243*

♦ **Medigesic®** *see* Butalbital Compound and Acetaminophen *on page 175*

- **Medihaler-Iso®** *see* Isoproterenol *on page 632*
- **Medilium®** *see* Chlordiazepoxide *on page 250*
- **Medimet®** *see* Methyldopa *on page 750*
- **Medipain 5®** *see* Hydrocodone and Acetaminophen *on page 568*
- **Mediplast® Plaster** *see page 1294*
- **Medipren® [OTC]** *see* Ibuprofen *on page 592*
- **Medi-Quick® Topical Ointment [OTC]** *see* Bacitracin, Neomycin, and Polymyxin B *on page 130*
- **Meditran®** *see* Meprobamate *on page 724*
- **Medi-Tuss® [OTC]** *see* Guaifenesin *on page 548*
- **Medium Chain Triglycerides** *see page 1294*
- **Medralone® Injection** *see* Methylprednisolone *on page 754*
- **Medrol® Oral** *see* Methylprednisolone *on page 754*


## Medroxyprogesterone (me DROKS ee proe JES te rone)

**U.S. Brand Names** Amen®; Curretab®; Cycrin®; Depo-Provera® Injection; Provera®

**Synonyms** Acetoxymethylprogesterone; Methylacetoxyprogesterone

**Therapeutic Category** Contraceptive; Progestin

**Pregnancy Risk Factor** X

**Lactation** Enters breast milk/compatible

**Use** Endometrial carcinoma or renal carcinoma as well as secondary amenorrhea or abnormal uterine bleeding due to hormonal imbalance; reduction of endometrial hyperplasia in postmenopausal women receiving 0.625 mg conjugated estrogens for 12-14 consecutive days per month; Depo-Provera® injection is used for the prevention of pregnancy

**Mechanism of Action/Effect** Inhibits secretion of pituitary gonadotropins, which prevents follicular maturation and ovulation, stimulates growth of mammary tissue

**Contraindications** Hypersensitivity to medroxyprogesterone or any component; pregnancy; thrombophlebitis; cerebral apoplexy; undiagnosed vaginal bleeding; liver dysfunction

**Warnings** Use with caution in patients with depression, diabetes, epilepsy, asthma, migraines, renal or cardiac dysfunction. Pretreatment exams should include Pap smear, physical exam of breasts and pelvic areas. May increase serum cholesterol, LDL, decrease HDL and triglycerides. Use of any progestin (progesterone and derivatives ie, medroxyprogesterone) during the first 4 months of pregnancy is not recommended. Monitor patient closely for loss of vision, sudden onset of proptosis, diplopia, migraine, and signs or symptoms of thromboembolic disorders.

**Drug Interactions**

**Decreased Effect:** Aminoglutethimide may decrease effects by increasing hepatic metabolism.

**Effects on Lab Values** Altered thyroid and liver function tests

**Adverse Reactions**

>10%:
- Cardiovascular: Swelling of face
- Central nervous system: Headache, mood changes, nervousness
- Endocrine & metabolic: Amenorrhea, irregular menstrual cycles, menorrhagia, spotting, ovarian enlargement, ovarian cyst formation
- Gastrointestinal: Abdominal pain

1% to 10%:
- Cardiovascular: Hot flashes
- Central nervous system: Dizziness, mental depression, insomnia
- Dermatologic: Dermatitis, acne, melasma, loss or gain of body, facial, or scalp hair
- Endocrine & metabolic: Hyperglycemia, galactorrhea, breast pain, libido decrease
- Gastrointestinal: Nausea, change in appetite, weight gain
- Genitourinary: Vaginitis, leukorrhea
- Local: Pain or itching at implant site
- Neuromuscular & skeletal: Myalgia

<1% (Limited to important or life-threatening symptoms): Thromboembolism

**Overdose/Toxicology** Toxicity is unlikely following single exposure of excessive doses. Supportive treatment is adequate in most cases.

**Pharmacodynamics/Kinetics**

**Half-life Elimination:** 30 days

**Metabolism:** Oral: Liver

**Excretion:** Oral: Urine and feces

**Formulations**

Medroxyprogesterone acetate:
- Injection, suspension: 100 mg/mL (5 mL); 150 mg/mL (1 mL); 400 mg/mL (1 mL, 2.5 mL, 10 mL)
- Tablet: 2.5 mg, 5 mg, 10 mg

**Dosing**

**Adults:**

Oral:
- Amenorrhea: 5-10 mg/day or 2.5 mg/day for 5-10 days
- Abnormal uterine bleeding: 5-10 mg for 5-10 days starting on day 16 or 21 of cycle
- Accompanying cyclic estrogen therapy, postmenopausal: 2.5-10 mg the last 10-13 days of estrogen dosing each month

I.M.:
- Endometrial or renal carcinoma: 400-1000 mg/week

Contraception: 150 mg every 3 months

**Elderly:** Refer to adult dosing.

**Hepatic Impairment:** Dose needs to be lowered in patients with alcoholic cirrhosis.

**Monitoring Laboratory Tests Must have pregnancy test prior to beginning therapy.**

**Additional Nursing Issues**

**Physical Assessment:** Monitor for effectiveness of therapy and adverse effects (see above). Instruct patient on appropriate dose scheduling (according to purpose of therapy), possible side effects, and symptoms to report. **Pregnancy risk factor X** - determine that patient is not pregnant before beginning treatment and do not give to women of childbearing age unless both male and female are capable of complying with barrier contraceptive measures during therapy and for 1 month following therapy.

**Patient Information/Instruction:** Follow dosage schedule and do not take more than prescribed. You may experience sensitivity to sunlight (use sunblock, wear protective clothing and eyewear, and avoid extensive exposure to direct sunlight); dizziness, anxiety, depression (use caution when driving or engaging in tasks that require alertness until response to drug is known); changes in appetite (maintain adequate hydration and diet - 2-3 L/day of fluids unless instructed to restrict fluid intake); decreased libido or increased body hair (reversible when drug is discontinued); hot flashes (cool clothes and environment may help). May cause discoloration of stool (green). Report swelling of face, lips, or mouth; absence or altered menses; abdominal pain; vaginal itching, irritation, or discharge; heat, warmth, redness, or swelling of extremities; or sudden onset change in vision. **Pregnancy precautions:** Inform prescriber if you are pregnant. Do not get pregnant during or for 1 month following therapy. Male/female: Consult prescriber for instruction on appropriate barrier contraceptive measures. This drug may cause severe fetal defects.

**Geriatric Considerations:** No specific recommendations for dosage adjustments. Monitor closely for adverse effects when starting therapy.

♦ **Medroxyprogesterone and Estrogens** *see* Estrogens and Medroxyprogesterone *on page 445*

## Medrysone (ME dri sone)

**U.S. Brand Names** HMS Liquifilm®

**Therapeutic Category** Corticosteroid, Ophthalmic

**Pregnancy Risk Factor** C

**Lactation** Excretion in breast milk unknown/use caution

**Use** Treatment of allergic conjunctivitis, vernal conjunctivitis, episcleritis, ophthalmic epinephrine sensitivity reaction

**Mechanism of Action/Effect** Decreases inflammation by suppression of migration of polymorphonuclear leukocytes and reversal of increased capillary permeability

**Contraindications** Fungal, viral, or untreated pus-forming bacterial ocular infections; not for use in iritis and uveitis

**Warnings** Prolonged use has been associated with the development of corneal or scleral perforation and posterior subcapsular cataracts. May mask or enhance the establishment of acute purulent untreated infections of the eye. Effectiveness and safety have not been established in children. Medrysone is a synthetic corticosteroid; structurally related to progesterone; if no improvement after several days of treatment, discontinue medrysone and institute other therapy. Duration of therapy: 3-4 days to several weeks dependent on type and severity of disease. Taper dose to avoid disease exacerbation. Pregnancy factor C.

**Adverse Reactions**

1% to 10%: Ocular: Temporary mild blurred vision

<1% (Limited to important or life-threatening symptoms): Stinging, burning eyes, corneal thinning, increased intraocular pressure, glaucoma, damage to the optic nerve, defects in visual activity, cataracts, secondary ocular infection

**Overdose/Toxicology** Systemic toxicity is unlikely from the ophthalmic preparation.

**Pharmacodynamics/Kinetics**

**Metabolism:** Liver

**Excretion:** Kidneys and feces

**Formulations** Solution, ophthalmic: 1% (5 mL, 10 mL)

**Dosing**

**Adults:** Ophthalmic: Instill 1 drop in conjunctival sac 2-4 times/day up to every 4 hours; may use every 1-2 hours during first 1-2 days.

**Elderly:** Refer to adult dosing.

**Administration**

**Other:** Ophthalmic: Shake well before using. Do not touch dropper to the eye.

**Additional Nursing Issues**

**Physical Assessment:** See Contraindications and Warnings/Precautions for cautious use. Assess knowledge/teach patient appropriate use, interventions to reduce side effects, and adverse symptoms to report (see Adverse Reactions). **Pregnancy risk factor C** - systemic absorption is unlikely or minimal. Note breast-feeding caution.

**Patient Information/Instruction:** For ophthalmic use only. Shake before using. Apply prescribed amount as often as directed. Wash hands before using and do not let tip of applicator touch eye or contaminate tip of applicator. Tilt head back and look upward. Gently pull down lower lid and put drop(s) in inner corner of eye. Close eye and roll eyeball in all directions. Do not blink for ½ minute. Apply gentle pressure to inner corner of eye for 30 seconds. Wipe away excess from skin around eye. Do not use any other eye preparation for at least 10 minutes. Do not touch tip of applicator to eye or contaminate tip of applicator. Do not share medication with anyone else. May cause sensitivity to bright light (dark glasses may help); temporary stinging or blurred vision

(Continued)

## Medrysone *(Continued)*

may occur. Inform prescriber if you experience eye pain, redness, burning, watering, dryness, double vision, puffiness around eye, vision disturbances, or other adverse eye response; worsening of condition or lack of improvement within 3-4 days. **Pregnancy/breast-feeding precautions:** Inform prescriber if you are pregnant. Consult prescriber if breast-feeding.

- **Medsaplatin** *see* Cisplatin *on page 273*
- **Medsaposide** *see* Etoposide *on page 463*
- **Medsaposide** *see* Etoposide Phosphate *on page 466*
- **Medsavorin** *see* Leucovorin *on page 662*

## Mefloquine (ME floe kwin)

**U.S. Brand Names** Lariam®

**Therapeutic Category** Antimalarial Agent

**Pregnancy Risk Factor** C

**Lactation** Enters breast milk/not recommended

**Use** Treatment of acute malarial infections and prevention of malaria

**Mechanism of Action/Effect** Mefloquine is a quinoline-methanol compound structurally similar to quinine; mefloquine's effectiveness in the treatment and prophylaxis of malaria is due to the destruction of the asexual blood forms of the malarial pathogens that affect humans, *Plasmodium falciparum, P. vivax, P. malariae, P. ovale*

**Contraindications** Hypersensitivity to mefloquine or any component

**Warnings** Discontinue if unexplained neuropsychiatric disturbances occur. Use caution in epilepsy patients or in patients with significant cardiac disease. If mefloquine is to be used for a prolonged period, periodic evaluations including liver function tests and ophthalmic examinations should be performed. (Retinal abnormalities have not been observed with mefloquine in humans; however, it has with long-term administration to rats). In cases of life-threatening, serious, or overwhelming malaria infections due to *Plasmodium falciparum*, patients should be treated with intravenous antimalarial drug. Mefloquine may be given orally to complete the course. Caution should be exercised with regard to driving, piloting airplanes, and operating machines since dizziness, disturbed sense of balance; neuropsychiatric reactions have been reported with mefloquine. Pregnancy factor C.

**Drug Interactions**

**Cytochrome P-450 Effect:** Unknown; potentially similar to quinidine.

**Decreased Effect:** Mefloquine may decrease the effect of valproic acid.

**Increased Effect/Toxicity:** Increased toxicity with beta-blockers. Increased toxicity/levels of chloroquine, quinine, and quinidine (hold treatment until at least 12 hours after these drugs).

**Adverse Reactions**

>10%:

Central nervous system: Difficulty concentrating, dizziness, headache, insomnia, lightheadedness, vertigo

Gastrointestinal: Vomiting, diarrhea, stomach pain, nausea, anorexia

Ocular: Visual disturbances

Otic: Tinnitus

<1% (Limited to important or life-threatening symptoms): Bradycardia, extrasystoles, syncope, seizures

**Overdose/Toxicology** Cardiotoxic symptoms of overdose include vomiting and diarrhea. Treatment is supportive.

**Pharmacodynamics/Kinetics**

**Distribution:** Concentrates in erythrocytes

**Half-life Elimination:** 21-22 days

**Metabolism:** Liver

**Excretion:** Urine

**Formulations** Tablet, as hydrochloride: 250 mg

**Dosing**

**Adults:** Oral:

Treatment of mild to moderate malaria infection: 5 tablets (1250 mg) as a single dose with at least 8 oz of water

Malaria prophylaxis: 1 tablet (250 mg) weekly starting 1 week before travel, continuing weekly during travel and for 4 weeks after leaving endemic area

**Elderly:** Refer to adult dosing.

**Administration**

**Oral:** Do not take drug on empty stomach. Take with food and at least 8 oz of water.

**Monitoring Laboratory Tests** When use is prolonged, periodically monitor liver function tests.

**Additional Nursing Issues**

**Physical Assessment:** When used for prophylaxis, begin treatment 1 week before entering endemic areas. Monitor for CNS disturbances and GI distress. Ophthalmic exams should be scheduled when used for long periods of time. **Pregnancy risk factor C** - benefits of use should outweigh possible risks. Breast-feeding is not recommended.

**Patient Information/Instruction:** Take on schedule as directed, with a full 8 oz of water. Ophthalmic exams will be necessary when used long-term. When taking for prophylaxis, begin 1 week before traveling to endemic areas, continue during travel period, and for 4 weeks following return. You may experience GI distress (frequent small meals may help). You may experience dizziness, changes in mentation, insomnia, headache, visual disturbances (use caution when driving or engaging in tasks that require alertness until response to drug is known). **Pregnancy/breast-feeding precautions:** Use reliable contraception during and for 2 months following treatment. Breast-feeding is not recommended.

- **Mefoxin®** *see* Cefoxitin *on page 224*
- **Mega-B® [OTC]** *see* Vitamin, Multiple *on page 1219*
- **MegaB®** *see page 1294*
- **Megace®** *see* Megestrol *on this page*
- **Megacillin® Suspension** *see* Penicillin G Benzathine *on page 896*
- **Megaton™** *see page 1294*

## Megestrol (me JES trole)

**U.S. Brand Names** Megace®

**Therapeutic Category** Antineoplastic Agent, Miscellaneous; Progestin

**Pregnancy Risk Factor** X

**Lactation** Enters breast milk/contraindicated

**Use** Palliative treatment of breast and endometrial carcinomas, appetite stimulation, and promotion of weight gain in cachexia

**Mechanism of Action/Effect** A synthetic progestin with antiestrogenic properties which disrupt the estrogen receptor cycle. May also have a direct effect on the endometrium. Megestrol is an antineoplastic progestin thought to act through an antileutenizing effect mediated via the pituitary.

**Contraindications** Hypersensitivity to megestrol or any component; pregnancy

**Warnings** The U.S. Food and Drug Administration (FDA) currently recommends that procedures for proper handling and disposal of antineoplastic agents be considered. Use with caution in patients with a history of thrombophlebitis. Elderly females may have vaginal bleeding or discharge and need to be forewarned of this side effect and inconvenience.

**Effects on Lab Values** Altered thyroid and liver function tests

**Adverse Reactions**

>10%:
- Cardiovascular: Swelling of face
- Central nervous system: Headache, mood changes, nervousness
- Endocrine & metabolic: Amenorrhea, irregular menstrual cycles, menorrhagia, spotting, ovarian enlargement, ovarian cyst formation
- Gastrointestinal: Abdominal pain

1% to 10%:
- Cardiovascular: Hot flashes
- Central nervous system: Dizziness, mental depression, insomnia
- Dermatologic: Dermatitis, acne, melasma, loss or gain of body, facial, or scalp hair
- Endocrine & metabolic: Hyperglycemia, galactorrhea, breast pain, libido decrease
- Gastrointestinal: Nausea, change in appetite, weight gain
- Genitourinary: Vaginitis, leukorrhea
- Local: Pain or itching at implant site
- Neuromuscular & skeletal: Myalgia

<1% (Limited to important or life-threatening symptoms): Thromboembolism

**Overdose/Toxicology** Toxicity is unlikely following single exposure of excessive doses.

**Pharmacodynamics/Kinetics**

**Half-life Elimination:** 15-20 hours

**Time to Peak:** Within 1-3 hours

**Metabolism:** Liver

**Excretion:** Urine, feces, and bile

**Onset:** At least 2 months of continuous therapy is necessary.

**Formulations**

Megestrol acetate:
- Suspension, oral: 40 mg/mL with alcohol 0.06% (240 mL)
- Tablet: 20 mg, 40 mg

**Dosing**

**Adults:** Oral (refer to individual protocols):
- Breast carcinoma: 40 mg 4 times/day
- Endometrial: 40-320 mg/day in divided doses; use for 2 months to determine efficacy; maximum doses used have been up to 800 mg/day.
- Uterine bleeding: 40 mg 2-4 times/day
- HIV-related cachexia (male/female): Initial: 800 mg/day; daily doses of 400 and 800 mg/day were found to be clinically effective.

**Elderly:** Refer to adult dosing.

**Additional Nursing Issues**

**Physical Assessment:** Monitor for effectiveness of therapy and adverse effects (see Adverse Reactions). Instruct patient on appropriate dose scheduling (according to purpose of therapy), possible side effects, and symptoms to report. **Pregnancy risk factor X** - determine that patient is not pregnant before beginning treatment and do not give to women of childbearing age unless both male and female are capable of complying with barrier contraceptive measures during therapy and 1 month following therapy. Breast-feeding is contraindicated.

**Patient Information/Instruction:** Follow dosage schedule and do not take more than prescribed. You may experience sensitivity to sunlight (use sunblock, wear protective clothing, and avoid extended exposure to direct sunlight); dizziness, anxiety, depression (use caution when driving or engaging in tasks that require alertness until

(Continued)

## Megestrol *(Continued)*

response to drug is known); change in appetite (maintain adequate hydration and diet - 2-3 L/day of fluids unless instructed to restrict fluid intake); decreased libido or increased body hair (reversible when drug is discontinued); hot flashes (cool clothes and environment may help). Report swelling of face, lips, or mouth; absence or altered menses; abdominal pain; vaginal itching, irritation, or discharge; heat, warmth, redness, or swelling of extremities; or sudden onset change in vision. **Pregnancy/breast-feeding precautions:** Inform prescriber if you are pregnant. Do not get pregnant during or for 1 month following therapy. Consult prescriber for instruction on appropriate contraceptive measures. This drug may cause severe fetal defects. Do not donate blood during or for 1 month following therapy (same reason). Do not breast-feed.

**Geriatric Considerations:** Elderly females may have vaginal bleeding or discharge and need to be forewarned of this side effect and inconvenience. No specific changes in dose are required for elderly. Megestrol has been used in the treatment of the failure to thrive syndrome in cachectic elderly in addition to proper nutrition.

- **Melanex®** *see* Hydroquinone *on page 583*
- **Mellaril®** *see* Thioridazine *on page 1123*
- **Mellaril-S®** *see* Thioridazine *on page 1123*
- **Melpaque HP®** *see* Hydroquinone *on page 583*

## Melphalan (MEL fa lan)

**U.S. Brand Names** Alkeran®

**Synonyms** L-PAM; L-Sarcolysin; Phenylalanine Mustard

**Therapeutic Category** Antineoplastic Agent, Alkylating Agent

**Pregnancy Risk Factor** D

**Lactation** Excretion in breast milk unknown/not recommended

**Use** Palliative treatment of multiple myeloma and nonresectable epithelial ovarian carcinoma; neuroblastoma, rhabdomyosarcoma, breast cancer; I.V. formulation: Use in patients in whom oral therapy is not appropriate

**Mechanism of Action/Effect** Alkylating agent which is a derivative of mechlorethamine that inhibits DNA and RNA synthesis via formation of carbonium ions; cross-links strands of DNA

**Contraindications** Hypersensitivity to melphalan or any component; severe bone marrow depression; patients whose disease was resistant to prior therapy; pregnancy

**Warnings** The U.S. Food and Drug Administration (FDA) currently recommends that procedures for proper handling and disposal of antineoplastic agents be considered.

Preparation of melphalan injection should be performed in a Class II laminar flow biologic safety cabinet. Personnel should be wearing surgical gloves and a closed front surgical gown with knit cuffs. Appropriate safety equipment is recommended for preparation, administration, and disposal of antineoplastics. If melphalan injection contacts the skin, wash and flush thoroughly with water. Melphalan is potentially mutagenic, carcinogenic, and teratogenic; produces amenorrhea. Reduce dosage or discontinue therapy if leukocyte count is $<3000/mm^3$ or platelet count is $<100,000/mm^3$; use with caution in patients with bone marrow suppression, impaired renal function, or who have received prior chemotherapy or irradiation; will cause amenorrhea. Toxicity to immunosuppressives is increased in the elderly. Start with lowest recommended adult doses. Signs of infection, such as fever and WBC rise, may not occur. Lethargy and confusion may be more prominent signs of infection.

**Drug Interactions**

**Decreased Effect:** Cimetidine and other $H_2$ antagonists: The reduction in gastric pH has been reported to decrease bioavailability of melphalan by 30%.

**Increased Effect/Toxicity:** Cyclosporine and melphalan increase the incidence of nephrotoxicity.

**Food Interactions** Food interferes with oral absorption.

**Effects on Lab Values** False-positive Coombs' test [direct]

**Adverse Reactions**

>10%

Hematologic: Myelosuppressive: Leukopenia and thrombocytopenia are the most common effects of melphalan. Irreversible bone marrow failure has been reported.
WBC: Moderate
Platelets: Moderate
Onset (days): 7
Nadir (days): 8-10 and 27-32
Recovery (days): 42-50

Second malignancies: Reported are melphalan more frequently

1% to 10%:

Cardiovascular: Vasculitis
Dermatologic: Vesiculation of skin, alopecia, pruritus, rash
Endocrine & metabolic: SIADH, sterility and amenorrhea
Gastrointestinal: Nausea and vomiting are mild; stomatitis and diarrhea are infrequent
Emetic potential: Low (<10%): $<100 mg/m^2$; high (>90%): $>100 mg/m^2$
Genitourinary: Bladder irritation, hemorrhagic cystitis
Hematologic: Anemia, agranulocytosis, hemolytic anemia
Respiratory: Pulmonary fibrosis, interstitial pneumonitis
Miscellaneous: Hypersensitivity

**BMT:**

Dermatologic: Alopecia

Gastrointestinal: Mucositis (severity increases with $Cl_{cr}$ ≤40 mL/minute), nausea and vomiting (moderate), diarrhea

Hematologic: Myelosuppression, secondary leukemia

Renal: Increased serum creatinine and azotemia possible without adequate hydration

Rare side effects: Abnormal LFTs, interstitial pneumonitis, secondary leukemia, SIADH, vasculitis

**Overdose/Toxicology** Symptoms of overdose include hypocalcemia, pulmonary fibrosis, nausea and vomiting, and bone marrow suppression. Treatment is symptomatic and supportive.

**Pharmacodynamics/Kinetics**

**Half-life Elimination:** 1.5 hours

**Time to Peak:** Reportedly within 2 hours

**Excretion:** Urine and feces

**Formulations**

Powder for injection: 50 mg

Tablet: 2 mg

**Dosing**

**Adults:**

Oral (refer to individual protocols); dose should always be adjusted to patient response and weekly blood counts:

Multiple myeloma: 6 mg/day initially adjusted as indicated **or** 0.15 mg/kg/day for 7 days **or** 0.25 mg/kg/day for 4 days; repeat at 4- to 6-week intervals.

Ovarian carcinoma: 0.2 mg/kg/day for 5 days, repeat every 4-5 weeks

I.V. (refer to individual protocols): Multiple myeloma: 16 mg/m$^2$ administered at 2-week intervals for 4 doses, then repeat monthly as per protocol for multiple myeloma.

High dose BMT: 140-240 mg/m$^2$ as a single dose or divided into 2-5 daily doses. Infuse over 20-60 minutes.

**Elderly:** Refer to adult dosing.

**Renal Impairment:**

$Cl_{cr}$ 10-50 mL/minute: Administer at 75% of normal dose.

$Cl_{cr}$ <10 mL/minute: Administer at 50% of normal dose.

**or**

BUN <30 mg/dL: Reduce dose by 50%.

Serum creatinine <1.5 mg/dL: Reduce dose by 50%.

Hemodialysis effects: Unknown

CAPD effects: Unknown

CAVH effects: Unknown

**Hepatic Impairment:** BUN <30 mg/dL: Reduce dose by 50%.

**Administration**

**Oral:** Administer on an empty stomach.

**I.V.:** I.V. dose should be administered as a single infusion over 15-30 minutes. Complete administration of I.V. dose within 60 minutes of reconstitution.

**I.V. Detail:** Avoid skin contact with I.V. formulation.

**BMT only:** Saline-based hydration (100-125 mg/m$^2$/hour) preceding (2-4 hours), during, and following (6-12 hours) administration reduces risk of drug precipitation in renal tubules. Hydrolysis causes loss of 1% melphalan injection per 10 minutes. Infusion of admixture must be completed within 100 minutes of preparation to deliver ordered dose. Reconstitute dose to 5 mg/mL in diluent provided by manufacturer. Dose may be infused via central or peripheral venous access without further dilution to minimize volume of infusion.

**Stability**

**Storage:** Tablets/injection: Protect from light. Store at room temperature (15°C to 30°C).

**Reconstitution:**

Injection: Preparation: **The time between reconstitution/dilution and administration of parenteral melphalan must be kept to a minimum (<60 minutes) because reconstituted and diluted solutions are unstable.** Dissolve powder initially with 10 mL of diluent to a concentration of 5 mg/mL. **Immediately** dilute dose in NS to a concentration ≥0.45 mg/mL. If the solution is **highly unstable**, administration should occur within 1 hour of dissolution. Do not refrigerate solution; precipitation occurs.

**Standard I.V. dilution:**

Dose/250-500 mL NS (concentration ≥0.45 mg/mL)

**Must be prepared fresh** - solution is stable for 1 hour after dilution and must be administered within that time period.

**Compatibility:** See the Chemotherapy Compatibility Chart *on page 1311.*

**Monitoring Laboratory Tests** CBC with differential, platelet count, serum electrolytes, serum uric acid

**Additional Nursing Issues**

**Physical Assessment:** Assess other medications patient may be taking (see Drug Interactions). Monitor results of all laboratory tests prior to each dose or cycle. Monitor infusion site closely; extravasation can cause serious tissue necrosis. Know and monitor for adverse effects of this medication (see Adverse Reactions). Institute and teach bleeding precautions (ie, avoid unnecessary injections, sharps, trauma, etc). Instruct patient about appropriate interventions to reduce side effects and symptoms to report. **Pregnancy risk factor D** - assess knowledge/teach appropriate use of barrier contraceptives. Breast-feeding is not recommended.

**Patient Information/Instruction:** Infusion: Report promptly any pain, irritation, or redness at infusion site. Oral: Preferable to take on an empty stomach, 1 hour prior to

(Continued)

## Melphalan *(Continued)*

or 2 hours after meals. Do not take alcohol, aspirin or aspirin-containing medications, and OTC medications without consulting prescriber. Inform prescriber of all prescription medication you are taking. Maintain adequate fluid balance (2-3 L/day of fluids unless instructed to restrict fluid intake). May cause hair loss (reversible); easy bleeding or bruising (use soft toothbrush or cotton swabs and frequent mouth care, use electric razor, avoid sharp knives or scissors); increased susceptibility to infection (avoid crowds or exposure to infection - do not have any vaccinations unless approved by prescriber). Report unusual bleeding or bruising or persistent fever or sore throat; blood in urine, stool, or vomitus; delayed healing of any wounds; skin rash; yellowing of skin or eyes; changes in color of urine or black stool; pain or burning on urination; respiratory difficulty; or other severe adverse reactions. **Pregnancy/breast-feeding precautions:** Do not get pregnant while taking this medication; use appropriate barrier contraceptive measures. Breast-feeding is not recommended.

**Geriatric Considerations:** Toxicity to immunosuppressives is increased in the elderly. Start with lowest recommended adult doses. Signs of infection, such as fever and WBC rise, may not occur. Lethargy and confusion may be more prominent signs of infection.

- **Melquin HP®** *see* Hydroquinone *on page 583*
- **Menadol® [OTC]** *see* Ibuprofen *on page 592*
- **Menest®** *see* Estrogens, Esterified *on page 449*
- **Meni-D®** *see* Meclizine *on page 712*
- **Meningococcal Polysaccharide Vaccine, Groups A, C, Y, and W-135** *see page 1256*
- **Menomune®-A/C/Y/W-135** *see page 1256*

## Menotropins (men oh TROE pins)

**U.S. Brand Names** Humegon™; Pergonal®

**Therapeutic Category** Gonadotropin; Ovulation Stimulator

**Pregnancy Risk Factor** X

**Lactation** Excretion in breast milk unknown/contraindicated (not likely to be used)

**Use** Sequentially with hCG to induce ovulation and pregnancy in the infertile woman with functional anovulation; used with hCG in men to stimulate spermatogenesis in those with primary hypogonadotropic hypogonadism

**Mechanism of Action/Effect** Actions occur as a result of both follicle stimulating hormone (FSH) effects and luteinizing hormone (LH) effects; menotropins stimulate the development and maturation of the ovarian follicle (FSH), cause ovulation (LH), and stimulate the development of the corpus luteum (LH); in males it stimulates spermatogenesis (LH)

**Contraindications** Primary ovarian failure; overt thyroid and adrenal dysfunction; abnormal bleeding; pregnancy; males with normal urinary gonadotropin concentrations, elevated gonadotropin levels indicating primary testicular failure

**Warnings** Advise patient of frequency and potential hazards of multiple pregnancy. To minimize the hazard of abnormal ovarian enlargement, use the lowest possible dose.

**Adverse Reactions**

**Male:**

>10%: Endocrine & metabolic: Gynecomastia

1% to 10%: Erythrocytosis (shortness of breath, dizziness, anorexia, syncope, epistaxis)

**Female:**

>10%:

Endocrine & metabolic: Ovarian enlargement
Gastrointestinal: Abdominal distention
Local: Pain/rash at injection site

1% to 10%: Ovarian hyperstimulation syndrome

<1% (Limited to important or life-threatening symptoms): Thromboembolism, pain, febrile reactions

**Overdose/Toxicology** Symptoms of overdose include ovarian hyperstimulation.

**Pharmacodynamics/Kinetics**

**Excretion:** Urine

**Formulations** Injection: Follicle stimulating hormone activity 75 units and luteinizing hormone activity 75 units per 2 mL ampul; follicle stimulating hormone activity 150 units and luteinizing hormone activity 150 units per 2 mL ampul

**Dosing**

**Adults:** I.M.:

Male: Following pretreatment with hCG, 1 ampul 3 times/week and hCG 2000 units twice weekly until sperm is detected in the ejaculate (4-6 months) then may be increased to 2 ampuls of menotropins (150 units FSH/150 units LH) 3 times/week

Female: 1 ampul/day (75 units of FSH and LH) for 9-12 days followed by 10,000 units hCG 1 day after the last dose; repeated at least twice at same level before increasing dosage to 2 ampuls (150 units FSH/150 units LH)

**Administration**

**I.M.:** I.M. administration only.

**Stability**

**Storage:** Lyophilized powder may be refrigerated or stored at room temperature.

**Reconstitution:** After reconstitution inject immediately, discard any unused portion.

**Additional Nursing Issues**

**Physical Assessment:** Female: Assess knowledge/teach appropriate method for measuring basal body temperature to indicate ovulation. Stress importance of following prescriber's instructions for timing intercourse. If self-administered, assess/teach appropriate injection technique and needle disposal. **Pregnancy risk factor X** - ascertain pregnancy status prior to beginning therapy.

**Patient Information/Instruction:** Self injection: Follow prescriber's recommended schedule for injections. Multiple ovulations resulting in multiple pregnancies have been reported. Male infertility and/or breast enlargement may occur. Report pain at injection site; enlarged breasts (male); difficulty breathing; nosebleeds; acute abdominal discomfort; or fever, pain, redness, or swelling of calves.

- **Mentax®** *see page 1247*
- **Mepergan®** *see* Meperidine and Promethazine *on next page*

## Meperidine (me PER i deen)

**U.S. Brand Names** Demerol®

**Synonyms** Isonipecaine Hydrochloride; Pethidine Hydrochloride

**Therapeutic Category** Analgesic, Narcotic

**Pregnancy Risk Factor** B/D (if used for prolonged periods or in high doses at term)

**Lactation** Enters breast milk/contraindicated

**Use** Management of moderate to severe pain; adjunct to anesthesia and preoperative sedation

**Mechanism of Action/Effect** Binds to opiate receptors in the CNS, causing inhibition of ascending pain pathways, altering the perception of and response to pain; produces generalized CNS depression

**Contraindications** Hypersensitivity to meperidine or any component; patients receiving MAO inhibitors presently or in the past 14 days; pregnancy (if used for prolonged periods or in high doses at term)

**Warnings** Use with caution in patients with pulmonary, hepatic, renal disorders, or increased intracranial pressure. Use with caution in patients with renal failure or seizure disorders or those receiving high-dose meperidine. Normeperidine (an active metabolite and CNS stimulant) may accumulate and precipitate twitches, tremors, or seizures. Some preparations contain sulfites which may cause allergic reaction. Not recommended as a drug of first choice for the treatment of chronic pain in the elderly due to the accumulation of normeperidine. For acute pain, its use should be limited to 1-2 doses.

**Drug Interactions**

**Cytochrome P-450 Effect:** CYP2D6 enzyme substrate

**Decreased Effect:** Phenytoin may decrease the analgesic effects of meperidine.

**Increased Effect/Toxicity:** May aggravate the adverse effects of isoniazid. MAO inhibitors, fluoxetine, and other serotonin uptake inhibitors greatly potentiate the effects of meperidine. Acute opioid overdosage symptoms can be seen, including severe toxic reactions. CNS depressants, tricyclic antidepressants, and phenothiazines may potentiate the effects of meperidine.

**Effects on Lab Values** ↑ amylase (S), BSP retention, CPK (I.M. injections)

**Adverse Reactions**

>10%:

Cardiovascular: Hypotension
Central nervous system: Fatigue, drowsiness, dizziness
Gastrointestinal: Nausea, vomiting, constipation
Neuromuscular & skeletal: Weakness
Miscellaneous: Histamine release

1% to 10%:

Cardiovascular: Tachycardia or bradycardia
Central nervous system: Nervousness, headache, convulsions, restlessness, malaise, confusion, false sense of well-being, nightmares
Gastrointestinal: Anorexia, stomach cramps, dry mouth, biliary spasm
Genitourinary: Ureteral spasms, decreased urination
Local: Pain at injection site
Neuromuscular & skeletal: Trembling
Ocular: Blurred vision
Respiratory: Dyspnea, shortness of breath

**Overdose/Toxicology** Symptoms of overdose include CNS depression, respiratory depression, mydriasis, bradycardia, pulmonary edema, chronic tremor, CNS excitability, and seizures. Treatment is symptomatic. Naloxone, 2 mg I.V. with repeat administration as necessary up to a total dose of 10 mg, can be used to reverse opiate effects. Naloxone should not be used to treat meperidine-induced seizures.

**Pharmacodynamics/Kinetics**

**Protein Binding:** 65% 75%

**Distribution:** Crosses the placenta

**Half-life Elimination:**

Parent drug: Terminal phase: Adults: 2.5-4 hours; Adults with liver disease: 7-11 hours
Normeperidine (active metabolite): 15-30 hours; is dependent on renal function and can accumulate with high doses or in patients with decreased renal function

**Metabolism:** Liver

**Excretion:** Urine

**Onset:**

Oral, S.C., I.M.: Onset of analgesic effect: Within 10-15 minutes; Peak effect: Within 1 hour
I.V.: Onset of effects: Within 5 minutes

(Continued)

## Meperidine *(Continued)*

**Duration:** 2-4 hours

**Formulations**

Meperidine hydrochloride:

Injection:

Multiple dose vials: 50 mg/mL (30 mL); 100 mg/mL (20 mL)

Single dose: 10 mg/mL (5 mL, 10 mL, 30 mL); 25 mg/dose (0.5 mL, 1 mL); 50 mg/dose (1 mL); 75 mg/dose (1 mL, 1.5 mL); 100 mg/dose (1 mL)

Syrup: 50 mg/5 mL (500 mL)

Tablet: 50 mg, 100 mg

**Dosing**

**Adults:** Doses should be titrated to necessary analgesic effect. When changing route of administration, note that oral doses are about half as effective as parenteral dose.

Oral, I.M., I.V.: S.C.: 50-150 mg/dose every 3-4 hours as needed; oral therapy is discouraged.

**Elderly:** Doses should be titrated to necessary analgesic effect, with adjustments for renal impairment; when changing route of administration, note that oral doses are about half as effective as parenteral dose.

Oral: 50 mg every 4 hours

I.M.: 25 mg every 4 hours

**Renal Impairment:**

$Cl_{cr}$ 10-50 mL/minute: Administer at 75% of normal dose.

$Cl_{cr}$ <10 mL/minute: Administer at 50% of normal dose.

**Hepatic Impairment:** Increased narcotic effect in cirrhosis; reduction in dose is more important for oral than I.V. route.

**Administration**

**I.V.:** Meperidine may be administered I.M. (preferably), S.C., or I.V. IVP should be given slowly, use of a 10 mg/mL concentration has been recommended.

**Stability**

**Storage:** Meperidine injection should be stored at room temperature and protected from light and freezing. Protect oral dosage forms from light.

**Compatibility:** Incompatible with aminophylline, heparin, phenobarbital, phenytoin, and sodium bicarbonate. See the Compatibility of Drugs Chart *on page 1315* and the Compatibility of Drugs in Syringe Chart *on page 1317.*

**Additional Nursing Issues**

**Physical Assessment:** Assess other medications patient may be taking for additive or adverse interactions (see Drug Interactions). Monitor for effectiveness of pain relief and monitor for signs of overdose (see above). Monitor blood pressure, CNS and respiratory status, and degree of sedation at beginning of therapy and at regular intervals with long-term use. May cause physical and/or psychological dependence. For inpatients, implement safety measures (eg, side rails up, call light within reach, instructions to call for assistance, etc). Assess knowledge/teach patient appropriate use (if self-administered). Teach patient to monitor for adverse reactions (see Adverse Reactions), adverse reactions to report, and appropriate interventions to reduce side effects. Discontinue slowly after prolonged use. **Pregnancy risk factor B/D** - see Pregnancy Risk Factor for cautious use. Breast-feeding is contraindicated.

**Patient Information/Instruction:** If self-administered, use exactly as directed (do not increase dose or frequency); may cause physical and/or psychological dependence. While using this medication, do not use alcohol and other prescription or OTC medications (especially sedatives, tranquilizers, antihistamines, or pain medications) without consulting prescriber. Maintain adequate hydration (2-3 L/day of fluids unless instructed to restrict fluid intake). May cause hypotension, dizziness, drowsiness, impaired coordination, or blurred vision (use caution when driving, climbing stairs, or changing position - rising from sitting or lying to standing, or when engaging in tasks requiring alertness until response to drug is known); loss of appetite, nausea, or vomiting (frequent mouth care, small frequent meals, chewing gum, or sucking lozenges may help); constipation (increased exercise, fluids, or dietary fruit and fiber may help - if constipation remains an unresolved problem, consult prescriber about use of stool softeners). Report chest pain, slow or rapid heartbeat, acute dizziness or persistent headache; changes in mental status; swelling of extremities or unusual weight gain; changes in urinary elimination; acute headache; back or flank pain or muscle spasms; blurred vision; skin rash; or shortness of breath. **Pregnancy/breast-feeding precautions:** Inform prescriber if you are or intend to be pregnant. Do not breast-feed.

**Geriatric Considerations:** Meperidine is not recommended as a drug of first choice for the treatment of chronic pain in the elderly due to the accumulation of its metabolite, normeperidine, which leads to serious CNS side effects (eg, tremor, seizures, etc). For acute pain, its use should be limited to 1-2 doses.

**Additional Information** The injection formulation contains sulfites.

Meperidine 75 mg I.M.; or 75-100 mg S.C. = meperidine 300 mg oral

**Related Information**

Narcotic/Opioid Analgesic Comparison *on page 1396*

## Meperidine and Promethazine (me PER i deen & proe METH a zeen)

**U.S. Brand Names** Mepergan®

**Synonyms** Promethazine and Meperidine

**Therapeutic Category** Analgesic, Combination (Narcotic)

**Pregnancy Risk Factor** B/D (if used for prolonged periods or in high doses at term)

**Lactation** Enters breast milk/contraindicated

**Use** Management of moderate to severe pain

**Formulations**

Capsule: Meperidine hydrochloride 50 mg and promethazine hydrochloride 25 mg

Injection: Meperidine hydrochloride 25 mg and promethazine hydrochloride 25 per mL (2 mL, 10 mL)

**Dosing**

**Adults:**

Oral: 1 capsule every 4-6 hours

I.M.: Inject 1-2 mL every 3-4 hours

**Elderly:** Refer to dosing in individual monographs.

**Additional Nursing Issues**

**Physical Assessment:** See individual components listed in Related Information. **Pregnancy risk factor B/D** - see Pregnancy Risk Factor - assess knowledge/instruct patient on need to use appropriate contraceptive measures and the need to avoid pregnancy. Breast-feeding is contraindicated.

**Patient Information/Instruction:** See individual components listed in Related Information. **Pregnancy/breast-feeding precautions:** Inform prescriber if you are or intend to be pregnant. Do not breast-feed.

**Related Information**

Meperidine *on page 721*

Promethazine *on page 978*

◆ **Mephentermine** *see page 1248*

◆ **Mephyton® Oral** *see* Phytonadione *on page 929*

## Mepivacaine (me PIV a kane)

**U.S. Brand Names** Carbocaine®; Isocaine® HCl; Polocaine®

**Therapeutic Category** Local Anesthetic

**Pregnancy Risk Factor** C

**Lactation** Excretion in breast milk unknown/compatible

**Use** Local anesthesia by nerve block; infiltration in dental procedures; **not** for use in spinal anesthesia

**Mechanism of Action/Effect** Mepivacaine is an amino amide local anesthetic similar to lidocaine; like all local anesthetics, mepivacaine acts by preventing the generation and conduction of nerve impulses

**Contraindications** Hypersensitivity to mepivacaine, any component, or other amide anesthetics; allergy to sodium bisulfate

**Warnings** Use with caution in patients with cardiac disease, renal disease, and hyperthyroidism. Convulsions due to systemic toxicity leading to cardiac arrest have been reported presumably due to intravascular injection. Pregnancy factor C.

**Drug Interactions**

**Increased Effect/Toxicity:** Beta-blockers could theoretically decrease clearance.

**Adverse Reactions** <1% (Limited to important or life-threatening symptoms): bradycardia, myocardial depression, hypotension, cardiovascular collapse, edema, seizures, respiratory arrest

**Overdose/Toxicology** Symptoms of overdose include dizziness, cyanosis, tremor, and bronchial spasm. Treatment is symptomatic and supportive. Termination of anesthesia by pneumatic tourniquet inflation should be attempted when mepivacaine is administered by infiltration or regional injection.

**Pharmacodynamics/Kinetics**

**Protein Binding:** 70% to 85%

**Half-life Elimination:** 1.9 hours

**Metabolism:** Liver

**Excretion:** Urine

**Onset:** Epidural: Within 7-15 minutes

**Duration:** 2-2.5 hours; similar onset and duration is seen following infiltration

**Formulations** Injection, as hydrochloride: 1% [10 mg/mL] (30 mL, 50 mL); 1.5% [15 mg/mL] (30 mL); 2% [20 mg/mL] (20 mL, 50 mL); 3% [30 mg/mL] (1.8 mL)

**Dosing**

**Adults:** Injectable local anesthetic: Varies with procedure, degree of anesthesia needed, vascularity of tissue, duration of anesthesia required, and physical condition of patient

**Elderly:** Refer to adult dosing.

**Additional Nursing Issues**

**Physical Assessment:** Monitor for effectiveness of anesthesia and adverse reactions (see Adverse Reactions). Monitor for return of sensation. Oral: Use caution to prevent gagging or choking and avoid food or drink for 1 hour. Teach patient adverse reactions to report; use and teach appropriate interventions to promote safety. **Pregnancy risk factor C** - benefits of use should outweigh possible risks.

**Patient Information/Instruction:** You will experience decreased sensation to pain, heat, or cold in the area and/or decreased muscle strength (depending on area of application) until effects wear off; use necessary caution to reduce incidence of possible injury until full sensation returns. Report irritation, pain, burning at injection site; chest pain or palpitations; or difficulty breathing.

Oral: This will cause numbness of your mouth. Do not eat or drink for 1 hour after use. Take small sips of water at first to ensure that you can swallow without difficulty. Your tongue and/or mouth may be numb - use caution to avoid biting yourself. Report

(Continued)

## Mepivacaine *(Continued)*

irritation, pain, burning at injection site; chest pain or palpitations; or difficulty breathing.

**Pregnancy precautions:** Inform prescriber if you are pregnant.

**Additional Information** The injection with levonordefrin formulation contains sulfites.

## Meprobamate (me proe BA mate)

**U.S. Brand Names** Equanil®; Miltown®; Neuramate®

**Therapeutic Category** Antianxiety Agent, Miscellaneous

**Pregnancy Risk Factor** D

**Lactation** Enters breast milk/not recommended

**Use** Management of anxiety disorders

**Unlabeled use:** Demonstrated value for muscle contraction, headache, premenstrual tension, external sphincter spasticity, muscle rigidity, opisthotonos-associated tetanus, insomnia, preprocedure sedation

**Mechanism of Action/Effect** Precise mechanism is not yet clear, but many effects have been ascribed to its CNS depressant actions

**Contraindications** Hypersensitivity to meprobamate or any component; acute intermittent porphyria; do not use in patients with pre-existing CNS depression, narrow-angle glaucoma, or severe uncontrolled pain; pregnancy

**Warnings** Physical and psychological dependence and abuse may occur. Allergic reaction may occur in patients with history of dermatological condition (usually by fourth dose). Use with caution in patients with renal or hepatic impairment, or with a history of seizures.

**Drug Interactions**

**Increased Effect/Toxicity:** CNS depressants when taken with meprobamate may result in increased CNS depression.

**Adverse Reactions**

>10%: Central nervous system: Drowsiness, ataxia

1% to 10%:

Central nervous system: Dizziness
Dermatologic: Rashes
Gastrointestinal: Diarrhea, vomiting
Ocular: Blurred vision
Respiratory: Wheezing

<1% (Limited to important or life-threatening symptoms): Purpura, Stevens-Johnson syndrome, thrombocytopenia, leukopenia, renal failure, dyspnea, bronchospasm

**Overdose/Toxicology** Symptoms of overdose include drowsiness, lethargy, ataxia, coma, hypotension, shock, and death. Treatment is supportive following attempts to enhance drug elimination.

**Pharmacodynamics/Kinetics**

**Distribution:** Crosses the placenta

**Half-life Elimination:** 10 hours

**Metabolism:** Liver

**Excretion:** Urine and feces

**Onset:** Onset of sedation: Oral: Within 1 hour

**Formulations**

Capsule, sustained release: 200 mg, 400 mg
Tablet: 200 mg, 400 mg, 600 mg

**Dosing**

**Adults:** Oral:

Tablet: 400 mg 3-4 times/day, up to 2400 mg/day
Capsule, sustained release: 400-800 mg twice daily

**Elderly:** Oral (use lowest effective dose): Initial: 200 mg 2-3 times/day

**Renal Impairment:**

$Cl_{cr}$ 10-50 mL/minute: Administer every 9-12 hours.
$Cl_{cr}$ <10 mL/minute: Administer every 12-18 hours.
Moderately dialyzable (20% to 50%)

**Hepatic Impairment:** Probably necessary in patients with liver disease; no specific recommendations.

**Additional Nursing Issues**

**Physical Assessment:** Assess other medications the patient may be taking for effectiveness and interactions (see Drug Interactions). See Contraindications and Warnings/Precautions for cautious use. Assess for history of addiction; long-term use can result in dependence, abuse, or tolerance; periodically evaluate need for continued use. Monitor therapeutic response (eg, mood, affect, anxiety level, sleep pattern) and adverse reactions at beginning of therapy and periodically with long-term use (see Adverse Reactions and Overdose/Toxicology). Taper dosage slowly when discontinuing. Assess knowledge/teach patient appropriate use, interventions to reduce side effects, and adverse symptoms to report. **Pregnancy risk factor D** - assess knowledge/teach appropriate use of barrier contraceptives. Breast-feeding is not recommended.

**Patient Information/Instruction:** Take exactly as directed (do not increase dose or frequency); may cause physical and/or psychological dependence. Do not chew or crush extended release capsule. Do not use excessive alcohol or other prescription or OTC medications (especially pain medications, sedatives, antihistamines, or hypnotics) without consulting prescriber. Maintain adequate hydration (2-3 L/day of fluids unless instructed to restrict fluid intake). You may experience drowsiness, lightheadedness, impaired coordination, dizziness, or blurred vision (use caution when driving or engaging in tasks requiring alertness until response to drug is known); nausea, vomiting, or dry mouth (small frequent meals, frequent mouth care, chewing gum, or sucking lozenges may help); or diarrhea (boiled milk, yogurt, or buttermilk may help). Report persistent CNS effects, skin rash or irritation, changes in urinary pattern, wheezing or respiratory difficulty, or worsening of condition. **Pregnancy/breast-feeding precautions:** Do not get pregnant while taking this medication; use appropriate barrier contraceptive measures. Breast-feeding is not recommended.

**Geriatric Considerations:** Meprobamate is not considered a drug of choice in the elderly because of its potential to cause physical and psychological dependence. Interpretive guidelines from the Health Care Financing Administration (HCFA) strongly discourage the use of meprobamate in residents of long-term care facilities.

**Breast-feeding Issues:** Breast milk concentrations are higher than plasma; effects are unknown. Breast-feeding is not recommended.

**Related Information**

Antipsychotic Medication Guidelines *on page 1436*

♦ **Meprobamate and Aspirin** *see* Aspirin and Meprobamate *on page 113*

♦ **Mepron™** *see* Atovaquone *on page 118*

♦ **Merbromin** *see page 1294*

## Mercaptopurine (mer kap toe PYOOR een)

**U.S. Brand Names** Purinethol®

**Synonyms** 6-Mercaptopurine; 6-MP

**Therapeutic Category** Antineoplastic Agent, Antimetabolite

**Pregnancy Risk Factor** D

**Lactation** Enters breast milk/contraindicated

**Use** Treatment of leukemias (ALL or AML) maintenance therapy

**Mechanism of Action/Effect** Purine antagonist which inhibits DNA and RNA synthesis

**Contraindications** Hypersensitivity to mercaptopurine or any component; patients whose disease showed prior resistance to mercaptopurine or thioguanine; severe liver disease; severe bone marrow depression; pregnancy (may cause birth defects, potentially carcinogenic)

**Warnings** The U.S. Food and Drug Administration (FDA) currently recommends that procedures for proper handling and disposal of antineoplastic agents be considered. Adjust dosage in patients with renal impairment or hepatic failure. Use with caution in patients with prior bone marrow suppression. Patients may be at risk for pancreatitis. Toxicity to immunosuppressives is increased in the elderly. Start with lowest recommended adult doses. Signs of infection, such as fever and WBC rise, may not occur. Lethargy and confusion may be more prominent signs of infection.

**Drug Interactions**

**Decreased Effect:** 6-MP inhibits the anticoagulation effect of warfarin by an unknown mechanism.

**Increased Effect/Toxicity:** Allopurinol can cause increased levels of 6-MP by inhibition of xanthine oxidase. Decrease dose of 6-MP by 75% when both drugs are used concomitantly. Seen only with oral 6-MP usage, not with I.V. May potentiate effect of bone marrow suppression (reduce 6-MP to 25% of dose).

Doxorubicin: Synergistic liver toxicity with 6-MP in >50% of patients, which resolved with discontinuation of the 6-MP.

Hepatotoxic drugs: Any agent which could potentially alter the metabolic function of the liver could produce higher drug levels and greater toxicities from either 6-MP or thioguanine (6-TG).

**Adverse Reactions**

>10%: Hepatic: 6-MP can cause an intrahepatic cholestasis and focal centrilobular necrosis manifested as hyperbilirubinemia, increased alkaline phosphatase, and increased AST. This may be dose related, occurring more frequently at doses >2.5 mg/kg/day; jaundice is noted 1-2 months into therapy, but has ranged from 1 week to 8 years.

1% to 10%:

- Dermatologic: Hyperpigmentation, rash
- Endocrine & metabolic: Hyperuricemia
- Gastrointestinal: Nausea, vomiting, diarrhea, stomatitis, anorexia, stomach pain, and mucositis may require parenteral nutrition and dose reduction; 6-TG is less GI toxic than 6-MP
- Hematologic: Leukopenia, thrombocytopenia, anemia may occur at high doses
- Myelosuppressive:
  - WBC: Moderate
  - Platelets: Moderate
  - Onset (days): 7-10
  - Nadir (days): 14
  - Recovery (days): 21
- Renal: Renal toxicity

<1% (Limited to important or life-threatening symptoms): Eosinophilia

**Overdose/Toxicology** Symptoms of overdose include nausea and vomiting (immediate); bone marrow suppression, hepatic necrosis, and gastroenteritis (delayed). Treatment is supportive.

(Continued)

## Mercaptopurine *(Continued)*

**Pharmacodynamics/Kinetics**

**Protein Binding:** 19%

**Distribution:** CNS penetration is poor

**Half-life Elimination:** 47 minutes

**Time to Peak:** Within 2 hours

**Metabolism:** Liver

**Excretion:** Urine

**Formulations** Tablet: 50 mg

**Dosing**

**Adults:** Oral (refer to individual protocols):
Induction: 2.5-5 mg/kg/day (100-200 mg)
Maintenance: 1.5-2.5 mg/kg/day **or** 80-100 mg/m²/day given once daily

**Elderly:** Oral (refer to individual protocols): Due to renal decline with age, start with lower recommended doses for adults.

**Renal Impairment:** Dose should be reduced to avoid accumulation, but specific guidelines are not available.

**Hepatic Impairment:** Dose should be reduced to avoid accumulation, but specific guidelines are not available.

**Monitoring Laboratory Tests** CBC with differential, platelet count, liver function, uric acid, urinalysis

**Additional Nursing Issues**

**Physical Assessment:** Monitor appropriate laboratory tests as ordered. Monitor for and teach patient to monitor for adverse effects as noted above: hepatic function, nutritional status, blood dyscrasias, renal status (eg, fluid balance, I & O ratio, signs of dehydration/edema, weight gain or loss), and opportunistic infection. **Pregnancy risk factor D** - assess knowledge/teach appropriate use of barrier contraceptives. Breast-feeding is contraindicated.

**Patient Information/Instruction:** Take daily dose at the same time each day. Preferable to take an on empty stomach (1 hour before or 2 hours after meals). Maintain adequate hydration (2-3 L/day of fluids unless instructed to restrict fluid intake). You may experience nausea and vomiting, diarrhea, or loss of appetite (frequent small meals may help/request medication) or weakness or lethargy (use caution when driving or engaging in tasks that require alertness until response to drug is known). Use good oral care to reduce incidence of mouth sores. You may be more susceptible to infection (avoid crowds or exposure to infection). May cause headache (request medication). Report signs of opportunistic infection (eg, fever, chills, sore throat, burning urination, fatigue); bleeding (eg, tarry stools, easy bruising); unresolved mouth sores, nausea, or vomiting; swelling of extremities, difficulty breathing, or unusual weight gain. **Pregnancy/breast-feeding precautions:** Do not get pregnant while taking this medication; use appropriate barrier contraceptive measures. Do not breast-feed.

**Geriatric Considerations:** Toxicity to immunosuppressives is increased in the elderly. Start with lowest recommended adult doses. Signs of infection, such as fever and WBC rise, may not occur. Lethargy and confusion may be more prominent signs of infection.

- **6-Mercaptopurine** *see* Mercaptopurine *on previous page*
- **Mercapturic Acid** *see* Acetylcysteine *on page 36*
- **Mercurochrome® Topical Solution** *see page 1294*
- **Meridia®** *see* Sibutramine *on page 1055*
- **Merlenate® Topical** *see page 1247*
- **Meronem®** *see* Meropenem *on this page*

## Meropenem (mer oh PEN em)

**U.S. Brand Names** Meronem®; Merrem® I.V.

**Therapeutic Category** Antibiotic, Carbapenem

**Pregnancy Risk Factor** B

**Lactation** Excretion in breast milk unknown/use caution

**Use** Meropenem is indicated as single agent therapy for the treatment of intra-abdominal infections including complicated appendicitis and peritonitis in adults and bacterial meningitis in pediatric patients >3 months of age caused by *S. pneumoniae*, *H. influenzae*, and *N. meningitidis* (penicillin-resistant pneumococci have not been studied in clinical trials); it is better tolerated than imipenem and highly effective against a broad range of bacteria

**Mechanism of Action/Effect** Inhibits cell wall synthesis in susceptible bacteria

**Contraindications** Hypersensitivity to meropenem or to other drugs in the same class or in patients who have experienced anaphylactic reactions to other beta-lactams

**Warnings** Seizures and other CNS events have been reported during treatment with meropenem. These experiences have occurred most commonly in patients with pre-existing CNS disorders, with bacterial meningitis, and/or decreased renal function. May cause pseudomembranous colitis.

**Drug Interactions**

**Decreased Effect:** Probenecid interferes with renal excretion of meropenem.

**Effects on Lab Values** ↑ SGPT, SGOT, alkaline phosphatase, LDH, bilirubin, platelets, eosinophils, BUN, creatinine; ↓ platelets, hemoglobin/hematocrit, WBC; prolonged or shortened PT; prolonged PTT; positive direct or indirect Coombs' test; presence of urine red blood cells

**Adverse Reactions**

1% to 10%:

Central nervous system: Headache
Dermatologic: Rash, pruritus
Gastrointestinal: Diarrhea, nausea, vomiting, constipation, oral moniliasis, glossitis
Local: Pain at injection site, phlebitis, thrombophlebitis
Respiratory: Apnea

<1% (Limited to important or life-threatening symptoms): Hypotension, heart failure (MI and arrhythmias), tachycardia, hypertension, edema, seizures, dysuria, RBCs in urine, cholestatic jaundice, hepatic failure, increase LFTs, anemia, hypo- and hypercytosis, bleeding events (epistaxis, melena, etc), renal failure, elevation of creatinine and BUN

**Overdose/Toxicology** No cases of acute overdose with resultant symptoms have been reported. Supportive therapy is recommended. Meropenem and metabolite are removable by dialysis.

**Pharmacodynamics/Kinetics**

**Protein Binding:** ~2%

**Distribution:** Meropenem penetrates well into most body fluids and tissues including the CSF

**Half-life Elimination:** ~1 hour

**Metabolism:** Minor, microbiologically inactive

**Excretion:** Urine

**Formulations**

Infusion: 500 mg (100 mL); 1 g (100 mL)
Infusion, ADD-vantage®: 500 mg (15 mL); 1 g (15 mL)
Injection: 25 mg/mL (20 mL); 33.3 mg/mL (30 mL)

**Dosing**

**Adults:** 1 g every 8 hours (see Administration)

**Elderly:** Refer to adult dosing.

**Renal Impairment:**

$Cl_{cr}$ 26-50 mL/minute: Administer 1 g every 12 hours.
$Cl_{cr}$ 10-25 mL/minute: Administer 500 mg every 12 hours.
$Cl_{cr}$ <10 mL/minute: Administer 500 mg every 24 hours.
Meropenem and its metabolites are readily dialyzable.
Continuous a-v hemofiltration (CAVH): Dose as for $Cl_{cr}$ 10-50 mL/minute

**Administration**

**I.V.:** Administer I.V. infusion over 15-30 minutes; I.V. bolus injection over 3-5 minutes.

**Stability**

**Storage:** Dry powder should be stored at controlled room temperature 20°C to 25°C (68°F to 77°F).

**Reconstitution:** Meropenem infusion vials reconstituted with sodium chloride are stable for up to 2 hours at room temperature or for 18 hours refrigerated; reconstituted with dextrose 5% injections are stable for 1 hour at room temperature and 8 hours refrigerated. Mini bags with normal saline are stable for up to 24 hours refrigerated; with dextrose stable for 6 hours.

**Compatibility:** Has not been established. Do not mix with or physically add to solutions containing other drugs.

**Monitoring Laboratory Tests** Perform culture and sensitivity testing prior to initiating therapy. Monitor renal function, liver function, CBC.

**Additional Nursing Issues**

**Physical Assessment:** Carefully assess history of previous drug allergies. Monitor appropriate laboratory results (renal, liver, blood). Monitor closely for CNS adverse effects, especially those patients with any history of seizures, head injuries, or other CNS events. Monitor for superinfections (eg, unhealed mouth sores). Check injection/infusion site carefully (phlebitis, thrombophlebitis). Note breast-feeding caution.

**Patient Information/Instruction:** Report pain at infusion/injection site, rash, or respiratory difficulty. You may experience gastric distress, diarrhea, mouth sores, respiratory difficulty, or headache (consult prescriber for appropriate medication). **Breast-feeding precautions:** Consult prescriber if breast-feeding.

**Geriatric Considerations:** Adjust dose based on renal function.

**Additional Information** Meropenem has a broad spectrum of activity similar to imipenem/cilastatin, but is currently only approved for complicated intra-abdominal infections and meningitis in patients >3 months of age. Data in other types of infections is accumulating and includes sepsis, bacteremia, febrile neutropenia, lower respiratory tract infections, and skin and skin structure infections. Adverse effects are similar between imipenem/cilastatin and meropenem, but meropenem appears to have a decreased risk of seizures. Meropenem should be reserved for patients with serious complicated or multiresistant organisms. However, cost may prohibit its use in many institutions and healthcare organizations.

1 g of meropenem contains 90.2 mg of sodium as sodium carbonate (3.92 mEq)
pH: 7.3-8.3

♦ **Merrem® I.V.** *see* Meropenem *on previous page*
♦ **Mersol®** *see page 1294*
♦ **Merthiolate®** *see page 1294*
♦ **Meruvax II** *see page 1256*

## Mesalamine (me SAL a meen)

**U.S. Brand Names** Asacol® Oral; Pentasa® Oral; Rowasa® Rectal

**Synonyms** 5-Aminosalicylic Acid; 5-ASA; Fisalamine; Mesalazine

(Continued)

## Mesalamine *(Continued)*

**Therapeutic Category** 5-Aminosalicylic Acid Derivative

**Pregnancy Risk Factor** B

**Lactation** Enters breast milk/use caution

**Use**

Oral: Remission and treatment of mildly to moderately active ulcerative colitis

Rectal: Treatment of active mild to moderate distal ulcerative colitis, proctosigmoiditis, or proctitis

**Mechanism of Action/Effect** Mesalamine (5-aminosalicylic acid) is the active component of sulfasalazine; the specific mechanism of action of mesalamine is unknown; however, it is thought that it modulates local chemical mediators of the inflammatory response, especially leukotrienes; action appears topical rather than systemic

**Contraindications** Hypersensitivity to mesalamine, sulfasalazine, sulfites, or salicylates

**Warnings** Pericarditis should be considered in patients with chest pain. Pancreatitis should be considered in any patient with new abdominal complaints. Use with caution in patients with impaired liver function. Elderly may have difficulty administering and retaining rectal suppositories. Given renal function decline with aging, monitor serum creatinine often during therapy.

**Drug Interactions**

**Decreased Effect:** Decreased digoxin bioavailability.

**Food Interactions** Oral: Mesalamine serum levels may be decreased if taken with food.

**Adverse Reactions**

**Oral:**

1% to 10%:

Central nervous system: Headache, Unusual drowsiness or weakness

Dermatologic: Alopecia, rash, heartburn

Gastrointestinal: Flatulence, gas, anorexia, nausea, vomiting, diarrhea, abdominal pain,

<1% (Limited to important or life-threatening symptoms): Pericarditis, palpitations, vasodilation, GI bleeding, duodenal ulcer, esophageal ulcer, albuminuria, thrombocytopenia, leukopenia, pancytopenia, anemia, hepatitis, elevated alkaline phosphatase, elevated SGOT/SGPT

**Rectal:**

>10%:

Central nervous system: Headache

Gastrointestinal: Abdominal pain, flatulence, gas, nausea

<1% (Limited to important or life-threatening symptoms): Pericarditis, alopecia, pancreatitis

**Overdose/Toxicology** Symptoms of overdose include decreased motor activity, diarrhea, vomiting, and renal function impairment. Treatment is supportive; emesis, gastric lavage, and follow with activated charcoal slurry.

**Pharmacodynamics/Kinetics**

**Half-life Elimination:** 5-ASA: 0.5-1.5 hours; Acetyl 5-ASA: 5-10 hours

**Time to Peak:** Within 4-7 hours

**Metabolism:** Liver (intestinal metabolism may also occur)

**Excretion:** Urine and feces

**Formulations**

Capsule, controlled release (Pentasa®): 250 mg

Suppository, rectal (Rowasa®): 500 mg

Suspension, rectal (Rowasa®): 4 g/60 mL (7s)

Tablet, enteric coated (Asacol®): 400 mg

**Dosing**

**Adults:** Usual course of therapy is 3-6 weeks:

Oral:

Capsule: 1 g 4 times/day

Tablet: 800 mg 3 times/day

Retention enema: 60 mL (4 g) at bedtime, retained overnight, approximately 8 hours

Rectal suppository: Insert 1 suppository in rectum twice daily.

Some patients may require rectal and oral therapy concurrently.

**Elderly:** Refer to adult dosing.

**Administration**

**Oral:** Swallow capsules or tablets whole, do not chew or crush.

**Other:**

Rectal enema: Shake bottle well. Retain enemas for 8 hours or as long as practical.

Suppositories: Remove foil wrapper; avoid excessive handling.

**Stability**

**Storage:** Unstable in presence of water or light. Once foil has been removed, unopened bottles have an expiration of 1 year following the date of manufacture.

**Additional Nursing Issues**

**Physical Assessment:** Assess effectiveness and interactions of other medications (see Drug Interactions). See Warnings/Precautions for use cautions. Assess for history of allergies (see Contraindications). Monitor effectiveness of therapy and adverse response (see Adverse Reactions and Overdose/Toxicology). Assess knowledge/teach patient appropriate use according to drug formulation (see above), possible side effects/interventions, and adverse symptoms to report. Note breast-feeding caution.

**Patient Information/Instruction:** Take as directed. Oral: Do not chew or break tablets. Enemas: Shake well before using, retain for 8 hours or as long as possible. Suppository: After removing foil wrapper, insert high in rectum without excessive handling (warmth will melt suppository). You may experience flatulence, headache, or hair loss (reversible). Report abdominal pain, unresolved diarrhea, severe headache, or chest pain. **Breast-feeding precautions:** Consult prescriber if breast-feeding.

**Geriatric Considerations:** Elderly may have difficulty administering and retaining rectal suppositories. Given renal function decline with aging, monitor serum creatinine often during therapy.

**Breast-feeding Issues:** Adverse effects (diarrhea) in a nursing infant have been reported while the mother received rectal administration of mesalamine within 12 hours after the first dose. The AAP recommends to monitor the infant stool for consistency and to use with caution.

**Additional Information** Some formulations may contain sulfites.

- **Mesalazine** *see* Mesalamine *on page 727*
- **M-Eslon®** *see* Morphine Sulfate *on page 790*

## Mesna (MES na)

**U.S. Brand Names** Mesnex™

**Synonyms** Sodium 2-Mercaptoethane Sulfonate

**Therapeutic Category** Antidote

**Pregnancy Risk Factor** B

**Lactation** Excretion in breast milk unknown/contraindicated

**Use** Detoxifying agent used as a protectant against hemorrhagic cystitis induced by ifosfamide and cyclophosphamide

**Mechanism of Action/Effect** Binds with and detoxifies urotoxic metabolites of ifosfamide and cyclophosphamide to prevent hemorrhagic cystitis induced by ifosfamide and cyclophosphamide

**Contraindications** Hypersensitivity to mesna or other thiol compounds

**Warnings** Examine morning urine specimen for hematuria prior to ifosfamide or cyclophosphamide treatment. If hematuria develops, reduce the ifosfamide/cyclophosphamide dose or discontinue the drug. Will not prevent or alleviate other toxicities associated with ifosfamide or cyclophosphamide and will not prevent hemorrhagic cystitis in all patients.

**Drug Interactions**

**Decreased Effect:** Warfarin: Questionable alterations in coagulation control.

**Effects on Lab Values** False-positive urinary ketones with Multistix® or Labstix®

**Adverse Reactions** 1% to 10%:

Cardiovascular: Hypotension

Central nervous system: Malaise, headache

Gastrointestinal: Diarrhea, nausea, vomiting, bad taste in mouth, soft stools

Neuromuscular & skeletal: Limb pain

**Pharmacodynamics/Kinetics**

**Distribution:** No tissue penetration; following glomerular filtration, mesna disulfide is reduced in renal tubules back to mesna

**Half-life Elimination:** Parent drug: 24 minutes; Mesna disulfide: 72 minutes

**Time to Peak:** 2-3 hours after administration

**Excretion:** Urine

**Formulations** Injection: 100 mg/mL (2 mL, 4 mL, 10 mL)

**Dosing**

**Adults:** Refer to individual protocols; oral dose is approximately equivalent to 2 times the I.V. dose.

I.V.:

Ifosfamide: 20% W/W of ifosfamide dose 15 minutes before ifosfamide administration and 4 and 8 hours after each dose of ifosfamide; **total daily dose is 60% to 100% of ifosfamide**. High-dose ifosfamide: 20% W/W 15 minutes before ifosfamide administration, and every 3 hours for 3-6 doses; some regimens use up to 160% of the total ifosfamide dose.

Cyclophosphamide: 20% W/W of cyclophosphamide dose 15 minutes prior to cyclophosphamide administration and 4 and 8 hours after each dose of cyclophosphamide; **total daily dose = 60% to 200% of cyclophosphamide dose**.

Oral: 40% W/W of the ifosfamide or cyclophosphamide agent dose in 3 doses at 4-hour intervals **or** 20 mg/kg/dose every 4 hours x 3 (oral mesna is not recommended for the first dose before ifosfamide or cyclophosphamide).

**Elderly:** Refer to adult dosing.

**Administration**

**Oral:** For oral administration, injection may be diluted in 1:1, 1:2, 1:10, 1:100 concentrations in carbonated beverages (cola, ginger ale, Pepsi®, Sprite®, Dr Pepper®, etc), juices (apple or orange), or whole milk (chocolate or white), and is stable 24 hours at refrigeration. Used in conjunction with ifosfamide. Examine morning urine specimen for hematuria prior to ifosfamide or cyclophosphamide treatment.

**I.V.:** Administer by I.V. infusion over 15-30 minutes or per protocol. Mesna can be diluted in $D_5W$ or NS to a final concentration of 1-20 mg/mL.

**Stability**

**Storage:** Diluted solutions are chemically and physically stable for 24 hours at room temperature. Polypropylene syringes are stable for 9 days at refrigeration or room temperature. Injection diluted for oral administration is stable 24 hours at refrigeration.

**Compatibility:** Incompatible with cisplatin. Compatible with cyclophosphamide, etoposide, lorazepam, potassium chloride, bleomycin, and dexamethasone. See the Chemotherapy Compatibility Chart *on page 1311*.

**Monitoring Laboratory Tests** Urinalysis

(Continued)

## Mesna *(Continued)*

**Additional Nursing Issues**

**Physical Assessment:** See Contraindications and Warnings/Precautions for use cautions. Monitor laboratory results (see above) and assess frequently for bladder hemorrhage. Breast-feeding is contraindicated.

**Patient Information/Instruction:** This drug is given (I.V.) to help prevent side effects of other chemotherapeutic agents you are taking. **Breast-feeding precautions:** Do not breast-feed.

**Related Information**

Ifosfamide *on page 597*

♦ **Mesnex™** *see* Mesna *on previous page*

## Mesoridazine (mez oh RID a zeen)

**U.S. Brand Names** Serentil®

**Therapeutic Category** Antipsychotic Agent, Phenothazine, Piperidine

**Pregnancy Risk Factor** C

**Lactation** Enters breast milk/contraindicated (AAP rates "of concern")

**Use** Symptomatic management of psychotic disorders, including schizophrenia, behavioral problems, alcoholism as well as reducing anxiety and tension occurring in neurosis

**Mechanism of Action/Effect** Blockade of postsynaptic CNS dopamine receptors

**Contraindications** Hypersensitivity to mesoridazine or any component (cross reactivity between phenothiazines may occur); severe CNS depression; coma

**Warnings** May cause hypotension, particularly with I.M. administration. Highly sedating, use with caution in disorders where CNS depression is a feature. Use with caution in Parkinson's disease. Use with caution in patients with hemodynamic instability; bone marrow suppression; predisposition to seizures; subcortical brain damage; or severe cardiac, hepatic, renal, or respiratory disease. May cause swallowing difficulties. Use with caution in breast cancer or other prolactin-dependent tumors (may elevate prolactin levels). May alter temperature regulation or mask toxicity of other drugs due to antiemetic effects. May alter cardiac conduction - life-threatening arrhythmias have occurred with therapeutic doses of phenothiazines. May cause orthostatic hypotension.

Phenothiazines may cause anticholinergic effects (eg, confusion, agitation, constipation, dry mouth, blurred vision, urinary retention); therefore, use with caution in patients with decreased gastrointestinal motility, urinary retention, BPH, xerostomia, or visual problems. Conditions which also may be exacerbated by cholinergic blockade include narrow-angle glaucoma (screening is recommended) and worsening of myasthenia gravis. Relative to other antipsychotics, mesoridazine has a high potency of cholinergic blockade.

May cause extrapyramidal reactions including pseudoparkinsonism, acute dystonic reactions, akathisia, and tardive dyskinesia (risk of these reactions is low relative to other neuroleptics). May be associated with neuroleptic malignant syndrome (NMS) or pigmentary retinopathy (particularly at doses >1 g/day).

Pregnancy factor C.

**Drug Interactions**

**Cytochrome P-450 Effect:** Unknown; metabolism may involve CYP isoenzymes.

**Decreased Effect:** Decreased effect with anticonvulsants and anticholinergics.

**Increased Effect/Toxicity:** Increased toxicity with CNS depressants, metrizamide (lowers seizure threshold), and propranolol.

**Effects on Lab Values** ↑ cholesterol (S), glucose; ↓ uric acid (S)

**Adverse Reactions**

>10%:

- Cardiovascular: Hypotension, orthostatic hypotension
- Central nervous system: Pseudoparkinsonism, akathisia, dystonias, tardive dyskinesia (persistent), dizziness
- Gastrointestinal: Constipation
- Ocular: Pigmentary retinopathy
- Respiratory: Nasal congestion
- Miscellaneous: Decreased sweating

1% to 10%:

- Dermatologic: Photosensitivity, rash
- Endocrine & metabolic: Changes in menstrual cycle, changes in libido, breast pain
- Gastrointestinal: Weight gain, nausea, vomiting, stomach pain
- Genitourinary: Dysuria, ejaculatory disturbances
- Neuromuscular & skeletal: Tremor

<1% (Limited to important or life-threatening symptoms): Neuroleptic malignant syndrome (NMS), lowering of seizures threshold, agranulocytosis, leukopenia, cholestatic jaundice, hepatotoxicity

**Overdose/Toxicology** Symptoms of overdose include deep sleep, coma, extrapyramidal symptoms, abnormal involuntary muscle movements, and hypotension. Treatment is symptomatic and supportive.

**Pharmacodynamics/Kinetics**

**Protein Binding:** 91% to 99%

**Half-life Elimination:** Time to steady-state serum: 4-7 days

**Time to Peak:** 2-4 hours

**Excretion:** Urine

**Duration:** 4-6 hours

**Formulations**

Mesoridazine besylate:

Injection: 25 mg/mL (1 mL)

Liquid, oral: 25 mg/mL (118 mL)

Tablet: 10 mg, 25 mg, 50 mg, 100 mg

**Dosing**

**Adults:**

Oral: 25-50 mg 3 times/day; maximum: 100-400 mg/day

I.M.: 25 mg initially, repeat in 30-60 minutes as needed; optimal dosage range: 25-200 mg/day

**Elderly:**

Nonpsychotic patients, dementia behavior: Oral: Initial: 10 mg 1-2 times/day; if <10 mg/day desires, consider administering 10 mg every other day (qod); increase dose at 4- to 7-day intervals by 10-25 mg/day; increase dose intervals (bid, tid, etc) as necessary to control response or side effects; maximum daily dose: 250 mg. Gradual increases (titration) may prevent some side effects or decrease their severity.

I.M.: Initial: 25 mg; repeat doses in 30-60 minutes if necessary; dose range: 25-200 mg/day. Elderly usually require less than maximal daily dose.

**Renal Impairment:** Not dialyzable (0% to 5%)

**Administration**

**Oral:** Dilute oral concentrate just prior to administration with distilled water, acidified tap water, orange or grape juice. Do not prepare and store bulk dilutions. Do not mix oral solutions of mesoridazine and lithium, these oral liquids are incompatible when mixed. **Note:** Avoid skin contact with oral medication; may cause contact dermatitis.

**I.V.:** Watch for hypotension when administering I.V.

**Monitoring Laboratory Tests** Baseline liver and kidney function, CBC prior to and periodically during therapy, ophthalmic screening

**Additional Nursing Issues**

**Physical Assessment:** Assess other medications patient is taking for effectiveness and interactions (see Drug Interaction). See Contraindications and Warnings/Precautions for cautious use. Has potential for psychological or physiological dependence, abuse, and tolerance. Review ophthalmic screening and monitor laboratory results (see above), therapeutic response (mental status, mood, affect), and adverse reactions at beginning of therapy and periodically with long-term use (eg, orthostatic hypotension, fluid balance, anticholinergic response, extrapyramidal effects, pigmentary retinopathy - see Adverse Reactions and Overdose). With I.M. or I.V. use, monitor closely for hypotension. **Note:** Avoid skin contact with oral or injection medication; may cause contact dermatitis (wash immediately with warm, soapy water). Initiate at lower doses (see Dosing) and taper dosage slowly when discontinuing. Assess knowledge/teach patient appropriate use, interventions to reduce side effects, and adverse symptoms to report (see below). **Pregnancy risk factor C** - instruct patient about appropriate contraceptive use. Breast-feeding is contraindicated.

**Patient Information/Instruction:** Use exactly as directed (do not increase dose or frequency); may cause physical and/or psychological dependence. It may take 2-3 weeks to achieve desired results; do not discontinue without consulting prescriber. Dilute oral concentration with water, orange or grape juice. Do not take within 2 hours of any antacid. Avoid excess alcohol or caffeine and other prescription or OTC medications not approved by prescriber. Maintain adequate hydration (2-3 L/day of fluids unless instructed to restrict fluid intake). Avoid skin contact with medication; may cause contact dermatitis (wash immediately with warm, soapy water). You may experience excess drowsiness, restlessness, dizziness, or blurred vision (use caution driving or when engaging in tasks requiring alertness until response to drug is known); dry mouth, nausea, vomiting (small frequent meals, frequent mouth care, chewing gum, or sucking lozenges may help); constipation (increased exercise, fluids, or dietary fruit and fiber may help); postural hypotension (use caution climbing stairs or when changing position from lying or sitting to standing); urinary retention (void before taking medication); photosensitivity (use sunscreen, wear protective clothing and eyewear, and avoid direct sunlight); decreased perspiration (avoid strenuous exercise in hot environments); or changes in menstrual cycle, libido, ejaculation (will resolve when medication is discontinued). Report persistent CNS effects (eg, trembling fingers, altered gait or balance, excessive sedation, seizures, unusual movements, anxiety, abnormal thoughts, confusion, personality changes); chest pain, palpitations, rapid heartbeat, severe dizziness; unresolved urinary retention or changes in urinary pattern; menstrual pattern, change in libido, swelling or pain in breasts (male or female); vision changes; skin rash or yellowing of skin; difficulty breathing; or worsening of condition. **Pregnancy/breast-feeding precautions:** Inform prescriber if you are or intend to be pregnant. Do not breast-feed.

**Geriatric Considerations:** (See Warnings/Precautions, Adverse Reactions, and Overdose/Toxicology.) Elderly patients have an increased risk of adverse response to side effects or adverse reactions to antipsychotics. These can include but are not limited to the following.

(Continued)

## Mesoridazine *(Continued)*

Anticholinergic effects: CNS toxicity with confusion, memory loss, psychotic behavior, and agitation.

Extrapyramidal effects (EPS): Parkinson's syndrome and akathisia may occur as often as 50% in patients >60 years of age. Tardive dyskinesia (motor restlessness) may be 40% in elderly; may be related to duration and total accumulated dose over time; may be somewhat reversible if diagnosed early enough.

Orthostatic hypotension: Increased risk for falls.

Sedation: In nonpsychotic patients, may result in feelings of depersonalization, derealization, and dysphoria.

Cardiac toxicity: Cardiac arrhythmias have occurred with therapeutic doses of antipsychotics.

Malignant neuroleptic syndrome: Development of hyperthermia, muscular rigidity, autonomic instability, and altered mental status.

Many elderly patients receive antipsychotic medications for inappropriate nonpsychotic behavior. Before initiating antipsychotic medication, all possible reversible causes should be investigated. Stress may cause acute "confusion" or worsening of baseline nonpsychotic behaviors; any changes in disease state (in any organ) may result in behavioral changes. Common acute changes in behavior may be due also to increases in drug dose addition, or addition of a new drug to the regimen; fluid/electrolyte alterations; infections; or changes in the environment.

Meta-analysis of controlled trials of antipsychotic (phenothiazines, butyrophenones) use with agitated, demented, elderly patients has concluded that the use of neuroleptics results in a response rate of 18%. Clearly, neuroleptic therapy for behavior control should be limited, with frequent attempts to withdraw the agent for behavior control. When use is indicated, initial doses should be lower to start and monitored closely.

**Additional Information** Some formulations may contain ethanol.

**Related Information**

Antipsychotic Agents Comparison *on page 1371*
Antipsychotic Medication Guidelines *on page 1436*


- **Mestatin®** *see* Nystatin *on page 843*
- **Mestinon®** *see* Pyridostigmine *on page 996*
- **Mestinon Time-Span®** *see* Pyridostigmine *on page 996*
- **Mestranol and Norethindrone** *see* Oral Contraceptives *on page 859*
- **Mestranol and Norethynodrel** *see* Oral Contraceptives *on page 859*
- **Metacortandralone** *see* Prednisolone *on page 960*
- **Metamucil® [OTC]** *see* Psyllium *on page 993*
- **Metamucil® Instant Mix [OTC]** *see* Psyllium *on page 993*
- **Metandren®** *see* Methyltestosterone *on page 756*
- **Metaprel® Syrup** *see* Metaproterenol *on this page*


## Metaproterenol (met a proe TER e nol)

**U.S. Brand Names** Alupent®; Arm-a-Med® Metaproterenol; Dey-Dose® Metaproterenol; Metaprel® Syrup; Prometa®

**Synonyms** Orciprenaline Sulfate

**Therapeutic Category** $Beta_2$ Agonist

**Pregnancy Risk Factor** C

**Lactation** Excretion in breast milk unknown

**Use** Bronchodilator in reversible airway obstruction due to asthma or COPD

**Mechanism of Action/Effect** Relaxes bronchial smooth muscle by action on $beta_2$-receptors with very little effect on heart rate

**Contraindications** Hypersensitivity to metaproterenol or any component; pre-existing cardiac arrhythmias associated with tachycardia

**Warnings** Use with caution in patients with hypertension, CHF, hyperthyroidism, CAD, diabetes, or sensitivity to sympathomimetics. Excessive prolonged use may result in decreased efficacy or increased toxicity and death. Use caution in patients with pre-existing cardiac arrhythmias associated with tachycardia. Metaproterenol has more $beta_1$ activity than other sympathomimetics such as albuterol and, therefore, may no longer be the beta-agonist of first choice. All patients should utilize a spacer device when using a metered dose inhaler. Oral use should be avoided due to the increased incidence of adverse effects. Because of its delayed onset of action (1 hour) and prolonged effect (4 or more hours), this may not be the drug of choice for assessing response to a bronchodilator. Pregnancy factor C.

**Drug Interactions**

**Decreased Effect:** Decreased effect of beta-blockers.

**Increased Effect/Toxicity:** Sympathomimetics, TCAs, MAO inhibitors taken with metaproterenol may result in toxicity to the patient.

**Effects on Lab Values** ↑ potassium (S)

**Adverse Reactions**

>10%:

Central nervous system: Nervousness, restlessness
Neuromuscular & skeletal: Tremor

1% to 10%:

Cardiovascular: Tachycardia, palpitations, hypertension, pounding heartbeat
Central nervous system: Headache, dizziness; lightheadedness

Gastrointestinal: Nausea, vomiting, bad taste

Neuromuscular & skeletal: Trembling, muscle cramps, weakness

Respiratory: Coughing

Miscellaneous: Sweating (increased)

<1% (Limited to important or life-threatening symptoms): Paradoxical bronchospasm

**Overdose/Toxicology** Symptoms of overdose include angina, arrhythmias, tremor, dry mouth, and insomnia. Beta-adrenergic stimulation can increase and cause increased heart rate, decreased blood pressure, and decreased CNS excitation. In cases of overdose, supportive therapy should be instituted.

**Pharmacodynamics/Kinetics**

**Onset:**

Oral: Onset of bronchodilation: Within 15 minutes; Peak effect: Within 1 hour

Inhalation: Onset of bronchodilation: Within 60 seconds

**Duration:** Oral or inhalation: ~1-5 hours, regardless of route administered

**Formulations**

Metaproterenol sulfate:

Aerosol, oral: 0.65 mg/dose (5 mL, 10 mL)

Solution for inhalation, preservative free: 0.4% [4 mg/mL] (2.5 mL); 0.6% [6 mg/mL] (2.5 mL); 5% [50 mg/mL] (10 mL, 30 mL)

Syrup: 10 mg/5 mL (480 mL)

Tablet: 10 mg, 20 mg

**Dosing**

**Adults:**

Oral: 20 mg 3-4 times/day

Inhalation: 2-3 inhalations every 3-4 hours, up to 12 inhalations in 24 hours

Nebulizer: 5-20 breaths of full strength 5% metaproterenol **or** 0.2 to 0.3 mL 5% metaproterenol in 2.5-3 mL normal saline until nebulized every 4-6 hours (can be given more frequently according to need)

**Elderly:** Oral: Initial: 10 mg 3-4 times/day, increasing as necessary up to 20 mg 3-4 times/day

**Administration**

**Oral:** Administer around-the-clock to promote less variation in peak and trough serum levels.

**Inhalation:** Do not use solutions for nebulization if they are brown or contain a precipitate. Shake inhaler well before using.

**Stability**

**Storage:** Store in a tight, light-resistant container. Do not use if brown solution or contains a precipitate.

**Additional Nursing Issues**

**Physical Assessment:** Assess effectiveness and interactions of other medications (see Drug Interactions). See Contraindications and Warnings/Precautions for use cautions. Monitor effectiveness of therapy (relief of airway obstruction) and adverse reactions (eg, cardiac and CNS changes - see Adverse Reactions) at beginning of therapy and periodically with long-term use. For inpatient care, monitor vital signs and lung sounds prior to and periodically during therapy. Assess knowledge/teach patient appropriate use, interventions to reduce side effects, and adverse symptoms to report. **Pregnancy risk factor C** - benefits of use should outweigh possible risk (especially with long-term use). Note breast-feeding caution.

**Patient Information/Instruction:** Use exactly as directed (see Administration below). Do not use more often than recommended. Maintain adequate hydration (2-3 L/day of fluids unless instructed to restrict fluid intake). You may experience nervousness, dizziness, or fatigue (use caution when driving or engaging in tasks requiring alertness until response to drug is known); dry mouth, unpleasant aftertaste, stomach upset (frequent small meals, frequent mouth care, chewing gum, or sucking hard candy may help); or increased perspiration. Report unresolved GI upset; dizziness or fatigue; vision changes; chest pain, rapid heartbeat, or palpitations; nervousness or insomnia; muscle cramping or tremor; or unusual cough. **Pregnancy/breast-feeding precautions:** Inform prescriber if you are or intend to be pregnant. Consult prescriber if breast-feeding.

**Administration:**

Self-administered inhalation: Store canister upside down; do not freeze. Shake canister before using. Sit when using medication. Close eyes when administering metaproterenol to avoid spray getting into eyes. Exhale slowly and completely through nose; inhale deeply through mouth while administering aerosol. Hold breath for 1-3 seconds after inhalation. Wait at least 1 full minute between inhalations. Wash mouthpiece between use. If more than one inhalation medication is used, use bronchodilator first and wait 5 minutes between medications.

Self-administered nebulizer: Wash hands before and after treatment. Wash and dry nebulizer after each treatment. Twist open the top of one unit dose vial and squeeze contents into nebulizer reservoir. Connect nebulizer reservoir to the mouthpiece or face-mask. Connect nebulizer to compressor. Sit in comfortable, upright position. Place mouthpiece in your mouth or put on face-mask and turn on compressor. If face-mask is used, avoid leakage around the mask to avoid mist getting into eyes which may cause vision problems. Breath calmly and deeply until no more mist is formed in nebulizer (about 5 minutes). At this point treatment is finished.

**Geriatric Considerations:** Metaproterenol has more $beta_1$ activity than other sympathomimetics such as albuterol and, therefore, may no longer be the beta agonist of first choice. The elderly may find it beneficial to utilize a spacer device when using a

(Continued)

## Metaproterenol *(Continued)*

metered dose inhaler. Oral use should be avoided due to the increased incidence of adverse effects.

**Related Information**

Inhalant (Asthma, Bronchospasm) Agents *on page 1388*

♦ **Metasep®** *see page 1294*

## Metformin (met FOR min)

**U.S. Brand Names** Glucophage®

**Therapeutic Category** Antidiabetic Agent (Biguanide)

**Pregnancy Risk Factor** B

**Lactation** Enters breast milk/not recommended

**Use** Management of noninsulin-dependent diabetes mellitus (Type II) as monotherapy when hyperglycemia cannot be managed on diet alone. May be used concomitantly with a sulfonylurea or insulin when diet and metformin or sulfonylurea alone do not result in adequate glycemic control.

Data suggests that some patients with NIDDM with secondary failure to sulfonylurea therapy may obtain significant improvement in metabolic control when metformin in combination with insulin and a sulfonylurea is used in lieu of insulin alone.

**Mechanism of Action/Effect** Decreases hepatic glucose production, decreasing intestinal absorption of glucose and improves insulin sensitivity (increases peripheral glucose uptake and utilization)

**Contraindications** Hypersensitivity to metformin or any component; renal disease or renal dysfunction (serum creatinine ≥1.5 mg/dL in males or ≥1.4 mg/dL in females or abnormal clearance) which may also result from conditions such as cardiovascular collapse, acute myocardial infarction, and septicemia; acute or chronic metabolic acidosis with or without coma (including diabetic ketoacidosis); should be temporarily discontinued for 48 hours in patients undergoing radiologic studies involving the intravascular administration of iodinated contrast materials (potential for acute alteration in renal function).

**Warnings** Administration of oral antidiabetic drugs has been reported to be associated with increased cardiovascular mortality as compared to treatment with diet alone or diet plus insulin. Metformin is substantially excreted by the kidney - the risk of accumulation and lactic acidosis increases with the degree of impairment of renal function. Patients with renal function below the limit of normal for their age should not receive metformin. In elderly patients, renal function should be monitored regularly. Use of concomitant medications that may affect renal function (ie, affect tubular secretion) may affect metformin disposition. Therapy should be suspended for any surgical procedures. Avoid use in patients with impaired liver function.

**Drug Interactions**

**Decreased Effect:** Drugs which tend to produce hyperglycemia (eg, diuretics, corticosteroids, phenothiazines, thyroid products, estrogens, oral contraceptives, phenytoin, nicotinic acid, sympathomimetics, calcium channel blocking drugs, isoniazid) may lead to a loss of glucose control.

**Increased Effect/Toxicity:** Furosemide increased the metformin plasma and blood $C_{max}$ without altering metformin renal clearance in a single dose study. Cationic drugs (eg, amiloride, digoxin, morphine, procainamide, quinidine, quinine, ranitidine, triamterene, trimethoprim, and vancomycin) which are eliminated by renal tubular secretion could have the potential for interaction with metformin by competing for common renal tubular transport systems. Cimetidine increases (by 60%) peak metformin plasma and whole blood concentrations.

**Adverse Reactions**

>10%:

Central nervous system: Headache

Gastrointestinal: Anorexia, nausea, vomiting, diarrhea, flatulence, constipation, heartburn, metallic taste, weight loss

<1% (Limited to important or life-threatening symptoms): Hypoglycemia, lactic acidosis, blood dyscrasias, aplastic anemia, hemolytic anemia, bone marrow suppression, thrombocytopenia, agranulocytosis

**Overdose/Toxicology** Hypoglycemia has not been observed with ingestion up to 85 g of metformin, although lactic acidosis has occurred in such circumstances. Metformin is dialyzable with a clearance of up to 170 mL/minute. Hemodialysis may be useful for removal of accumulated drug from patients in whom metformin overdose is suspected. Treatment is supportive.

**Pharmacodynamics/Kinetics**

**Protein Binding:** 92% to 99%

**Half-life Elimination:** 6.2 hours (prolonged in renal impairment)

**Excretion:** Renal; tubular secretion is major route

**Onset:** Within days; maximum effects up to 2 weeks

**Formulations** Tablet, as hydrochloride: 500 mg, 850 mg

**Dosing**

**Adults:** Oral (allow 1-2 weeks between dose titrations):

500 mg tablets: Initial: 500 mg twice daily (given with the morning and evening meals). Dosage increases should be made in increments of 1 tablet every week, given in divided doses, up to a maximum of 2500 mg/day. Doses of up to 2000 mg/day may be given twice daily. If a dose of 2500 mg/day is required, it may be better tolerated 3 times/day (with meals).

850 mg tablets: Initial: 850 mg once daily (given with the morning meal). Dosage increases should be made in increments of 1 tablet **every other** week, given in divided doses, up to a maximum of 2550 mg/day. The usual maintenance dose is 850 mg twice daily (with the morning and evening meals). Some patients may be given 850 mg 3 times/day (with meals).

**Transfer from other antidiabetic agents:** No transition period is generally necessary except when transferring from chlorpropamide. When transferring from chlorpropamide, care should be exercised during the first 2 weeks because of the prolonged retention of chlorpropamide in the body, leading to overlapping drug effects and possible hypoglycemia.

**Concomitant metformin and oral sulfonylurea therapy:** If patients have not responded to 4 weeks of the maximum dose of metformin monotherapy, consideration to a gradual addition of an oral sulfonylurea while continuing metformin at the maximum dose, even if prior primary or secondary failure to a sulfonylurea has occurred.

**Elderly:** The initial and maintenance dosing should be conservative, due to the potential for decreased renal function. Generally, elderly patients should **not** be titrated to the maximum dose of metformin.

**Renal Impairment:** The plasma and blood half-life of metformin is prolonged and the renal clearance is decreased in proportion to the decrease in creatinine clearance.

**Hepatic Impairment:** No studies have been conducted.

**Monitoring Laboratory Tests** Urine for glucose and ketones, fasting blood glucose, hemoglobin $A_{1c}$, and fructosamine. Initial and periodic monitoring of hematologic parameters (eg, hemoglobin/hematocrit and red blood cell indices) and renal function should be performed, at least annually. While megaloblastic anemia has been rarely seen with metformin, if suspected, vitamin $B_{12}$ deficiency should be excluded.

**Additional Nursing Issues**

**Physical Assessment:** Assess effectiveness and interactions of other medications (see Drug Interactions). See Warnings/Precautions and Contraindications for use cautions. Monitor effectiveness of therapy and monitor laboratory tests frequently during therapy (see above). Monitor for adverse response (eg, hypoglycemia - see Adverse Reactions and Overdose/Toxicology). Assess knowledge/teach patient or refer patient to diabetic educator for instruction in appropriate use, possible side effects and appropriate interventions, and adverse symptoms to report. Breast-feeding is not recommended.

**Patient Information/Instruction:** This medication is used to control diabetes; it is not a cure. Other components of treatment plan are important: follow prescribed diet, medication, and exercise regimen. Take exactly as directed; with meal(s) at the same time each day. Do not change dose or discontinue without consulting prescriber. Avoid alcohol while taking this medication; could cause severe reaction. Inform prescriber of all other prescription or OTC medications you are taking; do not introduce new medication without consulting prescriber. Do not take other medication within 2 hours of this medication unless so advised by prescriber. Maintain regular dietary intake and exercise routine and always carry quick source of sugar with you. You may experience side effects during first weeks of therapy (headache, nausea); consult prescriber if these persist. Report severe or persistent side effects, extended vomiting or flu-like symptoms, skin rash, easy bruising or bleeding, or change in color of urine or stool. **Breast-feeding precautions:** Breast-feeding is not recommended.

**Geriatric Considerations:** Limited data suggests that metformin's total body clearance may be decreased and AUC and half-life increased in older patients; presumably due to decreased renal clearance. Metformin has been well tolerated by the elderly but lower doses and frequent monitoring are recommended.

**Related Information**

Antidiabetic Oral Agents Comparison *on page 1370*

♦ **Methacholine** *see page 1248*

## Methadone (METH a done)

**U.S. Brand Names** Dolophine®

**Therapeutic Category** Analgesic, Narcotic

**Pregnancy Risk Factor** B/D (if used for prolonged periods or in high doses at term)

**Lactation** Enters breast milk/use caution (AAP rates "compatible")

**Use** Management of severe pain; used in narcotic detoxification maintenance programs

**Mechanism of Action/Effect** Binds to opiate receptors in the CNS, causing inhibition of ascending pain pathways, altering the perception of and response to pain; produces generalized CNS depression

**Contraindications** Hypersensitivity to methadone or any component; pregnancy (if used for prolonged periods or in high doses at term)

**Warnings** Tablets are to be used only for oral administration and **must not** be used for injection. Use with caution in patients with respiratory diseases including asthma, emphysema, or COPD and in patients with severe liver disease. Because methadone's effects on respiration last much longer than its analgesic effects, the dose must be titrated slowly. Because of its long half-life and risk of accumulation, it is not considered a drug of first choice in the elderly, who may be particularly susceptible to its CNS depressant and constipating effects.

**Drug Interactions**

**Cytochrome P-450 Effect:** CYP1A2, 2D6, and 3A3/4 enzyme substrate; CYP2D6 enzyme inhibitor

**Decreased Effect:** Phenytoin, pentazocine, and rifampin may increase the metabolism of methadone and may precipitate withdrawal.

(Continued)

## Methadone *(Continued)*

**Increased Effect/Toxicity:** CNS depressants, phenothiazines, tricyclic antidepressants, and MAO inhibitors may potentiate the adverse effects of methadone.

**Effects on Lab Values** ↑ thyroxine (S), aminotransferase [ALT (SGPT)/AST (SGOT)] (S)

**Adverse Reactions**

>10%:
- Cardiovascular: Hypotension
- Central nervous system: Fatigue, drowsiness, dizziness
- Gastrointestinal: Nausea, vomiting, constipation
- Neuromuscular & skeletal: Weakness
- Miscellaneous: Histamine release

1% to 10%:
- Cardiovascular: Tachycardia or bradycardia
- Central nervous system: Nervousness, headache, restlessness, malaise, confusion, false sense of well-being, insomnia
- Gastrointestinal: Anorexia, stomach cramps, dry mouth
- Genitourinary: Ureteral spasms, decreased urination
- Ocular: Blurred vision
- Respiratory: Dyspnea, shortness of breath

<1% (Limited to important or life-threatening symptoms): Paralytic ileus, biliary spasm, increased transaminases

**Overdose/Toxicology** Symptoms of overdose include respiratory depression, CNS depression, miosis, hypothermia, circulatory collapse, and convulsions. Treatment is supportive. Naloxone, 2 mg I.V. with repeat administration as necessary up to a total of 10 mg, can also be used to reverse toxic effects of the opiate.

**Pharmacodynamics/Kinetics**

**Protein Binding:** 80% to 85%

**Distribution:** Crosses the placenta

**Half-life Elimination:** 15-29 hours, may be prolonged with alkaline pH

**Metabolism:** Liver (N-demethylation)

**Excretion:** Urine (<10% as unchanged drug); increased renal excretion with urine pH <6

**Onset:**
- Oral: Onset of analgesia: Within 0.5-1 hour
- Parenteral: Onset of analgesia: Within 10-20 minutes; Peak effect: Within 1-2 hours

**Duration:** Oral: 6-8 hours, increases to 22-48 hours with repeated doses

**Formulations**

Methadone hydrochloride:
- Injection: 10 mg/mL (1 mL, 10 mL, 20 mL)
- Solution:
  - Oral: 5 mg/5 mL (5 mL, 500 mL); 10 mg/5 mL (500 mL)
  - Oral, concentrate: 10 mg/mL (30 mL)
- Tablet: 5 mg, 10 mg
- Tablet, dispersible: 40 mg

**Dosing**

**Adults:** Doses should be titrated to appropriate effects.
- Analgesia: Oral, I.M., I.V., S.C.: 2.5-10 mg every 3-8 hours as needed, up to 5-20 mg every 6-8 hours
- Detoxification: Oral: 15-40 mg/day; should not exceed 21 days and may not be repeated earlier than 4 weeks after completion of preceding course
- Maintenance of opiate dependence: Oral: 20-120 mg/day
- **Important note:** Methadone accumulates with repeated doses and dosage may need to be adjusted downward after 3-5 days to prevent toxic effects. Some patients may benefit from every 8- to 12-hour dosing interval (pain control).

**Elderly:** Doses should be titrated to appropriate effects: Oral, I.M.: 2.5 mg every 8-12 hours (see Geriatrics Considerations).

**Renal Impairment:**
- $Cl_{cr}$ <10 mL/minute: Administer at 50% to 75% of normal dose. **Important note:** Methadone accumulates with repeated doses and dosage may need to be adjusted downward after 3-5 days to prevent toxic effects. Some patients may benefit from every 8- to 12-hour dosing interval (pain control).

**Hepatic Impairment:** Avoid in severe liver disease.

**Stability**

**Compatibility:** Highly incompatible with all other I.V. agents when mixed together.

**Additional Nursing Issues**

**Physical Assessment:** Assess other medications patient may be taking for additive or adverse interactions (see Drug Interactions). Monitor for effectiveness of pain relief and monitor for signs of overdose (see above). Monitor blood pressure, CNS and respiratory status, and degree of sedation at beginning of therapy and at regular intervals with long-term use. May cause physical and/or psychological dependence. For inpatients, implement safety measures (eg, side rails up, call light within reach, instructions to call for assistance, etc). Assess knowledge/teach patient appropriate use (if self-administered). Teach patient to monitor for adverse reactions (see Adverse Reactions), adverse reactions to report, and appropriate interventions to reduce side effects. Discontinue slowly after prolonged use. **Pregnancy risk factor B/D** - see Pregnancy Risk Factor for cautious use. Note breast-feeding caution.

**Patient Information/Instruction:** If self-administered, use exactly as directed (do not increase dose or frequency); may cause physical and/or psychological dependence.

While using this medication, do not use alcohol and other prescription or OTC medications (especially sedatives, tranquilizers, antihistamines, or pain medications) without consulting prescriber. Maintain adequate hydration (2-3 L/day of fluids unless instructed to restrict fluid intake). May cause hypotension, dizziness, drowsiness, impaired coordination, or blurred vision (use caution when driving, climbing stairs, or changing position - rising from sitting or lying to standing, or when engaging in tasks requiring alertness until response to drug is known); loss of appetite, nausea, or vomiting (frequent mouth care, small frequent meals, chewing gum, or sucking lozenges may help); constipation (increased exercise, fluids, or dietary fruit and fiber may help - if constipation remains an unresolved problem, consult prescriber about use of stool softeners). Report chest pain, slow or rapid heartbeat, acute dizziness or persistent headache; changes in mental status; swelling of extremities or unusual weight gain; changes in urinary elimination; acute headache; back or flank pain or muscle spasms; blurred vision; skin rash; or shortness of breath. **Pregnancy/breast-feeding precautions:** Inform prescriber if you are or intend to be pregnant. If you are breast-feeding, take medication immediately after breast-feeding or 3-4 hours prior to next feeding.

**Geriatric Considerations:** Because of its long half-life and risk of accumulation, methadone is not considered a drug of first choice in the elderly. The elderly may be particularly susceptible to the CNS depressant and constipating effects of narcotics. Adjust dose for renal function.

**Additional Information** The oral solution formulation contains ethanol.

Methadone 10 mg I.M.; or 8-10 mg S.C. = methadone 10-20 mg oral

**Related Information**

Controlled Substances Comparison *on page 1379*

Narcotic/Opioid Analgesic Comparison *on page 1396*

♦ **Methadose®** *see* Methadone *on page 735*

♦ **Methaminodiazepoxide Hydrochloride** *see* Chlordiazepoxide *on page 250*

## Methamphetamine (meth am FET a meen)

**U.S. Brand Names** Desoxyn®; Desoxyn Gradumet®

**Synonyms** Desoxyephedrine Hydrochloride

**Therapeutic Category** Stimulant

**Pregnancy Risk Factor** C

**Lactation** Enters breast milk/contraindicated

**Use** Treatment of narcolepsy, exogenous obesity, attention-deficit/hyperactivity disorder (ADHD)

**Contraindications** Hypersensitivity to methamphetamine, amphetamine; patients with a history of drug abuse

**Warnings** Cardiovascular disease, nephritis, angina pectoris, hypertension, and glaucoma. Pregnancy factor C.

**Drug Interactions**

**Cytochrome P-450 Effect:** CYP2D6 enzyme substrate

**Increased Effect/Toxicity:** Increased toxicity with MAO inhibitors (hypertensive crisis).

**Adverse Reactions**

>10%:

Cardiovascular: Arrhythmia

Central nervous system: False feeling of well being, nervousness, restlessness, insomnia

1% to 10%:

Cardiovascular: Hypertension

Central nervous system: Mood or mental changes, dizziness, lightheadedness, headache

Endocrine & metabolic: Changes in libido

Gastrointestinal: Diarrhea, nausea, vomiting, stomach cramps, constipation, anorexia, weight loss, dry mouth

Ocular: Blurred vision

Miscellaneous: Sweating (increased)

<1% (Limited to important or life-threatening symptoms): Chest pain, CNS stimulation (severe), Tourette's syndrome, hyperthermia, seizures, paranoia

**Overdose/Toxicology** Symptoms of overdose include seizures, hyperactivity, coma, and hypertension. Treatment is supportive.

**Pharmacodynamics/Kinetics**

**Half-life Elimination:** 4-5 hours

**Metabolism:** Liver

**Excretion:** Urine

**Duration:** 12-24 hours

**Formulations**

Methamphetamine hydrochloride:

Tablet: 5 mg

Tablet, extended release (Gradumet®): 5 mg, 10 mg, 15 mg

**Dosing**

**Adults:** Exogenous obesity: Oral: 5 mg, 30 minutes before each meal; long-acting formulation: 10-15 mg in morning; treatment duration should not exceed a few weeks

**Elderly:** Not recommended for use in the elderly.

**Administration**

**Oral:** Dose should not be given in evening or at bedtime. Do not crush extended release tablet.

(Continued)

## Methamphetamine *(Continued)*

**Additional Nursing Issues**

**Physical Assessment:** Assess effectiveness and interactions of other medications patient may be taking (see Drug Interactions). Assess for history of psychopathology, homicidal or suicidal tendencies, or addiction; long-term use can result in dependence, abuse, or tolerance. Periodically evaluate the need for continued use. Monitor blood pressure, vital signs, and adverse reactions at start of therapy, when changing dosage, and at regular intervals during therapy (see Adverse Reactions). Monitor serum glucose closely with diabetic patients (amphetamines may alter antidiabetic requirements). Taper dosage slowly when discontinuing. Assess knowledge/teach patient appropriate use, possible side effects, and symptoms to report. **Pregnancy risk factor C** - benefits of use should outweigh possible risks. Breast-feeding is contraindicated.

**Patient Information/Instruction:** Take exactly as directed (do not increase dose or frequency without consulting prescriber); may cause physical and/or psychological dependence. Do not crush extended release tablets. Take early in day to avoid sleep disturbance, 30 minutes before meals. Avoid alcohol, caffeine, or OTC medications that act as stimulants. You may experience restlessness, false sense of euphoria, or impaired judgment (use caution when driving or engaging in tasks requiring alertness until response to drug is known); dry mouth (frequent small meals, frequent mouth care, sucking lozenges, or chewing gum may help); nausea or vomiting (small frequent meals, frequent mouth care may help); constipation (increased exercise, dietary fiber, fruit, or fluid may help); diarrhea (buttermilk, boiled milk, or yogurt may help); or altered libido (reversible). Diabetics need to monitor serum glucose closely (may alter antidiabetic medication requirements). Report chest pain, palpitations, or irregular heartbeat; extreme fatigue or depression; CNS changes (aggressiveness, restlessness, euphoria, sleep disturbances); severe unremitting abdominal distress or cramping; blackened stool; changes in sexual activity; or blurred vision. **Pregnancy/breast-feeding precautions:** Inform prescriber if you are or intend to be pregnant. Do not breast-feed.

**Additional Information** Some formulations may contain tartrazine.

## Methazolamide (meth a ZOE la mide)

**U.S. Brand Names** GlaucTabs®; Neptazane®

**Therapeutic Category** Carbonic Anhydrase Inhibitor; Diuretic, Carbonic Anhydrase Inhibitor; Ophthalmic Agent, Antiglaucoma

**Pregnancy Risk Factor** C

**Lactation** Excretion in breast milk unknown

**Use** Adjunctive treatment of open-angle or secondary glaucoma; short-term therapy of narrow-angle glaucoma when delay of surgery is desired

**Mechanism of Action/Effect** Noncompetitive inhibition of the enzyme carbonic anhydrase; thought that carbonic anhydrase is located at the luminal border of cells of the proximal tubule. When the enzyme is inhibited, there is an increase in urine volume and a change to an alkaline pH with a subsequent decrease in the excretion of titratable acid and ammonia.

**Contraindications** Hypersensitivity to methazolamide or any component; marked kidney or liver dysfunction; severe pulmonary obstruction

**Warnings** Sulfonamide-type reactions, melena, anorexia, nausea, vomiting, constipation, hematuria, glycosuria, urinary frequency, renal colic, renal calculi, crystalluria, polyuria, hepatic insufficiency, various CNS effects, transient myopia, bone marrow depression, thrombocytopenia/purpura, hemolytic anemia, leukopenia, pancytopenia, agranulocytosis, urticaria, pruritus, rash, Stevens-Johnson syndrome, weight loss, fever, acidosis. Use with caution in patients with respiratory acidosis and diabetes mellitus, impairment of mental alertness and/or physical coordination. Malaise and complaints of tiredness and myalgia are signs of excessive dosing and acidosis in the elderly. Pregnancy factor C.

**Drug Interactions**

**Decreased Effect:** Increased lithium excretion and altered excretion of other drugs by alkalinization of the urine, such as amphetamines, quinidine, procainamide, methenamine, phenobarbital, and salicylates.

**Increased Effect/Toxicity:** May induce hypokalemia which would sensitize a patient to digitalis toxicity. May increase the potential for salicylate toxicity. Hypokalemia may be compounded with concurrent diuretic use or steroids. Primidone absorption may be delayed.

**Adverse Reactions**

>10%:

Central nervous system: Malaise

Gastrointestinal: Metallic taste, anorexia

Genitourinary: Polyuria

Neuromuscular & skeletal: Weakness

1% to 10%:

Central nervous system: Mental depression, drowsiness, dizziness

Genitourinary: Crystalluria

<1% (Limited to important or life-threatening symptoms): Seizures, Stevens-Johnson syndrome, bone marrow suppression

**Pharmacodynamics/Kinetics**

**Protein Binding:** ~55%

**Distribution:** Distributes well into tissue

**Half-life Elimination:** ~14 hours

**Metabolism:** Slowly from GI tract

**Excretion:** Urine

**Onset:** Slow in comparison with acetazolamide (2-4 hours); Peak effect: 6-8 hours

**Duration:** 10-18 hours

**Formulations** Tablet: 25 mg, 50 mg

**Dosing**

**Adults:** Oral: 50-100 mg 2-3 times/day

**Elderly:** Refer to adult dosing.

**Additional Nursing Issues**

**Physical Assessment:** Assess allergy history (see Contraindication and Warnings/Precautions). Monitor blood pressure prior to beginning therapy and after first few doses, especially patients on another concomitant diuretic therapy. Monitor appropriate laboratory tests (WBC, electrolytes). Monitor for and/or teach patient to monitor and report adverse reactions (see Warnings/Precautions and Adverse Reactions). Use and teach patient postural hypotension precautions. **Pregnancy risk factor C** - benefits of use should outweigh possible risks. Note breast-feeding caution.

**Patient Information/Instruction:** Take with food; swallow whole, do not chew or crush. You may experience gastrointestinal upset and loss of appetite; frequent small meals are advised to reduce these effects and the metallic taste that sometimes occurs with this medication. You may experience lightheadedness, depression, dizziness, or weakness for a few days; use caution when driving or engaging in tasks that require alertness until response to drug is known. Report excessive tiredness; loss of appetite; cramping, pain, or weakness in muscles; acute GI symptoms; changes in CNS (depression, drowsiness); difficulty or pain on urination; visual changes; or skin rash. **Pregnancy/breast-feeding precautions:** Inform prescriber if you are or intend to be pregnant. Consult prescriber if breast-feeding.

**Geriatric Considerations:** Malaise and complaints of tiredness and myalgia are signs of excessive dosing and acidosis in the elderly.

**Related Information**

Glaucoma Drug Comparison *on page 1385*

## Methenamine (meth EN a meen)

**U.S. Brand Names** Hiprex®; Urex®

**Synonyms** Hexamethylenetetramine

**Therapeutic Category** Antibiotic, Miscellaneous

**Pregnancy Risk Factor** C

**Lactation** Enters breast milk/compatible

**Use** Prophylaxis or suppression of recurrent urinary tract infections; urinary tract discomfort secondary to hypermotility; should not be used to treat infections outside of urinary tract

**Mechanism of Action/Effect** Methenamine is hydrolyzed to formaldehyde and ammonia in acidic urine; formaldehyde has nonspecific bactericidal action

**Contraindications** Hypersensitivity to methenamine or any component; severe dehydration; renal insufficiency; hepatic insufficiency in patients receiving hippurate salt

**Warnings** Use with caution in patients with hepatic disease, gout, and the elderly. Doses of 8 g/day may cause bladder irritation, some products may contain tartrazine. Methenamine should not be used to treat infections outside of the lower urinary tract. Pregnancy factor C.

**Drug Interactions**

**Decreased Effect:** Sodium bicarbonate and acetazolamide will decrease effect secondary to alkalinization of urine.

**Increased Effect/Toxicity:** Sulfonamides may precipitate in the urine.

**Food Interactions** The therapeutic effect of methenamine may be decreased if taken with alkaline foods.

**Effects on Lab Values** ↑ catecholamines and VMA (U); ↓ HIAA (U)

**Adverse Reactions**

1% to 10%:

Dermatologic: Rash

Gastrointestinal: Nausea, vomiting, diarrhea, anorexia, abdominal cramping

<1% (Limited to important or life-threatening symptoms): Elevation in AST and ALT, hematuria

**Overdose/Toxicology** The drug is well tolerated. Treatment is supportive.

**Pharmacodynamics/Kinetics**

**Half-life Elimination:** 3-6 hours

**Metabolism:** Liver and gastric juices

**Excretion:** Urine

**Formulations**

Methenamine hippurate:

Tablet (Hiprex®, Urex®): 1 g (Hiprex® contains tartrazine dye)

Methenamine mandelate:

Tablet, enteric coated: 250 mg, 500 mg, 1 g

**Dosing**

**Adults:** Oral:

Hippurate: 0.5 to 1 g twice daily

(Continued)

## Methenamine *(Continued)*

Mandelate: 1 g 4 times/day after meals and at bedtime

**Elderly:** Refer to adult dosing.

**Renal Impairment:** $Cl_{cr}$ <50 mL/minute: Avoid use.

**Administration**

**Oral:** Administer around-the-clock to promote less variation in effect. Foods/diets which alkalinize urine pH >5.5 decrease activity of methenamine.

**Stability**

**Storage:** Protect from excessive heat

**Monitoring Laboratory Tests** Urinalysis, periodic liver function

**Additional Nursing Issues**

**Physical Assessment:** Assess effectiveness and interactions of other medications (see Drug Interactions). See Warnings/Precautions and Contraindications for use cautions. Monitor effectiveness of therapy, laboratory tests, and adverse response (see Adverse Reactions). Assess knowledge/teach patient possible side effects and interventions, and adverse symptoms to report. **Pregnancy risk factor C** - benefits of use should outweigh possible risks.

**Patient Information/Instruction:** Take per recommended schedule, at regular intervals around-the-clock. Complete full course of therapy; do not skip doses. Maintain adequate hydration (2-3 L/day of fluids unless instructed to restrict fluid intake). Avoid excessive citrus fruits, milk, or alkalizing medications. You may experience nausea or vomiting or GI upset (small frequent meals, frequent mouth care, sucking lozenges, or chewing gum may help). Report pain on urination or blood in urine, skin rash, other persistent adverse effects, or if condition does not improve. **Pregnancy precautions:** Inform prescriber if you are or intend to be pregnant.

**Geriatric Considerations:** Methenamine has little, if any, role in the treatment or prevention of infections in patients with indwelling urinary (Foley®) catheters. Furthermore, in noncatheterized patients, more effective antibiotics are available for the prevention or treatment of urinary tract infections. The influence of decreased renal function on the pharmacologic effects of methenamine results are unknown.

**Additional Information** The hippurate formulation contains tartrazine.

♦ **Methergine®** *see* Methylergonovine *on page 751*

## Methicillin (meth i SIL in)

**U.S. Brand Names** Staphcillin®

**Synonyms** Dimethoxyphenyl Penicillin Sodium

**Therapeutic Category** Antibiotic, Penicillin

**Pregnancy Risk Factor** B

**Lactation** Enters breast milk/use caution

**Use** Treatment of susceptible bacterial infections such as osteomyelitis, septicemia, endocarditis, and CNS infections due to penicillinase-producing strains of *Staphylococcus*; other antistaphylococcal penicillins are usually preferred

**Mechanism of Action/Effect** Inhibits bacterial cell wall synthesis in susceptible bacteria

**Contraindications** Hypersensitivity to methicillin, any component, penicillins, cephalosporins, or imipenem

**Warnings** Modify dosage in patients with renal impairment and in the elderly.

**Drug Interactions**

**Decreased Effect:** Efficacy of oral contraceptives may be reduced when taken with methicillin.

**Increased Effect/Toxicity:** Disulfiram or probenecid taken with methicillin may increase serum penicillin levels. Anticoagulants and methicillin may prolong bleeding times.

**Effects on Lab Values** Interferes with tests for urinary and serum proteins, uric acid, urinary steroids; may cause false-positive Coombs' test; may inactivate aminoglycosides *in vitro*

**Adverse Reactions**

1% to 10%:

Dermatologic: Rash

Renal: Acute interstitial nephritis

<1% (Limited to important or life-threatening symptoms): Hemorrhagic cystitis, eosinophilia, anemia, leukopenia, neutropenia, thrombocytopenia, phlebitis, serum sickness-like reactions

**Overdose/Toxicology** Symptoms of penicillin overdose include neuromuscular hypersensitivity (eg, agitation, hallucinations, asterixis, encephalopathy, confusion, and seizures). Electrolyte imbalance may occur if the preparation contains potassium or sodium salts, especially in renal failure. Hemodialysis may be helpful to aid in removal of the drug from blood; otherwise, treatment is supportive or symptom directed.

**Pharmacodynamics/Kinetics**

**Protein Binding:** 40%

**Distribution:** Crosses the placenta

**Half-life Elimination:** Normal renal function: 0.4-0.5 hour

**Time to Peak:** I.M.: 0.5-1 hour; I.V. infusion: Within 5 minutes

**Excretion:** Urine

**Formulations** Powder for injection, as sodium: 1 g, 4 g, 6 g, 10 g

**Dosing**

**Adults:** I.M., I.V.: 4-12 g/day in divided doses every 4-6 hours

**Elderly:** Refer to adult dosing.

**Renal Impairment:**

$Cl_{cr}$ 10-50 mL/minute: Administer every 6-8 hours.

$Cl_{cr}$ <10 mL/minute: Administer every 8-12 hours.

Not dialyzable (0% to 5%)

**Administration**

**I.M.:** Deep intragluteal; to avoid irritation, rotate sites.

**I.V.:** Can be administered IVP at a rate not to exceed 200 mg/minute or intermittent infusion over 20-30 minutes. Final concentration for administration should not exceed 20 mg/mL.

**Stability**

**Reconstitution:** Reconstituted solution is stable for 24 hours at room temperature and 4 days when refrigerated. Discard solutions if it has a distinctive hydrogen sulfide odor and/or color turns to a deep orange.

**Compatibility:** Incompatible with aminoglycosides and tetracyclines.

**Monitoring Laboratory Tests** Cultures should be obtained prior to administering first dose.

**Additional Nursing Issues**

**Physical Assessment:** Assess previous allergies. Monitor for adverse reactions (see above) and opportunistic infections (eg, fever, purulent vaginal discharge, oral plaques, or mouth sores). Note breast-feeding caution.

**Patient Information/Instruction:** This medication can only be administered by injection. Maintain adequate hydration (2-3 L/day of fluids unless instructed to restrict fluid intake). Small frequent meals, frequent mouth care, and adequate fluids may reduce the incidence of nausea or vomiting. If diabetic, drug may cause false tests with Clinitest® urine glucose monitoring; use of glucose oxidase methods (Clinistix®) or serum glucose monitoring is preferable. This drug may interfere with oral contraceptives; an alternate form of birth control should be used. Report difficulty breathing, acute diarrhea, systemic rash, fever, white plaques in mouth or mouth sores. **Breast-feeding precautions:** Consult prescriber if breast-feeding.

**Geriatric Considerations:** Because of its greater potential for interstitial nephritis, methicillin is not the parenteral antistaphylococcal agent of choice. Either nafcillin or oxacillin are preferred alternatives. Adjust dose for renal function.

**Additional Information**

Sodium content of 1 g: 2.6-3.1 mEq

pH: 6-8.5

## Methimazole (meth IM a zole)

**U.S. Brand Names** Tapazole®

**Synonyms** Thiamazole

**Therapeutic Category** Antithyroid Agent

**Pregnancy Risk Factor** D

**Lactation** Enters breast milk/use caution - see Breast-feeding Issues

**Use** Palliative treatment of hyperthyroidism

**Mechanism of Action/Effect** Inhibits the synthesis of thyroid hormones by blocking the oxidation of iodine in the thyroid gland, blocking iodine's ability to combine with tyrosine to form thyroxine and tri-iodothyronine ($T_3$), does not inactivate circulating $T_4$ and $T_3$

**Contraindications** Hypersensitivity to methimazole or any component; pregnancy

**Warnings** Use with extreme caution in patients receiving other drugs known to cause myelosuppression particularly agranulocytosis, patients >40 years of age. Avoid doses >40 mg/day (↑ myelosuppression). May cause acneiform eruptions or worsen the condition of the thyroid.

**Drug Interactions**

**Increased Effect/Toxicity:** Increased toxicity with lithium or potassium iodide. Anticoagulant activity is increased.

**Adverse Reactions**

>10%:

Central nervous system: Fever

Dermatologic: Rash

Hematologic: Leukopenia

1% to 10%:

Central nervous system: Dizziness

Gastrointestinal: Nausea, vomiting, stomach pain, abnormal taste

Hematologic: Agranulocytosis

Miscellaneous: SLE-like syndrome

<1% (Limited to important or life-threatening symptoms): Alopecia, nephrotic syndrome, thrombocytopenia, aplastic anemia, cholestatic jaundice

**Overdose/Toxicology** Symptoms of overdose include nausea, vomiting, epigastric distress, headache, fever, arthralgia, pruritus, edema, pancytopenia, and signs of hypothyroidism. Management of overdose is supportive.

(Continued)

## Methimazole *(Continued)*

**Pharmacodynamics/Kinetics**

**Protein Binding:** No plasma protein binding

**Distribution:** Crosses the placenta

**Half-life Elimination:** 4-13 hours

**Excretion:** Urine

**Onset:** Onset of antithyroid effect: Oral: Within 30-40 minutes

**Duration:** 2-4 hours

**Formulations** Tablet: 5 mg, 10 mg

**Dosing**

**Adults:** Oral: Administer in 3 equally divided doses at ~8-hour intervals.

Initial: 5 mg every 8 hours; maintenance dose: 5-15 mg/day up to 60 mg/day for severe hyperthyroidism

Adjust dosage as required to achieve and maintain serum $T_3$, $T_4$, and TSH levels in the normal range. An elevated $T_3$ may be the sole indicator of inadequate treatment. An elevated TSH indicates excessive antithyroid treatment.

**Elderly:** Refer to adult dosing.

**Stability**

**Storage:** Protect from light.

**Monitoring Laboratory Tests** $T_4$, $T_3$, CBC with differential, liver function (baseline and as needed), serum thyroxine, free thyroxine index

**Additional Nursing Issues**

**Physical Assessment:** Monitor all appropriate laboratory results and patient for signs or symptoms of hyper-/hypothyroidism. Assess for signs or symptoms of bleeding tendency. Monitor for skin rash or swelling of lymph nodes. **Pregnancy risk factor D** - assess knowledge/teach appropriate use of barrier contraceptives. Note breast-feeding caution.

**Patient Information/Instruction:** Take as directed, at the same time each day around-the-clock; do not miss doses or make up missed doses. This drug will need to be taken for an extended period of time to achieve appropriate results. You may experience nausea or vomiting (small frequent meals may help), dizziness or drowsiness (use caution when driving or engaging in tasks that require alertness until response to drug is known). Report rash, fever, unusual bleeding or bruising, unresolved headache, yellowing of eyes or skin, or changes in color of urine or feces, unresolved malaise. **Pregnancy/breast-feeding precautions:** Do not get pregnant while taking this medication; use appropriate barrier contraceptive measures. Consult prescriber if breast-feeding.

**Geriatric Considerations:** The use of antithyroid thioamides is as effective in the elderly as in younger adults; however, the expense, potential adverse effects, and inconvenience (compliance, monitoring) make them undesirable.

**Breast-feeding Issues:** American Academy of Pediatrics indicates a concern for thyroid effect in infants and warrants using caution and frequent monitoring (weekly or biweekly).

## Methocarbamol (meth oh KAR ba mole)

**U.S. Brand Names** Delaxin®; Marbaxin®; Robaxin®; Robomol®

**Therapeutic Category** Skeletal Muscle Relaxant

**Pregnancy Risk Factor** C

**Lactation** Enters breast milk/compatible

**Use** Treatment of muscle spasm associated with acute painful musculoskeletal conditions, supportive therapy in tetanus

**Mechanism of Action/Effect** Causes skeletal muscle relaxation by reducing the transmission of impulses from the spinal cord to skeletal muscle

**Contraindications** Hypersensitivity to methocarbamol or any component; renal impairment

**Warnings** Rate of injection should not exceed 3 mL/minute. Solution is hypertonic. Avoid extravasation. Use with caution in patients with a history of seizures. Pregnancy factor C.

**Drug Interactions**

**Increased Effect/Toxicity:** Increased effect/toxicity with CNS depressants.

**Adverse Reactions**

>10%: Central nervous system: Drowsiness, dizziness, lightheadedness

1% to 10%:

- Cardiovascular: Flushing of face, bradycardia, fever (allergic)
- Dermatologic: Allergic dermatitis
- Gastrointestinal: Nausea, vomiting
- Ocular: Nystagmus, conjunctivitis
- Respiratory: Nasal congestion

<1% (Limited to important or life-threatening symptoms): Syncope, convulsions, leukopenia, pain at injection site, thrombophlebitis

**Overdose/Toxicology** Symptoms of overdose include cardiac arrhythmias, nausea, vomiting, drowsiness, and coma. Treatment is supportive.

**Pharmacodynamics/Kinetics**

**Half-life Elimination:** 1-2 hours

**Time to Peak:** ~2 hours

**Metabolism:** Liver

**Excretion:** Urine

**Onset:** Onset of muscle relaxation: Oral: Within 30 minutes

**Formulations**

Injection: 100 mg/mL in polyethylene glycol 50% (10 mL)

Tablet: 500 mg, 750 mg

**Dosing**

**Adults:** Muscle spasm:

Oral: 1.5 g 4 times/day for 2-3 days, then decrease to 4-4.5 g/day in 3-6 divided doses

I.M., I.V.: 1 g every 8 hours if oral not possible

**Elderly:** Oral: Initial: 500 mg 4 times/day; titrate to response.

**Renal Impairment:** Do not administer parenteral formulation to patients with renal dysfunction.

**Administration**

**Oral:** Tablets may be crushed and mixed with food or liquid if needed. Avoid alcohol.

**I.V.:** Maximum rate is 3 mL/minute.

**I.V. Detail:** Monitor closely for extravasation. Administer I.V. while in recumbent position. Maintain position 15-30 minutes following infusion.

**Additional Nursing Issues**

**Physical Assessment:** Assess other medications for excess CNS depression. See Contraindications and Warnings/Precautions for use cautions. Monitor effectiveness of therapy (according to rational for therapy), and adverse reactions (see Adverse Reactions) at beginning and periodically during therapy. Monitor I.V. site closely to prevent extravasation. Assess knowledge/teach patient appropriate use, interventions to reduce side effects (postural hypotension precautions), and adverse symptoms to report. **Pregnancy risk factor C** - benefits of use should outweigh possible risks.

**Patient Information/Instruction:** Take exactly as directed. Do not increase dose or discontinue without consulting prescriber. Do not use alcohol, prescriptive or OTC antidepressants, sedatives, or pain medications without consulting prescriber. You may experience drowsiness, dizziness, lightheadedness (avoid driving or engaging in tasks requiring alertness until response to drug is known); or nausea or vomiting (small, frequent meals, frequent mouth care, or sucking hard candy may help). Report excessive drowsiness or mental agitation, chest pain, skin rash, swelling of mouth/face, difficulty speaking, or vision disturbances. **Pregnancy precautions:** Inform prescriber if you are or intend to be pregnant.

**Geriatric Considerations:** There is no specific information on the use of skeletal muscle relaxants in the elderly. Methocarbamol has a short half-life, so it may be considered one of the safer agents in this class.

## Methocarbamol and Aspirin (meth oh KAR ba mole & AS pir in)

**U.S. Brand Names** Robaxisal®

**Synonyms** Aspirin and Methocarbamol

**Therapeutic Category** Skeletal Muscle Relaxant

**Pregnancy Risk Factor** C/D (if full-dose aspirin in 3rd trimester)

**Lactation** Enters breast milk/use caution due to aspirin content

**Use** Adjunct to rest, physical therapy, and other measures for the relief of discomfort associated with acute, painful musculoskeletal disorders

**Formulations** Tablet: Methocarbamol 400 mg and aspirin 325 mg

**Dosing**

**Adults:** Oral: 2 tablets 4 times/day

**Elderly:** Refer to dosing in individual monographs.

**Additional Nursing Issues**

**Physical Assessment:** See individual components listed in Related Information. **Pregnancy risk factor C/D** - see Pregnancy Risk Factor - assess knowledge/instruct patient on need to use appropriate contraceptive measures and the need to avoid pregnancy. Note breast-feeding caution.

**Patient Information/Instruction:** See individual components listed in Related Information. **Pregnancy/breast-feeding precautions:** Inform prescriber if you are or intend to be pregnant. Consult prescriber if breast-feeding.

**Related Information**

Aspirin *on page 111*
Methocarbamol *on previous page*

## Methotrexate (meth oh TREKS ate)

**U.S. Brand Names** Folex® PFS; Rheumatrex®

**Synonyms** Amethopterin; MTX

**Therapeutic Category** Antimetabolite; Antineoplastic Agent, Antimetabolite; Antirheumatic, Disease Modifying

**Pregnancy Risk Factor** D

**Lactation** Enters breast milk/contraindicated

**Use** Treatment of trophoblastic neoplasms; leukemias; psoriasis; rheumatoid arthritis; breast, head, and lung carcinomas; osteosarcoma; sarcomas; carcinoma of gastric, esophagus, testes; lymphomas

**Mechanism of Action/Effect** An antimetabolite that inhibits DNA synthesis and cell reproduction in cancerous cells

(Continued)

## Methotrexate *(Continued)*

Folates must be in the reduced form ($FH_4$) to be active

Folates are activated by dihydrofolate reductase (DHFR)

DHFR is inhibited by MTX (by binding irreversibly), causing an increase in the intracellular dihydrofolate pool (the inactive cofactor) and inhibition of both purine and thymidylate synthesis (TS)

MTX enters the cell through an energy-dependent and temperature-dependent process which is mediated by an intramembrane protein; this carrier mechanism is also used by naturally occurring reduced folates, including folinic acid (leucovorin), making this a competitive process

At high drug concentrations (>20 μM), MTX enters the cell by a second mechanism which is not shared by reduced folates; the process may be passive diffusion or a specific, saturable process, and provides a rationale for high-dose MTX

A small fraction of MTX is converted intracellularly to polyglutamates, which leads to a prolonged inhibition of DHFR

**Contraindications** Hypersensitivity to methotrexate or any component; severe renal or hepatic impairment; pre-existing profound bone marrow depression in patients with psoriasis or rheumatoid arthritis, alcoholic liver disease, AIDS, pre-existing blood dyscrasias; pregnancy (do not use in women of childbearing age unless benefit outweighs risks)

**Warnings** The U.S. Food and Drug Administration (FDA) currently recommends that procedures for proper handling and disposal of antineoplastic agents be considered.

Preparation of methotrexate injection should be performed in a Class II laminar flow biologic safety cabinet. Personnel should be wearing surgical gloves and a closed front surgical gown with knit cuffs. Appropriate safety equipment is recommended for preparation, administration, and disposal of antineoplastics. If methotrexate contacts the skin, wash and flush thoroughly with water.

May cause photosensitivity type reaction; reduce dosage in patients with renal or hepatic impairment, ascites, and pleural effusion. Use with caution in patients with peptic ulcer disease, ulcerative colitis, or pre-existing bone marrow suppression. Monitor closely for pulmonary disease; use with caution in the elderly.

Because of the possibility of severe toxic reactions, fully inform patient of the risks involved. May cause hepatotoxicity, fibrosis and cirrhosis, along with marked bone marrow depression. Death from intestinal perforation may occur.

Toxicity to methotrexate or any immunosuppressive is increased in the elderly. Must monitor carefully. For rheumatoid arthritis and psoriasis, immunosuppressive therapy should only be used when disease is active and less toxic; traditional therapy is ineffective. Recommended doses should be reduced when initiating therapy in the elderly due to possible decreased metabolism, reduced renal function, and presence of interacting diseases and drugs.

**Drug Interactions**

**Cytochrome P-450 Effect:** Involvement with CYP isoenzymes not defined; may act as inhibitor of some isoenzymes.

**Decreased Effect:** Corticosteroids have been reported to decrease methotrexate entry into leukemia cells. Administration should be separated by 12 hours. Dexamethasone has been reported to not affect methotrexate entry. May decrease phenytoin and 5-FU activity.

**Increased Effect/Toxicity:**

Nonsteroidal anti-inflammatory drugs (NSAIDs): Decreased renal excretion of methotrexate and increased methotrexate toxicity.

Live virus vaccines may cause vaccinia infections.

Vincristine inhibits MTX efflux from the cell, leading to increased and prolonged MTX levels in the cell. The dose of VCR needed to produce this effect is not achieved clinically.

Salicylates, sulfonamides, probenecid, and high doses of penicillins compete with MTX for transport and reduce renal tubular secretion. Salicylates and sulfonamides may also displace MTX from plasma proteins, increasing MTX levels.

Increased formation of the Ara-C nucleotide can occur when MTX precedes Ara-C, thus promoting the action of Ara-C.

Cyclosporin and MTX interfere with each others renal elimination, which may result in increased toxicity.

**Food Interactions** Methotrexate peak serum levels may be decreased if taken with food.

**Adverse Reactions**

>10%:

Cardiovascular: Vasculitis

Central nervous system (with I.T. administration only):

Arachnoiditis: Acute reaction manifested as severe headache, nuchal rigidity, vomiting, and fever; may be alleviated by reducing the dose

Subacute toxicity: 10% of patients treated with 12-15 mg/m$^2$ of I.T. MTX may develop this in the second or third week of therapy; consists of motor paralysis of extremities, cranial nerve palsy, seizures, or coma. This has also been seen in pediatric cases receiving very high-dose I.V. MTX (when enough MTX can get across into the CSF).

Demyelinating encephalopathy: Seen months or years after receiving MTX; usually in association with cranial irradiation or other systemic chemotherapy

Dermatologic: Reddening of skin

Endocrine & metabolic: Hyperuricemia, defective oogenesis or spermatogenesis

Gastrointestinal: Ulcerative stomatitis, glossitis, gingivitis, nausea, vomiting, diarrhea, anorexia, intestinal perforation, mucositis (dose-dependent; appears in 3-7 days after therapy, resolving within 2 weeks)
Emetic potential:
<100 mg: Moderately low (10% to 30%)
≥100 mg or <250 mg: Moderate (30% to 60%)
≥250 mg: Moderately high (60% to 90%)
Hematologic: Leukopenia, thrombocytopenia
Renal: Renal failure, azotemia, nephropathy
Respiratory: Pharyngitis

1% to 10%:
Central nervous system: Dizziness, malaise, encephalopathy, seizures, fever, chills
Dermatitis: Alopecia, rash, photosensitivity, depigmentation or hyperpigmentation of skin
Endocrine & metabolic: Diabetes
Genitourinary: Cystitis
Hematologic: Hemorrhage
Myelosuppressive: This is the primary dose-limiting factor (along with mucositis) of MTX; occurs about 5-7 days after MTX therapy, and should resolve within 2 weeks
WBC: Mild
Platelets: Moderate
Onset (days): 7
Nadir (days): 10
Recovery (days): 21
Hepatic: Cirrhosis and portal fibrosis have been associated with chronic MTX therapy; acute elevation of liver enzymes are common after high-dose MTX, and usually resolve within 10 days
Neuromuscular & skeletal: Arthralgia
Ocular: Blurred vision
Renal: Renal dysfunction: Manifested by an abrupt rise in serum creatinine and BUN and a fall in urine output; more common with high-dose MTX, and may be due to precipitation of the drug. The best treatment is prevention: Aggressively hydrate with 3 L/m²/day starting 12 hours before therapy and continue for 24-36 hours; alkalinize the urine by adding 50 mEq of bicarbonate to each liter of fluid; keep urine flow over 100 mL/hour and urine pH >7.
Respiratory: Pneumonitis: Associated with fever, cough, and interstitial pulmonary infiltrates; treatment is to withhold MTX during the acute reaction
Miscellaneous: Anaphylaxis, decreased resistance to infection

**Overdose/Toxicology** Symptoms of overdose include nausea, vomiting, alopecia, melena, and renal failure.

Antidote: Leucovorin; administer as soon as toxicity is seen; administer 10 mg/m² orally or parenterally; follow with 10 mg/m² orally every 6 hours for 72 hours. After 24 hours following methotrexate administration, if the serum creatinine is ≥50% premethotrexate serum creatinine, increase leucovorin dose to 100 mg/m² every 3 hours until serum MTX level is $<5 \times 10^{-8}$M. Hydration and alkalinization may be used to prevent precipitation of MTX or MTX metabolites in renal tubules. Toxicity in low-dose range is negligible, but may present mucositis and mild bone marrow suppression; severe bone marrow toxicity can result from overdose. Neither peritoneal nor hemodialysis have been shown to ↑ elimination. Leucovorin should be administered intravenously, never intrathecally, for overdoses of intrathecal methotrexate.

**Pharmacodynamics/Kinetics**

**Protein Binding:** 50%

**Distribution:** Drug penetrates slowly into third space fluids, such as pleural effusions or ascites, and exits slowly from these compartments (slower than from plasma). Crosses the placenta. Does not achieve therapeutic concentrations in the CSF and must be given intrathecally if given for CNS prophylaxis or treatment. Sustained concentrations are retained in the kidney and liver.

**Half-life Elimination:** 8-12 hours with high doses and 3-10 hours with low doses

**Time to Peak:** Oral: 1-2 hours; Parenteral: 30-60 minutes

**Metabolism:** <10% metabolized; degraded by intestinal flora

**Excretion:** Urine and feces

**Onset:** Antirheumatic effects may require several weeks

**Formulations**

Methotrexate sodium:
Injection: 2.5 mg/mL (2 mL); 25 mg/mL (2 mL, 4 mL, 8 mL, 10 mL)
Injection, preservative free: 25 mg (2 mL, 4 mL, 8 mL, 10 mL)
Powder, for injection: 20 mg, 25 mg, 50 mg, 100 mg, 250 mg, 1 g
Tablet: 2.5 mg
Tablet, dose pack: 2.5 mg (4 cards with 2, 3, 4, 5, or 6 tablets each)

**Dosing**

**Adults:** Refer to individual protocols. May be administered orally, I.M., intra-arterially, intrathecally, I.V., or S.C.

Leucovorin may be administered concomitantly or within 24 hours of methotrexate.
I.V.: Range is wide from 30-40 mg/m²/week to 100-7500 mg/m² with leucovorin rescue
Doses not requiring leucovorin rescue range from 30-40 mg/m² I.V. or I.M. repeated weekly, or oral regimens of 10 mg/m² twice weekly
**High-dose MTX is considered to be >100 mg/m² and can be as high as 1500-7500 mg/m²**. These doses require leucovorin rescue. Patients receiving doses

(Continued)

## Methotrexate *(Continued)*

≥1000 mg/m$^2$ should have their urine alkalinized with bicarbonate or Bicitra® prior to and following MTX therapy.

Trophoblastic neoplasms: Oral, I.M.: 15-30 mg/day for 5 days; repeat in 7 days for 3-5 courses

Head and neck cancer: Oral, I.M., I.V.: 25-50 mg/m$^2$ once weekly

Rheumatoid arthritis: Oral: 7.5 mg once weekly **or** 2.5 mg every 12 hours for 3 doses/week; not to exceed 20 mg/week

Psoriasis: Oral: 2.5-5 mg/dose every 12 hours for 3 doses given once weekly

**or**

Oral, I.M.: 10-25 mg/dose given once weekly

Ectopic pregnancy: I.M./I.V.: 50 mg/m$^2$ single-dose without leucovorin rescue

**Elderly:** Refer to individual protocols; adjust for renal impairment.

May be administered orally, I.M., intra-arterially, intrathecally, I.V., or S.C.

**or**

Oral, I.M.: 10-25 mg/dose given once weekly

Rheumatoid arthritis/psoriasis: Oral:

Initial: 5 mg once weekly

If nausea occurs, split dose to 2.5 mg every 12 hours for the day of administration.

Dose may be increased to 7.5 mg/week based on response, not to exceed 20 mg/week.

Neoplastic disease: Refer to specific disease protocols.

**Renal Impairment:**

$Cl_{cr}$ 61-80 mL/minute: Reduce dose to 75%.

$Cl_{cr}$ 51-60 mL/minute: Reduce dose to 70%.

$Cl_{cr}$ 10-50 mL/minute: Reduce dose to 30% to 50%.

$Cl_{cr}$ <10 mL/minute: Avoid use.

Hemodialysis effects: Not dialyzable (0% to 5%)

Supplemental dose is not necessary.

Peritoneal dialysis effects: Supplemental dose is not necessary.

CAVH effects: Unknown

**Hepatic Impairment:**

Bilirubin 3.1-5 mg/dL or AST >180 units: Administer 75% of dose.

Bilirubin >5 mg/dL: Do not use.

**Administration**

**I.V.:** Methotrexate may be administered I.M., I.V., or I.T.; refer to Stability section for I.V. administration recommendations based on dosage.

**I.V. Detail:** Administration rates:

Doses <149 mg: Administer slow I.V. push.

Doses of 150-499 mg: Administer IVPB over 20-30 minutes.

Doses of 500-1500 mg: Administer IVPB over ≥60 minutes.

Doses >1500 mg: Administer IVPB over 1-6 hours.

Specific dosing schemes vary, but high doses should be followed by leucovorin calcium 24-36 hours after initiation of therapy to prevent toxicity.

Renal toxicity can be minimized/prevented by alkalinizing the urine (with sodium bicarbonate) and increasing urine flow (hydration therapy).

**Stability**

**Storage:** Store intact vials at room temperature (15°C to 25°C) and protect from light.

**Reconstitution:** Dilute powder with $D_5W$ or NS to a concentration ≤25 mg/mL (20 mg and 50 mg vials) and 50 mg/mL (1 g vial) as follows. Solution is stable for 7 days at room temperature.

20 mg = 20 mL (1 mg/mL)

50 mg = 5 mL (10 mg/mL)

1 g = 19.4 mL (50 mg/mL)

Further dilution in $D_5W$ or NS is stable for 24 hours at room temperature (21°C to 25°C).

**Standard I.V. dilution:** Maximum syringe size for IVP is a 30 mL syringe and syringe should be ≤75% full.

Doses <149 mg: Administer slow I.V. push

Dose/syringe (concentration ≤25 mg/mL)

Doses of 150-499 mg: Administer IVPB over 20-30 minutes

Dose/50 mL $D_5W$ or NS

Doses of 500-1500 mg: Administer IVPB over ≥60 minutes

Dose/250 mL $D_5W$ or NS

Doses >1500 mg: Administer IVPB over 1-6 hours

Dose/1000 mL $D_5W$ or NS

**Standard I.M. dilution:** Dose/syringe (concentration = 25 mg/mL)

I.V. dilutions are stable for 8 days at room temperature (25°C).

**Standard intrathecal dilution:**

Use preservative-free preparations for high-dose and intrathecal administration.

Dose/3-5 mL LR ± methotrexate (12 mg) ± hydrocortisone (15-25 mg)

Intrathecal dilutions are stable for 7 days at room temperature (25°C) but due to sterility issues, use within 24 hours.

**Compatibility:** Compatible with cytarabine and hydrocortisone in LR or NS for 7 days at room temperature (25°C). See the Chemotherapy Compatibility Chart *on page 1311.*

**Monitoring Laboratory Tests** For prolonged use (especially rheumatoid arthritis, psoriasis) a baseline liver biopsy, repeated at each 1-1.5 g cumulative dose interval, should be performed; WBC and platelet counts every 4 weeks; CBC and creatinine, LFTs every 3-4 months; chest x-ray

**Additional Nursing Issues**

**Physical Assessment:** Monitor laboratory results on a regular basis (see above). Assess other medications patients may be using to reduce incidence of serious drug interactions and/or toxicity (see Drug Interactions). Monitor closely for signs of adverse reactions (potential for severe toxic reactions - see Adverse Reactions, Warnings/ Precautions, and Overdose/Toxicology). Monitor knowledge/teach patient interventions to reduce adverse side effects and what to report to prescriber. **Pregnancy risk factor D** - assess knowledge/teach appropriate use of barrier contraceptives. Breast-feeding is contraindicated.

**Patient Information/Instruction:** Avoid alcohol to prevent serious side effects. Avoid intake of extra dietary folic acid, maintain adequate hydration (2-3 L/day of fluids unless instructed to restrict fluid intake) and adequate nutrition (frequent small meals may help). You may experience nausea and vomiting (small frequent meals may help or request antiemetic from prescriber); drowsiness, tingling, numbness, or blurred vision (avoid driving or engaging in tasks that require alertness until response to drug is known); mouth sores (frequent oral care is necessary); loss of hair; permanent sterility; skin rash; photosensitivity (use sunscreen, wear protective clothing and eyewear, and avoid direct sunlight). Report black or tarry stools, fever, chills, unusual bleeding or bruising, shortness of breath or difficulty breathing, yellowing of skin or eyes, dark or bloody urine, or acute joint pain or other side effects you may experience. **Pregnancy/breast-feeding precautions:** Do not get pregnant while taking this medication; use appropriate barrier contraceptive measures. The drug may cause permanent sterility and may cause birth defects. Do not breast-feed.

**Geriatric Considerations:** Toxicity to methotrexate or any immunosuppressive is increased in the elderly. Must monitor carefully. For rheumatoid arthritis and psoriasis, immunosuppressive therapy should only be used when disease is active and less toxic, traditional therapy is ineffective. Recommended doses should be reduced when initiating therapy in the elderly due to possible decreased metabolism, reduced renal function, and presence of interacting diseases and drugs. Adjust dose as needed for renal function ($Cl_{cr}$).

**Additional Information** Some formulations may contain benzyl alcohol. Cytotoxicity is determined by both drug concentration and duration of cell exposure. Extracellular drug concentrations of $1 \times 10^{-8}$M are required to inhibit thymidylate synthesis. Reduced folates are able to rescue cells and reverse MTX toxicity if given within 48 hours of the MTX dose. At concentrations >10 μM MTX, reduced folates are no longer effective.

**Related Information**

Leucovorin *on page 662*

## Methoxsalen (meth OKS a len)

**U.S. Brand Names** Oxsoralen® Topical; Oxsoralen-Ultra® Oral

**Synonyms** Methoxypsoralen; 8-MOP

**Therapeutic Category** Psoralen

**Pregnancy Risk Factor** C

**Lactation** Excretion in breast milk unknown

**Use**

Oral: Symptomatic control of severe, recalcitrant disabling psoriasis, not responsive to other therapy when to diagnosis has been supported by biopsy. Administer only in conjunction with a schedule of controlled doses of long-wave ultraviolet (UV) radiation; also used with long-wave ultraviolet (UV) radiation for repigmentation of idiopathic vitiligo.

Topical: Repigmenting agent in vitiligo, used in conjunction with controlled doses of UVA or sunlight

**Mechanism of Action/Effect** Bonds covalently to pyrimidine bases in DNA, inhibits the synthesis of DNA, and suppresses cell division. The augmented sunburn reaction involves excitation of the methoxsalen molecule by radiation in the long-wave ultraviolet light (UVA), resulting in transference of energy to the methoxsalen molecule producing an excited state ("triplet electronic state"). The molecule, in this "triplet state", then reacts with cutaneous DNA.

**Contraindications** Hypersensitivity to methoxsalen (psoralens); diseases associated with photosensitivity, cataract, invasive squamous cell cancer; children <12 years of age

**Warnings** Family history of sunlight allergy or chronic infections. Lotion should only be applied under direct supervision of a physician and should not be dispensed to the patient. For use only if inadequate response to other forms of therapy; serious burns may occur from UVA or sunlight even through glass if dose and or exposure schedule is not maintained. Some products may contain tartrazine. Use caution in patients with hepatic or cardiac disease. Pregnancy factor C.

**Drug Interactions**

**Increased Effect/Toxicity:** Concomitant therapy with other photosensitizing agents such as anthralin, coal tar, griseofulvin, phenothiazines, nalidixic acid, sulfanilamides, tetracyclines, and thiazide diuretics.

**Food Interactions** Methoxsalen serum concentrations may be increased if taken with food.

**Adverse Reactions**

**Systemic:**

>10%:

Dermatologic: Itching

Gastrointestinal: Nausea

1% to 10%:

Cardiovascular: Severe edema, hypotension

Central nervous system: Nervousness, vertigo, depression

(Continued)

## Methoxsalen *(Continued)*

Dermatologic: Painful blistering, burning, and peeling of skin; pruritus, freckling, hypopigmentation, rash, cheilitis, erythema

Neuromuscular & skeletal: Loss of muscle coordination

**Topical:**

1% to 10%: Dermatologic: Blistering and peeling of skin; reddened, sore skin

**Overdose/Toxicology** Symptoms of overdose include nausea and severe burns. Follow accepted treatment of severe burns. Keep room darkened until reaction subsides (8-24 hours or more).

**Pharmacodynamics/Kinetics**

**Time to Peak:** Oral: 2-4 hours

**Metabolism:** Liver

**Excretion:** Urine

**Formulations**

Capsule: 10 mg

Lotion: 1% (30 mL)

**Dosing**

**Adults:**

Psoriasis: Oral: 10-70 mg 1½-2 hours before exposure to ultraviolet light, 2-3 times at least 48 hours apart; dosage is based upon patient's body weight and skin type.

Vitiligo:

Oral: 20 mg 2-4 hours before exposure to UVA light or sunlight; limit exposure to 15-40 minutes based on skin basic color and exposure.

Topical: Apply lotion 1-2 hours before exposure to UVA light, no more than once weekly.

**Elderly:** Refer to adult dosing.

**Additional Nursing Issues**

**Physical Assessment:** See Warnings/Precautions and Drug Interactions - administered in conjunction with ultraviolet light or ultraviolet radiation therapy. Monitor knowledge/teach appropriate sunlight precautions. **Pregnancy risk factor C** - benefits of use should outweigh possible risks. Note breast-feeding caution.

**Patient Information/Instruction:** This medication is used in conjunction with specific ultraviolet treatment. Follow prescriber's directions exactly for oral medication which can be taken with food or milk to reduce nausea. Consult prescriber for specific dietary instructions. Avoid use of any other skin treatments unless approved by prescriber. Control exposure to direct sunlight as per prescriber's instructions. If sunlight cannot be avoided, use sunblock (consult prescriber for specific SPF level), wear protective clothing and wraparound protective eyewear. Consult prescriber immediately if burning, blistering, or skin irritation occur. **Pregnancy/breast-feeding precautions:** Inform prescriber if you are or intend to be pregnant. Consult prescriber if breast-feeding.

♦ **Methoxycinnamate and Oxybenzone** *see page 1294*

♦ **Methoxypsoralen** *see* Methoxsalen *on previous page*

## Methyclothiazide (meth i kloe THYR a zide)

**U.S. Brand Names** Aquatensen®; Enduron®

**Therapeutic Category** Diuretic, Thiazide

**Pregnancy Risk Factor** B

**Lactation** Excretion in breast milk unknown/use caution

**Use** Management of mild to moderate hypertension; treatment of edema in congestive heart failure and nephrotic syndrome

**Mechanism of Action/Effect** Inhibits sodium reabsorption in the distal tubules causing increased excretion of sodium and water, as well as, potassium and hydrogen ions

**Contraindications** Hypersensitivity to methyclothiazide, other thiazides or sulfonamides, or any component; anuria; pregnancy

**Warnings** Use with caution in renal disease, hepatic disease, gout, lupus erythematosus, and diabetes mellitus. Some products may contain tartrazine.

**Drug Interactions**

**Decreased Effect:** Bile acid sequestrants, methenamine, and NSAIDs may decrease effect of thiazides. Thiazides may decrease the effects of warfarin, antigout agents, and sulfonylureas.

**Increased Effect/Toxicity:** Increased toxicity/levels of lithium. May increase toxicity of allopurinol, anesthetics, antineoplastics, calcium salts, digitalis, loop diuretics, methyldopa, nondepolarizing neuromuscular blockers, and vitamin D. Amphotericin and anticholinergics may increase the toxicity of thiazides.

**Adverse Reactions**

1% to 10%:

Cardiovascular: Orthostatic hypotension

Endocrine & metabolic: Hypokalemia

Dermatologic: Photosensitivity

Gastrointestinal: Anorexia, epigastric distress

<1% (Limited to important or life-threatening symptoms): Necrotizing angiitis, vasculitis, cutaneous vasculitis, erythema multiforme, Stevens-Johnson syndrome, aplastic anemia, hemolytic anemia, leukopenia, agranulocytosis, thrombocytopenia, hepatic function impairment, respiratory distress

**Overdose/Toxicology** Symptoms of overdose include hypermotility, diuresis, and lethargy. Treatment is supportive.

**Pharmacodynamics/Kinetics**

**Distribution:** Crosses the placenta

**Excretion:** Urine

**Onset:** Onset of diuresis: Oral: 2 hours; Peak effect: 6 hours

**Duration:** ~1 day

**Formulations** Tablet: 5 mg

**Dosing**

**Adults:** Oral:

Edema: 2.5-10 mg/day

Hypertension: 2.5-5 mg/day

**Administration**

**Oral:** May be taken with food or milk. Take early in day to avoid nocturia. Take the last dose of multiple doses no later than 6 PM unless instructed otherwise.

**Monitoring Laboratory Tests** Serum potassium, renal function

**Additional Nursing Issues**

**Physical Assessment:** Monitor heart rate and positional blood pressure (standing and sitting/lying) and fluid balance (I & O, weight) on a regular basis. Monitor for signs of hypokalemia. If used to treat CHF, monitor for signs of effectiveness (eg, fluid balance, weight, edema, respiratory status). Monitor and teach patient to monitor for effectiveness of therapy, possible side effects, precautions, and symptoms to report. **Pregnancy risk factor D** - assess knowledge/teach appropriate use of barrier contraceptives. Note breast-feeding caution.

**Patient Information/Instruction:** Take exactly as directed - with meals. May take early in day to avoid nocturia. Include bananas or orange juice in daily diet but do not take dietary supplements without advice or consultation of prescriber. Do not use alcohol or OTC medication without consulting prescriber. Weigh weekly at the same time, in the same clothes. Report weight gain >5 lb/week. May cause dizziness or weakness; change position slowly when rising from sitting or lying position and avoid driving or tasks requiring alertness until response to drug is known. You may experience nausea or loss of appetite (small frequent meals may help), impotence (reversible), constipation (fluids, exercise, dietary fiber may help), photosensitivity (use sunscreen, wear protective clothing and eyewear, and avoid direct sunlight). This medication does not replace other antihypertensive interventions; follow instructions for diet and lifestyle changes. Report flu-like symptoms, headache, joint soreness or weakness, difficulty breathing, skin rash, or excessive fatigue, swelling of extremities, or difficulty breathing. **Pregnancy/breast-feeding precautions:** Do not get pregnant while taking this medication; use appropriate barrier contraceptive measures. Consult prescriber if breast-feeding.

## Methyclothiazide and Deserpidine

(meth i kloe THYE a zide & de SER pi deen)

**U.S. Brand Names** Enduronyl®; Enduronyl® Forte

**Synonyms** Deserpidine and Methyclothiazide

**Therapeutic Category** Antihypertensive Agent, Combination

**Pregnancy Risk Factor** C

**Lactation** Excretion in breast milk unknown

**Use** Management of mild to moderately severe hypertension

**Formulations** Tablet: Methyclothiazide 5 mg and deserpidine 0.25 mg; methyclothiazide 5 mg and deserpidine 0.5 mg

**Dosing**

**Adults:** Oral: Individualized, normally 1-4 tablets/day

**Additional Nursing Issues**

**Physical Assessment:** See individual components listed in Related Information. **Pregnancy risk factor C** - benefits of use should outweigh possible risks. Note breast-feeding caution.

**Patient Information/Instruction:** See individual components listed in Related Information. **Pregnancy/breast-feeding precautions:** Inform prescriber if you are on intend to get pregnant. Consult prescriber if breast-feeding.

**Related Information**

Methyclothiazide *on previous page*

## Methyclothiazide and Pargyline (meth i kloe THYE a zide & PAR gi leen)

**U.S. Brand Names** Eutron®

**Synonyms** Pargyline and Methyclothiazide

**Therapeutic Category** Antihypertensive Agent, Combination

**Pregnancy Risk Factor** C

**Lactation** Excretion in breast milk unknown

**Use** Management of hypertension

**Formulations** Tablet: Methyclothiazide 5 mg and pargyline hydrochloride 25 mg

**Dosing**

**Adults:** Oral: Individualized, normally 1-4 tablets/day

**Additional Nursing Issues**

**Physical Assessment:** See individual components listed in Related Information.

**Patient Information/Instruction:** See individual components listed in Related Information.

**Related Information**

Methyclothiazide *on previous page*

♦ **Methylacetoxyprogesterone** *see* Medroxyprogesterone *on page 714*

◆ **Methylbenzethonium Chloride** *see page 1294*

◆ **Methylcellulose** *see page 1294*

## Methyldopa (meth il DOE pa)

**U.S. Brand Names** Aldomet®

**Therapeutic Category** False Neurotransmitter

**Pregnancy Risk Factor** B

**Lactation** Enters breast milk/compatible

**Use** Management of moderate to severe hypertension

**Mechanism of Action/Effect** Stimulation of central alpha-adrenergic receptors by a false transmitter that results in a decreased sympathetic outflow to the heart, kidneys, and peripheral vasculature

**Contraindications** Hypersensitivity to methyldopa or any component (oral suspension contains benzoic acid and sodium bisulfite; injection contains sodium bisulfite); liver disease; pheochromocytoma

**Warnings** May rarely produce hemolytic anemia and liver disorders. Positive Coombs' test occurs in 10% to 20% of patients (perform periodic CBCs). Sedation, usually transient, may occur during initial therapy or whenever the dose is increased. Use with caution in patients with previous liver disease or dysfunction, the active metabolites of methyldopa accumulate in uremia. Patients with impaired renal function may respond to smaller doses. Elderly patients may experience syncope (avoid by giving smaller doses). Tolerance may occur usually between the second and third month of therapy. Adding a diuretic or increasing the dosage of methyldopa frequently restores blood pressure control. Because of its CNS effects, methyldopa is not considered a drug of first choice in the elderly.

**Drug Interactions**

**Decreased Effect:** Iron supplements can interact and cause a significant **increase** in blood pressure. Ferrous sulfate and ferrous gluconate decrease bioavailability.

**Increased Effect/Toxicity:** Lithium and methyldopa may increase lithium serum levels resulting in lithium toxicity. Levodopa and methyldopa may cause enhanced blood pressure lowering. Methyldopa may also potentiate the effect of levodopa. Tolbutamide and methyldopa may result in enhanced effects of tolbutamide due to decreased clearance.

**Effects on Lab Values** Methyldopa interferes with the following laboratory tests: urinary uric acid, serum creatinine (alkaline picrate method), AST (colorimetric method), and urinary catecholamines (falsely high levels)

**Adverse Reactions**

>10%: Cardiovascular: Peripheral edema

1% to 10%:

Central nervous system: Drug fever, mental depression, anxiety, nightmares, drowsiness, headache

Gastrointestinal: Dry mouth

<1% (Limited to important or life-threatening symptoms): Orthostatic hypotension, bradycardia (sinus), sodium retention, sexual dysfunction, gynecomastia, hyperprolactinemia, thrombocytopenia, hemolytic anemia, positive Coombs' test, leukopenia, transient leukopenia or granulocytopenia, cholestasis or hepatitis and heptocellular injury, increased liver enzymes, jaundice, cirrhosis, dyspnea, SLE-like syndrome

**Overdose/Toxicology** Symptoms of overdose include hypotension, sedation, bradycardia, dizziness, constipation or diarrhea, flatus, nausea, and vomiting. Treatment is supportive and symptomatic. Can be removed by hemodialysis.

**Pharmacodynamics/Kinetics**

**Protein Binding:** <15%

**Distribution:** Crosses the placenta

**Half-life Elimination:** 75-80 minutes; End-stage renal disease: 6-16 hours

**Metabolism:** Intestinally and in the liver

**Excretion:** Urine

**Onset:** Peak hypotensive effect: Oral, parenteral: Within 3-6 hours

**Duration:** 12-24 hours

**Formulations**

Suspension, oral: 250 mg/5 mL (5 mL, 473 mL)

Tablet: 125 mg, 250 mg, 500 mg

Methyldopate hydrochloride: Injection: 50 mg/mL (5 mL, 10 mL)

**Dosing**

**Adults:**

Oral: Initial: 250 mg 2-3 times/day; increase every 2 days as needed; usual dose: 1-1.5 g/day in 2-4 divided doses; maximum: 3 g/day

I.V.: 250-1000 mg every 6-8 hours; maximum: 1 g every 6 hours

**Elderly:** Oral: Initial: 125 mg 1-2 times/day; increase by 125 mg every 2-3 days as needed. Adjust for renal impairment. See Geriatric Considerations.

**Renal Impairment:**

$Cl_{cr}$ >50 mL/minute: Administer every 8 hours.

$Cl_{cr}$ 10-50 mL/minute: Administer every 8-12 hours.

$Cl_{cr}$ <10 mL/minute: Administer every 12-24 hours.

Slightly dialyzable (5% to 20%)

**Administration**

**I.V.:** Infuse over 30 minutes.

**Stability**

**Storage:** Injectable dosage form is most stable at acid to neutral pH. Stability of parenteral admixture at room temperature (25°C) is 24 hours. Stability of parenteral admixture at refrigeration temperature (4°C) is 4 days.

Standard diluent: 250-500 mg/100 mL $D_5W$

**Monitoring Laboratory Tests** CBC, liver enzymes, Coombs' test (direct)

**Additional Nursing Issues**

**Physical Assessment:** Assess effectiveness and interactions of other medications (see Drug Interactions). See Contraindications and Warnings/Precautions for use cautions. Continuous monitoring is recommended for I.V. therapy. For oral therapy, monitor for effectiveness of therapy (blood pressure supine and standing) and adverse reactions (see Adverse Reactions and Overdose/Toxicology) at beginning of therapy and on a regular basis with long-term therapy. Assess knowledge/teach patient appropriate use, possible side effects/interventions, and adverse symptoms to report.

**Patient Information/Instruction:** Take as directed. Do not skip dose or discontinue without consulting prescriber. Follow recommended diet and exercise program. Do not use OTC medications which may affect blood pressure (eg, cough or cold remedies, diet pills, stay-awake medications) without consulting prescriber. This medication may cause altered color of urine (normal); drowsiness, dizziness, or impaired judgment (use caution when driving or engaging in tasks that require alertness until response to drug is known); postural hypotension (use caution when rising from sitting or lying position or when climbing stairs); or dry mouth or nausea (frequent mouth care or sucking lozenges may help). Report altered CNS status (eg, nightmares, depression, anxiety, increased nervousness); sudden weight gain (weigh yourself in the same clothes at the same time of day once a week); unusual or persistent swelling of ankles, feet, or extremities; palpitations or rapid heartbeat; persistent weakness, fatigue, or unusual bleeding; or other persistent side effects.

**Geriatric Considerations:** Because of its CNS effects, methyldopa is not considered a drug of first choice in the elderly.

**Additional Information** The oral suspension formulation contains ethanol. The injection formulation contains sulfites.

## Methyldopa and Hydrochlorothiazide

(meth il DOE pa & hye droe klor oh THYE a zide)

**U.S. Brand Names** Aldoril®

**Synonyms** Hydrochlorothiazide and Methyldopa

**Therapeutic Category** Antihypertensive Agent, Combination

**Pregnancy Risk Factor** C

**Lactation** Enters breast milk/compatible

**Use** Management of moderate to severe hypertension

**Formulations**

Tablet:

- 15: Methyldopa 250 mg and hydrochlorothiazide 15 mg
- 25: Methyldopa 250 mg and hydrochlorothiazide 25 mg
- D30: Methyldopa 500 mg and hydrochlorothiazide 30 mg
- D50: Methyldopa 500 mg and hydrochlorothiazide 50 mg

**Dosing**

**Adults:** Oral: 1 tablet 2-3 times/day for first 48 hours, then decrease or increase at intervals of not less than 2 days until an adequate response is achieved

**Elderly:** Refer to dosing in individual monographs.

**Renal Impairment:** $Cl_{cr}$ 30 mL/minute: Thiazides are recommended; loops are preferred.

**Additional Nursing Issues**

**Physical Assessment:** See individual components listed in Related Information. **Pregnancy risk factor C** - benefits of use should outweigh possible risks.

**Patient Information/Instruction:** See individual components listed in Related Information. **Pregnancy precautions:** Inform prescriber if you are on intend to get pregnant.

**Related Information**

Hydrochlorothiazide *on page 566*
Methyldopa *on previous page*

♦ **Methylene Blue** *see page 1248*
♦ **Methylergometrine Maleate** *see* Methylergonovine *on this page*

## Methylergonovine (meth il er goe NOE veen)

**U.S. Brand Names** Methergine®

**Synonyms** Methylergometrine Maleate

**Therapeutic Category** Ergot Derivative

**Pregnancy Risk Factor** C

**Lactation** Excretion in breast milk unknown/not recommended

**Use** Prevention and treatment of postpartum and postabortion hemorrhage caused by uterine atony or subinvolution

**Mechanism of Action/Effect** Similar smooth muscle actions as seen with ergotamine; however, it affects primarily uterine smooth muscles producing sustained contractions and thereby shortens the third stage of labor

(Continued)

## Methylergonovine *(Continued)*

**Contraindications** Hypersensitivity to methylergonovine or any component; induction of labor; threatened spontaneous abortion; hypertension; toxemia

**Warnings** Use caution in patients with sepsis, obliterative vascular disease, hepatic or renal involvement, or hypertension. Give with extreme caution if using I.V. Pregnancy factor C.

**Adverse Reactions**

>10%:

Central nervous system: Headache, seizures

Genitourinary: Uterine cramping

1% to 10%: Gastrointestinal: Nausea, vomiting

<1% (Limited to important or life-threatening symptoms): Temporary chest pain, palpitations, bradycardia, coronary vasospasm, hypertension (sudden & severe), myocardial infarction, peripheral vasospasm, hematuria, dyspnea

**Overdose/Toxicology** Symptoms of overdose include prolonged gangrene, numbness in extremities, acute nausea, vomiting, abdominal pain, respiratory depression, hypotension, and seizures. Treatment is symptomatic and supportive.

**Pharmacodynamics/Kinetics**

**Distribution:** Rapidly distributed primarily to plasma and extracellular fluid following I.V. administration; distribution to tissues also occurs rapidly

**Half-life Elimination:** Biphasic: Initial: 1-5 minutes; Terminal: 30 minutes to 2 hours

**Time to Peak:** Within 30 minutes to 3 hours

**Metabolism:** Liver

**Excretion:** Urine and feces

**Onset:** Onset of oxytocic effect: Oral: 5-10 minutes; I.M.: 2-5 minutes; I.V.: Immediately

**Duration:** Oral: ~3 hours; I.M.: ~3 hours; I.V.: 45 minutes

**Formulations**

Methylergonovine maleate:

Injection: 0.2 mg/mL (1 mL)

Tablet: 0.2 mg

**Dosing**

**Adults:**

Oral: 0.2 mg 3-4 times/day for 2-7 days

I.M.: 0.2 mg after delivery of anterior shoulder, after delivery of placenta, or during puerperium; may be repeated as required at intervals of 2-4 hours

I.V.: Same dose as I.M., but should not be routinely administered I.V. because of possibility of inducing sudden hypertension and cerebrovascular accident

**Elderly:** Refer to adult dosing.

**Administration**

**I.V.:** Ampuls containing discolored solution should not be used. Administer over no less than 60 seconds.

**Additional Nursing Issues**

**Physical Assessment:** Monitor blood pressure, vaginal bleeding, and CNS status. Breast-feeding is not recommended.

**Patient Information/Instruction:** This drug will generally not be needed for more than a week. You may experience nausea and vomiting (small frequent meals may help), dizziness, headache, or ringing in the ears (will reverse when drug is discontinued). Report any respiratory difficulty, acute headache, or numb cold extremities, or severe abdominal cramping. **Breast-feeding precautions:** Breast-feeding is not recommended.

♦ **Methylmorphine** *see* Codeine *on page 299*

## Methylphenidate (meth il FEN i date)

**U.S. Brand Names** Ritalin®; Ritalin-SR®

**Therapeutic Category** Stimulant

**Pregnancy Risk Factor** C

**Lactation** Excretion in breast milk unknown

**Use** Treatment of attention-deficit/hyperactivity disorder (ADHD) and symptomatic management of narcolepsy; many unlabeled uses

**Mechanism of Action/Effect** Blocks the reuptake mechanism of dopaminergic neurons; appears to stimulate the cerebral cortex and subcortical structures similar to amphetamines

**Contraindications** Hypersensitivity to methylphenidate or any components; glaucoma; motor tics; Tourette's syndrome; patients with marked agitation, tension, and anxiety

**Warnings** Use with caution in patients with hypertension, dementia (may worsen agitation or confusion), or seizures. Has high potential for abuse. Treatment should include "drug holidays" or periodic discontinuation in order to assess the patient's requirements and to decrease tolerance and limit suppression of linear growth and weight. It is often useful in treating elderly patients who are discouraged, withdrawn, apathetic, or disinterested in their activities. In particular, it is useful in patients who are starting a rehabilitation program but have resigned themselves to fail. These patients may not have a major depressive disorder. Methylphenidate will not improve memory or cognitive function. Pregnancy factor C.

**Drug Interactions**

**Cytochrome P-450 Effect:** May inhibit CYP isoenzymes (profile not defined).

**Decreased Effect:** Effects of guanethidine, bretylium may be antagonized by methylphenidate.

**Increased Effect/Toxicity:** May increase serum concentrations of tricyclic antidepressants, warfarin, phenytoin, phenobarbital, and primidone. MAO inhibitors may potentiate effects of methylphenidate.

**Food Interactions** Food may increase oral absorption.

**Adverse Reactions**

>10%:

Cardiovascular: Tachycardia, hypertension

Central nervous system: Nervousness, insomnia

Gastrointestinal: Anorexia

1% to 10%:

Cardiovascular: Chest pain

Central nervous system: Dizziness, drowsiness

Dermatologic: Rash

Gastrointestinal: Stomach pain, nausea

Miscellaneous: Hypersensitivity reactions

<1% (Limited to important or life-threatening symptoms): Hypotension, palpitations, cardiac arrhythmias, movement disorders, precipitation of Tourette's syndrome and toxic psychosis (rare), headache, convulsions, thrombocytopenia, anemia, leukopenia, neuroleptic malignant syndrome

**Overdose/Toxicology** Symptoms of overdose include vomiting, agitation, tremor, hyperpyrexia, muscle twitching, hallucinations, tachycardia, mydriasis, sweating, and palpitations. There is no specific antidote; treatment is supportive.

**Pharmacodynamics/Kinetics**

**Half-life Elimination:** 2-4 hours

**Metabolism:** Liver

**Excretion:** Urine and feces

**Onset:** Immediate release tablet: Peak cerebral stimulation effect: Within 2 hours; Sustained release tablet: Peak effect: Within 4-7 hours

**Duration:** Immediate release tablet: 3-6 hours; Sustained release tablet: 8 hours

**Formulations**

Methylphenidate hydrochloride:

Tablet: 5 mg, 10 mg, 20 mg

Tablet, sustained release: 20 mg

**Dosing**

**Adults:** Oral (discontinue periodically to re-evaluate or if no improvement occurs within 1 month):

Narcolepsy: 10 mg 2-3 times/day, up to 60 mg/day

Depression: Initial: 2.5 mg every morning before 9 AM; dosage may be increased by 2.5-5 mg every 2-3 days as tolerated to a maximum of 20 mg/day. May be divided (eg, 7 AM and 12 noon), but should not be given after noon. Do not use sustained release product.

**Elderly:** Refer to adult dosing.

**Administration**

**Oral:** Do not crush or allow patient to chew sustained release dosage form. To effectively avoid insomnia, dosing should be completed by noon.

**Additional Nursing Issues**

**Physical Assessment:** Assess effectiveness and interactions of other medications (see Drug Interactions). See Contraindications and Warnings/Precautions for cautious use. Assess for history of addiction; long-term use can result in dependence, abuse, or tolerance. Evaluate periodically for need for continued use. After long-term use, taper dosage slowly when discontinuing. Monitor laboratory tests, effectiveness of therapy, and adverse reactions at beginning of therapy and periodically with long-term use. Assess knowledge/teach patient appropriate use, interventions to reduce side effects, and importance of reporting adverse symptoms promptly. **Pregnancy risk factor C** - benefits of use should outweigh possible risks. Note breast-feeding caution.

**Patient Information/Instruction:** Take exactly as directed; do not change dosage or discontinue without consulting prescriber. Response may take some time. Do not crush or chew sustained release tables. Avoid alcohol, caffeine, or other stimulants. Maintain adequate fluid intake (2-3 L/day of fluids unless instructed to restrict fluid intake). You may experience decreased appetite or weight loss (small frequent meals may help maintain adequate nutrition); restlessness, impaired judgment, or dizziness, especially during early therapy (use caution when driving or engaging in tasks requiring alertness until response to drug is known); Report unresolved rapid heartbeat; excessive agitation, nervousness, insomnia, tremors, or dizziness; blackened stool; skin rash or irritation; or altered gait or movement. **Pregnancy/breast-feeding precautions:** Inform prescriber if you are or intend to be pregnant. Consult prescriber if breast-feeding.

**Geriatric Considerations:** Methylphenidate is often useful in treating elderly patients who are discouraged, withdrawn, apathetic, or disinterested in their activities. In particular, it is useful in patients who are starting a rehabilitation program but have resigned themselves to fail; these patients may not have a major depressive disorder; will not improve memory or cognitive function; use with caution in patients with dementia who may have increased agitation and confusion (see Dosage and Adverse Reactions).

♦ **Methylphenyl Isoxazolyl Penicillin** *see* Oxacillin *on page 866*

♦ **Methylphytyl Napthoquinone** *see* Phytonadione *on page 929*

## Methylprednisolone (meth il pred NIS oh lone)

**U.S. Brand Names** Adlone® Injection; A-methaPred® Injection; depMedalone® Injection; Depoject® Injection; Depo-Medrol® Injection; Depopred® Injection; D-Med® Injection; Duralone® Injection; Medralone® Injection; Medrol® Oral; M-Prednisol® Injection; Solu-Medrol® Injection

**Synonyms** 6-α-Methylprednisolone

**Therapeutic Category** Corticosteroid, Parenteral

**Pregnancy Risk Factor** C

**Lactation** Excretion in breast milk unknown

**Use** Primarily as an anti-inflammatory or immunosuppressant agent in the treatment of a variety of diseases including those of hematologic, allergic, inflammatory, neoplastic, and autoimmune origin; prevention and treatment of graft-vs-host disease following allogeneic bone marrow transplantation

**Mechanism of Action/Effect** In a tissue-specific manner, corticosteroids regulate gene expression subsequent to binding specific intracellular receptors and translocation into the nucleus. Corticosteroids exert a wide array of physiologic effects, including modulation of carbohydrate, protein, and lipid metabolism, and maintenance of fluid and electrolyte homeostasis. Moreover, cardiovascular, immunologic, musculoskeletal, endocrine, and neurologic physiology are influenced by corticosteroids.

**Contraindications** Hypersensitivity to methylprednisolone; serious infections, except septic shock or tuberculous meningitis; known viral, fungal, or tubercular skin lesions; administration of live virus vaccines

**Warnings** Use with caution in patients with hyperthyroidism, cirrhosis, nonspecific ulcerative colitis, hypertension, osteoporosis, thromboembolic tendencies, CHF, convulsive disorders, myasthenia gravis, thrombophlebitis, peptic ulcer, or diabetes. Acute adrenal insufficiency may occur with abrupt withdrawal after long-term therapy or with stress. Because of the risk of adverse effects, systemic corticosteroids should be used cautiously in the elderly, in the smallest possible dose, and for the shortest possible time. Pregnancy factor C.

**Drug Interactions**

**Cytochrome P-450 Effect:** CYP3A enzyme inducer

**Decreased Effect:** Phenytoin, phenobarbital, rifampin increase clearance of methylprednisolone. Potassium-depleting diuretics enhance potassium depletion. Skin test antigens, immunizations decrease antibody response and increase potential infections.

**Increased Effect/Toxicity:** Methylprednisolone may increase circulating glucose levels → may need adjustments of insulin or oral hypoglycemics. Methylprednisolone increases cyclosporine and tacrolimus blood levels. Itraconazole increases corticosteroid levels.

**Effects on Lab Values** Interferes with skin tests

**Adverse Reactions** In chronic, long-term use, may result in cushingoid appearance, osteoporosis, muscle weakness (proximal), and suppression of the adrenal-hypothalmic pituitary axis.

>10%:
- Central nervous system: Insomnia, nervousness
- Gastrointestinal: Increased appetite, indigestion

1% to 10%:
- Central nervous system: Dizziness or lightheadedness, headache
- Dermatologic: Hirsutism, hypopigmentation
- Endocrine & metabolic: Diabetes mellitus, adrenal suppression, hyperlipidemia
- Hematologic: Transient leukocytosis
- Neuromuscular & skeletal: Arthralgia
- Ocular: Cataracts, glaucoma
- Miscellaneous: Sweating, infection

<1% (Limited to important or life-threatening symptoms): Seizures, pseudotumor cerebri, acne, skin atrophy, bruising, hyperpigmentation, Cushing's syndrome, arrhythmias, impaired wound healing, avascular necrosis, secondary malignancy, intractable hiccups

**Overdose/Toxicology** When consumed in high doses for prolonged periods, systemic hypercorticism and adrenal suppression may occur. In these cases, discontinuation should be done judiciously. Arrhythmias and cardiovascular collapse are possible with rapid intravenous infusion of high-dose methylprednisolone. May mask signs and symptoms of infection.

**Pharmacodynamics/Kinetics**

**Half-life Elimination:** 3-3.5 hours

**Onset:** Methylprednisolone sodium succinate is highly soluble and has a rapid effect by I.M. and I.V. routes. Methylprednisolone acetate has a low solubility and has a sustained I.M. effect.

**Duration:**
- Peak effect: Oral: 1-2 hours; I.M.: 4-8 days; Intra-articular: 1 week
- Duration: Oral: 30-36 hours; I.M.: 1-4 weeks; Intra-articular: 1-5 weeks

**Formulations**

Injection, as acetate: 20 mg/mL (5 mL, 10 mL); 40 mg/mL (1 mL, 5 mL, 10 mL); 80 mg/mL (1 mL, 5 mL)

Injection, as sodium succinate: 40 mg (1 mL, 3 mL); 125 mg (2 mL, 5 mL); 500 mg (1 mL, 4 mL, 8 mL, 20 mL); 1000 mg (1 mL, 8 mL, 50 mL); 2000 mg (30.6 mL)

Tablet: 2 mg, 4 mg, 8 mg, 16 mg, 24 mg, 32 mg

Tablet, dose pack: 4 mg (21s)

**Dosing**

**Adults: Only sodium succinate may be given I.V.;** methylprednisolone sodium succinate is highly soluble and has a rapid effect by I.M. and I.V. routes. Methylprednisolone acetate has a low solubility and has a sustained I.M. effect.

Anti-inflammatory or immunosuppressive: Oral: 2-60 mg/day in 1-4 divided doses to start, followed by gradual reduction in dosage to the lowest possible level consistent with maintaining an adequate clinical response.
I.M. (sodium succinate): 10-80 mg/day once daily
I.M. (acetate): 10-80 mg every 1-2 weeks
I.V. (sodium succinate): 10-40 mg over a period of several minutes and repeated I.V. or I.M. at intervals depending on clinical response; when high dosages are needed, give 30 mg/kg over a period ≥30 minutes and may be repeated every 4-6 hours for 48 hours.

Status asthmaticus: I.V. (sodium succinate): Loading dose: 2 mg/kg/dose, then 0.5-1 mg/kg/dose every 6 hours for up to 5 days
High-dose therapy for acute spinal cord injury: I.V. bolus: 30 mg/kg over 15 minutes, followed 45 minutes later by an infusion of 5.4 mg/kg/hour for 23 hours

Lupus nephritis: High-dose "pulse" therapy: I.V. (sodium succinate): 1 g/day for 3 days

Aplastic anemia: I.V. (sodium succinate): 1 mg/kg/day or 40 mg/day (whichever dose is higher), for 4 days. After 4 days, change to oral and continue until day 10 or until symptoms of serum sickness resolve, then rapidly reduce over approximately 2 weeks.

*Pneumocystis* pneumonia in AIDs patients: I.V.: 40-60 mg every 6 hours for 7-10 days

Intra-articular (acetate): Administer every 1-5 weeks.
Large joints: 20-80 mg
Small joints: 4-10 mg

Intralesional (acetate): 20-60 mg every 1-5 weeks

**Elderly:** Only sodium succinate salt may be given I.V. Use the lowest effective adult dose.

**Renal Impairment:**
Hemodialysis effects: Slightly dialyzable (5% to 20%)
Administer dose posthemodialysis.

**Administration**

**Oral:** Give oral formulation with meals to decrease GI upset. Give daily dose in the morning to mimic normal peak blood levels.

**I.V.:** Only sodium succinate formulation may be given I.V. Acetate salt should not be given I.V.

Parenteral: Methylprednisolone sodium succinate may be administered I.M. or I.V.; I.V. administration may be IVP over one to several minutes or IVPB or continuous I.V. infusion.

**I.V.: Succinate:**
Low dose: ≤1.8 mg/kg or ≤125 mg/dose: I.V. push over 3-15 minutes
Moderate dose: ≥2 mg/kg or 250 mg/dose: I.V. over 15-30 minutes
High dose: 15 mg/kg or ≥500 mg/dose: I.V. over ≥30 minutes
Doses >15 mg/kg or ≥1 g: Administer over 1 hour
Do **not** administer high-dose I.V. push; hypotension, cardiac arrhythmia, and sudden death have been reported in patients given high-dose methylprednisolone I.V. push over <20 minutes. Intermittent infusion over 15-60 minutes; maximum concentration: I.V. push 125 mg/mL.

**Topical:** For external use only. Apply sparingly.

**Stability**

**Storage:** Intact vials of methylprednisolone sodium succinate should be stored at controlled room temperature.

**Reconstitution:** Reconstituted solutions of methylprednisolone sodium succinate should be stored at room temperature (15°C to 30°C) and used within 48 hours. Stability of parenteral admixture at room temperature (25°C) and at refrigeration temperature (4°C) is 48 hours.

Standard diluent (Solu-Medrol®): 40 mg/50 mL $D_5W$; 125 mg/50 mL $D_5W$
Minimum volume (Solu-Medrol®): 50 mL $D_5W$

**Monitoring Laboratory Tests** Blood glucose, electrolytes

**Additional Nursing Issues**

**Physical Assessment:** Assess effectiveness and interactions of other medications (see Drug Interactions). See Contraindications and Warnings/Precautions for use cautions. Monitor for effectiveness of therapy and adverse reactions according to dose, route, and length of therapy (especially with systemic administration - see above). Assess knowledge/teach patient appropriate use, possible side effects/interventions, and adverse symptoms to report (ie, opportunistic infection, adrenal suppression - see Adverse Reactions and Overdose/Toxicology). Diabetics: Monitor serum glucose levels closely; corticosteroids can alter hypoglycemic requirements. Dose may need to be increased if patient is experiencing higher than normal levels of stress. When discontinuing, taper dose and frequency slowly. **Pregnancy risk factor C** - benefits of use should outweigh possible risks. Note breast-feeding caution.

**Patient Information/Instruction:** Maintain adequate nutritional intake; consult prescriber for possibility of special dietary instructions. If diabetic, monitor serum glucose closely and notify prescriber of any changes; this medication can alter hypoglycemic requirements. Inform prescriber if you are experiencing unusual stress; dosage may need to be adjusted. You will be susceptible to infection; avoid crowds or infected persons or persons with contagious diseases. You may experience insomnia or nervousness; use caution when driving or engaging in tasks requiring alertness until

(Continued)

## Methylprednisolone *(Continued)*

response to drug is known. Report increased pain, swelling, or redness in area being treated; excessive or sudden weight gain; swelling of extremities; difficulty breathing; muscle pain or weakness; change in menstrual pattern; vision changes; signs of hyperglycemia; signs of infection (eg, fever, chills, mouth sores, perianal itching, vaginal discharge); blackened stool; other persistent side effects; or worsening of condition. **Pregnancy/breast-feeding precautions:** Inform prescriber if you are or intend to be pregnant. Consult prescriber if breast-feeding.

Oral: Take as directed, with food or milk. Take once-a-day dose in the morning. Do not take more than prescribed or discontinue without consulting prescriber.

Intra-articular: Refrain from excessive use of joint following therapy, even if pain is gone.

**Geriatric Considerations:** Because of the risk of adverse effects, systemic corticosteroids should be used cautiously in the elderly, in the smallest possible dose, and for the shortest possible time.

**Additional Information**

Sodium content of 1 g sodium succinate injection: 2.01 mEq; 53 mg of sodium succinate salt is equivalent to 40 mg of methylprednisolone base

Methylprednisolone acetate: Depo-Medrol®

Methylprednisolone sodium succinate: Solu-Medrol®

**Related Information**

Antiemetics for Chemotherapy-Induced Nausea and Vomiting *on page 1307*
Corticosteroids Comparison, Systemic Equivalencies *on page 1383*
Corticosteroids Comparison, Topical *on page 1384*

♦ **6-α-Methylprednisolone** *see* Methylprednisolone *on page 754*

## Methyltestosterone (meth il tes TOS te rone)

**U.S. Brand Names** Android®; Metandren®; Oreton® Methyl; Testred®; Virilon®

**Therapeutic Category** Androgen

**Pregnancy Risk Factor** X

**Lactation** Excretion in breast milk unknown/contraindicated

**Use**

Male: Hypogonadism; delayed puberty; impotence and climacteric symptoms

Female: Palliative treatment of metastatic breast cancer; postpartum breast pain and/or engorgement

**Mechanism of Action/Effect** Male: Stimulates receptors in organs and tissues to promote growth and development of male sex organs and maintains secondary sex characteristics in androgen-deficient males.

**Contraindications** Hypersensitivity to methyltestosterone or any component; known or suspected carcinoma of the breast or the prostate; pregnancy

**Warnings** Use with extreme caution in patients with liver or kidney disease or serious heart disease. May accelerate bone maturation without producing compensatory gain in linear growth.

**Drug Interactions**

**Decreased Effect:** Decrease oral anticoagulant effect

**Adverse Reactions**

>10%:
- Cardiovascular: Edema
- Male: Virilism, priapism
- Female: Virilism, menstrual problems (amenorrhea), breast soreness
- Dermatologic: Acne

1% to 10%:
- Male: Prostatic hypertrophy, prostatic carcinoma, impotence, testicular
- Female: Hirsutism (increase in pubic hair growth) atrophy
- Gastrointestinal: GI irritation, nausea, vomiting
- Hepatic: Hepatic dysfunction

<1% (Limited to important or life-threatening symptoms): Leukopenia, polycythemia, hepatic necrosis, cholestatic hepatitis

**Overdose/Toxicology** Abnormal liver function tests

**Pharmacodynamics/Kinetics**

**Metabolism:** Liver

**Excretion:** Urine

**Formulations**

Capsule: 10 mg

Tablet: 10 mg, 25 mg

Tablet, buccal: 5 mg, 10 mg

**Dosing**

**Adults:** Buccal absorption produces twice the androgenic activity of oral tablets

Male:
- Oral: 10-40 mg/day
- Buccal: 5-25 mg/day

Female:
- Breast pain/engorgement:
  - Oral: 80 mg/day for 3-5 days
  - Buccal: 40 mg/day for 3-5 days
- Breast cancer:
  - Oral: 50-200 mg/day
  - Buccal: 25-100 mg/day

**Elderly:** Refer to adult dosing (buccal absorption produces twice the androgenic activity of oral tablets).

**Additional Nursing Issues**

**Physical Assessment:** (For use in children see pediatric reference.) Assess effectiveness and interactions of other medications (see Drug Interactions). See Warnings/Precautions and Contraindications for use cautions. Monitor effectiveness of therapy and adverse response (see Adverse Reactions and Overdose/Toxicology). Assess knowledge/teach patient appropriate use, possible side effects and appropriate interventions, and adverse symptoms to report. **Pregnancy risk factor X** - determine that patient is not pregnant before beginning treatment and do not give to women of childbearing age or males who may have intercourse with childbearing women unless both male and female are capable of complying with barrier contraceptive measures during therapy and for 1 month following therapy. Breast-feeding is contraindicated.

**Patient Information/Instruction:** Take as directed; do not discontinue without consulting prescriber. Diabetics should monitor serum glucose closely and notify prescriber of changes; this medication can alter hypoglycemic requirements. You may experience acne, growth of body hair, loss of libido, impotence, or menstrual irregularity (usually reversible); nausea or vomiting (small frequent meals, frequent mouth care, sucking lozenges, or chewing gum may help). Report changes in menstrual pattern; deepening of voice or unusual growth of body hair; fluid retention (swelling of ankles, feet, or hands, difficulty breathing, or sudden weight gain); change in color of urine or stool; yellowing of eyes or skin; unusual bruising or bleeding; or other adverse reactions. **Pregnancy/breast-feeding precautions:** Inform prescriber if you are pregnant. Do not get pregnant during or for 1 month following therapy. Male: Do not cause pregnancy. Male/female: Consult prescriber for instruction on appropriate contraceptive measures. This drug may cause severe fetal defects. Do not breast-feed.

**Geriatric Considerations:** Since elderly males have prostate changes with age, it would be best to obtain a PSA initially and periodically. Retention of sodium and water could be a problem in patients with CHF and hypertension.

## Methysergide (meth i SER jide)

**U.S. Brand Names** Sansert®

**Therapeutic Category** Ergot Derivative

**Pregnancy Risk Factor** X

**Lactation** Enters breast milk/contraindicated

**Use** Prophylaxis to reduce intensity or prevent vascular headaches

**Mechanism of Action/Effect** Ergotamine congener, however actions appear to differ; methysergide has minimal ergotamine-like oxytocic or vasoconstrictive properties, and has significantly greater serotonin-like properties

**Contraindications** Peripheral vascular disease; severe arteriosclerosis; pulmonary disease; severe hypertension; phlebitis; serious infections; pregnancy

**Warnings** Patients receiving long-term therapy may develop retroperitoneal fibrosis, pleuropulmonary fibrosis and fibrotic thickening of the cardiac valves. Fibrosis occurs rarely when therapy is interrupted for 3-4 weeks every 6 months. Use caution in patients with impairment of renal of hepatic function; some products may contain tartrazine.

**Adverse Reactions**

>10%:

- Cardiovascular: Postural hypotension, peripheral ischemia
- Central nervous system: Drowsiness
- Gastrointestinal: Nausea, vomiting, abdominal pain, diarrhea

1% to 10%:

- Cardiovascular: Peripheral edema, tachycardia, bradycardia
- Dermatologic: Rash
- Gastrointestinal: Heartburn, constipation

<1% (Limited to important or life-threatening symptoms): Fibrosis

**Overdose/Toxicology** Symptoms of overdose include hyperactivity, limb spasms, impaired mental function, and impaired circulation. Treatment is supportive.

**Pharmacodynamics/Kinetics**

**Half-life Elimination:** ~10 hours

**Metabolism:** Liver

**Excretion:** Not well defined

**Formulations** Tablet, as maleate: 2 mg

**Dosing**

**Adults:** Oral: 4-8 mg/day with meals; if no improvement is noted after 3 weeks, drug is unlikely to be beneficial. Must not be given continuously for longer than 6 months, and a drug-free interval of 3-4 weeks must follow each 6-month course.

**Elderly:** Refer to adult dosing; use with caution.

**Additional Nursing Issues**

**Physical Assessment:** Monitor effectiveness of therapy (see Dosing). Reduce dosage gradually to prevent "rebound" headache. Assess knowledge/teach postural hypotension precautions. **Pregnancy risk factor X** - determine that patient is not pregnant before beginning treatment and do not give to women of childbearing age unless female is capable of complying with barrier contraceptive measures during therapy and 1 month following therapy. Breast-feeding is contraindicated.

**Patient Information/Instruction:** This drug is meant to prevent migraine headaches, not treat acute attacks. Take as directed; do not take more than recommended and do not discontinue without consulting prescriber (must be discontinued slowly). You may experience weight gain (monitor dietary intake and exercise) or dizziness or vertigo (use caution when driving or engaging in tasks that require alertness until response to

(Continued)

## Methysergide *(Continued)*

drug is known). Small frequent meals may reduce nausea or vomiting. Diarrhea will lessen with use. Report cold, numb, tingling, or painful extremities or leg cramps, chest pain, difficulty breathing or shortness of breath, or pain on urination. **Pregnancy/breast-feeding precautions:** Inform prescriber if you are pregnant. Do not get pregnant during or for 1 month following therapy. Consult prescriber for instruction on appropriate barrier contraceptive measures. This drug may cause severe fetal defects. Do not breast-feed.

**Geriatric Considerations:** Use cautiously in the elderly, particularly since many elderly have cardiovascular disease which would put them at risk for cardiovascular adverse effects.

**Additional Information** Some formulations may contain tartrazine.

- **Meticorten®** *see* Prednisone *on page 962*
- **Metimyd®** *see page 1282*
- **Metipranolol** *see* Ophthalmic Agents, Glaucoma *on page 853*

## Metoclopramide (met oh kloe PRA mide)

**U.S. Brand Names** Clopra®; Maxolon®; Octamide®; Reglan®

**Therapeutic Category** Gastrointestinal Agent, Prokinetic

**Pregnancy Risk Factor** B

**Lactation** Enters breast milk/not recommended (AAP rates "of concern")

**Use** Symptomatic treatment of diabetic gastric stasis, gastroesophageal reflux; prevention of nausea associated with chemotherapy or postsurgery and facilitates intubation of the small intestine

**Mechanism of Action/Effect** Blocks dopamine receptors in chemoreceptor trigger zone of the CNS; enhances the response to acetylcholine of tissue in upper GI tract causing enhanced motility and accelerated gastric emptying without stimulating gastric, biliary, or pancreatic secretions

**Contraindications** Hypersensitivity to metoclopramide or any component; GI obstruction, perforation, or hemorrhage; pheochromocytoma; history of seizure disorder

**Warnings** Use with caution in patients with Parkinson's disease and in patients with a history of mental illness. Dosage and/or frequency of administration should be modified in response to degree of renal impairment, extrapyramidal reactions, depression. May exacerbate seizures in seizure patients. To prevent extrapyramidal reactions, patients may be pretreated with diphenhydramine. Elderly are more likely to develop dystonic reactions than younger adults. Use lowest recommended doses initially.

**Drug Interactions**

**Cytochrome P-450 Effect:** CYP1A2 and 2D6 enzyme substrate

**Decreased Effect:** Anticholinergic agents antagonize metoclopramide's actions.

**Increased Effect/Toxicity:** Opiate analgesics may increase CNS depression.

**Effects on Lab Values** ↑ aminotransferase [ALT (SGPT)/AST (SGOT)] (S), amylase (S)

**Adverse Reactions**

>10%:

Central nervous system: Restlessness, drowsiness
Gastrointestinal: Diarrhea
Neuromuscular & skeletal: Weakness

1% to 10%:

Central nervous system: Insomnia, depression
Dermatologic: Rash
Endocrine & metabolic: Breast tenderness, prolactin stimulation
Gastrointestinal: Nausea, dry mouth

<1% (Limited to important or life-threatening symptoms): Tachycardia, hypertension or hypotension, bradycardia, AV block, extrapyramidal reactions, tardive dyskinesia, methemoglobinemia,

Reference: Ganzini L, et al, *Arch Intern Med*, 1993, 153:1469-75.

**Overdose/Toxicology** Symptoms of overdose include drowsiness, ataxia, extrapyramidal reactions, seizures, methemoglobinemia (in infants). Disorientation, muscle hypertonia, irritability, and agitation are common. Metoclopramide often causes extrapyramidal symptoms (eg, dystonic reactions) requiring management with diphenhydramine 1-2 mg/kg (adults) up to a maximum of 50 mg I.M. or I.V. slow push followed by a maintenance dose for 48-72 hours. When these reactions are unresponsive to diphenhydramine, benztropine mesylate I.V. 1-2 mg (adults) may be effective. These agents are generally effective within 2-5 minutes.

**Pharmacodynamics/Kinetics**

**Protein Binding:** 30%

**Distribution:** Crosses the placenta

**Half-life Elimination:** Normal renal function: 4-7 hours (may be dose-dependent)

**Excretion:** Urine and feces

**Onset:** Oral: Within 0.5-1 hour; I.V.: Within 1-3 minutes

**Duration:** Duration of therapeutic effect: 1-2 hours, regardless of route administered

**Formulations**

Injection: 5 mg/mL (2 mL, 10 mL, 30 mL, 50 mL, 100 mL)
Solution, oral, concentrated: 10 mg/mL (10 mL, 30 mL)
Syrup, sugar free: 5 mg/5 mL (10 mL, 480 mL)
Tablet: 5 mg, 10 mg

**Dosing**

**Adults:**

Antiemetic (chemotherapy-induced emesis): I.V.: 1-2 mg/kg 30 minutes before chemotherapy and every 2-4 hours to every 4-6 hours (and usually given with diphenhydramine 25-50 mg I.V./oral)

Gastroesophageal reflux: Oral: 10-15 mg/dose up to 4 times/day 30 minutes before meals or food and at bedtime. Single doses of 20 mg are occasionally needed for provoking situations. Efficacy of continuing metoclopramide beyond 12 weeks in reflux has not been determined.

Gastrointestinal hypomotility (gastroparesis):

Oral: 10 mg 30 minutes before each meal and at bedtime for 2-8 weeks

I.V. (for severe symptoms): 10 mg over 1-2 minutes; 10 days of I.V. therapy may be necessary for best response.

Postoperative nausea and vomiting: I.M.: 10 mg near end of surgery; 20 mg doses may be used

Facilitate intubation: I.V.: 10 mg

**Elderly:**

Antiemetic (chemotherapy-induced emesis):

I.V.: 1-2 mg/kg/dose every 2-4 hours or (postsurgery); direct I.V. administration should be given slowly over 1-2 minutes.

I.M.: 10-20 mg (near end of surgery)

Diabetic gastroparesis:

Oral: Initial: 5 mg 30 minutes before meals and at bedtime for 2-8 weeks; increase if necessary to 10 mg doses.

I.V.: Initiate at 5 mg over 1-2 minutes; increase to 10 mg if necessary.

Gastroesophageal reflux: Oral: 5 mg 4 times/day, 30 minutes before meals and at bedtime; increase dose to 10 mg 4 times/day if no response at lower dose.

Postoperative nausea and vomiting: I.M.: 5 mg near end of surgery; may repeat dose if necessary.

**Renal Impairment:**

$Cl_{cr}$ 10-40 mL/minute: Administer at 50% of normal dose.

$Cl_{cr}$ <10 mL/minute: Administer at 25% of normal dose.

Not dialyzable (0% to 5%); supplemental dose is not necessary.

**Administration**

**I.V.:** Lower doses of metoclopramide can be given I.V. push undiluted over 1-2 minutes. Parenteral doses of up to 10 mg should be given I.V. push. Higher doses to be given IVPB. Infuse over at least 15 minutes.

**Stability**

**Storage:** Injection is a clear, colorless solution and should be stored at controlled room temperature and protected from freezing. Injection is photosensitive and should be protected from light during storage. Dilutions do not require light protection if used within 24 hours.

**Reconstitution:** Stability of parenteral admixture at room temperature (25°C) and at refrigeration temperature (4°C) is 24 hours.

**Standard diluent:** 10-150 mg/50 mL $D_5W$ or NS

Minimum volume: 50 mL $D_5W$ or NS; send 10 mg unmixed to nursing unit

**Compatibility:** Compatible with diphenhydramine.

**Monitoring Laboratory Tests** Periodic renal function

**Additional Nursing Issues**

**Physical Assessment:** Determine cause of vomiting prior to administration. Monitor vital signs (especially blood pressure) during I.V. administration. Monitor for extrapyramidal effects, parkinsonian-like reactions, adverse CNS changes. Inpatients should use safety measures (eg, side rails up, call light within reach, etc). Caution patient to call for assistance with ambulation. Breast-feeding is not recommended.

**Patient Information/Instruction:** Take this drug as prescribed, 30 minutes prior to eating. Do not increase dosage. Do not use alcohol or other CNS depressant or sleeping aids without consulting prescriber. May cause dizziness, drowsiness, or blurred vision; use caution when driving or engaging in tasks that require alertness until response to drug is known. May cause restlessness, anxiety, depression, or insomnia (will reverse when medication is discontinued). Report any CNS changes, involuntary movements, unresolved diarrhea. If diabetic, monitor serum glucose regularly. **Breast-feeding precautions:** Breast-feeding is not recommended.

**Geriatric Considerations:** Elderly are more likely to develop tardive dyskinesia syndrome (especially elderly females) reactions than younger adults. Use lowest recommended doses initially. Must consider renal function (estimate creatinine clearance). It is recommended to do involuntary movement assessments on elderly using this medication at high doses and for long-term therapy.

**Additional Information**

The injection formulation contains sulfites.

pH: 3.0-6.5

**Related Information**

Antiemetics for Chemotherapy-Induced Nausea and Vomiting *on page 1307*

♦ **Metocurine Iodide** *see page 1248*

## Metolazone (me TOLE a zone)

**U.S. Brand Names** Mykrox®; Zaroxolyn®

**Therapeutic Category** Diuretic, Thiazide

**Pregnancy Risk Factor** D

**Lactation** Enters breast milk/use caution

(Continued)

## Metolazone *(Continued)*

**Use** Management of mild to moderate hypertension; treatment of edema in congestive heart failure and nephrotic syndrome, impaired renal function

**Mechanism of Action/Effect** Inhibits sodium reabsorption in the distal tubules causing increased excretion of sodium and water, as well as, potassium and hydrogen ions

**Contraindications** Hypersensitivity to metolazone or any component, other thiazides, and sulfonamide derivatives; patients with hepatic coma, anuria; pregnancy

**Warnings** Use with caution in renal disease, hepatic disease, gout, lupus erythematosus, and diabetes mellitus. Some products may contain tartrazine. **Mykrox® is not bioequivalent to Zaroxolyn® and should not be interchanged for one another.**

**Drug Interactions**

**Increased Effect/Toxicity:** Concurrent administration with furosemide may cause excessive volume and electrolyte depletion. Increased digitalis glycosides toxicity. Increased lithium toxicity.

**Adverse Reactions**

>10%: Central nervousness: Dizziness

1% to 10%:

Cardiovascular: Orthostatic hypotension, palpitations, chest pain, cold extremities (rapidly acting), edema (rapidly acting), venous thrombosis (slow acting), syncope (slow acting)

Central nervous system: Headache, fatigue, lethargy, malaise, lassitude, anxiety, depression, nervousness, "weird" feeling (rapidly acting), chills (slow acting)

Endocrine & metabolic: Hypokalemia, impotence, reduced libido, excessive volume depletion (slow acting), hemoconcentration (slow acting), acute gouty attach (slow acting), weakness

Dermatologic: Rash, pruritus, dry skin (rapidly acting)

Gastrointestinal: Nausea, vomiting, abdominal pain, cramping, bloating, diarrhea or constipation, dry mouth

Genitourinary: Nocturia

Neuromuscular & skeletal: Muscle cramps, spasm

Ocular: Eye itching (rapidly acting)

Otic: Tinnitus (rapidly acting)

Respiratory: Cough (rapidly acting), epistaxis (rapidly acting), sinus congestion (rapidly acting), sore throat (rapidly acting),

<1% (Limited to important or life-threatening symptoms): Purpura, hyperglycemia, glycosuria, leukopenia, agranulocytosis, aplastic anemia, hepatitis

**Overdose/Toxicology** Symptoms of overdose include orthostatic hypotension, dizziness, drowsiness, syncope, hemoconcentration and hemodynamic changes due to plasma volume depletion. Treatment is symptomatic and supportive.

**Pharmacodynamics/Kinetics**

**Protein Binding:** 95%

**Distribution:** Crosses the placenta

**Half-life Elimination:** 6-20 hours, renal function dependent

**Excretion:** Enterohepatic recycling; 80% to 95% excreted in urine

**Onset:** Onset of diuresis: Within 60 minutes

**Duration:** 12-24 hours

**Formulations**

Tablet:

Zaroxolyn®: 2.5 mg, 5 mg, 10 mg

Mykrox®: 0.5 mg

**Dosing**

**Adults:** Oral:

Edema: 5-20 mg/dose every 24 hours

Hypertension: 2.5-5 mg/dose every 24 hours

Hypertension (Mykrox®): 0.5 mg/day; if response is not adequate, increase dose to maximum of 1 mg/day.

**Elderly:** Oral:

Zaroxolyn®: Initial: 2.5 mg/day or every other day

Mykrox®: 0.5 mg once daily; may increase to 1 mg if response is inadequate; do not use more than 1 mg/day.

**Renal Impairment:** Not dialyzable (0% to 5%)

**Administration**

**Oral:** May be taken with food or milk. Take early in day to avoid nocturia. Take the last dose of multiple doses no later than 6 PM unless instructed otherwise.

**Monitoring Laboratory Tests** Serum electrolytes (potassium, sodium, chloride, bicarbonate), renal function

**Additional Nursing Issues**

**Physical Assessment:** Monitor heart rate and positional blood pressure (standing and sitting/lying) and fluid balance (I & O, weight) on a regular basis. Monitor for signs of hypokalemia. If used to treat CHF, monitor for signs of effectiveness (eg, fluid balance, weight, edema, respiratory status). Monitor and teach patient to monitor for effectiveness of therapy, possible side effects, precautions, and symptoms to report. **Pregnancy risk factor D** - assess knowledge/teach appropriate use of barrier contraceptives. Note breast-feeding caution.

**Patient Information/Instruction:** Take exactly as directed - with meals. May take early in day to avoid nocturia. Include bananas or orange juice in daily diet but do not take dietary supplements without advice or consultation of prescriber. Do not use alcohol or OTC medication without consulting prescriber. Weigh weekly at the same time, in the same clothes. Report weight gain >5 lb/week. May cause dizziness or weakness (change position slowly when rising from sitting or lying, avoid driving or tasks requiring alertness until response to drug is known). You may experience nausea or loss of appetite (small frequent meals may help), impotence (reversible), constipation (fluids, exercise, dietary fiber may help), photosensitivity (use sunscreen, wear protective clothing and eyewear, and avoid direct sunlight). This medication does not replace other antihypertensive interventions; follow instructions for diet and lifestyle changes. Report flu-like symptoms, headache, joint soreness or weakness, difficulty breathing, skin rash, excessive fatigue, swelling of extremities, or difficulty breathing.

**Pregnancy/breast-feeding precautions:** Do not get pregnant while taking this medication; use appropriate barrier contraceptive measures. Consult prescriber if breast-feeding.

**Geriatric Considerations:** When metolazone is used in combination with other diuretics, there is an increased risk of azotemia and electrolyte depletion, particularly in the elderly, monitor closely. May be effective in patients with glomerular filtration rate <20 mL/minute. Metolazone is often used in combination with a loop diuretic in patients who are unresponsive to the loop diuretic alone.

**Additional Information** 5 mg of metolazone is approximately equivalent to 50 mg of hydrochlorothiazide.

## Metoprolol (me toe PROE lole)

**U.S. Brand Names** Lopressor®; Toprol XL®

**Therapeutic Category** Beta Blocker, $Beta_1$ Selective

**Pregnancy Risk Factor** C/D (2nd and 3rd trimesters)

**Lactation** Enters breast milk/use caution - see Breast-feeding Issues

**Use** Treatment of hypertension and angina pectoris; prevention of myocardial infarction, atrial fibrillation, flutter, symptomatic treatment of hypertrophic subaortic stenosis

**Unlabeled use:** Treatment of ventricular arrhythmias, atrial ectopy, migraine prophylaxis, essential tremor, aggressive behavior

**Mechanism of Action/Effect** Selective inhibitor of $beta_1$-adrenergic receptors; competitively blocks $beta_1$-receptors, with little or no effect on $beta_2$-receptors at doses <100 mg; does not exhibit any membrane stabilizing or intrinsic sympathomimetic activity

**Contraindications** Hypersensitivity to beta-blocking agents; uncompensated congestive heart failure; cardiogenic shock; bradycardia (heart rate <45 bpm) or heart block; sinus node dysfunction; A-V conduction abnormalities, systolic blood pressure <100 mm Hg; diabetes mellitus. Although metoprolol primarily blocks $beta_1$-receptors, high doses can result in $beta_2$-receptor blockage; therefore, use with caution in the elderly with bronchospastic lung disease. Pregnancy (2nd and 3rd trimesters).

**Warnings** Use with caution in patients with inadequate myocardial function, those undergoing anesthesia, patients with CHF, myasthenia gravis, impaired hepatic or renal function, severe peripheral vascular disease, bronchospastic disease, diabetes mellitus, or hyperthyroidism. Abrupt withdrawal of the drug should be avoided (may result in an exaggerated cardiac beta-adrenergic response, tachycardia, hypertension, ischemia, angina, myocardial infarction, and sudden death), drug should be discontinued over 1-2 weeks. Beta-blockers may impair glucose tolerance, potentiate hypoglycemia, and/or mask signs or symptoms of hypoglycemia in a diabetic patient. Sweating will continue. Pregnancy factor C/D (2nd and 3rd trimesters).

**Drug Interactions**

**Cytochrome P-450 Effect:** CYP2D6 enzyme substrate

**Decreased Effect:** Decreased effect of beta-blockers with aluminum salts, barbiturates, calcium salts, cholestyramine, colestipol, NSAIDs, penicillins (ampicillin), rifampin, salicylates, and sulfinpyrazone due to decreased bioavailability and plasma levels. Beta-blockers may decrease the effect of sulfonylureas.

**Increased Effect/Toxicity:** Pharmacologic effect of beta antagonists may be enhanced with concomitant use of calcium channel blockers, oral contraceptives, flecainide (bioavailability and effect of flecainide also enhanced), haloperidol (hypotensive effects of both drugs), $H_2$ antagonists (decreased metabolism), hydralazine (both drugs hypotensive effects increased), loop diuretics (increased serum levels of beta-blockers except atenolol), significant and fatal increases in blood pressure have occurred after decrease in dose or discontinuation of clonidine in patients receiving both clonidine and beta-blockers together (reduce doses of each cautiously with small decreases); peripheral ischemia of ergot alkaloids enhanced by beta-blockers. Beta-blockers increase serum concentration of lidocaine. Beta-blockers increase hypotensive effect of prazosin. Beta-blockers (metoprolol) may increase the action or serum levels of theophylline.

**Food Interactions** Metoprolol serum levels may be increased if taken with food.

**Adverse Reactions**

>10%:

Central nervous system: Drowsiness, insomnia

Endocrine & metabolic: Decreased sexual ability

1% to 10%:

Cardiovascular: Bradycardia, palpitations, edema, congestive heart failure, reduced peripheral circulation

Central nervous system: Mental depression

Gastrointestinal: Diarrhea or constipation, nausea, vomiting, stomach discomfort

Respiratory: Bronchospasm

Miscellaneous: Cold extremities

<1% (Limited to important or life-threatening symptoms): Chest pain, arrhythmias, orthostatic hypotension, nervousness, headache, depression, hallucinations, confusion (especially in the elderly), thrombocytopenia, leukopenia, shortness of breath, hepatitis, hepatic dysfunction, jaundice

(Continued)

## Metoprolol *(Continued)*

**Overdose/Toxicology** Symptoms of intoxication include cardiac disturbances, CNS toxicity, bronchospasm, hypoglycemia and hyperkalemia. The most common cardiac symptoms include hypotension and bradycardia. Atrioventricular block, intraventricular conduction disturbances, cardiogenic shock, and asystole may occur with severe overdose, especially with membrane-depressant drugs (eg, propranolol). CNS effects include convulsions, coma, and respiratory arrest. Treatment is symptom directed and supportive.

**Pharmacodynamics/Kinetics**

**Protein Binding:** 8%

**Half-life Elimination:** 3-4 hours; End-stage renal disease: 2.5-4.5 hours

**Metabolism:** Liver

**Excretion:** Urine

**Onset:** Peak antihypertensive effect: Oral: Within 1.5-4 hours

**Duration:** 10-20 hours

**Formulations**

Metoprolol tartrate:

Injection: 1 mg/mL (5 mL)

Tablet: 50 mg, 100 mg

Tablet, sustained release: 50 mg, 100 mg, 200 mg

**Dosing**

**Adults:**

Oral: 100-450 mg/day in 2-3 divided doses, begin with 50 mg twice daily and increase doses at weekly intervals to desired effect.

I.V.: 5 mg every 2 minutes for 3 doses in early treatment of myocardial infarction; thereafter give 50 mg orally every 6 hours 15 minutes after last I.V. dose and continue for 48 hours; then administer a maintenance dose of 100 mg twice daily.

**Elderly:**

Oral: Initial: 25 mg/day; usual dose range: 25-300 mg/day; increase at 1- to 2-week intervals.

Extended release: 50 mg/day initially as a single dose; increase at 1- to 2-week intervals.

**Renal Impairment:** Hemodialysis: Administer dose posthemodialysis or administer 50 mg supplemental dose. Supplemental dose is not necessary following peritoneal dialysis.

**Hepatic Impairment:** Reduced dose is probably necessary.

**Additional Nursing Issues**

**Physical Assessment:** Cardiac and blood pressure monitoring are required for I.V. use. Assess other medications the patient may taking for effectiveness and interactions (see Drug Interactions). Assess blood pressure and heart rate prior to and following first dose, any change in dosage, and periodically thereafter. Monitor or advise patient to monitor weight and fluid balance (I & O), assess for signs of CHF (edema, new cough or dyspnea, unresolved fatigue), and assess therapeutic effectiveness. Monitor serum glucose levels of diabetic patients since beta-blockers may alter glucose tolerance. Use/teach postural hypotension precautions. **Pregnancy risk factor C/D** - benefits of use should outweigh possible risks. Note breast-feeding caution.

**Patient Information/Instruction:** I.V. use in emergency situations - patient information is included in general instructions.

Oral: Take exactly as directed. Do not increase, decrease, or adjust dosage without consulting prescriber. Take pulse daily, prior to medication and follow prescriber's instruction about holding medication. Do not take with antacids. Do not use alcohol or OTC medications (eg, cold remedies) without consulting prescriber. If diabetic, monitor serum sugars closely (may alter glucose tolerance or mask signs of hypoglycemia). May cause fatigue, dizziness, or postural hypotension; use caution when changing position from lying or sitting to standing, when driving, or when climbing stairs until response to medication is known. May cause alteration in sexual performance (reversible). Report unresolved swelling of extremities, difficulty breathing or new cough, unresolved fatigue, unusual weight gain, unresolved constipation, or unusual muscle weakness. **Pregnancy/breast-feeding precautions:** Inform prescriber if you are pregnant. Consult prescriber if breast-feeding. **Pregnancy/breast-feeding precautions:** Inform prescriber if you are or intend to be pregnant. Consult prescriber if breast-feeding.

**Geriatric Considerations:** Due to alterations in the beta-adrenergic autonomic nervous system, beta-adrenergic blockade may result in less hemodynamic response than seen in younger adults.

**Breast-feeding Issues:** Metoprolol is considered compatible by the American Academy of Pediatrics. However, monitor the infant for signs of beta-blockade (hypotension, bradycardia, etc) with long-term use.

**Additional Information** Equivalent oral and I.V. dose: Ratio of approximately 2.5:1 (ie, 50 mg oral is equivalent to 20 mg I.V.).

**Related Information**

Beta-Blockers Comparison *on page 1376*

- **Metoxiprim** *see* Co-trimoxazole *on page 307*
- **Metreton® Ophthalmic** *see* Prednisolone *on page 960*
- **Metrodin® Injection** *see* Urofollitropin *on page 1195*
- **MetroGel® Topical** *see* Metronidazole *on next page*
- **MetroGel®-Vaginal** *see* Metronidazole *on next page*

♦ **Metro I.V.® Injection** *see* Metronidazole *on this page*

## Metronidazole (me troe NI da zole)

**U.S. Brand Names** Flagyl® Oral; MetroGel® Topical; MetroGel®-Vaginal; Metro I.V.® Injection; Protostat® Oral

**Therapeutic Category** Amebicide; Antibiotic, Topical; Antibiotic, Miscellaneous; Antiprotozoal

**Pregnancy Risk Factor** B (may be contraindicated in 1st trimester)

**Lactation** Enters breast milk/not recommended (AAP rates "of concern")

**Use** Treatment of susceptible anaerobic bacterial and protozoal infections in the following conditions: amebiasis, symptomatic and asymptomatic trichomoniasis; skin and skin structure infections; CNS infections; intra-abdominal infections; systemic anaerobic infections; topically for the treatment of acne rosacea; treatment of antibiotic-associated pseudomembranous colitis (AAPC)

**Mechanism of Action/Effect** Inhibits DNA synthesis in susceptible organisms

**Contraindications** Hypersensitivity to metronidazole or any component; pregnancy (1st trimester) (see Pregnancy Risk Factor)

**Warnings** Use with caution in patients with liver impairment, blood dyscrasias; history of seizures, congestive heart failure, or other sodium retaining states; reduce dosage in patients with severe liver impairment, CNS disease, and severe renal failure ($Cl_{cr}$ <10 mL/minute). Has been shown to be carcinogenic in rodents.

**Drug Interactions**

**Cytochrome P-450 Effect:** CYP2C9 enzyme substrate; CYP2C9, 3A3/4, and 3A5-7 enzyme inhibitor

**Decreased Effect:** Phenytoin, phenobarbital may decrease metronidazole half-life.

**Increased Effect/Toxicity:** Alcohol may cause a disulfiram-like reaction. Warfarin and metronidazole may increase bleeding times (PT) which may result in bleeding.

**Effects on Lab Values** May cause falsely decreased AST and ALT levels.

**Adverse Reactions**

**Systemic:**

>10%:

Central nervous system: Dizziness, headache

Gastrointestinal: Nausea, diarrhea, anorexia, vomiting

1% to 10%:

Central nervous system: Seizures

Neuromuscular & skeletal: Peripheral neuropathy

<1% (Limited to important or life-threatening symptoms): Ataxia, leukopenia, thrombophlebitis

**Topical:**

1% to 10%:

Dermatologic: Dry skin, redness or other signs of skin irritation not present before therapy, stinging or burning of the skin

Ocular: Watering of eyes

**Vaginal:**

>10%: Genitourinary: *Candida* cervicitis or vaginitis

1% to 10%:

Central nervous system: Dry mouth, furry tongue, diarrhea, nausea, vomiting, anorexia

Gastrointestinal: Altered taste sensation

Genitourinary: Burning or irritation of penis of sexual partner; burning or increased frequency of urination, vulvitis, dark urine

**Overdose/Toxicology** Symptoms of overdose include nausea, vomiting, ataxia, seizures, and peripheral neuropathy. Treatment is symptomatic and supportive.

**Pharmacodynamics/Kinetics**

**Protein Binding:** <20%

**Distribution:** Ratio of CSF to blood level (%): Normal meninges: 16-43; Inflamed meninges: 100

**Half-life Elimination:** 6-8 hours, increases with hepatic impairment; End-stage renal disease: 21 hours

**Time to Peak:** Within 1-2 hours

**Metabolism:** Liver

**Excretion:** Urine and feces

**Formulations**

Capsule: 375 mg

Gel, topical: 0.75% [7.5 mg/mL] (30 g)

Gel, vaginal: 0.75% (5 g applicator delivering 37.5 mg in 70 g tube)

Injection, ready to use: 5 mg/mL (100 mL)

Tablet: 250 mg, 500 mg

Metronidazole hydrochloride: Powder for injection: 500 mg

**Dosing**

**Adults:**

Amebiasis: Oral: 500-750 mg every 8 hours for 5-10 days

Trichomoniasis: Oral: 250 mg every 8 hours for 7 days or 2 g as a single dose

Anaerobic infections: Oral, I.V.: 500 mg every 6-8 hours, not to exceed 4 g/day

Antibiotic-associated pseudomembranous colitis: Oral: 250-500 mg 3-4 times/day for 10-14 days

*H. pylori*: 1 capsule with meals and at bedtime for 14 days in combination with other agents (eg, tetracycline, bismuth subsalicylate, and $H_2$-antagonist)

(Continued)

## Metronidazole *(Continued)*

Vaginosis: 1 applicatorful (~37.5 mg metronidazole) intravaginally once or twice daily for 5 days; apply once in morning and evening if using twice daily, if daily, use at bedtime

Topical (acne rosacea therapy): Apply and rub a thin film twice daily, morning and evening, to entire affected areas after washing. Significant therapeutic results should be noticed within 3 weeks. Clinical studies have demonstrated continuing improvement through 9 weeks of therapy.

**Elderly:** Use the lower end of the dosing recommendations for adults; do not administer as single dose as efficacy has not been established.

**Renal Impairment:**

$Cl_{cr}$ <10 mL/minute: Administer at 50% of dose or every 12 hours.

Hemodialysis effects: Extensively removed by hemodialysis and peritoneal dialysis (50% to 100%). Administer dose posthemodialysis. During peritoneal dialysis, dose as for $Cl_{cr}$ <10 mL/minute.

Continuous arteriovenous or venovenous hemofiltration (CAVH/CAVHD), dose as for normal renal function

**Hepatic Impairment:** Unchanged in mild liver disease; reduce dosage in severe liver disease.

**Administration**

**Oral:** May be taken with food to minimize stomach upset.

**I.V.:** Avoid contact between the drug and aluminum in the infusion set.

**Topical:** No Antabuse®-like reactions have been reported after **topical** application, although metronidazole can be detected in the blood.

**Stability**

**Storage:** Metronidazole injection should be stored at 15°C to 30°C and protected from light. Product may be refrigerated but crystals may form; crystals redissolve on warming to room temperature. Prolonged exposure to light will cause a darkening of the product. However, short-term exposure to normal room light does not adversely affect metronidazole stability. Direct sunlight should be avoided. Stability of parenteral admixture at room temperature (25°C): Out of overwrap stability: 30 days.

**Reconstitution:** Standard diluent: 500 mg/100 mL NS

**Additional Nursing Issues**

**Physical Assessment:** Assess effectiveness and interactions of other medications patient may be taking (see Drug Interactions). Monitor laboratory tests, therapeutic response and adverse, reactions (eg, CNS, neuromuscular, and dermatologic reactions - see Warnings/Precautions and Adverse Reactions) according to dose, route of administration, and purpose of therapy. Assess knowledge/teach patient appropriate use, interventions to reduce side effects, and adverse symptoms to report. Note Pregnancy Risk Factor. Breast-feeding is not recommended.

**Patient Information/Instruction:** Take exactly as directed, with meals. Avoid alcohol during and for 24 hours after last dose. With alcohol your may experience severe flushing, headache, nausea, vomiting, or chest and abdominal pain. May discolor urine (brown/black/dark) (normal). You may experience "metallic" taste disturbance or nausea or vomiting (small frequent meals, frequent mouth care, chewing gum, or sucking lozenges may help). Refrain from intercourse or use a barrier contraceptive if being treated for trichomoniasis. Report unresolved or severe fatigue; weakness; fever or chills; mouth or vaginal sores; numbness, tingling, or swelling of extremities; difficulty breathing; or lack of improvement or worsening of condition. **Pregnancy/breast-feeding precautions:** Inform prescriber if you are pregnant. Breast-feeding is not recommended.

Topical: Wash hands and area before applying and medication thinly. Wash hands after applying. Avoid contact with eyes. Do not cover with occlusive dressing. Report severe skin irritation or if condition does not improve.

**Geriatric Considerations:** Adjust dose based on renal function.

**Breast-feeding Issues:** Not compatible; resume breast-feeding 12-24 hours after last dose.

**Additional Information** Sodium content of 500 mg (I.V.): 322 mg (14 mEq)

◆ **Metubine® Iodide** *see page 1248*
◆ **Mevacor®** *see* Lovastatin *on page 695*
◆ **Meval®** *see* Diazepam *on page 355*
◆ **Mevinolin** *see* Lovastatin *on page 695*

## Mexiletine (MEKS i le teen)

**U.S. Brand Names** Mexitil®

**Therapeutic Category** Antiarrhythmic Agent, Class I-B

**Pregnancy Risk Factor** C

**Lactation** Enters breast milk/compatible

**Use** Management of serious ventricular arrhythmias; suppression of PVCs

**Unlabeled use:** Diabetic neuropathy

**Mechanism of Action/Effect** Class IB antiarrhythmic, structurally related to lidocaine, which inhibits inward sodium current, decreases rate of rise of Phase 0, increases effective refractory period/action potential duration ratio

**Contraindications** Hypersensitivity to mexiletine or any component; cardiogenic shock, second or third degree heart block

**Warnings** Exercise extreme caution in patients with pre-existing sinus node dysfunction. Mexiletine can worsen CHF, bradycardias, and other arrhythmias. Mexiletine, like other antiarrhythmic agents, is proarrhythmic. CAST study indicates a trend toward increased mortality with antiarrhythmics in the face of cardiac disease (myocardial infarction); elevation of AST/ALT; hepatic necrosis reported; leukopenia, agranulocytopenia, and thrombocytopenia; and seizures. Alterations in urinary pH may change urinary excretion. Electrolyte disturbances (eg, hypokalemia, hyperkalemia, etc) after drug response. Pregnancy factor C.

**Drug Interactions**

**Cytochrome P-450 Effect:** CYP2D6 enzyme substrate; CYP1A2 enzyme inhibitor

**Decreased Effect:** Decreased mexiletine plasma levels when used with phenobarbital, phenytoin, rifampin, cimetidine, other hepatic enzyme inducers, and drugs which make the urine acidic.

**Increased Effect/Toxicity:** Mexiletine and caffeine or theophylline may result in elevated levels of theophylline and caffeine.

**Effects on Lab Values** Abnormal liver function test, positive ANA, thrombocytopenia

**Adverse Reactions**

>10%:

- Central nervous system: Lightheadedness, dizziness, nervousness
- Gastrointestinal: Heartburn, nausea, vomiting
- Neuromuscular & skeletal: Trembling, unsteady gait

1% to 10%:

- Cardiovascular: Chest pain, premature ventricular contractions
- Central nervous system: Confusion, headache, insomnia
- Dermatologic: Rash
- Gastrointestinal: Constipation or diarrhea
- Hepatic: Increased LFTs
- Neuromuscular & skeletal: Weakness, numbness of fingers or toes
- Ocular: Blurred vision
- Otic: Tinnitus
- Respiratory: Shortness of breath

<1% (Limited to important or life-threatening symptoms): Leukopenia, agranulocytosis, thrombocytopenia, positive antinuclear antibody

**Overdose/Toxicology** Has a narrow therapeutic index and severe toxicity may occur slightly above the therapeutic range, especially with other antiarrhythmic drugs. Acute ingestion of twice the daily therapeutic dose is potentially life-threatening. Symptoms of overdose include sedation, confusion, coma, seizures, respiratory arrest and cardiac toxicity (sinus arrest, A-V block, asystole, and hypotension). The QRS and Q-T intervals are usually normal, although they may be prolonged after massive overdose. Other effects include dizziness, paresthesia, tremor, ataxia, and GI disturbance. Treatment is symptomatic and supportive.

**Pharmacodynamics/Kinetics**

**Protein Binding:** 50% to 70%

**Half-life Elimination:** 10-14 hours (average: 14.4 hours elderly, 12 hours in younger adults); increase in half-life with hepatic or heart failure

**Time to Peak:** 2-3 hours

**Metabolism:** Liver

**Excretion:** Urine

**Formulations** Capsule: 150 mg, 200 mg, 250 mg

**Dosing**

**Adults:** Oral: Initial: 200 mg every 8 hours (may load with 400 mg if necessary); adjust dose every 2-3 days; usual dose: 200-300 mg every 8 hours; maximum: 1.2 g/day (some patients respond to every 12-hour dosing). Patients with hepatic impairment or CHF may require dose reduction. When switching from another antiarrhythmic, initiate a 200 mg dose 6-12 hours after stopping former agents, 3-6 hours after stopping procainamide.

**Elderly:** Refer to adult dosing.

**Hepatic Impairment:** Patients with hepatic impairment or CHF may require dose reduction.

**Administration**

**Oral:** Take with food or antacid. Administer around-the-clock to promote less variation in peak and trough serum levels.

**Monitoring Laboratory Tests** Regular serum levels

**Additional Nursing Issues**

**Physical Assessment:** Assess other medications patient may be taking for effectiveness and interactions (see Drug Interactions). See Warnings/Precautions for cautious use. Monitor laboratory tests (see above), therapeutic response (cardiac status), and adverse reactions (see Warnings/Precautions and Adverse Reactions) at beginning of therapy, when titrating dosage, and on a regular basis with long-term therapy. **Note:** Mexiletine has a low toxic:therapeutic ratio and overdose may easily produce severe and life-threatening reactions (see Overdose/Toxicology). Assess knowledge/teach patient appropriate use, interventions to reduce side effects, and adverse symptoms to report. **Pregnancy risk factor C** - benefits of use should outweigh possible risks.

**Patient Information/Instruction:** Take exactly as directed, with food or antacids, around-the-clock. Do not take additional doses or discontinue without consulting prescriber. Do not change diet without consulting prescriber. You will need regular cardiac checkups and blood tests while taking this medication. You may experience drowsiness or dizziness, numbness, or visual changes (use caution when driving or engaging in tasks requiring alertness until response to drug is known); nausea, vomiting, or heartburn (small frequent meals, frequent mouth care, chewing gum, or sucking lozenges may help); or headaches or sleep disturbances (usually temporary, if

(Continued)

## Mexiletine *(Continued)*

persistent consult prescriber). Report chest pain, palpitation, or erratic heartbeat; increased weight or swelling of hands or feet; chills, fever, or persistent sore throat; numbness, weakness, trembling, or unsteady gait; blurred vision or ringing in ears; or difficulty breathing. **Pregnancy precautions:** Inform prescriber if you are or intend to be pregnant.

**Related Information**

Antiarrhythmic Drug Classification Comparison *on page 1366*

- **Mexitil®** *see* Mexiletine *on page 764*
- **Mezlin®** *see* Mezlocillin *on this page*

## Mezlocillin (mez loe SIL in)

**U.S. Brand Names** Mezlin®

**Therapeutic Category** Antibiotic, Penicillin

**Pregnancy Risk Factor** B

**Lactation** Enters breast milk (small amounts)/use caution

**Use** Treatment of infections caused by susceptible gram-negative aerobic bacilli (*Klebsiella, Proteus, Escherichia coli, Enterobacter, Pseudomonas aeruginosa, Serratia*) involving the skin and skin structure, bone and joint, respiratory tract, urinary tract, GI tract, as well as, septicemia

**Mechanism of Action/Effect** Interferes with bacterial cell wall synthesis during active multiplication causing cell death and resultant bactericidal activity against susceptible bacteria

**Contraindications** Hypersensitivity to mezlocillin, any component, penicillins, cephalosporins, or imipenem

**Warnings** If bleeding occurs during therapy, mezlocillin should be discontinued. Dosage modification required in patients with impaired renal function. Use with caution in patients with renal impairment or biliary obstruction.

**Drug Interactions**

**Decreased Effect:** Efficacy of oral contraceptives may be reduced by when taken with mezlocillin.

**Increased Effect/Toxicity:** Aminoglycosides (synergy), probenecid (decreased clearance), vecuronium (increased duration of neuromuscular blockade), heparin (increased risk of bleeding).

**Effects on Lab Values** False-positive direct Coombs'; false-positive urinary protein

**Adverse Reactions**

>10%:

Central nervous system: Headache

Gastrointestinal: Nausea (mild), vomiting

Miscellaneous: Oral candidiasis, vaginal candidiasis

1% to 10%:

Dermatologic: Urticaria, exfoliative dermatitis

Miscellaneous: Allergic reactions, specifically anaphylaxis; serum sickness-like reactions

<1% (Limited to important or life-threatening symptoms): Seizures, leukopenia, neutropenia, thrombocytopenia, jaundice, hepatotoxicity, interstitial nephritis, *Clostridium difficile* colitis

**Overdose/Toxicology** Symptoms of penicillin overdose include neuromuscular hypersensitivity (eg, agitation, hallucinations, asterixis, encephalopathy, confusion, and seizures). Electrolyte imbalance may occur if the preparation contains potassium or sodium salts, especially in renal failure. Hemodialysis may be helpful to aid in removal of the drug from blood; otherwise, treatment is supportive or symptom directed.

**Pharmacodynamics/Kinetics**

**Distribution:** Into bile, heart, peritoneal fluid, sputum, bone; does not cross the blood-brain barrier well unless meninges are inflamed; crosses the placenta

**Half-life Elimination:** Dose dependent: 50-70 minutes (prolonged in renal impairment)

**Time to Peak:** I.M.: 45-90 minutes after administration; I.V. infusion: Within 5 minutes

**Metabolism:** Liver

**Excretion:** Urine and bile

**Formulations** Powder for injection, as sodium: 1 g, 2 g, 3 g, 4 g, 20 g

**Dosing**

**Adults:** I.M., I.V.:

Uncomplicated urinary tract infection: 1.5-2 g every 6 hours

Serious infections: 3-4 g every 4-6 hours

**Elderly:** Refer to adult dosing.

**Renal Impairment:** I.M., I.V.:

$Cl_{cr}$ 10-30 mL/minute: Administer every 6-8 hours.

$Cl_{cr}$ <10 mL/minute: Administer every 8 hours.

Moderately dialyzable (20% to 50%)

**Hepatic Impairment:** Reduce dose by 50%.

**Administration**

**I.M.:** Administer I.M. injections in large muscle mass, not more than 2 g/injection. I.M. injections given over 12-15 seconds will be less painful. Alternate injection sites.

**I.V.:** Administer around-the-clock to promote less variation in peak and trough serum levels. Can administer IVP over 3-5 minutes. Rapid administration can result in seizures. If giving IVPB, administer over 30 minutes.

**Stability**

**Reconstitution:** Reconstituted solution is stable for 48 hours at room temperature and 7 days when refrigerated. For I.V. infusion in NS or $D_5W$, solution is stable for 48 hours at room temperature, 7 days when refrigerated, or 28 days when frozen. After freezing, thawed solution is stable for 48 hours at room temperature or 7 days when refrigerated. If precipitation occurs under refrigeration, warm in water bath (37°C) for 20 minutes and shake well.

**Monitoring Laboratory Tests** Perform culture and sensitivity testing prior to initiating therapy.

**Additional Nursing Issues**

**Physical Assessment:** Monitor and teach patient to monitor for adverse reactions (see above) and opportunistic infections (eg, fever, purulent vaginal discharge, oral plaques, or mouth sores). Note breast-feeding caution.

**Patient Information/Instruction:** This medication can only be administered by infusion or injection. Maintain adequate hydration (2-3 L/day of fluids unless instructed to restrict fluid intake). Small frequent meals, frequent mouth care, and adequate fluids may reduce incidence of nausea or vomiting. If diabetic, drug may cause false tests with Clinitest® urine glucose monitoring; use of glucose oxidase methods (Clinistix®) or serum glucose monitoring is preferable. This drug may interfere with oral contraceptives; an alternate form of birth control should be used. Report difficulty breathing, acute diarrhea, systemic rash, fever, white plaques in mouth, or mouth sores. **Breast-feeding precautions:** Consult prescriber if breast-feeding.

**Geriatric Considerations:** Mezlocillin and the other antipseudomonal infections should be used in combination with another antibiotic for the treatment of mixed infections or against gram-negative bacilli such as *P. aeruginosa* (ie, with an aminoglycoside). Sodium content is the lowest of the penicillins. Adjust dose for renal function.

**Additional Information**

Sodium content of 1 g: 42.6 mg (1.85 mEq)

pH: 4.5-8

- **Miacalcin® Injection** *see* Calcitonin *on page 182*
- **Miacalcin® Nasal Spray** *see* Calcitonin *on page 182*
- **Micardis®** *see* Telmisartan *on page 1099*
- **Micatin® Topical [OTC]** *see* Miconazole *on this page*

## Miconazole (mi KON a zole)

**U.S. Brand Names** Absorbine® Antifungal Foot Powder [OTC]; Breezee® Mist Antifungal [OTC]; Femizol-M® [OTC]; Fungoid® Creme; Fungoid® Tincture; Lotrimin® AF Powder [OTC]; Lotrimin® AF Spray Liquid [OTC]; Lotrimin® AF Spray Powder [OTC]; Maximum Strength Desenex® Antifungal Cream [OTC]; Micatin® Topical [OTC]; Monistat-Derm™ Topical; Monistat i.v.™ Injection; Monistat™ Vaginal; M-Zole® 7 Dual Pack [OTC]; Ony-Clear® Spray; Prescription Strength Desenex® [OTC]; Zeasorb-AF® Powder [OTC]

**Therapeutic Category** Antifungal Agent, Parenteral; Antifungal Agent, Topical; Antifungal Agent, Vaginal

**Pregnancy Risk Factor** C

**Lactation** Excretion in breast milk unknown/use caution

**Use**

I.V.: Treatment of severe systemic fungal infections and fungal meningitis that are refractory to standard treatment

Topical: Treatment of vulvovaginal candidiasis and a variety of skin and mucous membrane fungal infections

**Mechanism of Action/Effect** Inhibits biosynthesis of ergosterol, damaging the fungal cell wall membrane, which increases permeability causing leaking of nutrients

**Contraindications** Hypersensitivity to miconazole, fluconazole, ketoconazole, polyoxyl 35 castor oil, or any component

**Warnings** I.V.: Administer with caution to patients with hepatic insufficiency. The safety of miconazole in patients <1 year of age has not been established. Cardiorespiratory and anaphylaxis have occurred with excessively rapid administration. Pregnancy factor C.

**Drug Interactions**

**Cytochrome P-450 Effect:** CYP3A3/4 enzyme substrate; CYP2C enzyme inhibitor, CYP3A3/4 enzyme inhibitor (moderate), and CYP3A5-7 enzyme inhibitor

**Decreased Effect:** Amphotericin B may decrease antifungal effect of both agents.

**Increased Effect/Toxicity:** Miconazole coadministered with warfarin has increased the anticoagulant effect of warfarin. Phenytoin levels may be increased. Miconazole may inhibit the metabolism of oral sulfonylureas.

**Effects on Lab Values** ↑ protein

**Adverse Reactions**

1% to 10%: Genitourinary: Vulvar/vaginal burning

<1% (Limited to important or life-threatening symptoms): Vulvar itching, soreness, edema, or discharge; polyuria; burning or itching of penis of sexual partner

**Overdose/Toxicology** I.V.: Symptoms of overdose include nausea, vomiting, and drowsiness. Treatment is supportive.

**Pharmacodynamics/Kinetics**

**Protein Binding:** 91% to 93%

**Half-life Elimination:** I.V.: Multiphasic: Initial: 40 minutes; Secondary: 126 minutes; Terminal phase: 24 hours

(Continued)

## Miconazole *(Continued)*

**Metabolism:** Liver

**Excretion:** Feces and urine

**Formulations**

Cream:

Topical, as nitrate: 2% (15 g, 30 g, 56.7 g, 85 g)

Vaginal, as nitrate: 2% (45 g is equivalent to 7 doses)

Dual pack: Vaginal suppositories and external vulvar cream 2%

Injection: 1% [10 mg/mL] (20 mL)

Lotion, as nitrate: 2% (30 mL, 60 mL)

Powder, topical: 2% (45 g, 90 g, 113 g)

Spray, topical: 2% (105 mL)

Suppository, vaginal, as nitrate: 100 mg (7s); 200 mg (3s)

Tincture: 2% with alcohol (7.39 mL, 29.57 mL)

**Dosing**

**Adults:**

Topical: Apply twice daily for up to 1 month.

Intrathecal: Used in conjunction with I.V.: 20 mg every 1-2 days via a subcutaneous ventricular reservoirs; or every 3-7 days without using a reservoir

I.V.: Initial: 200 mg, then 1.2-3.6 g/day divided every 8 hours for up to 20 weeks

Bladder instillation for candidal infections: 200 mg diluted solution instilled in the bladder by continuous irrigation or 2-4 times per day

Vaginal: Insert contents of 1 applicator of vaginal cream (100 mg) or 100 mg suppository at bedtime for 7 days, or 200 mg suppository at bedtime for 3 days.

**Elderly:** Refer to adult dosing.

**Renal Impairment:** Not dialyzable (0% to 5%)

**Administration**

**I.V.:** Infuse I.V. dose over 30-60 minutes. Administer around-the-clock to promote less variation in peak and trough serum levels.

**Stability**

**Storage:** Protect from heat. Darkening of solution indicates deterioration.

**Reconstitution:** Stability of parenteral admixture at room temperature (25°C) is 2 days.

**Compatibility:** Dilute in normal saline or $D_5W$.

**Additional Nursing Issues**

**Physical Assessment:** See Contraindications and Warnings/Precautions for use cautions. Assess effectiveness and interactions of other medications (see Drug Interactions). I.V.: Monitor for phlebitis, pruritus, fever, rash, or chills. Monitor serum glucose in diabetic patients. Monitor fluid balance (I & O), and hydration status. Assess knowledge/teach patient appropriate use for formulation prescribed, possible side effects/interventions, and adverse symptoms to report. **Pregnancy risk factor C** - benefits of use should outweigh possible risks. Note breast-feeding caution.

**Patient Information/Instruction:** Take full course of therapy as directed; do not discontinue without consulting prescriber. Some infections may require long periods of therapy. Practice good hygiene measures to prevent reinfection.

Topical: Wash and dry area before applying medication; apply thinly. Do not get in or near eyes.

Vaginal: Insert high in vagina. Refrain from intercourse during treatment.

If you are diabetic you should test serum glucose regularly at the same time of day. You may experience nausea and vomiting (small, frequent meals may help) or headache, dizziness (use caution when driving). Report unresolved headache, rash, burning, itching, anorexia, unusual fatigue, diarrhea, nausea, or vomiting. **Pregnancy/breast-feeding precautions:** Inform prescriber if you are or intend to be pregnant. Consult prescriber if breast-feeding.

**Geriatric Considerations:** Assess patient's ability to self administer, may be difficult in patients with arthritis or limited range of motion.

**Additional Information**

Miconazole: Monistat i.v.™

Miconazole nitrate: Micatin®, Monistat™, Monistat-Derm™

- **Micostatin** *see* Nystatin *on page 843*
- **Micostyl** *see* Econazole *on page 412*
- **MICRhoGAM™** *see page 1256*
- **Microfibrillar Collagen Hemostat** *see page 1248*
- **Microgynon®** *see* Oral Contraceptives *on page 859*
- **Micro-K®** *see* Potassium Supplements *on page 952*
- **Micro-K® LS** *see* Potassium Supplements *on page 952*
- **Microlut®** *see* Levonorgestrel *on page 670*
- **Micronase®** *see* Glyburide *on page 538*
- **microNefrin®** *see* Epinephrine *on page 424*
- **Micronor®** *see* Norethindrone *on page 836*
- **Microrgan®** *see* Ciprofloxacin *on page 270*
- **Microsulfon®** *see* Sulfadiazine *on page 1081*
- **Microtid** *see* Ranitidine *on page 1008*
- ***Micrurus fluvius*** *see page 1246*
- **Midamor®** *see* Amiloride *on page 67*

## Midazolam (MID aye zoe lam)

**U.S. Brand Names** Versed®

**Therapeutic Category** Benzodiazepine

**Pregnancy Risk Factor** D

**Lactation** Enters breast milk/not recommended (AAP rates "of concern")

**Use** Preoperative sedation; provides conscious sedation prior to diagnostic or radiographic procedures; sedation for mechanically ventilated and intubated patients during anesthesia or in critical care (as continuous infusion)

Unlabeled use: Control of agitation in dementia, anxiety, status epilepticus

**Mechanism of Action/Effect** Depresses all levels of the CNS, including the limbic and reticular formation, probably through the increased action of gamma-aminobutyric acid (GABA), which is a major inhibitory neurotransmitter in the brain

**Contraindications** Hypersensitivity to midazolam or any component (cross-sensitivity with other benzodiazepines may occur); existing CNS depression; shock; acute narrow-angle glaucoma; pregnancy

**Warnings** Use with caution in patients with congestive heart failure, renal impairment, pulmonary disease, hepatic dysfunction, the elderly, and those receiving concomitant narcotics. Midazolam may cause respiratory depression/arrest. Serious respiratory reactions have also been reported after midazolam syrup, usually when used in combination with other sedative agents. Deaths and hypoxic encephalopathy have resulted when these reactions, regardless of the route of administration, were not promptly recognized and treated appropriately. Should only be used in settings where capabilities for adequate monitoring and resuscitative equipment are available.

**Drug Interactions**

**Cytochrome P-450 Effect:** CYP3A3/4 enzyme substrate

**Decreased Effect:** Theophylline may antagonize the sedative effects of midazolam.

**Increased Effect/Toxicity:** CNS depressants may increase sedation and respiratory depression. Doses of anesthetic agents should be reduced when used in conjunction with midazolam. Cimetidine may increase midazolam serum concentrations. **If narcotics or other CNS depressants are administered concomitantly, and age is <65 years, the midazolam dose should be reduced by 30%. If >65 years of age, reduce midazolam dose by at least 50%**

**Adverse Reactions**

>10%:

Cardiovascular: Hypotension

Local: Pain and local reactions at injection site (severity less than diazepam)

Miscellaneous: Hiccups

1% to 10%:

Cardiovascular: Cardiac arrest, bradycardia

Central nervous system: Drowsiness, ataxia, amnesia, dizziness, paradoxical excitement, sedation, headache

Gastrointestinal: Nausea, vomiting

Ocular: Blurred vision, diplopia

Respiratory: Respiratory depression, apnea, laryngospasm, bronchospasm

Miscellaneous: Physical and psychological dependence with prolonged use

<1% (Limited to important or life-threatening symptoms): Tachycardia, wheezing

**Overdose/Toxicology** Symptoms of overdose include respiratory depression, hypotension, coma, stupor, confusion, and apnea. Treatment for benzodiazepine overdose is supportive. Flumazenil has been shown to selectively block the binding of benzodiazepines to its receptor, resulting in reversal of CNS depression but not always respiratory depression.

**Pharmacodynamics/Kinetics**

**Protein Binding:** 97%

**Distribution:** Increased with congestive heart failure (CHF) and chronic renal failure

**Half-life Elimination:** 1-4 hours, increased with cirrhosis, CHF, obesity, elderly

**Metabolism:** Liver

**Excretion:** Metabolites in urine, ~2% to 10% excreted in feces

**Onset:**

I.M.: Within 15 minutes; Peak effect: 0.5-1 hour

I.V.: Within 1-5 minutes

**Duration:** I.M.: 2 hours mean, up to 6 hours

**Formulations**

Injection, as hydrochloride: 1 mg/mL (2 mL, 5 mL, 10 mL); 5 mg/mL (1 mL, 2 mL, 5 mL, 10 mL)

Syrup: 2 mg/mL (118 mL)

**Dosing**

**Adults:** The dose of midazolam needs to be individualized based on the patient's age, underlying diseases, and concurrent medications. Personnel and equipment needed for standard respiratory resuscitation should be immediately available during midazolam administration.

Preoperative sedation: I.M.: 0.07-0.08 mg/kg 30-60 minutes presurgery; usual dose: 5 mg

Conscious sedation: I.V.: Initial: 0.5-2 mg slow I.V. over at least 2 minutes; slowly titrate to effect by repeating doses every 2-3 minutes if needed; usual total dose: 2.5-5 mg. Use decreased doses in the elderly.

Healthy Adults <60 years: Some patients respond to doses as low as 1 mg. No more than 2.5 mg should be administered over a period of 2 minutes. Additional doses of midazolam may be administered after a 2-minute waiting period and evaluation of

(Continued)

## Midazolam *(Continued)*

sedation after each dose increment. A total dose >5 mg is generally not needed. If narcotics or other CNS depressants are administered concomitantly, the midazolam dose should be reduced by 30%.

Sedation in mechanically intubated patients: I.V. continuous infusion: 100 mg in 250 mL $D_5W$ or NS, (if patient is fluid-restricted, may concentrate up to a maximum of 0.5 mg/mL); initial dose: 0.01-0.05 mg/kg (~0.5-4 mg for a typical adult) initially and either repeated at 10-15 minute intervals until adequate sedation is achieved or continuous infusion rates of 0.02-0.1 mg/kg/hour (1-7 mg/hour) and titrate to reach desired level of sedation

**Elderly:** Conscious sedation: Titrate slowly, initial dose; 1 mg slow I.V. Administer no more than 1.5 mg in a 2-minute period. Wait 2 or more minutes for full effect, if additional titration is needed, administer no more than 1 mg over 2 minutes, waiting another 2 or more minutes to evaluate sedative effect. Total dose >3.5 mg is rarely necessary. **Note:** if other CNS depressants are used concomitantly, the midazolam dose may be at least 50% of the usual adult dose.

**Administration**

**I.M.:** Give deep I.M. into large muscle.

**Stability**

**Storage:** Stable for 24 hours at room temperature/refrigeration.

**Compatibility:** Compatible with NS, $D_5W$.

Standardized dose for continuous infusion: 100 mg/250 mL $D_5W$ or NS; maximum concentration: 0.5 mg/mL

See the Compatibility of Drugs in Syringe Chart *on page 1317.*

**Additional Nursing Issues**

**Physical Assessment:** Assess other medications the patient may be taking for effectiveness and interactions (see Drug Interactions). See Contraindications and Warnings/Precautions for cautious use. I.V. monitor cardiac and respiratory status continuously (see Dosing). Monitor I.V. infusion site carefully for extravasation.

I.V./I.M.: Monitor closely following administration. Provide bedrest and assistance with ambulation for several hours. **Note:** Full recovery usually occurs within 2-3 hours, but may take 6 hours.

**Pregnancy risk factor D** - ascertain pregnancy status. Benefits of use must outweigh possible risks for fetus. Breast-feeding is not recommended.

**Patient Information/Instruction:** Avoid use of alcohol or prescription or OTC sedatives or hypnotics for a minimum of 24 hours after administration. Avoid driving or engaging in any tasks that require alertness for 24 hours following administration. You may experience some loss of memory following administration. **Pregnancy/breast-feeding precautions:** Advise prescriber if you are pregnant; this medication is contraindicated for pregnant women. Breast-feeding is not recommended.

**Geriatric Considerations:** If concomitant CNS depressant medications are used in the elderly, the midazolam dose will be at least 50% less than doses used in healthy, young, unpremedicated patients (see Warnings/Precautions and Pharmacokinetics).

**Additional Information** Sodium content of 1 mL: 0.14 mEq

**Related Information**

Benzodiazepines Comparison *on page 1375*

## Midodrine (MI doe dreen)

**U.S. Brand Names** ProAmatine®

**Therapeutic Category** $Alpha_1$ Agonist

**Pregnancy Risk Factor** C

**Lactation** No data

**Use** Treatment of symptomatic orthostatic hypotension

**Unlabeled use:** Managing urinary incontinence

**Mechanism of Action/Effect** Midodrine forms an active metabolite, desglymidodrine that is an $alpha_1$-agonist. This agent increases arteriolar and venous tone resulting in a rise in standing, sitting, and supine systolic and diastolic blood pressure in patient with orthostatic hypotension.

**Contraindications** Hypersensitivity to midodrine or any component; severe organic heart disease, urinary retention, pheochromocytoma, thyrotoxicosis, persistent and significant supine hypertension; concurrent use of fludrocortisone

**Warnings** Only indicated for patients for whom orthostatic hypotension significantly impairs their daily life. Use is not recommended with supine hypertension and caution should be exercised in patients with diabetes, visual problems, urinary retention (reduce initial dose), or hepatic dysfunction. Monitor renal and hepatic function prior to and periodically during therapy. Safety and efficacy has not been established in children. Discontinue and re-evaluate therapy if signs of bradycardia occur. Pregnancy factor C.

**Drug Interactions**

**Increased Effect/Toxicity:** Concomitant fludrocortisone results in hypernatremia or an increase in intraocular pressure and glaucoma. Bradycardia may be accentuated with concomitant administration of cardiac glycosides, psychotherapeutics, and beta-blockers. Alpha-agonists may increase the pressure effects and alpha-antagonists may negate the effects of midodrine.

**Adverse Reactions**

>10%:

Dermatologic: Piloerection, pruritus

Genitourinary: Urinary urgency, retention, or polyuria

Neuromuscular & skeletal: Paresthesia

1% to 10%:
- Cardiovascular: Supine hypertension, facial flushing
- Central nervous system: Confusion, anxiety, dizziness, chills
- Dermatologic: Rash, dry skin
- Gastrointestinal: Xerostomia, nausea, abdominal pain
- Genitourinary: Dysuria
- Neuromuscular & skeletal: Pain

<1% (Limited to important or life-threatening symptoms): Flushing, headache, insomnia, leg cramps, visual changes

**Pharmacodynamics/Kinetics**

**Protein Binding:** Minimal

**Distribution:** Poorly distributed across membrane (eg, blood brain barrier)

**Half-life Elimination:** ~3-4 hours (active drug); 25 minutes (prodrug)

**Time to Peak:** 1-2 hours (active drug); 30 minutes (prodrug)

**Metabolism:** Rapid deglycination to desglymidodrine occurs in many tissues and plasma; further metabolism in the liver.

**Excretion:** Renal, minimal (2% to 4%); clearance of desglymidodrine: 385 mL/minute (predominantly by renal secretion)

**Onset:** Within 1 hour

**Duration:** May last for 2-3 hours

**Formulations** Tablet, as hydrochloride: 2.5 mg, 5 mg

**Dosing**

**Adults:** Oral: 10 mg 3 times/day during daytime hours (every 3-4 hours) when patient is upright (maximum: 40 mg/day)

**Elderly:** Refer to adult dosing.

**Renal Impairment:** 2.5 mg 3 times/day, gradually increasing as tolerated

**Administration**

**Oral:** Doses may be given in approximately 3- to 4-hour intervals (eg, shortly before or upon rising in the morning, at midday, in the late afternoon not later than 6 PM). Avoid dosing after the evening meal or within 4 hours of bedtime. Continue therapy only in patients who appear to attain symptomatic improvement during initial treatment. Standing systolic blood pressure may be elevated 15-30 mm Hg at 1 hour after a 10 mg dose. Some effect may persist for 2-3 hours.

**Monitoring Laboratory Tests** Kidney and liver function tests

**Additional Nursing Issues**

**Physical Assessment:** Assess effectiveness and interactions of other medications (see Drug Interactions). See Contraindications and Warnings/Precautions for use cautions (ie, use only for patients for whom orthostatic hypotension significantly impairs their daily life). Monitor for effectiveness of therapy (blood pressure supine and standing) and adverse reactions (see Adverse Reactions and Overdose/Toxicology) at beginning of therapy and on a regular basis with long-term therapy. Assess knowledge/teach patient appropriate use, possible side effects/interventions, and adverse symptoms to report. **Pregnancy risk factor C** - benefits of use should outweigh possible risks.

**Patient Information/Instruction:** This drug may relieve positional hypotension; effects must be evaluated regularly. Take prescribed amount 3 times daily (shortly before rising in the morning, at midday, and in late afternoon); do not take after 6 PM or within 4 hours of bedtime or when lying down for any length of time. Follow recommended diet and exercise program. Do not use OTC medications which may affect blood pressure (eg, cough or cold remedies, diet pills, stay-awake medications) without consulting prescriber. You may experience urinary urgency or retention (void before taking or consult prescriber if difficulty persists); or dizziness, drowsiness, or headache (use caution when driving or engaging in tasks that require alertness until response to drug is known). Report skin rash, severe gastric upset or pain, muscle weakness or pain, or other persistent side effects. **Pregnancy precautions:** Inform prescriber if you are or intend to be pregnant. Consult prescriber if breast-feeding.

♦ **Midol® 200 [OTC]** *see* Ibuprofen *on page 592*
♦ **Midol® PM Caplet** *see page 1294*
♦ **Midotens** *see* Labetalol *on page 649*

## Miglitol (MIG li tol)

**U.S. Brand Names** Glyset®

**Therapeutic Category** Antidiabetic Agent (Miscellaneous)

**Pregnancy Risk Factor** B

**Lactation** Excreted in breast milk (small amounts)/not recommended

**Use** Treatment of noninsulin-dependent diabetes mellitus (NIDDM); monotherapy adjunct to diet to improve glycemic control in patients with NIDDM whose hyperglycemia cannot be managed with diet alone; combination therapy with a sulfonylurea when diet plus either miglitol or a sulfonylurea alone do not result in adequate glycemic control. The effect of miglitol to enhance glycemic control is additive to that of sulfonylureas when used in combination.

**Mechanism of Action/Effect** In contrast to sulfonylureas, miglitol does not enhance insulin secretion. The antihyperglycemic action of miglitol results from a reversible inhibition of membrane-bound intestinal alpha-glucosidases which hydrolyze oligosaccharides and disaccharides to glucose and other monosaccharides in the brush border of the small intestine. In diabetic patients, this enzyme inhibition results in delayed glucose absorption and lowering of postprandial hyperglycemia.

**Contraindications** Hypersensitivity to miglitol or any component; diabetic ketoacidosis; inflammatory bowel disease; colonic ulceration; partial intestinal obstruction; patients
(Continued)

## Miglitol *(Continued)*

predisposed to intestinal obstruction, chronic intestinal diseases associated with marked disorders of digestion or absorption, or with conditions that may deteriorate as a result of increased gas formation in the intestine

**Warnings** GI symptoms are the most common reactions. The incidence of abdominal pain and diarrhea tend to diminish considerably with continued treatment. Long-term clinical trials in diabetic patients with significant renal dysfunction (serum creatinine >2 mg/dL) have not been conducted. Treatment of these patients is not recommended. Because of its mechanism of action, miglitol administered alone should not cause hypoglycemia in the fasting of postprandial state. In combination with a sulfonylurea will cause a further lowering of blood glucose and may increase the hypoglycemic potential of the sulfonylurea.

**Drug Interactions**

**Decreased Effect:** Miglitol may decrease the absorption and bioavailability of digoxin, propranolol, and ranitidine. Digestive enzymes (amylase, pancreatin, charcoal) may reduce the effect of miglitol and should **not** be taken concomitantly.

**Adverse Reactions**

>10%: Gastrointestinal: Flatulence (41.5%), diarrhea (28.7%), abdominal pain (11.7%)

1% to 10%: Dermatologic: Rash (4.3%)

**Overdose/Toxicology** An overdose of miglitol will not result in hypoglycemia. An overdose may result in transient increases in flatulence, diarrhea, and abdominal discomfort. No serious systemic reactions are expected in the event of an overdose.

**Pharmacodynamics/Kinetics**

**Protein Binding:** Negligible (<4%)

**Half-life Elimination:** ~2 hours

**Metabolism:** Not metabolized

**Excretion:** Renal as unchanged drug

**Formulations** Tablet: 25 mg, 50 mg, 100 mg

**Dosing**

**Adults:** Oral: 25 mg 3 times/day with the first bite of food at each meal; the dose may be increased to 50 mg 3 times/day after 4-8 weeks; maximum recommended dose: 100 mg 3 times/day

**Renal Impairment:** Miglitol is primarily excreted by the kidneys; there is little information of miglitol in patients with a $Cl_{cr}$ <25 mL/minute.

**Hepatic Impairment:** No adjustment necessary.

**Administration**

**Oral:** Should be taken orally at the start (with the first bite) of each main meal.

**Monitoring Laboratory Tests** Monitor therapeutic response by periodic blood glucose tests; measurement of glycosylated hemoglobin is recommended for the monitoring of long-term glycemic control.

**Additional Nursing Issues**

**Physical Assessment:** Assess effectiveness and interactions of other medications (see Drug Interactions). See Warnings/Precautions and Contraindications for use cautions. Monitor effectiveness of therapy and monitor laboratory tests during treatment (see above). Monitor for adverse response (eg, hypoglycemia - see Adverse Reactions and Overdose/Toxicology). Assess knowledge/teach patient or refer patient to diabetic educator for instruction in appropriate use, possible side effects and appropriate interventions, and adverse symptoms to report. Note breast-feeding caution.

**Patient Information/Instruction:** Take this medication exactly as directed, with the first bite of each main meal. Do not change dosage or discontinue without first consulting prescriber. Do not take other medications with or within 2 hours of this medication unless so advised by prescriber. It is important to follow dietary and lifestyle recommendations of prescriber. You will be instructed in signs of hypo-/hyperglycemia by prescriber or diabetic educator. If combining miglitol with other diabetic medication (eg, sulfonylureas, insulin), keep source of glucose (sugar) on hand in case hypoglycemia occurs. You may experience mild side effects during first weeks of therapy (eg, bloating, flatulence, diarrhea, abdominal discomfort); these should diminish over time. Report severe or persistent side effects, fever, extended vomiting or flu, or change in color of urine or stool. **Breast-feeding precautions:** Consult prescriber if breast-feeding.

**Related Information**

Antidiabetic Oral Agents Comparison *on page 1370*


- **Migranal® Nasal Spray** *see* Dihydroergotamine *on page 374*
- **MIH** *see* Procarbazine *on page 970*
- **Miles Nervine® Caplets [OTC]** *see* Diphenhydramine *on page 381*
- **Milezzol** *see* Metronidazole *on page 763*
- **Milkinol®** *see page 1294*
- **Milk of Magnesia (Magnesium Hydroxide)** *see* Magnesium Supplements *on page 703*
- **Milliequivalent Conversions** *see page 1358*
- **Milophene®** *see* Clomiphene *on page 286*


## Milrinone (MIL ri none)

**U.S. Brand Names** Primacor®

**Therapeutic Category** Phosphodiesterase Enzyme Inhibitor

**Pregnancy Risk Factor** C

**Lactation** Excretion in breast milk unknown

**Use** Short-term I.V. therapy of congestive heart failure; calcium antagonist intoxication

**Mechanism of Action/Effect** Phosphodiesterase inhibitor resulting in vasodilation

**Contraindications** Hypersensitivity to milrinone or amrinone or any component

**Warnings** Use with caution in patients with severe obstructive aortic or pulmonic valvular disease; history of ventricular arrhythmias, atrial fibrillation, flutter; or with renal dysfunction. Pregnancy factor C.

**Adverse Reactions**

1% to 10%:

Cardiovascular: Arrhythmias, hypotension

Central nervous system: Headache

<1% (Limited to important or life-threatening symptoms): Ventricular fibrillation, chest pain, hypokalemia, thrombocytopenia

**Overdose/Toxicology** Treatment is supportive and symptomatic.

**Pharmacodynamics/Kinetics**

**Protein Binding:** ~70% in plasma

**Distribution:**

$V_d$ at steady-state following I.V. administration as a single bolus: 0.32 L/kg; not significantly bound to tissues

In patients with severe congestive heart failure (CHF), $V_d$ has been 0.33-0.47 L/kg.

**Half-life Elimination:** I.V.: 136 minutes in patients with CHF; patients with severe CHF have a more prolonged half-life, with values ranging from 1.7-2.7 hours. Patients with CHF have a reduction in the systemic clearance of milrinone, resulting in a prolonged elimination half-life. Alternatively, one study reported that 1 month of therapy with milrinone did not change the pharmacokinetic parameters for patients with CHF despite improvement in cardiac function.

**Time to Peak:**

Serum level: I.V.: Following a 125 mcg/kg dose, peak plasma concentrations of ~1000 ng/mL were observed at 2 minutes postinjection, decreasing to <100 ng/mL in 2 hours.

Therapeutic effect: Oral: Following doses of 7.5-15 mg, peak hemodynamic effects occurred at 90 minutes

Drug concentration levels:

Therapeutic:

Serum levels of 166 ng/mL, achieved during I.V. infusions of 0.25-1 mcg/kg/minute, were associated with sustained hemodynamic benefit in severe congestive heart failure patients over a 24-hour period.

Maximum beneficial effects on cardiac output and pulmonary capillary wedge pressure following I.V. infusion have been associated with plasma milrinone concentrations of 150-250 ng/mL.

Toxic: Serum concentrations >250-300 ng/mL have been associated with marked reductions in mean arterial pressure and tachycardia; however, more studies are required to determine the toxic serum levels for milrinone.

**Metabolism:** 12% hepatic

**Excretion:** Urine

**Formulations** Injection, as lactate: 1 mg/mL (5 mL, 10 mL, 20 mL)

**Dosing**

**Adults:** I.V.: Loading dose: 50 mcg/kg administered over 10 minutes followed by a maintenance dose titrated according to the hemodynamic and clinical response, see table.

| Maintenance Dosage | Dose Rate (mcg/kg/min) | Total Dose (mg/kg/24 h) |
|---|---|---|
| Minimum | 0.375 | 0.59 |
| Standard | 0.500 | 0.77 |
| Maximum | 0.750 | 1.13 |

**Elderly:** Refer to adult dosing.

**Renal Impairment:**

$Cl_{cr}$ 50 mL/minute/1.73 m$^2$: Administer 0.43 mcg/kg/minute.
$Cl_{cr}$ 40 mL/minute/1.73 m$^2$: Administer 0.38 mcg/kg/minute.
$Cl_{cr}$ 30 mL/minute/1.73 m$^2$: Administer 0.33 mcg/kg/minute.
$Cl_{cr}$ 20 mL/minute/1.73 m$^2$: Administer 0.28 mcg/kg/minute.
$Cl_{cr}$ 10 mL/minute/1.73 m$^2$: Administer 0.23 mcg/kg/minute.
$Cl_{cr}$ 5 mL/minute/1.73 m$^2$: Administer 0.2 mcg/kg/minute.

**Administration**

**I.V.:** Infuse via infusion pump.

**Stability**

**Storage:** Colorless to pale yellow solution. Store at room temperature and protect from light.

**Reconstitution:** Stable at 0.2 mg/mL in 0.9% sodium chloride or $D_5W$ for 72 hours at room temperature in normal light.

**Standardized dose**: 20 mg in 80 mL of 0.9% sodium chloride or $D_5W$ (0.2 mg/mL)

**Compatibility:** Incompatible with furosemide and procainamide. Compatible with atropine, calcium chloride, digoxin, epinephrine, lidocaine, morphine, propranolol, and sodium bicarbonate.

**Monitoring Laboratory Tests** Serum potassium

(Continued)

## Milrinone *(Continued)*

**Additional Nursing Issues**

**Physical Assessment:** Use infusion pump. Monitor cardiac/hemodynamic status continuously during therapy and serum potassium at regular intervals. **Pregnancy risk factor C.** Note breast-feeding caution.

**Patient Information/Instruction:** This drug can only be given intravenously. If you experience increased voiding call for assistance. Report pain at infusion site, numbness or tingling of extremities, or difficulty breathing. **Pregnancy/breast-feeding precautions:** Inform prescriber if you are pregnant. Consult prescriber if breast-feeding.

**Related Information**

Inotropic and Vasoconstrictor Comparison *on page 1391*

- ♦ **Miltown®** *see* Meprobamate *on page 724*
- ♦ **Mineral Oil** *see page 1294*
- ♦ **Minidyne®** *see page 1294*
- ♦ **Mini-Gamulin® Rh** *see page 1256*
- ♦ **Minims® Pilocarpine** *see* Ophthalmic Agents, Glaucoma *on page 853*
- ♦ **Minims® Pilocarpine** *see* Pilocarpine *on page 931*
- ♦ **Minipress®** *see* Prazosin *on page 958*
- ♦ **Minirin** *see* Desmopressin *on page 345*
- ♦ **Minitran® Patch** *see* Nitroglycerin *on page 831*
- ♦ **Minizide®** *see* Prazosin and Polythiazide *on page 959*
- ♦ **Minocin® IV Injection** *see* Minocycline *on this page*
- ♦ **Minocin® Oral** *see* Minocycline *on this page*

## Minocycline (mi noe SYE kleen)

**U.S. Brand Names** Dynacin® Oral; Minocin® IV Injection; Minocin® Oral

**Therapeutic Category** Antibiotic, Tetracycline Derivative

**Pregnancy Risk Factor** D

**Lactation** Enters breast milk/not recommended

**Use** Treatment of susceptible bacterial infections of both gram-negative and gram-positive organisms; acne, meningococcal carrier state

**Mechanism of Action/Effect** Inhibits bacterial protein synthesis by binding with the 30S and possibly the 50S ribosomal subunit(s) of susceptible bacteria; cell wall synthesis is not affected

**Contraindications** Hypersensitivity to minocycline, other tetracyclines, or any component; children <8 years of age; pregnancy

**Warnings** Should be avoided in renal insufficiency. Photosensitivity reactions can occur with minocycline.

**Drug Interactions**

**Decreased Effect:** Decreased effect with antacids (aluminum, calcium, zinc, or magnesium), bismuth salts, sodium bicarbonate, barbiturates, carbamazepine, hydantoins. Decreased effect of oral contraceptives.

**Increased Effect/Toxicity:** Minocycline may increase the effect of warfarin.

**Food Interactions** Minocycline serum concentrations are not altered if taken with dairy products.

**Adverse Reactions**

>10%:

Central nervous system: Dizziness, lightheadedness, unsteadiness
Dermatologic: Photosensitivity
Gastrointestinal: Nausea, diarrhea
Miscellaneous: Discoloration of teeth in children

1% to 10%:

Gastrointestinal: Pancreatitis, hypertrophy of the papilla
Hepatic: Hepatotoxicity
Miscellaneous: Superinfections (fungal overgrowth)

<1% (Limited to important or life-threatening symptoms): Pericarditis, increased intracranial pressure, bulging fontanels in infants, exfoliative dermatitis, acute renal failure, azotemia

**Overdose/Toxicology** Symptoms of overdose include diabetes insipidus, nausea, anorexia, and diarrhea. Treatment is supportive.

**Pharmacodynamics/Kinetics**

**Protein Binding:** 70% to 75%
**Distribution:** Crosses placenta; majority of a dose deposits for extended periods in fat
**Half-life Elimination:** 15 hours
**Excretion:** Urine

**Formulations**

Minocycline hydrochloride:

Capsule: 50 mg, 100 mg
Capsule (Dynacin®): 50 mg, 100 mg
Capsule, pellet-filled (Minocin®): 50 mg, 100 mg
Injection (Minocin® IV): 100 mg
Suspension, oral (Minocin®): 50 mg/5 mL (60 mL)

**Dosing**

**Adults:**

Infection: Oral, I.V.: 200 mg stat, 100 mg every 12 hours not to exceed 400 mg/24 hours

Acne: Oral: 50 mg 1-3 times/day

**Elderly:** Refer to adult dosing.

**Renal Impairment:** Not dialyzable (0% to 5%)

**Administration**

**Oral:** May be taken with food or milk.

**I.V.:** Infuse I.V. minocycline slowly, usually over a 6-hour period.

**I.V. Detail:** Avoid extravasation.

**Monitoring Laboratory Tests** Perform culture and sensitivity testing prior to initiating therapy.

**Additional Nursing Issues**

**Physical Assessment:** Monitor and/or teach patient to monitor for adverse reactions (see above) and opportunistic infections (eg, fever, purulent vaginal discharge, oral plaques, or mouth sores). Monitor I.V. infusion site closely; can be very irritating. Avoid extravasation. **Pregnancy risk factor D** - assess knowledge/teach appropriate use of barrier contraceptives. Effectiveness of oral contraceptives may be reduced by minocycline. Breast-feeding is not recommended.

**Patient Information/Instruction:** Take as directed, at regular intervals around-the-clock. May be taken with food or milk. Complete full course of therapy; do not discontinue even if condition is resolved. You may experience sensitivity to sun; avoid sun, use sunblock, or wear protective clothing. Frequent small meals may help reduce nausea, vomiting or diarrhea. If diabetic, drug may cause false tests with Clinitest® urine glucose monitoring; use of glucose oxidase methods (Clinistix®) or serum glucose monitoring is preferable. Report rash or itching, respiratory difficulty, yellowing of skin or eyes, change in color of urine or stool, fever or chills, unusual bruising or bleeding, or unresolved diarrhea. **Pregnancy/breast-feeding precautions:** Do not get pregnant while taking this medication - Oral contraceptives effectiveness may be reduced; use appropriate barrier contraceptive measures. Breast-feeding is not recommended.

**Geriatric Considerations:** Minocycline has not been studied in the elderly but its CNS effects may limit its use (see Adverse Reactions). Dose reduction for renal function not necessary.

**Additional Information**

Some formulations may contain ethanol or sulfites.

pH: 2-2.8

- **Minodiab** *see* Glipizide *on page 535*
- **Minofen®** *see* Acetaminophen *on page 32*
- **Minoxidil, Topical** *see page 1294*
- **Mintezol®** *see* Thiabendazole *on page 1119*
- **Minute-Gel®** *see page 1294*
- **Miochol-E®** *see page 1282*
- **Miostat® Intraocular** *see* Ophthalmic Agents, Glaucoma *on page 853*
- **Mirapex®** *see* Pramipexole *on page 955*
- **Mircette™** *see* Oral Contraceptives *on page 859*
- **Mireze®** *see* Nedocromil *on page 811*

## Mirtazapine (mir TAZ a peen)

**U.S. Brand Names** Remeron®

**Therapeutic Category** Antidepressant, Alpha-2 Antagonist

**Pregnancy Risk Factor** C

**Lactation** Enters breast milk/not recommended

**Use** Treatment of depression, works through noradrenergic and serotonergic pharmacologic action

**Mechanism of Action/Effect** Mirtazapine is a tetracyclic antidepressant that increases release of norepinephrine and serotonin. It does not inhibit the reuptake of norepinephrine or serotonin.

**Contraindications** Hypersensitivity to mirtazapine; use during or within 14 days of monoamine oxidase inhibitor therapy

**Warnings** Use with caution in patients with hepatic or renal dysfunction, predisposition to conditions that could be exacerbated by hypotension, history of mania or hypomania, seizure disorders, immunocompromized patients, or the elderly. Pregnancy factor C.

**Drug Interactions**

**Cytochrome P-450 Effect:** CYP1A2, 2C9, 2D6, and 3A3/4 enzyme substrate

**Increased Effect/Toxicity:** Additive impairment of cognitive and motor skills when used in conjunction with alcohol, benzodiazepines, and other CNS depressants. Possibly serious or fatal reactions can occur when given with or within 14 days of a monoamine oxidase (MAO) inhibitor.

**Adverse Reactions**

>10%:

Central nervous system: Somnolence

Endocrine & metabolic: Increased cholesterol

Gastrointestinal: Constipation, dry mouth, increased appetite, weight gain

1% to 10%:

Cardiovascular: Hypertension, vasodilatation, peripheral edema, edema

Central nervous system: Dizziness, abnormal dreams, abnormal thoughts, confusion, malaise

Endocrine & metabolic: Increased triglycerides

Gastrointestinal: Vomiting, anorexia, eructation, glossitis, cholecystitis

Genitourinary: Polyuria

(Continued)

## Mirtazapine *(Continued)*

Neuromuscular & skeletal: Myalgia, back pain, arthralgia, tremor, weakness

Respiratory: Dyspnea

Miscellaneous: Flu-like symptoms, thirst

<1% (Limited to important or life-threatening symptoms): Orthostatic hypotension, seizures (1 case reported), agranulocytosis, neutropenia, lymphadenopathy, liver function test increases

**Pharmacodynamics/Kinetics**

**Protein Binding:** 85%

**Half-life Elimination:** 20-40 hours

**Time to Peak:** 2 hours

**Metabolism:** Liver

**Excretion:** Urine and feces

**Onset:** Therapeutic effects generally in >2 weeks

**Formulations** Tablet: 15 mg, 30 mg

**Dosing**

**Adults:** Oral: Initial: 15 mg nightly, titrate up to 15-45 mg/day with dose increases made no more frequently than every 1-2 weeks.

**Elderly:** Oral: Initial: 7.5 mg/day as a single bedtime dose; increase by 7.5-15 mg/day every 1-2 weeks; usual dose: 15-30 mg/day; maximum: 45 mg/day

**Additional Nursing Issues**

**Physical Assessment:** Assess other medications patient may be taking for effectiveness and interactions (see Drug Interactions). See Warnings/Precautions for cautious use. Has potential for psychological or physiological dependence, abuse, or tolerance. Monitor therapeutic response (ie, mood, affect, mental status) and adverse reactions at beginning of therapy and periodically with long-term use (see Adverse Reactions and Overdose/Toxicology). Taper dosage slowly when discontinuing. Assess knowledge/teach patient appropriate use, interventions to reduce side effects, and adverse symptoms to report. **Pregnancy risk factor C** - benefits of use should outweigh possible risks. Breast-feeding is not recommended.

**Patient Information/Instruction:** Take exactly as directed (do not increase dose or frequency); may take 2-3 weeks to achieve desired results; may cause physical and/or psychological dependence. Take once-a-day dose at bedtime. Avoid excessive alcohol, caffeine, and other prescription or OTC medications not approved by prescriber. Maintain adequate hydration (2-3 L/day of fluids unless instructed to restrict fluid intake). You may experience drowsiness, dizziness, or lightheadedness (use caution when driving or engaging in tasks requiring alertness until response to drug is known); nausea, vomiting, anorexia, or dry mouth (small frequent meals, frequent mouth care, chewing gum, or sucking lozenges may help); or orthostatic hypotension (use caution when climbing stairs or changing position from lying or sitting to standing). Report persistent insomnia, agitation, or confusion; muscle cramping, tremors, weakness, or change in gait; breathlessness or difficulty breathing; chest pain, palpitations, or rapid heartbeat; change in urinary pattern; vision changes or eye pain; yellowing of eyes or skin; pale stools/dark urine; or worsening of condition. **Pregnancy/breast-feeding precautions:** Inform prescriber if you are or intend to be pregnant. Breast-feeding is not recommended.

**Related Information**

Antidepressant Agents Comparison *on page 1368*

## Misoprostol (mye soe PROST ole)

**U.S. Brand Names** Cytotec®

**Therapeutic Category** Prostaglandin

**Pregnancy Risk Factor** X

**Lactation** Enters breast milk/contraindicated

**Use** Prevention of NSAID-induced gastric ulcers

**Mechanism of Action/Effect** Misoprostol is a synthetic prostaglandin $E_1$ analog that replaces the protective prostaglandins consumed with prostaglandin-inhibiting therapies eg, nonsteroidal anti-inflammatory drugs

**Contraindications** Hypersensitivity to misoprostol or any component; pregnancy

**Warnings** Use with caution in patients with renal impairment and the elderly. Therapy is normally begun on the second or third day of next normal menstrual period.

**Food Interactions** Misoprostol peak serum concentrations may be decreased if taken with food.

**Adverse Reactions**

>10%: Gastrointestinal: Diarrhea, abdominal pain

1% to 10%:

Central nervous system: Headache

Gastrointestinal: Constipation, flatulence

<1% (Limited to important or life-threatening symptoms): Uterine stimulation, vaginal bleeding

**Overdose/Toxicology** Symptoms of overdose include sedation, tremor, convulsions, dyspnea, abdominal pain, diarrhea, hypotension, and bradycardia. Treatment is symptom directed and supportive.

**Pharmacodynamics/Kinetics**

**Half-life Elimination:** Parent and metabolite combined: 1.5 hours

**Time to Peak:** Active metabolite: Within 15-30 minutes

**Metabolism:** Liver

**Excretion:** Urine and feces

**Formulations** Tablet: 100 mcg, 200 mcg

**Dosing**

**Adults:** Oral: 200 mcg 4 times/day with food; if not tolerated, may decrease dose to 100 mcg 4 times/day with food or 200 mcg twice daily with food

**Elderly:** Oral: 100-200 mcg 4 times/day with food; if 200 mcg 4 times/day not tolerated, reduce to 100 mcg 4 times/day or 200 mcg twice daily with food. **Note:** To avoid the diarrhea potential, doses can be initiated at 100 mcg/day and increased 100 mcg/day at 3-day intervals until desired dose is achieved; also, recommend administering with food to decrease diarrhea incidence (see Geriatric Considerations).

**Administration**

**Oral:** Incidence of diarrhea may be lessened by having patient take dose right after meals and at bedtime.

**Additional Nursing Issues**

**Physical Assessment:** Assess knowledge/teach appropriate antiulcer diet and life-style. Monitor renal function, fluid balance (I & O, weight gain, edema). **Pregnancy risk factor X** - determine that patient is not pregnant before beginning treatment and do not give to women of childbearing age unless female is capable of complying with barrier contraceptive measures during therapy and 1 month following therapy. Breast-feeding is contraindicated.

**Patient Information/Instruction:** Take as directed; continue taking your NSAIDs while taking this medication. Take with meals or after meals to prevent nausea, diarrhea, and flatulence. Avoid using antacids. You may experience increased menstrual pain, or cramping; request analgesics. Report abnormal menstrual periods, spotting (may occur even in postmenstrual women), or severe menstrual bleeding. **Pregnancy/breast-feeding precautions:** Inform prescriber if you are pregnant. Do not get pregnant during or for 1 month following therapy. Consult prescriber for instruction on appropriate barrier contraceptive measures. This drug may cause severe fetal defects. Do not breast-feed.

**Geriatric Considerations:** Elderly, due to extensive use of NSAIDs and the high percentage of asymptomatic hemorrhage and perforation from NSAIDs, are at risk for NSAID-induced ulcers and may be candidates for misoprostol use. However, routine use for prophylaxis is not justified. Patients must be selected upon demonstration that they are at risk for NSAID-induced lesions. Misoprostol should not be used as a first-line therapy for gastric or duodenal ulcers.

- **Misoprostol and Diclofenac** *see* Diclofenac and Misoprostol *on page 360*
- **Misostol** *see* Mitoxantrone *on page 780*
- **Mithracin®** *see* Plicamycin *on page 942*
- **Mithramycin** *see* Plicamycin *on page 942*

## Mitomycin (mye toe MYE sin)

**U.S. Brand Names** Mutamycin®

**Synonyms** Mitomycin-C; MTC

**Therapeutic Category** Antineoplastic Agent, Antibiotic

**Pregnancy Risk Factor** D

**Lactation** Enters breast milk/contraindicated

**Use** Therapy of disseminated adenocarcinoma of stomach or pancreas in combination with other approved chemotherapeutic agents; bladder cancer, colorectal cancer

**Mechanism of Action/Effect** Isolated from *Streptomyces caespitosus*; acts primarily as an alkylating agent and produces DNA cross-linking (primarily with guanine and cytosine pairs); cell-cycle nonspecific; inhibits DNA and RNA synthesis by alkylation and cross-linking the strands of DNA

**Contraindications** Hypersensitivity to mitomycin or any component; platelet counts $<75,000/mm^3$; leukocyte counts $<3000/mm^3$ or serum creatinine >1.7 mg/dL; thrombocytopenia; pregnancy

**Warnings** The U.S. Food and Drug Administration (FDA) currently recommends that procedures for proper handling and disposal of antineoplastic agents be considered.

Preparation of mitomycin injection should be performed in a Class II laminar flow biologic safety cabinet. Personnel should be wearing surgical gloves and a closed front surgical gown with knit cuffs. Appropriate safety equipment is recommended for preparation, administration, and disposal of antineoplastics. If mitomycin injection contacts the skin, wash and flush thoroughly with water.

Use with caution in patients with impaired renal or hepatic function, myelosuppression. Follow hemoglobin, hematocrit, BUN, and creatinine closely after therapy especially after second and subsequent cycles. Bone marrow depression, notably thrombocytopenia and leukopenia, may contribute to the development of a secondary infection; hemolytic uremic syndrome, a serious and often fatal syndrome, has occurred in patients receiving long-term therapy and is correlated with total dose and total duration of therapy. Mitomycin is potentially carcinogenic and teratogenic.

**Drug Interactions**

**Increased Effect/Toxicity:** *Vinca* alkaloids or doxorubicin may enhance cardiac toxicity when coadministered with mitomycin.

(Continued)

## Mitomycin *(Continued)*

### Adverse Reactions

>10%:

Gastrointestinal: **Nausea and vomiting (mild to moderate) seen in almost 100% of patients**; other toxicities include stomatitis, hepatic toxicity, diarrhea, anorexia
Emetic potential: Moderate (30% to 60%)
Time course of nausea/vomiting: Onset: 1-2 hours; Duration: 48-72 hours

Hematologic: Leukopenia, thrombocytopenia; Myelosuppressive: Dose-related toxicity and may be cumulative; related to both total dose (incidence higher at doses >50 mg) and schedule, may occur at anytime within 8 weeks of treatment.
WBC: Moderate
Platelets: Severe
Onset (days): 21
Nadir (days): 36
Recovery (days): 42-56

Local: **Vesicant chemotherapy**

1% to 10%:

Dermatologic: Discolored fingernails (violet), alopecia
Gastrointestinal: Mouth ulcers
Neuromuscular & skeletal: Extremity paresthesia
Renal: Elevation of creatinine seen in 2% of patients; hemolytic uremic syndrome observed in <10% of patients and is dose-dependent (doses ≥60 mg or >50 mg/m$^2$ have higher risk)
Respiratory: Interstitial pneumonitis or pulmonary fibrosis have been noticed in 7% of patients, and it occurs independent of dosing. Manifested as dry cough and progressive dyspnea; usually is responsive to steroid therapy.

<1% (Limited to important or life-threatening symptoms): Cardiac failure (in patients treated with doses >30 mg/m$^2$), bone marrow suppression (leukopenia, thrombocytopenia), microangiopathic hemolytic anemia, thrombophlebitis

**Overdose/Toxicology** Symptoms of overdose include bone marrow suppression, nausea, vomiting, and alopecia. Treatment is symptom directed and supportive.

### Pharmacodynamics/Kinetics

**Distribution:** High drug concentrations found in kidney, tongue, muscle, heart, and lung tissue; probably not distributed into the CNS

**Half-life Elimination:** 23-78 minutes; Terminal: 50 minutes

**Metabolism:** Liver

**Excretion:** Urine and bile

**Formulations** Powder for injection: 5 mg, 20 mg, 40 mg

### Dosing

**Adults:** Refer to individual protocols.

I.V.:
Single agent therapy: 20 mg/m$^2$ every 6-8 weeks
Combination therapy: 10 mg/m$^2$ every 6-8 weeks
Bone marrow transplant:
40-50 mg/m$^2$
2-40 mg/m$^2$/day for 3 days
Total cumulative dose should not exceed 50 mg/m$^2$; see table.

| Nadir After Prior Dose/mm$^3$ | | % of Prior Dose to Be Given |
|---|---|---|
| **Leukocytes** | **Platelets** | |
| 4000 | >100,000 | 100 |
| 3000-3999 | 75,000-99,999 | 100 |
| 2000-2999 | 25,000-74,999 | 70 |
| 2000 | <25,000 | 50 |

Intravesicular instillations for bladder carcinoma: 20-40 mg/dose (1 mg/mL in sterile aqueous solution) instilled into the bladder for 3 hours repeated up to 3 times/week for up to 20 procedures per course

**Elderly:** Refer to adult dosing.

**Renal Impairment:**
$Cl_{cr}$ <10 mL/minute: Administer 75% of normal dose.
Hemodialysis effects: Unknown
CAPD effects: Unknown
CAVH effects: Unknown

### Administration

**I.V.:** Vesicant. Administer slow I.V. push by central-line only.

**I.V. Detail:** Avoid extravasation - severe local tissue necrosis occurs. Flush with 5-10 mL of I.V. solution before and after drug administration. IVPB infusions should be closely monitored for adequate vein patency.

**Extravasation management:** Care should be taken to avoid extravasation. If extravasation occurs, the site should be observed closely. These injuries frequently cause necrosis. A plastic surgery consult may be required. Few agents have been effective as antidotes, but there are reports in the literature of some benefit with dimethylsulfoxide (DSMO). Delayed dermal reactions with mitomycin are possible, even in patients who are asymptomatic at time of drug administration.

**Stability**

**Storage:** Store intact vials of lyophilized powder at room temperature.

**Reconstitution:** Solution is stable for 7 days at room temperature and 14 days at refrigeration if protected from light. Dilute powder with SWI to a concentration of 0.5 mg/mL as follows:

5 mg = 10 mL

20 mg = 40 mL

Further dilution in NS is stable for 24 hours at room temperature

**Standard I.V. dilution:**

I.V. push: Dose/syringe (concentration = 0.5 mg/mL)

Maximum syringe size for IVP is a 30 mL syringe and syringe should be ≤75% full. Syringe is stable for 7 days at room temperature and 14 days at refrigeration if protected from light.

IVPB: Dose/100 mL NS

IVPB solution is stable for 24 hours at room temperature.

**Compatibility:** See the Chemotherapy Compatibility Chart *on page 1311*.

**Monitoring Laboratory Tests** Platelet count, CBC with differential, prothrombin time, renal and pulmonary function

**Additional Nursing Issues**

**Physical Assessment:** Monitor infusion site closely for extravasation (see above). Monitor laboratory results and respiratory status on a regular basis (be alert for dyspnea, abnormal lung sounds, nonproductive cough). Monitor fluid status (I & O, edema) and monitor for opportunistic infection. **Pregnancy risk factor D** - assess knowledge/teach appropriate use of barrier contraceptives. Breast-feeding is contraindicated.

**Patient Information/Instruction:** This drug can only be given I.V. Make note of scheduled return dates. Maintain adequate hydration (2-3 L/day of fluids unless instructed to restrict fluid intake) and nutrition. You may experience, rash, skin lesions, loss of hair, or permanent sterility. Small frequent meals may help if you experience nausea, vomiting, loss of appetite. Frequent mouth care will help reduce the incidence of mouth sores. Use caution when driving or engaging in tasks that require alertness because you may experience dizziness, drowsiness, syncope, or blurred vision. Report difficulty breathing, swelling of extremities, or sudden weight gain; burning, pain, or redness at infusion site; unusual bruising or bleeding; pain on urination; or other adverse effects. **Pregnancy/breast-feeding precautions:** Do not get pregnant while taking this medication; use appropriate barrier contraceptive measures. Do not breast-feed.

♦ **Mitomycin-C** *see* Mitomycin *on page 777*

## Mitotane (MYE toe tane)

**U.S. Brand Names** Lysodren®

**Synonyms** o,p′-DDD

**Therapeutic Category** Antineoplastic Agent, Miscellaneous

**Pregnancy Risk Factor** C

**Lactation** Enters breast milk/contraindicated

**Use** Treatment of inoperable adrenal cortical carcinoma

**Mechanism of Action/Effect** Causes adrenal cortical atrophy; drug affects mitochondria in adrenal cortical cells and decreases production of cortisol; also alters the peripheral metabolism of steroids

**Contraindications** Hypersensitivity to mitotane or any component

**Warnings** The U.S. Food and Drug Administration (FDA) currently recommends that procedures for proper handling and disposal of antineoplastic agents be considered. Patients should be hospitalized when mitotane therapy is initiated until a stable dose regimen is established. Discontinue temporarily following trauma or shock since the prime action of mitotane is adrenal suppression. Exogenous steroids may be indicated since adrenal function may not start immediately. Administer with care to patients with severe hepatic impairment. Observe patients for neurotoxicity with prolonged (2 years) use. Pregnancy factor C.

**Drug Interactions**

**Decreased Effect:** Mitotane may enhance the clearance of barbiturates and warfarin by induction of the hepatic microsomal enzyme system resulting in a decreased effect. Coadministration of spironolactone has resulted in negation of mitotane's effect. Mitotane may increase clearance of phenytoin by microsomal enzyme stimulation.

**Increased Effect/Toxicity:** CNS depressants taken with mitotane may enhance CNS depression.

**Adverse Reactions**

>10%:

Central nervous system: Vertigo, mental depression, dizziness; all are reversible with discontinuation of the drug and can occur in 15% to 26% of patients

Dermatologic: Rash (15%) which may subside without discontinuation of therapy, hyperpigmentation

Gastrointestinal: 75% to 80% will experience nausea, vomiting, and anorexia; diarrhea can occur in 20% of patients

Ocular: Diplopia, visual disturbances, blurred vision (reversible with discontinuation)

1% to 10%:

Cardiovascular: Orthostatic hypotension

Central nervous system: Fever

Endocrine & metabolic: Flushing of skin

Genitourinary: Hemorrhagic cystitis

(Continued)

## Mitotane *(Continued)*

Neuromuscular & skeletal: Myalgia

Ocular: Diplopia, lens opacities, toxic retinopathy

<1% (Limited to important or life-threatening symptoms): Hypertension, flushing, hypercholesterolemia, tremor, weakness, hypouricemia, hematuria, albuminuria, shortness of breath, wheezing

**Overdose/Toxicology** Symptoms of overdose include diarrhea, vomiting, numbness of limbs, and weakness. Treatment is symptom directed and supportive.

**Pharmacodynamics/Kinetics**

**Distribution:** Stored mainly in fat tissue but is found in all body tissues

**Half-life Elimination:** 18-159 days

**Time to Peak:** Within 3-5 hours

**Metabolism:** Liver and other tissues

**Excretion:** Urine and bile

**Formulations** Tablet: 500 mg

**Dosing**

**Adults:** Oral: Start at 1-6 g/day in divided doses, then increase incrementally to 8-10 g/day in 3-4 divided doses; dose is changed on basis of side effect with aim of giving as high a dose as tolerated; maximum daily dose: 18 g

**Hepatic Impairment:** Dose may need to be decreased in patients with liver disease.

**Stability**

**Storage:** Protect from light. Store at room temperature.

**Additional Nursing Issues**

**Physical Assessment:** Monitor for effectiveness of therapy and adverse reactions to drug (see Adverse Reactions). Assess knowledge/teach patient to maintain adequate nutrition and hydration, and to monitor and report changes in blood pressure, hepatic function, CNS, and signs of adrenal insufficiency (weakness, lethargy, anorexia, weight loss). **Pregnancy risk factor C** - contraceptive education is advisable. Breast-feeding is contraindicated.

**Patient Information/Instruction:** Desired effects of this drug may not be seen for 2-3 months. Wear identification that alerts medical personnel that you are taking this drug in event of shock or trauma. Maintain adequate hydration (2-3 L/day of fluids unless instructed to restrict fluid intake) and nutrition. Avoid alcohol or OTC medications unless approved by prescriber. May cause dizziness and vertigo (avoid driving or performing tasks requiring alertness until response to drug is known); nausea, vomiting, or loss of appetite (small frequent meals, frequent mouth care, sucking lozenges, or chewing gum may help); orthostatic hypotension (use caution when rising from sitting or lying position or climbing stairs); muscle aches or pain (if severe, request medication from prescriber). Report severe vomiting or acute loss of appetite, muscular twitching, fever or infection, blood in urine or pain on urinating, or darkening of skin. **Pregnancy/breast-feeding precautions:** Inform prescriber if you are or intend to be pregnant. Do not breast-feed.

## Mitoxantrone (mye toe ZAN trone)

**U.S. Brand Names** Novantrone®

**Synonyms** DHAD

**Therapeutic Category** Antineoplastic Agent, Antibiotic

**Pregnancy Risk Factor** D

**Lactation** Enters breast milk/contraindicated

**Use** FDA approved for the treatment of acute nonlymphocytic leukemia (ANLL) in adults; mitoxantrone is also found to be very active against various leukemias, lymphoma, and breast cancer, and moderately active against pediatric sarcoma

**Mechanism of Action/Effect** Analogue of the anthracyclines, but different in mechanism of action, cardiac toxicity, and potential for tissue necrosis; inhibits DNA and RNA synthesis

**Contraindications** Hypersensitivity to mitoxantrone or any component; pregnancy

**Warnings** Not for intra-arterial or intrathecal injection. The FDA currently recommends that procedures for proper handling and disposal of antineoplastic agents be considered.

Mitoxantrone preparation should be performed in a Class II laminar flow biologic safety cabinet. Personnel should be wearing surgical gloves and a closed front surgical gown with knit cuffs. Appropriate safety equipment is recommended for preparation, administration, and disposal of antineoplastics. If mitoxantrone contacts the skin, wash and flush thoroughly with water. Dosage should be reduced in patients with impaired hepatobiliary function; use with caution in patients with pre-existing myelosuppression. Predisposing factors for mitoxantrone-induced cardiotoxicity include prior anthracycline therapy, prior cardiovascular disease, and mediastinal irradiation. The risk of developing cardiotoxicity is <3% when the cumulative doses are <100-120 mg/m$^2$ in patients with predisposing factors and <160 mg/m$^2$ in patients with no predisposing factors.

**Adverse Reactions**

>10%:

Central nervous system: Headache

Dermatologic: Alopecia

Gastrointestinal: Nausea, vomiting, diarrhea, abdominal pain, mucositis, stomatitis, GI bleeding

Hematologic: Leukopenia

Emetic potential: Moderate (31% to 72%)

Genitourinary: Discoloration of urine (blue-green)

Hepatic: Abnormal LFTs

Respiratory: Coughing, shortness of breath

1% to 10%:

Cardiovascular: Arrhythmias, congestive heart failure, hypotension

Central nervous system: Seizures, fever

Dermatologic: Pruritus, skin desquamation

Hematologic: Myelosuppressive effects of chemotherapy:

WBC: Mild

Platelets: Mild

Onset (days): 7-10

Nadir (days): 14

Recovery (days): 21

Hepatic: Transient elevation of liver enzymes, jaundice

Ocular: Conjunctivitis

Renal: Renal failure

Local: Pain or redness at injection site

**Irritant chemotherapy** with blue skin discoloration

**BMT:**

Cardiovascular: Bradycardia (infusion-related), heart failure

Dermatologic: Alopecia

Gastrointestinal: Severe mucositis, skin discoloration

**Overdose/Toxicology** Symptoms of overdose include leukopenia, tachycardia, and marrow hypoplasia. No known antidote. Treatment is symptom directed and supportive.

**Pharmacodynamics/Kinetics**

**Protein Binding:** Protein binding: >95%; Albumin binding: 76%

**Distribution:** Distributes into pleural fluid, kidney, thyroid, liver, heart, and red blood cells

**Half-life Elimination:** 37 hours; may be prolonged with liver impairment

**Metabolism:** Liver

**Excretion:** Urine and bile

**Formulations** Injection, as base: 2 mg/mL (10 mL, 12.5 mL, 15 mL)

**Dosing**

**Adults:** Refer to individual protocols; I.V. (may dilute in $D_5W$ or NS):

ANLL leukemias: 12 mg/m²/day once daily for 3 days; acute leukemia in relapse: 8-12 mg/m²/day once daily for 4-5 days

Solid tumors: 12-14 mg/m² every 3-4 weeks **or** 2-4 mg/m²/day for 5 days

Maximum total dose: 80-120 mg/m² in patients with predisposing factor and <160 mg in patients with no predisposing factor

BMT high dose: I.V.: 24-48 mg/m² as a single dose; duration of infusion is 1-4 hours; generally combined with other high-dose chemotherapeutic drugs.

**Dose modifications are based on degree of leukopenia or thrombocytopenia.** See table.

| Granulocyte Count Nadir (cells/mm³) | Platelet Count Nadir (cells/mm³) | Total Bilirubin (mg/dL) | Dose Adjustment |
|---|---|---|---|
| >2000 | >150,000 | <1.5 | Increase by 1 mg/m² |
| 1000-2000 | 75,000-150,000 | <1.5 | Maintain same dose |
| <1000 | <75,000 | 1.5-3 | Decrease by 1 mg/m² |

**Elderly:** Refer to adult dosing.

**Hepatic Impairment:** Official dosage adjustment recommendations have not been established.

Moderate dysfunction (bilirubin 1.5-3 mg/dL): Some clinicians recommend a 50% dosage reduction.

Severe dysfunction (bilirubin >3.0 mg/dL) have a lower total body clearance and may require a dosage adjustment to 8 mg/m²; some clinicians recommend a dosage reduction to 25% of dose.

**Dose modifications based on degree of leukopenia or thrombocytopenia**; see table.

**Administration**

**I.V.:** Irritant. Do **not** give I.V. bolus over <3 minutes; can be administered I.V. intermittent infusion over 15-30 minutes.

**I.V. Detail:** Avoid extravasation - although has not generally been proven to be a vesicant.

**BMT only:** Extensive pretreatment with anthracyclines increases risk of cardiac toxicity.

**Stability**

**Storage:** Store intact vials at room temperature or refrigeration.

**Reconstitution:** Dilute in at least 50 mL of NS or $D_5W$. Solution is stable for 7 days at room temperature or refrigeration.

**Standard I.V. dilution:** IVPB: Dose/100 mL $D_5W$ or NS

Solution is stable for 7 days at room temperature and refrigeration.

**Compatibility:** Do not mix with any other drugs. Incompatible with heparin and hydrocortisone. See the Chemotherapy Compatibility Chart *on page 1311*.

**Monitoring Laboratory Tests** CBC, serum uric acid, liver function, ECHO

(Continued)

## Mitoxantrone *(Continued)*

**Additional Nursing Issues**

**Physical Assessment:** Monitor laboratory tests results on a regular basis (especially uric acid levels). Monitor infusion site for extravasation. Monitor EKG, peripheral circulation, blood pressure, and CNS status prior to and frequently during therapy. Assess for opportunistic infections (eg, persistent fever, malaise, sore throat, unusual bleeding or bruising). **Pregnancy risk factor D.** Breast-feeding is contraindicated.

**Patient Information/Instruction:** This drug can only be given I.V. Make note of scheduled return dates. Your urine may turn blue-green for 24 hours after infusion and the whites of your eyes may have a blue-green tinge; this is normal. Maintain adequate hydration (2-3 L/day of fluids unless instructed to restrict fluid intake) and nutrition. You may experience rash, skin lesions, or loss of hair. Small frequent meals may help if you experience nausea, vomiting, or loss of appetite. Frequent mouth care will help reduce the incidence of mouth sores. Use caution when driving or engaging in tasks that require alertness because you may experience dizziness, drowsiness, syncope, or blurred vision. Report chest pain or heart palpitations; difficulty breathing or constant cough; swelling of extremities or sudden weight gain; burning, pain, or redness at infusion site; persistent fever or chills; unusual bruising or bleeding; twitching or tremors; or pain on urination. **Pregnancy/breast-feeding precautions:** Do not get pregnant while taking this medication. Do not breast-feed.

- ♦ **Mitran® Oral** *see* Chlordiazepoxide *on page 250*
- ♦ **Mitroken** *see* Ciprofloxacin *on page 270*
- ♦ **Mitrolan® Chewable Tablet** *see page 1294*
- ♦ **MK383** *see* Tirofiban *on page 1141*
- ♦ **MK462** *see* Rizatriptan *on page 1033*
- ♦ **MK594** *see* Losartan *on page 693*
- ♦ **MMR** *see page 1256*
- ♦ **M-M-R® II** *see page 1256*
- ♦ **Moban®** *see* Molindone *on page 785*
- ♦ **Mobenol®** *see* Tolbutamide *on page 1146*

## Modafinil (moe DAF i nil)

**U.S. Brand Names** Provigil®

**Therapeutic Category** Central Nervous System Stimulant, Nonamphetamine

**Pregnancy Risk Factor** C

**Lactation** Excretion in breast milk unknown/use caution

**Use** Improve wakefulness in patients with excessive daytime sleepiness associated with narcolepsy

**Mechanism of Action/Effect** The mechanism(s) of action for modafinil have not been defined. It does not appear to stimulate receptors commonly associated with sleep/wake regulation (including norepinephrine, serotonin, melatonin, GABA, dopamine, adenosine, and histamine-3 receptors).

**Contraindications** Hypersensitivity to modafinil or any component; history of angina, ischemic EKG changes, left ventricular hypertrophy, or clinically significant mitral valve prolapse associated with CNS stimulant use

**Warnings** Caution when operating machinery or driving. Although functional impairment has not been demonstrated for modafinil, any agent affecting the CNS may alter judgment, thinking, or motor skills. Use with caution in patients with a recent history of myocardial infarction, unstable angina, hypertension, or history of psychosis. Efficacy of oral contraceptives may be reduced - use alternative contraceptive measures. Prolonged administration may lead to drug dependence.

**Drug Interactions**

**Cytochrome P-450 Effect:** CYP3A4 enzyme substrate; CYP1A2, CYP2B6, and CYP3A4 enzyme inducer

**Decreased Effect:** Modafinil may induce its own metabolism. Coadministration with other substrates of CYP3A4 such as oral contraceptives, cyclosporine, and (to a limited degree) theophylline may result in decreased serum concentrations/efficacy of these agents. Agents which induce CYP3A4, including phenobarbital, carbamazepine, and rifampin, may result in decreased concentrations of modafinil.

**Increased Effect/Toxicity:** Coadministration with drugs metabolized by CYP2C19, including diazepam, phenytoin, and propranolol, may result in increased serum concentrations/toxicity from these agents. In populations deficient in CYP2D6, where CYP2C19 acts as a secondary metabolic pathway, concentrations of agents such as tricyclic antidepressants and SSRIs may be increased during coadministration. Clomipramine concentrations may be increased.

Modafinil may suppress CYP2C9, potentially increasing the concentrations/toxicity of agents metabolized by this isoenzyme, including warfarin and phenytoin.

Agents which inhibit CYP3A4, including ketoconazole and itraconazole, may result in increased concentrations/toxicity of modafinil.

**Adverse Reactions** Limited to events which were equal to or greater than placebo:

1% to 10%:

Cardiovascular: Chest pain (2%), hypertension (2%), hypotension (2%), vasodilation (1%), arrhythmia (1%), syncope (1%)

Central nervous system: Nervousness (8%), dizziness (5%), depression (4%), anxiety (4%), cataplexy (3%), insomnia (3%), dyskinesia (2%), chills (2%), fever (1%), confusion (1%), amnesia (1%), emotional lability (1%), ataxia (1%)

Dermatologic: Dry skin (1%)

Endocrine & metabolic: Hyperglycemia (1%), albuminuria (1%)
Gastrointestinal: Diarrhea (8%), dry mouth (5%), anorexia (5%), vomiting (1%), mouth ulceration (1%), gingivitis (1%)
Genitourinary: Abnormal urine (1%), urinary retention (1%), ejaculatory disturbance (1%)
Hematologic: Eosinophilia (1%)
Hepatic: Abnormal liver function (3%), elevated GGT
Neuromuscular & skeletal: Neck pain (2%), hypertonia (2%), neck rigidity (1%), joint disorder (1%), tremor (1%), paresthesia (3%)
Ocular: Amblyopia (2%), abnormal vision (2%)
Respiratory: Pharyngitis (6%), lung disorder (4%), dyspnea (2%), asthma (1%), epistaxis (1%)

**Overdose/Toxicology** Symptoms of overdose include agitation, irritability, aggressiveness, confusion, nervousness, tremor, insomnia, palpitations, and elevations in hemodynamic parameters. Treatment is symptomatic and supportive. Cardiac monitoring is warranted.

**Pharmacodynamics/Kinetics**

**Protein Binding:** 60% (albumin)

**Half-life Elimination:** 15 hours

**Time to Peak:** 2-4 hours

**Metabolism:** Hepatic, multiple pathways including cytochrome P-450 isoenzyme 3A4; may induce its own metabolism

**Excretion:** Renal, as metabolites (<10% excreted unchanged)

**Formulations** Tablet: 100 mg, 200 mg

**Dosing**

**Adults:** Oral: Initial: 200 mg as a single daily dose

**Elderly:** Lower doses are recommended due to decreased metabolite elimination.

**Renal Impairment:** Data is not available for dosage recommendations in severe renal failure.

**Hepatic Impairment:** Reduce dose by 50%.

**Additional Nursing Issues**

**Physical Assessment:** See Contraindications and Warnings/Precautions for use cautions. Assess effectiveness and interactions of other medications, especially those that are metabolized by P-450 enzymes (see Drug Interactions). Note that modafinil has potential for abuse; caution patient about inappropriate or overuse. Assess knowledge/teach patient possible side effects/interventions, and adverse symptoms to report (see Adverse Reaction). **Pregnancy risk factor C** - benefits of use should outweigh possible risks. Note breast-feeding caution.

**Patient Information/Instruction:** Take exactly as prescribed; do not exceed recommended dosage without consulting prescriber. Maintain healthy sleep hygiene. Do not share medication with anyone else. Void before taking medication. You may experience headache, nervousness, confusion, or dizziness (use caution when driving or engaging in tasks requiring alertness until response to drug is known); diarrhea (yogurt or buttermilk may help); or dry mouth or sore mouth, loss of appetite, or vomiting (small frequent meals, frequent mouth care, chewing gum, or sucking lozenges may help). Diabetics should monitor glucose levels closely. Report chest pain or palpitations; difficulty breathing; excessive insomnia, CNS agitation, depression, or memory disturbances; vision changes; changes in urinary pattern or ejaculation disturbances; or persistent joint pain or stiffness. **Pregnancy/breast-feeding precautions:** Inform prescriber if you are or intend to be pregnant. Consult prescriber if breast-feeding.

**Pregnancy Issues:** Embryotoxicity has been observed in animal models (at threshold dosages above those employed therapeutically). There are no controlled studies in humans; should be used in pregnancy only if potential benefit exceeds risk.

- **Modane® Bulk [OTC]** *see* Psyllium *on page 993*
- **Modane® Plus Tablet** *see page 1294*
- **Modane® Soft [OTC]** *see* Docusate *on page 392*
- **Modecate®** *see* Fluphenazine *on page 505*
- **Modecate® Enanthate** *see* Fluphenazine *on page 505*
- **Modicon™** *see* Oral Contraceptives *on page 859*
- **Modified Dakin's Solution** *see* Sodium Hypochlorite Solution *on page 1063*
- **Modified Shohl's Solution** *see* Sodium Citrate and Citric Acid *on page 1063*
- **Moditen® Hydrochloride** *see* Fluphenazine *on page 505*
- **Moducal®** *see page 1294*
- **Moduret®** *see* Amiloride and Hydrochlorothiazide *on page 68*
- **Moduretic®** *see* Amiloride and Hydrochlorothiazide *on page 68*

## Moexipril (mo EKS i pril)

**U.S. Brand Names** Univasc®

**Therapeutic Category** Angiotensin-Converting Enzyme (ACE) Inhibitors

**Pregnancy Risk Factor** C/D (2nd and 3rd trimesters)

**Lactation** Excretion in breast milk unknown

**Use** Treatment of hypertension, alone or in combination with thiazide diuretics

**Mechanism of Action/Effect** Competitive inhibitor of angiotensin-converting enzyme (ACE); prevents conversion of angiotensin I to angiotensin II, a potent vasoconstrictor; results in lower levels of angiotensin II which causes an increase in plasma renin activity and a reduction in aldosterone secretion

(Continued)

## Moexipril *(Continued)*

**Contraindications** Hypersensitivity to moexipril, moexiprilat, or any component; hypersensitivity or allergic reactions or angioedema related to an ACE inhibitor; pregnancy (2nd and 3rd trimesters)

**Warnings** Use with caution and modify dosage in patients with renal impairment especially renal artery stenosis, severe congestive heart failure, or with coadministered diuretic therapy. Experience in children is limited. Severe hypotension may occur in patients who are sodium and/or volume depleted. Initiate lower doses and monitor closely when starting therapy in these patients. ACE inhibitors may be preferred agents in elderly patients with congestive heart failure and diabetes mellitus (diabetic proteinuria is reduced, minimal CNS effects, and enhanced insulin sensitivity), however, due to decreased renal function, tolerance must be carefully monitored. If possible, discontinue the diuretic 2-3 days prior to initiating moexipril in patients receiving them to reduce the risk of symptomatic hypotension. Pregnancy factor C/D (2nd and 3rd trimesters).

**Drug Interactions**

**Decreased Effect:** Rifampin may decrease the effect of ACE inhibitors. Antacids may decrease the bioavailability of ACE inhibitors, may be more likely to occur with captopril, separate administration times by 1-2 hours. NSAIDs, specifically indomethacin, may reduce the hypotensive effects of ACE inhibitors. More likely to occur in low renin or volume dependent hypertensive patients.

**Increased Effect/Toxicity:** Diuretics have additive hypotensive effects with ACE inhibitors. Probenecid increases blood levels of captopril which may occur in other ACE inhibitors. Phenothiazines taken with ACE inhibitors may increase the pharmacologic effects of the ACE inhibitor. Allopurinol and ACE inhibitors may cause a higher risk of hypersensitivity reaction when taken concurrently. Digoxin and ACE inhibitors may result in elevated serum digoxin levels. Lithium and ACE inhibitors may result in elevated serum levels of lithium with symptoms of toxicity. Potassium supplements or potassium-sparing diuretics with ACE inhibitors may result in elevated serum potassium levels.

**Effects on Lab Values** ↑ BUN, creatinine, potassium, positive Coombs' [direct]; ↓ cholesterol (S); may cause false-positive results in urine acetone determinations using sodium nitroprusside reagent

**Adverse Reactions**

1% to 10%:

Cardiovascular: Hypotension, peripheral edema
Central nervous system: Headache, dizziness, fatigue
Dermatologic: Rash, alopecia, flushing, rash
Endocrine & metabolic: Hyperkalemia
Gastrointestinal: Diarrhea, nausea, heartburn
Genitourinary: Polyuria
Neuromuscular & skeletal: Myalgia
Renal: Reversible increases in creatinine or BUN
Respiratory: Cough, pharyngitis, upper respiratory infection, sinusitis

<1% (Limited to important or life-threatening symptoms): Chest pain, myocardial infarction, palpitations, arrhythmias, syncope, cerebrovascular accident, orthostatic hypotension, hypercholesterolemia, anemia, elevated LFTs, hepatitis, oliguria, proteinuria, bronchospasm, dyspnea, eosinophilic pneumonitis

**Overdose/Toxicology** Mild hypotension has been the primary toxic effect seen with acute overdose. Bradycardia may also occur. Hyperkalemia occurs even with therapeutic doses, especially in patients with renal insufficiency and those taking NSAIDs. Treatment is symptom directed and supportive.

**Pharmacodynamics/Kinetics**

**Protein Binding:** Moexipril: 90%; Moexiprilat: 50% to 70%

**Half-life Elimination:** Moexipril: 1 hour; Moexiprilat: 2-10 hours

**Time to Peak:** 1-2 hours

**Metabolism:** Liver

**Excretion:** Feces

**Duration:** >24 hours

**Formulations** Tablet, as hydrochloride: 7.5 mg, 15 mg

**Dosing**

**Adults:** Oral: Initial: 7.5 mg once daily (in patients **not** receiving diuretics), 1 hour prior to a meal **or** 3.75 mg once daily (when combined with thiazide diuretics); maintenance dose: 7.5-30 mg/day in 1 or 2 divided doses 1 hour before meals

**Elderly:** Dose the same as adults; adjust for renal impairment. Tablet may be cut in half (3.75 mg) for starting therapy (see Renal Impairment and Additional Information).

**Renal Impairment:** $Cl_{cr}$ ≤40 mL/minute: Patients may be cautiously placed on 3.75 mg once daily, then upwardly titrated to a maximum of 15 mg/day.

**Administration**

**Oral:** Food may delay and reduce peak serum levels; take on an empty stomach, if possible.

**Monitoring Laboratory Tests** Electrolytes, CBC, renal function

**Additional Nursing Issues**

**Physical Assessment:** Assess effectiveness and interactions of other medications (see Drug Interactions). See Warnings/Precautions and Contraindications for use cautions. Monitor effectiveness of therapy, laboratory tests, and adverse response on a regular basis during therapy (see Adverse Reactions and Overdose/Toxicology). Assess knowledge/teach patient appropriate use, possible side effects and appropriate interventions, and adverse symptoms to report. **Pregnancy risk factor C/D** -

see Pregnancy Risk Factor - assess knowledge/teach patient use of barrier contraceptives. Note breast-feeding caution. See Pregnancy Issues.

**Patient Information/Instruction:** Take exactly as directed; do not discontinue without consulting prescriber. Take first dose at bedtime. This drug does not eliminate need for diet or exercise regimen as recommended by prescriber. Do not take potassium supplements or salt substitutes containing potassium without consulting prescriber. May cause dizziness, fainting, lightheadedness (use caution when driving or engaging in tasks that require alertness until response to drug is known); postural hypotension (use caution when rising from lying or sitting position or climbing stairs); nausea, vomiting, abdominal pain, dry mouth, or transient loss of appetite (small frequent meals, frequent mouth care, sucking lozenges, or chewing gum may help) - report if these persist. Report chest pain or palpitations; difficulty in breathing or unusual cough; or other persistent adverse reactions. **Pregnancy/breast-feeding precautions:** Do not get pregnant while taking this medication; use appropriate barrier contraceptive measures. If you are, or plan to be pregnant, notify your prescriber at once. Consult prescriber if breast-feeding.

**Geriatric Considerations:** Due to frequent decreases in glomerular filtration (also creatinine clearance) with aging, elderly patients may have exaggerated responses to ACE inhibitors. Differences in clinical response due to hepatic changes are not observed.

**Pregnancy Issues:** ACE inhibitors can cause fetal injury or death if taken during the 2nd or 3rd trimester. Discontinue ACE inhibitors as soon as pregnancy is detected. ACE inhibitors should not be used if patient is sexually active and not using contraceptives.

**Additional Information** The antihypertensive effect of moexipril may decrease towards the end of the dosing interval; blood pressure should be monitored prior to dosing. If blood pressure control is not adequate, an increased dose or divided dose may be attempted. Moexipril offers no therapeutic advantage over other ACE inhibitors. To reduce the risk of hypotension, discontinue therapy 2-3 days prior to starting moexipril if possible. If diuretics cannot be stopped for a short period, initiate dose at 3.75 mg/day.

**Related Information**

ACE Inhibitors and Angiotensin Antagonists Comparison *on page 1362*

## Moexipril and Hydrochlorothiazide

(mo EKS i pril & hye droe klor oh THYE a zide)

**U.S. Brand Names** Uniretic™

**Therapeutic Category** Antihypertensive Agent, Combination

**Pregnancy Risk Factor** C/D (2nd and 3rd trimesters)

**Lactation** Enters breast milk/use caution

**Use** Combination therapy for hypertension, however, not indicated for initial treatment of hypertension; replacement therapy in patients receiving separate dosage forms (for patient convenience); when monotherapy with one component fails to achieve desired antihypertensive effect, or when dose-limiting adverse effects limit upward titration of monotherapy

**Formulations** Tablet:

Moexipril hydrochloride 7.5 mg and hydrochlorothiazide 12.5 mg
Moexipril hydrochloride 15 mg and hydrochlorothiazide 25 mg

**Dosing**

**Adults:** Oral: A patient who is not adequately controlled on either medication alone may be started on either Uniretic™ 7.5/12.5 or Uniretic™ 15/25 once daily (taken 1 hour before a meal). Additional dosage titration may be based on clinical response. The maximum dose evaluated in clinical studies was 30 mg/50 mg.

**Note:** Patients receiving moexipril and hydrochlorothiazide in separate tablets may wish to receive Uniretic™ at equivalent dosages once daily.

**Elderly:** Overall safety and efficacy are not different in elderly patients, although a higher moexipril AUC was observed in elderly patients. Greater sensitivity to effects may be observed in some older individuals. See adult dosing.

**Additional Nursing Issues**

**Physical Assessment:** See individual components listed in Related Information. **Pregnancy risk factor C/D** - see Pregnancy Risk Factor - assess knowledge/instruct patient on need to use appropriate contraceptive measures and the need to avoid pregnancy. Note breast-feeding caution.

**Patient Information/Instruction:** See individual components listed in Related Information. **Pregnancy/breast-feeding precautions:** Inform prescriber if you are or intend to be pregnant. Consult prescriber if breast-feeding.

**Related Information**

Hydrochlorothiazide *on page 566*
Moexipril *on page 783*

♦ **Moi-Stir®** *see page 1294*

♦ **Moisture® Ophthalmic Drops** *see page 1294*

## Molindone (moe LIN done)

**U.S. Brand Names** Moban®

**Therapeutic Category** Antipsychotic Agent, Dihydoindoline

**Pregnancy Risk Factor** C

**Lactation** Excretion in breast milk unknown

**Use** Management of psychotic disorder

**Mechanism of Action/Effect** Mechanism of action mimics that of chlorpromazine; however, it produces more extrapyramidal effects and less sedation than chlorpromazine

(Continued)

## Molindone *(Continued)*

**Contraindications** Hypersensitivity to molindone or any component (cross reactivity between phenothiazines may occur); severe CNS depression; coma

**Warnings** May be sedating, use with caution in disorders where CNS depression is a feature. Use with caution in Parkinson's disease. Use with caution in patients with hemodynamic instability; bone marrow suppression; predisposition to seizures; subcortical brain damage; or severe cardiac, hepatic, renal, or respiratory disease. May cause swallowing difficulties. Use with caution in breast cancer or other prolactin-dependent tumors (may elevate prolactin levels). May alter temperature regulation or mask toxicity of other drugs due to antiemetic effects. May alter cardiac conduction - life-threatening arrhythmias have occurred with therapeutic doses of neuroleptics. May cause orthostatic hypotension.

May cause anticholinergic effects (eg, confusion, agitation, constipation, dry mouth, blurred vision, urinary retention); therefore, use with caution in patients with decreased gastrointestinal motility, urinary retention, BPH, xerostomia, or visual problems. Conditions which also may be exacerbated by cholinergic blockade include narrow-angle glaucoma (screening is recommended) and worsening of myasthenia gravis. Relative to other neuroleptics, molindone has a low potency of cholinergic blockade.

May cause extrapyramidal reactions including pseudoparkinsonism, acute dystonic reactions, akathisia, and tardive dyskinesia (risk of these reactions is high relative to other neuroleptics). May be associated with neuroleptic malignant syndrome (NMS) or pigmentary retinopathy.

Pregnancy factor C.

**Drug Interactions**

**Cytochrome P-450 Effect:** CYP2D6 enzyme substrate

**Increased Effect/Toxicity:** Increased toxicity with CNS depressants, antihypertensives, and anticonvulsants.

**Adverse Reactions**

>10%:

- Cardiovascular: Orthostatic hypotension
- Central nervous system: Akathisia, extrapyramidal effects, persistent tardive dyskinesia
- Gastrointestinal: Constipation, dry mouth
- Ocular: Blurred vision
- Miscellaneous: Decreased sweating

1% to 10%:

- Central nervous system: Mental depression, altered central temperature regulation
- Endocrine & metabolic: Change in menstrual periods, swelling of breasts

<1% (Limited to important or life-threatening symptoms): Tachycardia, arrhythmias, seizures, neuroleptic malignant syndrome (NMS), agranulocytosis (more often in women between fourth and tenth weeks of therapy), leukopenia (usually in patients with large doses for prolonged periods)

**Overdose/Toxicology** Symptoms of overdose include deep sleep, extrapyramidal symptoms, cardiac arrhythmias, seizures, and hypotension. Treatment is symptom directed and supportive.

**Pharmacodynamics/Kinetics**

**Half-life Elimination:** 1.5 hours

**Time to Peak:** 1.5 hours

**Metabolism:** Liver

**Excretion:** Urine and feces (90% within 24 hours)

**Formulations**

Molindone hydrochloride:

- Concentrate, oral: 20 mg/mL (120 mL)
- Tablet: 5 mg, 10 mg, 25 mg, 50 mg, 100 mg

**Dosing**

**Adults:** Oral: 50-75 mg/day increase at 3- to 4-day intervals up to 225 mg/day

**Elderly:** Oral: Nonpsychotic patients, dementia behavior: Initial: 5-10 mg 1-2 times/day; increase at 4- to 7-day intervals by 5-10 mg/day; increase dosing intervals (bid, tid, etc) as necessary to control response or side effects. Maximum daily dose: 112 mg; gradual increases (titration) may prevent some side effects or decrease their severity.

**Monitoring Laboratory Tests** Baseline liver and kidney function, CBC prior to and periodically during therapy, ophthalmic screening

**Additional Nursing Issues**

**Physical Assessment:** Assess other medications patient is taking for effectiveness and interactions (see Drug Interactions). See Contraindications and Warnings/Precautions for cautious use. Has potential for psychological or physiological dependence, abuse, and tolerance. Review ophthalmic screening and monitor laboratory results (see above), therapeutic response (mental status, mood, affect), and adverse reactions at beginning of therapy and periodically with long-term use (orthostatic hypotension, anticholinergic response, extrapyramidal effects - see Adverse Reactions and Overdose/Toxicology). Initiate at lower doses (see Dosing) and taper dosage slowly when discontinuing. Assess knowledge/teach patient appropriate use, interventions to reduce side effects, and adverse symptoms to report (see below). **Pregnancy risk factor C** - benefits of use should outweigh possible risks. Note breast-feeding caution.

**Patient Information/Instruction:** Use exactly as directed (do not increase dose or frequency); may cause physical and/or psychological dependence. It may take 2-3 weeks to achieve desired results; do not discontinue without consulting prescriber. Avoid excess alcohol or caffeine and other prescription or OTC medications not approved by prescriber. Maintain adequate hydration (2-3 L/day of fluids unless instructed to restrict fluid intake). You may experience excess drowsiness, restlessness, dizziness, or blurred vision (use caution driving or when engaging in tasks requiring alertness until response to drug is known); constipation (increased exercise, fluids, or dietary fruit and fiber may help); postural hypotension (use caution climbing stairs or when changing position from lying or sitting to standing); or decreased perspiration (avoid strenuous exercise in hot environments). Report persistent CNS effects (eg, trembling fingers, altered gait or balance, excessive sedation, seizures, unusual movements, anxiety, abnormal thoughts, confusion, personality changes); chest pain, palpitations, rapid heartbeat, severe dizziness; unresolved urinary retention or changes in urinary pattern; changes in menstrual pattern or breast tenderness; vision changes; skin rash or yellowing of skin; difficulty breathing; or worsening of condition. **Pregnancy/breast-feeding precautions:** Inform prescriber if you are or intend to be pregnant. Consult prescriber if breast-feeding.

**Geriatric Considerations:** (See Warnings/Precautions, Adverse Reactions, and Overdose/Toxicology.) Elderly patients have an increased risk of adverse response to side effects or adverse reactions to antipsychotics. These can include but are not limited to the following.

Anticholinergic effects: CNS toxicity with confusion, memory loss, psychotic behavior, and agitation.

Extrapyramidal effects (EPS): Parkinson's syndrome and akathisia may occur as often as 50% in patients >60 years of age. Tardive dyskinesia (motor restlessness) may be 40% in elderly; may be related to duration and total accumulated dose over time; may be somewhat reversible if diagnosed early enough.

Orthostatic hypotension: Increased risk for falls.

Sedation: In nonpsychotic patients, may result in feelings of depersonalization, derealization, and dysphoria.

Cardiac toxicity: Cardiac arrhythmias have occurred with therapeutic doses of antipsychotics.

Malignant neuroleptic syndrome: Development of hyperthermia, muscular rigidity, autonomic instability, and altered mental status.

Many elderly patients receive antipsychotic medications for inappropriate nonpsychotic behavior. Before initiating antipsychotic medication, all possible reversible causes should be investigated. Stress may cause acute "confusion" or worsening of baseline nonpsychotic behaviors; any changes in disease state (in any organ) may result in behavioral changes. Common acute changes in behavior may be due also to increases in drug dose addition, or addition of a new drug to the regimen; fluid/electrolyte alterations; infections; or changes in the environment.

Meta-analysis of controlled trials of antipsychotic (phenothiazines, butyrophenones) use with agitated, demented, elderly patients has concluded that the use of neuroleptics results in a response rate of 18%. Clearly, neuroleptic therapy for behavior control should be limited, with frequent attempts to withdraw the agent for behavior control. When use is indicated, initial doses should be lower to start and monitor closely.

**Additional Information** Some formulations may contain ethanol.

**Related Information**

Antipsychotic Agents Comparison *on page 1371*
Antipsychotic Medication Guidelines *on page 1436*


- **Mol-Iron® [OTC]** *see* Iron Supplements *on page 627*
- **Mollifene® Ear Wax Removal Formula** *see page 1291*
- **Mometasone** *see* Topical Corticosteroids *on page 1152*
- **MOM (Magnesium Hydroxide)** *see* Magnesium Supplements *on page 703*
- **Monacolin K** *see* Lovastatin *on page 695*
- **Monafed®** *see* Guaifenesin *on page 548*
- **Monafed® DM** *see* Guaifenesin and Dextromethorphan *on page 549*
- **Monazole-7®** *see* Miconazole *on page 767*
- **Monistat-Derm™ Topical** *see* Miconazole *on page 767*
- **Monistat i.v.™ Injection** *see* Miconazole *on page 767*
- **Monistat™ Vaginal** *see* Miconazole *on page 767*
- **Monitan®** *see* Acebutolol *on page 31*
- **Monocid®** *see* Cefonicid *on page 219*
- **Monocidur** *see* Cefonicid *on page 219*
- **Monoclate-P®** *see* Antihemophilic Factor (Human) *on page 99*
- **Monoclonal Antibody** *see* Muromonab-CD3 *on page 793*
- **Mono-Gesic®** *see* Salsalate *on page 1042*
- **Monoket®** *see* Isosorbide Mononitrate *on page 635*
- **Mono Mack** *see* Isosorbide Mononitrate *on page 635*
- **Monopril®** *see* Fosinopril *on page 518*


## Montelukast (mon te LOO kast)

**U.S. Brand Names** Singulair®

**Therapeutic Category** Leukotriene Receptor Antagonist

**Pregnancy Risk Factor** B

**Lactation** Excretion in breast milk unknown/use caution (zafirlukast is contraindicated)

**Use** Prophylaxis and treatment of asthma in adults or children ≥6 years of age

(Continued)

## Montelukast *(Continued)*

**Mechanism of Action/Effect** Montelukast is a selective leukotriene receptor antagonist which inhibits cysteinyl leukotriene that is responsible for edema, smooth muscle contraction that is felt to be associated with the signs and symptoms of asthma.

**Contraindications** Hypersensitivity to montelukast or any component

**Warnings** The chewable tablets contain 0.842 mg of phenylalanine per 5 mg tablet which should be avoided in phenylketonuric patients. Montelukast is only for prophylactic treatment and should **not** be used for acute asthma attacks, including status asthmaticus; neither should it be used as monotherapy for exercise-induced asthma. Has been associated with eosinophilic vasculitis (Churg-Strauss syndrome), usually following reduction or withdrawal of oral corticosteroids.

**Drug Interactions**

**Cytochrome P-450 Effect:** CYP2A6, and 2C9, 3A3/4 enzyme substrate

**Decreased Effect:** Phenobarbital decreases montelukast area under the curve by 40%. Clinical significance is uncertain. Rifampin may increase the metabolism of montelukast similar to phenobarbital. No dosage adjustment is recommended when taking phenobarbital with montelukast.

**Adverse Reactions**

<10%: Central nervous system: Headache

1% to 10%:

Central nervous system: Fatigue, asthenia, dizziness
Dermatologic: Rash
Gastrointestinal: Dyspepsia, gastroenteritis, abdominal pain
Hepatic: Elevated ALT, AST
Respiratory: Cough, nasal congestion, influenza
Miscellaneous: Dental pain

<1% (Limited to important or life-threatening symptoms): Anaphylaxis, angioedema, pruritus, eosinophilic vasculitis (Churg-Strauss syndrome)

**Pharmacodynamics/Kinetics**

**Protein Binding:** >99% protein bound

**Time to Peak:** Chewable tablet: 2-2.5 hours; Film-coated tablet: 4 hours

**Metabolism:** Liver

**Excretion:** Bile

**Duration:** >24 hours

**Formulations**

Tablet: 10 mg
Tablet, chewable: 5 mg

**Dosing**

**Adults:** Oral: One 10 mg tablet daily in the evening

**Elderly:** Refer to adult dosing.

**Renal Impairment:** No adjustment necessary.

**Hepatic Impairment:** No adjustment necessary in mild to moderate hepatic disease. Patients with severe hepatic disease were **not** studied.

**Administration**

**Oral:** Take dose in the evening.

**Additional Nursing Issues**

**Physical Assessment:** Not for use in acute asthma attacks, including status asthmaticus. Assess effectiveness and interactions of other medications (see Drug Interactions). See Contraindications and Warnings/Precautions for cautious use. Monitor effectiveness of therapy and adverse reactions (see Adverse Reactions) at beginning of therapy and periodically with long-term use. Assess knowledge/teach patient appropriate use, interventions to reduce side effects, and adverse symptoms to report. Note breast-feeding caution.

**Patient Information/Instruction:** This medication is not for an acute asthmatic attack; in acute attack, follow instructions of prescriber. Do not stop other asthma medication unless advised by prescriber. Take every evening on a continuous basis; do not discontinue even if feeling better (this medication may help reduce incidence of acute attacks). You may experience mild headache (mild analgesic may help); fatigue or dizziness (use caution when driving). Report skin rash or itching, abdominal pain or persistent GI upset, unusual cough or congestion, or worsening of asthmatic condition. **Breast-feeding precautions:** Consult prescriber if breast-feeding.

**Additional Information** Chewable tablets are sweetened with aspartame which contains 0.842 mg of phenylalanine per 5 mg tablet.

♦ **8-MOP** *see* Methoxsalen *on page 747*

♦ **More Attenuated Enders Strain** *see page 1256*

♦ **More-Dophilus® [OTC]** *see Lactobacillus acidophilus* and *Lactobacillus bulgaricus on page 651*

## Moricizine (mor I siz een)

**U.S. Brand Names** Ethmozine®

**Therapeutic Category** Antiarrhythmic Agent, Class I

**Pregnancy Risk Factor** B

**Lactation** Enters breast milk/not recommended

**Use** For treatment of ventricular tachycardia and life-threatening ventricular arrhythmias

**Unlabeled use:** PVCs, complete and nonsustained ventricular tachycardia

**Mechanism of Action/Effect** Class I antiarrhythmic agent; reduces the fast inward current carried by sodium ions, shortens Phase I and Phase II repolarization, resulting in decreased action potential duration and effective refractory period

**Contraindications** Hypersensitivity to moricizine or any component; pre-existing second or third degree A-V block and in patients with right bundle-branch block when associated with left hemiblock, unless pacemaker is present; cardiogenic shock

**Warnings** Considering the known proarrhythmic properties and lack of evidence of improved survival for any antiarrhythmic drug in patients without life-threatening arrhythmias, it is prudent to reserve the use for patients with life-threatening ventricular arrhythmias. CAST II trial demonstrated a trend towards decreased survival for patients treated with moricizine. Proarrhythmic effects occur as with other antiarrhythmic agents. Hypokalemia, hyperkalemia, hypomagnesemia may affect response to Class I agents. Use with caution in patients with sick-sinus syndrome, hepatic, and renal impairment.

**Drug Interactions**

**Cytochrome P-450 Effect:** May act as inhibitor of CYP1A2; may be a substrate for CYP isoenzymes

**Decreased Effect:** Decreased levels of theophylline (50%).

**Increased Effect/Toxicity:** Increased serum levels of moricizine by up to 50%, when taken with cimetidine.

**Food Interactions** Moricizine peak serum concentrations may be decreased if taken with food.

**Adverse Reactions**

>10%: Central nervous system: Dizziness

1% to 10%:

- Cardiovascular: Proarrhythmia, palpitations, cardiac death, EKG abnormalities, congestive heart failure
- Central nervous system: Headache, fatigue, insomnia
- Endocrine & metabolic: Decreased libido
- Gastrointestinal: Nausea, diarrhea, ileus
- Ocular: Blurred vision, periorbital edema
- Respiratory: Dyspnea

<1% (Limited to important or life-threatening symptoms): Ventricular tachycardia, cardiac chest pain, hypotension or hypertension, syncope, supraventricular arrhythmias, myocardial infarction, apnea

**Overdose/Toxicology** Has a narrow therapeutic index and severe toxicity may occur slightly above the therapeutic range, especially if combined with other antiarrhythmic drugs. Acute single ingestion of twice the daily therapeutic dose is life-threatening. Symptoms of overdose include increases in P-R, QRS, Q-T intervals and amplitude of the T wave, A-V block, bradycardia, hypotension, ventricular arrhythmias (monomorphic or polymorphic ventricular tachycardia), and asystole. Other symptoms include dizziness, blurred vision, headache, and GI upset.

Treatment is symptom directed and supportive. **Note:** Type 1A antiarrhythmic agents should not be used to treat cardiotoxicity caused by Type 1C drugs.

**Pharmacodynamics/Kinetics**

**Protein Binding:** 95% in plasma

**Half-life Elimination:** Normal patient: 3-4 hours; Cardiac disease patient: 6-13 hours

**Metabolism:** Liver

**Excretion:** Feces and urine; some enterohepatic recycling occurs

**Formulations** Tablet, as hydrochloride: 200 mg, 250 mg, 300 mg

**Dosing**

**Adults:** Oral: 200-300 mg every 8 hours, adjust dosage at 150 mg/day at 3-day intervals. See table for dosage recommendations of transferring from other antiarrhythmic agents to Ethmozine®. Hospitalization required to start therapy.

**Moricizine**

| Transferred From | Start Ethmozine® |
|---|---|
| Encainide, propafenone, tocainide, or mexiletine | 8-12 hours after last dose |
| Flecainide | 12-24 hours after last dose |
| Procainamide | 3-6 hours after last dose |
| Quinidine, disopyramide | 6-12 hours after last dose |

**Elderly:** Refer to adult dosing.

**Renal Impairment:** Start at 600 mg/day or less.

**Hepatic Impairment:** Start at 600 mg/day or less.

**Monitoring Laboratory Tests** Electrolytes (correct any imbalance) prior to beginning therapy

**Additional Nursing Issues**

**Physical Assessment:** Assess other medications patient may be taking for effectiveness and interactions (see Drug Interactions). See Warnings/Precautions for cautious use. Monitor laboratory tests (see above), therapeutic response (cardiac status), and adverse reactions (see Warnings/Precautions and Adverse Reactions) at beginning of therapy, when titrating dosage, and on a regular basis with long-term therapy. **Note:** Moricizine has a low toxic:therapeutic ratio and overdose may easily produce severe and life-threatening reactions (see Overdose/Toxicology). Assess knowledge/teach patient appropriate use, interventions to reduce side effects, and adverse symptoms to report. Breast-feeding is not recommended.

**Patient Information/Instruction:** Take exactly as directed; do not take additional doses or discontinue without consulting prescriber. You will need regular cardiac checkups and blood tests while taking this medication. You may experience dizziness

(Continued)

## Moricizine *(Continued)*

or visual changes (use caution when driving or engaging in tasks requiring alertness until response to drug is known); nausea or vomiting (small frequent meals, frequent mouth care, chewing gum, or sucking lozenges may help); or headaches, sleep disturbances, or decreased libido (usually temporary, if persistent consult prescriber). Report chest pain, palpitation, or erratic heartbeat; increased weight or swelling of hands or feet; blurred vision or facial swelling; acute diarrhea; changes in bowel or bladder patterns; or difficulty breathing. **Breast-feeding precautions:** Breast-feeding is not recommended.

**Geriatric Considerations:** Due to moricizine binding to plasma albumin and alpha-glycoprotein, other highly bound drugs may displace moricizine. Since elderly may require multiple drugs, caution with highly bound drugs is necessary. Consider changes in renal and hepatic function with age and monitor closely since half-life may be prolonged.

**Related Information**

Antiarrhythmic Drug Classification Comparison *on page 1366*

◆ **Morphine-HP®** *see* Morphine Sulfate *on this page*

## Morphine Sulfate (MOR feen SUL fate)

**U.S. Brand Names** Astramorph™ PF Injection; Duramorph® Injection; Kadian™; MS Contin® Oral; MSIR® Oral; MS/L®; MS/S®; OMS® Oral; Oramorph SR™ Oral; RMS® Rectal; Roxanol™ Oral; Roxanol SR™ Oral

**Synonyms** MS

**Therapeutic Category** Analgesic, Narcotic

**Pregnancy Risk Factor** B/D (if used for prolonged periods or in high doses at term)

**Lactation** Enters breast milk/use caution (AAP rates "compatible")

**Use** Relief of moderate to severe acute and chronic pain; pain of myocardial infarction; relieves dyspnea of acute left ventricular failure and pulmonary edema; preanesthetic medication

**Mechanism of Action/Effect** Binds to opiate receptors in the CNS, causing inhibition of ascending pain pathways, altering the perception of and response to pain; produces generalized CNS depression

**Contraindications** Hypersensitivity to morphine sulfate; increased intracranial pressure; severe respiratory depression; pregnancy (if used for prolonged periods or in high doses at term)

**Warnings** Some preparations contain sulfites which may cause allergic reactions. Infants <3 months of age are more susceptible to respiratory depression; use with caution and generally in reduced doses in this age group. Use with caution in patients with impaired respiratory function or severe hepatic dysfunction and in patients with hypersensitivity reactions to other phenanthrene derivative opioid agonists (codeine, hydrocodone, hydromorphone, levorphanol, oxycodone, oxymorphone). Morphine shares the toxic potential of opiate agonists and usual precautions of opiate agonist therapy should be observed. May cause hypotension in patients with acute myocardial infarction. Elderly may be particularly susceptible to the CNS depressant and constipating effects of narcotics.

**Drug Interactions**

**Cytochrome P-450 Effect:** CYP2D6 enzyme substrate

**Decreased Effect:** Phenothiazines may antagonize the analgesic effect of morphine and other opiate agonists.

**Increased Effect/Toxicity:** CNS depressants (phenothiazines, tranquilizers, anxiolytics, sedatives, hypnotics, or alcohol), tricyclic antidepressants may potentiate the effects of morphine and other opiate agonists. Dextroamphetamine may enhance the analgesic effect of morphine and other opiate agonists.

**Food Interactions** Oral: Morphine bioavailability may be increased if taken with food.

**Effects on Lab Values** ↑ aminotransferase [ALT (SGPT)/AST (SGOT)] (S)

**Adverse Reactions**

>10%:
- Cardiovascular: Hypotension
- Central nervous system: Fatigue, drowsiness, dizziness
- Gastrointestinal: Nausea, vomiting, constipation
- Neuromuscular & skeletal: Weakness
- Miscellaneous: Histamine release

1% to 10%:
- Cardiovascular: Tachycardia or bradycardia
- Central nervous system: Nervousness, headache, restlessness, malaise, confusion, false sense of well-being
- Dermatologic: Rash, urticaria
- Gastrointestinal: Anorexia, stomach cramps, dry mouth, biliary spasm
- Genitourinary: Ureteral spasms, decreased urination
- Local: Pain at injection site
- Neuromuscular & skeletal: Trembling
- Ocular: Blurred vision
- Respiratory: Dyspnea, shortness of breath

<1% (Limited to important or life-threatening symptoms): Increased ICP, biliary tract spasm, muscle rigidity, increased AST/ALT

**Overdose/Toxicology** Symptoms of overdose include respiratory depression, miosis, hypotension, bradycardia, apnea, and pulmonary edema. Treatment is symptomatic. Naloxone, 2 mg I.V. with repeat administration as necessary up to a total dose of 10 mg, can be used to reverse opiate effects.

**Pharmacodynamics/Kinetics**

**Half-life Elimination:** 2-4 hours

**Metabolism:** Liver

**Excretion:** Urine; up to 10% via bile in feces

**Onset:** Oral: 1 hour; I.V.: 5-10 minutes

**Duration:** 3-5 hours (up to 12 hours for extended release)

**Formulations**

Capsule (MSIR®): 15 mg, 30 mg

Capsule, sustained release (Kadian™): 20 mg, 50 mg, 100 mg

Injection: 0.5 mg/mL (10 mL); 1 mg/mL (10 mL, 30 mL, 60 mL); 2 mg/mL (1 mL, 2 mL, 60 mL); 3 mg/mL (50 mL); 4 mg/mL (1 mL, 2 mL); 5 mg/mL (1 mL, 30 mL); 8 mg/mL (1 mL, 2 mL); 10 mg/mL (1 mL, 2 mL, 10 mL); 15 mg/mL (1 mL, 2 mL, 20 mL); 25 mg/mL (4 mL, 10 mL, 20 mL, 40 mL); 50 mg/mL (10 mL, 20 mL, 40 mL)

Injection:

- Preservative free (Astramorph™ PF, Duramorph®): 0.5 mg/mL (2 mL, 10 mL); 1 mg/mL (2 mL, 10 mL); 10 mg/mL (20 mL); 25 mg/mL (20 mL)
- I.V. via PCA pump: 1 mg/mL (10 mL, 30 mL, 60 mL); 5 mg/mL (30 mL)
- I.V. infusion preparation: 25 mg/mL (4 mL, 10 mL, 20 mL)

Solution, oral: 10 mg/5 mL (5 mL, 10 mL, 100 mL, 120 mL, 500 mL); 20 mg/5 mL (5 mL, 100 mL, 120 mL, 500 mL)

- MSIR®: 10 mg/5 mL (5 mL, 120 mL, 500 mL); 20 mg/5 mL (5 mL 120 mL, 500 mL); 20 mg/mL (30 mL, 120 mL)
- MS/L®: 100 mg/5 mL (120 mL) 20 mg/5 mL
- OMS®: 20 mg/mL (30 mL, 120 mL)
- Roxanol™: 10 mg/2.5 mL (2.5 mL); 20 mg/mL (1 mL, 1.5 mL, 30 mL, 120 mL, 240 mL)

Suppository, rectal: 5 mg, 10 mg, 20 mg, 30 mg

- MS/S®, RMS®, Roxanol™: 5 mg, 10 mg, 20 mg, 30 mg

Tablet: 15 mg, 30 mg

- MSIR®: 15 mg, 30 mg
- Controlled release:
  - MS Contin®: 15 mg, 30 mg, 60 mg, 100 mg, 200 mg
  - Roxanol™ SR: 30 mg
- Soluble: 10 mg, 15 mg, 30 mg
- Sustained release (Oramorph SR™): 30 mg, 60 mg, 100 mg

**Dosing**

**Adults:** Doses should be titrated to appropriate effect; when changing routes of administration in chronically treated patients, please note that **oral doses are approximately 50% as effective as parenteral dose.**

Oral: Prompt release: 10-30 mg every 4 hours as needed; controlled release: 15-30 mg every 8-12 hours

I.M., I.V., S.C.: 2.5-20 mg/dose every 2-6 hours as needed; usual: 10 mg/dose every 4 hours as needed

I.V., S.C. continuous infusion: 0.8-10 mg/hour; may increase depending on pain relief/adverse effects; usual range: up to 80 mg/hour

Epidural: Initial: 5 mg in lumbar region; if inadequate pain relief within 1 hour, give 1-2 mg; maximum: 10 mg/24 hours.

Intrathecal (1/10 of epidural dose): 0.2-1 mg/dose; repeat doses are **not** recommended.

Rectal: 10-20 mg every 4 hours

**Elderly:** Refer to adult dosing.

**Renal Impairment:**

$Cl_{cr}$ 10-50 mL/minute: Administer at 75% of normal dose.

$Cl_{cr}$ <10 mL/minute: Administer at 50% of normal dose.

**Hepatic Impairment:** Unchanged in mild liver disease; substantial extrahepatic metabolism may occur. Excessive sedation may occur in cirrhosis.

**Administration**

**Oral:** Do not crush controlled release drug product, swallow whole. Administration of oral morphine solution with food may increase bioavailability.

**I.V.:** When giving morphine I.V. push, it is best to first dilute in 4-5 mL of sterile water, and then to administer slowly (eg, 15 mg over 3-5 minutes). Use preservative-free solutions for intrathecal or epidural use.

**Stability**

**Storage:**

Suppositories: Refrigerate suppositories; do not freeze.

Injection: Degradation depends on pH and presence of oxygen; relatively stable in pH ≤4; darkening of solutions indicate degradation.

**Reconstitution:** Usual concentration for continuous I.V. infusion = 0.1-1 mg/mL in $D_5W$.

**Compatibility:** See the Compatibility of Drugs Chart *on page 1315* and the Compatibility of Drugs in Syringe Chart *on page 1317*.

**Additional Nursing Issues**

**Physical Assessment:** Assess other medications patient may be taking for additive or adverse interactions (see Drug Interactions). Monitor for effectiveness of pain relief and monitor for signs of overdose (see above). Monitor blood pressure, CNS and respiratory status, and degree of sedation at beginning of therapy and at regular intervals with long-term use. May cause physical and/or psychological dependence. For inpatients, implement safety measures (eg, side rails up, call light within reach, instructions to call for assistance, etc). Assess knowledge/teach patient appropriate use (if self-administered). Teach patient to monitor for adverse reactions (see Adverse Reactions), adverse reactions to report, and appropriate interventions to reduce side

(Continued)

## Morphine Sulfate *(Continued)*

effects. Discontinue slowly after prolonged use. **Pregnancy risk factor B/D** - see Pregnancy Risk Factor for cautious use. Note breast-feeding caution.

**Patient Information/Instruction:** If self-administered, use exactly as directed (do not increase dose or frequency); may cause physical and/or psychological dependence. While using this medication, do not use alcohol and other prescription or OTC medications (especially sedatives, tranquilizers, antihistamines, or pain medications) without consulting prescriber. Maintain adequate hydration (2-3 L/day of fluids unless instructed to restrict fluid intake). May cause hypotension, dizziness, drowsiness, impaired coordination, or blurred vision (use caution when driving, climbing stairs, or changing position - rising from sitting or lying to standing, or when engaging in tasks requiring alertness until response to drug is known); loss of appetite, nausea, or vomiting (frequent mouth care, small frequent meals, chewing gum, or sucking lozenges may help); constipation (increased exercise, fluids, or dietary fruit and fiber may help - if constipation remains an unresolved problem, consult prescriber about use of stool softeners). Report chest pain, slow or rapid heartbeat, acute dizziness, or persistent headache; changes in mental status; swelling of extremities or unusual weight gain; changes in urinary elimination or pain on urination; acute headache; back or flank pain or muscle spasms; blurred vision; skin rash; or shortness of breath. **Pregnancy/breast-feeding precautions:** Inform prescriber if you are or intend to be pregnant. If you are breast-feeding, take medication immediately after breast-feeding or 3-4 hours prior to next feeding.

**Geriatric Considerations:** The elderly may be particularly susceptible to the CNS depressant and constipating effects of narcotics. For chronic administration of narcotic analgesics, morphine is preferable in the elderly due to its pharmacokinetics and side effect profile as compared to meperidine and methadone.

**Additional Information** Morphine I.M. or S.C. 10 mg = 30-60 mg oral

**Related Information**

Controlled Substances Comparison *on page 1379*
Hallucinogenic Drugs Comparison *on page 1386*
Narcotic/Opioid Analgesic Comparison *on page 1396*

- ♦ **Mosco® Liquid** *see page 1294*
- ♦ **Motofen®** *see* Difenoxin and Atropine *on page 367*
- ♦ **Motrin®** *see* Ibuprofen *on page 592*
- ♦ **Motrin® IB [OTC]** *see* Ibuprofen *on page 592*
- ♦ **Motrin® IB Sinus Caplets** *see page 1294*
- ♦ **6-MP** *see* Mercaptopurine *on page 725*
- ♦ **MPHO** *see* Amphotericin B *on page 83*
- ♦ **M-Prednisol® Injection** *see* Methylprednisolone *on page 754*
- ♦ **M-R-VAX® II** *see page 1256*
- ♦ **MS** *see* Morphine Sulfate *on page 790*
- ♦ **MS Contin® Oral** *see* Morphine Sulfate *on page 790*
- ♦ **MSD® Enteric Coated ASA** *see* Aspirin *on page 111*
- ♦ **MS-IR®** *see* Morphine Sulfate *on page 790*
- ♦ **MSIR® Oral** *see* Morphine Sulfate *on page 790*
- ♦ **MS/L®** *see* Morphine Sulfate *on page 790*
- ♦ **MS/S®** *see* Morphine Sulfate *on page 790*
- ♦ **MST Continus** *see* Morphine Sulfate *on page 790*
- ♦ **MTC** *see* Mitomycin *on page 777*
- ♦ **MTX** *see* Methotrexate *on page 743*
- ♦ **Muco-Fen-DM®** *see* Guaifenesin and Dextromethorphan *on page 549*
- ♦ **Muco-Fen-LA®** *see* Guaifenesin *on page 548*
- ♦ **Mucomyst®** *see* Acetylcysteine *on page 36*
- ♦ **Mucoplex®** *see page 1294*
- ♦ **Mucosil™** *see* Acetylcysteine *on page 36*
- ♦ **Multipax®** *see* Hydroxyzine *on page 588*
- ♦ **Multiple Vitamins** *see* Vitamin, Multiple *on page 1219*
- ♦ **Multitest CMI®** *see page 1248*
- ♦ **Multivitamins/Fluoride** *see* Vitamin, Multiple *on page 1219*
- ♦ **Multi Vit® Drops [OTC]** *see* Vitamin, Multiple *on page 1219*
- ♦ **Mumps Skin Test Antigen** *see page 1248*
- ♦ **Munobal** *see* Felodipine *on page 474*
- ♦ **Mupiban** *see* Mupirocin *on this page*

## Mupirocin (myoo PEER oh sin)

**U.S. Brand Names** Bactroban®; Bactroban® Nasal

**Synonyms** Pseudomonic Acid A

**Therapeutic Category** Antibiotic, Topical

**Pregnancy Risk Factor** B

**Lactation** Excretion in breast milk unknown

**Use** Topical treatment of impetigo due to *Staphylococcus aureus*, beta-hemolytic *Streptococcus*, and *S. pyogenes*

**Mechanism of Action/Effect** Binds to bacterial isoleucyl transfer-RNA synthetase resulting in the inhibition of protein and RNA synthesis

**Contraindications** Hypersensitivity to mupirocin or polyethylene glycol

**Warnings** Potentially toxic amounts of polyethylene glycol contained in the vehicle may be absorbed percutaneously in patients with extensive burns or open wounds. Prolonged use may result in over growth of nonsusceptible organisms. For external use only. Not for treatment of pressure sores.

**Adverse Reactions** 1% to 10%:

Dermatologic: Pruritus, rash, erythema, dry skin

Local: Burning, stinging, tenderness, edema, pain

**Pharmacodynamics/Kinetics**

**Protein Binding:** 95%

**Half-life Elimination:** 17-36 minutes

**Metabolism:** Liver and skin

**Excretion:** Urine

**Formulations**

Mupirocin calcium: Ointment:

Intranasal: 2% (1 g single use tube)

Topical: 2% (15 g, 30 g)

**Dosing**

**Adults:** Topical: Apply small amount to affected area 2-5 times/day for 5-14 days.

**Elderly:** Refer to adult dosing.

**Administration**

**Topical:** For external use only.

**Stability**

**Compatibility:** Do not mix with Aquaphor®, coal tar solution, or salicylic acid.

**Additional Nursing Issues**

**Physical Assessment:** See Warnings/Precautions and Contraindications for use cautions. Assess for effectiveness of therapy and symptoms of infection. Assess knowledge/teach patient appropriate application and use and adverse symptoms (see Adverse Reactions) to report. Note breast-feeding caution.

**Patient Information/Instruction:** For external use only. Wash hands before and after application. Apply this film over affected areas exactly as directed. Avoid getting in eyes. Report rash; persistent burning, stinging, swelling, itching, or pain. **Breast-feeding precautions:** Consult prescriber if breast-feeding.

**Geriatric Considerations:** Not for treatment of pressure sores; contains polyethylene glycol vehicle.

♦ **Murine® Ear Drops** *see page 1291*

♦ **Murine® Ear Drops** *see page 1294*

♦ **Murine® Plus Ophthalmic** *see page 1294*

♦ **Murine® Solution** *see page 1294*

♦ **Muro 128® Ophthalmic** *see page 1294*

♦ **Murocel® Ophthalmic Solution** *see page 1294*

## Muromonab-CD3 (myoo roe MOE nab see dee three)

**U.S. Brand Names** Orthoclone® OKT3

**Synonyms** Monoclonal Antibody; OKT3

**Therapeutic Category** Immunosuppressant Agent

**Pregnancy Risk Factor** C

**Lactation** Excretion in breast milk unknown/contraindicated

**Use** Treatment of acute allograft rejection in renal transplant patients; treatment of acute hepatic, cardiac, kidney, and pancreas rejection episodes resistant to conventional treatment; treatment of acute graft-versus-host disease following bone marrow transplantation resistant to conventional treatment

**Mechanism of Action/Effect** Reverses graft rejection by binding to T cells and interfering with their function

**Contraindications** Hypersensitivity to OKT3 or any murine product; patients in fluid overload or those with >3% weight gain within 1 week prior to start of OKT3; antimouse antibody titers >1:1000

**Warnings** It is imperative, especially prior to the first few doses, that there be no clinical evidence of volume overload, uncontrolled hypertension, or uncompensated heart failure, including a clear chest x-ray and weight restriction ≤3% above the patient's minimum weight during the week prior to injection. Pregnancy factor C.

May result in an increased susceptibility to infection. Dosage of concomitant immunosuppressants should be reduced during OKT3 therapy. Cyclosporine should be discontinued

**Suggested Prevention/Treatment of Muromonab-CD3 First-Dose Effects**

| Adverse Reaction | Effective Prevention or Palliation | Supportive Treatment |
|---|---|---|
| Severe pulmonary edema | Clear chest x-ray with in 24-hour preinjection; weight restriction to ≤3% gain over 7 days preinjection | Prompt intubation and oxygenation; 24-hour close observation |
| Fever, chills | 1 mg/kg methylprednisolone sodium succinate preinjection; fever reduction below 37.8°C (100°F) preinjection | Cooling blanket<br>Acetaminophen prn |
| Respiratory effects | 100 mg hydrocortisone sodium succinate 30-minute postinjection | Additional 100 mg hydrocortisone sodium succinate prn |

(Continued)

## Muromonab-CD3 *(Continued)*

or decreased to 50% usual maintenance dose and maintenance therapy resumed about 3 days before stopping OKT3.

Severe pulmonary edema has occurred in patients with fluid overload. **First-dose effect** (flu-like symptoms, anaphylactic-type reaction) may occur within 30 minutes to 6 hours, up to 24 hours after the first dose and may be minimized by using the recommended regimens. See table. Cardiopulmonary resuscitation may be needed. If the patient's temperature is >37.8°C, reduce before administering OKT3.

**Drug Interactions**

**Decreased Effect:** Decreased effect with immunosuppressive drugs.

**Increased Effect/Toxicity:** Recommend decreasing dose of prednisone to 0.5 mg/kg, azathioprine to 0.5 mg/kg (approximate 50% decrease in dose), and discontinuing cyclosporine while patient is receiving OKT3.

**Adverse Reactions** First-dose effect (cytokine release syndrome), onset 1-3 hours after dose, duration 12-16 hours, severity mild to life-threatening, signs and symptoms include fever, chilling, dyspnea, wheezing, chest pain, chest tightness, nausea, vomiting, and diarrhea. Hypervolemic pulmonary edema, nephrotoxicity, meningitis, and encephalopathy are possible. Reactions tend to decrease with repeated doses.

>10%:
- Cardiovascular: Tachycardia (including ventricular)
- Central nervous system: Dizziness, faintness
- Gastrointestinal: Diarrhea, nausea, vomiting
- Hematologic: Transient lymphopenia
- Neuromuscular & skeletal: Trembling
- Respiratory: Shortness of breath

1% to 10%:
- Central nervous system: Headache
- Neuromuscular & skeletal: Stiff neck
- Ocular: Photophobia
- Respiratory: Pulmonary edema

<1% (Limited to important or life-threatening symptoms): Hypertension, hypotension, chest pain or tightness, pancytopenia, secondary lymphoproliferative disorder or lymphoma, thrombosis of major vessels in renal allograft; increased BUN and creatinine, dyspnea, wheezing

**Pharmacodynamics/Kinetics**

**Half-life Elimination:** Time to steady-state: Trough level: 3-14 days; pretreatment levels are restored within 7 days after treatment is terminated.

**Formulations** Injection: 5 mg/5 mL

**Dosing**

**Adults:** I.V. (refer to individual protocols): 5 mg/day once daily for 10-14 days

**Elderly:** Refer to adult dosing.

**Renal Impairment:** Removal by dialysis: Molecular size of OKT3 is 150,000 daltons. Not dialyzed by most standard dialyzers; however, may be dialyzed by high flux dialysis. OKT3 will be removed by plasmapheresis. Administer following dialysis treatments.

**Administration**

**I.V.:** Give I.V. push over <1 minute at a final concentration of 1 mg/mL; **do not give I.M.**. Methylprednisolone sodium succinate 1 mg/kg I.V. given prior to first muromonab-CD3 administration, and I.V. hydrocortisone sodium succinate 50-100 mg, given 30 minutes after administration are strongly recommended to decrease the incidence of reactions to the first dose.

**I.V. Detail:** Filter each dose through a low protein-binding 0.22 micron filter (Millex GV) before administration. Patient temperature should not exceed 37.8°C (100°F) at time of administration.

**Stability**

**Storage:** Refrigerate; do not shake or freeze. Stable in Becton Dickinson syringe for 16 hours at room temperature or refrigeration.

**Monitoring Laboratory Tests** Chest x-ray, CBC with differential, immunologic monitoring of T cells, serum levels of OKT3

**Additional Nursing Issues**

**Physical Assessment:** Note Drug Interactions information. Monitor pretreatment laboratory results prior to beginning therapy. Monitor closely for acute adverse pulmonary and cardiac effects, and anaphylactic-type effects during and for 24 hours following first infusion (see Warnings/Precautions). Monitor vital signs, cardiac status, and respiratory status on a regular basis. Monitor/instruct patient on appropriate interventions to reduce side effects, to monitor for signs of opportunistic infection (eg, persistent fever, malaise, sore throat, unusual bleeding or bruising), and reactions to report. **Pregnancy risk factor C.** Breast-feeding is contraindicated.

**Patient Information/Instruction:** There may be a severe reaction to the first infusion of this medication. You may experience high fever, chills, difficulty breathing, or congestion. You will be closely monitored and comfort measures provided. Effects are substantially reduced with subsequent infusions. During the period of therapy and for some time after the regimen of infusions you will be susceptible to infection. People may wear masks and gloves while caring for you to protect you as much as possible from infection (avoid crowds and people with infections or contagious diseases). You may experience dizziness, faintness, or trembling (use caution until response to medication is known); nausea or vomiting (frequent small meals, frequent mouth care); sensitivity to direct sunlight (wear dark glasses, and protective clothing, use sunscreen, or avoid exposure to direct sunlight). Report chest pain or tightness; symptoms of respiratory infection, wheezing, or difficulty breathing; vision change; or muscular trembling. **Pregnancy/breast-feeding precautions:** Inform prescriber if you are or intend to be pregnant. Do not breast-feed.


- **Muroptic-5®** *see page 1294*
- **Muro's Opcon®** *see page 1282*
- **Muse® Pellet** *see* Alprostadil *on page 56*
- **Mustargen® Hydrochloride** *see* Mechlorethamine *on page 710*
- **Mustine** *see* Mechlorethamine *on page 710*
- **Mutamycin®** *see* Mitomycin *on page 777*
- **M.V.I.®** *see* Vitamin, Multiple *on page 1219*
- **M.V.I.®-12** *see* Vitamin, Multiple *on page 1219*
- **M.V.I.® Concentrate** *see* Vitamin, Multiple *on page 1219*
- **M.V.I.® Pediatric** *see* Vitamin, Multiple *on page 1219*
- **Myambutol®** *see* Ethambutol *on page 456*
- **Mycelex®** *see* Clotrimazole *on page 294*
- **Mycelex®-7** *see* Clotrimazole *on page 294*
- **Mycelex®-G** *see* Clotrimazole *on page 294*
- **Mycifradin® Sulfate Oral** *see* Neomycin *on page 815*
- **Mycifradin® Sulfate Topical** *see* Neomycin *on page 815*
- **Mycinettes® [OTC]** *see* Benzocaine *on page 141*
- **Mycitracin® Topical [OTC]** *see* Bacitracin, Neomycin, and Polymyxin B *on page 130*
- **Mycobutin®** *see* Rifabutin *on page 1018*
- **Mycogen II Topical** *see* Nystatin and Triamcinolone *on page 844*
- **Mycolog®-II Topical** *see* Nystatin and Triamcinolone *on page 844*
- **Myconel® Topical** *see* Nystatin and Triamcinolone *on page 844*


## Mycophenolate (mye koe FEN oh late)

**U.S. Brand Names** CellCept®

**Therapeutic Category** Immunosuppressant Agent

**Pregnancy Risk Factor** C

**Lactation** Excretion in breast milk unknown

**Use** Immunosuppressant used with corticosteroids and cyclosporine in prevention of organ rejection in patients receiving allogenic renal and cardiac transplants

**Mechanism of Action/Effect** Inhibition of purine synthesis of human lymphocytes and proliferation of human lymphocytes

**Contraindications** Hypersensitivity to mycophenolate mofetil, mycophenolic acid, or any component

**Warnings** Increased risk for infection and development of lymphoproliferative disorders. Patients should be monitored appropriately and given supportive treatment should these conditions occur. Increased toxicity in patients with renal impairment. Pregnancy factor C.

**Drug Interactions**

**Decreased Effect:** Antacids decrease $C_{max}$ and AUC, **do not administer together.** Cholestyramine resin decreases AUC, **do not administer together.**

**Increased Effect/Toxicity:** Acyclovir and ganciclovir levels may increase due to competition for tubular secretion of these drugs. Probenecid may increase mycophenolate levels due to inhibition of tubular secretion. High doses of salicylates may increase free fraction of mycophenolic acid.

**Adverse Reactions** 1% to 10%:

Cardiovascular: Hypertension

Central nervous system: Insomnia, dizziness, fever, headache

Dermatologic: Rash, acne

Endocrine & metabolic: Hypercholesteremia, hypophosphatemia, hypokalemia, hyperkalemia, hyperglycemia

Gastrointestinal: Diarrhea, constipation, nausea, vomiting, oral moniliasis, dyspepsia, GI tract hemorrhage

Hematologic: Leukopenia, neutropenia, anemia, thrombocytopenia

Neuromuscular & skeletal: Tremor, back pain, myalgia

Renal: Renal tubular necrosis, hematuria

Respiratory: Dyspnea, cough, pharyngitis

Miscellaneous: 1% incidence of lymphoproliferative disease

**Pharmacodynamics/Kinetics**

**Half-life Elimination:** 18 hours; Serum concentrations: Correlation of toxicity or efficacy is still being developed, however, one study indicated that 12-hour AUCs >40 mcg/mL/hour were correlated with efficacy and decreased episodes of rejection.

**Metabolism:** Mycophenolate mofetil is metabolized to the acid form which is pharmacologically active; mycophenolic acid is glucuronidated to an inactive form; enterohepatic cycling occurs

**Excretion:** Urine

**Formulations** Capsule, as mofetil: 250 mg

**Dosing**

**Adults:** Oral: 1 g twice daily within 72 hours of transplant (although 3 g/day has been given in some clinical trials, there was decreased tolerability and no efficacy advantage).

(Continued)

## Mycophenolate *(Continued)*

**Dosage adjustment for neutropenia**: Dose should be decreased or stopped in patients who develop severe neutropenia (ANC <1.3 x 10,000/μL).

**Elderly:** Refer to adult dosing.

**Renal Impairment:** Doses >2 g/day are not recommended due to the possibility for enhanced immunosuppression as well as toxicity.

**Monitoring Laboratory Tests** Renal and liver function, CBC

**Additional Nursing Issues**

**Physical Assessment:** Assess other medications patient may be taking for effectiveness and interactions (see Drug Interactions). Note Warnings/Precautions and Contraindications for cautious use. Monitor laboratory tests, response to therapy, and adverse reactions (see Warnings/Precautions and Adverse Reactions). Diabetic patients should monitor glucose levels closely (this medication may alter glucose levels). Monitor/instruct patient on appropriate interventions to reduce side effects, to monitor for signs of opportunistic infection (eg, persistent fever, malaise, sore throat, unusual bleeding or bruising), and adverse reactions to report. **Pregnancy risk factor C** - benefits of use should outweigh possible risks. Note breast-feeding caution.

**Patient Information/Instruction:** Take as directed, preferably 1 hour before or 2 hours after meals. Do not take within 1 hour before or 2 hours after antacids or cholestyramine medications. Do not alter dose and do not discontinue without consulting prescriber. Maintain adequate hydration (2-3 L/day of fluids unless instructed to restrict fluid intake) during entire course of therapy. You will be susceptible to infection (avoid crowds and people with infections or contagious diseases). If you are diabetic, monitor glucose levels closely (may alter glucose levels). You may experience dizziness or trembling (use caution until response to medication is known); nausea or vomiting (frequent small meals, frequent mouth care may help); diarrhea (boiled milk, yogurt, or buttermilk may help); sores or white plaques in mouth (frequent rinsing of mouth and frequent mouth care may help); or muscle or back pain (mild analgesics may be recommended). Report chest pain; acute headache or dizziness; symptoms of respiratory infection, cough, or difficulty breathing; unresolved gastrointestinal effects; fatigue, chills, fever unhealed sores, white plaques in mouth; irritation in genital area or unusual discharge; unusual bruising or bleeding; or other unusual effects related to this medication. **Pregnancy/breast-feeding precautions:** Inform prescriber if you are or intend to be pregnant. Consult prescriber if breast-feeding.


- ♦ **Mycostatin®** *see* Nystatin *on page 843*
- ♦ **Myco-Triacet® II** *see* Nystatin and Triamcinolone *on page 844*
- ♦ **Mydfrin®** *see page 1282*
- ♦ **Mydfrin® Ophthalmic Solution** *see* Phenylephrine *on page 920*
- ♦ **Mydriacyl®** *see page 1248*
- ♦ **Mydriacyl®** *see page 1282*
- ♦ **Mykrox®** *see* Metolazone *on page 759*
- ♦ **Mylanta®** *see page 1294*
- ♦ **Mylanta Gas®** *see page 1294*
- ♦ **Mylanta®-II** *see page 1294*
- ♦ **Mylanta® Soothing Antacids [OTC]** *see* Calcium Supplements *on page 185*
- ♦ **Myleran®** *see* Busulfan *on page 171*
- ♦ **Mylicon®** *see page 1294*
- ♦ **Myminic® Expectorant [OTC]** *see* Guaifenesin and Phenylpropanolamine *on page 550*
- ♦ **Myoflex® Cream** *see page 1294*
- ♦ **Myotonachol™** *see* Bethanechol *on page 151*
- ♦ **Myphetane DC®** *see* Brompheniramine, Phenylpropanolamine, and Codeine *on page 163*
- ♦ **Myphetapp®** *see page 1294*
- ♦ **Mysoline®** *see* Primidone *on page 964*
- ♦ **Mytelase® Caplets®** *see* Ambenonium *on page 63*
- ♦ **Mytrex® F Topical** *see* Nystatin and Triamcinolone *on page 844*
- ♦ **Mytussin® [OTC]** *see* Guaifenesin *on page 548*
- ♦ **Mytussin® AC** *see* Guaifenesin and Codeine *on page 549*
- ♦ **Mytussin® DAC** *see* Guaifenesin, Pseudoephedrine, and Codeine *on page 552*
- ♦ **Mytussin® DM [OTC]** *see* Guaifenesin and Dextromethorphan *on page 549*
- ♦ **M-Zole® 7 Dual Pack [OTC]** *see* Miconazole *on page 767*


## Nabumetone (na BYOO me tone)

**U.S. Brand Names** Relafen®

**Therapeutic Category** Nonsteroidal Anti-Inflammatory Agent (NSAID)

**Pregnancy Risk Factor** C

**Lactation** Enters breast milk/not recommended

**Use** Management of osteoarthritis and rheumatoid arthritis

**Mechanism of Action/Effect** Nabumetone is a nonacidic, nonsteroidal anti-inflammatory drug that inhibits the production of inflammation and pain during arthritis. The active metabolite of nabumetone is felt to be the compound primarily responsible for therapeutic effect. Comparatively, the parent drug is a poor inhibitor of prostaglandin synthesis.

**Contraindications** Hypersensitivity to nabumetone; should not be administered to patients with active peptic ulceration and those with severe hepatic impairment or in patients in whom nabumetone, aspirin, or other NSAIDs have induced asthma, urticaria, or other allergic-type reactions; fatal asthmatic reactions have occurred following NSAID administration

**Warnings** There is potential for GI ulceration, bleeding, or perforation with NSAID use. Elderly patients may sometimes require lower doses. Patients with impaired renal function may need a dose reduction. Use with caution in patients with severe hepatic impairment. Pregnancy factor C.

**Drug Interactions**

**Increased Effect/Toxicity:** Nabumetone may increase the hypoprothrombinemic effect of warfarin.

**Food Interactions** Nabumetone peak serum concentrations may be increased if taken with food or dairy products.

**Adverse Reactions**

1% to 10%:

Cardiovascular: Edema

Central nervous system: Dizziness, headache, fatigue, insomnia, nervousness, somnolence

Dermatologic: Pruritus, rash

Gastrointestinal: Constipation, flatulence, nausea, guaiac postive stool, stomatitis, gastritis, dry mouth, vomiting, diarrhea, heartburn, abdominal pain

Otic: Tinnitus

<1% (Limited to important or life-threatening symptoms): Chest pain, arrhythmia, hypertension, myocardial infarction, thrombophlebitis, toxic epidermal necrolysis, erythema multiforme, Stevens-Johnson syndrome, hyperglycemia, hypokalemia, albuminuria, azotemia, hyperuricemia, interstitial nephritis, nephrotic syndrome, vaginal bleeding, hematuria, anemia, leukopenia, granulocytopenia, thrombocytopenia, cholestatic jaundice, dyspnea, eosinophilic pneumonia, hypersensitivity pneumonitis

**Overdose/Toxicology** Symptoms of overdose include apnea, metabolic acidosis, coma, nystagmus, leukocytosis, and renal failure. Management of nonsteroidal anti-inflammatory (NSAID) intoxication is supportive and symptomatic.

**Pharmacodynamics/Kinetics**

**Protein Binding:** >99%

**Distribution:** Diffusion occurs readily into synovial fluid with peak concentrations in 4-12 hours

**Half-life Elimination:** Major metabolite: 24 hours

**Time to Peak:** Metabolite: Oral: Within 3-6 hours

**Metabolism:** A prodrug being rapidly metabolized to an active metabolite (6-methoxy-2-naphthylacetic acid); extensive first-pass hepatic metabolism

**Excretion:** 80% recovered in urine and 10% in feces, with very little excreted as unchanged compound

**Onset:** May require several days to maximum effect

**Formulations** Tablet: 500 mg, 750 mg

**Dosing**

**Adults:** Oral: 1000 mg/day; an additional 500-1000 mg may be needed in some patients to obtain more symptomatic relief; may be administered once or twice daily.

**Elderly:** Refer to adult dosing; do not exceed 2000 mg/day.

**Renal Impairment:** None necessary; however, adverse effects due to accumulation of inactive metabolites of nabumetone that are renally excreted have not been studied and should be considered.

**Additional Nursing Issues**

**Physical Assessment:** Assess effectiveness and interactions of other medications patient may be taking (see Contraindications and Drug Interactions). Monitor laboratory tests (see above) and therapeutic response (eg, relief of pain and inflammation, increased activity tolerance), and adverse reactions (eg, GI effects, hepatotoxicity, or ototoxicity) at beginning of therapy and periodically throughout therapy (see Warnings/Precautions, Adverse Reactions, and Overdose/Toxicology). Schedule ophthalmic evaluations for patients who develop eye complaints during long-term NSAID therapy. Assess knowledge/teach patient appropriate use, interventions to reduce side effects, and adverse symptoms to report. **Pregnancy risk factor C.** Breast-feeding is not recommended.

**Patient Information/Instruction:** Take this medication exactly as directed; do not increase dose without consulting prescriber. Do not crush tablets or break capsules. Take with food or milk to reduce GI distress. Maintain adequate fluid intake (2-3 L/day of fluids unless instructed to restrict fluid intake). Do not use alcohol, aspirin, or aspirin-containing medication, and all other anti-inflammatory medications without consulting prescriber. You may experience drowsiness, dizziness, nervousness, or headache (use caution when driving or engaging in tasks requiring alertness until response to drug is known); anorexia, nausea, vomiting, or heartburn (frequent small meals, frequent oral care, sucking lozenges, or chewing gum may help); fluid retention (weigh yourself weekly and report unusual (3-5 lb/week) weight gain). GI bleeding, ulceration, or perforation can occur with or without pain; discontinue medication and contact prescriber if persistent abdominal pain or cramping, or blood in stool occurs. Report breathlessness, difficulty breathing, or unusual cough; chest pain, rapid heartbeat, palpitations; unusual bruising/bleeding; blood in urine, stool, mouth, or vomitus; swollen extremities; skin rash or itching; acute fatigue; or changes in hearing or ringing in ears. **Pregnancy/breast-feeding precautions:** Inform prescriber if you are pregnant. Breast-feeding is not recommended.

**Geriatric Considerations:** In trials with nabumetone, no significant differences were noted between young and elderly in regards to efficacy and safety. However, elderly are at high risk for adverse effects from nonsteroidal anti-inflammatory agents. As

(Continued)

## Nabumetone *(Continued)*

much as 60% of elderly can develop peptic ulceration and/or hemorrhage asymptomatically. The concomitant use of $H_2$ blockers, omeprazole, and sucralfate is not effective as prophylaxis with the exception of NSAID-induced duodenal ulcers which may be prevented by the use of ranitidine. Misoprostol is the only prophylactic agent proven effective. Also, concomitant disease and drug use contribute to the risk for GI adverse effects. Use lowest effective dose for shortest period possible. Consider renal function decline with age. Use of NSAIDs can compromise existing renal function especially when $Cl_{cr}$ is ≤30 mL/minute. Tinnitus may be a difficult and unreliable indication of toxicity due to age-related hearing loss or eighth cranial nerve damage. CNS adverse effects such as confusion, agitation, and hallucination are generally seen in overdose or high-dose situations, but elderly may demonstrate these adverse effects at lower doses than younger adults.

**Related Information**

Nonsalicylate/Nonsteroidal Anti-inflammatory Comparison *on page 1401*


- **NAC** *see* Acetylcysteine *on page 36*
- ***N*-Acetylcysteine** *see* Acetylcysteine *on page 36*
- ***N*-Acetyl-L-Cysteine** *see* Acetylcysteine *on page 36*
- **N-Acetyl-P-Aminophenol** *see* Acetaminophen *on page 32*


## Nadolol (nay DOE lole)

**U.S. Brand Names** Corgard®

**Therapeutic Category** Beta Blocker, Nonselective

**Pregnancy Risk Factor** C

**Lactation** Enters breast milk/use caution (AAP rates "compatible")

**Use** Treatment of hypertension and angina pectoris; prevention of myocardial infarction; prophylaxis of migraine headaches

**Mechanism of Action/Effect** Competitively blocks response to $beta_1$- and $beta_2$-adrenergic stimulation; does not exhibit any membrane stabilizing or intrinsic sympathomimetic activity

**Contraindications** Hypersensitivity to nadolol or any component; uncompensated congestive heart failure; cardiogenic shock; bradycardia or heart block

**Warnings** Increase dosing interval in patients with renal dysfunction. Abrupt withdrawal of beta-blockers may result in an exaggerated cardiac beta-adrenergic responsiveness. Symptomatology has included reports of tachycardia, hypertension, ischemia, angina, myocardial infarction, and sudden death. It is recommended that patients be tapered gradually off of beta-blockers over a period of 1-2 weeks rather than via abrupt discontinuation. Use with caution in patients with bronchial asthma, bronchospasms, CHF, or diabetes mellitus. Beta-blockers may impair glucose tolerance, potentiate hypoglycemia, and/or mask symptoms of hypoglycemia in a diabetic patient. Pregnancy factor C.

**Drug Interactions**

**Decreased Effect:** Decreased effect of beta-blockers with aluminum salts, barbiturates, calcium salts, cholestyramine, colestipol, NSAIDs, penicillins (ampicillin), rifampin, salicylates, and sulfinpyrazone due to decreased bioavailability and plasma levels. Beta-blockers may decrease the effect of sulfonylureas.

**Increased Effect/Toxicity:** Other hypotensive agents, diuretics and phenothiazines may increase hypotensive effects of nadolol. Nadolol may enhance neuromuscular blocking agents and will antagonize beta-agonist drugs (albuterol, etc). Other drug interactions similar to propranolol may occur.

**Adverse Reactions**

>10%:

Central nervous system: Drowsiness, insomnia

Endocrine & metabolic: Decreased sexual ability

1% to 10%:

Cardiovascular: Bradycardia, palpitations, edema, congestive heart failure, reduced peripheral circulation

Central nervous system: Mental depression

Gastrointestinal: Diarrhea or constipation, nausea, vomiting, stomach discomfort

Respiratory: Bronchospasm

Miscellaneous: Cold extremities

<1% (Limited to important or life-threatening symptoms): Chest pain, arrhythmias, orthostatic hypotension, nervousness, headache, depression, hallucinations, confusion (especially in the elderly), thrombocytopenia, leukopenia, shortness of breath

**Overdose/Toxicology** Symptoms of intoxication include cardiac disturbances, CNS toxicity, bronchospasm, hypoglycemia and hyperkalemia. The most common cardiac symptoms include hypotension and bradycardia. Atrioventricular block, intraventricular conduction disturbances, cardiogenic shock, and asystole may occur with severe overdose. CNS effects include convulsions, coma, and respiratory arrest. Treatment is symptom directed and supportive. Glucagon has been used to reverse cardiac depression.

**Pharmacodynamics/Kinetics**

**Protein Binding:** 28%

**Distribution:** Concentration in human breast milk is 4.6 times higher than serum

**Half-life Elimination:** 10-24 hours; increased half-life with decreased renal function; End-stage renal disease: 45 hours

**Time to Peak:** Within 2-4 hours persisting for 17-24 hours

**Excretion:** Urine

**Duration:** 24 hours

**Formulations** Tablet: 20 mg, 40 mg, 80 mg, 120 mg, 160 mg

**Dosing**

**Adults:** Oral: Initial: 40-80 mg/day, increase dosage gradually by 40-80 mg increments at 3- to 7-day intervals until optimum clinical response is obtained with profound slowing of heart rate. Doses up to 160-240 mg/day in angina and 240-320 mg/day in hypertension may be necessary. Doses as high as 640 mg/day have been used.

**Elderly:** Oral: Initial: 20 mg/day; increase doses by 20 mg increments at 3- to 7-day intervals; usual dosage range: 20-240 mg/day. Adjust for renal impairment.

**Renal Impairment:**

$Cl_{cr}$ 31-40 mL/minute: Administer every 24-36 hours or administer 50% of normal dose.

$Cl_{cr}$ 10-30 mL/minute: Administer every 24-48 hours or administer 50% of normal dose.

$Cl_{cr}$ <10 mL/minute: Administer every 40-60 hours or administer 25% of normal dose.

Hemodialysis effects: Moderately dialyzable (20% to 50%) via hemodialysis. Administer dose postdialysis or administer 40 mg supplemental dose. Supplemental dose is not necessary following peritoneal dialysis.

**Hepatic Impairment:** Reduced dose is probably necessary.

**Additional Nursing Issues**

**Physical Assessment:** Assess other medications the patient may taking for effectiveness and interactions (see Drug Interactions). Assess blood pressure and heart rate prior to and following first dose, any change in dosage, and periodically thereafter. Monitor or advise patient to monitor weight and fluid balance (I & O), assess for signs of CHF (edema, new cough or dyspnea, unresolved fatigue), and assess therapeutic effectiveness. Monitor serum glucose levels of diabetic patients since beta-blockers may alter glucose tolerance. Use/teach postural hypotension precautions. **Pregnancy risk factor C** - benefits of use should outweigh possible risks. Note breast-feeding caution.

**Patient Information/Instruction:** Check pulse daily prior to taking medication. If pulse is <50, hold medication and consult prescriber. Do not adjust dosage without consulting prescriber. May cause dizziness, fatigue, blurred vision; change position slowly (lying/sitting to standing) and use caution when driving or engaging in tasks that require alertness until response to drug is known. Exercise and increasing bulk or fiber in diet may help resolve constipation. If diabetic, monitor serum glucose closely (the drug may mask symptoms of hypoglycemia). Report swelling in feet or legs, difficulty breathing or persistent cough, unresolved fatigue, unusual weight gain >5 lb/week, or unresolved constipation. **Pregnancy/breast-feeding precautions:** Inform prescriber if you are or intend to be pregnant. Consult prescriber if breast-feeding.

**Geriatric Considerations:** Due to alterations in the beta-adrenergic autonomic nervous system, beta-adrenergic blockade may result in less hemodynamic response than seen in younger adults. Studies indicate that despite decreased sensitivity to the chronotropic effects of beta blockade with age, there appears to be an increased myocardial sensitivity to the negative inotropic effect during stress (eg, exercise). See Warnings/Precautions.

**Breast-feeding Issues:** Considered compatible by the American Academy of Pediatrics. However, monitor the infant for signs of beta-blockade (hypotension, bradycardia, etc) with long-term use.

**Related Information**

Beta-Blockers Comparison *on page 1376*

♦ **Nadopen-V®** *see* Penicillin V Potassium *on page 900*

♦ **Nadostine®** *see* Nystatin *on page 843*

## Nafarelin (NAF a re lin)

**U.S. Brand Names** Synarel®

**Therapeutic Category** Hormone, Posterior Pituitary; Luteinizing Hormone-Releasing Hormone Analog

**Pregnancy Risk Factor** X

**Lactation** Enters breast milk/contraindicated

**Use** Treatment of endometriosis, including pain and reduction of lesions; treatment of central precocious puberty (gonadotropin-dependent precocious puberty) in children of both sexes

**Mechanism of Action/Effect** Potent synthetic decapeptide analogue of gonadotropin-releasing hormone (GnRH; LHRH) which is approximately 200 times more potent than GnRH in terms of pituitary release of luteinizing hormone (LH) and follicle-stimulating hormone (FSH)

**Contraindications** Hypersensitivity to GnRH, GnRH-agonist analogs, or any components; undiagnosed abnormal vaginal bleeding; pregnancy

**Warnings** Use with caution in patients with risk factors for decreased bone mineral content. Nafarelin therapy may pose an additional risk. Hypersensitivity reactions occur in 0.2% of the patients.

**Adverse Reactions**

>10%:

Central nervous system: Headache, emotional lability

Dermatologic: Acne

Endocrine & metabolic: Hot flashes, breakthrough bleeding, spotting, menorrhagia, decreased libido, decreased breast size, amenorrhea, hypoestrogenism

Genitourinary: Vaginal dryness

Respiratory: Nasal irritation

(Continued)

## Nafarelin *(Continued)*

1% to 10%:

Cardiovascular: Edema, chest pain

Central nervous system: Insomnia, mental depression

Dermatologic: Urticaria, rash, pruritus, seborrhea

Respiratory: Shortness of breath, rhinitis

**Pharmacodynamics/Kinetics**

**Protein Binding:** 80% bound to plasma proteins

**Time to Peak:** Maximum serum concentration: 10-45 minutes

**Formulations** Solution, nasal, as acetate: 2 mg/mL (10 mL)

**Dosing**

**Adults:** Endometriosis: 1 spray (200 mcg) in 1 nostril each morning and the other nostril each evening starting on days 2-4 of menstrual cycle for 6 months

**Administration**

**Inhalation:** Nasal spray: Do not give to pregnant or breast-feeding patients. Do not use topical nasal decongestant for at least 30 minutes after nafarelin use.

**Stability**

**Storage:** Store at room temperature. Protect from light.

**Additional Nursing Issues**

**Physical Assessment:** (For treatment of precocious puberty consult appropriate pediatric reference.) Endometriosis: Assess knowledge/teach correct administration and timing of nasal spray. Monitor and teach patient to monitor for effectiveness, possible adverse reactions (see above), and symptoms to report. **Pregnancy risk factor X.** Breast-feeding is contraindicated.

**Patient Information/Instruction:** You will begin this treatment between days 2-4 of your regular menstrual cycle. Use as directed - daily at the same time (arising and bedtime), and rotate nostrils. Maintain regular follow-up schedule. You may experience hot flashes, flushing or redness (cold clothes and cool environment may help), decreased or increased libido, emotional lability, weight gain, decreased breast size, or hirsutism. Report any breakthrough bleeding or continuing menstruation or musculoskeletal pain. Do not use a nasal decongestant within 30 minutes after nafarelin. **Pregnancy/breast-feeding precautions:** Consult prescriber about pregnancy. Do not breast-feed.

**Additional Information** Each spray delivers 200 mcg.

♦ **Nafazair®** *see page 1282*

♦ **Nafazair® Ophthalmic** *see page 1294*

♦ **Nafcil™ Injection** *see* Nafcillin *on this page*

## Nafcillin (naf SIL in)

**U.S. Brand Names** Nafcil™ Injection; Nallpen® Injection; Unipen® Injection; Unipen® Oral

**Synonyms** Ethoxynaphthamido Penicillin Sodium

**Therapeutic Category** Antibiotic, Penicillin

**Pregnancy Risk Factor** B

**Lactation** Excretion in breast milk unknown

**Use** Treatment of bacterial infections such as osteomyelitis, septicemia, endocarditis, and CNS infections caused by susceptible strains of *Staphylococcus*

**Mechanism of Action/Effect** Interferes with bacterial cell wall synthesis during active multiplication, causing cell wall death and resultant bactericidal activity against susceptible bacteria

**Contraindications** Hypersensitivity to nafcillin, any component, penicillins, cephalosporins, or imipenem

**Warnings** Extravasation of I.V. infusions should be avoided. Modification of dosage is necessary in patients with both severe renal and hepatic impairment. Elimination rate will be slow in neonates.

**Drug Interactions**

**Decreased Effect:** Chloramphenicol may decrease nafcillin levels. Oral contraceptives may have a decreased contraceptive effect when taken with nafcillin. If taken concomitantly with warfarin, nafcillin may inhibit the anticoagulant response to warfarin. This effect may persist for up to 30 days after nafcillin has been discontinued. Subtherapeutic cyclosporin levels may result when taken concomitantly with nafcillin.

**Increased Effect/Toxicity:** Probenecid may cause an increase in nafcillin levels.

**Food Interactions** Nafcillin serum concentrations may be decreased if taken with food.

**Effects on Lab Values** Positive Coombs' test (direct)

**Adverse Reactions**

Local: **Vesicant chemotherapy**

<1% (Limited to important or life-threatening symptoms): Neutropenia, thrombophlebitis (oxacillin is less likely to cause phlebitis and is often preferred in pediatric patients), acute interstitial nephritis

**Overdose/Toxicology** Symptoms of penicillin overdose include neuromuscular hypersensitivity (eg, agitation, hallucinations, asterixis, encephalopathy, confusion, and seizures). Electrolyte imbalance may occur if the preparation contains potassium or sodium salts, especially in renal failure. Hemodialysis may be helpful to aid in the removal of drug from blood; otherwise, treatment is supportive or symptom directed.

**Pharmacodynamics/Kinetics**

**Protein Binding:** 90%

**Distribution:** Crosses the placenta

**Half-life Elimination:** 0.5-1.5 hours, with normal hepatic function; End-stage renal disease: 1.2 hours

**Time to Peak:** Oral: Within 2 hours; I.M.: Within 0.5-1 hour

**Excretion:** Bile and urine; undergoes enterohepatic recycling

**Formulations**

Nafcillin sodium:

Capsule: 250 mg

Powder for injection: 500 mg, 1 g, 2 g, 4 g, 10 g

Solution: 250 mg/5 mL (100 mL)

Tablet: 500 mg

**Dosing**

**Adults:**

I.M.: 500 mg every 4-6 hours

I.V.: 500-2000 mg every 4-6 hours

Oral (serum levels are usually low):

250-500 mg every 4-6 hours; or 1 g every 4-6 hours

**Elderly:** Refer to adult dosing.

**Renal Impairment:**

Not necessary

Hemodialysis effects: Not dialyzable (0% to 5%) via hemodialysis; supplemental dosage is not necessary with hemo- or peritoneal dialysis or continuous arteriovenous or venovenous hemofiltration (CAVH/CAVHD).

**Administration**

**Oral:** Administer around-the-clock to promote less variation in peak and trough serum levels. Should be preferably administered on an empty stomach, since there is decreased absorption with food.

**I.M.:** Rotate injection sites.

**I.V.:** Vesicant. Administer around-the-clock to promote less variation in peak and trough serum levels. Infuse over 30-60 minutes.

**I.V. Detail: Extravasation management:** Use cold packs.

Hyaluronidase (Wydase®): Add 1 mL NS to 150 unit vial to make 150 units/mL of concentration; mix 0.1 mL of above with 0.9 mL NS in 1 mL syringe to make final concentration = 15 units/mL.

**Stability**

**Storage:** Refrigerate oral solution after reconstitution. Discard after 7 days. Reconstituted parenteral solution is stable for 3 days at room temperature, 7 days when refrigerated, or 12 weeks when frozen. For I.V. infusion in NS or $D_5W$, solution is stable for 24 hours at room temperature and 96 hours when refrigerated.

**Monitoring Laboratory Tests** Perform culture and sensitivity studies prior to initiating drug therapy. Monitor renal, hepatic, CBC with prolonged therapy.

**Additional Nursing Issues**

**Physical Assessment:** Assess patient reports of allergy or sensitivity before administering. Monitor infusion site for extravasation (see above). Monitor response to therapy; if no response, re-evaluate therapy. Advise females using oral contraceptives to use barrier contraception - nafcillin may reduce effect of oral contraceptives. Note breast-feeding caution.

**Patient Information/Instruction:** Oral: Take at regular intervals around-the-clock, preferably on and empty stomach with full glass of water. Take complete course of treatment as prescribed. You may experience nausea or vomiting; small frequent meals and good mouth care may help. If diabetic, drug may cause false tests with Clinitest® urine glucose monitoring; use of glucose oxidase methods (Clinistix®) or serum glucose monitoring is preferable. This drug may interfere with oral contraceptives; an alternate form of birth control should be used. Report persistent fever, sore throat, sores in mouth, diarrhea, unusual bleeding or bruising. Report difficulty breathing or skin rash. Notify prescriber if condition does not respond to treatment. **Breast-feeding precautions:** Consult prescriber if breast-feeding.

**Geriatric Considerations:** Nafcillin has not been studied exclusively in the elderly, however, given its route of elimination, dosage adjustments based upon age and renal function is not necessary.

**Additional Information**

Sodium content of 1 g: 66.7 mg (2.9 mEq)

pH: 6-8.5

♦ **Naftifine** *see page 1247*

♦ **Naftin®** *see page 1247*

♦ **$NaHCO_3$** *see* Sodium Bicarbonate *on page 1061*

## Nalbuphine (NAL byoo feen)

**U.S. Brand Names** Nubain®

**Therapeutic Category** Analgesic, Narcotic

**Pregnancy Risk Factor** B/D (if used for prolonged periods or in high doses at term)

**Lactation** Excretion in breast milk unknown/use caution

**Use** Relief of moderate to severe pain; preoperative analgesia, postoperative and surgical anesthesia, and obstetrical analgesia during labor and delivery

(Continued)

## Nalbuphine *(Continued)*

**Mechanism of Action/Effect** Binds to opiate receptors in the CNS, causing inhibition of ascending pain pathways, altering the perception of and response to pain; produces generalized CNS depression

**Contraindications** Hypersensitivity to nalbuphine or any component, including sulfites; pregnancy (if used for prolonged periods or in high doses at term)

**Warnings** Use with caution in patients with recent myocardial infarction, biliary tract surgery, or sulfite sensitivity. May produce respiratory depression. Use with caution in women delivering premature infants. Use with caution in patients with a history of drug dependence, head trauma or increased intracranial pressure, decreased hepatic or renal function.

**Drug Interactions**

**Increased Effect/Toxicity:** Barbiturate anesthetics may increase CNS depression.

**Adverse Reactions**

>10%:

Central nervous system: Fatigue, drowsiness
Miscellaneous: Histamine release

1% to 10%:

Cardiovascular: Hypotension
Central nervous system: Headache, nightmares, dizziness
Gastrointestinal: Anorexia, nausea, vomiting, dry mouth
Local: Pain at injection site
Neuromuscular & skeletal: Weakness

<1% (Limited to important or life-threatening symptoms): Tachycardia or bradycardia, hypertension, dyspnea, shortness of breath

**Overdose/Toxicology** Symptoms of overdose include CNS depression, respiratory depression, miosis, hypotension, and bradycardia. Treatment is symptomatic. Naloxone, 2 mg I.V. with repeat administration as necessary up to a total dose of 10 mg, can be used to reverse opiate effects.

**Pharmacodynamics/Kinetics**

**Half-life Elimination:** 3.5-5 hours

**Metabolism:** Liver

**Excretion:** Feces and urine

**Onset:** Peak effect: I.M.: 30 minutes; I.V.: 1-3 minutes

**Formulations** Injection, as hydrochloride: 10 mg/mL (1 mL, 10 mL); 20 mg/mL (1 mL, 10 mL)

**Dosing**

**Adults:** I.M., I.V., S.C.: 10 mg/70 kg every 3-6 hours; maximum single dose: 20 mg; maximum daily dose: 160 mg

**Elderly:** Refer to adult dosing; use with caution.

**Renal Impairment:** Use with caution and reduce dose.

**Hepatic Impairment:** Use with caution and reduce dose.

**Stability**

**Compatibility:** See the Compatibility of Drugs in Syringe Chart *on page 1317*.

**Additional Nursing Issues**

**Physical Assessment:** Note Drug Interactions. Monitor for effectiveness of pain relief and monitor for signs of overdose (see above). Monitor blood pressure, CNS and respiratory status, and degree of sedation at beginning of therapy and at regular intervals during use. For inpatients, implement safety measures (eg, side rails up, call light within reach, instructions to call for assistance, etc). Generally used in conjunction with surgical anesthesia or during labor and delivery; however, if self-administered for relief of pain, assess knowledge/teach patient appropriate use. Teach patient to monitor for adverse reactions (see Adverse Reactions), adverse reactions to report, and appropriate interventions to reduce side effects. **Pregnancy risk factor B/D** - see Pregnancy Risk Factor for cautious use. Note breast-feeding caution.

**Patient Information/Instruction:** If self-administered, use exactly as directed (do not increase dose or frequency); may cause physical and/or psychological dependence. While using this medication, do not use alcohol and other prescription or OTC medications (especially sedatives, tranquilizers, antihistamines, or pain medications) without consulting prescriber. Maintain adequate hydration (2-3 L/day of fluids unless instructed to restrict fluid intake). May cause hypotension, dizziness, drowsiness, impaired coordination, or blurred vision (use caution when driving, climbing stairs, or changing position - rising from sitting or lying to standing, or when engaging in tasks requiring alertness until response to drug is known); loss of appetite, nausea, or vomiting (frequent mouth care, small frequent meals, chewing gum, or sucking lozenges may help); constipation (increased exercise, fluids, or dietary fruit and fiber may help - if constipation remains an unresolved problem, consult prescriber about use of stool softeners). Report chest pain, slow or rapid heartbeat, acute dizziness or persistent headache; changes in mental status; swelling of extremities or unusual weight gain; changes in urinary elimination or pain on urination; acute headache; back or flank pain or muscle spasms; blurred vision; skin rash; or shortness of breath. **Pregnancy/breast-feeding precautions:** Inform prescriber if you are or intend to be pregnant. If you are breast-feeding, take medication immediately after breast-feeding or 3-4 hours prior to next feeding.

**Geriatric Considerations:** The elderly may be particularly susceptible to CNS effects; monitor closely.

**Additional Information** The injection formulation contains sulfites.

**Related Information**

Narcotic/Opioid Analgesic Comparison *on page 1396*

- ♦ **Naldecon®** *see page 1306*
- ♦ **Naldecon® DX Adult Liquid [OTC]** *see* Guaifenesin, Phenylpropanolamine, and Dextromethorphan *on page 551*
- ♦ **Naldecon-EX® Children's Syrup [OTC]** *see* Guaifenesin and Phenylpropanolamine *on page 550*
- ♦ **Naldecon® Senior DX [OTC]** *see* Guaifenesin and Dextromethorphan *on page 549*
- ♦ **Naldecon® Senior EX [OTC]** *see* Guaifenesin *on page 548*
- ♦ **Naldelate®** *see page 1306*
- ♦ **Nalfon®** *see* Fenoprofen *on page 476*
- ♦ **Nalgest®** *see page 1306*
- ♦ **Nallpen® Injection** *see* Nafcillin *on page 800*
- ♦ ***N*-Allylnoroxymorphone Hydrochloride** *see* Naloxone *on next page*


## Nalmefene (NAL me feen)

**U.S. Brand Names** Revex®

**Therapeutic Category** Antidote

**Pregnancy Risk Factor** B

**Lactation** Enters breast milk/use caution

**Use** Complete or partial reversal of opioid drug effects, including respiratory depression induced by natural or synthetic opioids; reversal of postoperative opioid depression; management of known or suspected opioid overdose (if opioid dependence is suspected, nalmefene should only be used in opioid overdose if the likelihood of overdose is high based on history or the clinical presentation of respiratory depression with concurrent pupillary constriction is present)

**Mechanism of Action/Effect** Nalmefene acts as a competitive antagonist at opioid receptor sites, preventing or reversing the respiratory depression, sedation, and hypotension induced by opiates; no pharmacologic activity of its own (eg, opioid agonist activity) has been demonstrated

**Contraindications** Hypersensitivity to nalmefene, naltrexone, or any component

**Warnings** May induce symptoms of acute withdrawal in opioid-dependent patients. Recurrence of respiratory depression is possible if the opioid involved is long-acting. Observe patients until there is no reasonable risk of recurrent respiratory depression. Dosage may need to be decreased in renal and hepatic impairment. Safety and efficacy have not been established in children. Avoid abrupt reversal of opioid effects in patients of high cardiovascular risk or who have received potentially cardiotoxic drugs. Animal studies indicate nalmefene may not completely reverse buprenorphine-induced respiratory depression.

**Drug Interactions**

**Increased Effect/Toxicity:** Potential increased risk of seizures exists with use of flumazenil and nalmefene coadministration.

**Adverse Reactions**

>10%: Gastrointestinal: Nausea

1% to 10%:

Cardiovascular: Tachycardia, hypertension

Central nervous system: Fever, dizziness

Gastrointestinal: Vomiting

Miscellaneous: Postoperative pain

<1% (Limited to important or life-threatening symptoms): Arrhythmia, bradycardia, increased AST

**Overdose/Toxicology** No reported symptoms with significant overdose. Large doses of opioids administered to overcome a full blockade of opioid antagonists, however, have resulted in adverse respiratory and circulatory reactions.

**Pharmacodynamics/Kinetics**

**Protein Binding:** 45%

**Distribution:** Rapid

**Half-life Elimination:** 10.8 hours

**Time to Peak:** 2.3 hours

**Metabolism:** Liver

**Excretion:** Urine and feces

**Onset:** I.M., S.C.: 5-15 minutes

**Formulations** Injection, as hydrochloride: 100 mcg/mL [blue label] (1 mL); 1000 mcg/mL [green label] (2 mL)

**Dosing**

**Adults:**

Reversal of postoperative opioid depression: Blue labeled product (100 mcg/mL): Titrate to reverse the undesired effects of opioids; initial dose for nonopioid dependent patient: 0.25 mcg/kg followed by 0.25 mcg/kg incremental doses at 2- to 5-minute intervals. After a total dose >1 mcg/kg, further therapeutic response is unlikely.

Management of known/suspected opioid overdose: Green labeled product (1000 mcg/mL): Initial: 0.5 mg/70 kg; may repeat with 1 mg/70 kg in 2-5 minutes. Further increase beyond a total dose of 1.5 mg/70 kg will not likely result in improved response and may result in cardiovascular stress and precipitated withdrawal syndrome. (If opioid dependency is suspected, administer a challenge dose of 0.1 mg/70 kg; if no withdrawal symptoms are observed in 2 minutes, the recommended doses can be administered).

(Continued)

## Nalmefene *(Continued)*

**Elderly:** Refer to adult dosing.

**Renal Impairment:** Not necessary with single uses.

**Hepatic Impairment:** Not necessary with single uses.

**Administration**

**I.V.:** Slow administration (over 60 seconds) of incremental doses is recommended to minimize hypertension and dizziness.

**I.V. Detail:** Check dosage strength carefully before use to avoid error. Dilute drug (1:1) with diluent and use smaller doses in patients known to be at increased cardiovascular risk. May be administered via I.M. or S.C. routes if I.V. access is not feasible.

**Additional Nursing Issues**

**Physical Assessment:** Assess patient for opioid dependency (see Warnings/Precautions). Monitor vital signs and cardiac status carefully during infusion and for some time thereafter (effects may continue for several days, use nonopioid analgesics for pain). Note breast-feeding caution.

**Patient Information/Instruction:** This drug can only be administered I.V. You may experience drowsiness, dizziness, or blurred vision for several days; use caution when driving or engaging in tasks requiring alertness until response to drug is known. Small frequent meals and good mouth care may reduce any nausea or vomiting. Report yellowing of eyes or skin, unusual bleeding, dark or tarry stools, acute headache, or palpitations. **Breast-feeding precautions:** Wait 4 hours before breast-feeding.

**Pregnancy Issues:** Limited information available

**Additional Information** Proper steps should be used to prevent use of the incorrect dosage strength; the goal of treatment in the postoperative setting is to achieve reversal of excessive opioid effects without inducing a complete reversal and acute pain

## Naloxone (nal OKS one)

**U.S. Brand Names** Narcan® Injection

**Synonyms** *N*-Allylnoroxymorphone Hydrochloride

**Therapeutic Category** Antidote

**Pregnancy Risk Factor** B

**Lactation** Excretion in breast milk unknown/not recommended

**Use** Reverses CNS and respiratory depression in suspected narcotic overdose; coma of unknown etiology

**Investigational use:** Refractory shock, alcoholic coma, Alzheimer dementia, schizophrenia

**Mechanism of Action/Effect** Competes and displaces narcotics at narcotic receptor sites

**Contraindications** Hypersensitivity to naloxone or any component

**Warnings** Use with caution in patients with cardiovascular disease. Excessive dosages should be avoided after use of opiates in surgery, because naloxone may cause an increase in blood pressure and reversal of anesthesia. May precipitate withdrawal symptoms in patients addicted to opiates, including pain, hypertension, sweating, agitation, irritability, shrill cry, and failure to feed.

**Adverse Reactions** 1% to 10%:

Cardiovascular: Hypertension, hypotension, tachycardia, ventricular arrhythmias
Central nervous system: Insomnia, irritability, anxiety, narcotic withdrawal
Dermatologic: Rash
Gastrointestinal: Nausea, vomiting
Ocular: Blurred vision
Miscellaneous: Sweating

**Overdose/Toxicology** Naloxone is the drug of choice for respiratory depression that is known or suspected to be caused by overdose of an opiate or opioid. **Caution:** Naloxone's effects are due to its action on narcotic reversal, not due to any direct effect upon opiate receptors. Therefore, adverse events occur secondarily to reversal (withdrawal) of narcotic analgesia and sedation, which can cause severe reactions.

**Pharmacodynamics/Kinetics**

**Distribution:** Crosses the placenta

**Half-life Elimination:** 1-1.5 hours

**Metabolism:** Liver

**Excretion:** Urine

**Onset:** Endotracheal, I.M., S.C.: Within 2-5 minutes; I.V.: Within 2 minutes

**Duration:** 20-60 minutes; since shorter than that of most opioids, repeated doses are usually needed

**Formulations** Injection, as hydrochloride: 0.4 mg/mL (1 mL, 2 mL, 10 mL); 1 mg/mL (2 mL, 10 mL)

**Dosing**

**Adults:** I.M., I.V. (preferred), intratracheal, S.C.:

Continuous infusion: I.V.: If continuous infusion is required, calculate dosage/hour based on effective intermittent dose used and duration of adequate response seen, titrate dose 0.04-0.16 mg/kg/hour for 2-5 days in children, up to 0.8 mg/kg/hour in adults. Alternatively, continuous infusion utilizes $^2/_3$ of the initial naloxone bolus on an hourly basis. Add 10 times this dose to each liter of $D_5W$ and infuse at a rate of 100 mL/hour. $^1/_2$ of the initial bolus dose should be readministered 15 minutes after initiation of the continuous infusion to prevent a drop in naloxone levels. Increase infusion rate as needed to assure adequate ventilation.

Narcotic overdose: I.V.: 0.4-2 mg every 2-3 minutes as needed; may need to repeat doses every 20-60 minutes, if no response is observed after 10 mg, question the diagnosis. **Note:** Use 0.1-0.2 mg increments in patients who are opioid dependent and in postoperative patients to avoid large cardiovascular changes.

**Elderly:** Refer to adult dosing.

**Stability**

**Storage:** Protect from light.

**Reconstitution:** Stable in 0.9% sodium chloride and $D_5W$ at 4 mcg/mL for 24 hours.

**Compatibility:** Do not mix with alkaline solutions.

**Additional Nursing Issues**

**Physical Assessment:** Assess patient for opioid dependency (see Warnings/Precautions). Monitor vital signs and cardiorespiratory status continuously during infusion, maintain patent airway. Breast-feeding is not recommended.

**Patient Information/Instruction:** If patient is responsive, instructions are individualized. This drug can only be administered I.V. Report difficulty breathing, palpitations, or tremors. **Breast-feeding precautions:** Breast-feeding is not recommended.

**Geriatric Considerations:** In small trials, naloxone has shown temporary improvement in Alzheimer's disease; however, is not recommended for treatment.

**Breast-feeding Issues:** No data reported. Since naloxone is used for opiate reversal the concern should be on opiate drug levels in a breast-feeding mother and transfer to the infant rather than naloxone exposure. The safest approach would be **not** to breast-feed.

**Related Information**

Narcotic/Opioid Analgesic Comparison *on page 1396*

♦ **Nalspan®** *see page 1306*

## Naltrexone (nal TREKS one)

**U.S. Brand Names** ReVia®

**Therapeutic Category** Antidote

**Pregnancy Risk Factor** C

**Lactation** Excretion in breast milk unknown

**Use** Adjunct to the maintenance of an opioid-free state in detoxified individual; alcoholism

**Mechanism of Action/Effect** Naltrexone is a cyclopropyl derivative of oxymorphone similar in structure to naloxone and nalorphine (a morphine derivative); it acts as a competitive antagonist at opioid receptor sites

**Contraindications** Hypersensitivity to naltrexone; opioid dependent patients, patients in acute opiate withdrawal, positive urine screen for opioids, acute hepatitis; liver failure

**Warnings** Dose-related hepatocellular injury is possible. The margin of separation between the apparent safe and hepatotoxic doses appear to be only fivefold or less. Pregnancy factor C.

**Adverse Reactions**

>10%:
- Central nervous system: Insomnia, anxiety, nervousness, headache
- Gastrointestinal: Abdominal cramping, nausea, vomiting
- Neuromuscular & skeletal: Arthralgia

1% to 10%:
- Central nervous system: Dizziness
- Dermatologic: Rash
- Endocrine & metabolic: Polydipsia
- Gastrointestinal: Anorexia
- Respiratory: Sneezing

<1% (Limited to important or life-threatening symptoms): Thrombocytopenia, agranulocytosis, hemolytic anemia

**Overdose/Toxicology** Symptoms of overdose include clonic-tonic convulsions and respiratory failure. Patients receiving up to 800 mg/day for 1 week have shown no toxicity. Seizures and respiratory failure have been seen in animals.

**Pharmacodynamics/Kinetics**

**Protein Binding:** 21%

**Distribution:** Distributed widely throughout the body but considerable interindividual variation exists

**Half-life Elimination:** 4 hours; active metabolite, 6-β-naltrexol: 13 hours

**Time to Peak:** Within 60 minutes

**Metabolism:** Liver

**Excretion:** Urine

**Duration:** 50 mg: 24 hours; 100 mg: 48 hours; 150 mg: 72 hours

**Formulations** Tablet, as hydrochloride: 50 mg

**Dosing**

**Adults:** Do not give until patient is opioid-free for 7-10 days as required by urine analysis; Adults: Oral:

25 mg; if no withdrawal signs within 1 hour give another 25 mg; maintenance regimen is flexible, variable and individualized (50 mg/day to 100-150 mg 3 times/week)

Adjunct in the management of alcoholism: A flexible approach to dosing is recommended by the manufacturer; the following are acceptable regimens:
- 50 mg once daily
- 50 mg once daily on weekdays and 100 mg on Saturdays
- 100 mg every other day
- 150 mg every third day

**Elderly:** Refer to adult dosing.

**Monitoring Laboratory Tests** Periodic LFTs

(Continued)

## Naltrexone *(Continued)*

**Additional Nursing Issues**

**Physical Assessment:** Do not use until patient has been opioid-free for 7-10 days. Assess carefully for several days following start of therapy for narcotic withdrawal symptoms or severe adverse reactions (see Adverse Reactions). Use non-narcotic analgesics for pain. **Pregnancy risk factor C** - benefits should outweigh possible risks. Note breast-feeding caution.

**Patient Information/Instruction:** This medication will help you achieve abstinence from opiates if taken as directed. Do not increase or change dose. Do not use opiates or any medications not approved by your prescriber during naltrexone therapy. You may experience drowsiness, dizziness, or blurred vision (use caution when driving or engaging in tasks requiring alertness until response to drug is known); nausea or vomiting (small frequent meals, frequent mouth care, chewing gum, or sucking lozenges may help); decreased sexual function (reversible when drug is discontinued). Report yellowing of skin or eyes, change in color of stool or urine, increased perspiration or chills, acute headache, palpitations, or unusual joint pain. **Pregnancy/breast-feeding precautions:** Inform prescriber if you are or intend to be pregnant. Consult prescriber if breast-feeding.

## Nandrolone (NAN droe lone)

**U.S. Brand Names** Anabolin® Injection; Androlone®-D Injection; Androlone® Injection; Deca-Durabolin® Injection; Durabolin® Injection; Hybolin™ Decanoate Injection; Hybolin™ Improved Injection; Neo-Durabolic Injection

**Therapeutic Category** Androgen

**Pregnancy Risk Factor** X

**Lactation** Excretion in breast milk unknown/contraindicated

**Use** Control of metastatic breast cancer; management of anemia of renal insufficiency

**Mechanism of Action/Effect** Promotes tissue-building processes, increases production of erythropoietin, causes protein anabolism; increases hemoglobin and red blood cell volume

**Contraindications** Hypersensitivity to nandrolone or any component; carcinoma of breast or prostate; nephrosis; pregnancy; infants

**Warnings** Monitor diabetic patients carefully. Anabolic steroids may cause peliosis hepatis, liver cell tumors, and blood lipid changes with increased risk of arteriosclerosis. Use with caution in elderly patients, they may be at greater risk for prostatic hypertrophy. Use with caution in patients with cardiac, renal, or hepatic disease or epilepsy.

**Drug Interactions**

**Increased Effect/Toxicity:** Nandrolone may increase the effect of oral anticoagulants, insulin, oral hypoglycemic agents, adrenal steroids, or ACTH when taken together.

**Effects on Lab Values** Altered glucose tolerance tests

**Adverse Reactions**

**Male: Postpubertal:**

>10%:
- Dermatologic: Acne
- Endocrine & metabolic: Gynecomastia
- Genitourinary: Bladder irritability, priapism

1% to 10%:
- Central nervous system: Insomnia, chills
- Endocrine & metabolic: Decreased libido, hepatic dysfunction,
- Gastrointestinal: Nausea, diarrhea
- Genitourinary: Prostatic hypertrophy (elderly)
- Hematologic: Iron deficiency anemia, suppression of clotting factors

<1% (Limited to important or life-threatening symptoms): Hepatic necrosis, hepatocellular carcinoma

**Male: Prepubertal:**

>10%:
- Dermatologic: Acne
- Endocrine & metabolic: Virilism

1% to 10%:
- Central nervous system: Chills, insomnia, factors
- Dermatologic: Hyperpigmentation
- Gastrointestinal: Diarrhea, nausea
- Hematologic: Iron deficiency anemia, suppression of clotting

<1% (Limited to important or life-threatening symptoms): Hepatocellular carcinoma, necrosis

**Female:**

>10%: Endocrine & metabolic: Virilism

1% to 10%:
- Central nervous system: Chills, insomnia
- Endocrine & metabolic: Hypercalcemia
- Gastrointestinal: Nausea, diarrhea
- Hematologic: Iron deficiency anemia, suppression of clotting factors
- Hepatic: Hepatic dysfunction

<1% (Limited to important or life-threatening symptoms): Hepatic necrosis, hepatocellular carcinoma

**Pharmacodynamics/Kinetics**

**Metabolism:** Liver

**Excretion:** Urine

**Formulations**

Nandrolone phenpropionate:

Injection in oil: 25 mg/mL (5 mL); 50 mg/mL (2 mL)

Nandrolone decanoate:

Injection in oil: 50 mg/mL (1 mL, 2 mL); 100 mg/mL (1 mL, 2 mL); 200 mg/mL (1 mL)

Injection, repository: 50 mg/mL (2 mL); 100 mg/mL (2 mL); 200 mg/mL (2 mL)

**Dosing**

**Adults:** Deep I.M. (into gluteal muscle):

Breast cancer (phenpropionate): Male/Female: 50-100 mg/week

Anemia of renal insufficiency (decanoate):

Male: 100-200 mg/week

Female: 50-100 mg/week

**Elderly:** Refer to adult dosing.

**Administration**

**I.M.:** Inject deeply I.M., preferably into the gluteal muscle.

**Monitoring Laboratory Tests** LFTs on a regular basis

**Additional Nursing Issues**

**Physical Assessment:** Assess effectiveness and interactions of other medications (see Drug Interactions, eg, hypoglycemic agents, anticoagulants). See Warnings/Precautions and Contraindications for use cautions. Monitor effectiveness of therapy, laboratory tests, and adverse response (see Adverse Reactions and Overdose/Toxicology). Assess knowledge/teach patient appropriate use, possible side effects and appropriate interventions, and adverse symptoms to report. **Pregnancy risk factor X** - determine that patient is not pregnant before beginning treatment and do not give to women of childbearing age or males who may have intercourse with childbearing women unless both male and female are capable of complying with barrier contraceptive measures during therapy and for 1 month following therapy. Breast-feeding is contraindicated.

**Patient Information/Instruction:** This drug can only be given I.M. Diabetics should monitor serum glucose closely and notify prescriber of changes; this medication can alter hypoglycemic requirements. You may experience acne, growth of body hair, loss of libido, impotence, or menstrual irregularity (usually reversible); nausea or vomiting (small frequent meals, frequent mouth care, sucking lozenges, or chewing gum may help); diarrhea (buttermilk, boiled milk, yogurt may help). Report changes in menstrual pattern; enlarged or painful breasts; deepening of voice or unusual growth of body hair; fluid retention (swelling of ankles, feet, or hands, difficulty breathing, or sudden weight gain); unresolved changes in CNS (nervousness, chills, insomnia); change in color of urine or stool; yellowing of eyes or skin; unusual bruising or bleeding; or other adverse reactions. **Pregnancy/breast-feeding precautions:** Inform prescriber if you are pregnant. Do not get pregnant during or for 1 month following therapy. Male: Do not cause pregnancy. Male/female: Consult prescriber for instruction on appropriate barrier contraceptive measures. This drug may cause severe fetal defects. Do not breast-feed.

**Additional Information** Both phenpropionate and decanoate are injections in oil.


- ♦ **Naphazoline** *see page 1282*
- ♦ **Naphazoline** *see page 1294*
- ♦ **Naphazoline and Antazoline** *see page 1294*
- ♦ **Naphazoline and Pheniramine** *see page 1294*
- ♦ **Naphcon-A® Ophthalmic Solution** *see page 1294*
- ♦ **Naphcon Forte®** *see page 1282*
- ♦ **Naphcon Forte® Ophthalmic** *see page 1294*
- ♦ **Naphcon® Ophthalmic** *see page 1294*
- ♦ **Naprelan®** *see* Naproxen *on this page*
- ♦ **Naprodil** *see* Naproxen *on this page*
- ♦ **Naprosyn®** *see* Naproxen *on this page*


## Naproxen (na PROKS en)

**U.S. Brand Names** Aleve® [OTC]; Anaprox®; Naprelan®; Naprosyn®

**Therapeutic Category** Nonsteroidal Anti-Inflammatory Agent (NSAID)

**Pregnancy Risk Factor** B/D (3rd trimester or near delivery)

**Lactation** Enters breast milk/compatible

**Use** Management of osteoarthritis and rheumatoid disorders (including juvenile arthritis, ankylosing spondylitis); treatment of acute gout, tendonitis and bursitis, mild to moderate pain, primary dysmenorrhea, fever

**Mechanism of Action/Effect** Inhibits prostaglandin synthesis by decreasing the activity of the enzyme, cyclo-oxygenase, which results in decreased formation of prostaglandin precursors

**Contraindications** Hypersensitivity to naproxen; should not be administered to patients with active peptic ulceration and those with severe hepatic impairment or in patients in whom naproxen, aspirin, or other NSAIDs have induced asthma, urticaria, or other allergic-type reactions; fatal asthmatic reactions have occurred following NSAID administration; pregnancy (3rd trimester or near delivery)

**Warnings** Use with caution in patients with GI disease (bleeding or ulcers), cardiovascular disease (CHF, hypertension), renal or hepatic impairment, and patients receiving anticoagulants. Perform ophthalmologic evaluation for those who develop eye complaints

(Continued)

## Naproxen *(Continued)*

during therapy (blurred vision, diminished vision, changes in color vision, retinal changes). NSAIDs may mask signs/symptoms of infections. Photosensitivity reported. Elderly are at especially high-risk for adverse effects.

**Drug Interactions**

**Cytochrome P-450 Effect:** CYP2C8, 2C9, and 2C18 enzyme substrate

**Decreased Effect:** Naproxen may decrease the effect of furosemide.

**Increased Effect/Toxicity:** Naproxen could displace other highly protein-bound drugs, such as oral anticoagulants, hydantoins, salicylates, sulfonamides, and sulfonylureas. Naproxen and warfarin may cause a slight increase in free warfarin. Naproxen and probenecid may cause increased plasma half-life of naproxen. Naproxen and methotrexate may significantly increase and prolong blood methotrexate concentration, which may be severe or fatal.

**Food Interactions** Naproxen absorption rate may be decreased if taken with food.

**Effects on Lab Values** ↑ chloride (S), sodium (S), bleeding time

**Adverse Reactions**

1% to 10%:

Cardiovascular: Edema, palpitations

Central nervous system: Headache, dizziness, drowsiness, lightheadedness, vertigo

Dermatologic: Pruritus, skin eruptions, ecchymoses, sweating, purpura

Gastrointestinal: Constipation, heartburn, abdominal pain, nausea, heartburn, diarrhea, stomatitis

Ocular: Visual disturbances

Otic: Tinnitus

Respiratory: Dyspnea

<1% (Limited to important or life-threatening symptoms): Congestive heart failure, aseptic meningitis, epidermal necrolysis, erythema multiforme, Stevens-Johnson syndrome, epidermolysis bullosa, agranulocytosis, eosinophilia, granulocytopenia, leukopenia, thrombocytopenia, aplastic anemia, hemolytic anemia, abnormal LFTs, jaundice, glomerular nephritis, hematuria, interstitial nephritis, nephrotic syndrome, renal failure, renal papillary necrosis, eosinophilic pneumonitis

**Overdose/Toxicology** Symptoms of overdose include drowsiness, heartburn, vomiting, CNS depression, leukocytosis, and renal failure. Management is supportive and symptomatic. Seizures tend to be very short-lived and often do not require drug treatment.

**Pharmacodynamics/Kinetics**

**Protein Binding:** Highly protein bound >99%; increased free fraction in the elderly

**Half-life Elimination:** Normal renal function: 12-15 hours; End-stage renal disease: Unchanged

**Time to Peak:** Within 1-2 hours and persisting for up to 12 hours

**Excretion:** Urine

**Onset:** Analgesia: 1 hour; Anti-inflammatory: Within 2 weeks

**Duration:** Analgesia: Up to 7 hours; Anti-inflammatory: Peak: 2-4 weeks

**Formulations**

Suspension, oral: 125 mg/5 mL (15 mL, 30 mL, 480 mL)

Tablet, as sodium (Anaprox®): 220 mg (200 mg base); 275 mg (250 mg base); 550 mg (500 mg base)

Tablet:

Aleve®: 200 mg

Naprosyn®: 250 mg, 375 mg, 500 mg

Tablet, controlled release (Naprelan®): 375 mg, 500 mg

**Dosing**

**Adults:** Oral:

Rheumatoid arthritis, osteoarthritis, and ankylosing spondylitis: 500-1000 mg/day in 2 divided doses; may increase to 1.5 g/day of naproxen base for limited time period.

Mild to moderate pain or dysmenorrhea: Initial: 500 mg, then 250 mg every 6-8 hours; maximum: 1250 mg/day naproxen base

**Elderly:** Refer to adult dosing and Geriatric Considerations.

**Hepatic Impairment:** Reduce dose to 50%.

**Administration**

**Oral:** Suspension: Shake well before administration. Administer with food, milk, or antacids to decrease GI adverse effects.

**Monitoring Laboratory Tests** Periodic liver function, CBC, BUN, serum creatinine

**Additional Nursing Issues**

**Physical Assessment:** Assess effectiveness and interactions of other medications patient may be taking (see Contraindications and Drug Interactions). Monitor laboratory tests (see above) and therapeutic response (eg, relief of pain and inflammation, increased activity tolerance), and adverse reactions (eg, GI effects, hepatotoxicity, or ototoxicity) at beginning of therapy and periodically throughout therapy (see Warnings/Precautions, Adverse Reactions, and Overdose/Toxicology). Schedule ophthalmic evaluations for patients who develop eye complaints during long-term NSAID therapy (see Warnings/Precautions). Assess knowledge/teach patient appropriate use, interventions to reduce side effects, and adverse symptoms to report. **Pregnancy risk factor B/D** - see Pregnancy Risk Factor for cautious use.

**Patient Information/Instruction:** Take this medication exactly as directed; do not increase dose without consulting prescriber. Do not crush tablets or break capsules. Take with food or milk to reduce GI distress. Maintain adequate fluid intake (2-3 L/day of fluids unless instructed to restrict fluid intake). Do not use alcohol, aspirin, or aspirin-containing medication, and all other anti-inflammatory medications without consulting prescriber. You may experience drowsiness, dizziness, lightheadedness, or headache (use caution when driving or engaging in tasks requiring alertness until response to drug is known); anorexia, nausea, vomiting, or heartburn (frequent small meals, frequent mouth care, sucking lozenges, or chewing gum may help); fluid retention (weigh yourself weekly and report unusual (3-5 lb/week) weight gain). GI bleeding, ulceration, or perforation can occur with or without pain; discontinue medication and contact prescriber if persistent abdominal pain or cramping, or blood in stool occurs. Report breathlessness, difficulty breathing, or unusual cough; chest pain, rapid heartbeat, palpitations; unusual bruising/bleeding; blood in urine, stool, mouth, or vomitus; swollen extremities; skin rash or itching; acute fatigue; or changes in eyesight (double vision, color changes, blurred vision), hearing, or ringing in ears. **Pregnancy/breast-feeding precautions:** Notify prescriber if you are or intend to be pregnant. Do not take this drug during last trimester of pregnancy.

**Geriatric Considerations:** Elderly are at high risk for adverse effects from nonsteroidal anti-inflammatory agents. As much as 60% of elderly can develop peptic ulceration and/or hemorrhage asymptomatically. The concomitant use of $H_2$ blockers, omeprazole, and sucralfate is not effective as prophylaxis with the exception of NSAID-induced duodenal ulcers which may be prevented by the use of ranitidine. Misoprostol is the only prophylactic agent proven effective. Also, concomitant disease and drug use contribute to the risk for GI adverse effects. Use lowest effective dose for shortest period possible. Consider renal function decline with age. Use of NSAIDs can compromise existing renal function especially when $Cl_{cr}$ is ≤30 mL/minute. Tinnitus may be a difficult and unreliable indication of toxicity due to age-related hearing loss or eighth cranial nerve damage. CNS adverse effects such as confusion, agitation, and hallucination are generally seen in overdose or high-dose situations, but elderly may demonstrate these adverse effects at lower doses than younger adults.

**Additional Information** Naprosyn®: naproxen; Anaprox®: naproxen sodium; 275 mg of Anaprox® equivalent to 250 mg of Naprosyn®

**Related Information**

Nonsalicylate/Nonsteroidal Anti-inflammatory Comparison *on page 1401*

## Naratriptan (NAR a trip tan)

**U.S. Brand Names** Amerge™

**Therapeutic Category** Serotonin 5-$HT_{1D}$ Receptor Agonist

**Pregnancy Risk Factor** C

**Lactation** Excretion in breast milk unknown/not recommended

**Use** Treatment of acute migraine headache with or without aura

**Mechanism of Action/Effect** The therapeutic effect for migraine is due to serotonin agonist activity.

**Contraindications** Hypersensitivity to naratriptan or any component; cerebrovascular, peripheral vascular disease (ischemic bowel disease), ischemic heart disease (angina pectoris, history of myocardial infarction, or proven silent ischemia), or in patients with symptoms consistent with ischemic heart disease, coronary artery vasospasm, or Prinzmetal's variant angina; uncontrolled hypertension or patients who have received within 24 hours another 5-HT agonist (sumatriptan, zolmitriptan) or ergotamine-containing product; patients with known risk factors associated with coronary artery disease; patients with severe hepatic or renal disease ($Cl_{cr}$ <15 mL/minute); do **not** administer naratriptan to patients with hemiplegic or basilar migraine

**Warnings** Use only if there is a clear diagnosis of migraine. Patients who are at risk of CAD but have had a satisfactory cardiovascular evaluation may receive naratriptan but with extreme caution (ie, in a physician's office where there are adequate precautions in place to protect the patient). Blood pressure may increase with the administration of naratriptan. Monitor closely, especially with the first administration of the drug. If the patient does not respond to the first dose, re-evaluate the diagnosis of migraine before trying a second dose. Pregnancy factor C.

**Drug Interactions**

**Decreased Effect:** Smoking increases the clearance of naratriptan.

**Increased Effect/Toxicity:** Ergot-containing drugs (dihydroergotamine or methysergide) may cause vasospastic reactions when taken with naratriptan. Avoid concomitant use with ergots; separate dose of naratriptan and ergots by at least 24 hours. Oral contraceptives taken with naratriptan reduced the clearance of naratriptan +30% which may contribute to adverse effects. Selective serotonin reuptake inhibitors (SSRIs) (eg, fluoxetine, fluvoxamine, paroxetine, sertraline) may cause lack of coordination, hyperreflexia, or weakness and should be avoided when taking naratriptan.

**Adverse Reactions**

1% to 10%:

Central nervous system: Dizziness, drowsiness, malaise/fatigue, paresthesias

Gastrointestinal: Nausea, vomiting

Miscellaneous: Pain or pressure in throat or neck

<1% (Limited to important or life-threatening symptoms): Coronary artery vasospasm, transient myocardial ischemia, myocardial infarction, ventricular tachycardia, ventricular fibrillation, palpitations, hypertension, EKG changes (PR prolongation, Q-$T_c$ prolongation, premature ventricular contractions, atrial flutter or atrial fibrillation) hypotension, heart murmurs, bradycardia, hyperlipidemia, hypercholesterolemia, hypothyroidism, hyperglycemia, glycosuria, ketonuria, eye hemorrhage, abnormal liver function tests, abnormal bilirubin tests, convulsions, allergic reaction, panic, hallucinations

(Continued)

## Naratriptan *(Continued)*

**Pharmacodynamics/Kinetics**

**Protein Binding:** Plasma: 28% to 31%

**Time to Peak:** 2-3 hours

**Metabolism:** Liver, cytochrome P-450 isoenzymes

**Excretion:** Urine

**Onset:** 30 minutes

**Formulations** Tablet: 1 mg, 2.5 mg

**Dosing**

**Adults:** Oral: 1 mg to 2.5 mg at the onset of headache. It is recommended to use the lowest possible dose to minimize adverse effects. If headache returns or dose not fully resolve, the dose may be repeated after 4 hours. Do not exceed 5 mg in 24 hours.

**Elderly:** Not recommended for use in the elderly.

**Renal Impairment:**

$Cl_{cr}$: 18-39 mL/minute: Initial: 1 mg; do not exceed 2.5 mg in 24 hours.

$Cl_{cr}$: <15 mL/minute: Do not use.

**Hepatic Impairment:** Contraindicated in patients with severe liver failure. The maximum dose is 2.5 mg in 24 hours for patients with mild or moderate liver failure. The recommended starting dose is 1 mg.

**Administration**

**Oral:** Do **not** crush or chew tablet; swallow whole with water.

**Additional Nursing Issues**

**Physical Assessment:** Note Warnings/Precautions (clear diagnosis of migraine) and Drug Interactions. Assess effectiveness of therapy. Assure patient knowledge of appropriate use, possible side effects (see Adverse Reactions), and symptoms to report. **Pregnancy risk factor C** - benefits of use should outweigh possible risks. Breast-feeding is not recommended.

**Patient Information/Instruction:** This drug is to be used to reduce your migraine, not to prevent or reduce the number of attacks. If headache returns or is not fully resolved, the dose may be repeated after 4 hours. If you have no relief with first dose, do not take a second dose without consulting prescriber. **Do not exceed 5 mg in 24 hours. Do not take within 24 hours of any other migraine medication without first consulting prescriber.** You may experience some dizziness, fatigue, or drowsiness; use caution when driving or engaging in tasks that require alertness until response to drug is known. Frequent mouth care and sucking on lozenges may relieve dry mouth. Report immediately any chest pain, heart throbbing, tightness in throat, skin rash or hives, hallucinations, anxiety, or panic. **Pregnancy/breast-feeding precautions:** Inform prescriber if you are or intend to be pregnant. Breast-feeding is not recommended.

**Geriatric Considerations:** Naratriptan was not studied in patients >65 years of age. Use in elderly patients is not recommended because of the presence of risk factors associated with adverse effects. These include the presence of coronary artery disease, decreased liver or renal function, and the risk of pronounced blood pressure increases.


- **Narcan® Injection** *see* Naloxone *on page 804*
- **Narcotic/Opioid Analgesic Comparison** *see page 1396*
- **Nardil®** *see* Phenelzine *on page 915*
- **Nasabid®** *see* Guaifenesin and Pseudoephedrine *on page 551*
- **Nasacort®** *see* Triamcinolone *on page 1171*
- **Nasacort® AQ** *see* Triamcinolone *on page 1171*
- **Nasahist B®** *see page 1294*
- **NāSal™** *see page 1294*
- **Nasalcrom® Nasal Solution** *see* Cromolyn Sodium *on page 309*
- **Nasalide® Nasal Aerosol** *see* Flunisolide *on page 497*
- **Nasal Moist®** *see page 1294*
- **Nasarel™** *see* Flunisolide *on page 497*
- **Nascobal®** *see* Cyanocobalamin *on page 311*
- **Nasonex® Nasal Spray** *see* Topical Corticosteroids *on page 1152*
- **Natabec® [OTC]** *see* Vitamin, Multiple *on page 1219*
- **Natabec® FA [OTC]** *see* Vitamin, Multiple *on page 1219*
- **Natabec® Rx** *see* Vitamin, Multiple *on page 1219*
- **Natacyn® Ophthalmic** *see* Natamycin *on this page*
- **Natalins® [OTC]** *see* Vitamin, Multiple *on page 1219*
- **Natalins® Rx** *see* Vitamin, Multiple *on page 1219*


## Natamycin (na ta MYE sin)

**U.S. Brand Names** Natacyn® Ophthalmic

**Synonyms** Pimaricin

**Therapeutic Category** Antifungal Agent, Ophthalmic

**Pregnancy Risk Factor** C

**Lactation** Excretion in breast milk unknown

**Use** Treatment of blepharitis, conjunctivitis, and keratitis caused by susceptible fungi (*Aspergillus, Candida*), *Cephalosporium, Curvularia, Fusarium, Penicillium, Microsporum, Epidermophyton, Blastomyces dermatitidis, Coccidioides immitis, Cryptococcus neoformans, Histoplasma capsulatum, Sporothrix schenckii,* and *Trichomonas vaginalis*

**Mechanism of Action/Effect** Increases cell membrane permeability in susceptible fungi

**Contraindications** Hypersensitivity to natamycin or any component

**Warnings** Failure to improve (keratitis) after 7-10 days of administration suggests infection caused by a microorganism not susceptible to natamycin. Inadequate as a single agent in fungal endophthalmitis. Pregnancy factor C.

**Adverse Reactions** <1% (Limited to important or life-threatening symptoms): Blurred vision, photophobia, eye pain, eye irritation not present before therapy

**Pharmacodynamics/Kinetics**

**Distribution:** Adheres to cornea and is retained in the conjunctival fornices

**Formulations** Suspension, ophthalmic: 5% (15 mL)

**Dosing**

**Adults:** Ophthalmic: Instill 1 drop in conjunctival sac every 1-2 hours, after 3-4 days reduce to 1 drop 6-8 times/day; usual course of therapy is 2-3 weeks.

**Elderly:** Refer to adult dosing.

**Administration**

**Topical:** Ophthalmic: Shake well before using, do not touch dropper to eye.

**Stability**

**Storage:** Store at room temperature (8°C to 24°C/46°F to 75°F). Protect from excessive heat and light. Do not freeze.

**Additional Nursing Issues**

**Physical Assessment:** Monitor effectiveness of therapy (see Warnings/Precautions). Assess knowledge/teach patient appropriate use, interventions to reduce side effects, and adverse symptoms to report (see Adverse Reactions). **Pregnancy risk factor C** - systemic absorption unlikely or minimal. Note breast-feeding caution.

**Patient Information/Instruction:** For ophthalmic use only. Store at room temperature. Shake before using. Apply prescribed amount as often as directed. Wash hands before using and do not let tip of applicator touch eye or contaminate tip of applicator. Tilt head back and look upward. Gently pull down lower lid and put drop(s) in inner corner of eye. Close eye and roll eyeball in all directions. Do not blink for ½ minute. Apply gentle pressure to inner corner of eye for 30 seconds. Wipe away excess from skin around eye. Do not use any other eye preparation for at least 10 minutes. Do not touch tip of applicator to eye or contaminate tip of applicator. Do not share medication with anyone else. May cause sensitivity to bright light (dark glasses may help); temporary stinging or blurred vision may occur. Inform prescriber if you experience eye pain, redness, burning, watering, dryness, double vision, puffiness around eye, vision disturbances, or other adverse eye response; worsening of condition or lack of improvement within 7-10 days. **Pregnancy/breast-feeding precautions:** Inform prescriber if you are pregnant. Consult prescriber if breast-feeding.

**Geriatric Considerations:** Assess patient's ability to self-administer ophthalmic drops.


- **Natulan** *see* Procarbazine *on page 970*
- **Nature's Tears® Solution** *see page 1294*
- **Naus-A-Way® Liquid** *see page 1294*
- **Nausetrol® Liquid** *see page 1294*
- **Navane®** *see* Thiothixene *on page 1127*
- **Navelbine®** *see* Vinorelbine *on page 1215*
- **Naxen®** *see* Naproxen *on page 807*
- **Naxifelar** *see* Cephalexin *on page 237*
- **Naxil** *see* Naproxen *on page 807*
- **Naxodol (Carisoprodol With Naproxen)** *see* Carisoprodol *on page 202*
- **Nazil® Ofteno** *see page 1294*
- **ND-Stat®** *see page 1294*
- **Nebcin® Injection** *see* Tobramycin *on page 1142*
- **NebuPent™ Inhalation** *see* Pentamidine *on page 901*


## Nedocromil (ne doe KROE mil)

**U.S. Brand Names** Tilade® Inhalation Aerosol

**Therapeutic Category** Mast Cell Stabilizer

**Pregnancy Risk Factor** B

**Lactation** Excretion in breast milk unknown/use caution

**Use** Maintenance therapy in patients with mild to moderate bronchial asthma

**Mechanism of Action/Effect** Inhibits the activation of and mediator release from a variety of inflammatory cell types associated with asthma including eosinophils, neutrophils, macrophages, mast cells, monocytes, and platelets; it inhibits the release of histamine, leukotrienes, and slow-reacting substance of anaphylaxis; it inhibits the development of early and late bronchoconstriction responses to inhaled antigen

**Contraindications** Hypersensitivity to nedocromil or any component

**Warnings** Safety and efficacy in children <12 years of age have not been established. If systemic or inhaled steroid therapy is at all reduced, monitor patients carefully. Nedocromil is **not** a bronchodilator and, therefore, should not be used for reversal of acute bronchospasm.

**Adverse Reactions**

>10%: Gastrointestinal: Unpleasant taste after inhalation

1% to 10%:

Cardiovascular: Chest pain

Central nervous system: Dizziness, dysphonia, headache, fatigue

Dermatologic: Rash

Gastrointestinal: Nausea, vomiting, heartburn, diarrhea, abdominal pain, dry mouth

(Continued)

## Nedocromil *(Continued)*

Hepatic: Increased ALT

Neuromuscular & skeletal: Arthritis, tremor

Respiratory: Cough, pharyngitis, rhinitis, bronchitis, upper respiratory infection, bronchospasm, increased sputum production

**Pharmacodynamics/Kinetics**

**Protein Binding:** 89%

**Half-life Elimination:** 1.5-2 hours

**Excretion:** Urine

**Duration:** 2 hours

**Formulations** Aerosol, as sodium: 1.75 mg/activation (16.2 g)

**Dosing**

**Adults:** Inhalation: 2 inhalations 4 times/day; may reduce dosage to 2-3 times/day once desired clinical response to initial dose is observed. Drug has no known therapeutic systemic activity when delivered by inhalation.

**Elderly:** Refer to adult dosing.

**Stability**

**Storage:** Store at 2°C to 30°C/36°F to 86°F. Do not freeze.

**Additional Nursing Issues**

**Physical Assessment:** Not for use during acute bronchospasm. Monitor effectiveness of therapy and adverse reactions (see Adverse Reactions) at beginning of therapy and periodically with long-term use. Assess knowledge/teach patient appropriate use, interventions to reduce side effects, and adverse symptoms to report. Note breast-feeding caution.

**Patient Information/Instruction:** Do not use during acute bronchospasm. Use exactly as directed; do not use more often than instructed or discontinue without consulting prescriber. You may experience drowsiness, dizziness, fatigue, especially during early therapy (use caution when driving or engaging in tasks requiring alertness until response to drug is known); dry mouth, nausea, or vomiting (small frequent meals, frequent mouth care, chewing gum, or sucking lozenges may help). Report persistent runny nose, cough, cold symptoms; unresolved gastrointestinal effects; skin rash; joint pain or tremor; or if breathing difficulty persists or worsens. **Breast-feeding precautions:** Consult prescriber if breast-feeding.

Use: Review use of inhalator with prescriber or follow package insert for directions. Prime with three activations prior to first use or if unused more than 7 days. Keep inhalator clean and unobstructed. Always rinse mouth and throat after use of inhaler to prevent advantageous infection. If you are also using a steroid bronchodilator, wait 10 minutes before using this aerosol.

**Geriatric Considerations:** Elderly may have difficulty using inhaler delivery system, especially if they have physical or medical impairment (ie, Parkinson's disease, stroke, etc). If this prophylactic modality is desired but patient cannot tolerate nedocromil inhalations, consider cromolyn sodium solution for nebulizer use.

**Related Information**

Inhalant (Asthma, Bronchospasm) Agents *on page 1388*

♦ **N.E.E.® 1/35** *see* Oral Contraceptives *on page 859*

## Nefazodone (nef AY zoe done)

**U.S. Brand Names** Serzone®

**Therapeutic Category** Antidepressant, Serotonin Reuptake Inhibitor/Antagonist

**Pregnancy Risk Factor** C

**Lactation** Enters breast milk/not recommended

**Use** Treatment of depression

**Mechanism of Action/Effect** Inhibits serotonin (5-HT) reuptake and is a potent antagonist at Type 2 serotonin (5-HT) receptors; minimal affinity for cholinergic, histaminic, or alpha$_1$-adrenergic receptors

**Contraindications** Hypersensitivity to nefazodone or any component; concomitant use of any MAO inhibitors, astemizole, or terfenadine

**Warnings** Monitor closely and use with extreme caution in patients with cardiac disease, cerebrovascular disease, or seizures. Very sedating and can be dehydrating. Therapeutic effect may take up to 4 weeks. Therapy is normally maintained for several months after optimum response is reached to prevent recurrence of depression. Discontinue therapy and re-evaluate if priapism occurs. Pregnancy factor C.

**Drug Interactions**

**Cytochrome P-450 Effect:** CYP3A3/4 enzyme substrate; CYP3A3/4 enzyme inhibitor

**Decreased Effect:** Decreased effect of nefazodone with clonidine, methyldopa, oral hypoglycemics, anticoagulants.

**Increased Effect/Toxicity:** Nefazodone may increase terfenadine and astemizole serum concentrations (which have been associated with serious ventricular arrhythmias and death). Nefazodone increases serum levels of fluoxetine, triazolam (reduce triazolam dose by 75%), alprazolam (reduce alprazolam dose by 50%), phenytoin, CNS depressants, MAO inhibitors (allow 14 days after MAO inhibitors are stopped or 7 days after nefazodone is stopped). Digoxin serum levels may increase. Potential for serotonin syndrome if combined with other serotonergic drugs.

**Food Interactions** Nefazodone absorption may be delayed and bioavailability may be decreased if taken with food.

**Adverse Reactions**

>10%:

Central nervous system: Headache, drowsiness, insomnia, agitation, dizziness, confusion

Gastrointestinal: Dry mouth, nausea

Neuromuscular & skeletal: Tremor

1% to 10%:

Cardiovascular: Postural hypotension

Central nervous system: Muscle weakness

Gastrointestinal: Constipation, vomiting

Ocular: Blurred vision, amblyopia

<1% (Limited to important or life-threatening symptoms): Tachycardia, hypertension, syncope, extrasystoles, chest pain, A-V block, CHF, hemorrhage, neuroleptic malignant syndrome, gastrointestinal hemorrhage, anemia, leukopenia, hepatitis, dyspnea, asthma, epistaxis

**Overdose/Toxicology** Symptoms of overdose include drowsiness, vomiting, hypotension, tachycardia, incontinence, and coma. Following initiation of essential overdose management, toxic symptoms should be treated.

**Pharmacodynamics/Kinetics**

**Half-life Elimination:** 2-4 hours (parent compound), active metabolites persist longer

**Time to Peak:** 30 minutes, prolonged in presence of food

**Metabolism:** Liver

**Excretion:** Urine and feces

**Onset:** Therapeutic effects take at least 2 weeks to appear

**Formulations** Tablet, as hydrochloride: 50 mg, 100 mg, 150 mg, 200 mg, 250 mg

**Dosing**

**Adults:** Oral: 200 mg/day, administered in two divided doses initially, with a range of 300-600 mg/day in two divided doses thereafter; dosage adjustments should be made at weekly intervals.

**Elderly:** Oral: Initial: 50 mg twice daily; increase dose to 100 mg twice daily in 2 weeks; usual maintenance dose: 200-400 mg/day

**Administration**

**Oral:** Dosing after meals may decrease lightheadedness and postural hypotension, but may also decrease absorption and therefore effectiveness.

**Additional Nursing Issues**

**Physical Assessment:** Assess other medications patient may be taking for effectiveness and interactions (see Drug Interactions). See Warnings/Precautions for cautious use. Has potential for psychological or physiological dependence, abuse, or tolerance. Monitor therapeutic response (ie, mental status, mood, affect, suicidal ideation), and adverse reactions at beginning of therapy and periodically with long-term use (see Adverse Reactions and Overdose/Toxicology). Taper dosage slowly when discontinuing. Assess knowledge/teach patient appropriate use, interventions to reduce side effects, and adverse symptoms to report. **Pregnancy risk factor C** - benefits of use should outweigh possible risks. Breast-feeding is not recommended.

**Patient Information/Instruction:** Take exactly as directed (do not increase dose or frequency); may take 2-3 weeks to achieve desired results; may cause physical and/or psychological dependence. Avoid excessive alcohol, caffeine, and other prescription or OTC medications not approved by prescriber. Maintain adequate hydration (2-3 L/day of fluids unless instructed to restrict fluid intake). You may experience drowsiness, dizziness, or lightheadedness (use caution when driving or engaging in tasks requiring alertness until response to drug is known); nausea or vomiting (small frequent meals, frequent mouth care, chewing gum, or sucking lozenges may help); or orthostatic hypotension (use caution when climbing stairs or changing position from lying or sitting to standing). Report persistent insomnia or excessive daytime sedation; muscle cramping, tremors, weakness, or change in gait; chest pain, palpitations, or rapid heartbeat; vision changes or eye pain; difficulty breathing or breathlessness; abdominal pain or blood in stool; or worsening of condition. **Pregnancy/breast-feeding precautions:** Inform prescriber if you are or intend to be pregnant. Breast-feeding is not recommended.

**Geriatric Considerations:** Data on nefazodone in the elderly is limited, specifically regarding efficacy. Clinical trials in adult patients have found it superior to placebo and similar to imipramine. Nefazodone's $C_{max}$ and AUC have been reported to be increased twofold in the elderly and women after a single dose compared to younger patients, however, these differences were markedly reduced with multiple dosing.

**Related Information**

Antidepressant Agents Comparison *on page 1368*

## Nelfinavir (nel FIN a veer)

**U.S. Brand Names** Viracept®

**Therapeutic Category** Antiretroviral Agent, Protease Inhibitor

**Pregnancy Risk Factor** B

**Lactation** Enters breast milk/contraindicated

**Use** Monotherapy or preferably in combination therapy with nucleoside analogs in the treatment of HIV infection when antiretroviral therapy is required

**Mechanism of Action/Effect** Inhibits HIV-1 protease enzyme; inhibition of the viral protease prevents cleavage of the gag-pol polyprotein resulting in the production of immature, noninfectious virions; cross-resistance with other protease inhibitors is possible, although, not known at this time

**Contraindications** Hypersensitivity to nelfinavir or product components

(Continued)

## Nelfinavir *(Continued)*

**Warnings** Avoid use of powder formulation in patients with phenylketonuria since it contains 11.2 mg phenylalanine per gram of powder. Use extreme caution when administered to patients with hepatic insufficiency since nelfinavir is metabolized in the liver and excreted predominantly in the feces. Due to potential serious and life-threatening drug interactions, the following drugs should not be coadministered with nelfinavir: terfenadine, astemizole, cisapride, triazolam, midazolam, ergot derivatives, amiodarone, or quinidine. Concurrent use with some anticonvulsants may significantly limit nelfinavir's effectiveness. Spontaneous bleeding episodes have been reported in patients with hemophilia A and B. New onset diabetes mellitus, exacerbation of diabetes, and hyperglycemia have been reported in HIV-infected patients receiving protease inhibitors.

**Drug Interactions**

**Cytochrome P-450 Effect:** CYP3A3/4 enzyme substrate; CYP3A3/4 enzyme inducer; CYP3A3/4 enzyme inhibitor

**Decreased Effect:** Rifampin decreases nelfinavir's plasma AUC by ~82%; the two drugs should not be administered concurrently. Serum levels of the hormones in oral contraceptives may decrease significantly with administration of nelfinavir. Patients should use alternative methods of contraceptives during nelfinavir therapy. Phenobarbital, phenytoin, and carbamazepine may decrease serum levels and consequently effectiveness of nelfinavir. Delaviradine concentrations may be decreased by up to 50% during nelfinavir treatment.

**Increased Effect/Toxicity:** Nelfinavir inhibits the metabolism of cisapride, terfenadine, astemizole, amiodarone, quinidine, ergot derivatives, midazolam, and triazolam, and should not be administered concurrently due to risk of life-threatening cardiac arrhythmias. A 20% increase in rifabutin plasma AUC has been observed when coadministered with nelfinavir (decrease rifabutin dose by 50%). An increase in midazolam and triazolam serum levels may occur resulting in significant oversedation when administered with nelfinavir. Indinavir and ritonavir may increase nelfinavir plasma concentrations resulting in potential increases in side effects (the safety of these combinations have not been established). concentrations of nelfinavir may be doubled during therapy with delaviradine.

**Food Interactions** Nelfinavir taken with food increases plasma concentration time curve (AUC) by two- to threefold. Do not administer with acidic food or juice (orange juice, apple juice, or applesauce) since the combination may have a bitter taste.

**Adverse Reactions**

>10%: Gastrointestinal: Diarrhea

1% to 10%:

Central nervous system: Decreased concentration
Dermatologic: Rash
Gastrointestinal: Nausea, flatulence, abdominal pain
Neuromuscular & skeletal: Weakness

<1% (Limited to important or life-threatening symptoms): Migraine, seizures, suicidal ideation, fever, hyperlipidemia, hyperuricemia, hypoglycemia, vomiting, GI bleeding, pancreatitis, leukopenia, thrombocytopenia, hepatitis, elevated LFTs, arthralgia, kidney calculus, dyspnea, allergic reaction

Protease inhibitors cause hyperglycemia and dyslipidemia (elevated cholesterol/triglycerides) and a redistribution of fat (protease paunch, buffalo hump, facial atrophy and breast engorgement)

**Pharmacodynamics/Kinetics**

**Protein Binding:** 98%

**Half-life Elimination:** 3.5-5 hours

**Time to Peak:** 2-4 hours

**Metabolism:** Liver

**Excretion:** Feces and urine

**Formulations**

Nelfinavir mesylate:

Powder, oral: 50 mg/g [144 g] (contains 11.2 mg phenylalanine)
Tablet: 250 mg

**Dosing**

**Adults:** 750 mg (3 tablets of 250 mg each) 3 times/day with meals

**Elderly:** Refer to adult dosing.

**Renal Impairment:** No adjustment necessary.

**Hepatic Impairment:** Use caution when administering to patients with hepatic impairment since nelfinavir is predominantly eliminated by the liver.

**Administration**

**Oral:** Oral powder: Mix powder in a small amount of water, milk, formula, soy milk, soy formula, or dietary supplement. Be sure entire contents is consumed to receive full dose. Do not use acidic food/juice to dilute due to bitter taste. Do not store dilution for longer than 6 hours.

**Stability**

**Storage:** Oral powder diluted in nonacidic liquid is stable for 6 hours at room temperature.

**Monitoring Laboratory Tests** Liver function tests, blood glucose levels, CBC with differential, CD4 cell count, plasma levels of HIV RNA

**Additional Nursing Issues**

**Physical Assessment:** Carefully assess effect and interactions of other medications patient may be taking (see Drug Interactions). Monitor laboratory results prior to beginning therapy and regularly thereafter. Monitor for adverse reactions as identified above. Instruct patient/caregiver in appropriate administration, scheduling, and adverse symptoms to report. Breast-feeding is contraindicated.

**Patient Information/Instruction:** This is not a cure for HIV and has not been shown to reduce the risk of transmitting HIV to others. The long-term effects of use are not known. Should be taken as scheduled with food (mix powder with nonacidic, noncitric fluids and do not store reconstituted powder mixture for longer than 6 hours). If you miss a dose, take as soon as possible and return to regular schedule (never take a double dose). Frequent blood tests may be required with prolonged therapy. You may experience nausea and vomiting (small frequent meals, frequent mouth care, sucking lozenges, or chewing gum may help). Report rash; respiratory difficulty; CNS changes (migraine, confusion, suicidal ideation); muscular or skeletal pain, weakness, or tremors; or other adverse reactions. Use appropriate barrier contraceptive measures (as alternative to oral contraceptives) to reduce risk of transmitting infection and potential pregnancy. **Breast-feeding precautions:** Do not breast-feed.

**Breast-feeding Issues:** The CDC recommends that mothers with the diagnosis of HIV **not** breast-feed to minimize the risk of infection transfer to the infant.

**Related Information**

Antiretroviral Agents Comparison *on page 1373*


- ♦ **Nelova™ 0.5/35E** *see* Oral Contraceptives *on page 859*
- ♦ **Nelova™ 1/35E** *see* Oral Contraceptives *on page 859*
- ♦ **Nelova™ 1/50M** *see* Oral Contraceptives *on page 859*
- ♦ **Nelova™ 10/11** *see* Oral Contraceptives *on page 859*
- ♦ **Nembutal®** *see* Pentobarbital *on page 905*
- ♦ **Neo-Calglucon® [OTC]** *see* Calcium Supplements *on page 185*
- ♦ **Neo-Codema®** *see* Hydrochlorothiazide *on page 566*
- ♦ **Neo-Cortef®** *see page 1282*
- ♦ **Neo-Cortef® Ophthalmic** *see* Neomycin and Hydrocortisone *on page 817*
- ♦ **Neo-Cultol®** *see page 1294*
- ♦ **NeoDecadron® Ophthalmic** *see* Neomycin and Dexamethasone *on next page*
- ♦ **NeoDecadron® Topical** *see* Neomycin and Dexamethasone *on next page*
- ♦ **NeoDexadron®** *see page 1282*
- ♦ **Neo-Dexameth®** *see page 1282*
- ♦ **Neo-Dexameth® Ophthalmic** *see* Neomycin and Dexamethasone *on next page*
- ♦ **Neodol** *see* Acetaminophen *on page 32*
- ♦ **Neo-Durabolic Injection** *see* Nandrolone *on page 806*
- ♦ **Neo-Estrone®** *see* Estrogens, Esterified *on page 449*
- ♦ **Neo-Estrone® Vaginal Cream** *see* Estrone *on page 451*
- ♦ **Neofed® [OTC]** *see* Pseudoephedrine *on page 992*
- ♦ **Neo-fradin® Oral** *see* Neomycin *on this page*
- ♦ **Neomicol®** *see* Miconazole *on page 767*
- ♦ **Neomixin® Topical [OTC]** *see* Bacitracin, Neomycin, and Polymyxin B *on page 130*


## Neomycin (nee oh MYE sin)

**U.S. Brand Names** Mycifradin® Sulfate Oral; Mycifradin® Sulfate Topical; Neo-fradin® Oral; Neo-Tabs® Oral

**Therapeutic Category** Ammonium Detoxicant; Antibiotic, Aminoglycoside; Antibiotic, Topical

**Pregnancy Risk Factor** C

**Lactation** Excretion in breast milk unknown

**Use** Prepares GI tract for surgery; treatment of minor skin infections; treatment of diarrhea caused by *E. coli*; adjunct in the treatment of hepatic encephalopathy, as irrigant during surgery

**Mechanism of Action/Effect** Interferes with bacterial protein synthesis by binding to 30S ribosomal subunits

**Contraindications** Hypersensitivity to neomycin or any component, or other aminoglycosides; patients with intestinal obstruction

**Warnings** Use with caution in patients with renal impairment, pre-existing hearing impairment (ototoxicity), neuromuscular disorders. Topical neomycin is a contact sensitizer with sensitivity occurring in 5% to 15% of patients treated with the drug. Symptoms include itching, reddening, edema, and failure to heal. Do not use as peritoneal lavage. Pregnancy factor C.

**Drug Interactions**

**Decreased Effect:** May decrease GI absorption of digoxin and methotrexate.

**Increased Effect/Toxicity:** Oral neomycin may potentiate the effects of oral anticoagulants. Neomycin may increase the adverse effects with other neurotoxic, ototoxic, or nephrotoxic drugs.

**Adverse Reactions**

**Oral:**

>10%: Gastrointestinal: Nausea, diarrhea, vomiting, irritation or soreness of the mouth or rectal area

<1% (Limited to important or life-threatening symptoms): Neurotoxicity, eosinophilia, ototoxicity (auditory), ototoxicity (vestibular), nephrotoxicity, dyspnea

**Topical:** >10%: Dermatologic: Contact dermatitis

**Overdose/Toxicology** Symptoms of overdose (rare due to poor oral bioavailability) include ototoxicity, nephrotoxicity, and neuromuscular toxicity. The treatment of choice following a single acute overdose appears to be maintenance of urine output of at least 3

(Continued)

## Neomycin *(Continued)*

mL/kg/hour during the acute treatment phase. Dialysis is of questionable value in enhancing aminoglycoside elimination. If required, hemodialysis is preferred over peritoneal dialysis in patients with normal renal function. Chelation with penicillin may be of benefit.

**Pharmacodynamics/Kinetics**

**Half-life Elimination:** 3 hours (age and renal function dependent)

**Time to Peak:** Oral: 1-4 hours; I.M.: Within 2 hours

**Metabolism:** Slightly hepatic

**Excretion:** Urine and feces

**Formulations**

Neomycin sulfate:

Cream: 0.5% (15 g)

Ointment, topical: 0.5% (15 g, 30 g, 120 g)

Solution, oral: 125 mg/5 mL (480 mL)

Tablet: 500 mg [base 300 mg]

**Dosing**

**Adults:**

Topical: Apply ointment 1-4 times/day; topical solutions containing 0.1% to 1% neomycin have been used for irrigation

Oral:

Preoperative intestinal antisepsis: 1 g each hour for 4 doses then 1 g every 4 hours for 5 doses; or 1 g at 1 PM, 2 PM, and 11 PM on day preceding surgery as an adjunct to mechanical cleansing of the bowel and oral erythromycin; or 6 g/day divided every 4 hours for 2-3 days

Hepatic coma: 500-2000 mg every 6-8 hours or 4-12 g/day divided every 4-6 hours for 5-6 days

Chronic hepatic insufficiency: 4 g/day for an indefinite period

**Elderly:** Refer to adult dosing.

**Renal Impairment:** Dialyzable (50% to 100%)

**Monitoring Laboratory Tests** Renal function; perform culture and sensitivity prior to initiating therapy.

**Additional Nursing Issues**

**Physical Assessment:** Assess effectiveness and interactions of other medications (see Drug Interactions). See Contraindications and Warnings/Precautions for use cautions. Monitor effectiveness of therapy, laboratory tests (see Monitoring Laboratory Tests), and adverse response (eg, ototoxicity, nephrotoxicity, neurotoxicity - see Adverse Reactions and Overdose/Toxicology). Assess knowledge/teach patient appropriate use (application of cream/ointment), possible side effects/interventions, and adverse symptoms to report. Pregnancy risk factor C - benefits of use should outweigh possible risks. Minimal absorption across GI mucosa or skin surfaces, however with ulceration, open or burned surfaces (especially large surfaces) absorption is possible. Note breast-feeding caution.

**Patient Information/Instruction:**

Oral: Take as directed. Maintain adequate hydration (2-3 L/day of fluids unless instructed to restrict fluid intake). You may experience nausea or vomiting (small frequent meals, frequent mouth care, sucking lozenges, or chewing gum may help); constipation (exercise, increased fluid or fiber in diet may help, or consult prescriber); or diarrhea (buttermilk, boiled milk, or yogurt may help). Report immediately any change in hearing,; ringing or sense of fullness in ears; persistent diarrhea; changes in voiding patterns; or numbness, tingling, or pain in any extremity. **Pregnancy/breast-feeding precautions:** Inform prescriber if you are or intend to be pregnant. Consult prescriber if breast-feeding.

Topical: Apply a thin film of cream or ointment; do not overuse. Report rash, itching, redness, or failure of condition to improve.

## Neomycin and Dexamethasone (nee oh MYE sin & deks a METH a sone)

**U.S. Brand Names** AK-Neo-Dex® Ophthalmic; NeoDecadron® Ophthalmic; NeoDecadron® Topical; Neo-Dexameth® Ophthalmic

**Synonyms** Dexamethasone and Neomycin

**Therapeutic Category** Antibiotic/Corticosteroid, Ophthalmic; Antibiotic/Corticosteroid, Topical

**Pregnancy Risk Factor** C

**Lactation** Excretion in breast milk unknown

**Use** Treatment of steroid responsive inflammatory conditions of the palpebral and bulbar conjunctiva, lid, cornea, and anterior segment of the globe

**Formulations**

Cream: Neomycin sulfate 0.5% [5 mg/g] and dexamethasone 0.1% [1 mg/g] (15 g, 30 g)

Ointment, ophthalmic: Neomycin sulfate 0.35% [3.5 mg/g] and dexamethasone 0.05% [0.5 mg/g] (3.5 g)

Solution, ophthalmic: Neomycin sulfate 0.35% [3.5 mg/mL] and dexamethasone 0.1% [1 mg/mL] (5 mL)

**Dosing**

**Adults:**

Ophthalmic: Instill 1-2 drops in eye(s) every 3-4 hours.

Topical: Apply thin coat 3-4 times/day until favorable response is observed, then reduce dose to 1 application/day.

**Elderly:** Refer to adult dosing.

**Additional Nursing Issues**

**Physical Assessment:** See individual components listed in Related Information. **Pregnancy risk factor C** - benefits of use should outweigh possible risks. Note breast-feeding caution.

**Patient Information/Instruction:** See individual components listed in Related Information. **Pregnancy/breast-feeding precautions:** Inform prescriber if you are on intend to get pregnant. Consult prescriber if breast-feeding.

**Related Information**

Dexamethasone *on page 346*
Neomycin *on page 815*
Ophthalmic Agents *on page 1282*

## Neomycin and Hydrocortisone (nee oh MYE sin & hye droe KOR ti sone)

**U.S. Brand Names** Neo-Cortef® Ophthalmic

**Synonyms** Hydrocortisone and Neomycin

**Therapeutic Category** Antibiotic/Corticosteroid, Ophthalmic; Antibiotic/Corticosteroid, Topical

**Pregnancy Risk Factor** C

**Lactation** For topical use

**Use** Treatment of susceptible topical bacterial infections with associated inflammation

**Formulations**

Cream: Neomycin sulfate 0.5% and hydrocortisone 1% (20 g)

Ointment, topical: Neomycin sulfate 0.5% and hydrocortisone 0.5% (20 g); neomycin sulfate 0.5% and hydrocortisone 1% (20 g)

Solution, ophthalmic: Neomycin sulfate 0.5% and hydrocortisone 0.5% (5 mL)

**Dosing**

**Adults:** Topical: Apply to area in a thin film 2-4 times/day

**Elderly:** Refer to adult dosing.

**Additional Nursing Issues**

**Physical Assessment:** See individual components listed in Related Information. **Pregnancy risk factor C** - benefits of use should outweigh possible risks.

**Patient Information/Instruction:** See individual components listed in Related Information. **Pregnancy precautions:** Inform prescriber if you are on intend to get pregnant.

**Related Information**

Hydrocortisone *on page 578*
Neomycin *on page 815*
Ophthalmic Agents *on page 1282*

## Neomycin and Polymyxin B (nee oh MYE sin & pol i MIKS in bee)

**U.S. Brand Names** Neosporin® Cream [OTC]; Neosporin® G.U. Irrigant

**Synonyms** Polymyxin B and Neomycin

**Therapeutic Category** Antibiotic, Topical

**Pregnancy Risk Factor** C/D (for G.U. irrigant)

**Lactation** Excretion in breast milk unknown

**Use** Short-term as a continuous irrigant or rinse in the urinary bladder to prevent bacteriuria and gram-negative rod septicemia associated with the use of indwelling catheters; to help prevent infection in minor cuts, scrapes, and burns; treatment of superficial ocular infections involving the conjunctiva or cornea

**Formulations**

Cream: Neomycin sulfate 3.5 mg and polymyxin B sulfate 10,000 units per g (0.94 g, 15 g)

Solution, irrigant: Neomycin sulfate 40 mg and polymyxin B sulfate 200,000 units per mL (1 mL, 20 mL)

**Dosing**

**Adults:**

Bladder irrigation: **Not for I.V. injection**; add 1 mL irrigant to 1 liter isotonic saline solution and connect container to the inflow of lumen of 3-way catheter. Continuous irrigant or rinse in the urinary bladder for up to a maximum of 10 days with administration rate adjusted to patient's urine output; usually no more than 1 L of irrigant is used per day.

Ophthalmic:

Ointment: Instill 1/2" ribbon into the conjunctival sac every 3-4 hours for acute infections or 2-3 times/day for mild to moderate infections for 7-10 days

Solution: Instill 1-2 drops every 15-30 minutes for acute infections; 1-2 drops every 3-6 hours for mild-moderate infections.

Topical: Apply cream 1-4 times/day to affected area.

**Elderly:** Refer to adult dosing.

**Additional Nursing Issues**

**Physical Assessment:** See individual components listed in Related Information. **Pregnancy risk factor C/D** - see Pregnancy Risk Factor - assess knowledge/instruct patient on need to use appropriate contraceptive measures and the need to avoid pregnancy. Note breast-feeding caution.

**Patient Information/Instruction:** See individual components listed in Related Information. **Pregnancy/breast-feeding precautions:** Inform prescriber if you are or intend to be pregnant. Consult prescriber if breast-feeding.

**Related Information**

Neomycin *on page 815*
Polymyxin B Sulfate *on page 946*

- **Neomycin, Bacitracin, and Polymyxin B** *see* Bacitracin, Neomycin, and Polymyxin B *on page 130*
- **Neomycin, Bacitracin, Polymyxin B, and Hydrocortisone** *see* Bacitracin, Neomycin, Polymyxin B, and Hydrocortisone *on page 131*
- **Neomycin, Polymyxin B, and Dexamethasone** *see page 1282*
- **Neomycin, Polymyxin B, and Gramicidin** *see page 1282*
- **Neomycin, Polymyxin B, and Hydrocortisone** *see page 1282*
- **Neomycin, Polymyxin B, and Hydrocortisone** *see page 1291*
- **Neomycin, Polymyxin B, and Prednisolone** *see page 1282*
- **Neopap® [OTC]** *see* Acetaminophen *on page 32*
- **Neoral® Oral** *see* Cyclosporine *on page 317*
- **Neosar® Injection** *see* Cyclophosphamide *on page 313*
- **Neosporin® Cream [OTC]** *see* Neomycin and Polymyxin B *on previous page*
- **Neosporin® G.U. Irrigant** *see* Neomycin and Polymyxin B *on previous page*
- **Neosporin® Ophthalmic Ointment** *see* Bacitracin, Neomycin, and Polymyxin B *on page 130*
- **Neosporin® Ophthalmic Ointment** *see page 1282*
- **Neosporin® Ophthalmic Solution** *see page 1282*
- **Neosporin® Topical Ointment [OTC]** *see* Bacitracin, Neomycin, and Polymyxin B *on page 130*

## Neostigmine (nee oh STIG meen)

**U.S. Brand Names** Prostigmin®

**Therapeutic Category** Acetylcholinesterase Inhibitor (Peripheral)

**Pregnancy Risk Factor** C

**Lactation** Excretion in breast milk unknown/not recommended

**Use** Diagnosis and treatment of myasthenia gravis; prevent and treat postoperative bladder distention and urinary retention; reversal of the effects of nondepolarizing neuromuscular blocking agents after surgery

**Mechanism of Action/Effect** Inhibits destruction of acetylcholine by acetylcholinesterase which facilitates transmission of impulses across myoneural junction

**Contraindications** Hypersensitivity to neostigmine, bromides, or any component; GI or GU obstruction

**Warnings** Does **not** antagonize and may prolong the Phase I block of depolarizing muscle relaxants (eg, succinylcholine). Use with caution in patients with epilepsy, asthma, bradycardia, hyperthyroidism, cardiac arrhythmias, or peptic ulcer. Adequate facilities should be available for cardiopulmonary resuscitation when testing and adjusting dose for myasthenia gravis. Have atropine and epinephrine ready to treat hypersensitivity reactions. Overdosage may result in cholinergic crisis, this must be distinguished from myasthenic crisis. Anticholinesterase insensitivity can develop for brief or prolonged periods. Pregnancy factor C.

**Drug Interactions**

**Decreased Effect:** Antagonizes effects of nondepolarizing muscle relaxants (eg, pancuronium, tubocurarine). Atropine antagonizes the muscarinic effects of neostigmine.

**Increased Effect/Toxicity:** Neuromuscular blocking agent effects are increased when combined with neostigmine.

**Effects on Lab Values** ↑ aminotransferase [ALT (SGPT)/AST (SGOT)] (S), amylase (S)

**Adverse Reactions**

Respiratory: Bronchoconstriction

>10%:

Gastrointestinal: Hyperperistalsis, nausea, vomiting, salivation, diarrhea, stomach cramps

Miscellaneous: Increased sweating

1% to 10%:

Genitourinary: Urge to urinate

Ocular: Small pupils, lacrimation

Respiratory: Increased bronchial secretions

<1% (Limited to important or life-threatening symptoms): A-V block, bradycardia, hypotension, bradyarrhythmias, asystole, seizures, thrombophlebitis, laryngospasm, respiratory paralysis

**Overdose/Toxicology** Symptoms of overdose include muscle weakness, blurred vision, excessive sweating, tearing and salivation, nausea, vomiting, diarrhea, hypertension, bradycardia, muscle weakness, and paralysis. Atropine sulfate injection should be readily available as an antagonist for the effects of neostigmine.

**Pharmacodynamics/Kinetics**

**Half-life Elimination:** Normal renal function: 0.5-2.1 hours; End-stage renal disease: Prolonged

**Metabolism:** Liver

**Excretion:** 50% excreted renally as unchanged drug

**Onset:** I.M.: Within 20-30 minutes; I.V.: Within 1-20 minutes

**Duration:** I.M.: 2.5-4 hours; I.V.: 1-2 hours

**Formulations**

Injection, as methylsulfate: 0.25 mg/mL (1 mL); 0.5 mg/mL (1 mL, 10 mL); 1 mg/mL (10 mL)

Tablet, as bromide: 15 mg

**Dosing**

**Adults:**

Myasthenia gravis:

Diagnosis: I.M.: 0.02 mg/kg as a single dose

Treatment:

Oral: 15 mg/dose every 3-4 hours up to 375 mg/day maximum

I.M., I.V., S.C.: 0.5-2.5 mg every 1-3 hours up to 10 mg/24 hours maximum

Reversal of nondepolarizing neuromuscular blockade after surgery in conjunction with atropine: I.V.: 0.5-2.5 mg; total dose not to exceed 5 mg

Bladder atony: I.M., S.C.:

Prevention: 0.25 mg every 4-6 hours for 2-3 days

Treatment: 0.5-1 mg every 3 hours for 5 doses after bladder has emptied

**Elderly:** Refer to adult dosing.

**Renal Impairment:**

$Cl_{cr}$ 10-50 mL/minute: Administer 50% of normal dose.

$Cl_{cr}$ <10 mL/minute: Administer 25% of normal dose.

**Administration**

**I.M.:** In the diagnosis of myasthenia gravis, all anticholinesterase medications should be discontinued for at least 8 hours before administering neostigmine.

**Additional Nursing Issues**

**Physical Assessment:** When using for MG diagnosis, see Warnings/Precautions. For bladder atony: Assess bladder adequacy prior to administering medication, monitor for therapeutic response, and adverse effects (eg, vital signs, respiratory and CNS response), and cholinergic crisis (DUMBELS - **d**iarrhea, **u**rination, **m**iosis, **b**roncho-spasm/**b**radycardia, **e**xcitability, **l**acrimation, and **s**alivation/excessive **s**weating) (see Adverse Reactions and Overdose/Toxicology). Teach patient symptoms to report. **Pregnancy risk factor C** - benefits of use should outweigh possible risks. Breast-feeding is not recommended.

**Patient Information/Instruction:** Take this drug exactly as prescribed. You may experience visual difficulty (eg, blurring and dark adaptation - use caution at night) or urinary frequency. Promptly report any muscle weakness, respiratory difficulty, severe or unresolved diarrhea, persistent abdominal cramping or vomiting, sweating, or tearing. **Pregnancy/breast-feeding precautions:** Inform prescriber if you are pregnant. Breast-feeding is not recommended.

**Geriatric Considerations:** Many elderly will have diseases which may influence the use of neostigmine. Also, many elderly will need doses reduced 50% due to creatinine clearances in the 10-50 mL/minute range (common in the aged). Side effects or concomitant disease may warrant use of pyridostigmine.

**Additional Information**

Neostigmine bromide: Prostigmin® tablet

Neostigmine methylsulfate: Prostigmin® injection

- **Neostrata™ HQ** *see* Hydroquinone *on page 583*
- **Neo-Synephrine®** *see page 1282*
- **Neo-Synephrine® 12 Hour Nasal Solution** *see page 1294*
- **Neo-Synephrine® Nasal Solution [OTC]** *see* Phenylephrine *on page 920*
- **Neo-Synephrine® Ophthalmic Solution** *see* Phenylephrine *on page 920*
- **Neo-Tabs® Oral** *see* Neomycin *on page 815*
- **Neotopic** *see* Bacitracin, Neomycin, and Polymyxin B *on page 130*
- **Neotricin HC® Ophthalmic Ointment** *see* Bacitracin, Neomycin, Polymyxin B, and Hydrocortisone *on page 131*
- **Neotricin HC® Ophthalmic Ointment** *see page 1282*
- **NeoVadrin® [OTC]** *see* Vitamin, Multiple *on page 1219*
- **NeoVadrin® B Complex** *see page 1294*
- **Nephro-Calci® [OTC]** *see* Calcium Supplements *on page 185*
- **Nephrocaps® [OTC]** *see* Vitamin, Multiple *on page 1219*
- **Nephrocaps®** *see page 1294*
- **Nephro-Fer™ [OTC]** *see* Iron Supplements *on page 627*
- **Nephronex®** *see* Nitrofurantoin *on page 829*
- **Nephrox Suspension [OTC]** *see* Aluminum Hydroxide *on page 60*
- **Neptazane®** *see* Methazolamide *on page 738*
- **Nervocaine®** *see* Lidocaine *on page 674*
- **Nesacaine®** *see* Chloroprocaine *on page 251*
- **Nesacaine®-MPF** *see* Chloroprocaine *on page 251*
- **Nestrex®** *see* Pyridoxine *on page 997*
- **Neucalm®** *see* Hydroxyzine *on page 588*
- **Neugal** *see* Ranitidine *on page 1008*
- **Neugeron** *see* Carbamazepine *on page 195*
- **Neupogen® Injection** *see* Filgrastim *on page 483*
- **Neuramate®** *see* Meprobamate *on page 724*
- **Neurontin®** *see* Gabapentin *on page 525*
- **Neurosine** *see* Buspirone *on page 170*
- **Neut® Injection** *see* Sodium Bicarbonate *on page 1061*
- **Neutra-Phos®-K** *see* Phosphate Supplements *on page 926*
- **Neutrexin® Injection** *see* Trimetrexate Glucuronate *on page 1182*

- ♦ **Neutrogena® Acne Mask** *see page 1294*
- ♦ **Neutrogena® T/Derm** *see page 1294*


## Nevirapine (ne VYE re peen)

**U.S. Brand Names** Viramune®

**Therapeutic Category** Antiretroviral Agent, Reverse Transcriptase Inhibitor (Non-Nucleoside)

**Pregnancy Risk Factor** C

**Lactation** Enters breast milk/contraindicated

**Use** In combination therapy with other antiretroviral agents in HIV-1 infected adults previously treated for whom current therapy is deemed inadequate

**Mechanism of Action/Effect** Blocks the RNA-dependent DNA polymerase activity

**Contraindications** Hypersensitivity to nevirapine or its components

**Warnings** Nevirapine should be discontinued in patients who develop a severe rash that may be accompanied with constitutional symptoms (eg, fever, blistering, oral lesions, conjunctivitis, swelling, muscle or joint aches, or general malaise). Severe hepatotoxic reactions may occur. Pregnancy factor C.

**Drug Interactions**

**Cytochrome P-450 Effect:** CYP3A3/4 enzyme substrate; CYP3A3/4 enzyme inducer; CYP3A3/4 enzyme inhibitor

**Decreased Effect:** Rifabutin and rifampin may decrease plasma concentration of nevirapine. Ketoconazole concentrations are decreased by nevirapine. Saquinavir and indinavir concentrations may decrease (clinical significance unknown).

**Increased Effect/Toxicity:** Cimetidine and macrolide antibiotics may increase nevirapine plasma concentrations. Increased toxicity when used concomitantly with protease inhibitors or oral contraceptives. Ketoconazole should not be coadministered.

**Adverse Reactions**

>10%:

- Central nervous system: Headache, fever
- Dermatologic: Rash
- Gastrointestinal: Nausea, diarrhea, abdominal pain
- Hematologic: Thrombocytopenia

1% to 10%:

- Gastrointestinal: Ulcerative stomatitis
- Hematologic: Anemia, thrombocytopenia
- Hepatic: Hepatitis, increased LFTs
- Neuromuscular & skeletal: Peripheral neuropathy, paresthesia, myalgia

<1% (Limited to important or life-threatening symptoms): Stevens-Johnson syndrome, hepatotoxicity, hepatic necrosis

**Overdose/Toxicology** No toxicities have been reported with acute ingestion of large sums of tablets.

**Pharmacodynamics/Kinetics**

**Metabolism:** Liver

**Excretion:** Urine

**Formulations**

- Suspension, oral: 50 mg/5 mL (240 mL)
- Tablet: 200 mg

**Dosing**

**Adults:** Oral: Initial: 200 mg/day for the first 14 days, followed by 200 mg twice daily in combination with nucleoside analogue antiretroviral agents

**Elderly:** Refer to adult dosing.

**Monitoring Laboratory Tests** Perform CBC. Monitor liver function tests in the first 6 months of therapy. Interrupt therapy in patients experiencing liver function test abnormalities until values return to baseline. Should be discontinued permanently if abnormalities recur on readministration.

**Additional Nursing Issues**

**Physical Assessment:** Monitor laboratory results carefully. Monitor for adverse reactions as identified above. **Pregnancy risk factor C** - benefits of use should outweigh possible risks. Breast-feeding is contraindicated.

**Patient Information/Instruction:** If rash develops, contact prescriber. **Pregnancy/breast-feeding precautions:** Inform prescriber if you are or intend to be pregnant. Do not breast-feed.

**Breast-feeding Issues:** The CDC recommends **not** to breast-feed if diagnosed with HIV to avoid postnatal transmission of the virus.

**Related Information**

Antiretroviral Agents Comparison *on page 1373*


- ♦ **New Decongestant®** *see page 1306*
- ♦ **N.G.T.® Topical** *see* Nystatin and Triamcinolone *on page 844*
- ♦ **Niacin** *see page 1294*


## Nicardipine (nye KAR de peen)

**U.S. Brand Names** Cardene®; Cardene® SR; Cardene® I.V.

**Therapeutic Category** Calcium Channel Blocker

**Pregnancy Risk Factor** C

**Lactation** Enters breast milk/not recommended

**Use** Management of essential hypertension

**Mechanism of Action/Effect** Inhibits calcium ion from entering the "slow channels" or select voltage-sensitive areas of vascular smooth muscle and myocardium during depolarization, producing a relaxation of coronary vascular smooth muscle and coronary vasodilation; increases myocardial oxygen delivery in patients with vasospastic angina

**Contraindications** Hypersensitivity to nicardipine or any component, calcium channel blockers; advanced aortic stenosis

**Warnings** Use with caution in patients with angina; may increase frequency, severity, and duration of angina during initiation of therapy. Titrate dosages for impaired renal or hepatic function patients with caution. Use cautiously with patients who have CHF and/or receiving beta-blockers. Do not abruptly withdraw (chest pain). Elderly may have a greater hypotensive effect. Pregnancy factor C.

**Drug Interactions**

**Cytochrome P-450 Effect:** CYP3A3/4 enzyme substrate

**Increased Effect/Toxicity:** $H_2$ blockers (cimetidine) and nicardipine may increase bioavailability of nicardipine. Nicardipine and propranolol or metoprolol may increase cardiac depressant effects on A-V conduction. Nicardipine and cyclosporine may increase cyclosporine levels.

**Food Interactions** Nicardipine average peak concentrations may be decreased if taken with food.

**Adverse Reactions**

**Oral:**

1% to 10%:

- Cardiovascular: Flushing, palpitations, tachycardia, pedal edema
- Central nervous system: Headache, dizziness, somnolence
- Gastrointestinal: Nausea
- Neuromuscular & skeletal: Weakness

<1% (Limited to important or life-threatening symptoms): Postural hypotension, atypical chest pain, ventricular extrasystoles, ventricular tachycardia, chest pain pectoris, abnormal LFTs

**I.V.:**

>10%: Central nervous system: Headache

1% to 10%:

- Cardiovascular: Hypotension, tachycardia, abnormal EKG, postural hypotension, ventricular extrasystoles
- Central nervous system: Dizziness
- Gastrointestinal: Nausea, vomiting

<1% (Limited to important or life-threatening symptoms): Chest pain, atrioventricular block, ST segment depression, inverted T wave, DVT, supraventricular tachycardia, ventricular tachycardia, syncope, hypophosphatemia, thrombocytopenia

**Overdose/Toxicology** The primary cardiac symptoms of calcium blocker overdose include hypotension and bradycardia. Noncardiac symptoms include confusion, stupor, nausea, vomiting, metabolic acidosis, and hyperglycemia. Following initial gastric decontamination, if possible, repeated calcium administration may promptly reverse the depressed cardiac contractility (but not sinus node depression or peripheral vasodilation). Glucagon and epinephrine may treat refractory hypotension. Glucagon and epinephrine also increase the heart rate (outside the U.S., 4-aminopyridine may be available as an antidote). Dialysis and hemoperfusion are not effective in enhancing elimination although repeat-dose activated charcoal may serve as an adjunct with sustained-release preparations.

**Pharmacodynamics/Kinetics**

**Protein Binding:** 95%

**Half-life Elimination:** 2-4 hours

**Time to Peak:** Peak serum levels occur within 20-120 minutes and an onset of hypotension occurs within 20 minutes

**Metabolism:** Liver

**Excretion:** Urine

**Onset:** Oral: 1-2 hours; I.V.: 10 minutes

**Duration:** 2-6 hours

**Formulations**

Nicardipine hydrochloride:

- Capsule: 20 mg, 30 mg
- Capsule, sustained release: 30 mg, 45 mg, 60 mg
- Injection: 2.5 mg/mL (10 mL)

**Dosing**

**Adults:**

- Oral: 40 mg 3 times/day (allow 3 days between dose increases)
- Oral, sustained release: Initial: 30 mg twice daily, titrate up to 60 mg twice daily
- I.V. (dilute to 0.1 mg/mL): Initial: 5 mg/hour increased by 2.5 mg/hour every 15 minutes to a maximum of 15 mg/hour
- Oral to I.V. dose equivalents:
  - 20 mg every 8 hours orally = 0.5 mg/hour I.V.
  - 30 mg every 8 hours orally = 1.2 mg/hour I.V.
  - 40 mg every 8 hours orally = 2.2 mg/hour I.V.

**Elderly:** Refer to adult dosing.

**Renal Impairment:** Titrate dose beginning with 20 mg 3 times/day (immediate release) or 30 mg twice daily (sustained release).

**Hepatic Impairment:** Starting dose: 20 mg twice daily (immediate release) with titration. See table.

(Continued)

## Nicardipine *(Continued)*

**Equivalent Oral vs I.V. Infusion Doses**

| Oral Dose | Equivalent I.V. Infusion |
|---|---|
| 20 mg q8h | 0.5 mg/h |
| 30 mg q8h | 1.2 mg/h |
| 40 mg q8h | 2.2 mg/h |

**Administration**

**Oral:** Do not chew or crush the sustained release formulation, swallow whole. Do not open or cut capsules.

**I.V.:** Ampuls must be diluted before use. Administer as a slow continuous infusion.

**I.V. Detail:** Avoid extravasation.

**Stability**

**Storage:** I.V.: Store at room temperature and protect from light. Freezing does not affect stability.

**Compatibility:** Compatible with $D_5W$, $D_5{}^1/_2NS$, $D_5NS$, and $D_5W$ with 40 mEq potassium chloride; 0.45% and 0.9% NS. Incompatible with sodium bicarbonate 5% or lactated Ringer's solution. Diluted solution is stable for 24 hours at room temperature.

**Additional Nursing Issues**

**Physical Assessment:** Monitor I.V. infusion site closely. Avoid extravasation. Monitor blood pressure, heart rate, and I & O ratio closely when starting or adjusting dosage. Monitor blood pressure closely when used in conjunction with nitrates. Use orthostatic precautions for inpatients; advise outpatients about orthostatic precautions. **Pregnancy risk factor C** - benefits of use should outweigh possible risks. Breast-feeding is not recommended.

**Patient Information/Instruction:** Take as directed; do not alter dosage regimen or increase, decrease, or discontinue without consulting prescriber. Do not crush or chew tablets or capsules. Take with nonfatty food. Avoid caffeine and alcohol. Consult prescriber before increasing exercise routine (decreased angina does not mean it is safe to increase exercise). Change position slowly to prevent orthostatic events. May cause dizziness or fatigue; use caution when driving or engaging in tasks that require alertness until response to drug is known. Frequent small meals, frequent mouth care, sucking lozenges, or chewing gum may reduce nausea. Report swelling, difficulty breathing or new cough, unresolved fatigue, unusual weight gain, or unresolved dizziness. **Pregnancy/breast-feeding precautions:** Inform prescriber if you are or intend to be pregnant. Breast-feeding is not recommended.

**Geriatric Considerations:** Elderly may experience a greater hypotensive response. Constipation may be more of a problem in the elderly.

**Additional Information** pH: 3.5

**Related Information**

Calcium Channel Blocking Agents Comparison *on page 1378*

- **N'ice® Vitamin C Drops [OTC]** *see* Ascorbic Acid *on page 108*
- **Nicobid®** *see page 1294*
- **Nicoderm® Patch** *see* Nicotine *on this page*
- **Nicolan** *see* Nicotine *on this page*
- **Nicolar®** *see page 1294*
- **Nicorette®** *see* Nicotine *on this page*
- **Nicorette® DS Gum** *see* Nicotine *on this page*
- **Nicorette® Gum** *see* Nicotine *on this page*
- **Nicorette® Plus** *see* Nicotine *on this page*

## Nicotine (nik oh TEEN)

**U.S. Brand Names** Habitrol™ Patch; Nicoderm® Patch; Nicorette® DS Gum; Nicorette® Gum; Nicotrol® NS Nasal Spray; Nicotrol® Patch [OTC]; ProStep® Patch

**Therapeutic Category** Smoking Cessation Aid

**Pregnancy Risk Factor** D (transdermal); X (chewing gum)

**Lactation** Excretion in breast milk unknown/contraindicated

**Use** Treatment aid to smoking cessation while participating in a behavioral modification program under medical supervision

**Mechanism of Action/Effect** Nicotine is one of two naturally-occurring alkaloids which exhibit their primary effects via autonomic ganglia stimulation. The other alkaloid is lobeline which has many actions similar to those of nicotine but is less potent. Nicotine is a potent ganglionic and central nervous system stimulant, the actions of which are mediated via nicotine-specific receptors. Biphasic actions are observed depending upon the dose administered. The main effect of nicotine in small doses is stimulation of all autonomic ganglia; with larger doses, initial stimulation is followed by blockade of transmission. Biphasic effects are also evident in the adrenal medulla; discharge of catecholamines occurs with small doses, whereas prevention of catecholamines release is seen with higher doses as a response to splanchnic nerve stimulation. Stimulation of the central nervous system (CNS) is characterized by tremors and respiratory excitation. However, convulsions may occur with higher doses, along with respiratory failure secondary to both central paralysis and peripheral blockade to respiratory muscles.

**Contraindications** Hypersensitivity or allergy to nicotine or any components used in the transdermal system; pregnancy; nonsmokers; patients who are smoking during the post-myocardial infarction period; patients with life-threatening arrhythmias, severe or worsening angina pectoris, active temporomandibular joint disease

**Warnings** Use with caution in oropharyngeal inflammation and in patients with history of esophagitis, peptic ulcer, coronary artery disease, vasospastic disease, angina, hypertension, hyperthyroidism, diabetes, and hepatic dysfunction. Nicotine is known to be one of the most toxic of all poisons. While the gum is being used to help the patient overcome a health hazard, it also must be considered a hazardous drug vehicle.

Nicotine nasal spray: Fatal dose: 40 mg

**Drug Interactions**

**Cytochrome P-450 Effect:** CYP2A6, 2B6 enzyme substrate; CYP1A2 enzyme inducer

**Adverse Reactions**

**Chewing gum:**

>10%:

- Cardiovascular: Tachycardia
- Central nervous system: Headache (mild)
- Gastrointestinal: Nausea, vomiting, indigestion, excessive salivation, belching, increased appetite, mouth or throat soreness
- Neuromuscular & skeletal: Jaw muscle ache
- Miscellaneous: Hiccups

1% to 10%:

- Central nervous system: Insomnia, dizziness, nervousness
- Endocrine & metabolic: Dysmenorrhea
- Gastrointestinal: GI distress, eructation
- Neuromuscular & skeletal: Myalgia
- Respiratory: Hoarseness
- Miscellaneous: Hiccups

<1% (Limited to important or life-threatening symptoms): Atrial fibrillation, erythema, itching, hypersensitivity reactions

**Transdermal systems:**

>10%:

- Cardiovascular: Tachycardia
- Central nervous system: Headache (mild)
- Dermatologic: Pruritus, erythema
- Gastrointestinal: Increased appetite

1% to 10%:

- Central nervous system: Insomnia, nervousness
- Endocrine & metabolic: Dysmenorrhea
- Neuromuscular & skeletal: Myalgia

<1% (Limited to important or life-threatening symptoms): Atrial fibrillation, itching, hypersensitivity reactions

**Overdose/Toxicology** Symptoms of overdose include nausea, vomiting, abdominal pain, mental confusion, diarrhea, salivation, tachycardia, respiratory and cardiovascular collapse. Treatment is symptomatic and supportive. Remove patch, rinse area with water, and dry. Do not use soap as this may increase absorption.

**Pharmacodynamics/Kinetics**

**Half-life Elimination:** 4 hours

**Time to Peak:** Transdermal: 8-9 hours

**Metabolism:** Liver

**Excretion:** Urine

**Onset:** Intranasal nicotine may more closely approximate the time course of plasma nicotine levels observed after cigarette smoking than other dosage forms.

**Duration:** Transdermal: 24 hours

**Formulations**

Patch, transdermal:

- Habitrol™: 21 mg/day; 14 mg/day; 7 mg/day (30 systems/box)
- Nicoderm®: 21 mg/day; 14 mg/day; 7 mg/day (14 systems/box)
- Nicotrol® [OTC]: 15 mg/day (gradually released over 16 hours)
- ProStep®: 22 mg/day; 11 mg/day (7 systems/box)

Pieces, chewing gum, as polacrilex: 2 mg/square [OTC] (96 pieces/box); 4 mg/square (96 pieces/box)

Spray, nasal: 0.5 mg/actuation [10 mg/mL - 200 actuations] (10 mL)

**Dosing**

**Adults:**

Gum: Chew 1 piece of gum when urge to smoke, up to 30 pieces/day; most patients require 10-12 pieces of gum/day.

Transdermal patch (patients should be advised to completely stop smoking upon initiation of therapy): Apply new patch every 24 hours to nonhairy, clean, dry skin on the upper body or upper outer arm; each patch should be applied to a different site.

- Initial starting dose: 21 mg/day for 4-8 weeks for most patients
- First weaning dose: 14 mg/day for 2-4 weeks
- Second weaning dose: 7 mg/day for 2-4 weeks
- Initial starting dose for patients <100 pounds, smoke <10 cigarettes/day, have a history of cardiovascular disease: 14 mg/day for 4-8 weeks followed by 7 mg/day for 2-4 weeks
- In patients who are receiving >600 mg/day of cimetidine: Decrease to the next lower patch size.

(Continued)

## Nicotine *(Continued)*

Benefits of use of nicotine transdermal patches beyond 3 months have not been demonstrated.

Spray: 1-2 sprays/hour; do not exceed more than 5 doses (10 sprays) per hour; each dose (2 sprays) contains 1 mg of nicotine. **Warning:** A dose of 40 mg can cause fatalities.

**Elderly:** Refer to adult dosing; use with caution.

**Administration**

**Oral:** Patients should be instructed to chew slowly to avoid jaw ache and to maximize benefit.

**Topical:** Patches cannot be cut. Use of an aerosol corticosteroid may diminish local irritation under patches.

**Additional Nursing Issues**

**Physical Assessment:** See Contraindications and Warnings/Precautions for use cautions. Monitor cardiac status and vital signs prior to, when beginning, and periodically during therapy. Monitor effectiveness of therapy (according to rational for therapy), and adverse reactions (see extensive list of Adverse Reactions) at beginning and periodically during therapy. Assess knowledge/teach patient appropriate use, interventions to reduce side effects, and adverse symptoms to report for prescribed form of drug. **Pregnancy risk factor D/X** - see Pregnancy Risk Factor - determine that patient is not pregnant before beginning treatment and do not give to women of childbearing age unless female is capable of complying with barrier contraceptive measures. Breast-feeding is contraindicated.

**Patient Information/Instruction:** Use exactly as directed; do not use more often than prescribed. Stop smoking completely during therapy.

Gum: Chew slowly for 30 minutes. Discard chewed gum away from access by children.

Transdermal patch: Follow directions in package for dosing schedule and use. Do not cut patches. Apply to clean, dry skin in different site each day. Do not touch eyes; wash hands after application. You may experience dizziness or lightheadedness; use caution driving or when engaging in tasks requiring alertness until response to drug is known. For nausea, vomiting or GI upset, small frequent meals, chewing gum, frequent oral care may help. Report persistent vomiting, diarrhea, chills, sweating, chest pain or palpitations, or burning or redness at application site.

Spray: Follow directions in package. Blow nose gently before use. Use 1-2 sprays/hour; do not exceed 5 doses (10 sprays) per hour. Excessive use can result in severe (even life-threatening) reactions. You may experience temporary stinging or burning after spray.

**Pregnancy/breast-feeding precautions:** Inform prescriber if you are pregnant. Do not get pregnant during or for 1 month following therapy. Consult prescriber for instruction on appropriate barrier contraceptive measures. This drug may cause severe fetal defects. Do not breast-feed.

**Geriatric Considerations:** Must evaluate benefit in the elderly who may have chronic diseases mentioned (see Warnings/Precautions and Contraindications). The transdermal systems are as effective in the elderly as they are in younger adults; however, complaints of body aches, dizziness, and asthenia were reported more often in the elderly.

♦ **Nicotinell TTS** *see* Nicotine *on page 822*

♦ **Nicotinex®** *see page 1294*

♦ **Nicotrol® NS Nasal Spray** *see* Nicotine *on page 822*

♦ **Nicotrol® Patch [OTC]** *see* Nicotine *on page 822*

♦ **Nico-Vert® [OTC]** *see* Meclizine *on page 712*

## Nifedipine (nye FED i peen)

**U.S. Brand Names** Adalat®; Adalat® CC; Procardia®; Procardia XL®

**Therapeutic Category** Calcium Channel Blocker

**Pregnancy Risk Factor** C

**Lactation** Enters breast milk/compatible

**Use** Angina, hypertension (sustained release only), pulmonary hypertension

**Mechanism of Action/Effect** Inhibits calcium ion from entering the "slow channels" or select voltage-sensitive areas of vascular smooth muscle and myocardium during depolarization, producing a relaxation of coronary vascular smooth muscle and coronary vasodilation; increases myocardial oxygen delivery in patients with vasospastic angina

**Contraindications** Hypersensitivity to nifedipine or any other calcium channel blocker and adenosine; sick-sinus syndrome; second or third degree A-V block; hypotension (<90 mm Hg systolic); advanced aortic stenosis, acute myocardial infarction within 4 weeks

**Warnings** Use with caution and titrate dosages for patients with impaired renal or hepatic function. Use caution when treating patients with congestive heart failure, sick-sinus syndrome, severe left ventricular dysfunction, hypertrophic cardiomyopathy (especially obstructive), hypotension (<90 mm Hg systolic), second or third degree A-V block, concomitant therapy with beta-blockers or digoxin, edema, or increased intracranial pressure with cranial tumors. Do not abruptly withdraw (may cause chest pain). Elderly may experience hypotension and constipation more readily. Pregnancy factor C.

**Drug Interactions**

**Cytochrome P-450 Effect:** CYP3A3/4 and 3A5-7 enzyme substrate

**Decreased Effect:** Phenobarbital and nifedipine may decrease nifedipine levels. Quinidine and nifedipine may decrease quinidine serum levels. Rifampin and nifedipine may decrease nifedipine serum levels.

**Increased Effect/Toxicity:** Beta-blockers and nifedipine may increase adverse effects. $H_2$-blockers and nifedipine may increase bioavailability and serum concentrations of nifedipine. Phenytoin and nifedipine may increase phenytoin levels. Nifedipine and quinidine may increase nifedipine serum levels. Theophylline and nifedipine may increase theophylline levels. Vincristine and nifedipine may increase vincristine levels. Nifedipine and digoxin may increase digoxin levels.

**Food Interactions** Nifedipine serum levels may be decreased if taken with food. Increased therapeutic and vasodilator side effects, including severe hypotension and myocardial ischemia, may occur if nifedipine is taken with grapefruit juice.

**Adverse Reactions**

>10%:
- Cardiovascular: Peripheral edema, flushing
- Central nervous system: Dizziness, lightheadedness, headache
- Gastrointestinal: Nausea

1% to 10%:
- Cardiovascular: Congestive heart failure, hypotension, tachycardia
- Gastrointestinal: Constipation, gingival hyperplasia
- Neuromuscular & skeletal: Weakness
- Respiratory: Dyspnea, cough, nasal congestion

<1% (Limited to important or life-threatening symptoms): Chest pain, hypotension (excessive), gingival hyperplasia, transient blindness, photosensitivity, myoclonus, gynecomastia

**Overdose/Toxicology** Primary cardiac symptoms of calcium blocker overdose include hypotension and bradycardia. Noncardiac symptoms include confusion, stupor, nausea, vomiting, metabolic acidosis, and hyperglycemia. Following initial gastric decontamination, treat symptomatically.

**Pharmacodynamics/Kinetics**

**Protein Binding:** 92% to 98% (concentration dependent)

**Half-life Elimination:** Adults, normal: 2-5 hours; Adults with cirrhosis: 7 hours

**Metabolism:** Liver

**Excretion:** Urine

**Onset:** Oral: Within 20 minutes; S.L.: Within 1-5 minutes

**Formulations**

Capsule, liquid-filled (Adalat®, Procardia®): 10 mg, 20 mg
Tablet, extended release (Adalat® CC): 30 mg, 60 mg, 90 mg
Tablet, sustained release (Procardia XL®): 30 mg, 60 mg, 90 mg

**Dosing**

**Adults:**
- Initial: 10 mg 3 times/day as capsules or 30 mg once daily as sustained release
- Usual dose: 10-30 mg 3 times/day as capsules or 30-60 mg once daily as sustained release
- Maximum: 120-180 mg/day
- **Increase sustained release at 7- to 14-day intervals**

**Elderly:** Refer to adult dosing.

**Hepatic Impairment:** Reduce oral dose by 50% to 60% in patients with cirrhosis.

**Administration**

**Oral:** Sustained release tablets should be swallowed whole; do not crush or chew.

**Additional Nursing Issues**

**Physical Assessment:** Monitor blood pressure, heart rate, and I & O ratio closely when starting or adjusting dosage. Monitor blood pressure closely when used in conjunction with other antihypertensives. Use orthostatic precautions for inpatients; advise outpatients about orthostatic precautions. Monitor serum glucose closely in diabetic patients. Monitor for gingival hyperplasia. **Pregnancy risk factor C** - benefits of use should outweigh possible risks.

**Patient Information/Instruction:** Take as directed; do not alter dosage regimen or increase, decrease, or discontinue without consulting prescriber. Do not crush or chew tablets or capsules. Consult prescriber before increasing exercise routine (decreased angina does not mean it is safe to increase exercise). Change position slowly to prevent orthostatic events. May cause dizziness or fatigue; use caution when driving or engaging in tasks that require alertness until response to drug is known. Maintain good oral care and inspect gums for swelling or redness. May cause frequent urination at night. Report irregular heartbeat, swelling, difficulty breathing or new cough, unresolved fatigue, unusual weight gain, unresolved dizziness or constipation, and swollen or bleeding gums. **Pregnancy precautions:** Inform prescriber if you are or intend to be pregnant.

**Geriatric Considerations:** Elderly may experience a greater hypotensive response. Theoretically, constipation may be more of a problem in elderly patients.

**Related Information**

Calcium Channel Blocking Agents Comparison *on page 1378*


- **Nifedipres** *see* Nifedipine *on previous page*
- **Niferex®** *see page 1294*
- **Niferex®-PN** *see* Vitamin, Multiple *on page 1219*
- **Nilandron™** *see* Nilutamide *on next page*

♦ **Nilstat®** *see* Nystatin *on page 843*

## Nilutamide (ni LU ta mide)

**U.S. Brand Names** Nilandron™

**Therapeutic Category** Antineoplastic Agent, Miscellaneous

**Pregnancy Risk Factor** C

**Lactation** Not indicated for use in women

**Use** Treatment of metastatic prostatic cancer

**Mechanism of Action/Effect** Nonsteroidal antiandrogen that inhibits androgen uptake or inhibits binding of androgen in target tissues

**Contraindications** Hypersensitivity to nilutamide or any component; severe hepatic impairment; severe respiratory insufficiency

**Warnings** Interstitial pneumonitis has been reported in 2% of patients exposed to nilutamide. Patients typically experienced progressive exertional dyspnea, and possibly cough, chest pain, and fever. X-rays showed interstitial or alveolo-interstitial changes. The suggestive signs of pneumonitis most often occurred within the first 3 months of nilutamide treatment.

Hepatitis or marked increases in liver enzymes leading to drug discontinuation occurred in 1% of nilutamide patients. There has been a report of elevated hepatic enzymes followed by death in a 65 year old patient treated with nilutamide.

Foreign postmarketing surveillance has revealed isolated cases of aplastic anemia in which a causal relationship with nilutamide could not be ascertained.

13% to 57% of patients receiving nilutamide reported a delay in adaptation to the dark, ranging from seconds to a few minutes. This effect sometimes does not abate as drug treatment is continued. Caution patients who experience this effect about driving at night or through tunnels. This effect can be alleviated by wearing tinted glasses.

Pregnancy factor C.

**Adverse Reactions**

>10%:

Central nervous system: Pain, headache, insomnia
Gastrointestinal: Nausea, constipation, anorexia
Genitourinary: Impotence, testicular atrophy, gynecomastia
Endocrine & metabolic: Loss of libido, hot flashes
Neuromuscular & skeletal: Weakness
Ocular: Impaired adaption to dark

1% to 10%:

Cardiovascular: Hypertension
Central nervous system: Flu syndrome, fever, dizziness, depression, hypesthesia
Dermatologic: Alopecia, dry skin, rash
Gastrointestinal: Heartburn, vomiting, abdominal pain
Genitourinary: Urinary tract infection, hematuria, urinary tract disorder, nocturia
Respiratory: Dyspnea, upper respiratory infection, pneumonia
Ocular: Chromatopsia, impaired adaption to light, abnormal vision
Miscellaneous: Sweating

**Overdose/Toxicology** One case of massive overdose has been published. A 79-year old man attempted suicide by ingesting 13 g of nilutamide. There were no clinical signs or symptoms, or changes in parameters such as transaminase or chest x-ray. Maintenance treatment (150 mg/day) was resumed 30 days later. Management is supportive. Dialysis is of no benefit.

**Pharmacodynamics/Kinetics**

**Distribution:** Moderately binds to plasma proteins and low binding to erythrocytes

**Half-life Elimination:** 38-59 hours

**Metabolism:** Extensive

**Excretion:** Urine

**Formulations** Tablet: 50 mg

**Dosing**

**Adults:** Oral: 6 tablets (50 mg each) once a day for a total daily dose of 300 mg for 30 days followed thereafter by 3 tablets (50 mg each) once a day for a total daily dose of 150 mg

**Elderly:** Refer to adult dosing.

**Stability**

**Storage:** Store at room temperature (15°C to 30°C/59°F to 86°F). Protect from light.

**Monitoring Laboratory Tests** Chest x-rays prior to and regularly during treatment. Measure serum hepatic enzyme levels at baseline and at regular intervals (3 months). If transaminases increase over 2-3 times the upper limit of normal, discontinue treatment. Perform appropriate laboratory testing at the first symptom/sign of liver injury (eg, jaundice, dark urine, fatigue, abdominal pain, or unexplained GI symptoms) and nilutamide treatment must be discontinued immediately if transaminases exceed 3 times the upper limit of normal.

**Additional Nursing Issues**

**Physical Assessment:** Monitor results of laboratory tests closely (notify prescriber immediately if transaminase levels exceed 2x normal). Monitor respiratory function on a regular basis and notify prescriber immediately at signs of adverse respiratory effects (interstitial pneumonia - see Warnings/Precautions). Instruct patient on appropriate use, possible side effects, and symptoms to report.

**Patient Information/Instruction:** Take as prescribed; do not change dosing schedule or stop taking without consulting prescriber. Avoid alcohol while taking this medication; may cause severe reaction. Periodic laboratory tests are necessary while taking this medication. You may experience dizziness, confusion, or blurred vision (avoid driving or engaging in tasks that require alertness until response to drug is known); loss of light accommodation (avoid night driving and use caution in poorly lighted or changing light situations); impotence; or loss of libido (discuss with prescriber). Report any decreased respiratory function (eg, dyspnea, increased cough); yellowing of skin or eyes; change in color of urine or stool; unusual bruising or bleeding; chest pain; difficulty or painful voiding.

## Nimodipine (nye MOE di peen)

**U.S. Brand Names** Nimotop®

**Therapeutic Category** Calcium Channel Blocker

**Pregnancy Risk Factor** C

**Lactation** Excretion in breast milk unknown

**Use** Improvement of neurological deficits due to spasm following subarachnoid hemorrhage from ruptured congenital intracranial aneurysms in patients who are in good neurological condition postictus

**Mechanism of Action/Effect** Nimodipine shares the pharmacology of other calcium channel blockers; animal studies indicate that nimodipine has a greater effect on cerebral arterials than other arterials; inhibits calcium ion from entering the "slow channels" or select voltage sensitive areas of vascular smooth muscle and myocardium during depolarization

**Contraindications** Hypersensitivity to nimodipine or any component

**Warnings** Use with caution and titrate dosages for patients with impaired renal or hepatic function. Nimodipine may lower blood pressure like other calcium channel blockers. Pregnancy factor C.

**Drug Interactions**

**Cytochrome P-450 Effect:** CYP3A3/4 enzyme substrate

**Increased Effect/Toxicity:** Calcium channel blockers and nimodipine may result in enhanced cardiovascular effects of other calcium channel blockers. Cimetidine and nimodipine may increase serum nimodipine levels. Nimodipine and omeprazole may increase the bioavailability of nimodipine. Nimodipine and valproic acid may increase nimodipine levels.

**Adverse Reactions**

1% to 10%:

Cardiovascular: Hypotension, peripheral edema

Central nervous system: Dizziness, lightheadedness, headache

Gastrointestinal: Diarrhea, nausea

<1% (Limited to important or life-threatening symptoms): Edema, abnormal EKG abnormalities, tachycardia, congestive heart failure, thrombocytopenia, anemia, palpitations, flushing, disseminated intravascular coagulation, hepatitis, jaundice, elevated SGPT (ALT) levels, dyspnea

**Overdose/Toxicology** Primary cardiac symptoms of calcium blocker overdose include hypotension and bradycardia. Noncardiac symptoms include confusion, stupor, nausea, vomiting, metabolic acidosis and hyperglycemia. Treat symptomatically.

**Pharmacodynamics/Kinetics**

**Protein Binding:** >95%

**Half-life Elimination:** 3 hours, increases with reduced renal function

**Time to Peak:** Oral: Within 1 hour

**Metabolism:** Liver

**Excretion:** Feces and urine

**Formulations** Capsule, liquid-filled: 30 mg

**Dosing**

**Adults:** Oral: 60 mg every 4 hours for 21 days, start therapy within 96 hours after subarachnoid hemorrhage.

**Elderly:** Refer to adult dosing.

**Renal Impairment:** Not removed by hemo- or peritoneal dialysis; supplemental dose is not necessary.

**Hepatic Impairment:** Reduce dosage to 30 mg every 4 hours in patients with liver failure.

**Administration**

**Oral:** If the capsules cannot be swallowed, the liquid may be removed by making a hole in each end of the capsule with an 18-gauge needle and extracting the contents into a syringe. If given via NG tube, follow with a flush of 30 mL NS.

**Additional Nursing Issues**

**Physical Assessment:** Monitor neurological response and vital signs, I & O ratio, weight, edema, signs or symptoms of adverse reactions (see above) at beginning of therapy and throughout therapy. Monitor closely if patient is also taking beta blockers, nitrates, or other antihypertensive medications (see Warnings/Precautions). **Pregnancy risk factor C** - benefits of use should outweigh possible risks. Note breast-feeding caution.

**Patient Information/Instruction:** Take as prescribed, for the length of time prescribed; do not discontinue without consulting prescriber. You may experience headache (if unrelieved, consult prescriber), nausea or vomiting (frequent small meals may help), constipation (increased dietary bulk and fluids may help). Promptly report any chest pain or swelling of hands or feet, respiratory distress, sudden weight gain, or unresolved constipation. **Pregnancy/breast-feeding precautions:** Inform prescriber if you are or intend to be pregnant. Consult prescriber if breast-feeding.

**Geriatric Considerations:** Elderly may experience a greater hypotensive response. Constipation may be more of a problem in the elderly.

- **Nimotop®** *see* Nimodipine *on previous page*
- **Nipent™ Injection** *see* Pentostatin *on page 906*

## Nisoldipine (NYE sole di peen)

**U.S. Brand Names** Sular®

**Therapeutic Category** Calcium Channel Blocker

**Pregnancy Risk Factor** C

**Lactation** Excretion in breast milk unknown

**Use** Management of hypertension, alone or in combination with other antihypertensive agents

**Mechanism of Action/Effect** As a dihydropyridine calcium channel blocker, structurally similar to nifedipine, nisoldipine impedes the movement of calcium ions into vascular smooth muscle and cardiac muscle. Dihydropyridines are potent vasodilators and are not as likely to suppress cardiac contractility and slow cardiac conduction as other calcium antagonists such as verapamil and diltiazem; nisoldipine is 5-10 times as potent a vasodilator as nifedipine.

**Contraindications** Hypersensitivity to nisoldipine, any component, or other dihydropyridine calcium channel blockers

**Warnings** Increased angina and/or myocardial infarction in patients with coronary artery disease. Use with caution in patients with hypotension, congestive heart failure, and hepatic impairment. Pregnancy factor C.

**Drug Interactions**

**Cytochrome P-450 Effect:** CYP3A3/4 enzyme substrate

**Increased Effect/Toxicity:** Grapefruit juice may increase the serum concentrations of nisoldipine. Propranolol and nisoldipine may increase cardiovascular adverse effects. $H_2$-antagonists or omeprazole may cause an increase in the serum concentrations of nisoldipine. Digoxin and nisoldipine may increase digoxin effect.

**Food Interactions** Nisoldipine bioavailability may be increased if taken with high-lipid foods or with grapefruit juice.

**Adverse Reactions**

>10%:

Cardiovascular: Peripheral edema, tachycardia

Central nervous system: Headache

1% to 10%:

Cardiovascular: Vasodilation, palpitation, chest pain

Central nervous system: Dizziness

Dermatologic: Rash

Gastrointestinal: Nausea

Respiratory: Pharyngitis, sinusitis

<1% (Limited to important or life-threatening symptoms): Atrial fibrillation, CHF, first degree A-V block, hypertension, hypotension, myocardial infarction, postural hypotension, ventricular extrasystoles, supraventricular tachycardia, syncope, systolic ejection murmur, T wave abnormalities, venous insufficiency, exfoliative dermatitis, gastrointestinal hemorrhage, vaginal hemorrhage, abnormal LFTs, hepatomegaly, elevated serum creatinine, elevated BUN, anemia, leukopenia, hematuria, dyspnea

**Overdose/Toxicology** Primary cardiac symptoms of calcium blocker overdose include hypotension and bradycardia. Noncardiac symptoms include confusion, stupor, nausea, vomiting, metabolic acidosis and hyperglycemia. Treat symptomatically.

**Pharmacodynamics/Kinetics**

**Half-life Elimination:** 7-12 hours

**Metabolism:** Intestine and liver

**Excretion:** Urine

**Duration:** >24 hours

**Formulations** Tablet, extended release: 10 mg, 20 mg, 30 mg, 40 mg

**Dosing**

**Adults:** Oral: Initial: 20 mg once daily, then increase by 10 mg/week (or longer intervals) to attain adequate control of blood pressure; doses >60 mg once daily are not recommended.

**Elderly:** Oral: 10 mg/day, increase by 10 mg/week (or longer intervals) to attain adequate blood pressure control. Those with hepatic disease should be started with 10 mg/day.

**Hepatic Impairment:** A starting dose not exceeding 10 mg/day is recommended for patients with hepatic impairment.

**Administration**

**Oral:** Administer at the same time each day to ensure minimal fluctuation of serum levels. Avoid high fat diet.

**Additional Nursing Issues**

**Physical Assessment:** Monitor blood pressure, cardiac rhythm, I & O ratio, weight, edema, signs or symptoms of adverse reactions (see above) at beginning of therapy or when titrating dose, and periodically throughout long-term therapy. Monitor closely if patient is also taking beta blockers, nitrates, or other antihypertensive medications (see Warnings/Precautions). When discontinuing, taper gradually (over 2 weeks). **Pregnancy risk factor C** - benefits of use should outweigh possible risks. Note breast-feeding caution.

**Patient Information/Instruction:** Take as prescribed - swallow whole (do not crush or break). May be taken with food but avoid grapefruit products and high fat foods. Do not stop abruptly without consulting prescriber. You may experience headache (if unrelieved, consult prescriber), nausea or vomiting (frequent small meals may help), constipation (increased dietary bulk and fluids may help), depression (should resolve when drug is discontinued). May cause dizziness or drowsiness; use caution when driving or engaging in tasks that require alertness until response to drug is known. Promptly report any chest pain or swelling of hands or feet, respiratory distress, sudden weight gain, or unresolved constipation. **Pregnancy/breast-feeding precautions:** Inform prescriber if you are or intend to be pregnant. Consult prescriber if breast-feeding.

**Geriatric Considerations:** Elderly may experience a greater hypotensive response. Constipation may be more of a problem in the elderly. Calcium channel blockers are no more effective in the elderly than other therapies; however, they do not cause significant CNS effects which is an advantage over some antihypertensive agents.

**Related Information**

Calcium Channel Blocking Agents Comparison *on page 1378*


- **Nistaken** *see* Propafenone *on page 981*
- **Nistaquim** *see* Nystatin *on page 843*
- **Nitalapram** *see* Citalopram *on page 276*
- **Nitradisc** *see* Nitroglycerin *on page 831*
- **Nitrek® Patch** *see* Nitroglycerin *on page 831*
- **Nitro-Bid® I.V. Injection** *see* Nitroglycerin *on page 831*
- **Nitro-Bid® Ointment** *see* Nitroglycerin *on page 831*
- **Nitroderm TTS** *see* Nitroglycerin *on page 831*
- **Nitrodisc® Patch** *see* Nitroglycerin *on page 831*
- **Nitro-Dur® Patch** *see* Nitroglycerin *on page 831*
- **Nitrofural** *see* Nitrofurazone *on next page*


## Nitrofurantoin (nye troe fyoor AN toyn)

**U.S. Brand Names** Furadantin®; Furalan®; Furan®; Furanite®; Macrobid®; Macrodantin®

**Therapeutic Category** Antibiotic, Miscellaneous

**Pregnancy Risk Factor** B

**Lactation** Enters breast milk/compatible

**Use** Prevention and treatment of urinary tract infections caused by susceptible gram-negative and some gram-positive organisms; *Pseudomonas*, *Serratia*, and most species of *Proteus* are generally resistant to nitrofurantoin

**Mechanism of Action/Effect** Inhibits several bacterial enzyme systems including acetyl coenzyme A interfering with metabolism and possibly cell wall synthesis

**Contraindications** Hypersensitivity to nitrofurantoin or any component; renal impairment; infants <1 month (due to the possibility of hemolytic anemia)

**Warnings** Use with caution in patients with G-6-PD deficiency, patients with anemia, vitamin B deficiency, diabetes mellitus, or electrolyte abnormalities. Therapeutic concentrations of nitrofurantoin are not attained in urine of patients with $Cl_{cr}$ <40 mL/minute (elderly). Use with caution if prolonged therapy is anticipated due to possible pulmonary toxicity.

**Drug Interactions**

**Decreased Effect:** Antacids decrease absorption of nitrofurantoin.

**Increased Effect/Toxicity:** Probenecid decreases renal excretion of nitrofurantoin.

**Food Interactions** Nitrofurantoin serum concentrations may be increased if taken with food.

**Effects on Lab Values** False-positive urine glucose with Clinitest®

**Adverse Reactions**

>10%:
- Cardiovascular: Chest pains
- Central nervous system: Chills, fever
- Gastrointestinal: Stomach upset, diarrhea, anorexia, vomiting
- Respiratory: Pneumonitis, cough, dyspnea

1% to 10%:
- Central nervous system: Fatigue, drowsiness, headache, dizziness
- Gastrointestinal: Sore throat
- Hematologic: Granulocytopenia, leukopenia, megaloblastic anemia
- Neuromuscular & skeletal: Weakness, paresthesia, numbness

<1% (Limited to important or life-threatening symptoms): Hypersensitivity, hemolytic anemia, hepatitis

**Overdose/Toxicology** Symptoms of overdose include vomiting. Treatment is supportive.

**Pharmacodynamics/Kinetics**

**Protein Binding:** 40%

**Distribution:** Crosses the placenta

**Half-life Elimination:** 20-60 minutes (prolonged in renal impairment)

**Metabolism:** Tissue

**Excretion:** Bile and urine

**Formulations**

Capsule: 50 mg, 100 mg

Capsule:
- Macrocrystal: 25 mg, 50 mg, 100 mg
- Macrocrystal/monohydrate: 100 mg

Suspension, oral: 25 mg/5 mL (470 mL)

**Dosing**

**Adults:** Oral: 50-100 mg/dose every 6 hours (not to exceed 400 mg/24 hours)

Prophylaxis: 50-100 mg/dose at bedtime

(Continued)

## Nitrofurantoin *(Continued)*

**Elderly:** Refer to adult dosing (see Geriatric Considerations).

**Renal Impairment:**

$Cl_{cr}$ <50 mL/minute: Avoid use.

Avoid use in hemo and peritoneal dialysis and continuous arteriovenous or venovenous hemofiltration (CAVH/CAVHD).

**Administration**

**Oral:** Suspension: Shake well before use. Higher peak serum levels may cause increased GI upset. Give with meals to slow the rate of absorption and decrease adverse effects.

**Monitoring Laboratory Tests** CBC, periodic liver function

**Additional Nursing Issues**

**Physical Assessment:** Assess effectiveness and interactions of other medications (see Drug Interactions). See Warnings/Precautions and Contraindications for use cautions. Monitor effectiveness of therapy, laboratory tests, and adverse response (see Adverse Reactions). Diabetics cannot use Clinitest® (see above); advise on another method of glucose testing. Assess knowledge/teach patient appropriate use, possible side effects and interventions, and adverse symptoms to report.

**Patient Information/Instruction:** Take per recommended schedule, at regular intervals around-the-clock. Complete full course of therapy; do not skip doses. Maintain adequate hydration (2-3 L/day of fluids unless instructed to restrict fluid intake). Diabetics should consult prescriber if using Clinitest® for glucose testing. Nitrofurantoin may discolor urine dark yellow or brown (normal). You may experience nausea or vomiting or GI upset (small frequent meals, frequent mouth care, sucking lozenges, or chewing gum may help); fatigue, drowsiness, blurred vision (use caution when driving or engaging in tasks that require alertness until response to drug is known). Report chest pains or palpitations; pain on urination or blood in urine; skin rash; muscle weakness, pain, or tremors; excessive fatigue or weakness; other persistent adverse effects; or if condition does not improve.

**Geriatric Considerations:** Because of nitrofurantoin's decreased efficacy in patients with a $Cl_{cr}$ <40 mL/minute and its side effect profile, it is not an antibiotic of choice for acute or prophylactic treatment of urinary tract infections in the elderly.

## Nitrofurazone (nye troe FYOOR a zone)

**U.S. Brand Names** Furacin® Topical

**Synonyms** Nitrofural

**Therapeutic Category** Antibiotic, Topical

**Pregnancy Risk Factor** C

**Lactation** Excretion in breast milk unknown

**Use** Antibacterial agent in second and third degree burns and skin grafting

**Mechanism of Action/Effect** A broad antibacterial spectrum; it acts by inhibiting bacterial enzymes involved in carbohydrate metabolism; effective against a wide range of gram-negative and gram-positive organisms; bactericidal against most bacteria commonly causing surface infections including *Staphylococcus aureus, Streptococcus, Escherichia coli, Enterobacter cloacae, Clostridium perfringens, Aerobacter aerogenes,* and *Proteus* sp; not particularly active against most *Pseudomonas aeruginosa* strains and does not inhibit viruses or fungi. Topical preparations of nitrofurazone are readily soluble in blood, pus, and serum and are nonmacerating.

**Contraindications** Hypersensitivity to nitrofurazone or any component

**Warnings** Use with caution in patients with renal impairment and patients with G-6-PD deficiency. Pregnancy factor C.

**Adverse Reactions** <1% (Limited to important or life-threatening symptoms): Rash, dermatologic reactions

**Formulations**

Cream: 0.2% (4 g, 28 g)

Ointment, soluble dressing: 0.2% (28 g, 56 g, 454 g, 480 g)

Solution, topical: 0.2% (480 mL, 3780 mL)

**Dosing**

**Adults:** Topical: Apply once daily or every few days to lesion or place on gauze.

**Elderly:** Refer to adult dosing.

**Administration**

**Topical:** Notify prescriber if area under soluble dressing becomes irritated or a rash develops.

**Stability**

**Storage:** Avoid exposure to direct sunlight, excessive heat, strong fluorescent lighting, and alkaline materials.

**Additional Nursing Issues**

**Physical Assessment:** Monitor and/or teach patient to monitor and report signs of sensitization reaction (eg, swelling, redness, itching, burning); failure to heal; and overgrowth of nonsusceptible organisms including fungi. Assess/teach patient appropriate application technique for prescribed formulation if used at home. **Pregnancy risk factor C** - benefits of use should outweigh possible risks. Note breast-feeding caution.

**Patient Information/Instruction:** Follow specific prescriber instructions for application. Protect skin around treated areas with vaseline or zinc ointment. Do not apply to skin around eyes. Report signs of sensitization reaction (eg, swelling, redness, itching, burning). **Pregnancy/breast-feeding precautions:** Inform prescriber if you think you are pregnant. Consult prescriber if breast-feeding.

♦ **Nitrogard® Buccal** *see* Nitroglycerin *on this page*
♦ **Nitrogen Mustard** *see* Mechlorethamine *on page 710*

## Nitroglycerin (nye troe GLI ser in)

**U.S. Brand Names** Deponit® Patch; Minitran® Patch; Nitrek® Patch; Nitro-Bid® I.V. Injection; Nitro-Bid® Ointment; Nitrodisc® Patch; Nitro-Dur® Patch; Nitrogard® Buccal; Nitroglyn® Oral; Nitrolingual® Translingual Spray; Nitrol® Ointment; Nitrong® Oral Tablet; Nitrostat® Sublingual; Nitro-time® Capsules; Transdermal-NTG® Patch; Transderm-Nitro® Patch; Tridil® Injection

**Synonyms** Glyceryl Trinitrate; Nitroglycerol; NTG

**Therapeutic Category** Vasodilator

**Pregnancy Risk Factor** C

**Lactation** Excretion in breast milk unknown

**Use** Treatment of angina pectoris; I.V. for congestive heart failure (especially when associated with acute myocardial infarction); pulmonary hypertension; hypertensive emergencies occurring perioperatively (especially during cardiovascular surgery)

**Mechanism of Action/Effect** Reduces cardiac oxygen demand by decreasing left ventricular pressure and systemic vascular resistance; dilates coronary arteries and improves collateral flow to ischemic regions; esophageal smooth muscle is relaxed by same mechanism

**Contraindications** Hypersensitivity to nitroglycerin or any component; closed-angle glaucoma; severe anemia, early myocardial infarction, head trauma, cerebral hemorrhage, allergy to adhesive (transdermal), uncorrected hypovolemia (I.V.), inadequate cerebral circulation, increased intracranial pressure, constrictive pericarditis and pericardial tamponade; transdermal NTG is not effective for immediate relief of angina

**Warnings** Do not use extended release preparations in patients with GI hypermotility or malabsorptive syndrome. Use with caution in patients with hepatic impairment. Available preparations of I.V. nitroglycerin differ in concentration or volume. Pay attention to dilution and dosage. I.V. preparations contain alcohol and/or propylene glycol. Pregnancy factor C.

**Drug Interactions**

**Decreased Effect:** I.V. nitroglycerin may antagonize the anticoagulant effect of heparin, monitor closely. May need to decrease heparin dosage when nitroglycerin is discontinued.

**Increased Effect/Toxicity:** Alcohol, aspirin, and calcium channel blockers may enhance nitroglycerin's hypotensive effect. Has been associated with severe reactions and death when sildenafil is given concurrently with nitrites.

**Adverse Reactions**

>10%:
- Cardiovascular: Flushing of face and neck, orthostatic hypotension, tachycardia
- Central nervous system: Headache, restlessness
- Gastrointestinal: Nausea or vomiting

1% to 10%: Dermatologic: Sore, reddened skin (topical dosage forms)

**Overdose/Toxicology** Symptoms of overdose include hypotension, throbbing headache, palpitations, bloody diarrhea, bradycardia, cyanosis, tissue hypoxia, metabolic acidosis, clonic convulsions, circulatory collapse, and methemoglobinemia with extremely large overdoses. Treatment is supportive and symptomatic.

**Pharmacodynamics/Kinetics**

**Protein Binding:** 60%

**Half-life Elimination:** 1-4 minutes

**Metabolism:** Liver

**Excretion:** Urine

**Onset:**
- Sublingual tablet: 1-3 minutes
- Translingual spray: 2 minutes
- Buccal tablet: 2-5 minutes
- Sustained release: 20-45 minutes
- Topical: 15-60 minutes
- Transdermal: 40-60 minutes
- I.V. drip: Immediate

**Duration:**
- Sublingual tablet: 30-60 minutes
- Translingual spray: 30-60 minutes
- Buccal tablet: 2 hours
- Sustained release: 4-8 hours
- Topical: 2-12 hours
- Transdermal: 18-24 hours
- I.V. drip: 3-5 minutes

**Formulations**

Capsule, sustained release: 2.5 mg, 6.5 mg, 9 mg

Injection: 0.5 mg/mL (10 mL); 0.8 mg/mL (10 mL); 5 mg/mL (1 mL, 5 mL, 10 mL, 20 mL); 10 mg/mL (5 mL, 10 mL)

Ointment, topical (Nitrol®): 2% [20 mg/g] (30 g, 60 g)

Patch, transdermal, topical: Systems designed to deliver 2.5, 5, 7.5, 10, or 15 mg NTG over 24 hours

Spray, translingual: 0.4 mg/metered spray (13.8 g)

Tablet:
- Buccal, controlled release: 1 mg, 2 mg, 3 mg
- Sublingual (Nitrostat®): 0.3 mg, 0.4 mg, 0.6 mg

(Continued)

## Nitroglycerin *(Continued)*

Sustained release: 2.6 mg, 6.5 mg, 9 mg

**Dosing**

**Adults: Note:** Hemodynamic and antianginal tolerance often develop within 24-48 hours of continuous nitrate administration.

Buccal: Initial: 1 mg every 3-5 hours while awake (3 times/day); titrate dosage upward if angina occurs with tablet in place.

Oral: 2.5-9 mg 2-4 times/day (up to 26 mg 4 times/day)

I.V.: 5 mcg/minute, increase by 5 mcg/minute every 3-5 minutes to 20 mcg/minute. If no response at 20 mcg/minute increase by 10 mcg/minute every 3-5 minutes, up to 200 mcg/minute.

Ointment: Include a nitrate free interval, ~10 to 12 hours; Apply 0.5" to 2" every 6 hours with a nitrate free interval.

Patch, transdermal: 0.2-0.4 mg/hour initially and titrate to doses of 0.4-0.8 mg/hour. Tolerance is minimized by using a patch-on period of 12-14 hours and patch-off period of 10-12 hours.

Sublingual: 0.2-0.6 mg every 5 minutes for maximum of 3 doses in 15 minutes; may also use prophylactically 5-10 minutes prior to activities which may provoke an attack.

Translingual: 1-2 sprays into mouth under tongue every 3-5 minutes for maximum of 3 doses in 15 minutes, may also be used 5-10 minutes prior to activities which may provoke an attack prophylactically.

May need to use nitrate-free interval (10-12 hours/day) to avoid tolerance development. Tolerance may possibly be reversed with acetylcysteine. Gradually decrease dose in patients receiving NTG for prolonged period to avoid withdrawal reaction.

**Elderly:** Refer to adult dosing.

**Administration**

**Oral:** Do not crush sublingual drug product.

**I.V.:** I.V. must be prepared in glass bottles and use special sets intended for nitroglycerin. glass I.V. bottles and administration sets provided by manufacturer.

**I.V. Detail:** Nitroglycerin can be absorbed by plastic (polyvinyl chloride) tubing or containers. Infusion pump may not infuse accurately with different tubing. Be alert to potential for unregulated flow.

**Topical:** Transdermal patches are labeled as mg/hour.

**Stability**

**Storage:** Doses should be made in glass bottles, Excel® or PAB® containers. Adsorption occurs to soft plastic (eg, PVC). Premixed bottles are stable according to the manufacturer's expiration dating. Store sublingual tablets and ointment in tightly closed containers at 15°C to 30°C.

**Reconstitution:** Doses should be made in glass bottles, Excel® or PAB® containers; adsorption occurs to soft plastic (eg, PVC). Nitroglycerin diluted in $D_5W$ or NS in glass containers is physically and chemically stable for 48 hours at room temperature and 7 days under refrigeration. In $D_5W$ or NS in Excel®/PAB® containers is physically and chemically stable for 24 hours at room temperature and 14 days under refrigeration.

Standard diluent: 50 mg/250 mL $D_5W$; 50 mg/500 mL $D_5W$

Minimum volume: 100 mg/250 mL $D_5W$; concentration should not exceed 400 mcg/mL.

**Compatibility:** Dose is variable and may require titration, therefore it is not advisable to mix with other agents. See the Compatibility of Drugs Chart *on page 1315*.

**Additional Nursing Issues**

**Physical Assessment:** Monitor blood pressure and heart rate on a regular basis (eg, hypotension, arrhythmias). Monitor for orthostatic hypotension. If therapy is being discontinued, reduce dosage gradually. **Pregnancy risk factor C** - benefits of use should outweigh possible risks. Note breast-feeding caution.

**Patient Information/Instruction:**

Oral: Take as directed. Do not chew or swallow sublingual tablets; allow to dissolve under tongue. Do not chew or crush extended release capsules; swallow with 8 oz of water.

Spray. Spray directly on mucous members; do not inhale.

Topical: Spread prescribed amount thinly on applicator; rotate application sites.

Transdermal: Place on hair-free area of skin, rotate sites.

Do not change brands without consulting prescriber. Do not discontinue abruptly. Keep medication in original container, tightly closed. Take medication while sitting down and use caution when changing position (rise from sitting or lying position slowly). May cause dizziness; use caution when driving or engaging in hazardous activities until response to drug is known. If chest pain is unresolved in 15 minutes, seek emergency medical help at once. Report acute headache, rapid heartbeat, unusual restlessness or dizziness, muscular weakness, or blurring vision. **Pregnancy/breast-feeding precautions:** Inform prescriber if you are or intend to be pregnant. Consult prescriber if breast-feeding.

**Geriatric Considerations:** Caution should be used when using nitrate therapy in the elderly due to hypotension. Hypotension is enhanced in the elderly due to decreased baroreceptor response, decreased venous tone, and often hypovolemia (dehydration) or other hypotensive drugs.

**Additional Information**

Some formulations may contain ethanol.

pH: 3.0-6.5

- **Nitroglycerol** *see* Nitroglycerin *on page 831*
- **Nitroglyn® Oral** *see* Nitroglycerin *on page 831*
- **Nitrolingual® Translingual Spray** *see* Nitroglycerin *on page 831*
- **Nitrol® Ointment** *see* Nitroglycerin *on page 831*
- **Nitrong® Oral Tablet** *see* Nitroglycerin *on page 831*
- **Nitropress®** *see* Nitroprusside *on this page*

## Nitroprusside (nye troe PRUS ide)

**U.S. Brand Names** Nitropress®

**Synonyms** Sodium Nitroferricyanide; Sodium Nitroprusside

**Therapeutic Category** Vasodilator

**Pregnancy Risk Factor** C

**Lactation** Excretion in breast milk unknown

**Use** Management of hypertensive crises; congestive heart failure; used for controlled hypotension to reduce bleeding during surgery

**Mechanism of Action/Effect** Causes peripheral vasodilation by direct action on venous and arteriolar smooth muscle, thus reducing peripheral resistance; will increase cardiac output by decreasing afterload; reduces aortal and left ventricular impedance

**Contraindications** Hypersensitivity to nitroprusside or any component; decreased cerebral perfusion; arteriovenous shunt or coarctation of the aorta (eg, compensatory hypertension)

**Warnings** Use with caution in patients with increased intracranial pressure (head trauma, cerebral hemorrhage), severe renal impairment, hepatic failure, hypothyroidism. Use only as an infusion with 5% dextrose in water. Continuously monitor patient's blood pressure. Excessive amounts of nitroprusside can cause cyanide toxicity (usually in patients with decreased liver function) or thiocyanate toxicity (usually in patients with decreased renal function, or in patients with normal renal function but prolonged nitroprusside use). Pregnancy factor C.

**Adverse Reactions** 1% to 10%:

Cardiovascular: Excessive hypotensive response, palpitations, substernal distress
Central nervous system: Disorientation, psychosis, headache, restlessness
Endocrine & metabolic: Thyroid suppression
Gastrointestinal: Nausea, vomiting
Neuromuscular & skeletal: Weakness, muscle spasm
Otic: Tinnitus
Respiratory: Hypoxia
Miscellaneous: Sweating, thiocyanate toxicity

**Overdose/Toxicology** Symptoms of overdose include hypotension, vomiting, hyperventilation, tachycardia, muscular twitching, hypothyroidism, cyanide or thiocyanate toxicity. Thiocyanate toxicity includes psychosis, hyper-reflexia, confusion, weakness, tinnitus, seizures, and coma; cyanide toxicity includes acidosis (decreased $HCO_3$, decreased pH, increased lactate), increase in mixed venous blood oxygen tension, tachycardia, altered consciousness, coma, convulsions, and almond smell on breath.

Nitroprusside has been shown to release cyanide *in vivo* with hemoglobin. Cyanide toxicity does not usually occur because of the rapid uptake of cyanide by erythrocytes and its eventual incorporation into thiocyanate in the liver. However, high doses, prolonged administration of nitroprusside, or reduced elimination can lead to cyanide poisoning or thiocyanate intoxication. Anemia and liver impairment pose a risk for cyanide accumulation, while renal impairment predisposes thiocyanate accumulation. If toxicity develops, airway support with oxygen therapy is germane, followed closely with antidotal therapy of amyl nitrate perles, sodium nitrate 300 mg I.V. for adults and sodium thiosulfate 12.5 g I.V.; nitrates should not be administered to neonates and small children. Thiocyanate is dialyzable. May be mixed with sodium thiosulfate in I.V. to prevent cyanide toxicity.

**Pharmacodynamics/Kinetics**

**Half-life Elimination:** Parent drug: <10 minutes; Thiocyanate: 2.7-7 days

**Metabolism:** Nitroprusside is converted to cyanide ions in the bloodstream; decomposes to prussic acid which in the presence of sulfur donor is converted to thiocyanate (liver and kidney rhodanase systems)

**Excretion:** Urine

**Onset:** Onset of hypotensive effect: <2 minutes

**Duration:** Within 1-10 minutes following discontinuation of therapy, effects cease

**Formulations** Injection, as sodium: 10 mg/mL (5 mL); 25 mg/mL (2 mL)

**Dosing**

**Adults:** Administration requires the use of an infusion pump. Average dose: 5 mcg/kg/minute.

I.V.: Initial: 0.3-0.5 mcg/kg/minute; increase in increments of 0.5 mcg/kg/minute, titrating to the desired hemodynamic effect or the appearance of headache or nausea; usual dose: 3 mcg/kg/minute; rarely need >4 mcg/kg/minute; maximum: 10 mcg/kg/minute. When >500 mcg/kg is administered by prolonged infusion of faster than 2 mcg/kg/minute, cyanide is generated faster than an unaided patient can handle.

**Elderly:** Refer to adult dosing.

**Administration**

**I.V.:** I.V. infusion only, use only as an infusion with 5% dextrose in water. Infusion pump required. Not for direct injection.

(Continued)

## Nitroprusside *(Continued)*

**I.V. Detail:** Continuously monitor patient's blood pressure.

**Stability**

**Reconstitution:** Brownish solution is usable, discard if bluish in color. Nitroprusside sodium should be reconstituted freshly by diluting 50 mg in 250-1000 mL of $D_5W$. Use only clear solutions; solutions of nitroprusside exhibit a color described as brownish, brown, brownish-pink, light orange, and straw. Solutions are highly sensitive to light. Exposure to light causes decomposition, resulting in a highly colored solution of orange, dark brown or blue. **A blue color indicates almost complete degradation and breakdown to cyanide. Solutions should be wrapped with aluminum foil or other opaque material to protect from light (do as soon as possible).** Stability of parenteral admixture at room temperature (25°C) and at refrigeration temperature (4°C) is 24 hours.

**Additional Nursing Issues**

**Physical Assessment:** Monitor blood pressure and heart rate continuously while infusing. Monitor infusion site for extravasation. Monitor acid/base balance; metabolic acidosis is early sign of cyanide toxicity (see Overdose/Toxicology). Monitor fluid balance (I & O). **Pregnancy risk factor C.** Note breast-feeding caution.

**Patient Information/Instruction:** Patient condition should indicate extent of education and instruction needed. This drug can only be given I.V. You will be monitored at all times during infusion. Promptly report any chest pain or pain/burning at site of infusion. **Breast-feeding precautions:** Consult prescriber if breast-feeding.

**Geriatric Considerations:** Elderly patients may have an increased sensitivity to nitroprusside possibly due to a decreased baroreceptor reflex, altered sensitivity to vasodilating effects or a resistance of cardiac adrenergic receptors to stimulation by catecholamines.

**Additional Information** pH: 3.5-6.0


- ♦ **Nitrostat® Sublingual** *see* Nitroglycerin *on page 831*
- ♦ **Nitro-time® Capsules** *see* Nitroglycerin *on page 831*
- ♦ **Nivoflox** *see* Ciprofloxacin *on page 270*
- ♦ **Nix™ Creme Rinse** *see* Permethrin *on page 911*
- ♦ **Niyaplat** *see* Cisplatin *on page 273*


## Nizatidine (ni ZA ti deen)

**U.S. Brand Names** Axid® AR [OTC]; Axid®

**Therapeutic Category** Histamine $H_2$ Antagonist

**Pregnancy Risk Factor** C

**Lactation** Enters breast milk/may be compatible

**Use** Treatment and maintenance of duodenal ulcer; treatment of gastroesophageal reflux disease (GERD); OTC tablet used for prevention of meal-induced heartburn, acid indigestion, and sour stomach

**Mechanism of Action/Effect** Nizatidine is an $H_2$-receptor antagonist.

**Contraindications** Hypersensitivity to nizatidine or any component; hypersensitivity to other $H_2$ antagonists

**Warnings** Use with caution in children <12 years of age. Use with caution in patients with liver and renal impairment. Dosage modification required in patients with renal impairment.

**Effects on Lab Values** False-positive urine protein using Multistix®, gastric acid secretion test, skin tests allergen extracts, serum creatinine and serum transaminase concentrations, urine protein test

**Adverse Reactions**

>10%: Central nervous system: Headache (16%)

1% to 10%:

Central nervous system: Dizziness, insomnia, somnolence, nervousness, anxiety

Dermatologic: Rash, pruritus

Gastrointestinal: Abdominal pain, constipation, diarrhea, nausea, flatulence, vomiting, heartburn, dry mouth, anorexia

<1% (Limited to important or life-threatening symptoms): Ventricular tachycardia, anemia, eosinophilia, thrombocytopenic purpura, elevated AST or ALT, elevated alkaline phosphatase, hepatitis, jaundice, bronchospasm, laryngeal edema

**Overdose/Toxicology** Symptoms of overdose include muscular tremor, vomiting, and rapid respiration. $LD_{50}$ ~80 mg/kg. Treatment is symptomatic and supportive.

**Pharmacodynamics/Kinetics**

**Protein Binding:** ~35%

**Half-life Elimination:** Normal renal function: 1-2 hours; End-stage renal disease: 3.5-11 hours

**Time to Peak:** 0.5-3 hours

**Excretion:** Urine

**Formulations**

Capsule: 150 mg, 300 mg

Tablet: 75 mg

**Dosing**

**Adults:** Oral:

Active duodenal ulcer:

Treatment: 300 mg at bedtime or 150 mg twice daily

Maintenance: 150 mg/day

Meal-induced heartburn, acid indigestion, and sour stomach: 75 mg tablet [OTC] twice daily, 30-60 minutes prior to consuming food or beverages

**Elderly:** Refer to adult dosing.

**Renal Impairment:**

$Cl_{cr}$ 50-80 mL/minute: Administer 75% of normal dose.

$Cl_{cr}$ 10-50 mL/minute: Administer 50% of normal dose or 150 mg/day for active treatment and 150 mg every other day for maintenance treatment.

$Cl_{cr}$ <10 mL/minute: Administer 25% of normal dose or 150 mg every other day for treatment and 150 mg every 3 days for maintenance treatment.

**Administration**

**Oral:** Giving dose at 6 PM may better suppress nocturnal acid secretion than taking dose at 10 PM.

**Additional Nursing Issues**

**Physical Assessment:** Evaluate effectiveness of treatment. Instruct patient on possible side effects (see Adverse Reactions) and symptoms to report. **Pregnancy risk factor C** - benefits of use should outweigh possible risks.

**Patient Information/Instruction:** Take as directed; do not increase dose. It may take several days before you notice relief. If antacids approved by prescriber, take 1 hour between antacid and nizatidine. Avoid OTC medications, especially cold or cough medication and aspirin or anything containing aspirin. Follow ulcer diet as prescriber recommends. May cause drowsiness; use caution when driving or engaging in tasks that require alertness until response to drug is known. Report fever, sore throat, tarry stools, changes in CNS, or muscle or joint pain. **Pregnancy precautions:** Inform prescriber if you are or intend to be pregnant.

**Geriatric Considerations:** $H_2$ blockers are the preferred drugs for treating peptic ulcer disorder (PUD) in the elderly due to cost and ease of administration. These agents are no less or more effective than any other therapy. The preferred agents (due to side effects and drug interaction profile and pharmacokinetics) are ranitidine, famotidine, and nizatidine. Treatment for PUD in the elderly is recommended for 12 weeks since their lesions are larger, and therefore, take longer to heal. Always adjust dose based upon creatinine clearance.


- ♦ **Nizoral®** *see* Ketoconazole *on page 643*
- ♦ **N-Methylhydrazine** *see* Procarbazine *on page 970*
- ♦ **Nobesine®** *see* Diethylpropion *on page 365*
- ♦ **Nolahist®** *see page 1294*
- ♦ **Nolamine® Tablet** *see page 1306*
- ♦ **Nolex® LA** *see* Guaifenesin and Phenylpropanolamine *on page 550*
- ♦ **Nolvadex®** *see* Tamoxifen *on page 1095*
- ♦ **Nonoxynol 9** *see page 1294*
- ♦ **Nonsalicylate/Nonsteroidal Anti-inflammatory Comparison** *see page 1401*
- ♦ **No Pain-HP®** *see page 1294*
- ♦ **Noradrenaline Acid Tartrate** *see* Norepinephrine *on this page*
- ♦ **Norboral** *see* Glyburide *on page 538*
- ♦ **Norcet®** *see* Hydrocodone and Acetaminophen *on page 568*
- ♦ **Norciden** *see* Danazol *on page 332*
- ♦ **Nordeoxyguanosine** *see* Ganciclovir *on page 526*
- ♦ **Nordet** *see* Oral Contraceptives *on page 859*
- ♦ **Nordette®** *see* Oral Contraceptives *on page 859*
- ♦ **Nordiol** *see* Oral Contraceptives *on page 859*
- ♦ **Nordryl® Injection** *see* Diphenhydramine *on page 381*
- ♦ **Nordryl® Oral** *see* Diphenhydramine *on page 381*


## Norepinephrine (nor ep i NEF rin)

**U.S. Brand Names** Levophed® Injection

**Synonyms** Levarterenol Bitartrate; Noradrenaline Acid Tartrate

**Therapeutic Category** Alpha/Beta Agonist

**Pregnancy Risk Factor** D

**Lactation** Excretion in breast milk unknown

**Use** Treatment of shock which persists after adequate fluid volume replacement

**Mechanism of Action/Effect** Stimulates $beta_1$-adrenergic receptors and alpha-adrenergic receptors causing increased contractility and heart rate as well as vasoconstriction, thereby increasing systemic blood pressure and coronary blood flow; clinically alpha effects (vasoconstriction) are greater than beta effects (inotropic and chronotropic effects)

**Contraindications** Hypersensitivity to norepinephrine or sulfites; pregnancy

**Warnings** Blood/volume depletion should be corrected, if possible, before norepinephrine therapy. Extravasation may cause severe tissue necrosis, give into a large vein. The drug should not be given to patients with peripheral or mesenteric vascular thrombosis because ischemia may be increased and the area of infarct extended. Use with caution during cyclopropane and halothane anesthesia. Use with caution in patients with occlusive vascular disease. Some products may contain sulfites.

**Drug Interactions**

**Increased Effect/Toxicity:** Increased effect with tricyclic antidepressants, MAO inhibitors, antihistamines (diphenhydramine, tripelennamine), guanethidine, ergot alkaloids, and methyldopa. Atropine sulfate may block the reflex bradycardia caused by norepinephrine and enhances the vasopressor response.

**Adverse Reactions**

>10%:

Central nervous system: Headache

(Continued)

## Norepinephrine *(Continued)*

Gastrointestinal: Nausea, vomiting

1% to 10%:

Cardiovascular: Premature ventricular beats, bradycardia, hypertension, hypotension, chest pain, palpitations, tachycardia, ventricular arrhythmias

Central nervous system: Nervousness or restlessness

Respiratory: Dyspnea

**Overdose/Toxicology** Symptoms of overdose include hypertension, sweating, cerebral hemorrhage, and convulsions. Infiltrate the area of extravasation with phentolamine 5-10 mg in 10-15 mL of saline solution.

**Pharmacodynamics/Kinetics**

**Metabolism:** By catechol-o-methyltransferase (COMT) and monoamine oxidase (MAO)

**Excretion:** Urine

**Onset:** I.V.: Very rapid-acting

**Duration:** Limited

**Formulations** Injection, as bitartrate: 1 mg/mL (4 mL)

**Dosing**

**Adults: Note:** Norepinephrine dosage is stated in terms of norepinephrine base and intravenous formulation is norepinephrine bitartrate.

**Norepinephrine bitartrate 2 mg = norepinephrine base 1 mg**

Continuous I.V. infusion:

Initiate at 4 mcg/minute and titrate to desired response; 8-12 mcg/minute is usual range

ACLS dosing range: 0.5-30 mcg/minute

**Rate of infusion: 4 mg in 500 mL $D_5W$**

2 mcg/minute = 15 mL/hour
4 mcg/minute = 30 mL/hour
6 mcg/minute = 45 mL/hour
8 mcg/minute = 60 mL/hour
10 mcg/minute = 75 mL/hour

**Elderly:** Refer to adult dosing.

**Administration**

**I.V.:** Administer into large vein to avoid the potential for extravasation; potent drug, must be diluted prior to use. Rate (mL/hour) = dose (mcg/kg/minute) x weight (kg) x 60 minutes/hour divided by concentration (mcg/mL). Central line administration is required. Do not administer $NaHCO_3$ through an I.V. line containing norepinephrine.

**I.V. Detail:** Administer into large vein to avoid the potential for extravasation. Potent drug, must be diluted prior to use.

**Extravasation management:** Use phentolamine as antidote. Mix 5 mg with 9 mL of NS. Inject a small amount of this dilution into extravasated area. Blanching should reverse immediately. Monitor site; if blanching should recur, additional injections of phentolamine may be needed.

**Stability**

**Storage:** Readily oxidized; protect from light. Do not use if brown coloration.

**Reconstitution:** Dilute with $D_5W$ or DS/NS, but not recommended to dilute in normal saline. Stability of parenteral admixture at room temperature (25°C) is 24 hours.

**Compatibility: Not** stable with alkaline solutions. Incompatible with many medications. Consult pharmacist for specific information. See the Compatibility of Drugs Chart *on page 1315.*

**Additional Nursing Issues**

**Physical Assessment:** Assess other medications patient may be taking (see Drug Interactions). Monitor blood pressure and cardiac status, CNS status, skin temperature and color during and following infusion. Monitor fluid status (I & O). Assess infusion site frequently for extravasation. Blanching along vein pathway is a preliminary sign of extravasation. **Pregnancy risk factor D.** Note breast-feeding caution.

**Patient Information/Instruction:** This drug is used in emergency situations. Patient information is based on patient condition.

**Additional Information**

The injection formulation contains sulfites.

pH: 3-4.5

**Related Information**

Inotropic and Vasoconstrictor Comparison *on page 1391*

- **Norethin™ 1/35E** *see* Oral Contraceptives *on page 859*
- **Norethin™ 1/50M** *see* Oral Contraceptives *on page 859*

## Norethindrone (nor eth IN drone)

**U.S. Brand Names** Aygestin®; Micronor®; Nor-QD®

**Synonyms** Norethisterone

**Therapeutic Category** Contraceptive; Progestin

**Pregnancy Risk Factor** X

**Lactation** Enters breast milk/use caution

**Use** Treatment of amenorrhea; abnormal uterine bleeding; endometriosis

**Mechanism of Action/Effect** Inhibits secretion of pituitary gonadotropin (LH) which prevents follicular maturation and ovulation; in the presence of adequate endogenous estrogen, transforms a proliferative endometrium to a secretory one

**Contraindications** Hypersensitivity to norethindrone; thromboembolic disorders; severe hepatic disease; breast cancer; undiagnosed vaginal bleeding; pregnancy

**Warnings** Use of any progestin during the first 4 months of pregnancy is not recommended. Discontinue if sudden partial or complete loss of vision, proptosis, diplopia, or migraine occur. **There is a higher rate of failure with progestin only contraceptives.** Progestin-induced withdrawal bleeding occurs within 3-7 days after discontinuation of drug. Use with caution in patients with asthma, diabetes, seizure disorder, migraine, cardiac or renal dysfunction, or psychic depression.

**Drug Interactions**

**Decreased Effect:** Rifampin decreases pharmacologic effect of norethindrone.

**Effects on Lab Values** Thyroid function test, metyrapone test, liver function tests, coagulation tests (prothrombin time, factors VII, VIII, IX, X)

**Adverse Reactions** 1% to 10%:

Cardiovascular: Edema, thromboembolic disorders, hypertension
Central nervous system: Mental depression, nervousness, dizziness, fatigue, headache
Dermatologic: Hirsutism, rash, melasma or chloasma, photosensitivity
Endocrine & metabolic: Breakthrough bleeding, spotting, changes in menstrual flow
Gastrointestinal: Weight gain or loss
Hepatic: Cholestatic jaundice

**Pharmacodynamics/Kinetics**

**Protein Binding:** 80%

**Half-life Elimination:** 10 hours

**Metabolism:** Liver

**Excretion:** Urine and feces

**Formulations**

Tablet: 0.35 mg, 5 mg
Tablet, as acetate: 5 mg

**Dosing**

**Adults:** Oral:

Amenorrhea and abnormal uterine bleeding: Norethindrone 5-20 mg or norethindrone acetate 2.5-10 mg on days 5-25 of menstrual cycle **or** to induce optimum secretory transformation of the endometrium; administer norethindrone acetate 2.5-10 mg/day for 5-10 days beginning during the latter half of the menstrual cycle.

Endometriosis: Norethindrone 10 mg/day for 14 days; increase at increments of 5 mg/day every 2 weeks up to 30 mg/day **or** using norethindrone acetate 5 mg/day for 14 days; increase at increments of 2.5 mg/day every 2 weeks up to 15 mg/day.

Contraception: Progesterone only: Norethindrone 0.35 mg every day of the year starting on first day of menstruation. If one dose is missed take as soon as remembered, then next tablet at regular time. If two doses are missed, take one of the missed doses, discard the other, and take daily dose at usual time. If three doses are missed, use another form of birth control until menses appear or pregnancy is ruled out.

**Administration**

**Oral:** Take with food.

**Monitoring Laboratory Tests** Long-term therapy, annual Pap tests, mammogram

**Additional Nursing Issues**

**Physical Assessment:** Assess patient knowledge/teach appropriate administration schedule, adverse signs to report. Teach appropriate breast self-exam and the need for regular breast self-exam and necessity of annual physical check-up with long-term use. **Pregnancy risk factor X** - determine that patient is not pregnant before beginning treatment. Note breast-feeding caution. See Breast-feeding Issues.

**Patient Information/Instruction:** Take according to prescribed schedule. Follow instructions for regular self-breast exam. You may experience dizziness or lightheadedness; use caution when driving or engaging in tasks that require alertness until response to drug is known. Limit intake of caffeine. Avoid high-dose vitamin C, folate, or pyridoxine. You may experience photosensitivity; use sunscreen, wear protective clothing and eyewear, and avoid direct sunlight. You may experience loss of hair (reversible), weight gain or loss. Report sudden severe headache or vomiting, disturbances of vision or speech, sudden blindness, numbness of weakness in an extremity, chest pain, calf pain, respiratory difficulty, depression or acute fatigue, unusual bleeding, spotting, or changes in menstrual flow. **Pregnancy/breast-feeding precautions:** Inform prescriber if pregnant. Consult prescriber if breast-feeding.

**Breast-feeding Issues:** Norethindrone can cause changes in milk production in the mother. Monitor infant growth. Use lowest possible dose of norethindrone for less effect on milk production.


- **Norethindrone Acetate and Ethinyl Estradiol** *see* Oral Contraceptives *on page 859*
- **Norethisterone** *see* Norethindrone *on previous page*
- **Norfenon®** *see* Propafenone *on page 981*
- **Norflex™** *see* Orphenadrine *on page 864*


## Norfloxacin (nor FLOKS a sin)

**U.S. Brand Names** Chibroxin™ Ophthalmic; Noroxin® Oral

**Therapeutic Category** Antibiotic, Quinolone

**Pregnancy Risk Factor** C

**Lactation** Enters breast milk/contraindicated

**Use** Uncomplicated urinary tract infections and cystitis caused by susceptible gram-negative and gram-positive bacteria; sexually transmitted disease (eg, uncomplicated urethral and cervical gonorrhea) caused by *N. gonorrhoeae*; prostatitis due to *E. coli*; ophthalmic solution for conjunctivitis

**Mechanism of Action/Effect** Norfloxacin is a DNA gyrase inhibitor. DNA gyrase is an essential bacterial enzyme that maintains the superhelical structure of DNA. DNA gyrase (Continued)

## Norfloxacin *(Continued)*

is required for DNA replication and transcription, DNA repair, recombination, and transposition; bactericidal

**Contraindications** Hypersensitivity to quinolones

**Warnings** Not recommended in children <18 years of age. Other quinolones have caused transient arthropathy in children. CNS stimulation may occur which may lead to tremor, restlessness, confusion, and very rarely to hallucinations or convulsive seizures. Use with caution in patients with known or suspected CNS disorders. Pregnancy factor C.

**Drug Interactions**

**Cytochrome P-450 Effect:** CYP1A2 and 3A3/4 enzyme inhibitor

**Decreased Effect:** Decreased absorption with antacids containing aluminum, magnesium, and/or calcium (by up to 98% if given at the same time).

**Increased Effect/Toxicity:** Quinolones cause increased levels of caffeine, warfarin, cyclosporine, and theophylline. Cimetidine, and probenecid may increase norfloxacin serum levels.

**Food Interactions** Norfloxacin average peak serum concentrations may be decreased if taken with dairy products.

**Adverse Reactions**

**Ophthalmic:**

>10%: Ocular: Burning or other discomfort of the eye, crusting or crystals in corner of eye

1% to 10%:

Gastrointestinal: Bad taste instillation

Ocular: Foreign body sensation, conjunctival hyperemia, itching of eye

**Systemic:**

>10%:

Central nervous system: Dizziness or lightheadedness, headache, nervousness, drowsiness, insomnia

Gastrointestinal: Nausea, diarrhea, vomiting, abdominal pain

1% to 10%: Dermatologic: Photosensitivity

<1% (Limited to important or life-threatening symptoms): Stevens-Johnson syndrome, anemia, increased liver enzymes, interstitial nephritis, shortness of breath

**Overdose/Toxicology** Symptoms of overdose include acute renal failure and seizures. Following GI decontamination, use supportive measures.

**Pharmacodynamics/Kinetics**

**Protein Binding:** 15%

**Distribution:** Crosses the placenta

**Half-life Elimination:** 4.8 hours (can be higher with reduced glomerular filtration rates)

**Time to Peak:** Within 1-2 hours

**Metabolism:** Liver

**Excretion:** Urine and feces

**Formulations**

Solution, ophthalmic: 0.3% [3 mg/mL] (5 mL)

Tablet: 400 mg

**Dosing**

**Adults:**

Ophthalmic: Instill 1-2 drops in affected eye(s) 4 times/day for up to 7 days

Oral:

Urinary tract infections: 400 mg twice daily for 3-21 days depending on severity of infection or organism sensitivity; maximum: 800 mg/day

Uncomplicated gonorrhea: 800 mg as a single dose (CDC recommends as an alternative regimen to ciprofloxacin or ofloxacin)

Prostatitis: 400 mg every 12 hours for 4 weeks

**Elderly:** Refer to adult dosing.

**Renal Impairment:** $Cl_{cr}$ ≤30 mL/minute: Administer 400 mg every 24 hours.

**Administration**

**Oral:** Hold antacids or sucralfate for 3-4 hours after giving norfloxacin; do not administer together. Best taken on an empty stomach with water.

**Monitoring Laboratory Tests** Perform culture and sensitivity prior to beginning therapy. Monitor CBC, renal and hepatic function periodically if therapy is prolonged.

**Additional Nursing Issues**

**Physical Assessment:** Monitor effectiveness of other medications patient may be taking (see Drug Interactions). Monitor response to therapy. Monitor for adverse reactions or teach patient adverse reactions and symptoms to report. If no improvement or relapse, therapy should be re-evaluated. **Pregnancy risk factor C** - benefits of use should outweigh possible risks. Breast-feeding is contraindicated.

**Patient Information/Instruction:**

Oral: Take per recommended schedule, preferably on empty stomach (1 hour before or 2 hours after meals). Maintain adequate hydration (2-3 L/day of fluids unless instructed to restrict fluid intake). Take complete prescription; do not skip doses. Do not take with antacids. You may experience dizziness, lightheadedness; use caution when driving or engaging in tasks that require alertness until response to drug is known. Small frequent meals and frequent mouth care may reduce nausea or vomiting. You may experience photosensitivity; use sunscreen, wear protective clothing and eyewear, and avoid direct sunlight. Report persistent diarrhea or GI disturbances; excessive sleepiness or agitation; tremors; rash; pain, inflammation, or rupture of tendon; or changes in vision. **Pregnancy/breast-feeding precautions:** Inform prescriber if you are or intend to be pregnant. Do not breast-feed.

Ophthalmic: Tilt head back and instill 1-2 drops in affected eye 4 times a day for length of time prescribed. Do not allow tip of applicator to touch eye or any contaminated surface.

**Geriatric Considerations:**

Ophthalmic: Assess ability to self-administer eye drops.

Oral: Adjust dose for renal function.

- **Norgesic®** *see* Orphenadrine, Aspirin, and Caffeine *on page 865*
- **Norgesic® Forte** *see* Orphenadrine, Aspirin, and Caffeine *on page 865*
- **Norgestimate and Ethinyl Estradiol** *see* Oral Contraceptives *on page 859*
- **Norgestrel** *see* Oral Contraceptives *on page 859*
- **Norgestrel and Ethinyl Estradiol** *see* Oral Contraceptives *on page 859*
- **Norinyl® 1+35** *see* Oral Contraceptives *on page 859*
- **Norinyl® 1+50** *see* Oral Contraceptives *on page 859*
- **Norisodrine®** *see* Isoproterenol *on page 632*
- **Normiflo®** *see* Ardeparin *on page 105*
- **Normodyne®** *see* Labetalol *on page 649*
- **Noroxin® Oral** *see* Norfloxacin *on page 837*
- **Norpace®** *see* Disopyramide *on page 386*
- **Norplant® Implant** *see* Levonorgestrel *on page 670*
- **Norpramin®** *see* Desipramine *on page 343*
- **Nor-QD®** *see* Norethindrone *on page 836*
- **Nor-tet® Oral** *see* Tetracycline *on page 1111*

## Nortriptyline (nor TRIP ti leen)

**U.S. Brand Names** Aventyl® Hydrochloride; Pamelor®

**Therapeutic Category** Antidepressant, Tricyclic (Secondary Amine)

**Pregnancy Risk Factor** D

**Lactation** Enters breast milk/contraindicated

**Use** Treatment of various forms of depression, often in conjunction with psychotherapy. Maximum antidepressant effect may not be seen for 2 or more weeks after initiation of therapy; has also demonstrated effectiveness for chronic pain.

**Mechanism of Action/Effect** Traditionally believed to increase the synaptic concentration of serotonin and/or norepinephrine in the central nervous system by inhibition of their reuptake by the presynaptic neuronal membrane. However, additional receptor effects have been found including desensitization of adenyl cyclase, down regulation of beta-adrenergic receptors, and down regulation of serotonin receptors.

**Contraindications** Hypersensitivity to tricyclic antidepressants; narrow-angle glaucoma; pregnancy

**Warnings** Use with caution in patients with cardiac conduction disturbances or with a history of hyperthyroidism. Should not be abruptly discontinued in patients receiving high doses for prolonged periods. Use with caution with renal or hepatic impairment.

**Drug Interactions**

**Cytochrome P-450 Effect:** CYP1A2 and 2D6 enzyme substrate

**Decreased Effect:** Blocks the uptake of guanethidine and thus prevents the hypotensive effect of guanethidine.

**Increased Effect/Toxicity:** Nortriptyline may potentiate the action of other CNS depressants such as sedatives or hypnotics. Nortriptyline may potentiate the vasopressor and cardiac effects of sympathomimetic agents such as isoproterenol, epinephrine, etc. With MAO inhibitors, hyperpyrexia, hypertension, tachycardia, confusion, seizures, and death have been reported. Additive anticholinergic effect is seen with other anticholinergic agents. Cimetidine reduces the metabolism of nortriptyline. May increase prothrombin time in patients stabilized on warfarin resulting in increased potential for bleeding. Potential for serotonin syndrome if combined with other serotonergic drugs.

**Effects on Lab Values** ↑ glucose

**Adverse Reactions** Anticholinergic effects may be pronounced; moderate to marked sedation can occur (tolerance to these effects usually occurs).

>10%:

Central nervous system: Dizziness, drowsiness, headache

Gastrointestinal: Dry mouth, constipation, increased appetite, nausea, unpleasant taste, weight gain

Neuromuscular & skeletal: Weakness

1% to 10%:

Cardiovascular: Hypotension, postural hypotension, arrhythmias, tachycardia

Central nervous system: Nervousness, restlessness, parkinsonian syndrome, insomnia, sedation, fatigue, anxiety, impaired cognitive function, seizures have occurred occasionally, extrapyramidal symptoms are possible

Gastrointestinal: Diarrhea, heartburn

Genitourinary: Sexual dysfunction, urinary retention

Neuromuscular & skeletal: Tremor

Ocular: Eye pain, blurred vision

Miscellaneous: Sweating (excessive)

<1% (Limited to important or life-threatening symptoms): Alopecia, leukopenia, eosinophilia, rarely agranulocytosis, cholestatic jaundice, increased liver enzymes, increased intraocular pressure, sudden death

**Overdose/Toxicology** Symptoms of overdose include agitation, confusion, hallucinations, urinary retention, hypothermia, hypotension, seizures, and ventricular tachycardia.

(Continued)

## Nortriptyline *(Continued)*

Treatment is symptomatic and supportive. Alkalinization by sodium bicarbonate and/or hyperventilation may limit cardiac toxicity.

**Pharmacodynamics/Kinetics**

**Protein Binding:** 93% to 95%

**Half-life Elimination:** 28-31 hours

**Time to Peak:** Within 7-8.5 hours

**Metabolism:** Liver

**Excretion:** Urine and bile (small amounts)

**Onset:** 1-3 weeks before therapeutic effects are seen

**Formulations**

Nortriptyline hydrochloride:

Capsule: 10 mg, 25 mg, 50 mg, 75 mg

Solution: 10 mg/5 mL (473 mL)

**Dosing**

**Adults:** Depression: Oral: 25 mg 3-4 times/day up to 150 mg/day

**Elderly:** Depression: Oral: Initial: 10-25 mg at bedtime; dosage can be increased by 25 mg every 3 days for inpatients and weekly for outpatients if tolerated. Usual maintenance dose: 75 mg as a single bedtime dose, however, lower or higher doses may be required to stay within the therapeutic window.

**Hepatic Impairment:** Lower doses and slower titration are recommended dependent on individualization of dosage.

**Stability**

**Storage:** Protect from light.

**Additional Nursing Issues**

**Physical Assessment:** Assess other medications patient may be taking for effectiveness and interactions (see Drug Interactions). See Contraindications and Warnings/Precautions for cautious use. Has potential for psychological or physiological dependence, abuse, or tolerance. Monitor therapeutic response (ie, mental status, mood, affect, suicidal ideation), and adverse reactions at beginning of therapy and periodically with long-term use (see Adverse Reactions and Overdose/Toxicology). Taper dosage slowly when discontinuing (allow 3-4 weeks between discontinuing nortriptyline and starting another antidepressant). Assess knowledge/teach patient appropriate use (capsule/solution), interventions to reduce side effects, and adverse symptoms to report. **Pregnancy risk factor D** - assess knowledge/teach appropriate use of barrier contraceptives. Breast-feeding is contraindicated.

**Patient Information/Instruction:** Oral: Take exactly as directed (do not increase dose or frequency); may take 2-3 weeks to achieve desired results; may cause physical and/or psychological dependence. Take once-a-day dose at bedtime. Avoid excessive alcohol, caffeine, and other prescription or OTC medications not approved by prescriber. Maintain adequate hydration (2-3 L/day of fluids unless instructed to restrict fluid intake). You may experience drowsiness, lightheadedness, impaired coordination, dizziness, or blurred vision (use caution when driving or engaging in tasks requiring alertness until response to drug is known); nausea, vomiting, altered taste, dry mouth (small frequent meals, frequent mouth care, chewing gum, sucking lozenges may help); constipation (increased exercise, fluids, or dietary fruit and fiber may help); diarrhea (buttermilk, yogurt, or boiled milk may help); increased appetite (monitor dietary intake to avoid excess weight gain); postural hypotension (use caution when climbing stairs or changing position from lying or sitting to standing); urinary retention (void before taking medication); or sexual dysfunction (reversible). Report persistent CNS effects (eg, insomnia, nervousness, restlessness, hallucinations, daytime sedation, impaired cognitive function); muscle cramping or tremors; chest pain, palpitations, rapid heartbeat, swelling of extremities, or severe dizziness; blurred vision or eye pain; yellowing of eyes or skin; pale stools/dark urine; or worsening of condition. **Pregnancy/breast-feeding precautions:** Do not get pregnant while taking this medication; use appropriate barrier contraceptive measures. Do not breast-feed.

**Geriatric Considerations:** Since nortriptyline is the least likely of the tricyclic antidepressants (TCAs) to cause orthostatic hypotension and one of the least anticholinergic and sedating TCAs, it is a preferred agent when a TCA is indicated. Data from a clinical trial comparing fluoxetine to tricyclics suggests that fluoxetine is significantly less effective than nortriptyline in hospitalized elderly patients with unipolar affective disorder, especially those with melancholia and concurrent cardiovascular disease.

**Related Information**

Antidepressant Agents Comparison *on page 1368*

Peak and Trough Guidelines *on page 1331*


- **Norvas** *see* Amlodipine *on page 76*
- **Norvasc®** *see* Amlodipine *on page 76*
- **Norvir®** *see* Ritonavir *on page 1030*
- **Norzine®** *see* Thiethylperazine *on page 1121*
- **Nositrol [Sodium Succinate]** *see* Hydrocortisone *on page 578*
- **Nōstrilla®** *see page 1294*
- **Nostril® Nasal Solution [OTC]** *see* Phenylephrine *on page 920*
- **Novacef** *see* Cefixime *on page 216*
- **Novacet® Topical** *see page 1306*
- **Novahistine® Decongestant** *see* Phenylephrine *on page 920*
- **Novahistine® DH Liquid** *see page 1306*
- **Novahistine® Elixir** *see page 1294*

- **Novahistine® Expectorant** *see* Guaifenesin, Pseudoephedrine, and Codeine *on page 552*
- **Novambarb®** *see* Amobarbital *on page 77*
- **Novamilor** *see* Amiloride and Hydrochlorothiazide *on page 68*
- **Novamoxin®** *see* Amoxicillin *on page 80*
- **Novantrone®** *see* Mitoxantrone *on page 780*
- **Novantrone®** *see* Mitoxantrone *on page 780*
- **Novasen** *see* Aspirin *on page 111*
- **Noviken-N** *see* Nifedipine *on page 824*
- **Novo-Alprazol** *see* Alprazolam *on page 55*
- **Novo-Atenol** *see* Atenolol *on page 115*
- **Novo-AZT** *see* Zidovudine *on page 1227*
- **Novo-Butamide** *see* Tolbutamide *on page 1146*
- **Novocain® Injection** *see* Procaine *on page 969*
- **Novo-Captopril** *see* Captopril *on page 192*
- **Novo-Carbamaz** *see* Carbamazepine *on page 195*
- **Novo-Chlorhydrate** *see* Chloral Hydrate *on page 245*
- **Novo-Chlorpromazine** *see* Chlorpromazine *on page 256*
- **Novo-Cimetine** *see* Cimetidine *on page 268*
- **Novo-Clonidine** *see* Clonidine *on page 289*
- **Novo-Clopate** *see* Clorazepate *on page 292*
- **Novo-Cloxin** *see* Cloxacillin *on page 295*
- **Novo-Cromolyn** *see* Cromolyn Sodium *on page 309*
- **Novo-Cycloprine** *see* Cyclobenzaprine *on page 312*
- **Novo-Difenac®** *see* Diclofenac *on page 358*
- **Novo-Difenac®-SR** *see* Diclofenac *on page 358*
- **Novo-Diflunisal** *see* Diflunisal *on page 368*
- **Novo-Digoxin** *see* Digoxin *on page 370*
- **Novo-Diltazem** *see* Diltiazem *on page 377*
- **Novo-Dipam** *see* Diazepam *on page 355*
- **Novo-Dipiradol** *see* Dipyridamole *on page 383*
- **Novo-Doparil** *see* Methyldopa and Hydrochlorothiazide *on page 751*
- **Novo-Doxepin** *see* Doxepin *on page 399*
- **Novo-Doxylin** *see* Doxycycline *on page 406*
- **Novo-Famotidine** *see* Famotidine *on page 470*
- **Novo-Fibrate** *see* Clofibrate *on page 285*
- **Novo-Flupam** *see* Flurazepam *on page 507*
- **Novo-Flurprofen** *see* Flurbiprofen *on page 509*
- **Novo-Flutamide** *see* Flutamide *on page 510*
- **Novo-Folacid** *see* Folic Acid *on page 515*
- **Novo-Furan** *see* Nitrofurantoin *on page 829*
- **Novo-Gesic-C8** *see* Acetaminophen and Codeine *on page 34*
- **Novo-Gesic-C15** *see* Acetaminophen and Codeine *on page 34*
- **Novo-Gesic-C30** *see* Acetaminophen and Codeine *on page 34*
- **Novo-Glyburide** *see* Glyburide *on page 538*
- **Novo-Hexidyl** *see* Trihexyphenidyl *on page 1179*
- **Novo-Hydrazide** *see* Hydrochlorothiazide *on page 566*
- **Novo-Hydroxyzin** *see* Hydroxyzine *on page 588*
- **Novo-Hylazin** *see* Hydralazine *on page 564*
- **Novo-Keto-EC** *see* Ketoprofen *on page 645*
- **Novo-Lexin** *see* Cephalexin *on page 237*
- **Novolin® 70/30** *see* Insulin Preparations *on page 609*
- **Novolin® L** *see* Insulin Preparations *on page 609*
- **Novolin® N** *see* Insulin Preparations *on page 609*
- **Novolin® R** *see* Insulin Preparations *on page 609*
- **Novo-Lorazepam** *see* Lorazepam *on page 691*
- **Novo-Medopa®** *see* Methyldopa *on page 750*
- **Novo-Medrone** *see* Medroxyprogesterone *on page 714*
- **Novo-Mepro** *see* Meprobamate *on page 724*
- **Novo-Metformin** *see* Metformin *on page 734*
- **Novo-Methacin** *see* Indomethacin *on page 606*
- **Novo-Metoprolol** *see* Metoprolol *on page 761*
- **Novo-Mucilax** *see* Psyllium *on page 993*
- **Novo-Naprox** *see* Naproxen *on page 807*
- **Novo-Nidazol** *see* Metronidazole *on page 763*
- **Novo-Nifedin** *see* Nifedipine *on page 824*
- **Novo-Oxazepam** *see* Oxazepam *on page 868*
- **Novo-Pen-VK®** *see* Penicillin V Potassium *on page 900*
- **Novo-Pindol** *see* Pindolol *on page 934*
- **Novo-Piroxicam** *see* Piroxicam *on page 940*
- **Novo-Poxide** *see* Chlordiazepoxide *on page 250*

- ♦ **Novo-Pramine** *see* Imipramine *on page 600*
- ♦ **Novo-Prazin** *see* Prazosin *on page 958*
- ♦ **Novo-Prednisolone** *see* Prednisolone *on page 960*
- ♦ **Novo-Prednisone** *see* Prednisone *on page 962*
- ♦ **Novo-Profen®** *see* Ibuprofen *on page 592*
- ♦ **Novo-Propamide** *see* Chlorpropamide *on page 259*
- ♦ **Novo-Propoxyn** *see* Propoxyphene *on page 984*
- ♦ **Novo-Propoxyn Compound (contains caffeine)** *see* Propoxyphene and Aspirin *on page 985*
- ♦ **Novo-Purol** *see* Allopurinol *on page 53*
- ♦ **Novo-Pyrazone** *see* Sulfinpyrazone *on page 1086*
- ♦ **Novo-Ranidine** *see* Ranitidine *on page 1008*
- ♦ **Novo-Reserpine** *see* Reserpine *on page 1013*
- ♦ **Novo-Ridazine** *see* Thioridazine *on page 1123*
- ♦ **Novo-Rythro Encap** *see* Erythromycin *on page 435*
- ♦ **Novo-Salmol** *see* Albuterol *on page 45*
- ♦ **Novo-Secobarb** *see* Secobarbital *on page 1049*
- ♦ **Novo-Selegiline** *see* Selegiline *on page 1050*
- ♦ **Novo-Semide** *see* Furosemide *on page 523*
- ♦ **Novo-Soxazole** *see* Sulfisoxazole *on page 1086*
- ♦ **Novo-Spiroton** *see* Spironolactone *on page 1070*
- ♦ **Novo-Spirozine** *see* Hydrochlorothiazide and Spironolactone *on page 568*
- ♦ **Novo-Sucralate** *see* Sucralfate *on page 1078*
- ♦ **Novo-Sundac** *see* Sulindac *on page 1088*
- ♦ **Novo-Tamoxifen** *see* Tamoxifen *on page 1095*
- ♦ **Novo-Tetra** *see* Tetracycline *on page 1111*
- ♦ **Novo-Thalidone** *see* Chlorthalidone *on page 260*
- ♦ **Novo-Timol** *see* Ophthalmic Agents, Glaucoma *on page 853*
- ♦ **Novo-Timol** *see* Timolol *on page 1138*
- ♦ **Novo-Tolmetin** *see* Tolmetin *on page 1149*
- ♦ **Novo-Triamzide** *see* Hydrochlorothiazide and Triamterene *on page 568*
- ♦ **Novo-Trimel** *see* Co-trimoxazole *on page 307*
- ♦ **Novo-Triolam** *see* Triazolam *on page 1174*
- ♦ **Novo-Tripramine** *see* Trimipramine *on page 1183*
- ♦ **Novo-Tryptin** *see* Amitriptyline *on page 73*
- ♦ **Novo-Veramil** *see* Verapamil *on page 1208*
- ♦ **Novo-Zolamide** *see* Acetazolamide *on page 34*
- ♦ **Nozolon** *see* Gentamicin *on page 531*
- ♦ **NPH Iletin® I** *see* Insulin Preparations *on page 609*
- ♦ **NPH Insulin** *see* Insulin Preparations *on page 609*
- ♦ **NPH-N** *see* Insulin Preparations *on page 609*
- ♦ **NTG** *see* Nitroglycerin *on page 831*
- ♦ **NTZ® Long Acting Nasal Solution** *see page 1294*
- ♦ **Nu-Alprax** *see* Alprazolam *on page 55*
- ♦ **Nu-Amilzide** *see* Amiloride and Hydrochlorothiazide *on page 68*
- ♦ **Nu-Amoxi** *see* Amoxicillin *on page 80*
- ♦ **Nu-Ampi Trihydrate** *see* Ampicillin *on page 90*
- ♦ **Nu-Atenol** *see* Atenolol *on page 115*
- ♦ **Nubain®** *see* Nalbuphine *on page 801*
- ♦ **Nu-Capto** *see* Captopril *on page 192*
- ♦ **Nu-Carbamazepine** *see* Carbamazepine *on page 195*
- ♦ **Nu-Cephalex** *see* Cephalexin *on page 237*
- ♦ **Nu-Cimet** *see* Cimetidine *on page 268*
- ♦ **Nu-Clonidine** *see* Clonidine *on page 289*
- ♦ **Nu-Cloxi** *see* Cloxacillin *on page 295*
- ♦ **Nucofed®** *see* Guaifenesin, Pseudoephedrine, and Codeine *on page 552*
- ♦ **Nucofed® Pediatric Expectorant** *see* Guaifenesin, Pseudoephedrine, and Codeine *on page 552*
- ♦ **Nu-Cotrimox** *see* Co-trimoxazole *on page 307*
- ♦ **Nucotuss®** *see* Guaifenesin, Pseudoephedrine, and Codeine *on page 552*
- ♦ **Nu-Diclo** *see* Diclofenac *on page 358*
- ♦ **Nu-Diflunisal** *see* Diflunisal *on page 368*
- ♦ **Nu-Diltiaz** *see* Diltiazem *on page 377*
- ♦ **Nu-Doxycycline** *see* Doxycycline *on page 406*
- ♦ **Nu-Famotidine** *see* Famotidine *on page 470*
- ♦ **Nu-Flurprofen** *see* Flurbiprofen *on page 509*
- ♦ **Nu-Gemfibrozil** *see* Gemfibrozil *on page 530*
- ♦ **Nu-Glyburide** *see* Glyburide *on page 538*
- ♦ **Nu-Hydral** *see* Hydralazine *on page 564*
- ♦ **Nu-Ibuprofen** *see* Ibuprofen *on page 592*
- ♦ **Nu-Indo** *see* Indomethacin *on page 606*
- ♦ **Nu-Iron®** *see page 1294*

- **Nu-Ketoprofen** *see* Ketoprofen *on page 645*
- **Nu-Ketoprofen-E** *see* Ketoprofen *on page 645*
- **Nullo®** *see page 1294*
- **Nu-Loraz** *see* Lorazepam *on page 691*
- **NuLytely®** *see* Polyethylene Glycol-Electrolyte Solution *on page 945*
- **Nu-Medopa** *see* Methyldopa *on page 750*
- **Nu-Metop** *see* Metoprolol *on page 761*
- **Numorphan®** *see* Oxymorphone *on page 875*
- **Numzitdent® [OTC]** *see* Benzocaine *on page 141*
- **Numzit Teething® [OTC]** *see* Benzocaine *on page 141*
- **Nu-Naprox** *see* Naproxen *on page 807*
- **Nu-Nifedin** *see* Nifedipine *on page 824*
- **Nu-Pen-VK** *see* Penicillin V Potassium *on page 900*
- **Nupercainal®** *see page 1294*
- **Nu-Pindol** *see* Pindolol *on page 934*
- **Nu-Pirox** *see* Piroxicam *on page 940*
- **Nu-Prazo** *see* Prazosin *on page 958*
- **Nuprin® [OTC]** *see* Ibuprofen *on page 592*
- **Nu-Prochlor** *see* Prochlorperazine *on page 971*
- **Nu-Propranolol** *see* Propranolol *on page 986*
- **Nuquin HP®** *see* Hydroquinone *on page 583*
- **Nu-Ranit** *see* Ranitidine *on page 1008*
- **Nuromax® Injection** *see page 1248*
- **Nu-Sulfinpyrazone** *see* Sulfinpyrazone *on page 1086*
- **Nu-Tears® II Solution** *see page 1294*
- **Nu-Tears® Solution** *see page 1294*
- **Nu-Tetra** *see* Tetracycline *on page 1111*
- **Nu-Timolol** *see* Ophthalmic Agents, Glaucoma *on page 853*
- **Nu-Timolol** *see* Timolol *on page 1138*
- **Nutracort®** *see* Hydrocortisone *on page 578*
- **Nutracort®** *see* Topical Corticosteroids *on page 1152*
- **Nutraplus® Topical [OTC]** *see* Urea *on page 1193*
- **Nu-Triazide** *see* Hydrochlorothiazide and Triamterene *on page 568*
- **Nu-Triazo** *see* Triazolam *on page 1174*
- **Nutrilipid®** *see* Fat Emulsion *on page 471*
- **Nu-Trimipramine** *see* Trimipramine *on page 1183*
- **Nutritional and Herbal Products** *see page 1268*
- **Nu-Verap** *see* Verapamil *on page 1208*
- **Nyaderm** *see* Nystatin *on this page*
- **Nydrazid®** *see* Isoniazid *on page 630*


## Nystatin (nye STAT in)

**U.S. Brand Names** Mycostatin®; Nilstat®; Nystat-Rx®; Nystex®; O-V Staticin®

**Therapeutic Category** Antifungal Agent, Oral Nonabsorbed; Antifungal Agent, Topical; Antifungal Agent, Vaginal

**Pregnancy Risk Factor** B/C (oral)

**Lactation** Does not enter breast milk/compatible

**Use** Treatment of susceptible cutaneous, mucocutaneous, and oral cavity fungal infections normally caused by the *Candida* species

**Mechanism of Action/Effect** Binds to sterols in fungal cell membrane, changing the cell wall permeability allowing for leakage of cellular contents and cell death

**Contraindications** Hypersensitivity to nystatin or any component

**Warnings** Pregnancy factor C (oral).

**Adverse Reactions**

**Oral:** 1% to 10%: Gastrointestinal: Nausea, vomiting, diarrhea, stomach pain

**Topical:** 1% to 10%: Dermatologic: Skin irritation not present before therapy

**Vaginal:** 1% to 10%: Genitourinary: Vaginal irritation not present before therapy

**Overdose/Toxicology** Symptoms of overdose include nausea, vomiting, and diarrhea. Treatment is supportive.

**Pharmacodynamics/Kinetics**

**Excretion:** Feces

**Onset:** Onset of symptomatic relief from candidiasis: Within 24-72 hours

**Formulations**

Cream: 100,000 units/g (15 g, 30 g)

Ointment, topical: 100,000 units/g (15 g, 30 g)

Powder, for preparation of oral suspension: 50 million units, 1 billion units, 2 billion units, 5 billion units

Powder, topical: 100,000 units/g (15 g)

Suspension, oral: 100,000 units/mL (5 mL, 60 mL, 480 mL)

Tablet:

Oral: 500,000 units

Vaginal: 100,000 units (15 and 30/box with applicator)

Troche: 200,000 units

(Continued)

## Nystatin *(Continued)*

**Dosing**

**Adults:**

Oral candidiasis: Suspension (swish and swallow orally): 400,000-600,000 units 4 times/day; troche: 200,000-400,000 units 4-5 times/day

Mucocutaneous infections: Topical: Apply 2-3 times/day to affected areas; very moist topical lesions are treated best with powder.

Intestinal infections: Oral tablets: 500,000-1,000,000 units every 8 hours

Vaginal infections: Vaginal tablets: Insert 1 tablet/day at bedtime for 2 weeks. (May also be given orally.)

**Elderly:** Refer to adult dosing.

**Administration**

**Oral:**

Suspension: Shake well before using. Should be swished about the mouth and retained in the mouth for as long as possible (several minutes) before swallowing.

Troches: Must be allowed to dissolve slowly and should not be chewed or swallowed whole.

**Stability**

**Storage:** Keep vaginal inserts in refrigerator. Protect from temperature extremes, moisture, and light.

**Additional Nursing Issues**

**Physical Assessment:** Ascertain that cause of infection is fungal. Avoid skin contact when applying. Monitor for therapeutic response, adverse reactions (see Adverse Reactions) at beginning of therapy and periodically throughout therapy. Assess knowledge/teach patient appropriate use, interventions to reduce side effects, and adverse symptoms to report. **Pregnancy risk factor B/C** - benefits of use should outweigh possible risks.

**Patient Information/Instruction:** Take as directed. Maintain adequate hydration (2-3 L/day of fluids unless instructed to restrict fluid intake). Do not allow medication to come in contact with eyes. Report persistent nausea, vomiting, or diarrhea; or if condition being treated worsens or does not improve. **Pregnancy precautions:** Inform prescriber if you are pregnant.

Oral tablets: Swallow whole; do not crush or chew.

Oral suspension: Shake well before using. Remove dentures, clean mouth (do not replace dentures until after using medications). Swish suspension in mouth for several minutes before swallowing.

Oral troches: Remove dentures, clean mouth (do not replace dentures until after using medication). Allow troche to dissolve in mouth; do not chew or swallow whole.

Topical: Wash and dry area before applying (do not reuse towels without washing, apply clean clothing after use). Report unresolved burning, redness, or swelling in treated areas.

Vaginal tablets: Wash hands before using. Lie down to insert high into vagina at bedtime.

**Geriatric Considerations:** For oral infections, patients who wear dentures must have them removed and cleaned in order to eliminate source of reinfection.

**Additional Information** Some formulations may contain ethanol.

## Nystatin and Triamcinolone (nye STAT in & trye am SIN oh lone)

**U.S. Brand Names** Mycogen II Topical; Mycolog®-II Topical; Myconel® Topical; Myco-Triacet® II; Mytrex® F Topical; N.G.T.® Topical; Tri-Statin® II Topical

**Synonyms** Triamcinolone and Nystatin

**Therapeutic Category** Antifungal Agent, Topical; Corticosteroid, Topical

**Pregnancy Risk Factor** C

**Lactation** Excretion in breast milk unknown

**Use** Treatment of cutaneous candidiasis

**Formulations**

Cream: Nystatin 100,000 units and triamcinolone acetonide 0.1% (15 g, 30 g, 45 g, 60 g, 240 g)

Ointment, topical: Nystatin 100,000 units and triamcinolone acetonide 0.1% (15 g, 30 g, 60 g, 120 g)

**Dosing**

**Adults:** Topical: Apply sparingly 2-4 times/day

**Elderly:** Refer to adult dosing.

**Additional Nursing Issues**

**Physical Assessment:** See individual components listed in Related Information. **Pregnancy risk factor C** - benefits of use should outweigh possible risks. Note breast-feeding caution.

**Patient Information/Instruction:** See individual components listed in Related Information. **Pregnancy/breast-feeding precautions:** Inform prescriber if you are on intend to get pregnant. Consult prescriber if breast-feeding.

**Related Information**

Nystatin *on previous page*

Triamcinolone *on page 1171*

- **Nystat-Rx®** *see* Nystatin *on previous page*
- **Nystex®** *see* Nystatin *on previous page*
- **Nytol® Extra Strength** *see* Diphenhydramine *on page 381*

- **Nytol® Oral [OTC]** *see* Diphenhydramine *on page 381*
- **Occlucort®** *see* Betamethasone *on page 148*
- **Occlusal-HP Liquid** *see page 1294*
- **Occucoat™** *see page 1248*
- **Ocean Nasal Mist** *see page 1294*
- **OCL®** *see* Polyethylene Glycol-Electrolyte Solution *on page 945*
- **Octamide®** *see* Metoclopramide *on page 758*
- **Octocaine®** *see* Lidocaine *on page 674*
- **Octocaine® With Epinephrine** *see* Lidocaine and Epinephrine *on page 677*
- **Octostim®** *see* Desmopressin *on page 345*


## Octreotide (ok TREE oh tide)

**U.S. Brand Names** Sandostatin®; Sandostatin LAR®

**Therapeutic Category** Antidiarrheal; Antisecretory Agent; Somatostatin Analog

**Pregnancy Risk Factor** B

**Lactation** Enters breast milk/contraindicated

**Use** Control of symptoms in patients with metastatic carcinoid and vasoactive intestinal peptide-secreting tumors (VIPomas); pancreatic tumors, gastrinoma, secretory diarrhea; Acromegaly

**Unlabeled use:** AIDS-associated secretory diarrhea, control of bleeding of esophageal varices, breast cancer, cryptosporidiosis, Cushing's syndrome, insulinomas, small bowel fistulas, postgastrectomy dumping syndrome, chemotherapy-induced diarrhea, GVHD-induced diarrhea, Zollinger-Ellison syndrome

**Mechanism of Action/Effect** Mimics natural somatostatin by inhibiting serotonin release, and the secretion of gastrin, VIP, insulin, glucagon, secretin, motilin, and pancreatic polypeptide

**Contraindications** Hypersensitivity to octreotide or any component

**Warnings** Dosage adjustment may be required to maintain symptomatic control. Insulin requirements may be reduced as well as sulfonylurea requirements. Monitor patients for cholelithiasis, hyper- or hypoglycemia. Use with caution in patients with renal impairment. Do not administer Sandostatin LAR® intravenously or subcutaneously.

**Drug Interactions**

**Cytochrome P-450 Effect:** CYP2D6 (high dose) and 3A enzyme inhibitor

**Decreased Effect:** Octreotide may lower cyclosporine serum levels (case report of a transplant rejection due to reduction of serum cyclosporine levels).

**Increased Effect/Toxicity:** May increase the effect of insulin or sulfonylurea agents which may result in hypoglycemia.

**Adverse Reactions**

1% to 10%:

Cardiovascular: Flushing, edema

Central nervous system: Fatigue, headache, dizziness, vertigo, anorexia, depression

Endocrine & metabolic: Hypoglycemia or hyperglycemia (1%), hypothyroidism, galactorrhea

Gastrointestinal: Nausea, vomiting, diarrhea, constipation, abdominal pain, cramping, discomfort, fat malabsorption, loose stools, flatulence

Hepatic: Jaundice, hepatitis, increase LFTs, cholelithiasis has occurred, presumably by altering fat absorption and decreasing the motility of the gallbladder

Local: Pain at injection site

Neuromuscular & skeletal: Weakness

<1% (Limited to important or life-threatening symptoms): Chest pain, hypertensive reaction, alopecia, thrombophlebitis, shortness of breath

**Overdose/Toxicology** Symptoms of overdose include hypo- or hyperglycemia, blurred vision, dizziness, drowsiness, and loss of motor function. Well tolerated bolus doses up to 1000 mcg have failed to produce adverse effects.

**Pharmacodynamics/Kinetics**

**Half-life Elimination:** 60-110 minutes

**Metabolism:** Liver

**Excretion:** Kidney

**Duration:** 6-12 hours

**Formulations**

Injection, as acetate: 0.05 mg/mL (1 mL); 0.1 mg/mL (1 mL); 0.2 mg/mL (5 mL); 0.5 mg/mL (1 mL); 1 mg/mL (5 mL)

Depot injection kit, microsphere suspension (Sandostatin LAR®): Vial with diluent and syringe: 10 mg, 20 mg, 30 mg powder

**Dosing**

**Adults:** S.C.: Initial: 50 mcg 1-2 times/day and titrate dose based on patient tolerance and response

Carcinoid: 100-600 mcg/day in 2-4 divided doses

VIPomas: 200-300 mcg/day in 2-4 divided doses

Diarrhea: Initial: I.V.: 50-100 mcg every 8 hours; increase by 100 mcg/dose at 48-hour intervals; maximum dose: 500 mcg every 8 hours

Esophageal varices bleeding: I.V. bolus: 25-50 mcg followed by continuous I.V. infusion of 25-50 mcg/hour

Acromegaly, carcinoid tumors, and VIPomas (depot injection): Patients must be stabilized on subcutaneous octreotide for at least 2 weeks before switching to the long-acting depot: Upon switch: 20 mg I.M. intragluteally every 4 weeks for 2-3 months, then the dose may be modified based upon response

(Continued)

## Octreotide *(Continued)*

**Dosage adjustment for acromegaly:** After 3 months of depot injections the dosage may be continued or modified as follows:

GH ≤2.5 ng/mL, IGF-1 is normal, symptoms are controlled: Maintain octreotide LAR® at 20 mg I.M. every 4 weeks

GH >2.5 ng/mL, IGF-1 is elevated, or symptoms: Increase octreotide LAR® to 10 mg I.M. every 4 weeks

GH ≤1 ng/mL, IGF-1 is normal, symptoms controlled: Reduce octreotide LAR® to 10 mg I.M. every 4 weeks

Dosages >40 mg are not recommended

**Dosage adjustment for carcinoid tumors and VIPomas:** After 2 months of depot injections the dosage may be continued or modified as follows:

Increase to 30 mg I.M. every 4 weeks if symptoms are inadequately controlled

Decrease to 10 mg I.M. every 4 weeks, for a trial period, if initially responsive to 20 mg dose

Dosage >30 mg is not recommended

**Elderly:** Refer to adult dosing.

**Renal Impairment:** Half-life may be increased, requiring adjustment of maintenance dose

**Administration**

**I.M.:** Sandostatin LAR®: Administer immediately after reconstitution; administer in gluteal muscle, avoid deltoid administration

**I.V.:** IVP should be administered undiluted over 3 minutes. IVPB should be administered over 15-30 minutes. Continuous I.V. infusion rates have ranged from 25-50 mcg/hour for the treatment of esophageal variceal bleeding.

**I.V. Detail:** Do not use if solution contains particles or is discolored. I.V. administration may be IVP, IVPB, or continuous I.V. infusion.

**Other:** Can be administered S.C.

**Stability**

**Storage:** Octreotide is a clear solution and should be stored under refrigeration. Ampuls may be stored at room temperature for up to 14 days when protected from light.

**Reconstitution:** Stability of parenteral admixture in NS at room temperature (25°C) and at refrigeration temperature (4°C) is 48 hours.

Common diluent: 50-100 mcg/50 mL NS; common diluent for continuous I.V. infusion: 1200 mcg/250 mL NS

Minimum volume: 50 mL NS

**Monitoring Laboratory Tests** Vitamin $B_{12}$ levels with chronic therapy

**Additional Nursing Issues**

**Physical Assessment:** Monitor effectiveness of therapy. Monitor on a regular basis for frequency and consistency of stools, for dehydration (skin turgor, urinary output, thirst). Diabetic patients should be monitored closely for symptoms of hyper-/hypoglycemia. Instruct patient on appropriate use, possible side effects (see Adverse Reactions), and symptoms to report. Breast-feeding is contraindicated.

**Patient Information/Instruction:** Schedule injections between meals to decrease GI effects. May affect dietary fat and vitamin $B_{12}$. Consult prescriber about appropriate diet. Diabetic patients should monitor serum glucose closely (this drug may increase the effects of insulin or sulfonylureas); report abnormal glucose levels so appropriate adjustment can be made. You may experience skin flushing; nausea or vomiting (small frequent meals, frequent mouth care, sucking lozenges, or chewing gum may help); dizziness, fatigue, or drowsiness (use caution when driving or engaging in tasks that require alertness until response to drug is known). Report weight gain, swelling of extremities, or respiratory difficulty; acute or persistent GI distress (eg, diarrhea, vomiting, constipation, abdominal pain); muscle weakness or tremors or loss of motor function; chest pain or palpitations; blurred vision; pain, redness, or swelling at injection site; or emotional depression. **Breast-feeding precautions:** Do not breast-feed.

**Administration:** Slowly warm solution to room temperature. Inject slowly to reduce local reaction. Rotate injection sites, using hip, thigh, or abdomen. Dispose of syringes in closed container away from access of other persons.

- **Ocu-Carpine® Ophthalmic** *see* Pilocarpine *on page 931*
- **OcuClear® Ophthalmic** *see page 1294*
- **OcuCoat® Ophthalmic Solution** *see page 1294*
- **OcuCoat® PF Ophthalmic Solution** *see page 1294*
- **Ocu-Dex®** *see* Dexamethasone *on page 346*
- **Ocufen®** *see page 1282*
- **Ocufen® Ophthalmic** *see* Flurbiprofen *on page 509*
- **Ocuflox®** *see page 1282*
- **Ocuflox™ Ophthalmic** *see* Ofloxacin *on next page*
- **OcuHist® [OTC]** *see page 1282*
- **Ocu-Pentolate®** *see page 1248*
- **Ocupress® Ophthalmic** *see* Carteolol *on page 206*
- **Ocupress® Ophthalmic** *see* Ophthalmic Agents, Glaucoma *on page 853*
- **Ocusert Pilo-20® Ophthalmic** *see* Ophthalmic Agents, Glaucoma *on page 853*
- **Ocusert Pilo-20® Ophthalmic** *see* Pilocarpine *on page 931*
- **Ocusert Pilo-40® Ophthalmic** *see* Ophthalmic Agents, Glaucoma *on page 853*
- **Ocusert Pilo-40® Ophthalmic** *see* Pilocarpine *on page 931*
- **Ocusulf-10®** *see page 1282*

- ♦ **Ocusulf-10® Ophthalmic** *see* Sulfacetamide *on page 1080*
- ♦ **Ocutricin® Topical Ointment** *see* Bacitracin, Neomycin, and Polymyxin B *on page 130*
- ♦ **Ocu-Tropine® Ophthalmic** *see* Atropine *on page 119*
- ♦ **Oestrilin®** *see* Estrone *on page 451*
- ♦ **Oestrogel** *see* Estradiol *on page 441*
- ♦ **Off-Ezy® Wart Remover** *see page 1294*


## Ofloxacin (oh FLOKS a sin)

**U.S. Brand Names** Floxin®; Ocuflox™ Ophthalmic

**Therapeutic Category** Antibiotic, Ophthalmic; Antibiotic, Otic; Antibiotic, Quinolone

**Pregnancy Risk Factor** C

**Lactation** Enters breast milk/contraindicated

**Use** Quinolone antibiotic for skin and skin structure, lower respiratory and urinary tract infections, and sexually transmitted diseases, bacterial conjunctivitis caused by susceptible organisms

**Mechanism of Action/Effect** Ofloxacin, a fluorinated quinolone, is a pyridine carboxylic acid derivative which exerts a broad spectrum bactericidal effect. It inhibits DNA gyrase inhibitor, an essential bacterial enzyme that maintains the superhelical structure of DNA. DNA gyrase is required for DNA replication and transcription, DNA repair, recombination, and transposition within the bacteria.

**Contraindications** Hypersensitivity to ofloxacin or other members of the quinolone group such as nalidixic acid, oxolinic acid, cinoxacin, norfloxacin, lomefloxacin, and ciprofloxacin; do not inject ophthalmic solution subconjunctivally or directly into anterior chamber of eye

**Warnings** Use with caution in patients with epilepsy or other CNS diseases which could predispose seizures. Use with caution in patients with renal impairment. Failure to respond to an ophthalmic antibiotic after 2-3 days may indicate the presence of resistant organisms, or another causative agent. Use caution with systemic preparation in children <18 years of age due to association of other quinolones with transient arthropathy. Pregnancy factor C.

**Drug Interactions**

**Decreased Effect:** Decreased absorption with antacids containing aluminum, magnesium, and/or calcium (by up to 98% if given at the same time).

**Increased Effect/Toxicity:** Quinolones can cause increased caffeine, warfarin, cyclosporine, and theophylline levels. Azlocillin, cimetidine, and probenecid may increase ofloxacin serum levels.

**Food Interactions** Ofloxacin average peak serum concentrations may be decreased by 20% if taken with food.

**Adverse Reactions**

**Ophthalmic:**

>10%: Ocular: Burning or other discomfort of the eye, crusting or crystals in corner of eye

1% to 10%:

Gastrointestinal: Bad taste instillation

Ocular: Foreign body sensation, conjunctival hyperemia, itching of eye

**Systemic:**

>10%:

Central nervous system: Dizziness or lightheadedness, headache, nervousness, drowsiness, insomnia

Gastrointestinal: Nausea, diarrhea, vomiting, abdominal pain

1% to 10%:

Dermatologic: Photosensitivity

Local: Pain at injection site

<1% (Limited to important or life-threatening symptoms): Stevens-Johnson syndrome, anemia, increased liver enzymes, interstitial nephritis, shortness of breath, vasculitis, Tourette's syndrome, hepatitis

**Overdose/Toxicology** Symptoms of overdose include acute renal failure, seizures, nausea, and vomiting. Treatment includes GI decontamination, if possible, and supportive care. Not removed by peritoneal or hemodialysis.

**Pharmacodynamics/Kinetics**

**Protein Binding:** 20%

**Half-life Elimination:** 5-7.5 hours (prolonged in renal impairment)

**Metabolism:** Primarily unchanged

**Excretion:** Urine

**Formulations**

Injection: 200 mg (50 mL); 400 mg (10 mL, 20 mL, 100 mL)

Solution, ophthalmic: 0.3% (5 mL)

Tablet: 200 mg, 300 mg, 400 mg

Solution, otic: 0.3% (5 mL)

**Dosing**

**Adults:**

Oral, I.V.: 200-400 mg every 12 hours for 7-10 days for most infections or for 6 weeks for prostatitis

Ophthalmic: Instill 1-2 drops in affected eye(s) every 2-4 hours for the first 2 days, then use 4 times/day for an additional 5 days.

Otic:

Otitis externa: 10 drops into affected ear twice daily for 10 days

Chronic otitis media with perforated tympanic membranes: 10 drops into affected ear twice daily for 14 days

(Continued)

## Ofloxacin *(Continued)*

**Elderly:** Oral, I.V.: 200-400 mg every 12-24 hours (based on estimated renal function) for 7 days to 6 weeks depending on indication.

**Renal Impairment:**

$Cl_{cr}$ 10-50 mL/minute: Administer 50% of normal dose or administer every 24 hours.

$Cl_{cr}$ <10 mL/minute: Administer 25% of normal dose or administer 50% of normal dose every 24 hours.

Continuous arteriovenous or venovenous hemofiltration (CAVH): 300 mg every 24 hours

**Administration**

**Oral:** Do not take within 2 hours of food or any antacids which contain zinc, magnesium, or aluminum.

**I.V.:** Administer over at least 60 minutes. Infuse separately.

**I.V. Detail:** Do not administer in same tubing with any solution containing metal ions (eg, calcium, copper, iron, magnesium, zinc). May chelate with metal ions.

**Monitoring Laboratory Tests** Perform culture and sensitivity studies before initiating therapy. Monitor CBC, renal and hepatic function periodically if therapy is prolonged.

**Additional Nursing Issues**

**Physical Assessment:** Assess allergy history before initiating therapy. Assess effectiveness and interactions of other medication (see Drug Interactions). See Warnings/Precautions and Contraindications for use cautions. Monitor effectiveness of therapy, laboratory tests, and adverse response (see Adverse Reactions and Overdose/Toxicology). Assess knowledge/teach patient appropriate use, possible side effects and appropriate interventions, and adverse symptoms to report. **Pregnancy risk factor C** - benefits of use should outweigh possible risks. Breast-feeding is contraindicated.

**Patient Information/Instruction:**

Oral: Take per recommended schedule; complete full course of therapy and do not skip doses. Take on an empty stomach (1 hour before or 2 hours after meals, dairy products, antacids, or other medication). Maintain adequate hydration (2-3 L/day of fluids unless instructed to restrict fluid intake).

Oral/I.V.: You may experience dizziness, lightheadedness (use caution when driving or engaging in tasks that require alertness until response to drug is known); nausea, vomiting, or taste perversion (small frequent meals, frequent mouth care, sucking lozenges, or chewing gum may help); photosensitivity (use sunscreen, wear protective clothing and eyewear, and avoid direct sunlight). Report GI disturbances, CNS changes (excessive sleepiness, agitation, or tremors), skin rash, changes in vision, difficulty breathing, signs of opportunistic infection (sore throat, chills, fever, burning, itching on urination, vaginal discharge, white plaques in mouth), or worsening of condition. **Pregnancy/breast-feeding precautions:** Inform prescriber if you are or intend to be pregnant. Do not breast-feed.

Ophthalmic: Tilt head back, instill 1-2 drops in affected eye as frequently as prescribed. Do not allow tip of applicator to touch eye or any contaminated surface. You may experience some stinging or burning or a bad taste in you mouth after instillation. Report persistent pain, burning, swelling, or visual disturbances.

**Geriatric Considerations:** Must adjust dose for renal function.

**Additional Information** pH: 3.5-5.5

**Related Information**

Ophthalmic Agents *on page 1282*
Otic Agents *on page 1291*
TB Drug Comparison *on page 1402*

♦ **Ogen® Oral** *see* Estropipate *on page 452*
♦ **Ogen® Vaginal** *see* Estropipate *on page 452*
♦ **OKT3** *see* Muromonab-CD3 *on page 793*

## Olanzapine (oh LAN za peen)

**U.S. Brand Names** Zyprexa™

**Synonyms** LY170053

**Therapeutic Category** Antipsychotic Agent, Thienobenzodiaepine

**Pregnancy Risk Factor** C

**Lactation** Enters breast milk/contraindicated

**Use** Treatment of the manifestations of psychotic disorders

**Mechanism of Action/Effect** Olanzapine is a thienobenzodiazepine neuroleptic; thought to work by antagonizing dopamine and serotonin activities. It is a selective monoaminergic antagonist with high affinity binding to serotonin $5-HT_{2A}$ and $5-HT_{2C}$, dopamine $D_{1-4}$, muscarinic $M_{1-5}$, histamine $H_1$, and alpha$_1$-adrenergic receptor sites.

**Contraindications** Hypersensitivity to olanzapine or any component

**Warnings** Moderately to highly sedating, use with caution in disorders where CNS depression is a feature. Use with caution in Parkinson's disease. Use with caution in patients with hemodynamic instability; bone marrow suppression; predisposition to seizures; subcortical brain damage; or severe cardiac, hepatic, renal, or respiratory disease. Neuroleptics may cause swallowing difficulties. Use with caution in breast cancer or other prolactin-dependent tumors (may elevate prolactin levels). May alter temperature regulation or mask toxicity of other drugs due to antiemetic effects. Life-threatening arrhythmias have occurred with therapeutic doses of some neuroleptics.

May cause anticholinergic effects (eg, constipation, dry mouth, blurred vision, urinary retention); therefore, use with caution in patients with decreased gastrointestinal motility, urinary retention, BPH, xerostomia, or visual problems. Conditions which also may be exacerbated by cholinergic blockade include narrow-angle glaucoma (screening is recommended) and worsening of myasthenia gravis. Relative to other neuroleptics, olanzapine has a moderate potency of cholinergic blockade.

May cause extrapyramidal reactions, including pseudoparkinsonism, acute dystonic reactions, akathisia, and tardive dyskinesia (risk of these reactions is low relative to other neuroleptics). May be associated with neuroleptic malignant syndrome (NMS) or pigmentary retinopathy.

Pregnancy factor C.

**Drug Interactions**

**Cytochrome P-450 Effect:** CYP1A2 enzyme substrate, CYP2C19 enzyme substrate (minor), and CYP2D6 enzyme substrate (minor)

**Decreased Effect:** Cigarette smoking, levodopa, pergolide, bromocriptine, and charcoal may reduce the effects of olanzapine. Reduction of effects may be seen with cytochrome P-450 enzyme inducers (eg, rifampin, omeprazole, carbamazepine, etc).

**Increased Effect/Toxicity:** Effects may be potentiated with cytochrome P-450 $1A_2$ inhibitors (eg, fluvoxamine). Increased sedation with alcohol or other CNS depressants. Increased risk of hypotension and orthostatic hypotension with antihypertensives.

**Adverse Reactions**

>10%: Central nervous system: Headache, somnolence, insomnia, agitation, nervousness, hostility, dizziness

1% to 10%:

- Central nervous system: Dystonic reactions, parkinsonian events, akathisia, anxiety, personality changes, fever
- Gastrointestinal: Dry mouth, constipation, abdominal pain, weight gain
- Neuromuscular & skeletal: Arthralgia
- Ocular: Amblyopia
- Respiratory: Rhinitis, cough, pharyngitis

<1% (Limited to important or life-threatening symptoms): Tardive dyskinesia, neuroleptic malignant syndrome

**Pharmacodynamics/Kinetics**

**Protein Binding:** 93%

**Half-life Elimination:** 21-54 hours (mean 30 hours)

**Time to Peak:** ~6 hours

**Metabolism:** Liver

**Excretion:** Urine and feces

**Formulations** Tablet: 2.5 mg, 5 mg, 7.5 mg, 10 mg

**Dosing**

**Adults:** Oral: Usual starting dose: 5-10 mg once daily; increase to 10 mg once daily within 5-7 days, thereafter adjust by 5 mg/day at 1-week intervals, up to a maximum of 20 mg/day. Doses as high as 30-50 mg per day have been used

**Elderly:** Oral: Initial: 5 mg/day with increases of 5 mg/day with 5-7 days to attain a target dose of 10 mg/day within first weeks of initiation. Thereafter, adjust by 5 mg/day at weekly intervals; maximum: 20 mg/day (see Geriatric Considerations).

**Hepatic Impairment:** Dosage adjustment may be necessary, however, there are no specific recommendations. Monitor closely.

**Monitoring Laboratory Tests** Ophthalmic screening

**Additional Nursing Issues**

**Physical Assessment:** Assess other medications patient is taking for effectiveness and interactions (especially with drugs that alter P-450 enzymes - see Drug Interactions). See Contraindications and Warnings/Precautions for cautious use. Has potential for psychological or physiological dependence, abuse, and tolerance. Review ophthalmic screening (see Monitoring Laboratory Tests) and monitor therapeutic response (eg, mental status, mood, affect) and adverse reactions at beginning of therapy and periodically with long-term use (sedation, CNS changes, extrapyramidal effects, neuroleptic malignant syndrome - see Adverse Reactions and Overdose). Initiate at lower doses (see Dosing) and taper dosage slowly when discontinuing. Assess knowledge/teach patient appropriate use, interventions to reduce side effects, and adverse symptoms to report (see below). **Pregnancy risk factor C** - benefits of use should outweigh possible risks. Breast-feeding is contraindicated.

**Patient Information/Instruction:** Use exactly as directed (do not increase dose or frequency); may cause physical and/or psychological dependence. It may take 2-3 weeks to achieve desired results; do not discontinue without consulting prescriber. Avoid excess alcohol or caffeine and other prescription or OTC medications not approved by prescriber. Maintain adequate hydration (2-3 L/day of fluids unless instructed to restrict fluid intake). You may experience excess drowsiness, restlessness, dizziness, or blurred vision (use caution driving or when engaging in tasks requiring alertness until response to drug is known); or constipation (increased exercise, fluids, or dietary fruit and fiber may help). Report persistent CNS effects (eg, trembling fingers, altered gait or balance, excessive sedation, seizures, unusual movements, anxiety, abnormal thoughts, confusion, personality changes); unresolved constipation or gastrointestinal effects; vision changes; difficulty breathing; unusual cough or flu-like symptoms; or worsening of condition. **Pregnancy/breast-feeding precautions:** Inform prescriber if you are or intend to be pregnant. Do not breast-feed.

**Geriatric Considerations:** (See Warnings/Precautions, Adverse Reactions, and Overdose/Toxicology.) Elderly patients have an increased risk of adverse response to side effects or adverse reactions to antipsychotics. These can include but are not limited to the following.

(Continued)

## Olanzapine *(Continued)*

Anticholinergic effects: CNS toxicity with confusion, memory loss, psychotic behavior, and agitation.

Extrapyramidal effects (EPS): Parkinson's syndrome and akathisia may occur as often as 50% in patients >60 years of age. Tardive dyskinesia (motor restlessness) may be 40% in elderly; may be related to duration and total accumulated dose over time; may be somewhat reversible if diagnosed early enough.

Orthostatic hypotension: Increased risk for falls.

Sedation: In nonpsychotic patients, may result in feelings of depersonalization, derealization, and dysphoria.

Cardiac toxicity: Cardiac arrhythmias have occurred with therapeutic doses of antipsychotics.

Malignant neuroleptic syndrome: Development of hyperthermia, muscular rigidity, autonomic instability, and altered mental status.

Many elderly patients receive antipsychotic medications for inappropriate nonpsychotic behavior. Before initiating antipsychotic medication, all possible reversible causes should be investigated. Stress may cause acute "confusion" or worsening of baseline nonpsychotic behaviors; any changes in disease state (in any organ) may result in behavioral changes. Common acute changes in behavior may be due also to increases in drug dose addition, or addition of a new drug to the regimen; fluid/electrolyte alterations; infections; or changes in the environment.

Meta-analysis of controlled trials of antipsychotic (phenothiazines, butyrophenones) use with agitated, demented, elderly patients has concluded that the use of neuroleptics results in a response rate of 18%. Clearly, neuroleptic therapy for behavior control should be limited, with frequent attempts to withdraw the agent for behavior control. When use is indicated, initial doses should be lower to start and monitored closely.

**Related Information**

Antipsychotic Agents Comparison *on page 1371*
Antipsychotic Medication Guidelines *on page 1436*

♦ **Oleovitamin A** *see* Vitamin A *on page 1217*
♦ **Olopatadine** *see page 1282*

## Olsalazine (ole SAL a zeen)

**U.S. Brand Names** Dipentum®

**Therapeutic Category** 5-Aminosalicylic Acid Derivative

**Pregnancy Risk Factor** C

**Lactation** Enters breast milk/use caution (monitor for diarrhea)

**Use** Maintenance of remission of ulcerative colitis in patients intolerant to sulfasalazine

**Mechanism of Action/Effect** The mechanism of action appears to be localized in color rather than systemic

**Contraindications** Hypersensitivity to salicylates

**Warnings** Diarrhea is a common adverse effect of olsalazine. Use with caution in patients with hypersensitivity to salicylates, sulfasalazine, or mesalamine. Pregnancy factor C.

**Drug Interactions**

**Increased Effect/Toxicity:** Olsalazine has been reported to increase the prothrombin time in patients taking warfarin.

**Effects on Lab Values** ↑ ALT, AST (S)

**Adverse Reactions**

>10%: Gastrointestinal: Diarrhea, cramps, abdominal pain

1% to 10%:

Central nervous system: Headache, fatigue, depression
Dermatologic: Rash, itching
Gastrointestinal: Nausea, heartburn, bloating, anorexia
Neuromuscular & skeletal: Arthralgia

<1% (Limited to important or life-threatening symptoms): Blood dyscrasias, hepatitis

**Overdose/Toxicology** Symptoms of overdose include decreased motor activity and diarrhea. Treatment is supportive.

**Pharmacodynamics/Kinetics**

**Protein Binding:** >99% bound to plasma proteins

**Time to Peak:** Within 1 hour

**Metabolism:** Mostly by colonic bacteria to the active drug, 5-aminosalicylic acid

**Excretion:** Feces

**Formulations** Capsule, as sodium: 250 mg

**Dosing**

**Adults:** Oral: 1 g/day in 2 divided doses

**Elderly:** Refer to adult dosing.

**Administration**

**Oral:** Take with food in evenly divided doses.

**Additional Nursing Issues**

**Physical Assessment:** Assess effectiveness and interactions of other medications (see Drug Interactions). See Warnings/Precautions for use cautions. Assess for history of allergies (see Contraindications). Monitor effectiveness of therapy and adverse response (see Adverse Reactions and Overdose/Toxicology). Assess knowledge/teach patient appropriate use according to drug formulation (see above), possible side effects/interventions, and adverse symptoms to report. **Pregnancy risk factor C** - benefits of use should outweigh possible risks. Note breast-feeding caution.

**Patient Information/Instruction:** Take as directed, with meals, in evenly divided doses. You may experience flu-like symptoms or muscle pain (a mild analgesic may help); diarrhea (boiled milk or yogurt may help); or nausea or loss of appetite (small frequent meals, frequent mouth care, sucking lozenges, or chewing gum may help). Report persistent diarrhea or abdominal cramping, skin rash or itching, or other adverse reactions. **Pregnancy/breast-feeding precautions:** Inform prescriber if you are or intend to be pregnant. Consult prescriber if breast-feeding.

**Geriatric Considerations:** No specific data is available on elderly to suggest the drug needs alterations in dose. Since so little is absorbed, dosing should not be changed for reasons of age. Diarrhea may pose a serious problem for elderly in that it may cause dehydration, electrolyte imbalance, hypotension, and confusion.

## Omeprazole (oh ME pray zol)

**U.S. Brand Names** Prilosec™

**Therapeutic Category** Proton Pump Inhibitor

**Pregnancy Risk Factor** C

**Lactation** Enters breast milk/contraindicated

**Use** Duodenal ulcer; gastric ulcer; eradication of *H. pylori* in patients with duodenal ulcer disease (when combined with clarithromycin and amoxicillin); gastroesophageal reflux disease (GERD) with erosive esophagitis; poorly responsive symptomatic gastroesophageal reflux disease (GERD); maintenance of healing of erosive esophagitis; pathological hypersecretory conditions

**Mechanism of Action/Effect** Suppresses gastric acid secretion by inhibiting the parietal cell H+/K+ ATP pump

**Contraindications** Hypersensitivity to omeprazole or any component

**Warnings** In long-term (2-year) studies in rats, omeprazole produced a dose-related increase in gastric carcinoid tumors. While available endoscopic evaluations and histologic examinations of biopsy specimens from human stomachs have not detected a risk from short-term exposure to omeprazole, further human data on the effect of sustained hypochlorhydria and hypergastrinemia is needed to rule out the possibility of an increased risk for the development of tumors in humans receiving long-term therapy. Bioavailability may be increased in the elderly. Pregnancy factor C.

**Drug Interactions**

**Cytochrome P-450 Effect:** CYP2C8, 2C9, 2C18, 2C19, and 3A3/4 enzyme substrate; CYP1A2 enzyme inducer CYP2C19, 2C8, 2C9, and 2C19 enzyme inhibitor, CYP3A3/4 enzyme inhibitor (weak)

**Decreased Effect:** The clinical effect of ketoconazole, itraconazole, and other drugs dependent upon acid for absorption is reduced. Theophylline clearance is increased slightly.

**Increased Effect/Toxicity:** Omeprazole may increase the half-life of diazepam, digoxin, phenytoin, warfarin, and other drugs metabolized by the liver.

**Adverse Reactions**

1% to 10%:

Cardiovascular: Chest pain, tachycardia, bradycardia, edema

Central nervous system: Headache (7%), dizziness, muscle weakness (muscle weakness occurred in more frequently than 1% of patients)

Dermatologic: Rash, urticaria, pruritus, dry skin, purpura, petechiae

Gastrointestinal: Diarrhea, nausea, abdominal pain, vomiting, constipation, anorexia, irritable colon, fecal discoloration, esophageal candidiasis, dry mouth, altered taste

Genitourinary: Testicular pain, urinary tract infection, urinary frequency

Neuromuscular & skeletal: Back pain, muscle cramps, myalgia, joint pain, leg pain

Renal: Pyuria, proteinuria, hematuria, glycosuria

Respiratory: Cough

<1% (Limited to important or life-threatening symptoms): Chest pain, anaphylaxis (rare)

**Overdose/Toxicology** Symptoms of overdose include hypothermia, sedation, and convulsions. Decreased respiratory rate demonstrated in animals only. Treatment is supportive. Not dialyzable.

**Pharmacodynamics/Kinetics**

**Protein Binding:** 95%

**Half-life Elimination:** 30-90 minutes

**Metabolism:** Liver

**Excretion:** Urine

**Onset:** Onset of antisecretory action: Oral: Within 1 hour; Peak effect: 2 hours

**Duration:** 72 hours

**Formulations** Capsule, delayed release: 10 mg, 20 mg

**Dosing**

**Adults:** Oral:

Active duodenal ulcer: 20 mg/day for 4-8 weeks

GERD or severe erosive esophagitis: 20 mg/day for 4-8 weeks

Pathological hypersecretory conditions: 60 mg once daily to start; doses up to 120 mg 3 times/day have been administered; administer daily doses >80 mg in divided doses.

*Helicobacter pylori*: Combination therapy with bismuth subsalicylate, tetracycline, clarithromycin, and $H_2$ antagonist; or clarithromycin and omeprazole; dose: 20 mg twice daily

Gastric ulcers: 40 mg/day for 4-8 weeks

(Continued)

## Omeprazole *(Continued)*

**Elderly:** Refer to adult dosing.

**Renal Impairment:** No adjustment necessary.

**Hepatic Impairment:** No adjustment necessary.

**Administration**

**Oral:** Capsule should be swallowed whole. Do not chew, crush, or open. Administration via NG tube should be in an acidic juice.

**Stability**

**Storage:** Omeprazole stability is a function of pH; it is rapidly degraded in acidic media, but has acceptable stability under alkaline conditions. Prilosec™ is supplied as capsules for oral administration; each capsule contains 20 mg of omeprazole in the form of enteric coated granules to inhibit omeprazole degradation by gastric acidity; therefore, the manufacturer recommends against extemporaneously preparing it in an oral liquid form for administration via an NG tube.

**Additional Nursing Issues**

**Physical Assessment:** Assess other medications patient may be taking, especially those dependent on cytochrome P-450 metabolism (eg, phenytoin, digoxin, warfarin), or those requiring an acid environment for absorption (eg, ketoconazole, ampicillin, digoxin). Monitor for CNS changes (eg, dizziness, asthenia), cardiac arrhythmias (tachycardia, bradycardia), and fluid balance (I & O ratio). **Pregnancy risk factor C** - benefits of use should outweigh possible risks. Breast-feeding is contraindicated.

**Patient Information/Instruction:** Take as directed, before eating. Do not crush or chew capsules. You may experience anorexia; small frequent meals may help to maintain adequate nutrition. Report changes in urination or pain on urination, unresolved severe diarrhea, testicular pain, or changes in respiratory status. **Pregnancy/breast-feeding precautions:** Inform prescriber if you are or intend to be pregnant. Discontinue breast-feeding prior to starting this medication.

**Geriatric Considerations:** The incidence of side effects in the elderly is no different than that of younger adults (≤65 years of age) despite slight decrease in elimination and increase in bioavailability. Bioavailability may be increased in the elderly (≥65 years of age), however, dosage adjustments are not necessary.


- **Omifin** *see* Clomiphene *on page 286*
- **OmniHIB®** *see page 1256*
- **Omnipen®** *see* Ampicillin *on page 90*
- **Omnipen®-N** *see* Ampicillin *on page 90*
- **OMS® Oral** *see* Morphine Sulfate *on page 790*
- **Oncaspar®** *see* Pegaspargase *on page 890*
- **Oncovin® Injection** *see* Vincristine *on page 1213*


## Ondansetron (on DAN se tron)

**U.S. Brand Names** Zofran®, Zofran® ODT

**Therapeutic Category** Selective 5-$HT_3$ Receptor Antagonist

**Pregnancy Risk Factor** B

**Lactation** Excretion in breast milk unknown/opportunity for use is minimal

**Use** May be prescribed for patients who are refractory to or have severe adverse reactions to standard antiemetic therapy. Ondansetron may be prescribed for young patients (ie, <45 years of age who are more likely to develop extrapyramidal reactions to high-dose metoclopramide) who are to receive highly emetogenic chemotherapeutic agents.

**Mechanism of Action/Effect** Selective 5-$HT_3$ receptor antagonist, blocking serotonin, both peripherally on vagal nerve terminals and centrally in the chemoreceptor trigger zone

**Contraindications** Hypersensitivity to ondansetron or any component

**Warnings** **Ondansetron should be used on a scheduled basis, not as an "as needed" (PRN) basis,** since data supports the use of this drug in the prevention of nausea and vomiting and not in the rescue of nausea and vomiting. Ondansetron should only be used in the first 24-48 hours of receiving chemotherapy. Data does not support any increased efficacy of ondansetron in delayed nausea and vomiting.

**Drug Interactions**

**Cytochrome P-450 Effect:** CYP1A2, 2D6, 2E1, and 3A3/4 enzyme substrate

**Decreased Effect:** Metabolized by the hepatic cytochrome P-450 enzymes; therefore, the drug's clearance and half-life may be changed with concomitant use of cytochrome P-450 inducers (eg, barbiturates, carbamazepine, rifampin, phenytoin, and phenylbutazone).

**Increased Effect/Toxicity:** Increased toxicity with inhibitors (eg, cimetidine, allopurinol, and disulfiram).

**Adverse Reactions**

>10%: Central nervous system: Headache, drowsiness,

1% to 10%:

Cardiovascular: Bradycardia, hypotension
Central nervous system: Dizziness, fatigue
Dermatologic: Pruritus
Gastrointestinal: Constipation, diarrhea, abdominal pain, dry mouth
Hepatic: Transient elevations of AST/ALT
Neuromuscular & skeletal: Weakness

<1% (Limited to important or life-threatening symptoms): Tachycardia, chest pain, EKG changes, seizures, bronchospasm, shortness of breath, wheezing

**Pharmacodynamics/Kinetics**

**Protein Binding:** 70% to 76%

**Half-life Elimination:** 4 hours

**Metabolism:** Liver

**Excretion:** Urine and feces

**Onset:** Within 30 minutes

**Formulations**

Ondansetron hydrochloride:

Injection: 2 mg/mL (20 mL); 32 mg (single-dose vials)

Oral Solution: 4 mg/5 mL (5 mg as HCl)

Tablet: 4 mg, 8 mg

Orally disintegrating tablets: 4 mg, 8 mg

**Dosing**

**Adults:** This drug should be administered on a scheduled basis (not prn) during the first 24-48 hours of chemotherapy.

Oral: 8 mg 30 minutes before chemotherapy; repeat 4 and 8 hours after initial dose or every 8 hours for a maximum of 48 hours.

I.V.: Administer either three 0.15 mg/kg doses or a single 32 mg dose. With the 3-dose regimen, the initial dose is given 30 minutes prior to chemotherapy with subsequent doses administered 4 and 8 hours after the first dose. With the single-dose regimen 32 mg is infused over 15 minutes beginning 30 minutes before the start of emetogenic chemotherapy. Dosage should be calculated based on weight:

>80 kg: 12 mg IVPB

45-80 kg: 8 mg IVPB

<45 kg: 0.15 mg/kg/dose IVPB

**Elderly:** Refer to adult dosing.

**Hepatic Impairment:** Maximum daily dose: 8 mg in cirrhotic patients with severe liver disease

**Administration**

**I.V.:** First dose should be given 30 minutes prior to beginning chemotherapy.

I.V.: Inject over 2-5 minutes.

IVPB: Inject over 15 minutes.

**Stability**

**Storage:** Injection may be stored between 36°F and 86°F.

**Reconstitution:** Stable when mixed in 5% dextrose or 0.9% sodium chloride for 48 hours at room temperature. Does not need protection from light.

**Additional Nursing Issues**

**Physical Assessment:** See Dosing for appropriate scheduling and administration. Monitor for effectiveness of therapy and adverse reactions (see above). Monitor and instruct patient to monitor possible side effects and symptoms to report. Caution patient to request assistance due to possible dizziness, hypotension, or muscular weakness. Note breast-feeding caution.

**Patient Information/Instruction:** This drug may cause drowsiness; use caution when driving or engaging in tasks that require alertness until response to drug is known. You may experience constipation and headache (request appropriate treatment from prescriber). Do not change position rapidly (rise slowly). Good mouth care and sucking on lozenges may help relieve nausea. Report persistent headache, excessive drowsiness, fever, numbness or tingling, or severe changes in elimination patterns (constipation or diarrhea), chest pain, or palpitations. **Breast-feeding precautions:** Consult prescriber if breast-feeding.

**Geriatric Considerations:** Elderly have a slightly decreased hepatic clearance rate. This does not, however, require a dose adjustment.

**Additional Information** pH: 3.3-4.0

**Related Information**

Antiemetics for Chemotherapy-Induced Nausea and Vomiting *on page 1307*

- **Ony-Clear® Nail Aerosol** *see page 1294*
- **Ony-Clear® Spray** *see* Miconazole *on page 767*
- **Onyvul®** *see* Urea *on page 1193*
- **OPC-17116** *see* Grepafloxacin *on page 545*
- **Opcon®** *see page 1282*
- **Opcon® Ophthalmic** *see page 1294*
- **o,p′-DDD** *see* Mitotane *on page 779*
- **Operand®** *see page 1294*
- **Ophthalgan® Ophthalmic** *see page 1294*
- **Ophthalmic Agents** *see page 1282*

## Ophthalmic Agents, Glaucoma (op THAL mik AY gents, glaw COE ma)

**U.S. Brand Names** Adsorbocarpine® Ophthalmic; Akarpine® Ophthalmic; AKBeta® Ophthalmic; AKPro® Ophthalmic; Alphagan® Ophthalmic; Azopt® Ophthalmic; Betagan® Liquifilm® Ophthalmic; Betimol® Ophthalmic; Betoptic® Ophthalmic; Betoptic® S Ophthalmic; Carbastat® Ophthalmic; Carboptic® Ophthalmic; Epifrin®; Epinal®; Floropryl® Ophthalmic; Glaucon®; Humorsol® Ophthalmic; Iopidine®; Isopto® Carbachol Ophthalmic; Isopto® Carpine Ophthalmic; Isopto® Eserine; Miostat® Intraocular; Ocupress® Ophthalmic; Ocusert Pilo-20® Ophthalmic; Ocusert Pilo-40® Ophthalmic; OptiPranolol® Ophthalmic; Phospholine Iodide® Ophthalmic; Pilagan® Ophthalmic; Pilocar® Ophthalmic; Pilopine HS® Ophthalmic; Piloptic® Ophthalmic; Pilostat® Ophthalmic; Propine® Ophthalmic; Timoptic® OcuDose®; Timoptic® Ophthalmic; Timoptic-XE® Ophthalmic; Trusopt® Ophthalmic; Xalatan® Ophthalmic

(Continued)

## Ophthalmic Agents, Glaucoma *(Continued)*

**Synonyms** Apraclonidine; Betaxolol; Brimonidine; Brinzolamide; Carbachol; Carteolol; Demercarium; Dipiverin; Dorzolamide; Echothiophate; Epinephrine; Eserine Sulfate; Isoflurophate; Latanoprost; Levobunolol; Metipranolol; Physostigmine; Pilocarpine; Timolol

**Therapeutic Category** Ophthalmic Agent

**Pregnancy Risk Factor** C/B (sympathomimetics)

**Use** Lowering intraocular pressure in patients with chronic, open-angle glaucoma or ocular hypertension

**Mechanism of Action/Effect**

Dirrect-acting cholinergic agents: Direct-acting cholinergic stimulation resulting in increased outflow of aqueous humor, and possibly some decrease in production. These effects decrease intraocular pressure.

Acetylcholinesterase inhibitors: Inhibition of acetylcholinesterase increases the persistence of local acetylcholine concentrations, resulting in cholinergic effects. These effects include an increase in the outflow of aqueous humor, reducing intraocular pressure.

Sympathomimetics: Stimulate alpha- or beta-adrenoreceptors to increase outflow of aqueous humor, reducing intraocular pressure.

Carbonic anhydrase inhibitors: Inhibition of carbonic anhydrase decreases production of aqueous humor secretion and results in a reduction in intraocular pressure.

Beta-blockers: Lowers intraocular pressure by reducing production of aqueous humor and possibly increases outflow of aqueous humor.

**Contraindications** Hypersensitivity to the individual drug or any component; individual formulations may contain sulfites or benzalkonium chloride

Direct-acting cholinergic agents and acetylcholinesterase inhibitors: Acute inflammatory disease of the anterior chamber, acute iritis

Sympathomimetics: Angle-closure glaucoma

Beta-blockers: Second and third degree A-V block, severe asthma, severe congestive heart failure, cardiogenic shock, severe COPD

**Warnings** Systemic absorption may lead to hypersensitivity reactions and/or systemic effects. Do not administer while wearing contact lenses.

Direct-acting cholinergic agents and acetylcholinesterase inhibitors: Use with caution in the presence of corneal abrasion or in patients undergoing general anesthesia, peptic ulcer, narrow-angle glaucoma, Parkinson's disease, or urinary tract obstruction.

Sympathomimetics: Use with caution in patients with hypertension, dysrhythmias, or cardiac disease. Dipiverin contains sodium metabisulfite.

Carbonic anhydrase inhibitors: Use with caution in renal or hepatic impairment (agents and metabolites may accumulate), sulfonamide allergy (due to cross-reactivity). Use with oral carbonic anhydrase inhibitors is not recommended. Dorzolamide contains benzalkonium chloride.

Beta-blockers: Use with caution in patients with congestive heart failure, asthma, diabetes mellitus, heart block, bradycardia, thyroid disease, or peripheral vascular disease.

**Adverse Reactions** Representative profiles of adverse effects are listed by pharmacologic category. Consult complete product prescribing information for individual products.

**Direct-acting cholinergic agents and acetylcholinesterase inhibitors:**

>10%:

Ocular: Blurred vision

1% to 10%:

Central nervous system: Headache

Genitourinary: Polyuria

Ocular: Burning, stinging, ciliary spasm, retinal detachment, photophobia, acute iritis, lacrimation, conjunctival and ciliary congestion (early in therapy)

<1% (Limited to important or life-threatening symptoms): Hypertension, tachycardia, nausea, vomiting, diarrhea, salivation, diaphoresis

**Sympathomimetic agents:**

>10%:

Central nervous system: Headache, fatigue, drowsiness

Gastrointestinal: Xerostomia

Ocular: Burning, stinging, ocular hyperemia, blurring, ocular allergic reactions, ocular pruritus

1% to 10%:

Central nervous system: Dizziness

Gastrointestinal: Taste disturbances

Ocular: Blepharitis, ocular irritation, corneal staining, photophobia, eyelid erythema, eyelid edema, ocular pain, ocular dryness, tearing, abnormal vision, lid crusting, conjunctival hemorrhage, ocular discharge, bulbar conjunctival follicles

Respiratory: Upper respiratory symptoms

<1% (Limited to important or life-threatening symptoms): Allergic reactions, diarrhea, tachycardia, hypotension, arrhythmias

**Carbonic anhydrase inhibitors:**

1% to 10%:

Gastrointestinal: Bitter taste

Ocular: Burning, stinging, discomfort, blurred vision, tearing, dryness, photophobia, superficial punctate, keratitis, ocular allergic irritation

<1% (Limited to important or life-threatening symptoms): Headache, fatigue, rash, nausea, urolithiasis, weakness, iridocyclitis, electrolyte disturbance

**Beta-blockers:**

>10%: Ocular: Burning, stinging

1% to 10%:

Cardiovascular: Bradycardia, arrhythmia, hypotension

Central nervous system: Dizziness, headache

Dermatologic: Alopecia, erythema

Ocular: Blepharoconjunctivitis, conjunctivitis

Respiratory: Bronchospasm

<1% (Limited to important or life-threatening symptoms): Rash, pruritus, visual disturbances, keratitis

### Pharmacodynamics/Kinetics

**Distribution:**

Brinzolamide and dorzolamide: Accumulate in red blood cells, binding to carbonic anhydrase (brinzolamide and metabolite)

**Half-life Elimination:**

Betaxolol: 12-22 hours (after oral administration)

Carteolol: 6 hours (after oral administration)

Dorzolamide: Terminal RBC half-life of 147 days

Latanoprost: 17 minutes

Metipranolol: ~3 hours

Physostigmine: 15-40 minutes

Timolol: 2-2.7 hours; prolonged with reduced renal function

**Onset:**

Apraclonidine: Ophthalmic: 1 hour; maximum IOP: 3-5 hours

Betaxolol: Ophthalmic: 30 minutes

Brimonidine: 1-4 hours

Carbachol: Ophthalmic instillation: Onset of miosis: 10-20 minutes; Intraocular administration: Onset of miosis: Within 2-5 minutes

Dipiverin: Ocular pressure effect: Within 30 minutes; Mydriasis: May occur within 30 minutes

Dorzolamide: Peak effect: 2 hours

Echothiophate: Miosis: 10-30 minutes; Intraocular pressure decrease: 4-8 hours; Peak intraocular pressure decrease: 24 hours

Epinephrine: Conjunctival instillation: Intraocular pressure falls within 1 hour; Peak effect: Within 4-8 hours

Isoflurophate: Peak IOP reduction: 24 hours; Onset of miosis: Within 5-10 minutes

Latanoprost: 3-4 hours; Maximum effect: 8-12 hours

Levobunolol: Decrease in intraocular pressure (IOP) can be noted within 1 hour; Peak effect: 2-6 hours

Metipranolol: ≤30 minutes; Maximum effect: ~2 hours

Pilocarpine:

Ophthalmic instillation: Miosis: Within 10-30 minutes; Intraocular pressure reduction: 1 hour required

Ocusert® Pilo application: Miosis: 1.5-2 hours; Reduced intraocular pressure: Within 1.5-2 hours; miosis within 10-30 minutes

Physostigmine: Within 2 minutes

**Duration:**

Betaxolol: 12 hours

Brimonidine: 12 hours

Brinzolamide: 8-12 hours

Carbachol: Duration of reduction in intraocular pressure: 4-8 hours; Intraocular administration: 24 hours

Carteolol: 12 hours

Dipiverin: Ocular pressure effect: ≥12 hours; Mydriasis: Several hours

Dorzolamide: 8-12 hours

Echothiophate: Up to 1-4 weeks

Epinephrine: Conjunctival instillation: Duration of ocular effect: 12-24 hours

Isoflurophate: IOP reduction: 1 week; Miosis: Up to 4 weeks

Levobunolol: 1-7 days

Metipranolol: Intraocular pressure reduction has persisted for 24 hours following ocular instillation.

Pilocarpine:

Ophthalmic instillation: Miosis: 4-8 hours; Intraocular pressure reduction: 4-12 hours

Ocusert® Pilo application: Reduced intraocular pressure: ~1 week

Physostigmine: 12-48 hours

Timolol: ~4 hours; intraocular effects persist for 24 hours after ophthalmic instillation

### Formulations

**Apraclonidine, hydrochloride:** 0.5% (5 mL); 1% (0.1 mL, 0.25 mL)

**Betaxolol, hydrochloride:**

Solution (Betoptic®): 0.5% (2.5 mL, 5 mL, 10 mL)

Suspension (Betoptic® S): 0.25% (2.5 mL, 10 mL, 15 mL)

**Brimonidine, tartrate:** Solution: 0.2% (5 mL, 10 mL)

**Brinzolamide:** Suspension: 1% (2.5 mL, 5 mL, 10 mL, 15 mL)

**Carbachol:**

Solution:

Intraocular (Carbastat®, Miostat®): 0.01% (1.5 mL)

Topical:

Carboptic®: 3% (15 mL)

Isopto® Carbachol: 0.75% (15 mL, 30 mL); 1.5% (15 mL, 30 mL); 2.25% (15 mL); 3% (15 mL, 30 mL)

**Carteolol, hydrochloride:** Solution (Ocupress®): 1% (5 mL, 10 mL)

(Continued)

## Ophthalmic Agents, Glaucoma *(Continued)*

**Demercarium, bromide:** Solution: 0.125% (5 mL); 0.25% (5 mL)
**Dipiverin, hydrochloride:** Solution: 0.1% (5 mL, 10 mL, 15 mL)
**Dorzolamide, hydrochloride:** Solution: 2%
**Echothiophate:** Powder for reconstitution: 1.5 mg [0.03%] (5 mL); 3 mg [0.06%] (5 mL); 6.25 mg [0.125%] (5 mL); 12.5 mg [0.25%] (5 mL)
**Epinephrine:**
Solution, as hydrochloride (Epifrin®, Glaucon®): 0.1% (1 mL, 30 mL); 0.5% (15 mL); 1% (1 mL, 10 mL, 15 mL); 2% (10 mL, 15 mL)
Solution, as borate (Epinal®): 0.5% (7.5 mL); 1% (7.5 mL)
**Isoflurophate:** Ointment: 0.025% in polyethylene mineral oil gel (3.5 g)
**Latanoprost:** 0.005% (2.5 mL)
**Levobunolol, hydrochloride:** Solution: 0.25% (5 mL, 10 mL, 15 mL); 0.5% (2 mL, 5 mL, 10 mL, 15 mL)
**Metipranolol, hydrochloride:** Solution: 0.3% (5 mL, 10 mL)
**Physostigmine, sulfate:** Ointment: 0.25% (3.5 g, 3.7 g)
**Pilocarpine, hydrochloride:**
Gel, as hydrochloride (Pilopine HS®): 4% (3.5 g)
Ocular therapeutic system (Ocusert® Pilo): Releases 20 or 40 mcg per hour for 1 week (8s)
Solution, as hydrochloride (Adsorbocarpine®, Akarpine®, Isopto® Carpine, Pilagan®, Pilocar®, Piloptic®, Pilostat®): 0.25% (15 mL); 0.5% (15 mL, 30 mL); 1% (1 mL, 2 mL, 15 mL, 30 mL); 2% (1 mL, 2 mL, 15 mL, 30 mL); 3% (15 mL, 30 mL); 4% (1 mL, 2 mL, 15 mL, 30 mL); 5% (15 mL); 6% (15 mL, 30 mL); 8% (2 mL); 10% (15 mL)
Solution, as nitrate (Pilagan®): 1% (15 mL); 2% (15 mL); 4% (15 mL)
**Timolol:**
Gel, as maleate (Timoptic-XE®): 0.25% (2.5 mL, 5 mL); 0.5% (2.5 mL, 5 mL)
Solution, as hemihydrate (Betimol®): 0.25% (2.5 mL, 5 mL, 10 mL, 15 mL); 0.5% (2.5 mL, 5 mL, 10 mL, 15 mL)
Solution, as maleate (Timoptic®): 0.25% (2.5 mL, 5 mL, 10 mL, 15 mL); 0.5% (2.5 mL, 5 mL, 10 mL, 15 mL)
Solution, as maleate, preservative free, single use (Timoptic® OcuDose®): 0.25%, 0.5%

### Dosing

**Adults:**

**Apraclonidine:** Instill 1 drop in operative eye 1 hour prior to laser surgery, second drop in eye upon completion of procedure.
**Betaxolol:** Instill 1 drop twice daily.
**Brimonidine:** Instill 1 drop in affected eye(s) 3 times/day (approximately every 8 hours).
**Brinzolamide:** Instill 1 drop in affected eye(s) 3 times/day.
**Carbachol:**
Ophthalmic: Instill 1-2 drops up to 3 times/day.
Intraocular: Instill 0.5 mL into anterior chamber before or after securing sutures.
**Carteolol:** Instill 1 drop in affected eye(s) twice daily.
**Demercarium:**
Glaucoma: Instill 1 drop into eyes twice weekly to a maximum dosage of 1 or 2 drops twice daily for up to 4 months.
Strabismus:
Diagnosis: Instill 1 drop daily for 2 weeks, then 1 drop every 2 days for 2-3 weeks. If eyes become straighter, an accommodative factor is demonstrated.
Therapy: Instill not more than 1 drop at a time in both eyes every day for 2-3 weeks. Then reduce dosage to 1 drop every other day for 3-4 weeks and re-evaluate. Continue at 1 drop every 2 days to 1 drop twice a week and evaluate the patient's condition every 4-12 weeks. If improvement continues, reduce dose to 1 drop once a week and eventually stop medication. Discontinue therapy after 4 months if control of the condition still requires 1 drop every 2 days.
**Dipiverin:** Instill 1 drop every 12 hours into the eyes.
**Dorzolamide:** Glaucoma: Instill 1 drop in the affected eye(s) 3 times/day.
**Echothiophate:**
Glaucoma: Instill 1 drop twice daily into eyes with 1 dose just prior to bedtime. Some patients have been treated with 1 dose/day or every other day
Accommodative esotropia:
Diagnosis: Instill 1 drop of 0.125% once daily into both eyes at bedtime for 2-3 weeks.
Treatment: Use lowest concentration and frequency which gives satisfactory response, with a maximum dose of 0.125% once daily, although more intensive therapy may be used for short periods of time.
**Epinephrine:** Instill 1-2 drops in eye(s) once or twice daily.
**Isoflurophate:**
Glaucoma: Instill 0.25" strip in eye every 8-72 hours.
Strabismus: Instill 0.25" strip to each eye every night for 2 weeks then reduce to 0.25" every other night to once weekly for 2 months.
**Latanoprost:** Instill 1 drop in the affected eye(s) once daily in the evening.
**Levobunolol:** Instill 1 drop in the affected eye(s) 1-2 times/day.
**Metipranolol:** Instill 1 drop in the affected eye(s) twice daily.
**Physostigmine:**
Ointment (eserine sulfate): Instill a small quantity to lower fornix up to 3 times/day.
Solution (Isopto® Eserine): Instill 1-2 drops into eye(s) up to 4 times/day.

**Pilocarpine:**
Nitrate solution: Shake well before using; instill 1-2 drops 2-4 times/day.
Hydrochloride solution:
Instill 1-2 drops up to 6 times/day; adjust the concentration and frequency as required to control elevated intraocular pressure.
To counteract the mydriatic effects of sympathomimetic agents: Instill 1 drop of a 1% solution in the affected eye.
Gel: Instill 0.5" ribbon into lower conjunctival sac once daily at bedtime.
Ocular systems: Systems are labeled in terms of mean rate of release of pilocarpine over 7 days; begin with 20 mcg/hour at night and adjust based on response.
**Timolol:** Initial: 0.25% solution, instill 1 drop twice daily; increase to 0.5% solution if response not adequate; decrease to 1 drop/day if controlled; do not exceed 1 drop twice daily of 0.5% solution.

**Administration**
**Other:** After instillation, apply finger pressure over nasolacrimal duct to decrease systemic absorption.

**Stability**
**Storage:** Store solutions at room temperature. Refrigerate pilocarpine gel.

**Additional Nursing Issues**
**Physical Assessment:** See Drug Interactions, Contraindications, and Warnings/Precautions for cautious use. Monitor for therapeutic effectiveness (periodic intraocular pressure, fundoscopic exam, or visual field testing) at regular intervals with long-term therapy. Assess knowledge/teach patient appropriate use, interventions to reduce side effects, and adverse symptoms to report (see Warnings/Precautions, Adverse Reactions, and Overdose/Toxicology). **Pregnancy risk factor C/B** - benefits of use should outweigh possible risks.
**Patient Information/Instruction:** For ophthalmic use only. Apply prescribed amount as often as directed. Wash hands before using and do not touch tip of applicator to eye or contaminate tip of applicator. Tilt head back and look upward. Gently pull down lower lid and put drop(s) inside lower eyelid at inner corner. Close eye and roll eyeball in all directions. Do not blink for ½ minute. Apply gentle pressure to inner corner of eye for 30 seconds. Wipe away excess from skin around eye. Do not use any other eye preparation for at least 10 minutes. Do not share medication with anyone else. Temporary stinging or blurred vision may occur. Immediately report any adverse cardiac or CNS effects (usually signifies overdose). Report persistent eye pain, redness, burning, watering, dryness, double vision, puffiness around eye, vision disturbances, other adverse eye response, or worsening of condition or lack of improvement. **Pregnancy/breast-feeding precautions:** Inform prescriber if you are or intend to be pregnant.
**Geriatric Considerations:** Because systemic absorption does occur with ophthalmic administration, the elderly with other disease states or syndromes that may be affected by an individual agent (cholinergic drugs with Parkinson's, beta-blockers in bradycardia, CHF, COPD, etc) should be monitored closely.

**Additional Information** Some formulations may contain sulfites. The salicylate injection contains benzyl alcohol.

Ocusert® 20 mcg is approximately equivalent to 0.5% or 1% drops.
Ocusert® 40 mcg is approximately equivalent to 2% or 3% drops.

**Related Information**
Glaucoma Drug Comparison *on page 1385*

♦ **Ophthetic®** *see page 1248*
♦ **Opium and Belladonna** *see* Belladonna and Opium *on page 136*

## Opium Tincture (OH pee um TING chur)

**Synonyms** Deodorized Opium Tincture; DTO
**Therapeutic Category** Analgesic, Narcotic; Antidiarrheal
**Pregnancy Risk Factor** B/D (if used for prolonged periods or in high doses at term)
**Lactation** Enters breast milk/use caution
**Use** Treatment of diarrhea or relief of pain
**Mechanism of Action/Effect** Contains many narcotic alkaloids including morphine; its mechanism for gastric motility inhibition is primarily due to this morphine content; it results in a decrease in digestive secretions, an increase in GI muscle tone, and therefore a reduction in GI propulsion
**Contraindications** Hypersensitivity to morphine sulfate; increased intracranial pressure; severe respiratory depression; severe liver or renal insufficiency; pregnancy (if used for prolonged periods or in high doses at term)
**Warnings** Opium shares the toxic potential of opiate agonists, and usual precautions of opiate agonist therapy should be observed. Some preparations contain sulfites which may cause allergic reactions. This is **not** paregoric, dose accordingly.

**Drug Interactions**
**Decreased Effect:** Phenothiazines may antagonize the analgesic effect of opiate agonists.
**Increased Effect/Toxicity:** Opium tincture and CNS depressants, MAO inhibitors, tricyclic antidepressants may potentiate the effects of opiate agonists (eg, codeine, morphine, etc). Dextroamphetamine may enhance the analgesic effect of opiate agonists.

**Effects on Lab Values** ↑ aminotransferase [ALT (SGPT)/AST (SGOT)] (S)

**Adverse Reactions**
>10%:
Cardiovascular: Hypotension
Central nervous system: Fatigue, drowsiness
(Continued)

## Opium Tincture *(Continued)*

Neuromuscular & skeletal: Weakness

1% to 10%:

Central nervous system: Nervousness, headache, restlessness, malaise, confusion, false sense of well-being

Gastrointestinal: Dry mouth

Genitourinary: Ureteral spasms, decreased urination

Local: Pain at injection site

Neuromuscular & skeletal: Trembling

Ocular: Blurred vision

Miscellaneous: Histamine release

<1% (Limited to important or life-threatening symptoms): Tachycardia or bradycardia, dyspnea, shortness of breath

**Overdose/Toxicology** Primary attention should be directed to ensuring adequate respiratory exchange. Naloxone, 2 mg I.V. with repeat administration as necessary up to a total of 10 mg, can also be used to reverse toxic effects of the opiate.

**Pharmacodynamics/Kinetics**

**Metabolism:** Liver

**Excretion:** Urine

**Duration:** 4-5 hours

**Formulations** Liquid: 10% [0.6 mL equivalent to morphine 6 mg] with alcohol 19%

**Dosing**

**Adults:** Oral:

Diarrhea: 0.3-1 mL/dose every 2-6 hours to maximum of 6 mL/24 hours

Analgesia: 0.6-1.5 mL/dose every 3-4 hours

**Additional Nursing Issues**

**Physical Assessment:** Assess other medications patient may be taking for additive or adverse interactions (see Drug Interactions). Monitor for effectiveness of pain relief and monitor for signs of overdose (see above). Monitor blood pressure, CNS and respiratory status, and degree of sedation at beginning of therapy and at regular intervals with long-term use. May cause physical and/or psychological dependence. For inpatients, implement safety measures (eg, side rails up, call light within reach, instructions to call for assistance, etc). Assess knowledge/teach patient appropriate use (if self-administered). Teach patient to monitor for adverse reactions (see Adverse Reactions), adverse reactions to report, and appropriate interventions to reduce side effects. Discontinue slowly after prolonged use. **Pregnancy risk factor B/D** - see Pregnancy Risk Factor for cautious use. Note breast-feeding caution.

**Patient Information/Instruction:** If self-administered, use exactly as directed (do not increase dose or frequency); may cause physical and/or psychological dependence. While using this medication, do not use alcohol and other prescription or OTC medications (especially sedatives, tranquilizers, antihistamines, or pain medications) without consulting prescriber. Maintain adequate hydration (2-3 L/day of fluids unless instructed to restrict fluid intake). May cause hypotension, dizziness, drowsiness, impaired coordination, or blurred vision (use caution when driving, climbing stairs, or changing position - rising from sitting or lying to standing, or when engaging in tasks requiring alertness until response to drug is known); dry mouth (frequent mouth care, small frequent meals, chewing gum, or sucking lozenges may help). Report slow or rapid heartbeat, acute dizziness, or persistent headache; changes in mental status; swelling of extremities or unusual weight gain; changes in urinary elimination or pain on urination; acute headache; trembling or muscle spasms; blurred vision; skin rash; or shortness of breath. **Pregnancy/breast-feeding precautions:** Inform prescriber if you are or intend to be pregnant. If you are breast-feeding, take medication immediately after breast-feeding or 3-4 hours prior to next feeding.

**Additional Information** Some formulations may contain ethanol.

- ♦ **Opthaflox** *see* Ciprofloxacin *on page 270*
- ♦ **Opticrom®** *see* Cromolyn Sodium *on page 309*
- ♦ **Opticrom® Ophthalmic Solution** *see* Cromolyn Sodium *on page 309*
- ♦ **Opticyl®** *see page 1248*
- ♦ **Opticyl®** *see page 1282*
- ♦ **Optigene® Ophthalmic** *see page 1294*
- ♦ **Optimine®** *see* Azatadine *on page 123*
- ♦ **OptiPranolol® Ophthalmic** *see* Ophthalmic Agents, Glaucoma *on page 853*
- ♦ **Optised® Ophthalmic** *see page 1294*
- ♦ **Orabase®-B [OTC]** *see* Benzocaine *on page 141*
- ♦ **Orabase® HCA** *see* Hydrocortisone *on page 578*
- ♦ **Orabase®-O [OTC]** *see* Benzocaine *on page 141*
- ♦ **Orabase® Plain** *see page 1294*
- ♦ **Orabase® With Benzocaine Paste** *see page 1294*
- ♦ **Oracit®** *see* Sodium Citrate and Citric Acid *on page 1063*
- ♦ **Orafen** *see* Ketoprofen *on page 645*
- ♦ **Orafer®** *see* Iron Supplements *on page 627*
- ♦ **Orajel® Brace-Aid Oral Anesthetic [OTC]** *see* Benzocaine *on page 141*
- ♦ **Orajel® Maximum Strength [OTC]** *see* Benzocaine *on page 141*
- ♦ **Orajel® Mouth-Aid [OTC]** *see* Benzocaine *on page 141*
- ♦ **Orajel® Perioseptic** *see page 1294*

## Oral Contraceptives (OR al kon tra SEP tivs)

**U.S. Brand Names** Alesse™; Brevicon®; CombiPatch®; Demulen®; Desogen®; Estrostep®; Estrostep® Fe; Genora® 0.5/35; Genora® 1/35; Genora® 1/50; Jenest-28™; Levlen®; Levora®; Loestrin®; Loestrin® Fe; Lo/Ovral®; Mircette™; Modicon™; N.E.E.® 1/35; Nelova™ 0.5/35E; Nelova™ 1/35E; Nelova™ 1/50M; Nelova™ 10/11; Nordette®; Norethin™ 1/35E; Norethin™ 1/50M; Norinyl® 1+35; Norinyl® 1+50; Ortho-Cept®; Ortho-Cyclen®; Ortho-Novum® 1/35; Ortho-Novum® 1/50; Ortho-Novum® 7/7/7; Ortho-Novum® 10/11; Ortho Tri-Cyclen®; Ovcon® 35; Ovcon® 50; Ovral®; Ovrette®; Tri-Levlen®; Tri-Norinyl®; Triphasil®; Zovia®

**Synonyms** Desogestrel and Ethinyl Estradiol; Ethinyl Estradiol and Ethynodiol Diacetate; Ethinyl Estradiol and Levonorgestrel; Ethinyl Estradiol and Norethindrone; Ethinyl Estradiol and Norgestrel; Ethynodiol Diacetate and Ethinyl Estradiol; Levonorgestrel and Ethinyl Estradiol; Mestranol and Norethindrone; Mestranol and Norethynodrel; Norethindrone Acetate and Ethinyl Estradiol; Norgestimate and Ethinyl Estradiol; Norgestrel; Norgestrel and Ethinyl Estradiol

**Therapeutic Category** Contraceptive, Oral

**Pregnancy Risk Factor** X

**Lactation** Enters breast milk/use caution

**Use** Prevention of pregnancy; treatment of hypermenorrhea, endometriosis, female hypogonadism; ethinyl estradiol and norgestrel formulations are also used for postcoital contraception

**Mechanism of Action/Effect** Combination oral contraceptives inhibit ovulation via a negative feedback mechanism on the hypothalamus, which alters the normal pattern of gonadotropin secretion of a follicle-stimulating hormone (FSH) and luteinizing hormone by the anterior pituitary. The follicular phase FSH and midcycle surge of gonadotropins are inhibited. In addition, oral contraceptives produce alterations in the genital tract, including changes in the cervical mucus rendering it unfavorable for sperm penetration even if ovulation occurs. Changes in the endometrium may also occur, producing an unfavorable environment for nidation. Oral contraceptive drugs may alter the tubal transport of the ova through the fallopian tubes. Progestational agents may also alter sperm fertility.

**Contraindications** Hypersensitivity to active ingredient (ethinyl estradiol, norgestrel, desogestrel, ethynodiol diacetate, levonorgestrel, norethindrone, mestranol, norethynodrel, or norgestimate) or any component; known or suspected pregnancy; thromboembolic disorders; cerebrovascular or coronary artery disease; carcinoma of the breast; estrogen-dependent tumor; undiagnosed abnormal vaginal bleeding; coronary artery disease; women smokers >35 years of age

**Warnings** Use of any progestin during the first 4 months of pregnancy is not recommended. Use with caution in patients with asthma, seizure disorders, migraine, cardiac, renal or hepatic impairment, cerebrovascular disorders or history of breast cancer, a history of thromboembolism, stroke, myocardial infarction, liver tumor, or hypertension. Risk of cardiovascular side effects increases in those women who smoke cigarettes or age >35 years. Use lowest estrogen content which produces satisfactory results. Use with caution in women >40 years of age. May increase the risk of breast, cervical, or hepatic cancer.

Progestin: Use with caution in patients with a history of mental depression.

**Drug Interactions**

**Decreased Effect:** Decreased effect (possible pregnancy) of oral contraceptives with barbiturates, hydantoins (phenytoin, rifampin), antibiotics (penicillins, tetracyclines, griseofulvin). Ritonavir may reduce the effect of ethinyl estradiol which may result in loss of contraception.

**Increased Effect/Toxicity:** Oral contraceptives may increase toxicity of acetaminophen, anticoagulants, benzodiazepines, caffeine, corticosteroids, metoprolol, theophylline, and tricyclic antidepressants.

**Food Interactions** CNS effects of caffeine may be enhanced if oral contraceptives are used concurrently with caffeine.

**Effects on Lab Values** ↑ platelet aggregation, thyroid binding globulin, total thyroid hormone ($T_4$), serum triglycerides/phospholipids; ↓ antithrombin III, serum folate concentration

**Adverse Reactions**

>10%:

- Cardiovascular: Peripheral edema
- Endocrine & metabolic: Enlargement of breasts, breast tenderness
- Gastrointestinal: Nausea, anorexia, bloating

1% to 10%:

- Central nervous system: Headache
- Endocrine & metabolic: Increased libido
- Gastrointestinal: Vomiting, diarrhea

<1% (Limited to important or life-threatening symptoms): Hypertension (greatest in older women with continued use), thromboembolism, stroke, myocardial infarction, edema, depression, anxiety, chloasma, melasma, rash, decreased glucose tolerance (greatest if estrogen dose is >75 mcg), amenorrhea, alterations in frequency and flow of menses, increased triglycerides and LDL, cholestatic jaundice, increased susceptibility to *Candida* infection, breast tumors

See tables.

**Overdose/Toxicology** Toxicity is unlikely following single exposure of excessive doses. Treatment following emesis and charcoal administration should be supportive and symptomatic.

(Continued)

## Oral Contraceptives *(Continued)*

### Achieving Proper Hormonal Balance in an Oral Contraceptive

| Estrogen | | Progestin | |
|---|---|---|---|
| **Excess** | **Deficiency** | **Excess** | **Deficiency** |
| Nausea, bloating<br>Cervical mucorrhea, polyposis<br>Melasma<br>Migraine headache<br>Breast fullness or tenderness<br>Edema | Early or midcycle breakthrough bleeding<br>Increased spotting<br>Hypomenorrhea | Increased appetite<br>Weight gain<br>Tiredness, fatigue<br>Hypomenorrhea<br>Acne, oily scalp*<br>Hair loss, hirsutism*<br>Depression<br>Monilial vaginitis<br>Breast regression | Late breakthrough bleeding<br>Amenorrhea<br>Hypermenorrhea |

*Result of androgenic activity of progestins.

### Pharmacological Effects of Progestins Used in Oral Contraceptives

| | Progestin | Estrogen | Antiestrogen | Androgen |
|---|---|---|---|---|
| Norgestrel/levonorgestrel | +++ | 0 | ++ | +++ |
| Ethynodiol diacetate | ++ | +* | +* | + |
| Norethindrone acetate | + | + | +++ | + |
| Norethindrone | + | +* | +* | + |
| Norethynodrel | + | +++ | 0 | 0 |

*Has estrogenic effect at low doses; may have antiestrogenic effect at higher doses.

+++ = pronounced effect

++ = moderate effect

+ = slight effect

0 = no effect

**Pharmacodynamics/Kinetics**

**Protein Binding:** Ethinyl estradiol: 95%; Desogestrel: 50% to 80%; Levonorgestrel: 75% to 90%; Norethindrone: 60% to 70%

**Half-life Elimination:**

Ethinyl estradiol: 6-26 hours
Ethynodiol diacetate: 5-14 hours
Levonorgestrel: 11-45 hours
Norethindrone: 5-14 hours
Norgestrel: 11-45 hours

**Time to Peak:** Levonorgestrel; Norgestrel Oral: 0.5-2 hours; Norethindrone: Oral: 0.5-4 hours

**Metabolism:** Liver

**Excretion:** Renal and feces

**Formulations**

Tablet:

Alesse™: Ethinyl estradiol 0.02 mg and levonorgestrel 0.1 mg (21s, 28s)

Brevicon®, Genora® 0.5/35, Modicon™, Nelova™ 0.5/35E:
Ethinyl estradiol 0.035 mg and norethindrone 0.5 mg (21s, 28s)

Demulen®; Zovia®
1/35: Ethinyl estradiol 0.035 mg and ethynodiol diacetate 1 mg (21s, 28s)
1/50: Ethinyl estradiol 0.05 mg and ethynodiol diacetate 1 mg (21s, 28s)

Desogen®; Ortho-Cept®
Ethinyl estradiol 0.03 mg and desogestrel 0.15 mg (21s, 28s)

Estrostep®:
Triangular tablet (white): Ethinyl estradiol 0.02 mg and norethindrone acetate 1 mg
Square tablet (white): Ethinyl estradiol 0.03 mg and norethindrone acetate 1 mg
Round tablet (white): Ethinyl estradiol 0.035 mg and norethindrone acetate 1 mg

Estrostep® Fe:
Triangular tablet (white): Ethinyl estradiol 0.02 mg and norethindrone acetate 1 mg
Square tablet (white): Ethinyl estradiol 0.03 mg and norethindrone acetate 1 mg
Round tablet (white): Ethinyl estradiol 0.035 mg and norethindrone acetate 1 mg
Brown tablet: Ferrous fumarate 75 mg

Genora® 1/35, N.E.E.® 1/35, Nelova® 1/35E, Norethin™ 1/35E, Norinyl® 1+35, Ortho-Novum® 1/35:
Ethinyl estradiol 0.035 mg and norethindrone 1 mg (21s, 28s)

Genora® 1/50, Nelova™ 1/50M, Norethin™ 1/50M, Ortho-Novum® 1/50: Mestranol 50 mcg and norethindrone 1 mg

Jenest-28™:
Phase 1 (7 white tablets): Ethinyl estradiol 0.035 mg and norethindrone 0.5 mg
Phase 2 (14 peach tablets): Ethinyl estradiol 0.035 mg and norethindrone 1 mg and 7 green inert tablets (28s)

Levlen®, Levora®, Nordette®
Ethinyl estradiol 0.03 mg and levonorgestrel 0.15 mg (21s, 28s)

Loestrin® 1.5/30:
Ethinyl estradiol 0.03 mg and norethindrone acetate 1.5 mg (21s)

Loestrin® Fe 1.5/30:
- Ethinyl estradiol 0.03 mg and norethindrone acetate 1.5 mg with ferrous fumarate 75 mg in 7 inert tablets (28s)

Loestrin® 1/20:
- Ethinyl estradiol 0.02 mg and norethindrone acetate 1 mg (21s)

Loestrin® Fe 1/20:
- Ethinyl estradiol 0.02 mg and norethindrone acetate 1 mg with ferrous fumarate 75 mg in 7 inert tablets (28s)

Lo/Ovral®:
- Ethinyl estradiol 0.03 mg and norgestrel 0.3 mg (21s and 28s)

Ortho-Cyclen®:
- Ethinyl estradiol 0.035 mg and norgestimate 0.25 mg (21s, 28s)

Ortho Tri-Cyclen®:
- Phase 1 (7 white tablets): Ethinyl estradiol 0.035 mg and norgestimate 0.18 mg
- Phase 2 (5 light blue tablets): Ethinyl estradiol 0.035 mg and norgestimate 0.215 mg
- Phase 3 (10 blue tablets): Ethinyl estradiol 0.035 mg and norgestimate 0.25 mg (21s, 28s)

Ortho-Novum® 7/7/7:
- Phase 1 (7 white tablets): Ethinyl estradiol 0.035 mg and norethindrone 0.5 mg
- Phase 2 (7 light peach tablets): Ethinyl estradiol 0.035 mg and norethindrone 0.75 mg
- Phase 3 (7 peach tablets): Ethinyl estradiol 0.035 mg and norethindrone 1 mg (21s, 28s)

Ortho-Novum® 10/11, Nelova® 10/11:
- Phase 1 (10 white tablets): Ethinyl estradiol 0.035 mg and norethindrone 0.5 mg
- Phase 2 (11 dark yellow tablets): Ethinyl estradiol 0.035 mg and norethindrone 1 mg (21s, 28s)

Ovcon® 35:
- Ethinyl estradiol 0.035 mg and norethindrone 0.4 mg (21s, 28s)

Ovcon® 50:
- Ethinyl estradiol 0.050 mg and norethindrone 1 mg (21s, 28s)

Ovral®:

Ovrette®, Norgestrel®: 0.075 mg
- Ethinyl estradiol 0.05 mg and norgestrel 0.5 mg (21s and 28s)

Preven™: Ethinyl estradiol 0.05 mg and levonorgestrel 0.25 mg

Tri-Levlen®, Triphasil®
- Phase 1 (6 brown tablets): Ethinyl estradiol 0.03 mg and levonorgestrel 0.05 mg
- Phase 2 (5 white tablets): Ethinyl estradiol 0.04 mg and levonorgestrel 0.075 mg
- Phase 3 (10 yellow tablets): Ethinyl estradiol 0.03 mg and levonorgestrel 0.125 mg (21s, 28s)

Tri-Norinyl®:
- Phase 1 (7 blue tablets): Ethinyl estradiol 0.035 mg and norethindrone 0.5 mg
- Phase 2 (9 green tablets): Ethinyl estradiol 0.035 mg and norethindrone 1 mg
- Phase 3 (5 blue tablets): Ethinyl estradiol 0.035 mg and norethindrone 0.5 mg (21s, 28s)

**Dosing**

**Adults:**

Oral contraception:

**Monophasic formulations** (Brevicon®, Demulen®, Genora®, Jenest-28™ Levlen®, Modicon™, Necon®, Nelova™, Nordette®, Norethin™, Norinyl®, Ortho-Novum®, Ovcon®, Zovia®):

1 tablet daily, beginning on day 5 of menstrual cycle (first day of menstrual flow is day 1). With 21-tablet packages, new dosing cycle begins 7 days after last tablet taken; with 28-tablet packages, dosage is 1 tablet daily without interruption; extra tablets are placebos or contain iron. If next menstrual period does not begin on schedule, rule out pregnancy before starting new dosing cycle; if menstrual period begins, start new dosing cycle 7 days after last tablet was taken; if all doses have been taken on schedule and one menstrual period is missed, continue dosing cycle; if two consecutive menstrual periods are missed, pregnancy test is required before new dosing cycle is started.

**Missed doses monophasic formulations** (refer to package insert for complete information):

One dose missed: Take as soon as remembered or take 2 tablets next day.

Two doses missed: Take 2 tablets as soon as remembered or 2 tablets next 2 days. Use a backup method of contraception (condom or spermicide foam) for 7 days after missed dose.

Three doses missed: Begin new compact of tablets starting on day 1 (for day 1 starters) of next cycle. Use a backup method of contraception (condom or spermicide foam) for 7 days after missed dose.

**Biphasic formulations** (Jenest™-28, Ortho-Novum™ 10/11, Nelova™ 10/11): With 21 tablet: 1 first color tablet/day for 10 days, then next color tablet for 11 days.

**Triphasic formulations** (Ortho-Novum™ 7/7/7, Tri-Norinyl®, Triphasil®): 1 tablet/day in the sequence specified by the manufacturer

**Missed doses biphasic/triphasic formulations (Necon® 10/11, Nelova™ 10/11, Ortho-Novum® 10/11, Ortho-Novum™ 7/7/7, Tri-Norinyl®, Triphasil®, Tri-Levlen®)** (refer to package insert for complete information):

One dose missed: Take as soon as remembered or take 2 tablets next day.

Two doses missed in week 1 or 2 of the pack: Take 2 tablets as soon as remembered and 2 tablets the next day. Resume taking 1 pill a day until you finish the pack. You may become pregnant if you have sex during the 7 days

(Continued)

## Oral Contraceptives *(Continued)*

after a missed dose. You **must** use another form of contraception, sponge or condom.

Two doses missed in week 3 of the pack (Day 1 Starter): Throw out the remaining pack and start a new pack of pills the same day. You may become pregnant if you have sex during the 7 days after a missed dose. You **must** use another form of contraception, sponge or condom.

Two doses missed in week 3 of the pack (Sunday Starter): Take 1 tablet every day until Sunday. Discard the remaining pack and start a new pack of pills on the same day. You may become pregnant if you have sex during the 7 days after a missed dose. You must use another form of contraception, sponge or condom.

Three or more doses missed (Day 1 Starter): Throw out rest of the pack and begin new compact of tablets starting on the same day.

Three or more doses missed (Sunday Starter): Take 1 pill every day until Sunday. On Sunday discard the pack and start a new pack. You may become pregnant if you have sex during the 7 days after a missed dose. Use another form of contraception, sponge or condom. Consult package labeling for additional information.

**Postcoital contraception "morning after" pill:**

Ovral®: 2 tablets within 72 hours of intercourse and 2 tablets 12 hours later

LoOvral®, Nordette®, Levlen®, Triphasil®, Tri-Levlen®: 4 tablets within 72 hours of intercourse and 4 tablets 12 hours later

Preven™: 2 tablets within 72 hours of intercourse and 2 tablets 12 hours later

**Monitoring Laboratory Tests** Pap smear and pregnancy tests prior to beginning therapy

**Additional Nursing Issues**

**Physical Assessment:** Monitor or teach patient to monitor blood pressure on a regular basis. Monitor or teach patient to monitor for occurrence of adverse effects and symptoms to report (eg, thromboembolic disease, visual changes, neuromuscular weakness - see above). Assess knowledge/teach importance of regular (monthly) blood pressure checks and annual physical assessment, Pap smear, and vision assessment. Teach importance of maintaining prescribed schedule of dosing (see Dosing for dosing and missed dose information). **Pregnancy risk factor X** - do not use if patient is pregnant. Note breast-feeding caution.

**Patient Information/Instruction:** Take exactly as directed by prescriber (also see package insert). You are at risk of becoming pregnant if doses are missed. If you miss a dose, take as soon as possible or double the dose next day. If more than three doses are missed, contact prescriber for restarting directions. Use additional form of contraception during first week of taking this medication. Detailed and complete information on dosing and missed doses can be found in the package insert. Be aware that some medications may reduce the effectiveness of oral contraceptives; an alternate form of contraception may be needed (see Drug Interactions).

It is important that you check your blood pressure monthly (on same day each month) and that you have an annual physical assessment, Pap smear, and vision assessment while taking this medication.

Avoid smoking while taking this medication; smoking increases risk or adverse effects, including thromboembolic events and heart attacks. You may experience loss of appetite (small frequent meals will help); constipation (increased fluids, exercise, and dietary fiber, or stool softeners may help). Diabetics should use accurate serum glucose testing to identify any changes in glucose tolerance; notify prescriber of significant changes so antidiabetic medication can be adjusted if necessary. Report immediately pain or muscle soreness; swelling, heat, or redness in calves; shortness of breath; sudden loss of vision; unresolved leg or foot swelling; change in menstrual pattern (unusual bleeding, amenorrhea, breakthrough spotting); breast tenderness that does not go away; acute abdominal cramping; signs of vaginal infection (drainage, pain, itching); changes in CNS (blurred vision, confusion, acute anxiety, or unresolved depression); or significant weight gain (>5 lb/week).

**Pregnancy/breast-feeding precautions:** This drug may cause severe fetal complication. If you suspect you may be pregnant, contact prescriber immediately. Consult prescriber if breast-feeding.


- **Oraminic® II** *see page 1294*
- **Oramorph SR™ Oral** *see* Morphine Sulfate *on page 790*
- **Oranor** *see* Norfloxacin *on page 837*
- **Orap™** *see* Pimozide *on page 932*
- **Orasept® [OTC]** *see* Benzocaine *on page 141*
- **Orasol® [OTC]** *see* Benzocaine *on page 141*
- **Orasone®** *see* Prednisone *on page 962*
- **Orazinc® [OTC]** *see* Zinc Supplements *on page 1230*
- **Orazinc® Oral** *see page 1294*
- **Orbenin®** *see* Cloxacillin *on page 295*
- **Orciprenaline Sulfate** *see* Metaproterenol *on page 732*
- **Ordrine AT® Extended Release Capsule** *see* Caramiphen and Phenylpropanolamine *on page 195*
- **Oretic®** *see* Hydrochlorothiazide *on page 566*
- **Oreton® Methyl** *see* Methyltestosterone *on page 756*
- **Orex®** *see page 1294*

- ♦ **Orexin**® *see page 1294*
- ♦ **Organidin**® **NR** *see* Guaifenesin *on page 548*
- ♦ **Orgaran**® *see* Danaparoid *on page 330*
- ♦ **Orinase**® **Diagnostic Injection** *see* Tolbutamide *on page 1146*
- ♦ **Orinase**® **Oral** *see* Tolbutamide *on page 1146*


## Orlistat (OR li stat)

**Therapeutic Category** Lipase Inhibitor

**Pregnancy Risk Factor** B (see Breast-feeding Considerations)

**Lactation** Excretion in breast milk unknown/not recommended

**Use** Management of obesity, including weight loss and weight management when used in conjunction with a reduced-calorie diet; reduce the risk of weight regain after prior weight loss; indicated for obese patients with an initial body mass index (BMI) ≥30 kg/m² or ≥27 kg/m² in the presence of other risk factors; see table

**Body Mass Index (BMI), kg/m²**
**Height (feet, inches)**

| Weight (lb) | 5'0" | 5'3" | 5'6" | 5'9" | 6'0" | 6'3" |
|---|---|---|---|---|---|---|
| 140 | 27 | 25 | 23 | 21 | 19 | 18 |
| 150 | 29 | 27 | 24 | 22 | 20 | 19 |
| 160 | 31 | 28 | 26 | 24 | 22 | 20 |
| 170 | 33 | 30 | 28 | 25 | 23 | 21 |
| 180 | 35 | 32 | 29 | 27 | 25 | 23 |
| 190 | 37 | 34 | 31 | 28 | 26 | 24 |
| 200 | 39 | 36 | 32 | 30 | 27 | 25 |
| 210 | 41 | 37 | 34 | 31 | 29 | 26 |
| 220 | 43 | 39 | 36 | 33 | 30 | 28 |
| 230 | 45 | 41 | 37 | 34 | 31 | 29 |
| 240 | 47 | 43 | 39 | 36 | 33 | 30 |
| 250 | 49 | 44 | 40 | 37 | 34 | 31 |

**Contraindications** Hypersensitivity to orlistat or any component; chronic malabsorption syndrome or cholestasis

**Warnings** Patients should be advised to adhere to dietary guidelines; gastrointestinal adverse events may increase if taken with a diet high in fat (>30% total daily calories from fat). The daily intake of fat should be distributed over three main meals. If taken with any one meal very high in fat, the possibility of gastrointestinal effects increases. Patients should be counseled to take a multivitamin supplement that contains fat-soluble vitamins to ensure adequate nutrition because orlistat has been shown to reduce the absorption of some fat-soluble vitamins and beta-carotene. The supplement should be taken once daily at least 2 hours before or after the administration of orlistat (ie, bedtime). Some patients may develop increased levels of urinary oxalate following treatment; caution should be exercised when prescribing it to patients with a history of hyperoxaluria or calcium oxalate nephrolithiasis. As with any weight-loss agent, the potential exists for misuse in appropriate patient populations (eg, patients with anorexia nervosa or bulimia).

**Drug Interactions**

**Increased Effect/Toxicity:** Vitamin K absorption may be decreased when taken with orlistat.

**Adverse Reactions**

Central nervous system: Headache, dizziness, sleep disorder, anxiety, depression

Dermatitis: Dry skin, rash

Gastrointestinal: Oily spotting, flatus with discharge, fecal urgency, fatty/oily stool, oily evacuation, increased defecation, fecal incontinence

Neuromuscular & skeletal: Back pain, pain of lower extremities, arthritis, myalgia, joint disorder, tendonitis

Otic: Otitis

Respiratory: Influenza; respiratory tract infection; ear, nose, and throat symptoms

**Overdose/Toxicology** Single doses of 800 mg and multiple doses of up to 400 mg 3 times daily for 15 days have been studied in normal weight and obese patients without significant adverse findings. In case of significant overdose, it is recommended that the patient be observed for 24 hours.

**Formulations** Capsule: 120 mg

**Dosing**

**Adults:** 120 mg 3 times daily with each main meal containing fat (during or up to 1 hour after the meal); omit dose if meal is occasionally missed or contains no fat.

**Elderly:** Refer to adult dosing.

**Monitoring Laboratory Tests** Changes in coagulation parameters

**Additional Nursing Issues**

**Physical Assessment:** Assess effectiveness of other medications (especially anticoagulants - see Drug Interactions). Monitor effectiveness of therapy, laboratory results, and adverse reactions at beginning of therapy and periodically during therapy (see Adverse Reactions). Assess knowledge/teach patient appropriate use, possible side effects and interventions, and adverse symptoms to report. Breast-feeding is not recommended.

(Continued)

## Orlistat *(Continued)*

**Patient Information/Instruction:** Take this medication exactly as ordered; do not alter prescribed dose without consulting prescriber. Maintain prescribed diet (high fat meals may result in GI distress), exercise regimen, and vitamin supplements as prescribed. You may experience dizziness or lightheadedness (use caution when driving or engaging in tasks requiring alertness until response to drug is known) or increased flatus and fecal urgency (this may lessen with continued use). Report persistent back, muscle, or joint pain; signs of respiratory tract infection or flu-like symptoms; skin rash or irritation; or other reactions. **Breast-feeding precautions:** Breast-feeding is not recommended.

**Breast-feeding Issues:** There are no adequate and well-controlled studies of orlistat in pregnant women. Because animal reproductive studies are not always predictive of human response, orlistat is not recommended for use during pregnancy. Teratogenicity studies were conducted in rats and rabbits at doses up to 800 mg/kg/day. Neither study showed embryotoxicity or teratogenicity. This dose is 23 and 47 times the daily human dose calculated on a body surface area basis for rats and rabbits, respectively.

- **Ormazine** *see* Chlorpromazine *on page 256*
- **Ornade® Spansule®** *see page 1294*
- **Ornex® No Drowsiness** *see page 1294*

## Orphenadrine (or FEN a dreen)

**U.S. Brand Names** Norflex™

**Therapeutic Category** Anti-Parkinson's Agent (Anticholinergic); Skeletal Muscle Relaxant

**Pregnancy Risk Factor** C

**Lactation** Excretion in breast milk unknown

**Use** Treatment of muscle spasm associated with acute painful musculoskeletal conditions; supportive therapy in tetanus

**Mechanism of Action/Effect** Indirect skeletal muscle relaxant thought to work by central atropine-like effects; has some euphorogenic and analgesic properties

**Contraindications** Hypersensitivity to orphenadrine or any component; glaucoma; GI obstruction; cardiospasm; myasthenia gravis

**Warnings** Use with caution in patients with CHF or cardiac arrhythmias. Some products contain sulfites. Pregnancy factor C.

**Drug Interactions**

**Cytochrome P-450 Effect:** CYP2B6, 2D6, and 3A3/4 enzyme substrate; CYP2B6 enzyme inhibitor

**Adverse Reactions**

1% to 10%:

Cardiovascular: Flushing of face, tachycardia, syncope, pounding heartbeat

Central nervous system: Confusion, dizziness, drowsiness, headache, stimulation (paradoxical)

Dermatologic: Rash

Gastrointestinal: Nausea, vomiting, constipation, stomach cramps

Genitourinary: Decreased urination

Neuromuscular & skeletal: Trembling

Ocular: Nystagmus, increased intraocular pressure, blurred vision

Respiratory: Nasal congestion

<1% (Limited to important or life-threatening symptoms): Aplastic anemia

**Overdose/Toxicology** Symptoms of overdose include blurred vision, tachycardia, confusion, seizures, respiratory arrest, and dysrhythmias. There is no specific treatment for antihistamine overdose. Clinical toxicity is due to blockade of cholinergic receptors. Lethal dose is 2-3 g; treatment is generally symptomatic. For anticholinergic overdose with severe life-threatening symptoms, physostigmine 1-2 mg I.V. slowly, may be given to reverse these effects.

**Pharmacodynamics/Kinetics**

**Protein Binding:** 20%

**Half-life Elimination:** 14-16 hours

**Metabolism:** Extensive

**Excretion:** Urine

**Onset:** Peak effect: Oral: Within 2-4 hours

**Duration:** 4-6 hours

**Formulations**

Orphenadrine citrate:

Injection: 30 mg/mL (2 mL, 10 mL)

Tablet: 100 mg

Tablet, sustained release: 100 mg

**Dosing**

**Adults:**

Oral: 100 mg twice daily

I.M., I.V.: 60 mg every 12 hours

**Elderly:** Not recommended for use in the elderly; see Geriatric Considerations.

**Administration**

**Oral:** Do not crush sustained release drug product.

**Additional Nursing Issues**

**Physical Assessment:** See Warnings/Precautions and Contraindications for use cautions. Monitor effectiveness of therapy (according to rational for therapy), and adverse reactions (see Adverse Reactions) at beginning of therapy and periodically with long-term use. Do not discontinue abruptly; taper dosage slowly. Assess knowledge/teach patient appropriate use, interventions to reduce side effects (postural hypotension precautions), and adverse symptoms to report. **Pregnancy risk factor C** - benefits of use should outweigh possible risks. Note breast-feeding caution.

**Patient Information/Instruction:** Take exactly as directed. Do not increase dose or discontinue without consulting prescriber. Do not chew or crush sustained release tablets. Do not use alcohol, prescriptive or OTC antidepressants, sedatives, or pain medications without consulting prescriber. You may experience drowsiness, dizziness, lightheadedness (avoid driving or engaging in tasks requiring alertness until response to drug is known); nausea or vomiting (small, frequent meals, frequent mouth care, or sucking hard candy may help); constipation (increased dietary fluids and fibers or increased exercise may help); or decreased urination (void before taking medication). Report excessive drowsiness or mental agitation, chest pain, skin rash, swelling of mouth/face, difficulty speaking, or vision disturbances. **Pregnancy/breast-feeding precautions:** Inform prescriber if you are or intend to be pregnant. Consult prescriber if breast-feeding.

**Geriatric Considerations:** Because of its anticholinergic side effects, orphenadrine is not a drug of choice in the elderly.

**Additional Information** The injection formulation contains sulfites.

## Orphenadrine, Aspirin, and Caffeine

(or FEN a dreen, AS pir in, & KAF een)

**U.S. Brand Names** Norgesic® Forte; Norgesic®

**Synonyms** Aspirin, Orphenadrine, and Caffeine; Caffeine, Orphenadrine, and Aspirin

**Therapeutic Category** Skeletal Muscle Relaxant

**Pregnancy Risk Factor** D

**Lactation** Enters breast milk/use caution due to aspirin content

**Use** Relief of discomfort associated with skeletal muscular conditions

**Formulations**

Tablet: Orphenadrine citrate 25 mg, aspirin 385 mg, and caffeine 30 mg

Tablet (Norgesic® Forte): Orphenadrine citrate 50 mg, aspirin 770 mg, and caffeine 60 mg

**Dosing**

**Adults:** Oral: 1-2 tablets 3-4 times/day

**Elderly:** Not recommended for use in the elderly; refer to individual monographs.

**Additional Nursing Issues**

**Physical Assessment:** See individual components listed in Related Information. **Pregnancy risk factor D** - assess knowledge/instruct patient on need to use appropriate contraceptive measures and the need to avoid pregnancy. Note breast-feeding caution.

**Patient Information/Instruction:** See individual components listed in Related Information. **Pregnancy/breast-feeding precautions:** Inform prescriber if you are or intend to be pregnant. Consult prescriber if breast-feeding.

**Related Information**

Aspirin *on page 111*
Orphenadrine *on previous page*

- **Ortho® 0.5/35** *see* Oral Contraceptives *on page 859*
- **Ortho-Cept®** *see* Oral Contraceptives *on page 859*
- **Orthoclone® OKT3** *see* Muromonab-CD3 *on page 793*
- **Ortho-Cyclen®** *see* Oral Contraceptives *on page 859*
- **Ortho® Dienestrol Vaginal** *see* Dienestrol *on page 365*
- **Ortho-Est® Oral** *see* Estropipate *on page 452*
- **Ortho-Novum® 1/35** *see* Oral Contraceptives *on page 859*
- **Ortho-Novum® 1/50** *see* Oral Contraceptives *on page 859*
- **Ortho-Novum® 7/7/7** *see* Oral Contraceptives *on page 859*
- **Ortho-Novum® 10/11** *see* Oral Contraceptives *on page 859*
- **Ortho Tri-Cyclen®** *see* Oral Contraceptives *on page 859*
- **Or-Tyl® Injection** *see* Dicyclomine *on page 362*
- **Orudis®** *see* Ketoprofen *on page 645*
- **Orudis® KT [OTC]** *see* Ketoprofen *on page 645*
- **Oruvail®** *see* Ketoprofen *on page 645*
- **Os-Cal® 500 [OTC]** *see* Calcium Supplements *on page 185*
- **Osmitrol® Injection** *see* Mannitol *on page 706*
- **Osmoglyn® Ophthalmic** *see page 1294*
- **Osteocalcin® Injection** *see* Calcitonin *on page 182*
- **Ostoforte®** *see* Ergocalciferol *on page 432*
- **Otic Agents** *see page 1291*
- **Oticair®** *see page 1291*
- **Otic-Care®** *see page 1291*
- **Otic Domeboro®** *see page 1291*
- **Oti Tricin®** *see page 1291*
- **Otobiotic® Otic** *see page 1291*
- **Otocalm®** *see page 1291*
- **Otocalm® Ear** *see page 1306*
- **Otocort®** *see page 1291*

- ♦ **Otomycin-HPN®** *see page 1291*
- ♦ **Otosporin®** *see page 1291*
- ♦ **Otrivin® Nasal** *see page 1294*
- ♦ **Otrozol** *see* Metronidazole *on page 763*
- ♦ **Ovcon® 35** *see* Oral Contraceptives *on page 859*
- ♦ **Ovcon® 50** *see* Oral Contraceptives *on page 859*
- ♦ **Overdose and Toxicology** *see page 1439*
- ♦ **Ovide™ Topical Lotion** *see page 1294*
- ♦ **Ovol®** *see page 1294*
- ♦ **Ovral®** *see* Oral Contraceptives *on page 859*
- ♦ **Ovrette®** *see* Oral Contraceptives *on page 859*
- ♦ **O-V Staticin®** *see* Nystatin *on page 843*


## Oxacillin (oks a SIL in)

**U.S. Brand Names** Bactocill®; Prostaphlin®

**Synonyms** Methylphenyl Isoxazolyl Penicillin; Sodium Oxacillin

**Therapeutic Category** Antibiotic, Penicillin

**Pregnancy Risk Factor** B

**Lactation** Enters breast milk/compatible

**Use** Treatment of bacterial infections such as osteomyelitis, septicemia, endocarditis, and CNS infections due to susceptible strains of *Staphylococcus*

**Mechanism of Action/Effect** Inhibits bacterial cell wall synthesis by binding to one or more of the penicillin binding proteins (PBPs); which in turn inhibits the final transpeptidation step of peptidoglycan synthesis in bacterial cell walls, thus inhibiting cell wall biosynthesis. Bacteria eventually lyse due to ongoing activity of cell wall autolytic enzymes (autolysins and murein hydrolases) while cell wall assembly is arrested.

**Contraindications** Hypersensitivity to oxacillin, any component, penicillins, cephalosporins, or imipenem

**Warnings** Modify dosage in patients with renal impairment and in the elderly.

**Drug Interactions**

**Decreased Effect:** Efficacy of oral contraceptives may be reduced when taken with oxacillin.

**Increased Effect/Toxicity:** Probenecid increases penicillin levels. Penicillins and anticoagulants may increase the effect of anticoagulants.

**Food Interactions** Oxacillin serum levels may be decreased if taken with food.

**Effects on Lab Values** May interfere with urinary glucose tests using cupric sulfate (Benedict's solution, Clinitest®); may inactivate aminoglycosides *in vitro*; false-positive urinary and serum proteins

**Adverse Reactions**

>10%:

- Central nervous system: Headache
- Gastrointestinal: Nausea (mild), vomiting
- Miscellaneous: Oral candidiasis, vaginal candidiasis

1% to 10%:

- Dermatologic: Urticaria, exfoliative dermatitis
- Miscellaneous: Allergic reactions, specifically anaphylaxis; serum sickness-like reactions

<1% (Limited to important or life-threatening symptoms): Seizures, leukopenia, neutropenia, thrombocytopenia, jaundice, hepatotoxicity, interstitial nephritis, *Clostridium difficile* colitis

**Overdose/Toxicology** Symptoms of penicillin overdose include neuromuscular hypersensitivity (eg, agitation, hallucinations, asterixis, encephalopathy, confusion, and seizures). Electrolyte imbalance may occur if the preparation contains potassium or sodium salts, especially in renal failure. Hemodialysis may be helpful to aid in removal of the drug from blood; otherwise, treatment is supportive or symptom directed.

**Pharmacodynamics/Kinetics**

**Distribution:** Into bile, synovial and pleural fluids, bronchial secretions; also distributes to peritoneal and pericardial fluids; crosses the placenta; penetrates the blood-brain barrier only when meninges are inflamed

**Half-life Elimination:** Absorption: Oral: 35% to 67%; Adults: 23-60 minutes (prolonged with reduced renal function and in neonates)

**Time to Peak:** Oral: Within 2 hours; I.M.: Within 30-60 minutes

**Metabolism:** Liver

**Excretion:** Urine and bile

**Formulations**

Oxacillin sodium:

- Capsule: 250 mg, 500 mg
- Powder for injection: 250 mg, 500 mg, 1 g, 2 g, 4 g, 10 g
- Powder for oral solution: 250 mg/5 mL (100 mL)

**Dosing**

**Adults:**

- Oral: 500-1000 mg every 4-6 hours for at least 5 days
- I.M., I.V.: 250 mg to 2 g/dose every 4-6 hours

**Elderly:** Refer to adult dosing.

**Renal Impairment:**

- $Cl_{cr}$ <10 mL/minute: Use lower range of the usual dosage.
- Not dialyzable (0% to 5%)

**Administration**

**Oral:** Take on an empty stomach 1 hour before meals or 2 hours after meals. Take all medication; do not skip doses.

**I.V.:** Administer around-the-clock to promote less variation in peak and trough serum levels. Administer IVP over 10 minutes. Administer IVPB over 30 minutes.

**I.V. Detail:** Rapid administration may result in seizures.

**Stability**

**Reconstitution:** Reconstituted parenteral solution is stable for 3 days at room temperature and 7 days when refrigerated. For I.V. infusion in NS or $D_5W$, solution is stable for 6 hours at room temperature.

**Monitoring Laboratory Tests** Perform culture and sensitivity studies prior to initiating therapy.

**Additional Nursing Issues**

**Physical Assessment:** Assess patient reports of allergy or sensitivity before administering. I.V. - monitor infusion site for extravasation. Monitor response to therapy; if no response, therapy should be re-evaluated. Advise females using oral contraceptives to use barrier contraception - oxacillin may reduce effect of oral contraceptives.

**Patient Information/Instruction:** Take at regular intervals around-the-clock, preferably on empty stomach with a full glass of water. Take complete course of treatment as prescribed. You may experience nausea or vomiting; small frequent meals and good mouth care may help. If diabetic, drug may cause false tests with Clinitest® urine glucose monitoring; use of glucose oxidase methods (Clinistix®) or serum glucose monitoring is preferable. This drug may interfere with oral contraceptives; an alternate form of birth control should be used. Report persistent fever, sore throat, sores in mouth, diarrhea, unusual bleeding or bruising, difficulty breathing, or skin rash. Notify prescriber if condition does not respond to treatment.

**Geriatric Considerations:** Oxacillin has not been studied in the elderly. Dosing adjustments are not necessary except in renal failure (eg, $Cl_{cr}$ <10 mL/minute).

**Breast-feeding Issues:** No adverse effects have been reported in the nursing infant. Theoretically, the antibiotic effect of oxacillin may appear in the infant and change the bowel flora or affect culture results.

**Additional Information**

Sodium content of 1 g: 2.8-3.1 mEq

pH: 6-8.5

## Oxaprozin (oks a PROE zin)

**U.S. Brand Names** Daypro™

**Therapeutic Category** Nonsteroidal Anti-Inflammatory Agent (NSAID)

**Pregnancy Risk Factor** C/D (3rd trimester or near delivery)

**Lactation** Excretion in breast milk unknown/not recommended

**Use** Acute and long-term use in the management of signs or symptoms of osteoarthritis and rheumatoid arthritis

**Mechanism of Action/Effect** Inhibits prostaglandin synthesis by decreasing the activity of the enzyme, cyclo-oxygenase, which results in decreased formation of prostaglandin precursors

**Contraindications** Hypersensitivity to oxaprozin; aspirin allergy; pregnancy (3rd trimester or near delivery); history of GI disease; renal or hepatic dysfunction; bleeding disorders; cardiac failure; elderly; debilitated

**Warnings** Pregnancy factor C (1st and 2nd trimesters).

**Drug Interactions**

**Increased Effect/Toxicity:** Increased toxicity with aspirin, oral anticoagulants, and diuretics.

**Adverse Reactions**

1% to 10%:

Central nervous system: Sleep disturbance, CNS inhibition

Dermatologic: Rash

Gastrointestinal: nausea, vomiting, abdominal cramps, dyspepsia, anorexia, flatulence

Genitourinary: Dysuria, frequency

Otic: Tinnitus

<1% (Limited to important or life-threatening symptoms): Anaphylaxis, serum sickness, edema blood pressure changes, peptic ulcer, GI bleeding, abnormal LFT's, stomatitis, rectal bleeding, pancreatitis, anemia, thrombocytopenia, leukopenia, ecchymosis, agranulocytosis, pancytopenia, weight gain, weight loss, weakness, malaise, pruritus, urticaria, photosensitivity, exfoliative dermatitis, erythema multiforme, Stevens-Johnson syndrome, toxic epidermal necrolysis, blurred vision, conjunctivitis, acute interstitial nephritis, nephrotic syndrome, renal insufficiency, decreased menstrual flow, shortness of breath, wheezing

**Overdose/Toxicology** Symptoms of overdose include acute renal failure, vomiting, drowsiness, and leukocytes. Management of nonsteroidal anti-inflammatory (NSAID) intoxication is supportive and symptomatic. Since many NSAIDs undergo enterohepatic cycling, multiple doses of charcoal may be needed to reduce the potential for delayed toxicities.

(Continued)

## Oxaprozin *(Continued)*

**Pharmacodynamics/Kinetics**

**Protein Binding:** >99%, bound to albumin

**Half-life Elimination:** 40-50 hours

**Metabolism:** Liver

**Excretion:** Urine and feces

**Onset:** Steady-state 4-7 days

**Duration:** Absorption: Almost completely; Protein binding: >99%; Half-life: 40-50 hours; Time to peak: 2-4 hours

**Formulations** Tablet: 600 mg

**Dosing**

**Adults:** Oral (individualize lowest effective dose to minimize adverse effects):

Osteoarthritis: 600-1200 mg once daily

Rheumatoid arthritis: 1200 mg once daily

Maximum: 1800 mg/day or 26 mg/kg (whichever is lower) in divided doses

**Elderly:** Refer to adult dosing; see Additional Information.

**Monitoring Laboratory Tests** CBC; hepatic, renal function

**Additional Nursing Issues**

**Physical Assessment:** Assess effectiveness and interactions of other medications patient may be taking (see Contraindications and Drug Interactions). Monitor laboratory tests (see above) and therapeutic response (eg, relief of pain and inflammation, increased activity tolerance), and adverse reactions (eg, GI effects, hepatotoxicity, or ototoxicity) at beginning of therapy and periodically throughout therapy (see Warnings/Precautions, Adverse Reactions, and Overdose/Toxicology). Schedule ophthalmic evaluations for patients who develop eye complaints during long-term NSAID therapy. Assess knowledge/teach patient appropriate use, interventions to reduce side effects, and adverse symptoms to report. **Pregnancy risk factor C/D** - see Pregnancy Risk Factor - benefits of use should outweigh possible risks. Breast-feeding is not recommended.

**Patient Information/Instruction:** Take this medication exactly as directed; do not increase dose without consulting prescriber. Do not crush tablets or break capsules. Take with food or milk to reduce GI distress. Maintain adequate fluid intake (2-3 L/day of fluids unless instructed to restrict fluid intake). Do not use alcohol, aspirin, or aspirin-containing medication, and all other anti-inflammatory medications without consulting prescriber. You may experience drowsiness, dizziness, or nervousness (use caution when driving or engaging in tasks requiring alertness until response to drug is known); anorexia, nausea, vomiting, or heartburn (frequent small meals, frequent mouth care, sucking lozenges, or chewing gum may help). GI bleeding, ulceration, or perforation can occur with or without pain; discontinue medication and contact prescriber if persistent abdominal pain or cramping, or blood in stool occurs. Report vaginal bleeding; breathlessness, difficulty breathing, or unusual cough; chest pain, rapid heartbeat, palpitations; unusual bruising/bleeding; blood in urine, stool, mouth, or vomitus; swollen extremities; skin rash or itching; acute fatigue; or swelling of face, lips, tongue, or throat. **Pregnancy/breast-feeding precautions:** Inform prescriber if you are or intend to be pregnant. Breast-feeding is not recommended.

**Geriatric Considerations:** Elderly are at high risk for adverse effects from nonsteroidal anti-inflammatory agents. As much as 60% of elderly can develop peptic ulceration and/or hemorrhage asymptomatically. The concomitant use of $H_2$ blockers, omeprazole, and sucralfate is not generally effective as prophylaxis with the exception of NSAID-induced duodenal ulcers which may be prevented by the use of ranitidine. Misoprostol is the only prophylactic agent proven effective. Also, concomitant disease and drug use contribute to the risk for GI adverse effects. Use lowest effective dose for shortest period possible. Consider renal function decline with age. Use of NSAIDs can compromise existing renal function especially when $Cl_{cr}$ is ≤30 mL/minute. Tinnitus may be a difficult and unreliable indication of toxicity due to age-related hearing loss or eighth cranial nerve damage. CNS adverse effects such as confusion, agitation, and hallucination are generally seen in overdose or high-dose situations, but elderly may demonstrate these adverse effects at lower doses than younger adults.

**Additional Information** There are no clinical guidelines to predict which NSAID will give response in a particular patient. Trials with each must be initiated until response determined; consider dose, patient convenience, and cost.

**Related Information**

Nonsalicylate/Nonsteroidal Anti-inflammatory Comparison *on page 1401*

## Oxazepam (oks A ze pam)

**U.S. Brand Names** Serax®

**Therapeutic Category** Benzodiazepine

**Pregnancy Risk Factor** D

**Lactation** Enters breast milk/not recommended

**Use** Treatment of anxiety and management of alcohol withdrawal

**Mechanism of Action/Effect** Benzodiazepine anxiolytic sedative that produces CNS depression at the subcortical level, except at high doses, whereby it works at the cortical level. Like other benzodiazepines it potentiates the actions of gamma amino butyric acid (GABA).

**Contraindications** Hypersensitivity to oxazepam or any component; cross-sensitivity with other benzodiazepines may exist; should not be used in patients with psychoses or severe hypotension; pregnancy

**Warnings** Use with caution in patients using other CNS depressants. Use caution in patients with renal or hepatic impairment. Use with caution in patients with a history of drug dependence. Administer with extreme caution to geriatric patients or patients with compromised pulmonary function.

**Drug Interactions**

**Increased Effect/Toxicity:** Increased toxicity with CNS depressants (eg, barbiturates, morphine), MAO inhibitors, tricyclic antidepressants, alcohol, narcotics, phenothiazines, and other sedative-hypnotics.

**Adverse Reactions**

>10%:

Central nervous system: Drowsiness, ataxia, lightheadedness, headache, dizziness, impaired coordination, anxiety, fatigue, slurred speech, irritability, nervousness, insomnia, memory impairment, cognitive disorder, dysarthria, anxiety

Gastrointestinal: Decreased salivation (dry mouth)

Genitourinary: Micturition difficulties

1% to 10%:

Cardiovascular: Tachycardia, syncope

Central nervous system: Confusion, depersonalization, mental depression, perceptual disturbances, akathisia, agitation, disinhibition, talkativeness, derealization, dream abnormalities, fear

Endocrine & metabolic: Increased libido, decreased libido

Gastrointestinal: Abdominal or stomach cramps, increased or decreased appetite, weight gain or loss, nausea, vomiting

Neuromuscular & skeletal: Muscle cramps, parethesias, weakness

Ocular: Photophobia, blurred vision

Otic: Tinnitus

Respiratory: Nasal congestion

Miscellaneous: Sweating

<1% (Limited to important or life-threatening symptoms): Agranulocytosis, anemia, leukopenia, neutropenia, thrombocytopenia, hepatic dysfunction, dystonic extrapyramidal effects

**Overdose/Toxicology** Symptoms of overdose include somnolence, confusion, coma, hypoactive reflexes, dyspnea, hypotension, slurred speech, and impaired coordination. Treatment for benzodiazepine overdose is supportive. Flumazenil has been shown to selectively block the binding of benzodiazepines to CNS receptors, resulting in a reversal of benzodiazepine-induced CNS depression, but not respiratory depression due to toxicity.

**Pharmacodynamics/Kinetics**

**Half-life Elimination:** 1-2 hours

**Time to Peak:** Within 2-4 hours

**Metabolism:** Liver (primarily as glucuronides)

**Excretion:** Excretion of unchanged drug (50%) and metabolites; excreted without need for liver metabolism

**Formulations**

Capsule: 10 mg, 15 mg, 30 mg

Tablet: 15 mg

**Dosing**

**Adults:** Oral:

Anxiety: 10-30 mg 3-4 times/day

Alcohol withdrawal: 15-30 mg 3-4 times/day

Hypnotic: 15-30 mg

**Elderly:** Oral: Anxiety: 10 mg 2-3 times/day; increase gradually as needed to a total of 30-45 mg/day.

**Renal Impairment:** Not dialyzable (0% to 5%)

**Additional Nursing Issues**

**Physical Assessment:** Assess other medications the patient may be taking for effectiveness and interactions (see Drug Interactions). See Contraindications and Warnings/Precautions for cautious use. Assess for history of addiction; long-term use can result in dependence, abuse, or tolerance; periodically evaluate need for continued use. Monitor therapeutic response (eg, mood, affect, anxiety level, sleep pattern) and adverse reactions at beginning of therapy and periodically with long-term use (see Adverse Reactions and Overdose/Toxicology). Taper dosage slowly when discontinuing. Assess knowledge/teach patient appropriate use, interventions to reduce side effects, and adverse symptoms to report. **Pregnancy risk factor D** - assess knowledge/teach appropriate use of barrier contraceptives. Breast-feeding is not recommended.

**Patient Information/Instruction:** Take exactly as directed (do not increase dose or frequency); may take 2-3 weeks to achieve desired results; may cause physical and/or psychological dependence. Do not use excessive alcohol or other prescription or OTC medications (especially pain medications, sedatives, antihistamines, or hypnotics) without consulting prescriber. Maintain adequate hydration (2-3 L/day of fluids unless instructed to restrict fluid intake). You may experience drowsiness, lightheadedness, impaired coordination, dizziness, or blurred vision (use caution when driving or engaging in tasks requiring alertness until response to drug is known); nausea, vomiting, or dry mouth (small frequent meals, frequent mouth care, chewing gum, or sucking lozenges may help); constipation (increased exercise, fluids, or dietary fruit and fiber may help); altered sexual drive or ability (reversible); or photosensitivity (use sunscreen, wear protective clothing and eyewear, and avoid direct sunlight). Report persistent CNS effects (eg, confusion, depression, increased sedation, excitation, headache, agitation, insomnia or nightmares, dizziness, fatigue, impaired coordination, changes in personality, or changes in cognition); changes in urinary pattern; muscle cramping, weakness, tremors, or rigidity; ringing in ears or visual disturbances; chest

(Continued)

## Oxazepam *(Continued)*

pain, palpitations, or rapid heartbeat; excessive perspiration, excessive GI symptoms (cramping, constipation, vomiting, anorexia); or worsening of condition. **Pregnancy/ breast-feeding precautions:** Do not get pregnant while taking this medication; use appropriate barrier contraceptive measures. Breast-feeding is not recommended.

**Geriatric Considerations:** Because of its relatively short half-life and its lack of active metabolites, oxazepam is recommended for use in the elderly when a benzodiazepine is indicated.

**Other Issues:** Taper dosage gradually after long-term therapy, especially in epileptic patients. Abrupt withdrawal may cause tremors, nausea, vomiting, abdominal and/or muscle cramps.

**Related Information**

Anxiolytic/Hypnotic Use in Long-Term Care Facilities *on page 1430*
Benzodiazepines Comparison *on page 1375*


- ♦ **Oxicanol** *see* Piroxicam *on page 940*
- ♦ **Oxiconazole** *see page 1247*
- ♦ **Oxifungol** *see* Fluconazole *on page 491*
- ♦ **Oxiken** *see* Dobutamine *on page 389*
- ♦ **Oxilapine Succinate** *see* Loxapine *on page 696*
- ♦ **Oxipor® VHC** *see page 1294*
- ♦ **Oxistat®** *see page 1247*
- ♦ **Oxitopisa** *see* Oxytocin *on page 877*
- ♦ **Oxitraklin** *see* Oxytetracycline *on page 876*
- ♦ **Oxpam®** *see* Oxazepam *on page 868*
- ♦ **Oxpentifylline** *see* Pentoxifylline *on page 908*
- ♦ **Oxsoralen® Topical** *see* Methoxsalen *on page 747*
- ♦ **Oxsoralen-Ultra® Oral** *see* Methoxsalen *on page 747*
- ♦ **Oxy-5® Advanced Formula for Sensitive Skin** *see page 1294*
- ♦ **Oxy-5® Tinted** *see page 1294*
- ♦ **Oxy-10® Advanced Formula for Sensitive Skin** *see page 1294*
- ♦ **Oxy 10® Wash** *see page 1294*


## Oxybutynin (oks i BYOO ti nin)

**U.S. Brand Names** Ditropan®; Ditropan XL®

**Therapeutic Category** Antispasmodic Agent, Urinary

**Pregnancy Risk Factor** B

**Lactation** Enters breast milk/contraindicated

**Use** Antispasmodic for neurogenic bladder (urgency, frequency, urge incontinence) and uninhibited bladder

**Mechanism of Action/Effect** Direct antispasmodic effect on smooth muscle, also inhibits the action of acetylcholine on smooth muscle (exhibits $1/5$ the anticholinergic activity of atropine, but is 4-10 times the antispasmodic activity); does not block effects at skeletal muscle or at autonomic ganglia; increases bladder capacity, decreases uninhibited contractions, and delays desire to void; therefore, decreases urgency and frequency

**Contraindications** Hypersensitivity to drug or specific component; glaucoma; myasthenia gravis; partial or complete GI obstruction; GU obstruction; ulcerative colitis (may cause ileus and toxic megacolon); intestinal atony; megacolon; toxic megacolon

**Warnings** Use with caution in patients with urinary tract obstruction, hyperthyroidism, reflux esophagitis, heart disease, hepatic or renal disease, prostatic hypertrophy, autonomic neuropathy, hypertension, hiatal hernia. Caution should be used in the elderly due to anticholinergic activity (eg, confusion, constipation, blurred vision, and tachycardia).

**Drug Interactions**

**Increased Effect/Toxicity:** Additive sedation with CNS depressants and alcohol. Additive anticholinergic effects with antihistamines and anticholinergic agents.

**Effects on Lab Values** May suppress the wheal and flare reactions to skin test antigens.

**Adverse Reactions**

>10%:
- Central nervous system: Drowsiness
- Gastrointestinal: Dry mouth, constipation
- Miscellaneous: Sweating (decreased)

1% to 10%:
- Cardiovascular: Tachycardia, palpitations
- Central nervous system: Dizziness, insomnia, fever, headache
- Dermatologic: Rash
- Endocrine & metabolic: Decreased flow of breast milk, decreased sexual ability, hot flashes
- Gastrointestinal: Nausea, vomiting
- Genitourinary: Urinary hesitancy or retention
- Neuromuscular & skeletal: Weakness
- Ocular: Blurred vision, mydriatic effect

<1% (Limited to important or life-threatening symptoms): Increased intraocular pressure

**Overdose/Toxicology** Symptoms of overdose include hypotension, circulatory failure, psychotic behavior, flushing, respiratory failure, paralysis, tremor, irritability, seizures, delirium, hallucinations, and coma. Treatment is symptomatic and supportive. For anticholinergic overdose with severe life-threatening symptoms, physostigmine 1-2 mg I.V. slowly, may be given to reverse these effects.

**Pharmacodynamics/Kinetics**

**Half-life Elimination:** 1-2.3 hours

**Time to Peak:** Within 60 minutes

**Metabolism:** Liver

**Excretion:** Urine

**Onset:** Oral: 30-60 minutes; Peak effect: 3-6 hours

**Duration:** 6-10 hours

**Formulations**

Oxybutynin chloride:

Syrup: 5 mg/5 mL (473 mL)

Tablet: 5 mg

Tablet, extended release: 5 mg, 10 mg

**Dosing**

**Adults:** Oral:

Adults: 5 mg 2-3 times/day up to maximum of 5 mg 4 times/day

Extended release: Initial: 5 mg once daily, may increase in 5-10 mg increments; maximum: 30 mg daily

**Note**: Should be discontinued periodically to determine whether the patient can manage without the drug and to minimize resistance to the drug

**Elderly:** Oral: 2.5-5 mg twice daily; increase by 2.5 mg increments every 1-2 days. **Note**: Should be discontinued periodically to determine whether the patient can manage without the drug and to minimize resistance to the drug.

**Administration**

**Oral:** Should be administered on an empty stomach with water.

**Additional Nursing Issues**

**Physical Assessment:** Note Contraindications and Warnings/Precautions. Assess other medications patient may be taking for interactions (see Drug Interactions). Assess voiding pattern, incontinent episodes, frequency, urgency, distention, and urinary retention prior to beginning therapy and periodically with long-term use. Assess knowledge/teach patient appropriate use, possible side effects, and symptoms to report. Breast-feeding is contraindicated.

**Patient Information/Instruction:** Take prescribed dose preferably on an empty stomach (1 hour before or 2 hours after meals). You may experience dizziness, lightheadedness, or drowsiness (use caution when driving or engaging in tasks requiring alertness until response to drug is known); dry mouth or changes in appetite (small frequent meals, frequent mouth care, sucking lozenges, or chewing gum may help); constipation (frequent exercise or increased dietary fiber, fruit, and fluid or stool softener may help); decreased sexual ability (reversible with discontinuance of drug); decreased sweating (use caution in hot weather, avoid extreme exercise or activity). Report rapid heartbeat, palpitations, or chest pain; difficulty voiding; or vision changes. Swallow extended-release tablets whole, do not chew or crush. **Breast-feeding precautions:** Do not breast-feed.

**Geriatric Considerations:** Caution should be used in the elderly due to anticholinergic activity (eg, confusion, constipation, blurred vision, and tachycardia). Start with lower doses. Oxybutynin may cause memory problems in the elderly. A study of 12 health volunteers with an average age of 69 showed cognitive decline while taking the drug (*J Am Geriatr Soc*, 1998, L46:8-13).

- **Oxycel®** *see page 1248*
- **Oxycocet** *see* Oxycodone and Acetaminophen *on page 873*
- **Oxycodan** *see* Oxycodone and Aspirin *on page 873*

# Oxycodone (oks i KOE done)

**U.S. Brand Names** OxyContin®; OxyIR™; Percolone™; Roxicodone™

**Synonyms** Dihydrohydroxycodeinone

**Therapeutic Category** Analgesic, Narcotic

**Pregnancy Risk Factor** B/D (if used for prolonged periods or in high doses at term)

**Lactation** Enters breast milk/use caution

**Use** Management of moderate to severe pain; normally used in combination with non-narcotic analgesics

**Mechanism of Action/Effect** Binds to opiate receptors in the CNS, causing inhibition of ascending pain pathways, altering the perception of and response to pain; produces generalized CNS depression

**Contraindications** Hypersensitivity to oxycodone or any component; pregnancy (if used for prolonged periods or in high doses at term)

**Warnings** Use with caution in patients with hypersensitivity reactions to other phenanthrene derivative opioid agonists (morphine, hydrocodone, hydromorphone, levorphanol, oxycodone, oxymorphone), respiratory diseases including asthma, emphysema, COPD, or severe liver or renal insufficiency. May be habit-forming. Some preparations contain sulfites which may cause allergic reactions. Dextromethorphan has equivalent antitussive activity but has much lower toxicity in accidental overdose.

Use with caution in the elderly, debilitated, severe hepatic or renal function, hypothyroidism, Addison's disease, prostatic hypertrophy, or urethral stricture. Respiratory depressant effects and capacity to elevate CSF pressure may be exaggerated in presence of head injury, other intracranial lesion, or pre-existing intracranial pressure.

**Drug Interactions**

**Cytochrome P-450 Effect:** CYP2D6 enzyme substrate

**Decreased Effect:** Phenothiazines may antagonize the analgesic effect of opiate agonists.

(Continued)

## Oxycodone *(Continued)*

**Increased Effect/Toxicity:** MAO inhibitors. may increase adverse symptoms. Cimetidine may increase narcotic analgesic serum levels resulting in toxicity. Alcohol may potentiate adverse effects of oxycodone. When used with methohexital, thiopental, thiamylal, may need to decrease dose to induce anesthesia when narcotic analgesics are also used. CNS depressants, tricyclic antidepressants may potentiate the effects of opiate agonists. Dextroamphetamine may enhance the analgesic effect of opiate agonists.

**Adverse Reactions**

>10%:
- Cardiovascular: Hypotension
- Central nervous system: Fatigue, drowsiness, dizziness
- Gastrointestinal: Nausea, vomiting
- Neuromuscular & skeletal: Weakness

1% to 10%:
- Central nervous system: Nervousness, headache, restlessness, malaise
- Gastrointestinal: Stomach cramps, dry mouth, biliary spasm, constipation
- Genitourinary: Ureteral spasms, decreased urination
- Ocular: Blurred vision
- Miscellaneous: Histamine release

<1% (Limited to important or life-threatening symptoms): Dyspnea, shortness of breath

**Overdose/Toxicology** Symptoms of toxicity include CNS depression, respiratory depression, and miosis. Naloxone, 2 mg I.V. with repeat administration as necessary up to a total of 10 mg, can also be used to reverse toxic effects of the opiate.

**Pharmacodynamics/Kinetics**

**Metabolism:** Liver

**Excretion:** Urine

**Onset:** Oral: Within 10-15 minutes

**Duration:** 4-5 hours; Controlled release: Up to 12 hours

**Formulations**

Oxycodone hydrochloride:
- Capsule, immediate release (OxyIR™): 5 mg
- Liquid, oral: 5 mg/5 mL (500 mL)
- Solution, oral concentrate: 20 mg/mL (30 mL)
- Tablet: 5 mg
  - Percolone™: 5 mg
- Tablet, controlled release (OxyContin®): 10 mg, 20 mg, 40 mg, 80 mg
- Tablet, sustained release (Roxicodone™): 10 mg, 30 mg

**Dosing**

**Adults:**

Oral: 2.5-5 mg every 6 hours as needed

Controlled release:

Opioid naive (not currently on opioid): 10 mg every 12 hours

Currently on opioid/ASA or acetaminophen or NSAID combination:
- 1-5 tablets: 10-20 mg every 12 hours
- 6-9 tablets: 20-30 mg every 12 hours
- 10-12 tablets: 30-40 mg every 12 hours
- May continue the nonopioid as a separate drug.

Currently on opioids: Use standard conversion chart to convert daily dose to oxycodone equivalent. Divide daily dose in 2 (for every 12-hour dosing) and round down to nearest dosage form.

**Elderly:** Refer to adult dosing.

**Hepatic Impairment:** Reduce dosage in patients with severe liver disease.

**Additional Nursing Issues**

**Physical Assessment:** Assess other medications patient may be taking for additive or adverse interactions (see Drug Interactions). Monitor for effectiveness of pain relief and monitor for signs of overdose (see above). Monitor blood pressure, CNS and respiratory status, and degree of sedation at beginning of therapy and at regular intervals with long-term use. May cause physical and/or psychological dependence. For inpatients, implement safety measures (eg, side rails up, call light within reach, instructions to call for assistance, etc). Assess knowledge/teach patient appropriate use (if self-administered). Teach patient to monitor for adverse reactions (see Adverse Reactions), adverse reactions to report, and appropriate interventions to reduce side effects. Discontinue slowly after prolonged use. **Pregnancy risk factor B/D** - see Pregnancy Risk Factor for cautious use. Note breast-feeding caution.

**Patient Information/Instruction:** If self-administered, use exactly as directed (do not increase dose or frequency); may cause physical and/or psychological dependence. While using this medication, do not use alcohol and other prescription or OTC medications (especially sedatives, tranquilizers, antihistamines, or pain medications) without consulting prescriber. Maintain adequate hydration (2-3 L/day of fluids unless instructed to restrict fluid intake). May cause hypotension, dizziness, drowsiness, impaired coordination, or blurred vision (use caution when driving, climbing stairs, or changing position - rising from sitting or lying to standing, or when engaging in tasks requiring alertness until response to drug is known); nausea, vomiting or dry mouth (frequent mouth care, small frequent meals, chewing gum, or sucking lozenges may help); constipation (increased exercise, fluids, or dietary fruit and fiber may help - if constipation remains an unresolved problem, consult prescriber about use of stool softeners). Report persistent dizziness or headache; excessive fatigue or sedation;

changes in mental status; changes in urinary elimination or pain on urination; weakness or trembling; blurred vision; or shortness of breath. **Pregnancy/breast-feeding precautions:** Inform prescriber if you are or intend to be pregnant. If you are breast-feeding, take medication immediately after breast-feeding or 3-4 hours prior to next feeding.

**Geriatric Considerations:** The elderly may be particularly susceptible to the CNS depressant and constipating effects of narcotics.

**Additional Information** Some formulations may contain ethanol. Prophylactic use of a laxative should be considered. Blood level of 5 mg/L has been associated with fatality.

**Related Information**

Controlled Substances Comparison *on page 1379*
Narcotic/Opioid Analgesic Comparison *on page 1396*

## Oxycodone and Acetaminophen (oks i KOE done & a seet a MIN oh fen)

**U.S. Brand Names** Percocet®; Roxicet® 5/500; Roxilox®; Tylox®

**Synonyms** Acetaminophen and Oxycodone

**Therapeutic Category** Analgesic, Combination (Narcotic)

**Pregnancy Risk Factor** C

**Lactation** Enters breast milk/use caution

**Use** Management of moderate to severe pain

**Formulations**

Caplet: Oxycodone hydrochloride 5 mg and acetaminophen 500 mg
Capsule: Oxycodone hydrochloride 5 mg and acetaminophen 500 mg
Solution, oral: Oxycodone hydrochloride 5 mg and acetaminophen 325 mg per 5 mL (5 mL, 500 mL)
Tablet: Oxycodone hydrochloride 5 mg and acetaminophen 325 mg

**Dosing**

**Adults:** Doses should be titrated to appropriate analgesic effects.
Oral: 1-2 tablets every 4-6 hours as needed for pain
Maximum daily dose of acetaminophen: 4 g/day

**Elderly:** Doses should be titrated to appropriate analgesic effects: Oral: 1 tablet or capsule every 6 hours as needed; do not exceed 4 g/day of acetaminophen.

**Hepatic Impairment:** Dose should be reduced in patients with severe liver disease.

**Additional Nursing Issues**

**Physical Assessment:** See individual components listed in Related Information. **Pregnancy risk factor C** - benefits of use should outweigh possible risks. Note breast-feeding caution.

**Patient Information/Instruction:** See individual components listed in Related Information. **Pregnancy/breast-feeding precautions:** Inform prescriber if you are on intend to get pregnant. Consult prescriber if breast-feeding.

**Additional Information** Some formulations may contain sulfites.

**Related Information**

Acetaminophen *on page 32*
Oxycodone *on page 871*

## Oxycodone and Aspirin (oks i KOE done & AS pir in)

**U.S. Brand Names** Codoxy®; Percodan®; Percodan®-Demi; Roxiprin®

**Synonyms** Aspirin and Oxycodone

**Therapeutic Category** Analgesic, Combination (Narcotic)

**Pregnancy Risk Factor** D

**Lactation** Enters breast milk/use caution particularly due to aspirin content

**Use** Relief of moderate to moderately severe pain

**Formulations**

Tablet:
Percodan®: Oxycodone hydrochloride 4.5 mg, oxycodone terephthalate 0.38 mg, and aspirin 325 mg
Percodan®-Demi: Oxycodone hydrochloride 2.25 mg, oxycodone terephthalate 0.19 mg, and aspirin 325 mg

**Dosing**

**Adults:** Oral (based on oxycodone combined salts): Percodan®: 1 tablet every 6 hours as needed for pain or Percodan®-Demi: 1-2 tablets every 6 hours as needed for pain

**Elderly:** Refer to adult dosing.

**Hepatic Impairment:** Dose should be reduced in patients with severe liver disease.

**Additional Nursing Issues**

**Physical Assessment:** See individual components listed in Related Information. **Pregnancy risk factor D** - assess knowledge/instruct patient on need to use appropriate contraceptive measures and the need to avoid pregnancy. Note breast-feeding caution.

**Patient Information/Instruction:** See individual components listed in Related Information. **Pregnancy/breast-feeding precautions:** Inform prescriber if you are on intend to get pregnant. Consult prescriber if breast-feeding.

**Related Information**

Aspirin *on page 111*
Oxycodone *on page 871*

♦ **OxyContin®** *see* Oxycodone *on page 871*
♦ **Oxydess® II** *see* Dextroamphetamine *on page 353*
♦ **OxyIR™** *see* Oxycodone *on page 871*
♦ **Oxymetazoline** *see page 1294*

## Oxymetholone (oks i METH oh lone)

**U.S. Brand Names** Anadrol®

**Therapeutic Category** Anabolic Steroid

**Pregnancy Risk Factor** X

**Lactation** Excretion in breast milk unknown

**Use** Anemias caused by the administration of myelotoxic drugs

**Mechanism of Action/Effect** Stimulates receptors in organs and tissues to promote growth and development of male sex organs and maintains secondary sex characteristics in androgen-deficient males

**Contraindications** Hypersensitivity to oxymetholone or any component; carcinoma of breast or prostate; nephrosis; pregnancy

**Warnings** Anabolic steroids may cause peliosis hepatis, liver cell tumors, and blood lipid changes with increased risk of arteriosclerosis. Monitor diabetic patients carefully. Use with caution in elderly patients, they may be at greater risk for prostatic hypertrophy. Use with caution in patients with cardiac, renal, or hepatic disease or epilepsy.

**Drug Interactions**

**Increased Effect/Toxicity:** Oxymetholone may increase prothrombin times with patients receiving warfarin leading to toxicity. Insulin effects may be enhanced leading to hypoglycemia.

**Effects on Lab Values** Altered glucose tolerance tests, altered thyroid function tests, altered metyrapone tests

**Adverse Reactions**

**Male: Postpubertal:**

>10%:
- Dermatologic: Acne
- Endocrine & metabolic: Gynecomastia
- Genitourinary: Bladder irritability, priapism

1% to 10%:
- Central nervous system: Insomnia, chills
- Endocrine & metabolic: Decreased libido
- Gastrointestinal: Nausea, diarrhea
- Genitourinary: Prostatic hypertrophy (elderly)
- Hematologic: Iron deficiency anemia, suppression of clotting factors
- Hepatic: Hepatic dysfunction

<1% (Limited to important or life-threatening symptoms): Hepatic necrosis, hepatocellular carcinoma

**Male: Prepubertal:**

>10%:
- Dermatologic: Acne
- Endocrine & metabolic: Virilism

1% to 10%:
- Central nervous system: Chills, insomnia
- Dermatologic: Hyperpigmentation
- Gastrointestinal: Diarrhea, nausea
- Hematologic: Iron deficiency anemia, suppression of clotting factors

<1% (Limited to important or life-threatening symptoms): Hepatic necrosis, hepatocellular carcinoma

**Female:**

>10%: Endocrine & metabolic: Virilism

1% to 10%:
- Central nervous system: Chills, insomnia
- Endocrine & metabolic: Hypercalcemia
- Gastrointestinal: Nausea, diarrhea
- Hematologic: Iron deficiency anemia, suppression of clotting factors
- Hepatic: Hepatic dysfunction

<1% (Limited to important or life-threatening symptoms): Hepatic necrosis, hepatocellular carcinoma

**Overdose/Toxicology** Symptoms include confusion and abnormal liver function tests. Treatment is supportive.

**Pharmacodynamics/Kinetics**

**Half-life Elimination:** 9 hours

**Excretion:** Urine

**Formulations** Tablet: 50 mg

**Dosing**

**Adults:** Erythropoietic effects: Oral: 1-5 mg/kg/day in 1 daily dose; maximum: 100 mg/day; give for a minimum trial of 3-6 months because response may be delayed

**Elderly:** Refer to adult dosing.

**Monitoring Laboratory Tests** Liver function

**Additional Nursing Issues**

**Physical Assessment:** See Warnings/Precautions and Contraindications for use cautions. Monitor effectiveness of therapy, laboratory tests, and adverse response (see Adverse Reactions and Overdose/Toxicology). Assess knowledge/teach patient appropriate use, possible side effects (eg, hypoglycemia)/interventions, and adverse symptoms to report. **Pregnancy risk factor X** - determine that patient is not pregnant before beginning treatment and do not give to women of childbearing age or males who may have intercourse with childbearing women unless both male and female are capable of complying with barrier contraceptive measures during therapy and for 1 month following therapy. Note breast-feeding caution.

**Patient Information/Instruction:** Take as directed; do not exceed recommended dosage. If diabetic, monitor serum glucose closely and notify prescriber of changes; this medication can alter hypoglycemic requirements. You may experience acne, growth of body hair or baldness, deepening of voice, loss of libido, impotence, swelling of breasts, menstrual irregularity, or priapism (most are reversible); drowsiness, dizziness, or blurred vision (use caution driving or engaging in tasks that require alertness until response to drug is known); or nausea or vomiting (small frequent meals and good mouth care may help). Report persistent GI distress or diarrhea; change in color of urine or stool; yellowing of eyes or skin; swelling of ankles, feet, or hands; unusual bruising or bleeding; or other adverse reactions. **Pregnancy/breast-feeding precautions:** Inform prescriber if you are pregnant. Do not get pregnant during or for 1 month following therapy. Male: Do not cause a pregnancy. Male/female: Consult prescriber for instruction on appropriate barrier contraceptive measures. This drug may cause severe fetal defects. Consult prescriber if breast-feeding.

## Oxymorphone (oks i MOR fone)

**U.S. Brand Names** Numorphan®

**Therapeutic Category** Analgesic, Narcotic

**Pregnancy Risk Factor** B/D (if used for prolonged periods or in high doses at term)

**Lactation** Excretion in breast milk unknown/use caution

**Use** Management of moderate to severe pain and preoperatively as a sedative and a supplement to anesthesia

**Mechanism of Action/Effect** Oxymorphone hydrochloride (Numorphan®) is a potent narcotic analgesic with uses similar to those of morphine. The drug is a semisynthetic derivative of morphine (phenanthrene derivative) and is closely related to hydromorphone chemically (Dilaudid®).

**Contraindications** Hypersensitivity to oxymorphone or any component; increased intracranial pressure; severe respiratory depression; pregnancy (if used for prolonged periods or in high doses at term)

**Warnings** Some preparations contain sulfites which may cause allergic reactions. Use with caution in patients with impaired respiratory function or severe hepatic dysfunction and in patients with hypersensitivity reactions to other phenanthrene derivative opioid agonists (codeine, hydrocodone, hydromorphone, levorphanol, oxycodone, oxymorphone).

**Drug Interactions**

**Decreased Effect:** Decreased effect with phenothiazines.

**Increased Effect/Toxicity:** Increased effect/toxicity with CNS depressants (phenothiazines, tranquilizers, anxiolytics, sedatives, hypnotics, or alcohol), tricyclic antidepressants, and dextroamphetamine.

**Adverse Reactions**

>10%:
- Cardiovascular: Hypotension
- Central nervous system: Fatigue, drowsiness, dizziness
- Gastrointestinal: Nausea, vomiting
- Neuromuscular & skeletal: Weakness

1% to 10%:
- Cardiovascular: Tachycardia or bradycardia
- Central nervous system: Nervousness, headache, restlessness, malaise, confusion, false sense of well-being
- Gastrointestinal: Anorexia, stomach cramps, dry mouth, biliary spasm, constipation
- Genitourinary: Ureteral spasms, decreased urination
- Local: Pain at injection site
- Neuromuscular & skeletal: Trembling
- Ocular: Blurred vision
- Respiratory: Dyspnea, shortness of breath
- Miscellaneous: Histamine release

**Overdose/Toxicology** Symptoms of overdose include respiratory depression, miosis, hypotension, bradycardia, apnea, and pulmonary edema. Treatment of overdose includes maintaining patent airway and establishing an I.V. line. Naloxone, 2 mg I.V., with repeat administration as necessary up to a total of 10 mg, can also be used to reverse toxic effects of the opiate.

**Pharmacodynamics/Kinetics**

**Metabolism:** Liver

**Excretion:** Urine

**Onset:** Onset of analgesia: I.V., I.M., S.C.: Within 5-10 minutes; Rectal: Within 15-30 minutes

**Duration:** Duration of analgesia: Parenteral, rectal: 3-4 hours

**Formulations**

Oxymorphone hydrochloride:
- Injection: 1 mg (1 mL); 1.5 mg/mL (1 mL, 10 mL)
- Suppository, rectal: 5 mg

**Dosing**

**Adults:**
- I.M., S.C.: 0.5 mg initially, 1-1.5 mg every 4-6 hours as needed
- I.V.: 0.5 mg initially
- Rectal: 5 mg every 4-6 hours

(Continued)

## Oxymorphone *(Continued)*

**Elderly:** Refer to adult dosing.

**Stability**

**Storage:** Refrigerate suppository.

**Additional Nursing Issues**

**Physical Assessment:** Assess other medications patient may be taking for additive or adverse interactions (see Drug Interactions). Monitor for effectiveness of pain relief and monitor for signs of overdose (see above). Monitor blood pressure, CNS and respiratory status, and degree of sedation at beginning of therapy and at regular intervals with long-term use. May cause physical and/or psychological dependence. For inpatients, implement safety measures (eg, side rails up, call light within reach, instructions to call for assistance, etc). Assess knowledge/teach patient appropriate use (if self-administered). Teach patient to monitor for adverse reactions (see Adverse Reactions), adverse reactions to report, and appropriate interventions to reduce side effects. **Pregnancy risk factor B/D** - see Pregnancy Risk Factor for cautious use. Note breast-feeding caution.

**Patient Information/Instruction:** If self-administered, use exactly as directed (do not increase dose or frequency); may cause physical and/or psychological dependence. While using this medication, do not use alcohol and other prescription or OTC medications (especially sedatives, tranquilizers, antihistamines, or pain medications) without consulting prescriber. Maintain adequate hydration (2-3 L/day of fluids unless instructed to restrict fluid intake). May cause hypotension, dizziness, drowsiness, impaired coordination, or blurred vision (use caution when driving, climbing stairs, or changing position - rising from sitting or lying to standing, or when engaging in tasks requiring alertness until response to drug is known); nausea, vomiting or dry mouth (frequent mouth care, small frequent meals, chewing gum, or sucking lozenges may help); constipation (increased exercise, fluids, or dietary fruit and fiber may help - if constipation remains an unresolved problem, consult prescriber about use of stool softeners). Report persistent dizziness or headache; excessive fatigue or sedation; changes in mental status; changes in urinary elimination or pain on urination; weakness or trembling; blurred vision; or shortness of breath. **Pregnancy/breast-feeding precautions:** Inform prescriber if you are or intend to be pregnant. If you are breast-feeding, take medication immediately after breast-feeding or 3-4 hours prior to next feeding.

**Geriatric Considerations:** The elderly may be particularly susceptible to the CNS depressant and constipating effects of narcotics.

**Related Information**

Narcotic/Opioid Analgesic Comparison *on page 1396*

## Oxytetracycline (oks i tet ra SYE kleen)

**U.S. Brand Names** Terramycin® I.M. Injection; Terramycin® Oral; Uri-Tet® Oral

**Therapeutic Category** Antibiotic, Tetracycline Derivative

**Pregnancy Risk Factor** D

**Lactation** Enters breast milk/not recommended

**Use** Treatment of susceptible bacterial infections; both gram-positive and gram-negative, as well as, *Rickettsia* and *Mycoplasma* organisms

**Mechanism of Action/Effect** Inhibits bacterial protein synthesis by binding with the 30S and possibly the 50S ribosomal subunit(s) of susceptible bacteria, cell wall synthesis is not affected

**Contraindications** Hypersensitivity to tetracycline or any component; pregnancy

**Warnings** Photosensitivity can occur with oxytetracycline. Avoid in children ≤8 years of age.

**Drug Interactions**

**Decreased Effect:** Decreased effect with antacids containing aluminum, calcium, or magnesium. Iron and bismuth subsalicylate may decrease doxycycline bioavailability.

**Increased Effect/Toxicity:** Oxytetracycline may increase the effect of warfarin.

**Food Interactions** Oxytetracycline serum concentrations may be decreased if taken with dairy products.

**Adverse Reactions Systemic:**

>10%:

- Central nervous system: Dizziness, lightheadedness, unsteadiness
- Dermatologic: Photosensitivity
- Gastrointestinal: Nausea, diarrhea
- Miscellaneous: Discoloration of teeth in children

1% to 10%:

- Gastrointestinal: Pancreatitis, hypertrophy of the papilla
- Hepatic: Hepatotoxicity
- Miscellaneous: Superinfections (fungal overgrowth)

<1% (Limited to important or life-threatening symptoms): Pericarditis, increased intracranial pressure, bulging fontanels in infants, paresthesia, acute renal failure, azotemia

**Overdose/Toxicology** Symptoms of overdose include nausea, anorexia, and diarrhea. Treatment is supportive.

**Pharmacodynamics/Kinetics**

**Distribution:** Crosses the placenta

**Half-life Elimination:** 8.5-9.6 hours (prolonged in renal impairment)

**Time to Peak:** Within 2-4 hours

**Metabolism:** Liver

**Excretion:** Urine, while much higher amounts can be found in bile

**Formulations**

Oxytetracycline hydrochloride:

Capsule: 250 mg

Injection with lidocaine 2%: 5% [50 mg/mL] (2 mL, 10 mL); 12.5% [125 mg/mL] (2 mL)

**Dosing**

**Adults:**

Oral: 250-500 mg/dose every 6 hours

I.M.: 250-500 mg every 24 hours or 300 mg/day divided every 8-12 hours

**Elderly:** Refer to adult dosing.

**Renal Impairment:** $Cl_{cr}$ <10 mL/minute: Administer every 24 hours or avoid use if possible.

**Hepatic Impairment:** Avoid use in patients with severe liver disease.

**Administration**

**Oral:** Do not give with antacids, iron products, or dairy products. Give 1 hour before or 2 hours after meals.

**I.M.:** Injection for intramuscular use only.

**Monitoring Laboratory Tests** Perform culture and sensitivity prior to beginning therapy.

**Additional Nursing Issues**

**Physical Assessment:** Assess history of allergies. Monitor response to therapy. Monitor and/or teach patient to monitor and report adverse reactions. **Pregnancy risk factor D** - assess knowledge/teach appropriate use of barrier contraceptives. Breast-feeding is not recommended.

**Patient Information/Instruction:** Take as directed, around-the-clock. Finish all doses; do not skip doses. May take with food to reduce GI upset. Do not take with antacids, iron products, or dairy products. You may be sensitive to sunlight; use sunblock, wear protective clothing, or avoid direct sun. If diabetic, drug may cause false tests with Clinitest® urine glucose monitoring; use of glucose oxidase methods (Clinistix®) or serum glucose monitoring is preferable. Report rash, difficulty breathing, yellowing of skin or eyes, change in color of urine or stool, easy bruising or bleeding, fever, chills, perianal itching, purulent vaginal discharge, white plaques in mouth, or persistent diarrhea. **Pregnancy/breast-feeding precautions:** Do not get pregnant while taking this medication - Oral contraceptives effectiveness may be reduced; use appropriate barrier contraceptive measures. Breast-feeding is not recommended.

**Geriatric Considerations:** Oxytetracycline has not been studied in the elderly, however, dose reduction for renal function is not necessary.

♦ **Oxytetracycline and Hydrocortisone** *see page 1282*

## Oxytocin (oks i TOE sin)

**U.S. Brand Names** Pitocin® Injection; Syntocinon® Injection; Syntocinon® Nasal Spray

**Synonyms** PIT

**Therapeutic Category** Oxytocic Agent

**Pregnancy Risk Factor** X

**Lactation** Excretion in breast milk unknown/contraindicated

**Use** Induces labor at term; controls postpartum bleeding; nasal preparation used to promote milk letdown in lactating females

**Mechanism of Action/Effect** Produces rhythmic uterine contractions characteristic of delivery and stimulates breast milk flow during nursing

**Contraindications** Hypersensitivity to oxytocin or any component; significant cephalo-pelvic disproportion; unfavorable fetal positions; fetal distress; hypertonic or hyperactive uterus; contraindicated vaginal delivery; prolapse; total placenta previa; vasa previa

**Warnings** To be used for medical rather than elective induction of labor. May produce antidiuretic effect (ie, water intoxication and excess uterine contractions). High doses or hypersensitivity to oxytocin may cause uterine hypertonicity, spasm, tetanic contraction, or rupture of the uterus. Severe water intoxication with convulsions, coma, and death has been associated with a slow oxytocin infusion over 24 hours.

**Adverse Reactions**

**Fetal:** <1% (Limited to important or life-threatening symptoms): Bradycardia, arrhythmias, intracranial hemorrhage, brain damage, neonatal jaundice, hypoxia, death

**Maternal:** <1% (Limited to important or life-threatening symptoms): Cardiac arrhythmias, premature ventricular contractions, hypotension, tachycardia, arrhythmias, seizures, coma, SIADH with hyponatremia, nausea, vomiting, pelvic hematoma, postpartum hemorrhage, increased uterine motility, fatal afibrinogenemia, increased blood loss, death, anaphylactic reactions

**Overdose/Toxicology** Symptoms of overdose include tetanic uterine contractions, impaired uterine blood flow, amniotic fluid embolism, uterine rupture, SIADH, and seizures. Treatment is symptom directed and supportive.

**Pharmacodynamics/Kinetics**

**Half-life Elimination:** 1-5 minutes

**Metabolism:** Rapid in the liver and plasma (by oxytocinase) and to a smaller degree the mammary gland

(Continued)

## Oxytocin *(Continued)*

**Excretion:** Renal

**Onset:** Onset of uterine contractions: I.V.: Within 1 minute

**Duration:** <30 minutes

**Formulations**

Injection: 10 units/mL (1 mL, 10 mL)

Solution, nasal: 40 units/mL (2 mL, 5 mL)

**Dosing**

**Adults:** I.V. administration requires the use of an infusion pump.

Induction of labor: I.V.: 0.001-0.002 units/minute; increase by 0.001-0.002 units every 15-30 minutes until contraction pattern has been established; maximum dose should not exceed 20 milliunits/minute.

Postpartum bleeding:

I.M.: Total dose of 10 units after delivery

I.V.: 10-40 units by I.V. infusion in 1000 mL of intravenous fluid at a rate sufficient to control uterine atony

Promotion of milk letdown: Intranasal: 1 spray or 3 drops in one or both nostrils 2-3 minutes before breast-feeding.

**Administration**

**I.V.:** Sodium chloride 0.9% (NS) and dextrose 5% in water ($D_5W$) have been recommended as diluents; dilute 10-40 units to 1 L in NS, LR, or $D_5W$.

**Stability**

**Storage:** Oxytocin should be stored at room temperature (15°C to 30°C) and protected from freezing.

**Compatibility:** Incompatible with norepinephrine and prochlorperazine.

**Additional Nursing Issues**

**Physical Assessment:**

I.V., I.M.: Monitor blood pressure, fluid intake and output, and labor closely if using oxytocin for induction; fetal monitoring is recommended (see Adverse Reactions).

Nasal spray for initial milk-letdown: Instruct in proper use of spray and adverse reactions to report.

Breast-feeding is contraindicated.

**Patient Information/Instruction:**

I.V., I.M.: Generally used in emergency situations. Drug teaching should be incorporated in other situational teaching.

Intranasal spray: While sitting up, hold bottle upright and squeeze into nostril.

**Breast-feeding precautions:** Do not breast-feed.


- ♦ **Oyst-Cal 500 [OTC]** *see* Calcium Supplements *on page 185*
- ♦ **Oystercal® 500** *see* Calcium Supplements *on page 185*
- ♦ **Ozoken** *see* Omeprazole *on page 851*
- ♦ **P-071** *see* Cetirizine *on page 242*
- ♦ **Pacerone®** *see* Amiodarone *on page 71*


## Paclitaxel (PAK li taks el)

**U.S. Brand Names** Taxol®

**Therapeutic Category** Antineoplastic Agent, Natural Source (Plant) Derivative

**Pregnancy Risk Factor** D

**Lactation** Enters breast milk/contraindicated

**Use** Treatment of metastatic carcinoma of the ovary after failure of first-line or subsequent chemotherapy; treatment of locally advanced or metastatic breast cancer; treatment of nonsmall cell lung cancer

**Mechanism of Action/Effect** Paclitaxel exerts its effects on microtubules and their protein subunits, tubulin dimers. Paclitaxel promotes microtubule assembly by enhancing the action of tubulin dimers, stabilizing existing microtubules, and inhibiting their disassembly. Maintaining microtubule assembly inhibits mitosis and affecting cell death. The $G_2$- and M-phases of the cell cycle are affected. In addition, the drug can distort mitotic spindles, resulting in the breakage of chromosomes.

**Contraindications** Hypersensitivity to paclitaxel or any component; pregnancy

**Warnings** The FDA currently recommends that procedures for proper handling and disposal of antineoplastic agents be considered. All patients should be premedicated prior to Taxol® administration to prevent severe hypersensitivity reactions. Current evidence indicates that prolongation of the infusion (to ≥6 hours) plus premedication may minimize this effect:

Dexamethasone 20 mg orally 14 and 7 hours before the infusion

Diphenhydramine 50 mg IVP 30 minutes before the infusion

Ranitidine 50 mg (or cimetidine 300 mg) IVPB 30 minutes before the infusion

Preparation of paclitaxel should be performed in a Class II laminar flow biologic safety cabinet. Personnel should be wearing surgical gloves and a closed front surgical gown with knit cuffs. Appropriate safety equipment is recommended for preparation, administration, and disposal of antineoplastics. If paclitaxel contacts the skin, wash and flush thoroughly with water.

**Drug Interactions**

**Cytochrome P-450 Effect:** CYP2C8 and 3A3/4 enzyme substrate

**Decreased Effect:** Paclitaxel metabolism is dependent on cytochrome P-450 isoenzymes. Inducers of these enzymes may decrease the effect of paclitaxel.

**Increased Effect/Toxicity:** In Phase I trials, myelosuppression was more profound when given after cisplatin than with alternative sequence. Pharmacokinetic data demonstrates a decrease in clearance of ~33% when administered following cisplatin. Possibility of an inhibition of metabolism in patients treated with ketoconazole.

**Adverse Reactions** Local: **Irritant chemotherapy**

>10%:
- Cardiovascular: Hypotension, abnormal EKG
- Dermatologic: Alopecia
- Gastrointestinal: Nausea, vomiting, diarrhea, mucositis
  - Emetic potential: Moderate: 30% to 60%
- Hematologic: Bleeding, neutropenia, leukopenia, thrombocytopenia, anemia, neutropenia is increased with longer infusions
- Hepatic: Abnormal liver function tests
- Neuromuscular & skeletal: Peripheral neuropathy, myalgia
- Miscellaneous: Hypersensitivity reactions, infections

1% to 10%:
- Cardiovascular: Bradycardia, severe cardiovascular events, hypotension
- Hepatic: Elevated serum hepatic enzymes

<1% (Limited to important or life-threatening symptoms): Radiation pneumonitis, rash, pruritus

**Pharmacodynamics/Kinetics**

**Protein Binding:** 89% to 98% bound to human serum proteins at concentrations of 0.1-50 μg/mL

**Distribution:** Initial rapid decline represents distribution to the peripheral compartment and significant elimination of the drug. Later phase is due to a relatively slow efflux of paclitaxel from the peripheral compartment. Mean steady state is 42-162 L/m$^2$, indicating extensive extravascular distribution and/or tissue binding.

**Half-life Elimination:** Administered by I.V. infusion and exhibits a biphasic decline in plasma concentrations. Mean: 5.3-17.4 hours after 1- and 6-hour infusions at dosing levels of 15-275 mg/m$^2$.

## Paclitaxel

**Drugs Which Are Visually Compatible With Taxol® via Y-Site**

Acyclovir (7 mg/mL)
Amikacin (5 mg/mL)
Bleomycin (1 unit/mL)
Calcium chloride (20 mg/mL)
Carboplatin (5 mg/mL)
Ceftazidime (40 mg/mL)
Ceftriaxone (20 mg/mL)
Cimetidine hydrochloride (12 mg/mL)
Cisplatin (1 mg/mL)
Cyclophosphamide (10 mg/mL)
Cytarabine (50 mg/mL)
Dexamethasone sodium phosphate (1 mg/mL)
Diphenhydramine hydrochloride (2 mg/mL)
Doxorubicin hydrochloride (2 mg/mL)
Etoposide (0.4 mg/mL)
Famotidine (2 mg/mL)
Fluconazole (2 mg/mL)
Fluorouracil (16 mg/mL)
Ganciclovir (20 mg/mL)
Gentamicin (5 mg/mL)
Haloperidol lactate (0.2 mg/mL)
Heparin (100 units/mL)
Hydrocortisone sodium succinate or hydrocortisone phosphate (1 mg/mL)
Hydromorphone (0.5 mg/mL)
Lorazepam (0.1 mg/mL)
Magnesium sulfate (100 mg/mL)
Mannitol (15%)
Meperidine (4 mg/mL)
Mesna (10 mg/mL)
Methotrexate sodium (15 mg/mL)
Metoclopramide hydrochloride (5 mg/mL)
Morphine sulfate (1 mg/mL)
Ondansetron (0.5 mg/mL)
Potassium chloride (0.1 mEq/mL)
Prochlorperazine edisylate (0.5 mg/mL)
Ranitidine hydrochloride (2 mg/mL)
Sodium bicarbonate (1 mEq/mL)
Vancomycin hydrochloride (10 mg/mL)

**Drugs Which Exhibit Turbidity Changes With Taxol® via Y-Site**
**(may be visually/chemically incompatible with Taxol®)**

Amphotericin B (0.6 mg/mL)
Chlorpromazine
Hydroxyzine
Methylprednisolone
Mitoxantrone

(Continued)

## Paclitaxel *(Continued)*

**Metabolism:** Hepatic metabolism in humans

**Excretion:**

Urinary recovery of unchanged drug: 1.3% to 12.6% following 1-, 6-, and 24-hour infusions of 15-275 mg/m$^2$

Mean total body clearance range:

After 1- and 6-hour infusions: 5.8-16.3 L/hour/m$^2$

After 24-hour infusions: 14.2-17.2 L/hour/m$^2$

**Formulations** Injection: 6 mg/mL (5 mL)

**Dosing**

**Adults:** Corticosteroids (dexamethasone), $H_1$ antagonists (diphenhydramine), and $H_2$ antagonists (cimetidine or ranitidine), should be administered prior to paclitaxel administration to minimize potential for anaphylaxis.

Adults: I.V. infusion: Refer to individual protocols.

Ovarian carcinoma: 135-175 mg/m$^2$ over 1-24 hours administered every 3 weeks

Metastatic breast cancer: Treatment is still undergoing investigation; most protocols have used doses of 175-250 mg/m$^2$ over 1-24 hours every 3 weeks

Nonsmall cell lung cancer: 135 mg/m$^2$ over 24 hours administered every 3 weeks (given in combination with cisplatin 75 mg/m$^2$)

AIDS-related Kaposi's sarcoma: 135 mg/m$^2$ over 3 hours every 3 weeks or 100 mg/m$^2$ over 3 hours every 2 weeks

**Hepatic Impairment:**

Total bilirubin ≤1.5 mg/dL and AST >2x normal limits: Total dose <135 mg/m$^2$

Total bilirubin 1.6-3.0 mg/dL: Total dose ≤75 mg/m$^2$

Total bilirubin ≥3.1 mg/dL: Total dose ≤50 mg/m$^2$

**Administration**

**I.V.:** Irritant. Manufacturer recommends administration over 2 hours. Other routes are being studied.

**I.V. Detail:** Should be administered in either glass or Excel®/PAB®. Should also use non-PVC tubing (eg, polyethylene) to minimize leaching. Administer through I.V. tubing containing an in-line (0.22 micron) filter. Formulated in a vehicle known as Cremophor® EL (polyoxyethylated castor oil). Cremophor® EL has been found to leach the plasticizer DEHP from polyvinyl chloride infusion bags or administration sets. Contact of the undiluted concentrate with plasticized polyvinyl chloride (PVC) equipment or devices is not recommended. Administer through IVEX-2® filters (which incorporate short inlet and outlet polyvinyl chloride-coated tubing) has not resulted in significant leaching of DEHP.

**Stability**

**Storage:** Store intact vials under refrigeration 2°C to 8°C.

**Reconstitution:** Further dilution in NS or $D_5W$ to a concentration of 0.3-1.2 mg/mL is stable for 48 hours at room temperature (25°C).

**Standard I.V. dilution:** IVPB: Dose/500-1000 mL $D_5W$ or NS

Solutions are stable for 48 hours at room temperature (25°C).

**Compatibility:** See the Chemotherapy Compatibility Chart *on page 1311*. See table for list of compatibilities.

**Monitoring Laboratory Tests** CBC, liver and kidney function

**Additional Nursing Issues**

**Physical Assessment:** Monitor appropriate laboratory tests as ordered. Monitor for adverse effects (eg, peripheral neuropathy, myelosuppression), opportunistic infection, and hypersensitivity (see above). **Pregnancy risk factor D.** Breast-feeding is contraindicated.

**Patient Information/Instruction:** This medication can only be administered by infusion, usually on a cyclic basis. Maintain adequate hydration (2-3 L/day of fluids unless instructed to restrict fluid intake) and nutrition (small frequent meals will help). You will most likely loss your hair (will grow back after therapy); experience some nausea or vomiting (request antiemetic); feel weak or lethargic (use caution when driving or engaging in tasks that require alertness until response to drug is known). Use good oral care to reduce incidence of mouth sores. You will be more susceptible to infection; avoid crowds or exposure to infection. Report numbness or tingling in fingers or toes (use care to prevent injury); signs of infection (fever, chills, sore throat, burning urination, fatigue); unusual bleeding (tarry stools, easy bruising, or blood in stool, urine, or mouth); unresolved mouth sores; nausea or vomiting; or skin rash or itching. **Pregnancy/breast-feeding precautions:** Do not get pregnant or breast-feed.

**Breast-feeding Issues:** Antineoplastic agents are generally contraindicated.

♦ **Pactens** *see* Naproxen *on page 807*

♦ **Palafer®** *see* Iron Supplements *on page 627*

♦ **Palmitate-A® 5000 [OTC]** *see* Vitamin A *on page 1217*

♦ **PALS®** *see page 1294*

♦ **2-PAM** *see* Pralidoxime *on page 954*

♦ **Pamelor®** *see* Nortriptyline *on page 839*

## Pamidronate (pa mi DROE nate)

**U.S. Brand Names** Aredia™

**Therapeutic Category** Antidote; Bisphosphonate Derivative

**Pregnancy Risk Factor** C

**Lactation** Excretion in breast milk unknown/use caution

**Use** FDA-approved: Treatment of hypercalcemia associated with malignancy; treatment of osteolytic bone lesions associated with multiple myeloma; moderate to severe Paget's disease of bone

**Mechanism of Action/Effect** A biphosphonate which inhibits bone resorption via actions on osteoclasts or on osteoclast precursors. Does not appear to produce any significant effects on renal tubular calcium handling and is poorly absorbed following oral administration (high oral doses have been reported effective); therefore, I.V. therapy is preferred.

**Contraindications** Hypersensitivity to pamidronate or other biphosphonates

**Warnings** Use caution in patients with renal impairment as the potential nephrotoxic effects of pamidronate are not known. Use caution in patients who are pregnant. Leukopenia has been observed with oral pamidronate and monitoring of white blood cell counts is suggested. Vein irritation and thrombophlebitis may occur with infusions. Has not been studied exclusively in the elderly. Monitor serum electrolytes periodically since elderly are often receiving diuretics which can result in decreases in serum calcium, potassium, and magnesium. Pregnancy factor C.

**Adverse Reactions**

1% to 10%:

- Central nervous system: Malaise, fever, convulsions
- Endocrine & metabolic: Hypomagnesemia, hypocalcemia, hypokalemia, fluid overload, hypophosphatemia
- Gastrointestinal: GI symptoms, nausea, diarrhea, constipation, anorexia
- Hematologic: Leukopenia, lymphopenia
- Hepatic: Abnormal hepatic function
- Neuromuscular & skeletal: Bone pain
- Respiratory: Dyspnea

<1% (Limited to important or life-threatening symptoms): Nephrotoxicity

**Overdose/Toxicology** Symptoms of overdose include hypocalcemia, EKG changes, seizures, bleeding, paresthesia, carpopedal spasm, and fever. Treat with I.V. calcium gluconate, and general supportive care; fever and hypotension can be treated with corticosteroids.

**Pharmacodynamics/Kinetics**

**Half-life Elimination:** Distribution half-life: 1.6 hours; Urinary (elimination) half-life: 2.5 hours; Bone half-life: 300 days

**Metabolism:** Not metabolized

**Excretion:** Biphasic; ~50% excreted unchanged in urine within 72 hours

**Onset:** Onset of effect: 24-48 hours; Maximum effect: 5-7 days

**Formulations** Powder for injection, lyophilized, as disodium: 30 mg, 60 mg, 90 mg

**Dosing**

**Adults:** Drug must be diluted properly before administration and infused slowly (over at least 1 hour). I.V.:

- Moderate cancer-related hypercalcemia (corrected serum calcium: 12-13 mg/dL): 60-90 mg given as a slow infusion over 2-24 hours
- Severe cancer-related hypercalcemia (corrected serum calcium: >13.5 mg/dL): 90 mg as a slow infusion over 2-24 hours
  - A period of 7 days should elapse before the use of second course. Repeat infusions every 2-3 weeks have been suggested, however, could be administered every 2-3 months according to the degree and of severity of hypercalcemia and/or the type of malignancy.
- Osteolytic bone lesions with multiple myeloma: 90 mg in 500 mL $D_5W$, 0.45% NaCl or 0.9% NaCl administered over 4 hours on a monthly basis
- Paget's disease: 30 mg in 500 mL 0.45% NaCl, 0.9% NaCl or $D_5W$ administered over 4 hours for 3 consecutive days

**Elderly:** Refer to adult dosing.

**Stability**

**Reconstitution:** Reconstitute by adding 10 mL of sterile water for injection to each 30 mg vial of lyophilized pamidronate disodium powder, the resulting solution will be 30 mg/10 mL. Pamidronate may be further diluted in 250-1000 mL of 0.45% or 0.9% sodium chloride or 5% dextrose. Pamidronate (reconstituted solution and infusion solution) is stable at room temperature and under refrigeration (36°F to 46°F or 2°C to 8°C) for 24 hours.

**Compatibility:** Pamidronate is incompatible with calcium-containing infusion solutions such as Ringer's injection.

**Monitoring Laboratory Tests** Serum electrolytes, monitor for hypocalcemia for at least 2 weeks after therapy; serum calcium, phosphate, magnesium, serum creatinine, CBC with differential

**Additional Nursing Issues**

**Physical Assessment:** Monitor laboratory results (see above) and assess for signs of hypocalcemia. Ensure adequate hydration. **Pregnancy risk factor C** - benefits of use should outweigh possible risks. Note breast-feeding caution.

**Patient Information/Instruction:** This medication can only be administered I.V. Avoid foods high in calcium or vitamins with minerals during infusion or for 2-3 hours after completion. You may experience nausea or vomiting (small frequent meals and good mouth care may help); or recurrent bone pain (consult prescriber for analgesic). Report unusual muscle twitching or spasms, severe diarrhea/constipation, or acute bone pain. **Pregnancy/breast-feeding precautions:** Inform prescriber if you are or intend to be pregnant. Consult prescriber if breast-feeding.

(Continued)

## Pamidronate *(Continued)*

**Geriatric Considerations:** Has not been studied exclusively in the elderly. Monitor serum electrolytes periodically since elderly are often receiving diuretics which can result in decreases in serum calcium, potassium, and magnesium.

- **Pamprin IB® [OTC]** *see* Ibuprofen *on page 592*
- **Panadol® [OTC]** *see* Acetaminophen *on page 32*
- **Panasal® 5/500** *see* Hydrocodone and Aspirin *on page 570*
- **Pan-B Antibodies** *see* Rituximab *on page 1031*
- **Pancrease®** *see* Pancrelipase *on this page*
- **Pancrease® MT 4** *see* Pancrelipase *on this page*
- **Pancrease® MT 10** *see* Pancrelipase *on this page*
- **Pancrease® MT 16** *see* Pancrelipase *on this page*

## Pancrelipase (pan kre LI pase)

**U.S. Brand Names** Cotazym®; Cotazym-S®; Creon 10®; Creon 20®; Ilozyme®; Ku-Zyme® HP; Pancrease®; Pancrease® MT 4; Pancrease® MT 10; Pancrease® MT 16; Protilase®; Ultrase® MT12; Ultrase® MT20; Viokase®; Zymase®

**Synonyms** Lipancreatin; Lipase, Protease, and Amylase

**Therapeutic Category** Enzyme

**Pregnancy Risk Factor** C

**Lactation** Enters breast milk/contraindicated

**Use** Replacement therapy in symptomatic treatment of malabsorption syndrome caused by pancreatic insufficiency

**Mechanism of Action/Effect** Replaces endogenous pancreatic enzymes to assist in digestion of protein, starch and fats

**Contraindications** Hypersensitivity to pancrelipase or any component, pork protein

**Warnings** Pancrelipase is inactivated by acids. Use microencapsulated products whenever possible, since these products permit better dissolution of enzymes in the duodenum and protect the enzyme preparations from acid degradation in the stomach. Pregnancy factor C.

**Drug Interactions**

**Decreased Effect:** Calcium carbonate, magnesium hydroxide may decrease the effect of pancrelipase.

**Adverse Reactions**

1% to 10%: High doses:
- Endocrine & metabolic: Hyperuricemia
- Gastrointestinal: Nausea, cramps, constipation, diarrhea
- Genitourinary: Hyperuricosuria
- Ocular: Lacrimation
- Respiratory: Sneezing, bronchospasm

<1% (Limited to important or life-threatening symptoms): Shortness of breath, bronchospasm

**Overdose/Toxicology** Symptoms of overdose include diarrhea, other transient intestinal upset, hyperuricosuria, and hyperuricemia. Treatment is supportive.

**Pharmacodynamics/Kinetics**

**Excretion:** Feces

**Formulations**

Capsule:
- Cotazym®: Lipase 8000 units, protease 30,000 units, amylase 30,000 units
- Ku-Zyme® HP: Lipase 8000 units, protease 30,000 units, amylase 30,000 units
- Ultrase® MT12: Lipase 12,000 units, protease 39,000 units, amylase 39,000 units
- Ultrase® MT20: Lipase 20,000 units, protease 65,000 units, amylase 65,000 units
- Enteric coated microspheres (Pancrease®): Lipase 4000 units, protease 25,000 units, amylase 20,000 units
- Enteric coated microtablets:
  - Pancrease® MT 4: Lipase 4500 units, protease 12,000 units, amylase 12,000 units
  - Pancrease® MT 10: Lipase 10,000 units, protease 30,000 units, amylase 30,000 units
  - Pancrease® MT 16: Lipase 16,000 units, protease 48,000 units, amylase 48,000 units
  - Pancrease® MT 20: Lipase 20,000 units, protease 44,000 units, amylase 56,000 units
- Enteric coated spheres:
  - Cotazym-S®: Lipase 5000 units, protease 20,000 units, amylase 20,000 units
  - Pancrelipase, Protilase®: Lipase 4000 units, protease 25,000 units, amylase 20,000 units
  - Zymase®: Lipase 12,000 units, protease 24,000 units, amylase 24,000 units
- Delayed release:
  - Creon 10®: Lipase 10,000 units, protease 37,500 units, amylase 33,200 units
  - Creon 20®: Lipase 20,000 units, protease 75,000 units, amylase 66,400 units

Powder (Viokase®): Lipase 16,800 units, protease 70,000 units, amylase 70,000 units per 0.7 g

Tablet:
- Ilozyme®: Lipase 11,000 units, protease 30,000 units, amylase 30,000 units
- Viokase®: Lipase 8000 units, protease 30,000 units, amylase 30,000 units

**Dosing**

**Adults:** Oral:

Powder: Actual dose depends on the digestive requirements of the patient.

0.7 g with meals

Enteric coated microspheres and microtablets: The following dosage recommendations are only an approximation for initial dosages. The actual dosage will depend on the digestive requirements of the individual patient.

4000-16,000 units of lipase with meals and with snacks or 1-3 tablets/capsules before or with meals and snacks; in severe deficiencies, dose may be increased to 8 tablets/capsules.

Occluded feeding tubes: 1 tablet of Viokase® crushed with one 325 mg tablet of sodium bicarbonate (to activate the Viokase®) in 5 mL of water can be instilled into the nasogastric tube and clamped for 5 minutes; then, flushed with 50 mL of tap water.

**Elderly:** Refer to adult dosing.

**Additional Nursing Issues**

**Physical Assessment:** If powder spills on skin, wash off immediately; do not inhale powder. Monitor for adverse effects and effectiveness of therapy. **Pregnancy risk factor C** - benefits of use should outweigh possible risks. Breast-feeding is contraindicated.

**Patient Information/Instruction:** Take before or with meals. Avoid taking with alkaline food. Do not chew, crush, or dissolve delayed release capsules; swallow whole. Do not inhale powder when preparing. You may experience some gastric discomfort. Report unusual joint pain or swelling, respiratory difficulty, or persistent GI upset. **Pregnancy/breast-feeding precautions:** Inform prescriber if your are or intend to be pregnant. Do not breast-feed.

**Geriatric Considerations:** No special considerations are necessary since drug is dosed to response; however, drug-induced diarrhea can result in unwanted side effects (confusion, hypotension, lethargy, fluid and electrolyte loss).


- **Pancuronium** *see page 1248*
- **Pandel®** *see* Hydrocortisone *on page 578*
- **Pandel®** *see* Topical Corticosteroids *on page 1152*
- **Panmycin® Oral** *see* Tetracycline *on page 1111*
- **PanOxyl®-AQ** *see page 1294*
- **PanOxyl® Bar** *see page 1294*
- **Panretin®** *see* Alitretinoin *on page 52*
- **Panscol®** *see page 1294*
- **Pantomicina** *see* Erythromycin *on page 435*


## Papaverine (pa PAV er een)

**U.S. Brand Names** Genabid®; Pavabid®; Pavatine®

**Therapeutic Category** Vasodilator

**Pregnancy Risk Factor** C

**Lactation** Excretion in breast milk unknown/not recommended

**Use**

Oral: Relief of peripheral and cerebral ischemia associated with arterial spasm; smooth muscle relaxant

Parenteral: Various vascular spasms associated with muscle spasms as in myocardial infarction, angina, peripheral and pulmonary embolism, peripheral vascular disease, angiospastic states, and visceral spasm (ureteral, biliary, and GI colic); testing for impotence

**Mechanism of Action/Effect** Smooth muscle spasmolytic producing a generalized smooth muscle relaxation including: vasodilatation, GI sphincter relaxation, bronchiolar muscle relaxation, and potentially a depressed myocardium (with large doses); muscle relaxation may occur due to inhibition or cyclic nucleotide phosphodiesterase, increasing cyclic AMP; muscle relaxation is unrelated to nerve innervation; papaverine increases cerebral blood flow in normal subjects; oxygen uptake is unaltered

**Contraindications** Complete atrioventricular block; Parkinson's disease

**Warnings** Use with caution in patients with glaucoma. Administer I.V. cautiously since apnea and arrhythmias may result. May, in large doses, depress cardiac conduction (eg, A-V node) leading to arrhythmias. May interfere with levodopa therapy of Parkinson's disease. Hepatic hypersensitivity has been noted with jaundice, eosinophilia, and abnormal LFTs. Pregnancy factor C.

**Drug Interactions**

**Cytochrome P-450 Effect:** CYP2D6 enzyme substrate

**Decreased Effect:** Papaverine decreases the effects of levodopa.

**Adverse Reactions** <1% (Limited to important or life-threatening symptoms): Flushing of the face, tachycardias, hypotension, arrhythmias with rapid I.V. use, depression, dizziness, vertigo, drowsiness, sedation, lethargy, headache, hepatic hypersensitivity, apnea with rapid I.V. use

**Overdose/Toxicology** Symptoms of overdose include nausea, vomiting, weakness, gastric distress, ataxia, hepatic dysfunction, drowsiness, nystagmus, hyperventilation, hypotension, and hypokalemia. Treatment is supportive.

**Pharmacodynamics/Kinetics**

**Protein Binding:** 90%

**Half-life Elimination:** 0.5-1.5 hours

**Metabolism:** Liver

**Excretion:** Urine

**Onset:** Oral: Rapid

**Formulations**

Capsule, sustained release, as hydrochloride: 150 mg

(Continued)

## Papaverine *(Continued)*

Tablet, as hydrochloride: 30 mg, 60 mg, 100 mg, 150 mg, 200 mg, 300 mg
Tablet, timed release, as hydrochloride: 200 mg

**Dosing**

**Adults:**

Oral: 100-300 mg 3-5 times/day
Oral, sustained release: 150-300 mg every 12 hours
I.M., I.V.: 30-120 mg every 3 hours as needed; for cardiac extrasystoles, give 2 doses 10 minutes apart I.V. or I.M.

**Elderly:** Refer to adult dosing.

**Administration**

**I.V.:** Rapid I.V. administration may result in arrhythmias and fatal apnea; administer no faster than over 1-2 minutes.

**Stability**

**Storage:** Protect from heat or freezing. Refrigerate injection at 2°C to 8°C (35°F to 46°F).

**Reconstitution:** Solutions should be clear to pale yellow. Precipitates with lactated Ringer's.

**Compatibility:** Physically incompatible with lactated Ringer's injection.

**Additional Nursing Issues**

**Physical Assessment:**

I.M., I.V.: Monitor blood pressure and heart rate.

Oral: Monitor blood pressure and heart rate prior to instituting therapy and at frequent intervals thereafter. Monitor effectiveness of treatment on a regular basis. Monitor and assess knowledge/teach patient possible side effects of treatment and adverse effects to report.

**Pregnancy risk factor C** - benefits of use should outweigh possible risks. Breast-feeding is not recommended.

**Patient Information/Instruction:** Oral: Take as directed; do not alter dosage without consulting prescriber. Do not chew, crush, or dissolve extended release tablets. Avoid alcohol while taking this medication. May cause dizziness, confusion, or blurred vision (avoid driving or engaging in tasks that require alertness until response to drug is known). Increased fiber in diet, exercise, and adequate hydration (2-3 L/day of fluids unless instructed to restrict fluid intake) may help if you experience constipation. Report rapid heartbeat or palpitations, CNS depression, persistent sedation or lethargy, or acute headache. **Pregnancy/breast-feeding precautions:** Inform prescriber if you are or intend to be pregnant. Breast-feeding is not recommended.

**Geriatric Considerations:** Vasodilators have been used to treat dementia upon the premise that dementia is secondary to a cerebral blood flow insufficiency. The hypothesis is that if blood flow could be increased, cognitive function would be increased. This hypothesis is no longer valid. The use of vasodilators for cognitive dysfunction is not recommended or proven by appropriate scientific study.

**Additional Information** pH: 3.0-4.5


- ♦ **Paracetaldehyde** *see* Paraldehyde *on this page*
- ♦ **Paracetamol** *see* Acetaminophen *on page 32*
- ♦ **Parachlorometaxylenol** *see page 1294*
- ♦ **Paraflex®** *see* Chlorzoxazone *on page 261*
- ♦ **Parafon Forte™ DSC** *see* Chlorzoxazone *on page 261*
- ♦ **Paral®** *see* Paraldehyde *on this page*


## Paraldehyde (par AL de hyde)

**U.S. Brand Names** Paral®

**Synonyms** Paracetaldehyde

**Therapeutic Category** Anticonvulsant, Miscellaneous

**Pregnancy Risk Factor** C

**Lactation** Not recommended

**Use** Treatment of status epilepticus and tetanus-induced seizures; sedative/hypnotic; treatment of alcohol withdrawal symptoms

**Mechanism of Action/Effect** Mechanism of action is unknown. Causes depression of CNS including ascending reticular activating system to exert sedative and anticonvulsant effects.

**Contraindications** Severe hepatic insufficiency, respiratory disease, GI inflammation or ulceration. Patients receiving disulfiram should not receive paraldehyde due to inhibition of paraldehyde metabolism.

**Warnings** Use with caution in patients with asthma or other bronchopulmonary disease. Imparts odor to exhaled air for as long as 24 hours after ingestion. Patient is unaware of odor. Flies may be attracted. May oxidize to form acetic acid. Under no circumstances use material that has a brownish color or a sharp, penetrating odor of acetic acid. Do not abruptly discontinue in patients receiving chronic therapy. Pregnancy factor C.

**Drug Interactions**

**Increased Effect/Toxicity:** Barbiturates and alcohol may enhance CNS depression; "disulfiram reaction" with disulfiram due to inhibition of acetaldehyde dehydrogenase by disulfiram; avoid concomitant use.

**Adverse Reactions**

>10%:

Central nervous system: Drowsiness
Dermatologic: Skin rash

Gastrointestinal: Strong and unpleasant breath, nausea, vomiting, stomach pain, irritation of mucous membrane

Respiratory: Coughing

1% to 10%:

Central nervous system: Clumsiness, dizziness, "hangover effect"

Local: Thrombophlebitis

<1% (Limited to important or life-threatening symptoms): Cardiovascular collapse, pulmonary edema, psychological and physical dependence with prolonged use, metabolic acidosis, hepatitis, respiratory depression

**Pharmacodynamics/Kinetics**

**Half-life Elimination:** 6-7.4 hours

**Metabolism:** Liver

**Excretion:** Renal: 3%; lung: 28%

**Onset:** Oral: 10-15 minutes

**Duration:** 6-8 hours

**Formulations** Liquid, oral or rectal: 1 g/mL (30 mL)

**Dosing**

**Adults:**

Oral, rectal:

Sedative: 5-10 mL

Hypnotic: 10-30 mL

Oral: Dilute in milk or iced fruit juice to mask taste and odor.

Rectal: Mix paraldehyde 2:1 with oil (cottonseed or olive).

**Elderly:** Refer to adult dosing.

**Hepatic Impairment:** Dosage may need to be reduced.

**Administration**

**Oral:** Dilute in milk or iced fruit juice. Do **not** use any plastic equipment for administration, use glass syringes and rubber tubing.

**Other:** Do **not** use any plastic equipment for administration, use glass syringes and rubber tubing. Rectal: Mix paraldehyde 2:1 with oil (cottonseed or olive).

**Stability**

**Storage:** Decomposes with exposure to air and light to acetaldehyde which then oxidizes to acetic acid. Store in tightly closed containers. Protect from light. Discards unused contents of any container which has been opened for >24 hours.

**Additional Nursing Issues**

**Physical Assessment:** Assess effectiveness and interactions of other medications patient may be taking (see Contraindications, Warnings/Precautions, and Drug Interactions). Long-term use can result in dependence, abuse, or tolerance; periodically evaluate need for continued use. Monitor for therapeutic response, laboratory values, and adverse reactions (see Adverse Reactions). Observe and teach seizure/safety precautions. Assess knowledge/teach patient appropriate use, interventions to reduce side effects, and adverse symptoms to report. **Pregnancy risk factor C** - benefits of use should outweigh possible risks. Breast-feeding is not recommended.

**Patient Information/Instruction:** Outpatients: Take exactly as directed (do not increase dose or frequency or discontinue without consulting prescriber). Oral: Dilute with milk or iced fruit juice to mask taste and odor; do not use plastic equipment for administration. While using this medication, do not use alcohol and other prescription or OTC medications (especially pain medications, sedatives, antihistamines, or hypnotics) without consulting prescriber. Do not use solution if it has a brown color. You may experience drowsiness, dizziness, or blurred vision (use caution when driving or engaging in tasks requiring alertness until response to drug is known); nausea, vomiting (small frequent meals, frequent mouth care, chewing gum, or sucking lozenges may help). Report chest pain or palpitation; difficulty breathing or unusual cough; sudden, severe headache; persistent GI symptoms (cramping, constipation, vomiting, anorexia); worsening of seizure activity, or loss of seizure control. **Pregnancy/breast-feeding precautions:** Inform prescriber if you are or intend to be pregnant. Breast-feeding is not recommended.

**Related Information**

Antipsychotic Medication Guidelines *on page 1436*

- **Paraplatin®** *see* Carboplatin *on page 199*
- **Parathar™ Injection** *see page 1248*
- **Paraxin** *see* Chloramphenicol *on page 248*
- **Par Decon®** *see page 1306*

## Paregoric (par e GOR ik)

**Synonyms** Camphorated Tincture of Opium

**Therapeutic Category** Analgesic, Narcotic

**Pregnancy Risk Factor** B/D (when used long-term or in high doses)

**Lactation** Enters breast milk/use caution - see Breast-feeding Issues

**Use** Treatment of diarrhea or relief of pain; neonatal opiate withdrawal

**Mechanism of Action/Effect** Increases smooth muscle tone in GI tract, decreases motility and peristalsis, diminishes digestive secretions

**Contraindications** Hypersensitivity to opium or any component; diarrhea caused by poisoning until the toxic material has been removed; pregnancy (long-term use or high doses)

(Continued)

## Paregoric *(Continued)*

**Warnings** Use with caution in patients with respiratory, hepatic or renal dysfunction, severe prostatic hypertrophy, or history of narcotic abuse. Opium shares the toxic potential of opiate agonists, and usual precautions of opiate agonist therapy should be observed. Some preparations contain sulfites which may cause allergic reactions.

**Drug Interactions**

**Increased Effect/Toxicity:** Increased effect/toxicity with CNS depressants (eg, alcohol, narcotics, benzodiazepines, tricyclic antidepressants, MAO inhibitors, phenothiazine).

**Effects on Lab Values** ↑ aminotransferase [ALT (SGPT)/AST (SGOT)] (S)

**Adverse Reactions**

>10%: (With higher doses)
- Cardiovascular: Hypotension
- Central nervous system: Drowsiness, dizziness
- Gastrointestinal: Constipation
- Neuromuscular & skeletal: Weakness

1% to 10%:
- Central nervous system: Restlessness, headache, malaise
- Genitourinary: Ureteral spasms, decreased urination
- Miscellaneous: Histamine release

<1% (Limited to important or life-threatening symptoms): Respiratory depression

**Overdose/Toxicology** Symptoms of overdose include hypotension, drowsiness, seizures, and respiratory depression. Naloxone, 2 mg I.V. with repeat administration as necessary up to a total of 10 mg, can be used to reverse opiate effects.

**Pharmacodynamics/Kinetics**

**Metabolism:** Liver

**Excretion:** Urine

**Formulations** Liquid: 2 mg morphine equivalent/5 mL [equivalent to 20 mg opium powder] (5 mL, 60 mL, 473 mL, 4000 mL)

**Dosing**

**Adults:** Oral: 5-10 mL 1-4 times/day

**Stability**

**Storage:** Store in light-resistant, tightly closed container

**Additional Nursing Issues**

**Physical Assessment:** Monitor for excessive sedation, respiratory depression, or hypotension. For inpatients, implement safety measures (ie, side rails up, call light within reach, patient instructions to call for assistance, etc). Has potential for psychological or physiological dependence. **Pregnancy risk factor B/D** - see Pregnancy Risk Factor for cautious use.

**Patient Information/Instruction:** Take exactly as directed; do not increase dosage. May cause dependence with prolonged or excessive use. Avoid alcohol and all other prescription and OTC that may cause sedation (sleeping medications, some cough/cold remedies, antihistamines, etc). You may experience drowsiness, dizziness, or impaired judgment (use caution when driving or engaging in tasks that require alertness until response to drug is known) or postural hypotension (use caution when rising from sitting or lying position or when climbing stairs). You may experience nausea or loss of appetite (frequent small meals may help) or constipation (a laxative may be necessary). Report unresolved nausea, vomiting, respiratory difficulty (shortness of breath or decreased respirations), chest pain, or palpitations. **Breast-feeding precautions:** If nursing, take immediately after feeding or 4-6 hour before next feeding.

**Breast-feeding Issues:** Information regarding use while breast-feeding is based on experience with morphine. Probably safe with low doses and by administering dose after breast-feeding to further minimize exposure to the drug. Monitor the infant for possible side effects related to opiates.

**Additional Information** Some formulations may contain ethanol. Contains morphine 0.4 mg/mL and alcohol 45%.


- ♦ **Paremyd® Ophthalmic** *see page 1248*
- ♦ **Parenteral Multiple Vitamin** *see* Vitamin, Multiple *on page 1219*
- ♦ **Parenteral Therapy Recommendations/Guidelines** *see page 1326*
- ♦ **Parepectolin®** *see* Kaolin and Pectin With Opium *on page 642*
- ♦ **Pargyline and Methyclothiazide** *see* Methyclothiazide and Pargyline *on page 749*
- ♦ **Parhist SR®** *see page 1294*


## Paricalcitol (par eh CAL ci tol)

**U.S. Brand Names** Zemplar™

**Therapeutic Category** Vitamin D Analog

**Pregnancy Risk Factor** C

**Lactation** Excretion in breast milk unknown/use caution

**Use** Prevention and treatment of secondary hyperparathyroidism associated with chronic renal failure; evaluation has been limited to patients on hemodialysis

**Mechanism of Action/Effect** Synthetic vitamin D analog which has been shown to reduce PTH serum concentrations

**Contraindications** Hypersensitivity to paricalcitol or any component; patients with evidence of vitamin D toxicity, hypercalcemia

**Warnings** Chronic administration can place patients at risk of hypercalcemia, elevated calcium-phosphorus product, and metastatic calcification. It should not be used in patients with evidence of hypercalcemia or vitamin D toxicity. Pregnancy factor C.

**Drug Interactions**

**Increased Effect/Toxicity:** Phosphate or vitamin D-related compounds should not be taken concurrently. Digitalis toxicity is potentiated by hypercalcemia.

**Adverse Reactions** The three most frequently reported events in the clinical studies were nausea, vomiting, and edema, which are commonly seen in hemodialysis patients.

>10%: Gastrointestinal: Nausea (13%)

1% to 10%:

Cardiovascular: Palpitations, peripheral edema (7%)

Central nervous system: Chills, malaise, fever, lightheadedness (5%)

Gastrointestinal: Vomiting (8%), GI bleeding (5%), xerostomia (3%)

Respiratory: Pneumonia (5%)

Miscellaneous: Flu-like symptoms, sepsis

**Overdose/Toxicology** Acute overdose may cause hypercalcemia. Monitor serum calcium and phosphorus closely during titration of paricalcitol. Dosage reduction/interruption may be required if hypercalcemia develops. Chronic use may predispose to metastatic calcification. Bone lesions may develop if parathyroid hormone is suppressed below normal.

**Pharmacodynamics/Kinetics**

**Protein Binding:** >99%

**Excretion:** Hepatobiliary excretion (74%) in healthy subjects; urinary excretion (16%), metabolites represent 51% to 59%

**Formulations** Injection: 5 mcg/mL (1 mL, 2 mL, 5 mL)

**Dosing**

**Adults:** I.V.: 0.04-0.1 mcg/kg (2.8-7 mcg) given as a bolus dose no more frequently than every other day at any time during dialysis; dose as high as 0.24 mcg/kg (16.8 mcg) have been administered safely. Usually start with 0.04 mcg/kg 3 times/week by I.V. bolus, increased by 0.04 mcg/kg every 2 weeks.

**Elderly:** Refer to adult dosing.

**Renal Impairment:** See adult dosing.

**Hepatic Impairment:** Kinetics have not been investigated in hepatically impaired patients.

**Monitoring Laboratory Tests** Serum calcium and phosphorus should be monitored closely (eg, twice weekly) during dose titration. Monitor serum PTH. In trials, a mean PTH level reduction of 30% was achieved within 6 weeks.

**Additional Nursing Issues**

**Physical Assessment:** Monitor laboratory results (see Monitoring Laboratory Tests). See Warnings/Precautions and Drug Interactions. Monitor patient response and adverse effects. Monitor for signs and symptoms of vitamin D intoxication. Assess knowledge/instruct patient on safe and appropriate use of paricalcitol and dietary requirements. **Pregnancy risk factor C** - benefits of use should outweigh possible risks. Note breast-feeding caution.

**Patient Information/Instruction:** Take as directed; do not increase dosage without consulting prescriber. Adhere to diet as recommended (do not take any other phosphate or vitamin D related compounds while taking paricalcitol). You may experience nausea or vomiting (small frequent meals, frequent mouth care, chewing gums, or sucking lozenges may help); swelling of extremities (elevate feet when sitting); lightheadedness or dizziness (use caution when driving or engaging in tasks requiring alertness until response to drug is known). Report persistent fever, gastric disturbances, abdominal pain or blood in stool, chest pain or palpitations, or signs of respiratory infection or flu. **Pregnancy/breast-feeding precautions:** Inform prescriber if you are or intend to be pregnant. Consult prescriber if breast-feeding.

**Geriatric Considerations:** Kinetics have not been investigated in geriatric patients.

♦ **Parlodel®** *see* Bromocriptine *on page 162*

♦ **Parnate®** *see* Tranylcypromine *on page 1164*

## Paromomycin (par oh moe MYE sin)

**U.S. Brand Names** Humatin®

**Therapeutic Category** Amebicide

**Pregnancy Risk Factor** C

**Lactation** Does not enter breast milk/compatible (see Breast-feeding)

**Use** Treatment of acute and chronic intestinal amebiasis; preoperatively to suppress intestinal flora; tapeworm infestations; rid bowel of nitrogen-forming bacteria in hepatic coma; treatment of *Cryptosporidium* diarrhea

**Mechanism of Action/Effect** Acts directly on ameba; has antibacterial activity against normal and pathogenic organisms in the GI tract; interferes with bacterial protein synthesis by binding to 30S ribosomal subunits

**Contraindications** Hypersensitivity to paromomycin or any component; intestinal obstruction; renal failure

**Warnings** Use with caution in patients with impaired renal function or possible or proven ulcerative bowel lesions. Pregnancy factor C.

**Drug Interactions**

**Decreased Effect:** Paromomycin may decrease the effect of digoxin and methotrexate.

**Increased Effect/Toxicity:** Paromomycin may increase the effect of oral anticoagulants.

**Food Interactions** Paromomycin may cause malabsorption of xylose, sucrose, and fats.

**Adverse Reactions**

1% to 10%: Gastrointestinal: Diarrhea, abdominal cramps, nausea, vomiting, heartburn

(Continued)

## Paromomycin *(Continued)*

<1% (Limited to important or life-threatening symptoms): Eosinophilia

**Overdose/Toxicology** Symptoms of overdose include nausea, vomiting, and diarrhea. Treatment is supportive and symptomatic.

**Pharmacodynamics/Kinetics**

**Excretion:** Feces

**Formulations** Capsule, as sulfate: 250 mg

**Dosing**

**Adults:** Oral:

Intestinal amebiasis: 25-35 mg/kg/day in 3 divided doses for 5-10 days

*Dientamoeba fragilis*: 25-30 mg/kg/day in 3 divided doses for 7 days

*Cryptosporidium*: Adults with AIDS: 1.5-2.25 g/day in 3-6 divided doses for 10-14 days (occasionally courses of up to 4-8 weeks may be needed)

Tapeworm (fish, dog, bovine, porcine): 1 g every 15 minutes for 4 doses

Hepatic coma: 4 g/day in 2-4 divided doses for 5-6 days

Dwarf tapeworm: 45 mg/kg/dose every day for 5-7 days

**Elderly:** Refer to adult dosing.

**Additional Nursing Issues**

**Physical Assessment:** Assess effectiveness and interactions of other medications (see Drug Interactions). See Contraindications and Warnings/Precautions for use cautions. Assess knowledge/teach patient appropriate use, reinfection prevention, possible side effects/interventions, and adverse symptoms to report (see Adverse Reactions and Overdose/Toxicology). **Pregnancy risk factor C** - benefits of use should outweigh possible risks.

**Patient Information/Instruction:** Take as directed, for full course of therapy. Do not skip doses. Maintain adequate hydration (2-3 L/day of fluids unless instructed to restrict fluid intake) and nutrition. If GI upset occurs, small frequent meals, frequent mouth care, sucking lozenges, or chewing gum may help. Report unresolved or severe nausea or vomiting, dizziness, ringing in ears, or loss of hearing. **Pregnancy precautions:** Inform prescriber if you are pregnant.

**Breast-feeding Issues:** Paromomycin is not expected to be excreted in breast milk since the drug is not systemically available after oral ingestion.

## Paroxetine (pa ROKS e teen)

**U.S. Brand Names** Paxil™

**Therapeutic Category** Antidepressant, Selective Serotonin Reuptake Inhibitor

**Pregnancy Risk Factor** C

**Lactation** Enters breast milk/not recommended

**Use** Treatment of depression; treatment of panic disorder and obsessive-compulsive disorder

**Mechanism of Action/Effect** Paroxetine is a selective serotonin reuptake inhibitor, chemically unrelated to tricyclic, tetracyclic, or other antidepressants; presumably, the inhibition of serotonin reuptake from brain synapse stimulated serotonin activity in the brain

**Contraindications** Hypersensitivity to SSRIs; do not use within 14 days of MAO inhibitors

**Warnings** Use cautiously in patients with a history of seizures, mania, renal disease, cardiac disease, suicidal ideation; or in children. Avoid ECT. Pregnancy factor C.

**Drug Interactions**

**Cytochrome P-450 Effect:** CYP2D6 enzyme substrate (minor); CYP1A2, 2D6, and 3A3/4 enzyme inhibitor

**Decreased Effect:** Decreased effect of paroxetine with phenobarbital and phenytoin.

**Increased Effect/Toxicity:** Increased toxicity with alcohol, cimetidine, and MAO inhibitors (hyperpyrexic crisis). Increased effect/toxicity of tricyclic antidepressants, fluoxetine, sertraline, phenothiazines, Class 1C antiarrhythmics, and warfarin. Potential for serotonin syndrome if combined with other serotonergic drugs.

**Effects on Lab Values** ↑ LFTs

**Adverse Reactions**

>10%:

Central nervous system: Headache, muscle weakness, somnolence, dizziness, insomnia

Gastrointestinal: Nausea, dry mouth, constipation, diarrhea

Genitourinary: Ejaculatory disturbances

Miscellaneous: Sweating

1% to 10%:

Cardiovascular: Palpitations, vasodilation, postural hypotension

Central nervous system: Nervousness, anxiety, agitation

Endocrine & metabolic: Decreased libido

Gastrointestinal: Anorexia, flatulence, vomiting, taste perversion

Genitourinary: Decreased libido

Neuromuscular & skeletal: Tremor, paresthesia

Ocular: Blurred vision

<1% (Limited to important or life-threatening symptoms): Bradycardia, hypotension, anemia, leukopenia, asthma

**Overdose/Toxicology** Symptoms of overdose include nausea, vomiting, drowsiness, sinus tachycardia, and dilated pupils. There are no specific antidotes. Treatment is supportive and symptomatic.

**Pharmacodynamics/Kinetics**

**Protein Binding:** 93% to 95%

**Half-life Elimination:** 21 hours

**Time to Peak:** 5.2 hours

**Metabolism:** Liver

**Excretion:** Hepatic and renal

**Onset:** Steady-state: ~10 days; therapeutic effects >2 weeks

**Formulations**

Suspension, oral: 10 mg/5 mL

Tablet: 10 mg, 20 mg, 30 mg, 40 mg

**Dosing**

**Adults:** Oral:

Depression: 20 mg once daily (maximum: 60 mg/day), preferably in the morning; in the elderly, in debilitated patients, or in patients with hepatic or renal impairment, start with 10 mg/day (maximum: 40 mg/day); adjust doses at 7-day intervals.

Obsessive compulsive disorder: Initial: 20 mg, then titrating upward, adjusting doses at intervals of 1 week minimum. Maximum daily dose: 60 mg

Panic attack: Initial: 10 mg every morning then titrating upward, adjusting doses of 10 mg at intervals of 1 week minimum; maximum: 60 mg/day

**Elderly:** Oral:

Depression: Initial: 10 mg once daily, preferably in the morning; usual dose: 20-30 mg/day; maximum: 40 mg/day

Obsessive compulsive disorder: Refer to adult dosing. Initial: 10 mg; maximum: 40 mg/day

Panic attack: Refer to adult dosing. Maximum: 40 mg/day.

**Renal Impairment:** Initial: 10 mg/day; maximum: 40 mg/day

**Hepatic Impairment:** Initial: 10 mg/day; maximum: 40 mg/day

**Monitoring Laboratory Tests** Hepatic and renal function

**Additional Nursing Issues**

**Physical Assessment:** Assess other medications patient may be taking for effectiveness and interactions (see Drug Interactions). See Warnings/Precautions for cautious use. Has potential for psychological or physiological dependence, abuse, or tolerance. Monitor laboratory tests, therapeutic response (ie, mental status, mood, affect, suicidal ideation), and adverse reactions at beginning of therapy and periodically with long-term use (see Adverse Reactions and Overdose/Toxicology). Taper dosage slowly when discontinuing. Assess knowledge/teach patient appropriate use, interventions to reduce side effects, and adverse symptoms to report. **Pregnancy risk factor C** - benefits of use should outweigh possible risks. Breast-feeding is not recommended.

**Patient Information/Instruction:** Take exactly as directed (do not increase dose or frequency); may take 2-3 weeks to achieve desired results; may cause physical and/or psychological dependence. Take in the morning to reduce the incidence of insomnia. Avoid excessive alcohol, caffeine, and other prescription or OTC medications not approved by prescriber. Maintain adequate hydration (2-3 L/day of fluids unless instructed to restrict fluid intake). You may experience drowsiness, dizziness, or light-headedness (use caution when driving or engaging in tasks requiring alertness until response to drug is known); nausea, vomiting, anorexia, or dry mouth (small frequent meals, frequent mouth care, chewing gum, or sucking lozenges may help); or orthostatic hypotension (use caution when climbing stairs or changing position from lying or sitting to standing). Report persistent insomnia or excessive daytime sedation; muscle cramping, tremors, weakness, or change in gait; chest pain, palpitations, or rapid heartbeat; vision changes or eye pain; difficulty breathing or breathlessness; abdominal pain or blood in stool; or worsening of condition. **Pregnancy/breast-feeding precautions:** Inform prescriber if you are or intend to be pregnant. Breast-feeding is not recommended.

**Geriatric Considerations:** Paroxetine's favorable side effect profile make it a useful alternative to traditional tricyclic antidepressants. Paroxetine is the most sedating of the currently available selective serotonin reuptake inhibitors. Paroxetine's half-life is approximately 21 hours and it has no active metabolites.

**Related Information**

Antidepressant Agents Comparison *on page 1368*

- **Partuss® LA** *see* Guaifenesin and Phenylpropanolamine *on page 550*
- **PAS** *see* Aminosalicylate Sodium *on page 70*
- **Patanol™** *see page 1282*
- **Pathocil®** *see* Dicloxacillin *on page 361*
- **Patient Factors That Influence Drug Therapy** *see page 19*
- **Pavabid®** *see* Papaverine *on page 883*
- **Pavatine®** *see* Papaverine *on page 883*
- **Paveral Stanley Syrup With Codeine Phosphate** *see* Codeine *on page 299*
- **Pavulon®** *see page 1248*
- **Paxil™** *see* Paroxetine *on previous page*
- **PBZ®** *see* Tripelennamine *on page 1186*
- **PBZ-SR®** *see* Tripelennamine *on page 1186*
- **PCE®** *see* Erythromycin *on page 435*
- **Peak and Trough Guidelines** *see page 1331*
- **Pebegal** *see* Benzonatate *on page 143*
- **Pectin With Opium and Kaolin** *see* Kaolin and Pectin With Opium *on page 642*
- **PediaCare® Oral** *see* Pseudoephedrine *on page 992*

- ♦ **Pediacof® Liquid** *see page 1306*
- ♦ **Pediaflor®** *see page 1294*
- ♦ **Pediapred® Oral** *see* Prednisolone *on page 960*
- ♦ **PediaProfen™** *see* Ibuprofen *on page 592*
- ♦ **Pediatric Dosage Estimation** *see page 1361*
- ♦ **Pediatric Triban®** *see* Trimethobenzamide *on page 1180*
- ♦ **Pediatrix** *see* Acetaminophen *on page 32*
- ♦ **Pediazole®** *see* Erythromycin and Sulfisoxazole *on page 438*
- ♦ **Pedi-Boro®** *see page 1294*
- ♦ **Pedi-Cort V® Topical** *see* Clioquinol and Hydrocortisone *on page 284*
- ♦ **Pedi-Dri® Topical** *see page 1247*
- ♦ **PediOtic®** *see page 1291*
- ♦ **Pedi-Pro® Topical** *see page 1247*
- ♦ **Pedituss® Liquid** *see page 1306*
- ♦ **PedvaxHIB™** *see page 1256*


## Pegaspargase (peg AS par jase)

**U.S. Brand Names** Oncaspar®

**Synonyms** PEG-L-Asparaginase

**Therapeutic Category** Antineoplastic Agent, Miscellaneous

**Pregnancy Risk Factor** C

**Lactation** Enters breast milk/contraindicated

**Use** Patients with acute lymphoblastic leukemia (ALL) who require L-asparaginase in their treatment regimen, but have developed hypersensitivity to the native forms of L-asparaginase. Use as a single agent should only be undertaken when multiagent chemotherapy is judged to be inappropriate for the patient.

**Mechanism of Action/Effect**

Pegaspargase is a modified version of the enzyme L-asparaginase; the L-asparaginase used in the manufacture of pegaspargase is derived from *Escherichia coli*

Some malignant cells (ie, lymphoblastic leukemia cells and those of lymphocyte derivation) must acquire the amino acid asparagine from surrounding fluid such as blood, whereas normal cells can synthesize their own asparagine. asparaginase is an enzyme that deaminates asparagine to aspartic acid and ammonia in the plasma and extracellular fluid and therefore deprives tumor cells of the amino acid for protein synthesis.

**Contraindications** Pancreatitis or a history of pancreatitis; patients who have had significant hemorrhagic events associated with prior L-asparaginase therapy; previous serious allergic reactions, such as generalized urticaria, bronchospasm, laryngeal edema, hypotension, or other unacceptable adverse reactions to pegaspargase.

**Warnings The U.S. Food and Drug Administration (FDA) currently recommends that procedures for proper handling and disposal of antineoplastic agents be considered.** Hypersensitivity reactions to pegaspargase, including life-threatening anaphylaxis, may occur during therapy, especially in patients with known hypersensitivity to the other forms of L-asparaginase. As a routine precaution, keep patients under observation for 1 hour with resuscitation equipment and other agents necessary to treat anaphylaxis (eg, epinephrine, oxygen, I.V. steroids) available. Use caution when treating patients with pegaspargase in combination with hepatotoxic agents, especially when liver dysfunction is present. Pregnancy factor C.

**Drug Interactions**

**Decreased Effect:** Asparaginase terminates methotrexate action by inhibition of protein synthesis and prevention of cell entry into the S Phase.

**Increased Effect/Toxicity:**

Aspirin, dipyridamole, heparin, warfarin, NSAIDs: Imbalances in coagulation factors have been noted with the use of pegaspargase - use with caution

Vincristine and prednisone: An increased toxicity has been noticed when asparaginase is administered with VCR and prednisone

Cyclophosphamide (decreased metabolism)

Mercaptopurine (increased hepatotoxicity)

Vincristine (increased neuropathy)

Prednisone (hyperglycemia)

**Adverse Reactions**

Overall, the adult patients had a somewhat higher incidence of L-asparaginase toxicities, except for hypersensitivity reactions, than the pediatric patients

>10%:

Cardiovascular: Edema

Central nervous system: Pain

Dermatologic: Urticaria, erythema

Gastrointestinal: Pancreatitis (sometimes fulminant and fatal); increased serum amylase and lipase

Hepatic: Elevations of AST, ALT and bilirubin (direct and indirect); jaundice, ascites and hypoalbuminemia, fatty changes in the liver, liver failure

Local: Induration, tenderness

Neuromuscular & skeletal: Arthralgia

Respiratory: Bronchospasm, dyspnea

Miscellaneous: Hypersensitivity: Acute or delayed, acute anaphylaxis, edema of the lips

1% to 10%:

Cardiovascular: Edema, hypotension, tachycardia, thrombosis

Central nervous system: Pain, fever, chills, malaise
Dermatologic: Rash, lip edema
Endocrine & metabolic: Hyperglycemia requiring insulin (3%)
Gastrointestinal: Emetic potential: Mild (>5%); abdominal pain, pancreatitis
Hematologic: Decreased anticoagulant effect, disseminated intravascular coagulation, decreased fibrinogen, hemolytic anemia, leukopenia, pancytopenia, thrombocytopenia, increased thromboplastin
Myelosuppressive effects:
WBC: Mild
Platelets: Mild
Onset (days): 7
Nadir (days): 14
Recovery (days): 21
Hepatic: ALT increase
Local: Injection site hypersensitivity
Respiratory: Dyspnea or bronchospasm

**Overdose/Toxicology** Symptoms of overdose include nausea and diarrhea.

**Pharmacodynamics/Kinetics**

**Distribution:** 70% to 80% of plasma volume; does not penetrate the CSF

**Half-life Elimination:** 5.73 days

**Metabolism:** Systemically degraded, only trace amounts are found in the urine

**Excretion:** Clearance unaffected by age, renal function, or hepatic function. L-asparaginase was measurable for at least 15 days following initial treatment with pegaspargase.

**Formulations** Injection, preservative free: 750 units/mL

**Dosing**

**Adults:** Dose must be individualized based upon clinical response and tolerance of the patient (refer to individual protocols). I.M. administration is **preferred** over I.V. administration; I.M. administration may decrease the incidence of hepatotoxicity, coagulopathy, and GI and renal disorders.
I.M., I.V.: 2500 units/m$^2$ every 14 days

**Administration**

**I.M.:** Must only be given as a deep intramuscular injection into a large muscle.
I.M.: limit the volume of a single injection site to 2 mL. If the volume to be administered is >2 mL, use multiple injection sites.

**I.V.:** Administer over a period of 1-2 hours in 100 mL of 0.9% sodium chloride or dextrose 5% in water.

**I.V. Detail:** Do not filter solution. Have available appropriate agents for maintenance of an adequate airway and treatment of a hypersensitivity reaction (antihistamine, epinephrine, oxygen, I.V. corticosteroids). Be prepared to treat anaphylaxis at each administration. Administer through an infusion that is already running.

**Stability**

**Storage:** Refrigerate at 2°C to 8°C (36°F to 46°F). Do not use of cloudy or if precipitate is present. Do not use if stored at room temperature for >48 hours. Do **not** freeze. Do not use product if it is known to have been frozen. Single-use vial; discard unused portions.

**Reconstitution:** Avoid excessive agitation; do **not** shake.
**Standard I.M. dilution:** Do not exceed 2 mL volume per injection site
**Standard I.V. dilution:** Dose/100 mL NS or $D_5W$; stable for 48 hours at room temperature.

**Monitoring Laboratory Tests** CBC, urinalysis, amylase, liver enzymes, prothrombin time, renal function, blood glucose

**Additional Nursing Issues**

**Physical Assessment:** Assess other medications patient may be taking for effectiveness and possible interactions (see Drug Interactions). Monitor infusion/injection site for extravasation. Be aware that anaphylactic reactions can occur with each administration (see Dosing). Monitor laboratory tests (pancreatic indicators), response to therapy, and possible adverse reactions (eg, EKG, peripheral circulation, serum glucose - hyperglycemia), CNS status, and opportunistic infections with each dose and on a regular basis (see Adverse Reactions). **Pregnancy risk factor C** - benefits of use must outweigh possible risk (see Pregnancy). Breast-feeding is contraindicated.

**Patient Information/Instruction:** This drug can only be given I.M. or I.V. Make note of scheduled return dates. Inform prescriber if you are using any other medications that may increase risk of bleeding. Possibility of hypersensitivity reactions includes anaphylaxis. Maintain adequate hydration (2-3 L/day of fluids unless instructed to restrict fluid intake) and nutrition (small frequent meals may help if you experience nausea, vomiting, or loss of appetite). Frequent mouth care may help reduce the incidence of mouth sores. You may experience dizziness, drowsiness, syncope, or blurred vision (use caution when driving or engaging in tasks that require alertness until response to drug is known). You may experience increased sweating, decreased sexual drive, or cough. Report immediately chest pain or heart palpitations; difficulty breathing or constant cough; rash, hives, or swelling of lips or mouth; or abdominal pain. Report swelling of extremities or sudden weight gain; burning, pain, or redness at infusion site; persistent fever or chills; unusual bruising or bleeding; twitching or tremors; pain on urination; or persistent nausea or diarrhea. **Pregnancy/breast-feeding precautions:** Inform prescriber if you are or intend to be pregnant. Do not breast-feed.

**Pregnancy Issues:** Based on limited reports in humans, the use of asparaginase does not seem to pose a major risk to the fetus when used in the 2nd and 3rd trimesters, or when exposure occurs prior to conception in either females or males. Because of the

(Continued)

## Pegaspargase *(Continued)*

teratogenicity observed in animals and the lack of human data after 1st trimester exposure, asparaginase should be used cautiously, if at all, during this period.

- **PEG-ES** *see* Polyethylene Glycol-Electrolyte Solution *on page 945*
- **PEG-L-Asparaginase** *see* Pegaspargase *on page 890*
- **Peglyte™** *see* Polyethylene Glycol-Electrolyte Solution *on page 945*

## Pemoline (PEM oh leen)

**U.S. Brand Names** Cylert®

**Synonyms** Phenylisohydantoin; PIO

**Therapeutic Category** Stimulant

**Pregnancy Risk Factor** B

**Lactation** Excretion in breast milk unknown/not recommended

**Use** Treatment of attention-deficit/hyperactivity disorder (ADHD); narcolepsy

**Mechanism of Action/Effect** Blocks the reuptake mechanism of dopaminergic neurons, appears to act at the cerebral cortex and subcortical structures; CNS and respiratory stimulant with weak sympathomimetic effects; actions may be mediated via increase in CNS dopamine

**Contraindications** Hypersensitivity to pemoline or any component; liver disease; psychosis

**Warnings** Use with caution in patients with renal dysfunction, hypertension, or a history of abuse.

**Drug Interactions**

**Decreased Effect:** Decreased effect of insulin.

**Increased Effect/Toxicity:** Pemoline taken with other CNS depressants, CNS stimulants or sympathomimetics may have additive therapeutic or side effects.

**Adverse Reactions**

>10%:

Central nervous system: Insomnia

Gastrointestinal: Anorexia, weight loss

1% to 10%:

Central nervous system: Dizziness, drowsiness, mental depression

Dermatologic: Rash

Gastrointestinal: Stomach pain, nausea

<1% (Limited to important or life-threatening symptoms): Seizures, precipitation of Tourette's syndrome, increased liver enzymes (usually reversible upon discontinuation), hepatitis, jaundice

**Overdose/Toxicology** Symptoms of overdose include tachycardia, hallucinations, and agitation. There is no specific antidote for intoxication and treatment is primarily supportive.

**Pharmacodynamics/Kinetics**

**Protein Binding:** 50%

**Half-life Elimination:** 12 hours

**Time to Peak:** Within 2-4 hours

**Metabolism:** Liver

**Excretion:** Urine; only negligible amounts can be detected in feces

**Onset:** Peak effect: 4 hours

**Duration:** 8 hours

**Formulations**

Tablet: 18.75 mg, 37.5 mg, 75 mg

Tablet, chewable: 37.5 mg

**Dosing**

**Adults:** Initial: 37.5 mg once daily; increase by 18.75 mg at 1-week intervals. Usual dose range: 56.25-75 mg; maximum daily dose: 112.5 mg; onset of effect within 3-4 weeks.

**Elderly:** Refer to adult dosing.

**Renal Impairment:** $Cl_{cr}$ <50 mL/minute: Avoid use.

**Administration**

**Oral:** Give medication in the morning.

**Monitoring Laboratory Tests** Liver enzymes

**Additional Nursing Issues**

**Physical Assessment:** Assess effectiveness and interactions of other medications (see Drug Interactions). See Contraindications and Warnings/Precautions for cautious use. After long-term use, taper dosage slowly when discontinuing. Monitor laboratory results (see above), effectiveness of therapy, and adverse reactions at beginning of therapy and periodically with long-term use. Assess knowledge/teach patient appropriate use, interventions to reduce side effects, and importance of reporting adverse symptoms promptly. Breast-feeding is not recommended.

**Patient Information/Instruction:** Take exactly as directed; do not change dosage or discontinue without consulting prescriber. Response may some time. Avoid alcohol, caffeine, or other stimulants. Maintain adequate fluid intake (2-3 L/day of fluids unless instructed to restrict fluid intake). You may experience nausea, decreased appetite, or altered taste sensation (small frequent meals may help maintain adequate nutrition); drowsiness, dizziness, or mental depression, especially during early therapy (use caution when driving or engaging in tasks requiring alertness until response to drug is known). Report unresolved rapid heartbeat; excessive agitation, nervousness, insomnia, tremors, dizziness, or seizures; skin rash or irritation; altered gait or movement; unusual mouth movements or vocalizations (Tourette's syndrome); or yellowing of skin or eyes, dark urine, or pale stools. **Breast-feeding precautions:** Breast-feeding is not recommended.

## Penbutolol (pen BYOO toe lole)

**U.S. Brand Names** Levatol®

**Therapeutic Category** Beta Blocker (with Intrinsic Sympathomimetic Activity)

**Pregnancy Risk Factor** C

**Lactation** Enters breast milk/use caution - see Breast-feeding Issues

**Use** Treatment of mild to moderate arterial hypertension

**Mechanism of Action/Effect** Blocks both $beta_1$- and $beta_2$-receptors and has mild intrinsic sympathomimetic activity. Has negative inotropic and chronotropic effects and can significantly slow A-V nodal conduction.

**Contraindications** Hypersensitivity to penbutolol; uncompensated congestive heart failure, cardiogenic shock, bradycardia or heart block, asthma

**Warnings** Negative myocardial inotropic and chronotropic effects may be additive to myocardial depressant effects of anesthetics. If undesirable, beta agonist (dopamine, isoproterenol) can reverse them. Beta-blockers may impair glucose tolerance, potentiate hypoglycemia, and/or mask signs or symptoms of hypoglycemia in a diabetic patient. Pregnancy factor C.

**Drug Interactions**

**Decreased Effect:** Penbutolol increases the volume of distribution for lidocaine, which could necessitate a larger loading dose.

**Adverse Reactions**

1% to 10%:

Cardiovascular: Congestive hea.t failure, arrhythmia

Central nervous system: Mental depression, headache, dizziness, fatigue

Gastrointestinal: Nausea, diarrhea, dyspepsia

Neuromuscular & skeletal: Arthralgia

<1% (Limited to important or life-threatening symptoms): Bradycardia, mesenteric arterial thrombosis, A-V block, persistent bradycardia, hypotension, edema, Raynaud's phenomena, cold extremities, insomnia, lethargy, nightmares, confusion, purpura, hypoglycemia, ischemic colitis, thrombocytopenia, bronchospasm, cough

**Overdose/Toxicology** Enhancement of elimination: Charcoal hemoperfusion can be used to lower serum levels. Treatment is symptom directed and supportive.

**Pharmacodynamics/Kinetics**

**Protein Binding:** 80% to 95%

**Half-life Elimination:** 22 hours

**Time to Peak:** 1.5-3 hours

**Metabolism:** Liver

**Excretion:** Urine

**Formulations** Tablet, as sulfate: 20 mg

**Dosing**

**Adults:** Oral: Initial: 20 mg once daily, full effect of a 20 or 40 mg dose is seen by the end of a 2-week period. Doses of 40-80 mg show little additional antihypertensive effects.

**Elderly:** Oral: Initial: 10 mg once daily

**Additional Nursing Issues**

**Physical Assessment:** Assess other medications the patient may taking for effectiveness and interactions (see Drug Interactions). Assess blood pressure and heart rate prior to and following first dose, any change in dosage, and periodically thereafter. Monitor or advise patient to monitor weight and fluid balance (I & O), assess for signs of CHF (edema, new cough or dyspnea, unresolved fatigue), and assess therapeutic effectiveness. Monitor serum glucose levels of diabetic patients since beta-blockers may alter glucose tolerance. Use/teach postural hypotension precautions. **Pregnancy risk factor C** - benefits of use should outweigh possible risks. Note breast-feeding caution (see Breast-feeding).

**Patient Information/Instruction:** Take exactly as directed. Do not increase, decrease, or adjust dosage without consulting prescriber. Take pulse daily, prior to medication and follow prescriber's instruction about holding medication. Do not take with antacids. Do not use alcohol or OTC medications (eg, cold remedies) without consulting prescriber. If diabetic, monitor serum sugars closely (may alter glucose tolerance or mask signs of hypoglycemia). May cause fatigue, dizziness, or postural hypotension; use caution when changing position from lying or sitting to standing, when driving, or when climbing stairs until response to medication is known. May cause alteration in sexual performance (reversible). Report unresolved swelling of extremities, difficulty breathing or new cough, unresolved fatigue, unusual weight gain, unresolved constipation, or unusual muscle weakness. **Pregnancy/breast-feeding precautions:** Inform prescriber if you are or intend to be pregnant. Consult prescriber if breast-feeding.

**Geriatric Considerations:** Due to alterations in the beta-adrenergic autonomic nervous system, beta-adrenergic blockade may result in less hemodynamic response than seen in younger adults. Studies indicate that despite decreased sensitivity to the chronotropic effects of beta blockade with age, there appears to be an increased myocardial sensitivity to the negative inotropic effect during stress (eg, exercise). Controlled trials have shown the overall response rate for propranolol to be only 20% to 50% in elderly populations. Therefore, all beta-adrenergic blocking drugs may result in a decreased response as compared to younger adults.

(Continued)

## Penbutolol *(Continued)*

**Breast-feeding Issues:** It is recommended that the infant be monitored for signs or symptoms of beta-blockade (hypotension, bradycardia, etc) with long-term use.

**Additional Information** A 10 mg dose reduces exercise-induced tachycardia by 50%. In the elderly, due to alterations in the beta-adrenergic autonomic nervous system, beta-blockade may result in less hemodynamic response in geriatric patients than seen in younger adults. Despite decreased sensitivity to the chronotropic effects of beta blockade with age, there appears to be an increased myocardial sensitivity to the negative inotropic effect during stress.

**Related Information**

Beta-Blockers Comparison *on page 1376*

## Penciclovir (pen SYE kloe veer)

**U.S. Brand Names** Denavir™

**Therapeutic Category** Antiviral Agent

**Pregnancy Risk Factor** B

**Lactation** Excretion in breast milk unknown

**Use** Topical treatment of herpes simplex labialis (cold sores); potentially used for Epstein-Barr virus infections; investigations are ongoing for immunocompromised patients with herpes

**Mechanism of Action/Effect** Phosphorylated in the virus-infected cells to penciclovir triphosphate, which competitively inhibits DNA polymerase in HSV-1 and HSV-2 strains. This prevents viral replication by inhibition of viral DNA synthesis. Some activity has been demonstrated against Epstein-Barr and varicella-zoster virus (VZV).

**Contraindications** Hypersensitivity to penciclovir or any of component; previous and significant adverse reactions to famciclovir

**Warnings** Apply only to herpes labialis on lips and face. Application to mucous membranes is not recommended. Effect has not been evaluated in immunocompromised patients.

**Adverse Reactions**

>10%: Dermatologic: Erythema (mild) (50%)

1% to 10%: Central nervous system: Headache (5.3%)

<1% (Limited to important or life-threatening symptoms): Local anesthesia

**Overdose/Toxicology** Penciclovir is poorly absorbed if ingested orally. Adverse reactions related to oral ingestion are unlikely.

**Pharmacodynamics/Kinetics**

**Protein Binding:** <20%

**Half-life Elimination:** 2 hours

**Metabolism:** Phosphorylated in virus-infected cells to active form

**Excretion:** Urine

**Formulations** Cream: 1% [10 mg/g] (2 g)

**Dosing**

**Adults:** Apply cream at the first sign or symptom of cold sore (eg, tingling, swelling); apply every 2 hours during waking hours for 4 days.

**Elderly:** Refer to adult dosing.

**Stability**

**Storage:** Store at or below 30°C. Do not freeze.

**Additional Nursing Issues**

**Physical Assessment:** See Warnings/Precautions and Contraindications for use cautions. Assess for effectiveness of therapy and symptoms of infection. Assess knowledge/teach patient appropriate application and use and adverse symptoms (see Adverse Reactions) to report. Note breast-feeding caution.

**Patient Information/Instruction:** This is not a cure for herpes (recurrences tend to appear within 3 months of original infection), nor will this medication reduce the risk of transmission to others when lesions are present. For external use only. Wash hands before and after application. Apply this film over affected areas at first sign of cold sore. Avoid use of other topical creams, lotions, or ointments unless approved by prescriber. You may experience headache, mild rash, or taste disturbances. **Breast-feeding precautions:** Consult prescriber if breast-feeding.


- **Penecort®** *see* Hydrocortisone *on page 578*
- **Penecort®** *see* Topical Corticosteroids *on page 1152*
- **Penetrex™** *see* Enoxacin *on page 420*
- **Penicil** *see* Penicillin G Procaine *on page 899*


## Penicillamine (pen i SIL a meen)

**U.S. Brand Names** Cuprimine®; Depen®

**Synonyms** D-3-Mercaptovaline; β,β-Dimethylcysteine; D-Penicillamine

**Therapeutic Category** Chelating Agent

**Pregnancy Risk Factor** D

**Lactation** Enters breast milk/contraindicated

**Use** Treatment of Wilson's disease, cystinuria, adjunct in the treatment of rheumatoid arthritis; lead, mercury, copper, and possibly gold poisoning. (**Note:** Oral DMSA is preferable for lead or mercury poisoning); primary biliary cirrhosis; as adjunctive therapy following initial treatment with calcium EDTA or BAL.

**Mechanism of Action/Effect** Chelates with lead, copper, mercury and other heavy metals to form stable, soluble complexes that are excreted in urine; depresses circulating

IgM rheumatoid factor, depresses T-cell but not B-cell activity; combines with cystine to form a compound which is more soluble, thus cystine calculi are prevented

**Contraindications** Hypersensitivity to penicillamine or any component; renal insufficiency; patients with previous penicillamine-related aplastic anemia or agranulocytosis; concomitant administration with other hematopoietic-depressant drugs (eg, gold, immunosuppressants, antimalarials, phenylbutazone); pregnancy

**Warnings** Cross-sensitivity with penicillin is possible; therefore, should be used cautiously in patients with a history of penicillin allergy. Patients on penicillamine for Wilson's disease or cystinuria should receive pyridoxine supplementation 25 mg/day. Once instituted for Wilson's disease or cystinuria, continue treatment on a daily basis. Interruptions of even a few days have been followed by hypersensitivity with reinstitution of therapy. Penicillamine has been associated with fatalities due to agranulocytosis, aplastic anemia, thrombocytopenia, Goodpasture's syndrome, and myasthenia gravis. Patients should be warned to report promptly any symptoms suggesting toxicity. Approximately 33% of patients will experience an allergic reaction. Since toxicity may be dose related, it is recommended not to exceed 750 mg/day in the elderly.

**Drug Interactions**

**Decreased Effect:** Decreased effect of penicillamine when taken with iron and zinc salts, antacids (magnesium, calcium, aluminum), and food. Digoxin levels may be decreased when taken with penicillamine.

**Increased Effect/Toxicity:** Increased effect or toxicity of gold, antimalarials, immunosuppressants, and phenylbutazone (hematologic, renal toxicity).

**Food Interactions** Penicillamine serum levels may be decreased if taken with food.

**Effects on Lab Values** Positive ANA

**Adverse Reactions**

>10%:

- Central nervous system: Fever
- Dermatologic: Rash, urticaria, itching
- Gastrointestinal: Hypogeusia, stomatitis, diarrhea, nausea, vomiting, anorexia, stomach pain
- Neuromuscular & skeletal: Arthralgia

1% to 10%:

- Cardiovascular: Edema of the face, feet, or lower legs
- Central nervous system: Fever, chills
- Gastrointestinal: Weight gain, sore throat
- Genitourinary: Bloody or cloudy urine
- Hematologic: Aplastic or hemolytic anemia, leukopenia, thrombocytopenia, agranulocytosis
- Miscellaneous: White spots on lips or mouth, positive ANA

<1% (Limited to important or life-threatening symptoms): Toxic epidermal necrolysis, pemphigus, increased friability of the skin, exfoliative dermatitis, cholestatic jaundice, hepatitis, nephrotic syndrome, wheezing

**Overdose/Toxicology** Symptoms of overdose include nausea and vomiting. Treatment is supportive.

**Pharmacodynamics/Kinetics**

**Protein Binding:** 80% bound to albumin

**Half-life Elimination:** 1.7-3.2 hours

**Time to Peak:** Within 2 hours

**Metabolism:** Liver

**Excretion:** Urine

**Formulations**

Capsule: 125 mg, 250 mg

Tablet: 250 mg

**Dosing**

**Adults:** Oral:

- Rheumatoid arthritis: 125-250 mg/day, may increase dose at 1- to 3-month intervals up to 1-1.5 g/day
- Wilson's disease (doses titrated to maintain urinary copper excretion >1 mg/day): 250 mg 4 times/day
- Cystinuria: 1-4 g/day in divided doses every 6 hours
- Lead poisoning (continue until blood lead level is <60 µg/dL): 25-35 mg/kg/d, administered in 3-4 divided doses; initiating treatment at 25% of this dose and gradually increasing to the full dose over 2-3 weeks may minimize adverse reactions.
- Primary biliary cirrhosis: 250 mg/day to start, increase by 250 mg every 2 weeks up to a maintenance dose of 1 g/day, usually given 250 mg 4 times/day.

**Elderly:** Refer to adult dosing.

**Renal Impairment:** $Cl_{cr}$ <50 mL/minute: Avoid use.

**Administration**

**Oral:** For patients who cannot swallow, contents of capsules may be administered in 15-30 mL of chilled purêed fruit or fruit juice. Give on an empty stomach (1 hour before meals and at bedtime).

**Stability**

**Storage:** Store in tight, well-closed containers.

**Monitoring Laboratory Tests** Urinalysis, CBC with differential, platelet count, liver function; weekly measurements of urinary and blood concentration of the intoxicating metal is indicated (3 months has been tolerated).

CBC: WBC <3500/mm$^3$, neutrophils <2000/mm$^3$, or monocytes >500/mm$^3$ indicate need to stop therapy immediately. Quantitative 24-hour urine protein at 1- to 2-week intervals

(Continued)

## Penicillamine *(Continued)*

initially (first 2-3 months); urinalysis, LFTs occasionally; platelet counts <100,000/mm³ indicate need to stop therapy until numbers of platelets increase.

**Additional Nursing Issues**

**Physical Assessment:** Assess effectiveness and interactions of other medications patient may be taking (see Contraindications, Warnings/Precautions, and Drug Interactions). Monitor laboratory tests (see above) and therapeutic response (dependent on purpose of therapy) and adverse reactions (especially opportunistic infections) at beginning of therapy and periodically throughout therapy (see Warnings/Precautions, Adverse Reactions, and Overdose/Toxicology). Schedule ophthalmic evaluations for patients who develop eye complaints during long-term NSAID therapy. Assess knowledge/teach patient appropriate use, interventions to reduce side effects, and adverse symptoms to report. **Pregnancy risk factor D** - assess knowledge/instruct patient on the need to use appropriate contraceptive measures and the need to avoid pregnancy. Breast-feeding is contraindicated.

**Patient Information/Instruction:** Take this medication exactly as directed; do not increase dose without consulting prescriber. Capsules may be opened and contents mixed in 15-30 mL of chilled fruit juice or puree; do not take with milk or milk products. Avoid alcohol or excess intake of vitamin A. It is preferable to take penicillamine on empty stomach (1 hour before or 2 hours after meals). Maintain adequate hydration (2-3 L/day of fluids unless instructed to restrict fluid intake).

Wilson's disease: Avoid chocolate, shellfish, nuts, mushrooms, liver, broccoli, molasses.

Lead poisoning: Decrease dietary calcium.

Cystinuria: Take with large amounts of water.

You may experience anorexia, nausea, vomiting (frequent small meals, frequent mouth care, sucking lozenges, or chewing gum may help). Report persistent fever or chills, unhealed sores, white spots or sores in mouth or vaginal area, extreme fatigue, or signs of infection; breathlessness, difficulty breathing, or unusual cough; unusual bruising/bleeding; blood in urine, stool, mouth, or vomitus; swollen face or extremities; skin rash or itching; muscle pain or cramping; or pain on urination. **Pregnancy/breast-feeding precautions:** Do not get pregnant while taking this medication; use appropriate barrier contraceptives. Do not breast-feed.

**Geriatric Considerations:** Close monitoring of elderly is necessary; since steady-state serum/tissue concentrations rise slowly, "go slow" with dose increase intervals; steady-state concentrations decline slowly after discontinuation suggesting extensive tissue distribution. Skin rashes and taste abnormalities occur more frequently in the elderly than in young adults; leukopenia, thrombocytopenia, and proteinuria occur with equal frequency in both younger adults and elderly. Since toxicity may be dose related, it is recommended not to exceed 750 mg/day in the elderly.

## Penicillin G Benzathine (pen i SIL in jee BENZ a theen)

**U.S. Brand Names** Bicillin® L-A; Permapen®

**Synonyms** Benzathine Benzylpenicillin; Benzathine Penicillin G; Benzylpenicillin Benzathine

**Therapeutic Category** Antibiotic, Penicillin

**Pregnancy Risk Factor** B

**Lactation** Enters breast milk/compatible

**Use** Active against some gram-positive organisms, few gram-negative organisms such as *Neisseria gonorrhoeae*, and some anaerobes and spirochetes; used only for the treatment of mild to moderately severe infections caused by organisms susceptible to low concentrations of penicillin G or for prophylaxis of infections caused by these organisms; used when patient cannot be kept in a hospital environment and neurosyphilis has been ruled out

The CDC and AAP do not currently recommend the use of penicillin G benzathine to treat congenital syphilis or neurosyphilis due to reported treatment failures and lack of published clinical data on its efficacy.

**Mechanism of Action/Effect** Interferes with bacterial cell wall synthesis during active multiplication, causing cell wall death and resultant bactericidal activity against susceptible bacteria

**Contraindications** Hypersensitivity to penicillins, any component, cephalosporins, or imipenem; history of hypersensitivity to other beta-lactams

**Warnings** Use with caution in patients with impaired renal function, seizure disorder. CDC and AAP do not currently recommend the use of penicillin G benzathine to treat congenital syphilis or neurosyphilis due to reported treatment failures and lack of published clinical data on its efficacy.

**Drug Interactions**

**Decreased Effect:** Tetracyclines may decrease penicillin effectiveness. Efficacy of oral contraceptives may be reduced when taken with penicillins.

**Increased Effect/Toxicity:** Probenecid increases penicillin levels. Aminoglycosides may lead to synergistic efficacy.

**Effects on Lab Values** Positive Coombs' [direct], false-positive urinary and/or serum proteins; false-positive or negative urinary glucose using Clinitest®

**Adverse Reactions**

1% to 10%: Local: Local pain

<1% (Limited to important or life-threatening symptoms): Convulsions, hemolytic anemia, positive Coombs' reaction, acute interstitial nephritis, Jarisch-Herxheimer reaction

**Overdose/Toxicology** Symptoms of penicillin overdose include neuromuscular hypersensitivity (eg, agitation, hallucinations, asterixis, encephalopathy, confusion, and seizures). Electrolyte imbalance may occur if the preparation contains potassium or sodium salts, especially in renal failure. Hemodialysis may be helpful to aid in removal of the drug from blood; otherwise, treatment is supportive or symptom directed.

**Pharmacodynamics/Kinetics**

**Time to Peak:** Within 12-24 hours; serum levels are usually detectable for 1-4 weeks depending on the dose. Larger doses result in more sustained levels rather than higher levels.

**Formulations** Injection: 300,000 units/mL (10 mL); 600,000 units/mL (1 mL, 2 mL, 4 mL)

**Dosing**

**Adults:** I.M.: Give undiluted injection; higher doses result in more sustained rather than higher levels. Use a penicillin G benzathine-penicillin G procaine combination to achieve early peak levels in acute infections.

Group A streptococcal upper respiratory infection: 1.2 million units as a single dose

Prophylaxis of recurrent rheumatic fever: 1.2 million units every 3-4 weeks or 600,000 units twice monthly

Early syphilis: 2.4 million units as a single dose in 2 injection sites

Syphilis of more than 1-year duration: 2.4 million units in 2 injection sites once weekly for 3 doses

Not indicated as single drug therapy for neurosyphilis, but may be given 1 time/week for 3 weeks following I.V. treatment (refer to Penicillin G monograph for dosing)

**Elderly:** Not indicated as single drug therapy for neurosyphilis, but may be given 1 time/week for 3 weeks following I.V. treatment (see Penicillin G for dosing). No adjustment for renal function or age is necessary. Following equal, simple I.M. injections, the elderly have serum penicillin concentrations approximately twice that of younger adults 48, 96, and 144 hours postadministration.

**Administration**

**I.M.:** Administer by deep I.M. injection in the upper outer quadrant of the buttock. Do **not** give I.V., intra-arterially, or S.C. When doses are repeated, rotate the injection site.

**Stability**

**Storage:** Store in refrigerator.

**Monitoring Laboratory Tests** Perform culture and sensitivity before administering first dose.

**Additional Nursing Issues**

**Physical Assessment:** Assess patient history for allergy. Monitor for hypersensitivity reaction and opportunistic infection.

**Patient Information/Instruction:** Take as directed, for full course of therapy. Maintain adequate hydration (2-3 L/day of fluids unless instructed to restrict fluid intake). If begin treated for sexually transmitted disease, partner will also need to be treated. Small frequent meals, frequent mouth care, sucking lozenges, or chewing gum may reduce nausea or dry mouth. Important to maintain good oral and vaginal hygiene to reduce incidence of opportunistic infection. If diabetic, drug may cause false tests with Clinitest® urine glucose monitoring; use of glucose oxidase methods (Clinistix®) or serum glucose monitoring is preferable. This drug may interfere with oral contraceptives; an alternate form of birth control should be used. Report persistent diarrhea, fever, chills, unhealed sores, bloody urine or stool, muscle pain, mouth sores, or difficulty breathing.

## Penicillin G, Parenteral, Aqueous

(pen i SIL in jee, pa REN ter al, AYE kwee us)

**U.S. Brand Names** Pfizerpen®

**Synonyms** Benzylpenicillin Potassium; Benzylpenicillin Sodium; Crystalline Penicillin; Penicillin G Potassium; Penicillin G Sodium

**Therapeutic Category** Antibiotic, Penicillin

**Pregnancy Risk Factor** B

**Lactation** Enters breast milk/compatible

**Use** Active against some gram-positive organisms, generally not *Staphylococcus aureus*; some gram-negative organisms such as *Neisseria gonorrhoeae*, and some anaerobes and spirochetes; although ceftriaxone is now the drug of choice for Lyme disease and gonorrhea

**Mechanism of Action/Effect** Interferes with bacterial cell wall synthesis during active multiplication, causing cell wall death and resultant bactericidal activity against susceptible bacteria

**Contraindications** Hypersensitivity to penicillins, any component, cephalosporins, or imipenem

**Warnings** Avoid intravascular or intra-arterial administration or injection into or near major peripheral nerves or blood vessels since such injections may cause severe and/or permanent neurovascular damage. Use with caution in patients with renal impairment (dosage reduction required), pre-existing seizure disorders.

**Drug Interactions**

**Decreased Effect:** Tetracyclines may decrease penicillin effectiveness. Efficacy of oral contraceptives may be reduced when taken with penicillins.

**Increased Effect/Toxicity:** Probenecid increases penicillin levels. Aminoglycosides may lead to synergistic efficacy.

**Effects on Lab Values** False-positive or negative urinary glucose determination using Clinitest®; positive Coombs' [direct]; false-positive urinary and/or serum proteins

(Continued)

## Penicillin G, Parenteral, Aqueous *(Continued)*

**Adverse Reactions** <1% (Limited to important or life-threatening symptoms): Convulsions, hemolytic anemia, positive Coombs' reaction, acute interstitial nephritis, Jarisch-Herxheimer reaction

**Overdose/Toxicology** Symptoms of penicillin overdose include neuromuscular hypersensitivity (eg, agitation, hallucinations, asterixis, encephalopathy, confusion, and seizures). Electrolyte imbalance may occur if the preparation contains potassium or sodium salts, especially in renal failure. Treatment is supportive or symptom directed.

**Pharmacodynamics/Kinetics**

**Protein Binding:** 65%

**Distribution:** Crosses the placenta; penetration across the blood-brain barrier is poor, despite inflamed meninges; relative diffusion of antimicrobial agents from blood into cerebrospinal fluid (CSF): Good only with inflammation (exceeds usual MICs)

Ratio of CSF to blood level (%): Normal meninges: <1; Inflamed meninges: 3-5

**Half-life Elimination:** Normal renal function: 20-50 minutes; End-stage renal disease: 3.3-5.1 hours

**Time to Peak:** I.M.: Within 30 minutes; I.V. Within 1 hour

**Metabolism:** Liver

**Excretion:** Urine

**Formulations**

Injection, as sodium: 5 million units

Injection:

Frozen premixed, as potassium: 1 million units, 2 million units, 3 million units

Powder, as potassium: 1 million units, 5 million units, 10 million units, 20 million units

**Dosing**

**Adults:** I.M., I.V.: 2-24 million units/day in divided doses every 4 hours

**Elderly:** Refer to adult dosing.

**Renal Impairment:** Dosage modification is required in patients with renal insufficiency.

$Cl_{cr}$ 30-50 mL/minute: Administer every 6 hours.

$Cl_{cr}$ 10-30 mL/minute: Administer every 8 hours.

$Cl_{cr}$ <10 mL/minute: Administer every 12 hours.

Moderately dialyzable (20% to 50%)

Continuous arteriovenous or venovenous hemofiltration (CAVH): Dose as $Cl_{cr}$ 10-50 mL/minute.

**Administration**

**I.M.:** Administer I.M. by deep injection in the upper outer quadrant of the buttock. Administer injection around-the-clock to promote less variation in peak and trough levels.

**I.V.:** While I.M. route is preferred route of administration, large doses should be administered by continuous I.V. infusion. Determine volume and rate of fluid administration required in a 24-hour period. Add appropriate daily dosage to this fluid. Rapid administration or excessive dosage can cause electrolyte imbalance, cardiac arrhythmias, and/or seizures.

**Stability**

**Storage:** Penicillin G potassium is stable at room temperature.

**Reconstitution:** Reconstituted parenteral solution is stable for 7 days when refrigerated (2°C to 15°C). Penicillin G potassium for I.V. infusion in NS or $D_5W$, solution is stable for 24 hours at room temperature.

**Compatibility:** Incompatible with aminoglycosides. Inactivated in acidic or alkaline solutions.

**Monitoring Laboratory Tests** Perform culture and sensitivity before administering first dose.

**Additional Nursing Issues**

**Physical Assessment:** Assess patient for allergy. Monitor for hypersensitivity reaction and opportunistic infection.

**Patient Information/Instruction:** This medication will be administered I.V. or I.M. Maintain adequate hydration (2-3 L/day of fluids unless instructed to restrict fluid intake). If being treated for sexually transmitted disease, partner will also need to be treated. Small frequent meals, frequent mouth care, sucking lozenges, or chewing gum may reduce nausea or dry mouth. Important to maintain good oral and vaginal hygiene to reduce incidence of opportunistic infection. If diabetic, drug may cause false tests with Clinitest® urine glucose monitoring; use of glucose oxidase methods (Clinistix®) or serum glucose monitoring is preferable. This drug may interfere with oral contraceptives; an alternate form of birth control should be used. Report persistent diarrhea, fever, chills, unhealed sores, bloody urine or stool, muscle pain, mouth sores, or difficulty breathing.

**Geriatric Considerations:** Despite a reported prolonged half-life, it is usually not necessary to adjust the dose of penicillin G or VK in the elderly to account for renal function changes with age, however, it is advised to calculate an estimated creatinine clearance and adjust dose accordingly.

**Additional Information**

Penicillin G potassium: 1.7 mEq of potassium and 0.3 mEq of sodium per 1 million units of penicillin G

Penicillin G sodium: 2 mEq of sodium per 1 million units of penicillin G

pH: 6-7.5

♦ **Penicillin G Potassium** *see* Penicillin G, Parenteral, Aqueous *on previous page*

## Penicillin G Procaine (pen i SIL in jee PROE kane)

**U.S. Brand Names** Crysticillin® A.S.; Wycillin®

**Synonyms** APPG; Aqueous Procaine Penicillin G; Procaine Benzylpenicillin; Procaine Penicillin G

**Therapeutic Category** Antibiotic, Penicillin

**Pregnancy Risk Factor** B

**Lactation** Enters breast milk/compatible

**Use** Moderately severe infections due to *Neisseria gonorrhoeae, Treponema pallidum* and other penicillin G-sensitive microorganisms that are susceptible to low but prolonged serum penicillin concentrations

**Mechanism of Action/Effect** Inhibits bacterial cell wall synthesis by binding to one or more of the penicillin binding proteins (PBPs); which in turn inhibits the final transpeptidation step of peptidoglycan synthesis in bacterial cell walls, thus inhibiting cell wall biosynthesis. Bacteria eventually lyse due to ongoing activity of cell wall autolytic enzymes (autolysins and murein hydrolases) while cell wall assembly is arrested.

**Contraindications** Hypersensitivity to penicillins, any component, cephalosporins, or imipenem; patients hypersensitive to procaine

**Warnings** May need to modify dosage in patients with severe renal impairment, seizure disorders. Avoid I.V., intravascular, or intra-arterial administration of penicillin G procaine since severe and/or permanent neurovascular damage may occur.

**Drug Interactions**

**Decreased Effect:** Tetracyclines may decrease penicillin effectiveness. Efficacy of oral contraceptives may be reduced when taken with penicillins.

**Increased Effect/Toxicity:** Probenecid increases penicillin levels. Aminoglycosides may lead to synergistic efficacy.

**Effects on Lab Values** Positive Coombs' [direct], false-positive urinary and/or serum proteins

**Adverse Reactions**

>10%: Local: Pain at injection site

<1% (Limited to important or life-threatening symptoms): Myocardial depression, vasodilation, conduction disturbances, seizures, hemolytic anemia, positive Coombs' reaction, interstitial nephritis, Jarisch-Herxheimer reaction

**Overdose/Toxicology** Symptoms of penicillin overdose include neuromuscular hypersensitivity (eg, agitation, hallucinations, asterixis, encephalopathy, confusion, and seizures). Electrolyte imbalance may occur if the preparation contains potassium or sodium salts, especially in renal failure. Hemodialysis may be helpful to aid in removal of the drug from blood; otherwise, treatment is supportive or symptom directed.

**Pharmacodynamics/Kinetics**

**Protein Binding:** ~65%

**Distribution:** Penetration across the blood-brain barrier is poor, despite inflamed meninges

**Time to Peak:** Within 1-4 hours; can persist within the therapeutic range for 15-24 hours

**Metabolism:** Liver

**Excretion:** Renal clearance is delayed in patients with impaired renal function; 60% to 90% of the drug is excreted unchanged via renal tubular excretion.

**Formulations** Injection, suspension: 300,000 units/mL (10 mL); 500,000 units/mL (1.2 mL); 600,000 units/mL (1 mL, 2 mL, 4 mL)

**Dosing**

**Adults:** I.M.:

Uncomplicated gonorrhea: 1 g probenecid orally, then 4.8 million units procaine penicillin divided into 2 injection sites 30 minutes later

Endocarditis caused by susceptible viridans *Streptococcus* (when used in conjunction with an aminoglycoside): 1.2 million units every 6 hours for 2-4 weeks

Neurosyphilis: 2-4 million units/day with 500 mg probenecid by mouth 4 times/day for 10-14 days; **penicillin G aqueous I.V. is the preferred agent**

**Elderly:** Refer to adult dosing.

**Renal Impairment:**

$Cl_{cr}$ 10-30 mL/minute: Administer every 8-12 hours.

$Cl_{cr}$ <10 mL/minute: Administer every 12-18 hours.

Moderately dialyzable (20% to 50%)

**Administration**

**I.M.:** Procaine suspension is for deep I.M. injection only. Rotate the injection site.

**Stability**

**Storage:** Store in refrigerator.

**Monitoring Laboratory Tests** Periodic renal and hematologic function with prolonged therapy; WBC count; perform culture and sensitivity before administering first dose.

**Additional Nursing Issues**

**Physical Assessment:** Assess patient history for allergy. Monitor for hypersensitivity reaction and opportunistic infection.

**Patient Information/Instruction:** Take as directed, for full course of therapy. Maintain adequate hydration (2-3 L/day of fluids unless instructed to restrict fluid intake). If being treated for sexually transmitted disease, partner will also need to be treated. Small frequent meals, frequent mouth care, sucking lozenges, or chewing gum may reduce nausea or dry mouth. Important to maintain good oral and vaginal hygiene to reduce incidence of opportunistic infection. If diabetic, drug may cause false tests with Clinitest® urine glucose monitoring; use of glucose oxidase methods (Clinistix®) or

(Continued)

## Penicillin G Procaine *(Continued)*

serum glucose monitoring is preferable. This drug may interfere with oral contraceptives; an alternate form of birth control should be used. Report persistent diarrhea, fever, chills, unhealed sores, bloody urine or stool, muscle pain, mouth sores, or difficulty breathing.

**Geriatric Considerations:** Dosage does not usually need to be adjusted in the elderly, however, if multiple doses are to be given, adjust dose for renal function.

♦ **Penicillin G Sodium** *see* Penicillin G, Parenteral, Aqueous *on page 897*

## Penicillin V Potassium (pen i SIL in vee poe TASS ee um)

**U.S. Brand Names** Beepen-VK®; Betapen®-VK; Pen.Vee® K; Robicillin® VK; Veetids®

**Synonyms** Pen VK; Phenoxymethyl Penicillin

**Therapeutic Category** Antibiotic, Penicillin

**Pregnancy Risk Factor** B

**Lactation** Enters breast milk (other penicillins are compatible with breast-feeding)

**Use** Treatment of moderate to severe susceptible bacterial infections; no longer recommended for dental procedure prophylaxis; prophylaxis in rheumatic fever; infections caused by susceptible organisms involving the respiratory tract, otitis media, sinusitis, skin, and urinary tract

**Mechanism of Action/Effect** Inhibits bacterial cell wall synthesis by binding to one or more of the penicillin binding proteins (PBPs); which in turn inhibits the final transpeptidation step of peptidoglycan synthesis in bacterial cell walls, thus inhibiting cell wall biosynthesis. Bacteria eventually lyse due to ongoing activity of cell wall autolytic enzymes (autolysins and murein hydrolases) while cell wall assembly is arrested.

**Contraindications** Hypersensitivity to penicillins, any component, cephalosporins, or imipenem

**Warnings** Use with caution in patients with severe renal impairment (modify dosage).

**Drug Interactions**

**Decreased Effect:** Tetracyclines may decrease penicillin effectiveness. Efficacy of oral contraceptives may be reduced when taken with penicillins.

**Increased Effect/Toxicity:** Probenecid increases penicillin levels. Aminoglycosides may cause synergistic efficacy.

**Food Interactions** May be administered with food, however, peak concentration may be delayed.

**Effects on Lab Values** False-positive or negative urinary glucose determination using Clinitest®; positive Coombs' [direct]; false-positive urinary and/or serum proteins

**Adverse Reactions**

>10%: Gastrointestinal: Mild diarrhea, vomiting, nausea, oral candidiasis

<1% (Limited to important or life-threatening symptoms): Convulsions, hemolytic anemia, positive Coombs' reaction, acute interstitial nephritis

**Overdose/Toxicology** Symptoms of penicillin overdose include neuromuscular hypersensitivity (eg, agitation, hallucinations, asterixis, encephalopathy, confusion, and seizures). Electrolyte imbalance may occur if the preparation contains potassium or sodium salts, especially in renal failure. Hemodialysis may be helpful to aid in removal of the drug from blood; otherwise, treatment is supportive or symptom directed.

**Pharmacodynamics/Kinetics**

**Protein Binding:** 80%, plasma protein

**Half-life Elimination:** 0.5 hours (prolonged in renal impairment)

**Time to Peak:** Oral: Within 0.5-1 hour

**Excretion:** Urine

**Formulations**

Powder for oral solution: 125 mg/5 mL (3 mL, 100 mL, 150 mL, 200 mL); 250 mg/5 mL (100 mL, 150 mL, 200 mL)

Tablet: 125 mg, 250 mg, 500 mg

**Dosing**

**Adults:** Oral:

Systemic infections: 125-500 mg every 6-8 hours

Prophylaxis of pneumococcal infections: 250 mg twice daily

Prophylaxis of recurrent rheumatic fever: 250 mg twice daily

**Elderly:** Refer to adult dosing.

**Renal Impairment:**

$Cl_{cr}$ 10-50 mL/minute: Administer every 8-12 hours.

$Cl_{cr}$ <10 mL/minute: Administer every 12-16 hours.

**Administration**

**Oral:** Administer around-the-clock to promote less variation in peak and trough serum levels. Take on an empty stomach 1 hour before or 2 hours after meals, to enhance absorption, take until gone, do not skip doses.

**Stability**

**Storage:** Refrigerate suspension after reconstitution; discard after 14 days.

**Monitoring Laboratory Tests** Periodic renal and hematologic function during prolonged therapy; perform culture and sensitivity before administering first dose.

**Additional Nursing Issues**

**Physical Assessment:** Assess patient history for allergy. Monitor for hypersensitivity reaction and opportunistic infection.

**Patient Information/Instruction:** Take at regular intervals around-the-clock, preferably on an empty stomach (1 hour before or 2 hours after meals) with 8 oz of water. Take entire prescription; do not skip doses or discontinue without consulting prescriber. Small frequent meals, frequent mouth care, sucking lozenges, or chewing gum may reduce nausea or dry mouth. Important to maintain good oral and vaginal hygiene to reduce incidence of opportunistic infection. If diabetic, drug may cause false tests with Clinitest® urine glucose monitoring; use of glucose oxidase methods (Clinistix®) or serum glucose monitoring is preferable. This drug may interfere with oral contraceptives; an alternate form of birth control should be used. Report persistent diarrhea, fever, chills, unhealed sores, bloody urine or stool, muscle pain, mouth sores, and difficulty breathing.

**Additional Information** 0.7 mEq of potassium per 250 mg penicillin V; 250 mg equals 400,000 units of penicillin. In Canada, a oral suspension is available as a benzathine salt in the strength of 180 mg/5 mL [300,000 units/5 mL] and 300 mg/5 mL [500,000 units/5 mL]. A Canadian tablet is available in 300 mg [500,000 units].


- **Penipot** *see* Penicillin G Procaine *on page 899*
- **Pennkinetic®** *see* Hydrocodone and Chlorpheniramine *on page 571*
- **Penprocilina** *see* Penicillin G Procaine *on page 899*
- **Pentacarinat®** *see* Pentamidine *on this page*
- **Pentacarinat® Injection** *see* Pentamidine *on this page*
- **Pentagastrin** *see page 1248*
- **Pentam-300® Injection** *see* Pentamidine *on this page*


## Pentamidine (pen TAM i deen)

**U.S. Brand Names** NebuPent™ Inhalation; Pentacarinat® Injection; Pentam-300® Injection

**Therapeutic Category** Antibiotic, Miscellaneous

**Pregnancy Risk Factor** C

**Lactation** Excretion in breast milk unknown/contraindicated

**Use** Treatment and prevention of pneumonia caused by *Pneumocystis carinii*; treatment of trypanosomiasis

**Mechanism of Action/Effect** Interferes with RNA/DNA synthesis and phospholipids leading to cell death in protozoa.

**Contraindications** Hypersensitivity to pentamidine isethionate or any component (inhalation and injection)

**Warnings** Use with caution in patients with diabetes mellitus, renal or hepatic dysfunction, hyper-/hypotension, leukopenia, thrombocytopenia, asthma, or hypo-/hyperglycemia. Pregnancy factor C.

**Drug Interactions**

**Cytochrome P-450 Effect:** CYP2C19 enzyme substrate

**Adverse Reactions**

**Inhalation:**

>10%:

Cardiovascular: Chest pain
Dermatologic: Rash
Respiratory: Wheezing, dyspnea, coughing, pharyngitis

1% to 10%: Gastrointestinal: Bitter or metallic taste

<1% (Limited to important or life-threatening symptoms): Hypoglycemia, renal insufficiency

**Systemic:**

>10%:

Cardiovascular: Hypotension
Dermatologic: Rash
Endocrine & metabolic: Hyperglycemia or hypoglycemia
Gastrointestinal: Nausea, vomiting, anorexia, diarrhea
Hematologic: Leukopenia or neutropenia, thrombocytopenia
Hepatic: Elevated LFTs
Renal: Nephrotoxicity

1% to 10%:

Hematologic: Anemia
Cardiovascular: Cardiac arrhythmias
Gastrointestinal: Pancreatitis, metallic taste
Local: Local reactions at injection site

<1% (Limited to important or life-threatening symptoms): Arrhythmias

**Overdose/Toxicology** Symptoms of overdose include hypotension, hypoglycemia, and cardiac arrhythmias. Treatment is supportive.

**Pharmacodynamics/Kinetics**

**Distribution:** Systemic accumulation of pentamidine does not appear to occur following inhalation therapy.

**Half-life Elimination:** 6.4-9.4 hours (prolonged in severe renal impairment)

**Excretion:** Urine

**Formulations**

Pentamidine isethionate:

Inhalation: 300 mg
Powder for injection, lyophilized: 300 mg

**Dosing**

**Adults:**

Treatment: I.M., I.V. (I.V. preferred): 4 mg/kg/day once daily for 14 days
Prevention: Inhalation: 300 mg every 4 weeks via Respirgard® II nebulizer

**Elderly:** Refer to adult dosing.

**Renal Impairment:**

$Cl_{cr}$ 10-50 mL/minute: Administer dose every 24-36 hours.

(Continued)

## Pentamidine *(Continued)*

$Cl_{cr}$ <10 mL/minute: Administer dose every 48 hours.

Not removed by hemo- or peritoneal dialysis or continuous arteriovenous or venovenous hemofiltration (CAVH/CAVHD). Supplemental dosage is not necessary.

**Administration**

**I.M.:** Deep I.M.

**I.V.:** Do not use NS as a diluent. Infuse I.V. slowly over a period of at least 60 minutes or administer deep I.M.

**I.V. Detail:** Patients receiving I.V. or I.M. pentamidine should be lying down.

**Inhalation:** Virtually undetectable amounts are transferred to healthcare personnel during aerosol administration.

**Stability**

**Storage:** Do not refrigerate due to the possibility of crystallization.

**Reconstitution:** Reconstituted solutions (60-100 mg/mL) are stable for 48 hours at room temperature and do not require light protection. Diluted solutions (1-2.5 mg/mL) in $D_5W$ are stable for at least 24 hours at room temperature.

**Compatibility:** Do not mix with any other drugs.

**Monitoring Laboratory Tests** Liver and renal function, blood glucose, serum potassium and calcium, EKG, CBC with platelets

**Additional Nursing Issues**

**Physical Assessment:** Monitor laboratory results. Monitor blood pressure, cardiac status, and respiratory function closely during I.V. administration or following I.M. injection. For inhalant use, instruct patient/caregiver on proper procedure for preparing solutions and use. **Pregnancy risk factor C** - benefits of use should outweigh possible risks. Breast-feeding is contraindicated.

**Patient Information/Instruction:** I.V. or I.M. preparations must be given every day. For inhalant use as directed. Prepare solution and nebulizer as directed. Protect medication from light. You will be required to have frequent laboratory tests and blood pressure monitoring while taking this drug. PCP pneumonia may still occur despite pentamidine use. Maintain adequate hydration (2-3 L/day of fluids unless instructed to restrict fluid intake). Frequent mouth care or sucking on lozenges may relieve the metallic taste. Diabetics should check glucose levels frequently. You may experience dizziness or weakness with posture changes; rise or change position slowly. Report unusual confusion or hallucinations, chest pain, unusual bleeding, or rash. **Pregnancy/breast-feeding precautions:** Inform prescriber if you are or intend to be pregnant. Do not breast-feed.

**Geriatric Considerations:** Ten percent of acquired immunodeficiency syndrome (AIDS) cases are in the elderly and this figure is expected to increase. Pentamidine has not as yet been studied exclusively in this population. Adjust dose for renal function.

**Additional Information** pH: 5.4 (sterile water); 4.09-4.38 ($D_5W$)

- **Pentamycetin®** *see* Chloramphenicol *on page 248*
- **Pentasa® Oral** *see* Mesalamine *on page 727*

## Pentazocine (pen TAZ oh seen)

**U.S. Brand Names** Talwin®; Talwin® NX

**Therapeutic Category** Analgesic, Narcotic

**Pregnancy Risk Factor** B/D (if used for prolonged periods or in high doses at term)

**Lactation** Enters breast milk/use caution

**Use** Relief of moderate to severe pain; a sedative prior to surgery and as a supplement to surgical anesthesia

**Mechanism of Action/Effect** Binds to opiate receptors in the CNS, causing inhibition of ascending pain pathways, altering the perception of and response to pain; produces generalized CNS depression; partial agonist-antagonist

**Contraindications** Hypersensitivity to pentazocine or any component; increased intracranial pressure (unless the patient is mechanically ventilated); pregnancy (if used for prolonged periods or in high doses at term)

**Warnings** Use with caution in seizure-prone patients, acute myocardial infarction, patients undergoing biliary tract surgery, patients with renal and hepatic dysfunction, head trauma, increased intracranial pressure, and patients with a history of prior opioid dependence or abuse. Pentazocine may precipitate opiate withdrawal symptoms in patients who have been receiving opiates regularly. Injection contains sulfites which may cause allergic reaction.

**Drug Interactions**

**Cytochrome P-450 Effect:** CYP2D6 enzyme substrate

**Decreased Effect:** May potentiate or reduce analgesic effect of opiate agonist (eg, morphine) depending on patients tolerance to opiates can precipitate withdrawal in narcotic addicts.

**Increased Effect/Toxicity:** Increased effect/toxicity with tripelennamine (can be lethal), CNS depressants (eg, phenothiazines, tranquilizers, anxiolytics, sedatives, hypnotics, or alcohol).

**Adverse Reactions**

>10%:

Central nervous system: Fatigue, drowsiness, false sense of well-being

Gastrointestinal: Nausea, vomiting

1% to 10%:

Cardiovascular: Tachycardia or bradycardia, hypertension or hypotension

Central nervous system: Nervousness, headache, restlessness, malaise, dizziness

Dermatologic: Rash, urticaria
Gastrointestinal: Dry mouth, biliary spasm, constipation
Genitourinary: Ureteral spasms, decreased urination
Local: Pain at injection site
Neuromuscular & skeletal: Weakness
Ocular: Blurred vision
Respiratory: Dyspnea, shortness of breath
Miscellaneous: Histamine release

<1% (Limited to important or life-threatening symptoms): Convulsions, increased intracranial pressure

**Overdose/Toxicology** Symptoms of overdose include drowsiness, sedation, respiratory depression, and coma. Naloxone, 2 mg I.V., with repeat administration as necessary up to a total of 10 mg, can also be used to reverse toxic effects of the opiate.

**Pharmacodynamics/Kinetics**

**Protein Binding:** 60%

**Half-life Elimination:** 2-3 hours; increased with decreased hepatic function

**Metabolism:** Liver

**Excretion:** Urine and feces

**Onset:** Oral, I.M., S.C.: Within 15-30 minutes; I.V.: Within 2-3 minutes

**Duration:** Oral: 4-5 hours; Parenteral: 2-3 hours

**Formulations**

Injection, as lactate: 30 mg/mL (1 mL, 1.5 mL, 2 mL, 10 mL)
Tablet: Pentazocine hydrochloride 50 mg and naloxone hydrochloride 0.5 mg

**Dosing**

**Adults:**

Oral: 50 mg every 3-4 hours; may increase to 100 mg/dose if needed, but should not exceed 600 mg/day
I.M., S.C.: 30-60 mg every 3-4 hours, not to exceed total daily dose of 360 mg
I.V.: 30 mg every 3-4 hours; do **not** exceed 30 mg/dose.

**Elderly:** Avoid use if possible (see Geriatric Considerations).

**Renal Impairment:**

$Cl_{cr}$ 10-50 mL/minute: Administer 75% of normal dose.
$Cl_{cr}$ <10 mL/minute: Administer 50% of normal dose.

**Hepatic Impairment:** Reduce dose or avoid use in patients with liver disease.

**Administration**

**I.V.:** Rotate injection site for I.M., S.C. use; avoid intra-arterial injection.

**Stability**

**Storage:** Injection: Store at room temperature, protect from heat and from freezing.

**Compatibility:** I.V. form is incompatible with aminophylline, amobarbital (and all other I.V. barbiturates), glycopyrrolate (same syringe), heparin (same syringe), nafcillin (Y-site). See the Compatibility of Drugs in Syringe Chart *on page 1317*.

**Additional Nursing Issues**

**Physical Assessment:** Assess other medications patient may be taking for additive or adverse interactions (see Drug Interactions). Monitor for effectiveness of pain relief and monitor for signs of overdose (see above). Monitor blood pressure, CNS and respiratory status, and degree of sedation at beginning of therapy and at regular intervals with long-term use. May cause physical and/or psychological dependence. For inpatients, implement safety measures (eg, side rails up, call light within reach, instructions to call for assistance, etc). Assess knowledge/teach patient appropriate use (if self-administered). Teach patient to monitor for adverse reactions (see Adverse Reactions), adverse reactions to report, and appropriate interventions to reduce side effects. **Pregnancy risk factor B/D** - see Pregnancy Risk Factor for cautious use. Note breast-feeding caution.

**Patient Information/Instruction:** If self-administered, use exactly as directed (do not increase dose or frequency); may cause physical and/or psychological dependence. While using this medication, do not use alcohol and other prescription or OTC medications (especially sedatives, tranquilizers, antihistamines, or pain medications) without consulting prescriber. Maintain adequate hydration (2-3 L/day of fluids unless instructed to restrict fluid intake). May cause hypotension, dizziness, drowsiness, impaired coordination, or blurred vision (use caution when driving, climbing stairs, or changing position - rising from sitting or lying to standing, or when engaging in tasks requiring alertness until response to drug is known); nausea, vomiting, loss of appetite, or dry mouth (frequent mouth care, small frequent meals, chewing gum, or sucking lozenges may help); constipation (increased exercise, fluids, or dietary fruit and fiber may help - if constipation remains an unresolved problem, consult prescriber about use of stool softeners). Report persistent dizziness or headache; excessive fatigue or sedation; changes in mental status; changes in urinary elimination or pain on urination; weakness or trembling; blurred vision; or shortness of breath. **Pregnancy/breast-feeding precautions:** Inform prescriber if you are or intend to be pregnant. Consult prescriber if breast-feeding.

**Geriatric Considerations:** Pentazocine is not recommended for use in the elderly because of its propensity to cause delirium and agitation. If pentazocine must be used, be sure to adjust dose for renal function.

**Additional Information** Hydrochloride formulation contains sulfites.

Pentazocine hydrochloride: Oral: Talwin® NX tablet (with naloxone); naloxone is used to prevent abuse by dissolving tablets in water and using as injection.

**Related Information**

Narcotic/Opioid Analgesic Comparison *on page 1396*

## Pentazocine Compound (pen TAZ oh seen KOM pownd)

**U.S. Brand Names** Talacen®; Talwin® Compound

**Therapeutic Category** Analgesic, Combination (Narcotic)

**Pregnancy Risk Factor** D/C (Talacen®)

**Lactation** Enters breast milk/contraindicated

**Use** Relief of moderate to severe pain; sedative prior to surgery; supplement to surgical anesthesia

**Contraindications** Hypersensitivity to pentazocine, aspirin, or acetaminophen; pregnancy

**Warnings** Contains sodium metasulfite as sulfite that may cause allergic-type reactions; potential for elevating CSF pressure due to respiratory effects which may be exaggerated in presence of head injury, intracranial lesions, or pre-existing increase in intracranial lesions. May experience hallucinations, disorientation, and confusion. May cause psychological and physical dependence. Use with caution in patients with myocardial infarction who have nausea or vomiting, patients with respiratory depression, severely limited respiratory reserve, severe bronchial asthma, other obstructive respiratory conditions or cyanosis, impaired renal or hepatic function, patients prone to seizures. Talwin®-ASA: Use with caution in patients with peptic ulcer or patients on anticoagulation therapy. Pregnancy factor C (Talacen®).

**Adverse Reactions**

>10%:

- Central nervous system: Fatigue, drowsiness, false sense of well-being
- Gastrointestinal: Nausea, vomiting

1% to 10%:

- Cardiovascular: Tachycardia or bradycardia, hypertension or hypotension
- Central nervous system: Nervousness, headache, restlessness, malaise, dizziness
- Dermatologic: Rash, urticaria
- Gastrointestinal: Dry mouth, biliary spasm, constipation
- Genitourinary: Ureteral spasms, decreased urination
- Local: Pain at injection site
- Neuromuscular & skeletal: Weakness
- Ocular: Blurred vision
- Respiratory: Dyspnea, shortness of breath
- Miscellaneous: Histamine release

<1% (Limited to important or life-threatening symptoms): Convulsions, increased intracranial pressure

**Pharmacodynamics/Kinetics**

**Half-life Elimination:** Pentazocine: 3.6 hours; acetaminophen: 2.8 hours

**Onset:** Pentazocine: 15-30 minutes; acetaminophen: 30 minutes

**Formulations**

Tablet:

- Talacen®: Pentazocine hydrochloride 25 mg and acetaminophen 650 mg
- Talwin® Compound: Pentazocine hydrochloride 12.5 mg and aspirin 325 mg

**Dosing**

**Adults:** Oral:

- Talwin®: 2 tablets 3-4 times/day
- Talacen®: 1 caplet every 4 hours up to maximum of 6 caplets

**Elderly:** Refer to adult dosing.

**Stability**

**Storage:** Controlled room temperature 15°C to 30°C (59°F to 86°F)

**Additional Nursing Issues**

**Physical Assessment: Assess patient for history of liver disease or alcohol abuse** (acetaminophen and excessive alcohol may have adverse liver effects). Assess other medications patient may be taking for additive or adverse interactions (see Drug Interactions). Monitor for effectiveness of pain relief and monitor for signs of overdose (see above). Monitor vital signs and signs of adverse reactions (see Adverse Reactions) at beginning of therapy and at regular intervals with long-term use. May cause physical and/or psychological dependence. Discontinue slowly after long-term use. For inpatients, implement safety measures (eg, side rails up, call light within reach, instructions to call for assistance, etc). Assess knowledge/teach patient appropriate use if self-administered. Teach patient to monitor for adverse reactions, adverse reactions to report, and appropriate interventions to reduce side effects. **Pregnancy risk factor C/D** - see Pregnancy Risk Factor - benefits of use should outweigh possible risks. Breast-feeding is contraindicated.

**Patient Information/Instruction:** If self-administered, use exactly as directed (do not increase dose or frequency); may cause physical and/or psychological dependence. Take with food or milk. While using this medication, do not use alcohol and other prescription or OTC medications (especially sedatives, tranquilizers, antihistamines, or pain medications) without consulting prescriber. Maintain adequate hydration (2-3 L/day of fluids unless instructed to restrict fluid intake). May cause hypotension, dizziness, drowsiness, confusion, or nervousness (use caution when driving, climbing stairs, or changing position - rising from sitting or lying to standing, or when engaging in tasks requiring alertness until response to drug is known); nausea, dry mouth, decreased appetite, or gastric distress (frequent mouth care, frequent sips of fluids, chewing gum, or sucking lozenges may help); constipation (increased exercise, fluids, or dietary fruit and fiber may help - if constipation remains an unresolved problem, consult prescriber about use of stool softeners). Report chest pain, rapid heartbeat or palpitations; persistent dizziness; change in mental status; shortness of breath or difficulty breathing; unusual bleeding (stool, mouth, urine) or bruising; unusual fatigue and weakness; pain on urination; change in elimination patterns or change in color of urine or stool; or unresolved nausea or vomiting. **Pregnancy/breast-feeding precautions:** Inform prescriber if you are or intend to be pregnant. Do not breast-feed.

**Pregnancy Issues:** Not known whether affects fetus. Use only if clearly needed.

**Additional Information** Some formulations may contain sulfites. Abrupt discontinuation after sustained use (generally >10 days) may cause withdrawal symptoms.

## Pentobarbital (pen toe BAR bi tal)

**U.S. Brand Names** Nembutal®

**Therapeutic Category** Anticonvulsant, Barbiturate; Barbiturate

**Pregnancy Risk Factor** D

**Lactation** Enters breast milk/contraindicated

**Use** Short-term treatment of insomnia; preoperative sedation; high-dose barbiturate coma for treatment of increased intracranial pressure or status epilepticus unresponsive to other therapy

**Mechanism of Action/Effect** Short-acting barbiturate with sedative, hypnotic, and anticonvulsant properties

**Contraindications** Hypersensitivity to barbiturates or any component; marked liver function impairment or latent porphyria; pregnancy

**Warnings** Tolerance to hypnotic effect can occur. Do not use for >2 weeks to treat insomnia. Taper dose to prevent withdrawal. Status epilepticus may result from abrupt discontinuation. Use of this agent as a hypnotic in the elderly is not recommended due to its long half-life and potential for physical and psychological dependence. Use with caution in patients with hypovolemic shock, congestive heart failure, hepatic impairment, respiratory dysfunction or depression, previous addiction to the sedative/hypnotic group, chronic or acute pain, or renal dysfunction. Tolerance or psychological and physical dependence may occur with prolonged use.

**Drug Interactions**

**Cytochrome P-450 Effect:** May induce P-450 isoenzymes in long-term use.

**Decreased Effect:** Decreased chloramphenicol. Decreased doxycycline effects.

**Increased Effect/Toxicity:** Increased effect with CNS depressants.

**Food Interactions** Food may decrease the rate but not the extent of oral absorption.

**Effects on Lab Values** ↑ ammonia (B); ↓ bilirubin (S)

**Adverse Reactions**

>10%:

Central nervous system: Dizziness, clumsiness or unsteadiness, lightheadedness, "hangover" effect, drowsiness

1% to 10%:

Central nervous system: Confusion, mental depression, unusual excitement, nervousness, faint feeling, headache, insomnia, nightmares

Gastrointestinal: Nausea, vomiting, constipation

<1% (Limited to important or life-threatening symptoms): Hypotension, exfoliative dermatitis, Stevens-Johnson syndrome, agranulocytosis, megaloblastic anemia, thrombocytopenia, laryngospasm, respiratory depression, apnea (especially with rapid I.V. use)

**Overdose/Toxicology** Symptoms of overdose include unsteady gait, slurred speech, confusion, jaundice, hypothermia, hypotension, respiratory depression, and coma. Treat symptomatically. Charcoal hemoperfusion may be beneficial in stage IV coma due to high serum concentration.

**Pharmacodynamics/Kinetics**

**Protein Binding:** 35% to 55%

**Half-life Elimination:** Adults, normal: 22 hours; range: 35-50 hours

**Metabolism:** Liver

**Excretion:** Kidney

**Onset:** Oral, rectal: 15-60 minutes; I.M.: Within 10-15 minutes; I.V.: Within 1 minute

**Duration:** Oral, rectal: 1-4 hours; I.V.: 15 minutes

**Formulations**

Pentobarbital sodium:

Capsule (C-II): 50 mg, 100 mg

Elixir (C-II): 18.2 mg/5 mL (473 mL, 4000 mL)

Injection (C-II): 50 mg/mL (1 mL, 2 mL, 20 mL, 50 mL)

Suppository, rectal (C-III): 30 mg, 60 mg, 120 mg, 200 mg

**Dosing**

**Adults:**

Hypnotic:

Oral: 100-200 mg at bedtime or 20 mg 3-4 times/day for daytime sedation

I.M.: 150-200 mg

I.V.: Initial: 100 mg, may repeat every 1-3 minutes up to 200-500 mg total dose

Rectal: 120-200 mg at bedtime

Preoperative sedation: I.M.: 150-200 mg

Barbiturate coma in head injury patient: I.V.: Loading dose: 5-10 mg/kg given slowly over 1-2 hours; Maintenance infusion: Initial: 1 mg/kg/hour; may increase to 2-3 mg/kg/hour; maintain burst suppression on EEG

**Elderly:** Not recommended for use in the elderly; see Geriatric Considerations.

**Hepatic Impairment:** Reduce dosage in patients with severe liver dysfunction.

**Administration**

**I.M.:** Pentobarbital may be administered by deep I.M.: No more than 5 mL (250 mg) should be injected at any one site because of possible tissue irritation.

(Continued)

## Pentobarbital *(Continued)*

**I.V.:** Pentobarbital must be administered by slow I.V. injection. I.V. push doses can be given undiluted, but should be administered no faster than 50 mg/minute. Avoid intra-arterial injection. Has many incompatibilities when given I.V.

**I.V. Detail:** Avoid extravasation. Institute safety measures to avoid injuries. Parenteral solutions are highly alkaline. Avoid rapid I.V. administration >50 mg/minute.

**Stability**

**Storage:** Protect from light. Aqueous solutions are not stable; a commercially available vehicle (containing propylene glycol) is more stable. When mixed with an acidic solution, precipitate may form. Use only clear solution.

**Compatibility:** See the Compatibility of Drugs in Syringe Chart *on page 1317*.

**Additional Nursing Issues**

**Physical Assessment:** Assess effectiveness and interactions of other medications patient may be taking (see Contraindications, Warnings/Precautions, and Drug Interactions). Assess for history of addiction; long-term use can result in dependence, abuse, or tolerance. Periodically evaluate the need for continued use.

I.V. (see Administration): Keep patient under observation (vital signs, CNS, cardiac and respiratory status), use safety precautions. Monitor effectiveness of therapy and adverse reactions (see above).

Oral: Monitor for therapeutic response and adverse reactions (see Adverse Reactions) at beginning of therapy and periodically with long-term use. Assess knowledge/teach patient appropriate use, possible side effects, and symptoms to report.

**Pregnancy risk factor D** - assess knowledge/instruct patient on need to use appropriate contraceptive measures and the need to avoid pregnancy. Breast-feeding is contraindicated.

**Patient Information/Instruction:** I.V./I.M.: Patient instructions and information are determined by patient condition and therapeutic purpose. If self-administered, use exactly as directed (do not increase dose or frequency); may cause physical and/or psychological dependence. While using this medication, do not use alcohol and other prescription or OTC medications (especially pain medications, sedatives, antihistamines, or hypnotics) without consulting prescriber. Maintain adequate hydration (2-3 L/day of fluids unless instructed to restrict fluid intake). You may experience drowsiness, dizziness, or blurred vision (use caution when driving or engaging in tasks requiring alertness until response to drug is known); nausea, vomiting, or loss of appetite (small frequent meals, frequent mouth care, chewing gum, or sucking lozenges may help); constipation (increased exercise, fluids, or dietary fruit and fiber may help). Report skin rash or irritation; CNS changes (confusion, depression, increased sedation, excitation, headache, insomnia, or nightmares); difficulty breathing or shortness of breath; changes in urinary pattern or menstrual pattern; muscle weakness or tremors; or difficulty swallowing or feeling of tightness in throat. **Pregnancy/breast-feeding precautions:** Do not get pregnant; use appropriate contraceptive measures to prevent possible harm to the fetus. Do not breast-feed.

**Dietary Issues:** High doses of pyridoxine may decrease drug effect. Barbiturates may increase the metabolism of vitamins D and K. Dietary requirements of vitamins D, K, C, $B_{12}$, folate, and calcium may be increased with long-term use.

**Geriatric Considerations:** Use of this agent as a hypnotic in the elderly is not recommended due to its long half-life and addiction potential.

**Additional Information** The injection formulation contains ethanol. Some formulations may contain tartrazine.

Pentobarbital: Nembutal® elixir pentobarbital sodium: Nembutal® capsule, injection, and suppository

Sodium content of 1 mL injection: 5 mg (0.2 mEq)

**Related Information**

Antipsychotic Medication Guidelines *on page 1436*

## Pentostatin (PEN toe stat in)

**U.S. Brand Names** Nipent™ Injection

**Synonyms** DCF; 2′-Deoxycoformycin

**Therapeutic Category** Antineoplastic Agent, Antibiotic

**Pregnancy Risk Factor** D

**Lactation** Enters breast milk/contraindicated

**Use** Treatment of adult patients with alpha-interferon-refractory hairy cell leukemia; non-Hodgkin's lymphoma, cutaneous T-cell lymphoma

**Mechanism of Action/Effect** Results in cell death, probably through inhibiting DNA or RNA synthesis. Following a single dose, pentostatin has the ability to inhibit ADA for periods exceeding 1 week.

**Contraindications** Limited or severely compromised bone marrow reserves (white blood cell count <3000 cells/mm$^3$); pregnancy

**Warnings** The FDA currently recommends that procedures for proper handling and disposal of antineoplastic agents be considered. Use extreme caution in the presence of renal insufficiency. Use with caution in patients with signs or symptoms of impaired hepatic function.

Preparation of pentostatin should be performed in a Class II laminar flow biologic safety cabinet. Personnel should be wearing surgical gloves and a closed front surgical gown with knit cuffs. Appropriate safety equipment is recommended for preparation, administration, and disposal of antineoplastics. If pentostatin contacts the skin, wash and flush thoroughly with water.

**Drug Interactions**

**Increased Effect/Toxicity:** Increased toxicity with vidarabine, fludarabine, and allopurinol.

**Adverse Reactions**

>10%:

Central nervous system: Headache, neurologic disorder, fever, fatigue, chills, pain
Dermatologic: Rash
Gastrointestinal: Vomiting, nausea, anorexia, diarrhea
Hematologic: Leukopenia, anemia, thrombocytopenia
Hepatic: Hepatic disorder, liver function tests (abnormal)
Neuromuscular & skeletal: Myalgia
Respiratory: Coughing
Miscellaneous: Allergic reaction

1% to 10%:

Cardiovascular: Chest pain, arrhythmia, peripheral edema, congestive heart failure, acute arrhythmias
Central nervous system: Anxiety, confusion, depression, dizziness, insomnia, lethargy, coma, seizures, malaise
Dermatologic: Dry skin, eczema, pruritus
Gastrointestinal: Constipation, flatulence, stomatitis, weight loss
Genitourinary: Dysuria
Hematologic: Myelosuppression
Hepatic: Liver dysfunction
Local: Thrombophlebitis
Neuromuscular & skeletal: Arthralgia, paresthesia, back pain, weakness
Ocular: Abnormal vision, eye pain, keratoconjunctivitis
Otic: Ear pain
Renal: Renal failure, hematuria
Respiratory: Bronchitis, dyspnea, lung edema, pneumonia
Miscellaneous: Death, opportunistic infections, sweating

**Overdose/Toxicology** Symptoms of overdose include severe renal, hepatic, pulmonary, and CNS toxicity. Treatment is supportive.

**Pharmacodynamics/Kinetics**

**Distribution:** I.V.: Distributes rapidly to body tissues and may obtain plasma concentrations ranging from 12-36 ng following doses of 250 mcg/kg for 4-5 days

**Half-life Elimination:** 5-15 hours

**Excretion:** Urine

**Formulations** Powder for injection: 10 mg/vial

**Dosing**

**Adults:** Refractory hairy cell leukemia: Adults (refer to individual protocols): 4 mg/m$^2$ every other week by I.V. bolus

**Elderly:** Refer to adult dosing.

**Renal Impairment:**

$Cl_{cr}$ <80 mL/minute: Use extreme caution.
$Cl_{cr}$ 50-60 mL/minute: 2 mg/m$^2$/dose

**Administration**

**I.V.:** I.V. bolus over ≥3-5 minutes in $D_5W$ or NS at concentrations ≥2 mg/mL

**Stability**

**Storage:** Vials are stable under refrigeration at 2°C to 8°C.

**Reconstitution:** Reconstituted vials or further dilutions, may be stored at room temperature exposed to ambient light. Diluted solutions are stable for 24 hours in $D_5W$ or 48 hours in NS or lactated Ringer's at room temperature. Infusion with 5% dextrose injection USP or 0.9% sodium chloride injection USP does not interact with PVC-containing administration sets or containers.

**Monitoring Laboratory Tests** CBC with differential, platelet count, liver function, serum uric acid

**Additional Nursing Issues**

**Physical Assessment:** Monitor appropriate laboratory tests as ordered. Monitor for adverse effects as noted above (eg, nutritional status, renal function, myelosuppression). Monitor I & O ratio, signs of fluid status changes (eg, edema, weight gain or loss). Monitor for opportunistic infection. **Pregnancy risk factor D** - assess knowledge/teach appropriate use of barrier contraceptives. Breast-feeding is contraindicated.

**Patient Information/Instruction:** This drug can only be administered by infusion on a specific schedule. Frequent blood tests and monitoring will be necessary. Maintain adequate hydration (2-3 L/day of fluids unless instructed to restrict fluid intake). You may experience nausea and vomiting, diarrhea, or loss of appetite (frequent small meals or frequent mouth care may help or request medication from prescriber); dizziness, weakness, or lethargy (use caution when driving); susceptibility to infections (avoid crowds and exposure to infection). Use frequent oral care with soft toothbrush or cotton swabs to reduce incidence of mouth sores. May cause headache (request medication). Report signs of infection (eg, fever, chills, sore throat, mouth sores, burning urination, perianal itching, or vaginal discharge); unusual bruising or bleeding (tarry stools, blood in urine, stool, or vomitus); vision changes or hearing; muscle tremors, weakness, or pain; CNS changes (eg, hallucinations, confusion, insomnia, seizures); or respiratory difficulty. **Pregnancy/breast-feeding precautions:** Do not get pregnant while taking this medication. Both male and female should use appropriate barrier contraceptive measures. Do not breast-feed.

## Pentoxifylline (pen toks I fi leen)

**U.S. Brand Names** Trental®

**Synonyms** Oxpentifylline

**Therapeutic Category** Blood Viscosity Reducer Agent

**Pregnancy Risk Factor** C

**Lactation** Enters breast milk/effect on infant unknown

**Use** Symptomatic management of peripheral vascular disease, mainly intermittent claudication

**Unapproved use:** AIDS patients with increased TNF, CVA, cerebrovascular diseases, diabetic atherosclerosis, diabetic neuropathy, gangrene, hemodialysis shunt thrombosis, vascular impotence, cerebral malaria, septic shock, sickle cell syndromes, and vasculitis

**Mechanism of Action/Effect** Mechanism of action remains unclear; is thought to reduce blood viscosity and improve blood flow by altering the rheology of red blood cells

**Contraindications** Hypersensitivity to pentoxifylline or any component and other xanthine derivatives (theophylline, caffeine, or theobromine); patients who exhibit intolerance, or with recent cerebral and/or retinal hemorrhage; recent cerebral or retinal hemorrhage

**Warnings** Use with caution in patients with renal impairment or chronic occlusive arterial disease of the limbs. Pregnancy factor C.

**Drug Interactions**

**Decreased Effect:** Blood pressure changes (decreases) have been observed with the addition of pentoxifylline therapy in patients receiving antihypertensives.

**Increased Effect/Toxicity:** Increased effect/toxic potential with cimetidine (increased levels) and other $H_2$ antagonists. May increase anticoagulation with warfarin. Pentoxifylline may increase the serum levels of theophylline.

**Food Interactions** Pentoxifylline peak serum levels may be decreased if taken with food.

**Effects on Lab Values** ↓ calcium (S), magnesium (S); false-positive theophylline levels

**Adverse Reactions**

1% to 10%:

Central nervous system: Dizziness, headache

Gastrointestinal: Heartburn, nausea, vomiting

<1% (Limited to important or life-threatening symptoms): Chest pain, arrhythmias, tremor, hallucinations, rash, hepatitis, jaundice, congestion, dyspnea

**Overdose/Toxicology** Symptoms of overdose include hypotension, flushing, convulsions, deep sleep, agitation, bradycardia, and A-V block. Treatment is supportive.

**Pharmacodynamics/Kinetics**

**Half-life Elimination:** Parent drug: 24-48 minutes; Metabolites: 60-96 minutes

**Time to Peak:** Within 2-4 hours

**Metabolism:** Liver

**Excretion:** Urine

**Formulations** Tablet, controlled release: 400 mg

**Dosing**

**Adults:** Oral: 400 mg 3 times/day with meals; may reduce to 400 mg twice daily if GI or CNS side effects occur

**Elderly:** Refer to adult dosing.

**Additional Nursing Issues**

**Physical Assessment:** Monitor effectiveness of treatment on a regular basis. Monitor cardiac status (eg, angina, arrhythmias) and blood pressure on a regular basis. Instruct patient about medication, possible adverse effects, and symptoms to report. **Pregnancy risk factor C** - benefits of use should outweigh possible risks. Note breast-feeding caution.

**Patient Information/Instruction:** Take as prescribed for full length of prescription. This may relieve pain of claudication, but additional therapy may be recommended. You may experience dizziness (use caution when driving); GI upset (small frequent meals may help). Report chest pain, persistent headache, nausea or vomiting. **Pregnancy/breast-feeding precautions:** Inform prescriber if you are or intend to be pregnant. Consult prescriber if breast-feeding.

**Geriatric Considerations:** Pentoxiphylline's value in the treatment of intermittent claudication is controversial. Walking distance improved statistically in some clinical trials, but the actual distance was minimal when applied to improving physical activity (see Usual Dosage and Monitoring Parameters).


- **Pentrax®** *see page 1294*
- **Pentrexyl** *see* Ampicillin *on page 90*
- **Pen.Vee® K** *see* Penicillin V Potassium *on page 900*
- **Pen-Vi-K** *see* Penicillin V Potassium *on page 900*
- **Pen VK** *see* Penicillin V Potassium *on page 900*
- **Pepcid®** *see* Famotidine *on page 470*
- **Pepcid® AC Acid Controller [OTC]** *see* Famotidine *on page 470*
- **Pepcidine®** *see* Famotidine *on page 470*
- **Peptavlon®** *see page 1248*
- **Pepto-Bismol® [OTC]** *see* Bismuth Subsalicylate *on page 154*
- **Pepto® Diarrhea Control [OTC]** *see* Loperamide *on page 688*
- **Peptol®** *see* Cimetidine *on page 268*
- **Percocet®** *see* Oxycodone and Acetaminophen *on page 873*
- **Percocet®-Demi** *see* Oxycodone and Acetaminophen *on page 873*

- ♦ **Percodan®** *see* Oxycodone and Aspirin *on page 873*
- ♦ **Percodan®-Demi** *see* Oxycodone and Aspirin *on page 873*
- ♦ **Percogesic® Tablet** *see page 1294*
- ♦ **Percolone™** *see* Oxycodone *on page 871*
- ♦ **Perdiem® Plain [OTC]** *see* Psyllium *on page 993*
- ♦ **Perfectoderm® Gel** *see page 1294*


## Pergolide (PER go lide)

**U.S. Brand Names** Permax®

**Therapeutic Category** Anti-Parkinson's Agent (Dopamine Agonist); Ergot Derivative

**Pregnancy Risk Factor** B

**Lactation** Excretion in breast milk unknown/not recommended

**Use** Adjunctive treatment to levodopa/carbidopa in the management of Parkinson's disease

**Mechanism of Action/Effect** Pergolide is a semisynthetic ergot alkaloid similar to bromocriptine but stated to be more potent and longer-acting; it is a centrally-active dopamine agonist stimulating both $D_1$ and $D_2$ receptors

**Contraindications** Hypersensitivity to pergolide mesylate or other ergot derivatives

**Warnings** Symptomatic hypotension occurs in 10% of patients. Use with caution in patients with a history of cardiac arrhythmias, hallucinations, or mental illness.

**Drug Interactions**

**Decreased Effect:** Dopamine antagonists, metoclopramide may have a decreased effect.

**Increased Effect/Toxicity:** Increased toxicity with highly plasma protein-bound drugs due to increased free drug.

**Adverse Reactions**

>10%:

Cardiovascular: Hypotension

Central nervous system: Dizziness, somnolence, insomnia, confusion, hallucinations, anxiety, dystonia

Gastrointestinal: Nausea, constipation

Genitourinary: Urinary tract infections

Neuromuscular & skeletal: Dyskinesia

Respiratory: Rhinitis

Miscellaneous: Flu syndrome

1% to 10%:

Cardiovascular: Arrhythmias, peripheral edema, vasodilation, palpitations, chest pain, hypertension, facial edema

Central nervous system: Chills

Gastrointestinal: Diarrhea, abdominal pain, vomiting, dry mouth, anorexia, weight gain

Neuromuscular & skeletal: Weakness, lower back pain

<1% (Limited to important or life-threatening symptoms): Cerebrovascular hemorrhage, myocardial infarction,

**Overdose/Toxicology** Symptoms of overdose include vomiting, hypotension, agitation, hallucinations, ventricular extrasystoles, and possible seizures. Data on overdose is limited. Treatment is supportive.

**Pharmacodynamics/Kinetics**

**Protein Binding:** 90% to plasma proteins

**Half-life Elimination:** 27 hours

**Metabolism:** Liver

**Excretion:** Urine and feces

**Formulations** Tablet, as mesylate: 0.05 mg, 0.25 mg, 1 mg

**Dosing**

**Adults:** When adding pergolide to levodopa/carbidopa, the dose of the latter can usually and should be decreased. Patients no longer responsive to bromocriptine may benefit by being switched to pergolide.

Oral: Start with 0.05 mg/day for 2 days, then increase dosage by 0.1 or 0.15 mg/day every 3 days over next 12 days, increase dose by 0.25 mg/day every 3 days until optimal therapeutic dose is achieved, up to 5 mg/day maximum; usual dosage range: 2-3 mg/day in 3 divided doses

**Elderly:** Refer to Geriatric Considerations.

**Additional Nursing Issues**

**Physical Assessment:** Assess effectiveness and interactions of other medications patient may be taking (see Contraindications and Drug Interactions). Monitor therapeutic response (eg, mental status, involuntary movements), and adverse reactions at beginning of therapy and periodically throughout therapy (see Warnings/Precautions, Adverse Reactions, and Overdose/Toxicology). Assess knowledge/teach patient appropriate use, interventions to reduce side effects, and adverse symptoms to report. Breast-feeding is not recommended.

**Patient Information/Instruction:** Take exactly as directed (may be prescribed in conjunction with levodopa/carbidopa); do not change dosage or discontinue without consulting prescriber. Therapeutic effects may take several weeks or months to achieve and you may need frequent monitoring during first weeks of therapy. Take with meals if GI upset occurs, before meals if dry mouth occurs, after eating if drooling or if nausea occurs. Take at the same time each day. Maintain adequate hydration (2-3 L/day of fluids unless instructed to restrict fluid intake); void before taking medication. Do not use alcohol and prescription or OTC sedatives or CNS depressants without consulting prescriber. You may experience drowsiness, dizziness, confusion, or vision

(Continued)

## Pergolide *(Continued)*

changes (use caution when driving, climbing stairs, or engaging in tasks requiring alertness until response to drug is known); orthostatic hypotension (use caution when changing position - rising to standing from sitting or lying); constipation (increased exercise, fluids, or dietary fruit and fiber may help); runny nose or flu-like symptoms (consult prescriber for appropriate relief); nausea, vomiting, loss of appetite, or stomach discomfort (small frequent meals, frequent mouth care, chewing gum, or sucking lozenges may help); photosensitivity (use sunscreen, wear protective clothing and eyewear, and avoid direct sunlight). Report unresolved constipation or vomiting; chest pain, palpitations, irregular heartbeat; ringing in ears; CNS changes (hallucination, loss of memory, seizures, acute headache, nervousness, etc); painful or difficult urination; increased muscle spasticity, rigidity, or involuntary movements; skin rash; or significant worsening of condition. **Breast-feeding precautions:** Breast-feeding is not recommended.

**Geriatric Considerations:** High incidence of syncope and orthostatic hypotension upon initiation of therapy. Use with caution in patients prone to cardiac dysrhythmias and in patients with a history of confusion or hallucinations.


- **Pergonal®** *see* Menotropins *on page 720*
- **Periactin®** *see* Cyproheptadine *on page 320*
- **Peri-Colace®** *see page 1294*
- **Peridane** *see* Pentoxifylline *on page 908*


## Perindopril Erbumine (per IN doe pril er BYOO meen)

**U.S. Brand Names** Aceon®

**Therapeutic Category** Angiotensin-Converting Enzyme (ACE) Inhibitors

**Pregnancy Risk Factor** D (especially during 2nd and 3rd trimesters)

**Lactation** Enters breast milk (small amounts)/effect on infant unknown

**Use** Treatment of stage I or II hypertension and congestive heart failure

**Mechanism of Action/Effect** Competitive inhibitor of angiotensin-converting enzyme (ACE); prevents conversion of angiotensin I to angiotensin II, a potent vasoconstrictor; results in lower levels of angiotensin II which, in turn, causes an increase in plasma renin activity and a reduction in aldosterone secretion

**Contraindications** Hypersensitivity to perindopril, perindoprilat, other ACE inhibitors, or any component; pregnancy; history of angioedema with other ACE inhibitors

**Warnings** Use with caution and modify dosage in patients with renal impairment (especially renal artery stenosis), severe congestive heart failure, or with coadministered diuretic therapy, valvular stenosis, or hyperkalemia (>5.7 mEq/L). Experience in children is limited. Severe hypotension may occur in patients who are sodium and/or volume depleted; initiate lower doses and monitor closely when starting therapy in these patients.

**Drug Interactions**

**Decreased Effect:** Rifampin may decrease the effect of ACE inhibitors. Antacids may decrease the bioavailability of ACE inhibitors. May be more likely to occur with captopril. Separate administration times by 1-2 hours. NSAIDs, specifically indomethacin, may reduce the hypotensive effects of ACE inhibitors. More likely to occur in low renin or volume dependent hypertensive patients.

**Increased Effect/Toxicity:** Diuretics have additive hypotensive effects with ACE inhibitors. Probenecid increases blood levels of captopril which may occur in other ACE inhibitors. Phenothiazines taken with ACE inhibitors may increase the pharmacologic effects of the ACE inhibitor. Allopurinol and ACE inhibitors may cause a higher risk of hypersensitivity reaction when taken concurrently. Digoxin, when taken with ACE inhibitors may result in elevated serum digoxin levels. Lithium, when taken with ACE inhibitors may result in elevated serum levels of lithium with symptoms of toxicity. Potassium supplements or potassium-sparing diuretics taken with ACE inhibitors may result in elevated serum potassium levels.

**Food Interactions** Perindopril active metabolite concentrations may be lowered if taken with food.

**Adverse Reactions**

1% to 10%

Central nervous system: Headache, dizziness, mood and sleep disorders, fatigue
Dermatologic: Rash, pruritus
Gastrointestinal: Nausea, epigastric pain, diarrhea, vomiting
Neuromuscular & skeletal: Muscle cramps
Respiratory: Cough (incidence is greater in women, 3:1)

<1% (Limited to important or life-threatening symptoms): Agranulocytosis for all ACE inhibitors (especially in patients with renal impairment or collagen vascular disease), possibly neutropenia; decreases in creatinine clearance in some elderly hypertensive patients or those with chronic renal failure, worsening of renal function in patients with bilateral renal artery stenosis, or furosemide therapy; proteinuria

**Overdose/Toxicology** Mild hypotension has been the primary toxic effect seen with acute overdose. Bradycardia may also occur. Hyperkalemia occurs even with therapeutic doses, especially in patients with renal insufficiency and those taking NSAIDs. Treatment is symptom directed and supportive.

**Pharmacodynamics/Kinetics**

**Protein Binding:** Perindopril: 10% to 20%; Perindoprilat: 60%

**Half-life Elimination:** Parent drug: 1.5-3 hours; Metabolite: 25-30 hours

**Time to Peak:** Occurs in 1 and 3-4 hours for perindopril and perindoprilat, respectively after chronic therapy; (maximum perindoprilat serum levels are 2-3 times higher and

$T_{max}$ is shorter following chronic therapy); in CHF, the peak of perindoprilat is prolonged to 6 hours

**Metabolism:** Liver

**Excretion:** Urine

**Formulations** Tablet: 2 mg, 4 mg, 8 mg

**Dosing**

**Adults:** Oral:

Congestive heart failure: 4 mg once daily

Hypertension: Initial: 4 mg/day but may be titrated to response; usual range: 4-8 mg/day, maximum: 16 mg/day

**Elderly:** Due to greater bioavailability and lower renal clearance of the drug in elderly subjects, dose reduction of 50% is recommended.

**Renal Impairment:**

$Cl_{cr}$ >60 mL/minute: Administer 4 mg/day.

$Cl_{cr}$ 30-60 mL/minute: Administer 2 mg/day.

$Cl_{cr}$ 15-29 mL/minute: Administer 2 mg every other day.

$Cl_{cr}$ <15 mL/minute: Administer 2 mg on the day of dialysis.

Perindopril and its metabolites are dialyzable.

**Monitoring Laboratory Tests** Serum creatinine, electrolytes, and WBC with differential initially and repeated at 2-week intervals for at least 90 days

**Additional Nursing Issues**

**Physical Assessment:** Note drug interactions above. Monitor blood pressure (standing and sitting), cardiac rate and rhythm, and fluid balance at beginning of therapy, when adjusting dosage and regularly with long-term therapy. Use and teach postural hypotension precautions and need for regular blood pressure monitoring. **Pregnancy risk factor D** - assess knowledge/teach appropriate use of barrier contraceptives. Note breast-feeding caution.

**Patient Information/Instruction:** This medication does not replace the to need to follow exercise and diet recommendations for hypertension. Take as directed; do not miss doses, alter dosage, or discontinue without consulting prescriber. Consult prescriber for appropriate diet. Change position slowly when rising from sitting or lying. May cause transient drowsiness; avoid driving or engaging in tasks that require alertness until response to drug is known. Small frequent meals may help reduce any nausea, vomiting, or epigastric pain. You may experience persistent cough; contact prescriber. Report unusual weight gain or swelling of ankles and hands; persistent fatigue; dry cough; difficulty breathing; palpitations; or swelling of face, eyes, or lips. **Pregnancy/breast-feeding precautions:** Do not get pregnant while taking this medication - use appropriate barrier contraceptive measures. Consult prescriber if breast-feeding.

♦ **Periostat™** *see* Doxycycline *on page 406*

♦ **Permapen®** *see* Penicillin G Benzathine *on page 896*

♦ **Permax®** *see* Pergolide *on page 909*

## Permethrin (per METH rin)

**U.S. Brand Names** Elimite™ Cream; Nix™ Creme Rinse

**Therapeutic Category** Antiparasitic Agent, Topical; Scabicidal Agent

**Pregnancy Risk Factor** B

**Lactation** Effect on infant unknown

**Use** Single application treatment of infestation with *Pediculus humanus capitis* (head louse) and its nits or *Sarcoptes scabiei* (scabies)

**Mechanism of Action/Effect** Inhibits sodium ion influx through nerve cell membrane channels in parasites resulting in delayed repolarization and thus paralysis and death of the pest

**Contraindications** Hypersensitivity to pyrethyroid, pyrethrin, or chrysanthemums

**Warnings** Treatment may temporarily exacerbate the symptoms of itching, redness, and swelling. For external use only.

**Adverse Reactions** 1% to 10%:

Dermatologic: Pruritus, erythema, rash of the scalp

Local: Burning, stinging, tingling, numbness or scalp discomfort, edema

**Pharmacodynamics/Kinetics**

**Metabolism:** Liver

**Excretion:** Urine

**Formulations**

Cream: 5% (60 g)

Creme rinse: 1% (60 mL with comb)

**Dosing**

**Adults:** Topical:

Head lice: After hair has been washed with shampoo, rinsed with water, and towel dried, apply a sufficient volume of topical liquid to saturate the hair and scalp. Leave on hair for 10 minutes before rinsing off with water; remove remaining nits; may repeat in 1 week if lice or nits still present.

Scabies: Apply cream from head to toe. Leave on for 8-14 hours before washing off with water. May reapply in 1 week if live mites appear.

**Elderly:** Refer to adult dosing.

**Administration**

**Topical:** Avoid contact with eyes and mucous membranes during application. Shake cream rinse well before using.

(Continued)

## Permethrin *(Continued)*

**Additional Nursing Issues**

**Physical Assessment:** See Warnings/Precautions and Contraindications for use cautions. Assess head, hair, and skin surfaces for presence of lice and nits. Assess knowledge/teach patient appropriate application and use and adverse symptoms (see Adverse Reactions above) to report. Note breast-feeding caution.

**Patient Information/Instruction:** For external use only. Do not apply to face and avoid contact with eyes or mucous membrane. Clothing and bedding must be washed in hot water or dry cleaned to kill nits. May need to treat all members of household and all sexual contacts concurrently. Wash all combs and brushes with permethrin and thoroughly rinse. **Breast-feeding precautions:** Consult prescriber if breast-feeding.

**Administration:** Cream rinse: Apply immediately after hair is shampooed and rinsed. Apply enough to saturate hair and scalp. Leave on hair for 10 minutes before rinsing with water. Remove nits with fine-tooth comb. May repeat in 1 week if lice or nits are still present.

Cream: Apply from neck to toes. Bathe to remove drug after 8-14 hours before washing off. Repeat in 7 days if lice or nits are still present. Report if condition persists or infection occurs.

**Geriatric Considerations:** Because of its minimal absorption, permethrin is a drug of choice and is preferred over lindane.

- ♦ **Permitil® Oral** *see* Fluphenazine *on page 505*
- ♦ **Pernox®** *see page 1294*
- ♦ **Peroxin A5®** *see page 1294*
- ♦ **Peroxin A10®** *see page 1294*

## Perphenazine (per FEN a zeen)

**U.S. Brand Names** Trilafon®

**Therapeutic Category** Antipsychotic Agent, Phenothazine, Piperazine

**Pregnancy Risk Factor** C

**Lactation** Enters breast milk/not recommended (AAP rates "of concern")

**Use** Management of manifestations of psychotic disorders, depressive neurosis, alcohol withdrawal, nausea and vomiting, nonpsychotic symptoms associated with dementia in the elderly, Tourette's syndrome, Huntington's chorea, spasmodic torticollis, and Reye's syndrome

**Mechanism of Action/Effect** Blocks postsynaptic mesolimbic dopaminergic receptors in the brain; exhibits a strong alpha-adrenergic blocking effect and depresses the release of hypothalamic and hypophyseal hormones

**Contraindications** Hypersensitivity to perphenazine or any component (cross reactivity between phenothiazines may occur); severe CNS depression; subcortical brain damage; bone marrow suppression; blood dyscrasias; coma

**Warnings** May cause hypotension, particularly with parenteral administration. May be sedating; use with caution in disorders where CNS depression is a feature. Use with caution in Parkinson's disease. Use with caution in patients with hemodynamic instability; predisposition to seizures; or severe cardiac, hepatic, renal, or respiratory disease. Neuroleptics may cause swallowing difficulty. Use with caution in breast cancer or other prolactin-dependent tumors (may elevate prolactin levels). May alter temperature regulation or mask toxicity of other drugs due to antiemetic effects. May alter cardiac conduction - life threatening arrhythmias have occurred with therapeutic doses of phenothiazines. May cause orthostatic hypotension.

Phenothiazines may cause anticholinergic effects (eg, confusion, agitation, constipation, dry mouth, blurred vision, urinary retention); therefore, use with caution in patients with decreased gastrointestinal motility, urinary retention, BPH, xerostomia, or visual problems. Conditions which also may be exacerbated by cholinergic blockade include narrow-angle glaucoma (screening is recommended) and worsening of myasthenia gravis. Relative to other neuroleptics, perphenazine has a low potency of cholinergic blockade.

May cause extrapyramidal reactions including pseudoparkinsonism, acute dystonic reactions, akathisia, and tardive dyskinesia (risk of these reactions is high relative to other neuroleptics). May be associated with neuroleptic malignant syndrome (NMS) or pigmentary retinopathy.

Pregnancy factor C.

**Drug Interactions**

**Cytochrome P-450 Effect:** CYP2D6 enzyme substrate; CYP2D6 enzyme inhibitor

**Decreased Effect:** Decreased effect of anticholinergics, anticonvulsants, guanethidine, and epinephrine.

**Increased Effect/Toxicity:** Increased toxicity with CNS depressants. Increased effect/toxicity of anticonvulsants.

**Effects on Lab Values** ↑ cholesterol (S), glucose; ↓ uric acid (S)

**Adverse Reactions**

>10%:

Cardiovascular: Hypotension, orthostatic hypotension

Central nervous system: Pseudoparkinsonism, akathisia, dystonias, tardive dyskinesia (persistent), dizziness

Gastrointestinal: Constipation

Ocular: Pigmentary retinopathy

Respiratory: Nasal congestion

Miscellaneous: Decreased sweating

1% to 10%:

Dermatologic: Photosensitivity, rash

Endocrine & metabolic: Changes in menstrual cycle, changes in libido, breast pain

Gastrointestinal: Weight gain, vomiting, stomach pain, nausea

Genitourinary: Difficulty in urination, ejaculatory disturbances

Neuromuscular & skeletal: Tremor

<1% (Limited to important or life-threatening symptoms): Neuroleptic malignant syndrome (NMS), lowering of seizures threshold, agranulocytosis, leukopenia, cholestatic jaundice, hepatotoxicity

**Overdose/Toxicology** Symptoms of overdose include deep sleep, dystonia, agitation, coma, abnormal involuntary muscle movements, hypotension, and arrhythmias. Treatment is symptom directed and supportive.

**Pharmacodynamics/Kinetics**

**Distribution:** Crosses the placenta

**Half-life Elimination:** 9 hours

**Time to Peak:** Within 4-8 hours

**Metabolism:** Liver

**Excretion:** Urine and bile

**Formulations**

Concentrate, oral: 16 mg/5 mL (118 mL)

Injection: 5 mg/mL (1 mL)

Tablet: 2 mg, 4 mg, 8 mg, 16 mg

**Dosing**

**Adults:**

Psychoses:

Oral: 4-16 mg 2-4 times/day not to exceed 64 mg/day

I.M.: 5 mg every 6 hours up to 15 mg/day in ambulatory patients and 30 mg/day in hospitalized patients

Nausea/vomiting:

Oral: 8-16 mg/day in divided doses up to 24 mg/day

I.M.: 5-10 mg every 6 hours as necessary up to 15 mg/day in ambulatory patients and 30 mg/day in hospitalized patients

I.V. (severe): 1 mg at 1- to 2-minute intervals up to a total of 5 mg

**Elderly:** Oral: Nonpsychotic patient; dementia behavior: Initial: 2-4 mg 1-2 times/day; increase at 4- to 7-day intervals by 2-4 mg/day. Increase dose intervals (bid, tid, etc) as necessary to control behavior response or side effects. Maximum daily dose: 32 mg; gradual increase (titration) may prevent some side effects or decrease their severity.

**Renal Impairment:** Not dialyzable (0% to 5%)

**Hepatic Impairment:** Dosage reductions should be considered in patients with liver disease although no specific guidelines are available.

**Administration**

**Oral:** Dilute oral concentration to at least 2 oz with water, juice, or milk only. Do not dilute with liquids containing coffee, tea, or apple juice. **Note:** Avoid skin contact with oral medication; may cause contact dermatitis.

**I.V.:** I.V. use, injection should be diluted to at least 0.5 mg/mL with NS and given at a rate of 1 mg/minute.

**Monitoring Laboratory Tests** Baseline liver and kidney function, CBC prior to and periodically during therapy, ophthalmic screening

**Additional Nursing Issues**

**Physical Assessment:** Assess other medications patient is taking for effectiveness and interactions (see Drug Interactions). See Contraindications and Warnings/Precautions for cautious use. Has potential for psychological or physiological dependence, abuse, and tolerance. Review ophthalmic screening and monitor laboratory results (see above), therapeutic response (mental status, mood, affect), and adverse reactions at beginning of therapy and periodically with long-term use (orthostatic hypotension, anticholinergic response, extrapyramidal effects, pigmentary retinopathy - see Adverse Reactions and Overdose/Toxicology). With I.M. or I.V., use monitor closely for hypotension. **Note:** Avoid skin contact with oral or injection medication; may cause contact dermatitis (wash immediately with warm, soapy water). Initiate at lower doses (see Dosing) and taper dosage slowly when discontinuing. Assess knowledge/teach patient appropriate use, interventions to reduce side effects, and adverse symptoms to report (see below). **Pregnancy risk factor C** - instruct patient about appropriate contraceptive use. Breast-feeding is not recommended.

**Patient Information/Instruction:** Use exactly as directed (do not increase dose or frequency); may cause physical and/or psychological dependence. It may take 2-3 weeks to achieve desired results; do not discontinue without consulting prescriber. Dilute oral concentration with milk, water, or citrus; do not dilute with liquids containing coffee, tea, or apple juice. Do not take within 2 hours of any antacid. Avoid excess alcohol or caffeine and other prescription or OTC medications not approved by prescriber. Maintain adequate hydration (2-3 L/day of fluids unless instructed to restrict fluid intake). Avoid skin contact with medication; may cause contact dermatitis (wash immediately with warm, soapy water). You may experience excess drowsiness, restlessness, dizziness, or blurred vision (use caution driving or when engaging in tasks requiring alertness until response to drug is known); dry mouth, nausea, vomiting (small frequent meals, frequent mouth care, chewing gum, or sucking lozenges may help); constipation (increased exercise, fluids, or dietary fruit and fiber may help); postural hypotension (use caution climbing stairs or when changing position from lying or sitting to standing); urinary retention (void before taking medication); or photosensitivity (use sunscreen, wear protective clothing and eyewear, and avoid direct sunlight);

(Continued)

## Perphenazine *(Continued)*

or decreased perspiration (avoid strenuous exercise in hot environments). Report persistent CNS effects (eg, trembling fingers, altered gait or balance, excessive sedation, seizures, unusual movements, anxiety, abnormal thoughts, confusion, personality changes); chest pain, palpitations, rapid heartbeat, severe dizziness; unresolved urinary retention or changes in urinary pattern; menstrual pattern, change in libido, or ejaculatory difficulty; vision changes; skin rash or yellowing of skin; difficulty breathing; or worsening of condition. **Pregnancy/breast-feeding precautions:** Inform prescriber if you are or intend to be pregnant. Breast-feeding is not recommended.

**Geriatric Considerations:** (See Warnings/Precautions, Adverse Reactions, and Overdose/Toxicology.) Elderly patients have an increased risk of adverse response to side effects or adverse reactions to antipsychotics. These can include but are not limited to the following.

Anticholinergic effects: CNS toxicity with confusion, memory loss, psychotic behavior, and agitation.

Extrapyramidal effects (EPS): Parkinson's syndrome and akathisia may occur as often as 50% in patients >60 years of age. Tardive dyskinesia (motor restlessness) may be 40% in elderly; may be related to duration and total accumulated dose over time; may be somewhat reversible if diagnosed early enough.

Orthostatic hypotension: Increased risk for falls.

Sedation: In nonpsychotic patients, may result in feelings of depersonalization, derealization, and dysphoria.

Cardiac toxicity: Cardiac arrhythmias have occurred with therapeutic doses of antipsychotics.

Malignant neuroleptic syndrome: Development of hyperthermia, muscular rigidity, autonomic instability, and altered mental status.

Many elderly patients receive antipsychotic medications for inappropriate nonpsychotic behavior. Before initiating antipsychotic medication, all possible reversible causes should be investigated. Stress may cause acute "confusion" or worsening of baseline nonpsychotic behaviors; any changes in disease state (in any organ) may result in behavioral changes. Common acute changes in behavior may be due also to increases in drug dose addition, or addition of a new drug to the regimen; fluid/electrolyte alterations; infections; or changes in the environment.

Meta-analysis of controlled trials of antipsychotic (phenothiazines, butyrophenones) use with agitated, demented, elderly patients has concluded that the use of neuroleptics results in a response rate of 18%. Clearly, neuroleptic therapy for behavior control should be limited, with frequent attempts to withdraw the agent for behavior control. When use is indicated, initial doses should be lower to start and monitored closely.

**Additional Information** Some formulations may contain ethanol. The injection formulation contains sulfites.

**Related Information**

Antiemetics for Chemotherapy-Induced Nausea and Vomiting *on page 1307*
Antipsychotic Agents Comparison *on page 1371*
Antipsychotic Medication Guidelines *on page 1436*


- **Perphenazine and Amitriptyline** *see* Amitriptyline and Perphenazine *on page 75*
- **Persa-Gel®** *see page 1294*
- **Persantine®** *see* Dipyridamole *on page 383*
- **Pertussin® CS** *see page 1294*
- **Pertussin® ES** *see page 1294*
- **Pethidine Hydrochloride** *see* Meperidine *on page 721*
- **PFA** *see* Foscarnet *on page 516*
- **Pfizerpen®** *see* Penicillin G, Parenteral, Aqueous *on page 897*
- **$PGE_1$** *see* Alprostadil *on page 56*
- **$PGE_2$** *see* Dinoprostone *on page 379*
- **Phanatuss® Cough Syrup [OTC]** *see* Guaifenesin and Dextromethorphan *on page 549*
- **Pharmaflur®** *see page 1294*
- **Phazyme®** *see page 1294*
- **Phenadex® Senior [OTC]** *see* Guaifenesin and Dextromethorphan *on page 549*
- **Phenameth® DM** *see* Promethazine and Dextromethorphan *on page 980*
- **Phenaphen® With Codeine** *see* Acetaminophen and Codeine *on page 34*
- **Phenazine®** *see* Promethazine *on page 978*
- **Phenazo** *see* Phenazopyridine *on this page*
- **Phenazodine®** *see* Phenazopyridine *on this page*


## Phenazopyridine (fen az oh PEER i deen)

**U.S. Brand Names** Azo-Standard® [OTC]; Baridium® [OTC]; Geridium®; Phenazodine®; Prodium® [OTC]; Pyridiate®; Pyridium®; Urodine®; Urogesic®

**Synonyms** Phenylazo Diamino Pyridine Hydrochloride

**Therapeutic Category** Analgesic, Urinary

**Pregnancy Risk Factor** B

**Lactation** Excretion in breast milk unknown

**Use** Symptomatic relief of urinary burning, itching, frequency and urgency in association with urinary tract infection or following urologic procedures

**Mechanism of Action/Effect** An azo dye which exerts local anesthetic or analgesic action on urinary tract mucosa through an unknown mechanism

**Contraindications** Hypersensitivity to phenazopyridine or any component; kidney or liver disease; patients with a $Cl_{cr}$ <50 mL/minute

**Warnings** Does not treat infection, acts only as an analgesic. Drug should be discontinued if skin or sclera develop a yellow color. Use with caution in patients with renal impairment. Use of this agent in the elderly is limited since accumulation of phenazopyridine can occur in patients with renal insufficiency.

**Effects on Lab Values** Phenazopyridine may cause delayed reactions with glucose oxidase reagents (Clinistix®); cupric sulfate tests (Clinitest®) are not affected; interference may also occur with urine ketone tests (Acetest®, Ketostix®) and urinary protein tests; tests for urinary steroids and porphyrins may also occur

**Adverse Reactions**

1% to 10%:

Central nervous system: Headache, dizziness

Gastrointestinal: Stomach cramps

<1% (Limited to important or life-threatening symptoms): Methemoglobinemia, hemolytic anemia, hepatitis, acute renal failure

**Overdose/Toxicology** Symptoms of overdose include methemoglobinemia, hemolytic anemia, skin pigmentation, and renal and hepatic impairment. For methemoglobinemia, the antidote is methylene blue 1-2 mg/kg I.V.

**Pharmacodynamics/Kinetics**

**Metabolism:** Liver and other tissues

**Excretion:** Urine (where it exerts its action); renal excretion (as unchanged drug) is rapid and accounts for 65% of the drug's elimination

**Formulations**

Phenazopyridine hydrochloride: Tablet:

Azo-Standard®, Prodium®: 95 mg

Baridium®, Geridium®, Pyridiate®, Pyridium®, Urodine®, Urogesic®: 100 mg

Geridium®, Phenazodine®, Pyridium®, Urodine®: 200 mg

**Dosing**

**Adults:** Oral: 100-200 mg 3 times/day after meals for 2 days when used concomitantly with an antibacterial agent

**Elderly:** Refer to adult dosing.

**Renal Impairment:**

$Cl_{cr}$ 50-80 mL/minute: Administer every 8-16 hours.

$Cl_{cr}$ <50 mL/minute: Avoid use.

**Additional Nursing Issues**

**Physical Assessment:** Monitor for effectiveness of therapy dependent on rational for administration. Monitor or instruct patient to monitor for adverse reactions and symptoms to report. Diabetics should use serum glucose monitoring (phenazopyridine may interfere with certain urine testing reagents - see Effects on Lab Values). Note breast-feeding caution.

**Patient Information/Instruction:** Take prescribed dose after meals. May discolor urine (orange/yellow) or feces (orange/red); this is normal but will stain fabric. Report persistent headache, dizziness, or stomach cramping. **Breast-feeding precautions:** Consult prescriber if breast-feeding.

**Geriatric Considerations:** Use of this agent in the elderly is limited since accumulation of phenazopyridine can occur in patients with renal insufficiency. It should not be used in patients with a $Cl_{cr}$ <50 mL/minute.

- **Phenazopyridine and Sulfamethoxazole** *see* Sulfamethoxazole and Phenazopyridine *on page 1083*
- **Phenazopyridine and Sulfisoxazole** *see* Sulfisoxazole and Phenazopyridine *on page 1088*
- **Phen DH® w/Codeine Liquid** *see page 1306*
- **Phendry® Oral [OTC]** *see* Diphenhydramine *on page 381*

## Phenelzine (FEN el zeen)

**U.S. Brand Names** Nardil®

**Therapeutic Category** Antidepressant, Monoamine Oxidase Inhibitor

**Pregnancy Risk Factor** C

**Lactation** Excretion in breast milk unknown/not recommended

**Use** Symptomatic treatment of atypical, nonendogenous, or neurotic depression

MAO inhibitors are usually reserved for patients who do not tolerate or respond to traditional "cyclic" or "second generation" antidepressants. Brain activity due to monoamine oxidase increases with age and even more so in patients with Alzheimer's disease. Therefore, MAO inhibitors may have an increased role in treating depressed patients with Alzheimer's disease. Phenelzine is less stimulating than tranylcypromine.

**Mechanism of Action/Effect** Thought to act by increasing endogenous concentrations of epinephrine, norepinephrine, dopamine and serotonin through inhibition of the enzyme (monoamine oxidase) responsible for the breakdown of these neurotransmitters

**Contraindications** Hypersensitivity to phenelzine or any component; pheochromocytoma; hepatic or renal disease; cerebrovascular defect; or cardiovascular disease. Do not use within 5 weeks of fluoxetine or 2 weeks of sertraline or paroxetine discontinuance.

**Warnings** Safety in children <16 years of age has not been established. Use with caution in patients who are hyperactive, hyperexcitable, or who have glaucoma. Avoid use of

(Continued)

## Phenelzine *(Continued)*

meperidine within 2 weeks of phenelzine use. Hypertensive crisis may occur with tyramine. Pregnancy factor C.

**Drug Interactions**

**Increased Effect/Toxicity:** Increased effect/toxicity of barbiturates, psychotropics, rauwolfia alkaloids, and CNS depressants. Increased toxicity with disulfiram (seizures), fluoxetine, sertraline, paroxetine, and other serotonin active agents (increased cardiac effect), tricyclic antidepressants, meperidine (increased cardiovascular instability), phenothiazines, sympathomimetics, or levodopa (hypertensive crisis), methyldopa, dopamine, tryptophan, tyramine-containing foods, furazolidone (increased blood pressure), and dextroamphetamine. Potential for serotonin syndrome if combined with other serotonergic drugs.

**Food Interactions** Clinically severe elevated blood pressure may occur if phenelzine is taken with tyramine-containing foods.

**Effects on Lab Values** ↓ glucose

**Adverse Reactions**

>10%:

Cardiovascular: Orthostatic hypotension
Central nervous system: Drowsiness, headache
Endocrine & metabolic: Decreased sexual ability
Neuromuscular & skeletal: Trembling, weakness
Ocular: Blurred vision

1% to 10%:

Cardiovascular: Tachycardia, peripheral edema
Central nervous system: Nervousness, chills
Gastrointestinal: Diarrhea, anorexia, dry mouth, constipation

<1% (Limited to important or life-threatening symptoms): Parkinsonism syndrome, leukopenia, hepatitis

**Overdose/Toxicology** Symptoms of overdose include tachycardia, palpitations, muscle twitching, seizures, insomnia, restlessness, transient hypertension, hypotension, drowsiness, hyperpyrexia, and coma. Treatment is symptom directed and supportive.

**Pharmacodynamics/Kinetics**

**Excretion:** Urine

**Onset:** Within 2-4 weeks

**Duration:** May continue to have a therapeutic effect and interactions 2 weeks after discontinuing therapy

**Formulations** Tablet, as sulfate: 15 mg

**Dosing**

**Adults:** Oral: 15 mg 3 times/day; may increase to 60-90 mg/day during early phase of treatment, then reduce to dose for maintenance therapy slowly after maximum benefit is obtained. Takes 2-4 weeks for a significant response to occur.

**Elderly:** Oral: Initial: 7.5 mg/day; increase by 7.5-15 mg/day every 3-4 days as tolerated; usual therapeutic dose: 15-60 mg/day in 3-4 divided doses.

**Stability**

**Storage:** Protect from light

**Additional Nursing Issues**

**Physical Assessment:** Assess other medications patient may be taking for effectiveness and interactions (see Drug Interactions). See Contraindications and Warnings/Precautions for cautious use. Has potential for psychological or physiological dependence, abuse, or tolerance. Monitor therapeutic response (ie, mental status, mood, affect, suicidal ideation), and adverse reactions at beginning of therapy and periodically with long-term use (see Adverse Reactions and Overdose/Toxicology). Taper dosage slowly when discontinuing (allow 3-4 weeks between discontinuing phenelzine and starting another antidepressant). Diabetics should monitor serum glucose closely (phenelzine may lower glucose level). Assess knowledge/teach patient appropriate use, interventions to reduce side effects (including tyramine-free diet), and adverse symptoms to report. See Tyramine Foods List *on page 1422.* **Pregnancy risk factor C** - benefits of use should outweigh possible risks. Breast-feeding is not recommended.

**Patient Information/Instruction:** Take exactly as directed (do not increase dose or frequency); may take 2-3 weeks to achieve desired results; may cause physical and/or psychological dependence. Avoid excessive alcohol, caffeine, and other prescription or OTC medications not approved by prescriber. Avoid tyramine-containing foods (eg, pickles, aged cheese, wine). Maintain adequate hydration (2-3 L/day of fluids unless instructed to restrict fluid intake). You may experience postural hypotension (use caution when climbing stairs or changing position from lying or sitting to standing); drowsiness, lightheadedness, dizziness (use caution when driving or engaging in tasks requiring alertness until response to drug is known); anorexia, dry mouth (small frequent meals, frequent mouth care, chewing gum, or sucking lozenges may help); constipation (increased exercise, fluids, or dietary fruit and fiber may help); or diarrhea (buttermilk, yogurt, or boiled milk may help). Diabetic patients should monitor serum glucose closely (Nardil® may effect glucose levels). Report persistent insomnia; chest pain, palpitations, irregular or rapid heartbeat, or swelling of extremities; muscle cramping, tremors, or altered gait; blurred vision or eye pain; yellowing of eyes or skin; pale stools/dark urine; or worsening of condition. **Pregnancy/breast-feeding precautions:** Inform prescriber if you are or intend to be pregnant. Breast-feeding is not recommended.

**Geriatric Considerations:** MAO inhibitors are effective and generally well tolerated by older patients. Potential interactions with tyramine- or tryptophan-containing foods (see Warnings/Precautions) and other drugs, and adverse effects on blood pressure have limited the use of MAO inhibitors. They are usually reserved for patients who do not tolerate or respond to traditional "cyclic" or "second generation" antidepressants. Brain activity due to monoamine oxidase increases with age and even more so in patients with Alzheimer's disease. Therefore, MAO inhibitors may have an increased role in treating depressed patients with Alzheimer's disease. Phenelzine is less stimulating than tranylcypromine.

**Related Information**

Antidepressant Agents Comparison *on page 1368*
Tyramine Foods List *on page 1422*


- ♦ **Pheneramine and Naphazoline** *see page 1282*
- ♦ **Phenerbel-S®** *see* Belladonna, Phenobarbital, and Ergotamine Tartrate *on page 137*
- ♦ **Phenergan®** *see* Promethazine *on page 978*
- ♦ **Phenergan® VC Syrup** *see* Promethazine and Phenylephrine *on page 980*
- ♦ **Phenergan® VC With Codeine** *see* Promethazine, Phenylephrine, and Codeine *on page 981*
- ♦ **Phenergan® With Codeine** *see* Promethazine and Codeine *on page 980*
- ♦ **Phenergan® With Dextromethorphan** *see* Promethazine and Dextromethorphan *on page 980*
- ♦ **Phenetron®** *see page 1294*
- ♦ **Phenhist® Expectorant** *see* Guaifenesin, Pseudoephedrine, and Codeine *on page 552*
- ♦ **Phenindamine** *see page 1294*


## Phenobarbital (fee noe BAR bi tal)

**U.S. Brand Names** Barbita®; Luminal®; Solfoton®

**Synonyms** Phenobarbitone; Phenylethylmalonylurea

**Therapeutic Category** Anticonvulsant, Barbiturate; Barbiturate

**Pregnancy Risk Factor** D

**Lactation** Enters breast milk/not recommended (AAP recommends "with caution")

**Use** Management of generalized tonic-clonic (grand mal) and partial seizures

**Mechanism of Action/Effect** Interferes with transmission of impulses from the thalamus to the cortex of the brain resulting in an imbalance in central inhibitory and facilitatory mechanisms

**Contraindications** Hypersensitivity to phenobarbital or any component; pre-existing CNS depression; severe uncontrolled pain; porphyria; severe respiratory disease with dyspnea or obstruction; pregnancy

**Warnings** Use with caution in patients with hypovolemic shock, congestive heart failure, hepatic impairment, respiratory dysfunction or depression, previous addiction to the sedative/hypnotic group, chronic or acute pain, renal dysfunction, and in the elderly, due to a long half-life and risk of dependence. Phenobarbital is not recommended as a sedative in the elderly; tolerance or psychological and physical dependence may occur with prolonged use. **Abrupt withdrawal in patients with epilepsy may precipitate status epilepticus.**

**Drug Interactions**

**Cytochrome P-450 Effect:** CYP1A2, 2B6, 2C, 2C8, 2C9, 2C18, 2C19, 2D6, 3A3/4, and 3A5-7 enzyme inducer

**Decreased Effect:** Phenobarbital is an enzyme inducer which increases the clearance rate of phenothiazines, haloperidol, quinidine, cyclosporine, tricyclic antidepressants, corticosteroids, theophylline, ethosuximide, warfarin, oral contraceptives, chloramphenicol, griseofulvin, doxycycline, and beta-blockers resulting in less-than-expected therapeutic effect.

**Increased Effect/Toxicity:** Phenobarbital in combination with propoxyphene, benzodiazepines, CNS depressants, valproic acid, methylphenidate, and chloramphenicol may have additive effects.

**Effects on Lab Values** ↑ ammonia (B), LFTs, copper (serum); ↓ bilirubin (S); assay interference of LDH

**Adverse Reactions**

>10%: Central nervous system: Dizziness, clumsiness or unsteadiness, lightheadedness, "hangover" effect, drowsiness

1% to 10%:

Central nervous system: Confusion, mental depression, unusual excitement, nervousness, faint feeling, headache, insomnia, nightmares

Gastrointestinal: Nausea, vomiting, constipation

<1% (Limited to important or life-threatening symptoms): Exfoliative dermatitis, Stevens-Johnson syndrome, agranulocytosis, megaloblastic anemia, thrombocytopenia, laryngospasm, respiratory depression, apnea (especially with rapid I.V. use)

**Overdose/Toxicology** Symptoms of overdose include unsteady gait, slurred speech, confusion, jaundice, hypothermia, hypotension, respiratory depression, and coma. In severe overdose, charcoal hemoperfusion may accelerate removal. Treatment is symptom directed and supportive.

**Pharmacodynamics/Kinetics**

**Protein Binding:** 20% to 45%

**Half-life Elimination:** 53-140 hours

**Time to Peak:** Oral: Within 1-6 hours

**Metabolism:** Liver

**Excretion:** Urine

**Onset:**

Oral: Onset of hypnosis: Within 20-60 minutes

I.V.: Onset of action: Within 5 minutes; Peak effect: Within 30 minutes

(Continued)

## Phenobarbital *(Continued)*

**Duration:** Oral: 6-10 hours; I.V.: 4-10 hours

**Formulations**

Phenobarbital sodium:

Capsule: 16 mg

Elixir: 15 mg/5 mL (5 mL, 10 mL, 20 mL); 20 mg/5 mL (3.75 mL, 5 mL, 7.5 mL, 120 mL, 473 mL, 946 mL, 4000 mL)

Injection: 30 mg/mL (1 mL); 60 mg/mL (1 mL); 65 mg/mL (1 mL); 130 mg/mL (1 mL)

Powder for injection: 120 mg

Tablet: 8 mg, 15 mg, 16 mg, 30 mg, 32 mg, 60 mg, 65 mg, 100 mg

**Dosing**

**Adults:**

Anticonvulsant: Status epilepticus: 300-800 mg initially followed by 120-240 mg/dose at 20-minute intervals until seizures are controlled or a total dose of 1-2 g

Anticonvulsant maintenance dose: Oral, I.V.: 1-3 mg/kg/day in divided doses or 50-100 mg 2-3 times/day

Sedation: Oral, I.M.: 30-120 mg/day in 2-3 divided doses

Hypnotic: Oral, I.M., I.V., S.C.: 100-320 mg at bedtime

Preoperative sedation: I.M.: 100-200 mg 1-1.5 hours before procedure

**Elderly:** Not recommended for use in the elderly.

**Renal Impairment:**

$Cl_{cr}$ <10 mL/minute: Administer every 12-16 hours.

Moderately dialyzable (20% to 50%)

**Hepatic Impairment:** Increased side effects may occur in severe liver disease. Monitor plasma levels and adjust dose accordingly.

**Administration**

**I.V.:** Avoid rapid I.V. administration >50 mg/minute. Avoid intra-arterial injection.

**I.V. Detail:** Parenteral solutions are highly alkaline. Avoid extravasation.

**Stability**

**Storage:** Protect elixir from light. Not stable in aqueous solutions. Use only clear solutions. Do not add to acidic solutions; precipitation may occur.

**Compatibility:** I.V. form is incompatible with benzquinamide (in syringe), cephalothin, chlorpromazine, hydralazine, hydrocortisone, hydroxyzine, insulin, levorphanol, meperidine, methadone, morphine, norepinephrine, pentazocine, prochlorperazine, promazine, promethazine, ranitidine (in syringe), and vancomycin. See the Compatibility of Drugs Chart *on page 1315.*

**Monitoring Laboratory Tests** Phenobarbital serum concentrations, CBC, LFTs

**Additional Nursing Issues**

**Physical Assessment:** Assess effectiveness and interactions of other medications patient may be taking (see Contraindications, Warnings/Precautions, and Drug Interactions). Assess for history of addiction; long-term use can result in dependence, abuse, or tolerance; periodically evaluate need for continued use.

I.V. (see Administration): Keep patient under observation (vital signs, neurologic, cardiac, and respiratory status), use safety precautions. Monitor effectiveness of therapy and adverse reactions (see above).

Oral: Monitor for therapeutic response and adverse reactions (see Adverse Reactions) at beginning of therapy and periodically with long-term use. Assess knowledge/teach patient appropriate use, possible side effects, and symptoms to report.

**Pregnancy risk factor D** - assess knowledge/instruct patient on need to use appropriate contraceptive measures and the need to avoid pregnancy. Breast-feeding is not recommended.

**Patient Information/Instruction:** I.V./I.M.: Patient instructions and information are determined by patient condition and therapeutic purpose. If self-administered, use exactly as directed (do not increase dose or frequency); may cause physical and/or psychological dependence. While using this medication, do not use alcohol and other prescription or OTC medications (especially pain medications, sedatives, antihistamines, or hypnotics) without consulting prescriber. Maintain adequate hydration (2-3 L/day of fluids unless instructed to restrict fluid intake). You may experience drowsiness, dizziness, or blurred vision (use caution when driving or engaging in tasks requiring alertness until response to drug is known); nausea, vomiting, or loss of appetite (small frequent meals, frequent mouth care, chewing gum, or sucking lozenges may help); constipation (increased exercise, fluids, or dietary fruit and fiber may help). Report skin rash or irritation; CNS changes (confusion, depression, increased sedation, excitation, headache, insomnia, or nightmares); difficulty breathing or shortness of breath; changes in urinary pattern or menstrual pattern; muscle weakness or tremors; or difficulty swallowing or feeling of tightness in throat. **Pregnancy/breast-feeding precautions:** Do not get pregnant while taking this medication; use appropriate barrier contraceptive measures. Breast-feeding is not recommended.

**Dietary Issues:** High doses of pyridoxine may decrease drug effect. Barbiturates may increase the metabolism of vitamins D and K. Dietary requirements of vitamins D, K, C, $B_{12}$, folate, and calcium may be increased with long-term use.

**Geriatric Considerations:** Due to its long half-life and risk of dependence, phenobarbital is not recommended as a sedative or hypnotic in the elderly. Interpretive guidelines from the Health Care Financing Administration discourage the use of this agent as a sedative/hypnotic in long-term care residents.

**Additional Information** Injectable solutions contain propylene glycol

Sodium content of injection (65 mg, 1 mL): 6 mg (0.3 mEq)

Phenobarbital: Barbita®, Solfoton®

Phenobarbital sodium: Luminal®

**Related Information**

Antipsychotic Medication Guidelines *on page 1436*
Peak and Trough Guidelines *on page 1331*

- ♦ **Phenobarbital, Belladonna, and Ergotamine Tartrate** *see* Belladonna, Phenobarbital, and Ergotamine Tartrate *on page 137*
- ♦ **Phenobarbital, Hyoscyamine, Atropine, and Scopolamine** *see* Hyoscyamine, Atropine, Scopolamine, and Phenobarbital *on page 591*
- ♦ **Phenobarbital, Theophylline, and Ephedrine** *see* Theophylline, Ephedrine, and Phenobarbital *on page 1118*
- ♦ **Phenobarbitone** *see* Phenobarbital *on page 917*
- ♦ **Phenol** *see page 1294*
- ♦ **Phenolsulfonphthalein** *see page 1248*
- ♦ **Phenoxine® [OTC]** *see* Phenylpropanolamine *on page 922*
- ♦ **Phenoxymethyl Penicillin** *see* Penicillin V Potassium *on page 900*

## Phentolamine (fen TOLE a meen)

**U.S. Brand Names** Regitine®

**Therapeutic Category** Alpha$_1$ Blockers

**Pregnancy Risk Factor** C

**Lactation** Excretion in breast milk unknown

**Use** Diagnosis of pheochromocytoma and treatment of hypertension associated with pheochromocytoma or other caused by excess sympathomimetic amines; as treatment of dermal necrosis after extravasation of drugs with alpha-adrenergic effects (norepinephrine, dopamine, epinephrine, dobutamine)

**Mechanism of Action/Effect** Competitively blocks alpha-adrenergic receptors to produce brief antagonism of circulating epinephrine and norepinephrine to reduce hypertension caused by alpha effects of these catecholamines; also has a positive inotropic and chronotropic effect on the heart

**Contraindications** Hypersensitivity to phentolamine or any component; renal impairment; coronary or cerebral arteriosclerosis

**Warnings** Myocardial infarction, cerebrovascular spasm and cerebrovascular occlusion have occurred following administration. Use with caution in patients with gastritis or peptic ulcer, tachycardia, or a history of cardiac arrhythmias. Pregnancy factor C.

**Drug Interactions**

**Decreased Effect:** Decreased effect with epinephrine and ephedrine.

**Increased Effect/Toxicity:** Increased toxicity with ethanol (disulfiram reaction).

**Effects on Lab Values** ↑ LFTs rarely

**Adverse Reactions**

>10%:

Cardiovascular: Hypotension, tachycardia, arrhythmias, reflex tachycardia, chest pain, orthostatic hypotension

Gastrointestinal: Nausea, vomiting, diarrhea, exacerbation of peptic ulcer, abdominal pain

Respiratory: Nasal congestion

1% to 10%:

Cardiovascular: Flushing of face

Central nervous system: Dizziness, fainting

Neuromuscular & skeletal: Weakness

Respiratory: Nasal stuffiness

<1% (Limited to important or life-threatening symptoms): Myocardial infarction

**Overdose/Toxicology** Symptoms of overdose include tachycardia, shock, vomiting, and dizziness. If fluid replacement is inadequate to treat hypotension, only alpha-adrenergic vasopressors such as norepinephrine should be used. Mixed agents such as epinephrine may cause more hypotension.

**Pharmacodynamics/Kinetics**

**Half-life Elimination:** 19 minutes

**Metabolism:** Liver

**Excretion:** Urine

**Onset:** I.M.: Within 15-20 minutes; I.V.: Immediate

**Duration:** I.M.: 30-45 minutes; I.V.: 15-30 minutes

**Formulations** Injection, as mesylate: 5 mg/mL (1 mL)

**Dosing**

**Adults:**

Treatment of alpha-adrenergic drug extravasation: S.C.:

Infiltrate area with small amount of solution made by diluting 5-10 mg of phentolamine in 10 mL 0.9% sodium chloride within 12 hours of extravasation.

If dose is effective, normal skin color should return to the blanched area within 1 hour.

Diagnosis of pheochromocytoma: I.M., I.V.: 5 mg

Surgery for pheochromocytoma: Hypertension: I.M., I.V.: 5 mg given 1-2 hours before procedure and repeated as needed every 2-4 hours

Hypertensive crisis: 5-20 mg

**Elderly:** Refer to adult dosing.

**Administration**

**I.V.:**

Vasoconstrictor (alpha-adrenergic agonist) extravasation: Infiltrate the area of extravasation with multiple small injections using only 27- or 30-gauge needles and

(Continued)

## Phentolamine *(Continued)*

changing the needle between each skin entry. Be careful not to cause so much swelling of the extremity or digit that a compartment syndrome occurs.

Pheochromocytoma: Inject each 5 mg over 1 minute.

**Stability**

**Reconstitution:** Reconstituted solution is stable for 48 hours at room temperature and 1 week when refrigerated.

**Additional Nursing Issues**

**Physical Assessment:** Check I.V. site frequently; extravasation needs immediate counteraction (see Administration). Monitor blood pressure and heart rate frequently. **Pregnancy risk factor C** - benefits of use should outweigh possible risks. Note breast-feeding caution.

**Patient Information/Instruction:** Immediately report pain at infusion site. Report any dizziness, feelings of faintness, or palpitations. Do not change position rapidly; rise slowly or ask for assistance. **Pregnancy/breast-feeding precautions:** Inform prescriber if you are or intend to be pregnant. Consult prescriber if breast-feeding.

**Additional Information** pH: 4.5-6.4

♦ **Phenylalanine Mustard** *see* Melphalan *on page 718*

♦ **Phenylazo Diamino Pyridine Hydrochloride** *see* Phenazopyridine *on page 914*

♦ **Phenyldrine® [OTC]** *see* Phenylpropanolamine *on page 922*

## Phenylephrine (fen il EF rin)

**U.S. Brand Names** AK-Dilate® Ophthalmic Solution; AK-Nefrin® Ophthalmic Solution; Alconefrin® Nasal Solution [OTC]; Doktors® Nasal Solution [OTC]; I-Phrine® Ophthalmic Solution; Isopto® Frin Ophthalmic Solution; Mydfrin® Ophthalmic Solution; Neo-Synephrine® Nasal Solution [OTC]; Neo-Synephrine® Ophthalmic Solution; Nostril® Nasal Solution [OTC]; Prefrin™ Ophthalmic Solution; Relief® Ophthalmic Solution; Rhinall® Nasal Solution [OTC]; Sinarest® Nasal Solution [OTC]; St. Joseph® Measured Dose Nasal Solution [OTC]; Vicks® Sinex® Nasal Solution [OTC]

**Therapeutic Category** Alpha/Beta Agonist; Ophthalmic Agent, Antiglaucoma; Ophthalmic Agent, Mydriatic

**Pregnancy Risk Factor** C

**Lactation** Excretion in breast milk unknown

**Use** Treatment of hypotension, vascular failure in shock; as a vasoconstrictor in regional analgesia; symptomatic relief of nasal and nasopharyngeal mucosal congestion; as a mydriatic in ophthalmic procedures and treatment of wide-angle glaucoma; supraventricular tachycardia

**Mechanism of Action/Effect** Potent, direct-acting alpha-adrenergic stimulator with weak beta-adrenergic activity; causes vasoconstriction of the arterioles of the nasal mucosa and conjunctiva; activates the dilator muscle of the pupil to cause contraction; produces vasoconstriction of arterioles in the body; produces systemic arterial vasoconstriction

**Contraindications** Hypersensitivity to phenylephrine or any component; pheochromocytoma; severe hypertension; bradycardia; ventricular tachyarrhythmias; narrow-angle glaucoma (ophthalmic preparation); acute pancreatitis; hepatitis; peripheral or mesenteric vascular thrombosis; myocardial disease; severe coronary disease

**Warnings** Injection may contain sulfites which may cause allergic reaction in some patients. Do not use if solution turns brown or contains a precipitate. Use with extreme caution in elderly patients, patients with hyperthyroidism, bradycardia, partial heart block, myocardial disease, or severe arteriosclerosis. Infuse into large veins to help prevent extravasation which may cause severe necrosis. The 10% ophthalmic solution has caused increased blood pressure in elderly patients and its use should, therefore, be avoided. Pregnancy factor C.

**Drug Interactions**

**Decreased Effect:** Alpha- and beta-adrenergic blocking agents may have a decreased effect if taken with phenylephrine.

**Increased Effect/Toxicity:** Phenylephrine taken with sympathomimetics, may induce tachycardia or arrhythmias. If taken with MAO inhibitors or oxytocic agents, actions may be potentiated.

**Adverse Reactions**

**Nasal:**

>10%: Burning, rebound congestion, sneezing

1% to 10%: Stinging, dryness

**Ophthalmic:**

>10%: Transient stinging

1% to 10%:

Central nervous system: Headache, browache

Ocular: Blurred vision, photophobia, lacrimation

**Parenteral** (cardiovascular use):

>10%:

Central nervous system: Headache

Gastrointestinal: Nausea, vomiting

1% to 10%:

Cardiovascular: Premature ventricular beats, bradycardia, hypertension, hypotension, chest pain, palpitations, tachycardia, ventricular arrhythmias

Central nervous system: Nervousness or restlessness

Respiratory: Dyspnea

**Overdose/Toxicology** Symptoms of overdose include vomiting, hypertension, palpitations, paresthesia, and ventricular extrasystoles. Treatment is supportive. In extreme cases, I.V. phentolamine may be used.

**Pharmacodynamics/Kinetics**

**Half-life Elimination:** 2.5 hours

**Metabolism:** Liver and intestine

**Excretion:** Urine

**Onset:** I.M., S.C.: Within 10-15 minutes; I.V.: Immediate

**Duration:** I.M.: 30 minutes to 2 hours; I.V.: 15-30 minutes; S.C.: 1 hour

**Formulations**

Injection, as hydrochloride (Neo-Synephrine®): 1% [10 mg/mL] (1 mL)

Nasal solution, as hydrochloride:

Drops:

Neo-Synephrine®: 0.125% (15 mL)

Alconefrin® 12: 0.16% (30 mL)

Alconefrin® 25, Neo-Synephrine®, Children's Nostril®, Rhinall®: 0.25% (15 mL, 30 mL, 40 mL)

Alconefrin®, Neo-Synephrine®: 0.5% (15 mL, 30 mL)

Spray:

Alconefrin® 25, Neo-Synephrine®, Rhinall®: 0.25% (15 mL, 30 mL, 40 mL)

Neo-Synephrine®, Nostril®, Sinex®: 0.5% (15 mL, 30 mL)

Neo-Synephrine®: 1% (15 mL)

Ophthalmic solution, as hydrochloride:

AK-Nefrin®, Isopto® Frin, Prefrin™ Liquifilm®, Relief®: 0.12% (0.3 mL, 15 mL, 20 mL)

AK-Dilate®, Mydfrin®, Neo-Synephrine®, Phenoptic®: 2.5% (2 mL, 3 mL, 5 mL, 15 mL)

AK-Dilate®, Neo-Synephrine®, Neo-Synephrine® Viscous: 10% (1 mL, 2 mL, 5 mL, 15 mL)

**Dosing**

**Adults:**

Nasal decongestant (therapy should not exceed 5 continuous days): Instill 1-2 sprays or instill 1-2 drops every 4 hours of 0.25% to 0.5% solution as needed; 1% solution may be used in adults in cases of extreme nasal congestion. Do not use nasal solutions more than 3 days.

Hypotension/shock:

I.M., S.C.: 2-5 mg/dose every 1-2 hours as needed (initial dose should not exceed 5 mg)

I.V. bolus: 0.1-0.5 mg/dose every 10-15 minutes as needed (initial dose should not exceed 0.5 mg)

I.V. infusion: 10 mg in 250 mL $D_5W$ or NS (1:25,000 dilution) (40 mcg/mL); start at 100-180 mcg/minute (2-5 mL/minute; 50-90 drops/minute) initially; when blood pressure is stabilized, maintenance rate: 40-60 mcg/minute (20-30 drops/minute).

Paroxysmal supraventricular tachycardia: I.V.: 0.25-0.5 mg/dose over 20-30 seconds

Ophthalmic procedures: Instill 1 drop of 2.5% or 10% solution, may repeat in 10-60 minutes as needed.

**Elderly:**

Nasal decongestant: Administer 2-3 drops or 1-2 sprays every 4 hours of 0.125% to 0.25% solution as needed; do not use more than 3 days.

Ophthalmic preparations for pupil dilation: Instill 1 drop of 2.5% solution, may repeat in 1 hour if necessary.

Refer to adult dosing for other uses and Geriatric Considerations for cautions on I.V. use.

**Administration**

**I.V.:** Concentration and rate of infusion can be calculated using the following formulas: Dilute 0.6 mg x weight (kg) to 100 mL; then the dose in mcg/kg/minute = 0.1 x the infusion rate in mL/hour.

**I.V. Detail:** May cause necrosis or sloughing tissue if extravasation occurs during I.V. administration or S.C. administration.

**Extravasation management:** Use phentolamine as antidote; mix 5 mg with 9 mL of NS. Inject a small amount of this dilution into extravasated area. Blanching should reverse immediately. Monitor site. If blanching should recur, additional injections of phentolamine may be needed.

**Stability**

**Reconstitution:** Stable for 48 hours in 5% dextrose in water at pH 3.5-7.5. Do not use brown colored solutions.

**Monitoring Laboratory Tests** Parenteral use: Monitor arterial blood gases

**Additional Nursing Issues**

**Physical Assessment:** Assess other medications patient may be taking for effectiveness and interactions (see Warnings/Precautions and Drug Interactions). This drug has multiple uses/doses (see above). Monitor therapeutic response and adverse reactions according to use (see Contraindications, Adverse Reactions, and Overdose/Toxicology).

Parenteral: Monitor arterial blood gases, adverse reactions (see Adverse Reactions and Overdose/Toxicology) and monitor infusion site frequently for patency (note extravasation treatment above).

Nasal or ophthalmic: Assess knowledge/teach patient appropriate use, interventions to reduce side effects, and adverse symptoms to report.

**Pregnancy risk factor C** - benefits of use should outweigh possible risks. Note breast-feeding caution. Systemic absorption from ophthalmic instillation is minimal.

(Continued)

## Phenylephrine *(Continued)*

**Patient Information/Instruction:**

Nasal decongestant: Do not use for more than 5 days in a row. Clear nose as much as possible before use. Tilt head back and instill recommended dose of drops or spray. Do not blow nose for 5-10 minutes. You may experience transient stinging or burning.

Ophthalmic: Open eye, look at ceiling, and instill prescribed amount of solution. Close eye and roll eye in all directions, and apply gentle pressure to inner corner of eye for 1-2 minutes after instillation. Do not let tip of applicator touch eye or contaminate tip of applicator. Temporary stinging or blurred vision may occur. Report persistent pain, burning, double vision, severe headache, or if condition worsens.

**Pregnancy/breast-feeding precautions:** Inform prescriber if you are pregnant. Consult prescriber if breast-feeding.

**Geriatric Considerations:** Phenylephrine I.V. should be used with extreme caution in the elderly. The 10% ophthalmic solution has caused increased blood pressure in elderly patients and its use should, therefore, be avoided. Since topical decongestants can be obtained OTC, elderly patients should be counseled about their proper use and in what disease states they should be avoided (see Warnings/Precautions).

**Additional Information** Some formulations may contain sulfites.

**Related Information**

Inotropic and Vasoconstrictor Comparison *on page 1391*
Ophthalmic Agents *on page 1282*

- **Phenylephrine and Isoproterenol** *see* Isoproterenol and Phenylephrine *on page 634*
- **Phenylephrine and Promethazine** *see* Promethazine and Phenylephrine *on page 980*
- **Phenylephrine and Zinc Sulfate** *see page 1294*
- **Phenylephrine, Guaifenesin, and Phenylpropanolamine** *see* Guaifenesin, Phenylpropanolamine, and Phenylephrine *on page 552*
- **Phenylephrine, Hydrocodone, Chlorpheniramine, Acetaminophen, and Caffeine** *see* Hydrocodone, Chlorpheniramine, Phenylephrine, Acetaminophen, and Caffeine *on page 576*
- **Phenylephrine, Promethazine, and Codeine** *see* Promethazine, Phenylephrine, and Codeine *on page 981*
- **Phenylethylmalonylurea** *see* Phenobarbital *on page 917*
- **Phenylfenesin® L.A.** *see* Guaifenesin and Phenylpropanolamine *on page 550*
- **Phenylisohydantoin** *see* Pemoline *on page 892*

## Phenylpropanolamine (fen il proe pa NOLE a meen)

**U.S. Brand Names** Acutrim® 16 Hours [OTC]; Acutrim® II, Maximum Strength [OTC]; Acutrim® Late Day [OTC]; Control® [OTC]; Dexatrim® Pre-Meal [OTC]; Maximum Strength Dex-A-Diet® [OTC]; Maximum Strength Dexatrim® [OTC]; Phenoxine® [OTC]; Phenyldrine® [OTC]; Prolamine® [OTC]; Propagest® [OTC]; Rhindecon®; Unitrol® [OTC]

**Synonyms** *dl*-Norephedrine Hydrochloride; PPA

**Therapeutic Category** Alpha/Beta Agonist

**Pregnancy Risk Factor** C

**Lactation** Excretion in breast milk unknown

**Use** Anorexiant and nasal decongestant

**Mechanism of Action/Effect** Releases tissue stores of epinephrine and thereby produces an alpha- and beta-adrenergic stimulation; this causes vasoconstriction and nasal mucosa blanching; also appears to depress central appetite centers

**Contraindications** Hypersensitivity to phenylpropanolamine

**Warnings** Use with caution in patients with high blood pressure, tachyarrhythmias, pheochromocytoma, bradycardia, cardiac disease, arteriosclerosis. Do not use for more than 3 weeks for weight loss. Pregnancy factor C.

**Drug Interactions**

**Decreased Effect:** Decreased effect of antihypertensives.

**Increased Effect/Toxicity:** Increased effect/toxicity with MAO inhibitors (hypertensive crisis), beta-blockers (increased vasopressor effects).

**Adverse Reactions**

>10%: Cardiovascular: Hypertension, palpitations

1% to 10%:

Central nervous system: Insomnia, restlessness, dizziness
Gastrointestinal: Xerostomia, nausea

<1% (Limited to important or life-threatening symptoms): Tightness in chest, bradycardia, arrhythmias, angina, severe headache

**Overdose/Toxicology** Symptoms of overdose include vomiting, hypertension, palpitations, paresthesia, excitation, and seizures. Treatment is supportive.

**Pharmacodynamics/Kinetics**

**Half-life Elimination:** 4.6-6.6 hours

**Metabolism:** Liver

**Excretion:** Urine

**Duration:** Timed release: Up to 24 hours

**Formulations**

Phenylpropanolamine hydrochloride:

Capsule: 37.5 mg
Capsule, timed release: 25 mg, 75 mg
Tablet: 25 mg, 50 mg
Tablet:
Precision release: 75 mg

Timed release: 75 mg

**Dosing**

**Adults:** Oral:

Decongestant: 25 mg every 4 hours or 50 mg every 8 hours, not to exceed 150 mg/day

Anorexic: 25 mg 3 times/day 30 minutes before meals or 75 mg (timed release) once daily in the morning

Precision release: 75 mg after breakfast

**Elderly:** See Geriatric Considerations. Oral:

Decongestant: 25 mg every 4-6 hours as needed

Urinary incontinence: 75 mg twice daily (use sustained release capsules)

**Administration**

**Oral:** Administer dose early in day to prevent insomnia. Observe for signs of nervousness, excitability.

**Additional Nursing Issues**

**Physical Assessment:** Assess other medications patient may be taking for effectiveness and interactions (see Drug Interactions). Note that this medication has both alpha- and beta-adrenergic effects. Monitor therapeutic response and adverse reactions (eg, blood pressure and heart rate, CNS status, and respiratory status - see Adverse Reactions and Overdose/Toxicology). Assess knowledge/teach patient appropriate use, interventions to reduce side effects, and adverse symptoms to report. **Pregnancy risk factor C** - benefits of use should outweigh possible risks. Note breast-feeding caution.

**Patient Information/Instruction:** Nasal decongestant: Do not use for longer than recommended (4-5 days in a row). Anorexiant: Do not use for longer than 3 weeks. With timed release form, take early in day; do not chew or crush. Do not use more often, or in greater dose than prescribed. You may experience dizziness or blurred vision (use caution when driving or engaging in tasks requiring alertness until response to drug is known). With nasal use you may experience burning or stinging (this will resolve). Report rapid heartbeat, chest pain, palpitations; persistent vomiting; excessive nervousness, trembling, or insomnia; difficult or painful urination; unresolved burning or stinging (eyes or nose); or acute headache. **Pregnancy/breast-feeding precautions:** Inform prescriber if you are or intend to be pregnant. Consult prescriber if breast-feeding.

**Geriatric Considerations:** Not recommended for use an as anorexiant in the elderly. Phenylpropanolamine is ~75% effective in controlling mild to moderate stress incontinence. Elderly patients should be counseled about the proper use of over-the-counter cough and cold preparations.

- **Phenylpropanolamine and Caramiphen** *see* Caramiphen and Phenylpropanolamine *on page 195*
- **Phenylpropanolamine and Guaifenesin** *see* Guaifenesin and Phenylpropanolamine *on page 550*
- **Phenylpropanolamine and Hydrocodone** *see* Hydrocodone and Phenylpropanolamine *on page 574*
- **Phenylpropanolamine, Brompheniramine, and Codeine** *see* Brompheniramine, Phenylpropanolamine, and Codeine *on page 163*
- **Phenylpropanolamine, Guaifenesin, and Dextromethorphan** *see* Guaifenesin, Phenylpropanolamine, and Dextromethorphan *on page 551*
- **Phenylpropanolamine, Guaifenesin, and Phenylephrine** *see* Guaifenesin, Phenylpropanolamine, and Phenylephrine *on page 552*
- **Phenyltoloxamine, Phenylpropanolamine, and Acetaminophen** *see page 1294*
- **Phenylzin® Ophthalmic** *see page 1294*

## Phenytoin (FEN i toyn)

**U.S. Brand Names** Dilantin®; Diphenylan Sodium®

**Synonyms** Diphenylhydantoin; DPH

**Therapeutic Category** Antiarrhythmic Agent, Class I-B; Anticonvulsant, Hydantoin

**Pregnancy Risk Factor** D

**Lactation** Enters breast milk/use caution (AAP rates "compatible")

**Use** Management of generalized tonic-clonic (grand mal), simple partial and complex partial seizures; prevention of seizures following head trauma/neurosurgery; ventricular arrhythmias, including those associated with digitalis intoxication, prolonged Q-T interval and surgical repair of congenital heart diseases in children; used for epidermolysis bullosa

**Mechanism of Action/Effect** Decreases seizure activity by increasing efflux or decreasing influx of sodium ions across cell membranes in the motor cortex during generation of nerve impulses; prolongs effective refractory period and suppresses ventricular pacemaker automaticity, shortens action potential in the heart

**Contraindications** Hypersensitivity to phenytoin, other hydantoins, or any component; heart block; sinus bradycardia; pregnancy

**Warnings** May increase frequency of petit mal seizures. I.V. form may cause hypotension, skin necrosis at I.V. site. Avoid I.V. administration in small veins. Use with caution in patients with porphyria. Discontinue if rash or lymphadenopathy occurs. Use with caution in patients with hepatic dysfunction, sinus bradycardia, S-A block, A-V block, or hepatic impairment. Elderly may have reduced hepatic clearance and low albumin levels, which will increase the free fraction of phenytoin in the serum and increase drug response.

**Drug Interactions**

**Cytochrome P-450 Effect:** CYP2C9 and 2C19 enzyme substrate; CYP1A2, 2B6, 2C, 2C9, 2C18, 2C19, 2D6, 3A3/4, and 3A5-7 enzyme inducer

(Continued)

## Phenytoin *(Continued)*

**Decreased Effect:** Decreased effect of phenytoin with rifampin, cisplatin, vinblastine, bleomycin, folic acid, theophylline, and continuous NG feedings. Phenytoin may decrease the effect of oral contraceptives, itraconazole, mebendazole, methadone, oral midazolam, valproic acid, cyclosporine, theophylline, doxycycline, quinidine, mexiletine, disopyramide. See Administration - Other.

**Increased Effect/Toxicity:** Amiodarone or disulfiram decreases metabolism of phenytoin. Isoniazid, chloramphenicol, or fluconazole may increase phenytoin serum concentrations. Valproic acid may increase, decrease or have no effect on phenytoin serum concentrations. Phenytoin may increase the effect of dopamine (enhanced hypotension), warfarin (enhanced anticoagulation), increase the rate of conversion of primidone to phenobarbital resulting in increased phenobarbital serum concentrations.

**Food Interactions** Phenytoin serum concentrations may be altered if taken with food. If taken with enteral nutrition, phenytoin serum concentrations may be decreased.

**Effects on Lab Values** ↑ glucose, alkaline phosphatase (S); ↓ thyroxine (S), calcium (S)

**Adverse Reactions** I.V. effects: Hypotension, bradycardia, cardiac arrhythmias, cardiovascular collapse (especially with rapid I.V. use), venous irritation and pain, thrombophlebitis, **vesicant chemotherapy**

**Effects not related to plasma phenytoin concentrations:** Hypertrichosis, gingival hypertrophy, thickening of facial features, carbohydrate intolerance, folic acid deficiency, peripheral neuropathy, vitamin D deficiency, osteomalacia, systemic lupus erythematosus

**Dose-related effects:** Nystagmus, blurred vision, diplopia, ataxia, slurred speech, dizziness, drowsiness, lethargy, coma, rash, fever, nausea, vomiting, gum tenderness, confusion, mood changes, folic acid depletion, osteomalacia, hyperglycemia

**Related to elevated concentrations:**
- >20 mcg/mL: Far lateral nystagmus
- >30 mcg/mL: 45° lateral gaze nystagmus and ataxia
- >40 mcg/mL: Decreased mentation
- >100 mcg/mL: Death

>10%:
- Central nervous system: Psychiatric changes, slurred speech, dizziness, drowsiness
- Gastrointestinal: Constipation, nausea, vomiting, gingival hyperplasia
- Neuromuscular & skeletal: Trembling

1% to 10%:
- Central nervous system: Headache, insomnia
- Dermatologic: Rash
- Gastrointestinal: Anorexia, weight loss
- Hematologic: Leukopenia
- Hepatic: Hepatitis
- Renal: Increase in serum creatinine

<1% (Limited to important or life-threatening symptoms): Hypotension, bradycardia, cardiac arrhythmias, cardiovascular collapse; rare: SLE-like syndrome, lymphadenopathy, hepatitis, Stevens-Johnson syndrome, blood dyscrasias, dyskinesias, pseudolymphoma, lymphoma

**Overdose/Toxicology** Symptoms of overdose include unsteady gait, slurred speech, confusion, nausea, hypothermia, fever, hypotension, respiratory depression, coma. Treatment is symptomatic.

**Pharmacodynamics/Kinetics**

**Protein Binding:**
- Adults: 90% to 95%
- Others: Increased free fraction (decreased protein binding)
- Patients with hyperbilirubinemia, hypoalbuminemia, uremia; see table.

| Disease States Resulting in a Decrease in Serum Albumin Concentration | Disease States Resulting in an Apparent Decrease in Affinity of Phenytoin for Serum Albumin |
|---|---|
| Burns | Renal failure<br>$Cl_{cr}$ <25 mL/min<br>(unbound fraction is increased two- to threefold in uremia) |
| Hepatic cirrhosis | Jaundice (severe) |
| Nephrotic syndrome | Other drugs (displacers) |
| Pregnancy | Hyperbilirubinemia<br>(total bilirubin >15 mg/dL) |
| Cystic fibrosis | |

**Half-life Elimination:** Oral: 22 hours (range: 7-42 hours); I.V.: 10-15 hours

**Time to Peak:** Oral: Extended-release capsule: Within 4-12 hours; Immediate release preparation: Within 2-3 hours

**Metabolism:** Follows dose-dependent capacity-limited (Michaelis-Menten) pharmacokinetics with increased $V_{max}$ in infants >6 months of age and children versus adults.

**Excretion:** Highly variable clearance dependent upon intrinsic hepatic function and dose administered; increased clearance and decreased serum concentrations with febrile illness; <5% excreted unchanged in urine; major metabolite (via oxidation) HPPA undergoes enterohepatic recycling and elimination in urine as glucuronides

**Onset:** I.V. Within 30 minutes to 1 hour; onset of fosphenytoin may be more rapid due to more rapid infusion

**Formulations**

Phenytoin sodium:

Capsule, extended release: 30 mg, 100 mg

Capsule, prompt: 30 mg, 100 mg

Injection: 50 mg/mL (2 mL, 5 mL)

Suspension, oral: 125 mg/5 mL (5 mL, 240 mL)

Tablet, chewable: 50 mg

**Dosing**

**Adults:**

Status epilepticus: I.V.: Loading dose: 15-20 mg/kg in a single or divided dose, followed by 100-150 mg/dose at 30-minute intervals up to a maximum of 1500 mg/24 hours; maintenance dose: 300 mg/day or 5-6 mg/kg/day in 3 divided doses or 1-2 divided doses using extended release

Anticonvulsant: Oral: Loading dose: 15-20 mg/kg; based on phenytoin serum concentrations and recent dosing history; administer oral loading dose in 3 divided doses given every 2-4 hours to decrease GI adverse effects and to ensure complete oral absorption; maintenance dose: same as I.V.

**Elderly:** Refer to adult dosing.

**Renal Impairment:** Phenytoin level in serum may be difficult to interpret in renal failure. Monitoring of free (unbound) concentrations or adjustment to allow interpretation is recommended.

**Hepatic Impairment:** Safe in usual doses in mild liver disease; clearance may be substantially reduced in cirrhosis and plasma level monitoring with dose adjustment advisable. Free phenytoin levels should be monitored closely.

**Administration**

**I.M.:** I.M. administration is not recommended due to erratic absorption, pain on injection and precipitation of drug at injection site.

**I.V.:** Vesicant. Phosphenytoin may be considered for loading in patients who are in status, or hemodynamically unstable or develop hypotension/bradycardia with I.V. administration of phenytoin. Phenytoin may be administered by IVP or IVPB administration. The maximum rate of I.V. administration is 50 mg/minute. Highly sensitive patients (eg, elderly, patients with pre-existing cardiovascular conditions) should receive phenytoin more slowly (eg, 20 mg/minute).

**I.V. Detail:** An in-line 0.22-5 micron filter is recommended for IVPB solutions due to the high potential for precipitation of the solution. Avoid extravasation. Following I.V. administration, NS should be injected through the same needle or I.V. catheter to prevent irritation.

**Other:** S.C. administration is not recommended because of the possibility of local tissue damage. Absorption is impaired when phenytoin suspension is given concurrently to patients who are receiving continuous nasogastric feedings. A method to resolve this interaction is to divide the daily dose of phenytoin and withhold the administration of nutritional supplements for 1-2 hours before and after each phenytoin dose.

**Stability**

**Storage:** Phenytoin is stable as long as it remains free of haziness and precipitation. Use only clear solutions. Parenteral solution may be used as long as there is no precipitate and it is not hazy, slightly yellowed solution may be used. Refrigeration may cause precipitate, sometimes the precipitate is resolved by allowing the solution to reach room temperature again. Drug may precipitate at a pH <11.5.

**Reconstitution:** May dilute with normal saline for I.V. infusion; stability is concentration dependent.

Standard diluent: Dose/100 mL NS

Minimum volume: Concentration should be maintained at 1-10 mg/mL secondary to stability problems (stable for 4 hours).

**Compatibility:** I.V. form is highly incompatible with many drugs and solutions such as dextrose in water, some saline solutions, amikacin, bretylium, dobutamine, cephapirin, insulin, levorphanol, lidocaine, meperidine, metaraminol, morphine, norepinephrine, heparin, potassium chloride, and vitamin B complex with C.

**Monitoring Laboratory Tests** Plasma phenytoin level, CBC, liver function. Note: Serum phenytoin concentrations should be interpreted in terms of the unbound concentration. Adjustment should be made in patients with renal impairment and/or hypoalbuminemia.

**Additional Nursing Issues**

**Physical Assessment:** Clearly identify class of seizures (note Warnings/Precautions). Note and monitor all other prescription and OTC medications patient may be taking (see Drug Interactions; phenytoin affects many other drugs). Monitor I.V. sites closely - phenytoin is highly alkaline and irritating. Administer I.V. slowly - monitor heart rate and blood pressure closely and monitor all patients for adverse/toxic results; phenytoin has narrow therapeutic range. Discontinue phenytoin dosage slowly; abrupt discontinuance can cause status epilepticus. Monitor CNS, condition of gums (ie, gingival hyperplasia), and liver function. Instruct diabetic patients to monitor serum glucose closely. **Pregnancy risk factor D** - assess knowledge/teach appropriate use of barrier contraceptives (phenytoin may interfere with effectiveness of oral contraceptives). Note breast-feeding caution.

**Patient Information/Instruction:** Take this drug as directed, with food. Do not change brands or discontinue without consulting prescriber. Follow good oral hygiene practices and have frequent dental checkups. If diabetic, monitor your serum glucose regularly as directed by prescriber; insulin dosage may need to be adjusted. You may experience dizziness, confusion, or vision changes; use caution when driving or engaging in tasks requiring alertness until response to drug is known. If GI upset occurs, frequent small meals may help. May discolor urine (red/pink). Report rash;

(Continued)

## Phenytoin *(Continued)*

unresolved nausea or vomiting; slurring speech or coordination difficulties; swollen glands; swollen, sore, or bleeding gums; yellowish color to skin or eyes; unusual bleeding and/or bruising; erection problems; difficulty breathing; or palpitations. Do not crush or open extended-release capsules. **Pregnancy/breast-feeding precautions:** Do not get pregnant; use barrier contraceptive measures to prevent possible harm to the fetus (effectiveness of oral contraceptives may be affected by phenytoin). Consult prescriber if breast-feeding.

**Geriatric Considerations:** Elderly may have low albumin which will increase free fraction and increase drug response. Monitor closely in those who are hypoalbuminemic. Free fraction measurements advised, also elderly may display a higher incidence of adverse effects (cardiovascular) when using the I.V. loading regimen; therefore, recommended to decrease loading I.V. dose to 25 mg/minute (see Warnings/Precautions).

**Additional Information** The injection formulation contains ethanol.

Phenytoin: Dilantin® chewable tablet and oral suspension
Phenytoin sodium, extended: Dilantin® Kapseal®
Phenytoin sodium, prompt: Diphenylan Sodium® capsule
Sodium content of 1 g injection: 88 mg (3.8 mEq)

**Related Information**

Peak and Trough Guidelines *on page 1331*

- ♦ **Pherazine® w/DM** *see* Promethazine and Dextromethorphan *on page 980*
- ♦ **Pherazine® With Codeine** *see* Promethazine and Codeine *on page 980*
- ♦ **Phicon®** *see page 1294*
- ♦ **Phillips® LaxCaps Capsule** *see page 1294*
- ♦ **Phillips'® Milk of Magnesia** *see* Magnesium Supplements *on page 703*
- ♦ **Phos-Ex®** *see* Calcium Supplements *on page 185*
- ♦ **Phos-Flur®** *see page 1294*
- ♦ **PhosLo®** *see* Calcium Supplements *on page 185*

## Phosphate Supplements (FOS fate SUP la ments)

**U.S. Brand Names** Fleet® Enema [OTC]; Fleet® Phospho®-Soda [OTC]; K-Phos® M.F.; K-Phos® Neutral; K-Phos® No. 2; K-Phos® Original; Neutra-Phos®-K; Uro-KP-Neutral®

**Synonyms** Potassium Acid Phosphate; Potassium Phosphate; Potassium Phosphate and Sodium Phosphate; Sodium Phosphate

**Therapeutic Category** Electrolyte Supplement

**Pregnancy Risk Factor** C

**Use** Treatment and prevention of hypophosphatemia; short-term treatment of constipation (oral/rectal); evacuation of the colon for rectal and bowel exams; source of phosphate in large volume I.V. fluids; urinary acidifier (potassium acid phosphate) for reduction in formation of calcium stones

**Mechanism of Action/Effect** Phosphorus participates in bone deposition, calcium metabolism, utilization of B complex vitamins, and as a buffer in acid-base equilibrium; as a laxative, exerts osmotic effect in the small intestine by drawing water into the lumen of the gut, producing distension, promoting peristalsis, and evacuation of the bowel

**Contraindications** Hyperphosphatemia, hyperkalemia (potassium salt form), hypocalcemia, hypomagnesemia, hypernatremia (sodium salt form), severe renal impairment, severe tissue trauma, heat cramps, CHF, abdominal pain (rectal forms), fecal impaction (rectal forms); patients with infected phosphate kidney stones

**Warnings** Use with caution in patients with renal impairment, patients receiving potassium-sparing drugs (potassium salt forms), patients with adrenal insufficiency, cirrhosis.

Parenteral **potassium** salt forms: should be administered only in patients with adequate urine flow. Must be diluted before I.V. use and infused slowly (see Drug Administration), and patients must be on a cardiac monitor during intermittent infusions.

**Drug Interactions**

**Decreased Effect:** Do not administer oral phosphate supplements at the same time as sucralfate, iron supplements, or antacids which contain aluminum, calcium, or magnesium, which may result in binding of the phosphate and reduced absorption.

**Increased Effect/Toxicity:** Potassium-containing preparations should be used with caution in patients receiving ACE-inhibitors, salt substitutes or potassium-sparing diuretics.

**Adverse Reactions**

Cardiovascular: Hypotension, edema; **potassium salt form:** arrhythmias, heart block, cardiac arrest
Central nervous system: Tetany, mental confusion, seizures, dizziness, headache
Endocrine & metabolic: Hyperphosphatemia, hyperkalemia **(potassium salt form)**, hypocalcemia, hypernatremia **(sodium salt form)**
Gastrointestinal: Nausea, vomiting, diarrhea, flatulence (oral use)
Local: Phlebitis (parenteral forms)
Neuromuscular & skeletal: Paresthesia, bone and joint pain, arthralgia, weakness, muscle cramps
Renal: Acute renal failure

**Pharmacodynamics/Kinetics**

**Half-life Elimination:** Oral forms excreted in feces; I.V. forms are excreted in the urine with over 80% of dose reabsorbed by the kidney

**Onset:** Catharsis: Oral: 3-6 hours; Rectal: 2-5 minutes

**Formulations**

Capsule:

Neutra-Phos®-K: Phosphorus 250 mg [8 mmol] and **potassium** 556 mg [14.25 mEq] per capsule

Neutra-Phos®: Phosphorus 250 mg [8 mmol], **potassium** 278 mg [7.125 mEq], and **sodium** 164 mg [7.125 mEq] per capsule

Enema (Fleet® Enema): **Sodium** phosphate 6 g and sodium biphosphate 16 g per 100 mL (67.5 mL pediatric enema unit, 135 mL adult enema unit)

Injection:

Phosphate **(as potassium phosphate)** 3 mmol and **potassium** 4.4 mEq per mL (15 mL)

Phosphate **(as sodium phosphate)** 3 mmol and **sodium** 4 mEq per mL (15 mL)

Powder:

Neutra-Phos®-K: Phosphorus 250 mg [8 mmol] and **potassium** 556 mg [14.25 mEq] per packet

Neutra-Phos®: Phosphorus 250 mg [8 mmol], **potassium** 278 mg [7.125 mEq], and **sodium** 164 mg [7.125 mEq] per packet

Solution, oral (Fleet® Phospho®-Soda): Phosphate 4 mmol/mL; **sodium** phosphate 18 g and sodium biphosphate 48 g per 100 mL (30 mL, 45 mL, 90 mL, 237 mL) (96.4 mEq sodium/20 mL)

Tablet:

K-Phos® M.F.: Phosphorus 125.6 mg [4 mmol], **potassium** 44.5 mg [1.1 mEq], and **sodium** 67 mg [2.9 mEq]

K-Phos® Neutral: Phosphorus 250 mg [8 mmol], **potassium** 45 mg [1.1 mEq], and **sodium** 298 mg [13 mEq] per tablet

K-Phos® No. 2: Phosphorus 250 mg [8 mmol], **potassium** 88 mg [2.3 mEq], and **sodium** 134 mg [5.8 mEq]

K-Phos® Original: Phosphorus 114 mg [3.7 mmol] and **potassium** 144 mg [3.7 mEq] per tablet

Uro-KP-Neutral®: Phosphorus 250 mg [8 mmol], **potassium** 49.4 mg [1.27 mEq], and **sodium** 250.5 mg [10.9 mEq]

**Dosing**

**Adults: Note:** Phosphate supplements are either sodium or potassium salt forms. Consider the contribution of these electrolytes also when determining appropriate phosphate replacement.

I.V. doses should be incorporated into the patient's maintenance I.V. fluids; intermittent I.V. infusion should be reserved for severe depletion situations; requires continuous cardiac monitoring (for potassium salts). It is difficult to determine total body phosphorus deficit, the following dosages are empiric guidelines: **Note:** Doses listed as mmol of **phosphate**:

Hypophosphatemia: Intermittent I.V. infusion: Varying dosages: 0.15-0.3 mmol/kg/dose over 12 hours; may repeat as needed to achieve desired serum level **or**

15 mmol/dose over 2 hours; use if serum phosphorus <2 mg/dL **or**

Low dose: 0.16 mmol/kg over 4-6 hours; use if serum phosphorus level 2.3-3 mg/dL

Intermediate dose: 0.32 mmol/kg over 4-6 hours; use if serum phosphorus level 1.6-2.2 mg/dL

High dose: 0.64 mmol/kg over 8-12 hours; use if serum phosphorus <1.5 mg/dL

Maintenance:

I.V.: 50-70 mmol/day

Oral: 50-150 mmol/day in divided doses

Laxative: Oral 1-2 capsules or packets (250-500 mg phosphorus/8-16 mmol) 4 times/day; dilute as instructed

Fleet® Phospho®-Soda:® Oral: 20-30 mL as a single dose

Laxative: Rectal: Enema: Contents of one 4.5 oz enema as a single dose, may repeat

Urinary acidification: Oral (K-Phos® Original): 2 tablets 4 times/day

**Administration**

**Oral:** Administer with food to reduce the risk of diarrhea. Do not swallow the capsule. Contents of 1 capsule or packet should be diluted in 75 mL water before administration. Administer tablets with a full glass of water. Maintain adequate fluid intake. Dilute oral solution with an equal volume of cool water. K-Phos® Original tablets (urinary acidifier) should be dissolved in 6-8 ounces of water before administration.

**I.V.:** For intermittent infusion, if peripheral line, dilute to a maximum concentration of 0.05 mmol/mL. If central line, dilute to a maximum concentration of 0.12 mmol/mL; maximum rate of infusion: 0.06 mmol/kg/hour; do **not** infuse with calcium containing I.V. fluids.

**Stability**

**Storage:** Phosphate salts may precipitate when mixed with calcium salts. Solubility is improved in amino acid parenteral nutrition solutions.

**Compatibility:** Check with a pharmacist to determine compatibility.

**Monitoring Laboratory Tests** Serum potassium (potassium salt forms), sodium (sodium salt forms), calcium, phosphorus, magnesium, renal function, reflexes; cardiac monitor (when intermittent infusion or high-dose I.V. replacement of potassium salts needed)

**Additional Nursing Issues**

**Physical Assessment:** Potassium salt forms: Assess other medications patient may be taking for effectiveness and interactions (eg, antacids and ACE inhibitors - see Drug Interactions). See Contraindications and Warnings/Precautions for cautious use. Monitor laboratory tests (serum K), therapeutic response, and adverse reactions at

(Continued)

## Phosphate Supplements *(Continued)*

beginning of therapy and periodically throughout therapy (see Adverse Reactions and Overdose/Toxicology). Assess knowledge/teach patient appropriate use, interventions to reduce side effects, and adverse symptoms to report. Note Breast-feeding caution.

I.V.: Monitor infusion site regularly and cardiac status on a regular basis (continuous EKG during highly concentrated infusions). Note Dosing instructions/information above. Instruct patient about adverse reactions to report.

**Patient Information/Instruction:** Take as directed; do not take more than directed. Swallow tablet whole with full glass of water or juice and stir before sipping slowly, with or after meals (do not take on an empty stomach). If taking potassium salt, take any antacids 2 hours before or after potassium. For capsules or packets, dissolve effervescent tablet or contents of packet or capsule in 4-6 ounces of water or juice. Consult prescriber about advisability of increasing dietary potassium. Report tingling of hands or feet; unresolved nausea or vomiting; chest pain or palpitations; persistent abdominal pain; feelings of weakness, dizziness, listlessness, confusion, acute muscle weakness or cramping; blood in stool or tarry stools; or easy bruising or unusual bleeding. **Breast-feeding precautions:** Consult prescriber if breast-feeding.

**Dietary Issues:** Avoid giving with oxalate (ie, berries, nuts, chocolate, beans, celery, tomato) or phytate-containing (ie, bran, whole wheat) foods.


- **Phospholine Iodide® Ophthalmic** *see* Ophthalmic Agents, Glaucoma *on page 853*
- **Phosphonoformic Acid** *see* Foscarnet *on page 516*
- **Phosphorated Carbohydrate Solution** *see page 1294*
- **Photofrin®** *see* Porfimer *on page 947*
- **Phrenilin®** *see* Butalbital Compound and Acetaminophen *on page 175*
- **Phrenilin Forte®** *see* Butalbital Compound and Acetaminophen *on page 175*
- ***p*-Hydroxyampicillin** *see* Amoxicillin *on page 80*
- **Phyllocontin®** *see* Theophylline *on page 1115*
- **Phylloquinone** *see* Phytonadione *on next page*


## Physostigmine (fye zoe STIG meen)

**U.S. Brand Names** Antilirium®; Isopto® Eserine

**Synonyms** Eserine Salicylate

**Therapeutic Category** Acetylcholinesterase Inhibitor (Peripheral); Ophthalmic Agent, Antiglaucoma

**Pregnancy Risk Factor** C

**Lactation** Excretion in breast milk unknown

**Use** Reverse toxic CNS effects caused by anticholinergic drugs; miotic in treatment of glaucoma

**Mechanism of Action/Effect** Inhibits destruction of acetylcholine by acetylcholinesterase which facilitates transmission of impulses across myoneural junction and prolongs the central and peripheral effects of acetylcholine

**Contraindications** Hypersensitivity to physostigmine or any component; GI or GU obstruction; physostigmine therapy for drug intoxications should be used with extreme caution in patients with asthma, gangrene, severe cardiovascular disease, or mechanical obstruction of the GI tract or urogenital tract. In these patients, physostigmine should be used only to treat life-threatening conditions.

**Warnings** Use with caution in patients with epilepsy, asthma, diabetes, gangrene, cardiovascular disease, bradycardia. Discontinue if excessive salivation or emesis, frequent urination or diarrhea occur. Reduce dosage if excessive sweating or nausea occurs. Administer I.V. slowly or at a controlled rate not faster than 1 mg/minute. Due to the possibility of hypersensitivity or overdose/cholinergic crisis, atropine should be readily available; ointment may delay corneal healing, may cause loss of dark adaptation; not intended as a first-line agent for anticholinergic toxicity or Parkinson's disease. Pregnancy factor C.

**Drug Interactions**

**Increased Effect/Toxicity:** Increased toxicity with bethanechol, methacholine. Succinylcholine may increase neuromuscular blockade with systemic administration.

**Effects on Lab Values** ↑ aminotransferase [ALT (SGPT)/AST (SGOT)] (S), amylase (S)

**Adverse Reactions**

**Ophthalmic:**

>10%:

Ocular: Lacrimation, marked miosis, blurred vision, eye pain
Miscellaneous: Sweating

1% to 10%:

Central nervous system: Headache, browache
Dermatologic: Burning, redness

**Systemic:**

>10%:

Gastrointestinal: Nausea, salivation, diarrhea, stomach pains
Ocular: Lacrimation
Miscellaneous: Sweating

1% to 10%:

Cardiovascular: Palpitations, bradycardia
Central nervous system: Restlessness, nervousness, hallucinations, seizures
Genitourinary: Frequent urge to urinate
Neuromuscular & skeletal: Muscle twitching
Ocular: Miosis

Respiratory: Dyspnea, bronchospasm, respiratory paralysis, pulmonary edema

**Overdose/Toxicology** Symptoms of overdose include muscle weakness, blurred vision, excessive sweating, tearing and salivation, nausea, vomiting, bronchospasm, and seizures. If physostigmine is used in excess or in the absence of an anticholinergic overdose, patients may manifest signs of cholinergic toxicity. At this point a cholinergic agent (eg, atropine 0.015-0.05 mg/kg) may be necessary.

**Pharmacodynamics/Kinetics**

**Distribution:** Crosses the blood-brain barrier readily and reverses both central and peripheral anticholinergic effects

**Half-life Elimination:** 15-40 minutes

**Metabolism:** Liver

**Excretion:** Via hydrolysis by cholinesterases

**Onset:** Ophthalmic instillation: Within 2 minutes; Parenteral: Within 5 minutes

**Duration:** Ophthalmic: 12-48 hours; Parenteral: 0.5-5 hours

**Formulations**

Injection, as salicylate: 1 mg/mL (2 mL)

Ointment, ophthalmic, as sulfate: 0.25% (3.5 g, 3.7 g)

**Dosing**

**Adults:**

Anticholinergic drug overdose:

I.M., I.V., S.C.: 0.5-2 mg to start; repeat every 20 minutes until response occurs or adverse effect occurs.

Repeat 1-4 mg every 30-60 minutes as life-threatening signs (arrhythmias, seizures, deep coma) recur; maximum I.V. rate: 1 mg/minute.

Ophthalmic:

Ointment: Instill a small quantity to lower fornix up to 3 times/day.

Solution: Instill 1-2 drops into eye(s) up to 4 times/day.

**Elderly:** Refer to adult dosing.

**Stability**

**Storage:** Do not use solution if cloudy or dark brown

**Additional Nursing Issues**

**Physical Assessment:** When used to reverse neuromuscular block (anesthesia or excessive acetylcholine), monitor patient safety until full return of neuromuscular functioning. Assess bladder and sphincter adequacy prior to administering medication. Assess other medications patient may be taking for effectiveness and interactions (see Drug Interactions). See Contraindications and Warnings/Precautions for cautious use. Monitor therapeutic effects, and adverse reactions: cholinergic crisis (DUMBELS - **d**iarrhea, **u**rination, **m**iosis, **b**ronchospasm/**b**radycardia, **e**xcitability, **l**acrimation, and **s**alivation/excessive **s**weating) (see Warnings/Precautions, Adverse Reactions, and Overdose/Toxicology). Assess knowledge/teach patient appropriate use of ophthalmic forms, interventions to reduce side effects, and adverse symptoms to report. **Pregnancy risk factor C** - benefits of use should outweigh possible risks. Note breast-feeding caution.

**Patient Information/Instruction:** Systemic: Maintain adequate hydration (2-3 L/day of fluids unless instructed to restrict fluid intake). May cause dizziness, drowsiness, or hypotension (rise slowly from sitting or lying position and use caution when driving or climbing stairs); vomiting or loss of appetite (frequent small meals, frequent mouth care, chewing gum, or sucking lozenges may help); or diarrhea (boiled milk, yogurt, or buttermilk may help). Report persistent abdominal discomfort; significantly increased salivation, sweating, tearing, or urination; flushed skin; chest pain or palpitations; acute headache; unresolved diarrhea; excessive fatigue, insomnia, dizziness, or depression; increased muscle, joint, or body pain; vision changes or blurred vision; or shortness of breath or wheezing. **Pregnancy/breast-feeding precautions:** Inform prescriber if you are or intend to be pregnant. Consult prescriber if breast-feeding.

Ophthalmic: For ophthalmic use only. Wash hands before using. Tilt head back and look upward. Put drops of suspension or apply thin ribbon of ointment inside lower eyelid. Close eye and roll eyeball in all directions. Do not blink for 1/2 minute. Apply gentle pressure to inner corner of eye for 30 seconds. Do not use any other eye preparation for at least 10 minutes. Do not touch tip of applicator to eye or contaminate tip of applicator. Do not share medication with anyone else. Wear sunglasses when in sunlight; you may be more sensitive to bright light. Inform prescriber if condition worsens or fails to improve or if you experience eye pain, vision disturbances, or other adverse eye response; excess sweating; urinary frequency; severe headache; or skin rash, redness, or burning.

**Geriatric Considerations:** Studies on the use of physostigmine in Alzheimer's disease have reported variable results. Doses generally were in the range of 2-4 mg 4 times/day. Limitations to the use of physostigmine include a short half-life requiring frequent dosing, variable absorption from the GI tract, and no commercially available oral product; therefore, not recommended for treatment of Alzheimer's disease.

**Additional Information** Some formulations may contain sulfites. The salicylate injection contains benzyl alcohol.

- ♦ **Physostigmine** *see* Ophthalmic Agents, Glaucoma *on page 853*
- ♦ **Phytomenadione** *see* Phytonadione *on this page*

## Phytonadione (fye toe na DYE one)

**U.S. Brand Names** AquaMEPHYTON® Injection; Konakion® Injection; Mephyton® Oral

**Synonyms** Methylphytyl Napthoquinone; Phylloquinone; Phytomenadione; Vitamin $K_1$

**Therapeutic Category** Vitamin, Fat Soluble

**Pregnancy Risk Factor** C

(Continued)

## Phytonadione *(Continued)*

**Lactation** Enters breast milk/compatible

**Use** Prevention and treatment of hypoprothrombinemia caused by drug-induced or anticoagulant-induced vitamin K deficiency, hemorrhagic disease of the newborn; phytonadione is more effective and is preferred to other vitamin K preparations in the presence of impending hemorrhage; oral absorption depends on the presence of bile salts

**Mechanism of Action/Effect** Promotes liver synthesis of clotting factors (II, VII, IX, X); however, the exact mechanism as to this stimulation is unknown. Menadiol is a water soluble form of vitamin K; phytonadione has a more rapid and prolonged effect than menadione; menadiol sodium diphosphate ($K_4$) is half as potent as menadione ($K_3$).

**Contraindications** Hypersensitivity to phytonadione or any component

**Warnings** Severe reactions resembling anaphylaxis or hypersensitivity have occurred rarely during or immediately after I.V. administration (even with proper dilution and rate of administration). Restrict I.V. administration for emergency use only. Ineffective in hereditary hypoprothrombinemia, hypoprothrombinemia caused by severe liver disease. Severe hemolytic anemia has been reported rarely in neonates following large doses (10-20 mg) of phytonadione. Pregnancy factor C.

**Drug Interactions**

**Decreased Effect:** The anticoagulant effects of warfarin, dicumarol, anisindione are reversed by phytonadione.

**Adverse Reactions** 1% to 10%:

Cardiovascular: Transient flushing reaction, rarely hypotension, cyanosis

Central nervous system: Dizziness (rarely), pain

Gastrointestinal: Abnormal taste, GI upset (oral)

Hematologic: Hemolysis in neonates and in patients with G-6-PD deficiency

Local: Tenderness at injection site

Respiratory: Dyspnea

Miscellaneous: Sweating, anaphylaxis, hypersensitivity reactions

**Pharmacodynamics/Kinetics**

**Metabolism:** Liver

**Excretion:** Bile and urine

**Onset:** Onset of increased coagulation factors: Oral: Within 6-12 hours; Parenteral: Within 1-2 hours; prothrombin may become normal after 12-14 hours

**Formulations**

Injection:

Aqueous colloidal: 2 mg/mL (0.5 mL); 10 mg/mL (1 mL, 2.5 mL, 5 mL)

Aqueous (I.M. only): 2 mg/mL (0.5 mL); 10 mg/mL (1 mL)

Tablet: 5 mg

**Dosing**

**Adults:** I.V. route should be restricted for emergency use only

Minimum daily requirement (not well established): 0.03 mcg/kg/day

Oral anticoagulant overdose: Oral, I.M., I.V., S.C.: 2.5-10 mg/dose; rarely up to 25-50 mg has been used; may repeat in 6-8 hours if given by I.M., I.V., S.C. route; may repeat 12-48 hours after oral route

Vitamin K deficiency: Due to drugs, malabsorption or decreased synthesis of vitamin K

Oral: 5-25 mg/24 hours

I.M., I.V.: 10 mg

**Elderly:** Refer to adult dosing.

**Administration**

**I.V.:** Dilute in normal saline, $D_5W$ or $D_5NS$ and infuse slowly; rate of infusion should not exceed 1 mg/minute. **This route should be used only if administration by another route is not feasible.** I.V. administration should not exceed 1 mg/minute; for I.V. infusion, dilute in PF (preservative free) $D_5W$ or normal saline.

**Stability**

**Storage:** Protect injection from light at all times; may be autoclaved.

**Monitoring Laboratory Tests** PT

**Additional Nursing Issues**

**Physical Assessment:** Monitor laboratory test results and bleeding response; inform prescriber if unusual bleeding continues. Caution patient about excessive intake of vitamin K containing foods. **Pregnancy risk factor C** - benefits of use should outweigh possible risks.

**Patient Information/Instruction:** Oral: Take only as directed; do not take more or more often than prescribed. Avoid excessive or increased intake of vitamin K containing food (eg, green leafy vegetables, dairy products, meats) unless recommended by prescriber. Avoid alcohol and any OTC or prescribed medications containing aspirin that are not approved by prescriber. Report bleeding gums; blood in urine, stool, or vomitus; unusual bruising of bleeding; or abdominal cramping. **Pregnancy precautions:** Inform prescriber if you are or intend to be pregnant.

**Additional Information** Injection contains benzyl alcohol 0.9% as preservative. Phytonadione is more effective and is preferred to other vitamin K preparations in the presence of impending hemorrhage. Oral absorption depends on the presence of bile salts.


- **Pilagan® Ophthalmic** *see* Ophthalmic Agents, Glaucoma *on page 853*
- **Pilagan® Ophthalmic** *see* Pilocarpine *on next page*
- **Pilocar® Ophthalmic** *see* Ophthalmic Agents, Glaucoma *on page 853*
- **Pilocar® Ophthalmic** *see* Pilocarpine *on next page*

## Pilocarpine (pye loe KAR peen)

**U.S. Brand Names** Adsorbocarpine® Ophthalmic; Akarpine® Ophthalmic; Isopto® Carpine Ophthalmic; Ocu-Carpine® Ophthalmic; Ocusert Pilo-20® Ophthalmic; Ocusert Pilo-40® Ophthalmic; Pilagan® Ophthalmic; Pilocar® Ophthalmic; Pilopine HS® Ophthalmic; Piloptic® Ophthalmic; Pilostat® Ophthalmic; Salagen® Oral

**Therapeutic Category** Cholinergic Agonist; Ophthalmic Agent, Antiglaucoma; Ophthalmic Agent, Miotic

**Pregnancy Risk Factor** C

**Lactation** Excretion in breast milk unknown

**Use**

Ophthalmic: Management of chronic simple glaucoma, chronic and acute angle-closure glaucoma; to counter effects of cycloplegics

Oral: Symptomatic treatment of xerostomia caused by salivary gland hypofunction resulting from radiotherapy for cancer of the head and neck or Sjögren's syndrome

**Mechanism of Action/Effect** Directly stimulates cholinergic receptors in the eye causing miosis (by contraction of the iris sphincter), loss of accommodation (by constriction of ciliary muscle), and lowering of intraocular pressure (with decreased resistance to aqueous humor outflow)

**Contraindications** Hypersensitivity to pilocarpine or any component; acute inflammatory disease of anterior chamber

**Warnings** Use with caution in patients with corneal abrasion, CHF, asthma, peptic ulcer, urinary tract obstruction, Parkinson's disease, or narrow-angle glaucoma. Pregnancy factor C.

**Adverse Reactions**

**Ophthalmic:**

>10%: Ocular: Blurred vision, miosis, decrease in night vision

1% to 10%:

- Central nervous system: Headache
- Genitourinary: Polyuria
- Local: Stinging, burning
- Ocular: Ciliary spasm, retinal detachment, browache, photophobia, acute iritis, lacrimation, conjunctival and ciliary congestion early in therapy
- Miscellaneous: Hypersensitivity reactions

<1% (Limited to important or life-threatening symptoms): Hypertension, tachycardia

**Systemic:** >10%: Miscellaneous: Sweating

1% to 10%:

- Cardiovascular: Edema, flushing, hypertension, tachycardia
- Central nervous system: Muscle weakness, headache, tremors, chills
- Gastrointestinal: Nausea, vomiting, heartburn, dysphagia
- Genitourinary: Polyuria
- Ocular: Amblyopia
- Respiratory: Epistaxis, rhinitis, voice change

**Overdose/Toxicology** Symptoms of overdose include bronchospasm, bradycardia, involuntary urination, vomiting, hypotension, and tremor. Atropine is the treatment of choice for intoxications manifesting with significant muscarinic symptoms. Atropine I.V. 2-4 mg every 3-60 minutes should be repeated to control symptoms and then continued as needed for 1-2 days following acute ingestion. Epinephrine 0.1-1 mg S.C. may be useful for reversing severe cardiovascular or pulmonary sequelae.

**Pharmacodynamics/Kinetics**

**Onset:**

Ophthalmic instillation: Miosis: Within 10-30 minutes; Intraocular pressure reduction: 1 hour required

Ocusert® Pilo application: Miosis: 1.5-2 hours; Reduced intraocular pressure: Within 1.5-2 hours; miosis within 10-30 minutes

**Duration:**

Ophthalmic instillation: Miosis: 4-8 hours; Intraocular pressure reduction: 4-12 hours

Ocusert® Pilo application: Reduced intraocular pressure: ~1 week

**Formulations**

Gel, ophthalmic, as hydrochloride (Pilopine HS®): 4% (3.5 g)

Ocular therapeutic system (Ocusert® Pilo): Releases 20 or 40 mcg per hour for 1 week (8s)

Solution, ophthalmic, as hydrochloride (Adsorbocarpine®, Akarpine®, Isopto® Carpine, Pilagan®, Pilocar®, Piloptic®, Pilostat®): 0.25% (15 mL); 0.5% (15 mL, 30 mL); 1% (1 mL, 2 mL, 15 mL, 30 mL); 2% (1 mL, 2 mL, 15 mL, 30 mL); 3% (15 mL, 30 mL); 4% (1 mL, 2 mL, 15 mL, 30 mL); 5% (15 mL); 6% (15 mL, 30 mL); 8% (2 mL); 10% (15 mL)

Solution, ophthalmic, as nitrate (Pilagan®): 1% (15 mL); 2% (15 mL); 4% (15 mL)

Tablet: 5 mg

**Dosing**

**Adults:**

Ophthalmic:

Nitrate solution: Shake well before using; instill 1-2 drops 2-4 times/day.

Hydrochloride solution:

Instill 1-2 drops up to 6 times/day; adjust the concentration and frequency as required to control elevated intraocular pressure.

To counteract the mydriatic effects of sympathomimetic agents: Instill 1 drop of a 1% solution in the affected eye.

Gel: Instill 0.5" ribbon into lower conjunctival sac once daily at bedtime.

Ocular systems: Systems are labeled in terms of mean rate of release of pilocarpine over 7 days; begin with 20 mcg/hour at night and adjust based on response.

(Continued)

## Pilocarpine *(Continued)*

Oral: 5 mg 3 times/day, titration up to 10 mg 3 times/day may be considered for patients who have not responded adequately.

**Elderly:** Refer to adult dosing.

**Stability**

**Storage:** Refrigerate gel. Store solution at room temperature of 8°C to 30°C (46°F to 86°F) and protect from light.

**Monitoring Laboratory Tests** Intraocular pressure, fundoscopic exam, visual field testing

**Additional Nursing Issues**

**Physical Assessment:** Monitor for adverse effects and response to treatment. Monitor results of intraocular pressure testing and visual field testing on a periodic basis. Teach patient appropriate administration of ophthalmic solution. **Pregnancy risk factor C.** Note breast-feeding caution.

**Patient Information/Instruction:** Use as often as recommended. Ophthalmic: Wash hands before using. Sit or lie down. Open eye, look at ceiling, and instill prescribed amount of solution. Do not blink for 30 seconds, close eye and roll eye in all directions, and apply gentle pressure to inner corner of eye for 1-2 minutes. Do not let tip of applicator touch eye or contaminate tip of applicator. Temporary stinging or blurred vision may occur. You may experience altered dark adaptation; use caution when driving at night or in poorly lit environments. Report persistent pain, redness, burning, double vision, or severe headache. **Breast-feeding precautions:** Consult prescriber if breast-feeding.

**Geriatric Considerations:** Assure the patient or a caregiver can adequately administer ophthalmic medication dosage form.

**Additional Information**

Ocusert® 20 mcg is approximately equivalent to 0.5% or 1% drops.

Ocusert® 40 mcg is approximately equivalent to 2% or 3% drops.

Oral: Avoid administering with high-fat meal. Fat decreases the rate of absorption, maximum concentration and increases the time it takes to reach maximum concentration.

♦ **Pilocarpine** *see* Ophthalmic Agents, Glaucoma *on page 853*

## Pilocarpine and Epinephrine (pye loe KAR peen & ep i NEF rin)

**U.S. Brand Names** E-Pilo-x® Ophthalmic; $P_xE_x$® Ophthalmic

**Synonyms** Epinephrine and Pilocarpine

**Therapeutic Category** Ophthalmic Agent, Antiglaucoma; Ophthalmic Agent, Miotic

**Pregnancy Risk Factor** C

**Lactation** Excretion in breast milk unknown

**Use** Treatment of glaucoma; counter effect of cycloplegics

**Formulations** Solution, ophthalmic: Epinephrine bitartrate 1% and pilocarpine hydrochloride 1%, 2%, 3%, 4%, 6% (15 mL)

**Dosing**

**Adults:** Ophthalmic: Instill 1-2 drops up to 6 times/day

**Elderly:** Refer to adult dosing.

**Additional Nursing Issues**

**Physical Assessment:** See individual components listed in Related Information. **Pregnancy risk factor C** - benefits of use should outweigh possible risks. Note breast-feeding caution.

**Patient Information/Instruction:** See individual components listed in Related Information. **Pregnancy/breast-feeding precautions:** Inform prescriber if you are on intend to get pregnant. Consult prescriber if breast-feeding.

**Additional Information** The ophthalmic solution contains sulfites.

**Related Information**

Epinephrine *on page 424*

Pilocarpine *on previous page*

♦ **Pilogrin** *see* Ophthalmic Agents, Glaucoma *on page 853*

♦ **Pilogrin** *see* Pilocarpine *on previous page*

♦ **Pilopine HS® Ophthalmic** *see* Ophthalmic Agents, Glaucoma *on page 853*

♦ **Pilopine HS® Ophthalmic** *see* Pilocarpine *on previous page*

♦ **Piloptic® Ophthalmic** *see* Ophthalmic Agents, Glaucoma *on page 853*

♦ **Piloptic® Ophthalmic** *see* Pilocarpine *on previous page*

♦ **Pilostat® Ophthalmic** *see* Ophthalmic Agents, Glaucoma *on page 853*

♦ **Pilostat® Ophthalmic** *see* Pilocarpine *on previous page*

♦ **Pima®** *see* Potassium Iodide *on page 951*

♦ **Pimaricin** *see* Natamycin *on page 810*

## Pimozide (PI moe zide)

**U.S. Brand Names** Orap™

**Therapeutic Category** Antipsychotic Agent, Diphenylbutylperidine

**Pregnancy Risk Factor** C

**Lactation** Excretion in breast milk unknown

**Use** Suppression of severe motor and phonic tics in patients with Tourette's disorder; management of psychosis

**Mechanism of Action/Effect** A potent centrally acting dopamine receptor antagonist resulting in its characteristic neuroleptic effects

**Contraindications** Hypersensitivity to pimozide or any component; severe CNS depression; coma; history of dysrhythmia; prolonged Q-T syndrome; concurrent use of macrolide antibiotics (such as erythromycin, clarithromycin); simple tics other than Tourette's

**Warnings** May cause hypotension; use with caution in patients with autonomic instability. Moderately sedating, use with caution in disorders where CNS depression is a feature. Use with caution in Parkinson's disease. Use with caution in patients with hemodynamic instability; bone marrow suppression; predisposition to seizures; subcortical brain damage; or severe cardiac, hepatic, renal, or respiratory disease. Neuroleptics may cause swallowing difficulty. Use with caution in breast cancer or other prolactin-dependent tumors (may elevate prolactin levels). May alter temperature regulation or mask toxicity of other drugs due to antiemetic effects. May alter cardiac conduction - life-threatening arrhythmias have occurred with therapeutic doses of phenothiazines. May cause orthostatic hypotension.

May cause anticholinergic effects (eg, confusion, agitation, constipation, dry mouth, blurred vision, urinary retention); therefore, use with caution in patients with decreased gastrointestinal motility, urinary retention, BPH, xerostomia, or visual problems. Conditions which also may be exacerbated by cholinergic blockade include narrow-angle glaucoma (screening is recommended) and worsening of myasthenia gravis. Relative to neuroleptics, pimozide has a moderate potency of cholinergic blockade.

May cause extrapyramidal reactions including pseudoparkinsonism, acute dystonic reactions, akathisia, and tardive dyskinesia (risk of these reactions is high relative to other neuroleptics). May be associated with neuroleptic malignant syndrome (NMS) or pigmentary retinopathy.

Because treatment with pimozide exposes the patient to serious risks, a decision to use pimozide chronically in Tourette's disorder is one that deserves full consideration by the patient (or patient's family) and prescriber. If the goal of treatment is symptomatic improvement of Tourette's, the patient's view of the need for treatment and assessment of response are critical in evaluating the impact of therapy and weighing its benefits against the risks.

Pregnancy factor C.

**Drug Interactions**

**Cytochrome P-450 Effect:** CYP3A3/4 enzyme substrate

**Increased Effect/Toxicity:** Increased effect/toxicity of alfentanil, CNS depressants, guanabenz (increased sedation), and MAO inhibitors.

**Effects on Lab Values** ↑ prolactin (S)

**Adverse Reactions**

>10%:

- Central nervous system: Akathisia, akinesia, extrapyramidal effects (parkinsonian), drowsiness
- Dermatologic: Rash
- Endocrine & metabolic: Edema of the breasts, unusual secretion of milk
- Gastrointestinal: Constipation, dry mouth
- Ocular: Blurred vision

1% to 10%:

- Cardiovascular: Facial edema
- Central nervous system: Tardive dyskinesia, mental depression, extrapyramidal effects (dystonic)
- Endocrine & metabolic: Decreased sexual ability
- Gastrointestinal: Diarrhea, anorexia

<1% (Limited to important or life-threatening symptoms): Ventricular arrhythmias, tachycardia, orthostatic hypotension, neuroleptic malignant syndrome (NMS), blood dyscrasias, jaundice

**Overdose/Toxicology** Symptoms of overdose include hypotension, respiratory depression, EKG abnormalities, extrapyramidal symptoms. Treatment is supportive and symptomatic.

**Pharmacodynamics/Kinetics**

**Protein Binding:** 99%

**Half-life Elimination:** 50 hours

**Time to Peak:** Within 6-8 hours

**Metabolism:** Liver

**Excretion:** Urine

**Formulations** Tablet: 2 mg

**Dosing**

**Adults:** Oral: Initial: 1-2 mg/day, then increase dosage as needed every other day; range is usually 7-16 mg/day; maximum: 20 mg/day or 0.3 mg/kg/day should not be exceeded.

**Elderly:** Recommend initial dose of 1 mg/day; periodically attempt gradual reduction of dose to determine if tic persists; follow up for 1-2 weeks before concluding the tic is a persistent disease phenomenon and not a manifestation of drug withdrawal. **Note:** Recommend obtaining a baseline EKG and done periodically, especially with dose increases or addition of drugs which may interact.

**Hepatic Impairment:** Reduction of dose is necessary in patients with liver disease.

**Monitoring Laboratory Tests** Baseline EKG and periodically during therapy, ophthalmic exam

(Continued)

## Pimozide *(Continued)*

**Additional Nursing Issues**

**Physical Assessment:** Assess other medications patient is taking for effectiveness and interactions (see Drug Interactions). See Contraindications and Warnings/Precautions for cautious use and assess patient/caregiver knowledge of rationale for therapy and risks involved. Has potential for psychological or physiological dependence, abuse, and tolerance. Review ophthalmic exam and monitor laboratory tests (see above), therapeutic response (mental status, mood, affect), and adverse reactions at beginning of therapy and periodically with long-term use (endocrine changes, extrapyramidal effects, neuroleptic malignant syndrome - see Adverse Reactions and Overdose). Initiate at lower doses (see Dosing) and decrease dosage slowly when discontinuing. Assess knowledge/teach patient appropriate use, interventions to reduce side effects, and adverse symptoms to report (see below). **Pregnancy risk factor C** - benefits of use should outweigh possible risks. Note breast-feeding caution.

**Patient Information/Instruction:** Use exactly as directed (do not increase dose or frequency); may cause physical and/or psychological dependence. It may take 2-3 weeks to achieve desired results; do not discontinue without consulting prescriber. Avoid excess alcohol or caffeine and other prescription or OTC medications not approved by prescriber. Maintain adequate hydration (2-3 L/day of fluids unless instructed to restrict fluid intake). You may experience excess drowsiness, restlessness, dizziness, or blurred vision (use caution driving or when engaging in tasks requiring alertness until response to drug is known); or constipation, dry mouth, anorexia (increased exercise, fluids, or dietary fruit and fiber may help). Report persistent CNS effects (eg, trembling fingers, altered gait or balance, excessive sedation, seizures, unusual muscle or facial movements, anxiety, abnormal thoughts, confusion, personality changes); unresolved constipation or gastrointestinal effects; breast swelling (male and female) or decreased sexual ability; vision changes; difficulty breathing; unusual cough or flu-like symptoms; or worsening of condition. **Pregnancy/breast-feeding precautions:** Inform prescriber if you are or intend to be pregnant. Consult prescriber if breast-feeding.

**Geriatric Considerations:** (See Warnings/Precautions, Adverse Reactions, and Overdose/Toxicology.) Elderly patients have an increased risk of adverse response to side effects or adverse reactions to antipsychotics. These can include but are not limited to the following.

Anticholinergic effects: CNS toxicity with confusion, memory loss, psychotic behavior, and agitation.

Extrapyramidal effects (EPS): Parkinson's syndrome and akathisia may occur as often as 50% in patients >60 years of age. Tardive dyskinesia (motor restlessness) may be 40% in elderly; may be related to duration and total accumulated dose over time; may be somewhat reversible if diagnosed early enough.

Orthostatic hypotension: Increased risk for falls.

Sedation: In nonpsychotic patients, may result in feelings of depersonalization, derealization, and dysphoria.

Cardiac toxicity: Cardiac arrhythmias have occurred with therapeutic doses of antipsychotics.

Malignant neuroleptic syndrome: Development of hyperthermia, muscular rigidity, autonomic instability, and altered mental status.

Many elderly patients receive antipsychotic medications for inappropriate nonpsychotic behavior. Before initiating antipsychotic medication, all possible reversible causes should be investigated. Stress may cause acute "confusion" or worsening of baseline nonpsychotic behaviors; any changes in disease state (in any organ) may result in behavioral changes. Common acute changes in behavior may be due also to increases in drug dose addition, or addition of a new drug to the regimen; fluid/electrolyte alterations; infections; or changes in the environment.

Meta-analysis of controlled trials of antipsychotic (phenothiazines, butyrophenones) use with agitated, demented, elderly patients has concluded that the use of neuroleptics results in a response rate of 18%. Clearly, neuroleptic therapy for behavior control should be limited, with frequent attempts to withdraw the agent for behavior control. When use is indicated, initial doses should be lower to start and monitored closely.

**Related Information**

Antipsychotic Agents Comparison *on page 1371*

## Pindolol (PIN doe lole)

**U.S. Brand Names** Visken®

**Therapeutic Category** Beta Blocker (with Intrinsic Sympathomimetic Activity)

**Pregnancy Risk Factor** B/D (2nd and 3rd trimesters)

**Lactation** Enters breast milk/use caution - see Breast-feeding Issues

**Use** Management of hypertension

**Unlabeled use:** Ventricular arrhythmias/tachycardia, antipsychotic-induced akathisia, situational anxiety; aggressive behavior associated with dementia; adjunct to SSRI antidepressant therapy

**Mechanism of Action/Effect** Blocks both beta$_1$- and beta$_2$-receptors and has mild intrinsic sympathomimetic activity; pindolol has negative inotropic and chronotropic effects and can significantly slow A-V nodal conduction

**Contraindications** Hypersensitivity to pindolol or any component; uncompensated congestive heart failure; cardiogenic shock; bradycardia or heart block; pregnancy (2nd and 3rd trimesters)

**Warnings** Use with caution in patients with inadequate myocardial function, undergoing anesthesia, bronchospastic disease, diabetes mellitus, hyperthyroidism, or impaired hepatic function. Use caution in patients with asthma, COPD. Abrupt withdrawal of the drug should be avoided (may exacerbate symptoms; discontinue over 1-2 weeks). Beta-blockers may impair glucose tolerance, potentiate hypoglycemia, and/or mask signs or symptoms of hypoglycemia in a diabetic patient.

**Drug Interactions**

**Cytochrome P-450 Effect:** CYP2D6 enzyme substrate

**Decreased Effect:** Decreased effect of beta-blockers with aluminum salts, barbiturates, calcium salts, cholestyramine, colestipol, NSAIDs, penicillins (ampicillin), rifampin, salicylates, and sulfinpyrazone due to decreased bioavailability and plasma levels. Beta-blockers may decrease the effect of sulfonylureas. Beta-blockers may affect the action or levels of ethanol, disopyramide, nondepolarizing muscle relaxants, and theophylline although the effects are difficult to predict.

**Increased Effect/Toxicity:** Increased effect with diuretics, other antihypertensives.

**Adverse Reactions**

>10%:

Central nervous system: Anxiety, dizziness, insomnia, fatigue
Endocrine & metabolic: Decreased sexual ability
Neuromuscular & skeletal: Arthralgia, weakness, back pain

1% to 10%:

Cardiovascular: Congestive heart failure, arrhythmia, reduced peripheral circulation
Central nervous system: Hallucinations, nightmares, vivid dreams
Dermatologic: Rash, itching
Gastrointestinal: Diarrhea, nausea, vomiting, stomach discomfort
Neuromuscular & skeletal: Numbness of extremities
Respiratory: Dyspnea

<1% (Limited to important or life-threatening symptoms): Bradycardia, chest pain, thrombocytopenia

**Overdose/Toxicology** Symptoms of intoxication include cardiac disturbances, CNS toxicity, bronchospasm, hypoglycemia, and hyperkalemia. The most common cardiac symptoms include hypotension and bradycardia. Atrioventricular block, intraventricular conduction disturbances, cardiogenic shock, and asystole may occur with severe overdose, especially with membrane-depressant drugs (eg, propranolol). CNS effects include convulsions, and coma. Respiratory arrest is commonly seen with propranolol and other membrane-depressant and lipid-soluble drugs. Treatment includes symptomatic treatment of seizures, hypotension, hyperkalemia, and hypoglycemia.

**Pharmacodynamics/Kinetics**

**Protein Binding:** 50%

**Half-life Elimination:** 2.5-4 hours; increased with renal insufficiency, age, and cirrhosis

**Time to Peak:** Within 1-2 hours

**Metabolism:** Liver

**Excretion:** Urine

**Duration:** ~12 hours

**Formulations** Tablet: 5 mg, 10 mg

**Dosing**

**Adults:** Oral: Initial: 5 mg twice daily, increase as necessary by 10 mg/day every 3-4 weeks; maximum daily dose: 60 mg.

**Elderly:** Oral: Initial: 5 mg once daily; increase as necessary by 5 mg/day every 3-4 weeks.

**Renal Impairment:** Reduction is necessary in severe impairment.

**Hepatic Impairment:** Reduction is necessary in severely impaired.

**Additional Nursing Issues**

**Physical Assessment:** Carefully assess all other medications patient may be taking for effectiveness/interaction (see Drug Interactions). Monitor cardiac, respiratory, hemodynamic status (including peripheral pulses), and CNS status prior to starting therapy, during first doses of therapy, when titrating dosage, and regularly thereafter. Monitor diabetic patients for serum glucose levels (may alter glucose tolerance, potentiate hypoglycemia, and mask symptoms of hypoglycemia). **Pregnancy risk factor B/D.** Note breast-feeding caution.

**Patient Information/Instruction:** Take as directed; do not discontinue without consulting prescriber. Avoid alcohol and do not take with antacids. You may experience nervousness, dizziness, or fatigue; use caution when driving or engaging in hazardous activities until response to drug is known. Frequent small meals may reduce incidence of nausea; adequate fluids and fiber intake may reduce constipation. Diabetic patients should monitor serum glucose regularly. Report chest pain, rapid heartbeat or palpitations, difficulty breathing, sudden increase in weight, swelling in ankles or hands, persistent dizziness or fatigue, trembling, increased anxiety, or sleeplessness. **Pregnancy/breast-feeding precautions:** Consult prescriber if pregnant or breast-feeding.

**Geriatric Considerations:** Due to alterations in the beta-adrenergic autonomic nervous system, beta-adrenergic blockade may result in less hemodynamic response than seen in younger adults. Studies indicate that despite decreased sensitivity to the chronotropic effects of beta blockade with age, there appears to be an increased myocardial sensitivity to the negative inotropic effect during stress (eg, exercise).

(Continued)

## Pindolol *(Continued)*

Controlled trials have shown the overall response rate for propranolol to be only 20% to 50% in elderly populations. Therefore, all beta-adrenergic blocking drugs may result in a decreased response as compared to younger adults (see Pharmacodynamics and Pharmacokinetics).

**Breast-feeding Issues:** There is not published experience with pindolol; however, other beta-blockers like metoprolol are considered compatible by the American Academy of Pediatrics. Monitor the infant for signs of beta-blockade (hypotension, bradycardia, etc) with long-term use.

**Related Information**

Beta-Blockers Comparison *on page 1376*

- **Pin-Rid®** *see page 1294*
- **Pin-X®** *see page 1294*
- **PIO** *see* Pemoline *on page 892*
- **Pipecuronium** *see page 1248*

## Piperacillin (pi PER a sil in)

**U.S. Brand Names** Pipracil®

**Therapeutic Category** Antibiotic, Penicillin

**Pregnancy Risk Factor** B

**Lactation** Enters breast milk (small amounts - other penicillins are compatible with breast-feeding)

**Use** Treatment of susceptible infections such as septicemia, acute and chronic respiratory tract infections, skin and soft tissue infections, and urinary tract infections due to susceptible strains of *Pseudomonas, Proteus,* and *Escherichia coli* and *Enterobacter*, normally used with other antibiotics (eg, aminoglycosides)

**Mechanism of Action/Effect** Inhibits bacterial cell wall synthesis by binding to one or more of the penicillin binding proteins (PBPs); which in turn inhibits the final transpeptidation step of peptidoglycan synthesis in bacterial cell walls, thus inhibiting cell wall biosynthesis. Bacteria eventually lyse due to ongoing activity of cell wall autolytic enzymes (autolysins and murein hydrolases) while cell wall assembly is arrested.

**Contraindications** Hypersensitivity to piperacillin, any component, penicillins, cephalosporins, or imipenem; patients with a history of beta-lactam allergy

**Warnings** Dosage modification is required in patients with impaired renal function. History of seizure activity.

**Drug Interactions**

**Decreased Effect:** Tetracyclines may decrease penicillin effectiveness. Efficacy of oral contraceptives may be reduced when taken with piperacillin. High concentrations of piperacillin may cause physical inactivation of aminoglycosides and lead to potential toxicity in patients with mild-moderate renal dysfunction.

**Increased Effect/Toxicity:** Probenecid may increase penicillin levels. Neuromuscular blockers may increase duration of blockade.

**Effects on Lab Values** May interfere with urinary glucose tests using cupric sulfate (Benedict's solution, Clinitest®); may inactivate aminoglycosides *in vitro*; false-positive urinary and serum proteins, positive Coombs' test [direct]

**Adverse Reactions**

>10%:

Central nervous system: Headache

Gastrointestinal: Nausea (mild), vomiting

Miscellaneous: Oral candidiasis, vaginal candidiasis

1% to 10%:

Dermatologic: Urticaria, exfoliative dermatitis

Miscellaneous: Allergic reactions, specifically anaphylaxis; serum sickness-like reactions

<1% (Limited to important or life-threatening symptoms): Seizures, leukopenia, neutropenia, thrombocytopenia, jaundice, hepatotoxicity, interstitial nephritis, *Clostridium difficile* colitis

**Overdose/Toxicology** Symptoms of penicillin overdose include neuromuscular hypersensitivity (eg, agitation, hallucinations, asterixis, encephalopathy, confusion, and seizures). Electrolyte imbalance may occur if the preparation contains potassium or sodium salts, especially in renal failure. Hemodialysis may be helpful to aid in removal of the drug from blood; otherwise, treatment is supportive or symptom directed.

**Pharmacodynamics/Kinetics**

**Distribution:** Crosses the placenta

**Half-life Elimination:** Dose-dependent; prolonged with moderately severe renal or hepatic impairment: 36-80 minutes

**Time to Peak:** I.M.: Within 30-50 minutes

**Excretion:** Urine and feces

**Formulations** Powder for injection, as sodium: 2 g, 3 g, 4 g, 40 g

**Dosing**

**Adults:**

I.M.: 2-3 g/dose every 6-12 hours; maximum: 24 g/24 hours

I.V.: 3-4 g/dose every 4-6 hours; maximum: 24 g/24 hours

**Elderly:** Adjust dose for renal impairment:

I.M.: 1-2 g every 8-12 hours

I.V.: 2-4 g every 6-8 hours

**Renal Impairment:**

$Cl_{cr}$ 10-50 mL/minute: Administer every 6-8 hours.

$Cl_{cr}$ <10 mL/minute: Administer every 8 hours.

Moderately dialyzable (20% to 50%)

Continuous arteriovenous or venovenous emofiltration (CAVH): Dose as for $Cl_{cr}$ 10-50 mL/minute.

**Administration**

**I.M.:** Do not administer more than 2 g per injection site.

**I.V.:** Administer around-the-clock to promote less variation in peak and trough serum levels. Give at least 1 hour apart from aminoglycosides. Rapid administration can lead to seizures. Administer direct I.V. over 3-5 minutes. Intermittently infusion over 30 minutes.

**Stability**

**Storage:** Reconstituted solution is stable (I.V. infusion) in NS or $D_5W$ for 24 hours at room temperature, 7 days when refrigerated, or 4 weeks when frozen. After freezing, thawed solution is stable for 24 hours at room temperature or 48 hours when refrigerated. 40 g bulk vial should **not** be frozen after reconstitution.

**Compatibility:** Piperacillin is incompatible with aminoglycosides.

**Monitoring Laboratory Tests** Perform culture and sensitivity before administering first dose.

**Additional Nursing Issues**

**Physical Assessment:** Assess patient history for allergy. Monitor for hypersensitivity reaction and opportunistic infection. Use serum glucose testing for diabetic patient (see Effects on Lab Values).

**Patient Information/Instruction:** This medication will be administered I.V. or I.M. Maintain adequate hydration (2-3 L/day of fluids unless instructed to restrict fluid intake). If being treated for sexually transmitted disease, partner will also need to be treated. Small frequent meals, frequent mouth care, sucking lozenges, or chewing gum may reduce nausea or dry mouth. Important to maintain good oral and vaginal hygiene to reduce incidence of opportunistic infection. Diabetics should use serum glucose testing while on this medication. If diabetic, drug may cause false tests with Clinitest® urine glucose monitoring; use of glucose oxidase methods (Clinistix®) or serum glucose monitoring is preferable. This drug may interfere with oral contraceptives; an alternate form of birth control should be used. Report persistent diarrhea, fever, chills, unhealed sores, bloody urine or stool, muscle pain, mouth sores, or difficulty breathing.

**Geriatric Considerations:** Antipseudomonal penicillins should not be used alone and are often combined with an aminoglycoside as empiric therapy for lower respiratory infection and sepsis in which gram-negative (including *Pseudomonas*) and/or anaerobes are of a high probability. Because of piperacillin's lower sodium content, it is preferred over ticarcillin in patients with a history of heart failure and/or renal or hepatic disease. Adjust dose for renal function.

**Additional Information**

Sodium content of 1 g: 1.85 mEq

pH: 5.5-7.5

## Piperacillin and Tazobactam Sodium

(pi PER a sil in & ta zoe BAK tam SOW dee um)

**U.S. Brand Names** Zosyn™

**Synonyms** Tazobactam and Piperacillin

**Therapeutic Category** Antibiotic, Penicillin

**Pregnancy Risk Factor** B

**Lactation** Enters breast milk/use caution (other penicillins are compatible)

**Use** Treatment of infections of lower respiratory tract, urinary tract, skin and skin structures, gynecologic, bone and joint infections, and septicemia caused by susceptible organisms. Tazobactam expands activity of piperacillin to include beta-lactamase producing strains of *S. aureus*, *H. influenzae*, Enterobacteriaceae, *Pseudomonas*, *Klebsiella*, *Citrobacter*, *Serratia*, *Bacteroides*, and other gram-negative anaerobes. Application to nosocomial infections may be limited by restricted activity against gram-negative organisms producing Class I beta-lactamases and inactivity against methicillin-resistant *Staphylococcus aureus*.

**Mechanism of Action/Effect** Piperacillin interferes with bacterial cell wall synthesis during active multiplication, causing cell wall death and resultant bactericidal activity against susceptible bacteria; tazobactam prevents degradation of piperacillin by binding to the active side on beta-lactamase; tazobactam inhibits many beta-lactamases, including staphylococcal penicillinase and Richmond and Sykes Types II, III, IV, and V, including extended spectrum enzymes; it has only limited activity against Class I beta-lactamases other than Class 1C

**Contraindications** Hypersensitivity to penicillins, any component, beta-lactamase inhibitors, cephalosporins, or imipenem

**Warnings** Due to sodium load and to the adverse effects of high serum concentrations of penicillins, dosage modification is required in patients with impaired or underdeveloped renal function. Use with caution in patients with seizures or in patients with history of beta-lactam allergy.

**Drug Interactions**

**Decreased Effect:** Tetracyclines may decrease penicillin effectiveness. Efficacy of oral contraceptives may be reduced when taken with piperacillin and tazobactam sodium. Aminoglycosides may cause physical inactivation of aminoglycosides in the presence of high concentrations of piperacillin and potential toxicity in patients with mild-moderate renal dysfunction.

**Increased Effect/Toxicity:** Probenecid may increase penicillin levels. Neuromuscular blockers may increase duration of blockade.

(Continued)

## Piperacillin and Tazobactam Sodium *(Continued)*

**Effects on Lab Values** Positive Coombs' [direct] test 3.8%, ALT, AST, bilirubin, and LDH

**Adverse Reactions**

>10%:

Central nervous system: Headache

Gastrointestinal: Nausea (mild), vomiting

Miscellaneous: Oral candidiasis, vaginal candidiasis

1% to 10%:

Dermatologic: Urticaria, exfoliative dermatitis

Miscellaneous: Allergic reactions, specifically anaphylaxis; serum sickness-like reactions

<1% (Limited to important or life-threatening symptoms): Seizures, leukopenia, neutropenia, thrombocytopenia, jaundice, hepatotoxicity, interstitial nephritis, *Clostridium difficile* colitis; several laboratory abnormalities have rarely been associated with piperacillin/tazobactam including reversible eosinophilia, and neutropenia (associated most often with prolonged therapy), positive direct Coombs' test, prolonged PT and PTT, transient elevations of LFT, increases in creatinine

**Overdose/Toxicology** Symptoms of penicillin overdose include neuromuscular hypersensitivity (eg, agitation, hallucinations, asterixis, encephalopathy, confusion, and seizures). Electrolyte imbalance may occur if the preparation contains potassium or sodium salts, especially in renal dysfunction. Hemodialysis may be helpful to aid in removal of the drug from blood; otherwise, treatment is supportive or symptom directed.

**Pharmacodynamics/Kinetics**

**Protein Binding:** Piperacillin: ~26% to 33%; Tazobactam: 31% to 32%

**Distribution:** Distributes well into lungs, intestinal mucosa, skin, muscle, uterus, ovary, prostate, gallbladder, and bile; penetration into CSF is low in subject with noninflamed meninges

**Half-life Elimination:** Piperacillin: 1 hour; Piperacillin (desethyl) metabolite: 1-1.5 hours; Tazobactam: 0.7-0.9 hour

**Metabolism:** Piperacillin: 6% to 9%; Tazobactam: ~26%

**Excretion:** Excretion of both piperacillin and tazobactam are directly proportional to renal function.

Piperacillin: 50% to 70% eliminated unchanged in urine, 10% to 20% excreted in bile

Tazobactam: Found in urine at 24 hours, with 26% as the inactive metabolite

**Formulations** Injection: Piperacillin sodium 2 g and tazobactam sodium 0.25 g; piperacillin sodium 3 g and tazobactam sodium 0.375 g; piperacillin sodium 4 g and tazobactam sodium 0.5 g (vials at an 8:1 ratio of piperacillin sodium to tazobactam sodium)

**Dosing**

**Adults:**

Severe infections: I.V.: Piperacillin/tazobactam 4/0.5 g every 8 hours or 3/0.375 g every 6 hours

Moderate infections: I.M.: Piperacillin/tazobactam 2/0.25 g every 6-8 hours; treatment should be continued for ≥7-10 days depending on severity of disease.

**Renal Impairment:**

$Cl_{cr}$ >40 mL/minute: No change

$Cl_{cr}$ 20-40 mL/minute: Administer 2/0.25 g every 6 hours.

$Cl_{cr}$ <20 mL/minute: Administer 2/0.25 g every 8 hours.

Hemodialysis: Administer 2/0.25 g every 8 hours with an additional dose of 0.75 g after each dialysis.

Hemodialysis removes 30% to 40% of piperacillin and tazobactam. Peritoneal dialysis removes 11% to 21% of tazobactam and 6% of piperacillin.

Continuous arteriovenous or venovenous hemofiltration (CAVH): Dose as for $Cl_{cr}$ 10-50 mL/minute.

**Hepatic Impairment:** Hepatic impairment does not affect the kinetics of piperacillin or tazobactam significantly.

**Administration**

**I.V.:** Administer by I.V. infusion over 30 minutes. Discontinue primary infusion, if possible, during infusion and administer aminoglycosides separately from Zosyn™.

**Stability**

**Storage:** Store at controlled room temperature. After reconstitution, solution is stable in NS or $D_5W$ for 24 hours at room temperature and 7 days when refrigerated.

**Reconstitution:** Use single dose vials immediately after reconstitution (discard unused portions after 24 hours at room temperature and 48 hours if refrigerated). Reconstitute with 5 mL of diluent per 1 g of piperacillin and then further dilute. Compatible diluents include NS, SW, dextran 6%, $D_5W$, $D_5W$ with potassium chloride 40 mEq, bacteriostatic saline and water.

**Compatibility:** Incompatible with lactated Ringer's solution. Temporarily discontinue other solutions infusing at the same site to avoid compatibility problems.

**Monitoring Laboratory Tests** LFTs, creatinine, BUN, CBC with differential, serum electrolytes, urinalysis, PT, PTT; perform culture and sensitivity before administering first dose.

**Additional Nursing Issues**

**Physical Assessment:** Assess patient history for allergy. Monitor for hypersensitivity reaction and opportunistic infection. Use serum glucose testing for diabetic patient. Note breast-feeding caution.

**Patient Information/Instruction:** This medication will be administered I.V. or I.M. Maintain adequate hydration (2-3 L/day of fluids unless instructed to restrict fluid intake). Small frequent meals, frequent mouth care, sucking lozenges, or chewing gum may reduce nausea or dry mouth. Important to maintain good oral and vaginal hygiene to reduce incidence of opportunistic infection. Diabetics should use serum glucose testing while receiving this medication. If diabetic, drug may cause false tests with Clinitest® urine glucose monitoring; use of glucose oxidase methods (Clinistix®) or serum glucose monitoring is preferable. This drug may interfere with oral contraceptives; an alternate form of birth control should be used. Report persistent diarrhea, fever, chills, unhealed sores, bloody urine or stool, muscle pain, mouth sores, or difficulty breathing, or skin rash. **Breast-feeding precautions:** Consult prescriber if breast-feeding.

**Geriatric Considerations:** Has not been studied exclusively in the elderly.

**Breast-feeding Issues:** Use by the breast-feeding mother may result in bowel flora change, or antibiotic effect on the infant. Use caution.

**Additional Information** Sodium content of 1 g: 2.35 mEq

**Related Information**

Piperacillin *on page 936*

- **Piperazine Estrone Sulfate** *see* Estropipate *on page 452*
- **Pipracil®** *see* Piperacillin *on page 936*

## Pirbuterol (peer BYOO ter ole)

**U.S. Brand Names** Maxair™ Autohaler™; Maxair™ Inhalation Aerosol

**Therapeutic Category** $Beta_2$ Agonist

**Pregnancy Risk Factor** C

**Lactation** Excretion in breast milk unknown

**Use** Prevention and treatment of reversible bronchospasm including asthma

**Mechanism of Action/Effect** Pirbuterol is a $beta_2$-adrenergic agonist with a similar structure to albuterol, specifically a pyridine ring has been substituted for the benzene ring in albuterol. The increased $beta_2$ selectivity of pirbuterol results from the substitution of a tertiary butyl group on the nitrogen of the side chain, which additionally imparts resistance of pirbuterol to degradation by monoamine oxidase and provides a lengthened duration of action in comparison to the less selective previous beta-agonist agents.

**Contraindications** Hypersensitivity to pirbuterol or albuterol

**Warnings** Excessive use may result in tolerance. Use with caution in patients with hyperthyroidism, diabetes mellitus. Cardiovascular disorders including coronary insufficiency or hypertension or sensitivity to sympathomimetic amines. Pregnancy factor C.

**Drug Interactions**

**Decreased Effect:** Decreased effect with beta-blockers.

**Increased Effect/Toxicity:** Increased toxicity with other beta agonists, MAO inhibitors, tricyclic antidepressants.

**Adverse Reactions**

>10%:

Central nervous system: Nervousness, restlessness

Neuromuscular & skeletal: Trembling

1% to 10%:

Cardiovascular: Tachycardia, pounding heartbeat

Central nervous system: Headache, dizziness, lightheadedness

Gastrointestinal: Taste changes, vomiting, nausea

<1% (Limited to important or life-threatening symptoms): Hypertension, arrhythmias, chest pain, insomnia, paradoxical bronchospasm

**Overdose/Toxicology** Symptoms of overdose include hypertension, tachycardia, angina, and hypokalemia. In cases of overdose, supportive therapy should be instituted, and prudent use of a cardioselective beta-adrenergic blocker (eg, atenolol or metoprolol) should be considered, keeping in mind the potential for induction of bronchoconstriction in an asthmatic individual. Dialysis has not been shown to be of value in the treatment of overdose with pirbuterol.

**Pharmacodynamics/Kinetics**

**Half-life Elimination:** 2-3 hours

**Metabolism:** Liver

**Excretion:** Kidney

**Onset:** Peak therapeutic effect: Inhalation: 0.5-1 hour

**Formulations**

Aerosol, oral, as acetate: 0.2 mg per actuation (25.6 g (300 inhalations))

Autohaler™: 0.2 mg per actuation (2.8 g (80 inhalations); 14 g (400 inhalations))

**Dosing**

**Adults:** Inhalation: 2 inhalations every 4-6 hours for prevention; 2 inhalations at an interval of at least 1-3 minutes, followed by a third inhalation in treatment of bronchospasm, not to exceed 12 inhalations/day

**Elderly:** Refer to adult dosing.

**Administration**

**Inhalation:** Shake inhaler well before use.

**Additional Nursing Issues**

**Physical Assessment:** Assess effectiveness and interactions of other medications (see Drug Interactions above). See Contraindications and Warnings/Precautions for use cautions. Monitor effectiveness of therapy (relief of airway obstruction) and adverse reactions (eg, cardiac and CNS changes - see Adverse Reactions) at beginning of therapy and periodically with long-term use. For inpatient care, monitor vital signs and lung sounds prior to and periodically during therapy. Assess knowledge/

(Continued)

## Pirbuterol *(Continued)*

teach patient appropriate use, interventions to reduce side effects, and adverse symptoms to report. **Pregnancy risk factor C** - benefits of use should outweigh possible risks. Note breast-feeding caution.

**Patient Information/Instruction:** Use exactly as directed (see Administration below). Do not use more often than recommended. Maintain adequate hydration (2-3 L/day of fluids unless instructed to restrict fluid intake). You may experience nervousness, dizziness, or fatigue (use caution when driving or engaging in tasks requiring alertness until response to drug is known); or dry mouth, stomach upset (frequent small meals, frequent mouth care, chewing gum, or sucking hard candy may help). Report unresolved GI upset; dizziness or fatigue; vision changes; chest pain, rapid heartbeat, or palpitations; nervousness or insomnia; muscle cramping or tremor; or unusual cough. **Pregnancy/breast-feeding precautions:** Inform prescriber if you are or intend to be pregnant. Consult prescriber if breast-feeding.

**Administration:** Self-administered inhalation: Store canister upside down; do not freeze. Shake canister before using. Sit when using medication. Close eyes when administering pirbuterol to avoid spray getting into eyes. Exhale slowly and completely through nose; inhale deeply through mouth while administering aerosol. Hold breath for 1-3 seconds after inhalation. Wait at least 1 full minute between inhalations. Wash mouthpiece between use. If more than one inhalation medication is used, use bronchodilator first and wait 5 minutes between medications.

**Geriatric Considerations:** Elderly patients may find it beneficial to utilize a spacer device when using a metered dose inhaler. Difficulty in using the inhaler often limits its effectiveness. The Autohaler™ may be easier for the elderly to use.

**Related Information**

Inhalant (Asthma, Bronchospasm) Agents *on page 1388*

♦ **Piroxan** *see* Piroxicam *on this page*

♦ **Piroxen** *see* Piroxicam *on this page*

## Piroxicam (peer OKS i kam)

**U.S. Brand Names** Feldene®

**Therapeutic Category** Nonsteroidal Anti-Inflammatory Agent (NSAID)

**Pregnancy Risk Factor** B/D (3rd trimester)

**Lactation** Enters breast milk (small amounts)/compatible

**Use** Symptomatic treatment of acute and chronic rheumatoid arthritis, osteoarthritis

**Mechanism of Action/Effect** Inhibits prostaglandin synthesis, acts on the hypothalamus heat-regulating center to reduce fever, blocks prostaglandin synthetase action which prevents formation of the platelet-aggregating substance thromboxane $A_2$; decreases pain receptor sensitivity. Other proposed mechanisms of action for salicylate anti-inflammatory action are lysosomal stabilization, kinin and leukotriene production, alteration of chemotactic factors, and inhibition of neutrophil activation. This latter mechanism may be the most significant pharmacologic action to reduce inflammation.

**Contraindications** Hypersensitivity to piroxicam, any component, aspirin or other nonsteroidal anti-inflammatory drugs (NSAIDs); active GI bleeding; patients who have experienced bronchospasm, nasal polyps, and angioedema caused by aspirin or other NSAIDs; pregnancy (3rd trimester)

**Warnings** Use with caution in patients with impaired cardiac function, hypertension, impaired renal function, GI disease (bleeding or ulcers), and patients receiving anticoagulants. Elderly have increased risk for adverse reactions to NSAIDs.

**Drug Interactions**

**Cytochrome P-450 Effect:** CYP2C9 and 2C18 enzyme substrate

**Decreased Effect:** Decreased effect of diuretics, beta-blockers. Decreased effect with aspirin, antacids, and cholestyramine.

**Increased Effect/Toxicity:** Increased effect/toxicity of lithium, warfarin, and methotrexate (controversial).

**Food Interactions** Onset of effect may be delayed if piroxicam is taken with food.

**Effects on Lab Values** ↑ chloride (S), sodium (S), bleeding time

**Adverse Reactions**

1% to 10%:

Cardiovascular: Edema

Central nervous system: Headache, dizziness, somnolence, vertigo

Dermatologic: Pruritus, rash

Gastrointestinal: Stomatitis, anorexia, epigastric distress, nausea, constipation, abdominal discomfort, flatulence, diarrhea, indigestion

Hematologic: Decreases in hemoglobin and hematocrit, anemia, leukopenia, eosinophilia

Renal: Elevated BUN, elevated serum creatinine, Polyuria, acute renal failure

Otic: Tinnitus

<1% (Limited to important or life-threatening symptoms): Congestive heart failure, hypertension, chest pain, erythema multiforme, toxic epidermal necrolysis, Stevens-Johnson syndrome, hypoglycemia, hyperglycemia, aplastic anemia, bone marrow depression, thrombocytopenia, hemolytic anemia, abnormal LFTs, jaundice, hepatitis, bronchospasm, dyspnea

**Overdose/Toxicology** Symptoms of overdose include nausea, epigastric distress, CNS depression, leukocytosis, and renal failure. Management of nonsteroidal anti-inflammatory (NSAID) intoxication is supportive and symptomatic. Multiple doses of activated charcoal may interrupt enterohepatic recycling of some NSAIDs.

**Pharmacodynamics/Kinetics**

**Protein Binding:** 99%

**Half-life Elimination:** 45-50 hours

**Metabolism:** Liver

**Excretion:** As unchanged drug (5%) and metabolites primarily in urine and to a small degree in feces

**Onset:** Onset of analgesia: Oral: Within 1 hour; Peak effect: 3-5 hours

**Formulations** Capsule: 10 mg, 20 mg

**Dosing**

**Adults:** Oral: 10-20 mg/day once daily; although associated with increase in GI adverse effects, doses >20 mg/day have been used (ie, 30-40 mg/day)

**Elderly:** Refer to adult dosing. **Note:** Some clinicians have used 10 mg every other day to initiate therapy in the elderly to help avoid side effects and produce therapeutic effect at minimal dose.

**Hepatic Impairment:** Reduction of dosage is necessary.

**Monitoring Laboratory Tests** Occult blood loss, hemoglobin, hematocrit, and periodic renal and hepatic function tests

**Additional Nursing Issues**

**Physical Assessment:** Assess effectiveness and interactions of other medications patient may be taking (see Contraindications and Drug Interactions). Monitor laboratory tests (see above) and therapeutic response (eg, relief of pain and inflammation, increased activity tolerance), and adverse reactions (eg, GI effects, hepatotoxicity, ototoxicity) at beginning of therapy and periodically throughout therapy (see Warnings/Precautions, Adverse Reactions, and Overdose/Toxicology). Schedule ophthalmic evaluations for patients who develop eye complaints during long-term NSAID therapy. Advise diabetic patients to use serum glucose testing (see Effects on Lab Values). Assess knowledge/teach patient appropriate use, interventions to reduce side effects, and adverse symptoms to report. **Pregnancy risk factor B/D** - see Pregnancy Risk Factor for cautious use.

**Patient Information/Instruction:** Take this medication exactly as directed; do not increase dose without consulting prescriber. Do not crush tablets or break capsules. Take with food or milk to reduce GI distress. Maintain adequate fluid intake (2-3 L/day of fluids unless instructed to restrict fluid intake). Do not use alcohol, aspirin, or aspirin-containing medication, and all other anti-inflammatory medications without consulting prescriber. You may experience drowsiness, dizziness, or nervousness (use caution when driving or engaging in tasks requiring alertness until response to drug is known); anorexia, nausea, vomiting, flatulence, or heartburn (frequent small meals, frequent mouth care, sucking lozenges, or chewing gum may help); fluid retention (weigh yourself weekly and report unusual (3-5 lb/week) weight gain). GI bleeding, ulceration, or perforation can occur with or without pain; discontinue medication and contact prescriber if persistent abdominal pain or cramping, or blood in stool occurs. Report unusual swelling of extremities or unusual weight gain; breathlessness, difficulty breathing, or unusual cough; chest pain, rapid heartbeat, palpitations; unusual bruising/bleeding; blood in urine, stool, mouth, or vomitus; unusual fatigue; changes in urinary pattern (polyuria or anuria); skin rash or itching; or change in hearing or ringing in ears. **Pregnancy precautions:** Inform prescriber if you are or intend to be pregnant.

**Geriatric Considerations:** Elderly are at high risk for adverse effects from nonsteroidal anti-inflammatory agents. As much as 60% of elderly can develop peptic ulceration and/or hemorrhage asymptomatically. The concomitant use of $H_2$ blockers, omeprazole, and sucralfate is not generally effective as prophylaxis with the exception of NSAID-induced duodenal ulcers which may be prevented by the use of ranitidine. Misoprostol is the only prophylactic agent proven effective. Also, concomitant disease and drug use contribute to the risk for GI adverse effects. Use lowest effective dose for shortest period possible. Consider renal function decline with age. Use of NSAIDs can compromise existing renal function especially when $Cl_{cr}$ is ≤30 mL/minute. Tinnitus may be a difficult and unreliable indication of toxicity due to age-related hearing loss or eighth cranial nerve damage. CNS adverse effects such as confusion, agitation, and hallucination are generally seen in overdose or high-dose situations, but elderly may demonstrate these adverse effects at lower doses than younger adults.

**Related Information**

Nonsalicylate/Nonsteroidal Anti-inflammatory Comparison *on page 1401*


- **Pisacaina** *see* Lidocaine *on page 674*
- **Pisacaina** *see* Lidocaine and Epinephrine *on page 677*
- ***p*-Isobutylhydratropic Acid** *see* Ibuprofen *on page 592*
- **PIT** *see* Oxytocin *on page 877*
- **Pitocin® Injection** *see* Oxytocin *on page 877*
- **Pitressin® Injection** *see* Vasopressin *on page 1205*
- **Pitrex®** *see page 1247*
- **Placidyl®** *see* Ethchlorvynol *on page 457*
- **Plantago Seed** *see* Psyllium *on page 993*
- **Plantain Seed** *see* Psyllium *on page 993*
- **Plaquenil®** *see* Hydroxychloroquine *on page 584*
- **Plaque Vaccine** *see page 1256*
- **Plasbumin®** *see* Albumin *on page 45*
- **Plasil** *see* Metoclopramide *on page 758*
- **Platinol®** *see* Cisplatin *on page 273*
- **Platinol®-AQ** *see* Cisplatin *on page 273*

- **Plavix®** *see* Clopidogrel *on page 291*
- **Plendil®** *see* Felodipine *on page 474*
- **Pletal®** *see* Cilostazol *on page 267*


## Plicamycin (plye kay MYE sin)

**U.S. Brand Names** Mithracin®

**Synonyms** Mithramycin

**Therapeutic Category** Antidote; Antineoplastic Agent, Antibiotic

**Pregnancy Risk Factor** X

**Lactation** Excretion in breast milk unknown/not recommended

**Use** Malignant testicular tumors, in the treatment of hypercalcemia and hypercalciuria of malignancy not responsive to conventional treatment; Paget's disease

**Mechanism of Action/Effect** Forms a complex with DNA in the presence of magnesium or other divalent cations inhibiting DNA-directed RNA synthesis

**Contraindications** Thrombocytopenia, bleeding diatheses, coagulation disorders; bone marrow function impairment; hypocalcemia; pregnancy (may cause permanent sterility and birth defects)

**Warnings** The U.S. Food and Drug Administration (FDA) currently recommends that procedures for proper handling and disposal of antineoplastic agents be considered. Use with caution in patients with hepatic or renal impairment. Reduce dosage in patients with renal impairment. Discontinue if bleeding or epistaxis occurs.

**Drug Interactions**

**Increased Effect/Toxicity:** Calcitonin, etidronate, or glucagon taken with plicamycin may result in additive hypoglycemic effects.

**Adverse Reactions**

>10%: Gastrointestinal: Anorexia, stomatitis, nausea, vomiting, diarrhea

Nausea and vomiting occur in almost 100% of patients within the first 6 hours after treatment; incidence increases with rapid injection; stomatitis has also occurred

Time course for nausea/vomiting: Onset 4-6 hours; Duration: 4-24 hours

1% to 10%:

Cardiovascular: Facial flushing

Central nervous system: Fever, headache, depression, drowsiness

Endocrine & metabolic: Hypocalcemia

Hematologic: Myelosuppressive: Mild leukopenia and thrombocytopenia

WBC: Moderate, but uncommon

Platelets: Moderate, rapid onset

Onset (days): 7-10

Nadir (days): 14

Recovery (days): 21

Clotting disorders: May also depress hepatic synthesis of clotting factors, leading to a form of coagulopathy; petechiae, increased prothrombin time, epistaxis, and thrombocytopenia may be seen and may require discontinuation of the drug. Epistaxis is frequently the first sign of this bleeding disorder.

Hepatic: Hepatotoxicity

Local: Pain at injection site

**Irritant chemotherapy**

Renal: Azotemia, nephrotoxicity

Miscellaneous: Hemorrhagic diathesis

**Overdose/Toxicology** Symptoms of overdose include bone marrow suppression, bleeding syndrome, and thrombocytopenia. Treatment is symptom directed and supportive.

**Pharmacodynamics/Kinetics**

**Protein Binding:** None

**Distribution:** Crosses blood-brain barrier in low concentrations

**Half-life Elimination:** Plasma: 1 hour

**Excretion:** Urine

**Onset:** Decreasing calcium levels: Onset of action: Within 24 hours; Peak effect: 48-72 hours

**Duration:** Decreasing calcium levels: 5-15 days

**Formulations** Powder for injection: 2.5 mg

**Dosing**

**Adults:** Refer to individual protocols. Dose should be diluted in 1 L of $D_5W$ or NS and administered over 4-6 hours.

**Dosage should be based on the patient's body weight. If a patient has abnormal fluid retention (eg, edema, hydrothorax, or ascites), the patient's ideal weight rather than actual body weight should be used to calculate the dose.**

I.V.:

Testicular cancer: 25-30 mcg/kg/day for 8-10 days

Blastic chronic granulocytic leukemia: 25 mcg/kg over 2-4 hours every other day for 3 weeks

Paget's disease: 15 mcg/kg/day once daily for 10 days

Hypercalcemia: 25 mcg/kg single dose which may be repeated in 48 hours if no response occurs

**or** 25 mcg/kg for 3-4 days

**or** 25-50 mcg/kg every other day for 3-8 doses

**Elderly:** Refer to adult dosing.

**Renal Impairment:**

$Cl_{cr}$ 10-50 mL/minute: Decrease dosage to 75% of normal dose.

$Cl_{cr}$ <10 mL/minute: Decrease dosage to 50% of normal dose.

Hemodialysis effects: Unknown
CAPD effects: Unknown
CAVH effects: Unknown

**Hepatic Impairment:** Treatment of hypercalcemia in patients with hepatic dysfunction: Reduce dose to 12.5 mcg/kg/day.

**Administration**

**I.V.:** Irritant. Rapid I.V. infusion has been associated with an increased incidence of nausea and vomiting; an antiemetic given prior to and during plicamycin infusion may be helpful. Administer I.V. infusion over 4-6 hours.

**I.V. Detail:** Avoid extravasation since plicamycin is a strong vesicant; local tissue irritation and cellulitis have been reported.

**Extravasation management:** Is an irritant; may produce local tissue irritation or cellulitis if infiltrated. If extravasation occurs, follow hospital procedure, discontinue I.V., and apply ice for 24 hours.

**Stability**

**Storage:** Store intact vials under refrigeration (2°C to 8°C). Vials are stable at room temperature (<25°C) for up to 3 months.

**Reconstitution:** Dilute powder in 4.9 mL SWI to result in a concentration of 500 mcg/mL which is stable for 24 hours at room temperature (25°C) and 48 hours under refrigeration (4°C). Further dilution in 1000 mL $D_5W$ or NS is stable for 24 hours at room temperature.

**Standard I.V. dilution:** Dose/1000 mL $D_5W$ or NS; solution is stable for 24 hours at room temperature (25°C).

**Compatibility:** See the Chemotherapy Compatibility Chart *on page 1311.*

**Monitoring Laboratory Tests** Hepatic and renal function, CBC, platelet count, prothrombin time, serum electrolytes

**Additional Nursing Issues**

**Physical Assessment:** Assess effectiveness and interactions of other medications (see Drug Interactions). See Warnings/Precautions, Contraindications, and Administration for use cautions. Monitor effectiveness of therapy and monitor laboratory tests frequently during therapy (see above). Monitor closely for adverse response (see Adverse Reactions and Overdose/Toxicology). Assess knowledge/teach patient possible side effects and appropriate interventions, and adverse symptoms to report. **Pregnancy risk factor D** - assess knowledge/teach appropriate use of barrier contraceptives. Breast-feeding is not recommended.

**Patient Information/Instruction:** This medication can only be administered I.V. and frequent blood tests will be necessary to monitor effects of the drug. Report pain, swelling, or irritation at infusion site. Do not take alcohol, and prescription or OTC medications containing aspirin or ibuprofen without consulting prescriber. Maintain adequate hydration (2-3 L/day of fluids unless instructed to restrict fluid intake). Maintain good oral hygiene (use soft toothbrush or cotton applicators several times a day and rinse mouth frequently). You will be susceptible to infection; avoid crowds and infected persons and do not receive any vaccinations unless approved by prescriber. Report persistent fever or chills, unhealed sores, oral or vaginal sores, foul-smelling urine, easy bruising or bleeding, yellowing of eyes or skin, or change in color of urine or stool. **Pregnancy/breast-feeding precautions:** Do not get pregnant while taking this medication - use appropriate barrier contraceptive measures. Breast-feeding is not recommended.


♦ **PMS-Amantadine** *see* Amantadine *on page 61*
♦ **PMS-Baclofen** *see* Baclofen *on page 131*
♦ **PMS-Benztropine** *see* Benztropine *on page 144*
♦ **PMS-Bethanechol Chloride** *see* Bethanechol *on page 151*
♦ **PMS-Carbamazepine** *see* Carbamazepine *on page 195*
♦ **PMS-Chloral Hydrate** *see* Chloral Hydrate *on page 245*
♦ **PMS-Cholestyramine** *see* Cholestyramine Resin *on page 262*
♦ **PMS-Clonazepam** *see* Clonazepam *on page 288*
♦ **PMS-Cyproheptadine** *see* Cyproheptadine *on page 320*
♦ **PMS-Desipramine** *see* Desipramine *on page 343*
♦ **PMS-Diazepam** *see* Diazepam *on page 355*
♦ **PMS-Docusate Calcium** *see* Docusate *on page 392*
♦ **PMS-Dopazide** *see* Methyldopa and Hydrochlorothiazide *on page 751*
♦ **PMS-Erythromycin** *see* Erythromycin *on page 435*
♦ **PMS-Ferrous Sulfate** *see* Iron Supplements *on page 627*
♦ **PMS-Flupam** *see* Flurazepam *on page 507*
♦ **PMS-Fluphenazine** *see* Fluphenazine *on page 505*
♦ **PMS-Hydromorphone** *see* Hydromorphone *on page 581*
♦ **PMS-Hydroxyzine** *see* Hydroxyzine *on page 588*
♦ **PMS-Imipramine** *see* Imipramine *on page 600*
♦ **PMS-Isoniazid** *see* Isoniazid *on page 630*
♦ **PMS-Ketoprofen** *see* Ketoprofen *on page 645*
♦ **PMS-Levazine** *see* Amitriptyline and Perphenazine *on page 75*
♦ **PMS-Levothyroxine Sodium** *see* Levothyroxine *on page 673*
♦ **PMS-Lidocaine Viscous** *see* Lidocaine *on page 674*
♦ **PMS-Lindane** *see* Lindane *on page 678*
♦ **PMS-Loperamine** *see* Loperamide *on page 688*
♦ **PMS-Lorazepam** *see* Lorazepam *on page 691*

- ♦ **PMS-Methylphenidate** *see* Methylphenidate *on page 752*
- ♦ **PMS-Nystatin** *see* Nystatin *on page 843*
- ♦ **PMS-Opium & Beladonna** *see* Belladonna and Opium *on page 136*
- ♦ **PMS-Oxazepam** *see* Oxazepam *on page 868*
- ♦ **PMS-Perphenazine** *see* Perphenazine *on page 912*
- ♦ **PMS-Prochlorperazine** *see* Prochlorperazine *on page 971*
- ♦ **PMS-Procyclidine** *see* Procyclidine *on page 973*
- ♦ **PMS-Progesterone** *see* Progesterone *on page 974*
- ♦ **PMS-Propranolol®** *see* Propranolol *on page 986*
- ♦ **PMS-Pseudoephedrine** *see* Pseudoephedrine *on page 992*
- ♦ **PMS-Pyrazinamide** *see* Pyrazinamide *on page 994*
- ♦ **PMS-Sodium Cromoglycate** *see* Cromolyn Sodium *on page 309*
- ♦ **PMS-Sulfasalazine** *see* Sulfasalazine *on page 1084*
- ♦ **PMS-Thioridazine** *see* Thioridazine *on page 1123*
- ♦ **PMS-Trihexyphenidyl** *see* Trihexyphenidyl *on page 1179*
- ♦ **Pneumococcal Vaccine** *see page 1256*
- ♦ **Pneumomist®** *see* Guaifenesin *on page 548*
- ♦ **Pneumovax® 23** *see page 1256*
- ♦ **Pnu-Imune® 23** *see page 1256*
- ♦ **Pod-Ben-25®** *see* Podophyllum Resin *on this page*
- ♦ **Podocon-25™** *see* Podophyllum Resin *on this page*
- ♦ **Podofilm®** *see* Podophyllum Resin *on this page*
- ♦ **Podofin®** *see* Podophyllum Resin *on this page*


## Podophyllum Resin (po DOF fil um REZ in)

**U.S. Brand Names** Pod-Ben-25®; Podocon-25™; Podofin®

**Synonyms** Mandrake; May Apple

**Therapeutic Category** Keratolytic Agent

**Pregnancy Risk Factor** X

**Lactation** Enters breast milk/contraindicated

**Use** Topical treatment of benign growths including external genital and perianal warts, papillomas, fibroids; compound benzoin tincture generally is used as the medium for topical application

**Mechanism of Action/Effect** Directly affects epithelial cell metabolism by arresting mitosis through binding to a protein subunit of spindle microtubules (tubulin)

**Contraindications** Not to be used on birthmarks, moles, or warts with hair growth; cervical, urethral, oral warts; not to be used by diabetic patient or patient with poor circulation; pregnancy

**Warnings** Use of large amounts of drug should be avoided. Avoid contact with the eyes as it can cause severe corneal damage; do not apply to moles, birthmarks, or unusual warts. To be applied by prescriber only. For external use only; 25% solution should not be applied to or near mucous membranes.

**Adverse Reactions**

1% to 10%:

Dermatologic: Pruritus

Gastrointestinal: Nausea, vomiting, abdominal pain, diarrhea

<1% (Limited to important or life-threatening symptoms): Renal failure, leukopenia, thrombocytopenia, hepatotoxicity, peripheral neuropathy

**Formulations** Liquid, topical: 25% in benzoin tincture (5 mL, 7.5 mL, 30 mL)

**Dosing**

**Adults:** Topical:

10% to 25% solution in compound benzoin tincture; apply drug to dry surface, use 1 drop at a time allowing drying between drops until area is covered. Total volume should be limited to <0.5 mL per treatment session.

Condylomata acuminatum: 25% solution is applied daily. Use a 10% solution when applied to or near mucous membranes.

Verrucae: 25% solution is applied 3-5 times/day directly to the wart.

**Elderly:** Refer to adult dosing.

**Administration**

**Topical:** Shake well before using. **Only to be applied by physician.** Solution should be washed off within 1-4 hours for genital and perianal warts and within 1-2 hours for accessible meatal warts. Use protective occlusive dressing around warts to prevent contact with unaffected skin. For external use only.

**Additional Nursing Issues**

**Physical Assessment:** See Contraindications, Warnings/Precautions, and Administration. **Pregnancy risk factor X** - determine that patient is not pregnant before beginning treatment and do not give to women of childbearing age or males who may have intercourse with childbearing women unless both male and female are capable of complying with barrier contraceptive measures during therapy and for 1 month following therapy. Breast-feeding is contraindicated.

**Patient Information/Instruction:** Cover with occlusive dressing to prevent contact with unaffected skin. Wash off medication as instructed by professional who applied the treatment. **Pregnancy/breast-feeding precautions:** Inform prescriber if you are pregnant. Do not get pregnant during or for 1 month following therapy. Male: Do not cause a pregnancy. Male/female: Consult prescriber for instruction on appropriate barrier contraceptive measures. This drug may cause severe fetal defects. Do not breast-feed.

- **Point-Two®** *see page 1294*
- **Poladex®** *see* Dexchlorpheniramine *on page 349*
- **Polaramine®** *see* Dexchlorpheniramine *on page 349*
- **Poliovirus Vaccine, Inactivated** *see page 1256*
- **Polocaine®** *see* Mepivacaine *on page 723*
- **Polycillin®** *see* Ampicillin *on page 90*
- **Polycillin-N®** *see* Ampicillin *on page 90*
- **Polycitra®-K** *see* Potassium Citrate and Citric Acid *on page 950*
- **Polycitra® Syrup** *see page 1306*
- **Polycose®** *see page 1294*
- **Polydine®** *see page 1294*


## Polyethylene Glycol-Electrolyte Solution

(pol i ETH i leen GLY kol ee LEK troe lite soe LOO shun)

**U.S. Brand Names** Colovage®; Colyte®; GoLYTELY®; NuLytely®; OCL®

**Synonyms** Electrolyte Lavage Solution; PEG-ES

**Therapeutic Category** Cathartic; Laxative, Bowel Evacuant

**Pregnancy Risk Factor** C

**Lactation** Excretion in breast milk unknown

**Use** Bowel cleansing prior to GI examination or following toxic ingestion

**Mechanism of Action/Effect** Induces catharsis by strong electrolyte and osmotic effects

**Contraindications** GI obstruction; gastric retention; bowel perforation; toxic colitis; megacolon

**Warnings** Safety and efficacy not established in children. Do not add flavorings as additional ingredients before use. Observe unconscious or semiconscious patients with impaired gag reflex or those who are otherwise prone to regurgitation or aspiration during administration. Use with caution in ulcerative colitis. Caution against the use of hot loop polypectomy. Pregnancy factor C.

**Drug Interactions**

**Decreased Effect:** Oral medications should not be administered within 1 hour of start of therapy.

**Adverse Reactions**

>10%: Gastrointestinal: Nausea, abdominal fullness, bloating

1% to 10%: Gastrointestinal: Abdominal cramps, vomiting, anal irritation

**Pharmacodynamics/Kinetics**

**Onset:** Oral: Within 1-2 hours

**Formulations** Powder, for oral solution: PEG 3350 236 g, sodium sulfate 22.74 g, sodium bicarbonate 6.74 g, sodium chloride 5.86 g and potassium chloride 2.97 g (2000 mL, 4000 mL, 4800 mL, 6000 mL)

**Dosing**

**Adults:** The recommended dose for adults is 4 L of solution prior to GI examination, as ingestion of this dose produces a satisfactory preparation in >95% of patients. Ideally the patient should fast for approximately 3-4 hours prior to administration, but in no case should solid food be given for at least 2 hours before the solution is given. The solution is usually administered orally, but may be given via nasogastric tube to patients who are unwilling or unable to drink the solution.

**Elderly:** Refer to adult dosing.

**Administration**

**Oral:**

Oral: At a rate of 240 mL (8 oz) every 10 minutes, until 4 liters are consumed or the rectal effluent is clear. Rapid drinking of each portion is preferred to drinking small amounts continuously. Do not add flavorings as additional ingredients before use.

Nasogastric tube: At a rate of 20-30 mL/minute (1.2-1.8 L/hour); the first bowel movement should occur approximately 1 hour after the start of administration.

**Stability**

**Storage:** Store at 59°F to 86°F before reconstitution.

**Reconstitution:** Use within 48 hours of preparation. Refrigerate reconstituted solution. Tap water may be used for preparation of the solution. Dissolution is facilitated by using lukewarm water. Shake container vigorously several times to ensure dissolution of powder.

**Monitoring Laboratory Tests** Electrolytes, serum glucose, BUN, urine osmolality

**Additional Nursing Issues**

**Physical Assessment:** Assess/instruct the patient on appropriate use of this medication. **Pregnancy risk factor C** - benefits of use should outweigh possible risks. Note breast-feeding caution.

**Patient Information/Instruction:** Chilled solution is often more palatable. Produces a watery stool which cleanses the bowel before examination. Prepare solution according to instructions on the bottle. For best results, no solid food should be consumed during the 3- to 4-hour period before drinking solution, but in no case should solid foods be eaten within 2 hours of taking. Drink 240 mL every 10 minutes. Rapid drinking of each portion is better than drinking small amounts continuously. The first bowel movement should occur approximately 1 hour after the start of administration. May experience some abdominal bloating and distention before bowel starts to move. If severe discomfort or distention occurs, stop drinking temporarily or drink each portion at longer intervals until these symptoms disappear. Continue drinking until the watery stool is clear and free of solid matter. This usually requires at least 3 L. It is best to drink all of the solutions. Discard any unused portion. **Pregnancy/breast-feeding precautions:**

(Continued)

## Polyethylene Glycol-Electrolyte Solution *(Continued)*

Inform prescriber if you are or intend to be pregnant. Consult prescriber if breast-feeding.


- **Polygam® S/D** *see* Immune Globulin, Intravenous *on page 602*
- **Poly-Histine CS®** *see* Brompheniramine, Phenylpropanolamine, and Codeine *on page 163*
- **Polymox®** *see* Amoxicillin *on page 80*
- **Polymyxin B and Bacitracin** *see* Bacitracin and Polymyxin B *on page 130*
- **Polymyxin B and Hydrocortisone** *see page 1291*
- **Polymyxin B and Neomycin** *see* Neomycin and Polymyxin B *on page 817*
- **Polymyxin B, Bacitracin, and Neomycin** *see* Bacitracin, Neomycin, and Polymyxin B *on page 130*
- **Polymyxin B, Bacitracin, Neomycin, and Hydrocortisone** *see* Bacitracin, Neomycin, Polymyxin B, and Hydrocortisone *on page 131*


## Polymyxin B Sulfate (pol i MIX in bee SUL fate)

**Therapeutic Category** Antibiotic, Irrigation; Antibiotic, Miscellaneous

**Pregnancy Risk Factor** B

**Lactation** Excretion in breast milk unknown

**Use**

Topical: Wound irrigation and bladder irrigation against *Pseudomonas aeruginosa*

Parenteral use of polymyxin B has mainly been replaced by less toxic antibiotics; it is reserved for life-threatening infections caused by organisms resistant to the preferred drugs

**Mechanism of Action/Effect** Binds to phospholipids, alters permeability, and damages the bacterial cytoplasmic membrane permitting leakage of intracellular constituents

**Contraindications** Concurrent use of neuromuscular blockers

**Warnings** Use with caution in patients with impaired renal function (modify dosage) neurotoxic reactions are usually associated with high serum levels, found in patients with impaired renal function. Avoid concurrent or sequential use of other nephrotoxic and neurotoxic drugs, particularly bacitracin, colistin, and the aminoglycosides. The drug's neurotoxicity can result in respiratory paralysis from neuromuscular blockade, especially when the drug is given soon after anesthesia or muscle relaxants. Polymyxin B sulfate is toxic when given parenterally; avoid parenteral use whenever possible.

**Drug Interactions**

**Increased Effect/Toxicity:** Increased/prolonged effect of neuromuscular blocking agents.

**Adverse Reactions** <1% (Limited to important or life-threatening symptoms): Neurotoxicity (irritability, drowsiness, ataxia, perioral paresthesia, numbness of the extremities, and blurring of vision), neuromuscular blockade, nephrotoxicity, respiratory arrest

**Overdose/Toxicology** Symptoms of overdose include respiratory paralysis, ototoxicity, and nephrotoxicity. Supportive care is indicated as treatment.

**Pharmacodynamics/Kinetics**

**Distribution:** Minimal distribution into the CSF; crosses the placenta

**Half-life Elimination:** 4.5-6 hours, increased with reduced renal function

**Time to Peak:** I.M.: Within 2 hours

**Excretion:** Urine

**Formulations**

Injection: 500,000 units (20 mL)

Powder for solution, ophthalmic: 500,000 units (20-50 mL diluent)

**Dosing**

**Adults:**

Otic: Instill 1-2 drops, 3-4 times/day; should be used sparingly to avoid accumulation of excess debris.

I.M.: 25,000-30,000 units/kg/day divided every 4-6 hours

I.V.: 15,000-25,000 units/kg/day divided every 12 hours or by continuous infusion

Intrathecal: 50,000 units/day for 3-4 days, then every other day for at least 2 weeks

Total daily dose should not exceed 2,000,000 units/day.

Bladder irrigation: Continuous irrigant or rinse in the urinary bladder for up to 10 days using 20 mg (equal to 200,000 units) added to 1 L of normal saline; usually no more than 1 L of irrigant is used per day unless urine flow rate is high; administration rate is adjusted to patient's urine output.

Topical irrigation or topical solution: 500,000 units/L of normal saline; topical irrigation should not exceed 2 million units/day in adults.

Ophthalmic: A concentration of 0.1% to 0.25% is administered as 1-3 drops every hour, then increasing the interval as response indicates to 1-2 drops 4-6 times/day.

**Elderly:** Refer to adult dosing.

**Renal Impairment:**

$Cl_{cr}$ 20-50 mL/minute: Administer 75% to 100% of normal dose every 12 hours.

$Cl_{cr}$ 5-20 mL/minute: Administer 50% of normal dose every 12 hours.

$Cl_{cr}$ <5 mL/minute: Administer 15% of normal dose every 12 hours.

**Administration**

**I.M.:** Administer into upper outer quadrant of gluteal muscle; however, I.M route is not recommended due to severe pain at injection site.

**I.V.:** Infuse over 60-90 minutes.

**I.V. Detail: Extravasation management:** Monitor I.V. site closely; extravasation may cause serious injury with possible necrosis and tissue sloughing. Rotate infusion site frequently.

**Stability**

**Storage:** Parenteral solutions stable for 7 days when refrigerated. Discard any unused portion after 72 hours.

**Compatibility:** Incompatible with calcium, magnesium, cephalothin, chloramphenicol, heparin, or penicillins. Aqueous solutions remain stable for 6-12 months under refrigeration.

**Monitoring Laboratory Tests** Perform culture and sensitivity prior to beginning therapy. Establish baseline renal function prior to initiating therapy. Monitor renal function closely.

**Additional Nursing Issues**

**Physical Assessment:** Assess allergy history before initiating therapy. Assess effectiveness and interactions of other medications (see Drug Interactions). See Warnings/Precautions and Contraindications for use cautions. Monitor effectiveness of therapy, laboratory tests, and adverse response (see Adverse Reactions and Overdose/Toxicology) during therapy. Assess knowledge/teach patient appropriate use according to drug form and purpose, possible side effects, and adverse symptoms to report. Note breast-feeding caution.

**Patient Information/Instruction:** Wound irrigation / bladder irrigation / gut sterilization / or I.V.: Immediately report numbness or tingling of mouth, tongue, or extremities; constant blurring of vision; increased nervousness or irritability; excessive drowsiness; or difficulty breathing.

Ophthalmic: tilt head back, place medication into eyes (as frequently as prescribed), close eyes, apply light pressure over inside corner of the eye for 1 minute. Do not touch medicine dropper to eye or contaminate tip of dropper. You may experience some stinging or burning or temporary blurring of vision - use caution driving or when engaging in hazardous tasks until vision clears. Report any adverse effects including respiratory difficulty or unusual numbness or tingling of mouth or tongue, increased nervousness or irritability, or excessive drowsiness.

**Breast-feeding precautions:** Consult prescriber if breast-feeding.

**Additional Information**

1 mg = 10,000 units

pH: 5-7.4

- **Poly-Pred® Ophthalmic Suspension** *see page 1282*
- **Polysaccharide-Iron Complex** *see page 1294*
- **Polysporin®** *see page 1282*
- **Polysporin® Ophthalmic** *see* Bacitracin and Polymyxin B *on page 130*
- **Polysporin® Topical** *see* Bacitracin and Polymyxin B *on page 130*
- **Polytar®** *see page 1294*
- **Polythiazide and Prazosin** *see* Prazosin and Polythiazide *on page 959*
- **Polytopic** *see* Bacitracin and Polymyxin B *on page 130*
- **Polytrim®** *see page 1282*
- **Poly-Vi-Flor®** *see* Vitamin, Multiple *on page 1219*
- **Poly-Vi-Sol® [OTC]** *see* Vitamin, Multiple *on page 1219*
- **Pontocaine®** *see* Tetracaine *on page 1110*
- **Porcelana® [OTC]** *see* Hydroquinone *on page 583*
- **Porcelana® Sunscreen [OTC]** *see* Hydroquinone *on page 583*

## Porfimer (POR fi mer)

**U.S. Brand Names** Photofrin®

**Therapeutic Category** Antineoplastic Agent, Miscellaneous

**Pregnancy Risk Factor** C

**Lactation** Enters breast milk/contraindicated

**Use** Esophageal cancer: Photodynamic therapy (PDT) with porfimer for palliation of patients with completely obstructing esophageal cancer, or of patients with partially obstructing esophageal cancer who cannot be satisfactorily treated with Nd:YAG laser therapy. Reduction of obstruction and palliation of symptoms in patients with completely or partially obstructing endobronchial nonsmall cell lung cancer

**Mechanism of Action/Effect** Photosensitizing agent used in the photodynamic therapy (PDT) of tumors: cytotoxic and antitumor actions of porfimer are light and oxygen dependent. Cellular damage caused by porfimer PDT is a consequence of the propagation of radical reactions.

**Contraindications** Porphyria or in patients with allergies to porphyrins; existing tracheoesophageal or bronchoesophageal fistula; tumors eroding into a major blood vessel

**Warnings** The U.S. Food and Drug Administration (FDA) currently recommends that procedures for proper handling and disposal of antineoplastic agents be considered.

Porfimer preparation should be performed in a Class II laminar flow biologic safety cabinet. Personnel should be wearing surgical gloves and a closed front surgical gown with knit cuffs. Appropriate safety equipment is recommended for preparation, administration, and disposal of antineoplastics. If porfimer contacts the skin, wash and flush thoroughly with water.

If the esophageal tumor is eroding into the trachea or bronchial tree, the likelihood of tracheoesophageal or bronchoesophageal fistula resulting from treatment is sufficiently high that PDT is not recommended. All patients who receive porfimer sodium will be photosensitive and must observe precautions to avoid exposure of skin and eyes to direct sunlight or bright indoor light for 30 days. The photosensitivity is due to residual drug which will be present in all parts of the skin. Exposure of the skin to ambient indoor light is, however, beneficial because the remaining drug will be inactivated gradually and

(Continued)

## Porfimer *(Continued)*

safely through a photobleaching reaction. Patients should not stay in a darkened room during this period and should be encouraged to expose their skin to ambient indoor light. Ocular discomfort has been reported; for 30 days, when outdoors, patients should wear dark sunglasses which have an average white light transmittance <4%.

Pregnancy factor C.

**Drug Interactions**

**Decreased Effect:** Compounds that quench active oxygen species or scavenge radicals (eg, dimethyl sulfoxide, beta-carotene, ethanol, mannitol) would be expected to decrease photodynamic therapy (PDT) activity. Allopurinol, calcium channel blockers and some prostaglandin synthesis inhibitors could interfere with porfimer. Drugs that decrease clotting, vasoconstriction, or platelet aggregation could decrease the efficacy of PDT. Glucocorticoid hormones may decrease the efficacy of the treatment.

**Increased Effect/Toxicity:** Concomitant administration of other photosensitizing agents (eg, tetracyclines, sulfonamides, phenothiazines, sulfonylureas, thiazide diuretics, griseofulvin) could increase the photosensitivity reaction.

**Adverse Reactions**

>10%:

- Cardiovascular: Atrial fibrillation, chest pain
- Central nervous system: Fever, pain, insomnia
- Dermatologic: Photosensitivity reaction
- Gastrointestinal: abdominal pain, constipation, dysphagia, nausea, vomiting
- Hematologic: Anemia
- Neuromuscular & skeletal: Back pain
- Respiratory: Dyspnea, pharyngitis, pleural effusion, pneumonia, respiratory insufficiency

1% to 10%:

- Cardiovascular: Hypertension, hypotension, edema, cardiac failure, tachycardia, chest pain (substernal)
- Central nervous system: Anxiety, confusion
- Endocrine & metabolic: Dehydration
- Gastrointestinal: Diarrhea, heartburn, eructation, esophageal edema, esophageal tumor bleeding, esophageal stricture, esophagitis, hematemesis, melena, weight loss, anorexia
- Genitourinary: Urinary tract infection
- Neuromuscular & skeletal: Weakness
- Respiratory: Coughing, tracheoesophageal fistula
- Miscellaneous: Moniliasis, surgical complication

**Overdose/Toxicology** Increased symptoms and damage to normal tissue might be expected with overdose of laser light following porfimer injection. Effects of overdose on the duration of photosensitivity are unknown. Laser treatment should not be given if an overdose of porfimer is administered. In the event of overdose, patients should protect their eyes and skin from direct sunlight or bright indoor lights for 30 days. At this time, patients should be tested for residual photosensitivity. Porfimer is not dialyzable.

**Pharmacodynamics/Kinetics**

**Protein Binding:** Plasma: 90%

**Half-life Elimination:** 250 hours

**Time to Peak:** Within 2 hours

**Excretion:** Total plasma clearance: 0.051 mL/minute/kg

**Formulations** Powder for injection, as sodium: 75 mg

**Dosing**

**Adults:** Refer to individual protocols.

I.V.: 2 mg/kg over 3-5 minutes

Photodynamic therapy is a two-stage process requiring administration of both drug and light. The first stage of PDT is the I.V. injection of porfimer. Illumination with laser light 40-50 hours following the injection with porfimer constitutes the second stage of therapy. A second laser light application may be given 90-120 hours after injection, preceded by gentle debridement of residual tumor.

Patients may receive a second course of PDT a minimum of 30 days after the initial therapy; up to three courses of PDT (each separated by a minimum of 30 days) can be given. Before each course of treatment, evaluate patients for the presence of a tracheoesophageal or bronchoesophageal fistula.

**Elderly:** Refer to adult dosing.

**Administration**

**I.V.:** Administer slow I.V. injection over 3-5 minutes.

**I.V. Detail:** Avoid extravasation. If extravasation occurs, take care to protect the area from light. There is no known benefit from injecting the extravasation site with another substance. Wipe up spills with a damp cloth. Avoid skin and eye contact due to the potential for photosensitivity reactions upon exposure to light; use of rubber gloves and eye protection is recommended.

**Stability**

**Storage:** Store intact vials at controlled room temperature of 20°C to 25°C/68°F to 77°F.

**Reconstitution:** Reconstitute each vial of porfimer with 31.8 mL of either 5% dextrose injection or 0.9% sodium chloride injection resulting in a final concentration of 2.5 mg/mL and a pH of 7-8. Shake well until dissolved. Protect the reconstituted product from bright light and use immediately. Reconstituted porfimer is an opaque solution in which detection of particulate matter by visual inspection is extremely difficult.

**Compatibility:** Do not mix porfimer with other drugs in the same solution.

**Additional Nursing Issues**

**Physical Assessment:** Monitor infusion site for extravasation (if extravasation occurs protect area from light). Monitor for adverse cardiac, CNS, respiratory, and photosensitivity reactions (see Warnings/Precautions and Adverse Reactions). Protect patient from exposure to light (cover eyes and skin for 30 days after treatment - sunblock is of no effect). Assess knowledge/teach patient or caregiver interventions to reduce side effects and adverse signs to report. **Pregnancy risk factor C.** Breast-feeding is contraindicated.

**Patient Information/Instruction:** This medication can only be administered I.V. and will be followed by laser light therapy. Avoid any exposure to sunlight or bright indoor light for 30 days following therapy (cover skin with protective clothing and wear dark sunglasses with light transmittance <4% when outdoors - severe blistering, burning, and skin/eye damage can result). After 30 days, test small area of skin (not face) for remaining sensitivity. Retest sensitivity if traveling to a different geographic area with greater sunshine. Exposure to indoor normal light is beneficial since it will help dissipate photosensitivity gradually. Maintain adequate hydration (2-3 L/day of fluids unless instructed to restrict fluid intake); maintain good oral hygiene (use soft toothbrush or cotton applicators several times a day and rinse mouth frequently). Small frequent meals, frequent mouth care, sucking lozenges, or chewing gum may reduce nausea or vomiting. Report rapid heart rate, chest pain or palpitations, difficulty breathing or air hunger, persistent fever or chills, foul-smelling urine or burning on urination, swelling of extremities, increased anxiety, confusion, or hallucination. **Pregnancy/breast-feeding precautions:** Inform prescriber if pregnant. Do not breast-feed.

- **Pork NPH Iletin® II** *see* Insulin Preparations *on page 609*
- **Pork Regular Iletin® II** *see* Insulin Preparations *on page 609*
- **Posipen** *see* Dicloxacillin *on page 361*
- **Posture® [OTC]** *see* Calcium Supplements *on page 185*
- **Posture®** *see page 1294*
- **Potasalan®** *see* Potassium Supplements *on page 952*
- **Potassium Acetate** *replaced by* Potassium Supplements *on page 952*
- **Potassium Acid Phosphate** *see* Phosphate Supplements *on page 926*
- **Potassium Bicarbonate** *replaced by* Potassium Supplements *on page 952*

## Potassium Bicarbonate and Potassium Chloride, Effervescent

(poe TASS ee um bye KAR bun ate & poe TASS ee um KLOR ide, ef er VES ent)

**U.S. Brand Names** Klorvess® Effervescent; K-Lyte/Cl® Tablet

**Therapeutic Category** Electrolyte Supplement, Oral

**Pregnancy Risk Factor** C

**Lactation** Enters breast milk/compatible

**Use** Treatment or prevention of hypokalemia

**Formulations**

Granules for oral solution, effervescent (Klorvess®): 20 mEq per packet

Tablet for oral solution, effervescent

Klorvess®: 20 mEq per packet

K/Lyte/Cl®: 25 mEq, 50 mEq per packet

**Dosing**

**Adults:** Oral:

Prevention: 16-24 mEq/day in 2-4 divided doses

Treatment: 40-100 mEq/day in 2-4 divided doses

**Elderly:** Refer to adult dosing.

**Additional Nursing Issues**

**Physical Assessment:** Assess for adequate kidney function, use of ACE inhibitors, or potassium-sparing diuretics prior to starting therapy. Monitor cardiac status and serum potassium levels on a regular basis. Instruct patient on appropriate diet and administration. **Pregnancy risk factor C.**

**Patient Information/Instruction:** Take as directed; do not take more than directed. Dissolve granules, powder, or tablets in 4-6 ounces of water or juice and stir before drinking. Do not take on an empty stomach; take with or after meals. Consult prescriber about increasing dietary potassium intake (eg, salt substitutes, orange juice, bananas, etc). Report tingling of hands or feet, unresolved nausea or vomiting, chest pain, palpitations, persistent abdominal pain, muscle cramping or weakness, tarry stools, easy bruising, or unusual bleeding. **Pregnancy precautions:** Inform prescriber if you are pregnant.

- **Potassium Chloride** *replaced by* Potassium Supplements *on page 952*

## Potassium Citrate (poe TASS ee um SIT rate)

**U.S. Brand Names** Urocit®-K

**Therapeutic Category** Alkalinizing Agent

**Pregnancy Risk Factor** No rating

**Lactation** Enters breast milk/compatible

**Use** Prevention of uric acid nephrolithiasis; prevention of calcium renal stones in patients with hypocitraturia; urinary alkalinizer when sodium citrate is contraindicated

**Contraindications** Severe renal insufficiency; sodium-restricted diet (sodium citrate); untreated Addison's disease; severe myocardial damage; acute dehydration; patients with hyperkalemia; patients with delayed gastric emptying, esophageal compression,

(Continued)

## Potassium Citrate *(Continued)*

intestinal obstruction or stricture, or those taking anticholinergic medication; patients with active urinary tract infection

**Warnings** Use caution in patients with congestive heart failure, hypertension, edema, or any condition sensitive to sodium or potassium intake. Citrate is converted to bicarbonate in the liver. This conversion may be blocked in patients who are severely ill, in shock, or in hepatic failure. Use caution with potassium-sparing diuretics and drugs that slow GI transit time.

**Drug Interactions**

**Increased Effect/Toxicity:** Concurrent administration with potassium-containing medications, potassium-sparing diuretics, ACE inhibitors, or cardiac glycosides could lead to toxicity.

**Adverse Reactions**

>10%: Gastrointestinal: Diarrhea, nausea, stomach pain, flatulence, vomiting (oral)

1% to 10%:

Cardiovascular: Bradycardia

Endocrine & metabolic: Hyperkalemia, metabolic alkalosis in patients with severe renal failure

Neuromuscular & skeletal: Weakness

Respiratory: Dyspnea

<1% (Limited to important or life-threatening symptoms): Chest pain, arrhythmias, heart block, hypotension

**Pharmacodynamics/Kinetics**

**Metabolism:** To bicarbonate in the liver

**Formulations** Tablet: 540 mg [5 mEq], 1080 mg [10 mEq]

**Dosing**

**Adults:** Oral: 10-20 mEq 3 times/day with meals up to 100 mEq/day

**Elderly:** Refer to adult dosing.

**Administration**

**Oral:** Swallow tablets whole with a full glass of water.

**Stability**

**Storage:** Store in a cool dry place.

**Additional Nursing Issues**

**Physical Assessment:** See Contraindications and Warnings/Precautions for use cautions. Assess effectiveness and interactions of other medications (see Drug Interactions). Assess kidney function prior to starting therapy. Monitor cardiac status and serum potassium at beginning of therapy and at regular intervals with long-term therapy. Assess knowledge/teach patient appropriate use, recommended diet, and adverse symptoms to report.

**Patient Information/Instruction:** Take as directed; do not take more than directed. Swallow tablet whole with full glass of water or juice and stir before sipping slowly, with or after meals (do not take on an empty stomach). Take any antacids 2 hours before or after potassium. Consult prescriber about advisability of increasing dietary potassium. Report tingling of hands or feet; unresolved nausea or vomiting; chest pain or palpitations; persistent abdominal pain; feelings of weakness, dizziness, listlessness, confusion, acute muscle weakness or cramping; blood in stool or tarry stools; or easy bruising or unusual bleeding.

**Additional Information** Parenteral $K_3PO_4$ contains 3 mmol of phosphorous/mL and 4.4 mEq of potassium/mL. If ordering by phosphorous content, use mmol instead of mEq since the mEq value for phosphorous varies with the pH of the solution due to valence changes of the phosphorus ion (1 mmol of phosphorous = 31 mg).

♦ **Potassium Citrate** *replaced by* Potassium Supplements *on page 952*

## Potassium Citrate and Citric Acid

(poe TASS ee um SIT rate & SI trik AS id)

**U.S. Brand Names** Polycitra®-K

**Synonyms** Citric Acid and Potassium Citrate

**Therapeutic Category** Alkalinizing Agent

**Pregnancy Risk Factor** A

**Lactation** Excretion in breast milk unknown/compatible

**Use** Treatment of metabolic acidosis; alkalinizing agent in conditions where long-term maintenance of an alkaline urine is desirable

**Contraindications** Severe renal insufficiency, oliguria or azotemia, potassium restricted diet, untreated Addison's disease, adynamia episodica hereditaria, acute dehydration, heat cramps, anuria, severe myocardial damage, hyperkalemia from any cause

**Warnings** Use with caution in patients with congestive heart failure, hypertension, pulmonary edema, or severe renal impairment. Large doses may cause hyperkalemia and alkalosis.

**Drug Interactions**

**Increased Effect/Toxicity:** Concurrent administration with potassium-containing medications, potassium-sparing diuretics, ACE inhibitors, or cardiac glycosides could lead to toxicity.

**Adverse Reactions**

>10%: Gastrointestinal: Diarrhea, nausea, stomach pain, flatulence, vomiting (oral)

1% to 10%:

Cardiovascular: Bradycardia

Endocrine & metabolic: Hyperkalemia, metabolic alkalosis in patients with severe renal failure

Neuromuscular & skeletal: Weakness
Respiratory: Dyspnea
<1% (Limited to important or life-threatening symptoms): Chest pain, arrhythmias, heart block, hypotension

**Pharmacodynamics/Kinetics**

**Metabolism:** To potassium bicarbonate; citric acid is metabolized to $CO_2$ and $H_2O$

**Formulations**

Crystals for reconstitution: Potassium citrate 3300 mg and citric acid 1002 mg per packet
Solution, oral: Potassium citrate 1100 mg and citric acid 334 mg per 5 mL

**Dosing**

**Adults:** Oral:

Mild to moderate hypocitraturia: 10 mEq 3 times/day with meals
Severe hypocitraturia: Initial: 20 mEq 3 times/day or 15 mEq 4 times/day with meals or within 30 minutes after meals; do not exceed 100 mEq/day

**Elderly:** Refer to adult dosing.

**Stability**

**Storage:** Protect from excessive heat or freezing.

**Additional Nursing Issues**

**Physical Assessment:** See Contraindications and Warnings/Precautions for use cautions. Assess kidney function prior to starting therapy. Monitor cardiac status and serum potassium at beginning of therapy and at regular intervals with long-term therapy. Assess knowledge/teach patient appropriate use, recommended diet, and adverse symptoms to report.

**Patient Information/Instruction:** Take as directed; do not take more than directed. Dilute crystals or solution in 4-6 ounces of juice or water; stir and drink. Swallow tablet whole with full glass of water or juice and stir before sipping slowly, with or after meals (do not take on an empty stomach). Take any antacids 2 hours before or after potassium. Consult prescriber about advisability of increasing dietary potassium. Report tingling of hands or feet; unresolved nausea or vomiting; chest pain or palpitations; persistent abdominal pain; feelings of weakness, dizziness, listlessness, confusion, acute muscle weakness or cramping; blood in stool or tarry stools; or easy bruising or unusual bleeding.

**Additional Information** Potassium citrate 3.4 mmol/5 mL and citric acid 1.6 mmol/5 mL = total of 5.0 mmol/5 mL citrate content

**Related Information**

Potassium Citrate *on page 949*
Sodium Citrate and Citric Acid *on page 1063*

♦ **Potassium Gluconate** *replaced by* Potassium Supplements *on next page*

## Potassium Iodide (poe TASS ee um EYE oh dide)

**U.S. Brand Names** Pima®; SSKI®; Thyro-Block®

**Synonyms** KI; Lugol's Solution; Strong Iodine Solution

**Therapeutic Category** Antithyroid Agent; Cough Preparation; Expectorant

**Pregnancy Risk Factor** D

**Lactation** Enters breast milk/use caution - see Breast-feeding Issues

**Use** Facilitate bronchial drainage and cough; reduce thyroid vascularity prior to thyroidectomy and management of thyrotoxic crisis; block thyroidal uptake of radioactive isotopes of iodine in a radiation emergency

**Mechanism of Action/Effect** Reduces viscosity of mucus by increasing respiratory tract secretions; inhibits secretion of thyroid hormone, fosters colloid accumulation in thyroid follicles

**Contraindications** Hypersensitivity to iodine; hyperkalemia; pulmonary tuberculosis; pulmonary edema; bronchitis; impaired renal function; pregnancy

**Warnings** Prolonged use can lead to hypothyroidism. Cystic fibrosis patients have an exaggerated response. Can cause acne flare-ups or dermatitis. Some preparations may contain sodium bisulfite (allergy). Use with caution in patients with a history of thyroid disease, patients with renal failure, or GI obstruction.

**Drug Interactions**

**Increased Effect/Toxicity:** Lithium may cause additive hypothyroid effects.

**Adverse Reactions** 1% to 10%:

Central nervous system: Fever, headache
Dermatologic: Urticaria, acne, angioedema, cutaneous hemorrhage
Endocrine & metabolic: Goiter with hypothyroidism
Gastrointestinal: Metallic taste, GI upset, nausea, vomiting, stomach pain, soreness of teeth and gums
Hematologic: Eosinophilia, hemorrhage (mucosal)
Neuromuscular & skeletal: Arthralgia
Respiratory: Rhinitis
Miscellaneous: Lymph node enlargement

**Overdose/Toxicology** Symptoms of overdose include angioedema, laryngeal edema in patients with hypersensitivity, muscle weakness, paralysis, peaked T waves, flattened P waves, prolongation of QRS complex, and ventricular arrhythmias. Removal of potassium can be accomplished by various means: removal through the GI tract with Kayexalate® administration; by way of the kidney through diuresis, mineralocorticoid administration, or increased sodium intake; by hemodialysis or peritoneal dialysis; or by shifting potassium back into the cells by insulin and glucose infusion or by administration of sodium bicarbonate. Calcium chloride reverses cardiac effects.

(Continued)

## Potassium Iodide *(Continued)*

**Pharmacodynamics/Kinetics**

**Excretion:** In euthyroid patient, renal clearance rate is 2 times that of the thyroid

**Onset:** 24-48 hours; Peak effect: 10-15 days after continuous therapy

**Formulations**

Solution, oral:

SSKI®: 1 g/mL (30 mL, 240 mL, 473 mL)

Lugol's solution, strong iodine: 100 mg/mL with iodine 50 mg/mL (120 mL)

Syrup: 325 mg/5 mL

Tablet: 130 mg

**Dosing**

**Adults:** Oral:

RDA: 130 mcg

Expectorant: 300-650 mg 2-3 times/day

Preoperative thyroidectomy: 50-250 mg (1-5 drops SSKI®) 3 times/day **or** 0.1-0.3 mL (3-5 drops) of strong iodine (Lugol's solution) 3 times/day; give for 10 days before surgery.

Thyrotoxic crisis: 300-500 mg (6-10 drops SSKI®) 3 times/day or 1 mL strong iodine (Lugol's solution) 3 times/day

Sporotrichosis:

Initial: 500 mg/dose 3 times/day

Oral increase: 50 mg/dose/day

Maximum: 1-2 g/dose 3 times/day

Continue treatment for 4-6 weeks after lesions have completely healed.

**Elderly:** Refer to adult dosing.

**Administration**

**Oral:** Dilute in 6 oz water, fruit juice, milk, or broth.

**Stability**

**Storage:** Store in tight, light-resistant containers at temperature <40°C. Freezing should be avoided.

**Monitoring Laboratory Tests** Thyroid function

**Additional Nursing Issues**

**Physical Assessment:** Assess/teach administration guidelines and adverse signs to report. **Pregnancy risk factor D** - assess knowledge/instruct patient on need to use appropriate contraceptive measures and the need to avoid pregnancy. Note breast-feeding caution.

**Patient Information/Instruction:** Take after meals. Dilute in 6 oz of water, fruit juice, milk, or broth. Do not chew tablets; swallow whole. Do not exceed recommended dosage. You may experience a metallic taste. Discontinue use and report stomach pain, severe nausea or vomiting, black or tarry stools, or unresolved weakness. **Pregnancy/breast-feeding precautions:** Use appropriate contraceptive measures; do not get pregnant while taking this drug (serious fetal damage has occurred). Consult prescriber if breast-feeding.

**Breast-feeding Issues:** American Academy of Pediatrics considers this drug compatible but iodine in breast milk may affect thyroid function.

**Additional Information** 10 drops of SSKI® = potassium iodide 500 mg

♦ **Potassium Phosphate** *see* Phosphate Supplements *on page 926*

♦ **Potassium Phosphate and Sodium Phosphate** *see* Phosphate Supplements *on page 926*

## Potassium Supplements (poe TASS ee um SUP la ments)

**U.S. Brand Names** Cena-K®; Effer-K™; Gen-K®; K+® 8; K+® 10; Kaochlor®; Kaochlor-Eff; Kaon-Cl®; Kato®; Kay Ciel®; Kaylixir®; K+ Care®; K+ Care® ET; K-Dur®; K-Electrolyte®; K-G® Elixir; K-Gen®; K-Lease®; K-Lor™; Klor-Con®; Klor-Con/25®; Klorvess®; Klorvess Klyte/Cl; Klotrix®; K-lyte®; K-Lyte/Cl®; K-lyte DS; K-Norm®; Kolyum®; K-Tab®; K-Vescent®; Micro-K®; Micro-K® LS; Potasalan®; Rum-K®; S-F Kaon®; Slow-K®; Ten-K®; Tri-K®; Trikates®; Twin-K®

**Synonyms** KCl (Potassium Chloride)

**Therapeutic Category** Electrolyte Supplement; Electrolyte Supplement, Oral; Electrolyte Supplement, Parenteral

**Pregnancy Risk Factor** A

**Lactation** Enters breast milk/compatible

**Use** Potassium deficiency; treatment or prevention of hypokalemia

**Mechanism of Action/Effect** Potassium is the major cation of intracellular fluid and is essential for the conduction of nerve impulses in heart, brain, and skeletal muscle; contraction of cardiac, skeletal, and smooth muscles; and maintenance of normal renal function, acid-base balance (acetate form), carbohydrate metabolism, and gastric secretion

**Contraindications** Severe renal impairment, untreated Addison's disease, heat cramps, hyperkalemia, severe tissue trauma; solid oral dosage forms are contraindicated in patients in whom there is a structural, pathological, and/or pharmacologic cause for delay or arrest in passage through the GI tract; an oral liquid potassium preparation should be used in patients with esophageal compression or delayed gastric emptying time

**Warnings** Use with caution in patients with cardiac disease, patients receiving potassium-sparing drugs. Patients must be on a cardiac monitor during intermittent infusions. Potassium injections should be administered only in patients with adequate urine flow. Injection must be diluted before I.V. use and infused slowly (see Administration). Some oral products contain the dye tartrazine (avoid use in sensitive individuals). Pregnancy factor C.

**Drug Interactions**

**Increased Effect/Toxicity:** Potassium-sparing diuretics, salt substitutes, ACE inhibitors such as captopril and enalapril may result in increased serum potassium.

**Adverse Reactions** Adverse reactions are usually dependent on rate of elimination or serum concentration.

Cardiovascular (with rapid I.V. administration or at high serum concentrations): Arrhythmias and cardiac arrest, heart block, hypotension, bradycardia, chest pain
Central nervous system: Mental confusion
Endocrine & metabolic: Hyperkalemia, metabolic alkalosis (acetate salt)
Gastrointestinal (with oral administration): Nausea, vomiting, diarrhea, abdominal pain, GI lesions, flatulence
Local: Pain at the site of injection, phlebitis, tissue necrosis with extravasation
Neuromuscular & skeletal: Muscle weakness, paresthesia, flaccid paralysis
Respiratory: Dyspnea

**Pharmacodynamics/Kinetics**

**Half-life Elimination:** Largely by the kidneys

**Formulations**

**Potassium acetate:** Injection: 2 mEq/mL

**Potassium chloride:**

Capsule, controlled release:
Micro-K®: 600 mg [8 mEq]
K-Lease®, K-Norm®, Micro-K® 10: 750 mg [10 mEq]
Injection, concentrate: 2 mEq/mL (5 mL, 10 mL, 20 mL, 50 mL, 100 mL)
Liquid:
Cena-K®, Kaochlor®, Kaochlor® SF, Kay Ciel®, Klorvess®, Potasalan®: 20 mEq/15 mL 10% (118 mL, 480 mL, 3840 mL)
Rum-K®: 30 mEq/15 mL 15% (480 mL, 3840 mL)
Cena-K®, Kaon-Cl®: 40 mEq/15 mL 20% (480 mL, 3840 mL)
Powder:
K + Care®: 15 mEq per packet
Gen-K®, Kato®, Kay Ciel®, K + Care®, K-Lor™, Klor-Con®, Micro-K® LS: 20 mEq per packet
K + Care®, Klor-Con/25®, K-Lyte/Cl®: 25 mEq per packet
Tablet, controlled release:
Kaon-Cl®: 500 mg [6.7 mEq]
Klor-Con® 8, K+® 8, Slow-K®: 600 mg [8 mEq]
K+® 10, Kaon-Cl® 10, K-Dur® 10, Klor-Con® 10, Klotrix®, K-Tab®, Ten-K®: 750 mg [10 mEq]
K-Dur® 20: 1500 mg [20 mEq]
Tablet, extended release: 750 mg [10 mEq]

**Potassium gluconate:**

Elixir: 20 mEq/15 mL (5 mL, 10 mL, 118 mL, 480 mL, 4000 mL) (K-G® Elixir, Kaon® Elixir)
Tablet: 500 mg, 595 mg

**Potassium bicarbonate:** Tablet for oral solution: 6.5 mEq potassium, 25 mEq bicarbonate (K+ Care®, K-Electrolyte®, K-Gen®, K-Lyte, Klor-Con/EF®); 25 mEq potassium (K+Care ET)

**Potassium bicarbonate and potassium chloride:**

Granules for solution: 20 mEq potassium per packet
Tablets for solution: 20 mEq potassium (Klorvess®), 25 mEq potassium (K-Lyte/CL), 50 mEq potassium (K-Lyte/CL® 50)

**Potassium bicarbonate and potassium citrate:** Tablet for solution: 50 mEq potassium (K-Lyte® DS)

**Potassium chloride and potassium gluconate:** Solution: 6.7 mEq potassium per 5 mL (Kolyum®)

**Potassium citrate and potassium gluconate:** Solution: 6.7 mEq potassium per 5 mL (Twin-K®)

**Potassium bicarbonate, potassium chloride, and potassium citrate:** Tablet for solution: 20 mEq potassium (Kaochlor-Eff®)

**Potassium acetate, potassium bicarbonate, and potassium citrate:** Solution: 15 mEq/5 mL (Tri-K®, Trikates®)

**Dosing**

**Adults:** I.V. doses should be incorporated into the patient's maintenance I.V. fluids; intermittent I.V. potassium administration should be reserved for severe depletion situations and requires EKG monitoring. Doses listed as mEq of **potassium**. When using microencapsulated or wax matrix formulations, use no more than 20 mEq as a single dose.

Normal daily requirement: Oral, I.V.: 40-80 mEq/day
Prevention of hypokalemia during diuretic therapy: Oral: 20-40 mEq/day in 1-2 divided doses
Treatment of hypokalemia: Oral, I.V.: 40-100 mEq/day in divided doses
Treatment of hypokalemia: I.V. intermittent infusion (must be diluted prior to administration): 10-20 mEq/dose (maximum dose: 40 mEq/dose) to infuse over 2-3 hours (maximum dose: 40 mEq over 1 hour)

**Administration**

**Oral:** Sustained release and wax matrix tablets should be swallowed whole; do not crush or chew. Effervescent tablets must be dissolved in water before use. Administer

(Continued)

## Potassium Supplements *(Continued)*

with food. Granules can be diluted or dissolved in water or juice. Do not administer liquid full strength, must be diluted in 2-6 parts of water or juice.

**I.V.:** Potassium must be diluted prior to parenteral administration. Maximum recommended concentration (peripheral line): 80 mEq/L; maximum recommended concentration (central line): 150 mEq/L or 15 mEq/100 mL. In severely fluid-restricted patients (with central lines): 200 mEq/L or 20 mEq/100 mL has been used. Maximum rate of infusion, see Dosage, I.V. intermittent infusion.

**Monitoring Laboratory Tests** Serum potassium, glucose, chloride, pH, urine output (if indicated), cardiac monitor (if intermittent I.V. infusion or potassium I.V. infusion rates >0.25 mEq/kg/hour)

**Additional Nursing Issues**

**Physical Assessment:** Assess other medications patient may be taking for effectiveness and interactions (eg, antacids and ACE inhibitors - see Drug Interactions). See Contraindications and Warnings/Precautions for cautious use. Monitor laboratory tests (serum K), therapeutic response, and adverse reactions at beginning of therapy and periodically throughout therapy (see Adverse Reactions). Assess knowledge/teach patient appropriate use, interventions to reduce side effects, and adverse symptoms to report.

I.V.: Monitor infusion site regularly and cardiac status on a regular basis (continuous EKG during highly concentrated infusions). Instruct patient about adverse reactions to report.

**Patient Information/Instruction:** Oral: Take as directed; do not take more than directed. Dissolve tablet or powder in 4-6 ounces of water or juice and stir drinking. Do not chew or crush extended release capsules. Take potassium with or after meals (do not take on empty stomach). Take any antacids 2 hours before or after potassium. Consult prescriber about advisability of increasing dietary potassium. Report tingling of hands or feet; unresolved nausea or vomiting; chest pain or palpitations; persistent abdominal pain; feelings of weakness, dizziness, listlessness, confusion, acute muscle weakness or cramping; blood in stool or black or tarry stools; or easy bruising or unusual bleeding.

**Geriatric Considerations:** Elderly may require less potassium than younger adults due to decreased renal function. For elderly who do not respond to replacement therapy, check serum magnesium. Due to long-term diuretic use, elderly may be hypomagnesemic.

- **Pounds/Kilograms Conversion** *see page 1351*
- **Povidone-Iodine** *see page 1294*
- **PPA** *see* Phenylpropanolamine *on page 922*

## Pralidoxime (pra li DOKS eem)

**U.S. Brand Names** Protopam®

**Synonyms** 2-PAM; Pralidoxime Chloride; 2-Pyridine Aldoxime Methochloride

**Therapeutic Category** Antidote

**Pregnancy Risk Factor** C

**Lactation** Excretion in breast milk unknown/not recommended

**Use** Reverse muscle paralysis with toxic exposure to organophosphate anticholinesterase pesticides and chemicals; control of overdose of drugs used to treat myasthenia gravis (ambenonium, neostigmine, pyridostigmine)

**Mechanism of Action/Effect** Reactivates cholinesterase that had been inactivated by phosphorylation due to exposure to organophosphate pesticides by displacing the enzyme from its receptor sites; removes the phosphoryl group from the active site of the inactivated enzyme

**Contraindications** Hypersensitivity to pralidoxime or any component; poisonings due to phosphorus, inorganic phosphates, or organic phosphates without anticholinesterase activity

**Warnings** Use with caution in patients with myasthenia gravis. Dosage modification required in patients with impaired renal function may not be effective for treating carbamate intoxication. Use with caution in patients receiving theophylline, succinylcholine, phenothiazines, and respiratory depressants (eg, narcotics, barbiturates). Pregnancy factor C.

**Drug Interactions**

**Decreased Effect:** Atropine, although often used concurrently with pralidoxime to offset muscarinic stimulation, these effects can occur earlier than anticipated

**Increased Effect/Toxicity:** Increased effect with barbiturates (potentiated). Avoid morphine, theophylline, succinylcholine, reserpine, and phenothiazines in patients with organophosphate poisoning.

**Adverse Reactions** >10%:

Cardiovascular: Tachycardia, hypertension
Central nervous system: Dizziness, headache, drowsiness
Dermatologic: Rash
Gastrointestinal: Nausea
Local: Pain at injection site after I.M. administration
Neuromuscular & skeletal: Muscle rigidity, weakness
Ocular: Blurred vision, diplopia
Respiratory: Hyperventilation, laryngospasm

**Overdose/Toxicology** Symptoms of overdose include blurred vision, nausea, tachycardia, and dizziness. Treatment is supportive.

**Pharmacodynamics/Kinetics**

**Half-life Elimination:** 0.8-2.7 hours

**Time to Peak:** I.V.: Within 5-15 minutes

**Metabolism:** Liver; not bound to plasma proteins

**Excretion:** Urine

**Formulations**

Injection: 20 mL vial containing 1 g each pralidoxime chloride with one 20 mL ampul diluent, disposable syringe, needle, and alcohol swab

Injection, as chloride: 300 mg/mL (2 mL)

Tablet, as chloride: 500 mg

**Dosing**

**Adults:**

Poisoning: I.M. (use in conjunction with atropine - atropine effects should be established before pralidoxime is administered), I.V.: 1-2 g; repeat in 1-2 hours if muscle weakness has not been relieved, then at 10- to 12-hour intervals if cholinergic signs recur.

Mild organophosphate poisoning: Oral: Initial: 1-3 g; repeat as needed in 5 hours.

Treatment of acetylcholinesterase inhibitor toxicity: Initial: 1-2 g followed by increments of 250 mg every 5 minutes until response is observed

**Elderly:** Refer to adult dosing.

**Renal Impairment:** Dose should be reduced.

**Administration**

**I.V.:** Infuse over 15-30 minutes at a rate not to exceed 200 mg/minute. May give I.M. or S.C. if I.V. is not accessible.

**I.V. Detail:** Reconstitute with 20 mL sterile water (preservative free) resulting in 50 mg/mL solution. Dilute in normal saline 20 mg/mL and infuse over 15-30 minutes. If a more rapid onset of effect is desired or in a fluid-restricted situation, the maximum concentration is 50 mg/mL. The maximum rate of infusion is over 5 minutes.

**Additional Nursing Issues**

**Physical Assessment:**

I.M.: Monitor vital signs, blood pressure, and respiratory status on a frequent basis.

I.V.: Continuous EKG and hemodynamic monitoring. Monitor fluid balance throughout therapy (oliguria). With organophosphate poisoning or anticholinesterase overdose, monitor closely for muscle weakness or twitching, reduction in respiratory function, or altered consciousness. Keep under observation for 24-48 hours.

**Pregnancy risk factor C.** Breast-feeding is not recommended.

**Patient Information/Instruction:** When administered in emergency situation, patient education and instruction should be appropriate to patient condition. **Breast-feeding precautions:** Breast-feeding is not recommended.


- **Pralidoxime Chloride** *see* Pralidoxime *on previous page*
- **PrameGel®** *see page 1294*
- **Pramet® FA** *see* Vitamin, Multiple *on page 1219*
- **Pramidal** *see* Loperamide *on page 688*
- **Pramilet® FA** *see* Vitamin, Multiple *on page 1219*


## Pramipexole (pra mi PEX ole)

**U.S. Brand Names** Mirapex®

**Therapeutic Category** Anti-Parkinson's Agent (Dopamine Agonist)

**Pregnancy Risk Factor** C

**Lactation** Excretion in breast milk unknown/not recommended

**Use** Treatment of the signs and symptoms of idiopathic Parkinson's disease; has been evaluated for use in the treatment of depression with positive results

**Mechanism of Action/Effect** Pramipexole is a nonergot dopamine agonist with specificity for the $D_2$ dopamine receptor, but has also been shown to bind to $D_3$ and $D_4$ receptors. By binding to these receptors, it is thought that pramipexole can stimulate dopamine activity on the nerves of the striatum and substantia nigra.

**Contraindications** Hypersensitivity to pramipexole or any component

**Warnings** Caution should be taken in patients with renal insufficiency and in patients with pre-existing dyskinesias. Pathologic degeneration and loss of photoreceptor cells were observed in the retinas of albino rats during studies, however, similar changes have not been observed in the retinas of pigmented rats, mice, monkeys, or minipigs. The significance of these data for humans remains unestablished. Pregnancy risk C.

**Drug Interactions**

**Increased Effect/Toxicity:** Cimetidine increases pramipexole AUC and half-life. Levodopa levels are increased with concurrent use of pramipexole.

**Adverse Reactions**

1% to 10%:

Cardiovascular: Edema, postural hypotension, syncope, tachycardia, chest pain

Central nervous system: Malaise, fever, dizziness, somnolence, insomnia, hallucinations, confusion, amnesia, dystonias, akathisia, thinking abnormalities, myoclonus, headache

Endocrine & metabolic: Decreased libido

Gastrointestinal: Nausea, constipation, anorexia, dysphagia, xerostomia

Genitourinary: Urinary frequency (up to 3%)

Neuromuscular & skeletal: Weakness, muscle twitching, leg cramps

Ocular: Vision abnormalities (3%)

<1% (Limited to important or life-threatening symptoms): Elevated liver transaminase levels

(Continued)

## Pramipexole *(Continued)*

**Pharmacodynamics/Kinetics**

**Protein Binding:** 15%

**Half-life Elimination:** ~8 hours (12-14 hours in the elderly)

**Time to Peak:** Within 2 hours

**Excretion:** Urine, 90% recovered as unmetabolized drug

**Formulations** Tablet: 0.125 mg, 0.25 mg, 1 mg, 1.5 mg

**Dosing**

**Adults:** Oral: Initial: 0.375 mg/day given in 3 divided doses, increase gradually by 0.125 mg/dose every 5-7 days; range: 1.5-4.5 mg/day.

**Elderly:** Refer to adult dosing.

**Administration**

**Oral:** Doses should be titrated gradually in all patients to avoid the onset of intolerable side effects. The dosage should be increased to achieve a maximum therapeutic effect, balanced against the side effects of dyskinesia, hallucinations, somnolence, and dry mouth.

**Additional Nursing Issues**

**Physical Assessment:** Monitor for improvement in symptoms of Parkinson's disease (eg, mentation, behavior, daily living activities, motor examinations), blood pressure, body weight changes, and heart rate. **Pregnancy risk factor C** - benefits of use should outweigh possible risks. Breast-feeding is not recommended.

**Patient Information/Instruction:** Do not take other medications, including over-the-counter products without consulting prescriber (especially important are other medicines that could make you sleepy such as sleeping pills, tranquilizers, some cold and allergy medicines, narcotic pain killers, or medicines that relax muscles). Avoid alcohol as this may increase the potential for drowsiness or sedation. **Pregnancy/breast-feeding precautions:** Inform prescriber if you are or intend to be pregnant. Breast-feeding is not recommended.

**Dietary Issues:** Food intake does not affect the extent of drug absorption, although the time to maximal plasma concentration is delayed by 60 minutes when taken with a meal

♦ **Pramotil** *see* Metoclopramide *on page 758*

♦ **Pramoxine** *see page 1294*

♦ **Prandin®** *see* Repaglinide *on page 1011*

♦ **Pravachol®** *see* Pravastatin *on this page*

## Pravastatin (PRA va stat in)

**U.S. Brand Names** Pravachol®

**Therapeutic Category** Antilipemic Agent (HMG-CoA Reductase Inhibitor)

**Pregnancy Risk Factor** X

**Lactation** Enters breast milk/contraindicated

**Use** Adjunct to diet for the reduction of elevated total and LDL cholesterol levels in patients with hypercholesterolemia (Type IIa, IIb, and IIc); used in hypercholesterolemic patients without clinically evident heart disease to reduce the risk of myocardial infarction, to reduce the risk for revascularization, and to reduce the risk of death due to cardiovascular causes with no increase in death from noncardiovascular diseases; reduce triglyceride levels; reduce risk of myocardial infarction, stroke, or revascularization in patients with previous MI and normal cholesterol levels

**Mechanism of Action/Effect** Pravastatin is a competitive inhibitor of 3-hydroxy-3-methylglutaryl coenzyme A (HMG-CoA) reductase, which is the rate-limiting enzyme involved in *de novo* cholesterol synthesis.

**Contraindications** Hypersensitivity to pravastatin; active liver disease or persistent, unexplained liver function enzyme elevations; pregnancy

**Warnings** May elevate aminotransferases. Can also cause myalgia and rhabdomyolysis. Use with caution in patients who consume large quantities of alcohol or who have a history of liver disease.

**Drug Interactions**

**Cytochrome P-450 Effect:** CYP3A3/4 enzyme substrate

**Increased Effect/Toxicity:** Cholestyramine in combination with pravastatin (separate administration times) may increase the therapeutic effect. Gemfibrozil or clofibrate in combination with pravastatin may increase adverse effects or toxicity. Itraconazole increases serum concentrations. No effect on prothrombin time was noted in patients stabilized on warfarin.

**Adverse Reactions**

1% to 10%:

Central nervous system: Headache, dizziness

Dermatologic: Rash

Gastrointestinal: Vomiting, flatulence, abdominal pain, diarrhea, constipation, nausea, heartburn

Neuromuscular & skeletal: Myalgia, elevated creatine phosphokinase (CPK)

Hepatic: Elevated ALT/AST

<1% (Limited to important or life-threatening symptoms): Chest pain

**Overdose/Toxicology** Very little adverse events. Treatment is symptomatic.

**Pharmacodynamics/Kinetics**

**Half-life Elimination:** ~77 hours for parent and metabolites

**Time to Peak:** 1-1.5 hours

**Metabolism:** Liver

**Excretion:** Up to 20% excreted in urine (8% unchanged); 70% in feces

**Onset:** Several days

**Formulations** Tablet, as sodium: 10 mg, 20 mg, 40 mg

**Dosing**

**Adults:** Oral: 10-20 mg once daily at bedtime, may increase to 40 mg/day at bedtime

**Elderly:** Refer to adult dosing.

**Administration**

**Oral:** May be taken without regard to meals. Take at bedtime.

**Monitoring Laboratory Tests** Obtain baseline LFTs and total cholesterol profile; creatine phosphokinase due to possibility of myopathy. Repeat tests 6 and 12 weeks after initiation of therapy and periodically thereafter.

**Additional Nursing Issues**

**Physical Assessment:** Assess other medications patient may be taking for effectiveness and/or interactions (see Drug Interactions). Assess knowledge/instruct patient on appropriate use, possible side effects (see Adverse Reactions), and symptoms to report. **Pregnancy risk factor X** - determine that patient is not pregnant before beginning treatment and do not give to women of childbearing age or to males who may have intercourse with women of childbearing age unless both male and female are capable of complying with barrier contraceptive measures during therapy and for 1 month following therapy. Breast-feeding is contraindicated.

**Patient Information/Instruction:** Take at bedtime since highest rate of cholesterol synthesis occurs between midnight and 5 AM. Do not change dosage without consulting prescriber. Maintain diet and exercise program as as prescribed. Have periodic ophthalmic exam while taking pravastatin (check for cataracts). You may experience mild GI disturbances (gas, diarrhea, constipation); inform prescriber if these are severe, or if you experience severe muscle pain or tenderness accompanied with malaise, blurred vision, or chest pain. **Pregnancy/breast-feeding precautions:** Inform prescriber if you are pregnant. Do not get pregnant during or for 1 month following therapy. Male: Do not cause a female to become pregnant. Male/female: Consult prescriber for instruction on appropriate barrier contraceptive measures. This drug may cause severe fetal defects. Do not breast-feed.

**Dietary Issues:** Before initiation of therapy, patients should be placed on a standard cholesterol-lowering diet for 3-6 months and the diet should be continued during drug therapy.

**Geriatric Considerations:** Effective and well tolerated in the elderly. The definition of and, therefore, when to treat hyperlipidemia in the elderly is a controversial issue. The National Cholesterol Education Program recommends that all adults 20 years of age and older maintain a plasma cholesterol <200 mg/dL. By this definition, 60% of all elderly would be considered to have a borderline high (200-239 mg/dL) or high (≥240 mg/dL) plasma cholesterol. However, plasma cholesterol has been shown to be a less reliable predictor of coronary heart disease in the elderly. Therefore, it is the authors' belief that pharmacologic treatment be reserved for those who are unable to obtain a desirable plasma cholesterol level by diet alone and for whom the benefits of treatment are believed to outweigh the potential adverse effects, drug interactions, and cost of treatment.

**Related Information**

Lipid-Lowering Agents Comparison *on page 1393*

♦ **Prax®** *see page 1294*

♦ **Prazidec** *see* Omeprazole *on page 851*

## Praziquantel (pray zi KWON tel)

**U.S. Brand Names** Biltricide®

**Therapeutic Category** Anthelmintic

**Pregnancy Risk Factor** B

**Lactation** Enters breast milk

**Use** All stages of schistosomiasis caused by all *Schistosoma* species pathogenic to humans; clonorchiasis, opisthorchiasis, cysticercosis, and many intestinal tapeworms

**Mechanism of Action/Effect** Increases the cell permeability to calcium in schistosomes, causing strong contractions and paralysis of worm musculature leading to detachment of suckers from the blood vessel walls and to dislodgment

**Contraindications** Hypersensitivity to praziquantel; ocular cysticercosis

**Warnings** Use caution in patients with severe hepatic disease. Patients with cerebral cysticercosis require hospitalization.

**Adverse Reactions** 1% to 10%:

Central nervous system: Dizziness, drowsiness, headache, malaise, CSF reaction syndrome in patients being treated for neurocysticercosis, fever

Gastrointestinal: Abdominal pain, anorexia, nausea, vomiting, diarrhea

Miscellaneous: Sweating

**Overdose/Toxicology** Symptoms of overdose include dizziness, drowsiness, headache, and liver function impairment. Treatment is supportive. Give fast-acting laxative.

(Continued)

## Praziquantel *(Continued)*

**Pharmacodynamics/Kinetics**

**Protein Binding:** ~80%

**Distribution:** CSF concentration is 14% to 20% of plasma concentration

**Half-life Elimination:** Parent drug: 0.8-1.5 hours; Metabolites: 4.5 hours

**Time to Peak:** Within 1-3 hours

**Metabolism:** Liver

**Excretion:** Urine

**Formulations** Tablet, tri-scored: 600 mg

**Dosing**

**Adults:** Oral:

Schistosomiasis: 20 mg/kg/dose 2-3 times/day for 1 day at 4- to 6-hour intervals
Flukes: 25 mg/kg/dose every 8 hours for 1-2 days
Cysticercosis: 50 mg/kg/day divided every 8 hours for 14 days
Tapeworms: 10-20 mg/kg as a single dose (25 mg/kg for *Hymenolepis nana*)

**Elderly:** Refer to adult dosing.

**Administration**

**Oral:** Tablets may be halved or quartered.

**Monitoring Laboratory Tests** Culture urine or feces for ova prior to instituting therapy.

**Additional Nursing Issues**

**Physical Assessment:** See Warnings/Precautions and Contraindications for use cautions. Worm infestations are easily transmitted, all close family members should be treated. Instruct patient/caregiver on appropriate use, transmission prevention, possible side effects and appropriate interventions, and adverse symptoms to report.

**Patient Information/Instruction:** Take exactly as directed for full course of medication. Tablets may be chewed, swallowed whole, or crushed and mixed with food. Increase dietary intake of fruit juices. All family members and close friends should also be treated. To reduce possibility of reinfection, wash hands and scrub nails carefully with soap and hot water before handling food, before eating, and before and after toileting. Keep hands out of mouth. Disinfect toilet daily and launder bed lines, undergarments, and nightclothes daily with hot water and soap. Do not go barefoot and do not sit directly on grass or ground. May cause dizziness, fainting, lightheadedness (use caution when driving or engaging in tasks that require alertness until response to drug is known); abdominal pain, nausea, or vomiting (frequent small meals, frequent mouth care, sucking lozenges, or chewing gum may help). Report unusual fatigue, persistent dizziness, CNS changes, change in color of urine or stool, or easy bruising or unusual bleeding.

## Prazosin (PRA zoe sin)

**U.S. Brand Names** Minipress®

**Synonyms** Furazosin

**Therapeutic Category** $Alpha_1$ Blockers

**Pregnancy Risk Factor** C

**Lactation** Excretion in breast milk unknown

**Use** Treatment of hypertension, severe congestive heart failure (in conjunction with diuretics and cardiac glycosides); reduce mortality in stable postmyocardial patients with left ventricular dysfunction (ejection fraction ≤40%)

**Unlabeled use:** Symptoms of benign prostatic hypertrophy

**Mechanism of Action/Effect** Competitively inhibits postsynaptic alpha-adrenergic receptors which results in vasodilation of veins and arterioles and a decrease in total peripheral resistance and blood pressure

**Contraindications** Hypersensitivity to prazosin, other alpha adrenergic antagonists, or any component

**Warnings** Marked orthostatic hypotension, syncope, and loss of consciousness may occur with first dose ("first dose phenomenon") and occurs more often in patients receiving beta-blockers, diuretics, low sodium diets, or larger first doses (ie, >1 mg/dose in adults). Avoid rapid increase in dose. Use with caution in patients with renal impairment. Pregnancy factor C.

**Drug Interactions**

**Decreased Effect:** Decreased antihypertensive effect if taken with NSAIDs.

**Increased Effect/Toxicity:** Increased hypotensive effect if taken with diuretics and antihypertensive medications (especially beta-blockers).

**Food Interactions** Food has variable effects on absorption.

**Effects on Lab Values** Increased urinary UMA 17%, norepinephrine metabolite 42%

**Adverse Reactions**

>10%:

Cardiovascular: Orthostatic hypotension
Central nervous system: Dizziness, lightheadedness, drowsiness, headache, malaise

1% to 10%:

Cardiovascular: Edema, palpitations
Central nervous system: Fatigue, nervousness
Gastrointestinal: Dry mouth
Genitourinary: Urinary incontinence

<1% (Limited to important or life-threatening symptoms): Chest pain, dyspnea

**Overdose/Toxicology** Symptoms of overdose include hypotension and drowsiness. Treatment is otherwise supportive and symptomatic.

**Pharmacodynamics/Kinetics**

**Protein Binding:** 92% to 97%

**Half-life Elimination:** 2-4 hours; increased with congestive heart failure

**Metabolism:** Liver

**Excretion:** 6% to 10% excreted renally as unchanged drug

**Onset:** Onset of hypotensive effect: Within 2 hours; Maximum decrease: 2-4 hours

**Duration:** 10-24 hours

**Formulations** Capsule, as hydrochloride: 1 mg, 2 mg, 5 mg

**Dosing**

**Adults:**

CHF, hypertension: Initial: 1 mg/dose 2-3 times/day; usual maintenance dose: 3-15 mg/day in divided doses 2-4 times/day; maximum daily dose: 20 mg

Hypertensive urgency: 10-20 mg once, may repeat in 30 minutes

Raynaud's: 0.5-3 mg twice daily

Benign prostatic hypertrophy: 2 mg twice daily

**Elderly:** Oral (first dose given at bedtime): Initial: 1 mg 1-2 times/day

**Additional Nursing Issues**

**Physical Assessment:** Assess effectiveness and interactions of other medications (see Drug Interactions). See Contraindications and Warnings/Precautions for use cautions. Monitor for effectiveness of therapy (blood pressure supine and standing) and adverse reactions (see Adverse Reactions and Overdose/Toxicology) at beginning of therapy and on a regular basis with long-term therapy. Assess knowledge/ teach patient appropriate use, possible side effects/interventions, and adverse symptoms to report. When discontinuing, monitor blood pressure and taper dose and frequency. **Pregnancy risk factor C** - contraceptive education may be indicated. Note breast-feeding caution.

**Patient Information/Instruction:** Take as directed (first dose at bedtime). Do not skip dose or discontinue without consulting prescriber. Follow recommended diet and exercise program. Do not use alcohol or OTC medications which may affect blood pressure (eg, cough or cold remedies, diet pills, stay-awake medications) without consulting physician. You may experience drowsiness, dizziness, or impaired judgment (use caution when driving or engaging in tasks that require alertness until response to drug is known); postural hypotension (use caution when rising from sitting or lying position or when climbing stairs); dry mouth or nausea (frequent mouth care or sucking lozenges may help); or urinary incontinence (void before taking medication). Report altered CNS status (eg, fatigue, lethargy, confusion, nervousness); sudden weight gain (weigh yourself in the same clothes at the same time of day once a week); unusual or persistent swelling of ankles, feet, or extremities; palpitations or rapid heartbeat; difficulty breathing; or other persistent side effects. **Pregnancy/breast-feeding precautions:** Inform prescriber if you are or intend to be pregnant - contraceptive use may be recommended. Consult prescriber if breast-feeding.

**Geriatric Considerations:** See Warnings/Precautions and Pharmacokinetics. Adverse effects such as dry mouth and urinary problems can be particularly bothersome in the elderly.

## Prazosin and Polythiazide (PRA zoe sin & pol i THYE a zide)

**U.S. Brand Names** Minizide®

**Synonyms** Polythiazide and Prazosin

**Therapeutic Category** Antihypertensive Agent, Combination

**Pregnancy Risk Factor** C

**Lactation** Excretion in breast milk unknown

**Use** Management of mild to moderate hypertension

**Formulations**

Capsule:

1: Prazosin 1 mg and polythiazide 0.5 mg

2: Prazosin 2 mg and polythiazide 0.5 mg

5: Prazosin 5 mg and polythiazide 0.5 mg

**Dosing**

**Adults:** Oral: Initial: 1 capsule 2-3 times/day; maintenance: May be slowly increased to a total daily dose of 20 mg. Therapeutic dosages often used range from 6-15 mg in divided doses.

**Elderly:** Refer to adult dosing.

**Additional Nursing Issues**

**Physical Assessment:** See individual components listed in Related Information. **Pregnancy risk factor C** - benefits of use should outweigh possible risks. Note breast-feeding caution.

**Patient Information/Instruction:** See individual components listed in Related Information. **Pregnancy/breast-feeding precautions:** Inform prescriber if you are on intend to get pregnant. Consult prescriber if breast-feeding.

**Related Information**

Prazosin *on previous page*


- **Precaptil** *see* Captopril *on page 192*
- **Precose®** *see* Acarbose *on page 29*
- **Pred Forte®** *see page 1282*
- **Pred Forte® Ophthalmic** *see* Prednisolone *on next page*
- **Pred-G®** *see page 1282*
- **Pred-G® SOP®** *see page 1282*
- **Pred Mild®** *see page 1282*

♦ **Pred Mild® Ophthalmic** *see* Prednisolone *on this page*

♦ **Prednicarbate** *see* Topical Corticosteroids *on page 1152*

♦ **Prednicen-M®** *see* Prednisone *on page 962*

## Prednisolone (pred NIS oh lone)

**U.S. Brand Names** AK-Pred® Ophthalmic; Articulose-50® Injection; Delta-Cortef® Oral; Econopred® Ophthalmic; Econopred® Plus Ophthalmic; Inflamase® Forte Ophthalmic; Inflamase® Mild Ophthalmic; Key-Pred® Injection; Key-Pred-SP® Injection; Metreton® Ophthalmic; Pediapred® Oral; Pred Forte® Ophthalmic; Pred Mild® Ophthalmic; Prednisol® TBA Injection; Prelone® Oral

**Synonyms** Deltahydrocortisone; Metacortandralone

**Therapeutic Category** Corticosteroid, Ophthalmic; Corticosteroid, Parenteral

**Pregnancy Risk Factor** C

**Lactation** Enters breast milk/compatible

**Use** Treatment of palpebral and bulbar conjunctivitis; corneal injury from chemical, radiation, thermal burns, or foreign body penetration; endocrine disorders, rheumatic disorders, collagen diseases, dermatologic diseases, allergic states, ophthalmic diseases, respiratory diseases, hematologic disorders, neoplastic diseases, edematous states, and GI diseases; useful in patients with inability to activate prednisone (liver disease)

**Mechanism of Action/Effect** Decreases inflammation by suppression of migration of polymorphonuclear leukocytes and reversal of increased capillary permeability; suppresses the immune system by reducing activity and volume of the lymphatic system

**Contraindications** Hypersensitivity to prednisolone or any component; acute superficial herpes simplex keratitis; systemic fungal infections; varicella

**Warnings** Use with caution in patients with hyperthyroidism, cirrhosis, nonspecific ulcerative colitis, hypertension, osteoporosis, thromboembolic tendencies, CHF, convulsive disorders, myasthenia gravis, thrombophlebitis, peptic ulcer, and diabetes. Acute adrenal insufficiency may occur with abrupt withdrawal after long-term therapy or with stress. Because of the risk of adverse effects, systemic corticosteroids should be used cautiously in the elderly, in the smallest possible dose, and for the shortest possible time. Pregnancy factor C.

**Drug Interactions**

**Cytochrome P-450 Effect:** CYP3A enzyme substrate; inducer of cytochrome P-450 enzymes

**Decreased Effect:** Systemic: Decreased effect or corticosteroids with barbiturates, aminoglutethimide, phenytoin, and rifampin. Decreased effect of salicylates, vaccines, and toxoids. Prednisolone may decrease the effect of isoniazid. Corticosteroids may decrease the effect of warfarin or IUD contraceptives.

**Increased Effect/Toxicity:** Systemic: The combined use of cyclosporine and prednisolone may result in elevated levels of both agents. Oral contraceptives may enhance the effect of prednisolone.

**Effects on Lab Values** Response to skin tests

**Adverse Reactions Systemic:**

>10%:
- Central nervous system: Insomnia, nervousness
- Gastrointestinal: Increased appetite, indigestion

1% to 10%:
- Central nervous system: Dizziness or lightheadedness, headache
- Dermatologic: Hirsutism, hypopigmentation
- Endocrine & metabolic: Diabetes mellitus
- Neuromuscular & skeletal: Arthralgia
- Ocular: Cataracts, glaucoma
- Respiratory: Epistaxis
- Miscellaneous: Sweating

<1% (Limited to important or life-threatening symptoms): Edema, hypertension, seizures pseudotumor cerebri, Cushing's syndrome, pituitary-adrenal axis suppression

**Overdose/Toxicology** When consumed in high doses for prolonged periods, systemic hypercorticism and adrenal suppression may occur, in those cases discontinuation of the corticosteroid should be done judiciously.

**Pharmacodynamics/Kinetics**

**Protein Binding:** I.V.: 65% to 91% (concentration dependent)

**Half-life Elimination:** I.V.: 3.6 hours; Biological: 18-36 hours; End-stage renal disease: 3-5 hours

**Metabolism:** Liver and tissue

**Excretion:** Urine

**Duration:** 18-36 hours

**Formulations**

Injection, as acetate (for I.M., intralesional, intra-articular, or soft tissue administration only): 25 mg/mL (10 mL, 30 mL); 50 mg/mL (30 mL)

Injection, as sodium phosphate (for I.M., I.V., intra-articular, intralesional, or soft tissue administration): 20 mg/mL (2 mL, 5 mL, 10 mL)

Injection, as tebutate (for intra-articular, intralesional, soft tissue administration only): 20 mg/mL (1 mL, 5 mL, 10 mL)

Liquid, oral, as sodium phosphate: 5 mg/5 mL (120 mL)

Solution, ophthalmic, as sodium phosphate: 0.125% (5 mL, 10 mL, 15 mL); 1% (5 mL, 10 mL, 15 mL)

Suspension, ophthalmic, as acetate: 0.12% (5 mL, 10 mL); 0.125% (5 mL, 10 mL, 15 mL); 1% (1 mL, 5 mL, 10 mL, 15 mL)

Syrup: 15 mg/5 mL (240 mL)

Tablet: 5 mg

**Dosing**

**Adults:** Dose depends upon condition being treated and response of patient. Consider alternate day therapy for long-term therapy. Discontinuation of long-term therapy requires gradual withdrawal by tapering the dose.

Oral, I.V., I.M. (sodium phosphate salt): 5-60 mg/day

I.M. (acetate salt): 4-60 mg/day

Rheumatoid arthritis: Oral: Initial: 5-7.5 mg/day, adjust dose as necessary

Multiple sclerosis (sodium phosphate): Oral: 200 mg/day for 1 week followed by 80 mg every other day for 1 month

Multiple sclerosis (acetate salt): I.M.: 200 mg/day for 1 week followed by 80 mg every other day for 1 month

Intra-articular, intralesional, soft-tissue administration:

Tebutate salt: 4-40 mg/dose

Acetate salt: 4-100 mg/dose

Sodium phosphate salt: 2-30 mg/dose

Ophthalmic suspension/solution: Instill 1-2 drops into conjunctival sac every hour during day, every 2 hours at night until favorable response is obtained, then use 1 drop every 4 hours.

**Elderly:** Use lowest effective adult dose. Dose depends upon condition being treated and response of patient; alternate day dosing may be attempted in some disease states.

**Renal Impairment:** Slightly dialyzable (5% to 20%)

**Administration**

**Oral:** Give oral formulation with food or milk to decrease GI effects.

**I.V.:** Do **not** give acetate or tebutate salt I.V.

**Monitoring Laboratory Tests** Blood glucose, electrolytes

**Additional Nursing Issues**

**Physical Assessment:** Assess other medications patient may be taking for effectiveness and interactions (see Drug Interactions). Note Contraindications and Warnings/Precautions for cautious use. Monitor laboratory tests, therapeutic response, and adverse effects according to indications for therapy, dose, route (systemic or topical), and duration of therapy (see Dosing, Warnings/Precautions, Adverse Reactions). With systemic administration, diabetics should monitor glucose levels closely (corticosteroids may alter glucose levels). Assess knowledge/teach patient appropriate use, interventions to reduce side effects, and adverse symptoms to report. When used for long-term therapy (longer than 10-14 days) do not discontinue abruptly; decrease dosage incrementally. **Pregnancy risk factor C** - benefits of use should outweigh possible risks.

**Patient Information/Instruction:** Take exactly as directed; do not increase dose or discontinue abruptly without consulting prescriber. Take oral medication with or after meals. Limit intake of caffeine or stimulants. Prescriber may recommend increased dietary vitamins, minerals, or iron. Diabetics should monitor glucose levels closely (antidiabetic medication may need to be adjusted). Inform prescriber if you are experiencing greater than normal levels of stress (medication may need adjustment). Some forms of this medication may cause GI upset (oral medication may be taken with meals to reduce GI upset; small frequent meals and frequent mouth care may reduce GI upset). You may be more susceptible to infection (avoid crowds and persons with contagious or infective conditions). Report promptly excessive nervousness or sleep disturbances; any signs of infection (sore throat, unhealed injuries); excessive growth of body hair or loss of skin color; changes in vision; excessive or sudden weight gain (>3 lb/week); swelling of face or extremities; difficulty breathing; muscle weakness; change in color of stools (black or tarry) or persistent abdominal pain; or worsening of condition or failure to improve. **Pregnancy precautions:** Inform prescriber if you are or intend to be pregnant.

Ophthalmic: For ophthalmic use only. Wash hands before using. Tilt head back and look upward. Put drops of suspension or apply thin ribbon of ointment inside lower eyelid. Close eye and roll eyeball in all directions. Do not blink for ½ minute. Apply gentle pressure to inner corner of eye for 30 seconds. Do not use any other eye preparation for at least 10 minutes. Do not touch tip of applicator to eye or contaminate tip of applicator. Do not share medication with anyone else. Wear sunglasses when in sunlight; you may be more sensitive to bright light. Inform prescriber if condition worsens or fails to improve or if you experience eye pain, disturbances of vision, or other adverse eye response.

**Geriatric Considerations:** Useful in patients with inability to activate prednisone (liver disease). Because of the risk of adverse effects, systemic corticosteroids should be used cautiously in the elderly, in the smallest possible dose, and for the shortest possible time.

**Additional Information** Some formulations may contain sulfites.

Sodium phosphate injection: For I.V., I.M., intra-articular, intralesional, or soft tissue administration

Tebutate injection: For intra-articular, intralesional, or soft tissue administration only

**Related Information**

Corticosteroids Comparison, Systemic Equivalencies *on page 1383*
Ophthalmic Agents *on page 1282*

- **Prednisolone and Gentamicin** *see page 1282*
- **Prednisol® TBA Injection** *see* Prednisolone *on previous page*

## Prednisone (PRED ni sone)

**U.S. Brand Names** Deltasone®; Liquid Pred®; Meticorten®; Orasone®; Prednicen-M®

**Synonyms** Deltacortisone; Deltadehydrocortisone

**Therapeutic Category** Corticosteroid, Oral

**Pregnancy Risk Factor** B

**Lactation** Enters breast milk/compatible

**Use** Treatment of a variety of diseases including adrenocortical insufficiency, hypercalcemia, rheumatic and collagen disorders; dermatologic, ocular, respiratory, gastrointestinal, and neoplastic diseases; organ transplantation and a variety of diseases including those of hematologic, allergic, inflammatory, and autoimmune in origin; not available in injectable form, prednisolone must be used

**Mechanism of Action/Effect** Decreases inflammation by suppression of migration of polymorphonuclear leukocytes and reversal of increased capillary permeability; suppresses the immune system by reducing activity and volume of the lymphatic system; suppresses adrenal function at high doses

**Contraindications** Hypersensitivity to prednisone or any component; serious infections, except septic shock or tuberculous meningitis; systemic fungal infections; varicella

**Warnings** Use with caution in patients with hypothyroidism, cirrhosis, hypertension, congestive heart failure, ulcerative colitis, thromboembolic disorders, and patients with an increased risk for peptic ulcer disease. May retard bone growth. Gradually taper dose to withdraw therapy. Because of the risk of adverse effects, systemic corticosteroids should be used cautiously in the elderly, in the smallest possible dose, and for the shortest possible time.

**Drug Interactions**

**Cytochrome P-450 Effect:** CYP3A3/4 enzyme substrate

**Decreased Effect:** Decreased effect with barbiturates, phenytoin, rifampin; decreased effect of salicylates, vaccines, and toxoids.

**Effects on Lab Values** Response to skin tests

**Adverse Reactions** In chronic, long-term use, may result in cushingoid appearance, osteoporosis, muscle weakness (proximal), and suppression of the adrenal-hypothalmic pituitary axis.

>10%:
- Central nervous system: Insomnia, nervousness
- Gastrointestinal: Increased appetite, indigestion

1% to 10%:
- Central nervous system: Dizziness or lightheadedness, headache
- Dermatologic: Hirsutism, hypopigmentation
- Endocrine & metabolic: Diabetes mellitus
- Neuromuscular & skeletal: Arthralgia
- Ocular: Cataracts, glaucoma
- Respiratory: Epistaxis
- Miscellaneous: Sweating

<1% (Limited to important or life-threatening symptoms): Edema, hypertension, seizures, Cushing's syndrome, pituitary-adrenal axis suppression

**Overdose/Toxicology** When consumed in high doses for prolonged periods, systemic hypercorticism and adrenal suppression may occur. In those cases, discontinuation of the corticosteroid should be done judiciously.

**Pharmacodynamics/Kinetics**

**Protein Binding:** 65% to 91% concentration dependent

**Half-life Elimination:** Normal renal function: 2.5-3.5 hours

**Metabolism:** Liver

**Excretion:** Urine

**Duration:** 24 hours

**Formulations**

Solution:
- Concentrate: 5 mg/mL (5 mL, 30 mL)
- Oral: 5 mg/5 mL (10 mL, 20 mL, 500 mL)

Syrup: 5 mg/5 mL (120 mL, 240 mL)

Tablet: 1 mg, 2.5 mg, 5 mg, 10 mg, 20 mg, 50 mg

**Dosing**

**Adults:** Dose depends upon condition being treated and response of patient; consider alternate day therapy for long-term therapy. Discontinuation of long-term therapy requires gradual withdrawal by tapering the dose.

Physiologic replacement: 4-5 mg/m²/day

5-60 mg/day in divided doses 1-4 times/day

**Elderly:** Refer to adult dosing; use the lowest effective dose. Oral dose depends upon condition being treated and response of patient. Alternate day dosing may be attempted.

**Renal Impairment:** Hemodialysis effects: Supplemental dose is not necessary.

**Administration**

**Oral:** Take with food to decrease GI upset.

**Monitoring Laboratory Tests** Blood glucose, electrolytes

**Additional Nursing Issues**

**Physical Assessment:** Assess effectiveness and interactions of other medications (see Drug Interactions). See Contraindications and Warnings/Precautions for use cautions. Monitor for effectiveness of therapy and adverse reactions according to dose and length of therapy. Assess knowledge/teach patient appropriate use, possible side effects/interventions, and adverse symptoms to report (ie, opportunistic infection, adrenal suppression - see Adverse Reactions and Overdose/Toxicology). Diabetics: Monitor serum glucose levels closely; corticosteroids can alter hypoglycemic requirements. Dose may need to be increased if patient is experiencing higher than normal levels of stress. When discontinuing, taper dose and frequency slowly.

**Patient Information/Instruction:** Take exactly as directed. Do not take more than prescribed dose and do not discontinue abruptly; consult prescriber. Take with or after meals. Take once-a-day dose with food in the morning. Limit intake of caffeine or stimulants. Maintain adequate nutrition; consult prescriber for possibility of special dietary recommendations. If diabetic, monitor serum glucose closely and notify prescriber of changes; this medication can alter hypoglycemic requirements. Notify prescriber if you are experiencing higher than normal levels of stress; medication may need adjustment. Periodic ophthalmic examinations will be necessary with long-term use. You will be susceptible to infection; avoid crowds or infected persons or persons with contagious diseases. You may experience insomnia or nervousness; use caution when driving or engaging in tasks requiring alertness until response to drug is known. Report weakness, change in menstrual pattern, vision changes, signs of hyperglycemia, signs of infection (eg, fever, chills, mouth sores, perianal itching, vaginal discharge), other persistent side effects, or worsening of condition.

**Geriatric Considerations:** Because of the risk of adverse effects, systemic corticosteroids should be used cautiously in the elderly, in the smallest possible dose, and for the shortest possible time.

**Related Information**

Corticosteroids Comparison, Systemic Equivalencies *on page 1383*

- **Prefrin®** *see page 1282*
- **Prefrin™ Liquifilm®** *see* Phenylephrine *on page 920*
- **Prefrin™ Ophthalmic Solution** *see* Phenylephrine *on page 920*
- **Pregnenedione** *see* Progesterone *on page 974*
- **Pregnyl®** *see* Chorionic Gonadotropin *on page 264*
- **Prelone® Oral** *see* Prednisolone *on page 960*
- **Premarin®** *see* Estrogens, Conjugated (Equine) *on page 446*
- **Premphase™** *see* Estrogens and Medroxyprogesterone *on page 445*
- **Prempro™** *see* Estrogens and Medroxyprogesterone *on page 445*
- **Prenatal Vitamins** *see* Vitamin, Multiple *on page 1219*
- **Prenavite® [OTC]** *see* Vitamin, Multiple *on page 1219*
- **Pre-Par®** *see* Ritodrine *on page 1029*
- **Prepidil® Vaginal Gel** *see* Dinoprostone *on page 379*
- **Prepulsid®** *see* Cisapride *on page 272*
- **Prescription Strength Desenex® [OTC]** *see* Miconazole *on page 767*
- **Presoken** *see* Diltiazem *on page 377*
- **Presoquim** *see* Diltiazem *on page 377*
- **Pressyn®** *see* Vasopressin *on page 1205*
- **PreSun® 29** *see page 1294*
- **Pretz®** *see page 1294*
- **Pretz-D® [OTC]** *see* Ephedrine *on page 422*
- **Prevacid®** *see* Lansoprazole *on page 655*
- **Prevalite®** *see* Cholestyramine Resin *on page 262*
- **PreviDent®** *see page 1294*
- **Prevpac®** *see* Lansoprazole, Amoxicillin, and Clarithromycin *on page 656*
- **Priftin®** *see* Rifapentine *on page 1022*
- **Prilocaine and Lidocaine** *see* Lidocaine and Prilocaine *on page 677*
- **Prilosec™** *see* Omeprazole *on page 851*
- **Primaclone** *see* Primidone *on next page*
- **Primacor®** *see* Milrinone *on page 772*

## Primaquine (PRIM a kween)

**Synonyms** Prymaccone

**Therapeutic Category** Aminoquinoline (Antimalarial)

**Pregnancy Risk Factor** C

**Lactation** Excretion in breast milk unknown

**Use** Provides radical cure of *P. vivax* or *P. ovale* malaria after a clinical attack has been confirmed by blood smear or serologic titer and postexposure prophylaxis

**Mechanism of Action/Effect** Eliminates the primary tissue exoerythrocytic forms of *P. falciparum*; disrupts mitochondria and binds to DNA

**Contraindications** Acutely ill patients who have a tendency to develop granulocytopenia (rheumatoid arthritis, SLE); patients receiving other drugs capable of depressing the bone marrow; patients receiving quinacrine

**Warnings** Use with caution in patients with G-6-PD deficiency, NADH methemoglobin reductase deficiency. Do not exceed recommended dosage. Pregnancy factor C.

**Drug Interactions**

**Increased Effect/Toxicity:** Increased toxicity/levels with quinacrine.

**Adverse Reactions**

>10%:

Gastrointestinal: Abdominal pain, nausea, vomiting

Hematologic: Hemolytic anemia

1% to 10%: Hematologic: Methemoglobinemia

(Continued)

## Primaquine *(Continued)*

<1% (Limited to important or life-threatening symptoms): Arrhythmias, leukopenia, agranulocytosis, leukocytosis

**Overdose/Toxicology** Symptoms of acute overdose include abdominal cramps, vomiting, cyanosis, methemoglobinemia (possibly severe), leukopenia, acute hemolytic anemia (often significant), and granulocytopenia. With chronic overdose, symptoms include ototoxicity and retinopathy. Treatment is supportive.

**Pharmacodynamics/Kinetics**

**Half-life Elimination:** 3.7-9.6 hours

**Time to Peak:** Within 1-2 hours

**Metabolism:** Liver

**Excretion:** Urine

**Formulations** Tablet, as phosphate: 26.3 mg [15 mg base]

**Dosing**

**Adults:** Oral: 15 mg/day (base) once daily for 14 days or 45 mg base once weekly for 8 weeks

**Administration**

**Oral:** Take with meals to decrease adverse GI effects. Drug has a bitter taste.

**Monitoring Laboratory Tests** Periodic CBC, visual color check of urine, glucose, electrolytes; if hemolysis suspected - CBC, haptoglobin, peripheral smear, urinalysis dipstick for occult blood

**Additional Nursing Issues**

**Physical Assessment:** See Contraindications and Warnings/Precautions for use cautions. Monitor effectiveness of therapy (according to purpose for therapy), laboratory tests (see Monitoring Laboratory Tests), and adverse response (see Adverse Reactions and Overdose/Toxicology). Assess knowledge/teach patient appropriate use, possible side effects/interventions, and adverse symptoms to report. **Pregnancy risk factor C** - benefits of use should outweigh possible risks. Note breast-feeding caution.

**Patient Information/Instruction:** It is important to complete full course of therapy for full effect. May be taken with meals to decrease GI upset and bitter aftertaste. Avoid alcohol. You should have regular ophthalmic exams (every 4-6 months) if using this medication over extended periods. You may experience nausea, vomiting, or loss of appetite (small frequent meals, frequent mouth care, sucking lozenges, or chewing gum may help). Report persistent GI disturbance, chest pain or palpitation, unusual fatigue, easy bruising or bleeding, visual or hearing disturbances, changes in urine (darkening, tinged with red, decreased volume), or any other persistent adverse reactions. **Pregnancy/breast-feeding precautions:** Inform prescriber if you are or intend to be pregnant, contraception may be recommended. Consult prescriber if breast-feeding.

**Additional Information** Primaquine phosphate 26.3 mg = primaquine base 15 mg

- **Primaquine and Chloroquine** *see* Chloroquine and Primaquine *on page 252*
- **Primatene® Mist [OTC]** *see* Epinephrine *on page 424*
- **Primaxin®** *see* Imipenem and Cilastatin *on page 599*

## Primidone (PRI mi done)

**U.S. Brand Names** Mysoline®

**Synonyms** Desoxyphenobarbital; Primaclone

**Therapeutic Category** Anticonvulsant, Miscellaneous; Barbiturate

**Pregnancy Risk Factor** D

**Lactation** Enters breast milk/not recommended (AAP recommends "with caution")

**Use** Management of grand mal, complex partial, and focal seizures

**Unlabeled use:** Benign familial tremor (essential tremor)

**Mechanism of Action/Effect** Decreases neuron excitability, raises seizure threshold similar to phenobarbital; primidone has two active metabolites, phenobarbital and phenylethylmalonamide (PEMA); PEMA may enhance the activity of phenobarbital

**Contraindications** Hypersensitivity to primidone, phenobarbital, or any component; porphyria; pregnancy

**Warnings** Use with caution in patients with renal or hepatic impairment, or pulmonary insufficiency. Abrupt withdrawal may precipitate status epilepticus.

**Drug Interactions**

**Cytochrome P-450 Effect:** CYP1A2, 2B6, 2C, 2C8, 3A3/4, and 3A5-7 enzyme inducer

**Decreased Effect:** Primidone may decrease serum concentrations of ethosuximide, valproic acid, or griseofulvin. Phenytoin may decrease primidone serum concentrations.

**Increased Effect/Toxicity:** Methylphenidate may increase primidone serum concentrations. Valproic acid may increase phenobarbital concentrations derived from primidone.

**Effects on Lab Values** ↑ alkaline phosphatase (S); ↓ calcium (S)

**Adverse Reactions**

>10%: Central nervous system: Dizziness, vertigo, ataxia, lethargy, behavior change, sedation, headache

1% to 10%:

Central nervous system: Drowsiness, mood changes
Gastrointestinal: Nausea, vomiting, anorexia
Genitourinary: Impotence

<1% (Limited to important or life-threatening symptoms): Leukopenia, malignant lymphoma-like syndrome, megaloblastic anemia, systemic lupus-like syndrome

**Overdose/Toxicology** Symptoms of overdose include unsteady gait, slurred speech, confusion, jaundice, hypothermia, fever, hypotension, coma, and respiratory arrest. Assure adequate hydration and renal function. Urinary alkalinization with I.V. sodium bicarbonate also helps to enhance elimination. Repeat oral doses of activated charcoal significantly reduce the half-life of primidone through nonrenal elimination. Hemodialysis or hemoperfusion is of uncertain value. Patients in stage IV coma due to high serum drug levels may require charcoal hemoperfusion.

**Pharmacodynamics/Kinetics**

**Protein Binding:** 99%

**Half-life Elimination:** Age dependent: Primidone: 10-12 hours; PEMA: 16 hours; Phenobarbital: 52-118 hours

**Time to Peak:** Oral: Within 4 hours

**Metabolism:** Liver

**Excretion:** Urine

**Formulations**

Suspension, oral: 250 mg/5 mL (240 mL)

Tablet: 50 mg, 250 mg

**Dosing**

**Adults:** Oral: Initial: 125-250 mg/day at bedtime; increase by 125-250 mg/day every 3-7 days; usual dose: 750-1500 mg/day in divided doses 3-4 times/day with maximum dosage of 2 g/day

**Elderly:** Refer to adult dosing.

**Renal Impairment:**

$Cl_{cr}$ 50-80 mL/minute: Administer every 8 hours.

$Cl_{cr}$ 10-50 mL/minute: Administer every 8-12 hours.

$Cl_{cr}$ <10 mL/minute: Administer every 12-24 hours.

Moderately dialyzable (20% to 50%)

Administer dose postdialysis or administer supplemental 30% dose.

**Hepatic Impairment:** Increased side effects may occur in severe liver disease. Monitor plasma levels and adjust dose accordingly.

**Stability**

**Storage:** Protect from light.

**Monitoring Laboratory Tests** Serum primidone and phenobarbital concentration, CBC. Monitor CBC at 6-month intervals to compare with baseline obtained at start of therapy. Since elderly patients metabolize phenobarbital at a slower rate than younger adults, it is suggested to measure both primidone and phenobarbital levels together.

**Additional Nursing Issues**

**Physical Assessment:** Assess effectiveness and interactions of other medications patient may be taking (see Contraindications and Drug Interactions). Monitor for therapeutic response (seizure activity, force, type, duration), laboratory values, and adverse reactions (see Adverse Reactions) at beginning of therapy and periodically with long-term use. Observe and teach seizure/safety precautions. Taper dosage slowly when discontinuing. Assess knowledge/teach patient appropriate use, interventions to reduce side effects, and adverse symptoms to report. **Pregnancy risk factor D** - assess knowledge/instruct patient on need to use appropriate contraceptive measures and the need to avoid pregnancy. Breast-feeding is not recommended.

**Patient Information/Instruction:** Take exactly as directed (do not increase dose or frequency or discontinue without consulting prescriber); may cause physical and/or psychological dependence. While using this medication, do not use alcohol and other prescription or OTC medications (especially pain medications, sedatives, antihistamines, or hypnotics) without consulting prescriber. Maintain adequate hydration (2-3 L/day of fluids unless instructed to restrict fluid intake). You may experience drowsiness, dizziness, or blurred vision (use caution when driving or engaging in tasks requiring alertness until response to drug is known); nausea, vomiting, or loss of appetite (small frequent meals, frequent mouth care, chewing gum, or sucking lozenges may help); impotence (reversible). Wear identification of epileptic status and medications. Report behavioral or CNS changes (confusion, depression, increased sedation, excitation, headache, insomnia, or lethargy); muscle weakness, or tremors; unusual bruising or bleeding (mouth, urine, stool); worsening of seizure activity, or loss of seizure control. **Pregnancy/breast-feeding precautions:** Do not get pregnant while taking this drug; use appropriate barrier contraceptive measures. Breast-feeding is not recommended.

**Geriatric Considerations:** Due to CNS effects, monitor closely when initiating drug in the elderly. Since elderly metabolize phenobarbital at a slower rate than younger adults, it is suggested to measure both primidone and phenobarbital levels together. Adjust dose for renal function in the elderly when initiating or changing dose.

**Related Information**

Peak and Trough Guidelines *on page 1331*

Phenobarbital *on page 917*

♦ **Primolut® Depot** *see* Hydroxyprogesterone *on page 585*

♦ **Principen®** *see* Ampicillin *on page 90*

♦ **Prinivil®** *see* Lisinopril *on page 681*

♦ **Prinzide® 10-12.5** *see* Lisinopril and Hydrochlorothiazide *on page 683*

♦ **Prinzide® 20-12.5** *see* Lisinopril and Hydrochlorothiazide *on page 683*

♦ **Prinzide® 20-25** *see* Lisinopril and Hydrochlorothiazide *on page 683*

♦ **Privine®** *see page 1282*

♦ **Privine® Nasal** *see page 1294*

- ♦ **ProAmatine®** *see* Midodrine *on page 770*
- ♦ **Pro-Amox®** *see* Amoxicillin *on page 80*
- ♦ **Pro-Ampi® Trihydrate** *see* Ampicillin *on page 90*
- ♦ **Proaqua®** *see* Benzthiazide *on page 144*
- ♦ **Proartinal** *see* Ibuprofen *on page 592*
- ♦ **Proavil** *see* Amitriptyline and Perphenazine *on page 75*
- ♦ **Probalan®** *see* Probenecid *on this page*
- ♦ **Pro-Banthine®** *see* Propantheline *on page 983*
- ♦ **Proben-C®** *see* Colchicine and Probenecid *on page 302*


## Probenecid (proe BEN e sid)

**U.S. Brand Names** Benemid®; Probalan®

**Therapeutic Category** Uricosuric Agent

**Pregnancy Risk Factor** B

**Lactation** Excretion in breast milk unknown

**Use** Prevention of gouty arthritis; hyperuricemia; prolongation of beta-lactam effect (eg, serum levels)

**Mechanism of Action/Effect** Competitively inhibits the reabsorption of uric acid at the proximal convoluted tubule, thereby promoting its excretion and reducing serum uric acid levels; increases plasma levels of weak organic acids (penicillins, cephalosporins, or other beta-lactam antibiotics) by competitively inhibiting their renal tubular secretion

**Contraindications** Hypersensitivity to probenecid or any component; high-dose aspirin therapy; moderate to severe renal impairment; children <2 years of age

**Warnings** Use with caution in patients with peptic ulcer. Use extreme caution in the use of probenecid with penicillin in patients with renal insufficiency. Probenecid may not be effective in patients with a creatinine clearance <30-50 mL/minute. May cause exacerbation of acute gouty attack.

**Drug Interactions**

**Decreased Effect:** Salicylates (high-dose) may decrease uricosuria. Decreased urinary levels of nitrofurantoin may decrease efficacy.

**Increased Effect/Toxicity:** Increases methotrexate toxic potential. Combination with diflunisal has resulted in 40% decrease in its clearance and as much as a 65% increase in plasma concentrations due to inhibition of diflunisal metabolism. Probenecid decreases clearance of beta-lactams such as penicillins and cephalosporins. Also increases acyclovir, thiopental, benzodiazepines, dapsone, sulfonylureas, zidovudine. Avoid concomitant use with ketorolac since its half-life is increased twofold with serum levels and toxicity significantly increased.

**Effects on Lab Values** False-positive glucosuria with Clinitest®

**Adverse Reactions**

>10%:
- Central nervous system: Headache
- Gastrointestinal: Anorexia, nausea, vomiting
- Neuromuscular & skeletal: Gouty arthritis (acute)

1% to 10%:
- Cardiovascular: Flushing of face
- Central nervous system: Dizziness
- Dermatologic: Rash, itching
- Gastrointestinal: Sore gums
- Genitourinary: Painful urination
- Renal: Renal calculi

<1% (Limited to important or life-threatening symptoms): Leukopenia, hemolytic anemia, aplastic anemia, hepatic necrosis, nephrotic syndrome

**Overdose/Toxicology** Symptoms of overdose include nausea, vomiting, tonic-clonic seizures, and coma. Activated charcoal is especially effective at binding probenecid, for GI decontamination.

**Pharmacodynamics/Kinetics**

**Half-life Elimination:** Normal renal function: 6-12 hours and is dose dependent

**Time to Peak:** 2-4 hours

**Metabolism:** Liver

**Excretion:** Urine

**Onset:** Effect on penicillin levels reached in about 2 hours

**Formulations** Tablet: 500 mg

**Dosing**

**Adults:** Oral:
- Hyperuricemia with gout: 250 mg twice daily for 1 week; increase to 250-500 mg/day; may increase by 500 mg/month, if needed, to maximum of 2-3 g/day (dosages may be increased by 500 mg every 6 months if serum urate concentrations are controlled)
- Prolong penicillin serum levels: 500 mg 4 times/day
- Gonorrhea: 1 g 30 minutes before penicillin, ampicillin, or amoxicillin

**Elderly:** Refer to adult dosing.

**Renal Impairment:** $Cl_{cr}$ <50 mL/minute: Avoid use.

**Monitoring Laboratory Tests** Uric acid, renal function, CBC

**Additional Nursing Issues**

**Physical Assessment:** Assess effectiveness and interactions of other medications patient may be taking (see Contraindications and Drug Interactions). Monitor for therapeutic response (eg, frequency and severity of gouty attacks), laboratory values, and adverse reactions (see Adverse Reactions and Overdose/Toxicology) at beginning of therapy and periodically with long-term use. Assess knowledge/teach patient appropriate use, interventions to reduce side effects, and adverse symptoms to report. Note breast-feeding caution.

**Patient Information/Instruction:** Take as directed; do not discontinue without consulting prescriber. May take 6-12 months to reduce gouty attacks (attacks may increase in frequency and severity for first few months of therapy). Take with food or antacids or alkaline ash foods (milk, nuts, beets, spinach, turnip greens). Maintain adequate hydration (2-3 L/day of fluids unless instructed to restrict fluid intake). Avoid aspirin, or aspirin-containing substances. Diabetics should use serum glucose monitoring. If you experience severe headache, contact prescriber for medication. You may experience dizziness or lightheadedness (use caution when driving, changing position, or engaging in tasks requiring alertness until response to drug is known); nausea, vomiting, indigestion, or loss of appetite (small frequent meals, frequent mouth care, chewing gum, or sucking lozenges may help). Report skin rash or itching, persistent headache, blood in urine or painful urination, excessive tiredness or easy bruising or bleeding, or sore gums. **Breast-feeding precautions:** Consult prescriber if breast-feeding.

**Geriatric Considerations:** Since probenecid loses its effectiveness when the $Cl_{cr}$ is <30 mL/minute, its usefulness in the elderly is limited.

♦ **Probenecid and Colchicine** *see* Colchicine and Probenecid *on page 302*

## Procainamide (proe kane A mide)

**U.S. Brand Names** Procanbid™; Promine®; Pronestyl®; Rhythmin®

**Synonyms** Procaine Amide Hydrochloride

**Therapeutic Category** Antiarrhythmic Agent, Class I-A

**Pregnancy Risk Factor** C

**Lactation** Enters breast milk/use caution - see Breast-feeding Issues (AAP rates "compatible")

**Use** Treatment of ventricular tachycardia, premature ventricular contractions, paroxysmal atrial tachycardia, and atrial fibrillation; prevent recurrence of ventricular tachycardia, paroxysmal supraventricular tachycardia, atrial fibrillation or flutter

**Mechanism of Action/Effect** Decreases myocardial excitability and conduction velocity and may depress myocardial contractility, by increasing the electrical stimulation threshold of ventricle, HIS-Purkinje system and through direct cardiac effects

**Contraindications** Hypersensitivity to procainamide, procaine, or related drugs; complete heart block; second or third degree heart block without pacemaker; torsade de pointes; myasthenia gravis; SLE

**Warnings** Use with caution in patients with marked A-V conduction disturbances, bundle-branch block or severe cardiac glycoside intoxication, ventricular arrhythmias with organic heart disease or coronary occlusion, supraventricular tachyarrhythmias unless adequate measures are taken to prevent marked increases in ventricular rates. May accumulate in patients with renal or hepatic dysfunction. Some tablets contain tartrazine. Injection may contain bisulfite (allergens). Long-term administration leads to the development of a positive antinuclear antibody test in 50% of patients which may result in a lupus erythematosus-like syndrome (in 20% to 30% of patients). Discontinue procainamide with SLE symptoms and choose an alternative agent. Elderly have reduced clearance and frequent drug interactions. Pregnancy factor C.

**Drug Interactions**

**Increased Effect/Toxicity:** Increased plasma/NAPA concentrations with cimetidine, ranitidine, beta-blockers, and amiodarone. Increased effect of skeletal muscle relaxants, quinidine and lidocaine, and neuromuscular blockers (succinylcholine). Increased NAPA levels/toxicity with trimethoprim.

**Adverse Reactions**

>10%: Gastrointestinal: Diarrhea, anorexia

1% to 10%:

Cardiovascular: Tachycardia, arrhythmias, A-V block, Q-T prolongation, widening QRS complex

Central nervous system: Dizziness, lightheadedness

Miscellaneous: SLE-like syndrome

<1% (Limited to important or life-threatening symptoms): Hemolytic anemia, agranulocytosis, neutropenia, leukopenia, thrombocytopenia, positive Coombs' test, pleural effusion

**Overdose/Toxicology** Procainamide has a low toxic:therapeutic ratio and may easily produce fatal intoxication (acute toxic dose: 5 g in adults). Symptoms of overdose include sinus bradycardia, sinus node arrest or asystole, P-R, QRS or Q-T interval prolongation, torsade de pointes (polymorphous ventricular tachycardia), and depressed myocardial contractility, which along with alpha-adrenergic or ganglionic blockade, may result in hypotension and pulmonary edema. Other effects are seizures, coma, and respiratory arrest. Treatment is symptomatic and effects usually respond to conventional therapies. **Note**: Do not use other Type 1A or 1C antiarrhythmic agents to treat ventricular tachycardia. Sodium bicarbonate may treat wide QRS intervals or hypotension. Markedly impaired conduction or high degree A-V block, unresponsive to bicarbonate, indicates consideration of a pacemaker.

**Pharmacodynamics/Kinetics**

**Protein Binding:** 15% to 20%

**Distribution:** Congestive heart failure of shock: Decreased $V_d$

**Half-life Elimination:**

Procainamide: (Dependent upon hepatic acetylator, phenotype, cardiac function, and renal function): Adults: 2.5-4.7 hours; Anephric: 11 hours

(Continued)

## Procainamide *(Continued)*

NAPA: (Dependent upon renal function): Adults: 6-8 hours; Anephric: 42 hours

**Time to Peak:** Capsule: Within 45 minutes to 2.5 hours; I.M.: 15-60 minutes

**Metabolism:** Liver

**Excretion:** Urine

**Onset:** I.M. 10-30 minutes

**Formulations**

Procainamide hydrochloride:

- Capsule: 250 mg, 375 mg, 500 mg
- Injection: 100 mg/mL (10 mL); 500 mg/mL (2 mL)
- Tablet: 250 mg, 375 mg, 500 mg
- Tablet, sustained release: 250 mg, 500 mg, 750 mg, 1000 mg
- Tablet, sustained release (Procanbid™): 500 mg, 1000 mg

**Dosing**

**Adults:** Must be titrated to patient's response.

Oral: 250-500 mg/dose every 3-6 hours or 500 mg to 1 g every 6 hours sustained release; usual dose: 50 mg/kg/24 hours; maximum: 4 g/24 hours

I.M.: 0.5-1 g every 4-8 hours until oral therapy is possible

I.V. (infusion requires use of an infusion pump): Loading dose: 15-18 mg/kg administered as slow infusion over 25-30 minutes or 100-200 mg/dose repeated every 5 minutes as needed to a total dose of 1 g; maintenance dose: 1-6 mg/minute by continuous infusion.

Infusion rate: 2 g/250 mL $D_5W$/NS (I.V. infusion requires use of an infusion pump):

- 1 mg/minute: 7 mL/hour
- 2 mg/minute: 15 mL/hour
- 3 mg/minute: 21 mL/hour
- 4 mg/minute: 30 mL/hour
- 5 mg/minute: 38 mL/hour
- 6 mg/minute: 45 mL/hour

Refractory ventricular fibrillation: 30 mg/minute, up to a total of 17 mg/kg; I.V. maintenance infusion: 1-4 mg/minute; monitor levels and do not exceed 3 mg/minute for >24 hours in adults with renal failure.

ACLS guidelines: I.V.: Infuse 20 mg/minute until arrhythmia is controlled, hypotension occurs, QRS complex widens by 50% of its original width, or total of 17 mg/kg is given

**Elderly:** Refer to adult dosing.

**Renal Impairment:**

$Cl_{cr}$ 10-50 mL/minute: Administer every 6-12 hours.

$Cl_{cr}$ <10 mL/minute: Administer every 8-24 hours.

Dialysis:

- Procainamide: Moderately hemodialyzable (20% to 50%): 200 mg supplemental dose posthemodialysis is recommended.
- N-acetylprocainamide: Not dialyzable (0% to 5%)
- Procainamide/N-acetylprocainamide: Peritoneal dialysis: Not dialyzable (0% to 5%)
- Procainamide/N-acetylprocainamide: Replace by blood level during continuous arteriovenous or venovenous hemofiltration (CAVH/CAVHD).

**Hepatic Impairment:** Reduce dose 50%.

**Administration**

**Oral:** Do **not** crush or chew sustained release drug product.

**I.V.:** Maximum rate: 50 mg/minute; give around-the-clock to promote less variation in peak and trough serum levels.

**Stability**

**Storage:** Procainamide may be stored at room temperature up to 27°C; however, refrigeration retards oxidation, which causes color formation. The solution is initially colorless but may turn slightly yellow on standing. Injection of air into the vial causes the solution to darken. Solutions darker than a light amber should be discarded.

**Reconstitution:** Minimum volume: 1 g/250 mL NS/$D_5W$

Stability of admixture at room temperature in $D_5W$ or NS is 24 hours. Some information indicates that procainamide may be subject to greater decomposition in $D_5W$ unless the admixture is refrigerated or the pH is adjusted. Procainamide is believed to form an association complex with dextrose - the bioavailability of procainamide in this complex is not known and the complex formation is reversible.

**Monitoring Laboratory Tests** CBC with differential, platelet count

**Additional Nursing Issues**

**Physical Assessment:** Assess other medications patient may be taking for effectiveness and interactions (see Drug Interactions). See Warnings/Precautions for cautious use. I.V. requires use of infusion pump and continuous cardiac and hemodynamic monitoring. Monitor laboratory tests (see above), therapeutic response (cardiac status), and adverse reactions (see Warnings/Precautions and Adverse Reactions) at beginning of therapy, when titrating dosage, and on a regular basis with long-term therapy. **Note:** Procainamide has a low toxic:therapeutic ratio and overdose may easily produce severe and life-threatening reactions (see Overdose/Toxicology). Assess knowledge/teach patient appropriate use, interventions to reduce side effects, and adverse symptoms to report. **Pregnancy risk factor C** - benefits of use should outweigh possible risks. Note breast-feeding caution.

**Patient Information/Instruction:** Oral: Take exactly as directed; do not take additional doses or discontinue without consulting prescriber. You will need regular cardiac checkups and blood tests while taking this medication. You may experience dizziness, lightheadedness, or visual changes (use caution when driving or engaging in tasks requiring alertness until response to drug is known); loss of appetite (small frequent meals, frequent mouth care, chewing gum, or sucking lozenges may help); headaches (prescriber may recommend mild analgesic); or diarrhea (exercise, yogurt, or boiled milk may help - if persistent consult prescriber). Report chest pain, palpitation, or erratic heartbeat; increased weight or swelling of hands or feet; acute diarrhea; or unusual fatigue and tiredness. **Pregnancy/breast-feeding precautions:** Inform prescriber if you are or intend to be pregnant. Consult prescriber if breast-feeding.

**Geriatric Considerations:** Monitor closely since clearance is reduced in those >60 years of age. If clinically possible, start doses at lowest recommended dose. Also, elderly frequently have drug therapy which may interfere with the use of procainamide. Adjust dose for renal function in the elderly.

**Breast-feeding Issues:** Considered compatible by the American Academy of Pediatrics. However, the AAP stated concern regarding long-term effects and potential for infant toxicity. Use caution and monitor closely if continuing to breast-feed while taking procainamide.

**Additional Information** Some formulations may contain benzyl alcohol or tartrazine. The injection formulation contains sulfites.

**Related Information**

Antiarrhythmic Drug Classification Comparison *on page 1366*

Peak and Trough Guidelines *on page 1331*

## Procaine (PROE kane)

**U.S. Brand Names** Novocain® Injection

**Therapeutic Category** Local Anesthetic

**Pregnancy Risk Factor** C

**Lactation** Excretion in breast milk unknown

**Use** Produces spinal anesthesia and epidural and peripheral nerve block by injection and infiltration methods

**Mechanism of Action/Effect** Blocks both the initiation and conduction of nerve impulses by decreasing the neuronal membrane's permeability to sodium ions, which results in inhibition of depolarization with resultant blockade of conduction

**Contraindications** Hypersensitivity to procaine, PABA, parabens, or other ester local anesthetics

**Warnings** Patients with cardiac diseases, hyperthyroidism, or other endocrine diseases may be more susceptible to toxic effects of local anesthetics. Some preparations contain metabisulfite. Pregnancy factor C.

**Drug Interactions**

**Decreased Effect:** Decreased effect of sulfonamides with the PABA metabolite of procaine, chloroprocaine, and tetracaine. Decreased/increased effect of vasopressors, ergot alkaloids, and MAO inhibitors on blood pressure when using anesthetic solutions with a vasoconstrictor.

**Adverse Reactions**

1% to 10%: Local: Burning sensation at site of injection, tissue irritation, pain at injection site

<1% (Limited to important or life-threatening symptoms): Aseptic meningitis resulting in paralysis can occur, CNS stimulation followed by CNS depression, chills

**Overdose/Toxicology** Treatment is symptomatic and supportive. Termination of anesthesia by pneumatic tourniquet inflation should be attempted when procaine is administered by infiltration or regional injection.

**Pharmacodynamics/Kinetics**

**Half-life Elimination:** 7.7 minutes

**Metabolism:** Rapidly hydrolyzed by plasma enzymes to para-aminobenzoic acid and diethylaminoethanol (80% conjugated before elimination)

**Excretion:** Urine

**Onset:** Onset of effect: Injection: Within 2-5 minutes

**Duration:** 0.5-1.5 hours (dependent upon patient, type of block, concentration, and method of anesthesia)

**Formulations** Injection, as hydrochloride: 1% [10 mg/mL] (2 mL, 6 mL, 30 mL, 100 mL); 2% [20 mg/mL] (30 mL, 100 mL); 10% (2 mL)

**Dosing**

**Adults:** Dose varies with procedure, desired depth, and duration of anesthesia, desired muscle relaxation, vascularity of tissues, physical condition, and age of patient.

**Elderly:** Refer to adult dosing.

**Additional Nursing Issues**

**Physical Assessment:** Monitor response; degree of pain sensation. Monitor site of injection for adverse reaction. Epidural: Monitor CNS status (see Adverse Reactions). **Pregnancy risk factor C.** Note breast-feeding caution.

**Patient Information/Instruction:** The purpose of this medication is to reduce pain sensation. Report local burning or pain at injection site. **Pregnancy/breast-feeding precautions:** Inform prescriber if your are pregnant. Consult prescriber if breast-feeding.

**Additional Information** The injection formulation contains sulfites.


- **Procaine Amide Hydrochloride** *see* Procainamide *on page 967*
- **Procaine Benzylpenicillin** *see* Penicillin G Procaine *on page 899*
- **Procaine Penicillin G** *see* Penicillin G Procaine *on page 899*
- **Pro-Cal-Sof® [OTC]** *see* Docusate *on page 392*
- **Procanbid™** *see* Procainamide *on page 967*

## Procarbazine (proe KAR ba zeen)

**U.S. Brand Names** Matulane®

**Synonyms** Ibenzmethyzin; MIH; N-Methylhydrazine

**Therapeutic Category** Antineoplastic Agent, Alkylating Agent

**Pregnancy Risk Factor** D

**Lactation** Excretion in breast milk unknown/not recommended

**Use** Treatment of Hodgkin's disease, non-Hodgkin's lymphoma, brain tumor, bronchogenic carcinoma

**Mechanism of Action/Effect** Mechanism of action is not clear, methylating of nucleic acids; inhibits DNA, RNA, and protein synthesis; may damage DNA directly and suppresses mitosis; metabolic activation required by host

**Contraindications** Hypersensitivity to procarbazine or any component; pre-existing bone marrow aplasia; alcohol ingestion; pregnancy

**Warnings** The U.S. Food and Drug Administration (FDA) currently recommends that procedures for proper handling and disposal of antineoplastic agents be considered. Use with caution in patients with pre-existing renal or hepatic impairment. Modify dosage in patients with renal or hepatic impairment or marrow disorders. Reduce dosage with serum creatinine >2 mg/dL or total bilirubin >3 mg/dL. Procarbazine possesses MAO inhibitor activity. Procarbazine is a carcinogen which may cause acute leukemia. Procarbazine may cause infertility.

**Drug Interactions**

**Increased Effect/Toxicity:** Procarbazine exhibits weak monoamine oxidase (MAO) inhibitor activity. Foods containing high amounts of tyramine should, therefore, be avoided (see related information and table in Appendix/Miscellaneous for a list of foods containing tyramine). When an MAO inhibitor is given with food high in tyramine, hypertensive crisis, intracranial bleeding, and headache have been reported.

Sympathomimetic amines (epinephrine and amphetamines) and antidepressants (tricyclics) should be used cautiously with procarbazine. Barbiturates, narcotics, phenothiazines, and other CNS depressants can cause somnolence, ataxia, and other symptoms of CNS depression. Alcohol has caused a disulfiram-like reaction with procarbazine. May result in headache, respiratory difficulties, nausea, vomiting, sweating, thirst, hypotension, and flushing.

**Food Interactions** Clinically severe and possibly life-threatening elevations in blood pressure may occur if procarbazine is taken with tyramine-containing foods.

**Adverse Reactions**

>10%:

Central nervous system: Mental depression, manic reactions, hallucinations, dizziness, headache, nervousness, insomnia, nightmares, ataxia, disorientation, confusion, seizure, CNS stimulation

Endocrine & metabolic: Amenorrhea

Gastrointestinal: Severe nausea and vomiting occur frequently and may be dose-limiting; anorexia, abdominal pain, stomatitis, dysphagia, diarrhea, and constipation; use a nonphenothiazine antiemetic, when possible

Emetic potential: Moderately high (60% to 90%)

Time course of nausea/vomiting: Onset: 24-27 hours; Duration: variable

Hematologic: Thrombocytopenia, hemolytic anemia, anemia

Myelosuppressive: May be dose-limiting toxicity; procarbazine should be discontinued if leukocyte count is <4000/mm$^3$ or platelet count <100,000/mm$^3$

WBC: Moderate

Platelets: Moderate

Onset (days): 14

Nadir (days): 21

Recovery (days): 28

Neuromuscular & skeletal: Weakness, paresthesia, neuropathies, decreased reflexes, foot drop, tremors

Ocular: Nystagmus

Respiratory: Pleural effusion, cough

1% to 10%:

Dermatologic: Alopecia, hyperpigmentation

Gastrointestinal: Diarrhea, stomatitis, constipation

Hepatic: Hepatotoxicity

Neuromuscular & skeletal: Peripheral neuropathy

<1% (Limited to important or life-threatening symptoms): Orthostatic hypotension, hypertensive crisis, pneumonitis

**Overdose/Toxicology** Symptoms of overdose include arthralgia, alopecia, paresthesia, bone marrow suppression, hallucinations, nausea, vomiting, diarrhea, seizures, and coma. Treatment is supportive. Adverse effects such as marrow toxicity may begin as late as 2 weeks after exposure.

**Pharmacodynamics/Kinetics**

**Distribution:** Crosses the blood-brain barrier and distributes into CSF

**Half-life Elimination:** 1 hour

**Metabolism:** Liver and kidney

**Excretion:** Urine

**Formulations** Capsule, as hydrochloride: 50 mg

**Dosing**

**Adults:** Refer to individual protocols.

Oral (dose based on patient's ideal weight if the patient has abnormal fluid retention):

Initial: 2-4 mg/kg/day in single or divided doses for 7 days then increase dose to 4-6 mg/kg/day until response is obtained or leukocyte count decreased <4000/mm$^3$ or the platelet count decreased. <100,000/mm$^3$; maintenance: 1-2 mg/kg/day

In MOPP, 100 mg/m$^2$/day on days 1-14 of a 28-day cycle

**Elderly:** Refer to adult dosing; adjust for renal impairment. Use with caution.

**Renal Impairment:** Use with caution, may result in increased toxicity.

**Hepatic Impairment:** Use with caution, may result in increased toxicity.

**Stability**

**Storage:** Protect from light

**Monitoring Laboratory Tests** CBC with differential, platelet and reticulocyte count, urinalysis, liver and renal function

**Additional Nursing Issues**

**Physical Assessment:** Monitor frequently for adverse CNS reactions, GI reactions and electrolyte imbalance (antiemetic generally required), opportunistic infection, and acute myelosuppression (see Adverse Reactions for specific symptoms). Assess knowledge/teach patient about dietary cautions (procarbazine had some MAO inhibitory effects). See Tyramine Foods List *on page 1422*. Teach interventions to reduce side effects and adverse effects to report. **Pregnancy risk factor D** - assess knowledge/teach both male and female appropriate use of barrier contraceptive measures. Breast-feeding is not recommended.

**Patient Information/Instruction:** Take as directed. Maintain adequate hydration (2-3 L/day of fluids unless instructed to restrict fluid intake). Avoid aspirin and aspirin-containing substances. Avoid alcohol; may cause acute disulfiram reaction - flushing, headache, acute vomiting, chest and/or abdominal pain. Avoid tyramine-containing foods (aged cheese, chocolate, pickles, aged meat, wine, etc). You may experience mental depression, nervousness, insomnia, nightmares, dizziness, confusion, or lethargy (use caution when driving or engaging in tasks that require alertness until response to drug is known); photosensitivity (use sunscreen, wear protective clothing and eyewear, and avoid direct sunlight). You may experience rash or hair loss (reversible), loss of libido, increased sensitivity to infection (avoid crowds and infected persons). Report persistent fever, chills, sore throat; unusual bleeding; blood in urine, stool (black stool), or vomitus; unresolved depression; mania; hallucinations; nightmares; disorientation; seizures; chest pain or palpitations; or difficulty breathing. **Pregnancy/breast-feeding precautions:** Do not get pregnant while taking this medication; use appropriate contraceptive measures. Breast-feeding is not recommended.

**Related Information**

Tyramine Foods List *on page 1422*

- **Procardia®** *see* Nifedipine *on page 824*
- **Procardia XL®** *see* Nifedipine *on page 824*
- **Procetofene** *see* Fenofibrate *on page 475*
- **ProChlorax** *see* Clidinium and Chlordiazepoxide *on page 281*

## Prochlorperazine (proe klor PER a zeen)

**U.S. Brand Names** Compazine®

**Therapeutic Category** Antipsychotic Agent, Phenothazine, Piperazine

**Pregnancy Risk Factor** C

**Lactation** Enters breast milk/not recommended

**Use** Management of nausea and vomiting; acute and chronic psychosis

**Mechanism of Action/Effect** Blocks postsynaptic mesolimbic dopaminergic $D_1$ and $D_2$ receptors in the brain, including the medullary chemoreceptor trigger zone; exhibits a strong alpha-adrenergic and anticholinergic blocking effect and depresses the release of hypothalamic and hypophyseal hormones; believed to depress the reticular activating system, thus affecting basal metabolism, body temperature, wakefulness, vasomotor tone and emesis

**Contraindications** Hypersensitivity to prochlorperazine or any component; cross-sensitivity with other phenothiazines may exist; avoid use in patients with narrow-angle glaucoma, bone marrow depression, severe liver or cardiac disease, or respiratory disorders

**Warnings** Injection contains sulfites which may cause allergic reactions. May impair ability to perform hazardous tasks requiring mental alertness or physical coordination. Some products contain tartrazine dye, avoid use in sensitive individuals.

Tardive dyskinesia: Prevalence rate may be 40% in the elderly; development of the syndrome and the irreversible nature are proportional to duration and total cumulative dose over time. May be reversible if diagnosed early in therapy.

High incidence of extrapyramidal reactions, especially in children or the elderly, so reserve use to those who are unresponsive to other antiemetics; incidence of extrapyramidal reactions is increased with acute illnesses such as chickenpox, measles, CNS infections, gastroenteritis, and dehydration.

Drug-induced **Parkinson's syndrome** occurs often. **Akathisia** is the most common extrapyramidal reaction in the elderly.

Increased confusion, memory loss, psychotic behavior, and agitation frequently occur as a consequence of anticholinergic effects.

**Lowers seizure threshold**, use cautiously in patients with seizure history.

Orthostatic hypotension is due to alpha-receptor blockade, the elderly are at greater risk for orthostatic hypotension.

Antipsychotic associated sedation in nonpsychotic patients is extremely unpleasant due to feelings of depersonalization, derealization, and dysphoria.

Life-threatening arrhythmias have occurred at therapeutic doses of antipsychotics.

(Continued)

## Prochlorperazine *(Continued)*

Pregnancy factor C.

**Drug Interactions**

**Cytochrome P-450 Effect:** Metabolism may involve CYP isoenzymes.

**Increased Effect/Toxicity:** Additive effects with other CNS depressants, anticonvulsants. Epinephrine may cause hypotension.

**Effects on Lab Values** False-positives for phenylketonuria, urinary amylase, uroporphyrins, urobilinogen

**Adverse Reactions** Incidence of extrapyramidal reactions are higher with prochlorperazine than chlorpromazine.

>10%:

- Cardiovascular: Hypotension (especially with I.V. use), orthostatic hypotension, tachycardia, arrhythmias
- Central nervous system: Pseudoparkinsonism, akathisia, tardive dyskinesia (persistent), dizziness, dystonias
- Gastrointestinal: Dry mouth, constipation
- Genitourinary: Urinary retention
- Ocular: Pigmentary retinopathy, blurred vision
- Respiratory: Nasal congestion
- Miscellaneous: Decreased sweating

1% to 10%:

- Dermatologic: Photosensitivity, rash
- Endocrine & metabolic: Changes in menstrual cycle, breast pain, changes in libido
- Gastrointestinal: Weight gain, nausea, vomiting, stomach pain
- Genitourinary: Dysuria, ejaculatory disturbances
- Neuromuscular & skeletal: Tremor

<1% (Limited to important or life-threatening symptoms): Neuroleptic malignant syndrome (NMS), lowering of seizures threshold, agranulocytosis, leukopenia, thrombocytopenia, cholestatic jaundice, hepatotoxicity

**Overdose/Toxicology** Symptoms of overdose include deep sleep, coma, extrapyramidal symptoms, abnormal involuntary muscle movements, and hypotension. Treatment is symptom directed and supportive.

**Pharmacodynamics/Kinetics**

**Distribution:** Crosses the placenta

**Half-life Elimination:** 23 hours

**Metabolism:** Hepatic

**Onset:** Oral: Within 30-40 minutes; I.M.: Within 10-20 minutes; Rectal: Within 60 minutes

**Duration:** Persists longest with I.M. and oral extended-release doses (12 hours); shortest following rectal and immediate release oral administration (3-4 hours)

**Formulations**

- Capsule, sustained action, as maleate: 10 mg, 15 mg, 30 mg
- Injection, as edisylate: 5 mg/mL (2 mL, 10 mL)
- Suppository, rectal: 2.5 mg, 5 mg, 25 mg (12/box)
- Syrup, as edisylate: 5 mg/5 mL (120 mL)
- Tablet, as maleate: 5 mg, 10 mg, 25 mg

**Dosing**

**Adults:**

Antiemetic:

- Oral: 5-10 mg 3-4 times/day; usual maximum: 40 mg/day
- I.M.: 5-10 mg every 3-4 hours; usual maximum: 40 mg/day
- I.V.: 2.5-10 mg; maximum 10 mg/dose or 40 mg/day; may repeat dose every 3-4 hours as needed
- Rectal: 25 mg twice daily

Antipsychotic:

- Oral: 5-10 mg 3-4 times/day; doses up to 150 mg/day may be required in some patients for treatment of severe disturbances
- I.M.: 10-20 mg every 4-6 hours may be required in some patients for treatment of severe disturbances; change to oral as soon as possible.

**Elderly:** Dementia behavior (nonpsychotic): Initial: 2.5-5 mg 1-2 times/day; increase dose at 4- to 7-day intervals by 2.5-5 mg/day. Increase dosing intervals (twice daily, 3 times/day, etc) as necessary to control response or side effects. Maximum daily dose should probably not exceed 75 mg in the elderly. Gradual increases (titration) may prevent some side effects or decrease their severity. See Geriatric Considerations.

**Renal Impairment:** Not dialyzable (0% to 5%)

**Administration**

**Oral:** Avoid skin contact with oral solution contact dermatitis has occurred.

**I.M.:** I.M. should be administered into the upper outer quadrant of the buttock. Avoid skin contact injection, contact dermatitis has occurred.

**I.V.:** IVP should be administered at a concentration of 1 mg/mL at a rate of 5 mg/minute.

**I.V. Detail:** Do not dilute with any diluent containing parabens as a preservative. Avoid skin contact injection, contact dermatitis has occurred. I.V. may be administered IVP or IVPB.

**Stability**

**Storage:** Protect from light. Clear or slightly yellow solutions may be used.

**Compatibility:** Incompatible when mixed with aminophylline, amphotericin B, ampicillin, calcium salts, cephalothin, foscarnet (Y-site), furosemide, hydrocortisone, hydromorphone, methohexital, midazolam, penicillin G, pentobarbital, phenobarbital, and thiopental. Do not mix in same syringe with other agents. See the Compatibility of Drugs in Syringe Chart *on page 1317.*

**Monitoring Laboratory Tests** Baseline liver and kidney function, CBC prior to and periodically during therapy

**Additional Nursing Issues**

**Physical Assessment:** Assess all other medications patient may be taking (see Drug Interactions and Warnings/Precautions). For I.V., continuously monitor blood pressure and heart rate during administration. Monitor blood pressure and heart rate, fluid balance (I & O ratio), and dehydration. Monitor for seizures, especially with known seizure disorder. Monitor for excessive sedation, neuromuscular malignant syndrome, autonomic instability (eg, anticholinergic effects, such as flushing, excessive sweating, constipation, urinary retention), and extrapyramidal effects (eg, tardive dyskinesia, akathisia, pseudoparkinsonism). **Pregnancy risk factor C** - benefits of use should outweigh possible risks. Breast-feeding is not recommended.

**Patient Information/Instruction:** Take exact amount as prescribed. Do not change brand names. Do not crush or chew tablets or capsules. Do not discontinue without consulting prescriber. Avoid alcohol or other sedatives or sleep-inducing drugs. Avoid skin contact with drug; wash immediately with warm soapy water. You may experience appetite changes; small frequent meals may help. Maintain adequate fluid intake (2-3 L/day of fluids unless instructed to restrict fluid intake). May cause dizziness, tremors, or visual disturbance (especially during early therapy); use caution when driving or engaging in tasks that require alertness until response to drug is known. Do not change position rapidly (rise slowly). May cause photosensitivity reaction; use sunscreen, wear protective clothing and eyewear, and avoid direct sunlight. Report immediately any changes in gait or muscular tremors. Report unresolved changes in voiding or elimination (constipation or diarrhea), acute dizziness or unresolved sedation, any vision changes, palpitations, yellowing of skin or eyes, and changes in color of urine or stool (pink or red brown urine is expected). **Pregnancy/breast-feeding precautions:** Inform prescriber if you are or intend to be pregnant. Breast-feeding is not recommended.

**Geriatric Considerations:** Due to side effect profile (dystonias, EPS) this is not a preferred drug in the elderly for antiemetic therapy.

**Additional Information** The edisylate injection formulation contains benzyl alcohol and sulfites.

Prochlorperazine: Compazine® suppository
Prochlorperazine edisylate: Compazine® oral solution and injection
Prochlorperazine maleate: Compazine® capsule and tablet
pH: 4.2-6.2

**Related Information**

Antiemetics for Chemotherapy-Induced Nausea and Vomiting *on page 1307*
Antipsychotic Medication Guidelines *on page 1436*

- **Procort® [OTC]** *see* Hydrocortisone *on page 578*
- **Procort® [OTC]** *see* Topical Corticosteroids *on page 1152*
- **Procrit®** *see* Epoetin Alfa *on page 426*
- **Proctocort™** *see* Hydrocortisone *on page 578*
- **Proctocort™** *see* Topical Corticosteroids *on page 1152*
- **Proctofene** *see* Fenofibrate *on page 475*
- **Proctofoam® NS** *see page 1294*
- **Procyclid** *see* Procyclidine *on this page*

## Procyclidine (proe SYE kli deen)

**U.S. Brand Names** Kemadrin®

**Therapeutic Category** Anticholinergic Agent; Anti-Parkinson's Agent (Anticholinergic)

**Pregnancy Risk Factor** C

**Lactation** Excretion in breast milk unknown/not recommended

**Use** Relieves symptoms of parkinsonian syndrome and drug-induced extrapyramidal symptoms

**Mechanism of Action/Effect** Thought to act by blocking excess acetylcholine at cerebral synapses; many of its effects are due to its pharmacologic similarities with atropine

**Contraindications** Angle-closure glaucoma; safe use in children not established

**Warnings** Use with caution in hot weather or during exercise. Elderly patients frequently develop increased sensitivity and require strict dosage regulation - side effects may be more severe in elderly patients with atherosclerotic changes. Use with caution in patients with tachycardia, cardiac arrhythmias, hypertension, hypotension, prostatic hypertrophy (especially in the elderly) or any tendency toward urinary retention, liver or kidney disorders and obstructive disease of the GI or GU tract. When given in large doses or to susceptible patients, may cause weakness and inability to move particular muscle groups. Pregnancy factor C.

**Drug Interactions**

**Decreased Effect:** Decreased effect of psychotropics.

**Increased Effect/Toxicity:** Increased toxicity with phenothiazines, meperidine, and tricyclic antidepressants.

**Adverse Reactions**

>10%:

Dermatologic: Dry skin
Gastrointestinal: Constipation, dry throat, dry mouth
Respiratory: Dry nose
Miscellaneous: Sweating (decreased)

(Continued)

## Procyclidine *(Continued)*

1% to 10%:
- Dermatologic: Increased sensitivity to light
- Endocrine & metabolic: Decreased flow of breast milk
- Gastrointestinal: Dysphagia

<1% (Limited to important or life-threatening symptoms): Tachycardia, orthostatic hypotension, ventricular fibrillation, palpitations, coma, drowsiness, nervousness, hallucinations; the elderly may be at increased risk for confusion and hallucinations, headache, loss of memory, fatigue, ataxia, false sense of well-being (especially with elderly or with high doses), loss of memory (elderly), hyperthermia, fever, heat stroke, toxic psychosis

**Overdose/Toxicology** Symptoms of overdose include disorientation, hallucinations, delusions, blurred vision, dysphagia, absent bowel sounds, hyperthermia, hypertension, and urinary retention. For anticholinergic overdose with severe life-threatening symptoms, physostigmine 1-2 mg S.C. or I.V. slowly, may be given to reverse these effects.

**Pharmacodynamics/Kinetics**

**Onset:** Oral: Within 30-40 minutes

**Duration:** 4-6 hours

**Formulations** Tablet, as hydrochloride: 5 mg

**Dosing**

**Adults:** Oral: 2.5 mg 3 times/day after meals; if tolerated, gradually increase dose, to a maximum of 20 mg/day if necessary.

**Elderly:** Oral: Initial: 2.5 mg once or twice daily, gradually increasing as necessary. Avoid use if possible (see Geriatric Considerations).

**Hepatic Impairment:** Decrease dose to a twice daily dosing regimen.

**Administration**

**Oral:** Should be administered after meals to minimize stomach upset. Avoid alcohol.

**Additional Nursing Issues**

**Physical Assessment:** Assess effectiveness and interactions of other medications patient may be taking (see Contraindications and Drug Interactions). Monitor renal function, therapeutic response (eg, Parkinsonian symptoms), and adverse reactions such as anticholinergic syndrome (dry mouth and mucous membranes, constipation, epigastric distress, CNS disturbances, paralytic ileus) at beginning of therapy and periodically throughout therapy (see Warnings/Precautions, Adverse Reactions, and Overdose/Toxicology). Assess knowledge/teach patient appropriate use, interventions to reduce side effects, and adverse symptoms to report. **Pregnancy risk factor C** - benefits of use should outweigh possible risks. Breast-feeding is not recommended.

**Patient Information/Instruction:** Take exactly as directed (after meals); do not increase, decrease, or discontinue without consulting prescriber. Take at the same time each day. Do not use alcohol and all prescription or OTC sedatives or CNS depressants without consulting prescriber. You may experience drowsiness, dizziness, confusion, and blurred vision (use caution when driving, climbing stairs, or engaging in tasks requiring alertness until response to drug is known); increased susceptibility to heat stroke, decreased perspiration (use caution in hot weather - maintain adequate fluids and reduce exercise activity); constipation (increased exercise, fluids, or dietary fruit and fiber may help); dry skin or nasal passages (consult prescriber for appropriate relief). Report unresolved constipation, chest pain or palpitations, difficulty breathing, CNS changes (hallucination, loss of memory, nervousness, etc), painful or difficult urination, increased muscle spasticity or rigidity, skin rash, or significant worsening of condition. **Pregnancy/breast-feeding precautions:** Inform prescriber if you are or intend to be pregnant. Breast-feeding is not recommended.

**Geriatric Considerations:** Anticholinergic agents are generally not well tolerated in the elderly and their use should be avoided when possible (see Warnings/Precautions, Adverse Reactions). In the elderly, anticholinergic agents should not be used as prophylaxis against extrapyramidal symptoms. Elderly patients frequently develop increased sensitivity and require strict dosage regulation - side effects may be more severe in elderly patients with atherosclerotic changes.

- **Procytox®** *see* Cyclophosphamide *on page 313*
- **Prodiem® Plain** *see* Psyllium *on page 993*
- **Prodium® [OTC]** *see* Phenazopyridine *on page 914*
- **Profasi® HP** *see* Chorionic Gonadotropin *on page 264*
- **Profenal® Ophthalmic** *see page 1248*
- **Profenid®** *see* Ketoprofen *on page 645*
- **Profenid® 200** *see* Ketoprofen *on page 645*
- **Profenid®-IM** *see* Ketoprofen *on page 645*
- **Profen II®** *see* Guaifenesin and Phenylpropanolamine *on page 550*
- **Profen-LA®** *see* Guaifenesin and Phenylpropanolamine *on page 550*
- **Profilate® OSD** *see* Antihemophilic Factor (Human) *on page 99*
- **Profilate® SD** *see* Antihemophilic Factor (Human) *on page 99*
- **Progestasert®** *see* Progesterone *on this page*

## Progesterone (proe JES ter one)

**U.S. Brand Names** Crinone™; Progestasert®

**Synonyms** Pregnenedione; Progestin

**Therapeutic Category** Progestin

**Pregnancy Risk Factor** X

**Lactation** Excretion in breast milk unknown

**Use** Intrauterine contraception in women who have had at least 1 child, are in a stable, mutually monogamous relationship, and have no history of pelvic inflammatory disease; amenorrhea; functional uterine bleeding

**Mechanism of Action/Effect** Natural steroid hormone that induces secretory changes in the endometrium, promotes mammary gland development, relaxes uterine smooth muscle, blocks follicular maturation and ovulation, and maintains pregnancy

**Contraindications** Hypersensitivity to progesterone or any component; pregnancy; thrombophlebitis; undiagnosed vaginal bleeding; carcinoma of the breast; cerebral apoplexy

**Warnings** Use with caution in patients with impaired liver function, depression, diabetes, and epilepsy. Use of any progestin during the first 4 months of pregnancy is not recommended. Monitor closely for loss of vision, proptosis, diplopia, migraine, and signs or symptoms of embolic disorders. Not a progestin of choice in the elderly for hormonal cycling.

**Drug Interactions**

**Cytochrome P-450 Effect:** CYP3A3/4 enzyme substrate; CYP3A3/4 enzyme inducer

**Decreased Effect:** Aminoglutethimide may decrease effect by increasing hepatic metabolism.

**Effects on Lab Values** Thyroid function, metyrapone, liver function, coagulation tests, endocrine function tests

**Adverse Reactions**

**Intrauterine device:**

>10%:

Cardiovascular: Edema

Endocrine & metabolic: Breakthrough bleeding, spotting, changes in menstrual flow, amenorrhea

Gastrointestinal: Anorexia

Neuromuscular & skeletal: Weakness

1% to 10%:

Cardiovascular: Embolism, central thrombosis

Central nervous system: Mental depression, fever, insomnia

Dermatologic: Melasma or chloasma, allergic rash with or without pruritus

Endocrine: Changes in cervical erosion and secretions, increased breast tenderness

Gastrointestinal: Weight gain or loss

Hepatic: Cholestatic jaundice

**Injection (I.M.):**

>10% Local: Pain at injection site

1% to 10%: Local: Thrombophlebitis

**Systemic:**

>10%:

Cardiovascular: Swelling of face

Central nervous system: Headache, mood changes, nervousness

Endocrine & metabolic: Amenorrhea, irregular menstrual cycles, menorrhagia, spotting, ovarian enlargement, ovarian cyst formation

Gastrointestinal: Abdominal pain

1% to 10%:

Cardiovascular: Hot flashes

Central nervous system: Dizziness, mental depression, insomnia

Dermatologic: Dermatitis, acne, melasma, loss or gain of body, facial, or scalp hair

Endocrine & metabolic: Hyperglycemia, galactorrhea, breast pain, libido decrease

Gastrointestinal: Nausea, change in appetite, weight gain

Genitourinary: Vaginitis, leukorrhea

Neuromuscular & skeletal: Myalgia

<1% (Limited to important or life-threatening symptoms): Thromboembolism, allergic reaction, hot flashes, migraine, tremor, aggressive reactions, forgetfulness, asthma

**Overdose/Toxicology** Toxicity is unlikely following single exposure of excessive doses. Supportive treatment is adequate in most cases.

**Pharmacodynamics/Kinetics**

**Half-life Elimination:** 5 minutes

**Excretion:** Urine

**Duration:** 24 hours

**Formulations**

Gel: 4% (45 mg), 8% (90 mg)

Intrauterine system, reservoir: 38 mg in silicone fluid

**Dosing**

**Adults:**

Gel:

Assisted reproductive technology: One applicatorful (90 mg) once daily; 90 mg twice daily with partial or complete ovarian failure. If pregnancy occurs, continue treatment for 10-12 weeks.

Secondary amenorrhea: One applicatorful (45 mg) every other day for 6 doses; may increase to 90 mg at same schedule if response is inadequate.

I.M.

Amenorrhea: 5-10 mg/day for 6-8 consecutive days

Functional uterine bleeding: 5-10 mg/day for 6 doses

Intrauterine device: Contraception: Female: Insert a single system into the uterine cavity; contraceptive effectiveness is retained for 1 year and system must be replaced 1 year after insertion

(Continued)

## Progesterone *(Continued)*

**Elderly:** Refer to adult dosing.

**Additional Nursing Issues**

**Physical Assessment:** Monitor blood pressure, mammogram, and results of Pap smears and pregnancy tests before beginning treatment and at least annually with vaginal insert. Monitor for adverse effects (see above) and effectiveness of therapy. Instruct patient about importance of annual physicals, Pap smears, and vision assessments. **Pregnancy risk factor X** - determine that patient is not pregnant before beginning treatment. Note breast-feeding caution.

**Patient Information/Instruction:** This drug can only be given I.M. on a daily basis for a specific number of days (or inserted vaginally to remain for 1 year as a contraceptive). It is important that you you have an annual physical assessment, Pap smear, and vision assessment while taking this medication. You may experience increased facial hair or loss of head hair (reversible); photosensitivity (use sunscreen, wear protective clothing and eyewear, and avoid direct sunlight); loss of appetite (small frequent meals will help); constipation (increased fluids, exercise, dietary fiber, or stool softeners may help). Diabetics should use accurate serum glucose testing to identify any changes in glucose tolerance. Report immediately pain or muscle soreness; swelling, heat, or redness in calves; shortness of breath; sudden loss of vision; unresolved leg or foot swelling; change in menstrual pattern (unusual bleeding, amenorrhea, breakthrough spotting); breast tenderness that does not go away; acute abdominal cramping; signs of vaginal infection (drainage, pain, itching); or changes in CNS (eg, blurred vision, confusion, acute anxiety, or unresolved depression). **Pregnancy/breast-feeding precautions:** This drug may cause severe fetal complication. If you suspect you may be pregnant contact prescriber immediately. Consult prescriber if breast-feeding.

**Geriatric Considerations:** Not a progestin of choice in the elderly for hormonal cycling.


- **Progesterone Oil** *see* Progesterone *on page 974*
- **Progestin** *see* Progesterone *on page 974*
- **Proglycem® Oral** *see* Diazoxide *on page 357*
- **Prograf®** *see* Tacrolimus *on page 1093*
- **ProHIBiT®** *see page 1256*
- **Pro-Indo®** *see* Indomethacin *on page 606*
- **Proken M** *see* Metoprolol *on page 761*
- **Prolaken** *see* Metoprolol *on page 761*
- **Prolamine® [OTC]** *see* Phenylpropanolamine *on page 922*
- **Proleukin®** *see* Aldesleukin *on page 47*
- **Prolixin Decanoate® Injection** *see* Fluphenazine *on page 505*
- **Prolixin Enanthate® Injection** *see* Fluphenazine *on page 505*
- **Prolixin® Injection** *see* Fluphenazine *on page 505*
- **Prolixin® Oral** *see* Fluphenazine *on page 505*
- **Proloprim®** *see* Trimethoprim *on page 1181*
- **Pro-Lorazepam®** *see* Lorazepam *on page 691*


## Promazine (PROE ma zeen)

**U.S. Brand Names** Sparine®

**Therapeutic Category** Antipsychotic Agent, Phenothiazine, Aliphatic

**Pregnancy Risk Factor** C

**Lactation** Excretion in breast milk unknown/not recommended

**Use** Management of manifestations of psychotic disorders; alcohol withdrawal; nausea and vomiting; behavioral symptoms associated with dementia in the elderly, Tourette's syndrome; Huntington's chorea; spasmodic torticollis and Reye's syndrome

**Mechanism of Action/Effect** Blocks postsynaptic mesolimbic dopaminergic $D_1$ and $D_2$ receptors in the brain; exhibits a strong alpha-adrenergic blocking and anticholinergic effect, depresses the release of hypothalamic and hypophyseal hormones; believed to depress the reticular activating system thus affecting basal metabolism, body temperature, wakefulness, vasomotor tone, and emesis

**Contraindications** Hypersensitivity to promazine or any component (cross reactivity between phenothiazines may occur); severe CNS depression; bone marrow suppression; coma; do not use intra-arterial injection of the parenteral formulation

**Warnings** Moderately sedating, use with caution in disorders where CNS depression is a feature. Use with caution in Parkinson's disease. Use with caution in patients with hemodynamic instability; bone marrow suppression; predisposition to seizures; subcortical brain damage; or severe cardiac, hepatic, renal, or respiratory disease. Neuroleptics may cause swallowing difficulty. Use with caution in breast cancer or other prolactin-dependent tumors (may elevate prolactin levels). May alter temperature regulation or mask toxicity of other drugs due to antiemetic effects. May alter cardiac conduction - life-threatening arrhythmias have occurred with therapeutic doses of phenothiazines. May cause orthostatic hypotension.

Phenothiazines may cause anticholinergic effects (eg, confusion, agitation, constipation, dry mouth, blurred vision, urinary retention); therefore, use with caution in patients with decreased gastrointestinal motility, urinary retention, BPH, xerostomia, or visual problems. Conditions which also may be exacerbated by cholinergic blockade include narrow-angle glaucoma (screening is recommended) and worsening of myasthenia gravis. Relative to other neuroleptics, promazine has a high potency of cholinergic blockade.

May cause extrapyramidal reactions including pseudoparkinsonism, acute dystonic reactions, akathisia, and tardive dyskinesia (risk of these reactions is moderate relative to other neuroleptics). May be associated with neuroleptic malignant syndrome (NMS) or pigmentary retinopathy.

Pregnancy factor C.

**Effects on Lab Values** ↑ cholesterol (S), glucose; ↓ uric acid (S)

**Adverse Reactions**

>10%:
- Cardiovascular: Hypotension, orthostatic hypotension
- Central nervous system: Pseudoparkinsonism, akathisia, dystonias, tardive dyskinesia (persistent), dizziness
- Gastrointestinal: Constipation
- Ocular: Pigmentary retinopathy
- Respiratory: Nasal congestion
- Miscellaneous: Decreased sweating

1% to 10%:
- Central nervous system: Dizziness
- Dermatologic: Photosensitivity, rash
- Endocrine & metabolic: Changes in menstrual cycle, changes in libido, breast pain
- Gastrointestinal: Weight gain, nausea, vomiting, stomach pain
- Genitourinary: Dysuria, ejaculatory disturbances
- Neuromuscular & skeletal: Tremor

<1% (Limited to important or life-threatening symptoms): Neuroleptic malignant syndrome (NMS), lowering of seizures threshold, agranulocytosis, leukopenia, cholestatic jaundice, hepatotoxicity

**Overdose/Toxicology** Symptoms of overdose include deep sleep, coma, extrapyramidal symptoms, abnormal involuntary muscle movements, and hypotension. Treatment is symptom directed and supportive.

**Pharmacodynamics/Kinetics**

**Half-life Elimination:** The specific pharmacokinetics of promazine are poorly established but probably resemble those of other phenothiazines. Most phenothiazines have long half-lives in the range of 24 hours or more.

**Metabolism:** Liver

**Formulations**

Promazine hydrochloride:
- Injection: 25 mg/mL (10 mL); 50 mg/mL (1 mL, 2 mL, 10 mL)
- Tablet: 25 mg, 50 mg, 100 mg

**Dosing**

**Adults:** Oral, I.M.:
- Psychosis: 10-200 mg every 4-6 hours not to exceed 1000 mg/day
- Antiemetic: 25-50 mg every 4-6 hours as needed

**Elderly:** Nonpsychotic patients; dementia behavior: Initial: 25 mg 1-2 times/day; increase dose at 4- to 7-day intervals by 25 mg/day. Increase dose intervals (bid, tid, etc) as necessary to control response or side effects. Maximum daily dose: 500 mg; gradual increases (titration) may prevent some side effects or decrease their severity.

**Renal Impairment:** Not dialyzable (0% to 5%)

**Administration**

**Oral:** Solutions may be diluted or mixed with fruit juices or other liquids, but must be administered immediately after mixing. Absorption is inhibited by antacids for about 1 hour. **Note:** Avoid skin contact with oral medications; may cause contact dermatitis.

**I.M.:** I.M. injections should be deep injections.

**I.V.:** I.V., dilute to at least 25 mg/mL and give slowly.

**Stability**

**Storage:** Protect all dosage forms from light, clear or slightly yellow solutions may be used. Should be dispensed in amber or opaque vials/bottles.

**Compatibility:** Injection is incompatible when mixed with aminophylline, dimenhydrinate, methohexital, nafcillin, penicillin G, pentobarbital, phenobarbital, sodium bicarbonate, and thiopental.

**Monitoring Laboratory Tests** Baseline liver and kidney function, CBC prior to and periodically during therapy, ophthalmic exam

**Additional Nursing Issues**

**Physical Assessment:** Assess other medications patient is taking for effectiveness and interactions (see Drug Interactions). See Contraindications and Warnings/Precautions for cautious use. Has potential for psychological or physiological dependence, abuse, and tolerance. Review ophthalmic exam and monitor laboratory results (see above), therapeutic response (mental status, mood, affect), and adverse reactions at beginning of therapy and periodically with long-term use (endocrine changes, orthostatic hypotension, anticholinergic response, extrapyramidal effects, pigmentary retinopathy, neuroleptic malignant syndrome - see Adverse Reactions and Overdose/Toxicology). With I.M. or I.V. use, monitor closely for hypotension. **Note:** Avoid skin contact with oral or injection medication; may cause contact dermatitis (wash immediately with warm, soapy water). Initiate at lower doses (see Dosing) and taper dosage slowly when discontinuing. Assess knowledge/teach patient appropriate use, interventions to reduce side effects, and adverse symptoms to report (see below). **Pregnancy risk factor C** - instruct patient about appropriate contraceptive use. Breast-feeding is not recommended.

**Patient Information/Instruction:** Use exactly as directed (do not increase dose or frequency); may cause physical and/or psychological dependence. It may take 2-3 weeks to achieve desired results; do not discontinue without consulting prescriber.

(Continued)

## Promazine *(Continued)*

Dilute oral concentration with milk, water, or citrus juice; drink immediately after mixing. Do not take within 2 hours of any antacid. Avoid excess alcohol or caffeine and other prescription or OTC medications not approved by prescriber. Maintain adequate hydration (2-3 L/day of fluids unless instructed to restrict fluid intake). Avoid skin contact with medication; may cause contact dermatitis (wash immediately with warm, soapy water). You may experience excess drowsiness, restlessness, dizziness, or blurred vision (use caution driving or when engaging in tasks requiring alertness until response to drug is known); dry mouth, nausea, vomiting (small frequent meals, frequent mouth care, chewing gum, or sucking lozenges may help); constipation (increased exercise, fluids, or dietary fruit and fiber may help); postural hypotension (use caution climbing stairs or when changing position from lying or sitting to standing); urinary retention (void before taking medication); photosensitivity (use sunscreen, wear protective clothing and eyewear, and avoid direct sunlight); or decreased perspiration (avoid strenuous exercise in hot environments). Report persistent CNS effects (eg, trembling fingers, altered gait or balance, excessive sedation, seizures, unusual muscle or skeletal movements, anxiety, abnormal thoughts, confusion, personality changes); chest pain, palpitations, rapid heartbeat, severe dizziness; unresolved urinary retention or changes in urinary pattern; menstrual pattern changes, change in libido or ejaculatory difficulty; vision changes; skin rash or yellowing of skin; difficulty breathing; or worsening of condition. **Pregnancy/breast-feeding precautions:** Inform prescriber if you are or intend to be pregnant. Breast-feeding is not recommended.

**Geriatric Considerations:** (See Warnings/Precautions, Adverse Reactions, and Overdose/Toxicology.) Elderly patients have an increased risk of adverse response to side effects or adverse reactions to antipsychotics. These can include but are not limited to the following.

Anticholinergic effects: CNS toxicity with confusion, memory loss, psychotic behavior, and agitation.

Extrapyramidal effects (EPS): Parkinson's syndrome and akathisia may occur as often as 50% in patients >60 years of age. Tardive dyskinesia (motor restlessness) may be 40% in elderly; may be related to duration and total accumulated dose over time; may be somewhat reversible if diagnosed early enough.

Orthostatic hypotension: Increased risk for falls.

Sedation: In nonpsychotic patients, may result in feelings of depersonalization, derealization, and dysphoria.

Cardiac toxicity: Cardiac arrhythmias have occurred with therapeutic doses of antipsychotics.

Malignant neuroleptic syndrome: Development of hyperthermia, muscular rigidity, autonomic instability, and altered mental status.

Many elderly patients receive antipsychotic medications for inappropriate nonpsychotic behavior. Before initiating antipsychotic medication, all possible reversible causes should be investigated. Stress may cause acute "confusion" or worsening of baseline nonpsychotic behaviors; any changes in disease state (in any organ) may result in behavioral changes. Common acute changes in behavior may be due also to increases in drug dose addition, or addition of a new drug to the regimen; fluid/electrolyte alterations; infections; or changes in the environment.

Meta-analysis of controlled trials of antipsychotic (phenothiazines, butyrophenones) use with agitated, demented, elderly patients has concluded that the use of neuroleptics results in a response rate of 18%. Clearly, neuroleptic therapy for behavior control should be limited, with frequent attempts to withdraw the agent for behavior control. When use is indicated, initial doses should be lower to start and monitored closely.

**Additional Information** Some formulations may contain ethanol, tartrazine, or sulfites.

**Related Information**

Antipsychotic Agents Comparison *on page 1371*
Antipsychotic Medication Guidelines *on page 1436*

♦ **Prometa®** *see* Metaproterenol *on page 732*

## Promethazine (proe METH a zeen)

**U.S. Brand Names** Phenazine®; Phenergan®; Prorex®

**Therapeutic Category** Antiemetic

**Pregnancy Risk Factor** C

**Lactation** Enters breast milk/not recommended

**Use** Symptomatic treatment of various allergic conditions, antiemetic, motion sickness, and as a sedative

**Mechanism of Action/Effect** Blocks postsynaptic mesolimbic dopaminergic receptors in the brain; exhibits a strong alpha-adrenergic blocking effect and depresses the release of hypothalamic and hypophyseal hormones; competes with histamine for the $H_1$-receptor; reduces stimuli to the brainstem reticular system

**Contraindications** Hypersensitivity to promethazine or any component; narrow-angle glaucoma

**Warnings** Do not give S.C. or intra-arterially, necrotic lesions may occur. Injection may contain sulfites which may cause allergic reactions in some patients. Use with caution in patients with cardiovascular disease, impaired liver function, asthma, sleep apnea, and seizures. Rapid I.V. administration may produce a transient fall in blood pressure; rate of administration should not exceed 25 mg/minute. Slow I.V. administration may produce a slightly elevated blood pressure. Because promethazine is a phenothiazine (and can, therefore, cause side effects such as extrapyramidal symptoms), it is not considered an antihistamine of choice in the elderly. Pregnancy factor C.

**Drug Interactions**

**Cytochrome P-450 Effect:** CYP2D6 enzyme substrate

**Increased Effect/Toxicity:** Epinephrine should not be used together with promethazine since blood pressure may decrease further. Additive effects with other CNS depressants.

**Effects on Lab Values** Alters the flare response in intradermal allergen tests

**Adverse Reactions**

>10%:

Central nervous system: Slight to moderate drowsiness

Respiratory: Thickening of bronchial secretions

1% to 10%:

Central nervous system: Headache, fatigue, nervousness, dizziness

Gastrointestinal: Dry mouth, abdominal pain, nausea, diarrhea, increased appetite, weight gain

Neuromuscular & skeletal: Arthralgia

Respiratory: Pharyngitis

<1% (Limited to important or life-threatening symptoms): Tachycardia, bradycardia, palpitations, hypotension, hepatitis, irregular respiration, bronchospasm

**Overdose/Toxicology** Symptoms of overdose include CNS depression, respiratory depression, possible CNS stimulation, dry mouth, fixed and dilated pupils, and hypotension. Treatment is symptom directed and supportive.

**Pharmacodynamics/Kinetics**

**Metabolism:** Liver

**Excretion:** Urine and feces

**Onset:** I.V.: Within 20 minutes (3-5 minutes with I.V. injection)

**Duration:** 2-6 hours

**Formulations**

Promethazine hydrochloride:

Injection: 25 mg/mL (1 mL, 10 mL); 50 mg/mL (1 mL, 10 mL)

Suppository, rectal: 12.5 mg, 25 mg, 50 mg

Syrup: 6.25 mg/5 mL (5 mL, 120 mL, 240 mL, 480 mL, 4000 mL); 25 mg/5 mL (120 mL, 480 mL, 4000 mL)

Tablet: 12.5 mg, 25 mg, 50 mg

**Dosing**

**Adults:**

Antihistamine (including allergic reactions to blood or plasma):

Oral, rectal: 12.5 mg 3 times/day and 25 mg at bedtime

I.M., I.V.: 25 mg, may repeat in 2 hours when necessary; switch to oral route as soon as feasible

Antiemetic: Oral, I.M., I.V., rectal: 12.5-25 mg every 4 hours as needed

Motion sickness: Oral, rectal: 25 mg 30-60 minutes before departure, then every 12 hours as needed

Sedation: Oral, I.M., I.V., rectal: 25-50 mg/dose

**Elderly:** Refer to adult dosing and Geriatric Considerations.

**Renal Impairment:** Not dialyzable (0% to 5%)

**Administration**

**I.M.:** Administer into deep muscle.

**I.V.:** Avoid I.V. use. If necessary, may dilute to a maximum concentration of 25 mg/mL and infuse at a maximum rate of 25 mg/minute.

**I.V. Detail:** Rapid I.V. administration may produce a transient fall in blood pressure.

**Stability**

**Storage:** Protect from light and from freezing.

**Compatibility:** Compatible (when comixed in the same syringe) with atropine, chlorpromazine, diphenhydramine, droperidol, fentanyl, glycopyrrolate, hydromorphone, hydroxyzine hydrochloride, meperidine, midazolam, nalbuphine, pentazocine, prochlorperazine, scopolamine. Incompatible when mixed with aminophylline, cefoperazone (Y-site), chloramphenicol, dimenhydrinate (same syringe), foscarnet (Y-site), furosemide, heparin, hydrocortisone, methohexital, penicillin G, pentobarbital, phenobarbital, and thiopental. See the Compatibility of Drugs in Syringe Chart *on page 1317*.

**Additional Nursing Issues**

**Physical Assessment:** Assess other medications patient may be taking for effectiveness and interactions (see Warnings/Precautions and Drug Interactions). Monitor therapeutic response and adverse reactions (eg, blood pressure, CNS depression, respiratory status - see Adverse Reactions and Overdose/Toxicology). When used as an antiemetic, determine cause of vomiting prior to administration. Use and teach sedation safety measures (side rails up, call light within reach, etc). Assess knowledge/teach patient appropriate use, interventions to reduce side effects, and adverse symptoms to report. **Pregnancy risk factor C** - benefits of use should outweigh possible risks. Breast-feeding is not recommended.

**Patient Information/Instruction:** Take this drug as prescribed; do not increase dosage. Do not use alcohol or other CNS depressants or sleeping aids without consulting prescriber. May cause dizziness, drowsiness, or blurred vision (use caution when driving or engaging in tasks requiring alertness until response to drug is known); nausea, dry mouth, appetite disturbances (small frequent meals, frequent mouth care, chewing gum, or sucking lozenges may help). Report unusual weight gain, unresolved nausea or diarrhea, chest pain or palpitations, excess sedation or stimulation, or sore

(Continued)

## Promethazine *(Continued)*

throat or difficulty breathing. **Pregnancy/breast-feeding precautions:** Inform prescriber if you are or intend to be pregnant. Breast-feeding is not recommended.

**Geriatric Considerations:** Because promethazine is a phenothiazine (and can, therefore, cause side effects such as extrapyramidal symptoms), it is not considered an antihistamine of choice in the elderly.

**Additional Information** Some formulations may contain benzyl alcohol. The injection formulation contains sulfites.

**Related Information**

Antiemetics for Chemotherapy-Induced Nausea and Vomiting *on page 1307*

## Promethazine and Codeine (proe METH a zeen & KOE deen)

**U.S. Brand Names** Phenergan® With Codeine; Pherazine® With Codeine; Prothazine-DC®

**Synonyms** Codeine and Promethazine

**Therapeutic Category** Antihistamine/Antitussive

**Pregnancy Risk Factor** C

**Lactation** Enters breast milk (codeine)/not recommended

**Use** Temporary relief of coughs and upper respiratory symptoms associated with allergy or the common cold

**Formulations** Syrup: Promethazine hydrochloride 6.25 mg and codeine phosphate 10 mg per 5 mL (120 mL, 180 mL, 473 mL)

**Dosing**

**Adults:** Oral: 10-20 mg/dose every 4-6 hours as needed; maximum: 120 mg codeine/day; or 5-10 mL every 4-6 hours as needed

**Elderly:** Refer to dosing in individual monographs.

**Additional Nursing Issues**

**Physical Assessment:** See individual components listed in Related Information. **Pregnancy risk factor C** - benefits of use should outweigh possible risks. Breast-feeding is not recommended.

**Patient Information/Instruction:** See individual components listed in Related Information. **Pregnancy/breast-feeding precautions:** Inform prescriber if you are on intend to get pregnant. Breast-feeding is not recommended.

**Related Information**

Codeine *on page 299*

Promethazine *on page 978*

## Promethazine and Dextromethorphan

(proe METH a zeen & deks troe meth OR fan)

**U.S. Brand Names** Phenameth® DM; Phenergan® With Dextromethorphan; Pherazine® w/DM

**Synonyms** Dextromethorphan and Promethazine

**Therapeutic Category** Antihistamine/Antitussive

**Pregnancy Risk Factor** C

**Lactation** Excretion in breast milk unknown/not recommended

**Use** Temporary relief of coughs and upper respiratory symptoms associated with allergy or the common cold

**Formulations** Syrup: Promethazine hydrochloride 6.25 mg and dextromethorphan hydrobromide 15 mg per 5 mL with alcohol 7% (120 mL, 480 mL, 4000 mL)

**Dosing**

**Adults:** Oral: 5 mL every 4-6 hours, up to 30 mL in 24 hours

**Elderly:** Refer to dosing in individual monographs.

**Additional Nursing Issues**

**Physical Assessment:** See individual components listed in Related Information. **Pregnancy risk factor C** - benefits of use should outweigh possible risks. Breast-feeding is not recommended.

**Patient Information/Instruction:** See individual components listed in Related Information. **Pregnancy/breast-feeding precautions:** Inform prescriber if you are on intend to get pregnant. Breast-feeding is not recommended.

**Related Information**

Promethazine *on page 978*

♦ **Promethazine and Meperidine** *see* Meperidine and Promethazine *on page 722*

## Promethazine and Phenylephrine (proe METH a zeen & fen il EF rin)

**U.S. Brand Names** Phenergan® VC Syrup; Prometh VC Plain Liquid

**Synonyms** Phenylephrine and Promethazine

**Therapeutic Category** Antihistamine/Decongestant Combination

**Pregnancy Risk Factor** C

**Lactation** Excretion in breast milk unknown/not recommended

**Use** Temporary relief of upper respiratory symptoms associated with allergy or the common cold

**Formulations** Liquid: Promethazine hydrochloride 6.25 mg and phenylephrine hydrochloride 5 mg per 5 mL (120 mL, 240 mL, 473 mL)

**Dosing**

**Adults:** Oral: 5 mL every 4-6 hours, not to exceed 30 mL in 24 hours

**Elderly:** Refer to dosing in individual monographs.

**Additional Nursing Issues**

**Physical Assessment:** See individual components listed in Related Information. **Pregnancy risk factor C** - benefits of use should outweigh possible risks. Breast-feeding is not recommended.

**Patient Information/Instruction:** See individual components listed in Related Information. **Pregnancy/breast-feeding precautions:** Inform prescriber if you are on intend to get pregnant. Breast-feeding is not recommended.

**Related Information**

Phenylephrine *on page 920*
Promethazine *on page 978*

## Promethazine, Phenylephrine, and Codeine

(proe METH a zeen, fen il EF rin, & KOE deen)

**U.S. Brand Names** Mallergan-VC® With Codeine; Phenergan® VC With Codeine

**Synonyms** Codeine, Promethazine, and Phenylephrine; Phenylephrine, Promethazine, and Codeine

**Therapeutic Category** Antihistamine/Decongestant/Antitussive

**Pregnancy Risk Factor** C

**Lactation** Enters breast milk/not recommended

**Use** Temporary relief of coughs and upper respiratory symptoms including nasal congestion

**Formulations** Liquid: Promethazine hydrochloride 6.25 mg, phenylephrine hydrochloride 5 mg, and codeine phosphate 10 mg per 5 mL with alcohol 7% (120 mL, 240 mL, 480 mL, 4000 mL)

**Dosing**

**Adults:** 5 mL syrup every 4-6 hours

**Elderly:** Refer to dosing in individual monographs.

**Additional Nursing Issues**

**Physical Assessment:** See individual components listed in Related Information. **Pregnancy risk factor C** - benefits of use should outweigh possible risks. Breast-feeding is not recommended.

**Patient Information/Instruction:** See individual components listed in Related Information. **Pregnancy/breast-feeding precautions:** Inform prescriber if you are on intend to get pregnant. Breast-feeding is not recommended.

**Related Information**

Codeine *on page 299*
Phenylephrine *on page 920*
Promethazine *on page 978*

- **Prometh VC Plain Liquid** *see* Promethazine and Phenylephrine *on previous page*
- **Promine®** *see* Procainamide *on page 967*
- **Promit®** *see* Dextran 1 *on page 352*
- **Pronaxil** *see* Naproxen *on page 807*
- **Pronestyl®** *see* Procainamide *on page 967*
- **Pronto® Shampoo** *see page 1294*
- **Propacet®** *see* Propoxyphene and Acetaminophen *on page 985*
- **Propaderm®** *see* Beclomethasone *on page 135*

## Propafenone (proe pa FEEN one)

**U.S. Brand Names** Rythmol®

**Therapeutic Category** Antiarrhythmic Agent, Class I-C

**Pregnancy Risk Factor** C

**Lactation** Excretion in breast milk unknown

**Use** Life-threatening ventricular arrhythmias

**Unlabeled use:** Supraventricular tachycardias, including those patients with Wolff-Parkinson-White syndrome

**Mechanism of Action/Effect** Propafenone is a Class 1C antiarrhythmic agent which possesses local anesthetic properties, blocks the fast inward sodium current, and slows the rate of increase of the action potential. prolongs conduction and refractoriness in all areas of the myocardium, with a slightly more pronounced effect on intraventricular conduction; it prolongs effective refractory period, reduces spontaneous automaticity and exhibits some beta-blockade activity.

**Contraindications** Hypersensitivity to propafenone or any component; uncontrolled congestive heart failure; bronchospastic disorders; cardiogenic shock; conduction disorders (A-V block, sick-sinus syndrome); bradycardia

**Warnings** Until evidence to the contrary, propafenone should be considered acceptable only for the treatment of life-threatening arrhythmias. Propafenone may cause new or worsened arrhythmias, worsen CHF, decrease A-V conduction and alter pacemaker thresholds. Use with caution in patients with recent myocardial infarction, congestive heart failure, or hepatic or renal dysfunction. Elderly may be at greater risk for toxicity. Pregnancy factor C.

**Drug Interactions**

**Cytochrome P-450 Effect:** CYP1A2, 2D6, 3A3/4 enzyme substrate; CYP2D6 enzyme inhibitor

(Continued)

## Propafenone *(Continued)*

**Decreased Effect:** Decreased propafenone levels with rifampin.

**Increased Effect/Toxicity:** Increased propafenone levels with cimetidine, quinidine, and beta-blockers. Increased effect/levels of warfarin, beta-blockers metabolized by the liver, local anesthetics, cyclosporine, and digoxin (**Note:** Reduce dose of digoxin by 25%).

**Food Interactions** Propafenone serum concentrations may be increased if taken with food.

**Adverse Reactions**

>10%:

Central nervous system: Dizziness, drowsiness

Gastrointestinal: Dry mouth

1% to 10%:

Cardiovascular: A-V block (first and second degree), cardiac conduction disturbances, palpitations, congestive heart failure, chest pain, bradycardia

Central nervous system: Headache, anxiety, loss of balance

Gastrointestinal: Abnormal taste, constipation, nausea, vomiting, abdominal pain, heartburn, anorexia, flatulence, diarrhea

Ocular: Blurred vision

Respiratory: Dyspnea

<1% (Limited to important or life-threatening symptoms): New or worsened arrhythmias (proarrhythmic effect), bundle-branch block, leukopenia, thrombocytopenia, agranulocytosis

**Overdose/Toxicology** Propafenone has a narrow therapeutic index and severe toxicity may occur slightly above the therapeutic range, especially if combined with other antiarrhythmic drugs. Acute single ingestion of twice the daily therapeutic dose is life-threatening. Symptoms of overdose include increased P-R, QRS, or Q-T intervals and amplitude of the T wave, A-V block, bradycardia, hypotension, ventricular arrhythmias (monomorphic or polymorphic ventricular tachycardia), and asystole. Other symptoms include dizziness, blurred vision, headache, and GI upset. Treatment is supportive. **Note:** Class 1A antiarrhythmic agents should not be used to treat cardiotoxicity caused by Class 1C drugs. Sodium bicarbonate may reverse QRS prolongation, bradycardia, and hypotension. Ventricular pacing may be needed. Hemodialysis is only of possible benefit for tocainide or flecainide overdose in patients with renal failure.

**Pharmacodynamics/Kinetics**

**Half-life Elimination:** After a single dose (100-300 mg): 2-8 hours; half-life after chronic dosing ranges from 10-32 hours

**Time to Peak:** Peak levels occur in 2 hours with a 150 mg dose and 3 hours after a 300 mg dose. This agent exhibits nonlinear pharmacokinetics. When dose is increased from 300-900 mg/day, serum concentrations increase tenfold. This nonlinearity is thought to be due to saturable first-pass hepatic enzyme metabolism.

**Metabolism:** Two genetically determined metabolism groups exist: fast or slow metabolizers; 10% of Caucasians are slow metabolizers

**Formulations** Tablet, as hydrochloride: 150 mg, 225 mg, 300 mg

**Dosing**

**Adults:** Oral: 150 mg every 8 hours, increase at 3- to 4-day intervals up to 300 mg every 8 hours. **Note:** Patients who exhibit significant widening of QRS complex or second or third degree A-V block may need dose reduction.

**Elderly:** Refer to adult dosing

**Hepatic Impairment:** Reduction is necessary.

**Additional Nursing Issues**

**Physical Assessment:** Assess other medications patient may be taking for effectiveness and interactions (see Drug Interactions). See Warnings/Precautions and Contraindications for cautious use. Monitor laboratory tests (see above), therapeutic response (cardiac status), and adverse reactions (see Warnings/Precautions and Adverse Reactions) at beginning of therapy, when titrating dosage, and on a regular basis with long-term therapy. **Note:** Propafenone has a low toxic:therapeutic ratio and overdose may easily produce severe and life-threatening reactions (see Overdose/Toxicology). Assess knowledge/teach patient appropriate use, interventions to reduce side effects, and adverse symptoms to report. **Pregnancy risk factor C** - benefits of use should outweigh possible risks. Note breast-feeding caution.

**Patient Information/Instruction:** Take exactly as directed; do not take additional doses or discontinue without consulting prescriber. You will need regular cardiac checkups and blood tests while taking this medication. You may experience dizziness, drowsiness, or visual changes (use caution when driving or engaging in tasks requiring alertness until response to drug is known); abnormal taste, nausea or vomiting, or loss of appetite (small frequent meals, frequent mouth care, chewing gum, or sucking lozenges may help); headaches (prescriber may recommend mild analgesic); or diarrhea (exercise, yogurt, or boiled milk may help - if persistent consult prescriber). Report chest pain, palpitation, or erratic heartbeat; difficulty breathing, increased weight or swelling of hands or feet; acute persistent diarrhea or constipation; or changes in vision. **Pregnancy/breast-feeding precautions:** Inform prescriber if you are or intend to be pregnant. Consult prescriber if breast-feeding.

**Geriatric Considerations:** Elderly may have age-related decreases in hepatic Phase I metabolism. Propafenone is dependent upon liver metabolism, therefore, monitor closely in the elderly and adjust dose more gradually during initial treatment (see Warnings/Precautions). No differences in clearance noted with impaired renal function and, therefore, no adjustment for renal function in the elderly is necessary.

**Related Information**

Antiarrhythmic Drug Classification Comparison *on page 1366*

♦ **Propagest® [OTC]** *see* Phenylpropanolamine *on page 922*

## Propantheline (proe PAN the leen)

**U.S. Brand Names** Pro-Banthine®

**Therapeutic Category** Anticholinergic Agent

**Pregnancy Risk Factor** C

**Lactation** Excretion in breast milk unknown

**Use** Adjunctive treatment of peptic ulcer, irritable bowel syndrome, pancreatitis, ureteral and urinary bladder spasm; reduce duodenal motility during diagnostic radiologic procedures

**Mechanism of Action/Effect** Competitively blocks the action of acetylcholine at postganglionic parasympathetic receptor sites

**Contraindications** Hypersensitivity to propantheline; narrow-angle glaucoma; ulcerative colitis; toxic megacolon; obstructive disease of the GI or urinary tract

**Warnings** Use with caution in patients with hyperthyroidism, hepatic, cardiac, or renal disease, hypertension, GI infections, or other endocrine diseases. Pregnancy factor C.

**Drug Interactions**

**Decreased Effect:** Decreased effect with antacids (decreased absorption). Decreased effect of sustained release dosage forms (decreased absorption).

**Increased Effect/Toxicity:** Increased effect/toxicity with anticholinergics, disopyramide, narcotic analgesics, bretylium, Type I antiarrhythmics, antihistamines, phenothiazines, tricyclic antidepressants, corticosteroids (increased IOP), CNS depressants (sedation), adenosine, amiodarone, beta-blockers, and amoxapine.

**Adverse Reactions**

>10%:

Dermatologic: Dry skin
Gastrointestinal: Constipation, dry mouth, dry throat
Respiratory: Dry nose
Miscellaneous: Sweating (decreased)

1% to 10%: Gastrointestinal: Dysphagia

<1% (Limited to important or life-threatening symptoms): Tachycardia, increased intraocular pressure

**Overdose/Toxicology** Symptoms of overdose include CNS disturbances, flushing, respiratory failure, paralysis, coma, urinary retention, and hyperthermia. For anticholinergic overdose with severe life-threatening symptoms, physostigmine 1-2 mg S.C. or I.V. slowly, may be given to reverse these effects.

**Pharmacodynamics/Kinetics**

**Metabolism:** Liver and GI tract

**Excretion:** Urine, bile, and other body fluids

**Onset:** Oral: Within 30-45 minutes

**Duration:** 4-6 hours

**Formulations** Tablet, as bromide: 7.5 mg, 15 mg

**Dosing**

**Adults:** Oral:

Antisecretory: 15 mg 3 times/day before meals or food and 30 mg at bedtime
Antispasmodic: 15 mg 3 times/day before meals or food and 30 mg at bedtime

**Elderly:** Antisecretory: Oral: 7.5 mg 3 times/day before meals and at bedtime

**Administration**

**Oral:** Give before meals so that the drug's peak (1-3 hours) occurs when food is no longer in the stomach offering a buffering effect.

**Additional Nursing Issues**

**Physical Assessment:** Assess effectiveness and interactions of other medications (see Drug Interactions). See Warnings/Precautions and Contraindications for use cautions (eg, GI or GU obstructions). Monitor effectiveness of therapy and adverse response (see Adverse Reactions and Overdose/Toxicology). Assess knowledge/teach patient appropriate use, possible side effects and appropriate interventions, and adverse symptoms to report. **Pregnancy risk factor C** - benefits of use should outweigh possible risks. Note breast-feeding caution.

**Patient Information/Instruction:** Take as directed before meals; do not increase dose and do not discontinue without consulting prescriber. Void before taking medication. You may experience constipation (increased dietary fruit, fluids, fiber, and exercise may help). Report chest pain or rapid heartbeat, or excessive and persistent anticholinergic effects (blurred vision, headache, flushing, tachycardia, nervousness, constipation, dizziness, insomnia, mental confusion or excitement, dry mouth, altered taste perception, dysphagia, palpitations, bradycardia, urinary hesitancy or retention, impotence, decreased sweating). **Pregnancy/breast-feeding precautions:** Inform prescriber if you are or intend to be pregnant. Consult prescriber if breast-feeding.

**Geriatric Considerations:** The primary use of propantheline in the geriatric population is for treatment of urinary incontinence due to detrusor instability. Even though it does not cross the blood-brain barrier, CNS effects have been reported. Orthostatic hypotension may also occur, therefore, avoid long-term use in the elderly.

♦ **Proparacaine** *see page 1248*
♦ **Proparacaine and Fluorescein** *see page 1248*
♦ **Propecia®** *see* Finasteride *on page 485*
♦ **Propine® Ophthalmic** *see* Ophthalmic Agents, Glaucoma *on page 853*
♦ **Pro-Piroxicam®** *see* Piroxicam *on page 940*

## Propoxyphene (proe POKS i feen)

**U.S. Brand Names** Darvon®; Darvon-N®; Dolene®

**Synonyms** Dextropropoxyphene

**Therapeutic Category** Analgesic, Narcotic

**Pregnancy Risk Factor** C/D (if used for prolonged periods)

**Lactation** Enters breast milk/use caution (AAP rates "compatible")

**Use** Management of mild to moderate pain

**Mechanism of Action/Effect** Binds to opiate receptors in the CNS, causing inhibition of ascending pain pathways, altering the perception of and response to pain; produces generalized CNS depression

**Contraindications** Hypersensitivity to propoxyphene or any component; pregnancy (if used for prolonged periods)

**Warnings** Give with caution in patients dependent on opiates. Substitution may result in acute opiate withdrawal symptoms. Use with caution in patients with severe renal or hepatic dysfunction. When given in excessive doses, either alone or in combination with other CNS depressants or propoxyphene products, propoxyphene is a major cause of drug-related deaths. **Do not exceed recommended dosage.** Pregnancy factor C/D (if prolonged use).

**Drug Interactions**

**Cytochrome P-450 Effect:** CYP3A3/4 enzyme inhibitor

**Decreased Effect:** Decreased effect with cigarette smoking.

**Increased Effect/Toxicity:** CNS depressants (phenothiazines, tranquilizers, anxiolytics, sedatives, hypnotics, or alcohol) may potentiate pharmacologic effects. Propoxyphene may inhibit the metabolism and increase the serum concentrations of carbamazepine, phenobarbital, MAO inhibitors, tricyclic antidepressants, and warfarin.

**Food Interactions** Onset of effect may be delayed if propoxyphene is taken with food.

**Effects on Lab Values** False-positive methadone test; ↑ LFTs; ↓ glucose (S), 17-OHCS (U)

**Adverse Reactions**

>10%:

Cardiovascular: Hypotension
Central nervous system: Fatigue, drowsiness, dizziness
Gastrointestinal: Nausea, vomiting
Neuromuscular & skeletal: Weakness

1% to 10%:

Central nervous system: Nervousness, headache, convulsions, restlessness, malaise, false sense of well-being, nightmares
Dermatologic: Rash, urticaria
Gastrointestinal: Dry mouth, constipation, increased LFT's
Genitourinary: Ureteral spasms, decreased urination
Neuromuscular & skeletal: Trembling
Ocular: Blurred vision
Otic: Tinnitus
Miscellaneous: Histamine release

<1% (Limited to important or life-threatening symptoms): Hypertension, hepatotoxicity

**Overdose/Toxicology** Symptoms of overdose include CNS disturbances, respiratory depression, hypotension, pulmonary edema, and seizures. Naloxone, 2 mg I.V. with repeat administration as necessary up to a total of 10 mg, can also be used to reverse toxic effects of the opiate. Charcoal is very effective (>95%) at binding propoxyphene.

**Pharmacodynamics/Kinetics**

**Half-life Elimination:** Parent drug: 8-24 hours (mean: ~15 hours); Norpropoxyphene: 34 hours

**Metabolism:** Liver

**Excretion:** Urine

**Onset:** Onset of effect: Oral: Within 0.5-1 hour

**Duration:** 4-6 hours

**Formulations**

Capsule, as hydrochloride: 65 mg
Tablet, as napsylate: 100 mg

**Dosing**

**Adults:** Oral:

Hydrochloride: 65 mg every 3-4 hours as needed for pain; maximum: 390 mg/day
Napsylate: 100 mg every 4 hours as needed for pain; maximum: 600 mg/day

**Elderly:** Oral:

Hydrochloride: 65 mg every 4-6 hours as needed for pain
Napsylate: 100 mg every 4-6 hours as needed for pain

**Renal Impairment:**

$Cl_{cr}$ <10 mL/minute: Avoid use.
Not dialyzable (0% to 5%)

**Hepatic Impairment:** Reduced doses should be used.

**Administration**

**Oral:** Should be administered with glass of water on empty stomach. Food may decrease rate of absorption, but may slightly increase bioavailability.

**Additional Nursing Issues**

**Physical Assessment:** Monitor for effectiveness of pain relief. Monitor blood pressure, mental and respiratory status, degree of sedation, and CNS changes. Monitor for signs of overdose (see above). **Pregnancy risk factor C/D** - see Pregnancy Risk Factor - assess knowledge/instruct patient on use of barrier contraceptive measures;

danger of use during pregnancy must outweigh risk to fetus. Note breast-feeding caution.

**Patient Information/Instruction:** Take as directed; do not take a larger dose or more often than prescribed. Do not use alcohol, other prescription or OTC sedatives, tranquilizers, antihistamines, or pain medications without consulting prescriber. May cause dizziness, drowsiness, or impaired judgment; avoid driving or engaging in tasks requiring alertness until response to drug is known. If you experience vomiting or loss of appetite, frequent mouth care, small frequent meals, chewing gum, or sucking lozenges may help. Increased fluid intake, exercise, fiber in diet may help with constipation (if unresolved consult prescriber). Report unresolved nausea or vomiting, difficulty breathing or shortness of breath, or unusual weakness. **Pregnancy/breast-feeding precautions:** Inform prescriber if you are or intend to be pregnant. Breast-feeding women should take this drug 4-5 hours before nursing.

**Geriatric Considerations:** The elderly may be particularly susceptible to the CNS depressant effects of narcotics.

**Additional Information** 100 mg of napsylate = 65 mg of hydrochloride

Propoxyphene hydrochloride: Darvon®

Propoxyphene napsylate: Darvon-N®

**Related Information**

Narcotic/Opioid Analgesic Comparison *on page 1396*

## Propoxyphene and Acetaminophen

(proe POKS i feen & a seet a MIN oh fen)

**U.S. Brand Names** Darvocet-N®; Darvocet-N® 100; Genagesic®; Propacet®; Wygesic®

**Synonyms** Acetaminophen and Propoxyphene

**Therapeutic Category** Analgesic, Combination (Narcotic)

**Pregnancy Risk Factor** C

**Lactation** Enters breast milk/compatible

**Use** Management of mild to moderate pain

**Formulations**

Tablet:

Darvocet-N®: Propoxyphene napsylate 50 mg and acetaminophen 325 mg

Darvocet-N® 100: Propoxyphene napsylate 100 mg and acetaminophen 650 mg

Genagesic®, Wygesic®: Propoxyphene hydrochloride 65 mg and acetaminophen 650 mg

**Dosing**

**Adults:** Oral:

Darvocet-N®: 1-2 tablets every 4 hours as needed; maximum: 600 mg propoxyphene napsylate/day

Darvocet-N® 100: 1 tablet every 4 hours as needed; maximum: 600 mg propoxyphene napsylate/day

**Elderly:** Refer to adult dosing.

**Additional Nursing Issues**

**Physical Assessment:** See individual components listed in Related Information. **Pregnancy risk factor C** - benefits of use should outweigh possible risks.

**Patient Information/Instruction:** See individual components listed in Related Information. **Pregnancy precautions:** Inform prescriber if you are on intend to get pregnant.

**Related Information**

Acetaminophen *on page 32*

Propoxyphene *on previous page*

## Propoxyphene and Aspirin (proe POKS i feen & AS pir in)

**U.S. Brand Names** Bexophene®; Darvon® Compound-65 Pulvules®

**Synonyms** Aspirin and Propoxyphene

**Therapeutic Category** Analgesic, Combination (Narcotic)

**Pregnancy Risk Factor** D

**Lactation** Enters breast milk/use caution due to aspirin content

**Use** Management of mild to moderate pain

**Formulations**

Capsule: Propoxyphene hydrochloride 65 mg and aspirin 389 mg with caffeine 32.4 mg

Tablet (Darvon-N® with A.S.A.): Propoxyphene napsylate 100 mg and aspirin 325 mg

**Dosing**

**Adults:** 1 capsule (propoxyphene 65 mg) every 4 hours; maximum: 390 mg/day

**Elderly:** Refer to dosing in individual monographs.

**Renal Impairment:** Dose reduction is recommended.

**Hepatic Impairment:** Dose reduction is recommended.

**Additional Nursing Issues**

**Physical Assessment:** See individual components listed in Related Information. **Pregnancy risk factor D** - assess knowledge/instruct patient on need to use appropriate contraceptive measures and the need to avoid pregnancy. Note breast-feeding caution.

**Patient Information/Instruction:** See individual components listed in Related Information. **Pregnancy/breast-feeding precautions:** Inform prescriber if you are on intend to get pregnant. Consult prescriber if breast-feeding.

**Related Information**

Aspirin *on page 111*

Propoxyphene *on previous page*

## Propranolol (proe PRAN oh lole)

**U.S. Brand Names** Betachron E-R®; Inderal®; Inderal® LA

**Therapeutic Category** Antiarrhythmic Agent, Class II; Beta Blocker, Nonselective

**Pregnancy Risk Factor** C

**Lactation** Enters breast milk/use caution (AAP rates "compatible")

**Use** Management of hypertension, angina pectoris, pheochromocytoma, essential tremor, tetralogy of Fallot cyanotic spells, and arrhythmias (such as atrial fibrillation and flutter, A-V nodal re-entrant tachycardias, and catecholamine-induced arrhythmias); prevention of myocardial infarction, migraine headache; symptomatic treatment of hypertrophic subaortic stenosis

**Unlabeled use:** Tremor due to Parkinson's disease, alcohol withdrawal, aggressive behavior, antipsychotic-induced akathisia, bleeding esophageal varices, anxiety, schizophrenia, acute panic, and gastric bleeding in portal hypertension

**Mechanism of Action/Effect** Nonselective beta-adrenergic blocker (Class II antiarrhythmic); competitively blocks response to $beta_1$- and $beta_2$-adrenergic stimulation which results in decreases in heart rate, myocardial contractility, blood pressure, and myocardial oxygen demand

**Contraindications** Hypersensitivity to beta-blockers; uncompensated congestive heart failure; cardiogenic shock; bradycardia or heart block; pulmonary edema; severe hyperactive airway disease or chronic obstructive lung disease; Raynaud's disease

**Warnings** Safety and efficacy in children have not been established. Administer very cautiously to patients with CHF, asthma, diabetes mellitus, and hyperthyroidism. Abrupt withdrawal of the drug should be avoided, drug should be discontinued over 1-2 weeks. May potentiate hypoglycemia in a diabetic patient and mask signs or symptoms. Pregnancy factor C.

**Drug Interactions**

**Cytochrome P-450 Effect:** CYP1A2, 2C18, 2C19, and 2D6 enzyme substrate

**Decreased Effect:**

Aluminum salts, barbiturates, calcium salts, cholestyramine, colestipol, NSAIDs, penicillins (ampicillin), rifampin, salicylates and sulfinpyrazone decrease effect of beta-blockers due to decreased bioavailability and plasma levels

Beta-blockers may decrease the effect of sulfonylureas

Ascorbic acid decreases propranolol $Cp_{max}$ and AUC and increases the $T_{max}$ significantly resulting in a greater decrease in the reduction of heart rate, possibly due to decreased absorption and first pass metabolism (n=5)

Nefazodone decreased peak plasma levels and AUC of propranolol and increases time to reach steady state; monitoring of clinical response is recommended

**Increased Effect/Toxicity:** Increased effect/toxicity of beta-blockers with calcium blockers (diltiazem, felodipine, nicardipine), contraceptives, flecainide, haloperidol (hypotensive effects), $H_2$-antagonists (cimetidine, possibly ranitidine), hydralazine, loop diuretics, possibly MAO inhibitors, phenothiazines, propafenone, quinidine (in extensive metabolizers), ciprofloxacin, thyroid hormones (when hypothyroid patient is converted to euthyroid state)

Beta-blockers may increase the effect/toxicity of flecainide, haloperidol (hypotensive effects), hydralazine, phenothiazines, acetaminophen, anticoagulants (warfarin), benzodiazepines, clonidine (hypertensive crisis after or during withdrawal of either agent), epinephrine (initial hypertensive episode followed by bradycardia), nifedipine and verapamil lidocaine, ergots (peripheral ischemia), prazosin (postural hypotension)

Beta-blockers may affect the action or levels of ethanol, disopyramide, nondepolarizing muscle relaxants and theophylline although the effects are difficult to predict

**Food Interactions** Propranolol serum levels may be increased if taken with food.

**Effects on Lab Values** ↑ thyroxine (S)

**Adverse Reactions**

>10%:

Central nervous system: Drowsiness, insomnia

Endocrine & metabolic: Decreased sexual ability

1% to 10%:

Cardiovascular: Bradycardia, palpitations, edema, congestive heart failure, reduced peripheral circulation

Central nervous system: Mental depression

Gastrointestinal: Diarrhea or constipation, nausea, vomiting, stomach discomfort

Respiratory: Bronchospasm

Miscellaneous: Cold extremities

<1% (Limited to important or life-threatening symptoms): Chest pain, arrhythmias, orthostatic hypotension, nervousness, headache, hallucinations, confusion (especially in the elderly), thrombocytopenia, leukopenia, shortness of breath

**Overdose/Toxicology** Symptoms of intoxication include cardiac disturbances, CNS toxicity, bronchospasm, hypoglycemia, and hyperkalemia. The most common cardiac symptoms include hypotension and bradycardia. Atrioventricular block, intraventricular conduction disturbances, cardiogenic shock, and asystole may occur with severe overdose, especially with membrane-depressant drugs (eg, propranolol). CNS effects include convulsions and coma. Respiratory arrest is commonly seen with propranolol and other membrane-depressant and lipid-soluble drugs. Treatment is symptom directed and supportive.

**Pharmacodynamics/Kinetics**

**Protein Binding:** 93%

**Distribution:** Crosses the placenta

**Half-life Elimination:** 4-6 hours

**Metabolism:** Liver

**Excretion:** Urine

**Onset:** Onset of beta blockade: Oral: Within 1-2 hours

**Duration:** ~6 hours

**Formulations**

Propranolol hydrochloride:

- Capsule, sustained action: 60 mg, 80 mg, 120 mg, 160 mg
- Injection: 1 mg/mL (1 mL)
- Solution, oral (strawberry-mint flavor): 4 mg/mL (5 mL, 500 mL); 8 mg/mL (5 mL, 500 mL)
- Solution, oral, concentrate: 80 mg/mL (30 mL)
- Tablet: 10 mg, 20 mg, 40 mg, 60 mg, 80 mg

**Dosing**

**Adults:**

Tachyarrhythmias:

- Oral: 10-30 mg/dose every 6-8 hours
- I.V.: 1 mg/dose slow IVP; repeat every 5 minutes up to a total of 5 mg.

Hypertension: Oral: Initial: 40 mg twice daily; increase dosage every 3-7 days; usual dose: ≤320 mg divided in 2-3 doses/day; maximum daily dose: 640 mg.

Migraine headache prophylaxis: Oral: Initial: 80 mg/day divided every 6-8 hours; increase by 20-40 mg/dose every 3-4 weeks to a maximum of 160-240 mg/day given in divided doses every 6-8 hours. If satisfactory response not achieved within 6 weeks of starting therapy, drug should be withdrawn gradually over several weeks.

Thyrotoxicosis:

- Oral: 10-40 mg/dose every 6 hours
- I.V.: 1-3 mg/dose slow IVP as a single dose

Oral:

- Angina: 80-320 mg/day in doses divided 2-4 times/day
- Pheochromocytoma: 30-60 mg/day in divided doses
- Myocardial infarction prophylaxis: 180-240 mg/day in 3-4 divided doses
- Hypertrophic subaortic stenosis: 20-40 mg 3-4 times/day
- Essential tremor: 40 mg twice daily initially; maintenance doses: usually 120-320 mg/day

**Elderly:** Arrhythmias: Initial: 10 mg twice daily or 60 mg once daily as sustained release capsules; increase dosage every 3-7 days; usual dose range: 10-320 mg given 1-2 times/day. Refer to adult dosing for additional uses.

**Renal Impairment:**

$Cl_{cr}$ 31-40 mL/minute: Administer every 24-36 hours or administer 50% of normal dose.

$Cl_{cr}$ 10-30 mL/minute: Administer every 24-48 hours or administer 50% of normal dose.

$Cl_{cr}$ <10 mL/minute: Administer every 40-60 hours or administer 25% of normal dose.

Not dialyzable (0% to 5%); supplemental dose is not necessary.

Peritoneal dialysis effects: Supplemental dose is not necessary.

**Hepatic Impairment:** Marked slowing of heart rate may occur in cirrhosis with conventional doses; low initial dose and regular heart rate monitoring.

**Administration**

**I.V.:** I.V. administration should not exceed 1 mg/minute. I.V. dose is much smaller than oral dose.

**Stability**

**Storage:** Protect injection from light. Solutions have maximum stability at pH of 3 and decompose rapidly in alkaline pH. Propranolol is stable for 24 hours at room temperature in $D_5W$ or NS.

**Compatibility:** Compatible in saline. Incompatible with $HCO_3^-$.

**Additional Nursing Issues**

**Physical Assessment:** Assess effectiveness and interactions of other medications patient may be taking (see Drug Interactions). Monitor therapeutic response and adverse reactions (cardiac status, vital signs, fluid status) when starting or adjusting dosage (see Warnings/Precautions and Adverse Reactions). I.V. infusion requires hemodynamic monitoring. Monitor serum glucose closely in diabetic patients. Beta-blockers may alter serum glucose levels. Use and teach orthostatic precautions. Assess knowledge/teach patient appropriate use, interventions to reduce side effects, and adverse symptoms to report. **Pregnancy risk factor C** - benefits of use should outweigh possible risks. See Breast-feeding note below.

**Patient Information/Instruction:** Take exactly as directed; do not increase, decrease, or discontinue without consulting prescriber. Take at the same time each day. Tablets may be crushed and taken with liquids. Do not alter dietary intake of protein or carbohydrates without consulting prescriber. You may experience orthostatic hypotension, dizziness, drowsiness, or blurred vision (use caution when driving, climbing stairs, or changing position - rising from sitting or lying to standing - or engaging in tasks requiring alertness until response to drug is known); nausea, vomiting, or stomach discomfort (small frequent meals, frequent mouth care, chewing gum, or sucking lozenges may help); decreased sexual ability (reversible). If diabetic, monitor serum glucose closely. Report unusual swelling of extremities, difficulty breathing, unresolved cough, or unusual weight gain, cold extremities, persistent diarrhea, confusion, hallucinations, headache, nervousness, lack of improvement, or worsening of condition. **Pregnancy/breast-feeding precautions:** Inform prescriber if you are or intend to be pregnant. Consult prescriber if breast-feeding.

(Continued)

## Propranolol *(Continued)*

**Geriatric Considerations:** Since bioavailability increased in the elderly, about twofold geriatric patients may require lower maintenance doses, therefore, as serum and tissue concentrations increase beta$_1$ selectivity diminishes; due to alterations in the beta-adrenergic autonomic nervous system, beta-adrenergic blockade may result in less hemodynamic response than seen in younger adults.

**Breast-feeding Issues:** Propranolol is excreted in breast milk and is considered compatible by the American Academy of Pediatrics. It is recommended that the infant be monitored for signs or symptoms of beta-blockade (hypotension, bradycardia, etc) with long-term use.

**Related Information**

Antiarrhythmic Drug Classification Comparison *on page 1366*
Beta-Blockers Comparison *on page 1376*

## Propranolol and Hydrochlorothiazide

(proe PRAN oh lole & hye droe klor oh THYE a zide)

**U.S. Brand Names** Inderide®

**Synonyms** Hydrochlorothiazide and Propranolol

**Therapeutic Category** Antihypertensive Agent, Combination

**Pregnancy Risk Factor** C

**Lactation** Enters breast milk/compatible

**Use** Management of hypertension

**Formulations**

Capsule, long-acting (Inderide® LA):
- 80/50 Propranolol hydrochloride 80 mg and hydrochlorothiazide 50 mg
- 120/50 Propranolol hydrochloride 120 mg and hydrochlorothiazide 50 mg
- 160/50 Propranolol hydrochloride 160 mg and hydrochlorothiazide 50 mg

Tablet (Inderide®):
- 40/25 Propranolol hydrochloride 40 mg and hydrochlorothiazide 25 mg
- 80/25 Propranolol hydrochloride 80 mg and hydrochlorothiazide 25 mg

**Dosing**

**Adults:** Dose is individualized

**Elderly:** Refer to dosing in individual monographs.

**Additional Nursing Issues**

**Physical Assessment:** See individual components listed in Related Information. **Pregnancy risk factor C** - benefits of use should outweigh possible risks.

**Patient Information/Instruction:** See individual components listed in Related Information. **Pregnancy precautions:** Inform prescriber if you are on intend to get pregnant.

**Related Information**

Hydrochlorothiazide *on page 566*
Propranolol *on page 986*


- **Progress** *see* Dinoprostone *on page 379*
- **Propulsid®** *see* Cisapride *on page 272*
- **Propylhexedrine** *see page 1294*
- **2-Propylpentanoic Acid** *see* Valproic Acid and Derivatives *on page 1198*


## Propylthiouracil (proe pil thye oh YOOR a sil)

**Synonyms** PTU

**Therapeutic Category** Antithyroid Agent

**Pregnancy Risk Factor** D

**Lactation** Enters breast milk/use caution (AAP rates as compatible)

**Use** Palliative treatment of hyperthyroidism as an adjunct to ameliorate hyperthyroidism in preparation for surgical treatment or radioactive iodine therapy and in the management of thyrotoxic crisis

**Mechanism of Action/Effect** Inhibits the synthesis of thyroid hormones by blocking the oxidation of iodine in the thyroid gland; blocks synthesis of thyroxine and tri-iodothyronine

**Contraindications** Hypersensitivity to propylthiouracil or any component; pregnancy

**Warnings** Use with caution in patients >40 years of age because PTU may cause hypoprothrombinemia and bleeding. Use with extreme caution in patients receiving other drugs known to cause agranulocytosis; may cause agranulocytosis, thyroid hyperplasia, thyroid carcinoma (usage >1 year). Enters breast milk.

**Drug Interactions**

**Increased Effect/Toxicity:** Propylthiouracil may increase the anticoagulant activity of warfarin.

**Food Interactions** Propylthiouracil serum levels may be altered if taken with food.

**Adverse Reactions**

>10%:
- Central nervous system: Fever
- Dermatologic: Skin rash
- Hematologic: Leukopenia

1% to 10%:
- Central nervous system: Dizziness
- Gastrointestinal: Nausea, vomiting, loss of taste perception, stomach pain
- Hematologic: Agranulocytosis
- Miscellaneous: SLE-like syndrome

<1% (Limited to important or life-threatening symptoms): Edema, cutaneous vasculitis, agranulocytosis, thrombocytopenia, bleeding, aplastic anemia, cholestatic jaundice, hepatitis, nephritis

**Overdose/Toxicology** Symptoms of overdose include nausea, vomiting, epigastric pain, headache, fever, arthralgia, pruritus, edema, pancytopenia, epigastric distress, headache, fever, CNS stimulation, or depression. Treatment is supportive. Monitor bone marrow response. Forced diuresis, dialysis, and charcoal hemoperfusion have been used to enhance elimination.

**Pharmacodynamics/Kinetics**

**Protein Binding:** 75% to 80%

**Half-life Elimination:** 1.5-5 hours; End-stage renal disease: 8.5 hours

**Time to Peak:** Oral: Within 1 hour; persists for 2-3 hours

**Metabolism:** Liver

**Excretion:** Urine

**Onset:** For significant therapeutic effects 24-36 hours are required. Peak effect: Remissions of hyperthyroidism do not usually occur before 4 months of continued therapy.

**Formulations** Tablet: 50 mg

**Dosing**

**Adults:** Oral: Administer in 3 equally divided doses at approximately 8-hour intervals. Adjust dosage to maintain $T_3$, $T_4$, and TSH levels in normal range; elevated $T_3$ may be sole indicator of inadequate treatment. Elevated TSH indicates excessive antithyroid treatment.

Initial: 300-450 mg/day in divided doses every 8 hours (severe hyperthyroidism may require 600-1200 mg/day); maintenance: 100-150 mg/day in divided doses every 8-12 hours

**Elderly:** Use lower dose recommendations; adjust for renal impairment.

Initial: 150-300 mg/day in divided doses every 8 hours

Maintenance: 100-150 mg/day in divided doses every 8-12 hours

**Renal Impairment:**

$Cl_{cr}$ 10-50 mL/minute: Administer at 75% of normal dose.

$Cl_{cr}$ <10 mL/minute: Administer at 50% of normal dose.

**Monitoring Laboratory Tests** CBC with differential, prothrombin time, liver and thyroid function ($T_4$, $T_3$, TSH); periodic blood counts are recommended for chronic therapy.

**Additional Nursing Issues**

**Physical Assessment:** Monitor all appropriate laboratory results and patient for signs or symptoms of hyper-/hypothyroidism. Assess for signs or symptoms of bleeding tendency. Monitor for skin rash or swelling of lymph nodes. **Pregnancy risk factor D** - assess knowledge/teach appropriate use of barrier contraceptives.

**Patient Information/Instruction:** Take as directed, at the same time each day around-the-clock; do not miss doses or make up missed doses. This drug will need to be taken for an extended period of time to achieve appropriate results. You may experience nausea or vomiting (small frequent meals may help), dizziness or drowsiness (use caution when driving or engaging in tasks that require alertness until response to drug is known). Report rash, fever, unusual bleeding or bruising, unresolved headache, yellowing of eyes or skin, or changes in color of urine or feces, unresolved malaise. **Pregnancy precautions:** Do not get pregnant; use appropriate contraceptive measures to prevent possible harm to the fetus.

**Geriatric Considerations:** The use of antithyroid thioamides is as effective in the elderly as they are in younger adults; however, the expense, potential adverse effects, and inconvenience (compliance, monitoring) make them undesirable.


- **Propyl-Thyracil®** *see* Propylthiouracil *on previous page*
- **2-Propylvaleric Acid** *see* Valproic Acid and Derivatives *on page 1198*
- **Prorazin®** *see* Prochlorperazine *on page 971*
- **Prorex®** *see* Promethazine *on page 978*
- **Proscar®** *see* Finasteride *on page 485*
- **Pro-Sof® Plus** *see page 1294*
- **ProSom™** *see* Estazolam *on page 440*
- **Prostaglandin $E_1$** *see* Alprostadil *on page 56*
- **Prostaglandin $E_2$** *see* Dinoprostone *on page 379*
- **Prostaphlin®** *see* Oxacillin *on page 866*
- **ProStep® Patch** *see* Nicotine *on page 822*
- **Prostigmin®** *see* Neostigmine *on page 818*
- **Prostin $E_2$® Vaginal Suppository** *see* Dinoprostone *on page 379*
- **Prostin $F_2$ Alpha®** *see page 1248*


## Protamine Sulfate (PROE ta meen SUL fate)

**Therapeutic Category** Antidote

**Pregnancy Risk Factor** C

**Lactation** Excretion in breast milk unknown

**Use** Treatment of heparin overdosage; neutralize heparin during surgery or dialysis procedures

**Mechanism of Action/Effect** Combines with strongly acidic heparin to form a stable complex (salt) neutralizing the anticoagulant activity of both drugs

**Contraindications** Hypersensitivity to protamine or any component

**Warnings** For I.V. use only. May not be totally effective in some patients following cardiac surgery despite adequate doses. May cause hypersensitivity reaction in patients with a history of allergy to fish (have epinephrine 1:1000 available) and in patients sensitized to

(Continued)

## Protamine Sulfate *(Continued)*

protamine (via protamine zinc insulin). Rapid administration can cause severe hypotensive and anaphylactoid-like reactions. Heparin rebound associated with anticoagulation and bleeding has been reported to occur occasionally. Symptoms typically occur 8-9 hours after protamine administration, but may occur as long as 18 hours later. Pregnancy factor C.

**Adverse Reactions**

>10%:

Cardiovascular: Sudden fall in blood pressure, bradycardia

Respiratory: Dyspnea

1% to 10%: Hemorrhage

<1% (Limited to important or life-threatening symptoms): Pulmonary hypertension

**Overdose/Toxicology** Symptoms of overdose include hypertension. May cause hemorrhage. Doses exceeding 100 mg may cause paradoxical anticoagulation.

**Pharmacodynamics/Kinetics**

**Onset:** I.V. injection: Heparin neutralization occurs within 5 minutes

**Formulations** Injection: 10 mg/mL (5 mL, 10 mL, 25 mL)

**Dosing**

**Adults:** Protamine dosage is determined by the dosage of heparin; 1 mg of protamine neutralizes 90 USP units of heparin (lung) and 115 USP units of heparin (intestinal); maximum: 50 mg

In the situation of heparin overdosage, since blood heparin concentrations decrease rapidly **after** administration, adjust the protamine dosage depending upon the duration of time since heparin administration as follows:

| Time Elapsed | Dose of Protamine (mg) to Neutralize 100 units of Heparin |
|---|---|
| Immediate | 1-1.5 |
| 30-60 min | 0.5-0.75 |
| >2 h | 0.25-0.375 |

If heparin administered by deep S.C. injection, use 1-1.5 mg protamine per 100 units heparin. This may be done by a portion of the dose (eg, 25-50 mg) given slowly I.V. followed by the remaining portion as a continuous infusion over 8-16 hours (the expected absorption time of the S.C. heparin dose).

**Elderly:** Refer to adult dosing.

**Administration**

**I.V.:** For I.V. use only. Administer slow IVP (50 mg over 10 minutes). Rapid I.V. infusion causes hypotension. Reconstitute vial with 5 mL sterile water. Resulting solution equals 10 mg/mL. Inject without further dilution over 1-3 minutes; maximum of 50 mg in any 10-minute period.

**Stability**

**Storage:** Refrigerate; avoid freezing. Remains stable for at least 2 weeks at room temperature; preservative-free formulation does not require refrigeration.

**Compatibility:** Incompatible with cephalosporins and penicillins.

**Monitoring Laboratory Tests** Coagulation test, APTT or ACT

**Additional Nursing Issues**

**Physical Assessment:** See Warnings/Precautions and Contraindications for use cautions. Monitor effectiveness of therapy by monitoring laboratory tests frequently during therapy (see above). Monitor closely for adverse response (eg, sudden hemodynamic changes - see Adverse Reactions and Overdose/Toxicology). Assess knowledge/teach patient possible side effects and adverse symptoms to report. **Pregnancy risk factor C.** Note breast-feeding caution.

**Patient Information/Instruction:** Report any difficulty breathing, rash or flushing, feeling of warmth, tingling or numbness, dizziness, or disorientation. **Pregnancy/breast-feeding precautions:** Inform prescriber if you are pregnant. Consult prescriber if breast-feeding.

**Related Information**

Heparin *on page 558*


- **Prothazine-DC®** *see* Promethazine and Codeine *on page 980*
- **Protilase®** *see* Pancrelipase *on page 882*
- **Protirelin** *see page 1248*
- **Protopam®** *see* Pralidoxime *on page 954*
- **Protostat® Oral** *see* Metronidazole *on page 763*
- **Pro-Trin®** *see* Co-trimoxazole *on page 307*


## Protriptyline (proe TRIP ti leen)

**U.S. Brand Names** Vivactil®

**Therapeutic Category** Antidepressant, Tricyclic (Secondary Amine)

**Pregnancy Risk Factor** C

**Lactation** Excretion in breast milk unknown/not recommended

**Use** Treatment of various forms of depression, often in conjunction with psychotherapy

**Mechanism of Action/Effect** Increases the synaptic concentration of serotonin and/or norepinephrine in the central nervous system by inhibition of reuptake by the presynaptic neuronal membrane

**Contraindications** Hypersensitivity to protriptyline or any component; narrow-angle glaucoma

**Warnings** Use with caution in patients with cardiac conduction disturbances, history of hyperthyroidism, seizure disorders, or decreased renal function. Protriptyline should not be abruptly discontinued in patients receiving high doses for prolonged periods. Pregnancy factor C.

**Drug Interactions**

**Cytochrome P-450 Effect:** Metabolism may involve CYP isoenzymes.

**Decreased Effect:** Decreased effect of guanethidine. Decreased effect with barbiturates, carbamazepine, and phenytoin.

**Increased Effect/Toxicity:** Increased toxicity of alcohol, MAO inhibitors, sympathomimetics, CNS depressants, and anticholinergics (paralytic ileus and hyperpyrexia). Increased toxicity with MAO inhibitors (hyperpyretic crisis, convulsions, and death), cimetidine (increased drug levels). Potential for serotonin syndrome if combined with other serotonergic drugs.

**Effects on Lab Values** ↑ glucose

**Adverse Reactions** Anticholinergic effects may be pronounced; moderate to marked sedation can occur (tolerance to these effects usually occurs).

>10%:
- Central nervous system: Dizziness, drowsiness, headache
- Gastrointestinal: Dry mouth, constipation, increased appetite, nausea, unpleasant taste, weight gain
- Neuromuscular & skeletal: Weakness

1% to 10%:
- Cardiovascular: Hypotension, postural hypotension, arrhythmias, tachycardia, sudden death
- Central nervous system: Nervousness, restlessness, parkinsonian syndrome, insomnia, sedation, fatigue, anxiety, impaired cognitive function, seizures have occurred occasionally, extrapyramidal symptoms are possible
- Gastrointestinal: Diarrhea, heartburn
- Genitourinary: Sexual dysfunction, urinary retention
- Neuromuscular & skeletal: Tremor
- Ocular: Eye pain, blurred vision
- Miscellaneous: Sweating (excessive)

<1% (Limited to important or life-threatening symptoms): Alopecia, testicular edema, leukopenia, eosinophilia, rarely agranulocytosis, cholestatic jaundice, increased liver enzymes, increased intraocular pressure

**Overdose/Toxicology** Symptoms of overdose include confusion, hallucinations, urinary retention, hypotension, tachycardia, seizures, and hyperthermia. Following initiation of essential overdose management, toxic symptoms should be treated. Ventricular arrhythmias often respond to systemic alkalinization (sodium bicarbonate 0.5-2 mEq/kg I.V.) Physostigmine (1-2 mg I.V. slowly for adults) may be indicated for reversing life-threatening cardiac arrhythmias.

**Pharmacodynamics/Kinetics**

**Protein Binding:** 92%

**Distribution:** Crosses the placenta

**Half-life Elimination:** 54-92 hours, averaging 74 hours

**Time to Peak:** Within 24-30 hours

**Metabolism:** Liver

**Excretion:** Urine

**Onset:** Maximum antidepressant effect: 2 weeks of continuous therapy is commonly required

**Formulations** Tablet, as hydrochloride: 5 mg, 10 mg

**Dosing**

**Adults:** Oral: 15-60 mg in 3-4 divided doses

**Elderly:** Oral: Initial: 5-10 mg/day; increase every 3-7 days by 5-10 mg; usual dose: 15-20 mg/day.

**Additional Nursing Issues**

**Physical Assessment:** Assess other medications patient may be taking for effectiveness and interactions (see Drug Interactions). See Contraindications and Warnings/Precautions for cautious use. Has potential for psychological or physiological dependence, abuse, or tolerance. Monitor therapeutic response (ie, mental status, mood, affect, suicidal ideation) and adverse reactions at beginning of therapy and periodically with long-term use (see Adverse Reactions and Overdose/Toxicology). Taper dosage slowly when discontinuing (allow 3-4 weeks between discontinuing protriptyline and starting another antidepressant). Assess knowledge/teach patient appropriate use, interventions to reduce side effects, and adverse symptoms to report. **Pregnancy risk factor C** - benefits of use should outweigh possible risks. Breast-feeding is not recommended.

**Patient Information/Instruction:** Take exactly as directed (do not increase dose or frequency); may take 2-3 weeks to achieve desired results; may cause physical and/or psychological dependence. Avoid excessive alcohol, caffeine, and other prescription or OTC medications not approved by prescriber. Maintain adequate hydration (2-3 L/day of fluids unless instructed to restrict fluid intake). You may experience drowsiness, lightheadedness, impaired coordination, dizziness, or blurred vision (use caution when driving or engaging in tasks requiring alertness until response to drug is known); nausea, vomiting, altered taste, dry mouth (small frequent meals, frequent mouth care, chewing gum, or sucking lozenges may help); constipation (increased exercise, fluids, or dietary fruit and fiber may help); diarrhea (buttermilk, yogurt, or boiled milk may

(Continued)

## Protriptyline *(Continued)*

help); increased appetite (monitor dietary intake to avoid excess weight gain); postural hypotension (use caution when climbing stairs or changing position from lying or sitting to standing); urinary retention (void before taking medication); or sexual dysfunction (reversible). Report persistent CNS effects (eg, insomnia, nervousness, restlessness, hallucinations, daytime sedation, impaired cognitive function); muscle cramping or tremors; chest pain, palpitations, rapid heartbeat, swelling of extremities, or severe dizziness; blurred vision or eye pain; yellowing of eyes or skin; pale stools/dark urine; or worsening of condition. **Pregnancy/breast-feeding precautions:** Inform prescriber if you are or intend to be pregnant. Breast-feeding is not recommended.

**Geriatric Considerations:** Little data on use in the elderly. Strong anticholinergic properties which may limit protriptyline's use; more often stimulating rather than sedating effects.

**Related Information**

Antidepressant Agents Comparison *on page 1368*


- **Proventil®** *see* Albuterol *on page 45*
- **Proventil® HFA** *see* Albuterol *on page 45*
- **Provera®** *see* Medroxyprogesterone *on page 714*
- **Provigil®** *see* Modafinil *on page 782*
- **Provocholine®** *see page 1248*
- **Proxigel® Oral** *see page 1294*
- **Prozac®** *see* Fluoxetine *on page 502*
- **Prozoladex** *see* Goserelin *on page 543*
- **PRP-D** *see page 1256*
- **Prymaccone** *see* Primaquine *on page 963*


## Pseudoephedrine (soo doe e FED rin)

**U.S. Brand Names** Actifed® Allergy Tablet (Day) [OTC]; Afrin® Tablet [OTC]; Cenafed® [OTC]; Children's Silfedrine® [OTC]; Decofed® Syrup [OTC]; Drixoral® Non-Drowsy [OTC]; Efidac/24® [OTC]; Neofed® [OTC]; PediaCare® Oral; Sudafed® [OTC]; Sudafed® 12 Hour [OTC]; Sufedrin® [OTC]; Triaminic® AM Decongestant Formula [OTC]

**Synonyms** *D*-Isoephedrine Hydrochloride

**Therapeutic Category** Alpha/Beta Agonist

**Pregnancy Risk Factor** C

**Lactation** Enters breast milk/use caution (AAP rates "compatible")

**Use** Temporary symptomatic relief of nasal congestion due to common cold, upper respiratory allergies, and sinusitis; also promotes nasal or sinus drainage

**Mechanism of Action/Effect** Directly stimulates alpha-adrenergic receptors of respiratory mucosa causing vasoconstriction; directly stimulates beta-adrenergic receptors causing bronchial relaxation, increased heart rate and contractility

**Contraindications** Hypersensitivity to pseudoephedrine or any component; MAO inhibitor therapy

**Warnings** Use with caution in patients >60 years of age. Administer with caution to patients with hypertension, hyperthyroidism, diabetes mellitus, cardiovascular disease, ischemic heart disease, increased intraocular pressure, or prostatic hypertrophy. Elderly patients are more likely to experience adverse reactions to sympathomimetics. Overdosage may cause hallucinations, seizures, CNS depression, and death. Pregnancy factor C.

**Drug Interactions**

**Decreased Effect:** Decreased effect of methyldopa, reserpine.

**Increased Effect/Toxicity:** MAO inhibitors may increase blood pressure effects of pseudoephedrine. Sympathomimetic agents may increase toxicity.

**Food Interactions** Onset of effect may be delayed if pseudoephedrine is taken with food.

**Effects on Lab Values** Interferes with urine detection of amphetamine (false-positive)

**Adverse Reactions**

>10%:

- Cardiovascular: Tachycardia, palpitations, arrhythmias
- Central nervous system: Nervousness, transient stimulation, insomnia, excitability, dizziness, drowsiness, headache
- Neuromuscular & skeletal: Tremor

1% to 10%:

- Neuromuscular & skeletal: Weakness
- Miscellaneous: Sweating

<1% (Limited to important or life-threatening symptoms): Convulsions, shortness of breath, dyspnea

**Overdose/Toxicology** Symptoms of overdose include seizures, nausea, vomiting, cardiac arrhythmias, hypertension, and agitation. There is no specific antidote for pseudoephedrine intoxication. Treatment is primarily supportive.

**Pharmacodynamics/Kinetics**

**Half-life Elimination:** 9-16 hours

**Metabolism:** Partially in the liver

**Excretion:** Urine

**Onset:** Decongestant effect: Oral: 15-30 minutes

**Duration:** 4-6 hours (up to 12 hours with extended release formulation administration)

**Formulations**

Pseudoephedrine hydrochloride:

Capsule: 60 mg

Capsule, timed release: 120 mg
Drops, oral: 7.5 mg/0.8 mL (15 mL)
Liquid: 15 mg/5 mL (120 mL); 30 mg/5 mL (120 mL, 240 mL, 473 mL)
Syrup: 15 mg/5 mL (118 mL)
Tablet: 30 mg, 60 mg
Tablet, timed release: 120 mg

Pseudoephedrine sulfate: Extended release: 120 mg, 240 mg

**Dosing**

**Adults:** Oral: 30-60 mg every 4-6 hours, sustained release: 120 mg every 12 hours; maximum: 240 mg/24 hours

**Elderly:** Nasal congestion: 30-60 mg every 6 hours as needed

**Renal Impairment:** Reduce dose.

**Administration**

**Oral:** Do not crush extended release drug product, swallow whole.

**Additional Nursing Issues**

**Physical Assessment:** Assess effectiveness and interactions of other medications (see Drug Interactions). See Contraindications and Warnings/Precautions for cautious use. Monitor effectiveness of therapy (relief of cough, lung sounds, and respiratory pattern) and adverse reactions (eg, cardiac and CNS changes - see Adverse Reactions) at beginning of therapy and periodically with long-term use. Assess knowledge/teach patient appropriate use, interventions to reduce side effects, and adverse symptoms to report. **Pregnancy risk factor C** - benefits of use should outweigh possible risks. Note breast-feeding caution.

**Patient Information/Instruction:** Take only as prescribed; do not exceed prescribed dose or frequency. Do not chew or crush timed release capsule. Maintain adequate hydration (2-3 L/day of fluids unless instructed to restrict fluid intake). You may experience nervousness, insomnia, dizziness, or drowsiness (use caution when driving or engaging in tasks requiring alertness until response to drug is known). Report persistent CNS changes (dizziness, sedation, tremor, agitation, or convulsions); difficulty breathing; chest pain, palpitations, or rapid heartbeat; muscle tremor; or lack of improvement or worsening or condition. **Pregnancy/breast-feeding precautions:** Inform prescriber if you are or intend to be pregnant. Consult prescriber if breast-feeding.

**Geriatric Considerations:** Elderly patients should be counseled about the proper use of over-the-counter cough and cold preparations. Elderly are more predisposed to adverse effects of sympathomimetics since they frequently have cardiovascular diseases and diabetes mellitus as well as multiple drug therapies. It may be advisable to treat with a short-acting/immediate-release formulation before initiating sustained-release/long-acting formulations.

**Additional Information**

Pseudoephedrine hydrochloride: Cenafed® syrup [OTC], Decofed® syrup [OTC], Neofed® [OTC], Sudafed® [OTC], Sudafed® 12 Hour [OTC], Sudafed® tablet [OTC], Sufedrin® [OTC]

Pseudoephedrine sulfate: Afrinol® [OTC]

- ♦ **Pseudoephedrine and Acrivastine** *see* Acrivastine and Pseudoephedrine *on page 38*
- ♦ **Pseudoephedrine and Azatadine** *see* Azatadine and Pseudoephedrine *on page 124*
- ♦ **Pseudoephedrine and Carbinoxamine** *see* Carbinoxamine and Pseudoephedrine *on page 198*
- ♦ **Pseudoephedrine and Dextromethorphan** *see page 1294*
- ♦ **Pseudoephedrine and Guaifenesin** *see* Guaifenesin and Pseudoephedrine *on page 551*
- ♦ **Pseudoephedrine and Ibuprofen** *see page 1294*
- ♦ **Pseudoephedrine and Loratadine** *see* Loratadine and Pseudoephedrine *on page 690*
- ♦ **Pseudoephedrine, Guaifenesin, and Codeine** *see* Guaifenesin, Pseudoephedrine, and Codeine *on page 552*
- ♦ **Pseudoephedrine, Hydrocodone, and Guaifenesin** *see* Hydrocodone, Pseudoephedrine, and Guaifenesin *on page 577*
- ♦ **Pseudo-Gest Plus® Tablet** *see page 1294*
- ♦ **Pseudomonic Acid A** *see* Mupirocin *on page 792*
- ♦ **Psor-a-set® Soap** *see page 1294*
- ♦ **Psorcon™** *see* Topical Corticosteroids *on page 1152*
- ♦ **psoriGel®** *see page 1294*
- ♦ **Psorion® Cream** *see* Betamethasone *on page 148*
- ♦ **P&S® Shampoo** *see page 1294*

## Psyllium (SIL i yum)

**U.S. Brand Names** Effer-Syllium® [OTC]; Fiberall® Powder [OTC]; Fiberall® Wafer [OTC]; Hydrocil® [OTC]; Konsyl-D® [OTC]; Konsyl® [OTC]; Metamucil® [OTC]; Metamucil® Instant Mix [OTC]; Modane® Bulk [OTC]; Perdiem® Plain [OTC]; Reguloid® [OTC]; Serutan® [OTC]; Syllact® [OTC]; V-Lax® [OTC]

**Synonyms** Plantago Seed; Plantain Seed

**Therapeutic Category** Laxative, Bulk-Producing

**Pregnancy Risk Factor** C

**Lactation** Excretion in breast milk unknown/compatible

**Use** Treatment of chronic atonic or spastic constipation and in constipation associated with rectal disorders; management of irritable bowel syndrome

**Mechanism of Action/Effect** Adsorbs water in the intestine to form a viscous liquid which promotes peristalsis and reduces transit time

(Continued)

## Psyllium *(Continued)*

**Contraindications** Hypersensitivity to psyllium or any component; fecal impaction; GI obstruction

**Warnings** May contain aspartame which is metabolized in the GI tract to phenylalanine which is contraindicated in individuals with phenylketonuria. Use with caution in patients with esophageal strictures, ulcers, stenosis, or intestinal adhesions. Elderly may have insufficient fluid intake which may predispose them to fecal impaction and bowel obstruction. Pregnancy factor C.

**Drug Interactions**

**Decreased Effect:** Decreased effect of warfarin, digitalis, potassium-sparing diuretics, salicylates, tetracyclines, nitrofurantoin when taken together. Separate administration times to reduce potential for drug-drug interaction.

**Adverse Reactions** 1% to 10%:

Gastrointestinal: Esophageal or bowel obstruction, diarrhea, constipation, abdominal cramps

Respiratory: Bronchospasm

Miscellaneous: Anaphylaxis upon inhalation in susceptible individuals, rhinoconjunctivitis

**Overdose/Toxicology** Symptoms of overdose include abdominal pain, diarrhea, and constipation.

**Pharmacodynamics/Kinetics**

**Onset:** 12-24 hour, but full effect may take 2-3 days; Peak effect: May take 2-3 days

**Formulations**

Granules: 4.03 g per rounded teaspoon (100 g, 250 g); 2.5 g per rounded teaspoon

Powder: Psyllium 50% and dextrose 50% (6.5 g, 325 g, 420 g, 480 g, 500 g)

Powder:

Effervescent: 3 g/dose (270 g, 480 g); 3.4 g/dose (single-dose packets)

Psyllium hydrophilic: 3.4 g per rounded teaspoon (210 g, 300 g, 420 g, 630 g)

Squares, chewable: 1.7 g, 3.4 g

Wafers: 3.4 g

**Dosing**

**Adults:** Oral (administer at least 3 hours before or after drugs): 1-2 rounded teaspoonfuls or 1-2 packets or 1-2 wafers in 8 oz glass of liquid 1-3 times/day.

**Elderly:** Refer to adult dosing.

**Administration**

**Oral:** Inhalation of psyllium dust may cause sensitivity to psyllium (eg, runny nose, watery eyes, wheezing). Must be mixed in a glass of water or juice. Drink a full glass of liquid with each dose. Separate dose from other drug therapies.

**Additional Nursing Issues**

**Physical Assessment:** Assess other medications patient may be taking and instruct patient about timing of all medications. **Pregnancy risk factor C** - benefits of use should outweigh possible risks.

**Patient Information/Instruction:** Mix in large (8 oz or more) glass of water or juice and drink immediately. Mix carefully; do not inhale powder. Report unresolved or persistent constipation, watery diarrhea, or respiratory difficulty. **Pregnancy precautions:** Inform prescriber if you are or intend to be pregnant.

**Geriatric Considerations:** Elderly may have insufficient fluid intake which may predispose them to fecal impaction and bowel obstruction. Patients should have a 1 month trial, with at least 14 g/day, before effects in bowel function are determined. Bloating and flatulence are mostly a problem in first 4 weeks of therapy.

**Additional Information** 3.4 g psyllium hydrophilic mucilloid per 7 g powder is equivalent to a rounded teaspoonful or one packet

Sodium content of Metamucil® Instant Mix (orange): 6 mg (0.27 mEq)

**Related Information**

Laxatives: Classification and Properties Comparison *on page 1392*

- **Pteroylglutamic Acid** *see* Folic Acid *on page 515*
- **PTU** *see* Propylthiouracil *on page 988*
- **Pulmicort®** *see* Budesonide *on page 164*
- **Pulmicort Turbuhaler®** *see* Budesonide *on page 164*
- **Pulmophylline** *see* Theophylline *on page 1115*
- **Pulmozyme®** *see* Dornase Alfa *on page 397*
- **Puralube® Tears Solution** *see page 1294*
- **Purge®** *see page 1294*
- **Puri-Clens™** *see page 1294*
- **Purinethol®** *see* Mercaptopurine *on page 725*
- **Purinol®** *see* Allopurinol *on page 53*
- **PVF® K** *see* Penicillin V Potassium *on page 900*
- **$P_xE_x$® Ophthalmic** *see* Pilocarpine and Epinephrine *on page 932*
- **Pyocidin-Otic®** *see page 1291*
- **Pyrantel Pamoate** *see page 1294*

## Pyrazinamide (peer a ZIN a mide)

**Synonyms** Pyrazinoic Acid Amide

**Therapeutic Category** Antitubercular Agent

**Pregnancy Risk Factor** C

**Lactation** Enters breast milk

**Use** Adjunctive treatment of tuberculosis in combination with other antituberculosis agents

**Mechanism of Action/Effect** Converted to pyrazinoic acid in susceptible strains of *Mycobacterium* which lowers the pH of the environment; bacteriostatic or bactericidal depending on the drug's concentration at the site of infection

**Contraindications** Hypersensitivity to pyrazinamide or any component; severe hepatic damage; acute gout

**Warnings** Administer with at least one other effective agent for tuberculosis; use with caution in patients with renal failure, chronic gout, diabetes mellitus, or porphyria. Pyrazinamide is used in the 2-month intensive treatment phase of a 6-month treatment plan. Pregnancy factor C.

**Effects on Lab Values** Reacts with Acetest® and Ketostix® to produce pinkish-brown color.

**Adverse Reactions**

1% to 10%:

Central nervous system: Malaise

Gastrointestinal: Nausea, vomiting, anorexia

Neuromuscular & skeletal: Arthralgia, myalgia

<1% (Limited to important or life-threatening symptoms): Porphyria, thrombocytopenia, hepatotoxicity, interstitial nephritis

**Overdose/Toxicology** Symptoms of overdose include gout, gastric upset, and hepatic damage (mild). Treatment is supportive.

**Pharmacodynamics/Kinetics**

**Distribution:** Widely distributed into body tissues and fluids including the liver, lung, and CSF

Relative diffusion of antimicrobial agents from blood into cerebrospinal fluid (CSF): Adequate with or without inflammation (exceeds usual MICs)

Ratio of CSF to blood level (%): Inflamed meninges: 100

**Half-life Elimination:** 9-10 hours, increased with reduced renal or hepatic function; End-stage renal disease: 9 hours

**Metabolism:** Liver

**Excretion:** Urine

**Formulations** Tablet: 500 mg

**Dosing**

**Adults:** Oral (calculate dose on ideal body weight rather than total body weight): **Note:** A four-drug regimen (isoniazid, rifampin, pyrazinamide, and either streptomycin or ethambutol) is preferred for the initial, empiric treatment of TB. When the drug susceptibility results are available, the regimen should be altered as appropriate.

**Patients with TB and without HIV infection:**

**OPTION 1:**

Isoniazid resistance rate <4%: Administer daily isoniazid, rifampin, and pyrazinamide for 8 weeks followed by isoniazid and rifampin daily or directly observed therapy (DOT) 2-3 times/week for 16 weeks.

If isoniazid resistance rate is not documented, ethambutol or streptomycin should also be administered until susceptibility to isoniazid or rifampin is demonstrated. Continue treatment for at least 6 months or 3 months beyond culture conversion.

**OPTION 2:** Administer daily isoniazid, rifampin, pyrazinamide, and either streptomycin or ethambutol for 2 weeks followed by DOT 2 times/week administration of the same drugs for 6 weeks, and subsequently, with isoniazid and rifampin DOT 2 times/week administration for 16 weeks.

**OPTION 3:** Administer isoniazid, rifampin, pyrazinamide, and either ethambutol or streptomycin by DOT 3 times/week for 6 months.

**Patients with TB and with HIV infection:**

Administer any of the above OPTIONS 1, 2 or 3, however, treatment should be continued for a total of 9 months and at least 6 months beyond culture conversion.

**Note:** Some experts recommend that the duration of therapy should be extended to 9 months for patients with disseminated disease, miliary disease, disease involving the bones or joints, or tuberculosis lymphadenitis.

Daily therapy: 15-30 mg/kg/day (maximum: 2 g/day)

Directly observed therapy (DOT): Twice weekly: 50-70 mg/kg (maximum: 4 g)

DOT: 3 times/week: 50-70 mg/kg (maximum: 3 g)

**Elderly:** Oral: Start with a lower daily dose (15 mg/kg) and increase as tolerated.

**Renal Impairment:**

$Cl_{cr}$ <50 mL/minute: Avoid use or reduce dose to 12-20 mg/kg/day.

Avoid use in hemo- and peritoneal dialysis as well as continuous. arteriovenous or venovenous hemofiltration (CAVH/CAVHD).

**Hepatic Impairment:** Reduce dose.

**Monitoring Laboratory Tests** Periodic liver function, serum uric acid, sputum culture, chest x-ray 2-3 months into treatment and at completion

**Additional Nursing Issues**

**Physical Assessment:** Monitor laboratory tests (LFTs) prior to and every 2-4 weeks during therapy. Monitor patient understanding of treatment protocol and necessity of laboratory tests. **Pregnancy risk factor C.**

**Patient Information/Instruction:** Take with food for full length of therapy. Do not miss doses and do not discontinue without consulting prescriber. You will need regular medical follow-up while taking this medication. You may experience nausea or loss of appetite; small frequent meals, frequent mouth care, sucking lozenges, or chewing gum may help. Report unusual fever, unresolved nausea or vomiting, change in color of urine, pale stools, easy bruising or bleeding, blood in urine or difficulty urinating,

(Continued)

## Pyrazinamide *(Continued)*

yellowing of skin or eyes, or extreme joint pain. **Pregnancy precautions:** Inform prescriber if you are or intend to be pregnant.

**Geriatric Considerations:** Pyrazinamide is used in the 2-month intensive treatment phase of a 6-month treatment plan. Most elderly acquired their *Mycobacterium tuberculosis* infection before effective chemotherapy was available; however, older persons with new infections (not reactivation), or who are from areas where drug-resistant *M. tuberculosis* is endemic, or who are HIV-infected should receive 3-4 drug therapies including pyrazinamide.

**Related Information**

TB Drug Comparison *on page 1402*

- **Pyrazinamide, Rifampin, and Isoniazid** *see* Rifampin, Isoniazid, and Pyrazinamide *on page 1021*
- **Pyrazinoic Acid Amide** *see* Pyrazinamide *on page 994*
- **Pyrethrins** *see page 1294*
- **Pyridiate®** *see* Phenazopyridine *on page 914*
- **2-Pyridine Aldoxime Methochloride** *see* Pralidoxime *on page 954*
- **Pyridium®** *see* Phenazopyridine *on page 914*

## Pyridostigmine (peer id oh STIG meen)

**U.S. Brand Names** Mestinon®; Mestinon Time-Span®; Regonol® Injection

**Therapeutic Category** Acetylcholinesterase Inhibitor (Peripheral)

**Pregnancy Risk Factor** C

**Lactation** Enters breast milk/compatible

**Use** Symptomatic treatment of myasthenia gravis; antidote for nondepolarizing neuromuscular blockers; not a cure; patient may develop resistance to the drug

**Mechanism of Action/Effect** Inhibits destruction of acetylcholine by acetylcholinesterase which facilitates transmission of impulses across myoneural junction

**Contraindications** Hypersensitivity to pyridostigmine, bromides, or any component; GI or GU obstruction

**Warnings** Use with caution in patients with epilepsy, asthma, bradycardia, hyperthyroidism, cardiac arrhythmias, or peptic ulcer. Adequate facilities should be available for cardiopulmonary resuscitation when testing and adjusting dose for myasthenia gravis. Have atropine and epinephrine ready to treat hypersensitivity reactions. Overdosage may result in cholinergic crisis, this must be distinguished from myasthenic crisis. Anticholinesterase insensitivity can develop for brief or prolonged periods. Pregnancy factor C.

**Drug Interactions**

**Increased Effect/Toxicity:** Increased effect of depolarizing neuromuscular blockers (succinylcholine). Increased toxicity with edrophonium.

**Effects on Lab Values** ↑ aminotransferase [ALT (SGPT)/AST (SGOT)] (S), amylase (S)

**Adverse Reactions**

>10%:
- Gastrointestinal: Diarrhea, nausea, stomach cramps, mouth watering
- Miscellaneous: Sweating (increased)

1% to 10%:
- Genitourinary: Urge to urinate
- Ocular: Small pupils, lacrimation
- Respiratory: Increased bronchial secretions

<1% (Limited to important or life-threatening symptoms): Bradycardia, A-V block, seizures, laryngospasm, respiratory paralysis

**Overdose/Toxicology** Symptoms of overdose include muscle weakness, blurred vision, excessive sweating, tearing and salivation, nausea, vomiting, diarrhea, hypertension, bradycardia, and paralysis. Atropine is the treatment of choice for intoxications manifesting significant muscarinic symptoms. Atropine I.V. 2-4 mg every 3-60 minutes should be repeated to control symptoms and then continued as needed for 1-2 days following acute ingestion.

**Pharmacodynamics/Kinetics**

**Metabolism:** Liver

**Onset:** Oral: 15-30 minutes; I.V.: 2-5 minutes; I.M.: 15-30 minutes

**Duration:** Oral: Up to 6-8 hours (due to slow absorption); I.V.: 2-3 hours

**Formulations**

Pyridostigmine bromide:
- Injection: 5 mg/mL (2 mL, 5 mL)
- Syrup (raspberry flavor): 60 mg/5 mL (480 mL)
- Tablet: 60 mg
- Tablet, sustained release: 180 mg

**Dosing**

**Adults:** Normally, sustained release dosage form is used at bedtime for patients who complain of morning weakness.

Myasthenia gravis:
- Oral: Initial: 60 mg 3 times/day with maintenance dose ranging from 60 mg to 1.5 g/day; sustained release formulation should be dosed at least every 6 hours (usually 12-24 hours)
- I.M., I.V.: 2 mg every 2-3 hours or 1/30th of oral dose

Reversal of nondepolarizing neuromuscular blocker: I.M., I.V.: 10-20 mg preceded by atropine

**Elderly:** Refer to adult dosing.

**Administration**

**Oral:** Do **not** crush sustained release drug product.

**Stability**

**Storage:** Protect from light.

**Additional Nursing Issues**

**Physical Assessment:** When used to reverse neuromuscular block (anesthesia or excessive acetylcholine), monitor patient safety until full return of neuromuscular functioning. Assess bladder and sphincter adequacy prior to administering medication. See Contraindications and Warnings/Precautions for cautious use. Monitor therapeutic effects, and adverse reactions: cholinergic crisis (DUMBELS - **d**iarrhea, **u**rination, **m**iosis, **b**ronchospasm/**b**radycardia, **e**xcitability, **l**acrimation, and **s**alivation/excessive **s**weating) (see Warnings/Precautions, Adverse Reactions, and Overdose/Toxicology). Assess knowledge/teach patient appropriate use (self injections, oral), interventions to reduce side effects, and adverse symptoms to report. **Pregnancy risk factor C** - benefits of use should outweigh possible risks.

**Patient Information/Instruction:** This drug will not cure myasthenia gravis, but may help reduce symptoms. Use as directed; do not increase dose or discontinue without consulting prescriber. Take extended release tablets at bedtime; do not chew or crush extended release tablets. Maintain adequate hydration (2-3 L/day of fluids unless instructed to restrict fluid intake). May cause dizziness, drowsiness, or hypotension (rise slowly from sitting or lying position and use caution when driving or climbing stairs); vomiting or loss of appetite (frequent small meals, frequent mouth care, chewing gum, or sucking lozenges may help); or diarrhea (boiled milk, yogurt, or buttermilk may help). Report persistent abdominal discomfort; significantly increased salivation, sweating, tearing, or urination; flushed skin; chest pain or palpitations; acute headache; unresolved diarrhea; excessive fatigue, insomnia, dizziness, or depression; increased muscle, joint, or body pain; vision changes or blurred vision; or shortness of breath or wheezing. **Pregnancy precautions:** Inform prescriber if you are or intend to be pregnant.

**Geriatric Considerations:** See Warnings/Precautions and Adverse Reactions.

**Additional Information** Some formulations may contain benzyl alcohol. The syrup formulation contains ethanol.

## Pyridoxine (peer i DOKS een)

**U.S. Brand Names** Nestrex®

**Synonyms** Vitamin $B_6$

**Therapeutic Category** Antidote; Vitamin, Water Soluble

**Pregnancy Risk Factor** A/C (if dose exceeds RDA recommendation)

**Lactation** Enters breast milk/compatible - see Breast-feeding Issues

**Use** Prevents and treats vitamin $B_6$ deficiency, pyridoxine-dependent seizures in infants, adjunct to treatment of acute toxicity from isoniazid, cycloserine, or hydralazine overdose

**Mechanism of Action/Effect** Precursor to pyridoxal, which functions in the metabolism of proteins, carbohydrates, and fats; pyridoxal also aids in the release of liver and muscle-stored glycogen and in the synthesis of GABA (within the central nervous system) and heme

**Contraindications** Hypersensitivity to pyridoxine or any component

**Warnings** Dependence and withdrawal may occur with doses >200 mg/day. Pregnancy factor C (if dose exceeds RDA recommendation).

**Drug Interactions**

**Decreased Effect:** Pyridoxine may decrease serum levels of levodopa, phenobarbital, and phenytoin (patients taking levodopa without carbidopa should avoid supplemental vitamin $B_6$ >5 mg per day, which includes multivitamin preparations).

**Effects on Lab Values** Urobilinogen

**Adverse Reactions** <1% (Limited to important or life-threatening symptoms): Seizures have occurred following I.V. administration of very large doses; increased AST

**Overdose/Toxicology** Symptoms of overdose include ataxia and sensory neuropathy with doses of 50 mg to 2 g daily over prolonged periods.

**Pharmacodynamics/Kinetics**

**Half-life Elimination:** 15-20 days

**Metabolism:** Metabolized in 4-pyridoxic acid (active form), and other metabolites

**Excretion:** Urine

**Formulations**

Pyridoxine hydrochloride:

- Injection: 100 mg/mL (10 mL, 30 mL)
- Tablet: 25 mg, 50 mg, 100 mg
- Tablet, extended release: 100 mg

**Dosing**

**Adults:**

Recommended daily allowance (RDA):
- Male: 1.7-2.0 mg
- Female: 1.4-1.6 mg

Dietary deficiency: Oral: 10-20 mg/day for 3 weeks

Drug-induced neuritis (eg, isoniazid, hydralazine, penicillamine, cycloserine): Oral:
- Treatment: 100-200 mg/24 hours
- Prophylaxis: 25-100 mg/24 hours

Treatment of seizures and/or coma from acute isoniazid toxicity, a dose of pyridoxine hydrochloride equal to the amount of INH ingested can be given I.M./I.V. in divided

(Continued)

## Pyridoxine *(Continued)*

doses together with other anticonvulsants; if the amount INH ingested is not known, administer 5 g I.V. pyridoxine.

Treatment of acute hydralazine toxicity, a pyridoxine dose of 25 mg/kg in divided doses I.M./I.V. has been used.

**Elderly:** Refer to adult dosing.

**Administration**

**I.M.:** Burning may occur at the injection site after I.M. or S.C. administration.

**I.V.:** Seizures have occurred following I.V. administration of very large doses.

**Stability**

**Storage:** Protect from light.

**Additional Nursing Issues**

**Physical Assessment:** See Contraindications and Warnings/Precautions for use cautions. Assess effectiveness and interactions of other medications (see Drug Interactions). Monitor effectiveness of therapy and adverse effects at beginning of therapy and regularly with long-term use (see Adverse Reactions). Assess knowledge/teach patient appropriate use, dietary instruction, possible side effects/interventions, and adverse symptoms to report. **Pregnancy risk factor A/C** - see Pregnancy Risk Factor for cautious use.

**Patient Information/Instruction:** Take exactly as directed. Do not take more than recommended. Do not chew or crush extended release tablets. Do not exceed recommended intake of dietary B6 (eg, red meat, bananas, potatoes, yeast, lima beans, and whole grain cereals). You may experience burning or pain at injection site; notify prescriber if this persists.

**Geriatric Considerations:** Use with caution in patients with Parkinson's disease treated with levodopa.

**Breast-feeding Issues:** The AAP considers pyridoxine compatible with nursing. However, very high doses 600 mg/day may decrease or inhibit lactation.

## Pyrimethamine (peer i METH a meen)

**U.S. Brand Names** Daraprim®

**Therapeutic Category** Antimalarial Agent

**Pregnancy Risk Factor** C

**Lactation** Enters breast milk/contraindicated (AAP rates "compatible")

**Use** Prophylaxis of malaria due to susceptible strains of plasmodia (not suitable for travelers to most areas); in conjunction with quinine and sulfadiazine for the treatment of uncomplicated attacks of chloroquine-resistant *P. falciparum* malaria; used in conjunction with fast-acting schizonticide to initiate transmission control and suppression cure; synergistic combination with sulfonamide in treatment of toxoplasmosis

**Mechanism of Action/Effect** Inhibits parasitic dihydrofolate reductase, resulting in inhibition of vital tetrahydrofolic acid synthesis

**Contraindications** Hypersensitivity to pyrimethamine, chloroguanide; megaloblastic anemia secondary to folate deficiency; resistant malaria; patients with seizure disorders

**Warnings** When used for more than 3-4 days, it may be advisable to give leucovorin to prevent hematologic complications. Use with caution in patients with impaired renal or hepatic function or with possible G-6-PD. Pregnancy factor C (may be carcinogenic).

**Drug Interactions**

**Decreased Effect:** Pyrimethamine effectiveness is decreased by acid.

**Increased Effect/Toxicity:** Increased effect with sulfonamides (synergy), methotrexate, and TMP/SMZ.

**Adverse Reactions**

1% to 10%: (More frequent with higher doses)

Central nervous system: Insomnia, lightheadedness, fever, malaise, seizures, depression

Gastrointestinal: Anorexia, abdominal cramps, vomiting, diarrhea, dry mouth, atrophic glossitis

Hematologic: Megaloblastic anemia, leukopenia, thrombocytopenia, agranulocytosis

<1% (Limited to important or life-threatening symptoms): Pulmonary eosinophilia, Stevens-Johnson syndrome, erythema multiforme, anaphylaxis

**Overdose/Toxicology** Symptoms of overdose include megaloblastic anemia, leukopenia, thrombocytopenia, anorexia, CNS stimulation, seizures, nausea, vomiting, and hematemesis. Following GI decontamination, leucovorin should be administered in an I.M. or I.V. dosage of 5-15 mg/day or orally for 5-7 days, or as required to reverse symptoms of folic acid deficiency. Provide other supportive treatment as required.

**Pharmacodynamics/Kinetics**

**Protein Binding:** 80%

**Half-life Elimination:** 80-95 hours

**Time to Peak:** Within 1.5-8 hours

**Formulations** Tablet: 25 mg

**Dosing**

**Adults:**

Malaria chemoprophylaxis (for areas where chloroquine-resistant *P. falciparum* exists):

Begin prophylaxis 2 weeks before entering endemic area: 25 mg once weekly.

Dosage should be continued for all age groups for at least 6-10 weeks after leaving endemic areas.

Chloroquine-resistant *P. falciparum* malaria (when used in conjunction with quinine and sulfadiazine): 25 mg twice daily for 3 days.

Toxoplasmosis: 50-75 mg/day together with 1-4 g of a sulfonamide for 1-3 weeks depending on patient's tolerance and response, then reduce dose by 50% and continue for 4-5 weeks **or** 25-50 mg/day for 3-4 weeks.

**Elderly:** Refer to adult dosing.

**Administration**

**Oral:** Take with meals to minimize GI distress.

**Stability**

**Storage:** Pyrimethamine tablets may be crushed to prepare oral suspensions of the drug in water, cherry syrup, or sucrose-containing solutions at a concentration of 1 mg/mL; stable at room temperature for 5-7 days.

**Monitoring Laboratory Tests** CBC, including platelet counts twice weekly; liver and renal function

**Additional Nursing Issues**

**Physical Assessment:** Monitor laboratory results and patient symptoms to assess for folic acid deficiency, hepatic and renal function. When used for prophylaxis, begin treatment 1 week before leaving for endemic areas. **Pregnancy risk factor C** (may be carcinogenic) - benefits of use should outweigh possible risks. Breast-feeding is contraindicated.

**Patient Information/Instruction:** Take on schedule as directed and take full course of therapy. If used for prophylaxis, begin 2 weeks before traveling to endemic areas, continue during travel period, and for 6-10 weeks following return. Regular blood tests will be necessary during therapy. You may experience GI distress (frequent small meals may help). You may experience dizziness, changes in mentation, insomnia, headache, or visual disturbances (use caution when driving or operating dangerous machinery). Report unresolved nausea or vomiting, anorexia, skin rash, fever, sore throat, unusual bleeding or bruising, yellowing of skin or eyes, and change in color of urine or stool. **Pregnancy precautions:** Inform prescriber if you are or intend to be pregnant. Do not breast-feed.

- ♦ **Pyrinex® Pediculicide Shampoo** *see page 1294*
- ♦ **Pyrinyl II® Liquid** *see page 1294*
- ♦ **Pyrinyl Plus® Shampoo** *see page 1294*
- ♦ **Pyrithione Zinc** *see page 1294*
- ♦ **Pyronium®** *see* Phenazopyridine *on page 914*
- ♦ **Quadra-Hist®** *see page 1306*
- ♦ **Quadrax** *see* Ibuprofen *on page 592*
- ♦ **Quelicin® Injection** *see page 1248*
- ♦ **Queltuss®** *see* Guaifenesin and Dextromethorphan *on page 549*
- ♦ **Quemicetina** *see* Chloramphenicol *on page 248*
- ♦ **Questran®** *see* Cholestyramine Resin *on page 262*
- ♦ **Questran® Light** *see* Cholestyramine Resin *on page 262*

## Quetiapine (kwe TYE a peen)

**U.S. Brand Names** Seroquel®

**Therapeutic Category** Antipsychotic Agent, Dibenzothiazepine

**Pregnancy Risk Factor** C

**Lactation** Excretion in breast milk unknown/not recommended

**Use** Treatment of acute exacerbations of schizophrenia or other psychotic disorders. Like other atypical antipsychotics, quetiapine is probably best tried in cases for which typical antipsychotic drugs have proven ineffective.

**Mechanism of Action/Effect** Antagonizes multiple receptor types in the central nervous system, including dopamine ($D_2$), serotonin (5-$HT_2$) receptors, which are believed to mediate antipsychotic activity

**Contraindications** Hypersensitivity to quetiapine or any component (cross reactivity between phenothiazines may occur); severe CNS depression; bone marrow suppression; blood dyscrasias; severe hepatic disease; coma

**Warnings** May be sedating, use with caution in disorders where CNS depression is a feature. Use with caution in Parkinson's disease. May cause orthostatic hypotension; use caution in patients predisposed to hypotension or with hemodynamic instability; prior myocardial infarction, cerebrovascular disease or ischemic heart disease. Caution in patients with hypercholesterolemia; thyroid disease; predisposition to seizures; subcortical brain damage; hepatic impairment; or severe cardiac, renal, or respiratory disease. May alter temperature regulation or mask toxicity of other drugs due to antiemetic effects. May alter cardiac conduction - life-threatening arrhythmias have occurred with therapeutic doses of neuroleptics.

May cause anticholinergic effects (eg, confusion, agitation, constipation, dry mouth, blurred vision, urinary retention); therefore, use with caution in patients with decreased gastrointestinal motility, urinary retention, BPH, xerostomia, or visual problems. Conditions which also may be exacerbated by cholinergic blockade include narrow-angle glaucoma (screening is recommended) and worsening of myasthenia gravis. Relative to other antipsychotics, quetiapine has a moderate potency of cholinergic blockade. Risk of neuroleptic malignant syndrome, extrapyramidal effects or tardive dyskinesias appears to be very low relative to other antipsychotics.

Has been noted to cause cataracts in animals, lens examination on initiation of therapy and every 6 months is recommended.

Pregnancy factor C.

(Continued)

## Quetiapine *(Continued)*

**Drug Interactions**

**Cytochrome P-450 Effect:** CYP2D6 and 3A3/4 enzyme substrate

**Decreased Effect:** Coadministration with enzyme-inducing drugs (phenytoin, carbamazepine, phenobarbital, corticosteroids, rifampin) may result in lower blood levels of quetiapine. Thioridazine increases clearance of quetiapine.

**Increased Effect/Toxicity:** Quetiapine reduces the metabolism of lorazepam. Inhibitors of cytochrome P-450 isoenzyme 3A (eg, ketoconazole, itraconazole, fluconazole, and erythromycin) may result in increased blood levels of quetiapine. Effects of alcohol and other sedatives may be potentiated.

**Adverse Reactions**

>10%:

Central nervous system: Somnolence (6% to 39%), agitation (6% to 28%), headache (5% to 31%), insomnia (4% to 15%), dizziness (6% to 11%)

Cardiovascular: Postural hypotension (4% to 14%)

Gastrointestinal: Xerostomia (8% to 19%)

Hepatic: Increased serum transaminases (5% to 17%)

<2%:

Increases in cholesterol and triglycerides, seizures, hypothyroidism, tachycardia, dyspepsia, constipation, weight gain. Lens changes have been observed in patients receiving long-term therapy.

**Pharmacodynamics/Kinetics**

**Protein Binding:** 83% bound to plasma proteins

**Half-life Elimination:** 6 hours

**Time to Peak:** 1.5 hours

**Metabolism:** Hepatic - primarily metabolized by cytochrome P-450 isoenzyme 3A4 to inactive metabolites

**Excretion:** As metabolites, in urine and feces

**Formulations** Tablet, as fumarate: 25 mg, 100 mg, 200 mg

**Dosing**

**Adults:** Oral: 25-100 mg 2-3 times/day; usual starting dose 25 mg twice daily, increased in increments of 25-50 mg 2-3 times/day on the second or third day. By the fourth day, the dose should be in the range of 300-400 mg/day in 2-3 divided doses. Further adjustments may be made, as needed, at intervals of at least 2 days in adjustments of 25-50 mg twice daily. Usual maintenance range: 150-750 mg/day. Maximum: 800 mg/day.

**Elderly:** Lower clearance in elderly patients (40%), resulting in higher concentrations. Dosage adjustment may be required.

**Hepatic Impairment:** Lower clearance in hepatic impairment (30%), may result in higher concentrations. Dosage adjustment may be required.

**Monitoring Laboratory Tests** Eye examination every 6 months while on this medication

**Additional Nursing Issues**

**Physical Assessment:** Assess other medications patient is taking for effectiveness and interactions (especially drugs affected by P-450 enzymes - see Drug Interactions). See Contraindications and Warnings/Precautions for cautious use. Has potential for psychological or physiological dependence, abuse, and tolerance. Review ophthalmic exam and monitor laboratory results (see above), therapeutic response (mental status, mood, affect), and adverse reactions at beginning of therapy and periodically with long-term use (CNS responses, orthostatic hypotension, seizure threshold - see Adverse Reactions and Overdose). Initiate at lower doses (see Dosing) and taper dosage slowly when discontinuing. Assess knowledge/teach patient appropriate use, interventions to reduce side effects, and adverse symptoms to report (see below). **Pregnancy risk factor C** - benefits of use should outweigh possible risks. Breast-feeding is not recommended.

**Patient Information/Instruction:** Use exactly as directed (do not increase dose or frequency); may cause physical and/or psychological dependence. It may take 2-3 weeks to achieve desired results; do not discontinue without consulting prescriber. Avoid excess alcohol or caffeine and other prescription or OTC medications not approved by prescriber. Maintain adequate hydration (2-3 L/day of fluids unless instructed to restrict fluid intake). You may experience excess drowsiness, restlessness, dizziness, or blurred vision (use caution driving or when engaging in tasks requiring alertness until response to drug is known); mouth sores or GI upset (small frequent meals, frequent mouth care, chewing gum, or sucking lozenges may help); constipation (increased exercise, fluids, or dietary fruit and fiber may help); or postural hypotension (use caution climbing stairs or when changing position from lying or sitting to standing). Report persistent CNS effects (eg, somnolence, agitation, insomnia); severe dizziness; vision changes; difficulty breathing; or worsening of condition. **Pregnancy/breast-feeding precautions:** Inform prescriber if you are or intend to be pregnant. Breast-feeding is not recommended.

**Geriatric Considerations:** (See Warnings/Precautions, Adverse Reactions, and Overdose/Toxicology.) Elderly patients have an increased risk of adverse response to side effects or adverse reactions to antipsychotics. These can include but are not limited to the following.

Anticholinergic effects: CNS toxicity with confusion, memory loss, psychotic behavior, and agitation.

Extrapyramidal effects (EPS): Parkinson's syndrome and akathisia may occur as often as 50% in patients >60 years of age. Tardive dyskinesia (motor restlessness) may be

40% in elderly; may be related to duration and total accumulated dose over time; may be somewhat reversible if diagnosed early enough.

Orthostatic hypotension: Increased risk for falls.

Sedation: In nonpsychotic patients, may result in feelings of depersonalization, derealization, and dysphoria.

Cardiac toxicity: Cardiac arrhythmias have occurred with therapeutic doses of antipsychotics.

Malignant neuroleptic syndrome: Development of hyperthermia, muscular rigidity, autonomic instability, and altered mental status.

Many elderly patients receive antipsychotic medications for inappropriate nonpsychotic behavior. Before initiating antipsychotic medication, all possible reversible causes should be investigated. Stress may cause acute "confusion" or worsening of baseline nonpsychotic behaviors; any changes in disease state (in any organ) may result in behavioral changes. Common acute changes in behavior may be due also to increases in drug dose addition, or addition of a new drug to the regimen; fluid/electrolyte alterations; infections; or changes in the environment.

Meta-analysis of controlled trials of antipsychotic (phenothiazines, butyrophenones) use with agitated, demented, elderly patients has concluded that the use of neuroleptics results in a response rate of 18%. Clearly, neuroleptic therapy for behavior control should be limited, with frequent attempts to withdraw the agent for behavior control. When use is indicated, initial doses should be lower to start and monitored closely.

**Additional Information** Quetiapine has a low incidence of extrapyramidal reactions.

**Related Information**

Antipsychotic Agents Comparison *on page 1371*

- ♦ **Quibron®** *see* Theophylline and Guaifenesin *on page 1118*
- ♦ **Quibron®-T** *see* Theophylline *on page 1115*
- ♦ **Quibron®-T/SR** *see* Theophylline *on page 1115*
- ♦ **Quick Dissolve Maalox® Maximum Strength** *see* Calcium Supplements *on page 185*
- ♦ **Quiess®** *see* Hydroxyzine *on page 588*
- ♦ **Quilagen** *see* Gentamicin *on page 531*
- ♦ **Quimocyclar** *see* Tetracycline *on page 1111*
- ♦ **Quinaglute® Dura-Tabs®** *see* Quinidine *on next page*
- ♦ **Quinalan®** *see* Quinidine *on next page*
- ♦ **Quinalbarbitone Sodium** *see* Secobarbital *on page 1049*

## Quinapril (KWIN a pril)

**U.S. Brand Names** Accupril®

**Therapeutic Category** Angiotensin-Converting Enzyme (ACE) Inhibitors

**Pregnancy Risk Factor** C/D (2nd and 3rd trimesters)

**Lactation** Excretion in breast milk unknown

**Use** Management of hypertension and treatment of congestive heart failure

**Mechanism of Action/Effect** Competitive inhibitor of angiotensin-converting enzyme (ACE); prevents conversion of angiotensin I to angiotensin II, a potent vasoconstrictor; results in lower levels of angiotensin II which causes an increase in plasma renin activity and a reduction in aldosterone secretion

**Contraindications** Hypersensitivity to quinapril; history of angioedema induced by other ACE inhibitors; pregnancy (2nd and 3rd trimesters)

**Warnings** Use with caution in patients with renal insufficiency, autoimmune disease, or renal artery stenosis. Excessive hypotension may be more likely in volume-depleted patients, the elderly, and following the first dose (first dose phenomenon). Quinapril should be discontinued if laryngeal stridor or angioedema of the face, tongue, or glottis is observed. Pregnancy factor C/D (2nd and 3rd trimesters).

**Drug Interactions**

**Decreased Effect:** Rifampin may decrease the effect of ACE inhibitors. Antacids may decrease the bioavailability of ACE inhibitors, may be more likely to occur with captopril, separate administration times by 1-2 hours. NSAIDs, specifically indomethacin, may reduce the hypotensive effects of ACE inhibitors. More likely to occur in low renin or volume dependent hypertensive patients.

**Increased Effect/Toxicity:** Diuretics have additive hypotensive effects with ACE inhibitors. Probenecid increases blood levels of captopril which may occur in other ACE inhibitors. Phenothiazines taken with ACE inhibitors may increase the pharmacologic effects of the ACE inhibitor. Allopurinol and ACE inhibitors may cause a higher risk of hypersensitivity reaction when taken concurrently.

**Adverse Reactions**

1% to 10%:

Cardiovascular: Hypotension
Central nervous system: Dizziness, headache, fatigue
Gastrointestinal: Diarrhea, vomiting, nausea, abdominal pain
Renal: Increased BUN/serum creatinine
Respiratory: Upper respiratory symptoms, cough

<1% (Limited to important or life-threatening symptoms): Myocardial infarction, chest pain pectoris, cerebrovascular accident, orthostatic hypotension, rhythm disturbances, tachycardia, peripheral edema, vasculitis, palpitations, syncope, vasodilation, heart failure, hypertensive crisis, cardiogenic shock, exfoliative dermatitis, dermatopolymyositis, agranulocytosis, thrombocytopenia, renal failure, asthma, bronchospasm, eosinophilic pneumonitis

(Continued)

## Quinapril *(Continued)*

**Overdose/Toxicology** Mild hypotension has been the primary toxic effect seen with acute overdose. Bradycardia may also occur. Hyperkalemia occurs even with therapeutic doses, especially in patients with renal insufficiency and those taking NSAIDs. Treatment is symptom directed and supportive.

**Pharmacodynamics/Kinetics**

**Protein Binding:** ~97%

**Half-life Elimination:** Quinapril: 0.8 hours; Quinaprilat: 2 hours

**Time to Peak:** Quinapril: 1 hour; Quinaprilat: ~2 hours

**Metabolism:** Liver

**Excretion:** Urine and feces

**Onset:** 1 hour

**Duration:** 24 hours

**Formulations** Tablet, as hydrochloride: 5 mg, 10 mg, 20 mg, 40 mg

**Dosing**

**Adults:** Oral: Initial: 10 mg once daily, adjust according to blood pressure response at peak and trough blood levels; in general, the normal dosage range is 20-80 mg/day.

**Elderly:** Oral: Initial: 2.5-5 mg/day; increase dosage at increments of 2.5-5 mg at 1- to 2-week intervals; adjust for renal impairment.

**Renal Impairment:**

$Cl_{cr}$ >60 mL/minute: Administer 10 mg/day.

$Cl_{cr}$ 30-60 mL/minute: Administer 5 mg/day.

$Cl_{cr}$ 10-30 mL/minute: Administer 2.5 mg/day.

**Hepatic Impairment:** In patients with alcoholic cirrhosis, hydrolysis of quinapril to quinaprilat is impaired; however, the subsequent elimination of quinaprilat is unaltered.

**Stability**

**Storage:** Store at room temperature.

**Reconstitution:** Unstable in aqueous solutions. To prepare solution for oral administration, mix prior to administration and use within 10 minutes.

**Monitoring Laboratory Tests** CBC, renal function tests, electrolytes

**Additional Nursing Issues**

**Physical Assessment:** Assess effectiveness and interactions of other medications (see Drug Interactions). See Warnings/Precautions and Contraindications for use cautions. Monitor effectiveness of therapy, laboratory tests, and adverse response on a regular basis during therapy (especially postural hypotension following first dose) (see Adverse Reactions and Overdose/Toxicology). Assess knowledge/teach patient appropriate use according to drug form and purpose of therapy, possible side effects and appropriate interventions, and adverse symptoms to report. **Pregnancy risk factor C/D** - see Pregnancy Risk Factor - assess knowledge/teach patient use of barrier contraceptive measures. See Pregnancy Issues. Note breast-feeding caution.

**Patient Information/Instruction:** Take exactly as directed; do not discontinue without consulting prescriber. Take first dose at bedtime. Take all doses on an empty stomach (30 minutes before or 2 hours after meals). This drug does not eliminate need for diet or exercise regimen as recommended by prescriber. May cause dizziness, fainting, lightheadedness (use caution when driving or engaging in tasks requiring alertness until response to drug is known); postural hypotension (use caution when rising from lying or sitting position or climbing stairs); nausea, vomiting, altered taste, abdominal pain, dry mouth, or transient loss of appetite (small frequent meals, frequent mouth care, sucking lozenges, or chewing gum may help) - report if these persist. Report chest pain or palpitations; mouth sores; fever or chills; swelling of extremities; skin rash; numbness, tingling, or pain in muscles; difficulty in breathing or unusual cough; or other persistent adverse reactions. **Pregnancy/breast-feeding precautions:** Do not get pregnant; use appropriate contraceptive measures. Consult prescriber if breast-feeding.

**Geriatric Considerations:** Due to frequent decreases in glomerular filtration (also creatinine clearance) with aging, elderly patients may have exaggerated responses to ACE inhibitors. Differences in clinical response due to hepatic changes are not observed.

**Pregnancy Issues:** ACE inhibitors can cause fetal injury or death if taken during the 2nd or 3rd trimester. Discontinue ACE inhibitors as soon as pregnancy is detected. ACE inhibitors should not be used if patient is sexually active and not using contraceptives.

**Additional Information** Patients taking diuretics are at risk for developing hypotension on initial dosing. To prevent this, discontinue diuretics 2-3 days prior to initiating quinapril. May restart diuretics if blood pressure is not controlled by quinapril alone.

**Related Information**

ACE Inhibitors and Angiotensin Antagonists Comparison *on page 1362*

♦ **Quinidex® Extentabs®** *see* Quinidine *on this page*

## Quinidine (KWIN i deen)

**U.S. Brand Names** Cardioquin®; Quinaglute® Dura-Tabs®; Quinalan®; Quinidex® Extentabs®; Quinora®

**Therapeutic Category** Antiarrhythmic Agent, Class I-A

**Pregnancy Risk Factor** C

**Lactation** Enters breast milk/compatible

**Use** Prophylaxis after cardioversion of atrial fibrillation and/or flutter to maintain normal sinus rhythm; prevent recurrence of paroxysmal supraventricular tachycardia, paroxysmal A-V junctional rhythm, paroxysmal ventricular tachycardia, paroxysmal atrial fibrillation, and atrial or ventricular premature contractions; has activity against *Plasmodium falciparum* malaria

**Mechanism of Action/Effect** Class 1A antiarrhythmic agent; depresses Phase 0 of the action potential; decreases myocardial excitability and conduction velocity, and myocardial contractility by decreasing sodium influx during depolarization and potassium efflux in repolarization; also reduces calcium transport across cell membrane

**Contraindications** Hypersensitivity to the drug or cinchona derivatives (eg, quinine); patients with complete A-V block with an A-V junctional or idioventricular pacemaker; patients with intraventricular conduction defects (marked widening of QRS complex); patients with cardiac-glycoside induced A-V conduction disorders

**Warnings** Use with caution in patients with myocardial depression, sick-sinus syndrome, incomplete A-V block, hepatic and/or renal insufficiency, and myasthenia gravis. Hemolysis may occur in patients with G-6-PD (glucose-6-phosphate dehydrogenase) deficiency. Quinidine-induced hepatotoxicity, including granulomatous hepatitis can occur, increased serum AST and alkaline phosphatase concentrations, and jaundice may occur. Use with caution in the elderly. Pregnancy factor C.

**Drug Interactions**

**Cytochrome P-450 Effect:** CYP3A3/4 and 3A5-7 enzyme substrate; CYP2D6 and 3A3/4 enzyme inhibitor

**Decreased Effect:** Phenobarbital, phenytoin, and rifampin may decrease quinidine serum concentrations (rifampin may decrease quinidine half-life by 50%, probably by inducing the CYP3A isozyme).

**Increased Effect/Toxicity:** Quinidine potentiates nondepolarizing and depolarizing muscle relaxants. Quinidine may increase plasma concentration of digoxin; closely monitor digoxin concentrations. Digoxin dosage may need to be reduced (by one-half) when quinidine is initiated; new steady-state digoxin plasma concentrations occur in 5-7 days. Quinidine may enhance coumarin anticoagulants. Beta-blockers and quinidine may increase bradycardia. Use with verapamil, diltiazem, amiodarone, alkalinizing agents, and cimetidine may increase quinidine serum concentrations.

**Food Interactions** Quinidine serum levels may be increased if taken with food. Food has a variable effect on absorption of sustained release formulation.

**Adverse Reactions**

>10%:

Cardiovascular: Flushing

Gastrointestinal: Bitter taste, diarrhea, anorexia, nausea, vomiting, stomach cramping

1% to 10%:

Cardiovascular: Hypotension, syncope

Central nervous system: Lightheadedness, severe headache, confusion, delirium, fever, vertigo

Dermatologic: Rash

Ocular: Blurred vision

Otic: Tinnitus

Respiratory: Wheezing

<1% (Limited to important or life-threatening symptoms): Tachycardia, heart block, ventricular fibrillation, vascular collapse, anemia, thrombocytopenic purpura, blood dyscrasias, respiratory depression, pneumonitis, bronchospasm

**Overdose/Toxicology** Has a low toxic:therapeutic ratio and may easily produce fatal intoxication (acute toxic dose: 1 g in adults). Symptoms of overdose include sinus bradycardia, sinus node arrest or asystole, P-R, QRS or Q-T interval prolongation, torsade de pointes (polymorphous ventricular tachycardia), and depressed myocardial contractility, which along with alpha-adrenergic or ganglionic blockade, may result in hypotension and pulmonary edema. Other effects are anticholinergic (dry mouth, dilated pupils, and delirium) as well as seizures, coma, and respiratory arrest. Treatment is symptomatic and effects usually respond to conventional therapies. **Note:** Do not use other Class 1A or 1C antiarrhythmic agents to treat ventricular tachycardia. Sodium bicarbonate may treat wide QRS intervals or hypotension. Markedly impaired conduction or high degree A-V block, unresponsive to bicarbonate, indicates consideration of a pacemaker.

**Pharmacodynamics/Kinetics**

**Protein Binding:** 80% to 90%

**Distribution:** Decreased with congestive heart failure, malaria; increased with cirrhosis; crosses the placenta

**Half-life Elimination:** 6-8 hours; increased half-life with elderly, cirrhosis, and congestive heart failure

**Metabolism:** Liver

**Excretion:** Urine

**Formulations**

Injection, as gluconate: 80 mg/mL (10 mL)

Tablet, as polygalacturonate: 275 mg

Tablet, as sulfate: 200 mg, 300 mg

Tablet:

Sustained action, as sulfate: 300 mg

Sustained release, as gluconate: 324 mg

**Dosing**

**Adults:** Dosage expressed in terms of the salt: 267 mg of quinidine gluconate = 275 mg of quinidine polygalacturonate = 200 mg of quinidine sulfate.

(Continued)

## Quinidine *(Continued)*

Test dose: Oral, I.M.: 200 mg administered several hours before full dosage (to determine possibility of idiosyncratic reaction)

Oral:

Sulfate: 100-600 mg/dose every 4-6 hours; begin at 200 mg/dose and titrate to desired effect (maximum daily dose: 3-4 g)

Gluconate: 324-972 mg every 8-12 hours

I.M.: 400 mg/dose every 4-6 hours

I.V.: 200-400 mg/dose diluted and given at a rate ≤10 mg/minute

**Elderly:** Refer to adult dosing.

**Renal Impairment:**

$Cl_{cr}$ <10 mL/minute: Administer 75% of normal dose.

Hemodialysis effects: Slightly hemodialyzable (5% to 20%); 200 mg supplemental dose posthemodialysis is recommended; not dialyzable (0% to 5%) by peritoneal dialysis.

**Hepatic Impairment:** Larger loading dose may be indicated; reduce maintenance doses by 50% and monitor serum levels closely.

**Administration**

**Oral:** Do not crush sustained release drug product. Give around-the-clock to promote less variation in peak and trough serum levels.

**I.V.:** Give around-the-clock to promote less variation in peak and trough serum levels. Maximum I.V. infusion rate: 10 mg/minute.

**Stability**

**Storage:** Do not use discolored parenteral solution.

**Monitoring Laboratory Tests** Routine CBC, liver and renal function during long-term administration

**Additional Nursing Issues**

**Physical Assessment:** Assess other medications patient may be taking for effectiveness and interactions (see Drug Interactions and Contraindications). See Warnings/Precautions and Contraindications for cautious use. I.V. requires use of infusion pump and continuous cardiac and hemodynamic monitoring. Monitor laboratory tests (see above), therapeutic response (cardiac status), and adverse reactions (see Warnings/Precautions and Adverse Reactions) at beginning of therapy, when titrating dosage, and on a regular basis with long-term therapy. **Note:** Quinidine has a low toxic:therapeutic ratio and overdose may easily produce severe and life-threatening reactions (see Overdose/Toxicology). Assess knowledge/teach patient appropriate use, interventions to reduce side effects, and adverse symptoms to report. **Pregnancy risk factor C** - benefits of use should outweigh possible risks.

**Patient Information/Instruction:** Take exactly as directed, around-the-clock; do not take additional doses or discontinue without consulting prescriber. Do not crush, chew, or break sustained release capsules. You will need regular cardiac checkups and blood tests while taking this medication. You may experience dizziness, drowsiness, or visual changes (use caution when driving or engaging in tasks requiring alertness until response to drug is known); abnormal taste, nausea or vomiting, or loss of appetite (small frequent meals, frequent mouth care, chewing gum, or sucking lozenges may help); headaches (prescriber may recommend mild analgesic); or diarrhea (exercise, yogurt, or boiled milk may help - if persistent consult prescriber). Report chest pain, palpitation, or erratic heartbeat; difficulty breathing or wheezing; CNS changes (confusion, delirium, fever, consistent dizziness); skin rash; sense of fullness or ringing in ears; or changes in vision. **Pregnancy precautions:** Inform prescriber if you are or intend to be pregnant.

**Geriatric Considerations:** Clearance may be decreased with a resultant increased half-life. Must individualize dose. Bioavailability and half-life are increased in the elderly due to decreases in both renal and hepatic function with age.

**Additional Information**

Quinidine gluconate: Duraquin®, Quinaglute® Dura-Tabs®, Quinalan®, Quinatime®

Quinidine polygalacturonate: Cardioquin®

Quinidine sulfate: Cin-Quin®, Quinidex® Extentabs®, Quinora®

**Related Information**

Antiarrhythmic Drug Classification Comparison *on page 1366*

Peak and Trough Guidelines *on page 1331*

♦ **Quini Durules®** *see* Quinidine *on page 1002*

## Quinine (KWYE nine)

**U.S. Brand Names** Formula Q®

**Therapeutic Category** Antimalarial Agent

**Pregnancy Risk Factor** X

**Lactation** Enters breast milk/compatible

**Use** Suppression or treatment of chloroquine-resistant *P. falciparum* malaria; treatment of *Babesia microti* infection; prevention and treatment of nocturnal recumbency leg muscle cramps

**Mechanism of Action/Effect** Depresses oxygen uptake and carbohydrate metabolism; intercalates into DNA, disrupting the parasite's replication and transcription; affects calcium distribution within muscle fibers and decreases the excitability of the motor end-plate region; cardiovascular effects similar to quinidine

**Contraindications** Hypersensitivity to quinine or any component; tinnitus; optic neuritis; G-6-PD deficiency; history of black water fever; thrombocytopenia with quinine or quinidine; pregnancy

**Warnings** Use with caution in patients with cardiac arrhythmias (quinine has quinidine-like activity) and in patients with myasthenia gravis.

**Drug Interactions**

**Cytochrome P-450 Effect:** CYP3A3/4 enzyme substrate; CYP3A3/4 enzyme inhibitor

**Decreased Effect:** Phenobarbital, phenytoin, and rifampin may decrease quinine serum concentrations.

**Increased Effect/Toxicity:** Beta-blockers + quinine may increase bradycardia. Quinine may enhance warfarin anticoagulant effect. Quinine potentiates nondepolarizing and depolarizing muscle relaxants. Quinine may increase plasma concentration of digoxin. Closely monitor digoxin concentrations. Digoxin dosage may need to be reduced (by one-half) when quinine is initiated. New steady-state digoxin plasma concentrations occur in 5-7 days. Verapamil, amiodarone, alkalinizing agents, and cimetidine may increase quinine serum concentrations.

**Effects on Lab Values** Positive Coombs' [direct]

**Adverse Reactions**

>10%:

Central nervous system: Severe headache

Gastrointestinal: Nausea, vomiting, diarrhea

Ocular: Blurred vision

Otic: Tinnitus

<1% (Limited to important or life-threatening symptoms): Chest pain hypoglycemia, hemolysis, thrombocytopenia, hepatitis

**Overdose/Toxicology** Symptoms of mild toxicity include nausea, vomiting, and cinchonism. Severe intoxication may cause ataxia, obtundation, convulsions, coma, and respiratory arrest. With massive intoxication quinidine-like cardiotoxicity (hypotension, QRS and Q-T interval prolongation, A-V block, and ventricular arrhythmias) may be fatal. Retinal toxicity occurs 9-10 hours after ingestion (blurred vision, impaired color perception, constriction of visual fields and blindness). Other toxic effects include hypokalemia, hypoglycemia, hemolysis, and congenital malformations when taken during pregnancy. Treatment includes symptomatic therapy with conventional agents. **Note:** Avoid Type 1A and 1C antiarrhythmic drugs. Treat cardiotoxicity with sodium bicarbonate. Dialysis and hemoperfusion procedures are ineffective in enhancing elimination.

**Pharmacodynamics/Kinetics**

**Protein Binding:** 70% to 95%

**Half-life Elimination:** 8-14 hours

**Time to Peak:** Within 1-3 hours

**Metabolism:** Liver

**Excretion:** Bile and saliva with <5% excreted unchanged in urine

**Formulations**

Quinine sulfate:

Capsule: 64.8 mg, 65 mg, 200 mg, 300 mg, 325 mg

Tablet: 162.5 mg, 260 mg

**Dosing**

**Adults:** Oral:

Treatment of chloroquine-resistant malaria: 650 mg every 8 hours for 3-7 days in conjunction with another agent

Suppression of malaria: 325 mg twice daily and continued for 6 weeks after exposure

Babesiosis: 650 mg every 6-8 hours for 7 days

Leg cramps: 200-300 mg at bedtime

**Elderly:** Refer to adult dosing.

**Renal Impairment:**

$Cl_{cr}$ 10-50 mL/minute: Administer every 8-12 hours or 75% of normal dose.

$Cl_{cr}$ <10 mL/minute: Administer every 24 hours or 30% to 50% of normal dose.

Not removed by hemo- or peritoneal dialysis; dose for $Cl_{cr}$ <10 mL/minute.

Continuous arteriovenous or venovenous hemofiltration (CAVH): Dose as for $Cl_{cr}$ 10-50 mL/minute.

**Administration**

**Oral:** Do not crush sustained release preparations. Avoid use of aluminum-containing antacids because of drug absorption problems. Swallow dose whole to avoid bitter taste. May be administered with food.

**Stability**

**Storage:** Protect from light.

**Additional Nursing Issues**

**Physical Assessment:** Determine if any previous allergy to quinine exists. Monitor effectiveness of other medications patient may be taking, especially digoxin (see Drug Interactions). Monitor hearing periodically. Teach necessity of following drug regimen and reporting adverse effects (see Overdose/Toxicology). **Pregnancy risk factor X** - assess knowledge/instruct patient on need to use appropriate contraceptive measures and the need to avoid pregnancy.

**Patient Information/Instruction:** Take on schedule as directed, with full 8 oz of water. Do not chew or crush sustained release tablets. You will need to return for follow-up blood tests. You may experience GI distress (taking medication with food, and frequent small meals may help). You may experience dizziness, changes in mentation, insomnia, headache, or visual disturbances (use caution when driving or engaging in tasks requiring alertness until response to drug is known). May discolor urine (black/brown/dark). Report persistent sore throat, fever, chills, flu-like signs, ringing in ears, vision disturbances, or unusual bruising or bleeding. Seek emergency help for palpitations or chest pain. **Pregnancy precautions:** Use reliable contraception during and for 2 months following treatment.

(Continued)

## Quinine *(Continued)*

**Geriatric Considerations:** Efficacy in nocturnal leg cramps is not well supported in the medical and pharmacy literature, however, some patients do respond. Nonresponders should be evaluated for other possible etiologies.

- **Quinol** *see* Hydroquinone *on page 583*
- **Quinora®** *see* Quinidine *on page 1002*
- **Quinsana Plus®** *see page 1247*
- **Rabies (Immune Globulin Human)** *see page 1256*
- **Rabies Virus Vaccine** *see page 1256*
- **Racet® Topical** *see* Clioquinol and Hydrocortisone *on page 284*
- **Racovel** *see* Levodopa and Carbidopa *on page 667*
- **Radiostol®** *see* Ergocalciferol *on page 432*

## Raloxifene (ral OX i feen)

**U.S. Brand Names** Evista®

**Synonyms** Keoxifene Hydrochloride

**Therapeutic Category** Selective Estrogen Receptor Modulator (SERM)

**Pregnancy Risk Factor** X

**Lactation** Contraindicated

**Use** Prevention of osteoporosis in postmenopausal women

**Mechanism of Action/Effect** A selective estrogen receptor modulator that if affects some, but not all of the estrogen receptors. In some instances, raloxifene blocks estrogen. It acts like estrogen to prevent bone loss and improve lipid profiles, but it has the potential to block some estrogen effects such as those that lead to breast or uterine cancer.

**Contraindications** Pregnancy; active or past history of venous thromboembolic events, including DVT, PE, and retinal vein thrombosis; not intended for use in premenopausal women

**Warnings** Severe hepatic insufficiency; lowered serum total and LDL cholesterol, but not total HDL or triglycerides; raloxifene should be stopped 72 hours prior to or during prolonged immobilization due to risk of thromboembolic events.

**Drug Interactions**

**Decreased Effect:** Ampicillin and cholestyramine reduce raloxifene absorption.

**Increased Effect/Toxicity:** Effects on highly protein-bound drugs are unclear. Use caution with highly protein-bound drugs, warfarin, clofibrate, indomethacin, naproxen, ibuprofen, diazepam, phenytoin, or tamoxifen.

**Adverse Reactions**

>10%:
- Cardiovascular: Hot flashes
- Neuromuscular & skeletal: Arthralgia
- Respiratory: Sinusitis
- Miscellaneous: Flu syndrome, infection

1% to 10%:
- Cardiovascular: Chest pain,
- Central nervous system: Fever, migraine, depression, insomnia
- Dermatologic: Rash, sweating
- Endocrine & metabolic: Weight gain, peripheral edema
- Gastrointestinal: Nausea, dyspepsia, vomiting, flatulence, GI disorder, Gastroenteritis
- Genitourinary: Urinary tract infection, vaginitis, cystitis, leukorrhea, endometrial disorder
- Neuromuscular & skeletal: Myalgia, leg cramps, arthritis
- Respiratory: Pharyngitis, cough, pneumonia, laryngitis

**Pharmacodynamics/Kinetics**

**Protein Binding:** 95% to albumin and alpha$_1$-acid glycoprotein

**Half-life Elimination:** 28-32.5 hours

**Metabolism:** Liver

**Excretion:** Feces (<6% in urine)

**Formulations** Tablet, as hydrochloride: 60 mg

**Dosing**

**Adults:** Oral: 1 tablet (60 mg) daily; may be administered any time of the day without regard to meals.

**Elderly:** Refer to adult dosing.

**Hepatic Impairment:** Avoid use, safety has not been established.

**Administration**

**Oral:** Raloxifene should be stopped 72 hours prior to or during prolonged immobilization due to risk of thromboembolic events.

**Monitoring Laboratory Tests** Monitor lipid profile, bone mineral density

**Additional Nursing Issues**

**Physical Assessment:** Monitor effectiveness of therapy on a regular basis. Inform patient about use of drug, possible adverse effects, and symptoms to report. **Pregnancy risk factor X** - determine that patient is not pregnant before beginning therapy. Breast-feeding is contraindicated.

**Patient Information/Instruction:** May be taken at any time of day without regard to meals. This medication is given to reduce incidence of osteoporosis; it will not reduce hot flashes or flushing. You may experience flu-like symptoms at beginning of therapy (these may resolve with use). Mild analgesics may reduce joint pain. Rest and cool environment may reduce hot flashes. Report fever; acute migraine; insomnia or emotional depression; unusual weight gain; unresolved gastric distress; urinary infection or vaginal burning or itching; chest pain; or swelling, warmth, or pain in calves. **Pregnancy/breast-feeding precautions:** Inform prescriber if you are pregnant. Do not breast-feed.

**Geriatric Considerations:** No need to cycle with progesterone.

**Additional Information** The decrease in estrogen-related adverse effects with the selective estrogen-receptor modulators in general and raloxifene in particular should improve compliance and decrease the incidence of cardiovascular events and fractures while not increasing breast cancer. However, raloxifene is also associated with increased cimacteric symptoms which may adversely effect compliance.

♦ **Ramace** *see* Ramipril *on this page*

## Ramipril (RAM i pril)

**U.S. Brand Names** Altace™

**Therapeutic Category** Angiotensin-Converting Enzyme (ACE) Inhibitors

**Pregnancy Risk Factor** C/D (2nd and 3rd trimesters)

**Lactation** Enters breast milk/not recommended

**Use** Treatment of hypertension, alone or in combination with thiazide diuretics; treatment of congestive heart failure after myocardial infarction.

**Mechanism of Action/Effect** Ramipril is an angiotensin-converting enzyme (ACE) inhibitor which prevents the formation of angiotensin II from angiotensin I and exhibits pharmacologic effects that are similar to captopril. Ramipril must undergo conversion in the liver to its biologically active metabolite, ramiprilat. The pharmacodynamic effects of ramipril result from the high-affinity, competitive, reversible binding of ramiprilat to angiotensin-converting enzyme thus preventing the formation of the potent vasoconstrictor angiotensin II.

**Contraindications** Hypersensitivity to ramipril or ramiprilat, or any other angiotensin-converting enzyme inhibitors; pregnancy (2nd and 3rd trimesters)

**Warnings** Use with caution and modify dosage in patients with renal impairment (decrease dosage) (especially renal artery stenosis), severe congestive heart failure, or with coadministered diuretic. Severe hypotension may occur in the elderly and patients who are sodium and/or volume depleted, initiate lower doses and monitor closely when starting therapy in these patients. Should be discontinued if laryngeal stridor or angioedema of the face, tongue, or glottis is observed. This isomerized enzyme-inhibitor complex has a slow rate of dissociation, which results in high potency and a long duration of action. Pregnancy factor C/D (2nd and 3rd trimesters).

**Drug Interactions**

**Decreased Effect:** Rifampin may decrease the effect of ACE inhibitors.

**Increased Effect/Toxicity:** Diuretics have additive hypotensive effects with ACE inhibitors. Probenecid increases blood levels of captopril which may occur in other ACE inhibitors. Lithium and ACE inhibitors may result in elevated serum levels of lithium with symptoms of toxicity. Potassium supplements or potassium-sparing diuretics with ACE inhibitors may result in elevated serum potassium levels.

**Effects on Lab Values** Increases BUN, creatinine, potassium, positive Coombs' [direct]; decreases cholesterol (S); may cause false-positive results in urine acetone determinations using sodium nitroprusside reagent

**Adverse Reactions**

>10% Respiratory: Cough

1% to 10%:

Central nervous system: Headache, dizziness, fatigue, syncope, vertigo, muscle weakness

Gastrointestinal: Vomiting, nausea, diarrhea

<1% (Limited to important or life-threatening symptoms): Hypotension, chest pain, palpitations, myocardial infarction, tachycardia, leukopenia, eosinophilia, proteinuria, increased BUN/serum creatinine, asthma, bronchospasm, dyspnea, upper respiratory infection, eosinophilic pneumonitis

**Overdose/Toxicology** Mild hypotension has been the primary toxic effect seen with acute overdose. Bradycardia may also occur. Hyperkalemia occurs even with therapeutic doses, especially in patients with renal insufficiency and those taking NSAIDs. Treatment is symptom directed and supportive.

**Pharmacodynamics/Kinetics**

**Distribution:** Plasma levels decline in a triphasic fashion. Rapid decline is a distribution phase to peripheral compartment, plasma protein, and tissue ACE (half-life 2-4 hours); 2nd phase is an apparent elimination phase representing the clearance of free ramiprilat (half-life: 9-18 hours).

**Half-life Elimination:** Ramiprilat: >50 hours

**Time to Peak:** ~1 hour

**Metabolism:** Liver

**Excretion:** Urine and feces

**Onset:** 1-2 hours

**Duration:** 24 hours

**Formulations** Capsule: 1.25 mg, 2.5 mg, 5 mg, 10 mg

**Dosing**

**Adults:**

Oral: 2.5-5 mg once daily, maximum: 20 mg/day

Congestive heart failure: Initial: 1.25-2.5 mg twice daily; titrate over several weeks to a "target dose" of 5 mg twice daily (see Renal Impairment adjustment below and Additional Information).

(Continued)

## Ramipril *(Continued)*

**Elderly:** Refer to adult dosing (see Geriatric Considerations); adjust for renal function for elderly since glomerular filtration rates are decreased; may see exaggerated hypotensive effects if renal clearance is not considered (see Additional Information).

**Renal Impairment:** $Cl_{cr}$ <40 mL/minute: Patients should be started on 1.25 mg/day and titrated up to 5 mg/day maximum.

**Monitoring Laboratory Tests** CBC, renal function tests, electrolytes

**Additional Nursing Issues**

**Physical Assessment:** Assess effectiveness and interactions of other medications (see Drug Interactions). See Warnings/Precautions and Contraindications for use cautions. Monitor effectiveness of therapy, laboratory tests, and adverse response on a regular basis during therapy (see Adverse Reactions and Overdose/Toxicology). Assess knowledge/teach patient appropriate use according to drug form and purpose of therapy, possible side effects and appropriate interventions, and adverse symptoms to report. **Pregnancy risk factor C/D** - see Pregnancy Risk Factor - assess knowledge/teach patient use of barrier contraceptive measures. See Pregnancy Issues. Breast-feeding is not recommended.

**Patient Information/Instruction:** Take exactly as directed; do not discontinue without consulting prescriber. Take first dose at bedtime. This drug does not eliminate need for diet or exercise regimen as recommended by prescriber. Do not take potassium supplements or salt substitutes containing potassium without consulting prescriber. May cause dizziness, fainting, lightheadedness (use caution when driving or engaging in tasks requiring alertness until response to drug is known); postural hypotension (use caution when rising from lying or sitting position or climbing stairs); nausea or vomiting (small frequent meals, frequent mouth care, sucking lozenges, or chewing gum may help) - report if these persist. Report chest pain or palpitations; difficulty in breathing or unusual cough; or other persistent adverse reactions. **Pregnancy/breast-feeding precautions:** Do not get pregnant; use appropriate contraceptive measures. If you are, or plan to be pregnant, notify your prescriber at once. Breast-feeding is not recommended.

**Geriatric Considerations:** Due to frequent decreases in glomerular filtration (also creatinine clearance) with aging, elderly patients may have exaggerated responses to ACE inhibitors. Differences in clinical response due to hepatic changes are not observed.

**Breast-feeding Issues:** The manufacturer states that after single dose studies, ramipril was not excreted in breast milk; however, since the amount excreted with daily dosing is unknown, nursing while taking ramipril is not recommended.

**Pregnancy Issues:** ACE inhibitors can cause fetal injury or death if taken during the 2nd or 3rd trimester. Discontinue ACE inhibitors as soon as pregnancy is detected. ACE inhibitors should not be used if patient is sexually active and not using contraceptives.

**Additional Information** Some patients may have a decreased hypotensive effect between 12 and 16 hours; consider dividing total daily dose into 2 doses 12 hours apart. If patient is receiving a diuretic, a potential for first-dose hypotension is increased. To decrease this potential, stop diuretic for 2-3 days prior to initiating ramipril. If diuretic cannot be stopped temporarily, then initiate therapy with 1.25 mg daily. Continue diuretic if needed to control blood pressure. Capsules should be swallowed whole; if this cannot be done, capsule contents may be mixed with applesauce; also, contents may be mixed with apple juice or water. Mixtures in juice and water are stable for 24 hours at room temperature or 48 hours with refrigeration.

**Related Information**

ACE Inhibitors and Angiotensin Antagonists Comparison *on page 1362*

- ♦ **Ramses®** *see page 1294*
- ♦ **Randikan** *see* Kanamycin *on page 641*
- ♦ **Ranifur** *see* Ranitidine *on this page*
- ♦ **Ranisen** *see* Ranitidine *on this page*

## Ranitidine (ra NI ti deen)

**U.S. Brand Names** Zantac®; Zantac® 75 [OTC]

**Therapeutic Category** Histamine $H_2$ Antagonist

**Pregnancy Risk Factor** B

**Lactation** Enters breast milk/may be compatible

**Use** Short-term treatment of active duodenal ulcers and benign gastric ulcers; long-term prophylaxis of duodenal ulcer and gastric hypersecretory states, gastroesophageal reflux, recurrent postoperative ulcer, upper GI bleeding, prevention of acid-aspiration pneumonitis during surgery, and prevention of stress-induced ulcers; causes fewer interactions than cimetidine

**Mechanism of Action/Effect** Competitive inhibition of histamine at $H_2$-receptors, gastric acid secretion, gastric volume and hydrogen ion concentration reduced

**Contraindications** Hypersensitivity to ranitidine or any component

**Warnings** Use with caution in children <12 years of age. Use with caution in patients with liver and renal impairment. Dosage modification is required in patients with renal impairment. Long-term therapy may cause vitamin $B_{12}$ deficiency.

**Drug Interactions**

**Cytochrome P-450 Effect:** CYP2D6 and 3A3/4 enzyme inhibitor

**Decreased Effect:** Variable effects on warfarin. Antacids may decrease absorption of ranitidine. Ketoconazole and itraconazole absorption is decreased by ranitidine. May produce altered serum levels of procainamide and ferrous sulfate. Decreased effect of nondepolarizing muscle relaxants, cefpodoxime, cyanocobalamin (decreased absorption), diazepam, and oxaprozin. Decreased toxicity of atropine.

**Increased Effect/Toxicity:** Increased toxicity of cyclosporine (increased serum creatinine), gentamicin (neuromuscular blockade), glipizide, glyburide, midazolam (increased concentrations), metoprolol, pentoxifylline, phenytoin, and quinidine.

**Effects on Lab Values** False-positive urine protein using Multistix®, gastric acid secretion test, skin test allergen extracts, serum creatinine and serum transaminase concentrations, urine protein test

**Adverse Reactions**

1% to 10%:

Central nervous system: Dizziness, sedation, malaise, headache, drowsiness
Dermatologic: Rash
Gastrointestinal: Constipation, nausea, vomiting, diarrhea

<1% (Limited to important or life-threatening symptoms): Bradycardia, tachycardia, asystole, A-V block, PVC, erythema multiforme, thrombocytopenia, granulocytopenia, leukopenia, pancytopenia, aplastic anemia, eosinophilia, elevated LFTs, hepatitis, jaundice, bronchospasm

**Overdose/Toxicology** Symptoms of overdose include muscular tremor, vomiting, rapid respiration, renal failure, and CNS depression. Treatment is symptomatic and supportive.

**Pharmacodynamics/Kinetics**

**Protein Binding:** 15%

**Distribution:** Minimally penetrates the blood-brain barrier

**Half-life Elimination:** Adults: 2-2.5 hours; End-stage renal disease: 6-9 hours

**Time to Peak:** Oral: Within 1-3 hours and persisting for 8 hours

**Metabolism:** Liver

**Excretion:** Urine and feces

**Onset:** 1-2 hours

**Duration:** 8-12 hours

**Formulations**

Ranitidine hydrochloride:

Capsule (GELdose™): 150 mg, 300 mg
Granules, effervescent (EFFERdose™): 150 mg
Infusion, preservative free, in NaCl 0.45%: 1 mg/mL (50 mL)
Injection: 25 mg/mL (2 mL, 10 mL, 40 mL)
Syrup (peppermint flavor): 15 mg/mL (473 mL)
Tablet: 75 mg [OTC]; 150 mg, 300 mg
Tablet, effervescent (EFFERdose™): 150 mg

**Dosing**

**Adults:**

Short-term treatment of ulceration: 150 mg/dose twice daily or 300 mg at bedtime
Prophylaxis of recurrent duodenal ulcer: Oral: 150 mg at bedtime
Gastric hypersecretory conditions:

Oral: 150 mg twice daily, up to 6 g/day
I.M., I.V.: 50 mg/dose every 6-8 hours (dose not to exceed 400 mg/day)
I.V.: 50 mg/dose IVPB every 6-8 hours (dose not to exceed 400 mg/day)
**or**
Continuous I.V. infusion: Initial: 50 mg IVPB, followed by 6.25 mg/hour titrated to gastric pH >4.0 for prophylaxis or >7.0 for treatment; **continuous I.V. infusion is preferred in patients with active bleeding.**

Gastric hypersecretory conditions: Doses up to 2.5 mg/kg/hour (220 mg/hour) have been used.

**Elderly:** Refer to adult dosing.

**Renal Impairment:**

$Cl_{cr}$ 10-50 mL/minute: Administer at 75% of normal dose or administer every 18-24 hours.

$Cl_{cr}$ <10 mL/minute: Administer at 50% of normal dose or administer every 18-24 hours.

Slightly dialyzable (5% to 20%)

**Hepatic Impairment:** Unchanged

**Administration**

**I.M.:** I.M. solution does not need to be diluted before use.

**I.V.:** Ranitidine injection may be administered I.M. or I.V.

IVP: Ranitidine (usually 50 mg) should be diluted to a total of 20 mL with NS or $D_5W$ and administered over at least 5 minutes.

IVPB: Administer over 15-20 minutes.

Continuous I.V. infusion: Administer at 6.25 mg/hour and titrate dosage based on gastric pH by continuous infusion over 24 hours.

**I.V. Detail:** I.V. must be diluted and may be administered IVP or IVPB or continuous I.V. infusion.

**Stability**

**Storage:** Ranitidine injection should be stored at 4°C to 30°C and protected from light. Injection solution is a clear, colorless to yellow solution. Slight darkening does not affect potency.

Stability at room temperature:

Prepared bags: 2 days
Premixed bags: Manufacturer expiration dating and out of overwrap stability: 15 days

(Continued)

## Ranitidine *(Continued)*

Stability of prepared bags at refrigeration temperature (4°C) is 10 days.

**Compatibility:** Solution for I.V. infusion in NS or $D_5W$ is stable for 30 days when frozen. I.V. form is incompatible with amphotericin B, clindamycin, diazepam (same syringe), hetastarch (Y-line), hydroxyzine (same syringe), midazolam (same syringe), pentobarbital (same syringe), phenobarbital (same syringe). See the Compatibility of Drugs in Syringe Chart *on page 1317*.

**Monitoring Laboratory Tests** AST, ALT, serum creatinine; when used to prevent stress-related GI bleeding, measure the intragastric pH and try to maintain pH >4; occult blood with GI bleeding; monitor renal function and adjust dosage as indicated.

**Additional Nursing Issues**

**Physical Assessment:** Assess other patient medications patient may be taking for effectiveness and interactions (see Drug Interactions). Monitor laboratory results and renal function. Observe for signs of GI bleeding. Evaluate effectiveness of treatment and possible side effects on a regular basis. Assess knowledge/teach patient appropriate use, possible adverse reactions, and symptoms to report.

**Patient Information/Instruction:** Take exactly as directed (at meals and bedtime); do not increase dose - may take several days before you notice relief. If antacids are approved by prescriber, allow 1 hour between antacid and ranitidine. Avoid OTC medications, especially cold or cough medication and aspirin or anything containing aspirin. Follow diet as prescriber recommends. You may experience constipation or diarrhea (request assistance from prescriber); nausea or vomiting (frequent small meals, frequent mouth care, sucking lozenges, or chewing gum may help); impotence or loss of libido (reversible when drug is discontinued); drowsiness, dizziness, or fatigue (use caution when driving or engaging in tasks requiring alertness until response to drug is known). Report skin rash, fever, sore throat, tarry stools, changes in CNS, muscle or joint pain, yellowing of skin or eyes, and change in color of urine or stool.

**Geriatric Considerations:** $H_2$ blockers are the preferred drugs for treating PUD in the elderly due to cost and ease of administration.

**Additional Information** pH: 6.7-7.3

## Ranitidine Bismuth Citrate (ra NI ti deen BIZ muth SIT rate)

**U.S. Brand Names** Tritec®

**Synonyms** RBC

**Therapeutic Category** Histamine $H_2$ Antagonist

**Pregnancy Risk Factor** C

**Lactation** Excretion in breast milk unknown

**Use** In combination with clarithromycin for the treatment of active duodenal ulcer associated with *H. pylori* infection; not to be used alone for the treatment of active duodenal ulcer

**Contraindications** Hypersensitivity to ranitidine or bismuth compounds or components; acute porphyria

**Warnings** Avoid use in patients with $Cl_{cr}$ <25 mL/minute. Do not use for maintenance therapy or for >16 weeks. Pregnancy factor C.

**Adverse Reactions**

>10%:

Central nervous system: Headache

Gastrointestinal: Darkening of the tongue and/or stool, taste disturbance

1% to 10%:

Gastrointestinal: Diarrhea, constipation, abdominal pain, gastric upset

Miscellaneous: Flu-like symptoms

<1% (Limited to important or life-threatening symptoms): Anemia, nausea, vomiting, flatulence, rash, dizziness, thrombocytopenia, elevated LFTs

**Pharmacodynamics/Kinetics**

**Protein Binding:** Bismuth: 90%; Ranitidine: 15%

**Half-life Elimination:** Bismuth: 11-28 days; Ranitidine: 3 hours; Complex: 5-8 days

**Time to Peak:** Bismuth: 1-2 hours; Ranitidine: 0.5-5 hours; Complex: 1 week

**Metabolism:** Ranitidine: Liver

**Excretion:** ~30% of ranitidine and <1% of bismuth excreted in the urine

**Formulations** Tablet: 400 mg (ranitidine 162 mg, trivalent bismuth 128 mg, and citrate 110 mg)

**Dosing**

**Adults:** Oral: 400 mg twice daily for 4 weeks with clarithromycin 500 mg 2-3 times daily for first 2 weeks

**Elderly:** Refer to adult dosing.

**Renal Impairment:** $Cl_{cr}$ <25 mL/minute: Not recommended

**Administration**

**Oral:** Take with food.

**Monitoring Laboratory Tests** $C^{13}$-urea breath tests to detect *H. pylori*, endoscopic evidence of ulcer healing, CBCs, LFTs, renal function

**Additional Nursing Issues**

**Physical Assessment:** Monitor for signs or symptoms of adverse effects as noted above. Monitor laboratory results as appropriate. Instruct patient on appropriate diet and activity regimen related to gastric and/or duodenal ulcers. **Pregnancy risk factor C** - benefits of use should outweigh possible risks. Note breast-feeding caution.

**Patient Information/Instruction:** Take as directed, with food. Do not supplement therapy with OTC medications. This drug may cause darkening of tongue or stool and may change your taste sensation. Report unresolved headache (prescriber may recommend something for relief), dizziness, diarrhea, constipation (prescriber may recommend something for relief), weakness, or loss of appetite. **Pregnancy/breast-feeding precautions:** Inform prescriber if you are or intend to be pregnant. Consult prescriber if breast-feeding.

- **Rastinon** *see* Tolbutamide *on page 1146*
- **Raxar®** *see* Grepafloxacin *on page 545*
- **Raxedin** *see* Loperamide *on page 688*
- **RBC** *see* Ranitidine Bismuth Citrate *on previous page*
- **R & C® Shampoo** *see page 1294*
- **Rea-Lo® [OTC]** *see* Urea *on page 1193*
- **Rebetrol®** *see* Ribavirin *on page 1016*
- **Rebetron™** *see* Interferon Alfa-2b and Ribavirin Combination Pack *on page 615*
- **Recombinant Hirudin** *see* Lepirudin *on page 659*
- **Recombinant Human Deoxyribonuclease** *see* Dornase Alfa *on page 397*
- **Recombinant Plasminogen Activator** *see* Reteplase *on page 1015*
- **Recombinate®** *see* Antihemophilic Factor (Recombinant) *on page 100*
- **Recombivac HB®** *see page 1256*
- **Redisol®** *see* Cyanocobalamin *on page 311*
- **Redoxon®** *see* Ascorbic Acid *on page 108*
- **Redoxon® Forte** *see* Ascorbic Acid *on page 108*
- **Reese's® Pinworm Medicine** *see page 1294*
- **Refludan®** *see* Lepirudin *on page 659*
- **Refresh® Ophthalmic Solution** *see page 1294*
- **Refresh® Plus Ophthalmic Solution** *see page 1294*
- **Regaine®** *see page 1294*
- **Regitine®** *see* Phentolamine *on page 919*
- **Reglan®** *see* Metoclopramide *on page 758*
- **Regonol® Injection** *see* Pyridostigmine *on page 996*
- **Regulace®** *see page 1294*
- **Regular (Concentrated) Iletin® II U-500** *see* Insulin Preparations *on page 609*
- **Regular Iletin® I** *see* Insulin Preparations *on page 609*
- **Regular Insulin** *see* Insulin Preparations *on page 609*
- **Regular Purified Pork Insulin** *see* Insulin Preparations *on page 609*
- **Regulax SS® [OTC]** *see* Docusate *on page 392*
- **Regulex®** *see* Docusate *on page 392*
- **Reguloid® [OTC]** *see* Psyllium *on page 993*
- **Rela®** *see* Carisoprodol *on page 202*
- **Relafen®** *see* Nabumetone *on page 796*
- **Relaxadon®** *see* Hyoscyamine, Atropine, Scopolamine, and Phenobarbital *on page 591*
- **Relefact® TRH Injection** *see page 1248*
- **Relief®** *see page 1282*
- **Relief® Ophthalmic Solution** *see* Phenylephrine *on page 920*
- **Remeron®** *see* Mirtazapine *on page 775*
- **Remicade™** *see* Infliximab *on page 608*
- **Renagel®** *see* Sevelamer *on page 1054*
- **Renedil®** *see* Felodipine *on page 474*
- **Renitec** *see* Enalapril *on page 416*
- **Rentamine® Liquid** *see page 1294*
- **ReoPro®** *see* Abciximab *on page 28*

## Repaglinide (re PAG li nide)

**U.S. Brand Names** Prandin®

**Therapeutic Category** Antidiabetic Agent (Miscellaneous)

**Pregnancy Risk Factor** C

**Lactation** Excretion in breast milk unknown/contraindicated

**Use** Management of noninsulin-dependent diabetes mellitus (Type II); an adjunct to diet and exercise to lower the blood glucose in patients with Type II diabetes mellitus whose hyperglycemia cannot be controlled satisfactorily by diet and exercise alone; in combination with metformin to lower blood glucose in patients whose hyperglycemia cannot be controlled by exercise, diet and either agent alone

**Mechanism of Action/Effect** Nonsulfonylurea hypoglycemic agent which blocks ATP-dependent potassium channels, depolarizing the membrane and facilitating calcium entry through calcium channels. Increased intracellular calcium stimulates insulin release from the pancreatic beta cells.

**Contraindications** Hypersensitivity to repaglinide or any component; diabetic ketoacidosis, with or without coma (treat with insulin); Type 1 diabetes

**Warnings** Use with caution in patients with hepatic impairment. As compared to treatment with diet alone or diet plus insulin, the administration of oral hypoglycemic drugs is associated with increased cardiovascular mortality. May cause hypoglycemia. Proper patient selection, dosage, and instructions to the patients are important to avoid hypoglycemic episodes. It may be necessary to discontinue repaglinide and administer insulin if the patient is exposed to stress (fever, trauma, infection, surgery). Caution when used in combination with another hypoglycemic agent (ie, metformin). Pregnancy factor C.

(Continued)

## Repaglinide *(Continued)*

### Drug Interactions

**Cytochrome P-450 Effect:** CYP3A4 enzyme substrate

**Decreased Effect:** Drugs which induce cytochrome P-450 isoenzyme 3A4 may increase metabolism of repaglinide (troglitazone, rifampin, barbiturates, carbamazepine). Certain drugs (thiazides, diuretics, corticosteroids, phenothiazines, thyroid products, estrogens, oral contraceptives, phenytoin, nicotinic acid, sympathomimetics, calcium channel blockers, isoniazid) tend to produce hyperglycemia and may lead to loss of glycemic control.

**Increased Effect/Toxicity:** Agents that inhibit cytochrome P-450 isoenzyme 3A4 (eg, ketoconazole, miconazole, erythromycin) may increase repaglinide concentrations. Hypoglycemic effect may be potentiated when given concomitantly with other highly protein-bound drugs (ie, phenylbutazone, oral anticoagulants, hydantoins, salicylates, NSAIDs, sulfonamides) Concurrent use of other hypoglycemic agents may increase risk of hypoglycemia.

### Adverse Reactions

>10%:

Central nervous system: Headache (9% to 11%)
Endocrine & metabolic: Hypoglycemia (16% to 31%)

1% to 10%:

Cardiovascular: Chest pain (2% to 3%)
Gastrointestinal: Nausea (3% to 5%), heartburn (2% to 4%), vomiting (2% to 3%) constipation (2% to 3%), diarrhea (4% to 5%), tooth disorder (<1% to 2%)
Respiratory: Upper respiratory tract infection (10% to 16%), sinusitis (3% to 6%), rhinitis (3% to 7%), bronchitis (2% to 6%)
Genitourinary: Urinary tract infection (2% to 3%)
Neuromuscular: Arthralgia (3% to 6%), back pain (5% to 6%), paresthesia (2% to 3%)
Miscellaneous: Allergy (1% to 2%)

<1% (Limited to important or life-threatening symptoms): Anaphylactoid reaction

**Overdose/Toxicology** Symptoms of severe hypoglycemia include seizures, cerebral damage, tingling of lips and tongue, nausea, yawning, confusion, agitation, tachycardia, sweating, convulsions, stupor, and coma. Management includes glucose administration (oral for milder hypoglycemia or by injection in more severe forms) and symptomatic treatment.

### Pharmacodynamics/Kinetics

**Protein Binding:** >98%

**Half-life Elimination:** 1 hour

**Time to Peak:** Within 1 hour

**Metabolism:** Extensive hepatic metabolism by cytochrome P-450. Isoenzyme 3A4 is a primary metabolic pathway.

**Excretion:** Feces

**Onset:** Insulin levels increase within 15-60 minutes after a dose

**Duration:** Up to 24 hours

**Formulations** Tablet: 0.5 mg, 1 mg, 2 mg

### Dosing

**Adults:** Oral: Should be taken within 15 minutes of the meal, but time may vary from immediately preceding the meal to as long as 30 minutes before the meal.

Initial: For patients not previously treated or whose Hb $A_{1c}$ is <8%, the starting dose is 0.5 mg. For patients previously treated with blood glucose-lowering agents whose Hb $A_{1c}$ is ≥8%, the initial dose is 1 or 2 mg before each meal.

Dose adjustment: Determine dosing adjustments by blood glucose response, usually fasting blood glucose. Double the preprandial dose up to 4 mg until satisfactory blood glucose response is achieved. At least 1 week should elapse to assess response after each dose adjustment.

Dose range: 0.5-4 mg taken with meals. Repaglinide may be dosed preprandial 2, 3 or 4 times/day in response to changes in the patient's meal pattern. Maximum recommended daily dose: 16 mg.

Patients receiving other oral hypoglycemic agents: When repaglinide is used to replace therapy with other oral hypoglycemic agents, it may be started the day after the final dose is given. Observe patients carefully for hypoglycemia because of potential overlapping of drug effects. When transferred from longer half-life sulfonylureas (eg, chlorpropamide), close monitoring may be indicated for up to ≥1 week.

Combination therapy: If repaglinide monotherapy does not result in adequate glycemic control, metformin may be added. Or, if metformin therapy does not provide adequate control, repaglinide may be added. The starting dose and dose adjustments for combination therapy are the same as repaglinide monotherapy. Carefully adjust the dose of each drug to determine the minimal dose required to achieve the desired pharmacologic effect. Failure to do so could result in an increase in the incidence of hypoglycemic episodes. Use appropriate monitoring of FPG and Hb $A_{1c}$ measurements to ensure that the patient is not subjected to excessive drug exposure or increased probability of secondary drug failure. If glucose is not achieved after a suitable trial of combination therapy, consider discontinuing these drugs and using insulin.

**Elderly:** Refer to adult dosing.

**Renal Impairment:** Initial dosage adjustment does not appear to be necessary, but make subsequent increases carefully in patients with renal function impairment or renal failure requiring hemodialysis.

**Hepatic Impairment:** Conservative initial and maintenance doses are recommended in moderate impairment. Avoid use in severe disease.

**Monitoring Laboratory Tests** Fasting blood glucose and glycosylated hemoglobin (Hb $A_{1c}$) levels

**Additional Nursing Issues**

**Physical Assessment:** Assess all other medications patient may be taking for possible interactions or alterations in effectiveness (especially anything that is metabolized via the cytochrome P-450 route - see Drug Interactions). Monitor laboratory tests and cardiovascular status before and during therapy (every 3 months) (see Warnings/Precautions). Monitor for effectiveness of therapy and adverse reactions on a regular basis. Assess/teach particulars of this medication, knowledge of disease, signs of hyper-/hypoglycemia, and refer patient to a diabetic educator as appropriate. **Pregnancy risk factor C** - benefits of use should outweigh possible risks. Breast-feeding is contraindicated.

**Patient Information/Instruction:** Take this medication exactly as directed - 3-4 times a day, 15-30 minutes prior to a meal. If you skip a meal (or add an extra meal) skip (or add) a dose for that meal. Do not change dosage or discontinue without first consulting prescriber. It is important to follow dietary and lifestyle recommendations of prescriber. You will be instructed in signs of hypo-/hyperglycemia by prescriber or diabetic educator; be alert for adverse hypoglycemia (tachycardia, profuse perspiration, tingling of lips and tongue, seizures, or change in sensorium) and follow prescriber's instructions for intervention. You may experience mild side effects during first weeks of therapy (eg, headache, diarrhea, constipation, bloating); if these do not diminish, notify prescriber. Increasing dietary fiber or fluids and increasing exercise may reduce constipation (for persistent diarrhea consult prescriber). Mild analgesics may reduce headaches. Frequent mouth care, small frequent meals, chewing gum, sucking lozenges may help reduce nausea, vomiting, or heartburn. Report chest pain, palpitations, or irregular heartbeat; respiratory difficulty or symptoms of upper respiratory infection; urinary tract infection (burning or itching on urination); muscle pain or back pain; or persistent GI problems. **Pregnancy/breast-feeding precautions:** Inform prescriber if you are or intend to be pregnant. Do not breast-feed.

**Geriatric Considerations:** Repaglinide has not been studied exclusively in the elderly; information from the manufacturer states that no differences in its effectiveness or adverse effects had been identified between persons younger than and older than 65 years of age. How "tightly" a geriatric patient's blood glucose should be controlled is controversial; however, a fasting blood glucose <150 mg/dL is now an acceptable end-point. Such a decision should be based on the patient's functional status, how well he/she recognizes hypoglycemic or hyperglycemic symptoms, and how to respond to them and their other disease states.

**Breast-feeding Issues:** It is not known whether repaglinide is excreted in breast milk. Because the potential for hypoglycemia in nursing infants may exist, decide whether to discontinue repaglinide or discontinue breast-feeding. If repaglinide is discontinued and if diet alone is inadequate for controlling blood glucose, consider insulin therapy.

**Pregnancy Issues:** Safety in pregnant women has not been established. Use during pregnancy only if clearly needed. Insulin is the drug of choice for the control of diabetes mellitus during pregnancy.

**Related Information**

Antidiabetic Oral Agents Comparison *on page 1370*


- **Repan®** *see* Butalbital Compound and Acetaminophen *on page 175*
- **Reposans-10® Oral** *see* Chlordiazepoxide *on page 250*
- **Resaid®** *see page 1294*
- **Rescaps-D® S.R. Capsule** *see* Caramiphen and Phenylpropanolamine *on page 195*
- **Rescon Liquid** *see page 1294*
- **Rescriptor®** *see* Delavirdine *on page 340*
- **Resectisol® Irrigation Solution** *see* Mannitol *on page 706*


## Reserpine (re SER peen)

**U.S. Brand Names** Serpalan®

**Therapeutic Category** Rauwolfia Alkaloid

**Pregnancy Risk Factor** C

**Lactation** Enters breast milk/use caution

**Use** Management of mild to moderate hypertension

**Unlabeled use:** Management of tardive dyskinesia

**Mechanism of Action/Effect** Reduces blood pressure via depletion of sympathetic biogenic amines (norepinephrine and dopamine); this also commonly results in sedative effects

**Contraindications** Hypersensitivity to reserpine or any component; any ulcerative condition; mental depression

**Warnings** Discontinue reserpine 7 days before electroshock therapy. Use with caution in patients with impaired renal function or peptic ulcer disease, gallstones, and the elderly. At high doses, significant mental depression may occur. Some products may contain tartrazine. Pregnancy factor C.

**Drug Interactions**

**Decreased Effect:** Decreased effect of indirect-acting sympathomimetics.

**Increased Effect/Toxicity:** If reserpine is taken with MAO inhibitors, direct-acting sympathomimetics, and tricyclic antidepressants, there may he increased effect or toxicity.

**Effects on Lab Values** ↓ catecholamines (U)

(Continued)

## Reserpine *(Continued)*

**Adverse Reactions**

>10%:

Central nervous system: Dizziness
Gastrointestinal: Anorexia, diarrhea, dry mouth, nausea, vomiting
Respiratory: Nasal congestion

1% to 10%:

Cardiovascular: Peripheral edema, arrhythmias, bradycardia, chest pain
Central nervous system: Headache
Gastrointestinal: Black stools
Genitourinary: Impotence
Miscellaneous: Bloody vomit

**Overdose/Toxicology** Symptoms of overdose include hypotension, bradycardia, CNS depression, sedation, coma, hypothermia, miosis, tremor, diarrhea, and vomiting. Treatment is symptom directed and supportive. Anticholinergic agents may be useful in reducing parkinsonian effects and bradycardia.

**Pharmacodynamics/Kinetics**

**Protein Binding:** 96%

**Distribution:** Crosses the placenta

**Half-life Elimination:** 50-100 hours

**Metabolism:** Liver

**Excretion:** Feces and urine

**Onset:** Onset of antihypertensive effect: Within 3-6 days

**Duration:** 2-6 weeks

**Formulations** Tablet: 0.1 mg, 0.25 mg

**Dosing**

**Adults:** Oral (full antihypertensive effects may take as long as 3 weeks): 0.1-0.25 mg/day in 1-2 doses; initial: 0.5 mg/day for 1-2 weeks; maintenance: reduce to 0.1-0.25 mg/day.

**Elderly:** Oral: Initial: 0.05 mg once daily increasing by 0.05 mg every week as necessary (full antihypertensive effects may take as long as 3 weeks).

**Renal Impairment:**

$Cl_{cr}$ <10 mL/minute: Avoid use.
Not removed by hemo- or peritoneal dialysis; supplemental dose is not necessary.

**Stability**

**Storage:** Protect oral dosage forms from light.

**Additional Nursing Issues**

**Physical Assessment:** Assess other medications patient may be taking for possible adverse reactions (see Drug Interactions). Monitor blood pressure and cardiac status prior to starting therapy, during first doses of therapy, when titrating dosage, and regularly thereafter. Instruct patient on use of medication, possible adverse effects, and symptoms to report. **Pregnancy risk factor C** - benefits of use should outweigh possible risks. Note breast-feeding caution.

**Patient Information/Instruction:** Take as directed; do not discontinue without consulting prescriber. May take up to 2 weeks to see effects of therapy. Avoid alcohol and maintain recommended diet. You may experience nervousness, dizziness, or fatigue; use caution when driving or engaging in hazardous activities until response to drug is known. Rise slowly from sitting or lying position until response to therapy is known. Small frequent meals or sucking lozenges may reduce nausea or loss of appetite; adequate dietary fruit, fluids, and fiber may reduce constipation. You may experience nasal stuffiness; avoid OTC medications, and consult prescriber. You may experience impotence; will resolve when medication is discontinued. Report chest pain, rapid heartbeat or palpitations, difficulty breathing, sudden increase in weight, swelling in ankles or hands, black tarry stools; or unusual feelings of depression. **Pregnancy/breast-feeding precautions:** Inform prescriber if you are or intend to be pregnant. Consult prescriber if breast-feeding.

**Geriatric Considerations:** Some studies advocate the use of reserpine because of its low cost, long half-life, and efficacy, but it is generally not considered a first-line drug. If it is to be used, doses should not exceed 0.25 mg and the patient should be monitored for depressed mood.


- **Reserpine and Hydrochlorothiazide** *see* Hydrochlorothiazide and Reserpine *on page 567*
- **Reserpine, Hydralazine, and Hydrochlorothiazide** *see* Hydralazine, Hydrochlorothiazide, and Reserpine *on page 565*
- **Respa-1st®** *see* Guaifenesin and Pseudoephedrine *on page 551*
- **Respa-DM®** *see* Guaifenesin and Dextromethorphan *on page 549*
- **Respa-GF®** *see* Guaifenesin *on page 548*
- **Respaire®-60 SR** *see* Guaifenesin and Pseudoephedrine *on page 551*
- **Respaire®-120 SR** *see* Guaifenesin and Pseudoephedrine *on page 551*
- **Respbid®** *see* Theophylline *on page 1115*
- **Respinol-G®** *see* Guaifenesin, Phenylpropanolamine, and Phenylephrine *on page 552*
- **Resporal®** *see page 1294*
- **Restoril®** *see* Temazepam *on page 1100*
- **Retavase™** *see* Reteplase *on next page*

## Reteplase (RE ta plase)

**U.S. Brand Names** Retavase™

**Synonyms** Recombinant Plasminogen Activator; r-PA

**Therapeutic Category** Thrombolytic Agent

**Pregnancy Risk Factor** C

**Lactation** Excretion in breast milk unknown/use caution

**Use** Management of acute myocardial infarction (AMI); improvement of ventricular function; reduction of the incidence of CHF and the reduction of mortality following AMI

**Mechanism of Action/Effect** Reteplase initiates local fibrinolysis by binding to fibrin in a thrombus (clot) and converting entrapped plasminogen to plasmin. Dissolution of thrombus occluding a coronary artery restores perfusion to ischemic myocardium. Reteplase is manufactured by recombinant DNA technology using *E. coli.*

**Contraindications** Active internal bleeding; history of cerebrovascular accident; recent intracranial or intraspinal surgery or trauma, intracranial neoplasm, arteriovenous malformations, or aneurysm; known bleeding diathesis; severe uncontrolled hypertension; history of severe allergic reactions to reteplase, alteplase, anistreplase, or streptokinase

**Warnings** Minimize venipuncture. Caution in readministration of reteplase (due to limited clinical experience).

An individualized consideration of risks and benefits must accompany a decision to use reteplase. factors which may increase risks include: recent major surgery (including CABG, organ biopsy, obstetrical delivery), previous puncture of noncompressible vessel, cerebrovascular disease, recent gastrointestinal or genitourinary bleeding, recent trauma, hypertension (systolic ≥180 mm Hg and/or diastolic ≥110 mm Hg), high liklihood of LV thrombus, acute pericarditis, subacute bacterial endocarditis, severe hepatic or renal dysfunction, hemostatic defects, hemorrhagic ophthalmologic conditions (including diabetic hemorrhagic retinopathy), septic thrombophlebitis, advanced age, patients receiving oral anticoagulants, or any condition where bleeding constitutes a particular hazard or would be difficult to manage due to its location.

Pregnancy factor C.

**Drug Interactions**

**Increased Effect/Toxicity:** Oral anticoagulants, heparin, and drugs which impair platelet aggregation (aspirin, nonsteroidal anti-inflammatory drugs, ticlopidine, clopidogrel, IIb/IIIa antagonists, and dipyridamole) may increase the risks of bleeding.

**Adverse Reactions** Bleeding is the most frequent adverse effect associated with reteplase. Heparin and aspirin have been administered concurrently with reteplase in clinical trials. The incidence of adverse events is a reflection of these combined therapies, and are comparable with comparison thrombolytics.

>10%: Local: Injection site bleeding (4.6% to 48.6%)

1% to 10%:
- Hematologic: Anemia (0.9% to 2.6%)
- Gastrointestinal: Bleeding (1.8% to 9.0%)
- Genitourinary: Bleeding (0.9% to 9.5%)

<1% (Limited to important or life-threatening symptoms): Intracranial hemorrhage (0.8%), allergic/anaphylactoid reactions, cholesterol embolization

Other adverse effects noted are frequently associated with myocardial infarction (and therefore may or may not be attributable to Retavase™) and include arrhythmias, hypotension, cardiogenic shock, pulmonary edema, cardiac arrest, reinfarction, pericarditis, tamponade, thrombosis, and embolism.

**Overdose/Toxicology** Symptoms of overdose include increased incidence of intracranial bleeding. Treatment is supportive.

**Pharmacodynamics/Kinetics**

**Half-life Elimination:** In serum, 13-16 minutes

**Metabolism:** Plasma clearance 250-450 mL/minute; cleared by hepatic and renal mechanisms

**Onset:** 30-90 minutes

**Formulations** Powder for injection, lyophilized: 10.8 units [reteplase 18.8 mg]

**Dosing**

**Adults:** 10 units I.V. over 2 minutes, followed by a second dose 30 minutes later of 10 units I.V. over 2 minutes; withhold second dose if serious bleeding or anaphylaxis occurs.

**Administration**

**I.V.:** Infuse over 2 minutes.

**I.V. Detail:** No other medications should be added to the injection solution.

**Stability**

**Storage:** Dosage kits should be stored at 2°C to 25°C (36°F to 77°F) and remain sealed until use in order to protect from light.

**Reconstitution:** Reteplase should be reconstituted using the diluent, syringe, needle, and dispensing pin provided with each kit.

**Additional Nursing Issues**

**Physical Assessment:** Monitor vital signs and laboratory results prior to, during, and after therapy. Assess infusion insertion site during and after therapy (every 15 minutes or as institutional policy). Observe and teach patient bleeding precautions (avoid invasive procedures and activities that could result in injury). Monitor closely for signs of excessive bleeding (eg, CNS changes; blood in urine, stool, or vomitus; unusual bruising or bleeding). Do not administer second bolus if patient experiences an adverse reaction to the initial bolus. **Pregnancy risk factor C** - benefits of use should outweigh possible risks. Note breast-feeding caution.

(Continued)

## Reteplase *(Continued)*

**Patient Information/Instruction:** This medication can only be administered I.V. You will have a tendency to bleed easily following this medication; use caution to prevent injury (use electric razor, use soft toothbrush, use caution with sharps). If bleeding occurs, apply pressure to bleeding spot until bleeding stops completely. Report unusual bruising or bleeding (eg, blood in urine, stool, or vomitus; bleeding gums; vaginal bleeding; nosebleeds); dizziness or changes in vision; back pain; skin rash; swelling of face, mouth, or throat; or difficulty breathing. **Pregnancy/breast-feeding precautions:** Inform prescriber if you are or intend to be pregnant. Consult prescriber if breast-feeding.

- **Retin-A™ Topical** *see* Tretinoin (Topical) *on page 1170*
- **Retinoic Acid** *see* Tretinoin (Topical) *on page 1170*
- **Retisol-A®** *see* Tretinoin (Topical) *on page 1170*
- **Retrovir®** *see* Zidovudine *on page 1227*
- **Retrovir-AZT** *see* Zidovudine *on page 1227*
- **Revapol** *see* Mebendazole *on page 709*
- **Reversol® Injection** *see* Edrophonium *on page 413*
- **Revex®** *see* Nalmefene *on page 803*
- **Rēv-Eyes™** *see page 1248*
- **ReVia®** *see* Naltrexone *on page 805*
- **Revitalose-C-1000®** *see* Ascorbic Acid *on page 108*
- **Rezine®** *see* Hydroxyzine *on page 588*
- **Rezulin®** *see* Troglitazone *on page 1187*
- **R-Gel®** *see page 1294*
- **RGM-CSF** *see* Sargramostim *on page 1045*
- **Rheaban®** *see page 1294*
- **Rheomacrodex®** *see* Dextran *on page 351*
- **Rheumatrex®** *see* Methotrexate *on page 743*
- **Rhinalar®** *see* Flunisolide *on page 497*
- **Rhinall® Nasal Solution [OTC]** *see* Phenylephrine *on page 920*
- **Rhinaris®-F** *see* Flunisolide *on page 497*
- **Rhinatate® Tablet** *see page 1306*
- **Rhindecon®** *see* Phenylpropanolamine *on page 922*
- **Rhinocort®** *see* Budesonide *on page 164*
- **Rhinosyn-DMX® [OTC]** *see* Guaifenesin and Dextromethorphan *on page 549*
- **Rhinosyn® Liquid** *see page 1294*
- **Rhinosyn-PD® Liquid** *see page 1294*
- **$Rh_o$(D) Immune Globulin** *see page 1256*
- **$Rh_o$(D) Immune Globulin (Intravenous-Human)** *see page 1256*
- **Rhodis™** *see* Ketoprofen *on page 645*
- **Rhodis-EC™** *see* Ketoprofen *on page 645*
- **RhoGAM™** *see page 1256*
- **Rhoprolene** *see* Betamethasone *on page 148*
- **Rhoprolene** *see* Topical Corticosteroids *on page 1152*
- **Rhoprosone** *see* Betamethasone *on page 148*
- **Rhoprosone** *see* Topical Corticosteroids *on page 1152*
- **Rhotral** *see* Acebutolol *on page 31*
- **Rhotrimine®** *see* Trimipramine *on page 1183*
- ***r*HuEPO-α** *see* Epoetin Alfa *on page 426*
- **Rhulicaine® [OTC]** *see* Benzocaine *on page 141*
- **Rhythmin®** *see* Procainamide *on page 967*
- **Ribavarin and Interferon Alfa-2b Combination Pack** *see* Interferon Alfa-2b and Ribavirin Combination Pack *on page 615*

## Ribavirin (rye ba VYE rin)

**U.S. Brand Names** Rebetrol®; Virazole® Aerosol

**Synonyms** RTCA; Tribavirin

**Therapeutic Category** Antiviral Agent

**Pregnancy Risk Factor** X

**Lactation** Excretion in breast milk unknown

**Use** Inhalation: Treatment of patients with respiratory syncytial virus (RSV) infections; may be used in other viral infections including influenza A and B and adenovirus; specially indicated for treatment of severe lower respiratory tract RSV infections in patients with an underlying compromising condition (prematurity, bronchopulmonary dysplasia and other chronic lung conditions, congenital heart disease, immunodeficiency, immunosuppression), and recent transplant recipients.

Oral capsule: Combination therapy with interferon alpha-2b, recombinant (Intron A®) injection is indicated for the treatment of chronic hepatitis c in patients with compensated liver disease who have relapsed after alpha interferon therapy.

**Mechanism of Action/Effect** Inhibits replication of RNA and DNA viruses; inhibits influenza virus RNA polymerase activity and inhibits the initiation and elongation of RNA fragments resulting in inhibition of viral protein synthesis

**Contraindications** Pregnancy; hypersensitivity to ribavirin; patients with autoimmune hepatitis

**Warnings** Use with caution in patients requiring assisted ventilation because precipitation of the drug in the respiratory equipment may interfere with safe and effective patient ventilation; monitor carefully in patients with COPD and asthma for deterioration of respiratory function. Ribavirin is potentially mutagenic, tumor-promoting, and gonadotoxic. **Healthcare professionals or family members who are pregnant or may become pregnant should be counseled about potential risks of exposure and counseled about risk reduction strategies.** Ribavirin may adhere to contact lenses. Anemia has been observed with the interferon/ribavirin combination; severe psychiatric events, including depression and suicidal behavior, during combination therapy. The combination should be avoided in patients with a psychiatric history.

**Drug Interactions**

**Decreased Effect:** Decreased effect of zidovudine.

**Adverse Reactions**

**Inhalation:**

1% to 10%:

Central nervous system: Fatigue, headache, insomnia
Gastrointestinal: Nausea, anorexia
Hematologic: Anemia

<1% (Limited to important or life-threatening symptoms): Hypotension, cardiac arrest, digitalis toxicity, mild bronchospasm, worsening of respiratory function, apnea

Oral (All adverse reactions documented while receiving combination therapy with interferon alpha-2b)

>10%

Central nervous system: Dizziness, headache, fatigue, insomnia, irritability, depression, emotional lability, impaired concentration, fever
Gastrointestinal: Nausea, anorexia, dyspepsia, vomiting
Musculoskeletal: Myalgia, arthralgia, asthenia
Respiratory: Dyspnea, sinusitis
Dermatologic: Alopecia, rash, pruritus
Cardiovascular: Chest pain
Hematologic: decreased hemoglobin, decreased WBC
Miscellaneous: Flu-like syndrome

1% to 10%:

Central nervous system: Nervousness
Gastrointestinal: Taste perversion
Endocrine and metabolic: Thyroid function test abnormalities

**Pharmacodynamics/Kinetics**

**Half-life Elimination:** 24 hours, much longer in the erythrocyte (16-40 days), which can be used as a marker for intracellular metabolism

**Time to Peak:** Inhalation: Within 60-90 minutes

**Metabolism:** Occurs intracellularly and may be necessary for drug action

**Excretion:** Hepatic metabolism is major route of elimination with 40% of the drug cleared renally as unchanged drug and metabolites.

**Formulations** See also Interferon Alfa-2b and Rebetron™ Combination Pack monograph.

Powder for aerosol: 6 g (100 mL)
Capsule: 200 mg (available only in Rebetron Combination Pack)

**Dosing**

**Adults:**

Aerosol inhalation: Use with Viratek® small particle aerosol generator (SPAG-2) at a concentration of 20 mg/mL (6 g reconstituted with 300 mL of sterile water without preservatives)

Aerosol only: 12-18 hours/day for 3 days, up to 7 days in length

**Elderly:** Refer to adult dosing.

**Stability**

**Reconstitution:** Do not use any water containing an antimicrobial agent to reconstitute drug. Reconstituted solution is stable for 24 hours at room temperature.

**Monitoring Laboratory Tests** CBC, reticulocyte count

**Additional Nursing Issues**

**Physical Assessment:** Monitor laboratory tests, respiratory status, and vital signs on a regular basis. Monitor (teach patient to monitor and report) adverse effects (eg, signs of opportunistic infection and anemia). Instruct patient on appropriate use of aerosol device. Dry precipitate can cause problems in ventilators and endotracheal tubes. Be alert to potential problems resulting in increased positive expiratory pressure and increased positive inspiratory pressure. **Pregnancy risk factor X** - Determine that patient is not pregnant before beginning treatment and do not give to women of childbearing age or males who may have intercourse with childbearing women unless both male and female are capable of complying with barrier contraceptive measures during therapy and 1 month following therapy. Note breast-feeding caution.

**Patient Information/Instruction:** Take as directed, for full course of therapy; do not discontinue even if feeling better. Use aerosol device as instructed. Maintain adequate fluid intake and report any swelling of ankles or feet, difficulty breathing, persistent lethargy, acute headache, insomnia, severe nausea or anorexia, confusion, fever, chills, sore throat, easy bruising or bleeding, mouth sores, or worsening of respiratory condition. **Pregnancy/breast-feeding precautions:** Inform prescriber if you are pregnant. Do not get pregnant during or for 1 month following therapy. Male: Do not cause a pregnancy. Male/female: Consult prescriber for instruction on appropriate barrier contraceptive measures. This drug may cause severe fetal defects. Consult prescriber if breast-feeding.

## Riboflavin (RYE boe flay vin)

**U.S. Brand Names** Riobin®

**Synonyms** Lactoflavin; Vitamin $B_2$; Vitamin G

**Therapeutic Category** Vitamin, Water Soluble

**Pregnancy Risk Factor** A/C (if dose exceeds RDA recommendation)

**Lactation** Enters breast milk/compatible

**Use** Prevent riboflavin deficiency and treat ariboflavinosis

**Mechanism of Action/Effect** Component of flavoprotein enzymes that work together, which are necessary for normal tissue respiration; also needed for activation of pyridoxine and conversion of tryptophan to niacin

**Warnings** Riboflavin deficiency often occurs in the presence of other B vitamin deficiencies. Pregnancy factor C (if dose exceeds RDA recommendation).

**Drug Interactions**

**Decreased Effect:** Decreased absorption with probenecid.

**Effects on Lab Values** Large doses may interfere with urinalysis based on spectrometry. May cause false elevations in fluorometric determinations of catecholamines and urobilinogen.

**Adverse Reactions** 1% to 10%: Genitourinary: Discoloration of urine (yellow-orange)

**Pharmacodynamics/Kinetics**

**Half-life Elimination:** Biologic: 66-84 minutes

**Metabolism:** Metabolic fate unknown

**Excretion:** Urine

**Formulations** Tablet: 25 mg, 50 mg, 100 mg

**Dosing**

**Adults:** Oral:

Riboflavin deficiency: 5-30 mg/day in divided doses

Recommended daily allowance: 1.2-1.7 mg

**Elderly:** Refer to adult dosing.

**Additional Nursing Issues**

**Physical Assessment:** Assess knowledge/teach patient appropriate use, dietary instruction, possible side effects, and adverse symptoms to report. **Pregnancy risk factor A/C** - see Pregnancy Risk Factor for cautious use.

**Patient Information/Instruction:** Take with food. Large doses may cause bright yellow or orange urine.

**Additional Information** Dietary sources of riboflavin include liver, kidney, dairy products, green vegetables, eggs, whole grain cereals, yeast, and mushroom.


- **Rid-A-Pain® [OTC]** *see* Benzocaine *on page 141*
- **Ridaura®** *see* Auranofin *on page 121*
- **Ridene** *see* Nicardipine *on page 820*
- **RID® Shampoo** *see page 1294*


## Rifabutin (rif a BYOO tin)

**U.S. Brand Names** Mycobutin®

**Synonyms** Ansamycin

**Therapeutic Category** Antibiotic, Miscellaneous; Antitubercular Agent

**Pregnancy Risk Factor** B

**Lactation** Excretion in breast milk unknown

**Use** Adjunctive therapy for the prevention of disseminated *Mycobacterium avium-intracellulare* complex (MAC) in patients with advanced HIV infection; studies have shown it to halve the risk of MAC bacteremia in patients with AIDS, to decrease the incidence of fever and fatigue, and prevent deterioration in performance status

**Mechanism of Action/Effect** Inhibits DNA-dependent RNA polymerase at the beta subunit which prevents chain initiation

**Contraindications** Hypersensitivity to rifabutin or any other rifamycins; rifabutin is contraindicated in patients with a WBC <1000/mm$^3$ or a platelet count <50,000 mm$^3$

**Warnings** Rifabutin as a single agent must not be administered to patients with active tuberculosis since its use may lead to the development of tuberculosis that is resistant to both rifabutin and rifampin. Rifabutin should be discontinued in patients with AST >500 units/L or if total bilirubin is >3 mg/dL. Use with caution in patients with liver impairment. Modification of dosage should be considered in patients with renal impairment.

**Drug Interactions**

**Cytochrome P-450 Effect:** CYP3A3/4 enzyme inducer

**Decreased Effect:** Decreased plasma concentration (due to induction of liver enzymes) of verapamil, methadone, digoxin, cyclosporine, corticosteroids, oral anticoagulants, theophylline, barbiturates, chloramphenicol, ketoconazole, oral contraceptives, quinidine, non-nucleoside reverse transcriptase inhibitors, halothane, and perhaps clarithromycin.

**Increased Effect/Toxicity:** Concentrations are increased by indinavir (reduce rifabutin to 50% of standard dose).

**Adverse Reactions**

>10%:

Dermatologic: Rash

Gastrointestinal: Vomiting, nausea, discolored feces, saliva (reddish orange)

Genitourinary: Discolored urine (reddish orange)

Miscellaneous: Discolored sputum, sweat, tears (reddish orange)

1% to 10%:

Central nervous system: Headache

Gastrointestinal: Abdominal pain, diarrhea, anorexia, flatulence, eructation
Hematologic: Anemia, thrombocytopenia

<1% (Limited to important or life-threatening symptoms): Chest pain, neutropenia, leukopenia, uveitis

**Overdose/Toxicology** Symptoms of overdose include nausea, vomiting, hepatotoxicity, lethargy, CNS disturbances, and depression. Treatment is supportive. Hemodialysis will remove rifabutin; however, its effect on outcome is unknown.

**Pharmacodynamics/Kinetics**

**Protein Binding:** 85%

**Distribution:** Distributes to body tissues including the lungs, liver, spleen, eyes, and kidneys

**Half-life Elimination:** 45 hours (range: 16-69 hours)

**Time to Peak:** Within 2-4 hours

**Metabolism:** To active and inactive metabolites

**Excretion:** Renal and biliary clearance of unchanged drugs is 10%; 30% excreted in feces; 53% in urine as metabolites

**Formulations** Capsule: 150 mg

**Dosing**

**Adults:** Oral: 300 mg once daily. For patients who experience GI upset, rifabutin can be administered 150 mg twice daily with food.

**Elderly:** Refer to adult dosing.

**Administration**

**Oral:** Rifabutin is best taken on an empty stomach but may be taken with meals to minimize nausea or vomiting.

**Monitoring Laboratory Tests** Periodic liver function, CBC with differential, platelet count

**Additional Nursing Issues**

**Physical Assessment:** Monitor laboratory tests. Assess other medications patient may be taking (see P-450 interactions above). Monitor for CNS changes (eg, confusion, ataxia). Inform patient that effect of oral contraceptives may by lessened; alternative contraceptive measures are recommended if a sexually active female wishes to avoid pregnancy. Note breast-feeding caution.

**Patient Information/Instruction:** May take with food if GI upset occurs. Will discolor urine, stool, saliva, tears, sweat, and other body fluid a red-brown color. Stains on clothing or contact lenses are permanent. Report skin rash, vomiting, fever, chills, flu-like symptoms, dark urine or pale stools, unusual bleeding or bruising, or unusual confusion, depression, or fatigue. **Breast-feeding precautions:** Consult prescriber if breast-feeding.

- ♦ **Rifadin®** *see* Rifampin *on this page*
- ♦ **Rifadin® Injection** *see* Rifampin *on this page*
- ♦ **Rifadin® Oral** *see* Rifampin *on this page*
- ♦ **Rifamate®** *see* Rifampin and Isoniazid *on page 1021*
- ♦ **Rifampicin** *see* Rifampin *on this page*

## Rifampin (RIF am pin)

**U.S. Brand Names** Rifadin® Injection; Rifadin® Oral; Rimactane® Oral

**Synonyms** Rifampicin

**Therapeutic Category** Antibiotic, Miscellaneous; Antitubercular Agent

**Pregnancy Risk Factor** C

**Lactation** Enters breast milk/compatible

**Use** Management of active tuberculosis; eliminate meningococci from asymptomatic carriers; prophylaxis of *Haemophilus influenzae* type b infection; in combination with other anti-infectives in the treatment of staphylococcal infections

**Mechanism of Action/Effect** Inhibits bacterial RNA synthesis by binding to the beta subunit of DNA-dependent RNA polymerase, blocking RNA transcription

**Contraindications** Hypersensitivity to rifampin or any component

**Warnings** Use with caution in patients with liver impairment. Modification of dosage should be considered in patients with severe liver impairment. Use with caution in patients with porphyria. Monitor closely if intermittent therapy is used. Hypersensitivity reactions and thrombocytopenia occur more frequently in this setting. Use rifampin with caution in patients receiving halothane or isoniazid due to increased risk of hepatotoxicity. Pregnancy factor C.

**Drug Interactions**

**Cytochrome P-450 Effect:** CYP3A3/4 enzyme substrate; CYP1A2, 2C9, 2C18, 2C19, 2D6, 3A3/4, and 3A5-7 enzyme inducer

**Decreased Effect:** Rifampin induces liver enzymes which may decrease the plasma concentration of calcium channel blockers (verapamil, diltiazem, nifedipine), methadone, digoxin, cyclosporine, corticosteroids, haloperidol, oral anticoagulants, theophylline, barbiturates, chloramphenicol, imidazole antifungals (ketoconazole), oral contraceptives, acetaminophen, benzodiazepines, hydantoins, sulfa drugs, enalapril, beta-blockers, clofibrate, dapsone, antiarrhythmics (disopyramide, mexilitine, quinidine, tocainide), doxycycline, fluoroquinolones, levothyroxine, nortriptyline, tacrolimus, zidovudine, protease inhibitors, and non-nucleoside reverse transcriptase inhibitors.

**Increased Effect/Toxicity:** Increased serum levels of rifampin when given with co-trimoxazole or probenecid. Rifampin given with halothane or isoniazid increases the potential for hepatotoxicity.

**Food Interactions** Rifampin concentrations may be decreased if taken with food.

(Continued)

## Rifampin *(Continued)*

**Effects on Lab Values** Positive Coombs' reaction [direct], inhibit standard assay's ability to measure serum folate and $B_{12}$

**Adverse Reactions**

>10%:

Gastrointestinal: Diarrhea, stomach cramps, fecal discoloration, discoloration of saliva (reddish orange)

Genitourinary: Discoloration of urine

Miscellaneous: Discoloration of sputum, sweat, and tears (reddish orange)

1% to 10%: Miscellaneous: Fungal overgrowth

<1% (Limited to important or life-threatening symptoms): Eosinophilia, blood dyscrasias (leukopenia, thrombocytopenia), hepatitis, renal failure (interstitial nephritis)

**Overdose/Toxicology** Symptoms of overdose include nausea, vomiting, hepatotoxicity, lethargy, and CNS depression. Treatment is supportive.

**Pharmacodynamics/Kinetics**

**Protein Binding:** 80%

**Distribution:**

Crosses the blood-brain barrier well

Relative diffusion of antimicrobial agents from blood into cerebrospinal fluid (CSF): Adequate with or without inflammation (exceeds usual MICs)

Ratio of CSF to blood level (%): Inflamed meninges: 25

**Half-life Elimination:** 3-4 hours, prolonged with hepatic impairment; End-stage renal disease: 1.8-11 hours

**Time to Peak:** Oral: 2-4 hours and persisting for up to 24 hours; food may delay or slightly reduce

**Metabolism:** Liver

**Excretion:** Feces and urine

**Formulations**

Capsule: 150 mg, 300 mg

Powder for injection: 600 mg (contains a sulfite)

**Dosing**

**Adults:** I.V. infusion dose is the same as for the oral route

Tuberculosis therapy: Oral: **Note:** A four-drug regimen (isoniazid, rifampin, pyrazinamide, and either streptomycin or ethambutol) is preferred for the initial, empiric treatment of TB. When the drug susceptibility results are available, the regimen should be altered as appropriate.

**Patients with TB and without HIV infection:**

**OPTION 1:**

Isoniazid resistance rate <4%: Administer daily isoniazid, rifampin, and pyrazinamide for 8 weeks followed by isoniazid and rifampin daily or directly observed therapy (DOT) 2-3 times/week for 16 weeks.

If isoniazid resistance rate is not documented, ethambutol or streptomycin should also be administered until susceptibility to isoniazid or rifampin is demonstrated. Continue treatment for at least 6 months or 3 months beyond culture conversion.

**OPTION 2:** Administer daily isoniazid, rifampin, pyrazinamide, and either streptomycin or ethambutol for 2 weeks followed by DOT 2 times/week administration of the same drugs for 6 weeks, and subsequently, with isoniazid and rifampin DOT 2 times/week administration for 16 weeks.

**OPTION 3:** Administer isoniazid, rifampin, pyrazinamide, and either ethambutol or streptomycin by DOT 3 times/week for 6 months.

**Patients with TB and with HIV infection:**

Administer any of the above OPTIONS 1, 2 or 3, however, treatment should be continued for a total of 9 months and at least 6 months beyond culture conversion.

**Note:** Some experts recommend that the duration of therapy should be extended to 9 months for patients with disseminated disease, miliary disease, disease involving the bones or joints, or tuberculosis lymphadenitis.

Oral:

Daily therapy: 10 mg/kg/day (maximum: 600 mg/day)

Directly observed therapy (DOT): Twice weekly: 10 mg/kg (maximum: 600 mg)

DOT: 3 times/week: 10 mg/kg (maximum: 600 mg)

*H. influenzae* prophylaxis: Oral: 600 mg every 24 hours for 4 days

Meningococcal prophylaxis: Oral: 600 mg every 12 hours for 2 days

Nasal carriers of *Staphylococcus aureus*: Oral: 600 mg/day for 5-10 days in combination with other antibiotics

Synergy for *Staphylococcus aureus* infections: Oral: Adults: 300-600 mg twice daily with other antibiotics

**Elderly:** Refer to adult dosing.

**Hepatic Impairment:** Dose reductions are necessary to reduce hepatotoxicity.

**Administration**

**Oral:** Should be administered 1 hour before or 2 hours after a meal on an empty stomach with a glass of water. Food may delay and reduce the amount of rifampin absorbed.

**I.M.:** Do not administer I.M. or S.C.

**I.V.:** Preferable administered at 500 mL over 3 hours. In selected situations, can be administered at 100 mL over 30 minutes.

**I.V. Detail:** Avoid extravasation.

**Stability**

**Storage:** Rifampin powder is reddish brown. Intact vials should be stored at room temperature and protected from excessive heat and light.

**Reconstitution:** Reconstituted vials are stable for 24 hours at room temperature. Stability of parenteral admixture at room temperature (25°C) is 4 hours in $D_5W$, 24 hours in NS.

**Monitoring Laboratory Tests** Periodic monitoring of liver function (AST, ALT), CBC; sputum culture, chest x-ray 2-3 months into treatment

**Additional Nursing Issues**

**Physical Assessment:** Assess effectiveness and interactions of other medications (see Drug Interactions - P-450 inducer). See Warnings/Precautions and Contraindications for use cautions. Monitor effectiveness of therapy, frequent laboratory tests (see above), and adverse response (see Adverse Reactions). Assess knowledge/teach patient appropriate use, possible side effects and interventions, and adverse symptoms to report. **Pregnancy risk factor C** - benefits of use should outweigh possible risks. **Note:** Rifampin may reduce effectiveness of oral contraceptives, therefore, alternative contraceptive methods should be used by women desiring to prevent pregnancy while taking rifampin.

**Patient Information/Instruction:** Take per recommended schedule. Complete full course of therapy; do not skip doses. Take on an empty stomach (1 hour before or 2 hours after meals). Maintain adequate hydration (2-3 L/day of fluids unless instructed to restrict fluid intake). Will discolor urine, stool, saliva, tears, sweat, and other body fluids red-brown. Stains on clothing or contact lenses are permanent. Report persistent vomiting; fever, chill, or flu-like symptoms; unusual bruising or bleeding; or other persistent adverse effects. **Pregnancy precautions:** Inform prescriber if you are or intend to be pregnant or if you are using oral contraceptives (rifampin may effect the effectiveness of certain oral contraceptives).

**Geriatric Considerations:** Rifampin, in combination with isoniazid, is the foundation of tuberculosis treatment. Since most older patients acquired their *Mycobacterium tuberculosis* infection before effective chemotherapy was available, either a 9-month regimen of isoniazid and rifampin or a 6-month regimen of isoniazid and rifampin with pyrazinamide (the first 2 months) should be effective.

**Related Information**

TB Drug Comparison *on page 1402*

## Rifampin and Isoniazid (RIF am pin & eye soe NYE a zid)

**U.S. Brand Names** Rifamate®

**Synonyms** Isoniazid and Rifampin

**Therapeutic Category** Antibiotic, Miscellaneous

**Pregnancy Risk Factor** C

**Lactation** Enters breast milk/compatible

**Use** Management of active tuberculosis; see individual monographs for additional information

**Formulations** Capsule: Rifampin 300 mg and isoniazid 150 mg

**Dosing**

**Adults:** Oral: 2 capsules/day

**Elderly:** Refer to dosing in individual monographs.

**Additional Nursing Issues**

**Physical Assessment:** See individual components listed in Related Information. **Pregnancy risk factor C** - benefits of use should outweigh possible risks.

**Patient Information/Instruction:** See individual components listed in Related Information. **Pregnancy precautions:** Inform prescriber if you are on intend to get pregnant.

**Related Information**

Isoniazid *on page 630*
Rifampin *on page 1019*

## Rifampin, Isoniazid, and Pyrazinamide

(RIF am pin, eye soe NYE a zid, & peer a ZIN a mide)

**U.S. Brand Names** Rifater®

**Synonyms** Isoniazid, Rifampin, and Pyrazinamide; Pyrazinamide, Rifampin, and Isoniazid

**Therapeutic Category** Antibiotic, Miscellaneous

**Pregnancy Risk Factor** C

**Lactation** Excretion in breast milk unknown

**Use** Management of active tuberculosis

**Formulations** Tablet: Rifampin 120 mg, isoniazid 50 mg, and pyrazinamide 300 mg

**Dosing**

**Adults:** Oral: Patients weighing:

≤44 kg: 4 tablets
45-54 kg: 5 tablets
≥55 kg: 6 tablets
Doses should be administered in a single daily dose

**Elderly:** Refer to dosing in individual monographs.

**Additional Nursing Issues**

**Physical Assessment:** See individual components listed in Related Information. **Pregnancy risk factor C** - benefits of use should outweigh possible risks. Note breast-feeding caution.

(Continued)

## Rifampin, Isoniazid, and Pyrazinamide *(Continued)*

**Patient Information/Instruction:** See individual components listed in Related Information. **Pregnancy/breast-feeding precautions:** Inform prescriber if you are on intend to get pregnant. Consult prescriber if breast-feeding.

**Related Information**

Isoniazid *on page 630*
Pyrazinamide *on page 994*
Rifampin *on page 1019*

## Rifapentine (RIF a pen teen)

**U.S. Brand Names** Priftin®

**Therapeutic Category** Antitubercular Agent

**Pregnancy Risk Factor** C

**Lactation** Excretion in breast milk unknown/contraindicated

**Use** Treatment of pulmonary tuberculosis (indication is based on the 6-month follow-up treatment outcome observed in controlled clinical trial). Rifapentine must always be used in conjunction with at least one other antituberculosis drug to which the isolate is susceptible; it may also be necessary to add a third agent (either streptomycin or ethambutol) until susceptibility is known.

**Mechanism of Action/Effect** Inhibits DNA-dependent RNA polymerase in susceptible strains of *Mycobacterium tuberculosis* (but not in mammalian cells). Rifapentine is bactericidal against both intracellular and extracellular MTB organisms. Strains which are resistant to other rifamycins including rifampin are likely to be resistant to rifapentine. Cross-resistance does not appear between rifapentine and other nonrifamycin antimycobacterial agents.

**Contraindications** Hypersensitivity to rifapentine, rifampin, rifabutin, and any rifamycin analog

**Warnings** Compliance with dosing regimen is absolutely necessary for successful drug therapy. Patients with abnormal liver tests and/or liver disease should only be given rifapentine when absolutely necessary and under strict medical supervision. Monitoring of liver function tests should be carried out prior to therapy and then every 2-4 weeks during therapy if signs of liver disease occur or worsen, rifapentine should be discontinued. Pseudomembranous colitis has been reported to occur with various antibiotics including other rifamycins. If this is suspected, rifapentine should be stopped and the patient treated with specific and supportive treatment. Experience in treating TB in HIV-infected patients is limited.

Rifapentine may produce a red-orange discoloration of body tissues/fluids including skin, teeth, tongue, urine, feces, saliva, sputum, tears, sweat, and cerebral spinal fluid. Contact lenses may become permanently stained.

Pregnancy factor C.

**Drug Interactions**

**Cytochrome P-450 Effect:** CYP3A4 and 2C8/9 enzyme inducer

**Decreased Effect:** Rifapentine may increase the metabolism of coadministered drugs that are metabolized by these enzymes. Enzymes are induced within 4 days after the first dose and returned to baseline 14 days after discontinuation of rifapentine. The magnitude of enzyme induction is dose and frequency dependent.

Rifampin has been shown to accelerate the metabolism and may reduce activity of the following drugs (therefore, rifapentine may also do the same): Phenytoin, disopyramide, mexiletine, quinidine, tocainide, chloramphenicol, clarithromycin, dapsone, doxycycline, fluoroquinolones, warfarin, fluconazole, itraconazole, ketoconazole, barbiturates, benzodiazepines, beta-blockers, diltiazem, nifedipine, verapamil, corticosteroids, cardiac glycoside preparations, clofibrate, oral or other systemic hormonal contraceptives, haloperidol, HIV protease inhibitors, sulfonylureas, cyclosporine, tacrolimus, levothyroxine, methadone, progestins, quinine, delavirdine, zidovudine, sildenafil, theophylline, amitriptyline, and nortriptyline.

Rifapentine should be used with extreme caution, if at all, in patients who are also taking protease inhibitors

Patients using oral or other systemic hormonal contraceptives should be advised to change to nonhormonal methods of birth control when receiving concomitant rifapentine.

**Increased Effect/Toxicity:** Rifapentine metabolism is mediated by esterase activity, therefore, there is minimal potential for rifapentine metabolism to be affected by other drug therapy.

**Adverse Reactions**

>10%: Endocrine & metabolic: Hyperuricemia (most likely due to pyrazinamide from initiation phase combination therapy)

1% to 10%:

Cardiovascular: Hypertension
Central nervous system: Headache, dizziness
Dermatologic: Rash, pruritus, acne
Gastrointestinal: Anorexia, nausea, vomiting, dyspepsia, diarrhea
Genitourinary: Pyuria, proteinuria, hematuria, urinary casts
Hematologic: Neutropenia, lymphopenia, anemia, leukopenia, thrombocytosis
Hepatic: Increased ALT, AST
Neuromuscular & skeletal: Arthralgia, pain
Respiratory: Hemoptysis

<1% (Limited to important or life-threatening symptoms): Aggressive reaction, hyperkalemia, pancreatitis, thrombocytopenia, purpura, hepatitis, gout, arthrosis

**Overdose/Toxicology** There is no experience with treatment of acute overdose with rifapentine; experience with other rifamycins suggests that gastric lavage followed by activated charcoal may help adsorb any remaining drug from the GI tract. Hemodialysis or forced diuresis is not expected to enhance elimination of unchanged rifapentine in an overdose.

**Pharmacodynamics/Kinetics**

**Protein Binding:** Rifapentine and 25-desacetyl metabolite were 97.7% and 93.2% protein bound (mainly to albumin). Rifapentine and metabolite accumulate in human monocyte-derived macrophages with intracellular/extracellular ratios of 24:1 and 7:1 respectively.

**Half-life Elimination:** Rifapentine: 14-17 hours; 25-desacetyl rifapentine: 13 hours

**Time to Peak:** 5-6 hours

**Metabolism:** Hydrolyzed by an esterase and esterase enzyme to form the active metabolite 25-desacetyl rifapentine

**Excretion:** Extent of renal excretion is unknown; excreted as parent drug and metabolite; 17% of administered dose is excreted via the kidneys

**Formulations** Tablet, film-coated: 150 mg

**Dosing**

**Adults: Rifapentine should not be used alone**; initial phase should include a 3- to 4-drug regimen.

Intensive phase of short-term therapy: 600 mg (four 150 mg tablets) given twice weekly (at intervals not less than 72 hours); following the intensive phase, treatment should continue with rifapentine 600 mg once weekly for 4 months in combination with INH or appropriate agent for susceptible organisms.

**Elderly:** Refer to adult dosing.

**Hepatic Impairment:** Unknown

**Stability**

**Storage:** Store at room temperature (15°C to 30°C; 59°F to 86°F). Protect from excessive heat and humidity.

**Monitoring Laboratory Tests** Perform baseline liver function tests at beginning of therapy. Patients with pre-existing hepatic problems should have liver function tests monitored every 2-4 weeks during therapy. Perform CBC monthly.

**Additional Nursing Issues**

**Physical Assessment:** Monitor laboratory tests and liver status frequently (see Adverse Reactions). Monitor blood pressure. Assess for allergic history related to other antitubercular medications. Assess other medications the patient may be taking. (Rifapentine is a P-450 enzyme inducer which may accelerate the metabolism and reduce the activity of drugs that that are metabolized by P-450 enzymes - see Drug Interactions). Monitor for adverse effects and effectiveness of therapy. Assess knowledge/teach patient appropriate use of rifapentine. **Pregnancy risk factor C** - benefits of use should outweigh risks. Instruct patient on use of nonhormonal contraception. Breast-feeding is contraindicated.

**Patient Information/Instruction:** Best to take on empty stomach (1 hour before or 2 hours after meals); however, may be taken with food if GI upset occurs. Follow recommended dosing schedule exactly; do not increase dose or skip doses. You will need to be monitored on a regular basis while taking this medication. This medication will stain urine, stool, saliva, tears, sweat, and other body fluids a red-brown color. Stains on clothing or contact lenses are permanent. Report vomiting; fever, chills or flu-like symptoms; muscle weakness or unusual fatigue; dark urine, pale stools, or unusual bleeding or bruising; yellowing skin or eyes; skin rash; swelling of extremities; chest pain or palpitations; or persistent gastrointestinal upset. **Pregnancy/breast-feeding precautions:** Inform prescriber if you are or intend to be pregnant - nonhormonal contraceptive use may be recommended. Do not breast-feed.

**Dietary Issues:** Food increases AUC and maximum serum concentration by 43% and 44% respectively as compared to fasting conditions.

**Pregnancy Issues:** Has been shown to be teratogenic in rats and rabbits. Rat offspring showed cleft palates, right aortic arch, and delayed ossification and increased number of ribs. Rabbits displayed ovarian agenesis, pes varus, arhinia, microphthalmia, and irregularities of the ossified facial tissues. Rat studies also show decreased fetal weight, increased number of stillborns, and decreased gestational survival. No adequate well-controlled studies in pregnant women are available. Rifapentine should be used during pregnancy only if the potential benefit justifies the potential risk to the fetus.

**Additional Information** Rifampin has been shown to inhibit standard microbiological assays for serum folate and vitamin $B_{12}$; this should be considered for rifapentine; therefore, alternative assay methods should be considered.

Rifapentine has only been studied in patients with tuberculosis receiving a 6-month short-course intensive regimen approval. Outcomes have been based on 6-month follow-up treatment observed in clinical trial 008 as a surrogate for the 2-year follow-up generally accepted as evidence for efficacy in the treatment of pulmonary tuberculosis.

◆ **Rifater®** *see* Rifampin, Isoniazid, and Pyrazinamide *on page 1021*

◆ **Rilutek®** *see* Riluzole *on this page*

## Riluzole (RIL yoo zole)

**U.S. Brand Names** Rilutek®

**Synonyms** 2-Amino-6-Trifluoromethoxy-Benzothiazole; RP54274

(Continued)

## Riluzole *(Continued)*

**Therapeutic Category** Glutamate Inhibitor

**Pregnancy Risk Factor** C

**Lactation** Excretion in breast milk unknown

**Use** Treatment of patients with amyotrophic lateral sclerosis (ALS); riluzole can extend survival or time to tracheostomy

**Mechanism of Action/Effect** Inhibitory effect on glutamate release, inactivation of voltage-dependent sodium channels; and ability to interfere with intracellular events that follow transmitter binding at excitatory amino acid receptors

**Contraindications** Severe hypersensitivity reactions to riluzole or any component

**Warnings** Among 4000 patients given riluzole for ALS, there were 3 cases of marked neutropenia (ANC <500/mm$^3$), all seen within the first 2 months of treatment. Use with caution in patients with concomitant renal insufficiency. Use with caution in patients with current evidence or history of abnormal liver function. Monitor liver chemistries. Pregnancy factor C.

**Drug Interactions**

**Cytochrome P-450 Effect:** CYP1A2 enzyme substrate

**Decreased Effect:** Drugs that induce CYP1A2 (eg, cigarette smoke, charbroiled food, rifampin, omeprazole) could increase the rate of riluzole elimination.

**Increased Effect/Toxicity:** Inhibitors of CYP1A2 (eg, caffeine, theophylline, amitriptyline, quinolones) could decrease the rate of riluzole elimination resulting in accumulation of riluzole.

**Adverse Reactions**

>10%:

Gastrointestinal: Nausea, vomiting, diarrhea, abdominal pain or gas, anorexia
Miscellaneous: Aggravation reaction

1% to 10%:

Cardiovascular: Peripheral edema
Central nervous system: Insomnia, headache, malaise
Dermatologic: Alopecia, eczema, pruritus
Gastrointestinal: Constipation, stomatitis
Neuromuscular & skeletal: Back pain, myalgia
Respiratory: Dyspnea, increased cough, pneumonia, rhinitis

<1% (Limited to important or life-threatening symptoms): Hypertension, tachycardia, seizures, exfoliative dermatitis, neutropenia

**Overdose/Toxicology** No specific antidote or treatment information is available. Treatment should be supportive and directed toward alleviating symptoms.

**Pharmacodynamics/Kinetics**

**Protein Binding:** 96% bound to plasma proteins, mainly albumin and lipoproteins

**Half-life Elimination:** 12 hours

**Metabolism:** Extensively to 6 major and a number of minor metabolites. Metabolism is mostly hepatic and consists of cytochrome P-450 dependent hydroxylation and glucuronidation; principle isozyme is CYP1A2.

**Formulations** Tablet: 50 mg

**Dosing**

**Adults:** Oral: 50 mg every 12 hours; no increased benefit can be expected from higher daily doses, but adverse events are increased.

**Dosage adjustment in smoking:** Cigarette smoking is known to induce CYP1A2; patients who smoke cigarettes would be expected to eliminate riluzole faster. There is no information, however, on the effect of, or need for, dosage adjustment in these patients.

**Dosage adjustment in special populations:** Females and Japanese patients may possess a lower metabolic capacity to eliminate riluzole compared with male and Caucasian subjects, respectively.

**Elderly:** Refer to adult dosing.

**Renal Impairment:** Use with caution in patients with concomitant renal insufficiency.

**Hepatic Impairment:** Use with caution in patients with current evidence or history of abnormal liver function indicated by significant abnormalities in serum transaminase, bilirubin or GGT levels. Baseline elevations of several LFTs (especially elevated bilirubin) should preclude use of riluzole.

**Stability**

**Storage:** Protect from bright light.

**Monitoring Laboratory Tests** Monitor serum aminotransferases including ALT levels before and during therapy. Evaluate serum ALT levels every month during the first 3 months of therapy, every 3 months during the remainder of the first year and periodically thereafter. Evaluate ALT levels more frequently in patients who develop elevations. Maximum increases in serum ALT usually occurred within 3 months after the start of therapy and were usually transient when <5 x ULN.

In trials, if ALT levels were <5 x ULN, treatment continued and ALT levels usually returned to below 2 x ULN within 2-6 months. Treatment in studies was discontinued, however, if ALT levels exceed 5 x ULN, so that there is no experience with continued treatment of ALS patients once ALT values exceed 5 x ULN.

If a decision is made to continue treatment in patients when the ALT exceeds 5 x ULN, frequent monitoring (at least weekly) of complete liver function is recommended. Discontinue treatment if ALT exceeds 10 x ULN or if clinical jaundice develops.

**Additional Nursing Issues**

**Physical Assessment:** Assess effectiveness and interactions of other medications patient may be taking (see Drug Interactions and Dosing). Monitor laboratory tests (see above), therapeutic response, and adverse reactions at beginning of therapy and periodically throughout therapy (see Warnings/Precautions, Adverse Reactions, and Overdose/Toxicology). Assess knowledge/teach patient appropriate use, interventions to reduce side effects, and adverse symptoms to report. **Pregnancy risk factor C** - benefits of use should outweigh possible risks. Note breast-feeding caution.

**Patient Information/Instruction:** This drug will not cure or stop disease but it may slow progression. Take as directed, at the same time each day, preferably on an empty stomach (1 hour before or 2 hours after meals). Avoid alcohol. You may experience increased spasticity, dizziness or sleepiness; use caution when driving or engaging in tasks requiring alertness until response to drug is known. Small frequent meals, frequent mouth care, chewing gum, or sucking lozenges may reduce nausea, vomiting, or anorexia. Report fever; severe vomiting, diarrhea, or constipation; change in color of urine or stool; yellowing of skin or eyes; acute back pain or muscle pain; or worsening of condition. **Pregnancy/breast-feeding precautions:** Inform prescriber if you are or intend to be pregnant. Consult prescriber if breast-feeding.

**Geriatric Considerations:** In clinical trials, no difference was demonstrated between elderly and younger adults. However, renal changes with age can be expected to result in higher serum concentrations of the parent drug and its metabolites.

**Additional Information** May be obtained through Rhone-Poulenc Rorer Inc (Collegeville, PA) for compassionate use (through treatment IND process) by calling 800-727-6737 for treatment of amyotrophic lateral sclerosis. May be more effective for amyotrophic lateral sclerosis of bulbar onset. In animal models, riluzole was a potent inhibitor of seizures induced by ouabain.

♦ **Rimactane®** *see* Rifampin *on page 1019*

♦ **Rimactane® Oral** *see* Rifampin *on page 1019*

## Rimantadine (ri MAN ta deen)

**U.S. Brand Names** Flumadine®

**Therapeutic Category** Antiviral Agent

**Pregnancy Risk Factor** C

**Lactation** Enters breast milk/contraindicated

**Use** Prophylaxis (adults and children >1 year) and treatment (adults) of influenza A viral infection

**Mechanism of Action/Effect** Exerts its inhibitory effect on three antigenic subtypes of influenza A virus (H1N1, H2N2, H3N2) early in the viral replicative cycle, possibly inhibiting the uncoating process; it has no activity against influenza B virus and is two- to eightfold more active than amantadine

**Contraindications** Hypersensitivity to drugs of the adamantine class, including rimantadine and amantadine

**Warnings** Use with caution in patients with renal and hepatic dysfunction. Avoid use, if possible, in patients with recurrent and eczematoid dermatitis, uncontrolled psychosis, or severe psychoneurosis. An increase in seizure incidence may occur in patients with seizure disorders. Discontinue drug if seizures occur. Consider the development of resistance during rimantadine treatment of the index case as likely if failure of rimantadine prophylaxis among family contact occurs and if index case is a child. Viruses exhibit cross-resistance between amantadine and rimantadine. Pregnancy factor C.

**Drug Interactions**

**Decreased Effect:**

Acetaminophen: Reduction in AUC and peak concentration of rimantadine.

Aspirin: Peak plasma and AUC concentrations of rimantadine are reduced.

**Increased Effect/Toxicity:** Cimetidine: Rimantadine clearance is decreased (~16%) which may result in an increased side effects by rimantadine.

**Food Interactions** Food does not affect rate or extent of absorption.

**Adverse Reactions** 1% to 10%:

Cardiovascular: Orthostatic hypotension, edema

Central nervous system: Dizziness, confusion, headache, insomnia, difficulty in concentrating, anxiety, restlessness, irritability, hallucinations; incidence of CNS side effects may be less than that associated with amantadine

Gastrointestinal: Nausea, vomiting, dry mouth, abdominal pain, anorexia

Genitourinary: Urinary retention

**Overdose/Toxicology** Agitation, hallucinations, ventricular cardiac arrhythmias (torsade de pointes and PVCs), slurred speech, anticholinergic effects (dry mouth, urinary retention and mydriasis), ataxia, tremor, myoclonus, seizures, and death have been reported with amantadine, a related drug. Treatment is symptomatic (do not use physostigmine). Tachyarrhythmias may be treated with beta-blockers such as propranolol. Dialysis is not recommended except possibly in renal failure.

**Pharmacodynamics/Kinetics**

**Half-life Elimination:** 25.4 hours (increased in the elderly)

**Metabolism:** Liver

**Excretion:** <25% of dose excreted in urine as unchanged drug; hemodialysis does not contribute to the clearance of rimantadine; no data exist establishing a correlation between plasma concentration and antiviral effect

**Formulations**

Rimantadine hydrochloride:

Syrup: 50 mg/5 mL (60 mL, 240 mL, 480 mL)

Tablet: 100 mg

(Continued)

## Rimantadine *(Continued)*

**Dosing**

**Adults:** Oral:

Prophylaxis: 100 mg twice daily

Treatment: 100 mg twice daily

**Elderly:** Prophylaxis and treatment: Oral: Decrease to 100 mg/day in elderly patients (see Geriatric Considerations).

**Renal Impairment:** $Cl_{cr}$ ≤10 mL/minute: Administer 50% normal dose.

**Hepatic Impairment:** Administer 50% normal dose with severe hepatic impairment.

**Administration**

**Oral:** Initiation of rimantadine within 48 hours of the onset of influenza A illness halves the duration of illness and significantly reduces the duration of viral shedding and increased peripheral airways resistance. Continue therapy for 5-7 days after symptoms begin.

**Additional Nursing Issues**

**Physical Assessment:** Monitor effectiveness of treatment and adverse reactions especially blood pressure and CNS changes. Utilize/teach postural hypotension precautions. **Pregnancy risk factor C** - benefits of use should outweigh possible risks. Breast-feeding is contraindicated.

**Patient Information/Instruction:** Take as directed, for full course of therapy. Use caution when changing position (rising from sitting or lying) until response is known. Report CNS changes (eg, confusion, insomnia, anxiety, restlessness, irritability, hallucinations), difficulty urinating, or severe nausea or vomiting. **Pregnancy/breast-feeding precautions:** Inform prescriber if you are or intend to be pregnant. Do not breast-feed.

**Geriatric Considerations:** Monitor GI effects in the elderly or patients with renal or hepatic impairment. Dosing must be individualized (100 mg 1-2 times/day). It is recommended that nursing home patients receive 100 mg/day (see Pharmacodynamics/Kinetics).


- ♦ **Rimexolone** *see page 1282*
- ♦ **Rimso®-50** *see* Dimethyl Sulfoxide *on page 379*
- ♦ **Riobin®** *see* Riboflavin *on page 1018*
- ♦ **Riopan® [OTC]** *see* Magaldrate *on page 702*
- ♦ **Riopan Plus® [OTC]** *see* Magaldrate and Simethicone *on page 703*
- ♦ **Riopan® Plus Extra Strength** *see* Magaldrate and Simethicone *on page 703*
- ♦ **Riphenidate** *see* Methylphenidate *on page 752*


## Risedronate (ris ED roe nate)

**U.S. Brand Names** Actonel®

**Therapeutic Category** Bisphosphonate Derivative

**Pregnancy Risk Factor** C

**Lactation** Enters breast milk/use caution

**Use** Treatment of Paget's disease of bone in patients who meet at least one of the following criteria: 1) serum alkaline phosphatase ≥2 times the upper limit of normal; 2) symptomatic; 3) to induce remission in those who are at risk for future complications

**Unlabeled use:** Prevention of bone loss in postmenopausal women (5 mg/day cyclically for 2 years then 1 year off therapy)

**Contraindications** Hypersensitivity to bisphosphonates or any component; hypocalcemia

**Warnings** Potential for accumulation in renal insufficiency; use with caution in patients with hyperphosphatemia (may increase renal tubular absorption of phosphate). Use with caution in pregnant patients. Use caution in hypocalcemic patients. Not recommended for patients with severe renal impairment ($Cl_{cr}$ <30 mL/minute). Hypocalcemia must be corrected before therapy initiation. Other disturbances of mineral metabolism (eg, vitamin D deficiency) should also be effectively treated. Ensure adequate calcium and vitamin D intake to provide for enhanced needs of serum calcium and phosphate. Pregnancy factor C.

**Drug Interactions**

**Decreased Effect:** Calcium supplements/salts decrease absorption of risedronate.

**Food Interactions** Mean oral bioavailability is decreased when given with food. Take ≥30 minutes before the first food or drink of the day other than water.

**Adverse Reactions**

>10%:

Central nervous system: Headache (18%)

Dermatologic: Rash (11.5%)

Gastrointestinal: Abdominal pain (11.5%), diarrhea (19.7%)

Neuromuscular & skeletal: Arthralgia (32.8%)

1% to 10%:

Cardiovascular: Chest pain (6.6%), edema (8.2%)

Central nervous system: Dizziness (6.6%)

Gastrointestinal: Belching (3.3%), colitis (3.3%), constipation (6.6%), nausea (9.8%)

Neuromuscular & skeletal: Bone pain (4.9%), leg cramps (3.3%), myasthenia (3.3%), asthenia (4.9%)

Ocular: Amblyopia (3.3%), dry eyes (3.3%)

Otic: Tinnitus (3.3%)

Respiratory: Bronchitis (3.3%), sinusitis (4.9%)

Miscellaneous: Flu-like syndrome (9.8%), neoplasm (3.3%)

<1% (Limited to important or life-threatening symptoms): Bilateral iritis

**Overdose/Toxicology** Decreases in serum calcium following substantial overdose may be expected in some patients. Signs and symptoms of hypocalcemia may also occur in some of these patients. Gastric lavage may remove unabsorbed drug. Administration of milk or antacids to chelate risedronate may be helpful. Standard procedures that are effective for treating hypocalcemia, including I.V. administration of calcium, would be expected to restore physiologic amounts of ionized calcium to relieve signs and symptoms of hypocalcemia.

**Pharmacodynamics/Kinetics**

**Half-life Elimination:** Terminal: 220 hours

**Onset:** May require weeks

**Formulations** Tablet: 30 mg

**Dosing**

**Adults:** Oral: 30 mg once daily for 2 months. Retreatment may be considered (following post-treatment observation ≥2 months) if relapse occurs or if treatment fails to normalize serum alkaline phosphatase. For retreatment, the dose and duration of therapy are the same as for initial treatment. No data available on more than one course of treatment.

**Elderly:** Refer to adult dosing.

**Renal Impairment:** $Cl_{cr}$ <30 mL/minute: Not recommended

**Administration**

**Oral:** Risedronate should be administered 30 or more minutes before the first food or drink of the day other than water. Risedronate should be taken in an upright position with a full glass (6-8 oz) of plain water and the patient should avoid lying down for 30 minutes to minimize the possibility of GI side effects.

**Monitoring Laboratory Tests** Serum calcium (adjusted to albumin); serum electrolytes, phosphate, magnesium, serum creatinine

**Additional Nursing Issues**

**Physical Assessment:** Monitor laboratory results on a regular basis during therapy (see Monitoring Laboratory Tests). Assess bone and joint pain (Paget's). Monitor for adverse reactions or instruct patient about signs of adverse reactions to report. Assess knowledge/instruct on proper administration of risedronate. **Pregnancy risk factor C** - benefits of use should outweigh risks. Note breast-feeding caution.

**Patient Information/Instruction:** In order to be effective, this drug must be taken exactly as prescribed. Take 30 minutes before first food of the day with 6-8 ounces of water and avoid lying down for 30 minutes after ingestion. You may experience headache (request analgesic); skin rash; or abdominal pain, diarrhea, or constipation (report if persistent). Report unresolved muscle or bone pain or leg cramps; acute abdominal pain; chest pain, palpitations, or swollen extremities; disturbed vision or excessively dry eyes; ringing in the ears; or persistent flu-like symptoms. **Pregnancy/breast-feeding precautions:** Inform prescriber if you are or intend to be pregnant. Consult prescriber if breast-feeding.

**Dietary Issues:** Food may reduce absorption (similar to other bisphosphonates).

♦ **Risperdal®** *see* Risperidone *on this page*

## Risperidone (ris PER i done)

**U.S. Brand Names** Risperdal®

**Therapeutic Category** Antipsychotic Agent, Benzisoxazole

**Pregnancy Risk Factor** C

**Lactation** Excretion in breast milk unknown/contraindicated

**Use** Management of psychotic disorders (eg, schizophrenia); nonpsychotic symptoms associated with dementia in the elderly

**Mechanism of Action/Effect** Risperidone is a benzisoxazole derivative, mixed serotonin-dopamine antagonist; binds to 5-$HT_2$ receptors in the CNS and in the periphery with a very high affinity; binds to dopamine-$D_2$ receptors with less affinity. Is thought to improve negative symptoms of psychoses and reduce the incidence of extrapyramidal side effects.

**Contraindications** Hypersensitivity to risperidone or any component

**Warnings** Low to moderately sedating, use with caution in disorders where CNS depression is a feature. Use with caution in Parkinson's disease. Use with caution in patients with hemodynamic instability; bone marrow suppression; predisposition to seizures; subcortical brain damage; or severe cardiac, hepatic, renal, or respiratory disease. Neuroleptics may cause swallowing difficulties. Use with caution in breast cancer or other prolactin-dependent tumors (may elevate prolactin levels). May alter temperature regulation or mask toxicity of other drugs due to antiemetic effects. May alter cardiac conduction (low risk relative to other neuroleptics) - life-threatening arrhythmias have occurred with therapeutic doses of neuroleptics. Avoid in patients with Q-T prolongation.

May cause anticholinergic effects (eg, confusion, agitation, constipation, dry mouth, blurred vision, urinary retention); therefore, use with caution in patients with decreased gastrointestinal motility, urinary retention, BPH, xerostomia, or visual problems. Conditions which also may be exacerbated by cholinergic blockade include narrow-angle glaucoma (screening is recommended) and worsening of myasthenia gravis. Relative to other neuroleptics, risperidone has a low potency of cholinergic blockade.

May cause extrapyramidal reactions including pseudoparkinsonism, acute dystonic reactions, akathisia, and tardive dyskinesia (risk of these reactions is low relative to other neuroleptics). May be associated with neuroleptic malignant syndrome (NMS) or pigmentary retinopathy.

Pregnancy factor C.

(Continued)

## Risperidone *(Continued)*

**Drug Interactions**

**Cytochrome P-450 Effect:** CYP2D6 enzyme substrate; CYP2D6 enzyme inhibitor (weak)

**Increased Effect/Toxicity:** Increased toxicity with quinidine and warfarin. May antagonize effects of levodopa. Carbamazepine decreases risperidone serum concentrations. Clozapine decreases clearance of risperidone.

**Adverse Reactions** Risperidone causes less tardive dyskinesia, extrapyramidal effects, anticholinergic effects, and hypotension than phenothiazine and butyrophenone classes of antipsychotics, especially when doses do not exceed 6 mg/day.

1% to 10%:

Cardiovascular: Hypotension (especially orthostatic), tachycardia, arrhythmias, abnormal T waves with prolonged ventricular repolarization, EKG changes, syncope

Central nervous system: Sedation (occurs at daily doses ≥20 mg/day), headache, dizziness, restlessness, anxiety, extrapyramidal reactions, dystonic reactions, pseudo-Parkinson signs and symptoms, tardive dyskinesia, neuroleptic malignant syndrome, altered central temperature regulation

Endocrine & metabolic: Amenorrhea, galactorrhea, gynecomastia sexual dysfunction (up to 60%)

Gastrointestinal: Constipation, adynamic ileus, GI upset, dry mouth (problem for denture user), nausea and anorexia, weight gain

Genitourinary: Urinary retention, overflow incontinence, priapism

Hematologic: Agranulocytosis, leukopenia (usually in patients with large doses for prolonged periods)

Hepatic: Cholestatic jaundice

Ocular: Blurred vision, retinal pigmentation, decreased visual acuity (may be irreversible)

<1% (Limited to important or life-threatening symptoms): Seizures, hypertension, A-V block, myocardial infarction

**Pharmacodynamics/Kinetics**

**Protein Binding:** Plasma: 90%

**Half-life Elimination:** 24 hours (risperidone and its active metabolite)

**Time to Peak:** 1 hour

**Metabolism:** Extensive by cytochrome P-450

**Excretion:** Urine and feces

**Formulations**

Solution, oral: 1 mg/mL (100 mL)

Tablet: 1 mg, 2 mg, 3 mg, 4 mg

**Dosing**

**Adults:** Recommended starting dose: 1 mg twice daily; slowly increase to the optimum range of 4-8 mg/day. Daily dosages >10 mg do not appear to offer any additional benefit, and the incidence of extrapyramidal reactions is higher than with lower doses.

**Elderly:** Oral: **Dosing adjustment in renal, hepatic impairment, and elderly:** Starting dose of 0.5 mg once or twice daily is advisable; dosages >6 mg/day increase incidence of extrapyramidal side effects; increase dose at 0.5 mg twice daily at weekly intervals if possible. If rapid escalation in dose is needed, then initial increases at 1 mg twice daily for 3 days may be used to achieve a target dose of 3 mg twice daily.

**Renal Impairment:** Starting dose of 0.5 mg twice daily is advisable.

**Hepatic Impairment:** Starting dose of 0.5 mg twice daily is advisable.

**Administration**

**Oral:** Mix solution with 4 ounces of water, orange juice, or milk. Not compatible with tea or cola.

**Monitoring Laboratory Tests** Ophthalmic exam

**Additional Nursing Issues**

**Physical Assessment:** Assess other medications patient is taking for effectiveness and interactions (see Drug Interactions). See Contraindications and Warnings/Precautions for cautious use. Has potential for psychological or physiological dependence, abuse, and tolerance. Review ophthalmic exam (see Monitoring Laboratory Tests) and monitor therapeutic response (mental status, mood, affect), and adverse reactions at beginning of therapy and periodically with long-term use (CNS responses, anticholinergic and extrapyramidal effects, orthostatic hypotension - see Adverse Reactions and Overdose/Toxicology). Initiate at lower doses (see Dosing) and taper dosage slowly when discontinuing. Assess knowledge/teach patient appropriate use, interventions to reduce side effects, and adverse symptoms to report (see below). **Pregnancy risk factor C** - benefits of use should outweigh possible risks. Breast-feeding is contraindicated.

**Patient Information/Instruction:** Use exactly as directed (do not increase dose or frequency); may cause physical and/or psychological dependence. It may take 2-3 weeks to achieve desired results; do not discontinue without consulting prescriber. Dilute solution with water, milk, orange or grapefruit juice; do not dilute with beverages containing caffeine, tannin, or pactinate (eg, coffee, colas, tea, or apple juice). Avoid excess alcohol or caffeine and other prescription or OTC medications not approved by prescriber. Maintain adequate hydration (2-3 L/day of fluids unless instructed to restrict fluid intake). You may experience excess sedation, drowsiness, restlessness, dizziness, or blurred vision (use caution driving or when engaging in tasks requiring alertness until response to drug is known); dry mouth, nausea, or GI upset (small frequent meals, frequent mouth care, chewing gum, or sucking lozenges may help); postural hypotension (use caution climbing stairs or when changing position from lying or sitting to standing); or urinary retention (void before taking medication). Report persistent

CNS effects (eg, trembling fingers, altered gait or balance, excessive sedation, seizures, unusual muscle or skeletal movements, anxiety, abnormal thoughts, confusion, personality changes); chest pain, palpitations, rapid heartbeat, severe dizziness; swelling or pain in breasts (male and female), altered menstrual pattern, sexual dysfunction; pain or difficulty on urination; vision changes; skin rash or yellowing of skin; difficulty breathing; or worsening of condition. **Pregnancy/breast-feeding precautions:** Inform prescriber if you are or intend to be pregnant. Do not breast-feed.

**Geriatric Considerations:** (See Warnings/Precautions, Adverse Reactions, and Overdose/Toxicology.) Elderly patients have an increased risk of adverse response to side effects or adverse reactions to antipsychotics. These can include but are not limited to the following.

Anticholinergic effects: CNS toxicity with confusion, memory loss, psychotic behavior, and agitation.

Extrapyramidal effects (EPS): Parkinson's syndrome and akathisia may occur as often as 50% in patients >60 years of age. Tardive dyskinesia (motor restlessness) may be 40% in elderly; may be related to duration and total accumulated dose over time; may be somewhat reversible if diagnosed early enough.

Orthostatic hypotension: Increased risk for falls.

Sedation: In nonpsychotic patients, may result in feelings of depersonalization, derealization, and dysphoria.

Cardiac toxicity: Cardiac arrhythmias have occurred with therapeutic doses of antipsychotics.

Malignant neuroleptic syndrome: Development of hyperthermia, muscular rigidity, autonomic instability, and altered mental status.

Many elderly patients receive antipsychotic medications for inappropriate nonpsychotic behavior. Before initiating antipsychotic medication, all possible reversible causes should be investigated. Stress may cause acute "confusion" or worsening of baseline nonpsychotic behaviors; any changes in disease state (in any organ) may result in behavioral changes. Common acute changes in behavior may be due also to increases in drug dose addition, or addition of a new drug to the regimen; fluid/electrolyte alterations; infections; or changes in the environment.

Meta-analysis of controlled trials of antipsychotic (phenothiazines, butyrophenones) use with agitated, demented, elderly patients has concluded that the use of neuroleptics results in a response rate of 18%. Clearly, neuroleptic therapy for behavior control should be limited, with frequent attempts to withdraw the agent for behavior control. When use is indicated, initial doses should be lower to start and monitored closely.

**Breast-feeding Issues:** No information describing the excretion of risperidone in breast milk has been located. However, the manufacturer recommends **not** to breast-feed while taking risperidone.

**Related Information**

Antipsychotic Agents Comparison *on page 1371*
Antipsychotic Medication Guidelines *on page 1436*

♦ **Ritalin®** *see* Methylphenidate *on page 752*
♦ **Ritalin-SR®** *see* Methylphenidate *on page 752*
♦ **Ritmolol** *see* Metoprolol *on page 761*

# Ritodrine (RI toe dreen)

**U.S. Brand Names** Pre-Par®; Yutopar®

**Therapeutic Category** $Beta_2$ Agonist

**Pregnancy Risk Factor** B (contraindicated before 20th week)

**Lactation** Excretion in breast milk unknown

**Use** Inhibits uterine contraction in preterm labor

**Mechanism of Action/Effect** Tocolysis due to its uterine $beta_2$-adrenergic receptor stimulating effects; this agent's $beta_2$ effects can also cause bronchial relaxation and vascular smooth muscle stimulation

**Contraindications** Do not use before 20th week of pregnancy, cardiac arrhythmias, pheochromocytoma

**Warnings** Monitor hydration status and blood glucose concentrations. Fatal maternal pulmonary edema has been reported, sometimes after delivery. Fluid overload must be avoided, hydration levels should be monitored closely. If pulmonary edema occurs, the drug should be discontinued. Use with caution in patients with moderate preeclampsia, diabetes, or migraine. Some products may contain sulfites. Maternal deaths have been reported in patients treated with ritodrine and concurrent corticosteroids (pulmonary edema).

**Drug Interactions**

**Decreased Effect:** Decreased effect with beta-blockers.

**Increased Effect/Toxicity:** Increased effect/toxicity with meperidine, sympathomimetics, diazoxide, magnesium, betamethasone (pulmonary edema), potassium-depleting diuretics, and general anesthetics.

**Adverse Reactions**

>10%:

Cardiovascular: Increases in maternal and fetal heart rates and maternal hypertension, palpitations, chest pain
Central nervous system: Headache
Dermatologic: Erythema
Endocrine & metabolic: Temporary hyperglycemia (maternal)

(Continued)

## Ritodrine *(Continued)*

Gastrointestinal: Nausea, vomiting
Neuromuscular & skeletal: Tremor (trembling)
Respiratory: Pulmonary edema

1% to 10%:
Central nervous system: Nervousness, anxiety, restlessness
Dermatologic: Rash

<1% (Limited to important or life-threatening symptoms): Ketoacidosis, impaired liver function, agranulocytosis, leukopenia

**Overdose/Toxicology** Symptoms of overdose include tachycardia, palpitations, hypotension, nervousness, nausea, vomiting, and tremor. Use an appropriate beta-blocker as an antidote.

**Pharmacodynamics/Kinetics**

**Protein Binding:** 32%

**Distribution:** Crosses the placenta

**Half-life Elimination:** 15 hours

**Time to Peak:** Within 0.5-1 hour

**Metabolism:** Liver

**Excretion:** Urine

**Formulations**

Ritodrine hydrochloride:
Injection: 10 mg/mL (5 mL); 15 mg/mL (10 mL)
Tablet: 10 mg

**Dosing**

**Adults:** I.V.: 50-100 mcg/minute; increase by 50 mcg/minute every 10 minutes; continue for 12 hours after contractions have stopped.

**Renal Impairment:** Hemodialysis effects: Removed by hemodialysis.

**Administration**

**I.V.:** Use microdrip chamber or I.V. pump to control infusion rate.

**I.V. Detail:** Monitor amount of I.V. fluid administered to prevent fluid overload. Place patient in left lateral recumbent position to reduce risk of hypotension.

**Stability**

**Storage:** Stable for 48 hours at room temperature after dilution in 500 mL of NS, $D_5W$, or LR I.V. solutions.

**Monitoring Laboratory Tests** Hematocrit, serum potassium, glucose, colloidal osmotic pressure

**Additional Nursing Issues**

**Physical Assessment:** Assess other medications patient may be taking for effectiveness and interactions (see Drug Interactions). Monitor heart rate (maternal and fetal), blood pressure, respiratory status, and uterine contractions during I.V. infusion and regularly with oral administration. Maintain patient in left lateral position during infusion (to reduce risk of hypotension) and avoid fluid overload. Monitor maternal serum glucose (temporary hyperglycemia). Assess knowledge/teach patient appropriate use, interventions to reduce side effects, and adverse symptoms to report.

**Patient Information/Instruction:**

I.V.: Remain in left lateral position during infusion; do not get out of bed. Report rapid heartbeat, dizziness, difficulty breathing, nervousness or restlessness, skin itching or rash.

Oral: Take as directed and follow instruction of prescriber for physical activity. Report palpitations or chest pain, acute nausea or vomiting, difficulty breathing, skin irritation or rash, abdominal cramping, vaginal discharge, or other signs of labor.

**Additional Information** The injection formulation contains sulfites.

## Ritonavir (rye TON a veer)

**U.S. Brand Names** Norvir®

**Therapeutic Category** Antiretroviral Agent, Protease Inhibitor

**Pregnancy Risk Factor** B

**Lactation** Enters breast milk/contraindicated

**Use** Treatment of HIV, especially advanced cases; usually is used as part of triple or double therapy with other nucleoside and protease inhibitors

**Mechanism of Action/Effect** Ritonavir prevents cleavage of protein precursors essential for HIV infection of new cells and viral replication. Saquinavir- and zidovudine-resistant HIV isolates are generally susceptible to ritonavir. Used in combination therapy, resistance to ritonavir develops slowly; strains resistant to ritonavir are cross-resistant to indinavir and saquinavir.

**Contraindications** Hypersensitivity to ritonavir or any component; avoid use with astemizole, terfenadine, ergot alkaloids and rifabutin

**Warnings** Use caution in patients with hepatic insufficiency. Avoid use with benzodiazepines, antiarrhythmics (flecainide, bepridil, amiodarone, quinidine), and certain analgesics (meperidine, piroxicam, propoxyphene).

**Drug Interactions**

**Cytochrome P-450 Effect:** CYP1A2, 2A6, 2C9, 2C19, 2E1, and 3A3/4 enzyme substrate, CYP2D6 enzyme substrate (minor); CYP1A2 and 2D6 enzyme inducer; CYP2A6, 2C9, 1A2, 2C19, 2D6, 2E1, and 3A3/4 enzyme inhibitor

**Decreased Effect:** Concurrent use of rifampin, rifabutin, dexamethasone, and many anticonvulsants lowers serum concentration of ritonavir. Ritonavir may reduce the concentration of ethinyl estradiol which may result in loss of contraception. Theophylline concentrations may be reduced in concurrent therapy.

**Increased Effect/Toxicity:** Ketoconazole increases ritonavir's plasma levels. Ritonavir may decrease metabolism of terfenadine and astemizole resulting in rare but serious cardiac arrhythmias. Enhanced cardiac effects when administered with flecainide, quinidine, amiodarone, and bepridil. Increased toxic effects also possible with coadministration with cisapride and benzodiazepines. Avoid administration with propoxyphene, meperidine, or piroxicam (acetaminophen or oxycodone as alternatives). Avoid use with ergot alkaloids, bupropion and clozapine. May cause an Antabuse® reaction with metronidazole or disulfuram. Ritonavir may significantly increase the AUC of the following drugs: fentanyl, methadone, lidocaine, erythromycin, clarithromycin, carbamazepine, nefazodone, sertraline, itraconazole, tricyclic antidepressants, some neuroleptics, ketoconazole, miconazole, loratadine, quinine, amlodipine, diltiazem, felodipine, isradipine, nicardipine, nifedipine, nimodipine, nisoldipine, nitrendipine, verapamil, tamoxifen, bromocriptine, indinavir, fluvastatin, lovastatin, simvastatin, cyclosporine, tacrolimus, dexamethasone, warfarin

**Adverse Reactions**

>10%:

Gastrointestinal: Diarrhea, nausea, vomiting, taste perversion

Endocrine & metabolic: Increased GGT, increased triglycerides

Hematologic: Anemia, decreased WBCs

Neuromuscular & skeletal: Weakness

1% to 10%:

Cardiovascular: Vasodilation

Central nervous system: Headache, fever, malaise, paresthesia, dizziness, insomnia, somnolence, thinking abnormally

Dermatologic: Rash

Gastrointestinal: Abdominal pain, anorexia, constipation, heartburn, flatulence, local throat irritation, increased CPK

Endocrine & metabolic: Hyperlipidemia, increased glucose, increased uric acid, increased CPK, increased potassium, increased calcium

Hematologic: Decreased neutrophils, increased eosinophils, increased, neutrophils, increased prothrombin time, increased WBC

Neuromuscular & skeletal: Myalgia

Respiratory: Pharyngitis

Hepatitis: Increased LFTs

Miscellaneous: Sweating

Protease inhibitors cause hyperglycemia and dyslipidemia (elevated cholesterol/triglycerides) and a redistribution of fat (protease paunch, buffalo hump, facial atrophy and breast engorgement)

**Pharmacodynamics/Kinetics**

**Protein Binding:** 98% to 99%

**Distribution:** High concentrations are produced in serum and lymph nodes

**Half-life Elimination:** 3-5 hours

**Metabolism:** Liver

**Excretion:** Renal clearance is negligible

**Formulations**

Capsule: 100 mg

Solution: 80 mg/mL (240 mL)

**Dosing**

**Adults:** Oral: 600 mg twice daily with meals

**Hepatic Impairment:** Not determined; caution is advised with severe impairment.

**Administration**

**Oral:** Take with food. Liquid formulations usually have an unpleasant taste. Consider mixing it with chocolate milk or a liquid nutritional supplement.

**Monitoring Laboratory Tests** Renal and liver function, CBC, electrolytes

**Additional Nursing Issues**

**Physical Assessment:** Monitor laboratory results. Monitor for adverse reactions. Diarrhea may be severe. Observe for signs of dehydration. Monitor effectiveness after long-term therapy. Monitor closely for opportunistic infections. Contraindicated for breast-feeding women; ritonavir is only used to treat patients with HIV and the CDC recommends that women with HIV not nurse to prevent transmission of HIV. Breast-feeding is contraindicated.

**Patient Information/Instruction:** Take with food. Mix liquid formulation with chocolate milk or liquid nutritional supplement. You may experience headache or confusion; if these persist notify prescriber. Diarrhea may be moderate to severe. Notify prescriber if problematic. Report swelling, numbness of tongue, mouth, lips, unresolved vomiting, fever, chills, or extreme fatigue. **Breast-feeding precautions:** Do not breast-feed while taking this drug. Do not breast-feed.

**Breast-feeding Issues:** The CDC recommends against breast-feeding if diagnosed with HIV to avoid postnatal transmission of the virus.

**Pregnancy Issues:** Administer during pregnancy only if benefits to mother outweigh risks to the fetus.

**Related Information**

Antiretroviral Agents Comparison *on page 1373*

♦ **Rituxan®** *see* Rituximab *on this page*

## Rituximab (ri TUK si mab)

**U.S. Brand Names** Rituxan®

**Synonyms** Anti-CD20 Monoclonal Antibodies; C2B8 Monoclonal Antibody; Pan-B Antibodies

(Continued)

## Rituximab *(Continued)*

**Therapeutic Category** Antineoplastic Agent, Miscellaneous

**Pregnancy Risk Factor** C

**Lactation** Excretion in breast milk unknown/contraindicated

**Use** Non-Hodgkin's lymphoma: Treatment of patients with relapsed or refractory low-grade or follicular, CD20 positive, B-cell non-Hodgkin's lymphoma

**Mechanism of Action/Effect** Binds to the CD20 antigen on B-lymphocytes and recruits immune effector functions to mediate B-cell lysis *in vitro*. The antibody induces cell death in the DHL-4 human B-cell lymphoma line.

**Contraindications** Type I hypersensitivity or anaphylactic reactions to murine proteins or to any component of this product

**Warnings** Rituximab is associated with hypersensitivity reactions which may respond to adjustments in the infusion rate. Hypotension, bronchospasm, and angioedema have occurred as part of an infusion-related symptom complex (see Administration). In most cases, patients who have experienced nonlife-threatening reactions have been able to complete the full course of therapy. Medications for the treatment of hypersensitivity reactions (eg, epinephrine, antihistamines, corticosteroids) should be available for immediate use in the event of such a reaction during administration.

Discontinue infusions in the event of serious or life-threatening cardiac arrhythmias. Patients who develop clinically significant arrhythmias should undergo cardiac monitoring during and after subsequent infusions of rituximab. Patients with pre-existing cardiac conditions including arrhythmias and angina have had recurrences of these events during rituximab therapy; monitor these patients throughout the infusion and immediate postinfusion periods.

Pregnancy factor C.

**Adverse Reactions**

>10%:

Central nervous system: Headache (14%)

Gastrointestinal: Nausea (18%)

Hematologic: Leukopenia (11%)

Miscellaneous: Fever (49%), chills (32%), asthenia (16%), angioedema (13%)

Immunologic: Rituximab-induced B-cell depletion occurred in 70% to 80% of patients and was associated with decreased serum immunoglobulins in a minority of patients. The incidence of infection does not appear to be increased. During the treatment period, 50 patients in the pivotal trial developed infectious events, including six grade 3 events (there were no grade 4 events. The six serious events were not associated with neutropenia).

Infusion-related: An infusion-related symptom complex consisting of fever and chills/rigors occurred in the majority of patients during the first rituximab infusion. Other frequent infusion-related symptoms included nausea, urticaria, fatigue, headache, pruritus, bronchospasm, dyspnea, sensation of tongue or throat swelling (angioedema), rhinitis, vomiting, hypotension, flushing, and pain at disease sites. These reactions generally occurred within 30 minutes to 2 hours of beginning the first infusion, and resolved with slowing or interruption of the infusion and with supportive care (I.V. saline, diphenhydramine, and acetaminophen). The incidence of infusion-related events decreased from 80% during the first infusion to ~40% with subsequent infusions. Mild to moderate hypotension requiring interruption of rituximab infusion, with or without the administration of I.V. saline, occurred in 10%. Isolated occurrences of severe reactions requiring epinephrine have been reported in patients receiving rituximab for other indications. Angioedema was reported in 13% and was serious in one patient.

1% to 10%:

Cardiovascular: Hypotension (10%)

Central nervous system: Myalgia (7%), dizziness (7%)

Dermatologic: Pruritus (10%), rash (10%), urticaria (8%)

Gastrointestinal: Vomiting (7%), abdominal pain (6%)

Hematologic: During the treatment period (up to 30 days following the last dose), the following occurred: Severe thrombocytopenia, severe neutropenia, and severe anemia

Respiratory: Bronchospasm occurred in 8%; 25% of these patients were treated with bronchodilators; rhinitis (8%)

Miscellaneous: Throat irritation (6%)

<1% (Limited to important or life-threatening symptoms): Four patients developed arrhythmias during rituximab infusion. One of the four discontinued treatment based on ventricular and supraventricular tachycardias. The other three patients experienced trigeminy and irregular pulses and did not require discontinuation of therapy. Angina was reported during infusion and myocardial infarction occurred 4 days postinfusion in one subject with a history of myocardial infarction. A single occurrence of transient aplastic anemia (pure red-cell aplasia) and two occurrences of hemolytic anemia were reported.

**Note:** Twenty-one patients have received more than one course of rituximab. The percentage of patients reporting any adverse event upon retreatment was similar to the percentage of patients reporting adverse events upon initial exposure. The following adverse events were reported more frequently in retreated patients: Asthenia, throat irritation, flushing, tachycardia, anorexia, leukopenia, thrombocytopenia, anemia, peripheral edema, dizziness, depression, respiratory symptoms, night sweats, pruritus.

**Pharmacodynamics/Kinetics**

**Half-life Elimination:** After first dose, half-life = 59.8 hours; 174 hours after fourth infusion. Detectable in serum 3-6 months after treatment.

**Onset:** Depletion of circulating B cells occurs within the first three doses (administered weekly)

**Duration:** Depletion was sustained in up to 83% of patients for up to 6-9 months. Median B-cell levels returned to normal by 12 months following completion of treatment.

**Formulations** Injection (preservative free): 100 mg (10 mL); 500 mg (10 mL)

**Dosing**

**Adults:** I.V. (refer to individual protocols): **Do not administer I.V. push or bolus** (hypersensitivity reactions may occur). Consider premedication (consisting of acetaminophen and diphenhydramine) before each infusion of rituximab. Premedication may attenuate infusion-related events. Because transient hypotension may occur during infusion, give consideration to withholding antihypertensive medications 12 hours prior to rituximab infusion.

I.V. infusion: 375 mg/m$^2$ once weekly for 4 doses (days 1, 8, 15, and 22).

First infusion: Initial infusion rate = 50 mg/hour. If hypersensitivity or infusion-related events do not occur, infusion may be increased by 50 mg/hour every 30 minutes, to a maximum of 400 mg/hour. Interrupt infusion if hypersensitivity or infusion-related effect occurs. After symptoms improve, infusion may be reinstituted at one-half the previous rate.

Subsequent infusions: Initial rate = 100 mg/hour. Increase by 50 mg/hour every 30 minutes, as tolerated, to a maximum of 400 mg/hour.

**Elderly:** Refer to adult dosing.

**Administration**

**I.V.:** Do **not** administer as an I.V. push or bolus. Rituximab is associated with hypersensitivity reactions which may respond to adjustments in the infusion rate. Hypotension, bronchospasm, and angioedema have occurred as part of an infusion-related symptom complex. Interrupt rituximab infusion for severe reactions and resume at a 50% reduction in rate (eg, from 100 to 50 mg/hour) when symptoms have completely resolved. Treatment of these symptoms with diphenhydramine and acetaminophen is recommended; additional treatment with bronchodilators or I.V. saline may be indicated. In most cases, patients who have experienced nonlife-threatening reactions have been able to complete the full course of therapy.

**I.V. Detail:** Discontinue infusions in the event of serious or life-threatening cardiac arrhythmias.

**Stability**

**Storage:** Store under refrigeration; protect vials from direct sunlight. Stable at room temperature for 12 hours. Stable at 2°C to 8°C for 24 hours.

**Reconstitution:** Withdraw necessary amount of rituximab and dilute to a final concentration of 1-4 mg/mL into an infusion bag containing either 0.9% sodium chloride or 5% dextrose in water.

**Monitoring Laboratory Tests** CBC w/differential, peripheral CD20+ cells. Patients with elevated HAMA/HACA titers may have an allergic reaction when treated with rituximab or other antibodies from a mouse genetic source.

**Additional Nursing Issues**

**Physical Assessment:** Prior to administering first dose, assess patient history for allergies (see Monitoring Laboratory Tests) and antihypertensive medications (see Dosing). Note Warnings/Precautions and Contraindications for cautious use. Monitor laboratory tests prior to, during, and following therapy (see Monitoring Laboratory Tests), response to therapy, and adverse reactions, especially infusion related (eg, chills, fever, nausea, angioedema, etc). See Warnings/Precautions, Adverse Reactions, and Dosing. Monitor/instruct patient on appropriate interventions to reduce side effects, to monitor for signs of opportunistic infection (eg, persistent fever, malaise, sore throat, unusual bleeding or bruising), and adverse reactions to report. **Pregnancy risk factor C** - benefits of use should outweigh possible risks. Breast-feeding is contraindicated.

**Patient Information/Instruction:** You may experience a reaction during the infusion of this medication including high fever, chills, difficulty breathing, or congestion. You will be closely monitored and comfort measures provided. Maintain adequate hydration (2-3 L/day of fluids unless instructed to restrict fluid intake) during entire course of therapy. You will be susceptible to infection and people may wear masks and gloves while caring for you to protect you as much as possible (ie, avoid crowds and people with infections or contagious diseases). You may experience dizziness or trembling (use caution until response to medication is known); or nausea or vomiting (frequent small meals, frequent mouth care may help). Report persistent dizziness, swelling of extremities, unusual weight gain, difficulty breathing, chest pain or tightness; symptoms of respiratory infection, wheezing or bronchospasms, or difficulty breathing; unresolved gastrointestinal effects; skin rash or redness; sore or irritated throat; fatigue, chills, fever, unhealed sores, white plaques in mouth or genital area; unusual bruising or bleeding; or other unusual effects related to this medication. **Pregnancy/breast-feeding precautions:** Inform prescriber if you are or intend to be pregnant. Do not breast-feed until approved by prescriber.

♦ **Rivotril®** *see* Clonazepam *on page 288*

## Rizatriptan (rye za TRIP tan)

**U.S. Brand Names** Maxalt®; Maxalt-MLT™

**Synonyms** MK462

(Continued)

## Rizatriptan *(Continued)*

**Therapeutic Category** Serotonin 5-$HT_{1D}$ Receptor Agonist

**Pregnancy Risk Factor** C

**Lactation** Excretion in breast milk unknown/not recommended

**Use** Acute treatment of migraine with or without aura

**Mechanism of Action/Effect** Selective agonist for serotonin (5-$HT_{-1D}$ receptor) in cranial arteries to cause vasoconstriction and reduce sterile inflammation associated with antidromic neuronal transmission correlating with relief of migraine

**Contraindications** Hypersensitivity to rizatriptan; documented ischemic heart disease or Prinzmetal's angina; uncontrolled hypertension; basilar or hemiplegic migraine; during or within 2 weeks of MAO inhibitors

**Warnings** Use only in patients with a clear diagnosis of migraine. Use with caution in the elderly or patients with hepatic or renal impairment, history of hypersensitivity to sumatriptan or adverse effects from sumatriptan, and in patients at risk of coronary artery disease. Do not use with ergotamines. May increase blood pressure transiently; may cause coronary vasospasm (less than sumatriptan); avoid in patients with signs/symptoms suggestive of reduced arterial flow (ischemic bowel, Raynaud's) which could be exacerbated by vasospasm. Phenylketonurics (tablets contain phenylalanine).

Patients who experience sensations of chest pain/pressure/tightness or symptoms suggestive of angina following dosing should be evaluated for coronary artery disease or Prinzmetal's angina before receiving additional doses.

Caution in dialysis patients or hepatically impaired. Reconsider diagnosis of migraine if no response to initial dose. Long-term effects on vision have not been evaluated.

Pregnancy factor C.

**Drug Interactions**

**Increased Effect/Toxicity:** Use within 24 hours of another selective 5-$HT_1$ antagonist or ergot-containing drug should be avoided due to possible additive vasoconstriction. Use with propranolol increased plasma concentration of rizatriptan by 70%. Rarely, concurrent use with SSRIs results in weakness and incoordination; monitor closely. MAO inhibitors and nonselective MAO inhibitors increase concentration of rizatriptan.

**Food Interactions** Food delays absorption.

**Adverse Reactions**

1% to 10%:

Cardiovascular: Systolic/diastolic blood pressure increases (5-10 mm Hg), chest pain (5%)

Central nervous system: Dizziness, drowsiness, fatigue (13% to 30% - dose related)

Dermatologic: Skin flushing

Endocrine & metabolic: Mild increase in growth hormone, hot flashes

Gastrointestinal: Nausea, vomiting, abdominal pain, dry mouth (<5%)

Respiratory: Dyspnea

<1% (Limited to important or life-threatening symptoms): Syncope, bradycardia, neurological/psychiatric abnormalities

**Pharmacodynamics/Kinetics**

**Protein Binding:** Minimal (14%)

**Half-life Elimination:** 2-3 hours

**Time to Peak:** 1-1.5 hours

**Metabolism:** Substantial nonrenal clearance by monoamine oxidase-A; undergoes first-pass metabolism

**Excretion:** 8% to 16% excreted unchanged in urine; parent and metabolites eliminated (82%)

**Onset:** Within 30 minutes

**Duration:** 14-16 hours

**Formulations** Tablet, as benzoate:

Maxalt®: 5 mg, 10 mg

Maxalt-MLT™ (orally disintegrating): 5 mg, 10 mg

**Dosing**

**Adults:** Oral: 5-10 mg, repeat after 2 hours if significant relief is not attained; maximum: 30 mg in a 24-hour period (use 5 mg dose in patients receiving propranolol 15 mg maximum in 24 hours)

**Elderly:** Refer to adult dosing.

**Stability**

**Storage:** Store in blister pack until administration.

**Monitoring Laboratory Tests** Consider monitoring vital signs and EKG with first dose in patients with liklihood of unrecognized coronary disease, such as patients with significant hypertension, hypercholesterolemia, obese patients, diabetics, smokers with other risk factors or strong family history of coronary artery disease

**Additional Nursing Issues**

**Physical Assessment:** Assess other medications patient may be taking for interactions (see Drug Interactions). Assess effectiveness of therapy on a regular basis and monitor for adverse reactions (especially symptoms of angina - see Adverse Reactions) and instruct patient on reactions to report. Assess knowledge/instruct patient on appropriate administration and cautions about use. **Pregnancy risk factor C** - benefits of use should outweigh possible risks. Breast-feeding is not recommended.

**Patient Information/Instruction:** Administration of orally disintegrating tablets: Do not open blister pack before using. Open with dry hands. Do not crush, chew, or swallow tablet; allow to dissolve on tongue. Take as prescribed; do not increase dosing schedule. May repeat one time after 2 hours, if first dose is ineffective. Do not ever take more than two doses without consulting prescriber. You may experience dizziness or drowsiness (use caution when driving, climbing stairs, or engaging in tasks requiring alertness until response to drug is known); skin flushing or hot flashes (cool clothes or a cool environment may help); mild abdominal discomfort or nausea or vomiting. Report severe dizziness, acute headache, chest pain or palpitation, stiff or painful neck or facial swelling, muscle weakness or pain, changes in mental acuity, blurred vision, eye pain, or excessive perspiration or urination. **Pregnancy/breast-feeding precautions:** Inform prescriber if you are or intend to be pregnant. Breast-feeding is not recommended.

- **rIFN-A** *see* Interferon Alfa-2a *on page 612*
- **rIFN-α2** *see* Interferon Alfa-2b *on page 614*
- **rIFN-b** *see* Interferon Beta-1a *on page 616*
- **rIFN-b** *see* Interferon Beta-1b *on page 617*
- **RMS® Rectal** *see* Morphine Sulfate *on page 790*
- **Robafen® AC** *see* Guaifenesin and Codeine *on page 549*
- **Robafen® CF [OTC]** *see* Guaifenesin, Phenylpropanolamine, and Dextromethorphan *on page 551*
- **Robafen DM® [OTC]** *see* Guaifenesin and Dextromethorphan *on page 549*
- **Robaxin®** *see* Methocarbamol *on page 742*
- **Robaxisal®** *see* Methocarbamol and Aspirin *on page 743*
- **Robicillin® VK** *see* Penicillin V Potassium *on page 900*
- **Robidrine®** *see* Pseudoephedrine *on page 992*
- **Robinul®** *see* Glycopyrrolate *on page 539*
- **Robinul® Forte** *see* Glycopyrrolate *on page 539*
- **Robitussin® [OTC]** *see* Guaifenesin *on page 548*
- **Robitussin® A-C** *see* Guaifenesin and Codeine *on page 549*
- **Robitussin-CF® [OTC]** *see* Guaifenesin, Phenylpropanolamine, and Dextromethorphan *on page 551*
- **Robitussin® Cough Calmers** *see page 1294*
- **Robitussin®-DAC** *see* Guaifenesin, Pseudoephedrine, and Codeine *on page 552*
- **Robitussin®-DM [OTC]** *see* Guaifenesin and Dextromethorphan *on page 549*
- **Robitussin-PE® [OTC]** *see* Guaifenesin and Pseudoephedrine *on page 551*
- **Robitussin® Pediatric** *see page 1294*
- **Robitussin® Severe Congestion Liqui-Gels® [OTC]** *see* Guaifenesin and Pseudoephedrine *on page 551*
- **Robomol®** *see* Methocarbamol *on page 742*
- **Rocaltrol®** *see* Calcitriol *on page 183*
- **Rocephin®** *see* Ceftriaxone *on page 232*
- **Rocuronium** *see page 1248*
- **Rofact™** *see* Rifampin *on page 1019*

## Rofecoxib (roe fe COX ib)

**U.S. Brand Names** Vioxx®

**Therapeutic Category** Nonsteroidal Anti-Inflammatory Agent (NSAID)

**Pregnancy Risk Factor** C (D after 34 weeks gestation or close to delivery)

**Lactation** Excretion in breast milk unknown/not recommended

**Use** Relief of the signs and symptoms of osteoarthritis; management of acute pain in adults; treatment of primary dysmenorrhea

**Mechanism of Action/Effect** Inhibits prostaglandin synthesis by decreasing the activity of the enzyme, cyclo-oxygenase-2 (COX-2), which results in decreased formation of prostaglandin precursors. Rofecoxib does not inhibit cyclo-oxygenase-1 (COX-1) at therapeutic concentrations.

**Contraindications** Hypersensitivity to rofecoxib or any component, aspirin, or other nonsteroidal anti-inflammatory drugs (NSAIDs); pregnancy (after 34 weeks gestation or close to delivery)

**Warnings** Gastrointestinal irritation, ulceration, bleeding, and perforation may occur with NSAIDs (it is unclear whether rofecoxib is associated with rates of these events which are similar to nonselective NSAIDs). Use with caution in patients with a history of GI disease (bleeding or ulcers), decreased renal function, hepatic disease, congestive heart failure, hypertension, or asthma. Anaphylactoid reactions may occur, even with no prior exposure to rofecoxib. Pregnancy risk C (D after 34 weeks gestation or close to delivery).

**Drug Interactions**

**Cytochrome P-450 Effect:** May be a mild inducer of cytochrome P-450 isoenzyme 3A4 (CYP3A4).

**Decreased Effect:** Efficacy of thiazide diuretics, loop diuretics (furosemide), or ACE-inhibitors may be diminished by rofecoxib. Rifampin reduces the serum concentration of rofecoxib by approximately 50%. Antacids may reduce rofecoxib absorption.

**Increased Effect/Toxicity:** Cimetidine increases AUC of rofecoxib by 23%. Rofecoxib may increase plasma concentrations of methotrexate and lithium. Rofecoxib may be used with low-dose aspirin, however, rates of gastrointestinal bleeding may be increased with coadministration. Rofecoxib may increase the INR in patients receiving warfarin and may increase the risk of bleeding complications.

**Food Interactions** Time to peak concentrations are delayed when taken with a high-fat meal, however peak concentration and AUC are unchanged. Rofecoxib may be taken without regard to meals.

(Continued)

## Rofecoxib *(Continued)*

**Adverse Reactions**

2% to 10%:

Cardiovascular: Peripheral edema (3.7%), hypertension (3.5%)

Central nervous system: Headache (4.7%), dizziness (3%), weakness (2.2%)

Gastrointestinal: Diarrhea (6.5%), nausea (5.2%), heartburn (4.2%), epigastric discomfort (3.8%), dyspepsia (3.5%), abdominal pain (3.4%)

Genitourinary: Urinary tract infection (2.8%)

Neuromuscular & skeletal: Back pain (2.5%)

Respiratory: Upper respiratory infection (8.5%), bronchitis (2.0%), sinusitis (2.7%)

Miscellaneous: Flu-like syndrome (2.9%)

0.1% to 2%:

Cardiovascular: Chest pain, upper extremity edema, atrial fibrillation, bradycardia, arrhythmia, palpitation, tachycardia, venous insufficiency, fluid retention

Central nervous system: Anxiety, depression, decreased mental acuity, hypesthesia, insomnia, neuropathy, migraine, paresthesia, somnolence, vertigo, fever, pain

Dermatologic: Alopecia, atopic dermatitis, basal cell carcinoma, contact dermatitis, pruritus, rash, erythema, urticaria, dry skin

Endocrine & metabolic: Weight gain, hypercholesteremia

Gastrointestinal: Reflux, abdominal distension, abdominal tenderness, constipation, dry mouth, esophagitis, flatulence, gastritis, gastroenteritis, hematochezia, hemorrhoids, oral ulceration, dental caries, aphthous stomatitis

Genitourinary: Breast mass, cystitis, dysuria, menopausal disorder, nocturia, urinary retention, vaginitis, pelvic pain

Hematologic: Hematoma

Neuromuscular & skeletal: Muscle spasm, sciatica, arthralgia, bursitis, cartilage trauma, joint swelling, muscle cramps, muscle weakness, myalgia, tendonitis, traumatic arthropathy, fracture (wrist)

Ocular: Blurred vision, conjunctivitis

Otic: Otic pain, otitis media, tinnitus

Respiratory: Asthma, cough, dyspnea, pneumonia, respiratory infection, pulmonary congestion, rhinitis, epistaxis, laryngitis, dry throat, pharyngitis, tonsillitis, diaphragmatic hernia

Miscellaneous: Allergy, fungal infection, insect bite reaction, syncope, viral syndrome, herpes simplex, herpes zoster, increased sweating

<0.1% (Limited to severe or life-threatening symptoms): Congestive heart failure, cerebrovascular accident, deep venous thrombosis, myocardial infarction, unstable angina, transient ischemic attack, colitis, colonic neoplasm, cholecystitis, duodenal ulcer, gastrointestinal bleeding, intestinal obstruction, pancreatitis, lymphoma, breast cancer, prostatic cancer, urolithiasis

**Overdose/Toxicology** Symptoms may include epigastric pain, drowsiness, lethargy, nausea, and vomiting. Gastrointestinal bleeding may occur. Rare manifestations include hypertension, respiratory depression, coma, and acute renal failure. Treatment is symptomatic and supportive. Hemodialysis does not remove rofecoxib.

**Pharmacodynamics/Kinetics**

**Protein Binding:** 87%

**Half-life Elimination:** 17 hours

**Time to Peak:** 2-3 hours

**Metabolism:** Hepatic (99%), minor metabolism by cytochrome P450 isoenzyme 3A4 (CYP3A4)

**Excretion:** In urine, as metabolites (<1% unchanged drug)

**Onset:** 45 minutes

**Duration:** Up to >24 hours

**Formulations**

Suspension, oral: 12.5 mg/5 mL, 25 mg/5 mL

Tablets: 12.5 mg, 25 mg

**Dosing**

**Adults:** Oral:

Osteoarthritis: 12.5 mg once daily; may be increased to a maximum of 25 mg once daily

Acute pain and management of dysmenorrhea: 50 mg once daily as needed (use for longer than 5 days is not recommended)

**Elderly:** No specific adjustment is recommended. However, the AUC in elderly patients may be increased by 34% as compared to younger subjects. Use the lowest recommended dose. See dosing for adults.

**Renal Impairment:** Use in advanced renal disease is not recommended.

**Hepatic Impairment:** No specific dosage adjustment is recommended (AUC may be increased by 69%).

**Additional Nursing Issues**

**Physical Assessment:** See Contraindications and Warnings/Precautions for use cautions. Assess effectiveness and interactions of other medications (see Drug Interactions, ie, monitor patients taking lithium closely). Assess allergy history (aspirin, NSAIDS, salicylates). Monitor effectiveness of therapy (pain, range of motion, mobility, ADL function, inflammation). Assess knowledge/teach patient appropriate use, possible side effects/interventions, and adverse symptoms to report (see Adverse Reaction and Overdose/Toxicology). **Pregnancy risk factor C/D** - see Pregnancy Risk Factor for cautious use. Breast-feeding is not recommended.

**Patient Information/Instruction:** Do not take more than recommended dose. May be taken with food to reduce GI upset. Do not take with antacids. Avoid alcohol, aspirin, and OTC medication unless approved by prescriber. You may experience dizziness, confusion, or blurred vision (avoid driving or engaging in tasks requiring alertness until response to drug is known); anorexia, nausea, vomiting, taste disturbance, gastric distress (small frequent meals, frequent mouth care, sucking lozenges, or chewing gum may help). GI bleeding, ulceration, or perforation can occur with or without pain; it is unclear whether rofecoxib has rates of these events which are similar to nonselective NSAIDs. Stop taking medication and report immediately stomach pain or cramping, unusual bleeding or bruising, or blood in vomitus, stool, or urine. Report persistent insomnia; skin rash; unusual fatigue or easy bruising or bleeding; muscle pain, tremors, or weakness; sudden weight gain; changes in hearing (ringing in ears); changes in vision; changes in urination pattern; or respiratory difficulty. **Pregnancy/breast-feeding precautions:** Inform prescriber if you are or intend to be pregnant. Breast-feeding is not recommended.

**Pregnancy Issues:** In late pregnancy may cause premature closure of the ductus arteriosus.


♦ **Roferon-A®** *see* Interferon Alfa-2a *on page 612*

♦ **Rogaine® for Men** *see page 1294*

♦ **Rogaine® for Women** *see page 1294*

♦ **Rogal** *see* Piroxicam *on page 940*

♦ **Rogitine®** *see* Phentolamine *on page 919*

♦ **Rolaids®** *see* Calcium Supplements *on page 185*

♦ **Rolaids® Chewable Tablet** *see page 1294*

♦ **Rolatuss® Plain Liquid** *see page 1294*

♦ **Romazicon™ Injection** *see* Flumazenil *on page 496*

♦ **Romir** *see* Captopril *on page 192*

♦ **Rondec® Drops** *see* Carbinoxamine and Pseudoephedrine *on page 198*

♦ **Rondec® Filmtab®** *see* Carbinoxamine and Pseudoephedrine *on page 198*

♦ **Rondec® Syrup** *see* Carbinoxamine and Pseudoephedrine *on page 198*

♦ **Rondec-TR®** *see* Carbinoxamine and Pseudoephedrine *on page 198*


## Rosiglitazone (ROSE i gli ta zone)

**U.S. Brand Names** Avandia®

**Therapeutic Category** Antidiabetic Agent (Thiazolidinedione)

**Pregnancy Risk Factor** C

**Lactation** Excretion in breast milk unknown/not recommended

**Use**

Type II diabetes, monotherapy: Improve glycemic control as an adjunct to diet and exercise

Type II diabetes, combination therapy: In combination with metformin when diet, exercise, and metformin alone or diet, exercise, and rosiglitazone alone do not result in adequate glycemic control.

**Mechanism of Action/Effect** Thiazolidinedione antidiabetic agent that lowers blood glucose by improving target cell response to insulin, without increasing pancreatic insulin secretion. It has a mechanism of action that is dependent on the presence of insulin for activity.

**Contraindications** Hypersensitivity to rosiglitazone or any component of the formulation; active liver disease (transaminases >2.5 times the upper limit of normal at baseline); with patients who experience jaundice during troglitazone therapy

**Warnings** Should not be used in diabetic ketoacidosis. Mechanism requires the presence of insulin, therefore, use in type I diabetes is not recommended. Use with caution in premenopausal, anovulatory women; may result in resumption of ovulation, increasing the risk of pregnancy. May result in hormonal imbalance; development of menstrual irregularities should prompt reconsideration of therapy. Use with caution in patients with anemia or depressed leukocyte counts (may reduce hemoglobin, hematocrit, and/or WBC). Use with caution in patients with heart failure or edema; may increase in plasma volume and/or increase cardiac hypertrophy. In general, use should be avoided in patients with NYHA class 3 or 4 heart failure. Use with caution in patients with elevated transaminases (AST or ALT); see Contraindications and Monitoring. Idiosyncratic hepatotoxicity has been reported with another thiazolidinedione agent (troglitazone). Monitoring should include periodic determinations of liver function. Pregnancy risk C.

**Drug Interactions**

**Cytochrome P-450 Effect:** Substrate for cytochrome P-450 isoenzyme 2C8 (CYP2C8); minor metabolism by CYP2C9

**Increased Effect/Toxicity:** When rosiglitazone was coadministered with glyburide, metformin, digoxin, warfarin, ethanol, or ranitidine, no significant pharmacokinetic alterations were observed.

**Food Interactions** Peak concentrations are lower by 28% and delayed when administered with food, but these effects are not believed to be clinically significant. Rosiglitazone may be taken without regard to meals.

**Adverse Reactions**

>10%: Endocrine and Metabolic: Weight gain, increase in total cholesterol, increased LDL cholesterol, decreased HDL cholesterol

1% to 10%:

Cardiovascular: Edema (4.8%)

Central nervous system: Headache (5.9%), fatigue (3.6%)

Endocrine & metabolic: Hyperglycemia (3.9%), hypoglycemia (0.5% to 1.6%)

Gastrointestinal: Diarrhea (2.3%)

Hematologic: Anemia (1.9%)

(Continued)

## Rosiglitazone *(Continued)*

Neuromuscular & skeletal: Back pain (4%)
Respiratory: Upper respiratory tract infection (9.9%), sinusitis (3.2%)
Miscellaneous: Injury (7.6%)

<1% (Limited to important or life-threatening symptoms): Elevated transaminases, increased bilirubin

**Overdose/Toxicology** Experience in overdose is limited. Symptoms may include hypoglycemia. Treatment is supportive.

**Pharmacodynamics/Kinetics**

**Protein Binding:** 99.8%

**Half-life Elimination:** 3.15-3.59 hours

**Time to Peak:** 1 hour

**Metabolism:** Hepatic (99%), metabolism by cytochrome P-450 isoenzyme 2C8 (CYP2C8), minor metabolism via CYP2C9

**Excretion:** As metabolites, in urine and feces

**Onset:** Delayed, may require up to 12 weeks to achieve maximal effect

**Formulations** Tablet: 2 mg, 4 mg

**Dosing**

**Adults:** Oral: Initial: 4 mg daily as a single daily dose or in divided doses twice daily. If response is inadequate after 12 weeks of treatment, the dosage may be increased to 8 mg daily as a single daily dose or in divided doses twice daily.

**Elderly:** Refer to adult dosing.

**Renal Impairment:** No dosage adjustment is required.

**Hepatic Impairment:** Clearance is significantly lower in hepatic impairment. Therapy should not be initiated if the patient exhibits active liver disease of increased transaminases (>2.5 times the upper limit of normal) at baseline. For patients with normal hepatic enzymes who are switched from troglitazone to rosiglitazone, a 1-week washout is recommended before initiating therapy with rosiglitazone.

**Monitoring Laboratory Tests** Hemoglobin $A_1c$, liver enzymes (prior to initiation of therapy, every 2 months for the first year of therapy, then periodically thereafter). Patients with an elevation in ALT >3 times the upper limit of normal should be rechecked as soon as possible. If the ALT levels remain >3 times the upper limit of normal, therapy with rosiglitazone should be discontinued.

**Additional Nursing Issues**

**Physical Assessment:** Monitor laboratory results closely. Assess other medications patient may be taking (see Warnings/Precautions and Drug Interactions) Monitor response to therapy closely until response is stable. Advise women using oral contraceptives about need for alternative method of contraception. Monitor closely for signs of liver failure (eg, nausea, vomiting, fatigue, loss of appetite, yellowing of eyes or skin, dark urine or pale stool). Assess knowledge/teach risks of hypoglycemia, its symptoms, treatment, and predisposing conditions. Refer patient to a diabetic educator, if possible. **Pregnancy risk factor C** - benefits of use should outweigh possible risks. Breast-feeding is not recommended.

**Patient Information/Instruction:** May be taken without regard to meals. Follow directions of prescriber. If dose is missed at the usual meal, take it with next meal. Do not double dose if daily dose is missed completely. Monitor urine or serum glucose as recommended by prescriber. More frequent monitoring is required during periods of stress, trauma, surgery, pregnancy, increased activity or exercise. Avoid alcohol. Report chest pain, rapid heartbeat or palpitations, abdominal pain, fever, rash, hypoglycemia reactions, yellowing of skin or eyes, dark urine or light stool, or unusual fatigue or nausea/vomiting. **Pregnancy/breast-feeding precautions:** Use alternate means of contraception if using oral contraceptives. Breast-feeding is not recommended.

**Dietary Issues:** Management of type 2 diabetes should include diet control.

**Pregnancy Issues:** Treatment during mid to late gestation was associated with fetal death and growth retardation in animal models.


- ♦ **RotaShield®** *see page 1256*
- ♦ **Rotavirus Vaccine** *see page 1256*
- ♦ **Roubac®** *see* Co-trimoxazole *on page 307*
- ♦ **Rowasa® Rectal** *see* Mesalamine *on page 727*
- ♦ **Roxanol™ Oral** *see* Morphine Sulfate *on page 790*
- ♦ **Roxanol SR™ Oral** *see* Morphine Sulfate *on page 790*
- ♦ **Roxicet® 5/500** *see* Oxycodone and Acetaminophen *on page 873*
- ♦ **Roxicodone™** *see* Oxycodone *on page 871*
- ♦ **Roxilox®** *see* Oxycodone and Acetaminophen *on page 873*
- ♦ **Roxiprin®** *see* Oxycodone and Aspirin *on page 873*
- ♦ **RP54274** *see* Riluzole *on page 1023*
- ♦ **r-PA** *see* Reteplase *on page 1015*
- ♦ **R-Tannamine® Tablet** *see page 1306*
- ♦ **R-Tannate® Tablet** *see page 1306*
- ♦ **RTCA** *see* Ribavirin *on page 1016*
- ♦ **Rubella and Measles Vaccines, Combined** *see page 1256*
- ♦ **Rubella and Mumps Vaccines, Combined** *see page 1256*
- ♦ **Rubella Virus Vaccine, Live** *see page 1256*
- ♦ **Rubeola Vaccine** *see page 1256*
- ♦ **Rubex®** *see* Doxorubicin *on page 401*

- ♦ **Rubidomycin Hydrochloride** *see* Daunorubicin Hydrochloride *on page 336*
- ♦ **Rubilem** *see* Daunorubicin Hydrochloride *on page 336*
- ♦ **Rubramin®** *see* Cyanocobalamin *on page 311*
- ♦ **Rubramin-PC®** *see* Cyanocobalamin *on page 311*
- ♦ **Rum-K®** *see* Potassium Supplements *on page 952*
- ♦ **Ru-Tuss® DE** *see* Guaifenesin and Pseudoephedrine *on page 551*
- ♦ **Ru-Tuss® Liquid** *see page 1294*
- ♦ **Ru-Vert-M®** *see* Meclizine *on page 712*
- ♦ **Rymed®** *see* Guaifenesin and Pseudoephedrine *on page 551*
- ♦ **Rymed-TR®** *see* Guaifenesin and Phenylpropanolamine *on page 550*
- ♦ **Ryna-C® Liquid** *see page 1306*
- ♦ **Rynacrom®** *see* Cromolyn Sodium *on page 309*
- ♦ **Ryna-CX®** *see* Guaifenesin, Pseudoephedrine, and Codeine *on page 552*
- ♦ **Ryna® Liquid** *see page 1294*
- ♦ **Rynatan® Pediatric Suspension** *see page 1306*
- ♦ **Rynatan® Tablet** *see page 1306*
- ♦ **Rynatuss® Pediatric Suspension** *see page 1294*
- ♦ **Rythmol®** *see* Propafenone *on page 981*
- ♦ **Sabulin®** *see* Albuterol *on page 45*

## Sacrosidase (sak RO se dase)

**U.S. Brand Names** Sucraid™

**Therapeutic Category** Enzyme, Gastrointestinal

**Pregnancy Risk Factor** C

**Lactation** Enters breast milk/compatible

**Use** Oral replacement therapy in sucrase deficiency, as seen in congenital sucrase-isomaltase deficiency (CSID)

**Mechanism of Action/Effect** Sacrosidase is a naturally occurring gastrointestinal enzyme which breaks down the disaccharide sucrose to its monosaccharide components. Hydrolysis is necessary to allow absorption of these nutrients.

**Contraindications** Hypersensitivity to yeast, yeast products, or glycerin

**Warnings** Hypersensitivity reactions to sacrosidase, including bronchospasm, have been reported. Administer initial doses in a setting where acute hypersensitivity reactions may be treated within a few minutes. Skin testing for hypersensitivity may be performed prior to administration to identify patients at risk. Pregnancy factor C.

**Drug Interactions**

**Increased Effect/Toxicity:** Drug-drug interactions have not been evaluated.

**Food Interactions** May be inactivated or denatured if administered with fruit juice, warm or hot food or liquids. Since isomaltase deficiency is not addressed by supplementation of sacrosidase, adherence to a low-starch diet may be required.

**Adverse Reactions**

Central nervous system: Insomnia, headache, nervousness
Gastrointestinal: Abdominal pain, vomiting, nausea, diarrhea, constipation
Endocrine and metabolic: Dehydration
Respiratory: Bronchospasm
Miscellaneous: Hypersensitivity reaction

**Overdose/Toxicology** Symptoms may include epigastric pain, drowsiness, lethargy, nausea, and vomiting. Gastrointestinal bleeding may occur. Rare manifestations include hypertension, respiratory depression, coma, and acute renal failure. Treatment is symptomatic and supportive. Forced diuresis, hemodialysis and/or urinary alkalinization are not likely to be useful.

**Formulations** Solution, oral: 8500 int. units per mL

**Dosing**

**Adults:** Oral: 17,000 int. units (2 mL) per meal or snack. Doses should be diluted with 2-4 ounces of water, milk or formula with each meal or snack. Approximately one-half of the dose may be taken before, and the remainder of a dose taken at the completion of each meal or snack.

**Elderly:** Refer to adult dosing.

**Stability**

**Storage:** Store under refrigeration at 4°C to 8°C (36°F to 46°F). Protect from heat or light.

**Additional Nursing Issues**

**Physical Assessment:** See Contraindications and Warnings/Precautions for use cautions (eg, skin testing). Monitor effectiveness of therapy and adverse reactions at beginning of therapy and periodically with long-term use (see Adverse Reactions). Assess knowledge/teach patient appropriate use, interventions to reduce side effects, and adverse symptoms to report. **Pregnancy risk factor C** - benefits of use should outweigh possible risks.

**Patient Information/Instruction:** Use exactly as directed. Dilute dose in 2-4 ounces of water, milk, or formula; do not dilute with fruit juice or warm or cold liquids. Take half the dose at beginning of meal and half the dose at end of meal. Maintain adequate fluid intake (2-3 L/day of fluids unless instructed to restrict fluid intake). Follow prescribers recommended diet exactly. You may experience headache or nervousness (use caution when driving or engaging in tasks requiring alertness until response to drug is known); nausea, vomiting, or GI disturbance (frequent small meals, frequent mouth care, chewing gum, or sucking hard candy may help). Report immediately skin rash or difficulty breathing; persistent vomiting, abdominal pain, or blood in stools;

(Continued)

## Sacrosidase *(Continued)*

change in CNS status (depression, agitation, lethargy); or other adverse response.

**Pregnancy precautions:** Inform prescriber if you are or intend to be pregnant.

**Dietary Issues:** Adherence to a low-starch diet may be required despite supplementation of sucrase activity since isomaltase deficiency is not addressed.

**Additional Information** The oral solution contains 50% glycerol.

- **Safe Tussin® 30 [OTC]** *see* Guaifenesin and Dextromethorphan *on page 549*
- **Sal-Acid® Plaster** *see page 1294*
- **Salactic® Film** *see page 1294*
- **Salagen® Oral** *see* Pilocarpine *on page 931*
- **Salazopyrin®** *see* Sulfasalazine *on page 1084*
- **Salazopyrin EN-Tabs®** *see* Sulfasalazine *on page 1084*
- **Salbulin** *see* Albuterol *on page 45*
- **Salbutalan** *see* Albuterol *on page 45*
- **Salbutamol** *see* Albuterol *on page 45*
- **Saleto-200® [OTC]** *see* Ibuprofen *on page 592*
- **Saleto-400®** *see* Ibuprofen *on page 592*
- **Salflex®** *see* Salsalate *on page 1042*
- **Salgesic®** *see* Salsalate *on page 1042*
- **Salicylazosulfapyridine** *see* Sulfasalazine *on page 1084*
- **Salicylic Acid** *see page 1294*
- **Salicylic Acid and Lactic Acid** *see page 1294*
- **Salicylic Acid and Propylene Glycol** *see page 1294*
- **SalineX®** *see page 1294*
- **Saliva Substitute** *see page 1294*

## Salmeterol (sal ME te role)

**U.S. Brand Names** Serevent®; Serevent® Diskus®

**Therapeutic Category** $Beta_2$ Agonist

**Pregnancy Risk Factor** C

**Lactation** Enters breast milk/not recommended

**Use** Maintenance treatment of asthma and in prevention of bronchospasm in patients >12 years of age with reversible obstructive airway disease, including patients with symptoms of nocturnal asthma, who require regular treatment with inhaled, short-acting $beta_2$ agonists; prevention of exercise-induced bronchospasm; long-term maintenance treatment of bronchospasm associated with COPD

**Mechanism of Action/Effect** Relaxes bronchial smooth muscle by selective action on $beta_2$-receptors with little effect on heart rate; because salmeterol acts locally in the lung, therapeutic effect is not predicted by plasma levels

**Contraindications** Hypersensitivity to salmeterol, adrenergic amines, or any ingredients; need for acute bronchodilation. Use within 2 weeks of MAO inhibitor

**Warnings** Salmeterol is not meant to relieve acute asthmatic symptoms. **Acute episodes should be treated with short-acting $beta_2$ agonist.** Do not increase the frequency of salmeterol. Patients receiving maintenance dosages should not use additional salmeterol for exercise-induced asthma prevention. Cardiovascular effects are not common with salmeterol when used in recommended doses. All beta agonists may cause elevation in blood pressure, heart rate, and result in excitement (CNS). Use with caution in patients with prostatic hypertrophy, diabetes, cardiovascular disorders, convulsive disorders, thyrotoxicosis, or others who are sensitive to the effects of sympathomimetic amines. Paroxysmal bronchospasm (which can be fatal) has been reported with this and other inhaled agents. If this occurs, discontinue treatment. The elderly may be at greater risk of cardiovascular side effects; safety and efficacy have not been established in children <12 years of age. Pregnancy factor C.

**Drug Interactions**

**Cytochrome P-450 Effect:** CYP3A3/4 enzyme substrate

**Decreased Effect:** Decreased toxicity (cardiovascular) with MAO inhibitors, tricyclic antidepressants. Decreased effect with beta-adrenergic blockers (eg, propranolol).

**Increased Effect/Toxicity:** (Cardiovascular): MAO inhibitors, tricyclic antidepressants

**Adverse Reactions**

>10%:

Central nervous system: Headache

Respiratory: Pharyngitis

1% to 10%:

Cardiovascular: Tachycardia, palpitations, elevation or depression of blood pressure, cardiac arrhythmias

Central nervous system: Nervousness, CNS stimulation, hyperactivity, insomnia, malaise, dizziness

Gastrointestinal: GI upset, diarrhea, nausea

Neuromuscular & skeletal: Tremors (may be more common in the elderly), myalgias, back pain, arthralgia

Respiratory: Upper respiratory infection, cough, bronchitis

<1% (Limited to important or life-threatening symptoms): Immediate hypersensitivity reactions (rash, urticaria, bronchospasm), paradoxical bronchospasms, laryngeal spasm, arrhythmias, atrial fibrillation

**Overdose/Toxicology** Decontamination: Lavage/activated charcoal. Prudent use of a cardioselective beta-adrenergic blocker (eg, atenolol or metoprolol). Keep in mind the potential for induction of bronchoconstriction in an asthmatic. Dialysis has not been shown to be of value in treatment of overdose with salmeterol.

**Pharmacodynamics/Kinetics**

**Protein Binding:** 94% to 98%

**Half-life Elimination:** 3-4 hours

**Metabolism:** Liver

**Onset:** 5-20 minutes (average 10 minutes); Peak effect: 2-4 hours

**Duration:** 12 hours

**Formulations**

Aerosol, oral, as xinafoate: 21 mcg/spray [60 inhalations] (6.5 g), [120 inhalations] (13 g)

Powder, for inhalation (Serevent® Diskus®): 50 mcg/inhalation (60 blisters)

**Dosing**

**Adults:**

Inhalation, aerosol: 42 mcg (2 puffs) twice daily (12 hours apart) for maintenance and prevention of symptoms of asthma

Prevention of exercise-induced asthma: 42 mcg (2 puffs) 30-60 minutes prior to exercise; additional doses should not be used for 12 hours. Maintenance treatment of bronchospasm associated with COPD: 42 micrograms (2 puffs) twice daily (morning and evening - 12 hours apart)

Inhalation, powder (Serevent® Diskus®): 50 mcg per inhalation twice daily for maintenance and prevention of symptoms of asthma symptoms

Prevention of exercise-induced asthma: One inhalation at least 30 minutes prior to exercise; additional doses should not be used for 12 hours.

Note: do not use spacer with inhalation powder

**Elderly:** Refer to adult dosing and Geriatric Considerations.

**Administration**

**Inhalation: Not** to be used for the relief of acute attacks.

**Stability**

**Storage:** Serovent® Diskus®: Stable for 6 weeks after removal from foil pouch. Store cannister with nozzle down. Protect from freezing temperature and direct sunlight. The therapeutic effect may decrease when the canister is cold therefore the canister should remain at room temperature. Store canister with nozzle end down. Do not store at temperatures >120°F.

**Monitoring Laboratory Tests** Pulmonary function

**Additional Nursing Issues**

**Physical Assessment:** Not for use to relieve acute asthmatic attacks. Assess effectiveness and interactions of other medications (see Drug Interactions). See Contraindications and Warnings/Precautions for use cautions. Monitor effectiveness of therapy (relief of airway obstruction) and adverse reactions (eg, cardiac and CNS changes - see Adverse Reactions) at beginning of therapy and periodically with long-term use. For inpatient care, monitor vital signs and lung sounds prior to and periodically during therapy. Assess knowledge/teach patient appropriate use, interventions to reduce side effects, and adverse symptoms to report. **Pregnancy risk factor C** - benefits of use should outweigh possible risks. Breast-feeding is not recommended.

**Patient Information/Instruction:** Use exactly as directed (see Administration below). Do not use more often than recommended (excessive use may result in tolerance, overdose may result in serious adverse effects) and do not discontinue without consulting prescriber. Do not use for acute attacks. Maintain adequate hydration (2-3 L/day of fluids unless instructed to restrict fluid intake). You may experience nervousness, dizziness, or fatigue (use caution when driving or engaging in tasks requiring alertness until response to drug is known); or dry mouth, stomach upset (frequent small meals, frequent mouth care, chewing gum, or sucking hard candy may help). Report unresolved GI upset; dizziness or fatigue; vision changes; chest pain, rapid heartbeat, or palpitations; insomnia; nervousness or hyperactivity; muscle cramping, tremors, or pain; unusual cough; or rash (hypersensitivity). **Pregnancy/breast-feeding precautions:** Inform prescriber if you are or intend to be pregnant. Breast-feeding is not recommended.

**Administration:** Self-administered inhalation: Store canister upside down; do not freeze. Shake canister before using. Sit when using medication. Close eyes when administering salmeterol to avoid spray getting into eyes. Exhale slowly and completely through nose; inhale deeply through mouth while administering aerosol. Hold breath for 1-3 seconds after inhalation. Wait at least 1 full minute between inhalations. Wash mouthpiece between use. If more than one inhalation medication is used, use bronchodilator first and wait 5 minutes between medications.

**Geriatric Considerations:** Geriatric patients were included in four clinical studies of salmeterol; no apparent differences in efficacy and safety were noted in geriatric patients compared to younger adults. Because salmeterol is only to be used for prevention of bronchospasm, patients also need a short-acting beta-agonist to treat acute attacks. Elderly patients should be carefully counseled about which inhaler to use and the proper scheduling of doses; a spacer device may be utilized to maximize effectiveness.

**Related Information**

Inhalant (Asthma, Bronchospasm) Agents *on page 1388*


- **Salmonine® Injection** *see* Calcitonin *on page 182*
- **Salofalk** *see* Aminosalicylate Sodium *on page 70*
- **Sal-Plant® Gel** *see page 1294*

## Salsalate (SAL sa late)

**U.S. Brand Names** Argesic®-SA; Artha-G®; Disalcid®; Marthritic®; Mono-Gesic®; Salflex®; Salgesic®; Salsitab®

**Synonyms** Disalicylic Acid

**Therapeutic Category** Salicylate

**Pregnancy Risk Factor** C

**Lactation** Enters breast milk/contraindicated

**Use** Treatment of minor pain or fever; arthritis

**Mechanism of Action/Effect** Inhibits prostaglandin synthesis, acts on the hypothalamus heat-regulating center to reduce fever, blocks prostaglandin synthetase action which prevents formation of the platelet-aggregating substance thromboxane $A_2$

**Contraindications** Hypersensitivity to salsalate

**Warnings** Use with caution in patients with platelet and bleeding disorders, renal dysfunction, erosive gastritis, or peptic ulcer disease. Previous nonreaction does not guarantee future safe taking of medication. Pregnancy factor C.

**Drug Interactions**

**Decreased Effect:** Decreased effect with urinary alkalinizers, antacids, and corticosteroids. Decreased effect of uricosurics and spironolactone.

**Increased Effect/Toxicity:** Increased effect/toxicity of oral anticoagulants, hypoglycemics, and methotrexate.

**Food Interactions** Salsalate peak serum levels may be delayed if taken with food.

**Effects on Lab Values** False-negative results for glucose oxidase urinary glucose tests (Clinistix®); false-positives using the cupric sulfate method (Clinitest®); also, interferes with Gerhardt test, VMA determination; 5-HIAA, xylose tolerance test and $T_3$ and $T_4$

**Adverse Reactions**

>10%: Gastrointestinal: Nausea, heartburn, stomach pains, heartburn

1% to 10%:

- Central nervous system: Drowsiness
- Dermatologic: Rash
- Gastrointestinal: Gastrointestinal ulceration
- Hematologic: Hemolytic anemia
- Neuromuscular & skeletal: Weakness
- Respiratory: Dyspnea
- Miscellaneous: Anaphylactic shock

<1% (Limited to important or life-threatening symptoms): Leukopenia, thrombocytopenia, iron deficiency anemia, does not appear to inhibit platelet aggregation, occult bleeding, hepatotoxicity, impaired renal function, bronchospasm

**Overdose/Toxicology** Symptoms of overdose include respiratory alkalosis, hyperpnea, tachypnea, tinnitus, headache, hyperpyrexia, metabolic acidosis, hypoglycemia, and coma. Nomograms, such as the "Done" nomogram, can be very helpful for estimating the severity of aspirin poisoning and for directing treatment using serum salicylate levels. Treatment can also be based upon symptomatology.

**Salicylates**

| Toxic Symptoms | Treatment |
|---|---|
| Overdose | Induce emesis with ipecac, and/or lavage with saline, followed with activated charcoal |
| Dehydration | I.V. fluids with KCl (no $D_5W$ only) |
| Metabolic acidosis (must be treated) | Sodium bicarbonate |
| Hyperthermia | Cooling blankets or sponge baths |
| Coagulopathy/hemorrhage | Vitamin K I.V. |
| Hypoglycemia (with coma, seizures, or change in mental status) | Dextrose 25 g I.V. |
| Seizures | Diazepam 5-10 mg I.V. |

**Pharmacodynamics/Kinetics**

**Half-life Elimination:** 7-8 hours

**Metabolism:** Hydrolyzed in the liver to salicylic acid (active)

**Excretion:** Renal

**Onset:** Therapeutic effects occur within 3-4 days of continuous dosing

**Formulations**

Capsule: 500 mg

Tablet: 500 mg, 750 mg

**Dosing**

**Adults:** Oral: 3 g/day in 2-3 divided doses

**Elderly:** Refer to adult dosing.

**Renal Impairment:** In patients with end-stage renal disease undergoing hemodialysis: 750 mg twice daily with an additional 500 mg after dialysis

**Additional Nursing Issues**

**Physical Assessment:** Assess effectiveness and interactions of other medications patient may be taking (see Contraindications and Drug Interactions). Monitor laboratory tests (see above) and therapeutic response (eg, relief of pain and inflammation, increased activity tolerance), and adverse reactions (eg, GI effects, hepatotoxicity) at beginning of therapy and periodically throughout therapy (see Warnings/Precautions, Adverse Reactions, and Overdose/Toxicology). Schedule ophthalmic evaluations for patients who develop eye complaints during long-term NSAID therapy. Assess knowledge/teach patient appropriate use, interventions to reduce side effects, and adverse symptoms to report. **Pregnancy risk factor C** - benefits of use must outweigh possible risks. Breast-feeding is contraindicated.

**Patient Information/Instruction:** Take this medication exactly as directed; do not increase dose without consulting prescriber. Do not crush tablets or break capsules. Take with food or milk to reduce GI distress. Maintain adequate fluid intake (2-3 L/day of fluids unless instructed to restrict fluid intake). Do not use alcohol, aspirin, or aspirin-containing medication, and all other anti-inflammatory medications without consulting prescriber. You may experience drowsiness (use caution when driving or engaging in tasks requiring alertness until response to drug is known); nausea or heartburn (frequent small meals, frequent mouth care, sucking lozenges, or chewing gum may help). GI bleeding, ulceration, or perforation can occur with or without pain; discontinue medication and contact prescriber if persistent abdominal pain or cramping, or blood in stool occurs. Report breathlessness or difficulty breathing; unusual bruising/bleeding; blood in urine, stool, mouth, or vomitus; unusual fatigue; skin rash or itching; change in urinary pattern; or change in hearing or ringing in ears. **Pregnancy/breast-feeding precautions:** Inform prescriber if you are or intend to be pregnant. Do not breast-feed.

**Geriatric Considerations:** Elderly are at high risk for adverse effects from nonsteroidal anti-inflammatory agents. As much as 60% of elderly can develop peptic ulceration and/or hemorrhage asymptomatically. The concomitant use of $H_2$ blockers, omeprazole, and sucralfate is not effective as prophylaxis with the exception of NSAID-induced duodenal ulcers which may be prevented by the use of ranitidine. Misoprostol is the only prophylactic agent proven effective. Also, concomitant disease and drug use contribute to the risk for GI adverse effects. Use lowest effective dose for shortest period possible. Consider renal function decline with age. Use of NSAIDs can compromise existing renal function especially when $Cl_{cr}$ is ≤30 mL/minute. Tinnitus may be a difficult and unreliable indication of toxicity due to age-related hearing loss or eighth cranial nerve damage. CNS adverse effects such as confusion, agitation, and hallucinations are generally seen in overdose or high-dose situations, but elderly may demonstrate these adverse effects at lower doses than younger adults.

**Breast-feeding Issues:** Salsalate is metabolized to salicylate which is contraindicated while breast-feeding.

**Related Information**

Nonsalicylate/Nonsteroidal Anti-inflammatory Comparison *on page 1401*

- **Salsitab®** *see* Salsalate *on previous page*
- **Sandimmune® Injection** *see* Cyclosporine *on page 317*
- **Sandimmune® Oral** *see* Cyclosporine *on page 317*
- **Sandimmun Neoral®** *see* Cyclosporine *on page 317*
- **Sandoglobulin®** *see* Immune Globulin, Intravenous *on page 602*
- **Sandoglobulina®** *see* Immune Globulin, Intravenous *on page 602*
- **Sandostatin®** *see* Octreotide *on page 845*
- **Sandostatina®** *see* Octreotide *on page 845*
- **Sandostatin LAR®** *see* Octreotide *on page 845*
- **Sang CyA®** *see* Cyclosporine *on page 317*
- **Sani-Supp® Suppository** *see page 1294*
- **Sanorex®** *see* Mazindol *on page 708*
- **Sansert®** *see* Methysergide *on page 757*
- **Santyl®** *see* Collagenase *on page 303*

## Saquinavir (sa KWIN a veer)

**U.S. Brand Names** Fortovase®; Invirase®

**Therapeutic Category** Antiretroviral Agent, Protease Inhibitor

**Pregnancy Risk Factor** B

**Lactation** Enters breast milk/contraindicated

**Use** In combination with other retroviral agents in the treatment of advanced HIV infection in selected patients based on changes in surrogate markers. In a randomized, double-blind study of 297 patients, a triple drug combination of saquinavir, zalcitabine, and zidovudine reduced HIV-1 replication, increased CD4+ cell counts, and decreased levels of activation markers in serum more than did treatment with zidovudine and either saquinavir or zalcitabine; postexposure chemoprophylaxis following occupational exposure to HIV

**Mechanism of Action/Effect** As an inhibitor of HIV protease, saquinavir prevents the cleavage of viral polyprotein precursors which are needed to generate functional proteins in and maturation of HIV-infected cells

**Contraindications** Hypersensitivity to saquinavir or any component; exposure to direct sunlight without sunblock or protective clothing; do not administer concurrently with terfenadine, cisapride, astemizole, triazolam, midazolam, or ergot derivatives

**Warnings** Spontaneous bleeding episodes have been reported in patients with hemophilia receiving an HIV protease inhibitor. New onset diabetes mellitus, exacerbation of diabetes, and hyperglycemia have been reported in HIV-infected patients receiving protease inhibitors. May exacerbate pre-existing hepatic dysfunction. Use caution in hepatitis B or C and cirrhosis.

**Drug Interactions**

**Cytochrome P-450 Effect:** CYP3A3/4 enzyme substrate; CYP3A3/4 enzyme inhibitor

**Decreased Effect:** Rifampin may decrease saquinavir's plasma levels and AUC by 40% to 80%. Nevirapine, rifabutin, phenobarbital, phenytoin, dexamethasone, or

(Continued)

## Saquinavir *(Continued)*

carbamazepine may decrease saquinavir concentrations. May decrease delavirdine concentrations.

**Increased Effect/Toxicity:** Ketoconazole significantly increases plasma levels and AUC of saquinavir. As a known, although not potent inhibitor of the cytochrome P-450 system, saquinavir may decrease the metabolism of terfenadine and astemizole resulting in rare but serious cardiac arrhythmias. Other drugs which may have increased serum levels and adverse effects if coadministered with saquinavir include calcium channel blockers, clindamycin, dapsone, quinidine, triazolam. Ketoconazole, clarithromycin, indinavir, delavirdine may increase saquinavir levels. Concurrent administration may increase nelfinavir (~18%) and substantially increase saquinavir (392%). Ritonavir increases AUC of saquinavir at least 17-fold. Avoid ergot alkaloids.

**Food Interactions** Administer within 2 hours of a meal (a high fat meal maximizes bioavailability). Saquinavir levels may increase if taken with grapefruit juice.

**Adverse Reactions**

1% to 10%:

Dermatologic: Rash

Endocrine & metabolic: Hyperglycemia, elevated CPK

Gastrointestinal: Diarrhea, abdominal discomfort, nausea, abdominal pain, buccal mucosa, ulceration

Neuromuscular & skeletal: Paresthesia, weakness

<1% (Limited to important or life-threatening symptoms): Seizures, fever, Stevens-Johnson syndrome, acute myeloblastic leukemia, hemolytic anemia, thrombocytopenia, jaundice, ascites, exacerbation of chronic liver disease, elevated LFTs, creatine phosphokinase; altered AST, ALT, bilirubin, hemoglobin, bullous skin eruption, polyarthritis, portal hypertension

Protease inhibitors cause hyperglycemia and lyslipidemia (elevated cholesterol/triglycerides) and a redistribution of fat (protease paunch, buffalo hump, facial atrophy and breast engorgement)

**Pharmacodynamics/Kinetics**

**Protein Binding:** 98%

**Distribution:** Widely distributed; minimal CSF penetration

**Half-life Elimination:** 13 hours

**Metabolism:** Liver

**Excretion:** Feces and urine

**Formulations**

Capsule, as mesylate: 200 mg

Capsule, soft gelatin (Fortovase®): 200 mg

**Dosing**

**Adults:** Oral

Invirase®: 600 mg 3 times/day; lower doses (<1800 mg/day) have not demonstrated effective antiviral therapy

Fortovase®: 1200 mg 3 times/day

Use in combination with a nucleoside analog (AZT or ddC)

**Administration**

**Oral:** Take saquinavir within 2 hours after a full meal. Avoid direct sunlight when taking saquinavir.

**Stability**

**Storage:**

Fortovase®: Store in refrigerator. Storage at room temperature is stable for 3 months.

Invirase®: Store at room temperature.

**Monitoring Laboratory Tests** CBC, renal and liver function, electrolytes, triglycerides, cholesterol, glucose, CD4 cell count, plasma levels of HIV RNA

**Additional Nursing Issues**

**Physical Assessment:** Monitor laboratory results on a regular basis. Assess effectiveness of other medications patient may be taking for possible decreased or toxic effects (see Drug Interactions). Monitor for effectiveness of therapy and adverse reactions, including opportunistic infections and glucose levels for diabetic patients (see Warnings/Precautions and Adverse Reactions). Contraindicated for breast-feeding women. Saquinavir is only used to treat patients with HIV and the CDC recommends that women with HIV not nurse to prevent transmission of HIV.

**Patient Information/Instruction:** Saquinavir is is not a cure for HIV nor has it been found to reduce transmission of HIV. Take as directed, with food. Diabetics will need to monitor glucose levels frequently while taking this medication; this medication may exacerbate diabetes and hyperglycemia. You may experience headache or confusion; if these persist notify prescriber. You may develop sensitivity to sunlight (wear protective clothing, use sunblock, or avoid direct sunlight); mouth sores (frequent oral care is necessary). Report persistent nausea, vomiting, abdominal pain, or diarrhea; skin rash or irritation; muscles weakness or tremors; easy bruising or bleeding; fever or chills; yellowing of eyes or skin; or dark urine or pale stools. **Breast-feeding precautions:** Do not breast-feed.

**Breast-feeding Issues:** The CDC recommends **not** to breast-feed if diagnosed with HIV to avoid postnatal transmission of the virus.

**Additional Information** The indication for saquinavir for the treatment of HIV infection is based on changes in surrogate markers. At present, there are no results from controlled clinical trials evaluating the effect of regimens containing saquinavir on patient survival or the clinical progression of HIV infection, such as the occurrence of opportunistic infections or malignancies. In cell culture, saquinavir is additive to synergistic with AZT, ddC, and DDI without enhanced toxicity.

**Related Information**

Antiretroviral Agents Comparison *on page 1373*

## Sargramostim (sar GRAM oh stim)

**U.S. Brand Names** Leukine™

**Synonyms** GM-CSF; Granulocyte-Macrophage Colony Stimulating Factor; RGM-CSF

**Therapeutic Category** Colony Stimulating Factor

**Pregnancy Risk Factor** C

**Lactation** Excretion in breast milk unknown

**Use**

**Myeloid reconstitution after autologous bone marrow transplantation:**

Non-Hodgkin's lymphoma (NHL)
Acute lymphoblastic leukemia (ALL)
Hodgkin's lymphoma
Metastatic breast cancer

**Peripheral stem cell transplantation**

Metastatic breast cancer
Non-Hodgkin's lymphoma
Hodgkin's lymphoma
Multiple myeloma

Although GM-CSF has been demonstrated to accelerate myeloid engraftment in autologous bone marrow transplant, decrease median duration of antibiotic administration, reduce the median duration of infectious episodes, and shorten the median duration of hospitalization, no difference in relapse rate or survival or disease response has been found in placebo-controlled trials. Safety and efficacy of GM-CSF given simultaneously with cytotoxic chemotherapy have not been established. Concurrent treatment may increase myelosuppression.

**Mechanism of Action/Effect** Stimulates proliferation, differentiation and functional activity of neutrophils, eosinophils, monocytes, and macrophages; see table.

| Proliferation/Differentiation | G-CSF (Filgrastim) | GM-CSF (Sargramostim) |
|---|---|---|
| Neutrophils | Yes | Yes |
| Eosinophils | No | Yes |
| Macrophages | No | Yes |
| Neutrophil migration | Enhanced | Inhibited |

**Contraindications** Hypersensitivity to GM-CSF, yeast-derived products, or any component; patients with excessive myeloid blasts (>30%) in the bone marrow or peripheral blood

**Warnings** Do **not** administer 24 hours prior to or after chemotherapy or 12 hours prior to or after radiation therapy. Use with caution in patients with pre-existing cardiac problems, hypoxia, fluid retention, pulmonary infiltrates or CHF, renal or hepatic impairment. rapid increase in peripheral blood counts. If ANC is >20,000/mm$^3$, or platelets >500,000/mm$^3$ decrease dose by 50% or discontinue drug (counts will fall to normal within 3-7 days after discontinuing drug). Growth factor potential: caution with myeloid malignancies. Precaution should be exercised in the usage of GM-CSF in any malignancy with myeloid characteristics. GM-CSF can potentially act as a growth factor for any tumor type, particularly myeloid malignancies. Tumors of nonhematopoietic origin may have surface receptors for GM-CSF. Pregnancy factor C.

**Drug Interactions**

**Increased Effect/Toxicity:** Lithium, corticosteroids may potentiate myeloproliferative effects.

**Adverse Reactions**

>10%:

"First-dose" effects: Fever, hypotension, tachycardia, rigors, flushing, nausea, vomiting, dyspnea
Central nervous system: Neutropenic fever
Dermatologic: Alopecia
Endocrine & metabolic: Polydipsia
Gastrointestinal: Nausea, vomiting, diarrhea, stomatitis, GI hemorrhage, mucositis
Neuromuscular & skeletal: Bone pain, myalgia

1% to 10%:

Cardiovascular: Chest pain, peripheral edema, capillary leak syndrome
Central nervous system: Headache
Dermatologic: Rash
Endocrine & metabolic: Fluid retention
Gastrointestinal: Anorexia, sore throat, constipation
Hematologic: Leukocytosis
Local: Pain at injection site
Neuromuscular & skeletal: Weakness
Respiratory: Dyspnea, cough

<1% (Limited to important or life-threatening symptoms): Hypotension, flushing, pericardial effusion, transient supraventricular arrhythmias, pericarditis

**Overdose/Toxicology** Symptoms of overdose include dyspnea, malaise, nausea, fever, headache, and chills. Discontinue drug and wait for levels to fall. Treatment is supportive. Monitor CBC, respiratory symptoms, and fluid status. Discontinue drug and wait for levels to fall, monitor for pulmonary edema. Toxicity of GM-CSF is dose-dependent.

(Continued)

## Sargramostim *(Continued)*

Severe reactions such as capillary leak syndrome are seen at higher doses (>15 mcg/kg/day).

**Pharmacodynamics/Kinetics**

**Half-life Elimination:** 2 hours

**Time to Peak:** S.C.: Within 1-2 hours

**Onset:** Increase in WBC in 7-14 days

**Duration:** WBC will return to baseline within 1 week after discontinuing drug.

**Formulations** Injection: 250 mcg, 500 mcg

**Dosing**

**Adults:**

I.V. infusion over ≥2 hours or S.C.:

Existing clinical data suggest that starting GM-CSF between 24 and 72 hours subsequent to chemotherapy may provide optimal neutrophil recover. Continue therapy until the occurrence of an absolute neutrophil count of 10,000/μL after the neutrophil nadir.

**The available data suggest that rounding the dose to the nearest vial size may enhance patient convenience and reduce costs without clinical detrement.**

**Myeloid reconstitution after peripheral stem cell, allogeneic or autologous bone marrow transplant:** I.V.: 250 mcg/m²/day for 21 days to begin 2-4 hours after the marrow infusion on day 0 of autologous bone marrow transplant or ≥24 hours after chemotherapy or 12 hours after last dose of radiotherapy.

If a severe adverse reaction occurs, reduce or temporarily discontinue the dose until the reaction abates.

If blast cells appear or progression of the underlying disease occurs, disrupt treatment.

Interrupt or reduce the dose by half if ANC is >20,000 cells/mm³

Patients should not receive sargramostim until the postmarrow infusion ANC is <500 cells/mm³.

**Neutrophil recovery following chemotherapy in AML:** I.V.: 250 mg/m²/day over a 4-hour period starting ~day 11 or 4 days following the completion of induction chemotherapy, if day 10 bone marrow is hypoblastic with <5% blasts.

If a second cycle of chemotherapy is necessary, administer ~4 days after the completion of chemotherapy if the bone marrow is hypoblastic with <5% blasts.

Continue sargramostim until ANC is >1500 cells/mm³ for consecutive days or a maximum of 42 days.

Discontinue sargramostim immediately if leukemic regrowth occurs.

If a severe adverse reaction occurs, reduce the dose by 50% or temporarily discontinue the dose until the reaction abates.

**Mobilization of peripheral blood progenitor cells:** I.V.: 250 mcg/m²/day over 24 hours or S.C. once daily.

Continue the same dose through the period of PBPC collection.

The optimal schedule for PBPC collection has not been established (usually begun by day 5 and performed daily until protocol specified targets are achieved).

If WBC >50,000 cells/mm³, reduce the dose by 50%.

If adequate numbers of progenitor cells are not collected, consider other mobilization therapy.

**Postperipheral blood progenitor cell transplantation:** I.V.: 250 mcg/m²/day over 24 hours or S.C. once daily beginning immediately following infusion of progenitor cells and continuing until ANC is >1500 for 3 consecutive days is attained.

**BMT failure or engraftment delay:** I.V.: 250 mcg/m²/day for 14 days as a 2-hour infusion.

The dose can be repeated after 7 days off therapy if engraftment has not occurred.

If engraftment still has not occurred, a third course of 500 mcg/m²/day for 14 days may be tried after another 7 days off therapy; if there is still no improvement, it is unlikely that further dose escalation will be beneficial.

If a severe adverse reaction occurs, reduce or temporarily discontinue the dose until the reaction abates.

If blast cells appear or disease progression occurs, discontinue treatment.

**Administration**

**I.V.:** I.V. infusion should be over at least 2 hours; incompatible with dextrose-containing solutions.

**Other:** Administer by S.C. (undiluted). Do not shake solution. When administering GM-CSF subcutaneously, rotate injection sites.

**Stability**

**Storage:** Sargramostim is available as a sterile, white, preservative-free, lyophilized powder. Sargramostim should be stored at 2°C to 8°C (36°F to 46°F). Vials should not be frozen or shaken.

**Reconstitution:** Sargramostim is stable after dilution in 1 mL of bacteriostatic or nonbacteriostatic sterile water for injection for 30 days at 2°C to 8°C or 25°C. Sargramostim may also be further diluted in 0.9% sodium chloride to a concentration ≥10 mcg/mL for I.V. infusion administration. This diluted solution is stable for 48 hours at room temperature and refrigeration. If the final concentration of sargramostim is <10 mcg/mL, human albumin should be added to the saline prior to the addition of sargramostim to prevent absorption of the components to the delivery system. It is recommended that 1 mg of human albumin per 1 mL of 0.9% sodium chloride (eg, 1 mL of 5% human albumin per 50 mL of 0.9% sodium chloride) be added.

**Standard diluent:** Dose ≥250 mcg/25 mL NS

**Compatibility:** Sargramostim is incompatible with dextrose-containing solutions.

**Monitoring Laboratory Tests** To avoid potential complications of excessive leukocytosis (WBC >50,000 cells/mm$^3$, ANC >20,000 cells/mm$^3$) a CBC with differential is recommended twice per week during therapy. Sargramostim therapy should be interrupted or the dose reduced by half if the ANC is >20,000 cells/mm$^3$. Monitoring of renal and hepatic function in patients displaying renal or hepatic dysfunction prior to initiation of treatment is recommended and at least biweekly during sargramostim administration.

**Additional Nursing Issues**

**Physical Assessment:** Monitor for "first dose effects" (see Dosing) and medicate appropriately. Monitor fluid balance (I & O ratio), weight, CNS response, and GI effects. **Pregnancy risk factor C** - benefits of use should outweigh possible risks. Note breast-feeding caution.

**Patient Information/Instruction:** You may experience bone pain (request analgesic), nausea and vomiting (small frequent meals may help), hair loss (reversible). Report fever, chills, unhealed sores, severe bone pain, difficulty breathing, swelling or pain at infusion site. Avoid crowds or exposure to infected persons; you will be susceptible to infection. **Pregnancy/breast-feeding precautions:** Inform prescriber if you are or intend to be pregnant. Consult prescriber if breast-feeding.

**Pregnancy Issues:** Animal reproduction studies have not been conducted. It is not known whether sargramostim can cause fetal harm when administered to a pregnant woman or can affect reproductive capability. Sargramostim should be given to a pregnant woman only if clearly needed.

**Additional Information**

Reimbursement Hotline (Leukine™): 1-800-321-4669
Professional Services (IMMUNEX): 1-800-334-6273

- **Sarna Topical Lotion** *see page 1294*
- **S.A.S™** *see* Sulfasalazine *on page 1084*
- **SAStid® Plain Therapeutic Shampoo and Acne Wash** *see page 1294*
- **Scabene®** *see* Lindane *on page 678*
- **Scabisan Shampoo** *see* Lindane *on page 678*
- **Scalpicin®** *see* Hydrocortisone *on page 578*
- **Scalpicin®** *see* Topical Corticosteroids *on page 1152*

## Scopolamine (skoe POL a meen)

**U.S. Brand Names** Isopto® Hyoscine Ophthalmic; Transderm Scop® Patch

**Synonyms** Hyoscine

**Therapeutic Category** Anticholinergic Agent

**Pregnancy Risk Factor** C

**Lactation** Enters breast milk/compatible

**Use** Preoperative medication to produce amnesia and decrease salivation and respiratory secretions to produce cycloplegia and mydriasis; treatment of iridocyclitis, prevention of nausea and vomiting by motion; produces more CNS depression, mydriasis, and cycloplegia but less effective in preventing reflex bradycardia and affects the intestines than atropine

**Mechanism of Action/Effect** Blocks the action of acetylcholine at parasympathetic sites in smooth muscle, secretory glands and the CNS; increases cardiac output, dries secretions, antagonizes histamine and serotonin

**Contraindications** Hypersensitivity to scopolamine or any component; narrow-angle glaucoma; acute hemorrhage, GI or GU obstruction; thyrotoxicosis; tachycardia secondary to cardiac insufficiency; paralytic ileus

**Warnings** Use with caution with hepatic or renal impairment since adverse CNS effects occur more often in these patients. Anticholinergic agents are not well tolerated in the elderly and their use should be avoided when possible. Pregnancy factor C.

**Drug Interactions**

**Decreased Effect:** Decreased effect of acetaminophen, levodopa, ketoconazole, digoxin, riboflavin, and potassium chloride in wax matrix preparations.

**Increased Effect/Toxicity:** Additive adverse effects with other anticholinergic agents.

**Adverse Reactions**

**Ophthalmic:**

>10%: Ocular: Blurred vision, photophobia

1% to 10%:
- Ocular: Local irritation, increased intraocular pressure
- Respiratory: Congestion

<1% (Limited to important or life-threatening symptoms): Vascular congestion, edema, drowsiness, eczematoid dermatitis, follicular conjunctivitis, exudate

**Systemic:**

>10%:
- Dermatologic: Dry skin
- Gastrointestinal: Constipation, dry mouth, dry throat
- Local: Irritation at injection site
- Respiratory: Dry nose
- Miscellaneous: Sweating (decreased)

1% to 10%:
- Dermatologic: Increased sensitivity to light
- Endocrine & metabolic: Decreased flow of breast milk
- Gastrointestinal: Dysphagia

<1% (Limited to important or life-threatening symptoms): Orthostatic hypotension, ventricular fibrillation, tachycardia, palpitations, confusion, drowsiness, headache, loss

(Continued)

## Scopolamine *(Continued)*

of memory, ataxia, fatigue, rash, bloated feeling, nausea, vomiting, dysuria, weakness, increased intraocular pain, blurred vision

**Note:** Systemic adverse effects have been reported following ophthalmic administration.

**Overdose/Toxicology** Symptoms of overdose include dilated pupils, flushed skin, tachycardia, hypertension, and EKG abnormalities. CNS manifestations resemble acute psychosis. CNS depression, circulatory collapse, respiratory failure, and death can occur. For a scopolamine overdose with severe life-threatening symptoms, physostigmine 1-2 mg S.C. or I.V. slowly should be given to reverse toxic effects.

**Pharmacodynamics/Kinetics**

**Time to Peak:** Peak effect: 20-60 minutes; it may take 3-7 days for full recovery

**Metabolism:** Liver

**Excretion:** Urine

**Onset:** Onset of effect: Oral, I.M.: 0.5-1 hour; I.V.: 10 minutes

**Duration:** Oral, I.M.: 4-6 hours; I.V.: 2 hours; Transdermal: 3 days

**Formulations**

Disc, transdermal: 1.5 mg/disc (4's)

Injection, as hydrobromide: 0.3 mg/mL (1 mL); 0.4 mg/mL (0.5 mL, 1 mL); 0.86 mg/mL (0.5 mL); 1 mg/mL (1 mL)

Solution, ophthalmic, as hydrobromide: 0.25% (5 mL, 15 mL)

**Dosing**

**Adults:**

Preoperatively: I.M., I.V., S.C.: 0.3-0.65 mg; may be repeated every 4-6 hours

Motion sickness: Transdermal: Apply 1 disc behind the ear at least 4 hours prior to exposure and every 3 days as needed; effective if applied as soon as 2-3 hours before anticipated need, best if 12 hours before.

Ophthalmic:

Refraction: Instill 1-2 drops of 0.25% to eye(s) 1 hour before procedure.

Iridocyclitis: Instill 1-2 drops of 0.25% to eye(s) up to 4 times/day.

**Elderly:** Avoid use; see Geriatric Considerations.

**Administration**

**I.V.:** Inject over 2-3 minutes.

**I.V. Detail:** Dilute with an equal volume of sterile water and give by direct I.V.

**Topical:** Topical disc is programmed to deliver *in vivo* 0.5 mg over 3 days. Once applied, do not remove the patch for 3 full days.

**Stability**

**Reconstitution:** Avoid acid solutions, because hydrolysis occurs at pH <3.

**Compatibility:** Physically compatible when mixed in the same syringe with atropine, butorphanol, chlorpromazine, dimenhydrinate, diphenhydramine, droperidol, fentanyl, glycopyrrolate, hydromorphone, hydroxyzine, meperidine, metoclopramide, morphine, pentazocine, pentobarbital, perphenazine, prochlorperazine, promazine, promethazine, or thiopental.

**Additional Nursing Issues**

**Physical Assessment:** Assess other medications patient may be taking for effectiveness and interactions (see Warnings/Precautions and Drug Interactions). When used preoperatively, advise patient about blurred vision, closely monitor patient safety (side rails up, call light within reach, etc), and monitor adverse effects.

Ophthalmic, transdermal, oral: Monitor therapeutic response and adverse reactions (see Adverse Reactions and Overdose/Toxicology). Assess knowledge/teach patient appropriate use, interventions to reduce side effects, and adverse symptoms to report.

**Pregnancy risk factor C** - benefits of use should outweigh possible risks. (Systemic effects have been reported following ophthalmic administration.)

**Patient Information/Instruction:** Take as directed (see Administration). You may experience drowsiness, confusion, impaired judgment, or vision changes (use caution when driving or engaging in tasks requiring alertness until response to drug is known); dry mouth, nausea, or vomiting (small frequent meals, frequent mouth care, chewing gum, or sucking lozenges may help); orthostatic hypotension (use caution when climbing stairs and when rising from lying or sitting position); constipation (increased exercise, fluid, or dietary fiber may reduce constipation, if not effective consult prescriber); increased sensitivity to heat and decreased perspiration (avoid extremes of heat, reduce exercise in hot weather); decreased milk if breast-feeding. Report hot, dry, flushed skin; blurred vision or vision changes; difficulty swallowing; chest pain, palpitations, or rapid heartbeat; painful or difficult urination; increased confusion, depression, or loss of memory; rapid or difficult respirations; muscle weakness or tremors; or eye pain.

**Administration:** Transdermal: Apply patch behind ear the day before traveling. Wash hands before applying and avoid contact with the eyes. Do not remove for 3 days.

Ophthalmic: Instill as often as recommended. Wash hands before using. Sit or lie down, open eye, look at ceiling, and instill prescribed amount of solution. Do not blink for 30 seconds, close eye and roll eye in all directions, and apply gentle pressure to inner corner of eye for 1-2 minutes. Do not let tip of applicator touch eye or contaminate tip of applicator. Temporary stinging or blurred vision may occur.

**Pregnancy precautions:** Inform prescriber if you are or intend to be pregnant.

**Geriatric Considerations:** Because of its long duration of action as a mydriatic agent, it should be avoided in elderly patients. Anticholinergic agents are not well tolerated in the elderly and their use should be avoided when possible.

**Related Information**

Antiemetics for Chemotherapy-Induced Nausea and Vomiting *on page 1307*

Ophthalmic Agents *on page 1282*

- **Scopolamine, Hyoscyamine, Atropine, and Phenobarbital** *see* Hyoscyamine, Atropine, Scopolamine, and Phenobarbital *on page 591*
- **Scot-Tussin® [OTC]** *see* Guaifenesin *on page 548*
- **Scot-Tussin DM® Cough Chasers** *see page 1294*
- **Scot-Tussin® Senior Clear [OTC]** *see* Guaifenesin and Dextromethorphan *on page 549*
- **SeaMist®** *see page 1294*
- **Sebizon® Topical Lotion** *see* Sulfacetamide *on page 1080*
- **Sebulex®** *see page 1294*
- **Sebulon®** *see page 1294*

## Secobarbital (see koe BAR bi tal)

**U.S. Brand Names** Seconal™ Injection

**Synonyms** Quinalbarbitone Sodium

**Therapeutic Category** Barbiturate

**Pregnancy Risk Factor** D

**Lactation** Enters breast milk/use caution (AAP rates "compatible")

**Use** Short-term treatment of insomnia and as preanesthetic agent

**Mechanism of Action/Effect** Interferes with transmission of impulses from the thalamus to the cortex of the brain resulting in an imbalance in central inhibitory and facilitatory mechanisms

**Contraindications** Hypersensitivity to secobarbital or any component; CNS depression; uncontrolled pain; pregnancy with toxemia or bleeding

**Warnings** Use with caution in patients with hypovolemic shock, congestive heart failure, hepatic impairment, respiratory dysfunction or depression, previous addiction to the sedative/hypnotic group, chronic or acute pain, renal dysfunction, and the elderly. Tolerance or psychological and physical dependence may occur with prolonged use.

**Drug Interactions**

**Decreased Effect:** Decreased effect of betamethasone and other corticosteroids, tricyclic antidepressants, chloramphenicol, estrogens, cyclophosphamide, oral anticoagulants, doxycycline, and theophylline.

**Increased Effect/Toxicity:** Increased effect/toxicity with CNS depressants, chloramphenicol, and chlorpropamide.

**Adverse Reactions**

>10%: Central nervous system: Dizziness, clumsiness or unsteadiness, lightheadedness, "hangover" effect, drowsiness

1% to 10%:

Central nervous system: Confusion, mental depression, unusual excitement, nervousness, faint feeling, headache, insomnia, nightmares

Gastrointestinal: Nausea, vomiting, constipation

<1% (Limited to important or life-threatening symptoms): Exfoliative dermatitis, Stevens-Johnson syndrome, agranulocytosis, megaloblastic anemia, thrombocytopenia, laryngospasm, respiratory depression, apnea (especially with rapid I.V. use)

**Overdose/Toxicology** Symptoms of overdose include unsteady gait, slurred speech, confusion, jaundice, hypothermia, fever, hypotension, respiratory depression, and coma. Charcoal hemoperfusion or hemodialysis may be useful, especially in the presence of very high serum barbiturate levels when the patient is in shock, coma, or renal failure. Forced alkaline diuresis is of no value in the treatment of intoxications with short-acting barbiturates.

**Pharmacodynamics/Kinetics**

**Protein Binding:** 45% to 60%

**Distribution:** Crosses the placenta

**Half-life Elimination:** 25 hours

**Time to Peak:** Within 2-4 hours

**Metabolism:** Liver

**Excretion:** Renally as inactive metabolites and small amounts as unchanged drug

**Onset:** Onset of hypnosis: Oral: Within 1-3 minutes; I.V. injection: Within 15-30 minutes

**Duration:** ~15 minutes

**Formulations** Injection, as sodium: 50 mg/mL (2 mL)

**Dosing**

**Adults:** Hypnotic:

I.M.: 100-200 mg/dose

I.V.: 50-250 mg/dose

**Elderly:** Not recommended for use in the elderly (see Geriatric Considerations).

**Renal Impairment:** Slightly dialyzable (5% to 20%)

**Administration**

**I.V.:** Maximum infusion rate: 50 mg/15 seconds; avoid intra-arterial injection.

**I.V. Detail:** Give undiluted or diluted with sterile water for injection, normal saline, or Ringer's injection.

**Stability**

**Reconstitution:** Do not shake vial during reconstitution, rotate ampul. Aqueous solutions are not stable, reconstitute with aqueous polyethylene glycol. Aqueous (sterile water) solutions should be used within 30 minutes. Do not use bacteriostatic water for injection or lactated Ringer's.

(Continued)

## Secobarbital *(Continued)*

**Compatibility:** I.V. form is incompatible when mixed with benzquinamide (in syringe), cimetidine (same syringe), codeine, erythromycin, glycopyrrolate (same syringe), hydrocortisone, insulin, levorphanol, methadone, norepinephrine, pentazocine, phenytoin, sodium bicarbonate, tetracycline, and vancomycin. See the Compatibility of Drugs in Syringe Chart *on page 1317*.

**Additional Nursing Issues**

**Physical Assessment:** Assess effectiveness and interactions of other medications (see Drug Interactions). See Contraindications and Warnings/Precautions for cautious use. Assess for history of addiction; long-term use can result in dependence, abuse, or tolerance. Evaluate periodically for need for continued use. After long-term use, taper dosage slowly when discontinuing.

I.V. (see Administration): Monitor infusion site frequently (keep patient under observation - monitor vital signs, CNS, cardiac and respiratory status), observe safety/seizure precautions, and monitor effectiveness and adverse reactions.

Oral: For inpatient use, institute safety measures (side rails, night light, call bell, assistance with ambulation). For outpatient use, monitor effectiveness and adverse reactions (see Adverse Reactions) at beginning of therapy and periodically with long-term use. Assess knowledge/teach patient appropriate use, interventions to reduce side effects, and adverse symptoms to report. **Pregnancy risk factor D** - assess knowledge/teach both male and female appropriate use of barrier contraceptives. Note breast-feeding caution.

**Patient Information/Instruction:** I.V.: Patient instruction and information is determined by patient condition and therapeutic purpose.

Oral: Use exactly as directed (do not increase dose or frequency or discontinue without consulting prescriber); may cause physical and/or psychological dependence. While using this medication, do not use alcohol or other prescription or OTC medications (especially, pain medications, sedatives, antihistamines, or hypnotics) without consulting prescriber. Maintain adequate hydration (2-3 L/day of fluids unless instructed to restrict fluid intake). You may experience drowsiness, dizziness, or blurred vision (use caution when driving or engaging in tasks requiring alertness until response to drug is known); nausea or vomiting (small frequent meals, frequent mouth care, chewing gum, or sucking lozenges may help); constipation (increased exercise, fluids, or dietary fruit and fiber may help). Report skin rash or irritation; CNS changes (confusion, depression, increased sedation, excitation, headache, insomnia, or nightmares); difficulty breathing or shortness of breath; difficulty swallowing or feeling of tightness in throat; unusual weakness or unusual bleeding in mouth, urine, or stool; or other unanticipated adverse effects. **Pregnancy/breast-feeding precautions:** Do not get pregnant while taking this medication. Use appropriate barrier contraceptive measures. Consult prescriber if breast-feeding.

**Geriatric Considerations:** Use of this agent in the elderly is not recommended due to its long half-life and addiction potential.

**Related Information**

Antipsychotic Medication Guidelines *on page 1436*

- **Secobarbital and Amobarbital** *see* Amobarbital and Secobarbital *on page 78*
- **Seconal®** *see* Secobarbital *on previous page*
- **Seconal™ Injection** *see* Secobarbital *on previous page*
- **Secran®** *see* Vitamin, Multiple *on page 1219*
- **Secretin** *see page 1248*
- **Secretin Ferring Powder** *see page 1248*
- **Sectral®** *see* Acebutolol *on page 31*
- **Sedapap-10®** *see* Butalbital Compound and Acetaminophen *on page 175*
- **Sefulken** *see* Diazoxide *on page 357*
- **Selax®** *see* Docusate *on page 392*
- **Selected Adverse Effects** *see page 1339*
- **Selected Over-the-Counter Products** *see page 1294*
- **Selected Prescription Combination Products** *see page 1306*

## Selegiline (seh LEDGE ah leen)

**U.S. Brand Names** Eldepryl®

**Synonyms** Deprenyl; L-Deprenyl

**Therapeutic Category** Antidepressant, Monoamine Oxidase Inhibitor; Anti-Parkinson's Agent (Monoamine Oxidase Inhibitor)

**Pregnancy Risk Factor** C

**Lactation** Excretion in breast milk unknown

**Use** Adjunct in the management of parkinsonian patients in which levodopa/carbidopa therapy is deteriorating

**Unlabeled use:** Early Parkinson's disease

**Investigational use:** Selegiline is being studied in Alzheimer's disease. Small studies have shown some improvement in behavioral and cognitive performance in patients, however, further study is needed.

**Mechanism of Action/Effect** Potent monoamine oxidase (MAO) Type B inhibitor; MAO-B plays a major role in the metabolism of dopamine; selegiline may also increase dopaminergic activity by interfering with dopamine reuptake at the synapse

**Contraindications** Hypersensitivity to selegiline; concomitant use of meperidine

**Warnings** Increased risk of nonselective MAO inhibition occurs with doses >10 mg/day. A monoamine oxidase inhibitor type "B", there should **not** be a problem with tyramine-containing products as long as the typical doses are employed. Pregnancy factor C.

**Drug Interactions**

**Cytochrome P-450 Effect:** CYP2D6 enzyme substrate

**Increased Effect/Toxicity:** Meperidine in combination with selegiline has caused agitation, delirium, and death; it may be prudent to avoid other opioids as well. MAO inhibitors or tricyclic antidepressants taken with selegiline have been associated with increased CNS toxicity. Selective serotonin reuptake inhibitors, like fluoxetine have increased vasopressor effect and should be avoided. Potential for serotonin syndrome if combined with other serotonergic drugs. Avoid tyramine-containing foods (potential for reactions).

**Food Interactions** Case reports of clinically severe blood pressure elevations have occurred if selegiline is taken with tyramine-containing foods. The risk is increased with higher doses of selegiline. Generally not a problem; however, it is possible and has been reported rarely.

**Adverse Reactions**

>10%:

Central nervous system: Mood changes, dizziness
Gastrointestinal: Nausea, vomiting, dry mouth, abdominal pain
Neuromuscular & skeletal: Dyskinesias

1% to 10%:

Cardiovascular: Orthostatic hypotension, arrhythmias, hypertension, chest pain, bradycardia, peripheral edema, tardive dyskinesia
Central nervous system: Hallucinations, confusion, depression, insomnia, agitation, loss of balance, headache, drowsiness, weakness
Dermatologic: Photosensitivity, rash
Gastrointestinal: GI bleeding, diarrhea or constipation, heartburn, circumoral paresthesias, taste changes
Genitourinary: Prostatic hypertrophy, dysuria, polyuria
Neuromuscular & skeletal: Increased involuntary movements, bradykinesia, muscle twitches, coordination difficulties
Ocular: Blepharospasm, blurred vision or diplopia
Otic: Tinnitus
Respiratory: Asthma
Miscellaneous: Bruxism, sweating

**Overdose/Toxicology** Symptoms of overdose include tachycardia, palpitations, muscle twitching, and seizures. Both hypertension or hypotension can occur with intoxication. While treating hypertension, care is warranted to avoid sudden drops in blood pressure, since this may worsen MAO inhibitor toxicity. Cardiac arrhythmias are best treated with phenytoin or procainamide. Treatment is generally symptom directed and supportive.

**Pharmacodynamics/Kinetics**

**Half-life Elimination:** 9 minutes

**Metabolism:** Liver

**Excretion:** Urine

**Onset:** Onset of therapeutic effects: Within 1 hour

**Duration:** 24-72 hours

**Formulations** Capsule, as hydrochloride: 5 mg

**Dosing**

**Adults:** Oral: 5 mg twice daily with breakfast and lunch or 10 mg in the morning

**Elderly:** Oral: Initial: 5 mg in the morning; may increase to a total of 10 mg/day.

**Additional Nursing Issues**

**Physical Assessment:** Assess effectiveness and interactions of other medications patient may be taking (see Warnings/Precautions and Drug Interactions). Monitor therapeutic response (eg, mental status, involuntary movements), and adverse reactions at beginning of therapy and periodically throughout therapy (see Warnings/Precautions, Adverse Reactions, and Overdose/Toxicology). Patient should be cautioned against eating foods high in tyramine. See Tyramine Foods List *on page 1422*. Assess knowledge/teach patient appropriate use, interventions to reduce side effects, and adverse symptoms to report. **Pregnancy risk factor C** - benefits of use should outweigh possible risks. Note breast-feeding caution.

**Patient Information/Instruction:** Take exactly as directed (may be prescribed in conjunction with levodopa/carbidopa); do not change dosage or discontinue without consulting prescriber. Therapeutic effects may take several weeks or months to achieve and you may need frequent monitoring during first weeks of therapy. Take with meals if GI upset occurs, before meals if dry mouth occurs, after eating if drooling or if nausea occurs. Take at the same time each day. Avoid tyramine-containing foods (low potential for reaction). Maintain adequate hydration (2-3 L/day of fluids unless instructed to restrict fluid intake); void before taking medication. Do not use alcohol and prescription or OTC sedatives or CNS depressants without consulting prescriber. You may experience drowsiness, dizziness, confusion, or vision changes (use caution when driving, climbing stairs, or engaging in tasks requiring alertness until response to drug is known); orthostatic hypotension (use caution when changing position - rising to standing from sitting or lying); constipation (increased exercise, fluids, or dietary fruit and fiber may help); runny nose or flu-like symptoms (consult prescriber for appropriate relief); nausea, vomiting, loss of appetite, or stomach discomfort (small frequent meals, frequent mouth care, chewing gum, or sucking lozenges may help). Report unresolved constipation or vomiting; chest pain, palpitations, irregular heartbeat; CNS changes (hallucination, loss of memory, seizures, acute headache, nervousness, etc);

(Continued)

## Selegiline *(Continued)*

painful or difficult urination; increased muscle spasticity, rigidity, or involuntary movements; skin rash; or significant worsening of condition. **Pregnancy/breast-feeding precautions:** Inform prescriber if you are or intend to be pregnant. Consult prescriber if breast-feeding.

**Geriatric Considerations:** Selegiline is also being studied in Alzheimer's disease, but further studies are needed to assess its usefulness. Do not use at daily doses exceeding 10 mg/day because of the risks associated with nonselective inhibition of MAO.

**Related Information**

Tyramine Foods List *on page 1422*

- **Selenium Sulfide** *see page 1294*
- **Seloken** *see* Metoprolol *on page 761*
- **Selopres** *see* Metoprolol *on page 761*
- **Selsun®** *see page 1294*
- **Selsun Blue®** *see page 1294*
- **Selsun Gold® for Women** *see page 1294*
- **Semicid®** *see page 1294*
- **Semprex®-D** *see* Acrivastine and Pseudoephedrine *on page 38*
- **Semprex-D® Capsule** *see page 1294*
- **Senexon®** *see page 1294*
- **Senna** *see page 1294*
- **Senna-Gen®** *see page 1294*
- **Senokot®** *see page 1294*
- **Senolax®** *see page 1294*
- **Sensibit** *see* Loratadine *on page 689*
- **Sensorcaine®** *see* Bupivacaine *on page 167*
- **Sensorcaine®-MPF** *see* Bupivacaine *on page 167*
- **Septa® Topical Ointment [OTC]** *see* Bacitracin, Neomycin, and Polymyxin B *on page 130*
- **Septra®** *see* Co-trimoxazole *on page 307*
- **Septra® DS** *see* Co-trimoxazole *on page 307*
- **Ser-A-Gen®** *see* Hydralazine, Hydrochlorothiazide, and Reserpine *on page 565*
- **Ser-Ap-Es®** *see* Hydralazine, Hydrochlorothiazide, and Reserpine *on page 565*
- **Serathide®** *see* Hydralazine, Hydrochlorothiazide, and Reserpine *on page 565*
- **Serax®** *see* Oxazepam *on page 868*
- **Serentil®** *see* Mesoridazine *on page 730*
- **Serevent®** *see* Salmeterol *on page 1040*
- **Serevent® Diskus®** *see* Salmeterol *on page 1040*
- **Sermorelin Acetate** *see page 1248*
- **Serocryptin®** *see* Bromocriptine *on page 162*
- **Seromycin® Pulvules®** *see* Cycloserine *on page 316*
- **Serophene®** *see* Clomiphene *on page 286*
- **Seroquel®** *see* Quetiapine *on page 999*
- **Serotonin Syndrome** *see page 1345*
- **Serozide®** *see* Etoposide *on page 463*
- **Serozide®** *see* Etoposide Phosphate *on page 466*
- **Serpalan®** *see* Reserpine *on page 1013*
- **Sertan®** *see* Primidone *on page 964*

## Sertraline (SER tra leen)

**U.S. Brand Names** Zoloft™

**Therapeutic Category** Antidepressant, Selective Serotonin Reuptake Inhibitor

**Pregnancy Risk Factor** C

**Lactation** Enters breast milk/not recommended

**Use** Treatment of major depression; also being studied for use in obesity and obsessive-compulsive disorder

**Mechanism of Action/Effect** Antidepressant with selective inhibitory effects on presynaptic serotonin (5-HT) reuptake

**Contraindications** Hypersensitivity to sertraline or any component; use of MAO inhibitors within 14 days of starting sertraline

**Warnings** Do not use in combination with monoamine oxidase inhibitors or within 14 days of discontinuing or initiating treatment with a monoamine oxidase inhibitor, due to the risk of serotonin syndrome. Use with caution in patients with pre-existing seizure disorders; patients in whom weight loss is undesirable; patients with recent myocardial infarction or unstable heart disease; patients with hepatic or renal impairment; patients taking other psychotropic medications; or agitated or hyperactive patients as the drug may produce or activate mania or hypomania. Because the risk of suicide is inherent in depression, patients should be closely monitored until depressive symptoms remit. Prescriptions should be written for minimum quantities to reduce the risk of overdose. Pregnancy factor C.

**Drug Interactions**

**Cytochrome P-450 Effect:** CYP3A3/4 enzyme substrate, CYP2D6 enzyme substrate (minor); CYP1A2 and 2D6 enzyme inhibitor (weak); CYP2C9, 2C18, 2C19, and 3A3/4 enzyme inhibitor

**Increased Effect/Toxicity:** May inhibits metabolism by CYP isoenzyme 3A4. Drugs metabolized by this system include astemizole, triazolam, and cisapride. Weak inhibitor of CYP2D6 isoenzyme. Drugs metabolized by this system include desipramine, dextromethorphan, haloperidol, imipramine, metoprolol, perphenazine, propafenone, and thioridazine.

MAO inhibitors and possibly use with lithium or tricyclic antidepressants → **serotonin syndrome** serotonergic hyperstimulation with the following clinical features: mental status changes, restlessness, myoclonus, hyper-reflexia, diaphoresis, diarrhea, shivering, and tremor. May decrease metabolism/plasma clearance of some drugs (diazepam, tolbutamide) resulting in increased duration and pharmacological effects. May displace highly plasma protein-bound drugs from binding sites (eg, warfarin) to resulting in an increased anticoagulant effect.

**Food Interactions** Sertraline average peak serum levels may be increased if taken with food.

**Effects on Lab Values** Minor ↑ triglycerides (S), LFTs; ↓ uric acid (S)

**Adverse Reactions** In clinical trials, dizziness and nausea were two of the most frequent side effects that led to discontinuation of therapy.

1% to 10%:

- Cardiovascular: Palpitations
- Central nervous system: Insomnia, agitation, dizziness, headache, somnolence, nervousness, fatigue, pain
- Dermatologic: Dermatological reactions
- Endocrine & metabolic: Sexual dysfunction in men
- Gastrointestinal: Dry mouth, diarrhea or loose stools, nausea, constipation
- Genitourinary: Micturition disorders
- Neuromuscular & skeletal: Tremors
- Ocular: Visual difficulty
- Otic: Tinnitus
- Miscellaneous: Sweating

<1% (Limited to important or life-threatening symptoms): Edema, hypertension, hypotension, postural hypotension, syncope, tachycardia, chest pain, myocardial infarction, coma, convulsions, anemia, elevated AST (SGOT)/ALT (SGPT), bronchospasm, dyspnea

**Overdose/Toxicology** Serious toxicity has not yet been reported. Monitor cardiovascular, gastrointestinal, and hepatic function. There are no specific antidotes for sertraline overdose; treatment should be aimed first at decontamination, then provide symptomatic and supportive care.

**Pharmacodynamics/Kinetics**

**Protein Binding:** 98%

**Half-life Elimination:** Parent: 24 hours; Metabolites: 66 hours

**Time to Peak:** 4.5-8.4 hours

**Metabolism:** Liver

**Excretion:** Renal and hepatic

**Onset:** Steady-state 7 days; therapeutic effects in >2 weeks

**Formulations** Tablet, as hydrochloride: 25 mg, 50 mg, 100 mg

**Dosing**

**Adults:** Oral: Initial: 50 mg/day in the morning; increase by 50 mg/day increments every 2-3 days if tolerated to 100 mg/day; additional increases may be necessary; maximum: 200 mg/day. If somnolence is noted, give at bedtime.

**Elderly:** Oral: Initial: 25 mg/day in the morning; increase by 25 mg/day increments every 2-3 days if tolerated to 75-100 mg/day; additional increases may be necessary; maximum: 200 mg/day.

**Renal Impairment:** Hemodialysis effect: Not removed by hemodialysis.

**Hepatic Impairment:** Sertraline is extensively metabolized by the liver. Caution should be used in patients with hepatic impairment.

**Additional Nursing Issues**

**Physical Assessment:** Assess other medications patient may be taking for effectiveness and interactions (see Drug Interactions). See Warnings/Precautions for cautious use. Has potential for psychological or physiological dependence, abuse, or tolerance. Monitor therapeutic response (ie, mental status, mood, affect, suicidal ideation), and adverse reactions at beginning of therapy and periodically with long-term use (see Adverse Reactions and Overdose/Toxicology). Taper dosage slowly when discontinuing. Assess knowledge/teach patient appropriate use, interventions to reduce side effects, and adverse symptoms to report. **Pregnancy risk factor C** - benefits of use should outweigh possible risks. Breast-feeding is not recommended.

**Patient Information/Instruction:** Take exactly as directed (do not increase dose or frequency); may take 2-3 weeks to achieve desired results; may cause physical and/or psychological dependence. Take in the morning to reduce the incidence of insomnia. Avoid excessive alcohol, caffeine, and other prescription or OTC medications not approved by prescriber. Maintain adequate hydration (2-3 L/day of fluids unless instructed to restrict fluid intake). You may experience drowsiness, dizziness, or lightheadedness (use caution when driving or engaging in tasks requiring alertness until response to drug is known); nausea, vomiting, anorexia, or dry mouth (small frequent meals, frequent mouth care, chewing gum, or sucking lozenges may help); postural hypotension (use caution when climbing stairs or changing position from sitting or lying

(Continued)

## Sertraline *(Continued)*

to standing); urinary pattern changes (void before taking medication); or male sexual dysfunction (reversible). Report persistent insomnia or daytime sedation, agitation, nervousness, fatigue; muscle cramping, tremors, weakness, or change in gait; chest pain, palpitations, or swelling of extremities; vision changes or eye pain; changes in hearing or ringing in ears; difficulty breathing or breathlessness; skin rash or irritation; or worsening of condition. **Pregnancy/breast-feeding precautions:** Inform prescriber if you are or intend to be pregnant. Breast-feeding is not recommended.

**Geriatric Considerations:** Sertraline's favorable side effect profile makes it a useful alternative to the traditional tricyclic antidepressants. Its potential stimulation effect and anorexia may be bothersome.

**Related Information**

Antidepressant Agents Comparison *on page 1368*

- **Serutan® [OTC]** *see* Psyllium *on page 993*
- **Servigenta** *see* Gentamicin *on page 531*
- **Serzone®** *see* Nefazodone *on page 812*

## Sevelamer (se VEL a mer)

**U.S. Brand Names** Renagel®

**Therapeutic Category** Phosphate Binder

**Pregnancy Risk Factor** C

**Lactation** Excretion in breast milk unknown/use caution (not absorbed systemically but may alter maternal nutrition)

**Use** Reduction of serum phosphorous in patients with end-stage renal disease

**Mechanism of Action/Effect** Sevalamer (a polymeric compound) binds phosphate within the intestinal lumen, limiting absorption and decreasing serum phosphate concentrations without altering calcium, aluminum, or bicarbonate concentrations.

**Contraindications** Hypersensitivity to sevelamer or any component; hypophosphatemia; bowel obstruction

**Warnings** Use with caution in patients with gastrointestinal disorders including dysphagia, swallowing disorders, severe gastrointestinal motility disorders, or major gastrointestinal surgery. May cause reductions in vitamin D, E, K, and folic acid absorption. Long-term studies of carcinogenic potential have not been completed. Capsules should not be taken apart or chewed. Pregnancy risk factor C.

**Drug Interactions**

**Decreased Effect:** No formal drug interaction studies have been undertaken. Sevelamer may bind to some drugs in the gastrointestinal tract and decrease their absorption. When changes in absorption of oral medications may have significant clinical consequences (such as antiarrhythmic and antiseizure medications), these medications should be taken at least 1 hour before or 3 hours after a dose of sevelamer.

**Adverse Reactions**

>10%:

Cardiovascular: Hypotension (11%), thrombosis (10%)
Central nervous system: Headache (10%)
Endocrine and metabolic: Decreased absorption of vitamins D, E, K and folic acid
Gastrointestinal: Diarrhea (16%), dyspepsia (5% to 11%), vomiting (12%)
Neuromuscular and skeletal: Pain (13%)
Miscellaneous: Infection (15%)

1% to 10%:

Cardiovascular: Hypertension (9%)
Gastrointestinal: Nausea (7%), flatulence (4%), diarrhea (4%), constipation (2%)
Respiratory: Cough (4%)

**Overdose/Toxicology** Sevelamer is not absorbed systemically. There are no reports of overdosage in patients.

**Pharmacodynamics/Kinetics**

**Excretion:** Feces

**Formulations** Capsule: 403 mg

**Dosing**

**Adults:** Oral: 2-4 capsules 3 times/day with meals; the initial dose may be based on serum phosphorous. Phosphorous: Initial:

>6.0 mg/dL and <7.5 mg/dL: 2 capsules 3 times/day
>7.5 mg/dL and <9.0 mg/dL: 3 capsules 3 times/day
≥9.0 mg/dL: 4 capsules 3 times/day

Dosage should be adjusted based on serum phosphorous concentration, with a goal of lowering to <6.0 mg/dL; maximum daily dose studied was 30 capsules/day.

**Elderly:** See Adult Dosing.

**Monitoring Laboratory Tests** Serum phosphorus

**Additional Nursing Issues**

**Physical Assessment:** See Contraindications and Warnings/Precautions for use cautions. Assess knowledge/teach patient appropriate use, possible side effects/interventions, and adverse symptoms to report. **Pregnancy risk factor C** - benefits of use should outweigh possible risks. Note breast-feeding caution.

**Patient Information/Instruction:** Take as directed, with meals. Do not break or chew capsule. You may experience headache or dizziness (use caution when driving or engaging in tasks requiring alertness until response to drug is known); upset stomach, nausea, or vomiting (frequent small meals, frequent mouth care, or sucking hard candy may help); diarrhea (yogurt or buttermilk may help); hypotension (use caution when rising from sitting or lying position or when climbing stairs or bending over); or mild neuromuscular pain or stiffness (mild analgesic may help). Report persistent adverse reactions. **Pregnancy/breast-feeding precautions:** Inform prescriber if you are or intend to be pregnant. Consult prescriber if breast-feeding.

- **S-F Kaon®** *see* Potassium Supplements *on page 952*
- **Shohl's Solution** *see* Sodium Citrate and Citric Acid *on page 1063*
- **Shur-Seal®** *see page 1294*

## Sibutramine (si BYOO tra meen)

**U.S. Brand Names** Meridia®

**Therapeutic Category** Anorexiant

**Pregnancy Risk Factor** C

**Lactation** Excretion in breast milk unknown/not recommended

**Use** In conjunction with diet resulting in weight loss for obese patients

**Mechanism of Action/Effect** Sibutramine inhibits norepinephrine, serotonin, and dopamine reuptake

**Contraindications** Hypersensitivity to sibutramine or any component; patients receiving MAO inhibitors or other centrally-acting appetite suppressants; sibutramine should not be taken in combination with serotonergic agents (eg, fluoxetine, fluvoxamine, paroxetine, sertraline, venlafaxine, sumatriptan, dihydroergotamine, dextromethorphan, meperidine, pentazocine, fentanyl, lithium, or tryptophan) due to the risk of the severe sometimes fatal reaction, "serotonin syndrome"; patients diagnosed with anorexia nervosa or those who have severe hepatic impairment should not receive sibutramine

**Warnings** Exclude other possible causes of obesity (ie, hypothyroidism) prior to starting therapy. Sibutramine may increase blood pressure or heart rate so use with caution in patients with cardiac diseases including coronary artery disease, arrhythmias, congestive heart failure, or stroke. Use with caution in patients with narrow angle glaucoma or with mild to moderate hepatic failure. Use caution in concomitant administration of sibutramine with decongestants, cough, cold, or allergy products that may raise blood pressure (eg, phenylpropanolamine, pseudoephedrine, ephedrine). Pregnancy factor C.

**Drug Interactions**

**Cytochrome P-450 Effect:** CYP3A3/4 enzyme substrate

**Decreased Effect:** Concomitant use of CNS active drugs with sibutramine has not been studied. Use with caution and (see Contraindications).

**Increased Effect/Toxicity:** Concomitant administration of ketoconazole has resulted in elevated serum concentrations of sibutramine. Smaller increases in serum sibutramine levels were seen with coadministration of erythromycin.

**Adverse Reactions**

>10%:
- Cardiovascular: Insomnia
- Central nervous system: Headache, constipation, dry mouth
- Respiratory: Rhinitis

1% to 10%:
- Cardiovascular: Chest pain, tachycardia, vasodilation, hypertension, palpitation, peripheral edema,
- Central nervous system: Migraine, dizziness, nervousness, anxiety, depression, paresthesia, somnolence
- Dermatologic: Rash, sweating, pruritus
- Gastrointestinal: Abdominal pain, increased appetite, nausea, dyspepsia, gastritis, vomiting, diarrhea, flatulence, gastroenteritis
- Genitourinary: Dysmenorrhea
- Hepatic: Elevated AST, ALT GGT, LDH, alkaline phosphate and bilirubin
- Neuromuscular & skeletal: Back pain, asthenia, arthralgia
- Respiratory: Sinusitis, cough, bronchitis, dyspnea
- Miscellaneous: Allergic reaction

<1% (Limited to important or life-threatening symptoms): Convulsions, acute interstitial nephritis (one case)

**Overdose/Toxicology** Symptoms of overdose include hypertension, tachycardia, headache, and palpitations. Treatment is supportive.

**Pharmacodynamics/Kinetics**

**Protein Binding:** 94% to 97%

**Time to Peak:** Within 3-4 hours

**Metabolism:** Liver, undergoes first-pass metabolism

**Excretion:** Urine and feces

**Formulations** Capsule, as hydrochloride: 5 mg, 10 mg, 15 mg (100s)

**Dosing**

**Adults:** Initial: 10 mg daily in the morning. The dose may be increased to 15 mg daily after 4 weeks of therapy if there is inadequate weight loss. The maximum dose is 15 mg daily. The 5 mg dosage form is reserved for patients who cannot tolerate the 10 mg dose.

**Elderly:** Use with caution; adjust dose based on renal or hepatic function.

**Hepatic Impairment:** No adjustment necessary for mild to moderate liver failure. Sibutramine is contraindicated in patients with severe liver failure.

**Administration**

**Oral:** May take with or without food.

**Additional Nursing Issues**

**Physical Assessment:** Assess effectiveness and interactions of other medications patient may be taking (see Contraindications, Warnings/Precautions, and Drug Interactions). Periodically evaluate the need for continued use. Monitor blood pressure,

(Continued)

## Sibutramine *(Continued)*

vital signs, and adverse reactions at start of therapy, when changing dosage, and at regular intervals during therapy (see Adverse Reactions). Assess knowledge/teach patient appropriate use, possible side effects, and symptoms to report. **Pregnancy risk factor C** - use only if benefits outweigh possible risks. Breast-feeding is not recommended.

**Patient Information/Instruction:** Take exactly as directed (do not increase dose or frequency without consulting prescriber). Take with or without meals; if gastric distress occurs, may be taken with meals (do not take at bedtime). Avoid alcohol, caffeine, or OTC medications that act as stimulants. You may experience restlessness, dizziness, sleepiness (use caution when driving or engaging in tasks requiring alertness until response to drug is known); experience insomnia (taking medication early in morning may help, warm milk and quiet environment at bedtime may help); increased appetite, nausea or vomiting (small frequent meals, frequent mouth care may help); constipation (increased exercise, dietary fiber, fruit, or fluid may help); diarrhea (buttermilk, boiled milk, or yogurt may help); or altered menstrual periods (reversible). Report chest pain, palpitations, or irregular heartbeat; excessive nervousness, excitation, or sleepiness; back pain, muscle weakness, or tremors; CNS changes (acute headache, aggressiveness, restlessness, excitation, sleep disturbances); menstrual pattern changes; rash; blurred vision; runny nose, sinusitis, cough, or difficulty breathing. **Pregnancy/breast-feeding precautions:** Inform prescriber if you are or intend to be pregnant. Breast-feeding is not recommended.

- **Sigafam** *see* Famotidine *on page 470*
- **Silace-C®** *see page 1294*
- **Siladryl® Oral [OTC]** *see* Diphenhydramine *on page 381*
- **Silafed® Syrup** *see page 1294*
- **Silain®** *see page 1294*
- **Silaminic® Cold Syrup** *see page 1294*
- **Silaminic® Expectorant [OTC]** *see* Guaifenesin and Phenylpropanolamine *on page 550*

## Sildenafil (sil DEN a fil)

**U.S. Brand Names** Viagra™

**Therapeutic Category** Phosphodiesterase Enzyme Inhibitor

**Pregnancy Risk Factor** B

**Lactation** Not indicated for use in women

**Use** Oral therapy for the treatment of erectile dysfunction

**Mechanism of Action/Effect** Sildenafil enhances the effect of nitric oxide by inhibiting phosphodiesterase type 5 (PDE5), resulting in smooth muscle relaxation and inflow of blood into the corpus cavernosum with sexual stimulation.

**Contraindications** Hypersensitivity to sildenafil or any component; contraindicated in patients taking nitrates, since it potentiates the hypotensive effect; age >65%; hepatic impairment; severe renal impairment; creatinine clearance <30 mL/minute

**Warnings** A thorough medical history and physical examination to diagnose erectile dysfunction should be undertaken to determine potential underlying causes and appropriate treatment. There is a potential cardiac risk associated with sexual activity which may need to be considered in patients with cardiovascular disease before starting sildenafil therapy. Use with caution in patients predisposed to priapism (ie, sickle cell anemia, multiple myeloma or leukemia). Use with caution in patients with anatomical deformation of the penis (ie, angulation, cavernosal fibrosis, or Peyronie's disease). Use of sildenafil with other approaches to treat erectile dysfunction is **not** recommended. May cause hypotension; use caution in patients with MI, stroke, or life-threatening arrhythmia (within last 6 months); resting hypotension or hypertension; history of unstable angina or cardiac failure; and retinitis pigmentosa.

**Drug Interactions**

**Cytochrome P-450 Effect:** CYP3A3/4 enzyme substrate (major); CYP2C9 enzyme substrate (minor)

**Decreased Effect:** May decrease the serum concentration and efficacy of sildenafil.

**Increased Effect/Toxicity:** Sildenafil potentiates the hypotensive effects of nitrates which in combination is contraindicated. May add to effect of other antihypertensives. Cytochrome P-450 (CYP3A4) enzyme inhibitors (erythromycin, itraconazole, mibefradil, and cimetidine) increase the serum concentrations of sildenafil. May potentiate bleeding in patients receiving heparin.

**Food Interactions** Amount and rate of absorption of sildenafil is reduced when taken with a high fat meal.

**Adverse Reactions**

>10%:

Central nervous system: Headache

**Note:** Dyspepsia and abnormal vision (blurred or increased sensitivity to light) occurred at an incidence of >10% with doses of 100 mg.

1% to 10%:

Cardiovascular: Flushing

Central nervous system: Dizziness

Dermatologic: Rash

Genitourinary: Urinary tract infection

Ophthalmic: Abnormal vision (blurred or increased sensitivity to light)

Respiratory: Nasal congestion

<2% (Limited to important of life-threatening symptoms): Shock, allergic reaction, chest pain, angina pectoris, AV block, migraine, syncope, tachycardia, palpitation, hypotension, postural hypotension, myocardial ischemia, cerebral thrombosis, cardiac arrest, heart failure, abnormal electrocardiogram, cardiomyopathy, colitis, abnormal liver function tests, rectal hemorrhage, anemia, leukopenia, edema, gout, unstable diabetes, hyperglycemia, peripheral edema, hyperuricemia, hypoglycemic reaction, hypernatremia, myalgia, bone pain, hypertonia, neuralgia, vertigo, asthma, dyspnea, sinusitis, bronchitis, contact dermatitis, exfoliative dermatitis, eye hemorrhage, cataract, cystitis, breast enlargement, genital edema, anorgasmia, seizures, priapism, diplopia

**Pharmacodynamics/Kinetics**

**Protein Binding:** ~96% bound to plasma proteins

**Time to Peak:** 30-120 minutes

**Metabolism:** Liver; also converts sildenafil to an active metabolite

**Excretion:** Feces and urine

**Onset:** ~60 minutes

**Duration:** 2-4 hours

**Formulations** Tablet, as citrate: 25 mg, 50 mg, 100 mg

**Dosing**

**Adults:** Oral: 50 mg tablet, approximately 1 hour before sexual activity. Adjust dose based on effectiveness or tolerance, decrease to 25 mg or increase to the maximum daily dose of 100 mg. Do not take more than once daily.

**Elderly:** Initial: 25 mg, 1 hour before sexual activity. Age >65 years was associated with increased serum sildenafil concentrations which may increase side effects and efficacy.

**Renal Impairment:** $Cl_{cr}$ <30 mL/minute: Initial: 25 mg, 1 hour before sexual activity.

**Hepatic Impairment:** Cirrhosis: Initial: 25 mg, 1 hour before sexual activity.

**Administration**

**Oral:** Take orally anywhere from 0.5-4 hours before sexual activity. Recommendations are to take 1 hour before sexual activity.

**Additional Nursing Issues**

**Physical Assessment:** Monitor other medications patient may be taking for effectiveness and interactions (see Drug Interactions and Contraindications). Instruct patient on appropriate use and cautions, possible side effects (see Adverse Reactions), and symptoms to report.

**Patient Information/Instruction:** Inform prescriber of all other medications you are taking; serious side effects can result when sildenafil is used with nitrates and some other medications. Do not combine sildenafil with other approaches to treating erectile dysfunction without consulting prescriber. Note that sildenafil provides no protection against sexually transmitted diseases, including HIV. You may experience headache, flushing, or abnormal vision (blurred or increased sensitivity to light); use caution when driving at night or in poorly lit environments. Report immediately acute allergic reactions, chest pain or palpitations, persistent dizziness, sign of urinary tract infection, rash, respiratory difficulties, genital swelling, or other adverse reactions.

**Breast-feeding Issues:** Sildenafil is not indicated for use in women.

**Pregnancy Issues:** Sildenafil is not indicated for use in women.

- **Sildicon-E® [OTC]** *see* Guaifenesin and Phenylpropanolamine *on page 550*
- **Silphen® Cough [OTC]** *see* Diphenhydramine *on page 381*
- **Silphen DM®** *see page 1294*
- **Siltussin® [OTC]** *see* Guaifenesin *on page 548*
- **Siltussin-CF® [OTC]** *see* Guaifenesin, Phenylpropanolamine, and Dextromethorphan *on page 551*
- **Siltussin DM® [OTC]** *see* Guaifenesin and Dextromethorphan *on page 549*
- **Silvadene®** *see* Silver Sulfadiazine *on page 1059*

## Silver Nitrate (SIL ver NYE trate)

**U.S. Brand Names** Dey-Drop® Ophthalmic Solution

**Synonyms** $AgNO_3$

**Therapeutic Category** Antibiotic, Ophthalmic; Antibiotic, Topical; Cauterizing Agent, Topical; Topical Skin Product, Antibacterial

**Pregnancy Risk Factor** C

**Lactation** For topical use

**Use** Prevention of gonococcal ophthalmia neonatorum; cauterization of wounds and sluggish ulcers, removal of granulation tissue and warts; aseptic prophylaxis of burns

**Mechanism of Action/Effect** Free silver ions precipitate bacterial proteins by combining with chloride in tissue forming silver chloride; coagulates cellular protein to form an eschar; silver ions or salts or colloidal silver preparations can inhibit the growth of both gram-positive and gram-negative bacteria. This germicidal action is attributed to the precipitation of bacterial proteins by liberated silver ions. Silver nitrate coagulates cellular protein to form an eschar, and this mode of action is the postulated mechanism for control of benign hematuria, rhinitis, and recurrent pneumothorax.

**Contraindications** Hypersensitivity to silver nitrate or any component; not for use on broken skin or cuts

**Warnings** Do not use applicator sticks on the eyes. Repeated applications of the ophthalmic solution into the eye can cause cauterization of the cornea and blindness. Pregnancy factor C.

(Continued)

## Silver Nitrate *(Continued)*

**Drug Interactions**

**Decreased Effect:** Sulfacetamide preparations are incompatible.

**Adverse Reactions**

>10%:

Dermatologic: Burning and skin irritation
Ocular: Chemical conjunctivitis

1% to 10%:

Dermatologic: Staining of the skin
Hematologic: Methemoglobinemia
Ocular: Cauterization of the cornea, blindness

**Overdose/Toxicology** Symptoms of overdose include pain and burning of the mouth, salivation, vomiting, diarrhea, shock, coma, convulsions, and death; blackening of skin and mucous membranes. Absorbed nitrate can cause methemoglobinemia. Fatal dose is as low as 2 g; administer sodium chloride in water (10 g/L) to cause precipitation of silver.

**Pharmacodynamics/Kinetics**

**Excretion:** Although the highest amounts of silver noted on autopsy have been in the kidneys, excretion in urine is minimal.

**Formulations**

Applicator, topical: 75% with potassium nitrate 25% (6")
Ointment, topical: 10% (30 g)
Solution:

Ophthalmic: 1% (wax ampuls)
Topical: 10% (30 mL); 25% (30 mL); 50% (30 mL)

**Dosing**

**Adults:**

Ointment: Apply in an apertured pad on affected area or lesion for approximately 5 days.

Sticks: Apply to mucous membranes and other moist skin surfaces only on area to be treated 2-3 times/week for 2-3 weeks.

Topical solution: Apply a cotton applicator dipped in solution on the affected area 2-3 times/week for 2-3 weeks.

**Elderly:** Refer to adult dosing.

**Administration**

**Other:** Applicators are **not** for ophthalmic use.

**Stability**

**Storage:** Must be stored in a dry place. Exposure to light causes silver to oxidize and turn brown, dipping in water causes oxidized film to readily dissolve.

**Monitoring Laboratory Tests** With prolonged use, monitor methemoglobin levels.

**Additional Nursing Issues**

**Physical Assessment:** Assess knowledge/teach appropriate technique for topical application. Monitor for overuse symptoms (see above). **Pregnancy risk factor C** - benefits of use should outweigh possible risks.

**Patient Information/Instruction:** Use as directed; do not use more often than instructed. Store container in dry, dark place.

Ointment: Apply on pad to affected area for 4-5 days.

Sticks: Apply to mucous membranes and other moist skin surfaces to be treated 2-3 times each week for 2-3 weeks.

Solution: Apply to affected area with cotton applicator dipped in solution 2-3 times each week for 2-3 weeks.

Handle with care; silver nitrate stains skin, clothing and utensils. Discontinue and contact prescriber if treated areas worsen or if redness, or irritation develops in surrounding area. **Pregnancy precautions:** Inform prescriber if you are or intend to be pregnant.

## Silver Protein, Mild (SIL ver PRO teen, mild)

**U.S. Brand Names** Argyrol® S.S. 20%

**Therapeutic Category** Antibiotic, Topical

**Pregnancy Risk Factor** C

**Lactation** For topical use

**Use** Used during eye surgery to stain and coagulate mucus which is then removed by irrigation; eye infections

**Formulations** Solution, ophthalmic: 20% (15 mL, 30 mL)

**Dosing**

**Adults:**

Preop in eye surgery: Place 2-3 drops into eye(s), then rinse out with sterile irrigating solution

Eye infections: 1-3 drops into the affected eye(s) every 3-4 hours for several days

**Elderly:** Refer to adult dosing.

**Additional Nursing Issues**

**Physical Assessment:** Assess knowledge/teach patient appropriate application and use and adverse symptoms to report. **Pregnancy risk factor C.**

**Patient Information/Instruction:** Instill as many times per day as directed. Wash hands before using. Gently pull lower eyelid forward and instill prescribed amount of ointment into lower eyelid. Close eye and roll eyeball in all directions. May cause blurred vision; use caution when driving or engaging in tasks that require clear vision.

Report any adverse reactions such as rash or itching, burning or pain in eye, worsening of condition, or if condition does not improve. **Pregnancy precautions:** Inform prescriber if you are or intend to be pregnant.

## Silver Sulfadiazine (SIL ver sul fa DYE a zeen)

**U.S. Brand Names** Silvadene®; SSD® AF; SSD® Cream; Thermazene®

**Therapeutic Category** Antibiotic, Topical

**Pregnancy Risk Factor** C/D (near term)

**Lactation** For external use

**Use** Prevention and treatment of infection in second and third degree burns

**Mechanism of Action/Effect** Acts upon the bacterial cell wall and cell membrane. Bactericidal for many gram-negative and gram-positive bacteria and is effective against yeast. Active against *Pseudomonas aeruginosa*, *Pseudomonas maltophilia*, *Enterobacter* species, *Klebsiella* species, *Serratia* species, *Escherichia coli*, *Proteus mirabilis*, *Morganella morganii*, *Providencia rettgeri*, *Proteus vulgaris*, *Providencia* species, *Citrobacter* species, *Acinetobacter calcoaceticus*, *Staphylococcus aureus*, *Staphylococcus epidermidis*, *Enterococcus* species, *Candida albicans*, *Corynebacterium diphtheriae*, and *Clostridium perfringens*

**Contraindications** Hypersensitivity to silver sulfadiazine or any component; pregnancy (at or near term)

**Warnings** Use with caution in patients with G-6-PD deficiency, renal impairment, or history of allergy to other sulfonamides. Sulfadiazine may accumulate in patients with impaired hepatic or renal function. Use of analgesic might be needed before application. Systemic absorption is significant and adverse reactions may be due to sulfa component. Pregnancy factor C/D (near term).

**Drug Interactions**

**Decreased Effect:** Topical proteolytic enzymes are inactivated by silver sulfadiazine.

**Adverse Reactions**

>10%: Local: Burning feeling on treated areas

1% to 10%: Dermatologic: Itching, rash, erythema multiforme, discoloration of skin

**Pharmacodynamics/Kinetics**

**Excretion:** Urine

**Formulations** Cream, topical: 1% [10 mg/g] (20 g, 50 g, 100 g, 400 g, 1000 g)

**Dosing**

**Adults:** Topical: Apply once or twice daily

**Elderly:** Refer to adult dosing.

**Administration**

**Topical:** Apply with a sterile-gloved hand. Apply to a thickness 1/16". Burned area should be covered with cream at all times.

**Stability**

**Storage:** Discard if cream is darkened (reacts with heavy metals resulting in release of silver).

**Monitoring Laboratory Tests** Serum electrolytes, urinalysis, renal function, CBC in patients with extensive burns on long-term treatment

**Additional Nursing Issues**

**Physical Assessment:** Monitor development of granulation. Observe for hypersensitivity reactions (eg, irritation, redness, burning or itching in unburned areas). Long-term use over large areas - monitor kidney function, and serum sulfa levels (significant absorption can occur). **Pregnancy risk factor C/D.**

**Patient Information/Instruction:** Usually applied by professional in burn care setting. Patient instruction should be appropriate to extent of burn, patient understanding, etc.

**Additional Information** Contains methylparaben and propylene glycol.

- **Simethicone** *see page 1294*
- **Simethicone and Magaldrate** *see* Magaldrate and Simethicone *on page 703*
- **Simethicone, Magnesium Hydroxide, Aluminum Hydroxide** *see page 1294*
- **Simron® [OTC]** *see* Iron Supplements *on page 627*
- **Simulect®** *see* Basiliximab *on page 133*

## Simvastatin (SIM va stat in)

**U.S. Brand Names** Zocor®

**Therapeutic Category** Antilipemic Agent (HMG-CoA Reductase Inhibitor)

**Pregnancy Risk Factor** X

**Lactation** Enters breast milk/contraindicated

**Use** Adjunct to dietary therapy to decrease elevated serum total and LDL cholesterol concentrations in primary hypercholesterolemia; treatment of homozygous familial hypercholesterolemia; reduce risk of myocardial infarction, stroke, or TIA

**Mechanism of Action/Effect** Simvastatin is a derivative of lovastatin that acts by competitively inhibiting 3-hydroxy-3-methylglutaryl-coenzyme A (HMG-CoA) reductase, the enzyme that catalyzes the rate-limiting step in cholesterol biosynthesis; lowers total and LDL cholesterol with increase in HDL

**Contraindications** Hypersensitivity to simvastatin or lovastatin or other HMG-CoA reductase inhibitors; active liver disease or unexplained elevations of serum transaminases; pregnancy; severe electrolyte or endocrine problems

**Warnings** Combination therapy with other hypolipidemic agents may be required to achieve optimal reductions of LDL cholesterol.

(Continued)

## Simvastatin *(Continued)*

**Drug Interactions**

**Cytochrome P-450 Effect:** CYP3A3/4 enzyme substrate

**Increased Effect/Toxicity:** Simvastatin may increased the effect or toxicity of warfarin, erythromycin, niacin, cyclosporin, gemfibrozil, or digoxin.

**Adverse Reactions**

1% to 10%:

Central nervous system: Headache

Dermatologic: Rash

Gastrointestinal: Flatulence, abdominal cramps, diarrhea, constipation, nausea, heartburn

Hepatic: Elevated serum transaminases

Neuromuscular & skeletal: Myalgia, elevated creatine phosphokinase (CPK)

<1% (Limited to important or life-threatening symptoms): Toxic epidermal necrolysis, erythema multiforme, Stevens-Johnson syndrome, thrombocytopenia, leukopenia, hemolytic anemia, eosinophilia, elevated EST, positive ANA, hepatitis, cholestatic jaundice, cirrhosis, hepatic necrosis, hepatoma, rhabdomyolysis, dyspnea, lupus-erythematosus-like syndrome

**Overdose/Toxicology** Very few adverse events. Treatment is symptomatic.

**Pharmacodynamics/Kinetics**

**Protein Binding:** ~95%

**Time to Peak:** 1.3-2.4 hours

**Metabolism:** Liver

**Excretion:** Urine and feces

**Onset:** >3 days; maximal effects after 2 weeks

**Formulations** Tablet: 5 mg, 10 mg, 20 mg, 40 mg, 80 mg

**Dosing**

**Adults:** Oral: Initial: 5-10 mg/day as a single bedtime dose. If LDL is ≤190 mg/dL (4.9 mmol/L), start with 5 mg; if LDL is >190 mg/dL (4.9 mmol/L), start with 10 mg/day. Increase every 4 weeks as needed. Maximum: 80 mg/day.

**Elderly:** Oral: Initial: 5 mg/day as a single bedtime dose. Increase as needed every 4 weeks by 5-10 mg. Maximum LDL lowering may be achieved with ≤20 mg/day.

**Renal Impairment:** Recommended starting dose: 5 mg. Patient should be closely monitored. In patients with severe renal insufficiency, high systemic levels may occur.

**Administration**

**Oral:** May be taken without regard to meals.

**Stability**

**Storage:** Tablets should be stored in well closed containers at temperatures between 5°C to 30°C (41°F to 86°F).

**Monitoring Laboratory Tests** Creatine phosphokinase levels due to possibility of myopathy; serum cholesterol (total and fractionated); obtain liver function tests prior to initiation, 6 and 12 weeks after initiation or first dose, and periodically thereafter (semiannually).

**Additional Nursing Issues**

**Physical Assessment:** Monitor laboratory test results. Assess other medications (prescriptive and OTC) patient may be taking; adjustment may be necessary. **Pregnancy risk factor X** - determine that patient is not pregnant before beginning treatment and do not give to women of childbearing age unless female is capable of complying with barrier contraceptive measures 1 month prior to therapy, during therapy, and for 1 month following therapy. Breast-feeding is contraindicated.

**Patient Information/Instruction:** Take this medication as directed, with meals, 1 hour prior to or after any other medications. You may experience nausea, flatulence, dyspepsia (small frequent meals may help), headache, muscle or joint pain (will probably lessen with continued use), and light sensitivity (use sunblock and wear protective clothing). Report severe and unresolved gastric upset, any vision changes, changes in color of urine or stool, yellowing of skin or eyes, and any unusual bruising. **Pregnancy/breast-feeding precautions:** Inform prescriber if you are pregnant. Do not get pregnant 1 month before, during, or for 1 month following therapy. Consult prescriber for instruction on appropriate contraceptive measures. This drug may cause severe fetal defects. Do not donate blood during or for 1 month following therapy (same reason). Do not breast-feed.

**Geriatric Considerations:** Effective and well tolerated in the elderly. The definition of and, therefore, when to treat hyperlipidemia in the elderly is a controversial issue. The National Cholesterol Education Program recommends that all adults 20 years of age and older maintain a plasma cholesterol <200 mg/dL. By this definition, 60% of all elderly would be considered to have a borderline high (200-239 mg/dL) or high (≥240 mg/dL) plasma cholesterol. However, plasma cholesterol has been shown to be a less reliable predictor of coronary heart disease in the elderly. Therefore, it is the authors' belief that pharmacologic treatment be reserved for those who are unable to obtain a desirable plasma cholesterol level by diet alone and for whom the benefits of treatment are believed to outweigh the potential adverse effects, drug interactions, and cost of treatment.

**Related Information**

Lipid-Lowering Agents Comparison *on page 1393*


- **Sinaplin** *see* Ampicillin *on page 90*
- **Sinarest® 12 Hour Nasal Solution** *see page 1294*
- **Sinarest® Nasal Solution [OTC]** *see* Phenylephrine *on page 920*
- **Sinarest® No Drowsiness** *see page 1294*

- **Sincalide** *see page 1248*
- **Sine-Aid® IB Caplets** *see page 1294*
- **Sine-Aid® Maximum Strength** *see page 1294*
- **Sinedol** *see* Acetaminophen *on page 32*
- **Sinedol 500** *see* Acetaminophen *on page 32*
- **Sinemet®** *see* Levodopa and Carbidopa *on page 667*
- **Sinemet® CR** *see* Levodopa and Carbidopa *on page 667*
- **Sine-Off® Maximum Strength No Drowsiness Formula** *see page 1294*
- **Sinequan® Oral** *see* Doxepin *on page 399*
- **Sinex® Long-Acting** *see page 1294*
- **Singulair®** *see* Montelukast *on page 787*
- **Sinuberase®** *see Lactobacillus acidophilus* and *Lactobacillus bulgaricus on page 651*
- **Sinubid® Tablet** *see page 1294*
- **Sinufed® Timecelles®** *see* Guaifenesin and Pseudoephedrine *on page 551*
- **Sinumist®-SR Capsulets®** *see* Guaifenesin *on page 548*
- **Sinus Excedrin® Extra Strength** *see page 1294*
- **Sinusol-B®** *see page 1294*
- **Sinus-Relief®** *see page 1294*
- **Sinutab® Tablets** *see page 1294*
- **Sinutab® Without Drowsiness** *see page 1294*
- **SK** *see* Streptokinase *on page 1074*
- **Skelid®** *see* Tiludronate *on page 1137*
- **SKF 104864** *see* Topotecan *on page 1157*
- **Skin Test Antigens, Multiple** *see page 1248*
- **Sleep-eze 3® Oral [OTC]** *see* Diphenhydramine *on page 381*
- **Sleepinal® [OTC]** *see* Diphenhydramine *on page 381*
- **Sleepwell 2-nite® [OTC]** *see* Diphenhydramine *on page 381*
- **Slim-Mint® [OTC]** *see* Benzocaine *on page 141*
- **Slo-bid™** *see* Theophylline *on page 1115*
- **Slo-Niacin®** *see page 1294*
- **Slo-Phyllin®** *see* Theophylline *on page 1115*
- **Slo-Phyllin GG®** *see* Theophylline and Guaifenesin *on page 1118*
- **Slow FE® [OTC]** *see* Iron Supplements *on page 627*
- **Slow-K®** *see* Potassium Supplements *on page 952*
- **Slow-Mag®** *see* Magnesium Supplements *on page 703*
- **Slow-Mag®** *see page 1294*
- **SMX-TMP** *see* Co-trimoxazole *on page 307*
- **SMZ-TMP** *see* Co-trimoxazole *on page 307*
- **Snaplets-EX® [OTC]** *see* Guaifenesin and Phenylpropanolamine *on page 550*
- **Sodium 2-Mercaptoethane Sulfonate** *see* Mesna *on page 729*
- **Sodium Acid Carbonate** *see* Sodium Bicarbonate *on this page*
- **Sodium Benzoate and Caffeine** *see* Caffeine and Sodium Benzoate *on page 179*

## Sodium Bicarbonate (SOW dee um bye KAR bun ate)

**U.S. Brand Names** Neut® Injection

**Synonyms** Baking Soda; $NaHCO_3$; Sodium Acid Carbonate; Sodium Hydrogen Carbonate

**Therapeutic Category** Alkalinizing Agent; Antacid; Electrolyte Supplement, Oral; Electrolyte Supplement, Parenteral

**Pregnancy Risk Factor** C

**Lactation** Enters breast milk/compatible

**Use** Management of metabolic acidosis; gastric hyperacidity; as an alkalinization agent for the urine; treatment and hyperkalemia

**Mechanism of Action/Effect** Dissociates to provide bicarbonate ion which neutralizes hydrogen ion concentration and raises blood and urinary pH

**Contraindications** Alkalosis, hypernatremia, severe pulmonary edema, hypocalcemia, unknown abdominal pain

**Warnings** **Use of I.V. $NaHCO_3$ should be reserved for documented metabolic acidosis and for hyperkalemia-induced cardiac arrest.** Routine use in cardiac arrest is not recommended. Avoid extravasation, tissue necrosis can occur due to the hypertonicity of $NaHCO_3$. May cause sodium retention especially if renal function is impaired; not to be used in treatment of peptic ulcer; use with caution in patients with CHF, edema, cirrhosis, or renal failure. Not the antacid of choice for the elderly because of sodium content and potential for systemic alkalosis. Pregnancy factor C.

**Drug Interactions**

**Decreased Effect:** Decreased effect/levels of lithium, chlorpropamide, and salicylates due to urinary alkalinization.

**Increased Effect/Toxicity:** Increased toxicity/levels of amphetamines, ephedrine, pseudoephedrine, flecainide, quinidine, and quinine due to urinary alkalinization.

**Food Interactions** Concurrent doses with iron may decrease iron absorption.

**Adverse Reactions** 1% to 10%:

Cardiovascular: Edema, cerebral hemorrhage, aggravation of congestive heart failure

Central nervous system: Tetany, intracranial acidosis

Gastrointestinal: Belching, gastric distension, flatulence

(Continued)

## Sodium Bicarbonate *(Continued)*

Endocrine & metabolic: Metabolic alkalosis, hypernatremia, hypokalemia, hypocalcemia, hyperosmolality

Local: **Vesicant chemotherapy**

Respiratory: Pulmonary edema

Miscellaneous: Increased affinity of hemoglobin for oxygen-reduced pH in myocardial tissue necrosis when extravasated

**Overdose/Toxicology** Symptoms of overdose include hypocalcemia, hypokalemia, hypernatremia, and seizures. Treatment is symptom directed and supportive.

**Pharmacodynamics/Kinetics**

**Excretion:** Reabsorbed by kidney and <1% is excreted by urine

**Onset:** Oral: Rapid; I.V.: 15 minutes

**Duration:** Oral: 8-10 minutes; I.V.: 1-2 hours

**Formulations**

Injection: 4% [40 mg/mL = 2.4 mEq/5 mL] (5 mL); 4.2% [42 mg/mL = 5 mEq/10 mL] (10 mL); 7.5% [75 mg/mL = 8.92 mEq/10 mL] (10 mL, 50 mL); 8.4% [84 mg/mL = 10 mEq/10 mL] (10 mL, 50 mL)

Powder: 120 g, 480 g

Tablet: 300 mg [3.6 mEq]; 325 mg [3.8 mEq]; 520 mg [6.3 mEq]; 600 mg [7.3 mEq]; 650 mg [7.6 mEq]

**Dosing**

**Adults:**

Cardiac arrest: **Routine use of $NaHCO_3$ is not recommended and should be given only after adequate alveolar ventilation has been established and effective cardiac compressions are provided.**

I.V.: Initial: 1 mEq/kg/dose one time; maintenance: 0.5 mEq/kg/dose every 10 minutes or as indicated by arterial blood gases

Metabolic acidosis: Dosage should be based on the following formula if blood gases and pH measurements are available:

$HCO_3^-$(mEq) = 0.2 x weight (kg) x base deficit (mEq/L) **or**

$HCO_3^-$(mEq) = 0.5 x weight (kg) x [24 - serum $HCO_3^-$ (mEq/L)]

If acid-base status is not available: 2-5 mEq/kg I.V. infusion over 4-8 hours; subsequent doses should be based on patient's acid-base status

Chronic renal failure: Oral: Initiate when plasma $HCO_3^-$ <15 mEq/L

Start with 20-36 mEq/day in divided doses, titrate to bicarbonate level of 18-20 mEq/L

Renal tubular acidosis: Oral: Distal: 0.5-2 mEq/kg/day in 4-5 divided doses

Urine alkalinization: Oral: Initial: 48 mEq (4 g), then 12-24 mEq (1-2 g) every 4 hours; dose should be titrated to desired urinary pH; doses up to 16 g/day (200 mEq) in patients <60 years and 8 g (100 mEq) in patients >60 years

Antacid: Oral: 325 mg to 2 g 1-4 times/day

**Elderly:** Not recommended for use in the elderly (see Geriatric Considerations).

**Administration**

**I.V.:** Vesicant. Advise patient of milk-alkali syndrome if use is long-term.

**I.V. Detail:** Observe for extravasation when giving I.V.

**Stability**

**Storage:** Store injection at room temperature. Protect from heat and from freezing. Use only clear solutions.

**Compatibility:** Incompatible with acids, acidic salts, alkaloid salts, calcium salts, catecholamines, and atropine. See the Compatibility of Drugs Chart *on page 1315.*

**Additional Nursing Issues**

**Physical Assessment:** Assess other medications patient may be taking for effectiveness and interactions (especially calcium channel blockers or cardiac glycosides - see Warnings/Precautions and Drug Interactions).

I.V.: Monitor therapeutic response (cardiac status, arterial blood gases, and electrolytes), and adverse reactions (eg, CHF, tetany, intracranial acidosis - see Adverse Reactions and Overdose/Toxicology). Monitor infusion site for patency (if extravasation occurs, elevate extravasation site and apply warm compresses). Teach patient adverse effects to report.

Oral: Monitor effectiveness of treatment and adverse response (see above). Assess knowledge/teach patient appropriate use, interventions to reduce side effects, and adverse symptoms to report.

**Pregnancy risk factor C** - benefits of use should outweigh possible risks.

**Patient Information/Instruction:** Do not use for chronic gastric acidity. Take as directed. Chew tablets thoroughly and follow with a full glass of water, preferably on an empty stomach (2 hours before or after food). Take at least 2 hours before or after any other medications. Report CNS effects (eg, irritability, confusion); muscle rigidity or tremors; swelling of feet or ankles; difficulty breathing; chest pain or palpitations; respiratory changes; or tarry stools. **Pregnancy precautions:** Inform prescriber if you are or intend to be pregnant.

**Geriatric Considerations:** Not the antacid of choice for the elderly because of sodium content and potential for systemic alkalosis (see maximum daily dose under Usual Dosage).

**Additional Information**

Sodium content of injection 50 mL, 8.4% = 1150 mg = 50 mEq; each 6 mg of $NaHCO_3$ contains 12 mEq sodium; 1 mEq $NaHCO_3$ = 84 mg

Each 84 mg of sodium bicarbonate provides 1 mEq of sodium and bicarbonate ions; each gram of sodium bicarbonate provides 12 mEq of sodium and bicarbonate ions

◆ **Sodium Chloride** *see page 1294*

## Sodium Citrate and Citric Acid (SOW dee um SIT rate & SI trik AS id)

**U.S. Brand Names** Bicitra®; Oracit®

**Synonyms** Citric Acid and Sodium Citrate; Modified Shohl's Solution; Shohl's Solution

**Therapeutic Category** Alkalinizing Agent

**Pregnancy Risk Factor** No rating

**Lactation** Excretion in breast milk unknown/compatible

**Use** Treatment of metabolic acidosis; alkalinizing agent in conditions where long-term maintenance of an alkaline urine is desirable

**Contraindications** Severe renal insufficiency, sodium-restricted diet

**Warnings** Conversion to bicarbonate may be impaired in patients with hepatic failure, in shock, or who are severely ill. Pregnancy factor C.

**Drug Interactions**

**Decreased Effect:** Decreased effect/levels of lithium, chlorpropamide, and salicylates due to urinary alkalinization.

**Increased Effect/Toxicity:** Increased toxicity/levels of amphetamines, ephedrine, pseudoephedrine, flecainide, quinidine, and quinine due to urinary alkalinization.

**Adverse Reactions** 1% to 10%:

Central nervous system: Tetany

Endocrine & metabolic: Metabolic alkalosis, hyperkalemia

Gastrointestinal: Diarrhea, nausea, vomiting

**Overdose/Toxicology** Symptoms of overdose include hypokalemia, hypernatremia, tetany, and seizures. Treatment is symptom directed and supportive.

**Formulations**

Solution, oral:

Bicitra®: Sodium citrate 500 mg and citric acid 334 mg per 5 mL (15 mL unit dose, 480 mL)

Oracit®: Sodium citrate 490 mg and citric acid 640 mg per 5 mL

Polycitra®: Sodium citrate 500 mg and citric acid 334 mg with potassium citrate 550 mg per 5 mL

**Dosing**

**Adults:** Oral: 15-30 mL with water after meals and at bedtime

**Elderly:** Refer to adult dosing.

**Administration**

**Oral:** Dilute with 30-90 mL of chilled water to enhance taste. Give after meals.

**Additional Nursing Issues**

**Physical Assessment:** See Contraindications and Warnings/Precautions for use cautions. Assess kidney function prior to starting therapy. Monitor cardiac status and serum potassium at beginning of therapy and at regular intervals with long-term therapy. Assess knowledge/teach patient appropriate use, possible side effects, and adverse symptoms to report.

**Patient Information/Instruction:** Take as often as directed, preferably on an empty stomach (1 hour before or 2 hours after meals) and at least 2 hours before or after any other medications. Dilute with 4-6 ounces of chilled water. You may experience diarrhea or nausea and vomiting; if severe, contact prescriber. Report changes in CNS status (eg, irritability, tremors, confusion), swelling of feet or ankles, difficulty breathing, palpitations, abdominal pain, or tarry stools.

**Additional Information** May be ordered as modified Shohl's solution. 1 mL of Bicitra® contains 1 mEq of sodium and the equivalent of 1 mEq of bicarbonate.

**Related Information**

Potassium Citrate and Citric Acid *on page 950*

◆ **Sodium Citrate and Potassium Citrate Mixture** *see page 1306*

◆ **Sodium Ethacrynate** *see* Ethacrynic Acid *on page 455*

◆ **Sodium Ferric Gluconate** *see* Ferric Gluconate *on page 481*

◆ **Sodium Hyaluronate** *see page 1248*

◆ **Sodium Hyaluronate** *see page 1282*

◆ **Sodium Hydrogen Carbonate** *see* Sodium Bicarbonate *on page 1061*

## Sodium Hypochlorite Solution

(SOW dee um hye poe KLOR ite soe LOO shun)

**Synonyms** Dakin's Solution; Modified Dakin's Solution

**Therapeutic Category** Disinfectant, Antibacterial (Topical)

**Pregnancy Risk Factor** C

**Lactation** For external use

**Use** Treatment of athlete's foot (0.5%); wound irrigation (0.5%); disinfect utensils and equipment (5%)

**Formulations**

Solution: 5% (4000 mL)

Solution (modified Dakin's solution):

Full strength: 0.5% (1000 mL)

Half strength: 0.25% (1000 mL)

Quarter strength: 0.125% (1000 mL)

(Continued)

## Sodium Hypochlorite Solution *(Continued)*

**Dosing**

**Adults:** Topical irrigation

**Elderly:** Refer to adult dosing.

**Administration**

**Topical:** For external use only; do **not** ingest.

**Additional Nursing Issues**

**Physical Assessment:** Assess knowledge/teach patient appropriate application and use and adverse symptoms to report. **Pregnancy risk factor C.**

**Patient Information/Instruction:** Use exactly as directed; do not overuse. Avoid contact with eyes. Report worsening of condition or lack of healing. **Pregnancy precautions:** Inform prescriber if you are or intend to be pregnant.

## Sodium Lactate (SOW dee um LAK tate)

**Therapeutic Category** Alkalinizing Agent

**Pregnancy Risk Factor** A

**Lactation** Excretion in breast milk unknown/compatible

**Use** Source of bicarbonate for prevention and treatment of mild to moderate metabolic acidosis

**Formulations**

Injection:

1.87 g/100 mL [sodium 16.7 mEq and lactate 16.7 mEq per 100 mL] (1000 mL)

560 mg/mL [sodium 5 mEq sodium and lactate 5 mEq per mL] (10 mL)

**Dosing**

**Adults:** Dosage depends on degree of acidosis

**Elderly:** Refer to adult dosing.


- **Sodium *L*-Triiodothyronine** *see* Liothyronine *on page 679*
- **Sodium Nitroferricyanide** *see* Nitroprusside *on page 833*
- **Sodium Nitroprusside** *see* Nitroprusside *on page 833*
- **Sodium Oxacillin** *see* Oxacillin *on page 866*
- **Sodium P.A.S.** *see* Aminosalicylate Sodium *on page 70*


## Sodium Phenylbutyrate (SOW dee um fen il BYOO ti rate)

**U.S. Brand Names** Buphenyl®

**Synonyms** Ammonapse

**Therapeutic Category** Urea Cycle Disorder (UCD) Treatment Agent

**Pregnancy Risk Factor** C

**Lactation** Excretion in breast milk unknown

**Use** Adjunctive therapy in the chronic management of patients with urea cycle disorder involving deficiencies of carbamoylphosphate synthetase, ornithine transcarbamylase, or argininosuccinic acid synthetase

**Formulations**

Powder: 3.2 g [sodium phenylbutyrate 3 g] per teaspoon (500 mL, 950 mL); 9.1 g [sodium phenylbutyrate 8.6 g] per **tablespoon** (500 mL, 950 mL)

Tablet: 500 mg

**Dosing**

**Adults:**

Powder: Patients weighing <20 kg: 450-600 mg/kg/day or 9.9-13 g/m²/day, administered in equally divided amounts with each meal or feeding, 4-6 times daily; safety and efficacy of doses >20 g/day has not been established.

Tablet: 450-600 mg/kg/day or 9.9-13 g/m²/day, administered in equally divided amounts with each meal; safety and efficacy of doses >20 g/day have not been established.

**Elderly:** Refer to adult dosing.


- **Sodium Phosphate** *see* Phosphate Supplements *on page 926*
- **Sodium Phosphate** *see page 1294*


## Sodium Polystyrene Sulfonate
(SOW dee um pol ee STYE reen SUL fon ate)

**U.S. Brand Names** Kayexalate®; SPS®

**Therapeutic Category** Antidote

**Pregnancy Risk Factor** C

**Lactation** Excretion in breast milk unknown/use caution

**Use** Treatment of hyperkalemia

**Mechanism of Action/Effect** Removes potassium by exchanging sodium ions for potassium ions in the intestine before the resin is passed from the body; exchange capacity is 1 mEq/g *in vivo*, and *in vitro* capacity is 3.1 mEq/g, therefore, a wide range of exchange capacity exists such that close monitoring of serum electrolytes is necessary

**Contraindications** Hypersensitivity to sodium polystyrene sulfonate or any component; hypernatremia

**Warnings** Use with caution in patients with severe congestive heart failure, hypertension, edema, or renal failure. Large oral doses may cause fecal impaction (especially in the elderly). Enema will reduce the serum potassium faster than oral administration, but the oral route will result in a greater reduction over several hours. Pregnancy factor C.

**Drug Interactions**

**Increased Effect/Toxicity:** Systemic alkalosis and seizure has occurred aftercation-exchange resins were administered with nonabsorbable cation-donating antacids and laxatives (eg, magnesium hydroxide, aluminum carbonate).

**Adverse Reactions**

>10%: Gastrointestinal: Constipation, anorexia, nausea, vomiting

1% to 10%:

Endocrine & metabolic: Hypokalemia, hypocalcemia, hypomagnesemia, sodium retention

Gastrointestinal: Fecal impaction

**Overdose/Toxicology** Symptoms of overdose include hypokalemia including cardiac dysrhythmias, confusion, irritability, EKG changes, muscle weakness, and GI effects. Treatment is supportive, limited to management of fluid and electrolytes.

**Pharmacodynamics/Kinetics**

**Excretion:** Feces

**Onset:** Within 2-24 hours

**Formulations**

Oral or rectal:

Powder for suspension: 454 g

Suspension: 1.25 g/5 mL with sorbitol 33% and alcohol 0.3% (60 mL, 120 mL, 200 mL, 500 mL)

**Dosing**

**Adults:**

Oral: 15 g (60 mL) 1-4 times/day

Rectal: 30-50 g every 6 hours

**Elderly:** Refer to adult dosing and Geriatric Considerations.

**Administration**

**Oral:** Administer oral (or NG) as ~25% sorbitol solution; never mix in orange juice. Chilling the oral mixture will increase palatability.

**Other:** Rectal: Enema route is less effective than oral administration. Administer cleansing enema first. Retain enema in colon for at least 30-60 minutes and for several hours, if possible. Enema should be followed by irrigation with normal saline to prevent necrosis.

**Monitoring Laboratory Tests** Serum electrolytes (potassium, sodium, calcium, magnesium), EKG

**Additional Nursing Issues**

**Physical Assessment:** Monitor laboratory tests (see above). Monitor EKG until potassium levels are normal. Monitor for adverse reactions (eg, fecal impaction - see Adverse Reactions) and teach patient interventions and importance of reporting adverse symptoms promptly. **Pregnancy risk factor C** - benefits of use should outweigh possible risks. Note breast-feeding caution.

**Patient Information/Instruction:** Emergency instructions depend on patient's condition. You will be monitored for effects of this medication and frequent blood tests may be necessary. Oral: Take as directed. Mix well with a full glass of liquid (not orange juice). You may experience nausea or vomiting (small frequent meals, frequent mouth care, chewing gum, or sucking lozenges may help); or constipation or fecal impaction (increased dietary fluids and exercise may help). Report persistent constipation or gastrointestinal distress; chest pain or rapid heartbeat; or mental confusion or muscle weakness. **Pregnancy/breast-feeding precautions:** Inform prescriber if pregnant. Consult prescriber if breast-feeding.

**Geriatric Considerations:** Large doses in the elderly may cause fecal impaction and intestinal obstruction. Best to administer using sorbitol 70% as vehicle.

**Additional Information** 1 g of resin binds approximately 1 mEq of potassium; sodium content of 1 g: 31 mg (1.3 mEq)


- **Sodium Sulamyd®** *see page 1282*
- **Sodium Sulamyd® Ophthalmic** *see* Sulfacetamide *on page 1080*
- **Sodium Sulfacetamide** *see* Sulfacetamide *on page 1080*
- **Sodium Thiosulfate** *see page 1246*
- **Sodol®** *see* Carisoprodol *on page 202*
- **SoFlax™** *see* Docusate *on page 392*
- **Solaquin® [OTC]** *see* Hydroquinone *on page 583*
- **Solaquin Forte®** *see* Hydroquinone *on page 583*
- **Solarcaine® [OTC]** *see* Benzocaine *on page 141*
- **Solarcaine® Aloe Extra Burn Relief [OTC]** *see* Lidocaine *on page 674*
- **Solfoton®** *see* Phenobarbital *on page 917*
- **Solium®** *see* Chlordiazepoxide *on page 250*
- **Soltric** *see* Mebendazole *on page 709*
- **Solu-Cortef®** *see* Hydrocortisone *on page 578*
- **Solu-Cortef®** *see* Topical Corticosteroids *on page 1152*
- **Solu-Medrol® Injection** *see* Methylprednisolone *on page 754*
- **Solurex L.A.®** *see* Dexamethasone *on page 346*
- **Soma®** *see* Carisoprodol *on page 202*
- **Soma® Compound** *see* Carisoprodol and Aspirin *on page 203*
- **Soma® Compound w/Codeine** *see* Carisoprodol, Aspirin, and Codeine *on page 203*
- **Sominex® Oral [OTC]** *see* Diphenhydramine *on page 381*
- **Somnol®** *see* Flurazepam *on page 507*

- **Som Pam**® *see* Flurazepam *on page 507*
- **Sopamycetin** *see* Chloramphenicol *on page 248*
- **Sophipren Ofteno** *see* Prednisolone *on page 960*
- **Sophixin Ofteno** *see* Ciprofloxacin *on page 270*
- **Soprodol**® *see* Carisoprodol *on page 202*

## Sorbitol (SOR bi tole)

**Therapeutic Category** Genitourinary Irrigant; Laxative, Miscellaneous

**Lactation** Excretion in breast milk unknown

**Use** GU irrigant in transurethral prostatic resection (or other transurethral resection) or other transurethral surgical procedures; diuretic; humectant; sweetening agent; hyperosmotic laxative; facilitate the passage of sodium polystyrene sulfonate through the intestinal tract

**Mechanism of Action/Effect** A polyalcoholic sugar with osmotic cathartic actions

**Contraindications** Anuria

**Warnings** Use with caution in patients with severe cardiopulmonary or renal impairment and in patients unable to metabolize sorbitol.

**Adverse Reactions** 1% to 10%:

Cardiovascular: Edema

Endocrine & metabolic: Fluid and electrolyte losses, lactic acidosis

Gastrointestinal: Diarrhea, nausea, vomiting, abdominal discomfort, dry mouth

**Overdose/Toxicology** Symptoms of overdose include nausea, diarrhea, fluid and electrolyte loss. Treatment is supportive to ensure fluid and electrolyte balance.

**Pharmacodynamics/Kinetics**

**Metabolism:** Liver

**Onset:** About 0.25-1 hour

**Formulations**

Solution: 70%

Solution, genitourinary irrigation: 3% (1500 mL, 3000 mL); 3.3% (2000 mL)

**Dosing**

**Adults:** Hyperosmotic laxative (as single dose, at infrequent intervals):

Oral: 30-150 mL (as 70% solution)

Rectal enema: 120 mL as 25% to 30% solution

Adjunct to sodium polystyrene sulfonate: 15 mL as 70% solution orally until diarrhea occurs (10-20 mL/2 hours) or 20-100 mL as an oral vehicle for the sodium polystyrene sulfonate resin

When administered with charcoal:

Oral: 4.3 mL/kg of 70% sorbitol with 1 g/kg of activated charcoal every 4 hours until first stool containing charcoal is passed

Topical: 3% to 3.3% as transurethral surgical procedure irrigation

**Elderly:** Refer to adult dosing.

**Additional Nursing Issues**

**Physical Assessment:** When used as cathartic, determine cause of constipation before use and patient knowledge of nonpharmacological treatment and prevention of constipation. Note breast-feeding caution.

**Patient Information/Instruction:** Cathartic: Use of cathartics on a regular basis will have adverse effects. Increased exercise, increased fluid intake, or increased dietary fruit and fiber may be effective in preventing and resolving constipation. **Breast-feeding precautions:** Consult prescriber if breast-feeding.

**Geriatric Considerations:** Causes for constipation must be evaluated prior to initiating treatment. Nonpharmacological dietary treatment should be initiated before laxative use. Sorbitol is as effective as lactulose but is much less expensive.

- **Sorbitrate**® *see* Isosorbide Dinitrate *on page 634*
- **Soridol**® *see* Carisoprodol *on page 202*
- **Sotacor**® *see* Sotalol *on this page*

## Sotalol (SOE ta lole)

**U.S. Brand Names** Betapace®

**Therapeutic Category** Antiarrhythmic Agent, Class II; Antiarrhythmic Agent, Class III; Beta Blocker, $Beta_1$ Selective

**Pregnancy Risk Factor** B

**Lactation** Enters breast milk/use caution - see Breast-feeding Issues

**Use** Treatment of documented ventricular arrhythmias, such as sustained ventricular tachycardia, that in the judgment of the physician are life-threatening

**Mechanism of Action/Effect**

Beta-blocker which contains both beta-adrenoreceptor-blocking (Vaughan Williams Class II) and cardiac action potential duration prolongation (Vaughan Williams Class III) properties

Class II effects: Increased sinus cycle length, slowed heart rate, decreased A-V nodal conduction, and increased A-V nodal refractoriness

Class III effects: Prolongation of the atrial and ventricular monophasic action potentials, and effective refractory prolongation of atrial muscle, ventricular muscle, and atrioventricular accessory pathways in both the antegrade and retrograde directions

Sotalol is a racemic mixture of *d*- and *l*-sotalol; both isomers have similar Class III antiarrhythmic effects while the *l*-isomer is responsible for virtually all of the beta-blocking activity

Sotalol has both $beta_1$- and $beta_2$-receptor blocking activity

The beta-blocking effect of sotalol is a noncardioselective [half maximal at about 80 mg/day and maximal at doses of 320-640 mg/day]. Significant beta blockade occurs at oral doses as low as 25 mg/day.

The Class III effects are seen only at oral doses ≥160 mg/day

**Contraindications** Hypersensitivity to sotalol; bronchial asthma; sinus bradycardia; second and third degree A-V block (unless a functioning pacemaker is present); congenital or acquired long Q-T syndromes; cardiogenic shock; uncontrolled congestive heart failure

**Warnings** Use with caution in patients with congestive heart failure, peripheral vascular disease, hypokalemia, hypomagnesemia, renal dysfunction, or sick-sinus syndrome. Abrupt withdrawal may result in return of life-threatening arrhythmias. Sotalol can provoke new or worsening ventricular arrhythmias.

**Drug Interactions**

**Decreased Effect:** Decreased effect of beta-blockers with aluminum salts, barbiturates, calcium salts, cholestyramine, colestipol, NSAIDs, penicillins (ampicillin), rifampin, salicylates, and sulfinpyrazone due to decreased bioavailability and plasma levels. Beta-blockers may decrease the effect of sulfonylureas. Beta-agonists such as albuterol, terbutaline may have less of a therapeutic effect when administered concomitantly. Beta-blockers may affect the action or levels of ethanol, disopyramide, nondepolarizing muscle relaxants, and theophylline although the effects are difficult to predict.

**Increased Effect/Toxicity:** Increased effect/toxicity of beta-blockers with calcium blockers since there may be additive effects on AV conduction or ventricular function. Sotalol in combination with Class I antiarrhythmic agents, phenothiazines, tricyclic antidepressants, terfenadine, or astemizole may contribute to further prolongation of Q-T interval. Beta-blockers and clonidine (hypertensive crisis after or during withdrawal of either agent). Beta-blocker and catecholamine depleting agents (reserpine or guanethidine) may result in additive hypotension or bradycardia. Beta-blockers may affect the action or levels of ethanol, disopyramide, nondepolarizing muscle relaxants, and theophylline although the effects are difficult to predict.

**Food Interactions** Sotalol peak serum concentrations may be decreased if taken with food.

**Adverse Reactions**

>10%:

- Central nervous system: Drowsiness, insomnia
- Endocrine & metabolic: Decreased sexual ability

1% to 10%:

- Cardiovascular: Bradycardia, palpitations, edema, congestive heart failure, reduced peripheral circulation
- Central nervous system: Mental depression
- Gastrointestinal: Diarrhea or constipation, nausea, vomiting, stomach discomfort
- Respiratory: Bronchospasm
- Miscellaneous: Cold extremities

<1% (Limited to important or life-threatening symptoms): Chest pain, arrhythmias, orthostatic hypotension, nervousness, headache, depression, hallucinations, confusion (especially in the elderly), thrombocytopenia, leukopenia, shortness of breath

**Overdose/Toxicology** Symptoms of intoxication include cardiac disturbances, CNS toxicity, bronchospasm, hypoglycemia and hyperkalemia. The most common cardiac symptoms include hypotension and bradycardia. Atrioventricular block, intraventricular conduction disturbances, cardiogenic shock, and asystole may occur with severe overdose, especially with membrane-depressant drugs (eg, propranolol). CNS effects include convulsions, and coma. Respiratory arrest is commonly seen with propranolol and other membrane-depressant and lipid-soluble drugs. Treatment is symptomatic.

**Pharmacodynamics/Kinetics**

**Protein Binding:** Not protein bound

**Distribution:** Low lipid solubility

**Half-life Elimination:** 12 hours

**Metabolism:** Not metabolized

**Excretion:** Renal

**Onset:** Rapid, 1-2 hours; Peak effect: 2.5-4 hours

**Duration:** 8-16 hours

**Formulations** Tablet, as hydrochloride: 80 mg, 120 mg, 160 mg, 240 mg

**Dosing**

**Adults:** Sotalol should be initiated and doses increased in a hospital with facilities for cardiac rhythm monitoring and assessment. Proarrhythmic events can occur after initiation of therapy and with each upward dosage adjustment.

Oral:

- Initial: 80 mg twice daily
- Dose may be increased (gradually allowing 2-3 days between dosing increments in order to attain steady-state plasma concentrations and to allow monitoring of Q-T intervals) to 240-320 mg/day
- Most patients respond to a total daily dose of 160-320 mg/day in 2-3 divided doses
- Some patients, with life-threatening refractory ventricular arrhythmias, may require doses as high as 480-640 mg/day; however, these doses should only be prescribed when the potential benefit outweighs the increased of adverse events

**Elderly:** Age does not significantly alter the pharmacokinetics of sotalol, but impaired renal function in elderly patients can increase the terminal half-life, resulting in increased drug accumulation. Adjust dose for renal impairment.

(Continued)

## Sotalol *(Continued)*

**Renal Impairment:**

Impaired renal function can increase the terminal half-life, resulting in increased drug accumulation.

$Cl_{cr}$ >60 mL/minute: Administer every 12 hours.

$Cl_{cr}$ 30-60 mL/minute: Administer every 24 hours.

$Cl_{cr}$ 10-30 mL/minute: Administer every 36-48 hours.

$Cl_{cr}$ <10 mL/minute: Individualize dose.

Hemodialysis effects: Hemodialysis would be expected to reduce sotalol plasma concentrations because sotalol is not bound to plasma proteins and does not undergo extensive metabolism. Administer dose postdialysis or administer supplemental 80 mg dose; peritoneal dialysis does not remove sotalol. Supplemental dose is not necessary.

**Monitoring Laboratory Tests** Serum magnesium, potassium

**Additional Nursing Issues**

**Physical Assessment:** Assess other medications patient may be taking for effectiveness and interactions (see Contraindications and Drug Interactions). See Warnings/Precautions and Contraindications for cautious use. Initiation of therapy and adjustment of dosage should be done as inpatient with close cardiac monitoring. Monitor laboratory tests, therapeutic response (cardiac status), and adverse reactions (see Warnings/Precautions and Adverse Reactions) at beginning of therapy, when titrating dosage, and on a regular basis with long-term therapy. Assess knowledge/teach patient appropriate use, interventions to reduce side effects, and adverse symptoms to report.

**Patient Information/Instruction:** Take exactly as directed; do not take additional doses or discontinue without consulting prescriber. You will need regular cardiac checkups and blood tests while taking this medication. You may experience dizziness, drowsiness, or visual changes (use caution when driving or engaging in tasks requiring alertness until response to drug is known); orthostatic hypotension (use caution when climbing stairs or when changing position - rising from lying or sitting position); abnormal taste, nausea or vomiting, or loss of appetite (small frequent meals, frequent mouth care, chewing gum, or sucking lozenges may help); decreased sexual ability (reversible); or constipation (increased exercise, dietary fiber, fruit, or fluid may help). Report chest pain, palpitation, or erratic heartbeat; difficulty breathing or unusual cough; mental depression or persistent insomnia (hallucinations); or changes in vision.

**Geriatric Considerations:** Since elderly frequently have $Cl_{cr}$ <60 mL/minute, attention to dose, creatinine clearance, and monitoring is important. Make dosage adjustments at 3-day intervals or after 5-6 doses at any dosage.

**Breast-feeding Issues:** Sotalol is considered compatible by the American Academy of Pediatrics. It is recommended that the infant be monitored for signs or symptoms of beta-blockade (hypotension, bradycardia, etc) with long-term use.

**Additional Information** Serum concentrations have not been systematically evaluated: Concentration effect curves for the beta-blocking and antiarrhythmic agents of sotalol are different. Serum levels of 340-3440 ng/mL have shown a 70% to 100% reduction in VPBs. Average serum concentrations associated with significant Q-T prolongation were 2550 ng/mL. Average serum concentrations associated with maximum heart reduction by 50% was 804 ng/mL.

**Related Information**

Antiarrhythmic Drug Classification Comparison *on page 1366*
Beta-Blockers Comparison *on page 1376*

♦ **Sound-Alike Comparison List** *see page 1448*
♦ **Soyacal®** *see* Fat Emulsion *on page 471*
♦ **Spancap® No. 1** *see* Dextroamphetamine *on page 353*
♦ **Span-FF® [OTC]** *see* Iron Supplements *on page 627*

## Sparfloxacin (spar FLOKS a sin)

**U.S. Brand Names** Zagam®

**Therapeutic Category** Antibiotic, Quinolone

**Pregnancy Risk Factor** C

**Lactation** Enters breast milk/contraindicated

**Use** Treatment of adults with community-acquired pneumonia caused by *C. pneumoniae, H. influenzae, H. parainfluenzae, M. catarrhalis, M. pneumoniae,* or *S. pneumoniae,* also for treatment of acute bacterial exacerbations of chronic bronchitis caused by *C. pneumoniae, E. cloacae, H. influenzae, H. parainfluenzae, K. pneumoniae, M. catarrhalis, S. aureus, S. pneumoniae*; offers potential advantage over other fluoroquinolones due to enhanced activity (particularly against gram-positive cocci and anaerobes) and a long half-life, allowing once-daily dosing.

**Mechanism of Action/Effect** Inhibits DNA-gyrase in susceptible organisms; inhibits relaxation of supercoiled DNA and promotes breakage of double-stranded DNA

**Contraindications** Hypersensitivity to sparfloxacin, other quinolones, or any component

**Warnings** CNS stimulation may occur (eg, tremor, restlessness, confusion, and very rarely hallucinations or seizures). Use with caution in patients with known or suspected CNS disorder or renal dysfunction. Prolonged use may result in superinfection. If an allergic reaction (eg, itching, urticaria, dyspnea, pharyngeal or facial edema, loss of consciousness, tingling, cardiovascular collapse) occurs, discontinue the drug immediately. Use caution to avoid possible photosensitivity reactions during and for several days following fluoroquinolone therapy. Pseudomembranous colitis may occur and should be considered in patients who present with diarrhea. Pregnancy factor C.

**Drug Interactions**

**Decreased Effect:** Decreased absorption with antacids containing aluminum, magnesium, zinc, iron and/or calcium (by up to 98% if given at the same time). Phenytoin serum levels may be reduced by quinolones. Antineoplastic agents may also decrease serum levels of fluoroquinolones.

**Increased Effect/Toxicity:** Quinolones cause increased levels of caffeine, warfarin, cyclosporine, and theophylline (although one study indicates that sparfloxacin may not affect theophylline metabolism), cimetidine, and probenecid increase quinolone levels. An increased incidence of seizures may occur with foscarnet.

**Adverse Reactions**

1% to 10%:

Cardiovascular: Q-$T_c$ interval prolongation (1.3%)

Central nervous system: Insomnia, dizziness, headache, agitation, sleep disorders, anxiety, delirium

Dermatologic: Photosensitivity reaction, pruritus, vasodilatation

Gastrointestinal: Diarrhea, dyspepsia, nausea, abdominal pain, vomiting, flatulence, taste perversion, dry mouth

Hematologic: Leukopenia, eosinophilia, anemia

Hepatic: Increased LFTs

<1% (Limited to important or life-threatening symptoms): Palpitations, hypertension, tachycardia, sinus bradycardia, arrhythmias, angina pectoris, atrial fibrillation, atrial flutter, complete AV block, supraventricular extrasystoles, ventricular extrasystoles, postural hypotension, cyanosis, migraine, ecchymosis, exfoliative dermatitis, angioedema, menorrhagia hematuria, polyuria, asthma, epistaxis, pneumonia, bronchitis, hemoptysis, sinusitis, dyspnea, lymphadenopathy

**Pharmacodynamics/Kinetics**

**Distribution:** Distributes into many tissues, including lung, skin, prostate, and gynecologic tissue; CSF penetration is limited

**Half-life Elimination:** 16 hours

**Time to Peak:** 3-5 hours

**Metabolism:** Liver

**Excretion:** Urine

**Formulations** Tablet: 200 mg

**Dosing**

**Adults:** Loading dose: 2 tablets (400 mg) on day 1

Maintenance dose: 1 tablet (200 mg) daily for 9 additional days (completes 10 days therapy with a total of 11 tablets)

**Elderly:** Refer to adult dosing.

**Renal Impairment:** $Cl_{cr}$ <50 mL/minute: Administer 400 mg on day 1 as a loading dose, then 200 mg every 48 hours for a total of 8 additional days of therapy (total 6 tablets).

**Administration**

**Oral:** May take without regard to meals.

**Monitoring Laboratory Tests** Perform culture and sensitivity prior to beginning therapy. Monitor CBC, renal and hepatic function periodically if therapy is prolonged.

**Additional Nursing Issues**

**Physical Assessment:** Monitor effectiveness of other medications patient may be taking (see Drug Interactions). Monitor adverse reactions and response to therapy. If no improvement or relapse occurs, treatment should be re-evaluated. Monitor for signs of opportunistic infection (eg, chills, fever, burning on urination, easy bleeding or bruising, unhealed wounds, vaginal discharge, fuzzy tongue). **Pregnancy risk factor C** - benefits of use should outweigh possible risks. Breast-feeding is contraindicated.

**Patient Information/Instruction:** Take per recommended schedule around-the-clock. Maintain adequate hydration (2-3 L/day of fluids unless instructed to restrict fluid intake). Take complete prescription and do not skip doses; if dose is missed take as soon as possible, do not double doses. Do not take with antacids. You may experience dizziness, lightheadedness, anxiety, insomnia, or confusion; use caution when driving or engaging in tasks that require alertness until response to drug is known. Small frequent meals, frequent mouth care, sucking lozenges, or chewing gum may reduce nausea, vomiting, or taste disturbances. You may experience photosensitivity; use sunscreen, wear protective clothing and eyewear, and avoid direct sunlight. Report palpitations or chest pain; persistent diarrhea or GI disturbances or abdominal pain; muscle tremor or pain; pain, inflammation, or rupture of tendon; yellowing of eyes or skin, easy bruising or bleeding; unusual fatigue; fever, chills, signs of infection; or worsening of condition. **Pregnancy/breast-feeding precautions:** Inform prescriber if pregnant. Do not breast-feed.

**Geriatric Considerations:** Adjust dose based on renal function; evaluate patient's drug regimen prior to initiating therapy to avoid or make allowances for possible drug interactions since elderly frequently have diseases requiring medications that can interact with quinolones.


- ♦ **Sparine®** *see* Promazine *on page 976*
- ♦ **Spaslin®** *see* Hyoscyamine, Atropine, Scopolamine, and Phenobarbital *on page 591*
- ♦ **Spasmolin®** *see* Hyoscyamine, Atropine, Scopolamine, and Phenobarbital *on page 591*
- ♦ **Spasmophen®** *see* Hyoscyamine, Atropine, Scopolamine, and Phenobarbital *on page 591*
- ♦ **Spasquid®** *see* Hyoscyamine, Atropine, Scopolamine, and Phenobarbital *on page 591*
- ♦ **Spec-T® [OTC]** *see* Benzocaine *on page 141*
- ♦ **Spectam®** *see* Spectinomycin *on next page*

♦ **Spectazole™ Topical** *see* Econazole *on page 412*

## Spectinomycin (spek ti noe MYE sin)

**U.S. Brand Names** Spectam®; Trobicin®

**Therapeutic Category** Antibiotic, Miscellaneous

**Pregnancy Risk Factor** B

**Lactation** Enters breast milk/effect on infant unknown

**Use** Treatment of uncomplicated gonorrhea (ineffective against syphilis)

**Mechanism of Action/Effect** A bacteriostatic antibiotic that selectively binds to the 30s subunits of ribosomes, and thereby inhibiting bacterial protein synthesis

**Contraindications** Hypersensitivity to spectinomycin or any component

**Warnings** Since spectinomycin is ineffective in the treatment of syphilis and may mask symptoms, all patients should be tested for syphilis at the time of diagnosis and 3 months later.

**Adverse Reactions** <1% (Limited to important or life-threatening symptoms): Dizziness, headache, chills, nausea, vomiting, abdominal cramps

**Pharmacodynamics/Kinetics**

**Half-life Elimination:** 1.7 hours

**Time to Peak:** Within 1 hour

**Excretion:** Urine

**Duration:** Up to 8 hours

**Formulations** Injection, as hydrochloride: 2 g, 4 g

**Dosing**

**Adults:** I.M.:

Uncomplicated urethral endocervical or rectal gonorrhea: 2 g deep I.M. or 4 g where antibiotic resistance is prevalent 1 time; 4 g (10 mL) dose should be given as two 5 mL injections, followed by doxycycline 100 mg twice daily for 7 days

Disseminated gonococcal infection: 2 g every 12 hours

**Elderly:** Refer to adult dosing.

**Renal Impairment:** Hemodialysis effects: 50% removed by hemodialysis

**Administration**

**I.M.:** For I.M. use only.

**Stability**

**Reconstitution:** Use reconstituted solutions within 24 hours; reconstitute with supplied diluent only.

**Monitoring Laboratory Tests** Test for syphilis before treatment and 3 months later (see Warnings/Precautions).

**Additional Nursing Issues**

**Physical Assessment:** Assess knowledge/teach patient sexually transmitted diseases precautions. Monitor effectiveness and evaluate laboratory results (see above). Note breast-feeding caution.

**Patient Information/Instruction:** This medication can only be administered I.M. You will need to return for follow-up blood tests. **Breast-feeding precautions:** Consult prescriber if breast-feeding.

**Additional Information** Some formulations may contain benzyl alcohol.

♦ **Spherulin®** *see page 1248*

♦ **Spironazide®** *see* Hydrochlorothiazide and Spironolactone *on page 568*

## Spironolactone (speer on oh LAK tone)

**U.S. Brand Names** Aldactone®

**Therapeutic Category** Diuretic, Potassium Sparing

**Pregnancy Risk Factor** D

**Lactation** Enters breast milk/compatible

**Use** Management of edema associated with excessive aldosterone excretion; hypertension; primary hyperaldosteronism; hypokalemia; treatment of hirsutism; cirrhosis of liver accompanied by edema or ascites

**Mechanism of Action/Effect** Competes with aldosterone for receptor sites in the distal renal tubules, increasing sodium chloride and water excretion while conserving potassium and hydrogen ions; may block the effect of aldosterone on arteriolar smooth muscle as well

**Contraindications** Hypersensitivity to spironolactone or any component; hyperkalemia; renal failure; anuria; patients receiving other potassium-sparing diuretics or potassium supplements; pregnancy

**Warnings** Use with caution in patients with dehydration, hepatic disease, hyponatremia, or renal sufficiency. It is recommended the drug may be discontinued several days prior to adrenal vein catheterization. Shown to be tumorigenic in toxicity studies using rats at 25-250 times the usual human dose.

**Drug Interactions**

**Increased Effect/Toxicity:** Potassium, potassium-sparing diuretics, indomethacin, and angiotensin-converting enzymes inhibitors may increase serum potassium levels.

**Food Interactions** Administration with food increases absorption.

**Effects on Lab Values** May cause false elevation in serum digoxin concentrations measured by RIA.

**Adverse Reactions**

1% to 10%:

Cardiovascular: Arrhythmia

Central nervous system: Confusion, nervousness, dizziness, drowsiness, lack of energy, clumsiness, unusual fatigue, headache, fever, chills

Endocrine & metabolic: Hyperkalemia, breast tenderness in females, deepening of voice in females, enlargement of breast in males, inability to achieve or maintain an erection, increased hair growth in females, decreased sexual ability, menstrual irregularities

Gastrointestinal: Diarrhea, nausea, vomiting, stomach cramps, dryness of mouth

Neuromuscular & skeletal: Weakness, numbness or paresthesia in hands, feet, or lips,

Miscellaneous: Increased thirst

<1% (Limited to important or life-threatening symptoms): Agranulocytosis, shortness of breath, dyspnea, renal dysfunction

**Overdose/Toxicology** Symptoms of overdose include drowsiness, confusion, clinical signs of dehydration and electrolyte imbalance, and hyperkalemia. Ingestion of large amounts of potassium-sparing diuretics may result in life-threatening hyperkalemia. This can be treated with I.V. glucose, with concurrent regular insulin. Sodium bicarbonate may also be used as a temporary measure. If needed, Kayexalate® oral or rectal solutions in sorbitol may also be used.

**Pharmacodynamics/Kinetics**

**Protein Binding:** 91% to 98%

**Half-life Elimination:** 78-84 minutes

**Time to Peak:** Within 1-3 hours (primarily as the active metabolite)

**Metabolism:** Liver

**Excretion:** Urinary and biliary excretion

**Formulations** Tablet: 25 mg, 50 mg, 100 mg

**Dosing**

**Adults:** To reduce delay in onset of effect, a loading dose of 2 or 3 times the daily dose may be administered on the first day of therapy. Oral:

Edema, hypertension, hypokalemia: 25-200 mg/day in 1-2 divided doses

Diagnosis of primary aldosteronism: 100-400 mg/day in 1-2 divided doses

**Elderly:** Oral: Initial: 25-50 mg/day in 1-2 divided doses, increasing by 25-50 mg every 5 days as needed; adjust for renal impairment.

**Renal Impairment:**

$Cl_{cr}$ 10-50 mL/minute: Administer every 12-24 hours.

$Cl_{cr}$ <10 mL/minute: Avoid use.

**Stability**

**Storage:** Protect from light.

**Monitoring Laboratory Tests** Serum electrolytes (potassium, sodium), renal function

**Additional Nursing Issues**

**Physical Assessment:** Monitor effectiveness of therapy and adverse reactions frequently when starting therapy and on a regular basis thereafter, especially fluid status, hyperkalemia (eg, arrhythmias, fatigue, muscle weakness, paresthesia, confusion), and hyponatremia (eg, anorexia, nausea/vomiting, diarrhea, headaches, lethargy, hyper-reflexia, seizures). Diuretic effect may be delayed 2-3 days and antihypertensive effect may be delayed 2-3 weeks. Teach patient effects to monitor and symptoms to report. **Pregnancy risk factor D** - assess knowledge/teach appropriate use of barrier contraceptives.

**Patient Information/Instruction:** Take as directed, with meals or milk. This diuretic does not cause potassium loss; avoid excessive potassium intake (eg, salt substitutes, low-salt foods, bananas, nuts). Weigh yourself weekly at the same time, in the same clothes, and report weight loss more than 5 lb/week. You may experience dizziness, drowsiness, headache; use caution when driving or engaging in tasks requiring alertness until response to drug is known. Small frequent meals, frequent mouth care, sucking lozenges, or chewing gum may reduce dry mouth, nausea, or vomiting. You may experience decreased sexual ability (reversible with discontinuing of medication). Report mental confusion; clumsiness; persistent fatigue, chills, numbness, or muscle weakness in hands, feet, or face; acute persistent diarrhea; breast tenderness or increased body hair in females; breast enlargement or inability to achieve erection in males; chest pain, rapid heartbeat or palpitations; or difficulty breathing. **Pregnancy precautions:** Do not get pregnant while taking this medication; use appropriate barrier contraceptive measures.

**Geriatric Considerations:** See Warnings/Precautions; monitor serum potassium.

- **Spironolactone and Hydrochlorothiazide** *see* Hydrochlorothiazide and Spironolactone *on page 568*
- **Spirozide®** *see* Hydrochlorothiazide and Spironolactone *on page 568*
- **Sporanox®** *see* Itraconazole *on page 639*
- **Sportscreme®** *see page 1294*
- **SPS®** *see* Sodium Polystyrene Sulfonate *on page 1064*
- **S-P-T** *see* Thyroid *on page 1130*
- **SRC® Expectorant** *see* Hydrocodone, Pseudoephedrine, and Guaifenesin *on page 577*
- **SSD® AF** *see* Silver Sulfadiazine *on page 1059*
- **SSD® Cream** *see* Silver Sulfadiazine *on page 1059*
- **SSKI®** *see* Potassium Iodide *on page 951*
- **Stadol®** *see* Butorphanol *on page 178*
- **Stadol® NS** *see* Butorphanol *on page 178*
- **Stagesic®** *see* Hydrocodone and Acetaminophen *on page 568*

## Stanozolol (stan OH zoe lole)

**U.S. Brand Names** Winstrol®

**Therapeutic Category** Anabolic Steroid

(Continued)

## Stanozolol *(Continued)*

**Pregnancy Risk Factor** X

**Lactation** Enters breast milk/contraindicated

**Use** Prophylactic use against hereditary angioedema

**Mechanism of Action/Effect** Synthetic testosterone derivative with similar androgenic and anabolic actions

**Contraindications** Hypersensitivity to stanozolol or any component; nephrosis; carcinoma of breast or prostate; pregnancy

**Warnings** Anabolic steroids may cause peliosis hepatis, liver cell tumors, and blood lipid changes with increased risk of arteriosclerosis. Monitor diabetic patients carefully. Use with caution in elderly patients, they may be at greater risk for prostatic hypertrophy. Use with caution in patients with cardiac, renal, or hepatic disease or epilepsy.

**Drug Interactions**

**Increased Effect/Toxicity:** ACTH, adrenal steroids may increase risk of edema and acne. Stanozolol enhances the hypoprothrombinemic effects of oral anticoagulants and enhances the hypoglycemic effects of insulin and sulfonylureas (oral hypoglycemics).

**Adverse Reactions**

**Male: Postpubertal:**

>10%:

Dermatologic: Acne

Endocrine & metabolic: Gynecomastia

Genitourinary: Bladder irritability, priapism

1% to 10%:

Central nervous system: Insomnia, chills

Endocrine & metabolic: Decreased libido, hepatic dysfunction,

Gastrointestinal: Nausea, diarrhea

Genitourinary: Prostatic hypertrophy (elderly)

Hematologic: Iron deficiency anemia, suppression of clotting factors

<1% (Limited to important or life-threatening symptoms): Hepatic necrosis, hepatocellular carcinoma

**Female:**

>10%: Endocrine & metabolic: Virilism

1% to 10%:

Central nervous system: Chills, insomnia

Endocrine & metabolic: Hypercalcemia

Gastrointestinal: Nausea, diarrhea

Hematologic: Iron deficiency anemia, suppression of clotting factors

Hepatic: Hepatic dysfunction

<1% (Limited to important or life-threatening symptoms): Hepatic necrosis, hepatocellular carcinoma

**Pharmacodynamics/Kinetics**

**Metabolism:** In an analogous fashion to testosterone

**Excretion:** In an analogous fashion to testosterone

**Formulations** Tablet: 2 mg

**Dosing**

**Adults:** Oral: Initial: 2 mg 3 times/day, may then reduce to a maintenance dose of 2 mg/day or 2 mg every other day after 1-3 months

**Elderly:** Refer to adult dosing.

**Hepatic Impairment:** Avoid use in patients with severe liver dysfunction.

**Additional Nursing Issues**

**Physical Assessment:** Assess effectiveness and interactions of other medications (see Drug Interactions, eg, anticoagulants and hypoglycemic agents). See Warnings/Precautions and Contraindications for use cautions. Monitor effectiveness of therapy and adverse response (see Adverse Reactions and Overdose/Toxicology). Assess knowledge/teach patient appropriate use, possible side effects/interventions, and adverse symptoms to report. **Pregnancy risk factor X** - determine that patient is not pregnant before beginning treatment and do not give to women of childbearing age unless patient and sexual partners are capable of complying with barrier contraceptive measures 1 month prior to therapy, during therapy, and for 1 month following therapy. Breast-feeding is contraindicated.

**Patient Information/Instruction:** Take as directed; do not exceed recommended dosage. Diabetics should monitor serum glucose closely and notify prescriber of changes; this medication can alter hypoglycemic requirements. You may experience decrease of libido or impotence (usually reversible); nausea, vomiting, or GI distress (frequent small meals, frequent mouth care, chewing gum, or sucking lozenges may help); or diarrhea (buttermilk, boiled milk, yogurt may help). Report persistent GI distress or diarrhea; change in color of urine or stool; unusual bruising, bleeding, or yellowing of eyes or skin; fluid retention (swelling of ankles, feet, or hands, difficulty breathing, or sudden weight gain); unresolved CNS changes (insomnia or chills); menstrual irregularity; excessive growth of body hair; or other adverse reactions. **Pregnancy/breast-feeding precautions:** Inform prescriber if you are pregnant. Do not get pregnant 1 month before, during, or for 1 month following therapy. Consult prescriber for instruction on appropriate contraceptive measures. This drug may cause severe fetal defects. Do not donate blood during or for 1 month following therapy (same reason). Do not breast-feed.

- **Staphcillin®** *see* Methicillin *on page 740*
- **Statex®** *see* Morphine Sulfate *on page 790*

## Stavudine (STAV yoo deen)

**U.S. Brand Names** Zerit®

**Synonyms** D4T

**Therapeutic Category** Antiretroviral Agent, Reverse Transcriptase Inhibitor (Nucleoside)

**Pregnancy Risk Factor** C

**Lactation** Enters breast milk/contraindicated

**Use** Treatment of adults with advanced HIV infection who are intolerant to approved therapies with proven clinical benefit or who have experienced significant clinical or immunologic deterioration while receiving these therapies, or for whom such therapies are contraindicated

**Mechanism of Action/Effect** Inhibits reverse transcriptase of the human immunodeficiency virus (HIV)

**Contraindications** Hypersensitivity to stavudine or any component

**Warnings** Use with caution in patients who demonstrate previous hypersensitivity to zidovudine, didanosine, zalcitabine, pre-existing bone marrow suppression, or renal insufficiency, or peripheral neuropathy. Peripheral neuropathy may be the dose-limiting side effect. Potentially fatal lactic acidosis and severe hepatomegaly have been reported; use with caution in patients at risk of hepatic disease. Pregnancy factor C.

**Adverse Reactions** All adverse reactions reported below were similar to comparative agent (zidovudine), except for peripheral neuropathy, which was greater with stavudine

>10%:
- Neuromuscular & skeletal: Peripheral neuropathy (dose related)
- Central nervous system: Headache, chills/fever, malaise, insomnia, anxiety, depression, pain
- Gastrointestinal: Nausea, vomiting, anorexia, diarrhea, abdominal pain

1% to 10%
- Hematologic: Neutropenia, thrombocytopenia
- Hepatic: increased bilirubin
- Neuromuscular & skeletal: Myalgia, arthralgia, back pain, weakness

<1% (Limited to important or life-threatening symptoms): Anemia, lactic acidosis, hepatomegaly, hepatic failure, pancreatitis

**Pharmacodynamics/Kinetics**

**Half-life Elimination:** 1-1.6 hours

**Time to Peak:** 1 hour after administration

**Excretion:** Renal

**Formulations**

Capsule: 15 mg, 20 mg, 30 mg, 40 mg

Powder for oral solution: 1 mg/mL (200 mL)

**Dosing**

**Adults:** Oral (Dose may be cut in half if symptoms of peripheral neuropathy occur):
- ≥60 kg: 40 mg every 12 hours
- <60 kg: 30 mg every 12 hours

**Elderly:** Refer to adult dosing.

**Renal Impairment:**

$Cl_{cr}$ >50 mL/minute:
- ≥60 kg: Administer 40 mg every 12 hours.
- <60 kg: Administer 30 mg every 12 hours.

$Cl_{cr}$ 26-50 mL/minute:
- ≥60 kg: Administer 20 mg every 12 hours.
- <60 kg: Administer 15 mg every 12 hours.

$Cl_{cr}$ 10-25 mL/minute:
- ≥60 kg: Administer 20 mg every 24 hours.
- <60 kg: Administer 15 mg every 24 hours.

Hemodialysis:
- ≥60 kg: Administer 20 mg every 24 hours.
- <60 kg: Administer 15 mg every 24 hours.

**Administration**

**Oral:** Take without regard to meals.

**Monitoring Laboratory Tests** Liver function

**Additional Nursing Issues**

**Physical Assessment:** Monitor on a regular basis for peripheral neuropathy. Assess knowledge/teach appropriate administration, effects to monitor, and symptoms to report. **Pregnancy risk factor C** - benefits of use should outweigh possible risks. Breast-feeding is contraindicated.

**Patient Information/Instruction:** This medication does not cure HIV. Use appropriate precautions to prevent transmission to others. Take as directed, around-the-clock, and take for full length of prescription. Maintain adequate hydration (2-3 L/day of fluids unless instructed to restrict fluid intake) and nutrition. Frequent small meals, frequent mouth care, sucking lozenges, or chewing gum may reduce nausea or vomiting. Buttermilk or yogurt may help reduce diarrhea. Report immediately any tingling, unusual pain, or numbness in extremities. Report fever, chills, unusual fatigue or acute depression, acute abdominal or back pain, persistent muscle pain or weakness, or unusual bruising or bleeding. **Pregnancy/breast-feeding precautions:** Inform prescriber if you are pregnant. Do not breast-feed.

**Breast-feeding Issues:** The CDC recommends **not** to breast-feed if diagnosed with HIV to avoid postnatal transmission of the virus.

**Related Information**

Antiretroviral Agents Comparison *on page 1373*

- **S-T Cort®** *see* Hydrocortisone *on page 578*
- **S-T Cort®** *see* Topical Corticosteroids *on page 1152*
- **Stelazine®** *see* Trifluoperazine *on page 1176*
- **Stemetil®** *see* Prochlorperazine *on page 971*
- **Stenox** *see* Fluoxymesterone *on page 504*
- **Stieva-A®** *see* Tretinoin (Topical) *on page 1170*
- **Stieva-A® 0.025%** *see* Tretinoin (Topical) *on page 1170*
- **Stieva-A® Forte** *see* Tretinoin (Topical) *on page 1170*
- **Stilbestrol** *see* Diethylstilbestrol *on page 366*
- **Stilphostrol®** *see* Diethylstilbestrol *on page 366*
- **Stimate® Nasal** *see* Desmopressin *on page 345*
- **St. Joseph® Cough Suppressant** *see page 1294*
- **St. Joseph® Measured Dose Nasal Solution [OTC]** *see* Phenylephrine *on page 920*
- **Stop®** *see page 1294*
- **Streptase®** *see* Streptokinase *on this page*


## Streptokinase (strep toe KYE nase)

**U.S. Brand Names** Kabikinase®; Streptase®

**Synonyms** SK

**Therapeutic Category** Thrombolytic Agent

**Pregnancy Risk Factor** C

**Lactation** Excretion in breast milk unknown

**Use** Thrombolytic agent used in treatment of recent severe or massive deep vein thrombosis, pulmonary emboli, myocardial infarction, and occluded arteriovenous cannulas

**Mechanism of Action/Effect** Activates the conversion of plasminogen to plasmin by forming a complex, exposing plasminogen-activating site, and cleaving a peptide bond that converts plasminogen to plasmin; plasmin degrades fibrin, fibrinogen and other procoagulant proteins into soluble fragments; effective both outside and within the formed thrombus/embolus

**Contraindications** Hypersensitivity to streptokinase or any component; recent streptococcal infection within the last 6 months; any internal bleeding; brain carcinoma; cerebrovascular accident or transient ischemic attack, GI bleeding, trauma or surgery, prolonged external cardiac massage, intracranial or intraspinal surgery or trauma within 1 month; arteriovenous malformation or aneurysm; bleeding diathesis; severe hepatic or renal disease; subacute bacterial endocarditis; pericarditis; hemostatic defects; suspected aortic dissection, severe uncontrolled hypertension (BP systolic ≥180 mm Hg, BP diastolic ≥110 mm Hg)

**Warnings** Avoid I.M. injections. Use with caution in patients with a history of cardiac arrhythmias, major surgery within last 10 days, GI bleeding, recent trauma, or severe hypertension. Antibodies to streptokinase remain for 3-6 months after initial dose; use another thrombolytic enzyme (eg, alteplase) if thrombolytic therapy is indicated in patients with prior streptokinase therapy. Pregnancy factor C.

**Drug Interactions**

**Decreased Effect:** Antifibrinolytic agents (aminocaproic acid) may decrease effectiveness.

**Increased Effect/Toxicity:** Increased toxicity with anticoagulants. Antiplatelet agents may increase risk of bleeding.

**Adverse Reactions**

>10%:

Cardiovascular: Hypotension, arrhythmias, trauma arrhythmias
Dermatologic: Angioneurotic edema
Hematologic: Surface bleeding, internal bleeding, cerebral hemorrhage
Ocular: Periorbital swelling
Respiratory: Bronchospasm
Miscellaneous: Anaphylaxis

<1% (Limited to important or life-threatening symptoms): Anemia, bronchospasm

**Overdose/Toxicology** Symptoms of overdose include epistaxis, bleeding gums, hematoma, spontaneous ecchymoses, and oozing at the catheter site. If uncontrollable bleeding occurs, discontinue infusion. Whole blood or blood products may be used to reverse bleeding.

**Pharmacodynamics/Kinetics**

**Half-life Elimination:** 83 minutes

**Excretion:** By circulating antibodies and via the reticuloendothelial system

**Onset:** Activation of plasminogen occurs almost immediately

**Duration:** Fibrinolytic effects last only a few hours, while anticoagulant effects can persist for 12-24 hours.

**Formulations** Powder for injection: 250,000 units (5 mL, 6.5 mL); 600,000 units (5 mL); 750,000 units (6 mL, 6.5 mL); 1,500,000 units (6.5 mL, 10 mL, 50 mL)

**Dosing**

**Adults:** I.V.:

Antibodies to streptokinase remain for at least 3-6 months after initial dose: See Warnings/Precautions.

An intradermal skin test of 100 units has been suggested to predict allergic response to streptokinase. If a positive reaction is not seen after 15-20 minutes, a therapeutic dose may be administered.

**Guidelines for acute myocardial infarction** (AMI): 1.5 million units over 60 minutes

Administration:

Dilute two 750,000 unit vials of streptokinase with 5 mL dextrose 5% in water ($D_5W$) each, gently swirl to dissolve.

Add this dose of the 1.5 million units to 150 mL $D_5W$.

This should be infused over 60 minutes; an in-line filter ≥0.45 micron should be used.

Monitor for the first few hours for signs of anaphylaxis or allergic reaction. **Infusion should be slowed if lowering of 25 mm Hg in blood pressure or terminated if asthmatic symptoms appear.**

Begin heparin 5000-10,000 unit bolus followed by 1000 units/hour approximately 3-4 hours after completion of streptokinase infusion or when PTT is <100 seconds.

**Guidelines for acute pulmonary embolism** (APE): 3 million unit dose over 24 hours

Administration:

Dilute four 750,000 unit vials of streptokinase with 5 mL dextrose 5% in water ($D_5W$) each, gently swirl to dissolve.

Add this dose of 3 million units to 250 mL $D_5W$, an in-line filter ≥0.45 micron should be used.

Administer 250,000 units (23 mL) over 30 minutes followed by 100,000 units/hour (9 mL/hour) for 24 hours.

Monitor for the first few hours for signs of anaphylaxis or allergic reaction. **Infusion should be slowed if blood pressure is lowered by 25 mm Hg or if asthmatic symptoms appear.**

Begin heparin 1000 units/hour about 3-4 hours after completion of streptokinase infusion or when PTT is <100 seconds.

**Guidelines for thromboses:** Administer 250,000 units to start, then 100,000 units/hour for 24-72 hours depending on location.

**Guidelines for cannula occlusion:** Administer 250,000 units into cannula, clamp for 2 hours, then aspirate contents and flush with normal saline.

**Elderly:** Refer to adult dosing.

**Administration**

**I.M.:** Do **not** administer by intramuscular injection.

**I.V.:** For I.V. or intracoronary use only. Infusion pump is required. Use in-line filter >0.8 micron.

**Stability**

**Storage:** Streptokinase, a white lyophilized powder, may have a slight yellow color in solution due to the presence of albumin. Intact vials should be stored at room temperature. Reconstituted solutions should be refrigerated and are stable for 24 hours. Stability of parenteral admixture at room temperature (25°C) is 8 hours and at refrigeration (4°C) is 24 hours.

**Monitoring Laboratory Tests** PT, APTT, platelet count, hematocrit, fibrinogen concentration

**Additional Nursing Issues**

**Physical Assessment:** Monitor for symptoms of bleeding, vital signs (including temperature) closely, and EKG continuously. Initiate bleeding precautions. Avoid all invasive procedures. If invasive procedures must be performed, maintain pressure on venous sites for at least 15 minutes and on arterial sites for at least 30 minutes. Do not mix with other drugs. **Pregnancy risk factor C.** Note breast-feeding caution.

**Patient Information/Instruction:** Following infusion, absolute bedrest is important; call for assistance changing position. You will have increased tendency to bleed; avoid razors, scissors or sharps, and use soft toothbrush or cotton swabs. Report back pain, abdominal pain, muscle cramping, acute onset headache, or chest pain. **Pregnancy/breast-feeding precautions:** Inform prescriber if you are pregnant or suspect you might be pregnant. Consult prescriber if breast-feeding.

**Geriatric Considerations:** Investigators applied analysis to data for patients ≥75 years of age from two large trials studying the impact of streptokinase on patient outcome after acute myocardial infarction. Their conclusion was that age alone is not a contraindication to the use of streptokinase and that thrombolytic therapy is cost-effective and is beneficial toward the survival of elderly patients. Additional studies are needed to determine if a weight-adjusted dose will maintain efficacy but decrease adverse events such as stroke.

## Streptomycin (strep toe MYE sin)

**Therapeutic Category** Antibiotic, Aminoglycoside; Antitubercular Agent

**Pregnancy Risk Factor** D

**Lactation** Enters breast milk/compatible

**Use** Combination therapy of active tuberculosis; in combination with other agents for treatment of streptococcal or enterococcal endocarditis, mycobacterial infections, plague, tularemia, and brucellosis. Streptomycin is indicated for persons from endemic areas of drug-resistant *Mycobacterium tuberculosis* or who are HIV infected.

**Mechanism of Action/Effect** Inhibits bacterial protein synthesis by binding directly to the 30S ribosomal subunits causing faulty peptide sequence to form in the protein chain

**Contraindications** Hypersensitivity to streptomycin, aminoglycosides, or any component; pregnancy

**Warnings** Use with caution in patients with pre-existing vertigo, tinnitus, hearing loss, neuromuscular disorders, or renal impairment. Modify dosage in patients with renal impairment. Aminoglycosides are associated with nephrotoxicity or ototoxicity. The ototoxicity may be proportional to the amount of drug given and the duration of treatment. Tinnitus or vertigo are indications of vestibular injury and impending hearing damage. Renal damage is usually reversible.

(Continued)

## Streptomycin *(Continued)*

**Drug Interactions**

**Increased Effect/Toxicity:** Increased/prolonged effect with depolarizing and nondepolarizing neuromuscular blocking agents. Concurrent use with amphotericin or loop diuretics may increase nephrotoxicity.

**Effects on Lab Values** False-positive urine glucose with Benedict's solution

**Adverse Reactions**

1% to 10%:

Neuromuscular & skeletal: Neuromuscular blockade

Otic: Ototoxicity (auditory), ototoxicity (vestibular)

Renal: Nephrotoxicity

<1% (Limited to important or life-threatening symptoms): Eosinophilia, anemia, dyspnea

**Overdose/Toxicology** Symptoms of overdose include ototoxicity, nephrotoxicity, and neuromuscular toxicity. The treatment of choice following a single acute overdose appears to be maintenance of urine output of at least 3 mL/kg/hour during the acute treatment phase. Dialysis is of questionable value in enhancing aminoglycoside elimination. If required, hemodialysis is preferred over peritoneal dialysis in patients with normal renal function. Chelation with penicillins is experimental.

**Pharmacodynamics/Kinetics**

**Protein Binding:** 34%

**Distribution:** To extracellular fluid including serum, abscesses, ascitic, pericardial, pleural, synovial, lymphatic, and peritoneal fluids; crosses the placenta

**Half-life Elimination:** 2-4.7 hours (prolonged in renal impairment)

**Time to Peak:** Within 1 hour

**Metabolism:** None

**Excretion:** Urine, bile, saliva, sweat, and tears

**Formulations** Injection, as sulfate: 400 mg/mL (2.5 mL)

**Dosing**

**Adults:** Intramuscular (may also be given intravenous piggyback):

Tuberculosis therapy: **Note:** A four-drug regimen (isoniazid, rifampin, pyrazinamide and either streptomycin or ethambutol) is preferred for the initial, empiric treatment of TB. When the drug susceptibility results are available, the regimen should be altered as appropriate.

**Patients with TB and without HIV infection:**

**OPTION 1:**

Isoniazid resistance rate <4%: Administer daily isoniazid, rifampin, and pyrazinamide for 8 weeks followed by isoniazid and rifampin daily or directly observed therapy (DOT) 2-3 times/week for 16 weeks.

If isoniazid resistance rate is not documented, ethambutol or streptomycin should also be administered until susceptibility to isoniazid or rifampin is demonstrated. Continue treatment for at least 6 months or 3 months beyond culture conversion.

**OPTION 2:** Administer daily isoniazid, rifampin, pyrazinamide, and either streptomycin or ethambutol for 2 weeks followed by DOT 2 times/week administration of the same drugs for 6 weeks, and subsequently, with isoniazid and rifampin DOT 2 times/week administration for 16 weeks.

**OPTION 3:** Administer isoniazid, rifampin, pyrazinamide, and either ethambutol or streptomycin by DOT 3 times/week for 6 months.

**Patients with TB and with HIV infection:** Administer any of the above OPTIONS 1, 2 or 3, however, treatment should be continued for a total of 9 months and at least 6 months beyond culture conversion.

**Note:** Some experts recommend that the duration of therapy should be extended to 9 months for patients with disseminated disease, miliary disease, disease involving the bones or joints, or tuberculosis lymphadenitis.

Daily therapy: 15 mg/kg/day (maximum: 1 g)

Directly observed therapy (DOT): Twice weekly: 25-30 mg/kg (maximum: 1.5 g)

DOT: 3 times/week: 25-30 mg/kg (maximum: 1 g)

Enterococcal endocarditis: 1 g every 12 hours for 2 weeks, 500 mg every 12 hours for 4 weeks in combination with penicillin

Streptococcal endocarditis: 1 g every 12 hours for 1 week, 500 mg every 12 hours for 1 week

Tularemia: 1-2 g/day in divided doses for 7-10 days or until patient is afebrile for 5-7 days

Plague: 2-4 g/day in divided doses until the patient is afebrile for at least 3 days

**Elderly:** Intramuscular: 10 mg/kg/day, not to exceed 750 mg/day; dosing interval should be adjusted for renal function. Some authors suggest not to give more than 5 days/week or give as 20-25 mg/kg/dose twice weekly.

**Renal Impairment:**

$Cl_{cr}$ 10-50 mL/minute: Administer every 24-72 hours.

$Cl_{cr}$ <10 mL/minute: Administer every 72-96 hours.

Removed by hemo- and peritoneal dialysis: Administer dose postdialysis.

**Administration**

**I.M.:** Inject deep I.M. into large muscle mass.

**I.V.:** I.V. administration is not recommended. Has been administered intravenously over 30-60 minutes.

**Stability**

**Storage:** Depending upon manufacturer, reconstituted solution remains stable for 2-4 weeks when refrigerated and 24 hours at room temperature. Exposure to light causes darkening of solution without apparent loss of potency.

**Monitoring Laboratory Tests** Hearing (audiogram), BUN, creatinine; serum concentration of the drug should be monitored. Perform culture and sensitivity prior to initiating therapy.

**Additional Nursing Issues**

**Physical Assessment:** Assess previous history of allergies. Assess effectiveness and interactions of other medication (see Drug Interactions). See Warnings/Precautions and Contraindications for use cautions. Monitor effectiveness of therapy, laboratory tests, and adverse response (hypersensitivity, ototoxicity, nephrotoxicity, neuromuscular blockade) on a regular basis during therapy (see Adverse Reactions and Overdose/Toxicology). Assess knowledge/teach patient appropriate use and administration if self-administered, possible side effects and appropriate interventions, and adverse symptoms to report. **Pregnancy risk factor D** - assess knowledge/teach appropriate use of barrier contraceptives.

**Patient Information/Instruction:** This medication can only be given by intramuscular injection. Therapy for TB or HIV will generally last several months. Do not discontinue even if you are feeling better. Maintain adequate hydration (2-3 L/day of fluids unless instructed to restrict fluid intake). You may experience headache or dizziness (use caution when driving or engaging in tasks requiring alertness until response to drug is known); nausea, vomiting, or loss of appetite (frequent small meals, frequent mouth care, sucking lozenges, or chewing gum may help). Report immediately any rash, joint or back pain, or difficulty breathing; swelling of extremities or weight gain greater than 5 lb/week; fever, chills, mouth sores, vaginal itching or drainage, or foul-smelling stool; change in hearing, ringing or sense of fullness in ears; numbness, loss of sensation, clumsiness, change in strength, or altered gait. **Pregnancy precautions:** Do not get pregnant while taking this medication; use appropriate barrier contraceptive measures.

**Geriatric Considerations:** Streptomycin is indicated for persons from endemic areas of drug-resistant *Mycobacterium tuberculosis* or who are HIV infected. Since most older patients acquired the *M. tuberculosis* infection prior to the availability of effective chemotherapy, isoniazid and rifampin are usually effective unless resistant organisms are suspected or the patient is HIV infected. Adjust dose interval for renal function.

**Additional Information** The injection formulation contains sulfites.

**Related Information**

TB Drug Comparison *on page 1402*

## Streptozocin (strep toe ZOE sin)

**U.S. Brand Names** Zanosar®

**Therapeutic Category** Antineoplastic Agent, Alkylating Agent

**Pregnancy Risk Factor** C

**Lactation** Enters breast milk/contraindicated

**Use** Treat metastatic islet cell carcinoma of the pancreas, carcinoid tumor and syndrome, Hodgkin's disease, palliative treatment of colorectal cancer

**Mechanism of Action/Effect** Interferes with the normal function of DNA by alkylation and cross-linking the strands of DNA, and by possible protein modification

**Warnings** The U.S. Food and Drug Administration (FDA) currently recommends that procedures for proper handling and disposal of antineoplastic agents be considered.

Preparation of streptozocin should be performed in a Class II laminar flow biologic safety cabinet. Personnel should be wearing surgical gloves and a closed front surgical gown with knit cuffs. Appropriate safety equipment is recommended for preparation, administration, and disposal of antineoplastics. If streptozocin contacts the skin, wash and flush thoroughly with water.

Renal toxicity is dose-related and cumulative and may be severe or fatal. Other major toxicities include liver dysfunction, diarrhea, nausea, and vomiting.

Discontinue treatment in the presence of significant renal toxicity. Do not use in combination with other nephrotoxic drugs.

Pregnancy factor C.

**Drug Interactions**

**Decreased Effect:** Phenytoin results in negation of streptozocin cytotoxicity.

**Increased Effect/Toxicity:** Doxorubicin prolongs half-life and thus prolonged leukopenia and thrombocytopenia.

**Adverse Reactions**

>10%:

- Gastrointestinal: Nausea and vomiting in all patients usually 1-4 hours after infusion; diarrhea in 10% of patients
  - Emetic potential: High (>90%)
  - Time course of nausea/vomiting: Onset 1-3 hours; Duration: 1-12 hours
- Hepatic: Increased LFTs and hypoalbuminemia
- Renal: Renal dysfunction occurs in 65% of patients; proteinuria, decreased $Cl_{cr}$, increased BUN, hypophosphatemia, and renal tubular acidosis; use caution with patients on other nephrotoxic agents; nephrotoxicity (25% to 75% of patients)

1% to 10%:

- Endocrine & metabolic: Hypoglycemia: Seen in 6% of patients; may be prevented with the administration of nicotinamide
- Local: Pain at injection site
  - **Vesicant chemotherapy**

<1% (Limited to important or life-threatening symptoms): Liver dysfunction, secondary malignancy, leukopenia, thrombocytopenia

- Myelosuppressive:
  - WBC: Mild

(Continued)

## Streptozocin *(Continued)*

Platelets: Mild
Onset (days): 7
Nadir (days): 14
Recovery (days): 21

**Overdose/Toxicology** Symptoms of overdose include bone marrow suppression, nausea, and vomiting. Treatment of bone marrow suppression is supportive.

**Pharmacodynamics/Kinetics**

**Distribution:** Concentrates in the liver, intestine, pancreas, and kidney

**Half-life Elimination:** 35-40 minutes

**Metabolism:** Liver and/or kidney

**Excretion:** Urine, bile, and expired air

**Formulations** Injection: 1 g

**Dosing**

**Adults:** I.V. (refer to individual protocols):

Single agent therapy: 1-1.5 g/m$^2$ weekly for 6 weeks followed by a 4-week observation period

Combination therapy: 0.5-1 g/m$^2$ for 5 consecutive days followed by a 4- to 6-week observation period

**Elderly:** Refer to adult dosing.

**Renal Impairment:**

$Cl_{cr}$ 10-50 mL/minute: Administer 75% of dose.

$Cl_{cr}$ <10 mL/minute: Administer 50% of dose.

**Hepatic Impairment:** Dose should be decreased in patients with severe liver disease.

**Administration**

**I.V.:** Vesicant. Slow I.V. infusion in ≥100 mL $D_5W$ or NS over 30-60 minutes; may be administered by rapid I.V. push.

**Stability**

**Storage:** Refrigerate vials. Protect from light.

**Reconstitution:** Solution is stable 48 hours at room temperature and 96 hours with refrigeration. May be diluted in $D_5W$ or sodium chloride.

**Monitoring Laboratory Tests** Liver function tests, CBC, renal function tests (BUN, serum creatinine) at baseline and weekly during therapy

**Additional Nursing Issues**

**Physical Assessment:** Monitor infusion site closely for extravasation (stop infusion and restart in another site). Monitor closely for signs of severe adverse gastrointestinal, nephrotic, or renal reactions (see Adverse Reactions). Antiemetic therapy should be instituted as per protocol prior to infusion. Monitor serum glucose frequently (sudden release of insulin may precipitate hypoglycemia). **Pregnancy risk factor C** - benefits of use should outweigh possible risks. Breast-feeding is contraindicated.

**Patient Information/Instruction:** This drug can only be given I.V. Maintain adequate hydration (2-3 L/day of fluids unless instructed to restrict fluid intake). Avoid aspirin and aspirin-containing substances. You may experience nervousness, dizziness, confusion, or lethargy (use caution when driving or engaging in tasks requiring alertness until response to drug is known); coagulopathy (use caution with knives or sharp objects, avoid injury, use electric razor, brush teeth with soft brush or cotton swabs). You may have increased sensitivity to infection (avoid crowds and exposure to infection). Report persistent fever; chills; sore throat; unusual bleeding; blood in urine, stool, vomitus, or stool; chest pain or palpitations, or difficulty breathing. **Pregnancy/breast-feeding precautions:** Inform prescriber if you are or intend to be pregnant - contraceptives may be recommended. Do not breast-feed.

- **Stresstabs® 600 Advanced Formula Tablets [OTC]** *see* Vitamin, Multiple *on page 1219*
- **Strong Iodine Solution** *see* Potassium Iodide *on page 951*
- **Stuartnatal® 1 + 1** *see* Vitamin, Multiple *on page 1219*
- **Stuart Prenatal® [OTC]** *see* Vitamin, Multiple *on page 1219*
- **Sublimaze® Injection** *see* Fentanyl *on page 478*
- **Succimer** *see page 1246*
- **Succinylcholine** *see page 1248*
- **Sucraid™** *see* Sacrosidase *on page 1039*

## Sucralfate (soo KRAL fate)

**U.S. Brand Names** Carafate®

**Synonyms** Aluminum Sucrose Sulfate, Basic

**Therapeutic Category** Gastrointestinal Agent, Miscellaneous

**Pregnancy Risk Factor** B

**Lactation** Enters breast milk/compatible

**Use** Short-term management of duodenal ulcers

**Unlabeled use:** Gastric ulcers; maintenance of duodenal ulcers; suspension may be used topically for treatment of stomatitis due to cancer chemotherapy and other causes of esophageal and gastric erosions; GERD, esophagitis, treatment of NSAID mucosal damage, prevention of stress ulcers, postsclerotherapy for esophageal variceal bleeding.

**Mechanism of Action/Effect** Forms a complex by binding with positively charged proteins in exudates, forming a viscous paste-like, adhesive substance, when combined with gastric acid adheres to the damaged mucosal area. This selectively forms a protective coating that protects the lining against peptic acid, pepsin, and bile salts.

**Contraindications** Hypersensitivity to sucralfate or any component

**Warnings** Successful therapy with sucralfate should not be expected to alter the posthealing frequency of recurrence or the severity of duodenal ulceration. Use with caution in patients with chronic renal failure who have an impaired excretion of absorbed aluminum. Because of the potential for sucralfate to alter the absorption of some drugs, take other medications 2 hours before sucralfate when alterations in bioavailability are believed to be critical. Do not give antacids within 30 minutes of administration.

**Drug Interactions**

**Decreased Effect:** Sucralfate may decrease the effect of digoxin, phenytoin, theophylline, ciprofloxacin, and itraconazole when coadministered. Because of the potential for sucralfate to alter the absorption of some drugs, take other medications 2 hours before sucralfate when alterations in bioavailability are believed to be critical.

**Adverse Reactions** 1% to 10%: Gastrointestinal: Constipation

**Overdose/Toxicology** Toxicity is minimal, may cause constipation

**Pharmacodynamics/Kinetics**

**Distribution:** Acts locally at ulcer sites; unbound in the GI tract to aluminum and sucrose octasulfate

**Metabolism:** Not metabolized

**Excretion:** Urine

**Onset:** Paste formation and ulcer adhesion occur within 1-2 hours.

**Duration:** Up to 6 hours

**Formulations**

Suspension, oral: 1 g/10 mL (420 mL)

Tablet: 1 g

**Dosing**

**Adults:** Oral:

Stress ulcer prophylaxis: 1 g 4 times/day

Stress ulcer treatment: 1 g every 4 hours

Duodenal ulcer:

Treatment: 1 g 4 times/day, 1 hour before meals or food and at bedtime for 4-8 weeks, or alternatively 2 g twice daily; treatment is recommended for 4-8 weeks in adults, the elderly will require 12 weeks.

Maintenance: Prophylaxis: 1 g twice daily

Stomatitis: 1 g/10 mL suspension; swish and spit or swish and swallow 4 times/day.

**Elderly:** Refer to adult dosing.

**Renal Impairment:** Aluminum salt is minimally absorbed (<5%), however, may accumulate in renal failure.

**Stability**

**Storage:** Suspension: Shake well. Refrigeration is **not** necessary; do **not** freeze.

**Additional Nursing Issues**

**Physical Assessment:** Assess other medications patient may be taking (see Drug Interactions). Instruct patient on appropriate timing of administration with regard to other medications and interventions to reduce constipation.

**Patient Information/Instruction:** Take recommended dose before meals or on an empty stomach. Take any other medications at least 2 hours before taking sucralfate. Do not take antacids within 30 minutes of taking sucralfate. May cause constipation; increased exercise, increased dietary fiber, fruit or fluids, or mild stool softener may be helpful. If constipation or gastric distress persists, consult prescriber.

**Dietary Issues:** Interferes with absorption of vitamin A, vitamin D, vitamin E, and vitamin K.

**Geriatric Considerations:** Caution should be used in the elderly due to reduced renal function. Patients with $Cl_{cr}$ <30 mL/minute may be at risk for aluminum intoxication. Due to low side effect profile, this may be an agent of choice in the elderly with PUD.


♦ **Sucrets® [OTC]** *see* Dyclonine *on page 411*

♦ **Sucrets® Cough Calmers** *see page 1294*

♦ **Sudafed® [OTC]** *see* Pseudoephedrine *on page 992*

♦ **Sudafed® 12 Hour [OTC]** *see* Pseudoephedrine *on page 992*

♦ **Sudafed Plus® Tablet** *see page 1294*

♦ **Sudafed® Severe Cold** *see page 1294*

♦ **Sudex®** *see* Guaifenesin and Pseudoephedrine *on page 551*

♦ **Sufedrin® [OTC]** *see* Pseudoephedrine *on page 992*

♦ **Sufisal** *see* Pentoxifylline *on page 908*

♦ **Sugar-Free Liquid Pharmaceuticals** *see page 1416*

♦ **Sular®** *see* Nisoldipine *on page 828*

♦ **Sulbactam and Ampicillin** *see* Ampicillin and Sulbactam *on page 92*

♦ **Sulconazole** *see page 1247*

♦ **Sulcrate®** *see* Sucralfate *on previous page*

♦ **Sulcrate® Suspension Plus** *see* Sucralfate *on previous page*

♦ **Sulf-10®** *see page 1282*

♦ **Sulf-10® Ophthalmic** *see* Sulfacetamide *on next page*


## Sulfabenzamide, Sulfacetamide, and Sulfathiazole

(sul fa BENZ a mide, sul fa SEE ta mide, & sul fa THYE a zole)

**U.S. Brand Names** Gyne-Sulf®; Sultrin™; Trysul®; Vagilia®; V.V.S.®

**Synonyms** Sulfacetamide, Sulfabenzamide, and Sulfathiazole; Sulfathiazole, Sulfacetamide, and Sulfabenzamide; Triple Sulfa

**Therapeutic Category** Antibiotic, Vaginal

(Continued)

## Sulfabenzamide, Sulfacetamide, and Sulfathiazole *(Continued)*

**Pregnancy Risk Factor** C (avoid if near term)

**Lactation** Excretion in breast milk unknown

**Use** Treatment of *Haemophilus vaginalis* vaginitis

**Mechanism of Action/Effect** Interferes with microbial folic acid synthesis and growth via inhibition of para-aminobenzoic acid metabolism

**Contraindications** Hypersensitivity to sulfabenzamide, sulfacetamide, sulfathiazole or any component; renal dysfunction; pregnancy (if near term)

**Warnings** Associated with Stevens-Johnson syndrome; if local irritation or systemic toxicity develops, discontinue therapy. Pregnancy factor C (avoid if near term).

**Adverse Reactions**

>10%: Dermatologic: Local irritation, pruritus, urticaria

<1% (Limited to important or life-threatening symptoms): Stevens-Johnson syndrome

**Pharmacodynamics/Kinetics**

**Metabolism:** Primarily by acetylation

**Excretion:** By glomerular filtration into urine

**Formulations**

Cream, vaginal: Sulfabenzamide 3.7%, sulfacetamide 2.86%, and sulfathiazole 3.42% (78 g with applicator, 90 g, 120 g)

Tablet, vaginal: Sulfabenzamide 184 mg, sulfacetamide 143.75 mg, and sulfathiazole 172.5 mg (20 tablets/box with vaginal applicator)

**Dosing**

**Adults:**

Cream: Insert 1 applicatorful in vagina twice daily for 4-6 days. Dosage may then be decreased to $\frac{1}{2}$ to $\frac{1}{4}$ of an applicatorful twice daily.

Tablet: Insert 1 tablet intravaginally twice daily for 10 days.

**Elderly:** Refer to adult dosing.

**Additional Nursing Issues**

**Physical Assessment:** Assess patient knowledge/teach appropriate administration and adverse symptoms to report. **Pregnancy risk factor C.** Note breast-feeding caution.

**Patient Information/Instruction:** This medication is to be inserted into vagina; do not ingest tablets. Complete full course of therapy. Wash hands before inserting applicator gently into vagina and releasing cream or tablet. Wash hands and applicator with soap and water following each application. Discontinue and notify prescriber immediately if burning, irritation, or signs of allergic reaction occur. **Pregnancy/breast-feeding precautions:** Inform prescriber if you are pregnant before use. Consult prescriber if breast-feeding.

## Sulfacetamide (sul fa SEE ta mide)

**U.S. Brand Names** AK-Sulf® Ophthalmic; Bleph®-10 Ophthalmic; Cetamide® Ophthalmic; Isopto® Cetamide® Ophthalmic; Ocusulf-10® Ophthalmic; Sebizon® Topical Lotion; Sodium Sulamyd® Ophthalmic; Sulf-10® Ophthalmic

**Synonyms** Sodium Sulfacetamide

**Therapeutic Category** Antibiotic, Ophthalmic; Antibiotic, Sulfonamide Derivative

**Pregnancy Risk Factor** C

**Lactation** Excretion in breast milk unknown

**Use** Treatment and prophylaxis of conjunctivitis due to susceptible organisms; corneal ulcers; adjunctive treatment with systemic sulfonamides for therapy of trachoma; topical application in scaling dermatosis (seborrheic); bacterial infections of the skin

**Mechanism of Action/Effect** Interferes with bacterial growth by inhibiting bacterial folic acid synthesis through competitive antagonism of PABA

**Contraindications** Hypersensitivity to sulfacetamide or any component, sulfonamides; infants <2 months of age

**Warnings** Inactivated by purulent exudates containing PABA. Use with caution in severe dry eye. Ointment may retard corneal epithelial healing. Sulfite in some products may cause hypersensitivity reactions. Cross-sensitivity may occur with previous exposure to other sulfonamides given by other routes. Pregnancy factor C.

**Drug Interactions**

**Decreased Effect:** Silver containing products are incompatible with sulfacetamide solutions.

**Adverse Reactions**

1% to 10%: Local: Irritation, stinging, burning

<1% (Limited to important or life-threatening symptoms): Stevens-Johnson syndrome, exfoliative dermatitis, toxic epidermal necrolysis

**Pharmacodynamics/Kinetics**

**Half-life Elimination:** 7-13 hours

**Excretion:** When absorbed, excreted primarily in urine as unchanged drug

**Formulations**

Sulfacetamide sodium:

Lotion: 10% (85 g)

Ointment, ophthalmic: 10% (3.5 g)

Solution, ophthalmic: 10% (1 mL, 2 mL, 2.5 mL, 5 mL, 15 mL); 15% (5 mL, 15 mL); 30% (15 mL)

**Dosing**

**Adults:**

Ophthalmic:

Ointment: Apply to lower conjunctival sac 1-4 times/day and at bedtime.

Solution: Instill 1-3 drops several times daily up to every 2-3 hours in lower conjunctival sac during waking hours and less frequently at night.

Topical:

Seborrheic dermatitis: Apply at bedtime and allow to remain overnight. In severe cases, may apply twice daily.

Secondary cutaneous bacterial infections: Apply 2-4 times/day until infection clears.

**Elderly:** Refer to adult dosing.

**Stability**

**Storage:** Protect from light. Discolored solution should not be used.

**Compatibility:** Incompatible with silver and zinc sulfate. Sulfacetamide is inactivated by blood or purulent exudates.

**Additional Nursing Issues**

**Physical Assessment:** Assess for previous sulfonamide allergic reactions (see Warnings/Precautions). Monitor effectiveness of therapy. Assess knowledge/teach patient appropriate use (ophthalmic/topical), interventions to reduce side effects, and adverse symptoms to report (see Adverse Reactions). **Pregnancy risk factor C** - benefits of use should outweigh possible risks. Note breast-feeding caution.

**Patient Information/Instruction:** Use as directed. Complete full course of therapy even if condition appears improved.

Topical: For topical use only. Apply a thin film of ointment to affected area as often as directed. Do not cover with occlusive dressing. Report increased skin redness, irritation, or development of open sores; or if condition worsens or does not improve.

Ophthalmic: For ophthalmic use only. Store at room temperature. Shake before using. Apply prescribed amount as often as directed. Wash hands before using and do not let tip of applicator touch eye or contaminate tip of applicator. Tilt head back and look upward. Gently pull down lower lid and put drop(s) in inner corner of eye. Close eye and roll eyeball in all directions. Do not blink for ½ minute. Apply gentle pressure to inner corner of eye for 30 seconds. Wipe away excess from skin around eye. Do not use any other eye preparation for at least 10 minutes. Do not touch tip of applicator to eye or contaminate tip of applicator. Do not share medication with anyone else. May cause sensitivity to bright light (dark glasses may help); temporary stinging or blurred vision may occur. Inform prescriber if you experience eye pain, redness, burning, watering, dryness, double vision, puffiness around eye, vision disturbances, or other adverse eye response; worsening of condition or lack of improvement within 3-4 days.

**Pregnancy/breast-feeding precautions:** Inform prescriber if you are pregnant. Consult prescriber if breast-feeding.

**Geriatric Considerations:** Assess whether patient can adequately instill drops or ointment.

**Breast-feeding Issues:** Systemic sulfonamides are excreted in breast milk. Sodium sulfacetamide is an eye drop and the extent of absorption is unknown.

**Related Information**

Ophthalmic Agents *on page 1282*


- **Sulfacetamide and Fluorometholone** *see page 1282*
- **Sulfacetamide and Prednisolone** *see page 1282*
- **Sulfacetamide, Sulfabenzamide, and Sulfathiazole** *see* Sulfabenzamide, Sulfacetamide, and Sulfathiazole *on page 1079*
- **Sulfacet-R® Topical** *see page 1306*


## Sulfadiazine (sul fa DYE a zeen)

**U.S. Brand Names** Microsulfon®

**Therapeutic Category** Antibiotic, Sulfonamide Derivative

**Pregnancy Risk Factor** B/D (at term)

**Lactation** Enters breast milk/contraindicated

**Use** Treatment of urinary tract infections and nocardiosis, rheumatic fever prophylaxis; adjunctive treatment in toxoplasmosis; uncomplicated attack of malaria

**Mechanism of Action/Effect** Interferes with bacterial growth by inhibiting bacterial folic acid synthesis through competitive antagonism of PABA

**Contraindications** Hypersensitivity to any sulfa drug or any component; porphyria; pregnancy (at term); sunblock containing PABA

**Warnings** Use with caution in patients with impaired hepatic function or impaired renal function, G-6-PD deficiency. Dosage modification required in patients with renal impairment. Fluid intake should be maintained ≥1500 mL/day, or give sodium bicarbonate to keep urine alkaline. More likely to cause crystalluria because it is less soluble than other sulfonamides.

**Drug Interactions**

**Decreased Effect:** Decreased effect with PABA or PABA metabolites of drugs (eg, procaine, proparacaine, tetracaine, sunblock).

**Increased Effect/Toxicity:** Increased effect of oral anticoagulants and oral hypoglycemic agents.

**Adverse Reactions**

>10%:

Central nervous system: Fever, dizziness, headache

Dermatologic: Itching, rash, photosensitivity

Gastrointestinal: Anorexia, nausea, vomiting, diarrhea

(Continued)

## Sulfadiazine *(Continued)*

1% to 10%:

Dermatologic: Lyell's syndrome, Stevens-Johnson syndrome

Hematologic: Granulocytopenia, leukopenia, thrombocytopenia, aplastic anemia, hemolytic anemia

Hepatic: Hepatitis

<1% (Limited to important or life-threatening symptoms): Jaundice, interstitial nephritis, acute nephropathy, hematuria

**Overdose/Toxicology** Symptoms of overdose include drowsiness, dizziness, anorexia, abdominal pain, nausea, vomiting, hemolytic anemia, acidosis, jaundice, fever, and agranulocytosis. Doses as little as 2-5 g/day may produce toxicity. The aniline radical is responsible for hematologic toxicity. High volume diuresis may aid in elimination and prevention of renal failure. Leucovorin 5-15 mg/day has been used to speed recovery of bone marrow.

**Pharmacodynamics/Kinetics**

**Distribution:** Throughout body tissues and fluids including pleural, peritoneal, synovial, and ocular fluids; distributed throughout total body water; readily diffused into CSF

**Half-life Elimination:** 10 hours

**Time to Peak:** Within 3-6 hours

**Metabolism:** By N-acetylation

**Excretion:** Urine

**Formulations** Tablet: 500 mg

**Dosing**

**Adults:** Oral: Toxoplasmosis: 2-8 g/day divided every 6 hours in conjunction with pyrimethamine 25 mg/day and with supplemental folinic acid

**Elderly:** Refer to adult dosing.

**Administration**

**Oral:** Tablets may be crushed to prepare oral suspension of the drug in water or with a sucrose-containing solution. Aqueous suspension with concentrations of 100 mg/mL should be stored in the refrigerator and used within 7 days. Administer around-the-clock to promote less variation in peak and trough serum levels.

**Monitoring Laboratory Tests** Perform culture and sensitivity prior to initiating therapy.

**Additional Nursing Issues**

**Physical Assessment:** Assess for history of previous allergies before first dose. Monitor (teach patient to monitor and report) adverse reactions (see above). Instruct patient on necessity to maintain adequate hydration and adverse symptoms to report. **Pregnancy Risk Factor B/D** - see Pregnancy Risk Factor for cautious use. Breast-feeding is contraindicated.

**Patient Information/Instruction:** Take as directed, at regular intervals around-the-clock. Take 1 hour before or 2 hours after meals with full glass of water. Complete full course of therapy even if you are feeling better. Avoid aspirin or aspirin-containing products and avoid large quantities of vitamin C. It is very important to maintain adequate hydration (2-3 L/day of fluids unless instructed to restrict fluid intake) to prevent kidney damage. You may experience dizziness or headache (use caution when driving or engaging in tasks requiring alertness until response to drug is known); photosensitivity (use sunblock, wear protective clothing and eyewear, and avoid direct sunlight); nausea, vomiting, or loss of appetite (small frequent meals, frequent mouth care, sucking lozenges, or chewing gum may help). Report skin rash, persistent diarrhea, persistent or severe sore throat, fever, vaginal itching or discharge, unusual bruising or bleeding, fatigue, persistent headache or abdominal pain, or difficulty breathing. **Pregnancy/breast-feeding precautions:** Inform prescriber if you are pregnant. Do not breast-feed.

**Dietary Issues:** Supplemental folinic acid should be administered to reverse symptoms or prevent problems due to folic acid deficiency. Avoid large quantities of vitamin C or acidifying agents (cranberry juice) to prevent crystalluria.

♦ **Sulfalax® [OTC]** *see* Docusate *on page 392*

## Sulfamethoxazole (sul fa meth OKS a zole)

**U.S. Brand Names** Gantanol®; Urobak®

**Therapeutic Category** Antibiotic, Sulfonamide Derivative

**Pregnancy Risk Factor** B/D (at term)

**Lactation** Enters breast milk/compatible

**Use** Treatment of urinary tract infections, nocardiosis, toxoplasmosis, acute otitis media, and acute exacerbations of chronic bronchitis due to susceptible organisms

**Mechanism of Action/Effect** Interferes with bacterial growth by inhibiting bacterial folic acid synthesis through competitive antagonism of PABA

**Contraindications** Hypersensitivity to any sulfa drug or any component; porphyria; pregnancy (at term); sunblock containing PABA

**Warnings** Maintain adequate fluid intake to prevent crystalluria. Use with caution in patients with renal or hepatic impairment, and patients with G-6-PD deficiency. Should not be used for group A beta-hemolytic streptococcal infections.

**Drug Interactions**

**Cytochrome P-450 Effect:** CYP2C9 enzyme inhibitor

**Decreased Effect:** Decreased effect with PABA or PABA metabolites of drugs (eg, procaine, proparacaine, tetracaine).

**Increased Effect/Toxicity:** Increased effect of oral anticoagulants, oral hypoglycemic agents, and methotrexate.

**Food Interactions** The presence of food delays but does not reduce absorption.

**Adverse Reactions**

>10%:

Central nervous system: Fever, dizziness, headache

Dermatologic: Itching, rash, photosensitivity

Gastrointestinal: Anorexia, nausea, vomiting, diarrhea

1% to 10%:

Dermatologic: Lyell's syndrome, Stevens-Johnson syndrome

Hematologic: Granulocytopenia, leukopenia, thrombocytopenia, aplastic anemia, hemolytic anemia

Hepatic: Hepatitis

<1% (Limited to important or life-threatening symptoms): Vasculitis, hematuria, acute nephropathy, interstitial nephritis

**Overdose/Toxicology** Symptoms of overdose include drowsiness, dizziness, anorexia, abdominal pain, nausea, vomiting, hemolytic anemia, acidosis, jaundice, fever, and agranulocytosis. The aniline radical is responsible for hematologic toxicity. High volume diuresis may aid in elimination and prevention of renal failure. Leucovorin 5-15 mg/day has been used to speed recovery of bone marrow.

**Pharmacodynamics/Kinetics**

**Protein Binding:** 70%

**Distribution:** Crosses the placenta; readily enters the CSF

**Half-life Elimination:** 9-12 hours (prolonged in renal impairment)

**Time to Peak:** Within 3-4 hours

**Metabolism:** Primarily in the liver, with 10% to 20% as the N-acetylated form in the plasma

**Excretion:** Urine

**Formulations**

Suspension, oral (cherry flavor): 500 mg/5 mL (480 mL)

Tablet: 500 mg

**Dosing**

**Adults:** Oral: 2 g stat, 1 g 2-3 times/day; maximum: 3 g/24 hours

**Elderly:** Oral: Same as adults unless $Cl_{cr}$ <30 mL/minute; see Renal Impairment. Single dose or 3-day dosing has not been shown to be reliable for treating urinary tract infections in the elderly.

**Renal Impairment:**

$Cl_{cr}$ 10-50 mL/minute: Administer every 18 hours.

$Cl_{cr}$ <10 mL/minute: Administer every 24 hours.

Moderately dialyzable (20% to 50%)

**Administration**

**Oral:** Administer around-the-clock to promote less variation in peak and trough serum levels.

**Stability**

**Storage:** Protect from light

**Monitoring Laboratory Tests** Perform culture and sensitivity prior to initiating therapy.

**Additional Nursing Issues**

**Physical Assessment:** Assess for history of previous allergies before first dose. Monitor (teach patient to monitor and report) adverse reactions (see above). Instruct patient on necessity to maintain adequate hydration. **Pregnancy Risk Factor B/D** - see Pregnancy Risk Factor for cautious use.

**Patient Information/Instruction:** Take as directed, at regular intervals around-the-clock. Take 1 hour before or 2 hours after meals with a full glass of water. Take full course of therapy even if you feeling better. Avoid aspirin or aspirin-containing products and avoid large quantities of vitamin C. It is very important to maintain adequate hydration (2-3 L/day of fluids unless instructed to restrict fluid intake) to prevent kidney damage. You may experience dizziness or headache (use caution when driving or engaging in tasks requiring alertness until response to drug is known); photosensitivity (use sunscreen, wear protective clothing and eyewear, and avoid direct sunlight); nausea, vomiting, or loss of appetite (small frequent meals, frequent mouth care, sucking lozenges, or chewing gum may help). Report skin rash, persistent diarrhea, persistent or severe sore throat, fever, vaginal itching or discharge, unusual bruising or bleeding, fatigue, persistent headache or abdominal pain, blackened stool, or difficulty breathing. **Pregnancy precautions:** Inform prescriber if you are pregnant.

**Geriatric Considerations:** Sulfamethoxazole is an effective anti-infective agent. Most prescribers prefer the combination of sulfamethoxazole and trimethoprim for its dual mechanism of action. Trimethoprim penetrates the prostate. Adjust dose for renal function.

**Related Information**

Co-trimoxazole *on page 307*

## Sulfamethoxazole and Phenazopyridine

(sul fa meth OKS a zole & fen az oh PEER i deen)

**Synonyms** Phenazopyridine and Sulfamethoxazole

**Therapeutic Category** Antibiotic, Sulfonamide Derivative

**Pregnancy Risk Factor** B/D (at term)

**Lactation** Excretion in breast milk unknown

**Use** Treatment of urinary tract infections complicated with pain

**Formulations** Tablet: Sulfamethoxazole 500 mg and phenazopyridine 100 mg

**Dosing**

**Adults:** Oral: 4 tablets to start, then 2 tablets twice daily for up to 2 days, then switch to sulfamethoxazole only

(Continued)

## Sulfamethoxazole and Phenazopyridine *(Continued)*

**Elderly:** Refer to adult dosing.

**Additional Nursing Issues**

**Physical Assessment:** See individual components listed in Related Information. **Pregnancy risk factor B/D** - see Pregnancy Risk Factor - assess knowledge/instruct patient on need to use appropriate contraceptive measures and the need to avoid pregnancy. Note breast-feeding caution.

**Patient Information/Instruction:** See individual components listed in Related Information. **Pregnancy/breast-feeding precautions:** Inform prescriber if you are on intend to get pregnant. Consult prescriber if breast-feeding.

**Related Information**

Phenazopyridine *on page 914*
Sulfamethoxazole *on page 1082*

- **Sulfamethoxazole and Trimethoprim** *see* Co-trimoxazole *on page 307*
- **Sulfamylon® Topical** *see* Mafenide *on page 702*

## Sulfanilamide (sul fa NIL a mide)

**U.S. Brand Names** AVC™ Cream; AVC™ Suppository; Vagitrol®

**Therapeutic Category** Antifungal Agent, Vaginal

**Pregnancy Risk Factor** C (avoid use after 7th month)

**Lactation** Contraindicated

**Use** Treatment of vulvovaginitis caused by *Candida albicans*

**Mechanism of Action/Effect** Interferes with microbial folic acid synthesis and growth via inhibition of para-aminiobenzoic acid metabolism

**Contraindications** Hypersensitivity to sulfanilamide, aminacrine, allantoin, or any component; pregnancy (avoid use after 7th month)

**Warnings** Pregnancy factor C (avoid after 7th month).

**Adverse Reactions**

1% to 10%:

Central nervous system: Kernicterus
Dermatologic: Itching, rash, burning, irritation, exfoliative dermatitis, Stevens-Johnson syndrome
Gastrointestinal: Nausea, vomiting
Genitourinary: Crystalluria
Hematologic: Agranulocytosis, hemolytic anemia in patients with severe G-6-PD deficiency
Hepatic: Hepatic toxicity

<1% (Limited to important or life-threatening symptoms): Irritation of penis of sexual partner

**Formulations**

Cream, vaginal (AVC™, Vagitrol®): 15% [150 mg/g] (120 g with applicator)
Suppository, vaginal (AVC™): 1.05 g (16s)

**Dosing**

**Adults:** Insert 1 applicatorful intravaginally once or twice daily through one complete menstrual cycle or insert 1 suppository intravaginally once or twice daily for 30 days.

**Elderly:** Refer to adult dosing.

**Administration**

**Other:** For vaginal use only.

**Additional Nursing Issues**

**Physical Assessment:** See Contraindications and Warnings/Precautions for use cautions. Assess knowledge/teach patient appropriate administration, possible side effects/interventions, and adverse symptoms to report (see Adverse Reactions). **Pregnancy risk factor C** - see Pregnancy Risk Factor for cautious use. Breast-feeding is contraindicated.

**Patient Information/Instruction:** Complete full course of therapy as directed. Insert vaginally as directed by prescriber or see package insert. You may be sensitive to direct sunlight (wear protective clothing, use sunblock, and avoid excessive exposure to direct sunlight). Sexual partner may experience irritation of penis; best to refrain from intercourse during period of treatment. Report persistent vaginal burning, itching, or irritation; rash; yellowing of eyes or skin, dark urine, or pale stool; unresolved nausea or vomiting; or painful urination. **Breast-feeding precautions:** Do not breast-feed.

## Sulfasalazine (sul fa SAL a zeen)

**U.S. Brand Names** Azulfidine®; Azulfidine® EN-tabs®

**Synonyms** Salicylazosulfapyridine

**Therapeutic Category** 5-Aminosalicylic Acid Derivative

**Pregnancy Risk Factor** B/D (at term)

**Lactation** Enters breast milk/use caution

**Use** Management of ulcerative colitis, rheumatoid arthritis

**Mechanism of Action/Effect** Acts locally in the colon to decrease the inflammatory response and systemically interferes with secretion by inhibiting prostaglandin synthesis

**Contraindications** Hypersensitivity to sulfasalazine, sulfa drugs, or any component; hypersensitivity to salicylates; porphyria; GI or GU obstruction; children <2 years of age; pregnancy (at term)

**Warnings** Use with caution in patients with renal impairment, impaired hepatic function or urinary obstruction, blood dyscrasias severe allergies or asthma, or G-6-PD deficiency. May cause folate deficiency (consider providing 1 mg/day folate supplement).

**Drug Interactions**

**Decreased Effect:** Decreased effect with iron, digoxin and PABA or PABA metabolites of drugs (eg, procaine, proparacaine, tetracaine). Decreased effect of oral anticoagulants, methotrexate, and oral hypoglycemic agents.

**Adverse Reactions**

>10%:

Central nervous system: Fever, dizziness, headache

Dermatologic: Itching, rash, photosensitivity, orange-yellow discoloration of skin

Gastrointestinal: Anorexia, nausea, vomiting, diarrhea

Genitourinary: Reversible oligospermia, orange-yellow discoloration of urine

1% to 10%:

Dermatologic: Lyell's syndrome, Stevens-Johnson syndrome

Hematologic: Granulocytopenia, leukopenia, thrombocytopenia, aplastic anemia, hemolytic anemia

Hepatic: Hepatitis

<1% (Limited to important or life-threatening symptoms): Interstitial nephritis, acute nephropathy, hematuria

**Overdose/Toxicology** Symptoms of overdose include drowsiness, dizziness, anorexia, abdominal pain, nausea, vomiting, hemolytic anemia, acidosis, jaundice, fever, and agranulocytosis. The aniline radical is responsible for hematologic toxicity. High volume diuresis may aid in elimination and prevention of renal failure. Leucovorin 5-15 mg/day has been used to speed recovery of bone marrow.

**Pharmacodynamics/Kinetics**

**Distribution:** Small amounts appear in feces

**Half-life Elimination:** 5.7-10 hours

**Metabolism:** Following absorption, both components are metabolized in the liver; split into sulfapyridine and 5-aminosalicylic acid (5-ASA) in the colon

**Excretion:** Urine

**Formulations**

Suspension, oral: 250 mg/5 mL (473 mL)

Tablet: 500 mg

Tablet, enteric coated: 500 mg

**Dosing**

**Adults:**

Ulcerative colitis: Oral: 1 g 3-4 times/day, 2 g/day maintenance in divided doses; not to exceed 6 g/day.

Rheumatoid arthritis: Initial: 500 mg increasing to 2 g per day in 2-4 divided doses.

**Elderly:** Refer to adult dosing.

**Renal Impairment:**

$Cl_{cr}$ 10-30 mL/minute: Administer twice daily.

$Cl_{cr}$ <10 mL/minute: Administer once daily.

**Hepatic Impairment:** Avoid use.

**Administration**

**Oral:** Shake suspension well. GI intolerance is common during the first few days of therapy (give with meals).

**Stability**

**Storage:** Protect from light.

**Additional Nursing Issues**

**Physical Assessment:** Assess effectiveness and interactions of other medications (see Drug Interactions). See Warnings/Precautions for use cautions. Assess for history of allergies (see Contraindications). Monitor effectiveness of therapy, and adverse response (see Adverse Reactions and Overdose/Toxicology). Assess knowledge/teach patient appropriate use, possible side effects/interventions, and adverse symptoms to report. **Pregnancy risk factor B/D** - see Pregnancy Risk Factor for cautious use. Note breast-feeding caution.

**Patient Information/Instruction:** Do not crush, chew, or dissolve coated tablets. Shake suspension well before use. Do not take on an empty stomach or with antacids. Maintain adequate hydration (2-3 L/day of fluids unless instructed to restrict fluid intake) to prevent kidney damage. Increased dietary iron may be recommended. You may experience nervousness or dizziness (use caution when driving or engaging in hazardous activities until response to drug is known). You may experience photosensitivity (use sunscreen, wear protective clothing and eyewear, and avoid direct sunlight). Orange-yellow color of urine, sweat, tears is normal and will stain contact lenses and clothing. Report rash, persistent nausea or anorexia, or lack of improvement in symptoms (after 1-2 months). **Pregnancy/breast-feeding precautions:** Inform prescriber if you are pregnant. Consult prescriber if breast-feeding.

**Dietary Issues:** Since sulfasalazine impairs folate absorption, consider providing 1 mg/day folate supplement.

**Geriatric Considerations:** Adjust dose for renal function (see Additional Information).

**Breast-feeding Issues:** The American Academy of Pediatrics classifies this agent to be used with caution since adverse effects have been reported in nursing infants.

**Additional Information** Sulfasalazine can be used as a disease modifying agent in the treatment of rheumatoid arthritis that has not responded adequately to anti-inflammatory agents.

- **Sulfathiazole, Sulfacetamide, and Sulfabenzamide** *see* Sulfabenzamide, Sulfacetamide, and Sulfathiazole *on page 1079*
- **Sulfatrim®** *see* Co-trimoxazole *on page 307*

## Sulfinpyrazone (sul fin PEER a zone)

**U.S. Brand Names** Anturane®

**Therapeutic Category** Uricosuric Agent

**Pregnancy Risk Factor** C/D (near term)

**Lactation** Excretion in breast milk unknown

**Use** Treatment of chronic gouty arthritis and intermittent gouty arthritis

**Unlabeled use:** To decrease the incidence of sudden death following myocardial infarction

**Mechanism of Action/Effect** Acts by increasing the urinary excretion of uric acid, thereby decreasing blood urate levels; this effect is therapeutically useful in treating patients with acute intermittent gout, chronic tophaceous gout, and acts to promote resorption of tophi; also has antithrombic and platelet inhibitory effects

**Contraindications** Hypersensitivity to sulfinpyrazone, phenylbutazone, or other pyrazolones; active peptic ulcers; GI inflammation; blood dyscrasias; pregnancy (at term)

**Warnings** Safety and efficacy are not established in children <18 years of age. Use with caution in patients with impaired renal function and urolithiasis. Pregnancy factor C/D (at term).

**Drug Interactions**

**Cytochrome P-450 Effect:** CYP2C and 3A3/4 enzyme inducer; CYP2C9 enzyme inhibitor

**Decreased Effect:** Decreased effect/levels of theophylline, verapamil. Decreased uricosuric activity with salicylates, niacins.

**Increased Effect/Toxicity:** Increased effect of oral hypoglycemics and anticoagulants. Risk of acetaminophen hepatotoxicity is increased, while therapeutic effects may be reduced.

**Effects on Lab Values** ↓ uric acid (S)

**Adverse Reactions**

>10%:

Gastrointestinal: Nausea, vomiting, stomach pain

Endocrine & metabolic: Gouty arthritis

Renal: Uric acid stones

1% to 10%: Dermatologic: Dermatitis, rash

<1% (Limited to important or life-threatening symptoms): GI bleeding, anemia, agranulocytosis, thrombocytopenia, aplastic anemia, leukopenia, increased bleeding time (decreased platelet aggregation), hepatic necrosis, renal failure

**Overdose/Toxicology** Symptoms of overdose include drowsiness, dizziness, anorexia, abdominal pain, nausea, vomiting, hemolytic anemia, acidosis, jaundice, fever, and agranulocytosis. The aniline radical is responsible for hematologic toxicity. High volume diuresis may aid in elimination and prevention of renal failure. Leucovorin 5-15 mg/day has been used to speed recovery of bone marrow.

**Pharmacodynamics/Kinetics**

**Half-life Elimination:** 2.7-6 hours

**Time to Peak:** 1.6 hours

**Metabolism:** Hepatic to two active metabolites

**Excretion:** Renal excretion with 22% to 50% as unchanged drug

**Formulations**

Capsule: 200 mg

Tablet: 100 mg

**Dosing**

**Adults:** Oral: 100-200 mg twice daily; maximum daily dose: 800 mg

**Elderly:** Refer to adult dosing (see Geriatric Considerations).

**Renal Impairment:** $Cl_{cr}$ <50 mL/minute: Avoid use.

**Monitoring Laboratory Tests** Serum and urinary uric acid, CBC

**Additional Nursing Issues**

**Physical Assessment:** Assess effectiveness and interactions of other medications patient may be taking (see Contraindications and Drug Interactions). Monitor for therapeutic response (eg, frequency and severity of gouty attacks), laboratory values, and adverse reactions (see Adverse Reactions and Overdose/Toxicology) at beginning of therapy and periodically with long-term use. Assess knowledge/teach patient appropriate use, interventions to reduce side effects, and adverse symptoms to report. **Pregnancy risk factor C/D** - benefits of use should outweigh possible risks. Note breast-feeding caution.

**Patient Information/Instruction:** Take as directed, with meals or antacids and a full glass of water. Avoid aspirin or acetaminophen products and avoid large quantities of vitamin C. It is very important to maintain adequate hydration (2-3 L/day of fluids unless instructed to restrict fluid intake) to prevent kidney damage. You may experience nausea or vomiting (small frequent meals, frequent mouth care, chewing gum, or sucking lozenges may help). Report skin rash, persistent stomach pain, painful urination or bloody urine, unusual bruising or bleeding, fatigue, or yellowing of eyes or skin. **Pregnancy/breast-feeding precautions:** Inform prescriber if you are or intend to be pregnant. Consult prescriber if breast-feeding.

**Geriatric Considerations:** Since sulfinpyrazone loses its effectiveness when the $Cl_{cr}$ is <50 mL/minute, its usefulness in the elderly is limited.

## Sulfisoxazole (sul fi SOKS a zole)

**Synonyms** Sulfisoxazole Acetyl; Sulphafurazole

**Therapeutic Category** Antibiotic, Sulfonamide Derivative

**Pregnancy Risk Factor** B/D (at term)

**Lactation** Enters breast milk/compatible

**Use** Treatment of urinary tract infections, otitis media, *Chlamydia*; nocardiosis; treatment of acute pelvic inflammatory disease in prepubertal children; often used in combination with trimethoprim

**Mechanism of Action/Effect** Interferes with bacterial growth by inhibiting bacterial folic acid synthesis through competitive antagonism of PABA

**Contraindications** Hypersensitivity to any sulfa drug or any component; porphyria; pregnancy (at term); patients with urinary obstruction; sunblock containing PABA

**Warnings** Use with caution in patients with G-6-PD deficiency (hemolysis may occur), hepatic or renal impairment. Dosage modification is required in patients with renal impairment. Risk of crystalluria should be considered in patients with impaired renal function.

**Drug Interactions**

**Decreased Effect:** Decreased effect with PABA or PABA metabolites of drugs (eg, procaine, proparacaine, tetracaine), thiopental.

**Increased Effect/Toxicity:** Increased effect of oral anticoagulants, methotrexate, and oral hypoglycemic agents.

**Food Interactions** Food interferes with folate absorption.

**Effects on Lab Values** False-positive protein in urine; false-positive urine glucose with Clinitest®

**Adverse Reactions**

>10%:

- Central nervous system: Fever, dizziness, headache
- Dermatologic: Itching, rash, photosensitivity
- Gastrointestinal: Anorexia, nausea, vomiting, diarrhea

1% to 10%:

- Dermatologic: Lyell's syndrome, Stevens-Johnson syndrome
- Hematologic: Granulocytopenia, leukopenia, thrombocytopenia, aplastic anemia, hemolytic anemia
- Hepatic: Hepatitis

<1% (Limited to important or life-threatening symptoms): Interstitial nephritis, acute nephropathy, hematuria

**Overdose/Toxicology** Symptoms of overdose include drowsiness, dizziness, anorexia, abdominal pain, nausea, vomiting, hemolytic anemia, acidosis, jaundice, fever, and agranulocytosis. Doses as little as 2-5 g/day may produce toxicity. The aniline radical is responsible for hematologic toxicity. High volume diuresis may aid in elimination and prevention of renal failure. Leucovorin 5-15 mg/day has been used to speed recovery of bone marrow.

**Pharmacodynamics/Kinetics**

**Protein Binding:** Within 2-3 hours

**Distribution:** Crosses the placenta

Relative diffusion of antimicrobial agents from blood into cerebrospinal fluid (CSF): Adequate with or without inflammation (exceeds usual MICs); routine alkalinization of urine is normally not required; not for use in patients <2 months of age

Ratio of CSF to blood level (%): Normal meninges: 50-80; Inflamed meninges: 80+

**Half-life Elimination:** 4-7 hours (prolonged in renal impairment)

**Time to Peak:** Within 2-3 hours

**Metabolism:** Liver

**Excretion:** Urine

**Formulations**

Suspension, oral, pediatric, as acetyl (raspberry flavor): 500 mg/5 mL (480 mL)

Tablet: 500 mg

**Dosing**

**Adults:**

Oral: 2-4 g stat, 4-8 g/day in divided doses every 4-6 hours

Pelvic inflammatory disease: 500 mg every 6 hours for 21 days; used in combination with ceftriaxone

*Chlamydia trachomatis*: 500 mg every 6 hours for 10 days

Ophthalmic:

Solution: Instill 1-2 drops to affected eye every 2-3 hours.

Ointment: Apply small amount to affected eye 1-3 times/day and at bedtime.

**Elderly:** Oral: Urinary tract infections: 2 g stat, 2-8 g/day every 6 hours; adjust dose for $Cl_{cr}$. Single and 3-day dosing for urinary tract infections in the elderly are not reliable.

**Renal Impairment:**

$Cl_{cr}$ 10-50 mL/minutes: Administer every 8-12 hours.

$Cl_{cr}$ <10 mL/minute: Administer every 12-24 hours.

Hemodialysis effects: >50% removed by hemodialysis

**Administration**

**Oral:** Administer around-the-clock to promote less variation in peak and trough serum levels.

**Stability**

**Storage:** Protect from light.

**Monitoring Laboratory Tests** CBC, urinalysis, renal function. Obtain specimen for culture prior to first dose.

**Additional Nursing Issues**

**Physical Assessment:** Assess for history of previous allergies before first dose. Monitor (teach patient to monitor and report) adverse reactions (see above). Instruct patient on necessity to maintain adequate hydration. Caution diabetic patients to use

(Continued)

## Sulfisoxazole *(Continued)*

something other than Clinitest® for glucose monitoring (sulfisoxazole may alter Clinitest® response). **Pregnancy risk factor B/D** - see Pregnancy Risk Factor for cautious use.

**Patient Information/Instruction:** Take as directed, at regular intervals around-the-clock. Take 1 hour before or 2 hours after meals with a full glass of water. Take full course of therapy even if you are feeling better. Avoid aspirin or aspirin-containing products and avoid large quantities of vitamin C. It is very important to maintain adequate hydration (2-3 L/day of fluids unless instructed to restrict fluid intake) to prevent kidney damage. You may experience dizziness or headache (use caution when driving or engaging in tasks requiring alertness until response to drug is known); photosensitivity (use sunscreen, wear protective clothing and eyewear, and avoid direct sunlight); nausea, vomiting, or loss of appetite (small frequent meals, frequent mouth care, sucking lozenges, or chewing gum may help). Diabetics: Drug may cause false tests with Clinitest® urine glucose monitoring; use of glucose oxidase methods (Clinistix®) or serum glucose monitoring is preferable. Report persistent nausea, vomiting, diarrhea, or abdominal pain; skin rash; persistent or severe sore throat, mouth sores, fever, or vaginal itching or discharge; unusual bruising or bleeding; blackened stool; fatigue; or difficulty breathing. **Pregnancy precautions:** Inform prescriber if you are pregnant.

Ophthalmic: Instill as often as recommended. Wash hands before using. Sit or lie down, open eye, look at ceiling, and instill prescribed amount of solution. Ointment: Pull lower lid down gently and instill thin ribbon of ointment inside lid. Close eye and roll eye in all directions, and apply gentle pressure to inner corner of eye for 1-2 minutes. Do not let tip of applicator touch eye or contaminate tip of applicator. Temporary stinging or blurred vision may occur. Report persistent pain, redness, burning, double vision, severe headache, or respiratory congestion.

**Geriatric Considerations:** Sulfisoxazole is an effective anti-infective agent. Most prescribers prefer the combination of sulfamethoxazole and trimethoprim for its dual mechanism of action. Trimethoprim penetrates the prostate. Adjust dose for renal function.

♦ **Sulfisoxazole Acetyl** *see* Sulfisoxazole *on page 1086*

♦ **Sulfisoxazole and Erythromycin** *see* Erythromycin and Sulfisoxazole *on page 438*

## Sulfisoxazole and Phenazopyridine

(sul fi SOKS a zole & fen az oh PEER i deen)

**Synonyms** Phenazopyridine and Sulfisoxazole

**Therapeutic Category** Antibiotic, Sulfonamide Derivative; Local Anesthetic

**Pregnancy Risk Factor** B/D (at term)

**Lactation** Excretion in breast milk unknown

**Use** Treatment of urinary tract infections and nocardiosis

**Formulations** Tablet: Sulfisoxazole 500 mg and phenazopyridine 50 mg

**Dosing**

**Adults:** Oral: 4-6 tablets to start, then 2 tablets 4 times/day for 2 days, then continue with sulfisoxazole only

**Elderly:** Refer to dosing in individual monographs.

**Renal Impairment:** $Cl_{cr}$ <50 mL/minute: Avoid use of phenazopyridine

**Additional Nursing Issues**

**Physical Assessment:** See individual components listed in Related Information. **Pregnancy risk factor B/D** - see Pregnancy Risk Factor - assess knowledge/instruct patient on need to use appropriate contraceptive measures and the need to avoid pregnancy. Note breast-feeding caution.

**Patient Information/Instruction:** See individual components listed in Related Information. **Pregnancy/breast-feeding precautions:** Inform prescriber if you are on intend to get pregnant. Consult prescriber if breast-feeding.

**Related Information**

Phenazopyridine *on page 914*
Sulfisoxazole *on page 1086*

♦ **Sulfizole®** *see* Sulfisoxazole *on page 1086*

♦ **Sulfur and Salicylic Acid** *see page 1294*

♦ **Sulfur and Sodium Sulfacetamide** *see page 1306*

## Sulindac (sul IN dak)

**U.S. Brand Names** Clinoril®

**Therapeutic Category** Nonsteroidal Anti-Inflammatory Agent (NSAID)

**Pregnancy Risk Factor** B/D (at term)

**Lactation** Excretion in breast milk unknown

**Use** Management of inflammatory disease, osteoarthritis; rheumatoid arthritis; acute gouty arthritis; ankylosing spondylitis; acute painful shoulder (bursitis or tendonitis); structurally similar to indomethacin but acts like aspirin; safest NSAID for use in mild renal impairment

**Mechanism of Action/Effect** Inhibits prostaglandin synthesis by decreasing the activity of the enzyme, cyclo-oxygenase, which results in decreased formation of prostaglandin precursors

**Contraindications** Hypersensitivity to sulindac, any component, aspirin or other nonsteroidal anti-inflammatory drugs (NSAIDs); patients in whom sulindac, aspirin, or other

NSAIDs have induced asthma, urticaria, or other allergic-type reactions; fatal asthmatic reactions have occurred following NSAID administration; pregnancy (at term)

**Warnings** Use with caution in patients with peptic ulcer disease, GI bleeding, bleeding abnormalities, impaired renal or hepatic function, congestive heart failure, hypertension, and patients receiving anticoagulants.

**Drug Interactions**

**Cytochrome P-450 Effect:** CYP2C9 enzyme inhibitor

**Decreased Effect:** Decreased effect of diuretics, beta-blockers, hydralazine, and captopril.

**Increased Effect/Toxicity:** Increased toxicity with probenecid, NSAIDs. Increased toxicity of digoxin, anticoagulants, methotrexate, lithium, aminoglycosides antibiotics (reported in neonates), cyclosporine (increased nephrotoxicity), and potassium-sparing diuretics (hyperkalemia).

**Food Interactions** The therapeutic effect of sulindac may be decreased if taken with food.

**Effects on Lab Values** ↑ chloride (S), sodium (S), bleeding time

**Adverse Reactions**

1% to 10%:

Cardiovascular: Edema

Central nervous system: Dizziness, headache, nervousness

Dermatologic: Pruritus, rash

Gastrointestinal: GI pain, heartburn, nausea, vomiting, diarrhea, constipation, flatulence, anorexia, abdominal cramps

Otic: Tinnitus

<1% (Limited to important or life-threatening symptoms): Congestive heart failure, hypertension, palpitation, arrhythmia, convulsions, aseptic meningitis, erythema multiforme, toxic epidermal necrolysis, Stevens-Johnson syndrome, exfoliative dermatitis, angioneurotic edema, peptic ulcer, GI bleeding, GI perforation, agranulocytosis, aplastic anemia, hemolytic anemia, bone marrow depression, leukopenia, thrombocytopenia, neutropenia, increased prothrombin time, abnormal LFTs, jaundice, hepatitis, hepatic failure, proteinuria, crystalluria, renal impairment, renal failure, nephrotic syndrome, interstitial nephritis, bronchial spasm, dyspnea

**Overdose/Toxicology** Symptoms of overdose include dizziness, vomiting, nausea, abdominal pain, hypotension, coma, stupor, metabolic acidosis, leukocytosis, and renal failure. Management of nonsteroidal anti-inflammatory (NSAID) intoxication is supportive and symptomatic. Seizures tend to be short-lived and often do not require drug treatment.

**Pharmacodynamics/Kinetics**

**Half-life Elimination:** Parent drug: 7 hours; Active metabolite: 18 hours

**Metabolism:** Sulindac is a prodrug and, therefore, requires metabolic activation; requires hepatic metabolism to sulfide metabolite (active) for therapeutic effects; also metabolized in the liver to sulfone metabolites (inactive)

**Excretion:** Principally in urine (50%) with some biliary excretion (25%)

**Onset:** Analgesic: ~1 hour

**Duration:** 12-24 hours

**Formulations** Tablet: 150 mg, 200 mg

**Dosing**

**Adults:** Maximum therapeutic response may not be realized for up to 3 weeks. Oral: 150-200 mg twice daily or 300-400 mg once daily; not to exceed 400 mg/day.

**Elderly:** Refer to adult dosing.

**Hepatic Impairment:** Dose reduction is necessary.

**Monitoring Laboratory Tests** Liver enzymes, BUN, serum creatinine, CBC, platelets

**Additional Nursing Issues**

**Physical Assessment:** Assess effectiveness and interactions of other medications patient may be taking (see Contraindications and Drug Interactions). Monitor laboratory tests (see above) and therapeutic response (eg, relief of pain and inflammation, increased activity tolerance), and adverse reactions (eg, GI and respiratory response, hepatotoxicity, ototoxicity) at beginning of therapy and periodically throughout therapy (see Warnings/Precautions, Adverse Reactions, and Overdose/Toxicology). Schedule ophthalmic evaluations for patients who develop eye complaints during long-term NSAID therapy. Assess knowledge/teach patient appropriate use, interventions to reduce side effects, and adverse symptoms to report. **Pregnancy risk factor B/D** - see Pregnancy Risk Factor for cautious use. Note breast-feeding caution.

**Patient Information/Instruction:** Take this medication exactly as directed; do not increase dose without consulting prescriber. Take with food or milk to reduce GI distress. Maintain adequate fluid intake (2-3 L/day of fluids unless instructed to restrict fluid intake). Do not use alcohol, aspirin, or aspirin-containing medication, and all other anti-inflammatory medications without consulting prescriber. You may experience dizziness, nervousness, or headache (use caution when driving or engaging in tasks requiring alertness until response to drug is known); nausea, vomiting, or heartburn (frequent small meals, frequent mouth care, sucking lozenges, or chewing gum may help); constipation (increased exercise, fluids, or dietary fruit and fiber may help). GI bleeding, ulceration, or perforation can occur with or without pain; discontinue medication and contact prescriber if persistent abdominal pain or cramping, or blood in stool occurs. Report breathlessness or difficulty breathing; unusual bruising/bleeding; blood in urine, stool, mouth, or vomitus; unusual fatigue; skin rash or itching; change in urinary pattern; or change in hearing or ringing in ears. **Pregnancy/breast-feeding precautions:** Inform prescriber if you are or intend to be pregnant. Consult prescriber if breast-feeding.

(Continued)

## Sulindac *(Continued)*

**Geriatric Considerations:** Elderly are at high risk for adverse effects from nonsteroidal anti-inflammatory agents. As much as 60% of elderly who develop GI complications can develop peptic ulceration and/or hemorrhage asymptomatically. The concomitant use of $H_2$ blockers, omeprazole, and sucralfate is not effective as prophylaxis with the exception of NSAID-induced duodenal ulcers which may be prevented by the use of ranitidine. Misoprostol is the only prophylactic agent proven effective. Also, concomitant disease and drug use contribute to the risk for GI adverse effects. Use lowest effective dose for shortest period possible. Consider renal function decline with age. Use of NSAIDs can compromise existing renal function especially when $Cl_{cr}$ is ≤30 mL/minute. Tinnitus may be a difficult and unreliable indication of toxicity due to age-related hearing loss or eighth cranial nerve damage. CNS adverse effects such as confusion, agitation, and hallucination are generally seen in overdose or high-dose situations, but elderly may demonstrate these adverse effects at lower doses than younger adults.

**Related Information**

Nonsalicylate/Nonsteroidal Anti-inflammatory Comparison *on page 1401*

- **Sulphafurazole** *see* Sulfisoxazole *on page 1086*
- **Sultrin™** *see* Sulfabenzamide, Sulfacetamide, and Sulfathiazole *on page 1079*
- **Sumacal®** *see page 1294*

## Sumatriptan Succinate (SOO ma trip tan SUKS i nate)

**U.S. Brand Names** Imitrex®

**Therapeutic Category** Serotonin 5-$HT_{1D}$ Receptor Agonist

**Pregnancy Risk Factor** C

**Lactation** Enters breast milk/use caution

**Use** Acute treatment of migraine with or without aura

**Unlabeled use:** Cluster headaches

**Mechanism of Action/Effect** Selective agonist for serotonin (5-$HT_{1D}$ receptor) in cranial arteries to cause vasoconstriction and reduces sterile inflammation associated with antidromic neuronal transmission correlating with relief of migraine

**Contraindications** Hypersensitivity to sumatriptan or any component; intravenous administration; use in patients with ischemic heart disease or Prinzmetal angina, patients with signs or symptoms of ischemic heart disease, uncontrolled hypertension; use with ergotamine derivatives; management of hemiplegic or basilar migraine

**Warnings** Sumatriptan is indicated only in patient populations with a clear diagnosis of migraine. Use with caution in the elderly, patients with hepatic or renal impairment. May cause mild, transient elevation of blood pressure. May cause coronary vasospasm. Pregnancy factor C.

**Drug Interactions**

**Increased Effect/Toxicity:** Increased toxicity with ergot-containing drugs, avoid use, wait 24 hours from last ergot containing drug (dihydroergotamine, or methysergide) before administering sumatriptan. MAO inhibitors decrease clearance of sumatriptan increasing the risk of systemic sumatriptan toxic effects. Sumatriptan may enhance CNS toxic effects when taken with selective serotonin reuptake inhibitors (SSRI) like fluoxetine, fluvoxamine, paroxetine, or sertraline.

**Adverse Reactions**

>10%:

Central nervous system: Dizziness
Endocrine & metabolic: Hot flashes
Gastrointestinal: Nausea, vomiting
Local: Injection site reaction
Neuromuscular & skeletal: Paresthesia

1% to 10%:

Cardiovascular: Tightness in chest
Central nervous system: Drowsiness, headache
Dermatologic: Burning sensation
Gastrointestinal: Abdominal discomfort, mouth discomfort
Neuromuscular & skeletal: Myalgia, numbness, weakness, neck pain, jaw discomfort
Miscellaneous: Sweating

<1% (Limited to important or life-threatening symptoms): Dyspnea

**Pharmacodynamics/Kinetics**

**Protein Binding:** 14% to 21%

**Half-life Elimination:** After S.C. administration: Distribution: 15 minutes; Terminal: 115 minutes

**Time to Peak:** Subcutaneous administration: 5-20 minutes

**Excretion:** After S.C. administration: Urine

**Onset:** Within 30 minutes

**Formulations**

Injection: 12 mg/mL (0.5 mL, 2 mL)
Spray, nasal: 5 mg (100 μL); 20 mg (100 μL)
Tablet: 25 mg, 50 mg

**Dosing**

**Adults:** Adults:

Oral: 25 mg (taken with fluids); maximum recommended dose is 100 mg. If a satisfactory response has not been obtained at 2 hours, a second dose of up to 100 mg may be given. Efficacy of this second dose has not been examined. If a headache returns, additional doses may be taken at intervals of at least 2 hours up to a daily maximum of 300 mg. There is no evidence that an initial dose of 100 mg provides substantially greater relief than 25 mg.

Intranasal: Single dose of 5, 10, or 20 mg administered in one nostril; a 10 mg dose may be achieved by administration of a single 5 mg dose in each nostril; if headache returns, the dose may be repeated once after 2 hours, not to exceed a total daily dose of 40 mg

S.C.: 6 mg; a second injection may be administered at least 1 hour after the initial dose, but not more than two injections in a 24-hour period

**Elderly:** Refer to adult dosing (see Geriatric Considerations and Warnings/Precautions).

**Administration**

**Oral:** Oral: Should be taken with fluids as soon as symptoms to appear.

**I.V.:** Do **not** administer I.V.; may cause coronary vasospasm.

**Other:** Administer subcutaneously.

**Stability**

**Storage:** Store at 2°C to 20°C (36°F to 86°F). Protect from light.

**Additional Nursing Issues**

**Physical Assessment:** For use only with a clear diagnosis of migraine. Assess other medications patient may be taking (See Drug Interactions). Monitor closely for effectiveness of therapy, vital signs, and adverse reactions, especially with first time administration. Instruct patient on proper administration (see Dosing), possible adverse effects, and symptoms to report. **Pregnancy risk factor C** - benefits of use should outweigh possible risks. Note breast-feeding caution.

**Patient Information/Instruction:** Take at first sign of migraine attack. This drug is to be used to reduce your migraine, not to prevent or reduce number of attacks. Oral: If headache returns or is not fully resolved after first dose, the dose may be repeated after 2 hours. **Do not exceed 300 mg in 24 hours.** S.C.: If headache returns or is not fully resolved after first dose, the dose may be repeated after 1 hour. **Do not exceed two injections in 24 hours. Do not take within 24 hours of any other migraine medication without first consulting prescriber.** You may experience some dizziness (use caution); hot flashes (cool room may help); nausea or vomiting (frequent small meals, frequent mouth care, sucking lozenges, or chewing gum may help); pain at injection site (lasts about 1 hour, will resolve); or excess sweating (will resolve). Report chest tightness or pain; excessive drowsiness; acute abdominal pain; skin rash or burning sensation; muscle weakness, soreness, or numbness; or respiratory difficulty. **Pregnancy/breast-feeding precautions:** Inform prescriber if you are or intend to be pregnant. Consult prescriber if breast-feeding.

**Geriatric Considerations:** Use cautiously in the elderly, particularly since many elderly have cardiovascular disease which would put them at risk for cardiovascular adverse effects. Safety and efficacy in the elderly (>65 years of age) have not been established. Pharmacokinetic disposition is, however, similar to that in young adults.

- **Summer's Eve® Medicated Douche** *see page 1294*
- **Sumycin® Oral** *see* Tetracycline *on page 1111*
- **Supeudol®** *see* Oxycodone *on page 871*
- **Suplena** *see* Vitamin, Multiple *on page 1219*
- **Supprelin™ Injection** *see* Histrelin *on page 561*
- **Suppress®** *see page 1294*
- **Suprax®** *see* Cefixime *on page 216*
- **Suprofen** *see page 1248*
- **Surbex®** *see page 1294*
- **Surbex-T® Filmtabs®** *see page 1294*
- **Surbex® With C Filmtabs®** *see page 1294*
- **Surfak® [OTC]** *see* Docusate *on page 392*
- **Surgicel®** *see page 1248*
- **Surmontil®** *see* Trimipramine *on page 1183*
- **Susano®** *see* Hyoscyamine, Atropine, Scopolamine, and Phenobarbital *on page 591*
- **Sus-Phrine®** *see* Epinephrine *on page 424*
- **Sustaire®** *see* Theophylline *on page 1115*
- **Sustiva™** *see* Efavirenz *on page 414*
- **Sween Cream®** *see page 1294*
- **Swim-Ear®** *see page 1291*
- **Swim-Ear® Otic** *see page 1294*
- **Sydolil** *see* Ergotamine Derivatives *on page 434*
- **Syllact® [OTC]** *see* Psyllium *on page 993*
- **Symadine®** *see* Amantadine *on page 61*
- **Symbols & Abbreviations Used in This Handbook** *see page 12*
- **Symmetrel®** *see* Amantadine *on page 61*
- **Synacol® CF [OTC]** *see* Guaifenesin and Dextromethorphan *on page 549*
- **Synacort®** *see* Hydrocortisone *on page 578*
- **Synacort®** *see* Topical Corticosteroids *on page 1152*
- **Synalar®** *see* Topical Corticosteroids *on page 1152*
- **Synalar-HP®** *see* Topical Corticosteroids *on page 1152*
- **Synalgos® [OTC]** *see* Aspirin *on page 111*
- **Synalgos®-DC** *see* Dihydrocodeine Compound *on page 373*
- **Synarel®** *see* Nafarelin *on page 799*

- ♦ **Syn-Captopril** *see* Captopril *on page 192*
- ♦ **Syn-Diltiazem** *see* Diltiazem *on page 377*
- ♦ **Synemol®** *see* Topical Corticosteroids *on page 1152*
- ♦ **Syn-Flunisolide** *see* Flunisolide *on page 497*
- ♦ **Syngestal** *see* Norethindrone *on page 836*
- ♦ **Syn-Minocycline** *see* Minocycline *on page 774*
- ♦ **Syn-Nadolol** *see* Nadolol *on page 798*
- ♦ **Synphasic®** *see* Oral Contraceptives *on page 859*
- ♦ **Syn-Pindol®** *see* Pindolol *on page 934*
- ♦ **Synthroid®** *see* Levothyroxine *on page 673*
- ♦ **Syntocinon®** *see* Oxytocin *on page 877*
- ♦ **Syntocinon® Injection** *see* Oxytocin *on page 877*
- ♦ **Syntocinon® Nasal Spray** *see* Oxytocin *on page 877*
- ♦ **Syprine®** *see page 1246*
- ♦ **Syracol-CF® [OTC]** *see* Guaifenesin and Dextromethorphan *on page 549*
- ♦ **Syraprim** *see* Co-trimoxazole *on page 307*
- ♦ **Syscor** *see* Nisoldipine *on page 828*
- ♦ **Systen** *see* Estradiol *on page 441*
- ♦ **Sytobex®** *see* Cyanocobalamin *on page 311*
- ♦ **$T_3$ Thyronine Sodium** *see* Liothyronine *on page 679*
- ♦ **$T_4$ Thyroxine Sodium** *see* Levothyroxine *on page 673*
- ♦ **Tabalon** *see* Ibuprofen *on page 592*
- ♦ **222® Tablets** *see* Aspirin and Codeine *on page 113*
- ♦ **282® Tablets** *see* Aspirin and Codeine *on page 113*
- ♦ **292® Tablets** *see* Aspirin and Codeine *on page 113*
- ♦ **624® Tablets** *see* Propoxyphene *on page 984*
- ♦ **Tablets That Cannot Be Crushed or Altered** *see page 1333*
- ♦ **Tac™-3** *see* Triamcinolone *on page 1171*
- ♦ **Tac™-40** *see* Triamcinolone *on page 1171*
- ♦ **TACE®** *see* Chlorotrianisene *on page 255*
- ♦ **Tacex** *see* Ceftriaxone *on page 232*


## Tacrine (TAK reen)

**U.S. Brand Names** Cognex®

**Synonyms** Tetrahydroaminoacrine; THA

**Therapeutic Category** Acetylcholinesterase Inhibitor (Central)

**Pregnancy Risk Factor** C

**Lactation** Excretion in breast milk unknown/not recommended

**Use** Treatment of mild to moderate dementia of the Alzheimer's type

**Contraindications** Hypersensitivity to tacrine or acridine derivatives; patients previously treated with the drug who developed jaundice

**Warnings** The use of tacrine has been associated with elevations in serum transaminases. Serum transaminases (specifically ALT) must be monitored throughout therapy. Use extreme caution in patients with current evidence of a history of abnormal liver function tests. Use caution in patients with bladder outlet obstruction, asthma, and sick-sinus syndrome (tacrine may cause bradycardia). Also, patients with cardiovascular disease, asthma, or peptic ulcer should use cautiously. Pregnancy factor C.

**Drug Interactions**

**Cytochrome P-450 Effect:** CYP1A2 enzyme substrate; CYP1A2 enzyme inhibitor

**Decreased Effect:** Tacrine may decrease the effect of anticholinergic (atropine) medications.

**Increased Effect/Toxicity:** Tacrine may increase the effect of theophylline, cimetidine, succinylcholine, fluvoxamine, cholinesterase inhibitors, or cholinergic agonists (bethanechol) when taken concomitantly.

**Adverse Reactions**

>10%:

Central nervous system: Ataxia, dizziness, headache

Gastrointestinal: Diarrhea, nausea, vomiting, heartburn, anorexia, abdominal pain, heartburn

Hepatic: Elevated transaminases

Musculoskeletal: Myalgia

1% to 10%:

Cardiovascular: Bradycardia, hypertension, hypotension, palpitation, syncope, flushing

Central nervous system: Insomnia, seizures

Dermatologic: Rash

Gastrointestinal: Belching, salivation

Ocular: Lacrimation

Musculoskeletal: Muscular weakness

Respiratory: Hyperventilation

Miscellaneous: Sweating

<1% (Limited to important or life-threatening symptoms): Tachycardia, parkinsonian extrapyramidal effects, asthma

**Overdose/Toxicology** Provide general supportive measures. Can cause cholinergic crisis characterized by severe nausea, vomiting, salivation, sweating, bradycardia, hypotension, collapse, and convulsions. Increased muscle weakness is a possibility and may result in death if respiratory muscles are involved.

Tertiary anticholinergics, such as atropine, may be used as an antidote for overdose. I.V. atropine sulfate titrated to effect is recommended at an initial dose of 1-2 mg I.V. with subsequent doses based upon clinical response. Atypical increases in blood pressure and heart rate have been reported with other cholinomimetics when coadministered with quaternary anticholinergics such as glycopyrrolate.

**Pharmacodynamics/Kinetics**

**Half-life Elimination:** 2-4 hours

**Onset:** May require weeks of treatment

**Formulations** Capsule, as hydrochloride: 10 mg, 20 mg, 30 mg, 40 mg

**Dosing**

**Adults:** Oral: Initial: 10 mg 4 times/day; may increase by 40 mg/day adjusted every 6 weeks; maximum: 160 mg/day; best administered separate from meal times; see table.

**Dose Adjustment Based Upon Transaminase Elevations**

| ALT | Regimen |
|---|---|
| ≤3 x ULN* | Continue titration |
| >3 to ≤5 x ULN | Decrease dose by 40 mg/day, resume when ALT returns to normal |
| >5 x ULN | Stop treatment, may rechallenge upon return of ALT to normal |

*ULN = upper limit of normal.

Patients with clinical jaundice confirmed by elevated total bilirubin (>3 mg/dL) should not be rechallenged with tacrine.

**Elderly:** Refer to adult dosing.

**Hepatic Impairment:** Patients with clinical jaundice confirmed by elevated total bilirubin (>3 mg/dL) should not be rechallenged with tacrine.

**Monitoring Laboratory Tests** ALT (SGPT) levels and other liver enzymes weekly for at least the first 18 weeks, then monitor once every 3 months

**Additional Nursing Issues**

**Physical Assessment:** Assess bladder and sphincter adequacy prior to administering medication. Assess other medications patient may be taking for effectiveness and interactions (see Drug Interactions). Monitor laboratory tests (ALT) throughout therapy (see above), therapeutic effect, and adverse reactions: cholinergic crisis (DUMBELS - **d**iarrhea, **u**rination, **m**iosis, **b**ronchospasm/**b**radycardia, **e**xcitability, **l**acrimation, and **s**alivation/excessive **s**weating) (see Warnings/Precautions, Adverse Reactions, and Overdose/Toxicology). Assess knowledge/teach patient appropriate use, interventions to reduce side effects, and adverse symptoms to report. **Pregnancy risk factor C** - benefits of use should outweigh possible risks. Breast-feeding is not recommended.

**Patient Information/Instruction:** This medication will not cure the disease, but may help reduce symptoms. Use as directed; do not increase dose or discontinue without consulting prescriber. Maintain adequate hydration (2-3 L/day of fluids unless instructed to restrict fluid intake). May cause dizziness, sedation, or hypotension (rise slowly from sitting or lying position and use caution when driving or climbing stairs); vomiting or loss of appetite (frequent small meals, frequent mouth care, or chewing gum, or sucking lozenges may help); or diarrhea (boiled milk, yogurt, or buttermilk may help). Report persistent abdominal discomfort; significantly increased salivation, sweating, tearing, or urination; flushed skin; chest pain or palpitations; acute headache; unresolved diarrhea; excessive fatigue, insomnia, dizziness, or depression; increased muscle, joint, or body pain; vision changes or blurred vision; shortness of breath or wheezing; or signs of jaundice (yellowing of eyes or skin, dark colored urine or light colored stool, abdominal pain, or easy fatigue). **Pregnancy/breast-feeding precautions:** Inform prescriber if you are or intend to be pregnant. Breast-feeding is not recommended.

**Geriatric Considerations:** Tacrine is currently FDA-approved for the treatment of Alzheimer's disease, it is clearly not a cure. At least 25% of patients may not tolerate the drug and only 50% of patients demonstrate some improvement in symptoms or a slowing of deterioration. While worth a trial in mild to moderate dementia of the Alzheimer's type, patients and their families must be counseled about the limitations of the drug and the importance of regular monitoring of liver function tests. No specific dosage adjustments are necessary due to age.

## Tacrolimus (ta KROE li mus)

**U.S. Brand Names** Prograf®

**Synonyms** FK506

**Therapeutic Category** Immunosuppressant Agent

**Pregnancy Risk Factor** C

**Lactation** Enters breast milk/contraindicated

**Use** Potent immunosuppressive drug used in liver, kidney, heart, lung, or small bowel transplant recipients

**Mechanism of Action/Effect** Suppressed humoral immunity (inhibits T-lymphocyte activation); produced by the fungus *Streptomyces tsukubaensis*

**Contraindications** Hypersensitivity to tacrolimus or any component (eg, hydrogenated castor oil, used in the parenteral dosage formulation)

**Warnings** Increased susceptibility to infection and the possible development of lymphoma may occur after administration of tacrolimus. It should not be administered simultaneously with cyclosporine. Since the pharmacokinetics show great inter- and intrapatient variability over time, monitoring of serum concentrations (trough for oral therapy) is

(Continued)

## Tacrolimus *(Continued)*

essential to prevent organ rejection and reduce drug-related toxicity. Injectable formulation contains small volume of ethanol. Pregnancy factor C.

**Drug Interactions**

**Cytochrome P-450 Effect:** CYP3A3/4 enzyme substrate

**Decreased Effect:**

Antacids: Impaired tacrolimus absorption (separate administration by at least 2 hours).

Agents which may decrease tacrolimus plasma concentrations and reduce the therapeutic effect include rifampin, rifabutin, phenytoin, phenobarbital, and carbamazepine.

**Increased Effect/Toxicity:** Amphotericin B and other nephrotoxic antibiotics have the potential to increase tacrolimus associated nephrotoxicity. Agents which may increase tacrolimus plasma concentrations resulting in toxicity are erythromycin, clarithromycin, clotrimazole, fluconazole, itraconazole, ketoconazole, diltiazem, nicardipine, verapamil, bromocriptine, cimetidine, danazol, metoclopramide, methylprednisolone, and cyclosporine (synergistic immunosuppression).

**Adverse Reactions**

>10%:

Cardiovascular: Hypertension, peripheral edema
Central nervous system: Headache, insomnia, pain, fever
Dermatologic: Pruritus
Endocrine & metabolic: Hypo-/hyperkalemia, hyperglycemia, hypomagnesemia
Gastrointestinal: Diarrhea, nausea, anorexia, vomiting, abdominal pain
Hematologic: Anemia, leukocytosis
Hepatic: LFT abnormalities, ascites
Neuromuscular & skeletal: Tremors, paresthesias, back pain, weakness
Renal: Nephrotoxicity, elevated BUN/creatinine
Respiratory: Pleural effusion, atelectasis, dyspnea

1% to 10%:

Central nervous system: Seizures
Dermatologic: Rash
Endocrine & metabolic: Hypophosphatemia, hyperuricemia
Gastrointestinal: Constipation
Genitourinary: Urinary tract infection
Hematologic: Thrombocytopenia
Neuromuscular & skeletal: Myoclonus
Renal: Oliguria
Miscellaneous: Infection

<1% (Limited to important of life-threatening symptoms): Hypertrophic cardiomyopathy, arthralgia, myalgia, hemolytic uremic syndrome, anaphylaxis, expressive aphasia, photophobia, secondary malignancy

**Overdose/Toxicology** Symptoms are extensions of immunosuppressive activity and adverse effects. Symptomatic and supportive treatment is required. Hemodialysis is not effective.

**Pharmacodynamics/Kinetics**

**Protein Binding:** Plasma: 77% (primarily alpha$_1$-glycoprotein); blood:plasma = >4:1

**Distribution:** Crosses placenta (placental plasma concentrations are 4 times greater than maternal plasma); breast milk concentrations = plasma concentrations

**Half-life Elimination:** 12 hours (range: 4-40 hours)

**Metabolism:** Liver

**Excretion:** <1% in urine as unchanged drug; elimination from the body is primarily via bile; clearance: 43 mL/kg/minute

**Formulations**

Capsule: 1 mg, 5 mg

Injection, with alcohol and surfactant: 5 mg/mL (1 mL)

**Dosing**

**Adults:**

I.V. continuous infusion: Initial (at least 6 hours after transplantation): 0.05-0.1 mg/kg/day; to prevent graft-vs-host disease, 0.03 mg/kg/day as continuous infusion

Oral (within 2-3 days): 0.15-0.3 mg/kg/day in divided doses every 12 hours; give 8-12 hours after discontinuation of I.V. infusion. May gradually adjust (decrease) maintenance dose via pharmacokinetic monitoring.

**Elderly:** Refer to adult dosing.

**Renal Impairment:** Administer the lowest recommended I.V./oral doses, adjusting downward if needed. Delay therapy for ≥48 hours in patients with postoperative oliguria.

Not dialyzable

**Hepatic Impairment:** Moderate-to-severe hepatic dysfunction may result in decreased clearance and accumulation of active metabolites. Adjust doses per pharmacokinetic monitoring and clinical evaluation.

**Administration**

**I.V.:** Administer by I.V. continuous infusion only (use infusion pump). Tacrolimus is dispensed in a 50 mL glass container with no overfill. It is intended to be infused over 12 hours. Polyolefin administration sets should be used. Dilute with 0.9% sodium chloride or D$_5$W to a concentration of 0.004-0.02 mg/mL prior to administration.

**I.V. Detail:** Do not mix with acyclovir or ganciclovir due to chemical degradation of tacrolimus (use different ports in multilumen lines). Do not alter dose with concurrent T-tube clamping. Adsorption of the drug to PVC tubing may become clinically significant with low concentrations.

**Stability**

**Storage:** Potency remains for 24 hours in dextrose 5% solutions or normal saline. Tacrolimus is completely available from plastic syringes, glass, or polyolefin containers, however, polyvinyl-containing sets (eg, Venoset®, Accuset®) adsorb significant amounts of the drug, and their use may lead to a lower dose being delivered to the patient.

**Monitoring Laboratory Tests** Renal function, hepatic function, serum electrolytes, glucose. Since pharmacokinetics show great inter- and intrapatient variability over time, monitoring of serum concentrations (trough for oral therapy) has proven helpful to prevent organ rejection and reduce drug-related toxicity. Measure 3 times/week for first few weeks, then gradually decrease frequency as patient stabilizes.

**Additional Nursing Issues**

**Physical Assessment:** Assess other medications patient may be taking for effectiveness and interactions (see Warnings/Precautions and Drug Interactions). Note Warnings/Precautions for cautious use. Monitor laboratory tests prior to, during, and following therapy (see Monitoring Laboratory Tests). Monitor response to therapy, and adverse reactions (see Warnings/Precautions, Adverse Reactions, and Dosing). Diabetic patients should monitor glucose levels closely (this medication may alter glucose levels). Monitor/instruct patient on appropriate use, interventions to reduce side effects, to monitor for signs of opportunistic infection (eg, persistent fever, malaise, sore throat, unusual bleeding or bruising), and adverse reactions to report. **Pregnancy risk factor C.** Breast-feeding is contraindicated.

**Patient Information/Instruction:** Take as directed, preferably 30 minutes hour before or 30 minutes after meals. Do not take within 2 hours before or after antacids. Do not alter dose and do not discontinue without consulting prescriber. Maintain adequate hydration (2-3 L/day of fluids unless instructed to restrict fluid intake) during entire course of therapy. You will be susceptible to infection (avoid crowds and people with infections or contagious diseases). If you are diabetic, monitor glucose levels closely (may alter glucose levels). You may experience nausea, vomiting, loss of appetite (frequent small meals, frequent mouth care may help); diarrhea (boiled milk, yogurt, or buttermilk may help); constipation (increased exercise or dietary fruit, fluid, or fiber may help, if not consult prescriber); muscle or back pain (mild analgesics may be recommended). Report chest pain; acute headache or dizziness; symptoms of respiratory infection, cough, or difficulty breathing; unresolved gastrointestinal effects; fatigue, chills, fever, unhealed sores, white plaques in mouth, irritation in genital area; unusual bruising or bleeding; pain or irritation on urination or change in urinary patterns; rash or skin irritation; or other unusual effects related to this medication. **Pregnancy/breast-feeding precautions:** Inform prescriber if you are or intend to be pregnant. Do not breast-feed.

**Additional Information** Each mL of injection contains polyoxyl 60 hydrogenated castor oil (HCO-60), 200 mg and dehydrated alcohol, USP, 80% v/v.

- **Tafil** *see* Alprazolam *on page 55*
- **Tagal** *see* Ceftazidime *on page 228*
- **Tagamet®** *see* Cimetidine *on page 268*
- **Tagamet® HB [OTC]** *see* Cimetidine *on page 268*
- **Talacen®** *see* Pentazocine Compound *on page 904*
- **Taloken** *see* Ceftazidime *on page 228*
- **Talpramin** *see* Imipramine *on page 600*
- **Talwin®** *see* Pentazocine *on page 902*
- **Talwin® Compound** *see* Pentazocine Compound *on page 904*
- **Talwin® NX** *see* Pentazocine *on page 902*
- **Tambocor™** *see* Flecainide *on page 487*
- **Tamine®** *see page 1294*
- **Tamofen®** *see* Tamoxifen *on this page*
- **Tamone®** *see* Tamoxifen *on this page*
- **Tamoxan** *see* Tamoxifen *on this page*

## Tamoxifen (ta MOKS i fen)

**U.S. Brand Names** Nolvadex®

**Therapeutic Category** Antineoplastic Agent, Miscellaneous

**Pregnancy Risk Factor** D

**Lactation** Enters breast milk/contraindicated

**Use** Palliative or adjunctive treatment of advanced breast cancer. Reduction of the incidence of breast cancer in women at high risk of breast cancer. Adjuvant therapy to reduce the occurrence of contralateral breast cancer

**Unlabeled use:** Treatment of mastalgia, gynecomastia, male breast cancer, and pancreatic carcinoma. Studies have shown tamoxifen to be effective in the treatment of primary breast cancer in elderly women. Comparative studies with other antineoplastic agents in elderly women with breast cancer had more favorable survival rates with tamoxifen. Initiation of hormone therapy rather than chemotherapy is justified for elderly patients with metastatic breast cancer who are responsive.

**Mechanism of Action/Effect** Competitively binds to estrogen receptors on tumors and other tissue targets, producing a nuclear complex that decreases DNA synthesis and inhibits estrogen effects; nonsteroidal agent with potent antiestrogenic properties which compete with estrogen for binding sites in breast and other tissues; cells accumulate in the $G_0$ and $G_1$ phases; therefore, tamoxifen is cytostatic rather than cytocidal.

(Continued)

## Tamoxifen *(Continued)*

**Contraindications** Hypersensitivity to tamoxifen; pregnancy

**Warnings** Use with caution in patients with leukopenia, thrombocytopenia, or hyperlipidemias. Ovulation may be induced. "Hot flashes" may be countered by Bellergal-S® tablets. Decreased visual acuity, retinopathy, and corneal changes have been reported with use for more than 1 year at doses above recommended. Hypercalcemia in patients with bone metastasis. Hepatocellular carcinomas have been reported in animal studies. Endometrial hyperplasia and polyps have occurred.

**Drug Interactions**

**Cytochrome P-450 Effect:** CYP1A2, 2A6, 2B6, 2C, 2D6, 2E1, and 3A3/4 enzyme substrate

**Increased Effect/Toxicity:** Allopurinol and tamoxifen results in exacerbation of allopurinol-induced hepatotoxicity. Cyclosporine serum levels may be increased when taken with tamoxifen. Significant enhancement of the anticoagulant effects of warfarin may occur with concomitant use of tamoxifen.

**Effects on Lab Values** $T_4$ elevations (no clinical evidence of hyperthyroidism)

**Adverse Reactions**

>10%:

Cardiovascular: Flushing (hot flashes)

Dermatologic: Skin rash

Gastrointestinal: Little to mild nausea (10%), vomiting, weight gain

Hematologic: Myelosuppressive: Transient thrombocytopenia occurs in ~24% of patients receiving 10-20 mg/day; platelet counts return to normal within several weeks in spite of continued administration; leukopenia has also been reported and does resolve during continued therapy; anemia has also been reported

WBC: Rare

Platelets: None

Hepatic: Hepatotoxicity

Neuromuscular & skeletal: Increased bone and tumor pain and local disease flare shortly after starting therapy; this will subside rapidly, but patients should be aware of this since many may discontinue the drug due to the side effects

1% to 10%:

Cardiovascular: Thromboembolism: Tamoxifen has been associated with the occurrence of venous thrombosis and pulmonary embolism; arterial thrombosis has also been described in a few case reports

Central nervous system: Lightheadedness, depression, dizziness, headache, lassitude, mental confusion

Endocrine & metabolic: Hypercalcemia may occur in patients with bone metastases; galactorrhea and vitamin deficiency, menstrual irregularities

Genitourinary: Vaginal bleeding or discharge, endometriosis, priapism, possible endometrial cancer

Neuromuscular & skeletal: Weakness

Ocular: Ophthalmologic effects (visual acuity changes, cataracts, or retinopathy), corneal opacities

**Overdose/Toxicology** Symptoms of overdose include hypercalcemia and edema. Provide general supportive care.

**Pharmacodynamics/Kinetics**

**Distribution:** High concentrations found in uterus, endometrial and breast tissue

**Half-life Elimination:** 7 days

**Time to Peak:** Within 4-7 hours

**Metabolism:** Liver

**Excretion:** Feces and urine

**Formulations** Tablet, as citrate: 10 mg, 20 mg

**Dosing**

**Adults:** Refer to individual protocols.

Oral: 10-20 mg twice daily in the morning and evening

High-dose therapy is under investigation.

**Elderly:** Refer to adult dosing.

**Monitoring Laboratory Tests** WBC and platelet counts

**Additional Nursing Issues**

**Physical Assessment:** Monitor adverse effects and response to therapy. Patient complaints of bone pain is usually an indication of a good therapeutic response and will usually subside as treatment continues. Assess or teach patient necessity of monitoring fluid balance (I & O, edema, weight) and hypercalcemia (insomnia, lethargy, nausea, dizziness). **Pregnancy risk factor D** - assess knowledge/teach both men and women appropriate use of barrier contraceptives. Breast-feeding is contraindicated.

**Patient Information/Instruction:** Take as directed, morning and night and maintain adequate hydration (2-3 L/day of fluids unless instructed to restrict fluid intake). You may experience menstrual irregularities, vaginal bleeding, hot flashes, hair loss, loss of libido (these will subside when treatment is completed). Bone pain may indicate a good therapeutic responses (consult prescriber for mild analgesics). For nausea, vomiting small, frequent meals, chewing gum, or sucking lozenges may help. You may experience photosensitivity (use sunscreen, wear protective clothing and eyewear, and avoid direct sunlight). Report unusual bleeding or bruising, severe weakness, sedation, mental changes, swelling or pain in calves, difficulty breathing, or any changes in vision. **Pregnancy/breast-feeding precautions:** Do not get pregnant while taking this medication; use appropriate contraceptive measures. Do not breast-feed.

**Geriatric Considerations:** Studies have shown tamoxifen to be effective in the treatment of primary breast cancer in elderly women. Comparative studies with other antineoplastic agents in elderly women with breast cancer had more favorable survival rates with tamoxifen. Initiation of hormone therapy rather than chemotherapy is justified for elderly patients with metastatic breast cancer who are responsive.

## Tamsulosin (tam SOO loe sin)

**U.S. Brand Names** Flomax®

**Therapeutic Category** Alpha$_1$ Blockers

**Pregnancy Risk Factor** B

**Lactation** Not indicated for use in women

**Use** Treatment of signs and symptoms of benign prostatic hyperplasia (BPH)

**Mechanism of Action/Effect** Antagonizes alpha$_{1A}$ adrenoreceptors in the prostate which mediate the dynamic component of urine flow obstruction by regulating smooth muscle tone of the bladder neck and prostate. When given to patients with BPH, blockade of alpha receptors leads to relaxation of these muscles, resulting in an improvement in urine flow rate and symptoms. Alpha blockade does not influence the static component of urinary obstruction, which is related to tissue proliferation.

**Contraindications** Hypersensitivity to tamsulosin or any component

**Warnings** Not intended for use as an antihypertensive drug. May cause orthostasis, syncope or dizziness. Patients should avoid situations where injury may occur as a result of syncope. Rule out prostatic carcinoma before beginning therapy with tamsulosin.

**Drug Interactions**

**Cytochrome P-450 Effect:** Extensice metabolism via CYP isoenzymes, profile not characterized

**Decreased Effect:** Metabolism by cytochrome P-450 isoenzymes may, in theory, be influenced by enzyme-inducing agents, resulting in decreased effects.

**Increased Effect/Toxicity:** Metabolized by cytochrome P-450 isoenzymes. Profile of involved isoenzymes has not been established. Concurrent cimetidine therapy increased AUC of tamsulosin by 44%. Use with caution in patients receiving concurrent warfarin therapy (may increase anticoagulant effect). Do not use in combination with other alpha-blocking drugs.

**Adverse Reactions** Incidences correspond to 0.4 mg and 0.8 mg doses, respectively.

>10%:

Central nervous system: Dizziness (14.9% to 17.1%), headache (19.3% to 21.1%)
Cardiovascular: Orthostatic hypotension (at least one occurrence) (16% to 19%)
Genitourinary: Ejaculatory disturbances (8.4% to 18.1%)
Respiratory: Rhinitis (13.1% to 17.9%)

1% to 10%:

Central nervous system: Somnolence (3% to 4.3%), insomnia (1.4% to 2.4%)
Cardiovascular: First-dose hypotension (0.4 mg dose only) (7%)
Endocrine and metabolic: Decreased libido (1% to 2%)
Gastrointestinal: Diarrhea (6.2% to 4.3%), nausea (2.6% to 3.9%)
Neuromuscular & skeletal: Back pain (7% to 8.3%)
Ocular: Amblyopia (0.2% to 2%)
Respiratory: Pharyngitis (5.8% to 5.1%), cough (3.4% to 4.5%), sinusitis (2.2% to 3.7%)
Miscellaneous: Infection (9% to 10.8%)

<1% (Limited to important or life-threatening symptoms): Skin rash, angioedema, urticaria

Signs and symptoms of orthostasis: In clinical trials, syncope and symptomatic hypotension were reported at incidences <1%, dizziness occurred at an incidence >10% (above). At least one orthostatic measurement was recorded in up to 19% of patients (at the 0.8 mg dose) versus 11% for placebo.

**Overdose/Toxicology** Symptoms of overdose include headache and hypotension. Treatment is supportive.

**Pharmacodynamics/Kinetics**

**Protein Binding:** 94% to 99%, primarily to alpha$_1$-acid glycoprotein (AAG)

**Half-life Elimination:** Healthy volunteers: 9-13 hours; target population: 14-15 hours

**Time to Peak:** Fasting: 4-5 hours; 6-7 hours when given with food

**Metabolism:** Metabolized by cytochrome P-450 isoenzymes. Individual isoenzyme profiles have not been established. Average clearance = 2.88 L/hour.

**Excretion:** Urine and feces

**Formulations** Capsule, as hydrochloride: 0.4 mg

**Dosing**

**Adults:** Oral: 0.4 mg once daily (approximately 30 minutes after the same meal each day). Dose may be increased to 0.8 mg daily after 2-4 weeks in patients who fail to respond to the lower dose. If dosing is interrupted for several days, reinitiate dosing at 0.4 mg daily.

**Elderly:** Although clearance may be decreased in the elderly, no dosage reduction is recommended. See adult dosing.

**Monitoring Laboratory Tests** Periodic lipid panels

**Additional Nursing Issues**

**Physical Assessment:** Assess effectiveness and interactions of other medications (see Drug Interactions). Monitor blood pressure. See Contraindications and Warnings/Precautions for use cautions (ie, not intended for use as an antihypertensive). Monitor for effectiveness of therapy (improvement of urine flow rate and symptoms) and adverse reactions (see Adverse Reactions and Overdose/Toxicology) at beginning of therapy and on a regular basis with long-term therapy. Assess knowledge/teach

(Continued)

## Tamsulosin *(Continued)*

patient appropriate use, possible side effects/interventions, and adverse symptoms to report.

**Patient Information/Instruction:** Take as directed 30 minutes, after same meal each day. Do not skip dose or discontinue without consulting prescriber. You may experience drowsiness, dizziness, or impaired judgment (use caution when driving or engaging in tasks that require alertness until response to drug is known); postural hypotension (use caution when rising from sitting or lying position or when climbing stairs); nausea (frequent mouth care or sucking lozenges may help); urinary incontinence (void before taking medication); ejaculatory disturbance (reversible, may resolve with continued use); diarrhea (boiled milk or yogurt may help); palpitations or rapid heartbeat; difficulty breathing, unusual cough, or sore throat; or other persistent side effects.

**Geriatric Considerations:** Metabolism of tamsulosin may be slower, and older patients may be more sensitive to the orthostatic hypotension caused by this medication. A 40% higher exposure (AUC) is anticipated in patients between 55 and 75 years of age as compared to younger subjects (20-32 years).

- **Tanac® [OTC]** *see* Benzocaine *on page 141*
- **Tanoral® Tablet** *see page 1306*
- **Tantaphen®** *see* Acetaminophen *on page 32*
- **Tapazole®** *see* Methimazole *on page 741*
- **Taporin** *see* Cefotaxime *on page 221*
- **Tarka®** *see* Trandolapril and Verapamil *on page 1163*
- **Taro-Ampicillin® Trihydrate** *see* Ampicillin *on page 90*
- **Taro-Atenol®** *see* Atenolol *on page 115*
- **Taro-Cloxacillin®** *see* Cloxacillin *on page 295*
- **Taro-Sone** *see* Betamethasone *on page 148*
- **Taro-Sone** *see* Topical Corticosteroids *on page 1152*
- **Tasedan** *see* Estazolam *on page 440*
- **Tasmar®** *see* Tolcapone *on page 1148*
- **TAT** *see page 1256*
- **Tavanic** *see* Levofloxacin *on page 669*
- **Tavist®** *see page 1294*
- **Tavist®-1** *see page 1294*
- **Tavist-D®** *see page 1294*
- **Taxol®** *see* Paclitaxel *on page 878*
- **Taxotere®** *see* Docetaxel *on page 390*
- **Taxus** *see* Tamoxifen *on page 1095*
- **Tazicef®** *see* Ceftazidime *on page 228*
- **Tazidime®** *see* Ceftazidime *on page 228*
- **Taziken** *see* Terbutaline *on page 1105*
- **Tazobactam and Piperacillin** *see* Piperacillin and Tazobactam Sodium *on page 937*
- **TB Drug Comparison** *see page 1402*
- **3TC** *see* Lamivudine *on page 652*
- **TCN** *see* Tetracycline *on page 1111*
- **Tear Drop® Solution** *see page 1294*
- **TearGard® Ophthalmic Solution** *see page 1294*
- **Teargen® Ophthalmic Solution** *see page 1294*
- **Tearisol® Solution** *see page 1294*
- **Tears Naturale® Free Solution** *see page 1294*
- **Tears Naturale® II Solution** *see page 1294*
- **Tears Naturale® Solution** *see page 1294*
- **Tears Plus® Solution** *see page 1294*
- **Tears Renewed® Solution** *see page 1294*
- **Tebamide®** *see* Trimethobenzamide *on page 1180*
- **Tebrazid** *see* Pyrazinamide *on page 994*
- **Tecnal** *see* Butalbital Compound and Aspirin *on page 176*
- **Tecnal C1/4, C1/2** *see* Butalbital Compound and Codeine *on page 177*
- **Tecprazin** *see* Praziquantel *on page 957*
- **Teczem®** *see* Enalapril and Diltiazem *on page 418*
- **Tedral®** *see* Theophylline, Ephedrine, and Phenobarbital *on page 1118*
- **Tega-Vert® Oral** *see page 1294*
- **Tegison®** *see* Etretinate *on page 468*
- **Tegopen®** *see* Cloxacillin *on page 295*
- **Tegretol®** *see* Carbamazepine *on page 195*
- **Tegretol®-XR** *see* Carbamazepine *on page 195*
- **Tegrin®-HC [OTC]** *see* Hydrocortisone *on page 578*
- **Tegrin®-HC [OTC]** *see* Topical Corticosteroids *on page 1152*
- **T.E.H.®** *see* Theophylline, Ephedrine, and Hydroxyzine *on page 1118*
- **Teladar®** *see* Betamethasone *on page 148*
- **Teladar®** *see* Topical Corticosteroids *on page 1152*
- **Teldrin®** *see page 1294*

♦ **Telechlor**® *see page 1294*

## Telmisartan (tel mi SAR tan)

**U.S. Brand Names** Micardis®

**Therapeutic Category** Angiotensin II Antagonists

**Pregnancy Risk Factor** C (1st trimester); D (2nd & 3rd trimester)

**Lactation** Enters breast milk/not recommended

**Use** Treatment of hypertension; may be used alone or in combination with other antihypertensive agents

**Mechanism of Action/Effect** Telmisartan is a nonpeptide angiotensin receptor antagonist. Angiotensin II acts as a vasoconstrictor. In addition to causing direct vasoconstriction, angiotensin II also stimulates the release of aldosterone. Once aldosterone is released, sodium as well as water are reabsorbed. The end result is an elevation in blood pressure. Telmisartan binds to the AT1 angiotensin II receptor. This binding prevents angiotensin II from binding to the receptor thereby blocking the vasoconstriction and the aldosterone secreting effects of angiotensin II.

**Contraindications** Hypersensitivity to telmisartan or any component; known sensitivity to other A-II receptor antagonists; pregnancy (2nd & 3rd trimesters); hyperaldosteronism (primary); renal artery stenosis (bilateral)

**Warnings** Avoid use or use smaller dose in volume-depleted patients. Use caution in patients with impaired hepatic function. Drugs which alter the renin-angiotensin system have been associated with deterioration in renal function, including oliguria, acute renal failure, and progressive azotemia. Use with caution in patients with renal artery stenosis (unilateral or bilateral) to avoid decrease in renal function; use caution in patients with pre-existing renal insufficiency (may decrease renal perfusion). Pregnancy risk factor C (1st trimester)/D (2nd and 3rd trimesters).

**Drug Interactions**

**Decreased Effect:** Telmisartan decreased the trough concentrations of warfarin during concurrent therapy, however INR was not changed.

**Increased Effect/Toxicity:** May increase serum digoxin concentrations.

**Adverse Reactions**

1% to 10%:

Cardiovascular: Hypertension (1%), chest pain (1%), peripheral edema (1%)

Central nervous system: Headache (1%), dizziness (1%), pain (1%), fatigue (1%)

Gastrointestinal: Diarrhea (3%), dyspepsia (1%), nausea (1%), abdominal pain (1%)

Genitourinary: Urinary tract infection (1%)

Neuromuscular & skeletal: Back pain (3%), myalgia (1%)

Respiratory: Upper respiratory infection (7%), sinusitis (3%), pharyngitis (1%), cough (1.6%)

Miscellaneous: Flu-like syndrome (1%)

<1% (Limited to important or life-threatening symptoms): Angioedema, allergic reaction, elevated liver enzymes, decrease in hemoglobin, increased serum creatinine and BUN, impotence, sweating, flushing, fever, malaise, palpitations, angina, tachycardia, abnormal EKG, insomnia, anxiety, nervousness, migraine, vertigo, depression, somnolence, paresthesia, involuntary muscle contractions, constipation, flatulence, dry mouth, hemorrhoids, gastroenteritis, enteritis, reflux, toothache, gout, hypercholesterolemia, diabetes mellitus, arthritis, arthralgia, leg cramps, fungal infection, abscess, otitis media, asthma, dyspnea, bronchitis, rhinitis, epistaxis, dermatitis, eczema, pruritus, rash, frequent urination, cystitis, abnormal vision, conjunctivitis, tinnitus, earache, cerebrovascular disorder

**Overdose/Toxicology** Symptoms of overdose may include hypotension, dizziness, and tachycardia. Vagal stimulation may result in bradycardia. Treatment is supportive.

**Pharmacodynamics/Kinetics**

**Protein Binding:** >99.5%

**Half-life Elimination:** Terminal: ~24 hours

**Time to Peak:** 0.5-1 hour

**Metabolism:** Hepatic, via conjugation to inactive metabolites

**Excretion:** Total body clearance 800 mL/minute; 97% of a dose is excreted in the feces due to extensive biliary secretion

**Onset:** 1-2 hours

**Duration:** Up to 24 hours

**Formulations** Tablet: 40 mg, 80 mg

**Dosing**

**Adults:** Oral: Initial: 40 mg once daily; usual maintenance dose range: 20-80 mg/day. Patients with volume depletion should be initiated on the lower dosage with close supervision.

**Elderly:** Refer to adult dosing.

**Hepatic Impairment:** Supervise patients closely.

**Monitoring Laboratory Tests** Monitor electrolytes, serum creatinine, BUN, urinalysis, symptomatic hypotension, and tachycardia

**Additional Nursing Issues**

**Physical Assessment:** See Contraindications and Warnings/Precautions for use cautions. Monitor laboratory results and blood pressure (supine and standing) at beginning of therapy and regularly during long-term therapy. Assess knowledge/teach patient appropriate use, need for regular blood pressure monitoring, possible side effects/interventions, and adverse symptoms to report. **Pregnancy risk factor C/D** - benefits of use should outweigh possible risks (see Pregnancy Risk Factor). Breast-feeding is not recommended.

(Continued)

## Telmisartan *(Continued)*

**Patient Information/Instruction:** Take exactly as directed. Do not miss doses, alter dosage, or discontinue without consulting prescriber. Do not alter salt or potassium intake without consulting prescriber. Monitor blood pressure on a regular basis as recommended by prescriber; at the same time each day. You may experience postural hypotension (change position slowly when rising from sitting or lying, when climbing stairs, or bending over); or transient nervousness, headache, or dizziness (use caution when driving or engaging in tasks requiring alertness until response to drug is known). Report unusual weight gain or swelling of ankles and hands; swelling of face, lips, throat, or tongue; persistent fatigue; dry cough or difficulty breathing; palpitations or chest pain; CNS changes; gastrointestinal disturbances; muscle or bone pain, cramping, or tremors; change in urinary pattern; or changes in hearing or vision. **Pregnancy/breast-feeding precautions:** Inform prescriber if you are or intend to be pregnant. Breast-feeding is not recommended.

**Related Information**

ACE Inhibitors and Angiotensin Antagonists Comparison *on page 1362*

## Temazepam (te MAZ e pam)

**U.S. Brand Names** Restoril®

**Therapeutic Category** Benzodiazepine

**Pregnancy Risk Factor** X

**Lactation** Enters breast milk/not recommended (AAP rates "of concern")

**Use** Short-term (7-10 days) treatment of insomnia

**Mechanism of Action/Effect** Benzodiazepine anxiolytic sedative that produces CNS depression at the subcortical level, except at high doses, whereby it works at the cortical level; causes minimal change in REM sleep patterns

**Contraindications** Hypersensitivity to temazepam or any component; pre-existing CNS depression or acute narrow-angle glaucoma; pregnancy

**Warnings** Safety and efficacy in children <18 years of age have not been established. May cause drug dependency. Avoid abrupt discontinuance in patients with prolonged therapy or seizure disorders. Use with caution in patients receiving other CNS depressants, in patients with renal or hepatic dysfunction, and the elderly.

**Drug Interactions**

**Cytochrome P-450 Effect:** CYP3A3/4 enzyme substrate

**Increased Effect/Toxicity:** Increased effect of CNS depressants.

**Adverse Reactions**

1% to 10%:

- Central nervous system: Drowsiness (9.1%), headache, fatigue, nervousness, lethargy, dizziness, hangover, anxiety depression, euphoria, confusion, nightmares, vertigo
- Gastrointestinal: Nausea, dry mouth, diarrhea, abdominal discomfort
- Neuromuscular & skeletal: Weakness
- Ocular: Blurred vision

<1% (Limited to important or life-threatening symptoms): Dyspnea, blood dyscrasias, abnormal LFTs

**Overdose/Toxicology** Symptoms of overdose include somnolence, confusion, coma, hypoactive reflexes, dyspnea, hypotension, slurred speech, and impaired coordination. Treatment for benzodiazepine overdose is supportive. Flumazenil has been shown to selectively block the binding of benzodiazepines to CNS receptors, resulting in a reversal of benzodiazepine-induced CNS depression but not always respiratory depression due to toxicity.

**Pharmacodynamics/Kinetics**

**Protein Binding:** 96%

**Half-life Elimination:** 9.5-12.4 hours

**Time to Peak:** Within 2-3 hours

**Metabolism:** Liver

**Excretion:** 80% to 90% excreted in urine as inactive metabolites

**Formulations** Capsule: 7.5 mg, 15 mg, 30 mg

**Dosing**

**Adults:** Oral: 15-30 mg at bedtime

**Elderly:** May be taken 30 minutes before the desired onset of sleep. Initial: 7.5 mg at bedtime; may need to increase to 15 mg.

**Additional Nursing Issues**

**Physical Assessment:** For short-term use. Assess effectiveness and interactions of other medications (see Drug Interactions). See Contraindications and Warnings/Precautions for cautious use. Assess for history of addiction; long-term use can result in dependence, abuse, or tolerance. Evaluate periodically for need for continued use. After long-term use, taper dosage slowly when discontinuing. For inpatient use, institute safety measures (side rails, night light, call bell, assistance with ambulation) and monitor effectiveness and adverse reactions. For outpatients, monitor for effectiveness of therapy and adverse reactions (see Adverse Reactions) at beginning of therapy and periodically with long-term use. Assess knowledge/teach patient appropriate use, interventions to reduce side effects, and adverse symptoms to report. **Pregnancy risk factor X** - determine that patient is not pregnant before beginning treatment and do not give to women of childbearing age or to males who may have intercourse with women of childbearing ages unless both male and female are capable of complying with barrier contraceptive measures 1 month prior to therapy and for 1 month following therapy. Breast-feeding is not recommended.

**Patient Information/Instruction:** Use exactly as directed (do not increase dose or frequency or discontinue without consulting prescriber); may cause physical and/or psychological dependence. May take with food to decrease GI upset. While using this medication, do not use alcohol or other prescription or OTC medications (especially, pain medications, sedatives, antihistamines, or hypnotics) without consulting prescriber. Maintain adequate hydration (2-3 L/day of fluids unless instructed to restrict fluid intake). You may experience drowsiness, dizziness, lightheadedness, or blurred vision (use caution when driving or engaging in tasks requiring alertness until response to drug is known); or dry mouth or gastrointestinal discomfort (small frequent meals, frequent mouth care, chewing gum, or sucking lozenges may help). Report CNS changes (confusion, depression, increased sedation, excitation, headache, abnormal thinking, insomnia, or nightmares, memory impairment, impaired coordination); muscle pain or weakness; difficulty breathing; persistent dizziness, chest pain, or palpitations; alterations in normal gait; vision changes; or ineffectiveness of medication. **Pregnancy/breast-feeding precautions:** Inform prescriber if you are pregnant. Do not get pregnant during or for 1 month following therapy. Male: Do not cause a female to become pregnant. Male/female: Consult prescriber for instruction on appropriate barrier contraceptive measures. This drug may cause severe fetal defects. Breast-feeding is not recommended.

**Geriatric Considerations:** Because of its lack of active metabolites, temazepam is recommended in the elderly when a benzodiazepine hypnotic is indicated. Hypnotic use should be limited to 10-14 days. If insomnia persists, the patient should be evaluated for etiology.

**Other Issues:** Taper dosage gradually after long-term therapy. Abrupt withdrawal may cause tremors, nausea, vomiting, abdominal and/or muscle cramps.

**Related Information**

Anxiolytic/Hypnotic Use in Long-Term Care Facilities *on page 1430*
Benzodiazepines Comparison *on page 1375*

♦ **Temazin® Cold Syrup** *see page 1294*
♦ **Temgesic®** *see* Buprenorphine *on page 168*
♦ **Temovate® Topical** *see* Topical Corticosteroids *on page 1152*
♦ **Temperal** *see* Acetaminophen *on page 32*
♦ **Tempra® [OTC]** *see* Acetaminophen *on page 32*

## Teniposide (ten i POE side)

**U.S. Brand Names** Vumon Injection

**Synonyms** EPT; VM-26

**Therapeutic Category** Antineoplastic Agent, Miscellaneous

**Pregnancy Risk Factor** D

**Lactation** Not recommended

**Use** Treatment of acute lymphocytic leukemia, small cell lung cancer

**Mechanism of Action/Effect** Inhibits mitotic activity; inhibits cells from entering mitosis

**Contraindications** Hypersensitivity to teniposide or Cremophor EL (polyoxyethylated castor oil) or any component; pregnancy

**Warnings** The U.S. Food and Drug Administration (FDA) currently recommends that procedures for proper handling and disposal of antineoplastic agents be considered.

Teniposide preparation should be performed in a Class II laminar flow biologic safety cabinet. Personnel should be wearing surgical gloves and a closed front surgical gown with knit cuffs. Appropriate safety equipment is recommended for preparation, administration, and disposal of antineoplastics. If teniposide contacts the skin, wash and flush thoroughly with water.

**Drug Interactions**

**Cytochrome P-450 Effect:** CYP3A3/4 enzyme substrate; CYP2C19 enzyme inhibitor

**Increased Effect/Toxicity:** Alteration of MTX transport has been found as a slow efflux of MTX and its polyglutamated form out of the cell, leading to intercellular accumulation of MTX. Sodium salicylate, sulfamethizole, and tolbutamide displace teniposide from protein-binding sites which could cause substantial increases in free drug levels, resulting in potentiation of toxicity.

**Adverse Reactions**

Local: **Irritant chemotherapy**

>10%:
- Gastrointestinal: Mucositis, nausea, vomiting, diarrhea
  - Emetic potential: Moderate (30% to 60%)
- Hematologic: Myelosuppression, leukopenia, neutropenia, thrombocytopenia
- Miscellaneous: Infection

1% to 10%:
- Cardiovascular: Hypotension
- Central nervous system: Fever
- Dermatologic: Alopecia, rash
- Hematologic: Hemorrhage
- Miscellaneous: Hypersensitivity

<1% (Limited to important or life-threatening symptoms): Hepatic dysfunction, peripheral neurotoxicity, renal dysfunction

**Overdose/Toxicology** Symptoms of overdose include bone marrow suppression, leukopenia, thrombocytopenia, nausea, and vomiting. Treatment is supportive.

(Continued)

## Teniposide *(Continued)*

**Pharmacodynamics/Kinetics**

**Protein Binding:** 99.4%

**Distribution:** Distributed mainly into liver, kidneys, small intestine, and adrenals; crosses blood-brain barrier to a limited extent

**Half-life Elimination:** 5 hours

**Metabolism:** Liver

**Excretion:** Urine and feces

**Formulations** Injection: 10 mg/mL (5 mL)

**Dosing**

**Adults:** I.V.:

50-180 mg/m$^2$ once or twice weekly for 4-6 weeks or 20-60 mg/m$^2$/day for 5 days

Acute lymphoblastic leukemia (ALL): 165 mg/m$^2$ twice weekly for 8-9 doses **or** 250 mg/m$^2$ weekly for 4-8 weeks

Small cell lung cancer: 80-90 mg/m$^2$/day for 5 days

**Dosage adjustment in Down syndrome patient:** Reduce initial dosing give the first course at half the usual dose. Patients with both Down syndrome and leukemia may be especially sensitive to myelosuppressive chemotherapy.

**Renal Impairment:** Data is insufficient, but dose adjustments may be necessary in patient with significant renal impairment.

**Hepatic Impairment:** Data is insufficient, but dose adjustments may be necessary in patient with significant hepatic impairment.

**Administration**

**I.V.:** Irritant. Slow I.V. infusion over ≥30 minutes.

**I.V. Detail:** Hypotension or increased nausea and vomiting can occur if infused rapidly. Flush thoroughly before and after administration. Do not use in-line filter during I.V. infusion.

Teniposide must be diluted with either $D_5W$ or 0.9% sodium chloride solutions to a final concentration of 0.1, 0.2, 0.4, or 1 mg/mL. In order to prevent extraction of the plasticizer DEHP, solutions should be prepared in non-DEHP-containing containers such as glass or polyolefin containers. **The use of polyvinyl chloride (PVC) containers is not recommended.**

**Stability**

**Storage:** Store ampuls in refrigerator at 2°C to 8°C (36°F to 46°F).

**Reconstitution:** Reconstituted solutions are stable at room temperature for up to 24 hours after preparation. Teniposide must be diluted with either $D_5W$ or 0.9% sodium chloride solutions to a final concentration of 0.1, 0.2, 0.4, or 1 mg/mL. In order to prevent extraction of the plasticizer DEHP, **solutions should be prepared in non-DEHP-containing containers such as glass or polyolefin containers.** The use of polyvinyl chloride (PVC) containers is not recommended. Administer 1 mg/mL solutions within 4 hours of preparation to reduce the potential for precipitation. Precipitation may occur at any concentration.

**Compatibility:** Incompatible with heparin.

**Monitoring Laboratory Tests** CBC, platelet count

**Additional Nursing Issues**

**Physical Assessment:** Monitor laboratory results before beginning each infusion. Monitor infusion site closely for extravasation; may cause local tissue necrosis. Monitor blood pressure during infusion (hypotension may require discontinuing infusion and administering supportive therapy) and monitor closely for possible anaphylactoid reaction (eg, chills, fever, tachycardia, dyspnea, hypotension). Monitor for opportunistic infection. **Pregnancy risk factor D** - assess knowledge/teach both male and female appropriate use of barrier contraceptives. Breast-feeding is not recommended.

**Patient Information/Instruction:** This drug can only be administered I.V. You will require regular blood tests to assess response to therapy. For nausea or vomiting, small frequent meals, frequent mouth care, chewing gum, or sucking lozenges may help, antiemetics may be prescribed. You may experience hair loss or loss of appetite (maintaining adequate nutrition is important). Report unusual bleeding or bruising, persistent fever or chills, sore throat, sores in mouth or vagina, or difficulty breathing. **Pregnancy/breast-feeding precautions:** Do not get pregnant while taking this medication; use appropriate barrier contraceptive measures. Breast-feeding is not recommended.

**Additional Information** May be available only through investigational protocols. Some formulations may contain benzyl alcohol.

**Related Information**

Antiemetics for Chemotherapy-Induced Nausea and Vomiting *on page 1307*


- **Ten-K®** *see* Potassium Supplements *on page 952*
- **Tenoretic®** *see* Atenolol and Chlorthalidone *on page 117*
- **Tenormin®** *see* Atenolol *on page 115*
- **Tensilon® Injection** *see* Edrophonium *on page 413*
- **Tenuate®** *see* Diethylpropion *on page 365*
- **Tenuate® Dospan®** *see* Diethylpropion *on page 365*
- **Tera-Cortril® Ophthalmic Suspension** *see page 1282*
- **Terazol® Vaginal** *see* Terconazole *on page 1106*


## Terazosin (ter AY zoe sin)

**U.S. Brand Names** Hytrin®

**Therapeutic Category** Alpha$_1$ Blockers

**Pregnancy Risk Factor** C

**Lactation** Excretion in breast milk unknown

**Use** Management of mild to moderate hypertension; alone or in combination with other agents such as diuretics or beta-blockers; benign prostate hypertrophy

**Mechanism of Action/Effect** Alpha$_1$-specific blocking agent with minimal alpha$_2$ effects; this allows peripheral postsynaptic blockade, with the resultant decrease in arterial tone, while preserving the negative feedback loop which is mediated by the peripheral presynaptic alpha$_2$-receptors; terazosin relaxes the smooth muscle of the bladder neck, thus reducing bladder outlet obstruction

**Contraindications** Hypersensitivity to terazosin, other alpha-adrenergic antagonists, or any component

**Warnings** Marked orthostatic hypotension, syncope, and loss of consciousness may occur with first dose ("first dose phenomenon"). This reaction is more likely to occur in patients receiving beta-blockers, diuretics, low sodium diets, or first doses >1 mg/dose in adults. Avoid rapid increase in dose. Use with caution in patients with renal impairment. Pregnancy factor C.

**Drug Interactions**

**Decreased Effect:** Decreased antihypertensive response with NSAIDs.

**Increased Effect/Toxicity:** Increased hypotensive effect with diuretics and antihypertensive medications (especially beta-blockers).

**Adverse Reactions**

>10%: Central nervous system: Dizziness, headache, muscle weakness

1% to 10%:

- Cardiovascular: Edema, palpitations, chest pain, peripheral edema, orthostatic hypotension, tachycardia
- Central nervous system: Fatigue, nervousness, drowsiness
- Gastrointestinal: Dry mouth
- Genitourinary: Urinary incontinence
- Ocular: Blurred vision
- Respiratory: Dyspnea, nasal congestion

<1% (Limited to important or life-threatening symptoms): Sexual dysfunction, priapism

**Overdose/Toxicology** Symptoms of overdose include hypotension, drowsiness, and shock. Treatment is supportive and symptomatic.

**Pharmacodynamics/Kinetics**

**Protein Binding:** 90% to 95%

**Half-life Elimination:** 9.2-12 hours

**Time to Peak:** Within 1 hour

**Metabolism:** Liver

**Excretion:** Feces and urine

**Onset:** 1-2 hours

**Formulations**

Capsule: 1 mg, 2 mg, 5 mg, 10 mg

Tablet: 1 mg, 2 mg, 5 mg, 10 mg

**Dosing**

**Adults:** Oral:

Hypertension: Initial: 1 mg at bedtime; slowly increase dose to achieve desired blood pressure, up to 20 mg/day; usual dose: 1-5 mg/day.

Dosage reduction may be needed when adding a diuretic or other antihypertensive agent. If drug is discontinued for more than several days, consider beginning with initial dose and retitrate as needed. Dosage may be given on a twice daily regimen if response is diminished at 24 hours and hypotensive is observed at 2-4 hours following a dose.

Benign prostatic hypertrophy: Initial: 1 mg at bedtime, increasing as needed; most patients require 10 mg day. If no response after 4-6 weeks of 10 mg/day, may increase to 20 mg/day.

**Elderly:** Refer to adult dosing.

**Additional Nursing Issues**

**Physical Assessment:** Assess effectiveness and interactions of other medications (see Drug Interactions). See Contraindications and Warnings/Precautions for use cautions. Monitor for effectiveness of therapy (blood pressure supine and standing) and adverse reactions (see Adverse Reactions and Overdose/Toxicology) at beginning of therapy and on a regular basis with long-term therapy. Assess knowledge/teach patient appropriate use, possible side effects/interventions, and adverse symptoms to report. When discontinuing, monitor blood pressure and taper dose and frequency. **Pregnancy risk factor C** - benefits of use should outweigh possible risks. Note breast-feeding caution.

**Patient Information/Instruction:** Take as directed, at bedtime. Do not skip dose or discontinue without consulting prescriber. Follow recommended diet and exercise program. Do not use alcohol or OTC medications which may affect blood pressure (eg, cough or cold remedies, diet pills, stay-awake medications) without consulting physician. You may experience drowsiness, dizziness, or impaired judgment (use caution when driving or engaging in tasks that require alertness until response to drug is known); postural hypotension (use caution when rising from sitting or lying position or when climbing stairs); dry mouth or nausea (frequent mouth care or sucking lozenges may help); urinary incontinence (void before taking medication); or sexual dysfunction (reversible, may resolve with continued use). Report altered CNS status (eg, fatigue, lethargy, confusion, nervousness); sudden weight gain (weigh yourself in the same clothes at the same time of day once a week); unusual or persistent swelling of ankles,

(Continued)

## Terazosin *(Continued)*

feet, or extremities; palpitations or rapid heartbeat; difficulty breathing; muscle weakness; or other persistent side effects. **Pregnancy/breast-feeding precautions:** Inform prescriber if you are or intend to be pregnant. Consult prescriber if breast-feeding.

**Geriatric Considerations:** Adverse reactions such as dry mouth and urinary problems can be particularly bothersome in the elderly.

♦ **Terbinafine** *see page 1247*

## Terbinafine, Oral (TER bin a feen, OR al)

**U.S. Brand Names** Lamisil® Oral

**Therapeutic Category** Antifungal Agent, Oral

**Pregnancy Risk Factor** B

**Lactation** Enters breast milk/contraindicated

**Use** Treatment of onychomycosis infections of the toenail or fingernail

**Mechanism of Action/Effect** Terbinafine is a synthetic allylamine derivative which inhibits squalene epoxidase which is a key enzyme in sterol biosynthesis in fungi. The resulting deficiency in ergosterol within the cell wall causes fungi death.

**Contraindications** Hypersensitivity to terbinafine or any component

**Warnings** Symptomatic hepatobiliary dysfunction including cholestatic hepatitis have been reported to occur rarely. Discontinue terbinafine if hepatobiliary dysfunction occurs. Isolated reports of serious skin reactions (ie, Stevens-Johnson syndrome and toxic epidermal necrolysis). Discontinue terbinafine treatment if progressive skin rash occurs.

Terbinafine therapy is not recommended in patients with liver disease or renal impairment (creatinine clearance <50 mL/minute). A decrease in terbinafine clearance by ~50% has been reported. Changes in ocular lens and retina have been reported, clinical significance is unknown. Neutropenia has been reported. If signs and symptoms of secondary infection occur, obtain a complete blood count. Discontinue therapy if neutrophil count is ≤1000 cells/mm$^3$ and start supportive therapy. Transient decreases in absolute lymphocyte count have been observed. Clinical significance is unknown.

**Drug Interactions**

**Decreased Effect:** Decreases clearance of I.V. administered caffeine.

**Increased Effect/Toxicity:** Increases clearance of cyclosporine by 15%. Terbinafine clearance increased by rifampin (100%), cimetidine (33%). Terbinafine clearance decreased by terfenadine (16%). Terbinafine clearance unaffected by cyclosporine.

**Adverse Reactions**

>10%: Central nervous system: Headache

1% to 10%:

- Dermatologic: Rash, pruritus, urticaria
- Gastrointestinal: Diarrhea, dyspepsia, abdominal pain, nausea, flatulence, abnormal taste
- Hepatic: Elevated liver enzyme ≥2 times upper limit of normal range
- Ocular: Visual disturbance

<1% (Limited to important or life-threatening symptoms): Serious skin reactions (toxic epidermal necrolysis, Stevens-Johnson syndrome), hepatobiliary dysfunction, transient decrease in absolute lymphocyte count neutropenia, cholestatic hepatitis, changes in ocular lens and retina

**Overdose/Toxicology** No information on human overdose. Symptomatic and supportive treatment is recommended.

**Pharmacodynamics/Kinetics**

**Time to Peak:** 2 hours

**Metabolism:** Liver

**Excretion:** Urine

**Formulations** Tablet: 250 mg

**Dosing**

**Adults:** Oral:

- Fingernail onychomycosis: 250 mg once daily for 6 weeks
- Toenail onychomycosis: 250 mg once daily for 12 weeks

**Elderly:** Refer to adult dosing.

**Stability**

**Storage:** Store at room temperature below 25°C (77°F) in tight container. Protect from light.

**Monitoring Laboratory Tests** Recommend baseline liver function tests, and repeat if therapy exceeds 6 weeks; consider monitoring CBC in patients with known or suspected immunodeficiency receiving terbinafine for more than 6 weeks

**Additional Nursing Issues**

**Physical Assessment:** Assess effectiveness and interactions of other medications (see Drug Interactions). See Warnings/Precautions and Contraindications for use cautions. Monitor effectiveness of therapy and laboratory tests (see above). Monitor adverse response (see Adverse Reactions and Overdose/Toxicology). Assess knowledge/teach patient possible side effects and appropriate interventions and adverse symptoms to report. Breast-feeding is contraindicated.

**Patient Information/Instruction:** Take as directed, around-the-clock, with food. Take full course of medication; do not discontinue without notifying prescriber. Practice good hygiene measures to prevent reinfection. Frequent blood tests may be required with prolonged therapy. You may experience nausea and vomiting (small frequent meals, frequent mouth care, sucking lozenges, or chewing gum may help). Report skin rash or other persistent adverse reactions. **Breast-feeding precautions:** Do not breast-feed.

**Breast-feeding Issues:** For nursing mothers, the ratio of terbinafine in milk to plasma is 7:1 after oral administration. Treatment with terbinafine is not recommended while nursing.

**Additional Information** Optimal clinical effect is seen some months after mycological cure and end of treatment due to the time required for healthy nail outgrowth. Meantime to overall success was approximately 10 months for toenails and 4 months for fingernails. When terbinafine is taken with food, absorption is increased by 20%. Terbinafine appears to be more effective than griseofulvin and at least as effective as itraconazole for the treatment of onychomycosis. Unlike itraconazole, terbinafine does not interact with drugs metabolized by cytochrome P-450 isoenzymes.

## Terbutaline (ter BYOO ta leen)

**U.S. Brand Names** Brethaire® Inhalation Aerosol; Brethine® Injection; Brethine® Oral; Bricanyl® Injection; Bricanyl® Oral

**Therapeutic Category** $Beta_2$ Agonist

**Pregnancy Risk Factor** B

**Lactation** Enters breast milk/compatible

**Use** Bronchodilator in reversible airway obstruction and bronchial asthma

**Unlabeled use:** For tocolysis, to inhibit premature uterine contractions

**Mechanism of Action/Effect** Relaxes bronchial smooth muscle by action on $beta_2$-receptors with less effect on heart rate

**Contraindications** Hypersensitivity to terbutaline or any component; cardiac arrhythmias associated with tachycardia; tachycardia caused by digitalis intoxication

**Warnings** Excessive or prolonged use may lead to tolerance. Paradoxical bronchoconstriction may occur with excessive use. If it occurs, discontinue terbutaline immediately. When used for tocolysis, there is some risk of maternal pulmonary edema, which has been associated with the following risk factors, excessive hydration, multiple gestation, occult sepsis and underlying cardiac disease. To reduce risk, limit fluid intake to 2.5-3 L/day, limit sodium intake, maintain maternal pulse to <130 beats/minute.

**Drug Interactions**

**Decreased Effect:** Decreased effect with beta-blockers.

**Increased Effect/Toxicity:** Increased toxicity with MAO inhibitors, tricyclic antidepressants.

**Adverse Reactions**

>10%:

Central nervous system: Nervousness, restlessness
Neuromuscular & skeletal: Trembling

1% to 10%:

Cardiovascular: Tachycardia, hypertension, pounding heartbeat
Central nervous system: Dizziness, lightheadedness, drowsiness, headache, insomnia
Gastrointestinal: Dry mouth, nausea, vomiting, bad taste in mouth
Neuromuscular & skeletal: Muscle cramps, weakness
Miscellaneous: Sweating

<1% (Limited to important or life-threatening symptoms): Chest pain, arrhythmias, paradoxical bronchospasm

**Overdose/Toxicology** Symptoms of overdose include seizures, nausea, vomiting, tachycardia, cardiac dysrhythmias, and hypokalemia. In cases of overdose, supportive therapy should be instituted. Prudent use of a cardioselective beta-adrenergic blocker (eg, atenolol or metoprolol) should be considered, keeping in mind the potential for induction of bronchoconstriction in an asthmatic. Dialysis has not been shown to be of value in the treatment of overdose with terbutaline.

**Pharmacodynamics/Kinetics**

**Protein Binding:** 25%

**Half-life Elimination:** 11-16 hours

**Metabolism:** Liver

**Excretion:** Urine

**Onset:** Oral: 30-45 minutes; S.C.: Within 6-15 minutes

**Formulations**

Terbutaline sulfate:
Aerosol, oral: 0.2 mg/actuation (10.5 g)
Injection: 1 mg/mL (1 mL)
Tablet: 2.5 mg, 5 mg

**Dosing**

**Adults:**

Oral:
12-15 years: 2.5 mg every 6 hours 3 times/day; not to exceed 7.5 mg in 24 hours
>15 years: 5 mg/dose every 6 hours 3 times/day; if side effects occur, reduce dose to 2.5 mg every 6 hours; not to exceed 15 mg in 24 hours.

S.C.: 0.25 mg/dose repeated in 15-30 minutes for one time only; a total dose of 0.5 mg should not be exceeded within a 4-hour period.

Nebulization: 0.1-0.3 mg/kg/dose every 4-6 hours

Inhalation: 2 inhalations every 4-6 hours; wait 1 minute between inhalations.

Tocolysis:
Acute: I.V. 2.5-10 mcg/minute; increased gradually every 10-20 minutes. Effective maximum dosages from 17.5-30 mcg/minute have been use with caution. Duration of infusion is at least 12 hours.
Oral: 2.5-10 mg every 4-6 hours for as long as necessary to prolong pregnancy depending on patient tolerance

(Continued)

## Terbutaline *(Continued)*

**Elderly:** Not recommended for use in the elderly (see Geriatric Considerations).

**Renal Impairment:**

$Cl_{cr}$ 10-50 mL/minute: Administer at 50% of normal dose.

$Cl_{cr}$ <10 mL/minute: Avoid use.

**Administration**

**Oral:** In oral administration, give around-the-clock to promote less variation in peak and trough serum levels.

**I.V.:** Use infusion pump.

**Other:** Inhalation: Use proper technique in using inhaler. Shake container, exhale slowly and completely through nose, inhale deeply through mouth while administering aerosol, hold breath for 2-3 seconds, then exhale slowly. Allow 1 minute between inhalations. Wash mouthpiece between use.

**Stability**

**Storage:** Store injection at room temperature. Protect from heat, light, and from freezing. Use only clear solutions.

**Monitoring Laboratory Tests** Serum potassium

Tocolysis: If patient receives therapy for more than 1 week, monitor serum glucose.

**Additional Nursing Issues**

**Physical Assessment:** Respiratory use: Assess effectiveness and interactions of other medications (see Drug Interactions). See Contraindications and Warnings/Precautions for use cautions. Monitor effectiveness of therapy (relief of airway obstruction) and adverse reactions (eg, cardiac and CNS changes - see Adverse Reactions) at beginning of therapy and periodically with long-term use. For inpatient care, monitor vital signs and lung sounds prior to and periodically during therapy. Assess knowledge/teach patient appropriate use, interventions to reduce side effects, and adverse symptoms to report.

Preterm labor use: Inpatient: Monitor maternal vital signs; respiratory, cardiac, and electrolyte status; frequency, duration, and intensity of contractions; and fetal heart rate. For outpatients, assess knowledge/teach patient appropriate use, interventions to reduce side effects, and adverse symptoms to report.

**Patient Information/Instruction:** Use exactly as directed (see Administration below). Do not use more often than recommended (excessive use may result in tolerance, overdose may result in serious adverse effects) and do not discontinue without consulting prescriber. Maintain adequate hydration (2-3 L/day of fluids unless instructed to restrict fluid intake). You may experience nervousness, dizziness, or fatigue (use caution when driving or engaging in tasks requiring alertness until response to drug is known); or dry mouth, stomach upset (frequent small meals, frequent mouth care, chewing gum, or sucking hard candy may help). Report unresolved GI upset; dizziness or fatigue; vision changes; chest pain, rapid heartbeat, or palpitations; insomnia, nervousness, or hyperactivity; muscle cramping, tremors, or pain; unusual cough; or rash (hypersensitivity).

Preterm labor: Notify prescriber immediately if labor resumes or adverse side effects are noted.

**Administration:** Self-administered inhalation: Store canister upside down; do not freeze. Shake canister before using. Sit when using medication. Close eyes when administering terbutaline to avoid spray getting into eyes. Exhale slowly and completely through nose; inhale deeply through mouth while administering aerosol. Hold breath for 1-3 seconds after inhalation. Wait at least 1 full minute between inhalations. Wash mouthpiece between use. If more than one inhalation medication is used, use bronchodilator first and wait 5 minutes between medications.

**Geriatric Considerations:** Oral terbutaline should be avoided in the elderly due to the increased incidence of adverse effects as compared to the inhaled form. Elderly patients may find it beneficial to utilize a spacer device when using the metered dose inhaler. Difficulty in using the inhaler often limits its effectiveness.

**Related Information**

Inhalant (Asthma, Bronchospasm) Agents *on page 1388*

## Terconazole (ter KONE a zole)

**U.S. Brand Names** Terazol® Vaginal

**Synonyms** Triaconazole

**Therapeutic Category** Antifungal Agent, Vaginal

**Pregnancy Risk Factor** C

**Lactation** Excretion in breast milk unknown

**Use** Local treatment of vulvovaginal candidiasis

**Mechanism of Action/Effect** Triazole ketal antifungal agent; involves inhibition of fungal cytochrome P-450

**Contraindications** Hypersensitivity to terconazole or components of the vaginal cream or suppository

**Warnings** Should be discontinued if sensitization or irritation occurs. Microbiological studies (KOH smear and/or cultures) should be repeated in patients not responding to terconazole in order to confirm the diagnosis and rule out other pathogens. Pregnancy factor C.

**Adverse Reactions**

1% to 10%: Genitourinary: Vulvar/vaginal burning

<1% (Limited to important or life-threatening symptoms): Vulvar itching, soreness, edema, or discharge; polyuria; burning or itching of penis of sexual partner

**Formulations**

Terazol® 7: Cream, vaginal: 0.4% (45 g)

Terazol® 3:

Suppository, vaginal: 80 mg (3's)

Cream, vaginal: 0.8% (20 g)

**Dosing**

**Adults:**

Terazol-7 vaginal cream: Insert 1 applicatorful intravaginally at bedtime for 7 consecutive days.

Terazol-3 vaginal suppository: Insert 1 suppository intravaginally at bedtime for 3 consecutive days.

Terazol-3 vaginal cream: Insert 1 applicatorful intravaginally at bedtime for 3 consecutive days.

**Elderly:** Refer to adult dosing.

**Stability**

**Storage:** Store at room temperature (13°C to 30°C/59°F to 86°F).

**Additional Nursing Issues**

**Physical Assessment:** See Contraindications and Warnings/Precautions for use cautions. Assess knowledge/teach patient appropriate administration, possible side effects/interventions, and adverse symptoms to report. **Pregnancy risk factor C** - benefits of use should outweigh possible risks. Note breast-feeding caution.

**Patient Information/Instruction:** Complete full course of therapy as directed. Insert vaginally as directed by prescriber or see package insert. Sexual partner may experience irritation of penis; best to refrain from intercourse during period of treatment. Report persistent vaginal burning, itching, irritation, or discharge. **Pregnancy/breast-feeding precautions:** Inform prescriber if you are or intend to be pregnant. Consult prescriber if breast-feeding.

**Geriatric Considerations:** Assess patient's ability to self-administer; may be difficult in patients with arthritis or limited range of motion.

- **Teriparatide** *see page 1248*
- **Terramicina** *see* Oxytetracycline *on page 876*
- **Terramycin® I.M. Injection** *see* Oxytetracycline *on page 876*
- **Terramycin® Oral** *see* Oxytetracycline *on page 876*
- **Terranumonyl** *see* Tetracycline *on page 1111*
- **Tesalon** *see* Benzonatate *on page 143*
- **Teslac®** *see* Testolactone *on this page*
- **TESPA** *see* Thiotepa *on page 1125*
- **Tessalon® Perles** *see* Benzonatate *on page 143*
- **Testex®** *see* Testosterone *on next page*
- **Testoderm® Transdermal System** *see* Testosterone *on next page*

## Testolactone (tes toe LAK tone)

**U.S. Brand Names** Teslac®

**Therapeutic Category** Androgen

**Pregnancy Risk Factor** C

**Lactation** Excretion in breast milk unknown

**Use** Palliative treatment of advanced disseminated breast carcinoma

**Mechanism of Action/Effect** Testolactone is a synthetic testosterone derivative without significant androgen activity. The drug inhibits steroid aromatase activity, thereby blocking the production of estradiol and estrone from androgen precursors such as testosterone and androstenedione. Unfortunately, the enzymatic block provided by testolactone is transient and is usually limited to a period of 3 months.

**Contraindications** Hypersensitivity to testolactone; in men for the treatment of breast cancer

**Warnings** The U.S. Food and Drug Administration (FDA) currently recommends that procedures for proper handling and disposal of antineoplastic agents be considered. Use with caution in hepatic, renal, or cardiac disease; prolonged use may cause drug-induced hepatic disease; or history of porphyria. Pregnancy factor C.

**Drug Interactions**

**Increased Effect/Toxicity:** Increased effects of oral anticoagulants.

**Effects on Lab Values** Plasma estradiol concentrations by RIA

**Adverse Reactions** 1% to 10%:

Cardiovascular: Edema

Dermatologic: Maculopapular rash

Endocrine & metabolic: Hypercalcemia,

Gastrointestinal: Anorexia, diarrhea, nausea, edema of the tongue

Neuromuscular & skeletal: Paresthesias, peripheral neuropathies

**Pharmacodynamics/Kinetics**

**Metabolism:** Liver

**Excretion:** Urine

**Formulations** Tablet: 50 mg

**Dosing**

**Adults:** Female: Oral: 250 mg 4 times/day for at least 3 months; desired response may take as long as 3 months.

**Elderly:** Refer to adult dosing.

**Monitoring Laboratory Tests** Plasma calcium levels

(Continued)

## Testolactone *(Continued)*

**Additional Nursing Issues**

**Physical Assessment:** Assess effectiveness and interactions of other medications (see Drug Interactions, eg, anticoagulants). See Warnings/Precautions and Contraindications for use cautions. Monitor effectiveness of therapy, laboratory tests (calcium levels), and adverse response (see Adverse Reactions and Overdose/Toxicology). Assess knowledge/teach patient appropriate use, possible side effects and appropriate interventions, and adverse symptoms to report. **Pregnancy risk factor C.** Note breast-feeding caution.

**Patient Information/Instruction:** Take as directed; do not discontinue without consulting prescriber. Effectiveness of therapy may take several months. Maintain adequate fluid intake (2-3 L/day of fluids unless instructed to restrict fluid intake) and diet and exercise program recommended by prescriber. You may experience nausea or vomiting (small frequent meals, frequent mouth care, sucking lozenges, or chewing gum may help). Report fluid retention (swelling of ankles, feet, or hands; difficulty breathing or sudden weight gain); numbness, tingling, or swelling of fingers, toes, or face; skin rash, redness, or irritation; or other adverse reactions. **Pregnancy/breast-feeding precautions:** Consult prescriber about pregnancy and breast-feeding.

♦ **Testopel® Pellet** *see* Testosterone *on this page*

## Testosterone (tes TOS ter one)

**U.S. Brand Names** Androderm® Transdermal System; Andro-L.A.® Injection; Andropository® Injection; Delatest® Injection; Delatestryl® Injection; depAndro® Injection; Depotest® Injection; Depo®-Testosterone Injection; Duratest® Injection; Durathate® Injection; Everone® Injection; Histerone® Injection; Testex®; Testoderm® Transdermal System; Testopel® Pellet

**Synonyms** Aqueous Testosterone

**Therapeutic Category** Androgen

**Pregnancy Risk Factor** X

**Lactation** Enters breast milk/contraindicated

**Use** Androgen replacement therapy in the treatment of delayed male puberty; postpartum breast pain and engorgement; inoperable breast cancer; male hypogonadism

**Mechanism of Action/Effect** Principal endogenous androgen responsible for promoting the growth and development of the male sex organs and maintaining secondary sex characteristics in androgen-deficient males

**Contraindications** Hypersensitivity to testosterone or any component; severe renal or cardiac disease; benign prostatic hypertrophy with obstruction; undiagnosed genital bleeding; males with carcinoma of the breast or prostate; pregnancy

**Warnings** Perform radiographic examination of the hand and wrist every 6 months to determine the rate of bone maturation. May accelerate bone maturation without producing compensating gain in linear growth. Has both androgenic and anabolic activity, the anabolic action may enhance hypoglycemia.

**Drug Interactions**

**Cytochrome P-450 Effect:** CYP3A3/4 and 3A5-7 enzyme substrate

**Increased Effect/Toxicity:** Warfarin and testosterone: Effects of oral anticoagulants may be enhanced.

**Effects on Lab Values** May cause a decrease in creatinine and creatine excretion and an increase in the excretion of 17-ketosteroids, thyroid function tests.

**Adverse Reactions**

>10%:

- Dermatologic: Acne
- Endocrine & metabolic: Menstrual problems (amenorrhea), virilism, breast soreness
- Genitourinary: Epididymitis, priapism, bladder irritability

1% to 10%:

- Cardiovascular: Flushing, edema
- Central nervous system: Excitation, aggressive behavior, sleeplessness, anxiety, mental depression, headache
- Dermatologic: Hirsutism (increase in pubic hair growth), skin irritation (transdermal patch)
- Gastrointestinal: Nausea, vomiting, GI irritation
- Genitourinary: Prostatic hypertrophy, prostatic carcinoma, impotence, testicular atrophy
- Hepatic: Hepatic dysfunction

<1% (Limited to important or life-threatening symptoms): Leukopenia, suppression of clotting factors, polycythemia, cholestatic hepatitis, hepatic necrosis

**Pharmacodynamics/Kinetics**

**Protein Binding:** 98% (to transcortin and albumin)

**Distribution:** Crosses the placenta

**Half-life Elimination:** 10-100 minutes

**Metabolism:** Liver

**Excretion:** Urine and feces via bile

**Duration:** Based upon the route of administration and which testosterone ester is used; cypionate and enanthate esters have the longest duration, up to 2-4 weeks after I.M. administration.

**Formulations**

Injection:

Aqueous suspension: 25 mg/mL (10 mL, 30 mL); 50 mg/mL (10 mL, 30 mL); 100 mg/mL (10 mL, 30 mL)

In oil, as cypionate: 100 mg/mL (1 mL, 10 mL); 200 mg/mL (1 mL, 10 mL)
In oil, as enanthate: 100 mg/mL (5 mL, 10 mL); 200 mg/mL (5 mL, 10 mL)
In oil, as propionate: 50 mg/mL (10 mL, 30 mL); 100 mg/mL (10 mL, 30 mL)
Pellet: 75 mg (1 pellet per vial)
Transdermal system:
Androderm® Transdermal System, Testoderm®: 4 mg/day; 6 mg/day
Testosterone: Androderm® 2.5 mg/day (60's); 5 mg/day (30's)

**Dosing**

**Adults:**

Male hypogonadism: I.M.: 50-400 mg every 2-4 weeks
Initiation of pubertal growth: 40-50 mg/m²/dose (cypionate or enanthate) monthly until the growth rate falls to prepubertal levels (~5 cm/year)
During terminal growth phase: 100 mg/m²/dose (cypionate or enanthate) monthly until growth ceases
Maintenance virilizing dose: 100 mg/m²/dose (cypionate or enanthate) twice monthly or 50-400 mg/dose every 2-4 weeks
Inoperable breast cancer: Adults: I.M.: 200-400 mg every 2-4 weeks
Hypogonadism: Male:
I.M.:
Testosterone or testosterone propionate: 10-25 mg 2-3 times/week
Testosterone cypionate or enanthate: 50-400 mg every 2-4 weeks
Postpubertal cryptorchism: Testosterone or testosterone propionate: 10-25 mg 2-3 times/week
Topical: Initial: 6 mg/day system applied daily applied on scrotal skin. If scrotal area is inadequate, start with a 4 mg/day system. Transdermal system should be worn for 22-24 hours. Determine total serum testosterone after 3-4 weeks of daily application. If patients have not achieved desired results after 6-8 weeks of therapy, another form of testosterone replacement therapy should be considered.

**Elderly:** Refer to adult dosing.

**Hepatic Impairment:** Reduce dose.

**Administration**

**I.M.:** Warm injection to room temperature and shaking vial will help redissolve crystals that have formed after storage. Administer by deep I.M. injection into the upper outer quadrant of the gluteus maximus.

**Topical:** Transdermal system should be applied on clean, dry, scrotal skin. Dry-shave scrotal hair for optimal skin contact. Do not use chemical depilatories. Applying a small amount of 0.1% triamcinolone to the skin under the drug reservoir of the transdermal system may reduce irritation.

**Monitoring Laboratory Tests** Periodic liver function, radiologic examination of wrist and hand every 6 months (when using in prepubertal children)

**Additional Nursing Issues**

**Physical Assessment:** (For use in children see pediatric reference.) Assess effectiveness and interactions of other medications (see Drug Interactions). See Warnings/Precautions and Contraindications for use cautions. Monitor effectiveness of therapy, laboratory tests, and adverse response (see Adverse Reactions and Overdose/Toxicology). Assess knowledge/teach patient appropriate use according to drug form and purpose of therapy, possible side effects and appropriate interventions, and adverse symptoms to report. **Pregnancy risk factor X** - determine pregnancy status before instituting therapy. Breast-feeding is contraindicated.

**Patient Information/Instruction:** Diabetics should monitor serum glucose closely and notify prescriber of changes; this medication may alter hypoglycemic requirements. You may experience acne, growth of body hair, loss of libido, impotence, or menstrual irregularity (usually reversible); nausea or vomiting (small frequent meals, frequent mouth care, sucking lozenges, or chewing gum may help). Report changes in menstrual pattern; enlarged or painful breasts; deepening of voice or unusual growth of body hair; persistent penile erection; fluid retention (swelling of ankles, feet, or hands, difficulty breathing or sudden weight gain); unresolved changes in CNS (nervousness, chills, insomnia, depression, aggressiveness); altered urinary patterns; change in color of urine or stool; yellowing of eyes or skin; unusual bruising or bleeding; or other persistent adverse reactions.

Topical: Apply to clean, dry scrotal skin. Dry shave scrotal hair for optimal skin contact. Do not use chemical depilatories.

**Pregnancy/breast-feeding precautions:** Inform prescriber if you are pregnant. Do not get pregnant during or for 1 month following therapy. Male: Do not cause a female to become pregnant. Male/female: Consult prescriber for instruction on appropriate barrier contraceptive measures. This drug may cause severe fetal defects. Do not breast-feed.

**Geriatric Considerations:** Geriatric patients may have an increased risk of prostatic hypertrophy or prostatic carcinoma.

**Additional Information**

Testosterone (aqueous): Histerone®, Tesanone®
Testosterone cypionate: Depotest®, Depo®-Testosterone, Duratest®
Testosterone enanthate: Andro-L.A.®, Andropository®, Delatestryl®, Durathate®, Everone®
Transdermal: Testosterone: Androderm®, Testoderm®

- **Testred®** *see* Methyltestosterone *on page 756*
- **Tetanus Antitoxin** *see page 1256*
- **Tetanus Immune Globulin** *see page 1256*

♦ **Tetra-Atlantis®** *see* Tetracycline *on next page*

## Tetracaine (TET ra kane)

**U.S. Brand Names** Pontocaine®

**Synonyms** Amethocaine Hydrochloride

**Therapeutic Category** Local Anesthetic

**Pregnancy Risk Factor** C

**Lactation** For topical use

**Use** Spinal anesthesia; local anesthesia in the eye for various diagnostic and examination purposes; topically applied to nose and throat for various diagnostic procedures; **approximately 10 times more potent than procaine**

**Mechanism of Action/Effect** Blocks both the initiation and conduction of nerve impulses by decreasing the neuronal membrane's permeability to sodium ions, which results in inhibition of depolarization with resultant blockade of conduction

**Contraindications** Hypersensitivity to tetracaine or any component; ophthalmic secondary bacterial infection; patients with liver disease, CNS disease, meningitis (if used for epidural or spinal anesthesia), myasthenia gravis

**Warnings** Ophthalmic preparations may delay wound healing. Use with caution in patients with cardiac disease and hyperthyroidism. Pregnancy factor C.

**Drug Interactions**

**Decreased Effect:** Aminosalicylic acid, sulfonamide effect may be antagonized.

**Adverse Reactions** 1% to 10%:

Cardiovascular: Cardiac arrest, hypotension, bradycardia, palpitations
Central nervous system: Seizures, restlessness, anxiety, dizziness
Gastrointestinal: Nausea, vomiting
Neuromuscular & skeletal: Weakness
Ocular: Blurred vision
Otic: Tinnitus
Respiratory: Apnea

**Overdose/Toxicology** Symptoms of overdose include seizures, respiratory depression, lacrimation, bradycardia, and hypotension. Treatment is supportive.

**Pharmacodynamics/Kinetics**

**Metabolism:** Liver

**Excretion:** Renal

**Onset:** Onset of anesthetic effect:

Ophthalmic instillation: Within 60 seconds

Topical or spinal injection: Within 3-8 minutes after applied to mucous membranes or when saddle block administered for spinal anesthesia

**Duration:** Topical: 1.5-3 hours

**Formulations**

Tetracaine hydrochloride:

- Cream: 1% (28 g)
- Injection: 1% [10 mg/mL] (2 mL)
- Injection, with dextrose 6%: 0.2% [2 mg/mL] (2 mL); 0.3% [3 mg/mL] (5 mL)
- Ointment:
  - Ophthalmic: 0.5% [5 mg/mL] (3.75 g)
  - Topical: 0.5% [5 mg/mL] (28 g)
- Powder for injection: 20 mg
- Solution, Ophthalmic: 0.5% [5 mg/mL] (1 mL, 2 mL, 15 mL, 59 mL)
- Solution, Topical: 2% [20 mg/mL] (30 mL, 118 mL)

**Dosing**

**Adults:** Maximum: 50 mg

Ophthalmic (not for prolonged use):

- Ointment: Apply ½" to 1" to lower conjunctival fornix
- Solution: Instill 1-2 drops.

Spinal anesthesia:

- High, medium, low, and saddle blocks: 0.2% to 0.3% solution
- Prolonged (2-3 hours): 1% solution
- Subarachnoid injection: 5-20 mg
- Saddle block: 2-5 mg; a 1% solution should be diluted with equal volume of CSF before administration.

Topical mucous membranes (2% solution): Apply as needed; dose should not exceed 20 mg.

Topical for skin: Ointment/cream: Apply to affected areas as needed.

**Elderly:** Refer to adult dosing.

**Stability**

**Storage:** Store solution in the refrigerator.

**Additional Nursing Issues**

**Physical Assessment: Note:** Tetracaine is 10 times as potent as procaine. Explain use, monitor vital signs, and monitor patient safety before, during, and following use according to formulation used and procedure being done. Caution patient that anesthetic effects of topical or ophthalmic preparation may last for some time after procedure (1-5 hours). Instruct in appropriate safety precautions (eg, heat/cold sensation, impaired vision and eye care, impaired swallowing sensation). **Pregnancy risk factor C.**

**Patient Information/Instruction:** Topical or ophthalmic anesthesia effects may last for some time following use; you will need to observe appropriate safety precautions to prevent injury (eg, do not rub or touch your eye, scratch your nose, or eat or drink (depending on use) until all sensation returns).

Ophthalmic: May cause temporary rash or stinging when used. Report any ringing in ears, feeling of weakness or faintness, chest pain or palpitation, or increased restlessness. **Pregnancy precautions:** Inform prescriber if you pregnant.

**Additional Information** The injection 1% formulation contains sulfites.

- **Tetracaine Hydrochloride, Benzocaine, Butyl Aminobenzoate, and Benzalkonium Chloride** *see* Benzocaine, Butyl Aminobenzoate, Tetracaine, and Benzalkonium Chloride *on page 142*
- **Tetracap® Oral** *see* Tetracycline *on this page*

## Tetracycline (tet ra SYE kleen)

**U.S. Brand Names** Achromycin® Ophthalmic; Achromycin® Topical; Nor-tet® Oral; Panmycin® Oral; Sumycin® Oral; Tetracap® Oral; Topicycline® Topical

**Synonyms** TCN

**Therapeutic Category** Antibiotic, Ophthalmic; Antibiotic, Tetracycline Derivative; Antibiotic, Topical

**Pregnancy Risk Factor** D/B (topical)

**Lactation** Enters breast milk/not recommended (AAP rates "compatible")

**Use** Treatment of susceptible bacterial infections of both gram-positive and gram-negative organisms; also infections due to *Mycoplasma*, *Chlamydia*, and *Rickettsia*; indicated for acne, exacerbations of chronic bronchitis, and treatment of gonorrhea and syphilis in patients that are allergic to penicillin; an NDA has been filed for its use concomitantly with metronidazole and bismuth subsalicylate for the treatment of peptic ulcer disease induced by *H. pylori*

**Mechanism of Action/Effect** Inhibits protein synthesis of susceptible bacteria; bacteriostatic - causes call death.

**Contraindications** Hypersensitivity to tetracycline or any component; pregnancy

**Warnings** Use with caution in patients with renal or hepatic impairment and in pregnancy. Dosage modification required in patients with renal impairment. Pseudotumor cerebri has been reported with tetracycline use. Outdated drug can cause nephropathy.

**Drug Interactions**

**Decreased Effect:** Calcium, magnesium- or aluminum-containing antacids, iron, zinc, sodium bicarbonate may decrease tetracycline absorption. Therapeutic effect of oral contraceptives and penicillins may be reduced with coadministration of tetracycline.

**Increased Effect/Toxicity:** Methoxyflurane anesthesia when concurrent with tetracycline may cause fatal nephrotoxicity. Warfarin with tetracyclines may cause increased anticoagulation.

**Food Interactions** Tetracycline serum concentrations may be decreased if taken with dairy products.

**Effects on Lab Values** False-negative urine glucose with Clinistix®

**Adverse Reactions**

**Systemic:**

>10%:

- Central nervous system: Dizziness, lightheadedness, unsteadiness
- Dermatologic: Photosensitivity
- Gastrointestinal: Nausea, diarrhea
- Miscellaneous: Discoloration of teeth in children

1% to 10%:

- Endocrine & metabolic: Diabetes insipidus syndrome
- Gastrointestinal: Pancreatitis, hypertrophy of the papilla
- Hepatic: Hepatotoxicity
- Miscellaneous: Superinfections (fungal overgrowth)

<1% (Limited to important or life-threatening symptoms): Pericarditis, increased intracranial pressure, exfoliative dermatitis, acute renal failure, azotemia

**Overdose/Toxicology** Symptoms of overdose include nausea, anorexia, and diarrhea. Treatment is supportive.

**Pharmacodynamics/Kinetics**

**Protein Binding:** 20% to 60%

**Distribution:** Small amount appears in bile

Relative diffusion of antimicrobial agents from blood into cerebrospinal fluid (CSF): Good only with inflammation (exceeds usual MICs)

Ratio of CSF to blood level (%): Inflamed meninges: 25

**Half-life Elimination:** Normal renal function: 8-11 hours; End-stage renal disease: 57-108 hours

**Time to Peak:** Oral: Within 2-4 hours

**Excretion:** Primary route is the kidney, with 60% of a dose excreted as unchanged drug in the urine

**Formulations**

Tetracycline hydrochloride:

- Capsule: 100 mg, 250 mg, 500 mg
- Ointment:
  - Ophthalmic: 1% [10 mg/mL] (3.5 g)
  - Topical: 3% [30 mg/mL] (14.2 g, 30 g)
- Solution, topical: 2.2 mg/mL (70 mL)
- Suspension:
  - Ophthalmic: 1% [10 mg/mL] (0.5 mL, 1 mL, 4 mL)
  - Oral: 125 mg/5 mL (60 mL, 480 mL)
- Tablet: 250 mg, 500 mg

(Continued)

## Tetracycline *(Continued)*

**Dosing**

**Adults:**

Ophthalmic:

Ointment: Instill every 2-12 hours.

Suspension: Instill 1-2 drops 2-4 times/day or more often as needed.

Topical: Apply to affected areas 1-4 times/day.

Oral: 250-500 mg/dose every 6 hours

*Helicobacter pylori*: Clinically effective treatment regimens include triple therapy with amoxicillin or tetracycline, metronidazole, and bismuth subsalicylate; amoxicillin, metronidazole, and $H_2$-receptor antagonist; or double therapy with amoxicillin and omeprazole. Adult dose: 850 mg 3 times/day to 500 mg 4 times/day.

**Elderly:** Refer to adult dosing.

**Renal Impairment:**

$Cl_{cr}$ 50-80 mL/minute: Administer every 8-12 hours.

$Cl_{cr}$ 10-50 mL/minute: Administer every 12-24 hours.

$Cl_{cr}$ <10 mL/minute: Administer every 24 hours.

Slightly dialyzable (5% to 20%) via hemo- and peritoneal dialysis nor via continuous arteriovenous or venovenous hemofiltration (CAVH/CAVHD); no supplemental dosage is necessary.

**Hepatic Impairment:** Avoid use or maximum dose is 1 g/day.

**Administration**

**Oral:** Oral should be given on an empty stomach (ie, 1 hour prior to, or 2 hours after meals) to increase total absorption. Administer at least 1-2 hours prior to, or 4 hours after antacid because aluminum and magnesium cations may chelate with tetracycline and reduce its total absorption. Administer around-the-clock to promote less variation in peak and trough serum levels.

**Stability**

**Storage:** Outdated tetracyclines have caused a Fanconi-like syndrome (nausea, vomiting, acidosis, proteinuria, glycosuria, aminoaciduria, polydipsia, polyuria, hypokalemia). Protect oral dosage forms from light.

**Compatibility:** See the Compatibility of Drugs Chart *on page 1315*.

**Monitoring Laboratory Tests** Renal, hepatic, and hematologic function; WBC. Perform culture and sensitivity studies prior to initiating therapy to determine the causative organism and its susceptibility to tetracycline.

**Additional Nursing Issues**

**Physical Assessment:** Assess effectiveness and interactions of other medications patient may be taking (see Drug Interactions). Monitor laboratory tests, therapeutic response, and adverse reactions (see Adverse Reactions) at beginning of therapy and periodically throughout therapy. Assess knowledge/teach patient appropriate use, interventions to reduce side effects, and adverse symptoms to report. **Pregnancy risk factor B/D** - assess knowledge/instruct patient on need to use appropriate barrier contraceptive measures (tetracycline may reduce effectiveness of oral contraceptives) and the need to avoid pregnancy. Breast-feeding is not recommended; may cause discoloration of infant's teeth.

**Patient Information/Instruction:** Take this medication exactly as directed. Take all of the prescription even if you see an improvement in your condition. Do not use more or more often than recommended.

Oral: Preferable to take on an empty stomach (1 hour before or 2 hours after meals). Take at regularly scheduled times, around-the-clock. Avoid antacids, iron, or dairy products within 2 hours of taking tetracycline. You may experience photosensitivity (use sunscreen, wear protective clothing and eyewear, and avoid direct sunlight); dizziness or lightheadedness (use caution when driving or engaging in tasks requiring alertness until response to drug is known); nausea/vomiting (frequent small meals, frequent mouth care, chewing gum, or sucking lozenges may help). Effect of oral contraceptives may be reduced; use barrier contraception. Report rash or intense itching, yellowing of skin or eyes, fever or chills, blackened stool, vaginal itching or discharge, foul-smelling stools, excessive thirst or urination, acute headache, unresolved diarrhea, difficulty breathing, condition does not improve, or worsening of condition.

**Pregnancy/breast-feeding precautions:** Do not get pregnant while taking this medication - effectiveness of oral contraceptives may be reduced; use appropriate barrier contraceptive measures. Breast-feeding is not recommended.

Ophthalmic: Sit down, tilt head back, instill solution or drops inside lower eyelid, and roll eyeball in all directions. Close eye and apply gentle pressure to inner corner of eye for 30 seconds. Do not touch tip of applicator to eye or any contaminated surface. May experience temporary stinging or blurred vision. Inform prescriber if condition worsens or does not improve in 3-4 days.

Topical: Wash area and pat dry (unless contraindicated). Avoid getting in mouth or eyes. You may experience temporary stinging or burning which will resolve quickly. Treated skin may turn yellow; this will wash off. May stain clothing (permanent). Report rash. Inform prescriber if condition worsens or does not improve in a few days.

**Dietary Issues:** Decreased absorption of magnesium, zinc, calcium, iron, and amino acids.

**Geriatric Considerations:** The role of tetracycline has decreased because of the emergence of resistant organisms. Doxycycline is the tetracycline of choice when one is indicated because of its better GI absorption, less interactions with divalent cations, longer half-life, and the fact that the majority is cleared by nonrenal mechanisms.

**Additional Information** Some formulations may contain sulfites.

**Related Information**

Ophthalmic Agents *on page 1282*

- **Tetrahydroaminoacrine** *see* Tacrine *on page 1092*
- **Tetrahydrocannabinol** *see* Dronabinol *on page 408*
- **Tetrahydrozoline** *see page 1294*
- **Tetramune®** *see page 1256*
- **Tetrasine® Extra Ophthalmic** *see page 1294*
- **Tetrasine® Ophthalmic** *see page 1294*
- **Texacort®** *see* Hydrocortisone *on page 578*
- **Texacort®** *see* Topical Corticosteroids *on page 1152*
- **TG** *see* Thioguanine *on page 1122*
- **6-TG** *see* Thioguanine *on page 1122*
- **T/Gel®** *see page 1294*
- **T-Gen®** *see* Trimethobenzamide *on page 1180*
- **T-Gesic®** *see* Hydrocodone and Acetaminophen *on page 568*
- **THA** *see* Tacrine *on page 1092*

## Thalidomide (tha LI doe mide)

**U.S. Brand Names** Contergan®; Distaval®; Kevadon®; Thalomid®

**Therapeutic Category** Immunosuppressant Agent

**Pregnancy Risk Factor** X

**Lactation** Excretion in breast milk unknown/not recommended

**Use** Thalidomide is approved for marketing only under a special distribution program. This program, called the "System for Thalidomide Education and Prescribing Safety" (STEPS), has been approved by the FDA. Prescribing and dispensing of thalidomide is restricted to prescribers and pharmacists registered with the program.

Acute treatment of cutaneous manifestations of moderate to severe erythema nodosum leprosum (ENL); maintenance therapy for suppression of cutaneous manifestations of ENL recurrence

Orphan drug status: Crohn's disease

**Investigational use:** Treatment or prevention of graft-versus-host reactions after bone marrow transplantation; in aphthous ulceration in HIV-positive patients; Langerhans cell histiocytosis, Behçet's syndrome; hypnotic agent; may be effective in rheumatoid arthritis, discoid lupus, and erythema multiforme; useful in Type 2 lepra reactions, but not Type 1; can assist in healing mouth ulcers in AIDS patients

**Mechanism of Action/Effect** A derivative of glutethimide; mode of action for immunosuppression is unclear; inhibition of neutrophil chemotaxis and decreased monocyte phagocytosis may occur; may cause 50% to 80% reduction of tumor necrosis factor - alpha.

**Contraindications** Hypersensitivity to thalidomide; pregnancy or women in childbearing years; neuropathy (peripheral)

**Warnings** Liver, hepatic, neurological disorders; constipation; congestive heart failure; hypertension

**Drug Interactions**

**Increased Effect/Toxicity:** Other medications known to cause peripheral neuropathy should be used with caution in patients receiving thalidomide; thalidomide may enhance the sedative activity of other drugs such as ethanol, barbiturates, reserpine, and chlorpromazine

**Adverse Reactions**

Controlled clinical trials: ENL:

>10%:

Central nervous system: Somnolence (37.5%), headache (12.5%)

Dermatologic: Rash (20.8%)

1% to 10%:

Cardiovascular: Peripheral edema

Central nervous system: Dizziness (4.2%), vertigo (8.3%), chills, malaise (8.3%)

Dermatologic: Dermatitis (fungal) (4.2%), nail disorder (4.2%), pruritus (8.3%), rash (maculopapular) (4.2%)

Gastrointestinal (4.2%): Constipation, diarrhea, nausea, moniliasis, tooth pain, abdominal pain

Genitourinary: Impotence (8.2%)

Neuromuscular & skeletal: Asthenia (8.3%), pain (8.3%), back pain (4.2%), neck pain (4.2%), neck rigidity (4.2%), tremor (4.2%)

Respiratory (4.2%): Pharyngitis, rhinitis, sinusitis

HIV-seropositive:

General: An increased viral load has been noted in patients treated with thalidomide. This is of uncertain clinical significance - see monitoring

>10%:

Central nervous system: Somnolence (36% to 37%), dizziness (18.7% to 19.4%), fever (19.4% to 21.9%), headache (16.7% to 18.7%)

Dermatologic: Rash (25%), maculopapular rash (16.7% to 18.7%), acne (3.1% to 11.1%)

Gastrointestinal: AST increase (2.8% to 12.5%), diarrhea (11.1% to 18.7%), nausea (≤12.5%), oral moniliasis (6.3% to 11.1%)

Hematologic: Leukopenia (16.7% to 25%), anemia (5.6% to 12.5%)

Neuromuscular & skeletal: Paresthesia (5.6% to 15.6%), weakness (5.6% to 21.9%)

(Continued)

## Thalidomide *(Continued)*

Miscellaneous: Diaphoresis (≤12.5%), lymphadenopathy (5.6% to 12.5%)

1% to 10%:

Cardiovascular: Peripheral edema (3.1% to 8.3%)

Central nervous system: Nervousness (2.8% to 9.4%), insomnia (≤9.4%), agitation (≤9.4%), chills (≤9.4%)

Dermatologic: Dermatitis (fungal) (5.6% to 9.4%), nail disorder (≤3.1%), pruritus (2.8% to 6.3%)

Gastrointestinal: Anorexia (2.8% to 9.4%), constipation (2.8% to 9.4%), xerostomia (8.3% to 9.4%), flatulence (8.3% to 9.4%), multiple abnormalities LFTs (≤9.4%), abdominal pain (2.8% to 3.1%)

Neuromuscular & skeletal: Back pain (≤5%), pain (≤3.1%)

Respiratory: Pharyngitis (6.3% to 8.3%), sinusitis (3.1% to 8.3%)

Miscellaneous: Accidental injury (≤5.6%), infection (6.3% to 8.3%)

Literature reports of other adverse reactions (Limited to important or life-threatening symptoms): Bradycardia, orthostatic hypotension, Raynaud's syndrome, erythema nodosum, myxedema, Hodgkin's disease, dyspnea, CML, lymphopenia, pancytopenia, acute renal failure, suicide attempt

**Pharmacodynamics/Kinetics**

**Half-life Elimination:** 8.7 hours

**Time to Peak:** 2-6 hours

**Metabolism:** Hepatic

**Formulations** Capsule: 50 mg (boxes contain 6 prescription packs of 14 capsules each)

**Dosing**

**Adults:**

Cutaneous ENL:

Initiate dosing at 100-300 mg/day taken once daily at bedtime (at least 1 hour after evening meal)

Patients weighing <50 kg: Initiate at lower dose

Severe cutaneous reaction or previously requiring high dose may be initiated at 400 mg/day; doses may be divided, but taken 1 hour after meals

Dosing should continue until active reaction subsides (usually at least 2 weeks), then tapered in 50 mg decrements every 2-4 weeks

Patients who flare during tapering or with a history or requiring prolonged maintenance should be maintained on the minimum dosage necessary to control the reaction. Efforts to taper should be repeated every 3-6 months.

Behçet's syndrome: 100-400 mg/day

Graft-vs-host reactions: 100-1600 mg/day; usual initial dose: 200 mg 4 times/day for use up to 700 days

AIDS-related aphthous stomatitis: 200 mg twice daily for 5 days, then 200 mg/day for up to 8 weeks

Discoid lupus erythematosus: 100-400 mg/day; maintenance dose: 25-50 mg

**Elderly:** Refer to adult dosing.

**Monitoring Laboratory Tests** Required pregnancy testing, WBC with differential. In HIV-seropositive patients: viral load after 1 and 3 months, then every 3 months.

**Additional Nursing Issues**

**Physical Assessment:** Patient must be capable of complying with STEPS program (see Use). Instruct patient on risks of pregnancy, appropriate contraceptive measures (see below), and necessity for frequent pregnancy testing (schedule pregnancy testing at time of dispensing and give patient schedule in writing). Assess other medications patient may be taking for possible interactions (see Drug Interactions). Monitor closely for adverse reactions (see above). Instruct patient on signs and symptoms to report and appropriate interventions for adverse reactions.

**Pregnancy risk factor X** - pregnancy test is required within 24 hours prior to beginning therapy, weekly during first month of therapy, and monthly thereafter for all women of childbearing age. Effective contraception with at least two reliable forms of contraception must be used for 1 month prior to beginning therapy, during therapy, and for 1 month following discontinuance of therapy. (Women who have undergone a hysterectomy or have been postmenopausal for at least 24 consecutive months are the only exception.) Do not prescribe, administer, or dispense to women of childbearing age or males who may have intercourse with women of childbearing age unless both female and male are capable of complying with contraceptive measures. (Even males who have undergone vasectomy must acknowledge these risks in writing.) Oral and written warnings concerning contraception and the hazards of thalidomide must be conveyed to females and males and they must acknowledge their understanding in writing. Parents or guardians must consent and sign acknowledgment for patients between 12 and 18 years of age following therapy. Breast-feeding is not recommended.

**Patient Information/Instruction:** You will be given oral and written instructions about the necessity of using two methods of contraception and and the necessity of keeping return visits for pregnancy testing. You may experience sleepiness, dizziness, lack of concentration (use caution when driving, climbing stairs, or engaging in tasks requiring alertness until response to drug is known); nausea or vomiting or loss of appetite (small frequent meals, frequent mouth care, chewing gum, or sucking lozenges may help); constipation or diarrhea; oral thrush (frequent mouth care is necessary); sexual dysfunction (reversible). Report any of the above if persistent or severe. Report chest pain or palpitations or swelling of extremities; back, neck, or muscle pain or stiffness; skin rash or eruptions; increased nervousness, anxiety, or insomnia; or any other symptom of adverse reactions. **Pregnancy/breast-feeding precautions:** Do not get pregnant. See Physical Assessment/Monitoring and Pregnancy. Breast-feeding is not recommended.

**Pregnancy Issues:** Embryotoxic with limb defects has been noted from the 27th to 40th gestational day of exposure. All cases of phocomelia occur from the 27th to 42nd gestational day. Fetal cardiac, gastrointestinal, and genitourinary tract abnormalities have also been described. Even a single dose of thalidomide taken during pregnancy can cause severe defects or fetal death. Mortality at or shortly after birth may be as high as 40%.

- **Thalitone®** *see* Chlorthalidone *on page 260*
- **Thalomid®** *see* Thalidomide *on page 1113*
- **THC** *see* Dronabinol *on page 408*
- **Theo-24®** *see* Theophylline *on this page*
- **Theobid®** *see* Theophylline *on this page*
- **Theochron®** *see* Theophylline *on this page*
- **Theoclear® L.A.** *see* Theophylline *on this page*
- **Theo-Dur®** *see* Theophylline *on this page*
- **Theo-G®** *see* Theophylline and Guaifenesin *on page 1118*
- **Theolair™** *see* Theophylline *on this page*
- **Theolate®** *see* Theophylline and Guaifenesin *on page 1118*

## Theophylline (thee OF i lin)

**U.S. Brand Names** Aerolate III®; Aerolate JR®; Aerolate SR® S; Aquaphyllin®; Asmalix®; Bronkodyl®; Elixicon®; Elixophyllin®; Quibron®-T; Quibron®-T/SR; Respbid®; Slo-bid™; Slo-Phyllin®; Sustaire®; Theo-24®; Theobid®; Theochron®; Theoclear® L.A.; Theo-Dur®; Theolair™; Theospan®-SR; Theovent®; Theo-X®; Uni-Dur®; Uniphyl®

**Therapeutic Category** Bronchodilator; Theophylline Derivative

**Pregnancy Risk Factor** C

**Lactation** Enters breast milk/compatible

**Use** Treatment of symptoms and reversible airway obstruction due to chronic asthma, chronic bronchitis, or COPD

**Mechanism of Action/Effect** Causes bronchodilatation, diuresis, CNS and cardiac stimulation, and gastric acid secretion by blocking phosphodiesterase which increases tissue concentrations of cyclic adenine monophosphate (cAMP) which in turn promotes catecholamine stimulation of lipolysis, glycogenolysis, and gluconeogenesis and induces release of epinephrine from adrenal medulla cells.

**Contraindications** Hypersensitivity to theophylline or any component

**Warnings** If a patient develops signs and symptoms of theophylline toxicity (eg, persistent, repetitive vomiting), a serum theophylline level should be measured and subsequent doses held. Due to potential saturation of theophylline clearance at serum levels in or (in some patients) less than the therapeutic range, dosage adjustment should be made in small increments (maximum: 25%). Due to wider interpatient variability, theophylline serum level measurements must be used to optimize therapy and prevent serious toxicity. Use with caution in patients with peptic ulcer, hyperthyroidism, seizure disorders, hypertension, and patients with cardiac arrhythmias (excluding bradyarrhythmias). Pregnancy factor C.

**Drug Interactions**

**Cytochrome P-450 Effect:** CYP1A2 enzyme substrate; also 2E enzyme substrate (minor)

**Decreased Effect:** Changes in diet may affect the elimination of theophylline. Charcoal-broiled foods may increase elimination, reducing half-life by 50%. The following factors decrease theophylline serum levels: Smoking (cigarettes, marijuana), high protein/low carbohydrate diet, charcoal, phenytoin, phenobarbital, carbamazepine, rifampin, I.V. isoproterenol, aminoglutethimide, barbiturates, hydantoins, ketoconazole, sulfinpyrazone, isoniazid, loop diuretics, and sympathomimetics.

**Increased Effect/Toxicity:** Changes in diet may affect the elimination of theophylline. The following factors cause increased serum theophylline levels: Hepatic cirrhosis, Cor pulmonale, congestive heart failure, fever/viral illness, propranolol, allopurinol (>600 mg/day), erythromycin, cimetidine, troleandomycin, ciprofloxacin (other quinolone antibiotics), oral contraceptives, beta-blockers, calcium channel blockers, corticosteroids, disulfiram, ephedrine, influenza virus vaccine, interferon, macrolides, mexiletine, thiabendazole, thyroid hormones, carbamazepine, isoniazid, and loop diuretics.

**Food Interactions** Food does not appreciably affect the absorption of liquid, fast-release products and most sustained release products; however, food may induce a sudden release (dose-dumping) of once-daily sustained release products resulting in an increase in serum drug levels and potential toxicity. Avoid excessive amounts of caffeine. Avoid extremes of dietary protein and carbohydrate intake. Limit charcoal-broiled foods.

| Theophylline Serum Levels (mcg/mL)* | Adverse Reactions |
|---|---|
| 15-25 | GI upset, diarrhea, N/V, abdominal pain, nervousness, headache, insomnia, agitation, dizziness, muscle cramp, tremor |
| 25-35 | Tachycardia, occasional PVC |
| >35 | Ventricular tachycardia, frequent PVC, seizure |

*Adverse effects do not necessarily occur according to serum levels. Arrhythmia and seizure can occur without seeing the other adverse effects.

(Continued)

## Theophylline *(Continued)*

**Adverse Reactions** See table.

**Uncommon at serum theophylline concentrations ≤20 mcg/mL**

1% to 10%:

Cardiovascular: Tachycardia

Central nervous system: Nervousness, restlessness

Gastrointestinal: Nausea, vomiting

<1% (Limited to important or life-threatening symptoms): Insomnia, irritability, seizures, tremor

**Overdose/Toxicology** Symptoms of overdose include nausea, vomiting, insomnia, irritability, tachycardia, seizures, tonic-clonic seizures, insomnia, and circulatory failure. If seizures have not occurred, induce vomiting; ipecac syrup is preferred. Do not induce emesis in the presence of impaired consciousness. Repeated doses of charcoal have been shown to be effective in enhancing the total body clearance of theophylline. Do not repeat charcoal doses if an ileus is present. Charcoal hemoperfusion may be considered if serum theophylline levels exceed 40 mcg/mL, the patient is unable to tolerate repeat oral charcoal administrations, or if severe toxic symptoms are present. Clearance with hemoperfusion is better than clearance from hemodialysis. Administer a cathartic, especially if sustained release agents were used. Phenobarbital administered prophylactically may prevent seizures.

**Pharmacodynamics/Kinetics**

**Protein Binding:** 40%; decreased protein binding in neonates (due to a greater percentage of fetal albumin), hepatic cirrhosis, uncorrected acidemia, women in 3rd trimester of pregnancy, and geriatric patients

**Distribution:** Crosses the placenta

**Half-life Elimination:** Mean half-life:

Acute pulmonary edema: 19 hours

Nonsmoker (healthy) 16-60 years: 8.2 hours

Nonsmoker (healthy) >60 years: 9.8 hours

Smoker: 4.4 hours

Cardiac compromised or liver failure: 20-30 hours

Hypothyroid: 11.6 hours

Hyperthyroid: 4.5 hours

**Metabolism:** Liver

**Excretion:** Urine

**Onset:** Oral: 1-2 hours; I.V.: <30 minutes

**Formulations**

Capsule:

Immediate release (Bronkodyl®, Elixophyllin®): 100 mg, 200 mg

Timed release:

8-12 hours (Aerolate®): 65 mg [III]; 130 mg [JR], 260 mg [SR]

8-12 hours (Slo-bid™): 50 mg, 75 mg, 100 mg, 125 mg, 200 mg, 300 mg

8-12 hours (Slo-Phyllin® Gyrocaps®): 60 mg, 125 mg, 250 mg

12 hours (Theobid® Duracaps®): 260 mg

12 hours (Theoclear® L.A.): 130 mg, 260 mg

12 hours (Theospan®-SR): 130 mg, 260 mg

12 hours (Theovent®): 125 mg, 250 mg

24 hours (Theo-24®): 100 mg, 200 mg, 300 mg

Elixir (Asmalix®, Elixomin®, Elixophyllin®, Lanophyllin®): 80 mg/15 mL (15 mL, 30 mL, 480 mL, 4000 mL)

Infusion, in $D_5W$: 0.4 mg/mL (1000 mL); 0.8 mg/mL (500 mL, 1000 mL); 1.6 mg/mL (250 mL, 500 mL); 2 mg/mL (100 mL); 3.2 mg/mL (250 mL); 4 mg/mL (50 mL, 100 mL);

Solution, oral:

Theolair™: 80 mg/15 mL (15 mL, 18.75 mL, 30 mL, 480 mL)

Syrup:

Aquaphyllin®, Slo-Phyllin®, Theoclear-80®, Theostat-80®: 80 mg/15 mL (15 mL, 30 mL, 500 mL)

Accurbron®: 150 mg/15 mL (480 mL)

Tablet: Immediate release:

Slo-Phyllin®: 100 mg, 200 mg

Theolair™: 125 mg, 250 mg

Quibron®-T: 300 mg

Tablet:

Controlled release (Theo-X®): 100 mg, 200 mg, 300 mg

Timed release:

12-24 hours: 100 mg, 200 mg, 300 mg, 450 mg

8-12 hours (Quibron®-T/SR): 300 mg

8-12 hours (Respbid®): 250 mg, 500 mg

8-12 hours (Sustaire®): 100 mg, 300 mg

8-12 hours (T-Phyl®): 200 mg

12-24 hours (Theochron®): 100 mg, 200 mg, 300 mg

8-24 hours (Theo-Dur®): 100 mg, 200 mg, 300 mg, 450 mg

8-24 hours (Theo-Sav®): 100 mg, 200 mg, 300 mg

24 hours (Theolair™-SR): 200 mg, 250 mg, 300 mg, 500 mg

24 hours (Uni-Dur®): 400 mg, 600 mg

24 hours (Uniphyl®): 400 mg

**Dosing**

**Adults:**

Initial dosage recommendation: Loading dose (to achieve a serum concentration of about 10 mcg/mL; loading doses should be given using a rapidly absorbed oral product **not** a sustained release product):

If no theophylline has been administered in the previous 24 hours: 4-6 mg/kg theophylline

If theophylline has been administered in the previous 24 hours: Administer ½ loading dose; 2-3 mg/kg theophylline can be given in emergencies when serum concentrations are not available

On the average, for every 1 mg/kg theophylline given, blood concentrations will rise 2 mcg/mL

Maintenance dose: See table.

**Maintenance Dose for Acute Symptoms**

| Population Group | Oral Theophylline (mg/kg/day) | I.V. Aminophylline |
|---|---|---|
| Healthy nonsmoking adults (including elderly patients) | 10<br>(not to exceed 900 mg/day) | 0.5 mg/kg/hour |
| Cardiac decompensation, cor pulmonale, and/or liver dysfunction | 5<br>(not to exceed 400 mg/day) | 0.25 mg/kg/hour |

*For continuous I.V. infusion divide total daily dose by 24 = mg/kg/hour.

Oral:

Nonsustained release: 16-20 mg/kg/day divided into 4 doses/day

Sustained release: 9-13 mg/kg/day divided into 2-3 doses/day

These recommendations, based on mean clearance rates for age or risk factors, were calculated to achieve a serum concentration of 10 mcg/mL. In healthy adults, a slow-release product can be used (9-13 mg/kg in divided dose). The total daily dose can be divided every 8-12 hours.

Use ideal body weight for obese patients. Dose should be adjusted further based on serum concentrations. Guidelines for obtaining theophylline serum concentrations are shown in the table under Monitoring Lab Tests.

**Elderly:** Elderly patients should be started with a 25% reduction in the adult dose.

**Administration**

**Oral:** Sustained release preparations should be taken with a full glass of water, swallowed whole, or cut in half if scored. Do **not** crush. Sustained release capsule forms may be opened and the contents sprinkled on soft foods; do **not** chew beads.

**Stability**

**Compatibility:** See the Compatibility of Drugs Chart *on page 1315*.

**Monitoring Laboratory Tests** Therapeutic levels:

Asthma: 10-15 mg/mL (peak level)

Toxic concentration: >20 mg/mL; see table.

**Guidelines for Drawing Theophylline Serum Levels**

| Dosage Form | Time to Draw Level* |
|---|---|
| I.V. bolus | 30 min after end of 30 min infusion |
| I.V. continuous infusion | 12-24 h after initiation of infusion |
| P.O. liquid, fast-release tab | Peak: 1 h post dose after at least 1 day of therapy<br>Trough: Just before a dose after at least 1 day of therapy |
| P.O. slow-release product | Peak: 4 h post dose after at least 1 day of therapy<br>Trough: Just before a dose after at least 1 day of therapy |

*The time to achieve steady-state serum levels is prolonged in patients with longer half-lives (eg, premature neonates, infants, and adults with cardiac or liver failure (see theophylline half-life table). In these patients, serum theophylline levels should be drawn after 48-72 hours of therapy; serum levels may need to be done prior to steady-state to assess the patients current progress or evaluate potential toxicity.

**Additional Nursing Issues**

**Physical Assessment:** Assess effectiveness and interactions of other medications (see Drug Interactions). See Contraindications and Warnings/Precautions for use cautions. Monitor effectiveness of therapy (respiratory rate, lung sounds, characteristics of cough and sputum) and adverse reactions (eg, cardiac and CNS changes - see Adverse Reactions) at beginning of therapy and periodically with long-term use. For inpatient care, monitor vital signs and lung sounds prior to and periodically during therapy. Assess knowledge/teach patient appropriate use, interventions to reduce side effects, and adverse symptoms to report. **Pregnancy risk factor C** - benefits of use should outweigh possible risks.

**Patient Information/Instruction:** Take exactly as directed; do not exceed recommended dosage. Avoid smoking (smoking may interfere with drug absorption as well as exacerbate condition for which medication is prescribed). If you are smoking when dosage is prescribed; inform prescriber if you stop smoking (dosage may need to be adjusted to prevent toxicity). Preferable to take on empty stomach (1 hour before or 2 hours after meals), with a full glass of water. Do not chew of crush sustained release forms; capsules may be opened and contents sprinkled on soft food (do not chew

(Continued)

## Theophylline *(Continued)*

beads). Avoid dietary stimulants (eg, caffeine, tea, colas, or chocolate - may increase adverse side effects). Maintain adequate hydration (2-3 L/day of fluids unless instructed to restrict fluid intake). You may experience nausea, vomiting, or lose of appetite (frequent small meals, frequent mouth care, chewing gum, or sucking lozenges may help). Report acute insomnia or restlessness, chest pain or rapid heartbeat, emotional lability or agitation, muscle tremors or cramping, acute headache, abdominal pain and cramping, blackened stool, or worsening of respiratory condition. **Pregnancy precautions:** Inform prescriber if you are or intend to be pregnant.

**Geriatric Considerations:** Although there is a great intersubject variability for half-lives of methylxanthines (2-10 hours), elderly as a group have slower hepatic clearance. Therefore, use lower initial doses and monitor closely for response and adverse reactions. Additionally, elderly are at greater risk for toxicity due to concomitant disease (eg, CHF, arrhythmias), and drug use (eg, cimetidine, ciprofloxacin, etc) (see Warnings/Precautions and Drug Interactions).

**Related Information**

Peak and Trough Guidelines *on page 1331*

## Theophylline and Guaifenesin (thee OF i lin & gwye FEN e sin)

**U.S. Brand Names** Bronchial®; Glycerol-T®; Lanophyllin-GG®; Quibron®; Slo-Phyllin GG®; Theo-G®; Theolate®

**Synonyms** Guaifenesin and Theophylline

**Therapeutic Category** Theophylline Derivative

**Pregnancy Risk Factor** C

**Lactation** Enters breast milk/compatible

**Use** Symptomatic treatment of bronchospasm associated with bronchial asthma, chronic bronchitis and pulmonary emphysema

**Formulations**

Capsule: Theophylline 150 mg and guaifenesin 90 mg; theophylline 300 mg and guaifenesin 180 mg

Elixir: Theophylline 150 mg and guaifenesin 90 mg per 15 mL (480 mL)

**Dosing**

**Adults:** Oral: 16 mg/kg/day or 400 mg theophylline/day in divided doses every 6-8 hours

**Elderly:** Refer to dosing in individual monographs.

**Additional Nursing Issues**

**Physical Assessment:** See individual components listed in Related Information. **Pregnancy risk factor C** - benefits of use should outweigh possible risks.

**Patient Information/Instruction:** See individual components listed in Related Information. **Pregnancy precautions:** Inform prescriber if you are on intend to get pregnant.

**Related Information**

Guaifenesin *on page 548*
Theophylline *on page 1115*

## Theophylline, Ephedrine, and Hydroxyzine

(thee OF i lin, e FED rin, & hye DROKS i zeen)

**U.S. Brand Names** Hydrophen®; Marax®; T.E.H.®

**Synonyms** Ephedrine, Theophylline, and Hydroxyzine; Hydroxyzine, Theophylline, and Ephedrine

**Therapeutic Category** Theophylline Derivative

**Pregnancy Risk Factor** C

**Lactation** Enters breast milk/contraindicated

**Use** Possibly effective for controlling bronchospastic disorders

**Formulations**

Syrup, dye free: Theophylline 32.5 mg, ephedrine 6.25 mg, and hydroxyzine 2.5 mg per 5 mL

Tablet: Theophylline 130 mg, ephedrine 25 mg, and hydroxyzine 10 mg

**Dosing**

**Adults:** Oral: 1 tablet 2-4 times/day

**Elderly:** Refer to dosing in individual monographs.

**Additional Nursing Issues**

**Physical Assessment:** See individual components listed in Related Information. **Pregnancy risk factor C** - benefits of use should outweigh possible risks. Breast-feeding is contraindicated.

**Patient Information/Instruction:** See individual components listed in Related Information. **Pregnancy/breast-feeding precautions:** Inform prescriber if you are on intend to get pregnant. Breast-feeding is contraindicated.

**Related Information**

Ephedrine *on page 422*
Hydroxyzine *on page 588*
Theophylline *on page 1115*

## Theophylline, Ephedrine, and Phenobarbital

(thee OF i lin, e FED rin, & fee noe BAR bi tal)

**U.S. Brand Names** Tedral®

**Synonyms** Ephedrine, Theophylline, and Phenobarbital; Phenobarbital, Theophylline, and Ephedrine

**Therapeutic Category** Theophylline Derivative

**Pregnancy Risk Factor** D

**Lactation** Enters breast milk/contraindicated

**Use** Prevention and symptomatic treatment of bronchial asthma; relief of asthmatic bronchitis and other bronchospastic disorders

**Formulations**

Suspension: Theophylline 65 mg, ephedrine sulfate 12 mg, and phenobarbital 4 mg per 5 mL

Tablet: Theophylline 118 mg, ephedrine sulfate 25 mg, and phenobarbital 11 mg; theophylline 130 mg, ephedrine sulfate 24 mg, and phenobarbital 8 mg

**Dosing**

**Adults:** Oral: 1-2 tablets or 10-20 mL every 4 hours

**Elderly:** Refer to dosing in individual monographs.

**Additional Nursing Issues**

**Physical Assessment:** See individual components listed in Related Information. **Pregnancy risk factor D** - assess knowledge/instruct patient on need to use appropriate contraceptive measures and the need to avoid pregnancy. Breast-feeding is contraindicated.

**Patient Information/Instruction:** See individual components listed in Related Information. **Pregnancy/breast-feeding precautions:** Inform prescriber if you are or intend to be pregnant. Do not breast-feed.

**Breast-feeding Issues:** Ephedrine, one of the ingredients, is contraindicated while nursing.

**Related Information**

Ephedrine *on page 422*
Phenobarbital *on page 917*
Theophylline *on page 1115*

♦ **Theospan®-SR** *see* Theophylline *on page 1115*
♦ **Theovent®** *see* Theophylline *on page 1115*
♦ **Theo-X®** *see* Theophylline *on page 1115*
♦ **Therabid® [OTC]** *see* Vitamin, Multiple *on page 1219*
♦ **Thera-Combex® H-P Kapseals®** *see page 1294*
♦ **TheraCys®** *see page 1256*
♦ **Theraflu® Non-Drowsy Formula Maximum Strength** *see page 1294*
♦ **Thera-Flur®** *see page 1294*
♦ **Thera-Flur-N®** *see page 1294*
♦ **Thera-Flur-N® ACT®** *see page 1294*
♦ **Theragran® [OTC]** *see* Vitamin, Multiple *on page 1219*
♦ **Theragran® Hematinic®** *see* Vitamin, Multiple *on page 1219*
♦ **Theragran® Liquid [OTC]** *see* Vitamin, Multiple *on page 1219*
♦ **Theragran-M® [OTC]** *see* Vitamin, Multiple *on page 1219*
♦ **Thera-Hist® Syrup** *see page 1294*
♦ **Theralax®** *see page 1294*
♦ **Theramine® Expectorant [OTC]** *see* Guaifenesin and Phenylpropanolamine *on page 550*
♦ **Therapeutic Multivitamins** *see* Vitamin, Multiple *on page 1219*
♦ **Therapeutic Nursing Management of Side Effects** *see page 22*
♦ **Theraplex Z®** *see page 1294*
♦ **Thermazene®** *see* Silver Sulfadiazine *on page 1059*
♦ **Theroxide® Wash** *see page 1294*

## Thiabendazole (thye a BEN da zole)

**U.S. Brand Names** Mintezol®

**Synonyms** Tiabendazole

**Therapeutic Category** Anthelmintic

**Pregnancy Risk Factor** C

**Lactation** Excretion in breast milk unknown

**Use** Treatment of strongyloidiasis, cutaneous larva migrans, visceral larva migrans, dracunculiasis, trichinosis, and mixed helminthic infections

**Mechanism of Action/Effect** Inhibits helminth-specific mitochondrial fumarate reductase

**Contraindications** Hypersensitivity to thiabendazole or any component

**Warnings** Use with caution in patients with renal or hepatic impairment, malnutrition or anemia, or dehydration. Pregnancy factor C.

**Drug Interactions**

**Increased Effect/Toxicity:** Increased levels of theophylline and other xanthines.

**Effects on Lab Values** ↑ glucose

**Adverse Reactions**

>10%:

Central nervous system: Hallucinations, delirium, dizziness, drowsiness, headache
Gastrointestinal: Anorexia, diarrhea, nausea, vomiting, drying of mucous membranes
Neuromuscular & skeletal: Numbness

1% to 10%: Dermatologic: Rash

<1% (Limited to important or life-threatening symptoms): Seizures, Stevens-Johnson syndrome, leukopenia, hepatotoxicity, nephrotoxicity

(Continued)

## Thiabendazole *(Continued)*

**Overdose/Toxicology** Symptoms of overdose include altered mental status and visual problems. Treatment is supportive.

**Pharmacodynamics/Kinetics**

**Time to Peak:** Within 1-2 hours

**Metabolism:** Rapid

**Excretion:** Feces and urine

**Formulations**

Suspension, oral: 500 mg/5 mL (120 mL)

Tablet, chewable (orange flavor): 500 mg

**Dosing**

**Adults:** Purgation is not required prior to use; drinking of fruit juice aids in expulsion of worms by removing the mucous to which the intestinal tapeworms attach themselves.

Oral: 50 mg/kg/day divided every 12 hours; maximum: 3 g/day

Strongyloidiasis: For 2 consecutive days

Cutaneous larva migrans: For 2-5 consecutive days

Visceral larva migrans: For 5-7 consecutive days

Trichinosis: For 2-4 consecutive days

Dracunculosis: 50-75 mg/kg/day divided every 12 hours for 3 days

**Renal Impairment:** Use with caution.

**Hepatic Impairment:** Use with caution.

**Additional Nursing Issues**

**Physical Assessment:** Assess effectiveness and interactions of other medications (see Drug Interactions). See Warnings/Precautions and Contraindications for use cautions. Worm infestations are easily transmitted, all close family members should be treated. Instruct patient/caregiver on appropriate use, transmission prevention, possible side effects and appropriate interventions, and adverse symptoms to report. **Pregnancy risk factor C** - benefits of use should outweigh possible risks. Note breast-feeding caution.

**Patient Information/Instruction:** Take exactly as directed for full course of medication. Tablets may be chewed, swallowed whole, or crushed and mixed with food. Increase dietary intake of fruit juices. All family members and close friends should also be treated. To reduce possibility of reinfection, wash hands and scrub nails carefully with soap and hot water before handling food, before eating, and before and after toileting. Keep hands out of mouth. Disinfect toilet daily and launder bed lines, undergarments, and nightclothes daily with hot water and soap. Do not go barefoot and do not sit directly on grass or ground. May cause dizziness, fainting, lightheadedness (use caution when driving or engaging in tasks requiring alertness until response to drug is known); abdominal pain, nausea, dry mouth, or vomiting (frequent small meals, frequent mouth care, sucking lozenges, or chewing gum may help). Report skin rash or itching, unresolved diarrhea or vomiting, CNS changes (hallucinations, delirium, acute headache), change in color of urine or stool, or easy bruising or unusual bleeding. **Pregnancy/breast-feeding precautions:** Inform prescriber if you are pregnant. Consult prescriber if breast-feeding.

- **Thiamazole** *see* Methimazole *on page 741*
- **Thiamilate®** *see* Thiamine *on this page*

## Thiamine (THYE a min)

**U.S. Brand Names** Thiamilate®

**Synonyms** Aneurine Hydrochloride; Thiaminium Chloride Hydrochloride; Vitamin $B_1$

**Therapeutic Category** Vitamin, Water Soluble

**Pregnancy Risk Factor** A/C (if dose exceeds RDA recommendation)

**Lactation** Enters breast milk/compatible

**Use** Treatment of thiamine deficiency including beriberi, Wernicke's encephalopathy syndrome, and peripheral neuritis associated with pellagra, alcoholic patients with altered sensorium; various genetic metabolic disorders

**Mechanism of Action/Effect** An essential coenzyme in carbohydrate metabolism by combining with adenosine triphosphate to form thiamine pyrophosphate

**Contraindications** Hypersensitivity to thiamine or any component

**Warnings** Use with caution with parenteral route (especially I.V.) of administration. Pregnancy factor C (if dose exceeds RDA recommendation).

**Food Interactions** High carbohydrate diets may increase thiamine requirement.

**Effects on Lab Values** False-positive for uric acid using the phosphotungstate method and for urobilinogen using the Ehrlich's reagent; large doses may interfere with the spectrophotometric determination of serum theophylline concentration

**Adverse Reactions** <1% (Limited to important or life-threatening symptoms): Cardiovascular collapse and death, paresthesia

**Pharmacodynamics/Kinetics**

**Excretion:** Renally as unchanged drug, and as pyrimidine after body storage sites become saturated

**Formulations**

Thiamine hydrochloride:

Injection: 100 mg/mL (1 mL, 2 mL, 10 mL, 30 mL); 200 mg/mL (30 mL)

Tablet: 50 mg, 100 mg, 250 mg, 500 mg

Tablet, enteric coated: 20 mg

**Dosing**

**Adults:**

Recommended daily allowance: >14 years: 1-1.5 mg

Thiamine deficiency (beriberi): 5-30 mg/dose I.M. or I.V. 3 times/day (if critically ill); then orally 5-30 mg/day in single or divided doses 3 times/day for 1 month

Wernicke's encephalopathy: Initial: 100 mg I.V., then 50-100 mg/day I.M. or I.V. until consuming a regular, balanced diet

Dietary supplement (depends on caloric or carbohydrate content of the diet): 1-2 mg/day

**Note:** The above doses can be found in multivitamin preparations.

Metabolic disorders: Oral: 10-20 mg/day (dosages up to 4 g/day in divided doses have been used)

**Elderly:** Refer to adult dosing.

**Administration**

**I.M.:** Parenteral form may be administered by I.M. or slow I.V. injection.

**I.V.:** Doses are usually administered over 1-2 minutes.

**Stability**

**Storage:** Protect oral dosage forms from light.

**Compatibility:** Incompatible with alkaline or neutral solutions and with oxidizing or reducing agents.

**Additional Nursing Issues**

**Physical Assessment:** Assess knowledge/teach patient appropriate administration (injection technique and needle disposal if I.M. self-administered) and dietary instruction. **Pregnancy risk factor A/C** - see Pregnancy Risk Factor for cautious use.

**Patient Information/Instruction:** Take exactly as directed; do not discontinue without consulting prescriber (deficiency state can occur in as little as 3 weeks). Follow dietary instructions (dietary sources include legumes, pork, beef, whole grains, yeast, fresh vegetables).

♦ **Thiaminium Chloride Hydrochloride** *see* Thiamine *on previous page*

## Thiethylperazine (thye eth il PER a zeen)

**U.S. Brand Names** Norzine®; Torecan®

**Therapeutic Category** Antiemetic

**Pregnancy Risk Factor** X

**Lactation** Excretion in breast milk unknown

**Use** Relief of nausea and vomiting

**Unlabeled use:** Treatment of vertigo

**Mechanism of Action/Effect** Blocks postsynaptic mesolimbic dopaminergic receptors in the brain; exhibits a strong alpha-adrenergic blocking effect and depresses the release of hypothalamic and hypophyseal hormones; acts directly on chemoreceptor trigger zone and vomiting center

**Contraindications** Hypersensitivity to thiethylperazine or any component; cross-sensitivity to other phenothiazines may exist; comatose states; pregnancy

**Warnings** Reduce or discontinue if extrapyramidal effects occur. Postural hypotension may occur after I.M. injection. The injectable form contains sulfite which may cause allergic reactions in some patients. Use caution in patients with narrow-angle glaucoma.

**Drug Interactions**

**Increased Effect/Toxicity:** Increased effect/toxicity with CNS depressants (eg, anesthetics, opiates, tranquilizers, alcohol), lithium, atropine, epinephrine, MAO inhibitors, tricyclic antidepressants

**Adverse Reactions**

>10%:

Central nervous system: Drowsiness, dizziness

Gastrointestinal: Dry mouth

Respiratory: Dry nose

1% to 10%:

Cardiovascular: Tachycardia, orthostatic hypotension

Central nervous system: Confusion, convulsions, extrapyramidal effects, tardive dyskinesia, fever, headache

Dermatologic: Rash

Hematologic: Agranulocytosis

Hepatic: Cholestatic jaundice

Otic: Tinnitus

**Overdose/Toxicology** Symptoms of overdose include deep sleep, coma, extrapyramidal symptoms, abnormal involuntary muscle movements, and hypotension. Treatment is symptom directed and supportive.

**Pharmacodynamics/Kinetics**

**Onset:** Onset of antiemetic effect: Within 30 minutes

**Duration:** ~4 hours

**Formulations**

Thiethylperazine maleate:

Injection: 5 mg/mL (2 mL)

Suppository, rectal: 10 mg

Tablet: 10 mg

**Dosing**

**Adults:**

Oral, I.M., rectal: 10 mg 1-3 times/day as needed

I.V. and S.C. routes of administration are not recommended

(Continued)

## Thiethylperazine *(Continued)*

**Elderly:** Refer to adult dosing.

**Renal Impairment:** Not dialyzable (0% to 5%)

**Hepatic Impairment:** Use with caution.

**Administration**

**I.M.:** Inject I.M. deeply into large muscle mass. Patient should be lying down and remain so for at least 1 hour after administration.

**I.V.:** I.V. injection is **not** recommended.

**Additional Nursing Issues**

**Physical Assessment:** Assess response (extrapyramidal effects, postural hypotension, abnormal muscle movements) and effectiveness of therapy at beginning of treatment and periodically thereafter.

I.M.: Patient should remain lying down for 1 hour following injection.

**Pregnancy risk factor X** - determine that patient is not pregnant before beginning treatment and do not give to women of childbearing age or males who may have intercourse with childbearing women unless both male and female are capable of complying with barrier contraceptive measures during therapy and for 1 month following therapy. Note breast-feeding caution.

**Patient Information/Instruction:** Take as directed; do not use more than recommended. Do not use alcohol and prescription or OTC depressant without consulting prescriber. May cause drowsiness, dizziness, stupor (use caution when driving or engaging in tasks requiring alertness until response to drug is known); dry mouth (frequent oral care and sucking on lozenges may help); photosensitivity (use sunscreen, wear protective clothing and eyewear, and avoid direct sunlight); postural hypotension (rise slowly from sitting or lying position and use caution when climbing stairs). Report abnormal or involuntary muscle movements or twitching or facial tics, acute drowsiness or restlessness, excessive fatigue or dizziness. **Pregnancy/breast-feeding precautions:** Inform prescriber if you are pregnant. Do not get pregnant during or for 1 month following therapy. Male: Do not cause a pregnancy. Male/female: Consult prescriber for instruction on appropriate contraceptive measures. This drug may cause severe fetal defects. Consult prescriber if breast-feeding.

**Geriatric Considerations:** Elderly are more likely to experience extrapyramidal reactions than younger adults. Dystonic reactions are possible but seen more often in younger adults. Confusion is also possible in the elderly.

**Additional Information**

Some formulations may contain sulfites.

pH: 3-4

**Related Information**

Antiemetics for Chemotherapy-Induced Nausea and Vomiting *on page 1307*

♦ **Thimerosal** *see page 1294*

## Thioguanine (thye oh GWAH neen)

**Synonyms** 2-Amino-6-Mercaptopurine; TG; 6-TG; 6-Thioguanine; Tioguanine

**Therapeutic Category** Antineoplastic Agent, Antimetabolite

**Pregnancy Risk Factor** D

**Lactation** Excretion in breast milk unknown

**Use** Remission induction in acute myelogenous (nonlymphocytic) leukemia; treatment of chronic myelogenous leukemia and granulocytic leukemia

**Mechanism of Action/Effect** Purine analog that is incorporated into DNA and RNA resulting in the blockage of synthesis and metabolism of purine nucleotides

**Contraindications** Hypersensitivity to thioguanine or any component; history of previous therapy resistance with either thioguanine or mercaptopurine (there is usually complete cross resistance between these two); pregnancy

**Warnings** The U.S. Food and Drug Administration (FDA) currently recommends that procedures for proper handling and disposal of antineoplastic agents be considered. Use with caution and reduce dose of thioguanine in patients with renal or hepatic impairment. Thioguanine is potentially carcinogenic and teratogenic. Myelosuppression may be delayed.

**Drug Interactions**

**Increased Effect/Toxicity:** Allopurinol can be used in full doses with 6-TG unlike 6-MP. Use with busulfan may cause hepatotoxicity and esophageal varices.

**Food Interactions** Enhanced absorption if administered between meals.

**Adverse Reactions**

>10%:

- Hematologic: Leukopenia; Thrombocytopenia; Myelosuppressive:
  - WBC: Moderate
  - Platelets: Moderate
  - Onset (days): 7-10
  - Nadir (days): 14
  - Recovery (days): 21

1% to 10%:

- Dermatologic: Skin rash
- Endocrine & metabolic: Hyperuricemia
- Gastrointestinal: Mild nausea or vomiting, anorexia, stomatitis, diarrhea
  - Emetic potential: Low (<10%)
- Neuromuscular & skeletal: Unsteady gait

<1% (Limited to important or life-threatening symptoms): Neurotoxicity, hepatitis, jaundice, veno-occlusive hepatic disease

**Overdose/Toxicology** Symptoms of overdose include bone marrow suppression, nausea, vomiting, malaise, hypertension, and sweating. Treatment is supportive. Dialysis is not useful.

**Pharmacodynamics/Kinetics**

**Distribution:** Crosses placenta

**Half-life Elimination:** 11 hours

**Time to Peak:** Within 8 hours

**Metabolism:** Liver

**Excretion:** Urine

**Formulations** Tablet, scored: 40 mg

**Dosing**

**Adults:** Total daily dose can be given at one time; offers little advantage over mercaptopurine; is sometimes ordered as 6-thioguanine, with 6 being part of the drug name and not some kind of unit or strength

Oral (**refer to individual protocols**): 2-3 mg/kg/day calculated to nearest 20 mg or 75-200 mg/m$^2$/day in 1-2 divided doses for 5-7 days or until remission is attained

**Renal Impairment:** Reduce dose.

**Hepatic Impairment:** Reduce dose.

**Monitoring Laboratory Tests** CBC with differential and platelet count, liver function, serum uric acid

**Additional Nursing Issues**

**Physical Assessment:** Monitor results of laboratory tests. Monitor for adverse effects as noted above (eg, nutritional status, renal function (fluid status, I & O ratio, edema/dehydration), myelosuppression, opportunistic infection). Instruct patient on safe use, possible side effects, and symptoms to report. **Pregnancy risk factor D** - assess knowledge/teach patient in appropriate barrier contraceptive measures. Note breast-feeding caution.

**Patient Information/Instruction:** You may experience nausea and vomiting, diarrhea, or loss of appetite (frequent small meals may help/request medication) or weakness or lethargy (use caution when driving or engaging in tasks requiring alertness until response to drug is known). Use good oral care to reduce incidence of mouth sores. Maintain adequate hydration (2-3 L/day of fluids unless instructed to restrict fluid intake). May cause headache (request medication). Report signs or symptoms of infection (eg, fever, chills, sore throat, burning urination, fatigue), bleeding (eg, tarry stools, easy bruising), vision changes, unresolved mouth sores, nausea or vomiting, CNS changes (hallucinations), or respiratory difficulty. Avoid crowds or exposure to infected persons; you will be susceptible to infection. **Pregnancy/breast-feeding precautions:** Do not get pregnant; use appropriate contraceptive measures to prevent possible harm to the fetus. The drug may cause permanent sterility and may cause birth defects. Consult prescriber if breast-feeding.

♦ **6-Thioguanine** *see* Thioguanine *on previous page*

## Thioridazine (thye oh RID a zeen)

**U.S. Brand Names** Mellaril®; Mellaril-S®

**Therapeutic Category** Antipsychotic Agent, Phenothazine, Piperidine

**Pregnancy Risk Factor** C

**Lactation** Excretion in breast milk unknown/not recommended

**Use** Management of manifestations of psychotic disorders; alcohol withdrawal; dementia in the elderly; behavioral problems in children

**Mechanism of Action/Effect** Blocks postsynaptic mesolimbic dopaminergic receptors in the brain; exhibits a strong alpha-adrenergic blocking effect and depresses the release of hypothalamic and hypophyseal hormones

**Contraindications** Hypersensitivity to thioridazine or any component (cross reactivity between phenothiazines may occur); severe CNS depression; circulatory collapse; severe hypotension; bone marrow suppression; blood dyscrasias; coma

**Warnings** Highly sedating, use with caution in disorders where CNS depression is a feature. Use with caution in Parkinson's disease. Use with caution in patients with hemodynamic instability; bone marrow suppression; predisposition to seizures; subcortical brain damage; severe cardiac, hepatic, renal, or respiratory disease. Neuroleptics may cause swallowing difficulty. Use with caution in breast cancer or other prolactin-dependent tumors (may elevate prolactin levels). May alter temperature regulation or mask toxicity of other drugs due to antiemetic effects. May alter cardiac conduction - life threatening arrhythmias have occurred with therapeutic doses of phenothiazines. May cause orthostatic hypotension.

Phenothiazines may cause anticholinergic effects (eg, confusion, agitation, constipation, dry mouth, blurred vision, urinary retention); therefore, use with caution in patients with decreased gastrointestinal motility, urinary retention, BPH, xerostomia, or visual problems. Conditions which also may be exacerbated by cholinergic blockade include narrow-angle glaucoma (screening is recommended) and worsening of myasthenia gravis. Relative to other neuroleptics, thioridazine has a high potency of cholinergic blockade.

May cause extrapyramidal reactions including pseudoparkinsonism, acute dystonic reactions, akathisia, and tardive dyskinesia (risk of these reactions is low relative to other neuroleptics). May be associated with neuroleptic malignant syndrome (NMS) or pigmentary retinopathy (particularly at doses >1g/day).

Pregnancy factor C.

(Continued)

## Thioridazine *(Continued)*

**Drug Interactions**

**Cytochrome P-450 Effect:** CYP1A2 and 2D6 enzyme substrate; CYP2D6 enzyme inhibitor

**Decreased Effect:** Decreased effect with anticholinergics. Decreased effect of guanethidine.

**Increased Effect/Toxicity:** Increased toxicity with CNS depressants, epinephrine (hypotension), lithium (rare), tricyclic antidepressants (cardiotoxicity), propranolol, pindolol.

**Effects on Lab Values** False-positives for phenylketonuria, urinary amylase, uroporphyrins, urobilinogen

**Adverse Reactions**

>10%:

- Central nervous system: Pseudoparkinsonism, akathisia, dystonias, tardive dyskinesia (persistent), dizziness
- Cardiovascular: Hypotension, orthostatic hypotension
- Gastrointestinal: Constipation
- Ocular: Pigmentary retinopathy
- Respiratory: Nasal congestion
- Miscellaneous: Decreased sweating

1% to 10%:

- Dermatologic: Photosensitivity, rash
- Endocrine & metabolic: Changes in menstrual cycle, changes in libido, breast pain
- Gastrointestinal: Weight gain, nausea, vomiting, stomach pain
- Genitourinary: Dysuria, ejaculatory disturbances
- Neuromuscular & skeletal: Tremor

<1% (Limited to important or life-threatening symptoms): Neuroleptic malignant syndrome (NMS), lowering of seizures threshold, agranulocytosis, leukopenia, cholestatic jaundice, hepatotoxicity

**Overdose/Toxicology** Symptoms of overdose include deep sleep, coma, extrapyramidal symptoms, abnormal involuntary muscle movements, hypotension, and arrhythmias. Treatment is symptom directed and supportive.

**Pharmacodynamics/Kinetics**

**Half-life Elimination:** 21-25 hours

**Time to Peak:** Within 1 hour

**Duration:** 4-5 days

**Formulations**

Thioridazine hydrochloride:

- Concentrate, oral, as hydrochloride: 30 mg/mL (120 mL); 100 mg/mL (3.4 mL, 120 mL)
- Suspension, oral, as hydrochloride: 25 mg/5 mL (480 mL); 100 mg/5 mL (480 mL)
- Tablet, as hydrochloride: 10 mg, 15 mg, 25 mg, 50 mg, 100 mg, 150 mg, 200 mg

**Dosing**

**Adults:** Oral:

- Psychosis: Initial: 50-100 mg 3 times/day with gradual increments as needed and tolerated; maximum: 800 mg/day in 2-4 divided doses; if >65 years, initial dose: 10 mg 3 times/day
- Depressive disorders, dementia: Initial: 25 mg 3 times/day; maintenance dose: 20-200 mg/day

**Elderly:** Oral: Nonpsychotic patient; dementia behavior: Initial: 10-25 mg 1-2 times/day; increase at 4- to 7-day intervals by 10-25 mg/day; increase dose intervals (qd, bid, etc) as necessary to control response or side effects. Maximum daily dose: 400 mg; gradual increases (titration) may prevent some side effects or decrease their severity.

**Renal Impairment:** Not dialyzable (0% to 5%)

**Administration**

**Oral:** Oral concentrate must be diluted in 2-4 oz of liquid (eg, water, fruit juice, carbonated drinks, milk, or pudding) before administration. Do not take antacid within 1 hour of taking drug. **Note:** Avoid skin contact with oral suspension or solution; may cause contact dermatitis.

**Stability**

**Storage:** Protect all dosage forms from light.

**Monitoring Laboratory Tests** Baseline liver and kidney function, CBC prior to and periodically during therapy, slit lamp ophthalmic exam before and during therapy

**Additional Nursing Issues**

**Physical Assessment:** Assess other medications patient is taking for effectiveness and interactions (see Drug Interactions). See Contraindications and Warnings/Precautions for cautious use. Has potential for psychological or physiological dependence, abuse, and tolerance. Review ophthalmic exam and monitor laboratory results (see above), therapeutic response (mental status, mood, affect, gait), and adverse reactions at beginning of therapy and periodically with long-term use (eg, excess sedation, extrapyramidal effects, tardive dyskinesia, CNS changes - see Adverse Reactions and Overdose/Toxicology). Avoid skin contact with liquid medication; may cause contact dermatitis (wash immediately with warm, soapy water). Initiate at lower doses (see Dosing) and taper dosage slowly when discontinuing. Assess knowledge/teach patient appropriate use, interventions to reduce side effects, and adverse symptoms to report (see below). **Pregnancy risk factor C** - benefits of use should outweigh possible risks. Breast-feeding is not recommended.

**Patient Information/Instruction:** Use exactly as directed (do not increase dose or frequency); may cause physical and/or psychological dependence. Do not discontinue without consulting prescriber. Tablets/capsules may be taken with food. Mix oral solution with 2-4 ounces of liquid (eg, juice, milk, water, pudding). Do not take within 2 hours of any antacid. Store away from light. Avoid excess alcohol or caffeine and other prescription or OTC medications not approved by prescriber. Maintain adequate hydration (2-3 L/day of fluids unless instructed to restrict fluid intake). Avoid skin contact with liquid medication; may cause contact dermatitis (wash immediately with warm, soapy water). May turn urine red-brown (normal). You may experience excess drowsiness, lightheadedness, dizziness, or blurred vision (use caution driving or when engaging in tasks requiring alertness until response to drug is known); nausea, vomiting, or dry mouth (small frequent meals, frequent mouth care, chewing gum, or sucking lozenges may help); constipation (increased exercise, fluids, or dietary fruit and fiber may help); postural hypotension (use caution climbing stairs or when changing position from lying or sitting to standing); urinary retention (void before taking medication); ejaculatory dysfunction (reversible); decreased perspiration (avoid strenuous exercise in hot environments); photosensitivity (use sunscreen, wear protective clothing and eyewear, and avoid direct sunlight). Report persistent CNS effects (eg, trembling fingers, altered gait or balance, excessive sedation, seizures, unusual movements, anxiety, abnormal thoughts, confusion, personality changes); chest pain, palpitations, rapid heartbeat, severe dizziness; unresolved urinary retention or changes in urinary pattern; altered menstrual pattern, change in libido, swelling or pain in breasts (male or female); vision changes; skin rash, irritation, or changes in color of skin (gray-blue); or worsening of condition. **Pregnancy/breast-feeding precautions:** Inform prescriber if you are or intend to be pregnant. Breast-feeding is not recommended.

**Dietary Issues:** Increase dietary intake of riboflavin. Liquid formulation is incompatible with enteral formulas.

**Geriatric Considerations:** (See Warnings/Precautions, Adverse Reactions, and Overdose/Toxicology.) Elderly patients have an increased risk of adverse response to side effects or adverse reactions to antipsychotics. These can include but are not limited to the following.

Anticholinergic effects: CNS toxicity with confusion, memory loss, psychotic behavior, and agitation.

Extrapyramidal effects (EPS): Parkinson's syndrome and akathisia may occur as often as 50% in patients >60 years of age. Tardive dyskinesia (motor restlessness) may be 40% in elderly; may be related to duration and total accumulated dose over time; may be somewhat reversible if diagnosed early enough.

Orthostatic hypotension: Increased risk for falls.

Sedation: In nonpsychotic patients, may result in feelings of depersonalization, derealization, and dysphoria.

Cardiac toxicity: Cardiac arrhythmias have occurred with therapeutic doses of antipsychotics.

Malignant neuroleptic syndrome: Development of hyperthermia, muscular rigidity, autonomic instability, and altered mental status.

Many elderly patients receive antipsychotic medications for inappropriate nonpsychotic behavior. Before initiating antipsychotic medication, all possible reversible causes should be investigated. Stress may cause acute "confusion" or worsening of baseline nonpsychotic behaviors; any changes in disease state (in any organ) may result in behavioral changes. Common acute changes in behavior may be due also to increases in drug dose addition, or addition of a new drug to the regimen; fluid/electrolyte alterations; infections; or changes in the environment.

Meta-analysis of controlled trials of antipsychotic (phenothiazines, butyrophenones) use with agitated, demented, elderly patients has concluded that the use of neuroleptics results in a response rate of 18%. Clearly, neuroleptic therapy for behavior control should be limited, with frequent attempts to withdraw the agent for behavior control. When use is indicated, initial doses should be lower to start and monitored closely.

**Additional Information** The oral concentration formulation contains ethanol.

Thioridazine: Mellaril-S® oral suspension

Thioridazine hydrochloride: Mellaril® oral solution and tablet

**Related Information**

Antipsychotic Agents Comparison *on page 1371*
Antipsychotic Medication Guidelines *on page 1436*

## Thiotepa (thye oh TEP a)

**Synonyms** TESPA; Triethylenethiophosphoramide; TSPA

**Therapeutic Category** Antineoplastic Agent, Alkylating Agent

**Pregnancy Risk Factor** D

**Lactation** Enters breast milk/not recommended

**Use** Treatment of superficial tumors of the bladder; palliative treatment of adenocarcinoma of breast or ovary; lymphomas and sarcomas; controlling intracavitary effusions caused by metastatic tumors

I.T. use: CNS leukemia/lymphoma

**Mechanism of Action/Effect** Alkylating agent that reacts with DNA phosphate groups to produce cross-linking of DNA strands leading to inhibition of DNA, RNA, and protein synthesis; mechanism of action has not been explored as thoroughly as the other alkylating agents, it is presumed that the aziridine rings open and react as nitrogen mustard; reactivity is enhanced at a lower pH

(Continued)

## Thiotepa *(Continued)*

**Contraindications** Hypersensitivity to thiotepa or any component; severe myelosuppression with leukocyte count <3000/mm$^3$ or platelet count <150,000/mm$^3$; pregnancy

**Warnings** The U.S. Food and Drug Administration (FDA) currently recommends that procedures for proper handling and disposal of antineoplastic agents be considered.

Preparation of thiotepa should be performed in a Class II laminar flow biologic safety cabinet. Personnel should be wearing surgical gloves and a closed front surgical gown with knit cuffs. Appropriate safety equipment is recommended for preparation, administration, and disposal of antineoplastics. If thiotepa contacts the skin, wash and flush thoroughly with water.

The drug is potentially mutagenic, carcinogenic, and teratogenic. Reduce dosage in patients with hepatic, renal, or bone marrow damage.

**Drug Interactions**

**Increased Effect/Toxicity:** Other alkylating agents or irradiation used concomitantly with thiotepa intensifies toxicity rather than enhancing therapeutic response. Prolonged muscular paralysis and respiratory depression may occur when neuromuscular blocking agents are administered. Succinylcholine and other neuromuscular blocking agents' action can be prolonged due to thiotepa inhibiting plasma pseudocholinesterase.

**Adverse Reactions**

>10%:

Hematopoietic: Dose-limiting toxicity which is dose-related and cumulative; moderate to severe leukopenia and severe thrombocytopenia have occurred. Anemia and pancytopenia may become fatal, so careful hematologic monitoring is required; intravesical administration may cause bone marrow suppression as well.

Hematologic: Myelosuppressive:
- WBC: Moderate
- Platelets: Severe
- Onset (days): 7-10
- Nadir (days): 14
- Recovery (days): 28

1% to 10%:
- Central nervous system: Dizziness, fever, headache
- Dermatologic: Alopecia, rash, pruritus, hyperpigmentation with high-dose therapy
- Endocrine & metabolic: Hyperuricemia
- Gastrointestinal: Anorexia, nausea and vomiting rarely occur
  - Emetic potential: Low (<10%)
- Genitourinary: Hemorrhagic cystitis
- Local: Pain at injection site
- Renal: Hematuria
- Miscellaneous: Tightness of the throat, allergic reactions

<1% (Limited to important or life-threatening symptoms): Carcinogenesis: Like other alkylating agents, this drug is carcinogenic.

**BMT:**
- Central nervous system: Confusion, inappropriate behavior, somnolence
- Dermatologic: Hyperpigmentation
- Gastrointestinal: Mucositis, mild nausea and vomiting
- Hepatic: Serum transaminitis, hyperbilirubinemia

**Overdose/Toxicology** Symptoms of overdose include nausea, vomiting, precipitation of uric acid in kidney tubules, bone marrow suppression, and bleeding. Therapy is supportive only. Thiotepa is dialyzable. Transfusions of whole blood or platelets have been proven beneficial.

**Pharmacodynamics/Kinetics**

**Half-life Elimination:** 109 minutes with dose-dependent clearance

**Metabolism:** Liver

**Excretion:** Urine

**Formulations** Powder for injection: 15 mg

**Dosing**

**Adults:** Refer to individual protocols. Dosing must be based on the clinical and hematologic response of the patient.

- I.M., I.V., S.C.: 30-60 mg/m$^2$ once per week
- I.V. doses of 0.3-0.4 mg/kg by rapid I.V. administration every 1-4 weeks, or 0.2 mg/kg or 6-8 mg/m$^2$/day for 4-5 days every 2-4 weeks
- High-dose therapy for bone marrow transplant: I.V.: 500 mg/m$^2$; up to 900 mg/m$^2$
- I.M. doses of 15-30 mg in various schedules have been given
- Intracavitary: 0.6-0.8 mg/kg
- Intrapericardial dose: Usually 15-30 mg
- Intravesical: Used for treatment of carcinoma of the bladder; patients should be dehydrated for 8-12 hours prior to treatment; instill 60 mg (in 30-60 mL of sterile water) into the bladder and retain for a minimum of 2 hours. Patient should be positioned every 15 minutes for maximal area exposure. Instillations usually once a week for 4 weeks.
- Intratumor: Use a 22-gauge needle to inject thiotepa directly into the tumor. Initial: 0.6-0.8 mg/kg (diluted to 10 mg/mL) are used every 1-4 weeks; maintenance dose: 0.07-0.8 mg/kg are administered at 1- to 4-week intervals
- Ophthalmic: 0.05% solution in LR has been instilled into the eye every 3 hours for 6-8 weeks for the prevention of pterygium recurrence

BMT high dose: I.V.: 360-1125 mg/m$^2$ as a single dose or divided into 2 daily doses; generally combined with other high-dose chemotherapeutic drugs.

**Administration**

**I.V.:** Administer I.V., intracavitary, and intrathecally.

**I.V. Detail:** Solutions should be filtered through a 0.22 micron filter prior to administration. A 1 mg/mL solution is considered isotonic; not a vesicant.

**BMT only:** Central nervous system effects increased with doses >1000 mg/m$^2$. Hyperpigmentation was most common on occluded areas of the skin.

**Stability**

**Storage:** Store intact vials under refrigeration (2°C to 8°C) and protect from light.

**Reconstitution:** Dilute powder 1.5 mL SWI to a concentration of 10 mg/mL which is stable for 8 hours at refrigeration. Further dilution in NS, $D_5W$, or lactated Ringer's should be used immediately (within 1 hour of preparation). Thiotepa is stable for 24 hours at a concentration of 5 mg/mL in NS at 8°C and 23°C; however, stability decreases significantly at concentrations <5 mg/mL (1 hour).

**Standard I.V. dilution:**

I.V. push: Dose/syringe (concentration = 10 mg/mL)

IVPB: Dose/250 mL $D_5W$

Further dilution in NS, $D_5W$, or lactated Ringer's should be used immediately (within one hour of preparation)

Continuous 24-hour I.V. infusion:

Dose ≥250 mg: qs to 50 mL (total volume) in NS

Dose 230-250 mg: qs to 45 mL (total volume) in NS

Dose 200-230 mg: qs to 40 mL (total volume) in NS

Thiotepa is stable for 24 hours at a concentration of 5 mg/mL in NS at 8°C and 23°C; however, stability decreases significantly at concentrations <5 mg/mL (1 hour).

**Standard intravesicular dilution:** 60 mg/30-60 mL SWI

Intravesicular doses should be prepared with 60 mg of drug diluted into 30-60 mL SWI. Solution is placed via catheter and retained for 2 hours for maximum effect.

**Standard intrathecal dilution:** 10-15 mg/3-5 mL lactated Ringer's

Intrathecal doses of 1-10 mg/m$^2$ should be diluted to 1-5 mg in lactated Ringer's.

All solutions should be **prepared fresh** and administered within 1 hour of preparation.

**Compatibility:** See the Chemotherapy Compatibility Chart *on page 1311*.

**Monitoring Laboratory Tests** CBC with differential, platelet count, uric acid, urinalysis

**Additional Nursing Issues**

**Physical Assessment:** Close monitoring of all blood tests is necessary to assess for adverse hematopoietic reaction (see Adverse Reactions). Be alert for unusual bleeding, petechia, blood in urine or stool, and avoid or use caution with any invasive procedures. Monitor for opportunistic infection and symptoms of gout (hyperuricemia). **Pregnancy risk factor D** - assess knowledge/teach both male and female appropriate use of barrier contraceptives. Breast-feeding is not recommended.

**Patient Information/Instruction:** This drug can only be administered I.V. You will require regular blood tests to assess response to therapy. Avoid alcohol and aspirin or aspirin-containing medications unless approved by prescriber. Maintain adequate hydration (2-3 L/day of fluids unless instructed to restrict fluid intake) to prevent kidney damage. For nausea and vomiting, small frequent meals, chewing gum, or sucking lozenges may help, antiemetics may be prescribed. You may experience amenorrhea or changed sperm production, rash, hair loss, or loss of appetite (maintaining adequate nutrition is important). You may have increased sensitivity to infection (avoid crowds and infected persons). Report unusual bleeding or bruising, persistent fever or chills, sore throat, sores in mouth or vagina, blackened stool, or difficulty breathing. **Pregnancy/breast-feeding precautions:** Do not get pregnant while taking this medication; both male and female should use appropriate barrier contraceptive measures. Breast-feeding is not recommended.

## Thiothixene (thye oh THIKS een)

**U.S. Brand Names** Navane®

**Synonyms** Tiotixene

**Therapeutic Category** Antipsychotic Agent, Thioxanthene Derivative

**Pregnancy Risk Factor** C

**Lactation** Excretion in breast milk unknown/not recommended

**Use** Management of psychotic disorders

**Mechanism of Action/Effect** Elicits antipsychotic activity by postsynaptic blockade of CNS dopamine receptors resulting in inhibition of dopamine-mediated effects; also has alpha-adrenergic blocking activity

**Contraindications** Hypersensitivity to trifluoperazine or any component (cross reactivity between phenothiazines may occur); severe CNS depression; circulatory collapse; blood dyscrasias; coma

**Warnings** May be sedating, use with caution in disorders where CNS depression is a feature. Use with caution in Parkinson's disease. Use with caution in patients with hemodynamic instability; predisposition to seizures; subcortical brain damage; bone marrow suppression; or severe cardiac, hepatic, renal, or respiratory disease. Neuroleptics may cause swallowing difficulty. Use with caution in breast cancer or other prolactin-dependent tumors (may elevate prolactin levels). May alter temperature regulation or mask toxicity of other drugs due to antiemetic effects. May alter cardiac conduction - life-threatening arrhythmias have occurred with therapeutic doses of neuroleptics. May cause orthostatic hypotension.

(Continued)

## Thiothixene *(Continued)*

Phenothiazines may cause anticholinergic effects (eg, confusion, agitation, constipation, dry mouth, blurred vision, urinary retention); therefore, use with caution in patients with decreased gastrointestinal motility, urinary retention, BPH, xerostomia, or visual problems. Conditions which also may be exacerbated by cholinergic blockade include narrow-angle glaucoma (screening is recommended) and worsening of myasthenia gravis. Relative to other neuroleptics, thiothixene has a low potency of cholinergic blockade.

May cause extrapyramidal reactions including pseudoparkinsonism, acute dystonic reactions, akathisia, and tardive dyskinesia (risk of these reactions is high relative to other neuroleptics). May be associated with neuroleptic malignant syndrome (NMS) or pigmentary retinopathy.

Pregnancy factor C.

**Drug Interactions**

**Cytochrome P-450 Effect:** CYP1A2 enzyme substrate

**Decreased Effect:** Decreased effect of guanethidine.

**Increased Effect/Toxicity:** Increased toxicity with CNS depressants, anticholinergics, and alcohol.

**Effects on Lab Values** ↑ cholesterol (S), glucose; ↓ uric acid (S); may cause false-positive pregnancy test

**Adverse Reactions**

>10%:

- Central nervous system: Pseudoparkinsonism, akathisia, dystonias, tardive dyskinesia (persistent), dizziness
- Gastrointestinal: Constipation
- Ocular: Pigmentary retinopathy
- Respiratory: Nasal congestion
- Miscellaneous: Decreased sweating

1% to 10%:

- Dermatologic: Photosensitivity, rash
- Endocrine & metabolic: Changes in menstrual cycle, changes in libido, breast pain
- Gastrointestinal: Weight gain, nausea, vomiting, stomach pain
- Genitourinary: Dysuria, ejaculatory disturbances
- Neuromuscular & skeletal: Tremor

<1% (Limited to important or life-threatening symptoms): Neuroleptic malignant syndrome (NMS), lowering of seizures threshold, agranulocytosis, leukopenia, cholestatic jaundice, hepatotoxicity, hypotension, orthostatic hypotension

**Overdose/Toxicology** Symptoms of overdose include muscle twitching, drowsiness, dizziness, rigidity, tremor, hypotension, and cardiac arrhythmias. Treatment is symptom directed and supportive.

**Pharmacodynamics/Kinetics**

**Protein Binding:** 91% to 99%

**Distribution:** Widely distributed

**Half-life Elimination:** >24 hours with chronic use

**Metabolism:** Liver

**Excretion:** Liver and kidney

**Formulations**

- Capsule: 1 mg, 2 mg, 5 mg, 10 mg, 20 mg
- Concentrate, as hydrochloride: 5 mg/mL
- Injection, as hydrochloride: 2 mg/mL (2 mL)
- Powder for injection, as hydrochloride: 5 mg/mL (2 mL)

**Dosing**

**Adults:** Mild to moderate psychosis:

- Oral: 2 mg 3 times/day, up to 20-30 mg/day; more severe psychosis: Initial: 5 mg 2 times/day, may increase gradually, if necessary; maximum: 60 mg/day
- I.M.: 4 mg 2-4 times/day, increase dose gradually; usual: 16-20 mg/day; maximum: 30 mg/day; change to oral dose as soon as able

**Elderly:** Nonpsychotic patients, dementia behavior: Initial: 1-2 mg 1-2 times/day; increase dose at 4- to 7-day intervals by 1-2 mg/day. Increase dosing intervals (bid, tid, etc) as necessary to control response or side effects; maximum daily dose: 30 mg. Gradual increases in dose may prevent some side effects or decrease their severity.

**Renal Impairment:** Not dialyzable (0% to 5%)

**Administration**

**Oral:** Oral concentration contains 7% alcohol. Dilute immediately before administration with water, fruit juice, milk, etc. **Note:** Avoid skin contact with oral medication; may cause contact dermatitis.

**Stability**

**Storage:** Refrigerate powder for injection.

**Reconstitution:** Reconstituted powder for injection is stable at room temperature for 48 hours.

**Monitoring Laboratory Tests** Baseline liver and kidney function, CBC prior to and periodically during therapy, ophthalmic exam

**Additional Nursing Issues**

**Physical Assessment:** Assess other medications patient is taking for effectiveness and interactions (see Drug Interactions). See Contraindications and Warnings/Precautions for cautious use. Has potential for psychological or physiological dependence, abuse, and tolerance. Review ophthalmic exam and monitor laboratory results (see above), therapeutic response (mental status, mood, affect, gait), and adverse reactions at beginning of therapy and periodically with long-term use (eg, excess sedation, extrapyramidal effects, tardive dyskinesia, CNS changes - see Adverse Reactions and Overdose/Toxicology). With I.M. use, monitor closely for hypotension. Avoid skin contact with liquid medication; may cause contact dermatitis (wash immediately with warm, soapy water). Initiate at lower doses (see Dosing) and taper dosage slowly when discontinuing. Assess knowledge/teach patient appropriate use, interventions to reduce side effects, and adverse symptoms to report (see below). **Note:** Thiothixene may cause false-positive pregnancy test (see Effects on Lab Values). **Pregnancy risk factor C** - benefits of use should outweigh possible risks. Breast-feeding is not recommended.

**Patient Information/Instruction:** Use exactly as directed (do not increase dose or frequency); may cause physical and/or psychological dependence. Do not discontinue without consulting prescriber. Tablets/capsules may be taken with food. Mix oral solution with 2-4 ounces of liquid (eg, juice, milk, water, pudding). Do not take within 2 hours of any antacid. Avoid excess alcohol or caffeine and other prescription or OTC medications not approved by prescriber. Maintain adequate hydration (2-3 L/day of fluids unless instructed to restrict fluid intake). May turn urine red-brown (normal). You may experience excess drowsiness, lightheadedness, dizziness, or blurred vision (use caution driving or when engaging in tasks requiring alertness until response to drug is known); nausea or vomiting (small frequent meals, frequent mouth care, chewing gum, or sucking lozenges may help); constipation (increased exercise, fluids, or dietary fruit and fiber may help); postural hypotension (use caution climbing stairs or when changing position from lying or sitting to standing); urinary retention (void before taking medication); ejaculatory dysfunction (reversible); decreased perspiration (avoid strenuous exercise in hot environments); photosensitivity (use sunscreen, wear protective clothing and eyewear, and avoid direct sunlight). Report persistent CNS effects (eg, trembling fingers, altered gait or balance, excessive sedation, seizures, unusual movements, anxiety, abnormal thoughts, confusion, personality changes); chest pain, palpitations, rapid heartbeat, severe dizziness; unresolved urinary retention or changes in urinary pattern; altered menstrual pattern, change in libido, swelling or pain in breasts (male or female); vision changes; skin rash, irritation, or changes in color of skin (gray-blue); or worsening of condition. **Pregnancy/breast-feeding precautions:** Inform prescriber if you are or intend to be pregnant. Breast-feeding is not recommended.

**Dietary Issues:** May cause increase in dietary riboflavin requirements.

**Geriatric Considerations:** (See Warnings/Precautions, Adverse Reactions, and Overdose/Toxicology.) Elderly patients have an increased risk of adverse response to side effects or adverse reactions to antipsychotics. These can include but are not limited to the following.

Anticholinergic effects: CNS toxicity with confusion, memory loss, psychotic behavior, and agitation.

Extrapyramidal effects (EPS): Parkinson's syndrome and akathisia may occur as often as 50% in patients >60 years of age. Tardive dyskinesia (motor restlessness) may be 40% in elderly; may be related to duration and total accumulated dose over time; may be somewhat reversible if diagnosed early enough.

Orthostatic hypotension: Increased risk for falls.

Sedation: In nonpsychotic patients, may result in feelings of depersonalization, derealization, and dysphoria.

Cardiac toxicity: Cardiac arrhythmias have occurred with therapeutic doses of antipsychotics.

Malignant neuroleptic syndrome: Development of hyperthermia, muscular rigidity, autonomic instability, and altered mental status.

Many elderly patients receive antipsychotic medications for inappropriate nonpsychotic behavior. Before initiating antipsychotic medication, all possible reversible causes should be investigated. Stress may cause acute "confusion" or worsening of baseline nonpsychotic behaviors; any changes in disease state (in any organ) may result in behavioral changes. Common acute changes in behavior may be due also to increases in drug dose addition, or addition of a new drug to the regimen; fluid/electrolyte alterations; infections; or changes in the environment.

Meta-analysis of controlled trials of antipsychotic (phenothiazines, butyrophenones) use with agitated, demented, elderly patients has concluded that the use of neuroleptics results in a response rate of 18%. Clearly, neuroleptic therapy for behavior control should be limited, with frequent attempts to withdraw the agent for behavior control. When use is indicated, initial doses should be lower to start and monitored closely.

**Additional Information** The concentration formulation contains ethanol.

**Related Information**

Antipsychotic Agents Comparison *on page 1371*
Antipsychotic Medication Guidelines *on page 1436*

♦ **Thorazine®** *see* Chlorpromazine *on page 256*
♦ **Thrombate III™** *see* Antithrombin III *on page 101*
♦ **Thrombinar®** *see page 1248*
♦ **Thrombin, Topical** *see page 1248*
♦ **Thrombogen®** *see page 1248*
♦ **Thrombostat®** *see page 1248*
♦ **Thypinone® Injection** *see page 1248*

♦ **Thyrar®** *see* Thyroid *on this page*

♦ **Thyro-Block®** *see* Potassium Iodide *on page 951*

## Thyroid (THYE royd)

**U.S. Brand Names** Armour® Thyroid; S-P-T; Thyrar®; Thyroid Strong®

**Synonyms** Desiccated Thyroid; Thyroid Extract

**Therapeutic Category** Thyroid Product

**Pregnancy Risk Factor** A

**Lactation** Enters breast milk/compatible

**Use** Replacement or supplemental therapy in hypothyroidism; pituitary TSH suppressants (thyroid nodules, thyroiditis, multinodular goiter, thyroid cancer), thyrotoxicosis, diagnostic suppression tests

**Mechanism of Action/Effect** The primary active compound is $T_3$ (tri-iodothyronine), which may be converted from $T_4$ (thyroxine) and then circulates throughout the body to influence growth and maturation of various tissues

**Contraindications** Hypersensitivity to beef or pork or any constituent; recent myocardial infarction or thyrotoxicosis uncomplicated by hypothyroidism uncorrected adrenal insufficiency

**Warnings** Ineffective for weight reduction. High doses may produce serious or even life-threatening toxic effects particularly when used with some anorectic drugs. Use cautiously in patients with pre-existing cardiovascular disease (angina, CHD), elderly since they may be more likely to have compromised cardiovascular function. Chronic hypothyroidism predisposes patients to coronary artery disease. Desiccated thyroid contains variable amounts of $T_3$, $T_4$, and other tri-iodothyronine compounds which are more likely to cause cardiac signs or symptoms due to fluctuating levels. Should avoid use in the elderly for this reason. Drug of choice is levothyroxine in the minds of many clinicians.

**Drug Interactions**

**Decreased Effect:** Thyroid hormones increase the therapeutic need for oral hypoglycemics or insulin. Cholestyramine can bind thyroid and reduce its absorption. Phenytoin may decrease thyroxine serum levels. Thyroid hormone may decrease effect of oral sulfonylureas.

**Increased Effect/Toxicity:** Thyroid may potentiate the hypoprothrombinemic effect of oral anticoagulants. Tricyclic antidepressants (TAD) coadministered with thyroid hormone may increase potential for toxicity of both drugs.

**Effects on Lab Values** Many drugs may have effects on thyroid function tests: para-aminosalicylic acid, aminoglutethimide, amiodarone, barbiturates, carbamazepine, chloral hydrate, clofibrate, colestipol, corticosteroids, danazol, diazepam, estrogens, ethionamide, fluorouracil, I.V. heparin, insulin, lithium, methadone, methimazole, mitotane, nitroprusside, oxyphenbutazone, phenylbutazone, PTU, perphenazine, phenytoin, propranolol, salicylates, sulfonylureas, and thiazides.

**Adverse Reactions** <1% (Limited to important or life-threatening symptoms): Palpitations, tachycardia, cardiac arrhythmias, chest pain, alopecia, excessive bone loss with overtreatment (excess thyroid replacement), tremor, hand tremors, myalgia, shortness of breath

**Overdose/Toxicology** Chronic excessive use results in signs and symptoms of hyperthyroidism, weight loss, nervousness, sweating, tachycardia, insomnia, heat intolerance, palpitations, vomiting, psychosis, fever, seizures, angina, arrhythmias, and CHF in those predisposed.

Reduce dose or temporarily discontinue therapy. Hypothalamic-pituitary-thyroid axis will return to normal in 6-8 weeks. Serum $T_4$ levels do not correlate well with toxicity. In massive acute ingestion, reduce GI absorption and give general supportive care.

**Pharmacodynamics/Kinetics**

**Protein Binding:** 99% (bound to albumin, thyroxine-binding globulin, and thyroxin-binding prealbumin)

**Half-life Elimination:** Liothyronine: 1-2 days; Thyroxine: 6-7 days

**Metabolism:** Liver and kidneys

**Excretion:** Urine

**Formulations**

Capsule, pork source in soybean oil (S-P-T): 60 mg, 120 mg, 180 mg, 300 mg

Tablet:

Armour® Thyroid: 15 mg, 30 mg, 60 mg, 90 mg, 120 mg, 180 mg, 240 mg, 300 mg

Thyrar® (bovine source): 30 mg, 60 mg, 120 mg

Thyroid Strong® (60 mg is equivalent to 90 mg thyroid USP):

Regular: 30 mg, 60 mg, 120 mg

Sugar coated: 30 mg, 60 mg, 120 mg, 180 mg

Thyroid USP: 15 mg, 30 mg, 60 mg, 120 mg, 180 mg, 300 mg

**Dosing**

**Adults:** Oral:

Initial: 15-30 mg; increase with 15 mg increments every 2-4 weeks; use 15 mg in patients with cardiovascular disease or myxedema. Maintenance dose: Usually 60-120 mg/day; monitor TSH and clinical symptoms.

Thyroid cancer: Requires larger amounts than replacement therapy.

**Elderly:** Not recommended for use in the elderly (see Geriatric Considerations).

**Monitoring Laboratory Tests** Monitor $T_4$ and TSH. TSH is the most reliable guide for evaluating adequacy of thyroid replacement dosage. TSH may be elevated during the first few months of thyroid replacement despite patients being clinically euthyroid. In cases where $T_4$ remains low and TSH is within normal limits, an evaluation of "free" (unbound) $T_4$ is needed to evaluate further increase in dosage.

**Additional Nursing Issues**

**Physical Assessment:** Assess other medications patient may be taking for effectiveness and/or interactions (see Drug Interactions). Assess appropriate laboratory tests prior to beginning therapy. **Important:** See Effects on Lab Values above when considering results of thyroid function tests. Monitor vital signs on a regular basis. Monitor for signs or symptoms of hypo-/hyperthyroidism (be aware of effects of aging on "typical" indications of hyper-/hypothyroidism).

**Patient Information/Instruction:** Thyroid replacement therapy is generally for life. Take as directed, in the morning before breakfast. Do not change brands and do not discontinue without consulting prescriber. Consult prescriber if drastically increasing or decreasing intake of goitrogenic food (eg, asparagus, cabbage, peas, turnip greens, broccoli, spinach, brussels sprouts, lettuce, soybeans). Report chest pain, rapid heart rate, palpitations, heat intolerance, excessive sweating, increased nervousness, agitation, or lethargy.

**Geriatric Considerations:** Desiccated thyroid contains variable amounts of $T_3$, $T_4$, and other triiodothyronine compounds which are more likely to cause cardiac signs or symptoms due to fluctuating levels. Should avoid use in the elderly for this reason. Many clinicians consider levothyroxine to be the drug of choice.

**Additional Information**

Equivalent levothyroxine dose: Thyroid USP 60 mg = levothyroxine 0.05-0.06 mg; liothyronine 0.015-0.0375 mg; liotrix 60 mg

Thyroid Strong® is 50% stronger than thyroid U.S.P.: each grain is equivalent to 1.5 grains of thyroid U.S.P.

Thyrar®: Bovine thyroid

S-P-T®: Pork thyroid suspended in soybean oil

**Related Information**

Levothyroxine *on page 673*


- **Thyroid Extract** *see* Thyroid *on previous page*
- **Thyroid-Stimulating Hormone** *see* Thyrotropin *on this page*
- **Thyroid Strong®** *see* Thyroid *on previous page*


## Thyrotropin (thye roe TROE pin)

**U.S. Brand Names** Thytropar®

**Synonyms** Thyroid-Stimulating Hormone; TSH

**Therapeutic Category** Diagnostic Agent, Hypothyroidism; Diagnostic Agent, Thyroid Function

**Pregnancy Risk Factor** C

**Lactation** Enters breast milk/compatible

**Use** Diagnostic aid to differentiate thyroid failure; diagnosis of decreased thyroid reserve, to differentiate between primary and secondary hypothyroidism and between primary hypothyroidism and euthyroidism in patients receiving thyroid replacement

**Mechanism of Action/Effect** Stimulates formation and secretion of thyroid hormone, increases uptake of iodine by thyroid gland

**Contraindications** Hypersensitivity to thyrotropin or any component; coronary thrombosis; untreated Addison's disease

**Warnings** Use with caution in patients with angina pectoris or cardiac failure, patients with hypopituitarism, or adrenal cortical suppression as may be seen with corticosteroid therapy. May cause thyroid hyperplasia. Pregnancy factor C.

**Adverse Reactions** <1% (Limited to important or life-threatening symptoms): Tachycardia, fever, anaphylaxis with repeated administration

**Overdose/Toxicology** Symptoms of overdose include weight loss, nervousness, sweating, tachycardia, insomnia, heat intolerance, menstrual irregularities, headache, angina pectoris, and CHF. Acute massive overdose may require cardiac glycosides for CHF. Fever should be controlled with the help of acetaminophen. Antiadrenergic agents, particularly propranolol 1-3 mg I.V. every 6 hours or 80-160 mg/day, can be used to treat increased sympathetic activity.

**Pharmacodynamics/Kinetics**

**Half-life Elimination:** 35 minutes, dependent upon thyroid state

**Excretion:** Urine

**Formulations** Injection: 10 units

**Dosing**

**Adults:** I.M., S.C.: 10 units/day for 1-3 days; follow by a radioiodine study 24 hours past last injection, no response in thyroid failure, substantial response in pituitary failure

**Elderly:** Refer to adult dosing.

**Stability**

**Reconstitution:** Refrigerate at 2°C to 8°C (36°F to 46°F) after reconstitution. Use within 2 weeks.

**Additional Nursing Issues**

**Physical Assessment:** Monitor for adverse reactions or overdose response. **Pregnancy risk factor C** - benefits of use should outweigh possible risks.

**Patient Information/Instruction:** You will receive this medication for 3 days prior to the radiologic studies. You may experience some nausea or vomiting. Report dizziness, faintness, palpitations, or any respiratory difficulties. **Pregnancy precautions:** Inform prescriber if you are or intend to be pregnant.


- **Thytropar®** *see* Thyrotropin *on this page*
- **Tiabendazole** *see* Thiabendazole *on page 1119*

## Tiagabine (tye AJ a bene)

**U.S. Brand Names** Gabitril®

**Therapeutic Category** Anticonvulsant, Miscellaneous

**Pregnancy Risk Factor** C

**Lactation** Enters breast milk/not recommended

**Use** Adjunctive therapy in adults and children 12 years and older in the treatment of partial seizures

**Mechanism of Action/Effect** The exact mechanism is not definitively known; however, *in vitro* experiments demonstrate that it enhances the activity of gamma aminobutyric acid (GABA), the major neuroinhibitory transmitter in the nervous system. Potentiation of GABA blocks the propagation of neural impulses which contribute to seizures.

**Contraindications** Hypersensitivity to tiagabine or any component

**Warnings** History of spike and wave EEG pattern - impairment of cognitive/neuropsychiatric function may occur. Caution in hepatic impairment and in patients not receiving enzyme-inducing drugs, such as patients on valproate monotherapy (lower dosages may be required). Do not discontinued abruptly; tiagabine should be withdrawn gradually to minimize the potential of increased seizure frequency, unless safety concerns require a more rapid withdrawal. May impair cognitive function. Pregnancy factor C.

**Drug Interactions**

**Cytochrome P-450 Effect:** CYP2D6 and 3A3/4 enzyme substrate

**Decreased Effect:** Modest decrease in valproate levels during concurrent therapy (10%). Carbamazepine, phenytoin, primidone, and phenobarbital decrease tiagabine blood levels.

**Increased Effect/Toxicity:** Unbound tiagabine levels increase with valproate; clinical significance is unknown.

**Food Interactions** Food reduces the rate but not the extent of absorption.

**Adverse Reactions** Frequency in trials where tiagabine was added to other anticonvulsants.

>10%:

Gastrointestinal: Nausea (11%)

Central nervous system: Dizziness (27%), weakness (20%), somnolence (18%), nervousness (10%)

1% to 10%:

Gastrointestinal: Abdominal pain (7%), diarrhea (7%), vomiting (7%), increased appetite (2%), mouth ulcer (2%)

Central nervous system: Concentration difficulty (6%), pain (5%), ataxia (5%), confusion (5%), speech disorder (4%), memory impairment (4%), aggressive behavior (2%), agitation (1%)

Neuromuscular and skeletal: Tremor (6%), paresthesia (4%), gait instability (3%)

Respiratory: Pharyngitis (7%), cough (4%)

Dermatologic: Rash (5%), pruritus (2%)

Ocular: Nystagmus (2%)

Moderately severe to incapacitating weakness may occur in approximately 1% of patients. Other effects noted during clinical trials (Limited to important or life-threatening symptoms) include allergic reaction, photosensitivity, sudden death, angina, dyspnea, apnea. Postmarketing reports of cognitive/neuropsychiatric effects, including nonconvulsive status epilepticus have occurred.

**Overdose/Toxicology** Somnolence, impaired consciousness, agitation, confusion, speech difficulty, hostility, depression, weakness, myoclonus, and seizures may occur. Treatment is supportive.

**Pharmacodynamics/Kinetics**

**Protein Binding:** 96%

**Half-life Elimination:** Volunteers: 7-9 hours; in patients receiving enzyme-inducing drugs: 4-7 hours

**Time to Peak:** 45 minutes

**Metabolism:** Hepatic, via cytochrome P-450 isoenzymes (primarily 3A4)

**Excretion:** Feces and urine

**Formulations** Tablet: 2 mg, 4 mg, 12 mg, 16 mg, 20 mg

**Dosing**

**Adults:** Oral: Starting dose: 4 mg once daily; the total daily dose may be increased in 4 mg increments beginning the second week of therapy; thereafter, the daily dose may be increased by 4-8 mg/day until clinical response is achieved, up to a maximum of 32 mg/day; the total daily dose at higher levels should be given in divided doses, 2-4 times/day.

**Elderly:** Refer to adult dosing.

**Monitoring Laboratory Tests** A therapeutic range for tiagabine has not been established. Monitor complete blood counts, renal function tests, liver function tests, and routine blood chemistry.

**Additional Nursing Issues**

**Physical Assessment:** Assess effectiveness and interactions of other medications patient may be taking (see Contraindications, Warnings/Precautions, and Drug Interactions). Monitor for therapeutic response (seizure activity, force, type, duration), laboratory values, and adverse reactions (see Adverse Reactions) at beginning of therapy and periodically with long-term use. Taper dosage slowly when discontinuing. Use and teach seizure/safety precaution. Assess knowledge/teach patient appropriate use, interventions to reduce side effects, and adverse symptoms to report. **Pregnancy risk factor C** - benefits of use should outweigh possible risks. Breast-feeding is not recommended.

**Patient Information/Instruction:** Take exactly as directed (do not increase dose or frequency or discontinue without consulting prescriber). While using this medication, do not use alcohol and other prescription or OTC medications (especially pain medications, sedatives, antihistamines, or hypnotics) without consulting prescriber. Maintain adequate hydration (2-3 L/day of fluids unless instructed to restrict fluid intake). You may experience drowsiness, dizziness, disturbed concentration, or blurred vision (use caution when driving or engaging in tasks requiring alertness until response to drug is known); nausea, vomiting, or loss of appetite (small frequent meals, frequent mouth care, chewing gum, or sucking lozenges may help). Wear identification of epileptic status and medications. Report behavioral or CNS changes; skin rash; muscle cramping, weakness, tremors, changes in gait; vision difficulties; persistent GI distress (cramping, pain, vomiting); chest pain, irregular heartbeat, or palpitations; cough or difficulty breathing; worsening of seizure activity, or loss of seizure control. **Pregnancy/breast-feeding precautions:** Inform prescriber if you are or intend to be pregnant. Breast-feeding is not recommended.

**Geriatric Considerations:** There has been limited clinical experience with geriatric patients during clinical evaluation - use with caution.

- **Tiamcinolone** *see* Topical Corticosteroids *on page 1152*
- **Tiazac™** *see* Diltiazem *on page 377*
- **Ticar®** *see* Ticarcillin *on this page*

## Ticarcillin (tye kar SIL in)

**U.S. Brand Names** Ticar®

**Therapeutic Category** Antibiotic, Penicillin

**Pregnancy Risk Factor** B

**Lactation** Enters breast milk/compatible

**Use** Treatment of susceptible infections such as septicemia, acute and chronic respiratory tract infections, skin and soft tissue infections, and urinary tract infections due to susceptible strains of *Pseudomonas*, *Proteus*, and *Escherichia coli* and *Enterobacter*, normally used with other antibiotics (eg, aminoglycosides)

**Mechanism of Action/Effect** Interferes with bacterial cell wall synthesis during active multiplication, causing cell wall death and resultant bactericidal activity against susceptible bacteria

**Contraindications** Hypersensitivity to ticarcillin, any component, penicillins, cephalosporins, or imipenem

**Warnings** Due to sodium load and adverse effects (anemia, neuropsychological changes), use with caution and modify dosage in patients with renal impairment. Serious and occasionally severe or fatal hypersensitivity (anaphylactoid) reactions have been reported in patients on penicillin therapy (especially with a history of beta-lactam hypersensitivity and/or a history of sensitivity to multiple allergens). Use with caution in patients with seizures.

**Drug Interactions**

**Decreased Effect:** Tetracyclines may decrease penicillin effectiveness. Efficacy of oral contraceptives may be reduced when taken with ticarcillin. Aminoglycosides may cause physical inactivation of aminoglycosides in the presence of high concentrations of ticarcillin and potential toxicity in patients with mild-moderate renal dysfunction.

**Increased Effect/Toxicity:** Probenecid may increase penicillin levels. Neuromuscular blockers may have an increased duration of action (neuromuscular blockade).

**Effects on Lab Values** False-positive urinary or serum protein, positive Coombs' test

**Adverse Reactions**

>10%:

Central nervous system: Headache

Gastrointestinal: Nausea (mild), vomiting

Miscellaneous: Oral candidiasis, vaginal candidiasis

1% to 10%:

Dermatologic: Urticaria, exfoliative dermatitis

Miscellaneous: Allergic reactions, specifically anaphylaxis; serum sickness-like reactions

<1% (Limited to important or life-threatening symptoms): Seizures, leukopenia, neutropenia, thrombocytopenia, jaundice, hepatotoxicity, interstitial nephritis, *Clostridium difficile* colitis

**Overdose/Toxicology** Symptoms of penicillin overdose include neuromuscular hypersensitivity (eg, agitation, hallucinations, asterixis, encephalopathy, confusion, and seizures). Electrolyte imbalance may occur if the preparation contains potassium or sodium salts, especially in renal failure. Hemodialysis may be helpful to aid in removal of the drug from blood; otherwise, treatment is supportive or symptom directed.

**Pharmacodynamics/Kinetics**

**Protein Binding:** 45% to 65%

**Distribution:** Attains high concentrations in bile; minimal concentrations attained in CSF with uninflamed meninges

**Half-life Elimination:** 1-1.3 hours (prolonged in renal or hepatic impairment)

**Time to Peak:** I.M.: Within 30-75 minutes

**Excretion:** Urine and feces

**Formulations** Powder for injection, as disodium: 1 g, 3 g, 6 g, 20 g, 30 g

**Dosing**

**Adults:** Ticarcillin is generally given I.M. only for the treatment of uncomplicated urinary tract infections.

I.V.: 1-4 g every 4-6 hours

(Continued)

## Ticarcillin *(Continued)*

**Elderly:** Ticarcillin is generally given I.M. only for the treatment of uncomplicated urinary tract infections.

I.V.: 3 g every 4-6 hours; adjust dosing interval for renal impairment.

**Renal Impairment:** I.V.:

$Cl_{cr}$ >60 mL/minute: Administer 3 g every 4 hours.
$Cl_{cr}$ 30-60 mL/minute: Administer 2 g every 4 hours.
$Cl_{cr}$ 10-30 mL/minute: Administer 2 g every 8 hours.
$Cl_{cr}$ <10 mL/minute: Administer 2 g every 12 hours.
$Cl_{cr}$ <10 mL/minute with hepatic dysfunction: Administer 2 g every 24 hours.
Peritoneal dialysis: Administer 3 g every 12 hours.
Hemodialysis: Administer 2 g every 12 hours; follow each dialysis with 3 g.

Moderately dialyzable (20% to 50%)

Continuous arteriovenous or venovenous hemofiltration (CAVH): Dose as for $Cl_{cr}$ 10-50 mL/minute.

**Administration**

**I.M.:** Do not give more than 2 g per injection.

**I.V.:** Administer around-the-clock. Administer 1 hour apart from aminoglycosides. Intermittently infusion over 30 minutes to 2 hours.

**I.V. Detail:** Too rapid of infusion may cause seizures.

**Stability**

**Storage:** Reconstituted solution is stable for 72 hours at room temperature and 14 days when refrigerated or 30 days when frozen. For I.V. infusion in NS or $D_5W$.

**Compatibility:** Incompatible with aminoglycosides.

**Monitoring Laboratory Tests** Serum electrolytes, bleeding time, and periodic tests of renal, hepatic, and hematologic function; perform culture and sensitivity before administering first dose.

**Additional Nursing Issues**

**Physical Assessment:** Assess patient history for allergy. Monitor for hypersensitivity reaction and opportunistic infection. Use serum glucose testing for diabetic patient.

**Patient Information/Instruction:** This medication will be administered I.V. or I.M. Maintain adequate hydration (2-3 L/day of fluids unless instructed to restrict fluid intake). Small frequent meals, frequent mouth care, sucking lozenges, or chewing gum may reduce nausea or dry mouth. Maintain good oral and vaginal hygiene to reduce incidence of opportunistic infection. If diabetic, drug may cause false tests with Clinitest® urine glucose monitoring; use of glucose oxidase methods (Clinistix®) or serum glucose monitoring is preferable. This drug may interfere with oral contraceptives; an alternate form of birth control should be used. Report persistent diarrhea or abdominal pain (do not use antidiarrhea medication without consulting prescriber), fever, chills, unhealed sores, bloody urine or stool, muscle pain, mouth sores, difficulty breathing, or skin rash.

**Geriatric Considerations:** When used as empiric therapy or for documented pseudomonal pneumonia, it is best to combine with an aminoglycoside such as gentamicin or tobramycin. High sodium may limit use in patients with congestive heart failure. Adjust dose for renal function.

**Additional Information**

Sodium content of 1 g: 5.2-6.5 mEq
pH: 6-8

## Ticarcillin and Clavulanate Potassium

(tye kar SIL in & klav yoo LAN ate poe TASS ee um)

**U.S. Brand Names** Timentin®

**Synonyms** Clavulanic Acid and Ticarcillin; Ticarcillin and Clavulanic Acid

**Therapeutic Category** Antibiotic, Penicillin

**Pregnancy Risk Factor** B

**Lactation** Enters breast milk (other penicillins are compatible with breast-feeding)

**Use** Treatment of infections of lower respiratory tract, urinary tract, skin and skin structures, bone and joint, and septicemia caused by susceptible organisms. Clavulanate expands activity of ticarcillin to include beta-lactamase producing strains of *S. aureus*, *H. influenzae*, Enterobacteriaceae, *Klebsiella*, *Citrobacter*, and *Serratia*

**Mechanism of Action/Effect** Ticarcillin interferes with bacterial cell wall synthesis during active multiplication, causing cell wall death and resultant bactericidal activity against susceptible bacteria; clavulanic acid prevents degradation of ticarcillin by binding to the active site on beta-lactamase

**Contraindications** Hypersensitivity to ticarcillin, clavulanate, penicillins, cephalosporins, or imipenem

**Warnings** Use with caution and modify dosage in patients with renal impairment. Serious and occasionally fatal hypersensitivity (anaphylactoid) reactions have been reported in patients on penicillin therapy. These reactions are more likely to occur in individuals with a history of cephalosporin hypersensitivity and/or a history of sensitivity to multiple allergens.

**Drug Interactions**

**Decreased Effect:** Tetracyclines may decrease penicillin effectiveness. Efficacy of oral contraceptives may be reduced when taken with ticarcillin and clavulanate potassium. Aminoglycosides may cause physical inactivation of aminoglycosides in the presence of high concentrations of ticarcillin and potential toxicity in patients with mild-moderate renal dysfunction.

**Increased Effect/Toxicity:** Probenecid may increase penicillin levels. Neuromuscular blockers may have an increased duration of action (neuromuscular blockade).

**Effects on Lab Values** Positive Coombs' test, false-positive urinary proteins

**Adverse Reactions**

>10%:

Central nervous system: Headache

Gastrointestinal: Nausea (mild), vomiting

Miscellaneous: Oral candidiasis, vaginal candidiasis

1% to 10%:

Dermatologic: Urticaria, exfoliative dermatitis

Miscellaneous: Allergic reactions, specifically anaphylaxis; serum sickness-like reactions

<1% (Limited to important or life-threatening symptoms): Seizures, leukopenia, neutropenia, thrombocytopenia, jaundice, hepatotoxicity, interstitial nephritis, *Clostridium difficile* colitis

**Overdose/Toxicology** Symptoms of overdose include neuromuscular hypersensitivity and seizures. Hemodialysis may be helpful to aid in removal of the drug from blood; otherwise, treatment is supportive or symptom directed.

**Pharmacodynamics/Kinetics**

**Protein Binding:** Ticarcillin: 45% to 65%; Clavulanic acid: 9%

**Distribution:** Low concentrations of ticarcillin distribute into the CSF and increase when meninges are inflamed

**Half-life Elimination:**

Clavulanate: 66-90 minutes

Ticarcillin: 66-72 minutes in patients with normal renal function; clavulanic acid does not affect the clearance of ticarcillin

Renal failure: Ticarcillin: ~13 hours

**Metabolism:** Clavulanic acid is metabolized in the liver

**Excretion:** Urine

**Formulations**

Infusion, premixed (frozen): Ticarcillin disodium 3 g and clavulanate potassium 0.1 g (100 mL)

Powder for injection: Ticarcillin disodium 3 g and clavulanate potassium 0.1 g (3.1 g, 31 g)

**Dosing**

**Adults:** I.V.: 3.1 g (ticarcillin 3 g plus clavulanic acid 0.1 g) every 4-6 hours; maximum: 18-24 g/day

Urinary tract infections: 3.1 g every 6-8 hours

**Elderly:** I.V.: (based on ticarcillin): 3 g every 4-6 hours; adjust for renal function.

**Renal Impairment:**

$Cl_{cr}$ >60 mL/minute: Administer 3.1 g every 4 hours.

$Cl_{cr}$ 30-60 mL/minute: Administer 2 g every 4 hours.

$Cl_{cr}$ 10-30 mL/minute: Administer 2 g every 8 hours.

$Cl_{cr}$ <10 mL/minute: Administer 2 g every 12 hours.

Peritoneal dialysis: Administer 3.1 g every 12 hours.

Hemodialysis: Administer 2 g every 12 hours; supplemented with 3.1 g after each dialysis.

Continuous arteriovenous or venovenous hemofiltration (CAVH): Dose as for $Cl_{cr}$ 10-50 mL/minute.

**Hepatic Impairment:** $Cl_{cr}$ <10 mL/minute with hepatic dysfunction: Administer 2 g every 24 hours.

**Administration**

**I.V.:** Infuse over 30 minutes. Administer 1 hour apart from aminoglycosides. Give around-the-clock. Rapid administration may lead to seizures.

**Stability**

**Storage:** Reconstituted solution is stable for 6 hours at room temperature and 72 hours when refrigerated. I.V. infusion in NS is stable for 24 hours at room temperature, 7 days when refrigerated, or 30 days when frozen. Darkening of solution indicates loss of potency of clavulanate potassium.

**Compatibility:** Incompatible with sodium bicarbonate, aminoglycosides.

**Monitoring Laboratory Tests** Serum electrolytes, bleeding time, and periodic tests of renal, hepatic, and hematologic function; perform culture and sensitivity before administering first dose.

**Additional Nursing Issues**

**Physical Assessment:** Assess patient history for allergy. Monitor for hypersensitivity reaction and opportunistic infection. Use serum glucose testing for diabetic patient.

**Patient Information/Instruction:** This medication will be administered I.V. or I.M. Maintain adequate hydration (2-3 L/day of fluids unless instructed to restrict fluid intake). Small frequent meals, frequent mouth care, sucking lozenges, or chewing gum may reduce nausea or dry mouth. Maintain good oral and vaginal hygiene to reduce incidence of opportunistic infection. If diabetic, drug may cause false tests with Clinitest® urine glucose monitoring; use of glucose oxidase methods (Clinistix®) or serum glucose monitoring is preferable. This drug may interfere with oral contraceptives; an alternate form of birth control should be used. Report persistent diarrhea or abdominal pain (do not use antidiarrhea medication without consulting prescriber), fever, chills, unhealed sores, bloody urine or stool, muscle pain, mouth sores, difficulty breathing, or skin rash.

(Continued)

## Ticarcillin and Clavulanate Potassium *(Continued)*

**Geriatric Considerations:** When used as empiric therapy or for a documented pseudomonal pneumonia, it is best to combine with an aminoglycoside such as gentamicin or tobramycin. High sodium content may limit use in patients with congestive heart failure. Adjust dose for renal function.

**Additional Information**

Sodium content of 1 g: 4.75 mEq
Potassium content of 1 g: 0.15 mEq
pH: 5.5-7.5

**Related Information**

Ticarcillin *on page 1133*

♦ **Ticarcillin and Clavulanic Acid** *see* Ticarcillin and Clavulanate Potassium *on page 1134*
♦ **TICE® BCG** *see page 1256*
♦ **Ticlid®** *see* Ticlopidine *on this page*

## Ticlopidine (tye KLOE pi deen)

**U.S. Brand Names** Ticlid®

**Therapeutic Category** Antiplatelet Agent

**Pregnancy Risk Factor** B

**Lactation** Excretion in breast milk unknown

**Use** Platelet aggregation inhibitor that reduces the risk of thrombotic stroke in patients who have had a stroke or stroke precursors

**Unlabeled use:** Protection of aortocoronary bypass grafts, diabetic microangiopathy, ischemic heart disease, prevention of postoperative DVT, reduction of graft loss following renal transplant

**Mechanism of Action/Effect** Ticlopidine is an inhibitor of platelet function with a mechanism which is different from other antiplatelet drugs. The drug significantly increases bleeding time. This effect may not be solely related to ticlopidine's effect on platelets. The prolongation of the bleeding time caused by ticlopidine is further increased by the addition of aspirin in *ex vivo* experiments. Although many metabolites of ticlopidine have been found, none have been shown to account for *in vivo* activity.

**Contraindications** Hypersensitivity to ticlopidine; active bleeding disorders; neutropenia or thrombocytopenia or a past history of TTP; severe liver impairment

**Warnings** Patients predisposed to bleeding such as those with gastric or duodenal ulcers; patients with underlying hematologic disorders; patients receiving oral anticoagulant therapy or nonsteroidal anti-inflammatory agents (including aspirin); liver disease; patients undergoing lumbar puncture or surgical procedure. May cause life-threatening neutropenia, agranulocytosis, and/or TTP. Ticlopidine should be discontinued if the absolute neutrophil count falls to $<1200/mm^3$ or if the platelet count falls to $<80,000/mm^3$. If possible, ticlopidine should be discontinued 10-14 days prior to surgery. Use caution when phenytoin or propranolol is used concurrently.

**Drug Interactions**

**Cytochrome P-450 Effect:** CYP2C19 enzyme inhibitor

**Decreased Effect:** Decreased effect with antacids (decreased absorption) and corticosteroids. Decreased effect of digoxin, cyclosporine.

**Increased Effect/Toxicity:** Increased effect/toxicity of aspirin, anticoagulants, theophylline, cimetidine (increased levels), and NSAIDs.

**Food Interactions** Ticlopidine bioavailability may be increased if taken with food.

**Effects on Lab Values** ↑ cholesterol (S), alkaline phosphatase, transaminases (S)

**Adverse Reactions**

>10%; Gastrointestinal: Abdominal pain, diarrhea

1% to 10%:
- Central nervous system: Dizziness
- Dermatologic: Rash
- Gastrointestinal: Nausea, vomiting, GI pain, gas pain

<1% (Limited to important or life-threatening symptoms): Stevens-Johnson syndrome, erythema multiforme, exfoliative dermatitis, neutropenia, thrombocytopenia, TTP, increased liver function tests, hematuria

**Overdose/Toxicology** Symptoms of overdose include ataxia, seizures, vomiting, abdominal pain, and hematologic abnormalities. Specific treatments are lacking. Treatment is symptomatic and supportive.

**Pharmacodynamics/Kinetics**

**Half-life Elimination:** 24 hours

**Metabolism:** Liver

**Onset:** Within 6 hours; Peak: Achieved after 3-5 days of oral therapy; serum levels do not correlate with clinical antiplatelet activity.

**Formulations** Tablet, as hydrochloride: 250 mg

**Dosing**

**Adults:**
- Oral: 1 tablet twice daily with food
- Stent implantation: Oral: 250 mg twice daily

**Elderly:** Oral: 250 mg twice daily with food; dosage in the elderly has not been determined; however, in two large clinical trials, the average age of subjects was 63 and 66 years; a dosage decrease may be necessary if bleeding abnormalities develop.

**Monitoring Laboratory Tests** CBC with differential and platelet counts every 2 weeks starting the second week through the third month of treatment; more frequent monitoring is recommended for patients whose absolute neutrophil counts have been consistently declining or are 30% less than baseline values. Liver function tests (alkaline phosphatase and transaminases) should be performed in the first 4 months of therapy if liver dysfunction is suspected.

**Additional Nursing Issues**

**Physical Assessment:** Monitor effectiveness of therapy (laboratory results) frequently at beginning of treatment and regularly thereafter (see Monitoring Laboratory Tests). Monitor and teach patient bleeding precautions, possible side effects, and adverse symptoms to report. Note breast-feeding caution.

**Patient Information/Instruction:** Take exact dosage prescribed, with food. Do not use aspirin or aspirin-containing medications and OTC medications without consulting prescriber. You may experience easy bleeding or bruising (use soft toothbrush or cotton swabs and frequent mouth care, use electric razor, avoid sharp knives or scissors). Report unusual bleeding or bruising or persistent fever or sore throat; blood in urine, stool, or vomitus; delayed healing of any wounds; skin rash; yellowing of skin or eyes; changes in color of urine of stool; pain or burning on urination; respiratory difficulty; or skin rash. **Breast-feeding precautions:** Consult prescriber if breast-feeding.

**Geriatric Considerations:** Because of the risk of neutropenia and its relative expense as compared with aspirin, ticlopidine should only be used in patients with a documented intolerance to aspirin.

♦ **Ticon®** *see* Trimethobenzamide *on page 1180*

♦ **Tienam®** *see* Imipenem and Cilastatin *on page 599*

♦ **Tigan®** *see* Trimethobenzamide *on page 1180*

♦ **Tilade® Inhalation Aerosol** *see* Nedocromil *on page 811*

♦ **Tilazem** *see* Diltiazem *on page 377*

## Tiludronate (tye LOO droe nate)

**U.S. Brand Names** Skelid®

**Synonyms** Tiludronic Acid

**Therapeutic Category** Bisphosphonate Derivative

**Pregnancy Risk Factor** C

**Lactation** Excretion in breast milk unknown

**Use** Treatment of Paget's disease of the bone in patients who have a level of serum alkaline phosphatase (SAP) at least twice the upper limit of normal, or who are symptomatic, or who are at risk for future complications of their disease

**Mechanism of Action/Effect** A biphosphonate which inhibits osteoclast activity, reducing enzymatic and transport processes that lead to resorption of bone. At least two possible mechanisms may be involved: detachment of osteoclasts from the bone surface (due to inhibition of protein-tyrosine-phosphatase) and inhibition of the osteoclastic proton pump, required to alter local pH to solubilize ions and bone matrix during resorption.

**Contraindications** Hypersensitivity to biphosphonates

**Warnings** Not recommended in severe renal impairment ($Cl_{cr}$ <30 mL/minute). May cause upper gastrointestinal problems (eg, dysphagia, esophageal diseases, gastritis, duodenitis, ulcers). Pregnancy factor C.

**Drug Interactions**

**Decreased Effect:** Concurrent administration of calcium salts, aluminum or magnesium containing antacids, and aspirin markedly decrease absorption/bioavailability (by 50% to 60%) of tiludronate if given within 2 hours of a dose.

**Increased Effect/Toxicity:** Administration of indomethacin increases bioavailability of tiludronate two- to fourfold.

**Food Interactions** Food ingested within 2 hours of a dose reduces absorption of tiludronate by 90%.

**Adverse Reactions** The following events occurred >2% and at a frequency > placebo:

1% to 10%:

Cardiovascular: Chest pain (2.7%), edema (2.7%)

Central nervous system: Dizziness (4.0%), paresthesia (4.0%)

Dermatologic: Rash (2.7%), skin disorder (2.7%)

Gastrointestinal: Nausea (9.3%), diarrhea (9.3%), heartburn (5.3%), vomiting (4.0%), flatulence (2.7%)

Neuromuscular & skeletal: Arthrosis (2.7%)

Ocular: cataract (2.7%), conjunctivitis (2.7%), glaucoma (2.7%)

Respiratory: Rhinitis (5.3%), sinusitis (5.3%), coughing (2.7%), pharyngitis (2.7%)

The following events occurred at a rate >2% but less than placebo: Pain, headache, infection, back pain, arthralgia, dyspepsia, flu-like symptoms. Other events reported <1% (Limited to important or life-threatening symptoms): Stevens-Johnson syndrome, abdominal pain, pathologic fractures, weakness, and increased sweating.

**Overdose/Toxicology** Hypocalcemia is a potential consequence of overdose. Treatment is supportive.

(Continued)

## Tiludronate *(Continued)*

**Pharmacodynamics/Kinetics**

**Protein Binding:** 90%

**Distribution:** Absorbed into bone matrix, steady-state not reached in 30 days of dosing

**Half-life Elimination:** Healthy volunteers: 50 hours; Pagetic patients: 150 hours

**Time to Peak:** Within 2 hours

**Metabolism:** Minimal, if any metabolism

**Excretion:** Urine

**Onset:** Delayed, may require several weeks

**Formulations** Tablet, as disodium: 240 mg [tiludronic acid 200 mg]; dosage is expressed in terms of tiludronic acid.

**Dosing**

**Adults:** Oral: 400 mg (2 tablets of tiludronic acid) daily for a period of 3 months

**Elderly:** Plasma concentrations of tiludronic acid are higher in elderly patients, but no dosage reduction is recommended. See adult dosing.

**Renal Impairment:** Tiludronate is excreted renally. It is not recommended for use in patients with severe renal impairment ($Cl_{cr}$ <30 mL/minute) and is not removed by dialysis.

**Administration**

**Oral:** Take with 6-8 oz of plain water. Do not take within 2 hours of food, aspirin, indomethacin, or calcium-, magnesium-, or aluminum-containing medications.

**Stability**

**Storage:** Do not remove tablet from foil strips until they are to be used.

**Monitoring Laboratory Tests** Serum calcium, alkaline phosphatase

**Additional Nursing Issues**

**Physical Assessment:** Monitor laboratory results on a regular basis during therapy (see Monitoring Laboratory Tests). Monitor for adverse reactions and instruct patient about signs of adverse reactions to report (see Adverse Reactions). **Pregnancy risk factor C** - benefits of use should outweigh possible risks. Note breast-feeding caution.

**Patient Information/Instruction:** In order to be effective this drug must be taken exactly as prescribed: Take 2 hours before or 2 hours after meals, aspirin, indomethacin, or calcium, magnesium, or aluminum containing medications such as antacids. Take with 6-8 oz. of water. Do not remove medication from foil strip until ready to be used. You may experience mild skin rash; abdominal pain, diarrhea, or constipation (report if persistent). Report unresolved muscle or bone pain or leg cramps; acute abdominal pain; chest pain, palpitations, or swollen extremities; disturbed vision or excessively dry eyes; ringing in the ears; persistent rash or skin disorder; unusual weakness or increased perspiration. **Pregnancy/breast-feeding precautions:** Inform prescriber if you are or intend to be pregnant. Consult prescriber if breast-feeding.

- **Tiludronic Acid** *see* Tiludronate *on previous page*
- **Timentin®** *see* Ticarcillin and Clavulanate Potassium *on page 1134*

## Timolol (TYE moe lole)

**U.S. Brand Names** Betimol® Ophthalmic; Blocadren® Oral; Timoptic® OcuDose®; Timoptic® Ophthalmic; Timoptic-XE® Ophthalmic

**Therapeutic Category** Beta Blocker, Nonselective; Ophthalmic Agent, Antiglaucoma

**Pregnancy Risk Factor** C/D (2nd and 3rd trimesters)

**Lactation** Enters breast milk/use caution - see Breast-feeding Issues

**Use** Ophthalmic dosage form used to treat elevated intraocular pressure such as glaucoma or ocular hypertension; oral dosage form used for treatment of hypertension and angina, to reduce mortality following myocardial infarction, and for prophylaxis of migraine

**Mechanism of Action/Effect** Blocks both $beta_1$- and $beta_2$-adrenergic receptors, reduces intraocular pressure by reducing aqueous humor production or possibly outflow; reduces blood pressure by blocking adrenergic receptors and decreasing sympathetic outflow, produces a negative chronotropic and inotropic activity through an unknown mechanism

**Contraindications** Hypersensitivity to beta-blockers; uncompensated congestive heart failure; cardiogenic shock; bradycardia or heart block; severe chronic obstructive pulmonary disease; asthma; pregnancy (2nd and 3rd trimesters)

**Warnings** Some products contain sulfites which can cause allergic reactions. Tachyphylaxis may develop. Use with a miotic in angle-closure glaucoma. Use with caution in patients with decreased renal or hepatic function (dosage adjustment required). Severe CNS, cardiovascular, and respiratory adverse effects have been seen following ophthalmic use. Patients with a history of asthma, congestive heart failure, or bradycardia appear to be at a higher risk. Pregnancy factor C/D (2nd and 3rd trimesters).

**Drug Interactions**

**Cytochrome P-450 Effect:** CYP2D6 enzyme substrate

**Decreased Effect:** Decreased effect of beta-blockers with aluminum salts, barbiturates, calcium salts, cholestyramine, colestipol, NSAIDs, penicillins (ampicillin), rifampin, salicylates, and sulfinpyrazone due to decreased bioavailability and plasma levels. Beta-blockers may decrease the effect of sulfonylureas. Beta-blockers may affect the action or levels of ethanol, disopyramide, nondepolarizing muscle relaxants and theophylline, although the effects are difficult to predict.

**Increased Effect/Toxicity:** Increased effect/toxicity of beta-blockers with calcium blockers (diltiazem, nifedipine, felodipine, nicardipine, verapamil, quinidine). Beta-blockers may increase the effect/toxicity of flecainide, haloperidol (hypotensive effects), hydralazine, phenothiazines, acetaminophen, clonidine (hypertensive crisis after or during withdrawal of either agent), epinephrine (initial hypertensive episode followed by bradycardia), lidocaine, and ergots (peripheral ischemia). Beta-blockers may affect the action or levels of ethanol, disopyramide, nondepolarizing muscle relaxants and theophylline, although the effects are difficult to predict.

**Adverse Reactions**

**Ophthalmic:**

>10%: Ocular: Conjunctival hyperemia

1% to 10%: Ocular: Anisocoria, corneal punctate keratitis, keratitis, corneal staining, decreased corneal sensitivity, eye pain, vision disturbances

**Systemic:**

>10%:

Central nervous system: Drowsiness, insomnia

Endocrine & metabolic: Decreased sexual ability

1% to 10%:

Cardiovascular: Bradycardia, palpitations, edema, congestive heart failure, reduced peripheral circulation

Central nervous system: Mental depression

Gastrointestinal: Diarrhea or constipation, nausea, vomiting, stomach discomfort

Respiratory: Bronchospasm

Miscellaneous: Cold extremities

<1% (Limited to important or life-threatening symptoms): Chest pain, arrhythmias, orthostatic hypotension, nervousness, headache, depression, hallucinations, confusion (especially in the elderly), thrombocytopenia, leukopenia, shortness of breath, nightmares, memory loss, Raynaud's phenomenon, rash, psoriasis

**Overdose/Toxicology** Symptoms of intoxication include cardiac disturbances, CNS toxicity, bronchospasm, hypoglycemia and hyperkalemia. The most common cardiac symptoms include hypotension and bradycardia. Atrioventricular block, intraventricular conduction disturbances, cardiogenic shock, and asystole may occur with severe overdose, especially with membrane-depressant drugs (eg, propranolol). CNS effects including convulsions, coma, and respiratory arrest are commonly seen with propranolol and other membrane-depressant and lipid-soluble drugs. Treatment is symptom directed and supportive.

**Pharmacodynamics/Kinetics**

**Protein Binding:** 60%

**Half-life Elimination:** 2-2.7 hours; prolonged with reduced renal function

**Metabolism:** Liver

**Excretion:** Urine

**Onset:** Onset of hypotensive effect: Oral: Within 15-45 minutes; Peak effect: Within 0.5-2.5 hours

**Duration:** ~4 hours; intraocular effects persist for 24 hours after ophthalmic instillation

**Formulations**

Gel, ophthalmic, as maleate (Timoptic-XE®): 0.25% (2.5 mL, 5 mL); 0.5% (2.5 mL, 5 mL)

Solution, ophthalmic, as hemihydrate (Betimol®): 0.25% (2.5 mL, 5 mL, 10 mL, 15 mL); 0.5% (2.5 mL, 5 mL, 10 mL, 15 mL)

Solution, ophthalmic, as maleate (Timoptic®): 0.25% (2.5 mL, 5 mL, 10 mL, 15 mL); 0.5% (2.5 mL, 5 mL, 10 mL, 15 mL)

Solution, ophthalmic, as maleate, preservative free, single use (Timoptic® OcuDose®): 0.25%, 0.5%

Tablet, as maleate (Blocadren®): 5 mg, 10 mg, 20 mg

**Dosing**

**Adults:**

Ophthalmic: Initial: 0.25% solution, instill 1 drop twice daily; increase to 0.5% solution if response not adequate; decrease to 1 drop/day if controlled; do not exceed 1 drop twice daily of 0.5% solution.

Oral:

Hypertension: Initial: 10 mg twice daily, increase gradually every 7 days, usual dosage: 20-40 mg/day in 2 divided doses; maximum: 60 mg/day.

Prevention of myocardial infarction: 10 mg twice daily initiated within 1-4 weeks after infarction.

Migraine headache: Initial: 10 mg twice daily, increase to maximum of 30 mg/day.

**Elderly:** Refer to adult dosing.

**Additional Nursing Issues**

**Physical Assessment:** See Contraindications and Warnings/Precautions for cautious use. Assess other medications patient may be taking for effectiveness and interactions (see Drug Interactions). Monitor for therapeutic effectiveness (appropriate for purpose of therapy, eg, migraine, ophthalmic, cardiac) and adverse reactions (eg, adrenergic blocking effects) (see Warnings/Precautions, Adverse Reactions, and Overdose/Toxicology) at beginning of therapy and regularly with long-term therapy. Assess knowledge/teach patient appropriate use, interventions to reduce side effects, and adverse symptoms to report. **Pregnancy risk factor C/D** - benefits of use should outweigh possible risks. Note breast-feeding caution.

**Patient Information/Instruction:**

Oral: Take exact dose prescribed; do not increase, decrease, or discontinue dosage without consulting prescriber. Take at the same time each day. Does not replace recommended diet or exercise program. If diabetic, monitor serum glucose closely. May cause postural hypotension (use caution when rising from sitting or lying position or climbing stairs); dizziness, drowsiness, or blurred vision (use caution when driving or engaging in tasks requiring alertness until response to drug is known); decreased sexual ability (reversible); or nausea or vomiting (small frequent meals or frequent mouth care may help). Report swelling of extremities, respiratory difficulty, or new

(Continued)

## Timolol *(Continued)*

cough; weight gain (>3 lb/week); unresolved diarrhea or vomiting; or cold blue extremities. **Pregnancy/breast-feeding precautions:** Inform prescriber if you are or intend to be pregnant. Consult prescriber if breast-feeding.

Ophthalmic: For ophthalmic use only. Apply prescribed amount as often as directed. Wash hands before using and do not touch tip of applicator to eye or contaminate tip of applicator. Tilt head back and look upward. Gently pull down lower lid and put drop(s) inside lower eyelid at inner corner. Close eye and roll eyeball in all directions. Do not blink for ½ minute. Apply gentle pressure to inner corner of eye for 30 seconds. Wipe away excess from skin around eye. Do not use any other eye preparation for at least 10 minutes. Do not share medication with anyone else. Temporary stinging or blurred vision may occur. Immediately report any adverse cardiac or CNS effects (usually signifies overdose). Report persistent eye pain, redness, burning, watering, dryness, double vision, puffiness around eye, vision disturbances, other adverse eye response, worsening of condition or lack of improvement. Inform prescriber if you are or intend to be pregnant. Consult prescriber if breast-feeding.

**Geriatric Considerations:** Due to alterations in the beta-adrenergic autonomic nervous system, beta-adrenergic blockade may result in less hemodynamic response than seen in younger adults.

**Breast-feeding Issues:** Timolol is excreted in breast milk and is considered compatible by the American Academy of Pediatrics. It is recommended that the infant be monitored for signs or symptoms of beta-blockade (hypotension, bradycardia, etc) with long-term use.


- **Timolol** *see* Ophthalmic Agents, Glaucoma *on page 853*
- **Timoptic® OcuDose®** *see* Ophthalmic Agents, Glaucoma *on page 853*
- **Timoptic® OcuDose®** *see* Timolol *on page 1138*
- **Timoptic® Ophthalmic** *see* Ophthalmic Agents, Glaucoma *on page 853*
- **Timoptic® Ophthalmic** *see* Timolol *on page 1138*
- **Timoptic-XE® Ophthalmic** *see* Ophthalmic Agents, Glaucoma *on page 853*
- **Timoptic-XE® Ophthalmic** *see* Timolol *on page 1138*
- **Timoptol®** *see* Ophthalmic Agents, Glaucoma *on page 853*
- **Timoptol®** *see* Timolol *on page 1138*
- **Timoptol® XE** *see* Ophthalmic Agents, Glaucoma *on page 853*
- **Timoptol® XE** *see* Timolol *on page 1138*
- **Tinactin®** *see page 1247*
- **Tinactin® for Jock Itch** *see page 1247*
- **Tinaderm®** *see page 1247*
- **TinBen®** *see page 1294*
- **TinCoBen®** *see page 1294*
- **Ting®** *see page 1247*
- **Tiniazol** *see* Ketoconazole *on page 643*
- **Tinver® Lotion** *see page 1246*


## Tioconazole (tye oh KONE a zole)

**U.S. Brand Names** Vagistat® Vaginal

**Therapeutic Category** Antifungal Agent, Vaginal

**Pregnancy Risk Factor** C

**Lactation** Excretion in breast milk unknown

**Use** Local treatment of vulvovaginal candidiasis

**Mechanism of Action/Effect** A 1-substituted imidazole derivative with a broad antifungal spectrum against a wide variety of dermatophytes and yeasts

**Contraindications** Hypersensitivity to tioconazole or any component

**Warnings** Not effective when applied to the scalp. Pregnancy factor C.

**Adverse Reactions**

1% to 10%: Genitourinary: Vulvar/vaginal burning

<1% (Limited to important or life-threatening symptoms): Vulvar itching, soreness, edema, or discharge; polyuria; burning or itching of penis of sexual partner

**Pharmacodynamics/Kinetics**

**Half-life Elimination:** 21-24 hours

**Excretion:** Urine and feces

**Formulations** Cream, vaginal: 6.5% with applicator (4.6 g)

**Dosing**

**Adults:** Vaginal: Insert 1 applicatorful in vagina, just prior to bedtime, as a single dose.

**Elderly:** Refer to adult dosing.

**Additional Nursing Issues**

**Physical Assessment:** Assess knowledge/teach patient appropriate administration, possible side effects/interventions, and adverse symptoms to report. **Pregnancy risk factor C** - 25% systemically absorbed. Note breast-feeding caution.

**Patient Information/Instruction:** Complete full course of therapy as directed. Insert vaginally as directed by prescriber or see package insert. Report persistent vaginal burning, itching, irritation, or discharge. **Breast-feeding precautions:** Consult prescriber if breast-feeding.


- **Tioguanine** *see* Thioguanine *on page 1122*
- **Tiotixene** *see* Thiothixene *on page 1127*

## Tirofiban (tye roe FYE ban)

**U.S. Brand Names** Aggrastat®

**Synonyms** MK383

**Therapeutic Category** Antiplatelet Agent, Glycoprotein IIb/IIIa Inhibitor

**Pregnancy Risk Factor** B

**Lactation** Excretion in breast milk unknown/contraindicated

**Use** In combination with heparin, is indicated for the treatment of acute coronary syndrome, including patients who are to be managed medically and those undergoing PTCA or atherectomy. In this setting, it has been shown to decrease the rate of a combined endpoint of death, new myocardial infarction or refractory ischemia/repeat cardiac procedure.

**Mechanism of Action/Effect** A reversible antagonist of fibrinogen binding to the GP IIb/IIIa receptor, the major platelet surface receptor involved in platelet aggregation. When administered intravenously, it inhibits *ex vivo* platelet aggregation in a dose- and concentration-dependent manner. When given according to the recommended regimen, >90% inhibition is attained by the end of the 30-minute infusion. Platelet aggregation inhibition is reversible following cessation of the infusion.

**Contraindications** Hypersensitivity to tirofiban or any component; history of intracranial/hemorrhagic intracranial neoplasm, A-V malformation or aneurysm; history of stroke in last 30 days, any history of hemorrhagic stroke, major surgery/trauma in last 30 days; history, symptoms, or findings which suggest aortic dissection; severe hypertension, acute pericarditis, concurrent use of other GP IIb/IIIa inhibitor, active bleeding (internal or history of bleeding diathesis); history of thrombocytopenia following prior exposure to tirofiban

**Warnings** Bleeding is the most common complication encountered during this therapy. Most major bleeding associated occurs at the arterial access site for cardiac catheterization. Use caution in patients with platelets <150,000/mm$^3$; patients with hemorrhagic retinopathy; when used in combination with other drugs impacting on coagulation. To minimize bleeding complications, care must be taken in sheath insertion/removal. Sheath hemostasis should be achieved at least 4 hours before hospital discharge. Other trauma and vascular punctures should be minimized. Avoid obtaining vascular access through a noncompressible site (eg, subclavian or jugular vein). Patients with severe renal insufficiency require dosage reduction.

**Drug Interactions**

**Increased Effect/Toxicity:** Use with aspirin and heparin is associated with an increase in bleeding over aspirin and heparin alone. Caution when used with other drugs which affect hemostasis - thrombolytics, oral anticoagulants, nonsteroidal anti-inflammatory drugs, dipyridamole, ticlopidine and clopidogrel. avoid concomitant use of other IIb/IIIa antagonists. Levothyroxine and omeprazole increase tirofiban clearance; however, the clinical significance of this interaction remains to be demonstrated.

**Adverse Reactions** Bleeding is the major drug-related adverse effect. Patients received background treatment with aspirin and heparin. Major bleeding was reported in 1.4% to 2.2%; minor bleeding in 10.5% to 12%; transfusion was required in 4.0% to 4.3%.

>1% (nonbleeding adverse events):

- Cardiovascular: Bradycardia (4%), coronary artery dissection (5%), edema (2%)
- Central nervous system: Dizziness (3%), fever (>1%), headache (>1%), vasovagal reaction (2%)
- Gastrointestinal: Nausea (>1%)
- Genitourinary: Pelvic pain (6%)
- Hematologic: Thrombocytopenia: <90,000/mm$^3$ (1.5%), <50,000/mm$^3$ (0.3%)
- Neuromuscular & skeletal: Leg pain (3%)
- Miscellaneous: Diaphoresis (2%)

<1% (Limited to important or life-threatening symptoms): Intracranial bleeding (0.0% to 0.1%), GI bleeding (0.1% to 0.2%), retroperitoneal bleeding (0.0% to 0.6%), GU bleeding (0.0% to 0.1%)

**Overdose/Toxicology** The most frequent manifestation of overdose is bleeding. Treatment is cessation of therapy and assessment of transfusion. Tirofiban is dialyzable.

**Pharmacodynamics/Kinetics**

**Distribution:** 35% unbound

**Metabolism:** Minimal

**Excretion:** Primarily unchanged drug; 65% in urine, 25% in feces clearance is reduced in elderly patients by 19% to 26%

**Formulations** Injection: 50 mcg/mL (500 mL); 250 mcg/mL (50 mL)

**Dosing**

**Adults:** I.V.: Initial rate of 0.4 mcg/kg/minute for 30 minutes and then continued at 0.1 mcg/kg/minute. Dosing should be continued through angiography and for 12-24 hours after angioplasty or atherectomy.

**Elderly:** Refer to adult dosing.

**Renal Impairment:** $Cl_{cr}$ <30 mL/minute: Reduce dose to 50% of normal rate.

**Administration**

**I.V.:** Infuse over 30 minutes. Tirofiban injection must be diluted to a concentration of 50 mcg/mL (premixed solution does not require dilution).

**I.V. Detail:** Intended for intravenous delivery using sterile equipment and technique. Do not add other drugs or remove solution directly from the bag with a syringe. Do not use plastic containers in series connections. Such use can result in air embolism by drawing air from the first container if it is empty of solution. Discard unused solution 24 hours following the start of infusion. May be administered through the same catheter as heparin.

(Continued)

## Tirofiban *(Continued)*

**Stability**

**Storage:** Store at 25°C (77°F); do not freeze. Protect from light during storage.

**Monitoring Laboratory Tests** Platelet count, persistent reductions <90,000/mm$^3$ may require interruption or discontinuation of infusion. Hemoglobin and hematocrit should be monitored prior to treatment, within 6 hours following loading infusion, and at least daily thereafter during therapy. Because tirofiban requires concurrent heparin therapy, aPTT levels should also be followed.

**Additional Nursing Issues**

**Physical Assessment:** Monitor vital signs and laboratory results prior to, during, and after therapy. Assess infusion insertion site during and after therapy (every 15 minutes or as institutional policy). Observe and teach patient bleeding precautions (avoid invasive procedures and activities that could result in injury). Monitor closely for signs of unusual or excessive bleeding (eg, CNS changes, blood in urine, stool, or vomitus; unusual bruising or bleeding). Breast-feeding is contraindicated.

**Patient Information/Instruction:** Emergency use may dictate depth of patient education. This medication can only be administered I.V. You will have a tendency to bleed easily following this medication. Use caution to prevent injury (use electric razor, use soft toothbrush, use caution with sharps). If bleeding occurs, apply pressure to bleeding spot until bleeding stops completely. Report unusual bruising or bleeding (eg, blood in urine, stool, or vomitus, bleeding gums, vaginal bleeding, nose bleeds); unusual and persistent fever; dizziness or changes in vision; back, leg, or pelvic pain; or persistent nausea or vomiting. **Breast-feeding precautions:** Do not breast-feed.


- **Tiroidine** *see* Levothyroxine *on page 673*
- **Ti-Screen®** *see page 1294*
- **Tisit® Blue Gel** *see page 1294*
- **Tisit® Liquid** *see page 1294*
- **Tisit® Shampoo** *see page 1294*
- **Tissue Plasminogen Activator, Recombinant** *see* Alteplase *on page 58*
- **Titralac® [OTC]** *see* Calcium Supplements *on page 185*
- **Titralac® Plus Liquid** *see page 1294*
- **TMP** *see* Trimethoprim *on page 1181*
- **TMP-SMX** *see* Co-trimoxazole *on page 307*
- **TMP-SMZ** *see* Co-trimoxazole *on page 307*
- **Tobra** *see* Tobramycin *on this page*
- **TobraDex®** *see page 1282*


## Tobramycin (toe bra MYE sin)

**U.S. Brand Names** AKTob® Ophthalmic; Nebcin® Injection; Tobrex® Ophthalmic

**Therapeutic Category** Antibiotic, Aminoglycoside; Antibiotic, Ophthalmic

**Pregnancy Risk Factor** C

**Lactation** Enters breast milk/compatible

**Use** Treatment of documented or suspected *Pseudomonas aeruginosa* infection; infection with a nonpseudomonal enteric bacillus which is more sensitive to tobramycin than gentamicin based on susceptibility tests; empiric therapy in cystic fibrosis and immunocompromised patients; topically used to treat superficial ophthalmic infections caused by susceptible bacteria

**Mechanism of Action/Effect** Interferes with bacterial protein synthesis by binding to 30S and 50S ribosomal subunits resulting in a defective bacterial cell membrane

**Contraindications** Hypersensitivity to tobramycin, other aminoglycosides, or any component

**Warnings** Use with caution in patients with renal impairment (dosage modification required), pre-existing auditory or vestibular impairment, and in patients with neuromuscular disorders. Aminoglycosides are associated with nephrotoxicity or ototoxicity. Ototoxicity may be proportional to the amount of drug given and the duration of treatment. Tinnitus or vertigo are indications of vestibular injury and impending hearing loss. Renal damage is usually reversible. Pregnancy factor C.

**Drug Interactions**

**Increased Effect/Toxicity:** Increased effect with extended spectrum penicillins (synergistic). Neuromuscular blockers may have an increased duration of action (neuromuscular blockade). Amphotericin B, cephalosporins, and loop diuretics may increase risk of nephrotoxicity.

**Effects on Lab Values** ↑ protein, BUN, aminotransferase [AST (SGOT)/ALT (SGPT)] (S), alkaline phosphatase, creatinine; ↓ magnesium, potassium, sodium, calcium (S)

**Adverse Reactions**

1% to 10%:

Renal: Nephrotoxicity

Neuromuscular & skeletal: Neurotoxicity (neuromuscular blockade)

Otic: Ototoxicity (auditory), ototoxicity (vestibular)

<1% (Limited to important or life-threatening symptoms): Eosinophilia, anemia, dyspnea

**Overdose/Toxicology** Symptoms of overdose include ototoxicity, nephrotoxicity, and neuromuscular toxicity. Treatment of choice following a single acute overdose appears to be maintenance of urine output of at least 3 mL/kg/hour during the acute treatment phase. Dialysis is of questionable value in enhancing aminoglycoside elimination. If required, hemodialysis is preferred over peritoneal dialysis in patients with normal renal function. Chelation with penicillins is investigational.

**Pharmacodynamics/Kinetics**

**Protein Binding:** 30%

**Distribution:** Crosses the placenta

Relative diffusion of antimicrobial agents from blood into cerebrospinal fluid (CSF): Minimal even with inflammation

Ratio of CSF to blood level (%): Normal meninges: Nil; Inflamed meninges: 14-23

**Half-life Elimination:** 2-3 hours, directly dependent upon glomerular filtration rate; Adults with impaired renal function: 5-70 hours

**Time to Peak:** I.M.: Within 30-60 minutes; I.V.: Within 30 minutes

**Excretion:** Urine

**Formulations**

Tobramycin sulfate:

Injection (Nebcin®): 10 mg/mL (2 mL); 40 mg/mL (1.5 mL, 2 mL)

Ointment, ophthalmic (Tobrex®): 0.3% (3.5 g)

Powder for injection (Nebcin®): 40 mg/mL (1.2 g vials)

Solution, ophthalmic: 0.3% (5 mL)

AKTob®, Tobrex®: 0.3% (5 mL)

**Dosing**

**Adults:** Individualization is critical because of the low therapeutic index.

**Use of ideal body weight (IBW) for determining the mg/kg/dose appears to be more accurate than dosing on the basis of total body weight (TBW).**

In morbid obesity, dosage requirement may best be estimated using a dosing weight of IBW + 0.4 (TBW - IBW).

Initial and periodic peak and trough plasma drug levels should be determined, particularly in critically ill patients with serious infections or in disease states known to significantly alter aminoglycoside pharmacokinetics (eg, cystic fibrosis, burns, or major surgery); 2-3 serum level measurements should be obtained after the initial dose to measure the half-life in order to determine the frequency of subsequent doses.

I.M., I.V.:

Severe life-threatening infections: 2-2.5 mg/kg/dose

Urinary tract infection: 1.5 mg/kg/dose

Synergy (for gram-positive infections): 1 mg/kg/dose

High-dose once-daily regimens: 5-7 mg/kg/dose once daily

Some clinicians suggest a daily dose of 4-7 mg/kg for all patients with normal renal function. This dose is at least as efficacious with similar, if not less, toxicity than conventional dosing.

Ophthalmic: Instill 1-2 drops of solution every 4 hours. Apply ointment 2-3 times/day. For severe infections, apply ointment every 3-4 hours or 2 drops of solution every 30-60 minutes initially, then reduce to less frequent intervals.

**Elderly:** Dosage should be based on an estimate of ideal body weight.

I.M., I.V.: 1.5-5 mg/kg/day in 1-2 divided doses

I.V.: Once daily or extended interval: 5-7 mg/kg/dose given every 24, 36, or 48 hours based on $Cl_{cr}$ (see Renal Impairment and Geriatric Considerations).

**Renal Impairment:**

$Cl_{cr}$ ≥60 mL/minute: Administer every 8 hours.

$Cl_{cr}$ 40-60 mL/minute: Administer every 12 hours.

$Cl_{cr}$ 20-40 mL/minute: Administer every 24 hours.

$Cl_{cr}$ 10-20 mL/minute: Administer every 48 hours.

$Cl_{cr}$ <10 mL/minute: Administer every 72 hours.

Dialyzable; 30% removal of aminoglycosides occurs during 4 hours of HD - administer dose after dialysis and follow levels.

Continuous arteriovenous or venovenous hemofiltration (CAVH/CAVHD): Dose as for $Cl_{cr}$ of 10-40 mL/minute and follow levels.

Administration in CAPD fluid:

Gram-negative infection: 4-8 mg/L (4-8 mcg/mL) of CAPD fluid

Gram-positive infection (ie, synergy): 3-4 mg/L (3-4 mcg/mL) of CAPD fluid

Administration IVPB/I.M.: Dose as for $Cl_{cr}$ <10 mL/minute and follow levels.

**Hepatic Impairment:** Monitor plasma concentrations.

**Administration**

**I.V.:** Infuse over 30-60 minutes. Give penicillins or cephalosporins at least 1 hour apart from tobramycin.

**Topical:** Eye solutions: Allow 5 minutes between application of "multiple-drop" therapy.

**Stability**

**Storage:** Tobramycin is stable at room temperature both as the clear, colorless solution and as the dry powder. Reconstituted solutions remain stable for 24 hours at room temperature and 96 hours when refrigerated.

**Reconstitution:** Stability of parenteral admixture at room temperature (25°C) and at refrigeration temperature (4°C) is 48 hours.

Standard diluent: Dose/100 mL NS

Minimum volume: 50 mL NS

**Compatibility:** Incompatible with penicillins.

**Monitoring Laboratory Tests** Urinalysis, BUN, serum creatinine, peak and trough plasma tobramycin levels. Obtain drug levels after the third dose. Peak levels are drawn 30 minutes after the end of a 30-minute infusion or 1 hour after initiation of infusion or I.M. injection. The trough is drawn just before the next dose. Perform culture and sensitivity studies prior to initiating therapy to determine the causative organism and its susceptibility to tobramycin.

(Continued)

## Tobramycin *(Continued)*

**Additional Nursing Issues**

**Physical Assessment:** Assess effectiveness and interactions of other medications patient may be taking (see Contraindications and Drug Interactions). Assess patient's hearing level before, during, and following therapy; report changes to prescriber immediately. Monitor for therapeutic response, laboratory values (see above) and adverse reactions: neurotoxicity (vertigo, ataxia), opportunistic infections (fever, mouth and vaginal sores or plaques, unhealed wounds, etc) (see Warnings/Precautions, Adverse Reactions, and Overdose/Toxicology) at beginning of therapy and periodically throughout therapy. Assess knowledge/ teach patient appropriate use, interventions to reduce side effects, and adverse symptoms to report. **Pregnancy risk factor C** - benefits of use should outweigh possible risks.

**Patient Information/Instruction:**

Systemic: Maintain adequate hydration (2-3 L/day of fluids unless instructed to restrict fluid intake). Report decreased urine output, swelling of extremities, difficulty breathing, vaginal itching or discharge, rash, diarrhea, oral thrush, unhealed wounds, dizziness, change in hearing acuity or ringing in ears, or worsening of condition. **Pregnancy precautions:** Inform prescriber if you are pregnant.

Ophthalmic: Use as frequently as recommended; do not overuse. Sit down, tilt head back, instill solution or drops inside lower eyelid, and roll eyeball in all directions. Close eye and apply gentle pressure to inner corner of eye for 30 seconds. Do not touch tip of applicator to eye or any contaminated surface. May experience temporary stinging or blurred vision. Do not use any other eye preparation for 10 minutes. Inform prescriber if condition worsens or does not improve in 3-4 days.

**Geriatric Considerations:** Aminoglycosides are important therapeutic interventions for susceptible organisms and as empiric therapy in seriously ill patients. Their use is not without risk of toxicity; however, these risks can be minimized if initial dosing is adjusted for estimated renal function and appropriate monitoring is performed. High-dose, once-daily aminoglycosides have been advocated as an alternative to traditional dosing regimens. To date, there is little information on the safety and efficacy of these regimens in persons with a creatinine clearance <60 mL/minute/70 kg. A dosing nomogram based upon creatinine clearance has been proposed. Additional studies comparing high-dose, once-daily aminoglycosides to traditional dosing regimens in the elderly are needed before once-daily aminoglycoside dosing can be routinely adopted to this patient population.

**Breast-feeding Issues:** Tobramycin is not absorbed orally, so any drug in breast milk is not available to the infant.

**Additional Information** Nebicin® injection formulation contains sulfites.

**Related Information**

Ophthalmic Agents *on page 1282*
Peak and Trough Guidelines *on page 1331*

♦ **Tobramycin and Dexamethasone** *see page 1282*
♦ **Tobrex®** *see page 1282*
♦ **Tobrex® Ophthalmic** *see* Tobramycin *on page 1142*

## Tocainide (toe KAY nide)

**U.S. Brand Names** Tonocard®

**Therapeutic Category** Antiarrhythmic Agent, Class I-B

**Pregnancy Risk Factor** C

**Lactation** Enters breast milk/contraindicated

**Use** Suppress and prevent symptomatic life-threatening ventricular arrhythmias

**Unlabeled use:** Trigeminal neuralgia

**Mechanism of Action/Effect** Class 1B antiarrhythmic agent; suppresses automaticity of conduction tissue by increasing electrical stimulation threshold of ventricle, HIS-Purkinje system, and spontaneous depolarization of the ventricles during diastole by a direct action on tissues; blocks both the initiation and conduction of nerve impulses by decreasing the neuronal membrane's permeability to sodium ions, which results in inhibition of depolarization with resultant blockade of conduction

**Contraindications** Hypersensitivity to tocainide, amide-type anesthetics, or any component; second or third degree A-V block without a pacemaker

**Warnings** May exacerbate some arrhythmias (eg, atrial fibrillation/flutter). Use with caution in CHF patients. Administer with caution in patients with pre-existing bone marrow failure, cytopenia, severe renal or hepatic disease. Pregnancy factor C.

**Drug Interactions**

**Decreased Effect:** Decreased tocainide plasma levels with cimetidine, phenobarbital, phenytoin, rifampin, and other hepatic enzyme inducers.

**Increased Effect/Toxicity:** Tocainide may increase serum levels of caffeine and theophylline.

**Adverse Reactions**

>10%:

Central nervous system: Nervousness, confusion, ataxia, dizziness
Gastrointestinal: Nausea, anorexia
Neuromuscular & skeletal: Tremor

1% to 10%:

Cardiovascular: Hypotension, tachycardia
Dermatologic: Rash
Gastrointestinal: Vomiting, diarrhea
Neuromuscular & skeletal: Arthralgia, myalgia, paresthesia

Ocular: Blurred vision

<1% (Limited to important or life-threatening symptoms): Bradycardia, palpitations, agranulocytosis, anemia, leukopenia, neutropenia, respiratory arrest

**Overdose/Toxicology** Tocainide has a narrow therapeutic index and severe toxicity may occur slightly above the therapeutic range, especially with other antiarrhythmic drugs. Acute ingestion of twice the daily therapeutic dose is potentially life-threatening. Symptoms of overdose include sedation, confusion, coma, seizures, respiratory arrest, and cardiac toxicity (sinus arrest, A-V block, asystole, and hypotension). The QRS and Q-T intervals are usually normal, although they may be prolonged after massive overdose. Other effects include dizziness, paresthesia, tremor, ataxia, and GI disturbance. Treatment is supportive.

**Pharmacodynamics/Kinetics**

**Protein Binding:** 10% to 20%

**Half-life Elimination:** 11-14 hours, prolonged with renal and hepatic impairment with half-life increased to 23-27 hours

**Time to Peak:** Peak serum levels occur within 30-160 minutes

**Metabolism:** Liver

**Excretion:** Urine

**Formulations** Tablet, as hydrochloride: 400 mg, 600 mg

**Dosing**

**Adults:** Oral: 1200-1800 mg/day in 3 divided doses, up to 2400 mg/day

**Elderly:** Refer to adult dosing.

**Renal Impairment:**

$Cl_{cr}$ <30 mL/minute: Administer 50% of normal dose or 600 mg once daily.

Moderately dialyzable (20% to 50%)

**Hepatic Impairment:** Maximum daily dose: 1200 mg

**Additional Nursing Issues**

**Physical Assessment:** Assess other medications patient may be taking for effectiveness and interactions (see Drug Interactions). See Warnings/Precautions and Contraindications for cautious use. Monitor therapeutic response (cardiac status) and adverse reactions (see Warnings/Precautions and Adverse Reactions) at beginning of therapy, when titrating dosage, and on a regular basis with long-term oral therapy. **Note:** Tocainide has a low toxic:therapeutic ratio and overdose may easily produce severe and life-threatening reactions (see Overdose/Toxicology). Assess knowledge/teach patient appropriate use, interventions to reduce side effects, and adverse symptoms to report. **Pregnancy risk factor C** - benefits of use should outweigh possible risks. Breast-feeding is contraindicated.

**Patient Information/Instruction:** Take exactly as directed, with food. If dose is missed, take as soon as possible, do not double next dose. Do not discontinue without consulting prescriber. You will need regular cardiac checkups while taking this medication. You may experience dizziness, nervousness, or visual changes (use caution when driving or engaging in tasks requiring alertness until response to drug is known); nausea or vomiting, or loss of appetite (frequent small meals, frequent mouth care, chewing gum, or sucking lozenges may help); mild muscle discomfort (analgesics may be recommended). Report chest pain, palpitations, or erratic heartbeat; difficulty breathing or unusual cough; mental confusion or depression; muscle tremor, weakness, or pain; or changes in vision. **Pregnancy/breast-feeding precautions:** Inform prescriber if you are or intend to be pregnant. Do not breast-feed.

**Geriatric Considerations:** Tocainide may cause confusion. Tremor indicates potential toxicity and should not be mistaken for age related changes. Renal and Phase I liver metabolism changes with age may affect clearance. Monitor closely since half-life may be prolonged.

**Related Information**

Antiarrhythmic Drug Classification Comparison *on page 1366*

♦ **Toesen®** *see* Oxytocin *on page 877*

♦ **Tofranil®** *see* Imipramine *on page 600*

♦ **Tofranil-PM®** *see* Imipramine *on page 600*

## Tolazamide (tole AZ a mide)

**U.S. Brand Names** Tolinase®

**Therapeutic Category** Antidiabetic Agent (Sulfonylurea)

**Pregnancy Risk Factor** D

**Lactation** Excretion in breast milk unknown

**Use** Adjunct to diet for the management of mild to moderately severe, stable, noninsulin-dependent (Type II) diabetes mellitus

**Mechanism of Action/Effect** Stimulates insulin release from the pancreatic beta cells; reduces glucose output from the liver; insulin sensitivity is increased at peripheral target sites

**Contraindications** Hypersensitivity to sulfonylureas; Type I diabetes therapy (IDDM); diabetes complicated by ketoacidosis; pregnancy

**Warnings** False-positive response has been reported in patients with liver disease, severe malnutrition, acute pancreatitis, renal dysfunction. Transferring a patient from one sulfonylurea to another does not require a priming dose; doses >1000 mg/day normally do not improve diabetic control.

**Drug Interactions**

**Increased Effect/Toxicity:** Monitor patient closely. Large number of drugs interact with sulfonylureas including salicylates, anticoagulants, $H_2$ antagonists, tricyclic antidepressants, MAO inhibitors, beta-blockers, and thiazide diuretics.

(Continued)

## Tolazamide *(Continued)*

**Adverse Reactions**

>10%:

Central nervous system: Headache, dizziness

Endocrine & metabolic: Hypoglycemia (mild)

Gastrointestinal: Constipation, diarrhea, heartburn, weight gain, anorexia, epigastric fullness, changes in sensation of taste

Renal: Polyuria

1% to 10%:

Dermatologic: Rash, urticaria, photosensitivity

Endocrine & metabolic: Hypoglycemia (severe)

<1% (Limited to important or life-threatening symptoms): Aplastic anemia, hemolytic anemia, bone marrow suppression, thrombocytopenia, agranulocytosis, cholestatic jaundice, hepatic porphyria

**Overdose/Toxicology** Symptoms of overdose include low blood sugar, tingling of lips and tongue, nausea, yawning, confusion, agitation, tachycardia, sweating, convulsions, stupor, and coma. Intoxication with sulfonylureas can cause hypoglycemia and is best managed with glucose administration (oral for milder hypoglycemia or by injection in more severe forms).

**Pharmacodynamics/Kinetics**

**Protein Binding:** >98% ionic/nonionic

**Half-life Elimination:** 7 hours

**Metabolism:** Liver

**Excretion:** Urine

**Onset:** Oral: Within 4-6 hours

**Duration:** 10-24 hours

**Formulations** Tablet: 100 mg, 250 mg, 500 mg

**Dosing**

**Adults:** Oral (doses >1000 mg/day normally do not improve diabetic control): Initial: 100 mg/day, increase at 2- to 4-week intervals; maximum: 1000 mg; give as a single or twice daily dose.

Conversion from insulin → tolazamide:

10 units day = 100 mg/day

20-40 units/day = 250 mg/day

>40 units/day = 250 mg/day and 50% of insulin dose

Doses >500 mg/day should be given in 2 divided doses

**Elderly:** Refer to adult dosing.

**Hepatic Impairment:** Initial and maintenance doses should be conservative.

**Monitoring Laboratory Tests** Urine glucose and ketones, fasting blood glucose, hemoglobin $A_{1c}$, fructosamine

**Additional Nursing Issues**

**Physical Assessment:** Assess effectiveness and interactions of other medications (see Drug Interactions). See Warnings/Precautions and Contraindications for use cautions. Monitor effectiveness of therapy and monitor laboratory tests frequently during therapy (see above). Monitor for adverse response (eg, hypoglycemia - see Adverse Reactions and Overdose/Toxicology). Assess knowledge/teach patient or refer patient to diabetic educator for instruction in appropriate use, possible side effects and appropriate interventions, and adverse symptoms to report. **Pregnancy risk factor D** - assess knowledge/teach patient use of barrier contraceptive measures. Note breast-feeding caution.

**Patient Information/Instruction:** This medication is used to control diabetes; it is not a cure. Other components of the treatment plan are important: follow prescribed diet, medication, and exercise regimen. Take exactly as directed; at the same time each day. Do not change dose or discontinue without consulting prescriber. Avoid alcohol while taking this medication; could cause severe reaction. Inform prescriber of all other prescription or OTC medications you are taking; do not introduce new medication without consulting prescriber. Do not take other medication within 2 hours of this medication unless so advised by prescriber. If you experience hypoglycemic reaction, contact prescriber immediately; maintain regular dietary intake and exercise routine and always carry quick source of sugar with you. You may be more sensitive to sunlight (use sunscreen, wear protective clothing and eyewear, and avoid direct sunlight). You may experience side effects during first weeks of therapy (headache, nausea, diarrhea, constipation, anorexia); consult prescriber if these persist. Report severe or persistent side effects, extended vomiting or flu-like symptoms, skin rash, easy bruising or bleeding, or change in color of urine or stool. **Pregnancy/breast-feeding precautions:** Do not get pregnant; use appropriate contraceptive measures to prevent possible harm to the fetus. Consult prescriber if breast-feeding.

**Geriatric Considerations:** Has not been studied in older patients, however, except for drug interactions it appears to have a safe profile and decline in renal function does not affect its pharmacokinetics.

**Related Information**

Antidiabetic Oral Agents Comparison *on page 1370*

## Tolbutamide (tole BYOO ta mide)

**U.S. Brand Names** Orinase® Diagnostic Injection; Orinase® Oral

**Therapeutic Category** Antidiabetic Agent (Sulfonylurea)

**Pregnancy Risk Factor** D

**Lactation** Enters breast milk/compatible - see Breast-feeding Issues

**Use** Adjunct to diet for the management of mild to moderately severe, stable, noninsulin-dependent (Type II) diabetes mellitus

**Mechanism of Action/Effect** A sulfonylurea hypoglycemic agent; its ability to lower elevated blood glucose levels in patients with functional pancreatic beta cells is similar to the other sulfonylurea agents; stimulates synthesis and release of endogenous insulin from pancreatic islet tissue. The hypoglycemic effect is attributed to an increased sensitivity of insulin receptors and improved peripheral utilization of insulin. Suppression of glucagon secretion may also contribute to the hypoglycemic effects of tolbutamide.

**Contraindications** Hypersensitivity to sulfonylureas; diabetes complicated by ketoacidosis; therapy of IDDM; pregnancy

**Warnings** False-positive response has been reported in patients with liver disease, idiopathic hypoglycemia of infancy, severe malnutrition, acute pancreatitis. Because of its low potency and short duration, it is a useful agent in the elderly if drug interactions can be avoided.

**Drug Interactions**

**Cytochrome P-450 Effect:** CYP2C8, 2C9, 2C18, and 2C19 enzyme substrate; CYP2C19 enzyme inhibitor

**Increased Effect/Toxicity:** Monitor patient closely. Large number of drugs interact with sulfonylureas including salicylates, anticoagulants, $H_2$ antagonists, tricyclic antidepressants, MAO inhibitors, beta-blockers, and thiazide diuretics. Chloramphenicol may increase half-life of tolbutamide.

**Adverse Reactions**

>10%:

Central nervous system: Headache, dizziness

Endocrine & metabolic: Hypoglycemia (mild)

Gastrointestinal: Constipation, diarrhea, heartburn, weight gain, anorexia, epigastric fullness, changes in sensation of taste

Renal: Polyuria

1% to 10%:

Dermatologic: Rash, urticaria, photosensitivity

Endocrine & metabolic: Hypoglycemia (severe)

<1% (Limited to important or life-threatening symptoms): Aplastic anemia, hemolytic anemia, bone marrow suppression, thrombocytopenia, agranulocytosis, cholestatic jaundice, hepatic porphyria

**Overdose/Toxicology** Symptoms of overdose include low blood sugar, tingling of lips and tongue, nausea, yawning, confusion, agitation, tachycardia, sweating, convulsions, stupor, and coma. Treatment includes I.V. glucose (12.5-25 g), epinephrine for anaphylaxis.

**Pharmacodynamics/Kinetics**

**Protein Binding:** 95% to 97% (principally to albumin) ionic/nonionic

**Half-life Elimination:** Plasma: 4-25 hours; Elimination: 4-9 hours

**Time to Peak:** Increased plasma concentrations and volume of distribution secondary to decreased albumin concentrations and less protein binding have been reported.

**Metabolism:** Hepatic metabolism to hydroxymethyltolbutamide (mildly active) and carboxytolbutamide (inactive) both rapidly excreted renally, <2% excreted in the urine unchanged; metabolism does not appear to be affected by age

**Onset:** Peak hypoglycemic action: Oral: 1-3 hours; I.V.: 30 minutes

**Duration:** Oral: 6-24 hours; I.V.: 3 hours

**Formulations**

Tolbutamide sodium:

Injection, diagnostic: 1 g (20 mL)

Tablet: 250 mg, 500 mg

**Dosing**

**Adults:** Divided doses may increase GI side effects.

Oral: Initial: 500-1000 mg 1-3 times/day; usual dose should not be more than 2 g/day.

I.V. bolus: 1 g over 2-3 minutes

**Elderly:** Oral: Initial: 250 mg 1-3 times/day; usual: 500-2000 mg; maximum: 3 g/day. Divided doses may increase GI side effects.

**Renal Impairment:** Not dialyzable (0% to 5%)

**Hepatic Impairment:** Dose reduction is necessary; start at 0.5 mg/day.

**Stability**

**Reconstitution:** Use parenteral formulation within 1 hour following reconstitution.

**Monitoring Laboratory Tests** Fasting blood glucose, hemoglobin $A_{1c}$, fructosamine

**Additional Nursing Issues**

**Physical Assessment:** Assess effectiveness and interactions of other medication (see Drug Interactions). See Warnings/Precautions and Contraindications for use cautions. Monitor effectiveness of therapy and monitor laboratory tests frequently during therapy (see above). Monitor for adverse response (hypoglycemia - see Adverse Reactions and Overdose/Toxicology). Assess knowledge/teach patient or refer patient to diabetic educator for instruction in appropriate use, possible side effects and appropriate interventions, and adverse symptoms to report. **Pregnancy risk factor D** - assess knowledge/teach appropriate use of barrier contraceptives.

**Patient Information/Instruction:** This medication is used to control diabetes; it is not a cure. Other components of treatment plan are important: follow prescribed diet, medication, and exercise regimen. Take exactly as directed; at the same time each day. Do not change dose or discontinue without consulting prescriber. Avoid alcohol while taking this medication; could cause severe reaction. Inform prescriber of all other prescription or OTC medications you are taking; do not introduce new medication without consulting prescriber. Do not take other medication within 2 hours of this

(Continued)

## Tolbutamide *(Continued)*

medication unless so advised by prescriber. If you experience hypoglycemic reaction, contact prescriber immediately. Maintain regular dietary intake and exercise routine and always carry quick source of sugar with you. You may be more sensitive to sunlight (use sunscreen, wear protective clothing and eyewear, and avoid direct sunlight). You may experience side effects during first weeks of therapy (headache, nausea, diarrhea, constipation, anorexia); consult prescriber is these persist. Report severe or persistent side effects, extended vomiting or flu-like symptoms, skin rash, easy bruising or bleeding, or change in color of urine or stool. **Pregnancy precautions:** Do not get pregnant; use appropriate contraceptive measures to prevent possible harm to the fetus.

**Geriatric Considerations:** Because of its low potency and short duration, it is a useful agent in the elderly if drug interactions can be avoided (see Pharmacodynamics and Pharmacokinetics).

**Breast-feeding Issues:** The American Academy of Pediatrics considers tolbutamide compatible with breast-feeding but recommends to monitor for possible jaundice in the infant.

**Additional Information** Sodium content of 1 g vial: 3.5 mEq

**Related Information**

Antidiabetic Oral Agents Comparison *on page 1370*

## Tolcapone (TOLE ka pone)

**U.S. Brand Names** Tasmar®

**Therapeutic Category** Anti-Parkinson's Agent (COMT Inhibitor)

**Pregnancy Risk Factor** C

**Lactation** Excretion in breast milk unknown/contraindicated

**Use** An adjunct to levodopa/carbidopa for the treatment of signs and symptoms of Parkinson's disease.

**Mechanism of Action/Effect** A reversible inhibitor of catechol-O-methyltransferase (COMT). COMT is the major route of metabolism for levodopa. When tolcapone is taken with levodopa the pharmacokinetics is altered, resulting in more sustained levodopa serum levels compared to when levodopa is taken alone.

**Contraindications** Hypersensitivity reactions to tolcapone or any component

**Warnings** Due to reports of fatal liver injury associated with use of this drug, the manufacturer is advising that tolcapone be reserved for use only in patients who do not have severe movement abnormalities and who do not respond to or who are not appropriate candidates for other available treatments. It is not recommended that patients receive tolcapone concomitantly with nonselective MAO inhibitors (see drug interactions). Selegiline is a selective MAO-B inhibitor and can be taken with tolcapone. Pregnancy factor C.

**Drug Interactions**

**Increased Effect/Toxicity:** Theoretically, nonselective MAO inhibitors (phenelzine and tranylcypromine) taken with tolcapone may inhibit the major metabolism pathways for catecholamines which may result in excessive adverse effects possibly due to levodopa accumulation. Concomitant therapy is not recommended.

**Food Interactions** Tolcapone taken with food within 1 hour before or 2 hours after the dose, decreases bioavailability by 10% to 20%

**Adverse Reactions** Patients receiving tolcapone are predisposed to orthostatic hypotension. Inform the patient and explain methods to manage the symptoms. Patients may experience diarrhea, most commonly 6-12 weeks after tolcapone is started. Diarrhea is sometimes associated with anorexia. Patients may experience hallucinations shortly after starting therapy, most commonly within the first 2 weeks. Hallucinations may diminish or resolve with a decrease in the levodopa dose. Hallucinations commonly accompany confusion and sometimes insomnia or excessive dreaming. Tolcapone may exacerbate or induce dyskinesia. Lowering the levodopa dose may help. Use tolcapone with caution in patients with severe renal or hepatic failure.

>10%:

Cardiovascular: Orthostasis

Central nervous system: Sleep disorder, excessive dreaming, headache, dizziness, somnolence, confusion

Gastrointestinal: Nausea, anorexia, diarrhea

Neuromuscular & skeletal: Dyskinesia, dystonia, muscle cramps

1% to 10%:

Cardiovascular: Hypotension, chest pain

Central nervous system: Hallucination, syncope, fatigue

Gastrointestinal: Vomiting, constipation, dry mouth, dyspepsia, abdominal pain, flatulence

Genitourinary: Urine discoloration

Neuromuscular & skeletal: Hyperkinesia, stiffness, arthritis

Respiratory: Dyspnea

<1% (Limited to important or life-threatening symptoms): Fatal liver injury, bradycardia, coronary artery disorder, heart arrest, angina pectoris, myocardial infarct, myocardial ischemia, arteriosclerosis, thrombosis, hypertension, vasodilation, amnesia, extrapyramidal syndrome, manic reaction, cerebrovascular accident, psychosis, myoclonus, delirium, encephalopathy, meningitis, cellulitis, hypercholesteremia, gastrointestinal hemorrhage, colitis, duodenal ulcer, uterine hemorrhage, anemia, leukemia, thrombocytopenia, cholecystitis, neuralgia, hemiplegia, hematuria, bronchitis, epistaxis, hyperventilation, allergic reaction

**Pharmacodynamics/Kinetics**

**Protein Binding:** >99.9%

**Half-life Elimination:** 2-3 hours

**Time to Peak:** Within 2 hours

**Metabolism:** Glucuronidation

**Excretion:** Urine and feces

**Formulations** Tablet: 100 mg, 200 mg

**Dosing**

**Adults:** Oral: Initial: 100 mg 3 times/day; may be increased to 200 mg 3 times/day; always with levodopa/carbidopa. Maximum recommended daily dose: 600 mg given in 3 divided doses (200 mg 3 times/day). **Note:** The levodopa dose may need to be decreased by 30% for a majority of patients receiving levodopa doses >600 mg/day.

**Elderly:** Refer to adult dosing.

**Renal Impairment:** Generally, no adjustment necessary; However, in patients with severe renal failure, treat with caution and do not exceed 100 mg three times daily.

**Hepatic Impairment:** Dose should be reduced in patients with cirrhotic liver disease since unbound drug increases by ~50%. Patients with severe liver failure should be treated with caution and receive doses no higher than 100 mg 3 times/day.

**Additional Nursing Issues**

**Physical Assessment:** Assess effectiveness and interactions of other medications patient may be taking (see Contraindications and Drug Interactions). Monitor therapeutic response (eg, mental status, involuntary movements), and adverse reactions (may exacerbate the adverse effects of levodopa including levodopa toxicity) at beginning of therapy and periodically throughout therapy (see Warnings/Precautions, Adverse Reactions, and Overdose/Toxicology). Assess knowledge/teach patient appropriate use, interventions to reduce side effects, and adverse symptoms to report. **Pregnancy risk factor C** - benefits of use should outweigh possible risks. Breast-feeding is contraindicated.

**Patient Information/Instruction:** Take exactly as directed (may be prescribed in conjunction with levodopa/carbidopa); do not change dosage or discontinue without consulting prescriber. Therapeutic effects may take several weeks or months to achieve and you may need frequent monitoring during first weeks of therapy. Best to take 2 hours before or after a meal; however, may be taken with meals if GI upset occurs. Take at the same time each day. Maintain adequate hydration (2-3 L/day of fluids unless instructed to restrict fluid intake). Do not use alcohol and prescription or OTC sedatives or CNS depressants without consulting prescriber. Urine or perspiration may appear darker. You may experience drowsiness, dizziness, confusion, or vision changes (use caution when driving, climbing stairs, or engaging in tasks requiring alertness until response to drug is known); orthostatic hypotension (use caution when changing position - rising to standing from sitting or lying); increased susceptibility to heat stroke, decreased perspiration (use caution in hot weather - maintain adequate fluids and reduce exercise activity); constipation (increased exercise, fluids, or dietary fruit and fiber may help); dry skin or nasal passages (consult prescriber for appropriate relief); nausea, vomiting, loss of appetite, or stomach discomfort (small frequent meals, frequent mouth care, chewing gum, or sucking lozenges may help). Report unresolved constipation or vomiting; chest pain or irregular heartbeat; difficulty breathing; acute headache or dizziness; CNS changes (hallucination, loss of memory, nervousness, etc); painful or difficult urination; abdominal pain or blood in stool; increased muscle spasticity, rigidity, or involuntary movements; skin rash; or significant worsening of condition. **Pregnancy/breast-feeding precautions:** Inform prescriber if you are or intend to be pregnant. Do not breast-feed.

♦ **Tolectin®** *see* Tolmetin *on this page*

♦ **Tolectin® DS** *see* Tolmetin *on this page*

♦ **Tolinase®** *see* Tolazamide *on page 1145*

## Tolmetin (TOLE met in)

**U.S. Brand Names** Tolectin®; Tolectin® DS

**Therapeutic Category** Nonsteroidal Anti-Inflammatory Agent (NSAID)

**Pregnancy Risk Factor** C/D (at term)

**Lactation** Enters breast milk/compatible

**Use** Treatment of rheumatoid arthritis and osteoarthritis

**Mechanism of Action/Effect** Inhibits prostaglandin synthesis by decreasing the activity of the enzyme, cyclo-oxygenase, which results in decreased formation of prostaglandin precursors

**Contraindications** Hypersensitivity to tolmetin or any component, aspirin, or other nonsteroidal anti-inflammatory drugs (NSAIDs); pregnancy (at term)

**Warnings** Use with caution in patients with upper GI disease, impaired renal function, congestive heart failure, hypertension, and patients receiving anticoagulants. If GI upset occurs with tolmetin, take with antacids other than sodium bicarbonate. Pregnancy factor C/D (at term).

**Drug Interactions**

**Decreased Effect:** Decreased effect with aspirin. Decreased effect of thiazides and furosemide.

**Increased Effect/Toxicity:** Increased toxicity of digoxin, methotrexate, cyclosporine, lithium, insulin, sulfonylureas, potassium-sparing diuretics, and aspirin.

**Food Interactions** Tolmetin peak serum concentrations may be decreased if taken with food.

**Effects on Lab Values** ↑ protein, bleeding time

(Continued)

## Tolmetin *(Continued)*

**Adverse Reactions**

1% to 10%:

Cardiovascular: Chest pain, hypertension, edema

Central nervous system: Headache, dizziness, drowsiness, depression

Dermatologic: Skin irritation

Endocrine & metabolic: Weight gain/loss

Gastrointestinal: Heartburn, abdominal pain, diarrhea, flatulence, vomiting, constipation, gastritis, peptic ulcer, nausea

Genitourinary: Urinary Tract Infection

Hematologic: Elevated BUN, transient decreases in hemoglobin/hematocrit

Ocular: Visual disturbances

Otic: Tinnitus

<1% (Limited to important or life-threatening symptoms): Congestive heart failure, erythema multiforme, toxic epidermal necrolysis, GI bleeding, agranulocytosis, hemolytic anemia, thrombocytopenia, granulocytopenia, hepatitis, abnormal LFTs, hematuria, renal failure, proteinuria

**Overdose/Toxicology** Symptoms of overdose include lethargy, mental confusion, dizziness, leukocytosis, and renal failure. Management of nonsteroidal anti-inflammatory (NSAID) intoxication is supportive and symptomatic. Since many NSAIDs undergo enterohepatic cycling, multiple doses of charcoal may be needed to reduce the potential for delayed toxicities.

**Pharmacodynamics/Kinetics**

**Half-life Elimination:** Biphasic: rapid: 2 hours; slow: 5 hours

**Time to Peak:** Within 30-60 minutes

**Excretion:** Urine

**Onset:** Analgesic: 1-2 hours; Anti-inflammatory: Days to weeks

**Formulations**

Tolmetin sodium:

Capsule (Tolectin® DS): 400 mg

Tablet (Tolectin®): 200 mg, 600 mg

**Dosing**

**Adults:** Oral: 400 mg 3 times/day; usual dose: 600 mg to 1.8 g/day; maximum: 2 g/day

**Elderly:** Oral: Initial: 200 mg 3 times/day; usual dose: 600 mg to 1.8 g/day; maximum: 2 g/day

**Monitoring Laboratory Tests** Occult blood loss, CBC, liver enzymes, BUN, serum creatinine, periodic liver function

**Additional Nursing Issues**

**Physical Assessment:** Assess effectiveness and interactions of other medications patient may be taking (see Contraindications and Drug Interactions). Monitor laboratory tests (see above) and therapeutic response (eg, relief of pain and inflammation, increased activity tolerance), and adverse reactions (eg, GI and CNS response, hepatotoxicity, ototoxicity) at beginning of therapy and periodically throughout therapy (see Warnings/Precautions, Adverse Reactions, and Overdose/Toxicology). Schedule ophthalmic evaluations for patients who develop eye complaints during long-term NSAID therapy. Assess knowledge/teach patient appropriate use, interventions to reduce side effects, and adverse symptoms to report. **Pregnancy risk factor C/D** - see Pregnancy Risk Factor for cautious use.

**Patient Information/Instruction:** Take this medication exactly as directed; do not increase dose without consulting prescriber. Do not crush tablets or break capsules. Take with food or milk to reduce GI distress. Maintain adequate fluid intake (2-3 L/day of fluids unless instructed to restrict fluid intake). Do not use alcohol, aspirin, or aspirin-containing medication, and all other anti-inflammatory medications without consulting prescriber. You may experience dizziness, nervousness, or headache (use caution when driving or engaging in tasks requiring alertness until response to drug is known); nausea, vomiting, or heartburn (frequent small meals, frequent mouth care, sucking lozenges, or chewing gum may help); constipation (increased exercise, fluids, or dietary fruit and fiber may help). GI bleeding, ulceration, or perforation can occur with or without pain; discontinue medication and contact prescriber if persistent abdominal pain or cramping, or blood in stool occurs. Report chest pain or palpitations; breathlessness or difficulty breathing; unusual bruising/bleeding; blood in urine, stool, mouth, or vomitus; unusual fatigue; skin rash or itching; unusual weight gain or swelling of extremities; change in urinary pattern; or change in vision or hearing or ringing in ears. **Pregnancy precautions:** Inform prescriber if you are or intend to be pregnant.

**Geriatric Considerations:** Elderly are at high risk for adverse effects from nonsteroidal anti-inflammatory agents. As much as 60% of elderly can develop peptic ulceration and/or hemorrhage asymptomatically. The concomitant use of $H_2$ blockers, omeprazole, and sucralfate is not effective as prophylaxis with the exception of NSAID-induced duodenal ulcers which may be prevented by the use of ranitidine. Misoprostol is the only prophylactic agent proven effective. Also, concomitant disease and drug use contribute to the risk for GI adverse effects. Use lowest effective dose for shortest period possible. Consider renal function decline with age. Use of NSAIDs can compromise existing renal function especially when $Cl_{cr}$ is ≤30 mL/minute. Tinnitus may be a difficult and unreliable indication of toxicity due to age-related hearing loss or eighth cranial nerve damage. CNS adverse effects such as confusion, agitation, and hallucination are generally seen in overdose or high-dose situations, but elderly may demonstrate these adverse effects at lower doses than younger adults.

**Additional Information** Sodium content of 200 mg: 0.8 mEq

**Related Information**
Nonsalicylate/Nonsteroidal Anti-inflammatory Comparison *on page 1401*

♦ **Tolnaftate** *see page 1247*

## Tolterodine (tole TER oh dine)

**U.S. Brand Names** Detrol™

**Therapeutic Category** Anticholinergic Agent

**Pregnancy Risk Factor** C

**Lactation** Excretion in breast milk unknown/contraindicated

**Use** Treatment of patients with an overactive bladder with symptoms of urinary frequency, urgency, or urge incontinence

**Mechanism of Action/Effect** Tolterodine is a competitive antagonist of muscarinic receptors. In animal models, tolterodine demonstrates selectivity for urinary bladder receptors over salivary receptors. Urinary bladder contraction is mediated by muscarinic receptors. Tolterodine increases residual urine volume and decreases detrusor muscle pressure.

**Contraindications** Hypersensitivity to tolterodine or any component; urinary retention or gastric retention; uncontrolled narrow-angle glaucoma

**Warnings** Use caution in patients with bladder flow obstruction, pyloric stenosis or other GI obstruction, narrow-angle glaucoma (controlled), or reduced hepatic/renal function. Pregnancy factor C.

**Drug Interactions**

**Cytochrome P-450 Effect:** CYP3A3/4 enzyme substrate, CYP2D6 enzyme substrate

**Increased Effect/Toxicity:** Fluoxetine, which inhibits cytochrome P-450 2D6, increases concentration 4.8 times. Other drugs which inhibit this isoenzyme may also interact. Studies with inhibitors of cytochrome isoenzyme 3A4 have not been performed. Macrolide antibiotics/azole antifungal agents may inhibit the metabolism of tolterodine. Doses of tolterodine >1 mg twice daily should not be exceeded.

**Adverse Reactions**

>10%: Central nervous system: Headache

1% to 10%:

Cardiovascular: Chest pain, hypertension (1.5%)

Central nervous system: Vertigo (8.6%), nervousness (1.1%), somnolence (3.0%)

Dermatologic: Pruritus (1.3%), rash (1.9%), dry skin (1.7%)

Gastrointestinal: Abdominal pain (7.6%), constipation (6.5%), diarrhea (4.0%), dyspepsia (5.9%), flatulence (1.3%), nausea (4.2%), vomiting (1.7%), weight gain (1.5%)

Genitourinary: Dysuria (2.5%), polyuria (1.1%), urinary retention (1.7%), urinary tract infection (5.5%)

Neuromuscular & skeletal: Back pain, falling (1.3%), paresthesia (1.1%)

Ocular: Vision abnormalities (4.7%), dry eyes (3.8%)

Respiratory: Bronchitis (2.1%), cough (2.1%), pharyngitis (1.5%), rhinitis (1.1%), sinusitis (1.1%), upper respiratory infection (5.9%)

Miscellaneous: Flu-like symptoms (4.4%), infection (2.1%)

**Pharmacodynamics/Kinetics**

**Distribution:** Highly bound to alpha$_1$-acid glycoprotein

**Metabolism:** Extensive hepatic metabolism primarily by hepatic cytochrome P-450 isoenzyme 2D6 (some metabolites share activity). Metabolism via isoenzyme 3A4 is a minor pathway in most patients. In patients with a genetic deficiency of isoenzyme 2D6, metabolism via isoenzyme 3A4 predominates.

**Excretion:** Primarily urinary excretion of parent drug and metabolites <1% excreted unchanged

**Formulations** Tablet, as tartrate: 1 mg, 2 mg

**Dosing**

**Adults:** Oral: Initial: 2 mg twice daily. The dose may be lowered to 1 mg twice daily based on individual response and tolerability.

Dosing adjustment in patients concurrently taking cytochrome P-450 3A4 inhibitors: 1 mg twice daily.

**Elderly:** Refer to adult dosing.

**Renal Impairment:** Use with caution.

**Hepatic Impairment:** Administer 1 mg twice daily.

**Additional Nursing Issues**

**Physical Assessment:** Assess patient's ability to void (see Contraindications). Monitor effectiveness of therapy and possible adverse effects. **Pregnancy risk factor C** - benefits of use should outweigh risks. Breast-feeding is contraindicated.

**Patient Information/Instruction:** Take as directed, preferably with food. You may experience headache (a mild analgesic may help); dizziness, nervousness, or sleepiness (use caution when driving, climbing stairs, or engaging in tasks requiring alertness until response to drug is known); abdominal discomfort, diarrhea, constipation, nausea or vomiting (small frequent meals, increased exercise, adequate fluid intake may help). Report back pain, muscle spasms, alteration in gait, or numbness of extremities; unresolved or persistent constipation, diarrhea, or vomiting; or symptoms of upper respiratory infection or flu. Report immediately any chest pain or palpitations; difficulty urinating or pain on urination. **Pregnancy/breast-feeding precautions:** Inform prescriber if you are or intend to be pregnant. Do not breast-feed.

**Dietary Issues:** Food increases bioavailability (~53% increase).

♦ **Tolu-Sed® DM [OTC]** *see* Guaifenesin and Dextromethorphan *on page 549*

♦ **Tonocard®** *see* Tocainide *on page 1144*

♦ **Topamax**® *see* Topiramate *on page 1155*

## Topical Corticosteroids (TOP i kal kor ti koe STER oyds)

**U.S. Brand Names** Aclovate® Topical; Ala-Cort®; Ala-Scalp®; Alphatrex®; Anucort-HC® Suppository; Anuprep HC® Suppository; Anusol® HC-1 [OTC]; Anusol® HC-2.5% [OTC]; Anusol-HC® Suppository; Aristocort®; Aristocort® A; Betatrex®; Beta-Val®; CaldeCORT®; CaldeCORT® Anti-Itch Spray; Cetacort®; Cloderm® Topical; Cordran®; Cordran® SP; CortaGel® [OTC]; Cortaid® Maximum Strength [OTC]; Cortaid® With Aloe [OTC]; Cort-Dome®; Cortef®; Cortef® Feminine Itch; Cortenema®; Corticaine®; Cortifoam®; Cortizone®-5 [OTC]; Cortizone®-10 [OTC]; Cutivate™; Decaspray®; Delta-Tritex®; Dermarest Dricort®; Derma-Smoothe/FS®; Dermatop®; DermiCort®; Dermolate® [OTC]; Dermtex® HC With Aloe; DesOwen® Topical; Diprolene®; Diprolene® AF; Diprosone®; Elocon® Topical; Florone®; Florone E®; Fluonid®; Flurosyn®; Flutex®; FS Shampoo®; Gynecort® [OTC]; Halog®; Halog®-E; Hemril-HC® Uniserts®; Hi-Cor-1.0®; Hi-Cor-2.5®; Hycort®; Hydrocort®; Hydro-Tex® [OTC]; Hytone®; Kenalog®; Kenalog® H; Kenalog® in Orabase®; Kenonel®; LactiCare-HC®; Lanacort® [OTC]; Lidex®; Lidex-E®; Locoid®; Maxiflor®; Maxivate®; Nasonex® Nasal Spray; Nutracort®; Pandel®; Penecort®; Procort® [OTC]; Proctocort™; Psorcon™; Scalpicin®; Solu-Cortef®; S-T Cort®; Synacort®; Synalar®; Synalar-HP®; Synemol®; Tegrin®-HC [OTC]; Teladar®; Temovate® Topical; Texacort®; Topicort®; Topicort®-LP; Triacet™; Triderm®; Tridesilon® Topical; U-Cort™; Ultravate™ Topical; Valisone®; Westcort®

**Synonyms** Alclometasone; Betamethasone; Clobetasol; Clocortolone; Corticosteroids, Topical; Desonide; Desoximetasone; Dexamethasone; Diflorasone; Fluocinolone; Fluocinonide; Flurandrenolide; Fluticasone; Halcinolide; Halobetasol; Hydrocortisone; Mometasone; Prednicarbate; Tiamcinolone

**Therapeutic Category** Corticosteroid, Topical

**Pregnancy Risk Factor** C

**Lactation** Excretion in breast milk unknown/use caution

**Use** Relief of inflammatory and pruritic manifestations of corticosteroid-responsive dermatologic conditions. Significant differences in potency are present within this class. The following list is designed to facilitate comparison.

**Lowest potency:**
- Alclometasone 0.05% cream, ointment (Aclovate®)
- Betamethasone 0.1% cream
- Betamethasone 0.2% cream
- Desonide 0.05% cream, ointment, lotion (Desowen™, Tridesilon®)
- Dexamethasone 0.04% aerosol (Decaspray®)
- Hydrocortisone 1% cream, ointment, lotion
- Hydrocortisone 2.5% cream, ointment
- Methylprednisolone acetate 0.25% ointment (Medrol®)
- Methylprednisolone acetate 1% ointment (Medrol®)

**Low potency:**
- Betamethasone valerate 0.025% cream (Valisone® reduced strength)
- Clocortolone 0.1% cream (Cloderm®)
- Fluocinolone acetonide 0.01% cream, solution (Synalar®)
- Flurandrenolide 0.025% cream, ointment (Cordran®, Cordran® SP)
- Hydrocortisone valerate 0.2% cream (Westcort®)
- Triamcinolone acetonide 0.025% cream, ointment (Kenalog®)

**Intermediate potency:**
- Betamethasone benzoate 0.025% cream, gel, lotion
- Betamethasone alerate 0.1% cream, ointment, lotion (Valisone®)
- Desoximetasone 0.05% cream, ointment (Topicort® LP)
- Fluocinolone acetonide 0.025% cream
- Flurandrenolide 0.05% cream, ointment, lotion (Cordran®, Cordran® SP)
- Fluticasone propionate 0.05% cream (Cutivate™)
- Halcinonide 0.025% cream, ointment (Halog®)
- Mometasone furoate 0.1% cream, ointment, lotion
- Triamcinolone acetonide 0.1% cream, ointment (Kenalog®)

**High potency:**
- Amcinonide 0.1% cream, ointment (Cyclocort®)
- Betamethasone dipropionate 0.05% cream, ointment, lotion (Diprosone®)
- Desoximetasone 0.25% cream, ointment (Topicort®)
- Flucinolone 0.2% cream (Synalar® HP)
- Flucinonide 0.05% cream, ointment (Lidex®)
- Halcinonide 0.1% cream, ointment, solution (Halog®)
- Triamcinolone acetonide 0.5% cream, ointment (Kenalog®)

**Very high potency:**
- Augmented betamethasone dipropionate 0.05% ointment (Diprolene®)
- Clobetasol propionate 0.05% cream, ointment (Temovate®)
- Diflorasone 0.05% gel, ointment (Fluorone®, Maxiflor®, Psorcon™)
- Halobetasol propionate 0.05% cream, ointment (Ultravate™)

**Mechanism of Action/Effect** Reverses capillary permeability and release of inflammatory mediators (leukotrienes and prostaglandins); suppresses migration of polymorphonuclear leukocytes; agents may be grouped by potency (see Use)

**Contraindications** Hypersensitivity to any specific agent or component; viral, fungal, or tubercular skin infection

**Warnings** May cause adrenal suppression or insufficiency, application to abraded or inflamed skin or large areas of the body may increase the risk of systemic absorption and adrenal suppression. Use only low-potency agents on or near the face. Pregnancy factor

C (however, exposure to fetus after topical application may be minimal due to low absorption).

**Adverse Reactions** When systemic absorption occurs, adrenocortical suppression may occur, as well as other systemic effects of steroids, including Cushing's syndrome, hypokalemia, glaucoma, and cataracts.

1% to 10%:

Dermatologic: Secondary infection, allergic contact dermatitis, dryness, rash, folliculitis, frurunculosis, pustules, pyoderma, hyperesthesia

Local: Burning, itching

<1% (Limited to important or life-threatening symptoms): Hypertrichosis, acneform eruptions, hypopigmentation, perioral dermatitis, bruising, maceration of skin, hirsuitism, skin atrophy, striae, telangectasia

**Pharmacodynamics/Kinetics**

**Metabolism:** Liver

**Formulations**

**Alclometasone dipropionate:**
- Cream: 0.05% (15 g, 45 g, 60 g)
- Ointment, topical: 0.05% (15 g, 45 g, 60 g)

**Betamethasone dipropionate (Diprosone®):**
- Aerosol: 0.1% (85 g)
- Cream: 0.05% (15 g, 45 g)
- Lotion: 0.05% (20 mL, 30 mL, 60 mL)
- Ointment: 0.05% (15 g, 45 g)

**Betamethasone dipropionate augmented (Diprolene®):**
- Cream: 0.05% (15 g, 45 g)
- Gel: 0.05% (15 g, 45 g)
- Lotion: 0.05% (30 mL, 60 mL)
- Ointment, topical: 0.05% (15 g, 45 g)

**Betamethasone valerate (Betatrex®, Valisone®):**
- Cream: 0.01% (15 g, 60 g); 0.1% (15 g, 45 g, 110 g, 430 g)
- Lotion: 0.1% (20 mL, 60 mL)
- Ointment: 0.1% (15 g, 45 g)

**Clobetasol propionate:**
- Cream: 0.05% (15 g, 30 g, 45 g)
- Cream in emollient base: 0.05% (15 g, 30 g, 60 g)
- Gel: 0.05% (15 g, 30 g, 45 g)
- Ointment,topical: 0.05% (15 g, 30 g, 45 g)
- Scalp application: 0.05% (25 mL, 50 mL)

**Clocortolone:** Cream, as pivalate: 0.1% (15 g, 45 g)

**Desonide:**
- Cream: 0.05% (15 g, 60 g)
- Lotion: 0.05% (60 mL, 120 mL)
- Ointment: 0.05% (15 g, 60 g)

**Desoximetasone:**
- Cream:
  - Topicort®: 0.25% (15 g, 60 g, 120 g)
  - Topicort®-LP: 0.05% (15 g, 60 g)
- Gel: 0.05% (15 g, 60 g)
- Ointment (Topicort®): 0.25% (15 g, 60 g)

**Dexamethasone:** Topical, aerosol: 0.01% (58 g); 0.04% (25 g)

**Diflorasone diacetate:**
- Cream: 0.05% (15 g, 30 g, 60 g)
- Ointment: 0.05% (15 g, 30 g, 60 g)

**Fluocinolone acetonide:**
- Cream: 0.01% (15 g, 60 g); 0.025% (15 g, 60 g)
  - Flurosyn®, Synalar®: 0.01% (15 g, 30 g, 60 g, 425 g)
  - Flurosyn®, Synalar®, Synemol®: 0.025% (15 g, 60 g, 425 g)
  - Synalar-HP®: 0.2% (12 g)
- Ointment: 0.025% (15 g, 60 g)
  - Flurosyn®, Synalar®: 0.025% (15 g, 30 g, 60 g, 425 g)
- Oil (Derma-Smoothe/FS®): 0.01% (120 mL)
- Shampoo (FS Shampoo®): 0.01% (180 mL)
- Solution: 0.01% (20 mL, 60 mL)
  - Fluonid®, Synalar®: 0.01% (20 mL, 60 mL)

**Fluocinonide:**
- Cream: 0.05% (15 g, 30 g, 60 g, 120 g)
  - Anhydrous, emollient (Lidex®): 0.05% (15 g, 30 g, 60 g, 120 g)
  - Aqueous, emollient (Lidex-E®): 0.05% (15 g, 30 g, 60 g, 120 g)
- Gel: 0.05% (15 g, 60 g)
  - Lidex®: 0.05% (15 g, 30 g, 60 g, 120 g)
- Ointment: 0.05% (15 g, 30 g, 60 g)
  - Lidex®: 0.05% (15 g, 30 g, 60 g, 120 g)
- Solution: 0.05% (20 mL, 60 mL)
  - Lidex®: 0.05% (20 mL, 60 mL)

**Flurandrenolide:**
- Cream, emulsified base (Cordran® SP): 0.025% (30 g, 60 g); 0.05% (15 g, 30 g, 60 g)
- Lotion (Cordran®): 0.05% (15 mL, 60 mL)
- Ointment, topical (Cordran®): 0.025% (30 g, 60 g); 0.05% (15 g, 30 g, 60 g)
- Tape (Cordran®): 4 mcg/cm$^2$ (7.5 cm x 60 cm, 7.5 cm x 200 cm rolls)

(Continued)

## Topical Corticosteroids *(Continued)*

**Fluticasone propionate:**
Cream (Cutivate™): 0.05% (15 g, 30 g, 60 g)
Ointment (Cutivate™): 0.005% (15 g, 60 g)
**Halcinolide:**
Cream (Halog®): 0.025% (15 g, 60 g, 240 g); 0.1% (15 g, 30 g, 60 g, 240 g)
Cream, emollient base (Halog®-E) : 0.1% (15 g, 30 g, 60 g)
Ointment, topical (Halog®): 0.1% (15 g, 30 g, 60 g, 240 g)
Solution (Halog®): 0.1% (20 mL, 60 mL)
**Halobetasol propionate:**
Cream: 0.05% (15 g, 45 g)
Ointment: 0.05% (15 g, 45 g)
**Hydrocortisone acetate:**
Aerosol, rectal (Cortifoam®): 10% [90 mg/applicatorful] 20 g
Cream (CaldeCORT®, Gynecort®, Cortaid® with Aloe, Cortef® Feminine Itch, Lanacort®): 0.5% (15 g, 22.5 g, 30 g)
Anusol-HC-1®, CaldeCORT®, Clocort® Maximum Strength, Cortaid® Maximum Strength, Dermarest Dricort®, U-Cort™: 1% (15 g, 21 g, 30 g, 120 g)
Ointment, topical:
Cortaid® with Aloe, Lanacort® 5: 0.5% (15 g, 30 g)
Gynecort® 10, Lanacort® 10: 1% (15 g, 30 g)
Solution, topical (Scalpicin®): 1%
Suppository, rectal (Anucort-HC®, Anuprep HC®, Anusol-HC®, Hemril-HC® Uniserts®): 25 mg
**Hydrocortisone, base:**
Aerosol, topical:
CaldeCORT® Anti-Itch Spray, Cortaid®: 0.5% (45 g, 58 g)
Cortaid® Maximum Strength: 1% (45 mL)
Cream:
Cort-Dome®, Corticaine®; Cortizone®-5, DermiCort®, Dermolate®, Dermtex® HC with Aloe, HydroSKIN®, Hydro-Tex®: 0.5% (15 g, 30 g, 120 g, 454 g)
Ala-Cort®, Cort-Dome®, DermiCort®, Hi-Cor-1.0®, Hycort®, Hytone®, Nutracort®, Penecort®, Synacort®: 1% (15 g, 20 g, 30 g, 60 g, 120 g, 240 g, 454 g)
Anusol-HC-2.5%®, Eldecort®, Hi-Cor-2.5®, Hydrocort®, Hytone®, Synacort®: 2.5% (15 g, 20 g, 30 g, 60 g, 120 g, 240 g, 454 g)
Rectal (Proctocort™): 1% (30 g)
Gel:
CortaGel®: 0.5% (15 g, 30 g)
CortaGel® Extra Strength: 1% (15 g, 30 g)
Lotion:
Cetacort®, DermiCort®, HydroSKIN®, S-T Cort®: 0.5% (60 mL, 120 mL)
Acticort 100®, Cetacort®, Cortizone-10®, Dermacort®, Hytone®, LactiCare-HC®, Nutracort®: 1% (60 mL, 120 mL)
Ala-Scalp®: 2% (30 mL)
Hytone®, LactiCare-HC®, Nutracort®: 2.5% (60 mL, 120 mL)
Ointment, topical:
Cortizone®-5, HydroSKIN®: 0.5% (30 g)
Cortizone®-10, Hycort®, HydroSKIN®, Hydro-Tex®, Hytone®, Tegrin®-HC: 1% (15 g, 20 g, 30 g, 60 g, 120 g, 240 g, 454 g)
Hytone®: 2.5% (20 g, 30 g)
Solution:
Pentecort®: 1% (30 mL, 60 mL)
Texacort®: 1% (30 mL)
Suspension, rectal (Cortenema®): 100 mg/60 mL (7s)
**Hydrocortisone, butyrate:**
Locoid®:
Cream: 0.1% (15 g, 45 g)
Ointment, topical: 0.1% (15 g, 45 g)
Solution, topical: 0.1% (20 mL, 60 mL)
Pandel®: Cream: 1% (15 g, 45 g)
**Hydrocortisone, valerate (Westcort®):**
Cream: 0.2% (15 g, 45 g, 60 g)
Ointment, topical: 0.2% (15 g, 45 g, 60 g, 120 g)
**Mometasone furoate:**
Cream: 0.1% (15 g, 45 g)
Lotion: 0.1% (30 mL, 60 mL)
Ointment: 0.1% (15 g, 45 g)
Nasal spray: 50 mcg (17 g)
**Prednicarbate:** Cream: 0.1% (15 g, 60 g)
**Triamcinolone:**
Aerosol, as acetonide (Kenalog®): 0.2 mg/2 second spray (23 g, 63 g)
Cream, as acetonide (Aristocort®, Flutex®, Kenalog®, Delta-Tritex®, Kenonel®, Triacet™, Triderm®): 0.025% (15 g, 60 g, 80 g, 240 g, 454 g); 0.1% (15 g, 30 g, 60 g, 80 g, 90 g, 120 g, 240 g); 0.5% (15 g, 20 g, 30 g, 240 g)
Lotion, as acetonide: 0.025% (60 mL); 0.1% (15 mL, 60 mL)
Ointment:
Oral (Kenalog® in Orabase®): 0.1% (5 g)
Topical, as acetonide (Flutex®, Kenalog®, Aristocort®): 0.025% (15 g, 30 g, 60 g, 80 g, 120 g, 454 g); 0.1% (15 g, 30 g, 60 g, 80 g, 120 g, 240 g, 454 g); 0.5% (15 g, 20 g, 30 g, 240 g)

**Dosing**

**Adults:**

**Alclometasone:** Apply a thin film to the affected area 2-3 times/day.

**Betamethasone:** Apply thin film 2-4 times/day.

**Clobetasol:** Apply twice daily for up to 2 weeks with no more than 50 g/week.

**Clocortolone:** Apply sparingly and gently; rub into affected area from 1-4 times/day.

**Desonide:** Apply 2-4 times/day sparingly.

**Desoximetasone:** Apply sparingly in a thin film twice daily.

**Dexamethasone:** Apply 1-4 times/day.

**Diflorasone:** Apply ointment sparingly 1-3 times/day; apply cream sparingly 2-4 times/day.

**Fluocinolone:** Apply a thin layer to affected area 2-4 times/day.

**Flurandrenolide:**

Ointment, cream: Apply sparingly 1-2 times/day.

Tape: Apply once daily.

Cream, lotion, ointment: Apply sparingly 2-3 times/day.

**Fluticasone:** Apply sparingly in a thin film twice daily.

**Halcinolide:** Apply sparingly 1-3 times/day, occlusive dressing may be used for severe or resistant dermatoses. A thin film of cream or ointment is effective; do not overuse.

**Halobetasol:** Apply sparingly to skin twice daily, rub in gently and completely. Treatment should not exceed 2 consecutive weeks and total dosage should not exceed 50 g/week.

**Hydrocortisone:** Apply to affected area 3-4 times/day.

**Mometasone:**

Topical: Apply sparingly to area once daily. Do not use occlusive dressings.

Nasal spray: One spray into each nostril daily.

**Prednicarbate:** Apply a thin film to affected area twice daily.

**Triamcinolone:** Apply a thin film 2-3 times/day.

**Administration**

**Topical:** For external use only. Do not use on open wounds, weeping lesions, or burns. Do not use occlusive dressings. Use only low-potency agents on or near the face.

**Stability**

**Storage:** Store at room temperature.

**Additional Nursing Issues**

**Physical Assessment:** See Contraindications and Warnings/Precautions for use cautions. When applied to large areas of skin or for extensive periods of time, monitor for adverse skin or systemic reactions. Assess knowledge/teach patient appropriate application and use and adverse symptoms (see Adverse Reactions) to report. **Pregnancy risk factor C** - systemic absorption may be minimal with appropriate use. Note breast-feeding caution.

**Patient Information/Instruction:** For external use only. Use exactly as directed; do not overuse. Do not apply to open wounds or weeping areas. Before using, wash and dry area gently. Apply a thin film to affected area and rub in gently. If dressing is necessary, use a porous dressing. Avoid contact with eyes. Avoid exposing treated area to direct sunlight; sunburn can occur. Report increased swelling, redness, rash, itching, signs of infection, worsening of condition, or lack of healing. **Pregnancy/breast-feeding precautions:** Inform prescriber if you are or intend to be pregnant. Consult prescriber if breast-feeding.

**Additional Information** Hydrocortisone base topical cream, lotion, and ointments in concentrations of 0.25%, 0.5%, and 1% may be OTC or prescriptive depending on the product labeling.

- **Topicort®** *see* Topical Corticosteroids *on page 1152*
- **Topicort®-LP** *see* Topical Corticosteroids *on page 1152*
- **Topicycline® Topical** *see* Tetracycline *on page 1111*
- **Topilene** *see* Betamethasone *on page 148*
- **Topilene** *see* Topical Corticosteroids *on page 1152*

## Topiramate (toe PYE ra mate)

**U.S. Brand Names** Topamax®

**Therapeutic Category** Anticonvulsant, Miscellaneous

**Pregnancy Risk Factor** C

**Lactation** Excretion in breast milk unknown/use caution

**Use** Adjunctive therapy for partial onset seizures in adults. Unlabeled use: bipolar disorder. Orphan drug status for Lennox-Gestaut syndrome

**Mechanism of Action/Effect** Mechanism is not fully understood. It is thought to decrease seizure frequency by blocking sodium channels in neurons, enhancing GABA activity and by blocking glutamate activity.

**Contraindications** Hypersensitivity to topiramate or any component

**Warnings** Avoid abrupt withdrawal of topiramate therapy, it should be withdrawn slowly to minimize the potential of increased seizure frequency; the risk of kidney stones is about 2-4 times that of the untreated population, the risk of this event may be reduced by increasing fluid intake. Use cautiously in patients with hepatic or renal impairment. Pregnancy factor C.

**Drug Interactions**

**Cytochrome P-450 Effect:** CYP2C19 enzyme substrate; CYP2C19 enzyme inhibitor

**Decreased Effect:** Phenytoin can decrease topiramate levels by as much as 48%, carbamazepine reduces it by 40%, and valproic acid reduces topiramate by 14%.

(Continued)

## Topiramate *(Continued)*

Digoxin levels and norethindrone blood levels are decreased when coadministered with topiramate.

**Increased Effect/Toxicity:** Concomitant administration with other CNS depressants will increase its sedative effects. Coadministration with other carbonic anhydrase inhibitors may increase the chance of nephrolithiasis.

**Adverse Reactions**

>10%:

Central nervous system: Fatigue, dizziness, ataxia, somnolence, psychomotor slowing, nervousness, memory difficulties, speech problems

Gastrointestinal: Nausea

Neuromuscular & skeletal: Paresthesia, tremor

Ocular: Nystagmus

Respiratory: Upper respiratory infection

1% to 10%:

Cardiovascular: Chest pain, edema

Central nervous system: Language problems, abnormal coordination, confusion, depression, difficulty concentrating, hypoesthesia

Endocrine & metabolic: Hot flashes

Gastrointestinal: Dyspepsia, abdominal pain, anorexia, constipation, xerostomia, gingivitis, weight loss

Neuromuscular & skeletal: Myalgia, weakness, back pain, leg pain, rigors

Otic: Decreased hearing

Renal: Nephrolithiasis

Respiratory: Pharyngitis, sinusitis, epistaxis

Miscellaneous: Flu-like symptoms

**Overdose/Toxicology** Activated charcoal has not been shown to adsorb topiramate and is therefore not recommended. Hemodialysis can remove the drug; however, most cases do not require removal and instead are best treated with supportive measures.

**Pharmacodynamics/Kinetics**

**Protein Binding:** 13% to 17%

**Half-life Elimination:** Mean: 21 hours

**Time to Peak:** ~2-4 hours

**Metabolism:** Minimal

**Excretion:** Urine (70%), as unchanged drug

**Formulations**

Tablet: 25 mg, 100 mg, 200 mg

Capsules, sprinkle: 15 mg, 25 mg, 50 mg

**Dosing**

**Adults:** Initial: 50 mg/day; titrate by 50 mg/day at 1-week intervals to target dose of 200 mg twice daily; usual maximum dose: 1600 mg/day

**Elderly:** Refer to adult dosing.

**Renal Impairment:** $Cl_{cr}$ <70 mL/minute: Administer 50% dose and titrate more slowly

Dialyzable: ~30%

**Hepatic Impairment:** Clearance may be minimally reduced.

**Additional Nursing Issues**

**Physical Assessment:** Assess effectiveness and interactions of other medications patient may be taking (see Drug Interactions). Monitor for therapeutic response (seizure activity, force, type, duration), laboratory values, and adverse reactions (see Adverse Reactions) at beginning of therapy and periodically with long-term use. Taper dosage slowly when discontinuing. Use and teach seizure/safety precautions. Assess knowledge/teach patient appropriate use, interventions to reduce side effects, and adverse symptoms to report. **Pregnancy risk factor C** - benefits of use should outweigh possible risks. Note breast-feeding caution.

**Patient Information/Instruction:** Take exactly as directed; do not increase dose or frequency or discontinue without consulting prescriber. While using this medication, do not use alcohol and other prescription or OTC medications (especially pain medications, sedatives, antihistamines, or hypnotics) without consulting prescriber. Maintain adequate hydration (2-3 L/day of fluids unless instructed to restrict fluid intake). You may experience drowsiness, dizziness, disturbed concentration, memory changes, or blurred vision (use caution when driving or engaging in tasks requiring alertness until response to drug is known); mouth sores, nausea, vomiting, or loss of appetite (small frequent meals, frequent mouth care, chewing gum, or sucking lozenges may help). Wear identification of epileptic status and medications. Report behavioral or CNS changes; skin rash; muscle cramping, weakness, tremors, changes in gait; chest pain, irregular heartbeat, or palpitations; hearing loss; cough or difficulty breathing; worsening of seizure activity, or loss of seizure control. **Pregnancy/breast-feeding precautions:** Inform prescriber if you are pregnant or intend to be pregnant. Consult prescriber if breast-feeding.

**Geriatric Considerations:** Since drug is renally excreted and most elderly will have creatinine clearance <70 mL/minute, doses must be reduced 50% and titrated more slowly. Obtain a serum creatinine and calculate creatinine clearance prior to starting therapy. Follow the recommended titration schedule and adjust time intervals to meet patient's needs.

♦ **Topisone** *see* Betamethasone *on page 148*

♦ **Topisone** *see* Topical Corticosteroids *on page 1152*

♦ **TOPO** *see* Topotecan *on next page*

♦ **Toposar® Injection** *see* Etoposide *on page 463*

## Topotecan (toe poe TEE kan)

**U.S. Brand Names** Hycamtin™

**Synonyms** Hycamptamine; SKF 104864; TOPO; TPT

**Therapeutic Category** Antineoplastic Agent, Natural Source (Plant) Derivative

**Pregnancy Risk Factor** D

**Lactation** Enters breast milk/contraindicated

**Use** Treatment of ovarian cancer after failure of first-line chemotherapy; treatment of small cell lung cancer sensitive disease after failure of first-line chemotherapy; experimentally in childhood solid tumors and leukemia resistant to standard therapies

**Contraindications** Hypersensitivity to topotecan or any component; pregnancy; severe bone marrow depression

**Warnings** The U.S. Food and Drug Administration (FDA) currently recommends that procedures for proper handling and disposal of antineoplastic agents be considered. Monitor bone marrow function. Should only administer to patients with adequate bone marrow reserves, baseline neutrophils at least 1,500 cells/mm$^3$ and platelet counts at least 100,000/mm$^3$.

**Drug Interactions**

**Decreased Effect:** Concurrent administration of TPT and G-CSF in clinical trials results in severe myelosuppression. Concurrent *in vitro* exposure to TPT and the topoisomerase II inhibitor etoposide results in no altered effect; sequential exposure results in potentiation. Concurrent exposure to TPT and 5-azacytidine results in potentiation both *in vitro* and *in vivo*. Myelosuppression was more severe when given in combination with cisplatin.

**Adverse Reactions**

>10%:

- Central nervous system: Headache
- Dermatologic: Alopecia (reversible)
- Gastrointestinal: Nausea, vomiting, diarrhea
  - Emetic potential: Moderately low (10% to 30%)
  - Hematologic: Myelosuppressive: Principle dose-limiting toxicity; white blood cell count nadir is 8-11 days after administration and is more frequent than thrombocytopenia (at lower doses); recover is usually within 21 days and cumulative toxicity has not been noted
  - WBC: Mild to severe
  - Platelets: Mild (at low doses)
  - Nadir (days): 8-11
  - Recovery (days): 14-21

1% to 10%:

- Neuromuscular & skeletal: Paresthesia
- Respiratory: Dyspnea

**Pharmacodynamics/Kinetics**

**Metabolism:** Topotecan (TPT) undergoes a rapid, pH-dependent opening of the lactone ring to yield a relatively inactive hydroxy acid in plasma.

**Excretion:** Plasma clearance fits a bi-exponential model.

**Formulations** Powder for injection, as hydrochloride, lyophilized: 4 mg (base)

**Dosing**

**Adults:** Most Phase II studies currently utilize topotecan at 1.5-2.0 mg/m$^2$/day for 5 days, repeated every 21-28 days. Alternative dosing regimens evaluated in Phase I studies have included 21-day continuous infusion (recommended Phase II dose: 0.53-0.7 mg/m$^2$/day) and weekly 24-hour infusions (recommended Phase II dose: 1.5 mg/m$^2$/week).

Dose modifications: Dosage modification may be required for toxicity

**Elderly:** Refer to adult dosing.

**Renal Impairment:**

$Cl_{cr}$ 40-60 mL/minute: No dosage adjustment with mild renal impairment.

$Cl_{cr}$ 20-39 mL/minute: Dosage adjustment to 0.75 mg/m$^2$ is recommended for moderate renal impairment.

Insufficient data available for severe renal impairment.

**Hepatic Impairment:** No dosage adjustment required.

**Administration**

**I.V.:** Each 4 mg vial is reconstituted with 4 mL sterile water for injection. Then the appropriate volume of the reconstitution solution is diluted in either 0.9% sodium chloride or 5% dextrose. Reconstituted product should be used immediately.

**Stability**

**Storage:** Intact vials should be stored in the refrigerator (2°C to 8°C) and protected from light. Shelf-life surveillance of the intact vials is ongoing. Unopened vials are stable until date indicated on package when stored between 20°C to 25°C (68°F to 77°F) and protected from light. Reconstituted vials diluted for infusion are stable at ~20°C to 25°C (68°F to 77°F) and ambient lighting for 24 hours.

**Reconstitution:** Final infusion preparation: Topotecan solutions further diluted to concentrations of 0.02 mg/mL, 0.1 mg/mL, or 6.7-330 mcg/mL in 5% dextrose injection, USP or 0.02 mg/mL, 0.1 mg/mL, or 10-500 mcg/mL in 0.9% sodium chloride injection, USP in plastic containers are stable for at least 24 hours at room temperature.

**Monitoring Laboratory Tests** CBC with differential and platelet count, renal function tests

(Continued)

## Topotecan *(Continued)*

**Additional Nursing Issues**

**Physical Assessment:** Monitor infusion site for extravasation. Monitor laboratory results before each cycle and regularly between cycles. Monitor and teach patient or caregiver to assess for possible reactions (especially signs and symptoms of myelosuppression), institute interventions to reduce side effects, and symptoms to report. **Pregnancy risk factor D.** Breast-feeding is contraindicated.

**Patient Information/Instruction:** This medication can only be administered I.V. and frequent blood tests may be necessary to monitor effects of the drug. Report pain, swelling, or irritation at infusion site. Do not use alcohol and prescription or OTC medications without consulting prescriber. Maintain adequate hydration (2-3 L/day of fluids unless instructed to restrict fluid intake); maintain good oral hygiene (use soft toothbrush or cotton applicators several times a day and rinse mouth frequently). You may experience nausea, vomiting, or loss of appetite (frequent small meals, frequent mouth care, sucking lozenges, or chewing gum may help, or consult prescriber). Hair loss may occur (reversible). You will be susceptible to infection; avoid crowds and infected persons and do not receive any vaccinations unless approved by prescriber. Report persistent fever or chills, unhealed sores, oral or vaginal sores, foul-smelling urine, painful urination, easy bruising or bleeding, yellowing of eyes or skin, and change in color of urine or stool. **Pregnancy/breast-feeding precautions:** Inform prescriber if you are pregnant. Do not breast-feed.

**Pregnancy Issues:** Animal studies found reduced fetal body weight, eye, brain, skull, and vertebrae malformations. May cause fetal harm in pregnant women.

**Additional Information** Topotecan preparation should be performed in a Class II laminar flow biologic safety cabinet. Personnel should be fully trained and wearing surgical gloves and a closed front surgical gown with knit cuffs. Appropriate safety equipment is recommended for preparation, administration, and disposal of topotecan. Accidental exposure to skin should be thoroughly washed with soap and water immediately.

♦ **Toprol XL®** *see* Metoprolol *on page 761*
♦ **Toradol® Injection** *see* Ketorolac Tromethamine *on page 646*
♦ **Toradol® Oral** *see* Ketorolac Tromethamine *on page 646*
♦ **Torecan®** *see* Thiethylperazine *on page 1121*

## Toremifene (TORE em i feen)

**U.S. Brand Names** Fareston®

**Therapeutic Category** Antineoplastic Agent, Miscellaneous

**Pregnancy Risk Factor** D

**Lactation** Excretion in breast milk unknown/contraindicated

**Use** Treatment of metastatic breast cancer in postmenopausal women with estrogen-receptor (ER) positive or ER unknown tumors

**Mechanism of Action/Effect** Nonsteroidal agent that competitively binds to estrogen receptors on tumors and other tissue targets (including breast and other tissues), producing a nuclear complex that decreases DNA synthesis and inhibits estrogen effects. Cells accumulate in the $G_0$ and $G_1$ phases; therefore, toremifene is cytostatic rather than cytocidal.

**Contraindications** Hypersensitivity to toremifene; pregnancy

**Warnings** Hypercalcemia and tumor flare have been reported in some breast cancer patients with bone metastases during the first weeks of treatment. Tumor flare is a syndrome of diffuse musculoskeletal pain and erythema with increased size of tumor lesions that later regress. It is often accompanied by hypercalcemia. Tumor flare does not imply treatment failure or represent tumor progression. Institute appropriate measures if hypercalcemia occurs, and if severe, discontinue treatment. Drugs that decrease renal calcium excretion (eg, thiazide diuretics) may increase the risk of hypercalcemia in patients receiving toremifene. Leukopenia and thrombocytopenia have been reported rarely.

Patients with a history of thromboembolic disease should generally not be treated with toremifene.

**Drug Interactions**

**Cytochrome P-450 Effect:** CYP3A3/4 enzyme substrate

**Decreased Effect:** Phenobarbital, phenytoin, and carbamazepine increase the rate of toremifene metabolism and lower blood levels.

**Increased Effect/Toxicity:** Inhibitors (such as ketoconazole or erythromycin) may increase blood levels of toremifene. Concurrent therapy with warfarin results in significant enhancement of anticoagulant effects; has been speculated that a ↓ in antitumor effect of tamoxifen may also occur due to alterations in the percentage of active tamoxifen metabolites.

**Adverse Reactions**

>10%:

Endocrine & metabolic: Hot flashes (35%), vaginal discharge (13%)
Gastrointestinal: Nausea (14%)
Miscellaneous: Diaphoresis (20%)

1% to 10%:

Cardiovascular: Thromboembolism: has been associated with the occurrence of venous thrombosis and pulmonary embolism; arterial thrombosis has also been described; cardiac failure, myocardial infarction, angina, edema
Central nervous system: Dizziness

Endocrine & metabolic: Hypercalcemia may occur in patients with bone metastases; galactorrhea and vitamin deficiency, menstrual irregularities

Gastrointestinal: Elevated transaminase levels, vomiting

Genitourinary: Vaginal bleeding or discharge, endometriosis, priapism, possible endometrial cancer

Ocular: Ophthalmologic effects (visual acuity changes, cataracts, or retinopathy), corneal opacities, dry eyes, blurred vision

Other events observed with unclear association with toremifene: Skin discoloration, pruritus, dermatitis, dyspnea, asthenia, paresis, tremor, anorexia, alopecia, jaundice, rigors.

**Overdose/Toxicology** Theoretically, overdose may manifest as an increase of antiestrogenic effects such as hot flashes; estrogenic effects such as vaginal bleeding; or nervous system disorders such as vertigo, dizziness, ataxia, and nausea. No specific antidote exists and treatment is symptomatic.

**Pharmacodynamics/Kinetics**

**Protein Binding:** >99% (primarily to albumin)

**Distribution:** Distribution half-life is 4 hours

**Half-life Elimination:** ~5 days

**Time to Peak:** Oral: Within 3 hours

**Metabolism:** Hepatic, primarily by cytochrome P-450 isoenzyme 3A4. Metabolite shares weak antiestrogenic activity.

**Excretion:** Feces and urine

**Formulations** Tablet: 60 mg

**Dosing**

**Adults:** Refer to individual protocols. Oral: 60 mg once daily, generally continued until disease progression is observed.

**Elderly:** Refer to adult dosing.

**Hepatic Impairment:** Toremifene is extensively metabolized in the liver and dosage adjustments may be indicated in patients with liver disease; however, no specific guidelines have been developed.

**Monitoring Laboratory Tests** Obtain periodic complete blood counts, calcium levels, and liver function tests. Closely monitor patients with bone metastases for hypercalcemia during the first few weeks of treatment. Leukopenia and thrombocytopenia have been reported rarely; monitor leukocyte and platelet counts during treatment.

**Additional Nursing Issues**

**Physical Assessment:** Assess pregnancy status prior to administration. Assess other medications patient may be taking for possible interactions or alterations in effectiveness (especially anything that is metabolized via the cytochrome P-450 route - see Drug Interactions). Monitor for adverse reactions (see Adverse Reactions). Instruct patient about signs of adverse reactions to report and possible interventions to address side effects. **Pregnancy risk factor D** - assess knowledge/teach appropriate use of barrier contraceptives. Breast-feeding is contraindicated.

**Patient Information/Instruction:** Take as directed, without regard to food. You may experience an initial "flare" of this disease (increased bone pain and hot flashes) which will subside with continued use. You may experience nausea, vomiting, or loss of appetite (frequent mouth care, frequent small meals, chewing gum, or sucking lozenges may help); dizziness (use caution when driving, climbing stairs, or engaging in tasks requiring alertness until response to drug is known); or loss of hair (will grow back). Report vomiting that occurs immediately after taking medication; chest pain, palpitations or swollen extremities; vaginal bleeding, hot flashes, or excessive perspiration; chest pain, unusual coughing, or difficulty breathing; or any changes in vision or dry eyes. **Pregnancy/breast-feeding precautions:** Do not get pregnant while taking this medication; use appropriate barrier contraceptive measures. Do not breast-feed.

♦ **Tornalate®** *see* Bitolterol *on page 157*

## Torsemide (TOR se mide)

**U.S. Brand Names** Demadex®

**Therapeutic Category** Diuretic, Loop

**Pregnancy Risk Factor** B

**Lactation** Excretion in breast milk unknown/use caution

**Use** Management of edema associated with congestive heart failure and hepatic or renal disease; used alone or in combination with antihypertensives in treatment of hypertension; I.V. form is indicated when rapid onset is desired

**Mechanism of Action/Effect** Inhibits reabsorption of sodium and chloride in the ascending loop of Henle and distal renal tubule, interfering with the chloride-binding cotransport system, thus causing increased excretion of water, sodium, chloride, magnesium, and calcium; does not alter GFR, renal plasma flow, or acid-base balance

**Contraindications** Hypersensitivity to torsemide or any component, or other sulfonylureas; anuria; safety in children <18 years has not been established

**Warnings** Excessive diuresis may result in dehydration, acute hypotensive or thromboembolic episodes and cardiovascular collapse. Rapid injection, renal impairment, or excessively large doses may result in ototoxicity. SLE may be exacerbated. Sudden alterations in electrolyte balance may precipitate hepatic encephalopathy and coma in patients with hepatic cirrhosis and ascites. Monitor carefully for signs of fluid or electrolyte imbalances, especially hypokalemia in patients at risk for such (eg, digitalis therapy, history of ventricular arrhythmias, elderly, etc), hyperuricemia, hypomagnesemia, or hypocalcemia. Use caution with exposure to ultraviolet light.

(Continued)

## Torsemide *(Continued)*

**Drug Interactions**

**Cytochrome P-450 Effect:** CYP2C9 enzyme substrate

**Decreased Effect:** Torsemide efficacy may be decreased with NSAIDs. Torsemide action may be reduced with probenecid. Diuretic action may be impaired in patients with cirrhosis and ascites if used with salicylates. Glucose tolerance may be decreased when used with sulfonylureas.

**Increased Effect/Toxicity:** Use with aminoglycosides may increase ototoxicity; anticoagulant activity is enhanced. Plasma concentrations of beta-blockers may be increased if used with beta-blockers. Ototoxicity may be increased with cisplatin. Arrhythmias may occur with diuretic-induced electrolyte disturbances in patients receiving digitalis. Plasma concentrations of lithium may be increased when used with lithium. Synergistic effects may result if used with thiazides.

**Adverse Reactions**

>10%:

Central nervous system: Headache, dizziness

Gastrointestinal: Constipation, upset stomach

1% to 10%:

Dermatologic: Photosensitivity, urticaria

Endocrine & metabolic: Electrolyte imbalance, dehydration, hyperuricemia

Gastrointestinal: Diarrhea, anorexia, pancreatitis

Ocular: Blurred vision

<1% (Limited to important or life-threatening symptoms): Orthostatic hypotension, hepatic dysfunction, agranulocytosis, leukopenia, anemia, thrombocytopenia, nephrocalcinosis, prerenal azotemia, interstitial nephritis

**Overdose/Toxicology** Symptoms include electrolyte depletion, volume depletion, hypotension, dehydration, and circulatory collapse. Electrolyte depletion may manifest as weakness, dizziness, mental confusion, anorexia, lethargy, vomiting, and cramps. Treatment is supportive.

**Pharmacodynamics/Kinetics**

**Protein Binding:** Plasma: ~97% to 99%

**Half-life Elimination:** 2-4; 7-8 hours in cirrhosis (dose modification appears unnecessary)

**Metabolism:** Hepatic by cytochrome P-450, 80%

**Excretion:** Urine

**Onset:** Onset of diuresis: 30-60 minutes; Peak effect: 1-4 hours

**Duration:** ~6 hours

**Formulations**

Injection: 10 mg/mL (2 mL, 5 mL)

Tablet: 5 mg, 10 mg, 20 mg, 100 mg

**Dosing**

**Adults:** Oral, I.V.: (The oral form may be given regardless of meal times. Patients may be switched from the I.V. form to the oral and vice-versa with no change in dose.)

Congestive heart failure: 10-20 mg once daily; may increase gradually for chronic treatment by doubling dose until the diuretic response is apparent (for acute treatment. I.V. dose may be repeated every 2 hours with double the dose as needed).

Chronic renal failure: 20 mg once daily; increase as described above.

Hepatic cirrhosis: 5-10 mg once daily with an aldosterone antagonist or a potassium-sparing diuretic; increase as described above.

Hypertension: 5 mg once daily; increase to 10 mg after 4-6 weeks if an adequate hypotensive response is not apparent. If still not effective, an additional antihypertensive agent may be added.

**Elderly:** Usual starting dose should be 5 mg, refer to adult dosing. No other dosage adjustment is needed.

**Administration**

**I.V.:** I.V. injections should be given over ≥2 minutes.

**I.V. Detail:** Ototoxicity has occurred with too rapid of injection.

**Monitoring Laboratory Tests** Renal function, electrolytes

**Additional Nursing Issues**

**Physical Assessment:** Monitor response and effectiveness of therapy; fluid balance (I & O ratio, edema, lung sounds, weight), blood pressures, and electrolyte status (weakness, fatigue, dizziness, vomiting, cramps). Assess knowledge/teach patient or caregiver interventions to reduce side effects and adverse signs to report. Note breast-feeding caution.

**Patient Information/Instruction:** Take recommended dosage with food or milk at the same time each day (preferably not in the evening to avoid sleep interruption). Do not miss doses, alter dosage, or discontinue without consulting prescriber. Include orange juice or bananas (or other potassium-rich foods) in daily diet; do not take potassium supplements without consulting prescriber. Do not use alcohol or OTC medications without consulting prescriber. You may experience postural hypotension; change position slowly when rising from sitting or lying. May cause transient drowsiness, blurred vision, or dizziness; avoid driving or engaging in tasks that require alertness until response to drug is known. You may have reduced tolerance to heat (avoid strenuous activity in hot weather or excessively hot showers). Increased exercise and increased dietary fiber, fruit, and fluids may reduce constipation. Report unusual weight gain or loss (>5 lb/week), swelling of ankles and hands, persistent fatigue, unresolved constipation or diarrhea, weakness, fatigue, dizziness, vomiting, cramps, change in hearing, or chest pain or palpitations. **Breast-feeding precautions:** Consult prescriber if breast-feeding.

**Pregnancy Issues:** A decrease in fetal weight, an increase in fetal resorption, and delayed fetal ossification has occurred in animal studies.

**Additional Information**

10-20 mg torsemide is approximately equivalent to furosemide 40 mg or bumetanide 1 mg.

pH: >8.3

- **Totacillin®** *see* Ampicillin *on page 90*
- **Totacillin®-N** *see* Ampicillin *on page 90*
- **Touro Ex®** *see* Guaifenesin *on page 548*
- **Touro LA®** *see* Guaifenesin and Pseudoephedrine *on page 551*
- **t-PA** *see* Alteplase *on page 58*
- **TPT** *see* Topotecan *on page 1157*
- **Tradol** *see* Tramadol *on this page*

## Tramadol (TRA ma dole)

**U.S. Brand Names** Ultram®

**Therapeutic Category** Analgesic, Non-narcotic

**Pregnancy Risk Factor** C

**Lactation** Excretion in breast milk unknown/not recommended

**Use** Relief of moderate to moderately severe pain

**Mechanism of Action/Effect** Binds to μ-opiate receptors in the CNS causing inhibition of ascending pain pathways, altering the perception of and response to pain; also inhibits the reuptake of norepinephrine and serotonin, which also modifies the ascending pain pathway

**Contraindications** Hypersensitivity to tramadol or any component; concurrent use of monoamine oxidase inhibitors; acute alcohol intoxication; concurrent use of centrally-acting analgesics, opioids, or psychotropic drugs

**Warnings** Elderly patients and patients with chronic respiratory disorders may be at greater risk of adverse events; liver disease. Patients with myxedema, hypothyroidism, or hypoadrenalism should use tramadol with caution and at reduced dosages. Do not use in opioid-dependent patients. Has been known to reinitiate physical dependence in those with a history of dependence on other opioids. Pregnancy factor C.

**Drug Interactions**

**Cytochrome P-450 Effect:** CYP2D6 enzyme substrate

**Decreased Effect:** Decreased effects with carbamazepine (decreases half-life by 33% to 50%).

**Increased Effect/Toxicity:** Increased toxicity with monoamine oxidase inhibitors (seizures). Quinidine inhibits cytochrome P-450 2D6, thereby increases tramadol serum concentrations. Tramadol half-life is increased 20% to 25% when used with cimetidine. Potential for serotonin syndrome if combined with other serotonergic drugs.

**Adverse Reactions**

1% to 10%

Central nervous system: Dizziness, headache, somnolence, stimulation, restlessness, confusion, insomnia

Endocrine & metabolic: Menopausal symptoms

Gastrointestinal: Nausea, diarrhea, constipation, vomiting, heartburn, stomach pain, anorexia, dry mouth

Genitourinary: Polyuria, dysuria

Neuromuscular & skeletal: Weakness

Ocular: Blurred vision

Miscellaneous: Sweating

<1% (Limited to important or life-threatening symptoms): Palpitations, orthostatic hypotension, syncope, tachycardia, seizures, cognitive dysfunction, respiratory depression, dyspnea, suicidal tendency

**Overdose/Toxicology** Symptoms of overdose include CNS and respiratory depression, GI cramping, and constipation. Naloxone, 2 mg I.V. with repeat administration as needed up to 10 mg, can also be used to reverse toxic effects of the opiate.

**Pharmacodynamics/Kinetics**

**Protein Binding:** 20%

**Half-life Elimination:** 6.3-7.4 hours

**Excretion:** Urine

**Onset:** 1 hour

**Formulations** Tablet, as hydrochloride: 50 mg

**Dosing**

**Adults:** Oral: 50-100 mg every 4-6 hours, not to exceed 400 mg/day

**Elderly:** Oral: >75 years: 50-100 mg every 4-6 hours not to exceed 300 mg/day; see renal or hepatic dosing.

**Renal Impairment:** $Cl_{cr}$ <30 mL/minute: Administer 50-100 mg dose every 12 hours; maximum: 200 mg/day

**Hepatic Impairment:** Cirrhosis: Recommended dose is 50 mg every 12 hours.

**Additional Nursing Issues**

**Physical Assessment:** Assess other medications patient may be taking for additive or adverse interactions (see Warnings/Precautions, Contraindications, and Drug Interactions). Monitor for therapeutic effectiveness. Monitor for signs of adverse reactions or overdose (see Adverse Reactions) at beginning of therapy and periodically during therapy. May cause physical and/or psychological dependence. Assess knowledge/teach patient appropriate use. Teach patient to monitor for adverse reactions, adverse reactions to report, and appropriate interventions to reduce side effects. **Pregnancy**

(Continued)

## Tramadol *(Continued)*

**risk factor C** - benefits of use should outweigh possible risks. Breast-feeding is not recommended.

**Patient Information/Instruction:** If self-administered, use exactly as directed (do not increase dose or frequency); may cause physical and/or psychological dependence. Take with food or milk. While using this medication, do not use alcohol and other prescription or OTC medications (especially pain medications, sedatives, antihistamines, or cough preparations) without consulting prescriber. Maintain adequate hydration (2-3 L/day of fluids unless instructed to restrict fluid intake). You may experience drowsiness, dizziness, or blurred vision (use caution when driving or engaging in tasks requiring alertness until response to drug is known); nausea, vomiting, or loss of appetite (small frequent meals, frequent mouth care, chewing gum, or sucking lozenges may help); constipation (increased exercise, fluids, or dietary fruit and fiber may help). Report severe unresolved constipation; difficulty breathing or shortness of breath; excessive sedation or increased insomnia and restlessness; changes in urinary pattern or menstrual pattern; muscle weakness or tremors; or chest pain or palpitations. **Pregnancy/breast-feeding precautions:** Inform prescriber if you are or intend to be pregnant. Do not breast-feed.

**Geriatric Considerations:** One study in the elderly found that tramadol 50 mg was similar in efficacy as acetaminophen 300 mg with codeine 30 mg.

♦ **Trandate®** *see* Labetalol *on page 649*

## Trandolapril (tran DOE la pril)

**U.S. Brand Names** Mavik®

**Therapeutic Category** Angiotensin-Converting Enzyme (ACE) Inhibitors

**Pregnancy Risk Factor** C/D (2nd and 3rd trimesters)

**Lactation** Enters breast milk/contraindicated

**Use** Management of hypertension alone or in combination with other antihypertensive agents

**Unlabeled use:** As a class, ACE inhibitors are recommended in the treatment of systolic congestive heart failure

**Mechanism of Action/Effect** Competitive inhibitor of angiotensin-converting enzyme (ACE); prevents conversion of angiotensin I to angiotensin II, a potent vasoconstrictor; results in lower levels of angiotensin II which causes an increase in plasma renin activity and a reduction in aldosterone secretion

**Contraindications** Hypersensitivity or angioedema to trandolapril, other ACE inhibitors, or any component; pregnancy (2nd and 3rd trimesters)

**Warnings** Use with caution and modify dosage in patients with renal impairment (decrease dosage) (especially renal artery stenosis), severe congestive heart failure, or with coadministered diuretic therapy. Severe hypotension may occur in patients who are sodium and/or volume depleted, initiate lower doses and monitor closely when starting therapy in these patients. ACE inhibitors may be preferred agents in elderly patients with congestive heart failure and diabetes mellitus (diabetic proteinuria is reduced, minimal CNS effects, and enhanced insulin sensitivity); however, due to decreased renal function, tolerance must be carefully monitored. Pregnancy factor C/D (2nd and 3rd trimesters).

**Drug Interactions**

**Decreased Effect:** Nonsteroidal anti-inflammatory agents may reduce effect of ACE-inhibition. Rifampin may decrease the effect of some ACE-inhibitors. Antacids may decrease absorption of some ACE-inhibitors. Absorption of tetracyclines may be reduced.

**Increased Effect/Toxicity:** Diuretics have additive hypotensive effects with ACE inhibitors. Lithium and trandolapril in combination have elevated serum levels of lithium with symptoms of toxicity. Potassium supplements or potassium-sparing diuretics with ACE inhibitors may result in elevated serum potassium levels. Allopurinol and trandolapril may cause neutropenia. Digoxin levels may be increased. Phenothiazines and probenecid may increase ACE-inhibitor effects.

**Adverse Reactions**

1% to 10%:

Central nervous system: Dizziness, headache, fatigue

Gastrointestinal: Diarrhea

Respiratory: Cough

<1% (Limited to important or life-threatening symptoms): Chest pain, AV first degree block, bradycardia, edema, flushing, hypotension, palpitations, increased potassium, leukopenia, neutropenia, increased AST/ALT, elevated creatinine, epistaxis, angioedema with laryngeal edema

**Overdose/Toxicology** Mild hypotension has been the primary toxic effect seen with acute overdose. Bradycardia may also occur. Hyperkalemia occurs even with therapeutic doses, especially in patients with renal insufficiency and those taking NSAIDs. Treatment is symptom directed and supportive.

**Pharmacodynamics/Kinetics**

**Protein Binding:** 80%

**Half-life Elimination:** Parent: 6 hours; Active metabolite trandolaprilat: 10 hours

**Time to Peak:** Parent: 1 hour; Active metabolite trandolaprilat: 4-10 hours

**Metabolism:** Liver

**Excretion:** Urine

**Onset:** 1-2 hours

**Duration:** Trandolaprilat (active metabolite) is very lipophilic in comparison to other ACE inhibitors which may contribute to its prolonged duration of action (72 hours after a single dose)

**Formulations** Tablet: 1 mg, 2 mg, 4 mg

**Dosing**

**Adults:** Initial dosage:

Patient not on diuretics: 1 mg/day; increase starting dose to 2 mg/day for African-American patients. Adjust dose at intervals ≥1 week based on clinical response. Usual dosage is 2-4 mg/day. Maximum recommended dose is 8 mg/day.

Patients on diuretics: If unable to first discontinue diuretic, proceed with caution and start at 0.5 mg/day and monitor patient closely for severe hypotension for several hours until blood pressure has stabilized.

**Elderly:** Refer to adult dosing.

**Renal Impairment:** $Cl_{cr}$ ≤30 mL/minute: Administer lowest doses, starting at 0.5 mg/day.

**Hepatic Impairment:** Patients with hepatic cirrhosis: Start dose at 0.5 mg.

**Monitoring Laboratory Tests** CBC, electrolytes, renal function, serum calcium

**Additional Nursing Issues**

**Physical Assessment:** Assess effectiveness and interactions of other medications (see Drug Interactions). See Warnings/Precautions and Contraindications for use cautions. Monitor effectiveness of therapy, laboratory tests, and adverse response on a regular basis during therapy (see Adverse Reactions and Overdose/Toxicology). Assess knowledge/teach patient appropriate use according to drug form and purpose of therapy, possible side effects and appropriate interventions, and adverse symptoms to report. **Pregnancy risk factor C/D** - see Pregnancy Risk Factor - assess knowledge/teach appropriate use of barrier contraceptives. Breast-feeding is contraindicated. See Pregnancy Issues.

**Patient Information/Instruction:** Take exactly as directed; do not discontinue without consulting prescriber. Take first dose at bedtime. This drug does not eliminate need for diet or exercise regimen as recommended by prescriber. May cause dizziness, fainting, lightheadedness (use caution when driving or engaging in tasks requiring alertness until response to drug is known); diarrhea (buttermilk, boiled milk, yogurt may help). Report chest pain or palpitations; swelling of extremities, mouth or tongue; skin rash; difficulty in breathing or unusual cough; or other persistent adverse reactions. **Pregnancy/breast-feeding precautions:** Do not get pregnant while taking this medication; use appropriate barrier contraceptive measures. Do not breast-feed.

**Geriatric Considerations:** Due to frequent decreases in glomerular filtration (also creatinine clearance) with aging, elderly patients may have exaggerated responses to ACE inhibitors. Differences in clinical response due to hepatic changes are not observed.

**Pregnancy Issues:** ACE inhibitors can cause fetal injury or death if taken during the 2nd or 3rd trimester. Discontinue ACE inhibitors as soon as pregnancy is detected. ACE inhibitors should not be used if patient is sexually active and not using contraceptives.

**Related Information**

ACE Inhibitors and Angiotensin Antagonists Comparison *on page 1362*

## Trandolapril and Verapamil (tran DOE la pril & ver AP a mil)

**U.S. Brand Names** Tarka®

**Therapeutic Category** Antihypertensive Agent, Combination

**Pregnancy Risk Factor** C/D (2nd and 3rd trimesters)

**Lactation** Enters breast milk/contraindicated

**Use** Combination drug for the treatment of hypertension, however, not indicated for initial treatment of hypertension; replacement therapy in patients receiving separate dosage forms (for patient convenience); when monotherapy with one component fails to achieve desired antihypertensive effect, or when dose-limiting adverse effects limit upward titration of monotherapy

**Formulations** Tablet:

Trandolapril 1 mg and verapamil hydrochloride 240 mg
Trandolapril 2 mg and verapamil hydrochloride 180 mg
Trandolapril 2 mg and verapamil hydrochloride 240 mg
Trandolapril 4 mg and verapamil hydrochloride 240 mg

**Dosing**

**Adults:** Oral: 1 tablet daily, individualize dose to achieve optimal effect. Patients receiving trandolapril (up to 8 mg) and verapamil (up to 240 mg) in separate tablets may wish to receive Tarka® at equivalent dosages once daily.

**Elderly:** Overall safety and efficacy are not different in elderly patients, although a greater sensitivity to effects may be observed in some older individuals.

**Renal Impairment:** Usual regimen need not be adjusted unless patient's creatinine clearance is <30 mL/minute. Titration of individual components must be done prior to switching to combination product

(Continued)

## Trandolapril and Verapamil *(Continued)*

**Hepatic Impairment:** Has not been evaluated in hepatic impairment. Verapamil is hepatically metabolized, adjustment of dosage in hepatic impairment is recommended.

**Additional Nursing Issues**

**Physical Assessment:** See individual components listed in Related Information. **Pregnancy risk factor C/D** - see Pregnancy Risk Factor - assess knowledge/instruct patient on need to use appropriate contraceptive measures and the need to avoid pregnancy. Breast-feeding is contraindicated.

**Patient Information/Instruction:** See individual components listed in Related Information. **Pregnancy/breast-feeding precautions:** Inform prescriber if you are or intend to be pregnant. Do not breast-feed.

**Related Information**

Trandolapril *on page 1162*
Verapamil *on page 1208*

♦ **Transamine Sulphate** *see* Tranylcypromine *on this page*
♦ **Transdermal-NTG® Patch** *see* Nitroglycerin *on page 831*
♦ **Transderm-Nitro® Patch** *see* Nitroglycerin *on page 831*
♦ **Transderm Scop® Patch** *see* Scopolamine *on page 1047*
♦ **Trans-Planta®** *see page 1294*
♦ **Trans-Ver-Sal® AdultPatch** *see page 1294*
♦ **Trans-Ver-Sal® PediaPatch** *see page 1294*
♦ **Trans-Ver-Sal® PlantarPatch** *see page 1294*
♦ **Tran-Ver-Sal®** *see page 1294*
♦ **Tranxene®** *see* Clorazepate *on page 292*

## Tranylcypromine (tran il SIP roe meen)

**U.S. Brand Names** Parnate®

**Synonyms** Transamine Sulphate

**Therapeutic Category** Antidepressant, Monoamine Oxidase Inhibitor

**Pregnancy Risk Factor** C

**Lactation** Excretion in breast milk unknown/not recommended

**Use** Symptomatic treatment of depressed patients refractory to or intolerant of tricyclic antidepressants or electroconvulsive therapy; has a more rapid onset of therapeutic effect than other MAO inhibitors, but causes more severe hypertensive reactions

**Mechanism of Action/Effect** Inhibits the enzymes monoamine oxidase A and B which are responsible for the intraneuronal metabolism of norepinephrine and serotonin, and increase their availability to postsynaptic neurons; decreased firing rate of the locus ceruleus, reducing norepinephrine concentration in the brain; agonist effects of serotonin

**Contraindications** Hypersensitivity to tranylcypromine; uncontrolled hypertension; pheochromocytoma; cardiovascular disease; severe renal or hepatic impairment

**Warnings** Safety in children <16 years of age has not been established. Use with caution in patients who are hyperactive, hyperexcitable, who have glaucoma, who have suicidal tendencies, who have diabetes, or are elderly. Hypertensive crisis may occur with tyramine. Pregnancy factor C.

**Drug Interactions**

**Cytochrome P-450 Effect:** CYP2A6 and 2C19 enzyme inhibitor

**Decreased Effect:** Decreased effect of antihypertensives.

**Increased Effect/Toxicity:** Increased toxicity with disulfiram (seizures), clomipramine, fluoxetine, and other serotonin-active agents (eg, fluvoxamine, paroxetine, sertraline, etc), tricyclic antidepressants (cardiovascular instability), meperidine (cardiovascular instability), phenothiazine (hypertensive crisis), sympathomimetics phenylephrine, phenylpropanolamine, pseudoephedrine (hypertensive crisis), sumatriptan (hypothetical), CNS depressants, levodopa (hypertensive crisis), tyramine-containing foods (eg, aged foods), and dextroamphetamine, methylphenidate (severe hypertensive reactions), dextromethorphan (serotonin syndrome).

**Effects on Lab Values** ↓ glucose

**Adverse Reactions**

>10%:

Cardiovascular: Orthostatic hypotension
Central nervous system: Drowsiness, headache
Endocrine & metabolic: Decreased sexual ability
Neuromuscular & skeletal: Trembling, weakness
Ocular: Blurred vision

1% to 10%:

Cardiovascular: Tachycardia, peripheral edema
Central nervous system: Nervousness, chills
Gastrointestinal: Diarrhea, anorexia, dry mouth, constipation

<1% (Limited to important or life-threatening symptoms): Parkinsonism syndrome, leukopenia, hepatitis

**Overdose/Toxicology** Symptoms of overdose include tachycardia, palpitations, muscle twitching, seizures, insomnia, transient hypotension, hypertension, hyperpyrexia, and coma. Treatment is symptom directed and supportive.

**Pharmacodynamics/Kinetics**

**Half-life Elimination:** 90-190 minutes

**Time to Peak:** Within 2 hours

**Excretion:** Urine

**Onset:** 2-3 weeks of continued dosing are required to obtain full therapeutic effect

**Duration:** May continue to have a therapeutic effect and interactions 2 weeks after discontinuing therapy

**Formulations** Tablet, as sulfate: 10 mg

**Dosing**

**Adults:** Oral: 10 mg twice daily for 2 weeks, increase by 10 mg increments at 1- to 3-week intervals; maximum: 60 mg/day

**Elderly:** Refer to adult dosing and Geriatric Considerations.

**Hepatic Impairment:** Use with care and monitor plasma levels and patient response closely.

**Monitoring Laboratory Tests** Blood glucose

**Additional Nursing Issues**

**Physical Assessment:** Assess other medications patient may be taking for effectiveness and interactions (see Drug Interactions). See Warnings/Precautions for cautious use. Has potential for psychological or physiological dependence, abuse, or tolerance. Monitor laboratory tests, therapeutic response (ie, mental status, mood, affect, suicidal ideation), and adverse reactions at beginning of therapy and periodically with long-term use (see Adverse Reactions and Overdose/Toxicology). Taper dosage slowly when discontinuing. Assess knowledge/teach patient appropriate use, interventions to reduce side effects, and adverse symptoms to report. See Tyramine Foods List *on page 1422*. **Pregnancy risk factor C** - benefits of use should outweigh possible risks. Breast-feeding is not recommended.

**Patient Information/Instruction:** Take exactly as directed (do not increase dose or frequency); may take 2-3 weeks to achieve desired results; may cause physical and/or psychological dependence. Take in the morning to reduce the incidence of insomnia. Avoid excessive alcohol, caffeine, and other prescription or OTC medications not approved by prescriber. Avoid tyramine-containing foods (eg pickles, aged cheese, wine); see prescriber for complete list of foods to be avoided. Maintain adequate hydration (2-3 L/day of fluids unless instructed to restrict fluid intake). You may experience drowsiness, dizziness, or blurred vision (use caution when driving or engaging in tasks requiring alertness until response to drug is known); anorexia or dry mouth (small frequent meals, frequent mouth care, chewing gum, or sucking lozenges may help); constipation (increased exercise, fluids, or dietary fruit and fiber may help); diarrhea (buttermilk, yogurt, or boiled milk may help); orthostatic hypotension (use caution when climbing stairs or changing position from lying or sitting to standing); or altered sexual ability (reversible). Report persistent excessive sedation; muscle cramping, tremors, weakness, or change in gait; chest pain, palpitations, rapid heartbeat, or swelling of extremities; vision changes; or worsening of condition. **Pregnancy/breast-feeding precautions:** Inform prescriber if you are or intend to be pregnant. Breast-feeding is not recommended.

**Geriatric Considerations:** MAO inhibitors are effective and generally well tolerated by older patients. Potential interactions with tyramine- or tryptophan-containing foods (see Warnings/Precautions), other drugs, and adverse effects on blood pressure have limited use of MAO inhibitors. They are usually reserved for patients who do not tolerate or respond to traditional "cyclic" or "second generation" antidepressants. Tranylcypromine is the preferred MAO inhibitor because its enzymatic-blocking effects are more rapidly reversed. The brain activity of monoamine oxidase increases with age and even more so in patients with Alzheimer's disease. Therefore, MAO inhibitors may have an increased role in treating depressed patients with Alzheimer's disease.

**Related Information**

Antidepressant Agents Comparison *on page 1368*
Tyramine Foods List *on page 1422*

## Trastuzumab (tras TU zoo mab)

**U.S. Brand Names** Herceptin®

**Therapeutic Category** Antineoplastic Agent, Miscellaneous

**Pregnancy Risk Factor** B

**Lactation** Excretion in breast milk unknown/not recommended

**Use** Treatment of patients with metastatic breast cancer whose tumors overexpress the HER-2 protein

**Mechanism of Action/Effect** Trastuzumab is a monoclonal antibody which binds to the extracellular domain of the human epidermal growth factor receptor 2 protein (HER-2). It mediates antibody-dependent cellular cytotoxicity against cells which overproduce HER-2.

**Contraindications** Hypersensitivity to hamster ovary cell proteins or any component

**Warnings** Congestive heart failure associated with trastuzumab may be severe and has been associated with disabling cardiac failure, death, mural thrombus, and stroke. Discontinuation should be strongly considered in patients who develop a clinically significant decrease in ejection fraction during therapy. Combination therapy which includes anthracyclines and cyclophosphamide increases the incidence and severity of cardiac dysfunction. Extreme caution should be used when treating patients with pre-existing cardiac disease or dysfunction, and in patients with previous exposure to anthracyclines. Advanced age may also predispose to cardiotoxicity. Do not administer as an I.V. bolus.

(Continued)

## Trastuzumab *(Continued)*

**Drug Interactions**

**Increased Effect/Toxicity:** Paclitaxel may result in a decrease in clearance of trastuzumab, increasing serum concentrations.

**Adverse Reactions** The most common reactions were infusion-associated, occurring in up to 40% of patients, consisting primarily of fever and/or chills which were mild to moderate in severity. These may be treated with acetaminophen, diphenhydramine, and meperidine with or without reduction of the infusion rate.

>10%:

Central nervous system: Pain (47%), fever (36%), chills (32%), headache (26%)
Dermatologic: Rash (18%)
Gastrointestinal: Nausea (33%), diarrhea (25%), vomiting (23%), abdominal pain (22%), anorexia (14%)
Neuromuscular & skeletal: Weakness (42%), back pain (22%)
Respiratory: Cough (26%), dyspnea (22%), rhinitis (14%), pharyngitis (12%)
Miscellaneous: Infection (20%)

1% to 10%:

Cardiovascular: Peripheral edema (10%), congestive heart failure (7%), tachycardia (5%)
Central nervous system: Insomnia (14%), dizziness (13%), paresthesia (9%), depression (6%), peripheral neuritis (2%), neuropathy (1%)
Dermatologic: Herpes simplex (2%), acne (2%)
Gastrointestinal: Nausea and vomiting (8%)
Genitourinary: Urinary tract infection (5%)
Hematologic: Anemia (4%), leukopenia (3%)
Neuromuscular & skeletal: Bone pain (7%), arthralgia (6%)
Respiratory: Sinusitis (9%)
Miscellaneous: Flu syndrome (10%), accidental injury (6%), allergic reaction (3%)

<1% (Limited to important or life-threatening symptoms): Cellulitis, anaphylactoid reaction, ascites, hydrocephalus, radiation injury, deafness, amblyopia, vascular thrombosis, pericardial effusion, cardiac arrest, hypotension, syncope, hemorrhage, shock, arrhythmia, hepatic failure, gastroenteritis, hematemesis, ileus, intestinal obstruction, colitis, esophageal ulcer, stomatitis, pancreatitis, hepatitis, hypothyroidism, pancytopenia, acute leukemia, coagulopathy, lymphangitis

**Overdose/Toxicology** There is no experience with overdose in human clinical trials. Treatment is supportive.

**Pharmacodynamics/Kinetics**

**Half-life Elimination:** Mean: 5.8 days (range: 1-32 days)

**Formulations** Powder for injection: 440 mg

**Dosing**

**Adults:** I.V.:

Loading dose: 4 mg/kg over 90 minutes; do not administer as an I.V. bolus or I.V. push.
Maintenance dose: 2 mg/kg once weekly (may be infused over 30 minutes if prior infusions are well tolerated).

**Elderly:** Refer to adult dosing.

**Renal Impairment:** No adjustment is necessary.

**Hepatic Impairment:** No adjustment is necessary.

**Administration**

**I.V.:** Administer loading dose over 90 minutes. Subsequent weekly doses can be infused over 30 minutes.

**I.V. Detail:** Observe patients closely during the infusion for fever, chills, or other infusion-related symptoms.

**Stability**

**Storage:** Store under refrigeration at 2°C to 8°C (36°F to 46°F) prior to reconstitution.

**Reconstitution:** Prepare each vial by reconstituting with 20 mL of bacteriostatic water for injection (supplied in carton). If patient has a known hypersensitivity to benzyl alcohol, it may be reconstituted with sterile water for injection. Stable for 28 days after reconstitution if refrigerated; do not freeze. If sterile water for injection without preservative is used for reconstitution, it must be used immediately. After dilution in 0.9% sodium chloride for injection in polyethylene bags, solution is stable for 24 hours.

**Additional Nursing Issues**

**Physical Assessment:** Monitor laboratory tests, response to therapy, and adverse reactions (eg, infusion related symptoms such as fever, chills, headache, CHF, CNS changes, or opportunistic infection - see Warnings/Precautions and Adverse Reactions). Assess knowledge/teach patient interventions to reduce side effects, and adverse symptoms to report. Breast-feeding is not recommended.

**Patient Information/Instruction:** This medication can only be administered by infusion. Report immediately any adverse reactions during infusion (eg, chills, fever, headache, backache, or nausea/vomiting) so appropriate medication can be administered. You will be susceptible to infection (avoid crowds or exposure to persons with infections or contagious diseases). You may experience dizziness or weakness (use caution when driving or engaging in tasks requiring alertness until response to drug is known); nausea or vomiting (small frequent meals, frequent mouth care, chewing gum, or sucking lozenges may help); diarrhea (boiled milk, yogurt, or buttermilk may help); or headache, back or joint pain (mild analgesics may offer relief). Report persistent gastrointestinal effects; sore throat, runny nose, or difficulty breathing; chest pain, irregular heartbeat, palpitations, swelling of extremities, or unusual weight gain; muscle or joint weakness, numbness, or pain; skin rash or irritation; itching or pain on urination; unhealed sores, white plaques in mouth or genital area, unusual bruising or bleeding; or other unusual effects related to this medication. **Breast-feeding precautions:** Breast-feeding is not recommended.

**Breast-feeding Issues:** It is not known whether trastuzumab is secreted in human milk. Because many immunoglobulins are secreted in milk, and the potential for serious adverse reactions exists, patients should discontinue nursing during treatment and for 6 months after the last dose.

- **Trasylol®** *see* Aprotinin *on page 104*
- **Trazil Ofteno/Ungena** *see* Tobramycin *on page 1142*

## Trazodone (TRAZ oh done)

**U.S. Brand Names** Desyrel®

**Therapeutic Category** Antidepressant, Serotonin Reuptake Inhibitor/Antagonist

**Pregnancy Risk Factor** C

**Lactation** Enters breast milk/contraindicated

**Use** Treatment of depression

**Mechanism of Action/Effect** Inhibits reuptake of serotonin and norepinephrine by the presynaptic neuronal membrane and desensitization of adenyl cyclase, down regulation of beta-adrenergic receptors, and down regulation of serotonin receptors

**Contraindications** Hypersensitivity to trazodone or any component

**Warnings** Monitor closely and use with extreme caution in patients with cardiac disease or arrhythmias. Very sedating, but little anticholinergic effect. Therapeutic effects may take up to 4 weeks. Therapy is normally maintained for several months after optimum response is reached to prevent recurrence of depression. Pregnancy factor C.

**Drug Interactions**

**Cytochrome P-450 Effect:** CYP2D6 and 3A3/4 enzyme substrate

**Decreased Effect:** Trazodone inhibits the hypotensive response to clonidine.

**Increased Effect/Toxicity:** Fluoxetine and other selective serotonin reuptake inhibitors, in combination with trazodone, may increase the clinical effect or side effects/toxicity. Increased effect/toxicity of phenytoin, CNS depressants, and MAO inhibitors. Digoxin serum levels are increased. Potential for serotonin syndrome if combined with other serotonergic drugs.

**Food Interactions** Time to peak serum levels may be increased if trazodone is taken with food.

**Adverse Reactions**

>10%:

Central nervous system: Dizziness, headache, confusion

Gastrointestinal: Nausea, bad taste in mouth, dry mouth

Neuromuscular & skeletal: Muscle tremors

1% to 10%:

Gastrointestinal: Diarrhea, constipation

Neuromuscular & skeletal: Weakness

Ocular: Blurred vision

<1% (Limited to important or life-threatening symptoms): Hypotension, tachycardia, bradycardia, seizures, extrapyramidal reactions, hepatitis

**Overdose/Toxicology** Symptoms of overdose include drowsiness, vomiting, hypotension, tachycardia, incontinence, coma, and priapism. Treatment is symptom directed and supportive.

**Pharmacodynamics/Kinetics**

**Protein Binding:** 85% to 95%

**Half-life Elimination:** 4-7.5 hours, 2 compartment kinetics

**Time to Peak:** Within 30-100 minutes, prolonged in the presence of food (up to 2.5 hours)

**Metabolism:** Liver

**Excretion:** Urine and feces

**Onset:** Therapeutic effects take 1-3 weeks to appear

**Formulations** Tablet, as hydrochloride: 50 mg, 100 mg, 150 mg, 300 mg

**Dosing**

**Adults:** Therapeutic effects may take up to 4 weeks. Therapy is normally maintained for several months after optimum response is reached to prevent recurrence of depression.

Oral: Initial: 150 mg/day in 3 divided doses (may increase by 50 mg/day every 3-7 days); maximum: 400 mg/day for outpatients; maximum for inpatients 600 mg/day.

**Elderly:** Therapeutic effects may take up to 4 weeks. Therapy is normally maintained for several months after optimum response is reached to prevent recurrence of depression.

Oral: 25-50 mg at bedtime with 25-50 mg/day dose increase every 3 days for inpatients and weekly for outpatients, if tolerated; usual dose: 75-150 mg/day, in 3 divided doses where practical (eg, dose of 75 mg/day as above should be divided into 2-3 doses).

**Administration**

**Oral:** Dosing after meals may decrease lightheadedness and postural hypotension.

**Monitoring Laboratory Tests** Baseline liver function prior to and periodically during therapy

**Additional Nursing Issues**

**Physical Assessment:** Assess other medications patient may be taking for effectiveness and interactions (see Drug Interactions). See Contraindications and Warnings/

(Continued)

## Trazodone *(Continued)*

Precautions for cautious use. Has potential for psychological or physiological dependence, abuse, or tolerance. Monitor laboratory tests, therapeutic response (ie, mental status, mood, affect, suicidal ideation), and adverse reactions at beginning of therapy and periodically with long-term use (see Adverse Reactions and Overdose/Toxicology). Taper dosage slowly when discontinuing (allow 3-4 weeks between discontinuing Desyrel® and starting another antidepressant). Assess knowledge/teach patient appropriate use, interventions to reduce side effects and adverse symptoms to report. **Pregnancy risk factor C** - benefits of use should outweigh possible risks. Breast-feeding is contraindicated.

**Patient Information/Instruction:** Take exactly as directed (do not increase dose or frequency); may take 2-4 weeks to achieve desired results; may cause physical and/or psychological dependence. Take after meals. Avoid excessive alcohol, caffeine, and other prescription or OTC medications not approved by prescriber. Maintain adequate hydration (2-3 L/day of fluids unless instructed to restrict fluid intake). You may experience drowsiness, lightheadedness, dizziness (use caution when driving or engaging in tasks requiring alertness until response to drug is known); postural hypotension (use caution when climbing stairs or changing position from lying or sitting to standing); nausea, dry mouth (small frequent meals, frequent mouth care, chewing gum, or sucking lozenges may help); constipation (increased exercise, fluids, or dietary fruit and fiber may help); or diarrhea (buttermilk, yogurt, or boiled milk may help). Report persistent dizziness or headache; muscle cramping, tremors, or altered gait; blurred vision or eye pain; chest pain or irregular heartbeat; or worsening of condition. **Pregnancy/breast-feeding precautions:** Inform prescriber if you are or intend to be pregnant. Do not breast-feed.

**Geriatric Considerations:** Very sedating, but little anticholinergic effects.

**Related Information**

Antidepressant Agents Comparison *on page 1368*

♦ **Trecator®-SC** *see* Ethionamide *on page 460*
♦ **Tremytoine®** *see* Phenytoin *on page 923*
♦ **Trendar® [OTC]** *see* Ibuprofen *on page 592*
♦ **Trental®** *see* Pentoxifylline *on page 908*

## Tretinoin (Oral) (TRET i noyn, oral)

**U.S. Brand Names** Vesanoid®

**Synonyms** All-*trans*-Retinoic Acid

**Therapeutic Category** Antineoplastic Agent, Miscellaneous

**Pregnancy Risk Factor** D

**Lactation** Enters breast milk/not recommended

**Use** Acute promyelocytic leukemia (APL): Induction of remission in patients with APL, French American British (FAB) classification M3 (including the M3 variant), characterized by the presence of the t(15;17) translocation or the presence of the PML/RARα gene who are refractory to or who have relapsed from anthracycline chemotherapy, or for whom anthracycline-based chemotherapy is contraindicated. Tretinoin is for the induction of remission only. All patients should receive an accepted form of remission consolidation or maintenance therapy for APL after completion of induction therapy with tretinoin.

**Mechanism of Action/Effect** Retinoid that induces maturation of acute promyelocytic leukemia (APL) cells in cultures; induces cytodifferentiation and decreased proliferation of APL cells

**Contraindications** Sensitivity to parabens, vitamin A, or other retinoids; pregnancy

**Warnings** Patients with acute promyelocytic leukemia (APL) are at high risk and can have severe adverse reactions to tretinoin. Administer under the supervision of a physician who is experienced in the management of patients with acute leukemia and in a facility with laboratory and supportive services sufficient to monitor drug tolerance and to protect and maintain a patient compromised by drug toxicity, including respiratory compromise.

About 25% of patients with APL, who have been treated with tretinoin, have experienced a syndrome called the retinoic acid-APL (RA-APL) syndrome which is characterized by fever, dyspnea, weight gain, radiographic pulmonary infiltrates and pleural or pericardial effusions. This syndrome has occasionally been accompanied by impaired myocardial contractility and episodic hypotension. It has been observed with or without concomitant leukocytosis. Endotracheal intubation and mechanical ventilation have been required in some cases due to progressive hypoxemia, and several patients have expired with multiorgan failure. The syndrome usually occurs during the first month of treatment, with some cases reported following the first dose.

Management of the syndrome has not been defined, but high-dose steroids given at the first suspicion of RA-APL syndrome appear to reduce morbidity and mortality. At the first signs suggestive of the syndrome, immediately initiate high-dose steroids (dexamethasone 10 mg I.V.) every 12 hours for 3 days or until resolution of symptoms, regardless of the leukocyte count. The majority of patients do not require termination of tretinoin therapy during treatment of the RA-APL syndrome.

During treatment, ~40% of patients will develop rapidly evolving leukocytosis. Rapidly evolving leukocytosis is associated with a higher risk of life-threatening complications.

If signs or symptoms of the RA-APL syndrome are present together with leukocytosis, initiate treatment with high-dose steroids immediately. Consider adding full-dose chemotherapy (including an anthracycline, if not contraindicated) to the tretinoin therapy on day 1 or 2 for patients presenting with a WBC count >5 x $10^9$/L or immediately, for patients presenting with a WBC count <5 x $10^9$/L, if the WBC count reaches ≥6 x $10^9$/L by day 5, or ≥10 x $10^9$/L by day 10 or ≥15 x $10^9$/L by day 28.

**Not to be used in women of childbearing potential** unless woman is capable of complying with effective contraceptive measures; therapy is normally begun on the second or third day of next normal menstrual period; two reliable methods of effective contraception must be used during therapy and for 1 month after discontinuation of therapy, unless abstinence is the chosen method. Within 1 week prior to the institution of tretinoin therapy, the patient should have blood or urine collected for a serum or urine pregnancy test with a sensitivity of at least 50 mIU/L. When possible, delay tretinoin therapy until a negative result from this test is obtained. When a delay is not possible, place the patient on two reliable forms of contraception. Repeat pregnancy testing and contraception counseling monthly throughout the period of treatment.

Initiation of therapy with tretinoin may be based on the morphological diagnosis of APL. Confirm the diagnosis of APL by detection of the t(15;17) genetic marker by cytogenetic studies. If these are negative, PML/RARα fusion should be sought using molecular diagnostic techniques. The response rate of other AML subtypes to tretinoin has not been demonstrated.

Retinoids have been associated with pseudotumor cerebri (benign intracranial hypertension), especially in children. Early signs or symptoms include papilledema, headache, nausea, vomiting and visual disturbances.

Up to 60% of patients experienced hypercholesterolemia or hypertriglyceridemia, which were reversible upon completion of treatment.

Elevated liver function test results occur in 50% to 60% of patients during treatment. Carefully monitor liver function test results during treatment and give consideration to a temporary withdrawal of tretinoin if test results reach >5 times the upper limit of normal.

**Drug Interactions**

**Cytochrome P-450 Effect:** CYP3A3/4 enzyme substrate

**Decreased Effect:** Metabolized by the hepatic cytochrome P-450 system: All drugs that induce this system would be expected to interact with tretinoin.

**Increased Effect/Toxicity:** Ketoconazole increases the mean plasma AUC of tretinoin. Other drugs which inhibit CYP3A4 would be expected to increase tretinoin concentrations, potentially increasing toxicity.

**Adverse Reactions** Virtually all patients experience some drug-related toxicity, especially headache, fever, weakness and fatigue. These adverse effects are seldom permanent or irreversible nor do they usually require therapy interruption

>10%:

- Cardiovascular: Arrhythmias, flushing, hypotension, hypertension, peripheral edema, chest discomfort, edema
- Central nervous system: Dizziness, anxiety, insomnia, depression, confusion, malaise, pain
- Dermatologic: Burning, redness, cheilitis, inflammation of lips, dry skin, pruritus, photosensitivity
- Endocrine & metabolic: Increased serum concentration of triglycerides
- Gastrointestinal: GI hemorrhage, abdominal pain, other GI disorders, diarrhea, constipation, heartburn, abdominal distention, weight gain or loss, anorexia, dry mouth
- Hematologic: Hemorrhage, disseminated intravascular coagulation
- Local: Phlebitis, injection site reactions
- Neuromuscular & skeletal: Bone pain, arthralgia, myalgia, paresthesia
- Ocular: Itching of eye
- Renal: Renal insufficiency
- Respiratory: Upper respiratory tract disorders, dyspnea, respiratory insufficiency, pleural effusion, pneumonia, rales, expiratory wheezing, dry nose
- Miscellaneous: Infections, shivering

1% to 10%:

- Cardiovascular: Cardiac failure, cardiac arrest, myocardial infarction, enlarged heart, heart murmur, ischemia, stroke, myocarditis, pericarditis, pulmonary hypertension, secondary cardiomyopathy, cerebral hemorrhage, pallor
- Central nervous system: Intracranial hypertension, agitation, hallucination, agnosia, aphasia, cerebellar edema, cerebellar disorders, convulsions, coma, CNS depression, encephalopathy, hypotaxia, no light reflex, neurologic reaction, spinal cord disorder, unconsciousness, dementia, forgetfulness, somnolence, slow speech, hypothermia
- Dermatologic: Skin peeling on hands or soles of feet, rash, cellulitis
- Endocrine & metabolic: Fluid imbalance, acidosis
- Gastrointestinal: Hepatosplenomegaly, ulcer, unspecified liver disorder
- Genitourinary: Dysuria, polyuria, enlarged prostate
- Hepatic: Ascites, hepatitis
- Neuromuscular & skeletal: Tremor, leg weakness, hyporeflexia, dysarthria, facial paralysis, hemiplegia, flank pain, asterixis, abnormal gait
- Ocular: Dry eyes, photophobia
- Renal: Acute renal failure, renal tubular necrosis
- Respiratory: Lower respiratory tract disorders, pulmonary infiltration, bronchial asthma, pulmonary/larynx edema, unspecified pulmonary disease
- Miscellaneous: Face edema, lymph disorders

<1% (Limited to important or life-threatening symptoms): Pseudomotor cerebri, alopecia, increase in erythrocyte sedimentation rate, decrease in hemoglobin and hematocrit, hepatitis

(Continued)

## Tretinoin (Oral) *(Continued)*

**Overdose/Toxicology** Symptoms of overdose include transient headache, facial flushing, cheilosis, abdominal pain, dizziness, and ataxia. All signs or symptoms have been transient and have resolved without apparent residual effects.

**Pharmacodynamics/Kinetics**

**Protein Binding:** >95%

**Half-life Elimination:** Parent drug: 0.5-2 hours

**Time to Peak:** Within 1-2 hours

**Metabolism:** Liver

**Excretion:** Urine and feces

**Formulations** Capsule: 10 mg

**Dosing**

**Adults:** Oral: 45 mg/m²/day administered as two evenly divided doses until complete remission is documented. Discontinue therapy 30 days after achievement of complete remission or after 90 days of treatment, whichever occurs first. If after initiation of treatment the presence of the t(15;17) translocation is not confirmed by cytogenetics or by polymerase chain reaction studies and the patient has not responded to tretinoin, consider alternative therapy.

**Note:** Tretinoin is for the induction of remission only. Optimal consolidation or maintenance regimens have not been determined. All patients should therefore receive a standard consolidation or maintenance chemotherapy regimen for APL after induction therapy with tretinoin unless otherwise contraindicated.

**Elderly:** Refer to adult dosing.

**Administration**

**Oral:** Administer with meals. Do not crush capsules.

**Monitoring Laboratory Tests** Monitor the patient's hematologic profile, coagulation profile, liver function results and triglyceride and cholesterol levels frequently.

**Additional Nursing Issues**

**Physical Assessment:** Assess other medications patient may be taking for interactions and effectiveness (see Drug Interactions). Monitor laboratory tests closely. Patient will require close monitoring; note Warnings/Precautions and extensive list of Adverse Reactions. Monitor cardiac, CNS, and respiratory status on a regular (frequent) basis during therapy. **Pregnancy risk factor D** - assess knowledge/teach both male and female appropriate use of barrier contraceptives during and for 1 month following therapy. See Warnings/Precautions. Breast-feeding is not recommended.

**Patient Information/Instruction:** Take with food. Do not crush, chew, or dissolve capsules. You will need frequent blood tests while taking this medication. Maintain adequate hydration (2-3 L/day of fluids unless instructed to restrict fluid intake), avoid alcohol and foods containing vitamin A, and foods with high fat content. You may experience lethargy, dizziness, visual changes, confusion, anxiety (avoid driving or engaging in tasks requiring alertness until response to drug is known). For nausea and vomiting, loss of appetite, or dry mouth small, frequent meals, chewing gum, or sucking lozenges may help. You may experience photosensitivity (use sunscreen, wear protective clothing and eyewear, and avoid direct sunlight). You may experience dry, itchy, skin, and dry or irritated eyes (avoid contact lenses). Report persistent vomiting or diarrhea, difficulty breathing, unusual bleeding or bruising, acute GI pain, bone pain, or vision changes immediately. **Pregnancy/breast-feeding precautions:** Do not get pregnant while taking this medication - both male and female should use appropriate barrier contraceptive measures. Do not give blood during this therapy or for 1 month following discontinuation of therapy. Breast-feeding is not recommended.

## Tretinoin (Topical) (TRET i noyn, TOP i kal)

**U.S. Brand Names** Retin-A™ Topical

**Synonyms** Retinoic Acid; Vitamin A Acid

**Therapeutic Category** Retinoic Acid Derivative

**Pregnancy Risk Factor** C

**Lactation** Enters breast milk/compatible

**Use** Treatment of acne vulgaris, photodamaged skin, and some skin cancers

**Mechanism of Action/Effect** Keratinocytes in the sebaceous follicle become less adherent which allows for easy removal; decreases microcomedone formation

**Contraindications** Hypersensitivity to tretinoin or any component; sunburn

**Warnings** Use with caution in patients with eczema. Avoid excessive exposure to sunlight and sunlamps. Avoid contact with abraded skin, mucous membranes, eyes, mouth, angles of the nose. Effects of chronic, long-term use are unknown. Safety in older individuals is not established. Pregnancy factor C.

**Drug Interactions**

**Cytochrome P-450 Effect:** CYP3A3/4 enzyme substrate

**Increased Effect/Toxicity:** Topical application of sulfur, benzoyl peroxide, salicylic acid, and resorcinol potentiates adverse reactions with tretinoin.

**Adverse Reactions** 1% to 10%:

Cardiovascular: Edema

Dermatologic: Excessive dryness, erythema, scaling of the skin, hyperpigmentation or hypopigmentation, photosensitivity, initial acne flare-up

Local: Stinging, blistering

**Overdose/Toxicology** Toxic signs of a topical overdose commonly respond to drug discontinuation, and generally resolve spontaneously within a few days to weeks.

**Pharmacodynamics/Kinetics**

**Metabolism:** Liver (small amount)

**Excretion:** Bile and urine

**Formulations**

Cream (Retin-A™): 0.025% (20 g, 45 g); 0.05% (20 g, 45 g); 0.1% (20 g, 45 g)

Gel, topical (Retin-A™): 0.01% (15 g, 45 g); 0.025% (15 g, 45 g)

Gel, topical (Retin-A™ Micro): 0.1% (20 g, 45 g)

Liquid, topical (Retin-A™): 0.05% (28 mL)

**Dosing**

**Adults:** Topical: Apply once daily before retiring; if stinging or irritation develops, decrease frequency of application. Relapses normally occur within 3-6 weeks after stopping medication.

**Additional Nursing Issues**

**Physical Assessment:** Assess knowledge/instruct patient on appropriate application, possible adverse effects, and symptoms to report. **Pregnancy risk factor C.**

**Patient Information/Instruction:** For once a day use, do not overuse. Avoid increased intake of vitamin A. Thoroughly wash hands before applying. Wash area to be treated at least 30 minutes before applying. Do not wash face more frequently than 2-3 times a day. Avoid using topical preparations that contain alcohol or harsh chemicals during treatment. You may experience increased sensitivity to sunlight; protect skin with sunblock, wear protective clothing, or avoid direct sunlight. Stop treatment and inform prescriber if rash, skin irritation, redness, scaling, or excessive dryness occurs. **Pregnancy precautions:** Inform prescriber if you are pregnant.

**Pregnancy Issues:** Oral tretinoin is teratogenic and fetotoxic in rats at doses 1000 and 500 times the topical human dose, respectively; however, tretinoin does not appear to be teratogenic when used topically since it is rapidly metabolized by the skin.

- **Triacet™** *see* Topical Corticosteroids *on page 1152*
- **Triacet™** *see* Triamcinolone *on this page*
- **Triacetin** *see page 1294*
- **Triaconazole** *see* Terconazole *on page 1106*
- **Triadapin®** *see* Doxepin *on page 399*
- **Triaken** *see* Ceftriaxone *on page 232*
- **Triam-A®** *see* Triamcinolone *on this page*

## Triamcinolone (trye am SIN oh lone)

**U.S. Brand Names** Amcort®; Aristocort®; Aristocort® A; Aristocort® Forte; Aristocort® Intralesional; Aristospan® Intra-Articular; Aristospan® Intralesional; Atolone®; Azmacort™; Delta-Tritex®; Flutex®; Kenacort®; Kenaject-40®; Kenalog®; Kenalog-10®; Kenalog-40®; Kenalog® H; Kenalog® in Orabase®; Kenonel®; Nasacort®; Nasacort® AQ; Tac™-3; Tac™-40; Triacet™; Triam-A®; Triam Forte®; Triderm®; Tri-Kort®; Trilog®; Trilone®; Tristoject®

**Therapeutic Category** Corticosteroid, Oral Inhaler; Corticosteroid, Nasal; Corticosteroid, Parenteral

**Pregnancy Risk Factor** C

**Lactation** Excretion in breast milk unknown

**Use**

Inhalation: Control of bronchial asthma and related bronchospastic conditions.

Systemic: Adrenocortical insufficiency, rheumatic disorders, allergic states, respiratory diseases, systemic lupus erythematosus, and other diseases requiring anti-inflammatory or immunosuppressive effects

Topical: Inflammatory dermatoses responsive to steroids

**Mechanism of Action/Effect** Decreases inflammation by suppression of migration of polymorphonuclear leukocytes and reversal of increased capillary permeability; suppresses the immune system by reducing activity and volume of the lymphatic system; suppresses adrenal function at high doses

**Contraindications** Hypersensitivity to triamcinolone; systemic fungal infections; serious infections (except septic shock or tuberculous meningitis); primary treatment of status asthmaticus

**Warnings** Use with caution in patients with hypothyroidism, cirrhosis, nonspecific ulcerative colitis, and patients at increased risk for peptic ulcer disease. Discontinue if skin irritation or contact dermatitis should occur. Do not use in patients with decreased skin circulation. Avoid the use of high potency steroids on the face. Fatalities have occurred due to adrenal insufficiency in asthmatic patients during and after transfer from systemic corticosteroids to aerosol steroids. Several months may be required for recovery from this syndrome. During this period, aerosol steroids do **not** provide the increased systemic steroid requirement needed to treat patients having trauma, surgery, or infections. Avoid using higher than recommended dose. Pregnancy factor C.

**Drug Interactions**

**Decreased Effect:** Decreased effect with barbiturates and phenytoin. Rifampin increased metabolism of triamcinolone. Vaccine and toxoid effects may be reduced.

**Increased Effect/Toxicity:** Salicylates or NSAIDs coadministered oral corticosteroids may increase risk of GI ulceration.

**Adverse Reactions**

**Systemic:**

>10%:

Central nervous system: Insomnia, nervousness

Gastrointestinal: Increased appetite, indigestion

(Continued)

## Triamcinolone *(Continued)*

1% to 10%:

Central nervous system: Dizziness or lightheadedness, headache
Dermatologic: Hirsutism, hypopigmentation
Endocrine & metabolic: Diabetes mellitus
Neuromuscular & skeletal: Arthralgia
Ocular: Cataracts, glaucoma
Respiratory: Epistaxis
Miscellaneous: Sweating

<1% (Limited to important or life-threatening symptoms): Edema, hypertension, seizures, Cushing's syndrome, pituitary-adrenal axis suppression

**Topical:**

1% to 10%:

Dermatologic: Itching, allergic contact dermatitis, erythema, dryness papular rashes, folliculitis, furunculosis, pustules, pyoderma, vesiculation, hyperesthesia, skin infection (secondary)
Local: Burning, irritation

<1% (Limited to important or life-threatening symptoms): Gastric ulcer, glaucoma, cataracts (posterior subcapsular)

**Overdose/Toxicology** When consumed in high doses for prolonged periods, systemic hypercorticism and adrenal suppression may occur. In those cases, discontinuation of the corticosteroid should be done judiciously.

**Pharmacodynamics/Kinetics**

**Half-life Elimination:** Biologic: 18-36 hours

**Duration:** Oral: 8-12 hours

**Formulations**

Aerosol:
Oral inhalation: 100 mcg/metered spray (2 oz)
Nasal: 55 mcg per actuation (15 mL)
Topical, as acetonide: 0.2 mg/2 second spray (23 g, 63 g)
Cream, as acetonide: 0.025% (15 g, 60 g, 80 g, 240 g, 454 g); 0.1% (15 g, 30 g, 60 g, 80 g, 90 g, 120 g, 240 g); 0.5% (15 g, 20 g, 30 g, 240 g)
Injection, as acetonide: 10 mg/mL (5 mL); 40 mg/mL (1 mL, 5 mL, 10 mL)
Injection, as diacetate: 25 mg/mL (5 mL); 40 mg/mL (1 mL, 5 mL, 10 mL)
Injection, as hexacetonide: 5 mg/mL (5 mL); 20 mg/mL (1 mL, 5 mL)
Lotion, as acetonide: 0.025% (60 mL); 0.1% (15 mL, 60 mL)
Ointment:
Oral: 0.1% (5 g)
Topical, as acetonide: 0.025% (15 g, 30 g, 60 g, 80 g, 120 g, 454 g); 0.1% (15 g, 30 g, 60 g, 80 g, 120 g, 240 g, 454 g); 0.5% (15 g, 20 g, 30 g, 240 g)
Spray, nasal, as acetonide: 55 mcg per actuation in aqueous base (16.5 g)
Syrup: 2 mg/5 mL (120 mL); 4 mg/5 mL (120 mL)
Tablet: 1 mg, 2 mg, 4 mg, 8 mg

**Dosing**

**Adults:** In general, single I.M. dose of 4-7 times oral dose will control patient from 4-7 days up to 3-4 weeks.

Intranasal: 2 sprays in each nostril once daily; may increase after 4-7 days up to 4 sprays once daily or 1 spray 4 times/day in each nostril.
Topical: Apply a thin film 2-3 times/day.
Oral: 4-48 mg/day
I.M.: Acetonide or hexacetonide: 60 mg (of 40 mg/mL), additional 20-100 mg doses (usual: 40-80 mg) may be given when signs or symptoms recur, best at 6-week intervals to minimize HPA suppression
Oral inhalation: 2 inhalations 3-4 times/day, not to exceed 16 inhalations/day
Intra-articular (hexacetonide): 2-20 mg every 3-4 weeks as hexacetonide salt
Intralesional (use 10 mg/mL) (diacetate or acetonide): 1 mg/injection site, may be repeated one or more times/week depending upon patients response; maximum; 30 mg at any one time; may use multiple injections if they are more than 1 cm apart
Intra-articular, intrasynovial, and soft-tissue injection (use 10 mg/mL or 40 mg/mL) (diacetate or acetonide): 2.5-40 mg depending upon location, size of joints, and degree of inflammation; repeat when signs or symptoms recur.
Sublesional (as acetonide): Up to 1 mg per injection site and may be repeated one or more times weekly; multiple sites may be injected if they are 1 cm or more apart, not to exceed 30 mg
See table.

**Triamcinolone Dosing**

<table>
<tr><th></th><th>Acetonide</th><th>Diacetate</th><th>Hexacetonide</th></tr>
<tr><td>Intrasynovial</td><td>2.5-40 mg</td><td>5-40 mg</td><td></td></tr>
<tr><td>Intralesional</td><td>2.5-40 mg</td><td rowspan="2">5-48 mg</td><td rowspan="2">Up to 0.5 mg/sq inch affected area</td></tr>
<tr><td>Sublesional</td><td>1-30 mg</td></tr>
<tr><td>Systemic I.M.</td><td>2.5-60 mg/d</td><td>~40 mg/wk</td><td>20-100 mg</td></tr>
<tr><td>Intra-articular</td><td></td><td>5-40 mg</td><td>2-20 mg average</td></tr>
<tr><td>large joints</td><td>5-15 mg</td><td></td><td>10-20 mg</td></tr>
<tr><td>small joints</td><td>2.5-5 mg</td><td></td><td>2-6 mg</td></tr>
<tr><td>Tendon sheaths</td><td>10-40 mg</td><td></td><td></td></tr>
<tr><td>Intradermal</td><td>1 mg/site</td><td></td><td></td></tr>
</table>

**Elderly:** Refer to adult dosing; use with caution (see Geriatric Considerations).

**Administration**

**Oral:** Once daily doses should be given in the morning.

**I.M.:** Inject I.M. dose deep in large muscle mass, avoid deltoid.

**Inhalation:** Inhaler: Rinse mouth and throat after use to prevent candidiasis. Use spacer device provided with Azmacort™.

**Topical:** Apply a thin film sparingly and avoid topical application on the face. Do not use on open skin or wounds. Do not occlude area unless directed.

**Other:** Avoid subcutaneous administration.

**Additional Nursing Issues**

**Physical Assessment:** Assess other medications patient may be taking for effectiveness and interactions (see Drug Interactions). Note Contraindications and Warnings/Precautions for cautious use. Monitor laboratory tests, therapeutic response, and adverse effects according to indications for therapy, dose, route (systemic or topical), and duration of therapy (see Dosing, Warnings/Precautions, Adverse Reactions). With systemic administration, diabetics should monitor glucose levels closely (corticosteroids may alter glucose levels). Assess knowledge/teach patient appropriate use, interventions to reduce side effects, and adverse symptoms to report. When used for long-term therapy (longer than 10-14 days) do not discontinue abruptly; decrease dosage incrementally. **Pregnancy risk factor C** - benefits of use should outweigh possible risks. Note breast-feeding caution.

**Patient Information/Instruction:** Take exactly as directed; do not increase dose or discontinue abruptly without consulting prescriber. Take oral medication with or after meals. Limit intake of caffeine or stimulants. Prescriber may recommend increased dietary vitamins, minerals, or iron. Diabetics should monitor glucose levels closely (antidiabetic medication may need to be adjusted). Inform prescriber if you are experiencing greater than normal levels of stress (medication may need adjustment). Some forms of this medication may cause GI upset (oral medication may be taken with meals to reduce GI upset; small frequent meals and frequent mouth care may reduce GI upset). You may be more susceptible to infection (avoid crowds and persons with contagious or infective conditions). Report promptly excessive nervousness or sleep disturbances; any signs of infection (sore throat, unhealed injuries); excessive growth of body hair or loss of skin color; changes in vision; excessive or sudden weight gain (>3 lb/week); swelling of face or extremities; difficulty breathing; muscle weakness; change in color of stools (black or tarry) or persistent abdominal pain; or worsening of condition or failure to improve. **Pregnancy/breast-feeding precautions:** Inform prescriber if you are or intend to be pregnant. Consult prescriber if breast-feeding.

Topical: For external use only. Not for eyes or mucous membranes or open wounds. Apply in very thin layer to occlusive dressing. Apply dressing to area being treated. Avoid prolonged or excessive use around sensitive tissues, genital, or rectal areas. Inform prescriber if condition worsens (swelling, redness, irritation, pain, open sores) or fails to improve.

Aerosol: Not for use during acute asthmatic attack. Follow directions that accompany product. Rinse mouth and throat after use to prevent candidiasis. Do not use intranasal product if you have a nasal infection, nasal injury, or recent nasal surgery. If using two products, consult prescriber in which order to use the two products. Inform prescriber if condition worsens or does not improve.

**Geriatric Considerations:** Because of the risk of adverse effects, systemic corticosteroids should be used cautiously in the elderly, in the smallest possible dose, and for the shortest possible time. Azmacort™ (metered dose inhaler) comes with its own spacer device attached and may be easier to use in older patients.

**Additional Information** 16 mg triamcinolone is equivalent to 100 mg cortisone (no mineralocorticoid activity)

**Related Information**

Corticosteroids Comparison, Systemic Equivalencies *on page 1383*
Corticosteroids Comparison, Topical *on page 1384*
Inhalant (Asthma, Bronchospasm) Agents *on page 1388*

- **Triamcinolone and Nystatin** *see* Nystatin and Triamcinolone *on page 844*
- **Triam Forte®** *see* Triamcinolone *on page 1171*
- **Triaminic® Allergy Tablet** *see page 1294*
- **Triaminic® AM Decongestant Formula [OTC]** *see* Pseudoephedrine *on page 992*
- **Triaminic® Cold Tablet** *see page 1294*
- **Triaminic® Expectorant [OTC]** *see* Guaifenesin and Phenylpropanolamine *on page 550*
- **Triaminicol® Multi-Symptom Cold Syrup** *see page 1294*
- **Triaminic® Syrup** *see page 1294*

## Triamterene (trye AM ter een)

**U.S. Brand Names** Dyrenium®

**Therapeutic Category** Diuretic, Potassium Sparing

**Pregnancy Risk Factor** D

**Lactation** Excretion in breast milk unknown

**Use** Alone or in combination with other diuretics to treat edema and hypertension; decreases potassium excretion caused by kaliuretic diuretics

**Mechanism of Action/Effect** Competes with aldosterone for receptor sites in the distal renal tubules, increasing sodium, chloride, and water excretion while conserving potassium and hydrogen ions; may block the effect of aldosterone on arteriolar smooth muscle as well

(Continued)

## Triamterene *(Continued)*

**Contraindications** Hypersensitivity to triamterene or any component; hyperkalemia; renal impairment; do not give to patients receiving spironolactone or amiloride; pregnancy

**Warnings** Use with caution in patients with severe hepatic encephalopathy, patients with diabetes, renal dysfunction, a history of renal stones, or those receiving potassium supplements or ACE inhibitors.

**Drug Interactions**

**Increased Effect/Toxicity:** Increased risk of hyperkalemia if given together with amiloride, spironolactone, and angiotensin-converting enzyme (ACE) inhibitors. Increased toxicity of amantadine (possibly by decreasing its renal excretion).

**Food Interactions** If triamterene is taken with foods high in potassium, hyperkalemia may result.

**Effects on Lab Values** Interferes with fluorometric assay of quinidine

**Adverse Reactions**

1% to 10%:

Cardiovascular: Hypotension, edema, congestive heart failure, bradycardia
Central nervous system: Dizziness, headache, fatigue
Gastrointestinal: Constipation, nausea
Respiratory: Dyspnea

<1% (Limited to important or life-threatening symptoms): Inability to achieve or maintain an erection, agranulocytosis, thrombocytopenia

**Overdose/Toxicology** Symptoms of overdose include drowsiness, confusion, clinical signs of dehydration, electrolyte imbalance, and hypotension. Ingestion of large amounts of potassium-sparing diuretics may result in life-threatening hyperkalemia. This can be treated with I.V. glucose, with concurrent regular insulin and I.V. sodium bicarbonate. If needed, Kayexalate® oral or rectal solutions in sorbitol may also be used.

**Pharmacodynamics/Kinetics**

**Onset:** Diuresis occurs within 2-4 hours

**Duration:** 7-9 hours

**Formulations** Capsule: 50 mg, 100 mg

**Dosing**

**Adults:** Oral: 100-300 mg/day in 1-2 divided doses; maximum: 300 mg/day

**Elderly:** Oral (when used alone; decrease total daily dose when combined with other diuretics or antihypotensives): Initial: 50 mg/day; maximum: 100 mg/day in 1-2 divided doses.

**Renal Impairment:** $Cl_{cr}$ <10 mL/minute: Avoid use.

**Hepatic Impairment:** Dose reduction is recommended in patients with cirrhosis.

**Administration**

**Oral:** If ordered once daily, dose should be given in the morning.

**Monitoring Laboratory Tests** Serum electrolytes, renal function

**Additional Nursing Issues**

**Physical Assessment:** Monitor effectiveness of therapy and adverse reactions frequently when starting therapy and on a regular basis thereafter, especially fluid status, hyperkalemia (eg, arrhythmias, fatigue, muscle weakness, paresthesia, confusion), and hyponatremia (eg, anorexia, nausea/vomiting, diarrhea, headaches, lethargy, hyper-reflexia, seizures). Teach patient effects to monitor and symptoms to report. **Pregnancy risk factor D** - assess knowledge/teach appropriate use of barrier contraceptives. Note breast-feeding caution.

**Patient Information/Instruction:** Take as directed, preferably after meals. This diuretic does not cause potassium loss; avoid excessive potassium intake (eg, salt substitutes, low-salt foods, bananas, nuts). Weigh yourself daily at the same time, in the same clothes, and report weight loss greater than 5 lb/week. Urine may appear blue (normal). You may experience dizziness, drowsiness, headache (use caution when driving or engaging in tasks requiring alertness until response to drug is known); nausea (small frequent meals, frequent mouth care, sucking lozenges, or chewing gum may help); decreased sexual ability (reversible with discontinuing of medication); or postural hypotension (change position slowly when rising from sitting or lying). Report persistent fatigue, muscle weakness, paresthesia, confusion, anorexia, headaches, lethargy, hyper-reflexia, seizures, swelling of extremities or respiratory difficulty (eg, chest pain, rapid heartbeat or palpitations). **Pregnancy/breast-feeding precautions:** Do not get pregnant while taking this medication; use appropriate barrier contraceptive measures. Consult prescriber if breast-feeding.

**Geriatric Considerations:** Monitor serum potassium (see Warnings/Precautions).

- ♦ **Triamterene and Hydrochlorothiazide** *see* Hydrochlorothiazide and Triamterene *on page 568*
- ♦ **Triapin®** *see* Butalbital Compound and Acetaminophen *on page 175*
- ♦ **Triavil®** *see* Amitriptyline and Perphenazine *on page 75*

## Triazolam (trye AY zoe lam)

**U.S. Brand Names** Halcion®

**Therapeutic Category** Benzodiazepine

**Pregnancy Risk Factor** X

**Lactation** Enters breast milk/not recommended

**Use** Short-term treatment of insomnia

**Mechanism of Action/Effect** Depresses all levels of the CNS, including the limbic and reticular formation, probably through the increased action of gamma-aminobutyric acid (GABA), which is a major inhibitory neurotransmitter in the brain

**Contraindications** Hypersensitivity to triazolam or any component; cross-sensitivity with other benzodiazepines may occur; pre-existing CNS depression; acute narrow-angle glaucoma; pregnancy

**Warnings** This drug may cause drug dependency. Avoid abrupt discontinuance in patients with prolonged therapy or seizure disorders. Not considered a drug of choice in the elderly.

**Drug Interactions**

**Cytochrome P-450 Effect:** CYP3A3/4 and 3A5-7 enzyme substrate

**Decreased Effect:** Decreased effect with phenytoin, phenobarbital.

**Increased Effect/Toxicity:** Increased effect/toxicity with CNS depressants, psychotropic medications, antihistamines, and alcohol. Coadministration with cimetidine or erythromycin may result in a longer half-life or effect of triazolam.

**Food Interactions** Food may decrease the rate of absorption.

**Adverse Reactions**

>10%:

Central nervous system: Drowsiness, ataxia, lightheadedness, headache, dizziness, impaired coordination, anxiety, fatigue, slurred speech, irritability, nervousness, insomnia, memory impairment, cognitive disorder, dysarthria, anxiety

Gastrointestinal: Decreased salivation (dry mouth)

Genitourinary: Micturition difficulties

1% to 10%:

Cardiovascular: Tachycardia, syncope

Central nervous system: Confusion, increased libido, depersonalization, mental depression, perceptual disturbances, parethesias, weakness, akathisia, agitation, disinhibition, talkativeness, derealization, dream abnormalities, fear, decreased libido

Gastrointestinal: Abdominal or stomach cramps, increased or decreased appetite, weight gain or loss, nausea, vomiting

Neuromuscular & skeletal: Muscle cramps

Ocular: Photophobia, blurred vision

Otic: Tinnitus

Respiratory: Nasal congestion

Miscellaneous: Sweating

<1% (Limited to important or life-threatening symptoms): Agranulocytosis, anemia, leukopenia, neutropenia, thrombocytopenia, hepatic dysfunction, dystonic extrapyramidal effects

**Overdose/Toxicology** Symptoms of overdose include somnolence, confusion, coma, diminished reflexes, dyspnea, and hypotension. Treatment for benzodiazepine overdose is supportive. Flumazenil has been shown to selectively block the binding of benzodiazepines to CNS receptors, resulting in reversal of benzodiazepine-induced CNS depression but not always respiratory depression.

**Pharmacodynamics/Kinetics**

**Protein Binding:** 89%

**Half-life Elimination:** 1.7-5 hours

**Metabolism:** Liver

**Excretion:** Urine

**Onset:** Onset of hypnotic effect: Within 15-30 minutes

**Duration:** 6-7 hours

**Formulations** Tablet: 0.125 mg, 0.25 mg

**Dosing**

**Adults:** Oral: 0.125-0.25 mg at bedtime

**Elderly:** Oral: Insomnia (short-term use): 0.0625-0.125 mg at bedtime (see Geriatric Considerations).

**Hepatic Impairment:** Reduce dose or avoid use in cirrhosis.

**Administration**

**Oral:** May take with food. Tablet may be crushed or swallowed whole. Onset of action is rapid, patient should be in bed when taking medication.

**Additional Nursing Issues**

**Physical Assessment:** Assess other medications patient may be taking for effectiveness and interactions (see Drug Interactions). See Contraindications and Warnings/Precautions for cautious use. Assess for history of addiction; long-term use can result in dependence, abuse, or tolerance; periodically evaluate need for continued use. Monitor therapeutic response (eg, mood, affect, anxiety level, sleep pattern) and adverse reactions at beginning of therapy and periodically with long-term use (see Adverse Reactions and Overdose/Toxicology). Taper dosage slowly when discontinuing. Assess knowledge/teach patient appropriate use, interventions to reduce side effects, and adverse symptoms to report. **Pregnancy risk factor X** - determine that patient is not pregnant before beginning treatment and do not give to women of childbearing age or males who may have intercourse with childbearing women unless both male and female are capable of complying with barrier contraceptive measures during therapy and for 1 month following therapy. Breast-feeding is not recommended.

**Patient Information/Instruction:** Take exactly as directed (do not increase dose or frequency); may take 2-3 weeks to achieve desired results; may cause physical and/or psychological dependence. Do not use excessive alcohol or other prescription or OTC medications (especially pain medications, sedatives, antihistamines, or hypnotics) without consulting prescriber. Maintain adequate hydration (2-3 L/day of fluids unless instructed to restrict fluid intake). You may experience drowsiness, lightheadedness, impaired coordination, dizziness, or blurred vision (use caution when driving or engaging in tasks requiring alertness until response to drug is known); nausea,

(Continued)

## Triazolam *(Continued)*

vomiting, or dry mouth (small frequent meals, frequent mouth care, chewing gum, or sucking lozenges may help); constipation (increased exercise, fluids, or dietary fruit and fiber may help); altered sexual drive or ability (reversible); or photosensitivity (use sunscreen, wear protective clothing and eyewear, and avoid direct sunlight). Report persistent CNS effects (eg, memory impairment, confusion, depression, increased sedation, excitation, headache, agitation, insomnia or nightmares, dizziness, fatigue, impaired coordination, changes in personality, or changes in cognition); changes in urinary pattern; muscle cramping, weakness, tremors, or rigidity; ringing in ears or visual disturbances; chest pain, palpitations, or rapid heartbeat; excessive perspiration; excessive GI symptoms (cramping, constipation, vomiting, anorexia); or worsening of condition. **Pregnancy/breast-feeding precautions:** Inform prescriber if you are pregnant. Do not get pregnant during or for 1 month following therapy. Male: Do not cause a pregnancy. Male/female: Consult prescriber for instruction on appropriate contraceptive measures. This drug may cause severe fetal defects. Breast-feeding is not recommended.

**Geriatric Considerations:** Due to the higher incidence of CNS adverse reactions and its short half-life, this benzodiazepine is not a drug of first choice. For short-term only.

**Related Information**

Anxiolytic/Hypnotic Use in Long-Term Care Facilities *on page 1430*
Benzodiazepines Comparison *on page 1375*


- **Tribakin** *see* Co-trimoxazole *on page 307*
- **Triban®** *see* Trimethobenzamide *on page 1180*
- **Tribavirin** *see* Ribavirin *on page 1016*
- **Trichloroacetaldehyde Monohydrate** *see* Chloral Hydrate *on page 245*
- ***Trichophyton* Skin Test** *see page 1248*
- **Tri-Clear® Expectorant [OTC]** *see* Guaifenesin and Phenylpropanolamine *on page 550*
- **Tricor®** *see* Fenofibrate *on page 475*
- **Tricosal®** *see* Choline Magnesium Trisalicylate *on page 263*
- **Triderm®** *see* Topical Corticosteroids *on page 1152*
- **Triderm®** *see* Triamcinolone *on page 1171*
- **Tridesilon® Topical** *see* Topical Corticosteroids *on page 1152*
- **Tridil® Injection** *see* Nitroglycerin *on page 831*
- **Trientine** *see page 1246*
- **Triethanolamine Polypeptide Oleate** *see page 1291*
- **Triethanolamine Salicylate** *see page 1294*
- **Triethylenethiophosphoramide** *see* Thiotepa *on page 1125*


## Trifluoperazine (trye floo oh PER a zeen)

**U.S. Brand Names** Stelazine®

**Therapeutic Category** Antipsychotic Agent, Phenothazine, Piperazine

**Pregnancy Risk Factor** C

**Lactation** Enters breast milk/not recommended

**Use** Treatment of psychoses and management of behavioral symptoms

**Mechanism of Action/Effect** Blocks postsynaptic mesolimbic dopaminergic receptors in the brain; exhibits alpha-adrenergic blocking effect and depresses the release of hypothalamic and hypophyseal hormones

**Contraindications** Hypersensitivity to trifluoperazine or any component (cross reactivity between phenothiazines may occur); severe CNS depression; bone marrow suppression; blood dyscrasias; severe hepatic disease; coma

**Warnings** May result in hypotension, particularly after I.M. administration. May be sedating, use with caution in disorders where CNS depression is a feature. Use with caution in Parkinson's disease. Use with caution in patients with hemodynamic instability; predisposition to seizures; subcortical brain damage; hepatic impairment; severe cardiac, renal, or respiratory disease. Neuroleptics may cause swallowing difficulty. Use with caution in breast cancer or other prolactin-dependent tumors (may elevate prolactin levels). May alter temperature regulation or mask toxicity of other drugs due to antiemetic effects. May alter cardiac conduction - life-threatening arrhythmias have occurred with therapeutic doses of phenothiazines. May cause orthostatic hypotension.

Phenothiazines may cause anticholinergic effects (eg, confusion, agitation, constipation, dry mouth, blurred vision, urinary retention); therefore, use with caution in patients with decreased gastrointestinal motility, urinary retention, BPH, xerostomia, or visual problems. Conditions which also may be exacerbated by cholinergic blockade include narrow-angle glaucoma (screening is recommended) and worsening of myasthenia gravis. Relative to other antipsychotics, trifluoperazine has a low potency of cholinergic blockade.

May cause extrapyramidal reactions, including pseudoparkinsonism, acute dystonic reactions, akathisia, and tardive dyskinesia (risk of these reactions is high relative to other neuroleptics). May be associated with neuroleptic malignant syndrome (NMS) or pigmentary retinopathy.

Pregnancy factor C.

**Drug Interactions**

**Cytochrome P-450 Effect:** CYP1A2 enzyme substrate

**Decreased Effect:** Decreased effect of anticonvulsants (increases requirements), guanethidine, and anticoagulants. Decreased effect of trifluoperazine with anticholinergics.

**Increased Effect/Toxicity:** Increased effect/toxicity with CNS depressants, metrizamide (increases seizures), propranolol, and lithium (rare encephalopathy).

**Effects on Lab Values** ↑ cholesterol (S), glucose; ↓ uric acid (S)

**Adverse Reactions**

>10%:

Central nervous system: Pseudoparkinsonism, akathisia, dystonias, tardive dyskinesia (persistent), dizziness
Gastrointestinal: Constipation
Ocular: Pigmentary retinopathy
Respiratory: Nasal congestion
Miscellaneous: Decreased sweating

1% to 10%:

Genitourinary: Dysuria
Dermatologic: Photosensitivity, rash
Endocrine & metabolic: Changes in menstrual cycle, changes in libido, breast pain
Gastrointestinal: Weight gain, nausea, vomiting, stomach pain
Neuromuscular & skeletal: Tremor

<1% (Limited to important or life-threatening symptoms): Neuroleptic malignant syndrome (NMS), lowering of seizures threshold, agranulocytosis, leukopenia, cholestatic jaundice, hepatotoxicity, hypotension, orthostatic hypotension

**Overdose/Toxicology** Symptoms of overdose include deep sleep, coma, extrapyramidal symptoms, abnormal involuntary muscle movements, hypo- or hypertension, and cardiac arrhythmias. Treatment is symptom directed and supportive.

**Pharmacodynamics/Kinetics**

**Half-life Elimination:** >24 hours with chronic use

**Metabolism:** Liver

**Formulations**

Trifluoperazine hydrochloride:

Concentrate, oral: 10 mg/mL (60 mL)
Injection: 2 mg/mL (10 mL)
Tablet: 1 mg, 2 mg, 5 mg, 10 mg

**Dosing**

**Adults:**

Psychoses:

Outpatients: Oral: 1-2 mg twice daily
Hospitalized or well supervised patient: Initial: 2-5 mg twice daily with optimum response in the 15-20 mg/day range; do not exceed 40 mg/day
I.M.: 1-2 mg every 4-6 hours as needed up to 10 mg/24 hours maximum

Nonpsychotic anxiety: Oral: 1-2 mg twice daily; maximum: 6 mg/day; therapy for anxiety should not exceed 12 weeks; do not exceed 6 mg/day for longer than 12 weeks when treating anxiety; agitation, jitteriness, or insomnia may be confused with original neurotic or psychotic symptoms.

**Elderly:** Oral: Nonpsychotic patients, dementia behavior: Initial: 0.5-1 mg 1-2 times/day; increase dose at 4- to 7-day intervals by 0.5-1 mg/day; increase dosing intervals (bid, tid, etc) as necessary to control response or side effects. Maximum daily dose: 40 mg. Gradual increases (titration) may prevent some side effects or decrease their severity.

I.M.: Initial: 1 mg every 4-6 hours; increase at 1 mg increments; do not exceed 6 mg/day

**Renal Impairment:** Not dialyzable (0% to 5%)

**Administration**

**Oral:** Oral concentrate must be diluted in 2-4 oz of liquid (water, carbonated drinks, fruit juices, tomato juice, milk, or pudding). Wash hands if undiluted concentrate is spilled on skin to prevent contact dermatosis. **Note:** Avoid skin contact with oral medication; may cause contact dermatitis.

**I.M.:** Give I.M. injection deep in upper outer quadrant of buttock.

**Stability**

**Storage:** Store injection at room temperature. Protect from heat and from freezing. Use only clear or slightly yellow solutions.

**Monitoring Laboratory Tests** Baseline liver and kidney function, CBC prior to and periodically during therapy, ophthalmic exam

**Additional Nursing Issues**

**Physical Assessment:** Assess other medications patient is taking for effectiveness and interactions (see Drug Interactions). See Contraindications and Warnings/Precautions for cautious use. Has potential for psychological or physiological dependence, abuse, and tolerance. Review ophthalmic exam and monitor laboratory results (see above), therapeutic response (mental status, mood, affect, gait), and adverse reactions at beginning of therapy and periodically with long-term use (eg, excess sedation, extrapyramidal effects, tardive dyskinesia, CNS changes - see Adverse Reactions and Overdose/Toxicology). With I.M. use, monitor closely for hypotension. **Note:** Avoid skin contact with liquid medication; may cause contact dermatitis (wash immediately with warm, soapy water). Initiate at lower doses (see Dosing) and taper dosage slowly when discontinuing. Assess knowledge/teach patient appropriate use, interventions to reduce side effects, and adverse symptoms to report (see below). **Pregnancy risk factor C** - benefits of use should outweigh possible risks. Breast-feeding is not recommended.

**Patient Information/Instruction:** Use exactly as directed (do not increase dose or frequency); may cause physical and/or psychological dependence. Do not discontinue without consulting prescriber. Tablets/capsules may be taken with food. Mix oral solution with 2-4 ounces of liquid (eg, juice, milk, water, pudding). Do not take within 2 hours of any antacid. Avoid excess alcohol or caffeine and other prescription or OTC

(Continued)

## Trifluoperazine *(Continued)*

medications not approved by prescriber. Maintain adequate hydration (2-3 L/day of fluids unless instructed to restrict fluid intake). Avoid skin contact with liquid medication; may cause contact dermatitis (wash immediately with warm, soapy water). You may experience excess drowsiness, lightheadedness, dizziness, or blurred vision (use caution driving or when engaging in tasks requiring alertness until response to drug is known); nausea or vomiting (small frequent meals, frequent mouth care, chewing gum, or sucking lozenges may help); constipation (increased exercise, fluids, or dietary fruit and fiber may help); postural hypotension (use caution climbing stairs or when changing position from lying or sitting to standing); urinary retention (void before taking medication); ejaculatory dysfunction (reversible); decreased perspiration (avoid strenuous exercise in hot environments); photosensitivity (use sunscreen, wear protective clothing and eyewear, and avoid direct sunlight). Report persistent CNS effects (eg, trembling fingers, altered gait or balance, excessive sedation, seizures, unusual movements, anxiety, abnormal thoughts, confusion, personality changes); chest pain, palpitations, rapid heartbeat, severe dizziness; unresolved urinary retention or changes in urinary pattern; altered menstrual pattern, changes in libido, swelling or pain in breasts (male or female); vision changes; skin rash, irritation, or changes in color of skin (gray-blue); or worsening of condition. **Pregnancy/breast-feeding precautions:** Inform prescriber if you are or intend to be pregnant. Breast-feeding is not recommended.

**Geriatric Considerations:** (See Warnings/Precautions, Adverse Reactions, and Overdose/Toxicology.) Elderly patients have an increased risk of adverse response to side effects or adverse reactions to antipsychotics. These can include but are not limited to the following.

Anticholinergic effects: CNS toxicity with confusion, memory loss, psychotic behavior, and agitation.

Extrapyramidal effects (EPS): Parkinson's syndrome and akathisia may occur as often as 50% in patients >60 years of age. Tardive dyskinesia (motor restlessness) may be 40% in elderly; may be related to duration and total accumulated dose over time; may be somewhat reversible if diagnosed early enough.

Orthostatic hypotension: Increased risk for falls.

Sedation: In nonpsychotic patients, may result in feelings of depersonalization, derealization, and dysphoria.

Cardiac toxicity: Cardiac arrhythmias have occurred with therapeutic doses of antipsychotics.

Malignant neuroleptic syndrome: Development of hyperthermia, muscular rigidity, autonomic instability, and altered mental status.

Many elderly patients receive antipsychotic medications for inappropriate nonpsychotic behavior. Before initiating antipsychotic medication, all possible reversible causes should be investigated. Stress may cause acute "confusion" or worsening of baseline nonpsychotic behaviors; any changes in disease state (in any organ) may result in behavioral changes. Common acute changes in behavior may be due also to increases in drug dose addition, or addition of a new drug to the regimen; fluid/electrolyte alterations; infections; or changes in the environment.

Meta-analysis of controlled trials of antipsychotic (phenothiazines, butyrophenones) use with agitated, demented, elderly patients has concluded that the use of neuroleptics results in a response rate of 18%. Clearly, neuroleptic therapy for behavior control should be limited, with frequent attempts to withdraw the agent for behavior control. When use is indicated, initial doses should be lower to start and monitored closely.

**Additional Information** Some formulations may contain benzyl alcohol. The concentrate formulation contains sulfites.

**Related Information**

Antipsychotic Agents Comparison *on page 1371*
Antipsychotic Medication Guidelines *on page 1436*

♦ **Trifluorothymidine** *see* Trifluridine *on this page*

## Trifluridine (trye FLURE i deen)

**U.S. Brand Names** Viroptic® Ophthalmic

**Synonyms** $F_3T$; Trifluorothymidine

**Therapeutic Category** Antiviral Agent, Ophthalmic

**Pregnancy Risk Factor** C

**Lactation** Excretion in breast milk unknown

**Use** Treatment of primary keratoconjunctivitis and recurrent epithelial keratitis caused by herpes simplex virus Types I and II

**Mechanism of Action/Effect** Interferes with viral replication by incorporating into viral DNA in place of thymidine, inhibiting thymidylate synthetase resulting in the formation of defective proteins

**Contraindications** Hypersensitivity to trifluridine or any component

**Warnings** Mild local irritation of conjunctiva and cornea may occur when instilled but usually is a transient effect. Pregnancy factor C.

**Adverse Reactions**

>10%: Local: Burning, stinging

<1% (Limited to important or life-threatening symptoms): Palpebral edema, epithelial keratopathy, keratitis, stromal edema, increased intraocular pressure

**Formulations** Solution, ophthalmic: 1% (7.5 mL)

**Dosing**

**Adults:** Ophthalmic: Instill 1 drop into affected eye every 2 hours while awake, to a maximum of 9 drops/day, until re-epithelialization of corneal ulcer occurs. Then use 1 drop every 4 hours for another 7 days. Do **not** exceed 21 days of treatment. If improvement has not taken place in 7-14 days, consider another form of therapy.

**Elderly:** Refer to adult dosing.

**Stability**

**Storage:** Refrigerate at 2°C to 8°C (36°F to 46°F). Storage at room temperature may result in a solution altered pH which could result in ocular discomfort upon administration and/or decreased potency.

**Additional Nursing Issues**

**Physical Assessment:** Monitor effectiveness of therapy, not for long-term use (see Dosing). Assess knowledge/teach patient appropriate use, interventions to reduce side effects, and adverse symptoms to report (see Adverse Reactions). **Pregnancy risk factor C** - systemic absorption minimal or unlikely. Note breast-feeding caution.

**Patient Information/Instruction:** For ophthalmic use only. Store in refrigerator; do not use discolored solution. Apply prescribed amount as often as directed. Wash hands before using and do not let tip of applicator touch eye or contaminate tip of applicator. Tilt head back and look upward. Gently pull down lower lid and put drop(s) in inner corner of eye. Close eye and roll eyeball in all directions. Do not blink for ½ minute. Apply gentle pressure to inner corner of eye for 30 seconds. Wipe away excess from skin around eye. Do not use any other eye preparation for at least 10 minutes. Do not touch tip of applicator to eye or contaminate tip of applicator. Do not share medication with anyone else. May cause sensitivity to bright light (dark glasses may help); temporary stinging or blurred vision may occur. Inform prescriber if you experience eye pain, redness, burning, watering, dryness, double vision, puffiness around eye, vision disturbances, or other adverse eye response; worsening of condition or lack of improvement within 7-14 days. **Pregnancy/breast-feeding precautions:** Inform prescriber if you are pregnant. Consult prescriber if breast-feeding.

**Geriatric Considerations:** Assess ability to self-administer.

- **Trihexy®** *see* Trihexyphenidyl *on this page*
- **Trihexyphen®** *see* Trihexyphenidyl *on this page*

## Trihexyphenidyl (trye heks ee FEN i dil)

**U.S. Brand Names** Artane®; Trihexy®

**Synonyms** Benzhexol Hydrochloride

**Therapeutic Category** Anticholinergic Agent; Anti-Parkinson's Agent (Anticholinergic)

**Pregnancy Risk Factor** C

**Lactation** Excretion in breast milk unknown

**Use** Adjunctive treatment of Parkinson's disease; treatment of drug-induced extrapyramidal effects and acute dystonic reactions

**Mechanism of Action/Effect** Thought to act by blocking excess acetylcholine at cerebral synapses; many of its effects are due to its pharmacologic similarities with atropine

**Contraindications** Hypersensitivity to trihexyphenidyl or any component; narrow-angle glaucoma; pyloric or duodenal obstruction; stenosing peptic ulcers; bladder neck obstructions; achalasia; myasthenia gravis

**Warnings** Use with caution in hot weather or during exercise. Elderly patients require strict dosage regulation. Use with caution in patients with tachycardia, cardiac arrhythmias, hypertension, hypotension, prostatic hypertrophy or any tendency toward urinary retention, liver or kidney disorders, and obstructive disease of the GI or GU tract. May exacerbate mental symptoms when used to treat extrapyramidal reactions. When given in large doses or to susceptible patients, may cause weakness. Pregnancy factor C.

**Drug Interactions**

**Decreased Effect:** Decreased effect of levodopa.

**Increased Effect/Toxicity:** Increased toxicity with narcotic analgesics, phenothiazines, tricyclic antidepressants, quinidine, levodopa, and anticholinergics.

**Adverse Reactions**

>10%:

Dermatologic: Dry skin
Gastrointestinal: Constipation, dry throat, dry mouth
Respiratory: Dry nose
Miscellaneous: Sweating (decreased)

1% to 10%:

Dermatologic: Increased sensitivity to light
Endocrine & metabolic: Decreased flow of breast milk
Gastrointestinal: Dysphagia

<1% (Limited to important or life-threatening symptoms): Tachycardia, orthostatic hypotension, ventricular fibrillation, palpitations, coma, drowsiness, nervousness, hallucinations, increased intraocular pain; the elderly may be at increased risk for confusion and hallucinations, headache, loss of memory, fatigue, ataxia, false sense of well-being (especially with elderly or with high doses), loss of memory (elderly), hyperthermia, fever, heat stroke, toxic psychosis, unusual excitement (high doses)

**Overdose/Toxicology** Symptoms of overdose include blurred vision, urinary retention, and tachycardia. For anticholinergic overdose with severe life-threatening symptoms, physostigmine 1-2 mg S.C. or I.V. slowly, may be given to reverse these effects.

(Continued)

## Trihexyphenidyl *(Continued)*

**Pharmacodynamics/Kinetics**

**Half-life Elimination:** 3.3-4.1 hours

**Time to Peak:** Within 1-1.5 hours

**Excretion:** Urine

**Onset:** Peak effect: Within 1 hour

**Formulations**

Trihexyphenidyl hydrochloride:

Capsule, sustained release: 5 mg

Elixir: 2 mg/5 mL (480 mL)

Tablet: 2 mg, 5 mg

**Dosing**

**Adults:** Oral:

Drug-induced extrapyramidal reaction: 1 mg on first day, increase as

Parkinsonism: Initial: 1-2 mg/day, increase by 2 mg increments at intervals of 3-5 days; usual dose: 5-15 mg/day in 3-4 divided doses needed; usual range: 5-15 mg/day in 3-4 divided doses

**Elderly:** Oral: Parkinsonism: 1 mg on first day, increase by 2 mg every 3-5 days as needed until a total of 6-10 mg/day (in 3-4 divided doses) is reached. If the patient is on concomitant levodopa therapy, the daily dose is reduced to 1-2 mg 3 times/day. Avoid use if possible (see Geriatric Considerations).

**Administration**

**Oral:** Tolerated best if given in 3 daily doses and with food. High doses may be divided into 4 doses, at meal times and at bedtime. Patients may be switched to sustained-action capsules when stabilized on conventional dosage forms.

**Monitoring Laboratory Tests** Intraocular pressure monitoring and gonioscopic evaluations should be performed periodically.

**Additional Nursing Issues**

**Physical Assessment:** Assess effectiveness and interactions of other medications patient may be taking (see Contraindications and Drug Interactions). Monitor renal function, therapeutic response (eg, parkinsonian symptoms), and adverse reactions such as anticholinergic syndrome (dry mouth and mucous membranes, constipation, epigastric distress, CNS disturbances, paralytic ileus) at beginning of therapy and periodically throughout therapy (see Warnings/Precautions, Adverse Reactions, and Overdose/Toxicology). Assess knowledge/teach patient appropriate use, interventions to reduce side effects, and adverse symptoms to report. **Pregnancy risk factor C** - benefits of use should outweigh possible risks. Note breast-feeding caution.

**Patient Information/Instruction:** Take exactly as directed; with meals if GI upset occurs, before meals if dry mouth occurs, after eating if drooling or if nausea occurs. Take at the same time each day. Maintain adequate hydration (2-3 L/day of fluids unless instructed to restrict fluid intake); void before taking medication. Do not use alcohol and all prescription or OTC sedatives or CNS depressants without consulting prescriber. You may experience drowsiness, confusion, or vision changes (use caution when driving, climbing stairs, or engaging in tasks requiring alertness until response to drug is known); increased susceptibility to heat stroke, decreased perspiration (use caution in hot weather - maintain adequate fluids and reduce exercise activity); constipation (increased exercise, fluids, or dietary fruit and fiber may help); dry skin or nasal passages (consult prescriber for appropriate relief). Report unresolved constipation, chest pain or palpitations, difficulty breathing, CNS changes (hallucination, loss of memory, nervousness, etc), painful or difficult urination, increased muscle spasticity or rigidity, skin rash, or significant worsening of condition. **Pregnancy/breast-feeding precautions:** Inform prescriber if you are or intend to be pregnant. Consult prescriber if breast-feeding.

**Geriatric Considerations:** Anticholinergic agents are generally not well tolerated in the elderly and their use should be avoided when possible. Elderly patients require strict dosage regulation. In the elderly, anticholinergic agents should not be used as prophylaxis against extrapyramidal symptoms.


- ♦ **Tri-Hydroserpine®** *see* Hydralazine, Hydrochlorothiazide, and Reserpine *on page 565*
- ♦ **Tri-Immunol®** *see page 1256*
- ♦ **Tri-K®** *see* Potassium Supplements *on page 952*
- ♦ **Trikates®** *see* Potassium Supplements *on page 952*
- ♦ **Tri-Kort®** *see* Triamcinolone *on page 1171*
- ♦ **Trilafon®** *see* Perphenazine *on page 912*
- ♦ **Tri-Levlen®** *see* Oral Contraceptives *on page 859*
- ♦ **Trilisate®** *see* Choline Magnesium Trisalicylate *on page 263*
- ♦ **Trilog®** *see* Triamcinolone *on page 1171*
- ♦ **Trilone®** *see* Triamcinolone *on page 1171*
- ♦ **Trimazide®** *see* Trimethobenzamide *on this page*
- ♦ **Trimesuxol** *see* Co-trimoxazole *on page 307*
- ♦ **Trimethaphan Camsylate** *see page 1248*


## Trimethobenzamide (trye meth oh BEN za mide)

**U.S. Brand Names** Arrestin®; Pediatric Triban®; Tebamide®; T-Gen®; Ticon®; Tigan®; Triban®; Trimazide®

**Therapeutic Category** Anticholinergic Agent; Antiemetic

**Pregnancy Risk Factor** C

**Lactation** Excretion in breast milk unknown

**Use** Control of nausea and vomiting (especially for long-term antiemetic therapy); less effective than phenothiazines but may be associated with fewer side effects

**Mechanism of Action/Effect** Acts centrally to inhibit the medullary chemoreceptor trigger zone

**Contraindications** Hypersensitivity to trimethobenzamide, benzocaine, or any component; injection contraindicated in children

**Warnings** May mask emesis due to Reye's syndrome or mimic CNS effects of Reye's syndrome in patients with emesis of other etiologies. Use in patients with acute vomiting should be avoided. Pregnancy factor C.

**Drug Interactions**

**Decreased Effect:** Antagonism of oral anticoagulants may occur.

**Adverse Reactions**

>10%: Central nervous system: Drowsiness

1% to 10%:

Cardiovascular: Hypotension

Central nervous system: Dizziness, headache

Gastrointestinal: Diarrhea

Neuromuscular & skeletal: Muscle cramps

Ocular: Blurred vision

<1% (Limited to important or life-threatening symptoms): Convulsions, blood dyscrasias, hepatic impairment

**Overdose/Toxicology** Symptoms of overdose include hypotension, seizures, CNS depression, cardiac arrhythmias, disorientation, and confusion. Treatment is symptom directed and supportive.

**Pharmacodynamics/Kinetics**

**Onset:** Onset of antiemetic effect: Oral: Within 10-40 minutes; I.M.: Within 15-35 minutes

**Duration:** 3-4 hours

**Formulations**

Trimethobenzamide hydrochloride:

Capsule: 100 mg, 250 mg

Injection: 100 mg/mL (2 mL, 20 mL)

Suppository, rectal: 100 mg, 200 mg

**Dosing**

**Adults:**

Oral: 250 mg 3-4 times/day

I.M., rectal: 200 mg 3-4 times/day

**Administration**

**I.M.:** Inject deep into upper outer quadrant of gluteal muscle.

**Stability**

**Storage:** Store injection at room temperature. Protect from heat and from freezing. Use only clear solutions.

**Additional Nursing Issues**

**Physical Assessment:** Assess effectiveness and interactions of other medications (see Drug Interactions). See Warnings/Precautions and Contraindications for use cautions (eg, GI or GU obstructions). Monitor effectiveness of therapy and adverse response (see Adverse Reactions and Overdose/Toxicology). Assess knowledge/teach patient appropriate use, possible side effects and appropriate interventions, and adverse symptoms to report. **Pregnancy risk factor C** - benefits of use should outweigh possible risks. Note breast-feeding caution.

**Patient Information/Instruction:** Take as directed before meals; do not increase dose and do not discontinue without consulting prescriber. You may experience drowsiness or blurred vision (use caution when driving or engaging in tasks that require alertness until response to drug is known) or diarrhea (buttermilk or yogurt may help). Report chest pain or palpitations, persistent dizziness or blurred vision, or CNS changes (disorientation, depression, confusion). **Pregnancy/breast-feeding precautions:** Inform prescriber if you are or intend to be pregnant. Consult prescriber if breast-feeding.

**Additional Information** pH: 5

**Related Information**

Antiemetics for Chemotherapy-Induced Nausea and Vomiting *on page 1307*

## Trimethoprim (trye METH oh prim)

**U.S. Brand Names** Proloprim®; Trimpex®

**Synonyms** TMP

**Therapeutic Category** Antibiotic, Miscellaneous

**Pregnancy Risk Factor** C

**Lactation** Enters breast milk/compatible

**Use** Treatment of urinary tract infections; acute otitis media in children; acute exacerbations of chronic bronchitis in adults; in combination with other agents for treatment of toxoplasmosis, *Pneumocystis carinii*

**Mechanism of Action/Effect** Inhibits folic acid reduction to tetrahydrofolate, and thereby inhibits microbial growth

**Contraindications** Hypersensitivity to trimethoprim or any component; megaloblastic anemia due to folate deficiency

**Warnings** Use with caution in patients with impaired renal or hepatic function or with possible folate deficiency. Pregnancy factor C.

(Continued)

## Trimethoprim *(Continued)*

**Drug Interactions**

**Cytochrome P-450 Effect:** Inhibits CYP isoenzymes (isoenzyme profile unknown)

**Increased Effect/Toxicity:** Increased effect/toxicity/levels of phenytoin. Concurrent use with ACE inhibitors increases risk of hyperkalemia. Increased myelosuppression with methotrexate. May increase levels of digoxin. Concurrent use with dapsone may increase levels of dapsone and trimethoprim. Concurrent use with procainamide may increase levels of procainamide and trimethoprim.

**Adverse Reactions**

1% to 10%:

Central nervous system: Headache

Gastrointestinal: Nausea, vomiting, epigastric distress

<1% (Limited to important or life-threatening symptoms): Aseptic meningitis, exfoliative dermatitis, Stevens-Johnson syndrome, blood dyscrasias, cholestatic jaundice, increased LFTs, methemoglobinemia, rash, hyperkalemia, hypersensitivity

**Overdose/Toxicology** Symptoms of acute toxicity include nausea, vomiting, confusion, and dizziness. Chronic overdose results in bone marrow suppression. Treatment of acute overdose is supportive following GI decontamination. Use oral leucovorin 5-15 mg/day for treatment of chronic overdose.

**Pharmacodynamics/Kinetics**

**Protein Binding:** 42% to 46%

**Half-life Elimination:** 8-14 hours (prolonged in renal impairment)

**Time to Peak:** Within 1-4 hours

**Metabolism:** Liver

**Excretion:** Urine

**Formulations** Tablet: 100 mg, 200 mg

**Dosing**

**Adults:** Oral: 100 mg every 12 hours or 200 mg every 24 hours

**Elderly:** Refer to adult dosing.

**Renal Impairment:**

$Cl_{cr}$ 15-30 mL/minute: Administer 100 mg every 18 hours or 50 mg every 12 hours.

$Cl_{cr}$ <15 mL/minute: Administer 100 mg every 24 hours or avoid use.

Moderately dialyzable (20% to 50%)

**Administration**

**Oral:** Take with milk or food.

**Monitoring Laboratory Tests** Periodic CBC during long-term therapy

**Additional Nursing Issues**

**Physical Assessment:** See Warnings/Precautions and Contraindications for use cautions. Monitor effectiveness of therapy, frequent laboratory tests (see above), and adverse response (see Adverse Reactions). Assess knowledge/teach patient appropriate use, possible side effects and interventions, and adverse symptoms to report. **Pregnancy risk factor C** - benefits of use should outweigh possible risks.

**Patient Information/Instruction:** Take per recommended schedule. Complete full course of therapy; do not skip doses. Do not chew or crush tablets; swallow whole with milk or food. Maintain adequate hydration (2-3 L/day of fluids unless instructed to restrict fluid intake). You may experience nausea, vomiting, or GI upset (small frequent meals, frequent mouth care, sucking lozenges, or chewing gum may help). Report skin rash, redness, or irritation; feelings of acute fatigue or weakness; unusual bleeding or bruising; or other persistent adverse effects. **Pregnancy precautions:** Inform prescriber if you are or intend to be pregnant.

**Dietary Issues:** May cause folic acid deficiency, supplements may be needed.

**Geriatric Considerations:** Trimethoprim is often used in combination with sulfamethoxazole; it can be used alone in patients who are allergic to sulfonamides; adjust dose for renal function (see Pharmacokinetics and Usual Dosage).


- **Trimethoprim and Polymyxin B** *see page 1282*
- **Trimethoprim and Sulfamethoxazole** *see* Co-trimoxazole *on page 307*
- **Trimethylpsoralen** *see* Trioxsalen *on page 1185*
- **Trimetoger** *see* Co-trimoxazole *on page 307*
- **Trimetox** *see* Co-trimoxazole *on page 307*


## Trimetrexate Glucuronate (tri me TREKS ate gloo KYOOR oh nate)

**U.S. Brand Names** Neutrexin® Injection

**Therapeutic Category** Antineoplastic Agent, Miscellaneous

**Pregnancy Risk Factor** D

**Lactation** Enters breast milk/contraindicated

**Use** Alternative therapy for the treatment of moderate-to-severe *Pneumocystis carinii* pneumonia (PCP) in immunocompromised patients, including patients with acquired immunodeficiency syndrome (AIDS), who are intolerant of, or are refractory to, co-trimoxazole therapy or for whom co-trimoxazole and pentamidine are contraindicated (concurrent folinic acid [leucovorin] must always be administered); not as effective as co-trimoxazole, however, much fewer treatment-limiting adverse effects

**Mechanism of Action/Effect** Exerts an antimicrobial effect through potent inhibition of the enzyme dihydrofolate reductase (DHFR)

**Contraindications** Hypersensitivity to trimetrexate or methotrexate; severe existing myelosuppression; pregnancy

**Warnings** The U.S. Food and Drug Administration (FDA) currently recommends that procedures for proper handling and disposal of antineoplastic agents be considered.

Preparation of trimetrexate should be performed in a Class II laminar flow biologic safety cabinet. Personnel should be wearing surgical gloves and a closed front surgical gown with knit cuffs. Appropriate safety equipment is recommended for preparation, administration, and disposal of antineoplastics. If trimetrexate contacts the skin, immediately wash with soap and water. **Must be administered with concurrent leucovorin to avoid potentially serious or life-threatening toxicities.** Leucovorin therapy must extend for 72 hours past the last dose of trimetrexate. Use with caution in patients with mild myelosuppression, severe hepatic or renal dysfunction, hypoproteinemia, hypoalbuminemia, or previous extensive myelosuppressive therapies.

**Drug Interactions**

**Cytochrome P-450 Effect:** Metabolized by CYP (isoenzyme unknown)

**Decreased Effect:** Trimetrexate is metabolized by cytochrome P-450 enzymes in the liver. Examples of drugs where this interaction may occur are erythromycin, rifampin, rifabutin, ketoconazole, and fluconazole.

**Increased Effect/Toxicity:** Cimetidine, clotrimazole, ketoconazole, and acetaminophen have been shown to decrease clearance of trimetrexate resulting in increased serum levels.

**Adverse Reactions**

>10%: Hematologic: Neutropenia

1% to 10%:

Central nervous system: Seizures, fever, confusion

Dermatologic: Rash

Gastrointestinal: Stomatitis, nausea, vomiting, stomach pain

Hematologic: Thrombocytopenia, anemia

Neuromuscular & skeletal: Peripheral neuropathy

Miscellaneous: Flu-like illness, hypersensitivity reactions

**Pharmacodynamics/Kinetics**

**Half-life Elimination:** 15-17 hours

**Metabolism:** Liver

**Formulations** Powder for injection: 25 mg

**Dosing**

**Adults:** I.V.: 45 mg/m$^2$ once daily for 21 days; it is necessary to reduce the dose in patients with liver dysfunction, although no specific recommendations exist

**Elderly:** Refer to adult dosing.

**Administration**

**I.V.:** Infuse over 60 minutes.

**I.V. Detail:** Reconstituted solution should be filtered (0.22 μM) prior to further dilution. Final solution should be clear, hue will range from colorless to pale yellow. Trimetrexate forms a precipitate instantly upon contact with chloride ion or leucovorin, therefore it should not be added to solutions containing sodium chloride or other anions. Trimetrexate and leucovorin solutions **must** be administered separately. Intravenous lines should be flushed with at least 10 mL of $D_5W$ between trimetrexate and leucovorin.

**Stability**

**Storage:** Intact vials should be refrigerated at 2°C to 8°C.

**Reconstitution:** Reconstituted I.V. solution is stable for 24 hours at room temperature or 7 days when refrigerated. Do not reconstitute with normal saline; precipitate will form.

**Monitoring Laboratory Tests** Absolute neutrophil counts (ANC), platelet count, renal function tests (serum creatinine, BUN), hepatic function (ALT, AST, alkaline phosphatase)

**Additional Nursing Issues**

**Physical Assessment:** Monitor laboratory results closely and notify prescriber of adverse changes. Monitor adverse reactions (see above) and patient response to therapy. See Warnings/Precautions. **Pregnancy risk factor D** - assess knowledge/teach both male and female appropriate use of barrier contraceptives during and for 1 month following therapy. Breast-feeding is contraindicated.

**Patient Information/Instruction:** This medication can only be administered I.V. Frequent blood tests will be required to assess effectiveness of therapy. Avoid aspirin, and aspirin-containing medication unless approved by prescriber. Report persistent fever, chills, joint pain, numbness or tingling of extremities, vomiting or nausea, acute abdominal pain, mouth sores, increased bruising or bleeding, blood in urine or stool, changes in sensorium (eg, confusion, hallucinations, seizures), increased difficulty breathing, or acute persistent malaise or weakness. **Pregnancy/breast-feeding precautions:** Do not get pregnant while taking this medication - both male and female should use appropriate barrier contraceptive measures. Do not give blood during this therapy or for 1 month following discontinuation of therapy. Do not breast-feed.

**Geriatric Considerations:** No specific recommendations are available for the elderly. Use with caution in patients with liver dysfunction (see Usual Dosage).

**Additional Information** Not a vesicant; methotrexate derivative.

pH: 3.5-5.5

## Trimipramine (trye MI pra meen)

**U.S. Brand Names** Surmontil®

**Therapeutic Category** Antidepressant, Tricyclic (Tertiary Amine)

**Pregnancy Risk Factor** C

**Lactation** Enters breast milk/contraindicated

**Use** Treatment of various forms of depression, often in conjunction with psychotherapy

(Continued)

## Trimipramine *(Continued)*

**Mechanism of Action/Effect** Increases the synaptic concentration of serotonin and/or norepinephrine in the central nervous system by inhibition of reuptake by the presynaptic neuronal membrane

**Contraindications** Narrow-angle glaucoma

**Warnings** Use with caution in patients with cardiovascular disease, conduction disturbances, seizure disorders, urinary retention, hyperthyroidism or those receiving thyroid replacement. Do not discontinue abruptly in patients receiving long-term high-dose therapy. Pregnancy factor C.

**Drug Interactions**

**Cytochrome P-450 Effect:** CYP2D6 enzyme substrate

**Decreased Effect:** Decreased effect of guanethidine and clonidine. Decreased effect with barbiturates, carbamazepine, and phenytoin.

**Increased Effect/Toxicity:** Increased effect/toxicity with MAO inhibitors (phenelzine, tranylcypromine), isocarboxazid (hyperpyretic crises), CNS depressants, alcohol (CNS depression), methylphenidate (increased levels), cimetidine (decreased clearance), and anticholinergics. Potential for serotonin syndrome if combined with other serotonergic drugs.

**Effects on Lab Values** ↑ glucose

**Adverse Reactions** Anticholinergic effects may be pronounced; moderate to marked sedation can occur (tolerance to these effects usually occurs)

>10%:

Central nervous system: Dizziness, drowsiness, headache

Gastrointestinal: Dry mouth, constipation, increased appetite, nausea, unpleasant taste, weight gain

Neuromuscular & skeletal: Weakness

1% to 10%:

Cardiovascular: Hypotension, postural hypotension, arrhythmias, tachycardia, sudden death

Central nervous system: Nervousness, restlessness, parkinsonian syndrome, insomnia, sedation, fatigue, anxiety, impaired cognitive function, seizures have occurred occasionally, extrapyramidal symptoms are possible

Gastrointestinal: Diarrhea, heartburn

Genitourinary: Sexual dysfunction, urinary retention

Neuromuscular & skeletal: Tremor

Ocular: Eye pain, blurred vision

Miscellaneous: Sweating (excessive)

<1% (Limited to important or life-threatening symptoms): Alopecia, testicular edema, leukopenia, eosinophilia, rarely agranulocytosis, cholestatic jaundice, increased liver enzymes, increased intraocular pressure

**Overdose/Toxicology** Symptoms of overdose include agitation, confusion, hallucinations, urinary retention, hypothermia, hypotension, tachycardia, and cardiac arrhythmias. Following initiation of essential overdose management, toxic symptoms should be treated.

Ventricular arrhythmias and EKG changes (QRS widening) often respond to systemic alkalinization (sodium bicarbonate 0.5-2 mEq/kg I.V.). Physostigmine (1-2 mg I.V. slowly for adults) may be indicated for reversing life-threatening cardiac arrhythmias. Treatment is symptomatic and supportive.

**Pharmacodynamics/Kinetics**

**Protein Binding:** 95%

**Half-life Elimination:** 20-26 hours

**Metabolism:** Liver

**Excretion:** Urine

**Onset:** Oral: Therapeutic effects require >2 weeks

**Formulations** Capsule, as maleate: 25 mg, 50 mg, 100 mg

**Dosing**

**Adults:** Oral: 50-150 mg/day as a single bedtime dose up to a maximum of 200 mg/day for outpatients and 300 mg/day for inpatients

**Elderly:** Oral: Initial: 25 mg at bedtime, increase by 25 mg/day every 3 days for inpatients and weekly for outpatients, as tolerated, to a maximum of 100 mg/day. See Geriatric Considerations.

**Additional Nursing Issues**

**Physical Assessment:** Assess other medications patient may be taking for effectiveness and interactions (see Drug Interactions). See Contraindications and Warnings/Precautions for cautious use. Has potential for psychological or physiological dependence, abuse, or tolerance. Monitor therapeutic response (ie, mental status, mood, affect, suicidal ideation), and adverse reactions at beginning of therapy and periodically with long-term use (see Adverse Reactions and Overdose/Toxicology). Taper dosage slowly when discontinuing (allow 3-4 weeks between discontinuing Surmontil® and starting another antidepressant). Assess knowledge/teach patient appropriate use, interventions to reduce side effects, and adverse symptoms to report. **Pregnancy risk factor C** - benefits of use should outweigh possible risks. Breast-feeding is contraindicated.

**Patient Information/Instruction:** Take exactly as directed (do not increase dose or frequency); may take 2-3 weeks to achieve desired results; may cause physical and/or psychological dependence. Take at bedtime. Avoid excessive alcohol, caffeine, and other prescription or OTC medications not approved by prescriber. Maintain adequate hydration (2-3 L/day of fluids unless instructed to restrict fluid intake). You may experience drowsiness, lightheadedness, dizziness, or blurred vision (use caution when driving or engaging in tasks requiring alertness until response to drug is known); nausea, altered taste, dry mouth (small frequent meals, frequent mouth care, chewing gum, or sucking lozenges may help); constipation (increased exercise, fluids, or dietary fruit and fiber may help); diarrhea (buttermilk, yogurt, or boiled milk may help); increased appetite (monitor dietary intake to avoid excess weight gain); postural hypotension (use caution when climbing stairs or changing position from lying or sitting to standing); urinary retention (void before taking medication); or sexual dysfunction (reversible). Report persistent CNS effects (eg, insomnia, restlessness, fatigue, anxiety, impaired cognitive function, seizures); muscle cramping or tremors; chest pain, palpitations, rapid heartbeat, swelling of extremities, or severe dizziness; unresolved urinary retention; vision changes or eye pain; yellowing of eyes or skin; pale stools/dark urine; or worsening of condition. **Pregnancy/breast-feeding precautions:** Inform prescriber if you are or intend to be pregnant. Do not breast-feed.

**Geriatric Considerations:** Similar to doxepin in its side effect profile. Has not been well studied in the elderly. Very anticholinergic and, therefore, not considered a drug of first choice in the elderly when selecting an antidepressant.

**Related Information**

Antidepressant Agents Comparison *on page 1368*

- **Trimox®** *see* Amoxicillin *on page 80*
- **Trimpex®** *see* Trimethoprim *on page 1181*
- **Trimzol** *see* Co-trimoxazole *on page 307*
- **Trinalin® Repetabs®** *see* Azatadine and Pseudoephedrine *on page 124*
- **TriNefrin® Extra Strength Tablet** *see page 1294*
- **Tri-Norinyl®** *see* Oral Contraceptives *on page 859*
- **Trinovum** *see* Oral Contraceptives *on page 859*
- **Triofed® Syrup** *see page 1294*
- **Triostat™ Injection** *see* Liothyronine *on page 679*
- **Triotann® Tablet** *see page 1306*

## Trioxsalen (trye OKS a len)

**U.S. Brand Names** Trisoralen®

**Synonyms** Trimethylpsoralen

**Therapeutic Category** Psoralen

**Pregnancy Risk Factor** C

**Lactation** Excretion in breast milk unknown

**Use** In conjunction with controlled exposure to ultraviolet light or sunlight for repigmentation of idiopathic vitiligo; increasing tolerance to sunlight with albinism; enhance pigmentation

**Mechanism of Action/Effect** Psoralens are thought to form covalent bonds with pyrimidine bases in DNA which inhibit the synthesis of DNA. This reaction involves excitation of the trioxsalen molecule by radiation in the long-wave ultraviolet light (UVA) resulting in transference of energy to the trioxsalen molecule producing an excited state. Binding of trioxsalen to DNA occurs only in the presence of ultraviolet light. The increase in skin pigmentation produced by trioxsalen and UVA radiation involves multiple changes in melanocytes and interaction between melanocytes and keratinocytes. In general, melanogenesis is stimulated but the size and distribution of melanocytes is unchanged.

**Contraindications** Hypersensitivity to psoralens; melanoma; history of melanoma or other diseases associated with photosensitivity; porphyria; acute lupus erythematosus; patients <12 years of age

**Warnings** Serious burns from UVA or sunlight can occur if dosage or exposure schedules are exceeded. Patients must wear protective eyewear to prevent cataracts. Use with caution in patients with severe hepatic or cardiovascular disease. Pregnancy factor C.

**Adverse Reactions**

>10%:

Dermatologic: Itching

Gastrointestinal: Nausea

1% to 10%:

Central nervous system: Dizziness, headache, mental depression, insomnia, nervousness

Dermatologic: Severe burns from excessive sunlight or ultraviolet exposure

Gastrointestinal: Gastric discomfort

**Pharmacodynamics/Kinetics**

**Half-life Elimination:** ~2 hours

**Onset:** Peak photosensitivity: 2 hours

**Duration:** Skin sensitivity to light remains for 8-12 hours

**Formulations** Tablet: 5 mg

**Dosing**

**Adults:** Oral: 10 mg/day as a single dose, 2-4 hours before controlled exposure to UVA (for 15-35 minutes) or sunlight. Do not continue for longer than 14 days.

**Elderly:** Refer to adult dosing.

**Administration**

**Oral:** To minimize gastric discomfort, tablets may be taken with milk or after a meal.

**Additional Nursing Issues**

**Physical Assessment:** See Warnings/Precautions - administered in conjunction with ultraviolet light of ultraviolet radiation therapy. Monitor knowledge/teach appropriate

(Continued)

## Trioxsalen *(Continued)*

safety measures and sunlight precautions. **Pregnancy risk factor C** - benefits of use should outweigh possible risks. Note breast-feeding caution.

**Patient Information/Instruction:** This medication is used in conjunction with specific ultraviolet treatment. Follow prescriber's directions exactly for oral medication which can be taken with food or milk to reduce nausea. Avoid use of any other skin treatments unless approved by prescriber. You must wear protective eyewear during treatments. Control exposure to direct sunlight as per prescriber's instructions. If sunlight cannot be avoided, use sunblock (consult prescriber for specific SPF level), wear protective clothing, and wraparound protective eyewear. Consult prescriber immediately if burning, blistering, or skin irritation occur. **Pregnancy/breast-feeding precautions:** Inform prescriber if you are or intend to be pregnant. Consult prescriber if breast-feeding.

♦ **Tripedia®** *see page 1256*

## Tripelennamine (tri pel EN a meen)

**U.S. Brand Names** PBZ®; PBZ-SR®

**Therapeutic Category** Antihistamine

**Pregnancy Risk Factor** B

**Lactation** Excretion in breast milk unknown/contraindicated

**Use** Perennial and seasonal allergic rhinitis and other allergic symptoms including urticaria

**Mechanism of Action/Effect** Competes with histamine for $H_1$-receptor sites on effector cells in the GI tract, blood vessels, and respiratory tract

**Contraindications** Hypersensitivity to tripelennamine or any component

**Warnings** Use with caution in patients with narrow-angle glaucoma, bladder neck obstruction, symptomatic prostate hypertrophy, asthmatic attacks, and stenosing peptic ulcer.

**Drug Interactions**

**Increased Effect/Toxicity:** Increased effect/toxicity with alcohol, CNS depressants, and MAO inhibitors.

**Adverse Reactions**

>10%:

Central nervous system: Slight to moderate drowsiness

Respiratory: Thickening of bronchial secretions

1% to 10%:

Central nervous system: Headache, fatigue, nervousness, dizziness

Gastrointestinal: Appetite increase, weight gain, nausea, diarrhea, abdominal pain, dry mouth

Neuromuscular & skeletal: Arthralgia

Respiratory: Pharyngitis

<1% (Limited to important or life-threatening symptoms): Edema, palpitations, hypotension, hepatitis, bronchospasm

**Overdose/Toxicology** Symptoms of overdose include CNS stimulation or depression, flushed skin, mydriasis, ataxia, athetosis, and dry mouth. There is no specific treatment for antihistamine overdose. Clinical toxicity is due to blockade of cholinergic receptors. For anticholinergic overdose with severe life-threatening symptoms, physostigmine 1-2 mg I.V. slowly, may be given to reverse these effects.

**Pharmacodynamics/Kinetics**

**Metabolism:** Liver

**Excretion:** Urine

**Onset:** Onset of antihistaminic effect: Within 15-30 minutes

**Duration:** 4-6 hours (up to 8 hours with PBZ-SR®)

**Formulations**

Tripelennamine hydrochloride:

Tablet: 25 mg, 50 mg

Tablet, extended release: 100 mg

**Dosing**

**Adults:** Oral: 25-50 mg every 4-6 hours, extended release tablets 100 mg morning and evening up to 100 mg every 8 hours

**Elderly:** Refer to adult dosing (see Geriatric Considerations).

**Administration**

**Oral:** Swallow extended release tablets whole; do not crush or chew.

**Additional Nursing Issues**

**Physical Assessment:** Assess effectiveness and interactions of other medications (see Drug Interactions). See Warnings/Precautions for cautious use. Monitor effectiveness of therapy and adverse reactions (see Adverse Reactions) at beginning of therapy and periodically with long-term use. Assess knowledge/teach patient appropriate use, interventions to reduce side effects, and adverse symptoms to report. Breast-feeding is contraindicated.

**Patient Information/Instruction:** Take as directed; do not exceed recommended dose. Avoid use of other depressants, alcohol, or sleep-inducing medications unless approved by prescriber. You may experience drowsiness or dizziness (use caution when driving or engaging in tasks requiring alertness until response to drug is known); or dry mouth, nausea, or abdominal discomfort (frequent small meals, frequent mouth care, chewing gum, or sucking hard candy may help). Report persistent dizziness, sedation, or agitation; chest pain, rapid heartbeat, or palpitations; difficulty breathing; changes in urinary pattern; yellowing of skin or eyes; dark urine or pale stool; or lack of improvement or worsening or condition. **Breast-feeding precautions:** Do not breast-feed.

**Geriatric Considerations:** Elderly are more likely to experience dizziness, syncope, confusion, hypotension, sedation, and paradoxical excitation than younger adults. Anticholinergic effects may cause constipation, urinary retention, and confusion. However, tripelennamine has lower anticholinergic effects than most antihistamines with the exception of second generation antihistamines.

- **Triphasil®** *see* Oral Contraceptives *on page 859*
- **Tri-Phen-Chlor®** *see page 1306*
- **Triphenyl® Expectorant [OTC]** *see* Guaifenesin and Phenylpropanolamine *on page 550*
- **Triphenyl® Syrup** *see page 1294*
- **Triple Antibiotic® Topical** *see* Bacitracin, Neomycin, and Polymyxin B *on page 130*
- **Triple Sulfa** *see* Sulfabenzamide, Sulfacetamide, and Sulfathiazole *on page 1079*
- **Triple X® Liquid** *see page 1294*
- **Triposed® Syrup** *see page 1294*
- **Triposed® Tablet** *see page 1294*
- **Triprolidine and Pseudoephedrine** *see page 1294*
- **Triptil®** *see* Protriptyline *on page 990*
- **TripTone® Caplets®** *see page 1294*
- **Trisoralen®** *see* Trioxsalen *on page 1185*
- **Tri-Statin® II Topical** *see* Nystatin and Triamcinolone *on page 844*
- **Tristoject®** *see* Triamcinolone *on page 1171*
- **Trisulfa®** *see* Co-trimoxazole *on page 307*
- **Trisulfa-S®** *see* Co-trimoxazole *on page 307*
- **Tritace** *see* Ramipril *on page 1007*
- **Tri-Tannate Plus® Liquid** *see page 1294*
- **Tri-Tannate® Tablet** *see page 1306*
- **Tritan® Tablet** *see page 1306*
- **Tritec®** *see* Ranitidine Bismuth Citrate *on page 1010*
- **Tri-Vi-Flor®** *see* Vitamin, Multiple *on page 1219*
- **Trixilem** *see* Daunorubicin Hydrochloride *on page 336*
- **Trobicin®** *see* Spectinomycin *on page 1070*
- **Trocaine® [OTC]** *see* Benzocaine *on page 141*
- **Trocal®** *see page 1294*

## Troglitazone (TROE gli to zone)

**U.S. Brand Names** Rezulin®

**Therapeutic Category** Antidiabetic Agent (Thiazolidinedione)

**Pregnancy Risk Factor** B

**Lactation** Excretion in breast milk unknown/not recommended

**Use** Type II diabetes: For use in patients with Type II diabetes currently on insulin therapy whose hyperglycemia is inadequately controlled (Hb $A_{1c}$ >8.5%) despite insulin therapy of over 30 units/day given as multiple injections.

Management of Type II diabetes should include diet control. Caloric restriction, weight loss and exercise are essential for the proper treatment of the diabetic patient. This is important not only the primary treatment of Type II diabetes but in maintaining the efficacy of drug therapy. Prior to initiation of troglitazone therapy, investigate secondary causes of poor glycemic control (eg, infection or poor injection technique).

Either monotherapy or combination therapy with sulfonylureas, for patients with Type II diabetes.

**Investigational:** A study showed troglitazone may be beneficial in the productive and metabolic consequences of polycystic ovary syndrome (PCOS) (400 mg/day) and less essential hypertension with NIDDM, but more studies are needed.

**Mechanism of Action/Effect** Thiazolidinedione antidiabetic agent that lowers blood glucose by improving target cell response to insulin, without increasing pancreatic insulin secretion. It has a unique mechanism of action that is dependent on the presence of insulin for activity. Troglitazone decreases hepatic glucose output and increases insulin-dependent glucose disposal in skeletal muscle and possible liver and adipose tissue.

**Contraindications** Hypersensitivity to troglitazone or any component; evidence of active liver disease or increased transaminase levels (>1.5 times upper limit of normal). Monitor transaminase levels and check liver function at the first suggestive symptoms of hepatic disease.

**Warnings** Caution is advised during the administration of troglitazone to patients with NYHA Class III or IV cardiac status (based on toxicities observed in rodent studies).

A total of 150 adverse event reports postmarketing have been reported to the FDA including 3 deaths from liver failure linked to the use of troglitazone. Approximately 600,000 patients in the U.S. and 200,000 patients in Japan have been treated with troglitazone.

Patients on troglitazone who develop jaundice or whose laboratory results indicate liver injury should stop taking the drug. Approximately 2% of patients can expect to stop taking the drug because of elevated liver enzymes.

Because of its mechanism of action, troglitazone is active only in the presence of insulin. Therefore, do not use in type I diabetes or for the treatment of diabetic ketoacidosis.
(Continued)

## Troglitazone *(Continued)*

Patients on troglitazone who develop jaundice or whose laboratory results indicate liver injury should stop taking the drug. Approximately 2% of patients can expect to stop taking the drug because of elevated liver enzymes.

Because of its mechanism of action, troglitazone is active only in the presence of insulin. Therefore, do not use in type I diabetes or for the treatment of diabetic ketoacidosis.

Patients receiving troglitazone in combination with insulin may be at risk for hypoglycemia, and a reduction in the dose of insulin may be necessary. Hypoglycemia has not been observed during the administration of troglitazone as monotherapy and would not be expected based on the mechanism of action.

Across all clinical studies, hemoglobin declined by 3% to 4% in troglitazone-treated patients compared with 1% to 2% with placebo. White blood cell counts also declined slightly in troglitazone-treated patients compared with those treated with placebo. These changes occurred within the first 4-8 weeks of therapy. Levels stabilized and remained unchanged for ≤2 years of continuing therapy. These changes may be due to the dilutional effects of increased plasma volume and have not been associated with any significant hematologic clinical effects.

**Drug Interactions**

**Cytochrome P-450 Effect:** CYP3A3/4 enzyme substrate; CYP3A3/4 enzyme inducer; CYP2C9, 2C19, and 3A3/4 enzyme inhibitor

**Decreased Effect:**

Cholestyramine: Concomitant administration of cholestyramine with troglitazone reduces the absorption of troglitazone by 70%. **Coadministration of cholestyramine and troglitazone is not recommended.**

Oral contraceptives: Administration of troglitazone with an oral contraceptive containing ethinyl estradiol and norethindrone reduced the plasma concentrations of both by 30%. These changes could result in loss of contraception.

Terfenadine: Coadministration of troglitazone with terfenadine decreases plasma concentrations of terfenadine and its active metabolite by 50% to 70% and may reduce the effectiveness of terfenadine.

**Increased Effect/Toxicity:** Coadministration of troglitazone with glyburide may further decrease plasma glucose levels.

**Adverse Reactions**

>10%:

Central nervous system: Headache, pain

Miscellaneous: Infection

1% to 10%:

Cardiovascular: Peripheral edema

Central nervous system: Dizziness

Gastrointestinal: Nausea, diarrhea, pharyngitis

Genitourinary: Urinary tract infection

Neuromuscular & skeletal: Neck pain, weakness

Respiratory: Rhinitis

Hepatic: Increased transaminase levels

<1% (limited to important or life-threatening symptoms): Hepatotoxicity

**Pharmacodynamics/Kinetics**

**Absorption:** Food increases absorption by 30% to 85%

**Bioavailability:** Absolute

**Protein Binding:** >99%, to serum albumin

**Half-life Elimination:** 16-34 hours

**Time to Peak:** 2-3 hours

**Metabolism:** Liver

**Excretion:** Feces and urine

**Onset:** Generally requires >3 weeks

**Formulations** Tablet: 200 mg, 400 mg

**Dosing**

**Adults:** Oral (take with meals):

Continue the current insulin dose upon initiation of troglitazone therapy.

Initiate therapy at 200 mg once daily in patients on insulin therapy. For patients not responding adequately, increase the dose after 2-4 weeks. The usual dose is 400 mg/day; maximum recommended dose: 600 mg/day.

It is recommended that the insulin dose be decreased by 10% to 25% when fasting plasma glucose concentrations decrease to <120 mg/dL in patients receiving concomitant insulin and troglitazone. Individualize further adjustments based on glucose-lowering response.

As monotherapy: Initial: 400 or 600 mg once daily; increase to 600 mg/day if inadequate response to 400 mg/day after 1 month. For patients with inadequate response to 600 mg/day after 1 month, alternative therapeutic options should be pursued.

In combination with sulfonylureas: Initiate troglitazone at 200 mg once daily; continue sulfonylurea at its current dose. The dose of troglitazone can be increased by 200 mg every 2-4 weeks to a maximum of 600 mg/day.

**Elderly:** Steady-state pharmacokinetics of troglitazone and metabolites in healthy elderly subjects were comparable to those seen in young adults. Refer to adult dosing.

**Renal Impairment:** Dose adjustment is not necessary. Do not use in active liver disease or increased transaminase levels.

**Hepatic Impairment:** Use with caution in patients with hepatic disease. Do not use in active liver disease or increased transaminase levels.

**Administration**

**Oral:** Patients who are NPO may need to have their dose held to avoid hypoglycemia.

**Monitoring Laboratory Tests** Urine for glucose and ketones, fasting blood glucose, hemoglobin $A_{1c}$, fructosamine

Target range:

Fasting blood glucose: <120 mg/dL

Glycosylated hemoglobin: <7%

**Serum transaminase levels should be monitored at the start of therapy, monthly for the first 8 months of treatment, every other month for the remainder of the first year, and periodically thereafter.** Additionally, liver function tests should be performed on any patient on troglitazone who develops symptoms of liver dysfunction, such as nausea, vomiting, abdominal pain, fatigue, loss of appetite, or dark urine.

**Additional Nursing Issues**

**Physical Assessment:** Monitor laboratory results closely. Assess other medications patient may be taking (see Warnings/Precautions and Drug Interactions) Monitor response to therapy closely until response is stable. Advise women using oral contraceptives about need for alternative method of contraception. Monitor closely for signs of liver failure (eg, nausea, vomiting, fatigue, loss of appetite, yellowing of eyes or skin, dark urine or pale stool). Assess knowledge/teach risks of hypoglycemia, its symptoms, treatment, and predisposing conditions. Refer patient to a diabetic educator, if possible. Breast-feeding is not recommended.

**Patient Information/Instruction:** Take with meals. Follow directions of prescriber. If dose is missed at the usual meal, take it with next meal. Do not double dose if daily dose is missed completely. Monitor urine or serum glucose as recommended by prescriber. More frequent monitoring is required during periods of stress, trauma, surgery, pregnancy, increased activity or exercise. Avoid alcohol. Report chest pain, rapid heartbeat or palpitations, abdominal pain, fever, rash, hypoglycemia reactions, yellowing of skin or eyes, dark urine or light stool, or unusual fatigue or nausea/vomiting. **Pregnancy/breast-feeding precautions:** Use alternate means of contraception if using oral contraceptives. Breast-feeding is not recommended.

**Related Information**

Antidiabetic Oral Agents Comparison *on page 1370*


- **Tromigal** *see* Erythromycin *on page 435*
- **Trompersantin** *see* Dipyridamole *on page 383*
- **Tronolane®** *see page 1294*
- **Tronothane® HCl** *see page 1294*
- **Tropicacyl®** *see page 1248*
- **Tropicacyl®** *see page 1282*
- **Tropicamide** *see page 1248*
- **Tropicamide** *see page 1282*
- **Tropyn Z** *see* Atropine *on page 119*


## Trovafloxacin (TROE va flox a sin)

**U.S. Brand Names** Trovan™

**Synonyms** Alatrovafloxacin Mesylate; CP-99,219-27

**Therapeutic Category** Antibiotic, Quinolone

**Pregnancy Risk Factor** C

**Lactation** Enters breast milk/contraindicated

**Use Should be used only in life- or limb-threatening infections.**

Treatment of nosocomial pneumonia, community-acquired pneumonia, complicated intra-abdominal infections, gynecologic/pelvic infections, complicated skin and skin structure infections

(Continued)

## Trovafloxacin *(Continued)*

**Mechanism of Action/Effect** Inhibits DNA gyrase and topoisomerase IV in susceptible organisms; blocks relaxation of supercoiled DNA and promoted breakage of double-stranded DNA. Activity *in vitro* includes atypical, gram-negative, gram-positive (including penicillin-resistant pneumococci), intra- and extracellular aerobic organisms.

**Contraindications** Hypersensitivity to trovafloxacin, alatrofloxacin, or other fluoroquinolones or components of formulations

**Warnings** For use only in serious life- or limb-threatening infections. Initiation of therapy must occur in an inpatient healthcare facility. May alter GI flora resulting in pseudomembranous colitis due to *Clostridium difficile*. Use with caution in patients with seizure disorders or severe cerebral atherosclerosis. Discontinue if skin rash or pain, inflammation, or rupture of a tendon occurs. May cause photosensitivity. CNS stimulation may occur which may lead to tremor, restlessness, confusion, hallucinations, paranoia, depression, nightmares, insomnia, or lightheadedness. Hepatic reactions have resulted in death. Risk of hepatotoxicity is increased if therapy exceeds 14 days. Pregnancy factor C.

**Drug Interactions**

**Decreased Effect:** Coadministration with antacids containing aluminum or magnesium, citric acid/sodium citrate, sucralfate, and iron markedly reduces absorption of trovafloxacin. Separate oral administration by at least 2 hours. Coadministration of intravenous morphine also reduces absorption. Separate I.V. morphine by 2 hours (when trovafloxacin is taken in fasting state) or 4 hours (when taken with food). Do not administer multivalent cations (eg, calcium, magnesium) through the same intravenous line.

**Food Interactions** Dairy products such as milk or yogurt may reduce absorption of oral trovafloxacin - avoid concurrent use. Enteral feedings may also limit absorption.

**Adverse Reactions Note:** Fatalities have occurred in patients developing hepatic necrosis.

1% to 10% (range reported in clinical trials):

Central nervous system: Dizziness (2% to 11%), lightheadedness (<1% to 4%), headache (1% to 5%)

Hepatic: Increased LFTs

Dermatologic: Rash (<1% to 2%), pruritus (<1% to 2%)

Gastrointestinal: Nausea (4% to 8%), abdominal pain (<1% to 1%), vomiting, diarrhea

Genitourinary: Vaginitis (<1% to 1%)

Local: Injection site reaction, pain, or inflammation

<1% (Limited to important or life-threatening symptoms): Phototoxicity, convulsions, dyskinesia, pseudomembranous colitis, allergic/anaphylactoid reaction, tendonitis, bronchospasm, interstitial nephritis, anaphylaxis, hepatic necrosis, pancreatitis, Stevens-Johnson syndrome

**Pharmacodynamics/Kinetics**

**Bioavailability:** 88%

**Protein Binding:** 76%

**Distribution:** Tissue concentrations are generally greater than serum concentrations

**Half-life Elimination:** 9.1-12.7 hours

**Time to Peak:** After oral dosing, within 2 hours

**Metabolism:** Hepatic conjugation (minimal involvement of cytochrome P-450)

**Excretion:** Feces and urine

**Formulations** See also Trovafloxacin/Azithromycin Compliance Pack.

Injection, as mesylate (alatrofloxacin): 5 mg/mL (40 mL, 60 mL)

Tablet, as mesylate (trovafloxacin): 100 mg, 200 mg

**Dosing**

**Adults & Elderly:**

Nosocomial pneumonia: I.V.: 300 mg single dose followed by 200 mg/day orally for a total duration of 10-14 days

Community-acquired pneumonia: Oral, I.V.: 200 mg/day for 7-14 days

Complicated intra-abdominal infections, including postsurgical infections/gynecologic and pelvic infections: I.V.: 300 mg as a single dose followed by 200 mg/day orally for a total duration of 7-14 days

Skin and skin structure infections, complicated, including diabetic foot infections: Oral, I.V.: 200 mg/day for 10-14 days

**Renal Impairment:** No adjustment is necessary. Trovafloxacin is not sufficiently removed by hemodialysis.

**Hepatic Impairment:**

Mild to moderate cirrhosis:

Initial dose for normal hepatic function: 300 mg I.V.; 200 mg I.V. or oral; 100 mg oral

Reduced dose: 200 mg I.V.; 100 mg I.V. or oral; 100 mg oral

Severe cirrhosis: No data available

**Administration**

**Oral:** Take without regard to meals.

**I.V.:** Not for I.M. or S.C. Administer over 60 minutes.

**Stability**

**Storage:** Store undiluted vials of solution at 15°C to 30°C (50°F to 86°F).

**Reconstitution:** Diluted solutions are stable for up to 7 days when refrigerated and up to 3 days at room temperature.

**Compatibility:** Dilute to a concentration of 0.5-2 mg/mL in dextrose 5% in water, 0.45% sodium chloride, dextrose 5% in water and 0.45% sodium chloride, dextrose 5% in water and 0.2% sodium chloride, or lactated Ringer's in dextrose 5% in water. Should not be diluted with 0.9% sodium chloride or lactated Ringer's.

**Monitoring Laboratory Tests** Perform culture and sensitivity testing prior to initiating therapy. Monitor CBC, liver function tests if therapy is longer than 21 days.

**Additional Nursing Issues**

**Physical Assessment:** Assess allergy history before initiating therapy. Assess effectiveness and interactions of other medications (see Drug Interactions). See Warnings/Precautions and Contraindications for use cautions. Monitor effectiveness of therapy, laboratory tests, and adverse response (see Adverse Reactions and Overdose/Toxicology). Assess knowledge/teach patient appropriate use, possible side effects and appropriate interventions, and adverse symptoms to report. **Pregnancy risk factor C** - benefits of use should outweigh possible risks. Breast-feeding is contraindicated.

**Patient Information/Instruction:** Take per recommended schedule; complete full course of therapy and do not skip doses. Take on an empty stomach (1 hour before or 2 hours after meals, dairy products, antacids, or other medication). Dizziness may be reduced if taken at bedtime with food. Maintain adequate hydration (2-3 L/day of fluids unless instructed to restrict fluid intake). You may experience dizziness or lightheadedness (use caution when driving or engaging in tasks that require alertness until response to drug is known); nausea or GI upset (small frequent meals, frequent mouth care, sucking lozenges, or chewing gum may help). Report CNS disturbances (hallucinations, gait disturbances); chest pain or palpitations; persistent GI disturbances; signs of opportunistic infection (sore throat, chills, fever, burning, itching on urination, vaginal discharge, white plaques in mouth); tendon pain, swelling, or redness; difficulty breathing, or worsening of condition. **Pregnancy/breast-feeding precautions:** Inform prescriber if you are or intend to be pregnant. Do not breast-feed.

## Trovafloxacin/Azithromycin Compliance Pak

(TROE va flox a sin/az ith roe MYE sin com PLY ance pak)

**U.S. Brand Names** Trovan®/Zithromax™ Compliance Pack

**Synonyms** Azithromycin/Trovafloxacin Compliance Pak

**Therapeutic Category** Antibiotic, Macrolide Combination; Antibiotic, Macrolide; Antibiotic, Quinolone

**Pregnancy Risk Factor** C

**Lactation** Enters breast milk/not recommended

**Formulations** Compliance Pak: Oral suspension (Zithromax™) 1 g and tablet (Trovan®) 100 mg

**Related Information**

Azithromycin *on page 126*

Trovafloxacin *on page 1189*

- **Trovan™** *see* Trovafloxacin *on page 1189*
- **Trovan®/Zithromax™ Compliance Pack** *see* Trovafloxacin/Azithromycin Compliance Pak *on this page*
- **Trusopt® Ophthalmic** *see* Ophthalmic Agents, Glaucoma *on page 853*
- **Tryptanol®** *see* Amitriptyline *on page 73*
- **Trysul®** *see* Sulfabenzamide, Sulfacetamide, and Sulfathiazole *on page 1079*
- **TSH** *see* Thyrotropin *on page 1131*
- **TSPA** *see* Thiotepa *on page 1125*
- **Tubasal®** *see* Aminosalicylate Sodium *on page 70*
- **Tucks® Cream/Gel/Pads** *see page 1294*
- **Tuinal®** *see* Amobarbital and Secobarbital *on page 78*
- **Tums® [OTC]** *see* Calcium Supplements *on page 185*
- **Tums® E-X Extra Strength Tablet [OTC]** *see* Calcium Supplements *on page 185*
- **Tums® Extra Strength Liquid [OTC]** *see* Calcium Supplements *on page 185*
- **Tums® Ultra® [OTC]** *see* Calcium Supplements *on page 185*
- **Tusibron® [OTC]** *see* Guaifenesin *on page 548*
- **Tusibron-DM® [OTC]** *see* Guaifenesin and Dextromethorphan *on page 549*
- **Tussafin® Expectorant** *see* Hydrocodone, Pseudoephedrine, and Guaifenesin *on page 577*

- **Tuss-Allergine® Modified T.D. Capsule** *see* Caramiphen and Phenylpropanolamine *on page 195*
- **Tussar® SF Syrup** *see* Guaifenesin, Pseudoephedrine, and Codeine *on page 552*
- **Tuss-DM® [OTC]** *see* Guaifenesin and Dextromethorphan *on page 549*
- **Tuss-Genade® Modified Capsule** *see* Caramiphen and Phenylpropanolamine *on page 195*
- **Tussigon®** *see* Hydrocodone and Homatropine *on page 572*
- **Tussionex®** *see* Hydrocodone and Chlorpheniramine *on page 571*
- **Tussi-Organidin® DM NR** *see* Guaifenesin and Dextromethorphan *on page 549*
- **Tussi-Organidin® NR** *see* Guaifenesin and Codeine *on page 549*
- **Tuss-LA®** *see* Guaifenesin and Pseudoephedrine *on page 551*
- **Tussogest® Extended Release Capsule** *see* Caramiphen and Phenylpropanolamine *on page 195*
- **Tusstat® Syrup** *see* Diphenhydramine *on page 381*
- **Twice-A-Day® Nasal** *see page 1294*
- **Twilite® Oral [OTC]** *see* Diphenhydramine *on page 381*
- **Twin-K®** *see* Potassium Supplements *on page 952*
- **Two-Dyne®** *see* Butalbital Compound and Acetaminophen *on page 175*
- **Tylenol® [OTC]** *see* Acetaminophen *on page 32*
- **Tylenol® Cold Effervescent Medication Tablet** *see page 1294*
- **Tylenol® Cold No Drowsiness** *see page 1294*
- **Tylenol® Flu Maximum Strength** *see page 1294*
- **Tylenol® Sinus Maximum Strength** *see page 1294*
- **Tylenol® With Codeine** *see* Acetaminophen and Codeine *on page 34*
- **Tylex 750** *see* Acetaminophen *on page 32*
- **Tylex CD** *see* Acetaminophen and Codeine *on page 34*
- **Tylox®** *see* Oxycodone and Acetaminophen *on page 873*
- **Tympangesic®** *see page 1291*
- **Typhoid Vaccine** *see page 1256*
- **Tyramine Foods List** *see page 1422*
- **Tyzine® Nasal** *see page 1294*
- **U-90152S** *see* Delavirdine *on page 340*
- **UAD Otic®** *see page 1291*
- **UAD® Topical** *see* Clioquinol and Hydrocortisone *on page 284*
- **UCB-P071** *see* Cetirizine *on page 242*
- **U-Cort™** *see* Hydrocortisone *on page 578*
- **U-Cort™** *see* Topical Corticosteroids *on page 1152*
- **UK** *see* Urokinase *on page 1195*
- **Ukidan®** *see* Urokinase *on page 1195*
- **Ulcedine** *see* Cimetidine *on page 268*
- **Ulcerease®** *see page 1294*
- **ULR®** *see* Guaifenesin, Phenylpropanolamine, and Phenylephrine *on page 552*
- **ULR-LA®** *see* Guaifenesin and Phenylpropanolamine *on page 550*
- **Ulsen** *see* Omeprazole *on page 851*
- **Ultracef®** *see* Cefadroxil *on page 211*
- **Ultram®** *see* Tramadol *on page 1161*
- **Ultra Mide® Topical** *see* Urea *on next page*
- **Ultraquin™** *see* Hydroquinone *on page 583*
- **Ultrase® MT12** *see* Pancrelipase *on page 882*
- **Ultrase® MT20** *see* Pancrelipase *on page 882*
- **Ultra Tears® Solution** *see page 1294*
- **Ultravate™ Topical** *see* Topical Corticosteroids *on page 1152*
- **Unamol** *see* Cisapride *on page 272*
- **Unasyn®** *see* Ampicillin and Sulbactam *on page 92*
- **Unasyna** *see* Ampicillin and Sulbactam *on page 92*
- **Unasyna Oral** *see* Ampicillin and Sulbactam *on page 92*
- **Undecylenic Acid and Derivatives** *see page 1247*
- **Undoguent® Topical** *see page 1247*
- **Unguentine® [OTC]** *see* Benzocaine *on page 141*
- **Uni-Bent® Cough Syrup** *see* Diphenhydramine *on page 381*
- **Unicap® [OTC]** *see* Vitamin, Multiple *on page 1219*
- **Uni-Decon®** *see page 1306*
- **Uni-Dur®** *see* Theophylline *on page 1115*
- **Unilax® Capsule** *see page 1294*
- **Unipen® Injection** *see* Nafcillin *on page 800*
- **Unipen® Oral** *see* Nafcillin *on page 800*
- **Uniphyl®** *see* Theophylline *on page 1115*
- **Uni-Pro® [OTC]** *see* Ibuprofen *on page 592*
- **Uniretic™** *see* Moexipril and Hydrochlorothiazide *on page 785*
- **Unitrol® [OTC]** *see* Phenylpropanolamine *on page 922*
- **Uni-Tussin® [OTC]** *see* Guaifenesin *on page 548*
- **Uni-Tussin® DM [OTC]** *see* Guaifenesin and Dextromethorphan *on page 549*

- **Univasc®** *see* Moexipril *on page 783*
- **Unizuric 300** *see* Allopurinol *on page 53*
- **Urabeth®** *see* Bethanechol *on page 151*

## Uracil Mustard (YOOR a sil MUS tard)

**Therapeutic Category** Antineoplastic Agent, Alkylating Agent

**Pregnancy Risk Factor** X

**Lactation** Enters breast milk/contraindicated

**Use** Palliative treatment in symptomatic chronic lymphocytic leukemia; non-Hodgkin's lymphomas, chronic myelocytic leukemia, mycosis fungoides, thrombocytosis, polycythemia vera, ovarian carcinoma

**Mechanism of Action/Effect** Polyfunctional alkylating agent. The basic reaction of uracil mustard, like that of any alkylating agent, is the replacement of the hydrogen in a reacting chemical with an alkyl group; cell cycle-phase nonspecific antineoplastic agent; exact site of drug action within the cell is not known, but the nucleoproteins of the cell nucleus are believed to be involved.

**Contraindications** Hypersensitivity to uracil mustard or any component; severe leukopenia; thrombocytopenia; aplastic anemia; patients whose bone marrow is infiltrated with malignant cells; pregnancy

**Warnings** The U.S. Food and Drug Administration (FDA) currently recommends that procedures for proper handling and disposal of antineoplastic agents be considered.

Use caution in patients with impaired kidney or liver function. The drug should be discontinued if intractable vomiting or diarrhea, precipitous falls in leukocyte or platelet count, or myocardial ischemia occurs. Use with caution in patients who have had high-dose pelvic radiation or previous use of alkylating agents. Patient should be hospitalized during initial course of therapy. May impair fertility in men and women. Use with caution in patients with pre-existing marrow depression.

**Adverse Reactions**

>10%:

Gastrointestinal: Nausea, vomiting, diarrhea

Hematologic: Myelosuppressive; leukopenia and thrombocytopenia nadir: 2-4 weeks, anemia

1% to 10%:

Central nervous system: Mental depression, nervousness

Dermatologic: Hyperpigmentation, alopecia

Endocrine & metabolic: Hyperuricemia

<1% (Limited to important or life-threatening symptoms): Hepatotoxicity

**Overdose/Toxicology** Symptoms of overdose include diarrhea, vomiting, and severe bone marrow suppression. No specific antidote to marrow toxicity is available.

**Pharmacodynamics/Kinetics**

**Excretion:** Urine

**Formulations** Capsule: 1 mg

**Dosing**

**Adults:** Oral (do not administer until 2-3 weeks after maximum effect of any previous x-ray or cytotoxic drug therapy of the bone marrow is obtained): 0.15 mg/kg in a single weekly dose for 4 weeks

Thrombocytosis: 1-2 mg/day for 14 days

**Monitoring Laboratory Tests** CBC

**Additional Nursing Issues**

**Physical Assessment:** Monitor laboratory tests, adverse reactions and patient response to therapy. Monitor closely for opportunistic infection. Assess knowledge/teach patient side effect precautions and adverse effects to report. **Pregnancy risk factor X** - determine that patient is not pregnant before beginning treatment and do not give to women of childbearing age or to males who may have intercourse with women of childbearing age unless both male and female are capable of complying with barrier contraceptive measures during therapy and for 1 month following therapy. Breast-feeding is contraindicated.

**Patient Information/Instruction:** This drug may take weeks or months for effectiveness to become apparent. Do not discontinue without consulting prescriber. Maintain adequate hydration (2-3 L/day of fluids unless instructed to restrict fluid intake). For nausea or vomiting, loss of appetite, or dry mouth, small frequent meals, chewing gum, or sucking lozenges may help. You may experience hair loss (reversible); diarrhea (if persistent, consult prescriber); nervousness, irritability, shakiness, amenorrhea, altered sperm production (usually reversible). Report persistent nausea or vomiting, fever, sore throat, chills, unusual bleeding or bruising, consistent feelings of tiredness or weakness, or yellowing of skin or eyes. **Pregnancy/breast-feeding precautions:** Inform prescriber if you are pregnant. Do not get pregnant during or for 1 month following therapy. Male: Do not cause a female to become pregnant. Male/female: Consult prescriber for instruction on appropriate barrier contraceptive measures. This drug may cause severe fetal defects. Do not breast-feed.

- **Urasal®** *see* Methenamine *on page 739*

## Urea (yoor EE a)

**U.S. Brand Names** Amino-Cerv™ Vaginal Cream; Aquacare® Topical [OTC]; Carmol® Topical [OTC]; Gormel® Creme [OTC]; Lanaphilic® Topical [OTC]; Nutraplus® Topical [OTC]; Rea-Lo® [OTC]; Ultra Mide® Topical; Ureacin®-20 Topical [OTC]; Ureaphil® Injection

**Synonyms** Carbamide

(Continued)

## Urea *(Continued)*

**Therapeutic Category** Diuretic, Osmotic; Keratolytic Agent; Topical Skin Product

**Pregnancy Risk Factor** C

**Lactation** Excretion in breast milk unknown

**Use** Reduces intracranial pressure and intraocular pressure; topically promotes hydration and removal of excess keratin in hyperkeratotic conditions and dry skin; mild cervicitis

**Mechanism of Action/Effect** Elevates plasma osmolality by inhibiting tubular reabsorption of water, thus enhancing the flow of water into extracellular fluid

**Contraindications** Severely impaired renal function, hepatic failure; active intracranial bleeding; sickle cell anemia; topical use in viral skin disease

**Warnings** Urea should not be used near the eyes. Use with caution if applied to face, broken, or inflamed skin. Use with caution in patients with mild hepatic or renal impairment. Pregnancy factor C.

**Drug Interactions**

**Decreased Effect:** Decreased effect/toxicity/levels of lithium.

**Adverse Reactions**

>10%: Gastrointestinal: Nausea, vomiting

1% to 10%:

Central nervous system: Headache

Local: Transient stinging, local irritation, tissue necrosis from extravasation of I.V. preparation

**Overdose/Toxicology** Increased BUN and decreased renal function are seen with toxicity. Treatment is supportive.

**Pharmacodynamics/Kinetics**

**Distribution:** Crosses the placenta

**Half-life Elimination:** 1 hour

**Excretion:** Urine

**Onset:** I.V.: Maximum effects within 1-2 hours

**Duration:** I.V.: 3-6 hours (diuresis can continue for up to 10 hours)

**Formulations**

Cream:

Topical: 2% [20 mg/mL] (75 g); 10% [100 mg/mL] (75 g, 90 g, 454 g); 20% [200 mg/mL] (45 g, 75 g, 90 g, 454 g); 30% [300 mg/mL] (60 g, 454 g); 40% (30 g)

Vaginal: 8.34% [83.4 mg/g] (82.5 g)

Injection: 40 g/150 mL

Lotion: 2% (240 mL); 10% (180 mL, 240 mL, 480 mL); 15% (120 mL, 480 mL); 25% (180 mL)

**Dosing**

**Adults:**

I.V. infusion: 1-1.5 g/kg by slow infusion (1-2½ hours); maximum: 120 g/24 hours

Topical: Apply 1-3 times/day.

Vaginal: Insert 1 applicatorful in vagina at bedtime for 2-4 weeks.

**Elderly:** Refer to adult dosing.

**Administration**

**Oral:** Injection dosage form may be used orally. Mix with carbonated beverages, jelly or jam, to mask unpleasant flavor.

**I.V.:** Do not infuse into leg veins.

**Additional Nursing Issues**

**Physical Assessment:**

I.V.: Monitor infusion site for extravasation (may cause tissue necrosis). Assess for effectiveness of therapy and adverse reactions.

Topical/vaginal: Assess knowledge/teach appropriate administration, possible side effects, symptoms to report.

**Pregnancy risk factor C.** Note breast-feeding caution.

**Patient Information/Instruction:**

Topical: For external use only. Best effect is obtained when applied to skin while still wet or moist after washing or bathing. Do not apply to broken, inflamed, or infected skin. Do not use near eyes. Report skin redness, irritation, or worsening of condition. **Breast-feeding precautions:** Consult prescriber if breast-feeding.

Vaginal: Wash hands before using. Insert full applicator into vagina gently and expel cream at bedtime. Wash applicator with soap and water following use. Remain lying down for 30 minutes following administration. Report if condition worsens or does not improve.

- **Urea and Hydrocortisone** *see page 1306*
- **Ureacin®-20 Topical [OTC]** *see* Urea *on previous page*
- **Ureaphil® Injection** *see* Urea *on previous page*
- **Urecholine®** *see* Bethanechol *on page 151*
- **Uremol™** *see* Urea *on previous page*
- **Urex®** *see* Methenamine *on page 739*
- **Uridon®** *see* Chlorthalidone *on page 260*
- **Urisec®** *see* Urea *on previous page*
- **Urispas®** *see* Flavoxate *on page 486*
- **Uri-Tet® Oral** *see* Oxytetracycline *on page 876*
- **Uritol®** *see* Furosemide *on page 523*
- **Urobak®** *see* Sulfamethoxazole *on page 1082*

♦ **Urocit®-K** *see* Potassium Citrate *on page 949*

♦ **Urodine®** *see* Phenazopyridine *on page 914*

## Urofollitropin (yoor oh fol li TROE pin)

**U.S. Brand Names** Metrodin® Injection

**Therapeutic Category** Ovulation Stimulator

**Pregnancy Risk Factor** X

**Lactation** Excretion in breast milk unknown/contraindicated

**Use** Induction of ovulation in patients with polycystic ovarian disease and to stimulate the development of multiple oocytes

**Mechanism of Action/Effect** Preparation of follicle-stimulating hormone 75 units with <1 unit of luteinizing hormone (LH) which is isolated from the urine of postmenopausal women. Follicle-stimulating hormone plays a role in the development of follicles. Elevated FSH levels early in the normal menstrual cycle are thought to play a significant role in recruiting a cohort of follicles for maturation. A single follicle is enriched with FSH receptors and becomes dominant over the rest of the recruited follicles. The increased number of FSH receptors allows it to grow despite declining FSH levels. This dominant follicle secretes low levels of estrogen and inhibin which further reduces pituitary FSH output. The ovarian stroma, under the influence of luteinizing hormone, produces androgens which the dominant follicle uses as precursors for estrogens.

**Contraindications** Hypersensitivity to urofollitropin; high levels of both LH and FSH indicating primary ovarian failure; uncontrolled thyroid or adrenal dysfunction; organic intracranial lesion such as a pituitary tumor; presence of any cause of infertility other than anovulation, unless the patient is a candidate for *in vitro* fertilization; abnormal bleeding of undetermined nature; ovarian cysts or enlargement not due to polycystic ovarian disease; pregnancy (may cause fetal harm)

**Warnings** Use lowest dose possible to avoid abnormal ovarian enlargement. If hyperstimulation occurs, discontinue use and hospitalize patient. Use with caution in patients with a history of thromboembolism.

**Adverse Reactions**

>10%:

Endocrine & metabolic: Ovarian enlargement or ovarian cysts

Local: Edema at injection site, pain at injection site

1% to 10%:

Cardiovascular: Arterial thromboembolism

Central nervous system: Fever, chills

Dermatologic: Rash or hives

Endocrine & metabolic: Breast tenderness

Gastrointestinal: Nausea, vomiting, abdominal pain, diarrhea

Miscellaneous: Hyperstimulation syndrome

**Overdose/Toxicology** Symptoms of overdose include possible hyperstimulation and multiple gestations. Supportive care to maintain fluid and electrolyte imbalance may be needed.

**Pharmacodynamics/Kinetics**

**Half-life Elimination:** 3.9 hours and 70.4 hours (FSH has two half-lives)

**Excretion:** Renal clearance: 0.75 mL/minute; Metabolic: 17.2 mL/minute

**Formulations** Injection: 0.83 mg [75 units FSH activity] (2 mL); 1.66 mg [150 units FSH activity]

**Dosing**

**Adults:** Female: S.C.: 75 units/day for 7-12 days; use with hCG may repeat course of treatment two more times.

**Administration**

**I.M.:** Reconstitute and administer immediately.

**Stability**

**Storage:** Protect from light. Refrigerate at 3°C to 25°C (37°F to 77°F).

**Additional Nursing Issues**

**Physical Assessment:** Arrange for pelvic exam prior to each treatment, frequently during each treatment period, and 1-2 weeks after treatment period. Teach patient about importance of 24-hour urine collection, self-injection (and needle disposal) procedures, and signs of ovulation. **Pregnancy risk factor X** - determine that patient is not pregnant before beginning treatment. Breast-feeding is contraindicated.

**Patient Information/Instruction:** This drug must be given according to a set schedule. Maintain a calendar of treatment days and ovulation days. Engage in intercourse daily beginning on the day prior to hCG administration until ovulation is apparent. Be aware that multiple births may result. You may experience flushing, abdominal distention, or breast tenderness. Report pain or heat in calves, fever, chills, rash, or difficulty breathing. **Pregnancy/breast-feeding precautions:** Inform prescriber if pregnant. Do not breast-feed.

♦ **Urogesic®** *see* Phenazopyridine *on page 914*

## Urokinase (yoor oh KIN ase)

**U.S. Brand Names** Abbokinase® Injection

**Synonyms** UK

**Therapeutic Category** Thrombolytic Agent

**Pregnancy Risk Factor** B

**Lactation** Excretion in breast milk unknown

**Use** Thrombolytic agent used in treatment of recent severe or massive deep vein thrombosis, pulmonary emboli, myocardial infarction, and occluded I.V. or dialysis cannulas; more expensive than streptokinase; not useful on thrombi over 1 week old

(Continued)

## Urokinase *(Continued)*

**Mechanism of Action/Effect** Promotes thrombolysis by directly activating plasminogen to plasmin, which degrades fibrin, fibrinogen, and other procoagulant plasma proteins

**Contraindications** Hypersensitivity to urokinase or any component; active internal bleeding; CVA (within 2 months); brain carcinoma; bacterial endocarditis; anticoagulant therapy; intracranial or intraspinal surgery; surgery or trauma within past 10 days

**Warnings** Use with caution in patients with severe hypertension, recent LP, patients receiving I.M. administration of medications, patients with trauma or surgery in the last 10 days.

**Drug Interactions**

**Increased Effect/Toxicity:** Increased toxicity (increased bleeding) with anticoagulants, antiplatelet drugs, aspirin, indomethacin, and dextran.

**Adverse Reactions**

>10%:

Cardiovascular: Hypotension, arrhythmias
Dermatologic: Angioneurotic edema
Hematologic: Bleeding at sites of percutaneous trauma
Ocular: Periorbital swelling
Respiratory: Bronchospasm
Miscellaneous: Anaphylaxis

<1% (Limited to important or life-threatening symptoms): Anemia, bronchospasm

**Overdose/Toxicology** Symptoms of overdose include epistaxis, bleeding gums, hematoma, spontaneous ecchymoses, and oozing at the catheter site. In the event of overdose, stop the infusion and reverse bleeding with blood products that contain clotting factors.

**Pharmacodynamics/Kinetics**

**Half-life Elimination:** 10-20 minutes

**Excretion:** Cleared by the liver with a small amount excreted in urine and bile

**Onset:** I.V.: Fibrinolysis occurs rapidly

**Duration:** 4 or more hours

**Formulations**

Powder for injection: 250,000 units (5 mL)
Powder for injection, catheter clear: 5000 units (1 mL)

**Dosing**

**Adults:**

Deep vein thrombosis: I.V.: Loading: 4400 units/kg over 10 minutes, then 4400 units/kg/hour for 12 hours

Myocardial infarction: Intracoronary: 750,000 units over 2 hours (6000 units/minute over up to 2 hours)

Occluded I.V. catheters:

5000 units (use only Abbokinase® Open Cath) in each lumen over 1-2 minutes, leave in lumen for 1-4 hours, then aspirate. May repeat with 10,000 units in each lumen if 5000 units fails to clear the catheter. **Do not infuse into the patient**. Volume to instill into catheter is equal to the volume of the catheter. Will not dissolve drug precipitate or anything other than blood products.

I.V. infusion: 200 units/kg/hour in each lumen for 12-48 hours at a rate of at least 20 mL/hour

Dialysis patient: 5000 units is administered in each lumen over 1-2 minutes; leave urokinase in lumen for 1-2 days, then aspirate.

Clot lysis (large vessel thrombi): Loading: I.V.: 4400 units/kg over 10 minutes, increase to 6000 units/kg/hour; maintenance: 4400-6000 units/kg/hour adjusted to achieve clot lysis or patency of affected vessel; doses up to 50,000 units/kg/hour have been used. **Note:** Therapy should be initiated as soon as possible after diagnosis of thrombi and continued until clot is dissolved (usually 24-72 hours).

Acute pulmonary embolism: Three treatment alternatives: 3 million unit dosage

Alternative 1: 12-hour infusion: 4400 units/kg (2000 units/lb) bolus over 10 minutes followed by 4400 units/kg/hour (2000 units/lb); begin heparin 1000 units/hour approximately 3-4 hours after completion of urokinase infusion or when PTT is <100 seconds.

Alternative 2: 2-hour infusion: 1 million unit bolus over 10 minutes followed by 2 million units over 110 minutes; begin heparin 1000 units/hour approximately 3-4 hours after completion of urokinase infusion or when PTT is <100 seconds.

Alternative 3: Bolus dose only: 15,000 units/kg over 10 minutes; begin heparin 1000 units/hour approximately 3-4 hours after completion of urokinase infusion or when PTT is <100 seconds.

**Elderly:** Refer to adult dosing.

**Administration**

**I.V.:** Use 0.22 or 0.45 micron filter during I.V. therapy. See Dosing for special instructions. Use infusion pump whenever possible.

**Stability**

**Storage:** Store in refrigerator.

**Reconstitution:** Reconstitute by gently rolling and tilting; do not shake. Contains no preservatives. Should not be reconstituted until immediately before using. Discard unused portion. Stable at room temperature for 24 hours after reconstitution.

**Monitoring Laboratory Tests** CBC, reticulocyte count, platelet count, DIC panel (fibrinogen, plasminogen, FDP, D-dimer, PT, PTT), thrombosis panel (AT-III, protein C), urinalysis, ACT

**Additional Nursing Issues**

**Physical Assessment:** Assess for bleeding. Avoid invasive procedures if possible. Apply pressure for extended period of time to control superficial bleeding. If signs of uncontrolled bleeding occur, stop infusion and notify prescriber immediately. Monitor vital signs closely during therapy. Monitor cardiac rhythm continually during coronary artery infusion. Maintain strict bedrest. Note breast-feeding caution.

**Patient Information/Instruction:** You will require frequent blood tests. Report any signs of unusual bleeding. Use electric razor and soft toothbrush. **Breast-feeding precautions:** Consult prescriber if breast-feeding.

- **Uro-KP-Neutral®** *see* Phosphate Supplements *on page 926*
- **Urolene Blue®** *see page 1248*
- **Uro-Mag®** *see* Magnesium Supplements *on page 703*
- **Urovalidin** *see* Phenazopyridine *on page 914*
- **Urozide®** *see* Hydrochlorothiazide *on page 566*
- **Ursodeoxycholic Acid** *see* Ursodiol *on this page*

## Ursodiol (ER soe dye ole)

**U.S. Brand Names** Actigall™

**Synonyms** Ursodeoxycholic Acid

**Therapeutic Category** Gallstone Dissolution Agent

**Pregnancy Risk Factor** B

**Lactation** Excretion in breast milk unknown

**Use** Gallbladder stone dissolution

**Mechanism of Action/Effect** Decreases the cholesterol content of bile and bile stones by reducing the secretion of cholesterol from the liver and the fractional reabsorption of cholesterol by the intestines

**Contraindications** Not to be used with cholesterol, radiopaque, bile pigment stones, or stones >20 mm in diameter; allergy to bile acids

**Warnings** Gallbladder stone dissolution may take several months of therapy. Complete dissolution may not occur and recurrence of stones within 5 years has been observed in 50% of patients. Use with caution in patients with a nonvisualizing gallbladder and those with chronic liver disease.

**Drug Interactions**

**Decreased Effect:** Decreased effect with aluminum-containing antacids, cholestyramine, colestipol, clofibrate, and oral contraceptives (estrogens).

**Adverse Reactions**

1% to 10%: Gastrointestinal: Diarrhea

<1% (Limited to important or life-threatening symptoms): Nausea, vomiting, heartburn, metallic taste, abdominal pain, biliary pain, constipation

**Overdose/Toxicology** Symptoms of overdose include diarrhea. No specific therapy for diarrhea or overdose.

**Pharmacodynamics/Kinetics**

**Half-life Elimination:** 100 hours

**Metabolism:** Undergoes extensive enterohepatic recycling. Following hepatic conjugation and biliary secretion, the drug is hydrolyzed to active ursodiol, where it is recycled or transformed to lithocholic acid by colonic microbial flora.

**Excretion:** Feces

**Formulations** Capsule: 300 mg

**Dosing**

**Adults:** Oral: 8-10 mg/kg/day in 2-3 divided doses; use beyond 24 months is not established. Obtain ultrasound images at 6-month intervals for the first year of therapy; 30% of patients have stone recurrence after dissolution.

**Elderly:** Refer to adult dosing; start at lowest dose.

**Administration**

**Oral:** Do not administer with aluminum-based antacids. If aluminum based antacids are needed, administer 2 hours after ursodiol.

**Monitoring Laboratory Tests** ALT, AST, sonogram

**Additional Nursing Issues**

**Physical Assessment:** Monitor bowel function. Can cause diarrhea. Note breast-feeding caution.

**Patient Information/Instruction:** Frequent blood work will be necessary to follow drug effects. Drug will need to be taken for 1-3 months after stone is dissolved. Stones may recur. Report any persistent nausea, vomiting, abdominal pain, or yellowing of skin or eyes. **Breast-feeding precautions:** Consult prescriber if breast-feeding.

**Geriatric Considerations:** No specific clinical studies in the elderly. Would recommend starting at lowest recommended dose with scheduled monitoring.

- **Ursofalk** *see* Ursodiol *on this page*
- **Utrogestan** *see* Progesterone *on page 974*
- **Uvega** *see* Lidocaine and Epinephrine *on page 677*
- **Vagilia®** *see* Sulfabenzamide, Sulfacetamide, and Sulfathiazole *on page 1079*
- **Vagistat® Vaginal** *see* Tioconazole *on page 1140*
- **Vagitrol®** *see* Sulfanilamide *on page 1084*

## Valacyclovir (val ay SYE kloe veer)

**U.S. Brand Names** Valtrex®

**Therapeutic Category** Antiviral Agent, Ophthalmic

**Pregnancy Risk Factor** B

(Continued)

## Valacyclovir *(Continued)*

**Lactation** Enters breast milk/compatible

**Use** Treatment of herpes zoster (shingles) in immunocompetent patients

**Mechanism of Action/Effect** Valacyclovir is rapidly converted to acyclovir before it exerts its antiviral activity against HSV-1, HSV-2, or VZV. It is most active against HSV-1 and least against VZV due to its varied affinity for thymidine kinase. Inhibits herpes viral DNA synthesis and replication.

**Contraindications** Hypersensitivity to valacyclovir, acyclovir, or any component

**Warnings**

Valacyclovir: Thrombotic thrombocytopenic purpura/hemolytic uremic syndrome has occurred in immunocompromised patients. Use caution and adjust the dose in elderly patients or those with renal insufficiency.

Acyclovir: Use with caution in patients with pre-existing renal disease or in those receiving other nephrotoxic drugs concurrently. Use with caution in patients with underlying neurologic abnormalities, serious hepatic or electrolyte abnormalities, or substantial hypoxia.

**Drug Interactions**

**Decreased Effect:** Cimetidine and/or probenecid has decreased the rate but not the extent of valacyclovir conversion to acyclovir leading to decreased effectiveness of valacyclovir.

**Increased Effect/Toxicity:** Valacyclovir and acyclovir have increased CNS side effects with zidovudine and probenecid.

**Adverse Reactions**

>10%: Gastrointestinal: Nausea, headache

1% to 10%:

Central nervous system: Dizziness, fatigue
Dermatologic: Pruritus
Gastrointestinal: Diarrhea, constipation, abdominal pain, anorexia
Neuromuscular & skeletal: Weakness
Ocular: Photophobia

**Overdose/Toxicology** Precipitation in renal tubules may occur. Treatment is symptomatic and includes hemodialysis, especially if compromised renal function develops.

**Pharmacodynamics/Kinetics**

**Protein Binding:** 17.9%; nonlinear relationship between dose and plasma concentrations

**Half-life Elimination:**

Normal renal function: 2.5-3.3 hours (acyclovir); ~30 minutes (valacyclovir)

End-stage renal disease: 14 hours removed partially by hemodialysis, half-life during dialysis: 4 hours; liver disease may decrease rate but not extent of conversion to acyclovir (half-life not affected)

**Metabolism:** Liver

**Excretion:** Urine

**Formulations** Caplets: 500 mg

**Dosing**

**Adults:** Oral: 1 g 3 times/day for 7 days

**Elderly:** Refer to adult dosing.

**Renal Impairment:**

$Cl_{cr}$ 30-49 mL/minute: Administer 1 g every 12 hours.
$Cl_{cr}$ 10-29 mL/minute: Administer 1 g every 24 hours.
$Cl_{cr}$ <10 mL/minute: Administer 500 mg every 24 hours.
Hemodialysis effects: 33% is removed during a 4-hour session.

**Administration**

**Oral:** If GI upset occurs, administer with meals.

**Additional Nursing Issues**

**Physical Assessment:** Monitor for signs or symptoms of adverse reactions indicated above. Observe for CNS changes. Avoid dehydration. Begin therapy at the earliest sign of zoster infection (within 48 hours of the rash).

**Patient Information/Instruction:** Begin use as soon as possible following development of signs of herpes zoster. Take with plenty of fluids. May take without regard to meals.

**Geriatric Considerations:** More convenient dosing and increased bioavailability, without increasing side effects, make valacyclovir a favorable choice compared to acyclovir. Has been shown to accelerate resolution of postherpetic pain. Adjust dose for renal impairment.

♦ **Valisone®** *see* Betamethasone *on page 148*
♦ **Valisone®** *see* Topical Corticosteroids *on page 1152*

## Valproic Acid and Derivatives (val PROE ik AS id & dah RIV ah tives)

**U.S. Brand Names** Depacon®; Depakene®; Depakote®

**Synonyms** Dipropylacetic Acid; Divalproex Sodium; DPA; 2-Propylpentanoic Acid; 2-Propylvaleric Acid

**Therapeutic Category** Anticonvulsant, Miscellaneous

**Pregnancy Risk Factor** D

**Lactation** Enters breast milk/compatible

**Use** Management of simple and complex absence seizures, mixed seizure types, myoclonic and generalized tonic-clonic (grand mal) seizures; may be effective in partial seizures and infantile spasms; prevention of migraine headaches

**Mechanism of Action/Effect** Suppression of absence seizures. Causes increased availability of gamma-aminobutyric acid (GABA), an inhibitory neurotransmitter, to brain neurons or may enhance the action of GABA or mimic its action at postsynaptic receptor sites.

**Contraindications** Hypersensitivity to valproic acid or derivatives or any component; hepatic dysfunction; pregnancy

**Warnings** Hepatic failure resulting in fatalities has occurred in patients. Monitor patients closely for appearance of malaise, weakness, facial edema, anorexia, jaundice, and vomiting. May cause severe thrombocytopenia or bleeding. Hepatotoxicity has been reported after 3 days to 6 months of therapy. Tremors may indicate overdosage. Use with caution in patients receiving other anticonvulsants or oral anticoagulants.

**Drug Interactions**

**Cytochrome P-450 Effect:** CYP2C19 enzyme substrate; CYP2C9 and 2D6 enzyme inhibitor, CYP3A3/4 enzyme inhibitor (weak)

**Decreased Effect:** Valproic acid may decrease effect of oral contraceptives, phenytoin, clonazepam, diazepam. Valproic acid effect may be decreased effect with phenobarbital, primidone, phenytoin, and carbamazepine.

**Increased Effect/Toxicity:** Valproic acid may increase effects of CNS depressants, alcohol, aspirin (bleeding), warfarin (bleeding), and MAO inhibitors. Potential for serotonin syndrome if combined with other serotonergic drugs.

**Food Interactions** Valproic acid serum concentrations may be decreased if taken with food.

**Effects on Lab Values** Valproic acid may cause abnormalities in liver function tests; false-positive result for urine ketones; accuracy of thyroid function tests

**Adverse Reactions**

1% to 10%:

Endocrine & metabolic: Change in menstrual cycle

Gastrointestinal: Abdominal cramps, anorexia, diarrhea, nausea, vomiting, weight gain

<1% (Limited to important or life-threatening symptoms): Alopecia, erythema multiforme, thrombocytopenia, prolongation of bleeding time, transient increased liver enzymes, liver failure

**Overdose/Toxicology** Symptoms of overdose include coma, deep sleep, motor restlessness, and visual hallucinations. Supportive treatment is necessary. Naloxone has been used to reverse CNS depressant effects, but may block the action of other anticonvulsants.

**Pharmacodynamics/Kinetics**

**Protein Binding:** 80% to 90%

**Half-life Elimination:** 8-17 hours

**Time to Peak:** Serum concentration: Within 1-4 hours; 3-5 hours after divalproex (enteric coated)

**Metabolism:** Liver

**Excretion:** Urine

**Formulations**

Capsule, sprinkle, as divalproex sodium (Depakote® Sprinkle®): 125 mg

Capsule, as valproic acid (Depakene®): 250 mg

Injection, as valproate sodium (Depacon®): 100 mg/mL (5 mL)

Syrup, as sodium valproate (Depakene®): 250 mg/5 mL (5 mL, 50 mL, 480 mL)

Tablet, delayed release, as divalproex sodium (Depakote®): 125 mg, 250 mg, 500 mg

**Dosing**

**Adults:**

Oral: Initial: 10-15 mg/kg/day in 1-3 divided doses; increase by 5-10 mg/kg/day at weekly intervals until therapeutic levels are achieved; maintenance: 30-60 mg/kg/day in 2-3 divided doses.

Rectal: Dilute syrup 1:1 with water for use as a retention enema; loading dose: 17-20 mg/kg one time; maintenance: 10-15 mg/kg/dose every 8 hours.

Injection: Administer by intravenous injection **only**, over 60 minutes at a rate ≤20 mg/minute. Use for longer than 14 days has not been studied.

**Elderly:** Refer to adult dosing.

**Renal Impairment:** Not dialyzable

**Hepatic Impairment:** Reduce dose.

**Administration**

**Oral:** Do not crush enteric coated drug product or capsules.

**I.V.:** Final concentration: ≤20 mg/minute over 60 minutes; use for longer than 14 days has not been studied.

**Monitoring Laboratory Tests** Liver enzymes, CBC with platelets, ammonium levels

**Additional Nursing Issues**

**Physical Assessment:** Assess effectiveness and interactions of other medications patient may be taking (see Drug Interactions). I.V.: Keep patient under observation (vital signs, NS, cardiac, respiratory status), observe safety/seizure precautions, and monitor for therapeutic response (seizure activity, force, type, duration). For outpatients, monitor therapeutic effect (seizure activity, frequency, force, type, duration) laboratory values, and adverse reactions (see Adverse Reactions) at beginning of therapy and periodically with long-term use. Taper dosage slowly when discontinuing. Assess knowledge/teach patient seizure safety precautions, appropriate use, interventions to reduce side effects, and adverse symptoms to report.

**Note:** Valproic acid will alter results of urine ketones (use serum glucose testing) and reduce effectiveness of oral contraceptives (use alternative form of contraception to prevent pregnancy). Some adverse reactions including hepatic failure and thrombocytopenia can occur 3 days to 6 months after beginning therapy.

(Continued)

## Valproic Acid and Derivatives *(Continued)*

**Pregnancy risk factor D** - assess knowledge/instruct patient on need to use appropriate contraceptive measures and the need to avoid pregnancy.

**Patient Information/Instruction:** When used to treat generalized seizures, patient instructions are determined by patient's condition and ability to understand.

Oral: Take as directed; do not alter dose or timing of medication. Do not increase dose or take more than recommended. Do not crush or chew capsule or enteric-coated pill. While using this medication, do not use alcohol and other prescription or OTC medications (especially pain medications, sedatives, antihistamines, or hypnotics) without consulting prescriber. Maintain adequate hydration (2-3 L/day of fluids unless instructed to restrict fluid intake). Diabetics should monitor serum glucose closely (valproic acid will alter results of urine ketones). Report alterations in menstrual cycle; abdominal cramps, unresolved diarrhea, vomiting, or constipation; skin rash; unusual bruising or bleeding; blood in urine, stool or vomitus; malaise; weakness; facial swelling; yellowing of skin or eyes; excessive sedation; or restlessness.

**Pregnancy precautions:** Do not get pregnant while taking this medication; use appropriate barrier contraceptive measures.

**Additional Information** Sodium content of valproate sodium syrup (5 mL): 23 mg (1 mEq)

Divalproex sodium: Depakote®

Valproate sodium: Depakene® syrup

Valproic acid: Depakene® capsule

**Related Information**

Peak and Trough Guidelines *on page 1331*

♦ **Valprosid®** *see* Valproic Acid and Derivatives *on page 1198*

## Valrubicin (val ru BYE cin)

**U.S. Brand Names** Valstar™

**Therapeutic Category** Antineoplastic Agent, Antibiotic

**Pregnancy Risk Factor** C

**Lactation** Excretion in breast milk unknown/not recommended

**Use** Intravesical therapy of BCG-refractory carcinoma *in situ* of the urinary bladder

**Mechanism of Action/Effect** Blocks function of DNA topoisomerase II; inhibits DNA synthesis, causes extensive chromosomal damage, and arrests cell development

**Contraindications** Hypersensitivity to anthracyclines, Cremophor® EL, or any component of this product; concurrent urinary tract infection or small bladder capacity (unable to tolerate a 75 mL instillation)

**Warnings** Complete response observed in only 1 of 5 patients, delay of cystectomy may lead to development of metastatic bladder cancer, which is lethal. If complete response is not observed after 3 months or disease recurs, cystectomy must be reconsidered. Do not administer if mucosal integrity of bladder has been compromised or bladder perforation is present. Following TURP, status of bladder mucosa should be evaluated prior to initiation of therapy. Administer under the supervision of a physician experienced in the use of intravesical chemotherapy. Aseptic technique must be used during administration. All patients of reproductive age should use an effective method of contraception during the treatment period. Irritable bladder symptoms may occur during instillation and retention. Caution in patients with severe irritable bladder symptoms. Do not clamp urinary catheter. Red-tinged urine is typical for the first 24 hours after instillation. Prolonged symptoms or discoloration should prompt contact with the physician.

Valrubicin preparation should be performed in a class II laminar flow biologic safety cabinet. Personnel should be wearing surgical gloves and a closed-front surgical gown with knit cuffs. Appropriate safety equipment is recommended for preparation, administration, and disposal of antineoplastics. If valrubicin contacts the skin, wash and flush thoroughly with water.

Pregnancy factor C.

**Drug Interactions**

**Decreased Effect:** No specific drug interactions studies have been performed. Systemic exposure to valrubicin is negligible, and interactions are unlikely.

**Increased Effect/Toxicity:** No specific drug interactions studies have been performed. Systemic exposure to valrubicin is negligible, and interactions are unlikely.

**Adverse Reactions**

>10%: Genitourinary: Frequency (61%), dysuria (56%), urgency (57%), bladder spasm (31%), hematuria (29%), bladder pain (28%), urinary incontinence (22%), cystitis (15%), urinary tract infection (15%)

1% to 10%:

Cardiovascular: Chest pain (2%), vasodilation (2%), peripheral edema (1%)

Central nervous system: Headache (4%), malaise (4%), dizziness (3%), fever (2%)

Dermatologic: Rash (3%)

Endocrine & metabolic: Hyperglycemia (1%)

Gastrointestinal: Abdominal pain (5%), nausea (5%), diarrhea (3%), vomiting (2%), flatulence (1%)

Genitourinary: Nocturia (7%), burning symptoms (5%), urinary retention (4%), urethral pain (3%), pelvic pain (1%), hematuria (microscopic) (3%)

Hematologic: Anemia (2%)

Neuromuscular & skeletal: Weakness (4%), back pain (3%), myalgia (1%)

Respiratory: Pneumonia (1%)

<1% (Limited to important or life-threatening symptoms): Tenesmus, pruritus, taste disturbance, skin irritation, decreased urine flow, urethritis

**Overdose/Toxicology** Inadvertent paravenous extravasation has not been associated with skin ulceration or necrosis. Myelosuppression is possible following inadvertent systemic administration, or following significant systemic absorption from intravesical instillation.

**Pharmacodynamics/Kinetics**

**Metabolism:** Negligible after intravesical instillation and 2 hour retention

**Excretion:** In urine, when expelled from urinary bladder

**Formulations** Injection: 200 mg/5mL

**Dosing**

**Adults:** Intravesical: 800 mg once weekly for 6 weeks

**Elderly:** Refer to adult dosing.

**Renal Impairment:** No adjustments are recommended.

**Hepatic Impairment:** No adjustments are recommended.

**Administration**

**I.V.:** Instill slowly via gravity flow through a urinary catheter (following sterile insertion). Withdraw the catheter and allow patient to retain solution for 2 hours. After 2 hours, the patient should void.

**Stability**

**Storage:** Store unopened vials under refrigeration at 2°C to 8°C (36°F to 48°F). Stable for 12 hours when diluted in 0.9% sodium chloride.

**Reconstitution:** Withdraw contents of four vials, each containing 200 mg in 5 mL (allowed to warm to room temperature without heating), and dilute with 55 mL of 0.9% sodium chloride injection, USP.

**Monitoring Laboratory Tests** Cystoscopy, biopsy, and urine cytology every 3 months for recurrence or progression

**Additional Nursing Issues**

**Physical Assessment:** This medication is administered by a physician through a urinary bladder catheter, using aseptic technique. Monitor patient response during and following instillation. Instruct patient on appropriate interventions to reduce side effects and adverse effects to report. **Pregnancy risk factor C** - benefits of use should outweigh possible risks (see Warnings). Breast-feeding is not recommended.

**Patient Information/Instruction:** This medication will be instilled into your bladder through a catheter to be retained for as long as possible. Your urine will be red tinged for the next 24 hours; report promptly if this continues for a longer period. You may experience altered urination patterns (frequency, dysuria, or incontinence), some bladder pain, pain on urination, or pelvic pain; report if these persist. Diabetics should monitor glucose levels closely (may cause hyperglycemia). It is important that you maintain adequate hydration (2-3 L/day of fluids unless instructed to restrict fluid intake). You may experience some dizziness or fatigue (use caution when driving or engaging in tasks requiring alertness until response to drug is known); or nausea, vomiting, or taste disturbance (small frequent meals, frequent mouth care, chewing gum, or sucking lozenges may help). Report chest pain or palpitations; persistent dizziness; swelling of extremities; persistent nausea, vomiting, diarrhea, or abdominal pain; muscle weakness, pain, or tremors; unusual cough or difficulty breathing; or other adverse effects related to this medication. **Pregnancy/breast-feeding precautions:** Inform prescriber if you are or intend to be pregnant. Breast-feeding is not recommended.

**Breast-feeding Issues:** It is not known whether valrubicin is secreted in human milk. Because many immunoglobulins are secreted in milk, and the potential for serious adverse reactions exists, a decision should be made whether to discontinue nursing or discontinue the drug, taking into account the importance of the drug to the mother.

## Valsartan (val SAR tan)

**U.S. Brand Names** Diovan™

**Therapeutic Category** Angiotensin II Antagonists

**Pregnancy Risk Factor** C/D (2nd and 3rd trimesters)

**Lactation** Excretion in breast milk unknown/contraindicated

**Use** Alone or in combination with other antihypertensive agents in treating essential hypertension; may have an advantage over losartan due to minimal metabolism requirements and consequent use in mild to moderate hepatic impairment

**Mechanism of Action/Effect** As a prodrug, valsartan produces direct antagonism of the angiotensin II (AT2) receptors. Valsartan blocks the vasoconstrictor and aldosterone-secreting effects of angiotensin II. It displaces angiotensin II from the AT1 receptor and produces its blood pressure lowering effects by antagonizing AT1-induced vasoconstriction, aldosterone release, catecholamine release, arginine vasopressin release, water intake, and hypertrophic responses. This action results in more efficient blockade of the cardiovascular effects of angiotensin II and fewer side effects than the ACE inhibitors.

**Contraindications** Hypersensitivity to valsartan or any component; pregnancy (2nd and 3rd trimesters); severe hepatic insufficiency; biliary cirrhosis or biliary obstruction; primary hyperaldosteronism; bilateral renal artery stenosis

**Warnings** Use extreme caution with concurrent administration of potassium-sparing diuretics or potassium supplements, in patients with mild-moderate hepatic dysfunction (adjust dose), in those who may be sodium/water depleted (eg, on high-dose diuretics), and in the elderly. Avoid use in patients with congestive heart failure, unilateral renal artery stenosis, aortic/mitral valve stenosis, coronary artery disease, or hypertrophic cardiomyopathy, if possible. Pregnancy factor C/D (2nd and 3rd trimesters).

(Continued)

## Valsartan *(Continued)*

**Drug Interactions**

**Decreased Effect:** Phenobarbital, ketoconazole, troleandromycin, sulfaphenazole

**Increased Effect/Toxicity:** Cimetidine, monoxidine

**Adverse Reactions**

1% to 10%:

Central nervous system: Headache, dizziness, drowsiness, ataxia
Endocrine & metabolic: Decreased libido
Gastrointestinal: Diarrhea, abdominal pain, nausea, abnormal taste
Genitourinary: Polyuria
Hematologic: Neutropenia
Hepatic: Elevated LFTs
Neuromuscular & skeletal: Arthralgia
Respiratory: Cough, upper respiratory infection, rhinitis, sinusitis, pharyngitis

<1% (Limited to important or life-threatening symptoms): Anemia, elevated creatinine, angioedema, hepatitis

**Overdose/Toxicology** Only mild toxicity (hypotension, bradycardia, hyperkalemia) has been reported with large overdoses (up to 5 g of captopril and 300 mg of enalapril). No fatalities have been reported. Treatment is symptomatic.

**Pharmacodynamics/Kinetics**

**Protein Binding:** 94% to 97%

**Half-life Elimination:** 9 hours

**Time to Peak:** 2 hours (maximal effect: 4-6 hours)

**Metabolism:** Liver

**Excretion:** Urine and feces

**Formulations** Capsule: 80 mg, 160 mg

**Dosing**

**Adults:** 80 mg/day; may be increased to 320 mg if needed (antihypertensive effect seen in 1-2 weeks with maximal effects observed in 4-6 weeks). See Additional Information.

**Elderly:** Refer to adult dosing and Additional Information.

**Renal Impairment:**

$Cl_{cr}$ >10 mL/minute: No dosage adjustment necessary.
Dialysis: Not significantly removed.

**Hepatic Impairment:** Mild to moderate liver disease: ≤80 mg/day

**Monitoring Laboratory Tests** Baseline and periodic electrolyte panels, renal and liver function, urinalysis

**Additional Nursing Issues**

**Physical Assessment:** Assess effectiveness and interactions of other medications (see Drug Interactions). See Warnings/Precautions and Contraindications for use cautions. Monitor effectiveness of therapy, laboratory tests, and adverse response on a regular basis during therapy (see Adverse Reactions and Overdose/Toxicology). Assess knowledge/teach patient appropriate use according to drug form and purpose of therapy, possible side effects and appropriate interventions, and adverse symptoms to report. **Pregnancy risk factor C/D** - see Pregnancy Risk Factor - assess knowledge/teach appropriate use of barrier contraceptives. Breast-feeding is contraindicated.

**Patient Information/Instruction:** Take exactly as directed; do not discontinue without consulting prescriber. Take first dose at bedtime. This drug does not eliminate need for diet or exercise regimen as recommended by prescriber. May cause dizziness, fainting, lightheadedness (use caution when driving or engaging in tasks requiring alertness until response to drug is known); mild hypotension use caution when changing position (rising from sitting or lying position) until response to therapy is established; decreased libido (will resolve). Report chest pain or palpitations; unrelenting headache; swelling of extremities, face, or tongue; muscle weakness or pain; difficulty in breathing or unusual cough; flu-like symptoms; or other persistent adverse reactions. **Pregnancy/breast-feeding precautions:** Do not get pregnant while taking this medication; use appropriate contraceptive measures. If you are, or plan to be pregnant, notify your prescriber at once. Do not breast-feed.

**Additional Information** Increasing dose beyond 80 mg/day has less antihypertensive effect than the addition of a diuretic to the 80 mg/day dose.

**Related Information**

ACE Inhibitors and Angiotensin Antagonists Comparison *on page 1362*

- **Valstar™** *see* Valrubicin *on page 1200*
- **Valtrex®** *see* Valacyclovir *on page 1197*
- **Vamate®** *see* Hydroxyzine *on page 588*
- **Vancenase® AQ Inhaler** *see* Beclomethasone *on page 135*
- **Vancenase® Nasal Inhaler** *see* Beclomethasone *on page 135*
- **Vanceril® Oral Inhaler** *see* Beclomethasone *on page 135*
- **Vancocin®** *see* Vancomycin *on this page*
- **Vancocin® CP** *see* Vancomycin *on this page*
- **Vancoled®** *see* Vancomycin *on this page*

## Vancomycin (van koe MYE sin)

**U.S. Brand Names** Lyphocin®; Vancocin®; Vancoled®

**Therapeutic Category** Antibiotic, Miscellaneous

**Pregnancy Risk Factor** C

**Lactation** Enters breast milk/use caution

**Use** Treatment of infections due to documented or suspected methicillin-resistant *S. aureus* or beta-lactam resistant coagulase negative *Staphylococcus*; serious or life-threatening infections (eg, endocarditis, meningitis) due to documented or suspected staphylococcal or streptococcal infections in patients who are allergic to penicillins and/or cephalosporins; empiric therapy of infections associated with gram-positive organisms; used orally for staphylococcal enterocolitis or for antibiotic-associated pseudomembranous colitis produced by *C. difficile* (see Additional Information)

**Mechanism of Action/Effect** Inhibits bacterial cell wall synthesis

**Contraindications** Hypersensitivity to vancomycin or any component; patients with previous severe hearing loss

**Warnings** Use with caution in patients with renal impairment or those receiving other nephrotoxic or ototoxic drugs. Dosage modification is required in patients with impaired renal function (especially elderly). Pregnancy factor C.

**Drug Interactions**

**Increased Effect/Toxicity:** Increased toxicity with other ototoxic or nephrotoxic drugs. Increased neuromuscular blockade with most neuromuscular blocking agents.

**Adverse Reactions**

**Oral:**

>10%: Gastrointestinal: Bitter taste, nausea, vomiting, stomatitis

1% to 10%:

Central nervous system: Chills, drug fever

Hematologic: Eosinophilia

<1% (Limited to important or life-threatening symptoms): Vasculitis, skin rash, thrombocytopenia, ototoxicity, renal failure, interstitial nephritis

**Parenteral:**

>10%:

Cardiovascular: Hypotension accompanied by flushing

Dermatologic: Erythematous rash on face and upper body (red neck or red man syndrome)

1% to 10%:

Central nervous system: Chills, drug fever

Hematologic: Eosinophilia

<1% (Limited to important or life-threatening symptoms): Vasculitis, ototoxicity, thrombocytopenia, renal failure

**Overdose/Toxicology** Symptoms of overdose include ototoxicity and nephrotoxicity. There is no specific therapy for overdose with vancomycin. Care is symptomatic and supportive. Peritoneal filtration and hemofiltration (not dialysis) have been shown to reduce the serum concentration of vancomycin. High flux dialysis may remove up to 25% of the drug.

**Pharmacodynamics/Kinetics**

**Protein Binding:** 10% to 50%

**Half-life Elimination:** Half-life (biphasic): Terminal: Adults: 5-11 hours, prolonged significantly with reduced renal function; End-stage renal disease: 200-250 hours

**Excretion:** Oral: Excreted primarily in the feces; I.V.: Urine

**Formulations**

Vancomycin hydrochloride:

Capsule: 125 mg, 250 mg

Powder for oral solution: 1 g, 10 g

Powder for injection: 500 mg, 1 g, 2 g, 5 g, 10 g

**Dosing**

**Adults:**

Initial dosage recommendation: I.V. (select dosage based on weight):

<60 kg: 750 mg

60-100 kg: 1 g

100-120 kg: 1.25 g

>120 kg: 1.5 g

Select interval based on estimated $Cl_{cr}$ >60 mL/minute every 12 hours, 40-60 mL/minute every 24 hours, <40 mL/minute every 24 hours; monitor levels.

**Antibiotic lock technique (for catheter infections):** 2 mg/mL in SWI/NS or $D_5W$; instill 3-5 mL into catheter port as a flush solution instead of heparin lock. (**Note:** Do not mix with any other solutions.)

Intrathecal: 20 mg/day; vancomycin is available as a powder for injection and may be diluted to 1-5 mg/mL concentration in preservative free 0.9% sodium chloride for administration into the CSF.

Oral: Pseudomembranous colitis produced by *C. difficile*: 125 mg 4 times/day

**Elderly:** See to adult dosing. Elderly may require greater dosage reduction than expected.

**Renal Impairment:** Vancomycin levels should be monitored in patients with any renal impairment.

$Cl_{cr}$ >60 mL/minute: Start with 1 g or 10-15 mg/kg/dose every 12 hours.

$Cl_{cr}$ 40-60 mL/minute: Start with 1 g or 10-15 mg/kg/dose every 24 hours.

$Cl_{cr}$ <40 mL/minute: Will need longer intervals; determine by serum concentration monitoring.

Hemodialysis: Not dialyzable (0% to 5%); generally not removed; exception minimal-moderate removal by some of the newer high-flux filters. Dose may need to be administered more frequently. Monitor serum concentrations.

Continuous ambulatory peritoneal dialysis (CAPD): Not significantly removed; administration via CAPD fluid: 15-30 mg/L (15-30 mcg/mL) of CAPD fluid.

Continuous arteriovenous hemofiltration: Dose as for $Cl_{cr}$ 10-40 mL/minute.

(Continued)

## Vancomycin *(Continued)*

**Antibiotic lock technique (for catheter infections):** 2 mg/mL in SWI/NS or $D_5W$; instill 3-5 mL into catheter port as a flush solution instead of heparin lock (**Note:** Do not mix with any other solutions).

**Hepatic Impairment:** Reduce dose by 60%.

**Administration**

**Oral:** May be administered with food. Shake well before administration.

**I.M.:** Do not administer I.M.

**I.V.:** Administer vancomycin by I.V. intermittent infusion over at least 60 minutes at a final concentration not to exceed 5 mg/mL. Administration of antihistamines just before the infusion may also prevent or minimize Red man syndrome.

**I.V. Detail:** If a maculopapular rash appears on the face, neck, trunk, and/or upper extremities (Red man syndrome), slow the infusion rate to over $1^1/_2$ to 2 hours and increase the dilution volume. Hypotension, shock, and cardiac arrest (rare) have also been reported with too rapid of infusion. Reactions are often treated with antihistamines and possibly steroids.

**Extravasation treatment:** Monitor I.V. site closely; extravasation will cause serious injury with possible necrosis and tissue sloughing. Rotate infusion site frequently.

**Stability**

**Storage:** Refrigerate oral solution.

**Reconstitution:** Vancomycin reconstituted intravenous solutions are stable for 14 days at room temperature or refrigeration. Stability of parenteral admixture at room temperature (25°C) or refrigeration temperature (4°C) is 7 days.

Standard diluent: 500 mg/150 mL $D_5W$; 750 mg/250 mL $D_5W$; 1 g/250 mL $D_5W$

Minimum volume: Maximum concentration is 5 mg/mL to minimize thrombophlebitis.

After the oral solution is reconstituted, it should be refrigerated and used within 2 weeks.

**Compatibility:** Incompatible with heparin, phenobarbital. See the Compatibility of Drugs Chart *on page 1315.*

**Monitoring Laboratory Tests** Perform culture and sensitivity studies prior to first dose. Periodic renal function, urinalysis, serum vancomycin concentrations, WBC, audiogram with prolonged use. Obtain drug levels after the third dose unless otherwise directed. Peaks are drawn 1 hour after the completion of a 1- to 2-hour infusion. Troughs are obtained just before the next dose.

**Additional Nursing Issues**

**Physical Assessment:** Assess effectiveness and interactions of other medications (see Drug Interactions). See Warnings/Precautions and Contraindications for use cautions. Monitor effectiveness of therapy, laboratory tests, and adverse response (eg, nephrotoxicity, ototoxicity - see Adverse Reactions and Overdose/Toxicology). Assess knowledge/teach patient appropriate use, possible side effects and appropriate interventions, and adverse symptoms to report.

I.V.: Monitor I.V. site closely and observe for Red man syndrome (see Administration).

**Pregnancy risk factor C** - benefits of use should outweigh possible risks. Note breast-feeding caution.

**Patient Information/Instruction:**

Oral: Take per recommended schedule. Complete full course of therapy; do not skip doses. Maintain adequate hydration (2-3 L/day of fluids unless instructed to restrict fluid intake). You may experience nausea, vomiting, or GI upset (small frequent meals, frequent mouth care, sucking lozenges, or chewing gum may help).

Oral or I.V.: Report chills or pain at infusion site, skin rash or redness, decrease in urine output, chest pain or palpitations, persistent GI disturbances, signs of opportunistic infection (sore throat, chills, fever, burning, itching on urination, vaginal discharge, white plaques in mouth), difficulty breathing, changes in hearing or fullness in ears, or worsening of condition.

**Pregnancy/breast-feeding precautions:** Inform prescriber if you are or intend to be pregnant. Consult prescriber if breast-feeding.

**Geriatric Considerations:** As a result of age-related changes in renal function and volume of distribution, accumulation and toxicity are a risk in the elderly. Careful monitoring and dosing adjustment is necessary.

**Breast-feeding Issues:** Vancomycin is excreted in breast milk but is poorly absorbed from the gastrointestinal tract. Therefore, systemic absorption would not be expected. Theoretically, vancomycin in the GI tract may affect the normal bowel flora in the infant, resulting in diarrhea.

**Additional Information** Vancomycin should **not** be used as first-line therapy to treat *C. difficile* induced diarrhea. To prevent or minimize resistance, it should be reserved for patients who do not respond to metronidazole.

pH: 2.4-4.5

**Related Information**

Peak and Trough Guidelines *on page 1331*

- **Vanex-LA®** *see* Guaifenesin and Phenylpropanolamine *on page 550*
- **Vanmicina®** *see* Vancomycin *on page 1202*
- **Vanoxide®** *see page 1294*
- **Vanoxide-HC®** *see* Benzoyl Peroxide and Hydrocortisone *on page 143*
- **Vantin®** *see* Cefpodoxime *on page 225*
- **Vapocet®** *see* Hydrocodone and Acetaminophen *on page 568*

- ♦ **Vapo-Iso®** *see* Isoproterenol *on page 632*
- ♦ **Vaponefrin®** *see* Epinephrine *on page 424*
- ♦ **Varicella Virus Vaccine** *see page 1256*
- ♦ **Varicella-Zoster Immune Globulin (Human)** *see page 1256*
- ♦ **Varivax®** *see page 1256*
- ♦ **Vascor®** *see* Bepridil *on page 146*
- ♦ **Vaseretic®** *see* Enalapril and Hydrochlorothiazide *on page 419*
- ♦ **Vaseretic® 5-12.5** *see* Enalapril and Hydrochlorothiazide *on page 419*
- ♦ **Vaseretic® 10-25** *see* Enalapril and Hydrochlorothiazide *on page 419*
- ♦ **Vasocidin®** *see page 1282*
- ♦ **Vaso Clear® [OTC]** *see page 1282*
- ♦ **VasoClear® Ophthalmic** *see page 1294*
- ♦ **Vasocon®-A [OTC]** *see page 1282*
- ♦ **Vasocon-A® Ophthalmic Solution** *see page 1294*
- ♦ **Vasocon Regular®** *see page 1282*
- ♦ **Vasocon Regular® Ophthalmic** *see page 1294*


## Vasopressin (vay soe PRES in)

**U.S. Brand Names** Pitressin® Injection

**Synonyms** Antidiuretic Hormone (ADH); 8-Arginine Vasopressin

**Therapeutic Category** Antidiuretic Hormone Analog; Hormone, Posterior Pituitary

**Pregnancy Risk Factor** B

**Lactation** Enters breast milk/compatible

**Use** Treatment of diabetes insipidus; prevention and treatment of postoperative abdominal distention; differential diagnosis of diabetes insipidus

**Unlabeled use:** Adjunct in the treatment of GI hemorrhage and esophageal varices

**Mechanism of Action/Effect** Increases cyclic adenosine monophosphate (cAMP) which increases water permeability at the renal tubule resulting in decreased urine volume and increased osmolality. Causes peristalsis by directly stimulating the smooth muscle in the GI tract.

**Contraindications** Hypersensitivity to vasopressin or any component; chronic nephritis; imminent labor

**Warnings** Use with caution in patients with seizure disorders, migraine, asthma, vascular disease, renal disease, cardiac disease, chronic nephritis with nitrogen retention, goiter with cardiac complications, arteriosclerosis. I.V. infiltration may lead to severe vasoconstriction and localized tissue necrosis, gangrene of extremities or tongue, and ischemic colitis. **Never use vasopressin if labor is imminent. May cause ruptured uterus if used in first stage labor.**

**Drug Interactions**

**Decreased Effect:** Lithium, epinephrine, demeclocycline, heparin, and alcohol block antidiuretic activity to varying degrees.

**Increased Effect/Toxicity:** Chlorpropamide, urea, clofibrate, carbamazepine, and fludrocortisone potentiate antidiuretic response.

**Adverse Reactions**

1% to 10%:

Cardiovascular: Increased blood pressure, bradycardia, arrhythmias, venous thrombosis, vasoconstriction with higher doses, chest pain

Central nervous system: Pounding in the head, fever, vertigo

Dermatologic: Urticaria, circumoral pallor

Gastrointestinal: Flatulence, abdominal cramps, nausea, vomiting

Neuromuscular & skeletal: Tremor

Miscellaneous: Sweating

<1% (Limited to important or life-threatening symptoms): Chest pain or myocardial infarction

**Overdose/Toxicology** Symptoms of overdose include drowsiness, weight gain, confusion, listlessness, and water intoxication. Water intoxication requires withdrawal of the drug. Severe intoxication may require osmotic diuresis and loop diuretics.

**Pharmacodynamics/Kinetics**

**Half-life Elimination:** Nasal: 15 minutes; Parenteral: 10-20 minutes

**Metabolism:** Liver and kidney

**Excretion:** Urine

**Onset:** Nasal: 1 hour

**Duration:** Nasal: 3-8 hours; Parenteral: I.M., S.C.: 2-8 hours

**Formulations** Injection, aqueous: 20 vasopressor units/mL (0.5 mL, 1 mL)

**Dosing**

**Adults:**

Diabetes insipidus (highly variable dosage; titrated based on serum and urine sodium and osmolality in addition to fluid balance and urine output):

I.M., S.C.: 5-10 units 2-4 times/day as needed (dosage range 5-60 units/day)

Abdominal distention: I.M.: 5 mg stat, 10 mg every 3-4 hours

GI hemorrhage:

Continuous I.V. infusion: 0.5 milliunits/kg/hour (0.0005 unit/kg/hour); double dosage as needed every 30 minutes to a maximum of 10 milliunits/kg/hour

I.V.: Initial: 0.2-0.4 unit/minute, then titrate dose as needed; if bleeding stops, continue at same dose for 12 hours, taper off over 24-48 hours.

(Continued)

## Vasopressin *(Continued)*

**Elderly:** Refer to adult dosing.

**Hepatic Impairment:** Some patients respond to much lower doses with cirrhosis.

**Administration**

**I.V.:** I.V. infusion administration requires the use of an infusion pump and should be administered in a peripheral line. Dilute aqueous in NS or $D_5W$ to 0.1-1 unit/mL.

Infusion rates:

100 units (aqueous) in 500 mL $D_5W$ rate
- 0.1 unit/minute: 30 mL/hour
- 0.2 units/minute: 60 mL/hour
- 0.3 units/minute: 90 mL/hour
- 0.4 units/minute: 120 mL/hour
- 0.5 units/minute: 150 mL/hour
- 0.6 units/minute: 180 mL/hour

**I.V. Detail:** Use extreme caution to avoid extravasation because of risk of necrosis and gangrene. Infusions are often supplemented with nitroglycerin infusions to minimize cardiac effects.

**Inhalation:** Administer on cotton plugs, nasal spray, or dropper.

**Stability**

**Storage:** Store injection at room temperature. Protect from heat and from freezing. Use only clear solutions.

**Monitoring Laboratory Tests** Serum and urine sodium, urine specific gravity, urine and serum osmolality

**Additional Nursing Issues**

**Physical Assessment:** Watch for signs of I.V. infiltration and gangrene. Monitor vital signs and blood pressure, I & O ratio, and weight. Assess for edema. Check nasal mucus membranes if used intranasally. Monitor for signs or symptoms of water intoxication, drowsiness, listlessness, headache, confusion, weight gain, seizures, and coma.

**Patient Information/Instruction:** Side effects such as abdominal cramps and nausea may be reduced by drinking a glass of water with each dose. Avoid alcohol use.

**Geriatric Considerations:** Elderly patients should be cautioned not to increase their fluid intake beyond that sufficient to satisfy their thirst in order to avoid water intoxication and hyponatremia. Under experimental conditions, the elderly have shown to have a decreased responsiveness to vasopressin with respect to its effects on water homeostasis.


- ♦ **Vasosulf®** *see page 1282*
- ♦ **Vasotec®** *see* Enalapril *on page 416*
- ♦ **Vasotec® I.V.** *see* Enalapril *on page 416*
- ♦ **Vatrix-S** *see* Metronidazole *on page 763*
- ♦ **VCR** *see* Vincristine *on page 1213*
- ♦ **V-Dec-M®** *see* Guaifenesin and Pseudoephedrine *on page 551*
- ♦ **Veetids®** *see* Penicillin V Potassium *on page 900*
- ♦ **Velban®** *see* Vinblastine *on page 1211*
- ♦ **Velosef®** *see* Cephradine *on page 239*
- ♦ **Velosulin® Human** *see* Insulin Preparations *on page 609*
- ♦ **Velsay** *see* Naproxen *on page 807*
- ♦ **Veltane®** *see page 1294*
- ♦ **Velvelan®** *see* Urea *on page 1193*


## Venlafaxine (VEN la faks een)

**U.S. Brand Names** Effexor®

**Therapeutic Category** Antidepressant, Serotonin/Norepinephrine Reuptake Inhibitor

**Pregnancy Risk Factor** C

**Lactation** Enters breast milk/contraindicated

**Use** Treatment of depression in adults, treatment of generalized anxiety disorder

**Unlabeled use:** Obsessive-compulsive disorder

**Mechanism of Action/Effect** Potentiates neurotransmitter activity in CNS. Venlafaxine and its active metabolite o-desmethylvenlafaxine (ODV) are potent inhibitors of neuronal serotonin and norepinephrine reuptake and weak inhibitors of dopamine reuptake. Causes beta-receptor down regulation and reduces adenylcyclase coupled beta-adrenergic systems in the brain.

**Contraindications** Hypersensitivity to venlafaxine or other components; do not use concomitantly with MAO inhibitors

**Warnings** Venlafaxine is associated with sustained increases in blood pressure (10-15 mm Hg SDBP). Venlafaxine may actuate mania or hypomania and seizures. Concurrent therapy with a monoamine oxidase inhibitor may result in serious or fatal reactions. At least 14 days should elapse between treatment with an MAO inhibitor and venlafaxine and at least 7 days should elapse after stopping venlafaxine and starting an MAO inhibitor. Patients with cardiovascular disorders or a recent myocardial infarction probably should only receive venlafaxine if the benefits of therapy outweigh the risks. Pregnancy factor C.

**Drug Interactions**

**Cytochrome P-450 Effect:** CYP2D6, 2E1, and 3A3/4 enzyme substrate; CYP2D6 enzyme inhibitor (weak)

**Increased Effect/Toxicity:** Increased toxicity with cimetidine, MAO inhibitors (hyperpyrexic crisis), tricyclic antidepressants, fluoxetine, paroxetine, fluvoxamine, sertraline, phenothiazine, class 1C antiarrhythmics, warfarin. Venlafaxine is a weak inhibitor of cytochrome P-450 2D6, which is responsible for metabolizing antipsychotics, antiarrhythmics, TCAs, and beta-blockers; therefore, toxic levels of these agents or interactions with these agents are possible, however, less likely than with more potent enzyme inhibitors. Potential for serotonin syndrome if combined with other serotonergic drugs.

**Effects on Lab Values** ↑ thyroid, uric acid, glucose, potassium, AST, cholesterol (S)

**Adverse Reactions**

>10%:

Central nervous system: Headache, somnolence, dizziness, insomnia, nervousness, abnormal dreams, anxiety
Endocrine & metabolic: Sexual dysfunction
Gastrointestinal: Nausea, anorexia, dry mouth, constipation, heartburn, weight loss, vomiting, diarrhea, taste perversion
Genitourinary: Abnormal ejaculation
Neuromuscular & skeletal: Weakness, neck pain, tremor
Ocular: Blurred vision, abnormal accommodation
Respiratory: Rhinitis
Miscellaneous: Increased sweating

1% to 10%:

Cardiovascular: Palpitations, hypertension, sinus tachycardia, chest pain, tachycardia
Central nervous system: Abnormal thinking, agitation, confusion, depersonalization, emotional lability, worsening depression,
Dermatologic: Skin rash
Gastrointestinal: Dysphagia
Genitourinary: Impotence, problems in urinating
Neuromuscular & skeletal: Tremor
Otic: Tinnitus
Miscellaneous: Yawning

<1% (Limited to important or life-threatening symptoms): Orthostatic hypotension, peripheral edema, seizures, dyspnea

**Overdose/Toxicology** Symptoms of overdose include somnolence and occasionally tachycardia. Most overdoses resolve with supportive treatment. Forced diuresis, dialysis, and hemoperfusion are not effective due to the large volume of distribution.

**Pharmacodynamics/Kinetics**

**Protein Binding:** Bound to human plasma 27% to 30%; steady-state achieved within 3 days of multiple dose therapy

**Half-life Elimination:** Active metabolite: 11-13 hours; Venlafaxine: 3-7 hours

**Metabolism:** Liver

**Excretion:** Urine

**Onset:** Therapeutic effects in >2 weeks

**Formulations** Tablet: 25 mg, 37.5 mg, 50 mg, 75 mg, 100 mg

**Dosing**

**Adults:** Oral: 75 mg/day, administered in 2 or 3 divided doses and taken with food. Dose may be increased in 75 mg/day increments at intervals of at least 4 days, up to 225-375 mg/day. Tapering to minimize symptoms of discontinuation is recommended when the drug is discontinued. Tapering should be over a 2-week period if the patient has received it longer than 6 weeks.

**Elderly:** When discontinuing this medication, it is imperative to taper the dose; if venlafaxine is used >6 weeks, the dose should be tapered over 2 weeks when discontinuing its use. No specific recommendations for elderly, but may be best to start lower at 25-50 mg twice daily and increase as tolerated by 25 mg/dose. Adjust dose for renal impairment (see Renal Impairment). Hold dose until a dialysis in dialysis patients.

**Renal Impairment:**

$Cl_{cr}$ 10-70 mL/minute: Decrease dose by 25%.
Hemodialysis: Decrease total daily dose by 50% given after completion of dialysis.

**Hepatic Impairment:** Reduce total dosage by 25%.

**Administration**

**Oral:** Should be administered with food.

**Additional Nursing Issues**

**Physical Assessment:** Assess other medications patient may be taking for effectiveness and interactions (see Drug Interactions). See Contraindications and Warnings/Precautions for cautious use. Has potential for psychological or physiological dependence, abuse, or tolerance. Monitor therapeutic response (ie, mental status, mood, affect, suicidal ideation), and adverse reactions at beginning of therapy and periodically with long-term use (see Adverse Reactions and Overdose/Toxicology). Taper dosage slowly when discontinuing. Assess knowledge/teach patient appropriate use, interventions to reduce side effects, and adverse symptoms to report. **Pregnancy risk factor C** - benefits of use should outweigh possible risks. Breast-feeding is contraindicated.

**Patient Information/Instruction:** Take exactly as directed (do not increase dose or frequency); may take 2-3 weeks to achieve desired results; may cause physical and/or psychological dependence. Take with food. Avoid excessive alcohol, caffeine, and other prescription or OTC medications not approved by prescriber. Maintain adequate hydration (2-3 L/day of fluids unless instructed to restrict fluid intake). You may experience excess drowsiness, lightheadedness, dizziness, or blurred vision (use caution when driving or engaging in tasks requiring alertness until response to drug is known); nausea, vomiting, anorexia, altered taste, dry mouth (small frequent meals, frequent

(Continued)

## Venlafaxine *(Continued)*

mouth care, chewing gum, or sucking lozenges may help); constipation (increased exercise, fluids, or dietary fruit and fiber may help); diarrhea (buttermilk, yogurt, or boiled milk may help); postural hypotension (use caution when climbing stairs or changing position from lying or sitting to standing); urinary retention (void before taking medication); or sexual dysfunction (reversible). Report persistent CNS effects (eg, insomnia, restlessness, fatigue, anxiety, abnormal thoughts, confusion, personality changes, impaired cognitive function); muscle cramping or tremors; chest pain, palpitations, rapid heartbeat, swelling of extremities, or severe dizziness; unresolved urinary retention; vision changes or eye pain; hearing changes or ringing in ears; skin rash or irritation; or worsening of condition. **Pregnancy/breast-feeding precautions:** Inform prescriber if you are or intend to be pregnant. Do not breast-feed.

**Geriatric Considerations:** Has not been studied exclusively in the elderly, however, its low anticholinergic activity, minimal sedation, and hypotension makes this a potentially valuable antidepressant in treating elderly with depression. No dose adjustment is necessary for age alone, additional studies are necessary; adjust dose for renal function in the elderly.

**Related Information**

Antidepressant Agents Comparison *on page 1368*

- **Venoglobulin®-I** *see* Immune Globulin, Intravenous *on page 602*
- **Venoglobulin®-S** *see* Immune Globulin, Intravenous *on page 602*
- **Ventolin®** *see* Albuterol *on page 45*
- **Ventolin® Rotocaps®** *see* Albuterol *on page 45*
- **VePesid® Injection** *see* Etoposide *on page 463*
- **VePesid® Oral** *see* Etoposide *on page 463*
- **Veracef** *see* Cephradine *on page 239*
- **Veraken** *see* Verapamil *on this page*

## Verapamil (ver AP a mil)

**U.S. Brand Names** Calan®; Calan® SR; Covera-HS®; Isoptin®; Isoptin® SR; Verelan®

**Synonyms** Iproveratril Hydrochloride

**Therapeutic Category** Antiarrhythmic Agent, Class IV; Calcium Channel Blocker

**Pregnancy Risk Factor** C

**Lactation** Enters breast milk (small amounts)/compatible

**Use** Orally used for treatment of angina pectoris (vasospastic, chronic stable, unstable) and hypertension; I.V. for supraventricular tachyarrhythmias (PSVT, atrial fibrillation, atrial flutter)

**Mechanism of Action/Effect** Inhibits calcium ion from entering the "slow channels" or select voltage-sensitive areas of vascular smooth muscle and myocardium during depolarization. Produces a relaxation of coronary vascular smooth muscle and coronary vasodilation. Increases myocardial oxygen delivery in patients with vasospastic (Prinzmetal's) angina. Slows automaticity and conduction of A-V node.

**Contraindications** Hypersensitivity to verapamil or any component; sinus bradycardia; advanced heart block; ventricular tachycardia; cardiogenic shock; atrial fibrillation or flutter associated with accessory conduction pathways; pregnancy

**Warnings** Use with caution in sick-sinus syndrome, severe left ventricular dysfunction, hepatic or renal impairment, hypertrophic cardiomyopathy (especially obstructive). Abrupt withdrawal may cause increased duration and frequency of chest pain. Use with caution in the elderly; they may experience more constipation and hypotension. Monitor EKG and blood pressure closely in patients receiving I.V. therapy particularly in patients with supraventricular tachycardia. Do not administer with oral or I.V. beta-adrenergic blocking drugs. Do not administer within 48 hours before or 24 hours after I.V. verapamil. Pregnancy factor C.

**Drug Interactions**

**Cytochrome P-450 Effect:** CYP1A2 and 3A3/4 enzyme substrate; CYP3A3/4 inhibitor

**Decreased Effect:** Rifampin or phenobarbital may decrease verapamil serum concentrations by increased hepatic metabolism. Lithium levels may be decreased.

**Increased Effect/Toxicity:** When verapamil is administered with carbamazepine, cyclosporine, digitalis, quinidine, and theophylline an increased risk of toxicity may occur. Additive hypotension may occur when used with other antihypertensive agents. Verapamil potentiates nondepolarizing muscle relaxants. Beta-blockers and verapamil may increase cardiac depressant effects on A-V conduction. $H_2$ blockers may increase bioavailability of verapamil. Use of fentanyl with verapamil may increase hypotension. Amiodarone and verapamil may increase cardiotoxicity. Aspirin and verapamil may cause bruising or prolong bleeding times beyond aspirin alone. Cimetidine and verapamil may cause increased bioavailability of verapamil. Carbamazepine and verapamil may cause increased serum carbamazepine levels. Cyclosporine and verapamil may cause increased serum cyclosporine levels. Digoxin and verapamil may cause increased digoxin levels. Doxorubicin and verapamil may cause increased doxorubicin levels and toxicity. Theophylline and verapamil may cause increased theophylline action secondary to decreased clearance of theophylline. Vecuronium and verapamil may cause increased vecuronium levels. Lithium levels may increase and sensitivity to neurotoxicity may be enhanced. May increase blood alcohol concentrations and prolong effects.

**Effects on Lab Values** ↑ alkaline phosphatase, CPK, LDH; aminotransferase [AST (SGOT)/ALT (SGPT)] (S)

**Adverse Reactions**

1% to 10%:

Cardiovascular: Bradycardia; first, second, or third degree A-V block; congestive heart failure, hypotension, peripheral edema

Central nervous system: Dizziness, lightheadedness, drowsiness, headache

Dermatologic: Rash

Gastrointestinal: Constipation, nausea

Neuromuscular & skeletal: Weakness

Respiratory: Dyspnea

<1% (Limited to important or life-threatening symptoms): Chest pain, hypotension (excessive), tachycardia, flushing, Stevens-Johnson syndrome, erythema multiforme, tinnitus

**Overdose/Toxicology** Primary cardiac symptoms of calcium blocker overdose include hypotension and bradycardia (second- or third-degree atrioventricular block, or sinus arrest with junctional rhythm). Intraventricular conduction is usually not affected so QRS duration is normal (verapamil does prolong the P-R interval).

Noncardiac symptoms include confusion, stupor, nausea, vomiting, metabolic acidosis and hyperglycemia. Following initial gastric decontamination, if possible, repeated calcium administration may promptly reverse depressed cardiac contractility (but not sinus node depression or peripheral vasodilation). Large doses of calcium chloride (up to 1 g/hour for 24 hours) have been used in refractory cases. Glucagon, epinephrine, and amrinone may treat refractory hypotension. Glucagon and epinephrine also increase heart rate (outside the U.S., 4-aminopyridine may be available as an antidote). Dialysis and hemoperfusion are not effective in enhancing elimination although repeat-dose activated charcoal may serve as an adjunct with sustained-release preparations.

**Pharmacodynamics/Kinetics**

**Protein Binding:** 90%

**Half-life Elimination:** Single dose: 2-8 hours, increased up to 12 hours with multiple dosing; increased half-life with hepatic cirrhosis

**Metabolism:** Liver

**Excretion:** Urine

**Onset:** Oral (nonsustained tablets): Peak effect: 2 hours; I.V.: Peak effect: 1-5 minutes

**Duration:** Oral (nonsustained tablets): 6-8 hours; I.V.: 10-20 minutes

**Formulations**

Verapamil hydrochloride:

Capsule, sustained release (Verelan®): 120 mg, 180 mg, 240 mg, 360 mg

Injection: 2.5 mg/mL (2 mL, 4 mL)

Isoptin®: 2.5 mg/mL (2 mL, 4 mL)

Tablet: 40 mg, 80 mg, 120 mg

Calan®, Isoptin®: 40 mg, 80 mg, 120 mg

Tablet sustained release: 180 mg, 240 mg

Calan® SR, Isoptin® SR: 120 mg, 180 mg, 240 mg

Covera-HS®: 180 mg, 240 mg

**Dosing**

**Adults:**

I.V.: SVT: 5-10 mg (approximately 0.075-0.15 mg/kg), second dose of 10 mg (~0.15 mg/kg) may be given 15-30 minutes after the initial dose if patient tolerates, but does not respond to initial dose

Oral:

Angina: Initial: 80-120 mg twice daily (elderly or small stature: 40 mg twice daily); range: 240-480 mg/day in 3-4 divided doses

Hypertension: Usual dose is 80 mg 3 times/day or 240 mg/day (sustained release); range 240-480 mg/day (no evidence of additional benefit in doses >360 mg/day)

**Elderly:**

Oral: 120-480 mg/24 hours divided 3-4 times/day

Sustained release: 120 mg/day; adjust dose after 24 hours by increases of 120 mg/day; when switching from immediate release forms, total daily dose may remain the same. Controlled onset: initiate therapy with 180 mg in the evening; titrate upward as needed to obtain desired response and avoiding adverse effects.

**Renal Impairment:** $Cl_{cr}$ <10 mL/minute: Administer at 50% to 75% of normal dose.

**Hepatic Impairment:** In cirrhosis, reduce dose to 20% to 50% of normal and monitor EKG.

**Administration**

**Oral:** Administer around-the-clock to promote less variation in peak and trough serum levels. Administer sustained release with food or milk. **Do not crush sustained release drug product.**

**I.V.:** Administer around-the-clock to promote less variation in peak and trough serum levels.

**Stability**

**Storage:** Store injection at room temperature. Protect from heat and from freezing. Use only clear solutions. Protect I.V. solution from light.

**Compatibility:** Compatible in solutions of pH of 3-6, but may precipitate in solutions having a pH ≥6. Incompatible with albumin, amphotericin B, ampicillin, dobutamine, hydralazine, mezlocillin, nafcillin sodium, oxacillin, sodium bicarbonate, sodium lactate in PVC bags, and trimethoprim-sulfamethoxazole. See the Compatibility of Drugs Chart *on page 1315*.

**Additional Nursing Issues**

**Physical Assessment:** Assess other medications patient may be taking for effectiveness and interactions (see Drug Interactions). I.V. requires use of infusion pump and

(Continued)

## Verapamil *(Continued)*

continuous cardiac and hemodynamic monitoring. Monitor laboratory tests (see above), therapeutic response (cardiac status), and adverse reactions (see Warnings/Precautions, Adverse Reactions, and Overdose/Toxicology) when beginning therapy, when titrating dosage, and periodically during long-term oral therapy. Assess knowledge/teach patient appropriate use (oral), interventions to reduce side effects, and adverse symptoms to report. **Pregnancy risk factor C** - benefits of use should outweigh possible risks.

**Patient Information/Instruction:** Oral: Take as directed, around-the-clock. Do not alter dosage or discontinue therapy without consulting prescriber. Do not crush or chew extended release form. Avoid (or limit) alcohol and caffeine. You may experience dizziness or lightheadedness (use caution when driving or engaging in tasks requiring alertness until response to drug is known); nausea or vomiting (small frequent meals, frequent mouth care, chewing gum, or sucking lozenges may help); constipation (increased exercise, dietary fiber, fruit, or fluids may help); diarrhea (buttermilk, boiled milk, or yogurt may help). Report chest pain, palpitations, or irregular heartbeat; unusual cough, difficulty breathing, or swelling of extremities (feet/ankles); muscle tremors or weakness; confusion or acute lethargy; or skin irritation or rash. **Pregnancy precautions:** Inform prescriber if you are or intend to be pregnant.

**Geriatric Considerations:** Elderly may experience a greater hypotensive response. Theoretically, constipation may be more of a problem in the elderly. Calcium channel blockers are no more effective in the elderly than other therapies, however, they do not cause significant CNS effects, which is an advantage over some antihypertensive agents. Generic verapamil products which are bioequivalent in young adults may not be bioequivalent in the elderly. Use generics cautiously.

**Related Information**

Antiarrhythmic Drug Classification Comparison *on page 1366*
Calcium Channel Blocking Agents Comparison *on page 1378*

- **Verazinc® [OTC]** *see* Zinc Supplements *on page 1230*
- **Verazinc® Oral** *see page 1294*
- **Verdilac** *see* Verapamil *on page 1208*
- **Verelan®** *see* Verapamil *on page 1208*
- **Vergon® [OTC]** *see* Meclizine *on page 712*
- **Vermicol** *see* Mebendazole *on page 709*
- **Vermox®** *see* Mebendazole *on page 709*
- **Versacaps®** *see* Guaifenesin and Pseudoephedrine *on page 551*
- **Versed®** *see* Midazolam *on page 769*
- **Versel™** *see page 1294*
- **Vertisal** *see* Metronidazole *on page 763*
- **Vesanoid®** *see* Tretinoin (Oral) *on page 1168*
- **Vexol®** *see page 1282*
- **Viagra™** *see* Sildenafil *on page 1056*
- **Vibazine®** *see* Buclizine *on page 163*
- **Vibramicina®** *see* Doxycycline *on page 406*
- **Vibramycin®** *see* Doxycycline *on page 406*
- **Vibra-Tabs®** *see* Doxycycline *on page 406*
- **Vicks® 44D Cough & Head Congestion Capsule** *see page 1294*
- **Vicks® 44D Non-Drowsy Cold & Cough Liqui-Caps** *see page 1294*
- **Vicks® 44E [OTC]** *see* Guaifenesin and Dextromethorphan *on page 549*
- **Vicks® Children's Chloraseptic® [OTC]** *see* Benzocaine *on page 141*
- **Vicks® Chloraseptic® Sore Throat [OTC]** *see* Benzocaine *on page 141*
- **Vicks® DayQuil® Allergy Relief 4 Hour Tablet** *see page 1294*
- **Vicks® DayQuil® Sinus Pressure & Congestion Relief [OTC]** *see* Guaifenesin and Phenylpropanolamine *on page 550*
- **Vicks Formula 44®** *see page 1294*
- **Vicks Formula 44® Pediatric Formula** *see page 1294*
- **Vicks® Pediatric Formula 44E [OTC]** *see* Guaifenesin and Dextromethorphan *on page 549*
- **Vicks® Sinex® Nasal Solution [OTC]** *see* Phenylephrine *on page 920*
- **Vicodin®** *see* Hydrocodone and Acetaminophen *on page 568*
- **Vicodin® ES** *see* Hydrocodone and Acetaminophen *on page 568*
- **Vicodin® HP** *see* Hydrocodone and Acetaminophen *on page 568*
- **Vicon-C®** *see page 1294*
- **Vicon Forte®** *see* Vitamin, Multiple *on page 1219*
- **Vicon® Plus [OTC]** *see* Vitamin, Multiple *on page 1219*
- **Vicoprofen®** *see* Hydrocodone and Ibuprofen *on page 573*

## Vidarabine (vye DARE a been)

**U.S. Brand Names** Vira-A® Ophthalmic

**Synonyms** Adenine Arabinoside; ARA-A; Arabinofuranosyladenine

**Therapeutic Category** Antiviral Agent, Ophthalmic

**Pregnancy Risk Factor** C

**Lactation** Excretion in breast milk unknown

**Use** Treatment of acute keratoconjunctivitis and epithelial keratitis due to herpes simplex virus; herpes simplex conjunctivitis

**Mechanism of Action/Effect** Inhibits viral DNA synthesis by blocking DNA polymerase

**Contraindications** Hypersensitivity to vidarabine or any component

**Warnings** Pregnancy factor C.

**Adverse Reactions** 1% to 10%: Ocular: Burning eyes, lacrimation, keratitis, photophobia, foreign body sensation, uveitis

**Formulations** Ointment, ophthalmic, as monohydrate: 3% [30 mg/mL = 28 mg/mL base] (3.5 g)

**Dosing**

**Adults:** Ophthalmic: Keratoconjunctivitis: Instill ½" of ointment in lower conjunctival sac every 3 hours up to 5 times/day while awake until complete re-epithelialization has occurred, then twice daily for an additional 7 days.

**Elderly:** Refer to adult dosing.

**Additional Nursing Issues**

**Physical Assessment:** Monitor effectiveness of therapy (for length of therapy see Dosing). Assess knowledge/teach patient appropriate use, interventions to reduce side effects, and adverse symptoms to report (see Adverse Reactions). **Pregnancy risk factor C** - benefits of use should outweigh possible risks. Note breast-feeding caution.

**Patient Information/Instruction:** For ophthalmic use only. Store in refrigerator. Apply prescribed amount as often as directed. Wash hands before using and do not let tip of applicator touch eye or contaminate tip of applicator. Tilt head back and look upward. Gently pull down lower lid and put drop(s) in inner corner of eye. Close eye and roll eyeball in all directions. Do not blink for ½ minute. Apply gentle pressure to inner corner of eye for 30 seconds. Wipe away excess from skin around eye. Do not use any other eye preparation for at least 10 minutes. Do not touch tip of applicator to eye or contaminate tip of applicator. Do not share medication with anyone else. May cause sensitivity to bright light (dark glasses may help); temporary stinging or blurred vision may occur. Inform prescriber if you experience eye pain, redness, burning, watering, dryness, double vision, puffiness around eye, vision disturbances, or other adverse eye response; worsening of condition or lack of improvement within 7-14 days. **Pregnancy/breast-feeding precautions:** Inform prescriber if you are pregnant. Consult prescriber if breast-feeding.

**Geriatric Considerations:** Assess ability to self-administer ophthalmic ointment.

- **Vi-Daylin® [OTC]** *see* Vitamin, Multiple *on page 1219*
- **Vi-Daylin/F®** *see* Vitamin, Multiple *on page 1219*
- **Videx®** *see* Didanosine *on page 363*
- **Viken** *see* Cefotaxime *on page 221*
- **Vilona** *see* Ribavirin *on page 1016*
- **Vilona Pediatrica** *see* Ribavirin *on page 1016*

## Vinblastine (vin BLAS teen)

**U.S. Brand Names** Alkaban-AQ®; Velban®

**Synonyms** Vincaleukoblastine; VLB

**Therapeutic Category** Antineoplastic Agent, Natural Source (Plant) Derivative

**Pregnancy Risk Factor** D

**Lactation** Enters breast milk/not recommended

**Use** Palliative treatment of Hodgkin's and non-Hodgkin's lymphoma, testicular, lung, head and neck, breast, and renal carcinomas, Kaposi's sarcoma, histiocytosis, choriocarcinoma, and idiopathic thrombocytopenic purpura

**Mechanism of Action/Effect** VLB arrests cell cycle growth in metaphase. Also inhibits RNA synthesis and amino acid metabolism resulting in inhibition of metabolic pathways and cell growth.

**Contraindications** Severe bone marrow suppression or presence of bacterial infection not under control prior to initiation of therapy; pregnancy

**Warnings** The U.S. Food and Drug Administration (FDA) currently recommends that procedures for proper handling and disposal of antineoplastic agents be considered.

Preparation of vinblastine should be performed in a Class II laminar flow biologic safety cabinet. Personnel should be wearing surgical gloves and a closed front surgical gown with knit cuffs. Appropriate safety equipment is recommended for preparation, administration, and disposal of antineoplastics. If vinblastine contacts the skin, wash and flush thoroughly with water.

Drug is a vesicant. Avoid extravasation. Dosage modification required in patients with impaired liver function and neurotoxicity. Using small amounts of drug daily for long periods may increase neurotoxicity and is therefore not advised. For I.V. use only. **Intrathecal administration results in death.** Use with caution in patients with cachexia or ulcerated skin. Monitor closely for shortness of breath or bronchospasm in patients receiving mitomycin C.

**Drug Interactions**

**Cytochrome P-450 Effect:** CYP3A3/4 and 3A5-7 enzyme substrate; CYP2D6 enzyme inhibitor

**Decreased Effect:** Phenytoin plasma levels may be reduced with concomitant combination chemotherapy with vinblastine. Alpha-interferon enhances interferon toxicity; phenytoin may ↓ plasma levels.

**Increased Effect/Toxicity:** Vinblastine levels may be increased when given with drugs that inhibit cytochrome P-450 3A enzyme substrate. Previous or simultaneous use with mitomycin-C has resulted in acute shortness of breath and severe bronchospasm within minutes or several hours after *Vinca* alkaloid injection and may occur up

(Continued)

## Vinblastine *(Continued)*

to 2 weeks after the dose of mitomycin. Mitomycin-C in combination with administration of VLB may cause acute shortness of breath and severe bronchospasm, onset may be within minutes or several hours after VLB injection.

**Adverse Reactions**

>10%:

Dermatologic: Alopecia

Gastrointestinal: Nausea and vomiting are most common and are easily controlled with standard antiemetics; constipation, diarrhea (less common), stomatitis, abdominal cramps, anorexia, metallic taste

Emetic potential: Moderate (30% to 60%)

Hematologic: Leukopenia; May cause severe bone marrow suppression and is the dose-limiting toxicity of VLB (unlike vincristine); severe granulocytopenia and thrombocytopenia may occur following the administration of VLB and nadir 7-10 days after treatment

Myelosuppressive:

WBC: Moderate - severe

Platelets: Moderate - severe

Onset (days): 4-7

Nadir (days): 4-10

Recovery (days): 17

1% to 10%:

Cardiovascular: Hypertension, Raynaud's phenomenon

Central nervous system: Depression, malaise, headache, seizures

Dermatologic: Rash, photosensitivity, dermatitis

Endocrine & metabolic: Hyperuricemia

Gastrointestinal: Paralytic ileus, stomatitis

Genitourinary: Urinary retention

Local: **Vesicant chemotherapy**

Neuromuscular & skeletal: Jaw pain, myalgia, paresthesia

Respiratory: Bronchospasm

<1% (Limited to important or life-threatening symptoms): Hemorrhagic colitis, rectal bleeding. Neurologic: VLB rarely produces neurotoxicity at clinical doses; however, neurotoxicity may be seen, especially at high doses; if it occurs, symptoms are similar to VCR toxicity (ie, peripheral neuropathy, loss of deep tendon reflexes, headache, weakness, urinary retention, and GI symptoms, tachycardia, orthostatic hypotension, convulsions)

**Overdose/Toxicology** Symptoms of overdose include bone marrow suppression, mental depression, paresthesia, loss of deep tendon reflexes, and neurotoxicity. There are no antidotes for vinblastine. Treatment is supportive and symptomatic, including fluid restriction or hypertonic saline (3% sodium chloride) for drug-induced secretion of inappropriate antidiuretic hormone (SIADH).

**Pharmacodynamics/Kinetics**

**Protein Binding:** 99% rapidly

**Half-life Elimination:** Half-life (biphasic): Initial 0.164 hours; Terminal: 25 hours

**Metabolism:** Liver

**Excretion:** Feces

**Formulations**

Vinblastine sulfate:

Injection: 1 mg/mL (10 mL)

Powder for reconstitution: 10 mg

**Dosing**

**Adults:** Refer to individual protocols. Varies depending upon clinical and hematological response. Give at intervals of at least 7 days and only after leukocyte count has returned to at least 4000/mm$^3$. Maintenance therapy should be titrated according to leukocyte count. Dosage should be reduced in patients with recent exposure to radiation therapy or chemotherapy. Single doses in these patients should not exceed 5.5 mg/m$^2$.

I.V.: 4-20 mg/m$^2$ (0.1-0.5 mg/kg) every 7-10 days **or** 5-day continuous infusion of 1.4-1.8 mg/m$^2$/day **or** 0.1-0.5 mg/kg/week

**Renal Impairment:** Not removed by hemodialysis

**Hepatic Impairment:**

Serum bilirubin 1.5-3.0 mg/dL or AST 60-180 units: Administer 50% of normal dose.

Serum bilirubin 3.0-5.0 mg/dL: Administer 25% of dose.

Serum bilirubin >5.0 mg/dL or AST >180 units: Omit dose.

**Administration**

**I.V.:** Vesicant. Drug is for I.V. administration only. **Fatal if given intrathecally.** May be administered by I.V. push or into a free flowing I.V. IVP over at least 1 minute is the desired route of administration because of potential for extravasation. However, has also been administered by continuous intravenous infusion - **central line only for continuous intravenous infusion administration.**

**I.V. Detail:** Follow guidelines for handling cytotoxic agents.

Avoid extravasation; may cause sloughing. Solution should be administered only by qualified personnel. Do not allow to come in contact with skin; if contact occurs, wash well with soap and water.

**Extravasation management:** Mix 250 units hyaluronidase with 6 mL of NS. Inject the hyaluronidase solution subcutaneously through 6 clockwise injections into the infiltrated area using a 25-gauge needle; change the needle with each new injection.

Apply heat immediately for 1 hour. Repeat 4 times/day for 3-5 days. Elevate extremity. Application of cold or hydrocortisone is contraindicated.

**Stability**

**Storage:** Store intact vials under refrigeration (2°C to 8°C) and protect from light.

**Reconstitution:** Standard I.V. dilution:

I.V. push: Dose/syringe (concentration = 1 mg/mL)

Maximum syringe size for IVP is a 30 mL syringe and syringe should be ≤75% full.

Continuous intravenous infusion: Dose = 250-1000 mL $D_5W$ or NS

Solutions are stable for 21 days at room temperature (25°C) and refrigeration (4°C). Protect from light.

**Compatibility:** See the Chemotherapy Compatibility Chart *on page 1311*.

**Monitoring Laboratory Tests** CBC with differential and platelet count, serum uric acid, hepatic function

**Additional Nursing Issues**

**Physical Assessment:** Monitor other medications patient may be taking for effectiveness and possible interactions, especially mitomycin-C (see Drug Interactions). Monitor laboratory results prior to each infusion. Monitor infusion site carefully; extravasation may cause tissue sloughing (see Administration). Monitor closely for extensive adverse reactions (see Adverse Reactions). Premedicate with antiemetic. Instruct patient on possible side effects, interventions, and symptoms to report. **Pregnancy risk factor D** - assess knowledge/teach both male and female appropriate use of barrier contraceptives. Breast-feeding is not recommended.

**Patient Information/Instruction:** This medication can only be administered by infusion, usually on a cyclic basis. Maintain adequate hydration (2-3 L/day of fluids unless instructed to restrict fluid intake) and nutrition (small frequent meals will help). You will most likely loss your hair (will grow back after therapy); experience nausea or vomiting (request antiemetic); photosensitivity (use sunscreen, wear protective clothing and eyewear, and avoid direct sunlight); or feel weak or lethargic (use caution when driving or engaging in tasks requiring alertness until response to drug is known). Use good oral care to reduce incidence of mouth sores. You will be more susceptible to infection; avoid crowds or exposure to infection. Report numbness or tingling in fingers or toes (use care to prevent injury); signs of infection (eg, fever, chills, sore throat, burning urination, fatigue); unusual bleeding (eg, tarry stools, easy bruising, blood in stool, urine, or mouth); unresolved mouth sores; skin rash or itching; or difficulty breathing. **Pregnancy/breast-feeding precautions:** Do not get pregnant. Breast-feeding is not recommended.

**Additional Information** Some formulations may contain benzyl alcohol.

♦ **Vincaleukoblastine** *see* Vinblastine *on page 1211*

♦ **Vincasar® PFS™ Injection** *see* Vincristine *on this page*

## Vincristine (vin KRIS teen)

**U.S. Brand Names** Oncovin® Injection; Vincasar® PFS™ Injection

**Synonyms** LCR; Leurocristine; VCR

**Therapeutic Category** Antineoplastic Agent, Natural Source (Plant) Derivative

**Pregnancy Risk Factor** D

**Lactation** Enters breast milk/not recommended

**Use** Treatment of leukemias, Hodgkin's disease, neuroblastoma, malignant lymphomas, Wilms' tumor, and rhabdomyosarcoma

**Mechanism of Action/Effect** Binds to microtubular protein of the mitotic spindle causing metaphase arrest; cell-cycle phase specific in the M and S phases

**Contraindications** Hypersensitivity to vincristine or any component; **for I.V. use only, never give intrathecally**; patients with demyelinating form of Charcot-Marie-Tooth syndrome; pregnancy

**Warnings** For I.V. use only. The U.S. Food and Drug Administration (FDA) currently recommends that procedures for proper handling and disposal of antineoplastic agents be considered.

Preparation of vincristine should be performed in a Class II laminar flow biologic safety cabinet. Personnel should be wearing surgical gloves and a closed front surgical gown with knit cuffs. Appropriate safety equipment is recommended for preparation, administration, and disposal of antineoplastics. If vincristine contacts the skin, wash and flush thoroughly with water.

Dosage modification required in patients with impaired hepatic function or who have preexisting neuromuscular disease. Drug is a vesicant. Avoid extravasation. Use with caution in the elderly. Avoid eye contamination. Observe closely for shortness of breath, bronchospasm, especially in patients treated with mitomycin C. Do not use with radiation.

**Drug Interactions**

**Cytochrome P-450 Effect:** CYP3A3/4 and 3A5-7 enzyme substrate; CYP2D6 enzyme inhibitor

**Decreased Effect:** Digoxin and phenytoin levels may decrease with combination chemotherapy.

**Increased Effect/Toxicity:** Vincristine levels may be increased when given with drugs that inhibit cytochrome P-450 3A enzyme substrate. Digoxin plasma levels and renal excretion may decrease with combination chemotherapy including vincristine. Vincristine should be given 12-24 hours before asparaginase to minimize toxicity (may decrease the hepatic clearance of vincristine). Acute pulmonary reactions may occur with mitomycin-C. Previous or simultaneous use with mitomycin-C has resulted in

(Continued)

## Vincristine *(Continued)*

acute shortness of breath and severe bronchospasm within minutes or several hours after *Vinca* alkaloid injection and may occur up to 2 weeks after the dose of mitomycin.

**Adverse Reactions**

>10%: Dermatologic: Alopecia occurs in 20% to 70% of patients

1% to 10%:

Cardiovascular: Orthostatic hypotension or hypertension, hypertension, hypotension

Central nervous system: Motor difficulties, seizures, headache, CNS depression, cranial nerve paralysis, fever

Dermatologic: Rash

Endocrine & metabolic: Hyperuricemia

SIADH: Rarely occurs, but may be related to the neurologic toxicity; may cause symptomatic hyponatremia with seizures; the increase in serum ADH concentration usually subsides within 2-3 days after onset

Gastrointestinal: Constipation and possible paralytic ileus secondary to neurologic toxicity; oral ulceration, abdominal cramps, anorexia, metallic taste, bloating, nausea, vomiting, weight loss, diarrhea

Emetic potential: Low (<10%)

Local: Phlebitis

**Vesicant chemotherapy**

Neurologic: Alterations in mental status such as depression, confusion, or insomnia; constipation, paralytic ileus, and urinary tract disturbances may occur. All patients should be on a prophylactic bowel management regimen. Cranial nerve palsies, headaches, jaw pain, optic atrophy with blindness have been reported. **Intrathecal administration of VCR has uniformly caused death; VCR should never be administered by this route.** Neurologic effects of VCR may be additive with those of other neurotoxic agents and spinal cord irradiation.

Neuromuscular & skeletal: Jaw pain, leg pain, myalgia, cramping, numbness, weakness

Peripheral neuropathy: Frequently the dose-limiting toxicity of VCR. Most frequent in patients >40 years of age; occurs usually after an average of 3 weekly doses, but may occur after just one dose. Manifested as loss of the deep tendon reflexes in the lower extremities, numbness, tingling, pain, paresthesias of the fingers and toes (stocking glove sensation), and "foot drop" or "wrist drop"

Ocular: Photophobia

<1% (Limited to important or life-threatening symptoms): Hematologic: Myelosuppressive: Occasionally mild leukopenia and thrombocytopenia may occur

WBC: Rare

Platelets: Rare

Onset (days): 7

Nadir (days): 10

Recovery (days): 21

**Overdose/Toxicology** Symptoms of overdose include bone marrow suppression, mental depression, paresthesia, loss of deep tendon reflexes, alopecia, and nausea. Severe symptoms may occur with 3-4 mg/m$^2$.

There are no antidotes for vincristine. Treatment is supportive and symptomatic, including fluid restriction or hypertonic saline (3% sodium chloride) for drug-induced secretion of inappropriate antidiuretic hormone (SIADH). Case reports suggest that folinic acid may be helpful in treating vincristine overdose. It is suggested that 100 mg folinic acid be given I.V. every 3 hours for 24 hours, then every 6 hours for 48 hours. This is in addition to supportive care. The use of pyridoxine, leucovorin factor, cyanocobalamin, or thiamine has been used with little success for drug-induced peripheral neuropathy.

**Pharmacodynamics/Kinetics**

**Protein Binding:** 75%

**Half-life Elimination:** Terminal: 24 hours

**Metabolism:** Liver

**Excretion:** Feces

**Formulations** Injection, as sulfate: 1 mg/mL (1 mL, 2 mL, 5 mL)

**Dosing**

**Adults:** Refer to individual protocols as dosages vary with protocol used. Adjustments are made depending upon clinical and hematological response and upon adverse reactions.

I.V.: 0.4-1.4 mg/m$^2$ (up to 2 mg maximum); may repeat every week. The average total dose per course of treatment should be around 2-2.5 mg. Some recommend capping the dose at 2 mg maximum to reduce toxicity; however, it is felt that this measure can reduce the efficacy of the drug.

**Hepatic Impairment:**

Serum bilirubin 1.5-3.0 mg/dL or AST 60-180 units: Administer 50% of normal dose.

Serum bilirubin 3.0-5.0 mg/dL: Administer 25% of dose.

Serum bilirubin >5.0 mg/dL or AST >180 units: Omit dose.

**Administration**

**I.V.:** Vesicant. For I.V. use only. **Fatal if given intrathecally.** IVP over at least 1 minute is the desired route of administration because of potential for extravasation. However, has also been administered IVPB over 15 minutes - **central line only for IVPB administration.**

**I.V. Detail:** Follow guidelines for handling cytotoxic agents. Drug should be administered by qualified personnel. Do not allow to come in contact with skin. If contact occurs, wash thoroughly with soap and water. Avoid extravasation; agent is a vesicant and will cause sloughing.

**Extravasation management:** Mix 250 units hyaluronidase with 6 mL of NS. Inject the hyaluronidase solution subcutaneously through 6 clockwise injections into the infiltrated area using a 25-gauge needle. Change the needle with each new injection. Elevate extremity. Apply heat immediately for 1 hour. Repeat 4 times/day for 3-5 days. Application of cold or hydrocortisone is contraindicated.

**Stability**

**Storage:** Store intact vials at refrigeration (2°C to 8°C) and protect from light.

**Reconstitution:** Further dilution in NS or $D_5W$ is stable for 21 days at room temperature (25°C) and refrigeration (4°C).

**Standard I.V. dilution:**

I.V. push: Dose/syringe (concentration = 1 mg/mL)

Maximum syringe size for IVP is 30 mL syringe and syringe should be ≤75% full

IVPB: Dose/50 mL $D_5W$

**Compatibility:** Compatible with doxorubicin, bleomycin, cytarabine, fluorouracil, methotrexate, and metoclopramide. See the Chemotherapy Compatibility Chart *on page 1311.*

**Monitoring Laboratory Tests** Serum electrolytes (sodium), hepatic function, neurologic examination, CBC, serum uric acid

**Additional Nursing Issues**

**Physical Assessment:** Assess other medications patient may be taking for effectiveness and possible interactions, especially mitomycin C (see Drug Interactions) Monitor laboratory results prior to each infusion. Monitor infusion site carefully; extravasation may cause tissue sloughing (see Administration). Monitor closely for extensive adverse reactions, especially central nervous system, neuromuscular and neurological reactions (see Adverse Reactions). Constipation is a potentially life-threatening complication; all patients should be on a prophylactic bowel management regimen. Instruct patient on possible side effects and interventions and symptoms to report. **Pregnancy risk factor D** - assess knowledge/teach both male and female appropriate use of barrier contraceptives during therapy. Breast-feeding is not recommended.

**Patient Information/Instruction:** This medication can only be administered by infusion, usually on a cyclic basis. Maintain adequate hydration (2-3 L/day of fluids unless instructed to restrict fluid intake) and nutrition (small frequent meals will help). You will most likely loss your hair (will grow back after therapy); experience constipation (request medication); or feel weak or lethargic (use caution when driving or engaging in tasks requiring alertness until response to drug is known). Use good oral care to reduce incidence of mouth sores. You will be more susceptible to infection; avoid crowds or exposure to infection. Report pain, numbness, or tingling in fingers or toes (use care to prevent injury); alterations in mental status (eg, confusion, insomnia, headaches, jaw pain, loss of vision); signs of infection (eg, fever, chills, sore throat, burning urination, fatigue); unusual bleeding (eg, tarry stools, easy bruising, or blood in stool, urine, or mouth), unresolved mouth sores; skin rash or itching; nausea; vomiting; abdominal pain; bloating; or difficulty breathing. **Pregnancy/breast-feeding precautions:** Do not get pregnant. Breast-feeding is not recommended.

## Vinorelbine (vi NOR el been)

**U.S. Brand Names** Navelbine®

**Therapeutic Category** Antineoplastic Agent, Natural Source (Plant) Derivative

**Pregnancy Risk Factor** D

**Lactation** Enters breast milk/contraindicated

**Use** Treatment of nonsmall cell lung cancer (as a single agent or in combination with cisplatin)

**Unlabeled use:** Breast cancer, ovarian carcinoma (cisplatin-resistant), Hodgkin's disease

**Mechanism of Action/Effect** Mitotic inhibition that causes metaphase arrest in neoplastic cells

**Contraindications** Severe bone marrow suppression (granulocyte counts <1000 cells/$mm^3$) or presence of bacterial infection not under control prior to initiation of therapy; pregnancy

**Warnings** For I.V. use only. The U.S. Food and Drug Administration (FDA) currently recommends that procedures for proper handling and disposal of antineoplastic agents be considered.

Preparation of vinorelbine should be performed in a Class II laminar flow biologic safety cabinet. Personnel should be wearing surgical gloves and a closed front surgical gown with knit cuffs. Appropriate safety equipment is recommended for preparation, administration, and disposal of antineoplastics. If vinorelbine contacts the skin, wash and flush thoroughly with water. Avoid extravasation. Dosage modification is required in patients with impaired liver function and neurotoxicity. Frequently monitor patients for myelosuppression both during and after therapy. Granulocytopenia is dose-limiting. **Intrathecal administration may result in death.** Use with caution in patients with cachexia or ulcerated skin.

**Drug Interactions**

**Cytochrome P-450 Effect:** CYP2D6 enzyme inhibitor

**Increased Effect/Toxicity:** Previous or simultaneous use with mitomycin-C has resulted in acute shortness of breath and severe bronchospasm within minutes or several hours after *Vinca* alkaloid injection and may occur up to 2 weeks after the dose of mitomycin.

(Continued)

## Vinorelbine *(Continued)*

Cisplatin: Incidence of granulocytopenia is significantly higher than with single-agent vinorelbine.

**Adverse Reactions**

>10%:

Dermatologic: Alopecia (12%)

Gastrointestinal: Nausea and vomiting are most common and are easily controlled with standard antiemetics; constipation, diarrhea, stomatitis, abdominal cramps, anorexia, metallic taste

Emetic potential: Moderate (30% to 60%)

Hematologic: May cause severe bone marrow suppression and is the dose-limiting toxicity of vinorelbine; severe granulocytopenia may occur following the administration of vinorelbine

Myelosuppressive:

WBC: Moderate - severe

Onset (days): 4-7

Nadir (days): 7-10

Recovery (days): 14-21

Neuromuscular and skeletal: Peripheral neuropathy (20% to 25%)

1% to 10%:

Central nervous system: Fatigue

Local: **Vesicant chemotherapy**

Neuromuscular & skeletal: Mild-moderate peripheral neuropathy manifested by paresthesia and hyperesthesia, loss of deep tendon reflexes; myalgia, arthralgia, jaw pain

<1% (Limited to important or life-threatening symptoms): Hemorrhagic colitis, severe peripheral neuropathy (generally reversible), vestibular and auditory toxicity

**Overdose/Toxicology** Symptoms of overdose include bone marrow suppression, mental depression, paresthesia, loss of deep tendon reflexes, and neurotoxicity. There are no antidotes for vinorelbine. Treatment is supportive and symptomatic, including fluid restriction or hypertonic saline (3% sodium chloride) for drug-induced secretion of inappropriate antidiuretic hormone (SIADH).

**Pharmacodynamics/Kinetics**

**Half-life Elimination:** Half-life (triphasic): Terminal: 27.7-43.6 hours; Mean plasma clearance: 0.97-1.26 L/hour/kg

**Metabolism:** Extensive hepatic metabolism to an active metabolite (deacetylvinorelbine)

**Excretion:** Urine and feces

**Formulations** Injection, as tartrate: 10 mg/mL (1 mL, 5 mL)

**Dosing**

**Adults:** Varies depending upon clinical and hematological response (refer to individual protocols).

I.V.: 30 mg/m$^2$ every 7 days

**Dosage adjustment in hematological toxicity (based on granulocyte counts):**

Granulocytes ≥1500 cells/mm$^3$ on day of treatment: Administer 30 mg/m$^2$.

Granulocytes 1000-1499 cells/mm$^3$ on day of treatment: Administer 15 mg/m$^2$.

Granulocytes <1000 cells/mm$^3$ on day of treatment: Do not administer. Repeat granulocyte count in 1 week. If 3 consecutive doses are held because granulocyte count is <1000 cells/mm$^3$, discontinue vinorelbine.

For patients who, during treatment, have experienced fever or sepsis while granulocytopenic or had 2 consecutive weekly doses held due to granulocytopenia, subsequent doses of vinorelbine should be:

22.5 mg/m$^2$ for granulocytes ≥1500 cells/mm$^3$

11.25 mg/m$^2$ for granulocytes 1000-1499 cells/mm$^3$

**Renal Impairment:** If moderate or severe neurotoxicity develops, discontinue vinorelbine.

**Hepatic Impairment:**

Serum bilirubin ≤2 mg/dL: Administer 30 mg/m$^2$.

Serum bilirubin 2.1-3 mg/dL: Administer 15 mg/m$^2$.

Serum bilirubin >3 mg/dL: Administer 7.5 mg/m$^2$.

In patients with concurrent hematologic toxicity and hepatic impairment, administer the lower doses determined from the above recommendations under Adult Dosing.

**Administration**

**I.V.:** Vesicant. For I.V. use only. **Fatal if given intrathecally.** Administer I.V. over 20-30 minutes; central line only for IVPB administration.

**I.V. Detail:** Do not administer in an extremity with poor circulation or repeatedly into the same vein. Avoid extravasation; may cause sloughing.

Extravasation management: Mix 250 units hyaluronidase with 6 mL of NS. Inject the hyaluronidase solution subcutaneously through 6 clockwise injections into the infiltrated area using a 25-gauge needle. Change the needle with each new injection. Elevate extremities. Apply heat immediately for 1 hour. Repeat 4 times/day for 3-5 days. Application of cold or hydrocortisone is contraindicated.

**Stability**

**Storage:** Store intact vials under refrigeration (2°C to 8°C). Vials are stable at room temperature for up to 72 hours.

**Reconstitution:** Further dilution in $D_5W$ or NS is stable for 24 hours at room temperature.

**Standard I.V. dilution:**

I.V. push: Dose/syringe (concentration = 1.5-3 mg/mL)

Maximum syringe size for IVP is a 30 mL syringe and syringe should be ≤75% full.

IVPB: Dose/50-250 mL $D_5W$ or NS (concentration = 0.5-2 mg/mL)

Solutions are stable for 24 hours at room temperature.

**Compatibility:** See the Chemotherapy Compatibility Chart *on page 1311.*

**Monitoring Laboratory Tests** CBC with differential and platelet count, serum uric acid, hepatic function

**Additional Nursing Issues**

**Physical Assessment:** Assess other medications patient may be taking for possible interactions, especially mitomycin C (see Drug Interactions). Monitor laboratory results prior to each infusion. Monitor infusion site carefully; extravasation may cause tissue sloughing (see Administration). Monitor closely for extensive adverse reactions (see Adverse Reactions). Premedicate with antiemetic. Instruct patient on possible side effects and interventions and symptoms to report. **Pregnancy risk factor D** - assess knowledge/teach both male and female appropriate use of barrier contraceptives during therapy. Breast-feeding is contraindicated.

**Patient Information/Instruction:** This medication can only be administered by infusion, usually on a cyclic basis. Maintain adequate hydration (2-3 L/day of fluids unless instructed to restrict fluid intake) and nutrition (small frequent meals will help). You will most likely loss your hair (will grow back after therapy); experience nausea or vomiting (request medication); feel weak or lethargic (use caution when driving or engaging in tasks requiring alertness until response to drug is known). Use good oral care to reduce incidence of mouth sores. You will be more susceptible to infection; avoid crowds or exposure to infection. Report weakness, skeletal pain, or tremors; signs of infection (eg, fever, chills, sore throat, burning urination, fatigue); unusual bleeding (eg, tarry stools, easy bruising, blood in stool, urine, or mouth); numbness, pain, or tingling of fingers or toes; unresolved mouth sores; skin rash or itching; uncontrolled nausea, vomiting, or abdominal pain; or difficulty breathing. **Pregnancy/breast-feeding precautions:** Do not get pregnant or breast-feed.

- **Vioform® [OTC]** *see page 1247*
- **Viokase®** *see* Pancrelipase *on page 882*
- **Viosterol** *see* Ergocalciferol *on page 432*
- **Vioxx®** *see* Rofecoxib *on page 1035*
- **Vira-A® Ophthalmic** *see* Vidarabine *on page 1210*
- **Viracept®** *see* Nelfinavir *on page 813*
- **Viramune®** *see* Nevirapine *on page 820*
- **Virazide** *see* Ribavirin *on page 1016*
- **Virazole® Aerosol** *see* Ribavirin *on page 1016*
- **Virilon®** *see* Methyltestosterone *on page 756*
- **Viroptic® Ophthalmic** *see* Trifluridine *on page 1178*
- **Viscoat®** *see page 1248*
- **Viscoat®** *see page 1282*
- **Visine® Extra Ophthalmic** *see page 1294*
- **Visine® L.R. Ophthalmic** *see page 1294*
- **Visken®** *see* Pindolol *on page 934*
- **Vistacon-50®** *see* Hydroxyzine *on page 588*
- **Vistaquel®** *see* Hydroxyzine *on page 588*
- **Vistaril®** *see* Hydroxyzine *on page 588*
- **Vistazine®** *see* Hydroxyzine *on page 588*
- **Vistide®** *see* Cidofovir *on page 265*
- **Vi-Syneral** *see* Vitamin, Multiple *on page 1219*
- **Vita-C® [OTC]** *see* Ascorbic Acid *on page 108*

## Vitamin A (VYE ta min aye)

**U.S. Brand Names** Aquasol A®; Del-Vi-A®; Palmitate-A® 5000 [OTC]

**Synonyms** Oleovitamin A

**Therapeutic Category** Vitamin, Fat Soluble

**Pregnancy Risk Factor** A/X (if dose exceeds RDA recommendation)

**Lactation** Enters breast milk/compatible at normal daily doses

**Use** Treatment and prevention of vitamin A deficiency

**Mechanism of Action/Effect** Needed for bone development, growth, visual adaptation to darkness, testicular and ovarian function, and as a cofactor in many biochemical processes

**Contraindications** Hypersensitivity to vitamin A or any component; hypervitaminosis A; pregnancy (in doses exceeding RDA recommendations)

**Warnings** Evaluate other sources of vitamin A while receiving this product. Patients receiving >25,000 units/day should be closely monitored for toxicity.

**Drug Interactions**

**Decreased Effect:** Cholestyramine resin decreases absorption of vitamin A. Neomycin and mineral oil may also interfere with vitamin A absorption.

**Increased Effect/Toxicity:** Retinoids may have additive adverse effects.

**Adverse Reactions Systemic:** 1% to 10%:

Central nervous system: Irritability, vertigo, lethargy, malaise, fever, headache

Dermatologic: Drying or cracking of skin

Endocrine & metabolic: Hypercalcemia

Gastrointestinal: Weight loss

Ocular: Visual changes

(Continued)

## Vitamin A *(Continued)*

Miscellaneous: Hypervitaminosis A

**Overdose/Toxicology** Symptoms of chronic overdose (adults: 25,000 units/day for 2-3 weeks) include increased intracranial pressure (headache, altered mental status, blurred vision), jaundice, ascites, and cutaneous desquamation. Symptoms of acute overdose (12,000 units/kg) include nausea, vomiting, and diarrhea. Toxic signs of overdose commonly respond to drug discontinuation and generally resolve spontaneously within a few days to weeks. When confronted with signs of increased intracranial pressure, treatment with dexamethasone (1.5 mg/kg I.V. load followed with 0.375 mg/kg every 6 hours for 5 days), and/or hyperventilation may be employed; forced diuresis, dialysis, and hemoperfusion are of no clinical benefit.

**Pharmacodynamics/Kinetics**

**Metabolism:** Conjugated with glucuronide, undergoes enterohepatic circulation

**Excretion:** In feces via biliary elimination

**Formulations**

Capsule: 10,000 units [OTC], 25,000 units, 50,000 units
Drops, oral (water miscible) [OTC]: 5000 units/0.1 mL (30 mL)
Injection: 50,000 units/mL (2 mL)
Tablet [OTC]: 5000 units

**Dosing**

**Adults:**

RDA:
Male: 1000 mcg
Female: 800 mcg

Severe deficiency with xerophthalmia: Oral: 500,000 units/day for 3 days, then 50,000 units/day for 14 days, then 10,000-20,000 units/day for 2 months

Deficiency (without corneal changes): Oral: 100,000 units/day for 3 days then 50,000 units/day for 14 days

Malabsorption syndrome (prophylaxis): Oral: 10,000-50,000 units/day of water miscible product

Dietary supplement: Oral: 4000-5000 units/day

**Elderly:** Refer to adult dosing.

**Administration**

**I.V.: Do not give by I.V. push.**

**Stability**

**Storage:** Protect from light.

**Additional Nursing Issues**

**Physical Assessment:** See Contraindications and Warnings/Precautions for use cautions. Assess effectiveness and interactions of other medications (see Drug Interactions). Assess knowledge/teach patient appropriate use and adverse symptoms to report (see Adverse Reaction and Overdose/Toxicology). **Pregnancy risk factor A/X** - see Pregnancy Risk Factor for cautious use.

**Patient Information/Instruction:** Take exactly as directed; do not take more than the recommended dose. Take with meals. Do not use mineral oil or other vitamin A supplements without consulting prescriber. Report persistent nausea, vomiting, or loss of appetite; excessively dry skin or lips; headache or CNS irritability; loss of hair; or changes in vision.

**Additional Information** •mcg retinol equivalent (0.3 mcg retinol = 1 unit vitamin A)

- **Vitamin A Acid** *see* Tretinoin (Topical) *on page 1170*
- **Vitamin A and D** *see page 1294*
- **Vitamin $B_1$** *see* Thiamine *on page 1120*
- **Vitamin $B_2$** *see* Riboflavin *on page 1018*
- **Vitamin $B_6$** *see* Pyridoxine *on page 997*
- **Vitamin $B_{12}$** *see* Cyanocobalamin *on page 311*
- **Vitamin $B_{12a}$** *see* Hydroxocobalamin *on page 583*
- **Vitamin B Complex** *see page 1294*
- **Vitamin B Complex With Vitamin C** *see page 1294*
- **Vitamin B Complex With Vitamin C and Folic Acid** *see page 1294*
- **Vitamin C** *see* Ascorbic Acid *on page 108*
- **Vitamin $D_2$** *see* Ergocalciferol *on page 432*

## Vitamin E (VYE ta min ee)

**U.S. Brand Names** Amino-Opti-E® [OTC]; Aquasol E® [OTC]; E-Complex-600® [OTC]; E-Vitamin® [OTC]; Vita-Plus® E Softgels® [OTC]; Vitec® [OTC]; Vite E® Creme [OTC]

**Synonyms** *d*-Alpha Tocopherol; *dl*-Alpha Tocopherol

**Therapeutic Category** Vitamin, Fat Soluble

**Pregnancy Risk Factor** A/C (if dose exceeds RDA recommendation)

**Lactation** Excretion in breast milk unknown/compatible

**Use** Prevention and treatment hemolytic anemia secondary to vitamin E deficiency; dietary supplement; antioxidant (used to decrease atherosclerotic risk); prevention and treatment of tardive dyskinesia

**Mechanism of Action/Effect** Prevents oxidation of vitamin A and C; protects polyunsaturated fatty acids in membranes from attack by free radicals and protects red blood cells against hemolysis

**Contraindications** Hypersensitivity to vitamin E or any component

**Warnings** May induce vitamin K deficiency. Pregnancy factor C (if dose exceeds RDA recommendation).

**Drug Interactions**

**Decreased Effect:** Decreased absorption with mineral oil. Delayed absorption of iron.

**Increased Effect/Toxicity:** Vitamin E may increase the effect of oral anticoagulants.

**Adverse Reactions** <1% (Limited to important or life-threatening symptoms) (with large doses): Nausea, diarrhea, intestinal cramps, gonadal dysfunction

**Pharmacodynamics/Kinetics**

**Distribution:** To all body tissues, especially adipose tissue, where it is stored

**Metabolism:** Liver

**Excretion:** Feces

**Formulations**

Capsule: 100 units, 200 units, 330 mg, 400 units, 500 units, 600 units, 1000 units
Capsule, water miscible: 73.5 mg, 147 mg, 165 mg, 330 mg, 400 units
Cream: 50 mg/g (15 g, 30 g, 60 g, 75 g, 120 g, 454 g)
Drops, oral: 50 mg/mL (12 mL, 30 mL)
Liquid, topical: 10 mL, 15 mL, 30 mL, 60 mL
Lotion: 120 mL
Oil: 15 mL, 30 mL, 60 mL
Ointment, topical: 30 mg/g (45 g, 60 g)
Tablet: 200 units, 400 units

**Dosing**

**Adults:** One unit of vitamin E = 1 mg *dl*-alpha-tocopherol acetate. Oral:
- Vitamin E deficiency: 60-75 units/day
- Prevention of vitamin E deficiency: 30 units/day
- Retinopathy prophylaxis: 15-30 units/kg/day to maintain plasma levels between 1.5-2 μg/mL (may need as high as 100 units/kg/day)
- Cystic fibrosis, beta-thalassemia, sickle cell anemia may require higher daily maintenance doses:
  - Cystic fibrosis: 100-400 units/day
  - Beta-thalassemia: 750 units/day
- Sickle cell: 450 units/day
- Recommended daily allowance:
  - Male: 10 mg (15 units)
  - Female: 8 mg (12 units)
- Topical: Apply a thin layer over affected area

**Elderly:** Refer to adult dosing.

**Administration**

**Oral:** Swallow capsules whole, do not crush or chew.

**Stability**

**Storage:** Protect from light.

**Additional Nursing Issues**

**Physical Assessment:** Assess effectiveness and interactions of other medications (see Drug Interactions). Assess knowledge/teach patient appropriate use (according to formulation prescribed) and adverse symptoms to report. **Pregnancy risk factor A/C** - see Pregnancy Risk Factor for cautious use.

**Patient Information/Instruction:** Take exactly as directed; do not take more than the recommended dose. Do not use mineral oil or other vitamin E supplements without consulting prescriber. Report persistent nausea, vomiting, or cramping; or gonadal dysfunction.

- ♦ **Vitamin G** *see* Riboflavin *on page 1018*
- ♦ **Vitamin $K_1$** *see* Phytonadione *on page 929*

## Vitamin, Multiple (VYE ta min, MUL ti pul)

**U.S. Brand Names** Adeflor®; Allbee® With C; Becotin® Pulvules®; Berocca®; Cefol® Filmtab®; Chromagen® OB [OTC]; Eldercaps® [OTC]; Filibon® [OTC]; Florvite®; Iberet-Folic-500®; LKV-Drops® [OTC]; Mega-B® [OTC]; Multi Vit® Drops [OTC]; M.V.I.®; M.V.I.®-12; M.V.I.® Concentrate; M.V.I.® Pediatric; Natabec® [OTC]; Natabec® FA [OTC]; Natabec® Rx; Natalins® [OTC]; Natalins® Rx; NeoVadrin® [OTC]; Nephrocaps® [OTC]; Niferex®-PN; Poly-Vi-Flor®; Poly-Vi-Sol® [OTC]; Pramet® FA; Pramilet® FA; Prenavite® [OTC]; Secran®; Stresstabs® 600 Advanced Formula Tablets [OTC]; Stuartnatal® 1 + 1; Stuart Prenatal® [OTC]; Therabid® [OTC]; Theragran® [OTC]; Theragran® Hematinic®; Theragran® Liquid [OTC]; Theragran-M® [OTC]; Tri-Vi-Flor®; Unicap® [OTC]; Vicon Forte®; Vicon® Plus [OTC]; Vi-Daylin® [OTC]; Vi-Daylin/F®

**Synonyms** B Complex; B Complex With C; Children's Vitamins; Hexavitamin; Multiple Vitamins; Multivitamins/Fluoride; Parenteral Multiple Vitamin; Prenatal Vitamins; Therapeutic Multivitamins; Vitamin, Multiple, Prenatal; Vitamin, Multiple, Therapeutic; Vitamin, Multiple With Iron

**Therapeutic Category** Vitamin

**Pregnancy Risk Factor** A/C (if dose exceeds RDA recommendation)

**Lactation** Enters breast milk/compatible

**Use** Dietary supplement

**Contraindications** Hypersensitivity to product components

**Warnings** RDA values are not requirements, but are recommended daily intakes of certain essential nutrients. Periodic dental exams should be performed to check for dental fluorosis. Use with caution in patients with severe renal or liver failure. Pregnancy factor C (if dose exceeds RDA recommendation).

**Adverse Reactions** 1% to 10%: Hypervitaminosis; refer to individual vitamin entries for individual reactions

**Formulations** See table in Appendix on page 1465.

(Continued)

## Vitamin, Multiple *(Continued)*

**Dosing**

**Adults:**

Oral: 1 tablet/day or 5 mL/day liquid

I.V.: >11 years: 5 mL of vials 1 and 2 (M.V.I.®-12)/one TPN bag/day

I.V. solutions: 10 mL/24 hours (M.V.I.®-12)

**Note:** Doses may be higher for burn or cystic fibrosis patients.

**Elderly:** Refer to adult dosing.

**Additional Nursing Issues**

**Physical Assessment:** Assess knowledge/teach patient appropriate use. **Pregnancy risk factor A/C** - see Pregnancy Risk Factor for cautious use.

**Patient Information/Instruction:** Do not take more than the recommended dose.

- **Vitamin, Multiple, Prenatal** *see* Vitamin, Multiple *on previous page*
- **Vitamin, Multiple, Therapeutic** *see* Vitamin, Multiple *on previous page*
- **Vitamin, Multiple With Iron** *see* Vitamin, Multiple *on previous page*
- **Vita-Plus® E Softgels® [OTC]** *see* Vitamin E *on page 1218*
- **Vitec® [OTC]** *see* Vitamin E *on page 1218*
- **Vite E® Creme [OTC]** *see* Vitamin E *on page 1218*
- **Vito Reins®** *see* Phenazopyridine *on page 914*
- **Vitrasert®** *see* Ganciclovir *on page 526*
- **Vivactil®** *see* Protriptyline *on page 990*
- **Viva-Drops® Solution** *see page 1294*
- **Vivelle® Transdermal** *see* Estradiol *on page 441*
- **Vivol®** *see* Diazepam *on page 355*
- **V-Lax® [OTC]** *see* Psyllium *on page 993*
- **VLB** *see* Vinblastine *on page 1211*
- **VM-26** *see* Teniposide *on page 1101*
- **Volmax®** *see* Albuterol *on page 45*
- **Voltaren®** *see page 1282*
- **Voltaren® Ophthalmic** *see* Diclofenac *on page 358*
- **Voltaren® Oral** *see* Diclofenac *on page 358*
- **Voltaren Rapide®** *see* Diclofenac *on page 358*
- **Voltaren-XR® Oral** *see* Diclofenac *on page 358*
- **VoSol HC®** *see page 1291*
- **VoSol® Otic** *see page 1291*
- **VP-16** *see* Etoposide *on page 463*
- **Vumon Injection** *see* Teniposide *on page 1101*
- **V.V.S.®** *see* Sulfabenzamide, Sulfacetamide, and Sulfathiazole *on page 1079*
- **Vytone® Topical** *see* Iodoquinol and Hydrocortisone *on page 620*

## Warfarin (WAR far in)

**U.S. Brand Names** Coumadin®

**Therapeutic Category** Anticoagulant, Coumarin Derivative

**Pregnancy Risk Factor** D

**Lactation** Enters breast milk/use caution (AAP rates "compatible")

**Use** Prophylaxis and treatment of venous thrombosis, pulmonary embolism and thromboembolic disorders; atrial fibrillation with risk of embolism and as an adjunct in the prophylaxis of systemic embolism after myocardial infarction

**Unlabeled use:** Prevention of recurrent transient ischemic attacks and to reduce risk of recurrent myocardial infarction

**Mechanism of Action/Effect** Interferes with hepatic synthesis of vitamin K-dependent coagulation factors (II, VII, IX, X)

**Contraindications** Hypersensitivity to warfarin or any component; severe liver or kidney disease; open wounds; uncontrolled bleeding; GI ulcers; neurosurgical procedures; malignant hypertension; pregnancy; brain trauma; TB; threatened abortion

**Warnings** **Do not switch brands** once desired therapeutic response has been achieved. Use with caution in patients with active tuberculosis or diabetes or in patients with heparin-induced thrombocytopenia and deep venous thrombosis. Concomitant use with vitamin K may decrease anticoagulant effect; monitor carefully. Concomitant use with NSAIDs or aspirin may cause severe GI irritation and also increase the risk of bleeding due to impaired platelet function. Salicylates may further increase warfarin's effect by displacing it from plasma protein binding sites. Patients with protein C or S deficiency are at increased risk of skin necrosis syndrome. The risk for bleeding complications decreases with the duration of therapy and may increase with advancing age (see Geriatric Considerations). If a patient is to undergo an invasive surgical procedure (dental to actual minor/major surgery), warfarin should be stopped 3 days before the scheduled surgery date and the INR/PT should be checked prior to the procedure.

**Drug Interactions**

**Cytochrome P-450 Effect:** CYP1A2 enzyme substrate (minor), CYP2C8, 2C9, 2C18, 2C19, and 3A3/4 enzyme substrate; CYP2C9 enzyme inhibitor

**Decreased Effect:** Decreased anticoagulant effect may occur when the drugs listed in the following table are administered with oral anticoagulants. See table.

**Increased Effect/Toxicity:** See tables.

**Food Interactions** The anticoagulant effects of warfarin may be decreased if taken with foods rich in vitamin K.

**Drugs That May Decrease Anticoagulant Effect When Administered With Oral Anticoagulants**

| Increased Warfarin Metabolism | Increased Procoagulant Factors | Decreased Drug Absorption | Other |
|---|---|---|---|
| Barbiturates<br>Carbamazepine<br>Glutethimide<br>Griseofulvin<br>Nafcillin<br>Phenytoin<br>Rifampin | Estrogens<br>Oral contraceptives<br>Vitamin K (including nutritional supplements) | Aluminum hydroxide<br>Cholestyramine*<br>Colestipol* | Ethchlorvynol<br>Griseofulvin<br>Spironolactone†<br>Sucralfate |

*Cholestyramine and colestipol may increase the anticoagulant effect by binding vitamin K in the gut; yet, the decreased drug absorption appears to be of more concern.

†Diuretic-induced hemoconcentration with subsequent concentration of clotting factors has been reported to decrease the effects of oral anticoagulants.

**Agents That May Increase Bleeding Tendency When Used With Oral Anticoagulants**

| Inhibit Platelet Aggregation | Inhibit Procoagulant Factors | Ulcerogenic Drugs |
|---|---|---|
| Cephalosporins<br>Clopidogrel<br>Dipyridamole<br>Indomethacin<br>Oxyphenbutazone<br>Penicillin, parenteral<br>Phenylbutazone<br>Salicylates<br>Sulfinpyrazone<br>Ticlopidine | Antimetabolites<br>Quinidine<br>Quinine<br>Salicylates | Adrenal corticosteroids<br>Indomethacin<br>Oxyphenbutazone<br>Phenylbutazone<br>Potassium products<br>Salicylates |

**Enhanced Anticoagulant Effects**

| Decrease Vitamin K | Displace Anticoagulant | Inhibit Metabolism | Other |
|---|---|---|---|
| Oral antibiotics: Can ↑/↓ INR Check INR 3 days after a patient begins antibiotics to see the INR value and adjust the warfarin dose accordingly | Chloral hydrate<br>Clofibrate<br>Diazoxide<br>Ethacrynic acid<br>Miconazole<br>Nalidixic acid<br>Phenylbutazone<br>Salicylates<br>Sulfonamides<br>Sulfonylureas<br>Triclofos | Alcohol (acute ingestion)*<br>Allopurinol<br>Amiodarone<br>Chloramphenicol<br>Chlorpropamide<br>Cimetidine<br>Ciprofloxacin<br>Co-trimoxazole<br>Disulfiram<br>Fluconazole<br>Flutamide<br>Isoniazid<br>Itraconazole<br>Metronidazole<br>Omperazole<br>Phenylbutazone<br>Phenytoin<br>Propafenone<br>Propoxyphene<br>Quinidine<br>Sulfinpyrazone<br>Sulfonamides<br>Tamoxifen<br>Tolbutamide<br>Zafirlukast<br>Zileuton | Acetaminophen<br>Anabolic steroids<br>Clofibrate<br>Danazol<br>Erythromycin<br>Gemfibrozil<br>Glucagon<br>Influenza vaccine<br>Ketoconazole<br>Piroxicam<br>Propranolol<br>Ranitidine<br>Sulindac<br>Tetracycline<br>Thyroid drugs |

* The hypoprothrombinemic effect of oral anticoagulants has been reported to be both increased and decreased during chronic and excessive alcohol ingestion. Data are insufficient to predict the direction of this interaction in alcoholic patients.

**Effects on Lab Values** Warfarin ↑ PTT

**Adverse Reactions**

1% to 10%:

Dermatologic: Skin lesions, alopecia, skin necrosis

Gastrointestinal: Anorexia, nausea, vomiting, stomach cramps, diarrhea

Hematologic: Hemorrhage, leukopenia, unrecognized bleeding sites (eg, colon cancer) may be uncovered by anticoagulation

Respiratory: Hemoptysis

<1% (Limited to important or life-threatening symptoms): Adrenal insufficiency, agranulocytosis, hepatotoxicity, renal damage

**Overdose/Toxicology** See table. Symptoms of overdose include internal or external hemorrhage and hematuria. Avoid emesis and lavage to avoid possible trauma and incidental bleeding. When an overdose occurs, the drug should be immediately discontinued and vitamin $K_1$ (phytonadione) may be administered, up to 25 mg I.V. for adults. (Continued)

## Warfarin *(Continued)*

When hemorrhage occurs, fresh frozen plasma transfusions can help control bleeding by replacing clotting factors. In urgent bleeding, prothrombin complex concentrates may be needed.

**Management of Elevated INR**

| INR | Patient Situation | Action |
|---|---|---|
| >3 and ≤5 | No bleeding or need for rapid reversal (ie, no need for surgery) | Omit next warfarin dose and/or restart at lower dose when INR approaches desired range. |
| >5 and <9 | No bleeding or need for rapid reversal | Omit next 1-2 doses, monitor INR more frequently and restart at lower dose when INR approaches target range **or** omit dose and give 1-2.5 mg vitamin K orally. |
| | No bleeding but reversal needed for surgery within 24 hours | Vitamin K 2-4 mg orally (expected reversal within 24 hours). Give additional 1-2 mg if INR remains high at 24 hours. |
| >9 and <20.0 | No bleeding | Stop warfarin, give phytonadione 3-5 mg orally. Check INR every 6-12 hours; repeat phytonadione if needed. Reassess need and dose of warfarin (reduction in 24-48 hours). |
| Rapid reversal required (ie, INR >20) | Serious bleeding or warfarin overdose | Stop warfarin, give phytonadione 10 mg I.V. Check INR every 6 hours, if needed, repeat phytonadione every 12 hours and give plasma transfusion or factor concentrate. Consider giving heparin if warfarin still indicated. |

From Fifth ACCP Consensus Conference on Antithrombotic Therapy.

**Pharmacodynamics/Kinetics**

**Half-life Elimination:** 3-5 days, highly variable among individuals

**Metabolism:** Liver

**Onset:** Onset of anticoagulation effect: Oral: Within 36-72 hours; Peak effect: Within 5-7 days; INR may increase within 36-72 hours; full therapeutic effect is not established until 5-7 days

**Formulations**

Warfarin sodium:

Powder for reconstitution, lyophilized: 2 mg, 5 mg

Tablet: 1 mg, 2 mg, 2.5 mg, 4 mg, 5 mg, 7.5 mg, 10 mg

**Dosing**

**Adults:**

Oral: 5-15 mg/day for 2-5 days, then adjust dose according to results of prothrombin time; usual maintenance dose ranges from 2-10 mg/day.

I.V. (administer as a slow bolus injection): 2-5 mg/day

**Elderly:** Oral: Usual maintenance dose: 2-5 mg/day

**Hepatic Impairment:** Monitor effect at usual doses. The response to oral anticoagulants may be markedly enhanced in obstructive jaundice, hepatitis, and cirrhosis. Prothrombin index should be closely monitored.

**Administration**

**Oral:** Do not take with food. Take at the same time each day.

**I.V.:** Administer as a slow bolus injection over 1-2 minutes. Avoid all I.M. injections.

**Stability**

**Storage:** Protect from light.

**Reconstitution:** Injection is stable for 4 hours at room temperature after reconstitution with 2.7 mL of sterile water.

**Monitoring Laboratory Tests** Prothrombin time (desirable range usually 1.5-2 times the control), hematocrit, INR (desirable range usually 2.0-3.0 with standard therapy, 2.5-3.5 with high-dose therapy)

**Additional Nursing Issues**

**Physical Assessment:** Assess effectiveness and interactions of other medications (see Drug Interactions). See Warnings/Precautions and Contraindications for use cautions. Monitor effectiveness of therapy, laboratory tests (see above) and adverse response (eg, thrombolytic reactions - see Adverse Reactions and Overdose/Toxicology). Assess knowledge/teach patient appropriate use, possible side effects and appropriate interventions (eg, bleeding precautions), and adverse symptoms to report. **Pregnancy risk factor D** - assess knowledge/teach appropriate use of barrier contraceptives. Note breast-feeding caution.

**Patient Information/Instruction:** Take exactly as directed; if dose is missed, take as soon as possible. Do not double doses. Do not take any medication your prescriber is not aware of and follow diet and activity as recommended by prescriber. You may have a tendency to bleed easily while taking this drug; brush teeth with soft brush, floss with waxed floss, use electric razor, and avoid scissors or sharp knives and potentially harmful activities. You may experience nausea or vomiting (small frequent meals, frequent mouth care, sucking lozenges, or chewing gum may help). May discolor urine or stool. Report skin rash or irritation, unusual fever, persistent nausea or GI upset, unusual bleeding or bruising (bleeding gums, nosebleed, blood in urine, dark stool, bloody emesis), pain in joints or back, swelling or pain at injection site.

**Pregnancy/breast-feeding precautions:** Do not get pregnant while taking this medication; use appropriate barrier contraceptive measures. Consult prescriber if breast-feeding.

**Dietary Issues:** Vitamin K can reverse the anticoagulation effects of warfarin. Large amounts of food high in vitamin K (such as green leafy vegetables) may reverse effects of warfarin, decrease prothrombin time, and lead to therapeutic failure. High doses of vitamin A, E, or C may alter PT.

**Geriatric Considerations:** Before committing an elderly patient to long-term anticoagulation therapy, their risk for bleeding complications secondary to falls, drug interactions, living situation, and cognitive status should be considered. A risk of bleeding complications has been associated with increased age.

**Related Information**

Peak and Trough Guidelines *on page 1331*


- **Warfilone®** *see* Warfarin *on page 1220*
- **Wart-Off®** *see page 1294*
- **4-Way® Long Acting Nasal Solution** *see page 1294*
- **Waytrax** *see* Ceftazidime *on page 228*
- **Wellbutrin®** *see* Bupropion *on page 169*
- **Wellcovorin®** *see* Leucovorin *on page 662*
- **Westcort®** *see* Hydrocortisone *on page 578*
- **Westcort®** *see* Topical Corticosteroids *on page 1152*
- **Whitfield's Ointment** *see page 1294*
- **Wigraine®** *see* Ergotamine Derivatives *on page 434*
- **Wimpred** *see* Prednisone *on page 962*
- **Winasorb** *see* Acetaminophen *on page 32*
- **40 Winks® [OTC]** *see* Diphenhydramine *on page 381*
- **WinRho SD®** *see page 1256*
- **Winstrol®** *see* Stanozolol *on page 1071*
- **Witch Hazel** *see page 1294*
- **Wyamine® Sulfate Injection** *see page 1248*
- **Wycillin®** *see* Penicillin G Procaine *on page 899*
- **Wydase® Injection** *see* Hyaluronidase *on page 563*
- **Wygesic®** *see* Propoxyphene and Acetaminophen *on page 985*
- **Wymox®** *see* Amoxicillin *on page 80*
- **Xalatan® Ophthalmic** *see* Ophthalmic Agents, Glaucoma *on page 853*
- **Xanax®** *see* Alprazolam *on page 55*
- **Xeloda™** *see* Capecitabine *on page 189*
- **Xenical®** *see* Orlistat *on page 863*
- **Xero-Lube®** *see page 1294*
- **Xitocin** *see* Oxytocin *on page 877*
- **X-Prep® Liquid** *see page 1294*
- **X-seb® T Shampoo** *see page 1294*
- **Xylocaina** *see* Lidocaine *on page 674*
- **Xylocaina** *see* Lidocaine and Epinephrine *on page 677*
- **Xylocaine®** *see* Lidocaine *on page 674*
- **Xylocaine® With Epinephrine** *see* Lidocaine and Epinephrine *on page 677*
- **Xylocard®** *see* Lidocaine *on page 674*
- **Xylometazoline** *see page 1294*
- **Xylo-Pfan® [OTC]** *see page 1248*
- **Yeast-Gard® Medicated Douche** *see page 1294*
- **Yectamicina** *see* Gentamicin *on page 531*
- **Yectamid** *see* Amikacin *on page 65*
- **Yellow Fever Vaccine** *see page 1256*
- **Yodoxin®** *see* Iodoquinol *on page 619*
- **Yutopar®** *see* Ritodrine *on page 1029*


## Zafirlukast (za FIR loo kast)

**U.S. Brand Names** Accolate®

**Synonyms** ICI 204, 219

**Therapeutic Category** Leukotriene Receptor Antagonist

**Pregnancy Risk Factor** B

**Lactation** Enters breast milk/contraindicated

**Mechanism of Action/Effect** Cysteinyl leukotriene production and receptor occupation have been correlated with the pathophysiology of asthma, including airway edema, smooth muscle constriction, and altered cellular activity associated with the inflammatory process, which contribute to the signs and symptoms of asthma. Leukotrienes are inflammatory mediators of asthma. Zafirlukast blocks leukotriene receptors and is able to reduce bronchoconstriction and inflammatory cell infiltration.

**Contraindications** Hypersensitivity to zafirlukast or any component

**Warnings** Not indicated for use in reversal of bronchospasm in acute asthma attacks, including status asthmaticus. Concomitant administration of zafirlukast and warfarin causes a clinically significant increase in prothrombin time (PT). Monitor patient's PT/INR closely. The clearance of zafirlukast is reduced in patients with stable alcoholic cirrhosis such that the $C_{max}$ and AUC are approximately 50% to 60% greater than those of normal

(Continued)

## Zafirlukast *(Continued)*

adults. May cause hepatitis/hyperbilirubinemia, which may progress to hepatic failure (rarely). Reduction of steroid dose in patients on zafirlukast has been associated with Churg-Strauss syndrome (eosinophilic vasculitis); use caution when reducing steroid dose.

**Drug Interactions**

**Cytochrome P-450 Effect:** CYP2C9 enzyme substrate; CYP2C9 and 3A3/4 enzyme inhibitor

**Decreased Effect:**

Aspirin: Coadministration with zafirlukast increased serum zafirlukast levels by ~45%.

Erythromycin: Coadministration of a single dose of zafirlukast with erythromycin to steady-state results in decreased mean plasma levels of zafirlukast by 40% due to a decrease in zafirlukast bioavailability.

Terfenadine: Coadministration of zafirlukast with terfenadine to steady-state results in a decrease in the mean $C_{max}$ (66%) and AUC (54%) of zafirlukast. No effect of zafirlukast on terfenadine plasma concentrations or EKG parameters was seen.

Theophylline: Coadministration of zafirlukast at steady-state with a single dose of liquid theophylline preparations results in decreased mean plasma levels of zafirlukast by 30%, but no effects on plasma theophylline levels were observed. However, postmarketing reports of increased theophylline levels have occurred.

**Increased Effect/Toxicity:** Zafirlukast is an inhibitor of the cytochrome P-450 2C9 and 3A4 isoenzyme pathways. Concomitant administration of zafirlukast and warfarin results in a 35% increase of PT. Studies with other drugs metabolized by the 2C9 or 3A4 pathways have not been studied and should be administered with caution in patients on zafirlukast. Postmarketing reports of increased theophylline levels after addition of zafirlukast to an existing regimen have been made.

**Adverse Reactions**

>10%: Central nervous system: Headache (12.9%)

1% to 10%:

Central nervous system: Dizziness, pain, fever
Gastrointestinal: Nausea, diarrhea, abdominal pain, vomiting, dyspepsia
Hepatic: SGPT elevation (1.5%)
Neuromuscular & skeletal: Myalgia, weakness, back pain

<1% (Limited to important or life-threatening symptoms): Elevated liver enzymes, hepatitis, hyperbilirubinemia, hepatic failure, eosinophilia, vasculitic rash, cardiac complications, neuropathy, hypersensitivity reactions as urticaria and rashes with or without blistering, angioedema, eosinophilic vasculitis (Churg-Strauss syndrome), agranulocytosis, bleeding, bruising, edema.

**Overdose/Toxicology** There is no experience with overdose in humans to date. Treatment is supportive.

**Pharmacodynamics/Kinetics**

**Protein Binding:** >99% bound, primarily to albumin

**Half-life Elimination:** 10 hours

**Time to Peak:** 3 hours

**Metabolism:** Liver

**Excretion:** Feces and urine

**Formulations** Tablet: Oral: 20 mg

**Dosing**

**Adults:** 20 mg twice daily

**Elderly:** The mean dose (mg/kg) normalized AUC and $C_{max}$ increase and plasma clearance decreases with increasing age. In patients >65 years of age, there is a two- to threefold greater $C_{max}$ and AUC compared to younger adults.

**Hepatic Impairment:** Clearance of zafirlukast is reduced with a greater $C_{max}$ and AUC of 50% to 60% in patients with alcoholic cirrhosis.

**Administration**

**Oral:** Take 1 hour before or 2 hours after meals.

**Additional Nursing Issues**

**Physical Assessment:** Not for use in acute asthma attack. Assess effectiveness and interactions of other medications (especially drugs affected by P-450 enzymes - see Drug Interactions). See Contraindications and Warnings/Precautions for cautious use. Monitor effectiveness of therapy and adverse reactions (see Adverse Reactions) at beginning of therapy and periodically with long-term use. Assess knowledge/teach patient appropriate use, interventions to reduce side effects, and adverse symptoms to report. Breast-feeding is contraindicated.

**Patient Information/Instruction:** Do not use during acute bronchospasm. Take regularly as prescribed, even during symptom-free periods. Do not take more than recommended or discontinue use without consulting prescriber. Do not stop taking other antiasthmatic medications unless instructed by prescriber. Avoid aspirin or aspirin-containing medications unless approved by prescriber. You may experience headache, drowsiness, dizziness, or blurred vision (use caution when driving or engaging in tasks requiring alertness until response to drug is known); gastric upset, nausea, or vomiting (small frequent meals, frequent mouth care, chewing gum, or sucking lozenges may help). Report persistent CNS or GI symptoms; muscle or back pain; weakness, fever, chills; yellowing of skin or eyes; dark urine, or pale stool; skin rash; or worsening of condition. **Breast-feeding precautions:** Do not breast-feed.

◆ **Zagam®** *see* Sparfloxacin *on page 1068*

## Zalcitabine (zal SITE a been)

**U.S. Brand Names** Hivid®

**Synonyms** ddC; Dideoxycytidine

**Therapeutic Category** Antiretroviral Agent, Reverse Transcriptase Inhibitor (Nucleoside)

**Pregnancy Risk Factor** C

**Lactation** Enters breast milk/contraindicated

**Use** Treatment in HIV-infected adults with advanced disease who cannot tolerate zidovudine or whose disease has progressed despite it; treatment of selected patients with advanced AIDS in combination with antiretroviral agents

**Mechanism of Action/Effect** Inhibits cell protein synthesis leading to cell death with viral replication.

**Contraindications** Hypersensitivity to zalcitabine or any component

**Warnings** Approved for use in combination with antiretroviral agents. Careful monitoring of pancreatic enzymes and liver function tests in patients with a history of pancreatitis, increased amylase, those on parenteral nutrition, or with a history of ethanol abuse is necessary. Discontinue use immediately if pancreatitis is suspected. Lactic acidosis and severe hepatomegaly and failure, possibly related to underlying hepatitis B, have rarely occurred with zalcitabine resulting in fatality. Use with caution in patients on digitalis, congestive heart failure, renal failure, hyperphosphatemia. Zalcitabine can cause severe peripheral neuropathy; avoid use, if possible, in patients with pre-existing neuropathy. Pregnancy factor C.

**Drug Interactions**

**Increased Effect/Toxicity:** Amphotericin, foscarnet, and aminoglycosides may potentiate the risk of developing peripheral neuropathy or other toxicities associated with zalcitabine by interfering with the renal elimination of zalcitabine. Other drugs associated with peripheral neuropathy include chloramphenicol, cisplatin, dapsone, disulfiram, ethionamide, glutethimide, gold, hydralazine, iodoquinol, isoniazid, metronidazole, nitrofurantoin, phenytoin, ribavirin, and vincristine. Concomitant use with zalcitabine may increase risk of peripheral neuropathy. Concomitant use of zalcitabine with didanosine is not recommended.

**Food Interactions** Food decreases peak plasma concentrations by 39%.

**Effects on Lab Values** May cause abnormalities in CBC, WBC, hemoglobin, platelet count, AST, ALT, or alkaline phosphatase.

**Adverse Reactions**

>10%:

Central nervous system: Fever (5% to 17%), malaise (2% to 13%)

Neuromuscular & skeletal: Peripheral neuropathy (28.3%)

1% to 10%:

Central nervous system: Headache (2.1%), dizziness (1.1%), fatigue (3.8%), seizures (1.3%)

Endocrine & metabolic: Hypoglycemia (1.8% to 6.3%), hyponatremia (3.5%), hyperglycemia (1% to 6%)

Hematologic: Anemia (occurs as early as 2-4 weeks), granulocytopenia (usually after 6-8 weeks)

Dermatologic: Rash (2% to 11%), pruritus (3% to 5%)

Gastrointestinal: Nausea (3%), dysphagia (1% to 4%), anorexia (3.9%), abdominal pain (3% to 8%), vomiting (1% to 3%), diarrhea (0.4% to 9.5%), weight loss, oral ulcers (3% to 7%), increased amylase (3% to 8%)

Hepatic: Abnormal hepatic function (8.9%), hyperbilirubinemia (2% to 5%)

Neuromuscular & skeletal: Myalgia (1% to 6%), foot pain

Respiratory: Pharyngitis (1.8%), cough (6.3%), nasal discharge (3.5%)

<1% (Limited to important or life-threatening symptoms): Edema, hypertension, palpitations, syncope, atrial fibrillation, tachycardia, heart racing, chest pain, night sweats, pain, hypocalcemia, constipation, pancreatitis, jaundice, hepatitis, hepatomegaly, hepatic failure, myositis, weakness, epistaxis

**Overdose/Toxicology** Symptoms of overdose include delayed peripheral neurotoxicity. Treatment is supportive.

**Pharmacodynamics/Kinetics**

**Protein Binding:** Minimal, 1% to 2%

**Half-life Elimination:** 2.9 hours

**Metabolism:** Intracellularly to active triphosphorylated agent; no significant hepatic metabolism

**Excretion:** Urine

**Formulations** Tablet: 0.375 mg, 0.75 mg

**Dosing**

**Adults:**

Combination therapy: 0.75 mg every 8 hours, given together with 200 mg of zidovudine (ie, total daily dose: 2.25 mg of zalcitabine and 600 mg of zidovudine). If zalcitabine is permanently discontinued or interrupted due to toxicities, decrease zidovudine dose to 100 mg every 4 hours.

**Dosing adjustment in peripheral neuropathy:** Zalcitabine should be discontinued in patients developing peripheral neuropathy. The drug may be restarted at 50% of the dose every 8 hours only if all findings related to the neuropathy improve to the point of classification as mild symptomatology. Therapy must be permanently discontinued if severe symptoms occur. **Note:** Zalcitabine-associated peripheral neuropathy may continue to worsen despite interruption of therapy.

**Dosing adjustment in hematologic toxicities:** Zalcitabine may need to be discontinued in patients with poor bone marrow reserve if significant anemia (Hgb = 7.5/dL

(Continued)

## Zalcitabine *(Continued)*

or a reduction >25% from baseline) or granulocytopenia (granulocyte count <750/ mm$^3$ or a reduction >50% from baseline) occur. Therapy should not be restarted until evidence of marrow recovery is obvious. For less severe blood dyscrasias, a reduction in the zidovudine dose may be adequate. Dose modification in patients who develop significant anemia, may not eliminate the need for transfusion. If recovery of the marrow does occur, however, gradual increases in dose may be tolerated.

**Renal Impairment:** Since renal excretion appears to be the major route of elimination, zalcitabine's elimination may be prolonged in patients with poor renal function.

$Cl_{cr}$ 10-40 mL/minute: Daily dose may be adjusted to 0.75 mg every 12 hours.
$Cl_{cr}$ <10 mL/minute: Further reduce dose to 0.75 mg every 24 hours.
Hemodialysis effects: Hemodialysis reduces plasma levels by 50%.

**Hepatic Impairment:**

Zalcitabine could possibly exacerbate existing liver dysfunction in patients with a previous history of liver disease or alcohol abuse. An elevation of liver function tests was observed in patients on zalcitabine therapy. Caution should be exercised in patients with hepatic impairment. Suspend treatment in patients who develop findings suggestive of lactic acidosis or hepatotoxicity. Hepatic failure and death have occurred possibly related to underlying hepatitis B.

If other moderate to severe adverse effects occur, such as increased LFTs, therapy with zalcitabine or both zalcitabine and zidovudine, in combination therapy, should be discontinued until the reaction resolves. Treatment may be restarted at lower doses. If the reaction recurs, discontinue therapy completely.

**Administration**

**Oral:** Food decreases absorption; take on an empty stomach. Administer around-the-clock. Do not take at the same time with dapsone.

**Stability**

**Storage:** Tablets should be stored in tightly closed bottles at room temperature (59°F to 86°F)

**Monitoring Laboratory Tests** CBC and serum chemistry (prior to initiation and appropriate intervals), renal function, CD4 counts, serum amylase, triglyceride, calcium (see Zidovudine monograph)

**Additional Nursing Issues**

**Physical Assessment:** Note Warnings/Precautions. Assess other medications patient may be taking for possible interactions (see Drug Interactions). Monitor for effectiveness of therapy and adverse reactions (see Adverse Reactions). Instruct patient on appropriate use, possible side effects and interventions, and symptoms to report. **Pregnancy risk factor C** - benefits of use should outweigh possible risks. Breast-feeding is contraindicated.

**Patient Information/Instruction:** Zalcitabine is not a cure for AIDS, nor has it been found to reduce transmission of AIDS. Take as directed, preferably on an empty stomach (1 hour before or 2 hours after meals). Take around-the-clock; do not take with other medications. You may experience headache or insomnia; if these persist notify prescriber. Report chest pain, palpitations, or rapid heartbeat; swelling of extremities; weight gain or loss >5 lb/week; signs of infection (eg, fever, chills, sore throat, burning urination, fatigue); unusual bleeding (eg, tarry stools, easy bruising, or blood in stool, urine, or mouth); pain, tingling, or numbness of toes or fingers; skin rash or irritation; or muscles weakness or tremors. **Pregnancy/breast-feeding precautions:** Inform prescriber if you are or intend to be pregnant. Do not breast-feed.

**Breast-feeding Issues:** The CDC recommends **not** to breast-feed if diagnosed with HIV to avoid postnatal transmission of the virus.

**Related Information**

Antiretroviral Agents Comparison *on page 1373*

- **Zamacort®** *see* Triamcinolone *on page 1171*
- **Zamtirel** *see* Salmeterol *on page 1040*
- **Zanosar®** *see* Streptozocin *on page 1077*
- **Zantac®** *see* Ranitidine *on page 1008*
- **Zantac® 75 [OTC]** *see* Ranitidine *on page 1008*
- **Zapex®** *see* Oxazepam *on page 868*
- **Zarontin®** *see* Ethosuximide *on page 461*
- **Zaroxolyn®** *see* Metolazone *on page 759*
- **Zeasorb-AF® Powder [OTC]** *see* Miconazole *on page 767*
- **Zebeta®** *see* Bisoprolol *on page 155*
- **Zefazone®** *see* Cefmetazole *on page 217*
- **Zemplar™** *see* Paricalcitol *on page 886*
- **Zemuron®** *see page 1248*
- **Zephiran®** *see page 1294*
- **Zephrex®** *see* Guaifenesin and Pseudoephedrine *on page 551*
- **Zephrex LA®** *see* Guaifenesin and Pseudoephedrine *on page 551*
- **Zerit®** *see* Stavudine *on page 1073*
- **Zestoretic® 10-12.5** *see* Lisinopril and Hydrochlorothiazide *on page 683*
- **Zestoretic® 20-12.5** *see* Lisinopril and Hydrochlorothiazide *on page 683*
- **Zestoretic® 20-25** *see* Lisinopril and Hydrochlorothiazide *on page 683*
- **Zestril®** *see* Lisinopril *on page 681*
- **Zetar®** *see page 1294*
- **Ziac™** *see* Bisoprolol and Hydrochlorothiazide *on page 156*

♦ **Ziagen®** *see* Abacavir *on page 28*

## Zidovudine (zye DOE vyoo deen)

**U.S. Brand Names** Retrovir®

**Synonyms** Azidothymidine; AZT; Compound S

**Therapeutic Category** Antiretroviral Agent, Reverse Transcriptase Inhibitor (Nucleoside)

**Pregnancy Risk Factor** C

**Lactation** Enters breast milk/contraindicated

**Use** Management of patients with HIV infections who have had at least one episode of *Pneumocystis carinii* pneumonia or who have CD4 cell counts ≤500/mm$^3$; patients who have HIV-related symptoms or who are asymptomatic with abnormal laboratory values indicating HIV-related immunosuppression; prevention of maternal/fetal HIV transmission in a subpopulation of HIV-infected women and their offspring (recommended for HIV-infected women with CD4+ cell counts >200/mm$^3$), no prior history of extensive zidovudine administration, no clinical indication for antiretroviral therapy and whose pregnancy is between 14 and 34 weeks' gestation when therapy is initiated; in combination therapy with other nucleosides such as zalcitabine

**Mechanism of Action/Effect** Zidovudine is a thymidine analog which interferes with the HIV virus that results in inhibition of viral replication.

**Contraindications** Life-threatening hypersensitivity to zidovudine or any component

**Warnings** Use with caution in patients with impaired renal or hepatic function. Reduce dosage or interrupt therapy in patients with anemia and/or granulocytopenia and myopathy. Often associated with hematologic toxicity including granulocytopenia, thrombocytopenia, and severe anemia requiring transfusions. Zidovudine has been shown to be carcinogenic in rats and mice. Pregnancy factor C.

**Drug Interactions**

**Cytochrome P-450 Effect:** CYP3A3/4 enzyme substrate

**Increased Effect/Toxicity:** Coadministration with drugs that are nephrotoxic (amphotericin B), cytotoxic (flucytosine, vincristine, vinblastine, doxorubicin, interferon), inhibit glucuronidation or excretion (acetaminophen, cimetidine, indomethacin, lorazepam, probenecid, aspirin), or interfere with RBC/WBC number or function (acyclovir, ganciclovir, pentamidine, dapsone). Although the AUC was unaffected, the rate of absorption and peak plasma concentrations were increased significantly when zidovudine was administered with clarithromycin (n=18). Valproic acid increased AZT's AUC by 80% and decreased clearance by 38% (believed due to inhibition first pass metabolism).

**Food Interactions** Zidovudine serum levels may be decreased if taken with food.

**Adverse Reactions**

>10%:

Central nervous system: Severe headache (42%), fever (16%)

Dermatologic: Rash (17%)

Gastrointestinal: Nausea (46% to 61%), anorexia (11%), diarrhea (17%), pain (20%), vomiting (6% to 25%)

Hematologic: Anemia (23% in children), leukopenia, granulocytopenia (39% in children)

Neuromuscular & skeletal: Weakness (19%)

1% to 10%:

Central nervous system: Malaise (8%), dizziness (6%), insomnia (5%), somnolence (8%)

Dermatologic: Hyperpigmentation of nails (bluish-brown)

Gastrointestinal: Dyspepsia (5%)

Hematologic: Changes in platelet count

Neuromuscular & skeletal: Paresthesia (6%)

<1% (Limited to important or life-threatening symptoms): Neurotoxicity, confusion, mania, seizures, bone marrow suppression, granulocytopenia, thrombocytopenia, pancytopenia, hepatotoxicity, cholestatic jaundice, tenderness, myopathy

**Overdose/Toxicology** Symptoms of overdose include nausea, vomiting, ataxia, and granulocytopenia. Erythropoietin, thymidine, and cyanocobalamin have been used experimentally to treat zidovudine-induced hematopoietic toxicity, yet none are presently specified as the agent of choice. Treatment is supportive.

**Pharmacodynamics/Kinetics**

**Protein Binding:** 25% to 38%

**Half-life Elimination:** Terminal: 60 minutes

**Metabolism:** Liver

**Excretion:** Urine

**Formulations**

Capsule: 100 mg

Injection: 10 mg/mL (20 mL)

Syrup (strawberry flavor): 50 mg/5 mL (240 mL)

Tablet: 300 mg

**Dosing**

**Adults:**

Prevention of maternal-fetal HIV transmission: Maternal (>14 weeks gestation): Oral: 100 mg 5 times/day until the start of labor. During labor and delivery, administer zidovudine I.V. at 2 mg/kg over 1 hour followed by a continuous I.V. infusion of 1 mg/kg/hour until the umbilical cord is clamped.

Asymptomatic HIV infection:

Oral: 100 mg every 4 hours while awake (500 mg/day)

(Continued)

## Zidovudine *(Continued)*

Symptomatic HIV infection:

Oral: Initial: 200 mg every 4 hours (1200 mg/day), then after 1 month, 100 mg every 4 hours (600 mg/day)

I.V.: 1-2 mg/kg/dose (infused over 1 hour) administered every 4 hours around-the-clock (6 doses/day)

**Patients should receive I.V. therapy only until oral therapy can be administered.**

Combination therapy with zalcitabine: Oral: 200 mg with zalcitabine 0.75 mg every 8 hours

**Dosage adjustment in anemia/granulocytopenia:**

Significant anemia (hemoglobin <7.5 g/dL or reduction >25% of baseline) or significant granulocytopenia (granulocyte count <750/mm$^3$ or reduction >50% from baseline) may require a dose interruption until evidence of marrow recovery is observed.

For less severe anemia or granulocytopenia, dose reduction may be adequate.

See also Zalcitabine monograph regarding dosage adjustment in combination therapy.

**Renal Impairment:**

$Cl_{cr}$ <10 mL/minute: May require minor dosing adjustment

Hemodialysis effects: At least partially removed by hemodialysis and peritoneal dialysis; administer dose after hemodialysis or administer 100 mg supplemental dose. During CAPD, dose as for $Cl_{cr}$ <10 mL/minute. During continuous arteriovenous or venovenous hemofiltration (CAVH/CAVHD), may require minor dosing adjustment (100 mg every 8 hours)

**Hepatic Impairment:** Reduce dose by 50% or double dosing interval in patients with cirrhosis.

**Administration**

**Oral:** Administer around-the-clock to promote less variation in peak and trough serum levels. Oral zidovudine should be administered 1 hour before or 2 hours after a meal with a glass of water.

**I.M.:** Do not give I.M.

**I.V.:** Infuse over 1 hour. Avoid rapid infusion or bolus injection.

**Stability**

**Storage:** Store undiluted vials at room temperature and protect from light.

**Reconstitution:** After dilution to ≤4 mg/mL, the solution is physically and chemically stable for 24 hours at room temperature and 48 hours if refrigerated. Attempt to administer diluted solution within 8 hours, if stored at room temperature or 24 hours if refrigerated to minimize potential for microbially contaminated solutions.

**Compatibility:** Incompatible with blood products and protein solutions.

**Monitoring Laboratory Tests** Monitor CBC and platelet count at least every 2 weeks, MCV, serum creatinine kinase, CD4 cell count

**Additional Nursing Issues**

**Physical Assessment:** Note Warnings/Precautions. Assess other medications patient may be taking for possible interactions (see Drug Interactions). Monitor for effectiveness of therapy and adverse reactions (see Adverse Reactions). Instruct patient on appropriate use, possible side effects and interventions, and symptoms to report. **Pregnancy risk factor C** - benefits of use should outweigh possible risks. Breast-feeding is contraindicated.

**Patient Information/Instruction:** Zidovudine is not a cure for AIDS, nor has it been found to reduce transmission of AIDS. Take as directed, preferably on an empty stomach (1 hour before or 2 hours after meals). Take around-the-clock; do not take with other medications. Take precautions to avoid transmission to others. You may experience headache or insomnia; if these persist notify prescriber. Report unresolved nausea or vomiting; signs of infection (eg, fever, chills, sore throat, burning urination, flu-like symptoms, fatigue); unusual bleeding (eg, tarry stools, easy bruising, or blood in stool, urine, or mouth); pain, tingling, or numbness of toes or fingers; skin rash or irritation; or muscles weakness or tremors. **Pregnancy/breast-feeding precautions:** Inform prescriber if you are or intend to be pregnant. Do not breast-feed.

**Dietary Issues:** Folate or vitamin $B_{12}$ deficiency increases zidovudine-associated myelosuppression.

**Breast-feeding Issues:** The CDC recommends **not** to breast-feed if diagnosed with HIV to avoid postnatal transmission of the virus.

**Other Issues:** Anemia occurs usually after 4-6 weeks of therapy. Dose adjustments and/or transfusions may be required.

**Related Information**

Antiretroviral Agents Comparison *on page 1373*


- **Zilactin-B® Medicated [OTC]** *see* Benzocaine *on page 141*
- **Zilactin-L® [OTC]** *see* Lidocaine *on page 674*
- **ZilaDent® [OTC]** *see* Benzocaine *on page 141*


## Zileuton (zye LOO ton)

**U.S. Brand Names** Zyflo™

**Therapeutic Category** 5-Lipoxygenase Inhibitor

**Pregnancy Risk Factor** C

**Lactation** Excretion in breast milk unknown

**Use** Prophylaxis and chronic treatment of asthma in adults and children ≥12 years of age

**Mechanism of Action/Effect** Specific inhibitor of 5-lipoxygenase and thus inhibits leukotriene (LTB1, LTC1, LTD1 and LTE1) formation. Leukotrienes are substances that induce numerous biological effects including augmentation of neutrophil and eosinophil migration, neutrophil and monocyte aggregation, leukocyte adhesion, increased capillary permeability and smooth muscle contraction.

**Contraindications** Hypersensitivity to zileuton or any component; active liver disease or transaminase elevations greater than or equal to three times the upper limit of normal (≥3 x ULN)

**Warnings** Elevations of one or more liver function tests may occur during therapy. These laboratory abnormalities may progress, remain unchanged or resolve with continued therapy. Use with caution in patients who consume substantial quantities of alcohol or have a past history of liver disease. Zileuton is not indicated for use in the reversal of bronchospasm in acute asthma attacks, including status asthmaticus. Zileuton can be continued during acute exacerbations of asthma. Pregnancy factor C.

**Drug Interactions**

**Cytochrome P-450 Effect:** CYP1A2, 2C9, and 3A3/4 enzyme substrate; CYP1A2 and 3A3/4 enzyme inhibitor

**Increased Effect/Toxicity:**

Propranolol: Doubling of propranolol AUC and consequent increased beta-blocker activity

Terfenadine: Decrease in clearance of terfenadine leading to increase in AUC

Theophylline: Doubling of serum theophylline concentrations - reduce theophylline dose and monitor serum theophylline concentrations closely.

Warfarin: Clinically significant increases in prothrombin time (PT) - monitor PT closely

**Adverse Reactions**

>10%:

Central nervous system: Headache (24.6%)

Hepatic: ALT elevation (12%)

1% to 10%:

Cardiovascular: Chest pain

Central nervous system: Pain, dizziness, fever, insomnia, malaise, nervousness, somnolence

Gastrointestinal: Dyspepsia, nausea, abdominal pain, constipation, flatulence

Hematologic: Low white blood cell count

Neuromuscular & skeletal: Myalgia, arthralgia, weakness

Ocular: Conjunctivitis

<1% (Limited to important or life-threatening symptoms): Rash, urticaria

**Overdose/Toxicology** Symptoms of overdose: Human experience is limited. Oral minimum lethal doses in mice and rats were 500-1000 mg/kg and 300-1000 mg/kg, respectively (providing >3 and 9 times the systemic exposure achieved at the maximum recommended human daily oral dose, respectively). No deaths occurred, but nephritis was reported in dogs at an oral dose of 1000 mg/kg. Treat symptomatically; institute supportive measures as required.

**Pharmacodynamics/Kinetics**

**Protein Binding:** 93%

**Distribution:** 1.2 L/kg

**Half-life Elimination:** 2.5 hours

**Time to Peak:** 1.7 hours

**Metabolism:** Liver (cytochrome P-450)

**Formulations** Tablet: 600 mg

**Dosing**

**Adults:** Oral: 600 mg 4 times/day with meals and at bedtime

**Elderly:** Zileuton pharmacokinetics were similar in healthy elderly subjects (>65 years) compared with healthy younger adults (18-40 years); refer to adult dosing.

**Renal Impairment:** Dosing adjustment is **not** necessary in renal impairment or renal failure (even during dialysis).

**Hepatic Impairment:** Contraindicated in patients with active liver disease.

**Administration**

**Oral:** Can be administered without regard to meals (ie, with or without food).

**Monitoring Laboratory Tests** Liver function tests

**Additional Nursing Issues**

**Physical Assessment:** Not for use to relieve acute asthmatic attacks. Assess effectiveness and interactions of other medications (see Drug Interactions). See Contraindications and Warnings/Precautions for use cautions. Monitor results of laboratory tests, effectiveness of therapy (relief of airway obstruction), and adverse reactions (see Adverse Reactions) at beginning of therapy and periodically with long-term use. For inpatient care, monitor vital signs and lung sounds prior to and periodically during therapy. Assess knowledge/teach patient appropriate use, interventions to reduce side effects, and adverse symptoms to report. **Pregnancy risk factor C** - benefits of use should outweigh possible risks. Note breast-feeding caution.

**Patient Information/Instruction:** This medication is not for an acute asthmatic attack; in acute attack, follow instructions of prescriber. Do not stop other asthma medication unless advised by prescriber. Take with meals and at bedtime on a continuous bases; do not discontinue even if feeling better (this medication may help reduce incidence of acute attacks). Avoid alcohol and other medications unless approved by your prescriber. You may experience mild headache (mild analgesic may help); fatigue or dizziness (use caution when driving); or nausea or heartburn (small frequent meals, frequent mouth care, sucking lozenges, or chewing gum may help). Report persistent headache, chest pain, rapid heartbeat, or palpitations; skin rash or itching; unusual bleeding (eg, tarry stools, easy bruising, or blood in stool, urine, or mouth); skin rash or irritation; muscle weakness or tremors; redness, irritation, or infections of the eye; or

(Continued)

## Zileuton *(Continued)*

worsening of asthmatic condition. **Pregnancy/breast-feeding precautions:** Inform prescriber if you are or intend to be pregnant. Consult prescriber if breast-feeding.

**Geriatric Considerations:** No differences in the pharmacokinetics found between younger adults and elderly; no dosage adjustments necessary. However, monitor liver effects closely as with any patient regardless of age.


- **Zinacef® Injection** *see* Cefuroxime *on page 233*
- **Zinca-Pak® Zincate®** *see* Zinc Supplements *on this page*
- **Zincate® Oral** *see page 1294*
- **Zinc Chloride** *see* Zinc Supplements *on this page*
- **Zincfrin® Ophthalmic** *see page 1294*
- **Zinc Gluconate** *see* Zinc Supplements *on this page*
- **Zincon® Shampoo** *see page 1294*
- **Zinc Oxide** *see page 1294*
- **Zinc Oxide, Cod Liver Oil, and Talc** *see page 1294*
- **Zinc Sulfate** *see* Zinc Supplements *on this page*
- **Zinc Sulfate** *see page 1294*


## Zinc Supplements (zink SUP la ments)

**U.S. Brand Names** Cold-eze® [OTC]; Eye-Sed® [OTC]; Orazinc® [OTC]; Verazinc® [OTC]; Zinca-Pak® Zincate®

**Synonyms** Zinc Chloride; Zinc Gluconate; Zinc Sulfate

**Therapeutic Category** Mineral, Oral; Mineral, Parenteral; Trace Element

**Pregnancy Risk Factor** A

**Lactation** Excretion in breast milk unknown/compatible

**Use** Cofactor for replacement therapy to different enzymes helps maintain normal growth rates, normal skin hydration and senses of taste and smell; zinc supplement (oral and parenteral); may improve wound healing in those who are deficient; promote wound healing in patients with pressure sores; lozenges are used to diminish symptoms and duration of the common cold

**Mechanism of Action/Effect** Provides for normal growth and tissue repair, is a cofactor for more than 70 enzymes; ophthalmic astringent and weak antiseptic due to precipitation of protein and clearing mucus from outer surface of the eye

**Contraindications** Hypersensitivity to zinc salts or any component

**Warnings** Do not take undiluted by direct injection into a peripheral vein because of potential for phlebitis, tissue irritation, and potential to increase renal loss of minerals from a bolus injection. Administration of zinc in absence of copper may decrease plasma levels. Excessive dose may increase HDL and impair immune system function.

**Drug Interactions**

**Decreased Effect:** Decreased penicillamine and tetracycline effect. Iron may decrease the uptake of zinc. Bran products, dairy products reduce absorption of zinc.

**Food Interactions** Zinc serum concentration may be decreased if taken with food, dairy products, or caffeine.

**Adverse Reactions** <1% (Limited to important or life-threatening symptoms): Hypotension, indigestion, nausea, vomiting, neutropenia, leukopenia, jaundice, pulmonary edema

**Overdose/Toxicology** Symptoms of overdose include hypotension, pulmonary edema, diarrhea, vomiting, oliguria, nausea, gastric ulcers, restlessness, dizziness, profuse sweating, decreased consciousness, blurred vision, tachycardia, hypothermia, hyperamylasemia, and jaundice.

This agent is corrosive and emesis or gastric lavage should be avoided, instead dilute rapidly with milk or water. Calcium disodium edetate or dimercaprol can be very effective at binding zinc. Supportive care should always be instituted.

**Pharmacodynamics/Kinetics**

**Excretion:** Feces and traces in urine

**Formulations**

Zinc carbonate, complex: Liquid: 15 mg/mL (30 mL)

Zinc chloride: Injection: 1 mg/mL (10 mL)

Zinc gluconate (14.3% zinc): Tablet: 10 mg (elemental zinc 1.4 mg), 15 mg (elemental zinc 2 mg), 50 mg (elemental zinc 7 mg), 78 mg (elemental zinc 11 mg)

Zinc sulfate (23% zinc):

Capsule: 110 mg (elemental zinc 25 mg), 220 mg (elemental zinc 50 mg)

Injection: 1 mg/mL (10 mL, 30 mL); 4 mg/mL (10 mL); 5 mg/mL (5 mL, 10 mL)

Tablet: 66 mg (elemental zinc 15 mg), 110 mg (elemental zinc 25 mg), 200 mg (elemental zinc 45 mg)

**Dosing**

**Adults:** Clinical response may not occur for up to 6-8 weeks.

RDA: Oral: Male: 15 mg **elemental** zinc/day; Female: 12 mg **elemental** zinc/day

Zinc deficiency: Oral: 25-50 mg **elemental** zinc/dose (110-220 mg zinc sulfate) 3 times/day

Supplement to parenteral nutrition solutions (clinical response may not occur for up to 6-8 weeks): I.V. (all doses are mcg of **elemental** zinc):

Stable metabolically: 2.5-4 mg **elemental** zinc/day; catabolic state: Increase by an additional 2 mg/day (eg, 4.5-6 mg **elemental** zinc/day)

Stable with fluid loss from small bowel: Additional 12.2 mg **elemental** zinc/L parenteral nutrition or 17.1 mg **elemental** zinc/kg of stool or ileostomy output

Wound healing: Oral: 50 mg **elemental** zinc (220 mg zinc sulfate) 3 times daily in patients with low serum zinc levels (<110 mcg/dL)

**Elderly:** Refer to adult dosing.

**Administration**

**Oral:** Administer with food if GI upset occurs.

**I.V.:** Dilute as component of daily parenteral nutrition or maintenance fluids. Do not give undiluted by direct injection into a peripheral vein due to potential for phlebitis and tissue irritation, and potential to increase renal losses of minerals from a bolus injection.

**Monitoring Laboratory Tests** Patients on TPN therapy should have periodic serum copper and serum zinc levels.

**Additional Nursing Issues**

**Physical Assessment:** See Contraindications and Warnings/Precautions for use cautions. Assess effectiveness and interactions of other medications (see Drug Interactions). Assess knowledge/teach patient appropriate use and adverse symptoms to report.

**Patient Information/Instruction:** Take as directed; do not take more than recommended. Take with food; however, avoid foods high in calcium, phosphorous, or phytate. Stop medication and contact prescriber if you develop severe nausea or vomiting or acute indigestion; easy bruising or bleeding; persistent dizziness; or unusual respiratory difficulty. Lozenges are to be dissolved slowly in mouth.


- **Zinecard®** *see* Dexrazoxane *on page 350*
- **Zinnat** *see* Cefuroxime *on page 233*
- **Zithromax™** *see* Azithromycin *on page 126*
- **ZNP® Bar** *see page 1294*
- **Zocor®** *see* Simvastatin *on page 1059*
- **Zofran®, Zofran® ODT** *see* Ondansetron *on page 852*
- **Zoladex® Implant** *see* Goserelin *on page 543*
- **Zoldan-A** *see* Danazol *on page 332*
- **Zolicef®** *see* Cefazolin *on page 214*


## Zolmitriptan (zohl mi TRIP tan)

**U.S. Brand Names** Zomig®

**Therapeutic Category** Serotonin 5-$HT_{1D}$ Receptor Agonist

**Pregnancy Risk Factor** C

**Lactation** Excretion in breast milk unknown

**Use** Acute treatment of migraine headaches with or without aura

**Mechanism of Action/Effect** Zolmitriptan is a selective 5-HT1B/1D agonist

**Contraindications** Hypersensitivity to zolmitriptan or any component; ischemic heart disease (angina pectoris, history of myocardial infarction, or proven silent ischemia) or in patients with symptoms consistent with ischemic heart disease, coronary artery vasospasm, or Prinzmetal's variant angina; uncontrolled hypertension or patients who have received within 24 hours another 5-HT agonist (sumatriptan) or ergotamine-containing product; patients within 2 weeks of discontinuing MAO inhibitors (ie, phenelzine); patients with known risk factors associated with coronary artery disease

**Warnings** Use only if there is a clear diagnosis of migraine. Patients who are at risk of CAD but have had a satisfactory cardiovascular evaluation may receive zolmitriptan but with extreme caution in a physician's office where adequate precautions to protect the patient. Blood pressure may increase with the administration of zolmitriptan, monitor closely, especially with the first administration of the drug. If the patient does not respond to the first dose, re-evaluate the diagnosis of migraine before trying a second dose. Pregnancy factor C.

**Drug Interactions**

**Increased Effect/Toxicity:** Ergot-containing drugs (dihydroergotamine or methysergide) may have additive effects when taken with zolmitriptan. Avoid concomitant use with ergots; separate dose of zolmitriptan and ergots by at least 24 hours.

**Effects on Lab Values** No interferences have been identified

**Adverse Reactions**

1% to 10%:

Cardiovascular: Chest pain

Central nervous system: Dizziness, somnolence, asthenia, paresthesia

Gastrointestinal: Dry mouth, dyspepsia, dysphagia, nausea

<1% (Limited to important or life-threatening symptoms): palpitations, hypertension, syncope, Q-T prolongation, tachycardia, cyanosis, hematemesis, pancreatitis, melena, ulcer, thrombocytopenia, eosinophilia, leukopenia, abnormal LFTs, elevated alkaline phosphatase, thrombophlebitis, hematuria, bronchospasm, epistaxis

**Pharmacodynamics/Kinetics**

**Half-life Elimination:** 3 hours

**Time to Peak:** Within 2 hours

**Excretion:** Urine and feces

**Formulations** Tablet: 2.5 mg and 5 mg

**Dosing**

**Adults:** Oral: Initial: 2.5 mg or lower (tablet is scored and can be split in half for a lower dose). If headache returns after 2 hours, re-evaluate diagnosis and repeat dose but do not exceed 10 mg over a 24-hour period.

**Elderly:** Refer to adult dosing.

**Hepatic Impairment:** It is recommended to use a lower dose in patients with moderate to severe liver failure. Monitor blood pressure after first dose is taken.

(Continued)

## Zolmitriptan *(Continued)*

**Additional Nursing Issues**

**Physical Assessment:** Note Warnings/Precautions (clear diagnosis of migraine) and Drug Interactions (avoid concomitant use with ergot containing drugs and MAO-A inhibitors). Assess effectiveness of therapy. Assure patient knowledge of appropriate use and symptoms to report. **Pregnancy risk factor C** - benefits of use should outweigh possible risks. Note breast-feeding caution.

**Patient Information/Instruction:** This drug is to be used to reduce your migraine, not to prevent or reduce number of attacks. If first dose brings relief, second dose may be taken anytime after 2 hours if migraine returns. If you have no relief with first dose, do not take a second dose without consulting prescriber. Do not exceed 10 mg in 24 hours. You may experience some dizziness or drowsiness; use caution when driving or engaging in tasks requiring alertness until response to drug is known. Frequent mouth care and sucking on lozenges may relieve dry mouth. Report immediately any chest pain, heart throbbing or tightness in throat; swelling of eyelids, face, or lips; skin rash or hives; easy bruising; blood in urine, stool, or vomitus; pain or itching with urination; or pain, warmth, or numbness in extremities. **Pregnancy/breast-feeding precautions:** Inform prescriber if you are or intend to be pregnant. Consult prescriber if breast-feeding.

**Geriatric Considerations:** Zolmitriptan use in the elderly patient has not been studied.

♦ **Zoloft™** *see* Sertraline *on page 1052*

## Zolpidem (zole PI dem)

**U.S. Brand Names** Ambien™

**Therapeutic Category** Hypnotic, Miscellaneous

**Pregnancy Risk Factor** B

**Lactation** Enters breast milk/use caution (AAP rates "compatible")

**Use** Short-term treatment of insomnia

**Mechanism of Action/Effect** Produces CNS depression at limbic, thalamic, and hypothalamic levels of the central nervous system. Structurally dissimilar to benzodiazepine, however, has much or all of its actions explained by its effects on benzodiazepine (BZD) receptors, especially the omega-1 receptor. Retains hypnotic and much of the anxiolytic properties of the BZD, but has reduced effects on skeletal muscle and seizure threshold.

**Warnings** Closely monitor elderly or debilitated patients for impaired cognitive or motor performance; not recommended for use in children <18 years of age.

**Drug Interactions**

**Cytochrome P-450 Effect:** CYP3A3/4 enzyme substrate

**Increased Effect/Toxicity:** Increased sedation and toxicity with alcohol, CNS depressants.

**Effects on Lab Values** ↑ aminotransferase [ALT (SGPT)/AST (SGOT)], bilirubin (S); ↓ RAI uptake

**Adverse Reactions**

1% to 10%:

- Central nervous system: Headache, drowsiness, dizziness
- Gastrointestinal: Nausea, diarrhea
- Neuromuscular & skeletal: Myalgia

<1% (Limited to important or life-threatening symptoms): Amnesia, confusion, falls, tremor

**Overdose/Toxicology** Symptoms of overdose include coma and hypotension. Treatment for overdose is supportive. Rarely is mechanical ventilation required. Flumazenil has been shown to selectively block binding to CNS receptors, resulting in a reversal of CNS depression, but not always respiratory depression.

**Pharmacodynamics/Kinetics**

**Protein Binding:** 92%

**Half-life Elimination:** 2-2.6 hours, in cirrhosis increased to 9.9 hours

**Metabolism:** Hepatic to inactive metabolites

**Onset:** 30 minutes

**Duration:** 6-8 hours

**Formulations** Tablet, as tartrate: 5 mg, 10 mg

**Dosing**

**Adults:** Duration of therapy should be limited to 7-10 days; oral: 10 mg immediately before bedtime; maximum: 10 mg

**Elderly:** Duration of therapy should be limited to 7-10 days: Oral: 5 mg immediately before bedtime.

**Renal Impairment:** Not dialyzable; decrease dose to 5 mg.

**Hepatic Impairment:** Not recommended

**Additional Nursing Issues**

**Physical Assessment:** For short-term use. Assess effectiveness and interactions of other medications (see Drug Interactions). See Contraindications and Warnings/Precautions for cautious use. Assess for history of addiction; long-term use can result in dependence, abuse, or tolerance. Evaluate periodically for need for continued use. After long-term use, taper dosage slowly when discontinuing. For inpatient use, institute safety measures (side rails, night light, call bell, assistance with ambulation) and monitor effectiveness and adverse reactions. For outpatients, monitor for effectiveness of therapy and adverse reactions (see Adverse Reactions) at beginning of therapy and periodically with long-term use. Assess knowledge/teach patient appropriate use, interventions to reduce side effects, and adverse symptoms to report. Note breast-feeding caution.

**Patient Information/Instruction:** Use exactly as directed (do not increase dose or frequency or discontinue without consulting prescriber); may cause physical and/or psychological dependence. While using this medication, do not use alcohol or other prescription or OTC medications (especially, pain medications, sedatives, antihistamines, or hypnotics) without consulting prescriber. Maintain adequate hydration (2-3 L/day of fluids unless instructed to restrict fluid intake). You may experience drowsiness, dizziness, or blurred vision (use caution when driving or engaging in tasks requiring alertness until response to drug is known); nausea (small frequent meals, frequent mouth care, chewing gum, or sucking lozenges may help); or diarrhea (buttermilk, boiled milk, yogurt may help). Report CNS changes (confusion, depression, increased sedation, excitation, headache, abnormal thinking, insomnia, or nightmares); muscle pain or weakness; difficulty breathing; chest pain or palpitations; or ineffectiveness of medication. **Breast-feeding precautions:** Consult prescriber if breast-feeding.

**Geriatric Considerations:** In doses >5 mg, there was subjective evidence of impaired sleep on the first post-treatment night. There have been few reports of increased hypotension and/or falls in the elderly with this drug. Can be considered a drug of choice in the elderly when a hypnotic is indicated.

**Related Information**

Anxiolytic/Hypnotic Use in Long-Term Care Facilities *on page 1430*

- **Zomig®** *see* Zolmitriptan *on page 1231*
- **Zonal** *see* Fluconazole *on page 491*
- **Zonalon® Topical Cream** *see* Doxepin *on page 399*
- **Zorbenal-G** *see* Tetracycline *on page 1111*
- **ZORprin®** *see* Aspirin *on page 111*
- **Zostrix®** *see page 1294*
- **Zostrix®-HP** *see page 1294*
- **Zosyn™** *see* Piperacillin and Tazobactam Sodium *on page 937*
- **Zovia®** *see* Oral Contraceptives *on page 859*
- **Zovirax®** *see* Acyclovir *on page 39*
- **Zyban™** *see* Bupropion *on page 169*
- **Zydone®** *see* Hydrocodone and Acetaminophen *on page 568*
- **Zyflo™** *see* Zileuton *on page 1228*
- **Zyloprim®** *see* Allopurinol *on page 53*
- **Zymase®** *see* Pancrelipase *on page 882*
- **Zymenol®** *see page 1294*
- **Zymerol** *see* Cimetidine *on page 268*
- **Zyprexa™** *see* Olanzapine *on page 848*
- **Zyrtec®** *see* Cetirizine *on page 242*

# CONTROLLED SUBSTANCE INDEX

## CONTROLLED SUBSTANCE II



## CONTROLLED SUBSTANCE III



## CONTROLLED SUBSTANCE IV



## CONTROLLED SUBSTANCE V

# APPENDIX TABLE OF CONTENTS

## APPENDIX TABLE OF CONTENTS *(Continued)*

## Overdose and Toxicology



## Miscellaneous

# ABBREVIATIONS & SYMBOLS COMMONLY USED IN MEDICAL ORDERS

| Abbreviation | From | Meaning |
|---|---|---|
| µg | | microgram |
| µmol | | micromole |
| °C | | degrees Celsius (Centigrade) |
| < | | less than |
| > | | greater than |
| ≤ | | less than or equal to |
| ≥ | | greater than or equal to |
| $\overline{aa}$, aa | ana | of each |
| ABG | | arterial blood gas |
| ac | ante cibum | before meals or food |
| ACE | | angiotensin-converting enzyme |
| ACLS | | adult cardiac life support |
| ad | ad | to, up to |
| a.d. | aurio dextra | right ear |
| ADH | | antidiuretic hormone |
| ad lib | ad libitum | at pleasure |
| AED | | antiepileptic drug |
| a.l. | aurio laeva | left ear |
| ALL | | acute lymphoblastic leukemia |
| ALT | | alanine aminotransferase (was SGPT) |
| AM | ante meridiem | morning |
| AML | | acute myeloblastic leukemia |
| amp | | ampul |
| amt | | amount |
| ANA | | antinuclear antibodies |
| ANC | | absolute neutrophil count |
| ANL | | acute nonlymphoblastic leukemia |
| aq | aqua | water |
| aq. dest. | aqua destillata | distilled water |
| APTT | | activated partial thromboplastin time |
| a.s. | aurio sinister | left ear |
| ASA (class I-IV) | | classification of surgical patients according to their baseline health (eg, healthy ASA I and II or increased severity of illness ASA III or IV) |
| ASAP | | as soon as possible |
| AST | | aspartate aminotransferase (was SGOT) |
| a.u. | aures utrae | each ear |
| A-V | | atrial-ventricular |
| bid | bis in die | twice daily |
| bm | | bowel movement |
| BMT | | bone marrow transplant |
| bp | | blood pressure |
| BSA | | body surface area |
| BUN | | blood urea nitrogen |
| c | cong | gallon |
| $\bar{c}$ | cum | with |
| cal | | calorie |
| cAMP | | cyclic adenosine monophosphate |
| cap | capsula | capsule |
| CBC | | complete blood count |
| cc | | cubic centimeter |
| CHF | | congestive heart failure |
| CI | | cardiac index |
| $Cl_{cr}$ | | creatinine clearance |
| cm | | centimeter |
| CNS | | central nervous system |
| comp | compositus | compound |
| cont | | continue |

| Abbreviation | From | Meaning |
|---|---|---|
| COPD | | chronic obstructive pulmonary disease |
| CSF | | cerebral spinal fluid |
| CT | | computed tomography |
| CVA | | cerebral vascular accident |
| CVP | | central venous pressure |
| d | dies | day |
| $D_5W$ | | dextrose 5% in water |
| $D_5 1/2 NS$ | | dextrose 5% in sodium chloride 0.45% |
| $D_{10}W$ | | dextrose 10% in water |
| d/c | | discontinue |
| DIC | | disseminated intravascular coagulation |
| dil | dilue | dilute |
| disp | dispensa | dispense |
| div | divide | divide |
| DNA | | deoxyribonucleic acid |
| dtd | dentur tales doses | give of such a dose |
| DVT | | deep vein thrombosis |
| EEG | | electroencephalogram |
| EKG | | electrocardiogram |
| elix, el | elixir | elixir |
| emp | | as directed |
| ESR | | erythrocyte sedimentation rate |
| E.T. | | endotracheal |
| et | et | and |
| ex aq | | in water |
| f, ft | fac, fiat, fiant | make, let be made |
| FDA | | Food and Drug Administration |
| $FEV_1$ | | forced expiratory volume |
| FVC | | forced vital capacity |
| g | gramma | gram |
| G-6-PD | | glucose-6-phosphate dehydrogenase |
| GA | | gestational age |
| GABA | | gamma-aminobutyric acid |
| GE | | gastroesophageal |
| GI | | gastrointestinal |
| gr | granum | grain |
| gtt | gutta | a drop |
| GU | | genitourinary |
| h | hora | hour |
| HIV | | human immunodeficiency virus |
| HPLC | | high performance liquid chromatography |
| hs | hora somni | at bedtime |
| IBW | | ideal body weight |
| ICP | | intracranial pressure |
| IgG | | immune globulin G |
| I.M. | | intramuscular |
| INR | | international normalized ratio |
| I.O. | | intraosseous |
| I & O | | input and output |
| IOP | | intraocular pressure |
| I.T. | | intrathecal |
| I.V. | | intravenous |
| IVH | | intraventricular hemorrhage |
| IVP | | intravenous push |
| JRA | | juvenile rheumatoid arthritis |
| kcal | | kilocalorie |
| kg | | kilogram |
| L | | liter |
| LDH | | lactate dehydrogenase |
| LE | | lupus erythematosus |
| liq | liquor | a liquor, solution |
| LP | | lumbar puncture |
| M | misce | mix |
| MAO | | monoamine oxidase |
| MAP | | mean arterial pressure |

## ABBREVIATIONS & SYMBOLS COMMONLY USED IN MEDICAL ORDERS *(Continued)*

| Abbreviation | From | Meaning |
|---|---|---|
| mcg | | microgram |
| m. dict | more dictor | as directed |
| mEq | | milliequivalent |
| mg | | milligram |
| MI | | myocardial infarction |
| min | | minute |
| mixt | mixtura | a mixture |
| mL | | milliliter |
| mm | | millimeter |
| mo | | month |
| mOsm | | milliosmols |
| MRI | | magnetic resonance image |
| ND | | nasoduodenal |
| NF | | National Formulary |
| ng | | nanogram |
| NG | | nasogastric |
| NMDA | | n-methyl-d-aspartate |
| nmol | | nanomole |
| no. | numerus | number |
| noc | nocturnal | in the night |
| non rep | non repetatur | do not repeat, no refills |
| NPO | | nothing by mouth |
| NSAID | | nonsteroidal anti-inflammatory drug |
| O, Oct | octarius | a pint |
| o.d. | oculus dexter | right eye |
| o.l. | oculus laevus | left eye |
| O.R. | | operating room |
| o.s. | oculus sinister | left eye |
| OTC | | over-the-counter (nonprescription) |
| o.u. | oculo uterque | each eye |
| PALS | | pediatric advanced life support |
| pc, post cib | post cibos | after meals |
| PCA | | postconceptional age |
| PCP | | *Pneumocystis carinii* pneumonia |
| PCWP | | pulmonary capillary wedge pressure |
| PDA | | patent ductus arteriosus |
| per | | through or by |
| PM | post meridiem | afternoon or evening |
| PNA | | postnatal age |
| P.O. | per os | by mouth |
| P.R. | per rectum | rectally |
| prn | pro re nata | as needed |
| PSVT | | paroxysmal supraventricular tachycardia |
| PT | | prothrombin time |
| PTT | | partial thromboplastin time |
| PUD | | peptic ulcer disease |
| pulv | pulvis | a powder |
| PVC | | premature ventricular contraction |
| q | | every |
| qd | | every day |
| qh | quiaque hora | every hour |
| qid | quater in die | four times a day |
| qod | | every other day |
| qs | quantum sufficiat | a sufficient quantity |
| qs ad | | a sufficient quantity to make |
| qty | | quantity |
| qv | quam volueris | as much as you wish |
| Rx | recipe | take, a recipe |
| RAP | | right atrial pressure |
| rep | repetatur | let it be repeated |
| $\bar{s}$ | sine | without |
| S-A | | sino-atrial |

| Abbreviation | From | Meaning |
|---|---|---|
| sa | secundum artem | according to art |
| sat | sataratus | saturated |
| S.C. | | subcutaneous |
| $S_{cr}$ | | serum creatinine |
| SIADH | | syndrome of inappropriate antidiuretic hormone |
| sig | signa | label, or let it be printed |
| S.L. | | sublingual |
| SLE | | systemic lupus erythematosus |
| sol | solutio | solution |
| solv | | dissolve |
| $\overline{ss}$, ss | semis | one-half |
| sos | si opus sit | if there is need |
| stat | statim | at once, immediately |
| supp | suppositorium | suppository |
| SVR | | systemic vascular resistance |
| SVT | | supraventricular tachycardia |
| SWI | | sterile water for injection |
| syr | syrupus | syrup |
| tab | tabella | tablet |
| tal | | such |
| tid | ter in die | three times a day |
| tr, tinct | tincture | tincture |
| trit | | triturate |
| tsp | | teaspoonful |
| TT | | thrombin time |
| u.d., ut dict | ut dictum | as directed |
| ung | unguentum | ointment |
| USAN | | United States Adopted Names |
| USP | | United States Pharmacopeia |
| UTI | | urinary tract infection |
| $V_d$ | | volume of distribution |
| $V_{dss}$ | | volume of distribution at steady-state |
| v.o. | | verbal order |
| w.a. | | while awake |
| x3 | | 3 times |
| x4 | | 4 times |
| y | | year |

# ANTIDOTES, ANTIVENINS, AND ANTITOXINS

| Agent | Use |
|---|---|
| Alcohol, ethyl<br>Lavacol® | Antidote for ethylene glycol overdose; antidote for methanol overdose |
| Antivenin<br>(*Crotalidae* polyvalent) | Neutralization of the venoms of North and South America crotalids: rattlesnakes, copperheads, tropical moccasins, fer-de-lance, bushmaster. Not effective against the venoms of coral snakes. |
| Antivenin<br>(*Latrodectus mactans*) | Treat patients with symptoms of black widow spider bites |
| Antivenin<br>(*Micrurus fluvius*) | Neutralization of the venom of Eastern coral snakes and Texas coral snakes but does not neutralize the venom of Arizona or Sonoran coral snakes |
| Cyanide antidote kit | Treatment of cyanide poisoning |
| Diphtheria antitoxin | Passive prevention and treatment of diphtheria |
| Insect sting kit<br>(Ana-Kit®) | Anaphylaxis emergency treatment of insect bites or stings by the sensitive patient that may occur within minutes of insect sting or exposure to an allergic substance |
| Sodium thiosulfate<br>(Tinver® Lotion) | Parenteral: Used alone or with sodium nitrite or amyl nitrite in cyanide poisoning or arsenic poisoning; reduce the risk of nephrotoxicity associated with cisplatin therapy. Topical: Treatment of tinea versicolor. |
| Succimer<br>(Chemet®) | Treatment of lead poisoning in children with blood levels higher than 45 μg/dL. Not indicated for prophylaxis of lead poisoning in a lead-containing environment. Oral: 10 mg/kg/dose every 8 hours for an additional 5 days followed by 10 mg/kg/dose every 12 hours for 14 days. |
| Trientine<br>(Syprine®) | Treatment of Wilson's disease in patients intolerant to penicillamine |

# ANTIFUNGAL AGENTS (TOPICAL)

| Generic Name | Comments |
|---|---|
| Butenafine (Mentax®) | Topical treatment of tinea pedis (athlete's foot) tinea cruris (jock itch). Apply once daily for 4 weeks. |
| Ciclopirox (Loprox®) | Treatment of tinea pedis (athlete's foot), tinea cruris (jock itch), tinea corporis (ringworm), cutaneous candidiasis, and tinea versicolor (pityriasis). Apply twice daily. Gently massage into affected area. If no improvement after 4 weeks, re-evaluate diagnosis. |
| Clioquinol (Vioform® OTC) | Topically used in the treatment of tinea pedis (athlete's foot), tinea cruris (jock itch), and skin infections caued by dermatophytic fungi (ringworm). Apply 2-3 times daily. Do not use for longer than 7 days. |
| Haloprogin (Halotex®) | Topical treatment of tinea pedis (athlete's foot), tinea cruris (jock itch), tinea corporis (ringworm), tinea manuum caused by *Trichophyton rubrum, Trichophyton tonsurans, Trichophyton mentagrophytes, Microsporum canis*, or *Epidermophyton floccosum*.. Topical treatment of *Malassezia furfur*. Apply liberally twice daily for 2-3 weeks. Intertriginous areas may require up to 4 weeks of treatment. |
| Naftifine (Naftin®) | Topical treatment of tinea cruris (jock itch), tinea corporis (ringworm), and tinea pedis (athlete's foot. Apply cream once daily and gel twice daily (morning and evening) for up to 4 weeks. |
| Oxiconazole (Oxistat®) | Treatment of tinea pedis (athlete's foot), tinea cruris (jock itch), and tinea corporis (ringworm). Apply once or twice daily to affected areas for 2 weeks for tinea corporis/tinea cruris and up to 1 month for tinea pedis. |
| Sulconazole (Exelderm®) | Treatment of superficial fungal infections of the skin, including tinea cruris (jock itch), tinea corporis (ringworm), tinea versicolor, and possible tinea pedis (athlete's foot - cream only). For tinea cruris, tinea corporis, and tinea versicolor, apply a small amount to the affected area and gently massage once or twice daily for 3 weeks (4 weeks for tinea pedis). |
| Terbinafine (Lamisil®) | Topical antifungal for the treatment of tinea pedis (athlete's foot), tinea cruris (jock itch), and tinea corporis (ringworm). **Unlabeled use:** Cutaneous candidiasis and pityriasis versicolor. For athlete's foot, apply to affected area twice daily for at least 1 week, not to exceed 4 weeks. For ringworm and jock itch, apply to affected area once or twice daily for at least 1 week, not to exceed 4 weeks. |
| Tolnaftate (Absorbine® Antifungal; Absorbine® Jock Itch; Absorbine Jr.® Antifungal; Aftate® for Athlete's Foot; Aftate® for Jock Itch; Blis-To-Sol®; Breezee® Mist Antifungal; Dr Scholl's® Athlete's Foot; Dr Scholl's® Maximum Strength Tritin; Genaspor®-NP-27®; Quinsana Plus®; Tinactin®; Tinactin® for Jock Itch; Ting®; Pitrex® (Canadian); Tinaderm® (Mexican)) | Treatment of tinea pedis (athlete's foot), tinea cruris (jock itch), tinea corporis (ringworm), tinea manuum, and tinea versicolor infections. Wash and dry affected area. Apply 1-2 drops of solution or small amount of cream or powder and rub into affected areas twice daily for 2-4 weeks. |
| Undecylenic acid and derivatives (Caldesene® Topical; Cruex® Topical; Fungoid® Topical Solution; Merlenate® Topical; Pedi-Dri® Topical; Pedi-Pro® Topical; Undoguent® Topical) | Treatment of athlete's foot (tinea pedis), ringworm (except nails and scalp), prickly heat, jock itch (tinea cruris), diaper rash, and other minor skin irritations due to superficial dermatophytes. Cleanse the affected area and apply as needed twice daily for 2-4 weeks. |

# DIAGNOSTICS AND SURGICAL AIDS

| Agent | Use |
|---|---|
| Apraclonidine (Iopidine®) | Prevention and treatment of postsurgical intraocular pressure elevation |
| Bentiromide (Chymex®) | Screening test for pancreatic exocrine insufficiency |
| *Candida albicans (Monilia)* (Dermatophytin-O) | Screen for the detection of nonresponsiveness to antigens in immunocompromised individuals |
| Cellulose, oxidized (Oxycel®; Surgicel®) | Temporary packing for the control of capillary, venous, or small arterial hemorrhage |
| Chondroitin sulfate - sodium hyaluronate (Viscoat®) | Surgical aid in anterior segment procedures, protects corneal endothelium and coats intraocular lens thus protecting it |
| Chymopapain (Chymodiactin®; Discase®) | Alternative to surgery in patients with herniated lumbar intervertebral disks |
| Coccidioidin skin test (Spherulin®) | Intradermal skin test in diagnosis of coccidioidomycosis; differential diagnosis of this disease from histoplasmosis, sarcoidosis, and other mycotic and bacterial infections. The skin test may be negative in severe forms of disease (anergy) or when prolonged periods of time have passed since infection. |
| Corticotropin (Acthar®; H.P. Acthar® Gel) | Diagnostic aid in adrenocortical insufficiency; repository dosage form is used for acute exacerbations of multiple sclerosis or severe muscle weakness in myasthenia gravis |
| Cosyntropin (Cortrosyn® Injection) | Diagnostic test to differentiate primary adrenal from secondary (pituitary) adrenocortical insufficiency |
| Cyclopentolate (AK-Pentolate®; Cyclogyl®; I-Pentolate®; Ocu-Pentolate®) | Diagnostic procedures requiring mydriasis and cycloplegia |
| Cyclopentolate and phenylephrine (Cyclomydril® Ophthalmic) | Induce mydriasis greater than that produced with cyclopentolate alone |
| Dapiprazole (Rē v-Eyes™) | Reverse dilation due to drugs (adrenergic or parasympathomimetic) after eye exams |
| Dimercaprol (BAL in Oil®) | Antidote to gold, arsenic, and mercury poisoning; adjunct to edetate calcium disodium in lead poisoning |
| Dinoprost tromethamine (Prostin $F_2$ Alpha®) | Abort 2nd trimester pregnancy |
| Doxacurium (Nuromax® Injection) | Adjunct to general anesthesia; provides skeletal muscle relaxation during surgery. Doxacurium is a long-acting nondepolarizing neuromuscular blocker with virtually no cardiovascular side effects. The characteristics of this agent make it especially useful in procedures requiring careful maintenance of hemodynamic stability for prolonged periods. |
| d-Xylose (Xylo-Pfan® [OTC]) | Also referred to as wood sugar; used in evaluating intestinal absorption and diagnosing malabsorptive states |
| Fluorescein sodium (AK-Fluor® Injection; Fluorescite® Injection; Fluorets® Ophthalmic Strips; Fluor-I-Strip®; Fluor-I-Strip-AT®; Flurate® Ophthalmic Solution; Fluress® Ophthalmic Solution; Ful-Glo® Ophthalmic Strips; Funduscein® Injection) | Demonstrates defects of corneal epithelium; diagnostic aid in ophthalmic angiography |
| Gelatin, absorbable (Gelfilm® Ophthalmic; Gelfoam® Topical) | Adjunct to provide hemostasis in surgery; used in oral and dental surgery; used in open prostatic surgery |
| Histoplasmin (Histolyn-CYL® Injection) | Diagnose histoplasmosis; assess cell-mediated immunity |
| Hydroxyamphetamine and tropicamide (Paremyd® Ophthalmic) | Diagnostic mydriasis with cycloplegia when short-term pupil dilation is desired |
| Hydroxypropyl methylcellulose (Gonak™; Goniosol®; Occucoat™) | Ophthalmic surgical aid in cataract extraction and intraocular implantation; gonioscopic examination |
| Indocyanine green (Cardio-Green®) | Determine hepatic function, cardiac output, and liver blood flow and for ophthalmic angiography |
| Mephentermine (Wyamine® Sulfate Injection) | Treatment of hypotension secondary to ganglionic blockade or spinal anesthesia; may be used as an emergency measure to maintain blood pressure until whole blood replacement becomes available |
| Methacholine (Provocholine®) | Diagnosis of bronchial airway hyperactivity in subjects who do not have clinically apparent asthma |
| Methylene blue (Urolene Blue®) | Antidote for cyanide poisoning and drug-induced methemoglobinemia, indicator dye, chronic urolithiasis. **Unlabeled use:** Has been used topically (0.1% solutions) in conjunction with polychromatic light to photoinactivate viruses such as herpes simplex; has been used alone or in combination with vitamin C for the management of chronic urolithiasis. |
| Metocurine iodide (Metubine® Iodide) | Adjunct ot anesthesia to induce skeletal muscle relaxation |
| Microfibrillar collagen hemostat (Avitene®; Helistat®; Hemotene®) | Adjunct to hemostasis when control of bleeding by ligature is ineffective or impractical |
| Mumps skin test antigen | Assess the status of cell-mediated immunity |

| Agent | Use |
|---|---|
| Pancuronium (Pavulon®) | Drug of choice for neuromuscular blockade except in patients with renal failure, hepatic failure, or cardiovascular instability. Produce skeletal muscle relaxation during surgery after induction of general anesthesia; increase pulmonary compliance during assisted respiration; facilitate endotracheal intubation; preferred muscle relaxant for neonatal cardiac patients, must provide artificial ventilation. |
| Pentagastrin (Peptavlon®) | Evaluate gastric acid secretory function in pernicious anemia, gastric carcinoma; used with suspected duodenal ulcer or Zollinger-Ellison tumor |
| Phenolsulfonphthalein | Evaluation of renal blood flow to aid in the determination of renal function |
| Pipecuronium (Arduan®) | Adjunct to general anesthesia; provide skeletal muscle relaxation during surgery and for endotracheal intubation; recommended only for procedures anticipated to last 90 minutes or longer. |
| Proparacaine (AK-Taine®; Alcaine®; I-Paracaine®; Ophthetic®) | Anesthesia for tonometry, gonioscopy; suture removal from cornea; removal of corneal foreign body; cataract extraction, glaucoma surgery; short operative procedure involving the cornea and conjunctiva |
| Proparacaine and fluorescein (Fluoracaine® Ophthalmic) | Anesthesia for tonometry, gonioscopy; suture removal from cornea; removal of corneal foreign body; cataract extraction, glaucoma surgery |
| Protirelin (Relefact® TRH Injection; Thypinone® Injection) | Adjunct in the diagnostic assessment of thyroid function, and an adjunct to other diagnostic procedures in assessment of patients with pituitary or hypothalamic dysfunction; causes release of prolactin from the pituitary and is used to detect defective control of prolactin secretion |
| Rocuronium (Zemuron®) | Inpatient and outpatient use as an adjunct to general anesthesia to facilitate both rapid-sequence and routine tracheal intubation; provide skeletal muscle relaxation during surgery or mechanical ventilation |
| Secretin (Secretin Ferring Powder) | Diagnose Zollinger-Ellison syndrome, chronic pancreatic dysfunction, and some hepatobiliary diseases such as obstructive jaundice resulting from cancer or stones in the biliary tract |
| Sermorelin acetate (Geref® Injection) | Evaluate ability of the somatotroph of the pituitary gland to secrete growth hormone |
| Sincalide (Kinevac®) | Postevacuation cholecystography; gallbladder bile sampling; stimulate pancreatic secretion for analysis |
| Skin test antigens, multiple (Multitest CMI®) | Detection of nonresponsiveness to antigens by means of delayed hypersensitivity skin testing |
| Sodium hyaluronate (AMO Vitrax®; Amvisc®; Amvisc® Plus; Healon®; Healon® GV) | Surgical aid in cataract extraction, intraocular implantation, corneal transplant, glaucoma filtration, and retinal attachment surgery |
| Succinylcholine (Anectine® Chloride Injection; Anectine® Flo-Pack®; Quelicin® Injection) | Produces skeletal muscle relaxation in procedures of short duration such as endotracheal intubation or endoscopic exams |
| Suprofen (Profenal® Ophthalmic) | Inhibition of intraoperative miosis |
| Teriparatide (Parathar™ Injection) | Diagnosis of hypocalcemia in either hypoparathyroidism or pseudohypoparathyroidism |
| Thrombin, topical (Thrombinar®; Thrombogen®; Thrombostat®) | Hemostasis whenever minor bleeding from capillaries and small venules is accessible; has been used in ocular surgery, upper GI hemorrhage, oral surgery, plastic surgery, orthopedic surgery, peripheral nerve repair, persistent lymphatic drainage, drainage of giant bulla in emphysemia, management of hemophiliacs, skin grafting, hemoptysis, hepatic trauma, and wound hematoma including hematoma in heparinized patients |
| *Trichophyton* skin test (Dermatophytin® Injection) | Assess cell-mediated immunity |
| Trimethaphan camsylate (Arfonad® Injection) | Hypertensive emergencies; controlled hypotension during surgery |
| Tropicamide (Mydriacyl®; Opticyl®; Tropicacyl®) | Short-acting mydriatic used in diagnostic procedures, as well as preoperatively and postoperatively; treatment of some cases of acute itits, iridocyclitis, and keratitis |

# IMMUNIZATION GUIDELINES

### Standards for Pediatric Immunization Practices

| | |
|---|---|
| Standard 1. | Immunization services are readily available. |
| Standard 2. | There are no barriers or unnecessary prerequisites to the receipt of vaccines. |
| Standard 3. | Immunization services are available free or for a minimal fee. |
| Standard 4. | Providers utilize all clinical encounters to screen and, when indicated, immunize children. |
| Standard 5. | Providers educate parents and guardians about immunizations in general terms. |
| Standard 6. | Providers question parents or guardians about contraindications and, before immunizing a child, inform them in specific terms about the risks and benefits of the immunizations their child is to receive. |
| Standard 7. | Providers follow only true contraindications. |
| Standard 8. | Providers administer simultaneously all vaccine doses for which a child is eligible at the time of each visit. |
| Standard 9. | Providers use accurate and complete recording procedures. |
| Standard 10. | Providers co-schedule immunization appointments in conjunction with appointments for other child health services. |
| Standard 11. | Providers report adverse events following immunization promptly, accurately, and completely. |
| Standard 12. | Providers operate a tracking system. |
| Standard 13. | Providers adhere to appropriate procedures for vaccine management. |
| Standard 14. | Providers conduct semiannual audits to assess immunization coverage levels and to review immunization records in the patient populations they serve. |
| Standard 15. | Providers maintain up-to-date, easily retrievable medical protocols at all locations where vaccines are administered. |
| Standard 16. | Providers operate with patient-oriented and community-based approaches. |
| Standard 17. | Vaccines are administered by properly trained individuals. |
| Standard 18. | Providers receive ongoing education and training on current immunization recommendations. |

Recommended by the National Vaccine Advisory Committee, April 1992.
Approved by the United States Public Health Service, May 1992.
Endorsed by the American Academy of Pediatrics, May 1992.

The Standards represent the consensus of the National Vaccine Advisory Committee (NVAC) and of a broad group of medical and public health experts about what constitutes the most desirable immunization practices. It is recognized by the NVAC that not all of the current immunization practices of public and private providers are in compliance with the Standards. Nevertheless, the Standards are expected to be useful as a means of helping providers to identify needed changes, to obtain resources if necessary, and to actually implement the desirable immunization practices in the future.

## Recommended Childhood Immunization Schedule
## United States, January - December 1999

Vaccines[1] are listed under the routinely recommended ages. [Bars] indicate range of recommended ages for immunization. Any dose not given at the recommended age should be given as a "catch up" immunization at any subsequent visit when indicated and feasible. (Ovals) indicate vaccines to be given if previously recommended doses were missed or given earlier than the recommended minimum age.

| Age ▶ / Vaccine ▼ | Birth | 1 mo | 2 mo | 4 mo | 6 mo | 12 mo | 15 mo | 18 mo | 4-6 y | 11-12 y | 14-16 y |
|---|---|---|---|---|---|---|---|---|---|---|---|
| Hepatitis B[2] | Hep B | | | | | | | | | | |
| | | Hep B | | | Hep B | | | | | (Hep B) | |
| Diphtheria, Tetanus, Pertussis[3] | | | DTaP | DTaP | DTaP | | DTaP[3] | | DTaP | Td | |
| *H. influenzae* type b[4] | | | Hib | Hib | Hib | Hib | | | | | |
| Polio[5] | | | IPV | IPV | Polio[5] | | | | Polio | | |
| Rotavirus[6] | | | *Rv*[6] | *Rv*[6] | *Rv*[6] | | | | | | |
| Measles, Mumps, Rubella[7] | | | | | | MMR | | | MMR[7] | (MMR[7]) | |
| Varicella[8] | | | | | | Var | | | | (Var[8]) | |

[1] This schedule indicates the recommended ages for routine administration of currently licensed childhood vaccines. Combination vaccines may be used whenever any components of the combination are indicated and its other components are not contraindicated. Providers should consult the manufacturers' package inserts for detailed recommendations.

[2] Infants born to HBsAg-negative mothers should receive the second dose of hepatitis B vaccine at least 1 month after the first dose. The third dose should be administered at least 4 months after the first dose and at least 2 months after the second dose, but not before 6 months of age for infants.

Infants born to HBsAg-positive mothers should receive hepatitis B vaccine and 0.5 mL hepatitis B immune globulin (HBIG) within 12 hours of birth at separate sites. The second dose is recommended at 1-2 months of age and the third dose at 6 months of age.

Infants born to mothers whose HBsAg status is unknown should receive hepatitis B vaccine within 12 hours of birth. Maternal blood should be drawn at the time of delivery to determine the mother's HBsAg status; if the HBsAg test is positive, the infant should receive HBIG as soon as possible (no later than 1 week of age).

All children and adolescents (through 18 years of age) who have not been immunized against hepatitis B may begin the series during any visit. Special efforts should be made to immunize children who were born in or whose parents were born in areas of the world with moderate or high endemicity of HBV infection.

[3] DTaP (diphtheria and tetanus toxoids and acellular pertussis vaccine) is the preferred vaccine for all doses in the immunization series, including completion of the series in children who have received 1 or more doses of whole-cell DTP vaccine. Whole-cell DTP is an acceptable alternative to DTaP. The fourth dose (DTP or DTaP) may be administered as early as 12 months of age, provided 6 months have elapsed since the third dose and if the child is unlikely to return at age 15-18 months. Td (tetanus and diphtheria toxoids) is recommended at 11-12 years of age if at least 5 years have elapsed since the last dose of DTP, DTaP, or DT. Subsequent routine Td boosters are recommended every 10 years.

[4] Three *H. influenzae* type b (Hib) conjugate vaccines are licensed for infant use. If PRP-OMP (PedvaxHIB® and COMVAX® [Merck]) is administered at 2 and 4 months of age, a dose at 6 months is not required. Because clinical studies in infants have demonstrated that using some combination products may induce a lower immune response to the Hib vaccine component, DTaP/Hib combination products should not be used for primary immunization in infants at 2, 4, or 6 months of age, unless FDA-approved for these ages.

[5] Two poliovirus vaccines currently are licensed in the United States: Inactivated poliovirus vaccine (IPV) and oral poliovirus vaccine (OPV). The ACIP, AAP, and AAFP now recommend that the first two doses of poliovirus vaccine should be IPV. The ACIP continues to recommend a sequential schedule of two doses of IPV administered at ages 2 and 4 months, followed by two doses of OPV at 12-18 months and 4-6 years. Use of IPV for all doses also is acceptable and is recommended for immunocompromised persons and their household contacts. OPV is no longer recommended for the first two doses of the schedule and is acceptable only for special circumstances such as: Children of parents who do not accept the recommended number of injections, late initiation of immunization which would require an unacceptable number of injections, and imminent travel to polio-endemic areas. OPV remains the vaccine of choice for mass immunization campaigns to control outbreaks due to wild poliovirus.

[6] Rotavirus vaccine(*Rv*) is italicized to indicate: 1) Health care providers may require time and resources to incorporate this new vaccine into practice; and 2) the AAFP feels that the decision to use rotavirus vaccine should be made by the parent or guardian in consultation with their physician or other health care provider. The first dose of Rv vaccine should not be administered before 6 weeks of age, and the minimum interval between doses is 3 weeks. The Rv vaccine series should not be initiated at 7 months of age or older, and all doses should be completed by the first birthday.

[7] The second dose of measles, mumps, and rubella vaccine (MMR) is recommended routinely at 4-6 years of age but may be administered during any visit, provided at least 4 weeks have elapsed since receipt of the first dose and that both doses are administered beginning at or after 12 months of age. Those who have not previously received the second dose should complete the schedule by the 11- to 12-year-old visit.

[8] Varicella vaccine is recommended at any visit on or after the first birthday for susceptible children, ie, those who lack a reliable history of chickenpox (as judged by a health care provider) and who have not been immunized. Susceptible persons 13 years of age or older should receive 2 doses, given at least 4 weeks apart.

Adapted from Advisory Committee on Immunization Practices (ACIP), the American Academy of Pediatrics (AAP), and the American Academy of Family Physicians (AAFP).

## IMMUNIZATION GUIDELINES *(Continued)*

# RECOMMENDATIONS OF THE ADVISORY COMMITTEE ON IMMUNIZATION PRACTICES (ACIP)

### Recommended Poliovirus Vaccination Schedules for Children

| Vaccine | Child's Age | | | |
|---|---|---|---|---|
| | 2 mo | 4 mo | 12-18 mo | 4-6 y |
| Sequential IPV*/OPV*/OPV† | IPV | IPV | OPV | OPV |
| OPV* | OPV | OPV | OPV‡ | OPV |
| IPV† | IPV | IPV | IPV | OPV |

*Inactivated poliovirus vaccine.

†Live, oral poliovirus vaccine.

‡For children who receive only OPV, the third dose of OPV may be administered as early as 6 months of age.

Adapted from *MMWR Morb Mortal Wkly Rep*, "Poliomyelitis Prevention in the United States: Introduction of a Sequential Vaccination Schedule of Inactivated Poliovirus Vaccine Followed by Oral Poliovirus Vaccine" 1997, 46(RR-3).

### Recommendations for Measles Vaccination*

| Category | Recommendations |
|---|---|
| Unvaccinated, no history of measles (12-15 mo) | A 2-dose schedule (with MMR) is recommended if born after 1956. The first dose is recommended at 12-15 mo; the second is recommended at 4-6 y |
| Children 12 mo in areas of recurrent measles transmission | Vaccinate; a second dose is indicated at 4-6 y (at school entry) |
| Children 6-11 mo in epidemic situations† | Vaccinate (with monovalent measles vaccine or, if not available, MMR); revaccination (with MMR) at 12-15 mo is necessary and a third dose is indicated at 4-6 y |
| Children 11-12 y who have received 1 dose of measles vaccine at ≥12 mo | Revaccinate (1 dose) |
| Students in college and other posthigh school institutions who have received 1 dose of measles vaccine at ≥12 mo | Revaccinate (1 dose) |
| History of vaccination before the first birthday | Consider susceptible and vaccinate (2 doses) |
| Unknown vaccine, 1963-1967 | Consider susceptible and vaccinate (2 doses) |
| Further attenuated or unknown vaccine given with IG | Consider susceptible and vaccinate (2 doses) |
| Egg allergy | Vaccinate; no reactions likely |
| Neomycin allergy, nonanaphylactic | Vaccinate; no reactions likely |
| Tuberculosis | Vaccinate; vaccine does not exacerbate infection |
| Measles exposure | Vaccinate or give IG, depending on circumstances |
| HIV-infected | Vaccinate (2 doses) unless severely compromised |
| Immunoglobulin or blood product received | Vaccinate at the appropriate interval |

*See text for details. MMR indicates measles-mumps-rubella vaccine; IG, immune globulin.

†See Outbreak Control.

Adapted from "Report of the Committee on Infectious Diseases," *1997 Red Book®*, 24th ed.

# HEPATITIS A INFORMATION

## Recommended Doses and Schedules for Hepatitis A Virus (HAV) Inactivated Vaccines

| Age | Vaccine* | Antigen Dose† | Volume per Dose (mL) | No. of Doses | Schedule |
|---|---|---|---|---|---|
| 2-18 y | Havrix‡ (SKB) | 360 ELU | 0.5 | 3 | Initial, 1, and 6-12 mo later |
| | Havrix (SKB) | 720 ELU | 0.5 | 2 | Initial and 6-12 mo later |
| | Vaqta (Merck) | 25 units§ | 0.5 | 2 | Initial and 6-18 mo later |
| ≥19 y | Havrix (SKB) | 1440 ELU | 1 | 2 | Initial and 6-12 mo later |
| | Vaqta (Merck) | 50 units§ | 1 | 2 | Initial and 6-12 mo later |

*SKB indicates SmithKline Beecham.

†ELU indicates enzyme-linked immunoassay units.

‡Children receiving 360 ELU for the first dose should receive two additional doses of either pediatric formulation (360 ELU or 720 ELU) to complete the schedule.

§Antigen units (each unit is equivalent to approximately 1 mg of viral protein).

Adapted from "Report of the Committee on Infectious Diseases," *1997 Red Book®*, 24th ed.

## Recommendations for Postexposure Immunoprophylaxis of Hepatitis A Infection

| Time Since Exposure (wk) | Future Exposure Likely | Age of Patient (y) | Recommended Prophylaxis |
|---|---|---|---|
| ≤2 | No | All ages | IG (0.02 mL/kg)* |
| | Yes | ≥2 | IG (0.02 mL/kg)* **and** HAV vaccine† |
| >2 | No | All ages | No prophylaxis |
| | Yes | ≥2 | HAV vaccine† |

*Immune globulin (IG) should be administered deep into a large muscle mass. Ordinarily no more than 5 mL should be administered in one site in an adult or large child; lesser amounts (maximum 3 mL) should be given to small children and infants.

†Dosage and schedule of hepatitis A virus vaccine as recommended according to age.

Adapted from "Report of the Committee on Infectious Diseases," *1997 Red Book®*, 24th ed.

## Recommendations for Pre-exposure Immunoprophylaxis of Hepatitis A Infection for Travelers*

| Age (y) | Likely Exposure (mo) | Recommended Prophylaxis |
|---|---|---|
| <2 | <3 | IG 0.02 mL/kg† |
| | 3-5 | IG 0.06 mL/kg† |
| | Long term | IG 0.06 mL/kg at departure and every 5 mo thereafter† |
| ≥2 | <3‡ | HAV vaccine§¶ **or** IG 0.02 mL/kg† |
| | 3-5‡ | HAV vaccine§¶ **or** IG 0.06 mL/kg† |
| | | HAV vaccine§¶ |

*HAV, hepatitis A virus; IG, immune globulin.

†IG should be administered deep into a large muscle mass. Ordinarily no more than 5 mL should be administered in one site in an adult or large child; lesser amounts (maximum 3 mL) should be given to small children and infants.

‡Vaccine is preferable, but IG is an acceptable alternative.

§Ensure protection in travelers whose departure is imminent, IG may also be given (see text).

¶Dose and schedule of HAV vaccine as recommended according to age.

Adapted from "Report of the Committee on Infectious Diseases," *1997 Red Book®*, 24th ed.

## IMMUNIZATION GUIDELINES *(Continued)*

## HEPATITIS B INFORMATION

### Persons Who Should Receive Pre-exposure Hepatitis B Immunization*

All infants†

Children at risk of acquisition of HBV by person-to-person (horizontal) transmission should be immunized

Adolescents‡: HBV vaccination should be given by or before 11-12 years of age; special efforts should be made to vaccinate **all** adolescents, not only those at high risk

Users of intravenous drugs

Sexually active heterosexual persons with more than one sex partner in the previous 6 months or who have a sexually transmitted disease

Sexually active homosexual or bisexual males

Healthcare workers and others at occupational risk of exposure to blood or blood-contaminated body fluid

Residents and staff of institutions for developmentally disabled persons

Staff of nonresidential child care and school programs for developmentally disabled persons if the program is attended by a known HBV carrier

Patients undergoing hemodialysis

Patients with bleeding disorders who receive clotting factor concentrates

Household contacts and sexual partners of HBV carriers

Members of households with adoptees who are $HB_sAg$-positive

International travelers to areas in which HBV infection is of high or intermediate endemicity

Inmates of long-term correctional facilities

*$Hb_sAg$ indicates hepatitis B surface antigen; HBIG, hepatitis B immune globulin; HBV, hepatitis virus.

†For those born to $Hb_sAg$-positive mothers, HBIG and vaccine is recommended for postexposure immunoprophylaxis (see text for specific recommendations).

‡Implementation can be initiated before children reach adolescence.

### Recommended Dosages of Hepatitis B Vaccines*

| | Vaccine† | | | |
|---|---|---|---|---|
| | Recombivax HB®‡ Dose | | Engerix-B®§♦ Dose | |
| | mcg | (mL) | mcg | (mL) |
| Infants of $HB_sAg$-negative mothers and children <11 y | 2.5 | (0.5)¶ | 10 | (0.5) |
| Infants of $HB_sAg$-positive mothers (HVIG 0.5 mL also is recommended) | 5 | (1)¶<br>(0.5)# | 10 | (0.5) |
| Children and adolescents 11-19 y | 5 | (0.5)# | 10 | (0.5) |
| Adults ≥20 y | 10 | (1)# | 20 | (1) |
| Patients undergoing dialysis and other immunosuppressed adults | 40 | (1)** | 40 | (2)† |

*Heptavax B (available from Merck and Co), a plasma-derived vaccine, is also licensed but no longer produced in the United States. $HB_sAg$ indicates hepatitis B surface antigen; HBIG, hepatitis B immune globulin.

†Vaccines should be stored at 2°C to 8°C. Freezing destroys effectiveness. Both vaccines are administered in a three-dose schedule.

‡Available from Merck and Co.

§Available from SmithKline Beecham.

♦The Food and Drug Administration has approved this vaccine for use in an optional four-dose schedule at 0, 1, 2, and 12 months.

¶Pediatric formulation

#Adult formulation.

**Special formulation for dialysis patients.

††Two 1 mL doses given in one site in a four-dose schedule at 0, 1, 2, and 6-12 months.

## Guide to Postexposure Immunoprophylaxis for Hepatitis B Infection*

| Type of Exposure | Immunoprophylaxis† |
|---|---|
| Accidental, percutaneous, or permucosal | Vaccination + HBIG |
| Household contact, chronic carrier | Vaccination |
| Household contact, acute case with identifiable blood exposure | Vaccination + HBIG |
| Perinatal | Vaccination + HBIG |
| Sexual, acute infection | Vaccination + HBIG |
| Sexual, chronic carrier | Vaccination |

*HBIG indicates hepatitis B immune globulin.

†For susceptible patients (eg, previously unvaccinated).

Adapted from "Report of the Committee on Infectious Diseases," *1997 Red Book®*, 24th ed.

# IMMUNIZATION GUIDELINES *(Continued)*

## IMMUNIZATIONS* (VACCINES)

| Drug | Use | Stability | Administration/ Patient Information |
|---|---|---|---|
| Anthrax vaccine adsorbed | Used for individuals who may come in contact with animal products which come from anthrax endemic areas and may be contaminated with *Bacillus anthracis* spores and for high-risk persons such as veterinarians and other handling potentially infected animals; Department of Defense is implementing an anthrax vaccination program for active duty and reserve personnel against the biological warfare agent anthrax | Refrigerate; do not freeze. | Injection may be deferred in patients with acute respiratory disease or other active infection. Persons receiving immunosuppressive agents may not have adequate response to immunization. If immunosuppression therapy is short-term, immunization should be delayed. If immunosuppression therapy is long-term, an extra dose of vaccine should be given a month or more after immunosuppressive therapy is discontinued. |
| Antirabies serum (equine) | Rabies prophylaxis | | I.M.: 1000 units/55 lb in a single dose; infiltrate up to 50% of dose around the wound. History of asthma, angioneurotic edema, or other allergies is important. |
| BCG vaccine (TheraCys®; TICE® BCG) | Immunization against tuberculosis; bladder instillation of vaccine as immunotherapy for treatment of bladder cancer (TheraCys®; TICE® BCG). BCG vaccine is not routinely recommended for use inthe U.S. for prevention of tuberculosis. BCG should be administered with caution to persons in groups at high risk for HIV infection or persons know to be severely immunocompromised. Although limited data suggests that the vaccine may be safe for use in asymptomatic children infected with HIV, BCG vaccination is not recommended for HIV infected adults or for persons with symptomatic disease. Vaccination should be restricted to persons at exceptionally high risk for tuberculosis infection. HIV infected persons thought to be infected with *Mycobacterium tuberculosis* should be strongly recommended for tuberculosis preventive therapy. | Refrigerate between 2°C and 8°C (35°F to 46°F) and protect from light. Use within 2 hours of mixing (TICE® BCG; TheraCys®). | Immunization against tuberculosis: 0.2-0.3 mL percutaneous; initial lesion usually appears after 10-14 days consisting of small red papule at injection site and reaches maximum diameter of 3 mm in 4-6 weeks; conduct postvaccinal tuberculin test in 2-3 months; if test is negative, repeat vaccination. Immunotherapy for bladder cancer: TICE® BCG vaccine 6 x $10^8$ viable organisms in 50 mL NS (preservative free) instilled into bladder and retained for 2 hours weekly for 6 weeks; refer to individual protocols. |
| Cholera vaccine | Primary immunization for cholera prophylaxis. The World Health Organization no longer recommends cholera vaccination for travel to or from cholera-endemic areas. Some countries may still require evidence of a complete primary series or a booster dose given within 6 months of arrival. Vaccination should not be considered as an alternative to continued careful selection of foods and water. | Refrigerate; avoid freezing. | 0.5 mL in two doses 1 week to 1 month or more apart. There is no data on the safety of cholera vaccination during pregnancy. Use in pregnancy should reflect actual increased risk. Persons who have had severe local or systemic reactions to a previous dose should not be revaccinated. Have epinephrine (1:1000) available for immediate use. Defer immunization in individuals with moderate or severe febrile illness. May cause malaise, fever, headache, pain, swelling, tenderness, erythema, and induration at the injection site. Local reaction can occur up to 7 days after injection. Review history of elderly to assure no drug or disease is contraindicated with use of this vaccine. |

## IMMUNIZATIONS* (VACCINES) *(continued)*

| Drug | Use | Stability | Administration/ Patient Information |
|---|---|---|---|
| Diphtheria and tetanus toxoid | Active immunity against diphtheria and tetanus when pertussis vaccine is contraindicated. Since protective tetanus and diphtheria antibodies decline with age, only 28% of persons >70 years of age in the U.S. are believed to be immune to tetanus, and most of the tetanus-induced deaths occur in people >60 years of age. It is advisable to offer Td especially to the elderly concurrent with their influenza and other immunization programs if history of vaccination is unclear. Boosters should be given at 10-year intervals; earlier for wounds. | Refrigerate. | Two primary doses of 0.5 mL each, administered at an interval of 4-6 weeks; third (reinforcing) dose of 0.5 mL 6-12 months later; boosters every 10 years. DT, Td, and T vaccines cause few problems (mild fever or soreness, swelling, and redness/ knot at the injection site). These problems usually last 1-2 days, but this does not happen nearly as often as with DTP vaccine. Td and T vaccines are not known to cause special problems for pregnant women or their unborn babies. A pregnant woman who needs Td vaccine should get it but wait until 2nd trimester if possible. |
| Diphtheria, tetanus toxoids, and acellular pertussis vaccine (Acel-Imune®; Tripedia®) | Fourth or fifth immunization of children 15 months to 7 years of age (period to seventh birthday) who have been previously immunized with 3 or 4 doses of whole-cell pertussis DTP vaccine. | Refrigerate at 2°C to 8°C (35°F to 46°F); do not freeze. | I.M.: After at least three doses of whole-cell DTP, administer 0.5 mL at 18 months (at least 6 months after third DTwP dose), then another dose at 4-5 years of age. DTaP should not be used in children <15 months of age and should not be used in children who have received fewer than 3 doses of DTP. |
| Diphtheria, tetanus toxoids, and whole-cell pertussis vaccine (Tri-Immunol®) | Active immunization of infants and children through 6 years of age (between 2 months and the seventh birthday) against diphtheria, tetanus, and pertussis. Recommended for both primary immunization and routine recall. Start immunization at once if whooping cough or diphtheria is present in the community. | | The primary immunization for children 2 months to 6 years of age, ideally beginning at the age of 2-3 months or at 6-week check-up. Administer 0.5 mL I.M. on three occasions at 4- to 8-week intervals with a re-enforcing dose administered 1 year after the third injection. The booster doses (0.5 mL I.M.) are administered when the child is 4-6 years of age. |
| Diphtheria, tetanus toxoids, whole-cell pertussis vaccine, and *Haemophilus* b conjugate vaccine (Tetramune®) | Active immunization of infants and children through 5 years of age (between 2 months and the sixth birthday) against diphtheria, tetanus, pertussis, and *Haemophilus* b disease when indications for immunization with DTP vaccine and HIB vaccine coincide. | Refrigerate. May be frozen (not diluent) without affecting potency. | The primary immunization for children 2 months to 5 years of age, ideally beginning at the age of 2-3 months or at 6-week checkup. Administer 0.5 mL I.M. on three occasions at 2-month intervals, followed by a fourth 0.5 mL dose at 15 months of age. If adverse reactions occurred with previous doses, immunization should be completed with diphtheria and tetanus toxoid absorbed (pediatric). Any febrile illness or active infection is reason for delaying use of *Haemophilus* b conjugate vaccine. |

# IMMUNIZATION GUIDELINES *(Continued)*

## IMMUNIZATIONS* (VACCINES) *(continued)*

| Drug | Use | Stability | Administration/ Patient Information |
|---|---|---|---|
| *Haemophilus* b conjugate vaccine (ActHIB®; HibTITER®; OmniHIB®; PedvaxHIB™; ProHIBiT®) | Routine immunization of children 2 months to 6 years of age against invasive disease caused by *H. influenzae* type b. Nonimmunized children ≥6 years of age with a chronic illness known to be associated with increased risk of *Haemophilus influenzae* type b disease, specifically, persons with anatomic or functional asplenia or sickle cell anemia or those who have undergone splenectomy, should receive Hib vaccine, as well as adults with specific dysfunction or certain complement deficiencies who are at especially high risk of *H. influenzae* type b infection (HIV-infected adults); patients with Hodgkin's disease or other hematologic neoplasms and immunosuppression (vaccinated at least 2 weeks before the initiation of chemotherapy or 3 months after the end of chemotherapy). *Haemophilus* b conjugate vaccines are not indicated for prevention of bronchitis or other infections due to *H. influenzae* in adults. | Store in refrigerator, may be frozen (not diluent) without affecting potency). Reconstituted Hib-Imune® remains stable for only 8 hours, whereas HibVAX® remains stable for 30 days when refrigerated. | Children: I.M.: 0.5 mL as a single dose. Have epinephrine 1:1000 available. |
| Hepatitis A vaccine (Havrix®) | For populations desiring protection against hepatitis A or for populations at high risk of exposure to hepatitis A virus (travelers to developing countries, household and sexual contacts of persons infected with hepatitis A), child day care employees, illicit drug users, male homosexuals, institutional workers (eg, institutions for the mentally and physically handicapped persons, prisons, etc), and healthcare workers who may be exposed to hepatitis A virus (eg, laboratory employees); protection lasts for approximately 15 years | | Inject I.M. into the deltoid muscle if possible. I.M.: 1 mL (1440 units), with a booster dose at 6-12 months. Use caution with patients with serious active infection, cardiovascular disease, or pulmonary disorders. Treatment for anaphylactic reactions should be immediately available. |
| Hepatitis B immune globulin (H-BIG®; HyperHep®) | Provide prophylactic passive immunity to hepatitis B infection to those individuals exposed; newborns of mothers known to be hepatitis B surface antigen positive; hepatitis B immune globulin is not indicated for treatment of active hepatitis B infections and is ineffective in the treatment of chronic active hepatitis B infection | Refrigerate at 2°C to 8°C (36°F to 46°F); do not freeze. | For I.M. injection (do not administer I.V.) only in gluteal or deltoid region. To prevent injury from injection, care should be taken when given to patients with thrombocytopenia or bleeding disorders. I.M.: Postexposure prophylaxis: 0.06 mL/kg; usual dose: 3-5 mL; repeat at 28-30 days after exposure. |
| Hepatitis B vaccine (Engerix-B®; Recombivax HB®) | Immunization against infection caused by all known subtypes of hepatitis B virus, in individuals considered at high risk of potential exposure to hepatitis B virus or $HB_sAg$-positive materials. | Refrigerate; do not freeze. | For I.M. injection (do not administer I.V.). The deltoid muscle is the preferred site (adults). Administer with caution in patients receiving anticoagulant therapy. S.C. injection may be administered in patients at risk of hemorrhage which may result in an increased incidence of local reactions and a reduced therapeutic effect. Patient will receive three doses of hepatitis B vaccine; immunity will last approximately 5-7 years. |

## IMMUNIZATIONS* (VACCINES) *(continued)*

| Drug | Use | Stability | Administration/ Patient Information |
|---|---|---|---|
| Immune globulin, intramuscular | Household and sexual contacts of persons with hepatitis A, measles, varicella, and possibly rubella; travelers to high-risk areas outside tourist routes. For travelers, IG is not an alternative to careful selection of foods and water; immune globulin can interfere with the antibody response to parenterally administered live virus vaccines. Frequent travelers should be tested for hepatitis A antibody, immune hemolytic anemia, and neutropenia (with TTP, I.V. route is usually used). | Refrigerate; do not freeze. | For I.M. injection only (do not administer I.V.); do not mix with other medications. Skin testing should not be performed as local irritation can occur and be misinterpreted as a positive reaction.<br>Hepatitis A: Pre-exposure prophylaxis upon travel into endemic areas (hepatitis A vaccine preferred); postexposure prophylaxis: 0.02 mL/kg given within 2 weeks of exposure.<br>Measles: Prophylaxis: 0.25 mL/kg/dose (max: 15 mL) given within 6 days of exposure followed by live attenuated measles vaccine in 3 months or at 15 months of age (whichever is later). For patients with leukemia, lymphoma, immunodeficiency disorders, generalized malignancy, or receiving immunosuppressive therapy: 0.5 mL/kg (max: 15 mL).<br>Poliomyelitis: Prophylaxis: 0.3 mg/kg/dose as a single dose<br>Rubella: Prophylaxis: 0.55 mL/kg/dose within 72 hours of exposure<br>Varicella: Prophylaxis: 0.6-1.2 mL/kg (varicella-zoster immune globulin preferred) within 72 hours of exposure<br>IgG deficiency: 1.3 mL/kg, then 0.66 mL/kg in 3-4 weeks<br>Hepatitis B: Prophylaxis: 0.06 mL/kg/dose (HBIG preferred) |
| Influenza virus vaccine (Flu-Imune®; Fluogen®; Fluzone®) | Provide active immunity to influenza virus strains contained in the vaccine; for high-risk persons, previous year vaccines do not prevent present year influenza. Those at risk for influenza injection include persons ≥65 years of age; institutionalized patients; persons of any age with chronic disorders of pulmonary and/or cardiovascular system; persons who have required medical follow-up following hospitalization for other chronic diseases such as diabetes, renal disease, immunodepressive disorders, etc; and travelers, especially those at risk. | Refrigerate | For I.M. administration only. I.M.: 0.5 mL each year of appropriate vaccine for the year, one dose is all that is necessary. Administer late in the fall to allow maximum titers to develop by peak epidemic periods usually occurring in early December. Waiting until the second or third trimester to vaccinate pregnant women with a high-risk condition may be reasonable. Antigenic response may not be as great as expected in patients requiring imunosuppressive drug. Hypersensitivity reactions may occur. Because of potential for febrile reactions, risks and benefits must carefully be considered in patients with a history of febrile convulsions. Influenza vaccines from previous seasons must not be used. Patients with sulfite sensitivity may be affected by this product. |

# IMMUNIZATION GUIDELINES *(Continued)*

## IMMUNIZATIONS* (VACCINES) *(continued)*

| Drug | Use | Stability | Administration/ Patient Information |
|---|---|---|---|
| Japanese encephalitis virus vaccine, inactivated | Active immunization against Japanese encephalitis for persons spending a month or longer in endemic areas, especially if travel will include rural areas | Refrigerate at 2°C to 8°C. Do not freeze. Discard 8 hours after reconstitution. | Three doses of 1 mL; booster doses of 1 mL may be administered 2 years after primary immunization series. Adverse reactions may occur shortly after vaccination or up to 17 days (usually within 10 days) after vaccination. If the patient has a past history of urticaria following hymenoptera envenomation, drugs, physical or other provocation, or of idiopathic origin, adverse reactions are more likely. Arm soreness and local redness can occur shortly after vaccination. International travel should not be initiated within 10 days of vaccination because of the possibility of delayed adverse reactions. Seek medical attention immediately upon onset of any adverse reactions. Epinephrine should be immediately available should an anaphylactic reaction occur. Precautions should be taken to avoid exposure to mosquito bites by use of insect repellants and protective clothing. Avoiding outdoor activity, especially during twilight periods and in the evening, will reduce risk further. Unknown whether the drug is excreted in breast milk. |
| Lyme disease vaccine (LYMErix®) | Active immunization against Lyme disease in individuals between 15-70 years of age | Store between 2°C and 8°C (36°F and 46°F. | I.M.: Vaccination with three doses of 30 mcg (0.5 mL), administered at 0, 1, and 12 months, is recommended for optimal protection. |
| Measles and rubella vaccines, combined (M-R-VAX® II) | Simultaneous immunization against measles and rubella | Refrigerate prior to use. Use as soon as possible. Discard if not used within 8 hours of reconstitution. | S.C.: Inject 0.5 mL into outer aspect of upper arm; no routine booster for rubella. |
| Measles, mumps, and rubella vaccines, combined (M-M-R® II) | Measles, mumps, and rubella prophylaxis in children (≥15 months) and adults; for HIV-infected children, MMR should routinely be administered at 15 months of age. | Refrigerate and protect from light prior to reconstitution. Use as soon as possible. Discard 8 hours after reconstitution. | Injection: 1000 $TCID_{50}$ each of measles virus vaccine and rubella virus vaccine, 5000 $TCID_{50}$ mumps virus vaccine |
| Measles virus vaccine, live (Attenuvax®) | Immunization for adults born after 1957 without documentation of live vaccine on or after first birthday, physician-diagnosed measles, or laboratory evidence of immunity should be vaccinated, ideally with two doses of vaccine separated by no less than 1 month. For those previously vaccinated with one dose of measles vaccine, revaccination is recommended for students entering colleges and other institutions of higher education, for healthcare workers at the time of employment, and for international travelers who visit endemic areas. | Refrigerate at 2°C to 8°C. Discard if left at room temperature for over 8 hours. Protect from light. | S.C.: Inject 0.5 mL into outer aspect of upper arm; no routine booster. |

## IMMUNIZATIONS* (VACCINES) *(continued)*

| Drug | Use | Stability | Administration/ Patient Information |
|---|---|---|---|
| Meningococcal polysaccharide vaccine, groups A, C, Y, and W-135 (Menomune®-A/ C/Y/W-135) | Immunization of persons 2 years of age and older in epidemic or endemic areas as might be determined in a population delineated by neighborhood, school, dormitory, or other reasonable boundary. The prevalent serogroup in such a situation should match a serogroup in the vaccine. Individuals at particular high-risk include persons with terminal component complement deficiencies and those with anatomic or function asplenia. For use with travelers visiting areas of a country that are recognized as having hyperendemic or epidemic meningococcal disease. Vaccinations should be considered for household or institutional contacts of persons with meningococcal disease as an adjunct to appropriate antibiotic chemoprophylaxis as well as medical and laboratory personnel at risk of exposure to meningococcal disease. | Discard remainder of vaccine within 5 days after reconstitution. Store reconstituted vaccine in refrigerator. | S.C.: 0.5 mL; do not inject intradermally or I.V. Have epinephrine 1:1000 available to control allergic reaction. Patients who undergo splenectomy secondary to trauma or nonlymphoid tumors respond well, however, those asplenic patients with lymphoid tumors who receive either chemotherapy or irradiation respond poorly. Avoid in pregnancy unless there is a substantial risk of infection. |
| Plague vaccine | Vaccinate selected travelers to countries where avoidance of rodents and fleas is impossible; laboratory and field personnel working with *Yersinia pestis* organisms possibly resistant to antimicrobials; those engaged in *Yersinia pestis* aerosol experiments or in field operations in areas with enzootic plague where regular exposure to potentially infected wild rodents, rabbits, or their fleas cannot be prevented. Prophylactic antibiotics may be indicated following definite exposure, whether or not the exposed persons have been vaccinated. | | Three I.M. doses: First dose 1 mL, second dose (0.2 mL) 1 month later, third dose (0.2 mL) 5 months after the second dose; booster doses (0.2 mL) at 1- to 2-year intervals if exposure continues. Do not use in pregnant females unless there is substantial and unavoidable risk of exposure. |
| Pneumococcal vaccine (Pneumovax® 23; Pnu-Imune® 23) | For children >2 years of age and adults who are at increased risk of pneumococcal disease and its complications because of underlying health conditions; older adults, including all those ≥65 years of age | Refrigerate | Administer S.C. or I.M. (deltoid muscle or lateral migthigh). Do not inject I.V. Have epinephrine injection (1:1000) available. I.M., S.C.: 0.5 mL. Revaccination should be considered if ≥6 years have elapsed since initial vaccination, for patients who received 14-valent pneumococcal vaccine and are at highest risk (asplenic) for fatal infection, or at ≥6 years in patients with nephrotic syndrome, renal failure, or transplant recipients. Use with caution in individuals who have had episodes of pneumococcal infection within the preceeding 3 years (pre-existing pneumococcal antibodies may result in increased reactions to vaccine). May cause relapse in patients with stable idiopathic thrombocytopenia purpura. Federal law requires that the date of administration, the vaccine manufacturer, lot number of vaccine, and the administering person's name, title, and address be entered into the patient's permanent medical record. |

# IMMUNIZATION GUIDELINES *(Continued)*

## IMMUNIZATIONS* (VACCINES) *(continued)*

| Drug | Use | Stability | Administration/ Patient Information |
|---|---|---|---|
| Poliovirus vaccine, inactivated (IPOL™) | Oral: Prevention of poliomyelitis for infants (6-12 weeks of age) and all nonimmunized children and adolescents through 18 years of age for routine prophylaxis. Persons traveling to areas where wild poliovirus is epidemic or endemic, and certain health personnel. Although a protective immune response to E-IPV cannot be assured in the immunocompromised individual, E-IPV is recommended because the vaccine is safe and some protection may result from its administration. | | Oral: Two 0.5 mL doses 6-8 weeks apart and a third dose of 0.5 mL 6-12 months after second dose. S.C.: Enhanced-potency inactivated poliovirus vaccine (E-IPV) is preferred for primary vaccination of adults, two doses 4-8 weeks apart, a third dose 6-12 months after the second. For adults with a completed primary series and for whom a booster is indicated, either OPV or E-IPV can be given. If immediate protection is needed, either OPV or E-IPV is recommended. |
| Rabies immune globulin (human) | Part of postexposure prophylaxis of persons with rabies exposure who lack a history of pre-exposure or postexposure prophylaxis with rabies vaccine or a recently documented neutralizing antibody response to previous rabies vaccination. It is preferable to give RIG with the first dose of vaccine, but it can be given up to 8 days after vaccination. | Refrigerate | I.M.: 20 units/kg in a single dose (RIG should always be administered in conjunction with rabies vaccine (DDCV)). Infiltrate half of the dose locally around the wound; administer the remainder I.M. Use with caution in individuals with thrombocytopenia, bleeding disorders, or prior allergic reactions to immune globulins. Severe adverse reactions can occur if the patient receives RIG I.V. |

## IMMUNIZATIONS* (VACCINES) *(continued)*

| Drug | Use | Stability | Administration/ Patient Information |
|---|---|---|---|
| Rabies virus vaccine | Pre-exposure rabies immunization for high-risk persons; postexposure antirabies immunization along with local treatment and immune globulin | Refrigerate. Reconstituted vaccine should be used immediately. | **Pre-exposure prophylaxis:** Two 1 mL doses I.M. or I.D. 1 week apart, third dose 3 weeks after second. If exposure continues, booster doses can be administered every 2 years, or an antibody titer determined and a booster dose administered if the titer is inadequate. **Postexposure prophylaxis:** All postexposure treatment should begin with immediate cleansing of the wound with soap and water. Persons not previously immunized should be given rabies immune globulin 20 units/kg body weight, half infiltrated at bite site if possible, remainder I.M. and 5 doses of rabies vaccine, 1 mL I.M. one each on days 0, 3, 7, 14, and 28. Persons who have previously received postexposure prophylaxis with rabies vaccine, received a recommended I.M. or I.D. pre-exposure series of rabies vaccine, or have a previously documented rabies antibody titer considered adequate should receive 2 doses of rabies vaccine, 1 mL I.M. one each on days 0 and 3. Complete pre-exposure prophylaxis does not eliminate the need for additional therapy with rabies vaccine after a rabies exposure. The FDA has not approved the I.D. use of rabies vaccine for postexposure prophylaxis. Recommendations for I.D. use of HDCV are currently being discussed. The decision for postexposure rabies vaccination depends on the species of biting animal, the circumstances of biting incident, and the type of exposure (bite, saliva contamination of wound, etc). The type of and schedule for postexposure prophylaxis depends upon the person's previous rabies vaccination status or the result of a previous or current serologic test for rabies antibody. Rabies vaccine is available only in I.M. form; it cannot be given intradermally. |
| $Rh_o$(D) immune globulin (Gamulin®, HypRho®-D; HypRho®-D Mini-Dose; MICRhoGAM™, Mini-Gamulin® Rh; RhoGAM™) | Prevention of isoimmunization in Rh-negative individuals exposed to Rh-positive blood during delivery of an Rh-positive infant, as a result of an abortion, following amniocentesis or abdominal trauma, or following a transfusion accident; prevention of hemolytic disease of the newborn if there is a subsequent pregnancy with an Rh-positive fetus | Reconstituted solution should be refrigerated and will remain stable for 30 days. Solutions that have been frozen should be discarded. | I.M. (administered I.M. to mothers not to infant): Obstetrical use: 1 vial (300 mcg) prevents maternal sensitization if fetal packed red blood cell volume that has entered the circulation is ≤15 mL; it if is more, give additional vials. The number of vials = RBC volume of the calculated fetomaternal hemorrhage divided by 15 mL. Postpartum prophylaxis: 300 mcg within 72 hours of delivery. Antepartum prophylaxis: 300 mcg at approximately 26-28 weeks gestation; followed by 300 mcg within 72 hours of delivery if infant is Rh-positive. Following miscarriage, abortion, or termination of ectopic pregnancy at up to 13 weeks gestation: 50 mcg ideally within 3 hours, but may be given up to 72 hours after. If pregnancy has been terminated at 13 or more weeks of gestation, administer 300 mcg. |

## IMMUNIZATION GUIDELINES *(Continued)*

### IMMUNIZATIONS* (VACCINES) *(continued)*

| Drug | Use | Stability | Administration/ Patient Information |
|---|---|---|---|
| $Rh_o(D)$ immune globulin (intravenous-human) (WinRho SD®) | Prevention of Rh isoimmunization in nonsensitized $Rh_o(D)$ antigen-negative women within 7 hours after spontaneous or induced abortion, amniocentesis, chorionic villus sampling, ruptured tubal pregnancy, abdominal trauma, transplacental hemorrhage, or in the normal course of pregnancy unless the blood type of the fetus or father is known to be $Rh_o(D)$ antigen-negative; suppression of Rh isoimmunization in $Rh_o(D)$ antigen-negative female children and female adults in their childbearing years transfused with $Rh_o(D)$ antigen-positive RBCs or blood components containing $Rh_o(D)$ antigen-positive RBCs; treatment of immune thrombocytopenia purpura in nonsplenectomized $Rh_o(D)$ antigen-positive patients | Store at 2°C to 8°C. Do not freeze. If not used immediately, store the product at room temperature for 4 hours. Discard unused portions. | Prevention of Rh isoimmunization: I.V.: 1500 units (300 mcg) at 28 weeks gestation or immediately after amniocentesis if before 34 weeks gestation or after chorionic villus sampling; repeat this dose every 12 weeks during the pregnancy, 600 units (120 mcg) at delivery (within 72 hours) and after invasive intrauterine procedures such as abortion, amniocentesis, or any other manipulation if at >34 weeks gestation. If the Rh status of the baby is not known at 72 hours, administer $Rh_o(D)$ immune globulin to the mother at 72 hours after delivery. If >72 hours have elapsed, do not withhold $Rh_o(D)$ immune globulin, but administer as soon as possible, up to 28 days after delivery.<br>I.M.: reconstitute vial with 1.25 mL and administer as above.<br>Transfusion: Administer within 72 hours after exposure for treatment of incompatible blood transfusions or massive fetal hemorrhage as follows: I.V.: 3000 units (600 mcg) every 8 hours until the total dose is administered (45 units [9 mcg] of Rh-positive blood/mL blood; 90 units [18 mcg] Rh positive red cells/mL cells). I.M.: 6000 units (1200 mcg) every 12 hours until the total dose is administered (60 units [12 mcg] of Rh-positive blood/mL blood; 120 units [24 mcg] Rh-positive red cells/mL cells).<br>Treatment of ITP: I.V.: Initial: 25-50 mcg/kg depending on the patient's Hg concentration; maintenance: 25-60 mcg/kg depending on the clinical response. |
| Rotavirus vaccine (RotaShield®) | Prevention of gastroenteritis caused by the rotavirus serotypes responsible for the majority of disease in infants and children in the U.S. (serotypes G 1,2,3, and 4. | Store lyophilized vaccine at room temperature below 25°C. Lyophilized vaccine (and diluent) may be refrigerated. Reconstituted vaccine is stable for 60 minutes at room temperature and 4 hours under refrigeration. | Children: Oral (for oral administration only): Three 2.5 mL doses. Recommended schedule for immunization is at 2, 4, and 6 months of age. Repeat dosing is not recommended if infant should regurgitate a dose. Not approved for administration to adults. |
| Rubella and mumps vaccines, combined (Biavax® II) | Promote active immunity to rubella and mumps by inducing production of antibodies | Refrigerate, discard unused portion within 8 hours. Protect from light. | Children >12 years and adults: 1 vial in outer aspect of the upper arm. Federal law requires that the date of administration, the vaccine manufacturer, lot number of vaccine, and the administering person's name, title, and address be entered into the patient's permanent medical record. |
| Rubella virus vaccine, live (Meruvax® II) | Provide vaccine-induced immunity to rubella | Refrigerate, discard reconstituted vaccine after 8 hours. | S.C.: 1000 $TCID_{50}$Federal law requires that the date of administration, the vaccine manufacturer, lot number of vaccine, and the administering person's name, title, and address be entered into the patient's permanent medical record. |

## IMMUNIZATIONS* (VACCINES) *(continued)*

| Drug | Use | Stability | Administration/ Patient Information |
|---|---|---|---|
| Tetanus antitoxin | Tetanus prophylaxis or treatment of active tetanus only when tetanus immune globulin (TIG) is not available. Tetanus immune globulin (Hyper-Tet®) is the preferred tetanus immunoglobulin for the treatment of active tetanus. May be given concomitantly with tetanus toxoid adsorbed when immediate treatment is required, but active immunization is desirable. | Refrigerate; do not freeze. | Inject 10,000-40,000 units into wound; administer 40,000-100,000 units I.V. Tetanus antitoxin is not the same as tetanus immune globulin. Sensitivity testing should be conducted in all individuals regardless of clinical history. Have epinephrine 1:1000 available. |
| Tetanus immune globulin (human) (Hyper-Tet®) | Passive immunization against tetanus; tetanus immune globulin is preferred over tetanus antitoxin for treatment of active tetanus; part of the management of an unclean wound in a person whose history of previous receipt of tetanus toxoid is unknown or who has received less than three doses of tetanus toxoid; elderly may require TIG more often than younger patients with tetanus infection due to declining antibody titers with age | Refrigerate at 2°C to 8°C (36°F to 46°F). | Administer I.M. 250 units for prophylaxis of tetanus; 3000-6000 units for treatment of tetanus. Do not give I.V. Never administer tetanus toxoid (Td) and TIG in the same syringe (toxoid will be neutralized). Toxoid may be given at a separate site. Have epinephrine 1:1000 available. Boosters will be necessary. |
| Tetanus toxoid (adsorbed) | Selective induction of active immunity against tetanus in selected patients. **Note:** Tetanus and diphtheria toxoids for adult use (Td) is the preferred immunizing agent for most adults and for children after 7 years of age. Young children should receive trivalent DTwP or DTaP (diphtheria/tetanus/pertussis – whole cell or acellular), as part of their childhood immunization program, unless pertussis is contraindicated, then TD is warranted. | Refrigerate; do not freeze. | Administer I.M. in the area of the vastus lateralis (midthigh laterally) or deltoid. Primary immunization: 0.5 mL; repeat 0.5 mL at 4-8 weeks after the first dose and at 6-12 months after the second dose. Routine booster doses are recommended only every 5-10 years. Have epinephrine 1:1000 available. Not equivalent to tetanus toxoid fluid. Tetanus toxoid adsorbed is the preferred toxoid for immunization and Td, TD, or DTaP/DTwP are the preferred adsorbed forms. Avoid injection into a blood vessel. |
| Tetanus toxoid (fluid) | Detection of delayed hypersensitivity and assessment of cell-mediated immunity; active immunization against tetanus in the rare adult or child who is allergic to the aluminum adjuvant (a product containing adsorbed tetanus toxoid is preferred) | Refrigerate | Do not administer I.V. Anergy testing: Intradermal: 0.1 mL. Primary immunization (**Note:** Td, TD, DTaP/DTwP are recommended): Inject three doses of 0.5 mL I.M. or S.C. at 4- to 8-week intervals. Give fourth dose 6-12 months after third dose. Booster doses: I.M., S.C.: 0.5 mL every 10 years. Have epinephrine 1:1000 available. |

# IMMUNIZATION GUIDELINES *(Continued)*

## IMMUNIZATIONS* (VACCINES) *(continued)*

| Drug | Use | Stability | Administration/ Patient Information |
|---|---|---|---|
| Typhoid vaccine | **Parenteral:** Promotes active immunity to typhoid fever for patients intimately exposed to a typhoid carrier or foreign travel to a typhoid fever endemic area. **Oral:** Immunize children older than 6 years and adults who expect intimate exposure of or household contact with typhoid fever, travelers to areas of the world with a risk of exposure to typhoid fever, and workers in microbiology laboratories with expected frequent contact with *S. typhi.* **Typhoid vaccine:** Live, attenuated TY21a typhoid vaccine should not be administered to immunocompromised persons, including those known to be infected with HIV. Parenteral inactivated vaccine is a theoretically safer alternative for this group. | Refrigerate. Do not freeze. Potency is not harmed if mistakenly placed in a freezer; however, remove from the freezer as soon as possible and place in refrigerator. Can be used if exposed to temperature ≤80°F. | Oral: Primary immunization: 1 capsule on alternate days (day 1, 3, 5, and 7); booster: Repeat full course of primary immunization every 5 years. S.C.: 0.5 mL; repeat dose in ≥4 weeks (total immunization is two doses). Booster: 0.5 mL every 3 years for. Postpone use in the presence of acute infection. Use during pregnancy only when clearly needed. Not all recipients of typhoid vaccine will be fully protected against typhoid fever. Travelers should take all necessary precautions to avoid contact or ingestion of potentially contaminated food or water sources. Unless a complete immunization schedule is followed, an optimum immune response may not be achieved. Doses of vaccine are different between S.C. and intradermal; only S.C. injection should be used. Oral capsule should be taken 1 hour before a meal with cold or lukewarm drink. Do not chew or swallow whole. Systemic adverse effects may persist for 1-2 days. Take all 4 doses exactly as directed on alternate days to obtain a maximal response. Vaccinating the elderly is often overlooked. If no record of immunization can be recalled, repeat primary series. |
| Varicella virus vaccine (Varicax®) | Immunization against chickenpox for healthy children between 12 months and 18 years (1 vaccination if 12 months to 13 years and not previously immunized; 2 vaccinations if 13-18 years 4-8 weeks apart); recommended to give with MMR vaccine | Store in freezer (-157°C). Store diluent separately at room temperature or in refrigerator. Discard if reconstituted vaccine is not used within 30 minutes. | S.C.: 2 doses of 0.5 mL separated by 4-8 weeks |

## IMMUNIZATIONS* (VACCINES) *(continued)*

| Drug | Use | Stability | Administration/ Patient Information |
|---|---|---|---|
| Varicella-zoster immune globulin (human) | Passive immunization of susceptible immunodeficient patients after exposure to varicella. Most effective if begun within 72 hours of exposure. There is no evidence that VZIG modifies established varicella-zoster infections. **Restrict administration to:** Patients with neoplastic disease (leukemia, lymphoma); congenital or acquired immunodeficiency; immunosuppressive therapy with steroids, antimetabolites, or other immunosuppressive treatment regimens; newborns or mothers who had onset of chickenpox within 5 days before delivery or within 48 hours after delivery; premature infant (≥28 weeks gestation) whose mother has no history of chickenpox; premature infants (<28 weeks gestation or ≤1000 g VZIG) regardless of maternal history. **One of the following types of exposure to chickenpox or zoster patients may warrant administration:** Continuous household contact; playmate contact (>1 hour play indoors); hospital contact (in same 2-4 bedroom or adjacent beds in a large ward or prolonged face-to-face contact with an infectious staff member of patient); susceptible to varicella-zoster; age <15 years (administer to immunocompromised adolescents and adults and to other older patients on an individual basis). An acceptable alternative to VZIG prophylaxis is to treat varicella, if it occurs, with high-dose I.V. acyclovir. | Refrigerate at 2°C to 8°C. | High-risk susceptible patients who are exposed again more than 3 weeks after a prior dose of VZIG should receive another full dose; there is no evidence VZIG modifies established varicella-zoster infections. I.M.: Administer by deep injection in the gluteal muscle or in another large muscle mass. Inject 125 units/10 kg (22 lb); maximum dose: 625 units (5 vials); minimum dose: 125 units; do not administer fractional doses. Do not inject I.V. VZIG is not indicated for prophylaxis or therapy of normal adults who are exposed to or who develop varicella. It is not indicated for treatment of herpes zoster. VZIG provides passive immunity for those susceptible to varicella, with neoplastic disease, in immunosuppressed elderly, or those institutionalized who are exposed to other patients with varicella. CDC provides specific guidelines for use. Age is the most important risk factor for reactivation of varicella-zoster. |
| Yellow fever vaccine | Vaccinate selected persons traveling or living in areas where yellow fever infection exists. | Ship vaccine on dry ice. Do not use vaccine unless shipping case contains some dry ice on arrival. Maintain vaccine continuously at a temperature between 0°C to 5°C. Sterilize and discard all unused rehydrated vaccine and containers after 1 hour. Avoid vigorous shaking. | Single dose S.C.: 0.5 mL. Immunity develops by the 10th day and WHO requires revaccination every 10 years to maintain travelers' vaccination certificate. If a pregnant woman is to be vaccinated only to satisfy an international requirement, efforts should be made to obtain a waiver letter. |

*Contact Poison Control Center.

# NUTRITIONAL AND HERBAL PRODUCTS

## TOP HERBAL PRODUCTS

This section contains general information on commonly encountered herbal or nutritional products. A more complete listing products follows.

### Chamomile

**Synonyms:** *Matricaria chamomilla*; *Matricaria recutita*

**Use:** Has been used for indigestion and its hypnotic properties; topical anti-inflammatory agent; used for hemorrhoids, irritable bowel, eczema, mastitis and leg ulcers; used to flavor cigarette tobacco

**Mechanism of Action/Effect:** Pharmacologic activities include antispasmodic, anti-inflammatory, antiulcer, and antibacterial effects; a sedative effect has also been documented

**Contraindications:** Hypersensitivity to *Asteraceae/Compositae* family

**Warnings:** Use with caution in asthmatics; cross sensitivity may occur in individuals allergic to ragweed pollens, asters, or chrysanthemums.

**Drug Interactions:** May increase effect of coumarin-type anticoagulants at high doses

**Adverse Reactions:** Contact dermatitis, immunologic contact urticaria, emesis (from dried flowering heads), anaphylaxis; while the toxicity of its main chemical constituent (Bisabolol) is low, the tea is essentially prepared from various allergens (ie, pollen-laden flower heads) which can cause hypersensitivity reactions especially in atopic individuals; contains various flavonoids (apigenin, herniarin)

**Dosing:**

Tea: ±150 mL $H_2O$ poured over heaping tablespoon (±3 g) of chamomile, covered and steeped 5-10 minutes; tea is used 3-4 times/day for GI upset

Liquid extract: 1-4 mL 3 times/day

**Pregnancy Implications:** Excessive use should be avoided due to potential teratogenicity.

### Chromium

**Use:** Improves glycemic control; increases lean body mass; reduces obesity; improves lipid profile by decreasing total cholesterol and triglycerides, increasing HDL

**Mechanism of Action/Effect:** Chromium picolinate is the only active form of chromium. It appears that chromium, in its trivalent form, increases insulin sensitivity and improves glucose transport into cells. The mechanism by which this happens could include one or more of the following: Increase the number of insulin receptors, enhance insulin binding to target tissues, promote activation of insulin-receptor tyrosine dinase activity, enhance beta-cell sensitivity in the pancreas.

**Drug Interactions:** Any medications that may also affect blood sugars (eg, beta-blockers, thiazides, medications prescribed to treat diabetes); discuss chromium use prior to initiating

**Adverse Reactions:** Nausea, loose stools, flatulence, changes in appetite; isolated reports of anemia, cognitive impairment, renal failure

**Dosing:** 50-600 mcg/day

### *Echinacea*

**Synonyms:** American Coneflower; Black Susans; Comb Flower; *Echinacea angustifolia*; Indian Head; Purple Coneflower; Scury Root; Snakeroot

**Use:** Prophylaxis and treatment of cold and flu; an immunostimulant in herbal medicine; treatment of minor upper respiratory tract infections, urinary tract infections, wound/skin infections, arthritis, vaginal yeast infections

**Mechanism of Action/Effect:** Contains a caffeic acid glycoside named echinacoside (0.1% concentration) which is bactericidal. Other caffeic acid glycosides and isolutylamides associated with the plant can cause immune stimulation by increasing leukocyte phagocytosis and promoting T-cell activation. Also has an antihyaluronidase and anti-inflammatory activity; constituents have been associated with antitumor, antispasmodic effects.

**Contraindications:** Autoimmune diseases, such as collagen vascular disease (lupus, RA), multiple sclerosis; allergy to sunflowers, daisies, ragweed; tuberculosis, HIV, AIDS, pregnancy (parenteral administration only contraindicated per Commission E, oral use of *Echinacea* is not contraindicated during pregnancy per Commission E)

**Warnings:** May alter immunosuppression; persons allergic to sunflowers may display cross-allergy potential

**Drug Interactions:** Theoretically may alter response to immunosuppressive therapy
**Adverse Reactions:** Tingling sensation of tongue, allergic reactions (rare), none known for oral and external use per Commission E; may become immunosuppressive with continuous use over 6-8 weeks
**Dosing:** Continuous use should not exceed 8 weeks.
Per Commission E: Expressed juice (of fresh herb): 6-9 mL/day
Capsule/tablet or tea form: 500 mg to 2 g 3 times/day
Liquid extract: 0.25-1 mL 3 times/day
Tincture: 1-2 mL 3 times/day
May be applied topically.

## Feverfew

**Synonyms:** Altamisa; Bachelor's Buttons; Featherfew; Featherfoil; Nosebleed; *Tanacetum parthenium*; Wild Quinine
**Lactation:** Contraindicated
**Use:** Prophylaxis and treatment of migraine headaches; treatment of menstrual complaints and fever
**Mechanism of Action/Effect:** Active ingredient is parthenolide (~0.2% concentration), a sesquiterpene which is a serotonin antagonist; also, the plant may be an inhibitor of prostaglandin synthesis and platelet aggregation; has spasmolytic effect on cerebral blood vessels; other anti-inflammatory effects, antimicrobial, antifungal
**Contraindications:** Pregnancy; children <2 years of age; allergies to feverfew and other members of Asteraceae, daisy, ragweed, chamomile
**Warnings:** Use with caution in patients taking medications with serotonergic properties.
**Drug Interactions:** Use with caution in patients taking aspirin or anticoagulants due to increased potential for bleeding.
**Adverse Reactions:** Mouth ulcerations, contact dermatitis, swelling of tongue or lips, abdominal pain, nausea, vomiting, loss of taste; postfeverfew syndrome: nervousness, insomnia, still joints, headache
**Dosing:** 125 mg of a preparation standardized to 0.2% parthenolide (250 mcg) once or twice daily

## Garlic

**Synonyms:** *Allium savitum*; Comphor of the Poor; Nectar of the Gods; Poor Mans Treacle; Rustic Treacle; Stinking Rose
**Use:** Lower LDL cholesterol and triglycerides and raise HDL cholesterol; protection against artherosclerosis, hypertension; antiseptic agent; may lower blood glucose and decrease thrombosis; potential anti-inflammatory and antitumor effects
**Mechanism of Action/Effect:** Garlic bulbs contain alliin, a parent to the substance allicin (after the bulb is ground), which is odoriferous and may have some antioxidant activity; ajoene (a byproduct of allicin) has potent platelet inhibition effects; garlic can also decrease LDL cholesterol levels and increase fibrinolytic activity
**Contraindications:** Pregnancy
**Warnings:** Cholesterol-lowering and hypotensive effects may require months. Use with caution in patients receiving treatment for hyperglycemia or hypertension.
**Drug Interactions:** Iodine uptake may be reduced with garlic ingestion; can exacerbate bleeding in patients taking aspirin or anticoagulant agents; may increase the risk of hypoglycemia; may increase response to antihypertensives
**Adverse Reactions:** Skin blistering, eczema, systemic contact dermatitis, immunologic contact urticaria, GI upset and changes in intestinal flora (rare) per Commission E, lacrimation, asthma (upon inhalation of garlic dust), allergic reactions (rare), change in odor of skin and breath (per Commission E)
**Half-Life Elimination:** N-acetyl-S-allyl-L-cysteine: 6 hours
**Excretion:** Pulmonary and renal
**Dosing:** Adults: 4-12 mg allicin/day
Average daily dose for cardiovascular benefit: 0.25-1 g/kg or 1-4 cloves daily in an 80 kg individual in divided doses
Toxic dose: >5 cloves or >25 mL of extract can cause GI symptoms
**Additional Information:** 1% as active as penicillin as an antibiotic; number one over-the-counter medication in Germany; enteric-coated products may demonstrate best results.

## Ginger

**Synonyms:** *Zingiber officinale*
**Pregnancy Risk Factor:** No administration for morning sickness during pregnancy per Commission E; however, literature does not support this caution. Indian

and Chinese women use large amounts routinely during pregnancy with no ill effects on pregnancy or fetus. High doses may be abortifacient.

**Use:** Digestive aid; treatment of nausea (antiemetic) and motion sickness; menstruation promoter in Chinese herbal medicine; treatment of headaches, colds, and flu; ginger oil is used as a flavoring agent in beverages and mouthwashes; may be useful in some forms of arthritis

**Mechanism of Action/Effect:** Unknown; may increase GI motility and thus block nausea feedback from the GI tract; appears to decrease prostaglandin synthesis; may have cardiotonic activity; may inhibit platelet aggregation

**Contraindications:** Gallstones (per Commission E)

**Warnings:** Use with caution in diabetics, patients on cardiac glycosides, and those receiving anticoagulants.

**Drug Interactions:** May alter response to cardiotonic, hypoglycemic, anticoagulant, and antiplatelet agents.

**Dosing:**

Prevention of motion sickness or digestive aid: 1-4 g/day (250 mg of ginger root powder 4 times/day)

Per Commission E: 2-4 g/day or equivalent preparations

## Ginkgo Biloba

**Synonyms:** Kew Tree; Maidenhair Tree

**Use:** Dilates blood vessels; plant/leaf extract has been used in Europe for intermittent claudication, arterial insufficiency, and cerebral vascular disease (dementia); tinnitus, visual disorders, traumatic brain injury, vertigo of vascular origin

Per Commission E: Demential syndromes including memory deficits, etc (tinnitus, headache); depressive emotional conditions, primary degenerative dementia, vascular dementia, or both

**Investigational:** Asthma, impotence (male)

**Mechanism of Action/Effect:** Inhibits platelet aggregation; ginkgo biloba leaf extract contain terpenoids and flavonoids which can allegedly inactivate oxygen-free radicals causing vasodilatation and antagonize effects of platelet activating factor (PAF); fruit pulp contains ginkolic acids which are allergens (seeds are not sensitizing)

**Contraindications:** Pregnancy; patients with clotting disorders; hypersensitivity to ginkgo biloba preparations (per Commission E)

**Warnings:** Use with caution following recent surgery or trauma. Effects may require 1-2 months.

**Drug Interactions:** Due to effects on PAF, use with caution in patients receiving anticoagulants or platelet inhibitors

**Adverse Reactions:** Palpitations, bilateral subdural hematomas, headache (very seldom per Commission E), dizziness, seizures (in children), restlessness, urticaria, cheilitis, nausea, diarrhea, vomiting, stomatitis, proctitis, stomach or intestinal upsets (very seldom per Commission E), hyphema, allergic skin reactions (very seldom per Commission E)

**Onset of Effect:** 1 hour

**Peak Absorption:** 2-3 hours

**Duration of Action:** 7 hours

**Bioavailability:** 70% to 100%

**Half-life:** Ginkgolide A: 4 hours; ginkgolide B: 10.6 hours; bilobalide: 3.2 hours

**Dosing:** Beneficial effects for cerebral ischemia in the elderly occur after 1 month of use.

Usual dosage: ~40 mg 3 times/day with meals; 60-80 mg twice daily to 3 times/day depending on indication; maximum dose: 360 mg/day

Cerebral ischemia: 120 mg/day in 2-3 divided doses (24% flavonoid-glycoside extract, 6% terpene glycosides)

**Additional Information:** Seeds and pulp are poisonous; beneficial effects for cerebral ischemia in the elderly occur after 1 month of use.

## Ginseng

**Synonyms:** *P. quinquefolium; P. trifolius*

**Lactation:** Not recommended

**Use:** Popular ingredient in herbal teas; has been advocated for its antistress and adaptogenic effects although these effects have not been scientifically confirmed, there is much suggestive scientific literature

**Mechanism of Action/Effect:** Active agent (ginsenosides) may have CNS stimulant and estrogen-like effect, anti-inflammatory, antiplatelet; adaptogen; may lower cholesterol; not effective as an aphrodisiac

**Contraindications:** Estrogen-receptor positive breast cancer

**Warnings:** Nervousness may occur during the first few days; use with caution with hypertensives, diabetes. Avoid long-term use. Not recommended in pregnancy.
**Drug Interactions:** May decrease effects of loop diuretics (furosemide); theoretically, may increase effect of antiplatelet agents, anticoagulants, hypoglycemics, and hypotensive agents
**Adverse Reactions:** Tachycardia, hypertension, sinus tachycardia, nervousness, agitation, mania, headache, sciatic nerve inflammation, Stevens-Johnson syndrome, hypoglycemia, vaginal bleeding, breast nodules
**Dosing:** Avoid long-term use.

Herbal tea: Usually about 1.75 g; 0.5-2 g/day
Dried root: 0.6-3 g/day of dried root or equivalent preparations
Ethanolic extract: 0.5-6 mL 1-3 times/day
Root: 1-2 g/day
Extract (7% ginsenosides): 100-300 mg 3 times/day

**Additional Information:** There are three forms of ginseng (American, Asian, and Siberian); each has slightly different properties.

## Glucosamine

**Use:** Osteoarthritis, rheumatoid arthritis, tendonitis, gout, bursitis
**Mechanism of Action/Effect:** Glucosamine is an amino sugar which is a key component in the synthesis of proteoglycans, a group of proteins found in cartilage. These proteoglycans are negatively charged, and attract water so they can produce synovial fluid in the joints. The theory is that supplying the body with these precursors will replenish important synovial fluid, and lead to production of new cartilage. Glucosamine also appears to inhibit cartilage-destroying enzymes (eg, collagenase and phospholipase A2), thus stopping the degenerative processes of osteoarthritis. A third mechanism may be glucosamine's ability to prevent production of damaging superoxide radicals, which may lead to cartilage destruction.
**Adverse Reactions:** Few effects (eg, flatulence, nausea)
**Drug Interactions:** May increase effect of oral anticoagulants.
**Dosing:** 500 mg of the sulfate form 3 times/day
**Additional Information:** Both a sulfate and a hydrochloride salt are available. Glucosamine appears more highly absorbed when administered in the sulfate form, and sulfate is also an important mineral in cartilage.

## Golden Seal

**Synonyms:** Eye Balm; Eye Root; *Hydrastis canadensis*; Indian Eye; Jaundice Root; Orange Root; Tumeric Root; Yellow Indian Paint; Yellow Root
**Lactation:** Contraindicated
**Use:** Gastrointestinal and peripheral vascular activity; used in sterile eyewashes; used as a mouthwash, laxative, to treat hemorrhoids, and to stop postpartum hemorrhage. Efficacy not established in clinical studies; has been used to treat mucosal inflammation/gastritis.
**Mechanism of Action/Effect:** Contains the alkaloids hydrastine (4%) and berberine (6%), which at higher doses can cause vasoconstriction, hypertension, and mucosal irritation; berberine can produce hypotension
**Contraindications:** Pregnancy
**Warnings:** Should not be used in patients with hypertension, glaucoma, diabetes, history of stroke, or heart disease.
**Drug Interactions:** May interfere with vitamin B absorption
**Adverse Reactions:** With high doses: Stimulation/agitation, nausea, vomiting, diarrhea, mouth and throat irritation, extremity numbness, respiratory failure
**Dosing:**

Root: 0.5-1 g 3 times/day
Solid form: Usual dose: 5-10 grains

## Hawthorn

**Synonyms:** *Crataegus laevigata; Crataegus monogyna; Crataegus oxyacantha; Crataegus pinnatifida*; English Hawthorn; Haw; Maybush; Whitehorn
**Lactation:** Contraindicated
**Use:** In herbal medicine, to treat cardiovascular abnormalities (arrhythmia, angina), Increased cardiac output, increased contractility of heart muscle; used as a sedative
**Mechanism of Action/Effect:** Contains flavonoids, catechin, and epicatechin which may be cardioprotective and have vasodilatory properties; shown to dilate coronary vessels
**Contraindications:** Pregnancy
**Drug Interactions:** Antihypertensives (effect enhanced), digoxin; effects with Viagra® are unknown

## NUTRITIONAL AND HERBAL PRODUCTS *(Continued)*

**Adverse Reactions:** Hypotension, bradycardia, hypertension, depression, fatigue, rash, nausea

**Dosing:** Daily dose of total flavonoids: 10 mg

Per Commission E: 160-900 mg native water-ethanol extract (ethanol 45% v/v or methanol 70% v/v, drug-extract ratio: 4-7:1, with defined flavonoid or procyanidin content), corresponding to 30-168.7 mg procyanidins, calculated as epicatechin, or 3.5-19.8 mg flavonoids, calculated as hyperoside in accordance with DAB 10 (German pharmacopoeia #10) in 2 or 3 individual doses; duration of administration: 6 weeks minimum

### Kava

**Synonyms:** Awa; Kew; *Piper methysticum*; Tonga

**Use:** Treatment of nervous anxiety, stress, and restlessness (per Commission E); used for sleep inducement and to reduce anxiety

**Restrictions:** Do not use for more than 3 months without medical advice per Commission E

**Mechanism of Action/Effect:** Contains alpha-pyrones in root extracts; may possess central dopaminergic antagonistic properties

**Contraindications:** Per Commission E: Pregnancy, endogenous depression. Extended continuous intake can cause a temporary yellow discoloration of skin, hair, and nails. In this case, further application must be discontinued. In rare cases, allergic skin reactions occur. Also, accommodative disturbances (eg, enlargement of the pupils and disturbances of the oculomotor equilibrium) have been described.

**Drug Interactions:** Coma can occur from concomitant administration of kava and alprazolam; may potentiate alcohol or CNS depressants, barbiturates, psychopharmacological agents

**Adverse Reactions:** Euphoria, depression, somnolence, skin discoloration (prolonged use), muscle weakness, eye disturbances

**Dosing:** Per Commission E: Herb and preparations equivalent to 60-120 mg kavalactones

### Melaleuca Oil

**Use:** Marketed as having fungicidal, bactericidal properties; used as a topical dermal agent for burns

**Mechanism of Action/Effect:** Consists of plant terpenes, pinenes, and cineole, derived from the *Melaleuca alternifolia* tree, the colorless or pale yellow oil can cause CNS depression; may be bacteriostatic

**Adverse Reactions:** Rarely causes allergic reactions or dermatitis

**Dosing:** Minimal toxic dose: Infant: <10 mL applied topically

### Melatonin

**Lactation:** Contraindicated

**Use:** Sleep disorders (eg, jet lag, insomnia, neurologic problems, shift work); aging; cancer; immune system support

**Mechanism of Action/Effect:** Melatonin is a hormone responsible for regulating the body's circadian rhythm and sleep patterns. Its release is prompted by darkness and inhibited by light. Secretion appears to peak during childhood, and declines gradually through adolescence and adulthood. Melatonin receptors have been found in blood cells, the brain, gut, and ovaries. This substance may also have a role in regulating cardiovascular and reproductive function through its antioxidant properties.

**Contraindications:** Immune disorders; pregnancy

**Drug Interactions:** Medications commonly used as sedatives or hypnotics, or those that induce sedation, drowsiness (g, benzodiazepines, narcotics); CNS depressants (prescription, supplements such as 5-HTP); other herbs known to cause sedation include kava kava, valerian

**Adverse Reactions:** Reduced alertness, headache, irritability, increased fatigue, drowsiness, sedation

**Dosing:** Sleep disturbances: 0.3-5 mg/day

### Sassafras Oil

**Synonyms:** *Sassafras albidum*

**Use:** Banned by FDA in food since 1960; used as a mild counterirritant on the skin (ie, for lice or insect bites); should not be ingested

**Mechanism of Action/Effect:** Contains safrole (up to 80%) which inhibits liver microsomal enzymes; its metabolite may cause hepatic tumors

**Adverse Reactions** (primarily related to sassafras oil and safrole): Tachycardia, flushing, hypotension, sinus tachycardia, anxiety, hallucinations, vertigo, aphasia, contact dermatitis, vomiting, fatty changes of liver, hepatic necrosis, mydriasis, diaphoresis; little documentation of adverse effects due to ingestion of herbal tea

**Absorption:** Orally

**Metabolism:** Hepatic

**Excretion:** Renal primarily

**Dosing:** Sassafras tea can contain as much as 200 mg (3 mg/kg) of safrole.

Lethal: ~5 mL

Toxic: 0.66 mg/kg (based on rodent studies)

**Patient Information:** Considered unsafe by the FDA.

## Saw Palmetto

**Synonyms:** Palmetto Scrub; *Sabal serrulata; Sabasilis serrulatae; Serenoa repens*

**Lactation:** Contraindicated

**Use:** Benign prostatic hyperplasia

**Mechanism of Action/Effect:** Liposterolic extract of the berries may inhibit the enzymes 5α-reductase, along with cyclo-oxygenase and 5-lipoxygenase, thus exhibiting antiandrogen and anti-inflammatory effects; does not reduce prostatic enlargement but may help increase urinary flow (not FDA approved)

**Contraindications:** Pregnancy

**Adverse Reactions:** Headache, gynecomastia, stomach problems (rare - per Commission E)

**Absorption:** Oral: Low

**Dosing:** Adults: Dried fruit: 0.5-1 g 3 times/day

**Patient Information:**

## Senna

**Synonyms:** *C. angustifolia; Cassia acutifolia*; Senna Alexandria

**Use:** Catharsis

**Mechanism of Action/Effect:** Contains up to 3% anthraquinone glycosides which can cause colonic stimulation

**Contraindications:** Per Commission E: Intestinal obstruction, acute intestinal inflammation (eg, Crohn's disease), colitis ulcerosa, appendicitis, abdominal pain of unknown origin, children <12 years, and pregnancy

**Drug Interactions:** Per Commission E: Potentiation of cardiac glycosides (with long-term use) is possible due to loss in potassium; effect on antiarrhythmics is possible; potassium deficiency can be increased by simultaneous application of thiazide diuretics, corticosteroids, and licorice root.

**Adverse Reactions:** Palpitations, tetany, dizziness, finger clubbing (reversible), hypokalemia, vomiting (with fresh plant leaves or pods), diarrhea, abdominal cramping, nausea, melanosis coli (reversible), cachexia, red discoloration in alkaline urine (yellow-brown in acidic urine), hepatitis, oliguria, proteinuria, dyspnea. Per Commission E: Long-term use/abuse can cause electrolyte imbalance; in single incidents, cramp-like discomforts of GI tract requiring a reduction in dosage

**Metabolism:** Hydrolyzed by bacteria in the colon thus releasing active sennosides

**Excretion:** Urine and feces

**Onset of Action:** Oral: 6-8 hours; Suppository: 0.5-2 hours

**Dosing:**

Sennosides:

Children >6 years: 20 mg at bedtime

Adults: 20-40 mg with water at bedtime

Senna granules: 2.5-5 mL (163-326 mg) at bedtime; maximum dose: 10 mL (652 mg)/day

Senna tablets:

Children >60 pounds: 1 tablet (187 mg) at bedtime; maximum daily dose: 2 tablets

Adults: 1-2 tablets (187-374 mg) at bedtime; maximum daily dose: 4 tablets (**Note:** Extra strength senna tablets contain 374 mg each.)

Senna syrup:

1 month to 1 year: 1.25-2.5 mL (55-109 mg) at bedtime, up to 5 mL/day

1-5 years: 2.5-5 mL (109-218 mg) at bedtime, up to 10 mL/day

5-15 years: 5-10 mL (218-436 mg) at bedtime, up to 20 mL/day

Adults: 10-15 mL (436-654 mg); maximum daily dose: 30 mL (1308 mg)

Senna suppositories:

Children >60 pounds: ½ suppository (326 mg)

Adults: 1 suppository (652 mg) at bedtime; can repeat in 2 hours

Tea: ½ to 2 teaspoons of leaves (0.5-4 g of the herb)

## NUTRITIONAL AND HERBAL PRODUCTS *(Continued)*

### St Johns Wort

**Synonyms:** Amber Touch-and-Feel; Goatweed; *Hypercium perforatum*; Klamath Weed; Rosin Rose

**Use:** Treatment of mild to moderate depression; traditionally for treatment of stress, anxiety, insomnia; topically for vitiligo; popular drug for AIDS patients due to possible antiretroviral activity; topically for wound healing. Per Commission E: Psychovegetative disorders, depressive moods, anxiety and/or nervous unrest; oily preparations for dyspeptic complaints; oily preparations externally for treatment of post-therapy of acute and contused injuries, myalgia, first degree burns

**Mechanism of Action/Effect:** Active ingredients are xanthones, flavonoids (hypericin) which can act as monoamine oxidase inhibitors, although *in vitro* activity is minimal; majority of activity appears to be related to GABA modulation; may be related to dopamine, serotonin, norepinephrine modulation also

**Contraindications:** Endogenous depression, pregnancy, children <2 years of age (not confirmed in animal models, *in vitro* only)

**Warnings:** May be photosensitizing

**Drug Interactions:** Avoid amphetamines or other stimulants. Use with caution in patients taking MAO inhibitors, levodopa, and 5-hydroxytryptophan. Avoid tyramine-containing foods due to presence of hypercin although human data of this potential drug interaction is lacking. Avoid concurrent use with SSRI or other antidepressants.

**Adverse Reactions:** Sinus tachycardia, photosensitization is possible especially in fair-skinned persons (per Commission E), stomach pains, abdominal pain

**Dosing:** Based on hypericin extract content

- Oral: 300 mg 3 times/day (not to be used longer than 8 weeks)
- Herb: 2-4 g 3 times/day
- Liquid extract: 2-4 mL 3 times/day
- Tincture: 2-4 mL 3 times/day
- Topical: Crushed leaves and flowers are applied to affected area after cleansing with soap and water
- Per Commission E: 2-4 g drug (dried herb) or 0.2-1 mg of total hypericin in other forms of drug application

### Valerian

**Synonyms:** Radix; Red Valerian; *Valeriana edulis; Valeriana wallichi*

**Use:** Sleep-promoting agent and minor tranquilizer (similar to benzodiazepines); used in anxiety, panic attacks, intestinal cramps, headache. Per Commission E: Restlessness, sleep disorders based on nervous conditions

**Mechanism of Action/Effect:** Most pharmacologic activity located in fresh root or dried rhizome; the plant contains essential oils (valerenic acid and valenol, valepotriates, and alkaloids <0.2% concentration) which may affect neurotransmitter levels (serotonin, GABA, and norepinephrine); also has antispasmodic properties

**Drug Interactions:** Not synergistic with alcohol; potentiation of other CNS depressants is possible

**Adverse Reactions:** Cardiac disturbances (unspecified), lightheadedness, restlessness, fatigue, nausea, tremor, blurred vision

**Dosing:**

- Sedative: 1-3 g (1-3 mL of tincture)
- Sleep aid: 1-3 mL of tincture at bedtime
- Dried root: 0.3-1 g

# HERBS AND COMMON NATURAL AGENTS

The authors have chosen to include this list of natural products and proposed medical claims. However, due to limited scientific investigation to support these claims, this list is not intended to imply that these claims have been scientifically proven.

## Proposed Medicinal Claims

| Herb | Medicinal Claim |
|---|---|
| Agrimony | Digestive disorders |
| Alfalfa | Source of carotene (vitamin A); contains natural fluoride |
| Allspice | General health |
| Aloe | Healing agent |
| Anise seed | Prevent gas |
| Astragalus | Enhance energy reserves; immune system modulation; adaptogen |
| Barberry bark | Treat halitosis |
| Bayberry bark | Relieve and prevent varicose veins |
| Bay leaf | Relieves cramps |
| Bee pollen | Renewal of enzymes, hormones, vitamins, amino acids, and others |
| Bergamot herb | Calming effect |
| Bilberry leaf | Increases night vision; reduces eye fatigue; antioxidant; circulation |
| Birch bark | Treat urinary problems; used for rheumatism |
| Blackberry leaf | Treat diarrhea |
| Black cohosh | Relieves menstrual cramps; phytoestrogen |
| Blueberry leaf | Diarrhea |
| Blue Cohosh | Regulate menstrual flow |
| Blue flag | Treatment of skin diseases and constipation |
| Boldo leaf | Stimulates digestion; treatment of gallstones |
| Boneset | Treatment of colds and flu |
| Bromelain | Digestive enzyme |
| Buchu leaf | Diuretic |
| Buckthorn bark | Expels worms; laxative |
| Burdock leaf and root | Treatment of severe skin problems; cases of arthritis |
| Butternut bark | Works well for constipation |
| Calendula flower | Mending and healing of cuts or wounds topically |
| Capsicum (Cayenne) | Normalizes blood pressure; circulation |
| Caraway seed | Aids digestion |
| Cascara sagrada bark | Remedies for chronic constipation |
| Catnip | Calming effect in children |
| Celery leaf and seed | Blood pressure; diuretic |
| Centaury | Stimulates the salivary gland |
| Chamomile flower | Excellent for a nervous stomach; relieves cramping associated with the menstrual cycle |
| Chickweed | Rich in vitamin C and minerals (calcium, magnesium, and potassium); diuretic; thyroid stimulant |
| Chicory root | Effective in disorders of the kidneys, liver, and urinary canal |
| Cinnamon bark | Prevents infection and indigestion; helps break down fats during digestion |
| Cleavers | Treatment of kidney and bladder disorders; useful in obstructions of the urinary organ |
| Cloves | General medicinal |
| Coriander seed | Stomach tonic |

## NUTRITIONAL AND HERBAL PRODUCTS *(Continued)*

### Proposed Medicinal Claims *(continued)*

| Herb | Medicinal Claim |
|---|---|
| Cornsilk | Diuretic |
| Cranberry | Urinary tract health |
| Cubeb berry | Chronic bladder trouble; increases flow of urine |
| Damiana leaf | Sexual impotency |
| Dandelion leaf | Diuretic |
| Dandelion root | Detoxify poisons in the liver; beneficial in lowering blood pressure |
| Dill weed | Digestive health |
| Dong Quai root | Female troubles; menopause and PMS symptoms; anemia; blood pressure |
| *Echinacea* root | Treat strep throat, lymph glands; immune modulating |
| Eucalyptus leaf | Mucolytic |
| Elder | Antiviral |
| Elecampane root | Cough with mucus |
| Eyebright herb | Eyesight |
| Fennel seed | Remedies for gas and acid stomach |
| Fenugreek seed | Allergies, coughs, digestion, emphysema, headaches, migraines, intestinal inflammation, ulcers, lungs, mucous membranes, and sore throat |
| Feverfew herb | Migraines; helps reduce inflammation in arthritis joints |
| Garlic capsules | Lowers blood cholesterol; anti-infective |
| Gentian | Digestive health |
| Ginger root | Antiemetic |
| Ginkgo biloba | Improves blood circulation to the brain; asthma; vertigo; tinnitus; impotence |
| Ginseng root, Siberian | Resistance against stress; slows the aging process; adaptogen |
| Goldenseal | Treatment of bladder infections, cankers, mouth sores, mucous membranes, and ulcers |
| Gota kola | "Memory herb"; nerve tonic; wound healing |
| Gravelroot (Queen of the Meadow) | Remedy for stones in the kidney and bladder |
| Green barley | Antioxidant |
| Hawthorn | Antioxidant; cardiotonic |
| Henna | External use only |
| Hibiscus flower | Diuretic |
| Hops flower | Insomnia; used to decrease the desire for alcohol |
| Horehound | Acute or chronic sore throat and coughs |
| Horsetail (Shavegrass) | Rich in minerals, especially silica; used to develop strong fingernails and hair, good for split ends; diuretic |
| Ho shou wu | Rejuvenator |
| Hydrangea root | Backaches |
| Juniper berry | Diuretic |
| Kava kava root | Calm nervousness; anxiety; pain |
| Kelp | High contents of natural plant iodine, for proper function of the thyroid; high levels of natural calcium, potassium, and magnesium |
| Lavender oil | Wound healing; decrease scarring (topical) |
| Lecithin | Break up cholesterol; prevent arteriosclerosis |
| Licorice root | Expectorant; used in peptic ulceration; adrenal exhaustion |

**Proposed Medicinal Claims** *(continued)*

| Herb | Medicinal Claim |
|---|---|
| Malva flower | Soothes inflammation in the mouth and throat; helpful for earaches |
| Marjoram | Beneficial for a sour stomach or loss of appetite |
| Marshmallow leaf | Demulcent |
| Milk thistle herb | Liver detoxifier; antioxidant |
| Motherwort | Nervousness |
| Mugwort | Used for rheumatism and gout |
| Mullein leaf | High in iron, magnesium, and potassium; sinuses; relieves swollen joints; soothing bronchial tissue |
| Mustard seed | General medicinal |
| Myrrh gum | Removes bad breath; sinus problems |
| Nettle leaf | Remedy for dandruff; antihistiminic qualities |
| Nettle root | Used in benign prostatic hyperplasia (BPH) |
| Nutmeg | Gas |
| Oregano leaf | Settles the stomach after meals; helps treat colds |
| Oregon grape root | Gallbladder problems |
| Papaya leaf | Digestive stimulant; contains the enzyme papain |
| Paprika (sweet) | Stimulates the appetite and gastric secretions |
| Passion flower | Mild sedative |
| Pau d'arco | Protects immune system; antifungal |
| Peppermint leaf | Excellent for headaches; digestive stimulation |
| Pleurisy root | Mucolytic |
| Poppy seed blue | Excellent in the making of breads and desserts |
| Prickly ash bark | Increases circulation |
| Psyllium seed | Lubricant to the intestinal tract |
| Red clover | Phytoestrogenic properties |
| Red raspberry leaf | Decreases menstrual bleeding |
| Rhubarb root | Powerful laxative |
| Rose hips | High content of vitamin C |
| Saw palmetto berry | Used in benign prostatic hyperplasia (BPH) |
| Scullcap | Nerve sedative |
| Seawrack (Bladderwrack) | Combat obesity; contains iodine |
| Senna leaf | Laxative |
| Shepherd's purse | Female reproductive health |
| Sheep sorrel | Diuretic |
| Slippery elm bark | Normalize bowel movement; beneficial for hemorrhoids and constipation |
| Solomon's seal root | Poultice for bruises |
| Spikenard | Skin ailments such as acne, pimples, blackheads, rashes, and general skin problems |
| Star anise | Promotes appetite and relieves flatulence |
| St John's wort | Mild to moderate depression |
| Summer savory leaf | Treats diarrhea, upset stomach, and sore throat |
| Thyme leaf | Ulcers (peptic) |
| Uva-ursi leaf | Diuretic; used in urinary tract health |
| Valerian root | Promotes sleep |
| Vervain | Remedy for fevers |
| White oak bark | Strong astringent |
| White willow bark | Used for minor aches and pains in the body; aspirin content |
| Wild alum root | Powerful astringent; used as rinse for sores in mouth and bleeding gums |

## NUTRITIONAL AND HERBAL PRODUCTS *(Continued)*

### Proposed Medicinal Claims *(continued)*

| Herb | Medicinal Claim |
|---|---|
| Wild cherry | Cough suppressant |
| Wild Oregon grape root | Chronic skin disease |
| Wild yam root | Used in female reproductive health |
| Wintergreen leaf | Valuable for colic and gas in the bowels |
| Witch hazel bark and leaf | Hemorrhoids |
| Wormwood | Antiparasitic |
| Yarrow root | Fevers |
| Yellow dock root | Good in all skin problems |
| Yerba santa | Bronchial congestion |
| Yohimbe | Natural aphrodisiac |
| Yucca root | Reduces inflammation of the joints |

# DRUG INTERACTIONS WITH HERBAL PRODUCTS

## Conventional Drugs and Other Substances That May Interact With Herbal Drugs Approved by the German Commission E

| Drug/Substance | Commission E Herbal Drug |
|---|---|
| Alcohol | Kava kava rhizome |
| Alkaline drugs | Oak bark |
| Alkaloids | Oak bark |
| Amantadine | Belladonna leaf and root<br>Henbane leaf<br>Pheasant's eye herb<br>Scopolia root |
| Antiarrhythmic agents | Aloe<br>Buckthorn bark/berry<br>Cascara sagrada bark<br>Senna fruit/leaves |
| Anticoagulants | Bromelain<br>Cinchona |
| Antihistamines | Henbane leaf |
| Barbiturates | Indian snakeroot<br>Kava kava rhizome |
| Caffeine-containing beverages | Cola |
| Calcium | Lily-of-the-valley<br>Pheasant's eye herb<br>Squill |
| Cardiac glycosides | Aloe<br>Buckthorn bark/berry<br>Cascara sagrada bark<br>Ephedra<br>Senna fruit/leaves |
| Corticosteroids | Aloe<br>Buckthorn bark/berry<br>Cascara sagrada bark<br>Senna fruit/leaves |
| CNS depressants | Kava kava<br>Melatonin<br>Valerian |
| Digitalis glycosides | Indian snakeroot<br>Licorice root |
| Dopamine receptor agonists | Chaste tree fruits (shown in animal experiments only) |
| Glucocorticoids | Lily-of-the-valley<br>Pheasant's eye herb<br>Squill |
| Guanethidine | Ephedra |
| Halothane | Ephedra |
| Laxatives | Lily-of-the-valley<br>Pheasant's eye herb<br>Squill |
| Levodopa | Indian snakeroot |
| Licorice root | Aloe<br>Buckthorn bark/berry<br>Cascara sagrada bark<br>Senna fruit/leaves |
| Lithium | Agave<br>Begolia<br>Borage<br>Broom<br>Buchu<br>Burdock<br>Calamus<br>Celery<br>Chicory<br>Dandelion<br>Ephedra<br>Foxglove<br>Guarana<br>Horsetail<br>Juniper<br>Lovage<br>Mate (yerba mate)<br>Onion<br>Saw palmetto<br>Uva ursi<br>Windflower |

## NUTRITIONAL AND HERBAL PRODUCTS *(Continued)*

### Conventional Drugs and Other Substances That May Interact With Herbal Drugs Approved by the German Commission E *(continued)*

| Drug/Substance | Commission E Herbal Drug |
|---|---|
| MAO inhibitors | Ephedra<br>Medicinal yeast |
| Oxytocin | Ephedra |
| Phenothiazines | Henbane leaf |
| Procainamide | Henbane leaf |
| Psychoaneleptic drugs | Cola |
| Psychopharmacological agents | Kava kava rhizome |
| Quinidine | Belladonna leaf and root<br>Henbane leaf<br>Lily-of-the-valley<br>Pheasant's eye herb<br>Scopolia root<br>Squill |
| Radioactive isotopes | Bugle weed |
| Saluretics | Lily-of-the-valley<br>Pheasant's eye herb<br>Squill |
| Secale alkaloid derivatives | Ephedra |
| Sympathomimetics | Indian snakeroot |
| Tetracycline | Bromelain |
| Thiazide diuretics | Aloe<br>Buckthorn bark/berry<br>Cascara sagrada bark<br>Licorice root<br>Senna fruit/leaves |
| Thyroid preparations | Bugle weed |
| Thrombocytic aggregation inhibitors | Bromelain |
| Tricyclic antidepressants | Belladonna leaf and root<br>Henbane leaf<br>Scopolia root |
| Urine-acidifying agents | Uva ursi leaf |

Adapted from Blumenthal M, Goldberg A, Gruenwald J, et al, *German Commission E Monographs: Therapeutic Monographs on Medicinal Plants for Human Use*, Austin, TX: American Botanical Council, 1997.

## Footnotes

1. Blumenthal M, "Herbal Monographs Initiated by Numerous Groups: WHO, USP, ESCOP, ABC, and AHP All Working Towards Similar Goals," *HerbalGram*, 1997, 40:30-7.
2. Bradley P, *British Herbal Compendium*, Vol 1, Bournemouth, England: British Herbal Medical Association, 1992.
3. Newell CA, Anderson LA, and Philippson JD, *Herbal Medicines: A Guide for Healthcare Professionals*, London, England: The Pharmaceutical Press, 1996.
4. Farnsworth NR, "The Relative Safety of Herbal Medicines," *HerbalGram*, 1993, 29:36A-H
5. McCaleb RS, "Food Ingredient Safety Evaluation," *Food Drug Law J*, 1992, 47:657-63.
6. Soloway R, *Personal Communication*, July 21, 1997.
7. Foster S, *Herbs of Commerce*, Austin, TX: American Herbal Products Association, 1992.

## References


Blumenthal M, Goldberg A, Gruenwald J, et al, *German Commission E Monographs: Therapeutic Monographs on Medicinal Plants for Human Use*, Austin, TX: American Botanical Council, 1997.

D'Arcy PF, "Adverse Reactions and Interactions With Herbal Medicines: Part 1. Adverse Reactions," *Adverse Drug Reaction Toxicol Rev*, 1991, 10(4):189-208.

D'Arcy PF, McEmay JC, and Welling PG, *Mechanisms of Drug Interactions*, New York, NY: Springer-Verlag, 1996.

DeSmet PA, "Health Risks of Herbal Remedies," *Drug Saf*, 1995, 13(2):81-93.

DeSmet PA, Keller K, Hansel R, et al, *Adverse Effects of Herbal Drugs*, Vol 3, New York, NY: Springer-Verlag, 1997.

DeSmet PA, Keller K, Hansel R, et al, *Adverse Effects of Herbal Drugs*, Vol 2, New York, NY: Springer-Verlag, 1993.

DeSmet PA, Keller K, Hansel R, et al, *Adverse Effects of Herbal Drugs*, Vol 1, New York, NY: Springer-Verlag.

Ernst E and DeSmet PA, "Risks Associated With Complementary Therapies," *Meyler's Side Effects of Drugs*, 13th ed, Dukes MN ed, New York, NY: Elsevier Science, 1996.

Fulder S and Tenne M, "Ginger as an Antinausea Remedy in Pregnancy: The Issue of Safety," *HerbalGram*, 1996, 36:47-50.

Keller K, "Therapeutic Use of Herbal Drugs and Their Potential Toxicity, Problems and Results of the Revision of Herbal Medicines in the EEC," *Proceedings of the 3rd International Conference on*

*Pharmacopoeias and Quality Control of Drugs*, Rome, November, 1992, published in Bologna, Fondazione Rhone-Poulenc Rorer per le Scienze Mediche, 1993.

McGuffin M, Hobbs C, Upton R, et al, *American Herbal Product Association's Botanical Safety Handbook: Guidelines for the Safe Use and Labeling for Herbs of Commerce*, Boca Raton, FL: CRC Press, 1997.

Siegers CP, "Anthranoid Laxatives and Colorectal Cancer," *Trends in Pharmaceutical Science*, 1992, 13:229-31.

## Herbs Contraindicated During Lactation According to German Commission E

Aloe (*Aloe vera*)

Basil (*Ocimum basillcum*)

Buckthorn bark and berry (*Rhamnus frangula, R. cathartica*)

Cascara sagrada (*Rhamnus purshiana*)

Coltsfoot leaf (*Tussilago farfara*)

Combinations of senna, peppermint oil and caraway oil

Kava kava root (*Piper methysticum*)

Petasite root (*Pefasites* spp)

Indian snakeroot (*Rauwolfia serpentina*)

Rhubarb root (*Rheum palmatum*)

Senna (*Cassia senna*)

## Herbs Contraindicated During Pregnancy According to German Commission E

Aloe (*Aloe vera*)

Autumn crocus (*Colchicum autumnale*)

Black cohosh root (*Cimicifuga racemosa*)

Buckthorn bark and berry (*Rhamnus frangula, R. cathartica*)

Cascara sagrada bark (*Rhamnus purshiana*)

Chaste tree fruit (*Vitex agnus-castus*)

Cinchona bark (*Cinchona* spp)

Cinnamon bark (*Cinnamomum zeylanicum*)

Coltsfoot leaf (*Tussliago farfara*)

*Echinacea purpurea* herb (*Echinacea purpurea*)

Fennel oil (*Foeniculum vulgare*)

Combination of licorice, peppermint, and chamomile

Combination of licorice, primrose, marshmallow, and anise

Combination of senna, peppermint oil, and caraway oil

Ginger root (*Zingiber officinale*)*

Indian snakeroot (*Rauwolfia serpentina*)

Juniper berry (*Juniperus comunis*)

Kava kava root (*Piper methysticum*)

Licorice root (*Glycyrrhiza glabra*)

Marsh tea (*Ledum palustre*)

Mayapple root (*Podophyllum peltatum*)

Petasite root (*Petasites* spp)

Rhubarb root (*Rheum palmatum*)

Sage leaf (*Salvia officinalis*)

Senna (*Cassia senna*)

*A subsequent review of the clinical literature could find no basis for the contraindication of ginger, a common spice, during pregnancy (Fulder and Tenne, 1996).

# OPHTHALMIC AGENTS

**Note:** Consult product literature for full prescribing information. See also, Ophthalmic Agents, Glaucoma in the Alphabetical Listing of Drugs section.

**Patient Instructions:** Wash hands before instilling. Sit or lie down to instill. Open eye, look at ceiling, and instill prescribed amount of medication. Close eye and apply gentle pressure to inner corner of eye. Do not let tip of applicator touch eye or contaminate tip of applicator. Temporary stinging or burning may occur. Report persistent pain, burning, vision disturbances, swelling, itching, rash, or worsening of condition.

## ANTIBACTERIAL

### Bacitracin

**Brand Names:** AK-Tracin®
**Use:** Treatment of susceptible bacterial infections
**Dose:** Instill 1/4" to 1/2" ribbon every 3-4 hours into conjunctival sac for acute infections, or 2-3 times/day for mild to moderate infections for 7-10 days.
**Strength:** Ointment: 500 units/g (3.5 g, 3.75 g)

### Bacitracin and Polymyxin B

**Brand Names:** AK-Poly-Bac®; Polysporin®
**Use:** Treatment of superficial infections caused by susceptible organisms
**Dose:** Instill 1/2" ribbon every 3-4 hours for acute infections or 2-3 times/day for mild to moderate infections for 7-10 days.
**Strength:** Ointment: Bacitracin 500 units and polymyxin B sulfate 10,000 units per g (3.5 g)

### Bacitracin, Neomycin, and Polymyxin B

**Brand Names:** AK-Spore® Ophthalmic Ointment; Neosporin® Ophthalmic Ointment
**Use:** Short-term treatment of superficial external ocular infections caused by susceptible organisms
**Dose:** Instill 1/2" ribbon into the conjunctival sac every 3-4 hours for acute infections or 2-3 times/day for mild to moderate infections for 7-10 days.
**Strength:** Ointment: Bacitracin 400 units, neomycin sulfate 3.5 mg, and polymyxin B sulfate 10,000 units per g

### Chloramphenicol

**Brand Names:** AK-Chlor®; Chlor-optic®
**Use:** Treatment of infection caused by susceptible organisms
**Dose:** Instill 1-2 drops or 1.25 cm (1/2") of ointment every 3-4 hours. Increase interval between applications after 48 hours to 2-3 times/day.
**Strength:**
- Ointment (AK-Chlor®; Chlor-optic®): 1% [10 mg/g] (3.5 g)
- Powder for ophthalmic solution (Chloromycetin®): 25 mg/vial (15 mL)

### Ciprofloxacin

**Brand Names:** Ciloxan™
**Use:** Treatment of infections caused by susceptible organisms
**Dose:**
- Solution: Instill 1-2 drops every 2 hours while awake for 2 days and 1-2 drops every 4 hours while awake for the next 5 days.
- Ointment: Instill one-half inch ribbon into the lower conjunctival sac 3 times/day for the first 2 days, the twice daily for the next 5 days.

**Strength:**
- Ointment: 0.3% (3.5 g)
- Solution: 3.5 mg/mL (2.5 mL, 5 mL)

### Erythromycin

**Brand Names:** Ilotycin®
**Use:** Treatment of infections caused by susceptible organisms
**Dose:** Apply 1/4" to 1/2" strip into conjunctival sac 3-4 times daily (up to 6 times daily).
**Strength:** Ointment: Erythromycin 0.5%

## Gentamicin

**Brand Names:** Genoptic®; Genoptic® S.O.P; Gentacidin®; Gentak®
**Use:** Treatment of infections caused by susceptible bacteria
**Dose:**

Ointment: Instill ½" (1.25 cm) 2-3 times/day to every 3-4 hours.
Solution: Instill 1-2 drops every 2-4 hours, up to 2 drops every hour for severe infections.

**Strength:**

Ointment: 0.3% [3 mg/g] (3.5 g)
Solution: 0.3% (1 mL, 5 mL, 15 mL)

## Neomycin, Polymyxin B, and Gramicidin

**Brand Names:** AK-Spore® Ophthalmic Solution; Neosporin® Ophthalmic Solution
**Use:** Treatment of superficial ocular infection
**Dose:** Instill 1-2 drops 4-6 times/day or more frequently as required for severe infections.
**Strength:** Solution: Neomycin sulfate 1.75 mg, polymyxin B sulfate 10,000 units, and gramicidin 0.025 mg per mL (2 mL, 10 mL)

## Ofloxacin

**Brand Names:** Ocuflox®
**Use:** Treatment of bacterial conjunctivitis caused by susceptible organisms
**Dose:** Instill 1-2 drops every 2-4 hours for the first 2 days, then use 4 times/day for an additional 5 days.
**Strength:** Solution: 0.3% (5 mL)

## Sulfacetamide

**Brand Names:** AK-Sulf®; Bleph®-10; Cetamide®; Isopto® Cetamide®; Ocusulf-10®; Sodium Sulamyd®; Sulf-10®
**Use:** Treatment and prophylaxis of conjunctivitis due to susceptible organisms; adjunctive treatment with systemic sulfonamides for therapy of trachoma
**Dose:** Do not use in patients with sulfonamide allergy.

Ointment: Apply to lower conjunctival sac 1-4 times/day and at bedtime.
Solution: Instill 1-3 drops several times daily up to every 2-3 hours in lower conjunctival sac during waking hours and less frequently at night.

**Strength:**

Ointment: 10% (3.5 g)
Solution: 10% (1 mL, 2 mL, 2.5 mL, 5 mL, 15 mL)

## Tetracycline

**Brand Names:** Achromycin®
**Use:** Treatment of susceptible bacterial infections
**Dose:**

Ointment: Instill every 2-12 hours.
Suspension: Instill 1-2 drops 2-4 times/day or more often as needed.

**Strength:**

Ointment: 1% [10 mg/mL] (3.5 g)
Suspension: 1% [10 mg/mL] (0.5 mL, 1 mL, 4 mL)

## Tobramycin

**Brand Names:** AKTob®; Tobrex®
**Use:** Treatment of superficial ophthalmic infections caused by susceptible bacteria
**Dose:**

Ointment: Apply 2-3 times/day. For severe infections, apply every 3-4 hours or 2 drops of solution every 30-60 minutes initially, then reduce to less frequent intervals.
Solution: Instill 1-2 drops every 4 hours.

**Strength:**

Ointment: 0.3% (3.5 g)
Solution: 0.3% (5 mL)

## Trimethoprim and Polymyxin B

**Brand Names:** Polytrim®
**Use:** Treatment of surface ocular bacterial infection
**Dose:** Instill 1-2 drops every 4-6 hours for 7-10 days.

## OPHTHALMIC AGENTS *(Continued)*

**Strength:** Solution: Trimethoprim sulfate 1 mg and polymyxin B sulfate 10,000 units per mL (10 mL)

## ANTIBIOTIC/ANTI-INFLAMMATORY

### Bacitracin, Neomycin, Polymyxin B, and Hydrocortisone

**Brand Names:** AK-Spore H.C.® Ophthalmic Ointment; Cortisporin® Ophthalmic Ointment; Neotricin HC® Ophthalmic Ointment
**Use:** Prevention and treatment of susceptible superficial topical infections
**Dose:** Ointment: Instill ½" ribbon to inside of lower lid every 3-4 hours until improvement occurs.
**Strength:** Ointment: Bacitracin 400 units, neomycin sulfate 3.5 mg, polymyxin B sulfate 10,000 units, and hydrocortisone 10 mg per g (3.5 g)

### Chloramphenicol and Prednisolone

**Brand Names:** Chloroptic-P®
**Use:** Topical anti-infective and corticosteroid for treatment of ocular infections
**Dose:** Instill 1-2 drops 2-4 times/day.
**Strength:** Ointment: Chloramphenicol 1% and prednisolone 0.5% (3.5 g)

### Neomycin and Dexamethasone

**Brand Names:** AK-Neo-Dex®; NeoDexadron®; Neo-Dexameth®
**Use:** Treatment of steroid responsive inflammatory conditions
**Dose:** Instill 1-2 drops every 3-4 hours.
**Strength:**
Ointment: Neomycin sulfate 0.35% [3.5 mg/g] and dexamethasone 0.05% [0.5 mg/g] (3.5 g)
Solution: Neomycin sulfate 0.35% [3.5 mg/mL] and dexamethasone 0.1% [1 mg/mL] (5 mL)

### Neomycin and Hydrocortisone

**Brand Names:** Cor-Oticin®; Neo-Cortef®
**Use:** Treatment of susceptible bacterial infections with associated inflammation
**Dose:** Instill 1-2 drops 3-4 times/day.
**Strength:** Solution: Neomycin sulfate 0.5% and hydrocortisone 0.5% (5 mL)

### Neomycin, Polymyxin B, and Dexamethasone

**Brand Names:** AK-Trol®; Dexacidin®; Maxitrol®
**Use:** Steroid-responsive inflammatory ocular conditions where bacterial infection or risk of bacterial infection exists
**Dose:**
Ointment: Place a small amount (~½") in the affected eye 3-4 times/day or apply at bedtime as an adjunct with drops.
Solution: Instill 1-2 drops into affected eye(s) every 3-4 hours. In severe disease, drops may be used hourly and tapered to discontinuation.
**Strength:**
Ointment: Neomycin sulfate 3.5 mg, polymyxin B sulfate 10,000 units, and and dexamethasone 0.1% per g (3.5 g)
Solution: Neomycin sulfate 3.5 mg, polymyxin B sulfate 10,000 units, and dexamethasone 0.1% per mL (5 mL)

### Neomycin, Polymyxin B, and Hydrocortisone

**Brand Names:** AK-Spore H.C.® Ophthalmic Suspension; Cortisporin® Ophthalmic Suspension
**Use:** Steroid-responsive inflammatory condition where bacterial infection or risk of bacterial infection exists
**Dose:** Instill 1-2 drops 2-4 times/day, or more frequently as required for severe infections. In acute infections, instill 1-2 drops every 15-30 minutes gradually reducing the frequency of administration as the infection is controlled.
**Strength:** Suspension: Neomycin sulfate 5 mg, polymyxin B sulfate 10,000 units, and hydrocortisone 10 mg per mL (7.5 mL)

## Neomycin, Polymyxin B, and Prednisolone

**Brand Names:** Poly-Pred® Ophthalmic Suspension
**Use:** Steroid-responsive inflammatory ocular conditions where bacterial infection or risk of bacterial infection exists
**Dose:** Instill 1-2 drops every 3-4 hours. Acute infections may require every 30-minute instillation initially with frequency of administration reduced as the infection is brought under control. To treat the lids: Instill 1-2 drops every 3-4 hours, close the eye, and rub the excess on the lids and lid margins.
**Strength:** Suspension: Neomycin sulfate 0.35%, polymyxin B sulfate 10,000 units, and prednisolone acetate 0.5% per mL (5 mL, 10 mL)

## Oxytetracycline and Hydrocortisone

**Brand Names:** Terra-Cortril® Ophthalmic Suspension
**Use:** Treatment of susceptible ophthalmic bacterial infections with associated inflammation
**Dose:** Instill 1 or 2 drops 3 times/day.
**Strength:** Suspension: Oxytetracycline hydrochloride 0.5% and hydrocortisone 0.5% (5 mL)

## Prednisolone and Gentamicin

**Brand Names:** Pred-G®; Pred-G® SOP®
**Use:** Treatment of steroid-responsive inflammatory conditions and superficial ocular infections
**Dose:**
- Ointment: Apply ½" ribbon to lower conjunctival sac 3 times/day.
- Solution: Instill 1 drop 2-4 times/day. During the initial 24-48 hours, the dosing frequency may be increased if necessary.

**Strength:**
- Ointment: Prednisolone acetate 0.6% and gentamicin sulfate 0.3% (3.5 g)
- Suspension: Prednisolone acetate 1% and gentamicin sulfate 0.3% (2 mL, 5 mL, 10 mL)

## Sulfacetamide and Fluorumetholone

**Brand Names:** FML-S® Ophthalmic Suspension
**Use:** Steroid-responsive inflammatory ocular conditions where infection is present or there is risk of infection
**Dose:** Instill 1-3 drops every 2-3 hours while awake. Do not use in sulfa-allergic patients.
**Strength:** Suspension: Sulfacetamide sodium 10% and fluorumetholone 0.1% (5 mL, 10 mL)

## Sulfacetamide and Prednisolone

**Brand Names:** AK-Cide®; Blephamide®; Cetapred®; Isopto® Cetapred®; Metimyd®; Vasocidin®
**Use:** Steroid-responsive inflammatory ocular conditions where infection is present or there is a risk of infection; ophthalmic suspension may be used as an otic preparation
**Dose:**
- Ointment: Apply to lower conjunctival sac 1-4 times/day.
- Solution: Instill 1-3 drops every 2-3 hours while awake.

**Strength:**
- Ointment:
  - AK-Cide®, Metimyd®, Vasocidin®: Sulfacetamide sodium 10% and prednisolone acetate 0.5% (3.5 g)
  - Blephamide®: Sulfacetamide sodium 10% and prednisolone acetate 0.2% (3.5 g)
  - Cetapred®: Sulfacetamide sodium 10% and prednisolone acetate 0.25% (3.5 g)
- Suspension: Sulfacetamide sodium 10% and prednisolone sodium phosphate 0.25% (5 mL)
- Suspension:
  - AK-Cide®, Metimyd®: Sulfacetamide sodium 10% and prednisolone acetate 0.5% (5 mL)
  - Blephamide®: Sulfacetamide sodium 10% and prednisolone acetate 0.2% (2.5 mL, 5 mL, 10 mL)
  - Isopto® Cetapred®: Sulfacetamide sodium 10% and prednisolone acetate 0.25% (5 mL, 15 mL)

## OPHTHALMIC AGENTS *(Continued)*

Vasocidin®: Sulfacetamide sodium 10% and prednisolone sodium phosphate 0.25% (5 mL, 10 mL)

**Tobramycin and Dexamethasone**

**Brand Names:** TobraDex®
**Use:** Treatment of external ocular infections caused by susceptible bacteria and steroid responsive inflammatory conditions
**Dose:** Instill 1-2 drops of solution every 4 hours. Apply ointment 2-3 times/day. For severe infections, apply ointment every 3-4 hours or 2 drops of solution every 30-60 minutes initially, then reduce to less frequent intervals.
**Strength:**
Ointment: Tobramycin 0.3%, dexamethasome 0.1% (3.5 g)
Suspension: Tobramycin 0.3%, dexamethasome 0.1% (2.5 mL, 5 mL, 10 mL)

## ANTIBIOTIC/VASOCONSTRICTOR

**Sulfacetamide and Phenylephrine**

**Brand Names:** Vasosulf®
**Use:** Treatment of superficial ocular infections due to susceptible microorganisms
**Dose:** Instill 1-2 drops into the lower conjunctival sac every 2-3 hours during the day, less often at night.
**Strength:** Solution: Sulfacetamide sodium 15% and phenylephrine hydrochloride 0.125% (5 mL, 15 mL)

## ANTIHISTAMINE AND ANTIHISTAMINE/DECONGESTANT

**Antazoline Phosphate and Naphazoline**

**Brand Names:** Vasocon®-A [OTC]
**Use:** Temporary relief of ocular itching due to seasonal allergic conjunctivitis
**Dose:** Instill 1-2 drops as needed up to 4 times/day.
**Strength:** Solution: Antazoline phosphate 0.5% and naphazoline 0.05%

**Levocabastine**

**Brand Names:** Liovistin™
**Use:** Temporary relief of ocular itching due to seasonal allergic conjunctivitis
**Dose:** Instill 1 drop 4 times/day.
**Strength:** Suspension: Levocabastine 0.05%

**Olopatadine**

**Brand Names:** Patanol™
**Use:**
**Dose:** Instill 1-2 drops 2 times/day at an interval of 6-8 hours.
**Strength:** Solution: Olopatadine 0.1%

**Pheneramine and Naphazoline**

**Brand Names:** OcuHist® [OTC]
**Use:** Temporary relief of ocular itching due to seasonal allergic conjunctivitis
**Dose:** Instill 1-2 drops up to 4 times/day.
**Strength:** Solution: Pheneramine maleate 0.3%, naphazoline 0.025%

## ANTI-INFLAMMATORY, STEROID

**Loteprednol**

**Brand Names:** Alrex™; Lotemax®
**Use:** Treatment relief of signs and symptoms of seasonal allergic conjunctivitis; treatment of steroid-responsive inflammatory condition of the eye
**Dose:**
Alrex™: Instill 1 drop 4 times/day.

Lotemax®: Inflammatory conditions: Apply 1-2 drops into the conjunctival sac 4 times/day. During the initial treatment within the first week, the dosing may be increased up to 2 drop every hour. Postoperative inflammation: Apply 1-2 drops into the conjunctival sac of the operated eye(s) 4 times/day beginning 24 hours after surgery and continuing throughout the first 2 weeks of the postoperative period.

**Strength:** Suspension, as etabonate: 0.2% (Alrex™): 5 mL, 10 mL; 0.5% (Lotemax®): 2.5 mL, 5 mL, 10 mL, 15 mL

### Prednisolone

**Brand Names:** Pred Forte®; Pred Mild®; Inflamase® Mlld
**Use:** Treatment of steroid-responsive inflammatory conditions
**Dose:** Instill 1-2 drops 2-4 times/day.
**Strength:** Solution: Prednisolone 0.12% (Pred Mild®); prednisolone 1% (Pred Forte®)

### Rimexolone

**Brand Names:** Vexol®
**Use:** Treatment of postoperative inflammation following ocular surgery; treatment of anterior uveitis
**Dose:**

Anterior uveitis: Instill 1-2 drops every hour during waking hours for the first week; then 1-2 drops every 2 hours during waking hours. Taper until uveitis is resolved.

Postoperative inflammation: Instill 1-2 drops 4 times/day beginning 24 hours after surgery and continuing for 2 weeks.

**Strength:** Solution: 1%

## ANTI-INFLAMMATORY, NONSTEROIDAL

### Diclofenac

**Brand Names:** Voltaren®
**Use:** Treatment of postoperative inflammation (following cataract surgery)
**Dose:** Cataract surgery: Instill 1 drop into affected eye 4 times/day beginning 24 hours after surgery and continuing for 2 weeks.
**Strength:** Solution: 0.1% (2.5 mL, 5 mL)

### Flurbiprofen

**Brand Names:** Ocufen®
**Use:** Inhibition of postoperative miosis
**Dose:** Instill 1 drop every 30 minutes for 2 hours prior to surgery (total of 4 drops).
**Strength:** Solution: 0.03% (2.5 mL)

### Ketorolac Tromethamine

**Brand Names:** Acular®
**Use:** Temporary relief of ocular itching due to seasonal allergic conjunctivitis
**Dose:** Instill 1 drop 4 times/day.
**Strength:** Solution: 0.5% (3 mL, 5 mL, 10 mL)

## ANTI-INFLAMMATORY, MAST CELL STABILIZER

### Cromolyn Sodium

**Brand Names:** Crolom™
**Use:** Treatment of inflammatory conditions of the eye caused by allergens
**Dose:** Instill 1-2 drops 4-6 times/day.
**Strength:** Solution: 4% (2.5 mL, 10 mL)

### Lodoxamide Tromethamine

**Brand Names:** Alomide®
**Use:** Treatment of inflammatory conditions of the eye caused by allergens
**Dose:** Instill 1-2 drops up to 4 times/day.
**Strength:** Solution: 0.1% (10 mL)

## OPHTHALMIC AGENTS *(Continued)*

### MIOTIC

#### Acetylcholine

**Brand Names:** Miochol-E®
**Use:** Produce complete miosis in cataract surgery, keratoplasty, iridectomy, and other anterior segment surgery where rapid miosis is required
**Dose:** Intraocular: 0.5-2 mL of 1% injection (5-20 mg) instilled into anterior chamber before or after securing one or more sutures
**Strength:** Solution: Intraocular: (1:100) 2 mL, 3 mL

### MYDRIATIC

#### Atropine

**Brand Names:** Atropair®; Atropine-Care®; Atropisol®; Isopto® Atropine; I-Tropine®
**Use:** Mydriasis and cycloplegia for examination of the retina and optic disc and accurate measurement of refractile errors; uveitis
**Dose:** Ophthalmic:

- Children: Solution 0.5%: Instill 1-2 drops twice daily for 1-3 days before procedure.
- Adults:
  - Ointment: Apply a small amount in the conjunctival sac up to 3 times/day.
  - Solution 1%: Instill 1-2 drops 1 hour before the procedure. Uveitis: Instill 1-2 drops 4 times/day.

**Strength:**

- Ointment: 1% (3.5 g)
- Solution: 0.5% (1 mL, 5 mL); 1% (5 mL, 15 mL)

#### Cyclopentolate

**Brand Names:** AK-Pentolate®; Cyclogyl®; I-Pentolate®
**Use:** For diagnostic procedures requiring mydriasis and cycloplegia
**Dose:**

- Infants: Instill 1 drop of 0.5% solution into each eye 5-10 minutes before examination.
- Children: Instill 1 drop of 0.5%, 1%, or 2% solution in eye followed by 1 drop of 0.5% or 1% solution in 5 minutes, if necessary.
- Adults: Instill 1 drop of 1% solution followed by another drop in 5 minutes; use 2% solution in heavily pigmented iris.

**Strength:** Solution: 0.5% (2 mL, 5 mL, 15 mL); 1% (2 mL, 5 mL, 15 mL); 2% (2 mL, 5 mL, 15 mL)

#### Homatropine

**Brand Names:** AK-Homatropine®; Isopto® Homatropine
**Use:** Cycloplegia and mydriasis for refraction; treatment of acute inflammatory conditions of the uveal tract
**Dose:**

- Children: Mydriasis and cycloplegia for refraction: Instill 1 drop of 2% solution immediately before the procedure. Repeat at 10-minute intervals as needed. Uveitis: Instill 1 drop of 2% solution 2-3 times/day.
- Adults: Mydriasis and cycloplegia for refraction: Instill 1-2 drops of 2% solution or 1 drop of 5% solution before the procedure. Repeat at 5- to 10-minute intervals as needed. Uveitis: Instill 1-2 drops of 2% or 5% solution 2-3 times/day up to every 3-4 hours as needed.

**Strength:** Solution: 2% (1 mL, 5 mL, 15 mL); 5% (1 mL, 5 mL, 15 mL)

#### Phenylephrine

**Brand Names:** AK-Dilate®; AK-Nefrin®; I-Phrine®; Mydfrin®; Neo-Synephrine®; Prefrin®; Relief®
**Use:** Mydriasis; treatment of wide-angle glaucoma

**Dose:**

Infants <1 year: Instill 1 drop of 2.5% solution 15-20 minutes before procedure.

Children and adults: Instill 1 drop of 2.5% or 10% solution. May repeat in 10-60 minutes, as needed.

**Strength:** Solution: 0.12% (0.3 mL, 15 mL, 20 mL); 2.5% (2 mL, 3 mL, 5 mL, 15 mL); 10% (1 mL, 2 mL, 5 mL, 15 mL)

## Scopolamine

**Brand Names:** Isopto® Scopolamine

**Use:** Cycloplegia and mydriasis; treatment of iridocyclitis

**Dose:**

Iridocyclitis:

Children: Instill 1 drop of 0.25% solution up to 3 times per day.

Adults: Instill 1-2 drops of 0.25% solution up to 4 times per day.

Refraction:

Children: Instill 1-2 drops of 0.25% solution twice daily for 2 days before procedure.

Adults: Instill 1-2 drops of 0.25% solution 1 hour before procedure.

**Strength:** Solution: 0.25% (5 mL, 15 mL)

## Tropicamide

**Brand Names:** Mydriacyl®; Opticyl®; Tropicacyl®

**Use:** Short-acting mydriatic used in diagnostic procedures as well as preoperatively; treatment of some cases of acute iritis; treatment of iridocyclitis and keratitis

**Dose:** Children and Adults (individuals with heavily pigmented eyes may require larger doses):

Cycloplegia: Instill 1-2 drops (1%). May repeat in 5 minutes. Exam must be performed within 30 minutes after the repeat dose. If the patient is not examined within 20-30 minutes, instill an additional drop.

Mydriasis: Instill 1-2 drops (0.5%) 15-20 minutes before exam; may repeat every 30 minutes as needed.

**Strength:** Solution: 0.5% (2 mL, 15 mL); 1% (2 mL, 3 mL, 15 mL)

# OSMOTIC

## Isosorbide

**Brand Names:** Ismotic®

**Use:** Short-term emergency treatment of acute angle-closure glaucoma and short-term reduction of intraocular pressure prior to and following intraocular surgery; may be used to interrupt an acute glaucoma attack; preferred agent when need to avoid nausea and vomiting.

**Dose:** Adults: Oral: Initial: 1.5 g/kg with a usual range of 1-3 g/kg 2-4 times/day, as needed.

**Strength:** Solution: 45% (15 mL, 30 mL)

# SURGICAL AID

## Chondroitin Sulfate - Sodium Hyaluronate

**Brand Names:** Viscoat®

**Use:** Surgical aid in anterior segment procedures; protects corneal endothelium and coats intraocular lens thus protecting it

**Dose:** Carefully introduce (using a 27-gauge needle or cannula) into anterior chamber after thoroughly cleaning the chamber with a balanced salt solution.

## Sodium Hyaluronate

**Brand Names:** AMO Vitrax®; Amvisc®; Amvisc® Plus; Healon®; Healon® GV

**Use:** Surgical aid in cataract extraction, intraocular implantation, corneal transplant, glaucoma filtration, and retinal attachment surgery

**Dose:** Depends upon procedure (slowly introduce a sufficient quantity into eye).

# OPHTHALMIC AGENTS *(Continued)*

## TOXIN

### Botulinum Toxin Type A

**Brand Names:** Botox®

**Use:** Treatment of strabismus and blepharospasms associated with dystonia (including benign essential blepharospasms or VII nerve disorders in patients >12 years of age

**Dose:**

Blepharospasm: 1.25-2.5 units (0.05-0.10 mL) injected into the orbicularis oculi muscle. Subsequent doses: Each treatment lasts approximately 3 months. At repeat treatment sessions, the dose may be increased up to twofold if the response from the initial treatment is considered insufficient (usually defined as an effect that does not last >2 months). There appears to be little benefit obtained from injecting >5 units per site. Some tolerance may be found if treatments are given any more frequently than every 3 months. The cumulative dose should not exceed 200 units in a 30-day period.

Strabismus: 1.25-5 units (0.05-0.15 mL) injected into any one muscle. Subsequent doses for residual/recurrent strabismus: Re-examine patient 7-14 days after each injection to assess the effects of that dose.

## VASOCONSTRICTOR

### Naphazoline

**Brand Names:** AK-Con®; Albalon®; Allerest® [OTC]; Clear Eyes® [OTC]; Comfort® [OTC]; Degest® [OTC]; Estivin II®; Liquifilm®; I-Naphline®; Muro's Opcon®; Nafazair®; Naphcon Forte®; Opcon®; Privine®; Vaso Clear® [OTC]; Vasocon Regular®

**Use:** Topical ocular vasoconstrictor; temporary relief of congestion, itching, and minor irritations; control hyperemia in patients with superficial corneal vascularity

**Dose:**

Children <6 years: Not recommended for use due to CNS depression (especially in infants).

Children >6 years and Adults: Instill 1-2 drops into conjunctival sac of affected eye(s) every 3-4 hours; therapy generally should not exceed 3-4 days.

**Strength:** Strengths ≤0.03% are OTC.

Solution: 0.012% (7.5 mL, 15 mL, 30 mL); 0.02% (15 mL); 0.03% (15 mL); 0.1% (15 mL)

# OTIC AGENTS

Consult product literature for full prescribing information.

**Patient Instructions:** Wash hands before instilling. Tilt head with affected ear upward. Gently grasp ear lobe and lift back and upward. Instill prescribed drops into ear canal. Do not push dropper into ear. Remain with head tilted for 2 minutes. Report ringing in ears, discharge, or worsening of condition.

## CERUMENOLYTICS

### Carbamide Peroxide [OTC]

**Brand Names:** Auro® Ear Drops; Debrox® Otic; ERO Ear; Mollifene® Ear Wax Removing Formula; Murine® Ear Drops

**Use:** Emulsify/disperse ear wax

**Dose:**

Children <12 years: Tilt head sideways and individualize the dose according to patient size; 3 drops (range: 1-5 drops) twice daily for up to 4 days. Tip of applicator should not enter ear canal. Keep drops in ear for several minutes by keeping head tilted and placing cotton in ear.

Children ≥12 years: Tilt head sideways and instill 5-10 drops twice daily up to 4 days. Tip of applicator should not enter ear canal. Keep drops in ear for several minutes by keeping head tilted and placing cotton in ear.

**Strengths:** 6.5% carbamide peroxide with various emulsifiers

### Triethanolamine Polypeptide Oleate [OTC]

**Brand Names:** Cerumenex®

**Use:** Emulsify/disperse ear wax

**Dose:** Children and Adults: Fill ear canal and insert cotton plug. Allow to remain 15-30 minutes. Flush ear with lukewarm water as a single treatment. If a second application is needed for unusually hard impactions, repeat the procedures.

**Strengths:** 10% triethanolamine oleate

## ANTIBIOTICS

### Chloramphenicol [Rx]

**Brand Names:** Chloromycetin®

**Use:** Treat infections

**Dose:** Instill 2-3 drops 3 times daily.

**Strengths:** Chloramphenicol 0.5%

### Ofloxacin [Rx]

**Brand Names:** Floxin®

**Use:** Treat otitis externa, otitis media with tympanostomy tubes, chronic suppurative otitis media with perforated tympanic membranes

**Dose:**

Acute otitis media with tympanostomy tubes: 1-12 years: Instill 5 drops twice daily for 10 days.

Chronic suppurative otitis media with perforated tympanic membranes: ≥12 years: Instill 10 drops twice daily for 14 days.

Otitis externa: 1-12 years: Instill 5 drops twice daily for 10 days; ≥12 years: Instill 10 drops twice daily for 10 days.

**Strengths:** Ofloxacin 0.3%

## OTIC AGENTS *(Continued)*

### ANTI-INFECTIVE/ANTI-INFLAMMATORY

**Acetic Acid and Hydrocortisone [Rx]**

**Brand Names:** Acetasol HC®; VoSol HC®

**Use:** Anti-inflammatory; drying agent

**Dose:** Insert saturated wick into ear. Leave in 24 hours, keeping moist with 3-5 drops every 4-6 hours. Keep moist for 24 hours. Remove wick and instill 5 drops 3 or 4 times/day.

**Strengths:** 1% hydrocortisone, 2% acetic acid, 3% propylene glycol diacetate

**Ciprofloxacin and Hydrocortisone [Rx]**

**Brand Names:** Cipro® HC Otic

**Use:** Acute otitis externa (swimmer's ear)

**Dose:** Instill 3 drops into affected ear twice daily for 7 days. Twice-daily dosing schedule is more convenient for patients than that of existing treatments with hydrocortisone, which are typically administered 3-4 times/day. A twice-daily dosage schedule may be especially helpful for parents and caregivers of young children.

**Strengths:** Ciprofloxacin hydrochloride 0.2% and hydrocortisone 1%

**Colistin, Neomycin, and Hydrocortisone [Rx]**

**Brand Names:** Coly-Mycin® S Otic Drops

**Use:** Superficial and susceptible bacterial infections of the external auditory canal; susceptible bacterial infections of mastoidectomy and fenestration cavities

**Dose:** Instill 4 drops into affected ear 3-4 times/day for 7-10 days.

**Strengths:** Colistin sulfate 0.3%, neomycin sulfate 0.47%, and hydrocortisone acetate 1% (5 mL, 10 mL)

**Cresyl Acetate [Rx]**

**Brand Names:** Cresylate®

**Use:** Acidifier; anti-infective; antifungal

**Dose:** Instill 2-4 drops as required.

**Strengths:** 25% m-cresyl acetate, 25% isopropanol

**Neomycin, Polymyxin B, and Hydrocortisone [Rx]**

**Brand Names:** AK-Spore H.C.® Otic; AntibiOtic® Otic; Bacticort® Otic; Cortatrigen® Otic; Cortisporin® Otic; Drotic® Otic; Ear-Eze® Otic; LazerSporin-C® Otic; Oticair® Otic; Otic-Care®; Otic Oti Tricin® Otic; Otocort® Otic; Otomycin-HPN® Otic; Otosporin® Otic; PediOtic® Otic; UAD® Otic

**Use:** Swimmer's ear (limited to 10 days)

**Dose:** Otic suspension is the preferred otic preparation.

Children: Instill 3 drops 3-4 times/day

Adults: Instill 4 drops 3-4 times/day

**Strengths:** Neomycin sulfate 5 mg, polymyxin B sulfate 10,000 units, and hydrocortisone 10 mg per mL (10 mL)

**Polymyxin B and Hydrocortisone [Rx]**

**Brand Names:** Otobiotic® Otic; Pyocidin-Otic®

**Use:** Superficial bacterial infections of the external ear canal

**Dose:** Instill 4 drops 3-4 times/day

**Strengths:** Polymyxin B sulfate 10,000 units and hydrocortisone 0.5%

## MISCELLANEOUS OTIC PREPARATIONS

### Acetic Acid and Aluminum Acetate [Rx]

**Brand Names:** Burrow's Otic®; Otic Domeboro®
**Use:** Local antibacterial; astringent
**Dose:** Insert saturated wick. Keep moist for 24 hours by instilling 4-6 drops every 2-3 hours.
**Strengths:** Acetic acid 2% in aluminum acetate solution

### Acetic Acid and Propylene Glycol [Rx]

**Brand Names:** Acetasol®; Acetic Acid Otic; VoSol® Otic
**Use:** Anti-infective; osmotic (antiedema)
**Dose:** Insert saturated wick and keep moist for 24 hours. Remove wick and instill 5 drops 4-3 times/day.
**Strengths:** Solution: 2% acetic acid with 3% propylene glycol diacetate, 0.02% benethonium chloride, 0.015% sodium acetate

### Alcohol [OTC]

**Brand Names:** Ear-Sol®
**Use:** Drying agent
**Dose:** Instill 6-8 drops twice daily.
**Strengths:** Alcohol 44%, propylene glycol and yerba santa (protective agent for skin)

### Alcohol and Hydrocortisone [OTC]

**Brand Names:** Ear-Sol® HC
**Use:** Drying agent; anti-inflammatory
**Dose:** Instill 4-6 drops less than 3-4 times daily.
**Strengths:** Alcohol 44%, hydrocortisone 1%, propylene glycol and yerba santa (protective agent for skin)

### Antipyrine and Benzocaine [Rx]

**Brand Names:** Allergan®; Auralgan Otic®; Auroto Otic®; Otocalm®
**Use:** Analgesic for swimmer's ear or otitis externa; facilitates ear wax removal
**Dose:** Fill ear canal. Moisten cotton pledget, place in ear canal, and repeat every 1-2 hours until pain and congestion are relieved. For ear wax removal, instill drops 3-4 times/day for 2-3 days.
**Strengths:** Solution: 1.4% benzocaine, 5.4% antipyrine

### Benzocaine [Rx]

**Brand Names:** Americaine®
**Use:** Local anesthetic; swimmer's ear
**Dose:** Instill 4-5 drops and insert cotton pledget.
**Strengths:** Solution: 20% benzocaine, 0.1% benethonium chloride, 1% glycerin PEG 300

### Benzocaine, Antipyrine, and Phenylephrine [Rx]

**Brand Names:** Tympangesic®
**Use:** Local anesthetic; analgesic
**Dose:** Fill ear canal and plug with saturated cotton. Repeat every 2-4 hours.
**Strengths:** Benzocaine 5%, antipyrine 5%, and phenylephrine 0.25%

### Boric Acid [OTC]

**Brand Names:** Dri/Ear®; Auro-Dri®; Ear-Dri®
**Use:** Prophylaxis of swimmer's ear
**Dose:** Instill 3-8 drops in each ear.
**Strengths:** Boric acid 2.7%, isopropyl alcohol

### Isopropyl Alcohol [OTC]

**Brand Names:** Swim-Ear®
**Use:** Drying agent
**Dose:** Instill 4-5 drops in affected ear after exposure to water.
**Strengths:** Isopropyl alcohol 95%, glycerin 5%

# SELECTED OVER-THE-COUNTER PRODUCTS

| Brand Name | Generic Name |
|---|---|
| 4-Way® Long Acting Nasal Solution | Oxymetazoline |
| 5-Benzagel® | Benzoyl peroxide |
| 10-Benzagel® | Benzoyl peroxide |
| A and D™ Ointment | Vitamin A and vitamin D |
| A.R.M.® Caplet | Chlorpheniramine and phenylpropanolamine |
| A-200™ Shampoo | Pyrethrins |
| Acnex® (Canadian) | Salicylic acid |
| Acnomel® (Canadian) | Salicylic acid |
| ACT® | Fluoride |
| Actagen® Syrup | Triprolidine and pseudoephedrine |
| Actagen® Tablet | Triprolidine and pseudoephedrine |
| Actifed® Allergy Tablet (Night) | Diphenhydramine and pseudoephedrine |
| ACU-dyne® | Povidone-iodine |
| Adsorbonac® Ophthalmic | Sodium chloride |
| Adsorbotear® Ophthalmic Solution | Artificial tears |
| Advanced Formula Oxy® Sensitive Gel | Benzoyl peroxide |
| Advil® Cold & Sinus Caplets | Pseudoephedrine and ibuprofen |
| Aeroaid® | Thimerosal |
| Aerodine® | Povidone-iodine |
| AeroZoin® | Benzoin |
| Afrin® Children's Nose Drops | Oxymetazoline |
| Afrin® Nasal Solution | Oxymetazoline |
| Afrin® Saline Mist | Sodium chloride |
| AK-Con® Ophthalmic | Naphazoline |
| AK-NaCl® | Sodium chloride |
| Akwa Tears® Solution | Artificial tears |
| Albalon® Liquifilm® Ophthalmic | Naphazoline |
| Albalon-A® Ophthalmic Solution | Naphazoline and antazoline |
| Alka-Seltzer® Plus Cold Liqui-Gels Capsules | Acetaminophen, chlorpheniramine, and pseudoephedrine |
| Alka-Seltzer® Plus Flu & Body Aches Non-Drowsy Liqui-Gels® | Acetaminophen, dextromethorphan, and pseudoephedrine |
| Allbee® With C | Vitamin B complex with vitamin C |
| Aller-Chlor® | Chlorpheniramine |
| Allercon® Tablet | Triprolidine and pseudoephedrine |
| Allerest® 12 Hour Capsule | Chlorpheniramine and phenylpropanolamine |
| Allerest® Eye Drops | Naphazoline |
| Allerest® Maximum Strength | Chlorpheniramine and pseudoephedrine |
| Allerest® No Drowsiness | Acetaminophen and pseudoephedrine |
| Allerest® 12 Hour Nasal Solution | Oxymetazoline |
| Allerfrin® Syrup | Triprolidine and pseudoephedrine |
| Allerfrin® Tablet | Triprolidine and pseudoephedrine |
| Allerphed Syrup | Triprolidine and pseudoephedrine |
| Alphamul® | Castor oil |
| AL-R® | Chlorpheniramine |
| Aludrox® | Aluminum hydroxide and magensium hydroxide |
| Ambi 10® | Benzoyl peroxide |
| Amesec® Capsules | Aminophylline, amobarbital, and ephedrine |
| Anamine® Syrup | Chlorpheniramine and pseudoephedrine |
| Anaplex® Liquid | Chlorpheniramine and pseudoephedrine |
| Antazoline-V® Ophthalmic Solution | Naphazoline and antazoline |
| Antihist-1® | Clemastine |
| Antiminth® | Pyrantel pamoate |
| Anusol® Ointment | Pramoxine |
| Apatate® | Vitamin B complex |
| Apo®-Gain (Canadian) | Minoxidil, topical |
| Aprodine® Syrup | Triprolidine and pseudoephedrine |
| Aprodine® Tablet | Triprolidine and pseudoephedrine |
| AquaSite® Ophthalmic Solution | Artificial tears |
| AquaTar® | Coal tar |
| Arthritis Foundation® NightTime Max Strength Caplet | Acetaminophen and diphenhydramine |

| Brand Name | Generic Name |
|---|---|
| Arthropan® | Choline salicylate |
| Aspirin-Free Bayer® Select® Allergy Sinus Caplets | Acetaminophen, chlorpheniraine, and pseudoephedrine |
| Aveeno® Cleansing Bar | Sulfur and salicylic acid |
| Ayr® Saline | Sodium chloride |
| Baker's P&S Topical | Phenol |
| Balnetar® Bath Oil | Coal tar, lanolin, and mineral oil |
| Banophen® Decongestant Capsule | Diphenhydramine and pseudoephedrine |
| Barc™ Liquid | Pyrethrins |
| Basaljel® | Aluminum carbonate |
| Bayer® Select® Chest Cold Caplets | Acetaminophen and dextromethorphan |
| Bayer® Select® Head Cold Caplets | Acetaminophen and pseudoephedrine |
| B-D Glucose® | Glucose, instant |
| Because® | Nonoxynol 9 |
| Benadryl® Decongestant Allergy Tablet | Diphenhydramine and pseudoephedrine |
| Ben-Aqua® | Benzoyl peroxide |
| Benoxyl® | Benzoyl peroxide |
| Benylin DM® | Dextromethorphan |
| Benza® | Benzalkonium chloride |
| Benzac AC® Gel | Benzoyl peroxide |
| Benzac AC® Wash | Benzoyl peroxide |
| Benzac W® Gel | Benzoyl peroxide |
| Benzac W® Wash | Benzoyl peroxide |
| Benzashave® Cream | Benzoyl peroxide |
| Benzedrex® Inhaler | Propylhexedrine |
| Berocca® | Vitamin B complex with vitamin C and folic acid |
| Betadine® | Povodine-iodine |
| Betadine® 5% Sterile Ophthalmic Prep Solution | Povidone-iodine |
| Betagen | Povodine-iodine |
| Biodine | Povodine-iodine |
| Bion® Tears Solution | Artificial tears |
| Bisac-Evac® | Bisacodyl |
| Bisacodyl Uniserts® | Bisacodyl |
| Bisco-Lax® | Bisacodyl |
| Black Draught® | Senna |
| BlemErase® Lotion | Benzoyl peroxide |
| Bluboro® | Aluminum acetate and calcium acetate |
| Borofax® Topical | Boric acid |
| Boropak® | Aluminum acetate and calcium acetate |
| BQ® Tablet | Chlorpheniramine, phenylpropanolamine, and acetaminophen |
| Breathe Free® | Sodium chloride |
| Brevoxyl® Gel | Benzoyl peroxide |
| Brofed® Elixir | Brompheniramine and pseudoephedrine |
| Bromaline® Elixir | Brompheniramine and phenylpropanolamine |
| Bromanate® Elixir | Brompheniramine and phenylpropanolamine |
| Bromarest® | Brompheniramine |
| Bromatapp® | Brompheniramine and phenylpropanolamine |
| Brombay® | Brompheniramine |
| Bromfed® Syrup | Brompheniramine and pseudoephedrine |
| Bromfed® Tablet | Brompheniramine and pseudoephedrine |
| Bromfenex® PD | Brompheniramine and pseudoephedrine |
| Bromphen® | Brompheniramine |
| Bromphen® Tablet | Brompheniramine and phenylpropanolamine |
| Brotane® | Brompheniramine |
| BSS® Ophthalmic | Balanced salt solution |
| Calm-X® Oral | Dimenhydrinate |
| Campho-Phenique® Liquid | Camphor and phenol |
| Capitrol® Shampoo | Chloroxine |
| Capsin® | Capsaicin |
| Capzasin-P® | Capsaicin |
| Carter's Little Pills® | Bisacodyl |
| Ceepryn® | Cetylpyridinium |
| Cellufresh® Ophthalmic Solution | Carboxymethylcellulose sodium |
| Celluvisc® Ophthalmic Solution | Carboxymethylcellulose sodium |

## SELECTED OVER-THE-COUNTER PRODUCTS *(Continued)*

| Brand Name | Generic Name |
|---|---|
| Cenafed® Plus Tablet | Triprolidine and pseudoephedrine |
| Cē pacol® Anesthetic Troches | Cetylpyridinium and benzocaine |
| Cē pacol® Troches | Cetylpyridinium |
| Cē pastat® | Phenol |
| Cerose-DM® Liquid | Chlorpheniramine, phenylephrine, and dextromethorphan |
| Chelated Manganese® | Manganese |
| Children's Hold® | Dextromethorphan |
| Children's Kaopectate® | Attapulgite |
| Chlo-Amine® | Chlorpheniramine |
| Chlorafed® Liquid | Chlorpheniraine and pseudoephedrine |
| Chloraseptic® Oral | Phenol |
| Chlorate® | Chlorpheniramine |
| Chloresium® | Chlorophyll |
| Chlorphed® | Brompheniramine |
| Chlorphed®-LA Nasal Solution | Oxymetazoline |
| ChlorPro® | Chlorpheniramine |
| Chlor-Rest® Tablet | Chlorpheniramine and phenylpropanolamine |
| Chlor-Trimeton® | Chlorpheniramine |
| Chlor-Trimeton® 4 Hour Relief Tablet | Chlorpheniraine and pseudoephedrine |
| Citracal® | Calcium citrate |
| Citrucel® Powder | Methylcellulose |
| Clear Away® Disc | Salicylic acid |
| Clear By Design® Gel | Benzoyl peroxide |
| Clear Eyes® | Naphazoline |
| Clearsil® Maximum Strength | Benzoyl peroxide |
| Clomycin® | Bacitracin, neomycin, polymyxin B, and lidocaine |
| Clysodrast® | Bisacodyl |
| Co-Hist® | Acetaminophen, chlorpheniramine, and pseudoephedrine |
| Colax® Tablet | Docusate and phenolphthalein |
| Cold & Allergy® Elixir | Brompheniramine and phenylpropanolamine |
| Coldrine® | Acetaminophen and pseudoephedrine |
| Collyrium Fresh® Ophthalmic | Tetrahydrozolone |
| Comfort® Ophthalmic | Naphazoline |
| Comfort® Tears Solution | Artificial tears |
| Comhist® LA Capsule | Chlorpheniramine, phenylephrine, and phenyltoloxamine |
| Comhist® Tablet | Chlorpheniramine, phenylephrine, and phenyltoloxamine |
| Compound W® | Salicylic acid |
| Comtrex® Maximum Strength Non-Drowsy | Acetaminophen, dextromethorphan, and pseudoephedrine |
| Congestant D® | Chlorpheniramine, phenylpropanolamine, and acetaminophen |
| Cophene-B® | Brompheniramine |
| Co-Pyronil® 2 Pulvules® | Chlorpheniramine and pseudoephedrine |
| Coricidin D'® | Chlorpheniramine, phenylpropanolamine, and acetaminophen |
| Coricidin® Tablet | Chlorpheniraine and acetaminophen |
| Corticaine® Topical Cream | Dibucaine and hydrocortisone |
| Creo-Terpin® | Dextromethorphan |
| Dacodyl® | Bisacodyl |
| Dairy Ease® | Lactase enzyme |
| Dakrina® Ophthalmic Solution | Artificial tears |
| Dallergy-D® Syrup | Chlorpheniramine and phenylephrine |
| Dapacin® Cold Capsule | Chlorpheniramine, phenylpropanolamine, and acetaminophen |
| Debrox® Otic | Carbamide peroxide |
| Deconamine® SR | Chlorpheniramine and pseudoephedrine |
| Deconamine® Tablet | Chlorpheniramine and pseudoephedrine |
| Deconamine® Syrup | Chlorpheniramine and pseudoephedrine |
| Deficol® | Bisacodyl |
| Degas® | Simethicone |
| Degest® 2 Ophthalmic | Naphazoline |
| Del Aqua-10® Gel | Benzoyl peroxide |
| Del Aqua-5® Gel | Benzoyl peroxide |

| Brand Name | Generic Name |
|---|---|
| Delfen® | Nonoxynol 9 |
| Delsym® | Dextromethorphan |
| Demazin® Syrup | Chlorpheniramine and phenylpropanolamine |
| Denorex® | Coal tar |
| Derifil® | Chlorophyll |
| Desitin® Ointment | Zinc oxide, cod liver oil, and talc |
| Desquam-E® Gel | Benzoyl peroxide |
| Desquam-X® Gel | Benzoyl peroxide |
| Desquam-X® Wash | Benzoyl peroxide |
| Devrom® Chewable Tablet | Bismuth subgallate |
| DHS® Tar | Coal tar |
| DHS Zinc® | Pyrithione zinc |
| Dialose® Plus Capsule | Docusate and casanthranol |
| Dialose® Plus Tablet | Docusate and phenolphthalein |
| Diamine T.D.® | Brompheniramine |
| Diaparene® | Methylbenzethonium chloride |
| Diasorb® | Attapulgite |
| Di-Gel® | Aluminum hydroxide, magnesium hydroxide, and simethicone |
| Dimaphen® Elixir | Brompheniramine and phenylpropanolamine |
| Dimaphen® Tablet | Brompheniramine and phenylpropanolamine |
| Dimetabs® Oral | Dimenhydrinate |
| Dimetane® Decongestant Elixir | Brompheniramine and phenylephrine |
| Dimetane® Extentabs® | Brompheniramine |
| Dimetapp® 4-Hour Liqui-Gel Capsule | Brompheniramine and phenylpropanolamine |
| Dimetapp® Elixir | Brompheniramine and phenylpropanolamine |
| Dimetapp® Extentabs® | Brompheniramine and phenylpropanolamine |
| Dimetapp® Sinus Caplets | Pseudoephedrine and ibuprofen |
| Dimetapp® Tablet | Brompheniramine and phenylpropanolamine |
| Diocto C® | Docusate and casanthranol |
| Diocto-K Plus® | Docusate and casanthranol |
| Dioctolose Plus® | Docusate and casanthranol |
| Disanthrol® | Docusate and casanthranol |
| Disobrom® | Dexbrompheniramine and pseudoephedrine |
| Disolan® Capsule | Docusate and phenolphthalein |
| Disophrol® Chronotabs® | Dexbrompheniramine and pseudoephedrine |
| Disophrol® Tablet | Dexbrompheniramine and pseudoephedrine |
| Docucal-P® Capsule | Docusate and phenolphthalein |
| Domeboro® Topical | Aluminum acetate and calcium acetate |
| Doxidan® Capsule | Docusate and phenolphthalein |
| Dr Scholl's® Disk | Salicylic acid |
| Dr Scholl's® Wart Remover | Salicylic acid |
| Dramamine® Oral | Dimenhydrinate |
| Dri-Ear® Otic | Boric acid |
| Dristan® Cold Caplets | Acetaminophen and pseudoephedrine |
| Dristan® Sinus Caplets | Pseudoephedrine and ibuprofen |
| Dristan® Long Lasting Nasal Solution | Oxymetazoline |
| Dristan® Saline Spray | Sodium chloride |
| Drixomed® | Dexbrompheniramine and pseudoephedrine |
| Drixoral® | Dexbrompheniramine and pseudoephedrine |
| Drixoral® Cough & Congestion Liquid Caps | Pseudoephedrine and dextromethorphan |
| Drixoral® Cough & Sore Throat Liquid Caps | Acetaminophen and dextromethorphan |
| Drixoral® Cough & Liquid Caps | Dextromethorphan |
| Drixoral® Nasal (Canadian) | Oxymetazoline |
| Drixoral® Syrup | Brompheniramine and pseudoephedrine |
| Dry Eye® Therapy Solution | Artificial tears |
| Dry Eyes® Solution | Artificial tears |
| Dryox® Gel | Benzoyl peroxide |
| Dryox® Wash | Benzoyl peroxide |
| DSMC Plus® | Docusate and casanthranol |
| D-S-S Plus® | Docusate and casanthranol |
| Duadacin® Capsule | Chlorpheniramine, phenylpropanolamine, and acetaminophen |
| Dulcolax® | Bisacodyl |
| DuoFilm® | Salicylic acid |

## SELECTED OVER-THE-COUNTER PRODUCTS *(Continued)*

| Brand Name | Generic Name |
|---|---|
| Duofilm® Solution | Salicylic acid and lactic acid |
| DuoPlant® Gel | Salicylic acid |
| Duplex® T | Coal tar |
| Duramist® Plus® | Oxymetazoline |
| Duration® Nasal Solution | Oxymetazoline |
| Dwelle® Ophthalmic Solution | Artificial tears |
| Dynafed® Maximum Strength | Acetaminophen and pseudoephedrine |
| E*R*O Ear | Carbamide peroxide |
| Ed A-Hist® Liquid | Chlorpheniramine and phenylephrine |
| Efodine® | Povidone-iodine |
| Emecheck® Liquid | Phosphorated carbohydrate solution |
| Emetrol® Liquid | Phosphorated carbohydrate solution |
| Emko® | Nonoxynol 9 |
| Emulsoil® | Castor oil |
| Encare® | Nonoxynol 9 |
| End Lice® Liquid | Pyrethrins |
| Equalactin® Chewable Tablet | Calcium polycarbophil |
| Estar® | Coal tar |
| Estivin® II Ophthalmic | Naphazoline |
| Exact® Cream | Benzoyl peroxide |
| Excedrin® Extra Strength Tablet | Acetaminophen and aspirin |
| Excedrin P.M.® | Acetaminophen and diphenhydramine |
| Ex-Lax® Extra Gentle Pills | Docusate and phenophthalein |
| Exsel® | Selenium sulfide |
| Eye-Lube-A® Solution | Artificial tears |
| Eye-Sed® Ophthalmic | Zinc sulfate |
| Eyesine® Ophthalmic | Tetrahydrozoline |
| Fedahist® Tablet | Chlorpheniramine and pseudoephedrine |
| Feen-a-Mint® Pills | Docusate and phenophthalein |
| Femilax® Tablet | Docusate and phenophthalein |
| Ferancee® | Ferrous salt and ascorbic acid |
| Fero-Grad 500® | Ferrous salt and ascorbic acid |
| Ferromar® | Ferrous salt and ascorbic acid |
| Fiberall® Chewable Tablet | Calcium polycarbophil |
| FiberCon® Tablet | Calcium polycarbophil |
| Fiber-Lax® Tablet | Calcium polycarbophil |
| Flatulex® | Simethicone |
| Fleet® Babylax® Rectal | Glycerin |
| Fleet® Enema | Sodium phosphate |
| Fleet® Flavored Castor Oil | Castor oil |
| Fleet® Laxative | Bisacodyl |
| Fleet® Mineral Oil Enema | Mineral oil |
| Fleet® Pain Relief | Pramoxine |
| Fleet® Phospho®-Soda | Sodium phosphate |
| Fluorigard® | Fluoride |
| Fluorinse® | Fluoride |
| Fluoritab® | Fluoride |
| Flura® | Fluoride |
| Flura-Drops® | Fluoride |
| Flura-Loz® | Fluoride |
| Folbesyn® | Vitamin B complex with vitamin C and folic acid |
| Fostex® | Sulfur and salicylic acid |
| Fostex® 10% BPO Gel | Benzoyl peroxide |
| Fostex® 10% Wash | Benzoyl peroxide |
| Fostex® Bar | Benzoyl peroxide |
| Fototar® | Coal tar |
| Freezone® Solution | Salicylic acid |
| Fungoid® | Triacetin |
| Gas-Ban DS® | Aluminum hydroxide, magnesium hydroxide, and simethicone |
| Gas-X® | Simethicone |
| Gaviscon® Liquid | Aluminum hydroxide and magnesium carbonate |
| Gaviscon® Tablet | Aluminum hydroxide and magnesium trisilicate |
| Gaviscon®-2 Tablet | Aluminum hydroxide and magnesium trisilicate |

| Brand Name | Generic Name |
|---|---|
| Gel Kam® | Fluoride |
| Gelpirin® Geltabs | Acetaminophen and aspirin |
| Gel-Tin® | Fluoride |
| Gelusil® | Aluminum hydroxide, magnesium hydroxide, and simethicone |
| Genac® Tablet | Triprolidine and pseudoephedrine |
| Genamin® Cold Syrup | Chlorpheniramine and phenylpropanolamine |
| Genasoft® Plus | Docusate and casanthranol |
| Genatap® Elixir | Brompheniramine and phenylpropanolamine |
| Geneye® Ophthalmic | Tetrahydrozoline |
| Gen-Minoxidil® (Canadian) | Minoxidil, topical |
| Gevrabon® | Vitamin B complex |
| Glutose® | Glucose, instant |
| Gly-Oxide® Oral | Carbamide peroxide |
| Goody's® Headache Powders | Acetaminophen and aspirin |
| Gordofilm® Liquid | Salicylic acid |
| Gynol II® | Nonoxynol 9 |
| Haley's M-O® Oral Suspension | Magnesium hydroxide and mineral oil emulsion |
| Hayfebrol® Liquid | Chlorpheniramine and pseudoephedrine |
| Head & Shoulders® Shampoo | Pyrithione zinc |
| Head & Shoulders® Intensive Treatment | Selenium sulfide |
| Histalet® Syrup | Chlorpheniramine and pseudoephedrine |
| Histatab® Plus Tablet | Chlorpheniramine and phenylephrine |
| Hista-Vadrin® Tablet | Chlorpheniramine, phenylephrine, and phenylpropanolamine |
| Histor-D® Syrup | Chlorpheniramine and phenylephrine |
| Histrodrix® | Dexbrompheniramine and pseudoephedrine |
| Hold® DM | Dextromethorphan |
| HuMist® Nasal Mist | Sodium chloride |
| HypoTears PF Solution | Artificial tears |
| HypoTears Solution | Artificial tears |
| Hytinic® | Polysaccharide-iron complex |
| Iberet®-Liquid | Ferrous sulfate, ascorbic acid, and vitamin B complex |
| I-Naphline® Ophthalmic | Naphazoline |
| Insta-Glucose® | Glucose, instant |
| Intercept™ | Nonoxynol 9 |
| Iodex® | Povidone-iodine |
| Iodex-p® | Povidone-iodine |
| Isodine® | Povidone-iodine |
| Isopto® Plain Solution | Artificial tears |
| Isopto® Tears Solution | Artificial tears |
| Itch-X® | Pramoxine |
| Just Tears® Solution | Artificial tears |
| Kaodene® | Kaolin and pectin |
| Kaopectate® Advanced Formula | Attapulgite |
| Kaopectate® Maximum Strength Caplets | Attapulgite |
| Kao-Spen® | Kaolin and pectin |
| Kapectolin® | Kaolin and pectin |
| Karidium® | Fluoride |
| Karigel® | Fluoride |
| Karigel®-N | Fluoride |
| Keralyt® Gel | Salicylic acid and propylene glycol |
| Klerist-D® Tablet | Chlorpheniramine and pseudoephedrine |
| Kloromin® | Chlorpheniraine |
| Kondremul® | Mineral oil |
| Koromex® | Nonoxynol 9 |
| Lac-Hydrin® Lotion | Lactic acid with ammonium hydroxide |
| Lacril® Ophthalmic Solution | Artificial tears |
| Lactaid® | Lactase enzyme |
| LactiCare® Lotion | Lactic acid and sodium-PCA |
| Lactrase® | Lactase enzyme |
| Lederplex® | Vitamin B complex |
| Legatrin PM® Caplet | Acetaminophen and diphenhydramine |
| Lice-Enz® Shampoo | Pyrethrins |
| Lipovite® | Vitamin B complex |

## SELECTED OVER-THE-COUNTER PRODUCTS *(Continued)*

| Brand Name | Generic Name |
|---|---|
| Liquifilm® Forte Solution | Artificial tears |
| Liquifilm® Tears Solution | Artificial tears |
| Listermint® With Fluoride | Fluoride |
| Loroxide® | Benzoyl peroxide |
| Lubriderm® Lotion | Lanolin, cetyl alcohol, glycerin, and petrolatum |
| LubriTears® Solution | Artificial tears |
| Luride® | Fluoride |
| Luride® Lozi-Tab | Fluoride |
| Luride®-SF Lozi-Tab® | Fluoride |
| Maalox® Anti-Gas | Simethicone |
| Maalox® | Aluminum hydroxide and magnesium hydroxide |
| Maalox® Plus | Aluminum hydroxide, magnesium hydroxide, and simethicone |
| Maalox® Therapeutic Concentrate | Aluminum hydroxide and magnesium hydroxide |
| Magalox Plus® | Aluminum hydroxide, magnesium hydroxide, and simethicone |
| Magonate® | Magnesium gluconate |
| Mallazine® Eye Drops | Tetrahydrozoline |
| Mallisol® | Povidone-iodine |
| Maltsuprex® | Malt soup extract |
| Marezine® | Cyclizine |
| Marmine® Oral | Dimenhydrinate |
| Massé® Breast Cream | Glycerin, lanolin, and peanut oil |
| Massengil® Medicated Douche w/ Cepticin | Povidone-iodine |
| MCT Oil® | Medium chain triglycerides |
| Mediplast® Plaster | Salicylic acid |
| Mega-B® | Vitamin B complex |
| Megaton™ | Vitamin B complex |
| Mercurochrome® Topical Solution | Merbromin |
| Mersol® | Thimerosal |
| Merthiolate® | Thimerosal |
| Metasep® | Parachlorometaxylenol |
| Midol® PM Caplet | Acetaminophen and diphenhydramine |
| Milkinol® | Mineral oil |
| Minidyne® | Povidone-iodine |
| Minute-Gel® | Fluoride |
| Mitrolan® Chewable Tablet | Calcium polycarbophi |
| Modane® Plus Tablet | Docusate and phenolphthalein |
| Moducal® | Glucose polymers |
| Moi-Stir® | Saliva substitute |
| Moisture® Ophthalmic Drops | Artificial tears |
| Mollifene® Ear Wax Removing Formula | Carbamide peroxide |
| Mosco® Liquid | Salicylic acid |
| Motrin® IB Sinus Caplets | Pseudoephedrine and ibuprofen |
| Mucoplex® | Vitamin B complex |
| Murine® Ear Drops | Carbamide peroxide |
| Murine® Plus Ophthalmic | Tetrahydrozoline |
| Murine® Solution | Artificial tears |
| Muro 128® Ophthalmic | Sodium chloride |
| Murocel® Ophthalmic Solution | Artificial tears |
| Muroptic-5® | Sodium chloride |
| Mylanta® | Aluminum hydroxide, magnesium hydroxide, and simethicone |
| Mylanta Gas® | Simethicone |
| Mylanta®-II | Aluminum hydroxide, magnesium hydroxide, and simethicone |
| Mylicon® | Simethicone |
| Myoflex® Cream | Triethanolamine salicylate |
| Myphetapp® | Brompheniramine and phenylpropanolamine |
| Nafazair® Ophthalmic | Naphazoline |
| Naphcon Forte® Ophthalmic | Naphazoline |
| Naphcon® Ophthalmic | Naphazoline |
| Naphcon-A® Ophthalmic Solution | Naphazoline and pheniramine |

| Brand Name | Generic Name |
|---|---|
| Nasahist B® | Brompheniramine |
| Nā Sal™ | Sodium chloride |
| Nasal Moist® | Sodium chloride |
| Nature's Tears® Solution | Artificial tears |
| Naus-A-Way® Liquid | Phosphorated carbohydrate solution |
| Nausetrol® Liquid | Phosphorated carbohydrate solution |
| Nazil® Ofteno (Mexican) | Naphazoline |
| ND-Stat® | Brompheniramine |
| Neo-Cultol® | Mineral oil |
| Neoloid® | Castor oil |
| Neo-Synephrine® 12 Hour Nasal Solution | Oxymetazoline |
| NeoVadrin® B Complex | Vitamin B complex |
| Nephrocaps® | Vitamin B complex with vitamin C and folic acid |
| Neutrogena® Acne Mask | Benzoyl peroxide |
| Neutrogena® T/Derm | Coal tar |
| Nicobid® | Niacin |
| Nicolar® | Niacin |
| Nicotinex | Niacin |
| Niferex® | Polysaccharide-iron complex |
| No Pain-HP® | Capsaicin |
| Nolahist® | Phenindamine |
| Nō strilla® | Oxymetazoline |
| Novahistine® Elixir | Chlorpheniramine and phenylephrine |
| NTZ® Long Acting Nasal Solution | Oxymetazoline |
| Nu-Iron® | Polysaccharide-iron complex |
| Nullo® | Chlorophyll |
| Nupercainal® | Dibucaine |
| Nu-Tears® Solution | Artificial tears |
| Nu-Tears® II Solution | Artificial tears |
| Occlusal-HP Liquid | Salicylic acid |
| Ocean Nasal Mist | Sodium chloride |
| OcuClear® Ophthalmic | Oxymetazoline |
| OcuCoat® Ophthalmic Solution | Artificial tears |
| OcuCoat® PF Ophthalmic Solution | Artificial tears |
| Off-Ezy® Wart Remover | Salicylic acid |
| Ony-Clear® Nail Aerosol | Triacetin |
| Opcon® Ophthalmic | Naphazoline |
| Operand® | Povidone-iodine |
| Ophthalgan® Ophthalmic | Glycerin |
| Ophthalmic Prep Solution | Povidone-iodine |
| Optigene® Ophthalmic | Tetrahydrozoline |
| Optised® Ophthalmic | Phenylephrine and zinc sulfate |
| Orabase® Plain | Gelatin, pectin, and methylcellulose |
| Orabase® With Benzocaine Paste | Benzocaine, gelatin, pectin, and sodium carboxymethylcellulose |
| Orajel® Perioseptic | Carbamide peroxide |
| Oraminic ® II | Brompheniramine |
| Orazinc® Oral | Zinc sulfate |
| Orex® | Saliva substitute |
| Orexin® | Vitamin B complex |
| Ornade® Spansule® | Chlorpheniramine and phenylpropanolamine |
| Ornex® No Drowsiness | Acetaminophen and pseudoephedrine |
| Osmoglyn® Ophthalmic | Glycerin |
| Otrivin® Nasal | Xylometazoline |
| Ovide™ Topical Lotion | Malathion |
| Ovol® (Canadian) | Simethicone |
| Oxipor® VHC | Coal tar |
| Oxy-5® Advanced Formula for Sensitive Skin | Benzoyl peroxide |
| Oxy-5® Tinted | Benzoyl peroxide |
| Oxy-10® Advanced Formula for Sensitive Skin | Benzoyl peroxide |
| Oxy 10® Wash | Benzoyl peroxide |
| PALS® | Chlorophyll |
| P&S® Shampoo | Salicylic acid |
| PanOxyl® Bar | Benzoyl peroxide |

## SELECTED OVER-THE-COUNTER PRODUCTS *(Continued)*

| Brand Name | Generic Name |
|---|---|
| PanOxyl®-AQ | Benzoyl peroxide |
| Panscol® | Salicylic acid |
| Parhist SR® | Chlorpheniramine and phenylpropanolamine |
| Pediaflor® | Fluoride |
| Pedi-Boro® | Aluminum acetate and calcium acetate |
| Pentrax® | Coal tar |
| Percogesic® Tablet | Acetaminophen and phenyltolaxamine |
| Perfectoderm® Gel | Benzoyl peroxide |
| Peri-Colace® | Docusate and casanthranol |
| Pernox® | Sulfur and salicylic acid |
| Peroxin A5® | Benzoyl peroxide |
| Peroxin A10® | Benzoyl peroxide |
| Persa-Gel® | Benzoyl peroxide |
| Pertussin® CS | Dextromethorphan |
| Pertussin® ES | Dextromethorphan |
| Pharmaflur® | Fluoride |
| Phazyme® | Simethicone |
| Phenetron® | Chlorpheniramine |
| Phenylzin® Ophthalmic | Phenylephrine and zinc sulfate |
| Phicon® | Pramoxine |
| Phillips'® LaxCaps® Capsule | Docusate and phenolphthalein |
| Phos-Flur® | Fluoride |
| Pin-Rid® | Pyrantel pamoate |
| Pin-X® | Pyrantel pamoate |
| Point-Two® | Fluoride |
| Polycose® | Glucose polymers |
| Polydine® | Povidone-iodine |
| Polytar® | Coal tar |
| Posture® | Calcium phosphate, dibasic |
| PrameGel® | Pramoxine |
| Prax® | Pramoxine |
| PreSun® 29 | Methoxycinnamate and oxybenzone |
| Pretz® | Sodium chloride |
| PreviDent® | Fluoride |
| Privine® Nasal | Naphazoline |
| Proctofoam® NS | Pramoxine |
| Pronto® Shampoo | Pyrethrins |
| Pro-Sof® Plus | Docusate and casanthranol |
| Proxigel® Oral | Carbamide peroxide |
| Pseudo-Gest Plus® Tablet | Chlorpheniramine and pseudoephedrine |
| Psor-a-set® Soap | Salicylic acid |
| psoriGel® | Coal tar |
| Puralube® Tears Solution | Artificial tears |
| Purge® | Castor oil |
| Puri-Clens™ | Methylbenzethonium chloride |
| Pyrinex® Pediculicide Shampoo | Pyrethrins |
| Pyrinyl II® Liquid | Pyrethrins |
| Pyrinyl Plus® Shampoo | Pyrethrins |
| R & C® Shampoo | Pyrethrins |
| Ramses® | Nonoxynol 9 |
| Reese's® Pinworm Medicine | Pyrantel pamoate |
| Refresh® Ophthalmic Solution | Artificial tears |
| Refresh® Plus Ophthalmic Solution | Artificial tears |
| Regaine® (Mexican) | Minoxidil, topical |
| Regulace® | Docusate and casanthranol |
| Rentamine® Liquid | Chlorpheniraine, ephedrine, phenylephrine, and carbetapentane |
| Resaid® | Chlorpheniramine and phenylpropanolamine |
| Rescon Liquid | Chlorpheniramine and phenylpropanolamine |
| Resporal® | Dexbrompheniramine and pseudoephedrine |
| R-Gel® | Capsaicin |
| Rheaban® | Attapulgite |
| Rhinosyn® Liquid | Chlorpheniraine and pseudoephedrine |
| Rhinosyn-PD® Liquid | Chlorpheniraine and pseudoephedrine |

| Brand Name | Generic Name |
|---|---|
| RID® Shampoo | Pyrethrins |
| Robitussin® Cough Calmers | Dextromethorphan |
| Robitussin® Pediatric | Dextromethorphan |
| Rogaine® for Men | Minoxidil, topical |
| Rogaine® for Women | Minoxidil, topical |
| Rolaids® Chewable Tablet | Dihydroxyaluminum sodium carbonate |
| Rolatuss® Plain Liquid | Chlorpheniramine and phenylephrine |
| Ru-Tuss® Liquid | Chlorpheniramine and phenylephrine |
| Ryna® Liquid | Chlorpheniramine and pseudoephredrine |
| Rynatuss® Pediatric Suspension | Chlorpheniramine, ephedrine, phenylephrine, and carbetapentane |
| Sal-Acid® Plaster | Salicylic acid |
| Salactic® Film | Salicylic acid |
| SalineX® | Sodium chloride |
| Sal-Plant® Gel | Salicylic acid |
| Sani-Supp® Suppository | Glycerin |
| Sarna Topical Lotion | Camphor, menthol, and phenol |
| SAStid® Plain Therapeutic Shampoo and Acne Wash | Sulfur and salicylic acid |
| Scot-Tussin DM® Cough Chasers | Dextromethorphan |
| SeaMist® | Sodium chloride |
| Sebulex® | Sulfur and salicylic acid |
| Sebulon® | Pyrithione zinc |
| Selsun® | Selenium sulfide |
| Selsun® Blue | Selenium sulfide |
| Selsun® Gold for Women | Selenium sulfide |
| Semicid® | Nonoxynol 9 |
| Semprex-D® Capsule | Acrivastine and pseudoephedrine |
| Senexon® | Senna |
| Senna-Gen® | Senna |
| Senokot® | Senna |
| Senolax® | Senna |
| Shur-Seal® | Nonoxynol 9 |
| Silace-C® | Docusate and casanthranol |
| Silafed® Syrup | Triprolidine and pseudoephedrine |
| Silain® | Simethicone |
| Silaminic® Cold Syrup | Chlorpheniramine and phenylpropanolamine |
| Silphen DM® | Dextromethorphan |
| Sinarest® 12 Hour Nasal Solution | Oxymetazoline |
| Sinarest® No Drowsiness | Acetaminophen and pseudoephedrine |
| Sine-Aid® IB Caplets | Pseudoephedrine and ibuprofen |
| Sine-Aid® Maximum Strength | Acetaminophen and pseudoephedrine |
| Sine-Off® Maximum Strength No Drowsiness | Acetaminophen and pseudoephedrine |
| Sinex® Long-Acting | Oxymetazoline |
| Sinubid® Tablet | Phenyltoloxamine, phenylpropanolamine, and acetaminophen |
| Sinus Excedrin® Extra Strength | Acetaminophen and pseudoephedrine |
| Sinusol-B® | Brompheniramine |
| Sinus-Relief® | Acetaminophen and pseudoephedrine |
| Sinutab® Tablet | Acetaminophen, chlorpheniramine, and pseudoephedrine |
| Sinutab® Without Drowsiness | Acetaminophen and pseudoephedrine |
| Slo-Niacin® | Niacin |
| Slow-Mag® | Magnesium chloride |
| Sportscreme® | Triethanolamine salicylate |
| St. Joseph® Cough Suppressant | Dextromethorphan |
| Stop® | Fluoride |
| Sucrets® Cough Calmers | Dextromethorphan |
| Sudafed Plus® Tablet | Chlorpheniramine and pseudoephedrine |
| Sudafed® Severe Cold | Acetaminophen, dextromethorphan, and pseudoephedrine |
| Sumacal® | Glucose polymers |
| Summer's Eve® Medicated Douche | Povidone-iodine |
| Suppress® | Dextromethorphan |
| Surbex® | Vitamin B complex |
| Surbex® With C Filmtabs® | Vitamin B complex with vitamin C |

## SELECTED OVER-THE-COUNTER PRODUCTS *(Continued)*

| Brand Name | Generic Name |
|---|---|
| Surbex-T® Filmtabs® | Vitamin B complex with vitamin C |
| Sween Cream® | Methylbenzethonium chloride |
| Swim-Ear® Otic | Boric acid |
| T/Gel® | Coal tar |
| Tamine® | Brompheniramine and phenylpropanolamine |
| Tavist® | Clemastine |
| Tavist-1® | Clemastine |
| Tavist-D® | Clemastine and phenylpropanolamine |
| Tear Drop® Solution | Artificial tears |
| TearGard® Ophthalmic Solution | Artificial tears |
| Teargen® Ophthalmic Solution | Artificial tears |
| Tearisol® Solution | Artificial tears |
| Tears Naturale® Free Solution | Artificial tears |
| Tears Naturale® Solution | Artificial tears |
| Tears Naturale® II Solution | Artificial tears |
| Tears Plus® Solution | Artificial tears |
| Tears Renewed® Solution | Artificial tears |
| Tega-Vert® Oral | Dimenhydrinate |
| Teldrin® | Chlorpheniramine |
| Telechlor® | Chlorpheniramine |
| Temazin® Cold Syrup | Chlorpheniramine and phenylpropanolamine |
| Tetrasine® Extra Ophthalmic | Tetrahydrozoline |
| Tetrasine® Ophthalmic | Tetrahydrozoline |
| Thera-Combex® H-P Kapseals® | Vitamin B complex with vitamin C |
| Theraflu® Non-Drowsy Formula Maximum Strength | Acetaminophen, dextromethorphan, and pseudoephedrine |
| Thera-Flur® | Fluoride |
| Thera-Flur-N® | Fluoride |
| Thera-Flur-N® ACT® | Fluoride |
| Thera-Hist® Syrup | Chlorpheniramine and phenylpropanolamine |
| Theralax® | Bisacodyl |
| Theraplex Z® | Pyrithione zinc |
| Theroxide® Wash | Benzoyl peroxide |
| TinBen® | Benzoin |
| TinCoBen® | Benzoin |
| Ti-Screen® | Methoxycinnamate and oxybenzone |
| Tisit® Blue Gel | Pyrethrins |
| Tisit® Liquid | Pyrethrins |
| Tisit® Shampoo | Pyrethrins |
| Titralac® Plus Liquid | Calcium carbonate and simethicone |
| Trans-Planta® (Canadian) | Salicylic acid |
| Trans-Ver-Sal® (Canadian) | Salicylic acid |
| Trans-Ver-Sal® AdultPatch | Salicylic acid |
| Trans-Ver-Sal® PediaPatch | Salicylic acid |
| Trans-Ver-Sal® PlantarPatch | Salicylic acid |
| Triaminic® Allergy Tablet | Chlorpheniraine and phenylpropanolamine |
| Triaminic® Cold Tablet | Chlorpheniraine and phenylpropanolamine |
| Triaminic® Syrup | Chlorpheniraine and phenylpropanolamine |
| Triaminicol® Multi-Symptom Cold Syrup | Chlorpheniramine, phenylpropanolamine, and dextromethorphan |
| Tri-Nefrin® Extra Strength Tablet | Chlorpheniraine and phenylpropanolamine |
| Triofed® Syrup | Triprolidine and pseudoephedrine |
| Triphenyl® Syrup | Chlorpheniramine and phenylpropanolamine |
| Triple X® Liquid | Pyrethrins |
| Triposed® Syrup | Triprolidine and pseudoephedrine |
| Triposed® Tablet | Triprolidine and pseudoephedrine |
| TripTone® Caplets® | Dimenhydrinate |
| Tri-Tannate Plus® Liquid | Chlorpheniramine, ephedrine, phenylephrine, and carbetapentane |
| Trocal® | Dextromethorphan |
| Tronolane® | Pramoxine |
| Tronothane® HCl | Pramoxine |
| Tucks® Cream/Gel/Pads | Witch hazel |
| Twice-A-Day® Nasal | Oxymetazoline |

| Brand Name | Generic Name |
|---|---|
| Tylenol® Cold Effervescent Medication Tablet | Chlorpheniramine, phenylpropanolamine, and acetaminophen |
| Tylenol® Cold No Drowsiness | Acetaminophen, dextromethorphan, and pseudoephedrine |
| Tylenol® Flu Maxumum Strength | Acetaminophen, dextromethorphan, and pseudoephedrine |
| Tylenol® Sinus Maximum Strength | Acetaminophen and pseudoephedrine |
| Tyzine® Nasal | Tetrahydrozoline |
| Ulcerease® | Phenol |
| Ultra Tears® Solution | Artificial tears |
| Unilax® Capsule | Docusate and phenolphthalein |
| Vanoxide® | Benzoyl peroxide |
| Vaso Clear® Ophthalmic | Naphazoline |
| Vasocon Regular® Ophthalmic | Naphazoline |
| Vasocon-A® Ophthalmic Solution | Naphazoline and antazoline |
| Veltane® | Brompheniramine |
| Verazinc® Oral | Zinc sulfate |
| Versel™ (Canadian) | Selenium sulfide |
| Vicks® 44D Cough & Head Congestion Capsule | Pseudoephedrine and dextromethorphan |
| Vicks® 44D Non-Drowsy Cold & Cough Liqui-Caps | Pseudoephedrine and dextromethorphan |
| Vicks Formula 44® | Dextromethorphan |
| Vicks Formula 44® Pediatric Formula | Dextromethorphan |
| Vicks® DayQuil® Allergy Relief 4 Hour Tablet | Brompheniramine and phenylpropanolamine |
| Vicon-C® | Vitamin B complex with vitamin C |
| Visine® Extra Ophthalmic | Tetrahydrozoline |
| Visine® L.R. Ophthalmic | Oxymetazoline |
| Viva-Drops® Solution | Artificial tears |
| Wart-Off® | Salicylic acid |
| Whitfield's Ointment | Benzoic acid and salicylic acid |
| Xero-Lube® | Saliva substitute |
| X-Prep® Liquid | Senna |
| X-seb® T Shampoo | Coal tar and salicyclic acid |
| Yeast-Gard® Medicated Douche | Povidone-iodine |
| Zephiran® | Benzalkonium chloride |
| Zetar® | Coal tar |
| Zincate® Oral | Zinc sulfate |
| Zincfrin® Ophthalmic | Phenylephrine and zinc sulfate |
| Zincon® Shampoo | Pyrithione zinc |
| ZNP® Bar | Pyrithione zinc |
| Zostrix® | Capsaicin |
| Zostrix®-HP | Capsaicin |
| Zymenol® | Mineral oil |

# SELECTED PRESCRIPTION COMBINATION PRODUCTS*

| Brand Name | Generic Name |
|---|---|
| Alersule Forte® | Chlorpheniramine, phenylephrine, and methscopolamine |
| Allergan® Ear Drops | Antipyrine and benzocaine |
| Ambenyl® Cough Syrup | Bromodiphenhydramine and codeine |
| Amgenal® Cough Syrup | Bromodiphenhydramine and codeine |
| Auroto® | Antipyrine and benzocaine |
| Bromanyl® Cough Syrup | Bromodiphenhydramine and codeine |
| Bromotuss® w/Codeine Cough Syrup | Bromodiphenhydramine and codeine |
| Carmol-HC® Topical | Urea and hydrocortisone |
| Codehist® DH Liquid | Chlorpheniramine, pseudoephedrine, and codeine |
| D.A.II® Tablet | Chlorpheniramine, phenylephrine, and methscopolamine |
| Dallergy® | Chlorpheniramine, phenylephrine, and methscopolamine |
| Decohistine® DH Liquid | Chlorpheniramine, pseudoephedrine, and codeine |
| Dihistine® DH Liquid | Chlorpheniramine, pseudoephedrine, and codeine |
| Dura-Vent/DA® | Chlorpheniramine, phenylephrine, and methscopolamine |
| Extendryl® SR | Chlorpheniramine, phenylephrine, and methscopolamine |
| Histalet Forte® Tablet | Chlorpheniramine, pyrilamine, phenylephrine, and phenylpropanolamine |
| Histor-D® Timescelles® | Chlorpheniramine, phenylephrine, and methscopolamine |
| Iberet-Folic-500® CR Tablet | Ferrous sulfate, ascorbic acid, vitamin B complex, and folic acid |
| Naldecon® | Chlorpheniramine, phenyltoloxamine, phenylpropanolamine, and phenylephrine |
| Naldelate® | Chlorpheniramine, phenyltoloxamine, phenylpropanolamine, and phenylephrine |
| Nalgest® | Chlorpheniramine, phenyltoloxamine, phenylpropanolamine, and phenylephrine |
| Nalspan® | Chlorpheniramine, phenyltoloxamine, phenylpropanolamine, and phenylephrine |
| New Decongestant® | Chlorpheniramine, phenyltoloxamine, phenylpropanolamine, and phenylephrine |
| Nolamine® Tablet | Chlorpheniramine, phenindamine, and phenylpropanolamine |
| Novacet® Topical | Sulfur and sodium sulfacetamide |
| Novahistine® DH Liquid | Chlorpheniramine, pseudoephedrine, and codeine |
| Otocalm® Ear | Antipyrine and benzocaine |
| Par Decon® | Chlorpheniramine, phenyltoloxamine, phenylpropanolamine, and phenylephrine |
| Pediacof® Liquid | Chlorpheniramine, phenylephrine, and codeine |
| Pedituss® Liquid | Chlorpheniramine, phenylephrine, and codeine |
| Phen DH® w/Codeine | Chlorpheniramine, pseudoephedrine, and codeine |
| Polycitra® Syrup | Sodium citrate and potassium citrate mixture |
| Quadra-Hist® | Chlorpheniramine, phenyltoloxamine, phenylpropanolamine, and phenylephrine |
| Rhinatate® Tablet | Chlorpheniramine, pyrilamine, and phenylephrine |
| R-Tannamine® Tablet | Chlorpheniramine, pyrilamine, and phenylephrine |
| R-Tannate® Tablet | Chlorpheniramine, pyrilamine, and phenylephrine |
| Ryna-C® Liquid | Chlorpheniramine, pseudoephedrine, and codeine |
| Rynatan® Pediatric Suspension | Chlorpheniramine, pyrilamine, and phenylephrine |
| Rynatan® Tablet | Chlorpheniramine, pyrilamine, and phenylephrine |
| Sulfacet-R® Topical | Sulfur and sodium sulfacetamide |
| Tanoral® Tablet | Chlorpheniramine, pyrilamine, and phenylephrine |
| Triotann® Tablet | Chlorpheniramine, pyrilamine, and phenylephrine |
| Tri-Phen-Chlor® | Chlorpheniramine, phenyltoloxamine, phenylpropanolamine, and phenylephrine |
| Tri-Tannate® Tablet | Chlorpheniramine, pyrilamine, and phenylephrine |
| Tritan® Tablet | Chlorpheniramine, pyrilamine, and phenylephrine |
| Uni-Decon® | Chlorpheniramine, phenyltoloxamine, phenylpropanolamine, and phenylephrine |

*See individual monographs for detailed information.

# ANTIEMETICS FOR CHEMOTHERAPY-INDUCED NAUSEA AND VOMITING

## Basic Principles of Antiemetic Therapy

1. Rule out other causes of nausea and vomiting before prescribing antiemetics.
2. Evaluate the relative emetic potential of antineoplastic drugs and choose antiemetics accordingly.
3. Treat delayed nausea and vomiting with **scheduled antiemetics** for a period of several days.
4. **Combination antiemetic regimens** provide greater protection against chemotherapy induced emesis than do single agents.
5. Head off trouble before it starts by initiating an aggressive antiemetic regimen before giving highly emetogenic chemotherapy.

### Time Course of Nausea and Vomiting

| Drug | Onset (h) | Duration (h) |
|---|---|---|
| Azacitidine | 1-3 | 3-4 |
| Carboplatin | 2-6 | 1-48 |
| Carmustine | 2-6 | 4-6 |
| Cisplatin | 1-4 | 12-96 |
| Cyclophosphamide | 6-8 | 8-24 |
| Cytarabine | 1-3 | 3-8 |
| Dacarbazine | 1-2 | 2-4 |
| Dactinomycin | 2-5 | 4-24 |
| Daunorubicin | 1-3 | 4-24 |
| Doxorubicin | 1-3 | 4-24 |
| Ifosfamide | 2-3 | 12-72 |
| Lomustine | 2-6 | 4-6 |
| Mechlorethamine | 1-3 | 2-8 |
| Mitomycin | 1-2 | 3-4 |
| Plicamycin | 4-6 | 4-24 |
| Streptozocin | 1-3 | 1-12 |

### Potency of Antiemetic Drugs

| Potency | Antiemetic Drug Class |
|---|---|
| Low | Anticholinergic<br>Antihistamine<br>Benzodiazepine<br>Cannabinoid<br>Corticosteroid<br>Phenothiazine |
| Low to moderate | Butyrophenone |
| High | Serotonin antagonist<br>Substituted benzamide (high dose) |

# ANTIEMETICS FOR CHEMOTHERAPY-INDUCED NAUSEA AND VOMITING *(Continued)*

### Types of Antiemetic Drugs

| Drug Class | Name |
|---|---|
| Anticholinergic drugs | Scopolamine (Transderm-Scop®) |
| Antihistamines | Diphenhydramine (Benadryl®) |
| Benzodiazepines | Alprazolam (Xanax®)<br>Lorazepam (Ativan®) |
| Butyrophenones | Domperidone (Motilium®) (investigational)<br>Droperidol (Inapsine®)<br>Haloperidol (Haldol®) |
| Cannabinoids | Dronabinol (Marinol®)<br>Nabilone (Cesamet®) |
| Corticosteroids | Dexamethasone (Decadron®)<br>Methylprednisolone (Medrol®) |
| Phenothiazines | Chlorpromazine (Thorazine®)<br>Perphenazine (Trilafon®)<br>Prochlorperazine (Compazine®)<br>Promethazine (Phenergan®)<br>Thiethylperazine (Torecan®) |
| Serotonin antagonists | Dolasetron (Anzemet®)<br>Granisetron (Kytril®)<br>Ondansetron (Zofran®)<br>Tropisetron (Navoban®) (investigational) |
| Substituted benzamides | Alizapride (Plitican®) (investigational)<br>Metoclopramide (Reglan®)<br>Trimethobenzamide (Tigan®) |

### Combinations of Antiemetic Drugs Resulting in Decreased Toxicity of the Primary Drug

| Primary Antiemetic Drug | Effective Secondary Drug |
|---|---|
| Phenothiazine | Antihistamine |
| Butyrophenone | Antihistamine |
| Substituted benzamide | Antihistamine<br>Corticosteroid<br>Benzodiazepine |
| Cannabinoid | Phenothiazine |

### Combinations of Antiemetic Drugs Resulting in Improved Efficacy of the Primary Antiemetic Drug

| Primary Antiemetic Drug | Effective Secondary Drug |
|---|---|
| Serotonin antagonist | Corticosteroid<br>Phenothiazine<br>Butyrophenone |
| Substituted benzamide | Corticosteroid<br>Corticosteroid with anticholinergic drug |
| Phenothiazine | Corticosteroid |
| Butyrophenone | Corticosteroid |
| Cannabinoid | Corticosteroid |
| Corticosteroid | Benzodiazepine |

## Emetogenic Potential of Single Chemotherapeutic Agents

### Class I
### Low (<10%)

Asparaginase
Bleomycin
Busulfan
Busulfan (oral)
Chlorambucil
Cladribine
Cyclophosphamide (oral)
Cytarabine
Docetaxel
Etoposide
Floxuridine
Fludarabine
Melphalan <100 mg/m$^2$
Mercaptopurine
Paclitaxel
Thioguanine (oral)
Thiotepa <60 mg
Vincristine

### Class II
### Moderately Low (10% to 30%)

Bleomycin
Busulfan 1 mg/kg (oral)
Cytarabine ≤20 mg
Doxorubicin ≤20 mg
Etoposide
Fluorouracil <1000 mg
Methotrexate <100 mg
Thiotepa >200 mg
Topotecan

### Class III
### Moderate (30% to 60%)

Azacitidine
Capecitabine
Carboplatin
Cisplatin ≤25 mg/m$^2$/day
Cyclophosphamide <1 g
Daunorubicin
Doxorubicin <75 mg or >20 mg
Fluorouracil ≥1000 mg
Gemcitabine
Idarubicin
Methotrexate <250 mg or ≥100 mg
Mitoxantrone
Paclitaxel
Teniposide
Vinblastine
Vinorelbine

### Class IV
### Moderately High (60% to 90%)

Carmustine <200 mg
Cisplatin <75 mg
Cyclophosphamide 1 g
Cytarabine 250 mg to 1 g
Dacarbazine <500 mg
Doxorubicin ≥75 mg
Hexamethyl melamine
Ifosfamide
Irinotecan (dose-limiting_
Lomustine <60 mg
Methotrexate ≥250 mg
Mitomycin
Procarbazine

### Class V
### High (>90%)

Carmustine ≥200 mg
Cisplatin ≥75 mg
Cyclophosphamide >1 g
Cytarabine >1 g
Dacarbazine ≥500 mg
Dactinomycin
Lomustine ≥60 mg
Mechlorethamine
Melphalan ≥100 mg/m$^2$
Pentostatin
Streptozocin
Thiotepa ≥100 mg/m$^2$

# ANTIEMETICS FOR CHEMOTHERAPY-INDUCED NAUSEA AND VOMITING *(Continued)*

**Initial Doses in Selected Antiemetic Regimens***

| Antiemetic Regimen | Adult Dose | Pediatric Dose |
|---|---|---|
| **For moderately emetogenic chemotherapy** | | |
| Dexamethasone | I.V.: 10-20 mg | I.V.: 10 mg/m$^2$/dose for the first dose, then 5 mg/m$^2$/dose q6h as needed |
| Dronabinol | P.O.: 10 mg | P.O.: 5 mg/m$^2$ starting 6-8 hours before chemotherapy and q4-6 hours after; to be continued for 12 hours after therapy discontinuation |
| Ondansetron | P.O.: 8 mg or I.V.: 10 mg | P.O.: 4-12 y: 4 mg 30 minutes before treatment; repeat 4 and 8 hours after initial dose<br>>12 y: See adult dose<br>I.V.: 10 mg/m$^2$/dose for the first dose, then 5 mg/m$^2$/dose q6h as needed |
| Prochlorperazine | P.O.: 5-10 mg; I.V.: 5-10 mg, or 25 mg by rectal suppository | P.O./P.R.: 0.4 mg/kg/24 hours in 3-4 divided doses<br>I.M.: 0.1-0.15 mg/kg/dose |
| **For highly emetogenic chemotherapy†** | | |
| Dexamethasone | I.V.: 20 mg | I.V.: 20 mg/m$^2$/dose for the first dose, then 5-10 mg/m$^2$/dose q6h as needed |
| Diphenhydramine | I.V.: 25-50 mg q2h x 2 | I.V.: ≤50 mg/m$^2$ q2h x 2 |
| Lorazepam | I.V.: 1-2 mg | I.V.: 2-15 y: 0.05 mg/kg (≤2 mg/dose) prior to chemotherapy |
| Metoclopramide | I.V.: 3 mg/kg of body weight q2h x 2 | I.V.: 1-2 mg/kg 30 minutes before chemotherapy q2-4h |
| Ondansetron | I.V.: 32 mg (in divided doses) | I.V.: 0.45 mg/kg as single dose 30 minutes prior to chemotherapy or 0.15 mg/kg 30 minutes before and 0.15 mg/kg at 4 and 8 hours after treatment |

Adapted with revisions from *N Engl J Med*, 1993, 329:1790-6.

*Antiemetic regimens for moderately emetogenic chemotherapy consist of single drugs; regimens for highly emetogenic chemotherapy consist of drugs given in combination (denoted by brackets).

†Use combination therapy.

# CHEMOTHERAPY COMPATIBILITY

LEGEND
C = Physically & chemically compatible
P = Physically compatible for at least two hours at room temperature
Y = Physically compatible for Y-site administration
I = Incompatible
BLANK Information not available

| | Amifostine | Amphotericin B | Bleomycin | Calcium Gluconate | Carboplatin | Carmustine | Cefazolin | Chlorpromazine | Cisplatin | Cyclophosphamide | Cytarabine | Dacarbazine | Dactinomycin | Daunorubicin | Dexamethasone | Diphenhydramine |
|---|---|---|---|---|---|---|---|---|---|---|---|---|---|---|---|---|
| Amifostine | | I | Y | Y | Y | P | Y | I | I | P | P | P | P | P | P | P |
| Amphotericin B | I | | | I | | | | I | | | | | | | | I |
| Bleomycin | Y | | | | | | I | | Y | Y | | P | | | C | C |
| Calcium Gluconate | Y | I | | | | | P | | | | | | | | | |
| Carboplatin | Y | | | | | | | | | | | | | | | |
| Carmustine | P | | | | | | | | | | | P | | | | |
| Cefazolin | Y | | I | P | | | | | | P | | | | | | |
| Chlorpromazine | I | I | | | | | | | P | P | P | | | | | Y |
| Cisplatin | I | | Y | | | | | P | | P | | | | | P | P |
| Cyclophosphamide | P | | Y | | | | P | P | P | | | P | | | P | P |
| Cytarabine | P | | | | | | | P | | | | P | | C | P | P |
| Dacarbazine | P | | P | | | P | | | | P | P | | P | | | |
| Dactinomycin | P | | | | | | | | | | | P | | | | |
| Daunorubicin | P | | | | | | | | | | C | | | | I | |
| Dexamethasone | P | | C | | | | | | P | P | P | | | I | | I |
| Diphenhydramine | P | I | C | | | | | Y | P | P | P | | | | I | |
| Doxorubicin | P | Y | Y | | | | | P | Y | Y | | P | | | I | P |
| Droperidol | P | | Y | | | | | Y | Y | Y | P | | | | | Y |
| Etoposide | P | | | | C | | | | P | C | C | | | C | | |
| Famotidine | P | | | P | | | P | | P | P | P | | | | P | |
| Fentanyl | | | | | | | | Y | | | | | | | | Y |
| Filgrastim | | I | Y | P | P | P | P | P | P | P | P | P | I | P | P | P |
| Floxuridine | P | | | | C | | | | P | | | | | | | |
| Fluconazole | P | I | | I | | | P | P | | | | | | | P | P |
| Fludarabine | P | I | P | | P | P | P | I | P | P | P | P | P | I | P | P |
| Fluorouracil | P | | P | | I | | | | I | C | I | P | | | | |
| Furosemide | P | | Y | P | | | | I | Y | Y | P | | | | P | |
| Gentamicin | P | I | P | | | | I | | | P | I | | | | | |
| Haloperidol | P | | | | | | | | | | | | | | | |
| Heparin | P | Y | P | P | | | P | I | Y | Y | I | I | | I | P | P |
| Hydrocortisone | P | P | I | P | | | | P | | | I | | | P | P | I |
| Hydromorphone | P | | | | | | I | Y | Y | P | P | | | | I | Y |
| Idarubicin | P | | | | | | I | | | P | P | | | | I | P |
| Ifosfamide | | | | | C | | | | C | | | | | | | |
| Insulin, Regular | | | | | | | P | | | | I | | | | | |
| Leucovorin | P | | Y | | | | | | C | Y | | | | | | |
| Lorazepam | P | | | | | | | | P | P | P | | | | | |
| Magnesium Sulfate | P | I | | P | | | P | | C | | | | | | | |
| Mannitol | Y | | | | | | | | P | | | | | | | |
| Mechlorethamine | P | | | | | | | | | | | | | | | |
| Melphalan | | I | P | P | P | P | P | I | P | P | P | P | P | P | P | P |
| Meperidine | P | | | | | | P | Y | | | | | | | P | Y |
| Mesna | P | | | | I | | | | I | P | | | | | | |
| Methotrexate | P | | Y | | | | I | I | Y | P | P | P | | | P | P |
| Methylprednisolone | P | | | I | | | | | Y | P | I | | | | | |
| Metoclopramide | P | | Y | I | | | | P | Y | Y | P | | | | P | P |
| Mitomycin | P | | Y | | | | | | Y | Y | | | | | | |
| Mitoxantrone | P | | | | | | | | | P | P | | | | | |
| Morphine | P | | | | | | P | Y | P | P | P | | | | P | Y |
| Ondansetron | P | I | P | P | P | P | P | P | P | P | P | P | P | P | P | P |
| Paclitaxel | | I | P | | P | | | I | P | P | P | P | | | P | P |
| Plicamycin | P | | | | | | | | | | | | | | | |
| Potassium Chloride | P | I | | P | | | | P | P | | P | | | | P | P |
| Prochlorperazine | I | I | | I | | | | Y | P | P | P | | | | P | Y |
| Promethazine | P | | | | | | | Y | P | P | P | | | | | Y |
| Sargramostim | | I | Y | P | P | P | P | I | P | P | P | P | P | | P | P |
| Sodium Bicarbonate | P | P | | | I | I | | | I | | P | | | | | |
| Thiotepa | P | | | | | | | | I | | | | | | | |
| Total Parenteral Nutrition | | | | P | | | P | | | | P | | | | | |
| Vancomycin | P | | | P | | | | | | P | | | | | | |
| Vinblastine | P | | C | | | | | | Y | Y | P | P | | | | |
| Vincristine | P | | C | | | | | | Y | Y | P | | | | | |
| Vinorelbine | | I | P | P | P | P | I | P | P | P | P | P | P | P | P | P |

# CHEMOTHERAPY COMPATIBILITY *(Continued)*

**LEGEND**
C = Physically & chemically compatible
P = Physically compatible for at least two hours at room temperature
Y = Physically compatible for Y-site administration
I = Incompatible
BLANK Information not available

| | Doxorubicin | Droperidol | Etoposide | Famotidine | Fentanyl | Filgrastim | Floxuridine | Fluconazole | Fludarabine | Fluorouracil | Furosemide | Gentamicin | Haloperidol | Heparin | Hydrocortisone | Hydromorphone |
|---|---|---|---|---|---|---|---|---|---|---|---|---|---|---|---|---|
| Amifostine | P | P | P | P | | | P | P | P | P | P | P | P | P | P | P |
| Amphotericin B | Y | | | | | I | | I | I | | | I | | | | |
| Bleomycin | Y | Y | | | | Y | | | P | P | Y | P | | P | I | |
| Calcium Gluconate | | | | P | | P | | I | | | P | | | P | P | |
| Carboplatin | | | C | | | P | C | | P | I | | | | | | |
| Carmustine | | | | | | P | | | P | | | | | | | |
| Cefazolin | | | | P | | P | | P | P | | | I | | P | | I |
| Chlorpromazine | P | Y | | | Y | P | | P | I | | I | | | I | P | Y |
| Cisplatin | Y | Y | P | P | | P | P | | P | I | Y | | | Y | | Y |
| Cyclophosphamide | Y | Y | C | P | | P | | | P | C | Y | P | | Y | | P |
| Cytarabine | | P | C | P | | P | | | P | I | P | I | | I | I | P |
| Dacarbazine | P | | | | | P | | | P | P | | | | I | | |
| Dactinomycin | | | | | | I | | | P | | | | | | | |
| Daunorubicin | | | C | | | P | | | I | | | | | I | P | |
| Dexamethasone | I | | | P | | P | | P | P | | P | | | P | P | I |
| Diphenhydramine | P | Y | | | Y | P | | P | P | | | | | P | I | Y |
| Doxorubicin | | Y | | P | | P | | | P | I | I | | | I | I | P |
| Droperidol | Y | | | | Y | P | | P | P | I | I | | | I | P | |
| Etoposide | | | | | | I | C | | P | C | | | | | | |
| Famotidine | P | | | | | P | | P | P | | P | P | | P | P | |
| Fentanyl | | Y | | | | | | | | I | | | | P | P | Y |
| Filgrastim | P | P | I | P | | | P | P | P | I | I | P | P | I | P | P |
| Floxuridine | | | C | | | P | | | P | C | | | | C | | |
| Fluconazole | | P | | P | | P | | | P | | I | P | I | P | P | |
| Fludarabine | P | P | P | P | | P | P | P | | P | P | P | P | P | P | P |
| Fluorouracil | I | I | C | | I | I | C | | P | | Y | | | Y | P | |
| Furosemide | I | I | | P | | I | | I | P | Y | | I | | P | Y | |
| Gentamicin | I | | I | | | P | | P | | I | P | | I | P | P | I |
| Haloperidol | | | | P | | P | | P | P | | I | | | I | | P |
| Heparin | | | | P | | P | | I | P | | | | P | I | | |
| Hydrocortisone | I | I | | P | P | I | C | P | P | Y | P | I | I | | I | |
| Hydromorphone | I | P | | P | P | P | | P | P | P | P | | | I | | |
| Idarubicin | P | | | | Y | P | | | P | | | P | | | | |
| Ifosfamide | | P | I | | | P | | | | | I | I | | I | I | |
| Insulin, Regular | | | C | | | P | | | P | C | | | | | | |
| Leucovorin | | | | P | | | | | | | | P | | P | P | |
| Lorazepam | Y | I | | | | P | C | P | | C | Y | | | Y | | |
| Magnesium Sulfate | P | | | | | P | | | P | | | | | | | |
| Mannitol | | | | P | | | | | P | | | P | | P | P | P |
| Mechlorethamine | | | | | | I | | | P | C | | P | | | | |
| Melphalan | | | | | | P | | | P | | | | | | | |
| Meperidine | P | P | P | P | | P | P | P | P | P | P | P | P | P | P | P |
| Mesna | | Y | | P | Y | P | | P | P | | I | P | | I | P | |
| Methotrexate | | | | | | P | | | P | | | | | | | |
| Methylprednisolone | P | I | | P | | P | | | P | C | Y | | | Y | | P |
| Metoclopramide | P | | | P | | I | | | P | | | | | P | Y | |
| Mitomycin | Y | Y | | P | Y | P | | P | P | Y | I | | | Y | P | |
| Mitoxantrone | Y | Y | | | | I | | | | Y | Y | | | Y | | |
| Morphine | | | | | | P | | | P | P | | | | I | P | |
| Ondansetron | P | Y | | P | Y | P | | P | P | | I | P | P | I | P | |
| Paclitaxel | P | P | P | P | | P | P | P | P | I | I | P | P | P | P | P |
| Plicamycin | P | P | P | P | | P | P | P | | P | P | P | P | P | P | P |
| Potassium Chloride | | | | | | P | | | | | | | | | | |
| Prochlorperazine | | P | Y | P | P | P | | P | P | P | P | | | P | P | |
| Promethazine | P | Y | | | Y | I | | P | I | | I | | | P | I | I |
| Sargramostim | P | Y | | | Y | P | | P | P | | I | | | I | I | I |
| Sodium Bicarbonate | P | P | P | P | P | | P | P | | | P | P | I | P | I | I |
| Thiotepa | | | | P | | P | | | P | | P | | | P | P | I |
| Total Parenteral Nutrition | | | | P | | I | | P | | P | P | P | | P | | |
| Vancomycin | | | | | | P | | P | P | | | | | I | P | P |
| Vinblastine | P | Y | | | | P | | | P | Y | I | | | I | | |
| Vincristine | Y | Y | | | | P | | | P | Y | I | | | Y | | |
| Vinorelbine | P | P | P | P | | P | P | P | P | I | I | P | P | P | P | P |

LEGEND
C = Physically & chemically compatible
P = Physically compatible for at least two hours at room temperature
Y = Physically compatible for Y-site administration
I = Incompatible
BLANK Information not available

| | Idarubicin | Ifosfamide | Insulin, Regular | Leucovorin | Lorazepam | Magnesium Sulfate | Mannitol | Mechlorethamine | Melphalan | Meperidine | Mesna | Methotrexate | Methylprednisolone | Metoclopramide | Mitomycin | Mitoxantrone |
|---|---|---|---|---|---|---|---|---|---|---|---|---|---|---|---|---|
| Amifostine | P | | | P | P | P | Y | P | | P | P | P | P | P | P | P |
| Amphotericin B | | | | | | I | | | I | | | | | | | |
| Bleomycin | | | | Y | | | | | P | | | Y | | Y | Y | |
| Calcium Gluconate | | | | | | P | | | P | | | | I | I | | |
| Carboplatin | | C | | | | | | | P | | I | | | | | |
| Carmustine | | | | | | | | | P | | | | | | | |
| Cefazolin | I | | P | | | P | | | P | P | | I | | | | |
| Chlorpromazine | | | | | | | | | I | Y | | I | | P | | |
| Cisplatin | | C | | C | P | C | P | | P | | I | Y | Y | Y | Y | |
| Cyclophosphamide | P | | | Y | P | | | | P | | P | P | P | Y | Y | P |
| Cytarabine | P | | I | | P | | | | P | | | P | I | P | | P |
| Dacarbazine | | | | | | | | | P | | | P | | | | |
| Dactinomycin | | | | | | | | | P | | | | | | | |
| Daunorubicin | | | | | | | | | P | | | | | | | |
| Dexamethasone | I | | | | | | | | P | P | | P | | P | | |
| Diphenhydramine | P | | | | | | | | P | Y | | P | | P | | |
| Doxorubicin | | | | Y | P | | | | P | | | P | P | Y | Y | |
| Droperidol | P | | | I | | | | | P | Y | | I | | Y | Y | |
| Etoposide | I | C | | | | | | | P | | | | | | | |
| Famotidine | | | P | | | P | | | P | P | | P | P | P | | |
| Fentanyl | | | | | | | | | | Y | | | | Y | | |
| Filgrastim | P | P | | P | P | | I | P | P | P | P | P | I | P | I | P |
| Floxuridine | | | | C | | | | | P | | | | | | | |
| Fluconazole | | | | P | | | | | P | P | | | | P | | |
| Fludarabine | | P | | | P | P | P | P | P | P | P | P | P | P | | P |
| Fluorouracil | | C | | C | | | C | | P | | | C | | Y | Y | P |
| Furosemide | I | | | Y | | | | | P | I | | Y | | I | Y | |
| Gentamicin | I | | P | | | P | P | | P | P | | | | | | |
| Haloperidol | | | | | | | | | P | | | | | | | |
| Heparin | I | | P | Y | | P | | | P | I | | Y | P | Y | Y | I |
| Hydrocortisone | I | | P | | | P | | | P | P | | | Y | P | | P |
| Hydromorphone | | | | | | P | | | P | | | P | | | | |
| Idarubicin | | | | | I | P | P | | P | I | | I | | P | | |
| Ifosfamide | | | | | | | | | P | | C | | | | | |
| Insulin, Regular | | | | | | P | | | | P | | | | P | | |
| Leucovorin | | | | | | | | | | | | Y | Y | Y | Y | |
| Lorazepam | I | | | | | | | | P | | | P | | | | |
| Magnesium Sulfate | P | | P | | | | | | | P | | | | P | | |
| Mannitol | P | | | | | | | | P | | | | | P | | |
| Mechlorethamine | | | | | | | | | P | | | | | | | |
| Melphalan | P | P | | | P | | P | P | | P | P | P | P | P | P | P |
| Meperidine | I | | P | | | P | | | P | | | | P | Y | | |
| Mesna | | C | | | | | | | P | | | | | | | |
| Methotrexate | I | | | Y | P | | | | P | | | | P | I | Y | |
| Methylprednisolone | | | | Y | | | | | P | P | | P | | Y | | |
| Metoclopramide | P | | P | Y | | P | P | | P | Y | | I | Y | | Y | |
| Mitomycin | | | | Y | | | | | P | | | Y | | Y | | |
| Mitoxantrone | | | | | | | | | P | | | | | | | |
| Morphine | | | P | | | P | | | P | I | | P | P | Y | | |
| Ondansetron | | P | | | I | P | C | P | P | P | P | P | I | P | P | P |
| Paclitaxel | | P | | | P | P | P | | | P | P | P | I | P | | I |
| Plicamycin | | | | | | | | | P | | | | | | | |
| Potassium Chloride | P | | P | | | P | Y | | P | P | | | I | P | | P |
| Prochlorperazine | | | | | | | | | P | Y | | P | | Y | | |
| Promethazine | | | | | | | | | P | Y | | I | | Y | | |
| Sargramostim | P | P | | | I | P | P | P | | P | P | P | I | P | I | P |
| Sodium Bicarbonate | I | | I | | | I | | | P | I | | P | | I | | |
| Thiotepa | | | | | | | | | P | | | | | | | |
| Total Parenteral Nutrition | P | | P | | | | | | | P | | | | P | | |
| Vancomycin | I | | P | | | P | | | P | P | | P | | | | |
| Vinblastine | I | | | Y | | | | | P | | | P | | Y | Y | |
| Vincristine | I | | | Y | | | | | P | | | P | | Y | Y | |
| Vinorelbine | P | P | | | P | | P | P | P | P | P | P | I | P | I | P |

# CHEMOTHERAPY COMPATIBILITY *(Continued)*

**LEGEND**

C = Physically & chemically compatible
P = Physically compatible for at least two hours at room temperature
Y = Physically compatible for Y-site administration
I = Incompatible
BLANK Information not available

| | Morphine | Ondansetron | Paclitaxel | Plicamycin | Potassium Chloride | Prochlorperazine | Promethazine | Sargramostim | Sodium Bicarbonate | Thiotepa | Total Parenteral Nutrition | Vancomycin | Vinblastine | Vincristine | Vinorelbine |
|---|---|---|---|---|---|---|---|---|---|---|---|---|---|---|---|
| Amifostine | P | P | | P | P | I | P | | P | P | | P | P | P | |
| Amphotericin B | | I | I | | I | I | | I | P | | | | | | I |
| Bleomycin | | P | P | | | | | Y | | | | | C | C | P |
| Calcium Gluconate | | | | | P | I | | P | | | P | P | | | P |
| Carboplatin | | Y | P | | | | | P | I | | | | | | P |
| Carmustine | | P | | | | | | P | I | | | | | | P |
| Cefazolin | P | P | | | | | | P | | | P | | | | I |
| Chlorpromazine | Y | P | I | | P | Y | Y | I | | | | | | | P |
| Cisplatin | P | P | P | | P | P | P | P | I | I | | | Y | Y | P |
| Cyclophosphamide | P | P | P | | | P | P | P | | | | P | Y | Y | P |
| Cytarabine | P | P | P | | P | P | P | P | P | | P | | P | P | P |
| Dacarbazine | | P | P | | | | | P | | | | | P | | P |
| Dactinomycin | | P | | | | | | P | | | | | | | P |
| Daunorubicin | | P | | | | | | | | | | | | | P |
| Dexamethasone | P | P | P | | P | P | | P | | | | I | | | P |
| Diphenhydramine | Y | P | P | | P | Y | Y | P | | | | | | | P |
| Doxorubicin | P | P | P | | | P | P | P | | | | | P | Y | P |
| Droperidol | Y | P | P | | P | Y | Y | P | | | | | Y | Y | P |
| Etoposide | | P | P | | Y | | | P | | | | | | | P |
| Famotidine | P | P | P | | P | | | P | P | | P | | | | P |
| Fentanyl | Y | | | | P | Y | Y | P | | | | | | | |
| Filgrastim | P | P | P | P | P | I | P | | P | I | | P | P | P | P |
| Floxuridine | | P | P | | | | | P | | | | | | | P |
| Fluconazole | P | P | P | | P | P | P | P | | | P | P | | | P |
| Fludarabine | P | P | | | P | I | P | | P | | | P | P | P | P |
| Fluorouracil | | I | P | | P | | | P | | | P | | Y | P | I |
| Furosemide | I | I | P | | P | I | I | P | P | | P | | I | I | I |
| Gentamicin | P | P | P | | P | | | P | | | P | | | | P |
| Haloperidol | P | P | P | | | | | I | | | | | | | P |
| Heparin | I | P | P | | P | P | I | P | P | | P | I | I | Y | P |
| Hydrocortisone | P | P | P | | P | I | I | I | P | | | P | | | P |
| Hydromorphone | | P | P | | | I | I | I | I | | | P | | | P |
| Idarubicin | | | | | P | | | P | I | | P | I | I | I | P |
| Ifosfamide | | P | P | | | | | P | | | | | | | P |
| Insulin, Regular | P | | | | P | | | | I | | P | P | | | |
| Leucovorin | | | | | | | | | | | | | S | S | |
| Lorazepam | | I | P | | | | | I | | | | | | | P |
| Magnesium Sulfate | P | P | P | | P | | | P | I | | | P | | | |
| Mannitol | | C | P | | S | | | P | | | | | | | P |
| Mechlorethamine | | P | | | | | | P | | | | | | | P |
| Melphalan | P | P | | P | P | P | P | | P | P | | P | P | P | P |
| Meperidine | I | P | P | | P | S | S | P | I | | P | P | | | P |
| Mesna | | P | P | | | | | P | | | | | | | P |
| Methotrexate | P | P | P | | | P | I | P | P | | | P | P | P | P |
| Methylprednisolone | P | I | I | | I | | | I | | | | | | | I |
| Metoclopramide | S | P | P | | P | S | S | P | I | | P | | S | S | P |
| Mitomycin | | P | | | | | | I | | | | | S | S | I |
| Mitoxantrone | | P | I | | P | | | P | | | | | | | P |
| Morphine | | P | P | | P | I | S | I | I | | P | P | | | P |
| Ondansetron | P | | P | | P | P | P | I | I | | | P | P | P | P |
| Paclitaxel | P | P | | | P | P | | | P | | | P | P | P | P |
| Plicamycin | P | P | P | | | P | I | P | P | | | P | | | P |
| Potassium Chloride | I | P | P | | P | | S | P | P | | | | | | P |
| Prochlorperazine | S | P | | | I | S | | P | | | | | | | P |
| Promethazine | I | I | | | P | P | P | | I | | P | P | P | P | |
| Sargramostim | I | I | P | | P | P | | I | | | P | I | | | I |
| Sodium Bicarbonate | | | | | | | | | | | | | | | I |
| Thiotepa | P | | | | | | | P | P | | | P | | | |
| Total Parenteral Nutrition | | | P | | P | | | P | I | | P | | | | P |
| Vancomycin | P | P | | | | | | | | | | | | | |
| Vinblastine | | P | P | | | | | P | | | | | | S | P |
| Vincristine | | P | P | | | | | P | | | | | S | | P |
| Vinorelbine | P | P | P | P | P | P | P | | I | I | | P | P | P | |

# COMPATIBILITY OF DRUGS

**KEY**

**Y** = Compatible
**N** = Incompatible
Blank = Information about compatibility was not available

| | aminophylline | amphotericin B | ampicillin | atropine | calcium gluconate | carbenicillin | cefazolin | cimetidine | clindamycin | diazepam | dopamine | epinephrine | erythromycin | fentanyl | furosemide | gentamicin |
|---|---|---|---|---|---|---|---|---|---|---|---|---|---|---|---|---|
| aminophylline | ■ | | Y | | Y | N | N | | N | Y | Y | N | N | | | |
| amphotericin B | | ■ | N | | N | N | | N | | | N | | | | | N |
| ampicillin | Y | N | ■ | N | N | Y | Y | | N | | N | | N | | | N |
| atropine | | | N | ■ | | | | Y | | N | | N | | Y | | |
| calcium gluconate | Y | N | N | | ■ | | N | | N | | Y | N | Y | | | |
| carbenicillin | N | N | Y | | | ■ | | Y | Y | | Y | N | N | | | N |
| cefazolin | N | | Y | | N | | ■ | N | | Y | | | N | | | N |
| cimetidine | | N | | Y | | Y | N | ■ | Y | | | Y | Y | | Y | Y |
| clindamycin | N | | N | | N | Y | | Y | ■ | | | | | | | Y |
| diazepam | Y | | | N | | | Y | | | ■ | | N | | | N | |
| dopamine | Y | N | N | | Y | Y | | | | | ■ | | | | | N |
| epinephrine | N | | | N | N | N | | Y | | N | | ■ | N | | N | |
| erythromycin | N | | N | | Y | N | N | Y | | | | N | ■ | | | |
| fentanyl | | | | Y | | | | | | | | | | ■ | | |
| furosemide | | | | | | | | Y | | N | | N | | | ■ | N |
| gentamicin | | N | N | | | N | N | | Y | | Y | | | | N | ■ |
| glycopyrrolate | | | | Y | | | | | | N | | | | | | |
| heparin sodium | Y | Y | Y | N | Y | | | Y | Y | N | Y | Y | N | | Y | N |
| hydrocortisone | Y | Y | N | | Y | Y | Y | | Y | | Y | | Y | | | |
| hydroxyzine | N | | | Y | | | | | | N | | | | Y | | |
| levarterenol | N | | | N | Y | N | N | Y | | N | | N | | | N | |
| lidocaine | Y | N | Y | | Y | Y | N | Y | | N | Y | N | Y | | | |
| meperidine | N | | | Y | | | | | | N | | Y | | Y | | |
| morphine | N | | | Y | | | | | | N | | | | Y | | |
| nitroglycerin | Y | | | | | | | | | | Y | | | | Y | |
| pentobarbital | Y | | | N | | | N | N | N | N | | | N | N | | |
| potassium chloride | Y | N | Y | Y | Y | Y | Y | Y | Y | N | Y | N | Y | | Y | |
| sodium bicarbonate | Y | Y | | N | N | | | | Y | N | | N | Y | | | |
| tetracycline | N | N | N | | N | N | N | Y | | | Y | | N | | N | |
| vancomycin | N | | | | Y | | | Y | | | | | Y | | | |
| verapamil | Y | N | Y | Y | Y | Y | Y | Y | Y | Y | Y | Y | Y | | Y | Y |
| vitamin B & C complex | N | | Y | Y | Y | N | Y | Y | Y | N | Y | Y | N | | Y | Y |

**NOTE:** Because the compatibility of two or more drugs in solution depends on several variables such as the solution itself, drug concentration and the method of mixing (bottle, syringe, or Y-site), this table is intended to be used solely as a guide to general drug compatibilities. Before mixing any drugs, the healthcare professional should ascertain if a potential incompatibility exists by referring to an appropriate information source.

## COMPATIBILITY OF DRUGS *(Continued)*

**KEY**

**Y** = Compatible
**N** = Incompatible
Blank = Information about compatibility was not available

| | glycopyrrolate | heparin sodium | hydrocortisone | hydroxyzine | levarterenol | lidocaine | meperidine | morphine | nitroglycerin | pentobarbital | potassium chloride | sodium bicarbonate | tetracycline | vancomycin | verapamil | vitamin B & C complex |
|---|---|---|---|---|---|---|---|---|---|---|---|---|---|---|---|---|
| aminophylline | | Y | Y | N | N | Y | N | N | Y | Y | Y | Y | N | N | Y | N |
| amphotericin B | | Y | Y | | | N | | | | | N | Y | N | | N | |
| ampicillin | | Y | N | | | Y | | | | | Y | | N | | Y | Y |
| atropine | Y | N | | Y | N | | Y | Y | | N | Y | N | | | Y | Y |
| calcium gluconate | | Y | Y | | Y | Y | | | | | Y | N | N | Y | Y | Y |
| carbenicillin | | | Y | | N | Y | | | | | Y | | N | | Y | N |
| cefazolin | | | Y | | N | N | | | | N | Y | | N | | Y | Y |
| cimetidine | | Y | | | Y | Y | | | | N | Y | | Y | Y | Y | Y |
| clindamycin | | Y | Y | | | | | | | N | Y | Y | | | Y | Y |
| diazepam | N | N | | N | N | N | N | N | | N | N | N | | | Y | N |
| dopamine | | Y | Y | | | Y | | | Y | | Y | | Y | | Y | Y |
| epinephrine | | Y | | | N | N | Y | | | | N | N | | | Y | Y |
| erythromycin | | N | Y | | | Y | | | | N | Y | Y | N | Y | Y | N |
| fentanyl | | | | Y | | | Y | Y | | N | | | | | | |
| furosemide | | Y | | | N | | | | Y | | Y | | N | | Y | Y |
| gentamicin | | N | | | | | | | | | | | | | Y | Y |
| glycopyrrolate | ■ | | | Y | | Y | Y | Y | | N | | N | | | | |
| heparin sodium | | ■ | N | N | Y | Y | N | N | | | Y | Y | N | N | Y | Y |
| hydrocortisone | | N | ■ | | Y | Y | | | | N | Y | Y | N | Y | Y | Y |
| hydroxyzine | Y | N | | ■ | | Y | Y | Y | | N | | | | | | N |
| levarterenol | | Y | Y | | ■ | | | | | N | Y | | Y | | Y | Y |
| lidocaine | Y | Y | Y | Y | | ■ | | | Y | Y | Y | Y | Y | | Y | Y |
| meperidine | Y | N | | Y | | | ■ | N | | N | | N | | | Y | |
| morphine | Y | N | | Y | | | N | ■ | | N | Y | N | | | Y | Y |
| nitroglycerin | | | | | | Y | | | ■ | | | | | | Y | |
| pentobarbital | N | | N | N | N | Y | N | N | | ■ | | N | N | N | Y | |
| potassium chloride | | Y | Y | | Y | Y | | Y | | | ■ | Y | Y | Y | Y | |
| sodium bicarbonate | N | Y | Y | | | Y | N | N | | N | Y | ■ | N | N | Y | N |
| tetracycline | | N | N | | Y | Y | | | | N | Y | N | ■ | | | Y |
| vancomycin | | N | Y | | | | | | | N | Y | N | | ■ | Y | Y |
| verapamil | | Y | Y | | Y | Y | Y | Y | Y | Y | Y | Y | | Y | ■ | Y |
| vitamin B & C complex | | Y | Y | N | Y | Y | | Y | | | | N | Y | Y | Y | ■ |

Reprinted from Malseed RT, Goldstein FJ, & Balkon N, *Pharmacology: Drug Therapy and Nursing Management* (4th ed), Philadelphia: JB Lippincott Co (1995). Used with permission.

# COMPATIBILITY OF DRUGS IN SYRINGE

| | atropine | butorphanol | chlorpromazine | cimetidine | dimenhydrinate | diphenhydramine | fentanyl | glycopyrrolate | heparin | hydroxyzine | meperidine |
|---|---|---|---|---|---|---|---|---|---|---|---|
| atropine | ■ | Y | Y | Y | M | M | M | Y | M | Y | Y |
| butorphanol | Y | ■ | Y | Y | N | Y | Y | | | Y | M |
| chlorpromazine | Y | Y | ■ | N | N | M | M | Y | N | M | M |
| cimetidine | Y | Y | N | ■ | | Y | Y | Y | Y | Y | Y |
| dimenhydrinate | M | N | N | | ■ | M | M | N | M | N | M |
| diphenhydramine | M | Y | | Y | M | ■ | | Y | | M | M |
| fentanyl | M | Y | M | | M | M | ■ | | M | Y | M |
| glycopyrrolate | Y | | Y | Y | N | Y | | ■ | | Y | Y |
| heparin | M | | N | | M | | M | | ■ | | N |
| hydroxyzine | Y | Y | M | Y | N | M | Y | Y | | ■ | M |
| meperidine | Y | M | M | Y | M | M | M | Y | N | M | ■ |
| metoclopramide | M | | M | | M | Y | M | | M | M | M |
| midazolam | Y | Y | Y | Y | N | Y | Y | Y | | Y | Y |
| morphine | M | Y | M | Y | M | M | M | Y | N | Y | N |
| nalbuphine | Y | | | Y | | | | | | Y | |
| pentazocine | M | Y | M | Y | M | M | M | N | N | Y | M |
| pentobarbital | M | N | N | N | N | N | N | N | | N | N |
| prochlorperazine | M | Y | Y | Y | N | M | M | Y | | M | M |
| promethazine | M | Y | M | Y | N | M | M | Y | N | M | Y |
| ranitidine | Y | | Y | | Y | Y | Y | Y | | N | Y |
| secobarbital | | | | N | | | | N | | | |
| thiopental | | | N | | N | N | | N | | | N |

**KEY**
**Y** = Compatible in a syringe
M = Moderately compatible, inject immediately after combining
**N** = Incompatible, do not mix in syringe
Blank = Information about compatibility is not currently available

## COMPATIBILITY OF DRUGS IN SYRINGE *(Continued)*

| | metoclopramide | midazolam | morphine | nalbuphine | pentazocine | pentobarbital | prochlorperazine | promethazine | ranitidine | secobarbital | thiopental |
|---|---|---|---|---|---|---|---|---|---|---|---|
| atropine | M | Y | M | Y | M | M | M | M | Y | | |
| butorphanol | | Y | Y | | Y | N | Y | Y | | | |
| chlorpromazine | M | Y | M | | M | N | Y | M | Y | | N |
| cimetidine | | Y | Y | Y | Y | N | Y | Y | | N | |
| dimenhydrinate | M | N | M | | M | N | N | N | Y | | N |
| diphenhydramine | Y | Y | M | | M | N | M | M | Y | | N |
| fentanyl | M | Y | M | | M | N | M | M | Y | | |
| glycopyrrolate | | Y | Y | | N | N | Y | Y | Y | N | N |
| heparin | M | | N | | N | | | N | | | |
| hydroxyzine | M | Y | Y | Y | Y | N | M | M | N | | |
| meperidine | M | Y | N | | M | N | M | Y | Y | | N |
| metoclopramide | ■ | Y | M | | M | | M | M | Y | | |
| midazolam | Y | ■ | Y | Y | | N | N | Y | N | | |
| morphine | M | Y | ■ | | M | N | M | M | Y | | N |
| nalbuphine | | Y | | ■ | | N | Y | Y | Y | | |
| pentazocine | M | | M | | ■ | N | M | Y | Y | | |
| pentobarbital | N | N | N | N | N | ■ | N | N | | | Y |
| prochlorperazine | M | N | M | Y | M | N | ■ | M | Y | | N |
| promethazine | M | Y | M | Y | Y | N | M | ■ | Y | | N |
| ranitidine | Y | N | Y | Y | Y | | Y | Y | ■ | | |
| secobarbital | | | | | | | | | | ■ | |
| thiopental | | | N | | | Y | N | N | | | ■ |

# EXTRAVASATION MANAGEMENT OF CHEMOTHERAPEUTIC AGENTS

## Risk Factors for Extravasation

- Vascular disease
- Elderly patients
- Vascular obstruction
- Vascular ischemia
- Prior radiation
- Small vessel diameter
- Venous spasms
- Traumatic catheter or needle insertion
- Decreased lymphatic drainage in mastectomy patients

## Purpose

To minimize harm caused to the patient by the extravasation of vesicant chemotherapeutic agents through prompt detection and treatment.

## Procedure

1. Stop administration of the chemotherapeutic agent.
2. Leave the needle in place.
3. Aspirate any residual drug and blood in the I.V. tubing, needle, and suspected extravasation site.
4. For all drugs except mechlorethamine (nitrogen mustard), remove the needle.
5. Apply cold pack if the extravasated drug is amsacrine, doxorubicin, daunorubicin, or mechlorethamine. Apply a hot pack if the extravasated drug is etoposide, teniposide, navelbine, vinblastine, vincristine, or vindesine. Refer to individual drug in Alphabetical Listing of Drugs for appropriate management.
6. Notify the physician who ordered the chemotherapy of the suspected extravasation. Institute the attached recommended interventions unless countermanded by the physician.
7. Document the date, time, needle size and type, insertion site, drug sequence, drug administration technique, approximate amount of drug extravasated, management, patient complaints, appearance of site, physician notification, and follow-up measures.
8. The extravasation site should be evaluated by the physician as soon as possible after the extravasation and periodically thereafter as indicated by symptoms.
9. For inpatients, assess the site every day for pain, erythema, induration, or skin breakdown. For outpatients, contact the patient daily for 3 days for assessment of the site, and weekly thereafter until the problem is resolved.
10. The plastic surgery service should be consulted by the physician if pain and/or tissue breakdown occur.

## Amsacrine/Daunorubicin/Doxorubicin/Epirubacin/Idarubicin

1. Apply cold pack immediately for 1 hour; repeat qid for 3-5 days.[1,2]
2. Dimethyl sulfoxide (DMSO) 50% to 99% (w/v) solution: Apply 1.5 mL to site every 6 hours for 14 days; allow to air dry, do not cover.[3]
3. Injection of sodium bicarbonate is contraindicated.[4]
4. Injection of hydrocortisone is of doubtful benefit.[4,5]

# EXTRAVASATION MANAGEMENT OF CHEMOTHERAPEUTIC AGENTS *(Continued)*

## Mechlorethamine (nitrogen mustard)

1. Mix 4 mL of 10% sodium thiosulfate with 6 mL of sterile water for injection.
2. Inject 4 mL of this solution into the existing I.V. line.
3. Remove the needle.
4. Inject 2-3 mL of the solution subcutaneously clockwise into the infiltrated area using a 25-gauge needle. Change the needle with each new injection.
5. Apply ice immediately for 6-12 hours.

## Mitomycin

1. Data is not currently available regarding potential antidotes and the application of heat or cold.
2. The site should be observed closely. These injuries frequently cause necrosis. A plastic surgery consult may be required.
3. Dimethyl sulfoxide (DMSO) 50% to 99% (w/v) solution: Apply 1.5 mL to site every 6 hours for 14 days; allow to air dry, do not cover.[3]

## Etoposide/Teniposide/Vinblastine/Vincristine/Vindesine/Vinorelbine[6]

1. Inject 3-5 mL of hyaluronidase (150 units/mL) subcutaneously clockwise into the infiltrated area using a 25-gauge needle. Change the needle with each injection.
2. Apply heat immediately for 1 hour; repeat qid for 3-5 days.
3. Application of cold is contraindicated.
4. Injection of hydrocortisone is contraindicated.

## Footnotes


1. Dorr RT, Alberts DS, and Stone A, "Cold Protection and Heat Enhancement of Doxorubicin Skin Toxicity in the Mouse," *Cancer Treat Rep*, 1985, 69:431-7.
2. Larson D, "What Is the Appropriate Management of Tissue Extravasation by Antitumor Agents?" *Plastic & Reconstr Surg*, 1985, 75:397-402.
3. Oliver IW, Aisner J, Hament A, et al, "A Prospective Study of Topical Dimethyl Sulfoxide for Treating Anthracycline Extravasation," *J Clin Onc*, 1988, 6:1732-5.
4. Dorr RT, Alberts DS, and Chen HS, "Limited Role of Corticosteroids in Ameliorating Experimental Doxorubicin Skin Toxicity in the Mouse," *Canc Chemother and Pharmacol*, 1980, 5:17-20.
5. Coleman JJ, Walker AP, and Didolkar MS, "Treatment of Adriamycin Induced Skin Ulcers: A Prospective Controlled Study," *J Surg Oncol*, 1983, 22:129-35.
6. Dorr RT and Alberts DS, "Vinca Alkaloid Skin Toxicity Antidote and Drug Disposition Studies in the Mouse," *JNCI*, 1985, 74:113-20.

# EXTRAVASATION TREATMENT OF OTHER DRUGS

| Medication Extravasated | Cold/ WarmPack | Antidote |
|---|---|---|
| **Vasopressors** | | |
| Dobutamine<br>Dopamine<br>Epinephrine<br>Norepinephrine<br>Phenylephrine | None | Phentolamine (Regitine®)<br>Mix 5 mg with 9 mL of NS<br>Inject a small amount of this dilution into extravasated area. Blanching should reverse immediately. Monitor site. If blanching should recur, additional injections of phentolamine may be needed. |
| **I.V. Fluids and Other Medications** | | |
| Aminophylline<br>Calcium<br>Dextrose, 10%<br>Electrolyte solutions<br>Esmolol<br>Magnesium sulfate<br>Metoprolol<br>Nafcillin<br>Parenteral nutrition preparations<br>Phenytoin<br>Potassium<br>Radiocontrast media<br>Sodium solutions | Cold | Hyaluronidase (Wydase®)<br>1. Add 1 mL NS to 150-unit vial to make 150 units/mL<br>2. Mix 0.1 mL of above with 0.9 mL NS in 1 mL syringe to make final concentration = 15 units/mL<br>3. Inject 5 injections of 0.2 mL each with a 25-gauge needle into area of extravasation |

# FOOD/ANTIBIOTIC INTERACTIONS

Many antibiotics need to be taken on an empty stomach (1 hour before or 2 hours after a meal). Following is a list of antibiotics and their relationship to food.

| Drug | Effect | Comment |
|---|---|---|
| Amoxicillin | Peak concentrations may be delayed with food | OK with food |
| Ampicillin | ↓ absorption with food | On empty stomach |
| Augmentin | Not affected by food | OK with food |
| Bacampicillin | Not affected by food | OK with food |
| Cephalosporins | Delayed absorption with food | OK with food |
| Cefadroxil | Not affected by food | OK with food |
| Cefuroxime | Bioavailability ↑ with food | OK with food |
| Ciprofloxacin | Not affected by food (nondairy) | OK with food (nondairy) |
| Clindamycin | Peak concentrations may be delayed with food | OK with food |
| Cloxacillin | ↓ absorption with food | On empty stomach |
| Colistin | Not affected by food | OK with food |
| Cyclacillin | Not affected by food | OK with food |
| Cycloserine | Not affected by food | OK with food |
| Dicloxacillin | ↓ absorption with food | On empty stomach |
| Erythromycin | ↓ absorption with food | Ethylsuccinate, estolate, and enteric coated are not affected by food |
| Ethambutol | Not affected by food | May cause gastric irritation; take with food |
| Griseofulvin | Enhanced absorption with high fat meals | For enhanced absorption; take with high fat meal |
| Isoniazid | ↓ absorption with food | On empty stomach |
| Lincomycin | ↓ absorption with food | On empty stomach |
| Metronidazole | Delayed absorption with food | May cause gastric irritation; take with food |
| Nafcillin | ↓ absorption with food | On empty stomach |
| Nitrofurantoin | Food ↑ bioavailability | Take with food; food also decreases gastric irritation |
| Norfloxacin | ↓ absorption with food | On empty stomach |
| Novobiocin | Peak concentrations may be delayed with food | OK with food |
| Oxacillin | ↓ absorption with food | On empty stomach |
| Penicillin G | ↓ absorption with food | On empty stomach |
| Penicillin VK | Peak concentration may be delayed with food | OK with food |
| Rifampin | Delayed absorption with food | On empty stomach |
| Sulfonamides | Delayed absorption with food | On empty stomach |
| Tetracyclines | Food and dairy products reduce serum concentrations | On empty stomach; doxycycline and minocycline may be taken with food |
| Trimethoprim | Not affected by food | OK with food |
| Troleandomycin | Not affected by food | OK with food |
| Vancomycin | Not affected by food | OK with food |

# FOOD/WATER DRUG ADMINISTRATION RECOMMENDATIONS

| Generic/Brand Name | Empty Stomach* | With Food | With Full Glass of Water |
|---|---|---|---|
| Acarbose (Precose) | | X (with first bite of meal) | |
| Acetazolamide (Diamox) | | X | |
| Alendronate (Fosamax) | X | | X |
| Allopurinol (Zyloprim) | | X | |
| Amiodarone (Cordarone) | | X | |
| Amoxicillin | | | |
| Ampicillin | X | | |
| Astemizole (Hismanal) | X | | |
| Augmentin | | | |
| Azathioprine (Imuran) | | X | |
| Azithromycin (Zithromax) | X | | |
| Bacampicillin (Spectrobid Suspension) | X | | |
| Bacampicillin (Spectrobid Tablet) | | | |
| Baclofen (Lioresal) | X | | |
| Benazepril (Lotensin) | X | | |
| Bromocriptine (Parlodel) | | X | |
| Buspirone (BuSpar) | | | |
| Captopril (Capoten) | X | | |
| Carbamazepine (Tegretol) | | X | |
| Carbenicillin (Geocillin) | X | | |
| Cefaclor (Ceclor) | X | | |
| Cefadroxil (Duricef, Ultracef) | | | |
| Cefixime (Suprax) | | | |
| Cefpodoxime (Vantin) | | X | |
| Cefprozil (Cefzil) | | | |
| Cefuroxime (Ceftin) | | X | |
| Cephalexin (Keflex) | | | |
| Cephradine (Anspor, Velosef) | | | |
| Chloramphenicol | X | | |
| Cholestyramine (Questran) | X | | |
| Cimetidine (Tagamet) | | X | |
| Cinoxacin (Cinobac) | | | |
| Ciprofloxacin (Cipro) | | | X |
| Cisapride (Propulsid) | X (15 minutes before meals) | | |
| Clarithromycin (Biaxin) | | | |
| Clindamycin HCl (Cleocin) | | X | X |
| Cloxacillin (Cloxapen, Tegopen) | X | X | |
| Codeine | | | |
| Corticosteroids (prednisone and others) | | X | |
| Co-trimoxazole (Bactrim, Septra) | X | | X |
| Demeclocycline (Declomycin) | X | | |
| Dicloxacillin (Dynapen) | X | | |
| Dicyclomine (Bentyl) | X | | |
| Diltiazem (Cardizem, Dilacor) | | | X |
| Dirithromycin (Dynabac) | | | |
| Docusate (Colace) | | | X |
| Doxycycline coated pellets | | | |
| Doxycycline (Vibramycin) | | | |
| Enalapril (Vasotec) | | | |
| Enoxacin (Penetrex) | X | | |
| Erythromycin (E-Mycin, Ilosone) | | | |
| Erythromycin (Eryc, PCE) | X | | |
| Erythromycin ethyl succinate (EES) | | | |
| Erythromycin (nonenteric coated) | X | | |
| Erythromycin estolate | | | |
| Erythromycin stearate | X | | |
| Erythromycin/sulfisoxazole (Pediazole) | | | |
| Ethambutol | | X | |

# FOOD/WATER DRUG ADMINISTRATION RECOMMENDATIONS *(Continued)*

| Generic/Brand Name | Empty Stomach* | With Food | With Full Glass of Water |
|---|---|---|---|
| Ethosuximide (Zarontin) | | X | |
| Etidronate (Didronel) | X | | |
| Felodipine | X | | |
| Fiorinal with codeine | | X | |
| Fluconazole (Diflucan) | | | |
| Flucytosine (Ancobon) | | X | |
| Fluvoxamine (Luvox) | | X | |
| Fosinopril (Monopril) | | X | |
| Gemfibrozil (Lopid) | X (30 minutes before meals) | | |
| Glipizide (Glucotrol) | X (before meals) | | |
| Glipizide (Glucotrol XL) | | X | |
| Glyburide (DiaBeta, Micronase) | | X | |
| Griseofulvin | | X | |
| Hydralazine (Apresoline) | | X | |
| Hydrochlorothiazide | | | |
| Hypoglycemics (oral) | standard-release glipizide | X (except standard glipizide) | |
| Iron | X (take with food if GI distress) | | |
| Isoniazid (INE) | X | | |
| Isosorbide dinitrate (Isordil) | X | | |
| Isosorbide mononitrate (Imdur) | X | | |
| Itraconazole (Sporanox) | | X | |
| Ketoconazole (Nizoral) | | X | |
| Lansoprazole (Prevacid) | X | | |
| Levodopa/carbidopa (Sinemet, Sinemet CR) | | X | |
| Lincomycin (Lincocin) | X | | X |
| Lithium | | X | |
| Lomefloxacin (Maxaquin) | | | X |
| Loracarbef (Lorabid) | X | | |
| Loratadine (Claritin) | X | | |
| Loratadine (Claritin-D 24-Hour) | X | | X |
| Lovastatin (Mevacor) | | X | |
| Melphalan (Alkeran) | X | | |
| Medroxyprogesterone (Cycrin, Provera) | | X | |
| Metformin (Glucophage) | | X | |
| Methacycline (Rondomycin) | | | |
| Methenamine mandelate and hippurate | | X | X |
| Methylphenidate (Ritalin) | X (30 minutes before meals) | | |
| Metoclopramide (Reglan) | X (15 minutes before meals) | | |
| Metoprolol (Lopressor) | X (take consistently with or without food) | | |
| Metronidazole (Flagyl) | | X | |
| Mexilitene (Mexitil) | | X | |
| Minocycline (Minocin) | | | |
| Misoprostil (Cytotec) | | X | |
| Mycelex troche 10 mg | | | |
| Nafcillin (Unipen) | X | | |
| Nalidixic acid (NegGram) | X | | |
| Nefazodone (Serzone) | X | | |
| Neomycin sulfate | | X | |
| Niacin | | X | |
| Nifedipine (Adalat CC) | X | | |
| Nifedipine immediate release | | X | |

| Generic/Brand Name | Empty Stomach* | With Food | With Full Glass of Water |
|---|---|---|---|
| Nifedipine sustained release (except Adalat CC) | X | | |
| Nitrofurantoin (Macrodantin, Macrobid) | | X | |
| Nitroglycerin (Nitro-Bid) | X | | |
| Nonsteroidal anti-inflammatory agents (ibuprofen and others) | | X | |
| Norfloxacin (Noroxin) | X | | X |
| Ofloxacin (Floxin) | X | | X |
| Omeprazole (Prilosec) | X | | |
| Oxacillin | X | | |
| Penicillin G | X | | |
| Penicillin V potassium (VK) | X | | |
| Pentoxifylline (Trental) | | X | |
| Pergolide (Permax) | | X | |
| Potassium supplements (oral) | | X | X |
| Pravastatin (Pravachol) | | | |
| Prednisone (Deltasone) | | X | |
| Probenecid (Benemid) | | X | X |
| Probucol (Lorelco) | | X | |
| Propafenone (Rythmol) | X | | |
| Propoxyphene + APAP (Darvocet) | | X | |
| Propranolol (Inderal) | X (take consistently with or without food) | | |
| Psyllium (Metamucil, Unifiber, others) | | X (or after meal) with full glass of water | |
| Rifampin (Rifadin, Rimactane) | X | | |
| Selegiline (Eldepryl) | | X | |
| Simvastatin (Zocor) | | | |
| Sucralfate (Carafate) | X | | |
| Sulfamethoxazole (Gantanol) | X | | X |
| Sulfasalazine (Azulfidine) | | X | X |
| Sulfisoxazole (Gantrisin) | X | | X |
| Sulfonamides | X | | X |
| Tacrine (Cognex) | X | | |
| Terramycin | X | | |
| Tetracycline | X | | X |
| Theophylline (TheoDur, others) | | | X |
| Thiazides | | | |
| Ticlopidine (Ticlid) | | X | |
| Trazodone (Desyrel) | | X | |
| Triamterene (Dyrenium) | | X | |
| Trimethoprim (Proloprim) | | | |
| Troleandomycin (TAO) | X | | |
| Valproate (Depakene, Depakote) | | X | |
| Vancomycin (Vancocin) | | | |
| Verapamil (Calan, Isoptin, Verelan) | | X | |
| Vitamin C (Ascorbic Acid) | | | X |
| Warfarin (Coumadin) | X | | |
| Zidovudine (Retrovir) | X | | |
| Zolpidem (Ambien) | X | | |

*Take 1 hour before or 2 hours after food.

# PARENTERAL THERAPY RECOMMENDATIONS/GUIDELINES

## I.V. Medication Recommendations

| Medication | Strength/Solution | Ref Exp | Infusion Time | Filtered | Comments |
|---|---|---|---|---|---|
| ALL MEDICATIONS HAVE A 24-HOUR ROOM TEMPERATURE EXPIRATION UNLESS NOTED IN COMMENT SECTION. | | | | | |
| Acyclovir (Zovirax®) | 500 mg in 100 mL NS or $D_5W$<br>1000 mg in 250 mL NS or $D_5W$ | 24 h after nurse admix | 60 min | Yes | May precipitate upon refrigeration, but resolves at room temperature |
| Amikacin (Amikin®) | All strengths in 100 mL NS or $D_5W$ | 30 d | 60 min | Yes | Monitor serum levels |
| Aminophylline | Various strengths in NS or $D_5W$ | 48 h | 0.25 mg/min | Yes | May place in volumes ranging from 250-1000 mL |
| Amphotericin B (Fungizone®) | All strengths in 500 mL $D_5W$ | 7 d | 6 h Protect from light | No | Incompatible in NS (may use a 5 micron filter) |
| Ampicillin | 500 mg - 1 g in 50 mL NS<br>>1 g in 100 mL NS | 3 d | 15-30 min | Yes | Incompatible in $D_5W$ |
| Ampicillin/ sulbactam (Unasyn®) | All strengths in 100 mL NS only | 3 d | 30-60 min | Yes | Incompatible in $D_5W$ |
| Aztreonam (Azactam®) | 500 mg - 1 g in 50 mg NS or $D_5W$<br>1 g in 100 mg NS or $D_5W$ | 7 d | 30-60 min | Yes | |
| Cefamandole (Mandol®) | 500 mg - 1 g in 50 mL NS or $D_5W$<br>>1 g in 100 mL NS or $D_5W$ | 4 d | 30-60 min | Yes | |
| Cefazolin (Ancef®, Kefzol®) | 500 mg - 1 g in 50 mL NS or $D_5W$<br>>1 g in 100 mL NS or $D_5W$ | 7 d | 30-60 min | Yes | |
| Cefepime (Maxipime®) | 0-1 g in 50 mL NS or $D_5W$<br>>1 g in 100 mL NS or $D_5W$ | 7 d | 30-60 min | Yes | |
| Cefonicid (Monocid®) | 500 mg in 50 mL NS or $D_5W$<br>1 g in 100 mL NS or $D_5W$ | 3 d | 30-60 min | Yes | |
| Cefoperazone (Cefobid®) | 1 g in 50 mL NS or $D_5W$<br>>1 g in 100 mL NS or $D_5W$ | 5 d | 30-60 min | Yes | |
| Cefotaxime (Claforan®) | All strengths in 100 mL NS or $D_5W$ | 5 d | 30-60 min | Yes | |
| Cefotetan (Cefotan®) | 1 g in 50 mL NS or $D_5W$<br>>1 g in 100 mL NS or $D_5W$ | 4 d | 30 min | Yes | |
| Cefoxitin (Mefoxin®) | 1 g in 50 mL NS or $D_5W$<br>>1 g in 100 mL NS or $D_5W$ | 7 d | 30-60 min | Yes | |
| Ceftazidime (Fortaz®, Tazidime®) | 1 g in 50 mL NS or $D_5W$<br>>1 g in 100 mL NS or $D_5W$ | 7 d | 30-60 min | Yes | |
| Ceftizoxime (Cefizox®) | 1 g in 50 mL NS or $D_5W$<br>>1 g in 100 mL NS or $D_5W$ | 7 d | 30-60 min | Yes | |
| Ceftriaxone (Rocephin®) | 1 g in 50 mL NS or $D_5W$<br>>1 g in 100 mL NS or $D_5W$ | 10 d | 30-60 min | Yes | |
| Cefuroxime (Zinacef®) | 750 mg - 1.5 g in 100 mL NS or $D_5W$ | 7 d | 30-60 min | Yes | I.V. equivalent to Ceftin® |

## I.V. Medication Recommendations *(continued)*

| Medication | Strength/Solution | Ref Exp | Infusion Time | Filtered | Comments |
|---|---|---|---|---|---|
| Cimetidine (Tagamet®) | 300 mg in 50 mL NS or $D_5W$ >300 mg in 100 mL NS or $D_5W$ | 7 d | 15-30 min | Yes | Incompatible with aminophylline and barbiturates |
| Ciprofloxacin (Cipro™) | 200 mg in 100 mL NS or $D_5W$ 400 mg in 250 mL NS or $D_5W$ | 14 d | 60 min | Yes | Do not exceed 2 mg/mL concentration |
| Clindamycin (Cleocin®) | 300-900 mg in 100 mL NS or $D_5W$ | 30 d | 30 mg/min | Yes | |
| Dobutamine (Dobutrex®) | 250 mg in 250 mL NS or $D_5W$ 500 mg in 500 mL NS or $D_5W$ | 7 d | 2.5-10 mcg/kg/min | Yes | May exhibit a pink color with no loss in potency |
| Doxycycline (Vibramycin®) | 50-100 mg in 250 mL NS or $D_5W$ | 3 d | 60 min | Yes | Protect from light; causes phlebitis |
| Erythromycin | 500 mg in 250 mL NS 1 g in 500 mL NS | 24 h after nurse admix | 60 min | Yes | Incompatible in $D_5W$ |
| Famotidine (Pepcid®) | 20-40 mg in 50 mL NS or $D_5W$ | 14 d | 15-30 min | Yes | |
| Fluconazole (Diflucan®) | 200 mg in 100 mL Viaflex® bag 400 mg in 200 mL Viaflex® bag | Mfg expired | 60 min 120 min | Yes | Maximum rate is 200 mg/h |
| Foscarnet (Foscavir®) | 24 mg/mL for central line mixed in 0-500 mL Viaflex® bag | 14 d | Must use I.V. pump at rate ordered | Yes | Must dilute with $D_5W$ or NS to 12 mg/mL for peripheral adm |
| Ganciclovir (Cytovene®) | 0-500 mg in 100 mL NS or $D_5W$ | 7 d | 60 min | Yes | Use procedures for cytotoxic agents |
| Gentamicin (Garamycin®) | All strengths in 100 mL NS or $D_5W$ | 30 d | 60 min | Yes | Monitor serum levels |
| Heparin | All strengths in NS or $D_5W$ | 7 d | As directed by physician | Yes | Can be compounded in volumes from 250-1000 mL |
| Imipenem/ cilastatin (Primaxin®) | 500 mg in 100 mL NS 1 g in 250 mL NS | 48 h | 30-60 min 60 min | No | Incompatible in $D_5W$ |
| Iron dextran (InFed™) | All strengths in 500 mL NS | 72 h | 1-6 h | No | Must give 0.5 mL test dose; incompatible in $D_5W$ |
| Levofloxacin (Levaquin®) | 0-500 mg in 100 ml NaCl or $D_5W$ | 14 d | Not < 60 min | Yes | Stable 72 hours at 77° in compatible I.V. solution. Final dilution 5mg/ml |
| Methicillin (Staphcillin®) | 500 mg - 1 g in 100 mL NS or $D_5W$ | 4 d | 30-60 min | Yes | Only stable at room temperature for 8 hours |
| Methyldopa (Aldomet®) | 250-500 mg in 100 mL $D_5W$ | 72 h | 30-60 min | Yes | 24-hour stability in NS |
| Metoclopramide (Reglan®) | >10 mg in 50 mL NS or $D_5W$ | 48 h | 15-30 min Protect from light | Yes | Only make IVPB for doses that exceed 10 mg |
| Metronidazole (Flagyl®) | 500 mg in 100 mL NS RTU | Mfg | 60 min | Yes | Incompatible in $D_5W$; do not refrigerate |
| Mezlocillin (Mezlin®) | 1-4 g in 100 mL NS or $D_5W$ | 7 d | 30-60 min | Yes | |
| Nafcillin (Nafcil™, Unipen®) | ≤2 g in 50 mL NS or $D_5W$ >2 g in 100 mL NS or $D_5W$ | 7 d | 15-30 min | Yes | |
| Ofloxacin (Floxin®) | 200 mg in 50 mL $D_5W$ RTU 400 mg in 100 mL $D_5W$ RTU | Mfg | 60 mg | Yes | May use 10 or 20 mL vials to admix with 14-day exp |

# PARENTERAL THERAPY RECOMMENDATIONS/GUIDELINES *(Continued)*

## I.V. Medication Recommendations *(continued)*

| Medication | Strength/Solution | Ref Exp | Infusion Time | Filtered | Comments |
|---|---|---|---|---|---|
| Penicillin G | 2-4 million units in 100 mL $D_5W$ | 7 d | 15-30 min | Yes | May use NS, but PCN is more stable in nonalkaline pH |
| Piperacillin (Pipracil®) | 1-4 g in 100 mL NS or $D_5W$ | 7 d | 30-60 min | Yes | |
| Piperacillin/ tazobactam (Zosyn™) | 2.25-4.5 g in 100 mL NS or $D_5W$ | 7 d | 30-60 min | Yes | |
| Potassium chloride | 0-40 mEq/L in NS or $D_5W$ and various solutions | 14 d | At rate ordered by physician | Yes | **Do not give undiluted KCl by direct I.V. injection** |
| Ranitidine (Zantac®) | 50 mg in 50 mL NS or $D_5W$ | 14 d | 30 min | Yes | |
| Ticarcillin (Ticar®) | 1-3 g in 50 mL NS or $D_5W$ | 72 h | 30-60 min | Yes | |
| Ticarcillin/ clavulanate (Timentin®) | 3.1 g in 100 mL NS | 7 d | 30-60 min | Yes | 72-hour stability in $D_5W$ |
| Tobramycin (Nebcin®) | All strengths in 100 mL NS or $D_5W$ | 30 d | 60 min | Yes | Monitor serum levels |
| Trimethoprim/ sulfamethoxazole (Bactrim™) | 80/400 mg SS or 160/ 800 mg DS in 250 mL $D_5W$ | 6 h after admix | 60-90 min | Yes | Incompatible in NS<br>Protect from light |
| Vancomycin (Vancocin®, Vancoled®) | 0-500 mg in 100 mL NS or $D_5W$<br>500 mg - 1.5 g in 250 mL NS or $D_5W$<br>>1.5 mg in 500 mL NS or $D_5W$ | 7 d | 90 min<br>120 min | Yes | Monitor serum levels; red-neck or red-man syndrome if administration too rapid |

NS = normal saline.

*Ref Exp = Refrigerator expiration.

## I.V. Push Recommended Guidelines

| Medication | Rate of Administration | Considerations |
|---|---|---|
| Acetazolamide (Diamox®) | 250-500 mg/min | Pain on injection |
| Aminophylline | 25 mg/min | Continuous I.V. infusion preferred |
| Atropine sulfate | 0.5 mg/min | |
| Benztropine (Cogentin®) | No restrictions | |
| Bretylium (Bretylol®) | 5 mg/kg over 1-2 min | |
| Bumetanide (Bumex®) | Given slowly, over 1-2 min | |
| Butorphanol (Stadol®) | 1 mg over 1 min | |
| Calcium gluconate | 1.5-2 mL/min | |
| Chlordiazepoxide (Librium®) | 50-100 mg given slowly over 1 min | Dilute with sterile $H_2O$ for injection |
| Chlorpromazine (Thorazine®) | 1 mg/mL given at 1 mg/min | |
| Codeine phosphate | 5 mg/min over 3-5 min | Causes respiratory depression |
| Dexamethasone (Decadron®) | Diluted with 10 mL NS over 3-5 min | Burning and tingling after administration |
| Dextrose 50% | 20-50 mL slowly at 3 mL/min | Administer into large peripheral or CVC |
| Diazepam (Valium®) | 5 mg/mL given at 5 mg/min | **Do not dilute!!!** |
| Diazoxide (Hyperstat®) | 15 mg/mL; must be infused within 30 sec | |
| Digoxin (Lanoxin®) | 500 mcg/mL given over 5 min | Pain on injection |
| Diltiazem (Cardizem®) | Over 2 min | Causes hypotension |
| Diphenhydramine (Benadryl®) | 10 mg/min | |
| Droperidol (Inapsine®) | Slowly over 5-10 min | |
| Epinephrine (Adrenalin®) | 0.1 mg/min | Diluted 1:10,000=0.1 mg/mL |
| Famotidine (Pepcid®) | 10 mg/min | Dilute 20 mg to 5-10 mL with NS |
| Fosphenytoin (Cerebyx®) | 100-150 mg PE/min not to exceed 150 mg PE/min | **Flush with NS before and after administration; EKG monitoring** |
| Furosemide (Lasix®) | 80 mg over 1-2 min | High dose not >4 mg/min |
| Glucagon | 1 mg/mL at rate of 1 mg/min | Admix with diluent supplied |
| Haloperidol (Haldol®) | 5 mg over 1 min | |
| Heparin sodium | 1000-10,000 units/over 1 min maximum | |
| Hydrocortisone (Solu-Cortef®) | 50 mg/min (30 sec up to 10 min) | |
| Hydromorphone (Dilaudid®) | Slowly over 3-5 min | Causes respiratory depression |
| Insulin regular | 5-30 units over 1 min | Only use regular insulin |
| Iron dextran (InFed™) | Give undiluted at 1 mL/min | Give test dose of 0.5 mL for first administration |
| Ketorolac (Toradol®) | 15 mg/mL or 30 mg/mL over 1 min | |
| Labetalol (Normodyne®) | 20 mg over 2 min | |
| Levothyroxine (Synthroid®) | Over 3-5 min or 50 mcg/min | |
| Lorazepam (Ativan®) | Rate should not exceed 2 mg/min | May be given diluted or undiluted |
| Meperidine (Demerol®) | 10 mg/mL given slowly over 3-5 min | Causes respiratory depression |
| Methylprednisolone | Over 1 to several min | For higher doses give by IVPB |

# PARENTERAL THERAPY RECOMMENDATIONS/GUIDELINES *(Continued)*

## I.V. Push Recommended Guidelines *(continued)*

| Medication | Rate of Administration | Considerations |
|---|---|---|
| Metoclopramide (Reglan®) | 10 mg/2 mL over 1-2 min | >10 mg give IVPB |
| **Note:** When using a glass ampul, withdraw with a filter needle then change to a regular needle for administration. | | |
| Metoprolol (Lopressor®) | Given over 1 min | |
| Morphine sulfate | Given slowly over 4-5 min | Dilute in 4-5 mL NS or sterile $H_2O$ |
| Nalbuphine (Nubain®) | 10 mg over 2-5 min | |
| Naloxone (Narcan®) | 0.4-2 mg over 15 seconds | May repeat dose every 3-6 hours |
| Ondansetron (Zofran®) | 4 mg given over 2-5 min | Doses >4 mg give IVPB |
| Phenobarbital | 60 mg/min | |
| Procainamide (Pronestyl®) | 20 mg/min | |
| Prochlorperazine (Compazine®) | 1 mg/mL given at 5 mg/min | |
| Promethazine (Phenergan®) | 25 mg/mL given at 25 mg/min | Concentration not >25 mg/mL |
| Propranolol (Inderal®) | 1 mg/min | |
| Protamine sulfate | 10 mg/mL very slowly over 1-3 min | Use for heparin overdose |
| Ranitidine (Zantac®) | Give over 5 min | Dilute to 20 mL with NS |
| Sodium bicarbonate | Rapidly over 1-2 min | |
| Torsemide (Demadex®) | Administer over 2 min | Oral dose and I.V. dose therapeutically equivalent |
| Verapamil (Isoptin®, Calan®) | 2.5-10 mg over 3 min | |

**Note:** When using a glass ampul, withdraw with a filter needle then change to a regular needle for administration.

# PEAK AND TROUGH GUIDELINES

| Drug | When to Sample | Therapeutic Levels* | Usual Half-Life | Steady State (Ideal Sampling Time) | Potentially Toxic Levels* |
|---|---|---|---|---|---|
| **Antibiotics** | | | | | |
| Gentamicin<br>Tobramycin | 30 min after 30 min infusion<br>Trough: <0.5 h before next dose | Peak: 4-10 mcg/mL<br>Trough: <2.0 mcg/mL | 2 h | 15 h | Peak: >12 mcg/mL<br>Trough: >2 mcg/mL |
| Amikacin | | Peak: 20-35 mcg/mL<br>Trough: <8 mcg/mL | 2 h | 15 h | Peak: >35 mcg/mL<br>Trough: >8 mcg/mL |
| Vancomycin | Peak: 1 h after 1 h infusion<br>Trough: <0.5 h before next dose | Peak: 30-40 mcg/mL<br>Trough: 5-10 mcg/mL | 6-8 h | 24 h | Peak: >80 mcg/mL<br>Trough: >13 mcg/mL |
| **Anticonvulsants** | | | | | |
| Carbamazepine | Trough: Just before next oral dose<br>In combination with other anticonvulsants | 4-12 mcg/mL<br>4-8 mcg/mL | 15-20 h | 7-12 d | >12 mcg/mL |
| Ethosuximide | Trough: Just before next oral dose | 40-100 mcg/mL | 30-60 h | 10-13 d | >100 mcg/mL |
| Phenobarbital | Trough: Just before next dose | 15-40 mcg/mL | 40-120 h | 20 d | >40 mcg/mL |
| Phenytoin<br>Free phenytoin | Trough: Just before next dose<br>Draw at same time as total level | 10-20 mcg/mL<br>1-2 mcg/mL | Concentration dependent | 5-14 d | >20 mcg/mL |
| Primidone | Trough: Just before next dose<br>(**Note:** Primidone is metabolized to phenobarb, order levels separately) | 5-12 mcg/mL | 10-12 h | 5 d | >12 mcg/mL |
| Valproic acid | Trough: Just before next dose | 50-100 mcg/mL | 5-20 h | 4 d | >150 mcg/mL |
| **Bronchodilators** | | | | | |
| Aminophylline (I.V.) | 18-24 h after starting or changing a maintenance dose given as a constant infusion | 10-20 mcg/mL | Nonsmoking adult: 8 h<br>Children and smoking adults: 4 h | 2 d | >20 mcg/mL |
| Theophylline (P.O.) | Peak levels: Not recommended<br>Trough level: Just before next dose | 10-20 mcg/mL | | 2 d | |

## PEAK AND TROUGH GUIDELINES *(Continued)*

*(continued)*

| Drug | When to Sample | Therapeutic Levels* | Usual Half-Life | Steady State (Ideal Sampling Time) | Potentially Toxic Levels* |
|---|---|---|---|---|---|
| **Cardiovascular Agents** | | | | | |
| Digoxin | Trough: Just before next dose (levels drawn earlier than 6 h after a dose will be artificially elevated) | 0.5-2 ng/mL | 36 h | 5 d | >2 ng/mL |
| Lidocaine | Steady-state levels are usually achieved after 6-12 h | 1.2-5.0 mcg/mL | 1.5 h | 5-10 h | >6 mcg/mL |
| Procainamide | Trough: Just before next oral dose<br>I.V.: 6-12 h after infusion started<br>Combined procainamide plus NAPA | 4-10 mcg/mL<br>NAPA: 6-10 h<br>5-30 mcg/mL | Procain: 2.7-5 h<br>>30 (NAPA + procain) | 20 h | >10 mcg/mL |
| Quinidine | Trough: Just before next oral dose | 2-5 mcg/mL | 6 h | 24 h | >10 mcg/mL |
| Warfarin | Same time of day each draw | See Warfarin monograph | 42 h | 5-7 d | See Warfarin monograph |
| **Other Agents** | | | | | |
| Amitriptyline plus nortriptyline | Trough: Just before next dose | 120-250 ng/mL | | 4-80 d | |
| Cyclosporine | Trough: Just before next dose | Months post-transplant:<br>Plasma: 50-150 ng/mL<br>Whole blood: 150-450 ng/mL | | Variable | |
| Desipramine | Trough: Just before next dose | 50-300 ng/mL | 12-54 h | 3-11 d | |
| Imipramine plus desipramine | Trough: Just before next dose | 150-300 ng/mL | 9-24 h | 2-5 d | |
| Lithium | Trough: Just before next dose | 0.6-1.2 mEq/mL (acute) | 18-20 h | 2-7 d | >3 mEq/mL |
| Nortriptyline | Trough: Just before next dose | 50-140 ng/mL | | 4-19 d | |

*Due to methodology differences, reference ranges may vary from laboratory to laboratory; check with the laboratory service used for their appropriate levels.

# TABLETS THAT CANNOT BE CRUSHED OR ALTERED

There are a variety of reasons for crushing tablets or capsule contents prior to administering to the patient. Patients may have nasogastric tubes which do not permit the administration of tablets or capsules; an oral solution for a particular medication may not be available from the manufacturer or readily prepared by pharmacy; patients may have difficulty swallowing capsules or tablets; or mixing of powdered medication with food or drink may make the drug more palatable.

Generally, medications which should not be crushed fall into one of the following categories.

- **Extended-Release Products.** The formulation of some tablets is specialized as to allow the medication within it to be slowly released into the body. This is sometimes accomplished by centering the drug within the core of the tablet, with a subsequent shedding of multiple layers around the core. Wax melts in the GI tract. Slow-K® is an example of this. Capsules may contain beads which have multiple layers which are slowly dissolved with time.
- **Medications Which Are Irritating to the Stomach.** Tablets which are irritating to the stomach may be enteric-coated which delays release of the drug until the time when it reaches the small intestine. Enteric-coated aspirin is an example of this.
- **Foul-Tasting Medication.** Some drugs are quite unpleasant to taste so the manufacturer coats the tablet in a sugar coating to increase its palatability. By crushing the tablet, this sugar coating is lost and the patient tastes the unpleasant tasting medication.
- **Sublingual Medication.** Medication intended for use under the tongue should not be crushed. While it appears to be obvious, it is not always easy to determine if a medication is to be used sublingually. Sublingual medications should indicate on the package that they are intended for sublingual use.
- **Effervescent Tablets.** These are tablets which, when dropped into a liquid, quickly dissolve to yield a solution. Many effervescent tablets, when crushed, lose their ability to quickly dissolve.

## Recommendations

1. It is not advisable to crush certain medications.
2. Consult individual monographs prior to crushing capsule or tablet.
3. If crushing a tablet or capsule is contraindicated, consult with your pharmacist to determine whether an oral solution exists or can be compounded.

| Drug Product | Dosage Forms | Reasons/Comments |
|---|---|---|
| Accutane® | Capsule | Mucous membrane irritant |
| Actifed 12® Hour | Capsule | Slow release† |
| Acutrim® | Tablet | Slow release |
| Adalat® CC | Tablet | Slow release |
| Aerolate® SR, JR, III | Capsule | Slow release*† |
| Allerest® 12-Hour | Tablet | Slow release |
| Artane® Sequels® | Capsule | Slow release*† |
| Arthritis Bayer® Time Release | Capsule | Slow release |
| A.S.A.® Enseals® | Tablet | Enteric-coated |
| Atrohist® Plus | Tablet | Slow release* |
| Atrohist® Sprinkle | Capsule | Slow release |
| Azulfidine® EN-tabs® | Tablet | Enteric-coated |
| Baros | Tablet | Effervescent tablet¶ |
| Bayer® Aspirin, low adult 81 mg strength | Tablet | Enteric-coated |
| Bayer® Aspirin, regular strength 325 mg caplet | Tablet | Enteric-coated |
| Bayer® Aspirin, regular strength EC caplet | Tablet | Enteric-coated |
| Betachron E-R® | Capsule | Slow release |
| Betapen®-VK | Tablet | Taste†† |
| Biohist® LA | Tablet | Slow release♦ |
| Bisacodyl | Tablet | Enteric-coated‡ |
| Bisco-Lax® | Tablet | Enteric-coated‡ |
| Bontril® Slow-Release | Capsule | Slow release |

# TABLETS THAT CANNOT BE CRUSHED OR ALTERED *(Continued)*

| Drug Product | Dosage Forms | Reasons/Comments |
|---|---|---|
| Breonesin® | Capsule | Liquid filled§ |
| Brexin® L.A. | Capsule | Slow release |
| Bromfed® | Capsule | Slow release† |
| Bromfed-PD® | Capsule | Slow release† |
| Calan® SR | Tablet | Slow release♦ |
| Cama® Arthritis Pain Reliever | Tablet | Multiple compressed tablet |
| Carbiset-TR® | Tablet | Slow release |
| Cardizem® | Tablet | Slow release |
| Cardizem® CD | Capsule | Slow release* |
| Cardizem® SR | Capsule | Slow release* |
| Carter's Little Pills® | Tablet | Enteric-coated |
| Ceftin® | Tablet | Taste<br>**Note:** Use suspension for children |
| Charcoal Plus® | Tablet | Enteric-coated |
| Chloral Hydrate | Capsule | **Note:** Product is in liquid form within a special capsule† |
| Chlorpheniramine Maleate Time Release | Capsule | Slow release |
| Chlor-Trimeton® Repetab® | Tablet | Slow release† |
| Choledyl® SA | Tablet | Slow release† |
| Cipro™ | Tablet | Taste†† |
| Claritin-D® | Tablet | Slow release |
| Codimal-L.A.® | Capsule | Slow release |
| Codimal-L.A.® Half | Capsule | Slow release |
| Colace® | Capsule | Taste†† |
| Comhist® LA | Capsule | Slow release* |
| Compazine® Spansule® | Capsule | Slow release† |
| Congess SR, JR | Capsule | Slow release |
| Contac® | Capsule | Slow release* |
| Cotazym-S® | Capsule | Enteric-coated* |
| Covera-HS™ | Tablet | Slow release |
| Creon® 10 Minimicrospheres™ | Capsule | Enteric-coated* |
| Creon® 20 | Capsule | Enteric-coated* |
| Cytospaz-M® | Capsule | Slow release |
| Cytoxan® | Tablet | **Note:** Drug may be crushed, but maker recommends using injection |
| Dallergy® | Capsule | Slow release† |
| Dallergy-D® | Capsule | Slow release |
| Dallergy-JR® | Capsule | Slow release |
| Deconamine® SR | Capsule | Slow release† |
| Deconsal® II | Tablet | Slow release |
| Deconsal® Sprinkle® | Capsule | Slow release* |
| Defen L.A.® | Tablet | Slow release♦ |
| Demazin® Repetabs® | Tablet | Slow release† |
| Depakene® | Capsule | Slow-release-mucous membrane irritant† |
| Depakote® | Capsule | Enteric-coated |
| Desoxyn® Gradumets® | Tablet | Slow release |
| Desyrel® | Tablet | Taste†† |
| Dexatrim® Max Strength | Tablet | Slow release |
| Dexedrine® Spansule® | Capsule | Slow release |
| Diamox® Sequels® | Capsule | Slow release |
| Dilatrate-SR® | Capsule | Slow release |
| Disobrom® | Tablet | Slow release |
| Disophrol® Chronotab® | Tablet | Slow release |
| Dital® | Capsule | Slow release |
| Donnatal® Extentab® | Tablet | Slow release† |
| Donnazyme® | Tablet | Enteric-coated |
| Drisdol® | Capsule | Liquid filled§ |
| Drixoral® | Tablet | Slow release† |
| Drixoral® Sinus | Tablet | Slow release |
| Dulcolax® | Tablet | Enteric-coated‡ |

| Drug Product | Dosage Forms | Reasons/Comments |
|---|---|---|
| Dynabac® | Tablet | Enteric-coated |
| Easprin® | Tablet | Enteric-coated |
| Ecotrin® | Tablet | Enteric-coated |
| E.E.S.® 400 | Tablet | Enteric-coated† |
| Efidac/24® | Tablet | Slow release |
| Efidac® 24 Chlorpheniramine | Tablet | Slow release |
| E-Mycin® | Tablet | Enteric-coated |
| Endafed® | Capsule | Slow release |
| Entex® LA | Tablet | Slow release† |
| Equanil® | Tablet | Taste†† |
| Eryc® | Capsule | Enteric-coated* |
| Ery-Tab® | Tablet | Enteric-coated |
| Erythrocin Stearate | Tablet | Enteric-coated |
| Erythromycin Base | Tablet | Enteric-coated |
| Eskalith CR® | Tablet | Slow release |
| Exgest® LA | Tablet | Slow release |
| Fedahist® Timecaps® | Capsule | Slow release† |
| Feldene® | Capsule | Mucous membrane irritant |
| Feocyte | Tablet | Slow release |
| Feosol® | Tablet | Enteric-coated† |
| Feosol® Spansule® | Capsule | Slow release*† |
| Feratab® | Tablet | Enteric-coated† |
| Fero-Grad 500® | Tablet | Slow release |
| Fero-Gradumet® | Tablet | Slow release |
| Ferralet S.R.® | Tablet | Slow release |
| Feverall™ Sprinkle Caps | Capsule | Taste* **Note:** Capsule contents intended to be placed in a teaspoonful of water or soft food. |
| Fumatinic® | Capsule | Slow release |
| Gastrocrom® | Capsule | **Note:** Contents should be dissolved in water for administration. |
| Geocillin® | Tablet | Taste |
| Glucotrol® XL | Tablet | Slow release |
| Gris-PEG® | Tablet | **Note:** Crushing may result in precipitation of larger particles. |
| Guaifed® | Capsule | Slow release |
| Guaifed®-PD | Capsule | Slow release |
| Guaifenex® LA | Tablet | Slow release♦ |
| Guaifenex® PSE | Tablet | Slow release♦ |
| GuaiMAX-D® | Tablet | Slow release |
| Humibid® DM | Tablet | Slow release |
| Humibid® DM Sprinkle | Capsule | Slow release* |
| Humibid® LA | Tablet | Slow release |
| Humibid® Sprinkle | Capsule | Slow release* |
| Hydergine® LC | Capsule | **Note:** Product is in liquid form within a special capsulet† |
| Hydergine® Sublingual | Tablet | Sublingual route† |
| Hytakerol® | Capsule | Liquid filled§† |
| Iberet® | Tablet | Slow release† |
| Iberet-500® | Tablet | Slow release† |
| ICAPS® Plus | Tablet | Slow release |
| ICAPS® Time Release | Tablet | Slow release |
| Ilotycin® | Tablet | Enteric-coated |
| Imdur™ | Tablet | Slow release♦ |
| Inderal® LA | Capsule | Slow release |
| Inderide® LA | Capsule | Slow release |
| Indocin® SR | Capsule | Slow release*† |
| Ionamin® | Capsule | Slow release |
| Isoptin® SR | Tablet | Slow release |
| Isordil® Sublingual | Tablet | Sublingual form• |
| Isordil® Tembid® | Tablet | Slow release |
| Isosorbide Dinitrate Sublingual | Tablet | Sublingual form• |

# TABLETS THAT CANNOT BE CRUSHED OR ALTERED *(Continued)*

| Drug Product | Dosage Forms | Reasons/Comments |
|---|---|---|
| Isosorbide Dinitrate SR | Tablet | Slow release |
| K+ 8® | Tablet | Slow release† |
| K+ 10® | Tablet | Slow release† |
| Kaon-Cl® 6.7 | Tablet | Slow release† |
| Kaon-Cl® 10 | Tablet | Slow release† |
| K+ Care® ET | Tablet | Effervescent tablet†¶ |
| K-Lease® | Capsule | Slow release*† |
| Klor-Con® | Tablet | Slow release† |
| Klor-Con/EF® | Tablet | Effervescent tablet†¶ |
| Klorvess® | Tablet | Effervescent tablet†¶ |
| Klotrix® | Tablet | Slow release† |
| K-Lyte® | Tablet | Effervescent tablet¶ |
| K-Lyte®/Cl | Tablet | Effervescent tablet¶ |
| K-Lyte DS® | Tablet | Effervescent tablet¶ |
| K-Tab® | Tablet | Slow release† |
| Levsinex® Timecaps® | Capsule | Slow release |
| Lexxel® | Tablet | Slow release |
| Lodrane LD® | Capsule | Slow release* |
| Mag-Tab® SR | Tablet | Slow release |
| Mestinon® | Tablet | Slow release† |
| Mi-Cebrin® | Tablet | Enteric-coated |
| Mi-Cebrin® T | Tablet | Enteric-coated |
| Micro-K® | Capsule | Slow release*† |
| Monafed® | Tablet | Slow release |
| Monafed® DM | Tablet | Slow release |
| Motrin® | Tablet | Taste†† |
| MS Contin® | Tablet | Slow release† |
| Muco-Fen-LA® | Tablet | Slow release♦ |
| Naldecon® | Tablet | Slow release† |
| Naprelan® | Tablet | Slow release |
| Nasatab LA® | Tablet | Slow release |
| Niaspan® | Tablet | Slow release |
| Nico-400® | Capsule | Slow release |
| Nicobid® | Capsule | Slow release |
| Nitro-Bid® | Capsule | Slow release* |
| Nitroglyn® | Capsule | Slow release* |
| Nitrong® | Tablet | Sublingual route• |
| Nitrostat® | Tablet | Sublingual route• |
| Nolamine® | Tablet | Slow release |
| Nolex® LA | Tablet | Slow release |
| Norflex® | Tablet | Slow release |
| Norpace CR® | Capsule | Slow release form within a special capsule |
| Novafed® A | Capsule | Slow release |
| Ondrox® | Tablet | Slow release |
| Optilets-500® | Tablet | Enteric-coated |
| Optilets-M-500® | Tablet | Enteric-coated |
| Oragrafin® | Capsule | **Note:** Product is in liquid form within a special capsule |
| Ordrine® SR | Capsule | Slow release |
| Oramorph SR™ | Tablet | Slow release† |
| Ornade® Spansule® | Capsule | Slow release |
| OxyContin® | Tablet | Slow release |
| Pabalate® | Tablet | Enteric-coated |
| Pabalate-SF® | Tablet | Enteric-coated |
| Pancrease® | Capsule | Enteric-coated* |
| Pancrease® MT | Capsule | Enteric-coated* |
| Panmycin® | Capsule | Taste |
| Papaverine Sustained Action | Capsule | Slow release |
| Pathilon® Sequels® | Capsule | Slow release* |
| Pavabid® Plateau® | Capsule | Slow release* |
| PBZ-SR® | Tablet | Slow release† |

| Drug Product | Dosage Forms | Reasons/Comments |
|---|---|---|
| Pentasa® | Capsule | Slow release |
| Perdiem® | Granules | Wax coated |
| Permitil® Chronotab® | Tablet | Slow release† |
| Phazyme® | Tablet | Slow release |
| Phazyme® 95 | Tablet | Slow release |
| Phenergan® | Tablet | Taste††† |
| Phyllocontin® | Tablet | Slow release |
| Plendil® | Tablet | Slow release |
| Pneumomits® | Tablet | Slow release♦ |
| Polaramine® Repetabs® | Tablet | Slow release† |
| Posicor® | Tablet | Mucus membrane irritant |
| Prelu-2® | Capsule | Slow release |
| Prevacid® | Capsule | Slow release |
| Prilosec™ | Capsule | Slow release |
| Pro-Banthine® | Tablet | Taste |
| Procainamide HCl SR | Tablet | Slow release |
| Procanbid® | Tablet | Slow release |
| Procardia® | Capsule | Delays absorption§# |
| Procardia XL® | Tablet | Slow release<br>**Note:** AUC is unaffected. |
| Profen® II | Tablet | Slow release♦ |
| Profen LA® | Tablet | Slow release♦ |
| Pronestyl-SR® | Tablet | Slow release |
| Proscar® | Tablet | **Note:** Crushed tablets should not be handled by women who are pregnant or who may become pregnant |
| Proventil® Repetabs® | Tablet | Slow release† |
| Prozac® | Capsule | Slow release* |
| Quibron-T/ SR® | Tablet | Slow release† |
| Quinaglute® Dura-Tabs® | Tablet | Slow release |
| Quinidex® Extentabs® | Tablet | Slow release |
| Quin-Release® | Tablet | Slow release |
| Respa-1st® | Tablet | Slow release♦ |
| Respa-DM® | Tablet | Slow release♦ |
| Respa-GF® | Tablet | Slow release♦ |
| Respahist® | Capsule | Slow release* |
| Respaire® SR | Capsule | Slow release |
| Respbid® | Tablet | Slow release |
| Ritalin-SR® | Tablet | Slow release |
| Robimycin® Robitab® | Tablet | Enteric-coated |
| Rondec-TR® | Tablet | Slow release† |
| Roxanol SR™ | Tablet | Slow release† |
| Ru-Tuss® DE | Tablet | Slow release |
| Sinemet CR® | Tablet | Slow release♦ |
| Singlet for Adults® | Tablet | Slow release |
| Slo-bid™ Gyrocaps® | Capsule | Slow release* |
| Slo-Niacin® | Tablet | Slow release |
| Slo-Phyllin GG® | Capsule | Slow release† |
| Slo-Phyllin® Gyrocaps® | Capsule | Slow release*† |
| Slow FE® | Tablet | Slow release† |
| Slow FE® With Folic Acid | Tablet | Slow release |
| Slow-K® | Tablet | Slow release† |
| Slow-Mag® | Tablet | Slow release |
| Sorbitrate SA® | Tablet | Slow release |
| Sorbitrate® Sublingual | Tablet | Sublingual route |
| Sparine® | Tablet | Taste†† |
| S-P-T | Capsule | **Note:** Liquid gelatin thyroid suspension. |
| Sudafed® 12-Hour | Capsule | Slow release† |
| Sudal® 60/500 | Tablet | Slow release |
| Sudal® 120/600 | Tablet | Slow release |
| Sudafed® 12-Hour | Tablet | Slow release† |
| Sudex® 60/500 | Tablet | Slow release♦ |

# TABLETS THAT CANNOT BE CRUSHED OR ALTERED *(Continued)*

| Drug Product | Dosage Forms | Reasons/Comments |
|---|---|---|
| Sustaire® | Tablet | Slow release† |
| Syn™-Rx | Tablet | Slow release |
| Syn™-Rx DM | Tablet | Slow release |
| Tavist-D® | Tablet | Multiple compressed tablet |
| Teczam® | Tablet | Slow release |
| Tegretol XR® | Tablet | Slow release |
| Teldrin® | Capsule | Slow release* |
| Tessalon® Perles | Capsule | Slow release |
| Theo-24® | Tablet | Slow release† |
| Theobid® Duracaps® | Capsule | Slow release*† |
| Theoclear® L.A | Capsule | Slow release† |
| Theochron® | Tablet | Slow release |
| Theo-Dur® | Tablet | Slow release†♦ |
| Theolair SR® | Tablet | Slow release† |
| Theo-Sav® | Tablet | Slow release♦ |
| Theo-Time® SR | Tablet | Slow release |
| Theovent® | Capsule | Slow release† |
| Theo-X® | Tablet | Slow release |
| Thorazine® Spansule® | Capsule | Slow release |
| Toprol XL® | Tablet | Slow release♦ |
| Touro A&H® | Capsule | Slow release* |
| Touro Ex® | Tablet | Slow release♦ |
| Touro LA® | Tablet | Slow release♦ |
| T-Phyl® | Tablet | Slow release |
| Trental® | Tablet | Slow release |
| Triaminic® | Tablet | Enteric-coated† |
| Triaminic®-12 | Tablet | Slow release† |
| Triaminic® TR | Tablet | Multiple compressed tablet† |
| Trilafon® Repetabs® | Tablet | Slow release† |
| Tri-Phen-Chlor® Time Release | Tablet | Slow release |
| Tri-Phen-Mine® SR | Tablet | Slow release |
| TripTone® Caplets | Tablet | Slow release |
| Tuss-LA® | Tablet | Slow release |
| Tylenol® Extended Relief Caplets | Tablet | Slow release |
| ULR-LA® | Tablet | Slow release |
| Uni-Dur® | Tablet | Slow release |
| Uniphyl® | Tablet | Slow release |
| Verelan® | Capsule | Slow release* |
| Volmax® | Tablet | Slow release† |
| Wellbutrin® | Tablet | Anesthetize mucus membrane |
| Wygesic® | Tablet | Taste |
| ZORprin® | Tablet | Slow release |
| Zyban™ | Tablet | Slow release |
| Zymase® | Capsule | Enteric-coated |

*Capsule may be opened and the contents taken without crushing or chewing; soft food such as applesauce or pudding may facilitate administration; contents may generally be administered via nasogastric tube using an appropriate fluid, provided entire contents are washed down the tube.

†Liquid dosage forms of the product are available; however, dose, frequency of administration, and manufacturers may differ from that of the solid dosage form.

‡Antacids and/or milk may prematurely dissolve the coating of the tablet.

§Capsule may be opened and the liquid contents removed for administration.

††The taste of this product in a liquid form would likely be unacceptable to the patient; administration via nasogastric tube should be acceptable.

¶Effervescent tablets must be dissolved in the amount of diluent recommended by the manufacturer.

#If the liquid capsule is crushed or the contents expressed, the active ingredient will be, in part, absorbed sublingually.

•Tablets are made to disintegrate under the tongue.

♦Tablet is scored and may be broken in half without affecting release characteristics.

Adapted from Mitchell JF and Pawlicki KS, "Oral Solid Dosage Forms That Should Not Be Crushed: 1998 Revision," *Hosp Pharm*, 1994, 29(7):666-75.

# SELECTED ADVERSE EFFECTS

Adverse drug reactions can range from inconvenient to life-threatening. The type of effects, the severity, and frequency of occurrence is dependent on the medication and dosage of the medication being used, as well as the individual's response to the therapy. Early recognition by healthcare providers or patients of these adverse side effects is a major factor if appropriate intervention is to implemented. The following are definitions of selected adverse effects, and examples of some (by no means all) medications associated with these adverse effects.

| Name | Description |
|---|---|
| Acute tubular necrosis | Acute renal failure characterized by direct toxicity to tubular cells. Cellular debris (casts) are a prominent feature of urinary sediment. Usually requires several days of treatment.<br>**Examples of associated drugs:** Aminoglycosides |
| Ageusia | Loss of sense of taste<br>**Examples of associated drugs:** Bleomycin, cisplatin, diltiazem |
| Akathisia | Evidenced by an uncontrollable constant need for motion, pacing, and squirming or restlessness; usually develops within first 2 months of antipsychotic treatment<br>**Examples of associated drugs:** Phenergan, haldo |
| Alopecia | Loss of body hair<br>**Examples of associated drugs:** Chemotherapeutic agents, beta-blockers |
| Anemia | A condition in which the number of red blood cells, the amount of hemoglobin, and the volume of packed red blood cells of blood is less than normal; manifested by pallor of the skin and mucus membranes, shortness of breath, palpitation of the heart, soft systolic murmurs, lethargy, fatigability, nose bleeds, bleeding gums, easy bruising, hematuria or blood in stool<br>**Examples of associated drugs:** Amoxicillin, warfarin |
| Angioedema | Localized swelling of the subcutaneous tissue of face, hands, feet, and genitalia<br>**Examples of associated drugs:** Ace inhibitors |
| Anhidrosis | Deficiency of or absence of sweat; since sweating is necessary for cooling, persons with anhidrosis are at increased risk for hyperthermia |
| Anorexia | Loss of desire for food<br>**Examples of associated drugs:** CNS stimulants |
| Anticholinergic effects | Usually used to describe blockade of muscarinic receptors. Symptoms include blurred vision, mydriasis, increased intraocular pressure, headache, flushing, tachycardia, nervousness, constipation, dizziness, insomnia, mental confusion or excitement, dry mouth, altered taste perception, dysphagia, constipation, palpitations, bradycardia, urinary hesitancy or retention, impotence, decreased sweating, susceptibility to heat prostration, thickening or drying of bronchial secretions.<br>**Examples of associated drugs:** Tricyclic antidepressants, antihistamines |
| Anticoagulant skin necrosis | Occurs early in therapy (3-5) days with oral anticoagulants (eg, warfarin). A paradoxical effect of oral anticoagulant therapy which involves micorembolization and necrosis of skin often localized to the abdomen, breast, buttock, and thigh regions. Genetic deficiency of protein C appears to be a risk factor.<br>**Examples of associated drugs:** Oral anticoagulants (eg, warfarin) |
| Cushing's syndrome | Usually a response to excess levels of circulating glucocorticoids; resembles Cushing's disease (pituitary tumor); characterized by obesity, hyperglycemia, glycosuria, muscle weakness, menstrual irregularities, fluid and electrolyte disturbances, hirsutism, myopathy, and decreased resistance to infection<br>**Examples of associated drugs:** Prednisone |

## SELECTED ADVERSE EFFECTS *(Continued)*

| Name | Description |
|---|---|
| Disulfiram reaction | Many drugs will produce a disulfiram-type reaction when the patient ingests alcohol. Symptoms includes nausea and/or vomiting, pounding or throbbing headache, systemic flushing, respiratory difficulties (dyspnea, hyperventilation), sweating, excessive thirst, cardiac disturbances (chest pain, palpitations), vertigo, visual disturbances (blurred or double vision), and CNS disturbances (confusion, convulsions). **Examples of associated drugs:** Metronidazole, cephalosporins with MTT side chains |
| Drug fever | Persistent fever which may be associated with low-grade allergic reaction to a drug entity. Often develops several days after initial defervescence from antibiotics. Other causes of fever related to drugs may be due to dopamine inhibition (see neuroleptic malignant syndrome). **Examples of associated drugs:** Beta-lactams, macrolides |
| Dysgeusia | Impairment of or perversion of sense of taste |
| Dystonia | Develops early in therapy – sometimes within hours of first dose. Typically, appears as severe spasms of the muscles of face, neck, tongue, and back. Oculogyric crisis (upward deviation of the eyes) and opisthotonus (tetanic spasm of back muscles cause trunk to arch forward, with head and lower extremities thrown backward. Acute cramping can cause dislocation of joints and laryngeal dystonia can impair respiration (can be fatal, requires emergency treatment). **Examples of associated drugs:** Haldol, phenothiazines |
| Eosinophilic pneumonitis | Development of interstitial penumonitis due to eosinophilic infiltrates. Shortness of breath and inflammation are prominent features. **Examples of associated drugs:** Mesalamine |
| Erythema multiforme | Cutaneous eruption of macules, papules, and/or subdermal vessicles (multiform appearance), including characteristic "target" or "iris" lesions over the dorsal aspect of the hands and forearms. Self-limiting eruptions are termed "minor", while major erruptions may be referred to as Stevens-Johnson syndrome. **Examples of associated drugs:** Phenytoin, sulfonamides |
| Extrapyramidal movemement disorders | Movement disorders associated with antipsychotic effects: Dystonia, pseudoparkinsonism, akathisia, tardive dyskinesia **Examples of associated drugs:** Metoclopramide, haldol, phenothiazines |
| Hallucinations | **Examples of associated drugs:** Opiates |
| Hepatotoxicity | Hepatocellular damage or multilobular hepatic necrosis can result in liver dysfunction manifested as jaundice or hepatitis; yellowing of skin or eyes is usually a later manifestation; anorexia, fatigue or malaise, nausea, darkening in color of urine or light colored stool may occur first **Examples of associated drugs:** Troglitazone |
| Interstitial nephritis | Acute renal failure characterized by localized inflammatory/allergic reaction, pronounced eosinophilic collection in interstitial cells of kidney. Eosinophils may appear in urine. Usually develops after several days of therapy. **Examples of associated drugs:** Beta-lactams, NSAIDs |
| Leukopenia/neutropenia | **Examples of associated drugs:** Beta-lactams, procainamide |
| Methemoglobinemia | Rare reaction in which the hemoglobin molecule is altered, rendering it unable to effectively carry oxygen after exposure to a chemical initiator. Cyanosis, respiratory distress, lactic acidosis, and shock may progress rapidly after exposure. May occur with any route of administration, including topical. **Examples of associated drugs:** Nitrates, local anesthetics |
| Myositis/rhabdomyolysis | Inflammation/toxicity to muscle cells characterized by muscle pain/stiffness. Pronounced lysis of muscle cells leads to dramatic incerase in serum CPK and possible precipitation of myoglobin in urine. **Examples of associated drugs:** HMG CoA reductase inhibitors (particularly when combined with drugs like erythomycin or cyclosporin) |

| Name | Description |
|---|---|
| Neuroleptic malignant syndrome | Rare, but may cause 30% to 50% fatality, response to antipsychotic therapy – usually with high-potency drugs. Manifests as extremely rigid musculoskeletal posturing, extremely high fevers, sweating, dysrhythmias, and acute fluctuations of blood pressure and consciousness, respiratory failure and/or cardiac collapse (requires immediate supportive care and withdrawal of antipsychotic medication). **Examples of associated drugs:** Haldol, phenothiazines |
| Neuromuscular blockade | Weakness, respiratory failure as neuromuscular transmission may be interrupted. Patients with decreased neuromuscular transmission (ie, myasthenia gravis) are at particular risk. **Examples of associated drugs:** Aminoglycosides, macrolides |
| Neutropenia | Usually associated with antineoplastic medications. A reduction in circulating neutrophils (white blood cells that are essential in fighting infection) means that both severity and incidence of infections are significantly increased. Usually, benign infections such as candidiasis can become systemically life-threatening. **Examples of associated drugs:** Beta-lactams, procainamide, carbamazepine |
| Opportunistic infection | Many medications reduce the natural resistance to infection and/or mask the more obvious indications of an infection when persons are receiving antineoplastics, antivirals, antibiotics, and glucocorticoids. Symptoms include sore throat, fever, chills, unhealed sores, purulent vaginal discharge, white plaques in mouth, fatigue, and joint pain. **Examples of associated drugs:** Chemotherapeutic agents, broad-spectrum antibiotics, immunosuppressants |
| Optic neuritis | Blurred vision, altered color discrimination, and constriction of visual fields **Examples of associated drugs:** Quinidine, cisplatin |
| Orthostatic hypotension | Reduced muscle tone in the venous wall which causes blood to pool in lower extremity veins when the person assumes an erect position from lying or sitting; blood return to the heart is decreased because of this pooling, resulting in decreased cardiac output, and abrupt fall in blood pressure **Examples of associated drugs:** Tricyclic antidepressants, beta-blockers |
| Paradoxical response | A response to a medication that is opposite of the anticipated response or side effects (eg, a paradoxical response to CNS depressants may be CNS excitation such as hyperactivity, aggression, decreased ability to concentrate, etc) **Examples of associated drugs:** Benzodiazepines, phenobarbital |
| Photophobia | Blocking muscarinic receptors on the sphincter of the iris decreases ability to adapt to bright light with intolerance for any bright light; both artificial lighting and outside sunlight **Examples of associated drugs:** Anticholinergics |
| Photosensitization/ phototoxicity | Phototoxic and photoallergic reactions result from a combination of a sensitizing agent and ultraviolet light. The sensitizing agent in photoxic reactions may be systemically ingested or locally applied. The reaction occurs within hours of exposure. Photoallergy results from chemical change to the structure of a sensitizing agent, and may require several days before symptoms appear. **Examples of associated drugs:** Fluoroquinolones, tetracyclines |
| Postural hypotension | See orthostatic hypotension. |
| Pseudoparkinsonism | Blocking of dopamine receptors produces symptoms that resemble Parkinson's disease: Bradycardia, facies, drooling, tremors, rigidity, gait disturbance, and stooped posture (usually develops within first month of therapy) **Examples of associated drugs:** Antipsychotic medications, haldol |
| Pulmonary fibrosis | Restrictive airway disease due to fibrous changes in the lungs, often manifest only after long-term drug administration. **Examples of associated drugs:** Nitrofurantoin, melphalan, amiodarone |

## SELECTED ADVERSE EFFECTS *(Continued)*

| Name | Description |
|---|---|
| Purple toes syndrome | Peripheral ischemia and cyanosis generally localized to the plantar surfaces and sides of the toes which may occasionally progress to necrosis or gangrene. The effect is believed to be caused by cholesterol microemboli. Effects are noted after weeks to months of therapy.<br>**Examples of associated drugs:** Oral anticoagulants |
| Seizures (drug-induced) | An infrequent, nonspecific effect of a variety of medications, particularly at high concentrations. Drug-induced seizures may occur due to lowering of seizure threshold, blockade of inhibitory neurotransmitters (GABA) or direct neuroexcitatory effects.<br>**Examples of associated drugs:** Tricyclic antidepressants (lower seizure threshold), high-dose beta-lactam or fluoroquinolone antibiotics (GABA blockade); theophylline or accumulation of normeperidine (neuroexcitation) |
| Serotonin syndrome | Presence of three or more of the following: Altered mental status (40% – primarily confusion or hypomania), agitation, tremor (50%), shivering, diarrhea, hyperreflexia (pronounced) in lower extremities, myoclonus (50%), ataxia or incoordination, fever (50% incidence; temperature >105°F associated with grave prognosis), diaphoresis<br>**Examples of associated drugs:** Serotonin reuptake inhibitors, MOMA (ecstasy), clomipramine, combinations of many drugs |
| Stevens-Johnson syndrome (SJS) | Rare reaction; symptoms include widespread lesions of the skin and mucous membranes, fever, malaise, and toxemia; reducing or discontinuing the sulfonamide at the first sign of skin rash may reduce the incidence of SJS<br>**Examples of associated drugs:** Associated primarily with sulfonamides and associated compounds such as sulfonylureas, thiazide diuretics, and loop diuretics; anticonvulsants |
| Stomatitis | **Examples of associated drugs:** Chemotherapeutic agents |
| Sulfite hypersensitivity | Reactions occur within 2-15 minutes after ingestion of inhalation and include nasal pruritus, rhinorrhea, conjunctivitis, generalized urticaria, dyspnea, wheezing, angioedema, flushing, weakness, and anaphylaxis; patients frequently have underlying allergies or asthmatic disease.<br>**Examples of associated drugs:** Sulfite derivatives are common antioxidant preservatives used in foods and medications. Sulfite derivatives include sodium bisulfite, potassium bisulfite, sodium metabisulfite, sodium sulfites, potassium metabisulfite, and sulfur dioxide. Most common food sources are fresh fruits and vegetables, shellfish, soft drinks, beer, wine, dried foods, and fruit drinks. Sympathomimetic medications are very susceptible to oxidation and frequently contain bisulfites in concentrations of 0.3% to 0.75%. |
| Tardive dyskinesia | Usually develops with long-term therapy – symptoms may be irreversible. Characterized by wormlike, writhing movements of tongue and facial muscles, lip-smacking, or flicking tongue movements; can progress to involuntary movements of digits or limbs.<br>**Examples of associated drugs:** Haldol, phenothiazines |
| Tendonitis/Achilles' tendon rupture | Pain associated with tendon area, most commonly in the Achilles' region, which may progress to tendon rupture, particularly if the effect is not recognized and therapy is continued.<br>**Examples of associated drugs:** Fluoroquinolone antibiotics |
| Teratogenic effects | Neonatal abnormalities (physical and mental) that result from impaired development at some stage in the fetal development; specificity of defects depends on several factors, including the period of fetal development when the medication was used (eg, some drugs are teratogenic during the early period of fetal development, some are teratogenic during later periods of development, and some have negative impact on fetal development during any period of the pregnancy)<br>**Examples of associated drugs:** Phenytoin, metronidazole |
| Thrombocytopenia | **Examples of associated drugs:** $H_2$ antagonists, beta-lactams |

| Name | Description |
|---|---|
| Tyramine reaction | Specific foods in the presence of MAO inhibitors; see Food/Drug Interactions for a list of tyramine-containing foods which the patient taking MAO inhibitors should be advised to avoid. Normally, dietary tyramine is inactivated by MAO (monamine oxidase) in the intestinal wall and by hepatic MAO. In the presence of MAO inhibitors, dietary tyramine is not inactivated, passes without metabolism into the circulation to promote the release of accumulated norepinephrine stores in the sympathetic nerve terminals, thereby causing massive vasoconstriction and acute stimulation of the heart. Reactions can be severe and usually require emergency treatment. **Examples of associated drugs:** MAO inhibitors |
| Vestibulotoxicity | Form of ototoxicity which affects vestibular function, as opposed to hearing. Primary symptom is ataxia or difficulty maintaining balance. **Examples of associated drugs:** Aminoglycosides |
| Virilization | Acne, deepening of voice, increased body and facial hair, baldness, clitoral enlargement, increased libido, menstrual irregularities (Hair loss, voice changes, and enlargement of clitoris may be irreversible.) **Examples of associated drugs:** Minoxidil, phenytoin |
| Xerostomia | Dry mouth results from blockade of muscarinic receptors on salivary glands. Decreased salivation and excessively dry mouth are extremely uncomfortable but also interfere with mastication and swallowing, resulting in poor nutrition. **Examples of associated drugs:** Clonidine, anticholinergics |

# DISCOLORATION OF FECES DUE TO DRUGS

**Black**
Acetazolamide
Aluminum hydroxide
Aminophylline
Amphetamine
Amphotericin B
Bismuth salts
Chlorpropamide
Clindamycin
Corticosteroids
Cyclophosphamide
Cytarabine
Digitalis
Ethacrynic acid
Ferrous salts
Fluorouracil
Hydralazine
Hydrocortisone
Iodide-containing drugs
Melphalan
Methotrexate
Methylprednisolone
Phenylephrine
Potassium salts
Prednisolone
Procarbazine
Sulfonamides
Tetracycline
Theophylline
Thiotepa
Triamcinolone
Warfarin

**Blue**
Chloramphenicol
Methylene blue

**Green**
Indomethacin
Medroxyprogesterone

**Yellow/Yellow-Green**
Senna

**Orange-Red**
Phenazopyridine
Rifampin

**Pink/Red**
Anticoagulants
Aspirin
Barium
Heparin
Oxyphenbutazone
Phenylbutazone
Tetracycline syrup

**White/Speckling**
Antibiotics (oral)
Barium

# DISCOLORATION OF URINE DUE TO DRUGS

**Black/Brown/Dark**
Cascara
Chloroquine
Ferrous salts
Metronidazole
Nitrofurantoin
Quinine
Senna

**Blue**
Triamterene

**Blue-Green**
Amitriptyline
Methylene blue

**Orange/Yellow**
Heparin
Phenazopyridine
Rifampin
Sulfasalazine
Warfarin

**Red/Pink**
Daunorubicin
Doxorubicin
Heparin
Ibuprofen
Oxyphenbutazone
Phenylbutazone
Phenytoin
Rifampin
Senna

# FEVER DUE TO DRUGS

**Most Common**
Cephalosporins
Iodides
Isoniazid
Methyldopa
Penicillins
Phenytoin
Procainamide
Quinidine
Streptomycin
Sulfas
Vancomycin

**Less Common**
Allopurinol
Antihistamines
Azathioprine
Barbiturates
Bleomycin
Carbamazepine
Cimetidine
Cisplatin
Clofibrate
Colistimethate
Diazoxide
Folic acid
Hydralazine
Hydroxyurea
Ibuprofen
Mercaptopurine
Nitrofurantoin
Para-aminosalicylic acid
Pentazocine
Procarbazine
Propylthiouracil
Sulindac
Streptozocin
Triamterene

*Drug Intell Clin Pharm*, Table 2, "Drugs Implicated in Causing a Fever," 1986, 20:416.

# SEROTONIN SYNDROME

### Diagnostic Criteria for Serotonin Syndrome

- Recent addition or dosage increase of any agent increasing serotonin activity or availability (usually within 1 day).
- Absence of abused substances, metabolic infectious etiology, or withdrawal.
- No recent addition or dosage increase of a neuroleptic agent prior to onset of signs and symptoms.
- Presence of three or more of the following: Altered mental status (seen in 40% of patients, primarily confusion or hypomania); agitation; tremor (50% incidence); shivering; diarrhea; hyperreflexia (pronounced in lower extremities; myoclonus (50% incidence); ataxia or incoordination; fever (50% incidence; temperature >105°F associated with grave prognosis); diaphoresis

### Drugs (as Single Causative Agent) Which Can Induce Serotonin Syndrome

Specific serotonin reuptake inhibitors (SSRI)
MDMA (Ectasy)
Clomipramine

### Drug Combinations Which Can Induce Serotonin Syndrome*

Alprazolam – Clomipramine

Bromocriptine – Levodopa/carbidopa

Buspirone – Trazodone

Citalopram – Moclobemide

Clomipramine – Clorgiline

Clomipramine – Lithium

Clomipramine – Monoamine oxidase inhibitor

Dihydroergotamine – Sertraline

Dihydroergotamine – Amitriptyline

Fentanyl – Sertraline

Fluoxetine – Carbamazepine

Fluoxetine – Lithium

Fluoxetine – Remoxipride

Fluoxetine – Tryptophan

Lithium – Fluvoxamine

Lithium – Paroxetine

Lysergic acid diethylamide (LSD) – Fluoxetine

Moclobemide – Citalopram

Moclobemide – Clomipramine

Moclobemide – Fluoxetine

Moclobemide – Pethidine

Monoamine oxidase inhibitor – Dextromethorphan

Monoamine oxidase inhibitor – Fluoxetine

Monoamine oxidase inhibitor – Fluvoxamine

Monoamine oxidase inhibitor – Meperidine

Monoamine oxidase inhibitor – Sertraline

Monoamine oxidase inhibitor – Tricyclic antidepressants

Monoamine oxidase inhibitor – Tryptophan

Monoamine oxidase inhibitor – Venlafaxine

Nefazodone – Paroxetine

Nortriptyline – Trazodone

Paroxetine – Dextromethorphan

Paroxetine – Dihydroergotamine

Paroxetine – Trazodone

Phenelzine – Trazodone – Dextropropoxyphene

S-adenosylmethionine – Clomipramine

Sertraline – Amitriptyline

Sumatriptan – Sertraline

Tranylcypromine – Clomipramine

Tramadol – Sertraline

Trazodone – Lithium – Amitriptyline

Trazodone – Fluoxetine

Valproic acid – Nefazodone

Venlafaxine – Tranylcypromine

Venlafaxine – Selegiline

*When administered within 2 weeks of each other.

## SEROTONIN SYNDROME *(Continued)*

### Guidelines for Treatment of Serotonin Syndrome

Therapy is primarily supportive with intravenous crystalloid solutions utilized for hypotension and cooling blankets for mild hyperthermia. Norepinephrine is the preferred vasopressor. Chlorpromazine (25 mg I.M.) or dantrolene sodium (1 mg/kg I.V. – maximum dose 10 mg/kg) may have a role in controlling fevers, although there is no proven benefit. Benzodiazepines are the first-line treatment in controlling rigors and thus, limiting fever and rhabdomyolysis, while clonazepam may be specifically useful in treating myoclonus. Endotracheal intubation and paralysis may be required to treat refractory muscular contractions. Tachycardia or tremor can be treated with beta-blocking agents; although due to its blockade of 5-HTIA receptors, the syndrome may worsen. Serotonin blockers such as diphenhydramine (50 mg I.M.), cyproheptadine (adults: 4-8 mg every 2-4 hours up to 0.5 mg/kg/day; children: up to 0.25 mg/kg/day), or chlorpromazine (25 mg I.M.) have been used with variable efficacy. Methysergide (2-6 mg/day) and nitroglycerin (I.V. infusion of 2 mg/kg/minute with lorazepam) also has been utilized with variable efficacy in case reports. It appears that cyproheptadine is most consistently beneficial.

Recovery seen within 1 day in 70% of cases; mortality rate is about 11%.

### Pharmacokinetics of Selective Serotonin-Reuptake Inhibitors (SSRIs)

| SSRI | Half-life (h) | Metabolite Half-life | Peak Plasma Level (h) | % Protein Bound | Bioavailability (%) |
|---|---|---|---|---|---|
| Citalopram | 35 | N/A | 4 | 80 | 80 |
| Fluoxetine | Initial: 24-72 Chronic: 96-144 | Norfluoxetine 4-16 days | 6-8 | 95 | 72 |
| Fluvoxamine | 16 | N/A | 3 | 80 | 53 |
| Paroxetine | 21 | N/A | 5 | 95 | >90 |
| Sertraline | 26 | N-desmethyl-sertraline 2-4 days | 5-8 | 98 | — |

### References


Gitlin MJ, "Venlafaxine, Monoamine Oxidase Inhibitors, and the Serotonin Syndrome," *J Clin Psychopharmacol*, 1997, 17:66-7.

Heisler MA, Guidery JR, and Arnecke B, "Serotonin Syndrome Induced by Administration of Venlafaxine and Phenelzine," *Ann Pharmacother*, 1996, 30:84.

Hodgman MJ, Martin TG, and Krenzelok EP, "Serotonin Syndrome Due to Venlafaxine and Maintenance Tranylcypromine Therapy," *Hum Exp Toxicol*, 1997, 16:14-7.

John L, Perreault MM, Tao T, et al, "Serotonin Syndrome Associated With Nefazodone and Paroxetine," *Ann Emerg Med*, 1997, 29:287-9.

LoCurto MJ, "The Serotonin Syndrome," *Emerg Clin North Am*, 1997, 15(3):665-75.

Martin TG, "Serotonin Syndrome," *Ann Emerg Med*, 1996, 28:520-6.

Mills K, "Serotonin Toxicity: A Comprehensive Review for Emergency Medicine," *Top Emerg Med*, 1993, 15:54-73.

Mills KC, "Serotonin Syndrome: A Clinical Update," *Crit Care Clin*, 1997, 13(4):763-83.

Nisijima K, Shimizu M, Abe T, et al, "A Case of Serotonin Syndrome Induced by Concomitant Treatment With Low-Dose Trazodone, and Amitriptyline and Lithium," *Int Clin Psychopharmacol*, 1996, 11:289-90.

Sobanski T, Bagli M, Laux G, et al, "Serotonin Syndrome After Lithium Add-On Medication to Paroxetine," *Pharmacopsychiatry*, 1997, 30:106-7.

Sporer, "The Serotonin Syndrome: Implicated Drugs, Pathophysiology and Management," *Drug Safety*, 1995, 13(2):94-104.

Sternbach H, "The Serotonin Syndrome," *Am J Psychiatry*, 1991, 146:705-7.

Van Berkum MM, Thiel J, Leikin JB, et al, "A Fatality Due to Serotonin Syndrome," *Medical Update for Psychiatrists*, 1997, 2:55-7.

# CALCULATIONS/CONVERSIONS/ LABORATORY VALUES

## APOTHECARY/METRIC CONVERSIONS

### Approximate Liquid Measures

Basic equivalent: 1 fluid ounce = 30 mL

Examples:

| | | | |
|---|---|---|---|
| 1 gallon | 3800 mL | 1 gallon | 128 fluid ounces |
| 1 quart | 960 mL | 1 quart | 32 fluid ounces |
| 1 pint | 480 mL | 1 pint | 16 fluid ounces |
| 8 fluid ounces | 240 mL | 15 minims | 1 mL |
| 4 fluid ounces | 120 mL | 10 minims | 0.6 mL |

### Approximate Household Equivalents

Basic equivalents:

| | | | |
|---|---|---|---|
| 1 teaspoonful | 5 mL | 1 tablespoonful | 15 mL |

### Weights

Basic equivalents:

| | | | |
|---|---|---|---|
| 1 ounce | 30 g | 15 grains | 1 g |

Examples:

| | | | |
|---|---|---|---|
| 4 ounces | 120 g | 1 grain | 60 mg |
| 2 ounces | 60 g | 1/100 grain | 600 mcg |
| 16 ounces | 1 lb | 1/150 grain | 400 mcg |
| 10 grains | 600 mg | 1/200 grain | 300 mcg |
| 7 1/2 grains | 500 mg | | |

### Metric Conversions

Basic equivalents:

| | | | |
|---|---|---|---|
| 1 g | 1000 mg | 1 mg | 1000 mcg |

Examples:

| | | | |
|---|---|---|---|
| 5 g | 5000 mg | 5 mg | 5000 mcg |
| 0.5 g | 500 mg | 0.5 mg | 500 mcg |
| 0.05 g | 50 mg | 0.05 mg | 50 mcg |

### Exact Equivalents

| | | | |
|---|---|---|---|
| 1 gram (g) | 15.43 grains | 0.1 mg | 1/600 gr |
| 1 milliliter (mL) | 16.23 minims | 0.12 mg | 1/500 gr |
| 1 minim | 0.06 milliliter | 0.15 mg | 1/400 gr |
| 1 grain (gr) | 64.8 milligrams | 0.2 mg | 1/300 gr |
| 1 pint (pt) | 473.2 mL | 0.3 mg | 1/200 gr |
| 1 ounce (oz) | 28.35 | 0.4 mg | 1/150 gr |
| 1 pound (lb) | 453.6 grams | 0.5 mg | 1/120 gr |
| 1 kilogram (kg) | 2.2 pounds | 0.6 mg | 1/100 gr |
| 1 quart (qt) | 946.4 mL | 0.8 mg | 1/80 gr |
| | | 1 mg | 1/65 gr |

### Solids*

| | | | |
|---|---|---|---|
| 1/4 grain | 15 mg | 1 1/2 grain | 100 mg |
| 1/2 grain | 30 mg | 5 grains | 300 mg |
| 1 grain | 60 mg | 10 grains | 600 mg |

*Use exact equivalents for compounding and calculations requiring a high degree of accuracy.

# CALCULATIONS/CONVERSIONS/LABORATORY VALUES *(Continued)*

## BODY SURFACE AREA OF ADULTS AND CHILDREN

### Calculating Body Surface Area in Children

In a child of average size, find weight and corresponding surface area on the boxed scale to the left; or, use the nomogram to the right. Lay a straightedge on the correct height and weight points for the child, then read the intersecting point on the surface area scale.

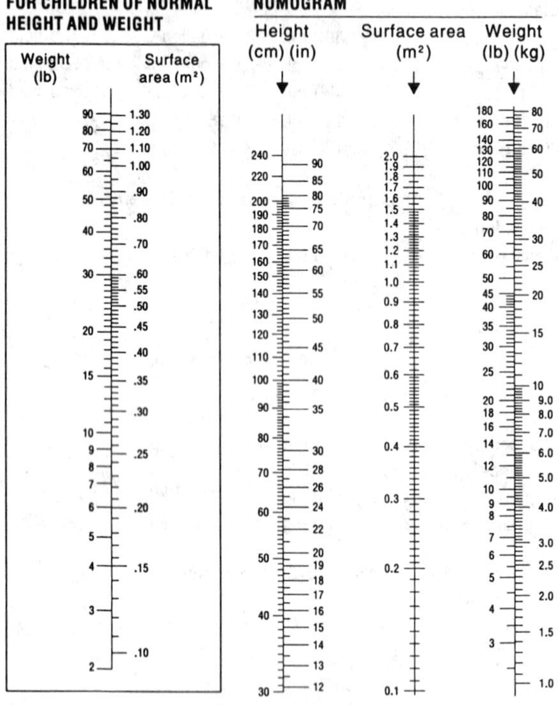

### BODY SURFACE AREA FORMULA (Adult and Pediatric)

$$\text{BSA (m}^2\text{)} = \sqrt{\frac{\text{Ht (in)} \times \text{Wt (lb)}}{3131}} \quad \text{or, in metric: BSA (m}^2\text{)} = \sqrt{\frac{\text{Ht (cm)} \times \text{Wt (kg)}}{3600}}$$

**References**

Lam TK and Leung DT, "More on Simplified Calculation of Body Surface Area," *N Engl J Med*, 1988, 318(17):1130 (Letter).

Mosteller RD, "Simplified Calculation of Body Surface Area", *N Engl J Med*, 1987, 317(17):1098 (Letter).

## IDEAL BODY WEIGHT CALCULATION

**Adults (18 years and older) (IBW is in kg)**

IBW (male) = 50 + (2.3 x height in inches over 5 feet)

IBW (female) = 45.5 + (2.3 x height in inches over 5 feet)

**Children (IBW is in kg; height is in cm)**

a. 1-18 years

$$\text{IBW} = \frac{(\text{height}^2 \times 1.65)}{1000}$$

b. 5 feet and taller

IBW (male) = 39 + (2.27 x height in inches over 5 feet)

IBW (female) = 42.2 + (2.27 x height in inches over 5 feet)

# CREATININE CLEARANCE ESTIMATING METHODS IN PATIENTS WITH STABLE RENAL FUNCTION

These formulas provide an acceptable estimate of the patient's creatinine clearance **except** in the following instances.

- Patient's serum creatinine is changing rapidly (either up or down).
- Patients are markedly emaciated.

In above situations, certain assumptions have to be made.

- In patients with rapidly rising serum creatinines (ie, >0.5-0.7 mg/dL/day), it is best to assume that the patient's creatinine clearance is probably <10 mL/minute.
- In emaciated patients, although their actual creatinine clearance is less than their calculated creatinine clearance (because of decreased creatinine production), it is not possible to easily predict how much less.

## Infants

**Estimation of creatinine clearance using serum creatinine and body length** (to be used when an adequate timed specimen cannot be obtained). **Note:** This formula may not provide an accurate estimation of creatinine clearance for infants younger than 6 months of age and for patients with severe starvation or muscle wasting.

$Cl_{cr} = K \times L/S_{cr}$

where:

$Cl_{cr}$ = creatinine clearance in mL/minute/1.73 $m^2$
K = constant of proportionality that is age specific

| Age | K |
|---|---|
| Low birth weight ≤1 y | 0.33 |
| Full-term ≤1 y | 0.45 |
| 2-12 y | 0.55 |
| 13-21 y female | 0.55 |
| 13-21 y male | 0.70 |

L = length in cm
$S_{cr}$ = serum creatinine concentration in mg/dL

### Reference

Schwartz GJ, Brion LP, and Spitzer A, "The Use of Plasma Creatinine Concentration for Estimating Glomerular Filtration Rate in Infants, Children and Adolescents," *Ped Clin N Amer*, 1987, 34:571-90.

## Children (1-18 years)

Method 1: (Traub SL, Johnson CE, *Am J Hosp Pharm*, 1980, 37:195-201)

$$Cl_{cr} = \frac{0.48 \times (\text{height}) \times BSA}{S_{cr} \times 1.73}$$

where:

BSA = body surface area in $m^2$
$Cl_{cr}$ = creatinine clearance in mL/min
$S_{cr}$ = serum creatinine in mg/dL
Height = in cm

## CALCULATIONS/CONVERSIONS/LABORATORY VALUES *(Continued)*

Method 2: Nomogram (Traub SL and Johnson CE, *Am J Hosp Pharm*, 1980, 37:195-201)

**Children 1-18 Years**

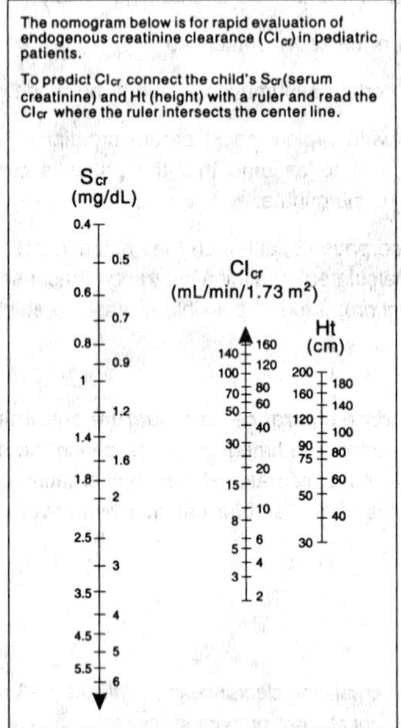

The nomogram below is for rapid evaluation of endogenous creatinine clearance ($Cl_{cr}$) in pediatric patients.
To predict $Cl_{cr}$, connect the child's $S_{cr}$ (serum creatinine) and Ht (height) with a ruler and read the $Cl_{cr}$ where the ruler intersects the center line.
$S_{cr}$ (mg/dL)
$Cl_{cr}$ (mL/min/1.73 m$^2$)
Ht (cm)


**Adults (18 years and older)**

Method: (Cockroft DW and Gault MH, *Nephron*, 1976, 16:31-41)

Estimated creatinine clearance ($Cl_{cr}$) (mL/min):

$$\text{Male} = \frac{(140 - \text{age})\ \text{IBW (kg)}}{72 \times S_{cr}}$$

$$\text{Female} = \text{estimated } Cl_{cr} \text{ male} \times 0.85$$

**Note:** The use of the patient's ideal body weight (IBW) is recommended for the above formula except when the patient's actual body weight is less than ideal. Use of the IBW is especially important in obese patients.

## POUNDS/KILOGRAMS CONVERSION

**1 pound = 0.45359 kilograms**
**1 kilogram = 2.2 pounds**

| lb | = kg | lb | = kg | lb | = kg |
|---|---|---|---|---|---|
| 1 | 0.45 | 70 | 31.75 | 140 | 63.50 |
| 5 | 2.27 | 75 | 34.02 | 145 | 65.77 |
| 10 | 4.54 | 80 | 36.29 | 150 | 68.04 |
| 15 | 6.80 | 85 | 38.56 | 155 | 70.31 |
| 20 | 9.07 | 90 | 40.82 | 160 | 72.58 |
| 25 | 11.34 | 95 | 43.09 | 165 | 74.84 |
| 30 | 13.61 | 100 | 45.36 | 170 | 77.11 |
| 35 | 15.88 | 105 | 47.63 | 175 | 79.38 |
| 40 | 18.14 | 110 | 49.90 | 180 | 81.65 |
| 45 | 20.41 | 115 | 52.16 | 185 | 83.92 |
| 50 | 22.68 | 120 | 54.43 | 190 | 86.18 |
| 55 | 24.95 | 125 | 56.70 | 195 | 88.45 |
| 60 | 27.22 | 130 | 58.91 | 200 | 90.72 |
| 65 | 29.48 | 135 | 61.24 | | |

## FAHRENHEIT/CENTIGRADE CONVERSIONS

**Celsius to Fahrenheit = (°C x 9/5) + 32 = °F**
**Fahrenheit to Celsius = (°F – 32) x 5/9 = °C**

| °C | = °F | °C | = °F | °C | = °F |
|---|---|---|---|---|---|
| 100.0 | 212.0 | 39.0 | 102.2 | 36.8 | 98.2 |
| 50.0 | 122.0 | 38.8 | 101.8 | 36.6 | 97.9 |
| 41.0 | 105.8 | 38.6 | 101.5 | 36.4 | 97.5 |
| 40.8 | 105.4 | 38.4 | 101.1 | 36.2 | 97.2 |
| 40.6 | 105.1 | 38.2 | 100.8 | 36.0 | 96.8 |
| 40.4 | 104.7 | 38.0 | 100.4 | 35.8 | 96.4 |
| 40.2 | 104.4 | 37.8 | 100.1 | 35.6 | 96.1 |
| 40.0 | 104.0 | 37.6 | 99.7 | 35.4 | 95.7 |
| 39.8 | 103.6 | 37.4 | 99.3 | 35.2 | 95.4 |
| 39.6 | 103.3 | 37.2 | 99.0 | 35.0 | 95.0 |
| 39.4 | 102.9 | 37.0 | 98.6 | 0 | 32.0 |
| 39.2 | 102.6 | | | | |

# CALCULATIONS/CONVERSIONS/LABORATORY VALUES *(Continued)*

## LABORATORY REFERENCE VALUES FOR ADULTS

### Automated Chemistry (CHEMISTRY A)

| Test | Values | Remarks |
|---|---|---|
| **Serum/Plasma** | | |
| Acetone | Negative | |
| Albumin | 3.2-5 g/dL | |
| Alcohol, ethyl | Negative | |
| Aldolase | 1.2-7.6 IU/L | |
| Ammonia | 20-70 mcg/dL | Specimen to be placed on ice as soon as collected |
| Amylase | 30-110 units/L | |
| Bilirubin, direct | 0-0.3 mg/dL | |
| Bilirubin, total | 0.1-1.2 mg/dL | |
| Calcium | 8.6-10.3 mg/dL | |
| Calcium, ionized | 2.24-2.46 mEq/L | |
| Chloride | 95-108 mEq/L | |
| Cholesterol, total | ≤220 mg/dL | Fasted blood required – normal value affected by dietary habits<br>This reference range is for a general adult population |
| HDL cholesterol | 40-60 mg/dL | Fasted blood required – normal value affected by dietary habits |
| LDL cholesterol | 65-170 mg/dL | LDLC calculated by Friewald formula... which has certain inaccuracies and is invalid at trig levels >300 mg/dL |
| $CO_2$ | 23-30 mEq/L | |
| Creatine kinase (CK) isoenzymes | | |
| CK-BB | 0% | |
| CK-MB (cardiac) | 0%-3.9% | |
| CK-MM (muscle) | 96%-100% | |
| CK-MB levels must be both ≥4% and 10 IU/L to meet diagnostic criteria for CK-MB positive result consistent with myocardial injury. | | |
| Creatine phosphokinase (CPK) | 8-150 IU/L | |
| Creatinine | 0.5-1.4 mg/dL | |
| Ferritin | 13-300 ng/mL | |
| Folate | 3.6-20 ng/dL | |
| GGT (gamma-glutamyltranspeptidase) | | |
| male | 11-63 IU/L | |
| female | 8-35 IU/L | |
| GLDH | To be determined | |
| Glucose (2-h postprandial) | Up to 140 mg/dL | |
| Glucose, fasting | 60-110 mg/dL | |
| Glucose, nonfasting (2-h postprandial) | 60-140 mg/dL | |
| Hemoglobin $A_{1c}$ | 8 | |
| Hemoglobin, plasma free | <2.5 mg/100 mL | |
| Hemoglobin, total glycosolated (Hb $A_1$) | 4%-8% | |
| Iron | 65-150 mcg/dL | |
| Iron binding capacity, total (TIBC) | 250-420 mcg/dL | |
| Lactic acid | 0.7-2.1 mEq/L | Specimen to be kept on ice and sent to lab as soon as possible |
| Lactate dehydrogenase (LDH) | 56-194 IU/L | |
| Lactate dehydrogenase (LDH) isoenzymes | | |
| $LD_1$ | 20%-34% | |
| $LD_2$ | 29%-41% | |
| $LD_3$ | 15%-25% | |
| $LD_4$ | 1%-12% | |
| $LD_5$ | 1%-15% | |
| Flipped $LD_1/LD_2$ ratios (>1 may be consistent with myocardial injury) particularly when considered in combination with a recent CK-MB positive result | | |
| Lipase | 23-208 units/L | |
| Magnesium | 1.6-2.5 mg/dL | Increased by slight hemolysis |
| Osmolality | 289-308 mOsm/kg | |

## Automated Chemistry (CHEMISTRY A) *(continued)*

| Test | Values | Remarks |
|---|---|---|
| Phosphatase, alkaline | | |
| adults 25-60 y | 33-131 IU/L | |
| adults 61 y or older | 51-153 IU/L | |
| infancy-adolescence | Values range up to 3-5 times higher than adults | |
| Phosphate, inorganic | 2.8-4.2 mg/dL | |
| Potassium | 3.5-5.2 mEq/L | Increased by slight hemolysis |
| Prealbumin | >15 mg/dL | |
| Protein, total | 6.5-7.9 g/dL | |
| SGOT (AST) | <35 IU/L (20-48) | |
| SGPT (ALT) (10-35) | <35 IU/L | |
| Sodium | 134-149 mEq/L | |
| Transferrin | >200 mg/dL | |
| Triglycerides | 45-155 mg/dL | Fasted blood required |
| Urea nitrogen (BUN) | 7-20 mg/dL | |
| Uric acid | | |
| male | 2.0-8.0 mg/dL | |
| female | 2.0-7.5 mg/dL | |
| **Cerebrospinal Fluid** | | |
| Glucose | 50-70 mg/dL | |
| Protein | | |
| adults and children | 15-45 mg/dL | CSF obtained by lumbar puncture |
| newborn infants | 60-90 mg/dL | |

On CSF obtained by cisternal puncture: About 25 mg/dL

On CSF obtained by ventricular puncture: About 10 mg/dL

**Note:** Bloody specimen gives erroneously high value due to contamination with blood proteins

**Urine**

**(24-hour specimen is required for all these tests unless specified)**

| Test | Values | Remarks |
|---|---|---|
| Amylase | 32-641 units/L | The value is in units/L and **not** calculated for total volume |
| Amylase, fluid (random samples) | | Interpretation of value left for physician, depends on the nature of fluid |
| Calcium | Depends upon dietary intake | |
| Creatine | | |
| male | 150 mg/24 h | Higher value on children and during pregnancy |
| female | 250 mg/24 h | |
| Creatinine | 1000-2000 mg/24 h | |
| Creatinine clearance (endogenous) | | |
| male | 85-125 mL/min | A blood sample must accompany urine specimen |
| female | 75-115 mL/min | |
| Glucose | 1 g/24 h | |
| 5-hydroxyindoleacetic acid | 2-8 mg/24 h | |
| Iron | 0.15 mg/24 h | Acid washed container required |
| Magnesium | 146-209 mg/24 h | |
| Osmolality | 500-800 mOsm/kg | With normal fluid intake |
| Oxalate | 10-40 mg/24 h | |
| Phosphate | 400-1300 mg/24 h | |
| Potassium | 25-120 mEq/24 h | Varies with diet; the interpretation of urine electrolytes and osmolality should be left for the physician |
| Sodium | 40-220 mEq/24 h | |
| Porphobilinogen, qualitative | Negative | |
| Porphyrins, qualitative | Negative | |
| Proteins | 0.05-0.1 g/24 h | |
| Salicylate | Negative | |
| Urea clearance | 60-95 mL/min | A blood sample must accompany specimen |
| Urea N | 10-40 g/24 h | Dependent on protein intake |
| Uric acid | 250-750 mg/24 h | Dependent on diet and therapy |

# CALCULATIONS/CONVERSIONS/LABORATORY VALUES *(Continued)*

## Automated Chemistry (CHEMISTRY A) *(continued)*

| Test | Values | Remarks |
|---|---|---|
| Urobilinogen | 0.5-3.5 mg/24 h | For qualitative determination on random urine, send sample to urinalysis section in Hematology Lab |
| Xylose absorption test | | |
| children | 16%-33% of ingested xylose | |
| adults | >4 g in 5 h | |
| **Feces** | | |
| Fat, 3-day collection | <5 g/d | Value depends on fat intake of 100 g/d for 3 days preceding and during collection |
| **Gastric Acidity** | | |
| Acidity, total, 12 h | 10-60 mEq/L | Titrated at pH 7 |

### Blood Gases

| | Arterial | Capillary | Venous |
|---|---|---|---|
| pH | 7.35-7.45 | 7.35-7.45 | 7.32-7.42 |
| $pCO_2$ (mm Hg) | 35-45 | 35-45 | 38-52 |
| $pO_2$ (mm Hg) | 70-100 | 60-80 | 24-48 |
| $HCO_3$ (mEq/L) | 19-25 | 19-25 | 19-25 |
| $TCO_2$ (mEq/L) | 19-29 | 19-29 | 23-33 |
| $O_2$ saturation (%) | 90-95 | 90-95 | 40-70 |
| Base excess (mEq/L) | -5 to +5 | -5 to +5 | -5 to +5 |

## HEMATOLOGY

### Complete Blood Count

| Age | Hgb (g/dL) | Hct (%) | RBC (mill/$mm^3$) | RDW |
|---|---|---|---|---|
| 0-3 d | 15.0-20.0 | 45-61 | 4.0-5.9 | <18 |
| 1-2 wk | 12.5-18.5 | 39-57 | 3.6-5.5 | <17 |
| 1-6 mo | 10.0-13.0 | 29-42 | 3.1-4.3 | <16.5 |
| 7 mo to 2 y | 10.5-13.0 | 33-38 | 3.7-4.9 | <16 |
| 2-5 y | 11.5-13.0 | 34-39 | 3.9-5.0 | <15 |
| 5-8 y | 11.5-14.5 | 35-42 | 4.0-4.9 | <15 |
| 13-18 y | 12.0-15.2 | 36-47 | 4.5-5.1 | <14.5 |
| Adult male | 13.5-16.5 | 41-50 | 4.5-5.5 | <14.5 |
| Adult female | 12.0-15.0 | 36-44 | 4.0-4.9 | <14.5 |

| Age | MCV (fL) | MCH (pg) | MCHC (%) | Plts (x $10^3/mm^3$) |
|---|---|---|---|---|
| 0-3 d | 95-115 | 31-37 | 29-37 | 250-450 |
| 1-2 wk | 86-110 | 28-36 | 28-38 | 250-450 |
| 1-6 mo | 74-96 | 25-35 | 30-36 | 300-700 |
| 7 mo to 2 y | 70-84 | 23-30 | 31-37 | 250-600 |
| 2-5 y | 75-87 | 24-30 | 31-37 | 250-550 |
| 5-8 y | 77-95 | 25-33 | 31-37 | 250-550 |
| 13-18 y | 78-96 | 25-35 | 31-37 | 150-450 |
| Adult male | 80-100 | 26-34 | 31-37 | 150-450 |
| Adult female | 80-100 | 26-34 | 31-37 | 150-450 |

## WBC and Diff

| Age | WBC ($\times 10^3/mm^3$) | Segs | Bands | Lymphs | Monos |
|---|---|---|---|---|---|
| 0-3 d | 9.0-35.0 | 32-62 | 10-18 | 19-29 | 5-7 |
| 1-2 wk | 5.0-20.0 | 14-34 | 6-14 | 36-45 | 6-10 |
| 1-6 mo | 6.0-17.5 | 13-33 | 4-12 | 41-71 | 4-7 |
| 7 mo to 2 y | 6.0-17.0 | 15-35 | 5-11 | 45-76 | 3-6 |
| 2-5 y | 5.5-15.5 | 23-45 | 5-11 | 35-65 | 3-6 |
| 5-8 y | 5.0-14.5 | 32-54 | 5-11 | 28-48 | 3-6 |
| 13-18 y | 4.5-13.0 | 34-64 | 5-11 | 25-45 | 3-6 |
| Adults | 4.5-11.0 | 35-66 | 5-11 | 24-44 | 3-6 |

| Age | Eosinophils | Basophils | Atypical Lymphs | No. of NRBCs |
|---|---|---|---|---|
| 0-3 d | 0-2 | 0-1 | 0-8 | 0-2 |
| 1-2 wk | 0-2 | 0-1 | 0-8 | 0 |
| 1-6 mo | 0-3 | 0-1 | 0-8 | 0 |
| 7 mo to 2 y | 0-3 | 0-1 | 0-8 | 0 |
| 2-5 y | 0-3 | 0-1 | 0-8 | 0 |
| 5-8 y | 0-3 | 0-1 | 0-8 | 0 |
| 13-18 y | 0-3 | 0-1 | 0-8 | 0 |
| Adults | 0-3 | 0-1 | 0-8 | 0 |

Segs = segmented neutrophils
Bands = band neutrophils
Lymphs = lymphocytes
Monos = monocytes

## Erythrocyte Sedimentation Rates and Reticulocyte Counts

| | | |
|---|---|---|
| Sedimentation rate, Westergren | Children | 0-20 mm/hour |
| | Adult male | 0-15 mm/hour |
| | Adult female | 0-20 mm/hour |
| Sedimentation rate, Wintrobe | Children | 0-13 mm/hour |
| | Adult male | 0-10 mm/hour |
| | Adult female | 0-15 mm/hour |
| Reticulocyte count | Newborns | 2%-6% |
| | 1-6 mo | 0%-2.8% |
| | Adults | 0.5%-1.5% |

# CALCULATIONS/CONVERSIONS/LABORATORY VALUES *(Continued)*

## LABORATORY REFERENCE VALUES FOR CHILDREN

### Chemistry

| | | |
|---|---|---|
| Albumin | 0-1 y | 2-4 g/dL |
| | 1 y to adult | 3.5-5.5 g/dL |
| Ammonia | Newborns | 90-150 μg/dL |
| | Children | 40-120 μg/dL |
| | Adults | 18-54 μg/dL |
| Amylase | Newborns | 0-60 units/L |
| | Adults | 30-110 units/L |
| Bilirubin, conjugated, direct | Newborns | <1.5 mg/dL |
| | 1 mo to adult | 0-0.5 mg/dL |
| Bilirubin, total | 0-3 d | 2-10 mg/dL |
| | 1 mo to adult | 0-1.5 mg/dL |
| Bilirubin, unconjugated, indirect | | 0.6-10.5 mg/dL |
| Calcium | Newborns | 7-12 mg/dL |
| | 0-2 y | 8.8-11.2 mg/dL |
| | 2 y to adult | 9-11 mg/dL |
| Calcium, ionized, whole blood | | 4.4-5.4 mg/dL |
| Carbon dioxide, total | | 23-33 mEq/L |
| Chloride | | 95-105 mEq/L |
| Cholesterol | Newborns | 45-170 mg/dL |
| | 0-1 y | 65-175 mg/dL |
| | 1-20 y | 120-230 mg/dL |
| Creatinine | 0-1 y | ≤0.6 mg/dL |
| | 1 y to adult | 0.5-1.5 mg/dL |
| Glucose | Newborns | 30-90 mg/dL |
| | 0-2 y | 60-105 mg/dL |
| | Children to adults | 70-110 mg/dL |
| Iron | Newborns | 110-270 μg/dL |
| | Infants | 30-70 μg/dL |
| | Children | 55-120 μg/dL |
| | Adults | 70-180 μg/dL |
| Iron binding | Newborns | 59-175 μg/dL |
| | Infants | 100-400 μg/dL |
| | Adults | 250-400 μg/dL |
| Lactic acid, lactate | | 2-20 mg/dL |
| Lead, whole blood | | <30 μg/dL |
| Lipase | Children | 20-140 units/L |
| | Adults | 0-190 units/L |
| Magnesium | | 1.5-2.5 mEq/L |
| Osmolality, serum | | 275-296 mOsm/kg |
| Osmolality, urine | | 50-1400 mOsm/kg |
| Phosphorus | Newborns | 4.2-9 mg/dL |
| | 6 wk to ≤18 mo | 3.8-6.7 mg/dL |
| | 18 mo to 3 y | 2.9-5.9 mg/dL |
| | 3-15 y | 3.6-5.6 mg/dL |
| | >15 y | 2.5-5 mg/dL |
| Potassium, plasma | Newborns | 4.5-7.2 mEq/L |
| | 2 d to 3 mo | 4-6.2 mEq/L |
| | 3 mo to 1 y | 3.7-5.6 mEq/L |
| | 1-16 y | 3.5-5 mEq/L |
| Protein, total | 0-2 y | 4.2-7.4 g/dL |
| | >2 y | 6-8 g/dL |
| Sodium | | 136-145 mEq/L |
| Triglycerides | Infants | 0-171 mg/dL |
| | Children | 20-130 mg/dL |
| | Adults | 30-200 mg/dL |
| Urea nitrogen, blood | 0-2 y | 4-15 mg/dL |
| | 2 y to adult | 5-20 mg/dL |

## Chemistry *(continued)*

| | | |
|---|---|---|
| Uric acid | Male | 3-7 mg/dL |
| | Female | 2-6 mg/dL |

### Enzymes

| | | |
|---|---|---|
| Alanine aminotransferase (ALT) | 0-2 mo | 8-78 units/L |
| (SGPT) | >2 mo | 8-36 units/L |
| Alkaline phosphatase (ALKP) | Newborns | 60-130 units/L |
| | 0-16 y | 85-400 units/L |
| | >16 y | 30-115 units/L |
| Aspartate aminotransferase (AST) | Infants | 18-74 units/L |
| (SGOT) | Children | 15-46 units/L |
| | Adults | 5-35 units/L |
| Creatine kinase (CK) | Infants | 20-200 units/L |
| | Children | 10-90 units/L |
| | Adult male | 0-206 units/L |
| | Adult female | 0-175 units/L |
| Lactate dehydrogenase (LDH) | Newborns | 290-501 units/L |
| | 1 mo to 2 y | 110-144 units/L |
| | >16 y | 60-170 units/L |

### Blood Gases

| | Arterial | Capillary | Venous |
|---|---|---|---|
| pH | 7.35-7.45 | 7.35-7.45 | 7.32-7.42 |
| $pCO_2$ (mm Hg) | 35-45 | 35-45 | 38-52 |
| $pO_2$ (mm Hg) | 70-100 | 60-80 | 24-48 |
| $HCO_3$ (mEq/L) | 19-25 | 19-25 | 19-25 |
| $TCO_2$ (mEq/L) | 19-29 | 19-29 | 23-33 |
| $O_2$ saturation (%) | 90-95 | 90-95 | 40-70 |
| Base excess (mEq/L) | -5 to +5 | -5 to +5 | -5 to +5 |

### Thyroid Function Tests

| | | |
|---|---|---|
| $T_4$ (thyroxine) | 1-7 d | 10.1-20.9 μg/dL |
| | 8-14 d | 9.8-16.6 μg/dL |
| | 1 mo to 1 y | 5.5-16 μg/dL |
| | >1 y | 4-12 μg/dL |
| FTI | 1-3 d | 9.3-26.6 |
| | 1-4 wks | 7.6-20.8 |
| | 1-4 mo | 7.4-17.9 |
| | 4-12 mo | 5.1-14.5 |
| | 1-6 y | 5.7-13.3 |
| | >6 y | 4.8-14 |
| $T_3$ by RIA | Newborns | 100-470 ng/dL |
| | 1-5 y | 100-260 ng/dL |
| | 5-10 y | 90-240 ng/dL |
| | 10 y to adult | 70-210 ng/dL |
| $T_3$ uptake | | 35%-45% |
| TSH | Cord | 3-22 μU/mL |
| | 1-3 d | <40 μU/mL |
| | 3-7 d | <25 μU/mL |
| | >7 d | 0-10 μU/mL |

# CALCULATIONS/CONVERSIONS/LABORATORY VALUES *(Continued)*

## MILLIEQUIVALENT CONVERSIONS

To convert mg/100 mL to mEq/L the following formula may be used:

$$\frac{(\text{mg}/100\ \text{mL}) \times 10 \times \text{valence}}{\text{atomic weight}} = \text{mEq/L}$$

To convert mEq/L to mg/100 mL the following formula may be used:

$$\frac{(\text{mEq/L}) \times \text{atomic weight}}{10 \times \text{valence}} = \text{mg}/100\ \text{mL}$$

To convert mEq/L to volume of percent of a gas the following formula may be used:

$$\frac{(\text{mEq/L}) \times 22.4}{10} = \text{volume percent}$$

### Valences and Atomic Weights of Selected Ions

| Substance | Electrolyte | Valence | Molecular Wt |
|---|---|---|---|
| Calcium | $Ca^{++}$ | 2 | 40 |
| Chloride | $Cl^{-}$ | 1 | 35.5 |
| Magnesium | $Mg^{++}$ | 2 | 24 |
| Phosphate | $HPO_4^{--}$ (80%) | 1.8 | 96* |
| pH = 7.4 | $H_2PO_4^{-}$ (20%) | 1.8 | 96* |
| Potassium | $K^{+}$ | 1 | 39 |
| Sodium | $Na^{+}$ | 1 | 23 |
| Sulfate | $SO_4^{--}$ | 2 | 96* |

*The molecular weight of phosphorus only is 31, and sulfur only is 32.

### Approximate Milliequivalents — Weights of Selected Ions

| Salt | mEq/g Salt | Mg Salt/mEq |
|---|---|---|
| Calcium carbonate [$CaCO_3$] | 20 | 50 |
| Calcium chloride [$CaCl_2 \cdot 2H_2O$] | 14 | 74 |
| Calcium gluceptate [$Ca(C_7H_{13}O_8)_2$] | 4 | 245 |
| Calcium gluconate [$Ca(C_6H_{11}O_7)_2 \cdot H_2O$] | 5 | 224 |
| Calcium lactate [$Ca(C_3H_5O_3)_2 \cdot 5H_2O$] | 7 | 154 |
| Magnesium gluconate [$Mg(C_6H_{11}O_7)_2 \cdot H_2O$] | 5 | 216 |
| Magnesium oxide [$MgO$] | 50 | 20 |
| Magnesium sulfate [$MgSO_4$] | 17 | 60 |
| Magnesium sulfate [$MgSO_4 \cdot 7H_2O$] | 8 | 123 |
| Potassium acetate [$K(C_2H_3O_2)$] | 10 | 98 |
| Potassium chloride [$KCl$] | 13 | 75 |
| Potassium citrate [$K_3(C_6H_5O_7) \cdot H_2O$] | 9 | 108 |
| Potassium iodide [$KI$] | 6 | 166 |
| Sodium acetate [$Na(C_2H_3O_2)$] | 12 | 82 |
| Sodium acetate [$Na(C_2H_3O_2) \cdot 3H_2O$] | 7 | 136 |
| Sodium bicarbonate [$NaHCO_3$] | 12 | 84 |
| Sodium chloride [$NaCl$] | 17 | 58 |
| Sodium citrate [$Na_3(C_6H_5O_7) \cdot 2H_2O$] | 10 | 98 |
| Sodium iodine [$NaI$] | 7 | 150 |
| Sodium lactate [$Na(C_3H_5O_3)$] | 9 | 112 |
| Zinc sulfate [$ZnSO_4 \cdot 7H_2O$] | 7 | 144 |

## Millimoles and Millequivalents

| **Definitions** | | |
|---|---|---|
| mole | = | gram molecular weight of a substance (aka molar weight) |
| millimole (mM) | = | milligram molecular weight of a substance (a millimole is 1/1000 of a mole) |
| equivalent weight | = | gram weight of a substance which will combine with or replace 1 gram (1 mole) of hydrogen; an equivalent weight can be determined by dividing the molar weight of a substance by its ionic valence |
| milliequivalent (mEq) | = | milligram weight of a substance which will combine with or replace 1 milligram (1 millimole) of hydrogen (a milliequivalent is 1/1000 of an equivalent) |
| **Calculations** | | |
| moles | = | $\frac{\text{weight of a substance (grams)}}{\text{molecular weight of that substance (grams)}}$ |
| millimoles | = | $\frac{\text{weight of a substance (milligrams)}}{\text{molecular weight of that substance (milligrams)}}$ |
| equivalents | = | moles x valence of ion |
| milliequivalents | = | millimoles x valence of ion |
| moles | = | $\frac{\text{equivalents}}{\text{valence of ion}}$ |
| millimoles | = | $\frac{\text{milliequivalents}}{\text{valence of ion}}$ |
| millimoles | = | moles x 1000 |
| milliequivalents | = | equivalents x 1000 |

**Note:** Use of equivalents and milliequivalents is valid only for those substances which have fixed ionic valences (eg, sodium, potassium, calcium, chlorine, magnesium bromine, etc). For substances with variable ionic valences (eg, phosphorous), a reliable equivalent value cannot be determined. In these instances, one should calculate millimoles (which are fixed and reliable) rather than milliequivalents.

# I.V. TO ORAL CONVERSION

1. **Consider drug class and indication. Conversion is acceptable only if the risk and benefit evaluation justifies conversion. Conversion should never be made only because of drug costs. The cost of failed therapy is much higher.**

   Assuming access is available, intravenous dosing rapidly produces effective serum concentrations, suitable when this benefit outweighs the risk of venous irritation/trauma, infection, and cost. Conversion from I.V. to oral is often dependent on the patient's specific clinical situation. As the clinical situation improves, oral administration may be acceptable. In general, changing the route of administration for a drug treating the patient's primary problem is to be approached with more caution than a drug which is a continuation of prior therapy.

2. **Consider pharmaceutical and pharmacokinetic issues.**

   Specifically, adjustments for bioavailability or to standard oral dosing must be made. It should be recognized that standard oral dosing is often a much lower total daily dose as compared to oral dosing (this is particularly true for some antibiotics. In addition, the patient must be able to ingest or receive the drug in the dosage form available. Drugs not available in a liquid dosage form may be difficult to convert.

3. **Consider the patient's ability to absorb drug.**

   The reliability of swallowing or enteral access should be considered. If the patient is receiving medications by an enteral access device such as an enteral feeding tube (eg, PEG, PEJ, or nasogastric), the function of these tubes should be assured. In addition, the functional status of the gastrointestinal tract must be evaluated. Obviously, NPO status normally precludes conversion to oral therapy. However, gastrointestinal motility should be assessed in all patients when a conversion is planned. The presence or suspicion of obstruction, use of multiple promotility agents, or problems with nausea/emesis should be assessed. Agents with complete absorption in ambulatory patients may not be well absorbed in acute illness. For patients receiving continuous enteral feedings, conversion should not be attempted until the patient has demonstrated an ability to tolerate feedings up to their

## CALCULATIONS/CONVERSIONS/LABORATORY VALUES *(Continued)*

goal rate. In addition, the presence or absence of diarrhea should be assessed as indicators of the patient's potential to absorb medications.

4. **Prospectively identify potential interferences with absorption.**

   Absorption of some medications may be dramatically altered in the presence of enteral feedings or specific electrolytes in the gastrointestinal tract. For example, sucralfate may reduce the absorption of fluoroquinolones to ineffective levels. In this instance, one may consider the replacement with an $H_2$antagonist to eliminate potential interferences or selection of comparable nonquinolone antibiotic coverage. Other drug binding agents include bile acid sequestrants and activated charcoal.

5. **Monitoring**

   With any change in the route of administration, consider that a recurrence may require reconsideration of the route.

### SPECIFIC MEDICATION GROUPS

#### Antibiotics

May be readily converted to oral therapy in most situations. Most institutions encourage evaluation of an initial response (3- to 5-day period) prior to oral therapy. In most cases, a lack of clinical improvement over the evaluation period or a recent change in the status should delay prompting to oral therapy.

| I.V. Agent | Usual I.V. Dose | Oral Agent | Common Oral Dose |
|---|---|---|---|
| Ampicillin | 1 g q6h | Amoxicillin | 500 mg q6h† |
| Ampicillin/ Sulbactam | 1.5-3 g q6h | Amoxicillin/ clavulanate | 500 mg q8h or 875 mg q12h |
| Azithromycin | 250 mg qd | | 250 mg qd |
| Cefazolin | 1 g q8h | Cephalexin | 500 mg q6h |
| Cefuroxime | 750 mg | Cefuroxime axetil | 250-500 mg q12h*† |
| Ciprofloxacin | 400-600 mg q12h | | 500-750 mg q12h |
| Clindamycin | 300-600 mg q8h | | 300-450 mg orally q6h |
| Co-trimoxazole | 7.5-20 mg/kg | | Equivalent # tablets (divide q6h or q12h) |
| Doxycycline | 100 mg q12h | | 100 mg q12h |
| Erythromycin | 500-1000 mg q6h | | 500 mg q6h |
| Fluconazole | 100 mg qd | | 100 mg qd |
| Levofloxacin | 500 mg q24h | | 500 mg q24h |
| Metronidazole | 500 mg q8-12h | | 500 mg q8h or 250 mg q6h |
| Ofloxacin | 200-400 mg q12h | | 200-400 mg q12h |
| Trovafloxacin | 100-200 mg qd | | 100-200 mg qd |

*Poor oral absorption.
Dose reduction.

#### Others

- $H_2$ antagonists – generally converted 1:1 to equivalent dose and scheduled orally.
- Methylprednisolone – may be converted to oral prednisone (each 4 mg methylprednisolone = 5 mg prednisone).
- Aminophylline – must be calculated based on infusion rate. However, a simple conversion calculation is possible: dose in mg/h x 10 = dose of sustained release product to be given every 12 hours (ie, a typical infusion of 30 mg/h = 300 mg of sustained release theophylline q12h or 150 mg q6h of nonsustained release product.

# PEDIATRIC DOSAGE ESTIMATIONS

Augsberger's rule:

(1.5 x weight in kg + 10) = child's approximate dose
% of adult dose

Clark's rule:

$$\frac{\text{weight (in pounds)}}{150} \times \text{adult dose} = \text{child's approximate dose}$$

## Dosage Estimations Based on Age

Augsberger's rule:

(4 x age in years + 20) = child's approximate dose
% of adult dose

Bastedo's rule:

$$\frac{\text{age in years} + 3}{30} \times \text{adult dose} = \text{child's approximate dose}$$

Cowling's rule:

$$\frac{\text{age at next birthday (in years)}}{24} \times \text{adult dose} = \text{child's approximate dose}$$

Dilling's rule:

$$\frac{\text{age (in years)}}{20} \times \text{adult dose} = \text{child's approximate dose}$$

Fried's rule for infants (younger than 1 year):

$$\frac{\text{age (in months)}}{150} \times \text{adult dose} = \text{infant's approximate dose}$$

Young's rule:

$$\frac{\text{age (in years)}}{\text{age} + 12} \times \text{adult dose} = \text{child's approximate dose}$$

# ACE INHIBITORS AND ANGIOTENSIN ANTAGONISTS COMPARISON*

| | Benazepril (Lotensin®) | Captopril (Capoten®) | Enalapril (Vasotec®) | Enalaprilat (Vasotec®) | Fosinopril (Monopril®) | Lisinopril (Prinvil®, Zestril®) | Moexipril (Univasc®) | Quinapril (Accupril®) | Ramipril (Altace™) | Trandolapril (Mavik®) |
|---|---|---|---|---|---|---|---|---|---|---|
| Route | P.O. | P.O. | P.O. | I.V. | P.O. | P.O. | P.O. | P.O. | P.O. | P.O. |
| Dosage forms (mg) | 5<br>10<br>20<br>40 | 12.5<br>25<br>50<br>100 | 2.5<br>5<br>10<br>20 | 1.25 mg/mL | 10<br>20 | 2.5<br>5.0<br>10<br>20<br>40 | 7.5<br>15 | 5<br>10<br>20<br>40 | 1.25<br>2.5<br>5<br>10 | 1<br>2<br>4 |
| Usual starting dose (mg) | 10 | 12.5-25 | 5 | 1.25 mg/mL | 10 | 5 | 7.5 | 10 | 2.5 | 1-2 |
| Starting dose in renal impairment (<30 mL/min) | 5 mg/d | 50%-75% | 2.5 mg/d | 0.625 | No adjustment | 2.5-5 | 3.75 | 2.5-5 | 1.25 | 1 mg |
| Dosing interval | qd | tid | qd | q6h over 5 min | qd | qd | qd | qd | qd | qd |
| Indications and starting dose | | | | | | | | | | |
| HTN | 10 mg qd<br>5 mg qd# | 12.5-25 mg bid-tid | 5 mg qd<br>2.5 mg qd# | x | 10 mg qd | 10 mg qd<br>5 mg qd# | 7.5 mg qd<br>3.75 mg qd• | 10 mg qd<br>5 mg qd¶ | 2.5 mg qd<br>1.25 mg qd• | 1 mg nonblack patient<br>2 mg black patient |
| CHF | | 12.5-25 mg tid | 2.5 mg qd-bid | | 10 mg qd | 5 mg qd | | 5 mg bid¶<br>2.5 mg bid# | 2.5 mg bid<br>1.25 mg qd• | |
| Protein binding | >95% | 25%-30% | | 50%-60% | ~95% | — | ~50% | <97% | ~73% ramipril<br>56% ramiprilat | 80% |
| Absorption (%) | 37 | 75 | 60 | I.V. | 36 | 25 | No | 60 | 50-100 | 10-70 |
| Prodrug | Y | N | Y | N | Y | N | Y | Y | Y | Y |
| Active metabolites | Benazeprilat | | Enalaprilat | | Fosinoprilat | | Moexiprilat | Quinaprilat | Ramiprilat | Trandolaprilat |
| Half-life normal renal function (h) | 10-11† | <2 | 1.3 | 11 | 12‡ | 12 | 2-9 (moexiprilat) | 2 | 13-17 | 6-10 |
| Half-life impaired renal function (h) | Prolonged | 3.5-32 | No data | Prolonged | Prolonged | Prolonged | Prolonged | Prolonged | Prolonged | Prolonged |
| Onset (h) | 0.5-1 | <0.5 | 4-6 | 0.25 | 1 | 1 | 1 | 1 | 1-2 | 0.5 |
| Peak (h) | 0.5-1 | 0.5-1.5 | 4-6 | 3-4 | ~3 | ~7 | | 1 | 1 | 2-4 |

| | Benazepril (Lotensin®) | Captopril (Capoten®) | Enalapril (Vasotec®) | Enalaprilat (Vasotec®) | Fosinopril (Monopril®) | Lisinopril (Prinvil®, Zestril®) | Moexipril (Univasc®) | Quinapril (Accupril®) | Ramipril (Altace™) | Trandolapril (Mavik®) |
|---|---|---|---|---|---|---|---|---|---|---|
| Duration | 24 | 6-12 | 24 | ~6 | 24 | 24 | 24 | 24 | 24 | >24 |
| Elimination | | | | | | | | | | |
| Total | No data | >95% | 94% urine and feces | No data | 50% urine 50% feces | No data | 13% urine 53% feces | 60% urine 37% feces | 60% urine 40% feces | 33% urine 66% feces |
| Unchanged | Trace | 40%-50% urine | 54% urine (40% enalapril) | >90% urine | Negligible | 100% urine§ | 1% urine 1% feces | Trace | <2§ | - |
| Incidence of side effects (%) | | | | | | | | | | |
| Cough | 1.9-3.4 | 0.5-2 | 1.3-2.2 | | 2.2 | 2.9-4.5 | 6.1 | 2 | 12 | 1.9 |
| Angioedema | 0.5 | 0.1 | 0.2 | | ≤1 | 0.1 | <1 | 0.1 | 0.3 | <1 |
| Rash | x | 4-7 | 1.3-1.4 | | ≤1 | 1.5 | 1.6 | x | x | <1 |
| Headache | 5 | 0.5-2 | 1.8-5.2 | | 3.2 | 5.3 | >1 | 5.6 | 5.4 | 1.3 |
| Dizziness | 3.3 | 0.5-2 | 4.3-7.9 | | 1.6 | 6.3 | 4.3 | 3.9 | 2.2 | <1 |
| Chest pain | | 1 | 2.1 | | ≤1 | 1.3 | >1 | x | <1 | <1 |
| Hypotension | 0.3 | x | 6.7 | | ≤1 | 1.2-5 | 0.5 | x | 0.5 | <1 |
| Diarrhea | | 0.5-2 | 1.4-2.1 | | 1.5 | 3.2 | 3.1 | x | <1 | 1 |

*All doses listed are oral and assume patient is **not** on a diuretic. See specific drug monograph for dosing concurrently with diuretics to avoid adverse reactions.

†Half-life accumulates after multiple dosing.

‡Fosinoprilat, after I.V. administration.

§Time frame undefined.

¶$Cl_{cr}$ 30-60 mL/min.

#$Cl_{cr}$ 10-30 mL/min.

•$Cl_{cr}$ <40 mL/min.

x — reported, no incidence given.

# ACE INHIBITORS AND ANGIOTENSIN ANTAGONISTS COMPARISON* *(Continued)*

**Comparisons of Indications and Adult Dosages**

| Drug | Hypertension | CHF | Renal Dysfunction | Dialyzable | Strengths (mg) |
|---|---|---|---|---|---|
| Benazepril | 20-80 mg qd<br>qd-bid<br>Maximum: 80 mg qd | Not FDA approved | $Cl_{cr}$ <30 mL/min: 5 mg/day initially<br>Maximum: 40 mg qd | Yes | Tablets<br>5, 10, 20, 40 |
| Candesartan | 8-32 mg qd<br>qd-bid<br>Maximum: 32 mg qd | Not approved | No adjustment necessary | No | Tablets<br>4, 8, 16, 32 |
| Captopril | 25-150 mg qd<br>bid-tid<br>Maximum: 450 mg qd | 6.25-100 mg tid<br>Maximum: 450 mg qd | $Cl_{cr}$ 10-50 mL/min: 75% of usual dose<br>$Cl_{cr}$ <10 mL/min: 50% of usual dose | Yes | Tablets<br>12.5, 25, 50, 100 |
| Enalapril | 5-40 mg qd<br>qd-bid<br>Maximum: 40 mg qd | 2.5-20 mg bid<br>Maximum: 20 mg bid | $Cl_{cr}$ 30-80 mL/min: 5 mg/day initially<br>$Cl_{cr}$ <30 mL/min: 2.5 mg/day initially | Yes | Tablets<br>2.5, 5, 10, 20 |
| (Enalaprilat*) | (0.625 mg, 1.25 mg, 2.5 mg<br>q6h<br>Maximum: 5 mg q6h) | (Not FDA approved) | $Cl_{cr}$ <30 mL/min: 0.625 mg) | (Yes) | (2.5 mg/2 mL vial) |
| Fosinopril | 10-40 mg qd<br>Maximum: 80 mg qd | 10-40 mg qd | No dosage reduction necessary | Not well dialyzed | Tablets<br>10, 20 |
| Irbesartan† | 150 mg qd<br>Maximum: 300 mg qd | Not FDA approved | No dosage reduction necessary | No | Tablets<br>75, 150, 300 |
| Lisinopril | 10-40 mg qd<br>Maximum: 80 mg qd | 5-20 mg qd | $Cl_{cr}$ 10-30 mL/min: 5 mg/day initially<br>$Cl_{cr}$ <10 mL/min: 2.5 mg/day initially | Yes | Tablets<br>5, 10, 20, 40 |
| Losartan† | 25-100 mg qd or bid | | No adjustment needed | No | Tablets<br>25, 50 |
| Moexipril | 7.5-30 mg qd<br>qd-bid<br>Maximum: 30 mg qd | Not FDA approved | $Cl_{cr}$ <30 mL/min: 3.75 mg/day initially<br>Maximum: 15 mg/day | Unknown | Tablets<br>7.5, 15 |
| Quinapril | 10-80 mg qd<br>qd-bid | 5-20 mg bid | $Cl_{cr}$ 30-60 mL/min: 5 mg/day initially<br>$Cl_{cr}$ <10 mL/min: 2.5 mg qd initially | Not well dialyzed | Tablets<br>5, 10, 20, 40 |
| Ramipril | 2.5-20 mg qd<br>qd-bid | 2.5-20 mg qd | $Cl_{cr}$ <40 mL/min: 1.25 mg/day<br>Maximum: 5 mg qd | Unknown | Capsules<br>1.25, 2.5, 5 |

## Comparisons of Indications and Adult Dosages *(continued)*

| Drug | Hypertension | CHF | Renal Dysfunction | Dialyzable | Strengths (mg) |
|---|---|---|---|---|---|
| Telmisartan | 20-80 mg qd | Not FDA approved | No dosage reduction necessary | No | Tablets<br>40, 80 |
| Trandolapril | 2-4 mg qd<br>maximum: 8 mg/d<br>qd-bid | Not FDA approved | $Cl_{cr}$ <30 mL/min: 0.5 mg/day initially | No | Tablets<br>1 mg, 2 mg, 4 mg |
| Valsartan† | 80-160 mg qd | Not FDA approved | Decrease dose only if $Cl_{cr}$ <10 mL/minute | No | Capsules<br>80, 160 |

*Enalaprilat is the only available ACEI in a parenteral formulation.

†Angiotensin II antagonist

Dosage is based on 70 kg adult with normal hepatic and renal function.

# ANTIARRHYTHMIC DRUG CLASSIFICATION COMPARISON

## Vaughan Williams Classification of Antiarrhythmic Agents and Their Indications/Adverse Effects

| Drug(s) | Indication | Route of Administration | Adverse Effects |
|---|---|---|---|
| Adenosine | SVT, PSVT | I.V. | Flushing, dizziness, bradycardia, syncope |
| Amiodarone | VT | P.O. | CNS, GI, thyroid, pulmonary fibrosis, liver, corneal deposits |
| Bretylium | VT, VF | I.V. | GI, orthostatic hypotension, CNS |
| Digoxin | AF, PSVT | P.O./I.V. | GI, CNS, arrhythmias |
| Diltiazem | AF, PSVT | P.O./I.V. | Hypotension, GI, liver |
| Disopyramide | AF, VT | P.O. | Anticholinergic effects, CHF |
| Esmolol | VT, SVT | I.V. | CHF, CNS, lupus-like syndrome, hypotension, bradycardia, bronchospasm |
| Flecainide | VT | P.O. | CHF, GI, CNS, blurred vision |
| Ibutilide | VT, VF | I.V. | Torsade de pointes, hypotension, branch bundle block, AV block, nausea, headache |
| Lidocaine | VT, VF, PVC | I.V. | CNS, GI |
| Magnesium | VT, VF | I.V. | Hypotension, CNS, hypothermia, myocardial depression |
| Mexiletine | VT | P.O. | GI, CNS |
| Moricizine | VT | P.O. | Dizziness, nausea, rash, seizures |
| Procainamide | AF, VT, WPW | P.O./I.V. | GI, CNS, lupus, fever, hematological, anticholinergic effects |
| Propafenone | VT | P.O. | GI, blurred vision, dizziness |
| Propranolol | SVT, VT, PVC, digoxin toxicity | P.O./I.V. | CHF, bradycardia, hypotension, CNS, fatigue |
| Quinidine | AF, PSVT, VT, WPW | P.O./I.V. | Hypotension, GI, thrombocytopenia, cinchonism |
| Sotalol | VT | P.O. | Bradycardia, hypotension, CHF, CNS, fatigue |
| Tocainide | VT | P.O. | GI, CNS, pulmonary, agranulocytosis |
| Verapamil | AF, PSVT | P.O./I.V. | Hypotension, CHF, bradycardia, vertigo, constipation |

AF = atrial fibrillation; PSVT = paroxysmal supraventricular tachycardia; VT = ventricular tachycardia; WPW = Wolf-Parkinson-White arrhythmias; VF = ventricular fibrillation; SVT = supraventricular tachycardia.

## Comparative Pharmacokinetic Properties of Antiarrhythmic Agents

| Drug(s) | Bioavailability (%) | Primary Route of Elimination | Volume of Distribution (L/kg) | Protein Binding (%) | Half-Life | Therapeutic Range (mcg/mL) |
|---|---|---|---|---|---|---|
| Amiodarone | 22-28 | Hepatic | 70-150 | 95-97 | 15-100 d | 1-2.5 |
| Bretylium | 15-20 | Renal | 4-8 | Negligible | 5-10 h | 0.5-2 |
| Diltiazem | 80-90 | Hepatic/Renal | 1.7 | 77-85 | 4-6 h | 0.05-0.2 |
| Disopyramide | 70-95 | Hepatic/Renal | 0.8-2 | 50-80 | 4-8 h | 2-6 |
| Esmolol | Refer to Beta-Blocker Comparison Chart | | | | | |
| Flecainide | 90-95 | Hepatic/Renal | 8-10 | 35-45 | 12-30 h | 0.3-2.5 |
| Ibutilide | – | Renal | 11 L/kg | 40% | 2-12 h | – |
| Lidocaine | 20-40 | Hepatic | 1-2 | 65-75 | 60-180 min | 1.5-5 |
| Mexiletine | 80-95 | Hepatic | 5-12 | 60-75 | 6-12 h | 0.75-2 |
| Moricizine | 34-38 | Hepatic | 6-11 | 92-95 | 1-6 h | — |
| Procainamide | 75-95 | Hepatic/Renal | 1.5-3 | 10-20 | 2.5-5 h | 4-15 |
| Propafenone* | 11-39 | Hepatic | 2.5-4 | 85-95 | 12-32 h<br>2-10 h | — |
| Propranolol | Refer to Beta-Blocker Comparison Chart | | | | | |
| Quinidine | 70-80 | Hepatic | 2-3.5 | 80-90 | 5-9 h | 2-6 |
| Sotalol | 90-95 | Renal | 1.6-2.4 | Negligible | 12-15 h | — |
| Tocainide | 90-95 | Hepatic | 1.5-3 | 10-30 | 12-15 h | 4-10 |
| Verapamil | 20-40 | Hepatic | 1.5-5 | 95-99 | 4-12 h | >50 ng/mL |

*__Top__ numbers reflect **poor** metabolizers and **bottom** numbers reflect **extensive** metabolizers

# ANTIDEPRESSANT AGENTS COMPARISON

| Drug | Class | Anticholinergic Side Effects | Cardiac Arrhythmia | Sedation | Orthostatic Hypotension | Time to Reach Steady State (d) | Half-life (h) | Dosage Range* (mg/d) |
|---|---|---|---|---|---|---|---|---|
| Amitriptyline (Elavil®) | TCA | ++++ | +++ | ++++ | ++ | 4-10 | 31-46 | 50-300 |
| Amoxapine (Asendin®) | TCA | +++ | ++ | ++ | + | 2-7 | 8 | 50-600 |
| Bupropion (Wellbutrin®) | Amino ketone | ++ | + | ++ | + | 1.5-5 | 8-24 | 200-450 |
| Citalopram (Celexa®) | SRI | 0 | 0 | 0 | 0 | 5-10 | 24-48 | 20-60 |
| Clomipramine (Anafranil®) | TCA | +++ | +++ | +++ | ++ | 7-14 | 19-37 | 25-250 |
| Desipramine (Norpramin®) | TCA | + | ++ | + | + | 2-11 | 12-24 | 25-300 |
| Doxepin (Sinequan®) | TCA | ++ | ++ | +++ | ++ | 2-8 | 8-24 | 25-300 |
| Fluoxetine (Prozac®) | SRI | 0/+ | 0 | 0/+ | 0/+ | 28-35 | 48-216 | 20-80 |
| Fluvoxamine (Luvox®) | SRI | + | 0 | — | + | 4-7 | 15 | 50-300 |
| Imipramine (Tofranil®) | TCA | ++ | +++ | ++ | +++ | 2-5 | 11-25 | 30-300 |
| Maprotiline (Ludiomil®) | Tetracyclic | ++ | ++ | ++ | + | 6-10 | 21-25 | 50-225 |
| Mirtazapine (Remeron®) | Tetracyclic | ++ | + | ++++ | + | 5 | 20-40 | 15-45 |
| Nefazodone (Serzone®) | Phenylpiperazine | + | + | + | + | 4-5 | 2-4 | 50-600 |

| Drug | Class | Anticholinergic Side Effects | Cardiac Arrhythmia | Sedation | Orthostatic Hypotension | Time to Reach Steady State (d) | Half-life (h) | Dosage Range* (mg/d) |
|---|---|---|---|---|---|---|---|---|
| Nortriptyline (Pamelor®, Aventyl®) | TCA | ++ | ++ | ++ | + | 4-19 | 18-44 | 30-100 |
| Paroxetine (Paxil™) | SRI | 0 | 0 | 0/+ | 0 | ~10 | 10-24 | 10-50 |
| Phenelzine (Nardil®) | MAO inhibitor | + | — | + | + | — | 2.4-2.8 | 45-90 |
| Protriptyline (Vivactil®) | TCA | +++ | +++ | + | + | 14-19 | 67-89 | 15-60 |
| Sertraline (Zoloft®) | SRI | 0 | 0 | + | 0 | 7 | 26 to >100 | 50-200 |
| Tranylcypromine (Parnate®) | MAO inhibitor | + | — | + | 0 | — | — | 30-60 |
| Trazodone (Desyrel®) | Triazalopyridine | + | + | ++ | ++ | 3-7 | 4-9 | 150-600 |
| Trimipramine (Surmontil®) | TCA | ++ | +++ | +++ | ++ | 2-6 | 7-30 | 50-300 |
| Venlafaxine (Effexor®) | Phenylethylamine | 0 | + | 0 | 0 | 3-4 | 5-11 | 75-375 |

TCA = tricyclic antidepressant.
SRI = serotonin reuptake inhibitor.
*This dosage range represents manufacturer guidelines and must be individualized for age, indication, and concurrent disease states.

# ANTIDIABETIC ORAL AGENTS COMPARISON

| | (Onset) Duration (h) | Usual Starting Dose | Equivalent Dose |
|---|---|---|---|
| **Sulfonylureas** | | | |
| ***First Generation*** | | | |
| Acetohexamide (Dymelor®) | (1) 12-24 | 250-1500 mg bid | 500 mg |
| Chlorpropamide (Diabinese®) | (1) May be >60 | 100-500 mg qd | 250 mg |
| Tolazamide (Tolinase®) | (4-6) 10-24 | 100-1000 mg qd-bid | 250 mg |
| Tolbutamide (Orinase®) | (1) 6-24 | 500-2000 mg qid-tid | 1000 mg |
| ***Second Generation*** | | | |
| Glimepiride (Amaryl®) | (2-3) 24 | 1-4 mg qd | ND |
| Glipizide (Glucotrol®) | (1) 12-24 | 2.5-40 mg qd or bid | 10 mg |
| Glipizide (Glucotrol® XL sustained release) | 24 | 5-10 mg qd | |
| Glyburide, nonmicronized (Diaβeta®, Micronase®) | (1) 24 | 1.25-20 mg qd or bid | 5 mg |
| Glyburide, micronized (Glynase™, PresTab™) | 24 | 0.75 mg qd | 3 mg |
| **Biguanides** | | | |
| Metformin (Glucophage®) | (1-3) 12 | 500 mg bid | ND |
| **Alpha Glucosidase Inhibitors** | | | |
| Acarbose (Precose™) | | 25 mg tid with each meal | ND |
| Miglitol (Glyset™) | | 25 mg tid with each meal | ND |
| **Thiazolidinedione** | | | |
| Troglitazone (Rezulin®) | 8 wk | 200-600 mg qd | ND |
| **Meglitinides** | | | |
| Repaglinide (Prandin®) | <1 | 0.5-1 mg before each meal | ND |

*See monograph for renal impairment.

ND = no data.

## Comparison of Contraindications and Adverse Effects

| | Sulfonylureas | Metformin | Acarbose | Troglitazone |
|---|---|---|---|---|
| | **Contraindications** | | | |
| Insulin dependency | A | A | A* | |
| Pregnancy/lactation | A | A | A | |
| Hypersensitivity to the agent | A | A | A | A |
| Hepatic impairment | R | A | R | A |
| Renal impairment | R | A | R | |
| Congestive heart failure | | A | | R |
| Chronic lung disease | | A | | |
| Peripheral vascular disease | | A | | |
| Steroid-induced diabetes | R | R | | |
| Inflammatory bowel disease | | A | A | |
| Major recurrent illness | R | A | | |
| Surgery | R | A | | |
| Alcoholism | R | A | | |
| | **Adverse Effects** | | | |
| Hypoglycemia | Yes | No | No | N |
| Body weight gain | Yes | No | No | N |
| Hypersensitivity | Yes | No | No | |
| Drug interactions | Yes | No | No | Y |
| Lactic acidosis | No | Yes | No | |
| Gastrointestinal disturbances | No | Yes | No | N |

*Can be used in conjunction with insulin. A = absolute; R = relative.

# ANTIPSYCHOTIC AGENTS COMPARISON

| Antipsychotic Agent | I.M./P.O. Potency | Equivalent Dosages (approx) (mg) | Usual Adult Daily Maintenance Dose (mg) | Sedation (Incidence) | Extrapyramidal Side Effects | Anticholinergic Side Effects | Cardiovascular Side Effects | Comments |
|---|---|---|---|---|---|---|---|---|
| Acetophenazine (Tindal®) | | 20 | 60-120 | Moderate | High | Low | Low | |
| Chlorpromazine (Thorazine®) | 4:1 | 100 | 200-1000 | High | Moderate | Moderate | Moderate/high | |
| Chlorprothixine* (Taractan®) | | 100 | 75-600 | High | Moderate | Moderate | Moderate | |
| Clozapine (Clozaril®) | | 50 | 75-900 | High | Very Low | High | High | <1% incidence of agranulocytosis; weekly-biweekly CBC required |
| Fluphenazine (Prolixin®, Permitil®) | 2:1 | 2 | 0.5-40 | Low | High | Low | Low | |
| Haloperidol (Haldol®) | 2:1 | 2 | 1-15 | Low | High | Low | Low | |
| Loxapine (Loxitane®) | | 10 | 25-250 | Moderate | Moderate | Low | Low | |
| Mesoridazine (Serentil®) | 3:1 | 50 | 30-400 | High | Low | High | Moderate | |
| Molindone (Moban®) | | 15 | 15-225 | Low | Moderate | Low | Low | May cause less weight gain |
| Olanzapine (Zyprexa™) | | 2 | 5-20 | Moderate/ High | Low | Moderate/High | Moderate/High | |
| Perphenazine (Trilafon®) | | 10 | 16-64 | Low | Moderate | Low | Low | |
| Pimozide (Orap™) | | 0.3-0.5 | 1-20 | Moderate | High | Moderate | Low | Contraindicated with macrolide antibiotics |
| Promazine (Sparine®) | | 200 | 40-1000 | Moderate | Moderate | High | Moderate | |
| Quetiapine (Seroquel®) | | N/A | 75-750 | Moderate | Very Low | Moderate | Moderate | |

## ANTIPSYCHOTIC AGENTS COMPARISON *(Continued)*

| Antipsychotic Agent | I.M./P.O. Potency | Equivalent Dosages (approx) (mg) | Usual Adult Daily Maintenance Dose (mg) | Sedation (Incidence) | Extrapyramidal Side Effects | Anticholinergic Side Effects | Cardiovascular Side Effects | Comments |
|---|---|---|---|---|---|---|---|---|
| Risperidone (Risperdal®) | | 1 | 1-16 | Low/ Moderate | Low | Low | Low | Target dose: 4-6 mg/d |
| Thioridazine (Mellaril®) | | 100 | 200-800 | High | Low | High | Moderate/high | May cause irreversible retinitis; pigmentosis at doses >800 mg/d |
| Thiothixene (Navane®) | 4:1 | 4 | 5-40 | Low | High | Low | Low/moderate | |
| Trifluoperazine (Stelazine®) | | 5 | 2-40 | Low | High | Low | Low | |

NA = not available

*Withdrawn from market

# ANTIRETROVIRAL AGENTS COMPARISON

## Renal Dosing Adjustment, Dosage Forms, and Adverse Reactions

| Chemical and Generic Names | Brand Name (company) | Dose (renal adjustment) | Dosage Forms | Adverse Reaction |
|---|---|---|---|---|
| **NRTIs (Nucleoside Reverse Transcriptase Inhibitors)** | | | | |
| Zidovudine (AZT) | Retrovir® (Glaxo-Wellcome) | 200 mg tid or 300 mg bid on empty stomach<br>(ESRD: 100 mg q6-8 h) | Tablet: 300 mg<br>Capsule: 100 mg<br>Syrup: 50 mg/mL (240 mL)<br>Injection: 10 mg/mL (20 mL) | Anemia, neutropenia, thrombocytopenia, headache, nausea, vomiting, myopathy, hepatitis, hyperpigmentation of nails |
| Zidovudine/ lamivudine | Combivir® (Glaxo-Wellcome) | 1 tablet bid (see lamivudine for dose adjustment) | Tablet: 300 mg zidovudine, 150 mg lamivudine | See individual agents |
| Didanosine (ddI) | Videx® (Bristol-Myers Squibb) | ≥60 kg: 200 mg bid on empty stomach<br><60 kg: 125 mg bid (adjust for $Cl_{cr}$ <60) | Tablet, chewable: 25 mg, 50 mg, 100 mg, 150 mg<br>Powder, oral: 100 mg, 167 mg, 250 mg, 375 mg<br>Powder, pediatric: 2 g, 4 g | Peripheral neuropathy, pancreatitis, abdominal pain, nausea, diarrhea, retinal depigmentation, anxiety, insomnia |
| Zalcitabine (ddC) | Hivid® (Roche) | 0.75 mg tid on empty stomach<br>$Cl_{cr}$ 10-40: bid<br>$Cl_{cr}$ <10: qd | Tablet: 0.375 mg, 0.75 mg | Peripheral neuropathy, oral/esophageal ulceration, rash, nausea, vomiting, diarrhea, abdominal pain, myalgia, pancreatitis |
| Stavudine (d4T) | Zerit® (Bristol-Myers Squibb) | ≥60 kg: 40 mg bid<br>$Cl_{cr}$ 26-50: 20 mg bid<br>$Cl_{cr}$ 10-25: 20 mg qd<br><60 kg: 30 mg bid<br>$Cl_{cr}$ 26-50: 15 mg bid<br>$Cl_{cr}$ 10-25: 15 mg qd | Capsule: 15 mg, 20 mg, 30 mg, 40 mg<br>Solution, oral: 1 mg/mL (200 mL) | Peripheral neuropathy, headache, abdominal or back pain, asthenia, nausea, vomiting, diarrhea, myalgia, anxiety, depression, pancreatitis, less frequently hepatotoxicity |
| Lamivudine (3TC) | Epivir® (Glaxo-Wellcome) | ≥50 kg: 150 mg bid<br><50 kg: 2 mg/kg bid<br>$Cl_{cr}$ 30-49: 150 mg qd<br>$Cl_{cr}$ 15-29: 150 mg first dose, then 100 mg qd<br>$Cl_{cr}$ 5-14: 150 mg first dose, then 50 mg qd<br>$Cl_{cr}$ <5: 50 mg first dose, then 25 mg qd | Tablet: 150 mg<br>Solution, oral: 10 mg/mL (240 mL) | Headache, insomnia, nausea, vomiting, diarrhea, abdominal pain, myalgia, arthralgia, pancreatitis in children |
| Abacavir | Ziagen® (Glaxo-Wellcome) | 300 mg bid | Tablet: 300 mg<br>Solution, oral: 20 mg/mL (240 mL) | Hypersensitivity syndrome (fever, fatigue, GI symptoms, ±rash); **do not restart abacavir in patients who have experienced this**; GI symptoms |

## ANTIRETROVIRAL AGENTS COMPARISON *(Continued)*

### Renal Dosing Adjustment, Dosage Forms, and Adverse Reactions *(continued)*

| Chemical and Generic Names | Brand Name (company) | Dose (renal adjustment) | Dosage Forms | Adverse Reaction |
|---|---|---|---|---|
| **NNRTIs (Non-nucleoside Reverse Transcriptase Inhibitors)** | | | | |
| Nevirapine | Viramune® (Roxane) | 200 mg qd for 14 days, then 200 mg bid | Tablet: 200 mg | Rash (severe), abnormal liver function tests, fever, nausea, headache |
| Delavirdine | Rescriptor® (Pharmacia/Upjohn) | 400 mg tid | Tablet: 100 mg | Rash |
| Efavirenz | Sustiva™ (DuPont) | 600 mg qd | Capsule: 50 mg, 100 mg, 200 mg | Dizziness, psychiatric symptoms (hallucinations, confusion, depersonalization, others), agitation, vivid dreams, rash, GI intolerance |
| **PIs (Protease Inhibitors)** | | | | |
| Saquinavir | Invirase® (Roche)<br>Fortavase® (Roche) | 600 mg tid with a full meal<br>1200 mg tid with a full meal | Capsule: 200 mg<br>Gelcap: 200 mg | Diarrhea, abdominal discomfort, nausea, headache, hyperglycemia/diabetes, dyslipidemia |
| Ritonavir | Norvir® (Abbott) | 600 mg bid with food (titrate) | Capsule: 100 mg<br>Solution, oral: 80 mg/mL (240 mL) | Asthenia, nausea, diarrhea, vomiting, anorexia, abdominal pain, circumoral and peripheral paresthesia, taste perversion, headache, hyperglycemia/diabetes, dyslipidemia |
| Indinavir | Crixivan® (Merck) | 800 mg q8h with water<br>(Hepatic insufficiency: 600 mg tid) | Capsule: 200 mg, 400 mg | Hyperbilirubinemia, nephrolithiasis, elevated AST/ALT, abdominal pain, nausea, vomiting, diarrhea, taste perversion, hyperglycemia/diabetes, dyslipidemia |
| Nelfinavir | Viracept® (Agouron) | 750 mg tid with food | Tablet: 250 mg<br>Powder, oral: 50 mg/g (144 g) | Diarrhea, nausea, hyperglycemia/diabetes, dyslipidemia |
| Amprenavir | Agenerase (Glaxo-Wellcome) | 1200 mg bid (avoid high fat meal) | Capsule: 150 mg<br>Solution, oral: 15 mg/mL (240 mL) | Rash (life-threatening), paresthesias (perioral), depression, nausea, diarrhea, vomiting, hyperglycemia/diabetes, dyslipidemia |

# BENZODIAZEPINES COMPARISON

| Agent | Relative Potency | Peak Blood Levels (oral) (h) | Protein Binding (%) | Volume of Distribution (L/kg) | Major Active Metabolite | Half-Life (parent) (h) | Half-Life* (metabolite) (h) | Usual Initial Dose | Adult Oral Dosage Range |
|---|---|---|---|---|---|---|---|---|---|
| **Anxiolytic** | | | | | | | | | |
| Alprazolam (Xanax®) | 0.5 | 1-2 | 80 | 0.9-1.2 | No | 12-15 | — | 0.25-0.5 tid | 0.75-4 mg/d |
| Chlordiazepoxide (Librium®) | 10 | 2-4 | 90-98 | 0.3 | Yes | 5-30 | 24-96 | 5-25 mg tid-qid | 15-100 mg/d |
| Diazepam (Valium®) | 5 | 0.5-2 | 98 | 1.1 | Yes | 20-80 | 50-100 | 2-10 mg bid-qid | 4-40 mg/d |
| Halazepam (Paxipam®) | 20 | | | | Yes | 14 | 50-100 | 20-40 mg tid-qid | 80-160 mg/d |
| Lorazepam (Ativan®)** | 1 | 1-6 | 88-92 | 1.3 | No | 10-20 | — | 0.5-2 mg tid-qid | 2-4 mg/d |
| Oxazepam (Serax®) | 15-30 | 2-4 | 86-99 | 0.6-2 | No | 5-20 | — | 10-30 mg tid-qid | 30-120 mg/d |
| Prazepam (Centrax®) | 10 | | | | Yes | 1.2 | 30-100 | 10 mg tid | 30 mg/d |
| **Sedative/Hypnotic** | | | | | | | | | |
| Estazolam (ProSom™) | 0.3 | 2 | 93 | — | No | 10-24 | — | 1 mg qhs | 1-2 mg |
| Flurazepam (Dalmane®) | 5 | 0.5-2 | 97 | — | Yes | Not significant | 40-114 | 15 mg qhs | 15-60 mg |
| Quazepam (Doral®) | 5 | 2 | 95 | 5 | Yes | 25-41 | 28-114 | 15 mg qhs | 7.5-15 mg |
| Temazepam (Restoril®) | 5 | 2-3 | 96 | 1.4 | No | 10-40 | — | 15-30 mg qhs | 15-30 mg |
| Triazolam (Halcion®) | 0.1 | 1 | 89-94 | 0.8-1.3 | No | 2.3 | — | 0.125-0.25 qhs | 0.125-0.25 mg |
| **Miscellaneous** | | | | | | | | | |
| Clonazepam (Klonopin™) | 0.25-0.5 | 1-2 | 86 | 1.8-4 | No | 18-50 h | — | 0.5 mg tid | 1.5-20 mg/d |
| Clorazepate (Tranxene®) | 7.5 | 1-2 | 80-95 | — | Yes | Not significant | 50-100 h | 7.5-15 mg bid-qid | 15-60 mg |
| Midazolam (Versed®) | 1.5 | 0.4-0.7† | 95 | 0.8-6.6 | No | 2-5 h | — | Individualized | NA |

* = significant metabolite.
**Reliable bioavailability when given I.M.
† = I.V. only.
NA = not available.

# BETA-BLOCKERS COMPARISON

| Agent* | Adrenergic Receptor Blocking Activity | Lipid Solubility | Protein Bound (%) | Half-life (h) | Bioavailability (%) | Primary (Secondary) Route of Elimination | Starting Oral Daily Dose | Indications | Usual Dosage |
|---|---|---|---|---|---|---|---|---|---|
| Acebutolol (Sectral®) | $beta_1$ | Low | 15-25 | 3-4 | 40<br>7-fold† | Hepatic (renal) | 400 mg | Hypertension<br>Arrhythmias | P.O.: 400-1200 mg/d |
| Atenolol (Tenormin®) | $beta_1$ | Low | <5-10 | 6-9‡ | 50-60<br>4-fold† | Renal (hepatic) | 50 mg | Hypertension<br>Angina pectoris<br>Acute MI | P.O. 50-200 mg/d<br>I.V.: 5 mg x 2 doses |
| Betaxolol (Kerlone®) | $beta_1$ | Low | 50 | 14-22 | 89 | Hepatic (renal) | 10 mg | Hypertension | P.O.: 10-20 mg |
| Bisoprolol (Zebeta™) | $beta_1$ | Low | 30 | 9-12 | 80 | Renal | 5 mg | Hypertension | P.O.: 10-20 mg |
| Carteolol (Cartrol®) | $beta_1$<br>$beta_2$ | Low | 23-30 | 6 | 85 | Renal | 2.5 mg | Hypertension | P.O.: 2.5-10 mg |
| Carvedilol (Coreg®) | $beta_1$<br>$beta_2$<br>$alpha_1$ | High | 95-98 | 6-10 | 25-35 | Hepatic (bile) | 6.25 mg bid | Hypertension<br>CHF: Class II, III | Hypertension: 12.5-50 mg/d<br>CHF: 3.125-25 mg bid<br>(weight >85 kg: 50 mg bid) |
| Esmolol (Brevibloc®) | $beta_1$ | Low | 55 | 0.15 | NA<br>5-fold† | Red blood cell | NA | Supraventricular tachycardia<br>Sinus tachycardia | I.V. infusion: 50-200 mcg/kg/min |
| Labetalol (Trandate®, Normodyne®) | $alpha_1$<br>$beta_1$<br>$beta_2$ | Moderate | 50 | 5.5-8 | 18-30<br>10-fold† | Renal (hepatic) | 200 mg | Hypertension | P.O.: 400-800 mg/d<br>I.V.: 20-80 mg at 10-min intervals up to a maximum of 300 mg **or** continuous infusion of 2 mg/min |
| Metoprolol (Lopressor®) | $beta_1$ | Moderate | 10-12 | 3-7 | 50<br>10-fold† | Hepatic (renal) | 50 mg | Hypertension<br>Angina pectoris<br>Acute MI | P.O.: 100-450 mg/d<br>I.V.: Post-MI 15 mg<br>Angina: 15 mg then 2-5 mg/h<br>Arrhythmias: 0.2 mg/kg |
| Metoprolol (long-acting) | | | | | 77 | | | | |
| Nadolol (Corgard®) | $beta_1$<br>$beta_2$ | Low | 25-30 | 20-24 | 30<br>5-8-fold† | Renal | 80 mg | Hypertension<br>Angina pectoris | P.O.: 40-320 mg/d |

| Agent* | Adrenergic Receptor Blocking Activity | Lipid Solubility | Protein Bound (%) | Half-life (h) | Bioavailability (%) | Primary (Secondary) Route of Elimination | Starting Oral Daily Dose | Indications | Usual Dosage |
|---|---|---|---|---|---|---|---|---|---|
| Penbutolol (Levatol®) | $beta_1$ $beta_2$ | High | 80-98 | 5 | 100 | Hepatic (renal) | 20 mg | Hypertension | P.O.: 20-40 mg |
| Pindolol (Visken®) | $beta_1$ $beta_2$ | Moderate | 40 | 3-4§ | 90 4-fold† | Hepatic (renal) | 20 mg | Hypertension | P.O.: 20-60 mg/d |
| Propranolol (Inderal®, various) | $beta_1$ $beta_2$ | High | 90 | 3-5 | 30 20-fold† | Hepatic | 80 mg | Hypertension Angina pectoris Arrhythmias | P.O.: 40-320 mg/d I.V.: 1-5 mg |
| Propranolol long-acting (Inderal-LA®) | | | | 8-11 | | | | Hypertrophic subaortic stenosis Prophylaxis (post-MI) | P.O.: 180-240 mg/d |
| Sotalol (Betapace®) | $beta_1$ $beta_2$ | Low | 0 | 12 | 90-100 | Urine | 160 mg | Ventricular arrhythmias | P.O.: 160-320 mg |
| Timolol (Blocadren®) | $beta_1$ $beta_2$ | Low to moderate | <10 | 4 | 75 7-fold† | Hepatic (renal) | 20 mg | Hypertension Prophylaxis (post-MI) | P.O.: 20-40 mg/d P.O.: 20 mg/d |

†Interpatient variations in plasma levels.

‡Half-life increased to 16-27 hours in creatinine clearances of 15-35 mL/min and >27 hours in $Cl_{cr}$ <15 mL/min.

§Half-life variable: 7-15 hours.

# CALCIUM CHANNEL BLOCKING AGENTS COMPARISON

| | Amlodipine | Bepridil | Diltiazem | Felodipine | Isradipine | Nicardipine | Nifedipine | Nisoldipine | Verapamil |
|---|---|---|---|---|---|---|---|---|---|
| Bioavailability (%) | 60-65 | 59 | 40 | 15 | 15-24 | 35 | 60-75 | 5 | 20-35 |
| Protein binding (%) | 95-98 | >99 | 77-85 | 99 | 95 | 95 | 95 | >99 | 83-92 |
| Half-life | 35-50 h | 24 h | 3.5-6 h (5-7 h in sustained released preparations) | 10-16 h | 8 h | 2-4 h | 2-5 h | 7-12 h | Oral: One dose: 2.8-7.4 h<br>Rep dose: 4.5-12 h<br>I.V. (biphasic)<br>Short phase: 4 min<br>Long phase: 2-5 h |
| Onset of action | — | 60 min | Oral: 60 min | 2-5 h | 120 min | 20 min | Oral: 10-20 min | — | Oral: 30 min<br>I.V.: 1-5 min |
| Peak | 6-12 h | 2-3 h | Oral: 2-3 h | 2-4 h | 1.5 h | 0.5-2 h | Oral: 0.5-6 h | 6-12 h | Oral: 1-2.2 h<br>Oral, ext release: 5-7 h<br>I.V.: 2 h |
| Duration of action | 24 h | — | Ext release: 12 h<br>Tablet: 6-8 h | 24 h | — | 8 h | 12-24 h | — | Oral, ext release: 24 h<br>Tablet: 8-10 h<br>I.V.: 2 h |
| Elimination | Renal; fecal | Renal | Biliary/renal: 96%-98% (2%-4% unchanged) | Renal: 70%<br>Biliary: 30% | Renal | Renal: 60%<br>Biliary/fecal 35% | Renal: 80%<br>Biliary/fecal 20% | Renal | Renal: 70%<br>Biliary/fecal: 9%-16% |
| Solubility in water | — | — | Yes | — | — | Slightly | No | — | Yes |
| Maximum tolerated dosage (adult) | 250 mg | — | 12 g | — | — | 600 mg (standard) 2160 mg (sustained) | 900 mg | — | 16 g (standard)<br>9.6 g (sustained) |
| Therapeutic dose | 5-10 mg/day | 200-400 mg/day | 30-60 mg tid or qid for standard 180-400 mg daily for sustained release | 2-10 mg/day | 5-20 mg/day | 20-40 mg tid for standard 30-60 mg bid for sustained release | 10-40 mg tid or qid for standard 90-180 mg once daily for sustained release | 20-60 mg/day | 80-160 mg qid for standard 120-240 mg once daily for sustained release |
| Actions | | | | | | | | | |
| contractility | 0 | ↓ | ↓ | 0/↑ | 0 | ↓ | ↑ | 0 | ↓↓ |
| heart rate | 0 | ↓ | ↓ | ↑ | +/– | ↑ | ↑ | +/– | ↓ |
| cardiac output | 0 | 0 | ↑ | ↑ | ↑ | ↑↑ | ↑ | 0 | ↓↑ |
| peripheral vascular resistance | ↓↓ | ↓ | ↓ | ↓↓ | ↓↓↓ | ↓↓↓ | ↓↓↓ | ↓↓↓ | ↓↓ |

ND = no data in humans. ++ = most frequent; + = less frequent; – = rare; 0 = no effect.

# CONTROLLED SUBSTANCES COMPARISON

| Drugs | CSA Schedules | Trade or Other Names | Medical Uses | Physical Dependence | Psychological Dependence | Tolerance | Duration (h) | Usual Method | Possible Effects | Effects of Overdose | Withdrawal Syndrome |
|---|---|---|---|---|---|---|---|---|---|---|---|
| **Narcotics** | | | | | | | | | | | |
| Heroin | I | Diacetylmorphine, horse, smack | None in U.S; analgesic, antitussive | High | High | Yes | 3-6 | Injected, sniffed, smoked | Euphoria, drowsiness, respiratory depression, constricted pupils, nausea | Slow and shallow breathing, clammy skin, convulsions, coma, possible death | Watery eyes, runny nose, yawning, lose of appetite, irritability, tremors, panic, cramps, nausea, chills and sweating |
| Morphine | II | Duramorph, MS-Contin, Roxanol, Oramorph SR | Analgesic | High | High | Yes | 3-6 | Oral, smoked, injected | | | |
| Codeine | II, III, V | Tylenol w/codeine, Empirin w/codeine, Robitussin A-C, Fiorinal w/codeine, APAP w/codeine | Analgesic, antitussive | Moderate | Moderate | Yes | 3-6 | Oral, injected | | | |
| Hydrocodone | II, III | Tussionex, Vicodin, Hycodan, Lorcet | Analgesic, antitussive | High | High | Yes | 3-6 | Oral | | | |
| Hydromorphone | II | Dilaudid | Analgesic | High | High | Yes | 3-6 | Oral, injected | | | |
| Oxycodone | II | Percodan, Percocet, Tylox, Roxicet, Roxicodone | Analgesic | High | High | Yes | 4-5 | Oral | | | |
| Methadone and LAAM | I, II | Dolophine, methadone, levo-alpha-acetylmethadol, levomethadyl acetate | Analgesic, treatment of dependence | High | High | Yes | 12-72 | Oral, injected | | | |
| Fentanyl and analogs | I, II | Innovar, Sublimaze, Alfenta, Sufenta, Duragesic | Analgesic, adjunct to anesthesia, anesthetic | High | High | Yes | 0.1-72 | Injected, transdermal patch | | | |
| Other narcotics | II, III, IV, V | Percodan, Percocet, Tylox, opium, Darvon, Talwin,* buprenorphine, meperdine (pethidine), Demerol | Analgesic, antidiarrheal | High-low | High-low | Yes | Variable | Oral, injected | | | |

# CONTROLLED SUBSTANCES COMPARISON *(Continued)*

| Drugs | CSA Schedules | Trade or Other Names | Medical Uses | Physical Dependence | Psychological Dependence | Tolerance | Duration (h) | Usual Method | Possible Effects | Effects of Overdose | Withdrawal Syndrome |
|---|---|---|---|---|---|---|---|---|---|---|---|
| **Depressants** | | | | | | | | | | | |
| Chloral hydrate | IV | Noctec Somnos, Felsules | Hypnotic | Moderate | Moderate | Yes | 5-8 | Oral | Slurred speech, disorientation, drunken behavior without odor of alcohol | Shallow respiration, clammy skin, dilated pupils, weak and rapid pulse, coma, possible death | Anxiety, insomnia, tremors, delirium, convulsions, possible death |
| Barbiturates | II, III, IV | Amytal, Fiorinal, Nembutal, Seconal, Tuinal, phenobarbital, pentobarbital | Anesthetic, anticonvulsant, sedative, hypnotic, veterinary euthanasia agent | High-moderate | High-moderate | Yes | 1-16 | Oral, injected | | | |
| Benzodiazepines | IV | Ativan, Dalmane, Diazepam, Librium, Xanax, Serax, Valium, Tranxene, Verstran, Versed, Halcion, Paxipam, Restoril | Antianxiety, sedative, anticonvulsant, hypnotic | Low | Low | Yes | 4-8 | Oral, injected | | | |
| Glutethimide | II | Doriden | Sedative, hypnotic | High | Moderate | Yes | 4-8 | Oral | | | |
| Other depressants | I, II, III, IV | Equanil, Miltown, Noludar, Placidyl, Valmid, methaqualone | Antianxiety, sedative, hypnotic | Moderate | Moderate | Yes | 4-8 | Oral | | | |

| Drugs | CSA Schedules | Trade or Other Names | Medical Uses | Physical Dependence | Psychological Dependence | Tolerance | Duration (h) | Usual Method | Possible Effects | Effects of Overdose | Withdrawal Syndrome |
|---|---|---|---|---|---|---|---|---|---|---|---|
| **Stimulants** | | | | | | | | | | | |
| Cocaine† | II | Coke, flake, snow, crack | Local anesthetic | Possible | High | Yes | 1-2 | Sniffed, smoked, injected | Increased alertness, excitation, euphoria, increased pulse rate and blood pressure, insomnia, loss of appetite | Agitation, increased body temperature, hallicinations, convulsions, possible death | Apathy, long periods of sleep, irritability, depression, disorientation |
| Amphetamine/ methamphetamine | II | Biphetamine, Desoxyn, Dexedrine, Obetrol, ice | Attention deficit disorder, narcolepsy, weight control | Possible | High | Yes | 2-4 | Oral, injected, smoked | | | |
| Methylphenidate | II | Ritalin | Attention deficit disorder, narcolepsy | Possible | High | Yes | 2-4 | Oral, injected | | | |
| Other stimulants | I, II, III, IV | Adipex, Didrex, Ionamin, Melfiat, Plegine, Captagon, Sanorex, Tenuate, Tepanil, Prelu-2, Preludin | Weight control | Possible | High | Yes | 2-4 | Oral, injected | | | |
| **Cannabis** | | | | | | | | | | | |
| Marijuana | I | Pot, Acapulco gold, grass, Reefer, Sinsemilla, Thai sticks | None | Unknown | Moderate | Yes | 2-4 | Smoked, oral | Euphoria, relaxed inhibitions, increased appetite, disorientation | Fatigue, paranoia, possible psychosis | Occasional reports of insomnia, hyperactivity, decreased appetite |
| Tetrahydro-cannabinol | I, II | THC, Marinol | Antinauseant | Unknown | Moderate | Yes | 2-4 | Smoked, oral | | | |
| Hashish and hashish oil | I | Hash, hash oil | None | Unknown | Moderate | Yes | 2-4 | Smoked, oral | | | |

## CONTROLLED SUBSTANCES COMPARISON *(Continued)*

| Drugs | CSA Schedules | Trade or Other Names | Medical Uses | Physical Dependence | Psychological Dependence | Tolerance | Duration (h) | Usual Method | Possible Effects | Effects of Overdose | Withdrawal Syndrome |
|---|---|---|---|---|---|---|---|---|---|---|---|
| **Hallucinogens** | | | | | | | | | | | |
| LSD | I | Acid, Microdot | None | None | Unknown | Yes | 8-12 | Oral | Illusions and hallucinations, altered perception of time and distance | Longer, more intense "trip" episodes, psychosis, possible death | Unknown |
| Mescaline and peyote | I | Mescal, buttons, cactus | None | None | Unknown | Yes | 8-12 | Oral | | | |
| Amphetamine variants | I | 2,5-DMA, STP, MDA, MDMA, ecstasy, DOM, DOB | None | Unknown | Unknown | Yes | Variable | Oral, injected | | | |
| Phencyclidine and analogs | I, II | PCE, PCPy, TCP, PCP, hog, loveboat, angel dust | None | Unknown | High | Yes | Days | Oral, smoked | | | |
| Other hallucinogens | I | Bufotenine, Ibogaine, DMT, DET, Psilocybin, Psilocyn | None | None | Unknown | Possible | Variable | Smoked, oral, injected, sniffed | | | |
| **Anabolic Steroids** | | | | | | | | | | | |
| Testosterone (Cypionate, Enanthate) | III | Depo-testosterone, Delatestryl | Hypogonadism | Unknown | Unknown | Unknown | 14-28 days | Injected | Virilization, acne, testicular atrophy, gynecomastia, agressive behavior, edema | Unknown | Possible depression |
| Nandrolone (Decanoate, Phenpropionate) | III | Nortestosterone, Durabolin, Deca-durabolin, Deca | Anemia, breast cancer | Unknown | Unknown | Unknown | 14-21 days | Injected | | | |
| Oxymetholone | III | Anadrol-50 | Anemia | Unknown | Unknown | Unknown | 24 | Oral | | | |

*Not designated a narcotic under the CSA.

†Designated a narcotic under the CSA.

From U.S. Department of Justice Drug Enforcement Administration, *Drugs of Abuse*, 1996, with permission.

# CORTICOSTEROIDS COMPARISON

## Corticosteroids, Systemic Equivalencies

| Glucocorticoid | Pregnancy Category | Approximate Equivalent Dose (mg) | Routes of Administration | Relative Anti-inflammatory Potency | Relative Mineralocorticoid Potency | Protein Binding (%) | Half-life | |
|---|---|---|---|---|---|---|---|---|
| | | | | | | | Plasma (min) | Biologic (h) |
| | | | Short-Acting | | | | | |
| Cortisone | D | 25 | P.O., I.M. | 0.8 | 2 | 90 | 30 | 8-12 |
| Hydrocortisone | C | 20 | I.M., I.V. | 1 | 2 | 90 | 80-118 | 8-12 |
| | | | Intermediate-Acting | | | | | |
| Methylprednisolone* | — | 4 | P.O., I.M., I.V. | 5 | 0 | — | 78-188 | 18-36 |
| Prednisolone | B | 5 | P.O., I.M., I.V., intra-articular, intradermal, soft tissue injection | 4 | 1 | 90-95 | 115-212 | 18-36 |
| Prednisone | B | 5 | P.O. | 4 | 1 | 70 | 60 | 18-36 |
| Triamcinolone* | C | 4 | P.O., I.M., intra-articular, intradermal, intrasynovial, soft tissue injection | 5 | 0 | — | 200+ | 18-36 |
| | | | Long-Acting | | | | | |
| Betamethasone | C | 0.6-0.75 | P.O., I.M., intra-articular, intradermal, intrasynovial, soft tissue injection | 25 | 0 | 64 | 300+ | 36-54 |
| Dexamethasone | C | 0.75 | P.O., I.M., I.V., intra-articular, intradermal, soft tissue injection | 25-30 | 0 | — | 110-210 | 36-54 |
| | | | Mineralocorticoids | | | | | |
| Fludrocortisone | C | — | P.O. | 10 | 125 | 42 | 210+ | 18-36 |

*May contain propylene glycol as an excipient in injectable forms.

# CORTICOSTEROIDS COMPARISON *(Continued)*

## Corticosteroids, Topical

| Steroid | | Vehicle |
|---|---|---|
| **Very High Potency** | | |
| 0.05% | Augmented betamethasone dipropionate (Diprolene®) | Ointment |
| 0.05% | Clobetasol propionate (Temovate®) | Cream, ointment |
| 0.05% | Diflorasone diacetate (Florone®, Maxiflor®, Psorcon®) | Gel, ointment |
| 0.05% | Halobetasol propionate (Ultravate®) | Cream, ointment |
| **High Potency** | | |
| 0.1% | Amcinonide (Cyclocort®) | Cream, ointment |
| 0.05% | Betamethasone dipropionate (Diprosone®) | Cream, ointment, lotion |
| 0.25% | Desoximetasone (Topicort®) | Cream, ointment |
| 0.2% | Fluocinolone (Synalar-HP®) | Cream |
| 0.05% | Fluocinonide (Lidex®) | Cream, ointment |
| 0.1% | Halcinonide (Halog®) | Cream, ointment, solution |
| 0.5% | Triamcinolone acetonide | Cream, ointment |
| **Intermediate Potency** | | |
| 0.025% | Betamethasone benzoate | Cream, gel, lotion |
| 0.1% | Betamethasone valerate (Valisone®) | Cream, ointment, lotion |
| 0.05% | Desoximetasone (Topicort® LP) | Cream |
| 0.025% | Fluocinolone acetonide | Cream, ointment |
| 0.05% | Flurandrenolide (Cordran®, Cordran® SP) | Cream, ointment, lotion |
| 0.05% | Fluticasone propionate (Cutivate®) | Cream |
| 0.025% | Halcinonide (Halog®) | Cream, ointment |
| 0.1% | Mometasone furoate | Cream, ointment, lotion |
| 0.1% | Triamcinolone acetonide (Kenalog®) | Cream, ointment |
| **Low Potency** | | |
| 0.01% | Betamethasone valerate (Valisone®, reduced strength) | Cream |
| 0.1% | Clocortolone (Cloderm®)† | Cream |
| 0.01% | Fluocinolone acetonide (Synalar®) | Cream, solution, shampoo, oil |
| 0.025% | Flurandrenolide (Cordran®, Cordran® SP) | Cream, ointment |
| 0.2% | Hydrocortisone valerate (Westcort®)† | Cream |
| 0.025% | Triamcinolone acetonide (Kenalog®) | Cream, ointment |
| **Lowest Potency** (may be ineffective for some indications) | | |
| 0.05% | Alclometasone (Aclovate®) | Cream, ointment |
| 0.1% | Betamethasone | Cream |
| 0.2% | Betamethasone | Cream |
| 0.05% | Desonide (Desowen®, Tridesilon®)† | Cream, ointment, lotion |
| 0.04% | Dexamethasone (Decaspray®) | Aerosol |
| 0.1% | Dexamethasone (Decadron® Phosphate, Decaderm®) | Cream |
| 1% | Hydrocortisone† | Cream, ointment, lotion |
| 2.5% | Hydrocortisone† | Cream, ointment |
| 0.25% | Methylprednisolone acetate (Medrol®)† | Ointment |
| 1% | Methylprednisolone acetate (Medrol®)† | Ointment |

†Fluorinated.

# GLAUCOMA DRUG COMPARISON

| Ophthalmic Agent | Reduces Aqueous Humor Production | Increases Aqueous Humor Outflow | Average Duration of Action | Strengths Available |
|---|---|---|---|---|
| **Cholinesterase Inhibitors*** | | | | |
| Demecarium | No data | Significant | 7 d | 0.125%-0.25% |
| Echothiophate | No data | Significant | 2 wk | 0.03%-0.25% |
| Isoflurophate | No data | Significant | 2 wk | 0.025% |
| Physostigmine | No data | Significant | 24 h | 0.25% |
| **Direct-Acting Cholinergic Agents** | | | | |
| Carbachol | Some activity | Significant | 8 h | 0.75%-3% |
| Pilocarpine | Some activity | Significant | 5 h | 0.5%, 1%, 2%, 3%, 4% |
| **Sympathomimetics** | | | | |
| Dipivefrin | Some activity | Moderate | 12 h | 0.1% |
| Epinephrine | Some activity | Moderate | 18 h | 0.25%-2% |
| **Beta-Blockers** | | | | |
| Betaxolol | Significant | Some activity | 12 h | 0.5% |
| Carteolol | Yes | No | 12 h | 1% |
| Levobunolol | Significant | Some activity | 18 h | 0.5% |
| Metipranolol | Significant | Some activity | 18 h | 0.3% |
| Timolol | Significant | Some activity | 18 h | 0.25%, 0.5% |
| **Carbonic Anhydrase Inhibitors** | | | | |
| Acetazolamide | Significant | No data | 10 h | 250 mg tab, 500 mg cap |
| Brinzolamide | Yes | No data | 8 h | 1% |
| Dorzolamide | Yes | No | 8 h | 2% |
| Methazolamide | Significant | No data | 14 h | 50 mg |
| **Prostaglandin Agonist** | | | | |
| Latanoprost | | Yes | 8-12 h | 0.005% |

Also see Ophthalmic Agents, Glaucoma in the Alphabetical Listing of Drugs section.

*All miotic drugs significantly affect accommodation.

# HALLUCINOGENIC DRUGS COMPARISON

**Principal Pharmacological Properties of Hallucinogenic Drugs**

| Drug; Chemical Structure | Duration of Acute Effect (h) | pKa | Route of Metabolism/ Excretion | Half-Life | Protein Binding (%) | $V_d$ (L/kg) | Urine Screen Positive for | Duration of Psychotropic Effects | Doses of Abuse | Fatal Dose |
|---|---|---|---|---|---|---|---|---|---|---|
| Phencyclidine (PCP); arylcyclohexylamine | 4-6 | 8.5 | Hepatic/urine | 1 h | 65 | 6.2-0.3 | 2 wk | Up to 1 mo | 1-9 mg | 1 mg/kg |
| Cocaine; tropane alkaloid | 0.5 | 5.6 | Plasma hydrolysis* | 48-75 min | 9-90 | 1.2-1.9 | 4 days (benzoylecgonine) | ≤5-7 d | 20-200 mg (intranasally) | 1-1.2 g |
| Cannabis; monoterpenoid | 0.5-3 | 10.6 | Hepatic hydroxylation | 25-57 h | 97-99 | 10 | Up to 4 d | ≤6 h | 5-15 mg THC | |
| LSD; indole alkylamine | 0.7-8 | 7.8 | Hepatic hydroxylation | 2.5 h | | 0.27 | 120 h | May last for days | 100-300 mcg | 0.2 mg/kg |
| Psilocybin; tryptamine | 0.5-6 | | | | | | Not detected | 12 h | 20-100 mushrooms | 5-15 mg of psilocybin |
| Mescaline; phenylalkylamine | 4.6 | Not known | Hepatic/urine† | 6 h | None | Not known | | 12 h | 5 mg/kg | 20 mg/kg |
| Morphine; alkaloid/ derivative of opium | 4-5 | 8.05 | Glucuronidation/ urine | 1.9-3.1 h | 35 | 3.2 | 48 h | ≤6 h | 2-20 mg | Variable – dependent on tolerance, nontolerant fatal dose is 120 mg orally or 30 mg parenterally |

**Principal Pharmacological Properties of Hallucinogenic Drugs** *(continued)*

| Drug; Chemical Structure | Duration of Acute Effect (h) | pKa | Route of Metabolism/ Excretion | Half-Life | Protein Binding (%) | $V_d$ (L/kg) | Urine Screen Positive for | Duration of Psychotropic Effects | Doses of Abuse | Fatal Dose |
|---|---|---|---|---|---|---|---|---|---|---|
| Heroin; diacetylmorphine | 3.4 | 7.6 | Hepatic‡ | 3-20 min | 40 | 25 | ~40 h | ≤6 h | 2.2 mg | Variable – dependent on tolerance |
| Amphetamine; β-(phenylisopropyl)-amine | Variable | 9.93 | Hepatic§ | 12 h¶ | 16-20 | 3-6 | 2-4 d | Delusions may remain for months | 100-1000 mg/d | Variable – dependent on tolerance |

*By serum cholinesterase.

†60% excreted unchanged.

‡Converted to morphine.

§Converted to phenylacetone.

¶Urine pH-dependent.

Reprinted with permission from Leikin JB, Krantz AJ, Zell-Kanter M, et al, "Clinical Features and Management of Intoxication Due to Hallucinogenic Drugs," *Med Toxicol Adverse Drug Exp*, 1989, 4(5):328.

# INHALANT (ASTHMA, BRONCHOSPASM) AGENTS COMPARISON

## Medications Commonly Used for Asthma, Bronchospasm, and COPD

| Agent | Indications | Onset | Duration | Frequency | Comments |
|---|---|---|---|---|---|
| | | **Anticholinergics** | | | |
| Ipratropium bromide (Atrovent®) | Bronchospasm associated with COPD | | 6 h | 2 puffs qid | Additive bronchodilating effects used with α-, $\beta_2$-adrenergic agonists |
| | | **Bronchodilators** | | | |
| Albuterol (Proventil®, Proventil® HFA, Ventolin®) | Prevent exercise-induced bronchospasm; relief and prevention of bronchospasm | 5 min | 6-8 h | 2 puffs q4-6h | |
| Bitolterol mesylate (Tornalate®) | Prevent and treat bronchial asthma and reversible bronchospasm | 5 min | 8 h | 2 puffs q8h | Contains a high alcohol content that may irritate the airway |
| Epinephrine (Bronkaid® Mist, Primatene® Mist) | Acute paroxysms of bronchial asthma; treatment of postintubation and infectious croup | 1-5 min | Individualize dosing | | OTC; shorter-acting and less effective than prescription β-agonists |
| Ipratropium bromide and albuterol sulfate (Combivent®) | Patients with chronic obstructive pulmonary disease (COPD) on a regular aerosol bronchodilator who continue to have evidence of bronchospasm and who require a second bronchodilator | | | 2 puffs qid | Additional doses may be administered; however, total doses should not exceed 12 in 24 hours |
| Isoetharine HCl (Bronkometer) | Bronchial asthma and reversible bronchospasm with bronchitis and emphysema | 5 min | 1-3 h | 1-2 puffs q4h | May cause cardiac stimulation |
| Isoproterenol (Medihaler-ISO®) | Bronchospasm associated with acute/chronic bronchial asthma, pulmonary emphysema, bronchitis, bronchiectasis | 2-5 min | 1-2 h | 1-2 puffs q4-6h | May cause cardiac stimulation; may cause saliva to turn pinkish-red |
| Isoproterenol HCl and phenylephrine bitartrate (Duo-Medihaler®) | Bronchospasm with acute/chronic bronchial asthma; reversible bronchospasm with emphysema and bronchitis | 2-5 min | 4-6 h | 1-2 puffs q4-6h | May cause cardiac stimulation |
| Metaproterenol sulfat (Alupent®, Metaprel®) | Bronchial asthma and reversible bronchospasm; acute asthmatic attacks in children ≥6 years of age | 5-30 min | 4-6 h | 2-3 puffs q3-4h (max 12 puffs/d) | Contraindicated in patients with arrhythmias; should not be used with other β-adrenergic aerosol inhalers because of additive effects |

## Medications Commonly Used for Asthma, Bronchospasm, and COPD *(continued)*

| Agent | Indications | Onset | Duration | Frequency | Comments |
|---|---|---|---|---|---|
| Pirbuterol acetate (Maxair™) | Prevent and reverse bronchospasm with reversible bronchospasm | Within 5 min | 4-6 h | 2 puffs q4-6h | |
| Salmeterol (Serevent®) | Long-term maintenance treatment of asthma and prevention of bronchospasm in patients >12 years of age | 20 min | 12 h | 2 puffs q12h | Not meant to relieve acute asthmatic symptoms |
| Terbutaline sulfate (Brethaire®) | Bronchial asthma and reversible bronchospasm with bronchitis or emphysema | 5-30 min | 6-8 h | 2 puffs q4-6h | |
| | | **Corticosteroids*** | | | |
| Beclomethasone dipropionate (Beclovent®, Vanceril®) | Bronchial asthma | | 6-8 h | 2 puffs q6-8h | Coughing and wheezing are more common |
| Dexamethasone Na phosphate (Decadron® phosphate respihaler) | Bronchial asthma | | 6-8 h | 3 puffs q6-8h (max 12 puffs/d) | |
| Flunisolide (AeroBid®) | Bronchial asthma | | 12 h | 2 puffs bid (max 4 puffs bid) | |
| Triamcinolone acetonide (Azmacort™) | Bronchial asthma | | 6-8 h | 2 puffs q6-8h (max 16 puffs/d) | Asthma should be reasonably stable before Azmacort™ treatment |
| | | **Miscellaneous** | | | |
| Cromolyn (Intal®) | Severe bronchial asthma; prevent exercise-induced bronchospasm | | 6 h | 2 puffs qid | Only useful in prophylaxis; has low toxicity and is as effective as theophylline in many patients |
| Nedocromil sodium (Tilade®) | Mild to moderate bronchial asthma | | 6 h | 2 puffs qid | Must be taken regularly for benefit — even during symptom-free periods |

*Not indicated for rapid relief of bronchospasm. Dysphonia and oral candidiasis can occur. Long-term use is associated with cataract formation.

# INHALANT (ASTHMA, BRONCHOSPASM) AGENTS COMPARISON *(Continued)*

## Estimated Comparative Daily Dosages for Children

| Drug | Low Dose | Medium Dose | High Dose |
|---|---|---|---|
| Beclomethasone dipropionate<br>42 mcg/puff<br>84 mcg/puff | 84-336 mcg<br>(2-8 puffs) | 336-672 mcg<br>(8-16 puffs) | >672 mcg<br>(>16 puffs) |
| Budesonide Turbuhaler<br>200 mcg/dose | 100-200 mcg | 200-400 mcg<br>(1-2 inhalations — 200 mcg) | >400 mcg<br>(>2 inhalations — 200 mcg) |
| Flunisolide<br>250 mcg/puff | 500-750 mcg<br>(2-3 puffs) | 1000-1250 mcg<br>(4-5 puffs) | >1250 mcg<br>(>5 puffs) |
| Fluticasone<br>MDI: 44, 110, 220 mcg/puff<br>DPI: 50, 100, 250 mcg/dose | 88-176 mcg<br>(2-4 puffs — 44 mcg)<br>(2-4 inhalations — 50 mcg) | 176-440 mcg<br>(4-10 puffs — 44 mcg)<br>or<br>(2-4 puffs — 110 mcg)<br>(2-4 inhalations — 100 mcg) | >440 mcg<br>(>4 puffs — 110 mcg)<br>(>4 inhalations — 100 mcg) |
| Triamcinolone acetonide<br>100 mcg/puff | 400-800 mcg<br>(4-8 puffs) | 800-1200 mcg<br>(8-12 puffs) | >1200 mcg<br>(>12 puffs) |

# INOTROPIC AND VASOCONSTRICTOR COMPARISON

## Cardiovascular Comparison

| Drug | Hemodynamic Effects | | | |
|---|---|---|---|---|
| | CO | TPR | Mean BP | Renal Perfusion |
| Amrinone (Inocor®) | ↑ | ↓ | — | ↑ |
| Dobutamine (Dobutrex®) | ↑ | ↓ | ↑ | — |
| Dopamine (Intropin®) | ↑ | +/—* | —/↑* | ↑* |
| Epinephrine (Adrenalin®) | ↑ | ↓ | ↑ | ↓ |
| Isoproterenol (Isuprel®) | ↑ | ↓ | ↓ | +/—† |
| Mephentermine (Wyamine®) | ↑ | —/↑ | ↑ | +/— |
| Metaraminol (Aramine®) | ↓ | ↑ | ↑ | ↓ |
| Methoxamine | —/↓ | ↑ | ↑ | ↓ |
| Milrinone (Primacor®) | ↑ | ↓ | — | ↑ |
| Norepinephrine (Levophed®) | —/↓ | ↑ | ↑ | ↓ |
| Phenylephrine (Neo-Synephrine®) | ↓ | ↑ | ↑ | ↓ |

↑ = increase ↓ = decrease, — = no change, * = dose dependent

†In patients with cardiogenic or septic shock, renal perfusion commonly increases, however, in the normal patient, renal perfusion may be reduced with isoproterenol.

# LAXATIVES: CLASSIFICATION AND PROPERTIES COMPARISON

| Laxative | Onset of Action | Site of Action | Mechanism of Action |
|---|---|---|---|
| **Saline** | | | |
| Magnesium citrate (Citroma®)<br>Magnesium hydroxide (Milk of Magnesia) | 30 min to 3 h | Small and large intestine | Attract/retain water in intestinal lumen increasing intraluminal pressure; cholecystokinin release |
| Sodium phosphate/ biphosphate enema (Fleet® Enema) | 2-15 min | Colon | |
| **Irritant/Stimulant** | | | |
| Cascara<br>Casanthranol<br>Senna (Senokot®) | 6-10 h | Colon | Direct action on intestinal mucosa; stimulate myenteric plexus; alter water and electrolyte secretion |
| Bisacodyl (Dulcolax®) tablets, suppositories | 15 min to 1 h | Colon | |
| Castor oil | 2-6 h | Small intestine | |
| Cascara aromatic fluid extract | 6-10 h | Colon | |
| **Bulk-Producing** | | | |
| Methylcellulose<br>Psyllium (Metamucil®)<br>Malt soup extract (Maltsupex®)<br>Calcium polycarbophil (Mitrolan®, FiberCon®) | 12-24 h (up to 72 h) | Small and large intestine | Holds water in stool; mechanical distention; malt soup extract reduces fecal pH |
| **Lubricant** | | | |
| Mineral oil | 6-8 h | Colon | Lubricates intestine; retards colonic absorption of fecal water; softens stool |
| **Surfactants/Stool Softener** | | | |
| Docusate sodium (Colace®)<br>Docusate calcium (Surfak®)<br>Docusate potassium (Dialose®) | 24-72 h | Small and large intestine | Detergent activity; facilitates admixture of fat and water to soften stool |
| **Miscellaneous and Combination Laxatives** | | | |
| Glycerin suppository | 15-30 min | Colon | Local irritation; hyperosmotic action |
| Lactulose (Cephulac®) | 24-48 h | Colon | Delivers osmotically active molecules to colon |
| Docusate/casanthranol (Peri-Colace®) | 8-12 h | Small and large intestine | Casanthranol – mild stimulant; docusate – stool softener |

# LIPID-LOWERING AGENTS COMPARISON

### Possible Effects on Lipoproteins

| Drug | Total Cholesterol % | LDL % | HDL % | TG % |
|---|---|---|---|---|
| Bile-acid resins | ↓20-25 | ↓20-35 | → | ↑5-20 |
| Fibric acid derivatives | ↓10 | ↓10 (↑) | ↑10-25 | ↓40-55 |
| HMG-CoA RI (statins) | ↓15-45 | ↓20-60 | ↑2-15 | ↓7-37 |
| Nicotinic acid | ↓25 | ↓20 | ↑20 | ↓40 |

### Comparative Dosages* of Agents Used to Treat Hyperlipidemia

| Antilipemic Agent | Usual Total Daily Dose | Average Dosing Interval |
|---|---|---|
| **HMG-CoA Reductase Inhibitors** | | |
| Atorvastatin | 10-80 mg/day | qd |
| Cerivastatin | 0.2-0.3 mg/day | qd |
| Fluvastatin | 20-40 mg/day | qd hs |
| Lovastatin | 20-40 mg/day | qd hs |
| Pravastatin | 20-40 mg/day | qd hs |
| Simvastatin | 10-20 mg/day | qd hs |
| **Fibric Acid Derivatives** | | |
| Clofibrate | 2000 mg/day | qid |
| Fenofibrate | 67-201 mg/day | qd |
| Gemfibrozil | 1200 mg/day | bid |
| **Miscellaneous Agents** | | |
| Niacin | 1.5-6 g/day | tid |
| **Bile Acid Sequestrants** | | |
| Colestipol | 30 g/day | bid |
| Cholestyramine | 24 g/day | tid-qid |

*Dosage is based on 70 kg adult with normal hepatic and renal function.

# LIPID-LOWERING AGENTS COMPARISON *(Continued)*

## Antihyperlipidemic Drugs: Effects

| Drug | Effects on Serum Lipids | | | Total Chol % | Side Effects/Monitoring Notes |
|---|---|---|---|---|---|
| | LDL % | HDL % | Trig % | | |
| Atorvastatin (Lipitor®) | 40-60 ↓ | 5-8 ↑ | 19-37 ↓ | 25-45 ↓ | GI, hepatic dysfunction, myositis; monitor LFTs, CPK if muscle pain. |
| Cerivastatin (Baycol®) | 25-28 ↓ | 10 ↑ | 11-13 ↓ | 17-20 ↓ | GI, hepatic dysfunction, myositis; monitor LFTs, CPK if muscle pain. |
| Colestipol (Colestid®) **or** Cholestyramine (Prevalite®) | 15-30 ↓ | 3-5 ↑ | No change ↑ | 17 ↓ | Possible increased TG, dose-dependent upper/ lower GI distress; may inhibit absorption of coadministered drugs |
| Fluvastatin (Lescol®) | 22-35 ↓ | — | — | — | GI, hepatic dysfunction, myositis; monitor LFTs, CPK if muscle pain. |
| Gemfibrozil (Lopid®) | 0-15 ↓ | 10-15 ↑ | 20-50 ↓ | | GI rashes, hepatic dysfunction, gallstones; potentiates warfarin; monitor LFTs |
| Lovastatin (Mevacor®) | 20-40 ↓ | 5-15 ↑ | 10-20 ↓ | 27-34 ↓ | GI, hepatic dysfunction, myositis; monitor LFTs, CPK if muscle pain. |
| Niacin | 10-25 ↓ | 15-30 ↑ | 20-50 ↓ | | Flushing, upper GI distress, hepatic dysfunction, hyperglycemia, increased uric acid |
| Niacin, sustained release | 10-25 ↓ | 15-30 ↑ | 20-50 ↓ | | Monitor LFTs, FBS; use with caution in patients with PUD, diabetes, history of liver disease, or gout. |
| Pravastatin (Pravachol®) | 22-34 ↓ | 7-12 ↑ | 15-24 ↓ | 16-25 ↓ | GI, hepatic dysfunction, myositis; monitor LFTs, CPK if muscle pain. |
| Simvastatin (Zocor®) | 30-40 ↓ | 5-15 ↑ | 10-20 ↓ | 17-28 ↓ | GI, hepatic dysfunction, myositis; monitor LFTs, CPK if muscle pain. |

# LOW MOLECULAR WEIGHT HEPARINS COMPARISON

| Name | Type | Limitation | Dose | Average MW |
|---|---|---|---|---|
| Ardeparin | Prophylaxis | Knee replacement | 50 units/kg q12h | 5500-6500 |
| Dalteparin | Prophylaxis | Abdominal surgery*<br>Abdominal surgery† | 2500 units/d<br>5000 units/d | 4000-6000 |
| | Prophylaxis | Hip surgery* | 5000 units/d | |
| | Treatment‡ | DVT | 100 units/kg bid<br>200 units/kg qd | |
| Danaproid | Prophylaxis | Hip replacement | 750 units bid | 6500 |
| | Treatment‡ | | 2000 units q12h | |
| Enoxaparin | Prophylaxis | Hip or knee replacement | 30 mg# | 3500-5500 |
| | Prophylaxis | High-risk hip replacement or abdominal surgery | 40 mg once daily | |
| | Treatment | DVT or PE | 1 mg/kg q12h | |
| | Treatment | Acute coronary | 1 mg/kg q12h | |

*Patients with low risk of DVT.

†Patients with high risk of DVT.

‡Not FDA approved.

#Patients weighing <100 lb or ?65 years of age may receive 0.5 mg/kg/dose every 12 hours.

# NARCOTIC/OPIOID ANALGESIC COMPARISON

I.V. administration is most reliable and rapid; I.M. or S.C. use may cause delayed absorption and peak effect, especially with impaired tissue perfusion. Many agents undergo a significant first-pass effect. All are metabolized by the liver and excreted primarily in urine.

### Dose Equivalents for Opioid Analgesics in Opioid-Naive Adults ≥50 kg*

| Drug | Approximate Equianalgesic Dose | | Usual Starting Dose for Moderate to Severe Pain | |
|---|---|---|---|---|
| | Oral | Parenteral | Oral | Parenteral |
| **Opioid Agonist** | | | | |
| Morphine† | 30 mg q3-4h (repeat around-the-clock dosing) 60 mg q3-4h (single dose or intermittent dosing) | 10 mg q3-4h | 30 mg q3-4h | 10 mg q3-4h |
| Codeine | 130 mg q3-4h | 75 mg q3-4h | 60 mg q3-4h | 60 mg q2h (I.M./S.C.) |
| Hydromorphone† (Dilaudid®) | 7.5 mg q3-4h | 1.5 mg q3-4h | 6 mg q3-4h | 1.5 mg q3-4h |
| Levorphanol (Levo-Dromoran®) | 4 mg q6-8h | 2 mg q6-8h | 4 mg q6-8h | 2 mg q6-8h |
| Meperidine (Demerol®) | 300 mg q2-3h | 100 mg q3h | NR | 100 mg q3h |
| Methadone (Dolophine®, others) | 20 mg q6-8h | 10 mg q6-8h | 20 mg q6-8h | 10 mg q6-8h |
| Oxymorphone† (Numorphan®) | NA | 1 mg q3-4h | NA | 1 mg q3-4h |
| **Combination Opioid/NSAID Preparations#** | | | | |
| Hydrocodone (in Lorcet®, Lortab®, Vicodin®, others) | 30 mg q3-4h | NA | 10 mg q3-4h | NA |
| Oxycodone (Roxicodone®, also in Percocet®, Percodan®, Tylox®, others) | 30 mg q3-4h | NA | 10 mg q3-4h | NA |
| **Opioid Agonist-Antagonist and Partial Agonist** | | | | |
| Buprenorphine (Buprenex®) | NA | 0.3-0.4 mg q6-8h | NA | 0.4 q6-8h |
| Butorphanol (Stadol®) | NA | 2 mg q3-4h | NA | 2 mg q3-4h |
| Nalbuphine (Nubain®) | NA | 10 mg q3-4h | NA | 10 mg q3-4h |
| Pentazocine (Talwin®, others) | 150 mg q3-4h | 60 mg q3-4h | 50 mg q4-6h | NR |

**Note:** Tables vary in the suggested doses that are equianalgesic to morphine. Clinical response is the criterion that must be applied for each patient; titration to clinical response is necessary. Because there is not complete cross tolerance among these drugs, it is usually necessary to use a lower than equianalgesic dose when changing drugs and to retitrate to response.

**Caution:** Recommended doses do not apply to patients with renal or hepatic insufficiency or other conditions affecting drug metabolism and kinetics.

***Caution:** Recommended doses do not apply for adult patients with body weight <50 kg. For recommended starting doses for adults <50 kg body weight, see following table.

†**Caution:** For morphine, hydromorphone, and oxymorphone, rectal administration is an alternate route for patients unable to take oral medications. Equianalgesic doses may differ from oral and parenteral doses because of pharmacokinetic differences. **Note:** A short-acting opioid should normally be used for initial therapy of moderate to severe pain.

‡**Caution:** Codeine doses >65 mg often are not appropriate because of diminishing incremental analgesia with increasing doses but continually increasing nausea, constipation, and other side effects.

NA = not available; NR = not recommended.

## Dose Equivalents for Opioid Analgesics in Opioid-Naive Adults <50 kg*

| Drug | Approximate Equianalgesic Dose | | Usual Starting Dose for Moderate to Severe Pain | |
|---|---|---|---|---|
| | Oral | Parenteral | Oral | Parenteral |
| **Opioid Agonist** | | | | |
| Morphine† | 30 mg q3-4h (repeat around-the-clock dosing) 60 mg q3-4h (single dose or intermittent dosing) | 10 mg q3-4h | 0.3 mg/kg q3-4h | 0.1 mg/kg q3-4h |
| Codeine‡ | 130 mg q3-4h | 75 mg q3-4h | 1 mg/kg q3-4h# | NR |
| Hydromorphone† (Dilaudid®) | 7.5 mg q3-4h | 1.5 mg q3-4h | 0.06 mg/kg q3-4h | 0.015 mg/kg q3-4h |
| Levorphanol (Levo-Dromoran®) | 4 mg q6-8h | 2 mg q6-8h | 0.04 mg/kg q6-8h | 0.02 mg/kg q6-8h |
| Meperidine (Demerol®) | 300 mg q2-3h | 100 mg q3h | NR | 0.75 mg/kg q2-3h |
| Methadone (Dolophine®, others) | 20 mg q6-8h | 10 mg q6-8h | 0.2 mg/kg q6-8h | 0.1 mg/kg q6-8h |
| Oxymorphone† (Numorphan®) | NA | 1 mg q3-4h | NR | NR |
| **Combination Opioid/NSAID Preparations** | | | | |
| Hydrocodone (in Lorcet®, Lortab®, Vicodin®, others) | 30 mg q3-4h | NA | 0.2 mg/kg q3-4h# | NA |
| Oxycodone (Roxicodone®, also in Percocet®, Percodan®, Tylox®, others) | 30 mg q3-4h | NA | 0.2 mg/kg q3-4h# | NA |
| **Opioid Agonist-Antagonist and Partial Agonist** | | | | |
| Buprenorphine (Buprenex®) | NA | 0.3-0.4 mg q6-8h | NA | 0.4 q6-8h |
| Butorphanol (Stadol®) | NA | 2 mg q3-4h | NA | 2 mg q3-4h |
| Nalbuphine (Nubain®) | NA | 10 mg q3-4h | NA | 10 mg q3-4h |
| Pentazocine (Talwin®, others) | 150 mg q3-4h | 60 mg q3-4h | 50 mg q4-6h | NR |

**Note:** Tables vary in the suggested doses that are equianalgesic to morphine. Clinical response is the criterion that must be applied for each patient; titration to clinical response is necessary. Because there is not complete cross tolerance among these drugs, it is usually necessary to use a lower than equianalgesic dose when changing drugs and to retitrate to response.

**Caution:** Recommended doses do not apply to patients with renal or hepatic insufficiency or other conditions affecting drug metabolism and kinetics.

***Caution:** Doses listed for patients with body weight <50 kg cannot be used as initial starting doses in babies younger than 6 months of age.

†**Caution:** For morphine, hydromorphone, and oxymorphone, rectal administration is an alternate route for patients unable to take oral medications. Equianalgesic doses may differ from oral and parenteral doses because of pharmacokinetic differences. **Note:** A short-acting opioid should normally be used for initial therapy of moderate to severe pain.

‡**Caution:** Codeine doses >65 mg often are not appropriate because of diminishing incremental analgesia with increasing doses but continually increasing nausea, constipation, and other side effects.

#**Caution:** Doses of aspirin and acetaminophen in combination opioid/NSAID preparations must also be adjusted to the patient's body weight.

NA = not available; NR = not recommended.

# NARCOTIC/OPIOID ANALGESIC COMPARISON
*(Continued)*

## Comparative Pharmacokinetics

| Drug | Onset (min) | Peak (h) | Duration (h) | Half-Life (h) | Average Dosing Interval (h) | | Equianalgesic Doses* (mg) | |
|---|---|---|---|---|---|---|---|---|
| | | | | | Median | Range | I.M. | Oral |
| Alfentanil | Immediate | ND | ND | 1-2 | — | — | ND | NA |
| Buprenorphine | 15 | 1 | 4-8 | 2-3 | | | 0.4 | — |
| Butorphanol | I.M.: 30-60<br>I.V.: 4-5 | 0.5-1 | 3-5 | 2.5-3.5 | 3 | (3-6) | 2 | — |
| Codeine | P.O.: 30-60<br>I.M.: 10-30 | 0.5-1 | 4-6 | 3-4 | 3 | (3-6) | 120 | 200 |
| Fentanyl | I.M.: 7-15<br>I.V.: Immediate | ND | 1-2 | 1.5-6 | 1 | (0.5-2) | 0.1 | NA |
| Hydrocodone | ND | ND | 4-8 | 3.3-4.4 | 6 | (4-8) | ND | ND |
| Hydromorphone | P.O.: 15-30 | 0.5-1 | 4-6 | 2-4 | 4 | (3-6) | 1.5 | 7.5 |
| Levorphanol | P.O.: 10-60 | 0.5-1 | 4-8 | 12-16 | 6 | (6-24) | 2 | 4 |
| Meperidine | P.O./I.M./S.C.: 10-15<br>I.V.: ≤5 | 0.5-1 | 2-4 | 3-4 | 3 | (2-4) | 75 | 300 |
| Methadone | P.O.: 30-60<br>I.V.: 10-20 | 0.5-1 | 4-6 (acute)<br>>8 (chronic) | 15-30 | 8 | (6-12) | 10 | 20 |
| Morphine | P.O.: 15-60<br>I.V.: ≤5 | P.O./I.M./<br>S.C.: 0.5-1<br>I.V.: 0.3 | 3-6 | 2-4 | 4 | (3-6) | 10 | 60† (acute)<br>30 (chronic) |
| Nalbuphine | I.M.: 30<br>I.V.: 1-3 | 1 | 3-6 | 5 | | — | 10 | — |
| Naloxone‡ | 2-5 | 0.5-2 | 0.5-1 | 0.5-1.5 | | — | — | — |
| Oxycodone | P.O.: 10-15 | 0.5-1 | 4-6 | 3-4 | 4 | (3-6) | NA | 30 |
| Oxymorphone | 5-15 | 0.5-1 | 3-6 | | | | 1 | 10§ |

## Comparative Pharmacokinetics *(continued)*

| Drug | Onset (min) | Peak (h) | Duration (h) | Half-Life (h) | Average Dosing Interval (h) | | Equianalgesic Doses* (mg) | |
|---|---|---|---|---|---|---|---|---|
| | | | | | Median | Range | I.M. | Oral |
| Pentazocine | 15-20 | 0.25-1 | 3-4 | 2-3 | 3 | (3-6) | | |
| Propoxyphene | P.O.: 30-60 | 2-2.5 | 4-6 | 3.5-15 | 6 | (4-8) | ND | 130¶-200# |
| Remifentanil | 1-3 | <0.3 | 0.1-0.2 | 0.15-0.3 | — | — | ND | ND |
| Sufentanil | 1.3-3 | ND | ND | 2.5-3 | — | — | 0.02 | NA |

ND = no data available. NA = not applicable.

*Based on acute, short-term use. Chronic administration may alter pharmacokinetics and decrease the oral parenteral dose ratio. The morphine oral-parenteral ratio decreases to ~ 1.5-2.5:1 upon chronic dosing.

†Extensive survey data suggest that the relative potency of I.M.:P.O. morphine of 1:6 changes to 1:2-3 with chronic dosing.

‡Narcotic antagonist

§Rectal.

¶HCl salt.

#Napsylate salt.

## NARCOTIC/OPIOID ANALGESIC COMPARISON
*(Continued)*

### Comparative Pharmacology

| Drug | Analgesic | Antitussive | Constipation | Respiratory Depression | Sedation | Emesis |
|---|---|---|---|---|---|---|
| **Phenanthrenes** | | | | | | |
| Codeine | + | +++ | + | + | + | + |
| Hydrocodone | + | +++ | | + | | |
| Hydromorphone | ++ | +++ | + | ++ | + | + |
| Levorphanol | ++ | ++ | ++ | ++ | ++ | + |
| Morphine sulfate | ++ | +++ | ++ | ++ | ++ | ++ |
| Oxycodone | ++ | +++ | ++ | ++ | ++ | ++ |
| Oxymorphone | ++ | + | ++ | +++ | | +++ |
| **Phenylpiperidines** | | | | | | |
| Alfentanil | ++ | | | | | |
| Fentanyl | ++ | | | + | | + |
| Meperidine | ++ | + | + | ++ | + | |
| Sufentanil | +++ | | | | | |
| **Diphenylheptanes** | | | | | | |
| Methadone | ++ | ++ | ++ | ++ | + | + |
| Propoxyphene | + | | | + | + | + |
| **Agonist/Antagonist** | | | | | | |
| Buprenorphine | ++ | N/A | +++ | +++ | ++ | ++ |
| Butorphanol | ++ | N/A | +++ | +++ | ++ | + |
| Dezocine | ++ | | + | ++ | + | ++ |
| Nalbuphine | ++ | N/A | +++ | +++ | ++ | ++ |
| Pentazocine | ++ | N/A | + | ++ | ++ or stimulation | ++ |

# NONSALICYLATE/NONSTEROIDAL ANTI-INFLAMMATORY AGENTS COMPARISON

| Name | Plasma Half-Life (h) | Time to Peak (h)* | Usual Duration (h) | Maximum Recommended Daily Dose (mg) | Considerations |
|---|---|---|---|---|---|
| Celecoxib (Celebrex®) | 11 | 2-3 | 12 | 400 | Selective COX-1 inhibitor |
| Choline magnesium salicylate (Trilisate®) | 2-30 | 2 | 8-24 | 4.5 g | Nonacetylated salicylates: limited antiplatelet effects |
| Diclofenac potassium immediate release (Cataflam®) | 1-2 | 1 | 8 | 200 | Less GI distress, less CNS depression |
| Diclofenac sodium delayed release (Voltaren®) | 1-2 | 2-3 | 8-12 | 225 | Less GI distress, less CNS depression |
| Diflunisal (Dolobid®) | 8-12 | 2-3 | 8-12 | 1.5 g | |
| Etodolac (Lodine®) | 7 | 1-2 | 6-8 | 1200 | Less GI distress |
| Fenoprofen (Nalfon®) | 2-3 | 1-2 | 4-6 | 3200 | Increased nephrotoxicity, increased antiplatelet activity |
| Flurbiprofen (Ansaid®) | 3-6 | 1.5-2 | | 300 | Increased GI distress |
| Ibuprofen (Motrin®) | 2 | 1-2 | 4-6 | 3200 | Less GI distress, moderately increased nephrotoxicity |
| Indomethacin (Indocin®) | 4.5 | 3-4 | 4-6 | 200 | Increased nephrotoxicity, GI distress, and CNS depression |
| Indomethacin SR | 4.5-6 | 2-4 | 6-12 | 150 | |
| Ketoprofen (Orudis®) | 1-4 | 0.5-2 | 4-6 | 300 | |
| Ketorolac (Toradol®) | 5-6 | 1 | 6-8 | P.O.: 40†<br>I.M.: 120 | Increased nephrotoxicity and GI distress |
| Meclofenamate (Meclomen®) | 2-3 | 0.5-1.5 | 2-4 | 400 | Less hepatic injury, increased GI distress |
| Mefenamic acid (Ponstel®) | 3.5 | 2-4 | 2-6 | 1000 | |
| Nabumetone (Relafen®) | 24 | 3-6 | >24 | 2000 | Less GI distress |
| Naproxen (Naprosyn®) | 9-20 | 1-2 | 2-7 | 1500 | Less GI distress |
| Naproxen sodium (Anaprox®) | 12-13 | 1-2 | 8-12 | 1375 | |
| Oxaprozin (Daypro™) | 42-50 | 3-5 | >24 | 1800 | Less GI distress |
| Piroxicam (Feldene®) | 30-86 | P.O.: 3-5 | 24 | 40 | Less hepatic injury |
| Salsalate (Disalcid®) | 7-8 | 2 | 8-24 | 3 g | Nonacetylated salicylates: limited antiplatelet effects |
| Sulindac (Clinoril®) | 7 (16)‡ | 2-4 | 12 | 400 | |
| Tolmetin (Tolectin®) | 5 | 0.5-1 | 6-8 | 1800 | |

Dosage is based on a 70 kg adult with normal hepatic and renal function.

*Food decreases the rate of absorption and may delay the time to peak levels.

†150 mg on the first day.

‡Half-life of active sulfide metabolite.

# TB DRUG COMPARISON

## TB Drugs in Special Situations

| Drug | Pregnancy | CNS TB Disease | Renal Insufficiency |
|---|---|---|---|
| Isoniazid | Safe | Good penetration | Normal clearance |
| Rifampin | Safe | Fair penetration<br>Penetrates inflamed meninges (10% to 20%) | Normal clearance |
| Pyrazinamide | Avoid | Good penetration | Clearance reduced<br>Decrease dose or prolong interval |
| Ethambutol | Safe | Penetrates inflamed meninges only (4% to 64%) | Clearance reduced<br>Decrease dose or prolong interval |
| Streptomycin | Avoid | Penetrates inflamed meninges only | Clearance reduced<br>Decrease dose or prolong interval |
| Capreomycin | Avoid | Penetrates inflamed meninges only | Clearance reduced<br>Decrease dose or prolong interval |
| Kanamycin | Avoid | Penetrates inflamed meninges only | Clearance reduced<br>Decrease dose or prolong interval |
| Ethionamide | Do not use | Good penetration | Normal clearance |
| Para-aminosalicylic acid | Safe | Penetrates inflamed meninges only (10% to 50%) | Incomplete data on clearance |
| Cycloserine | Avoid | Good penetration | Clearance reduced<br>Decrease dose or prolong interval |
| Ciprofloxacin | Do not use | Fair penetration (5% to 10%)<br>Penetrates inflamed meninges (50% to 90%) | Clearance reduced<br>Decrease dose or prolong interval |
| Ofloxacin | Do not use | Fair penetration (5% to 10%)<br>Penetrates inflamed meninges (50% to 90%) | Clearance reduced<br>Decrease dose or prolong interval |
| Amikacin | Avoid | Penetrates inflamed meninges only | Clearance reduced<br>Decrease dose or prolong interval |
| Clofazimine | Avoid | Penetration unknown | Clearance probably normal |

Safe = The drug has not been demonstrated to have teratogenic effects.

Avoid = Data on the drug's safety are limited, or the drug is associated with mild malformations (as in the aminoglycosides).

Do not use = Studies show an association between the drug and premature labor, congenital malformations, or teratogenicity.

## Second-Line TB Drugs

| Drug | Daily Dose (Maximum Dose) | Adverse Reactions |
|---|---|---|
| Capreomycin | 15-30 mg/kg (1 g) | Toxicity<br>–auditory<br>–vestibular<br>–renal |
| Kanamycin | 15-30 mg/kg (1 g) | Toxicity<br>–auditory<br>–vestibular<br>–renal |
| Ethionamide | 15-20 mg/kg (1 g) | GI upset<br>Hepatotoxicity<br>Hypersensitivity<br>Metallic taste<br>Bloating |
| Para-aminosalicylic acid (PAS) | 150 mg/kg (12 g) | GI upset<br>Hepatotoxicity<br>Hypersensitivity<br>Sodium load |
| Cycloserine | 15-20 mg/kg (1 g) | Psychosis<br>Convulsions<br>Depression<br>Headaches<br>Rash<br>Drug interactions |
| Ciprofloxacin | 500-1000 mg/day | GI upset<br>Dizziness<br>Hypersensitivity<br>Drug interactions<br>Headaches<br>Restlessness |
| Ofloxacin | 400-800 mg/day | GI upset<br>Dizziness<br>Hypersensitivity<br>Drug interactions<br>Headaches<br>Restlessness |
| Amikacin | 15 mg/kg | Renal toxicity<br>Vestibular dysfunction<br>Hearing loss<br>Chemical imbalance<br>Dizziness |
| Clofazimine | 100-300 mg/day | GI upset<br>Discoloration of skin<br>Severe abdominal pain and organ damage due to crystal deposition |

**Note**: Doses for children are the same as for adults. Use these drugs only in consultation with a clinician experienced in the management of drug-resistant TB.

## TB DRUG COMPARISON *(Continued)*

| Monitoring | Comments |
|---|---|
| Assess<br>–vestibular function<br>–hearing function<br>Measure<br>–blood urea nitrogen<br>–creatinine | Alter bacteriologic conversion, dosage may be reduced to 2-3 times/week |
| Assess<br>–vestibular function<br>–hearing function<br>Measure<br>–blood urea nitrogen<br>–creatinine | Alter bacteriologic conversion, dosage may be reduced to 2-3 times/week |
| Measure hepatic enzymes | Start with low dosage and increase as tolerated<br>May cause hypothyroid condition, especially if used with PAS |
| Measure hepatic enzymes<br>Assess volume status | Start with low dosage and increase as tolerated<br>Monitor cardiac patients for sodium load |
| Assess mental status<br>Measure serum drug levels | Start with low dosage and increase as tolerated<br>Pyridoxine may decrease CNS effects |
| Drug interactions | Not approved by FDA for TB treatment<br>Should not be used in children<br>Avoid<br>–antacids<br>–iron<br>–zinc<br>–sucralfate |
| Drug interactions | Not approved by FDA for TB treatment<br>Should not be used in children<br>Avoid<br>–antacids<br>–iron<br>–zinc<br>–sucralfate |
| Assess<br>–hearing function<br>Measure<br>–renal function<br>–serum drug levels | Not approved by FDA for TB treatment |
| Drug interactions | Not approved by FDA for TB treatment<br>Avoid sunlight<br>Consider dosing at mealtime<br>Efficacy unproven |

*Adjust weight-based dosages as weight changes

# CYTOCHROME P-450 ENZYMES AND DRUG METABOLISM

## BACKGROUND

There are five distinct groups of drug metabolizing which account for the majority of drug metabolism in humans. These enzymes "families", known as isoenzymes, are localized primarily in the liver. The nomenclature of this system has been standardized. Isoenzyme families are identified as a cytochrom (CYP prefix), followed by their numerical designation (eg, 1A2).

Enzymes may be inhibited (slowing metabolism through this pathway) or induced (increased in activity or number). Individual drugs metabolized by a specific enzyme are identified as substrates for the isoenzyme. Considerable effort has been expended in recent years to classify drugs metabolized by this system as either an inhibitor, inducer, or substrate of a specific isoenzyme. It should be noted that a drug may demonstrate complex activity within this scheme, acting as an inhibitor of one isoenzyme while serving as a substrate for another.

By recognizing that a substrate's metabolism may be dramatically altered by concurrent therapy with either an inducer or inhibitor, potential interactions may be identified and addressed. For example, a drug which inhibits CYP1A2 is likely to block metabolism of theophylline (a substrate for this isoenzyme). Because of this interaction, the dose of theophylline required to maintain a consistent level in the patient should be reduced when an inhibitor is added. Failure to make this adjustment may lead to supratherapeutic theophylline concentrations and potential toxicity.

This approach does have limitations. For example, the metabolism of specific drugs may have primary and secondary pathways. The contribution of secondary pathways to the overall metabolism may limit the impact of any given inhibitor. In addition, there may be up to a tenfold variation in the concentration of an isoenzyme across the broad population. In fact, a complete absence of an isoenzyme may occur in some genetic subgroups. Finally, the relative potency of inhibition, relative to the affinity of the enzyme for its substrate, demonstrates a high degree of variability. These issues make it difficult to anticipate whether a theoretical interaction will have a clinically relevant impact in a specific patient.

The details of this enzyme system continue to be investigated, and information is expanding daily. However, to be complete, it should be noted that other enzyme systems also influence a drug's pharmacokinetic profile. For example, a key enzyme system regulating the absorption of drugs is the p-glycoprotein system. Recent evidence suggests that some interaction originally attributed to the cytochrome system may, in fact, have been the result of inhibition of this enzyme.

The following tables represent an attempt to detail the available information with respect to isoenzyme activities. Within certain limits, they may be used to identify potential interactions. Of particular note, an effort has been made in each drug monograph to identify involvement of a particular isoenzyme in the drug's metabolism. These tables are intended to supplement the limited space available to list drug interactions in the monograph. Consequently, they may be used to define a greater range of both actual and potential drug interactions.

## CYTOCHROME P-450 ENZYMES AND DRUG METABOLISM *(Continued)*

## CYTOCHROME P-450 ENZYMES AND RESPECTIVE METABOLIZED DRUGS

### CYP1A2

#### Substrates

Acetaminophen
Acetanilid
Aminophylline
Amitriptyline (demethylation)
Antipyrine
Betaxolol
Caffeine
Chlorpromazine
Clomipramine (demethylation)
Clozapine
Cyclobenzaprine (demethylation)
Desipramine (demethylation)
Diazepam
Estradiol
Fluvoxamine
Grepafloxacin
Haloperidol
Imipramine (demethylation)
Levopromazine
Maprotiline
Methadone
Metoclopramide
Mirtazapine (hydroxylation)
Nortriptyline
Olanzapine (demethylation, hydroxylation)
Ondansetron
Phenacetin
Phenothiazines
Propafenone
Propranolol
Riluzole
Ritonavir
Ropinirole
Ropivacaine
Tacrine
Tamoxifen
Theophylline
Thioridazine
Thiothixene
Trifluoperazine
Verapamil
Warfarin (R-warfarin, minor pathway)
Zileuton
Zopiclone

#### Inducers

Carbamazepine
Charbroiled foods
Cigarette smoke
Cruciferous vegetables (cabbage, brussels sprouts, broccoli, cauliflower)
Nicotine
Omeprazole
Phenobarbital
Phenytoin
Primidone
Rifampin
Ritonavir

#### Inhibitors

Anastrozole
Cimetidine
Ciprofloxacin
Citalopram (weak)
Clarithromycin
Diethyldithiocarbamate
Diltiazem
Enoxacin
Erythromycin
Ethinyl estradiol
Fluvoxamine
Fluoxetine (high dose)
Grapefruit juice
Isoniazid
Ketoconazole
Levofloxacin
Mexiletine
Norfloxacin
Paroxetine (high dose)
Ritonavir
Sertraline (weak)
Tacrine
Tertiary TCAs
Zileuton

## CYP2A6

### Substrates

Letrozole
Montelukast
Nicotine
Ritonavir
Tamoxifen

### Inducers

Barbiturates

### Inhibitors

Diethyldithiocarbamate
Letrozole
Ritonavir
Tranylcypromine

## CYP2B6

### Substrates

Antipyrine
Bupropion (hydroxylation)
Cyclophosphamide
Ifosfamide
Nicotine
Orphenadrine
Tamoxifen

### Inducers

Phenobarbital
Phenytoin
Primidone

### Inhibitors

Diethyldithiocarbamate
Orphenadrine

## CYP2C
## (Specific isozyme has not been identified)

### Substrates

Antipyrine
Carvedilol
Clozapine (minor)
Mestranol
Mephobarbital
Tamoxifen
Ticrynafen

### Inducers

Carbamazepine
Phenobarbital
Phenytoin
Primidone
Sulfinpyrazone

### Inhibitors

Isoniazid
Ketoconazole
Ketoprofen

## CYP2C8

### Substrates

Carbamazepine
Diazepam
Diclofenac
Ibuprofen
Mephobarbital
Naproxen (5-hydroxylation)
Omeprazole
Paclitaxel
Retinoic acid
Tolbutamide
Warfarin (S-warfarin)

### Inducers

Phenobarbital
Primidone

### Inhibitors

Anastrozole
Omeprazole

## CYTOCHROME P-450 ENZYMES AND DRUG METABOLISM *(Continued)*

### CYP2C9

#### Substrates

Amitriptyline (demethylation)
Clomipramine
Dapsone
Diazepam
Diclofenac
Flurbiprofen
Fluvastatin
Glimepiride
Hexobarbital
Ibuprofen
Imipramine (demethylation)
Indomethacin
Irbesartan
Losartan
Mefenamic acid
Metronidazole
Mirtazapine
Montelukast
Naproxen (5-hydroxylation)
Omeprazole
Phenytoin
Piroxicam
Ritonavir
Sildenafil citrate
Tenoxicam
Tetrahydrocannabinol
Tolbutamide
Torsemide
Warfarin (S-warfarin)
Zafirlukast (hydroxylation)
Zileuton

#### Inducers

Carbamazepine
Fluconazole
Fluoxetine
Phenobarbital
Phenytoin
Rifampin

#### Inhibitors

Amiodarone
Anastrozole
Chloramphenicol
Cimetidine
Diclofenac
Disulfiram
Flurbiprofen
Fluoxetine
Fluvastatin
Fluvoxamine (potent)
Isoniazid
Ketoconazole (weak)
Ketoprofen
Metronidazole
Omeprazole
Phenylbutazone
Ritonavir
Sertraline
Sulfamethoxazole-trimethoprim
Sulfaphenazole
Sulfinpyrazone
Sulfonamides
Troglitazone
Valproic acid
Warfarin (R-warfarin)
Zafirlukast

### CYP2C18

#### Substrates

Amitriptyline
Clomipramine
Dronabinol
Imipramine
Naproxen
Omeprazole
Piroxicam
Proguanil
Propranolol
Retinoic acid
Tolbutamide
Warfarin

#### Inducers

Carbamazepine
Phenobarbital
Phenytoin
Rifampin

#### Inhibitors

Cimetidine
Fluconazole
Fluoxetine
Fluvastatin
Ketoconazole (weak)
Isoniazid
Sertraline

## CYP2C19

### Substrates

Amitriptyline (demethylation)
Barbiturates
Carisoprodol
Citalopram
Clomipramine (demethylation)
Desmethyldiazepam
Diazepam (N-demethylation, minor pathway)
Divalproex sodium
Hexobarbital
Imipramine (demethylation)
Lansoprazole
Mephenytoin
Mephobarbital
Moclobemide
Olanzapine (minor)
Omeprazole
Pentamidine
Phenytoin
Proguanil
Propranolol
Ritonavir
Tolbutamide
Topiramate
Valproic acid
Warfarin (R-warfarin)

### Inducers

Carbamazepine
Phenobarbital
Phenytoin
Rifampin

### Inhibitors

Cimetidine
Citalopram (weak)
Felbamate
Fluconazole
Fluoxetine
Fluvastatin
Fluvoxamine
Isoniazid
Ketoconazole (weak)
Letrozole
Omeprazole
Proguanil
Ritonavir
Sertraline
Teniposide
Tolbutamide
Topiramate
Tranylcypromine
Troglitazone

# CYTOCHROME P-450 ENZYMES AND DRUG METABOLISM *(Continued)*

## CYP2D6

### Substrates

Amitriptyline (hydroxylation)
Amphetamine
Betaxolol
Bisoprolol
Brofaromine
Bufurolol
Bupropion
Captopril
Carvedilol
Chlorpheniramine
Chlorpromazine
Cinnarizine
Clomipramine (hydroxylation)
Clozapine (minor pathway)
Codeine (hydroxylation, o-demethylation)
Cyclobenzaprine (hydroxylation)
Cyclophosphamide
Debrisoquin
Delavirdine
Desipramine
Dexfenfluramine
Dextromethorphan (o-demethylation)
Dihydrocodeine
Diphenhydramine
Dolasetron
Donepezil
Doxepin
Encainide
Fenfluramine
Flecainide
Fluoxetine (minor pathway)
Fluphenazine
Halofantrine
Haloperidol (minor pathway)
Hydrocodone
Hydrocortisone
Hydroxyamphetamine
Imipramine (hydroxylation)
Labetalol
Loratadine
Maprotiline
m-Chlorophenylpiperazine (m-CPP)
Meperidine
Methadone
Methamphetamine
Metoclopramide
Metoprolol
Mexiletine
Mianserin
Mirtazapine (hydroxylation)
Molindone
Morphine
Nortriptyline (hydroxylation)
Olanzapine (minor, hydroxymethylation)
Ondansetron
Orphenadrine
Oxycodone
Papaverine
Paroxetine (minor pathway)
Penbutolol
Pentazocine
Perhexiline
Perphenazine
Phenformin
Pindolol
Promethazine
Propafenone
Propranolol
Quetiapine
Remoxipride
Risperidone
Ritonavir (minor)
Ropivacaine
Selegiline
Sertindole
Sertraline (minor pathway)
Sparteine
Tamoxifen
Thioridazine
Tiagabine
Timolol
Tolterodine
Tramadol
Trazodone
Trimipramine
Tropisetron
Venlafaxine (o-desmethylation)
Yohimbine

### Inducers

Carbamazepine
Phenobarbital
Phenytoin
Rifampin
Ritonavir

### Inhibitors

Amiodarone
Chloroquine
Chlorpromazine
Cimetidine
Citalopram
Clomipramine
Codeine
Delavirdine
Desipramine
Dextropropoxyphene
Diltiazem
Doxorubicin
Fluoxetine
Fluphenazine
Fluvoxamine
Haloperidol
Labetalol
Lobeline
Lomustine
Methadone
Moclobemide
Norfluoxetine
Paroxetine
Perphenazine
Propafenone
Quinacrine
Quinidine
Ranitidine
Risperidone (weak)
Ritonavir
Sertindole
Sertraline (weak)
Thioridazine
Valproic acid
Venlafaxine (weak)
Vinblastine
Vincristine
Vinorelbine
Yohimbine

## CYP2E1

### Substrates

Acetaminophen
Acetone
Aniline
Benzene
Caffeine
Chlorzoxazone
Clozapine
Dapsone
Dextromethorphan
Enflurane
Ethanol
Halothane
Isoflurane
Isoniazid
Methoxyflurane
Nitrosamine
Ondansetron
Phenol
Ritonavir
Sevoflurane
Styrene
Tamoxifen
Theophylline
Venlafaxine

### Inducers

Ethanol
Isoniazid

### Inhibitors

Diethyldithiocarbamate (disulfiram metabolite)
Dimethyl sulfoxide
Disulfiram
Ritonavir

## CYTOCHROME P-450 ENZYMES AND DRUG METABOLISM *(Continued)*

### CYP3A3/4

**Substrates**

Acetaminophen
Alfentanil
Alprazolam**
Amiodarone
Amitriptyline (minor)
Amlodipine
Anastrozole
Androsterone
Antipyrine
Astemizole**
Atorvastatin
Benzphetamine
Bepridil
Budesonide
Bupropion (minor)
Buspirone
Busulfan
Bromazepam
Bromocriptine
Busulfan
Caffeine
Cannabinoids
Carbamazepine
Cerivastatin
Chlorpromazine
Cimetidine
Cisapride**
Citalopram
Clarithromycin
Clindamycin
Clomipramine
Clonazepam
Clozapine
Cocaine
Codeine (demethylation)
Cortisol
Cortisone
Cyclobenzaprine (demethylation)
Cyclophosphamide
Cyclosporine
Dapsone
Dehydroepiandrostendione
Delavirdine
Desmethyldiazepam
Dexamethasone
Dextromethorphan (minor, N-demethylation)
Diazepam (minor; hydroxylation, N-demethylation)
Digitoxin
Diltiazem
Disopyramide
Docetaxel
Dolasetron
Donepezil
Doxorubicin
Doxycycline
Dronabinol
Enalapril
Erythromycin
Estradiol
Ethinyl estradiol
Ethosuximide
Etoposide
Felodipine
Fentanyl
Fexofenadine
Finasteride
Fluoxetine
Flutamide
Glyburide
Granisetron
Halofantrine
Hydrocortisone
Hydroxyarginine
Ifosfamide
Imipramine
Indinavir
Isradipine
Itraconazole
Ketoconazole
Lansoprazole (minor)
Letrozole
Lidocaine
Loratadine
Losartan
Lovastatin
Methadone
Miconazole
Midazolam
Mifepristone
Mirtazapine (N-demethylation)
Montelukast
Navelbine
Nefazodone
Nelfinavir**
Nevirapine
Nicardipine
Nifedipine
Niludipine
Nimodipine
Nisoldipine
Nitrendipine
Omeprazole (sulfonation)
Ondansetron
Oral contraceptives
Orphenadrine
Paclitaxel
Pimozide**
Pravastatin
Prednisone
Progesterone
Proguanil
Propafenone
Quercetin
Quetiapine
Quinidine
Quinine
Repaglinide
Retinoic acid
Rifampin
Ritonavir**
Salmeterol
Saquinavir
Sertindole
Sertraline

Sibutramine##
Sildenafil citrate
Simvastatin
Sufentanil
Tacrolimus
Tamoxifen
Temazepam
Teniposide
Terfenadine**
Testosterone
Tetrahydrocannabinol
Theophylline
Tiagabine
Tolterodine
Toremifene
Trazodone
Tretinoin
Triazolam**
Troglitazone
Troleandomycin
Venlafaxine (N-demethylation)
Verapamil
Vinblastine
Vincristine
Warfarin (R-warfarin)
Yohimbine
Zatoestron
Zileuton
Ziprasidone
Zolpidem**
Zonisamide

**Inducers**

Carbamazepine
Dexamethasone
Ethosuximide
Glucocorticoids
Griseofulvin
Nafcillin
Nelfinavir
Nevirapine
Phenobarbital
Phenylbutazone
Phenytoin
Primidone
Progesterone
Rifabutin
Rifampin
Sulfadimidine
Sulfinpyrazone
Troglitazone

**Inhibitors**

Amiodarone
Anastrozole
Azithromycin
Cannabinoids
Cimetidine
Clarithromycin**
Clotrimazole
Cyclosporine
Danazol
Delavirdine
Dexamethasone
Diethyldithiocarbamate
Diltiazem
Dirithromycin
Disulfiram
Erythromycin**
Ethinyl estradiol
Fluconazole (weak)
Fluoxetine
Fluvoxamine**
Gestodene
Grapefruit juice
Indinavir
Isoniazid
Itraconazole**
Ketoconazole**
Metronidazole
Miconazole (moderate)
Nefazodone**
Nelfinavir
Nevirapine
Norfloxacin
Norfluoxetine
Omeprazole (weak)
Oxiconazole
Paroxetine (weak)
Propoxyphene
Quinidine
Quinine**
Ranitidine
Ritonavir**
Saquinavir
Sertindole
Sertraline
Troglitazone
Troleandomycin
Valproic acid (weak)
Verapamil
Zafirlukast
Zileuton

****Contraindications:**

Terfenadine, astemizole, cisapride, and triazolam contraindicated with nefazodone

Pimozide contraindicated with macrolide antibiotics

Alprazolam and triazolam contraindicated with ketoconazole and itraconazole

Terfenadine, astemizole, and cisapride contraindicated with fluvoxamine

Terfenadine contraindicated with ketoconazole, erythromycin, clarithromycin, troleandomycin

Ritonavir contraindicated with triazolam, zolpidem, astemizole, rifabutin, quinine, clarithromycin, troleandomycin

Nelfinavir contraindicated with rifabutin

##Do not use with SSRIs, sumatriptan, lithium, meperidine, fentanyl, dextromethorphan, or pentazocine within 2 weeks of a MAOI.

# CYTOCHROME P-450 ENZYMES AND DRUG METABOLISM *(Continued)*

## CYP3A5-7

### Substrates

Cortisol
Ethinyl estradiol
Lovastatin
Nifedipine
Quinidine
Terfenadine
Testosterone
Triazolam
Vinblastine
Vincristine

### Inducers

Phenobarbital
Phenytoin
Primidone
Rifampin

### Inhibitors

Clotrimazole
Ketoconazole
Metronidazole
Miconazole
Troleandomycin

## References


Baker GB, Urichuk CJ, and Coutts RT, "Drug Metabolism and Metabolic Drug-Drug Interactions in Psychiatry," *Child Adolescent Psychopharm News (Suppl)*.

DeVane CL, "Pharmacogenetics and Drug Metabolism of Newer Antidepressant Agents," *J Clin Psychiatry*, 1994, 55(Suppl 12):38-45.

*Drug Interactions Analysis and Management. Cytochrome (CYP) 450 Isozyme Drug Interactions*, Vancouver, WA: Applied Therapeutics, Inc, 523-7.

Ereshefsky L, "Drug-Drug Interactions Involving Antidepressants: Focus on Venlafaxine," *J Clin Psychopharmacol*, 1996, 16(3 Suppl 2):375-535.

Ereshefsky L, *Psychiatr Annal*, 1996, 26:342-50.

Fleishaker JC and Hulst LK, "A Pharmacokinetic and Pharmacodynamic Evaluation of the Combined Administration of Alprazolam and Fluvoxamine," *Eur J Clin Pharmacol*, 1994, 46(1):35-9.

Flockhart DA, et al, *Clin Pharmacol Ther*, 1996, 59:189.

Ketter TA, Flockhart DA, Post RM, et al, "The Emerging Role of Cytochrome P-450 3A in Psychopharmacology," *J Clin Psychopharmacol*, 1995, 15(6):387-98.

Michalets EL, "Update: Clinically Significant Cytochrome P-450 Drug Interactions," *Pharmacotherapy*, 1998, 18(1):84-112.

Nemeroff CB, DeVane CL, and Pollock BG, "Newer Antidepressants and the Cytochrome P450 System," *Am J Psychiatry*, 1996, 153(3):311-20.

Pollock BG, "Recent Developments in Drug Metabolism of Relevance to Psychiatrists," *Harv Rev Psychiatry*, 1994, 2(4):204-13.

Richelson E, "Pharmacokinetic Drug Interactions of New Antidepressants: A Review of the Effects on the Metabolism of Other Drugs," *Mayo Clin Proc*, 1997, 72(9):835-47.

Riesenman C, "Antidepressant Drug Interactions and the Cytochrome P450 System: A Critical Appraisal," *Pharmacotherapy*, 1995, 15(6 Pt 2):84S-99S.

Schmider J, Greenblatt DJ, von Moltke LL, et al, "Relationship of *In Vitro* Data on Drug Metabolism to *In Vivo* Pharmacokinetics and Drug Interactions: Implications for Diazepam Disposition in Humans," *J Clin Psychopharmacol*, 1996, 16(4):267-72.

Slaughter RL, *Pharm Times*, 1996, 7:6-16.

Watkins PB, "Role of Cytochrome P450 in Drug Metabolism and Hepatotoxicity," *Semin Liver Dis*, 1990, 10(4):235-50.

# CIGARETTE SMOKING AND EFFECTS ON DRUGS/TOXINS

| Drug | Effect |
|---|---|
| Amitriptyline | Possible decrease in tricyclic antidepressant drug levels due to increased hepatic metabolism |
| Arsenic | Possible increase in lung cancer |
| Asbestos | Increased risk of lung cancer |
| Ascorbic acid | Increased recommended dietary allowance (to 100 mg/day) |
| Beta-carotene | Increased risk of lung cancer |
| Caffeine | Increased metabolism |
| Chlordiazepoxide | Larger dose required to achieve sedative effects |
| Chromium (hexavalent) | Increased risk of lung cancer |
| Cocaine | Enhances (additively) cocaine-induced vasoconstriction in areas of atherosclerosis |
| Cotton dust | Exacerbation of respiratory effects of byssinosis |
| Desipramine | Possible decrease in tricyclic antidepressant drug levels due to increased hepatic metabolism |
| Diazepam | Larger dose required to achieve sedative effects |
| Diesel exhaust | Possible added effect for lung cancer |
| Estrogen | Increased risk of cardiovascular events |
| Ethyl alcohol | Increased risk for oral and esophageal cancer |
| Flecainide | Reduction of serum flecainide levels (by possibly increasing hepatic metabolism) |
| Fluvoxamine | Increased metabolism of fluvoxamine by 25%; lower serum concentrations of fluvoxamine |
| Heparin | Shorter heparin half-life |
| Imipramine | Possible decrease in tricyclic antidepressant drug levels due to increased hepatic metabolism |
| Mineral oil (cutting oil) mists | Synergistic effect of reduced lung function and chronic cough |
| Mustard gas | Possible increase in lung cancer |
| Neuroleptics | Increased risk for tardive dyskinesia |
| Nicotine | Increased metabolism |
| Nortriptyline | Possible decrease in tricyclic antidepressant drug levels due to increased hepatic metabolism |
| Pentazocine | Decreased analgesic effect |
| Propoxyphene | Decreased analgesic effect |
| Propranolol | Decreased therapeutic effect |
| Radiation | Possible increased risk of lung cancer |
| Radon | Increased risk of lung cancer |
| Ritonavir | Decreased ritonavir levels |
| Silica | Possible increased risk of lung cancer |
| Tacrine | Decreased insulin absorption; heavy smokers may require a 15% to 30% increase in insulin dosage than nonsmokers |
| Theophylline | Decreased theophylline levels with decreased effect |
| Uranium | Probable increase in lung cancer |
| Vinyl acetate | Enhanced respiratory impairment |
| Warfarin | |

From Schein JR, "Cigarette Smoking and Clinically Significant Drug Interactions", *Ann Pharmacother,* 1995, 29:1129-48.

Spigset O, Carleborg L, Hedenmalm K, et al, "Effect of Cigarette Smoking on Fluvoxamine Pharmacokinetics in Humans," *Clin Pharmacol Ther*, 1995, 58:399-403.

# SUGAR-FREE LIQUID PHARMACEUTICALS

The following sugar-free liquid preparations are listed by therapeutic category and alphabetically within each category. Please note that product formulations are subject to change by the manufacturer. Some of these products may contain sorbitol, xylitol, or other sweeteners which may be partially metabolized to provide calories.

## Analgesics

Acetaminophen Elixir (various)
APAP/APAP Plus
Aspirin/Buffered Aspirin (Medique®)
Bufferin® A/F Nite Time
Children's Anacin-3® Infants Drops
Children's Myapap® Elixir
Children's Panadol® Drops, Liquid, and Chewable Tablets
Children's Tylenol® Chewable Tablets
Conex® Liquid
Conex® With Codeine Liquid
Dolanex® Elixir
Extra Strength Tylenol® PM
Febrol® and Febrol® EX
I-Prin®
Methadone Hydrochloride Intensol
MS-Aid®
Myapap® Drops
No Drowsiness Tylenol®
Pain-Off®
Paregoric USP (Abbott)
Sep-A-Soothe® II
St Joseph® Aspirin-Free Liquid and Drops
Tempra® Chewable Tablets
Tylenol® Drops

## Antacids/Antiflatulents

Alcalak®
Aldroxicon®
Almag® Suspension
Aludrox® Suspension
Aluminum Hydroxide Suspension
Calglycine® Tablets
Camalox® Suspension
Citrocarbonate® Granules
Creamalin® Suspension
Delcid®
Di-Gel® Liquid (mint, lemon & orange flavored)
Digestamic®
Dimacid®
Gaviscon® Liquid
Gelusil® II
Gelusil® Liquid
Gelusil® Liquid Flavor Pack
Gelusil-M® Liquid
Kolantyl® Gel
Maalox® Plus Suspension
Maalox® Suspension
Maalox® Therapeutic Concentrate
Magnatril® Suspension
Magnesia and Alumina Oral Suspension USP (Abbott, Phillips Roxane)
Mallamint® Chewable Tablets
Marblen® Suspension and Tablets
Medi-Seltzer®/Plus
Milk of Bismuth
Milk of Magnesia USP
Mylanta® Liquid
Mylanta®-II Liquid
Mylicon® Drops
Nephrox® Suspension
Nutrajel®
Nutramag®

Pepto-Bismol® Liquid and Tablets
Phosphaljel® Suspension
Riopan Plus®
Riopan® Suspension
Silain-Gel® Liquid
Trisogel®
Titralac® Liquid
Titralac® Plus Liquid
WinGel® Liquid and Tablets

**Antiasthmatics**

Aerolate® Liquid
Alupent® Syrup
Choledyl® Pediatric Syrup
Droxine®
Elixophyllin® Elixir
Elixophyllin®-GG Liquid
Lanophyllin® Elixir
Lixolin® Liquid
Lufyllin® Elixir
Metaprel® Syrup
Mucomyst®-10
Mucomyst®-20
Mudrane® GG Elixir
Neothylline® Elixir
Neothylline® G
Organidin® Solution
Slo-Phyllin® 80 Syrup
Somophyllin® Oral Liquid
Somophyllin®-DF Oral Liquid
Tedral® Elixir and Suspension
Theolair™ 80 Syrup
Theolixir®
Theon® Syrup
Theo-Organidin® Elixir
Theophylline Elixir (Phillips Roxane)

**Antidepressants**

Sinequan® Oral Concentrate

**Antidiarrheals**

Corrective Mixture With Paregoric
Diasorb® Liquid and Tablets
Di-Gon® II
Diotame®
Donnagel®
Infantol® Pink
Kalicon® Suspension
Kaolin Mixture With Pectin NF (Abbott)
Kaolin-Pectin Suspension (Phillips Roxane)
Konsyl® Powder
Lomanate®
Lomotil® Liquid
Paregoric USP (various)
Parepectolin® (various)
Pepto-Bismol®
St Joseph® Antidiarrheal

**Antiepileptics**

Mysoline® Suspension
Paradione® Solution

**Antihistamine-Decongestants**

Actifed® With Codeine
Actifed® Syrup
Actidil® Syrup
Bromphen® Elixir
Dimetane® Decongestant Elixir
Dimetapp® Elixir
Hay-Febrol® Liquid
Isoclor® Liquid and Capsules
Naldecon® Pediatric Drops and Syrup
Naldecon® Syrup
Novahistine® Elixir
Phenergan® Fortis Syrup

## SUGAR-FREE LIQUID PHARMACEUTICALS *(Continued)*

Phenergan® Syrup
Rondec® DM Drops
Ryna® Liquid
S-T® Forte® Liquid
Tavist® Syrup
Trind® Liquid
Veltap® Elixir
Vistaril® Oral Suspension

**Anti-Infectives**

Augmentin® Suspension
Furadantin® Oral Suspension
Furoxone® Suspension
Humatin®
Mandelamine® Suspension/Forte®
Minocin® Suspension
Mycifradin® Sulfate Oral Solution
NegGram® Suspension
Proklar® Suspension
Sulfamethoxazole and Trimethoprim Suspension (Biocraft, Beecham, Burroughs Wellcome)
Vibramycin® Syrup

**Antiparkinsonism Agents**

Artane® Elixir

**Antispasmodics**

Antrocol® Elixir
Spasmophen® Elixir

**Corticosteroids**

Decadron® Elixir
Dexamethasone Solution (Roxane)
Dexamethasone Intensol Solution
Pediapred® Oral Liquid

**Cough Medicines**

Anatuss® With Codeine Syrup
Anatuss® Syrup
Brown Mixture NF (Lannett)
CCP® Caffeine Free
CCP® Cough/Cold Tablets
Cerose-DM®
Chlorgest-HD®
Codagest® Expectorant
Codiclear® DH Syrup
Codimal® DM
Colrex® Compound Elixir
Colrex® Expectorant
Conar® Syrup
Conar® Expectorant Syrup
Conex® Liquid
Conex® With Codeine Syrup
Contac Jr® Liquid
Day-Night Comtrex®
Decoral® Forte®
Dexafed® Cough Syrup
Dimetane®-DC Cough Syrup
Dimetane®-DX Cough Syrup
Entuss® Expectorant Liquid
Fedahist® Expectorant Syrup and Pediatric Drops
Guaificon®-DMS
Histafed® Pediatric Liquid
Hycomine® Syrup and Pediatric Syrup
Lanatuss® Expectorant
Medicon® D
Medi-Synal®
Naldecon-DX® Pediatric Drops and Syrup
Naldecon-DX® Adult Liquid
Non-Drowsy Comtrex®
Noratuss®-II Expectorant and Liquid
Organidin® Solution
Potassium Iodide Solution (various)

Prunicodeine®
Queltuss® Tablets
Robitussin-CF® Liquid
Robitussin® Night Relief Liquid
Rondec®-DM Drops
Rondec®-DM Syrup
Ryna® Liquid
Ryna-C® Liquid
Ryna-CX® Liquid
Scot-Tussin® DM Syrup
Scot-Tussin® Expectorant
Scot-Tussin® DM Cough Chasers
Silexin® Cough Syrup
Sorbutuss®
S-T® Expectorant, SF/D-F
S-T® Forte®, Sugar-Free
Sudodrin®/Sudodrin® Forte®
Terpin® Hydrate With Codeine Elixir (various)
Toclonol® Expectorant
Toclonol® Expectorant With Codeine
Tolu-Sed® Cough Syrup
Tolu-Sed® DM
Tricodene® Liquid
Trind-DM® Liquid
Tuss-Ornade®
Tussar® SF
Tussionex® Extended Release Suspension
Tussi-Organidin® Liquid
Tussirex® Sugar-Free

**Dental Preparations and Fluoride Preparations**

Cepacol® Mouthwash
Cepastat® Mouthwash and Gargle
Chloraseptic® Mouthwash and Gargle
Fluorigard® Mouthrinse
Fluorinse®
Flura-Drops®
Flura-Loz®
Flura® Tablets
Gel-Kam®
Karigel®
Karigel® N
Luride® Drops
Luride® SF Lozi-Tabs
Luride® 0.25 and 0.5 Lozi-Tabs
Luride® Lozi-Tabs
Pediaflor® Drops
Phos-Flur® Rinse/Supplement
Point-Two® Mouthrinse
Prevident® Disclosing Drops
Thera-Flur® Gel and Drops

**Diagnostic Agents**

Gastrografin®

**Dietary Substitutes**

Co-Salt®

**Iron Preparations/Blood Modifiers**

Amicar® Syrup
Beminal® Stress Plus With Iron
Chel-Iron® Drops
Chel-Iron® Liquid
Geritol® Complete Tablets
Geritonic™ Liquid
Hemo-Vite® Liquid
Iberet® Liquid
Iberet®-500 Liquid
Incremin® With Iron Syrup
Kovitonic® Liquid
Niferex®
Nu-Iron® Elixir
Vita-Plus H® Half Strength, Sugar-Free
Vita-Plus H®, Sugar-Free

## SUGAR-FREE LIQUID PHARMACEUTICALS *(Continued)*

**Laxatives**

Agoral® (plain, marshmallow, and raspberry)
Aromatic Cascara Fluidextract USP
Castor Oil
Castor Oil (flavored)
Castor Oil USP
Colace®, Liquid
Cologel®
Disonate™ Liquid
Doxinate® Solution
Emulsoil®
Fiberall® Powder
Haley's MO®
Hydrocil® Instant Powder
Hypaque® Oral Powder
Kondremul®
Kondremul® With Cascara
Kondremul® With Phenolphthalein
Konsyl® Powder
Liqui-Doss®
Magnesium Citrate Solution NF
Metamucil® Instant Mix (lemon-lime or orange)
Metamucil® SF Powder
Milk of Magnesia
Milk of Magnesia/Cascara Suspension
Milk of Magnesia/Mineral Oil Emulsion (various)
Milkinol® Liquid
Mineral Oil (various)
Neoloid® Liquid
Nu-LYTELY®
Phospho-Soda®
Sodium Phosphate & Biphosphate Oral Solution USP (Phillips Roxane)
Zymenol® Emulsion

**Potassium Products**

Cena-K® Solution
EM-K®-10% Liquid
K-G® Elixir
Kaochlor-Eff® Tablets for Solution
Kaochlor® S-F Solution
Kaon® Elixir (grape and lemon-lime flavor)
Kaon-Cl® 20% Liquid
Kay Ciel® Elixir
Kay Ciel® Powder
Kaylixir®
Klor-Con®/25 Powder
Klor-Con® EF Tablets
Klor-Con® Liquid 20%
Klor-Con® Powder
Klorvess® Effervescent Tablets
Klorvess® Granules
Kolyum® Liquid and Powder
Potachlor® 10% and 20% Liquid
Potasalan® Elixir
Potassine® Liquid
Potassium Chloride Oral Solution USP 5%, 10%, and 20% (various)
Potassium Gluconate Elixir NF
Rum-K® Solution
Tri-K® Liquid
Trikates® Solution

**Sedatives-Tranquilizers-Antipsychotics**

Butabarbital Sodium Elixir
Butisol Sodium® Elixir
Haldol® Concentrate
Loxitane® C Drops
Mellaril® Concentrate
Serentil® Concentrate
Thorazine® Concentrate

## Vitamin Preparations-Nutritionals

- Aquasol A® Drops
- BioCal® Tablets
- Bugs Bunny™ Chewable Tablets
- Bugs Bunny™ Plus Iron Chewable Tablets
- Bugs Bunny™ With Extra C Chewable Tablets
- Bugs Bunny™ Plus Minerals Chewable Tablets
- Calciferol™ Drops
- Caltrate® 600 Tablets
- Ce-Vi-Sol® Drops
- Cod Liver Oil (various)
- Decagen® Tablets
- DHT™ Intensol Solution (Roxane)
- Drisdol® in Propylene Glycol
- Flintstones™ Complete Chewable Tablets
- Flintstones™ With Extra C Chewable Tablets
- Flintstones™ Plus Iron Chewable Tablets
- Incremin® With Iron Liquid
- Kandium® Drops Tablets
- Lanoplex® Elixir
- Lycolan® Elixir
- Oyst-Cal® 500 Tablets
- Pediaflor®
- PMS® Relief
- Poly-Vi-Flor® Drops
- Poly-Vi-Flor®/Iron Drops
- Poly-Vi-Sol® Drops
- Poly-Vi-Sol®/Iron Drops
- Posture® Tablets
- Spiderman™ Children's Chewable Vitamin Tablets
- Spiderman™ Children's Plus Iron Tablets
- Theragran® Jr Children's Chewable Tablets
- Tri-Vi-Flor® Drops
- Tri-Vi-Sol® Drops
- Tri-Vi-Sol®/Iron Drops
- Vi-Daylin® ADC Drops
- Vi-Daylin® ADC/Fluoride Drops
- Vi-Daylin® ADC Plus Iron Drops
- Vi-Daylin® Drops
- Vi-Daylin®/Fluoride Drops
- Vi-Daylin® Plus Iron Drops
- Vitalize®

## Miscellaneous

- Altace™ Capsules
- Bicitra® Solution
- Cibalith-S® Syrup
- Colestid® Granules
- Dayto® Himbin® Liquid
- Digoxin® Elixir (Roxane)
- Duvoid®
- Glandosane®
- Lipomul®
- Lithium Citrate Syrup
- Nicorette® Chewing Gum
- Polycitra®-K Solution
- Polycitra®-LC Solution
- Tagamet® Liquid

## References

Hill EM, Flaitz CM, and Frost GR, "Sweetener Content of Common Pediatric Oral Liquid Medications," *Am J Hosp Pharm*, 1988, 45(1):135-42.

Kumar A, Rawlings RD, and Beaman DC, "The Mystery Ingredients: Sweeteners, Flavorings, Dyes, and Preservatives in Analgesic/Antipyretic, Antihistamine/Decongestant, Cough and Cold, Antidiarrheal, and Liquid Theophylline Preparations," *Pediatrics*, 1993, 91(5):927-33.

"Sugar Free Products," *Drug Topics Red Book*, 1992, 17-8.

# TYRAMINE FOODS LIST

| Food Types* | Allowed | Minimize Intake | Not Allowed |
|---|---|---|---|
| Beverages | Milk, decaffeinated coffee, tea, soda | Chocolate beverage, caffeine-containing drinks, clear spirits | Acidophilus milk, beer, ale, wine, malted beverages, alcohol-free and reduced alcohol beer and wine products |
| Breads/cereals | All except those containing cheese | None | Cheese bread and crackers |
| Dairy products | Cottage cheese, farmers or pot cheese, cream cheese, ricotta cheese, all milk, eggs, ice cream, pudding (except chocolate) | Yogurt (limit to 4 oz per day) | All other cheeses (aged cheese, American, Camembert, cheddar, Gouda, gruyere, mozzarella, parmesan, provolone, romano, Roquefort, stilton |
| Meat, fish, and poultry | All fresh or frozen | Aged meats, hot dogs, canned fish and meat | Chicken and beef liver, dried and pickled fish, pickled herring, summer or dry sausage, pepperoni, dried meats (ie, Genoa salami, hard salami, pepperoni, Lebanon bologna), meat extracts, bologna, liverwurst |
| Starches — potatoes/rice | All | None | Soybean (including paste) |
| Vegetables | All fresh, frozen, canned, or dried vegetable juices except those not allowed | Chili peppers, Chinese pea pods | Fava beans, sauerkraut, pickles, olives, Italian broad beans |
| Fruit | Fresh, frozen, or canned fruits and fruit juices | Avocado, banana, raspberries, figs | Banana peel extract |
| Soups | All soups not listed to limit or avoid | Commercially canned soups | Soups which contain broad beans, fava beans, cheese, beer, wine, any made with flavor cubes or meat extract, miso soup |
| Fats | All except fermented | Sour cream | Packaged gravy |
| Sweets | Sugar, hard candy, honey, molasses, syrups | Chocolate candies | None |
| Desserts | Cakes, cookies, gelatin, pastries, sherbets, sorbets | Chocolate desserts | Cheese-filled desserts |
| Miscellaneous | Salt, nuts, spices, herbs, flavorings, Worcestershire sauce | Soy sauce, peanuts | Brewer's yeast, yeast concentrates, all aged and fermented products, monosodium glutamate, vitamins with Brewer's yeast |

*Foods high in tyramine.

# MATERNAL/FETAL MEDICATIONS

Adapted from Briggs GG, "Medication Use During the Perinatal Period," *J Am Pharm Assoc*, 1998, 38:717-27.

## Antibiotics in Pregnancy

| Antibiotics Which Are Generally Regarded as Safe | |
|---|---|
| **Antibiotic** | **Comments** |
| Aminoglycosides (limited use) | |
| Penicillins | |
| Cephalosporins | |
| Clindmycin | |
| Erythromycin | |
| **Antibiotics to Be Avoided** | |
| Tetracyclines | Staining of deciduous teeth (4th month through term) |
| Aminoglycosides (prolonged use) | Eighth cranial nerve damage (hearing loss, vestibulotoxicity) |
| Fluoroquinolones | Potentially mutagenic, cartilage damage, arthropathy, and teratogenicity |
| Erythromycin estolate | Hepatotoxic in mother |
| Ribavirin | Possibly fetotoxic |

## Treatment and Prevention of Infection

| Prophylaxis | |
|---|---|
| Preterm premature rupture of membranes | Ampicillin, amoxicillin, cefazolin, amoxicillin/ clavulanate, ampicillin/sulbactam, erythromycin |
| Prevention of bacterial endocarditis | Ampicillin 2 g and gentamicin 1.5 mg/kg (max 120 mg) within 30 min of delivery, followed by 1 g ampicillin (I.V.) or amoxicillin (oral) 6 hours later |
| Cesarean section | Cefazolin (I.V. or uterine irrigation) or clindamycin/ gentamicin |
| **Treatment** | |
| Bacterial vaginosis | Clindamycin (oral or gel) in first trimester (gel has been associated with higher rate of preterm deliveries)<br>Metronidazole (oral) for 7 days or gel for 5 days (after first trimester) |
| Chorioamnionitis | Ampicillin plus gentamicin (clindamycin, erythromycin, or vancomycin if PCN allergic) |
| Genital herpes | First episode: Oral acyclovir<br>Near term treatment may reduce Cesarian sections<br>I.V. therapy for disseminated infection |
| Group B streptococci | Penicillin G 5 million units once, then 2.5 million units q4h<br>Ampicillin 2 g once, then 1 g q4h<br>Clindamycin or erythromycin if PCN allergic |
| HIV | Zidovudine (limits maternal-fetal transmission)<br>Oral dosing during pregnancy/I.V. prior to delivery<br>Other antiretroviral agents - effects unknown |
| Postpartum endometritis | Ampicillin (vancomycin if PCN allergic) plus clindamycin (or metronidazole) plus gentamicin until afebrile |
| Pyelonephritis | Ampicillin-gentamicin<br>Cefazolin<br>Co-trimoxazole |

## MATERNAL/FETAL MEDICATIONS *(Continued)*

### Treatment and Prevention of Infection *(continued)*

| | Prophylaxis |
|---|---|
| Urinary tract infection | Amoxicillin/ampicillin (resistance has increased)<br>Co-trimoxazole<br>Nitrofurantoin<br>Cephalexin |
| Vaginal candidiasis | Buconizole for 7 days<br>Clotrimazole for 7 days<br>Miconazole for 7 days<br>Terconazole for 7 days |

### Preterm Labor: Tocolytic Agents

| Drug Class | Route | Fetal/Neonatal Toxicities | Maternal Toxicities |
|---|---|---|---|
| Beta-adrenergic agonists | | | |
| Ritodrine, terbutaline | Oral, I.V., S.C. | Fetal tachycardia, intraventricular septal hypertrophy, neonatal hyperinsulinemia/ hypoglycemia | Pulmonary, edema, myocardial infarction, hypokalemia, hypotension, hyperglycemia, tachycardia |
| Magnesium | I.V. | Neurologic depression in newborn (loss of reflexes, hypotonia, respiratory depression(; fetal hypocalcemia and hypercalcuria; abnormal fetal bone mineralization and enamel hypoplasia | Hypotension, respiratory depression, ileus/constipation, hypocalcemia, pulmonary edema, hypotension, headache/ dizziness |
| NSAIDs | | | |
| Indomethacin | Oral, P.R. | Ductus arteriosis: premature closure, ricuspid regurgitation, primary pulmonary hypertension of the newborn, PDA; intraventricular hemorrhage, necrotizing enterocolitis, renal failure | GI bleeding, oligohydramnios, pulmonary edema, acute renal failure |
| Calcium channel blockers | | | |
| Nifedipine | Oral | Hypoxia secondary to maternal hypotension | Hypotension, flushing, tachycardia, headache |
| Nitrates | | | |
| Nitroglycerin | I.V./ S.L. | Hypoxia secondary to maternal hypotension | Hypotension, headache, dizziness |

## Pregnancy-Induced Hypertension*

| Drug Class | Maternal/Fetal Effects |
|---|---|
| **Antihypertensives Contraindicated in PIH** | |
| Diuretics | Reduction of maternal plasma volume exacerbates disease; use in chronic hypertension acceptable (if no superimposed pregnancy-induced hypertension) |
| ACE-inhibitors | Teratogenic in second and third trimester; fetal/ newborn anuria and hypotension, fetal oligohydramnios; neonatal death (congenital abnormalities of skull and renal failure) |
| **Hypertension Treatment†** | |
| Central-acting<br>Methyldopa | Relatively safe in second/third trimester |
| Beta-blockers<br>Acebutolol, atenolol, metoprolol, pindolol, propranolol | Increased risk of IUGR |
| Alpha-/beta-blocking<br>Labetolol | See beta-blockers |
| Vasodilators<br>Hydralazine | Relatively safe in second/third trimester |
| Nitrates<br>Nitroglycerin | Relatively safe in second/third trimester |
| Calcium channel blockers<br>Nifedipine | Relatively safe in second/third trimester |

*Includes management of pre-eclampsia/eclampsia and HELLP syndrome. **Note:** Prevention may include low-dose aspirin (81 mg/day) or calcium supplementation (2 g/day).

†All agents must be carefully titrated to avoid fetal hypoxia.

## Other Maternal-Fetal Drug Therapy

| Drug | Dose/Route |
|---|---|
| **Fetal Lung Maturation** | |
| Betamethasone | Two 12 mg doses I.M. at a 24-hour interval |
| Dexamethasone | Four 6 mg doses I.M. at 12-hour intervals |
| Doses repeated weekly up to 34 weeks gestation | |
| **Cervical Ripening** | |
| Oxytocin | I.V. dosing - often ineffective |
| Hygroscopic cervical dilators | |
| Dinoprostone (prostaglandin E2) | Gel (0.5 mg) or vaginal insert (10 mg, releasing 0.3 mg/h) |
| Misoprotil (prostaglandin E1) | Oral tablets inserted intravaginally 25-50 mcg q3-4h for up to 24 hours; oral dosing is investigational |
| **Analgesia During Labor** | |
| Meperidine | 25-50 mg I.V. q1-2h or 50-100 mg I.M. q2-4h |
| Fentanyl | 50-100 mcg q1h |
| Butorphanol | No advantage over other agents |
| Nalbuphine | No advantage over other agents |
| Tramadol | No advantage over other agents |
| **Postpartum Hemorrhage** | |
| Oxytocin | I.V. usually; also I.M. or intramyometrially (IMM) |
| Methylergonovine | I.M. or I.M.M.; contraindicated in hypertension |
| Carboprost (PG F2 alpha) | Pyrexia is common; contraindicated in cardiac, pulmonary, renal, or hepatic disease |
| Misoprostil | Rectal administration has been investigated |

# MATERNAL/FETAL TOXICOLOGY

## Drugs and Chemicals Proven to Be Teratogenic in Humans

| Drug/ Chemical | Fetal Adverse Effects | Relative Risk for Teratogenicity | Clinical Intervention |
|---|---|---|---|
| Alcohol | **Fetal alcohol syndrome:** Mental retardation, microcephaly, poor coordination, hypotonia, hyperactivity, short upturned nose, micrognathia or retrognathia (infancy) or prognathia (adolescence), short palpebral fissures, hypoplastic philtrum, thinned upper lips, microphthalmia, antenatal/postnatal growth retardation, occasional pathologies of eyes, mouth, heart, kidneys, gonads, skin, muscle, and skeleton | In alcoholic women consuming >2 g/kg/d ethanol over first trimester: 2- to 3-fold higher risk for congenital malformations (about 10%) | To calculate accurate dose of alcohol: **Prospective:** To discontinue exposure; if woman is alcoholic, refer to addiction center **During pregnancy:** To alleviate fears in mild or occasional drinkers who may terminate pregnancy based on unrealistic perception of risk, level 2 ultrasound to rule out visible malformation |
| Alkylating agents (busulfan, chlorambucil, cyclophosphamide, mechlorethamine) | Growth retardation, cleft palate, microphthalmia hypoplastic ovaries, cloudy corneas, agenesis of kidney, malformations of digits, cardiac defects, multiple other anomalies | Based on case reports, between 10% and 50% of cases were malformed for different drugs. It is possible that adverse outcome was overrepresented. | Level 2 ultrasound to rule out visible malformations. Supplement folic acid to women receiving antifolates (eg, methotrexate). |
| Antimetabolite agents (aminopterin azauridine, cytarabine, 5-FU, 6-MP, methotrexate) | Hydrocephalus, meningoencephalocele, anencephaly, malformed skull, cerebral hypoplasia, growth retardation, eye and ear malformations, malformed nose and cleft palate, malformed extremities and fingers **Aminopterin syndrome:** Cranial dysostosis, hydrocephalus, hypertelorism, anomalies of external ear, micrognathia, posterior cleft palate | Based on case reports 7%-75% of cases were malformed. It is possible that adverse outcome was overrepresented. | Level 2 ultrasound to rule out visible malformations. |
| Carbamazepine | Increased risk for neural tube defects (NTDs) | NTDs estimated at 1% with carbamazepine | Periconceptional folate; maternal and/or amniotic α-fetoprotein; ultrasound to rule out NTD. |

## Drugs and Chemicals Proven to Be Teratogenic in Humans *(continued)*

| Drug/ Chemical | Fetal Adverse Effects | Relative Risk for Teratogenicity | Clinical Intervention |
|---|---|---|---|
| Carbon monoxide | Cerebral atrophy, mental retardation, microcephaly, convulsions, spastic disorders, intrauterine or postnatal death | Based on case reports, when mother is severely poisoned, high risk for neurological sequelae; no increased risk in mild accidental exposures | Measure maternal carboxyhemoglobin levels. Treat with 100% oxygen for 5 hours after maternal carboxyhemoglobin returns to normal because fetal equilibration takes longer. If hyperbaric chamber available, should be used, as elimination half-life of CO is more rapid. Fetal monitoring by an obstetrician; sonographic follow-up. |
| Diethylstilbestrol (DES) | **Female offspring:** Clear cell vaginal or cervical adenocarcinoma in young female adults exposed in utero (before 18th week); irregular menses (oligomenorrhea), reduced pregnancy rates, increased rate of preterm deliveries, increased perinatal mortality and spontaneous abortion **Male offspring:** Cysts of epididymis, cryptorchidism, hypogonadism, diminished spermatogenesis | Exposure before 18 weeks of gestation: ≤1.4/1000 of exposed female with carcinoma. Congenital morphological changes in vaginal epithelium in 39% of exposures. | **Diagnosis:** Direct observation of mucosa and Shiller's test. **Treatment:** Mechanical excision or destruction in relatively confined area. Surgery and radiotherapy for diffused tumor. |
| Lead | Lower scores in developmental tests | Higher risk when maternal lead is >10 μg/dL | **Maternal lead levels >10 μg/dL:** Investigate for possible source of contamination. **Levels >25 μg/dL:** Consider chelation |
| Lithium carbonate | Possibly higher risk for Ebstein's anomaly; no detectable higher risk for other malformations | | Women who need lithium should continue therapy, with sonographic follow-up. Patients may need higher doses because of increased clearance rate. |

## MATERNAL/FETAL TOXICOLOGY *(Continued)*

### Drugs and Chemicals Proven to Be Teratogenic in Humans *(continued)*

| Drug/ Chemical | Fetal Adverse Effects | Relative Risk for Teratogenicity | Clinical Intervention |
|---|---|---|---|
| Methyl mercury, mercuric sulfide | Microcephaly, eye malformations, cerebral palsy, mental retardation, malocclusion of teeth | Women of affected babies consumed 9-27 ppm mercury; greater risk when ingested at 6-8 gestational months. Relative risk was not elucidated, but 13/220 babies born in Minamata, Japan, at time of contamination had severe disease. | Good correlation between mercury concentrations in maternal hair follicles and neurological outcome of the fetus. Hair mercury content >50 ppm was used successfully as a cut point for termination.<br>In acute poisoning, the fetus is 4-10 times more sensitive than the adult to methylmercury toxicity. |
| PCBs | **Stillbirth**<br>**Signs at birth:** White eye discharge, 30% (32/108); teeth present, 8.7% (11/127); irritated/ swollen gums, 11% (11/99); hyperpigmentation ("cola" staining), 42.5% (54/127); deformed/ small nails, 24.6% (30/ 122); acne, 12.8% (16/ 125)<br>**Subsequent history:** Bronchitis or pneumonia, 27.2% (30/ 124); chipped or broken teeth, 35.5% (38/107); hair loss, 12.2% (14/115); acne scars, 9.6% (11/115); generalized itching, 27.8% (32/1150)<br>**Developmental:** Do not meet milestones; lower scores than unexposed controls; evidence of CNS damage | 4%-20% (6/159-8/ 39) | These figures, which are from cases poisoned by high consumption of PCB-contaminated rice oil, cannot be extrapolated to cases in which maternal poisoning has not been verified.<br>Women working near PCBs (eg, hydroelectric facilities) should use effective protection. |
| Penicillamine | Skin hyperelastosis | Few case reports; risk unknown | |
| Phenytoin | **Fetal hydantoin syndrome:** Low nasal bridge, inner epicanthal folds, ptosis, strabismus, hypertelorism, low set or abnormal ears, wide mouth, large fontanels, anomalies and hypoplasia of distal phalanges and nails, skeletal abnormalities, microcephaly and mental retardation, growth deficiency, neuroblastoma, cardiac defects, cleft palate/lip | 5%-10% of typical syndrome; about 30% of partial picture.<br>Relative risk of 7 for offspring IQ ≤84. | Neurologist should consider changing to other medications. Keep phenytoin concentrations at lower effective levels. Level 2 ultrasound to rule out visible malformations, vitamin K to neonate. Epilepsy itself increases teratogenic risk. |

## Drugs and Chemicals Proven to Be Teratogenic in Humans *(continued)*

| Drug/ Chemical | Fetal Adverse Effects | Relative Risk for Teratogenicity | Clinical Intervention |
|---|---|---|---|
| Systemic retinoids (isotretinoin, etretinate) | Spontaneous abortions; deformities of cranium, ears, face, heart, limbs, liver; hydrocephalus, microcephalus, heart defects.<br>Cognitive defects even without dysmorphology | For isotretinoin: 38% risk. 80% of malformation are CNS. | Treated women should have an effective method of contraception. Pregnancy termination. If diagnosed too late, sonographic follow-up to rule out confirmed malformations. |
| Tetracycline | Yellow, gray-brown, or brown staining of deciduous teeth, destruction of enamel | From 4 months of gestation and on, occurs in 50% of fetuses exposed to tetracycline; 12.5% to oxytetracycline | If exposure before 14-16 weeks of gestation, no known risk |
| Thalidomide | Limb phocomelia, amelia, hypoplasia, congenital heart defects, renal malformations, cryptorchidism, abducens paralysis, deafness, microtia, anotia | About 20% risk when exposure to drug occurs in days 34-50 of gestation. | Thalidomide is an effective drug for some forms of leprosy. Treated women should have an effective mode of contraception. |
| Trimethadione | **Fetal trimethadione syndrome:** Intrauterine growth retardation, cardiac anomalies, microcephaly, cleft palate and lip, abnormal ears, dysmorphic face, mental retardation, tracheoesophageal fistula, postnatal death | Based on case reports: 83% risk; 32% infantile or neonatal death | No need for this antiepileptic to date |
| Valproic acid | Lumbosacral spina bifida with meningomyelocele; CNS defects, microcephaly, cardiac defects | 1.2% risk of neural tube defects | Level 2 ultrasound and maternal α-fetoproteins or amniocentesis to rule out neural tube defects. Epilepsy itself increases teratogenic risk. |
| Warfarin | **Fetal warfarin syndrome:** Nasal hypoplasia, chondrodysplasia punctata, branchydactyly, skull defects, abnormal ears, malformed eyes, CNS malformations, microcephaly, hydrocephalus, skeletal deformities, mental retardation, optic atrophy, spasticity, Dandy Walker malformations | 16% of exposed fetuses have malformation; another 3% hemorrhages; 8% stillbirths | **Prospective:** Switch to heparin for the first trimester. Deliver by a cesarean section. Women should be followed up in a high-risk perinatal unit. |

Reprinted with permission from "Drugs and Chemicals Proven to Be Teratogenic in Humans," *Maternal-Fetal Toxicology: A Clinician's Guide*, 2nd ed, Koren G, ed, New York, NY: Marcel Dekker, Inc, 1994, 37-43.

# ANXIOLYTIC/HYPNOTIC USE IN LONG-TERM CARE FACILITIES

One of the regulations regarding medication use in long-term care facilities concerns "unnecessary drugs." The regulation states, "Each resident's drug regimen must be free from unnecessary drugs." Recently, the Health Care Financing Administration (HCFA) issued the final interpretive guidelines on this regulation. The following is a summary of these guidelines as they pertain to anxiolytic/hypnotic agents.

A. **Long-Acting Benzodiazepines**

Long-acting benzodiazepine drugs should not be used in residents unless an attempt with a shorter-acting drug has failed. If they are used, the doses must be no higher than the listed dose, unless higher doses are necessary for maintenance or improvement in the resident's functional status. Daily use should be less then 4 continuous months unless an attempt at a gradual dose reduction is unsuccessful. Residents on diazepam for seizure disorders or for the treatment of tardive dyskinesia are exempt from this restriction. Residents on clonazepam for bipolar disorder, tardive dyskinesia, nocturnal myoclonus, or seizure disorder are also exempt. Residents on long-acting benzodiazepines should have a gradual dose reduction at least twice within 1 year before it can be concluded that the gradual dose reduction is "clinically contraindicated."

**Long-Acting Benzodiazepines**

| Generic | Brand | Maximum Daily Geriatric Dose (mg) |
|---|---|---|
| Chlordiazepoxide | Librium® | 20 |
| Clonazepam | Klonopin™ | 1.5 |
| Clorazepate | Tranxene® | 15 |
| Diazepam | Valium® | 5 |
| Flurazepam | Dalmane® | 15 |
| Halazepam | Paxipam® | 40 |
| Quazepam | Doral® | 7.5 |

**Benzodiazepine or Other Anxiolytic/Sedative Drugs**

Anxiolytic/sedative drugs should be used for purposes other than sleep induction only when other possible causes of the resident's distress have been ruled out and the use results in maintenance or improvement in the resident's functional status. Daily use should not exceed 4 continuous months unless an attempt at gradual dose reduction has failed. Anxiolytics should only be used for generalized anxiety disorder, dementia with agitated states that either endangers the resident or others, or is a source of distress or dysfunction; panic disorder or symptomatic anxiety associated with other psychiatric disorders. The dose should not exceed those listed below unless a higher dose is needed as evidenced by the resident's response. Gradual dosage reductions should be attempted at least twice within 1 year before it can be concluded that a gradual dose reduction is "clinically contraindicated."

**Short-Acting Benzodiazepines**

| Generic | Brand | Maximum Daily Geriatric Dose (mg) |
|---|---|---|
| Alprazolam | Xanax® | 0.75 |
| Estazolam* | ProSom® | 0.5 |
| Lorazepam | Ativan® | 2 |
| Oxazepam | Serax® | 30 |

*Primarily used as a hypnotic agent.

**Other Anxiolytic and Sedative Drugs**

| Generic | Brand | Maximum Daily Geriatric Dose (mg) |
|---|---|---|
| Chloral hydrate | Noctec®, etc | 750 |
| Diphenhydramine | Benadryl® | 50 |
| Hydroxyzine | Atarax®, Vistaril® | 50 |

**Note:** Chloral hydrate, diphenhydramine, and hydroxyzine are not necessarily drugs of choice for treatment of anxiety disorders. HCFA lists them only in the event of their possible use.

B. **Drugs Used for Sleep Induction**

Drugs for sleep induction should only be used when all possible reasons for insomnia have been ruled out (ie, pain, noise, caffeine). The use of the drug must result in the maintenance or improvement of the resident's functional status. Daily use of a hypnotic should not exceed 10 consecutive days unless an attempt at a gradual dose reduction is unsuccessful. The dose should not exceed those listed below unless a higher dose has been deemed necessary. Gradual dose reductions should be attempted at least three times within 6 months before it can be concluded that a gradual dose reduction is "clinically contraindicated."

**Hypnotic Drugs**

| Generic | Brand | Daily Geriatric Dose (mg) |
|---|---|---|
| Alprazolam* | Xanax® | 0.25 |
| Chloral hydrate | Noctec® | 500 |
| Diphenhydramine | Benadryl® | 25 |
| Estazolam | ProSom™ | 0.5 |
| Hydroxyzine | Atarax®, Vistaril® | 50 |
| Lorazepam* | Ativan® | 1 |
| Oxazepam* | Serax® | 15 |
| Temazepam | Restoril® | 7.5 |
| Triazolam | Halcion® | 0.125 |
| Zolpidem | Ambien® | 5 |

*Not officially indicated as a hypnotic agent.

**Note:** Chloral hydrate, diphenhydramine, and hydroxyzine are not necessarily drugs of choice for sleep disorders. HCFA lists them only in the event of their possible use.

C. **Miscellaneous Hypnotic/Sedative/Anxiolytic Drugs**

The initiation of the following medications should not occur in any dose in any resident. Residents currently using these drugs or residents admitted to the facility while using these drugs should receive gradual dose reductions. Newly admitted residents should have a period of adjustment before attempting reduction. Dose reductions should be attempted at least twice within 1 year before it can be concluded that it is "clinically contraindicated."

**Examples of Barbiturates**

| Generic | Brand |
|---|---|
| Amobarbital | Amytal® |
| Amobarbital/Secobarbital | Tuinal® |
| Butabarbital | Butisol Sodium® |
| Combinations | Fiorinal®, etc |
| Pentobarbital | Nembutal® |
| Secobarbital | Seconal™ |

**Miscellaneous Hypnotic/Sedative/Anxiolytic Agents**

| Generic | Brand |
|---|---|
| Ethchlorvynol | Placidyl® |
| Glutethimide | Doriden® |
| Meprobamate | Equanil®, Miltown® |
| Methyprylon | Noludar® |
| Paraldehyde | Paral® |

# FEDERAL OBRA REGULATIONS RECOMMENDED MAXIMUM DOSES

## Antidepressants

| Drug | Brand Name | Usual Max Daily Dose for Age ≥65 | Usual Max Daily Dose |
|---|---|---|---|
| Amitriptyline | Elavil® | 150 mg | 300 mg |
| Amoxapine | Asendin® | 200 mg | 400 mg |
| Desipramine | Norpramin® | 150 mg | 300 mg |
| Doxepin | Adapin®, Sinequan® | 150 mg | 300 mg |
| Imipramine | Tofranil® | 150 mg | 300 mg |
| Maprotiline | Ludiomil® | 150 mg | 300 mg |
| Nortriptyline | Aventyl®, Pamelor® | 75 mg | 150 mg |
| Protriptyline | Vivactil® | 30 mg | 60 mg |
| Trazodone | Desyrel® | 300 mg | 600 mg |
| Trimipramine | Surmontil® | 150 mg | 300 mg |

## Antipsychotics

| Drug | Brand Name | Usual Max Daily Dose for Age ≥65 | Usual Max Daily Dose | Daily Oral Dose for Residents With Organic Mental Syndromes |
|---|---|---|---|---|
| Acetophenazine | Tindal® | 150 mg | 300 mg | 20 mg |
| Chlorpromazine | Thorazine® | 800 mg | 1600 mg | 75 mg |
| Clozapine | Clozaril® | 25 mg | 450 mg | 50 mg |
| Fluphenazine | Prolixin® | 20 mg | 40 mg | 4 mg |
| Haloperidol | Haldol® | 50 mg | 100 mg | 4 mg |
| Loxapine | Loxitane® | 125 mg | 250 mg | 10 mg |
| Mesoridazine | Serentil® | 250 mg | 500 mg | 25 mg |
| Molindone | Moban® | 112 mg | 225 mg | 10 mg |
| Perphenazine | Trilafon® | 32 mg | 64 mg | 8 mg |
| Promazine | Sparine® | 50 mg | 500 mg | 150 mg |
| Risperidone | Risperdal® | 1 mg | 16 mg | 4 mg |
| Thioridazine | Mellaril® | 400 mg | 800 mg | 75 mg |
| Thiothixene | Navane® | 30 mg | 60 mg | 7 mg |
| Trifluoperazine | Stelazine® | 40 mg | 80 mg | 8 mg |
| Trifluopromazine | Vesprin® | 100 mg | 20 mg | – |

## Anxiolytics*

| Drug | Brand Name | Usual Daily Dose for Age ≥65 | Usual Daily Dose for Age ≤65 |
|---|---|---|---|
| Alprazolam | Xanax® | 2 mg | 4 mg |
| Chlordiazepoxide | Librium® | 40 mg | 100 mg |
| Clorazepate | Tranxene® | 30 mg | 60 mg |
| Diazepam | Valium® | 20 mg | 60 mg |
| Halazepam | Paxipam® | 80 mg | 160 mg |
| Lorazepam | Ativan® | 3 mg | 6 mg |
| Meprobamate | Miltown® | 600 mg | 1600 mg |
| Oxazepam | Serax® | 60 mg | 90 mg |
| Prazepam | Centrax® | 30 mg | 60 mg |

*__Note:__ HCFA-OBRA guidelines strongly urge clinicians not to use barbiturates, glutethimide, and ethchlorvynol due to their side effects, pharmacokinetics, and addiction potential in the elderly. Also, HCFA discourages use of long-acting benzodiazepines in the elderly.

## Hypnotics
## (Should not be used for more than 10 continuous days*)

| Drug | Brand Name | Usual Max Single Dose for Age ≥65 | Usual Max Single Dose |
|---|---|---|---|
| Alprazolam | Xanax® | 0.25 mg | 1.5 mg |
| Amobarbital | Amytal® | 105 mg | 300 mg |
| Butabarbital | Butisol® | 100 mg | 200 mg |
| Chloral hydrate | Noctec® | 750 mg | 1500 mg |
| Chloral hydrate | Various | 500 mg | 1000 mg |
| Diphenhydramine | Benadryl® | 25 mg | 50 mg |
| Ethchlorvynol | Placidyl® | 500 mg | 1000 mg |
| Flurazepam | Dalmane® | 15 mg | 30 mg |
| Glutethimide | Doriden® | 500 mg | 1000 mg |
| Halazepam | Paxipam® | 20 mg | 40 mg |
| Hydroxyzine | Atarax® | 50 mg | 100 mg |
| Lorazepam | Ativan® | 1 mg | 2 mg |
| Oxazepam | Serax® | 15 mg | 30 mg |
| Pentobarbital | Nembutal® | 100 mg | 200 mg |
| Secobarbital | Seconal® | 100 mg | 200 mg |
| Temazepam | Restoril® | 15 mg | 30 mg |
| Triazolam | Halcion® | 0.125 mg | 0.5 mg |

*__Note:__ HCFA-OBRA guidelines strongly urge clinicians not to use barbiturates, glutethimide, and ethchlorvynol due to their side effects, pharmacokinetics, and addiction potential in the elderly. Also, HCFA discourages use of long-acting benzodiazepines in the elderly and also discourages the use of diphenhydramine and hydroxyzine.

# HCFA GUIDELINES FOR UNNECESSARY DRUGS IN LONG-TERM CARE FACILITIES

**Procedures: §483.25(1)(1)**

Consider drug therapy "unnecessary" only after determining that the facility's use of the drug is:

- in excessive dose (including duplicate drug therapy)
- for excessive duration
- without adequate monitoring
- without adequate indications of use
- in the presence of adverse consequences which indicate the dose should be reduced or discontinued, or
- any combination of the reasons above

Allow the facility the opportunity to provide a rationale for the use of drugs prescribed outside the preceding guidelines. The facility may not justify the use of a drug prescribed outside the proceeding guidelines solely on the basis of "the doctor ordered it." This justification would render the regulation meaningless. The rationale must be based on sound risk-benefit analysis of the resident's symptoms and potential adverse effects of the drug.

Examples of evidence that would support a justification of why a drug is being used outside these guidelines but in the best interests of the resident may include, but are not limited to:

- a physician's note indicating for example, that the dosage, duration, indication, and monitoring are clinically appropriate, **and the reasons why they are clinically appropriate**; this note should demonstrate that the physician has carefully considered the risk/benefit to the resident in using drugs outside the guidelines
- a medical or psychiatric consultation or evaluation (eg, geriatric depression scale) that confirms the physician's judgment that use of a drug outside the guidelines is in the best interest of the resident
- physician, nursing, or other health professional documentation indicating that the resident is being monitored for adverse consequences or complications of the drug therapy
- documentation confirming that previous attempts at dosage reduction have been unsuccessful
- documentation (including MDS documentation) showing resident's subjective or objective improvement, or maintenance of function while taking the medication
- documentation showing that a resident's decline or deterioration is evaluated by the interdisciplinary team to determine whether a particular drug, or a particular dose, or duration of therapy, may be the cause
- documentation showing why the resident's age, weight, or other factors would require a unique drug dose or drug duration, indication, monitoring, and
- other evidence the survey team may deem appropriate

If the survey team determines that there is a deficiency in the use of antipsychotics, cite the facility under either the "unnecessary drug" regulation or the "antipsychotic drug" regulation, but not both.

**Note:** The unnecessary drug criterion of "adequate indications for use" does not simply mean that the **physician's order** must include a reason for using the drug (although such order writing is encouraged). It means that the **resident** lacks a valid clinical reason for use of the drug as evidenced by the survey team's evaluation of some, but not necessarily all, of the following: resident assessment, plan of care, reports of significant change, progress notes, laboratory reports, professional consults, drug orders, observation and interview of the resident, and other information.

# ANTIDEPRESSANT MEDICATION GUIDELINES

The under diagnosis and under treatment of depression in nursing homes has been documented in a *Journal of the American Medical Association* paper entitled "Depression and Mortality in the Nursing home" (*JAMA*, February 27, 1991, 265(8)). HCFA continues to support the accurate identification and treatment of depression in nursing homes.

The surveyor should not urge a facility to use behavioral monitoring charts (eg, documenting quantitatively (number of episodes) and objectively (eg, withdrawn behavior such as staying in their room, refusal to speak, etc)) when antidepressant drugs are used in nursing homes. Such charts are promoted in the interpretative guidelines for antipsychotic and benzodiazepine and other anxiolytic/sedative drugs, but **not** for antidepressant drugs. These charts may be helpful for monitoring the effects of antidepressant drugs in nursing homes, but they may place additional paperwork burden on the facility and thus act as a deterrent to the appropriate diagnosis and treatment of this condition.

The following is a list of commonly used antidepressant drugs.

| Generic Name | Brand Name |
|---|---|
| Amitriptyline* | Elavil® |
| Amoxapine | Asendin® |
| Bupropion | Wellbutrin® |
| Butriptyline* | Evadene® |
| Citalopram* | Celexa® |
| Clomipramine* | Anafranil® |
| Desipramine | Norpramin® |
| Dibenzepin* | Noveril® |
| Doxepin* | Sinequan® |
| Fluoxetine | Prozac® |
| Fluvoxamine | Luvox® |
| Imipramine* | Tofranil |
| Isocarboxazid* | Marplan® |
| Maprotiline | Ludiomil® |
| Mirtazapine | Remeron® |
| Nefazodone | Serzone® |
| Nortriptyline | Aventyl®, Pamelor® |
| Paroxetine | Paxil™ |
| Phenelzine* | Nardil® |
| Protriptyline | Vivactil® |
| Sertraline | Zoloft™ |
| Tranylcypromine* | Parnate® |
| Trazodone | Desyrel® |
| Trimipramine* | Surmontil® |
| Venlafaxine | Effexor® |

*These are not necessarily drugs of choice for depression in the elderly. They are listed here only in the event of their potential use.

# ANTIPSYCHOTIC MEDICATION GUIDELINES

Appropriate indications for use of antipsychotic medications are outlined in the Health Care Finance Administration's Omnibus Reconciliation Act (OBRA) of 1987. These regulations require that antipsychotics be used to treat specific conditions (listed below) and not solely for behavior control.

**Approved indications include:**

- acute psychotic episode
- atypical psychosis
- brief reactive psychosis
- delusional disorder
- Huntington's disease
- psychotic mood disorder (including manic depression and depression with psychotic features)
- schizo-affective disorder
- schizophrenia
- schizophrenic form disorder
- Tourette's disease
- short-term (7 days) for hiccups, nausea, vomiting, or pruritus
- organic mental syndrome with psychotic or agitated features:
    - behaviors are quantitatively and objectively documented
    - behaviors must be **persistent**
    - behaviors are not caused by preventable reasons
    - patient presents a danger to self or others
    - continuous crying or screaming if this impairs functional status
    - psychotic symptoms (hallucinations, paranoia, delusions) which cause resident distress or impaired functional capacity

"Clinically contraindicated" means that a resident with a "specific condition" who has had a history of recurrence of psychotic symptoms (eg, delusions, hallucinations) which have been stabilized with a maintenance dose of an antipsychotic drug without incurring significant side effects (eg, tardive dyskinesia) **should not receive gradual dose reductions**. In residents with organic mental syndromes (eg, dementia, delirium), "clinically contraindicated" means that a gradual dose reduction has been attempted **twice** in 1 year and that attempt resulted in the return of symptoms for which the drug was prescribed to a degree that a cessation in the gradual dose reduction, or a return to previous dose levels was necessary.

If the medication is being used outside the guidelines, the physician must provide justification why the continued use of the drug and the dose of the drug is clinically appropriate.

Antipsychotics should not be used if one or more of the following is/are the **only** indication:

- wandering
- poor self care
- restlessness
- impaired memory
- anxiety
- depression (without psychotic features)
- insomnia
- unsociability
- indifference to surroundings
- fidgeting
- nervousness
- uncooperativeness
- agitated behaviors which do **not** represent danger to the resident or others

Selection of an antipsychotic agent should be based on the side effect profile since all antipsychotic agents are equally effective at equivalent doses. Coadministration of two or more antipsychotics does not have any pharmacological basis or clinical advantage and increases the potential for side effects. See Antipsychotic Agents table in Comparison Charts.

## DOSING GUIDELINES

1. Daily dosages should be equal to or less than those listed below, unless documentation exists to support the need for higher doses to maintain or improve functional status.

| Generic | Brand | Daily Dose for Patients With Organic Mental Syndrome |
|---|---|---|
| Acetophenazine | Tindal® | 20 mg |
| Chlorpromazine | Thorazine® | 75 mg |
| Clozapine | Clozaril® | 50 mg |
| Fluphenazine | Prolixin® | 4 mg |
| Haloperidol | Haldol® | 4 mg |
| Loxapine | Loxitane® | 10 mg |
| Mesoridazine | Serentil® | 25 mg |
| Molindone | Moban® | 10 mg |
| Olanzapine | Zyprexa® | 5 mg |
| Perphenazine | Trilafon® | 8 mg |
| Pimozide | Orap™ | 4 mg |
| Prochlorperazine | Compazine® | 10 mg |
| Promazine | Sparine® | 150 mg |
| Quetiapine | Seroquel® | 100 mg |
| Risperidone | Risperdal® | 2 mg |
| Thioridazine | Mellaril® | 75 mg |
| Thiothixene | Navane® | 7 mg |
| Trifluoperazine | Stelazine® | 8 mg |

2. The dose of prochlorperazine may be exceeded for short-term (up to 7 days) for treatment of nausea and vomiting. Residents with nausea and vomiting secondary to cancer or cancer chemotherapy can also be treated with higher doses for longer periods of time.
3. The residents must receive adequate monitoring for significant side effects such as tardive dyskinesia, postural hypotension, cognitive-behavioral impairment, akathisia, and parkinsonism.
4. Gradual dosage reductions are to be attempted twice in 1 year if prescribed for OMS. If symptoms for which the drug has been prescribed return and both reduction attempts have proven unsuccessful, the physician may indicate further reductions are clinically contraindicated.
5. "Clinically contraindicated" means that a resident **need not undergo** a "gradual dose reduction" or "behavioral interventions" if:
   - The resident has a "specific condition" and has a history of recurrence of psychotic symptoms (eg, delusions, hallucinations), which have been stabilized with a maintenance dose of an antipsychotic drug without incurring significant side effects.
   - The resident has organic mental syndrome (now called "delirium, dementia, and amnestic and other cognitive disorders" by DSM IV) and has had a gradual dose reduction attempted **twice** in 1 year and that attempt resulted in the return of symptoms for which the drug was prescribed to a degree that a cessation in the gradual dose reduction, or a return to previous dose reduction was necessary.
   - The resident's physician provides a justification why the continued use of the drug and the dose of the drug is clinically appropriate. This justification should include: a) a diagnosis, but not simply a diagnostic label or code, but the description of symptoms, b) a discussion of the differential psychiatric and medical diagnosis (eg, why the resident's behavioral symptom is thought to be a result of a dementia with associated psychosis and/or agitated behaviors, and not the result of an unrecognized painful medical condition or a psychosocial or environmental stressor), c) a description of the justification for the choice of a particular treatment, or treatments, and d) a discussion of why the present dose is necessary to manage the symptoms of the resident. This information need not necessarily be in the physician's progress notes, but must be a part of the resident's clinical record.

Examples of evidence that would support a justification of why a drug is being used outside these guidelines but in the best interests of the resident may include, but are not limited to the following.

## ANTIPSYCHOTIC MEDICATION GUIDELINES *(Continued)*

1. A physician's note indicating for example, that the dosage, duration, indication, and monitoring are clinically appropriate, **and the reasons why they are clinically appropriate**; this note should demonstrate that the physician has carefully considered the risk/benefit to the resident in using drugs outside the guidelines.
2. A medical or psychiatric consultation or evaluation (eg, Geriatric Depression Scale) that confirms the physician's judgment that use of a drug outside the guidelines is in the best interest of the resident.
3. Physician, nursing, or other health professional documentation indicating that the resident is being monitored for adverse consequences or complications of the drug therapy.
4. Documentation confirming that previous attempts at dosage reduction have been unsuccessful.
5. Documentation (including MDS documentation) showing resident's subjective or objective improvement, or maintenance of function while taking the medication.
6. Documentation showing that a resident's decline or deterioration is evaluated by the interdisciplinary team to determine whether a particular drug, or a particular dose, or duration of therapy, may be the cause.
7. Documentation showing why the resident's age, weight, or other factors would require a unique drug dose or drug duration, indication, or monitoring.
8. Other evidence you may deem appropriate.

# OVERDOSE AND TOXICOLOGY

## GENERAL STABILIZATION OF THE PATIENT

The recommended treatment plan for the poisoned patient is not unlike general treatment plans taught in advanced cardiac life support (ACLS) or advanced trauma life support (ATLS) courses. In this manner, the initial approach to the poisoned patient should be essentially similar in every case, irrespective of the toxin ingested, just as the initial approach to the trauma patient is the same, irrespective of the mechanism of injury. This approach, which can be termed as routine poison management, essentially includes the following aspects.

- Stabilization: ABCs (airway, breathing, circulation; administration of glucose, thiamine, oxygen, and naloxone)
- History, physical examination leading toward the identification of class of toxin (toxidrome recognition)
- Prevention of absorption (decontamination)
- Specific antidote, if available
- Removal of absorbed toxin (enhancing excretion)
- Support and monitoring for adverse effects

| Drug | Effect | Comment |
|---|---|---|
| 25-50 g **dextrose** ($D_{50}W$) intravenously to reverse the effects of drug-induced hypoglycemia (adult) 1 mL/kg $D_{50}W$ diluted 1:1 (child) | This can be especially effective in patients with limited glycogen stores (ie, neonates and patients with cirrhosis) | Extravasation into the extremity of this hyperosmolar solution can cause Volkmann's contractures |
| 50-100 mg intravenous **thiamine** | Prevent Wernicke's encephalopathy | A water-soluble vitamin with low toxicity; rare anaphylactoid reactions have been reported |
| Initial dosage of **naloxone** should be 2 mg in adult patients preferably by the intravenous route, although intramuscular, subcutaneous, intralingual, and endotracheal routes may also be utilized. Pediatric dose is 0.1 mg/kg from birth until 5 years of age | Specific opioid antagonist without any agent properties | It should be noted that some semisynthetic opiates (such as meperidine or propoxyphene) may require higher initial doses for reversal, so that a total dose of 6-10 mg is not unusual for the adults. If the patient responds to a bolus dose and then relapses to a lethargic or comatose state, a naloxone drip can be considered. This can be accomplished by administering two-thirds of the bolus dose that revives the patient per hour or injecting 4 mg naloxone in 1 L crystalloid solution and administering at a rate of 100 mL/hour 0.4 mg/hour) |
| Oxygen, utilized in 100% concentration | Useful for carbon monoxide, hydrogen, sulfide, and asphyxiants | While oxygen is antidotal for carbon monoxide intoxication, the only relative toxic contraindication is in paraquat intoxication (in that it can promote pulmonary fibrosis) |
| Flumazenil | Benzodiazepine antagonist | Not routinely recommended due to increased risk of seizures |

## OVERDOSE AND TOXICOLOGY *(Continued)*

## LABORATORY EVALUATION OF OVERDOSE

**Unknown ingestion:** Electrolytes, anion gap, serum osmolality, arterial blood gases, serum drug concentration

**Known ingestion:** Labs tailored to agent

## ANION GAP

**Definition:** The difference in concentration between unmeasured cation and anion equivalents in serum.

Anion gap = $Na^+ - Cl^- - HCO_3^-$
(The normal anion gap is 10-14 mEq/L)

### Differential Diagnosis of Increased Anion Gap Acidosis

Organic anions

- Lactate (sepsis, hypovolemia, seizures, large tumor burden)
- Pyruvate
- Uremia
- Ketoacidosis (β-hydroxybutyrate and acetoacetate)
- Amino acids and their metabolites
- Other organic acids

Inorganic anions

- Hyperphosphatemia
- Sulfates
- Nitrates

### Differential Diagnosis of Decreased Anion Gap

Organic cations

- Hypergammaglobulinemia

Inorganic cations

- Hyperkalemia
- Hypercalcemia
- Hypermagnesemia

Medications and toxins

- Lithium

Hypoalbuminemia

### Toxins Affecting the Anion Gap

### Drugs Causing Increased Anion Gap (>12 mEq/L)

Nonacidotic

- Carbenicillin
- Sodium salts

Metabolic Acidosis

- Acetaminophen (ingestion >75-100 g)
- Acetazolamide
- Amiloride
- Ascorbic acid
- Benzalkonium chloride
- Benzyl alcohol
- Beta-adrenergic drugs
- Bialaphos
- 2-butanone
- Carbon monoxide
- Centrimonium bromide
- Chloramphenicol
- Colchicine
- Cyanide
- Dapsone
- Dimethyl sulfate
- Dinitrophenol
- Endosulfan
- Epinephrine (I.V. overdose)
- Ethanol
- Ethylene dibromide
- Ethylene glycol
- Fenoprofen
- Fluoroacetate
- Formaldehyde
- Fructose (I.V.)
- Glycol ethers
- Hydrogen sulfide
- Ibuprofen (ingestion >300 mg/kg)
- Inorganic acid
- Iodine
- Iron
- Isoniazid
- Ketamine
- Ketoprofen
- Metaldehyde
- Metformin

Methanol
Methenamine mandelate
Monochloracetic acid
Nalidixic acid
Naproxen
Niacin
Papaverine
Paraldehyde
Pennyroyal oil
Pentachlorophenol
Phenelzine
Phenformin (off the market)
Phenol
Phenylbutazone
Phosphoric acid
Potassium chloroplatinite
Propylene glycol
Salicylates
Sorbitol (I.V.)
Strychnine
Surfactant herbicide
Tetracycline (outdated)
Theophylline
Tienilic acid
Toluene
Tranylcypromine
Vacor
Verapamil

### Drugs Causing Decreased Anion Gap (<6 mEq/L)

Acidosis

Ammonium chloride
Bromide
Iodide
Lithium
Polymyxin B
Tromethamine

## OSMOLALITY

**Definition:** The summed concentrations of all osmotically active solute particles.

Predicted serum osmolality =
2 $Na^+$ + glucose (mg/dL) / 18 + BUN (mg/dL) / 2.8

The normal range of serum osmolality is 285-295 mOsm/L.

Differential diagnosis of increased serum osmolal gap (>10 mOsm/L)

Medications and toxins
- Alcohols (ethanol, methanol, isopropanol, glycerol, ethylene glycol)
- Mannitol
- Paraldehyde

### Calculated Osm

Osmolal gap = measured Osm − calculated Osm

0 to +10: Normal
>10: Abnormal
<0: Probable lab or calculation error

### Drugs Causing Increased Osmolar Gap

(by freezing-point depression, gap is >10 mOsm)

Ethanol*
Ethylene glycol*
Glycerol
Hypermagnesemia (>9.5 mEq/L)
Isopropanol* (acetone)
Iodine (questionable)
Mannitol
Methanol*
Propylene glycol
Severe alcoholic ketoacidosis or lactic acidosis
Sorbitol*

*Toxins increasing both anion and osmolar gap.

### Toxins Associated With Oxygen Saturation Gap

(>5% difference between measured and calculated value)

Carbon monoxide
Cyanide (questionable)
Hydrogen sulfide (possible)
Methemoglobin

### Toxins Eliminated by Multiple Dosing of Activated Charcoal

Acetaminophen
Amitriptyline
Atrazine (?)
Baclofen (?)
Bupropion (?)
Carbamazepine
Chlordecone
Cyclosporine
Dapsone
Dextropropoxyphene
Diazepam (desmethyldiazepam)
Digitoxin
Digoxin (with renal impairment)
Disopyramide
Glutethimide
Maprotiline
Meprobamate
Methotrexate

## OVERDOSE AND TOXICOLOGY *(Continued)*

- Methyprylon
- Nadolol
- Nortriptyline
- Phencyclidine (?)
- Phenobarbital
- Phenylbutazone
- Phenytoin (?)
- Piroxicam
- Propoxyphene
- Propranolol (?)
- Salicylates (?)
- Theophylline
- Valproic acid
- Vancomycin (?)

The following agents have been studied and have not been demonstrated to result in enhanced elimination.

- Amiodarone
- Chlopropamide
- Imipramine
- Tobramycin

### Toxins Eliminated by Forced Saline Diuresis

- Barium
- Bromides
- Chromium
- Cimetidine (?)
- Cis-platinum
- Cyclophosphamide
- Hydrazine
- Iodide
- Iodine
- Isoniazid (?)
- Meprobamate
- Methyl iodide
- Mushrooms (Group I)
- Nickel
- Potassium chloroplatinite
- Thallium
- Valproic acid (?)

### Toxins Eliminated by Alkaline Diuresis

- 2,4-D-chlorophenoxyacetic acid
- Barbital (serum levels >10 mg/dL)
- Chlorpropamide
- Fluoride
- Iopanoic Acid (?)
- Isoniazid (?)
- Mephobarbital
- Methotrexate
- 2-Methyl-4-chlorophenoxyacetic acid (MCPA)
- Orellanine (?)
- Phenobarbital
- Primidone
- Quinolones antibiotic
- Salicylates
- Sulfisoxazole
- Uranium

A urine flow of 3-5 mL/kg/hour should be achieved with a combination of isotonic fluids or diuretics. Alkalinization can be achieved by administration of 44-88 mEq of sodium bicarbonate per liter to titrate a urine pH of 7.5; 20-40 mEq/L of potassium chloride may also be required (potassium should not be administered in patients with renal insufficiency). It should be noted that the efficacy of forced diuresis has only been studied for salicylates and phenobarbital. Although several drugs can exhibit enhanced elimination through an acidic urine (tranylcypromine, quinine, chlorpheniramine, fenfluramine, strychnine, cathinone or khat, amphetamines, phencyclidine, nicotine, bismuth, diethylcarbamazine citrate, ephedrine, flecainide, local anesthetics), the practice of acidifying the urine should be discouraged in that it can produce metabolic acidosis and promote renal failure in the presence of rhabdomyolysis.

### Drugs and Toxins Removed by Hemoperfusion (Charcoal)

- *Amanita phalloides* (?)
- Atenolol (?)
- Bromisoval
- Bromoethylbutyramide
- Caffeine
- Carbamazepine
- Carbon tetrachloride (?)
- Carbromal
- Chloral hydrate (trichloroethanol)
- Chloramphenicol
- Chlorfenvinfos (?)
- Chlorpropamide
- Clonidine
- Colchicine (?)
- Creosote (?)
- Dapsone
- Demeton-S-methyl sulfoxide
- Diltiazem (?)
- Dimethoate
- Disopyramide
- Ethchlorvynol
- Ethylene oxide
- Glutethimide
- Levothyroxine (?)
- Lindane
- Liotrix
- Meprobamate
- Methaqualone
- Methotrexate
- Methsuximide
- Methyprylon (?)
- Metoprolol (?)

Nadolol (?)
Orellanine (?)
Oxalic acid (?)
Paraquat
Parathion (?)
Pentamidine
Phenelzine (?)
Phenobarbital
Phenol
Phenytoin
Podophyllin (?)
Procainamide (?)
Quinidine (?)
Rifabutin (?)
Sotalol (?)
Thallium
Thyroglobulin/thyroid hormone
Theophylline
Valproic acid
Verapamil (?)

Continuous arteriovenous hemofiltration has been used to treat lithium, paraquat, N-acetyl-procainamide and vancomycin ingestions with varying results. It is capable of filtering molecules with a molecular weight up to 50,000 but some substances such as thallium and formaldehyde cannot be removed by this method despite their low molecular weight.

Exchange transfusion is a useful modality to enhance drug elimination in neonatal or infant drug toxicity. Usually double or triple volume exchanges are performed. It has been utilized to treat barbiturate, acetaminophen, iron, caffeine, methyl salicylate, propafenone, ganciclovir, sodium nitrite, lead, phenazopyridine hydrochloride, pine oil, theophylline overdose, and nitrate exposure in pediatric patients. Exchange transfusions (500-2000 mL) volume replacement have also been used to treat adults with 80-150 g ingestions of parathion.

## TREATMENTS

| Drug or Drug Class | Signs/Symptoms | Treatment/Comments |
|---|---|---|
| Acetaminophen | Generally asymptomatic | Assess severity of ingestion; adult doses ≥140 mg/kg are thought to be toxic. Obtain serum concentration ≥4 hours postingestion and use acetaminophen nomogram to evaluate need for acetylcysteine. Gastric decontamination within 2-4 hours after ingestion. May administer activated charcoal for one dose, this may decrease absorption of acetylcysteine if given within 1 hour of acetylcysteine. For unknown ingested quantities and for significant ingestion give acetylcysteine orally (diluted 1:4 with juice or carbonated beverage); initial: 140 mg/kg then give 70 mg/kg every 4 hours for 17 doses. I.V. protocols are used in some institutions. |
| Alpha-adrenergic blocking agents | Hypotension, drowsiness | Give activated charcoal, additional treatment if symptomatic; use I.V. fluids, dopamine, or norepinephrine to treat hypotension. Epinephrine may worsen hypotension due to beta effects. |
| Aminoglycosides | Ototoxicity, nephrotoxicity, neuromuscular toxicity | Hemodialysis or peritoneal dialysis may be useful in patients with decreased renal function; calcium may reverse the neuromuscular toxicity. |

# OVERDOSE AND TOXICOLOGY *(Continued)*

## TREATMENTS *(continued)*

| Drug or Drug Class | Signs/Symptoms | Treatment/Comments |
|---|---|---|
| Anticholinergics, antihistamines | Coma, hallucinations, delirium, tachycardia, dry skin, urinary retention, dilated pupils | For life-threatening arrhythmias or seizures. Adults: 2 mg/dose physostigmine, may repeat 1-2 mg in 20 minutes and give 1-4 mg slow I.V. over 5-10 minutes if signs and symptoms recur (relatively contraindicated if QRS >0.1 msec). |
| Barbiturates | Respiratory depression, circulatory collapse, bradycardia, hypotension, hypothermia, slurred speech, confusion, coma | Repeated oral doses of activated charcoal given every 3-6 hours will increase clearance. Adults: 30-60 g. Assure GI motility, adequate hydration, and renal function. Urinary alkalinization with I.V. sodium bicarbonate will increase renal elimination of longer-acting barbiturates (eg, phenobarbital). Charcoal hemoperfusion may be required in severe overdose. |
| Benzodiazepines | Respiratory depression, apnea (after rapid I.V.), hypoactive reflexes, hypotension, slurred speech, unsteady gait, coma | Dialysis is of limited value; support blood pressure and respiration until symptoms subside. Flumazenil: Initial dose: 0.2 mg given I.V. over 30 seconds. If further response is desired after 30 seconds, give 0.3 mg over another 30 seconds. Further doses of 0.5 mg can be given over 30 seconds at 1-minute intervals up to a total of 3 mg. Continuous infusions may be used in rare instances since duration of benzodiazepines is longer than flumazenil. |
| Beta-adrenergic blockers | Hypotension, bronchospasm, bradycardia, hypoglycemia, seizures | Activated charcoal; treat symptomatically; glucagon, atropine, isoproterenol, dobutamine, or cardiac pacing may be needed to treat bradycardia, conduction defects, or hypotension. |
| Carbamazepine | Dizziness, drowsiness, ataxia, involuntary movements, opisthotonos, seizures, nausea, vomiting, agitation, nystagmus, coma, urinary retention, respiratory depression, tachycardia, arrhythmias | Use supportive therapy, general poisoning management as needed. Use repeated oral doses of activated charcoal given every 3-6 hours to decrease serum concentrations. Charcoal hemoperfusion may be needed. Treat hypotension with I.V. fluids, dopamine, or norepinephrine. Monitor EKG. Diazepam may control convulsions but may exacerbate respiratory depression. |

**TREATMENTS** *(continued)*

| Drug or Drug Class | Signs/Symptoms | Treatment/Comments |
|---|---|---|
| Cardiac glycosides | Hyperkalemia may develop rapidly and result in life-threatening cardiac arrhythmias, progressive bradyarrhythmias, second or third degree heart block unresponsive to atropine, ventricular fibrillation, asystole | Obtain serum drug level, induce emesis or perform gastric lavage. Give activated charcoal to reduce further absorption. Atropine may reverse heart block. Digoxin immune Fab (digoxin specific antibody fragments) is used in serious cases. Each 40 mg of digoxin immune Fab binds with 0.6 mg of digoxin. |
| Cholinergic | Nausea, vomiting, diarrhea, miosis, CNS depression, excessive salivation, excessive sweating, muscle weakness | Suction oral secretions, decontaminate skin, atropinize patient. Atropine dose must be individualized. Adults: Initial atropine dose: 1 mg; titrate dose upward. Pralidoxime (2-PAM) may need to be added for moderate to severe intoxications. |
| Cyanide | Myocardial depression, lactic acidosis, hypotension, respiratory depression, shock and cyanosis despite high oxygen saturation | Cyanide antidote kit: 1) Inhale vapor from 0.3 mL amyl nitrate ampul until I.V. sodium nitrite available; 2) sodium nitrite 300 mg I.V. then 3) sodium thiosulfate 12.5 g I.V. over 10 minutes |
| Heparin | Severe hemorrhage | 1 mg of protamine sulfate will neutralize approximately 90 units of heparin sodium (bovine) or 115 units of heparin sodium (porcine) or 100 units of heparin calcium (porcine). |
| Hydantoin derivatives | Nausea, vomiting, nystagmus, slurred speech, ataxia, coma | Gastric lavage or emesis; repeated oral doses of activated charcoal may increase clearance of phenytoin. Use 0.5-1 g/kg (30-60 g/dose) activated charcoal every 3-6 hours until nontoxic serum concentration is obtained. Assure adequate GI motility, supportive therapy. |
| Iron | Lethargy, nausea, vomiting, green or tarry stools, hypotension, weak rapid pulse, metabolic acidosis, shock, coma, hepatic necrosis, renal failure, local GI erosions | If immediately after ingestion and not already vomiting, give ipecac or lavage with saline solution. Give deferoxamine mesylate I.V. at 15 mg/kg/hour in cases of severe poisoning (serum iron >350 µg/mL) until the urine color is normal, the patient is asymptomatic, or a maximum daily dose of 8 g is reached. Urine output should be maintained >2 mL/kg/hour to avoid hypovolemic shock. |
| Isoniazid | Nausea, vomiting, blurred vision, CNS depression, intractable seizures, coma, metabolic acidosis | Control seizures with diazepam. Give pyridoxine I.V. equal dose to the suspected overdose of isoniazid or up to 5 g empirically. Give activated charcoal. |

## OVERDOSE AND TOXICOLOGY *(Continued)*

### TREATMENTS *(continued)*

| Drug or Drug Class | Signs/Symptoms | Treatment/Comments |
|---|---|---|
| Nonsteroidal anti-inflammatory drugs | Dizziness, abdominal pain, sweating, apnea, nystagmus, cyanosis, hypotension, coma, seizures (rarely) | Induce emesis. Give activated charcoal via NG tube. Fluid therapy is commonly effective in managing the hypotension that may occur following an acute NSAIDs overdose, except when this is due to an acute blood loss. Seizures tend to be very short-lived and often do not require drug treatment; although, recurrent seizures should be treated with I.V. diazepam. Since many of the NSAIDs undergo enterohepatic cycling, multiple doses of charcoal may be needed to reduce the potential for delayed toxicities. Provide symptomatic and supportive care. |
| Opioids and morphine analogs | Respiratory depression, miosis, hypothermia, bradycardia, circulatory collapse, pulmonary edema, apnea | Establish airway and adequate ventilation. Give naloxone 0.4 mg and titrate to a maximum of 10 mg. Additional doses may be needed every 20-60 minutes. May need to institute continuous infusion, as duration of action of opiates can be longer than duration of action of naloxone. |
| Organophosphates (insecticides, pyridostigmine, neostigmine) | Bronchospasm, diarrhea, diaphoresis, ventricular dysrhythmia, fasiculations, flacid paralysis, lethargy, coma | Atropine 2-5 mg every 15 minutes until symptoms abate (0.05 mg/kg children). If severe, may add pralidoxime 1-2 g over 15-30 minutes (20-50 mg/kg children); may repeat every 8-12 hours or continuous infusion 0.5 g/hour (10-20 mg/kg/hour children). |
| Phenothiazines | Deep, unarousable sleep, anticholinergic symptoms, extrapyramidal signs, diaphoresis, rigidity, tachycardia, cardiac dysrhythmias, hypotension | Activated charcoal; do **not** dialyze. Use I.V. benztropine mesylate 1-2 mg/dose slowly over 3-6 minutes for extrapyramidal signs. Use I.V. fluids and norepinephrine to treat hypotension. Avoid epinephrine which may cause hypotension due to phenothiazine-induced alpha-adrenergic blockade and unopposed epinephrine $B_2$ action. Use benzodiazepines for seizure management and to decrease rigidity. |

**TREATMENTS** *(continued)*

| Drug or Drug Class | Signs/Symptoms | Treatment/Comments |
|---|---|---|
| Salicylates | Nausea, vomiting, respiratory alkalosis, hyperthermia, dehydration, hyperapnea, tinnitus, headache, dizziness, metabolic acidosis, coma, hypoglycemia, seizures | Induce emesis or gastric lavage immediately. Give several doses of activated charcoal, rehydrate, and use sodium bicarbonate to correct metabolic acidosis and enhance renal elimination by alkalinizing the urine. Control hyperthermia by cooling blankets or sponge baths. Correct coagulopathy with vitamin K I.V. and platelet transfusions as necessary. Hypoglycemia may be treated with I.V. dextrose. Seizures should be treated with I.V. benzodiazepines (diazepam 5-10 mg I.V.). Give supplemental potassium after renal function has been determined to be adequate. Monitor electrolytes; obtain stat serum salicylate level and follow. |
| Tricyclic antidepressants | Agitation, confusion, hallucinations, urinary retention, hypothermia, hypotension, tachycardia, arrhythmias, seizures | Give activated charcoal ± lavage. Use sodium bicarbonate for QRS >0.1 msec; alkalinization by hyperventilation has been used in patients on mechanical ventilation; I.V. fluids and norepinephrine may be used for hypotension; benzodiazepines may be used for seizure management. |
| Warfarin | Internal or external hemorrhage, hematuria | For moderate overdoses, give oral, S.C., or I.D., or slow I.V. (I.V. associated with anaphylactoid reactions) phytonadione; usual dose: 2.5-10 mg, adjust per prothrombin time. For severe hemorrhage, give fresh frozen plasma or whole blood. See Warfarin monograph. |
| Xanthine derivatives | Vomiting, abdominal pain, bloody diarrhea, tachycardia, extrasystoles, tachypnea, tonic/clonic seizures | Give activated charcoal orally. Repeated oral doses of activated charcoal increase clearance. Use 0.5-1 g/kg (30-60 g/dose) of activated charcoal every 1-4 hours (depending on the severity of ingestion) until nontoxic serum concentrations are obtained. Assure adequate GI motility, supportive therapy. Charcoal hemoperfusion or hemodialysis can also be effective in decreasing serum concentrations and should be used if the serum concentration approaches 90-100 mcg/mL in acute overdoses. |

# SOUND-ALIKE COMPARISON LIST

The following list contains over 960 pairs of sound-alike drugs accompanied by a subjective pronunciation of each drug name. Any such list can only suggest possible pronunciation or enunciation miscues and is by no means meant to be exhaustive.

New or rarely used drugs are likely to cause the most problems related to interpretation. Healthcare workers should be made aware of the existence of both drugs in a sound-alike pair in order to avoid (or minimize) the potential for error. Drug companies attempt to avoid naming different drugs with similar-sounding names; however, mix-ups do occur. Reading current drug advertisements, professional literature, and drug handbooks is a good way to avert or surely lessen such sound-alike drug errors at all levels of the healthcare industry.

| Drug Name | Pronunciation |
|---|---|
| Accolate® | (ak' cue late) |
| Accutane® | (ak' yu tane) |
| Accolate® | (ak' cue late) |
| Accupril® | (ak' yu pril) |
| Accubron® | (ak' cue bron) |
| Accutane® | (ak' yu tane) |
| Accupril® | (ak' cue pril) |
| Accolate® | (ak' cue late) |
| Accupril® | (ak' cue pril) |
| Accutane® | (ak' yu tane) |
| Accutane® | (ak' yu tane) |
| Accubron® | (ak' cue bron) |
| Accutane® | (ak' yu tane) |
| Accolate® | (ak' cue late) |
| Accutane® | (ak' yu tane) |
| Accupril® | (ak' cue pril) |
| Accutane® | (ak' yu tane) |
| Acutrim® | (ak' yu trim) |
| acetazolamide | (a set a zole' a mide) |
| acetohexamide | (a set o heks' a mide) |
| acetohexamide | (a set o heks' a mide) |
| acetazolamide | (a set a zole' a mide) |
| Achromycin® | (ak roe mye' sin) |
| Adriamycin™ | (ade rya mye' sin) |
| Achromycin® | (ak roe mye' sin) |
| actinomycin | (ak ti noe mye' sin) |
| Actidil® | (ak' tee dill) |
| Actifed® | (ak' tee fed) |
| Actifed® | (ak' tee fed) |
| Actidil® | (ak' tee dill) |
| actinomycin | (ak ti noe mye' sin) |
| Achromycin® | (ak roe mye' sin) |
| Actron® | (ak' tron) |
| Acutrim® | (ak' yu trim) |
| Acutrim® | (ak' yu trim) |
| Accutane® | (ak' yu tane) |
| Acutrim® | (ak' yu trim) |
| Actron® | (ak' tron) |
| Adalat® | (ad' da lat) |
| Adapin® | (ad' da pin) |
| Adapin® | (ad' da pin) |
| Adalat® | (ad' da lat) |
| Adapin® | (ad' da pin) |
| Adipex-P® | (ad' di pex pea) |
| Adapin® | (ad' da pin) |
| Ativan® | (at' tee van) |
| Adderall® | (ad' der all) |
| Inderal® | (in' der al) |
| Adipex-P® | (ad' di pex pea) |
| Adapin® | (ad' da pin) |
| Adriamycin™ | (ade rya mye' sin) |
| Achromycin® | (ak roe mye' sin) |
| Adriamycin™ | (ade rya mye' sin) |
| Idamycin® | (eye da mye' sin) |
| Aerolone® | (air' o lone) |
| Aralen® | (air' a len) |
| Afrin® | (aye' frin or af' rin) |
| aspirin | (as' pir in) |
| Afrinol® | (af' ree nol) |
| Arfonad® | (arr' foe nad) |
| Agoral® | (ag' a ral) |
| Argyrol® | (ar' gee roll) |
| AK-Mycin® | (aye kay mye' sin) |
| Akne-Mycin® | (ak nee mye' sin) |
| Akne-Mycin® | (ak nee mye' sin) |
| AK-Mycin® | (aye kay mye' sin) |
| AKTob® | (ak' tobe) |
| AK-Trol® | (aye' kay trol) |
| AK-Trol® | (aye' kay trol) |
| AKTob® | (ak' tobe) |
| Alazide® | (al' a zide) |
| Alazine® | (al' a zine) |
| Alazine® | (al' a zine) |
| Alazide® | (al' a zide) |
| Aldactazide® | (al dak' ta zide) |
| Aldactone® | (al' dak tone) |
| Aldactone® | (al' dak tone) |
| Aldactazide® | (al dak' ta zide) |
| Aldomet® | (al' doe met) |
| Aldoril® | (al' doe ril) |
| Aldoril® | (al' doe ril) |
| Aldomet® | (al' doe met) |
| Aldoril® | (al' doe ril) |
| Elavil® | (el' a vil) |
| Alfenta® | (al fen' tah) |
| Sufenta® | (sue fen' tah) |
| alfentanil | (al fen' ta nill) |
| Anafranil® | (a naf' ra nil) |
| alfentanil | (al fen' ta nil) |
| remifentanil | (rem i fen' ta nil) |
| Alferon® | (al' fer on) |
| Alkeran® | (al' ker an) |
| Allegra® | (al leg' ra) |
| Viagra® | (vye ag' ra) |
| Alkeran® | (al' ker an) |
| Alferon® | (al' fer on) |
| Allerfrin® | (al' er frin) |
| Allergan® | (al' er gan) |
| Allergan® | (al' er gan) |
| Allerfrin® | (al' er frin) |
| Allergan® | (al' er gan) |
| Auralate® | (ahl' a late) |
| Altace™ | (al' tase) |
| alteplase | (al' te place) |
| alprazolam | (al pray' zoe lam) |
| triazolam | (trye ay' zoe lam) |

| Drug Name | Pronunciation |
|---|---|
| alteplase | (al' te place) |
| Altace™ | (al' tase) |
| alteplase | (al' te place) |
| anistreplase | (a nis' tre place) |
| Alupent® | (al' yu pent) |
| Atrovent® | (at' troe vent) |
| Alupent® | (al' yu pent) |
| Atrovent® | (at' troe vent) |
| amantadine | (a man' ta deen) |
| rimantadine | (ri man' to deen) |
| Amaryl® | (am' ah ril) |
| Ambenyl® | (am' ba nil) |
| Ambenyl® | (am' ba nil) |
| Amaryl® | (am' ah ril) |
| Ambenyl® | (am' ba nil) |
| Aventyl® | (a ven' til) |
| Ambi 10® | (am' bee ten') |
| Ambien™ | (am' bee en) |
| Ambien™ | (am' bee en) |
| Ambi 10® | (am' bee ten') |
| amiodarone | ((a mee' oh da rone) |
| amrinone | (am' ri none) |
| amitripyline | (a mee trip' ti leen) |
| imipramine | (im ip' ra meen) |
| ampicillin | (am pi sil' in) |
| bacampicillin | (ba kam pi sil' in) |
| amrinone | (am' ri none) |
| amiodarone | (a mee' oh da rone) |
| Anafranil® | (a naf' ra nil) |
| alfentanil | (al fen' ta nill) |
| Anafranil® | (a naf' ra nil) |
| enalapril | (e nal' a pril) |
| Anaprox® | (an' a prox) |
| Anaspaz® | (an' a spaz) |
| Anaspaz® | (an' a spaz) |
| Anaprox® | (an' a prox) |
| Anaspaz® | (an' a spaz) |
| Antispas® | (an' te spaz) |
| Anatrast® | (an' a trast) |
| Anatuss® | (an' a tuss) |
| Anatuss® | (an' a tuss) |
| Anatrast® | (an' a trast) |
| Ancobon® | (an' coe bon) |
| Oncovin® | (on' coe vin) |
| anistreplase | (a nis' tre place) |
| alteplase | (al' te place) |
| Ansaid® | (an' said) |
| Axid® | (aks' id) |
| Antispas® | (an' te spaz) |
| Anaspaz® | (an' a spaz) |
| Anturane® | (ann' chu rane) |
| Artane® | (ar' tane) |
| Aplisol® | (ap' lee sol) |
| A.P.L.® | (aye pee el') |
| A.P.L.® | (aye pee el') |
| Aplisol® | (ap' lee sol) |
| Apresoline® | (aye press' sow leen) |
| Priscoline® | (pris' coe leen) |
| AquaTar® | (ah' kwa tar) |
| Aquatag® | (ah' kwa tag) |
| Aquatag® | (ah' kwa tag) |
| AquaTar® | (ah' kwa tar) |
| Aralen® | (air' a len) |
| Aerolone® | (air' o lone) |
| Aralen® | (air' a len) |
| Arlidin® | (ar' le din) |
| Aramine® | (air' a meen) |
| Artane® | (ar' tane) |

| Drug Name | Pronunciation |
|---|---|
| Arfonad® | (arr' foe nad) |
| Afrinol® | (af' ree nol) |
| Argyrol® | (ar' gee roll) |
| Agoral® | (ag' a ral) |
| Arlidin® | (ar' le din) |
| Aralen® | (air' a len) |
| Arrestin® | (aye res' tin) |
| Aygestin® | (aye ges' tin) |
| Artane® | (ar' tane) |
| Anturane® | (an' chu rane) |
| Artane® | (ar' tane) |
| Aramine® | (air' a meen) |
| Asbron® | (as' bron) |
| aspirin | (as' pir in) |
| aspirin | (as' pir in) |
| Afrin® | (aye' frin or af' rin) |
| aspirin | (as' pir in) |
| Asbron® | (as' bron) |
| Atarax® | (at' a raks) |
| Ativan® | (at' tee van) |
| Atarax® | (at' a raks) |
| Marax® | (may' raks) |
| atenolol | (a ten' oh lole) |
| Tylenol® | (tye' le nole) |
| Atgam® | (at' gam) |
| Ativan® | (at' tee van) |
| Ativan® | (at' tee van) |
| Adapin® | (add' da pin) |
| Ativan® | (at' tee van) |
| Atarax® | (at' a raks) |
| Ativan® | (at' tee van) |
| Atgam® | (at' gam) |
| Ativan® | (at' tee van) |
| ATnativ® | (aye tee nay' tif) |
| Ativan® | (at' tee van) |
| Avitene® | (aye' va teen) |
| ATnativ® | (aye tee nay' tif) |
| Ativan® | (at' tee van) |
| Atrovent® | (at' troe vent) |
| Alupent® | (al' yu pent) |
| Augmentin® | (aug men' tin) |
| Azulfidine' | (ay zul' fi deen) |
| Auralate® | (ahl' a late) |
| Allergan® | (al' er gan) |
| Auralgan® | (a ral' gan) |
| Larylgan® | (la ril' gan) |
| Auralgan® | (a ral' gan) |
| Ophthalgan® | (opp thal' gan) |
| Aventyl® | (a ven' til) |
| Ambenyl® | (am' ba nil) |
| Aventyl® | (a ven' til) |
| Bentyl® | (ben' till) |
| Avitene® | (aye' va teen) |
| Ativan® | (at' tee van) |
| Axid® | (aks' id) |
| Ansaid® | (an' said) |
| Aygestin® | (aye ges' tin) |
| Arrestin® | (aye res' tin) |
| Azulfidine' | (ay zul' fi deen) |
| Augmentin® | (aug men' tin) |
| bacampicillin | (ba kam pi sil' in) |
| ampicillin | (am pi sil' in) |
| baclofen | (bak' loe fen) |
| Bactroban® | (bak' troe ban) |
| baclofen | (bak' loe fen) |
| Beclovent® | (bec' lo vent) |
| Bactocill® | (bak' tow sill) |
| Pathocil® | (path' o sill) |

## SOUND-ALIKE COMPARISON LIST *(Continued)*

| Drug Name | Pronunciation |
|---|---|
| Bactroban® | (bak' troe ban) |
| baclofen | (bak' loe fen) |
| Banophen® | (ban' o fen) |
| Barophen® | (bear' o fen) |
| Banthine® | (ban' theen) |
| Brethine® | (breath' een) |
| Banthine® | (ban' theen) |
| Pro-Banthine® | (pro ban' theen) |
| Barophen® | (bear' o fen) |
| Banophen® | (ban' o fen) |
| Beclovent® | (bec' lo vent) |
| baclofen | (bak' loe fen) |
| Beconase® | (beck' o nase) |
| Bexophene® | (beks' o feen) |
| Beminal® | (bem' eh nall) |
| Benemid® | (ben' a mid) |
| Benadryl® | (ben' a drill) |
| Bentyl® | (ben' till) |
| Benemid® | (ben' a mid) |
| Beminal® | (bem' eh nall) |
| Benoxyl® | (ben ox' ill) |
| Brevoxyl® | (brev ox' il) |
| Bentyl® | (ben' till) |
| Aventyl® | (a ven' til) |
| Bentyl® | (ben' till) |
| Benadryl® | (ben' a drill) |
| Bentyl® | (ben' till) |
| Cantil® | (can' til) |
| Bentyl® | (ben' til) |
| Trental® | (tren' tal) |
| Benylin® | (ben' eh lin) |
| Ventolin® | (ven' tow lin) |
| Benza® | (ben' zah) |
| Benzac® | (ben' zak) |
| Benzac® | (ben' zak) |
| Benza® | (ben' zah) |
| Betadine® | (bay' ta deen) |
| Betagan® | (bay' ta gan) |
| Betagan® | (bay' ta gan) |
| Betadine® | (bay' ta deen) |
| Betapace® | (bay' ta pace) |
| Betapen® | (bay' ta pen) |
| Betapen® | (bay' ta pen) |
| Betapace® | (bay' ta pace) |
| Bexophene® | (beks' o feen) |
| Beconase® | (beck' o nase) |
| Bicillin® | (bye sil' lin) |
| V-Cillin K® | (vee sil' lin kay) |
| Bicillin® | (bye sil' lin) |
| Wycillin® | (wye sil' lin) |
| bleomycin | (blee o mye' sin) |
| Cleocin® | (klee' o sin) |
| Bleph®-10 | (blef ten') |
| Blephamide® | (blef' a mide) |
| Blephamide® | (blef' a mide) |
| Bleph®-10 | (blef ten') |
| Borofax® | (boroe' faks) |
| Boropak® | (boroe' pak) |
| Boropak® | (boroe' pak) |
| Borofax® | (boroe' faks) |
| Brethine® | (breath' een) |
| Banthine® | (ban' theen) |
| Bretylol® | (brett' tee loll) |
| Brevital® | (brev' i tall) |
| Brevital® | (brev' i tall) |
| Bretylol® | (brett' tee loll) |

| Drug Name | Pronunciation |
|---|---|
| Brevoxyl® | (brev ox' il) |
| Benoxyl® | (ben ox' ill) |
| Bromfed® | (brom' fed) |
| Bromphen® | (brom' fen) |
| Bromphen® | (brom' fen) |
| Bromfed® | (brom' fed) |
| bumetanide | (byoo met' a nide) |
| Buminate® | (byoo' mi nate) |
| Bumex® | (byoo' mex) |
| Buprenex® | (byoo' pre nex) |
| Buprenex® | (byoo' pre nex) |
| Bumex® | (byoo' mex) |
| Buminate® | (byoo' mi nate) |
| bumetanide | (byoo met' a nide) |
| bupivacaine | (byoo piv' a kane) |
| mepivacaine | (me piv' a kane) |
| butabarbital | (byoo ta bar' bi tal) |
| butalbital | (byoo tal' bi tal) |
| butalbital | (byoo tal' bi tal) |
| butabarbital | (byoo ta bar' bi tal) |
| Byclomine® | (bye' clo meen) |
| Bydramine® | (bye' dra meen) |
| Byclomine® | (bye' clo meen) |
| Hycomine® | (hye' coe meen) |
| Bydramine® | (bye' dra meen) |
| Byclomine® | (bye' clo meen) |
| Bydramine® | (bye' dra meen) |
| Hydramyn® | (hye' dra min) |
| Cepastat® | (sea' pa stat) |
| Capastat® | (kap' a stat) |
| Cankaid® | (kan' kaid) |
| Enkaid® | (enn' kaid) |
| Cantil® | (can' til) |
| Bentyl® | (ben' till) |
| Capastat® | (kap' a stat) |
| Cepastat® | (sea' pa stat) |
| Capital® | (kap' i tal) |
| Capitrol® | (kap' i trol) |
| Capitrol® | (kap' i trol) |
| Capital® | (kap' i tal) |
| Capitrol® | (kap' i trol) |
| captopril | (kap' toe pril) |
| captopril | (kap' toe pril) |
| Capitrol® | (kap' i trol) |
| carboplatin | (kar' boe pla tin) |
| cisplatin | (sis' pla tin) |
| Cardio-Green® | (kar' dee yo green') |
| Cardioquin® | (kar' dee yo kwin) |
| Cardioquin® | (kar' dee yo kwin) |
| Cardio-Green® | (kar' dee yo green') |
| Cardura® | (kar dur' ah) |
| Cordarone® | (kor da rone') |
| Cardura® | (kar dur' ah) |
| Cordran® | (kor' dran) |
| Catapres® | (kat' a pres) |
| Catarase® | (kat' a race) |
| Catapres® | (kat' a pres) |
| Combipres® | (kom' bee pres) |
| Catapres® | (kat' a pres) |
| Ser-Ap-Es® | (ser ap' ess) |
| Catarase® | (kat' a race) |
| Catapres® | (kat' a pres) |
| cefazolin | (sef a' zoe lin) |
| cephalexin | (sef a leks' in) |
| cefazolin | (sef a' zoe lin) |
| cephalothin | (sef a' loe thin) |

| Drug Name | Pronunciation |
|---|---|
| cefotaxime | (sef o taks' eem) |
| cefoxitin | (se fox' i tin) |
| cefoxitin | (se fox' i tin) |
| cefotaxime | (sef o taks' eem) |
| ceftizoxime | (sef ti zoks' eem) |
| cefuroxime | (se fyoor ox' eem) |
| cefuroxime | (se fyoor ox' eem) |
| ceftizoxime | (sef ti zoks' eem) |
| Celexa® | (se lex' a) |
| Zyprexa® | (zye preks' a) |
| cephalexin | (sef a leks' in) |
| cefazolin | (sef a' zoe lin) |
| cephalothin | (sef a' loe thin) |
| cefazolin | (sef a' zoe lin) |
| cephapirin | (sef a pye' rin) |
| cephradine | (sef' ra deen) |
| cephradine | (sef' ra deen) |
| cephapirin | (sef a pye' rin) |
| chloroxine | (klor ox' een) |
| Choloxin® | (koe lox' in) |
| Choloxin® | (koe lox' in) |
| chloroxine | (klor ox' een) |
| chlorpropamide | (klor proe' pa mide) |
| chlorpromazine | (klor proe' ma zeen) |
| chlorpromazine | (klor proe' ma zeen) |
| chlorpropamide | (klor proe' pa mide) |
| Chorex® | (ko' reks) |
| Chymex® | (kye' meks) |
| Chymex® | (kye' meks) |
| Chorex® | (ko' reks) |
| cisplatin | (sis' pla tin) |
| carboplatin | (kar' boe pla tin) |
| Citracal® | (sit' tra cal) |
| Citrucel® | (sit' tru cel) |
| Citrucel® | (sit' tru cel) |
| Citracal® | (sit' tra cal) |
| clarithromycin | (kla rith' roe mye sin) |
| erythromycin | (er ith roe mye' sin) |
| Cleocin® | (klee' o sin) |
| bleomycin | (blee o mye' sin) |
| Cleocin® | (klee' o sin) |
| Lincocin® | (link' o sin) |
| Clinoxide® | (klin ox' ide) |
| Clipoxide® | (kleh pox' ide) |
| Clipoxide® | (kleh pox' ide) |
| Clinoxide® | (klin ox' ide) |
| Clocort® | (klo' kort) |
| Cloderm® | (klo' derm) |
| Cloderm® | (klo' derm) |
| Clocort® | (klo' kort) |
| clomiphene | (kloe' mi feen) |
| clomipramine | (kloe mi' pra meen) |
| clomiphene | (kloe' mi feen) |
| clonidine | (kloe' ni deen) |
| clomipramine | (kloe mi' pra meen) |
| clomiphene | (kloe' mi feen) |
| clonidine | (kloe' ni deen) |
| clomiphene | (kloe' mi feen) |
| clonidine | (kloe' ni deen) |
| clozapine | (kloe' za peen) |
| clonidine | (kloe' ni deen) |
| Klonopin™ | (klon' o pin) |
| clonidine | (kloe' ni deen) |
| Loniten® | (lon' eh ten) |
| clonidine | (kloe' ni deen) |
| quinidine | (kwin' i deen) |
| clotrimazole | (kloe trim' a zole) |
| co-trimoxazole | (koe-trye moks' a zole) |

| Drug Name | Pronunciation |
|---|---|
| Cloxapen® | (klox' a pen) |
| clozapine | (kloe' za peen) |
| Cozaar® | (koe' zar) |
| Zocor® | (zoe' cor) |
| clozapine | (kloe' za peen) |
| clonidine | (kloe' ni deen) |
| clozapine | (kloe' za peen) |
| Cloxapen® | (klox' a pen) |
| Co-Lav® | (koe' lav) |
| Colax® | (koe' laks) |
| co-trimoxazole | (koe-trye moks' a zole) |
| clotrimazole | (kloe trim' a zole) |
| CodAphen® | (kod' a fen) |
| Codafed® | (kode' a fed) |
| Codafed® | (kode' a fed) |
| CodAphen® | (kod' a fen) |
| codeine | (koe' deen) |
| Cophene® | (koe' feen) |
| codeine | (koe' deen) |
| Lodine® | (low' deen) |
| Colax® | (koe' laks) |
| Co-Lav® | (koe' lav) |
| Colestid® | (koe les' tid) |
| colistin | (koe lis' tin) |
| colistin | (koe lis' tin) |
| Colestid® | (koe les' tid) |
| Combipres® | (kom' bee pres) |
| Catapres® | (kat' a pres) |
| Congestac® | (kon ges' tak) |
| Congestant® | (kon ges' tant) |
| Congestant® | (kon ges' tant) |
| Congestac® | (kon ges' tak) |
| Cophene® | (koe' feen) |
| codeine | (koe' deen) |
| Cordarone® | (kor da rone') |
| Cardura® | (kar dur' ah) |
| Cordran® | (kor' dran) |
| Cardura® | (kar dur' ah) |
| Cort-Dome® | (kort' dome) |
| Cortone® | (kor' tone) |
| cortisone | (kor' ti sone) |
| Cortizone® | (kor' ti zone) |
| Cortizone® | (kor' ti zone) |
| cortisone | (kor' ti sone) |
| Cortone® | (kor' tone) |
| Cort-Dome® | (kort' dome) |
| Coumadin® | (ku' ma din) |
| Kemadrin® | (kem' a drin) |
| Crysticillin® | (kris ta sil' lin) |
| Crystodigin® | (kris toe dig' in) |
| Crystodigin® | (kris toe dig' in) |
| Crysticillin® | (kris ta sil' lin) |
| cycloserine | (sye kloe ser' een) |
| cyclosporine | (sye' kloe spor een) |
| Cyclospasmol® | (sye kloe spas' mol) |
| cyclosporine | (sye' kloe spor een) |
| cyclosporine | (sye' kloe spor een) |
| Cyclospasmol® | (sye kloe spas' mol) |
| cyclosporine | (sye' kloe spor een) |
| Cyklokapron® | (sye kloe kay' pron) |
| cyclosporine | (sye' kloe spor een) |
| cycloserine | (sye kloe ser' een) |
| Cyklokapron® | (sye kloe kay' pron) |
| cyclosporine | (sye' kloe spor een) |
| cytarabine | (sye tare' a been) |
| vidarabine | (vye dare' a been) |
| Cytotec® | (sye' toe tek) |
| Cytoxan® | (sye tox' an) |

## SOUND-ALIKE COMPARISON LIST *(Continued)*

| Drug Name | Pronunciation |
|---|---|
| Cytotec® | (sye' toe tek) |
| Sytobex® | (sye' toe beks) |
| Cytoxan® | (sye tox' an) |
| Cytotec® | (sye' toe tek) |
| dacarbazine | (da kar' ba zeen) |
| Dicarbosil® | (dye kar' bow sil) |
| dacarbazine | (da kar' ba zeen) |
| procarbazine | (proe kar' ba zeen) |
| dactinomycin | (dak ti noe mye' sin) |
| daunorubicin | (daw noe roo' bi sin) |
| Daranide® | (dare' a nide) |
| Daraprim® | (dare' a prim) |
| Daraprim® | (dare' a prim) |
| Daranide® | (dare' a nide) |
| Daricon® | (dare' eh kon) |
| Darvon® | (dar' von) |
| Darvon® | (dar' von) |
| Daricon® | (dare' eh kon) |
| Darvon® | (dar' von) |
| Devrom® | (dev' rom) |
| Darvon® | (dar' von) |
| Diovan® | (dye oh' van) |
| daunorubicin | (daw noe roo' bi sin) |
| dactinomycin | (dak ti noe mye' sin) |
| daunorubicin | (daw noe roo' bi sin) |
| doxorubicin | (dox o roo' bi sin) |
| Daypro® | (day' pro) |
| Deprol® | (deh' prol) |
| Decadron® | (dek' a dron) |
| Decholin® | (dek' o lin) |
| Decadron® | (dek' a dron) |
| Percodan® | (per' coe dan) |
| Decholin® | (dek' o lin) |
| Decadron® | (dek' a dron) |
| Deconal® | (dek' o nal) |
| Deconsal® | (dek' on sal) |
| Deconsal® | (dek' on sal) |
| Deconal® | (dek' o nal) |
| Delacort® | (del' a kort) |
| Delcort® | (del' kort) |
| Delcort® | (del' kort) |
| Delacort® | (del' a kort) |
| Delfen® | (del' fen) |
| Delsym® | (del' sim) |
| Delsym® | (del' sim) |
| Delfen® | (del' fen) |
| Demadex® | (dem' a deks) |
| Denorex® | (den' o reks) |
| Demerol® | (dem' eh rol) |
| dicumarol | (dye koo' ma role) |
| Demerol® | (dem' eh rol) |
| Dymelor® | (dye' meh lor) |
| Demerol® | (dem' eh rol) |
| Temaril® | (tem' a ril) |
| Denorex® | (den' o reks) |
| Demadex® | (dem' a deks) |
| Depakene® | (dep' a keen) |
| Depakote® | (dep' a kote) |
| Depakote® | (dep' a kote) |
| Depakene® | (dep' a keen) |
| Depogen® | (dep' o gen) |
| Depoject® | (dep' o ject) |
| Depoject® | (dep' o ject) |
| Depogen® | (dep' o gen) |
| Depo-Testadiol® | (dep o tes ta dye' ol) |
| Depotestogen® | (dep o tes' tow gen) |

| Drug Name | Pronunciation |
|---|---|
| Depogen® | (dep' o gen) |
| Depoject® | (dep' o ject) |
| Depoject® | (dep' o ject) |
| Depogen® | (dep' o gen) |
| Depotestogen® | (dep o tes' tow gen) |
| Depo-Testadiol® | (dep o tes ta dye' ol) |
| Deprol® | (deh' prol) |
| Daypro® | (day' pro) |
| Dermacort® | (der' ma kort) |
| DermiCort® | (der' meh kort) |
| Dermatop® | (der' ma top) |
| DermiCort® | (der' meh kort) |
| DermiCort® | (der' meh kort) |
| Dermacort® | (der' ma kort) |
| DermiCort® | (der' meh kort) |
| Dermatop® | (der' ma top) |
| deserpidine | (de ser' pi deen) |
| desipramine | (dess ip' ra meen) |
| Desferal® | (des' fer al) |
| Disophrol® | (dye' so frol) |
| Desferal® | (des' fer al) |
| desflurane | (des flu' rane) |
| desflurane | (des flu' rane) |
| Desferal® | (des' fer al) |
| desipramine | (dess ip' ra meen) |
| deserpidine | (de ser' pi deen) |
| desoximetasone | (des ox i met' a sone) |
| dexamethasone | (deks a meth' a sone) |
| Devrom® | (dev' rom) |
| Darvon® | (dar' von) |
| dexamethasone | (deks a meth' a sone) |
| desoximetasone | (des ox i met' a sone) |
| Diaβeta® | (dye a bay' tah) |
| Diabinese® | (dye ab' beh neese) |
| Diabinese® | (dye ab' beh neese) |
| Diaβeta® | (dye a bay' tah) |
| Diamox® | (dye' a moks) |
| Trimox® | (trye' moks) |
| Dicarbosil® | (dye kar' bow sil) |
| dacarbazine | (da kar' ba zeen) |
| diclofenac | (dye kloe' fen ak) |
| Diflucan® | (dye flu' can) |
| dicumarol | (dye koo' ma role) |
| Demerol® | (dem' eh rol) |
| Diflucan® | (dye flu' can) |
| diclofenac | (dye kloe' fen ak) |
| Diflucan® | (dye flu' can) |
| Diprivan® | (dye' pri van) |
| digitoxin | (di ji tox' in) |
| digoxin | (di jox' in) |
| digoxin | (di jox' in) |
| digitoxin | (di ji tox' in) |
| Dilantin® | (dye lan' tin) |
| Dilaudid® | (dye law' did) |
| Dilantin® | (dye lan' tin) |
| diltiazem | (dil tye' a zem) |
| Dilantin® | (dye lan' tin) |
| Dipentum® | (dye pen' tum) |
| Dilaudid® | (dye law' did) |
| Dilantin® | (dye lan' tin) |
| diltiazem | (dil tye' a zem) |
| Dilantin® | (dye lan' tin) |
| dimenhydrinate | (dye men hye' dri nate) |
| diphenhydramine | (dye fen hye' dra meen) |
| Dimetabs® | (dime' tabs) |
| Dimetapp® | (dime' tap) |

| Drug Name | Pronunciation |
|---|---|
| Dimetapp® | (dime' tap) |
| Dimetabs® | (dime' tabs) |
| Diovan® | (dye oh' van) |
| Darvon® | (dar' von) |
| Dipentum® | (dye pen' tum) |
| Dilantin® | (dye lan' tin) |
| diphenhydramine | (dye fen hye' dra meen) |
| dimenhydrinate | (dye men hye' dri nate) |
| Diphenatol® | (dye fen' ah tol) |
| diphenidiol | (dye fen' i dole) |
| diphenidiol | (dye fen' i dole) |
| Diphenatol® | (dye fen' ah tol) |
| Diphenylan® | (dye fen' eh lan) |
| dyphenylan | (dye fen' eh lan) |
| Diprivan® | (dye' pri van) |
| Diflucan® | (dye flu' can) |
| Diprivan® | (dip' riv an) |
| Ditropan® | (di troe' pan) |
| dipyridamole | (dye peer id' a mole) |
| disopyramide | (dye soe peer' a mide) |
| Disophrol® | (dye' so frol) |
| Desferal® | (des' fer al) |
| disopyramide | (dye soe peer' a mide) |
| dipyridamole | (dye peer id' a mole) |
| Ditropan® | (di troe' pan) |
| Diprivan® | (dip' riv an) |
| Ditropan® | (di troe' pan) |
| Intropin® | (in troe' pin) |
| Diutensin® | (dye yu ten' sin) |
| Salutensin® | (sal yu ten' sin) |
| dobutamine | (doe byoo' ta meen) |
| dopamine | (doe' pa meen) |
| docusate | (dok' yoo sate) |
| Doxinate® | (dox' eh nate) |
| Donnapine® | (don' a peen) |
| Donnazyme® | (don' a zime) |
| Donnazyme® | (don' a zime) |
| Donnapine® | (don' a peen) |
| dopamine | (doe' pa meen) |
| dobutamine | (doe byoo' ta meen) |
| dopamine | (doe' pa meen) |
| Dopram® | (doe' pram) |
| Dopar® | (doe' par) |
| Dopram® | (doe' pram) |
| Dopram® | (doe' pram) |
| dopamine | (doe' pa meen) |
| Dopram® | (doe' pram) |
| Dopar® | (doe' par) |
| doxepin | (dox' e pin) |
| Doxidan® | (dox' e dan) |
| Doxidan® | (dox' e dan) |
| doxepin | (dox' e pin) |
| Doxinate® | (dox' eh nate) |
| docusate | (dok' yoo sate) |
| doxorubicin | (dox o roo' bi sin) |
| daunorubicin | (daw noe roo' bi sin) |
| Duo-Cyp® | (du' o sip) |
| DuoCet™ | (du' o set) |
| DuoCet™ | (du' o set) |
| Duo-Cyp® | (du' o sip) |
| Dura-Gest® | (dur' a gest) |
| Duragen® | (dur' a gen) |
| Duragen® | (dur' a gen) |
| Dura-Gest® | (dur' a gest) |
| Dyazide® | (dye' a zide) |
| Dynacin® | (dye' na sin) |
| Dymelor® | (dye' meh lor) |
| Demerol® | (dem' eh rol) |
| Dymelor® | (dye' meh lor) |
| Pamelor® | (pam' meh lor) |
| Dynabac® | (dye' na bac) |
| Dynapen® | (dye' na pen) |
| Dynacin® | (dye' na sin) |
| Dyazide® | (dye' a zide) |
| Dynacin® | (dye' na sin) |
| Dynapen® | (dye' ne pen) |
| Dynapen® | (dye' na pen) |
| Dynabac® | (dye' na bac) |
| Dynapen® | (dye' ne pen) |
| Dynacin® | (dye' na sin) |
| dyphenylan | (dye fen' eh lan) |
| Diphenylan® | (dye fen' eh lan) |
| Dyrenium® | (dye ren' e um) |
| Pyridium® | (pye rid' dee um) |
| Dwelle® | (dwell) |
| Kwell® | (kwell) |
| Ecotrin® | (eh' ko trin) |
| Edecrin® | (ed' eh crin) |
| Edecrin® | (ed' eh crin) |
| Ecotrin® | (eh' ko trin) |
| Edecrin® | (ed' eh crin) |
| Ethaquin® | (eth' a kwin) |
| Elavil® | (el' a vil) |
| Aldoril® | (al' doe ril) |
| Elavil® | (el' a vil) |
| Eldepryl® | (el' de pril) |
| Elavil® | (el' a vil) |
| Equanil® | (eh' kwa nil) |
| Elavil® | (el' a vil) |
| Mellaril® | (mel' la ril) |
| Elavil® | (el' a vil) |
| Oruvail® | (or' yu vale) |
| Eldepryl® | (el' de pril) |
| Elavil® | (el' a vil) |
| Elixicon® | (eh lix' i con) |
| Elocon® | (ee' lo con) |
| Elocon® | (ee' lo con) |
| Elixicon® | (eh lix' i con) |
| emetine | (em' eh teen) |
| Emetrol® | (em' eh trol) |
| Emetrol® | (em' eh trol) |
| emetine | (em' eh teen) |
| enalapril | (e nal' a pril) |
| Anafranil® | (a naf' ra nil) |
| Endal® | (en' dal) |
| Intal® | (in' tal) |
| Enduron® | (en' du ron) |
| Imuran® | (im' yu ran) |
| Enduron® | (en' du ron) |
| Inderal® | (in' der al) |
| Enduronyl® | (en dur' o nil) |
| Inderal® | (in' der al) |
| Enduronyl® Forte | (en dur' o nil for' tay) |
| Inderal® 40 | (in' der al for' tee) |
| enflurane | (en' floo rane) |
| isoflurane | (eye soe flure' ane) |
| Enkaid® | (enn' kaid) |
| Cankaid® | (kan' kaid) |
| ephedrine | (e fed' rin) |
| Epifrin® | (ep' eh frin) |
| EpiPen® | (ep' eh pen) |
| Epifrin® | (ep' eh frin) |
| Epifrin® | (ep' eh frin) |
| ephedrine | (e fed' rin) |
| Epifrin® | (ep' eh frin) |
| EpiPen® | (ep' eh pen) |

## SOUND-ALIKE COMPARISON LIST *(Continued)*

| Drug Name | Pronunciation |
|---|---|
| Epinal® | (ep' eh nal) |
| Epitol® | (ep' eh tol) |
| Epitol® | (ep' eh tol) |
| Epinal® | (ep' eh nal) |
| Equanil® | (eh' kwa nil) |
| Elavil® | (el' a vil) |
| erythromycin | (er ith roe mye' sin) |
| clarithromycin | (kla rith' roe mye sin) |
| Esimil® | (es' eh mil) |
| Estinyl® | (es' teh nil) |
| Esimil® | (es' eh mil) |
| Ismelin® | (is' meh lin) |
| Esimil® | (es' eh mil) |
| F.M.L.® | (ef' em el) |
| Estinyl® | (es' teh nil) |
| Esimil® | (es' eh mil) |
| Estratab® | (es' tra tab) |
| Ethatab® | (eth' a tab) |
| Eskalith® | (es' ka lith) |
| Estratest® | (es' tra test) |
| Estratest® | (es' tra test) |
| Eskalith® | (es' ka lith) |
| Ethaquin® | (eth' a kwin) |
| Edecrin® | (ed' eh crin) |
| Ethatab® | (eth' a tab) |
| Estratab® | (es' tra tab) |
| ethosuximide | (eth o sux' i mide) |
| methsuximide | (meth sux' i mide) |
| etidocaine | (e ti' doe kane) |
| etidronate | (e ti droe' nate) |
| etidronate | (e ti droe' nate) |
| etidocaine | (e ti' doe kane) |
| etidronate | (e ti droe' nate) |
| etretinate | (e tret' i nate) |
| etretinate | (e tret' i nate) |
| etidronate | (e ti droe' nate) |
| Eurax® | (yoor' aks) |
| Serax® | (sear' aks) |
| Eurax® | (yoor' aks) |
| Urex® | (yu' eks) |
| Factrel® | (fak' trel) |
| Sectral® | (sek' tral) |
| fenoprofen | (fen o proe' fen) |
| flurbiprofen | (flure bi' proe fen) |
| Feosol® | (fee' o sol) |
| Fer-In-Sol® | (fehr' in sol) |
| Feosol® | (fee' o sol) |
| Festal® | (fes' tal) |
| Feosol® | (fee' o sol) |
| Fluosol® | (flu' o sol) |
| Fer-In-Sol® | (fehr' in sol) |
| Feosol® | (fee' o sol) |
| Festal® | (fes' tal) |
| Feosol® | (fee' o sol) |
| Feverall™ | (fee' ver all) |
| Fiberall® | (fye' ber all) |
| Fiberall® | (fye' ber all) |
| Feverall™ | (fee' ver all) |
| Fioricet® | (fee oh' reh set) |
| Lorcet® | (lor' set) |
| Fiorinal® | (fee or' reh nal) |
| Florinef® | (flor' eh nef) |
| Flaxedil® | (flaks' eh dil) |
| Flexeril® | (fleks' eh ril) |
| Flexeril® | (fleks' eh ril) |
| Flaxedil® | (flaks' eh dil) |

| Drug Name | Pronunciation |
|---|---|
| Flomax™ | (flo' maks) |
| Fosamax® | (fos' a maks) |
| Flomax® | (flo' maks) |
| Volmax® | (vol' maks) |
| Florinef® | (flor' eh nef) |
| Fiorinal® | (fee or' reh nal) |
| flunisolide | (floo nis' o lide) |
| fluocinonide | (floo o sin' o nide) |
| fluocinolone | (floo o sin' o lone) |
| fluocinonide | (floo o sin' o nide) |
| fluocinonide | (floo o sin' o nide) |
| flunisolide | (floo nis' o lide) |
| fluocinonide | (floo o sin' o nide) |
| fluocinolone | (floo o sin' o lone) |
| Fluosol® | (flu' o sol) |
| Feosol® | (fee' o sol) |
| flurbiprofen | (flure bi' proe fen) |
| fenoprofen | (fen o proe' fen) |
| F.M.L.® | (ef' em el) |
| Esimil® | (es' eh mil) |
| Fosamax® | (fos' a maks) |
| Flomax™ | (flo' maks) |
| Fostex® | (fos' teks) |
| pHisoHex® | (fye' so heks) |
| Fulvicin® | (ful' vi sin) |
| Furacin® | (fur' a sin) |
| Furacin® | (fur' a sin) |
| Fulvicin® | (ful' vi sin) |
| Gamastan® | (gam' a stan) |
| Garamycin® | (gar a mye' sin) |
| Gantanol® | (gan' ta nol) |
| Gantrisin® | (gan' tri sin) |
| Gantrisin® | (gan' tri sin) |
| Gantanol® | (gan' ta nol) |
| Gantrisin® | (gan' tri sin) |
| Gastrosed™ | (gas' troe sed) |
| Garamycin® | (gar a mye' sin) |
| Gamastan® | (gam' a stan) |
| Garamycin® | (gar a mye' sin) |
| kanamycin | (kan a mye' sin) |
| Garamycin® | (gar a mye' sin) |
| Terramycin® | (tehr a mye' sin) |
| Gastrosed™ | (gas' troe sed) |
| Gantrisin® | (gan' tri sin) |
| Genapap® | (gen' a pap) |
| Genapax® | (gen' a paks) |
| Genapap® | (gen' a pap) |
| Genatap® | (gen' a tap) |
| Genapax® | (gen' a paks) |
| Genapap® | (gen' a pap) |
| Genatap® | (gen' a tap) |
| Genapap® | (gen' a pap) |
| gentamicin | (jen ta mye' sin) |
| kanamycin | (kan a mye' sin) |
| Glucophage® | (glue' co faagsch) |
| Glucotrol® | (glue' co trol) |
| Glucotrol® | (glue' co trol) |
| Glucophage® | (glue' co faagsch) |
| Glycotuss® | (glye' co tuss) |
| Glytuss® | (glye' tuss) |
| Glytuss® | (glye' tuss) |
| Glycotuss® | (glye' co tuss) |
| gonadorelin | (goe nad o rell' in) |
| guanadrel | (gwahn' a drel) |
| Gonak™ | (gon' ak) |
| Gonic® | (gon' ik) |

| Drug Name | Pronunciation |
|---|---|
| Gonic® | (gon' ik) |
| Gonak™ | (gon' ak) |
| Granulex® | (gran' u lecks) |
| Regranex® | (re gra' neks) |
| guaifenesin | (gwye fen' e sin) |
| guanfacine | (gwahn' fa seen) |
| guanadrel | (gwahn' a drel) |
| gonadorelin | (goe nad o rell' in) |
| guanethidine | (gwahn eth' i deen) |
| guanidine | (gwahn' i deen) |
| guanfacine | (gwahn' fa seen) |
| guaifenesin | (gwye fen' e sin) |
| guanidine | (gwahn' i deen) |
| guanethidine | (gwahn eth' i deen) |
| Haldol® | (hal' dol) |
| Halenol® | (hal' e nol) |
| Haldol® | (hal' dol) |
| Halog® | (hay' log) |
| Halenol® | (hal' e nol) |
| Haldol® | (hal' dol) |
| Halfan® | (hal' fan) |
| Halfprin® | (half' prin) |
| Halfprin® | (half' prin) |
| Halfan® | (hal' fan) |
| Halfprin® | (half' prin) |
| Haltran® | (hal' tran) |
| Halog® | (hay' log) |
| Haldol® | (hal' dol) |
| Halotestin® | (hay lo tes' tin) |
| Halotex® | (hay' lo teks) |
| Halotestin® | (hay lo tes' tin) |
| Halotussin® | (hay lo tus' sin) |
| Halotex® | (hay' lo teks) |
| Halotestin® | (hay lo tes' tin) |
| Halotussin® | (hay lo tus' sin) |
| Halotestin® | (hay lo tes' tin) |
| Haltran® | (hal' tran) |
| Halfprin® | (half' prin) |
| Herplex® | (her' pleks) |
| Hiprex® | (hi' preks) |
| Hespan® | (hes' pan) |
| Histaspan® | (his' ta span) |
| Hexadrol® | (heks' a drol) |
| Hexalol® | (heks' a lol) |
| Hexalol® | (heks' a lol) |
| Hexadrol® | (heks' a drol) |
| Hiprex® | (hi' preks) |
| Herplex® | (her' pleks) |
| Histaspan® | (his' ta span) |
| Hespan® | (hes' pan) |
| Hycamtin® | (hye cam' tin) |
| Hycomine® | (hye' co meen) |
| Hycodan® | (hye' co dan) |
| Hycomine® | (hye' co meen) |
| Hycodan® | (hye' co dan) |
| Vicodin® | (vye' co din) |
| Hycomine® | (hye' co meen) |
| Byclomine® | (bye' clo meen) |
| Hycomine® | (hye' co meen) |
| Hycamtin® | (hye cam' tin) |
| Hycomine® | (hye' co meen) |
| Hycodan® | (hye' co dan) |
| Hydergine® | (hye' der geen) |
| Hydramyn® | (hye' dra min) |
| hydralazine | (hye dral' a zeen) |
| hydroxyzine | (hye drox' i zeen) |
| Hydramyn® | (hye' dra min) |
| Hydergine® | (hye' der geen) |
| Hydramyn® | (hye' dra min) |
| Bydramine® | (bye' dra meen) |
| Hydrocet® | (hye' dro set) |
| Hydrocil® | (hye' dro sil) |
| Hydrocil® | (hye' dro sil) |
| Hydrocet® | (hye' dro set) |
| hydroxyurea | (hye drox ee yoor ee' a) |
| hydroxyzine | (hye drox' i zeen) |
| hydroxyzine | (hye drox' i zeen) |
| hydralazine | (hye dral' a zeen) |
| hydroxyzine | (hye drox' i zeen) |
| hydroxyurea | (hye drox ee yoor ee' a) |
| Hygroton® | (hye gro' ton) |
| Regroton® | (reg' ro ton) |
| Hyper-Tet® | (hye' per tet) |
| HyperHep® | (hye' per hep) |
| Hyper-Tet® | (hye' per tet) |
| Hyperstat® | (hye' per stat) |
| HyperHep® | (hye' per hep) |
| Hyperab® | (hye' per ab) |
| HyperHep® | (hye' per hep) |
| Hyper-Tet® | (hye' per tet) |
| Hyperab® | (hye' per ab) |
| HyperHep® | (hye' per hep) |
| Hyperstat® | (hye' per stat) |
| Hyper-Tet® | (hye' per tet) |
| Hyperstat® | (hye' per stat) |
| Nitrostat® | (nye' troe stat) |
| Hytone® | (hye' tone) |
| Vytone® | (vye' tone) |
| Idamycin® | (eye da mye' sin) |
| Adriamycin™ | (ade rya mye' sin) |
| Imferon® | (im' fer on) |
| interferon | (in ter fer' on) |
| imipramine | (im ip' ra meen) |
| Norpramin® | (nor pray' min) |
| Imuran® | (im' yu ran) |
| Enduron® | (en' du ron) |
| Inapsine® | (i nap' seen) |
| Nebcin® | (neb' sin) |
| Inderal® | (in' der al) |
| Adderall® | (ad' der all) |
| Inderal® | (in' der al) |
| Enduron® | (en' du ron) |
| Inderal® | (in' der al) |
| Enduronyl® | (en dur' o nil) |
| Inderal® | (in' der al) |
| Isordil® | (eye' sor dil) |
| Inderal® | (in' der al) |
| Medrol® | (meh' drol) |
| Inderal® 40 | (in' der al for' tee) |
| Enduronyl® Forte | (en dur' o nil for' tay) |
| Indocin® | (in' doe sin) |
| Lincocin® | (lin' coe sin) |
| Indocin® | (in' doe sin) |
| Minocin® | (min' o sin) |
| Intal® | (in' tal) |
| Endal® | (en' dal) |
| interferon | (in ter fer' on) |
| Imferon® | (im' fer on) |
| Intropin® | (in tro' pin) |
| Isoptin® | (eye sop' tin) |
| Intropin® | (in troe' pin) |
| Ditropan® | (di troe' pan) |
| Ismelin® | (is' meh lin) |

## SOUND-ALIKE COMPARISON LIST *(Continued)*

| Drug Name | Pronunciation |
|---|---|
| Esimil® | (es' eh mil) |
| Ismelin® | (is' meh lin) |
| Ritalin® | (ri' ta lin) |
| isoflurane | (eye soe flure' ane) |
| enflurane | (en' floo rane) |
| isoflurane | (eye soe flure' ane) |
| isoflurophate | (eye soe flure' o fate) |
| isoflurophate | (eye soe flure' o fate) |
| isoflurane | (eye soe flure' ane) |
| Isoptin® | (eye sop' tin) |
| Intropin® | (in tro' pin) |
| Isoptin® | (eye sop' tin) |
| Isopto® Tears | (eye sop' tow tears) |
| Isopto® Tears | (eye sop' tow tears) |
| Isoptin® | (eye sop' tin) |
| Isordil® | (eye' sor dil) |
| Inderal® | (in' der al) |
| Isordil® | (eye' sor dil) |
| Isuprel® | (eye' sue prel) |
| Isordil® | (eye' sor dil) |
| Plendil® | (plen' dil) |
| Isuprel® | (eye' sue prel) |
| Isordil® | (eye' sor dil) |
| K-Lor™ | (kay' lor) |
| Kaochlor® | (kay' o klor) |
| kanamycin | (kan a mye' sin) |
| Garamycin® | (gar a mye' sin) |
| kanamycin | (kan a mye' sin) |
| gentamicin | (jen ta mye' sin) |
| Kaochlor® | (kay' o klor) |
| K-Lor™ | (kay' lor) |
| Kaopectate® | (kay oh pek' tate) |
| Kayexelate® | (kay eks' e late) |
| Kayexelate® | (kay eks' e late) |
| Kaopectate® | (kay oh pek' tate) |
| Keflex® | (keh' fleks) |
| Keflin® | (keh' flin) |
| Keflin® | (keh' flin) |
| Keflex® | (keh' fleks) |
| Kemadrin® | (kem' a drin) |
| Coumadin® | (ku' ma din) |
| Klonopin™ | (klon' o pin) |
| clonidine | (kloe' ni deen) |
| Komex® | (koe' meks) |
| Koromex® | (kor' o meks) |
| Koromex® | (kor' o meks) |
| Komex® | (koe' meks) |
| Kwell® | (kwell) |
| Dwelle® | (dwell) |
| Lamictal® | (la mic' tal) |
| Lamisil® | (lam' eh sil) |
| Lamisil® | (lam' eh sil) |
| Lamictal® | (la mic' tal) |
| lamotrigine | (la moe' tri jeen) |
| lamivudine | (la mi' vyoo deen) |
| lamivudine | (la mi' vyoo deen) |
| lamotrigine | (la moe' tri jeen) |
| Lanoxin® | (lan ox' in) |
| Levoxine® | (lev ox een) |
| Lanoxin® | (lan ox' in) |
| Levsinex® | (lev' si neks) |
| Lanoxin® | (lan ox' in) |
| Mefoxin® | (me fox' in) |
| Larylgan® | (la ril' gan) |
| Auralgan® | (a ral' gan) |
| Lasix® | (lay' siks) |

| Drug Name | Pronunciation |
|---|---|
| Lidex® | (lye' deks) |
| leucovorin | (loo koe vor' in) |
| Leukeran® | (lu' keh ran) |
| Leukeran® | (lu' keh ran) |
| leucovorin | (loo koe vor' in) |
| levodopa | (lee voe doe' pa) |
| methyldopa | (meth ill doe' pa) |
| levothyroxine | (lee voe thye rox' een) |
| liothyronine | (lye o thye' roe neen) |
| Levoxine® | (lev ox een) |
| Lanoxin® | (lan ox' in) |
| Levsinex® | (lev' si neks) |
| Lanoxin® | (lan ox' in) |
| Lidex® | (lye' deks) |
| Lasix® | (lay' siks) |
| Lidex® | (lye' deks) |
| Lidox® | (lye' dox) |
| Lidex® | (lye' deks) |
| Videx® | (vye' deks) |
| Lidex® | (lye' deks) |
| Wydase® | (wye' dase) |
| Lidox® | (lye' dox) |
| Lidex® | (lye' deks) |
| Lincocin® | (link' o sin) |
| Cleocin® | (klee' o sin) |
| Lincocin® | (lin' coe sin) |
| Indocin® | (in' doe sin) |
| Lincocin® | (link' o sin) |
| Minocin® | (min' o sin) |
| Lioresal® | (lye or' reh sal) |
| lisinopril | (lyse in' o pril) |
| liothyronine | (lye o thye' roe neen) |
| levothyroxine | (lee voe thye rox' een) |
| lisinopril | (lyse in' o pril) |
| Lioresal® | (lye or' reh sal) |
| Lithane® | (lith' ane) |
| Lithonate® | (lith' o nate) |
| Lithonate® | (lith' o nate) |
| Lithane® | (lith' ane) |
| Lithostat® | (lith' o stat) |
| Lithotabs® | (lith' o tabs) |
| Lithotabs® | (lith' o tabs) |
| Lithostat® | (lith' o stat) |
| Lodine® | (low' deen) |
| codeine | (koe' deen) |
| Lomodix® | (lo' mo dix) |
| Lovenox® | (lo' ve nox) |
| Loniten® | (lon' eh ten) |
| clonidine | (kloe' ni deen) |
| Lopressor® | (lo pres' sor) |
| Lopurin® | (lo pure' in) |
| Lopurin® | (lo pure' in) |
| Lopressor® | (lo pres' sor) |
| Lopurin® | (lo pure' in) |
| Lupron® | (lu' pron) |
| Lorcet® | (lor' set) |
| Fioricet® | (fee oh' reh set) |
| Lotrimin® | (low' tri min) |
| Otrivin® | (oh' tri vin) |
| Lovenox® | (lo' ve nox) |
| Lomodix® | (lo' mo dix) |
| Loxitane® | (loks' e tane) |
| Soriatane® | (sor' e ah tane) |
| Luminal® | (lu' mi nal) |
| Tuinal® | (tu' i nal) |
| Lupron® | (lu' pron) |

| Drug Name | Pronunciation |
|---|---|
| Lopurin® | (lo pure' in) |
| Lupron® | (lu' pron) |
| Nuprin® | (nu' prin) |
| Maalox® | (may' loks) |
| Monodox® | (mon' o doks) |
| Maltsupex® | (malt' su peks) |
| Manoplax® | (man' o laks) |
| Mandol® | (man' dole) |
| nadolol | (nay doe' lole) |
| Manoplax® | (man' o laks) |
| Maltsupex® | (malt' su peks) |
| Maox® | (may' oks) |
| Maalox® | (may' loks) |
| Maox® | (may' oks) |
| Marax® | (may' raks) |
| Marax® | (may' raks) |
| Maalox® | (may' loks) |
| Marax® | (may' raks) |
| Atarax® | (at' a raks) |
| Marax® | (may' raks) |
| Maox® | (may' oks) |
| Marcaine® | (mar' kane) |
| Narcan® | (nar' kan) |
| Marinol® | (mare' i nole) |
| Marnal® | (mar' nal) |
| Marnal® | (mar' nal) |
| Marinol® | (mare' i nole) |
| Matulane® | (mat' chu lane) |
| Modane® | (moe' dane) |
| Maxidex® | (maks' i deks) |
| Maxzide® | (maks' zide) |
| Maxzide® | (maks' zide) |
| Maxidex® | (maks' i deks) |
| Mebaral® | (meb' a ral) |
| Medrol® | (med' role) |
| Mebaral® | (meb' a ral) |
| Mellaril® | (mel' a ril) |
| Mebaral® | (meb' a ral) |
| Tegretol® | (teg' ree tol) |
| mecamylamine | (mek a mill' a meen) |
| mesalamine | (me sal' a meen) |
| Meclan® | (me' klan) |
| Meclomen® | (meh' klo men) |
| Meclan® | (me' klan) |
| Mezlin® | (mes' lin) |
| Meclomen® | (meh' klo men) |
| Meclan® | (me' klan) |
| Medrol® | (med' role) |
| Mebaral® | (meb' a ral) |
| Medrol® | (meh' drol) |
| Inderal® | (in' der al) |
| Mefoxin® | (me fox' in) |
| Lanoxin® | (lan ox' in) |
| Mellaril® | (mel' la ril) |
| Elavil® | (el' a vil) |
| Mellaril® | (mel' a ril) |
| Mebaral® | (meb' a ral) |
| melphalan | (mel' fa lan) |
| Mephyton® | (meh fye' ton) |
| mephenytoin | (me fen' i toyn) |
| Mephyton® | (meh fye' ton) |
| mephenytoin | (me fen' i toyn) |
| Mesantoin® | (meh san' toyn) |
| mephenytoin | (me fen' i toyn) |
| phenytoin | (fen' i toyn) |
| mephobarbital | (me foe bar' bi tal) |
| methocarbamol | (meth o kar' ba mole) |
| Mephyton® | (meh fye' ton) |

| Drug Name | Pronunciation |
|---|---|
| melphalan | (mel' fa lan) |
| Mephyton® | (meh fye' ton) |
| mephenytoin | (me fen' i toyn) |
| Mephyton® | (meh fye' ton) |
| methadone | (meth' a done) |
| mepivacaine | (me piv' a kane) |
| bupivacaine | (byoo piv' a kane) |
| Meprospan® | (meh' pro span) |
| Naprosyn® | (na' pro sin) |
| mesalamine | (me sal' a meen) |
| mecamylamine | (mek a mill' a meen) |
| Mesantoin® | (meh san' toyn) |
| mephenytoin | (me fen' i toyn) |
| Mesantoin® | (meh san' toyn) |
| Mestinon® | (meh' sti non) |
| Mestinon® | (meh' sti non) |
| Mesantoin® | (meh san' toyn) |
| Metahydrin® | (me ta hye' drin) |
| Metandren® | (me tan' dren) |
| Metandren® | (me tan' dren) |
| Metahydrin® | (me ta hye' drin) |
| metaproterenol | (met a proe ter' e nol) |
| metoprolol | (me toe' proe lole) |
| metaxalone | (me taks' a lone) |
| metolazone | (me tole' a zone) |
| methadone | (meth' a done) |
| Mephyton® | (meh fye' ton) |
| methazolamide | (meth a zoe' la mide) |
| metolazone | (me tole' a zone) |
| methenamine | (meth en' a meen) |
| methionine | (me thye' o neen) |
| methicillin | (meth i sill' in) |
| mezlocillin | (mez loe sill' in) |
| methionine | (me thye' o neen) |
| methenamine | (meth en' a meen) |
| methocarbamol | (meth o kar' ba mole) |
| mephobarbital | (me foe bar' bi tal) |
| methsuximide | (meth sux' i mide) |
| ethosuximide | (eth o sux' i mide) |
| methyldopa | (meth ill doe' pa) |
| levodopa | (lee voe doe' pa) |
| metolazone | (me tole' a zone) |
| metaxalone | (me taks' a lone) |
| metolazone | (me tole' a zone) |
| methazolamide | (meth a zoe' la mide) |
| metolazone | (me tole' a zone) |
| minoxidil | (mi nox' i dill) |
| metoprolol | (me toe' proe lole) |
| metaproterenol | (met a proe ter' e nol) |
| metyrapone | (me teer' a pone) |
| metyrosine | (me tye' roe seen) |
| metyrosine | (me tye' roe seen) |
| metyrapone | (me teer' a pone) |
| Mexitil® | (meks' i til) |
| Mezlin® | (mes' lin) |
| Mezlin® | (mes' lin) |
| Meclan® | (me' klan) |
| Mezlin® | (mes' lin) |
| Mexitil® | (meks' i til) |
| mezlocillin | (mez loe sill' in) |
| methicillin | (meth i sill' in) |
| miconazole | (mi kon' a zole) |
| Micronase® | (mye' croe nase) |
| Micronase® | (mye' croe nase) |
| Micronor® | (mye' croe nor) |
| Micronase® | (mye' croe nase) |
| miconazole | (mi kon' a zole) |
| Micronor® | (mye' croe nor) |

## SOUND-ALIKE COMPARISON LIST *(Continued)*

| Drug Name | Pronunciation |
|---|---|
| Micronase® | (mye' croe nase) |
| Midrin® | (mid' rin) |
| Mydfrin® | (mid' frin) |
| Milontin® | (mi lon' tin) |
| Miltown® | (mil' town) |
| Milontin® | (mi lon' tin) |
| Mylanta® | (mye lan' tah) |
| Miltown® | (mil' town) |
| Milontin® | (mi lon' tin) |
| Minizide® | (min' i zide) |
| Minocin® | (min' o sin) |
| Minocin® | (min' o sin) |
| Indocin® | (in' doe sin) |
| Minocin® | (min' o sin) |
| Lincocin® | (link' o sin) |
| Minocin® | (min' o sin) |
| Minizide® | (min' i zide) |
| Minocin® | (min' o sin) |
| Mithracin® | (mith' ra sin) |
| Minocin® | (min' o sin) |
| niacin | (nye' a sin) |
| minoxidil | (mi nox' i dill) |
| metolazone | (me tole' a zone) |
| Mithracin® | (mith' ra sin) |
| Minocin® | (min' o sin) |
| mitomycin | (mye toe mye' sin) |
| Mutamycin® | (mute a mye' sin) |
| Moban® | (moe' ban) |
| Modane® | (moe' dane) |
| Modane® | (moe' dane) |
| Matulane® | (mat' chu lane) |
| Modane® | (moe' dane) |
| Moban® | (moe' ban) |
| Modicon® | (mod' i kon) |
| Mylicon® | (mye' li kon) |
| moexipril | (mo ex' i pril) |
| Monopril® | (mon' oh pril) |
| Monodox® | (mon' o doks) |
| Maalox® | (may' loks) |
| Monopril® | (mon' oh pril) |
| moexipril | (mo ex' i pril) |
| Mutamycin® | (mute a mye' sin) |
| mitomycin | (mye toe mye' sin) |
| Myambutol® | (mya am' byoo tol) |
| Nembutal® | (nem' byoo tal) |
| Mycelex® | (mye' si leks) |
| Myoflex® | (mye' o fleks) |
| Mycifradin® | (mye ce fray' din) |
| Mycitracin® | (mye ce tray' sin) |
| Mycitracin® | (mye ce tray' sin) |
| Mycifradin® | (mye ce fray' din) |
| Mydfrin® | (mid' frin) |
| Midrin® | (mid' rin) |
| Mylanta® | (mye lan' tah) |
| Milontin® | (mi lon' tin) |
| Myleran® | (mye' leh ran) |
| Mylicon® | (mye' li kon) |
| Mylicon® | (mye' li kon) |
| Modicon® | (mod' i kon) |
| Mylicon® | (mye' li kon) |
| Myleran® | (mye' leh ran) |
| Myochrysine® | (mye o kris' seen) |
| vincristine | (vin kris' teen) |
| Myoflex® | (mye' o fleks) |
| Mycelex® | (mye' si leks) |
| nadolol | (nay doe' lole) |

| Drug Name | Pronunciation |
|---|---|
| Mandol® | (man' dole) |
| Naldecon® | (nal' dee kon) |
| Nalfon® | (nal' fon) |
| Nalfon® | (nal' fon) |
| Naldecon® | (nal' dee kon) |
| Nallpen® | (nall' pen) |
| Nalspan® | (nal' span) |
| naloxone | (nal ox' one) |
| naltrexone | (nal treks' one) |
| Nalspan® | (nal' span) |
| Nallpen® | (nall' pen) |
| naltrexone | (nal treks' one) |
| naloxone | (nal ox' one) |
| Naprosyn® | (na' pro sin) |
| Meprospan® | (meh' pro span) |
| Naprosyn® | (na' pro sin) |
| naproxen | (na prox' en) |
| Naprosyn® | (na' pro sin) |
| Natacyn® | (na' ta sin) |
| Naprosyn® | (na' pro sin) |
| Nebcin® | (neb' sin) |
| naproxen | (na prox' en) |
| Naprosyn® | (na' pro sin) |
| Narcan® | (nar' kan) |
| Norcuron® | (nor' ku ron) |
| Narcan® | (nar' kan) |
| Marcaine® | (mar' kane) |
| Nardil® | (nar' dil) |
| Norinyl® | (nor' eh nil) |
| Nasacort® | (nay' sa cort) |
| Nasalcrom® | (nay' sal crome) |
| Nasalcrom® | (nay' sal crome) |
| Nasacort® | (nay' sa cort) |
| Natacyn® | (na' ta sin) |
| Naprosyn® | (na' pro sin) |
| Navane® | (nav' ane) |
| Norvasc® | (nor' vask) |
| Nebcin® | (neb' sin) |
| Inapsine® | (i nap' seen) |
| Nebcin® | (neb' sin) |
| Naprosyn® | (na' pro sin) |
| nelfinavir | (nel fin' a vir) |
| nevirapine | (ne vir' a peen) |
| Nembutal® | (nem' byoo tal) |
| Myambutol® | (mya am' byoo tol) |
| Neptazane® | (nep' ta zane) |
| Nesacaine® | (nes' a kane) |
| Nesacaine® | (nes' a kane) |
| Neptazane® | (nep' ta zane) |
| Neupogen® | (nu' po gen) |
| Nutramigen® | (nu' tra gen) |
| nevirapine | (ne vir' a peen) |
| nelfinavir | (nel fin' a vir) |
| niacin | (nye' a sin) |
| Minocin® | (min' o sin) |
| nicardipine | (nye kar' de peen) |
| nifedipine | (nye fed' i peen) |
| Nicobid® | (nye' ko bid) |
| Nitro-Bid® | (nye' troe bid) |
| Nicoderm® | (nye' co derm) |
| Nitroderm® | (nye' tro derm) |
| Nicorette® | (nik' o ret) |
| Nordette® | (nor det') |
| nifedipine | (nye fed' i peen) |
| nicardipine | (nye kar' de peen) |
| nifedipine | (nye fed' i peen) |

| Drug Name | Pronunciation |
|---|---|
| nimodipine | (nye moe' di peen) |
| nifedipine | (nye fed' i peen) |
| nisoldipine | (nye' sole di peen) |
| Nilstat® | (nil' stat) |
| Nitrostat® | (nye' troe stat) |
| Nimodipine | (nye moe' di peen) |
| nifedipine | (nye fed' i peen) |
| nisoldipine | (nye' sole di peen) |
| nifedipine | (nye fed' i peen) |
| Nitro-Bid® | (nye' troe bid) |
| Nicobid® | (nye' ko bid) |
| Nitroderm® | (nye' tro derm) |
| Nicoderm® | (nye' co derm) |
| Nitroglycerin | (nye troe gli' ser in) |
| Nitroglyn® | (nye' troe glin) |
| Nitroglyn® | (nye' troe glin) |
| nitroglycerin | (nye troe gli' ser in) |
| Nitrostat® | (nye' troe stat) |
| Hyperstat® | (hye' per stat) |
| Nitrostat® | (nye' troe stat) |
| Nilstat® | (nil' stat) |
| Norcuron® | (nor' ku ron) |
| Narcan® | (nar' can) |
| Nordette® | (nor det') |
| Nicorette® | (nik' o ret) |
| Norinyl® | (nor' eh nil) |
| Nardil® | (nar' dil) |
| Norlutate® | (nor' lu tate) |
| Norlutin® | (nor lu' tin) |
| Norlutin® | (nor lu' tin) |
| Norlutate® | (nor' lu tate) |
| Norpramin® | (nor pray' min) |
| imipramine | (im ip' ra meen) |
| Norvasc® | (nor' vask) |
| Navane® | (nav' ane) |
| Norvasc® | (nor' vask) |
| Norvir® | (nor' vir) |
| Norvir® | (nor' vir) |
| Norvasc® | (nor' vask) |
| Novafed® | (nove' a fed) |
| Nucofed® | (nu' co fed) |
| Nucofed® | (nu' co fed) |
| Novafed® | (nove' a fed) |
| Nuprin® | (nu' prin) |
| Lupron® | (lu' pron) |
| Nutramigen® | (nu' tra gen) |
| Neupogen® | (nu' po gen) |
| olanzapine | (oh lan' za peen) |
| olsalazine | (ole sal' a zeen) |
| olsalazine | (ole sal' a zeen) |
| olanzapine | (oh lan' za peen) |
| Omnipaque® | (om' ni pak) |
| Omnipen® | (om' ni pen) |
| Omnipen® | (om' ni pen) |
| Omnipaque® | (om' ni pak) |
| Omnipen® | (om' ni pen) |
| Unipen® | (yu' ni pen) |
| Oncovin® | (on' coe vin) |
| Ancobon® | (an' coe bon) |
| Ophthaine® | (op' thane) |
| Ophthetic® | (op thet' ik) |
| Ophthalgan® | (opp thal' gan) |
| Auralgan® | (a ral' gan) |
| Ophthetic® | (op thet' ik) |
| Ophthaine® | (op' thane) |
| Ophthochlor® | (op' tho klor) |
| Ophthocort® | (op' tho kort) |
| Ophthocort® | (op' tho kort) |

| Drug Name | Pronunciation |
|---|---|
| Ophthochlor® | (op' tho klor) |
| oprelvekin | (op rel' ve kin) |
| Proleukin® | (pro lu' kin) |
| Orabase® | (or' a base) |
| Orinase® | (or' in ase) |
| Orasol® | (or' a sol) |
| Orasone® | (or' a sone) |
| Orasone® | (or' a sone) |
| Orasol® | (or' a sol) |
| Oretic® | (or et' ik) |
| Oreton® | (or' eh ton) |
| Oreton® | (or' eh ton) |
| Oretic® | (or et' ik) |
| Orinase® | (or' in ase) |
| Orabase® | (or' a base) |
| Orinase® | (or' in ase) |
| Ornade® | (or' nade) |
| Orinase® | (or' in ase) |
| Tolinase® | (tole' i nase) |
| Ornade® | (or' nade) |
| Orinase® | (or' in ase) |
| Otrivin® | (oh' tri vin) |
| Lotrimin® | (low' tri min) |
| Oruvail® | (or' yu vale) |
| Elavil® | (el' a vil) |
| oxymetazoline | (ox i met az' o leen) |
| oxymetholone | (ox i meth' o lone) |
| oxymetholone | (ox i meth' o lone) |
| oxymetazoline | (ox i met az' o leen) |
| oxymetholone | (ox i meth' o lone) |
| oxymorphone | (ox i mor' fone) |
| oxymorphone | (ox i mor' fone) |
| oxymetholone | (ox i meth' o lone) |
| Pamelor® | (pam' meh lor) |
| Dymelor® | (dye' meh lor) |
| Pathilon® | (path' i lon) |
| Pathocil® | (path' o sil) |
| Pathocil® | (path' o sil) |
| Pathilon® | (path' i lon) |
| Pathocil® | (path' o sil) |
| Placidyl® | (pla' ce dil) |
| Pathocil® | (path' o sill) |
| Bactocill® | (bak' tow sill) |
| Pavabid® | (pav' a bid) |
| Pavased® | (pav' a sed) |
| Pavased® | (pav' a sed) |
| Pavabid® | (pav' a bid) |
| Paxil® | (packs' ol) |
| Taxol® | (tacks' ol) |
| pentobarbital | (pen toe bar' bi tal) |
| phenobarbital | (fee noe bar' bi tal) |
| Percodan® | (per' coe dan) |
| Decadron® | (dek' a dron) |
| Perdiem® | (per dee' em) |
| Pyridium® | (pye rid' dee um) |
| Persantine® | (per san' teen) |
| Pertofrane® | (per' toe frane) |
| Pertofrane® | (per' toe frane) |
| Persantine® | (per san' teen) |
| Phazyme® | (fay' zeem) |
| Pherazine® | (fer' a zeen) |
| Phenergan® | (fen' er gan) |
| Phrenilin® | (fren' ni lin) |
| Phenergan® | (fen' er gan) |
| Theragran® | (ther' a gran) |
| phenobarbital | (fee noe bar' bi tal) |
| pentobarbital | (pen toe bar' bi tal) |
| phentermine | (fen' ter meen) |

## SOUND-ALIKE COMPARISON LIST *(Continued)*

| Drug Name | Pronunciation |
|---|---|
| phentolamine | (fen tole' a meen) |
| phentolamine | (fen tole' a meen) |
| phentermine | (fen' ter meen) |
| phentolamine | (fen tole' a meen) |
| Ventolin® | (ven' to lin) |
| phenytoin | (fen' i toyn) |
| mephenytoin | (me fen' i toyn) |
| Pherazine® | (fer' a zeen) |
| Phazyme® | (fay' zeem) |
| pHisoHex® | (fye' so heks) |
| Fostex® | (fos' teks) |
| Phos-Flur® | (fos' flur) |
| PhosLo® | (fos' lo) |
| PhosLo® | (fos' lo) |
| Phos-Flur® | (fos' flur) |
| PhosLo® | (fos' lo) |
| ProSom™ | (pro' som) |
| Phosphaljel® | (fos' fal gel) |
| Phospholine® | (fos' fo leen) |
| Phospholine® | (fos' fo leen) |
| Phosphaljel® | (fos' fal gel) |
| Phrenilin® | (fren' ni lin) |
| Phenergan® | (fen' er gan) |
| Phrenilin® | (fren' ni lin) |
| Trinalin® | (tri' na lin) |
| physostigmine | (fye zoe stig' meen) |
| Prostigmin® | (pro stig' min) |
| physostigmine | (fye zoe stig' meen) |
| pyridostigmine | (peer id o stig' meen) |
| Pitocin® | (pi toe' sin) |
| Pitressin® | (ph tres' sin) |
| Pitressin® | (ph tres' sin) |
| Pitocin® | (pi toe' sin) |
| Placidyl® | (pla' ce dil) |
| Pathocil® | (path' o sil) |
| Plaquenil® | (pla' kwe nil) |
| Platinol® | (pla' tee nol) |
| Platinol® | (pla' tee nol) |
| Plaquenil® | (pla' kwe nil) |
| Plendil® | (plen' dill) |
| Isordil® | (eye' sor dil) |
| Ponstel® | (pon' stel) |
| Pronestyl® | (pro nes' til) |
| Posicor® | (pos' e cor) |
| Proscar® | (pros' car) |
| pralidoxime | (pra li dox' eem) |
| pramoxine | (pra moks' een) |
| pralidoxime | (pra li dox' eem) |
| pyridoxine | (peer i dox' een) |
| Pramosone® | (pra' mo sone) |
| prednisone | (pred' ni sone) |
| pramoxine | (pra moks' een) |
| pralidoxime | (pra li dox' eem) |
| prazepam | (pra' ze pam) |
| prazosin | (pra' zoe sin) |
| prazosin | (pra' zoe sin) |
| prazepam | (pra' ze pam) |
| Precare® | (pre' kare) |
| Precose® | (pre' kose) |
| Precose® | (pre' kose) |
| Precare® | (pre' kare) |
| Predalone® | (pred' a lone) |
| prednisone | (pred' ni sone) |
| prednisolone | (pred nis' o lone) |
| prednisone | (pred' ni sone) |
| prednisone | (pred' ni sone) |
| Pramosone® | (pra' mo sone) |
| prednisone | (pred' ni sone) |
| Predalone® | (pred' a lone) |
| prednisone | (pred' ni sone) |
| prednisolone | (pred nis' o lone) |
| prednisone | (pred' ni sone) |
| primidone | (pri' mi done) |
| Premarin® | (prem' a rin) |
| Primaxin® | (pri maks' in) |
| prilocaine | (pril' o kane) |
| Prilosec™ | (pre' lo sek) |
| Prilosec™ | (pre' lo sek) |
| Prozac® | (proe' zak) |
| Prilosec™ | (pre' lo sek) |
| prilocaine | (pril' o kane) |
| Primaxin® | (pri maks' in) |
| Premarin® | (prem' a rin) |
| primidone | (pri' mi done) |
| prednisone | (pred' ni sone) |
| Priscoline® | (pris' coe leen) |
| Apresoline® | (aye press' sow leen) |
| Pro-Banthine® | (pro ban' theen) |
| Banthine® | (ban' theen) |
| Proleukin® | (pro lu' kin) |
| oprelvekin | (op rel' ve kin) |
| Pro-Sof® | (proe' sof) |
| ProSom™ | (pro' som) |
| ProSom™ | (pro' som) |
| PhosLo® | (fos' lo) |
| ProSom™ | (pro' som) |
| Pro-Sof® Plus | (proe' sof) |
| ProStep® | (proe' step) |
| Prozac® | (proe' zak) |
| procarbazine | (proe kar' ba zeen) |
| dacarbazine | (da kar' ba zeen) |
| promazine | (proe' ma zeen) |
| promethazine | (proe meth' a zeen) |
| Prometh® | (proe' meth) |
| Promit® | (proe' mit) |
| promethazine | (proe meth' a zeen) |
| promazine | (proe' ma zeen) |
| Promit® | (proe' mit) |
| Prometh® | (proe' meth) |
| Pronestyl® | (pro nes' til) |
| Ponstel® | (pon' stel) |
| Propacet® | (proe' pa set) |
| Propagest® | (proe' pa gest) |
| Propagest® | (proe' pa gest) |
| Propacet® | (proe' pa set) |
| Proscar® | (pros' car) |
| Posicor® | (pos' e cor) |
| Prostigmin® | (pro stig' min) |
| physostigmine | (fye zoe stig' meen) |
| protamine | (proe' ta meen) |
| Protopam® | (proe' toe pam) |
| Protopam® | (proe' toe pam) |
| protamine | (proe' ta meen) |
| Protopam® | (proe' toe pam) |
| Protropin® | (proe tro' pin) |
| Protropin® | (proe tro' pin) |
| Protopam® | (proe' toe pam) |
| Prozac® | (proe' zak) |
| Prilosec™ | (pre' lo sek) |
| Prozac® | (proe' zak) |
| ProStep® | (proe' step) |
| Pyridium® | (pye rid' dee um) |

| Drug Name | Pronunciation |
|---|---|
| Dyrenium® | (dye ren' e um) |
| Pyridium® | (pye rid' dee um) |
| Perdiem® | (per dee' em) |
| Pyridium® | (pye rid' dee um) |
| pyridoxine | (peer i dox' een) |
| Pyridium® | (pye rid' dee um) |
| pyrithione | (peer i thye' one) |
| pyridostigmine | (peer id o stig' meen) |
| physostigmine | (fye zoe stig' meen) |
| pyridoxine | (peer i dox' een) |
| Pyridium® | (pye rid' dee um) |
| pyridoxine | (peer i dox' een) |
| pralidoxime | (pra li dox' eem) |
| pyrithione | (peer i thye' one) |
| Pyridium® | (pye rid' dee um) |
| quinidine | (kwin' i deen) |
| clonidine | (kloe' ni deen) |
| quinidine | (kwin' i deen) |
| quinine | (kwye' nine) |
| quinine | (kwye' nine) |
| quinidine | (kwin' i deen) |
| Reglan® | (reg' lan) |
| Regonol® | (reg' o nol) |
| Regonol® | (reg' o nol) |
| Reglan® | (reg' lan) |
| Regonol® | (reg' o nol) |
| Regutol® | (reg' yu tol) |
| Regranex® | (re gra' neks) |
| Granulex® | (gran' u lecks) |
| Regroton® | (reg' ro ton) |
| Hygroton® | (hye gro' ton) |
| Regutol® | (reg' yu tol) |
| Regonol® | (reg' o nol) |
| remifentanil | (rem i fen' ta nil) |
| alfentanil | (al fen' ta nil) |
| Repan® | (ree' pan) |
| Riopan® | (rye' o pan) |
| Restore® | (res tore') |
| Restoril® | (res' tor ril) |
| Restoril® | (res' tor ril) |
| Restore® | (res tore') |
| Restoril® | (res' tor ril) |
| Vistaril® | (vis' tar ril) |
| Retrovir® | (re' tro vir) |
| ritonavir | (ri ton' o vir) |
| Revex® | (rev' ex) |
| Revia® | (rev' ve ah) |
| Revia® | (rev' ve ah) |
| Revex® | (rev' ex) |
| Rhythmin® | (rith' min) |
| Rythmol® | (rith' mol) |
| ribavirin | (rye ba vye' rin) |
| riboflavin | (rye' boe flay vin) |
| riboflavin | (rye' boe flay vin) |
| ribavirin | (rye ba vye' rin) |
| Rifadin® | (rif' a din) |
| Ritalin® | (ri' ta lin) |
| Rimactane® | (ri mak' tane) |
| rimantadine | (ri man' to deen) |
| rimantadine | (ri man' to deen) |
| Rimactane® | (ri mak' tane) |
| rimantadine | (ri man' to deen) |
| amantadine | (a man' ta deen) |
| Riobin® | (rye' o bin) |
| Riopan® | (rye' o pan) |
| Riopan® | (rye' o pan) |
| Repan® | (ree' pan) |
| Riopan® | (rye' o pan) |

| Drug Name | Pronunciation |
|---|---|
| Riobin® | (rye' o bin) |
| Ritalin® | (ri' ta lin) |
| Ismelin® | (is' meh lin) |
| Ritalin® | (ri' ta lin) |
| Rifadin® | (rif' a din) |
| Ritalin® | (ri' ta lin) |
| ritodrine | (ri' toe dreen) |
| ritodrine | (ri' toe dreen) |
| Ritalin® | (ri' ta lin) |
| ritonavir | ri ton' o vir) |
| Retrovir® | (re' tro vir) |
| Rocephin® | (roe sef' fen) |
| Roferon® | (roe fer' on) |
| Roferon® | (roe fer' on) |
| Rocephin® | (roe sef' fen) |
| Rynatan® | (rye' na tan) |
| Rynatuss® | (rye' na tuss) |
| Rynatuss® | (rye' na tuss) |
| Rynatan® | (rye' na tan) |
| Rythmol® | (rith' mol) |
| Rhythmin® | (rith' min) |
| Salacid® | (sal as' sid) |
| Salagen® | (sal' a gen) |
| Salagen® | (sal' a gen) |
| Salacid® | (sal as' sid) |
| Salutensin® | (sal yu ten' sin) |
| Diutensin® | (dye yu ten' sin) |
| saquinavir | (sa kwin' a veer) |
| Sinequan® | (si' ne kwan) |
| Seconal™ | (sek' o nal) |
| Sectral® | (sek' tral) |
| Sectral® | (sek' tral) |
| Factrel® | (fak' trel) |
| Sectral® | (sek' tral) |
| Seconal™ | (sek' o nal) |
| Septa® | (sep' tah) |
| Septra® | (sep' trah) |
| Septra® | (sep' trah) |
| Septa® | (sep' tah) |
| Ser-Ap-Es® | (ser ap' ess) |
| Catapres® | (kat' a pres) |
| Serax® | (sear' aks) |
| Eurax® | (yoor' aks) |
| Serax® | (sear' aks) |
| Urex® | (yu' eks) |
| Serax® | (sear' aks) |
| Zyrtec® | (zir' tec) |
| Serentil® | (su ren' til) |
| Surital® | (su' ri tal) |
| Silace® | (sye' lace) |
| Silain® | (sye' lain) |
| Silain® | (sye' lain) |
| Silace® | (sye' lace) |
| Sinequan® | (si' ne kwan) |
| saquinavir | (sa kwin' a veer) |
| Sinequan® | (si' ne kwan) |
| Seroquel® | (seer' oh kwel) |
| Seroquel® | (seer' oh kwel) |
| Sinequan® | (si' ne kwan) |
| Solarcaine® | (sole' ar kane) |
| Solatene® | (sole' a teen) |
| Solatene® | (sole' a teen) |
| Solarcaine® | (sole' ar kane) |
| Soriatane® | (sor' e ah tane) |
| Loxitane® | (loks' e tane) |
| Staphcillin® | (staf sil' lin) |
| Staticin® | (stat' i sin) |
| Staticin® | (stat' i sin) |

## SOUND-ALIKE COMPARISON LIST *(Continued)*

| Drug Name | Pronunciation |
|---|---|
| Staphcillin® | (staf sil′ lin) |
| streptomycin | (strep toe mye′ sin) |
| streptozocin | (strep toe zoe′ sin) |
| streptozocin | (strep toe zoe′ sin) |
| streptomycin | (strep toe mye′ sin) |
| Sudafed® | (sue′ da fed) |
| Sufenta® | (sue fen′ tah) |
| Sufenta® | (sue fen′ tah) |
| Alfenta® | (al fen′ tah) |
| Sufenta® | (sue fen′ tah) |
| Sudafed® | (sue′ da fed) |
| sulfasalazine | (sul fa sal′ a zeen) |
| sulfisoxazole | (sul fi sox′ a zole) |
| sulfisoxazole | (sul fi sox′ a zole) |
| sulfasalazine | (sul fa sal′ a zeen) |
| sumatriptan | (soo ma trip′ tan) |
| zolmitriptan | (zohl mi trip′ tan) |
| Suprax® | (su′ prax) |
| Surbex® | (sur′ beks) |
| Surbex® | (sur′ beks) |
| Suprax® | (su′ prax) |
| Surbex® | (sur′ beks) |
| Surfak® | (sur′ fak) |
| Surfak® | (sur′ fak) |
| Surbex® | (sur′ beks) |
| Surital® | (su′ ri tal) |
| Serentil® | (su ren′ til) |
| Sytobex® | (sye′ toe beks) |
| Cytotec® | (sye′ toe tek) |
| Tacaryl® | (tak′ a ril) |
| tacrine | (tak′ reen) |
| tacrine | (tak′ reen) |
| Tacaryl® | (tak′ a ril) |
| Tagamet® | (tag′ a met) |
| Tegopen® | (teg′ o pen) |
| Talacen® | (tal′ a sen) |
| Tegison® | (teg′ i son) |
| Talacen® | (tal′ a sen) |
| Tinactin® | (tin ak′ tin) |
| Taxol® | (tacks′ ol) |
| Paxil® | (packs′ ol) |
| Tedral® | (ted′ ral) |
| Teldrin® | (tel′ drin) |
| Tegison® | (teg′ i son) |
| Talacen® | (tal′ a sen) |
| Tegopen® | (teg′ o pen) |
| Tagamet® | (tag′ a met) |
| Tegopen® | (teg′ o pen) |
| Tegretol® | (teg′ ree tol) |
| Tegopen® | (teg′ o pen) |
| Tegrin® | (teg′ rin) |
| Tegretol® | (teg′ ree tol) |
| Mebaral® | (meb′ a ral) |
| Tegretol® | (teg′ ree tol) |
| Tegopen® | (teg′ o pen) |
| Tegrin® | (teg′ rin) |
| Tegopen® | (teg′ o pen) |
| Teldrin® | (tel′ drin) |
| Tedral® | (ted′ ral) |
| Temaril® | (tem′ a ril) |
| Demerol® | (dem′ eh rol) |
| Temaril® | (tem′ a ril) |
| Tepanil® | (tep′ a nil) |
| Tenex® | (ten′ eks) |
| Xanax® | (zan′ aks) |
| Tepanil® | (tep′ a nil) |

| Drug Name | Pronunciation |
|---|---|
| Temaril® | (tem′ a ril) |
| Tepanil® | (tep′ a nil) |
| Tofranil® | (toe fray′ nil) |
| terbinafine | (ter′ bin a feen) |
| terfenadine | (ter fen′ na deen) |
| terbinafine | (ter′ bin a feen) |
| terbutaline | (ter byoo′ ta leen) |
| terbutaline | (ter byoo′ ta leen) |
| terbinafine | (ter′ bin a feen) |
| terbutaline | (ter byoo′ ta leen) |
| tolbutamide | (tole byoo′ ta mide) |
| terconazole | (ter kone′ a zole) |
| tioconazole | (tye o kone′ a zole) |
| terfenadine | (ter fen′ na deen) |
| terbinafine | (ter′ bin a feen) |
| Terramycin® | (tehr a mye′ sin) |
| Garamycin® | (gar a mye′ sin) |
| testolactone | (tess toe lak′ tone) |
| testosterone | (tess toss′ ter one) |
| testosterone | (tess toss′ ter one) |
| testolactone | (tess toe lak′ tone) |
| Theelin® | (thee′ lin) |
| Theolair™ | (thee′ o lare) |
| Theoclear® | (thee′ o clear) |
| Theolair™ | (thee′ o lare) |
| Theolair™ | (thee′ o lare) |
| Theelin® | (thee′ lin) |
| Theolair™ | (thee′ o lare) |
| Theoclear® | (thee′ o clear) |
| Theolair™ | (thee′ o lare) |
| Thiola™ | (thye oh′ la) |
| Theolair™ | (thee′ o lare) |
| Thyrolar® | (thye′ roe lar) |
| Theragran® | (ther′ a gran) |
| Phenergan® | (fen′ er gan) |
| Theramin® | (there′ a min) |
| thiamine | (thye′ a min) |
| thiamine | (thye′ a min) |
| Theramin® | (there′ a min) |
| Thiola™ | (thye oh′ la) |
| Theolair™ | (thee′ o lare) |
| thioridazine | (thye o rid′ a zeen) |
| thiothixene | (thye o thix′ een) |
| thiothixene | (thye o thix′ een) |
| thioridazine | (thye o rid′ a zeen) |
| Thyrar® | (thyer′ are) |
| Thyrolar® | (thye′ roe lar) |
| Thyrar® | (thyer′ are) |
| Ticar® | (tye′ kar) |
| Thyrolar® | (thye′ roe lar) |
| Theolair™ | (thee′ o lare) |
| Thyrolar® | (thye′ roe lar) |
| Thyrar® | (thyer′ are) |
| Thyrolar® | (thye′ roe lar) |
| Thytropar® | (thye′ troe par) |
| Thytropar® | (thye′ troe par) |
| Thyrolar® | (thye′ roe lar) |
| Ticar® | (tye′ kar) |
| Thyrar® | (thyer′ are) |
| Ticar® | (tye′ kar) |
| Tigan® | (tye′ gan) |
| Ticon® | (tye′ kon) |
| Tigan® | (tye′ gan) |
| Tigan® | (tye′ gan) |
| Ticar® | (tye′ kar) |
| Tigan® | (tye′ gan) |

| Drug Name | Pronunciation |
|---|---|
| Ticon® | (tye' kon) |
| timolol | (tye' moe lole) |
| Tylenol® | (tye' le nole) |
| Timoptic® | (tim op' tik) |
| Viroptic® | (vir op' tik) |
| Tinactin® | (tin ak' tin) |
| Talacen® | (tal' a sen) |
| Tindal® | (tin' dal) |
| Trental® | (tren' tal) |
| tioconazole | (tye o kone' a zole) |
| terconazole | (ter kone' a zole) |
| TobraDex® | (toe' bra deks) |
| Tobrex® | (toe' breks) |
| tobramycin | (toe bra mye' sin) |
| Trobicin® | (troe' bi sin) |
| Tobrex® | (toe' breks) |
| TobraDex® | (toe' bra deks) |
| Tofranil® | (toe fray' nil) |
| Tepanil® | (tep' a nil) |
| tolazamide | (tole az' a mide) |
| tolazoline | (tole az' o leen) |
| tolazamide | (tole az' a mide) |
| tolbutamide | (tole byoo' ta mide) |
| tolazoline | (tole az' o leen) |
| tolazamide | (tole az' a mide) |
| tolbutamide | (tole byoo' ta mide) |
| terbutaline | (ter byoo' ta leen) |
| tolbutamide | (tole byoo' ta mide) |
| tolazamide | (tole az' a mide) |
| Tolinase® | (tole' i nase) |
| Orinase® | (or' in ase) |
| tolnaftate | (tole naf' tate) |
| Tornalate® | (tor' na late) |
| Tonocard® | (ton' o kard) |
| Torecan® | (tor' e kan) |
| Torecan® | (tor' e kan) |
| Tonocard® | (ton' o kard) |
| Tornalate® | (tor' na late) |
| tolnaftate | (tole naf' tate) |
| Trandate® | (tran' date) |
| Trendar® | (tren' dar) |
| Trandate® | (tran' date) |
| Trental® | (tren' tal) |
| Trendar® | (tren' dar) |
| Trandate® | (tran' date) |
| Trental® | (tren' tal) |
| Bentyl® | (ben' til) |
| Trental® | (tren' tal) |
| Tindal® | (tin' dal) |
| Trental® | (tren' tal) |
| Trandate® | (tran' date) |
| tretinoin | (tret' i noyn) |
| trientine | (trye' en teen) |
| Tri-Levlen® | (trye' lev len) |
| Trilafon® | (tri' la fon) |
| triacetin | (trye a see' tin) |
| Triacin® | (trye' a sin) |
| Triacin® | (trye' a sin) |
| triacetin | (trye a see' tin) |
| triamterene | (trye am' ter een) |
| trimipramine | (trye mi' pra meen) |
| Triapin® | (trye a pin) |
| Triban® | (trye' ban) |
| triazolam | (trye ay' zoe lam) |
| alprazolam | (al pray' zoe lam) |
| Triban® | (trye' ban) |
| Triapin® | (trye a pin) |
| trientine | (trye' en teen) |

| Drug Name | Pronunciation |
|---|---|
| tretinoin | (tret' i noyn) |
| Trilafon® | (tri' la fon) |
| Tri-Levlen® | (trye' lev len) |
| trimeprazine | (trye mep' ra zeen) |
| trimipramine | (trye mi' pra meen) |
| trimethaphan | (trye meth' a fan) |
| trimethoprim | (trye meth' o prim) |
| trimethoprim | (trye meth' o prim) |
| trimethaphan | (trye meth' a fan) |
| trimipramine | (trye mi' pra meen) |
| triamterene | (trye am' ter een) |
| trimipramine | (trye mi' pra meen) |
| trimeprazine | (trye mep' ra zeen) |
| Trimox® | (trye' moks) |
| Diamox® | (dye' a moks) |
| Trimox® | (trye' moks) |
| Tylox® | (tye' loks) |
| Trinalin® | (tri' na lin) |
| Phrenilin® | (fren' ni lin) |
| Triofed® | (trye' o fed) |
| Triostat™ | (tree' o stat) |
| Triostat™ | (tree' o stat) |
| Triofed® | (trye' o fed) |
| Trisoralen® | (trye sore' a len) |
| Trysul® | (trye' sul) |
| Trobicin® | (troe' bi sin) |
| tobramycin | (toe bra mye' sin) |
| Tronolane® | (tron' o lane) |
| Tronothane® | (tron' o thane) |
| Tronothane® | (tron' o thane) |
| Tronolane® | (tron' o lane) |
| Trysul® | (trye' sul) |
| Trisoralen® | (trye sore' a len) |
| Tuinal® | (tu' i nal) |
| Luminal® | (lu' mi nal) |
| Tuinal® | (tu' i nal) |
| Tylenol® | (tye' le nole) |
| Tussafed® | (tus' a fed) |
| Tussafin® | (tus' a fin) |
| Tussafin® | (tus' a fin) |
| Tussafed® | (tus' a fed) |
| Tylenol® | (tye' le nole) |
| atenolol | (a ten' oh lole) |
| Tylenol® | (tye' le nole) |
| timolol | (tye' moe lole) |
| Tylenol® | (tye' le nole) |
| Tuinal® | (tu' i nal) |
| Tylenol® | (tye' le nole) |
| Tylox® | (tye' loks) |
| Tylox® | (tye' loks) |
| Trimox® | (trye' moks) |
| Tylox® | (tye' loks) |
| Tylenol® | (tye' le nole) |
| Tylox® | (tye' loks) |
| Wymox® | (wye' moks) |
| Uni-Bent® | (yu' ni bent) |
| Unipen® | (yu' ni pen) |
| Unipen® | (yu' ni pen) |
| Uni-Bent® | (yu' ni bent) |
| Unipen® | (yu' ni pen) |
| Omnipen® | (om' ni pen) |
| Urex® | (yu' eks) |
| Eurax® | (yoor' aks) |
| Urex® | (yu' eks) |
| Serax® | (sear' aks) |
| V-Cillin K® | (vee sil' lin kay) |
| Bicillin® | (bye sil' lin) |
| V-Cillin K® | (vee' sil lin kay) |

## SOUND-ALIKE COMPARISON LIST *(Continued)*

| Drug Name | Pronunciation |
|---|---|
| Wycillin® | (wye sil' lin) |
| Vamate® | (vam' ate) |
| Vancenase® | (van' sen ase) |
| Vancenase® | (van' sen ase) |
| Vamate® | (vam' ate) |
| Vanceril® | (van' ser il) |
| Vansil™ | (van' sil) |
| Vansil™ | (van' sil) |
| Vanceril® | (van' ser il) |
| Vasocidin® | (vay so sye' din) |
| Vasodilan® | (vay so di' lan) |
| Vasodilan® | (vay so di' lan) |
| Vasocidin® | (vay so sye' din) |
| Vasosulf® | (vay' so sulf) |
| Velosef® | (vel' o sef) |
| VePesid® | (veh' pe sid) |
| Versed® | (ver' sed) |
| Velosef® | (vel' o sef) |
| Vasosulf® | (vay' so sulf) |
| Ventolin® | (ven' to lin) |
| phentolamine | (fen tole' a meen) |
| Ventolin® | (ven' tow lin) |
| Benylin® | (ben' eh lin) |
| Verelan® | (ver' e lan) |
| Voltaren® | (vo tare' en) |
| Versed® | (ver' sed) |
| VePesid® | (veh' pe sid) |
| Viagra® | (vye ag' ra) |
| Allegra® | (al leg' ra) |
| Vicodin® | (vye' co din) |
| Hycodan® | (hye' co dan) |
| vidarabine | (vye dare' a been) |
| cytarabine | (sye tare' a been) |
| Videx® | (vye' deks) |
| Lidex® | (lye' deks) |
| vinblastine | (vin blas' teen) |
| vincristine | (vin kris' teen) |
| vincristine | (vin kris' teen) |
| Myochrysine® | (mye o kris' seen) |
| vincristine | (vin kris' teen) |
| vinblastine | (vin blas' teen) |
| Viroptic® | (vir op' tik) |
| Timoptic® | (tim op' tik) |
| Visine® | (vye' seen) |
| Visken® | (vis' ken) |
| Visken® | (vis' ken) |
| Visine® | (vye' seen) |
| Vistaril® | (vis' tar ril) |
| Restoril® | (res' tor ril) |
| Volmax® | (vol' maks) |
| Flomax® | (flo' maks) |
| Voltaren® | (vo tare' en) |
| Verelan® | (ver' e lan) |
| Voltaren® | (vo tare' en) |
| Vontrol® | (von' trole) |
| Vontrol® | (von' trole) |
| Voltaren® | (vo tare' en) |
| Vytone® | (vye' tone) |
| Hytone® | (hye' tone) |
| Vytone® | (vye' tone) |
| Zydone® | (zye' doan) |
| Wycillin® | (wye sil' lin) |
| Bicillin® | (bye sil' lin) |
| Wycillin® | (wye sil' lin) |
| V-Cillin K® | (vee' sil lin kay) |
| Wydase® | (wye' dase) |
| Lidex® | (lye' deks) |
| Wymox® | (wye' moks) |
| Tylox® | (tye' loks) |
| Xanax® | (zan' aks) |
| Tenex® | (ten' eks) |
| Xanax® | (zan' aks) |
| Zantac® | (zan' tak) |
| Xalatan® | (za lan' tan) |
| Zarontin® | (za ron' tin) |
| Xylo-Pfan® | (zye' lo fan) |
| Zyloprim® | (zye' lo prim) |
| Yocon® | (yo' con) |
| Zocor® | (zoe' cor) |
| Zantac® | (zan' tak) |
| Xanax® | (zan' aks) |
| Zarontin® | (za ron' tin) |
| Xalatan® | (za lan' tan) |
| Zarontin® | (za ron' tin) |
| Zaroxolyn® | (za roks' o lin) |
| Zaroxolyn® | (za roks' o lin) |
| Zarontin® | (za ron' tin) |
| Zerit® | (zer' it) |
| Ziac™ | (zye' ak) |
| Ziac™ | (zye' ak) |
| Zerit® | (zer' it) |
| Zocor® | (zoe' cor) |
| Cozaar® | (koe' zar) |
| Zocor® | (zoe' cor) |
| Yocon® | (yo' con) |
| Zofran® | (zoe' fran) |
| Zosyn™ | (zoe' sin) |
| zolmitriptan | (zohl mi trip' tan) |
| sumatriptan | (soo ma trip' tan) |
| Zosyn™ | (zoe' sin) |
| Zofran® | (zoe' fran) |
| Zydone® | (zye' doan) |
| Vytone® | (vye' tone) |
| Zyloprim® | (zye' lo prim) |
| Xylo-Pfan® | (zye' lo fan) |
| Zyprexa® | (zye preks' a) |
| Celexa® | (se lex' a) |
| Zyrtec® | (zir' tec) |
| Serax® | (sear' aks) |

# MULTIPLE VITAMIN FORMULATIONS

| Product | A (IU) | D (IU) | E (IU) | $B_1$ (mg) | $B_2$ (mg) | $B_3$ (mg) | $B_5$ (mg) | $B_6$ (mg) | $B_{12}$ (mg) | C (mg) | Ca (mg) | F.A. (mg) | Fe | Other |
|---|---|---|---|---|---|---|---|---|---|---|---|---|---|---|
| Advanced Formula Centrum Liquid | 2500 | 400 | 30 | 1.5 | 1.7 | 20 | 10 | 2 | 6 | 60 | | | 9 | 300 mcg biotin, Cr, I, Mn, Mo, Zn |
| Certagen Liquid (15 mL) | 2500 | 400 | 30 | 1.5 | 1.7 | 20 | 10 | 2 | 6 | 60 | | | 9 | 3 mg Zn, Cr, Mn, Mo 300 mcg biotin |
| Theragran® Liquid (5 mL) | 5000 | 400 | | 10 | 10 | 100 | 21.4 | 4.1 | 5 | 200 | | | | |
| Thera Multi-Vitamin Liquid (5 mL) | 10,000 | 400 | | 10 | 10 | 100 | 21.4 | 4.1 | 5 | 200 | | | | |
| Theravite Liquid (5 mL) | 10,000 | 400 | | 10 | 10 | 100 | 21.4 | 4.1 | 5 | 200 | | | | |
| Allee C-800 Tablets | | | 45 | 15 | 17 | 100 | 25 | 25 | 12 | 800 | | | | |
| Cefol® Tablets | | | 30 | 15 | 10 | 100 | 20 | 5 | 6 | 750 | | 0.5 | | |
| Marnatal-F Tablets | 4000 | 400 | 30 | 3 | 3.4 | 20 | | 5 | 12 | 100 | 250 | 1 | 60 | Cu, I, Mg, Zn |
| Materna® Tablets | 5000 | 400 | 30 | 3 | 3.4 | 20 | 10 | 10 | 12 | 100 | 250 | 1 | 60 | |
| Multivitamins Capsules | 5000 | 400 | 10 | 2.5 | 2.5 | 20 | 5 | 0.5 | 2 | 50 | | | | |
| Mynatal Capsules | 5000 | 400 | 30 | 3 | 3 | 20 | | 10 | 12 | 80 | 300 | 1 | 65 | 30 mcg biotin, Cr, Cu, I, Mg, Mn, Mo, Zn |
| Mynatal P.N. Forte Caplets | 5000 | 400 | 30 | 3 | 3.4 | 20 | | 4 | 12 | 80 | 250 | 1 | 60 | I, Mg, Cu, Zn |
| Natalins® Tablets | 4000 | 400 | 15 | 1.5 | 1.6 | 17 | | 2.6 | 2.5 | 70 | 200 | 0.5 | 30 | Mg, Cu, Zn |
| Niferex®-P.N. Forte Tablets | 5000 | 400 | 30 | 3 | 3.4 | 20 | | 4 | 12 | 80 | 250 | 1 | 60 | |
| Os-Cal® Fortified Tablets | 1688 | 125 | 0.8 | 1.7 | 1.7 | 15 | | 2 | | 50 | 250 | | 5 | Mg, Mn, Zn |
| Pramiles FA Tablets | 4000 | 400 | | 3 | 2 | 10 | 1 | 3 | 3 | 60 | 250 | 1 | 40 | |
| Prenatal Maternal Tablets | 5000 | 400 | 30 | 2.9 | 3.4 | 20 | 10 | 12.2 | 12 | 100 | 250 | 1 | 60 | Cr, Cu, I, Mg, Mn, Mo, Zn, 30 mcg biotin |
| Prenatal Z Tablets | 5000 | 400 | 30 | 3 | 3 | 20 | | 12.2 | 12 | 80 | 300 | 1 | 65 | I, Mg, Zn |
| Prenate® 90 Tablets | 4000 | 400 | 30 | 3 | 3.4 | 20 | | 20 | 12 | 120 | 250 | | 90 | Cu, I, Zn |
| Stress Formula w/Zinc Tablets | | | 30 | 10 | 10 | 100 | 20 | 5 | 12 | 500 | | 0.4 | | 45 mg biotin, 23.9 mg Zn, Cu |
| Stress Formula Vitamins Tablets/Capsules | | | 30 | 10 | 10 | 100 | 20 | 5 | 12 | 500 | | 0.4 | | 45 mg biotin |
| Stresstabs Tablets | | | 30 | 10 | 10 | 100 | 20 | 5 | 12 | 500 | | 0.4 | | 45 mg biotin |
| Stuartnatal Plus Tablets | 4000 | 400 | 11 | 1.5 | 3 | 20 | | 10 | 12 | 120 | 200 | 1 | 65 | Cu, Zn |
| Theragran® Caplets | 5000 | 400 | 30 | 3 | 3.4 | 20 | 10 | 3 | 9 | 90 | | 0.4 | | 30 mcg biotin |
| Theragran®-M Caplets | 5000 | 400 | 30 | 3 | 3.4 | 20 | 10 | 3 | 9 | 90 | 40 | 0.4 | 27 | Cl, Cr, Cu, I, K, Mg, Mn, Mo, P, Se, Zn, 30 mcg biotin |
| Therapeutic-M Tablets | 5000 | 400 | 30 | 3 | 3.4 | 20 | 10 | 3 | 9 | 90 | | 0.4 | 27 | Ca, Cl, Cr, Cu, I, K, Mg, Mn, Mo, P, Se, Zn, biotin 30 mcg |
| Vicon Forte® Capsules | 8000 | | 50 | 10 | 5 | 25 | 10 | 2 | 10 | 150 | | 1 | | Mg, Mn, Zn |

F.A. = Folic Acid

# NOTES

# NOTES

# NOTES

# NOTES

# Other titles offered by Lexi-Comp . . .

## *DRUG INFORMATION HANDBOOK FOR ADVANCED PRACTICE NURSING 1999/2000*

by Beatrice B. Turkoski, RN, PhD; Brenda R. Lance, RN, MSN; Mark F. Bonfiglio, PharmD

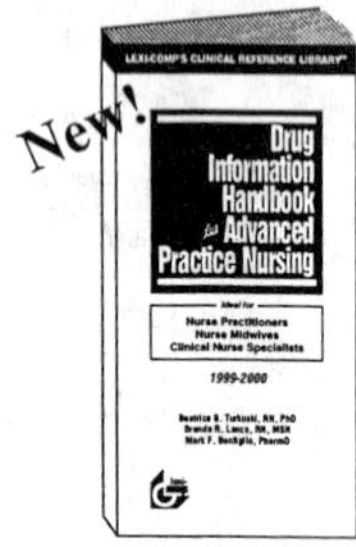


This handbook was designed specifically to meet the needs of Nurse Practitioners, Clinical Nurse Specialists, Nurse Midwives and graduate nursing students. The handbook is a unique resource for detailed, accurate information, which is vital to support the advanced practice nurse's rule in patient drug therapy management.

A concise introductory section reviews topics related to Pharmacotherapeutics.

Over 4750 U.S., Canadian, and Mexican medications are covered in the 1055 monographs. Drug data is presented in an easy-to-use, alphabetically organized format covering up to 46 key points of information including Adult, Pediatric and Geriatric Dosing (with adjustments for renal/hepatic impairment), Laboratory Tests used to monitor drug therapy, Pregnancy/Breast feeding implications, Physical Assessment/Monitoring Guidelines and Patient Education/Instruction. Monographs are cross-referenced to an appendix of over 230 pages of valuable comparison tables and additional information. Also included are two indices, Pharmacologic Category and Controlled Substance which facilitate comparison between agents.

## *DRUG INFORMATION HANDBOOK 7th Edition 1999-2000*

by Charles Lacy, PharmD; Lora L. Armstrong, BSPharm; Morton P. Goldman, PharmD; and Leonard L. Lance, BSPharm

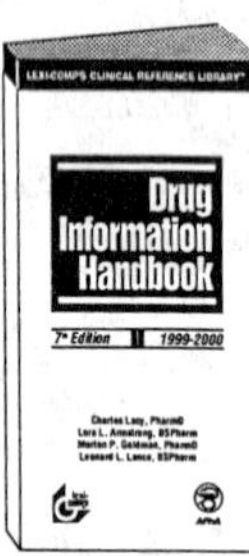


Specifically compiled and designed for the healthcare professional requiring quick access to concisely stated comprehensive data concerning clinical use of medications.

*The Drug Information Handbook* is an ideal portable drug information resource, containing 1250 drug monographs. Each monograph typically provides the reader with up to 29 key points of data concerning clinical use and dosing of the medication. Material provided in the Appendix section is recognized by many users to be, by itself, well worth the purchase of the handbook.

## *DRUG INFORMATION HANDBOOK POCKET 1999-2000*

by Charles Lacy, PharmD; Lora L. Armstrong, BSPharm; Morton P. Goldman, PharmD; and Leonard L. Lance, BSPharm

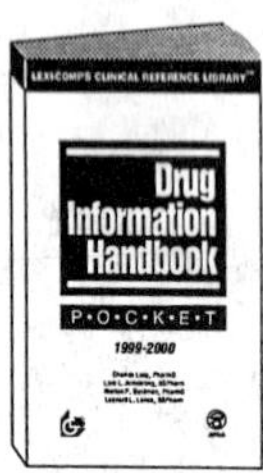


All medications found in the Drug Information Handbook, 7th Edition are included in this abridged pocket edition. It is specifically compiled and designed for the healthcare professional requiring quick access to concisely stated comprehensive data concerning clinical use of medications.

The outstanding cross-referencing allows the user to quickly locate the brand name, generic name, synonym, and related information found in the Appendix making this a useful quick reference for medical professionals at any level of training or experience.

**To order call toll free: 1-800-837-LEXI (5394)**

## *PEDIATRIC DOSAGE HANDBOOK* *6th Edition 1999-2000*

by Carol K. Taketomo, PharmD; Jane Hurlburt Hodding, PharmD; and Donna M. Kraus, PharmD

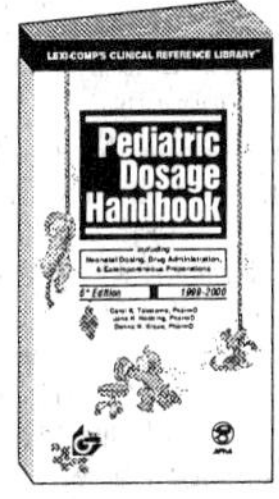


Special considerations must frequently be taken into account when dosing medications for the pediatric patient. This highly regarded quick reference handbook is a compilation of recommended pediatric doses based on current literature as well as the practical experience of the authors and their many colleagues who work every day in the pediatric clinical setting.

*The Pediatric Dosage Handbook* 6th Edition includes neonatal dosing, drug administration, and extemporaneous preparations for 640 medications used in pediatric medicine.

## *GERIATRIC DOSAGE HANDBOOK* *4th Edition 1998/99*

by Todd P. Semla, PharmD; Judith L. Beizer, PharmD; and Martin D. Higbee, PharmD

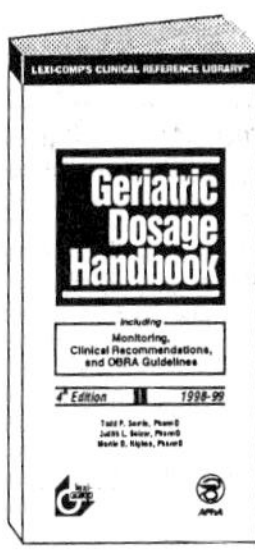


Many physiologic changes occur with aging, some of which affect the pharmacokinetics or pharmacodynamics of medications. Strong consideration should also be given to the effect of decreased renal or hepatic functions in the elderly as well as the probability of the geriatric patient being on multiple drug regimens.

Healthcare professionals working with nursing homes and assisted living facilities will find the 745 drug monographs contained in this handbook to be an invaluable source of helpful information.

## *DRUG INFORMATION HANDBOOK FOR THE ALLIED HEALTH PROFESSIONAL* *6th Edition 1999-2000*

by Leonard L. Lance, BSPharm; Charles Lacy, PharmD; and Morton P. Goldman, PharmD

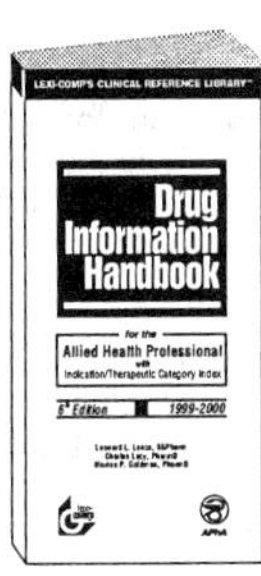


Working with clinical pharmacists, hospital pharmacy and therapeutics committees, and hospital drug information centers, the authors have assisted hundreds of hospitals in developing institution specific formulary reference documentation.

The most current basic drug and medication data from those clinical settings have been reviewed, coalesced, and cross-referenced to create this unique handbook. The handbook offers quick access to abbreviated monographs for 1384 generic drugs.

This is a great tool for physician assistants, medical records personnel, medical transcriptionists and secretaries, pharmacy technicians, and other allied health professionals.

**To order call toll free: 1-800-837-LEXI (5394)**

## *DRUG-INDUCED NUTRIENT DEPLETION HANDBOOK* 1999-2000

by Ross Pelton, RPh, PhD, CCN; James B. LaValle, RPh, DHM, NMD, CCN; Ernest B. Hawkins, RPh, MS; Daniel L. Krinsky, RPh, MS

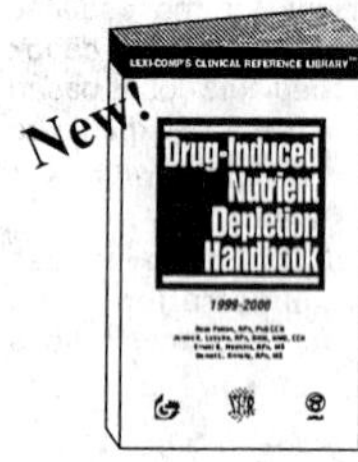


A complete and up-to-date listing of all drugs known to deplete the body of nutritional compounds.

Alphabetically organized and provides extensive cross-referencing to related information in the various sections of the book. Nearly 150 generic drugs that cause nutrient depletion are identified which are also cross-referenced to more detailed descriptions of the nutrients depleted and their actions. Symptoms of deficiencies, and sources of repletion are also included. This book also contains Studies and Abstracts section, a valuable Appendix, and Alphabetical & Pharmacological Indices.

## *ANESTHESIOLOGY & CRITICAL CARE DRUG HANDBOOK* 2nd Ed

***1999-2000*** by Andrew J. Donnelly, PharmD; Francesca E. Cunningham, PharmD; and Verna L. Baughman, MD

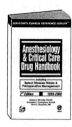


Contains over 512 generic medications with up to 25 fields of information presented in each monograph. It also contains the following Special Issues and Topics: Allergic Reaction, Anesthesia for Cardiac Patients in Noncardiac Surgery, Anesthesia for Obstetric Patients in Nonobstetric Surgery, Anesthesia for Patients With Liver Disease, Chronic Pain Management, Chronic Renal Failure, Conscious Sedation, Perioperative Management of Patients on Antiseizure Medication, Substance Abuse and Anesthesia.

The Appendix includes: Abbreviations & Measurements, Anesthesiology Information, Assessment of Liver & Renal Function, Comparative Drug Charts, Infectious Disease-Prophylaxis & Treatment, Laboratory Values, Therapy Recommendation, Toxicology, *and much more . . .*

## *DRUG INFORMATION HANDBOOK FOR PHYSICIAN ASSISTANTS*

***1999-2000*** by Michael J. Rudzinski, RPA-C, RPh; J. Fred Bennes, RPA, RPh

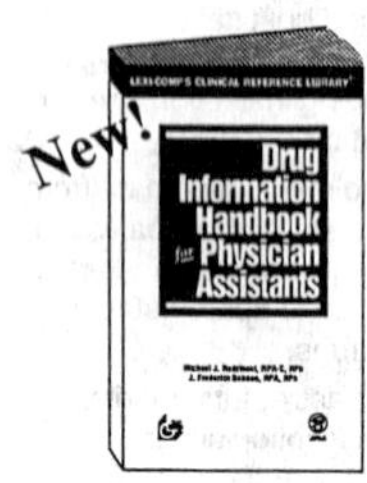


This comprehensive and easy-to-use handbook covers over 3,600 drugs and also includes monographs on commonly used herbal products. There are up to 24 key fields of information per monograph, such as; Pediatric and adult dosing with adjustments for renal/hepatic impairment, Labeled and unlabeled uses, Pregnancy & breast-feeding precautions, and Special PA issues. Brand (U.S. and Canadian) and generic names listed alphabetically for rapid access. It is fully cross-referenced by page number and includes alphabetical & pharmacologic indices.

**To order call toll free: 1-800-837-LEXI (5394)**

## *DRUG INFORMATION HANDBOOK FOR ONCOLOGY* ***1999-2000***

by Dominic A. Solimando, Jr, MA; Linda R. Bressler, PharmD, BCOP; Polly E. Kintzel, PharmD, BCPS, BCOP; Mark C. Geraci, PharmD, BCOP

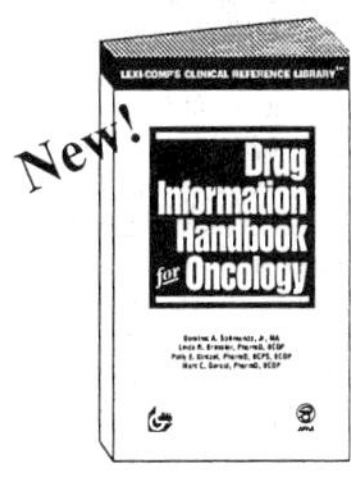


This comprehensive and easy-to-use oncology handbook was designed specifically to meet the needs of anyone who provides, prescribes, or administers therapy to cancer patients.

Presented in a concise and uniform format, this book contains the most comprehensive collection of oncology-related drug information available. Organized like a dictionary for ease of use, drugs can be found by looking up the *brand or generic name*!

This book contains 253 monographs, including over 1100 Antineoplastic Agents and Ancillary Medications.

Also containing up to 33 fields of information per monograph including: Use, U.S. Investigational, Bone Marrow/Blood Cell Transplantation, Vesicant, Emetic Potential. A Special Topics Section, Appendix, and Therapeutic Category & Key Word Index are valuable features to this book as well.

## *DRUG INFORMATION HANDBOOK FOR PSYCHIATRY* ***1999-2000***

by Matthew A. Fuller, PharmD; Martha Sajatovic, MD

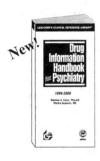


The source for comprehensive and clinically relevant drug information for the mental health professional. Alphabetically arranged by generic and brand name for ease-of-use. Containing monographs on 1,063 generic drugs and up to 34 key fields of information including; effect on mental status and effect on psychiatric treatment.

A special topics/issues section includes; psychiatric assessment, overview of selected major psychiatric disorders, clinical issues in the use of major classes of psychotropic medications, psychiatric emergencies, special populations, diagnostic and statistical manual of mental disorders (DSM-IV), and suggested reading. Also contains a valuable appendix section as well as a therapeutic category index and a alphabetical index.

## *DRUG INFORMATION HANDBOOK FOR DENTISTRY* ***5th Ed 1999-2000***

by Richard L. Wynn, BSPharm, PhD; Timothy F. Meiller, DDS, PhD; and Harold L. Crossley, DDS, PhD

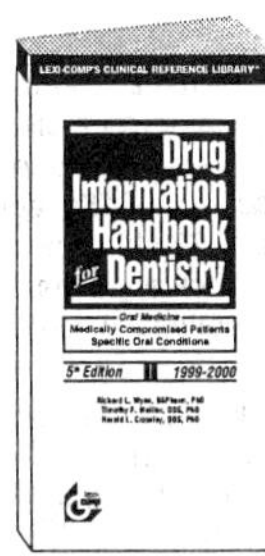


This handbook presents dental management and therapeutic considerations in medically compromised patients. Issues covered include oral manifestations of drugs, pertinent dental drug interactions, and dosing of drugs in dental treatment.

Selected oral medicine topics requiring therapeutic intervention include: managing the patient with acute or chronic pain including TMD, managing the patient with oral bacterial or fungal infections, current therapeutics in periodontal patients, managing the patient receiving chemotherapy or radiation for the treatment of cancer, managing the anxious patient, managing dental office emergencies, and treatment of common oral lesions.

**To order call toll free: 1-800-837-LEXI (5394)**

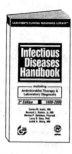

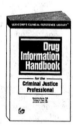

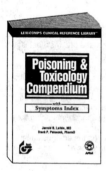

## *LABORATORY TEST HANDBOOK* *4th Edition*

by David S. Jacobs MD, FACP; Wayne R. DeMott, MD, FACP; Harold J. Grady, PhD; Rebecca T. Horvat, PhD; Douglas W. Huestis, MD; and Bernard L. Kasten Jr., MD, FACP

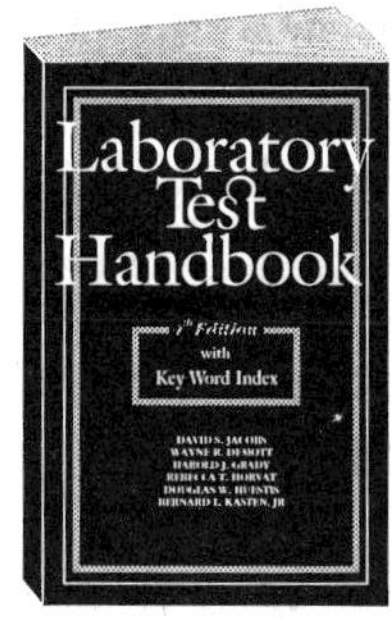


Contains over 900 clinical laboratory tests and is an excellent source of laboratory information for physicians of all specialties, nurses, laboratory professionals, students, medical personnel, or anyone who needs quick access to most the routine and many of the more specialized testing procedures available in today's clinical laboratory.

Including updated AMA CPT coding, each monograph contains test name, synonyms, patient care, specimen requirements, reference ranges, and interpretive information with footnotes and references.

## *LABORATORY TEST HANDBOOK CONCISE version*

by David S. Jacobs MD, FACP; Wayne R. DeMott, MD, FACP; Harold J. Grady, PhD; Rebecca T. Horvat, PhD; Douglas W. Huestis, MD; and Bernard L. Kasten Jr., MD, FACP

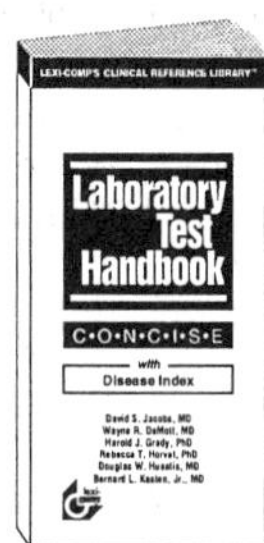


The authors of Lexi-Comp's highly regarded *Laboratory Test Handbook, 4th Edition* have selected and extracted key information for presentation in this portable abridged version.

The *Laboratory Test Handbook Concise* contains more than 800 tests entries for quick reference and is ideal for residents, nurses, and medical students or technologists requiring information concerning patient preparation, specimen collection and handling, and test result interpretation.

## *DIAGNOSTIC PROCEDURE HANDBOOK* by Joseph A. Golish, MD

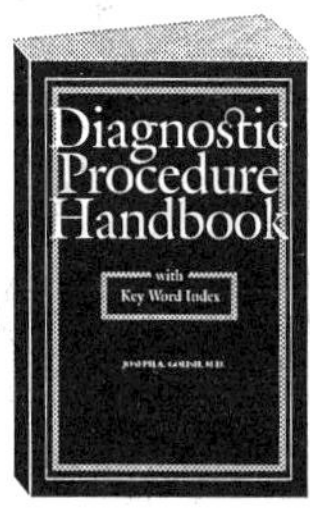


An ideal companion to the Laboratory Test Handbc k this publication details 295 diagnostic procedures including: Allergy, Immunology/Rheumotology, Infectious Disease, Cardiology, Critical Care, G stro-enterology, Nephrology, Urology, Hematolog Neurology, Ophthalmology, Pulmonary Func n, Pulmonary Medicine, Computed Tomograp Diagnostic Radiology, Invasive Radiology agnetic Resonance Imaging, Nuclear Medicine, Ultra-sound. A great reference handbook fo althcare professionals at any level of training a xperience.

**To order call toll free: 1-80 7-LEXI (5394)**

*NEW* titles targeted for release in print and on CD-ROM will include:

- ***Natural Therapeutics Pocket Guide***
- ***Natural Products Information Handbook***
- ***Drug Information Handbook for Cardiology***

## *"Lexi-Comp's Clinical Reference Library™ (CRL™) has established the new standard for quick reference information"*

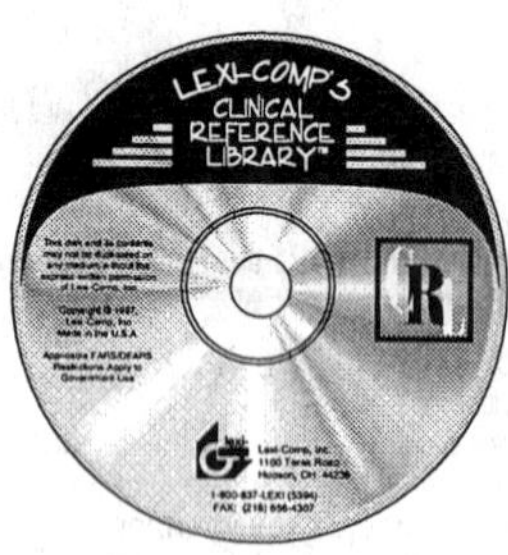


Lexi-Comp offers the Clinical Reference Library™ (CRL™), a series of clinical databases, as portable handbooks or integrated as part of a CD-ROM that also includes clinical decision support modules. CRL™ is delivered with a powerful search engine on a single CD-ROM and can be used with Microsoft® Windows™ release 3.1 or higher. In addition to our CD-ROM for Windows™, Lexi-Comp's databases can also be licensed for distribution on your Intranet, or used with your palmtop, Newton, or Windows™ CE device.

### *Clinical Decision Support Modules*

The Clinical Decision Support Modules are unique and significant to the power offered by Lexi-Comp's Clinical Reference Library™ on CD-ROM. These modules are also directly linked to CRL™'s databases.

**Patient Analysis** - Users can specify a patient's drug profile and automatically analyze the data for drug interactions, duplicate therapy, and drug allergy alerts. Printing this medication summary report for review by the physician will help decrease adverse drug events, increase productivity, and improve patient care.

**Stedman's Electronic Medical Dictionary™** - Instant access to he full functionality of a medical dictionary, including over 100,000 edical definitions, phrases, pronunciations, and related terms.

**C ulations** - Instant access to the following calculations: Body Su ce Area, Ideal Body Mass for Pediatrics and Adults, Esti ted Creatinine Clearance (Cockroft & Gault), and Tem ature Conversion.

**Drug I tification** - This powerful module allows rapid identific n of medications based on one or more of the following criptors: use, pattern, shape, scoring, markings, form, coat color, generic name, and manufacturer name. Color imag e displayed for visual verification.

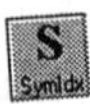


**Symptoms A sis** - Enter symptoms presented by a patient to receive sep lists of medicinal, nonmedicinal, and biological agen ociated with the selected symptoms.

**To order call to e: 1-800-837-LEXI (5394)**

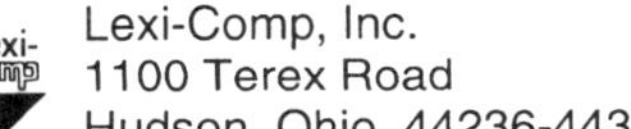

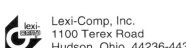

Lexi-Comp, Inc.
1100 Terex Road
Hudson, Ohio 44236-4438

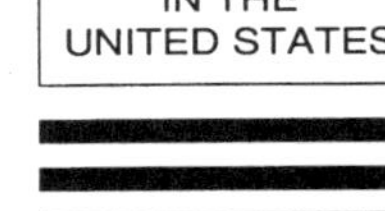

NO POSTAGE
NECESSARY
IF MAILED
IN THE
UNITED STATES

BUSINESS REPLY MAIL

FIRST-CLASS MAIL PERMIT NO 689 HUDSON, OH

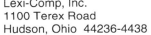

POSTAGE WILL BE PAID BY ADDRESSEE

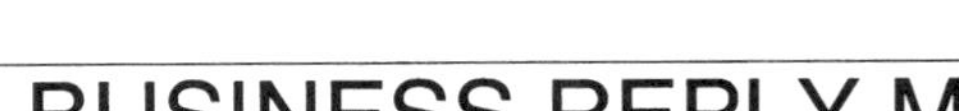

LEXI-COMP, INC.
*Drug Information Handbook for Nursing* Reply Card
1100 Terex Road
Hudson, OH 44236-9915

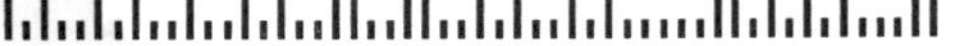